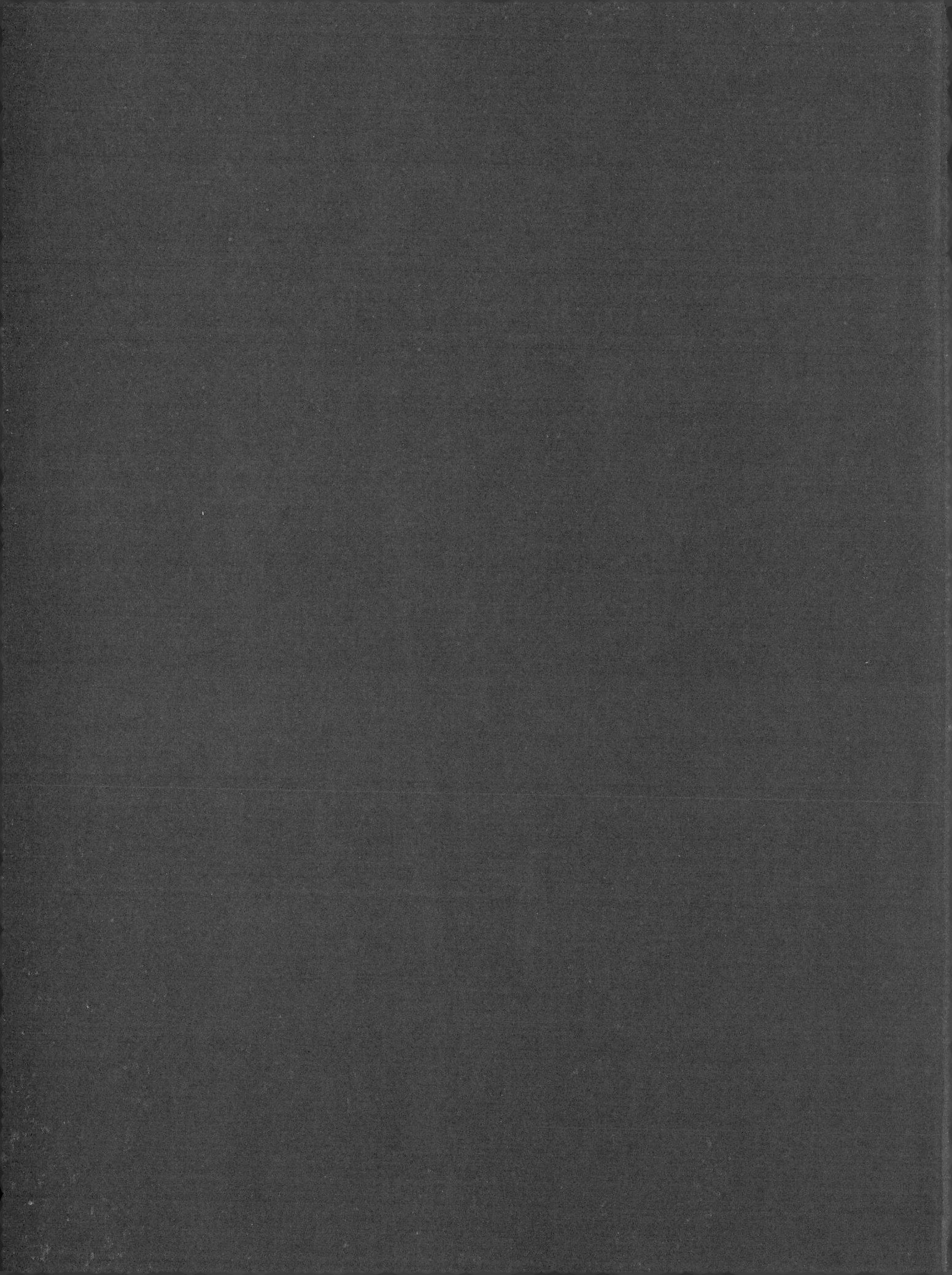

THE NEW AIRD'S COMPANION IN **Surgical Studies**

THIRD EDITION

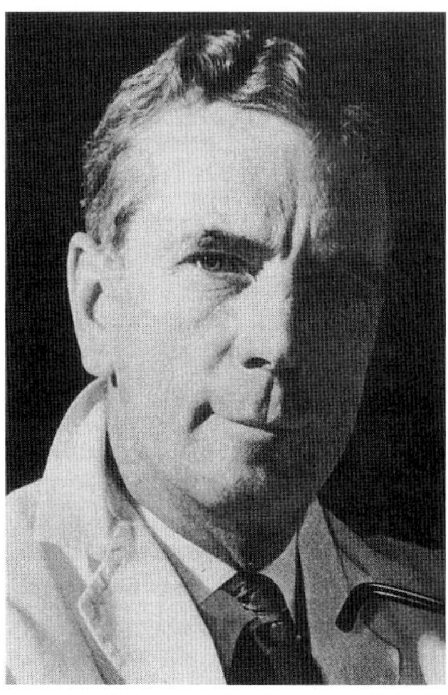

‘Surgery is learnt by apprenticeship and not from textbooks, not even from one profusely illustrated. The surgical student’s illustration is the living patient and his blackboard is the operation wound. Yet to make the most of his clinical opportunities, the student must have ready and rapid access to the ever growing canon of established surgical fact; he should be aware of the surgical conquests of the past, the tactics of the present and the strategy of the immediate future. When he examines a patient he should be armed already with a vicarious experience gained from reading and should be able to distinguish between the symptoms and signs which illustrate, and those which contradict, the observations of his clinical predecessors.’

Ian Aird,
Companion in Surgical Studies;
Ch. 1, p. 1, first edition 1949

Commissioning Editor: Michael J Houston
Project Development Manager: Hilary Hewitt
Project Manager: Rory MacDonald
Illustration Manager: Mick Ruddy
Design Manager: Jayne Jones
Marketing Manager: Ethel Cathers (USA), Gaynor Jones (UK & Rest of World)

THE NEW AIRD'S COMPANION IN **Surgical Studies**

THIRD EDITION

Edited by

Kevin G Burnand MS FRCS

Professor and Chairman of Surgery
Guys, Kings, St. Thomas' Medical School of King's College
London
UK

Anthony E Young MA MChir FRCS

Consultant Surgeon
Surgical Directorate
St. Thomas' Hospital
London
UK

Jonathan Lucas MBBS FRCS(Orth)

Consultant Orthopaedic Surgeon
Orthopaedic Department
Guy's Hospital
London
UK

Brian J Rowlands MD FRCS FACS

Professor of Surgery
Division of Gastrointestinal Surgery
University of Nottingham
Queen's Medical Centre
Nottingham
UK

John Scholefield MBChB FRCS(Eng) ChM

Reader in Surgery
University Hospital
Queen's Medical Centre
Nottingham
UK

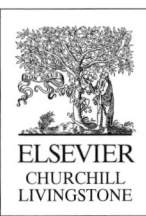

ELSEVIER
CHURCHILL
LIVINGSTONE
An imprint of Elsevier Ltd.

First published 1992
Second edition 1998
Third edition 2005

ISBN 0 443 07211 6

British Library Cataloguing in Publication Data
A catalogue record for this book is available from the British Library

Library of Congress Cataloging in Publication Data
A catalog record for this book is available from the Library of Congress

Notice
Medical knowledge is constantly changing. Standard safety precautions must be followed, but as new research and clinical experience broaden our knowledge, changes in treatment and drug therapy may become necessary or appropriate. Readers are advised to check the most current product information provided by the manufacturer of each drug to be administered to verify the recommended dose, the method and duration of administration, and contraindications. It is the responsibility of the practitioner, relying on experience and knowledge of the patient, to determine dosages and the best treatment for each individual patient. Neither the Publisher nor the editors/contributors assume any liability for any injury and/or damage to persons or property arising from this publication.
The Publisher

Printed in China

The Publisher's policy is to use **paper manufactured from sustainable forests**

Last digit is the print number : 9 8 7 6 5 4 3 2 1

Contents

Contributors

Paul Abrams MBChB MRCOY
Professor of Urology
Bristol Urological Institute
Southmead Hospital
Bristol, UK

Simon P Allison MD FRCP
Head, Clinical Nutrition and Investigation Unit
University Hospital
Nottingham, UK

John B Anderson ChM FRCS
Consultant Urological Surgeon
Department of Urology
Royal Hallamshire Hospital
Sheffield, UK

Roger M Atkins MA DM FRCS
Consultant Orthopaedic Surgeon and Reader in Orthopaedics
Department of Orthopaedic Surgery
Bristol Royal Infirmary
Bristol, UK

L Christopher Bainbridge MBChB FRCS
Consultant Hand Surgeon
Pulvertaft Hand Centre
Derbyshire Royal Infirmary
Derby, UK

John Bancewicz BSc ChM FRCS FRCS(Glas)
Reader in Surgery
Department of Surgery
Hope Hospital
Salford, UK

Marcus Bankes BSc FRCS(Orth)
Consultant Orthopaedic Surgeon
Department of Orthopaedics
Guy's Hospital
London, UK

Ian J Beckingham MBBJ FRCS MD
Consultant Hepatobiliary & Laparoscopic Surgeon
Department of Surgery
Queen's Medical Centre
Nottingham University Hospital
Nottingham, UK

Stephen J Beningfield MBChB FFRad(D)SA
Professor of Radiology
Division of Radiology
New Groote Schuur Hospital
Western Cape, South Africa

Sarah L Benyon MRCS MBBS(Hons) BSc(Hons)
Specialist Registrar, Plastic Surgery
Wexham Park Hospital
London, UK

Christopher Blake MBBS FRCS
Specialist Registrar, Urology
Bristol Urological Institute
Bristol, UK

James Bliss FRCS(Eng) FRCS(Orth)
Consultant Orthopaedic Surgeon
Orthopaedic Department
Guy's Hospital
London, UK

Kenneth D Boffard BSc(Hons) FRCS FRCS(Edin) FRCPS(Glas) FCS(SA) FACS
Professor of Surgery
Department of Surgery
Johannesburg Hospital
University of the Witwatersrand
Johannesburg, South Africa

Philippus C Bornman MBChB FRCS(Ed) FCS(SA) MMED
Professor of Surgery
Department of Surgery
Groote Schuur Hospital
Cape Town, South Africa

Douglas MG Bowley FRCS(Gen surgery)
Honorary Lecturer
Department of Surgery
University of Witswatersrand
Johannesburg, South Africa

Andrew W Bradbury BSc MD FRCSEd
Professor and Head of Surgery
Lincoln House (Research Institute)
University of Birmingham
Birmingham, UK

Adam Brooks MB ChB FRCS(Gen Surg) DMCC
Fellow in Trauma & Surgical Critical Care
Division of Trauma & Surgical Critical Care
University of Pennsylvania
Philadelphia, PA, USA

Peter Bullock MBChB FRCS
Consultant Neurosurgeon
King's College Hospital
London, UK

Frank D Burke MBBS FRCS
Professor of Hand Surgery
Pulvertaft Hand Centre
Derbyshire Royal Infirmary
Derby, UK

Kevin G Burnand MS FRCS
Professor and Chairman of Surgery
Guy's, Kings, St. Thomas' Medical School of King's College
London, UK

Gordon L Carlson BSc MD FRCS
Senior Lecturer in Surgery
Department of Colorectal Surgery
University of Manchester
Manchester, UK

Sean Carrie FRCS FRCS(orl)
Consultant Otolaryngologist
Freeman Hospital
Newcastle upon Tyne, UK

Aabir Chakraborty BSc MRCS
Specialist Registrar and Research Fellow
Department of Neurosurgery
Royal Free Hospital
London, UK

Christopher R Chapple BSc MD FRCS(Urol)
Consultant Urologist
Department of Urology
Royal Hallamshire Hospital
Sheffield, UK

Richard M Charnley DM FRCS
Consultant Hepato-Pancreato-Biliary Surgeon
Department of Surgery
Freeman Hospital
Newcastle upon Tyne, UK

Justin Cobb BM BCh MCh FRCS
Consultant in Trauma & Orthopaedics
UCH and Middlesex Hospital
London, UK

Mike Corrigan FDS(Eng) FDSRCPS(Glas) FRCS(Edin)
Formerly Consultant Oral and Maxillofacial Surgeon
The Leeds Teaching Hospitals NHS Trust
Leeds, UK

Prokar Dasgupta MSc(Urol) MD DLS FRCS(Urol) FEBU
Consultant and Honorary Senior Lecturer in Urology
Department of Urology
Guy's Hospital
London, UK

Mark S Davies BA(Oxon) MBBS FRCS FRCS(Orth)
Consultant Orthopaedic Surgeon
Department of Orthopaedics
Guy's & St Thomas' Hospitals NHS Trust
London, UK

J Michael Dixon BSc(Hons) MBChB MD FRCS FRCSEd
Consultant Surgeon & Honorary Senior Lecturer
Academic Office
Edinburgh Breast Unit
Western General Hospital
Edinburgh, UK

Peter Dziewulski FRCS FRCS(Plast.)
Consultant Plastic Surgeon
St Andrews Centre for Plastic Surgery and Burns
Chelmsford, UK

Peter H Earnshaw FRCS FRCSC
Consultant in Orthopaedics
Guy's Hospital
London, UK

Roger J H Emery MS FRCS(Ed)
Consultant Orthopaedic Surgeon
Department of Orthopaedics
St Mary's Hospital
London, UK

John WL Fielding MD FRCS FRCS MBChB
Consultant Surgeon
Queen Elizabeth Hospital
Birmingham, UK

Paul A Fields MBChB MRCP MRCPath PhD
Consultant Haematologist
Department of Haematology
Guy's and St Thomas' Hospital
London, UK

Ian M Franklin MBChB
Professor of Tranfusion Medicine
Academic Transfusion Unit
Department of Medicine
Glasgow, UK

Brian JC Freeman FRCS(Orth)
Consultant Spinal Surgeon
Centre for Spinal Studies and Surgery
University Hospital
Nottingham, UK

Paul V Gallagher FRCS
Consultant Surgeon
Wansbeck District Hospital
Ashington, UK

David T Gault MBChB FRCS
Consultant Plastic Surgeon
Mount Vernon Hospital
Middlesex, UK

Michael Gleeson MD FRCS
Consultant ENT Surgeon
Guy's Hospital
London, UK

James C Halstead MA(Cantab) MB BChir MRCS(Eng)
Specialist Registrar in Cadiothoracic Surgery
Department of Cardiothoracic Surgery
Papworth Hospital
Cambridge, UK

John RW Hardy BSc MBBS MD FRCS(Eng) FRCS(Ed) FRCS(Orth)
Orthopaedic Consultant
University of Bristol
Bristol, UK

Alexander G Heriot MD FRCS
Colorectal Fellow
Cleveland Clinic
Cleveland, OH, USA

Beverley Hunt MD FRCP FRCPath
Consultant Haematologist
Guy's and St Thomas' Hospital
London, UK

Sir Barry T Jackson MS FRCS FRCP
Past President of the Royal College of Surgeons of England
Consultant Emeritus
Guy's and St Thomas' Hospital
London, UK

David N James MBBS FRCA
Consultant Anaesthetist
Guy's and St Thomas' Hospital
London, UK

Robert W G Johnson MB MS FRCS FRCSEd
Consultant Surgeon; Honorary Reader in Surgery
Manchester Royal Infirmary
Manchester, UK

Simon E Kenny BsC ChB(Hons) MD FRCS
Consultant Paediatric Surgeon
Department of Paediatric Surgery
Institute of Child Health
Liverpool, UK

Andrew N Kingsnorth BSc MS FRCS FACS
Professor of Surgery
Postgraduate Medical School
Plymouth, UK

Jake EJ Krige FRCS FACS RCS(SA)
Principal Specialist and Associate Professor
Department of Surgery
University of Cape Town Medical School
Cape Town, South Africa

Vivek Kumar MS FRCS
Specialist Registrar
Department of Urology
Royal Hallamshire Hospital
Sheffield, UK

Anne L Lennard MBBS MRCPath
Senior Lecturer and Consultant in Hematology
Royal Victoria Infirmary
Newcastle Upon Tyne, UK

Thomas WJ Lennard MD FRCS
Professor of Surgery
Head of School of Surgical and Reproductive Sciences
The Medical School
University of Newcastle upon Tyne
Newcastle upon Tyne, UK

David A Lloyd MChir FRCS FC(SA)
Professor of Paediatric Surgery
Institute of Child Health
Alder Hey Children's Hospital
Liverpool, UK

Dileep N Lobo MS DM FRCS(Gen Surg)
Senior Lecturer in Gastrointestinal Surgery
University Hospital
Queen's Medical Centre
Nottingham, UK

Peter J Lodge MD FRCS
Consultant
Transplant Surgery
St James' & Seacroft University Hospital
Leeds, UK
United Kingdom

Jonathan D Lucas MBBS FRCS(Orth)
Consultant Orthopaedic Surgeon
Orthopaedic Department
Guy's Hospital
London, UK

Paul R Maddox MBBCh BSc FRCS
Consultant Surgeon
Royal United Hospital
Bath, UK

Robert C Mason BSc (Hons) MBChB (Hons) ChM MD FRCS
Consultant Upper GI Surgeon
Department of Surgery
St Thomas' Hospital
London, UK

Catharine L McGuinness MBBS FRCS
Consultant Vascular Surgeon
Royal Surrey County Hospital
Guildford, UK

Mark McGurk MD FRCS DLO FDS RCS
Professor of Maxillofacial Surgery
St Thomas' Hospital
London, UK

Radu Mihai FRCS
Research Fellow
Division of Surgery
Bristol Royal Infirmary
Bristol, UK

Catherine J Milroy BM BCh MA FRCS
Specialist Registrar in Plastic Surgery
Pan-Thames Rotation
London, UK

Neil J Mortensen MD FRCS
Professor of Colorectal Surgery
Department of Colorectal Surgery
John Radcliffe Hospital
Oxford, UK

John A Murie MA BSc MD FRCS
Consultant Vascular Surgeon
Department of Surgery
Royal Infirmary of Edinburgh
Edinburgh, UK

James E Nicholl MA FRCS(Orth)
Consultant Orthopaedic Surgeon
Kent and Sussex Hospital
Tunbridge Wells, UK

Patrick J O'Dwyer FRCS(I) MC FRCS(Glasg)
Professor of Surgery
University Department of Surgery
Western Infirmary
Glasgow, UK

William J Owen (Deceased) BSc MS FRCS
Formerly Consultant Surgeon and Senior Lecturer in Surgery
Guy's Hospital
London, UK

Simon Paterson-Brown MBBS MPhil MS FRCS
Consultant General and Upper Gastro-intestinal Surgeon
Clinical & Surgical Sciences (Surgery)
Royal Infirmary of Edinburgh
Edinburgh, UK

John Pepper MA MChir FRCS
Professor of Cardiothoracic Surgery
Royal Brompton Hospital
London, UK

Kumar Ravi MD
Fellow in Cardiology
Department of Medicine
Beth Israel Medical Center
New York, NY, USA

David A Ross MD FRCS(Plast)
Consultant Plastic Surgeon
Department of Surgery
Guy's & St Thomas' Hospital NHS Trust
London, UK

Gregory P Sadler MD FRCS(Ed) FRCS Gen Surg(Eng)
Consultant Endocrine Surgeon
Department of Endocrine Surgery
John Radcliffe Hospital
Oxford, UK

Rachel C Sam MBChB MA MRCS(Eng)
Specialist Registrar and Honorary Research Fellow
Lincoln House (Research Institute)
University of Birmingham
Birmingham, UK

Ann Sandison BSc MPhil MBChB FRCPath
Consultant Histopathologist
Department of Histopathology
Charing Cross Hospital
London, UK

Julian Scott MD MB ChB FRCS FRCSEd EBSOVasc
Professor of Vascular Surgery
Leeds Teaching Hospitals NHS Trust;
Molecular Vascular Medicine Unit
The Light Laboratories
University of Leeds
Leeds, UK

David Scott-Coombes MS FRCS
Consultant Endocrine Surgeon
Department of Endocrine Surgery
University Hospital of Wales
Cardiff, UK

Nicholas Screaton FRCR
Consultant Thoracic Radiologist
Papworth Hospital
Cambridge, UK

David P Shipstone MBChB FRCS(Urol)
Consultant Urological Surgeon
Department of Urology
Chesterfield Royal Hospital
Chesterfield, UK

Dominic AJ Slade MBChB FRCS
Specialist Registrar in General Surgery
Manchester Royal Infirmary
Manchester, UK

Michael A Smith BChir MB
Consultant Orthopaedic Surgeon
Orthopaedic Department
Guy's Hospital
London, UK

Paul J Smith MBBS RCSPG FRCPS FRCS
Consultant Plastic & Hand Surgeon
Mount Vernon Hospital
Northwood, UK

Helen Sweetland MBChB MD FRCS
Senior Lecturer, Consultant Surgeon
Department of Surgery
University of Wales College of Medicine
Cardiff, UK

Peter R Taylor MA MChir FRCS
Consultant Vascular Surgeon
Department of Vascular Surgery
Guy's and St Thomas's Hospital
London, UK

Kay Thomas MBBS MD FRCS
Specialist Registrar in Urology
Department of Urology
St George's Hospital
London, UK

Matthew M Thompson MD FRCS
Professor of General Surgery
St George's Hospital
London, UK

Benjamin NJ Thomson MBBS FRACS
Consultant Hepatobiliary Surgeon
Department of Surgical Oncology
Peter MacCallum Cancer Centre
Melbourne, Australia

Adrian R Timothy MBBS FRCP
Consultant Clinical Oncologist
Cancer Management Offices
Guy's Hospital
London, UK

Richard C Tiptaft BSc FRCS
Consultant Urologist
Guy's Hospital
London, UK

Tom Treasure MD MS FRCS
Professor of Cardiothoracic Surgery
St George's Hospital Medical School;
Consultant Cardiothoracic Surgeon
St George's Hospital
London, UK

Matthew G Tytherleigh FRCS
Clinical Research Fellow
Department of Colorectal Surgery
The John Radcliffe Hospital
Oxford

Anthony J Ward BMedSci(Hons) BMBS FRCS
Consultant Orthopaedic Surgeon
Department of Orthopaedic Surgery
Frenchay Hospital
Bristol, UK

Victoria MM Ward FRCS
Specialist Registrar in ENT
Guy's Hospital
London, UK

Peter Ward Booth MBChB
Department of Maxillofacial Surgery
The Queen Victoria Hospital
East Grinstead, UK

Nicholas A Watkin MA MChir FRCS (Urol)
Consultant Urological Surgeon
Department of Urology
London, UK

Francis (Frank) Wells MS BSc(Hons) FRCS(Emg) MBBS
Consultant Cardiothoracic Surgeon
Papworth Hospital
Cambridge, UK

Alastair CJ Windsor MD FRCS
Consultant Colorectal Surgeon
St Mark's Hospital
Harrow, UK

Shoo Yee Wong BMBS MRCSEd
Consultant Physician
University Hospitals
Conventry and Warwickshire
Coventry, UK

Anthony E Young MA MChir FRCS
Consultant Surgeon
Surgical Directorate
St. Thomas' Hospital
London, UK

Christopher Paul Young MD FRCS
Consultant Cardiothoracic Surgeon
Department of Cardiothoracic Surgery
St Thomas' Hospital
London, UK

Preface

This is the fifth edition of a book whose first editions appeared in 1949 and 1957 and which began a new life under our joint authorship in 1992. Aird's original book was unusual in that he was the sole author, a daunting role then but now clearly outside the powers of even a small group. The new editions have therefore been unashamedly multi-authored. Readers of the previous two editions may wonder why the authors of many of the chapters change between editions; this is not though ageing or lack of competence on their part, but simply reflects our desire for each edition to give a fresh view of topics which are for the most part in rapid evolution. We are grateful for the knowledge and enthusiasm that all the authors have shown and for their patience with our editorial style. Our intention has been to ensure that Aird's style of direct and simple writing is retained together with the practice of organising the chapters in a straightforward and familiar sequence. We also hope that we have held true to Aird's intention that a textbook should indeed be a "companion" during postgraduate studies and be a ready reference for trained surgeons needing to expand their knowledge of the general or the particular. For this reason we have continued the habit of extensive referencing.

Orthopedics was added to the last edition for completeness and to reduce the number of textbooks that trainees need to purchase; feedback shows this was a welcome change so it continues here and we are very grateful to Jonathan Lucas for having joining us as editor for the orthopaedic chapters.

We are grateful to all those at Elsevier who have helped bring this new edition to fruition and to our colleagues, surgical registrars and lecturers at St. Thomas' who have reviewed and corrected proofs.

AEY
KGB
London, 2005

Ian Aird: Historical Note

Ian Aird was born in Edinburgh in 1902. He showed early brilliance in school and later in university there, where he studied medicine. He went on to postgraduate medical studies in Paris, Vienna and St Louis, USA, before returning as Assistant Surgeon to the Royal Hospital for Sick Children in Edinburgh.

It was at this time, in the early 1930s, that what was later to be the Companion first began to take embryonic shape. To accompany his lectures to postgraduate students for their examination for the Edinburgh Fellowship, he prepared sets of duplicated lecture notes. These notes, treasured by past students, proved of such value that copies changed hands for substantial sums of money.

After war service in the Royal Army Medical Corps in North Africa, he returned to Edinburgh, and then in 1947 moved to London as Professor of Surgery at London University's Postgraduate Medical School, Hammersmith Hospital. He held his post until his death by his own hand in 1962.

Those 15 years saw a prodigious research and educational output from him as he put his department and particularly its research unit at the leading edge of world surgical progress.

An outstanding communicator, he was particularly concerned with the international dissemination of surgical knowledge. He lectured and examined widely on every continent except Antarctica.

He published a constant stream of articles in the medical journals of many countries. But his teaching reached its pinnacle and its widest audience in his Companion in Surgical Studies.

Margaret Aird
1992

An introduction to the history of surgery

1

Barry Jackson

INTRODUCTION

This chapter offers only a glimpse into 2000 years or more of surgical history. Biographical details have largely been avoided and many famous names are missing. Instead, important ideas and key developments in surgery are described, especially those of the last hundred years, for it is during this time that surgery as we know it today has evolved.

EARLY HISTORY

The craft of surgery is as old as mankind. It is reasonable to believe that the drainage of abscesses, the dressing of wounds, and the staunching of haemorrhage were practised by early humans, although our knowledge of prehistoric surgery is largely conjectural. The setting of fractures may also have been performed but there is no firm evidence of this. The one operation that is known with certainty to have been carried out by neolithic man is trephination of the skull.[1] Hundreds of skulls with trephine holes, some multiple, have been discovered in Europe and America, and from the evidence of callus formation it is known that many individuals survived. The indication for the operation, which is thought to have been performed with a sharpened flint, was probably to release supposed evil spirits from the skull of those with headache, vertigo, epilepsy or similar disorders. Other operations that may have been performed before written or pictorial records began are amputation of limbs and digits, and circumcision.[2]

THE ANCIENT EAST

Firm knowledge of early surgery relies on documentary evidence, of which there is a large amount regarding the practice of surgery in ancient Egypt, Babylon and India. The Edwin Smith papyrus, discovered in Luxor in 1862, contains descriptions of injuries, wounds, fractures, dislocations and tumours.[3] It is the oldest-known surgical text, having been compiled about 1700 BC.

The well-known code of Hammurabi, one of the earliest kings of Babylon, is engraved on a 2.5 metres tall pillar of polished black stone and may be seen in the Louvre.[4] It records various laws relating to medicine and surgery of the time: 'if a physician shall make a severe wound with a bronze lancet and kill him [the patient] or shall open an eye socket with a bronze lancet and destroy the eye, his hand shall be cut off'. If the patient was cured, or the eye preserved, the physician received 10 shekels of silver!

Ancient Hindu surgery was well advanced by the time of Susruta in the fifth century AD.[5] He advocated dissection of dead bodies, described the manual skills necessary for surgery, and suggested practising incisions on watermelons and cucumbers. He described over a hundred surgical instruments and many operations. In the treatment of perforating wounds of the abdomen he advised that any protrusion of the intestines should be washed with milk, lubricated with butter and reintroduced into the abdomen. If the intestine was perforated, the defect should be closed by applying black ants, of which the powerful jaws acted like pincers and held the edges of the wound in apposition.[6] The body of the ant was then removed (Fig. 1.1). Perhaps the best-known operation practised in India at that time was rhinoplasty. This was performed to reconstruct a nose that had been amputated either in battle or as a punishment.

GREEKS AND ROMANS

Most of the operations performed by Greek and Roman surgeons of classical times had been known and practised for centuries and few technical innovations were made. The two best-known names are Hippocrates, who practised around 400 BC, and Celsus, who practised in AD 30.[7]

The Hippocratic writings, many of which were not written by Hippocrates himself but by pupils and followers, cover many surgical problems such as fractures, dislocations, head injuries, varicose veins, leg ulcers, and rectal and anal disorders. Celsus, a cultured Roman, wrote an eight-volume medical treatise, of which the last two volumes were on surgery. He suggested that a surgeon should be young, have a strong and steady hand, be ambidextrous, have clear vision and not be moved by the cries of his patient. Celsus is still remembered today for his description of the four cardinal features of inflammation—*rubor, tumor, calor et dolor*—to which a hundred years later Galen added loss of function. Many surgical instruments from the time of Celsus were found in the ruins of Pompeii and are now preserved in the National Archaeological Museum in Naples (Fig. 1.2).

THE MIDDLE AGES

After the fall of the Roman Empire there was very little progress in the art or science of medicine until the advent of the Renaissance nearly a thousand years later. The practice of surgery fell into the hands of the uneducated; the itinerant operator for

REFERENCES

1. Parry TW. Br Med J 1923; 1: 457
2. Bishop WJ. The Early History of Surgery. Hale, London, 1960
3. Breasted JH. The Edwin Smith Surgical Papyrus. University Press, Chicago, 1930
4. Majno G. The Healing Hand: Man and Wound in the Ancient World. Harvard University Press, Cambridge, Massachusetts, 1975
5. Prakash UBS. Surg Gynecol Obstet 1978; 146: 263
6. Gudger EW. JAMA 1925; 84: 1861
7. Garrison FH. An Introduction to the History of Medicine. 4th edn. WB Saunders, Philadelphia, 1929

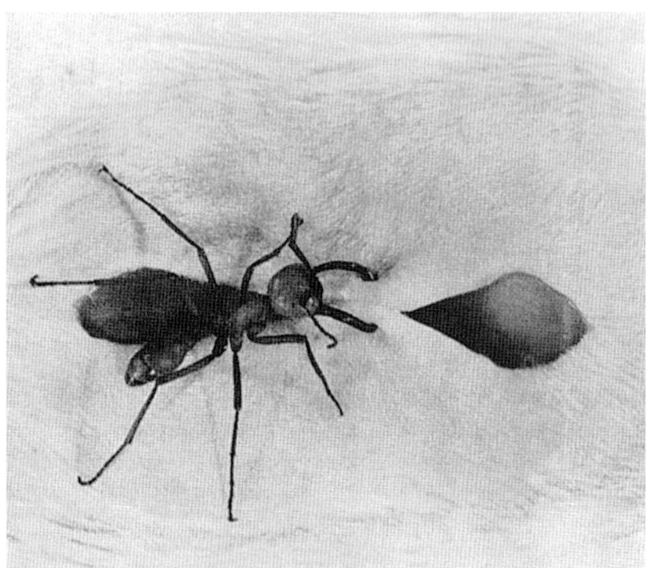

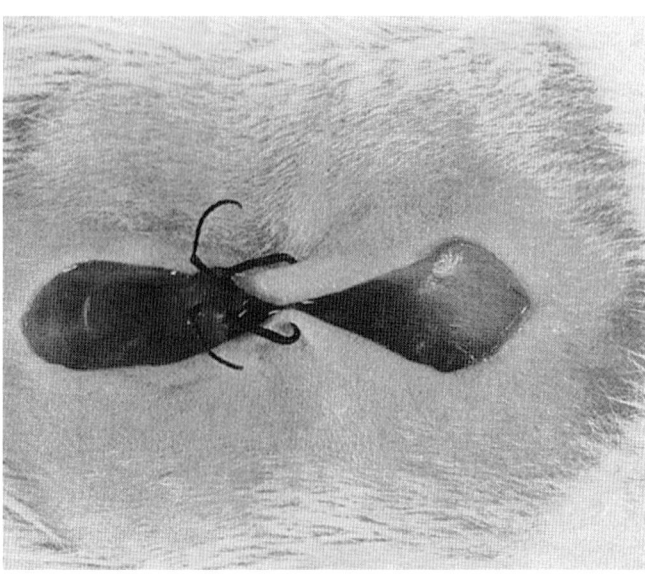

Figure 1.1 (**a**) The jaws of a dead South American soldier ant *Eciton burchelli* holding together the edges of a skin wound in a dead rat in a laboratory experiment. (**b**) The body of the ant has been removed. (From Majno 1975,[4] Harvard University Press.)

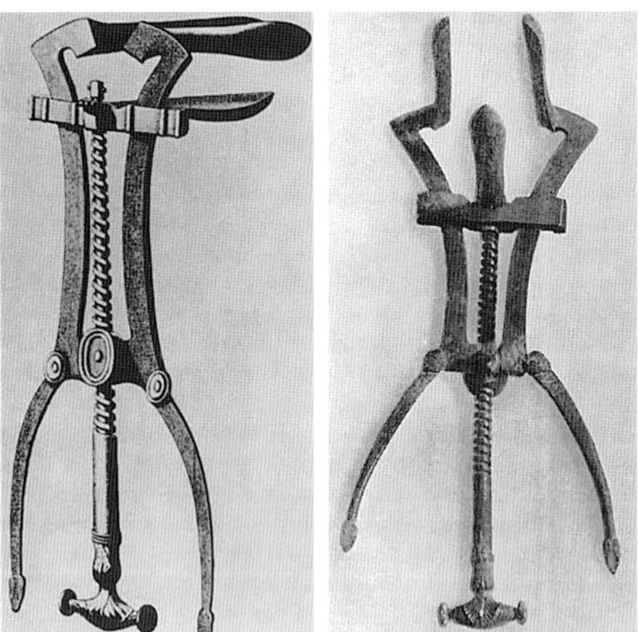

Figure 1.2 (**a**) A vaginal speculum from AD 79 excavated at Pompeii, showing one of the earliest-known applications of the screw; about one-third actual size (23 cm). (**b**) Photograph of the same speculum showing the remarkable state of preservation after nearly 2000 years. (a, From Vulpes 1847;[8] b, from Milne 1907.[9])

hernia, stone and cataract flourished. The use of the ligature to control haemorrhage, widely practised by the Greeks, was virtually abandoned, and the use of the red-hot cautery and the application of boiling oil to wounds became standard practice.

The 11th and 12th centuries, however, saw the establishment of the great universities of western Europe, among which were Salerno, Paris, Bologna, Montpellier, Padua, Oxford and Cambridge. Medical schools were present in these universities but little attention was paid to the teaching of surgery, which was considered an inferior discipline when compared with internal medicine. The physician was a learned graduate while the surgeon, with few exceptions, was an ill-educated artisan. Theodoric of Bologna, who lived around 1250, was such an exception.[10] He wrote a textbook of surgery in which he stressed the use of simple wound dressings. He maintained that pus was not always laudable and described the use of soporific sponges to induce sleep during operations. These sponges, which were used by several surgeons of the Middle Ages, were soaked in a decoction of herbs such as mandragora and are the forerunners of modern anaesthetic agents. Another noteworthy surgeon of this period was Guy de Chauliac of France, who wrote the definitive *Chirurgia Magna*, in which he recorded the history of surgery, described many instruments and operations, and insisted on the importance of anatomy. He opposed quacks, and suggested that a good surgeon 'should be courteous, sober, pious, merciful, not greedy of gain and with a sense of his own dignity'.[11]

THE RENAISSANCE

During the 200 years or so of the Renaissance there were profound changes in the theory and practice of surgery, both of which had remained more or less static since classical times. The new wave of scholasticism that occurred at this time had its origin in Italy, especially Florence, and spread throughout Europe. It was in Italy too that artists such as Michelangelo, Raphael and Leonardo da Vinci were among the first to take up the scientific study of human anatomy, a key advance necessary for the progression of surgery. These artists engaged in dissection of

REFERENCES

8. Vulpes B. Illustrazione di tutti gli instrument chirurgici scaveti in Ércolano e in Pompeii. Stamperia Reale, Naples, 1847
9. Milne JS. Surgical Instruments in Greek and Roman Times. Clarendon Press, Oxford, 1907.
10. Edwards H. Proc R Soc Med 1976; 69: 553
11. Ogden MS (ed). The Cyrurgie of Guy de Chauliac. Early English Text Society, London, 1971

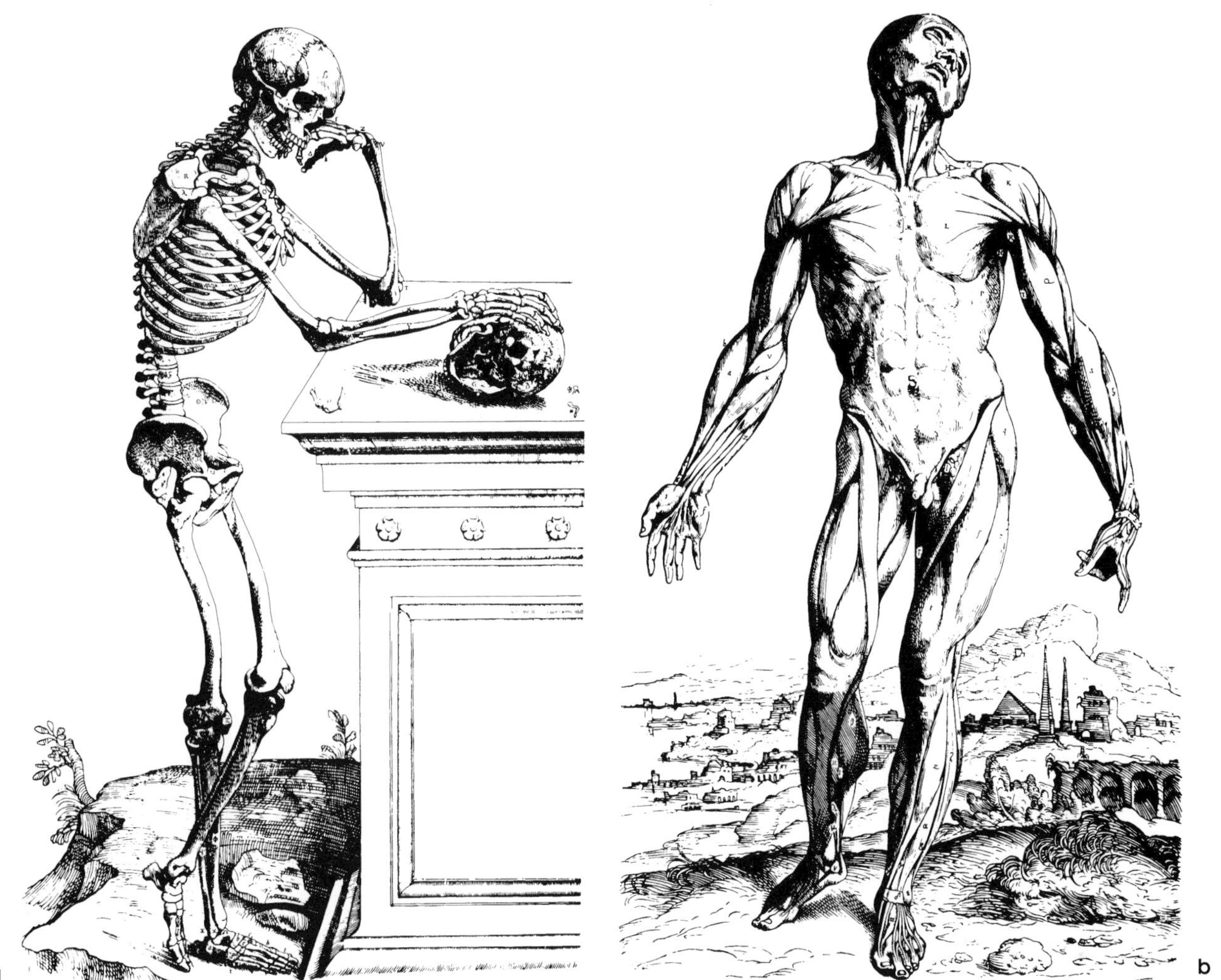

Figure 1.3 Two plates from Vesalius's *De Humani Corporis Fabrica* (1543). **(a)** A plate from the osteology series. Note the hyoid on the left and two of the ossicles on the right of the separate skull. Although this depiction of the skeleton is far more accurate than any earlier anatomical illustration, some errors of proportion are present. **(b)** One of the 16 plates from the myology series. These were designed for the use of artists and sculptors as well as physicians. The background is real and has been identified as being just outside Padua.

the human body, a practice that had been non-existent since the ancient dissections of a thousand years earlier. A transformation occurred with the publication in 1543 of *De Humani Corporis Fabrica* by Andreas Vesalius of Padua, then a 28-year-old surgeon and anatomist.[12] This book, illustrated by a pupil of Titian, is the foundation of modern topographical human anatomy and one of the most important books in the history of science (Fig. 1.3). In the same year the astronomer Copernicus, who was also qualified in medicine, suggested for the first time that the sun rather than the earth was the centre of the planetary system in *De Revolutionibus Orbium Coelestium*, another book that is an accepted landmark in the history of ideas. The introduction of printing from movable type by Gutenberg in Germany a hundred years earlier and the ability to reproduce woodcuts not only made these two great books possible but also had a profound influence on the diffusion of learning generally as well as the spread of surgical knowledge.

Another factor that had a major influence on the development of surgery at this time was the introduction of gunpowder and the resultant change in the nature and surgery of war wounds, best exemplified by the writings of Ambroise Paré of France, one of the greatest military surgeons of all time.[13] A one-time barber's apprentice who was unschooled in Latin, Paré reintroduced ligation of blood vessels to stop haemorrhage after amputation and abandoned the use of cautery and boiling oil. He wrote voluminously and his books reached a wide audience because they were written in the vernacular rather than in Latin. His famous aphorism 'I dressed the wound but God healed it' gives a measure of his sound common sense.

In England, Thomas Gale wrote the first surgical textbook in the English language in 1563 (Fig. 1.4),[14] although some years earlier an English translation of a German text had been published (Fig. 1.5). William Clowes wrote on gunshot wounds in 1588,[15] the year of the great Armada, and John Woodall advocated lemon juice as a cure for scurvy in 1617, some 300 years

REFERENCES

12. Simeone FA. Am J Surg 1984; 147: 432
13. Bagwell CE. Surg Gynecol Obstet 1981; 152: 350
14. Gale T. Certaine Workes of Chirurgerie. Hall, London, 1563. Reproduced in facsimile by De Capo Press, New York, 1971
15. Poynter FNL. Selected Writings of William Clowes 1544–1604. Harvey & Blythe, London, 1948

CERTAINE VVORKES
of Chirurgerie, nevvly compiled and
published by Thomas Gale, Maister in Chirurgerie.

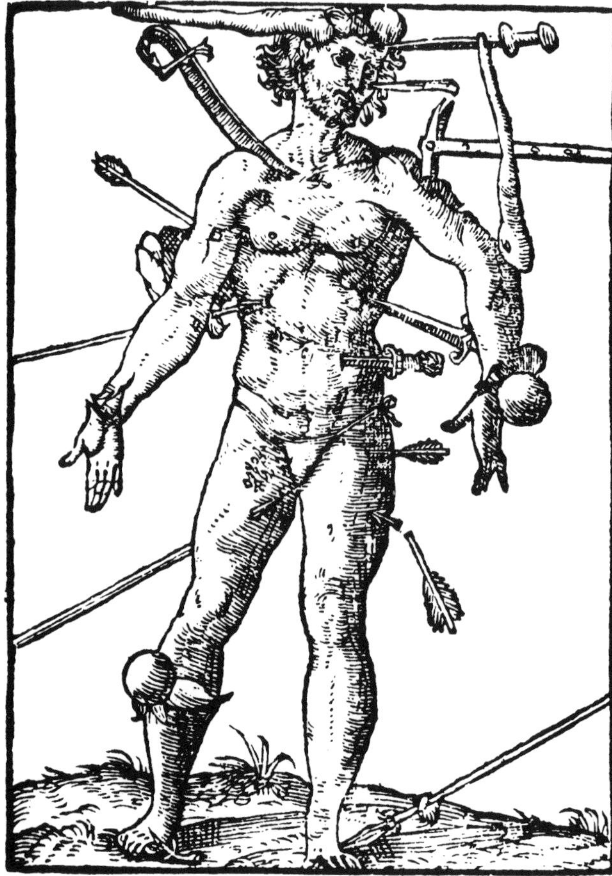

Figure 1.4 The title page of Gale's *Certaine Workes of Chirurgerie* (1563),[14] the first book on surgery written in English. It comprises four parts and contains several illustrations of surgical instruments. The wound man of the title page is seen in many early printed medical books and depicts the injuries that may have confronted a surgeon of the time.

¶ The noble experyence of the vertuous
handy warke of surgeri/practysyd & compyled by the moost experte mayster Iherome of Bruynswyke/borne in Straeßborowe in Almayne/ y which hath it fyrst proued/and trewly founde by his awne dayly experyenge. ¶ Item there after he hath authoryzed and done it to vnderstande thrugh the trewe sentences of the olde doctours and maysters very experte in the scyence of Surgery/As Galienus/Ipocras/Auicenna/Gwydo/Haly abbas/Lancfrancus of myllen/Iamericus/Rogerius/Albucasis/Placetinus/Brunus/Gwylhelmus de saliceto/& by many other maysters whose names be wrytten in this same boke. ¶ Here also shall ye fynde for to cure & hele all wounded mẽbres/and other swellynges. ¶ Item yf ye fynde ony names of herbes or of other thynges wherof ye haue no knowlege/y shall ye knowe playnly by the potecarys. ¶ Item Here shall you fynde also for to make salues/plasters/powders/oyles/and drynkes for woundes. ¶ Item who so desyreth of this science y playne knowlege let hym oftentymes rede this boke/ and than he shall gette perfyte vnderstandynge of the noble surgery.

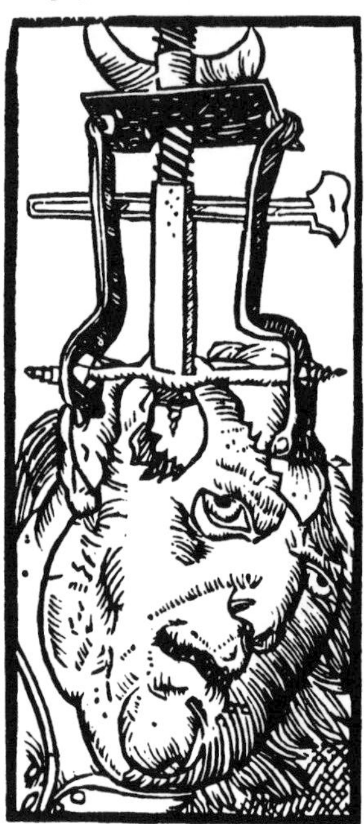

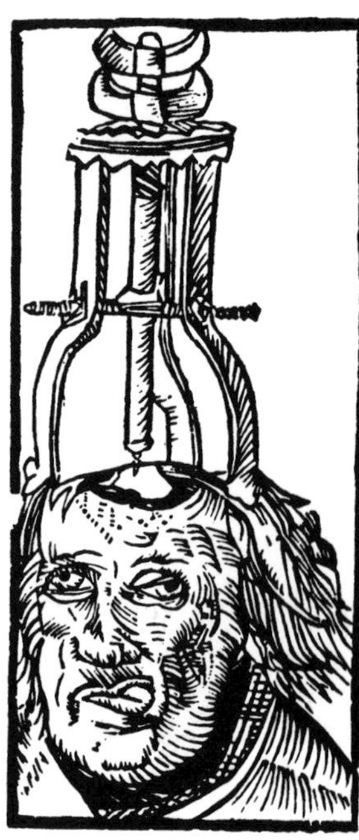

Figure 1.5 The title page of the English translation of *Das Buch der Cirurgie* (1525) by Hieronymous Brunschwig. The translator is unknown. Originally published in Strasburg in 1497, the English version is notable for its many dramatic woodcut illustrations. The text is mainly concerned with military surgery.

before the discovery of vitamin C.[16] But quackery abounded and to improve standards, Henry VIII assented to the union of barbers and surgeons. In 1540 the Barber-Surgeon's Company was founded, the forerunner of the Royal College of Surgeons of England.[17] The Company laid down strict rules both for barbers and for surgeons and imposed fines on unlicensed surgical practitioners in London as well as introducing an examination for surgeons at the end of their apprenticeship. This represented the start of formal surgical education.

THE 17TH AND 18TH CENTURIES

The 250 years after the Renaissance were marked by the consolidation and refinement of techniques and knowledge rather than by spectacular advances. For example, the use of skin flaps in amputation was introduced in 1679 by a naval surgeon from Plymouth,[18] and this technique gradually became more widely used, although in military practice the old circular method remained in favour, when the raw stump was allowed to heal by secondary intention.

Harvey's publication of *De Motu Cordis* in 1628 provided a major impetus to the understanding of circulatory physiology, although this work had no immediate impact on the practice of surgery.[19] Before this time, blood had been thought to ebb and flow through the heart but Harvey observed that the venous, aortic and pulmonary valves allowed blood to flow in only one direction. He reasoned that the blood must circulate through the body even though the capillaries were unknown to him and were not discovered until after his death.

Early attempts at blood transfusion, first in dogs and sheep and then between animals and humans, took place in Oxford and Paris in the mid 17th century.[20] Samuel Pepys makes reference to

REFERENCES

16. Appleby JH. Med Hist 1981; 25: 51
17. Dobson J, Walker RM. Barbers and Barber-Surgeons of London. Blackwell, Oxford, 1979
18. Poynter FNL (ed). The Journal of James Yonge (1647–1721) Plymouth Surgeon. Longmans, London, 1963
19. Keynes G. The Life of William Harvey. Clarendon Press, Oxford, 1966
20. Farr AD. Med Hist 1980; 24: 143

these experiments in his diary for 1667, when he writes of meeting a 32-year-old Bachelor of Divinity at Cambridge who had been transfused with the blood of a sheep by Fellows of the Royal Society and paid 20 shillings for the experience. Pepys comments that the patient was 'cracked a little in his head, though he speaks very reasonably and very well'.[21]

Lithotomy was perhaps the elective operation most often performed at this time.[22] Vesical calculus was common and exceptionally painful owing to the associated cystitis and trigonitis. For this reason many patients submitted themselves to the ordeal of the operation and, although most survived, many were left with a urinary fistula. William Cheselden of London, the author of the foremost anatomical textbook of the time, was a noted lithotomist and could perform the operation in a minute or less.[23] In 1740, he published his results in 213 patients cut publicly in front of an audience;[24] 105 were under the age of 10 years. Of the first 50 only three died; of the second 50, three; of the third 50, eight; and of the last 63, six. Cheselden explained that the reason so few died in the early part of the series was because at that time only good-risk patients came forward for the operation. Later, when the good results became known, poor-risk patients volunteered. This account is a noteworthy early example of honest surgical audit.

Many well-known names in the history of surgery date from the 18th century, with John Hunter being arguably the most famous and certainly the most important.[25] He was a man with an original mind, astonishing industry and a colourful character. Hunter was the first surgeon to apply experimental method to surgery, especially with his work on inflammation and ligature of arteries in cases of aneurysm. He brought the study of pathology and physiology to surgery, which previously had been based almost exclusively on anatomy. He dissected animals as well as humans, examined diseased parts as well as normal anatomy, and built up a vast collection of specimens of comparative anatomy and pathology that forms the basis of the Hunterian Museum in the Royal College of Surgeons of England. He influenced the development of surgery for decades after his death, not only by his writings but also through the work of his pupils, many of whom became leading surgeons.

One of Hunter's best-known pupils was Sir Astley Cooper, who wrote classic texts on hernias, dislocation and fractures of joints, diseases of the testis and breast, and the anatomy of the thymus gland.[26] He was the first surgeon to ligate the aorta for iliac aneurysm (Fig. 1.6), the first to perform a through-hip amputation, and one of the last great surgeons who felt the necessity to dissect the human body on a regular daily basis. He stated, 'if I laid my head upon my pillow at night without having dissected something that day I should think I had lost that day'. Unfortunately the supply of cadavers for such dissections was limited to the bodies of executed criminals, and this shortage of material led to the rise of the body snatcher or resurrectionist, who dug up freshly buried bodies at night from churchyard graves.[27] However, when the notorious Burke and Hare murders in Scotland started to supply the surgeon's dissecting room, public outcry led to the introduction of the Anatomy Act of 1832 in Great Britain and Ireland, and this regularized the supply of bodies for anatomical study.[28]

ANAESTHESIA AND ANTISEPSIS

The introduction of general anaesthesia in 1846[29] in the USA and the expounding of the principles of antisepsis by Lister in Scotland in 1867[30] were two of the most fundamental advances in the history of surgery and transformed the image of the profession. In the early 19th century, operations were infrequently performed because they were dangerous, painful, and had a high complication rate.[31] Although we can read of the triumphs of a few great surgeons, we read little of their disasters or the poor results of many lesser surgeons. Sepsis was almost universal. The surgeon had to operate rapidly to minimize shock and reduce excessive haemorrhage. Operations took place only once a week at most hospitals, when two or three operations would be performed before a large audience. For example, in 1831 a surgeon at Guy's Hospital in London excised a tumour weighing 56 lb (25 kg) in front of an audience of 680 onlookers. The death of the patient was ascribed by the *Lancet* to prolonged exposure in an atmosphere so poisoned by human exhalations that many onlookers were pale as death and near to fainting.[32]

The range of operative procedures was limited: tuberculosis, aneurysms, surface tumours, cataracts and abscesses accounted for most of the operations. Contrary to popular belief, a major amputation was unusual. Mortality was high, sometimes amounting to 60% for more extensive procedures. The surgeon needed to be a man of special demeanour and courage, and to have great physical strength in order to reduce dislocations, set fractures, and operate with great speed on the conscious patient. Surgery was universally considered to be of lower status than medicine, and physicians and surgeons did not rank equal in the eyes of society or each other. By the end of the 19th century, however, this picture had changed profoundly.

ANAESTHESIA

The early history of anaesthesia is long and convoluted, and has been admirably described elsewhere.[33] Soporific sponges soaked in herbs were used by the ancients to deaden pain, as were alcohol and opium. Morphine, named after Morpheus, the god of dreams, was discovered in 1805.[34] Humphrey Davy, later of chemistry fame, discovered the anaesthetic properties of nitrous oxide in 1799, and in the following year suggested that this gas might be used with advantage in surgical operations,[35] but his

REFERENCES

21. Latham R (ed). The Shorter Pepys. Bell and Hyman, London, 1986
22. Ellis HA. History of Bladder Stone. Blackwell, Oxford, 1969
23. Cope Z. William Cheselden. Livingstone, Edinburgh, 1953
24. Cheselden W. The Anatomy of the Human Body. 5th edn. Bowyer, London, 1740
25. Qvist G. John Hunter 1728–1793. Heinemann, London, 1981
26. Brock RC. The Life and Work of Astley Cooper. Livingstone, Edinburgh, 1952
27. Ball JM. The Sack-'em-up Men: An Account of the Rise and Fall of the Modern Resurrectionists. Oliver and Boyd, Edinburgh, 1928
28. Richardson R. Death, Dissection and the Destitute. Routledge & Kegan Paul, London, 1987
29. Bigelow HJ. Boston Med Surg J 1846; 35: 309
30. Lister J. Lancet 1867; i: 326
31. Jackson BT. Guy's Hosp Rep 1971; 120: 229
32. Leading article. Lancet 1830–1831; ii: 83
33. Duncum BM. The Development of Inhalational Anaesthesia. Oxford University Press, London, 1947
34. Sertürner FWA. J Pharm (Lpz) 1805; 14: 47
35. Davy H. Researches, Chemical and Philosophical, Chiefly Concerning Nitrous Oxide. Johnson, London, 1800. Reprinted by Butterworths, London, 1972

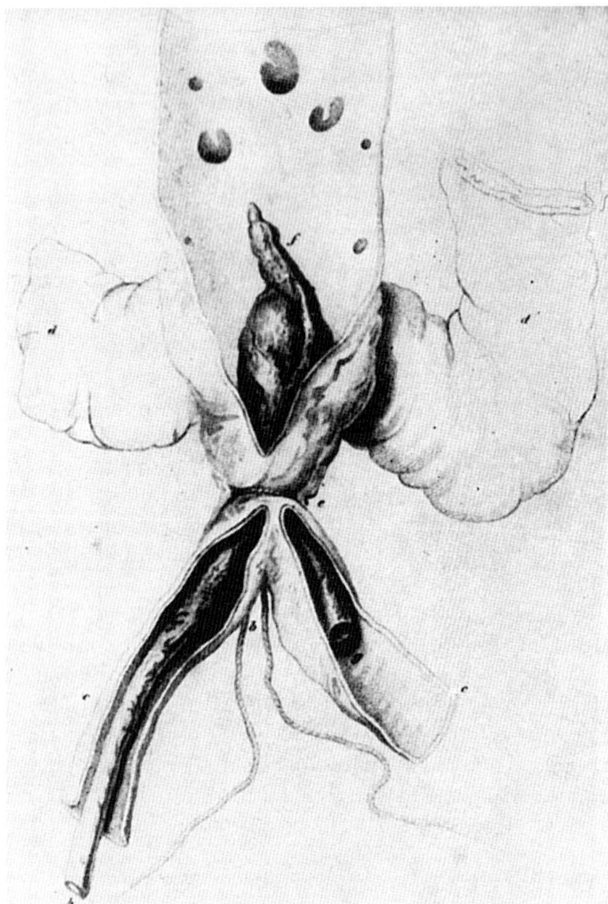

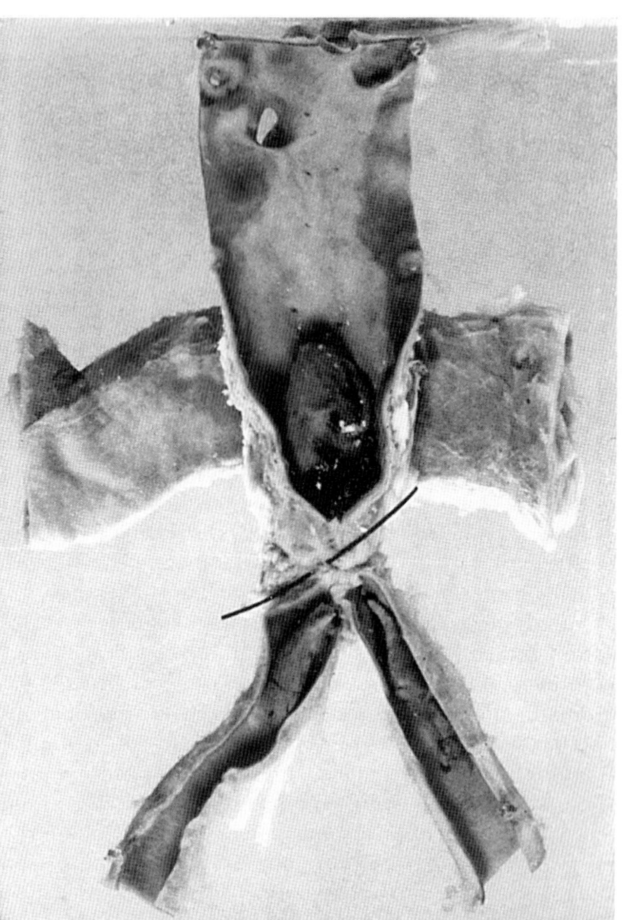

Figure 1.6 **(a)** A plate from *Surgical Essays* (1818) by Astley Cooper and Benjamin Travers, in which Cooper reported the first ligation of the human aorta. The operation was performed by Cooper in Guy's Hospital in 1817 on a 38-year-old man with a ruptured aneurysm extending from the left common iliac artery to the femoral artery. The patient survived for 40 hours. **(b)** The original specimen now preserved in the Astley Cooper pathological collection at Guy's Hospital, London.

suggestion was not followed up. Instead, nitrous oxide was used as laughing gas to enliven parties and dull lectures.

Inhalational anaesthesia was probably first used some 40 years later in 1842, when an American medical student, William Clark, administered ether to enable a tooth to be painlessly extracted. In the same year, Crawford Long of Georgia removed a small cyst from the neck of a patient under the influence of ether. Neither of these events was written up at the time, however, and the wider introduction of anaesthesia had to wait a little longer.

Horace Wells, a dentist, used nitrous oxide to extract teeth in 1844, but the credit for the true realization of the importance of inhalational ether as an anaesthetic agent is now generally credited to William Morton, another dentist, who on 16 October 1846 in Boston administered ether to a young man named Gilbert Abbott, while John Collins Warren, surgeon at the Massachusetts General Hospital, removed a vascular malformation from his neck. Several more painless operations were performed in Boston in the next few days, and a month later the discovery was published.[29] Within another month the news had crossed the Atlantic, and Robert Liston performed an above-knee amputation under ether anaesthetic at University College Hospital, London, on 21 December 1846.[36] By February 1847, the *Lancet* and other journals were reporting operations performed under ether from all parts of Britain, and most European centres were also using the technique. Chloroform, introduced by James Young Simpson of Edinburgh in the same year,[37] rapidly superseded ether as the most widely used anaesthetic. Despite the rapid spread of the technique, however, anaesthesia was slow to develop as a specialty. For years it was considered sufficient for the house surgeon to give the anaesthetic, and most hospitals did not appoint a consultant anaesthetist until well into the 20th century.

The rapid acceptance of anaesthesia perhaps stemmed in part from the general trend towards humanitarianism that was taking place in the mid-19th century. Reforms in public health, education, the prisons, and the almshouses, and the drive against drunkenness all had their origin in the wish to improve the human condition. Florence Nightingale, the founder of the modern nursing profession, was largely inspired by the desire to improve the lot of the common soldier after seeing at first hand the appalling conditions under which soldiers lived and fought during the Crimean war.[38]

ANTISEPSIS

Anaesthesia was speedily accepted; the greater advance of antisepsis and the germ theory of infection had a more difficult

REFERENCES

36. Cock FW. Am J Surg (Anaesthesia Suppl) 1915; 29: 98
37. Simpson JY. Lancet 1847; ii: 549
38. Goldie SM (ed). Florence Nightingale in the Crimean War 1854–56. Manchester University Press, Manchester, 1987

and lengthy gestation. Before Lister, surgeons and patients alike accepted that almost all wounds became septic and visible pus was called 'laudable', for if the wound was draining freely, infection was less likely to loculate and cause septicaemia. The cause of the sepsis was unknown. As early as 1546, Fracastoro of Verona, now better known for his naming and recognition of syphilis, had postulated the presence in the air of invisible particles that carried disease.[39] As there was no objective evidence that such particles existed, his theory was not accepted. The development of microscopy in the 17th century[40] enabled micro-organisms to be seen, but it still took some time for these to be accepted as the cause of infection, largely because of the theory of spontaneous generation, which postulated that the micro-organisms present in diseased and necrotic tissue had arisen *de novo*.

In 1846, the same year that general anaesthesia was discovered, Ignaz Semelweiss, an Austrian obstetrician working in Vienna, noted that there was a higher incidence of puerperal fever in the ward where medical students examined patients without washing their hands than in another ward where midwives, who had a higher standard of personal hygiene, attended the patient.[41] In the following year, he observed that the post-mortem appearance of one of his colleagues, who died after cutting his finger during a necropsy, was similar to that of the cadaver his colleagues had been examining. Semelweiss realized that a transmissible agent was responsible for the infection and instituted a rigorous policy of hand-washing in calcium chloride solution, after which the maternal mortality dropped from 10% to 1.2% within a year. Regrettably, his views were not accepted by the majority of his colleagues; he met with strong personal criticism, became mentally ill, and died at the age of 47.

Joseph Lister, later Lord Lister, the first surgical peer, held the chair of surgery in Glasgow when he began his work on the use of carbolic acid in the prevention of infection. He was influenced in his research by the work of Louis Pasteur, published in the early 1860s, which showed that putrefaction and fermentation were caused by micro-organisms carried in the air and on dust.[42] Lister reasoned that sepsis might be prevented if these micro-organisms could be killed. After preliminary experiments with other chemicals, Lister learned that in Carlisle the obnoxious smell of sewage had been notably reduced by treatment with carbolic acid, and that an outbreak of typhoid in the city had rapidly subsided at the same time. He therefore tried out carbolic acid as a topical dressing in patients with compound fractures of the leg, a condition that hitherto had usually been treated by amputation. Lister published his results in the *Lancet* in 1867 (Fig. 1.7).[30] Eleven patients were described: nine did well, one needed amputation, and one died. Lister followed up this first report with numerous lectures and further publications, continually refining the technical details of his method. He was a perfectionist and it is generally believed that it was his scrupulous attention to detail that enabled his results to be better than those of some of his detractors.

The acceptance of Lister's work was not universal. Some surgeons quickly became converts to his teaching (Fig. 1.8), while others were sceptical.[44] By and large, his British contemporaries were slow to adapt while overseas surgeons, especially those in Germany, were rapid converts. The reasons for hesitation were several: the method relied on great attention to detail and therefore was slow; carbolic acid was unpleasant, causing irritation to the wounds and carboluria if contact was prolonged; the method was expensive; and probably most importantly there was a failure by many surgeons to understand fully the theory of infection.

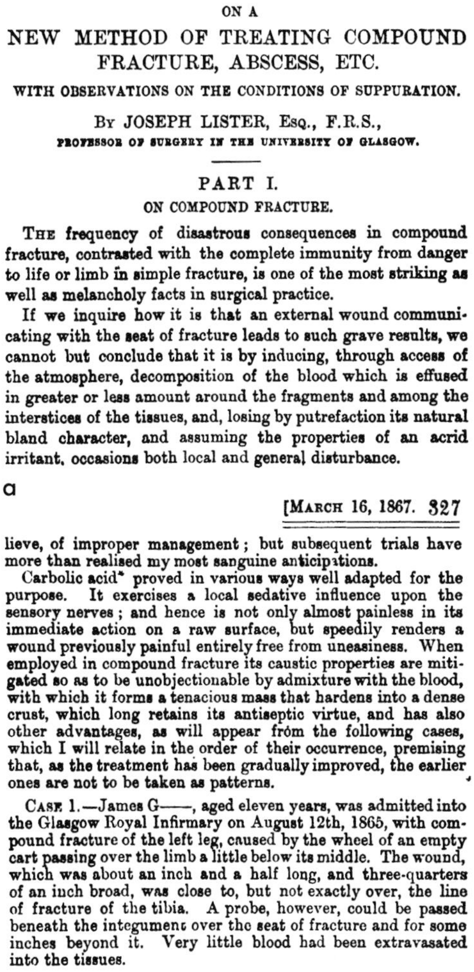

ON A
NEW METHOD OF TREATING COMPOUND FRACTURE, ABSCESS, ETC.
WITH OBSERVATIONS ON THE CONDITIONS OF SUPPURATION.
BY JOSEPH LISTER, ESQ., F.R.S.,
PROFESSOR OF SURGERY IN THE UNIVERSITY OF GLASGOW.

PART I.
ON COMPOUND FRACTURE.

THE frequency of disastrous consequences in compound fracture, contrasted with the complete immunity from danger to life or limb in simple fracture, is one of the most striking as well as melancholy facts in surgical practice.

If we inquire how it is that an external wound communicating with the seat of fracture leads to such grave results, we cannot but conclude that it is by inducing, through access of the atmosphere, decomposition of the blood which is effused in greater or less amount around the fragments and among the interstices of the tissues, and, losing by putrefaction its natural bland character, and assuming the properties of an acrid irritant, occasions both local and general disturbance.

a

[MARCH 16, 1867. 327

lieve, of improper management; but subsequent trials have more than realised my most sanguine anticipations.

Carbolic acid* proved in various ways well adapted for the purpose. It exercises a local sedative influence upon the sensory nerves; and hence is not only almost painless in its immediate action on a raw surface, but speedily renders a wound previously painful entirely free from uneasiness. When employed in compound fracture its caustic properties are mitigated so as to be unobjectionable by admixture with the blood, with which it forms a tenacious mass that hardens into a dense crust, which long retains its antiseptic virtue, and has also other advantages, as will appear from the following cases, which I will relate in the order of their occurrence, premising that, as the treatment has been gradually improved, the earlier ones are not to be taken as patterns.

CASE 1.—James G——, aged eleven years, was admitted into the Glasgow Royal Infirmary on August 12th, 1865, with compound fracture of the left leg, caused by the wheel of an empty cart passing over the limb a little below its middle. The wound, which was about an inch and a half long, and three-quarters of an inch broad, was close to, but not exactly over, the line of fracture of the tibia. A probe, however, could be passed beneath the integument over the seat of fracture and for some inches beyond it. Very little blood had been extravasated into the tissues.

b

Figure 1.7 (a) The beginning of Lister's historic article in the *Lancet* of 16 March 1867, in which he introduced the theory of antisepsis. (b) The first reference in the article to carbolic acid and details of the injury of the first patient to be treated by the new method. Arguably the most important patient of the 19th century, young James Greenlees made an uncomplicated infection-free recovery from a condition that normally necessitated amputation.

Over a period of 20 years, however, Lister's contributions became widely accepted and antisepsis gradually gave way to asepsis, a technique particularly associated with the name of von Bergmann of Berlin, who introduced steam sterilization of gowns and dressings in the 1880s and who tried to make the operating theatre germ-free.[45] The introduction of rubber surgical gloves is popularly credited to William Halsted,[46] but rubber gloves were being used in the operating theatre by a number of others before this time.[47] Gauze face-masks were probably first worn by Berger in Paris in 1897.[48] By the turn of the century, operating theatres were designed according to aseptic principles, with easily washable walls and floors, absence of awkward angles, a reduced spectator area, running water, sterilizers and filtered air ventila-

REFERENCES

39. Meade RH. An Introduction to the History of General Surgery. WB Saunders, Philadelphia, 1968
40. Clay RS, Court TH. The History of the Microscope. Griffiths, London, 1932
41. Wheeler ES. Am J Surg 1974; 127: 573
42. Guthrie D. Lord Lister, His Life and Doctrine. Livingstone, Edinburgh, 1949
43. Jackson BT. Ann R Coll Surg Eng 1974; 54: 189
44. Leading article. Lancet 1882; i: 1088
45. von Bergmann E. Ther Mh 1887; 1: 41
46. Halsted WS. Johns Hopkins Hosp Rep 1890–1891; 2: 308
47. Miller JM. Surgery 1982; 92: 541
48. Berger P. Bull Soc Chirurgiens Paris 1899; 25: 187

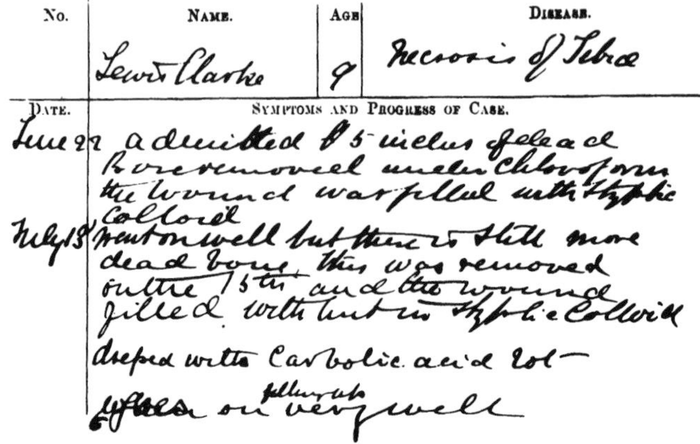
No. | Name. | Age | Disease.
Lewis Clarke | 9 | Necrosis of Tibia
Date. | Symptoms and Progress of Case.
dead bone this was removed
dressed with Carbolic acid Sol—

Figure 1.8 An extract dated 13 July (1867) from the case book of Thomas Kendall, surgeon in King's Lynn, Norfolk, describing the use of carbolic acid dressings some 4 months after Lister's paper had been published. Kendall is believed to be one of the first converts to Lister's antiseptic method. (From Jackson 1974,[43] copyright The Royal College of Surgeons of England. Reproduced with permission.)

tion (Fig. 1.9).[49] Lister lived to declare open some of these new theatres; when he died in 1912 he was internationally famous.

THE POST-LISTERIAN ERA

The general acceptance of asepsis marks a watershed in the history of surgery. The several thousand years of surgical knowledge before Lister can be summarized reasonably easily, but the hundred years after Lister have encompassed such an explosion of knowledge and scientific advance that greater selection and condensation of the developments become inevitable. By the turn of the 19th century the practice of surgery had been transformed, not only by Lister but also by developments in other scientific disciplines. Most of today's standard operations in abdominal surgery were regularly performed, while operations on the brain, the lungs and the heart had all been recorded. Elective hernia repair was starting to replace the truss. Electric lighting not only gave better illumination in the operating theatre but also enabled inspection of body cavities through primitive endoscopes such as the electric cystoscope, an instrument introduced by Nitze (Fig. 1.10).[51] Diagnostic imaging had begun with the discovery of X-rays by Röntgen in 1895,[53] and therapeutic radiology was introduced soon afterwards, first for benign skin conditions[54] and subsequently in the treatment of cancer.[55] Microscopy had been used to study and classify the resected surgical specimens and the science of bacteriology was in its infancy. Publicity for these advances had been aided by the increased speed of transmission of scientific information: telegraphy was widely used, scientific journals were increasing in number, photography was applied to medicine (Fig. 1.11), and the age of steam enabled easy travel for surgeons to visit clinics and colleagues in different countries.

ABDOMINAL SURGERY

Various operations on the contents of the abdominal cavity were occasionally reported before the last quarter of the 19th century, but only colostomy and ovariotomy were performed with any regularity. Littré of Paris was the first to suggest elective colostomy after he performed a necropsy on an infant with congenital anal atresia in 1710,[57] but the operation was not carried out

REFERENCES

49. Wangensteen OH, Wangensteen SD. Surgery 1975; 77: 403
50. Jackson BT. St Thomas's Hosp Gazette 1978; 76: 8
51. Nitze M. Wien Med Wochenschr 1879; 29: 649
52. Nitze M. Lehrbuch der Kystoskopie. Bergmann, Wiesbaden, 1889
53. Röntgen WC. SB Phys-Med Ges Würzburg 1895; 137: 132. English translation Nature 1896; 53: 274
54. Freund L. Wien Klin Wochenschr 1897; 10: 73
55. Lazarus-Barlow WS. Br Med J 1909; 1: 1465
56. Nitze M. Kystophotographischer Atlas. Bergmann, Wiesbaden, 1894
57. Dinnick T. Br J Surg 1934; 22: 142

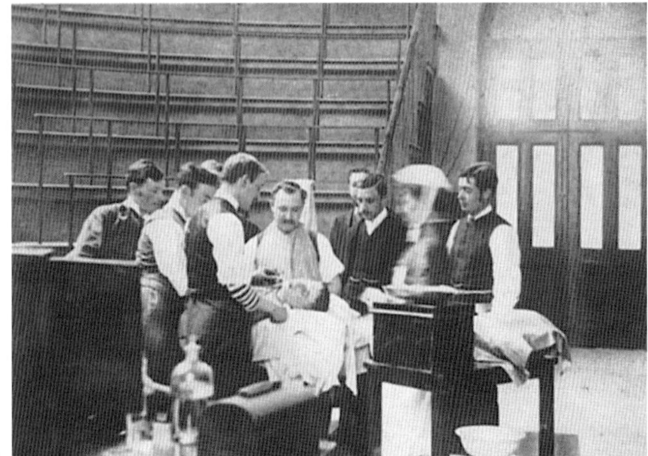
a

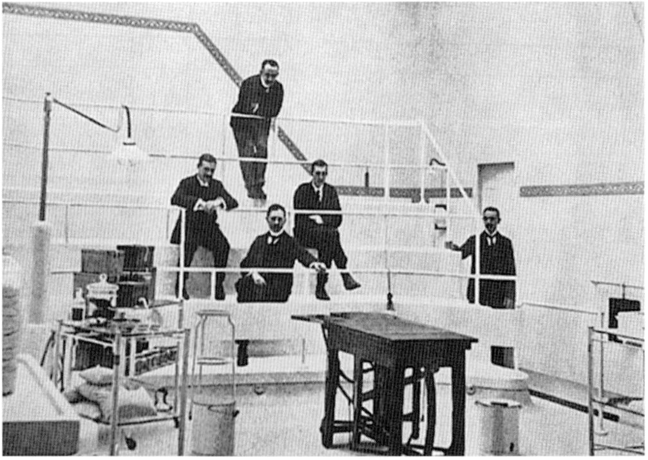
b

Figure 1.9 The operating theatre of St Thomas's Hospital, London, before and after the acceptance of Lister's teachings. **(a)** In the 1880s: the doors opened directly on to the main hospital corridor and the wooden spectator standings could accommodate 200 visitors. Wooden beams supported the roof 13.5 metres above the floor and the lighting was by gas. The theatre was regularly used by medical students for entertainment! **(b)** The same theatre in 1901, after conversion to incorporate the principles of asepsis. It was declared open by Lister himself. The floor and walls were tiled, the small spectator area was made of white marble, and positive-pressure ventilation was present throughout. Note that the wooden operating table had not yet been upgraded. (From Jackson BT 1978,[50] with permission.)

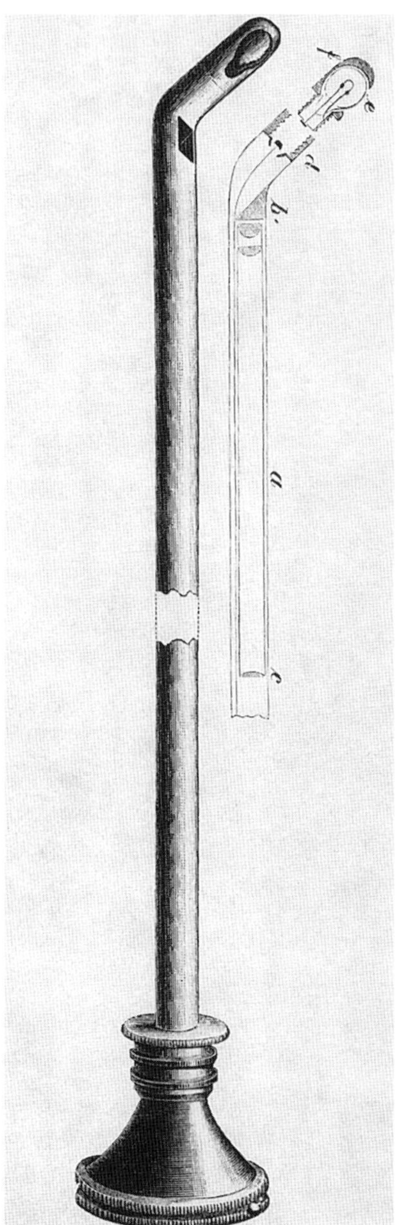

Figure 1.10 Max Nitze of Berlin demonstrated the forerunner of the modern cystoscope at a meeting in Dresden. The illumination was by means of an incandescent platinum loop, which required a cumbersome cooling system. This was soon replaced by a small carbon-filament bulb, which gave a much improved view of the bladder. Earlier instruments had been illuminated by reflected light, usually from a candle, down a silvered hollow tube. This illustration from Nitze's book on cystoscopy is designed to show the electrical features of his instrument rather than the cystoscope itself. (From Nitze 1889.[52])

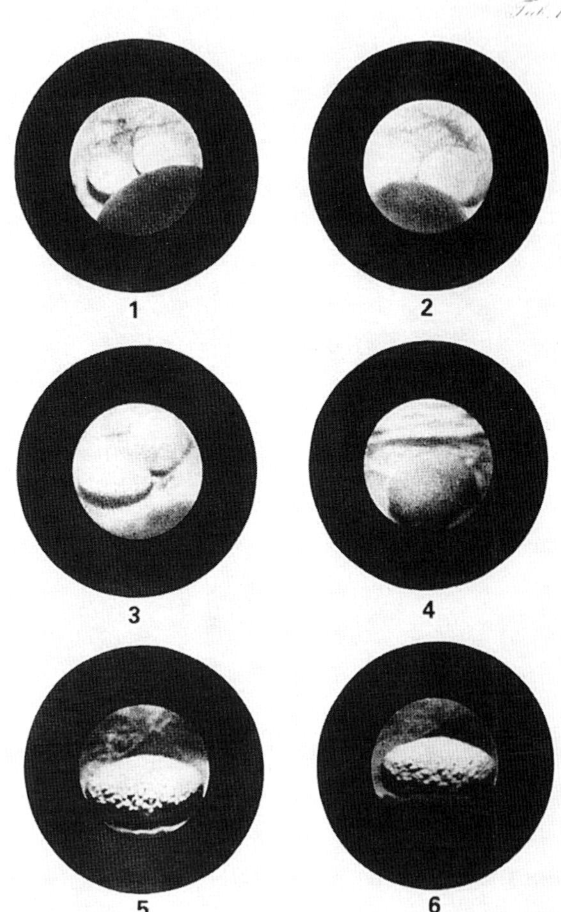

Figure 1.11 Photography was utilized in the teaching of clinical medicine from the early 1850s but did not have widespread use in surgical books and articles until towards the end of the century; most Victorian publications were illustrated by wood or steel engravings. These photographs of stones in the human urinary bladder are from an early atlas of endoscopy and were the first published photographs taken through a cystoscope. (From Nitze 1894.[56])

successfully until 1793.[58] During the next 50 years colostomy was performed through a transperitoneal approach by a number of surgeons, notably in France, but with few survivors. In 1839 Amussat of Paris reviewed the literature and, not unexpectedly, found that most of the deaths resulted from peritonitis.[59] This led him to devise an extraperitoneal colostomy fashioned in the lumbar region, which soon became the standard technique and was practised for the next 40 years until transperitoneal operations became safe with the introduction of antisepsis.

Ovariotomy, now called ovarian cystectomy, was first performed by a general practitioner surgeon named Ephraim McDowell of Kentucky in 1809.[60] A giant cyst weighing over 3 kg was removed after preliminary incision and drainage of nearly 7 kg of gelatinous content. The operation took 25 minutes, during which time the patient sang hymns and recited psalms to boost her morale. Amazingly, she lived for 32 years after her ordeal. In the UK the most notable ovariotomist was Thomas Spencer Wells. His results, published in 1880,[61] showed that his operative mortality dropped dramatically after the adoption of Lister's techniques. In his first 500 cases there was a 25.4% mortality; in the next 300 a mortality of 25.6%; and in his final 100, when antisepsis had been introduced, a mortality of 11%. Spencer Wells is now best known for his artery forceps, the final design of which he introduced in 1879.[62]

A large number of surgeons contributed to the rapid development of abdominal surgery during the last three decades of the 19th century. One name, Theodore Billroth, must be singled out as, by common consent, he is regarded as the father of abdominal surgery.[63] A graduate of Berlin University, Billroth was not only an outstanding surgical innovator but also a man of culture and an able musician. A pianist and violinist, he played

REFERENCES

58. Duret C. Rec Périod Soc Med Paris 1798; 4: 45
59. Amussat JZ. Mémoire sur la Possibilité d'établir un Anus artificiel dans la Région lombaire sans pénétrer dans le Péritoine. Baillière, Paris, 1839
60. Ellis H. Famous Operations. Harval, Pennsylvania, 1984
61. Leading article. Br Med J 1880; 1: 931
62. Wells TS. Br Med J 1879; 1: 926
63. Rutledge RH. Surgery 1979; 86: 672

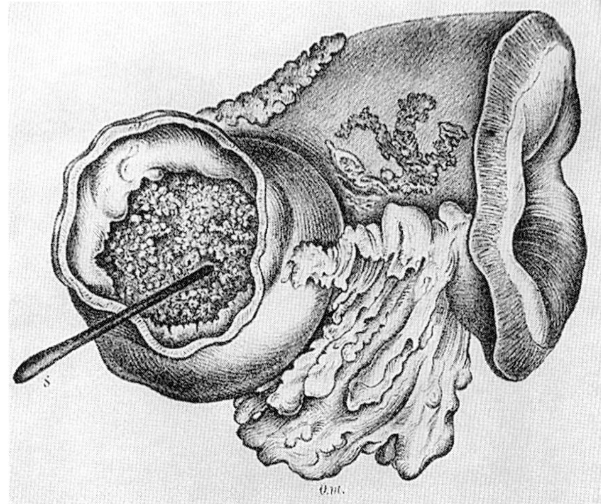

a

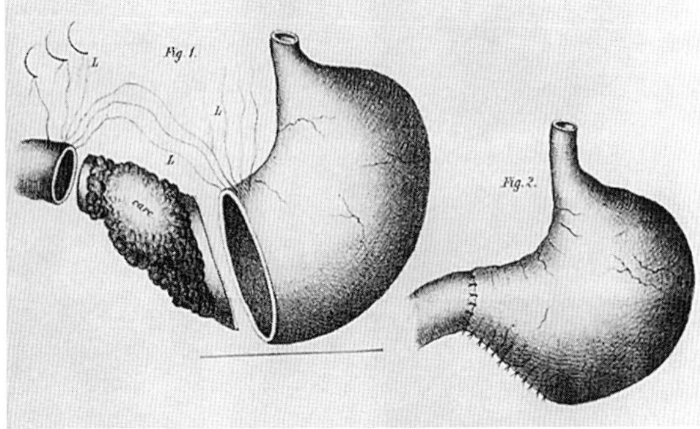

b

Figure 1.12 The first successful partial gastrectomy. This was performed by Billroth on 29 January 1881 on a 43-year-old woman with pyloric stenosis caused by a carcinoma. (**a**) The resected specimen showing the carcinoma almost totally obstructing the antrum. A probe passes through the lumen. (**b**) The method of reconstruction. Sixty-four carbolized silk sutures were used, most being serosa to serosa as described by Lembert but a few including the mucosa. No drain was inserted but carbolic acid–soaked swabs were used throughout. The operation lasted 1$^1/_2$ hours. Wine enemas were given during the first 2 weeks after operation, but by 3 weeks the patient was able to eat a cutlet and a beefsteak. Sadly, the patient died of recurrent disease 4 months later. (From Billroth 1881.[67])

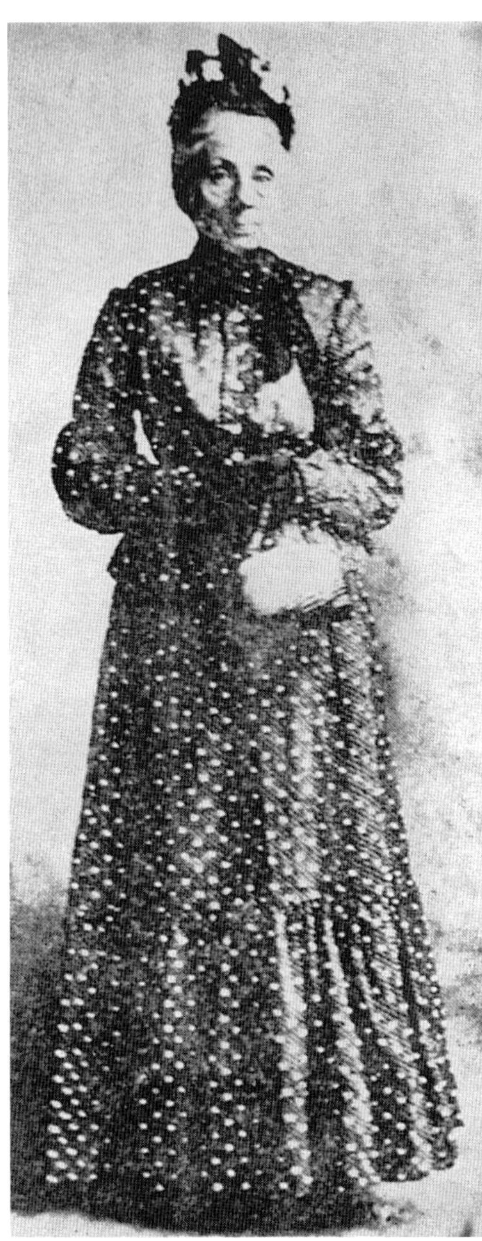

Figure 1.13 Mary Wiggins Burnsworth aged 68. In 1867, 38 years before this photograph was taken, Mrs Burnsworth was the first patient to undergo cholecystotomy and removal of gallstones. About 50 stones were removed, but one was left behind and was the cause of occasional abdominal discomfort in succeeding years. The operation was performed under chloroform anaesthesia by John Bobbs and was carried out on the third floor of a local drugstore in Indianapolis. It was not performed again for another 11 years. Mrs Burnsworth died in 1913, aged 77. (From Sparkman RS. Bobbs centennial: the first cholecystotomy. Surgery 1967; 61: 965. Reproduced with permission from Elsevier.[69])

chamber music with Brahms, who dedicated two of his string quartets to him. Appointed Professor of Surgery in Vienna in 1867, his voluminous writings contributed to his fame. In 1872 he was the first to perform total resection of the oesophagus,[64] and 2 years later the first to perform a total laryngectomy.[65] He is best known, however, for the first successful partial gastrectomy for cancer of the pylorus, which he performed in 1881 (Fig. 1.12).[66] Paradoxically, he at first resisted the introduction of Lister's methods on his unit, although he later adopted them enthusiastically.

Surgery of the gallbladder was developing alongside surgery of the stomach and intestine. In 1867 a little-known surgeon in Indianapolis, John Bobbs, was the first to perform a cholecystotomy and remove gallstones,[68] although it must be recorded that during the same operation he was also the first surgeon known to leave a stone behind! Nevertheless, the patient lived virtually symptom-free for a further 46 years (Fig. 1.13).[69] The first successful cholecystectomy was performed 15 years later, in 1882, by Carl Langenbuch of Berlin.[70]

The first elective appendicectomy was almost certainly that performed in 1880 by Lawson Tait of Birmingham but not recorded until 10 years later.[71] In 1886 the pathologist Reginald Fitz of Harvard classified the pathology of appendicitis, a name he coined, and distinguished it unequivocally from inflammation of the caecum.[72] Important as these details are, it is for another

REFERENCES

64. Billroth T. Arch Klin Chir 1872; 13: 65
65. Gussenbauer C. Arch Klin Chir Berl 1874; 17: 343
66. Billroth T. Wien Med Wochenschr 1881; 31: 161. English translation in Hurwitz A, Degenshein GA (eds). Milestones in Modern Surgery. Hoeber, New York, 1958
67. Billroth T. Clinical Surgery, translated by Dent CT. The New Sydenham Society, London, 1881.
68. Bobbs JS. Trans Med Soc Indiana 1868; 18: 68
69. Sparkman RS. Surgery 1967; 61: 965
70. Langenbuch CJA. Berl Klin Wochenschr 1882; 19: 725. English translation Gastroenterology 1983; 85: 1430
71. Tait RL. Birmingham Med Rev 1890; 27: 27
72. Fitz RH. Trans Assoc Am Physicians 1886; 1: 107

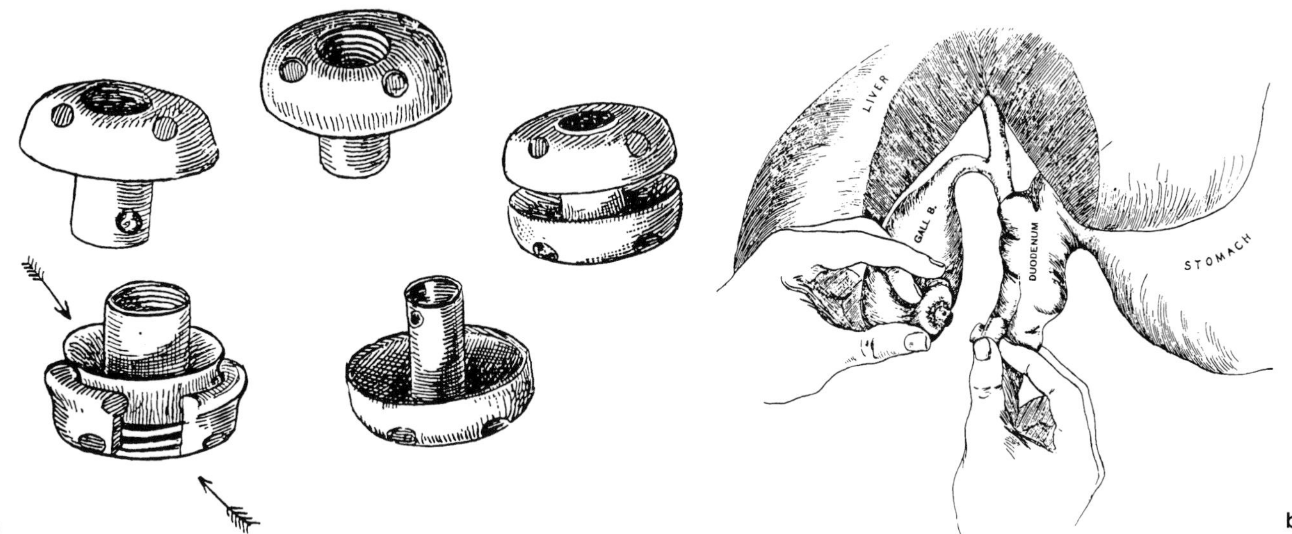

Figure 1.14 (a) The Murphy anastomotic button shown open and assembled. (b) The button in use during a cholecystoduodenostomy. This technique was popular for many years for all types of intestinal anastomosis despite some cases of intestinal obstruction caused by impaction of the device in the ileum. (From Murphy 1892.[76])

reason that acute appendicitis holds a special place in the history of surgery. Despite the enormous advance in the range of operations and the techniques employed, surgery in the early 20th century was still generally looked on with fear and trepidation by the public and not without misgiving by many surgeons. The mortality rate was still high for major operations, and it needed something more than surgical ingenuity to alter public attitude and for surgery to gain widespread acceptance. In the UK this change came about in 1902, with the drainage of an appendix abscess by Frederick Treves of the London Hospital. The patient was King Edward VII and the operation took place 2 days before his intended coronation.[73] The publicity that this operation received probably did more to promote the advance of surgery and to increase the esteem of the surgeon in the mind of patients than any of the far more dramatic events of the previous three decades; public confidence was gained.

ANASTOMOSES, SUTURES AND STAPLES

An early problem in the development of gastrointestinal surgery was to devise a satisfactory method of suturing so as to lessen the likelihood of anastomotic leakage. Antoine Lembert described his well-known seromuscular technique as early as 1826.[74] As gastric and intestinal operations became routine there was renewed interest in surgical technique and many different methods of anastomosis were described, some involving the placement of up to 200 sutures. Various mechanical splinting devices were introduced,[75] including the famous Murphy button, which worked on the principle of a male and a female half being inserted into the open ends to be anastomosed, snapped together by means of a spring, and the serosa lightly closed over the device (Fig. 1.14).[76] A few days later it became detached as a result of pressure necrosis and was passed per rectum. In the late 20th century a similar device made of biofragmentable material was introduced,[77] and mechanical aids for anastomosis in the form of surgical staplers were again to become popular.

A vast assortment of suture and ligature material has been used by surgeons past and present.[78] Two thousand years ago horsehair, cotton, animal sinews, strips of leather, and fibres from the bark of trees were used. Galen refers to the use of catgut and other Roman authors suggested human hair. Silk has been used for a thousand years or more. During the last century surgeons and suture makers have sought the ideal suture material and a succession of synthetic materials, both absorbable and non-absorbable, have been introduced, each one supposedly better than the last.

Just as there are some surgeons today who avoid cutaneous sutures and close the skin with strips of adhesive plaster, so there were similar advocates in the past (Fig. 1.15).

Wire sutures of gold were used in the 16th century and silver wire was used extensively in the 19th century. In the 1930s wires made of annealed iron, aluminium and bronze were available but met with little favour. Stainless steel, although used in the manufacture of some instruments from 1918, was not used as a suture material until the 1950s. The eyeless atraumatic needle with the suture material attached to the end of the needle also dates from this time.

Although first used by Hültl in Budapest in 1908[80] and refined by von Petz in 1924[81] and Friedrich in 1934,[82] stapling instruments have become popular only in the last few decades. This was stimulated by the development of modern instruments by Russian technologists in the 1950s and 1960s. Initially introduced for making end-to-end anastomoses of blood vessels without any narrowing, they were subsequently refined to enable side-to-side

REFERENCES

73. Trombley S. Sir Frederick Treves: The Extra-ordinary Edwardian. Routledge, London, 1989
74. Lembert A. Repert gén Anat Physiol Pathol 1826; 2: 100
75. Ravitch MM. South Med J 1982; 75: 1520
76. Murphy JB. Med Rec (NY) 1892; 42: 665
77. Hardy TG, Pace WG, Maney JW et al. Dis Colon Rectum 1985; 28: 484
78. Goldenberg IS. Surgery 1959; 46: 908
79. Bernard C, Huette C. Illustrated Manual of Operative Surgery and Surgical Anatomy, translated by Van Buren W, Isaacs C. New York, 1857.
80. Hültl H. Pester Med-Chir Presse 1909; 45: 108
81. von Petz A. Zentralbl Chir 1924; 51: 179
82. Friedrich H. Zentralbl Chir 1934; 61: 504

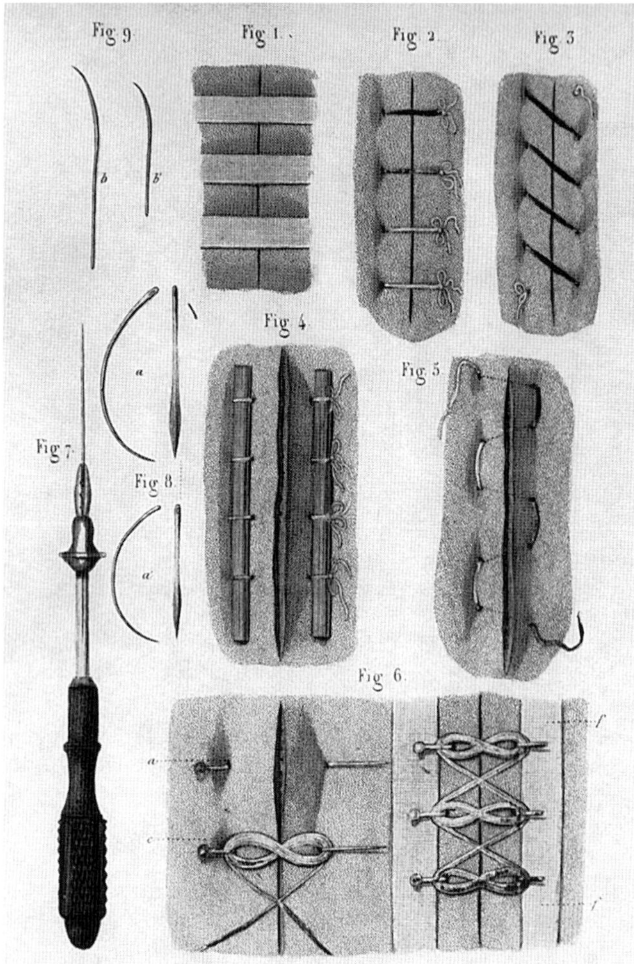

Figure 1.15 Methods of skin approximation used in the mid 19th century. Note that adhesive plaster strips were used as an alternative to sutures. The instrument is an early design of needle holder. (From Bernard and Huette, 1857.[79])

and tangential vascular anastomoses. Instruments for gastrointestinal stapling soon followed and were taken up by instrument makers in other parts of the world, notably the USA.[83]

In the past three decades there have been sporadic attempts to obviate the need for both sutures and staples by substituting fast-acting cyanoacrylate adhesives. These have been used on blood vessels, intestine and skin. The first account of an anastomosis effected by glue was in 1960.[84]

PHYSIOLOGY AND SURGERY

Until the introduction of antisepsis, the successful practice of surgery largely depended on a sound knowledge of anatomy. This was now complemented by advances in physiology, a science that developed rapidly in the 19th century. William Beaumont, an army surgeon in the USA, made important contributions to gastric physiology in the 1820s when he analysed the gastric juice of Alexis St Martin, a patient who had developed a gastrocutaneous fistula after a gunshot wound to the abdomen.[85] Claude Bernard, working in Paris, developed the concept of the *milieu intérieur* in 1859, and made important contributions to the understanding of exocrine pancreatic function, glycogenesis and the vasomotor system.[86] In 1877 the Russian Nicholas Eck described his method of anastomosing the portal vein to the inferior vena cava,[87] the first recorded successful anastomosis between blood vessels. However, Rudolph Virchow arguably eclipsed all these famous names. Although now remembered by surgeons mainly for his eponymous supraclavicular lymph node enlargement and the triad of factors predisposing to vascular thrombosis, Virchow's major importance lies in his being the founder of cellular pathology.[88] He showed that cells were essential components of all living tissues and that each cell had a physiological function. This concept allowed the development of histopathology and enabled surgeons to understand better such fundamental problems as inflammation and wound healing. He also clarified the nature of embolism, was the first to observe and define leukocytosis, and founded an influential medical journal that is still published today (*Virchows Archiv*).[89]

In the early part of the 20th century an understanding of shock was gradually unravelled,[90,91] and the concept of homeostasis was introduced.[92] In the 1950s, Francis Moore in Boston contributed greatly to the realization that metabolism was important in the management of the surgical patient,[93] and this work laid the foundation for the subsequent development of total parenteral nutrition.[94]

NEUROSURGERY

The beginnings of neurosurgery depended greatly on advances in physiology. Apart from trephination, elective surgery on the brain and spinal cord could not develop until accurate anatomical localization of the diseased area could be obtained. This advance depended on the meticulous correlation of neurological physical signs with subsequent post-mortem studies of the underlying disease and, more especially, on physiological experiments in animals when various areas of the brain were electrically stimulated and the resulting effects observed. By the 1870s these studies had advanced sufficiently for several publications detailing the physiological anatomy of the brain to appear.[95]

REFERENCES

83. Steichen FM, Ravitch MM. Curr Probl Surg 1982; 19: 4
84. Nathan HS, Nachlas MM, Soloman RD et al. Ann Surg 1960; 152: 648
85. Beaumont W. Experiments and Observations on the Gastric Juice and the Physiology of Digestion. Allen, Plattsburgh, 1833
86. Franklin KJ. A Short History of Physiology. 2nd edn. Staples Press, London, 1949
87. Eck NV. Voyenno Med J 1877; 130: 2. English translation Surg Gynecol Obstet 1953; 96: 375
88. Virchow RLK. Die Cellularpathologie. Hirschwald, Berlin, 1858. English translation Chance F (tr). Cellular Pathology. Churchill, London, 1860
89. Ackerknecht EH. Rudolf Virchow: Doctor, Statesman, Anthropologist. University of Wisconsin Press, Madison, 1953
90. Crile GW. An Experimental and Clinical Research into Certain Problems Relating to Surgical Operations. JB Lippincott, Philadelphia, 1901
91. Blalock A. Arch Surg (Chicago) 1927; 15: 762
92. Cannon WB. Physiol Rev 1929; 9: 399
93. Moore FD. Metabolic Care of the Surgical Patient. WB Saunders, Philadelphia, 1959
94. Dudrick SJ, Wilmore DW, Vars HM et al. Surgery 1968; 64: 138
95. Walker AE (ed). A History of Neurological Surgery. Williams & Wilkins, Baltimore, 1951

Applying this knowledge, William Macewen of Glasgow was able accurately to diagnose, localize and remove a meningioma from the left frontal lobe of a 14-year-old girl.[96] This operation, performed in 1879, was the first successful excision of a cerebral tumour. Victor Horsley of London was the first to remove successfully an accurately localized tumour of the spinal cord.[97] Enormous interest was generated by these reports, and during the decade 1886–96 more than 500 different surgeons reported operations on the brain, but few were as successful as Macewen or Horsley. Tumours were enucleated roughly with the fingers and haemorrhage from both the brain and the skull was difficult to control, with the result that the mortality was high, probably averaging around 40%.

It was Harvey Cushing of Boston who recognized the need for careful and gentle handling of tissues and the importance of ensuring haemostasis—two fundamental concepts in the prevention of shock, which extended far beyond neurosurgery. Cushing introduced silver clips to control bleeding from the cerebral vessels,[98] and stressed that speed in operating was of itself no virtue. His results justified his slow and bloodless techniques, for in 1915 he was able to publish a series of 130 excisions of brain tumours with a mortality of only 8%.[99] In the mid 1920s Cushing encouraged W. T. Bovie, a physicist, to develop the forerunner of modern electrocautery and introduced the technique into clinical practice, thus reducing blood loss even more.[100] This was perhaps the first application of physics leading to advances in operative technique.

Further developments in neurosurgery depended on advances in radiology, with the introduction of air ventriculography in 1918[101] followed in later years by pneumoencephalography,[102] myelography[103] and cerebral arteriography (Fig. 1.16).[104] Computerized tomography[105] and MRI[106] have now superseded earlier imaging methods.

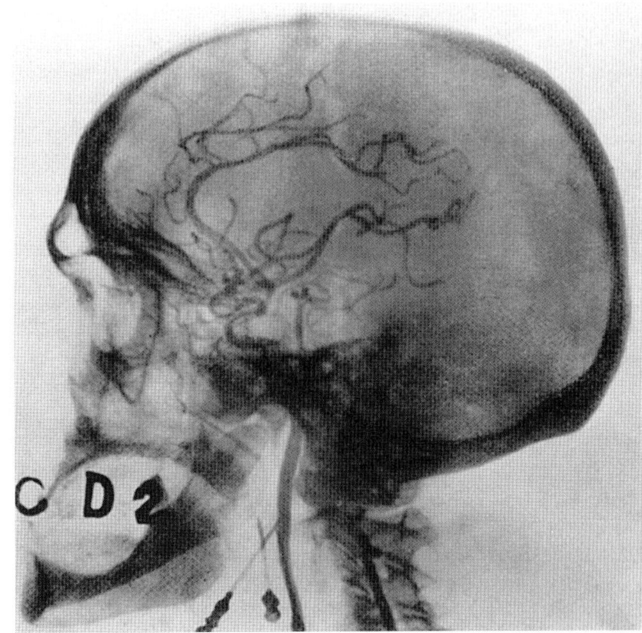

Figure 1.16 Carotid arteriography was introduced by Egas Moniz of Portugal in 1927 as a means of localizing cerebral tumours. He practised the technique in animals and human cadavers before obtaining his first images in the living patient. Nine years later he introduced the operation of prefrontal leucotomy, and in 1949 was awarded a Nobel Prize for his contributions to medicine. This illustration from his first paper on arteriography shows a carotid arteriogram in a cadaver head obtained using a 30% solution of sodium iodide. (From Moniz E: L'encephalographie arterielle: Son importance dans la localisation des tumeurs cerebrales Rev Neurol 2: 72–90, 1927, with permission from Masson Editeur.[104])

THORACIC SURGERY

An understanding of physiology was essential before elective operations on the thoracic contents could be undertaken, for if the pleural cavity was opened the lung collapsed, causing respiratory distress. Early attempts at overcoming this problem were made at the beginning of the 20th century, with the development of endotracheal insufflation anaesthesia.[107] By 1910, primitive positive-pressure anaesthetic apparatus was in use for operations on pulmonary tuberculosis, but there were still difficulties with the risk of over-distension of the lung and also with the build-up of carbon dioxide. A soda-lime absorber was first devised in 1915 but was not widely applied in clinical practice until 10 years later. Some years earlier, Ferdinand Sauerbruch, working in the department of Mikulicz in Breslau, had ingeniously tried a different approach. He devised a large negative-pressure operation chamber that accommodated the patient and the entire surgical team; the patient's head projected to the exterior through a snugly fitting collar, thus allowing atmospheric pressure to inflate the lung.[108] Not surprisingly, the practical difficulties of performing operations in these circumstances limited its acceptance. Sauerbruch also utilized physiological knowledge when in 1913 he was one of the first to describe section of the phrenic nerve to paralyse the diaphragm and so rest the lung in pulmonary tuberculosis.[109]

The surgery of tuberculosis and bronchiectasis accounted for almost all early thoracic operations. Operations for cancer of the lung were not widely practised until the 1930s. The first successful pneumonectomy for carcinoma was performed by Evarts Graham of Washington in 1933.[110]

CARDIAC SURGERY

The development of cardiac surgery provides another example of the interdependence and interaction of many different fields of technology and science leading to surgical advance. Physiology, radiology, haematology, perfusion techniques, engineering, physics, chemistry, mathematics and immunology are just some of the disciplines that have contributed to the development of cardiac surgery. Until the Second World War, surgery of the heart had largely been confined to the suturing of stab and gunshot wounds and resection of the pericardium.[111] The occasional attempt at valve surgery had also been made. In 1923, Cutler

REFERENCES

96. Macewen W. Glasgow Med J 1879; 12: 210
97. Gowers WR, Horsley V. Med Chir Trans 1888; 71: 377
98. Cushing H. Ann Surg 1911; 54: 1
99. Cushing H. JAMA 1915; 64: 189
100. Cushing H, Bovie WT. Surg Gynecol Obstet 1928; 47: 751
101. Dandy WE. Ann Surg 1918; 68: 5
102. Dandy WE. Ann Surg 1919; 70: 397
103. Sicard JA, Forestier J. Rev Neurol (Paris) 1921; 28: 1264
104. Moniz E. Rev Neurol (Paris) 1927; 34: 72. English translation J Neurosurg 1964; 21: 15
105. Ambrose J, Hounsfield G. Br J Radiol 1973; 46: 148, 1016
106. Hinshaw WS, Bottomley PA, Holland GN. Nature 1977; 270: 722
107. Meade RH. A History of Thoracic Surgery. Thomas, Springfield, Illinois, 1960
108. Sauerbruch F. Verh Dtsch Ges Chir 1904; 32: 105
109. Sauerbruch F. München Med Wochenschr 1913; 60: 625
110. Graham EA, Singer JJ. JAMA 1933; 101: 1371
111. Johnson SL. The History of Cardiac Surgery 1896–1955. Johns Hopkins Press, Baltimore, 1970

of Boston performed the first successful mitral valvotomy when he used a tenotomy knife introduced blindly through the left ventricle.[112] Two years later Souttar, working in London, performed the same operation by introducing his finger through the left atrium and dilating the stenosed valve.[113] Both operations were on children and both patients survived, but conservative medical opinion of the time was critical of such bold and innovative operations and they were rarely repeated. The next major advance was 13 years later, when a patent ductus arteriosus was successfully ligated.[114] In 1944, Crafoord of Stockholm excised a coarctation of the aorta and reunited the cut ends by direct suture.[115]

Another major advance in closed cardiac surgery was the systemic pulmonary bypass operation introduced by Blalock and Taussig in 1945 in cases of Fallot's tetralogy.[116] Many regard this operation as the beginning of modern heart surgery, as it showed that cyanotic congenital heart disease, previously nearly always fatal, could be cured.

Until 1952, all cardiac surgery was performed on the closed heart. The first open heart operation was closure of an atrial septal defect, carried out with the patient rendered hypothermic by surface cooling of the body to 30°C.[117] This allowed some 6–10 minutes of safe circulatory arrest. At the end of the decade, profound hypothermia was introduced,[118] with the patient being cooled to 10–15°C, giving safe circulatory arrest for up to 60 minutes, but this technique did not gain wide appeal. Extracorporeal circulation, allowing surgery on the dry heart, had been a goal for many years and during the 1950s and 1960s, several different heart–lung machines were devised, each using a different design of oxygenator.[119,120] These enabled more complex procedures to be carried out with relative safety, such as the first successful human mitral valve replacement, which was reported in 1961.[121]

In recent years, operations on the coronary circulation have become a major part of cardiac surgery. Coronary endarterectomy was introduced in 1957,[122] but this was superseded within a few years by coronary artery bypass grafting, first performed in 1962 but not reported until several years later.[123] In the 1970s, percutaneous transluminal coronary balloon angioplasty was introduced as a method of dilating atherosclerotic plaques in patients with angina,[124] and this has been extended by the use of intraluminal metallic stents that hold the vessel open. The success of these techniques depended on the accurate pre-operative localization of the stenoses by coronary arteriography, a procedure first used clinically in the early 1950s and refined a few years later by Sones,[125] who was the first to cannulate selectively the coronary vessels.

PERIPHERAL VASCULAR SURGERY

Simple ligation of peripheral arteries proximal and distal to an aneurysm had been practised for centuries, but reconstructive peripheral vascular surgery did not develop until the 1950s. Although Alexis Carrel had devised a satisfactory technique for vascular anastomosis at the turn of the century,[126] further advancement could not be made until accurate localization of atheromatous plaques within blood vessels was possible, until blood coagulation could be reliably controlled, and until satisfactory arterial substitutes had been introduced. These three advances were made over a period of some two decades.

Arteriography originated almost simultaneously in Germany[127] and the USA[128] in the early 1920s. In 1927 Egas Moniz of Portugal introduced carotid arteriography (Fig. 1.16)[104] and 2 years later R. dos Santos, also of Portugal, performed translumbar aortography;[129] radiology of the vascular system then advanced steadily. Seldinger introduced his technique of catheter angiography in 1953.[130]

Although heparin had been purified in 1918,[131] it did not come into general clinical use for several years. By the end of the Second World War, however, safe anticoagulation of patients was possible and contrast radiology enabled accurate assessment of atherosclerotic plaques.

The first superficial femoral thromboendarterectomy was performed in 1947,[132] and this new technique was soon used to remove atheromatous plaques in other vessels. It became apparent, however, that endarterectomy was not a satisfactory treatment for all arterial lesions, and this realization led to much research into the replacement of arteries using homografts as well as methods of preservation using freeze-drying techniques. The first abdominal aortic aneurysm to be resected, by Dubost in Paris in 1951, was replaced by an arterial homograft.[133] Despite the early good results, however, the long-term outcome of arterial homografting was unsatisfactory because of aneurysm formation, and synthetic arterial grafts were soon developed. Originally made of cloth, materials subsequently evaluated included nylon, Ivalon, Marlex, Dacron and Teflon®.[134] The use of reversed autogenous vein for bypassing atherosclerotic small-calibre arteries was first reported in France by Kunlin in 1949.[135]

The surgery of arterial embolism was revolutionized by the introduction of a narrow-gauge balloon catheter by Fogarty in 1963.[136]

A new approach for the treatment of stenosed arteries began in 1964, when transluminal dilatation of the femoral artery was reported using graded dilators made of Teflon®.[137] Grüntzig, working in Zurich, refined this technique by introducing the

REFERENCES

112. Cutler EC, Levine SA. Boston Med Surg J 1923; 188: 1023
113. Souttar HS. Br Med J 1925; 2: 603
114. Gross RE, Hubbard JP. JAMA 1939; 112: 729
115. Crafoord C, Nylin GJ. Thorac Surg 1945; 14: 347
116. Blalock A, Taussig HB. JAMA 1945; 128: 189
117. Lewis FJ, Taufic M. Surgery 1953; 33: 52
118. Drew CE, Anderson IM. Lancet 1959; i: 748
119. DeWall RA, Grage TB, Mcfee AS et al. Surgery 1961; 50: 931
120. DeWall RA, Grage TB, Mcfee AS et al. Surgery 1962; 51: 251
121. Starr A, Edwards ML. Ann Surg 1961; 154: 726
122. Bailey CP, May A, Lemmon WM. JAMA 1957; 164: 641
123. Sabiston DC Jr. Johns Hopkins Med J 1974; 134: 314
124. Grüntzig A. Lancet 1978; i: 263
125. Sones FM, Shirey EK, Proudfit WL et al. Circulation 1959; 20: 773
126. Carrel A. Lyon Méd 1902; 98: 859
127. Berberich J, Hirsch S. Klin Wochenschr 1923; 2: 2226
128. Brooks B. JAMA 1924; 82: 1016
129. dos Santos R, Lamas A, Caldas J. Bull Soc Med Chir Paris 1929; 55: 587
130. Seldinger S. Acta Radiol 1953; 39: 368
131. Howell WH, Holt LE. Am J Physiol 1918–1919; 47: 328
132. dos Santos JC. Mém Acad Chir (Paris) 1947; 73: 409
133. Dubost C, Allary M, Oeconomos N. Arch Surg 1952; 65: 405
134. Harrison JH. Am J Surg 1958; 95: 16
135. Kunlin J. Arch Mal Coeur 1949; 42: 371
136. Fogarty TJ, Cranley JJ, Krause RJ et al. Surg Gynecol Obstet 1963; 116: 241
137. Dotter CT, Judkins MP. Circulation 1964; 30: 654

coaxial low-profile strong plastic balloon catheter,[138] an innovation that led to modern angioplasty techniques. More recently, endoluminal stenting has been used to improve angioplasty results and covered stents have been used to treat aneurysms.

In recent years, the introduction of the operating microscope and the manufacture of ultrafine suture materials have enabled microvascular anastomosis to allow replantation of severed digits and limbs. This procedure was first successfully performed in a human in 1962, when a 12-year-old boy sustained a traumatic amputation of the right arm below the shoulder.[139]

SURGERY AND WAR

Advances in surgery have regularly been made during times of war. For example, the management of trauma and the treatment of shock have been heavily influenced by the knowledge gained during two world wars and in later conflicts. The specialty of plastic surgery began in the First World War with the work of Harold Gillies, a New Zealander, who introduced facial reconstruction using bone and soft tissue tube pedicle grafts.[140] During the Second World War another New Zealander, Archibald McIndoe, made important contributions on the treatment and rehabilitation of severely burned aircrew.[141] Two major advances particularly associated with war, and that have had widespread surgical application, have been the use of blood transfusion and the introduction of antibiotics.

BLOOD TRANSFUSION

Early experiments in the transfusion of blood took place in the 17th century. Several transfusions from animals to humans were reported, but the procedure rapidly fell into disrepute because of the severe reactions and occasional death that resulted. Interest in transfusion was not revived until the 19th century, when James Blundell, a lecturer in physiology and midwifery at Guy's and St Thomas's Hospitals in London, described the transfusion of 12–14 oz (336–392 mL) of blood collected from several donors into a patient moribund from gastric outlet obstruction.[142] This is the first authenticated record of transfusion of blood from human to human. Although this patient died soon afterwards, Blundell recorded several other human transfusions, with a success rate of 40%.

There were a number of other successful transfusions performed in the 19th century, the main indication being post-partum haemorrhage. Throughout the century the main use of transfusion was in the practice of obstetrics, but the results were poor because of the practical difficulties of transfusion as well as the frequent untoward reactions. The transfusion apparatus was crude and cumbersome (Fig. 1.17), and the donor blood often clotted within it while the transfusion was taking place. The problem of clotting was not overcome until 1914, when more or less simultaneously in Buenos Aires,[145] Belgium[146] and the USA[147] it was discovered that sodium citrate mixed with the donor blood was an effective anticoagulant and was not toxic to the recipient.

Landsteiner discovered agglutinins and isoagglutinins in blood in 1901[148]—an advance for which he was later awarded a Nobel Prize—and within a few years the ABO grouping had been formalized and cross-matching could be performed before transfusion. Despite the knowledge of blood groups and effective means of anticoagulation, blood transfusion was used infrequently until towards the end of the First World War. Battle casualties were more often treated with intravenous saline, and blood transfusion was only used as a desperate life-saving measure.

During the two decades after the First World War, however, enormous advances were made in the design of transfusion apparatus as well as in the discovery of many minor blood groups. It was about this time also that experiments into blood preservation were made that enabled the establishment of blood banks.[149] At the beginning of the Second World War the rhesus system was discovered,[150] and blood increasingly began to be transfused on a large scale to injured civilians and service personnel. During this war it was realized that large volumes of blood could be safely transfused into an individual patient, thus paving the way for the advances in surgical techniques made in the post-war years.

ANTIBIOTICS

Topical antiseptics of varying types were in widespread use at the beginning of the 20th century. The first systemic antiseptic, an arsenical named Salvarsan, was introduced by Ehrlich[151] and became widely used against spirochaetal infections, especially during the First World War. Ehrlich called this drug his 'magic bullet'. In 1935 Domagk discovered Prontosil,[152] a drug that killed streptococci in mice; its active constituent was soon afterwards found to be sulphanilamide. This, the first of the sulphonamides, could be given orally or parenterally, and was of special value in the treatment of gonorrhoea. Within a few years numerous other sulphonamides were synthesized and were widely used in the early part of the Second World War.[153]

Disappointment with the results of sulphonamide treatment of war wounds led to intensified research into a more potent chemotherapeutic agent by Florey and Chain in Oxford. These workers had already started to study the mould *Penicillium notatum*, the bactericidal effect of which had been described in 1929 by Alexander Fleming of St Mary's Hospital, London.[154] A year earlier, Fleming had noticed by chance that *Penicillium* mould, which had contaminated a culture plate, killed staphylococci, and in a series of laboratory experiments using a filtrate of the mould he showed that other pathogenic organisms were also killed. He named the filtrate penicillin. Although Fleming suggested that his findings might have clinical application, penicillin's potential was not appreciated at the time.

REFERENCES

138. Grüntzig A. Fortschr Röntgenst 1976; 124: 80
139. Malt RA, McKhann CF. JAMA 1964; 189: 716
140. Gillies HD. Plastic Surgery of the Face. Oxford University Press, London, 1920
141. McIndoe AH. Postgrad Med 1949; 6: 187
142. Blundell J. Med Chir Trans 1819; 10: 296
143. Blundell J. Researches Physiological and Pathological. Cox, London, 1824.
144. Blundell J. Lancet 1828–1829; ii: 321.
145. Agote L. An Inst Mod Clin Med (B Aires) 1914–1915; 1: 24
146. Hustin A. Bull Soc R Sci Med Brux 1914; 72: 104
147. Lewisohn R. Med Rec (NY) 1915; 87:141
148. Landsteiner K. Wien Klin Wochenschr 1901; 14: 1132
149. Fantus B. JAMA 1937; 109: 128
150. Landsteiner K, Wiener AS. Proc Soc Exp Biol NY 1940; 43: 223
151. Ehrlich P, Hata S. Die Experimentelle Chemotherapie der Spirillosen. Springer, Berlin, 1910
152. Domagk G. Dtsch Med Wochenschr 1935; 61: 250
153. Lockwood JS. Surg Gynecol Obstet 1941; 72: 307
154. Fleming A. Br J Exp Pathol 1929; 10: 226

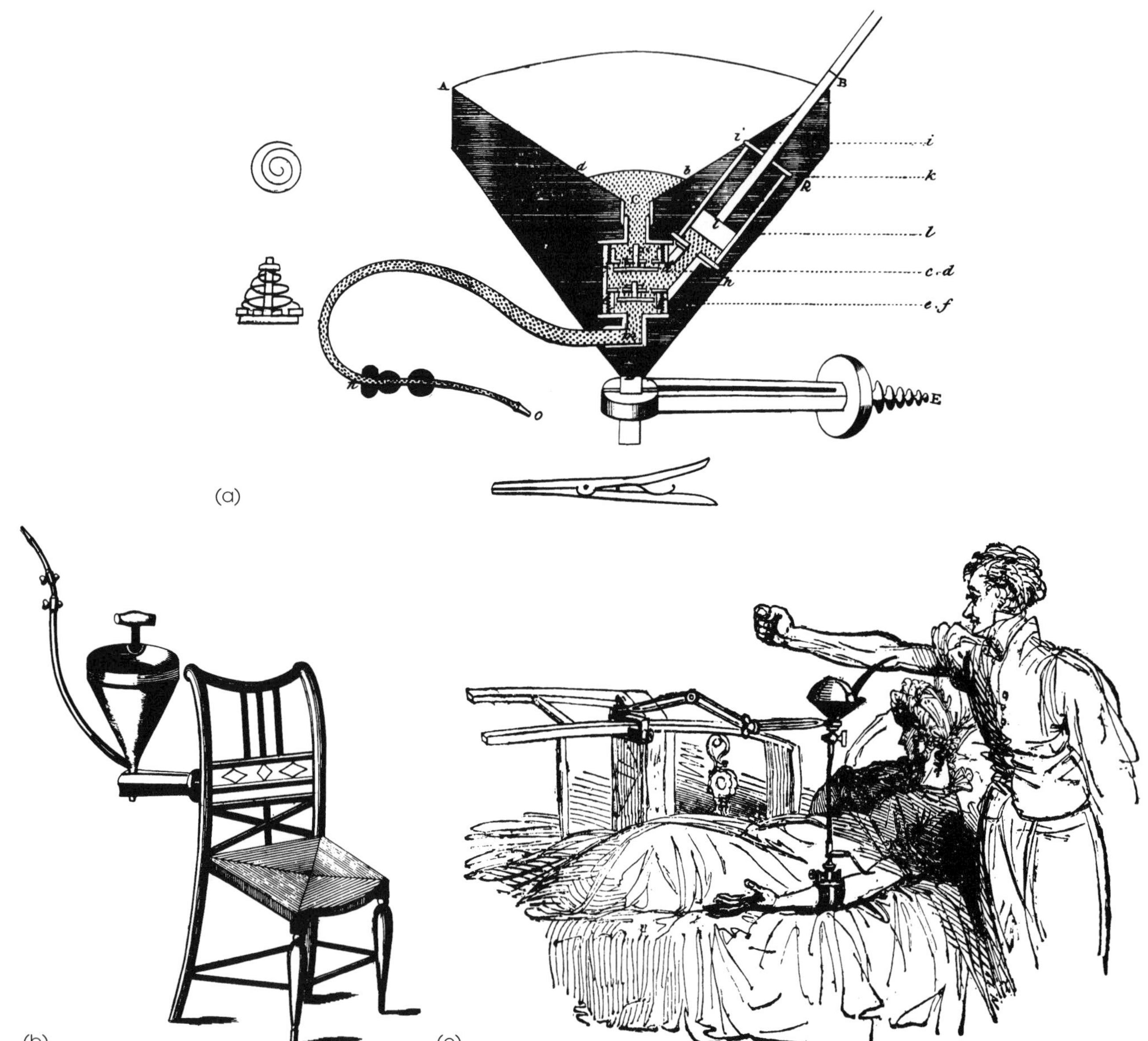

Figure 1.17 Blood transfusion apparatus used by James Blundell, lecturer in physiology and midwifery at Guy's and St Thomas's Hospitals, London, the first person to transfuse blood from human to human. (**a**) Blundell's 'impellor'. The outer (shaded) compartment was filled with warm water. The donor's blood flowed into the funnel-shaped part above, and the action of the pump forced the blood along a tube by means of two oppositely acting spring valves to the cannula inserted in the recipient's vein. (**b**) When in use the impellor was screwed to the back of a chair to give it stability. The blood donor sat on the chair while blood was flowing from his arm into the funnel. (**c**) Blundell's 'gravitator' superseded his impellor. There were fewer moving parts and the blood flowed by gravity. Again the apparatus was fixed to a chair but this time the donor had to stand while he watched his blood gushing into the funnel. (b, From Blundell 1824;[143] c, from Blundell 1828–1829.[144])

Florey and Chain produced a crude extract of penicillin in 1940 and showed that it was active in vivo. In the following year the drug was given to six human patients, the first being a policeman with septicaemia arising from an infected cut on his face. When the small supply of penicillin available ran out, the treatment was interrupted while the drug was recovered from the patient's urine for reinjection. Even though the first patient died, an exceedingly favourable therapeutic response was obtained.[155] By 1943 sufficient quantities of the new drug had been produced to allow its use under the strict control of doctors of the allied forces. Other antibiotics were quickly developed, including streptomycin in 1943, a drug that within a year was shown to be active against tuberculosis.[156]

ORGAN TRANSPLANTATION

Transplantation of the cornea was successfully performed in animals in the early 19th century[157] and in humans from 1906.[158] The cornea was a special case, however, and early attempts using

REFERENCES

155. Abraham EP, Chain E, Fletcher CM et al. Lancet 1941; ii: 177
156. Hinshaw HC, Feldman WH. Proc Mayo Clin 1945; 20: 313
157. Bigger SL. Dublin J Med Sci 1837; 11: 408
158. Zirm EK. v Graefes Arch Ophthalmol 1906; 64: 580

other tissues were failures. For example, John Hunter grafted human teeth into a cock's comb and the spur of a young cock into the comb of a hen without success,[159] and several workers, including Victor Horsley, unsuccessfully transplanted human thyroid in patients with myxoedema.[160]

Transplantation of organs with revascularization began to be practised in experimental animals soon after a reliable technique for vascular anastomosis had been devised by Carrel at the turn of the century.[126] Carrel himself, working with Guthrie first in Chicago and later in New York, transplanted kidney, heart, lung, thyroid and ovary in dogs, but in every instance the organ was rejected.[161] The explanation for this rejection remained obscure until the pioneer work of Medawar during the Second World War, which showed that the rejection of grafts was an immunological phenomenon.[162] This realization led to extensive research into immunosuppression.

RENAL TRANSPLANTATION

The first human renal allograft was in 1936 by Voronoy in the Ukraine in a patient with mercury poisoning,[163] but this, like all the few other human transplants performed around this time, was a failure. In the early 1950s two groups, one in Paris and the other in Boston, simultaneously restarted human kidney allografts. The French surgeons used no immunosuppression but Hume and his colleagues in Boston reported nine human renal transplants, of which four functioned between 37 and 180 days with the use of low-dose steroids for immunosuppression.[164] Although hardly a success, these results gave impetus to further human studies, and fully successful transplants—first between identical twins[165] and then between unrelated subjects using cadaveric donor kidneys[166]—were reported within a few years.

During the 1960s, three major developments changed the course of clinical transplantation. First, the understanding of tissue typing;[167] second, improved methods of obtaining vascular access were devised, thus enabling regular haemodialysis;[168,169] third, and most importantly, better methods of immunosuppression were introduced. Whole-body irradiation had earlier been shown to be useful but had a high incidence of severe toxic effects and 6-mercaptopurine was only moderately effective. After its introduction in 1961,[170] azathioprine quickly became the mainstay of treatment, usually used in combination with other drugs. A more powerful immunosuppressant was not discovered until 1976, when Borel introduced cyclosporin A.[171]

LIVER TRANSPLANTATION

In a brief communication published in 1955,[172] C. S. Welch of New York was the first to report liver transplantation. He transplanted an auxiliary liver into the abdomen of a dog, leaving the original liver in place. The following year he described 49 such canine auxiliary liver transplants.[173] The first human liver transplant was attempted by Starzl in Denver in 1963 on a 3-year-old child with biliary atresia.[174] This was unsuccessful. The first successful liver transplant was performed, again by Starzl, in 1967.[175] By this time immunosuppressive techniques had improved considerably and the patient, an 18-month-old child with a hepatoma, survived 13 months before dying of metastatic disease.

HEART, LUNG AND PANCREATIC TRANSPLANTATION

Transplantation of the heart and lungs in animals dates back nearly a hundred years.[176] During the 1940s, Demikhov of the Soviet Union performed 250 heterotopic and 67 orthotopic canine heart–lung transplants, with some animals surviving for several days; his work was largely unrecognized as it was not translated into English until 1962.[177] The technique of orthotopic cardiac transplantation was developed in painstaking animal experiments by Shumway and his team in the USA,[178] although Barnard in Cape Town was the first to carry out a human heart transplant.[179] The patient was a 54-year-old dentist who lived for 17 days after the operation.

Isolated lung transplantation in a human was first reported in 1963[180] and combined heart–lung transplantation in 1969;[181] both these operations were performed in the USA. Around this time, too, the first human pancreatic transplant was reported.[182]

SURGERY TODAY

The post-Listerian era, during which ever greater and more complex open operations were devised and perfected, is now being superseded by a new epoch in which there is an increasing trend towards less invasive, less painful, and less mutilating procedures. The introduction of histamine H_2-receptor antagonists in the treatment of peptic ulcer,[183] extracorporeal shockwave lithotripsy to fragment renal stones,[184] balloon dilatation of

REFERENCES

159. Dobson J. John Hunter. Livingstone, Edinburgh, 1969
160. Paget S. Sir Victor Horsley. A Study of his Life and Work. Constable, London, 1919
161. Carrel A, Guthrie CC. JAMA 1908; 51: 1662
162. Gibson T, Medawar PB. J Anat 1943; 77: 299
163. Voronoy YY. El Siglo Med 1936; 97: 296
164. Hume DM, Merrill JP, Miller BF et al. Clin Invest 1955; 34: 327
165. Merrill JP, Murray JE, Harrison JH et al. JAMA 1956; 160: 277
166. Merrill JP, Murray JE, Takacs FJ et al. JAMA 1963; 185: 347
167. Dausset J. Immunogenetics 1980; 10: 1
168. Quinton WE, Dillard DH, Scribner BH. Trans Am Soc Artif Intern Organs 1960; 6: 104
169. Brescia MJ, Cimino JE, Appel K et al. N Engl J Med 1966; 275: 1089
170. Calne RY, Murray JES. Forum 1961; 12: 118
171. Borel JF, Feurer C, Gubler HU et al. Agents Actions 1976; 6: 468
172. Welch CS. Transplant Bull 1955; 2: 54
173. Goodrich EO, Welch HF, Nelson JA et al. Surgery 1956; 39: 244
174. Starzl TE, Marchioro TL, von Kaulla KN et al. Surg Gynecol Obstet 1963; 117: 659
175. Starzl TE, Groth CG, Brettschneider L et al. Ann Surg 1968; 168: 392
176. Carrel A, Guthrie CC. Am Med 1905; 10: 1101
177. Demikhov VP. Experimental Transplantation of Vital Organs, translated by Haigh B Consultants Bureau, New York, 1962
178. Shumway NE, Lower RR, Stofer RC. Transplantation of the heart. In: Advances in Surgery. Year Book Medical Publishers, Chicago, 1966
179. Barnard C. S Afr Med 1967; 41: 1271
180. Hardy JD, Webb WR, Dalton ML et al. JAMA 1963; 186: 1065
181. Cooley DA, Bloodwell RD, Hallman GL et al. Ann Thorac Surg 1969; 8: 30
182. Kelly WD, Lillehei RC, Merkel FK et al. Surgery 1967; 61: 827
183. Wyllie JH, Hesselbo T, Black JW. Lancet 1972; ii: 1117
184. Chaussy C, Brendel W, Schmidt E. Lancet 1980; ii: 1265

pyloric stenosis,[185] and ultrasonically guided percutaneous drainage of abscesses[186] are just a few examples of the application of modern technology, which has begun to obviate the need for open surgical operations. This concept of minimally invasive surgery is well illustrated by developments in therapeutic endoscopy.

ENDOSCOPY

Throughout its history, endoscopy has been largely dependent on advances in optical technology. In 1806, Bozzini demonstrated the first primitive endoscope in Vienna.[187] The instrument comprised a silver cylinder containing a wax candle, the light of which was reflected along the cylinder by a concave mirror. The instrument was warmed, lubricated and inserted into various body cavities. Very poor illumination prevented its widespread adoption. In 1853 Desormeaux in Paris devised an instrument consisting of a polished tube, lenses and mirrors illuminated by a lamp burning a mixture of alcohol and turpentine.[188] He named it an endoscope. The invention of the carbon-filament lamp by Edison allowed Nitze to introduce, in 1879,[51] an electric-lighted cystoscope that for the first time provided satisfactory illumination of the interior of a body cavity (Fig. 1.10).

In the field of gastroenterology, the first attempts at gastroscopy were made in 1868,[189] but again the poor illumination precluded the technique from general use. Even after the introduction of electric bulbs, the illumination remained poor for many years because of the continued use of proximal lighting sources for both gastroscopy and sigmoidoscopy (Fig. 1.18). It was not until the 1920s that gastroscopy became an established diagnostic technique, largely owing to the work of Schindler.[191]

The development of fibre optics in the 1950s revolutionized the delivery of light and also enabled the transmission of ultra-clear images through flexible instruments. Hopkins, working in England, developed the forerunner of the modern flexible fibrescope,[192] and 3 years later, in 1957, Hirschowitz in the USA passed a much-improved version into the stomach of a young woman in Ann Arbor.[193]

The next decade saw the emergence of therapeutic endoscopy as technical advances enabled instruments of increasingly sophisticated design to be passed alongside the fibre-optic bundle. Endoscopic dilatation of oesophageal strictures in the USA,[194] endoscopic biliary sphincterotomy simultaneously in Germany[195] and Japan,[196] and endoscopic percutaneous nephrolithotomy (also in the USA)[197] were introduced in the early 1970s. Each of these techniques became rapidly accepted and refined as improved instrumentation became available. In 1973, a laser beam was successfully passed down an endoscope,[198] and within a year or so laser endoscopy was being used to control upper gastrointestinal haemorrhage.[199] By the end of the decade endoscopic biliary stenting was introduced.[200]

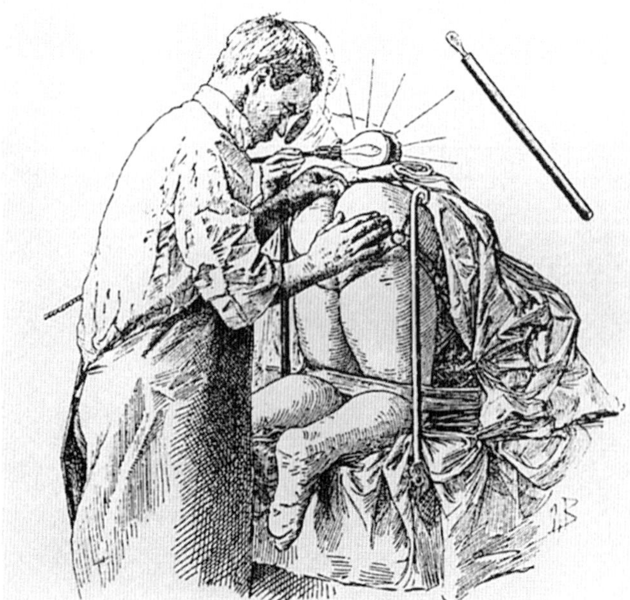

Figure 1.18 The technique of sigmoidoscopy using reflected electric light, popularized by Kelly at the beginning of the 20th century. Distal lighted instruments that allowed much-improved views were later introduced by Strauss in Germany and by J. P. Lockhart-Mummery in England. (From Kelly HA. Ann Surg 1895; 21: 468. Lippincott Williams & Wilkins.[190])

MINIMAL ACCESS SURGERY

Traditional practice in almost all surgical specialties has been transformed by advances in camera technology that enable the transmission of high-definition magnified images of endoscopic views to a television screen. Minimal access operations are now widely performed aided by specially designed endoscopic instruments.

SURGICAL RESEARCH

Operations common until recently, such as vagotomy procedures for peptic ulcer, are now rarely performed. Change in surgical practice is not new, however. Gastrorrhaphy, nephropexy, splanchnicectomy and cardio-omentopexy were operations often performed in the years between the two world wars; today they are historical curiosities. This is, in large measure, the outcome of research, a discipline without which surgery would stagnate. A multiplicity of different sciences now interacts within the broad title of surgical research, including genetics, immunology,

REFERENCES

185. Benjamin SB, Cattau EL, Glass RL. Gastrointest Endosc 1982; 28: 253
186. Smith EH, Bartrum RJ. Am J Roentgenol Radium Ther Nucl Med 1974; 122: 308
187. Bozzini PJ. Pract Heilk 1806; 24: 107. English translation Urology 1974; 3: 119
188. Desormeaux AJ. De l'Endoscope et de Ses Applications. Baillière, Paris, 1865
189. Kussmaul A. Dtsch Arch Klin Med 1869; 6: 456
190. Kelly HA. Ann Surg 1895; 21: 468
191. Schindler R. Münch Med Wochenschr 1932; 79: 1268
192. Hopkins HH, Kapany NS. Nature 1954; 173: 39
193. Hirschowitz BI, Curtiss LE, Peters CW et al. Gastroenterology 1958; 35: 50
194. Lilly JO, McCaffery TD. Am J Dig Dis 1971; 16: 1137
195. Classen M, Demling L. Dtsch Med Wochenschr 1974; 99: 496
196. Kawai K, Akasaka Y, Murakami K et al. Gastrointest Endosc 1974; 20: 148
197. Bissada NK, Meachum KR, Redman JF. J Urol 1974; 112: 414
198. Nath G, Gorisch W, Kreitmair A et al. Endoscopy 1973; 5: 213
199. Frümorgen P, Bodem F, Reidenbach HD et al. Gastrointest Endosc 1976; 23: 73
200. Soehendra N, Reijnders-Frederix V. Dtsch Med Wochenschr 1979; 104: 106

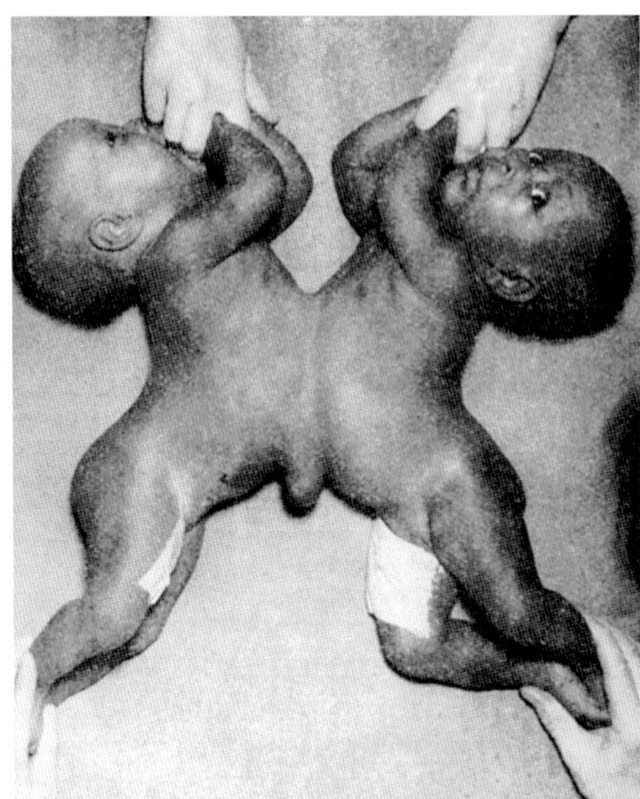

Figure 1.19 The conjoined twins of Kano. These twins were born in Kano, Nigeria, and shared a common liver and peritoneal cavity. They were separated by Ian Aird at the Hammersmith Hospital, London, in November 1953, in an operation that received widespread publicity. It was the first surgical separation of conjoined twins who shared a liver. There are many examples of conjoined twins in history, the most famous being the brothers Chang and Eng, who were born in Siam in 1811, who emigrated to the USA, became exhibits in Barnum's circus, married English sisters, fathered 19 children between them, and lived as farmers in later life. Unseparated, they died at the age of 63 within an hour of each other. (From Aird I. The conjoined twins of Kano. Br Med J 1954 Apr 10; 4866: 831–7, by permission of BMJ Publishing Group.[204])

physiology, biochemistry, radiology, pharmacology and engineering. Surgical research has flourished, stimulated by the founding of surgical research societies throughout the world. There is an ever-increasing trend towards specialization, particularly in the USA. First written in 1926,[201] the far-sighted words of Lord Moynihan are even more true today: 'surgery in days to come will be advanced by men [and women] trained in the methods and imbued with the spirit of experimental research, though it will no doubt continue to be practised to their profit by those who are merely craftsmen'. Ian Aird, the progenitor of this *Companion*, was one such surgeon who pursued research and advanced scientific knowledge. He made important contributions to surgical pathology with the discovery of the relationship between blood groups and carcinoma of the stomach[202] and peptic ulcer,[203] and became a public figure when he helped to separate the conjoined twins of Kano in 1953 (Fig. 1.19).[204]

The history of surgery has been a story of steady but uneven progress. It seems reasonable to suggest that the scientific training of young surgeons today, if combined with an intellectual curiosity and the facility for interdisciplinary collaboration, will ensure continuing surgical advances and therefore a continued and an ever-evolving history.

REFERENCES

201. Moynihan B. Lancet 1926; ii: 789
202. Aird I, Bentall HH, Roberts JAF. Br Med J 1953; 1: 799
203. Aird I, Bentall HH, Mehigan J et al. Br Med J 1954; 2:315
204. Aird I. Br Med J 1954; 1: 831

Fluid, electrolyte and nutrient replacement

2

Dileep N. Lobo, Simon P. Allison

Few subjects cause more confusion or lead to more difficulties in management than fluid and electrolyte balance,[1–4] yet at a practical level the concepts are straightforward and, if clearly understood, should enable the surgeon to manage most common situations in an effective and appropriate way. The basic physiology must be understood and can then be applied to the common situations encountered in daily surgical practice. There is a need to differentiate clearly between the requirements for volume replacement and resuscitation, and those for maintenance. It is important to achieve external balance between the body and its environment and internal balance between fluid compartments, because the normal fluxes and equilibria between them may be disturbed by disease.

TERMINOLOGY

Patients are often described loosely as 'wet' or 'dry' (or 'dehydrated') in a way that conveys different meanings to different people. The term *dehydration* means, in its strict sense, lack of water; yet it is used colloquially and variously to mean water lack, salt and water depletion, and even intravascular fluid deficit. Accurate diagnosis and precise terminology are the first steps to appropriate treatment (Table 2.1)

NORMAL ANATOMY AND PHYSIOLOGY OF BODY FLUIDS

The intracellular environment of early life forms in the sea was isotonic with the external environment, because these unicellular organisms had no means of regulating their internal osmotic pressure.[5] As life evolved, organisms became more complex, left the sea, and colonized land, facing the physiological challenges of thermoregulation, gas exchange, nutrition, and water and electrolyte balance. John Gamble summarized this beautifully when he wrote, 'Before our extremely remote ancestors could come ashore to enjoy their Eocene Eden or their Palaeozoic Palm Beach, it was necessary for them to establish an enclosed aqueous medium which would carry on the role of sea water.' Claude Bernard also described this concept when he introduced the idea of a stable *milieu interieur* maintained in part by the function of the kidney and its need to produce a *volume obligatoire*, the minimum volume of urine needed to excrete waste products and maintain internal stability.

Table 2.1 Terminology

Ambiguous term	Clear terms
Dehydration or 'dry' (includes salt?)	Water deficit Salt and water depletion
Hypovolaemia (which volume?)	Plasma/blood or extracellular fluid volume deficit
'Wet'	Peripheral/trunk oedema Pulmonary oedema Congestive heart failure Salt and water overload/excess
'Fluid' (which?)	Water/dextrose Salt and water (specify concentration) Colloid (specify) Red cells Whole blood

EXTERNAL BALANCE AND THE KIDNEY

In a state of equilibrium, water intake must equal water loss. The daily water balance in health is summarized in Table 2.2. The ability to excrete urine with different osmolality from plasma plays a central role in the regulation of water balance and the maintenance of plasma osmolality. Antidiuretic hormone (ADH) secretion is inhibited if the plasma osmolality is decreased, causing excretion of dilute urine and the return of the plasma osmolality to normal. When the plasma osmolality is increased, ADH release and thirst are stimulated, and the combination of decreased urinary water loss and increased water intake results in water retention and a decrease in plasma osmolality.

Table 2.2 Approximate daily water balance in health

	Intake (mL/day)	Output (mL/day)	
Water from beverages	400–1400	Urine	500–1500
Water from solid food	850	Skin and respiratory tract	900
Water from oxidation	350	Stool	200
Total	1600–2600	Total	1600–2600

REFERENCES

1. Stoneham MD, Hill EL. Variability in post-operative fluid and electrolyte prescription. Br J Clin Pract 1997; 51: 82–84
2. Callum KG, Gray AJG, Hoile RW et al. Extremes of Age: The 1999 Report of the National Confidential Enquiry into Perioperative Deaths. National Confidential Enquiry into Perioperative Deaths, London, 1999
3. Lobo DN, Dube MG, Neal KR et al. Clin Nutr 2001; 20: 125–130
4. Lobo DN, Dube MG, Neal KR et al. Ann R Coll Surg Engl 2002; 84: 156–160
5. Thompson WT. Va Med Mon (1918) 1968; 95: 587–590
6. Rose BD, Post TW. Clincal Physiology of Acid–Base and Electrolyte Disorders. McGraw-Hill, New York, 2001

Table 2.3 Renal filtration and normal daily excretion of water and electrolytes

Substance	Filtered	Excreted	Net reabsorption (%)
Water	180 L	0.5–3 L	98–99
Na^+	26 000 mmol	100–250 mmol	> 99
Cl^-	21 000 mmol	100–250 mmol	> 99
HCO_3^-	4800 mmol	0	~100
K^+	800 mmol	40–120 mmol	85–95
Urea	54 g	27–32 g	40–50

The obligatory renal water loss is directly related to the need for solute excretion. A minimum of 670 mL/day of urine is the *volume obligatoire*[6] if 800 mOsm of solute have to be excreted per day to maintain the steady state and the maximum urinary osmolality is 1200 mOsm/kg. In a catabolic state, or with excessive protein intake, the osmolar load is increased and the *volume obligatoire* is likewise increased. Similarly, if the maximum concentrating capacity of the kidney is impaired by disease, a larger volume of urine is required to excrete the same osmolar load (e.g. polyuric renal failure).

The renal handling of water and electrolytes is summarized in Table 2.3. The kidney responds to water or sodium excess or deficit via osmoreceptors and volume receptors, acting through ADH and the renin–angiotensin system to restore osmolality and volume of the extracellular fluid to normal (Fig. 2.1). Atrial natriuretic peptide (ANP) is secreted in response to intravascular volume expansion that causes stretching of receptors in the right atrium. Maintenance of volume always overrides the maintenance of osmolality if hypovolaemia and hypo-osmolality coincide.

The mechanisms that control salt and water balance in healthy people ensure maintenance of a sodium concentration of 135–145 mmol/L and an osmolality of the extracellular and intracellular fluid of close to 280 mOsm/kg despite wide variations in water intake. (As water passes freely across the cell membrane, there is osmotic equilibrium between the extracellular fluid and intracellular fluid.) Any effect of disease, such as the response to injury, which interferes with these control mechanisms alters sodium concentration unless care is taken to avoid excess or deficit of either water or salt.

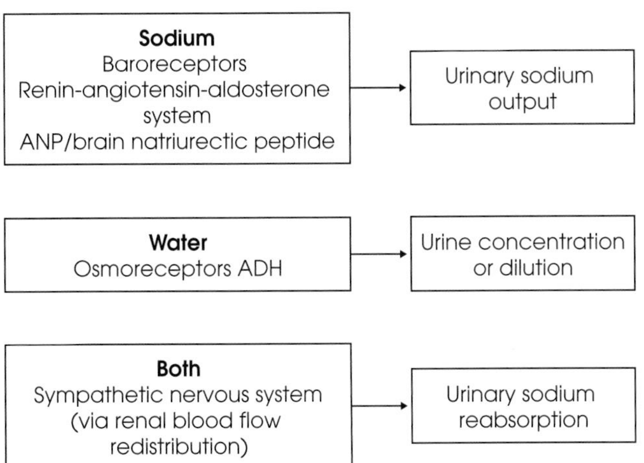

Figure 2.1 Pathways for response to changes in water and sodium in the extracellular fluid.

PHYSIOLOGICAL AND ENDOCRINE RESPONSES OF NORMAL SUBJECTS TO CRYSTALLOID INFUSIONS

To understand the altered responses of patients to changes in fluid and electrolyte balance, it is important to understand the changes that occur in normal subjects. Water deficit or excess results in an increase or decrease in plasma osmolality, with corresponding changes in ADH secretion and in the urinary volume and concentration. Salt deficiency induces a reduction in extracellular fluid volume, including the plasma volume, and stimulation of the renin–angiotensin–aldosterone system and ADH secretion, thereby reducing salt and water excretion in an attempt to preserve intravascular volume. As hypovolaemia also stimulates ADH release, hyponatraemia may result from a high water intake or excessive intravenous administration of hypotonic fluid. These mechanisms are extremely efficient, presumably because during evolution animals have been repeatedly exposed to these circumstances. Humans have, however, been exposed to salt excess only recently, and it is not surprising that mechanisms for excreting an excess saline load, even in health, are relatively inefficient.

This is illustrated by studies comparing the response of normal subjects to 0.9% saline and to 5% dextrose infusions. Infusion of 5% dextrose produces an abrupt diuresis, with restoration to normal water balance within 1–2 h of stopping the infusion. In contrast, 60% of the saline is still retained 6 h later.[7] Levels of ADH fall after infusion of both solutions, reflecting not only the influence of the osmoreceptors but also of the volume receptors on its secretion. During the infusion of both solutions, ANP rises abruptly from activation of the stretch receptors, but falls to baseline when the infusion is stopped, despite a residual extracellular fluid overload. Therefore ANP seems to be involved in the acute control of intravascular volume but not in the continuing excretion of excess sodium load in the interstitial space. The renin–angiotensin–aldosterone system is switched off after saline and aldosterone levels remain low, suggesting that normal excretion of a salt load may be largely dependent on the slow permissive effects of reduced renin–angiotensin–aldosterone system activity.[8] The problem may be exacerbated in situations when salt and water overload is combined with a low effective blood volume or cardiac output, as the volume receptors of the cardiovascular system activate the renin–angiotensin–aldosterone system to cause further salt retention, despite interstitial overload and oedema.

The chloride component of saline may also be a problem, because it has a sodium:chloride ratio of 1:1 compared with plasma, which has a ratio of 1.25–1.45:1. Saline therefore causes a rise in plasma chloride, leading to hyperchloraemic acidosis. Hyperchloraemia also causes renal vasoconstriction and reduced glomerular filtration rate, contributing further to the retention of a saline load. In contrast, the more physiological Ringer's lactate

REFERENCES

7. Lobo DN, Stanga Z, Simpson JAD et al. Clin Sci (Lond) 2001; 101: 173–179
8. Lobo DN, Myhill DJ, Stanga Z et al. Clin Nutr 2002; 21 (S1): 9–10

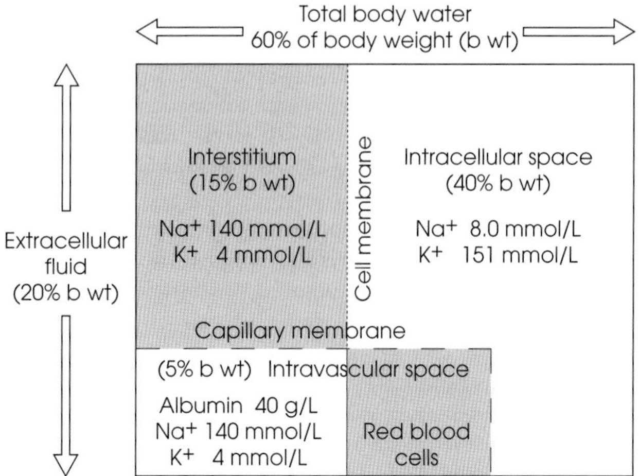

Figure 2.2 Distribution of body fluids and the sodium and potassium concentrations in the body water compartments.

Table 2.4 Electrolyte and mineral concentrations in body water compartments

Electrolyte	Extracellular fluid (mmol/L)	Intracellular fluid (mmol/L)	Total in body (mmol)
Sodium	140–155	10–18	3000–4000
Potassium	4.0–5.5	120–145	3000–4000
Calcium	2.2–2.5	–	25 000–27 000
Ionized calcium	0.9–1.3	–	–
Magnesium	0.7–1.2	15–25	900–1200
Chloride	98–106	2–6	3000–4000
Phosphate	0.7–1.3	8–20	30 000–32 000

or Hartmann's solution has a sodium:chloride ratio of 1.18:1 and does not cause hyperchloraemia. Sodium excretion following infusion of Hartmann's solution is also more rapid, reflecting the influence of chloride on renal sodium handling.[9] These observations are of practical importance in the management of patients.

BODY FLUID COMPARTMENTS, INTERNAL BALANCE AND FLUXES

The anatomy and composition of the body fluid compartments are shown in Fig. 2.2 and Table 2.4. In addition to internal balances between the extracellular and intracellular fluid and intravascular and interstitial spaces, the daily flux of fluid through the gastrointestinal tract will be considered.

COMPOSITION OF BODY FLUIDS

The concentrations of electrolytes and minerals in the body water compartments are summarized in Fig. 2.2 and Table 2.4. The total body sodium is 3000–4000 mmol, of which 44% is in the extracellular fluid, 9% in the intracellular fluid, and the remaining 47% in bone. A little more than half the bone sodium requires acid for its solution and is osmotically inactive; the rest is water-soluble and therefore exchangeable. The daily sodium intake is variable, but is on average 1 mmol/kg, which is equivalent to the amount excreted in the urine and faeces. Sodium loss in the sweat is negligible, except in those not acclimatized to heat.

Almost 98% of potassium is intracellular, 75% being in skeletal muscle. The normal daily intake of potassium, like that of sodium, is approximately 1 mmol/kg, and is matched by the urinary excretion, which increases in catabolic states.

EXTRACELLULAR FLUID AND INTRACELLULAR FLUID

In the average normal person, the body water comprises 60% of the body weight and 73% of the lean mass.[10] Fat and bone being relatively anhydrous, fatter individuals have a lower percentage of body water. Body water (Fig. 2.2) is functionally divided into the extracellular fluid (20% of body weight) and the intracellular fluid (40% of body weight), separated from each other by the cell membrane, the sodium–potassium adenosine triphosphatase pump of which ensures that sodium is the main extracellular cation maintaining the osmolality of the extracellular fluid. The negative charges on large intracellular molecules such as

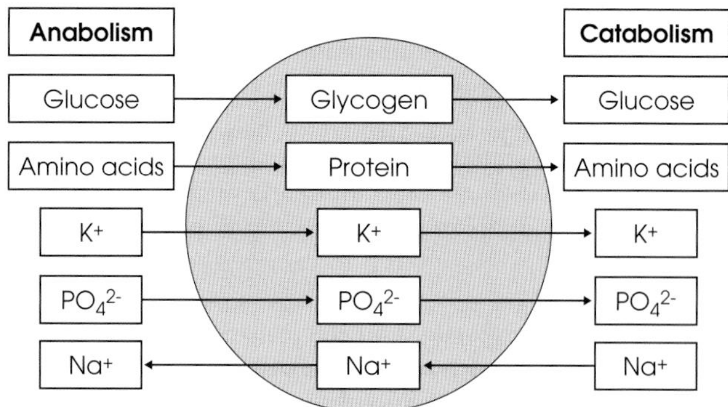

Figure 2.3 The metabolic tide of the cell. PO_4^{2-}, phosphate.

protein cause potassium to be retained within the cell to maintain electrical neutrality (the Donnan equilibrium). In catabolic states such as starvation or injury, glycogen and protein are broken down to glucose and amino acids, which escape from the cell with potassium. In severe illness, sodium pumping may also be impaired. As anabolism returns during feeding or convalescence, the metabolic tide of the cells turns to the synthesis of glycogen and protein. This necessitates cellular reuptake of potassium and phosphate, precipitating a fall in extracellular concentration of these ions (refeeding syndrome), which may need to be replaced (Fig. 2.3). The cell membrane is freely permeable to water, which shifts in and out of the cell in response to changes in the osmotic gradient.

INTRAVASCULAR VERSUS INTERSTITIAL COMPARTMENTS

The extracellular fluid is further divided by the capillary membrane into an intravascular and an interstitial compartment (Fig. 2.2). The equilibrium between these two compartments is determined by the membrane pore size, which is increased with inflammation; the relative concentration and hence oncotic pressure of proteins on the two sides of the membrane; and the

REFERENCES

9. Reid F, Lobo DN, Williams RN et al. Clin Sci (Lond) 2003; 104: 17–24
10. Moore FD. Metabolic Care of the Surgical Patient. WB Saunders, Philadelphia, 1959

capillary hydrostatic pressure.[11] Starling's equation, now known as the Law of the Capillary, indicates that the extravascular flux of water is inversely related to the capillary oncotic pressure as long as other factors in the equation remain constant:

$$F_{H_2O} = K_c \times SA\ [p_c - p_i) - (Op_i - Op_c)]$$

F_{H_2O} is the flux of water across the capillary; K_c the capillary hydraulic conductivity; SA the capillary surface area; p_c the capillary hydraulic pressure; p_i the interstitial hydraulic pressure; Op_i the interstitial oncotic pressure; and Op_c the capillary oncotic pressure.

The integrity of the intravascular volume is maintained by the oncotic pressure of the plasma proteins and the integrity of the capillary membrane. In health, albumin escapes through pores in the capillary membrane into the interstitial space at the rate of 5–7%/h, 10 times the rate of albumin synthesis. Albumin is then returned to the intravascular compartment by the lymphatic system and a steady state is achieved (Fig. 2.4).

FLUX THROUGH THE GASTROINTESTINAL TRACT

Although 8–9 L of fluid cross the duodenum, only about 150 mL are excreted in the faeces (Fig. 2.5). The reabsorptive capacity of the gut may fail when patients have diarrhoea, intestinal fistulae or the short bowel syndrome. In patients with a paralytic ileus or intestinal obstruction, as much as 6 L of water may be pooled in the gut and be effectively lost from the extracellular fluid. It is important for the surgeon to remember the content of the various gastrointestinal fluids when replacing fluid and electrolytes in patients with gastrointestinal losses (Table 2.5).

Transcapillary escape rate 4-5% of IVS albumin per hour

ISS

Capillary membrane

IVS

Albumin 40g/L

ISS albumin exceeds the IVS albumin by 30%

Flux 10 times the rate of albumin synthesis

Lymph Albumin 35g/L

Thoracic duct

Figure 2.4 Capillary permeability and albumin flux in health. ISS, interstitial space; IVS, intravascular space.

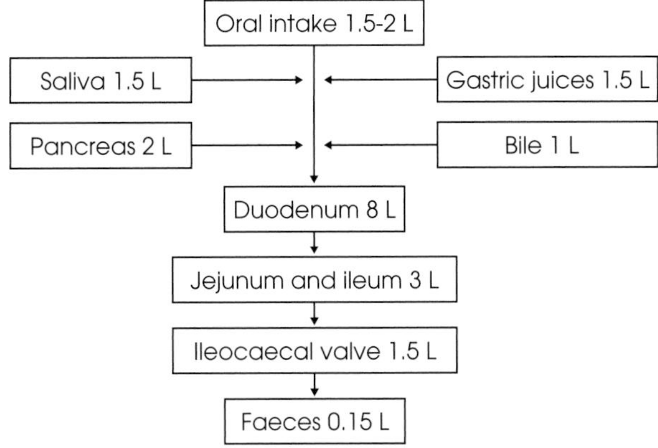

Figure 2.5 Flux of fluid across the gastrointestinal tract.

EFFECTS OF INJURY AND STARVATION AND THEIR THERAPEUTIC IMPLICATIONS

Many diseases and pathological states cause derangements in both internal and external fluid and electrolyte balance, which in turn can cause problems. In clinical practice, treatment should be directed towards maintaining normal balance by avoiding excess or deficit. It is important to understand the underlying pathophysiological changes to achieve this.

EFFECTS ON EXTERNAL BALANCE

The response of humans to starvation, stress and trauma is teleologically designed to preserve vital functions. John Hunter, in 1794, recognized that although these responses were designed to provide some advantage in the recovery process, when taken to the extreme they could threaten survival. He wrote, 'Impressions are capable of producing or increasing natural actions and are then called stimuli, but they are likewise capable of producing too much action, as well as depraved, unnatural action, or what we commonly call diseased action.'[12]

As well as the metabolic responses to injury (see *Nutrition* section), there are important changes in fluid and electrolyte physiology with retention of water and sodium and loss of potassium. Pringle et al.[13] demonstrated in 1905 that both anaesthesia and surgery produced a reduction in urine volume. The use of intravenous hydration gained acceptance in surgical practice[14] when it was recognized that the intravenous infusion of saline to restore losses in patients recovering from major surgery lessened both morbidity and mortality, mainly from renal failure. These authors recommended that patients should receive a litre

Table 2.5 Approximate electrolyte content of gastrointestinal secretions

Secretion	Sodium (mmol/L)	Potassium (mmol/L)	Chloride (mmol/L)
Saliva	44	20	–
Gastric juice	70–120	10	100
Bile	140	5	100
Pancreatic juice	140	5	75
Small intestine	110–120	5–10	105
Diarrhoea (adult)	120	15	90

REFERENCES

11. Starling EH. J Physiol 1896; 19: 312–326
12. Hunter JA. Treatise on the Blood, Inflammation and Gunshot Wounds. G Nicol, London, 1794
13. Pringle H, Maunsell RCB, Pringle S. Br Med J 1905; ii: 542–543
14. Coller FA, Dick VS, Maddock WG. JAMA 1936; 107: 1522–1527

of isotonic saline on the day of the operation, in addition to the replacement of abnormal losses with equivalent volumes of isotonic saline.[15] Subsequently, they withdrew their guidelines because of the high incidence of postoperative oedema and electrolyte imbalance. They found that postoperative patients were less able to excrete a salt and water load than those who had not undergone surgery,[16] describing this as postoperative 'salt intolerance' and suggesting that isotonic sodium-containing solutions should be avoided on the day of the operation and during the subsequent 2 days. They recommended replacement of water losses with dextrose solutions over this period.

Others have found postoperative oedema to be common in patients receiving sodium-containing intravenous fluids. A study published in 1942 suggested that the administration of sodium chloride and water was satisfactory therapy for patients in good or fair condition who had suffered acute gastrointestinal fluid losses.[17] These authors also found that patients with chronic illness and those in a poor general condition commonly accumulated the administered salt and water in the extravascular compartment and developed oedema.

Wilkinson et al.[18] studied the effects of surgery on the excretion of sodium and chloride, and found that the excretion of both ions was reduced for the first 6 days after surgery. They thought initially that this may have been a result of lack of salt intake during the usual period of postoperative starvation, but the findings persisted even when the salt intake was maintained by the intravenous or oral routes. This led them to conclude that the decrease in sodium and chloride excretion is 'an expression not merely of a failure of intake but also of some active process leading to a retention of sodium and chloride'. A year later, the same authors documented an increase in urinary potassium excretion in the early postoperative period despite a reduction in the potassium intake.[19] This resulted from the fact that potassium and protein exist in muscle in a ratio of 3:1, so that when protein is catabolized, potassium passes from the intracellular fluid to the extracellular fluid and is excreted by the kidneys.[20] Potassium is similarly linked to glycogen, being released during glycogenolysis and taken up during glycogen synthesis. These effects and the action of mineralocorticoids account for the increase in potassium excretion. There is often no fall in serum potassium concentration despite a reduction in total body potassium, because potassium is lost only in proportion to protein and passes continuously into the extracellular fluid.[20] Once feeding recommences, the cells begin to take up potassium as glycogen and protein are synthesized, resulting in a sudden fall in the serum potassium concentration revealing the underlying potassium deficit.

These findings of Wilkinson and colleagues were confirmed by Le Quesne and Lewis,[21] who attributed them to the fusion of three separate events: primary water retention, early sodium retention and late sodium retention. They found that primary water retention is independent of sodium retention and is rarely maintained after the first 24 h. In contrast, in a study of patients undergoing laparotomy,[22] who received 3 L of dextrose saline (30 mmol/L sodium) daily for 6 days postoperatively, there was persistence of a low plasma and high urinary osmolality as late as the sixth postoperative day, reflecting continuing impairment of free water clearance (Table 2.6). This emphasizes the ease with which excessive administration of hypotonic fluids to patients, particularly children and the elderly, may render them hyponatraemic, with the risk of developing potentially fatal cerebral oedema.

Table 2.6 Plasma and urinary osmolality in postoperative patients receiving hypotonic crystalloid infusions

	Osmolality (mOsm/kg) Postoperative day					
	0	1	2	3	4	5
Plasma	282	279	273	273	270	270
Urine	579	696	610	358	489	611

(Reproduced from Allison SP. Metabolic aspects of intensive care. Br J Hosp Med 1974; 11: 860–71, with permission.)

Postoperative patients may excrete less than 100 mmol of sodium during the first 4 or 5 days after surgery without postoperative fluids.[23] In patients given intravenous saline, however, the amount of sodium retained increases in proportion to the quantity infused. Intakes of 300 and 1000 mmol sodium during the first 4 days after surgery were associated with retention of 200 and 600 mmol respectively.[23]

In further studies, Tindall and Clarke observed the effects of two different postoperative fluid regimens on postoperative antidiuresis.[24] The group of patients who received high sodium intakes (450 mmol sodium in 3000 mL water per day) did not develop hyponatraemia, but had marked sodium (over 1023 mmol) and water retention (over 3509 mL) by the fourth day. Patients who were given 3 L of dextrose per day became hyponatraemic on the first day, but subsequently excreted the excess water as the plasma sodium concentration returned to normal.

Patients undergoing uncomplicated colonic surgery have been randomized to receive postoperative intravenous fluids according to the current hospital practice, i.e. at least 3 L of water and 154 mmol sodium per day (standard group), or 2 L or less of water and 77 mmol sodium per day (restricted group).[25] There was 3 kg greater weight gain in the patients receiving standard fluid replacement, reflecting positive salt and water balance, compared with a zero balance in the restricted group (Fig. 2.6). There was no significant difference in urine output, urinary sodium excretion, or blood urea concentration, but solid-phase and liquid-phase gastric emptying times were significantly

REFERENCES

15. Coller FA, Bartlett RM, Bingham DLC et al. Ann Surg 1938; 108: 769–782
16. Coller FA, Campbell KN, Vaughan HH et al. Ann Surg 1944; 119: 533–541
17. Power FH, Pedersen S, Maddock WG. Surgery 1942; 12: 438–444
18. Wilkinson AW, Billing BH, Nagy G et al. Lancet 1949; 1: 640–644
19. Wilkinson AW, Billing BH, Nagy G et al. Lancet 1950; 2: 135–137
20. Allison SP. Nutrition in Medicine: A Physician's View. Institut Danone, Brussels, 1996
21. Le Quesne LP, Lewis AAG. Lancet 1953; 1: 153–158
22. Allison SP. Br J Hosp Med 1974; 11: 860–871
23. Clark RG. In: Stoner HB, Clark RG, Frayn KN et al (eds). Folia Traumatologica Geigy: Metabolic Responses to Trauma. CIBA-Geigy, Basle, 1977: 5–8
24. Tindall SF, Clark RG. Br J Surg 1981; 68: 639–644
25. Lobo DN, Bostock KA, Neal KR et al. Lancet 2002; 359: 1812–1818

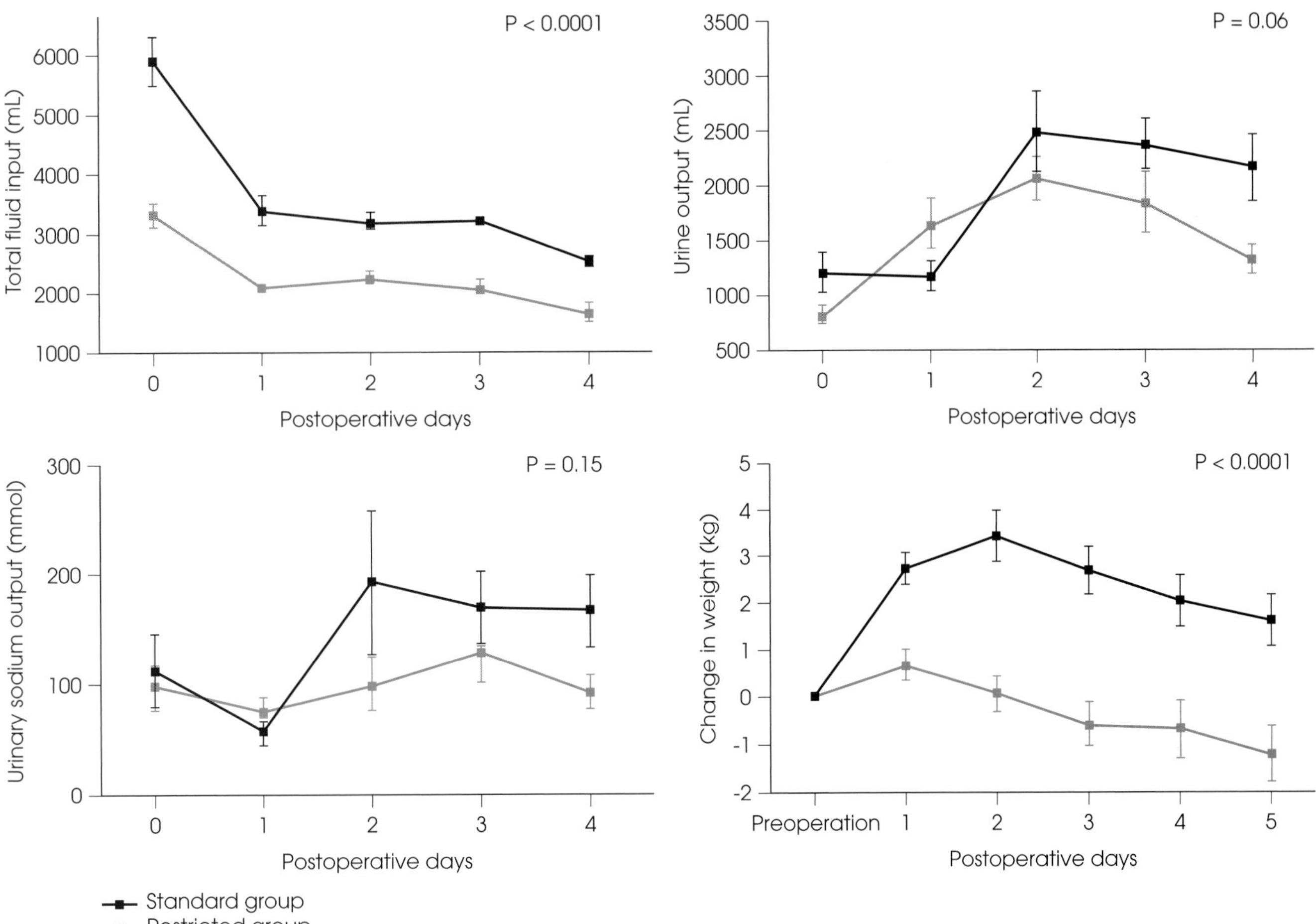

Figure 2.6 Total fluid input, urinary output, urinary sodium excretion, and change in body weight in patients receiving at least 3 L water and 154 mmol sodium per day (standard group) or 2 L water or less and 75 mmol sodium per day (restricted group) after uncomplicated colonic surgery. (After Lobo et al. The Lancet, 2002; 359: 1812–18, reprinted with permission from Elsevier[25].)

different, flatus was passed a day later, and stools were passed 2 days later. The restricted group also had fewer side effects and complications, and were able to be discharged 3 days earlier. These results show that salt and water retention is not a harmless and inevitable epiphenomenon, and should be avoided where possible by restricting maintenance fluids to the amount necessary to achieve zero balance. This is not to deny the need for adequate replacement of additional losses of intravascular or extracellular fluid.

The capacity to excrete an excess salt and water load returns as the flow phase of injury gives way to the recovery or anabolic phase. Moore coined the terms the *sodium retention phase of injury* and the *sodium diuresis phase of injury* to describe these two periods in the response to trauma or acute illness, and suggested that sodium and water retention may be part of an obligatory reaction mediated directly by the hormonal response to injury itself.[10] The sodium retention and diuresis phases are illustrated in Fig. 2.7, showing the fall in urinary sodium over the first 4 days after an uncomplicated 20% burn injury, despite positive salt and water balance, with a steady return of sodium excretion after the fourth day.[26] In contrast, early potassium excretion remains high, falling after the fourth day. Increased secretion of ADH, mineralocorticoids and catecholamines are described even in the presence of positive fluid balance.

The renin–angiotensin–aldosterone system is also stimulated by injury. Angiotensin is a powerful vasoconstrictor and promotes adrenal production of aldosterone, which in turn enhances sodium conservation by the kidneys and the gastrointestinal tract.[27] The catecholamines, adrenaline (epinephrine) and noradrenaline (norepinephrine), released by the adrenal medulla produce vasoconstriction of selected vascular beds, such as the skin and splanchnic circulation, resulting in redistribution of blood from non-essential to essential territories such as the coronary and cerebrovascular circulation. These changes are exacerbated by any additional deficit in effective blood volume.

EFFECTS ON INTERNAL BALANCE

Intravascular versus interstitial space

Although these responses to injury or starvation occur despite salt and water excess, they are exacerbated by intravascular hypovolaemia when blood or plasma has been lost. In the severely injured and critically ill, with a major inflammatory response there is leukocyte activation and increased microvascular

REFERENCES

26. Hinton P, Allison SP, Littlejohn S et al. Lancet 1973; 2: 218–221
27. Dick M, Dasta JF, Choban PS et al. Ann Pharmacother 1994; 28: 837–841

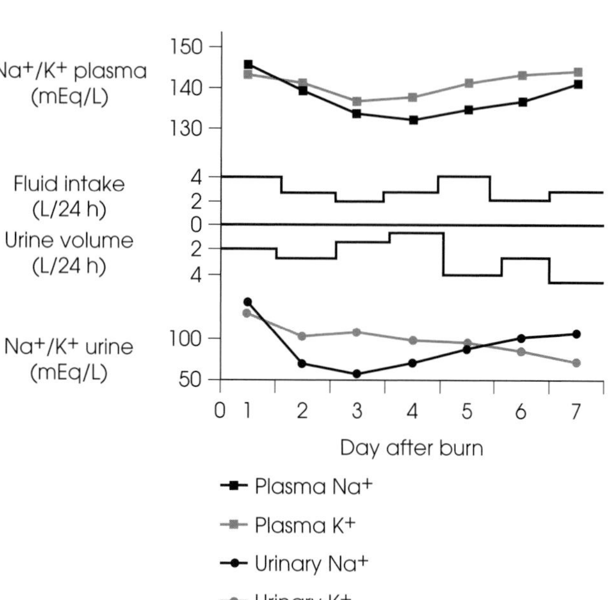

Figure 2.7 The sodium retention phase and sodium diuresis phase following moderate burn injury. (Redrawn from Hinton P, Allison SP, Littlejohn S, Lloyd J. Electrolyte changes after burn injury and effect of treatment. Lancet, 1973; 2: 218–21, with permission from Elsevier[26].)

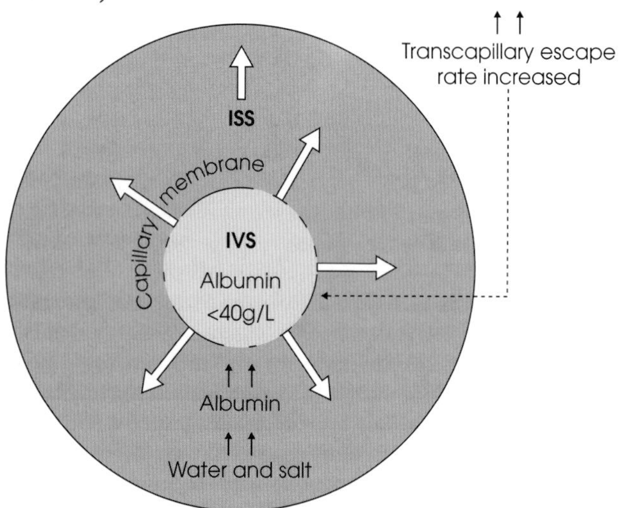

Figure 2.8 Capillary permeability and albumin flux in illness and after injury and stress. ISS, interstitial space; IVS, intravascular space.

permeability.[28–30] The transcapillary escape of albumin increases threefold or more,[30] causing redistribution of fluid into the interstitial space and hypoalbuminaemia (Fig. 2.8), which is further exacerbated by dilution caused by administered crystalloids. This response may be partly protective in that it allows immune mediators to cross the capillary barrier and reach the site of injury or infection. Increased capillary permeability also leads to intravascular hypovolaemia and an expansion of the interstitial space.

Severely injured and critically ill patients may require large amounts of sodium-containing crystalloids or colloids to maintain their intravascular volume and oxygen delivery to the cells, although artificial colloids allow the use of lower fluid volumes (as

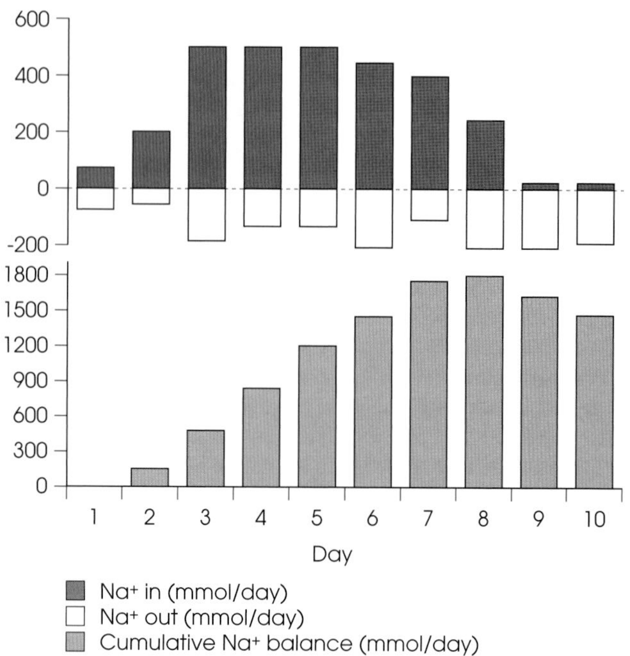

Figure 2.9 The daily and cumulative salt balance in a ventilated patient with a crushed chest when more than 2 L of saline per day was prescribed.

discussed later in this chapter). Resuscitation is therefore achieved, but at the expense of overexpansion of the interstitial space, which may be an inevitable price paid for adequate intravascular volume replacement. Continuing to give large volumes of salt-containing fluids for 'maintenance' may cause unnecessary and increasing fluid overload (Fig. 2.9). In one study on patients with peritonitis, the average extracellular fluid overload after the first 2 days of resuscitation exceeded 12 L, which took 3 weeks to mobilize and excrete.[31,32] Increased capillary permeability and a positive fluid balance may encourage multiorgan failure,[28,33–35] and attempts to limit interstitial oedema have shown benefit.[34,36]

The objective is to restore normal physiology and normal organ function, with a normal blood volume, body water, and electrolytes. This can never be achieved by inundation.[37]

Extracellular fluid versus intracellular fluid

Severe illness may be associated with impaired sodium pumping, the so-called *sick cell syndrome*.[38] This can be confirmed by

REFERENCES

28. Plante GE, Chakir M, Lehoux S et al. Can J Cardiol 1995; 11: 788–802
29. Ballmer-Weber BK, Dummer R, Kung E et al. Br J Cancer 1995; 71: 78–82
30. Fleck A, Raines G, Hawker F et al. Lancet 1985; 1: 781–784
31. Plank LD, Connolly AB, Hill GL. Ann Surg 1998; 228: 146–158
32. Plank LD, Hill GL. Ann N Y Acad Sci 2000; 904: 592–602
33. Gosling P. Care Crit Ill 1999; 15:11–16
34. Alsous F, Khamiees M, DeGirolamo A et al. Chest 2000; 117: 1749–1754
35. Arieff AI. Chest 1999; 115: 1371–1377
36. Mitchell JP, Schuller D, Calandrino FS et al. Am Rev Respir Dis 1992; 145: 990–998
37. Moore FD, Shires G. Ann Surg 1967; 166: 300–301
38. Flear CT, Singh CM. Br J Anaesth 1973; 45: 976–994

Table 2.7 Changes in muscle glycogen, sodium, potassium and creatine in patients with multiple organ failure

	Glycogen (μmol/100μmol creatine)	Sodium (μmol/100μmol creatine)	Potassium (μmol/100μmol creatine)	Total creatine (μmol/g dry weight)
Patients: median (range)	164 (78–407)	201 (125–507)	274 (175–485)	95 (43–121)
Normal range	151–383	40–132	319–415	18–159

(From Campbell IT et al. Proc Nutr Soc 1998; S7: 117A with permission.[39])

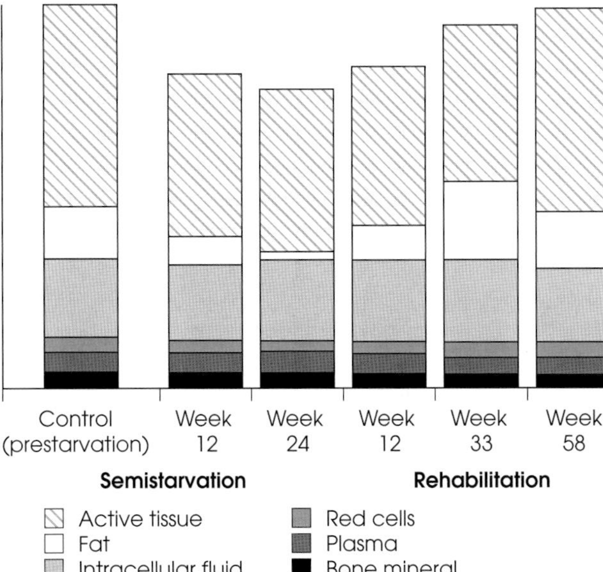

Figure 2.10 Major body compartments, as body weight, in young men in the state of normal nutrition, and in semistarvation and subsequent rehabilitation. (After Keys A, Brozek J et al. The Biology of Human Starvation (Vol 1, p. iv). © 1950 University of Minnesota Press: Minneapolis, with permission.[42])

measuring electrolyte and metabolite concentrations in muscle biopsies from critically ill patients (see Table 2.7),[39] and may be reversed by correcting the underlying condition (e.g. sepsis), by ensuring adequate cellular perfusion by restoring effective blood volume, and by manipulating metabolism by the use of insulin, glucose and potassium.[26]

EFFECTS OF STARVATION

Patients may also suffer from starvation and weight loss, leading to famine and refeeding oedema.[40–42] In semistarved normal volunteers who were then refed,[42] the fat and lean compartments of the body were found to shrink, but the extracellular fluid volume remained either at its prestarvation level or it decreased very slightly (Fig. 2.10). The extracellular fluid volume therefore occupies an increasing proportion of the body mass as starvation progresses. The degree of oedema may be related to the patient's sodium and water access and may be exacerbated by refeeding. Sodium and water balance may also be affected by the diarrhoea that afflicts famine victims, as well as cardiovascular decompensation from the effects of starvation on the myocardium.

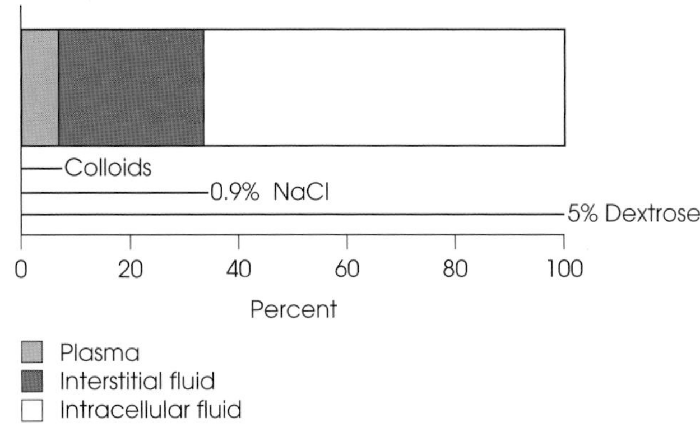

Figure 2.11 Distribution of infused fluids in the body water compartments.

PHARMACOLOGY OF FLUIDS

Salt-containing crystalloid and colloidal solutions are used during resuscitation to expand the intravascular volume. The properties of some commonly used crystalloids are summarized in Table 2.8.

The ability of a solution to expand the plasma volume is dependent on its volume of distribution and the metabolic fate of the solute. Colloids are mainly distributed in the intravascular compartment, but once the dextrose is metabolized, dextrose-containing solutions are distributed through the total body water and hence have a limited and transient blood volume-expanding capacity (Fig. 2.11, Table 2.9). Isotonic sodium-containing crystalloids are distributed throughout the whole extracellular fluid, including the plasma. Normal saline infusions were thought to expand the blood volume by a third of the volume of crystalloid infused.[43] In practice, the efficiency of these solutions to expand the plasma volume is between 20 and 25%, the remainder being sequestered in the interstitial space.[44,45] The price paid for

REFERENCES

39. Campbell IT, Green CJ, Jackson MJ. Proc Nutr Soc 1998; 57: 111A
40. Winick M. Hunger Disease: Studies by the Jewish Physicians in the Warsaw Ghetto. Wiley, New York, 1979
41. Shizgal HM. Surg Gynecol Obstet 1981; 152: 22–26
42. Keys A, Brozek J, Henschel A et al. The Biology of Human Starvation, Vol 1. University of Minnesota Press, Minneapolis, 1950
43. Kaye AD, Grogono AW. In: Miller RD, Cucchiara RF, Miller ED Jr et al (eds). Anesthesia, Vol 1. Churchill Livingstone, Philadelphia, 2000: 1586–1612
44. Lamke LO, Liljedahl SO. Resuscitation 1976; 5: 93–102
45. Svensen C, Hahn RG. Anesthesiology 1997; 87: 204–212

Table 2.8 Properties of commonly prescribed crystalloids

	Plasma*	0.9% Sodium chloride	Hartmann's	0.18% Sodium chloride/ 4% dextrose	5% Dextrose
Sodium (mmol/L)	135–145	154	131	31	0
Chloride (mmol/L)	95–105	154	111	31	0
$[Na^+]:[Cl^-]$ ratio	1.28–1.45:1	1:1	1.18:1	1:1	–
Potassium (mmol/L)	3.5–5.3	0	5	0	0
Bicarbonate (mmol/L)	24–32	0	29	0	0
Ca^{2+} (mmol/L)	2.2–2.6	0	4	0	0
Glucose (mmol/L)	3.5–5.5	0	0	222.2 (40 g)	277.8 (50 g)
pH	7.35–7.45	5.0–5.5	6.5	4.5	4.0
Osmolality (mOsm/L)	275–295	308	274	286	280

*Normal laboratory range from Queen's Medical Centre, Nottingham, UK.

Table 2.9 Volume of infusion required to expand the plasma volume by 1 L

	Infused volume (mL)	Δ Interstitial volume (mL)	Δ Intracellular volume (mL)
5% Albumin	1000	–	–
25% Albumin	250	– 750*	–
5% Dextrose	14 000	+ 3700	+ 9300
Hartmann's solution/ 0.9% saline	4700	+ 3700	–

*Fluid is drawn into the intravascular compartment from the interstitial compartment.

Table 2.10 Volume effects of some colloidal solutions

Colloidal solution	Initial plasma-expanding effect (%)
Long-acting (5–6 h)	
6% Dextran 60	120
6% HES 450/0.7	100
6% HES 200/0.62	100
Medium-acting (3–4 h)	
10% Dextran 40	200
6% HES 200/0.5	100
10% HES 200/0.5	130
Short-acting (1–2 h)	
6% HES 70/0.5	70
3% Gelatin	70
5% Albumin	70–90

HES, hydroxyl ethyl starch. Properties are dependent on concentration, the weight-averaged mean molecular weight, the number-averaged molecular weight, the molar substitution, and the degree of substitution.
(From Boldt J. Volume replacement in the surgical patient – does the type of solution make a difference? Br J Anaesth 2000; 84: 783–793, with permission of Oxford University Press.[47])

adequate intravascular filling is overexpansion of the interstitial space and tissue oedema, which has to be excreted once the shock phase has passed. Solutions of dextrose or hypotonic saline can cause significant hyponatraemia (sodium less than 130 mmol/L) and care should be taken to avoid this potentially harmful effect, particularly in children and the elderly.

Colloids are fluids that contain large particles that are retained within the circulation for some time, therefore exerting an oncotic pressure across the capillary membrane. Albumin solutions disperse at a similar time because they contain particles of uniform molecular weight, while synthetic colloids contain particles of varying sizes and molecular weights in an attempt to optimize the half-life and plasma volume-expanding capacities of the solutions.[46,47] The intravascular volume-expanding effects of commonly used colloids are summarized in Table 2.10.

METHODS OF ADMINISTRATION

ORAL OR ENTERAL

Patients with intact gastrointestinal function and moderate degrees of water and/or salt depletion may be rehydrated orally or enterally; for example, in the management of diarrhoeal diseases in children (see the *British National Formulary*).

INTRAVENOUS CANNULAE

Peripheral

Most fluids are infused through a peripheral venous cannula. Peripheral cannulae should be inserted and maintained with meticulous care and good technique using established protocols, because their potential for causing morbidity and even mortality from infection is often underestimated. Every hospital should have clear guidelines to ensure optimal care of peripheral cannulae as part of clinical governance. Insertion sites should be inspected daily, and cannulae removed or resited at the earliest sign of any inflammation. Cannulae should be resited at least every 72 h.

REFERENCES

46. Nolan J. Br Med Bull 1999; 55: 821–843
47. Boldt J. Br J Anaesth 2000; 84: 783–793

Central

Modern single or multilumen polyurethane or silastic cannulae inserted into the internal jugular or subclavian vein have even greater potential than peripheral cannulae to cause morbidity and mortality unless inserted and maintained by skilled staff observing strict protocols.

Subcutaneous

Either 0.9% saline (500–2000 mL daily) or 5% dextrose (500 mL) containing up to 34 mmol/L KCl and/or 4 mmol/L $MgSO_4$ can be infused via a fine butterfly cannula into the subcutaneous fat. This can be useful in the elderly or very young, and has been used safely in hospital and at home in patients with excessive gastrointestinal fluid losses.

Table 2.11 Clinical features and consequences of salt and water overload

- Peripheral oedema.
- Gastrointestinal oedema.
- Pulmonary oedema.
- Congestive cardiac failure.
- Possible hyperchloraemic acidosis.
- Confusion.
- Delayed return of gastrointestinal function to normal.
- Impaired wound healing, anastomotic oedema and anastomotic dehiscence.
- Pressure sores.
- Increased incidence of deep vein thrombosis.
- Delayed mobilization.

DIAGNOSIS

The diagnosis of fluid and electrolyte disorders is made from history, examination and investigations. It is important to consider the internal balance between the body fluid compartments as well as the external balance between the body and its environment.

HISTORY

A history of vomiting, diarrhoea, nasogastric aspirate, fistula losses or pooling in the gut from ileus or obstruction indicates the likelihood of a fluid deficit, and a knowledge of the electrolyte content (Table 2.5) of the fluid loss predicts the type of fluid required for replacement.

Table 2.12 Clinical features and consequences of salt and water depletion

- Reduced extracellular fluid and plasma volume.
- Dry mouth, reduced saliva or parotitis.
- Sunken facies.
- Diminished skin turgor.
- Postural hypotension.
- Tachycardia.
- Reduced stroke volume.
- Impaired renal perfusion.
- Increased viscosity of pulmonary mucus.
- Increased blood viscosity.

EXAMINATION

Fluid excess

The presence of oedema of the limbs or trunk, in the absence of venous or lymphatic obstruction, indicates expansion of the interstitial space (Table 2.11). Oedema is apparent only if the extracellular fluid is expanded by 2–3 L, although the patient's skin may show the indentation marks of clothes with more modest excess. When the jugular venous pressure is raised, it is usually indicative of heart failure or intravascular fluid overload. If the jugular veins do not fill with the patient horizontal, this suggests blood or plasma volume deficit, despite interstitial oedema.

Fluid deficit

Loss of blood or plasma can be recognized by the autonomic responses of pallor, sweating, tachycardia, hypotension, oliguria, and a low jugular venous pressure (Table 2.12).

Loss of extracellular fluid in the form of salt and water is usually called *dehydration*, which is a woolly and imprecise term. True dehydration, which is a pure water deficit, has to be extreme to produce any signs, although minor degrees of water lack cause marked thirst. The term *salt and water depletion* is more precise and is therefore to be preferred (Table 2.1). A firm diagnosis of this condition can be made only after consideration of all the symptoms and signs. A dry mouth may be present, but is more commonly caused by mouth breathing. Sunken facies may be present, but are more commonly associated with cachexia. A diminished skin turgor is apparent with a modest salt and water deficit of as little as 1–2 L, but is also a feature of aging and severe weight loss. With extreme deficits the blood pressure falls, but postural hypotension is a much earlier feature. A postural fall of more than 10 mmHg is usually present, and other cardiovascular signs include a tachycardia and a low central venous pressure.

INVESTIGATIONS AND THEIR INTERPRETATION

Urine

A low volume of concentrated urine, confirmed by finding a raised urine-to-plasma urea or osmolality ratio, is associated with a pure water deficit and with a salt and water deficit. When there is associated sepsis or renal failure, there may be small or large volumes of urine that are poorly concentrated.

Blood biochemistry

Creatinine and urea concentration

Concentrations of creatinine and urea are affected by muscle mass and protein turnover, respectively. Elevated values are compatible with prerenal failure from a fluid deficit, but intrinsic renal and postrenal failure may also be responsible.

Plasma sodium concentration

The plasma sodium concentration provides only a ratio of sodium to water in the extracellular fluid. Low plasma sodium may be caused by water excess, sodium lack, or a combination of both. When there are signs of fluid overload, a low serum sodium indicates that both water and sodium are present in excess, but water more so than sodium. In severely ill patients, the presence of the sick cell syndrome must be considered; this is caused by a failure of cellular sodium pumping producing an increase in the intracellular sodium. Conversely, a high plasma sodium may indicate water lack, sodium excess, or both. The interpretation of this finding again depends on the associated clinical features.

Plasma potassium

Because less than 2% of the body potassium is in the extracellular fluid, the plasma level is an indicator of deficit or excess, and also of the flux between the extracellular fluid and intracellular fluid, which is affected by cellular catabolism or anabolism. It is also dependent on acid–base changes and on renal function.

Plasma bicarbonate and chloride

Most biochemistry laboratories have stopped providing these values routinely but they are helpful where there are clinical indications of significant abnormalities of fluid balance.

Plasma, calcium, magnesium, other minerals, and trace elements

These should be measured where clinically appropriate.

MONITORING

WEIGHT

Weighing on admission and daily thereafter provides one of the most important measures of water balance. It is compromised by severe loss of fluid into the bowel, with ileus or obstruction, which are functionally outside the extracellular fluid but are included in the weight. Its interpretation as always needs to be tempered by clinical judgment. The changes in water balance that weight change assesses allows interpretation of changes in plasma sodium (in the absence of sick cell syndrome) and the correct prescription of the next day's fluids.

FLUID BALANCE CHARTS

The cumulative errors in fluid balance calculation can be large, because the insensible loss can only be estimated and there are often errors in measurement and recording. When checked against weight, however, these charts are invaluable in providing information on changes in the urine volume, the gastric aspirate, and the output from a fistula or stoma, which helps to guide replacement.

URINE

Oliguria and a low sodium output are part of the normal physiological response to surgery and acute illness or injury. An uncritical protocol that states that a postoperative urine output of less than 30 mL/h is an indication for giving saline is an important factor responsible for the postoperative fluid overload from which many patients suffer. It is important to recognize that if the blood urea concentration is not rising, the patient is passing enough urine to excrete waste products (*volume obligatoire*). Saline should be given only to replace a salt deficit or the projected losses over the next 24 h. In the absence of an intravascular or total extracellular fluid deficit, water given enterally, or 5% dextrose given intravenously, produce a much better diuresis than saline, which is mainly retained. Healthy kidneys, in the presence of dehydration, concentrate urine 100 times. The criteria for diagnosing intrinsic and oliguric renal failure are a urine volume of less than 400 mL and a urine:plasma urea ratio of less than 14.1.[48] A rising blood urea associated with poor urinary concentration and a urinary volume of less than a litre suggests polyuric renal failure.

BLOOD BIOCHEMISTRY

In most patients undergoing elective surgery, repeated biochemical measurements are unnecessary, but in complex cases they may need to be performed more frequently. Interpretation of these tests has already been discussed, but any changes should always be assessed in the light of the other measures and an understanding of the pathophysiology of the patient's condition.

TREATMENT

Fluid management can be considered in three phases: acute, postacute and maintenance.

THE ACUTE PHASE: RESUSCITATION AND TREATMENT OF HYPOVOLAEMIC SHOCK

Hypovolaemic shock is the most common type of shock occurring in the surgical patient, and the principles of resuscitation are covered in Chapter 7. The effective blood volume is the volume of blood in the arterial system at any given time, which provides perfusion of vital organs. It may be diminished by haemorrhage or by redistribution and pooling from loss of venomotor tone caused by sepsis.

Haemorrhage must be controlled and resuscitation started. Venous access should be established with two 16-G venous cannulae, and patients should receive a 2-L fluid bolus, preferably in the form of Hartmann's solution to avoid the hyperchloraemic acidosis caused by saline. Hypotonic solutions such as dextrose saline or dextrose should not be given. Colloids are theoretically ideal, but there is no clear evidence that colloids are better than crystalloids and a mixture of the two is often used. The stomach is decompressed with a nasogastric tube to avoid acute gastric dilatation and aspiration, and a urinary catheter should be inserted to assess the urinary output. Blood transfusion is usually required if the estimated blood loss is more than 30% of the blood volume.

The further management of patients with shock is dependent on the initial response (Fig. 2.12, Table 2.13). Patients who have lost less than 20% of their blood volume respond rapidly and remain haemodynamically stable provided there are no continuing losses. Those with a blood loss of between 20 and 40% who have a transient response to the initial fluid bolus require more fluid and usually require blood. Those who have a minimal response to the initial fluid bolus require early surgical control of blood loss. Occasionally, lack of response may be the result of direct cardiac injury, cardiac tamponade, or a tension pneumothorax.[49]

The use of albumin solutions to treat circulatory hypovolaemia is felt to be unjustified because of its expense and its rapid leakage from the circulation. Plasma substitutes, which normally have a shorter half-life than albumin in the circulation, may have a longer half-life in acute illness and injury[50] and are generally preferred for volume expansion. Alternatives include crystalloids (preferably Ringer's lactate or Hartmann's solution) or a combination of a crystalloid and a colloid. The relative effectiveness

REFERENCES

48. Luke RG, Kennedy AC. Postgrad Med J 1967; 43: 280–289
49. American College of Surgeons Committee on Trauma. Advanced Trauma Life Support for Doctors Student Course Manual. 6th edn. American College of Surgeons, Chicago, 1997
50. Salmon JB, Mythen MG. Blood Rev 1993; 7: 114–120

Table 2.13 Is my patient getting better?

- Improved blood pressure or less tachycardia.
- Better thermoregulation: patients with cardiogenic shock warm up, those with septic shock cool down.
- Increased urine output.
- Improved P_AO_2 oxygen saturation.
- Reduced base deficit and lactate.
- Shift of mixed venous oxygen concentration towards normal.
- Improved gastric mucosal pH (i.e. less acidic).
- The core peripheral temperature gradient narrows.
- Cardiac index or output returns to normal.
- The patient looks better.

Table 2.14 The postacute phase

- Salt and water overload.
- Increased interstitial volume.
- Oedema.
- May have low, normal or raised plasma volume and hypoalbuminaemia.
- Capillary permeability has probably returned to normal.
- Aim of treatment is to get rid of excess salt and water.
- Treat with salt and water restriction.
- May need a diuretic.
- Patients with a low plasma volume may benefit from salt-poor albumin infusion.

of these solutions, used separately or in combination, has been much debated.[51–56] The primary concern in the acute phase is to maintain the intravascular volume and ensure the circulation to vital organs rather than to address the albumin concentration.[26] Profound falls in albumin concentration may, however, predispose to systemic and pulmonary oedema[57] unless excessive administration of salt and water is avoided. Albumin solutions are still widely used in children to treat shock associated with meningococcal septicaemia, and to treat septic shock from spontaneous bacterial peritonitis in adults with liver cirrhosis.[58] Albumin infusions are, however, usually unnecessary.[59]

THE POSTACUTE PHASE

Salt and water overload is occasionally an inevitable consequence of resuscitation (Table 2.14). This can, however, take up to 3 weeks to excrete,[31] and if this is delayed by complications,[10,26] particularly in the elderly,[60] can cause persistent oedema. Additional overload must be avoided by sensible prescribing of maintenance fluids after the need for resuscitation has passed. It is important not to forget that salt and water are contained in antibiotic infusions and infusions used to maintain the patency of arterial and venous cannulae. Many antibiotics are sodium salts! A low serum albumin concentration, which can be the result of redistribution from inflammation, also follows dilution from fluid infusions.[61–63] Salt and water retention with oedema has erroneously been thought to be innocuous and with the patients rapidly able to excrete any excess that has been administered. There is now increasing evidence that suggests that salt and water accumulation is associated with inhibition of gastrointestinal function, pulmonary complications and prolonged recovery.[25,35,64–67]

In this phase, oedema associated with an elevated jugular venous pressure should be treated by salt and water restriction, which can be combined with diuretics in some cases. When there are persistent serous losses from wounds or into inflamed tissues, this can cause a gradual fall in blood volume evident by poor filling of the jugular veins even in the horizontal position. This is usually associated with a low blood pressure, tachycardia and oliguria. As the transcapillary escape of albumin may have returned to normal, it is logical to provide a low-salt concentrated colloid with a long half-life, i.e. 20% salt-poor albumin. Between 200 and 400 mL of this solution given over 48 h results in prompt improvement in, and the tachycardia and blood pressure with, a salt and water diuresis, thus avoiding the need for repeated infusions.[59] A diuretic should also be given if oedema is severe.

The use of concentrated salt-poor albumin with or without diuretics in the postacute period is illustrated in Fig. 2.12. Albumin infusions must be carefully monitored by direct measurement of the jugular venous pressure,[68] because inappropriate or excessive administration can be dangerous. Albumin infusions are used in this situation to treat plasma hypovolaemia in the presence of an interstitial salt and water overload, not to correct hypoalbuminaemia.

MAINTENANCE

Uncomplicated postoperative patients may inadvertently be prescribed an excess of both sodium and water, because maintenance requirements are not equivalent to those for resuscitation. Oliguria and salt and water retention are almost universal after surgery, stress and trauma, and most patients require no more than 2–2.5 L of water and 60–100 mmol of sodium per day. Potassium is best avoided on the first and second postoperative days, unless the serum potassium is low. Regular potassium supplements should, however, be prescribed from the second day onwards (Table 2.15).

Patients with excessive losses from nasogastric aspirate, diarrhoea, and intestinal fistulae must be prescribed equivalent replacements in addition to their maintenance requirements (Table 2.5).

REFERENCES

51. Schierhout G, Roberts I. Br Med J 1998; 316: 961–964
52. Cochrane Injuries Group Albumin Reviewers. Br Med J 1998; 317: 235–240
53. Choi PTL, Yip G, Quinonez LG et al. Crit Care Med 1999; 27: 200–210
54. Webb AR. Crit Care 1999; 3: R25–R28
55. Allison SP, Lobo DN. Crit Care 2000; 4: 147–150
56. Pulimood TB, Park GR. Crit Care 2000; 4: 151–155
57. Guyton AC. Circ Res 1959; 7: 649–657
58. Sort P, Navasa M, Arroyo V et al. N Engl J Med 1999; 341: 403–409
59. Allison SP, Lobo DN, Stanga Z. Clin Nutr 2001; 20: 275–279
60. Cheng AT, Plank LD, Hill GL. Arch Surg 1998; 133: 745–751
61. Marik PE. Heart Lung 1993; 22: 166–170
62. Mullins RJ, Garrison RN. Ann Surg 1989; 209: 651–659, discussion 659–661
63. Sitges-Serra A, Franch-Arcas G. Curr Opin Clin Nutr Metab Care 1998; 1: 9–14
64. Mecray PM, Barden RP, Ravdin IS. Surgery 1937; 1: 53–64
65. Starker PM, Lasala PA, Askanazi J et al. Ann Surg 1983; 198: 720–724
66. Gil MJ, Franch G, Guirao X et al. Nutrition 1997; 13: 26–31
67. Holte K, Sharrock NE, Kehlet H. Br J Anaesth 2002; 89: 622–632
68. Lucas CE, Weaver D, Higgins RF et al. J Trauma 1978; 18: 564–570

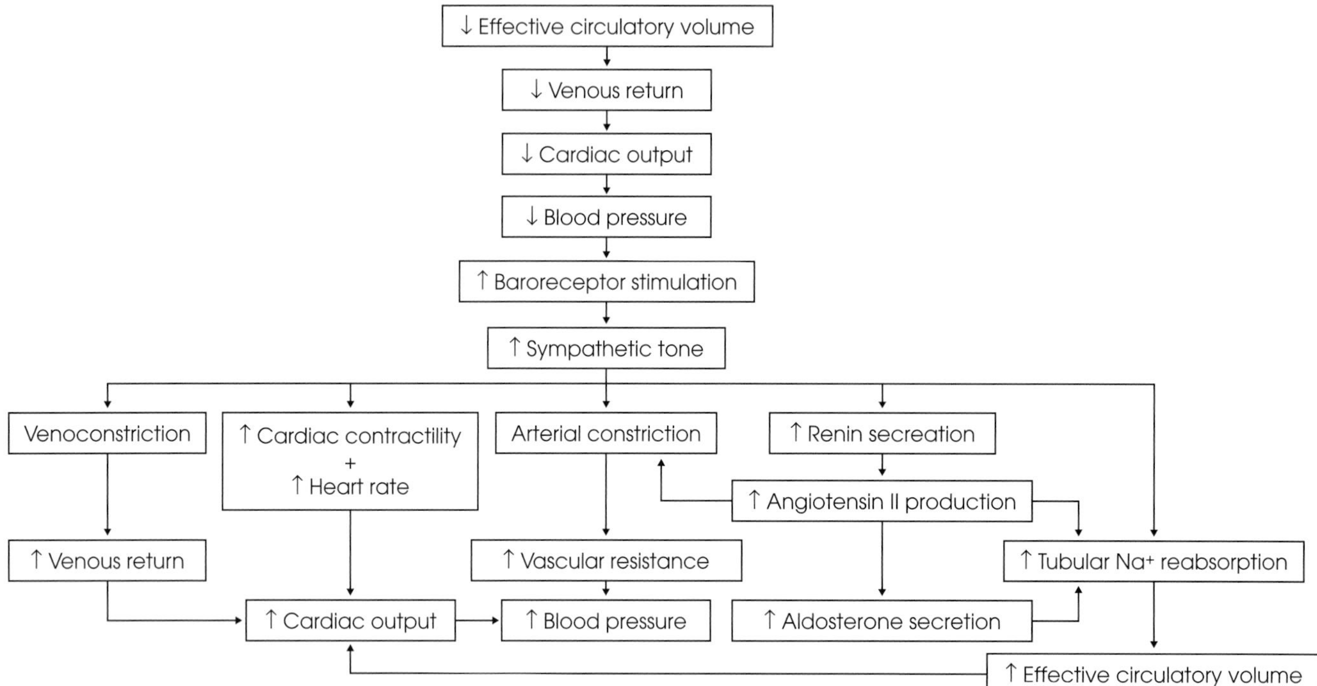

Figure 2.12 Haemodynamic responses to hypovolaemia. (After Rose BD, Post TW. Clinical physiology of acid-base and electrolyte disorders. © 2001, McGraw-Hill: New York, with permission of The McGraw-Hill Companies.[6])

Table 2.15 Maintenance: requirements and provision for a 70-kg man

	24-h requirement	Provided by 2.5 L dextrose (4%)/ saline (0.18%)
Water	25–35 mL/kg (1.7–2.5 L)	2.5 L
Sodium	1–1.2 mmol/kg (70–85 mmol)	75 mmol
Potassium	0.8–1 mmol/kg (56–70 mmol)	Must be added
Dextrose	100 g (400 cal) to prevent ketosis	100 g

Table 2.16 Normal arterial acid-base measurements

pH	7.35–7.45
P_AO_2 (kPa)	10.7–16.0
P_ACO_2 (kPa)	4.7–6.0
Bicarbonate (mmol/L)	22–26
Base excess (mmol/L)	− 2 to + 2
Anion gap (mmol/L)	10–14

In the early postoperative period, the daily urine output may be only slightly greater than the *volume obligatoire*, but if the blood urea concentration does not rise a fluid challenge is unnecessary. In the presence of a normal intravascular and extracellular fluid volume, it is inappropriate to give more isotonic sodium-containing fluids.

ACID–BASE BALANCE

The normal acid–base composition of the *milieu interieur* (Table 2.16) must be maintained within narrow limits for the optimal cellular function. This section will focus on the clinically important acid–base disturbances likely to be encountered in surgical practice; a more detailed description of the condition and its treatment can be found elsewhere.[6]

A normal blood pH of 7.4 is maintained by buffering systems in the blood. The pH of the extracellular fluid is controlled by the relative proportions of carbonic acid (derived from carbon dioxide) and bicarbonate defined by the Henderson–Hasselbalch equation,

$$\text{pH} = 6.10 + \log([\text{HCO}_3^-]/0.03\ p\text{CO}_2)$$

and also by phosphate according to the reaction,

$$\text{HPO}_4^{2-} + \text{H}^+ \rightleftharpoons \text{H}_2\text{PO}_4$$

The pH of intracellular fluid is dependent on haemoglobin and both organic and inorganic phosphate. It is also influenced by bone and its calcium salts.

In addition, three main organs play a vital role in acid–base control. First, the kidney, by controlling hydrogen and bicarbonate excretion and reabsorption; it also converts ammonia NH_3 to ammonium NH_4^+ in the urine.

The lung controls carbon dioxide levels in the blood, increasing expired carbon dioxide when more is produced or to compensate for metabolic acidosis.

The liver removes and recycles large amounts of lactate produced by anaerobic respiration (the Cori cycle).

These systems may be challenged by any condition in which acid losses are excessive, such as vomiting, and also when there are excessive alkaline losses of bicarbonate from pancreatic or upper small intestinal fistulae. Equally, increased production of

Table 2.17 Acid-base measurements: clinical disturbances

		Uncompensated			Compensated		
Disturbance	Type	pH	P_ACO_2	Bicarbonate	pH	P_ACO_2	Bicarbonate
Acidosis	Metabolic	↓↓	Normal	↓↓	↓	↓	↓
	Respiratory	↓↓	↑↑	Normal	↓	↑↑	↓
Alkalosis	Metabolic	↑↑	Normal	↑↑	↑	↑	↑
	Respiratory	↑↑	↓↓	Normal	↑	↓↓	↓

acids in lactic acidosis or ketoacidosis in diabetic patients whose condition is out of control can cause the acid–base balance to fail.

CLASSIFICATION OF ACID-BASE DISTURBANCES

Any disease that impairs renal, pulmonary or hepatic function can lead to disturbances in the acid–base balance that may be classified under the following headings (see also Table 2.17).

Respiratory acidosis

Respiratory acidosis is characterized by a rise in arterial carbon dioxide from alveolar hypoventilation. This may occur acutely from respiratory depression caused by drugs or neurological damage, from respiratory muscle weakness, from chest injury, or from acute airways obstruction. The partial pressure of carbon dioxide may also be permanently elevated in some cases of chronic obstructive airways disease, when it may be partially compensated for by an increase in plasma bicarbonate. The problem may be exacerbated in the perioperative period by atelectasis, respiratory infection, retained sputum, abdominal distension, splinting of the diaphragm, wound pain and high doses of opiates. Epidural analgesia may help to reduce some of these problems. In severe cases, particularly in those with prior lung disease, bronchial suction and mechanical ventilation may be necessary. Good chest physiotherapy in the postoperative period should, however, reduce the necessity for these more drastic measures.

Respiratory alkalosis

Respiratory alkalosis is the result of hyperventilation causing a low carbon dioxide and, in chronic cases, some compensatory reduction in the bicarbonate. It may be iatrogenic from deliberate or mistakenly overenthusiastic artificial ventilation, or it may be secondary to anxiety or distress. It can cause paraesthesiae, tetany and chest pain, and it may be relieved by reducing ventilation or by rebreathing expired air.

Metabolic acidosis

Metabolic acidosis is characterized by a low bicarbonate with a compensatory fall in the carbon dioxide from hyperventilation. Patients may complain of shortness of breath and hyperventilate with deep sighing respirations (Kussmaul's respiration). It may be caused by excess production of acid, which occurs in diabetic ketoacidosis, or lactic acidosis from tissue anoxia. Renal and liver failure—failure of the organs responsible for clearing organic acids—also cause metabolic acidosis, as does excessive loss of bicarbonate from pancreatic fistulae or intestinal fluid losses. Diarrhoea and purgative abuse may also give rise to acidosis accompanied by hypokalaemia, although a low potassium is usually accompanied by alkalosis. A hyperchloraemic acidosis may also result from the administration of large amounts of saline, as discussed earlier. The treatment of metabolic acidosis is primarily that of the underlying cause, although the administration of appropriate amounts of sodium bicarbonate orally or intravenously may be necessary. In metabolic acidosis potassium leaves the cell, but when the acidosis is corrected by a sodium bicarbonate infusion this effect is reversed, causing a fall in the serum potassium.

Metabolic alkalosis

Metabolic alkalosis is characterized by a pH of greater than 7.4 and an elevated bicarbonate. It is often accompanied by hypokalaemia from excretion of potassium or sodium in exchange for hydrogen in the distal tubule. This creates a vicious cycle of hypokalaemic alkalosis, in which the urine paradoxically becomes acidic as the kidney tries to retain potassium and sodium in preference to the hydrogen ions. This requires correction by a combination of potassium and sodium chloride solutions, which must be sufficient to raise plasma concentrations and also to allow the kidney sufficient cation to exchange for hydrogen in the distal tubule. These solutions also correct the chloride deficit. The commonest cause of alkalosis in surgical patients is loss of gastric acid from vomiting or nasogastric aspiration.

CLINICAL EVALUATION

It can be seen that the history gives clues to the likely problem. Acidosis is usually accompanied by hyperventilation, while alkalosis may cause tetany and muscle weakness. Investigations should include an arterial blood gas analysis and measurement of venous bicarbonate and chloride. The serum creatinine, urea and electrolytes should also be measured. An abnormally high anion gap is said to exist when the sum of the concentration of chloride and bicarbonate plus eight is less than the serum sodium concentration. This indicates a metabolic acidosis. Direct measurement of acid–base values should always be carried out when an abnormality is suspected.

MINERALS

MAGNESIUM

Half of the total body magnesium of 100–1400 mmol is in bone and half in the intracellular fluid. Only 12–20 mmol are present in the extracellular fluid at a concentration of 0.7–1.2 mmol/L. The normal daily intake is 12–15 mmol. Hypomagnesaemia, if severe or prolonged, causes hypoparathyroidism, which in turn causes hypocalcaemia. Many patients seem to tolerate levels of magnesium as low as 0.3–0.5 mmol/L without symptoms, suggesting that neuromuscular irritability, convulsions, peripheral vasodilatation, and cardiac arrhythmias are secondary to hypocalcaemia or to combined deficiency of calcium and magnesium. Hypocalcaemic patients should always have their magnesium level measured.

Most severe cases of hypomagnesaemia are the result of intestinal fluid losses, particularly from the distal gut.

Magnesium levels must be interpreted in the light of changes in serum albumin, to which it is bound. Oral supplements of magnesium oxide, glycerophosphate or chelate can be administered, although these may not be able to keep the serum magnesium above 0.5 mmol/L in severe cases of short bowel syndrome. Providing that symptoms do not develop, oral supplementation may suffice. The true extent of the magnesium depletion can be assessed by giving an intravenous magnesium load of 0.1 mmol/kg in 4 h. Normally, less than a quarter of the load is excreted in the urine over 24 h, reflecting the efficient renal conservation of magnesium in the face of deficiency. Administration of 1600 mmol of magnesium sulphate in saline over 2–3 days may be needed to replace the deficit in severe cases of deficiency.

CALCIUM

The body contains 33 000 mmol of calcium, mainly in bone. The normal concentration in plasma is 2.2–2.5 mmol/L, all except 0.01 mmol of which is bound to protein. The measured concentration, therefore, has to be adjusted upwards by 0.02 mmol for every 1-g fall in serum albumin between 40 and 25 g/L. Calcium is vital for nerve conduction, muscle contraction, hormone secretion, and many other metabolic processes. A low level of free calcium is associated with tetany, fits, unconsciousness and even death. Absorption, concentration and excretion are regulated by vitamin D, parathormone and calcitonin (see Ch. 18). Most filtered calcium is reabsorbed by the kidney, 240 mmol being filtered each day and only 2–10 mmol excreted. Vitamin D, from the diet or produced by the effect of sunlight on the skin, is hydroxylated in the liver and in the kidney to form its most active principle, 1–25$(OH)_2D_3$. Renal failure therefore causes bone disease in the same way as deficiencies of vitamin D and calcium deficiency.

Hypercalcaemia is usually the result of hyperparathyroidism or malignancy, and is less commonly caused by sarcoidosis or vitamin D intoxication. Hypercalcaemia impairs distal renal tubular concentration, giving rise to polyuria, salt and water depletion, and renal failure. Treatment is initially by crystalloid administration and rehydration, which may be sufficient to lower the calcium to normal, although the use of an intravenous bisphosphonate such as pamidronate may be necessary (See Ch. 18).

PHOSPHATE

The body contains 25 000–27 000 mmol of phosphate, mostly in bone, with 4500–5000 mmol in the intracellular fluid and only 12–20 mmol in the extracellular fluid, where its normal concentration is 0.7–1.4 mmol/L. It plays a vital role in many metabolic processes. Administration of excess glucose or refeeding after prolonged starvation without adequate phosphate intake may cause significant falls in the phosphate concentration in the extracellular fluid, leading to muscle weakness, cardiac and respiratory failure, coma and death. Because potassium levels often fall in similar circumstances, phosphate is usually replaced by intravenous administration of KH_2PO_4, with careful biochemical monitoring.

About 30 mmol of phosphate are excreted each day by the kidney, which is 20% of the filtered load. Renal failure may result in hyperphosphataemia requiring treatment to reduce phosphate absorption. Phosphate also plays an important part in acid–base control, as discussed earlier in this chapter.

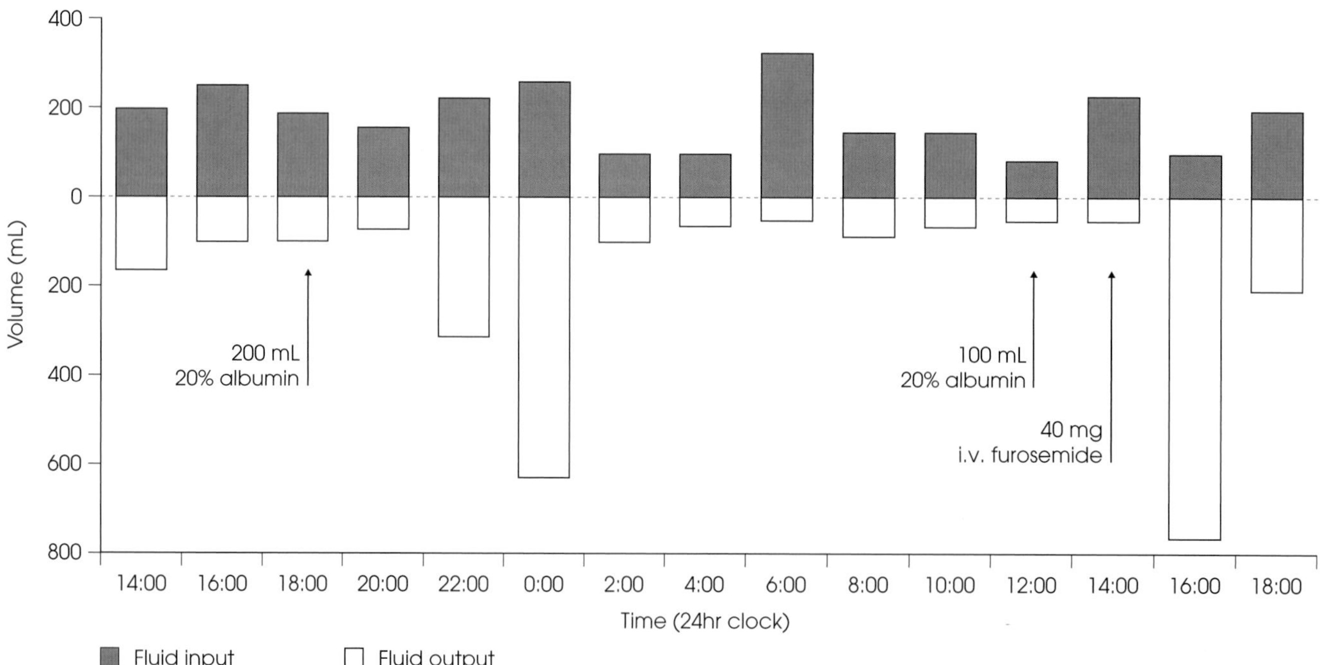

Figure 2.13 An example of the effects of concentrated salt-poor albumin, with and without furosemide, on urinary output in a patient with fluid overload in the postacute phase. Fluid balance is charted at 2-h intervals over a period of 28 h. (From Allison et al. 2001,[59] with permission.)

NUTRITION CASE

Although obesity and overnutrition certainly present risks to the surgical patient, malnutrition also adversely affects surgical outcome. Because many surgical conditions also influence nutritional status, a practical understanding of nutrition is essential.

MALNUTRITION

Incidence

Assessed by changes in weight and body composition, 10–40% of patients are undernourished on admission to hospital, depending on age and case mix 5–20% seriously so, and the majority deteriorate nutritionally during their hospital stay.[69,70] Involuntary loss of body tissue associated with illness is termed *protein-energy malnutrition,* but other single or multiple mineral or micronutrient deficiencies can occur without weight loss. A fifth of all surgical patients are significantly overweight or obese (body mass index, BMI, greater than 30) to an extent that increases the respiratory, cardiovascular and thromboembolic complications of surgery, as well as impairing mobilization and recovery.

Consequences

Fasting for more than 2 months induces weight loss in excess of 35%, with a progressive increase in mortality beyond this point (Fig. 2.14).[42,71–73] The more gradual weight loss described in studies of semistarvation, and the accelerated weight loss when starvation is accompanied by injury, are also shown in Fig. 2.14. The decision box indicates the level of 5–10% involuntary weight loss, at which significant impairment of function and clinical outcome begins and becomes progressively more severe as further tissue is lost. Many surgical patients have a minor degree of perioperative weight loss (2–3 kg) with no ill effect and, as appetite returns, they quickly regain normal function and any lost tissue. Some patients, however, with prior malnutrition or when complications of surgery occur, continue to lose weight without nutritional support. A low initial BMI (less than 20) or weight for height indicates a reduced reserve with which to meet catabolic illness, resulting in higher risk. Wound healing is particularly sensitive to recent nutritional intake.[74]

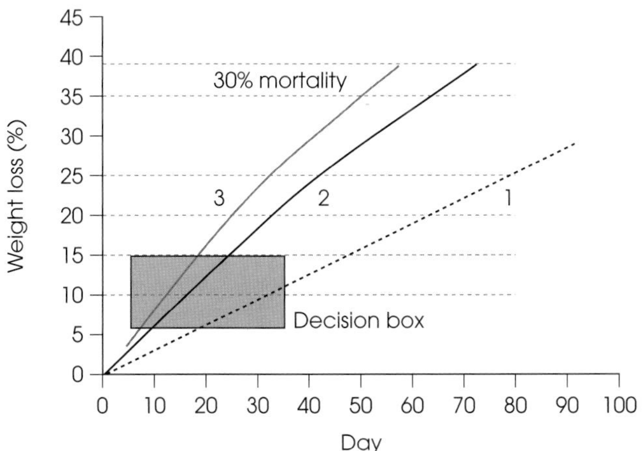

Figure 2.14 Percentage weight loss against time with 1, semistarvation at 20% energy;[42] 2, total starvation (Irish Republican Army) hunger strikers; and 3, during starvation after injury or during illness.[71] The decision box indicates the level of 5–10% involuntary weight loss, at which significant impairment of function and clinical outcome begins and becomes progressively more severe as further tissue is lost. (From Allison 1992,[72] with permission.)

Patients with fractured femurs were categorized into three nutritional groups on admission, normal, thin and very thin, using anthropometric indices.[75,76] The latter two groups were then randomized to receive hospital food only or the hospital food with an overnight nasogastric feed to provide additional energy and protein. Undernutrition was associated with increased mortality, prolonged rehabilitation, and longer hospital stay, and nasogastric feeding reversed these outcomes most strikingly in those with the most severe prior undernutrition. (Table 2.18). The important functional and clinical consequences of undernutrition are shown in Table 2.19.

Definition

Malnutrition can be defined as an excess, deficit or imbalance of nutrients sufficient to cause measurable changes in physiological function and clinical outcome. It should be responsive to nutritional treatment to achieve improvements in function and clinical outcome.

Diagnosis

Although malnutrition is common in hospital, it remains largely undetected and inadequately treated. Elective surgical patients should be screened for malnutrition in the surgical assessment clinic, and appropriate measures taken prior to hospital admission. Patients admitted as emergencies should have their nutrition assessed as soon as possible after admission. A history of loss of stamina or weakness going upstairs is indicative of malnutrition. Changes in anthropometric indices are useful and easily measured indicators of nutritional risk. Diagnosis may be considered in two stages: first rapid screening and second, if necessary, more detailed assessment.[70]

Rapid screening

This process takes less than 3 min and indicates the probability of current or potential nutritional risk. Some screening tools are scored numerically, while others are qualitative. One example of a screening tool is shown in Fig. 2.15. All screening tools should address the following questions:

- What is the BMI (weight in kg/(height in m)^2)?
- Is the patient obese (BMI > 30)?
- Is the patient's weight within the normal range (BMI 20–26)?
- Is the patient undernourished (BMI 18.5–20)?
- Is the patient severely undernourished? (BMI < 18.5)

It is, however, impossible to measure height and weight of all emergency admissions, although these should be measured at the

REFERENCES

69. McWhirter JP, Pennington CR. Br Med J 1994; 308: 945–948
70. Stratton RJ, Green CJ, Elia M. Disease-related Malnutrition: An Evidence-based Approach to Treatment. Cabi Publishing, Wallingford, 2003
71. Kinney JM. Br J Clin Pract Suppl 1988; 63: 114–120
72. Allison SP. Clin Nutr 1992; 11: 319–330
73. Hill GL. Disorders of Nutrition and Metabolism in Clinical Surgery: Understanding and Management. Churchill Livingstone, Edinburgh, 1992
74. Windsor JA, Hill GL. Ann Surg 1988; 207: 290–296
75. Bastow MD, Rawlings J, Allison SP. Lancet 1983; 1: 143–146
76. Bastow MD, Rawlings J, Allison SP. Br Med J 1983; 287: 1589–1592

Table 2.18 Effect of nutritional status and supplementary enteral nutrition on outcome after fractured femur

Group	Mortality (%)	Median rehabilitation time (days)	Hospital stay (days)
Well nourished: food only	4.8	10	–
Thin: control tube–fed	11.4	12	–
	12.8	10 (P = 0.04)	
Very thin: control tube-fed	21	23	38
	8	16 (P = 0.02)	29 (P = 0.04)

(From Bostow Md et al. Br Med J 1983; 287: 1589–1592, with permission from the BMJ Publishing Group.[76])

Table 2.19 Functional and clinical consequences of undernutrition

Function
- Muscle weakness, including the respiratory muscles.
- Impaired immunity and resistance to infection.
- Diminished wound healing.
- Depression and mood change.
- Impaired thermoregulation, predisposition to hypothermia.
- In severe cases, pancreatic, gut, cardiovascular responses are impaired.

Clinical
- Increased mortality.
- Increased surgical complications.
- Prolonged convalescence.
- Increased length of hospital stay.

Economic
- Increased costs.

earliest possible opportunity. The patient or family may be able to provide recent values, but as a last resort a subjective bedside impression of overweight, normal weight or thinness may suffice. A useful surrogate is a tape measurement of midarm circumference, taken midway between the olecranon and acromion with the arm hanging loosely by the side. Values may be compared with normal tables for age and sex and correlate well with other measures. Inadvertent weight loss of 5–10% over the previous 3 months is significant and gives an indication of the direction of recent change. Changes in appetite and food intake can be scored as mild, moderate or severe, and indicate the likely future direction of weight change. The catabolic effects of injury, surgery or complications, and the interference with food ingestion and absorption by disease, predict likely nutritional changes during illness. This allows appropriate measures to be taken to anticipate and prevent deterioration in nutritional status, even in patients who are well nourished on admission. All screening tools should be linked to a protocol for action, as shown in Fig. 2.15.

Detailed assessment

This longer process should be carried out by an experienced clinician, dietitian or nutrition nurse, who will have the screening data and will consider to what extent malnutrition has impaired function. Formal measurement of limb strength by hand dynamometry, or of respiratory muscle strength using peak expiratory flow, provide a valuable baseline for monitoring the response to treatment as improved nutrition produces a rapid improvement in muscle function long before any tissue gain. Depression, apathy and pain are also associated with diminished food intake. Formal enquiry concerning dentition, swallowing and gastrointestinal function is also important. Undernutrition causes mental changes of depression and apathy, creating a vicious circle.

METABOLIC EFFECTS OF INJURY

A rise of 13% in metabolic requirements for every degree rise in temperature above 37°C was first described by Dubois during the First World War.[77] In the 1930s, David Cuthbertson showed that injury caused an increase in metabolic rate, proportional to its severity, as well as a negative nitrogen balance from net breakdown of muscle protein.[78] These changes could have some teleological advantages as they enable injured animals to mobilize body substrates to meet the demands of injury and repair. They do, however, accelerate weight loss (Fig. 2.14) to a level where deleterious effects are soon apparent.

MECHANISM OF THE RESPONSE

The response can be divided into a very brief shock or 'ebb' phase, followed by the 'flow' phase of increased metabolism, and a third phase of convalescence, when inflammation subsides and lost tissue mass and function can be restored.

Neuroendocrine response

The hypothalamus receives efferent signals from the injured part from the nervous system and the circulation through cytokines. This stimulates an increase in catecholamine and cortisol production.[79,80] Glucagon secretion is also increased,[81] and in the shock phase there is an alpha-adrenergic suppression of insulin release, followed by a period of insulin resistance during the flow phase and beyond.[82] This hormonal pattern (Fig. 2.16) ensures

REFERENCES

77. DuBois D, DuBois EF. Arch Intern Med 1916; 17: 863–871
78. Cuthbertson DP. Q J Med 1932; 1: 233–246
79. Cope C, Nathanson IT, Rourke GM et al. Ann Surg 1943; 117: 937
80. Birke G, Duner H, Liljedahl SO et al. Acta Chir Scand 1957; 114: 87
81. Meguid MM, Brennan MF, Muller WA et al. Lancet 1972; 2: 1145
82. Martinez-Riquelme AE, Allison SP. Clin Nutr 2003; 22: 7–15

Is YOUR patient at nutritional risk

Q1a **Height** □.□□ meters
Q1b □ Estimated or □ measured

Q2a **Weight** □.□□ kg
Q2b □ Estimated or □ measured

Q3 **Body mass index** (BMI) = kg/m² (refer to ready-reckoner) □□

		Score
Greater than 20	□	0
18 to 20	□	2
less than 18	□	3

Q4 **Food intake** – has this decreased over the last month

Prior to admission or since the last review? (or is the patient NBM?)			Score
	Greater than 20	□	0
	18 to 20	□	1
	less than 18	□	2

Q5 Has the patient **unintentionally lost weight** over the

Last 3 months or since the last review?			Score
	No	□	0
Up to $^1/_2$ stone (3 kg)	A little	□	1
More than $^1/_2$ stone (3 kg)	Alot	□	2

Q6 **Stress factor/severity of illness**

				Score
None		None	□	0
Moderate	Minor or uncomplicated surgery, minor infection, Chromic disease, pressure sores, CVA, inflammatory bowel disease, other gastrointestinal disease, cirrhosis, renal failure, COPD, diabetes.	Moderate	□	1
Severe	Multiple injuries, multiple fractures, burns, head injury, multiple deep pressure sores, severe sepsis, malignant disease, severe dysphagia, pancreatitis, post-op complications.	Severe	□	2

Q7 **TOTAL SCORE** □

Review patient in 3 days

Q8 **Action**

If score 0–2	Repeat screening within 7 days	□
If score 3–4	Keep food record charts and start supplements if food intake poor	□
If score ≥5	Refer for expert advice	□

Figure 2.15 Example of a screening tool used at Queen's Medical Centre, Nottingham, UK.

an immediate mobilization of glycogen to release glucose, as well as lipolysis of triglyceride to free fatty acids and glycerol, to meet energy demands. Similar changes may be induced by catabolic hormone infusions.[83] There is diminished synthesis and increased catabolism of muscle protein, with release of amino acids, which are used by the liver as a source of new glucose,[84, 85] and for synthesis of acute-phase proteins.

Wounds have an obligatory requirement for glucose, which is broken down anaerobically, with recirculation of lactate through the Cori cycle.[86–89] A wound can therefore be regarded as an acquired organ with its own special demands for amino acids and energy substrates. Deprived of these, wound healing is impaired. After injury there is accelerated metabolism and protein loss, which is in contrast to the response to starvation, in which the metabolic rate falls and protein is conserved.

REFERENCES

83. Bessey PQ, Watters JM, Aoki TT et al. Ann Surg 1984; 200: 264–281
84. Long CL, Spencer JL, Kinney JM et al. J Appl Physiol 1971; 31: 110–116
85. Gump FE, Long C, Killian P et al. J Trauma 1974; 14: 378–388
86. Wilmore DW, Mason AD Jr, Pruitt BA Jr. Ann Surg 1976; 183: 314–320
87. Wilmore DW, Aulick LH, Mason AD et al. Ann Surg 1977; 186: 444–458
88. Wilmore DW, Aulick HL, Goodwin CW. Acta Chir Scand Suppl 1980; 498: 43–47
89. Black PR, Brooks DC, Bessey PQ et al. Ann Surg 1982; 196: 420–435

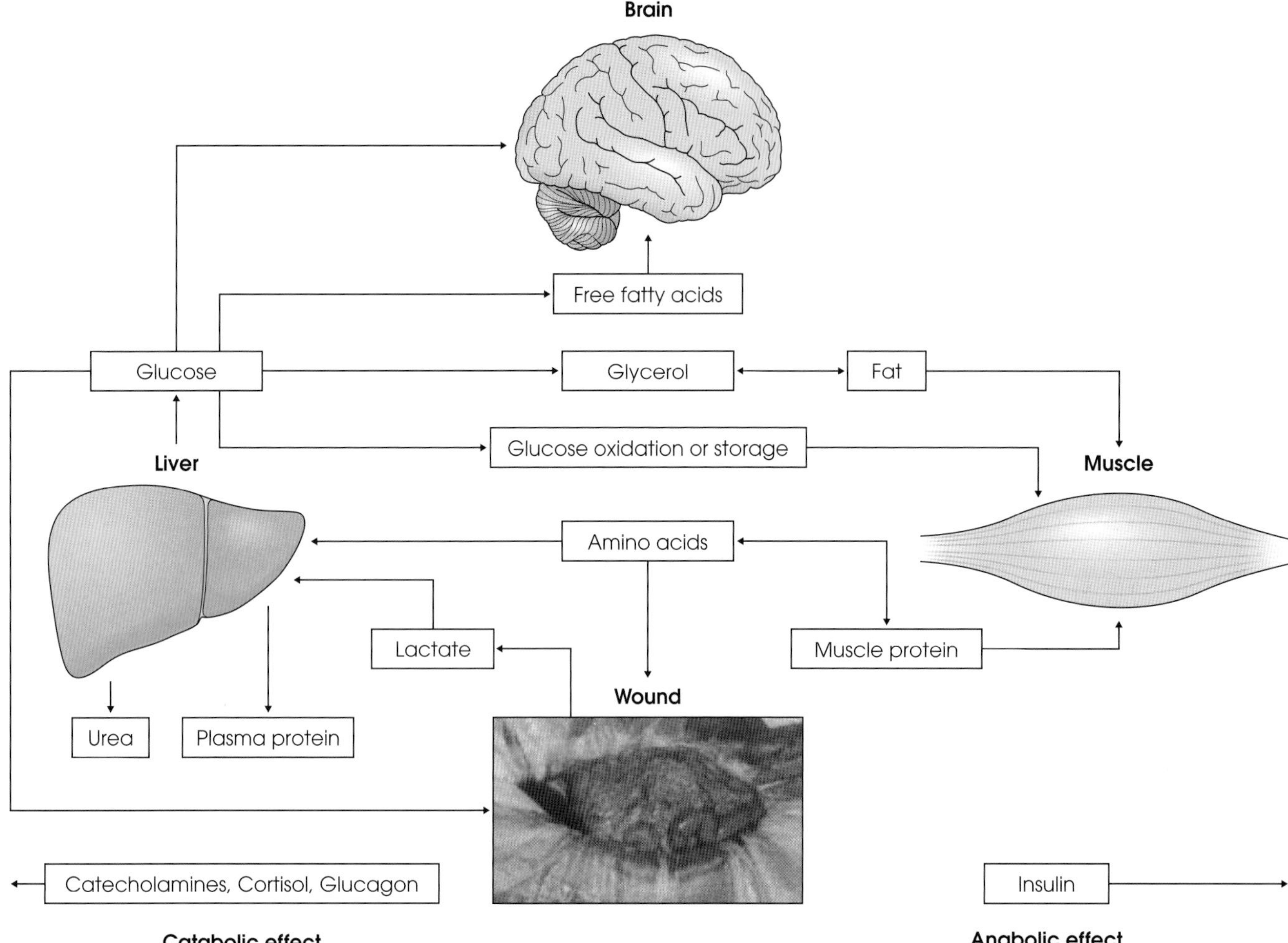

Figure 2.16 Neuroendocrine and metabolic responses to injury.

It has been known for many years that this process can be ameliorated but not reversed by nutrition. Nutritional support during the flow phase has therefore become more conservative, concentrating on removing factors such as pain, sepsis and fluid depletion that exacerbate the catabolic response. Insulin administered during critical illness not only controls the blood glucose but improves protein economy and outcome.[82,90] The supply of substrates such as glutamine,[91] normally plentiful in the body, may become rate-limiting or conditionally essential in severe illness. Glutamine forms an important substrate for immune cells and rapidly dividing tissues such as intestinal mucosal. 'Immune-enhancing diets' containing arginine, omega-3 fatty acids, and nucleotides are beneficial in some cases of major injury[92] and in cancer surgery.[93] Some loss of lean body mass from the metabolic response exacerbated by immobility is inevitable, but can be reduced by appropriate nutrition.

Cytokine response

Release of inflammatory cytokines, including interleukins 1 and 6 and tumour necrosis factor, causes inflammation at the site of injury, and stimulates catabolism by direct effects on tissue and indirect effects from the hypothalamus. This response is balanced during recovery by secretion of counter-inflammatory cytokines, limiting and terminating inflammation and fever. The intensity of the acute cytokine release and its counter-regulation are determined by the severity of the insult and by the genetic make-up of the individual.[94]

NUTRITIONAL REQUIREMENTS

ENERGY

The total energy expenditure is the sum of the resting expenditure and that from activity, which is variable but is about one and a half times the resting expenditure in the average normal subject and a 10–15% increase following meals, which is from diet-induced thermogenesis.[95] Although patients have decreased physical activity, the stress response to illness increases the resting expenditure in proportion to its severity. The stress factor is only 10% after uncomplicated surgery, which is more than offset by inactivity, but at the other extreme, major injury,

REFERENCES

90. van den Berghe G, Wouters P, Weekers F et al. N Engl J Med 2001; 345: 1359–1367
91. Pichard C, Kudsk KA. In: Vincent J-L (ed). Update in Intensive Care Medicine, Vol 34. Springer Verlag, Berlin, 2000
92. Kudsk KA, Minard G, Croce MA et al. Ann Surg 1996; 224: 531–540, discussion 540–543
93. Bozzetti F, Braga M, Gianotti L et al. Lancet 2001; 358: 1487–1492
94. Grimble RF. Clin Nutr 2001; 20: 469–476
95. Bursztein S, Elwyn DH, Askanazi J et al. Energy Metabolism, Indirect Calorimetry and Nutrition. Williams and Wilkins, Baltimore, 1993

Table 2.20 Calculation of energy expenditure using Schofield equations[20]

Weight (wt) in kg, resting metabolic rate (RMR) in kcal/24 h

Age (years)	RMR (male)	RMR (female)
15–18	17.6 × wt + 656	13.3 × wt + 690
18–30	15.0 × wt + 690	14.8 × wt + 485
30–60	11.4 × wt + 870	8.1 × wt + 842
> 60	11.7 × wt + 585	9.0 × wt + 656
'Fudge factors': add to RMR		
1. Add stress factor*	Postoperative	+ 10%
	Multiple injury	+ 25–30%
	Sepsis, for each 1° C rise	+ 10%
2. Add activity factor	Bed-bound awake	+ 10%
	Sitting out	+ 20%
	Mobile in ward	+ 30%
3. Add for thermogenic action of food (enteral or parenteral)		+ 10%
4. Reduce if on ventilator		− 15%

*If the stress factor has been added, do not also add factor for fever; this is double-accounting.

burns, acute pancreatitis, and sepsis may increase the energy expenditure by 30–50%. Conversely, prolonged starvation and weight loss reduce energy expenditure by 10%.

The resting expenditure may be accurately measured using indirect calorimetry[95] or estimated approximately from the Harris-Benedict[96] or Schofield equations[97] (Table 2.20). Although there is reasonable agreement between measured and estimated energy expenditure in most patients, this is less true in critically ill patients. The provision of one and a third to one and a half times the estimated resting expenditure, or 30 kcal/kg/day, meets the needs of most surgical patients.[98] In calculating the energy intake, it is useful to remember that fat gives 9 kcal/g and carbohydrate and protein approximately 4 kcal/g.

NITROGEN

In health, assuming their energy needs are satisfied, the majority of individuals are in nitrogen balance with an intake of 0.8 g/kg/day protein (0.13 g/kg/day nitrogen), whereas sick individuals need between 1 and 1.5 g/kg/day protein (0.15–0.25 g/kg/day nitrogen).

MICRONUTRIENTS

Patients should receive at least the recommended daily allowances for all vitamins and trace elements. There may be increased requirements for folate and other micronutrients, such as thiamine in individuals with alcoholism.

NUTRITIONAL TREATMENT

A group of Scandinavian surgeons carrying out colorectal surgery make a careful preoperative assessment, avoid starvation by administration of a glucose drink or infusion 2–4 h before surgery, rarely insert nasogastric tubes, use postoperative epidural analgesia, and encourage oral intake and mobilization on the first day postoperatively. This approach encouraging early oral food intake has greatly enhanced the clinical outcome and halved the length of hospital stay. Similar regimens are being used in other groups of surgical patients. Nasogastric tubes are still overused. Postoperative nausea and retching are common and do not require insertion of a nasogastric tube unless gastric emptying is impaired, when there is a serious risk of reflux and bronchial aspiration.

There is considerable evidence that nutritional support is of value in certain groups of patients, particularly where prior malnutrition exists.[70]

FOOD

When appetite is impaired, or the patient is elderly, small amounts of appetizing food, high in energy and protein density, meet nutritional needs. Milk is a cheap and effective nutrient and alcoholic drinks not only provide energy but also enhance appetite. Food stimulates the cephalic phase of digestion and the production of saliva, which contains many antibacterial agents, while intravenous nutrition bypasses this process.

SUPPLEMENTS

Snacks and milk-based drinks should be available on the ward, but palatable proprietary oral supplements have an important place in patients whose intake remains inadequate, and can improve outcome.[70]

ENTERAL NUTRITION

Routes of administration

Liquid feed can be administered via a tube into the stomach or small bowel. Although bolus feeding has its place in long-term enteral nutrition, there are advantages for hospital patients in giving the feed slowly by gravity drip, or preferably by a continuous infusion pump to avoid accidental administration of large boluses. For short periods, fine-bore nasogastric tube feeding should be employed where gastric emptying is satisfactory. Nasojejunal and nasoduodenal tubes can be used when gastric emptying is impaired. A gastrostomy or jejunostomy inserted surgically or endoscopically (percutaneous endoscopic gastrostomy) is used when prolonged enteral feeding is required in cases of mechanical or neurological dysphagia, or upper gastric intestinal obstruction.

Complications

Complications include distension, bloating, diarrhoea, and reflux with aspiration into the lungs, especially in unconscious patients. Reflux may be reduced by nursing the patient in a semirecumbent position and slowing the infusion rate. Diarrhoea may be caused by large bolus feeding or too-rapid administration, but most cases of enteral feed-induced diarrhoea are associated with antibiotic therapy. Loperamide or codeine should be given to slow peristalsis if the antibiotics cannot be stopped. It is advisable in most cases to take a plain abdominal radiograph to confirm the position of a nasoenteric tube before infusing feed, particularly in patients with impaired consciousness or gag reflex. Tube feeding

REFERENCES

96. Harris JA, Benedict FG. A Biometric Study of Basal Metabolism in Man (Publication 279). Carnegie Institute, Washington, 1919
97. Schofield WN. Hum Nutr Clin Nutr 1985; 39 (Suppl 1): 5–41
98. Kondrup J, Bak L, Hansen BS et al. Nutrition 1998; 14: 319–321

Table 2.21 Categories of feed

Polymeric	Contains whole protein, polysaccharides and fat with an energy density of 1.0 and 1.5 kcal/mL, and a range of protein concentrations from 40 to 60 g/L
Elemental	Predigested to amino acids and sugars: now rarely used
Peptide	Nitrogen in the form of peptides, carbohydrate as polysaccharide, fat as medium-chain triglycerides
Fibre	As polymeric with the addition of soluble fibre
'Immune-enhancing'	Containing glutamine, arginine, nucleotides and omega-3 fatty acids
Others	Variations in electrolyte content

should always be started slowly, i.e. at 20–30 mL/h, and increased gradually over 3 or 4 days until maximum tolerance is achieved or nutritional needs are met.

Composition of feed

Feeds may be divided into the categories shown in Table 2.21.

Parenteral nutrition

Parenteral nutrition, by whatever route it is given, requires skill and technique. In inexpert hands the risks outweigh the benefits because complications, particularly sepsis, are unacceptably high (in excess of 30%). All hospitals should have a skilled nutrition support team, with nurses trained in aseptic techniques to manage central lines. Feed should only be given intravenously where it is not possible to administer sufficient nutrients by the oral or enteral route. Parenteral nutrition can be regarded as the management of gastrointestinal failure, when it can be a life-saving treatment if gastrointestinal dysfunction is prolonged for several weeks. It may also be beneficial in patients who are unable to take feed by oral or enteral means for more than 7–10 days because of the effects of surgery or illness.

Unlike enteral feeding, parenteral nutrition has to be given in a predigested form, with nitrogen being given as amino acids and carbohydrate as glucose, while triglycerides are administered as a fat emulsion of long-chain, medium-chain or omega-3 fatty acids. The preparation should also include the daily requirements for minerals and micronutrients, and a quantity of water and electrolytes to maintain fluid and electrolyte balance. Parenteral nutrition has been greatly simplified in recent years by the provision of commercially available all-in-one bags, to which only the micronutrients have to be added in the pharmacy. These preparations can be administered peripherally or centrally.

Peripheral

Providing that there is adequate venous access, peripheral intravenous feeding has been used successfully for up to 2 or 3 weeks using Venflon cannulae changed daily, or a 15-cm sialastic or polyurethane paediatric cannulae. Peripherally inserted central cannulae (PICC lines) are also popular in some centres. The addition of cortisone and heparin may minimize damage to peripheral veins, and the use of nitroglycerine patches distally may also be of benefit. Isotonic and moderately hypertonic feeds may be safely administered by this route.

Central route

Central lines may be inserted via the subclavian or jugular route, ensuring that the tip of the cannula is at the junction of the superior vena cava and right atrium to minimize the risk of superior vena caval thrombosis. Modern cannulae are made of polyurethane and rarely cause this problem. A cuffed Hickman or Broviac catheter should be used for long-term parenteral nutrition, because these are well anchored in the tissues and less likely to be displaced. The central route is usually preferred when feeding is required for more than 2 or 3 weeks, or when peripheral veins are poor. Central lines should in theory be used exclusively for parenteral nutrition, but in skilled hands, multilumen lines are valuable for taking blood samples, and for the administration of other fluids, antibiotics and drugs in critically ill patients. Sepsis rates can be kept low by the assiduous use of aseptic techniques by skilled nurses.

WHOM TO FEED AND HOW

Excessive administration of intravenous fluids delays the return of gastrointestinal function and prevents early oral intake. Nutritional support of surgical patients can be considered in five situations: preoperative, perioperative, postoperative, in the critical care unit, and during convalescence.

Preoperative

There is no evidence that the normally nourished or slightly undernourished patient derives any benefit from preoperative nutrition, although bringing the patient to operation in a metabolically fed state (by administration of glucose orally or intravenously) not only reduces the metabolic response to injury but appears to improve outcome. There is, however, some evidence that patients with more than 10% recent weight loss may benefit from a short period of preoperative feeding, preferably by the oral or enteral route. Treatment of 5–10 days is sufficient to produce significant functional improvements and seems to enhance the postoperative recovery in malnourished patients. Evidence also suggests that immune-enhancing diets given enterally during this period may be of benefit in patients undergoing major surgery for upper gastrointestinal cancer.

Perioperative

In severe catabolic conditions, such as burns, requiring repeated surgical procedures, it has become the practice to continue the administration of nutrition enterally or parenterally during operations to avoid the reduction in overall nutritional intake that may accompany frequent dressings and surgery.

Postoperative

The objective should be to return to oral intake as early as possible. This is usually on the first day postoperatively if excessive opiates, fluids, and other drugs that impair gastrointestinal function are avoided. Oral supplements may also help to fill the gap between intake and requirements. Some studies of early enteral feeding by the gastric or jejunal route in the postoperative period have also shown benefit, especially in patients with prior malnutrition. Postoperative parenteral nutrition should be reserved for patients in whom it had been started preoperatively for prior malnutrition, or in whom gastrointestinal malfunction persists for more than 7–10 days postoperatively.

In the critical care unit

The average length of stay of most patients in intensive care units is too short for nutrition to have much impact, although it is desirable to begin enteral nutrition in those who stay for more than 5 days as soon as possible, and to supplement this with parenteral feeding where necessary. High metabolic rates are now rarely seen, and total energy intakes of more than 35 kcal/kg or nitrogen intakes more than 0.25 g/kg are almost never required. Excessive nutrients can be toxic, and glucose administration should not exceed 5 mg/kg/min as oxygen consumption and carbon dioxide production rise. Similarly, excessive nitrogen merely enhances urea production, which increases the demands on renal function. Insulin may have protein anabolic effects, and recent data shows that giving sufficient insulin to maintain the blood sugar within normal limits improves the clinical outcome.[90] The use of growth hormone has been shown to be deleterious.[99]

Convalescence

Patients given extra oral supplements to take after discharge have all gained weight compared with those taking normal food.[100] Functional, clinical, and quality-of-life benefits were, however, only seen in those with significant malnutrition prior to discharge.[101] Weight gain during acute illness is from fluid or fat, but lean body mass is slowly restored over 2–3 months with return to normal activity and home food, accompanied by further functional improvement.

REFERENCES

99. Ruokonen E, Takala J. Curr Opin Clin Nutr Metab Care 2002; 5: 199–209
100. Hessov I. Nutrition 2000; 16: 776
101. Beattie AH, Prach AT, Baxter JP et al. Gut 2000; 46: 813–818

Blood: haemostasis and transfusion

3

Beverley J. Hunt, Ian M. Franklin

INTRODUCTION

The arrest of bleeding and the rational use of blood products are critical to successful surgery. In the past few years, our understanding of haemostasis has improved; this is slowly changing the clinical management of bleeding. In blood transfusion, the challenge of transfusion-transmitted disease has altered practice, and the rationale for using blood products has been modified.

The modern era of blood transfusion began with Landsteiner's discovery of the ABO blood group system in 1902. This advance made compatible blood transfusion possible, although the technique of delivering the intravenous infusion was problematic. The first major advances occurred in the First World War (1914–18), during which it became clear that prompt availability of blood for transfusion could save life.

Specific developments occurred before blood transfusion could enter regular medical practice. These were the development of safe and effective citrate-based anticoagulant systems and the availability of improved systems for delivering the intravenous infusions. By the 1920s, the principles of safe blood donor selection were becoming established,[1] but the logistics of organizing the necessary donors, as well as the storage of blood and its delivery to patients, had to wait until the end of the Second World War. In the early post-war years, there was a ready supply of motivated people who had experienced the camaraderie and horrors of war and were prepared to be blood donors. Improved surgical techniques, anaesthesia and antibiotics enabled patients to survive more major surgery that needed blood transfusion to make a difference to both the outcome and the feasibility of surgery.

The early organization of the UK blood services was, not surprisingly, along military lines. The ready availability of safe blood in the new National Health Service hospitals led to the acceptance of blood transfusion as a major benefit. No trials were performed to test the value of blood transfusion in routine surgery if there was no clear and immediate life-threatening indication. Nor were there trials of albumin therapy, or of its precursors of purified protein fraction or freeze-dried plasma. There was a similar failure to conduct clinical trials of platelet concentrates when these were introduced in the late 1960s and early 1970s; this is less easy to forgive.

These omissions led to the use of blood, albumin, and fresh frozen plasma becoming automatic in certain clinical and surgical situations, accompanied by a casual approach to the prescribing of these biological products. By the first years of the 21st century, an awareness of the historical transmission by blood transfusion of human immunodeficiency virus and hepatitis B and C, as well as the uncertainty over the potential transmission of variant Creutzfeldt–Jakob disease, made this relaxed approach untenable. The new millennium has been characterized by an increasing caution in the prescription of blood and blood derivatives, and by their replacement, where possible, with recombinant or synthetic agents. Blood avoidance strategies have been introduced, and evidence is being assembled that will inform the future use of blood-based therapy.

HAEMOSTASIS

Haemostasis is a general term describing all the activities of blood and related tissues that are directed towards the control of haemorrhage and thrombosis; the process involves endothelial, vascular, hepatic, lymphatic and myeloid cells. Haemostasis involves the interaction of the blood vessel, platelets, coagulation factors, physiological inhibitors and fibrinolysis. A disruption of any of these factors can produce a bleeding or thrombotic disorder. The physiological clotting pathways in the blood have been largely elucidated, but much remains unexplored and highly complex. The haemostatic system has two diametrically opposed functions: the need to maintain fluidity in the circulation and the need to provide rapid clotting to prevent excessive blood loss when a blood vessel is damaged.

PLATELET–ENDOTHELIAL INTERACTION

A lacerated blood vessel almost immediately constricts, preventing blood loss (see Ch. 10). Damage to the endothelium exposes the subendothelium, which is rich in collagen and other factors that facilitate platelet adhesion. Platelet adhesion results in platelet activation and the release of the platelet granular contents, which activates other platelets, thus stimulating the process of platelet aggregation (Table 3.1).

Platelets are produced in the bone marrow by megakaryocytes, and are present in the blood at a concentration of $140–400 \times 10^9$/L.[2] In their resting state, they are biconvex discs with mean volumes of about 8.5 fL. Acute haemorrhage or inflammation leads to an increase in platelet count by increasing the production of the specific growth factor thrombopoietin.

Platelets have a number of glycoprotein receptors on their surface, each with a unique function. The two most important receptors for adhesion and aggregation are glycoproteins Ib and IIb/IIIa. Von Willebrand factor is secreted both by the endothelium and by platelets, and is the main ligand for platelet

REFERENCES

1. Keynes G. Blood Transfusion, Vol vii. Oxford Medical Publications, London, 1922: 166
2. Crawford N, Scrutton M. In: Bloom AL, Thomas DP, Tuddenham EGD (eds). Haemostasis and Thrombosis. Churchill Livingstone, Edinburgh, 1994: 89–114

Table 3.1 Platelet activation and sequelae

Event	Timescale	Consequences
Initial stimulus (e.g. collagen, ADP, thrombin)	Seconds	Shape changes: spherical with protrusions. Membrane activation with prostaglandin and thromboxane production.
Reversible aggregation	1–2 min	Secretion of amines, e.g. serotonin (with capillary vasoconstriction) and von Willebrand factor. Further membrane activity exposing platelet factor, with subsequent clot promotion.
Irreversible aggregation via von Willebrand factor and fibrin(ogen), producing the haemostatic plug	2–5 min	Further secretion of proteins (e.g. platelet factor 4, fibrinogen and factor V). Clot formation.
Clot retraction	5–20 min	Consolidation of haemostatic plug. Fibrin cross-linking.

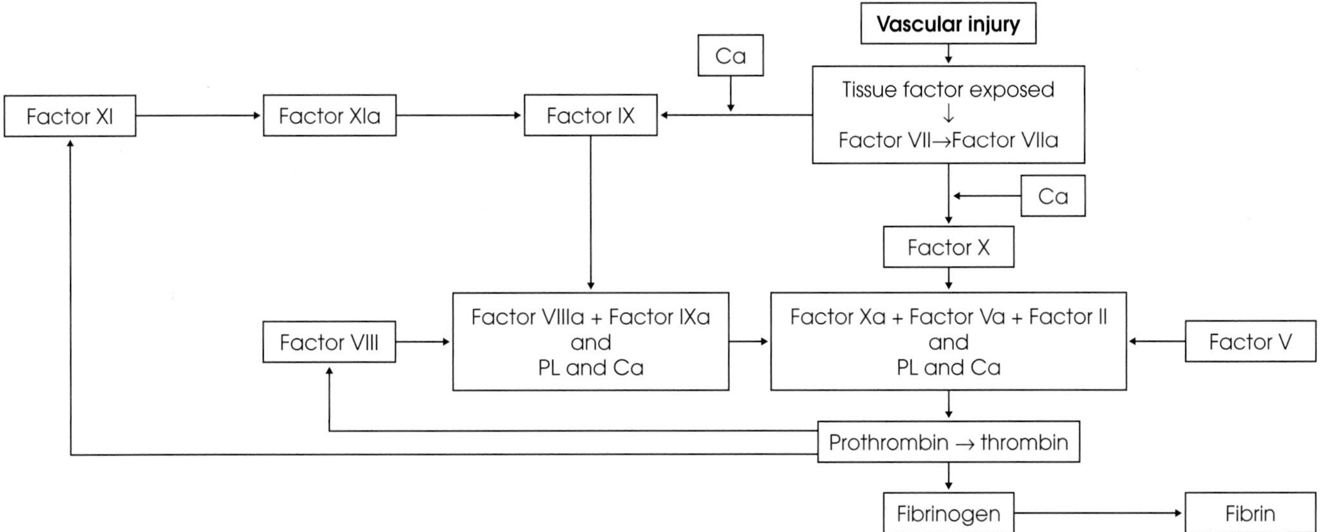

Figure 3.1 A simplified version of the coagulation cascade incorporating current concepts of haemostasis.

adhesion to exposed collagen in the subendothelium. During activation, the platelet granules discharge and the membrane molecules 'flip-flop', exposing the inner lipids (called platelet factor 3). Other factors – such as thromboxane (Fig. 3.1) and platelet activating factor – also cause platelet aggregation. The discharged granular contents enhance platelet aggregation; thus an amorphous mass of irreversibly aggregated platelets called the haemostatic plug is produced. Actin in the platelet cytoplasm causes retraction and consolidation of the plug after some minutes. Platelets are activated through many mechanisms, which explains why individual antiplatelet drugs are generally disappointing when used singly for preventing thrombosis.

VON WILLEBRAND FACTOR

Von Willebrand factor has two functions: to mediate platelet adhesion to damaged subendothelium, and to carry and stabilize plasma factor VIII.[3] It is synthesized and stored in the endothelium and megakaryocytes, and is secreted into the plasma as very large multimers. Von Willebrand factor binds to factor VIIIC and protects it from enzymatic destruction. Von Willebrand factor is highly mutable, as shown by the many abnormal forms, which cause lack of Von Willebrand factor activity resulting in a bleeding state; this is known as von Willebrand disease.

COAGULATION

At the same time as platelet activation, the coagulation cascade is activated by the exposure of tissue factor in the subendothelium; this cascade leads to thrombin generation and the conversion of soluble fibrinogen to insoluble fibrin. The mesh of platelets and fibrin eventually forms a stable haemostatic plug.[4] The activation of factor XII is not important in in vivo coagulation. Factor XI is now thought to be mainly activated by thrombin, and it is understood that the old intrinsic pathway is an amplification loop to thrombin generation (see Fig. 3.1).

Tissue factor, previously known as thromboplastin, is now considered the main activator of coagulation.[5] Active tissue factor is not normally present in the endothelium or cellular blood components, but is present in the subendothelium, adventia of the endothelium, and other cells of the body. Thus when a vessel wall is damaged, and the subendothelium containing tissue factor is exposed, the coagulation process is initiated. Tissue factor

REFERENCES

3. Ruggeri Z. Thromb Haemost 1999; 82: 576–584
4. Mann K. Thromb Haemost 1999; 82: 165–174
5. Morrissey J. Thromb Haemost 2001; 86: 66–74

binds to and activates factor VII, and a cascade of zymogens (factors II and X) are converted into their active serine proteases that lead to fibrin generation. Fibrin polymerization is stabilized by cross-linking under the action of factor XIII.

The coagulation cascade, through its amplification system, has the ability to transduce a small stimulus into a massive effect. The size of the local thrombus is limited by a complex interplay with the physiological anticoagulants.

PHYSIOLOGICAL ANTICOAGULANTS

The main physiological anticoagulants are antithrombin, the protein C system, and tissue factor pathway inhibitor.

Antithrombin

Antithrombin, previously called antithrombin III, is potentiated 10 000-fold by the heparinoids coating the endothelium. Unfractionated and low-molecular-weight heparins also potentiate the anticoagulant effect of antithrombin.

The protein C system

Thrombin, when bound to the endothelial surface molecule thrombomodulin, activates proteins C and S. Activated protein C inactivates factors Va and VIIIa, and also boosts fibrinolysis.

Tissue factor pathway inhibitor

Tissue factor pathway inhibitor, one of the serine protease inhibitors, inhibits the activation of factor X by tissue factor–factor VIIa complexes.[6] Tissue factor pathway inhibitor is primarily synthesized by the endothelium and is secreted into the plasma. This inhibits the first step in the coagulation cascade, and is one of the dominant regulatory signals that inhibit coagulation.

FIBRINOLYSIS

Circulating plasminogen is activated mainly by tissue plasminogen activator to form plasmin, a powerful serine protease that breaks down cross-linked fibrin to form fibrin degradation products. These products include many fragments, some of which are known as D-dimers.[7] Urokinase-type plasminogen activator is the main activator of plasminogen in solid tissues and in cells that organize the thrombus.

THE ENDOTHELIUM AND HAEMOSTASIS

The endothelium controls local haemostasis.[8] Normally the endothelium provides a thromboresistant surface that prevents platelet or leukocyte adhesion and activation of the coagulation system. Some of the activities of the endothelial cells, which promote the maintenance of the fluidity of blood by anticoagulation, fibrinolysis and vasodilatation, are listed in Box 3.1. The endothelium can, however, undergo a series of changes known as endothelial cell activation when exposed to cytokines, growth factors, mechanical forces and neighbouring cells. This results in the surface changing from 'antithrombotic' to 'prothrombotic'. Surface anticoagulant molecules such as thrombomodulin are lost. There is also loss of heparin sulphate, a reduced fibrinolytic potential, and a loss of platelet antiaggregatory effects.

Box 3.1 The normal effects of the endothelium on haemostasis

Anticoagulation
- Directly, by synthesizing antithrombin and tissue factor pathway inhibitor; also, by binding glycosaminoglycans (heparans), which potentiate antithrombin.
- Indirectly, by expressing thrombomodulin, a cofactor in the thrombin-induced activation of protein C.

Fibrinolysis
- Directly, by synthesizing and secreting tissue plasminogen activator.

Coagulation
- Directly, by synthesizing and secreting von Willebrand factor.

Antifibrinolysis
- Directly, by synthesizing and secreting plasminogen activator inhibitor type 1.

Vasodilatation
- Directly, by synthesizing nitric oxide and prostacyclin, which cause vasodilatation and inhibit platelet aggregation.

ASSAYS FOR ASSESSING HAEMOSTASIS

Assessing platelet function

The platelet counts, the appearance of platelets on a standard blood smear, and the platelet size from the automated counters are helpful in assessing coagulation.

The bleeding time provides an in vivo test of platelet endothelial interaction,[9] but it has fallen into disrepute because it is poorly reproducible and operator-dependent. The platelet function analyzer (PFA-100) produces a rapid in vitro screening test of platelet function, and is now superseding the classical bleeding time because it is reproducible and reliable in detecting the extent of platelet dysfunction.[10,11] There are congenital or acquired causes of platelet dysfunction; the use of aspirin being the most common cause of the latter. Further more complex tests of platelet aggregation may be necessary to identify the underlying platelet defect if an abnormality is detected.

Laboratory tests of coagulation

All coagulation tests are performed on citrated blood: 9 vol. of venous blood (i.e. 5 vol. of plasma) are added to 1 vol. of 3.2% sodium citrate. Allowance is made for patients with very abnormal haematocrits. Normal venous blood has an intrinsic tendency to clot within 5–10 min when taken into a glass tube, depending on the temperature and the type of glass. This is the whole blood clotting time as described by Lee and White.[12] Clotting occurs in seconds if tissue factor is added to activate the extrinsic pathway.

The activated clotting time is a refinement in which 2 mL of native venous blood is placed into a glass tube with kaolin particles to stimulate activation of the intrinsic pathway. The blood is incubated at 37°C and clotting normally occurs within 120 s. This assay is used by anaesthetists to monitor anticoagulation in extracorporeal circuits.

REFERENCES

6. Golino P. Thromb Res 2002; 106: 257–265
7. Colleen D. Thromb Haemost 1999; 82: 165–178
8. Hunt BJ, Jurd K. In: Hunt BJ, Poston L, Schachter M et al (eds). An Introduction to Vascular Biology: From Basic Science to Clinical Practice. Cambridge University Press, Cambridge, 2002: 186–215
9. Duke W. Arch Intern Med 1912; 10: 145
10. Favaloro E. Curr Opin Hematol 2002; 9: 407–415
11. Jilma B. J Lab Clin Med 2001; 138: 152–163
12. Lee R, White P. Am J Med Sci 1913; 145: 495–503

Prothrombin time and the international normalized ratio

The measurement of the prothrombin time is unchanged in principle from the technique described by Quick.[13] The method is simply the time taken for plasma to clot in a container after adding a source of tissue factor and calcium chloride. The result is expressed as a ratio against the time taken to clot by normal plasma, known as the prothrombin time.

The international normalized ratio is a modification of the prothrombin time, which allows comparison of the patient's time with an internationally defined control plasma clotting time.[14] Prolonged international normalized ratios may be caused by low levels of prothrombin and by other proteins in the extrinsic system (i.e. factor VII, X or V), either singly or in combination. It is now used most commonly to monitor the effects of oral anticoagulants, and is also a useful test of liver function.

Activated partial thromboplastin time (kaolin cephalin clotting time)

This test is virtually unchanged since it was first described as the one-stage procedure in 1953,[15] and forms the basis for assays of intrinsic clotting factors and common pathway. The partial thromboplastin is a procoagulant phospholipid (such as cephalin) that is added to citrated plasma prior to calcification. The added agents activate factor XII, and fibrin generation occurs normally in 30–45 s. Activated partial thromboplastin time is usually used as a routine screening test, and detects abnormalities of the intrinsic and common pathways. It is the best test for monitoring unfractionated heparin therapy.

Thrombin time, reptilase time and fibrinogen estimations

Plasma clots directly on the addition of thrombin or reptilase because of the direct conversion of fibrinogen to fibrin. The amount added is adjusted to give normal times of 12–15 s for the thrombin time, and 18–22 s for the reptilase time. These reagents are commonly used to check fibrinogen quality and quantity; the thrombin time may be used to check heparin therapy. Reptilase is extracted from the venom of the snake *Bothrops atrox*, and initiates formation of fibrin by releasing fibrinopeptide A only.

Prolongation of the clotting time by more than 2 s is abnormal and indicates low fibrinogen levels and/or dysfibrinogenaemia. A prolonged thrombin time with a normal reptilase time indicates the presence of heparin. Dysfibrinogenaemia may result from rare inherited abnormalities, or more commonly from severe liver disease.

Interpretation of clotting screens

Isolated prolongation of either the international normalized ratio or the activated partial thromboplastin time indicates a specific protein deficiency; factor VII deficiency for the former, and factor VIII, factor IX, factor XI or factor XII deficiency for the latter. If the prolongation of a patient's clotting time is corrected with 1:1 mixing with normal plasma, then this indicates that the abnormality is the result of a deficiency of one or more clotting factors. When a prolonged activated partial thromboplastin time is corrected with mixing with normal plasma, this is indicative of the presence of an inhibitor, such as a lupus anticoagulant, or antibodies to factor VIII or IX. Prolongation of both tests with a normal thrombin time indicates a deficiency of factors II, V or X, or a more general deficiency, which could be the result of liver failure, warfarin therapy, or disseminated intravascular coagulation.

Most coagulation assays are now performed on complex, dedicated, robotic machines. Near-patient testing devices are also being increasingly used in units distant to the general coagulation laboratory, and by patients for self-monitoring of anticoagulation. The key to successful use of all equipment is close adherence to quality control, which should be monitored by suitably qualified laboratory staff.

Fibrin and fibrinogen degradation products

When fibrinogen or fibrin is degraded by plasmin, a series of successively smaller fragments—X, Y, D and E—result. The earlier fragments, X and Y, are strong antagonists of thrombin (and reptilase), thus prolonging the thrombin time. Specific detection of fibrin degradation is offered by a monoclonal antibody that detects a fibrin degradation product formed by a dimer of two D fragments: a Dimer. D-dimer testing is now used widely to indicate the presence of thromboembolic disease, but increased levels of fibrin degradation products can also occur in a number of states, including disseminated intravascular coagulation, recent surgery, pregnancy, and inflammatory disorders. Thus although it is highly sensitive, D dimer testing is not specific.[16]

PREVENTING AND MANAGING SURGICAL BLEEDING AND THE NEED FOR TRANSFUSION

There is active debate about the optimal methods for managing surgical bleeding. In the past, attempts at perioperative blood conservation have been driven by fears of transfusion-transmitted infection, concerns about the clinical efficacy, and cost. The current concerns in the UK about variant Creutzfeldt–Jakob disease have stimulated interest in transfusion triggers, blood conservation techniques, and the use of pharmacological agents to obviate the need for transfusion. The use of blood should be minimized, but not at the risk of increasing patient morbidity and mortality. Near-patient haemostatic assessment in the operating theatre may enhance the future appropriate use of blood products. The use of the thromboelastograph has developed to such an extent that it is a prerequisite in orthotopic liver transplantation anaesthesia, and its use is being explored in other surgical fields.[17,18]

THE CAUSES OF PERIOPERATIVE BLEEDING

Excessive bleeding can be from surgical causes or a derangement of haemostasis. Blood loss is highly variable between operations performed by different surgeons. A surgeon's attention to careful haemostatic control may avoid a necessity of taking a patient back to theatre for surgical re-exploration to find a bleeding point.

REFERENCES

13. Quick A. J Biol Chem 1935; 109: 73–74
14. British Committee for Standards in Haematology, Haemostasis and Thrombosis Task Force. J Clin Pathol 1990; 43: 177–183
15. Langdell R, Wagner R, Brinkhous K. J Lab Clin Med 1953; 41: 637–647
16. Kelly J, Hunt B. Lancet 2002; 359: 456–458
17. Mallet S, Cox D. Br J Anaesth 1992; 69: 307–313
18. Vig S, Chitolie A, Bevan DH et al. Blood Coagul Fibrinolysis 2001; 12: 555–561

Control of haemostasis could also prevent the development of a dilutional coagulopathy associated with continued bleeding, requiring the use of blood products that are associated with a greater morbidity and mortality.

There is a subset of patients in whom generalized oozing occurs in the surgical field, which cannot be attributed to demonstrable bleeding vessels. There are no adequate definitions of an 'excessive bleeder'. In the past, non-surgical perioperative bleeding has been poorly understood and poorly managed. There are several reasons for this, which include a failure to recognize the limitations of laboratory tests and the recognition that there are no quick and reliable laboratory assays to look at some components of haemostasis that may be causing the problem (e.g. excessive fibrinolysis).

Perioperative haemostatic changes have not been extensively studied, although haemostatic activation is thought to occur as a result of high levels of catecholamines induced by complex surgery. In abdominal aortic aneurysm repairs and in total hip replacements, typical perioperative changes include a decrease in the platelet count and levels of factor VIII and von Willebrand factor, as well as an increase in antithrombin and protein C measurements.[19–21] The acute-phase reaction, which starts intraoperatively, further stimulates production of these factors.

Increased levels of tissue plasminogen activator and its main inhibitor, plasminogen activator inhibitor-1, have been found to cause a net increase in free tissue plasminogen activator during and after surgery.

PREOPERATIVE ASSESSMENT: IDENTIFYING THOSE AT RISK OF EXCESSIVE BLEEDING

A careful preoperative assessment identifies the majority of candidates at risk of bleeding, and thus minimizes the need for blood transfusion. A history of previous bleeding problems in the patient and their family, together with coexisting drug therapy (advice about withdrawing aspirin and warfarin follows later in this section) and any predisposing condition such as liver or renal disease, should be carefully noted. A personal or family history of a bleeding tendency may indicate a congenital bleeding abnormality, such as mild von Willebrand disease. Mild haemostatic defects that are not associated with active bleeding do not usually need treatment, but can cause torrential bleeding problems intraoperatively.

The most important determinants of the haemorrhagic risk are the patient's diagnosis, the operation planned, and whether previous surgery has been performed.

Prior to complex major surgery, a full blood count and baseline screening tests, including the prothrombin time, the partial thromboplastin time, and fibrinogen levels, should be measured. No other assays have been shown to be of value, unless an underlying congenital bleeding disorder is suspected.[22] Sometimes a bleeding tendency is suggested by a derangement of these baseline screening tests. More exact and sophisticated tests can be performed, and usually require advice from a haematologist.

Ideally patients should have normal haemostasis at the time of operation. If patients are receiving aspirin, this should be stopped at least 7 days prior to surgery to allow new unaffected platelets to be produced.

A series of options are available for patients who are receiving oral anticoagulation from coumarins, such as warfarin, prior to surgery. Warfarin should be stopped at least 3 days preoperatively if the patient can stop warfarin without the need for any perioperative thromboprophylaxis. Patients can be switched to heparin in the perioperative period if they still require thromboprophylaxis. Depending on the underlying prothrombotic state, the patient can switch to full-dose intravenous unfractionated heparin to maintain an activated partial thromboplastin time ratio of 2–2.5. This is desirable for patients with artificial heart valves.

Because the half-life of heparin is approximately 2 h, it can be stopped 2 h preoperatively and restarted as the patient's incision is being closed. The modern alternative is to switch to a low-molecular-weight heparin the day after stopping warfarin. The dose used depends on the patient's underlying prothrombotic state. A treatment dose can be given in those with severe prothrombotic states, and thromboprophylaxis doses to those with lesser prothrombotic states. If the patient is taught how to administer subcutaneous injections, this regime will allow the patient to remain at home and be admitted the day before surgery.

BLOOD AVOIDANCE STRATEGIES

It is important to minimize the need for donor blood products, and the following strategies may be helpful in individual patients: any pre-existing anaemia should be corrected if possible; antithrombotic therapy should be stopped or modified as discussed earlier in this chapter; and recombinant human erythropoietin can stimulate red cell production in some circumstances. Cell salvage can be used in the intraoperative or postoperative period. Autologous transfusion can be deposited in the blood bank preoperatively if the operation is elective and the patient fit enough. A unit of blood can be collected each week.[23] Intraoperative haemodilution can be used, but can interfere with coagulation.

Although transfusion carries risks, and some of these are specifically due to the use of allogeneic blood, risks are also associated with the use of autologous blood; these include giving the wrong blood (discussed further later in this chapter) and bacterial contamination.

The management of Jehovah's Witnesses requires careful discussion with the patient. Some Witnesses will accept autologous transfusion and cell salvage, some will not, but all will accept recombinant products. Preoperative assessment to treat anaemia due to haematinic deficiency, and preoperative treatment with recombinant erythropoietin, can reduce the need to transfuse.[24]

TRANSFUSION TRIGGERS

Previously, anaesthetists have tended to transfuse patients when their haemoglobin level has fallen below 10 g/dL or haematocrit has fallen below 30%. There is evidence that much

REFERENCES

19. Jorgensen KA, Stoffersen E, Sorensen PJ et al. Scand J Haematol 1980; 24: 101–104
20. Seyfer A. Ann Surg 1981; 193: 210
21. Gibbs NM, Crawford GP, Michalopoulos N. J Cardiothorac Vasc Anesth 1992; 6: 680–685
22. Francis C, Kaplan K. In: Hoffman R, Shattil SJ, Furie B (eds). Haematology: Basic Principles and Practice. Churchill Livingstone, Edinburgh, 2000: 2381–2391
23. Goodnough LT, Brecher ME. Intern Med 1998; 37: 238–245
24. Marsh JCW, Bevan DH. Br J Haematol 2002; 119: 25–37

lower levels of haemoglobin can be tolerated without adverse effects. In a healthy human the cardiac output does not increase until haemoglobin falls to less than 7 g/dL. In critically ill patients, a recent randomized trial indicated that a threshold as low as 7 g/dL is safe and possibly superior to a haemoglobin threshold of 9 g/dL.[25] Moderate haemodilution is well tolerated by young, healthy individuals undergoing elective surgery and in whom there are greater concerns about the potential long-term effects of transfusion. Moderate haemodilution may, however, be harmful in those patients with compromised respiratory or myocardial function.[26]

The 'transfusion trigger' should be a composite of variables specific for an individual patient. The large variability in use of blood transfusion between different units and surgeons needs to be addressed.[27,28] This is one of the focuses of the UK National Health Service *Better Blood Transfusion* Health Service Circulars 1998–9 and 2002. Each hospital must have a hospital transfusion committee that develops local protocols to assess the trigger for transfusion of red cells. Practice must be based on transfusion thresholds and targets that are set by local guidelines, because only in this way can important local factors be taken into account.[29] Current concerns over the unknown risk of variant Creutzfeldt–Jakob disease from blood transfusion should be taken seriously.

MANAGEMENT OF ACUTE BLOOD LOSS AND MASSIVE BLOOD LOSS

Blood loss may be profuse for a limited period or it may be massive. Massive blood loss is arbitrarily defined as the replacement of the patient's total blood volume in less than 24 h; these patients usually present as an emergency in the accident and emergency department, delivery suite, or operating theatre. After liver transplantation, massive blood loss can be predicted, and sophisticated monitoring and replacement protocols exist.

Continued oozing from venepuncture and injection sites, pressure sites, and postoperative drainage tubes is a sign of haemostatic failure. Management is aimed at prompt resuscitation, because the most frequent cause of death after massive transfusion is tissue hypoxia from inadequate replacement of circulating volume and red cells.[30] Shock must be treated and bleeding controlled (see Ch. 7). Managing the developing coagulopathy is a secondary issue. Intravascular filling is required to achieve an acceptable systolic blood pressure, and good venous access is essential. One or two large-bore intravenous cannulae should be inserted, and if possible a central line. Initially this replacement can be done by using crystalloid or colloid until red cell transfusion is available (see Ch. 7). No study has shown an advantage in using fresh whole blood, and the use of whole blood from 'walk in' donors is now considered an unacceptable and dangerous practice because of the risks of transfusion-transmitted disease.

It is not known whether crystalloid or colloid should be used as initial replacement therapy (see Ch. 7).[31,32] Larger volumes are required if crystalloids are used. Dextrans, and to a lesser extent hydroxyl ethyl starch, in large volumes have detrimental effects on coagulation, for they alter the formation of fibrin, making clots more amenable to fibrinolysis; both are absorbed on to the platelet surfaces and von Willebrand factor, causing decreased platelet function and an acquired von Willebrand syndrome.[33]

When blood is required urgently, it is possible to provide ABO group and rhesus (Rh) D group-specific blood within 5 min. In emergency cases, group O Rh-negative red cells can be used until the patient's ABO and Rh groups are known. Blood of the same ABO and Rh groups as the patient's should be used as soon as possible to avoid the inappropriate use of group O Rh-negative red cells, which are always in very short supply. Haemostatic blood components should be given based on the results of the regular coagulation screens, full blood counts, or thromboelastography. The aim is to maintain a platelet count greater than 50×10^9/L by administering platelet concentrates, and an international normalized ratio and an activated partial thromboplastin time ratio of less than 1.5 times the control value by giving fresh frozen plasma in doses of 15 mL/kg. It is important to repeat coagulation tests before giving additional quantities of plasma. Fibrinogen can be given if the fibrinogen is very low (less than 1.0 g/L) in the form of either cryoprecipitate or fibrinogen concentrates; the latter are unlicensed.

The use of pharmacological haemostatic agents can be considered. Persistent bleeding is known to stimulate fibrinolytic activity, and thromboelastography can provide a useful guide in this situation. The use of an intravenously administered anti-fibrinolytic agent, such as aprotinin 500 000 kIU or tranexamic acids 1 g, can be beneficial in reducing blood loss if an abnormality is confirmed.

ORDERING A RED CELL TRANSFUSION

From the time that a blood transfusion is requested to its infusion, patients may be exposed to error and receive the wrong blood component, either because the patient was not supposed to receive blood or because the patient receives a component intended for someone else.[34] The risk of errors begins with the request form, which must be correctly filled out and include all the patient identifiers, including their date of birth and hospital number. The sample for blood grouping and compatibility testing must be fully completed. The use of adhesive patient-identifying labels significantly increases the risk of errors in sample identification and is not recommended.

REFERENCES

25. Hebert PC, Wells G, Blajchman MA et al. N Engl J Med 1999; 340: 409–417
26. Hebert PC, Yetisir E, Martin C et al. Crit Care Med 2001; 29: 227–234
27. McClelland DBLE. Optimal Use of Donor Blood. Clinical Resource and Audit Group, Scottish Office, Edinburgh, 1995
28. Sanguis TSSG. Transfus Med 1994; 4: 251–268
29. McClelland DBLE (ed). Handbook of Transfusion Medicine. 3rd edn. The Stationery Office, London, 2001: 142. Also online. Available: http://www.transfusionguidelines.org.uk/transfusion_handbook/index.html
30. British Committee for Standardization in Haematology, Blood Transfusion Task Force. Clin Lab Haematol 1988; 10: 265–273
31. Cochrane Injuries Group Albumin Reviewers. Br Med J 1998; 317: 235–240
32. McClelland B. Br Med J 1998; 317: 829–830
33. de Jonge E, Levi M. Crit Care Med 2001; 29: 1261–1267.
34. Serious Hazards of Transfusion Reporting Scheme. Annual Report 2000–2001. Online. Available: http://www.shot.demon.co.uk/

ADMINISTRATION OF RED CELL TRANSFUSIONS

When blood is administered, the patient's identity must be checked against the blood pack, not the paperwork. Clear records must be kept in the patient's notes, giving the reason for the transfusion, what was given, any adverse events, and whether the transfusion had the desired effect. The time limits for transfusion and the temperature requirements of the component used must be observed, and the correct giving sets, infusion pumps, and blood warmers must be used.

THE BENEFITS AND HAZARDS OF BLOOD TRANSFUSION

Blood transfusions save life, and do so regularly in the patients experiencing a massive haemorrhage. The lives of many patients with chronic anaemia syndromes are also prolonged and improved by the ready availability of concentrated red cells. The majority of blood transfusions are used to support patients through surgery that is not life-saving or especially major in its scope.

It had been known for many years that the use of blood transfusion in elective operations varied between surgical teams and between hospitals. The pan-European Sanguis study,[28] published in 1994, provided clear evidence of disparities in transfusion practice in the absence of differences in outcome. At about the same time, a consensus conference on red cell transfusion in Edinburgh was unable to come forward with clear recommendations because of the absence of evidence on what constituted best practice.[35] Since then, a number of groups have established working parties or task forces to produce guidelines for blood transfusion, usually concentrating on the haemoglobin levels that should trigger the administration of blood.[36,37] Until recently, these trigger levels were selected empirically.

In 1999, Hebert and colleagues published an important study on two transfusion strategies in adults on intensive care units.[25] This showed that a restrictive transfusion policy produced a superior survival outcome than a more liberal regimen. The Hebert paper was published at almost the same time as evidence suggesting that albumin therapy might well cause excess deaths in patients with severe burns when compared with the use of crystalloid fluids.[31] Red cell transfusion studies have been reviewed recently by the Cochrane Database.[38] Ten trials were identified and analysed, which included around 1800 patients. The review concluded:

> '...limited published evidence supports the use of restrictive transfusion triggers in patients who are free of serious cardiac disease. However, most of the data on clinical outcomes were generated by a single trial.'

The authors of the review also pointed out that most of the trials were of poor quality, and that more trials were required. In the meantime, surgeons, blood bank consultants, and blood services should work together to implement currently available transfusion guidelines, using a more conservative transfusion policy in patients free of major cardiac disease and who do not have evidence of major haemorrhage.

IMMUNE COMPLICATIONS OF BLOOD TRANSFUSION

Acute haemolytic transfusion reaction

Incompatible transfused red cells react with the patient's own IgM anti-A and anti-B antibodies. This produces complement activation and acute intravascular haemolysis, with the potential clinical consequences of acute renal failure and disseminated intravascular coagulation. Infusion of ABO-incompatible blood arises most commonly from errors in taking or labelling the sample, collecting the wrong blood from the blood bank refrigerator, or inadequate checking when the transfusion is being started.

Severe allergic reaction (anaphylaxis)

Severe allergic reaction, or anaphylaxis, is a rare but life-threatening complication usually occurring in an early part of a transfusion, often one containing large volumes of plasma. Signs include hypotension, bronchospasm, oedema, vomiting, erythema, urticaria and conjunctivitis. It is caused by the presence of an IgE antibody to an infused allergen.

A few patients with IgA deficiency develop antibodies to IgA. Some of these patients have severe anaphylaxis if exposed to IgA by transfusion. These patients require saline-washed red cells or, if available, blood components from IgA-deficient donors.

FEBRILE NON-HAEMOLYTIC TRANSFUSION

Fevers or rigors occur in up to 2% of recipients, who are mainly multitransfused, previously pregnant patients. These reactions are probably less frequent with leukodepleted components. The fever that develops is usually associated with shivering and general discomfort. Most can be managed by slowing down the transfusion or by giving paracetamol. These reactions are unpleasant but not life-threatening.

Delayed transfusion reaction

Delayed transfusion reaction develops some days after red cell transfusion, suggesting that the transfused red cells are being destroyed abnormally quickly. There is a rapid fall in haemoglobin, a rise in bilirubin, and a positive direct antiglobulin test. This rare type of reaction usually occurs in patients who have developed red cell antibodies in the past, from transfusion or pregnancy. They may be undetectable when the patient is tested months or years later. However, a subsequent red cell transfusion can quickly boost the antibody. Antibodies of the Kidd (Jk) system are often the cause of such delayed haemolytic reactions.

Post-transfusion purpura or alloimmune thrombocytopenia

The unusual complication of post-transfusion purpura, or alloimmune thrombocytopenia, is now recognized more frequently. Recipients are usually multiparous women who receive a perioperative transfusion some years after their last pregnancy. Five to ten days after transfusion, they develop a profound thrombocytopenic purpura caused by the presence of alloantibodies to transfused platelets, which cross-react with the patient's own platelets. Severely affected patients usually respond to high doses of intravenous gamma globulin (2 g/kg over 2–3 days).

REFERENCES

35. Royal College of Physicians of Edinburgh. Transfus Med 1994; 4: 177–178
36. Spence RK. Am J Surg 1995; 170 (Suppl 6A): 3S–15S
37. American Society of Anesthesiologists Task Force on Blood Component Therapy. Anesthesiology 1996; 84: 732–747
38. Hill SR, Carless PA, Henry DA et al. Cochrane Database Syst Rev 2002; 2: CD002042

Previously, steroids and plasma exchange were used but were not effective in all cases. The use of platelet transfusion in raising the platelet count is largely ineffective.

Transfusion-related acute lung injury

Transfusion is followed by rapid onset of breathlessness and a non-productive cough. The chest radiograph characteristically shows bilateral infiltrates. Treatment is as for adult respiratory distress syndrome from any cause (see Ch. 21). In transfusion-related acute lung injury, an antibody is usually found in one of the donor plasmas that reacts very strongly with the patient's leukocytes. The implicated donors are almost always parous women.

Transfusion-associated graft-versus-host disease

Transfusion-associated graft-versus-host disease is extremely rare and nearly always fatal. It is caused by the donor lymphocytes in transfused blood engrafting in the bone marrow of the recipient and prohibiting normal cellular production. The patient presents with a pancytopenia that is resistant to most treatments. It is therefore vital that blood components from close relatives are either prohibited (as it is in the UK) or that the blood is irradiated prior to transfusion. Similarly, in immunosuppressed recipients, irradiated blood products must be given to prevent this fatal complication.[39]

Immunosuppressive effects of blood transfusion

The immunosuppressive effects of blood transfusion have been of theoretical concern for some years. Despite this, trials have been unable to confirm or refute whether blood transfusion predisposes recipients to an increased risk of cancer recurrence or perioperative bacterial infection.[40]

OTHER COMPLICATIONS OF TRANSFUSION

Acute complications in large-volume transfusions

Hypothermia impairs haemostasis and shifts the Bohr curve to the left, reducing red cell oxygen delivery to the tissues. A blood warmer should be used in adults receiving large volumes of blood.

Hypocalcaemia occurs from the presence of citrate anti-coagulant in fresh frozen plasma and platelets. In theory, infused citrate could lower plasma ionized calcium, but in practice rapid liver metabolism of citrate usually prevents this unless the patient has liver immaturity (neonates) or liver damage. Calcium gluconate can be given by slow intravenous injection if there is electrocardiographic or clinical evidence of hypocalcaemia.

The plasma or additive solution in a unit of red cells stored for 4–5 weeks may contain 5–10 mmol of potassium. In the presence of acidaemia and hypothermia, this additional potassium can lead to hyperkalaemia and consequently to cardiac arrhythmia. The situation is best avoided by keeping the patient warm.

Resuscitation usually improves acidosis in a shocked patient, despite the lactic acid content of transfused blood (1–2 mmol/unit of red cells).

Iron overload

Transfusion-dependent patients receiving red cells over a long period become overloaded with iron. Each unit of red cells contains 250 mg of iron, and tissue accumulation can cause liver and cardiac damage. Chelation therapy with desferrioxamine is used to minimize accumulation of iron in patients likely to receive long-term transfusions.

BLOOD COMPONENTS

RED CELL CONCENTRATES

Red cell concentrates are prepared by removing approximately 200 mL of plasma for fractionation, leaving the haematocrit of the residue at about 70%. The red cell viability is not compromised, but red cell concentrates with higher haematocrits are too viscous for easy transfusion. Supplementations of red cell concentrates are used increasingly. The available plasma is removed and the cells are supplemented by 100 mL of a crystalloid nutritive solution. The average haematocrit of this preparation is close to 60%, and has a better consistency and flow characteristics. The diluents are crystalloid solutions of saline, glucose, adenine and mannitol; some formulations have additional nutrients. These can extend the shelf-life of the red cells. Paediatric packs are available in which a single donation is partitioned into several packs containing less than 100 mL of red cell product. This allows a child to get blood from a limited number of donors, or for several patients to benefit from one donation within a few days of collection. Red cell preparations can be washed by successive changes of crystalloid solutions to be used in patients who have sensitivity to foreign proteins. The shelf-life of these transfusions is only 24 h. Red cells can also be frozen, and when thawed they are washed so that leukocyte and plasma contamination are minimized. There are now several international frozen stocks of rare types of blood.

Indications for use of red cells in surgery

There are a number of published guidelines for perioperative transfusion. The most recent UK version was produced by the Scottish Intercollegiate Guidelines Network.[41] The *Handbook of Transfusion Medicine* also contains detailed information.[29] Transfusion in this situation is rarely indicated if the haemoglobin is above 70 g/L, and almost never at haemoglobin greater than 100 g/L, unless serious cardiac disease is present.

PLATELET CONCENTRATES

In the past, standard concentrates were obtained from individual units of blood, and usually contained little more than 6×10^{11} platelets suspended in 60 mL plasma. Many platelet pools are now obtained from platelet donors by platelet pheresis, and contain sufficient numbers of platelets to increase an adult's platelet count by 50×10^9/L. Plastic packs with special plasticizers are used for storage, which allow efficient gaseous exchange to sustain oxidative metabolism in the platelets while they are in the packs. This enables platelets to be stored for up to 5 days at 22°C. Currently, platelet pools in the UK undergo prestorage leukocyte depletion as a precaution against the theoretical risk of variant Creutzfeldt–Jakob disease. This has had the benefit of reducing the risk of reactions to platelet transfusions.

REFERENCES

39. Janatpour K, Holland PV. Curr Hematol Rep 2002; 1: 149–155
40. Blajchman MA. Am J Ther 2002; 9: 389–395
41. Scottish Intercollegiate Guidelines Network. Perioperative blood transfusion for elective surgery. Online. Available: http://www.sign.ac.uk/guidelines/fulltext/54/index.html

FRESH FROZEN PLASMA

Freshly separated plasma is rapidly frozen to −30°C or even colder. Although the proteins of the prothrombin complex remain intact in liquid-stored plasma, factors V and VIII are labile. Factor VIII activity is reduced by half after 24 h at 20°C. Methylene blue-treated fresh frozen plasma is available that may reduce the risk of transfusion-transmitted viruses. A commercially available pathogen reduction process is also in use that provides a licensed, pooled, solvent detergent-treated product. Plans exist to import US fresh frozen plasma for children born after 31 December 1995, as a further precaution against variant Creutzfeldt–Jakob disease.

CRYOPRECIPITATE

Cryoprecipitate is prepared from fresh frozen plasma by careful cooling to 4°C, which allows a white gelatinous precipitate, rich in factor VIII, von Willebrand factor, fibrinogen and fibronectin, to be retained after recentrifugation. Five to ten donations of 10–30 mL are usually given to adults. Cryoprecipitate was used to treat haemophilia, but in view of the high number of units required, which increased risks of transfusion-transmitted infection, patients are now treated with recombinant or high-purity factors VIII and IX.

MONITORING PATIENTS FOR ADVERSE EVENTS OF TRANSFUSION

The blood pressure, pulse and temperature should be recorded before starting a transfusion, and the pulse and temperature should be checked again 15 min after beginning each blood pack. All patients should be observed throughout any transfusion. Blood pressure, pulse and temperature should be checked again when the transfusion is completed. Providing the patient is conscious, further recordings are only required if the patient becomes unwell or has symptoms or signs of a reaction. Unconscious patients should have their pulse and temperature checked at intervals during the transfusion.

THE PRINCIPLES OF SAFE BLOOD TRANSFUSION

Donor selection criteria

The donation procedure should be safe for the donor, and donors who may be considered high risk for a transmitted infection or other hazard are excluded. The reasons for exclusion relate to high-risk behaviours, such as intravenous drug abuse, a recent tattoo, recent travel to a malarious area, or taking a drug that would impair the performance of the blood donation (e.g. aspirin, which affects platelet function). A tick-box questionnaire and a personal interview are conducted for new donors or those who have not donated in the previous few years. Donors who are rejected are informed of the reason, if necessary provided with advice, and sometimes referred to other specialities. Many countries exclude donors who have lived in the UK for more than 6 months since 1980, because of the unknown risk of variant Creutzfeldt–Jakob disease being transmitted by blood transfusion.

Blood donation testing

In the UK, blood donations are tested for the following infections: human immunodeficiency viruses 1 and 2, hepatitis B, hepatitis C, syphilis and, since the end of 2002, human T cell lymphotrophic viruses 1 and 2. Other countries may test for other agents depending on the risks within their own donor populations. For example, US authorities are considering whether to test donations for West Nile virus.

Current tests for infection are highly specific and sensitive but are not perfect. Residual risks of virus transmission remain despite testing, and although small they never reach zero. The risk of transmission of variant Creutzfeldt–Jakob disease by blood transfusion is not known, and no test to exclude this risk from blood donations is likely to be available in the next few years. All UK blood supplies have had white cells removed (leukocyte depletion) since 1999 as a precaution. The current estimated risks of blood transfusion are shown in Table 3.2.

Blood is also tested for the ABO blood group, and for the Rh D group. Some blood for special purposes, for example transfusion to people with sickle cell disease, will be tested for other blood groups, such as Rh C and D, as well as Kell and Duffy types. The accuracy of the ABO/Rh D type as displayed on the blood pack is crucial to blood transfusion safety. Many blood banks now use a computer compatibility confirmation system, which does not require a donor–recipient cross-match.

Blood component processing

Whole blood is separated into red cell concentrates, platelets, and the plasma fraction. The latter is either used as single-donor fresh frozen plasma or sent to a fractionation facility for the manufacture of plasma-derived products such as albumin, immunoglobulins, or coagulation factors. Plasma collected in the UK is made into fresh frozen plasma for clinical use only, and the rest is destroyed as a precaution against variant Creutzfeldt–Jakob disease. Plasma for fractionation is imported from the USA.

Table 3.2 Known risks of red cell transfusion (per unit of red cells transfused)

Agent	Risk	No. of people affected
Hepatitis B	~ 1:80 000	Estimated 30 per year in UK
Hepatitis C	1:250 000	Estimated 10 annually in UK
HIV/AIDS		
England and Wales	< 1:2 000 000	Less than one in 10 years
Scotland and Northern Ireland	< 1:700 000	Less than one in 3 years
Human T-cell leukaemia/lymphoma virus I or II	1:80 000*	
Variant Creutzfeldt–Jakob disease	–	Unknown; transmits in sheep
Bacterial contamination	–	Low (less than three per year) but life-threatening; more common with platelets

*Pretesting and pre-leukocyte depletion.

During *leukocyte depletion*, white cells are removed from donated blood by filtration from all blood components, as a precaution against transmitting variant Creutzfeldt–Jakob disease. This has the additional advantage of reducing sensitization to white cell antigens and decreasing the incidence of febrile, non-haemolytic, transfusion reactions.

Pathogen inactivation strategies are also becoming available to treat the component in the bag to further reduce the risk of viruses and other adverse events. Fresh frozen plasma can be treated to reduce the risk of virus transmission using methylene blue treatment or a solvent detergent system to reduce virus contamination; this is also available as a licensed pharmaceutical. All these processes considerably increase the cost of blood components.

Security of blood matching and delivery to the patient

The most common hazard of blood transfusion is giving the wrong component. This error can be from a mistake in patient identity at the time of sampling, a laboratory error in the interpretation of the blood grouping findings, or more usually the result of bedside mistakes over patient identification. These mistakes can be addressed, in part, by technology. The identification of patients and blood packs can be improved by the use of using portable barcode readers. In France, a final check crossmatch is performed at the bedside. Staff education remains important.

Education of staff in the correct process for blood transfusion

Medical staff must always consider whether transfusion is necessary, and whether there are any alternatives. The bedside safety check is the final safeguard, and it is essential that this be carried out by checking the patient's wristband information against the blood pack, *not* against the transfusion documentation. Operating theatre staff must be especially vigilant because they are usually dealing with patients receiving blood while under general anaesthesia or in recovery.

PHARMACOLOGICAL AGENTS TO REDUCE BLEEDING

Pharmaceutical agents are used either to prevent bleeding or to treat established bleeding, the major indication being to prevent bleeding after cardiopulmonary bypass.[42] Drugs can be broadly classified into four groups: antifibrinolytics, desmopressin, fibrin sealants and recombinant VIIa.

ANTIFIBRINOLYTICS

Aprotinin

Aprotinin is a basic polypeptide extracted from bovine lung.[43,44] It inhibits certain serine proteases by binding to their active site. In low concentrations, aprotinin is a powerful inhibitor of plasmin, its molar potency in vitro being between a hundred and a thousand times that of tranexamic acid. Its main mechanism of action is through an antiplasmin effect, but in high doses (150–200 kIU/mL) it also inhibits kallikrein. It is licensed for use in cardiopulmonary bypass surgery, where it reduces bleeding and blood transfusion requirements by 60%.[43] Aprotinin can also be used in established fibrinolytic bleeding. 500 000 kIU is administered intravenously. A test dose should, however, be given first because it is a bovine protein and can provoke an immunological reaction.

Lysine analogues

The lysine analogues epsilon aminocaproic acid and tranexamic acid are competitive inhibitors of plasmin binding to fibrin. Both can be given to treat established fibrinolysis.[45] The recommended dose for tranexamic acid is up to 1 g by slow intravenous infusion.

DESMOPRESSIN ACETATE (DDAVP)

Desmopressin acetate is a synthetic vasopressin analogue that is relatively devoid of vasoconstrictor activity. It increases the plasma concentrations and activity of von Willebrand factor, probably by causing the release of von Willebrand factor from Weibel–Palade bodies in the endothelium. Plasma levels increase from two to five times above the baseline within an hour, and it also improves platelet function. Desmopressin causes shortening of the bleeding time in patients with von Willebrand disease, platelet function defects, and uraemia.[46] It also has a place in reducing bleeding in patients with functional platelet disorders, notably those who have received aspirin preoperatively. Side effects include flushing and an antidiuretic effect.[47]

FIBRIN SEALANTS

Fibrin sealants mimic the final part of the coagulation cascade, in that a source of thrombin is added to fibrinogen concentrates in the presence of calcium to form a clot. A 'gun' that mixes the reagents can administer them. They appear efficacious but generally trials are small and large methodological trials with clinical outcomes are required.[48]

RECOMBINANT ACTIVATED FACTOR VII

Recombinant activated factor VII is a novel agent that has been successfully used to treat haemophiliacs with inhibitors. It seems to cause clotting in areas where tissue factor is expressed, without causing generalized thrombosis. Following several anecdotal reports of its ability to reduce bleeding in patients with massive blood loss, a study in a small group of patients undergoing prostatectomy showed that preoperative recombinant factor VIIa prevented the need for blood transfusion and reduced blood loss by over half in those treated.[49] Safety is a major concern with this agent, because it could theoretically precipitate thrombosis on unstable atherosclerotic plaque. Future studies are awaited with interest.

SPECIAL SITUATIONS

DISSEMINATED INTRAVASCULAR COAGULATION

Disseminated intravascular coagulation is defined as the widespread activation of the haemostatic mechanism with formation

REFERENCES

42. Porte RJ, Leebeeek FW. Drugs 2002; 62: 2193–2211
43. Royston D, Bidstrup BP, Taylor KM et al. Lancet 1987; 2: 1289–1291
44. Segal H, Hunt BJ. Lancet 2000; 355: 1289–1290
45. Vinnicombe J, Shuttelworth K. Lancet 1996; 1: 230–232
46. Mannucci P. New Engl J Med 1983; 303: 8–12
47. Hunt B. Eur J Surg 1997; 14: 42–49
48. Carless P, Anthony D, Henry D. Br J Surg 2002; 89: 695–703
49. Frederich P, Henny C, Messelink E. Lancet 2003; 361: 201–205

of soluble or insoluble fibrin within the circulation in response to a noxious stimulus.[50] The coagulopathy can cause haemorrhage as well as thrombosis, and it is the result of an underlying condition, such as sepsis, activating the coagulation system. Microvascular and macrovascular thrombi cause peripheral ischaemia and end-organ damage particularly in the heart, kidneys, brain and skin. The formation of the fibrin and platelet meshwork partially blocks the microvasculature, causing fragmentation of the erythrocytes as they pass through the vessel. Half those affected develop a microangiopathic haemolytic anaemia.

Thrombin and bradykinin stimulate the release of tissue plasminogen activator from the endothelium, and there is simultaneous activation of plasminogen by the contact system. The fibrinolysis produced may lead to further bleeding, but by dissolving the inappropriately placed thrombi it is eventually beneficial.

Disseminated intravascular coagulation is accompanied by laboratory evidence of the consumption of platelets, coagulation factors and their inhibitors. This is measured by a prolonged prothrombin time and activated partial thromboplastin time. The fibrinogen level is reduced (often less than 1 g/L) and the platelet count is low. The increase in fibrinolytic activity is demonstrated by finding increased levels of fibrin degradation products and decreased fibrinogen. The peripheral blood film may show red cell fragmentation, which is evidence of a microangiopathic haemolytic anaemia. More sophisticated assays show reductions in the levels of the physiological anticoagulants, such as antithrombin, protein C and protein S.

Disseminated intravascular coagulation is potentiated by liver disease where haemostasis is already in a precarious balance, and by pregnancy, which induces a prothrombotic state. Haemorrhagic complications are the most common, but about 10% of patients develop severe thrombotic problems, which can lead to tissue necrosis and end-organ failure. Thrombosis usually causes skin infarcts, although purpura fulminans and haemorrhagic bullae can also occur.

The shocked patient must be vigorously resuscitated, and it is vital to treat the underlying cause. Broad-spectrum antibiotics should be given if septicaemia is suspected, even if it is not proven. The prothrombin time, activated partial thromboplastin time, fibrinogen level, platelet count, and fibrin degradation products must be measured to guide the replacement of blood components. The prothrombin time and activated partial thromboplastin time should be kept within a ratio of 1.5 of the control values, fibrinogen levels should be greater than 1 g/L, and the haematocrit kept above 0.30. After haemostatic replacement, the screening tests should be repeated. Clinical trials show that activated protein C is beneficial in systemic inflammatory response syndrome and disseminated intravascular coagulation.[51]

HYPERFIBRINOLYSIS

Bleeding occurs when there is excessive generation of plasmin secondary to the release of tissue and urokinase plasminogen activators.[52] Plasmin is a non-specific proteolytic enzyme and will split peptides with arginyl-lysyl amino acid sequences. These include fibrinogen, factors V and VIII, and the first component of complement.

Prostatic and pelvic tissues are especially rich in plasminogen activators, and they may be liberated during pelvic and prostatic surgery, especially operations on carcinoma of the prostate. They may also be released in any extensive operation, such as cardiopulmonary bypass or liver transplantation. Extremely high levels of plasminogen activators are found during the anhepatic phase of orthotopic liver transplantation, as a consequence of increased endothelial release and decreased hepatic clearance. Iatrogenic fibrinolytic bleeding can also occur through the use of exogenous fibrinolytic activators, such as streptokinase, urokinase or tissue plasminogen activator, used to lyse thrombus (see Chs 10 and 11).

Where hyperfibrinolysis is suspected, a global test of fibrinolytic activity, such as the thromboelastograph, should be available. Levels of fibrin degradation products (D-dimers) are greatly increased, and the prothrombin time, activated partial thromboplastin time, and thrombin time are mildly prolonged. The clinical and laboratory pictures are very similar to those found in disseminated intravascular coagulation. Treatment with an antifibrinolytic agent should be considered if fibrinolytic bleeding is suspected, but must not be used in disseminated intravascular coagulation. One gram of tranexamic acid or 500 000 units of aprotinin can be given intravenously.

HAEMOPHILIA A AND B

The sex-linked recessive disorder haemophilia A results in low levels of coagulation factor VIII. This disorder may arise from a spontaneous mutation in up to one-third of cases. The clinical picture depends on patients' factor VIII levels, and patients' conditions are classified as mild, moderate or severe according to their factor VIII level. Severe haemophilia occurs when levels of factor VIII are less than 1% and this condition is associated with spontaneous bleeding, especially haemarthrosis, muscle haematomas, and haematuria. Postoperative haemorrhage is life-threatening without treatment. Moderate haemophilia (factor VIII levels of 1–5%) and mild haemophilia (factor VIII levels of 6–40%) are not associated with spontaneous bleeds but marked bruising and bleeding occurs after trauma and surgery.

Laboratory abnormalities include a prolongation of the activated partial thromboplastin time and a reduction in factor VIII coagulant activity with normal von Willebrand factor levels. It is important to measure von Willebrand factor activity to exclude von Willebrand disease, which will also produce low levels of factor VIII.

Another sex-linked recessive disorder, haemophilia B, results in a deficiency of factor IX. The clinical features of this disorder and its classification are identical to those of haemophilia A, but laboratory investigations show a reduction in factor IX coagulant activity.

All haemophilia patients should be under the care of a haemophilia centre, which should be consulted before any planned or emergency operations. The aim is to prevent spontaneous bleeding by maintaining the levels of factor VIII or factor IX above 1% by regular intravenous injections.[53] These compounds should be self-administered or given by the patient's family. During surgery, the aim is to restore haemostasis to normal for the perioperative period. Haemophiliacs are given factor VIII or

REFERENCES

50. Hambleton J, Leung L, Levi M. Hematology (Am Soc Hematol Edu Program) 2002: 335–352
51. Griffin J, Zlokovic B, Fernandez J. Semin Hematol 2002; 39: 197–205
52. Hunt B, Segal H. J Clin Pathol 1996; 49: 958
53. Sanatagostino E, Gringeri A, Mannucci PM. Paediatr Drugs 2002; 4: 149–157

factor IX infusions so that the deficient factor is restored to 100% during the surgery and in the immediate postoperative period.

VON WILLEBRAND DISEASE

Heterozygous von Willebrand disease is the commonest congenital bleeding disorder, and is the result of a deficiency of von Willebrand factor. This factor is the ligand for platelet adhesion and also the carrier for factor VIII. Rarely, patients are homozygotes or mixed heterozygotes for von Willebrand disease and have no detectable von Willebrand factor. They can have spontaneous bleeding episodes in the same way as severe haemophiliacs.

Von Willebrand disease responds to intermediate-purity factor VIII preparations because these contain von Willebrand factor. Von Willebrand factor concentrates are also available but unlicensed. Mild haemophiliacs and patients with von Willebrand disease with basal levels of factor VIII greater than 0.05 IU/mL (5%) usually respond to intravenous desmopressin 0.3 μg/kg infused over 20 min. As tissue plasminogen activator is also released, reversal of the increased fibrinolysis with 500 mg to 1 g of tranexamic acid three to four times per day is advisable, particularly for procedures such as dental clearance. Antifibrinolytics are not indicated during surgery. Unfortunately, the response to desmopressin declines with daily use, so it does not provide prolonged cover after major surgery and infusions of specific factors may become necessary.[54]

PLATELET DISORDERS

Congenital platelet disorders do not usually cause severe problems, but surgery in affected patients requires special haemostatic precautions. Dental surgery can generally be managed well with careful haemostasis and 500 mg of tranexamic acid administered three to four times a day for 7 days. Platelet concentrates may be required in patients undergoing major surgery. Platelet antibodies may develop, however, and therefore concentrates should be used judiciously. Some patients respond to the use of desmopressin.

SICKLE CELL DISEASE AND THALASSAEMIA

The term *sickle cell disease* includes patients with SS, double heterozygotes for haemoglobin S and C and other variants. Patients with compensated sickle cell disease often have a haemoglobin level of about 80 g/L, but do not require transfusion. Splenic sequestration in children and in haemolytic or aplastic crises may, however, require transfusion. Prior to surgery, exchange transfusion may be beneficial to reduce the level of haemoglobin S to that of a heterozygote (i.e. less than 30%). Good hydration and oxygenation are essential perioperatively. Unusual red cell alloantibodies may have developed as a consequence of previous blood transfusions, making the task of finding compatible blood very difficult.[55]

The thalassaemia syndromes require a very different approach. People with β-thalassaemia minor (heterozygotes) have a mild anaemia that is microcytic but does not respond to iron therapy; indeed, iron is usually contraindicated because it can cause siderosis. Individuals with β-thalassaemia major (homozygotes) have a severe anaemia that develops from a few months after birth and is incompatible with life unless they receive regular transfusion. Inadequate blood transfusion results in gross bony distortion through marrow overgrowth. A regular hypertransfusion regimen is now advocated, and this is combined with chelating agents to try to prevent transfusion-induced siderosis. After some years, it may be necessary to remove the spleen, which inevitably becomes hypersplenic, causing increased transfusion requirements (see Ch. 32). This is also necessary for many patients with thalassaemia intermedia, a group of thalassaemics with a miscellaneous genetic background, some of whom have haemoglobin H disease, a form of α-thalassaemia in which only one out of the usual four genes is functional.

REFERENCES

54. Mannucci PM, Federici AB. Best Pract Res Clin Haematol 2001; 14: 455–462

Surgical infections and the use of antibiotics

4

Dominic A.J. Slade, Gordon L. Carlson

INTRODUCTION

Infection is defined as the inflammatory response to invasion and multiplication of micro-organisms within the (normally sterile) living tissues of a host.[1] Infection is distinguished from contamination, which is defined as the soiling of living or inanimate structures with potentially infectious material, and colonization, where the host response is minimal or non-existent. Common to all infections is the presence of an infecting agent within a susceptible host. A frequent feature of surgical infections is the presence of a closed unperfused or ischaemic tissue space.

An infection may arise endogenously from the vast population of micro-organisms that colonize our bodies, or exogenously from other humans, animals, or the environment in which we live. This chapter concentrates on diseases and aspects of infection with particular relevance to the practice of surgery.

BASIC SCIENCE SUMMARY

ACUTE INFECTION

The tissue response to infection is acute inflammation, with the classical signs of dolor (pain), rubor (redness), tumour (swelling), and calor (heat) initially described by Celsus in the first century AD, and functio laesa (loss of function), added later by Virchow. If well regulated and controlled, acute inflammation leads directly to tissue repair and remodelling, allowing the elimination of pathogenic microbes and the removal of necrotic tissue.

The pathophysiology of this response involves vascular, humoral and cellular mechanisms. These responses are coordinated by cytokines, which are small molecules capable of signalling between immune cells or behaving in a paracrine fashion. Inflammation starts with increased microvascular permeability to plasma proteins such as fibrinogen, and arteriolar and capillary vasodilatation, producing a protein-rich exudate in the surrounding tissues from release of local mediators such as prostaglandins, bradykinin and histamine. The inflamed vascular endothelium up-regulates adhesion molecules and proinflammatory mediators, which lead to the capture, rolling, margination and, ultimately, extravasation of neutrophils and later macrophages into the infected tissues. These effector cells travel along chemotactic gradients derived from complement and leukotrienes to their targets. The resultant cellular infiltrate not only produces further prostaglandins, but also generates cytokines and colony-stimulating factors that drive the systemic response to infection with mobilization of further neutrophils and macrophages to the infection site. Localized infection can lead to formation of abscesses containing a mixture of necrotic host tissues, bacteria, and effete neutrophils walled off by a fibrin capsule. Resolution of acute inflammation requires the removal of the infecting agent, pus (if present), and the resultant inflammatory exudate, allowing the tissues to return to their original state.

CHRONIC INFECTION

Chronic inflammation is said to exist when acute inflammation and tissue destruction coexist at the same time as attempts at healing. When chronic inflammation develops due to a microbial infection, this is termed *chronic infection*. Certain micro-organisms, such as *Mycobacterium tuberculosis* or *Actinomyces israelii*, have a propensity to produce chronic infection because, although they are of low intrinsic aggressiveness, the body has only limited defences against them. Chronic infection also occurs when bacteria live beyond the body's defence mechanisms, such as within dead bone in chronic osteomyelitis, and with infection involving materials such as sutures, prosthetic grafts or foreign bodies. Infection involving prostheses often resolves only on removal of the foreign material, with potentially devastating consequences if this happens to be a prosthetic cardiac valve or joint.

GENERALIZED INFECTION

SYSTEMIC INFLAMMATORY RESPONSE SYNDROME

A number of insults, including infection, can lead to a life-threatening condition called systemic inflammatory response syndrome, which comprises two or more of the following features:[2]

- temperature greater than 38°C or less than 36°C;
- heart rate greater than 90 beats/min;
- respiratory rate greater than 20 breaths/min;
- white blood cell count greater than 12×10^3 cells/mm^3, or less than 4×10^3 cells/mm^3, or greater than 10% immature neutrophils ('band forms').

The various causative pathologies are shown in Fig. 4.1.

SEPSIS

When systemic inflammatory response syndrome occurs as the result of a confirmed infection, it is known as sepsis. This distinction is made because many critically ill patients may develop systemic inflammatory response syndrome as a conse-

REFERENCES

1. Walter J, Israel M. General Pathology. 6th edn. Churchill Livingstone, Edinburgh, 1987: 97
2. Bone RC, Balk RA, Cerra FB et al. Chest 1992; 101: 1644–1655

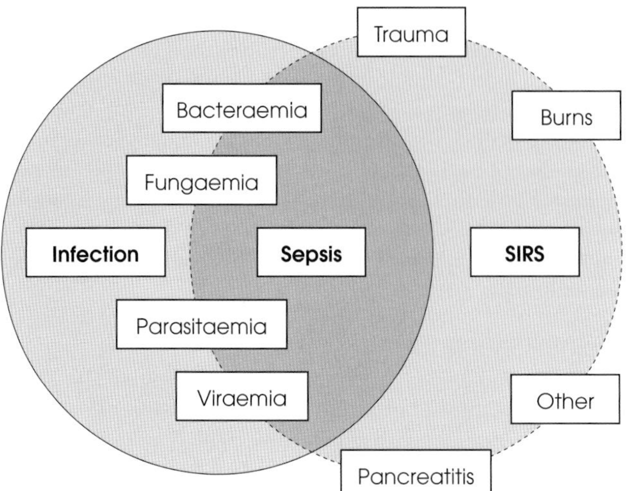

Figure 4.1 The relationships of systemic inflammatory response syndrome (SIRS), sepsis and infection, American College of Chest Physicians consensus, 1992. (After Bone R et al. Chest. 1992; 101: 1644–55, with permission.[2])

quence of such diverse insults as pancreatitis, burns, or trauma, without a primary infective cause.

Severe sepsis (sepsis syndrome) is characterized by organ dysfunction, lactic acidosis, abnormal mentation and oliguria. Criteria for diagnosis of sepsis syndrome involve evidence of dysfunction of one or more organs:[2]

- Cardiovascular system: lactate greater than 1.2 mmol/L or systemic vascular resistance less than 800 dyne/s/cm^3.
- Respiratory: P_AO_2/F_iO_2 less than 30 or P_AO_2 less than 9.3 kPa.
- Renal: urine output less than 120 mL over 4 h.
- Central nervous system: Glasgow Coma Scale score less than 15 in absence of sedation or neurological lesion.

The importance of these conditions is their capacity to progress to multiple organ dysfunction syndrome, which remains the commonest cause of death on intensive care units, with a mortality rate of 30–100% depending on the number of organs involved.[3] In the USA, there are 750 000 cases of severe sepsis every year, and approximately 30% of patients die, despite the advent of newer supportive therapies and better antibiotics.[4]

PREDISPOSING FACTORS TO INFECTION

Factors that influence the development of infections may be classified as surgical, patient, or bacterial.

SURGICAL FACTORS

Preoperative factors

Shaving of the operative site just before the start of surgery instead of the day before, and the use of clippers or depilatory creams instead of razors, reduce wound infection rates from 8–10% to 0.6–3%.[5] There is evidence that prolonged preoperative hospitalization increases the risk of wound infection to as much as 3.4% after a stay of more than 2 weeks.[6]

Perioperative factors

Host defences such as epithelial barriers are disrupted during surgery by incision, cessation of gastrointestinal motility through gut handling, and gut barrier function through perioperative starvation. Other factors, such as long operations (duration greater than 2 h), excessive use of diathermy, bringing drains out through operative wounds, poor apposition of tissues with resultant dead space, the consequent development of haematomas or seromas, and indelicate tissue handling, have all been identified with an increased risk of infection.

PATIENT FACTORS

Local

Tissue ischaemia may occur directly due to damage or ligation of blood vessels, or indirectly due to excessively tight sutures.

Foreign bodies may be forcibly implanted at the time of injury. These include clothing or dirt fragments from a gunshot wound, or foreign material placed deliberately during surgery, such as sutures, drains, and prosthetic graft materials. Foreign bodies adversely affect wound healing because of the reduced oxygen tension surrounding them, which interferes with neutrophil killing and local tissue metabolism. Foreign bodies have also been shown to substantially reduce the number of bacteria required to establish an infection following experimental inoculation.

Tissue necrosis may result from mechanical (crush injury), chemical (acid or alkali burns), ionizing radiation (radiotherapy), electrical or thermal (burns) injuries. Unchecked local infection, especially with abscess formation, may lead to further tissue necrosis.

Systemic

Tissue ischaemia from systemic illness, such as occlusive vascular disease, or low-flow states, such as hypovolaemic shock, predisposes to wound infection.

Pre-existing infections remote from the site of surgery more than double the risk of wound infection. This is especially true in the case of prostheses, for example urinary tract infection in the presence of a urinary catheter.

The rate of wound infection is increased in diabetes mellitus, liver cirrhosis, and severe systemic infections; with the administration of drugs such as glucocorticoids and immunosuppressive agents; and following radiotherapy and cancer chemotherapy, particularly in the presence of neutropenia.

Disease states associated with an increased risk of infection include uraemia, jaundice, malignancy, malnutrition and obesity. It has been shown that as a single predictor of wound infection risk, the American Society of Anesthesiologists (ASA) preoperative assessment score was at least as good as the traditional wound classification system.[7] The ASA scores of I and II (indicating no, or at worst minor, systemic illness) were associated with wound infection rates of 1.5–2.1%, whereas ASA scores of III and IV (indicating severe and life-threatening systemic illness) were associated with infection rates of 3.7–5.5%.

REFERENCES

3. Carrico CJ, Meakins JL, Marshall JC et al. Arch Surg 1986; 121: 196–208
4. Angus D, Linde-Zwirbe W, Lidicker J. Crit Care Med 2001; 20: 1303–1310
5. Alexander JW, Fischer JE, Boyajian M et al. Arch Surg 1983; 118: 347–352
6. Cruse P, Foord R. Surg Clin North Am 1980; 60: 27–40
7. Culver DH, Horan TC, Gaynes RP et al. Am J Med 1991; 91 (Suppl 3B): S152–S157

BACTERIAL FACTORS

Certain bacteria promote disease through the generation of toxins. These can be broadly classified into exotoxins, endotoxins and aggressins.

Exotoxins are usually secreted by actively dividing Gram-positive bacteria, the best-known examples being the neurotoxins of the clostridial species *tetani* and *botulinum*. Sometimes these toxins enhance the ability to cause infection, where they are referred to as aggressins.

Aggressins include hyaluronidase, streptokinase, coagulase, leukocidins and proteases that facilitate the breaching of host defences by digesting key tissue proteins and disabling components of the host's immune system.

Endotoxins are components of the outer leaflet of Gram-negative cell walls, which during life help to protect the organism from noxious substances. The molecule responsible for the toxicity of endotoxin is the heat-stable oligosaccharide lipid A moiety that is released by actively dividing bacteria and also on cell death. Endotoxins are capable of directly stimulating the coagulation and complement cascades, as well as stimulating macrophages to release pyrogenic cytokines. The resulting mediator response accounts for many of the manifestations of sepsis.

Synergy

Bacterial species can enhance each other's pathogenicity, a concept known as synergy. This may be as simple as one organism, such as *Escherichia coli*, lowering oxygen tension in a wound and creating the optimum conditions for a facultative anaerobe such as *Bacteroides fragilis*. A more complex synergism occurs in some variants of necrotizing fasciitis, where polymicrobial infections spread rapidly through tissues by the production of aggressins, such as streptokinase, and through lowered oxygen tensions, allowing colonies of anaerobic species to thrive (discussed further later in this chapter). Bacteria also behave synergistically in the generation of drug resistance. Through the exchange of transposons, small portions of extranuclear genetic material, commensal bacteria are capable of passing on genes for drug resistance to unrelated and potentially pathogenic species.

PATHOGENESIS

ENDOGENOUS INFECTION

Infections that occur after surgery are often derived from the 10^{14} bacteria that normally colonize our bodies. These infections are called endogenous or autogenous. A working knowledge of the organisms that colonize our various organs may allow us to predict which infections are likely to occur, and to plan appropriate antibiotic therapy, whether prophylactic or therapeutic. The most important organisms are discussed below by system.

Skin

Healthy skin has a large resident bacterial flora. The Gram-positive cocci include *Staphylococcus aureus*, which can be isolated from at least 30% of the general population, and coagulase-negative staphylococci. Important Gram-negative bacilli include *Pseudomonas aeruginosa* and *Acinetobacter* spp., while coliforms are frequently isolated from the skin of the perineum. Obligate anaerobes include peptostreptococci, often found in soft tissue infections, and *Propionibacterium* and coryneforms. The skin of the perineum and upper thigh may harbour the spores of *Clostridium perfringens* (*welchii*). *Candida albicans*, a yeast, is also present.

Respiratory tract

Most organisms are to be found in the nasopharynx and oral cavity, and include Gram-positive cocci such as *Staph. aureus* and *Streptococcus pneumoniae* along with several species of α-haemolytic *Viridans* streptococci. A rich flora of obligate anaerobes includes several species of each of the following: *Bacteroides*, peptostreptococci, *Prevotella*, and *Fusobacterium*. The actinomycete *A. israelii* is also present. The Gram-negative bacillus *E. coli* is a transient commensal, the numbers of which have been shown to increase on hospitalization.

Gastrointestinal tract

The stomach and biliary tract are sterile in health. The small intestinal flora is scanty, but includes Gram-positive cocci (such as enterococci), Gram-negative bacilli (especially *E. coli*), and yeasts such as *Ca. albicans*.

The colon carries almost 1.3 kg wet weight of commensal bacteria composed mostly of anaerobes. These include *B. fragilis*, clostridial species including *Cl. perfringens* and *Cl. difficile* and peptostreptococci. Of the aerobes, *E. coli* and enterococci predominate. Again, *Ca. albicans* is present.

Genitourinary tract

Only the lower urinary tract, principally the urethra, is colonized with coryneforms, coagulase-negative staphylococci, and group B streptococci and yeasts (*Ca. albicans*). The vagina is colonized with lactobacilli, *Bacteroides* spp., and small numbers of *Gardnerella vaginalis* and *Ca. albicans*.

Impact of commensal flora on health

The balance of normal flora can change as a result of hospitalization and especially following therapeutic interventions. The use of drugs that interfere with host defences, such as inhibitors of gastric acid secretion, the presence of intravenous or urethral catheters or nasogastric tubes, and the prolonged use of broad-spectrum antibiotics, are all known to derange the distribution and composition of the commensal flora. An important concept only recently appreciated has been termed *colonization resistance*; this is the ability of the commensal flora to resist the multiplication of pathogenic or invading organisms through competition for substrates and sites of attachment.

Probiotics

It has long been appreciated that commensal organisms, especially the gut flora, may be beneficial to humans by aiding digestion and through the production of useful substrates, such as vitamins. It has, however, only recently been appreciated that support of particular strains of colonic commensal flora, most notably lactobacilli, may help prevent disease. Probiotics, as these organisms are called, appear capable of modulating the immune system through the production of short-chain fatty acids, amino acids, antioxidants such as flavonoids and carotenoids, and bacterial cytokines known as bacteriokines. Commensal organisms can kill pathogenic bacteria through the production of bacteriocins and metabolic end-products toxic to other species, as well as by altering environmental conditions, such as pH, to interfere with reproduction.[8] A large amount of research interest

REFERENCES

8. Hentges D. Clin Infect Dis 1993; 16 (Suppl 4): S175–S180

has been focused on the therapeutic use of probiotics through feed additives, particularly in critically ill patients.

EXOGENOUS INFECTION

Exogenous infection is defined as infection acquired from other humans, animals, or the environment.

Human transmission of infection may be vertical (from mother to fetus) or horizontal. This may involve transmission of infection by the faecal–oral route, by expired droplets, by direct contact (including sexual intercourse), or by indirect contact (e.g. via blankets and clothing). Infections may be acquired from animals (zoonoses) by direct contact or through ingestion of animal products, such as meat or milk. Environmentally acquired infection may result from contact with infected water sources (including air-conditioning) or contaminated soil. Infection acquired in the hospital environment is termed *nosocomial*, and is frequently multiply antibiotic-resistant, due to the exposure of the relevant organisms to selection pressure.

ANTIBIOTICS AND THEIR USE

MECHANISMS OF ACTION

Antibiotics exploit the differences between mammalian and microbial cells. They may kill bacteria (in which case they are bactericidal), or arrest division and multiplication (where they are called bacteriostatic). Bacterial cells have a rigid cell wall to provide osmotic stability, differently structured and smaller ribosomes than mammals, lack of a nuclear membrane, and a particular dependence on certain metabolic pathways, especially those involving folate metabolism, for growth and multiplication.

The largest class of antibiotics, which includes penicillins and cephalosporins, is characterized by their common chemical structure, the β-lactam ring. β-Lactams are bactericidal through inhibition of cell wall synthesis. They are consequently ineffective against bacteria, such as mycoplasma, that lack cell walls. Bacteria resistant to penicillins produce β-lactamases; these enzymes hydrolyse these antibiotics to a harmless by-product. Therapeutic strategies for overcoming resistant species are the addition of specific β-lactamase inhibitors, such as clavulanic acid and tazobactam, or the use of a β-lactamase-resistant penicillin such as flucloxacillin. Glycopeptides such as vancomycin and teicopleinin inhibit cell wall synthesis but are bulky molecules and cannot penetrate the outer membrane of Gram-negative bacteria, thus confining their spectrum of activity to Gram-positive species.

Bacteriostatic agents include aminoglycosides and tetracyclines, which target the smaller bacterial ribosomal subunit, inhibiting or disrupting protein synthesis, while erythromycin, clarithromycin, clindamycin and chloramphenicol bind to the larger subunit, with similar consequences.

Inhibition of folate synthesis or DNA replication is the respective mode of action of sulphonamides and quinolones. Nitroimidazoles such as metronidazole work by breaking nucleic acid strands, whereas rifampicin inhibits RNA formation.

GENERAL PRINCIPLES UNDERLYING ANTIBIOTIC CHOICE AND PRESCRIPTION

Antibiotic prescription may be prophylactic or therapeutic. Before prescribing an antibiotic in either scenario it is important that as much evidence as possible is available to support the final choice. Most hospitals now employ guidelines for antibiotic prescribing to reduce costs and limit inappropriate prescribing. In established infection, the clinical history and examination should be supplemented with appropriate microbiological samples (blood, pus, urine, sputum, or cerebrospinal fluid if appropriate) for culture, sensitivity, and occasionally Gram stain. This may take several days; in the future, rapid (within hours) identification of bacterial species using gene microarrays may be possible. Initial antibiotic prescription is usually empirical, however, and it is unreasonable to delay treatment for a sick patient because of this.

The choice and dosage of antibiotic should be determined by two principle sets of factors. The first are patient characteristics, such as age, history of allergy, impaired renal or hepatic function, immune status, the severity of illness (which may determine the route of administration), and in women, whether the patient is pregnant, breastfeeding, or taking the oral contraceptive pill.[9] The second set of factors requires a sound working knowledge of microbiology to determine the likely range of pathogens, based on the putative site of infection, and their antibiotic sensitivity. In nosocomial infection, guidance on local antibiotic resistance may be important in determining the choice of antibiotic. Initial treatment can be modified in the light of later laboratory results. The clinician should be prepared to work closely with the local microbiology department to adjust treatment in response to new information, especially where infection with multiresistant organisms is concerned.

Whenever possible, in a proven infection with a documented pattern of sensitivity, it is sensible to use the most appropriate narrow-spectrum antibiotic available, and to limit its duration to the shortest time required to reduce the likelihood of unwanted effects, the development of resistant organisms, and superinfection with organisms such as *Cl. difficile* (discussed further later in this chapter). In some circumstances, careful interpretation of laboratory results in consideration of clinical information is required, for example in urinary tract contamination associated with a catheter, where the best treatment may be catheter removal and not antibiotic therapy.

MULTIPLY RESISTANT ORGANISMS

METHICILLIN-RESISTANT *STAPHYLOCOCCUS AUREUS*

The multiply resistant organism MRSA is usually resistant to two or more antibiotics, and is mostly responsible for nosocomial infection, although community outbreaks may also occur. Strains of MRSA are intrinsically no more virulent than methicillin-sensitive strains, but are resistant to commonly employed antibiotics. Active infection with MRSA, like *Staph. aureus*, is intimately related to increased host susceptibility. Some strains have a particular propensity to cause outbreaks of infection, and are referred to as epidemic MRSA. As well as being carried in the anterior nares of both patients and staff, MRSA colonizes the perineum, axillae, and chronic skin lesions (e.g. open wounds). Patients most commonly colonized with the organism are elderly, infirm, nursing home residents with skin lesions such as leg ulcers or pressure sores. Significant risk factors for MRSA colonization and infection include prolonged hospital stay and treatment

REFERENCES

9. British Medical Association and Royal Pharmaceutical Society of Great Britain. British National Formulary. BMJ Books, London, 2002

involving multiple antibiotics. Outbreaks most frequently occur on wards receiving such patients, especially large, open-plan, geriatric wards and high-intensity areas such as intensive care units.

Infection control procedures for MRSA depend on the perceived risk to patients, according to the type of ward, the MRSA strain, and the presence of active infection. Although some countries, such as the Netherlands, seem to have successfully adopted an approach designed to eliminate MRSA carriage in hospitals, the current policy in the UK is based on containment. A high-risk outbreak, such as epidemic MRSA in a hospital intensive care unit, requires isolation and treatment of patients with active infection, and screening of all staff and patients, followed by eradication with mupirocin and antiseptic baths. Units in which MRSA infection may be disastrous (e.g. orthopaedic wards) may need to be closed pending the adoption of measures to eliminate MRSA. In contrast, on a medical ward with MRSA colonization but no evidence of acute infection, general control measures involving hand-washing, use of gloves and aprons, careful disposal of infected bed linen, and decontamination of equipment used on an infected or colonized patient may be sufficient. Patients in whom there has been previous evidence of MRSA colonization or infection are treated as if they had continued colonization on subsequent hospital admissions and, if at all possible, should not be admitted to units in which the consequences of MRSA infection are particularly grave.

Treatment of active infection depends on individual sensitivities, but vancomycin and teicopleinin are common first-line agents, whereas rifampicin combined with ciprofloxacin or fusidic acid may be used when treatment of colonized lesions is necessary. Newer antibiotics, such as linezolid, may be of value in life-threatening MRSA infection.

VANCOMYCIN-RESISTANT ENTEROCOCCI

Enterococcal infection with strains resistant to vancomycin, VRE, is of considerable concern, particularly on renal and intensive care units. Because enterococci are part of the normal gut flora, they can acquire resistance to quinolones and third-generation cephalosporins through prolonged exposure to these agents. Strains of VRE are thus usually found in patients with long-standing urinary tract or intra-abdominal infections following multiple courses of antibiotics, and there are correspondingly few antibiotics available to treat them. Spread is thought to occur mainly on the hands of healthcare workers, but also through faecal contamination of equipment. Infection control measures include isolation of patients, institutional reduction in the use of antibiotics that select out resistant strains, and rapid detection of epidemics through stool culture surveillance.

The remainder of this section outlines some of the more common surgical infections, with suggested treatments and advice regarding prophylactic antibiotic regimens. It is not intended to be exhaustive, but merely to provide a framework for dealing with various conditions.

SKIN AND SOFT TISSUE INFECTION

FURUNCLE (BOIL)

A furuncle (or boil) is a focal infection of a hair follicle; the causative organism is usually *Staph. aureus*. Treatment other than incision and drainage for the acute condition is unnecessary in an otherwise healthy patient, unless there is evidence of surrounding cellulitis (see later).

CARBUNCLE

Carbuncles are characterized by poorly localized infection of a group of hair follicles with an associated cellulitis resulting in multiple discharging sinuses. They are most commonly found on the back of the neck in patients with diabetes, renal failure or malnutrition. Treatment requires both incision and drainage or laying open of the lesion along with penicillin and flucloxacillin therapy.

CELLULITIS

Certain organisms, notably *Strep. pyogenes* but occasionally anaerobes and polymicrobial infections, produce an acute, diffuse, poorly localized infection of the skin, and are capable of spreading through the subcutaneous tissues by secretion of aggressins such as hyaluronidase, streptokinase and proteases. Cellulitis is best treated with a combination of penicillin and flucloxacillin, or co-amoxiclav as a single agent, although associated abscesses will require incision and drainage.

ERYSIPELAS

The term *erysipelas* describes a cellulitis confined to the dermis, usually due to a group A β-haemolytic streptococcus. Erysipelas affects the face and limbs, and can be distinguished clinically from cellulitis and deep venous thrombosis by a palpable raised edge. Treatment initially involves parenteral penicillin with the addition of flucloxacillin if staphylococcal infection is suspected.

LYMPHANGITIS

Localized staphylococcal infection of a limb can lead to tracking, thin, red lines representing infection within the lymphatics, and may also be associated with tender lymphadenopathy. Treatment is that of the underlying infection.

INFECTED EPIDERMOID (SEBACEOUS) CYST

Epidermoid or sebaceous cysts occur commonly on hair-bearing skin, such as that of the face, neck, chest and shoulders. Infection of one of these retention cysts is best treated with incision and drainage, with later definitive excision of the cyst.

ABSCESS

A localized purulent infection that engenders acute inflammation in the surrounding tissues and a fibrin-rich 'pyogenic' membrane is called an abscess. The environment common to all abscesses is their acidic pH, low oxygen tension, and a high internal pressure. These features explain why systemic antibiotics have little effect on the localized infection, why they are painful, and why facultative anaerobic species often predominate within a polymicrobial infection. The treatment of established abscesses is thorough drainage, by either surgical or radiological means.

BREAST ABSCESS

Breast abscesses can be either lactational or non-lactational. Non-lactational abscesses are often associated with an underlying condition such as periductal mastitis, other suppurative processes, or trauma (see Ch. 22), whereas lactational breast abscesses are more often due to milk stasis or non-infectious inflammation. Indeed, bacterial infection, usually with *Staph. aureus*, and abscess formation occur in only 11% of cases of puerperal mastitis. Traditionally, breast abscesses were treated with dependent drainage, but in many cases abscesses will resolve with aspiration (which may require repeating) and, if infection is confirmed, antibiotic therapy. Cessation of breast feeding is frequently required.

Non-lactational breast abscesses are commonly periareolar, recurrent, and frequently develop as a consequence of periductal mastitis, although consideration should be given to the possibility of an inflammatory carcinoma. Incision and drainage with biopsy of the cavity wall is often necessary, but definitive treatment in periductal mastitis may also involve excision of the affected duct. Clues to the presence of chronic underlying periductal disease include nipple inversion, non-cyclical mastalgia, a history of nipple discharge, a subareolar mass, or the presence of a mammillary fistula. When infection occurs it is usually polymicrobial, with *Staph. aureus* occurring acutely and coagulase-negative staphylococci in the chronic form. Common to both forms are α-haemolytic streptococci. *Prevotella* spp., *Bacteroides* spp. and peptostreptococci are among the usual anaerobes isolated.

PILONIDAL ABSCESS

Infection of a pre-existing pilonidal sinus can lead to abscess formation, usually with coliforms and anaerobes such as *B. fragilis*. Treatment is initially by incision and drainage. A considerable proportion of sinuses require no further treatment, but excision of the sinus (preferably between episodes) may be necessary if recurrent infection occurs.

PERIANAL ABSCESS

Perianal abscesses usually arise secondary to infection of intersphincteric anal glands. Owing to the distinct anatomy of the region, infection may track through adjoining tissues to create ischiorectal or perianal abscesses. Recurrent abscesses are characteristic of the presence of fistula-in-ano and, occasionally, Crohn's disease (see Chs 27 and 28). The causative organisms are generally mixed colonic flora, such as coliforms and *Bacteroides* species. Less commonly, infection of skin adnexae may give rise to abscess formation in this region and may involve skin organisms, including *Staph. aureus*. Treatment requires incision and drainage.

PSOAS ABSCESS

Osteomyelitis of the spine or infection involving the kidneys, pancreas or colon may spread into the space bounded by the psoas fascia, ultimately presenting as a groin lump. Tuberculous osteomyelitis may present with vague back pain, night sweats and fevers, and eventually with a non-tender groin mass (or 'cold abscess'). Conversely, staphylococcal, *Strep. milleri* or coliform infection presents with the typical swinging pyrexia associated with abscess formation, and excruciating pain with the patient holding the leg in forced hip flexion on the affected side. Psoas abscess arising secondary to colonic pathology generally occurs as a complication of fistulating conditions (diverticular disease, Crohn's disease and occasionally carcinoma). The diagnosis can confidently be made by CT or sometimes ultrasound scanning.

Treatment is by drainage—either percutaneously under CT or ultrasound control, or surgically by incision above the inguinal ligament and into the retroperitoneal space—followed by definitive treatment of the underlying cause. Prolonged antibiotic or antituberculous chemotherapy may be necessary.

HYDRADENITIS SUPPURATIVA

Hydradenitis suppurativa, an inflammatory suppurative condition involving the apocrine sweat glands following puberty, deserves mention because it most frequently affects the axillae and perineum, but it is also seen in the inframammary creases, mons, scrotum, groin, umbilicus or anus. In time, it develops a characteristic appearance of scarring, sinus tract formation and recurrent abscesses. Secondary infection with staphylococci (*Staph. aureus* in 50% of patients) and streptococci characterize axillary disease, whereas perineal disease is more often associated with *Klebsiella*, *Proteus*, *E. coli*, and anaerobes such as *Bacteroides*.

Treatment modalities involve diagnosis of the condition, incision and drainage of abscesses when necessary, and even long-term metronidazole therapy for mild cases. Severe relapsing disease is best treated with radical excision and skin-grafting if required.

NECROTIZING SOFT TISSUE INFECTIONS

Necrotizing soft tissue infections are a group of rare and diverse disease processes characterized by rapid spread of infection through subfascial planes, as well as a marked systemic disturbance and pain, which are both often disproportionate to the clinical signs. These conditions are often difficult to diagnose, and are associated with a high morbidity and mortality. They have rejoiced under a number of eponyms, including Fournier's gangrene and Meleney's synergistic gangrene, and have also been described as hospital gangrene, gas gangrene and necrotizing fasciitis. None of these terms are particularly helpful, and it is important to realize that not all infections are gas-forming. Fournier's gangrene specifically refers to a synergistic mixed facultative anaerobic infection of the perineum arising from an underlying condition, in one series most commonly urogenital (45%) but also anorectal (33%) or dermal (21%).[10]

Recognition of necrotizing soft tissue infections requires a high index of suspicion, especially in patients with predisposing conditions, which include diabetes mellitus, occlusive vascular disease, renal failure, malnutrition, malignancy, immunosuppression and parenteral drug abuse. Necrotizing infections may develop in devitalized tissues, arising within areas of widespread trauma, but may also occur after relatively minor trauma (including elective surgery).

The classic features of necrotizing infections are severe pain at the infection site and deceptively minor cutaneous signs, ranging from bronzing to skin cyanosis. Gas-forming organisms produce crepitation and, as the infection establishes itself, dermal gangrene or epidermolysis becomes evident. Systemic features are particularly striking and include fever, tachycardia, abnormal mentation, oliguria, leukocytosis, and even shock or multiple organ dysfunction syndrome. Plain radiographs are usually not particularly helpful, but may reveal the presence of a foreign body, osteomyelitis, or free gas in the tissues suggestive of severe infection (Fig. 4.2). Ultrasound or CT scanning may demonstrate deep infection with free gas or surrounding tissue oedema.

Early diagnosis, with vigorous resuscitation and aggressive intravenous antibiotic therapy, together with radical surgical debridement of all affected tissues with a wide margin, is the key to successful treatment. There is some evidence to suggest the therapeutic benefit of hyperbaric oxygen therapy, although this is not widely available. Surgical management should include a low threshold for repeated examination under anaesthesia every 12–24 h, with further debridement of devitalized tissues

REFERENCES

10. Clayton MD, Fowler JE, Sharifi R et al. Surg Gynecol Obstet 1990; 170: 49–55

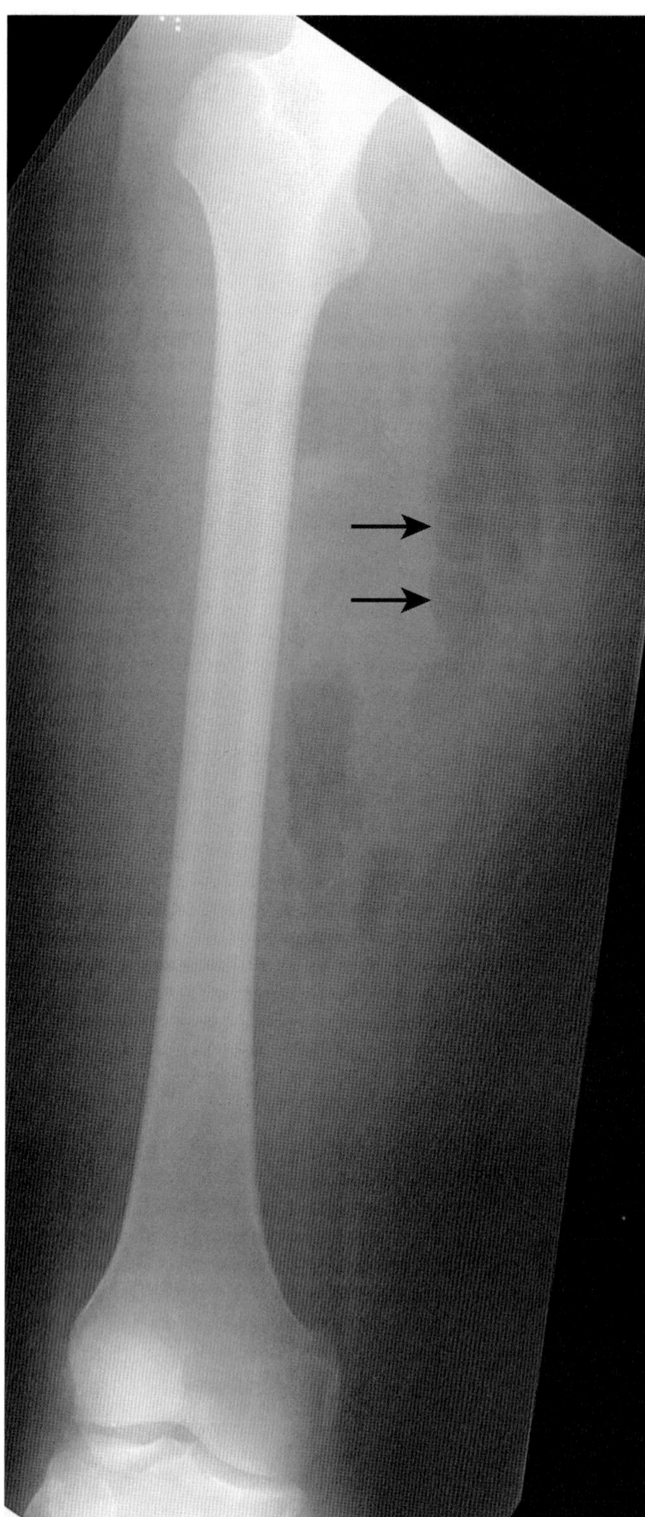

Figure 4.2 Radiograph showing gas in the soft tissues of the medial thigh (arrows) in a patient with necrotizing soft tissue infection of the right leg.

if necessary. Extensive plastic surgical reconstruction may be required at a later date. The usual pathogens include the group A streptococcus (*Strep. pyogenes*) and *Staph. aureus*. In synergistic infection, anaerobic organisms including *B. fragilis* and occasionally clostridia are isolated, in particular *Cl. perfringens* and *Cl. septicum*.

IMPORTANT NOSOCOMIAL INFECTIONS

WOUND INFECTION

Wound infection, also referred to as superficial incisional infection, is defined as a surgical site infection that occurs within 30 days of surgery, and involves only the skin or subcutaneous tissues of the incision with at least one of the following:[11]

- Purulent drainage from the superficial incision.
- Organisms found on culture of aseptically aspirated fluid or tissue, or from a swab and pus cells.
- At least two signs of inflammation are present (pain or tenderness, localized swelling, redness or heat), and either the incision is deliberately opened for management or a diagnosis of infection is made on clinical grounds.

Wound infection is one of the commonest causes of postoperative morbidity and greatly influences time to discharge from hospital as well as healthcare costs.

Altemeier demonstrated that the risk of wound infection varies according to the formula:[6]

$$\frac{\text{Dose of bacterial contamination} \times \text{virulence}}{\text{Resistance of host}}$$

Prevention of wound infection should entail the maintenance of normal resistance to bacterial invasion, prevention of bacterial wound contamination, and supplementation of the host resistance to infection.[12] It can be readily appreciated from the predisposing factors listed earlier that adequate tissue oxygenation and perfusion, tissue preservation through gentle handling and appropriate use of diathermy, and anticipation of those wounds at risk of infection are important maxims in the delivery of high-quality surgical care. Studies have shown that keeping the patient warm, reducing postoperative pain, and improving global oxygenation may all reduce the rate of postoperative wound infection, possibly by improving local tissue defence mechanisms against bacterial invasion.

Surgical wounds are classified into four groups according to their potential for subsequent infection.[13] Cruse and Foord have added infection rates for each category from their 10-year epidemiological study of almost 63 000 wounds, 2960 of which were infected (Table 4.1).[6] The incidence of infection after clean surgery is, and should be, very low indeed (less than 2%), because wound infection under these circumstances usually indicates a breach in aseptic technique. The majority of such infections involve *Staph. aureus*. The rates of wound infection are clearly higher when a wound is made involving an organ system with a significant resident pathogenic flora (e.g. the gut), or when the area incised is already infected.

The management of the infected wound depends on the type and severity of the infection and the associated systemic disturbance. In general, minor and common wound infections are best treated by removal of staples or sutures and packing. Pus should be sent for culture, but antibiotic therapy is not indicated in the absence of evidence of spreading infection (i.e. cellulitis and signs of sepsis). Antibiotic therapy should be reserved for

REFERENCES

11. Crowe M, Cooke E. J Hosp Infect 1998; 39: 3–11
12. Burke J (ed). Surgical Physiology. WB Saunders, Edinburgh, 1983: 270–283
13. National Academy of Sciences Ad Hoc Committee on Trauma. Ann Surg 1964; 160 (Suppl 2): 1

Table 4.1 Wound infection rates by class

	Clean	Clean contaminated	Contaminated	Dirty
Features	Elective Non-traumatic No acute inflammation No breach of sterile technique Primary closure No drains	Non-elective Clean, controlled Respiratory/gastrointestinal tract involved No entry into biliary/ urinary tract No contamination	Acute purulent inflammation *or* penetrating trauma < 4 h old *or* gastrointestinal tract spillage *or* major breach in sterile technique	Penetrating trauma > 4 h old *or* purulence/abscess formation *or* preoperative perforated viscus
Examples	Hernia repair Varicose vein surgery	Uncomplicated small bowel resection Pneumonectomy	Appendicectomy (non-perforated) Compound fracture	Bullet wound Perforated peptic ulcer
Infection rate without prophylaxis	Less than 1.5%	Less than 7%	Approximately 15%	As high as 40%

(After Cruse PJ, Foord R. Surg Clin North Am. 1980; 60: 27–40, with permission.[6])

wound infection associated with signs of cellulitis, or where there are clear signs of a systemic host response (e.g. pyrexia and tachycardia). Wounds with tissue necrosis should be debrided and left open. In all cases where a wound has been packed and allowed to heal by secondary intention, follow-up by a tissue viability or wound nurse is recommended.

PSEUDOMEMBRANOUS COLITIS

Pseudomembranous colitis is characterized by severe watery (occasionally bloody) diarrhoea, abdominal pain, and the presence of a pseudomembrane of mucosal plaques on sigmoidoscopy. The condition results from colonic proliferation of the pathogen *Cl. difficile* and the secretion of its cytopathic endotoxin. It is thought that *Cl. difficile* is responsible for virtually all episodes of antibiotic-associated colitis in adults, whether or not associated with a pseudomembrane[14] (see Ch. 28).

Elderly hospital patients prescribed prolonged courses of broad-spectrum antibiotics, particularly third-generation cephalosporins, broad-spectrum penicillins, or clindamycin, are especially at risk. Infection in a susceptible individual can occur via faecal–oral spread, or from environmental contamination from heat-resistant spores. These are found in abundance in hospital wards and rooms where other *Cl. difficile*-infected patients have been nursed. Children very rarely get the disease despite high carriage rates, and it has been suggested that they lack a colonic receptor essential to development of the condition. Normal host resistance to infection wanes with increasing age.

When severe, the disease may present with fulminant colitis, toxic dilatation and perforation as in ulcerative colitis, and an appreciable mortality rate.[14] Prompt diagnosis and treatment are therefore essential. The diagnosis is usually confirmed by stool cytotoxin testing (not culture), with a sensitivity of 94–100% and a specificity of 100%. Lower gastrointestinal endoscopy may be helpful but is not reliable because a pseudomembrane is not always present. Treatment involves resuscitation (fluid loss may be considerable), stopping the offending antibiotics if possible, and metronidazole or vancomycin (the latter usually reserved for more serious infections).

Occasionally patients present with an acute abdomen, and may even undergo laparotomy before the diagnosis is certain. In one series of 13 patients with *Cl. difficile* infection who required laparotomy, mortality was reduced to 14% by subtotal colectomy and ileostomy.

CENTRAL LINE INFECTION

Life-threatening infection related to the use of indwelling central venous catheters carries significant morbidity and mortality. The risk is particularly high in lines used for parenteral nutrition, where bacterial infection rates of up to 8% have been reported.[15] The causative organisms are usually skin commensals, most frequently coagulase-negative *Staphylococcus*, *Staph. aureus*, and less often multiply resistant organisms including *Candida*, enterococci and *Klebsiella* spp. Virtually all infection follows initial colonization of the catheter hub, frequently from the hands of medical attendants. Organisms rapidly become established in the fibrin sheath around the intravascular portion of the catheter, and gain access directly to the bloodstream and cardiac valves. Haematogenous spread to the central line from remote sites of infection is a theoretical but uncommon event.

Factors known to increase the risk of catheter colonization and subsequent infection are lines with multiple lumens, poor aseptic technique during insertion and subsequent care, multiple attempts at line placement, occlusive catheter dressings, loss of catheter patency through thrombosis, long duration of catheter use, and catheter site. In particular, groin lines are more likely to become infected.

Guidelines on the prevention of catheter sepsis suggest planning the likely duration of treatment, and using a tunnelled or totally implantable vascular device for patients requiring more than 30 days of vascular access.[16] Unless medically contraindicated, subclavian lines should be used in preference to other sites because the risk of infection may be lower. Peripherally inserted central catheters placed in the antecubital fossa with the tip lying in the subclavian vein have been shown to carry the lowest risk of infection, possibly because the arm has low counts of skin commensals and also because of the considerable distance between the hub and the intravascular portion of the catheter. Important aspects of catheter care shown to reduce colonization and sepsis rates include routine flushing with an anticoagulant,

REFERENCES

14. Bradbury A, Barrett S. Br J Surg 1997; 84: 150–159
15. Wilson M, Garrison R. In: Fry D (ed). Infections of Intravascular Devices in Surgical Infections. Little, Brown, New York, 1995: 541–549
16. Pratt RJ, Pellowe C, Loveday HP et al. J Hosp Infect 2001; 47 (Suppl): S21–S37

rigid adherence to aseptic handling protocols (which frequently requires a dedicated nursing team), and disinfection of the catheter hub before every access to the line. One strategy advocated for the reduction of catheter colonization is regular exchange of the catheter over a guide wire or insertion at a new site, but current evidence suggests that the risk of colonization remains constant over time and is not reduced by catheter replacement without a clinical indication.

Catheter infection should be borne in mind in any patient with a central line in whom there is evidence of sepsis. The diagnosis may be made on clinical grounds and treatment (see later) initiated immediately, although in some cases (e.g. in patients with permanent intravenous lines for home parenteral nutrition), the necessity of life-long venous access may make achieving a definitive diagnosis essential prior to line removal.

The diagnosis of catheter infection is usually confirmed by isolating an organism in blood withdrawn from the central line in greater numbers than those found on simultaneous peripheral blood culture, although a number of other techniques have been used, including the use of catheter brushes (to 'chimney sweep' the catheter and sample the fibrin sleeve), and acridine orange leukocyte cytospin (in which samples taken from the catheter are stained for organisms within the leukocytes).

In the face of sepsis due to proven catheter infection, it is logical to remove the line and insert a new one at a different site if required. If the diagnosis is in doubt then it is acceptable to exchange the catheter over a guide wire. Because catheter infection may be life-threatening and can have an alarmingly sudden onset, there is a place for antibiotic therapy once peripheral and central blood cultures have been taken, the line removed, and the tip sent for culture and sensitivity. In permanent feeding lines, an attempt may be made to salvage the catheter by administering, in addition to systemic therapy, antibiotic solutions directly down the catheter, together with urokinase to disrupt the fibrin sheath. This may be effective for infection with coagulase-negative staphylococci, but infection with *Staph. aureus* or *Candida*, or which is polymicrobial, should necessitate catheter removal.

INTRA-ABDOMINAL INFECTION

PERITONITIS

Inflammation of the parietal peritoneum results in peritonitis that may be primary, secondary or tertiary (see Ch. 25).

Primary peritonitis

Primary peritonitis occurs as a spontaneous infection, most commonly in patients with pre-existing hepatic ascites, but may also occur with intraperitoneal catheters used for peritoneal dialysis. Primary bacterial peritonitis also rarely occurs in immunosuppressed patients. Infection results from either catheter colonization or by haematogenous or lymphatic spread. Primary bacterial peritonitis is relatively rare, accounting for less than 1% of all peritonitis.[17] The causative organisms are often single Gram-negative bacilli, such as *E. coli*, *K. pneumoniae*, *Strep. pneumoniae*, *Strep. pyogenes*, and staphylococci, most commonly coagulase-negative species but also *Staph. aureus*.

Antibiotic treatment is usually effective, although loculated collections seen on ultrasound or CT scanning may require percutaneous drainage. Surgery may be required to remove prosthetic devices (e.g. peritoneal dialysis catheters) and, occasionally, to facilitate adequate peritoneal lavage and drain abscesses between loops of small intestine.

Secondary peritonitis

Secondary peritonitis may result from intra-abdominal pathologies as diverse as visceral perforation, inflammation of an intraperitoneal organ, blunt or penetrating abdominal trauma, surgery, malignancy or ischaemic necrosis. The infection is usually polymicrobial and synergistic between an aerobe capable of lowering the oxygen tension and facultative anaerobic species. Common causative organisms include *E. coli*, enterococci, *P. aeruginosa* and *Klebsiella* spp., along with *Bacteroides* spp., especially *B. fragilis* and peptostreptococci.

The management of secondary peritonitis is drainage and, wherever possible, surgical extirpation of the primary source of infection, followed by appropriate antibiotic and supportive therapy. Failure to eradicate the primary source of infection—which may occur, for example, when perforation is sited in the proximal gastrointestinal tract—is associated with a bad prognosis.

Tertiary peritonitis

Tertiary peritonitis is a condition confined to critically ill patients in whom infection persists after initial incomplete treatment. The causative organisms are frequently hospital-acquired, multiply resistant Gram-negative bacilli and yeasts.

INTRA-ABDOMINAL ABSCESS

Perforated appendicitis or diverticulitis are two of the commonest precipitants of intra-abdominal sepsis, accounting for a quarter of all intra-abdominal abscesses in one 10-year study[18] (see Ch. 25). Abscess formation may be promoted by limitation of infection to certain sites and by the anatomical arrangement of the organs within the peritoneal cavity, along with the extraordinary capacity for the omentum to contain and localize infection. Other factors, such as the migration of peritoneal fluid towards the subphrenic space by the relative negative pressure produced by the diaphragm and the site of the infecting focus, favour certain defined anatomical spaces, as outlined in Fig. 4.3.

In stable patients, the anatomy of infection should be delineated before planning treatment. Intraperitoneal abscesses are increasingly managed by percutaneous drainage under ultrasound or CT control, but eradication of the primary source of infection (e.g. an anastomotic leak) usually requires laparotomy. When a defect in the bowel is found in association with an abscess in a critically ill patient, consideration should be given to exteriorizing the bowel, rather than performing an anastomosis, because anastomotic healing is frequently impaired under these circumstances. Surgery is also likely to be required when the anatomy is unfavourable to percutaneous drainage, such as with multiple interloop abscesses. Patients should also receive broad-spectrum antibiotic therapy until pus from the abscess has been analysed to determine the causative organism's pattern of antibiotic sensitivity.

When extensive contamination of the peritoneal cavity has occurred with multiple abscesses, it may be better to leave the abdomen open, simply packed gently with gauze following

REFERENCES

17. Conn H. Gastroenterology 1976; 70: 455–457
18. Altemeier WA, Culbertson WR, Fullen WD et al. Am J Surg 1973; 125: 70–79

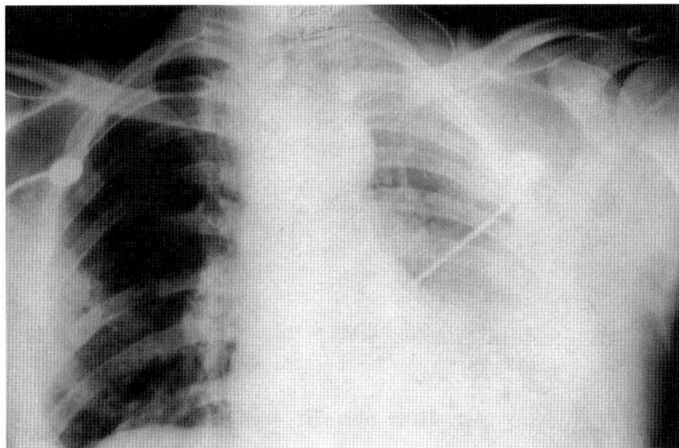
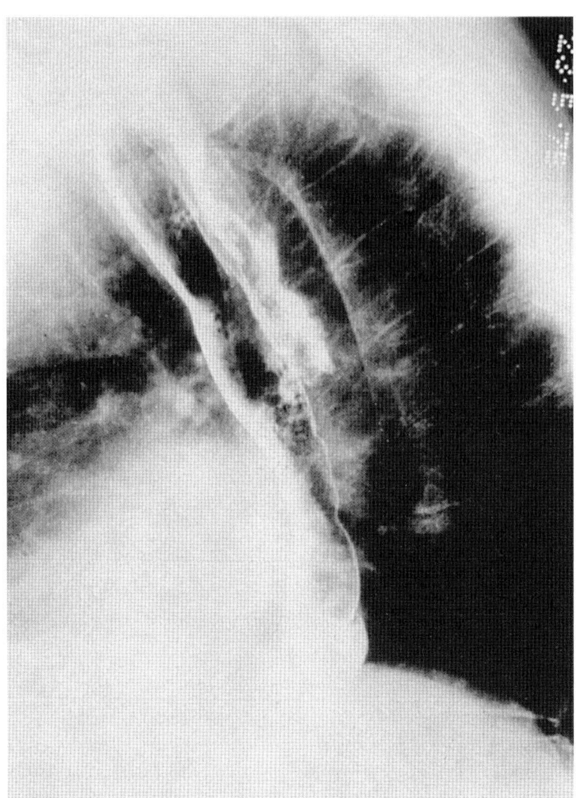

Figure 4.3 Lateral (**a**) and ventral (**b**) views of the peritoneal cavity showing potential sites for sepsis.

surgical intervention, a technique known as laparostomy.[19] This approach, combined usually with parenteral feeding, may obviate the need for multiple laparotomies and allows treatment of the whole peritoneal cavity as one large abscess cavity.

HEPATOBILIARY INFECTION

ACUTE CHOLECYSTITIS

Acute cholecystitis frequently results from obstruction of the cystic duct by a gallstone (see Ch. 30). A chemical cholecystitis develops from the action of phospholipase on the gallbladder mucosa. Secondary bacterial infection then occurs, principally by the Gram-negative aerobes *E. coli*, enterococci and *Klebsiella* spp. The pathogenicity of enterococci in biliary infections remains unclear. In up to 15% of cases the infection is complicated by anaerobes, but rarely as a sole isolate. The most commonly isolated anaerobic species are *Bacteroides* but clostridia are also found.

The condition is self-limiting and treated successfully in most cases with intravenous fluids, analgesics, and antibiotics if there is evidence of bacterial infection (as indicated by a rising leukocyte count, pyrexia and increasing abdominal tenderness). A small percentage of cases (15–25%) fail to settle, and open or laparoscopic cholecystectomy is reserved for those patients with either peritonitis, an inflammatory mass, or failure to improve despite maximal conservative therapy. Occasionally it is necessary to drain the gallbladder percutaneously to resolve the infection, and surgery can then be planned electively.

In some cases, cholecystitis develops in the absence of gallstone disease; this is known as acalculous cholecystitis and is usually associated with a vasculitis. It has also been described following primary infection by *Salmonella* spp., and may occur, usually in elderly men, as a consequence of critical illness. In 30–60% of patients it follows a systemic infection of either gastrointestinal or genitourinary origin, or after scarlet or typhoid fevers.[20] Acalculous cholecystitis may occasionally be precipitated by hypersensitivity to certain drugs, such as ceftriaxone, erythromycin, ampicillin, and thiazide diuretics, where the condition resolves on withdrawal of the agent.

EMPHYSEMATOUS CHOLECYSTITIS

Emphysematous cholecystitis is a rare condition affecting elderly diabetic men, comprising fulminant infection of the gallbladder with gas-forming clostridial and *Bacteroides* spp (see Ch. 30). The risk of perforation and associated mortality is approximately 15%.

ACUTE CHOLANGITIS

First described by Charcot, the classical features of ascending cholangitis are the triad of fever, hepatic pain, and jaundice (see Ch. 30). The condition is characterized by ascending infection within an obstructed biliary tree, and the most commonly isolated organisms are similar to those of cholecystitis, namely *E. coli*, enterococci and *Klebsiella* spp. Obstruction secondary to gallstone disease remains an important risk factor, but of increasing importance are malignant biliary obstruction treated by indwelling stents and receipt of an orthotopic liver transplant.[21]

REFERENCES

19. Mughal M, Bancewicz J, Irving M. Br J Surg 1986; 73: 253–259
20. Jennings W, Drabek G, Miller K. Surg Gynecol Obstet 1992; 174: 394–398
21. Lipsett P, Pitt H. Surg Clin North Am 1990; 70: 1297–1312

The mainstays of treatment are rapid use of appropriate empirical antibiotics and drainage of the biliary tree, usually achieved by endoscopic or percutaneous means.

PYOGENIC LIVER ABSCESS

Liver abscesses may form from direct, lymphatic, or rarely haematogenous spread (see Ch. 29). The most common causes are ascending cholangitis as a result of biliary tract pathology and secondary to portal pyaemia. Abscesses arising from cholangitis are often multiple and affect both lobes of the liver. Direct spread from empyema of the gallbladder may also lead to abscess formation. Causative organisms are coliforms, occasional anaerobes, but most commonly *Strep. milleri*. Amoebic liver abscess is rare but should be borne in mind in those with a history of travel to the tropics. Treatment is by percutaneous drainage under radiological control and broad-spectrum antibiotics. If *Strep. milleri* is isolated a prolonged course of treatment (3–6 months) with amoxicillin is usually recommended, because recrudescent infection is common.

Surprisingly, appropriate antibiotic therapy in hepatobiliary sepsis has been poorly examined in prospective clinical trials. Antibiotic choice should be based on the severity of illness and the suspected pathogens. In mild cholecystitis cephalosporins may be effective, but should be combined with metronidazole to cover anaerobes in severe infections. Single agents such as ciprofloxacin or piperacillin cover all the common pathogens effectively. Second-line single-agent therapy in severe infections can be with imipenem or meropenem, or combined tazobactam and piperacillin preparations.

PANCREATIC INFECTION

Severe pancreatitis carries a significant mortality, 10–15%, in part from multiple organ dysfunction syndrome but also to infectious complications, particularly infected necrosis and pancreatic abscess formation. Almost 10% of patients with acute pancreatitis develop some form of pancreatic infection, usually with colonic organisms that have been hypothesized to translocate across the intestinal wall.

Whatever the initiating event, it is the release of proteolytic enzymes and subsequent autolytic necrosis of pancreatic tissue that provide the ‘culture medium’ for subsequent infection. If the autodigestive process disrupts major pancreatic ducts then a lesser sac pancreatic pseudocyst can develop, and this may also become subsequently infected.

Pancreatic abscess carries a mortality of 100% when untreated, and up to 40% even when aggressively managed.[22] The essence of treatment is a high index of suspicion and early diagnosis. This can prove difficult, because features of infection such as fever, abdominal mass, and a neutrophil leukocytosis are also those of inflammation from acute pancreatitis. While sterile necrosis can be treated conservatively, infected necrosis carries a high risk of mortality, and aggressive surgical intervention is warranted. Contrast-enhanced CT scanning with aseptic diagnostic aspiration of areas of necrosis is therefore a useful diagnostic aid, and may need repeating to determine the need for surgery; CT-guided percutaneous drainage of an infected pseudocyst may also be effective.

Established pancreatic abscess or infected necrosis requires surgical debridement of all necrotic tissue and drainage of peripancreatic fluid (see also Ch. 31). Antibiotics may be useful for the associated sepsis. Microbiological examination of pancreatic aspirates may direct antibiotic choice, but carbepenems, which penetrate the pancreas and have an appropriate spectrum of activity for patients who are usually in intensive care units, are generally recommended.

GENITOURINARY INFECTIONS

SURGICAL URINARY TRACT INFECTION

The urinary tract is sterile in health. Infection frequently occurs when urine flow is disturbed, as it is in cases of urinary stasis, ureteric reflux or obstruction (see Chs 35 and 36). The portal of entry is usually the urethra. The vast majority of nosocomial urinary tract infections in surgical patients is associated with indwelling urinary catheters, which provide a direct access route to the external environment.[23] All urinary catheters eventually become colonized with pathogens derived from the patient’s perineum or nosocomial cross-infection from healthcare workers’ hands. These hospital organisms are frequently multiply antibiotic-resistant. Bacteriuria, defined as the presence of bacteria in the urine, occurs in more than 20% of catheterized patients, but only 2–6% develop symptoms of urinary tract infection. Of these, 1–4% develop positive blood cultures, with a 13–30% mortality.[16]

Causative organisms are most commonly *E. coli*, *Klebsiella*, *Pseudomonas*, *Proteus* and *Enterobacter* spp. The risk of developing bacteriuria correlates with the duration of catheterization, and may be reduced (or at least delayed) by using the smallest gauge catheter appropriate to the indication, good aseptic technique on insertion, maintenance of a closed drainage system, fixation of the catheter to prevent urethral reflux of urine, and good hygiene. The risk of infection is not influenced by catheter material, antiseptic cleansing of the meatus, addition of antiseptic solutions to the drainage bag, or regular bladder irrigation.

Patients with indwelling catheters are at increased risk of infection on catheter change or urinary tract instrumentation, and it is sensible to cover these interventions with an appropriate prophylactic antibiotic such as gentamycin.

ACUTE PYELONEPHRITIS

Acute bacterial infection of the kidney is far more likely to occur in the face of urinary obstruction or structurally abnormal urinary tracts (see Ch. 35). Pyelonephritis frequently presents with chills, fevers, dysuria and renal angle tenderness, but if severe may also present with sepsis and renal dysfunction. Urine culture commonly grows a single Gram-negative bacteria such as *E. coli*.

Treatment should be immediate, using blind antibiotic therapy with cefuroxime or co-amoxiclav until sensitivities are available. In the presence of obstruction to the collecting system, pyelonephritis may lead to suppuration and the presence of pus under high pressure, known as pyonephrosis. For this reason it is imperative that urinary tract obstruction is excluded by urgent ultrasound scanning and, if present, treated by emergency drainage with percutaneous nephrostomy or ureteric stenting. This has the advantage of relieving both the infection and the obstruction, allowing renal function to return to normal so that

REFERENCES

22. Bradley E. Ann Surg 1987; 206: 542–550
23. Asher E, Oliver B, Fry D. Am Surg 1988; 54: 466–469

the cause of the obstruction can be dealt with at a later stage. If an unusual organism is cultured, or if the patient suffers recurrent episodes of pyelonephritis, then it is prudent to look for an underlying cause such as aberrant renal tract anatomy.

PERINEPHRIC ABSCESS

Very rarely severe pyelonephritis may lead to intrarenal, cortical or even perinephric abscess formation (see Ch. 35). Predisposing conditions are urinary tract calculi with obstruction and diabetes mellitus. Historically, before the advent of antibiotics the commonest cause of renal abscess was haematogenous seeding of *Staph. aureus* from cutaneous infection; the condition was known as renal carbuncle. Nowadays, the commonest aetiology is ascending infection by Gram-negative bacteria such as *E. coli*. However, over a quarter of infections are polymicrobial, and infection with Gram-positive cocci, anaerobes and *Candida* have all been documented.[24]

Perinephric abscesses usually result from rupture of a renal parenchymal abscess through the renal fascia into the perinephric space. Presentations vary but may involve high swinging fevers, rigors and severe renal angle pain. Examination reveals marked loin tenderness or 'bogginess' in the presence of perinephric abscess, and with signs of systemic sepsis. Treatment includes a high index of suspicion for the condition and appropriate radiological imaging; CT scanning is considered to be the investigation of choice, with the advantage that prompt percutaneous drainage under radiological control can be carried out at the same time. Perinephric abscesses may require formal surgical drainage because they can be extensive. Broad-spectrum antibiotic therapy covering anaerobes as well as aerobes is also indicated. As with pyelonephritis, if the renal tract is obstructed it should be relieved immediately. Patients with very severe disease coupled with extensive destruction, obstruction or a non-functioning kidney may require nephrectomy.

BALANOPOSTHITIS

Infection of the glans penis (balanitis) and foreskin (posthitis) frequently occur together (see Ch. 35). The causative organisms are usually *Candida* spp., *Trichomonas vaginalis* and streptococci. Phimosis and diabetes mellitus are common predisposing conditions. Treatment with antifungal or broad-spectrum antibiotics along with simple hygiene is usually all that is required.

PROSTATITIS

True prostatitis as a result of bacterial infection residing in the prostate, proximal urethra and seminal vesicles may be either acute or chronic (see Ch. 37). Acute prostatitis is characterized by a systemic illness involving fever, rigors, myalgia and usually painful micturition, sometimes with pain on defecation. Rectal examination reveals an acutely tender, sometimes swollen, prostate gland. Chronic prostatitis is frequently more difficult to characterize, but the diagnosis can be made on finding pus cells in prostatic secretions after prostatic massage. It is thought to arise as a result of inadequately treated acute prostatitis. In both forms of the condition the commonest pathogen is *E. coli*, which rapidly responds to antibiotic treatment with trimethoprim or a quinolone such as ciprofloxacin. Whichever antibiotic is used, treatment should be continued for 4 weeks.

EPIDIDYMO-ORCHITIS

Acute infection of the epididymis that spreads to involve the testicle is commonest in men between 19 and 35 years of age, but also occurs in men over the age of 60 (see Ch. 39). *Chlamydia trachomatis* or, less commonly, *Neisseria gonorrhoeae* are found in sexually active young men, sometimes in association with a congenital anomaly. Infection with *E. coli* is more common in older men, and may occur in association with prostatitis, bladder outlet obstruction, and urethral stricture, or after any instrumentation of the urinary tract including catheterization. The condition may progress to abscess formation, especially when *E. coli* is involved.

Treatment should be with analgesia, bed rest, scrotal support, and doxycycline (in the case of chlamydial infection) or ampicillin (for gonococcal infection), and should be continued in both incidences for 2 weeks.

MUSCULOSKELETAL INFECTIONS

Historically, bone and joint infection was acquired by haematogenous spread, and was related to poor nutrition and hygiene. Today a more common aetiology, especially for chronic osteomyelitis, is traumatic contamination of a wound, including elective surgery. The pathogens responsible for musculoskeletal infection vary according to age and predisposing condition. In osteomyelitis, *Staph. aureus* remains the most common pathogen across all age groups, accounting for over 90% of cases. However, other organisms, such as *Haemophilus influenzae* in patients under the age of five and *Salmonella* spp., may less frequently be isolated, for example in patients with sickle cell disease. The majority of postoperative and traumatic bone and joint infections are due to *Staph. aureus*, but occasionally Gram-negative bacilli, including coliforms and *Pseudomonas*, are responsible.

Suitable antibiotics include flucloxacillin and fusidic acid for most situations. *H. influenzae* and coliform infections are better treated by cefuroxime with fusidic acid.

OSTEOMYELITIS

Osteomyelitis may occur as a result of haematogenous spread from a distant site of infection or from direct spread (see Ch. 41). In its acute form patients, usually children, develop severely painful bony lesions usually overlying metaphyses with sepsis. The suppurative process strips periosteum from the bone and may rupture into the soft tissues. Bone scans may be useful because they demonstrate bony changes long before plain radiographs.

Treatment involves analgesia, antibiotics and, in the presence of abscess formation or limited response to antimicrobials, surgical drainage.

CHRONIC OSTEOMYELITIS

Chronic osteomyelitis arises from bony necrosis following infective thrombosis of the bone or stripping of the periosteum from suppuration (see Ch. 41). This creates sequestrae, fragments of necrotic bone, which predispose to the sinus formation and discharge characteristic of chronic osteomyelitis. At the same time, new bone forms from the deep layers of the periosteum, creating an enveloping layer or *involucrum*. These features can be appreciated on a plain radiograph showing rarefaction of the metaphysis with widening of the bone where

REFERENCES

24. Borden T, Gibel L. In: Fry D (ed). Surgical Infections. Little, Brown, New York, 1995: 515–522

the involucrum has formed. Bacteria may lie dormant within chronic osteomyelitis and then flare up. Patients usually present with pain, fever and sometimes a discharging sinus.

Treatment depends on the clinical features but includes drainage if an acute abscess is present, and antibiotics and surgical excision of the sequestrae.

SEPTIC ARTHRITIS

Acute joint infection occurs following direct puncture, haematogenous spread from a distant site, or (rarely) rupture of a bone abscess into the synovial cavity (see Ch. 41). The clinical features are those of sepsis associated with an acutely painful, swollen joint, often the hip in children or the knee in adults.

Treatment involves diagnostic aspiration under anaesthesia, followed by exploration (if positive) and thorough lavage of the joint cavity. Untreated joint infection rapidly results in irreversible damage to the cartilage and permanent joint injury. Antibiotic choice is similar to that for osteomyelitis because over 80% of cases involve *Staph. aureus*, but modifications should be made as necessary on receipt of positive blood and pus culture results. Reactive arthritis in children and gouty arthritis in adults are important diagnostic pitfalls.

SPECIFIC INFECTIONS

TETANUS

Infection with the spore-forming, Gram-positive, anaerobic organism *Cl. tetani* is now a rare event in the developed world, due in part to successful immunization programmes. Infection results very rarely from surgical operations (particularly cholecystectomy) and accidental penetrating injury contaminated by spores found in the soil. The mean incubation period is 7–8 days.

The characteristic features of the disease result from release of the exotoxins tetanospasmin and tetanolysin. The former causes the characteristic tonic contraction of skeletal muscle followed by convulsions in the fully established disease, and is second only in potency to botulinum toxin. The latter, a haemolytic toxin, also binds to neuromuscular junctions. Together they lead to neuromuscular irritability at the site of inoculation, followed by lockjaw and facial grimace (risus sardonicus), and powerful spasms of the spinal extensors leading to excruciatingly painful arching of the back (opisthotonus). There may be spasm of the laryngeal and respiratory muscles that can lead to asphyxiation. Cardiac arrhythmias are common and may be fatal.

Management of the condition is by prophylaxis, including passive immunization with human tetanus immunoglobulin following injury more than 10 years after the last immunization. In the rare event of established disease, intravenous benzylpenicillin should be coupled with high-dose human anti-tetanus immunoglobulin and wound debridement. In severe cases, supportive measures such as sedation, tracheostomy, or even mechanical ventilation may be necessary.

ACTINOMYCOSIS

Actinomycosis results from endogenous infection with the microaerophilic, Gram-positive, branching bacillus *Actinomyces israelii*, although related microbes of the genus *Arachnia* are also described. Actinomycetes normally colonize the mouth and oropharynx, and have a very low virulence. They require two conditions to cause infection: first, injury that disrupts the epithelium; and second, an aerobic symbiont to maintain a low tissue redox potential and possibly provide factors necessary for growth and replication. Active infection tends to follow one of three patterns: pulmonary, cervicofacial or abdominal. Chronic inflammation with sinus formation discharging thin pus-containing, yellow, gritty specks ('sulphur granules') is characteristic. Microscopic examination after crushing these granules shows that they are made of the branching filaments of the organism.

Cervicofacial disease, the commonest form, occurs in conjunction with dental disease, following dental procedures or trauma. It presents with a chronic, indurated, non-tender, submandibular or parotid swelling that may go on to form discharging sinuses in the neck. Treatment includes dealing with the underlying dental condition as well as drainage of the infection.

Pulmonary disease may be suspected when there are similar discharging sinuses on the chest wall, and is usually preceded by aspiration, sometimes of a foreign body, or oesophageal trauma.

Abdominal infection is rare and may follow appendicectomy or abdominal trauma. It is associated with fibrosis or stricture formation, and it may be complicated by sinus formation or even be misdiagnosed as a colonic malignancy. Infection may spread to involve the liver via the portal circulation. Less commonly, pelvic infection occurs, particularly in women with an intrauterine contraceptive device.

Penicillins, such as amoxicillin, are effective against actinomycetes, and are usually given orally for cervicofacial disease and intravenously for abdominal or pulmonary disease. In patients allergic to penicillin, tetracyclines, fusidic acid and clindamycin are suitable alternatives.

ANTIBIOTIC PROPHYLAXIS

GENERAL PRINCIPLES

There is a wealth of evidence from published studies to support the routine use of prophylactic antibiotics in reducing postoperative infection.[25] Prophylactic antibiotics are now used in almost all branches of surgery for diverse reasons. The requirement is obvious in clean-contaminated wounds, such as in colonic surgery, where the risk of infection is inherent in the endogenous bowel flora. Sometimes it is to cover clean wounds, such as those in joint-replacement surgery, where although the infection risk is small, the consequences of infection are so grave as to warrant prophylaxis. There is no clear evidence that antibiotic prophylaxis in clean surgery, in a patient with a normal immune system, and in the absence of prosthetic implantation is of benefit.

The main principles of antibiotic prophylaxis are to achieve high target-tissue concentrations of appropriate drugs within 2 h of a skin incision, and for those levels to be maintained until wound closure. Most prophylactic antibiotics are given parenterally, achieving their optimal tissue concentrations in 20 min, in which case administration on induction of anaesthesia is adequate. When antibiotics with short plasma half-lives have been used in operations lasting more than 2 h, or where there has been blood loss in excess of 2 L, further doses may be given every 2 h, with timing of the last dose as close to wound closure as possible.

REFERENCES

25. Sandusky W. Surg Clin North Am 1980; 60: 83–92

Studies suggest that a single dose of antibiotic(s) is sufficient, but many surgeons continue treatment for a further 24 h. A distinction should be made in certain conditions between prophylaxis and treatment. For example, in acute non-perforated appendicitis a single dose of preoperative metronidazole, given either rectally or intravenously, is sufficient. In the case of perforated appendicitis the condition is now complicated by peritonitis, in which case parenteral treatment doses of cefuroxime and metronidazole may be necessary for 72 h or more.

Finally, it should be stressed that prophylactic antibiotics are adjuncts to reducing postoperative infection, and do not in any way make up for sloppy or careless surgery, poor application of sterile technique, rough tissue handling, or the wholesale devascularization of tissues.

ABDOMINAL SURGERY

All abdominal surgery carries the risk of wound infection with *Staph. aureus* and additionally, in the case of colonic surgery, the possibility of synergistic infections involving coliforms and facultative anaerobes (especially *B. fragilis*). Upper gastrointestinal surgery, particularly emergency surgery, may carry similar infection risks. Prophylactic regimens, providing cover of all these species, that are in common use include:

- one to three doses of intravenous cefuroxime with metronidazole started at induction; *or*
- one dose of intravenous co-amoxiclav, repeated if the operation lasts more than 2 h or if there is greater than 2 L of blood loss.

In the case of biliary tract surgery, even in the presence of infected bile, the use of antibiotics that are concentrated in the bile and cover appropriate organisms include:

- one to three doses of intravenous cefuroxime; *or*
- a single dose of intravenous co-amoxiclav.

ORTHOPAEDIC SURGERY

In the case of prosthetic joint-replacement surgery, antibiotic regimens mainly cover skin commensals, for example:

- A single dose of intravenous co-amoxiclav on induction, repeated if blood loss is greater than 2 L or if the procedure is longer than 2 h; *or*
- One to three doses of intravenous cefuroxime.

If the surgery involves a tourniquet, as in total knee replacement, then the antibiotic(s) should be given intravenously 5 min before cuff inflation. In compound fractures the requirement is for drugs with suitable staphylococcal activity, such as cephalosporins with or without flucloxacillin. For the open reduction of closed fractures, a single dose of ceftriaxone is appropriate.

VASCULAR SURGERY

In surgery involving prosthetic aortic or limb arterial bypass grafts, one to three doses of intravenous cefuroxime or co-amoxiclav will cover the significant pathogens, namely staphylococci and coliforms. For amputations and surgery on ischaemic or diabetic limbs, the main risk is clostridial gas gangrene. Intravenous penicillin and metronidazole at induction are recommended. Skin preparation with iodine-containing solutions may help destroy clostridial spores on the skin of the upper thigh.

CARDIOTHORACIC SURGERY

There is no proven requirement for prophylaxis in pulmonary surgery. Prophylactic antibiotics tend to be given in cardiac surgery not because of any proven benefit, but because of the significance of postoperative endocarditis or wound infection in this group of patients. Suitable agents should be those that cover coagulase-negative staphylococci and *Staph. aureus*, along with broad Gram-negative activity. Regimens include one or two doses of intravenous cefuroxime or single doses of co-amoxiclav, repeated if procedure length or intraoperative blood losses dictate.

UROLOGICAL SURGERY

The urinary tract is normally sterile, and it is only in prostatic surgery or in the face of an obstruction or malignancy that a broad-spectrum antibiotic, such as gentamycin or ciprofloxacin, is necessary. In transurethral ultrasound-guided prostatic biopsy, it is logical to cover the procedure with oral ciprofloxacin 1 h before and for two subsequent doses after the procedure.

Urinary tract infection should be treated on the basis of urine culture.

ASPLENIA

Patients undergoing splenectomy are at increased risk of infection from encapsulated bacteria, especially *Strep. pneumoniae*, *N. meningitidis* and *H. influenzae*. These patients should have pneumococcal and *H. influenzae* vaccinations before surgery in elective splenectomy or immediately following traumatic splenectomy. The pneumococcal vaccine should be repeated at intervals of 5–10 years. Meningococcal vaccines A and C are recommended only if the patient is travelling to endemic areas. Influenza vaccines should be given annually. Prophylactic phenoxymethylpenicillin should be given up to the age of 16 in children and for at least 2 years in adults. Patients should be given a supply of amoxicillin to be started in the event of any febrile illness or non-blanching rash. Most hospitals now supply asplenic patients with cards containing details of their condition and their vaccination status.

HOSPITAL-ACQUIRED INFECTION

Nosocomial infections are assuming epidemic proportions; a UK survey suggested that 9% of in-patients suffer hospital-acquired infections.[26] It has been suggested that almost 30% of these infections are preventable. Because many of the causative organisms are multiresistant bacteria, it is essential for hospitals to develop an infection control policy implemented by a dedicated team. Outbreaks of infection should be notified to the infection control team so that policies for the containment and treatment of that infection can be implemented.

PRINCIPLES OF INFECTION CONTROL

Hospital hygiene

There is a large body of evidence to implicate poor hospital hygiene and the subsequent transmission of causative pathogens in hospital-acquired infection.[16] General principles for maintenance of a clean ward environment should be adhered to. All healthcare workers should be included in education and training related to the reduction and prevention of hospital-acquired infection.

REFERENCES

26. Emmerson AM, Enstone JE, Griffin M et al. J Hosp Infect 1996; 32: 175–190

Patients with documented infection should ideally be nursed separately from other ward patients, and a treatment area separate from the main ward area should be available for dressings and dirty procedures. Procedures involving the insertion of intravenous and arterial catheters should be carried out in dedicated units or, even in the operating theatre.

Operating theatres should be clearly separate from the rest of the hospital, with standard ventilation systems and air filters. Theatre lists should be planned with 'dirty' cases last and adequate turnaround time for the theatre disinfection procedures following.

It is sensible to have limitations on the number and movement of staff during an operation, with exclusion of staff with active skin sepsis. During operations with established hepatitis B or human immunodeficiency virus-infected patients, procedures such as double gloving, use of disposable gowns and drapes, eye protection, and the avoidance of practices such as simultaneous suturing all decrease the risk of infection to the operating theatre staff.

Healthcare worker hygiene

Hand-washing

There is clear evidence to show that cross-infection, the transfer of nosocomial infection from one patient to another via the contaminated hands of the healthcare worker, can be reduced by simple measures such as effective hand-washing. Consensus opinion is that effective hand-washing between patients reduces the risk of hand-mediated transmission, which remains a major factor in the spread of multiresistant bacteria, most notably in high-risk areas such as intensive care units.[16] Interestingly, no one preparation is any better than soap and water for decontaminating hands and removing transient organisms, whereas alcohol-based hand rubs are better at destroying transient organisms, giving a greater initial reduction in flora but are incapable of removing dirt or soiling.

Patient hygiene

Patients should be screened on admission for pre-existing infection, especially MRSA, and treated immediately, including isolation if appropriate. Surgical intervention should be avoided or deferred if possible in these patients until they are proven on microbiological swabbing to be infection-free. Prolonged preoperative hospitalization should be avoided to reduce the risk of infection from hospital-acquired multiresistant organisms.

Anaesthesia and analgesia

5

David N. James

ANAESTHESIA: PERIOPERATIVE CARE

INTRODUCTION

This chapter cannot hope to cover the vast subject of anaesthesia and analgesia; instead we provide an outline of the more important elements that may be useful to the surgeon.

Compared with events in everyday life,[1] anaesthesia is safe; the risk of death directly attributable to anaesthesia is unknown, principally because anaesthesia and surgery are so intimately linked that the relative contributions that each make to this adverse outcome are difficult to unravel.

About 5 million operations are performed annually in the UK. The prevalence of death solely attributable to anaesthesia has been estimated as between 0.5 and 0.8 per 100 000 anaesthetics,[2] with human error featuring prominently as the cause in the majority of these cases. Studies from other countries have put a much higher figure on this outcome.[3] The intraoperative death of anaesthetized patients has an estimated prevalence of between one and 30 per 100 000 operations.[3]

Despite technological advances in clinical investigations, anaesthesia and surgery, the numbers of perioperative deaths remain remarkably constant;[4] about 20 000 deaths occurring within 30 days of operation are reported annually to the National Confidential Enquiry into Perioperative Deaths (NCEPOD). Of these, 2000 occur within 24 h of surgery and 100 intraoperatively. These figures probably are a slight underestimate of the true figure due to under-reporting; also, the lack of a denominator figure makes estimation of the national mortality rates for any group of patients difficult to calculate. A large proportion of these deaths are of elderly patients with significant comorbidities, especially cardiac, with low expectation of survival in the long run. The NCEPOD data indicate that there are disproportionately large numbers of general, colorectal, vascular, and orthopaedic (fractured neck of femur) surgical patients dying perioperatively.

The term *high risk* according to NCEPOD means a high chance of death occurring within 30 days of operation, and this organization has made many recommendations intended to improve clinical practice in the perioperative period;[5] in essence these may be summarized as:

- Preoperative recognition and management of coexisting medical problems in the surgical patient is essential.
- Adequate resuscitation with appropriate intravenous fluids is an essential part of the preoperative preparation.
- High-risk patients require access to postoperative critical care (intensive and high-dependency care), a limited resource.
- The need for the direct involvement in these patients' care by experienced surgeons and anaesthetists working alongside nurses and other professions allied to medicine as a team.

Box 5.1 Some factors contributing to the safety of modern anaesthesia

- Application of technological solutions to clinical problems
  Real-time physiological monitoring
  Engineered safety devices that physically prevent errors from being made (e.g. safety features of modern anaesthetic machines)
  Devices for managing the patient's airway (e.g. fibre-optic laryngoscopy and the laryngeal mask airway)
- Standards and guidelines promulgated by, for example, the Royal College of Anaesthetists and Association of Anaesthetists of Great Britain and Ireland
- Assessment of the human factor in adverse incidents and the systems approach to patient safety
- Use of patient simulation in training and development

Anaesthetists by nature tend to be risk-averse and focused on patient safety because anaesthesia carries risk and has no therapeutic benefit. It is widely believed that anaesthesia is much safer today, at least for healthy patients, than it was 25 or 50 years ago, although the extent of and reasons for the improvement are still open to debate.[6] Some of the features of modern-day anaesthesia that contribute to patient safety are outlined in Box 5.1.

It has been said that, in a 30-year career as a consultant, a surgeon spends 10 years learning when to operate and a further 20 years learning when not to operate. There is wisdom in this joke, for when a patient is critically ill and likely to die from a surgical condition, it is very difficult to decide not to operate. Nevertheless, it is an extremely important decision that needs to be made in consultation with patients, their family, and colleagues in both anaesthesia and surgery, and with other healthcare professionals, emphasizing the role of teamwork. When making the difficult decision not to operate, the extent to which a patient's comorbidities limit their functional ability and quality of life need to be considered in addition to the surgical

REFERENCES

1. Jones HJ, de Cossart L. Br J Surg 1999; 86: 149–157
2. Buck N, Devlin HB, Lunn JN. Report on the Confidential Enquiry into Perioperative Deaths. Nuffield Provincial Hospitals Trust, London, 1988
3. Pedersen T. Baillières Clin Anaesthesiol 1996; 10: 237–250
4. Gray AJG, Hoile RW, Ingram GS et al. The Report of the National Confidential Enquiry into Perioperative Deaths 1996–1997. NCEPOD, London, 1998
5. NCEPOD. Available: http://www.ncepod.org.uk
6. Gaba DM. Br Med J 2000; 320: 785–788

pathology. Patients' GPs can often give an invaluable insight into their normal medical condition and their wishes. To decide not to operate 'because the patient is going to die anyway' is avoiding the issue and may deprive the patient and family of their final hours or days together.

PREOPERATIVE RISK ASSESSMENT

RISK CLASSIFICATION

There is great interest in developing preoperative scoring systems to quantity the risk of an adverse postoperative outcome. The development of such systems is hampered by the complexity of inter-related factors, i.e. patient comorbidities; surgical procedure, technique and expertise; anaesthetic technique and expertise; and the resources of the healthcare environment. Many such systems have been shown to work well when applied to groups of patients, but are less satisfactory when applied to individuals because they lack sensitivity and specificity. Scoring systems should be used as adjuncts to the information obtained by clinicians at preoperative assessment of individual patients. Preoperative anaesthetic assessment should follow the traditional systematic format of history and examination followed by appropriate investigations. The first objective of preoperative assessment is to identify the risks to the patient of developing an adverse postoperative outcome (mortality or morbidity). The second objective is to identify any concurrent clinical problems (comorbidities) that may be brought under better control (optimized) prior to surgery. The third objective, given the completion of the first two objectives, is to formulate a perioperative management plan that attempts to minimize the remaining risk of an adverse outcome.

Review of the NCEPOD reports reveals that adverse outcomes occur more often in patients over 60 years of age, operated on as urgent or emergency cases, and classified using the American Society of Anesthesiologists (ASA) system[7] as III or higher (Tables 5.1 and 5.2). Over 80% had at least one comorbidity, commonly cardiorespiratory disease.

Preadmission clinics – involving assessment by an anaesthetist, surgeon or nurse – represent an attempt to reduce the rate of delay and cancellation of surgical procedures caused by inadequate preoperative assessment and preparation of patients.

Table 5.1 American Society of Anesthesiologists classification of physical status

Class	Definition
1	A normal healthy patient
2	A patient with a mild systemic disease
3	A patient with severe systemic disease that is not incapacitating
4	A patient with an incapacitating systemic disease that is a constant threat to life
5	A moribund patient who is not expected to survive for 24 h with or without operation
E	Emergency operation: the letter 'E' is appended to the appropriate classification

(After Marx et al 1973.[8])

Table 5.2 American Society of Anesthesiologists classification of mortality rates

ASA rating	Overall operative mortality rate (%)	Anaesthetic mortality rate (%)
I	0.06	0.01
II	0.04	0.01
III	4.3	0.29
IV	23.40	0.75
V	50.70	1.55
Total	1.80	0.08

(After Marx et al 1973.[8])

Use of strict protocols may be helpful if non-anaesthetic staff assess the patients.

CARDIAC RISK ASSESSMENT

We know that ischaemic heart disease is probably the biggest cause of serious adverse cardiac outcome after surgery. It is, therefore, important to be able to predict which patients are at risk of perioperative cardiac complications. Numerous researchers have attempted to develop tools for predicting the risk of an adverse cardiac outcome, using clinical and investigational data to develop multifactorial scoring systems. Postoperative cardiac morbidity has been defined as 'the occurrence of myocardial infarction, unstable angina, congestive cardiac failure, serious arrhythmias or cardiac death during the [perioperative] period'.[9]

Age

It is difficult to assess age as a risk factor independent of associated diseases, and several studies have shown it to be a risk factor for postoperative cardiac morbidity and mortality.[10] There are, however, an equal number of studies to refute these findings, many of which found age to be a risk factor only when other factors were present.[11]

Comorbidities

Many authors have reported a higher incidence of perioperative myocardial infarction in patients who have had prior myocardial infarction. The risk has been repeatedly shown to be greater if the operation is performed within 6 months of the myocardial infarction and greater still if performed within 3 months (Table 5.3).

Mortality associated with myocardial infarction is higher if it occurs during the perioperative period.[9,12] However, other data

REFERENCES

7. American Society of Anesthesiologists. Anesthesiology 1963; 24: 111
8. Marx GF, Mateo CV, Orkin LR. Anesthesiology 1973; 39: 54-58
9. Mangano DT. Anesthesiology 1990; 72: 153–184
10. Goldman L, Caldera DL, Southwick FS et al. Medicine (Baltimore) 1978; 57: 357–370
11. von Knorring J. Surgery 1981; 90: 55–60
12. Nettleman MD, Banitt L, Barry W et al. Am J Med 1997; 103: 357–362

Table 5.3 Rates of new perioperative myocardial infarctions

Time from infarction	Rate of new infarction
Within 3 months	37%
3–6 months	15%
More than 6 months	5%

from patients with previous myocardial infarction showed that – with invasive monitoring and aggressive therapy throughout the perioperative period – the reinfarction rates can be significantly reduced.[13] It is widely accepted that postoperative myocardial infarction is a major contributor to perioperative mortality, but only recently has anaesthesia been regarded as a culprit.[14] Myocardial infarction is a relatively uncommon occurrence when considered in relation to the incidence of perioperative ischaemia, but there is a clear relationship between the two.[15] The plethora of published works relating to outcome in patients with cardiovascular disease illustrates the multifactorial nature of the problem and the reader is referred to an excellent review by Coriat Preiz.[16] One of the problems with these multifactorial risk indices is that, while providing highly sensitive and specific information when applied to a large unselected population, they may not be as reliable when applied to a population already at high risk for postoperative complications, such as patients undergoing major vascular surgery.

Despite the association of angina with angiographically significant coronary artery disease, several studies have refuted stable angina as a risk factor or have found it to be a risk factor only when coexisting with congestive cardiac failure.

The presence and extent of preoperative congestive cardiac failure has consistently been shown to be associated with development of postoperative cardiac morbidity, both in isolation and when coexisting with angina.[10] Goldman's cardiac risk index weights the signs of congestive cardiac failure higher than any other cardiac risk factor.[17]

Peripheral vascular disease is widely accepted as being a high-risk factor for cardiac morbidity. Significant coronary artery disease has been shown to be present in up to 60% of patients screened prior to major vascular surgery and accounts for over 50% of the postoperative mortality in this group.[18]

Hypertension is a major risk factor for coronary artery disease, stroke and cardiac failure. Patients with hypertensive disease are more prone to perioperative haemodynamic instability, arrhythmias and myocardial ischaemia. A number of studies have shown hypertensive patients (with diastolic blood pressure greater than 110 mmHg) to be prone to postoperative hypertension and morbidity.[11] It is generally accepted that non-urgent surgery should not be undertaken in the presence of untreated hypertension above this level.

Despite the association of diabetes mellitus with atherosclerosis and (often silent) ischaemic heart disease, most studies have not found it to be a risk factor for cardiac morbidity or surgical complications when other variables are excluded.[10,11]

The presence of a rhythm other than sinus or the presence of more than five premature ventricular contractions in a minute on a preoperative ECG have been found to be independent risk factors for cardiac morbidity.

In patients with heart disease the results of the history and physical examination may be quite misleading, and it is helpful to use the Canadian Cardiovascular Society classification of the severity of angina (Table 5.4). Unstable angina is defined as new onset angina, angina increasing in intensity, or rest angina. It is important to recognize that myocardial ischaemia can present as acute dyspnoea rather than chest pain. Silent ischaemia (i.e. coronary artery disease in the absence of angina) may simply represent subclinical disease or that the patient's activity is restricted enough (usually by peripheral vascular disease) such that angina is not evoked. True silent ischaemia notoriously occurs in the presence of conditions that induce autonomic neuropathy (severe diabetes or uraemia) or where the cardiac nerves have been transected (transplanted heart).

Table 5.4 Canadian Cardiovascular Society grading of angina of effort

Grade	Definition
I	Ordinary physical activity does not cause angina (strenuous physical activity provokes angina)
II	Slight limitations of ordinary physical activity (climbing more than one flight of stairs or walking uphill provokes angina)
III	Marked limitation of ordinary physical activity (walking on the level or climbing one flight of stairs provokes angina)
IV	Inability to carry on any physical activity (angina may be present at rest)

Specialized investigations

There is a vast array of tests available for assessing patients at risk of perioperative cardiac morbidity. The specialized investigations in vogue for preoperative cardiac assessment are as follows:

Resting electrocardiogram

The resting ECG seldom provides an assessment of risk because in most patients the induction of myocardial ischaemia requires the presence of stress (i.e. increased myocardial oxygen demand in the face of fixed supply). Stress testing implies the creation of increased oxygen demand through exercise or inotropic stimulation with dobutamine, or decreased oxygen supply through the creation of a coronary steal syndrome with vasodilators such as dipyridamole or adenosine.

Exercise electrocardiogram

The exercise ECG has become a mainstay of assessment of cardiac risk. However, in approximately one-third of cases it may provide a false negative test, and it does not give information regarding the potential for revascularization. The sensitivity of the exercise

REFERENCES

13. Wells P, Kaplan JA. Am Heart J 1981; 102: 1029–1037
14. Lowenstein E. Anesthesiology 1985; 62, 103–106
15. Mangano DT, Browner WS, Hollenberg M et al. N Engl J Med 1990; 323: 1781–8
16. Coriat Preiz S. In: Desmonts JM (ed). Outcome after Anaesthesia and Surgery: Clinical Anaesthesiology, Vol 6. Ballière Tindall, London, 1992: 463–476
17. Goldman L, Caldera DL, Nussbaum SR et al. N Engl J Med 1977; 297: 845–850
18. Hertzer NR, Beven EG, Young JR et al. Ann Surg 1984; 199: 223–233

ECG as a predictor of diffuse or left main coronary artery disease is markedly enhanced if angina occurs at a low intensity of exercise, if there are diffuse ST changes, if angina persists after the cessation of exercise, if hypotension develops, or if angina occurs in the presence of ventricular dysfunction at rest.[19]

Certain conditions limit or prevent interpretation of the exercise ECG, including left bundle branch block, ventricular pacing, pre-excitation syndromes (e.g. Wolff–Parkinson–White), pre-existing ST depression more than 1 mm at rest, or exercise restriction through peripheral vascular disease. Others, such as recurrent angina after revascularization, mandate more detailed investigation. Both sets of conditions warrant non-invasive studies such as radionuclide imaging or dobutamine stress echocardiography.[19]

Radionuclide imaging

Radionuclide imaging usually involves creation of a coronary steal syndrome with a coronary vasodilator such as dipyridamole, which will reveal areas of impaired perfusion as a defect on a thallium scan. The scan is repeated in 4 h, after dipyridamole 'washout'. A fixed defect suggests an area of scarring; resolution implies reversible ischaemia that might benefit from revascularization.

Dobutamine stress echocardiogram

The dobutamine stress echocardiogram is the most popular non-invasive stress test because it is simple, reproducible, and requires no radioactive tracer. It enables assessment of a baseline ejection fraction and its response to inotropic stress (a decrease in ejection fraction implies diffuse coronary artery disease), or the presence of new or worsened wall motion abnormality in response to inotropy. Fifty-six of 184 patients undergoing vascular surgery had a positive dobutamine stress echo. Perioperative cardiac events (ischaemia, infarction, etc.) occurred in 18 patients, all of whom had had a positive stress test; no events occurred in patients who had a negative stress test. The odds ratio of an event with a new wall motion abnormality was 45:1.[20]

Multifactorial cardiac risk index

Using single risk factors, such as hypertension, has failed to correlate with an adverse cardiac outcome.[21] Numerous multifactorial risk indices have been suggested[22–24] since Goldman's seminal research.[17] Goldman and coworkers identified nine variables that correlated with an increased risk of an adverse cardiac outcome. Subsequent studies indicate that the cardiac risk index has high specificity and low sensitivity.[25] The incidence of myocardial infarction, fatal myocardial infarction, and overall mortality rate has been shown to be significantly higher in Goldman classes 3 and 4 after carotid endarterectomy.[26] Detsky subsequently modified the Goldman cardiac risk index,[27] incorporating the Canadian Cardiovascular Society angina score (Table 5.4), unstable angina, and a history of pulmonary oedema. The total point score of this modified risk index has been shown to correlate with the incidence of perioperative cardiac morbidity.

A multifactorial analysis of a large at-risk population revealed the following significant cardiac risk factors: ischaemic heart disease (i.e. angina, previous myocardial infarction, or congestive heart failure), diabetes mellitus, renal insufficiency with raised serum creatinine, and poor cardiopulmonary functional status.[28] Patients with recent non-Q wave (subendocardial) myocardial infarction with new onset of dyspnoea appear to be at particularly high risk.

Preoperative assessment and management of cardiac patients

Figure 5.1 provides a rational approach to the preoperative cardiac assessment of high-risk patient.[28] Care must be exercised in timing elective surgery after percutaneous transluminal coronary angioplasty, because patients are placed on antithrombotic therapy for about a month and on aspirin indefinitely; there is an increased bleeding risk if surgery is undertaken during this period.

There is mounting evidence that perioperative beta blockade provides myocardial protection. These drugs are recommended for high-risk cardiac patients.[29] This recommendation is partly based on the startling results of a study in which high-risk patients undergoing vascular surgery were randomized to the beta blocker bisoprolol or placebo. Treatment was started more than 7 days preoperatively with the goal of achieving a resting heart rate of less than 60 beats/min, and continued for 30 days postoperatively. In patients who received the beta blocker there was a 91% reduction in myocardial infarction or cardiac death.[30] There is also some evidence that the administration of α_2 agonists such as mivazerol may also provide perioperative cardiac protection.[31]

Site of surgery and type of anaesthesia

There have been a large number of studies indicating that intra-abdominal, thoracic or aortic vascular surgery are significant risk factors for perioperative myocardial infarction and other cardiorespiratory complications.[10,17] The majority of studies have found anaesthetic technique to have surprisingly little influence on postoperative outcome when either looking at general anaesthetic techniques or comparing general and regional anaesthesia provided that other preoperative risk factors are controlled.[10]

Postoperative multiple organ dysfunction

There seem to be two groups of high cardiac risk patients presenting for anaesthesia and surgery: those at risk of perioperative myocardial ischaemia and those whose hearts are at risk of failing to meet the physiological demands of surgery, resulting in suboptimal organ perfusion and ultimately in multiple organ

REFERENCES

19. Lee TH, Boucher CA. N Engl J Med 2001; 344: 1840–1845
20. Poldermans D, Fioretti PM, Forster T et al. Eur J Vasc Surg 1994; 8: 286–293
21. Forrest JB, Rehder K, Cahalan MK et al. Anesthesiology 1992; 76: 3–15
22. Tiret L, Hatton F. Stat Med 1998; 7: 947–954
23. Pedersen T, Eliasen K, Henriksen E. Acta Anaesthesiol Scand 1990; 34: 176–182
24. Cohen MM, Pope WDB, Tweed WA et al. Can J Anaesth 1992; 39: 430–439
25. Carliner NH, Fischer ML, Plotnick GD et al. Am J Cardiol 1985; 56: 51
26. Musser DJ, Nicholas GG, Reed JF. J Vasc Surg 1994; 19: 615–622
27. Detsky AS, Abrams HB, Forbath N et al. Arch Intern Med 1986; 146: 2131–2134
28. Fleisher LA, Eagle KA. N Engl J Med 2001; 345: 1677–1682
29. Eagle KA, Berger PB, Calkins H et al. Anesth Analg 2002; 94:1052–1064
30. Poldermans D, Boersma E, Bax JJ et al. N Engl J Med 1999; 341: 1789–1794
31. Oliver ME, Goldman L, Julian DG et al. Anesthesiology 1999; 91: 951–961

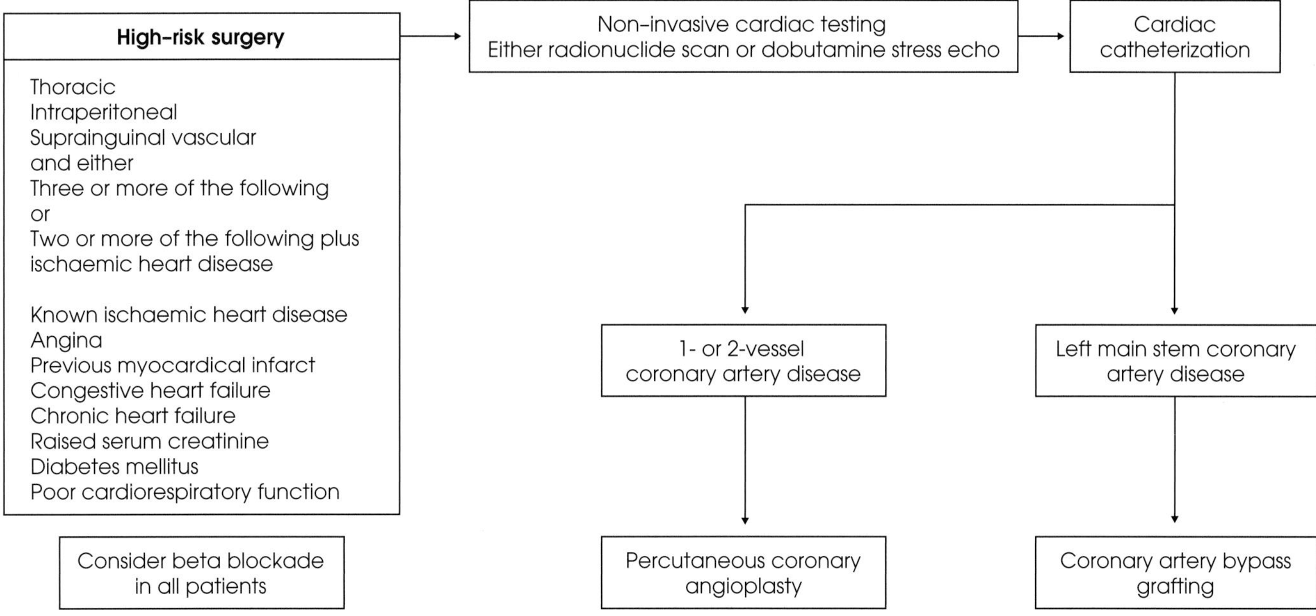

Figure 5.1 Strategy for the assessment and management of high-risk cardiac patients.

dysfunctions.[32] Cardiopulmonary exercise testing, or pharmacological stress testing in those patients unable to exercise, has demonstrated that patients with a lower anaerobic threshold and therefore less cardiopulmonary reserve have a higher perioperative mortality.[33] Shoemaker and colleagues noted that although only 7% of general surgical patients were preoperatively identified as being at high risk on clinical grounds, this group accounted for over 80% of mortality.[34] When comparing preoperative cardiovascular parameters with predicted values, Older and Smith revealed that many patients had cardiovascular function below what would be considered normal for their age.[35] Analysis of cardiovascular parameters of patients who survived surgery revealed that they mounted better compensatory increases in mean arterial pressure, cardiac index, left ventricular stroke work index, oxygen delivery and oxygen consumption than those who did not survive.[36] Not surprisingly, it was suggested that if this haemodynamic dysfunction could be corrected preoperatively then the magnitude of intraoperative compensatory haemodynamic changes could be reduced. By comparing cardiovascular status preoperatively with predicted values and correcting preoperative dysfunction it was possible to improve outcome. Del Guercio and Cohn demonstrated this by stratifying preoperative patients into one of four categories by means of invasive monitoring.[37] These groups strongly predicted postoperative mortality.

Extending this concept to its logical conclusion, Shoemaker proposed goal-directed therapy, by which haemodynamic and oxygen transport parameters were increased to supranormal values preoperatively, and demonstrated startling improvements in mortality rates in those patients able to attain these indicators.[34] In a randomized controlled prospective study of 107 high-risk patients, Boyd and coworkers produced a 75% reduction in mortality in patients treated with a deliberate perioperative increase of cardiac index and oxygen delivery.[38] Further analysis of the data suggested that this improvement was greater in patients who were sicker and/or those who required urgent surgery. Hayes and colleagues, however, demonstrated no benefit of aggressive optimization using high doses of dobutamine if patients failed to show improvement with simple fluid replacement;[39] indeed, attempts at aggressive optimization may even have been detrimental.

RESPIRATORY RISK ASSESSMENT

Patients with pulmonary compromise are at risk of perioperative complications that include hyper-reactive airways and postoperative ventilator dependence as a consequence of retained secretions, atelectasis, pneumonia, respiratory failure, pneumothorax or bronchopleural fistula. The site of the surgical incision plays an important role in determining the risk of these complications: likelihood increases from median sternotomy to upper abdominal, to thoracotomy and ultimately thoracoabdominal surgery, which imposes the greatest risk. After thoracotomy, functional residual capacity of the lung, is decreased by 30–40% for up to 3 weeks.

At one extreme of the spectrum of chronic obstructive pulmonary disease is chronic bronchitis, characterized by excessive sputum production, predisposition to atelectasis, intrapulmonary shunting, and hypoxaemia. In these patients, positive end expiratory pressure is helpful in maintaining functional residual capacity and improving oxygenation. At the other end of the spectrum is emphysema, characterized by expiratory airway

REFERENCES

32. Juste RN, Lawson AD, Soni N. Anaesthesia 1996; 51: 255–262
33. Older P, Smith R, Courtney P et al. Chest 1993; 104: 701–704
34. Shoemaker WC, Appel PL, Kram HB et al. Chest 1988; 94: 1176–1186
35. Older P, Smith R. Anaesth Intensive Care 1988; 16: 389–395
36. Boyd O. Clin Intensive Care 1997; 8: 9–13
37. Del Guercio LRM, Cohn JD. JAMA 1980; 243: 1350–1355
38. Boyd O, Grounds RM, Bennett ED. JAMA 1993; 270: 2699–2707
39. Hayes MA, Timmins AC, Yau EHS et al. N Engl J Med 1994; 330: 1717–1722

collapse and air trapping, increased dead space, and hypercarbia. Positive end expiratory pressure is not helpful and may exacerbate dead space effect. Many patients fall somewhere between the two extremes. The spectrum of airway obstruction includes:

- Extrinsic, allergic asthma with its onset in childhood, usually with well-defined allergies, which responds to prophylaxis with sodium cromoglycate, a mast cell stabilizer.
- Intrinsic asthma, which is of adult onset, with poorly defined allergies; cromoglycate is ineffective but airway obstruction responds to bronchodilators.
- Chronic obstructive pulmonary disease with superadded acute airway obstruction, which is resistant to cromoglycate and responds poorly to bronchodilators; steroids are usually required for perioperative protection or relief.

A clinical caveat is that audible wheezing may be absent with the most severe bronchospasm, as a result of slow expiratory flow. A simple method for a semiquantitative estimate of expiratory airflow is the forced expiratory time. The patient is asked to provide a maximal exhalation while the observer listens over the trachea. A forced expiratory time greater than 6 s implies a forced expiratory volume less than 1 L and the potential for carbon dioxide retention.

Pulmonary function tests have long been the principal investigational tool for lung dysfunction, but there is increasing interest in the prognostic value of exercise testing to assess predicted postoperative pulmonary function. A multifactorial pulmonary risk index is able to stratify patients as functionally inoperable or operable, and this more selective approach results in a substantial decrease in their postoperative complication rate.[40]

There are several preoperative interventions that may improve the patient's functional pulmonary reserve and decrease the risk of perioperative complications. Patients with severe lung disease may have pulmonary hypertension and right-sided heart failure. Transthoracic echocardiography may provide an assessment of this and allow optimization of cardiac status (e.g. using digoxin or diuretics).

Cessation of active smoking is the ideal but is seldom accomplished. To restore normal ciliary function, smoking must be stopped at least 6–8 weeks before anaesthesia. However, even stopping 24–48 h before surgery may allow a decrease in carboxyhaemoglobin, which impedes haemoglobin oxygen off-loading and which may reach levels of 10% in heavy smokers. If there are signs of infection (cough or altered sputum) a course of appropriate antibiotics should be administered for at least 1 week before elective surgery. Elective surgery should not be performed in patients who are actively wheezing without a trial of β_2-agonist, anticholinergic and/or steroid inhalers. Fixed airway obstruction or emphysema warrants the use of oral and intravenous steroid perioperative prophylaxis. If at all possible, patients should be taught how to use incentive spirometry before they come to surgery.

Perioperative respiratory risk has received relatively less investigation than cardiac risk. For non-cardiac surgery, pulmonary complications are significantly more frequent, associated with longer hospital stay, and occur in combination with cardiac complications in a substantial proportion of patients.[41] It has also been shown that abnormal results of clinical lung examination and chest radiography are important independent preoperative variables associated with pulmonary complications.[42] These studies indicated that simple clinical data have more predictive value than specialized pulmonary tests (Box 5.2).

Box 5.2 Respiratory risk assessment: poor prognostic clinical signs

General

- Rapid shallow breathing
- Alae nasi movement
- Cyanosis
- Cough and sputum before abdominal or thoracic surgery
- Pyrexia
- Anaemia

Pulmonary function measurements

- Partial pressure of oxygen in arterial blood (P_AO_2) < 9 kPa breathing air
- Partial pressure of carbon oxygen in arterial blood (P_ACO_2) > 6.5 kPa
  < 50% of predicted or 70 L/min will have 50% mortality
- Forced expiratory volume < 2 L: high risk
  < 1 L: exclude from general anaesthetic
- Forced vital capacity < 2 L: postoperative respiratory dysfunction
  < 1.5 L: ineffective cough
  < 1 L: likely to need postoperative respiratory support

Other independent risk factors for postoperative pulmonary complications include age of 60 years or over, body mass index of 27 or over, history of cancer, smoking within 8 weeks prior to surgery, upper abdominal incision, and impaired preoperative cognitive function.[43] The best preoperative predictors of postoperative complications in patients with severe chronic obstructive pulmonary disease undergoing non-cardiothoracic operations appear to be composite scoring systems such as the ASA physical status grading,[44] which consider non-pulmonary as well as pulmonary factors. Likewise, it has been shown that the best combination of predictors for developing pulmonary complications after intra-abdominal surgery was an age over 59 years and ASA classification higher than 1.[45]

Several studies have demonstrated that patients who smoke up till the time of surgery suffer significantly more postoperative pulmonary complications than non-smokers or ex-smokers, and new evidence suggests that reduction of smoking within 1 month prior to surgery is not associated with a decreased risk.[46] Recommendations for the optimum duration of cessation of smoking preoperatively vary, but most commonly accepted is a period of abstinence of longer than 2 months.

It must not be forgotten that there are other aspects of anaesthetic intervention that carry risk. Difficult tracheal intubation may increase anaesthetic morbidity and mortality in otherwise low-risk individuals. This has been well documented, with particular emphasis on obstetric and ear, nose and throat surgery. Most clinical methods and investigations used to predict difficulty of tracheal intubation suffer from low sensitivity and low

REFERENCES

40. Wyser C, Stutz P, Soler M et al. Am J Respir Crit Care Med 1999; 159: 1450–1456
41. Lawrence VA, Hilsenback SG, Mulrow CD et al. J Gen Intern Med 1995; 10: 671–678
42. Lawrence VA, Dhanda R, Hilsenback SG et al. Chest 1996; 110: 744–750
43. Brooks-Brunn JA. Chest 1997; 111: 564–571
44. Wong DH, Weber EC, Schell MJ et al. Anesth Analg 1995; 80: 276–284
45. Hall JC, Tarala RA, Hall JL et al. Chest 1991; 99: 923–927
46. Bluman LG, Mosca L, Newman N et al. Chest 1998; 113: 883–889

positive predictive values.[47] A multivariate analysis of predictors of difficult tracheal intubation has managed to produce not only good positive predictive value but, arguably of more clinical importance, a reduction in false negative prediction compared with many previous studies.[48]

RENAL RISK ASSESSMENT

When acute renal failure occurs after surgical procedures, the mortality rate is reported to be as high as 58%.[49] Acute renal failure in surgical patients is caused by an ischaemic renal insult that is the sum of multiple causes. Acute tubular necrosis is the most common mechanism of renal failure in these circumstances. A common scenario for the development of postoperative acute renal failure is one of a high-risk patient having a high-risk surgical procedure with simultaneous exposure to one or more nephrotoxic substances.

HEPATIC RISK ASSESSMENT

Experience shows that even minor surgery on cirrhotic patients results in high postoperative mortality. Liver dysfunction has multisystem sequelae, and improved perioperative care has not significantly reduced operative mortality. Any surgery on these patients should be undertaken at specialist centres. The Child–Pugh classification of liver disease (Table 5.5)[50,51] was originally described to assess operative risk in cirrhotic patients undergoing surgery for variceal bleeding. Its use has been extended to predict outcome in cirrhotic patients for all types of surgery. The mortalities of patients with cirrhosis and other risk factors have been estimated (Table 5.6). The causes of death in these patients are usually systemic sepsis, renal failure, bleeding, hepatic failure and encephalopathy. Poor nutrition, portal hypertension with ascites, and encephalopathy herald poor prognosis for any surgery in these patients.

NEUROLOGICAL RISK ASSESSMENT

Cerebrovascular accidents, delirium and cognitive dysfunction are the commonest neurological sequelae to surgery under general anaesthesia.

Cerebrovascular accidents

Risk factors associated with an increased incidence of postoperative cerebrovascular accidents include age,[52] cerebrovascular disease, hypertension, atrial fibrillation, type of surgery, snoring and carotid bruits. Conflicting evidence exists for the role of hypotension causing stroke in the postoperative period.

Table 5.5 Pugh's modification of the Child classification of severity of liver disease

Variable	1	2	3
Encephalopathy	None	Grade 1 or 2	Grade 3 or 4
Ascites	None	Slight	Moderate
Bilirubin (mmol/L)	< 35	35–60	> 60
Prothrombin (s prolonged)	1–4	4–10	> 10
Albumin (g/L)	> 35	28–35	< 28

The points for the five variables are added to give a score ranging from 5 to 15; patients with scores 5 or 6, 7–9, and 10–15 are classified as grade A (low risk: 5% mortality), grade B (moderate risk: 10% mortality), and grade C (high risk: mortality > 50%), respectively.

Table 5.6 Preoperative variables and mortality in cirrhotic patients

Variable	Mortality, if present (%)
Pulmonary failure	100
Cardiac failure	92
Gastrointestinal bleeding[86]	86
More than two antibiotics[82]	82
Second operation required[81]	81
Renal failure	73
More than 2 units of blood required	69
Hepatic decompensation	66
Positive blood or urine culture	61
Albumin < 30 g/L	58
Ascites	58
Less than 2 units of blood required	22

Box 5.3 Risk factors for postoperative delirium

Age
- Patients older than 75 years have a threefold increase in risk.

Comorbidities
- Neurological (structural): dementia, cerebrovascular disease and Parkinson disease
- Neurological (traumatic): cerebral hypoxia from any cause, head injury
- Psychological: affective dysfunction (anxiety–depression)
- Metabolic: severe hypo- and hypernatraemia
- Nutritional: thiamin deficiency (notably in alcoholic patients), hypo- and hyperglycaemia, hypoalbuminaemia, hypercalcaemia, hypophosphataemia, and acid–base disturbance

Comedications
- Withdrawal of, for example, alcohol, benzodiazepines or barbiturates
- Administration of, for example, centrally acting anticholinergics or opioid drugs

Delirium

Risk factors associated with an increased incidence of postoperative delirium[53] include age, multiple comorbidities and comedications (Box 5.3).

MULTIFACTORIAL SCORING SYSTEMS

To be able to draw meaningful conclusions from a scoring system designed to classify risk, the system must be highly specific and sensitive, and must exhibit good predictive value. Sensitivity is the

REFERENCES

47. Tse JC, Rimm EB, Hussain A. Anesth Analg 1995; 81: 254–258
48. Arne J, Descoins P, Fusciardi J et al. Br J Anaesth 1998; 80: 140–146
49. Brivet FG, Kleinknecht DJ, Loirat P et al. Crit Care Med 1996; 24: 192–198
50. Friedman LS. Hepatology 1999; 29: 1617–1623
51. Ziser A, Plevak DJ, Wiesner RH et al. Anesthesiology 1999; 90: 42–53
52. Kam PCA, Calcroft RM. Anaesthesia 1997; 52: 879–883
53. O'Keefe ST, Chonchubhair AN. Br J Anaesth 1994; 73: 673–687

ability of a classification system, applied preoperatively, to identify correctly patients who subsequently will have adverse events, specificity is the ability of the system to identify preoperatively patients who will not develop adverse events. For a positive response, predictive value is the probability that a patient identified by the scoring system as one who will have an adverse reaction really has it. None of the following scoring systems, used in isolation, fulfils all these criteria.

American Society of Anesthesiologists system

The ASA classification of physical status was introduced in 1941 as a means of standardizing preoperative evaluation of physical status to make patient comparison easier. It was not intended as a method of defining operative risk because it was recognized that this was also dependent on the nature of the surgery. The five-class system was introduced in the 1960s.[7] Although there may be discrepancy in classification of the same patient by different anaesthetists, the ASA rating, along with age and sex, remains one of the few truly prospective and widely applied preoperative descriptions. The ASA physical status rating has been shown to correlate well with overall surgical mortality (Tables 5.1 and 5.2).[54]

APACHE II

Although widely used in intensive care, the acute physiology, age and chronic health evaluation (APACHE) II system requires a 24-h sampling period for its 12 physiological variables, making it an unwieldy tool for preoperative risk assessment. Despite this, it has been found to have predictive value for risk of postoperative morbidity and mortality in a small study of patients undergoing elective major hepatic surgery.[55]

POSSUM

The physiological and operative severity score for the enumeration of mortality and morbidity (POSSUM) system uses both physiological and operative parameters. It is a tool for comparing the outcome (morbidity and mortality) of operative surgical patients. Patients are scored before operating (using measures of physiological derangement) and at operation (using an operative severity score) to give predictions of morbidity and hospital mortality. Like the APACHE II system, however, this system was designed for audit. It is unsuitable for preoperative risk evaluation because final outcome is required to generate the total score.[56]

HYBRID SCORING SYSTEMS

Prediction of overall risk of an adverse outcome should take account of not just age, comorbidities and physiological measurements, but all sources of risk, including the type and extent of surgery, the choice of anaesthetic technique, and the experience of both surgeon and anaesthetist. Classifying patients according to ASA class, age, procedure magnitude, and a global perception of risk expressed on a visual analogue scale (risk-VAS), Arvidsson and coworkers showed that although all four classifications were seen to correlate, the risk-VAS was the most efficient predictor of severe postoperative adverse events.[57] By combining ASA grade and Goldman's cardiac risk index in patients scheduled for elective non-cardiac surgery, it was possible to increase the accuracy of prediction of perioperative mortality.[58]

PAEDIATRIC ANAESTHESIA RISK

In 1954, Beecher and Todd found the anaesthesia death rate in the first year of life to be 'disproportionately high'. While children under the age of 10 years made up only 9% of a sample surgical population, they accounted for 20% of anaesthesia deaths. This mortality rate was five times that of young adults and higher than that of any other age group. In 1960, Schapira and colleagues found that babies under 1 year old made up 0.6% of their surgical population but 4.7% of the deaths. Also in 1960, the Baltimore Anesthesia Committee reported the anaesthesia mortality rate in the under-15 age group to be three per 10 000 operations, nearly three times that in the 15–24-year age group.[59]

The disturbing findings prompted a further study by this group to look more closely at the factors that affected paediatric anaesthesia mortality. Seventeen per cent of paediatric operative deaths were judged to have been wholly or partly due to anaesthesia, and over 20% of anaesthetic-contributory deaths occurred in infants in the first week of life. Most of these deaths were associated with major cardiac surgery. Over 82% of the deaths ascribed to anaesthesia were caused by postoperative respiratory complications; of those, drug-induced respiratory depression and aspiration of vomitus or blood were the two most common problems. A decade later, a review of cardiac arrest related to paediatric anaesthesia identified 73 cases in which anaesthesia was considered to have played an important role or to have been directly responsible for the arrest.[60] One-third of patients who suffered cardiac arrest died, and these deaths were attributed equally to cardiovascular and respiratory causes. Blood loss was the commonest cause of circulatory arrest, and preoperative anaemia was considered to be a contributory factor in seven patients.

In a further study of cardiac arrest associated with anaesthesia, children under the age of 12 years had an incidence three times that of the adult population.[61] A study showing a high rate of anaesthetic complications in children under 1 year old[62] led the authors to re-examine the data of patients less than 15 years of age. From a total of 40 240 anaesthetics there was only one death, but the incidence of major complications was 0.7 per 1000 anaesthetics. There were 12 cardiac arrests and half of these occurred in the group under 1 year of age. Although this group accounted for only 5% of the anaesthetized population, they suffered half of all complications. Complications were more frequent if the duration of preoperative fasting was less than 8 h.

The NCEPOD report published in 1990 collected data from all UK hospitals (except those in Scotland) identifying all deaths occurring within 30 days of surgery in children under the age of 10 years. Eighty per cent of deaths in the cardiac surgical group and 72% in the non-cardiac surgical group were in children classified as ASA class IV or V; only three deaths occurred in the

REFERENCES

54. Vacanti CJ, Van Houten RJ, Hill RC. Anesth Analg 1970; 49: 564
55. Gagner M, Franco D, Vons C et al. Surgery 1991; 110: 487–492
56. Copeland GP, Jones D, Walters M. Br J Surg 1991; 78: 355–360
57. Arvidsson S, Ouchterlony J, Sjostedt L et al. Acta Anaesthesiol Scand 1996; 40: 783–791
58. Prause G, Ratzenhofer-Comenda B, Pierer G et al. Anaesthesia 1997; 52: 203–206
59. Graff TD, Phillips OC, Benson DW et al. Anesth Analg 1964; 43: 40–47
60. Salem MR, Bennett EJ, Schweiss JF et al. JAMA 1975; 233: 238–241
61. Keehan RL, Boyan P. JAMA 1985; 253: 2373–2377
62. Tiret L, Hatton F. Can Anaesthesiol Soc 1986; 33: 336–344

non-cardiac group during elective surgery. Among the recommendations made was one that surgeons and anaesthetists should not undertake occasional paediatric practice, and that no trainee should be allowed to undertake surgery or anaesthesia on a child of any age without consultation with a consultant.

OPERATIVE RISK IN THE ELDERLY

Advances in modern medicine have seen the proportion of the elderly population grow, although the definition of the term *elderly* is arbitrary; 65 years and over is popular in the current medical literature. Our attitudes to anaesthesia and surgery in the elderly patient have changed enormously over the past century, as has our understanding of the physiology of ageing. Epidemiological studies show that we cannot evaluate a patient solely on the grounds of age, but must consider associated medical conditions prior to surgery and remember that 'elderly patients are a lot sicker than they appear'.[63]

The mortality rate in elderly patients is considered to be two to five times higher than that of young people following major operations,[64] particularly when advanced age is associated with coexisting medical disease. The original NCEPOD report, published in 1987, noted that 79% of perioperative deaths occurred in the over-65s, although this age group comprised only 22% of the surgical population; this fact was confirmed in later reports. Although perioperative complications may be related more closely to the number of pre-existing diseases and the type of surgery than to the age of the patient,[22,23,37] it has been suggested that old age per se should be included in the ASA classification, but this has not been accepted universally.[54] Interestingly, in a study of 148 patients over the age of 65 years declared fit for major surgery by standard criteria, only 13.5% on invasive monitoring had normal haemodynamic, respiratory and oxygen transport values.[63]

PREOPERATIVE PREPARATION

PREOPERATIVE OPTIMIZATION[65-67]

Evidence suggests that attention to cardiovascular and respiratory function in the preoperative period may improve postoperative outcome of high-risk patients undergoing major surgery. It has been suggested that haemodynamic monitoring should start in the preoperative period using central venous or pulmonary artery catheters to assess the fluid requirement and cardiac output. Most hospitals in the UK do not have the resources to admit all such patients preoperatively to an intensive care unit, but close monitoring of fluid status and replacing fluids more aggressively, especially in emergency patients, may be all that is needed to improve outcome.

PROPHYLAXIS OF VENOUS THROMBOEMBOLISM[68-71]

Venous thromboembolism is a significant perioperative problem, with pulmonary embolism accounting for about 10% of all hospital deaths and deep vein thromboses causing significant morbidity in the form of chronic leg swelling, skin changes, and ulceration. Calf vein deep vein thromboses are detectable in up to 10% of 'low-risk' patients but seldom extend into proximal veins. The aetiology of venous thromboembolism is outlined in Box 5.4. The risk of developing venous thromboembolism can be stratified as low, medium or high, depending on the type of operation, patient factors, and associated comorbidities.

Box 5.4 Aetiological factors in the development of perioperative venous thromboemboli

- Hypercoagulability caused by surgery or other factors (cancer or hormone therapy)
- Stasis of blood in the venous plexuses of the leg:
  Preoperatively (anaesthetized)
  Postoperatively (bed-bound)
- Damage to veins at the time of surgery
- Interference with venous return: pregnancy, pelvic surgery or pneumoperitoneum
- Dehydration
- Low cardiac output

Prophylaxis against the development of venous thromboembolism should involve a combination of general, pharmacological and mechanical measures. Subcutaneous heparin reduces the incidence of deep vein thromboses and fatal pulmonary embolism by about two-thirds. Traditionally, unfractionated heparin has been used, but there are advantages to the newer low-molecular-weight heparins. Giving low-molecular-weight heparin on the evening before surgery can minimize the small risk of bleeding when using epidural analgesia, because 12 h or more have elapsed before the epidural is inserted. Subcutaneous heparin is usually stopped when patients are fully mobile or when they leave hospital. However, the incidence of late deep vein thromboses in orthopaedic practice can be reduced by extended prophylaxis (up to 35 days). Warfarin is used most often in orthopaedic practice, where there is good evidence of its efficacy in relation to hip operations. Dextran 70 or 40 is as effective as subcutaneous heparin in preventing deep vein thromboses and pulmonary embolism, but is not often used because it requires intravenous infusion, may be associated with fluid overload, and anaphylaxis can occasionally occur. Aspirin provides some protection against venous thromboembolism but is less effective than other methods.

Antiembolic stockings reduce the risk of deep vein thromboses but are not proven to reduce the incidence of pulmonary embolism; they may give enhanced protection when used in combination with subcutaneous heparin. Below-the-knee stockings are probably as effective as above-the-knee stockings. Intermittent pneumatic calf compression devices compress the leg to 35–40 mmHg for about 10 s every minute, promoting venous flow. They are as effective as heparin in reducing the incidence of deep vein thromboses. The role of locoregional anaesthesia in the prevention of thromboembolism is complex; spinal and epidural anaesthesia appears to be protective in certain kinds of surgery, especially hip or knee replacement.

REFERENCES

63. Cole WH. Ann Surg 1968; 168: 310
64. Djokovic JL, Hedley-White J. JAMA 1979; 242: 2301–2306
65. Boyd O, Grounds RM, Bennett ED. JAMA 1993; 270: 2699–2707
66. Sinclair S, James S, Singer M. Br Med J 1997; 315: 909–912
67. Wilson J, Woods I, Fawcett J et al. Br Med J 1999; 318: 1099–1103
68. Clagett GP, Anderson FA, Heit I et al. Chest 1995; 108: 31S–34S
69. (Anonymous). Drugs Ther Bull 1999; 37: 78–80
70. (Anonymous). Drugs Ther Bull 1998; 36: 25–32
71. Thromboembotic Risk Factors (THRIFT) Consensus Group. Br Med J 1992; 305: 567–574

The oral contraceptive pill is considered a significant risk factor (possibly up to three to four times the risk) for the development of venous thromboembolism, particularly third-generation pills containing desogestrel or gestodene. Progestogen-only oral contraceptive pills (and injectable progestogen contraceptives) have not been associated with an increased risk of deep vein thromboses or pulmonary embolism. Advice on perioperative management is conflicting. Manufacturers and the British National Formulary recommend stopping the combined oral contraceptive pill for 4 weeks before major operations, and restarting after the next menstrual period and at least 2 weeks following full mobilization. By contrast, others advise that the oral contraceptive pill should not routinely be stopped because of insufficient evidence of risk and the danger of unwanted pregnancy.

The incidence of spontaneous venous thromboembolism is increased from three to 10 women per 10 000 per annum by hormone replacement therapy, but there are no good data on perioperative risk of venous thromboembolism. Stopping hormone replacement therapy may cause recurrence of troublesome menopausal symptoms and so therapy should not be stopped perioperatively as a routine. Women having major operations while on hormone replacement therapy should receive subcutaneous low-molecular-weight heparin combined with antiembolism stockings.

PREMEDICATION

It is well recognized that a clear explanation of anticipated events and a rapport with the anaesthetic team provides more effective anxiolysis than drugs. Premedication is much less commonly prescribed than a few years ago but is still indicated in anxious patients and those in whom there is an increased risk of gastro-oesophageal reflux. Some patients may benefit from sedation the night before surgery.

FASTING

Pulmonary aspiration of gastric contents is associated with significant morbidity and mortality. Factors predisposing to regurgitation and pulmonary aspiration include inadequate anaesthesia, pregnancy, obesity, difficult airway, emergency surgery, full stomach, and altered gastrointestinal motility. Aspiration of 30–40 mL of gastric contents can cause serious pulmonary damage; fasting before anaesthesia aims to reduce the volume of gastric contents.[72]

The preoperative fasting period depends on the type of food and fluids consumed; clear fluids are emptied from the stomach in an exponential manner with a half-life of 10–20 min, resulting in complete clearance within 2 h of ingestion. Examples of clear fluids are generally liquids that newsprint can be read through and include water, fruit juices without pulp, carbonated beverages, clear tea and black coffee, but not alcoholic drinks. Gastric emptying of solids is much slower than for fluids and varies depending on the type of food ingested. Foods with a high fat or meat content require at least 8 h to be emptied from the stomach, whereas a light meal such as toast is usually cleared in 4 h. Milk is considered a solid, because when mixed with gastric juice it thickens and congeals. However, a small amount of milk (10 mL) added to tea or coffee does not cause any increase in gastric volume or acidity. Cow's milk takes up to 5 h to empty from the stomach. Human breast milk has a lower fat and protein content and is emptied at a faster rate. Guidelines are outlined in Table 5.7.[73]

Table 5.7 American Society of Anesthesiologists fasting guidelines

Ingested material	Minimum fast (h)
Clear liquids	2
Breast milk	4
Infant formula milk	4–6
Non-human milk	6
Light meal	6

The above recommendations on preoperative fasting apply to elective, healthy patients.

The time interval between the last oral intake and any injury is considered as the fasting period, and thereafter the patient is at risk if this interval is short. The time taken to return to normal gastric emptying after trauma has not been established, and varies depending on the degree of trauma and the level of pain. The best indicators are probably signs of normal gastric motility, such as normal bowel sounds and patient hunger. There are a number of ways to control gastric acidity and volume that are used clinically, including antacids, H_2-receptor blockers, proton pump inhibitors and metoclopramide. The ASA do not recommend routine use of these agents in healthy, elective patients.

ROUTINE PREOPERATIVE INVESTIGATIONS

A system of routine preoperative investigations for in-patients prior to elective surgery is suggested in Table 5.8.

CONDUCT OF ANAESTHESIA

Only current general principles and concepts are presented. The selection of anaesthetic technique should take into account the nature of the intended surgery, the physical status of the patient, the experience of the anaesthetist, and the resources available. In general, patients for locoregional technique should be treated as if they were to receive general anaesthesia.

CLINICAL CONCEPT OF ANAESTHESIA

Figure 5.2 shows a clinical concept of anaesthesia.[74] Trauma causes stimulation of nociceptive pathways that project via the spinal cord to the brain, causing:

- Psychological arousal.
- The experience of pain, a signal to do something to stop the traumatizing process; the pain is remembered to help the organism to avoid the same kind of trauma in the future.
- Activation of reflexes: *sympathetic*, causing, among other things, increased heart rate and contractility to maintain blood pressure and blood flow to vital organs in case of blood loss, and *skeletal muscular*, causing increasing muscle tone around the traumatized area (intended to protect the tissues

REFERENCES

72. Maltby R. Can J Anaesth 1993; 40: R113–Rl17
73. American Society of Anesthesiologists Task Force on Preoperative Fasting. Anesthesiology 1999; 90: 896–905
74. Raeder JC. Acta Anaesthesiol Scand 1996; 40: 1068–1072

Table 5.8 Routine preoperative investigations

Investigation	Patient group
Urinalysis for sugar, blood and protein	All patients
ECG	Patients over 50 years old Patients with a history of heart disease, hypertension or chronic lung disease (A normal previous trace within 1 year is acceptable unless there is a recent cardiac history)
Full blood count	All females Men over 40 years old All patients undergoing major surgery Patients in whom anaemia is suspected
Creatinine and electrolytes	Patients over 60 years old All patients undergoing major surgery Patients receiving diuretic drugs Patients in whom renal disease is suspected
Blood glucose	Diabetic patients Patients with glycosuria
Coagulation screen	Patients with a history of bleeding tendency (some units measured before major surgery)
Sickle cell test	Black patients with unknown sickle status; if positive then haemoglobin electrophoresis should be performed
Pregnancy test	All women for whom there is any chance of pregnancy
Chest radiograph	Not routine Patients with acute cardiac or chest disease Patients with chronic cardiac or chest disease that has worsened in the past year Patients with a risk of pulmonary tuberculosis (recent arrival from a developing country or immunocompromise) Patients with malignant disease

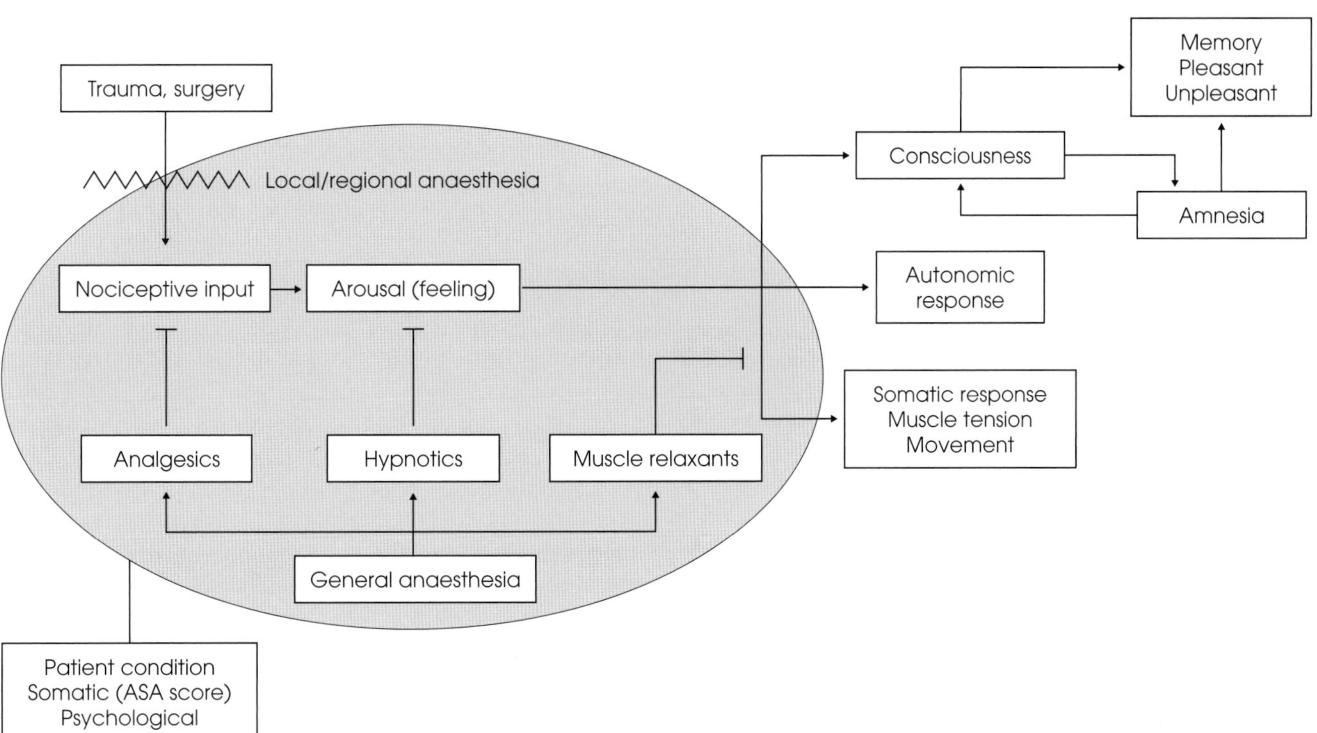

Figure 5.2 A concept of anaesthesia. (After Raeder JC. Basis of anaesthesia – what do we know after 150 years? Acta Anaesthesiol Scand 1996; 40: 1068–1072, with permission from Blackwell Publishing Ltd.[74])

from further penetration of traumatizing agents) and forceful movement (intended to withdraw the tissue from the source of trauma).

These primitive responses are to maximize the chances of survival; they protect the body against further harm and maximize the chances of short-term survival in the wild. Unfortunately, the body is unable to distinguish surgical trauma from any other cause of trauma, all causes bringing about the same series of physiological and psychological responses. On this basis major surgery represents massive trauma from which, if occurring in the wild, the individual is unlikely to survive.

This stress response to surgery may itself be harmful if not managed appropriately. With locoregional anaesthesia, the nociceptive impulses are blocked before reaching the central nervous system. With general anaesthesia, the responses within the central nervous system are controlled by drug action at different locations. Analgesics act in the spinal cord and deep cerebral structures (and possibly peripherally) to suppress the nociceptive input before consciousness, and autonomic and somatic responses are activated. Hypnotics act on the same responses, although predominantly on consciousness and amnesia. Neuromuscular blockers act by blocking transmission in the neuromuscular junction to control the somatic response of the striated muscles.

The inhalation anaesthetic agents provide all three actions – analgesia, hypnosis or amnesia, and muscle relaxation – in a dose-dependent manner. Ketamine has an analgesic action at a lower dose than its hypnotic action. This is quite different from the other intravenous anaesthetics, which do not have analgesic actions in ordinary induction doses. However, it has been shown that large doses of, for instance, propofol may provide complete anaesthesia in terms of control of all three major responses to trauma. It is not possible to achieve anaesthesia reliably by using intravenous analgesics alone (e.g. opioids) in high doses, because consciousness is not always diminished and the muscle tension may even be increased.

GENERAL ANAESTHESIA

The precise mechanisms of general anaesthesia are unclear, but a number of theories exist, none of which completely explain the phenomenon. The term *anaesthesia* literally means 'without feeling', and the model of balanced anaesthesia, while old, is a useful concept. This involves using combinations of drugs that work by different mechanisms, each drug reducing the requirement for the others, thereby reducing the effect of any single agent; a physical state comprising hypnosis (with amnesia), analgesia and skeletal muscle relaxation can be achieved (the triad of anaesthesia). This physical state allows a patient to undergo surgery without awareness of pain and provides the surgeon with the best operating conditions.

It may surprise some to learn that the process of anaesthesia entails much more than just 'keeping patients asleep for operations'. Since the processes of surgery and anaesthesia themselves represent profound physiological stressors, it is the role of the anaesthetist not just to provide anaesthesia, but to maintain physiological normality in the face of controlled trauma of varying magnitude (i.e. surgery) in patients with varying degrees of physiological reserve (i.e. comorbidities causing organ dysfunction). Once that is achieved, the anaesthetist then has to plan for the postoperative recovery of the patient.

The process of general anaesthesia has distinct phases as follows:

Preparation

Preparation and monitoring should be consistent with the amount of information required to ensure cardiovascular and respiratory stability during the surgery. Monitoring temperature, cardiovascular function, and level of oxygenation and ventilation is essential during the use of all general anaesthetics.

Induction

General anaesthetic agents differ qualitatively and quantitatively with regard to their pharmacological actions. The choice of agent for the production of general anaesthesia depends on a number of factors, including patient physical status, the operative procedure, need for rapid recovery and discharge, and the availability of appropriate equipment for anaesthetic delivery, respiratory support, and patient monitoring. The type of induction of anaesthesia can be determined by the age and physical status of the patient, the risk of gastric aspiration, the general anaesthetic agent(s) to be used, and whether intubation of the trachea is required. Tracheal intubation ensures control of ventilation and decreases the risk of pulmonary aspiration. If tracheal intubation is not required, a laryngeal mask airway, face mask, or nasal airway can be used. If problems arise (airway obstruction, hypoventilation or aspiration) it may become necessary to intubate the trachea.

Maintenance

The choice of anaesthetic agent depends on assessment of the cardiovascular and pulmonary status of the patient as well as the absence of factors contraindicating use of a particular agent. Unique aspects of the agents should be considered to avoid deleterious responses and potential morbidity, for example the use of barbiturates in the patient with acute intermittent porphyria and propofol in the patient with egg allergy. Maintenance of a stable course of anaesthesia with minimal alteration in physiological status requires constant assessment of the level of consciousness, muscle relaxation, and cardiorespiratory stability. Adjustment of the anaesthetic dose (inhalational or intravenous) and the addition of an analgesic agent and a neuromuscular blocking agent ensure this stable course. If amnestic agents are required as a component of the anaesthetic regimen, benzodiazepines or butyrophenones can be added. In some instances, ketamine can be used to produce anaesthesia and analgesia in which the patient is inattentive to sensory input and free of pain.

Emergence and recovery

The postoperative course after general anaesthesia is related to the operative procedure and the technique and agents used. The incidence of airway and oropharyngeal irritation is higher in patients who have been 'intubated'. Monitoring of respiration is essential, especially in patients who have been given muscle relaxants or opioids during the surgery. Nausea and vomiting are common after prolonged anaesthesia with inhalational anaesthetics and analgesic agents.

LOCOREGIONAL ANAESTHESIA

It is a commonly held belief that locoregional anaesthesia techniques are reserved for those patients too ill or frail to tolerate the effects of general anaesthesia; this is not the case. Certainly, locoregional anaesthetic techniques can offer advantages to certain patients, but they are techniques with their own side effects.

Box 5.5 Locoregional anaesthesia and coagulopathies

- Full (therapeutic) anticoagulation with oral warfarin or standard unfractionated heparin is an absolute contraindication to central neuraxial blockade and a relative contraindication to peripheral nerve blockade.
- Partial (prophylactic) anticoagulation with low-molecular-weight heparin or low-dose warfarin (international normalized ratio < 1.5) is a relative contraindication to central neural blockade and each patient should be assessed individually, with respect to risk and benefit.
- 'Minihep' (low-dose standard heparin 5000 units twice daily subcutaneously) is not associated with an increased risk of spinal or epidural haematoma. Wait for 4 h after a dose before performing epidural or spinal injection. Minihep should not be given until 1 h following spinal or epidural injection. These guidelines also apply for removal of epidural or spinal catheters.
- Low-molecular-weight heparin (< 40 mg enoxaparin): allow a 12-h interval between low-molecular-weight heparin administration and epidural or spinal injection. Avoid any further dose for 4 h post block. This also applies for removal of epidural or spinal catheters.
- Non-steroidal anti-inflammatory drugs (including aspirin) do not increase the risk of epidural or spinal haematoma.
- Intraoperative anticoagulation using 5000 units intravenous heparin following epidural or spinal injection appears safe, but careful postoperative observations are recommended. Bloody tap or blood in the epidural catheter is controversial. Some recommend delaying surgery for 12 h, others (if preoperative coagulation is normal) delay an intravenous bolus of heparin for 1 h.
- Fibrinolytic and thrombolytic drugs (streptokinase and tissue plasminogen activator): avoid neuraxial blocks for at least 24 h.
- Thrombocytopenia: epidurals are relatively contraindicated below platelet counts of 100 000 and a single intrathecal injection below 50 000.

Advantages

Locoregional anaesthesia using local anaesthetic agents reduces the nociceptive impulses from reaching the central nervous system during and after surgical procedures. Efferent signals to blood vessels, muscle and viscera are thus blocked, protecting against reflex responses to operative pain. Advantages of locoregional anaesthesia include reduced physiological derangement associated with surgery, less risk of pulmonary aspiration (airway reflexes are not obtunded), and the provision of postoperative analgesia. For some operative procedures locoregional anaesthesia is preferred over general anaesthesia (e.g. transurethral prostatectomy).

Contraindications

Contraindications include sepsis, anticoagulation, infection or tumour at needle placement site, and lack of patient cooperation or consent. Pre-existing neurological deficit, although not an absolute contraindication, dissuades some anaesthetists from the use of locoregional anaesthesia because of medicolegal considerations.

ANTICOAGULATION AND REGIONAL ANAESTHESIA

Bleeding and compression neuropraxia is a potential complication of regional anaesthesia in patients who are anticoagulated or have clotting abnormalities. Peripheral nerve blockade may still be used where compression due to bleeding is less likely (superficial nerves). More proximal or perivascular techniques are best avoided. Guidelines on performing locoregional techniques in the presence of coagulapathies are found in Box 5.5.

An epidural haematoma should be suspected in patients who complain of severe back pain a few hours or days following any central neuraxial block or with any prolonged or abnormal neurological deficit. An immediate MRI scan and neurosurgical referral is indicated.

Commonly used techniques

- Axillary brachial plexus and Bier's blocks are used for surgery on the distal forearm, hand and wrist.
- Subclavian perivascular brachial plexus and supraclavicular brachial plexus blocks are most suitable for the midportion of the upper extremity.
- Interscalene brachial plexus block is best for the proximal upper extremity and shoulder, although it may not block the C8 or T1 dermatomes.
- Spinal anaesthesia: motor block level is usually two dermatomal segments below the sensory level and sympathetic block is two above.
- Epidural anaesthesia: motor block may be about six dermatomal segments below the sensory level, with sympathetic block the same as sensory.

Adjuvants

Patients may receive premedication to alleviate anxiety; benzodiazepines are frequently used for this purpose and they have the additional advantage of raising the seizure threshold. Patients should not be so heavily sedated that their cooperation is lost. Addition of adrenaline (epinephrine) to the local anaesthetics produces more profound anaesthesia because it often shortens the time of onset, prolongs duration of many local anaesthetic agents, and serves as a marker of inadvertent intravenous injection. It also causes a reduction in peak blood levels and toxicity. Systemic absorption of adrenaline can occur and so should be avoided in patients who may be sensitive to its effects, i.e. hypertensive, hyperthyroid or beta-blocked patients or those prone to arrhythmias. It should not be used for blocks of the finger, toe or penis.

Complications (Box 5.6)

Systemic effects of toxic blood levels of local anaesthetic agents proceed from dizziness, metallic taste, tinnitus, nystagmus, facial twitching and seizures to respiratory depression and cardiovascular collapse. If toxic levels are rapidly reached (as with intravenous injection), central nervous, respiratory and cardiovascular depression may occur immediately without premonitory symptoms. Intravenous injection may be avoided by using proper technique, aspiration in all quadrants, and test doses. True allergic reactions to local anaesthetic agents are rare and are far more common with esters (cocaine) than with amide drugs such as lidocaine (lignocaine), bupivacaine and ropivacaine. Some reactions may be caused by the presence of methylparaben or similar preservatives and can be avoided by using preservative-free preparations.

Bupivacaine binds to myocardium and has been associated with the need for prolonged cardiopulmonary resuscitation. Maximum safe doses of common local anaesthetics are listed in

Box 5.6 Clinical features and treatment of local anaesthetic toxicity

Clinical features

- Mild toxicity: circumoral tingling
- Moderate toxicity: metallic taste
- Severe toxicity: tinnitus, visual disturbance, slurred speech, altered level of consciousness, convulsions, coma, respiratory arrest, cardiac arrhythmias and cardiovascular collapse

Treatment

- Stop injection or infusion as appropriate.
- Assess airway, breathing and circulation.
- Mild symptoms may be best treated by oxygen plus judicious doses of midazolam (1–4 mg) to increase the convulsion threshold.
- For moderate to severe toxicity, cardiovascular collapse is normally preceded by convulsions and is related to drug overdose in the presence of hypoxia, therefore prevent convulsions and maintain oxygenation.
- If the conscious level is deteriorating or if there are convulsions, intubate the trachea using thiopentone and suxamethonium for preference because this will decrease or stop convulsions.
- Start cardiopulmonary resuscitation if cardiovascular collapse ensues.

Table 5.9. Cardiac arrest has been estimated as occurring in six to seven per 10 000 spinal anaesthetics and one per 10 000 for all other techniques.

EPIDURALS AND OUTCOME AFTER MAJOR SURGERY

Postoperative pain may be a potent cause of adverse events in many organ systems.[75] It has been suggested that conducting surgery under epidural anaesthesia, either alone or in combination with general anaesthesia, may reduce perioperative morbidity and mortality compared with general anaesthesia alone.[76] This is thought to occur by their ability to attenuate the stress response to surgery.

Benefits include improved quality of postoperative analgesia in comparison with systemic opioids.

Lower cardiac morbidity was seen in high-risk patients undergoing major vascular surgery under combined general and epidural anaesthesia with postoperative epidural analgesia,[77] but subsequent studies have failed to confirm this finding and the study has been criticized on study design and size.

A meta-analysis showed a significant reduction in venous thromboembolism in patients undergoing surgery for hip fracture under regional (epidural or spinal) anaesthesia compared with general anaesthesia, but showed only a marginally better effect on early mortality.[78] Another meta-analysis found that thoracic epidural anaesthesia and analgesia using opioids and local anaesthetics was associated with a decreased incidence of atelectasis, pulmonary infections, and hypoxaemia compared with systemic opioids;[79] this may be related to improved diaphragmatic function.[80]

In a randomized controlled trial of patients undergoing major abdominal surgery using combined general and thoracic epidural anaesthesia, patients had earlier recovery of gut function than those receiving general anaesthesia alone followed by standard systemic opioid analgesia.[81] Optimum results are achieved when the epidural regimen combines local anaesthetics and opioids, because sole use of epidural morphine may delay recovery of gut motility and cause pruritus and nausea.[82] This may operate by

Table 5.9 Maximum recommended doses of common local anaesthetic agents

Agent	Maximum recommended dose of plain solution (mg/kg)	Maximum recommended dose of solution with adrenaline (epinephrine)
Bupivacaine	2 mg/kg	2 mg/kg
Levobupivacaine	2 mg/kg	6 mg/kg
Ropivacaine	3 mg/kg	8 mg/kg
Lidocaine (lignocaine)	3 mg/kg	–
Prilocaine	6 mg/kg	–
Cocaine	3 mg/kg	–

blocking the sympathetically mediated peristaltic inhibition while preserving vagal and sacral parasympathetic outflow.

A prospective, double-blind study of patients undergoing radical prostatectomy with pre-emptive epidural anaesthesia showed earlier resumption of oral nutrition, earlier mobilization, earlier discharge from hospital or intensive care units, improved patient activity at 3½ weeks and less pain enduring to 9½ weeks after operation.[83]

A retrospective study in patients undergoing oesophagectomy showed that those who received intraoperative and postoperative thoracic epidural anaesthesia and analgesia achieved earlier tracheal extubation and, with intensive physiotherapy, were mobilized and discharged from intensive care more rapidly than those receiving conventional management.[84]

The combination of epidurals, laparoscopic surgery, and a multimodal approach to aggressive postoperative rehabilitation may dramatically reduce hospital stay, as shown in nine elderly patients who stayed in hospital for only 2–3 days after colonic surgery, compared with the normal 10 days.[85] Clearly, larger studies are necessary for proper evaluation of this multimodal approach.

A systematic review of all relevant randomized trials published before 1997 was undertaken to obtain estimates of the effects of neuraxial blockade with epidural or spinal anaesthesia on

REFERENCES

75. Mangano DT, Siliciano D, Hollenberg M et al. Anesthesiology 1992; 76: 342–353
76. Kehlet H. Br J Anaesth 1997; 78: 606–617
77. Yeager MP, Glass DD, Neff RK et al. Anesthesiology 1987; 66: 729–736
78. Sorenson RM, Pace NL. Anesthesiology 1992; 77: 1095–1104
79. Ballantyne JC, Carr DB, deFerranti S et al. Anesth Analg 1998; 86: 598–612
80. Manikian B, Cantineau JP, Bertrand M et al. Anesthesiology 1988; 68: 379–386
81. Liu SS, Carpenter RL, Mackey DC et al. Anesthesiology 1995; 83: 757–765
82. Smith G, Power I, Cousins MJ. Br J Anaesth 1999; 82: 817–819
83. Gottschalk A, Smith DS, Jobes DR et al. JAMA 1998; 279: 1076–1082
84. Brodner G, Pogatski E, Van Aken H et al. Anesth Analg 1998; 86: 228–234
85. Bardram L, Funch-Jensen P, Jensen P et al. Lancet 1995; 345: 763–764

postoperative morbidity and mortality. Outcomes considered were deep vein thrombosis, pulmonary embolism, myocardial infarction, transfusion requirements, pneumonia, other infections, respiratory depression and renal failure. Overall mortality was reduced by about a third in patients allocated to neuraxial blockade. Neuraxial blockade reduced the odds of deep vein thrombosis by 44%, pulmonary embolism by 55%, transfusion requirements by 50%, pneumonia by 39%, and respiratory depression by 59%. There were also reductions in myocardial infarction and renal failure, although there was limited power to assess these subgroup effects. The proportional reductions in mortality did not clearly differ by surgical group, type of blockade (epidural or spinal), or in those trials in which neuraxial blockade was combined with general anaesthesia compared with trials in which neuraxial blockade was used alone.[86]

It must be remembered that epidurals carry risks of serious neurological complications, which are fortunately rare. Vigilance in the postoperative period is required to detect the triad of back pain, progressive motor weakness, and incontinence that may herald an epidural haematoma or abscess formation. Modern practice, using dilute concentrations of local anaesthetics or opioids in epidural infusions (thereby reducing motor weakness), is helpful in aiding diagnosis of this potentially devastating complication. If suspected, immediate radiological investigation (with MRI) and surgery are required to relieve spinal cord compression.

POSTOPERATIVE CARE

Within this chapter it would be impossible to provide detailed practical descriptions of the assessment and management of the myriad potential complications that can occur postoperatively, so the reader is instead referred to standard texts; a recommended text has been produced by the Advanced Life Support group.[87] We will, however, describe a few common complications that fall outside the remit of standard non-anaesthetic texts, such as postoperative nausea and vomiting, post-dural puncture headache, and the neurological sequelae of locoregional anaesthesia.

IMPROVING POSTOPERATIVE MORTALITY

The NCEPOD reports indicate that only about 10% of perioperative deaths occur on the day of surgery, which is not surprising, because the patient is under the direct continuous clinical supervision of an anaesthetist who takes great care to not only ensure anaesthesia but also to support vital organ function. Because the operation forms a small part of the perioperative period, it would seem that the postoperative period is the time when the patient is most at risk of developing complications. Not all patients who die are from high-risk groups, but surgical mortality increases as ASA rating increases.[88] Again, NCEPOD indicates that approximately 50% of postoperative deaths are in patients rated ASA IV or V, with about 30% of deaths in patients rated ASA III and 20% in patients rated ASA I or II. This may be partially explained by our inability to reliably identify patients at risk of adverse outcome.

RECOVERY AREAS

Patients recovering from the effects of anaesthesia and surgery benefit from specialist observation, because vital organ function is easily compromised at this time. The immediate postoperative period should occur in a dedicated clinical area, variously described as the recovery room or ward, the postoperative care unit or the postanaesthetic care unit. In the USA, recovery rooms were established in most hospitals between 1940 and 1950,[89] but the UK was slow to follow, establishing purpose-built recovery areas, open 24 h per day, only within the 1990s! Similarly, expertise in caring for critically ill patients has developed rapidly, particularly over the past 40 years. For the majority of patients, the immediate postoperative recovery period is the time when they are continuously closely monitored in recovery areas as they emerge from the anaesthetized state and recover protective reflexes and cardiorespiratory stability. For healthy patients undergoing relatively brief procedures with few postoperative sequelae, recovery is swift and major postoperative problems rare.

INTENSIVE CARE UNIT AND HIGH-DEPENDENCE UNIT

Selected patients who are recognized to be high risk should ideally be admitted to the intensive care unit or high-dependence unit, so that close continuous monitoring with or without organ support can be continued into the postoperative period. Critical care services have decreased the mortality for a range of critical illnesses.[90–92] Just as even the most minor surgery would not be contemplated without the use of an appropriately equipped and staffed recovery area, it has been argued that surgery for high-risk patients should not be undertaken without an appropriately equipped and staffed intensive care unit and high-dependence unit. Most high-risk patients admitted to an intensive care unit following surgery who die, do so after they have been discharged from the intensive care unit.[93] Again, NCEPOD tells us that 78% of surgical deaths occur 2 or more days after the operation, with over 60% taking place more than 4 days postsurgery. Sixty per cent of those who died were sent to a ward after the immediate recovery period. Most patients appear to have died from cardiorespiratory complications, renal failure, or infection. It is a fact that once returned to the ward from the recovery area, intensive care unit or high-dependence unit, the patient is no longer as closely supervised or monitored; this may be the time when many patients are most at risk.

Having emphasized the importance of recovery, the intensive care unit and the high-dependence unit, it should be remembered that it is not where the care is delivered that is important but what care is delivered; different intensive care unit protocols may influence the outcome of high-risk surgical patients.[94]

REFERENCES

86. Rodgers A, Walker N, Schug S et al. Br Med J 2000; 321: 1493
87. Advanced Life Support Group. Acute Medical Emergencies: the Practical Approach. BMJ Books, London, 2001
88. Wolters U, Wolf T, Stutzer H et al. Br J Anaesth 1996; 77: 217–222
89. Frost EAM, Thomson DA. In: Frost EAM, Thomson DA (eds). Post-Anaesthetic Care. Baillière Tindall, London, 1994: 749–754
90. Brown JJ, Sullivan G. Chest 1989; 96: 127–129
91. Pollack MM, Katz RW, Ruttimann UE et al. Crit Care Med 1988; 16: 11–17
92. Pollack MM, Patel KM, Ruttimann E. Crit Care Med 1997; 25: 1637–1642
93. Goldhill DR, Sumner A. Crit Care Med 1998; 26: 1337–1345
94. Sandison AJP, Wyncoll DLA, Edmondson RC et al. Eur J Vasc Endovasc Surg 1998; 16: 356–361

Intensive care units and high-dependence units should have defined admission criteria, and it is not surprising that the mortality of patients refused intensive care unit admission is high.[95] It was demonstrated some time ago that postoperative outcome can be improved by maintaining physiological values within narrow limits. It has also been demonstrated that patients with 'supranormal' values for cardiac output, oxygen delivery and oxygen consumption have an improved postoperative outcome.[96] More controversially, the same investigator went on to show that when 'supranormal' values of tissue perfusion were attained in a selected group of surgical patients, mortality was reduced from 33 to 4%; however, many doubt whether optimizing physiological values improves outcome.[39] It probably is true that patients who easily achieve and maintain excellent cardiorespiratory values do well and that patients who fail to achieve adequate organ perfusion do badly. A concept of accelerated recovery, consisting of optimal pain relief, early mobilization and nutrition, is in vogue because it may speed recovery and reduce hospital stays after major abdominal surgery.[97]

Graduated care means that the surgical patients should be cared for in the most appropriate location; this may be an intensive care unit, a high-dependence unit or a general ward. It is essential that there is regular re-evaluation, because the patients' requirements may change. High-risk patients should be identified preoperatively and from events occurring during the procedure and in the postoperative period. It should be possible to agree goals for the management of these patients, and for care to be organized to ensure that these goals are met. This may require intensive care unit or high-dependence unit admission, or additional support on the wards with a postoperative care team.[98] The NCEPOD Joint Report indicated that an average of 6.8% of the patients should have been on a high-dependence unit. In addition, more than 50% of surgical patients in an intensive care unit could have been in a high-dependence unit if one had been available.

Guidelines for admission to intensive care units and high-dependence units have been published.[99,100] They apply to patients with potentially recoverable conditions who can benefit from more detailed observations and treatment than can safely be provided on the wards. Intensive care is usually reserved for patients with threatened or established organ failure. High-dependency care is designed to monitor and support patients with, or likely to develop, acute (or acute on chronic) single-organ failure. There is some evidence that the UK lags behind much of Europe and the USA in the provision of facilities for caring for these critically ill patients,[98,101] with fewer intensive care unit beds per head of populations,[102] existing beds containing sicker patients,[103] and with relatively fewer high-dependence units.[104] Therefore preventing postoperative complications is likely to cost money.

IDENTIFYING POSTOPERATIVE PATIENTS AT RISK

The concept of the patient at risk team is being developed in many hospitals,[105] and has been shown to significantly decrease the need for cardiopulmonary resuscitation in critically ill patients admitted from the wards to the intensive care unit.

One study asserted that patients that develop poor postsurgical outcomes can usually be identified early in the postoperative period, often within the first 24 h following surgery.[106] These patients' outcomes might have been improved if their initial deterioration had been prevented or managed more aggressively.

Box 5.7 Risk factors for the pulmonary aspiration of gastric contents

- Full stomach
- Known reflux
- Raised intragastric pressure: intestinal obstruction, pregnancy, laparoscopic surgery
- Recent trauma
- Perioperative opioids
- Diabetes mellitus
- Topically anaesthetized airway

The study indicated that some types of surgery seem to be associated with a particularly high risk of instability in the postoperative period, notably emergency general, vascular and urological surgery. It was also found that at least 0.2% of surgical patients had a potentially serious postoperative event. Another study found that postoperative emergencies occurred at a median time of 15 h after surgery, with 79% occurring within the first 24 h. They included cardiac and respiratory arrests, airway and breathing problems, tachycardia, hypotension, and decreased levels of consciousness. Compared with controls, the emergencies were commoner in sicker patients and with surgery performed outside normal working hours.[107]

Many adverse events, such as silent ischaemia, deep venous thrombosis, or renal or hepatic dysfunction are not manifest for several days after surgery. Routine ward observations, such as blood pressure and heart rate, may not be sensitive enough to detect a patient at risk of developing postoperative complications.[108,109] In high-risk patients it may be better to monitor markers of inadequate perfusion, such as gastric intramucosal pH, serum lactate, serum base excess, or tissue oxygen tension.

SOME COMMON POSTOPERATIVE COMPLICATIONS

Aspiration of gastric contents

Risk factors for the pulmonary aspiration of gastric contents are listed in Box 5.7. The clinical presentation can vary but chest

REFERENCES

95. Metcalfe MA, Sloggett A, McPherson K. Lancet 1997; 350: 7–12
96. Shoemaker WC, Czer LSC. Crit Care Med 1979; 7: 424–429
97. Moiniche S, Bulow S, Hesselfeldt P et al. Eur J Surg 1995; 161: 283–288
98. Goldhill DR. Br Med J 1997; 314: 389
99. National Health Service Executive. Admission to Intensive Care and High Dependency Care Units. NHS Executive, London, 1996
100. Nasraway SA, Cohen IL, Dennis RC et al. Crit Care Med 1998; 26: 607–610
101. Vincent J-L, Thijs L, Cerny V. Crit Care Clin 1997; 13: 245–254
102. Angus DC, Sirio CA, Clermont G et al. Crit Care Clin 1997; 13: 389–407
103. Vincent J-L, Bihari DSP. JAMA 1995; 274: 639–644
104. Thompson F-J, Singer M. Postgrad Med J 1995; 71: 217–221
105. Lee A, Bishop G, Hillman KM et al. Anaesth Intensive Care 1995; 23: 183–186
106. Gamil M, Fanning A. Anaesthesia 1991; 46: 712–715
107. Lee A, Lum ME, O'Regan WJ et al. Anaesthesia 1998; 53: 529–535
108. Hamilton-Davies C, Mythen MG, Salmon JB et al. Intensive Care Med 1997; 23: 276–281
109. Mythen MG, Webb AR. Intensive Care Med 1994; 20: 99–104

Box 5.8 Suggested management for suspected pulmonary aspiration of gastric contents

Immediate management

- Administer 100% oxygen.
- Minimize the risk of further aspirate contaminating the airway.
- If the patient can be roused, suction the oro- or nasopharynx and place in the left lateral head-down position (recovery position).
- If the patient is unconscious but breathing spontaneously, apply cricoid pressure (avoid if patient actively vomiting) and place patient in the recovery position; intubate the trachea if bronchial lavage is indicated.
- If the patient is unconscious and apnoeic, intubate trachea immediately and commence ventilation (minimize positive-pressure ventilation until the endotracheal tube and airway have been suctioned and all aspirates are clear).

Subsequent management

- Empty the stomach with a large-bore nasogastric tube prior to attempting tracheal extubation.
- Monitor respiratory function and arrange a chest radiograph and measurement of arterial blood gases.
- Signs of respiratory failure warrant transfer to an intensive care unit.

signs include a wheeze and crackles, and tracheal aspiration may be acidic (but a negative finding does not exclude aspiration). Chest radiograph may show diffuse infiltrative pattern, especially in right lower lobe distribution (but often not acutely). In high-risk situations avoidance of general anaesthesia is the preferable option; where surgery under general anaesthesia is unavoidable, a rapid sequence induction should be undertaken. When aspiration is suspected the subsequent management is outlined in Box 5.8. There is no evidence that corticosteroids alter the outcome, and prophylactic antibiotics are not generally given routinely.

For patients at risk, a rapid induction sequence involves speedy tracheal intubation using a very short-acting neuromuscular blocker (usually suxamethonium) immediately following preoxygenation of the lungs and induction of anaesthesia, with posterior pressure on the cricoid cartilage to occlude the upper oesophagus. If intubation fails the drugs should wear off rapidly and the patient restart spontaneous ventilation before hypoxia intervenes. Meticulous preliminary assessment of the airway is mandatory to look for likely difficulties with tracheal intubation. If preoperative evaluation suggests a problem with tracheal intubation, alternative techniques should be considered, such as surgery under local or regional anaesthesia or awake fibre-optic tracheal intubation. The anaesthetist must have a management plan should tracheal intubation fail.

Malignant hyperthermia

Malignant hyperthermia is a disorder of skeletal muscle, inherited as an autosomal dominant condition.[110] It is associated with loss of normal calcium homeostasis at some point in the excitation–contraction coupling system. An abnormality anywhere along this complex process can cause the clinical features seen in malignant hyperthermia. This explains why differing chemical agents trigger malignant hyperthermia and also the heterogeneity seen in DNA studies. Worldwide, about 50% of malignant hyperthermia families have been shown to be linked to the ryanodine receptor on chromosome 19q. This controls a calcium efflux channel on the sarcoplasmic reticulum. Fifteen causative ryanodine receptor mutations have been found to date. Three other probable sites on chromosomes 1, 3 and 7 have also been linked to malignant hyperthermia. The incidence is about one in 10 000 to 15 000 of the general population, and it occurs in all races.

The mortality from malignant hyperthermia has fallen from 80–90 to 2–3%. This is due to better monitoring and awareness of malignant hyperthermia as well as the availability of sodium dantrolene for its treatment. Malignant hyperthermia is most commonly seen in young adults, especially men, and occurs more frequently in minor surgical procedures, for example dental or ear, nose and throat, when suxamethonium and inhalational anaesthetic agents are regularly used. A previously uneventful anaesthesia does not preclude malignant hyperthermia occurring, even when trigger agents must have been used before.

The clinical presentation is variable, often making the diagnosis difficult. It can be a florid, dramatic, life-threatening event or have an insidious onset. The clinical signs fall into three groups:

- Core temperature rising at over 2°C/h.
- Muscle effects, including muscle rigidity, hyperkalaemia, high creatinine kinase and myoglobinuria.
- Increased metabolism, including tachycardia, increased carbon dioxide production, and metabolic acidosis.

Although prevention is the ideal treatment, providing anaesthesia is often unavoidable; the key to anaesthetic management is a high degree of suspicion and preparedness.

Local anaesthetic toxicity

Local anaesthetic toxicity is related to high plasma levels of local anaesthetic found in drug overdose, direct intravascular injection, rapid absorption or injection into a highly vascular area (e.g. intercostal nerve block), cumulative effect of multiple injections, or continuous infusion. The recommended maximum doses quoted by manufacturers' data sheets (Table 5.9) are a guide only. Equally important are the site of injection, with relation to vascularity and absorption, and metabolic status, because acidosis, hypoxia and hypercarbia all potentiate the negative inotropic or chronotropic effects of local anaesthetics. Whenever possible, keep within the maximum dosing recommendations, aspirate carefully before injection, and divide large-volume injections into smaller aliquots. Clinical features and treatment are outlined in Box 5.6.

Postdural puncture headache

Postdural puncture headache is a complication of inadvertent breach of the dura mater and subarachnoid mater by an epidural or spinal needle;[111,112] its incidence should be less than 1%. The proposed mechanism is cerebrospinal fluid loss, at a rate greater than its rate of production, through a dural tear. The pressure in the subarachnoid space thus falls and the brain 'sinks' within the skull, stretching the meninges and causing a typical 'low-pressure' headache. Compensatory vasodilatation of intracranial vessels may further worsen the symptoms. The symptoms may not develop for several days. If untreated the headache is not only very unpleasant, but on rare occasions can be life-threatening, usually as a result of intracranial haemorrhage or coning of the brainstem.

REFERENCES

110. Hopkins PM. Br J Anaesth 2000; 85: 118–128
111. Reynolds F. Br Med J 1993; 306: 874–875
112. Carrie LE. Br J Anaesth 1993; 71: 179–180

Box 5.9 Presentation and management of postdural puncture headache

Common features of postdural puncture headache

- Typical onset 24–48 h after dural puncture
- Usually lasts 7–10 days if untreated
- Characteristically worse on standing, and often absent after overnight bed rest but returns after mobilizing
- Usually fronto-occipital, radiating to the neck, and with associated neck stiffness
- Photophobia, diplopia and difficulty in accommodation
- Hearing loss, tinnitus and cranial nerve VI palsy are possible
- Nausea (in up to 60% of cases)

Symptomatic management

- Bed rest
- Simple analgesics are unlikely to completely relieve severe postdural puncture headache
- Encourage fluid intake, although evidence of its clinical effectiveness is lacking
- Caffeine or theophyllines reduce intracranial vasodilatation and improve symptoms
- Sumatriptan (a cerebral vasoconstrictor) is reserved for those in whom blood patching is contraindicated
- Anecdotal evidence suggests that adrenocorticotropic hormone can alleviate symptoms
- Abdominal binders probably increase epidural vein blood flow, compressing dural sac and raising cerebrospinal fluid pressure
- Autologous epidural blood patching

Following a dural puncture with a 16–18-G Tuohy needle, the incidence of postdural puncture headache is approximately 70%; it is less likely in patients over the age of 65 years. Not all dural punctures are recognized at the time of needle insertion. Although it must be remembered that headaches are common, a headache in a patient who has had an epidural or a spinal should not automatically be assumed to be of a low-pressure type. The key differentiating feature of a postdural puncture headache is its positional nature: the headache is worse on standing. Abdominal compression can be used to assess a patient; if abdominal pressure effectively relieves a headache, it suggests that the headache is due to a dural tear.

Typical clinical features and a management plan are outlined in Box 5.9. Treatment is either to wait for the symptoms to resolve when the dural tear heals, or by epidural autologous blood patching to seal the dural tear. Neurosurgical closure has also been reported!

Postoperative nausea and vomiting

Although rarely life-threatening, morbidity associated with postoperative nausea and vomiting[113,114] may be the most unpleasant memory associated with a patient's hospital stay. Postoperative nausea and vomiting have been described as 'as or more debilitating than the after-effects of the surgery itself'.[115] Severe vomiting can result in hypokalaemia, hypochloraemia, hyponatremia, alkalosis and dehydration, pulmonary aspiration, and wound disruption,[116] and it can lead to increased length of hospital stay, increased bleeding, incisional hernias, and aspiration pneumonia. The incidence is between 5 and 75% in published series. If no prophylaxis is used, the incidence is probably around 30% for postoperative nausea and vomiting within 6 h[117] and 30% for postoperative nausea and vomiting within 24 h.

Some antiemetic drugs have multiple actions. In paediatric practice, where the extrapyramidal effects of the antidopaminergic drugs can be a serious problem, ondansetron is the drug of first choice. There is increased interest in using combinations of antiemetics to increase efficacy. The logical approach is to combine two drugs with different actions (and presumably different side effects). Studies with the combination of dexamethasone and ondansetron, or ondansetron and droperidol, showed clear improvements over monotherapy.

Postoperative nausea and vomiting have many causes, including presence of an oral airway; metabolic, vestibular, psychogenic or gastrointestinal disorders; intracranial hypertension; and emetic drugs. Postoperative nausea and vomiting are particularly distressing in ambulatory patients, because discharge may be delayed or admission may be required. It is important to identify patients at risk preoperatively (Box 5.10).

Patients receiving regional anaesthesia have a lower incidence of postoperative nausea and vomiting than those receiving general anaesthesia.[118] Only 10% of patients complain of postoperative nausea and vomiting without accompanying pain.[119] Other factors that need to be addressed in the management of postoperative nausea and vomiting include correcting hypotension and dehydration, providing analgesia, and administrating 'rescue' antiemetic agent.

Neurological sequelae following regional anaesthesia[120–122]

It has been reported that transient neurological sequelae occur in six or seven per 10 000 following spinal anaesthesia and one or two per 10 000 for all other techniques. Permanent neurological damage (neurological dysfunction lasting longer than 3 months) occurs in 12 per 10 000 following spinal anaesthesia and less than one per 10 000 for peripheral nerve blocks. Postoperative neurological dysfunction is strongly associated with paraesthesia on needle placement or pain on injection of local anaesthetic. Anaesthetized or heavily sedated patients are unable to respond to paraesthesia or intraneural injection. However, regional analgesia performed in such patients has never been demonstrated to produce an increased incidence of neurological sequelae. Paediatric regional anaesthesia is almost exclusively performed following a general anaesthetic. In over 24 000 central and peripheral blocks in paediatric patients, the complication rate was 1.5 per 1000 (all associated with central blocks), with no permanent neurological damage. Nerve injury is an important source of patient morbidity and medicolegal claims. The true incidence is unknown due to significant under-reporting. Many of the data presented below are from the ASA Closed Claims Project Database (1975–95).[123]

REFERENCES

113. Fisher DM. Anesthesiology 1997: 87: 1271–1273
114. Tramer MR. In: Tramer MR (ed). Evidence Based Resource in Anaesthesia and Analgesia. BMJ Books, London, 2000
115. Kovac AL, Pearman MH, Khalil SN et al. J Clin Anesth 1996; 8: 644
116. Palazzo MGA, Strunin L. Can Anaesth Soc J 1984; 31: 178
117. Macrae WA. Br J Anaesth 2001; 87: 88–98
118. Jellish WS, Thalji Z, Stevenson K et al. Anesth Analg 1996; 83: 559
119. Anderson R, Krohg K. Can Anaesth Soc J 1976; 23: 366
120. Sawyer RJ et al. Anaesthesia 2000; 55: 980–991
121. Prielipp RC et al. Anesthesiology 1999; 91: 345–354
122. Wheatley RG, Schug SA, Watson D. Br J Anaesth 2001; 87: 47–61
123. Cheney FW et al. Anesthesiology 1999; 90: 1062–1069

Box 5.10 Some risk factors for postoperative nausea and vomiting

All the risk factors below have been described as contributing to postoperative nausea and vomiting.

Surgery
- Gynaecological (especially ovarian) surgery
- Bowel or gallbladder surgery
- Head and neck surgery, including tonsillectomy and adenoidectomy
- Ophthalmic (especially squint) surgery
- Prolonged surgery

Anaesthesia
- Induction with methohexitone, etomidate or ketamine (compared with propofol or thiopental)
- Maintenance with nitrous oxide; avoidance reduces risk with an number needed to treat of 5
- Opioids increases the incidence of postoperative nausea and vomiting, but untreated pain is also emetogenic
- Spinal anaesthesia high blocks (above T5), hypotension, and the use of adrenaline (epinephrine) in the local anaesthetic
- Intraoperative dehydration
- Gastric dilatation from inexperienced bag and mask ventilation
- 'Motion' sickness due to fast or careless patient movement during emergence from anaesthesia

Patient factors
- Previous history of postoperative nausea and vomiting
- Children experience postoperative nausea and vomiting more than adults do
- Women experience postoperative nausea and vomiting more than men do, until after 70 years of age
- Obesity may be a risk factor
- History of motion sickness

Organizational
- Failure to audit and set up appropriate treatment protocols
- Poor education of medical and nursing staff, leading to under-use of effective treatment

The commonest nerve injuries encountered postoperatively are ulnar nerve (28%), brachial plexus (20%), lumbosacral root (16%) and spinal cord (13%). Less commonly affected nerves are sciatic, median, radial and femoral nerves. Many cases of perioperative nerve damage have no identifiable cause, but the mechanism for spinal cord injury is determined in 48% of claims and a regional anaesthetic has been found to have been administered in 68% of cases of spinal cord injury.

Neuropraxia (myelin sheath damaged but axon intact) usually recovers in weeks to months, with a good prognosis; axonotmesis (axon disrupted) has a variable prognosis; and neurotmesis (nerve completely severed) may require surgery repair and has a poor prognosis. Symptoms can occur within a day but may not present for 2–3 weeks, and the intensity and duration of symptoms vary with severity of injury, from numbness and mild paraesthesia lasting a few weeks to persistent painful paraesthesia, sensory loss, and motor loss lasting years and developing into reflex sympathetic dystrophy.

Ulnar neuropathy

Ulnar neuropathy occurs more commonly in males (3:1), in the obese, and with prolonged hospitalization. It is uncommon in young patients. It has been suggested to occur with frequency of between one in 200 to one in 350 patients. Eighty-five per cent of cases occur in association with general anaesthesia and 15% occur after regional block (6% after spinal), indicating the unclear aetiology. Injuries occur at the superficial condylar groove of the elbow. It has been suggested that there is less ulnar nerve compression with the arm in supination. Abduction of the arm is beneficial to the ulnar nerve, but this must be offset against possible stretch at the brachial plexus. Additional padding was explicitly stated to have been used in 27% of closed claims. In 62%, onset of symptoms was delayed to more than 1 day postoperatively. Abnormal nerve conduction is common in the contralateral unaffected arm, indicating subclinical neuropathy.

Brachial plexus injury

Causal factors include excessive stretch (arm abduction with lateral rotation of the head to the opposite side), compression (upward movement of the clavicle and sternal retraction), and associated regional block (only 16% of closed claims for brachial plexus injury). Pain and paraesthesiae were noted in 50% of claims associated with a regional technique. Lesions affecting the upper roots are commoner.

Lumbosacral root injury

Radiculopathy due to this cause occurs in association with a neuraxial block in 90% of cases (55% secondary to spinals and 37% to epidurals). Persistent postoperative radicular pain may occur in up to 0.2% of cases but will almost always resolve in weeks or months. Persisting paraesthesia, with or without motor symptoms, is the most common complaint.

Spinal cord injury

About 58% of cases of spinal cord injury are associated with previous regional anaesthesia in the closed claims data. The commonest mechanisms were epidural haematoma, chemical injury, anterior spinal artery syndrome, and meningitis, respectively. Lumbar epidural was the commonest regional technique implicated, four times more frequently than subarachnoid block and eight times more than thoracic epidural. Injury was more common in blocks performed for chronic pain management and in the presence of systemic anticoagulation. Delays in the diagnosis of cord or nerve compression are not uncommon, because persistent weakness or numbness is often presumed to be secondary to effects of epidural local anaesthetic infusions. Investigation in all suspected cases, after appropriate history and examination, is by spinal MRI.

The true incidence of major neurological injury after spinal or epidural anaesthesia is hard to estimate. An incidence of one in 100 000 for permanent disability has been proposed in obstetric patients.[124] Epidural haematoma in the presence of low-molecular-weight heparin may be as high as one in 1000 to one in 10 000, but others estimate the risk to be nearer one in 150 000 to one in 220 000 (following epidural and spinal, respectively).[125]

Epidural abscess

Epidural abscess is less common but should be suspected when long-term epidural catheters are used, and in immunocompromised or anticoagulated patients.

REFERENCES

124. Scott DB, Hibbard BM. Br J Anaesth 1990; 64: 537–541
125. Horlocker T et al. Anesth Analg 1998; 86: 1153–1156

Anterior spinal artery syndrome

Anterior spinal artery syndrome typically causes a lower limb spastic paralysis below the level of the lesion, flaccid paralysis at the level of the lesion, variable sensory loss, and sphincter impairment. It can be associated with general or locoregional anaesthesia and is usually related to prolonged hypotension, aortic cross-clamping, thrombosis, embolus, dissecting aortic aneurysm, polyarteritis nodosa, systemic lupus erythematosus and vertebral surgery.

Arachnoiditis

Arachnoiditis is a rare cause of paraplegia and there is no effective treatment. It typically presents as a gradual, progressive weakness and sensory loss beginning days to months after spinal anaesthetic, sometimes leading to complete paraplegia or death. Causes include meningitis, haemorrhage, spinal surgery, and secondary to substances introduced into the spinal or epidural space, for example accidental administration of the wrong drug.

Transient neurological symptoms

Transient neurological symptoms are defined as back pain or dysaesthesia radiating bilaterally to the legs or buttocks after total recovery from spinal anaesthesia and beginning within 24 h. Usually no objective neurological signs can be demonstrated. Pain is usually moderate and may be relieved by non-steroidal anti-inflammatory drugs (NSAIDs). Symptoms usually resolve over a few days. It appears to occur more frequently following the use of spinal 5% hyperbaric lidocaine (lignocaine) with adrenaline (epinephrine). Some studies also suggest a high incidence following spinal plain lidocaine.

Cauda equina syndrome

Cauda equina syndrome is characterized by lower back pain, saddle anaesthesia, sphincter impairment, and motor or sensory symptoms below the knees. Cauda equina syndrome has been reported in association with the use of spinal microcatheters (28-G) and 5% hyperbaric lidocaine (lignocaine). This was presumed secondary to pooling of hyperbaric local anaesthetic, leading to a subsequent ban in the USA on spinal catheters thinner than 24-G.

Prevention, diagnosis and treatment

Neurological sequelae of anaesthesia are becoming an increasing medicolegal problem.[117] Each regional technique has a unique set of potential risks and complications. Complications can arise as a result of medication or dosage errors, poor patient selection, or poor block technique.

Postoperative nerve injuries can be prevented by awareness of potential causes (e.g. careful positioning). A thorough history, examination, documentation of preoperative nerve lesions, and careful anaesthetic records of all aspects of regional techniques (including type of needle, paraesthesia, agent used, etc.) should be made. Performance of these blocks in awake or lightly sedated patients should be considered (this is not practical in children). It is advisable to avoid locoregional techniques in unwilling patients, and never continue injecting if there is pain or paraesthesiae. Neurophysiological tests such as electromyography and nerve conduction studies coupled with MRI can often diagnose specific sites of a lesion. Treatment and prognosis will depend on the severity of the lesion; treatment is best left to neurologists and neurosurgeons. Spinal cord compression or the cauda equina syndrome require urgent neurosurgical referral and decompression.[126]

ANALGESIA: PERIOPERATIVE PAIN MANAGEMENT

INTRODUCTION

Current perioperative pain management still leaves a significant number of patients suffering from moderate to severe pain. Pain assessment and reassessment are needed. Pain research has generated numerous systematic reviews on which to base clinical practice. Optimal perioperative pain management should help reduce postoperative complications and reduce hospital stay.

The International Association for the Study of Pain defines pain as 'an unpleasant sensory and emotional experience associated with actual or potential tissue damage or described in terms of such damage'.[127] This definition reflects the complex nature of pain, which is modulated by many factors (biological, psychological and sociological), and explains why assessment is difficult. The effects of different management strategies are difficult to predict and there is wide variability in individuals' expression of their pain and distress. This has been termed the biopsychosocial model of pain, all the elements of which must be considered when helping a patient manage their pain.

PHYSIOLOGICAL AND PSYCHOLOGICAL EFFECTS OF ACUTE INJURY

From a young age we learn to associate pain with injury. The normal human response to injury is first to remove oneself from harm's way, and then to protect the injured area while healing occurs. This injury response is the collected alterations of physiological and psychological processes, and aims to benefit the individual's short-term survival.[128] If prolonged, these altered processes may slow or even prevent recovery.[129] Biological systems are largely unable to distinguish the cause of the tissue injury, the body responding physiologically and psychologically in a similar way.[130] Although safe and effective postoperative pain relief is principally provided for humanitarian reasons, it may be possible to reduce organ dysfunctions and improve postoperative patient outcome by reducing the physiological and psychological responses to tissue injury.[131]

CARDIOVASCULAR EFFECTS

Severe acute pain increases heart rate, blood pressure, systemic and coronary vascular resistances, and cardiac output, mediated by the sympathetic nervous system. Cardiac work and myocardial oxygen consumption increase, while myocardial oxygen delivery decreases. The imbalance of myocardial oxygen supply and demand may result in myocardial ischaemia, infarction and

REFERENCES

126. Kroll DA, Caplan RA, Posner K et al. Anesthesiology 1990; 73: 202
127. Merskey H. Pain 1986; 3: S216–S222
128. Kehlet H. In: Cousins MJ, Brudenbaugh PO (eds). Neural Blockade in Clinical Anesthesia and Management of Pain. 2nd edn. JB Lippincott, Philadelphia, 1988: 145–188
129. Van den Berghe G, de Zegher F, Bouillon R. J Clin Endocrinol Metab 1998; 83: 1827–1834
130. Cousins MJ. Reg Anesth 1989; 16: 162–176
131. Kehlet H. Br J Anaesth 1994; 72: 365

failure, a situation worsened by coexistent hypoxaemia, coronary artery disease and anxiety. These adverse effects may be reduced by epidural blockade of the cardiac sympathetic fibres (T1 to 5) with local anaesthetic.[133] Clinical evidence that epidural blockade reduces the risk of adverse cardiac outcomes in 'high-risk' surgical patients is controversial,[133,134] although myocardial ischaemia has been noted on cessation of epidural analgesia in this group of patients.[135] Thoracic epidural blockade has, however, been shown to improve the myocardial oxygen supply, reducing myocardial ischaemia in both animal models[136,137] and clinically,[138] and has been associated with improved indices of myocardial function in patients with unstable angina.[139,140] It is unknown if epidural blockade is able to influence the incidence of adverse cardiovascular outcome in the longer term as does beta adrenoreceptor blockade with atenolol.[141]

RESPIRATORY EFFECTS

The pain associated with chest and abdominal surgery can cause significant postoperative respiratory dysfunction. Involuntary spinal reflexes cause increased skeletal muscle tone around the injury site. The effects of this 'muscle splinting' are worsened by voluntary reductions in thoracic and abdominal respiratory muscle excursions that, coupled with diaphragmatic dysfunction, cause reductions in lung volumes (tidal volumes, vital capacity and functional residual capacity) with regional lung collapse (atelectasis) and reduced alveolar ventilation, culminating in hypoxaemia and hypercapnia. Likewise, the patient's ability to cough is reduced, secretions are retained, and chest infection may ensue.[142] The increasing respiratory rate, in an attempt to maintain normal gas exchange, significantly increases metabolic rate, with consequent increased requirement for oxygen and metabolic substrates; hypoxaemia is worsened and respiratory muscle supervenes. This vicious circle accelerates the patient towards respiratory failure.[143] A meta-analysis of randomized controlled trials showed that when compared with conventional analgesic delivery, epidural opioid analgesia produced clinically significant beneficial effects on arterial oxygen saturation and on the incidence of atelectasis.[144] Epidural blockade with local anaesthetics has the potential to improve pulmonary function, but confirmatory data are insufficient to confirm this.

THROMBOEMBOLIC EFFECTS

Epidural blockade may reduce the incidences of both vascular graft occlusion after peripheral arterial surgery,[134,145] and deep venous thrombosis and pulmonary embolism following hip surgery.[146] These effects may be related to improved arterial and venous lower limb blood flow,[147] changes in blood coagulability, fibrinolysis and earlier postoperative mobilization. The systemic absorption of local anaesthetic agents used for neural blockade may themselves have an antithrombotic effect.[148]

GASTROINTESTINAL AND GENITOURINARY EFFECTS

Sympathetic activity, associated with severe pain, may increase intestinal secretions and smooth muscle sphincter tone, and decrease gastrointestinal motility (gastric stasis and paralytic ileus). Opioids may contribute significantly to gastric stasis,[149] while epidural blockade may significantly reduce gut transit time,[150] notably when using local anaesthetic agents but not epidural opioid.[151] The ability to provide early enteral feeding has been shown to reduce the surgical stress response, reduce post-operative septic complications, and improve wound healing.[152] Maximum benefit is likely to be gained if epidural blockade with local anaesthetic is continued for several days postoperatively and opioid dose minimized by using a multimodal analgesic regimen. Interestingly, intravenous lidocaine (lignocaine) appears to speed the return of bowel function after radical prostatectomy, as well as reducing pain and shortening hospital stay.[148] Sympathetic activity increases bladder sphincter tone and possibly urinary retention; unfortunately, opioids have the same effect. We could find no evidence that pain is associated with reductions in renal and hepatic blood.

NEUROENDOCRINE AND METABOLIC EFFECTS

Along with sympathetic nervous system stimulation,[153] tissue injury leads to a metabolic response with increased secretion of catabolic hormones and decreased secretion or action of anabolic hormones and cytokines. A transient hypometabolic phase ('ebb phase') is characterized by elevated metabolic rate, with consequent increases in oxygen consumption, cardiac output and catabolism. The last of these causes a negative nitrogen balance due to loss of muscle protein.[154,155] The 'flow phase' may last from days to weeks, depending on not just the magnitude of the surgery but the occurrence of complications such as infection, blood loss, tissue hypoxia and acidosis, hypothermia, pre-existing protein calorie deficits, and anxiety.

REFERENCES

132. Meissner A, Rolf N, Van Aken H. Anesth Analg 1997; 85: 517–528
133. Yeager MP, Glass DD, Neff RK et al. Anesthesiology 1987; 66: 729–736
134. Tuman KJ, McCarthy RJ, March RJ et al. Anesth Analg 1991; 73: 696–704
135. Garnett RL, MacIntyre A, Lindsay P et al. Can J Anaesth 1996; 43: 769–777
136. Vik-Mo H, Ottesen S, Renck H. Scand J Clin Lab Invest 1978; 38: 737–746
137. Klassen GA, Bramwell RS, Bromage PR et al. Anesthesiology 1980; 52: 8–15
138. Reiz S, Ostman M. Reg Anesth 1982; 7: S8–S18
139. Olausson K, Magnusdottir H, Lurje L et al. Circulation 1997; 96: 2178–2182
140. Blomberg S, Emmanuelsson H, Kvist H et al. Anesthesiology 1990; 73: 840–847
141. Mangano DT, Layug EL, Wallace A et al. N Engl J Med 1996; 335: 1713–1720
142. Craig DB. Anesth Analg 1981; 60: 46
143. Modig J et al. Acta Anaesthesiol Scand 1976; 20: 225–236
144. Ballantyne JC, Carr DB, deFerranti S et al. Anesth Analg 1998; 86: 598–612
145. Christopherson R, Beattie C, Frank SM et al. Anesthesiology 1993; 79: 422–434
146. Modig J, Borg T, Karlstrom G et al. Anesth Analg 1983; 62: 174–180
147. Modig J, Malmberg P, Karlstrom G. Acta Anaesthesiol Scand 1980; 24: 305–309
148. Groudine SB, Fisher HA, Kaufman RP Jr et al. Anesth Analg 1998; 86: 235–239
149. Nimmo WS. Br J Anaesth 1984; 56; 29–37
150. Ahn H, Bronge A, Johanson D et al. Br J Surg 1988; 75: 1176–1178
151. Thorn SE, Wattwil M, Naslund I. Reg Anesth 1992; 17: 91–94
152. Liu S, Carpenter RL, Mackey DC et al. Anesthesiology 1995; 83: 757–765
153. Riles TS, Fisher FS, Schaefer S et al. Ann Vasc Surg 1993; 7: 213–219
154. Weissman C. Anesthesiology 1990; 73: 308–327
155. Wilmore DW. J Am Coll Nutr 1983; 2: 3

It has been suggested that epidural block with local anaesthetic agents is the most effective way of reducing the metabolic response to surgery, postoperative morbidity and mortality, and speed of recovery.[156–159] The reduced metabolic response, using this technique, is more pronounced following lower abdomen and lower limb procedures than following upper abdominal and thoracic procedures; this is possibly due to our inability to completely block afferent neural impulses in the latter. To gain the maximum effect, the epidural block probably needs to be maintained for at least 48–72 h postoperatively.[128] Neuraxial opioids used alone appear to be less efficient in reducing the metabolic response. Conventional systemic analgesia, with the exception of high-dose opioids, has little or no modifying influence on the metabolic response to surgery.

IMMUNOLOGICAL EFFECTS

Surgical injury is known to be associated with immune dysfunction and expression of acute-phase proteins. Neural blockade appears to exert a slight influence on immunocompetence, although the mechanisms involved are unclear.[160]

PERSISTENT POSTOPERATIVE PAIN

Neuropathic pain as a cause of acute postoperative pain is frequently overlooked and often untreated.[161] This pain may persist long after apparent tissue healing and present as an array of clinical syndromes,[162] which broadly divide into neuralgias, complex regional pain syndromes, and deafferentation syndromes. It may be possible to reduce the incidence of the persistent pains that are associated with the deliberate transection of large nerves that occurs when limbs are amputated.[163] Surgical incisions are invariably associated with damage to small peripheral nerves, the damage ranging from neuropraxia to complete nerve transection. Many surgical interventions have been associated with persistent pain that can be long-lasting, severe, debilitating for the sufferer, difficult to manage, and consume considerable healthcare resources. Notorious procedures include lateral thoracotomy,[164] cholecystectomy, nephrectomy, radical mastectomy, varicose vein stripping, inguinal herniorrhaphy, episiotomy, and upper limb and facial procedures. Predisposing patient factors may include genetics, middle and old age, and pre-existing pain.[163,165]

PSYCHOLOGICAL RESPONSES

Adverse psychological effects[166,167] may not be in sharp focus in the postoperative period. Typical behavioural responses include self-absorption and concern, withdrawal from interpersonal contact, increased sensitivity to all external stimuli, grimacing, posturing, reduced activity, moaning, and seeking help and attention. Extremes of behaviour can occur in response to other social or environmental factors, often for some 'gain' from family, work, community and healthcare systems. Change in affect is also commonly observed. Initially feelings of fear (exacerbated by uncertainty, inappropriate beliefs and expectations) and anxiety predominate, followed by feelings of helplessness, loss of control, and depression if the pain remains unrelieved. Anger and resentment may supervene if it is believed that pain relief is being withheld. These effects are exacerbated by the sleep deprivation that accompanies unrelieved severe acute pain. This state may also unmask premorbid tendencies for anxiety, depression, or preoccupation with health and may occasionally provoke an acute psychotic reaction.

CONTEMPORARY ISSUES IN PAIN MANAGEMENT

Pain is the commonest symptom in clinical practice, yet is generally not well managed. A large audit of UK hospital patients found that up to 87% of patients reported severe or moderate pain at some time during their admission.[168] Another prospective audit found that in a UK hospital setting around 58% of patients had moderate to severe pain.[169] These surveys also indicate that many patients believe postoperative pain to be inevitable, significantly increasing their preoperative fear and anxiety. In 1990, a seminal report on pain after surgery highlighted the deficiencies in this area.[170] Some progress has been made since then, for example the widespread commissioning of acute pain services, which can organize educational programmes for staff and develop systems for formally assessing pain and pain guidelines; this has been shown capable of reducing moderate or severe pain from 37 to 13%.[171]

Pain can be classified in a number of ways:

- physiological, clinical, nociceptive or neuropathic;
- somatic or visceral; and
- acute or chronic.

The traditional division of pain into acute and chronic is not helpful; it may be more useful to view pain as a continuum (Fig. 5.3). One end of the continuum may be termed *complex pain* and may be a mixture of nociceptive (inflammatory) pain and neuropathic pain, exacerbated or improved by psychosocial factors. The other end of the continuum may be termed *simple pain*, being predominantly nociceptive pain again exacerbated or improved by psychosocial factors. That being said, the factors predisposing patients to developing persistent pain states are not yet fully understood.[117] The incidence of persistent pain after surgery is probably underestimated, with only a minority of sufferers attending a chronic pain clinic. One study found that about 20% of patients attending pain clinics did so because of pain related to surgery.[172]

REFERENCES

156. Kehlet H. Reg Anesth 1996; 21: 37–37
157. Bromage PR. Reg Anesth 1996; 21: 1–4
158. Brandt MR, Fernades A, Mordhorst R et al. Br Med J 1978; 1: 1106–1108
159. Jorgensen LN, Rasmussen LS, Nielsen PT et al. Br J Anaesth 1991; 66: 8–12
160. Kehlet H. Surg Clin North Am 1999; 79: 431–443
161. Hayes C, Molloy AR. Int Anesthesiol Clin 1997; 35: 67–81
162. Mersky H. Pain 1986; 3: S1–S225
163. Back S, Noreng MF, Tjellden NU. Pain 1988; 33: 287–301
164. Katz J, Jackson M, Kavanagh BP et al. Clin J Pain 1996; 12: 50–55
165. Cousins MJ, Reeve TS, Glynn CJ et al. Anaesth Intensive Care 1979; 7: 121–135
166. Peck C. In: Cousins MJ, Phillips GD (eds). Acute Pain Management. Churchill Livingstone, Edinburgh, 1986: 251–274
167. Chapman CR, Turner JA. J Pain Symptom Management 1985; 1: 9–20
168. Bruster S, Jarman B, Bosanquet N et al. Br Med J 1994; 309: 1542–1546
169. Straw P, Bruster S, Richards N et al. Health Serv J 2000; 5704: 24–26
170. Justins DM. Ann R Coll Surg Engl 1992; 74: 78–79
171. Harmer M, Davies KA. Anaesthesia 1998; 53: 424–430
172. Davies HTO, Crombie IK, Macrae WA et al. Pain Clin 1992; 5: 129–135

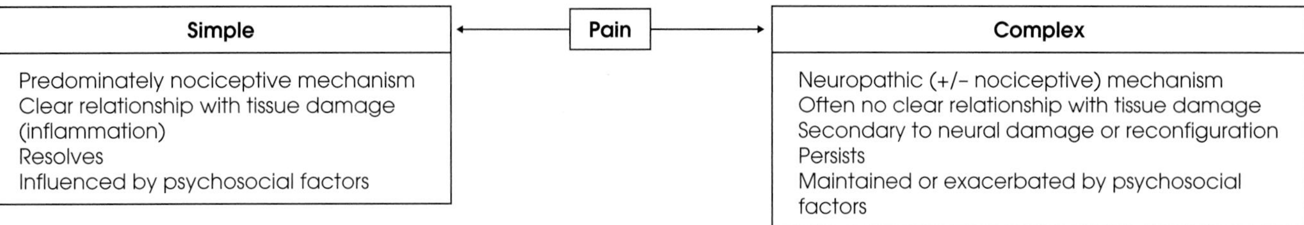

Simple
Pain
Complex
Predominately nociceptive mechanism
Clear relationship with tissue damage (inflammation)
Resolves
Influenced by psychosocial factors
Neuropathic (+/- nociceptive) mechanism
Often no clear relationship with tissue damage
Secondary to neural damage or reconfiguration
Persists
Maintained or exacerbated by psychosocial factors

Figure 5.3 The pain continuum.

Table 5.10 Simple scores that should be included on the ward patient observation chart

Score	Definition
Pain severity (scored by patient)	
0	None
1	Mild
2	Moderate
3	Severe
Sedation	
0	Awake
1	Can be roused
2	Mostly sleeping
3	Difficult to awaken
Nausea and vomiting	
0	None
1	Nausea
2	Vomiting

Box 5.11 Basic principles of acute postoperative pain management

- Assess pain regularly as part of standard ward observations.
- Use one opioid at a time, prescribed appropriately.
- Use a multimodal approach – i.e. a combination of paracetamol plus NSAIDs plus opioid and local anaesthetic – when there are no contraindications.
- Prescribe analgesics regularly rather than 'as required'.
- Administer analgesics pre-emptively where pain is expected.
- Plan your technique preoperatively and discuss this with the patient, especially with patient-controlled analgesia.
- Ensure that staff caring for the patient have the knowledge and skills (including clinical guidelines) required to manage postoperative pain.
- Non-pharmacological techniques, such as relaxation techniques, education and positioning, are important in helping to reduce pain and may reduce the dose of drugs required.
- Unexpected pain or increasing pain should be investigated.

In developing strategies to improve management of acute pain, it is important to base these on the best evidence available, with careful assessment of both safety and efficacy for any intervention.[173]

ASSESSMENT OF ACUTE POSTOPERATIVE PAIN

Poor pain assessment is a major barrier to good pain management,[174] while regular pain assessment using pain charts has been shown to increase the quality of analgesia.[175,176] Research and detailed audit assessment of pain often uses complex tools to study all aspects of the pain experience (cognitive, affective, etc.); these tools are not practical for daily clinical practice, so a much simpler assessment tool is required (Table 5.10).[177] Because pain is a uniquely subjective experience varying between individuals, it has been argued that attempting to quantify pain is misleading.[178] To be useful a rating scale must be simple, with minimal reassessment variability, and be sensitive enough to reflect responses to treatment. A 100-mm drawn line, called a visual analogue scale, is commonly used. It has been shown to be reliable over time, with little to choose between it and an 11-point numerical rating scale. Both have been shown to be more robust in clinical use than a four-point verbal rating scale also commonly used.[179,180] It has been found that a visual analogue scale score for pain severity of over 30 mm was equivalent to moderate or greater pain.[181] The use of simple global rating scales has received attention as a means of comparing treatment efficacy.

TRENDS IN ACUTE POSTOPERATIVE PAIN MANAGEMENT (Box 5.11)

Multimodal analgesia

There is good evidence of the benefits of employing multimodal analgesia after surgery.[182] This involves combining analgesic drugs that work by different mechanisms; NSAIDs, paracetamol, local anaesthetics, other non-opioid analgesics and opioids given in combination improve analgesia and reduce side effects.[183] In this scheme, the non-opioid drugs contribute significantly to the recovery of the patient by minimizing opioid side effects (e.g. ileus) by reducing the total opioid consumption. Evidence suggests that multimodal analgesia after major surgery can hasten recovery and reduce costs.[184] From this concept has grown the notion of *accelerated recovery* or *acute rehabilitation*. This approach requires superb postoperative pain management to facilitate early mobilization and oral feeding.[182] The inclusion of a locoregional technique using local anaesthetic agents can provide excellent

REFERENCES

173. McQuay H, Moore A. An Evidence-based Resource for Pain Relief. Oxford University Press, Oxford, 1998
174. Von Roenn JH, Cleeland CS, Gonin R et al. Ann Intern Med 1993; 119: 121–126
175. Rawal N, Berggren L. Pain 1994; 57: 117–123
176. Gould TH, Crosby DL, Harmer M et al. Br Med J 1992; 305: 1187–1193
177. McQuay H, Moore A, Justins DM. Br Med J 1997; 314: 1531–1535
178. Cox P. Anaesthesia 2001; 56: 499–500
179. DeLoach LJ, Higgins MS, Caplan AB et al. Anesth Analg 1998; 86: 102–106
180. Hartrick CT. Clin J Pain 2001; 17: 104–105
181. Collins SL, Moore RA, McQuay HJ. Pain 1997; 72: 95–97
182. Kehlet H, Dahl JB. Anesth Analg 1993; 77: 1048–1056
183. Cousins MJ, Power I. In: Wall PD, Melzack R (eds). Textbook of Pain. 4th edn. Churchill Livingstone, London, 1999
184. Brodner G, Van Aken H, Hertle L et al. Anesth Analg 2001; 92: 1594–1600

pain relief on movement, allowing early mobilization, and is therefore a fundamental component of 'fast-track' surgery.

NOTES ON INDIVIDUAL DRUGS

Paracetamol

Systematic reviews have found that paracetamol is effective when taken alone or in combination with NSAIDs for mild to moderate pain or as an adjunct to opioids.[185,186] It is a drug with a good safety record when used in recommended doses.

Non-steroidal anti-inflammatory drugs

Systematic reviews have found that NSAIDs are effective for mild to moderate pain and are useful adjuncts for severe pain.[173,185] However, NSAID use is restricted by side effects: peptic ulceration, antiplatelet actions, aspirin-induced asthma, and renal dysfunction. A review has indicated that new agents that selectively inhibit the inducible form of cyclo-oxygenase (COX-2) and spare the constitutive COX-1 that provides various physiological tissue functions (e.g. prostaglandin protection of the gastroduodenal mucosa and thromboxane-induced platelet aggregation) could represent a significant safety advance and permit their more widespread use for acute pain relief.[187]

Opioids

Opioids are the mainstay of the management of moderate to severe pain, but they have significant side effects: sedation, respiratory depression, nausea and vomiting, depression of gastrointestinal motility, and disruption of sleep patterns to name but a few.[176] Possibly the most serious limitation of opioid use is inability to control movement-associated pain after surgery. Generally, patients given systemic opioids after major surgery achieve adequate analgesia at rest but not during movement, when they may suffer severe discomfort. As a result, the patient minimizes any movement, but modern postoperative rehabilitation regimens following major surgery are dependent on analgesia that encourages mobilization.[188]

Tramadol is a synthetic analgesic with both opioid agonist and central nervous system effects through noradrenergic and serotonergic pathways. It has been reported to produce minimal sedation, respiratory depression and gastrointestinal stasis, and does not appear to have any abuse potential. Tramadol has been shown to be as effective as morphine in providing postoperative analgesia while permitting more rapid psychomotor recovery.[189]

Opioids may be administered by many routes. The secret to their successful use is as follows.

- Choose one opioid (e.g. morphine) and stick with it! More than one opioid prescribed simultaneously usually means that not enough of any single opioid has been given.
- Choose a route to administer the opioid. On general wards use either the oral (p.o.), intramuscular or subcutaneous (i.m./s.c.), or intravenous patient-controlled (i.v.-PCA) routes. Intravenous (i.v.) opioid infusions and boluses should generally not be undertaken outside critical care areas. The route used to administer the opioid does not affect the potency of the drug, merely the dose required and time taken to achieve pain relief.
- Choose the mode of opioid delivery, either bolus injection or continuous infusion.
- Achieve pain relief by 'titrating' small aliquots of opioid to the pain.
- Convert to oral opioids as soon as gastric and small bowel function return to normal and the patient can tolerate oral fluids.

Traditionally, the intramuscular route has been used to treat postoperative pain because of its simplicity and widespread applicability, the fixed dose of drug being given on a pro re nata (as necessary) basis. This method of postoperative analgesia is frequently unsatisfactory for many reasons, the most obvious being that administration of a standard dose of opioid ignores the wide between-patient and even within-patient variability in opioid requirements. There is little flexibility with this method, and frequently the postoperative analgesia it provides is inadequate. If the intramuscular route is to be more effectively used, frequent patient assessment is needed, with adjustments of dose and frequency to achieve optimal pain relief. Ideally opioid administration should start with an appropriate prescription (agent, dose, frequency and route of administration) individualized for each patient. The patient's response (pain relief and adverse effects) should then be repeatedly monitored, and the prescription altered accordingly to maximize analgesia and minimize side effects: titration of drug against clinical effect. Individual opioid requirements in the postoperative period vary considerably (up to 10-fold), and in adults age has been shown to be a better predictor of opioid requirements in the first 24 h after surgery than weight. This relationship can be used as a guide to prescribing opioids by either parenteral or enteral routes.

Patient-controlled analgesia

Patient-controlled analgesia is a technique whereby patients self-administer small doses of usually intravenous opioids, thereby titrating the opioid to achieve their pain needs. The danger of the system is related mainly to third-person intervention (e.g. clinical staff and relatives) rather than to equipment malfunction or incorrect prescribing, although these have been reported. Most patient-controlled analgesia devices consist of a microprocessor-controlled syringe pump triggered by depressing a button. A preset bolus dose of opioid is then delivered into a dedicated intravenous line. Alternatively, the intravenous patient-controlled analgesia may be attached to a pre-existing intravenous fluid infusion, provided a one-way valve is placed to prevent retrograde passage of the opioid up the drip set. A timer prevents further bolus doses being delivered until a specified period has elapsed (the lockout period). The prescriber sets the bolus dose and the lockout period, and may additionally set an overall dose limit for a longer period of time, usually a 4-h total dose limit. Some devices can deliver a continuous background infusion, although it is better to avoid this when constant surveillance is not available. If a continuous infusion is added to patient-controlled analgesia, it offers no advantage over patient-controlled analgesia alone.

REFERENCES

185. McQuay HJ. In: Tramer MJ (ed). Evidence Based Resource in Anaesthesia and Analgesia. BMJ Books, London, 2000: 87–103
186. Schug SA, Sidebotham DA, Mcguinnety M et al. Anesth Analg 1998; 87: 368–372
187. Kam PCA, Power I. Pain Rev 2000; 7: 3–13
188. Kehlet H. Reg Anesth 1996; 21: 149–151
189. Coetzee JF, Vanloggerenberg H. Br J Anaesth 1998; 81: 737–741

Patient-controlled analgesia does not cause more opioid side effects than pro re nata intramuscular opioid regimens and has a good safety record, except when excessive doses are prescribed or a background infusion included. Intravenous patient-controlled analgesia satisfies the needs of both patients and staff because it provides a perception of patient autonomy, eliminates time delays in providing analgesia, avoids painful intramuscular injections, and increases ease of nursing. Morphine remains the most popular opioid administered by this route. Use of the intravenous patient-controlled analgesia pump should be preceded by the administration of a loading dose of the drug by the anaesthetist giving the anaesthetic. Patient-controlled analgesia opioids may also be administered by the subcutaneous route using the same equipment but with a more concentrated solution of the drug to minimize the volume required.

The effectiveness of the system depends on the dose of drug given and the lockout period. Too low a dose may result in poor pain control and loss of confidence by the patient and ward staff, too high a dose produces unacceptable side effects. Too long a lockout period results in poor pain control, while too short a period may lead to overdosage. Patients also need preoperative instruction on how to use the device.

Local anaesthetic techniques

Systematic reviews have found that the use of local anaesthetics for central neural blockade is effective for the relief of postoperative pain, is opioid sparing, and therefore facilitates earlier rehabilitation. In addition, neural components of the stress response to acute injury are blunted by epidural local anaesthesia, and this can be associated with a reduction in perioperative complications.[184,190] A cumulative meta-analysis of randomized, controlled trials on the comparative effects of postoperative analgesic therapies on pulmonary outcome confirmed that the use of epidural analgesia is associated with less postoperative respiratory morbidity.[190] Multimodal perioperative management after major urological surgery, employing thoracic epidural analgesia to enable mobilization and oral nutrition, reduces hormonal and metabolic stress and aids convalescence.[184] Epidural local anaesthetics are often used in combination with low doses of epidural opioids, which are added to improve the analgesia. Unfortunately, even small opioid doses given spinally produce urinary retention, urticaria, nausea and vomiting, and a reduction in gut motility. For example, epidural morphine but not bupivacaine inhibits gastric motility on the day after cholecystectomy.[191]

Ketamine

The value of low-dose ketamine in the management of acute postoperative pain was confirmed in a 1999 review: ketamine reduces postoperative morphine requirements.[192] Unfortunately, even low doses of ketamine can produce side effects such as hallucinations, and alternative NMDA antagonists (e.g. dextramethorphan) are being assessed.[193] Low-dose ketamine is also effective for the relief of neuropathic pain.

Clonidine

Clonidine and other α_2 adrenergic receptor agonists can provide effective postoperative analgesia,[194] although side effects of sedation and hypotension limit their general use. Traditional use has concentrated on spinal or epidural administration of clonidine to take advantage of the known attenuating effect of stimulating spinal α_2 adrenergic receptors on pain perception.

Box 5.12 Some features of neuropathic pain

Clinical features suggestive of neuropathic pain include:

- A precipitating event that may have caused nerve damage.
- A delay between the precipitating event and the onset of pain.
- Little or no obvious tissue damage discernible at presentation.
- Pain variously described as spontaneous or paroxysmal, or burning, stabbing, pulsing, electric shock-like, or dysaesthetic (an unpleasant, abnormal sensation).
- Secondary hyperalgesia, allodynia and hyperpathia (increased pain threshold and repetitive stimulation causing a summation of pain) may be present.
- Sensory loss in the painful area.
- Pain provocation by tapping neuromas (radiating electric shock-like), for example Tinel sign
- Lack of effectiveness of opioid drugs, often with escalating doses, does not specifically identify neuropathic pain but is an indication.

Antidepressants and anticonvulsants

Systematic reviews confirm that tricyclic antidepressants and anticonvulsants are effective for the relief of neuropathic pain.[173]

Acute postoperative neuropathic pain

Neuropathic pain is common after some surgical operations, and attempts must be made to prevent chronicity.[195,196] The problem is dysfunction in the peripheral or central nervous system. Possible causes include nerve damage by surgical section, compression, stretching, ischaemia or infection. Changes in the spinal processing of nociceptive signals can take place in only days and could explain the lack of efficacy of pre-emptive analgesia. Neuropathic pain is more likely in the postoperative period, when persistent central changes may be favoured (e.g. inadequate analgesia in the perioperative period, large operations and pre-existing pain).[195] Some common features of neuropathic pain are outlined in Box 5.12. Perioperative neuropathic pain can be managed initially with systemic lidocaine (lignocaine; 1 mg/kg per hour) or ketamine (5–10 mg/h), and later with an oral tricyclic antidepressant or anticonvulsant.

Pre-emptive analgesia

It has been proposed that effective analgesia given prior to an insult can act pre-emptively and reduce central neural sensitization and postoperative pain.[197] Evidence of this from animal experiments is convincing, but clinical studies are less impressive. Pre-emptive therapy with a single agent given before surgery is likely to fail, as afferent neuronal activity into the spinal cord continues for some time afterwards. To have any chance of producing a clinically significant effect, pre-emptive analgesia

REFERENCES

190. Ballantyne JC, Carr DB, Deferranti S et al. Anesth Analg 1998; 86: 598–612
191. Thorn SE, Wattwil M, Naslund I. Reg Anesth 1992; 17: 91–94
192. Schmid RL, Sandler AN, Katz J. Pain 1999; 82: 111–125
193. Grace RF, Power I, Zammit A et al. Anesth Analg 1998; 87: 1135–1138
194. Sandler AN. Canadian J Anaesthesia 1996; 43: 1191–1194
195. Cousins MJ, Power I, Smith G. Reg Analg Pain Med 2000; 25: 6–21
196. Perkins FM, Kehlet H. Anesthesiology 2000; 93: 1123–1133
197. Woolf Q, Chong MS. Anesth Analg 1993; 77: 362–379

must include a strategy for modulating the sustained neuronal input into the spinal cord into the postoperative period.[195]

THE PROBLEMS OF AMPUTEES[200]

Amputation of limbs and removal of viscera are sometimes associated with painful sequelae, which are commonly described as phantom pains. Other painful and non-painful neurological phenomena are also associated with amputated limbs, for example stump pain.

As many as 60–80% of amputees may complain of phantom limb pain shortly after limb removal, with about 10% suffering persistent, severe, often incapacitating pain. The syndrome is not influenced by age, gender, or the pathology necessitating amputation. It is less common in young children. There are conflicting reports associating preamputation pain with phantom pain. The onset of the pain is often within a week of amputation and is believed to gradually diminish with time (often years). The pain is usually intermittent, often occurring at least daily, and only a few patients are in constant pain. The duration of attacks is usually measured in seconds, minutes or hours, rarely days. The character of the pain is variously described as shooting, pricking, boring, stabbing, squeezing, throbbing and burning. The pain is usually located distally in the amputated limb. The experience of pain can be modulated by attention distraction, anxiety, autonomic events and environmental conditions. Rarely, appearance of the pain has been reported following spinal anaesthesia in previously pain-free patients.

Almost all amputees experience stump pain immediately after amputation. Between 5 and 21% of patients' pain may persist. Stimulating the stump, for example pressing on tender neuromata, easily precipitates these pains. Spontaneous stump movements that are painful are reported. There may be an association between stump and phantom pain.

The underlying mechanisms are not fully defined, but clearly amputation is the severest form of nerve injury and involves a combination of peripheral, spinal and supraspinal mechanisms, which is reflected in the fact that persisting phantom limb pain is difficult to manage, causes significant distress to the sufferer, and consumes significant amounts of healthcare resources. A discussion of the management of chronic phantom pain is beyond the scope of this chapter, but perioperative neuraxial (notably epidural) and peripheral neural blockade may help to reduce the incidence of phantom limb and stump pains, but unfortunately the evidence is conflicting.

MANAGEMENT OF ACUTE PAIN IN OPIOID-TOLERANT PATIENTS[199]

This is a difficult area of clinical practice that challenges the personal values and beliefs of clinical staff. The fact remains that patients who, for whatever reason, consume opioids in their daily lives do suffer acutely painful episodes and are no less deserving of appropriate treatment than anyone else. Opioid users fall into one of the three categories described below.

- Addicted: addiction is a psychological state that translates into drug-seeking behaviours and is marked by compulsion, loss of control over use, and ongoing use despite physical or social harm.
- Physically dependent: withdrawal phenomena develop after cessation or antagonism of a drug.
- Pseudoaddicted: the term *pseudoaddiction* has been coined to describe patients who exhibit drug-seeking behaviour, resembling addiction, in response to unrelieved pain.

Confusing the terminology can lead to catastrophic breakdowns of patient–healthcarer relationships, to the detriment of all concerned. The term *pseudoaddiction* is very relevant to pain arising after surgery. It describes those patients who demand opioids and can exhibit other drug-seeking behaviours, invariably entering into conflict with their healthcarers. This arises simply because their prescribed pain relief is inadequate for their needs. This situation is not infrequently observed among cancer patients, who develop tolerances just as addicts do.

This 'physical dependence' on opioids will be manifested as a withdrawal (or abstinence) syndrome if the drug is acutely ceased or antagonized. The clinical features of an opioid withdrawal syndrome include yawning, sweating, lacrimation, rhinorrhoea, anxiety, papillary dilatation, piloerection and chills ('cold turkey'), tachycardia, hypertension, nausea and vomiting, cramping abdominal pains, and diarrhoea. Development of opioid withdrawal syndrome postoperatively can potentially seriously affect patient outcome. This is not the time for healthcarers to indulge in moral indignation and deprive these patients of their continuing 'baseline' opioid requirements and additional opioids to relieve the acute postoperative pain. This is also not the time to embark on an 'opioid addiction rehabilitation programme'.

Generally the management plan should include the following:

- Involve local drug and alcohol services or liaison psychiatry early in the management of opioid abusers.
- Identify the group to which the patient belongs and the extent of the problem.
- Accept that any pain-scoring system is not likely to be reliable; opioid abusers in particular often have very unrealistic expectations of what constitutes pain relief and report high pain scores while heavily sedated.
- Design a management plan (to which all staff should adhere) with ward staff and the patient as soon as possible preoperatively. The patient should be assured that the staff aim to give good pain relief but that patient safety is paramount. Pethidine should be avoided at ever-higher doses because it may precipitate norpethidine toxicity.
- Calculate the baseline opioid requirements of cancer and chronic pain sufferers from all oral opioids used.
- Transfer back to oral opioid as soon as is practical, using a long-acting opioid. Opioid abusers can recommence their preoperative methadone dosage with oral morphine for residual acute pain.
- Set expected goals of dosage, route of administration, and time frame with the patient.
- The goal for opioid abusers should be discharge on methadone into the care of a drug and alcohol service. Unfortunately, not all opioid abusers will want to enter a methadone programme.

Intravenous patient-controlled analgesia opioids are regarded as useful for both groups of patients. Baseline opioid requirements can be provided by a background infusion (to prevent withdrawal), and additional opioid required to manage the acute postoperative pain can be provided by an increased bolus

REFERENCES

198. Jensen TS, Nikolajsen L. In: Wall PD, Melzack R (eds). Textbook of Pain. 4th edn. Churchill Livingstone, London, 1999: 799–814
199. Macintyre P, Ready LB. Acute Pain Management: a Practical Guide. WB Saunders, London, 1996

requirement with the usual lockout period. The baseline and acute pain requirements can be provided by the oral route once it is re-established. Patients given high doses of opioids for as little as 7 to 10 days for any reason may exhibit a withdrawal syndrome on acute cessation of the drug. In the context of acute postoperative pain, as the acute pain subsides a natural opioid 'weaning' process occurs as less opioid is required day by day. The clinical features of withdrawal can be prevented by dose reductions of 10–25% daily depending on the chronicity of the usage.

DAY-STAY SURGERY

Good recovery after day surgery requires a swift return to 'street fitness' and ongoing freedom from pain, nausea, vomiting and other complications. Good pain management in this context is challenging and has not always been satisfactory. Surveys have found that about 30% of patients suffer moderate to severe pain in the first 24 h after day-stay surgery.[200,201] Other studies have shown that pain is a common reason for delayed discharge and unplanned hospital admission after day surgery,[202] as well as a common reason for patients subsequently to consult a general practitioner. Analgesic techniques used in day surgery should ideally be safe (especially when administered at home), effective, devoid of side effects, and cost-effective. No single technique exists that will satisfy these requirements, and in practice analgesia is best achieved by a combination of drugs and techniques.

ACUTE PAIN SERVICES

There are three ways to deal with the problem of globally poor acute postoperative pain management: pin our hopes to magic pharmacological bullets, ignore the problem, or maximize the effectiveness of our existing resources. The logical way of achieving the last of these is by developing acute pain services. The aim of acute pain services is to provide safe and effective postoperative pain management for all patients. The organization of acute pain services requires a reappraisal of the traditional approach to managing postoperative pain.[203] Adoption of a high-tech approach will benefit only a small number of patients,[204] and if unsupervised may increase the rates of adverse incidents. The new multidisciplinary approach of acute pain services is being developed by increasing numbers of hospitals across Europe, North America and Australasia[205,206] following the recommendations from many governmental and non-governmental bodies.[207–209]

MANAGEMENT OF PAIN ASSOCIATED WITH PAEDIATRIC SURGERY

The management of acute postoperative pain in children has also been reported to need improvement.[210] Once again, the problem revolves around the same myths and fears that have thwarted adult patients, with a few extra for good measure, including 'children experience less pain than adults', 'neonates don't experience or remember pain', 'children cannot localize or describe their pain' and 'pain is character-building for children'. As in adults, there is no evidence that the use of opioids for treatment of severe pain in children leads to opioid dependence or addiction.

Managing acute postoperative pain management in children is challenging. As in adults, pain management should encompass pharmacological and non-pharmacological strategies. Good pain relief needs to be attained in recovery before the child is discharged to the ward or the home. As in adult practice, postoperative analgesia using the oral route is preferable.

CLINICAL ASSESSMENT OF PAIN IN CHILDREN

The pain rating scale chosen should be appropriate for the age and cognitive development of the child. Self-reporting scales of pain intensity appear to be reliable in children over 4 years of age,[211,212] and numerous pain rating scales have been devised for children of all ages, from neonates[213] to older children; the latter usually involve a modified visual analogue scale, for example Poker Chip Tool[214] and Wong–Baker Faces.[215]

Valuable information can be gleaned by observing non-verbal behavioural cues, remembering that a quiet, withdrawn child may be in severe pain. Physiological signs, such as tachycardia, may play a key role in very young children but need to be interpreted in the clinical context. Pain ratings provided by parents or regular carers can be valid and reliable,[216] and the ability to console children may help to distinguish pain from other causes of distress, such as parental separation, an unfamiliar environment, and hunger and thirst with fasting.

PHARMACOLOGICAL STRATEGIES

The choice of drug therapy for managing postoperative pain is influenced by the child's age, type of surgery, presence of comorbidities, and postoperative care environment. Generally:

- Pain following minor surgery can usually be managed with oral paracetamol and NSAIDs. If paracetamol is used as the sole analgesic, higher doses are required.[217] For day-stay surgery, parents need to be given sufficient information to manage residual pain.
- For major surgery, parenteral opioids remain the mainstay of postoperative pain management. Local anaesthetic blocks

REFERENCES

200. Audit Commission of England and Wales. A Short Cut to Better Services: Day Surgery in England and Wales. HMSO, London, 1990
201. Hawkshaw D. Br J Nurs 1994; 3: 348–350
202. Gold BS, Kitz DS, Lecky H et al. JAMA 1989; 262: 3008–3010
203. Rawal N, Berggren L. Pain 1994; 57: 117–123
204. Ready LB et al. Anesthesiology 1988; 68: 100–106
205. Rawal N, Allvin R. Eur J Anaesthesiol 1998; 15: 354–363
206. Semple P, Jackson IJB. Anaesthesia 1991; 46: 1074–1076
207. Ready LB, Ashburn M, Caplan RA et al. Anesthesiology 1995; 82: 1071–1081
208. Wheatley RG, Madej TH, Jackson IJB et al. Br J Anaesth 1991; 67: 353–359
209. Cartwright PD, Helfinger RG, Howell JJ et al. Anaesthesia 1991; 46: 188–191
210. Mather L, Mackie J. Pain 1983; 15: 271–282
211. Maunuksela EL, Olkkola KT, Korpela R. Clin Pharmacol Ther 1987; 42: 137–141
212. Finley GA, McGrath PJ. Prog Pain Res Manage, Vol 10. IASP, Seattle, 1998
213. Krechel SW, Bildner J. Paediatric Anaesthesia 1995; 5: 53–61
214. Hester NO, Foster RL. In: Tyler DC, Krane EJ (eds). Advances in Pain Research and Therapy: Pediatric Pain, Vol 15. Raven Press, New York, 1990: 79–84
215. Whaley L, Wong D. Nursing Care of Infants and Children. 4th edn. Mosby-Yearbook, St Louis, 1991
216. Wilson GA, Doyle E. Anaesthesia 1996; 51: 1005–1007
217. Anderson BJ, Woolard GA, Holford NHG. Paediatr Anaesth 1996; 24: 669–673

initiated preoperatively and intraoperatively are being increasingly used for pain management following major surgery.

Paracetamol

Paracetamol is a safe and effective agent in children and infants (including neonates for short courses at recommended doses),[218] administered orally or rectally. For acute postoperative pain it can be used as part of a multimodal approach. It has a good safety record and appears to be safe up to 100 mg/kg per day in children and up to 60 mg/kg per day in neonates.

Non-steroidal anti-inflammatory drugs

Diclofenac (0.5–1 mg/kg, 8-hourly, orally) or ibuprofen (4–10 mg/kg, every 6–8 h, orally) are frequently used to manage pain in children. The contraindications to their use are the same as those for adult patients. Aspirin should be used with caution because of the risk of precipitating Reye's syndrome. Little data are available on the parenteral use of NSAIDs in children.

Opioids

Opioid administration in children requires routine repeated monitoring, including a pain score and sedation score in addition to the traditional routine ward observation of heart rate, respiratory rate (and effort), blood pressure and temperature.[219] As in adults, a decrease in respiratory rate may be a late sign of opioid-induced respiratory depression. Pulse oximetry is a valuable adjunct to clinical observation. Respiratory depression may be greater with pethidine than with morphine at equianalgesic doses.[220] As in adults, morphine is the drug of first choice, with fentanyl as an alternative when morphine is absolutely or relatively contraindicated. The neurotoxicity of pethidine's metabolite norpethidine should eliminate its use in children and adults. Side effects should be managed with similar agents to those used in adults, remembering that young children may have difficulty expressing subjective symptoms such as pruritus, nausea and constipation.

In the past, minimal amounts of opioids were administered to infants intraoperatively due to concerns about respiratory and haemodynamic side effects. The pharmacokinetics of opioids are widely variable among preterm and full-term neonates and infants, with increased elimination half-life,[221–223] so the initial and infusion dose for infants up to 6 months of age should be reduced.[224] Where opioid analgesia is administered to infants, they should be cared for and monitored by experienced staff in an appropriate environment, operating within clear clinical guidelines and with access to immediate respiratory support facilities and resuscitation equipment. The long-term effects of opioids on pain pathway development are unknown.[225]

Oral route

Codeine is commonly used for mild to moderate pain and when converting from parenteral to enteral routes of administration at a dose of 0.3–1.0 mg/kg every 4–6 h. Codeine has good oral bioavailability, and it is converted to morphine except in the 10% of adults who lack the converting enzyme. Constipation is a frequent complaint with regular dosing and should be treated prophylactically. Ideally codeine should be used in conjunction with non-opioid analgesics such as paracetamol and NSAIDs (multimodal analgesia). Morphine sulphate may be used in the management of continuing acute pain states, for example burns. Slow-release morphine preparations may be used in these situations when the daily morphine dose is stable, using the normal preparation for breakthrough pain.

Intramuscular route

Parenteral administration may be needed in the postoperative period, but intermittent intramuscular injections provide poor analgesia, and are painful and frightening to children. This route may be of use for a single dose of opioid if the pain is severe and no other route of administration is available.

Subcutaneous route

Morphine has similar absorption characteristics if given by either subcutaneous or intramuscular routes. Morphine administered via an indwelling subcutaneous cannula (inserted while the child is anaesthetized)[226] offers advantages for postoperative pain management in children because it seems to satisfy nurses, patients and parents alike, and is flexible (it may be used for intermittent injections and continuous infusion).[227] This route requires adequate peripheral perfusion and is not recommended in a shocked or hypothermic child.

Intravenous route

Opioids can be administered by the intravenous route but only in critical care areas as:

- intermittent boluses of morphine in a dose of 0.03–0.05 mg/kg, until the child is comfortable; or
- continuous infusion of morphine (0.01–0.04 mg/kg per hour) for children over 6 months of age,[228–230] which avoids the plasma morphine variations associated with intermittent boluses.

PATIENT-CONTROLLED ANALGESIA

Intravenous patient-controlled analgesia provides safe and effective analgesia in children as young as 5 years of age[231] and is possibly more effective than intermittent intramuscular injections in the older child.[232] It can be used as it is with adults, for example an intravenous bolus dose of morphine 0.01–0.02 mg/kg with a 5-min lockout period. Postoperative analgesia may be improved, without increasing the side effects, by including a small background infusion (e.g. morphine 5 μg/kg per hour.[233] As with

REFERENCES

218. Berde CB. Pediatr Clin North Am 1989; 36: 921–940
219. Morton NS. Paediatr Anaesth 1993; 3: 179–184
220. Hamunen K. Br J Anaesth 1993; 70: 414–418
221. Lynn AM, Slattery JT. Anesthesiology 1987; 66: 136–139
222. Choonara I, Ekbom Y, Lindstrom B et al. Br J Clin Pharmacol 1990; 30: 897–900
223. Barrett DA, Elias-Jones AC, Rutter N et al. Br J Clin Pharmacol 1991; 32: 31–37
224. McRorie TI, Lynn AM, Nespeca MK et al. Am J Dis Child 1992; 146: 972–976
225. Aynsley-Green A. Paediatr Anaesth 1996; 6: 167–172
226. Lamacraft G, Cooper MG, Cavaletto BP. J Pain Symptom Manage 1997; 13: 43–49
227. McNicol LR. Br J Anaesth 1993; 71: 396–399
228. Bray RJ. Anaesthesia 1983; 38: 1075–1078
229. Hendrickson M, Myre L, Johnson DG et al. J Pediatr Surg 1990; 25: 185–191
230. Lynn AM, Opein KE, Tyler DC. Crit Care Med 1984; 12: 863–866
231. Caukroger PB, Chapman MJ, Davey RB. Burns 991; 17: 396–399
232. Berde CB, Lehn BM, Yee JD et al. J Pediatri 1991; 118: 460–466
233. Doyle E, Harper I, Morton NS. Br J Anaesth 1993; 71: 818–822

adults, the safety and effectiveness of the technique is likely to be maximized if clear and repeated instruction in its use is provided, the patient alone activates the patient-controlled analgesia machine, and regular assessment of pain and side effects is undertaken. Patient-controlled analgesia may be unsuitable for children less than 5 years old, older children with developmental delay, those with altered levels of consciousness, and those unable to understand the idea of patient-controlled analgesia. Care must be exercised in children who have renal failure, using a lower bolus dose, close monitoring and no background infusion. Side effects are managed in a similar way to those in adults.

LOCOREGIONAL ANALGESIA

Locoregional techniques are increasingly used in children and infants (including neonates) for anaesthesia and postoperative analgesia. The anatomical differences of children must be borne in mind when performing locoregional techniques, with close adherence to mass of local anaesthetic agent used if toxicity is to be avoided. The volume of local anaesthetic solution required to achieve a satisfactory locoregional block in children is relatively larger (on a body weight basis) than with adults. Generally there are no special requirements for the postoperative care of patients receiving routine locoregional single-shot analgesia, although parents need to be made aware of the likely duration of blockade and any precautions that may be required. However, audal blocks may prevent discharge after day-stay surgery, due to the problem of leg weakness and inability to void urine.

Peripheral nerve blocks

Wound filtration with local anaesthetic agents may be used as an adjunct to postoperative analgesia after many surgical procedures in children and adults, and as the sole analgesic technique for many minor day-case procedures. Bupivacaine 0.25% is frequently used for this purpose, there being no evidence that higher concentrations achieve better or prolonged analgesia. Ropivacaine may become the agent of choice by virtue of its lower potential for cardiotoxicity and lesser motor blockade. Ilio-inguinal and iliohypogastric block provides good postoperative analgesia after groin surgery.[234] EMLA cream can do much to reduce the pain and fear of injections for painful procedures such as lumbar puncture, combined if necessary with sedation. It should be applied generously under an occlusive dressing at least an hour before the procedure. EMLA should be used with care in the newborn infant, and application restricted to one site per day because there is potential for methaemoglobinaemia secondary to prilocaine absorption. Its use in the first week of life in premature neonates of less than 32 weeks' gestation is not recommended.[235]

Epidural analgesia

Continuous epidural infusions are safe and effective for postoperative analgesia in children after thoracic, abdominal, urological and orthopaedic procedures, provided there is close monitoring by experienced staff, operating with clear clinical guidelines, in an appropriate environment. The haemodynamic and respiratory effects appear minimal compared with those in adults.[236] There is limited information on the pharmacokinetics of such infusions, but maximum local anaesthetic doses must be adhered to.[237,238] Infants under 1 year of age should have continuous cardiorespiratory monitoring, and regular observation should include pain score, sedation score, extent of motor blockade, and cardiorespiratory parameters, as well as checking of the infusion rate. All infusions should be delivered with an appropriate volumetric pump, and ideally solutions for epidural infusion should be prepared within a central sterile suite under the supervision of a pharmacist. An anaesthetist should be available on site to deal with any problems, in particular inadequate analgesia due to block regression. The overall management should remain under the care of the anaesthetist initiating the block, with appropriate on-call anaesthetic cover after hours, preferably within the context of an acute pain service.

Caudal analgesia

The approach to the epidural space is a versatile technique for providing both operative and postoperative analgesia for a wide variety of procedures. Prolonged sacral analgesia in in-patients can be achieved by supplementation with caudal morphine 20–30 μg/kg, provided that appropriate facilities are available for respiratory monitoring. The analgesic blockade can be extended by placement of a caudal epidural catheter and the use of an infusion, as for lumbar epidural analgesia. The addition of adrenaline (epinephrine) to bupivacaine does not appear to reduce absorption, as it does for lidocaine (lignocaine), and therefore does not permit a larger dose to be used; however, adrenaline has been shown to significantly prolong caudal blockade in infants and younger children.[239]

PSYCHOLOGICAL STRATEGIES

Children's fear and anxiety of impending surgical procedures may be reduced by psychological preparation.[240,241] It would also seem sensible to familiarize the child with environments, equipment and procedures preoperatively and to maintain the child in contact with parents or carers up to the induction of anaesthesia, which may decrease postoperative pain.[242] The least painful route, when possible along with use of EMLA patches, should give premedication.

REFERENCES

234. Trotter C, Martin P, Youngson G et al. Paediatr Anaesth 1995; 5; 363–367
235. Gourrier E, Karoubi P, El Hanache A et al. Pain 1996; 68: 431–434
236. Murat I, Delleur MM, Esteve C et al. Br J Anaesth 1987; 69: 1441
237. Berde CB. Anesth Analg 1992; 75; 164–166
238. Eyres RI. Paediatr Anaesth 1995; 22: 213–218
239. Warner MA, Kunkel SE, Offord SO et al. Anesth Analg 1987; 66: 995–998
240. Ferguson BF. Pediatrics 1979; 64: 656–664
241. Woffer J, Visintainer M. Pediatrics 1979; 64: 646–655
242. Schofield N, White J. Br Med J 1989; 299: 1371–1375

Burns

6

Peter Dziewulski

INTRODUCTION

The skin is the largest organ in the body, and burn injury to the skin can range from being relatively trivial to one of the most severe injuries that humans can sustain. Major burn injury often requires admission to intensive care, multiple surgical procedures to achieve wound healing followed by prolonged rehabilitation, and possibly a lifetime of reconstructive procedures to achieve psychosocial, aesthetic and functional recovery.

HISTORY

Neanderthal cave paintings have been found depicting burn treatment. Hippocrates (400 BC), Celsus (first century AD) and Galen (second century AD) all wrote on burn wound care. Ambroise Paré (1510–90) described burn wound excision. Dupuytren (1832) described six degrees of burn depth that remain in use today. The 20th century has brought great advances in burn care. These include the scientific understanding of fluid loss and resuscitation (Underhill 1920, Evans 1952), the hypermetabolic response to trauma (Sneve 1905, Wilmore 1974), and the control of infection with topical antimicrobial agents (Moyer 1965, Fox 1969). In 1870, Pollock first described skin grafting of a burn. In 1960, Jackson and colleagues pioneered excision and grafting. Janzekovic (1970) developed the technique of tangential excision of deep partial-thickness burns. Further advances in wound resurfacing, such as the use of cultured skin and the development of artificial skin, are more recent innovations.[1]

INCIDENCE

It is estimated that burn injury affects approximately a quarter of a million people in the UK each year. About 175 000 of these attend accident and emergency departments, and 13 000 patients with burn injuries require hospital admission. Approximately 1000 patients per year are severely burnt and require formal fluid resuscitation. There are an average of 300 deaths from burns per year in the UK.[2] The UK figures are representative of most of the developed world, although the USA has an even higher incidence. Burns are an even more major problem in developing countries, with a much higher incidence and mortality.

About half of all admissions to burn units in the UK are of children between the ages of 1 and 5 years, and sadly the incidence of injury in this age group remains static. The other vulnerable group is the elderly, and the incidence of burns in this cohort of patients is increasing. The incidence of major burn injury in the UK is, however, decreasing.[2]

PREVENTION

Ninety per cent of burn injuries are preventable. Prevention has traditionally been dependent on education or legislation. There have been numerous educational campaigns that have successfully modified people's behaviour. Legislation has also been effective; examples include laws that demand sprinkler systems and smoke detectors in public and commercial buildings, and those that ensure safe transport and storage of flammable materials.

CLASSIFICATION

A burn is defined as coagulative destruction of the surface layers of the body. Burn injuries can be classified according to their aetiology, depth, and the percentage of body surface area involved.

The skin is made up of the epidermis and dermis, with the adnexal structures such as the hair follicles, sweat and sebaceous glands residing in the deeper layers of the dermis. These adnexal structures are important because they are the source of proliferating epithelial cells (keratinocytes), which resurface wounds when the skin has been injured. Loss of the barrier function of the skin allows invasion of micro-organisms and systemic sepsis. Increased fluid losses from the injured skin continue until re-epithelialization occurs.

Burn injury to the skin can be classified as partial or full thickness (Fig. 6.1). The majority of adnexal structures are preserved and epithelialization is rapid (10–14 days) if only the epidermis and the superficial part of the dermis have been injured (superficial partial-thickness injury), and the risk of hypertrophic scarring is low. When the burn extends down into the deeper parts of the dermis, more adnexal structures are destroyed, epithelialization is slower (3–6 weeks), and there is a high incidence of hypertrophic scarring. Full-thickness burns involve destruction of all the constituents of the skin and usually require surgical intervention to achieve wound healing.

REFERENCES

1. Thomas S, Barrow RE, Herndon DN. In: Herndon DN (ed). Total Burn Care. 2nd edn. Saunders, Edinburgh, 2002: 1–10
2. National Burn Care Review Committee. Standards and Strategy for Burn Care: A Review of Burn Care in the British Isles. British Association of Plastic Surgeons, London

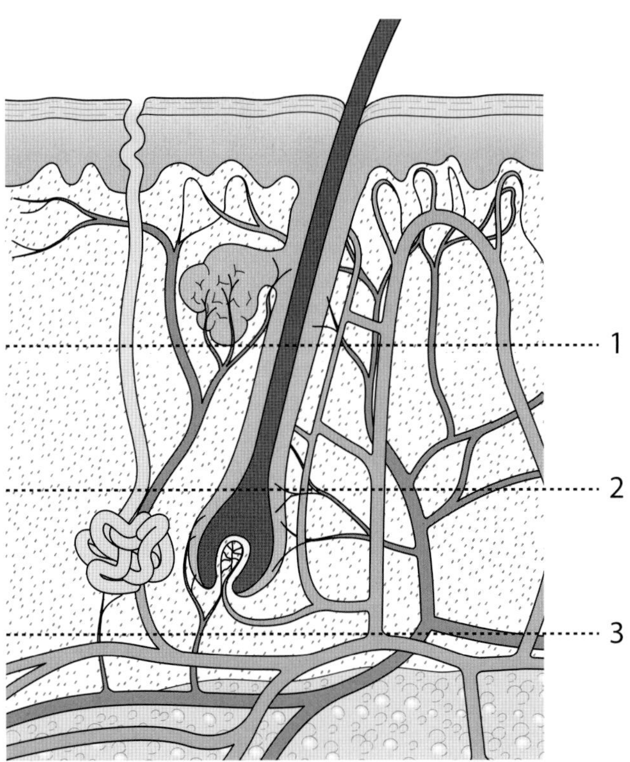

Figure 6.1 Depth of burn wound. (**a**) Superficial partial-thickness burn; most adnexal structures intact. (**b**) Deep partial-thickness burn; only deep adnexal structures intact. (**c**) Full-thickness burn; all structures damaged.

AETIOLOGY

Burn injury can be thermal, electrical or chemical. Cold injury has a similar pathophysiology, and radiation injury can also damage the skin.

Thermal injury accounts for approximately 90% of all burns. The depth of thermal tissue injury is related to the temperature and its duration of application.

Wet-heat injuries, such as scalds from hot liquids, are the commonest type of injury. They account for 70% of burns seen in children and are also common in the elderly. Scald injuries tend to cause partial-thickness burns that heal when treated conservatively.

Dry thermal injuries are caused by flame, direct contact or radiant heat. Flame burns are common in adults and are often associated with smoke inhalation injuries. They tend to cause deep partial-thickness or full-thickness skin loss and usually require surgical intervention. Radiant heat injuries tend to occur in house fires, where patients are confined in a hot environment. Contact injuries occur by direct contact with a hot object. Prolonged contact with a moderately hot object, such as a radiator, can cause injury. These contact burns occur in people such as the elderly, epileptics, drug addicts and alcoholics, who may have been unconscious or suffered a blackout for a period of time. Contact burns tend to be deep and require surgical intervention.

ELECTRICAL INJURY

Electrical injury accounts for approximately 5% of patients admitted to a burn unit. There are often 'entry' and 'exit' points where the electric current has travelled from one part of the body to another. The electric current disrupts cell membranes and produces direct tissue damage. The tissues also act as a conductor and generate heat that is related to the voltage of the electricity. These injuries can be further classified into high- and low-voltage injuries.

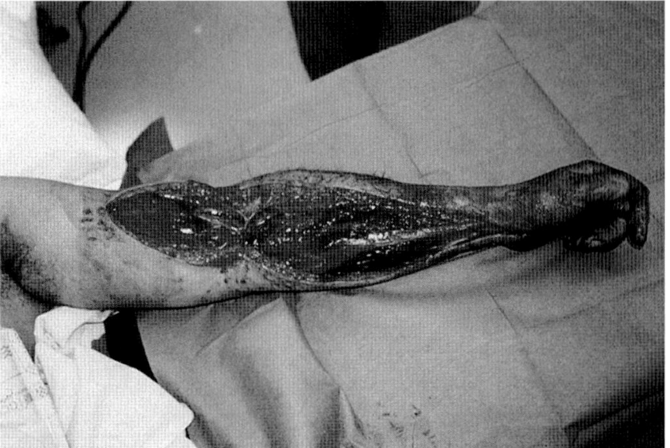

Figure 6.2 High-voltage electrical injury; this injury initially required a fasciotomy and subsequently a midhumeral amputation.

Low-voltage injuries from domestic electricity tend to cause small, deep contact burns at the points of entry and exit. The alternating current can also interfere with cardiac conduction and lead to arrhythmias. High-voltage injuries (greater than 1000 V) lead to extensive tissue damage and often to limb loss (Fig. 6.2). Cardiac asystole and arrhythmias can occur. Muscle injury leads to rhabdomyolysis, compartment syndromes and renal failure. This type of injury has a high mortality.

Flash injuries occur when current arcs from a high-voltage source. No current passes through the body, but the heat from the arc can cause flash burns to exposed parts of the body such as the hands and face. The burn is usually partial thickness unless the clothes catch fire and cause a flame burn.

Electrocardiographic monitoring is required for high-voltage injuries or if a low-voltage injury has given rise to an arrhythmia or a period of loss of consciousness. Cardiac monitoring is not required if the initial ECG is normal and there has been no history of loss of consciousness.[3]

CHEMICAL INJURIES

Chemical injuries are responsible for approximately 5% of patients seen in a burn unit. They mainly occur as household or industrial accidents. Acid burns cause damage by coagulative necrosis, which tends to be local and short-lived. Alkali burns tend to cause progressive liquefactive necrosis. They penetrate deeper, and their effects are prolonged. Cement burns are alkali burns.

The management of chemical burns is the same whatever the agent involved. The area must be thoroughly irrigated with water after removing all the patient's clothing. This dilutes the chemical and limits tissue damage. The process is usually performed by putting the patient in a drench shower, which is present in most emergency departments. Ocular injuries also require copious irrigation followed by referral to an ophthalmologist.

REFERENCES

3. Blackwell N, Hayllar J. Postgrad Med J 2002; 78: 283–285

Hydrofluoric acid is widely used for glass etching and is also used in the electronics industry. It is very corrosive and toxic. The fluoride ion rapidly penetrates through the skin, causing progressive tissue damage and intense pain. It chelates calcium ions and can lead to hypocalcaemia, which can be fatal. After initial irrigation, calcium gluconate gel is applied topically to chelate the fluoride ions.

PATHOPHYSIOLOGY

Tissue necrosis is directly related to the temperature and duration of the burn. Boiling water can cause partial-thickness injury in 0.1 s and full-thickness skin injury in 1 s.

Domestic water at 75°C can cause partial-thickness injury in 1 s and full-thickness injury in 10 s. Thus a fall into a domestic bath can have serious consequences. Prolonged contact with an object at a temperature of only 50°C can still cause a deep burn.[4]

Burn injury results in a local and a systemic response.

LOCAL RESPONSE

The initial local effect of a burn injury can be divided histologically into three differential zones of tissue damage and blood flow.[5]

1. The zone of necrosis: tissue necrosis centrally, caused by direct destruction of tissue by the burn.
2. The zone of ischaemia, which surrounds the zone of necrosis and can progress. This leads to an apparent increase in the area of skin necrosis or in the depth of injury.
3. The zone of inflammation (hyperaemia), which surrounds the zone of ischaemia and is associated with increased vascular permeability.

Following burn injury to the skin, inflammatory mediators are released via the arachidonic acid pathway and inflammatory cells. These mediators include histamine, prostaglandins (prostaglandin E_2), prostacyclins (prostaglandin I_2), leukotrienes, thromboxanes, kinins, serotonin, catecholamines, free oxygen radicals and platelet-activating factor. The local action of these inflammatory mediators causes an increase in microvascular permeability and oedema formation, microvascular stasis, and thrombosis. These actions can lead to progressive injury and cell death, leading to an increase in the depth of the burn wound.

SYSTEMIC RESPONSE

In burns of greater than 25 or 30% of the total body surface area (TBSA), the release of mediators into the circulation causes a systemic response. Tumour necrosis factor-α, interferon-γ, and interleukins 1, 6, 8, 12 and 18, together with the other mediators described earlier, stimulate the systemic response.[6]

These effects may be reduced by early aggressive wound excision and closure.

MANAGEMENT

Management depends on many variables, including the age of the patient, comorbid factors, and the size, depth and anatomical location of the burn.

In general the aims are to restore form, function and feeling. This requires early aesthetic wound closure, rehabilitation and psychosocial recovery. The criteria for referral to a burn unit are summarized in Box 6.1.

Box 6.1 Criteria for referral of burn patients

Complex*

A burn injury is more likely to be complex if associated with the following criteria:

- Age under 5 years or over 60 years.
- Site involvement (with dermal or full-thickness loss): face, hands, perineum, feet, neck or circumferential.
- Inhalation injury: any significant such injury, excluding pure carbon monoxide poisoning.
- Mechanism of injury: chemical injury (> 5% of TBSA), exposure to ionizing radiation injury, high-pressure steam injury, high-tension electrical injury, hydrofluoric acid injury (> 1% TBSA) or suspicion of non-accidental burn injury (adult or paediatric).

A complex burn injury is also suggested by one involving:

- Size of skin injury (with dermal or full-thickness loss): paediatric (younger than 16 years) > 5% of TBSA or adult (16 years old or over) > 10% TBSA.

A burn injury may also be deemed complex if it occurs alongside:

- Existing conditions, for example cardiac limitation and/or myocardial infarction within 5 years, decreased exercise tolerance, diabetes, pregnancy, immunosuppression for any reason, hepatic impairment or cirrhosis.
- Associated injuries: crush injuries, fractures, head injury or penetrating injuries.

Non-complex†

All burn injuries felt not to be complex may be referred for assessment and admission according to the skin surface area involved.

- Size of skin injury: paediatric, 2–5% of TBSA if dermal or any smaller injury if full-thickness loss; adult, 5–10% of TBSA if dermal or any smaller injury if full-thickness loss.

Non-acute referrals

Non-acute referrals from accident and emergency, GP, practice nurse or district nurse in the postacute phase include:

- Wound healing: any wound unhealed at 14 days postinjury.
- Complications: any significant infection, septic episode or suggestion of a toxic shock-like illness.
- Rehabilitation: any healed wound where the scarring suggests there will be a significant aesthetic impact and/or psychological disturbance; the need to consider skin camouflage; a significant functional limitation; the need to consider pressure therapy or other forms of scar modification; or the need to consider surgical reconstruction.

*All injuries deemed to be complex need referral to the local burn centre or burn unit.

†All non-complex injuries referrals should be made to a local plastic surgery unit (burn facility).

MANAGEMENT OF MINOR BURNS

Fortunately, the vast majority of burns are relatively small and can be managed on an outpatient basis. Small blisters can be left but larger ones should be deroofed and the fluid evacuated.[7] Numerous dressings are advocated for small burns and these are described later in this chapter.

REFERENCES

4. Lawrence JC, Bull JP. J Mech Inst Eng 1976; 5: 61–63
5. Jackson DM. Br J Plast Surg 1953; 40: 588–596
6. Vindenes HA, Ulvestad E, Bjerknes R. Eur J Surg 1998; 164: 647–656
7. Rockwell WB, Ehrlich HP. J Burn Care Rehabil 1990; 11: 93–95

Box 6.2 Emergency management of burn injury

First aid
- Stop the burning process.
- Cool the burn wound.

Primary survey
A: airway and cervical spine control
- Clear airway, then open airway with jaw thrust or chin lift.
- Stabilize cervical spine.

B: breathing and ventilation
- Expose chest and ensure equal and adequate expansion.
- Ventilate or intubate if necessary.
- ALWAYS PROVIDE SUPPLEMENTAL OXYGEN.
- Carbon monoxide poisoning may give a cherry pink, non-breathing patient.
- Beware a respiratory rate greater than 20 breaths/min.
- Beware circumferential chest burns – may require escharotomy.

C: circulation with haemorrhage control
- Check pulse.
- Capillary refill test – over 2 s is abnormal – check other limbs.
- Hypovolaemia or need for escharotomy.
- Stop bleeding with direct pressure.
- Mental obtundation occurs with 50% loss of total blood volume.
- Pallor occurs with 30% loss of total blood volume.

D: disability – neurological status
- Establish level of consciousness: A, alert; V, responds to vocal stimuli; P, responds to painful stimuli; U, unresponsive.
- Examine pupillary response to light.
- Hypoxaemia and shock give a restless patient with decreased level of consciousness.

E: Exposure and environmental control
- Remove all clothing and jewellery.
- Estimate burn surface area.
- Keep patient warm.

F: fluid resuscitation proportional to burn size
- Insert a large-bore i.v. line through unburned skin.
- Take blood samples: full blood count, urea and electrolytes, coagulation, arterial blood gases and carboxyhaemoglobin.

Fluids
Start fluids using a modified Parkland formula: quarter TBSA per kg/h for the first 8 h (2–4 mL/kg per % TBSA: half in first 8 h; rest in next 16 h) from the time of injury.
- Add maintenance for children.
- Warm Hartmann's solution.
- Replace blood losses with blood.

Monitor adequacy of resuscitation
- Urinary catheter.
- Pulse, blood pressure and respiratory rate.
- ECG, pulse oximetry and arterial blood gases.
- Insert nasogastric tube.

Baseline investigations
- X ray: lateral C spine, chest X-ray and pelvis

Pain relief
- Intravenous morphine titrated incrementally.

Wound management
- 'Cling' film – no Flamazine.

Secondary survey
- History: AMPLE (allergies, medications, past history, last ate and event).
- Mechanism of injury.
- Examination: head to toe.
- Records.
- Re-evaluate.
- Support and reassure patients, relatives and staff.

IMMEDIATE MANAGEMENT OF MAJOR BURNS

The immediate management of the major burn (Box 6.2) follows the guidelines of standard trauma care systems such as Advanced Trauma Life Support® or Emergency Management of the Severe Burn® courses.

Burn wound assessment

Estimation of depth

Determining the depth of the burn wound can be difficult (Fig. 6.3). In general, superficial partial-thickness wounds are pink, moist and blistered; they blanche on pressure and are very painful. Deep partial-thickness burns are either white or red with fixed staining; they do not blanche on pressure. Full-thickness burns characteristically have a leathery appearance and are insensate. It is usually easy to diagnose a very superficial burn or a full-thickness burn. Deep dermal burns can be more difficult to assess and are often classified as indeterminate on first assessment (Box 6.3). Techniques such as laser Doppler scanning can give an estimate of dermal blood flow and the depth of burn injury.

Estimation of burn size

The size of the burn can be estimated using a Lund and Browder chart. The rule of nines is useful for rapid estimation of size and the rule of tens is used in children. In the rule of tens, the head and the anterior and posterior trunk all account for 20% of the patient's TBSA (2 × 10), with the limbs each accounting for 10%, and the hand for 1% (Fig. 6.4).

Escharotomy

Escharotomies are required for circumferential full-thickness burns of the chest, limbs or digits. In limbs or digits, such burns impair the circulation and cause distal ischaemia. Circumferential full-thickness chest burns can restrict chest wall excursion and impair ventilation. Because full-thickness burns are anaesthetic, midaxial escharotomies can be performed either at the bedside or in the operating room. Fasciotomies are required only when burns are very deep and extend into muscle, or to limit muscle necrosis in high-voltage electrical injuries (Fig. 6.5).

Inhalation injury

Smoke inhalation is the most serious associated injury that complicates cutaneous burns and accounts for a significant number of deaths.[8] Smoke contains numerous noxious products of combustion, including soot, hydrocarbons, aldehydes, cyanides and carbon monoxide. Carbon monoxide has a 300 times greater affinity than oxygen to bind to haemoglobin (forming carboxyhaemoglobin), and can seriously impair oxygen carriage and delivery in the blood. Carboxyhaemoglobin has an elimination half-life of 4 h on room air, but on inspiration of 100% oxygen

REFERENCES

8. Smith DL, Cairns BA, Ramadan F et al. J Trauma 1994; 37: 655–659

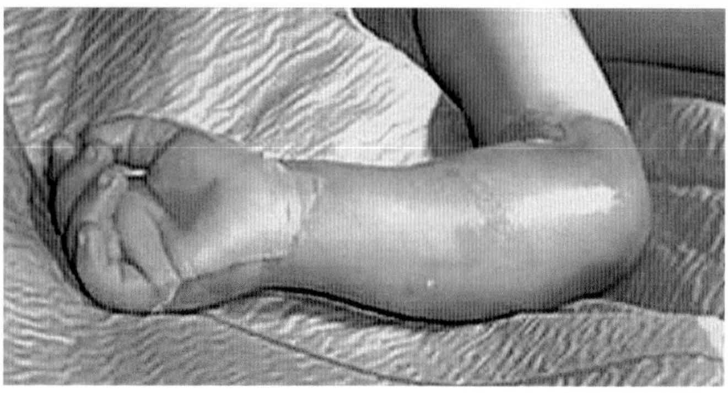

a

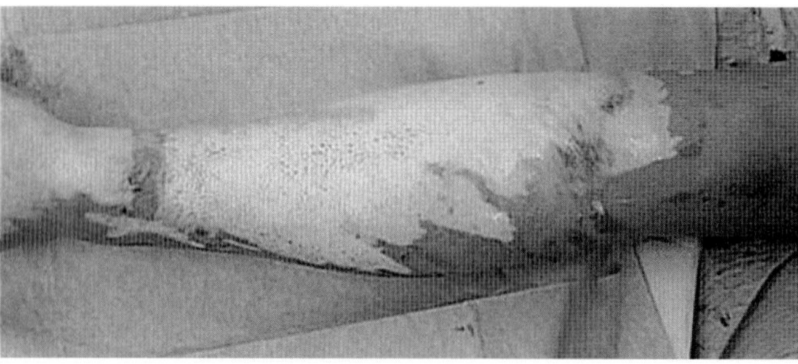

b

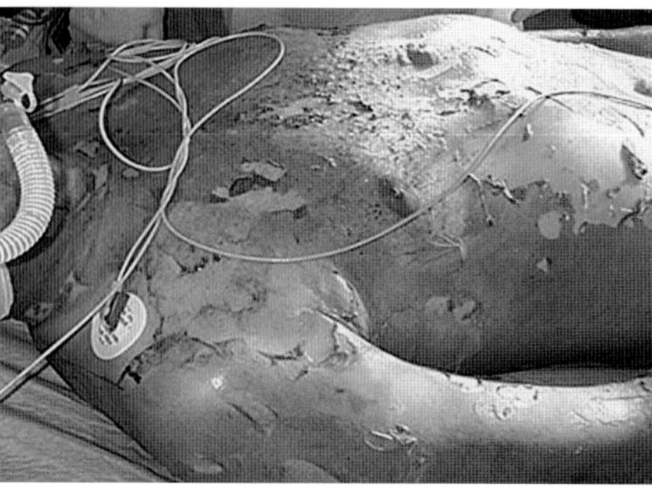

c

Figure 6.3 Clinical examples of burns of different depths: (**a**) superficial partial-thickness burn, (**b**) deep partial-thickness burn, and (**c**) full-thickness burn.

Ignore simple erythema

Superficial

Deep

Region	**%**
Head	
Neck	
Anterior trunk	
Posterior trunk	
Right arm	
Left arm	
Buttocks	
Genitalia	
Right leg	
Left leg	
Total burn	

Relative percentage of body surface area affected by growth						
Area	**Age 0**	**1**	**5**	**10**	**15**	**Adult**
A - $\frac{1}{2}$ of head	$9\frac{1}{2}$	$8\frac{1}{2}$	$6\frac{1}{2}$	$5\frac{1}{2}$	$4\frac{1}{2}$	$3\frac{1}{2}$
B - $\frac{1}{2}$ of one thigh	$2\frac{3}{4}$	$3\frac{1}{4}$	4	$4\frac{1}{2}$	$4\frac{1}{2}$	$9\frac{3}{4}$
C - $\frac{1}{2}$ of one leg	$2\frac{1}{2}$	$2\frac{1}{2}$	$2\frac{3}{4}$	3	$3\frac{1}{4}$	$3\frac{1}{2}$

Figure 6.4 Estimating burn size: the Lund and Browder chart. (Redrawn from Smith & Nephew Ltd.)

Box 6.3 Clinical determination of burn depth

Partial thickness
- Blistered
- Pink and moist underneath blisters
- Wound blanches under pressure
- Demonstrates capillary refill
- Sensation intact

Deep dermal
- Some blistering
- Wound moist or dry
- Wound white or fixed staining (red)
- No blanching or capillary refill
- Sensation diminished

Full thickness
- No blisters
- Wound dry
- Leathery appearance to eschar: feels hard
- Charring
- Fixed staining and haemorrhage areas
- Insensate

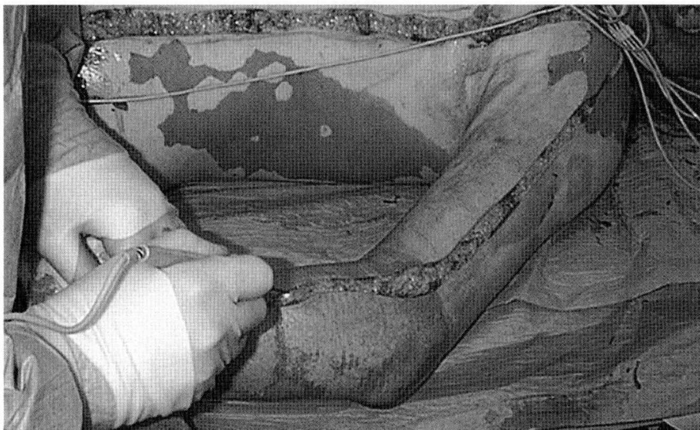

Figure 6.5 Escharotomy: a midaxial incision is made with a cutting diathermy.

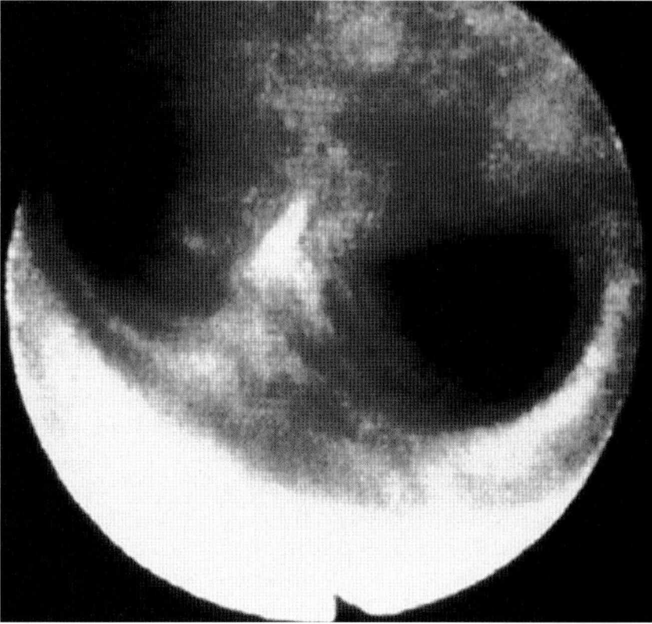

Figure 6.6 Bronchoscopy: typical bronchoscopic appearance following smoke inhalation, with erythematous, friable, ulcerating mucosa.

this drops to 30 min. Carbon monoxide poisoning is managed by high-flow (100%) oxygen therapy.

Inhalation injury can be divided into upper airway injuries above the vocal cords (supraglottic) and injuries of the entire airway below the cords, including the trachea, bronchi and lung parenchyma (subglottic). The site of injury determines the diagnosis, treatment and outcome.[9]

Supraglottic injuries are usually caused by heat and oedema, and may cause rapid obstruction of the upper airway. These injuries usually resolve spontaneously as the oedema subsides after 3–5 days. Affected patients may require intubation and mechanical ventilation if the airway is compromised.

Subglottic injuries tend to be chemical in nature and usually have a more prolonged course. The tracheobronchial mucociliary apparatus is damaged and functions poorly. Necrotic cellular debris, fibrinous exudate and mucus form 'casts' that can obstruct bronchi, causing distal atelectasis, collapse and secondary infection.[9] Damage to the respiratory epithelium is usually self-limiting and takes approximately 14 days to recover unless infection occurs. Patients often develop respiratory failure and require mechanical ventilation. Smoke inhalation injury causes hypoxia, ventilation perfusion mismatching, increased airway resistance, increased alveolar epithelial permeability, decreased pulmonary compliance and increased pulmonary vascular resistance. Increased airway pressures and barotrauma can then develop during positive-pressure ventilation.[10]

Inhalation injury is usually diagnosed from the clinical symptoms and signs, which include evidence of facial burns, facial swelling, burnt nasal hairs, soot in the nose or mouth, intraoral swelling, oedema visible on laryngoscopy, hoarseness of the voice, and stridor. Lower airway injuries are suggested by a history of a fire in an enclosed space, loss of consciousness, obtundation, anxiety, facial or intraoral burns, soot in the mouth or nostrils, cough, dyspnoea, wheeze and carbonaceous sputum. There are also signs and symptoms of respiratory distress, such as tachypnoea, use of the accessory muscles of respiration, cyanosis, and evidence of impaired gas exchange.

Investigations such as a chest X-ray and arterial blood gases are often initially normal.

Carboxyhaemoglobin levels are useful, although normal levels do not exclude smoke inhalation injury. Fibre-optic examination of the lower trachea and bronchi is the most useful investigation and may demonstrate characteristic appearances. These include soot present below the cords, hyperaemia, oedema, and ulceration of the mucosa (Fig. 6.6). Bronchoscopy allows either endo- or nasotracheal intubation in patients whose airways are at risk.

Treatment of inhalation injuries is mainly supportive after the diagnosis is made and the airway is controlled. It is always safer to intubate a patient with an upper airway injury if obstruction is a possibility, rather than having to perform an emergency intubation, which can be hazardous.

REFERENCES

9. Pruitt BA Jr, Cioffi WG. J Intensive Care Med 1995; 10: 117–127
10. Fitzpatrick JC, Cioffi WG Jr. Respir Care Clin North Am 1997; 3: 21–49

Patients with a significant lower airway injury may require more fluid replacement for resuscitation, as hypovolaemia can exacerbate the pulmonary injury.[11] Regular chest physiotherapy, tracheobronchial suction and positioning are useful in clearing secretions. Nebulized heparin, acetylcysteine and salbutamol have been shown to be helpful in smoke inhalation injury.[12] The heparin prevents cast formation, acetylcysteine is a mucolytic agent, and salbutamol is a bronchodilator.

Therapeutic bronchoscopy may be required for stubborn plugs and secretions not responding to other treatments.

Prolonged ventilation may require tracheostomy. Prolonged endotracheal intubation and tracheostomy have similar long-term complication rates.[13] Patients with extensive and deep facial, head and neck burns, and those with a severe smoke inhalation injury requiring prolonged ventilation are candidates for early tracheostomy.

Complications of inhalation injury include pneumothorax following mechanical ventilation. Uncontrolled degradation of extracellular matrix proteins by proteases released by activated neutrophils can lead to acute respiratory distress syndrome. Persistence of the inflammatory response, worsening gas exchange, and inability to ventilate the patient can progress to multiple organ failure and death. Late complications are associated with mechanical damage from endotracheal or tracheostomy tubes, leading to tracheomalacia and stenosis (see Ch. 21). Lung fibrosis following an inhalation injury can lead to emphysema and bronchiectasis.

In patients requiring mechanical ventilation, the airway pressures may be reduced by using pressure-controlled ventilation with settings adjusted to higher flow rates (15–20 mL/min), smaller tidal volumes (6–8 mL/kg), and physiological positive end-expiratory pressures (5 mmH_2O). Permissive hypercapnia should be employed and lower oxygen saturations (greater than 92%) should be accepted.[10] High-frequency positive-pressure ventilation has been shown to reduce mortality and infection.[14,15]

Fluid resuscitation

Effective fluid resuscitation is vital if a victim of a major thermal injury is to survive. Modern fluid resuscitation formulae have been developed from both experimental and clinical studies that have examined the pathophysiology of burn oedema and shock.

Following burn injury there is loss of capillary integrity, with leakage of fluid and proteins from the intravascular to the interstitial compartment. Burn shock is characterized by specific haemodynamic changes, including an initial decrease in cardiac output, decrease in plasma volume and oliguria. The primary goal of resuscitation is to restore circulating volume and preserve tissue perfusion to avoid ischaemia. Resuscitation is complicated by and accentuates burn oedema.

The best resuscitation fluid and formula are still disputed. The principles of fluid replacement therapy can be summarized as a modification of the seven principles described by J.A.D. Settle in 1996.[16]

1. To achieve survival, patients with extensive burns need to be given large quantities of fluid, which must contain sodium salts.
2. The total volume of salt-containing fluid required to satisfy obligatory burn oedema and make good urine losses is between 2 and 4 mL/kg per % burn, but the actual volume is to some extent dependent on the type of salt solution used.
3. Compared with the use of an isotonic salt solution, the use of fluid-containing colloid is associated with less generalized oedema, a reduced total fluid volume requirement, and a reduced period of plasma volume deficit.
4. The quantity of sodium ions required for effective resuscitation is of the order of 0.5 mmol/kg per % burn.
5. The resuscitation fluid should preferably be a balanced salt solution with chloride content not exceeding 100 mmol/L and with bicarbonate and/or lactate as the secondary anion.
6. The total water requirement and sodium concentration of the resuscitation fluid varies depending on the treatment of the burn wound; the amount of sodium-free water should be minimized, with only enough being given to prevent hypernatraemia.
7. Methods of monitoring the effectiveness of resuscitation should be selected for the particular patient and should take into account the fluid regimen in use; effective resuscitation should result in an hourly urine output of 0.5–1 mL/kg body weight.

Burns greater than 15% of the TBSA in an adult and 10% in a child require formal fluid resuscitation. Larger burns can be resuscitated with oral rehydration using Dioralyte or Moyer's solution (4 g NaCl plus 1.5 g $NaHCO_3$ per litre of water), but this is recommended only in exceptional circumstances such as armed conflict or for the management of mass casualties.

The optimal fluid and formula for resuscitation is still debated, and the value of colloid is still unclear. A recent systematic review of randomized controlled trials on the use of human albumin solution in critically ill patients suggested that albumin administration might be deleterious and increase mortality (see Ch. 2).[17]

The choice of formula depends on local circumstances, experience and expertise. A formula should be easy to understand, and regular use leads to familiarity and confidence. Commonly used resuscitation formulae are given in Box 6.4.

Resuscitation is a dynamic process, and the endpoints differ for different patients and for different burns. The pulse, blood pressure, respiratory rate, capillary refill, core–peripheral temperature gradient, urine output, and osmolality are routinely recorded in patients undergoing resuscitation. Invasive haemodynamic monitoring of blood pressure, central venous pressure, pulmonary artery wedge pressure, and cardiac output can also be used to assess resuscitation in patients with larger injuries and if there is concomitant smoke inhalation. Oesophageal echo-Doppler measurement is a minimally invasive technique that is routinely used to monitor adequacy of fluid therapy in larger burns. Serial arterial blood gas estimation, which allows the

REFERENCES

11. Navar PD, Saffle JR, Warden GD. Am J Surg 1985; 150: 716–720
12. Desai MH, Mlcak R, Richardson J et al. J Burn Care Rehabil 1998; 19: 210–212, erratum J Burn Care Rehabil 1999; 20: 49
13. Moylan JA, Alexander LG Jr. World J Surg 1978; 2: 185–191
14. Rue LW III, Cioffi WG, Mason AD et al. Arch Surg 1993; 128: 772–778
15. Cortiella J, Mlcak R, Herndon D. J Burn Care Rehabil 1999; 20: 232–235
16. Settle JAD. In: Settle JAD (ed). Principles and Practice of Burns Management. Churchill Livingstone, Edinburgh, 1996: 217–222
17. Cochrane Injuries Group Albumin Reviewers. Br Med J 1998; 317: 235–240

Box 6.4 Formulae for fluid resuscitation and ongoing metabolic requirements

Crystalloid resuscitation: Parkland formula

Adults

4 mL × weight (kg) × burn % TBSA = volume given in first 24 h

- Equates to 0.25 mL/kg per % TBSA per h in first 8 h.
- Using Hartmann's solution or Ringer's lactate.
- Half given in first 8 h, remainder in subsequent 16 h.
- Includes metabolic requirement in adults.

Children

As above but add maintenance requirements as dextrose saline or feed:

- 4 mL/kg per hour for first 10 kg
- 2 mL/kg per hour for second 10 kg
- 1 mL/kg per hour for third 10 kg

Colloid resuscitation: Muir and Barclay formula

Adults and children

0.5 mL × weight (kg) × burn % TBSA = volume of aliquot

- Use human albumin solution (4.5%).
- Give one aliquot over 4, 4, 4, 6, 6 and 12 h.
- Add maintenance fluid requirement.

Continuing fluid requirements (after 24 h)

Adults

1500 mL/m^2 burn surface area (BSA) (maintenance) + 3000 mL/m^2 burn BSA (burn losses) per 24 h

Children

1500 mL/m^2 BSA (maintenance) + 3750 mL/m^2 burn BSA (burn losses) per 24 h

base excess and serum lactate to be measured, provides useful additional information on the adequacy of resuscitation.[18]

Monitoring and constant re-evaluation of the resuscitation process are essential. The formulae are only guides and can be unreliable in the young and the old, and in patients with larger burn injuries, other injuries, or concomitant medical problems.

Fluid requirements are increased in patients who have delayed or inadequate resuscitation, deep burns, petrol burns, electrical burns or inhalation injury (5.7 mL/kg per % burn)[11] and in children (5.8 mL/kg per % burn).[19] Under-resuscitation causes hypovolaemia, shock, renal failure, ischaemia–reperfusion injury and multiple organ failure, while over-resuscitation can cause generalized and pulmonary oedema, and worsens compartment syndromes of the limbs and abdomen.

After fluid resuscitation, burn patients require nutrition and continuing fluid replacement to counteract hypermetabolism, pyrexia and evaporative wound losses. The daily fluid and nutritional requirements can be calculated (Boxes 6.4 and 6.5) and should be given enterally if possible.

ONGOING MANAGEMENT

Hypermetabolism and nutrition

Cuthbertson recognized nearly a century ago that injury is associated with increased energy expenditure, accelerated metabolism of protein, and loss of body nitrogen.[20] Burn patients experience an 'ebb' phase immediately after the injury for approximately 48 h, when their metabolic rate is decreased. This is followed by a 'flow' or hypermetabolic phase characterized by a hyperdynamic circulation, hyperthermia, and increased oxygen consumption and carbon dioxide production.[21] This is associated with increased glucose consumption, glycogenolysis, proteolysis, lipolysis and futile substrate cycling. This response occurs days after injury and continues for up to a year after the burn. It causes weight loss, muscle weakness, immunosuppression and impaired wound healing. Weight loss of greater than 20% is associated with increased mortality.[22]

The hypermetabolic response following burn injury is greater than that seen in any other disease state. A patient with a burn of 40% of body surface area or more has basal metabolic requirements that are twice normal. This response is temperature-sensitive but not temperature-dependent, and it can be attenuated but not abolished by environmental heating. Patients with large burns maintain a core temperature of 1–2°C above normal.

Burn injury causes increased production of catabolic stress hormones, especially the catecholamines, cortisol and glucagons, which increase gluconeogenesis, glycogenolysis and muscle proteolysis. Insulin is less effective when the blood sugar is elevated and there is inhibition of protein synthesis, lipogenesis and glycogenesis.

The hypermetabolic response can be modulated by environmental changes, by nutrition, and by hormonal manipulation.

Increasing the ambient temperature attenuates the hypermetabolic response, abolishes shivering, reduces evaporative heat loss, and improves patient comfort.[23]

Enteral feeding is also valuable because excessive protein breakdown can be limited by adequate carbohydrate intake. Immediate enteral nutrition can also limit hypermetabolism, preserve gut mucosal integrity (reducing bacterial translocation), and prevent stress ulceration (see Ch. 26).[24]

Nutritional requirements can be calculated using formulae (Box 6.5) or by indirect calorimetry. Most formulae overestimate calorific requirements.[25]

The major source of calories should be carbohydrate given as glucose, which may require supplemental insulin to control the blood sugar. Increased amounts of protein must be given to satisfy continuing demands and to provide essential amino acids for enzymes, wound healing and immune function. The calculated energy requirements should be given as non-protein calories. The non-protein calorie:nitrogen ratio should be 100:1 or less in burns that are greater than 10%.

Lipids are poorly utilized for energy in burn patients and therefore only about 30% of non-protein calories are given as fat. Omega-3 fatty acids present in fish oils may have some immune benefits.[26] Vitamins and trace elements, such as vitamins A and C, should be given in addition to iron, zinc and selenium.

REFERENCES

18. Cartotto R, Choi J, Gomez M et al. J Burn Care Rehabil 2003; 24: 75–84
19. Merrell SW, Saffle JR, Sullivan JJ et al. Am J Surg 1986; 152: 664–669
20. Cuthbertson DP. J Parenter Enteral Nutr 1979; 3: 108–129
21. Wilmore DW, Long JM, Mason AD Jr et al. Ann Surg 1974; 180: 653–669
22. Wilmore DW. Clin Plast Surg 1974; 1: 603–619
23. Wilmore DW, Mason AD Jr, Johnson DW et al. J Appl Physiol 1975; 38: 593–597
24. McDonald WS, Sharp CW Jr, Deitch EA. Ann Surg 1991; 213: 177–183
25. Curreri PW, Richmond D, Marvin J et al. J Am Diet Assoc 1974; 65: 415–417
26. Saffle JR, Medina E, Raymond J et al. J Trauma 1985; 25: 32–39

Box 6.5 Formulae for nutritional requirements of burned patients

Adults

Step 1: calculate body mass requirement (BMR)

Patient's age (years)	Males (kcal/day)	Females (kcal/day)
15–18	17.6 W* + 656	13.3 W* + 690
18–30	15.0 W* + 690	14.8 W* + 485
30–60	11.4 W* + 870	8.1 W* + 842

*W, weight in kg.

Step 2: adjust BMR for stress

Multiply by a factor for burn size:

- Partial-thickness burn: add 1% for each 1% BSA, e.g. for 40% partial thickness × 1.4.*
- Full-thickness burn: add 2% for each 1% BSA, e.g. for 40% full thickness × 1.8.*

*To a maximum of 50% BSA.

Step 3: add a combined factor for activity and diet-induced thermogenesis

- Ventilated patient: × 1.1
- Bed-bound but not ventilated: × 1.2
- Mobile on ward: × 1.25

Children

The recommended formulae are based on body surface area.

Child's age (years)	Daily requirements (kcal/day)
0–1	2100 kcal/m^2 (SA)* + 2100 kcal/m^2 (BSA)†
1–11	1800 kcal/m^2 (SA)* + 1300 kcal/m^2 (BSA)†
12–18	1500 kcal/m^2 (SA)* + 1500 kcal/m^2 (BSA)†

*Formula for body surface area (SA): SA (m^2) = √{height (cm) × weight (kg) ÷ 3600} (or use surface area nomogram).
†Formula for BSA in calculation: BSA = (% burn × SA)/100

Enteral feeding consisting of about 20% protein, 70% carbohydrate and 10% fat should be started as soon as possible after the burn injury. The feed is administered either through a nasogastric or a nasojejunal tube.

Postpyloric jejunal feeding can be continuous in the perioperative phase.[27] Gastric residual volumes should be recorded as increasing values indicate intolerance, which may be an early indicator of splanchnic hypoperfusion and sepsis.

Parenteral nutrition is to be avoided if possible in burn patients because it has been shown to increase their mortality.[28]

Hormonal modulation of the hypermetabolic response has been achieved in both experimental and clinical studies. A variety of methods have been employed, including blocking catecholamines with beta blockers, and administration of counter-regulatory agents (such as insulin and insulin-like growth factor 1) and anabolic agents (such as growth hormone, testosterone and oxandrolone).[29]

Sepsis, antibiotics and topical antimicrobials

Infection has characteristically been the major complication following burn injury.

The burn wound is usually sterile for the first 6–12 h following the injury. It then becomes contaminated and colonized with bacteria. The source of these micro-organisms can be exogenous (from the environment or cross-infection from the staff) or endogenous (from adjacent colonized uninjured skin, bacterial translocation from the gut, or direct faecal self-contamination). The wound can become colonized despite the most fastidious care, because it is a perfect culture medium for micro-organisms. The burn patient is often immunocompromised and is unable to deal with the colonizing micro-organisms effectively.

In the initial stages, Gram-positive organisms such as *Staphylococcus aureus* predominate, with Gram-negative organisms becoming more prevalent a week or so after injury. As bacteria are eliminated from the wound, fungi (such as *Candida albicans*) predominate, and as these organisms are removed viruses can cause problems.

Regular swabs provide essential microbiological surveillance of the burn wound, although these do not necessarily indicate what is happening at the interface between the eschar and viable tissue. Quantitative microbiology, which gives the numbers of organisms per gram of tissue, can be very useful.[30] It is common to find between 10^3 and 10^5 organisms per gram of burn tissue, and bacterial counts greater than 10^5 are indicative of invasive infection, although this should be interpreted with caution.[30]

It is difficult to diagnose sepsis in a burnt patient. Such patients are invariably hypermetabolic, with a raised temperature, pulse, respiratory rate and white cell count. Thus the normal markers of systemic infection are already present. Examination of the burn wound may give valuable clues. Surrounding erythema, progressive focal necrosis with black or brown patches, rapid eschar separation, punctate haemorrhagic subeschar lesions, conversion of the burn to full thickness, odour and purulence are all indicative of infection. Black lesions in the surrounding skin are indicative of an aggressive pseudomonal infection (ecthyma gangrenosum).[31]

Persistent hyperpyrexia (over 39.5°C) or hypothermia (under 36.5°C), a sudden change in the white cell count (greater than 15 000 or less than 5000), tachypnoea (greater than 30 breaths/min), hyperglycaemia, thrombocytopenia (platelets less than 100 000), or ileus demonstrated by increased gastric residual volumes[32,33] are all valuable indicators of infection in a patient with burns. Positive blood cultures can be difficult to interpret because of commensal growth and the low yield.

A diagnosis of sepsis can be made in the presence of a source using the above clinical criteria.

Burn patients who have indwelling urinary catheters and are ventilated are very susceptible to nosocomial infection. Infection associated with intravenous and intra-arterial catheters is also a particular problem in burnt patients. These infections arise from migration of bacteria along the catheter, and peripheral lines should be changed every 72 h. Central venous lines and arterial

REFERENCES

27. Gottschlich MM, Jenkins M, Warden GD et al. J Parenter Enteral Nutr 1990; 14: 225–236
28. Jenkins ME, Gottschlich MM, Warden GD. J Burn Care Rehabil 1994; 15: 199–205
29. Spies M, Muller MJ, Herndon DN. In: Herndon DN (ed). Total Burn Care. 2nd edn. Saunders, Edinburgh, 2002: 363–381
30. McManus AT, Kim SH, McManus WF et al. Arch Surg 1987; 122: 74–76
31. Heggers JP, Robson MC. Clin Plast Surg 1986; 13: 39–47
32. Heggers JP, Hawkins H, Edgar P et al. In: Herndon DN (ed). Total Burn Care. 2nd edn. Saunders, Edinburgh, 2002: 120–169
33. Wolf SE, Jeschke MG, Rose JK et al. Arch Surg 1997; 132: 1310–1313

catheters can be left in place for 7 days.[34] Line sepsis can be difficult to diagnose and is often a diagnosis of exclusion. Suppurative thrombophlebitis must be suspected in patients who persistently grow organisms on blood cultures. Pus can be milked from the affected vein, which may have to be excised.

A patient with the symptoms and signs of sepsis should be immediately started on antibiotics. The choice of antibiotic should be guided by previous cultures and sensitivities, and close liaison with a microbiologist is essential. It is preferable to use a narrow-spectrum bactericidal antibiotic. The use of multiple broad-spectrum antibiotics should be avoided if possible, because these encourage the emergence of resistant organisms. Antibiotics are used only prophylactically after major wound excision, which can produce a significant bacteraemia. Multiresistant *Pseudomonas* species, *Acinetobacter* species, vancomycin-resistant *Enterococcus* and methicillin-resistant *S. aureus* all occur in burns. Methicillin-resistant *S. aureus* colonization of patients can serve as a useful measure of the adequacy of a unit's infection control.

Toxic shock syndrome, which is caused by toxins from specific *S. aureus* phage types, can be alarming and rapidly fatal. It is rare but unfortunately affects young children with small burn injuries. There is rapid onset and progression of symptoms including vomiting, diarrhoea, hyperpyrexia, tachycardia, tachypnoea, a rash that leads to desquamation, oliguria, convulsions and coma. There is an associated drop in the haemoglobin and leukocytes. Treatment consists of resuscitation, organ support, anti-staphylococcal antibiotic therapy, and administration of whole blood or fresh frozen plasma.[35]

Infection control is vital in every burn unit. Cross-infection can be reduced or eliminated by effective infection control and cohort nursing.

Washing a wound in a shower significantly reduces quantitative culture counts, and topical antimicrobials are used to limit bacterial growth within the wound. A large eschar can limit penetration of the topical agents and prevent contact with the bacteria.

Topical antimicrobial agents are used in an attempt to limit colonization and keep bacterial numbers in the wound at low levels. The introduction of topical antimicrobial agents resulted in a significant reduction in burn mortality.[32]

Topical agents currently used include silver-containing products such as 0.5% silver nitrate solution, 1% silver sulphadiazine (Flamazine) and colloidal silver (Acticoat®). Silver products are active against *S. aureus*, *Pseudomonas aeruginosa*, enteric organisms and *C. albicans*. Flamazine is the commonest antimicrobial agent used in burn care in the UK. It does not penetrate eschar very well, but it is effective for up to 24 h, allowing once-daily application. It can, however, delay epithelialization.

Povidone iodine has a broad antibacterial and antifungal activity but a short duration of activity. Mupirocin (Bactroban®) is effective against Gram-positive organisms, especially methicillin-resistant *S. aureus*, and has some activity against Gram-negative organisms.[36] Nystatin is an effective antifungal agent that can be used topically to reduce fungal wound infection and orally to prevent gut colonization.

Hypochlorite used at lower concentrations (0.025%) is toxic to bacteria but not to human cells. It has a broad spectrum and is bactericidal against *P. aeruginosa* and *S. aureus* as well as other Gram-positive and Gram-negative organisms.[37]

Analgesia and sedation

Burn injury causes significant pain and anxiety, and in major burns these problems can be intense and prolonged. It is vital that adequate pain relief is given, particularly before wound care. Similarly, anxiety about pain or procedures can be equally as debilitating and should be controlled. Most burn units now employ an escalating pain and anxiety protocol.[38] Obviously requirements for pain relief, sedation and anxiolysis will vary depending on the stage after the burn. Opiates should be used for pain and benzodiazepines for sedation and anxiolysis. Ketamine, a neuroleptic agent, is useful for procedures such as dressing changes, especially in children. Centrally acting agents such as the tricyclic antidepressants, clonidine and gabapentin have a role to play in modulating the pain response.[39] Non-steroidal anti-inflammatory agents are useful but care must be taken in prescribing these in the acute phase, especially in elderly patients who are susceptible to renal impairment and gastrointestinal haemorrhage.

Pain and anxiety can be measured using scoring systems. Children can pose a particularly difficult problem. Large doses of analgesics and sedatives are sometimes required, because hypermetabolism reduces the potency of the drugs and tolerance unfortunately develops. Relaxation therapy, hypnotherapy and other non-pharmacological techniques can be useful in helping to control pain and anxiety.

Complications

Most patients with major burn injury are at risk of developing complications. The majority are related to sepsis and the systemic inflammatory response, although specific complications can occur in every system.

Systemic inflammatory response syndrome and organ failure

Patients with a significant burn injury, with or without smoke inhalation, develop a clinical picture of systemic inflammation. The systemic inflammatory response syndrome has been defined as the presence of two or more of the following: a core temperature over 38°C or under 36°C; a heart rate over 90 beats/min; a respiratory rate over 20 breaths/min; and a white blood cell count greater than 12 000 cells/μL or less than 4000 cells/μL.[40]

The systemic inflammatory response syndrome encompasses a broad clinical spectrum ranging from tachypnoea, tachycardia, fever and leucocytosis to shock and multisystem organ failure.

Tissue damage caused by direct thermal injury or by ischaemia–reperfusion is the precipitating event for systemic inflammation. Tissue injury results in the release of pro-inflammatory cytokines such as tumour necrosis factor-α; interleukins 1, 6, 8, 12, and 18; and interferon-gamma.[41] Sepsis, ischaemia–reperfusion injury, multiple trauma and acute pancreatitis are other well-recognized causes.

REFERENCES

34. Sheridan RL, Weber JM, Peterson HF et al. Burns 1995; 21: 127–129
35. Cole RP, Shakespeare PG. Burns 1990; 16: 221–224
36. Strock LL, Lee MM, Rutan RL et al. J Burn Care Rehabil 1990; 11: 454–459
37. Heggers JP, Sazy JA, Stenberg BD et al. J Burn Care Rehabil 1991; 12: 420–424
38. Sheridan RL, Hinson M, Nackel A et al. J Burn Care Rehabil 1997; 18: 455–459
39. Hedderich R, Ness TJ. Crit Care Clin 1999; 15: 167–184
40. Bone RC, Balk RA, Cerra FB et al. Chest 1992; 101: 1644–1655
41. Sherwood ER, Traber DL. In: Herndon DN (ed). Total Burn Care. 2nd edn. Saunders, Edinburgh, 2002: 257–270

Some patients with systemic inflammatory response syndrome develop multiple organ dysfunction syndrome with the development of renal insufficiency and inotrope or ventilator dependence. Some of these patients go on to full multiple system organ failure, which is often fatal.[42] It is not clear what factors escalate this chain of events, but intestinal failure with repeated bouts of bacterial translocation has been postulated as one possible cause.[43]

Cardiovascular system

Major burn injury affects cardiac function in a number of ways. Initially the preload is reduced, and myocardial depression occurs, leading to a decrease in cardiac output.[44] This is followed by a hyperdynamic phase characterized by increased cardiac output and decreased afterload because of a lowered systemic vascular resistance. Depending on the clinical picture, fluid administration to increase the intravascular volume and/or inotropic support is required.

In the early phase after burn injury, coagulation factors are diluted and depleted, but later there is a tendency for patients to be hypercoagulable. Deep vein thrombosis and pulmonary embolism are a recognized risk after the early stage of burn injury, and prophylaxis should be given.[45] The presence of femoral venous catheters, which are often the only available vascular access site in a patient with major burns, has been associated with a significant incidence of thrombosis.[46]

Respiratory system

Mechanical ventilation may be required for upper and lower airway inhalation injury, but respiratory failure and hypoxia from acute lung injury can also occur in burn patients without inhalation injury. This can lead to acute respiratory distress syndrome, which presents with dyspnoea, severe hypoxia and decreased lung compliance. There are usually bilateral diffuse pulmonary infiltrates on chest radiography.

Patients with a severe burn, with or without inhalation, will require intubation for airway compromise or for operation. At 4–5 days after the burn, their oxygenation deteriorates and they require higher inspired oxygen concentrations. Lung compliance increases, requiring higher inflation pressures, and at 7 days after the burn lung infiltrates appear on the chest X-ray.[47]

Burn patients develop lung injury from smoke inhalation and from acute respiratory distress syndrome brought on by systemic inflammation. Treatment is mainly supportive until the process ceases. Steroid treatment does not prevent these problems after smoke inhalation injury.[48]

Gastrointestinal system and stress ulcer prophylaxis

Splanchnic hypoperfusion, mucosal atrophy, altered absorption and increased intestinal permeability occur after burns and lead to diminished gut barrier function. This is seen as feeding intolerance, mucosal ulceration, and bleeding from the stomach and duodenum. This may also lead to bacterial translocation, which stimulates the systemic inflammatory response.

These changes can be attenuated by aggressive fluid resuscitation and early enteral nutrition. These two therapies have reduced the incidence of gastrointestinal haemorrhage in burn patients.[49] Gastric acid production is reduced by histamine-2 receptor blockers (ranitidine) or proton pump inhibitors (omeprazole), or by improving the gastric mucus barrier (sucralfate), and these treatments may reduce the risk of 'distress ulcers' (see Ch. 26).

Renal system and electrolyte disturbance

Renal failure can occur as single organ failure or as part of a multiple organ failure syndrome. Renal failure caused by a failure of initial resuscitation is uncommon.[50]

After major full-thickness burns or high-voltage electrical burns, red blood cell and muscle destruction can lead to haemoglobinuria, myoglobinuria and acute tubular necrosis. This can be avoided by aggressive fluid resuscitation maintaining a urine output of 1–2 mL/kg per hour. Alkalinization of the urine and the use of an osmotic diuretic such as mannitol may also be helpful.

Later-onset renal failure can occur 2–14 days after the burn and is usually part of multiple organ failure secondary to sepsis and the systemic inflammatory response. It can also occur following administration of nephrotoxic drugs.

The underlying cause must if possible be treated, but patients may require haemofiltration or dialysis. The mortality associated with renal failure remains high, especially in the patients who develop multiple organ failure.[51]

Electrolyte disturbances are common following major burn injury. Hyponatraemia is not uncommon after resuscitation of children and is usually the result of overzealous administration of hypotonic solutions such as 5% dextrose or dextrose saline. It can lead to hyperpyrexia, cerebral oedema and convulsions.[52] In the late phase, hypernatraemia may occur because of excessive water losses and inadequate replacement.

It is important to ensure that nutrition following a burn is given enterally and that particular attention is paid to fluid balance.

Nervous system

Patients surviving major burn injury can develop a generalized critical care neuropathy characterized by global weakness that can prolong ventilator dependence, mobilization and rehabilitation. Isolated peripheral neuropathy from entrapment can also hinder functional outcome.[53]

Bones and joints

Patients surviving major burn injury can become osteopenic as the result of prolonged immobilization and hypermetabolism, and this increases the risk of fracture.[54]

REFERENCES

42. Deitch EA, Goodman ER. Surg Clin North Am 1999; 79: 1471–1488
43. Swank GM, Deitch EA. World J Surg 1996; 20: 411–417
44. Agarwal N, Petro J, Salisbury RE. J Trauma 1983; 23: 577–583
45. Harrington DT, Mozingo DW, Cancio L et al. J Trauma 2001; 50: 495–499
46. Joynt GM, Kew J, Gomersall CD et al. Chest 2000; 117: 178–183
47. Wolf S, Prough D, Herndon DN. In: Herndon DN (ed). Total Burn Care. 2nd edn. Saunders, Edinburgh, 2002: 399–420
48. Nieman GF, Clark WR, Hakim T. Burns 1991; 17: 384–390
49. Pruitt BA Jr, Goodwin CW Jr. World J Surg 1981; 5: 209–222
50. Jeschke MG, Barrow RE, Wolf SE et al. Arch Surg 1998; 133: 752–756
51. Chrysopoulo MT, Jeschke MG, Dziewulski P et al. J Trauma 1999; 46: 141–144
52. Mukhdomi GJ, Desai MH, Herndon DN. Burns 1996; 22: 316–319
53. Kowalske K, Holavanahalli R, Helm P. J Burn Care Rehabil 2001; 22: 353–357
54. Klein GL, Herndon DN, Langman CB et al. J Pediatr 1995; 126: 252–256

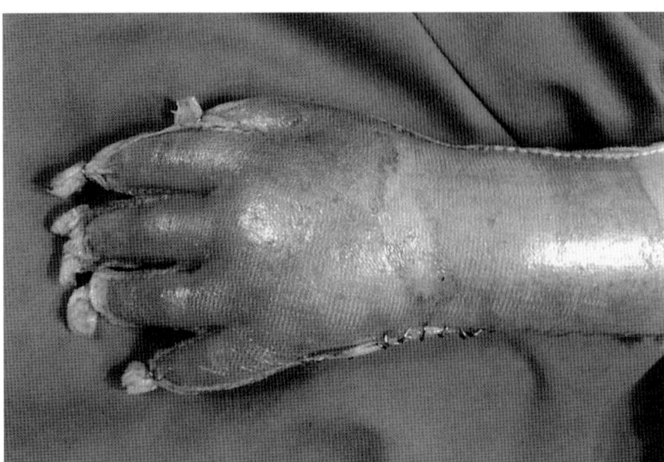

Figure 6.7 Superficial partial-thickness burn treated with Biobrane© glove.

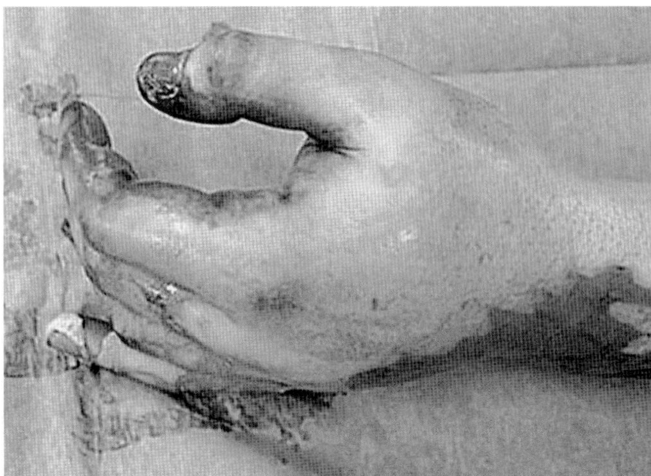

a

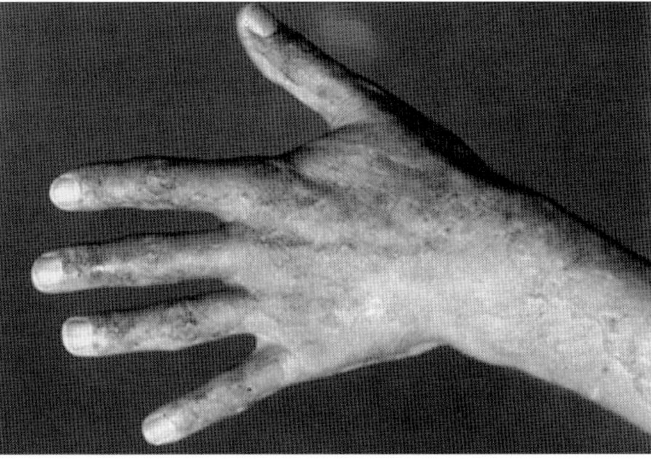

b

Figure 6.8 Tangential excision and sheet split-skin grafting; a deep partial-thickness burn hand (**a**) before and (**b**) after.

In the recovery phase, heterotopic or periarticular ossification may limit movement.[55] This complication is rare.

WOUND MANAGEMENT

Treatment planning

Once the size, site and depth of the burn wound have been estimated and initial resuscitation has been completed, a plan must be formulated to treat the burn. Early aggressive surgical intervention in deeper burns limits the duration of admission and reduces the associated morbidity and mortality. The treatment plan for the burn depends on the following factors: the patient's general condition and age, the burn depth, the burn size and the site of the burn.

Superficial partial-thickness wounds

In superficial partial-thickness burns, rapid spontaneous re-epithelialization should be encouraged, with the minimum number of painful dressing changes. Infection should if possible be prevented, because this can convert a superficial burn to a deeper one that requires skin grafting.

A partial-thickness burn needs cleaning, with the removal of loose epidermis and deroofing of blisters. The wound can then be covered with a semibiological dressing such as Biobrane®, conventional dressings such as Vaseline® gauze, or a silicone sheet (Mepitel®). Conventional dressings need frequent changes, which can be painful but are useful for small burns of less than 5%.

A topical antimicrobial such as Flamazine (silver sulphadiazine 1%) can be used with the conventional dressing to try to limit bacterial colonization. Biological dressings consist of allograft skin, xenograft skin (porcine), and human amnion. These products are not always available, they have to be collected and stored, and there are other concerns over the transmission of infection and their cost. Synthetic dressings such as Duoderm®, Omniderm®, Tegaderm® and hydrocolloids have all been used with anecdotal success. Patients treated with newer dressings such as Biobrane® appear to have lower pain scores, shorter in-patient stays, and a reduced time to healing compared with those treated with conventional dressings (Fig. 6.7).[56]

Deep partial-thickness wounds

Deep partial-thickness injuries have a significant morbidity. They take a long time to heal, often become infected, and heal with unsightly scars. Conservative management, which aims to achieve spontaneous healing, usually requires prolonged and painful dressing changes and the resultant scar is invariably hypertrophic, leading to cosmetic and functional debility. An early surgical approach that tries to preserve dermis and achieve prompt wound healing is therefore preferred (Fig. 6.8).

Full-thickness wounds

Full-thickness burns will not heal spontaneously unless they are very small. They invariably require skin grafting. Necrotic tissue is excised and the resultant wound is then closed to reduce the risks of infection and systemic sepsis. Prompt excision and wound closure reduce the morbidity and mortality in patients with full-thickness burns.

Modern surgical approach

Deep burns are best excised and the resultant wounds covered with autologous split-skin grafts. Meshed grafts are usually used, and the amount of wound that can be closed depends on the donor sites available and the mesh ratio used (Fig. 6.9). Operative

REFERENCES

55. Evans EB. Clin Orthop 1991; 263: 94–101
56. Barret JP, Dziewulski P, Ramzy PI et al. Plast Reconstr Surg 2000; 105: 62–65

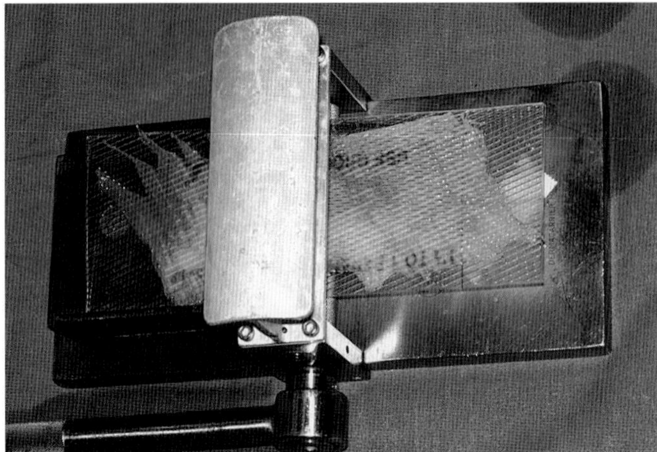

Figure 6.9 A split-skin graft being meshed.

Table 6.1 Estimated approximate blood loss in patients with > 30% TBSA burn

Days post injury	Estimated blood loss (mL/cm² burn excised)*
0–1	0.4
1–2	0.6
2–16	0.75
> 16	0.5

*To estimate blood requirements preoperatively, the burn size in cm² should be estimated; a calculation can then be made if the time post injury is known. (Desai MH, Herndon DN et al. Early burn wound excision significantly reduces blood loss. Ann Surg. 1990; 211: 753–9.[57])

blood loss varies with the time of excision post burn (Table 6.1). This is preferably done as early as possible.

Cosmetically and functionally sensitive areas such as the face and hands need thicker autografts for wound closure. In general it is preferable to use sheet grafts in children, because they give a better aesthetic result. When the size of the burn is large or if there is a lack of donor sites, it may be possible to obtain temporary wound closure with allograft, xenograft, and other biological or semibiological dressings, or with synthetic skin substitutes, while the donor sites heal. Patients with larger burns need to return to the operating room for further grafting when their donor sites have healed. This is usually done on a weekly basis.

Serial wound excision and grafting is commonly practised in the UK. This method is employed for larger burns where donor sites are scarce. The surgical technique is similar to that described earlier, but the amount of burn wound excised is only equivalent to the amount that can be covered by meshed split-skin grafts from the available donor sites. Unexcised areas are treated with topical antimicrobials until donor sites have healed and can be reharvested. This is usually 7–14 days later. The unexcised, unhealed areas of burn wound are susceptible to invasive wound infection, and this treatment method has a higher morbidity and mortality than early excision.[58,59] The use of the topical antimicrobial Flamacerium (silver sulphadiazine and cerium nitrate) has been reported to decrease episodes of invasive wound infection, and to reduce the morbidity and mortality of re-excision.[60]

An early aggressive surgical approach has been shown to improve the mortality of patients with large full-thickness burns. In addition, early excision reduces the time to wound healing, shortening the in-patient stay.[58,59]

Techniques of wound excision

A deep partial-thickness burn wound can be excised in a 'tangential' fashion by repeated shaving of the wound as originally described by Janzekovic. This preserves a viable dermal bed and minimizes scarring.[61] A similar technique can be used to treat full-thickness burns. Fascial excision is reserved for very deep or infected burns. It consists of surgical excision of the full thickness of the integument, including the subcutaneous fat down to fascia. This is done with electrocautery, which affords excellent haemostasis. Unfortunately, fascial excision leaves a permanent contour defect. Occasionally a primary limb amputation must be considered, but this is usually reserved for high-voltage electrical injuries or very deep thermal injuries with extensive muscle involvement and rhabdomyolysis, which is life-threatening.

Wound closure

Following wound excision it is vital to obtain wound closure. This is permanent if autologous split-skin grafts are used, or temporary when allograft or skin substitutes are applied. Closure of the burn wound reduces invasive infection, evaporative water loss, heat loss and pain; it also promotes wound healing.

Temporary skin substitutes are often used to achieve temporary wound closure following excision until donor sites have regenerated and are ready for harvesting.

Autologous skin grafts are still the best way of resurfacing burns. These can be harvested as either split-thickness or full-thickness grafts. Split-skin grafts take more easily. Full-thickness grafts tend not to be used for acute burns but are extremely useful for later reconstruction. Split-skin grafts can be harvested either with a hand knife or with a powered dermatome. Skin grafts can be used as sheet grafts or they can be meshed. The grafts can be meshed at varying ratios: 1:1, 1.5:1, 2:1, 3:1, 4:1, 6:1 or 9:1. In practice, grafts meshed with an expansion ratio more than 3:1 are prone to allow desiccation of the interstices, with subsequent graft loss. Narrowly meshed allograft can be placed on top of the widely meshed autograft in a 'sandwich' technique to protect the interstices.[62]

Donor sites

A donor site is in essence a superficial partial-thickness skin wound and should heal within 7 days, depending on the thickness of the graft harvested. Care of the donor site is equally as important as the care of the grafted area. In larger burns with limited donor sites that require repeated harvesting, recombinant human growth hormone (0.2 mg/kg per day) has been shown to increase donor site healing by up to 25%.[63]

REFERENCES

57. Herndon DN et al. Ann Surg 1990; 211: 753–762
58. Herndon DN, Parks DH. J Trauma 1986; 26: 149–152
59. Herndon DN, Barrow RE, Rutan RL et al. Ann Surg 1989; 209: 547–552
60. de Gracia CG. Burns 2001; 27: 67–74
61. Janzekovic Z. J Trauma 1970; 10: 1103–1108
62. Alexander JW, MacMillan BG, Law E et al. J Trauma 1981; 21: 433–438
63. Herndon DN, Hawkins HK, Nguyen TT et al. Ann Surg 1995; 221: 649–656

Allograft, xenograft and skin substitute

Allograft skin is used for temporary wound closure, and its use has been a key factor in improving the mortality associated with extensive burns. Porcine skin is commonly used and is commercially available. Its main use is as a biological dressing for partial-thickness wounds. Other biological dressings that have been mainly used on partial-thickness wounds include human placenta and potato skins, which adhere to the wound, promoting and protecting re-epithelialization.

Transcyte® is a commercially available, bilayered, temporary skin substitute that contains screened allogeneic human dermal fibroblasts that produce biologically active wound-healing factors when in contact with the burn wound. Recent clinical studies have been promising.[64]

Integra® is an acellular, bilaminar skin substitute that is designed to provide permanent wound closure and to replace dermis. It is made up of a disposable upper layer of Silastic that acts as a temporary epidermis. The lower layer is a cross-linked matrix of bovine collagen and chondroitin-6-sulphate, which is incorporated into the wound and becomes a 'neodermis'. After this matrix is vascularized by host cells over 3 weeks or so, the silastic covering can be removed before thin epidermal autografts are applied. Integra® has been extensively studied and has produced encouraging results both in single-centre studies and in a multicentre randomized controlled trial.[65–67]

Epidermal cells (keratinocytes) can be grown in a tissue culture laboratory and then used to assist wound closure. From a 1-cm^2 biopsy enough cells can be cultured in approximately 3–4 weeks to cover 1 m^2 of body surface area. These cells can be cultured commercially for patients with large burn injuries; however, the cost is significant. After successful take, the grafted areas remain fragile and blister easily because of poor and delayed basement membrane formation. In general, the use of cultured endothelial cells should be reserved for patients with massive full-thickness burns (greater than 80%).[68]

Rehabilitation

Rehabilitation of the burn patient begins on admission, with the short-term goal of preserving the patient's range of motion and function. This is attained by positioning, splinting and physiotherapy. Longer-term rehabilitation should provide functional and psychosocial training to reintegrate the patient to independent living and preinjury activities if possible.

SCAR MANAGEMENT

The hypertrophic scar is, unfortunately, a common sequel of burn injury. It is common in wounds treated conservatively that take longer than 3 weeks to heal and in skin-grafted areas. These scars are typically thick, red, raised and lumpy, and they cause significant aesthetic, functional and psychosocial morbidity. They can also cause pain and itching.

Scar maturation can be modulated by scar massage, pressure, and the use of topical silicone. Custom-made pressure garments are effective but expensive. Scars tend to take 18–24 months to mature, and scar management must be undertaken during this period. Patients must be supervised regularly on a 3-monthly basis in an outpatient clinic. The scars should be moisturized with creams and protected from excessive sun exposure.

Reconstruction

Postburn reconstruction must be undertaken by a multidisciplinary team. Hypertrophic burn scars can cause contractures when located near joints and other functionally and aesthetically important areas. It is useful to identify the patient's reconstructive requirements and available donor sites at the beginning of treatment.[69] Function takes preference over aesthetic appearance, although improving cosmesis often leads to improved function, confidence and psychosocial well-being. Reconstruction can be subdivided into release of contractures, resurfacing of unstable or unsightly scars, and reconstruction of missing parts. Many techniques are available but simplicity is often a virtue.[70]

THE BURN TEAM

Burn injury can lead to profound physiological, aesthetic, psychological and social sequelae. A multidisciplinary team approach is therefore essential. The core members of the team include surgeons, anaesthetists, intensivists, paediatricians, nurses, physiotherapists, occupational therapists, microbiologists, nutritionists, psychologists or psychotherapists, and social workers. It must not be forgotten that patients and their family are vitally important and contribute significantly to the final outcome and recovery.

OUTCOME

Outcome following burn injury has always been assessed in terms of morbidity and mortality. The old rule that the age of the patient added to the percentage area of the burn equals the mortality is now invalid, and survival rates have improved dramatically over the past 25 years.[71] Patients with major burn injury now survive, and in certain specialist centres a child with a 96% full-thickness burn has a 50% chance of survival.[72] Unfortunately these improvements have not occurred in burn injury of the elderly, where the mortality remains high.

Following survival, the morbidity and complications of treatment, the time to complete healing, and the length of the in-patient stay determine the process of burn care. Following discharge, the functional, aesthetic and psychosocial outcome must be assessed. A good overall outcome measure of functional and psychosocial recovery is return to work.[73]

Despite the long-term functional and aesthetic damage that often persists after a burn injury, many burn patients achieve a very satisfactory quality of life.

REFERENCES

64. Noordenbos J, Dore C, Hansbrough JF. J Burn Care Rehabil 1999; 20: 275–281
65. Heimbach DM, Warden GD, Luterman A et al. J Burn Care Rehabil 2003; 24: 42–48
66. Ryan CM, Schoenfeld DA, Malloy M et al. J Burn Care Rehabil 2002; 23: 311–317
67. Dantzer E, Braye FM. Br J Plast Surg 2001; 54: 659–664
68. Barret JP, Wolf SE, Desai MH et al. Ann Surg 2000; 231: 869–876
69. Brou JA, Robson MC, McCauley RL et al. J Burn Care Rehabil 1989; 10: 555–560
70. Robson MC, Barnett RA, Leitch IO et al. World J Surg 1992; 16: 87–96
71. Ryan CM, Schoenfeld DA, Thorpe WP et al. N Engl J Med 1998; 338: 362–366
72. Spies M, Herndon DN, Rosenblatt JI et al. Lancet 2003; 361: 989–994
73. Saffle JR, Tuohig GM, Sullivan JJ et al. J Burn Care Rehabil 1996; 17: 353–361

Principles in the management of major trauma

7

Kenneth D. Boffard, Douglas M. G. Bowley, Adam Brooks

INTRODUCTION

There are few areas of surgery where a coordinated response, rapid assessment, and early intervention have such a dramatic effect on outcome as in the management of major trauma. The first-known medical text, the Smith Papyrus (c.1500 BC), documented attempts to treat wounded patients. It was, however, only in the early 1970s that the American College of Surgeons first formally recognized trauma as a surgical disease.[1]

In the UK, a retrospective study of 1000 trauma deaths in 1988 concluded that, of those who reached hospital alive, one-third of deaths occurring after major injury were preventable,[2] most through missed or inadequately managed haemorrhage. Data from the UK Trauma Audit and Research Network have suggested that there has been an improvement in trauma care in the UK,[3] perhaps as a consequence of initiatives such as the Advanced Trauma Life Support™ (ATLS®) course and the increased provision of accident and emergency services. Trauma continues to be an important cause of mortality, morbidity and permanent disability throughout the world. New concepts and techniques have been introduced in the management of injury, and several of the principles of trauma management are changing.

HISTORY OF TRAUMA MANAGEMENT

Wars have always been great stimulators of progress in trauma care. Numerous advances have come about as a result, including the ligation of wounds in place of cautery by Ambroise Paré in 1631, the introduction of the ambulance by Volant and battlefield triage by Baron Jean Larrey, and the recognition that survival could be improved by early evacuation to medical care with the development of helicopter evacuation in the Korean and Vietnam conflicts; this was a major factor in the reduced mortality of those admitted within about an hour of wounding. War also influenced the structure of civilian trauma care. In 1941, the Queen's Hospital in Birmingham (later known as the Birmingham Accident Hospital), under the directorship of William Gissane, became the first British accident hospital dedicated to the management of air-raid casualties and industrial injuries. This hospital was the first trauma unit of its kind and the forerunner of many similar institutions.

The development of the ATLS® course through the American College of Surgeons in 1978 was a major milestone.[1] More than 300 000 doctors in 37 countries have been trained, leading to a fundamental change in the approach to the injured patient. The introduction of ATLS® has been shown to significantly reduce the mortality from trauma.

Until recently, the improvements in training in resuscitation were not mirrored by changes in the surgical response to trauma. Initiatives by the International Association for the Surgery of Trauma and Surgical Intensive Care (IATSIC), in centres in Australia, Europe, South Africa, the UK and the USA, have led to the development of the Definitive Surgical Trauma Care (DSTC™) course, directed towards improving training in the technical aspects of surgical care of the trauma patient.[4]

In 1978, Trunkey described the trimodal distribution of death following trauma, which was another major milestone in the development of the organized response to trauma. The first peak of deaths after trauma occurs within minutes of injury, from irreversible (non-survivable) injury or airway problems; a second peak of death occurs from a few minutes to within a few hours, from potentially reversible causes such as haemorrhage; and a third peak occurs days to weeks after the primary injury, from sepsis and multiple organ failure. The second peak or 'golden hour' is where most benefit from emergency intervention can be achieved, and ATLS® is directed primarily at this peak. A systems approach to regional care of major trauma was introduced at the Maryland Institute for Emergency Medical Services in Baltimore,[5] and at the Cook County Hospital, Chicago.[6] Concurrent successes observed at these hospitals applying structured protocols have since served as models for trauma centres elsewhere.

EPIDEMIOLOGY

PATTERNS AROUND THE WORLD

It is estimated that, by the year 2020, 8.4 million people will die every year from injury and injuries from road traffic accidents, which will be the third most common cause of disability worldwide.[7] The prevalence of trauma is distributed unequally, and falls most heavily on developing countries. For example, there is a direct relationship between the degree of poverty and

REFERENCES

1. Committee on Trauma of the American College of Surgeons. Advanced Trauma Life Support Student Course Manual. American College of Surgeons, Chicago, 1997
2. Anderson ID, Woodford M, de Dombal FT et al. Br Med J 1988; 296: 1305–1308
3. Lecky F, Woodford M, Yates DW. Lancet 2000; 355: 1771–1775.
4. Boffard KD (ed). Manual of Definitive Surgical Trauma Care. Arnold, London, 2003
5. Boyd DR, Cowley RA. World J Surg 1983; 7:149–157
6. Lowe RJ, Baker RJ. J Trauma 1973; 13: 285–290
7. Murray CJL, Lopez AD. Lancet 1997; 349: 1498–1504

deprivation and child pedestrian accident rates;[8] school-age children are at particular risk because they often live in crowded urban areas with few alternatives for play but the street and inadequate parental supervision.[9] In the developing world, overcrowded urban slums, mass unemployment, and obvious disparities between the 'haves' and 'have nots' lead to overall social dysfunction, crime and violence.[10]

The incidence of road fatalities varies widely throughout the world. In developed countries, increased legislation has led to the successful reduction in deaths from road trauma. Australia in particular has introduced successful primary and secondary prevention programmes that have led to a dramatic fall in death and serious injury on the roads. The USA has seen a decrease in road traffic–related deaths and also in the firearm-related injury rate. The annual firearm-related death rate declined by 21% between 1993 and 1997.[11] Safer vehicles and improved driving practices, coupled with improvements in emergency medical services, have been credited with the reduction in motor vehicle-related injuries and deaths.[12] Improved economic conditions, an aging population, violence prevention programmes, and changes in law enforcement practices and sentencing are believed to have made a significant contribution.

Despite advances in the management of major trauma, it remains the cause of 7–10% of the world's mortality, and injury remains the leading cause of death in young adults in the UK. The annual incidence of major trauma in the UK is 27 cases per 100 000 of the population.

COSTS

The economic impact of trauma is immense. The overall cost of gun violence in the USA in 1998 was estimated at US$100 billion.[13] The cost of traffic accidents to society is even higher; the American National Highway Traffic Safety Administration has calculated that for each individual killed in a car crash, 45 require emergency department treatment and nine require hospital admission.[14] Costs of car crashes are estimated to be almost three times higher than those associated with gunshot wounds.[15] In the UK alone, the cost of treating these injuries has been estimated at £1.2 billion a year,[16] while the World Health Organization has estimated that the price in economic terms paid by society is equivalent to 15 times the gross national product of the country.

ALCOHOL AND SUBSTANCE ABUSE

In the Middle Ages, alcohol was considered to be the elixir of life, but it has more recently been described as 'an ancient plague and a modern poison'.[17] There is a strong association between drinking alcohol and high-risk behaviour, such as dangerous driving, violent and aggressive behaviour, crime and suicide.[18,19] This gives alcohol a central role in the aetiology of traumatic injury.[15,20] Injured patients who test positive for alcohol are 3.5 times more likely to be readmitted for a second injury compared with other patients.[21] Illicit drug use appears to be increasing,[22] and may also be a root cause of trauma, either because of the intoxicating effects or the crime that surrounds obtaining drugs.

INJURY PREVENTION

Primary injury prevention aims to stop an injury from occurring, using education and enforcement. These measures include anti-drink-driving campaigns and enforcement of speed limits.

Secondary injury prevention attempts to lessen the consequences of injury, and can be active or passive. Active secondary preventive measures include bicycle helmets and seat belts. Correct use of seat belts is thought to reduce the risk of death or serious injury for front-seat occupants of cars involved in road traffic accidents by approximately 45%.[23] The risk of fatal head injury to motorcyclists is reduced by about one-third by the use of helmets.[24] Helmets have been shown to reduce the risk of brain injury for bicyclists by 88%.[25] Passive secondary measures may be more effective because active prevention measures are successful only if the individual chooses to employ them. Air bags, which deploy automatically, are an example of passive secondary measures. In purely frontal road traffic accidents, air bags provide a reduced risk of fatality of approximately one-third. In all crashes, the reduction in risk of death has been estimated at 11%.[26]

Tertiary injury prevention accepts that injury has occurred, but aims to maximize the outcome by improving delivery of healthcare, both by individuals and by systems. Tertiary injury prevention attempts to improve the delivery of care to wounded patients. The ATLS® and DSTC™ programmes are examples of this form of injury prevention.

MECHANISMS OF TRAUMA

BLUNT TRAUMA

Blunt injury can occur as a result of motor vehicle accidents, pedestrian accidents, falls or blunt assault. In the UK, road traffic

REFERENCES

8. Kendrick D. Arch Dis Child 1993; 68: 669–672
9. Rivara FP, Grossman DC, Cummings P. N Engl J Med 1997; 337: 543–548
10. Bowley DM, Khavandi A, Boffard KD et al. S Afr Med J 2002; 92: 798–802
11. Centers for Disease Control and Prevention. Morb Mortal Wkly Rep 1999; 48: 45
12. Engelhardt S, Hoyt D, Coimbra R et al. J Trauma 2001; 51: 633–638
13. Cook PJ, Ludwig J. Gun Violence: The Real Costs. Oxford University Press, New York, 2000
14. National Highway Traffic Safety Administration. National Automotive Sampling System Crash Worthiness Data System: 1992–1994. Publication DOT HS 808 538. US Department of Transportation, Washington, 1997
15. Soderstrom CA, Cole FJ, Porter JM. J Trauma 2001; 50: 1–12
16. Department of Health. Our Healthier Nation—A Contract for Health. HMSO, London, 1998
17. Lundberg GD. JAMA 1984; 252: 1911–1912
18. Field CA, Claassen CA, O'Keefe G. J Trauma 2001; 50: 13–19
19. Allan A, Roberts MC, Allan MM et al. S Afr Med J 2001; 91: 145–150
20. Hadfield RJ, Mercer M, Parr MJ. Resuscitation 2001; 48: 25–36
21. Rivara FP, Koepsell TD, Jurkovich GJ et al. JAMA 1993; 270: 1962–1964
22. Soderstrom CA, Dischinger PC, Kerns TJ et al. J Trauma 2001; 51: 557–564
23. Rivara FP, Grossman DC, Cummings P. New Engl J Med 1997; 337: 543–548
24. Evans L, Frick MC. Accid Anal Prev 1988; 20: 447–458
25. Thompson RS, Rivara FP, Thompson DC. N Engl J Med 1989; 320: 1361–1367
26. National Highway Traffic Safety Administration. Effectiveness of Occupant Protection Systems and their Use: Third Report to Congress. US Department of Transportation, Washington, 1996

accidents are the main mechanism of trauma leading to serious injury. The mechanism of injury means that the multiple body systems are frequently involved and complicate the evaluation, investigation, management and coordination of surgical specialities. The pathophysiology of blunt injury results from direct impact, rapid deceleration, acceleration, or rotational forces on the organs.

Direct impact with the body and compression of the tissues is the commonest mechanism of injury. This direct pressure affects the superficial tissues more than deeper structures and frequently causes extremity bony injury, with the limbs being injured in 85% of victims. Direct forces on the abdomen may cause rupture of the solid organs, especially the liver and spleen, and may lead to devastating haemorrhage. The bowel can be crushed against the spinal column or may rupture as a result of the sudden increase in intraluminal pressure. The bony rib cage surrounding the thorax provides some limited protection from direct forces on the thorax in blunt trauma (see Ch. 21). In the young especially, the flexibility of the ribs may absorb some of the impact and can mislead the unwary because they may not fracture but spring back into position, hiding the underlying lung contusion, which can be severe. Laceration of the lung by fractured ribs or tearing of the intercostal vessels may lead to overwhelming haemorrhage from the injured vessels and the development of a haemothorax. An air leak will cause a pneumothorax, which may tension if a one-way valve is formed at the site of injury.

Rapid deceleration leads to shearing forces as the organs and tissues move relative to each other. These forces are most marked at the interface between mobile and fixed structures, such as the duodenojejunal flexure or the ligamentum arteriosum in the chest. Movement at these points leads to the tearing of blood vessels at the junctions, and aortic transection or dissection of the intima and a thoracic aortic dissection (see Ch. 22). In the abdomen, serosal or full-thickness tears of the bowel wall can occur.

Rotational injuries are similar to shearing forces and are common in the limbs, leading to spiral fractures of long bones (see Ch. 55) or diffuse axonal brain injury (see Ch. 15). Direct blunt injury to the head can cause direct injury at the site, contusion and bleeding of the cerebral tissue, or a *contrecoup* injury where the brain moves separately to the bony box of the skull and strikes the skull at a point opposite to the initial force, causing further injury.

PENETRATING TRAUMA

In civilian trauma, penetrating injury occurs either from a stab injury or from a gunshot wound. In military injuries, fragment wounds are the most common cause of penetrating trauma. Modern fragmentation devices are designed to deliver hundreds of preformed fragments, leading to multiple penetrating injuries; the intention is to maim rather than kill.

Stab wounds

Stab wounds can be caused by a wide variety of weapons, from simple knives or sharpened bicycle spokes to samurai swords (Fig. 7.1). Tissues are incised in the path of the weapon, and the damage is limited to this track.

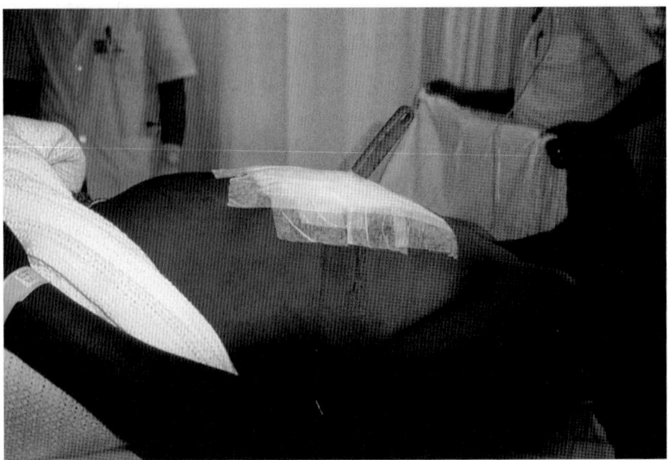

Figure 7.1 Stab wound to the abdomen.

Gunshot wounds

The wounding potential of a gunshot depends on the path of the bullet through the tissues, the structures that it passes through, and the energy that it transfers. Rounds from handguns tend to be associated with lower energy transfer than those from military weapons, and it is more appropriate to refer to *high-energy* or *low-energy* injuries. The energy that is transferred from the projectile to the body tissues depends on the relationship between the energy of the missile, the surface area presented to the tissue, and the retardation of the missile in the tissue. When the bullet penetrates the body, the transfer of energy expands the tissues, creating a temporary cavity. High-energy missiles produce greater cavitation; this causes tissue destruction remote from the missile path, and the creation of a temporary vacuum that sucks debris and contaminants into the wound track. Solid, inelastic organs such as bone and liver retard the bullet significantly, causing increased transfer of energy to these tissues and significant destruction. Less dense, elastic organs such as the lungs are less affected by cavitation.

All gunshot wounds are contaminated with bacteria,[27] and while there is little debate that surgical treatment is appropriate for high-energy, contaminated wounds in war,[28] the judgement of how much tissue has been damaged, and what to remove, is complex.[29] The authors of a study of over 4000 wounded in the Second World War noted, 'it is surprising to see how much apparently non-vital tissue recovered'.[30] The exposure to large numbers of civilian gunshot wounds around the world has enabled surgeons to relearn that some gunshot wounds can be treated conservatively.[31,32] Not all wounds to the extremity caused by handguns can be treated conservatively,[30] and mature surgical judgment must be exercised and each wound treated on its individual merits.

Shotgun blast at ranges less than 5 m are fatal in 90% of cases,[33] because the multiple lead shot acts as a single mass on impact, and therefore presents a large surface area to the tissues; consequently the energy transfer is great. The individual shot then spreads out, leading to multiple permanent and temporary cavitation, and massive tissue destruction and loss. Repair does

REFERENCES

27. Fackler ML. Ann Emerg Med 1996; 28: 194–203
28. Cooper GJ, Ryan JM. Br J Surg 1990; 77: 606–610
29. Fackler ML, Breteau JP, Courbil LJ et al. Surgery 1989; 105: 576–584
30. Fackler ML. JAMA 1988; 259: 2730–2736
31. MacFarlane C. Int Surg 1999; 84: 93–98
32. Brunner RG, Fallon WF Jr. Am Surg 1990; 56: 104–107
33. Ordog GJ (ed). Management of Gunshot Wounds. Elsevier, New York, 1988

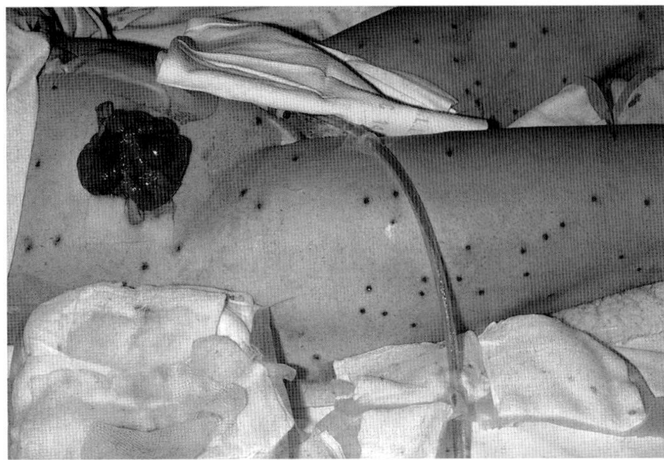

Figure 7.2 Shotgun wound.

not involve removal of individual pellets unless the pellet itself is causing an immediate problem (Fig. 7.2).

Blast

Bombs and blast produce their damaging effect through the integration of the blast wave, blast wind, fragments and flash burns. Fragments cause the majority of injuries.

Explosions occur as a result of the rapid chemical transformation of materials into gaseous products that rapidly expand to occupy a large volume. This expanding gas becomes a high-pressure sphere, within which the pressure greatly exceeds atmospheric pressure. A blast wave is formed at the edge of this sphere, and surrounds and compresses victims, causing organ contusion, disturbance at tissue interfaces, tissue disruption and haemorrhage. The blast wave is followed by a powerful blast wind produced by the displaced air. Close to the point of explosion the wind can displace the victim, avulse limbs, and disrupt the torso. Fragments can take many forms and cause the majority of injuries in bomb blast. Primary missiles arise from the bomb, and may be part of the bomb casing or can arise from nails or ball-bearings wrapped around the explosive in terrorist devices. Secondary missiles are fragments of the immediate surroundings carried by the blast wind.

Blast is associated with specific injuries, some of which, for example tympanic membrane rupture, should raise suspicion that there could be a significant blast injury (Table 7.1). Injuries such as blast lung may be lethal, and are the result of disturbance at the air–lung interface, intra-alveolar haemorrhage, and alveolar disruption with pulmonary oedema. Disruption of the alveolae may result in pneumothorax, haemothorax, or air embolism into the pulmonary circulation. Air embolism can also present with air entrapment in the coronary arteries, and leads to arrhythmias, ischaemia and sudden death. In the retinal and cerebral circulation it can cause blindness, neurological deficits, and loss of consciousness. Blast can also cause momentary compression then re-expansion of gas trapped within the bowel, and may lead to bowel perforation.

CRUSH INJURY

Crush injury can occur in entrapment following motor vehicle crashes (Fig. 7.3), explosions or natural disasters, when the victim is trapped by debris and masonry from a collapsed building. Crush injury to limbs is relatively common, and a rapid restoration of the circulation may result in pronounced

Table 7.1 Relative effects of various overpressures lasting for 4ms

Overpressure (psi)	Effect
1	Damage to ordinary structures – flying glass and debris
2	Slight chance of perforation of tympanic membrane
15	50% chance of perforation of tympanic membrane
40	Serious damage to reinforced concrete structures
70	50% chance of severe pulmonary damage
130	50% mortality

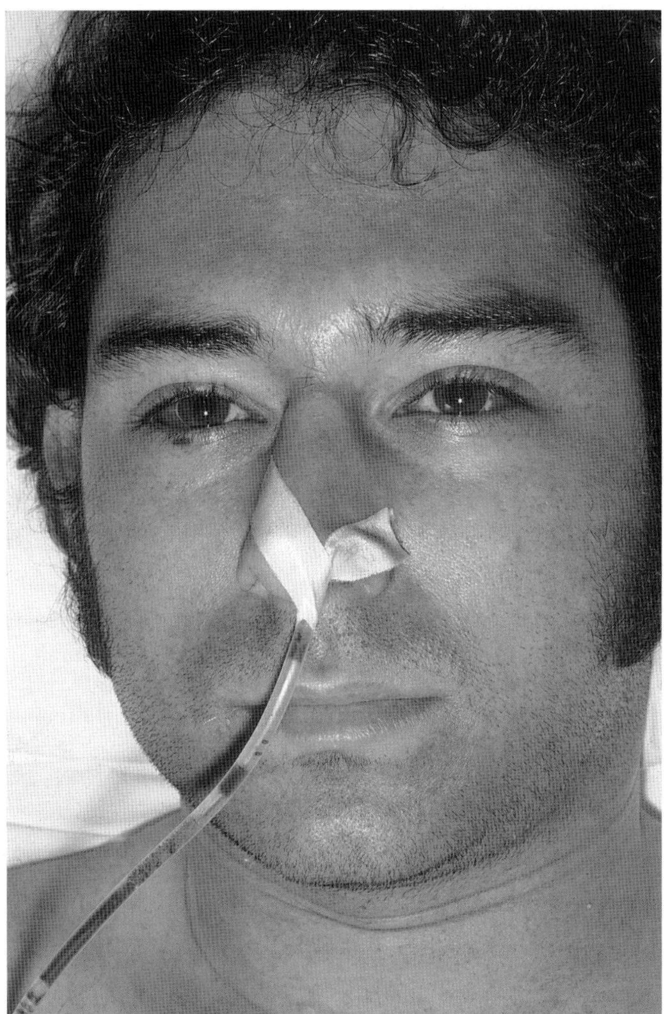

Figure 7.3 Crush injury.

hyperkalaemia from reperfusion. Release of myoglobin from these damaged muscles can cause acute renal failure. Crush injury may lead to the development of limb compartment syndrome, requiring fasciotomy to reduce the compartmental pressure and allow capillary perfusion (see Ch. 10).

THERMAL INJURY

Burns are relatively common in trauma and may occur in isolation or in conjunction with multiple injuries, for example vehicle fires and explosions following a crash. The time of exposure and the burn agent are important factors in the severity of the burn, as is evidence of airway and inhalational burns. Burn victims should be resuscitated according to ATLS® guidelines and other injuries looked for (for further information see Ch. 6).

RESUSCITATION

Resuscitation for trauma follows the principles of the ATLS® course.[1] The objective is to identify and treat immediate threats to life. Universal precautions are essential. As a minimum, all members of the trauma team should wear gloves, masks with visors, and aprons, and also protect themselves from radiation; ideally the resuscitation process and any key radiographs should take place simultaneously.

HANDOVER FROM PREHOSPITAL PERSONNEL

Information from paramedics can be vital, and the *MIST* handover should be used:

- Mechanism of injury.
- Injuries identified.
- Signs at scene.
- Treatment administered.

PRIMARY SURVEY AND RESUSCITATION

Airway

Evaluation of the airway is the first priority. If a patient can speak, the airway is not immediately threatened; however, if the patient does not reply to a simple question, then measures to establish an airway must be taken while protecting the cervical spine. Injury to the cervical spine is assumed in the presence of multisystem injury, especially if there is alteration of the conscious level or blunt injury above the clavicle.

Breathing

All trauma patients should receive high-flow oxygen. Respiratory effort is assessed and the rate recorded. The patient's neck and chest are inspected for wounds, tracheal deviation and surgical emphysema; chest percussion and auscultation are undertaken.

Circulation

The commonest cause of shock after trauma is hypovolaemia; there are five places that a patient can lose a large volume of blood:

- externally into the environment;
- into the chest;
- into the abdomen;
- into the retroperitoneum and pelvis; and
- into the external muscle compartments.

This can be summarized by the aphorism 'blood on the floor and four more'.

External bleeding must be controlled and intravenous access obtained. Blood is drawn for cross-match and a bolus of warmed crystalloid commenced. Other causes of shock after trauma that are not hypovolaemic should be excluded.

Disability

The level of consciousness is assessed by the Glasgow Coma Scale (GCS) (see Ch. 15) and the pupils are assessed.

Exposure with control of the environment

Clothing is removed, and the back of the patient examined by 'log-rolling' the individual while protecting spinal alignment. Trauma patients can rapidly become cold, and warming with warm air blankets is vital.

Adjuncts to the primary survey are listed below.

- Monitoring. ECG, non-invasive blood pressure, and pulse oximetry should be the minimum standard of monitoring in the resuscitation area. End tidal CO_2 and central venous pressure monitoring may be helpful.
- Urinary and gastric catheters. A gastric catheter should not be placed via the nose in the presence of maxillofacial injury or suspected base of skull fracture. Inspection of the genitalia and rectum must always precede urinary catheterization; a urinary catheter should not be inserted if a urethral injury is suspected (see Ch. 38).
- Diagnostic studies.

The following X-rays are routinely obtained: a lateral cervical spine, an anteroposterior chest; and an anteroposterior pelvis. The need for more sophisticated imaging—focused abdominal sonography for trauma (FAST) scan, CT, or diagnostic peritoneal lavage—should be considered.

SECONDARY SURVEY

The secondary survey phase comprises an AMPLE history and a head-to-toe examination of the patient:

- Allergy.
- Medication.
- Past medical history.
- Last meal.
- Events of the incident.

DEFINITIVE CARE

After identifying the injuries, initiating resuscitation, and obtaining diagnostic studies, definitive care should begin.

SYSTEMS INJURY

HEAD INJURY (see Ch. 15)

The most common cause of death after trauma is severe brain injury; head injury also causes major morbidity in survivors.[34,35] There are two major categories of brain injury: focal injuries and diffuse injuries. An understanding of the concept of secondary brain injury, caused by hypotension and hypoxia, is fundamental, and the treatment of a head-injured patient should emphasize early control of the airway (while immobilizing the cervical spine), ensuring adequate ventilation and oxygenation, correcting hypovolaemia, and prompt imaging by CT. Recent guidelines have attempted to improve the management of severe traumatic brain injury.[36,37]

REFERENCES

34. Finfer SR, Cohen J. Resuscitation 2001; 48: 77–90
35. McKenzie EJ, Siegel JH, Shapiro S et al. J Trauma 1988; 28: 281–297
36. Brain Trauma Foundation, American Association of Neurological Surgeons, Joint Section on Neurotrauma and Critical Care. J Neurotrauma 1996; 13: 641–734
37. Maas AI, Dearden M, Teasdale GM et al. Acta Neurochir (Wien) 1997; 139: 286–294

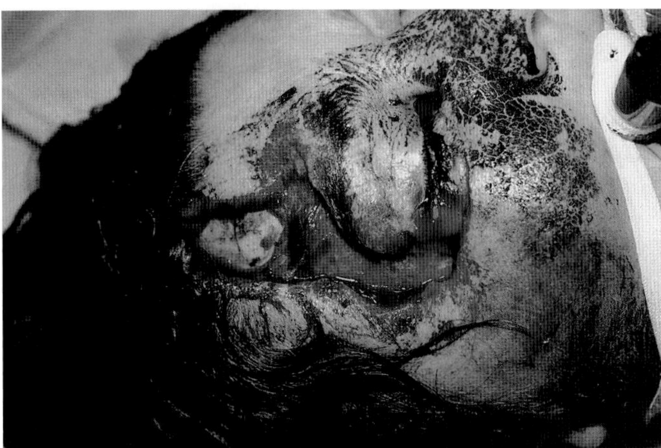

Figure 7.4 Injury due to impact with car windscreen.

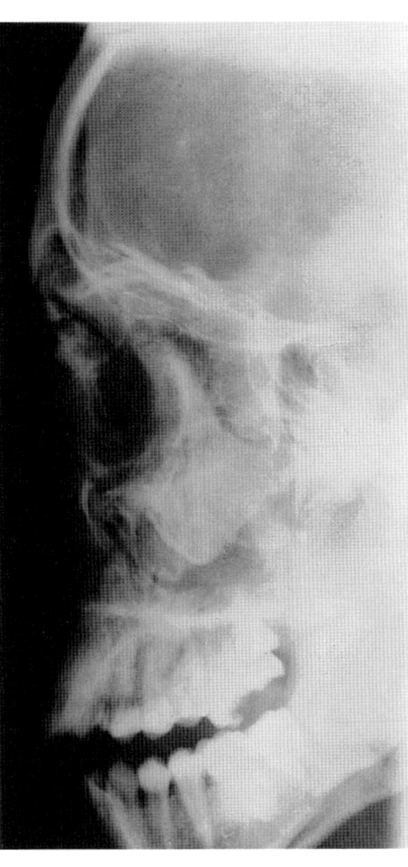

Figure 7.5 Lateral radiograph of anterior head and face shows fracture of frontonasal process, aerocele in frontal area, disruption or orbit and elements of Le Fort III fracture of mid-third of face.

Penetrating head injury

The management of penetrating head injury follows the ATLS® template, and early involvement of a neurosurgeon is vital.[36] Classical treatment of compound depressed skull fractures includes debridement and closure of all scalp wounds to minimize the risk of delayed intracranial infection. A non-surgical approach may prove to be equally safe for selected patients with blunt, compound, depressed skull fractures without significant intracranial haematomas or dural damage.[38]

Seizures in the early post-traumatic period following head injury may cause secondary brain damage as a result of increased metabolic demands, raised intracranial pressure, and excess neurotransmitter release. Prophylactic anti-epileptics are effective in reducing early seizures, but guidance from a neurosurgeon should be sought.[39] Broad-spectrum antibiotics are recommended for all penetrating craniocerebral injuries,[40] but are not given for closed fracture of the skull base.

Emergency craniotomy is required for patients with missile injuries if there is significant mass effect from a haematoma or bullet track. Removal of fragments of the projectile or in-driven bone fragments should not be pursued at the expense of damaging normal brain tissue. Patients with penetrating craniocerebral gunshot injuries with a GCS score of 5 or less after resuscitation, or a score of 8 or less with CT findings of transventricular or bihemispheric injury, have such poor outcome that conservative treatment may be indicated.[41] Notification of the local organ transplant coordinator may be appropriate (see Ch. 8).

Maxillofacial injury (see Ch. 13)

Blunt trauma to the face produces soft tissue and bony injury, and may arise as a result of assault or motor vehicle crashes (Fig. 7.4). Midface fractures are common; fracture is at one of three levels as described by Le Fort (Fig. 7.5). The loss of bony integrity of the midface, mandibular fractures, broken teeth, and soft tissue bleeding can jeopardize the airway, especially in the unconscious patient. Attention must be directed towards maintenance of the airway—through simple measures, intubation, or provision of a surgical airway—in the resuscitation of these patients. Avulsed teeth, broken dentures, and other inhaled foreign bodies can also be a source of pulmonary complications. It is also important to recognize that maxillofacial injury and head trauma is associated with cervical spine injury, and appropriate measures should be undertaken to immobilize the spine. Ocular trauma can also occur in facial trauma, and must be managed appropriately.

NECK

The management of penetrating neck injuries, which penetrates the platysma by mandatory surgical exploration, has been challenged in recent years; a more conservative approach in selected stable patients associated with improvements in diagnostic imaging, arteriography and endoscopy has shown similar results.

Classically, the neck is divided into three anatomic zones:

- Zone I: at the thoracic outlet.
- Zone II: between the cricoid and the angle of the mandible.
- Zone III: extending from the angle of mandible to the base of the skull.

Surgical exposure of injuries in zones I and III is more difficult. Arteriography and interventional radiology may play a role in the diagnosis and management of these injuries, and endoscopic evaluation of the trachea and digestive tracts provides further information. Patients in whom these investigations are negative may be managed conservatively.

CERVICAL VASCULAR INJURY (see Ch. 10)

Blunt injury to the vessels of the neck may occur as a result of a direct blow to the neck, or with acute hyperextension. Contusion or intimal damage of the vessels can occur as the vessels are stretched over the cervical vertebrae. Potential vascular injury must

REFERENCES

38. Heary RF, Hunt CD, Krieger AJ et al. J Trauma 1993; 35: 441–447
39. Schierhout G, Roberts I. Cochrane Database Syst Rev 2001; 4: CD000173
40. Bayston R, de Louvois J, Brown EM et al. Lancet 2000; 355: 1813–1817
41. Semple PL, Domingo Z. S Afr Med J 2001; 91: 141–145

Table 7.2 Indications for thoracotomy after penetrating chest injury

Immediate (emergency room thoracotomy)	Urgent	Delayed (consider minimally invasive techniques)
Penetrating chest wound with cardiovascular collapse or cardiac arrest in the casualty area	Cardiac tamponade	Retained haemothorax
Shock (< 60 mmHg) despite resuscitation, with high likelihood of intrathoracic injury	Massive haemothorax or significant ongoing blood loss	Empyema
	Massive air leak from chest tube	Diaphragmatic injury
	Injury demonstrated to major airway or oesophagus	
	Vascular injury low in the neck	

be evaluated by pulses, palpation, the presence of bruits, and an expanding haematoma. An acute neurological deficit suggestive of a hemispheric stroke is a clear indication of vascular injury. Arteriography is the best investigation, but may be replaced by duplex Doppler. The management of these injuries may be augmented by interventional radiology; however, bleeding vessels and intimal tears usually require operative repair by an experienced surgeon. Patency should be restored wherever possible.

CHEST INJURY

Blunt injury to the chest (see Ch. 21)

Pulmonary contusion is the most commonly diagnosed intrathoracic injury in victims of blunt trauma; it is an independent risk factor for pneumonia and adult respiratory distress syndrome, and is associated with a mortality rate of 10–25%.[42] Significant contusion is often not diagnosed until 24 h after admission, because chest radiographic signs are typically delayed and often underestimate the degree of pulmonary injury.[43] Early CT scan is often helpful, and if the injury is bilateral and associated with pneumothorax or haemothorax the outcome is likely to be worse.[43,44] Respiratory dysfunction arises from a combination of pulmonary dysfunction in the contused segment and remote lung injury mediated by cytokines released by the injury to the lung parenchyma.[44]

Blunt chest trauma in adults often results in fractured ribs, which may lead to a flail chest, defined as fracture of two or more ribs in two or more places with resultant paradoxical movement of a segment of the chest wall (see Ch. 21). The force required to disrupt the integrity of the thoracic cage typically produces an underlying pulmonary contusion. Traditional treatment has been the use of mechanical ventilation to internally splint the chest until fibrous union of the broken ribs occurred. This treatment requires significant resources, with many days on a ventilator, and is often at the cost of significant morbidity associated with tracheostomy and hospital-acquired pneumonia. Careful conservative treatment, with supplemental oxygen, aggressive physiotherapy, and effective use of analgesia can often avoid the need for ventilation.[45]

Although not indicated for all flail chests, selected patients with greatly unstable or displaced chest wall segments having operative fixation of rib fractures have been shown to have reduced ventilator requirement, reduced requirement for tracheostomy, and reduced rates of ventilator-associated pulmonary barotraumas, pneumonia, intensive care stay and mortality.[46]

Penetrating injury

The chest is situated between two important anatomical areas: the neck and the abdomen. All patients with penetrating injury below the nipples anteriorly, or below the tip of the scapula posteriorly, should be assumed to have an intra-abdominal injury in addition to a thoracic injury. All patients with penetrating injuries of the neck must be considered to have an associated intrathoracic injury, until proven otherwise. Gunshot wounds can cause injuries across anatomical boundaries irrespective of the position of the entrance wound.

Most patients with chest trauma are successfully managed by tube thoracostomy with careful monitoring of drainage and vital signs. Indications for immediate thoracotomy are based on physical findings combined with information from radiological imaging of the chest (Table 7.2).[47] An indication for thoracotomy is often given as the drainage of 1.5 L of blood from the chest tube; however, the amount of blood loss from the tube is not always a reliable guide to the severity of intrathoracic injury. The amount of blood loss must be considered in the light of the clinical condition of the patient, but if blood loss is greater than 1 L, thoracotomy should be considered. Minimally invasive techniques may be valuable (see Ch. 21).[48,49]

Tracheobronchial injury

Many patients with blunt tracheobronchial injuries die before they reach hospital.[50,51] Patients surviving to reach hospital can be classified into two broad groups. In the first group, subcutaneous emphysema and dyspnoea are the most common initial signs,[52] as free communication between the injury and the pleural space results in mediastinal and subcutaneous emphysema and a large air leak from the intercostal drain. Chest radiographs may reveal pneumothorax, pneumomediastinum, and the fallen lung sign, where the apex of the lung is seen at the level of the carina.

REFERENCES

42. Cohn SM. J Trauma 1997; 42: 973–979
43. Pape HC, Remmers D, Rice J et al. J Trauma 2000; 49: 496–504
44. Miller PR, Croce MA, Bee TK et al. J Trauma 2001; 51: 223–228
45. Richardson JD, Adams L, Flint LM. Ann Surg 1982; 196: 481–487
46. Ahmed Z, Mohyuddin Z. J Thorac Cardiovasc Surg 1995; 110: 1676–1680
47. Demetriades D, Velmahos GC. Scand J Surg 2002; 91: 41–45
48. Murray JA, Demetriades D, Asensio JA et al. J Am Coll Surg 1998; 187: 626–630
49. Lang-Lazdunski L, Mouroux J, Pons F et al. Ann Thorac Surg 1997; 63: 327–333.
50. Martin de Nicolas JL, Gamez AP, Cruz F et al. Ann Thorac Surg 1996; 62: 269–272
51. Bertelsen S, Howitz P. Thorax 1972; 27: 188–194
52. Lin M-Y, Wu M-H, Chan CS et al. Ann Emerg Med 1995; 25: 412–415

In the second group of patients, peribronchial connective tissue remains intact and allows distal lung ventilation.[53] Signs are correspondingly less obvious, and the diagnosis is frequently missed. Correctly identifying these injuries relies on a high index of suspicion combined with endoscopic examination of the tracheobronchial tree. The location of the lesions appears to be constant: 80% occur within 2.5 cm of the carina, 80% involve the main stem of the bronchi, 15% are tracheal, and 5% are distal bronchial lesions. Treatment is primarily surgical, although if the transection is less than one-third of the circumference of the airway and the lung is fully expanded, then conservative treatment may be applied successfully (see Ch. 21).

Cardiac injury

Blunt cardiac injury refers to a spectrum of injuries that range from simple electrocardiogram changes to cardiac wall rupture. Blunt cardiac trauma is only of clinical significance when associated with significant symptoms, because it is these patients who are at risk of developing complications. The diagnosis of this condition has been the subject of some debate; however, data now suggest that the combination of a normal electrocardiograph and cardiac troponin I effectively excludes significant blunt cardiac trauma.[54] Unfortunately, the positive predictive value of this combination is less reliable. Patients with abnormal results or evidence of clinical sequelae should undergo echocardiography and monitoring (see Ch. 22).

Aortic injury

Traumatic aortic injuries cause or contribute to 15% of fatalities following road traffic accident.[55] Most patients with traumatic aortic injuries die before they reach hospital, and the vast majority have major coexisting thoracic and extrathoracic injuries.[56]

Three mechanisms are thought to contribute to aortic rupture:

- shearing stress generated by differential movement between a fixed portion of the aorta and a relatively more mobile portion;
- a very high peak of intraluminal pressure occurring during the moment of the accident; and
- crushing of the aorta between the chest wall and the spinal column (the so-called osseous pinch).[57]

Approximately 90% of traumatic aortic injuries occur at the aortic isthmus, defined as the proximal descending aorta within 1 cm of the origin of the left subclavian artery.[56]

The most sensitive chest radiographic findings of aortic injury are widening of the mediastinum (greater than 8 cm at the arch) and an abnormal or indistinct aortic contour (Fig. 7.6).[57] The initial chest radiograph may be reported as normal in up to 44% of patients.[58] Aortography is still the best diagnostic tool, with a sensitivity of almost 100% and a specificity of 98% for detecting traumatic aortic injury (Fig. 7.7).[57] Helical CT has been reported to have 100% sensitivity,[58] and it has the advantages of being non-invasive and able to demonstrate injuries other than traumatic aortic injury.[59]

Traumatic aortic injuries must be repaired. The traditional method has been called clamp and sew. The risk of paraplegia increases dramatically after a clamp time of 30 min,[60] and a recent review of the literature has confirmed that paraplegia is less likely if a shunt or bypass technique is used (see Ch. 56).[61]

The increasing sophistication of endovascular techniques has led to attempts to treat traumatic aortic injuries by stents, thus avoiding the considerable morbidity of open repair.[62] This approach holds great promise for the future (see Ch. 10).

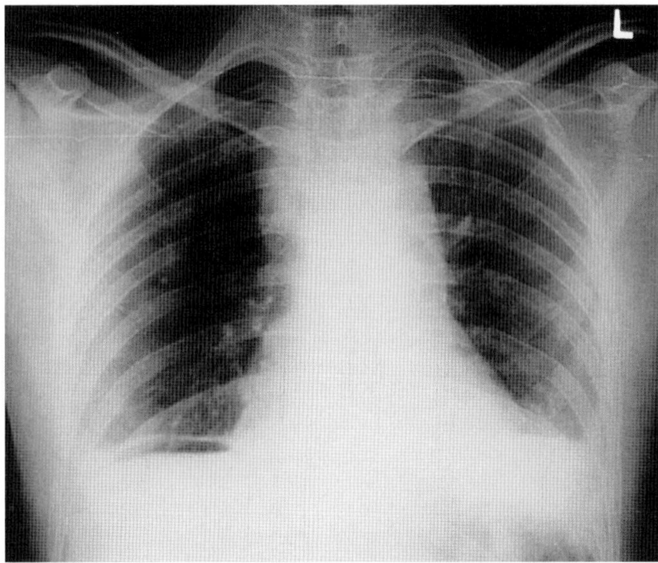

Figure 7.6 Chest radiograph of patient who suffered sudden deceleration of the isthmus of the thoracic aorta showing widening of superior mediastinum, opacification between aorta and pulmonary artery and loss of clarity of left upper lung field ('apical capping'). Aortic injury suspected only after laparotomy for visceral injuries which accounts for air under the diaphragm.

Diaphragmatic injury

Blunt diaphragmatic injury is not uncommon, although it may be unrecognized initially and only present later, when it is associated with greater morbidity and mortality (see Ch. 21). It is therefore important to have a high index of suspicion for this injury. Diagnosis may be difficult. Chest radiographs may show the gastric bubble and nasogastric tube in the stomach above the diaphragm, but this is not always the case, and both ultrasound and CT can miss the injury if the abdominal organs are not herniated into the chest at the time of imaging. Laparoscopy is the most sensitive technique for diagnosing diaphragm rupture. Rupture is reportedly more common on the left because the liver acts to protect the right hemidiaphragm; blunt trauma tends to cause large defects and is frequently associated with significant other abdominal injuries. Repair of these injuries can be undertaken through a laparotomy, and there are reports of

REFERENCES

53. Singh N, Narasimhan KL, Rao KLN et al. J Trauma 1999; 46: 962–964
54. Salim A, Velmahos GC, Jindal A et al. J Trauma 2001; 50: 237–243
55. Pretre R, Chilcott M. N Engl J Med 1997; 336: 626–632
56. Dosios TJ, Salemis N, Angouras D et al. J Trauma 2000; 49: 696–703
57. Fishman JE. J Thorac Imaging 2000; 15: 97–103
58. Demetriades D, Gomez H, Velmahos GC et al. Arch Surg 1998; 133: 1084–1088
59. Beese RC, Allan R, Treasure T. Ann R Coll Surg Engl 2001; 83: 10–13
60. Fabian TC, Richardson JD, Croce MA et al. J Trauma 1997; 42: 374–380
61. Jahromi AS, Kazemi K, Safar HA et al. J Vasc Surg 2001; 34: 1029–1034
62. Gan JP, Campbell WA. J Trauma 2002; 52: 154–157

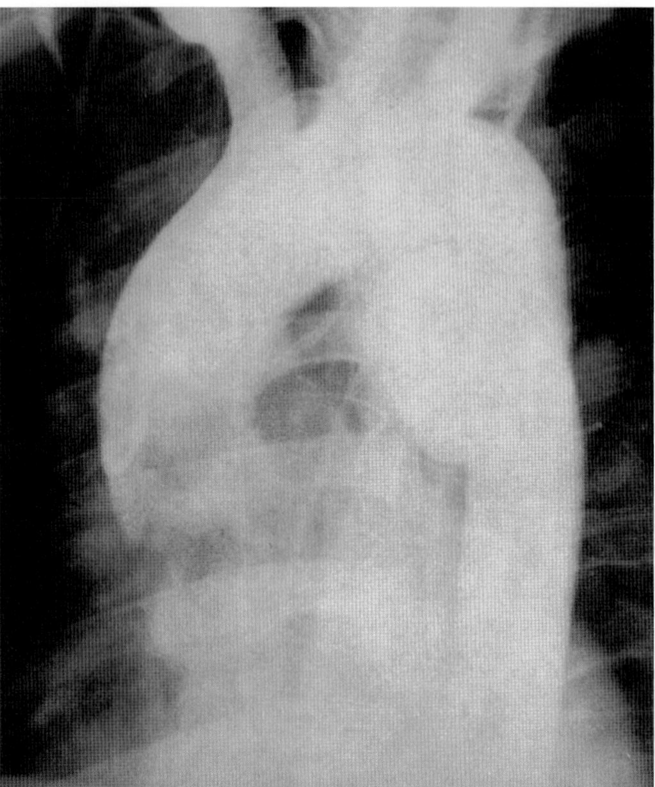

Figure 7.7 Aortogram showing isthmic rupture of the thoracic aorta resulting in false aneurysm formation. At operation, haematoma extended from the root of the thoracic aorta down to the mid descending aorta. The femoral artery and left atrium were cannulated for bypass, the aorta was cross-clamped proximal and distal to the rupture, and after excising the edges, a Dacron graft was successfully interposed.

laparoscopic repair although long-term follow-up data are still required.

ABDOMINAL INJURY

The pathophysiology of penetrating torso injury and diagnosis of these injuries have been discussed elsewhere in this chapter. Most hospitals continue with a policy of mandatory laparotomy in gunshot wounds of the abdomen, because of the high incidence of organ injury; however, some centres follow a conservative or expectant approach in stable patients with abdominal stab wounds, or perform laparoscopy to determine peritoneal penetration. At operation specific organ injuries are addressed; this may include resection and anastomosis of small-bowel injury and the management of large-bowel injury as discussed previously. Some patients who are critically unstable may benefit from damage control procedures[63] and delayed definitive surgery after further resuscitation. Limited antibiotic prophylaxis is used.[64]

SOLID VISCUS INJURY

Splenic injury

During the past two decades, there has been growing enthusiasm for preservation of the injured spleen, which reflects concerns for the postoperative complications of splenectomy as well as physiological risks to the asplenic patient (see Ch. 32). Patients who undergo splenectomy after trauma display overall immunosuppression, and are at increased risk of overwhelming postsplenectomy infection (OPSI). The risk of OPSI appears to vary according to the patient's age, with the rate of serious infection in asplenic children less than 5 years old exceeding 10%, and although the risk for OPSI in adults is much less, it is approximately 1%.[65]

The ideal candidates for non-operative management are haemodynamically stable. Patients with mild hypotension with a systolic blood pressure greater than 90 mmHg on arrival, who respond quickly to infusion of crystalloid, and who remain haemodynamically stable thereafter may also be considered for conservative management.[66,67] When more than 1 unit of blood has been transfused, surgical repair is usually required,[68] and an increasing grade of injury is also likely to result in failure, although relying on CT grade of splenic injuries alone frequently does not predict the clinical outcome.[69] Patients with grade I injuries may fail, and patients with high-grade (IV and V) injuries may be successfully managed conservatively.[70,71] A dynamic CT showing blushing of contrast material implies the presence of a contained pseudoaneurysm or active bleeding, when embolization may be valuable (Fig. 7.8).[72]

In detecting bowel injury CT has an overall sensitivity of approximately 94%.[73] The presence of a moderate (GCS 9–13) or severe (GCS less than 8) closed head injury is no longer considered a contraindication to non-operative management in appropriately monitored patients.[74]

Elderly patients have been considered poor candidates for non-operative management, and a large multicentre trial has documented that patients aged more than 55 years failed non-operative management more frequently than patients aged less than 55 (19% versus 10%). Some centres report no difficulties in managing older patients conservatively.[75,76]

Liver injury (see Ch. 29)

Over the past decade, increasing understanding of the healing potential of the liver and the increasing sophistication of CT scanning has meant that non-operative management has come to dominate the management of blunt liver injuries. Approximately

REFERENCES

63. Johnson JW, Gracias VH, Schwab CW et al. J Trauma 2001; 51: 261–269, discussion 269–271
64. Luchette FA, Borzotta AP, Croce MA et al. J Trauma 2000; 48: 508–518
65. Potoka DA, Schall LC, Ford HR. J Pediatr Surg 2002; 37: 294–299
66. Davis KA, Fabian TC, Croce MA et al. J Trauma 1998; 44: 1008–1013
67. Pachter HL, Guth AA, Hofstetter SR et al. Ann Surg 1998; 227: 708–717
68. Velmahos GC, Chan LS, Kamel E et al. Arch Surg 2000; 135: 674–679
69. Gavant ML, Schurr M, Flick PA et al. Am J Roentgenol 1997; 168: 207–212
70. Peitzman AB, Heil B, Rivera L et al. J Trauma 2000; 49: 177–187
71. Goan YG, Huang MS, Lin JM. J Trauma 1998; 45: 360–364
72. Yao DC, Jeffrey RB Jr, Mirvis SE et al. Am J Roentgenol 2002; 178: 17–20
73. Killeen KL, Shanmuganathan K, Poletti PA et al. J Trauma 2001; 51: 26–36
74. Archer LP, Rogers FB, Shackford SR. Arch Surg 1996; 131: 309–315
75. Cocanour CS, Moore FA, Ware DN et al. J Trauma 2000; 48: 606–610
76. Albrecht RM, Schermer CR, Morris A. Am Surg 2002; 68: 227–230

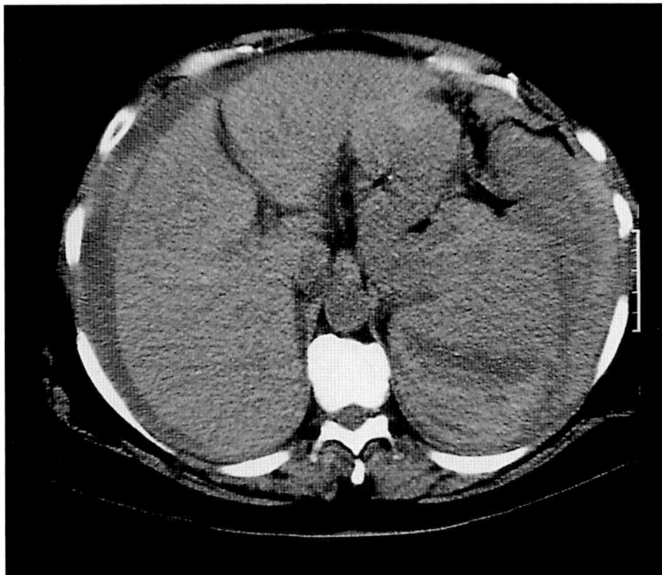

Figure 7.8 CT scan of a patient with a ruptured spleen.

85% of all patients with blunt hepatic trauma are stable. In this group, non-operative management significantly improves outcomes over operative management, because of decreased infections, transfusion, and length of hospital stay.[77]

In a recent study of 119 patients with blunt hepatic injuries, 61 were selected for non-operative management. Six of the 61 required delayed surgery; however, all six patients were successfully managed using minimally invasive surgery, including laparoscopic application of fibrin glue as a haemostatic agent.[78]

Higher-grade liver injuries are more likely to fail a trial of conservative management; nevertheless, the non-operative approach has been extended to include grade IV and grade V injuries by use of aggressive resuscitation and adjunctive therapies, such as angioembolization, laparoscopic haemostasis, and CT-guided drainage of perihepatic collections. In a series of 25 patients with grade III to grade V liver lacerations, intra-abdominal pressure evaluation was used to guide a protocol of laparoscopic abdominal decompression and hepatic evaluation. Five patients required decompression and 60% were treated solely through the laparoscope, avoiding laparotomy.[79] As well as drainage of large haemoperitoneum, biliary peritonitis can be controlled via the laparoscope, and this may be combined with endoscopic retrograde cholangiopancreatography to achieve control of biliary leaks.[80]

Contrast-enhanced CT scanning is the mainstay of diagnosis for hepatic injuries after blunt trauma in the stable patient; the initial CT findings help to determine suitability for non-operative treatment.

For unstable patients, investigation is not appropriate and laparotomy is indicated, with the damage control approach now accepted as the standard of care.[81]

Pancreaticoduodenal injury

Pancreaticoduodenal injuries are relatively rare because their retroperitoneal location confers a degree of relative protection to these organs (see Ch. 27). This location also makes them relatively inaccessible to diagnostic techniques. In blunt trauma these organs are often injured in association with other structures, and injury may be suspected only at laparotomy, when bile staining of the retroperitoneum is found. Surgical management depends on the stability of the patient, and ranges from repair with pyloric exclusion techniques for the duodenum to drainage or resection of the pancreatic tail. A Whipple procedure (pancreaticoduodenectomy) is rarely required at the initial operation because massive pancreatoduodenal trauma usually occurs in patients who are critically unstable from other injuries, making them candidates for damage control rather than a prolonged operation.

Renal injury (see Ch. 35)

Over 90% of injuries to the kidneys are as a result of blunt trauma.[82] Over recent years, as with injuries to the liver and spleen, there has been a progressive trend towards non-operative management, unless the patient is haemodynamically unstable.[83] Even high-grade renal injuries can be treated non-operatively, and patients treated in this manner have been shown to have fewer days in intensive care, significantly lower transfusion requirements, and fewer complications compared with patients undergoing surgical exploration.[82] Although intravenous urography can demonstrate renal injury, CT scans accurately document the severity of the renal injury and enable assessment of associated injuries. The incidence of urinary complications correlates significantly with an increasing grade of injury. Complications may be delayed and, therefore, repeat imaging several days after significant renal injury is important to document functioning renal parenchyma and identify delayed complications that may require intervention.[84]

HOLLOW VISCUS INJURY

Blunt trauma can rupture the bowel as a result of an acute rise in the intraluminal pressure or shear forces, especially at the duodenojejunal flexure or ileocaecal junction. Rapid deceleration may also cause tearing of the mesentery and its vessels, leading to bleeding and bowel ischaemia. It is vital to fully assess both the small and large bowel when performing a laparotomy, to look for perforations and to explore haematomas on the mesenteric border. Small-bowel injuries can be repaired either directly or by resection and anastomosis when more significant. There has, however, been more debate on the management of large-bowel trauma (see Ch. 27). Traditional surgical technique was to exteriorize the bowel as a stoma, with later anastomosis. This approach has been challenged, and recent publications have shown that the majority of large-bowel injuries can be safely repaired, or an anastomosis fashioned at the initial surgery, without a marked increase in morbidity or mortality (see Ch. 28).[85]

REFERENCES

77. Malhotra AK, Fabian TC, Croce MA et al. Ann Surg 2000; 231: 804–813
78. Chen RJ, Fang JF, Lin BC et al. J Trauma 1998; 44: 691–695
79. Chen RJ, Fang JF, Chen MF. J Trauma 2001; 51: 44–50
80. Carrillo EH, Spain DA, Wohltmann CD et al. J Trauma 1999; 46: 619–622
81. Shapiro MB, Jenkins DH, Schwab CW et al. J Trauma 2000; 49: 969–978
82. Kuo RL, Eachempati SR, Makhuli MJ et al. World J Surg 2002; 26: 416–419
83. Altman AL, Haas C, Dinchman KH et al. J Urol 2000; 164: 27–30
84. Blankenship JC, Gavant ML, Cox CE et al. World J Surg 2001; 25: 1561–1564
85. Cayten CG, Fabian TC, Garcia VF et al. In: Trauma Practice Guidelines. Online. Available: http://www.east.org 2002

PELVIC INJURY

The mechanism of injury and fracture pattern in pelvic fracture from blunt trauma may provide some guide as to the blood loss (see Ch. 54). These injuries can be devastating, with extremely high mortality and massive blood loss. During resuscitation, simple measures to reduce the pelvic volume, such as tying a sheet around the pelvis and internally rotating the legs, should be undertaken. An external fixator, clamp, or other compressive device can be applied to close and stabilize the pelvis. Arteriography and embolization[86] have a major role in the management of pelvic bleeding and should be incorporated into management protocols.

VASCULAR INJURY (see Ch. 10)

Vascular injury can occur through direct injury of the vessel by a bullet or knife. Vessels can also be damaged through energy transfer as a missile passes close to a vessel, producing contusion of the vessel wall or the formation of an intimal flap. Both peripheral and major vessels can be injured, and unstable patients require immediate surgical exploration, resection of the vessel to healthy tissue, and patching, anastomosis, or grafting—preferably with native vessels. It is ideal to repair both artery and vein when they are both injured. Occasionally, in a very unstable patient, it may be necessary to ligate or shunt vessels. Where the patient is more stable, further investigation can be undertaken to provide information before surgery, and radiological intervention provides definitive treatment. At the end of a vascular procedure, a completion-on-table angiogram should always be obtained to assess the repair.

SPINAL INJURY (see Ch. 56)

The US Major Trauma Outcome Study estimated that the incidence of acute spinal-cord injury was 2.6% of blunt trauma patients.[87] The average lifetime cost of treating an individual with traumatic spinal-cord injury is estimated to be between US$500 000 and US$2 million.[88]

Initial treatment for spinal injury should focus on the airway, breathing and circulation. In addition, the National Acute Spinal Cord Injury Study phase 3 trial showed that high-dose steroids given within 8 h of injury reduced disability.[89] Rehabilitation after spinal injury requires a multidisciplinary approach to reduce morbidity from the psychological and physical problems attendant with spinal cord injury.[88]

EXTREMITY INJURY

The priority for patients with extremity injury is resuscitation according to ATLS® protocols. Although no improvement in survival has been shown for polytrauma patients undergoing stabilization of long-bone fractures within 48 h of injury compared with those receiving later stabilization, early mobility is improved and pulmonary morbidity is decreased.[90,91]

Early long-bone stabilization in patients with brain or chest injury appears to neither enhance nor worsen outcome. Current recommendations support management on an individual basis, with the important caveat to avoid any operative procedure that might lead to hypotension or hypoxia and cause a secondary insult.[90]

PSYCHOLOGICAL TRAUMA: POST-TRAUMATIC STRESS DISORDER

An individual's reaction to a traumatic situation or experience may vary along a continuum from a normal reaction to an abnormal, excessive or prolonged reaction. Even a normal reaction may comprise a wide range of responses, from numbness and denial to anger and guilt. Flashbacks are also a normal reaction to trauma, and are usually visual but may involve any of the sensory modalities. It is important that victims suffering such responses are reassured that these are normal reactions to their experiences. Emotions may follow the natural sequence associated with loss: denial, anger, depression and acceptance. The acute stress reaction has a limited 2-day to 4-week course and is similar to post-traumatic stress disorder. A few individuals and healthcare providers exposed to acutely traumatic situations may suffer from excessive or prolonged emotional reaction. These symptoms must last 30 days to meet criteria for post-traumatic stress disorder, which is defined by re-experiencing the traumatic event, numbing of responsiveness, and disturbances of arousal. These patients need continuing psychological support.

TRAUMA IN SPECIAL SITUATIONS

TRAUMA IN THE ELDERLY

Improved health, medical intervention, and changing demographics mean that the older age group is set to increase in both numbers and overall percentage of the population. Defining this group by age alone is difficult, because many in their seventies or eighties may enjoy full and active lifestyles while younger patients may suffer from chronic ill health and disability. The mechanisms of injury are similar in the older age groups, with blunt trauma most common, particularly from falls and road traffic accidents (especially as pedestrians).

Although trauma resuscitation should proceed according to ATLS® guidelines, it is important to consider any coexisting medical conditions and medications because these factors may further complicate the clinical picture. Elderly patients compensate poorly for blood loss, and even a relatively small haemorrhage may lead to hypotension because of an impaired sympathetic response. Patients on beta blockers or with pacemakers may fail to produce a tachycardic response. Pre-existing renal impairment may reduce the value of urinary output as an indicator of perfusion, and elderly patients are also more susceptible to hypothermia and its complications.

REFERENCES

86. Velmahos GC, Toutouzas KG, Vassiliu P et al. J Trauma 2002; 53: 303–308, discussion 308
87. Burney RE, Maio RF, Maynard F et al. Arch Surg 1993; 128: 596–599
88. McDonald JW, Sadowsky C. Lancet 2002; 359: 417–425
89. Bracken MB, Shepard MJ, Holford TR et al. JAMA 1997; 277: 1597–1604
90. Dunham CM, Bosse MJ, Clancy TV et al. J Trauma 2001; 50: 958–967
91. Robinson CM. J Bone Joint Surg Br 2001; 83: 781–791

TRAUMA IN CHILDREN (see Ch. 40)

Injury is the primary cause of death and disability among children and adolescents,[92] and socioeconomic disadvantage is associated with both the increased rate and severity of injury.[93]

The sequence of resuscitation for children is the same as that for adults; the first priority is the airway, with provision of oxygen and protection of the cervical spine. Infants breathe through their noses, so the nostrils should be cleared and gastric tubes should not be placed through the nose. Cuffed endotracheal tubes are not used until the child weighs around 30 kg, because the paediatric trachea is short and soft, and cuffed tubes provoke mucosal oedema, ulceration and stenosis.

Thoracic trauma is the second leading cause of death in children, after head injury, and the presence of thoracic injury in addition to other injuries in a child increases the probability of death by three to four times.[94] The chest wall of a child is very compliant, and therefore significant intrathoracic injuries can be present without rib fractures. Infants and small children breathe primarily with their diaphragm and when injured tend to cry and swallow air, which causes gastric distension, limiting movement of the diaphragm and compromising respiration; all severely injured children should have gastric decompression tubes.

Intravenous access can be difficult in injured children, and if this route is unsuccessful intraosseous access in the proximal tibia of an uninjured leg is the preferred alternative for children younger than 6 years. A surgical cut-down is a good alternative.

Head injury is the commonest cause of death and disability among injured children.[95] The management of head injury in children follows the same principles as that for adults, with avoidance of the secondary insults of hypoxia and hypotension, and early involvement of specialists.

The vast majority of serious abdominal injuries are caused by blunt trauma, and more than 90% of injuries to solid organs can be managed non-operatively.[96] Helical (spiral) CT is the ideal to document the severity of blunt organ injury. The consistently high success rates for non-operative management in children can lull the surgical team into a false sense of security; approximately 3% of children with blunt abdominal injuries have a hollow viscus injury, and delay causes significant morbidity and mortality. Surgeons must have a high index of suspicion to diagnose these injuries.[97] Injury in children may be the result of abuse or neglect; child abuse is the second leading cause of death of children in the USA.[98] Future fatal injuries may be avoided if a doctor acts on suspicion that injuries are non-accidental and alerts the child protection services.

TRAUMA IN WOMEN

Although there are many different forms of violence against women, they often share certain characteristics. Most forms, including intimate partner violence and child sexual abuse, do not occur as unique incidents, but are ongoing over time, even over decades. Often the woman not only knows the perpetrator before the first incident, but might live with him.[99]

Physical and sexual violence by an intimate partner may have a profound impact on the physical and mental health of those who experience it. This form of violence affects 20–50% of women at some stage in life in most populations surveyed globally.[100] Violence is frequently used to resolve a crisis of male identity. Poverty and heavy alcohol consumption increase the risk of violence against women, and educational, economical and social empowerment are protective.[101]

Trauma to a pregnant woman is an injury with a double impact. Serious trauma during pregnancy is relatively rare; in North America, approximately 0.4% of all pregnant women require admission to hospital for the treatment of injuries.[102] From 1990 to 1999 in the USA, injuries caused one-third of pregnancy-associated deaths. The leading cause of pregnancy-associated death was homicide.[103]

The initial priorities in managing an injured pregnant patient are the same as for any other patient; however, normal pregnancy causes significant physiological changes in the mother that can confound resuscitation. Early involvement of obstetricians is important, and the key to fetal survival is successful treatment of the mother.

SURGICAL DECISION-MAKING IN TRAUMA

DIAGNOSTIC TECHNIQUES

Clinical

Investigation of the injured patient begins during the primary survey, and is solely directed towards finding any source of hypovolaemic shock. This initial clinical examination may provide sufficient information to demand urgent surgical intervention without the need for delaying investigations. Resuscitation room investigations can rapidly locate the source of bleeding in unstable, multiply injured patients or exclude the torso as a site of major haemorrhage. In less severely injured patients, selective investigations may provide information on the site of the injuries, allowing a more considered approach and occasionally selection of a non-operative policy.

The clinical assessment of the patient during the primary and later secondary survey is a vital aspect of the investigation of the trauma patient, although the percentage of even experienced trauma specialists who are able to detect intra-abdominal injury may be only 65%.[104] It is important that all subsequent investigations are reviewed in the light of this clinical assessment. A detailed knowledge of the incident and prehospital events is vital in the assessment, and can be obtained from prehospital personnel or the patient. Information on the use and deployment of seat belts and air bags, as well as knowledge of speeds and injuries to other passengers, provide an idea of likely injury patterns.

The secondary survey includes a thorough examination of the patient from top to toe, and should include rectal and penile or vaginal examination. Clinical examination can be hampered; it

REFERENCES

92. Smith R, Pless IB. Br Med J 1994; 308: 1312–1313
93. Roberts I, Power C. Br Med J 1996; 313: 784–786
94. Eichelberger MR, Randolph JG. Surg Clin North Am 1981; 61: 1181–1197
95. Lescohier I, DiScala C. Pediatrics 1993; 91: 721–725
96. Siplovich L, Kawar B. J Pediatr Surg 1997; 32: 1464–1465
97. Nance ML, Keller MS, Stafford PW. J Pediatr Surg 2000; 35: 1300–1303
98. Felzen Johnson C. Pediatr Int 2002; 44: 554–560
99. Watts C, Zimmerman C. Lancet 2002; 359: 1232–1237
100. Jewkes R. Br Med J 2002; 324: 253–254
101. Jewkes R. Lancet 2002; 359: 1423–1429
102. Lavery JP, Staten-McCormick M. Obstet Gynecol Clin North Am 1995; 22: 69–90
103. Nannini A, Weiss J, Goldstein R et al. J Am Med Womens Assoc 2002; 57: 140–143
104. Powell DC, Bivins BA, Bell RM. Surg Gynecol Obstet 1982; 155: 257–264

has been reported that half of the injured patients have an altered mental state on admission as a consequence of alcohol, drugs or head injury. It is vital to have a high index of suspicion to detect early physical signs, especially when associated with distracting injuries in the multiply injured patient. Serial clinical examination is required to detect changes and clinical deterioration if sophisticated imaging is not available. There should be a low threshold for investigation.

Wound exploration and probing

Exploration of potentially penetrating abdominal wounds in the emergency room is inappropriate, because it is an imprecise technique with an accuracy of only 55% and a false-positive rate of 88%.[105] It is not an alternative to laparotomy and is contraindicated in patients with generalized abdominal signs. If other investigations are not available, it should be carried out in theatre, by a surgeon, as a formal procedure, because there is a small risk of precipitating torrential haemorrhage. The wound should be extended surgically if necessary to identify any penetration of the peritoneum.

Plain radiographs

Plain X-rays of the cervical spine, chest and pelvis should be obtained in severely injured patients. The pelvic and spine views are primarily used to assess bony integrity and misalignment that suggests ligament rupture. A pelvic radiograph is preferred over clinical examination, which may cause disruption of clot and increase haemorrhage. In addition, recognition of specific fracture patterns is a useful guide to the anticipated blood loss. The lateral cervical spine view is only 85% sensitive for fractures, and therefore must be augmented by other imaging. A plain supine chest radiograph taken during the primary survey is vital in the initial evaluation of chest trauma to display a haemothorax, a pneumothorax and mediastinal widening. The supine film can be difficult to interpret, and the addition of an erect film at a later stage can be useful to demonstrate thoracic pathology more clearly.

Bullet markers (simple opened-out paper clips), applied over penetrating wounds before radiographs are taken, provide significant further information regarding the path of a penetrating missile or track of a stab wound through the body.

Ultrasound

The earliest reports of ultrasound in the assessment of the abdomen were published in the 1970s,[106] and described its use in the evaluation of splenic haematomas. The research that followed concentrated on the detection of organ injury, and demonstrated a sensitivity of only 80% for the detection of splenic injury.[107] Haemoperitoneum can be more reliably detected than organ injury and became the focus of trauma ultrasound. Rozycki and colleagues assessed the ability of surgeons (non-radiologists) to use ultrasound in the emergency room to diagnose abdominal bleeding.[108,109] It soon became apparent that the technique had wider application than just the investigation of the injured abdomen, and therefore the term *focused abdominal sonography for trauma* was accepted at the International Consensus Conference on FAST in 1997.[110]

A focused technique, FAST attempts to detect only blood in a body cavity. Ultrasound images of three dependent abdominal regions are visualized: the right upper quadrant (perihepatic), left upper quadrant (perisplenic), and the pelvis. The pericardium is assessed to detect cardiac tamponade. Radiologists, accident and emergency staff, or surgeons can successfully perform this technique—as long as they have been adequately trained and maintain a sufficient level of experience—with a sensitivity of 81–88.2% and a specificity of 90–99.7%.[109,111–114]

Being a rapid investigation, FAST can be performed in the resuscitation room and can be applied as a screening tool in all injured patients. In the unstable trauma patient, the presence of blood can be detected within seconds and will indicate the need for a laparotomy. In more stable patients, a CT scan can be obtained following FAST to provide further anatomical information and provide an opportunity for non-operative management. The limitations of the technique must be recognized and clinical evaluation of the patient must prevail in the face of an apparently negative scan, because a single normal ultrasound examination cannot be taken as a guarantee that there is no intra-abdominal injury. In this situation the scan must either be repeated after a short period of time or an alternative investigation employed. In penetrating trauma, FAST is less sensitive because ultrasound may be able to detect blood volumes only in excess of 100 mL in the abdomen; however, a positive examination mandates laparotomy without further investigation. Alternative diagnostic imaging is required after a negative scan.

It is possible to employ FAST in the evaluation of thoracic injuries, and it has been shown to be rapid and accurate in the assessment of the pericardium for cardiac tamponade (see Ch. 22).[115,116] In detecting traumatic effusions, FAST has been shown to be faster than and as sensitive as conventional X-ray,[117] and in experienced hands pneumothorax has been detected with a sensitivity of 95%.[118]

Diagnostic peritoneal lavage

Diagnostic peritoneal lavage was considered the investigation of first choice for blunt abdominal trauma since its introduction by Root and coworkers in 1965.[119] Despite the introduction of ultrasound and CT, diagnostic peritoneal lavage has remained the investigation of choice in many hospitals.

REFERENCES

105. Oreskovich SR. Ann Surg 1983; 198: 411–419
106. Kristensen JK, Buemann B, Kuhl E. Acta Chir Scand 1971; 137: 653–657
107. Asher WM, Parvin S, Virgilio RW et al. Radiology 1976; 118: 411–415
108. Rozycki GS, Ochsner MG, Jaffin JH et al. J Trauma 1993; 34: 516–526, discussion 526–527
109. Rozycki GS, Ochsner MG, Schmidt JA et al. J Trauma 1995; 39: 492–498, discussion 498–500
110. Scalea TM, Rodriguez A, Chiu WC et al. J Trauma 1999; 46: 466–472
111. Dolich MO, McKenney MG, Varela JE et al. J Trauma 2001; 50: 108–112
112. Healey MA, Simons RK, Winchell RJ et al. J Trauma 1996; 40: 875–885
113. McKenney KL, McKenney MG, Nunez DB et al. Emerg Radiol 1996; 3: 113–117
114. Boulanger BR, Brenneman FD, McLellan BA et al. J Trauma 1995; 39: 325–330
115. Rozycki GS, Feliciano DV, Davis TP. Surg Clin North Am 1998; 78: 295–310
116. Rozycki GS, Feliciano DV, Schmidt JA et al. Ann Surg 1996; 223: 737–746
117. Sisley AC, Rozycki GS, Ballard RB et al. J Trauma 1998; 44: 291–297
118. Dulchavsky SA, Schwarz KL, Kirkpatrick AW et al. J Trauma 2001; 50: 201–205
119. Root HD, McKinley CR, Lafave JW et al. Surgery 1965; 57: 633–637

Table 7.3 Criteria for positive peritoneal lavage following infusion of 1 litre of normal saline

Red blood cell count	>50 000/ml
White cell blood count	> 500/ml
Bile	Present
Bacteria	Present on Gram stain
Vegetable fibre	Present

Lavage cell counts of 100 000 red cells per mm^3 and 500 white cells per mm^3 have been shown (Table 7.3) to produce reliable and reproducible results,[120] with a sensitivity of 90% and accuracy of 97% for intraperitoneal bleeding.[104] These measurements provide an appropriate balance between sensitivity and non-therapeutic laparotomy, which has been estimated at 10–15%. Equivocal results (red cell count 50 000–100 000 cells/mm^3 and white cell count 10–50 cells/mm^3) must be interpreted after clinical evaluation of the patient, and alternative investigations such as CT used to improve the diagnostic accuracy in stable patients. The role of lavage in penetrating trauma is less clear and lavage counts between 1000 and 10 000 red cells per mm^3 have been used to provide an appropriate sensitivity, because of the small amounts of blood that may be associated with isolated punctures of the bowel. In patients with a pelvic fracture, a supra-umbilical site is recommended to avoid the pelvic haematoma, and cell counts of 200 000 red cells per mm^3 are used as a threshold.

The open and closed percutaneous techniques have been described for the performance of lavage. Both have equal sensitivity and specificity, although the closed technique is faster.[121,122] There is a small incidence of iatrogenic injury with both techniques. There are a number of relative contraindications to lavage, including obesity, pregnancy, and multiple abdominal scars.

Computerized tomography

The contrast-enhanced helical CT scan is the investigation of choice in the haemodynamically stable injured patient. Modern machines acquire a 'trauma scan', with 1-cm cuts from the top of the diaphragm to the pubic symphysis, within 3–5 min once the patient is in the machine. Many CT protocols include imaging of the thorax, and in patients with significant head injury the upper and lower cervical spine.

Compared with alternative methods of investigation, CT has a number of advantages. It images individual organs and the retroperitoneal structures can be seen. The grade of organ injury and the degree of haemoperitoneum have been shown to be useful predictive factors for the success of non-operative management, but the final decision should be made on clinical grounds. In the evaluation of abdominal injury, CT has a sensitivity of 88% and a negative predictive value of 97%,[123] but may be limited in the diagnosis of small intestinal[124] and pancreatic injuries.[125]

Thoracic CT is more sensitive for the detection of parenchymal and pleural injuries than a chest radiograph; however, many of the injuries detected are minor and may require no treatment.[126] Occult pneumothoraces have also been diagnosed on abdominal CT scan;[127] however, the clinical significance of these is low, and the majority of small anterior pneumothoraces can be managed without drainage if the patient does not require positive-pressure ventilation.[126,128] Contrast-enhanced CT is becoming the first investigation in the evaluation of traumatic thoracic aortic disruption.[129]

For the unstable patient, CT is not appropriate.

Diagnostic laparoscopy

The role of laparoscopy in the evaluation of blunt abdominal trauma is limited in the majority of patients.[130] It has been shown that the technique does not improve outcome compared with lavage in blunt abdominal injury and is time-consuming, resource-intensive and expensive.[131,132] Technically, trauma laparoscopy may be limited by the presence of significant volumes of blood, and it is difficult to fully assess the small bowel and the retroperitoneal structures. Laparoscopy is, however, valuable in the assessment of diaphragm rupture in selected stable patients where there is clinical suspicion.[133]

Laparoscopic evaluation of patients with penetrating stab wounds in the thoracoabdominal region is useful. The technique has a sensitivity of 100% for the identification of peritoneal penetration,[134] and confirmation of penetration should be followed by formal laparotomy to assess for intra-abdominal injury. Laparoscopy has occasionally been employed in the assessment of gunshot wounds where there is real doubt about peritoneal penetration when the course of the bullet appears to be tangential.

Magnetic resonance imaging

Technical and logistic factors mean that there is a very limited role for MRI in the acute assessment of the trauma patient. Magnetic resonance cholangiography for assessing the biliary and pancreatic system in the stable acute trauma patient has not yet been adequately assessed.

Multimodality investigation

Because no single diagnostic technique is ideal in the investigation of every patient with abdominal or thoracic trauma, the clinician should adopt a selective policy towards investigation dependent on individual patients, their cardiovascular status, and the likely injuries. It has been shown that in the evaluation

REFERENCES

120. Feliciano DV. Surg Clin North Am 1991; 71: 241–256
121. Velmahos GC, Demetriades D, Stewart M et al. J R Coll Surg Edinb 1998; 43: 235–238
122. Cue JI, Miller FB, Cryer HG et al. J Trauma 1990; 30: 880–883
123. Catre MG. Can J Surg 1995; 38: 117–122
124. Sherck JP. J Trauma 1990; 30: 1–7
125. Ahkrass R, Brandt CP. Am Surg 1996; 62: 647–651
126. Marts B, Durham R, Shapiro M et al. Am J Surg 1994; 168: 688–692
127. Neff MA, Monk JS, Peters K et al. J Trauma 2000; 49: 281–285
128. Wolfman NT, Myers WS, Glauser SJ et al. Am J Roentgenol 1998; 171: 1317–1320
129. Beese RC, Allan R, Treasure T. Ann R Coll Surg Engl 2001; 83: 10–13
130. Brooks A, Boffard KD. Trauma 1999; 1: 150–160
131. Salvino CK, Esposito TJ, Marshall WJ et al. J Trauma 1993; 34: 506–515
132. Leppaniemi AK, Elliot DC. Ann Med 1996; 28: 483–489
133. Townsend MC, Flancbaum L, Choban PS et al. J Trauma 1993; 35: 647–651
134. Zantut LF, Ivatury RR, Smith S et al. J Trauma 1997; 42: 825–831

of abdominal injury the investigations are complementary, and that their use in combination with clinical evaluation will improve the overall accuracy and organ specificity of abdominal investigation.[135]

Selective conservatism

Non-operative management of solid-organ injury is a technique that has become progressively accepted over recent years. First embraced by paediatric surgeons, the widespread use of CT has allowed accurate assessment of the grade or extent of the organ injury and the volume of the haemoperitoneum. Interventional radiology has added much to the success of this technique and can be used to embolize bleeding vessels.

Early reports on the successful conservative management of adult splenic injuries suggested that non-operative management should only be attempted when there are minimal physical signs, cardiovascular stability, and less than 2 units of transfused blood required.[136] The prognostic value of CT has also been questioned, and although accurate determination of injury grade was possible, it was felt that clinical criteria should be used.[137] Up to half the blunt liver injuries in adults can be managed non-operatively,[138] with success rates of up to 80%. Most renal injuries in stable patients can be managed non-operatively unless there is evidence of renal pedicle injury on CT.

In children, non-operative management has been recommended in lesser grades of splenic and liver injuries,[139] and possibly in pancreatic trauma as well.

EMERGENCY ROOM THORACOTOMY

For patients presenting *in extremis*, desperate measures are required to save life. A left anterolateral thoracotomy can be performed in the casualty area to control bleeding by compression, clamps or simple sutures. Patients undergoing emergency room thoracotomy for anything other than isolated penetrating cardiac injury rarely survive; however, this surgery can be used to release tamponade, or to control torrential bleeding, air embolism or bronchopleural fistula, and allow open cardiac massage and occlusion of the descending thoracic aorta. Patients with a high likelihood of isolated, penetrating intrathoracic injury associated with severe hypotension (less than 60 mmHg) or a witnessed cardiac arrest may benefit from an emergency thoracotomy. Less clear benefits are apparent in patients with profound hypotension and extrathoracic or blunt injury.[140,141]

Emergency thoracotomy exposes the trauma team to considerable risk from the rapid use of sharp instruments in an uncontrolled situation. Clear indications need to be present and attempts at resuscitation should not be unduly prolonged. If patients respond, they should be moved promptly to the operating theatre for definitive care, and the exercise should be terminated if the efforts to save the patient are futile.[140,141]

DAMAGE CONTROL SURGERY

Exsanguinating haemorrhage after severe injury leads to metabolic acidosis, profound hypothermia and a coagulopathy (see Ch. 3). These inter-related factors reinforce each other to create 'a bloody vicious cycle', which leads to death as a consequence of an irreversible metabolic insult.[142]

Damage control is a term used in the US Navy to describe the capacity of a ship to absorb damage and maintain mission integrity.[143] In trauma surgery, damage control describes the concept of saving life by using surgery as a tool of resuscitation, rather than as an end in itself.[142,144] Damage control is a three-phase surgical approach to injured patients at the limit of their physiological reserves, most usually applied in the abdomen, but also in other settings, such as thoracic or vascular trauma.[142,144]

Phase 1

Phase 1 is the initial surgical procedure, when only the minimum is done to stop haemorrhage and limit or contain contamination before the operation is aborted.

Phase 2

In phase 2, resuscitation continues in the intensive care unit, where attempts are made to restore normal physiological functions before returning to the operating theatre.

Phase 3

In phase 3, definitive surgery is undertaken as soon as the patient has been fully resuscitated, when the patient is returned to the operating room for removal of packs and completion of definitive surgical procedures. A thorough search is made for missed injuries; these potent causes of morbidity and mortality have been described as 'the nemesis of the trauma surgeon'.[145]

ABDOMINAL COMPARTMENT SYNDROME

Trauma patients who may have been packed, or have retroperitoneal haematoma or visceral oedema, are at high risk for the development of the abdominal compartment syndrome. This condition can result in renal, respiratory and cardiovascular impairment,[146,147] and may lead to multiple organ dysfunction and death. A high index of suspicion is required, and bladder pressure measurements must be recorded on a regular basis.[148] A bladder pressure greater than 30 mmHg is an indication for further laparotomy or a laparostomy (leaving the abdominal wall open). Avoiding primary closure of the abdominal fascia at the initial laparotomy reduces the risk of compartment syndrome.

Temporary closure of the defect should be achieved using either the Bogota bag or OpSite™ sandwich technique to cover

REFERENCES

135. Liu M, Lee CH, P'eng FK. J Trauma 1993; 35: 267–270
136. Mucha P, Daly RC, Farnell MB. J Trauma 1986; 26: 970–979
137. Becker CD, Spring P, Glattli A et al. Am J Roentgenol 1994; 162: 343–347
138. Carrillo EH, Platz A, Miller FB et al. Br J Surg 1998; 85: 461–468
139. Losty PD, Okoye BO, Walter DP et al. Br J Surg 1997; 84: 1006–1008
140. Aihara R, Millham FH, Blansfield J et al. J Trauma 2001; 50: 1027–1030
141. Grove CA, Lemmon G, Anderson G et al. Am Surg 2002; 68: 313–316
142. Kashuk JL, Moore EE, Millikan JS et al. J Trauma 1982; 22: 672–679
143. Johnson JW, Gracias VH, Schwab CW et al. J Trauma 2001; 51: 261–269
144. Moore EE, Burch JM, Franciose RJ et al. World J Surg 1998; 22: 1184–1190
145. Scalea TM, Phillips TF, Goldstein AS et al. J Trauma 1988; 28: 962–967
146. Offner PJ, de Souza AL, Moore EE et al. Arch Surg 2001; 136: 676–681
147. Sugrue M, Buist MD, Hourihan F et al. Br J Surg 1995; 82: 235–238
148. Kron IL, Harman PK, Nolan SP. Ann Surg 1984; 199: 28–30

the abdominal contents, and a 'vacuum-pack' closure of the abdomen is the method of choice.[149] Definitive closure of the abdominal wall is obtained at a later stage if necessary.

POST-INJURY CRITICAL CARE AND MULTIPLE ORGAN FAILURE

Severely injured patients require management in the intensive therapy unit, where organ support, invasive monitoring, and a high level of nursing care can be provided. These patients make significant demands on the intensive therapy unit resources for the management of sepsis and multiple organ failure. The introduction of the damage control philosophy has extended the role of the intensive therapy unit to providing secondary resuscitation following damage control. This resuscitation phase is directed at the reversal of acidosis, treatment of hypothermia, and correction of coagulopathy—the triad that defines these patients (see *Damage control surgery* section, p. 13).

The immediate management of the traumatized patient in the intensive therapy unit is directed to the re-evaluation and management of the airway, breathing and circulation. Many trauma patients require intubation and ventilatory support. Numerous ventilatory strategies have been attempted in trauma patients to provide adequate oxygenation while limiting lung injury, and are beyond the scope of this chapter. Circulatory support should initially be provided by adequate fluid resuscitation using warm fluids with blood and coagulation products as appropriate. Inotropic support of the circulation may be necessary if sepsis and organ failure supervene. Patients with a head injury should be managed by protocol to achieve appropriate cerebral oxygenation and cerebral perfusion pressure.

After the initial resuscitation and stabilization of the trauma patient, it is important that the potential for missed injury in this group of patients is recognized. A formal tertiary survey and review of all diagnostic imaging should be undertaken.

The critical care management of severely injured patients following resuscitation or damage control procedures is directed towards maintenance of the body systems, support through the metabolic response to trauma, and the management (preferably prevention) of complications and sepsis.[150]

The systemic inflammatory response syndrome forms part of the response to trauma; the diagnostic criteria are listed in the next section of this chapter. Sepsis may supervene, especially in injured patients, where bowel injury and contamination may have occurred and there is prolonged ventilation of damaged and contused lungs. Antibiotic therapy should be directed against proven organisms following culture, and there should be a raised awareness of the potential for fungal infection.

SYSTEMIC INFLAMMATORY RESPONSE SYNDROME

Systemic inflammatory response syndrome is commonly found in the intensive therapy unit, and is differentiated from the normal metabolic response to trauma. It consists of:

- temperature above 38°C or below 36°C;
- heart rate more than 90 beats/min;
- respiratory rate more than 20 breaths/min or P_ACO_2 less than 4.3 kPa; and
- white blood cell count more than 12 000 cells/mm^3.

Some patients continue to deteriorate despite intensive care support, and the condition progresses to multiple organ dysfunction and then death.

BLOOD TRANSFUSION IN TRAUMA

Trauma is a disease of bleeding. Approximately 40% of the 11 million units of blood transfused in the USA every year are utilized for emergency resuscitation.[151] Recognition of acute blood loss after injury, haemostasis, and restoration of intravascular volume are fundamental to the care of injured patients. Untreated haemorrhage leads to diminished cardiac output and inadequate peripheral oxygen delivery, which may lead to death or triggering of the cytokine cascade, ultimately leading to multiple organ failure.

Provision of blood for trauma patients plays a central role in their care, and although allogeneic (donated) blood is life-saving, its use may be associated with serious adverse effects, such as transfusion reactions, alloimmunization, and immunomodulation, which can lead to increased postoperative infections and organ dysfunction, and transmission of diseases such as viral hepatitis and human immunodeficiency virus. In addition, donated blood is unacceptable to Jehovah's Witnesses.[152,153]

Current evidence supports restrictive blood transfusion protocols in place of more liberal transfusion strategies (see Ch. 3).[154]

Alternatives to allogeneic blood in trauma are limited to autotransfusion and blood substitutes. Autotransfusion can be used safely; however, logistic and clinical problems remain.[155,156] Blood substitutes, known as haemoglobin oxygen carriers, can be made from outdated human blood cells, from other animal species, or using recombinant technology.[157] The ideal blood substitute remains elusive;[158] however, trials are ongoing and these products appear to have tremendous potential.

VENOUS THROMBOEMBOLISM (see Ch. 11)

Venous thromboembolism is a common, life-threatening complication of major trauma. Deep venous thrombosis has been reported in up to 60% of seriously injured patients, with a fatal pulmonary embolism rate of up to 2% in the absence of prophylaxis.[159] A recent consensus report concluded that the use of low-molecular-weight heparin, started when primary hemostasis has occurred, is the simplest and most efficacious option for

REFERENCES

149. Barker DE, Kaufman HJ, Smith LA et al. J Trauma 2000; 48: 201–206
150. Hotchkiss RS, Karl IE. New Engl J Med 2003; 348: 138–150
151. Schulman CI, Nathe K, Brown M et al. J Trauma 2002; 52: 1224–1225
152. Aiboshi J, Moore EE, Ciesla DJ et al. Shock 2001; 15: 302–306
153. Regan F, Taylor C. Br Med J 2002; 325: 143–147
154. Hebert PC, Wells G, Blajchman MA et al. N Engl J Med 1999; 340: 409
155. Smith LA, Barker DE, Burns RP. Am J Surg 1997; 63: 47–49
156. Hughes LG, Thomas DW, Wareham K et al. Anaesthesia 2001; 56: 217–220
157. Chang TMS. Trends Biotechnol 1999; 17: 61–67
158. Sloan EF, Koneigsburg M, Gens D. JAMA 1999; 282: 1857–1864
159. Norwood SH, McAuley CE, Berne JD et al. Arch Surg 2002; 137: 696–701

high-risk trauma patients. The presence of non-bleeding solid injury is not considered a contraindication to the use of low-molecular-weight heparin prophylaxis.[160] There are limited level-1 evidence-based guidelines.[161]

ORGAN DONATION (see Ch. 8)

Trauma patients with brain stem death are a vital source of organs for organ donation programmes. Strict criteria exist and must be adhered to for the diagnosis of brain stem death, and the process must be managed compassionately. The inclusion of the transplant coordinator at an early stage is imperative, and frequent discussion with the relatives to gain their consent and to keep them informed throughout the process is vital.

REHABILITATION

Significant numbers of trauma patients, especially those with head, spinal, and extremity injury, suffer functional impairment after their injuries. Rehabilitation aims to restore function as much as possible to minimize the disadvantages experienced by the individual. Effective management requires coordination between the patient, medical carers and social services.

Rehabilitation also addresses the impact of the consequences of postinjury impairment, and attempts to achieve maximum potential independent and productive living for disabled persons within the community. Organization of services has been shown to enhance recovery and lower overall costs.[162,163] Nevertheless, there are few comparative trials to support the efficacy of rehabilitation in improving outcomes after trauma.[164] Rehabilitation is a somewhat neglected area in trauma care, and holds the promise to greatly improve quality of life for the victims of serious injury.

MASS CASUALTY INCIDENTS

In a mass casualty incident, a hospital is challenged with a large number of casualties within a short period of time.[165] To deal with this, hospitals will implement a prearranged plan so that appropriate personnel and resources can be mobilized. Mass casualty incidents must be differentiated from disasters, when an event (such as an earthquake) causes social and medical infrastructure to fail.[166]

In a typical incident, about 10–15% of survivors are severely injured and the rest have moderate or mild trauma;[167] patients cannot all be attended to at once. Casualties have to be sorted into groups according to their clinical needs; otherwise severely wounded patients may be neglected while resources are used to treat less severely injured patients. The process of matching patients to available resources is called triage. Typically, casualties are triaged as:

- Priority 1: critical; requires immediate action to save life.
- Priority 2: urgent; severe injury, but some delay will be tolerated.
- Priority 3: less serious injury; delay acceptable.
- Priority 4: dead on arrival, or injury so severe that survival is unlikely despite full treatment.

Triage is the most important phase of an incident,[168] and this duty is usually delegated to an experienced clinician. The purpose of triage is initially to preserve scarce resources for the relatively few seriously injured casualties by filtering out the others.[165,166] Overtriage occurs when patients with relatively minor injuries are incorrectly assigned to be assessed and treated in a sophisticated trauma area. A direct relationship has been identified between overtriage and mortality of the critically injured. Overtriage rates of approximately 50% have been reported,[165] and it has been suggested that this level of overtriage is acceptable to minimize undertriage.[166]

SCORING SYSTEMS IN TRAUMA

Trauma scoring is a tool to allow the analysis and comparison of individual patients and patient groups for research, outcome prediction, and evaluation of care. These scoring systems have become increasingly sophisticated, but all rely heavily on the quality and completeness of the data that are used. Scoring systems are based on either anatomical data (such as the injury severity score), where data are taken from clinical examination, surgery or post-mortem results, or physiological data (such as the GCS and the revised trauma score), usually taken at the time of the resuscitation. Other scoring systems combine both anatomical and physiological data, and attempt to provide accurate estimates of the probability of survival. These systems, such as trauma score–injury severity score, use coefficients derived from large patient groups collated in the Major Trauma Outcome Study in the USA or from the UK Trauma Audit and Research Network database to improve their accuracy. The American Association for the Surgery of Trauma has devised individual organ injury scores running from 1 to 6 (6 being a mortal injury) to allow accurate comparison of results.[169]

FURTHER READING

American Association for the Surgery of Trauma. Organ Injury Scaling. Online. Available: http://www.aast.org

Boffard KD (ed). Manual of Definitive Surgical Trauma Care. Arnold, London, 2003.

Eastern Association for the Surgery of Trauma. Trauma Practice Guidelines. Online. Available: http://www.east.org/tpg.html 2003

Committee on Trauma of the American College of Surgeons. Advanced Trauma Life Support® Student Course Manual. American College of Surgeons, Chicago, 1997.

Committee on Trauma of the American College of Surgeons. Resources for Optimal Care of the Injured Patient. American College of Surgeons, Chicago, 1999.

Trauma resource. Online. Available: http://www.trauma.org

REFERENCES

160. Geerts WH, Heit JA, Clagett GP et al. Chest 2001; 119 (Suppl): 132S–175S
161. Rogers FB, Cipolle MD, Velmahos G et al. J Trauma 2002; 53: 142–164
162. Khan S, Khan A, Feyz M. Brain Inj 2002; 16: 537–554
163. Beaulieu CL. Surg Clin North Am 2002; 82: 393–408
164. Hawkins ML, Lewis FD, Medeiros RS. J Trauma 1996; 41: 257–263
165. Hirshberg A, Holcomb JB, Mattox KL. Ann Emerg Med 2001; 37: 647–652
166. Ryan J, Gavalas M. Hosp Med 1998; 59: 944–946
167. Frykberg ER, Tepas JJ III. Ann Surg 1988; 208: 569–576
168. Kennedy K, Aghababian RV, Gans L et al. Ann Emerg Med 1996; 28: 136–144
169. American Association for the Surgery of Trauma. Organ Injury Scaling Systems. Online. Available: www.aast.org 2000

Transplantation

8

Robert W.G. Johnson, Peter Lodge

INTRODUCTION

The last 50 years have seen incredibly rapid progress in clinical transplantation, moving from experimental concept to an established place in clinical practice. It has become the treatment of choice for vital organ failure: the ultimate form of constructive surgery. Progress has occurred as a result of the ability to manipulate the immune response using powerful immunosuppressive drugs. With that has come a greater knowledge of the immune system.

The original concept was to avoid unnecessary death from failure of a single vital organ such as the kidney, the liver or the heart. That concept has been progressively modified with time from the simple ambition to save life to the determination to improve quality of life. Other organs and tissues have been embraced: the cornea for vision, the pancreas or pancreatic islets for diabetes, small bowel, arteries, tendons and bone.

HISTORICAL REVIEW

Organ transplantation became a technical possibility through the pioneering experimental work of Alexis Carrel in the early years of the twentieth century. Carrel left his native France to work in the USA and, in collaboration with Charles Guthrie, established a technique for sewing blood vessels together that led ultimately to the transplantation of several solid organs in animals, including the kidney, liver and heart.[1,2] Carrel and Guthrie reported that these allografted organs failed to sustain good function in the long term but they could not explain why. More than 30 years elapsed before the term *rejection* was coined, together with an explanation of the mechanism of rejection. In 1943, Gibson and Medawar deduced that the rapid destruction of a second set of skin allografts applied to a patient with severe burns was due to an active immune process.[3]

Returning to the experimental laboratory, Medawar established that stimulation of the recipient's immune system by donor antigen caused the development of a new colony of lymphocytes capable of invading and destroying grafted tissue.[4,5] Sensitized lymphoid cells from an animal that had rejected a graft could then be used to passively transfer transplant immunity. This cell transfer produced accelerated rejection of a graft in a previously unsensitized recipient.[6]

In January 1951 two French surgeons, Charles Dubost and Marceau Servelle, each carried out a renal transplant from the same cadaver donor, who had been executed on the guillotine; although both kidneys functioned for a while, the recipients both died from uraemia within a few days. Rene Küss performed a third cadaver renal transplant at the end of January 1951 but the renal artery thrombosed. A further six transplants were attempted in France during 1952, including the first live related donor transplant, carried out by Michon and Hamburger on Christmas Eve. Unfortunately, all transplants failed to function for more than a few days. The unique feature of this French experience was the fact that all these kidneys were transplanted into the iliac fossa, attached to the iliac vessels, and drained into the bladder. Previous transplants had been attached to the arm or groin.

The first successful cadaver transplant, which was placed in the groin, was achieved by David Hume in 1953.[7] His patient, a physician, survived for 6 months without rejection and then died of an unrelated cause. This was the first of a series of eight unrelated cadaver transplants carried out without matching or immunosuppression; all the other transplants that he attempted were rejected.

The earliest series of successful human renal transplants with prolonged survival was achieved by John Merrill and Joe Murray in 1954.[8] They avoided the problem of rejection by transplanting kidneys between identical twins. Their excellent results led Murray and others to the search for methods to prevent graft rejection in unrelated recipients by modifying the immune response. Whole body and subsequently lymphoid irradiation were used at first but without success.

The major breakthrough came with the introduction of the anticancer drug 6-mercaptopurine[9] and its prodrug azathioprine. The possibility of azathioprine inducing 'pharmacological immunosuppression' was first conceived by Roy Calne who, while working with Murray in Boston, proved the concept in the laboratory in 1960 by successfully transplanting kidneys between mongrel dogs treated with azathioprine.[10,11] Azathioprine was eventually introduced into clinical practice by Murray in 1963.[12] It was the combination of azathioprine with prednisolone that formed the drug regimen that allowed the establishment of clinical renal transplant programmes in the late 1960s. The jigsaw

REFERENCES

1. Carrel A, Guthrie CC. Science 1905; 22: 473
2. Carrel A, Guthrie CC. Science 1906; 23: 394
3. Gibson T, Medawar PB. J Anat 1943; 77: 299
4. Medawar PB. J Anat 1944; 78: 176
5. Medawar PB. J Anat 1945; 79: 157
6. Mitchison NA. Nature 1953; 171: 267
7. Hume DM, Merrill JP, Miller BF et al. J Clin Invest 1955; 34: 327
8. Merrill JP, Murray JE, Harrison JE et al. JAMA 1956; 160: 277–282
9. Schwartz R, Dameshek W. Nature 1959; 183: 1682–1683
10. Calne RY. Lancet 1960; 1: 417–418
11. Calne RY, Alexandre GPJ, Murray JE. Ann NY Acad Sci 1962; 99: 743–761
12. Murray JE, Merrill JP, Harrison JH et al. N Engl J Med 1963; 268: 1315–1323

was completed by Belzer in 1967, with the discovery of a method to store kidneys ex vivo for up to 3 days using continuous hypothermic perfusion.[13]

The immunosuppressive cocktail of azathioprine and prednisolone developed in the 1960s remained the standard for more than 20 years. Minor modifications were introduced, such as the use of low-dose prednisolone to reduce morbidity[14] and the introduction of antilymphocyte globulin, but the results of clinical renal transplantation remained disappointing: mortality rates in the UK, Europe and the USA remained around 25% and average 1-year graft survival was only 55%. The search for newer and more specific immunosuppressive drugs proved frustrating. Antilymphocyte globulin was a popular addition to conventional immunosuppression; it could be used either as an initial induction therapy[15] or as a treatment for rejection.[16] However, the use of antilymphocyte globulin was associated with an increased risk of viral and fungal infection, as well as malignancies such as lymphoma.

The discovery of cyclosporine by Borel in 1976[17] changed the whole approach to transplantation. Once again it was Calne who first realized its importance from reports of Borel's in vitro work and applied it to transplantation, at first in the laboratory[18] and subsequently in the clinic.[19] Cyclosporine was the first precision immunosuppressive agent blocking the cytokine interleukin-2 and preventing proliferation of sensitized lymphocytes. Cyclosporine improved graft survival after renal transplantation by 30% and dramatically reduced morbidity, especially when used as a monotherapy without steroids. The greatest impact, however, was on non-renal transplants. Graft and patient survival after liver transplantation increased from 30 to 70%. Results for heart, lung and intestinal transplant also improved substantially. In 1984, with the release of cyclosporine on to the market, clinical transplantation became respectable.

PRINCIPLES OF CLINICAL ORGAN TRANSPLANTATION

ORGAN DONATION

Organ donors may be either living or cadaveric. In the UK the vast majority of donated organs are retrieved from cadaveric donors, and most (80%) are multiorgan donors, allowing retrieval of kidneys, liver, heart and lungs, cornea and pancreas. Retrieval of so many disparate organs, often from hospitals far removed from the transplant centre, requires sensitive, skilful coordination and military precision because time is of the essence. Clear guidelines are necessary for donor selection, consent, donor preparation and coordinated organ removal.

Cadaver donor selection

Withdrawal of life support from a prospective donor requires the confident diagnosis of brain stem infarction by an independent physician, preferably a neurologist. The legal requirement is that the patient shall be ventilator-dependent with absent brain stem reflexes. The relevant reflexes are craniofacial: the gag reflex, the corneal reflex, the iris light reflex and the oculogyric reflex. Absence of all these reflexes, which have their central connections in the brain stem alongside the respiratory centre, signifies infarction of the brain stem.[20]

Consent for organ donation must been obtained from the next of kin. This should be sought even in the presence of a signed donor card. It is also wise to seek agreement from the coroner. In the absence of any known relative, the duty hospital manager has legal custody of the body and can give consent when satisfied that a proper search has been made and all the statutory conditions have been met.

Potential donors should be judged on physiological rather than calendar age; nonetheless, as a general rule the majority will be between 4 and 65 years old and have normal function of the organs to be donated. There is no absolute age limit because recipients are now accepted who are very young and indeed much older.

Finally, the donor must be free from any transmissible infection or malignancy.

Donor management

The management of organ donors is aimed at avoiding failure of potentially transplantable organs after brain stem infarction. The approach is therefore similar to that offered to any intensive care patient with the potential for multiple organ failure, but it differs substantially from the management of a head injury patient.

Hydration is very important, especially if the head injury has been complicated by diabetes insipidus. Vigorous fluid loading is likely to benefit the kidney but may cause pulmonary oedema and even oedema of the liver, making those organs unusable. Fluid management should be guided by invasive pressure and volume monitoring. Pulmonary artery catheterization is a reasonable way to approach this; a suitable pulmonary artery occlusion pressure to aim for would be 12–14 torr. Colloid solutions are more suitable than crystalloids for this purpose. Cardiac output and tissue oxygen delivery need to be maintained as for the critically ill. Tissue oxygen delivery needs to be at least 650 mL/m^2 per minute, with a cardiac index of 4.5 L/m^2 per minute. This may require vigorous inotropic support that, together with the catecholamine release at the time of brain stem death, may result in damage to the contractile mechanism of the heart. Nonetheless, low-dose infusion of noradrenaline (norepinephrine) is commonly used to maintain arterial pressure between 65 and 70 torr. The hormonal and metabolic consequences of brain stem death play an important role in organ viability. Novitsky has shown that infusion of 100 mg of hydrocortisone, 2 μg/h of thyroxine and 5–10 units of insulin leads to a restoration of cardiac function, aerobic metabolism and energy stores.[21] Renal function is also improved.

REFERENCES

13. Belzer OF, Ashby BS, Dunphy JE. Lancet 1967; 2: 536–538
14. McGeown MG, Kennedy JA et al. Lancet 1977; ii: 648–651
15. Sheil AGR, Kelly GE et al. Lancet 1971; i: 359–363
16. Hoitsma AJ, van Lier HJ et al. Transplantation 1985; 39: 274–279
17. Borel JF, Feurer C, Gubler HU et al. Agents Actions 1976; 6: 468–475
18. Calne RY, White DJG. IRCS Med Sci: Cardiovasc Syst 1977; 5: 595
19. Calne RY, White DJG, Thiru S et al. Lancet 1978; 2: 1323–1327
20. Pallis C. In: Morris PJ (ed). Kidney Transplantation, Principles and Practice. 3rd edn. WB Saunders, Philadelphia, 1988
21. Novitsky D, Cooper DKC, Richard B. Transplantation 1987; 43; 852–854

Organ retrieval

The transplant coordinator is crucial to the success of multiorgan retrieval. At least two surgical teams and sometimes up to four are involved, often from distant centres; all are convinced that their role is paramount. Maintenance of discipline and good manners is essential, if only to preserve the confidence and good will of the local hospital and to ensure future organ donations. The coordinator conducts the orchestra, collects the essential donor data, talks to the relatives and to the local medical and nursing staff. The coordinator also plays a key role in education about the whole process, both at the time of donation and on educational visits to hospitals in between donations.

Order of procedure

The abdominal retrieval team has the most preparatory work to do, and therefore they begin before the arrival of the cardiothoracic team. A skilled anaesthetist is essential to maintain cardiopulmonary stability and to coordinate the delivery of the drugs required by the two teams; these would include a single-shot, broad-spectrum antibiotic and heparinization.

The liver is mobilized to divide the ligaments and determine whether or not there is an aberrant hepatic artery. The aorta and vena cava are cannulated ready to infuse cardioplegia and cold preservation fluid for the abdominal organs. Cannulation of the superior mesenteric vein is often performed to increase the perfusion of the liver; this should be avoided if the pancreas is to be collected because it causes oedema of the pancreas.

Once the liver has been adequately cooled it can be fully mobilized. The time taken to cool the liver is usually more than sufficient for the cardiothoracic team to complete the removal of the heart and lungs. The liver and pancreas are then removed en bloc, taking care to preserve the short right renal vein and the coeliac axis. The liver and pancreas can then be separated in ice on the work bench. The aim is to obtain the whole pancreas together with the duodenum.

The kidneys are usually removed using an en bloc technique (Fig. 8.1), taking segments of aorta and vena cava above and below the renal vessels. This ensures that if there are multiple renal arteries they can be included on a Carrel patch of aorta for subsequent anastomosis to the external iliac artery (Fig. 8.2). There are no collateral connections on the arterial side of the renal circulation, and failure to revascularize a polar artery will result in an area of infarction in the donor kidney. It is vital that lower polar vessels are kept intact because they are the main source of blood supply to the renal pelvis and ureter. To further protect the ureteric blood supply, the loose connective tissue around the ureter should also be kept intact, especially in the triangle between the gonadal veins, the renal vein and the lower pole of the kidney.

Principles of organ preservation

The viability of solid organs for transplantation is entirely dependent on rapid cooling. This is achieved by rapid per aortic perfusion with a cold, non-penetrant solution. Kidneys in particular are very prone to injury by under-perfusion as a result of hypotension in the donor's agonal phase; this is exacerbated by the release of large quantities of catecholamines at the time of brain stem infarction. Untreated, vasospasm of the renal microcirculation will result. This leads to entrapment of hypoxic, rigid, deformed red cells, giving the kidney a characteristic blotchy, cyanosed appearance. This can be avoided by maintaining a profuse donor diuresis during the surgical procedure and achieving rapid intra-arterial cooling aided by an i.v. injection

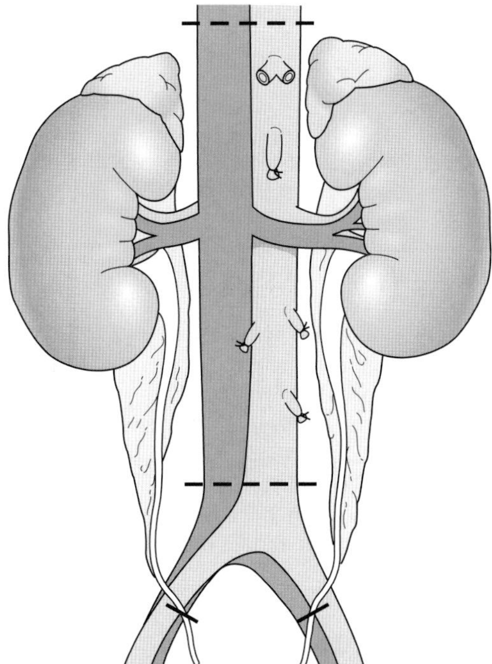

Figure 8.1 En bloc removal of the two kidneys when cold and together with the aorta and vena cava avoids the danger of damaging polar blood vessels. Careful separation of the two kidneys with appropriate cuffs of aorta or vena cava can then be achieved in ice on the work bench.

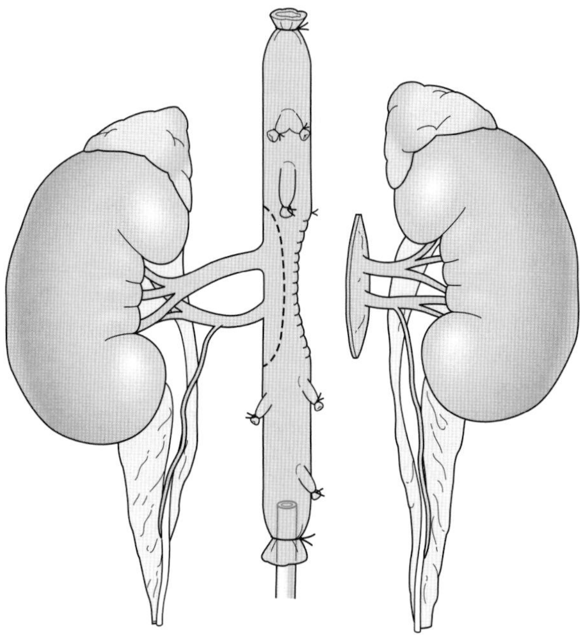

Figure 8.2 The left kidney has two arteries preserved on a cuff of aorta (a Carrel patch) to facilitate implantation.

of 250 mg of chlorpromazine and 100 mg of phenoxybenzamine to the donor before cardiac arrest.

Cooling of solid organs slows the rate of metabolism and reduces the need for oxygen; as a consequence essential cellular processes such as the sodium pump are switched off. This would inevitably lead to mass migration of sodium ions and water molecules into the cells, which would then be disrupted when the organ is eventually reperfused at body temperature. To avoid this, cooling fluids need to be specially formulated with a high colloid oncotic pressure, high potassium and magnesium concentration, and low sodium content. A number of suitable preservation fluids are available; of these, Belzer's University of Wisconsin solution is probably the most universally applicable for liver, pancreas and kidney, whereas Ross and Marshall's mannitol-based hyperosmolar citrate solution[22] is primarily for the kidney.

Organs for transplantation are aseptically packed in two sterile plastic bags containing a generous amount of preservation fluid. The bags containing the organs are then stored in insulated boxes containing ice. These precautions are designed to keep the organ away from the surface of the ice, which is of indeterminate temperature down to −20°C and can cause thermal injury by direct contact. Separated from the ice by the preservation fluid, the organ remains at the temperature of melting ice, 0°C.

RECIPIENT SELECTION

Careful recipient selection is important, first to avoid subjecting recipients to a major procedure for which they are unsuited because of comorbid disease, and second to avoid wastage of scarce organs. Recipients need, therefore, to be selected on both clinical and immunological grounds. Clinical selection is dealt with later in relation to specific organ transplantation.

Immunological selection

Blood group and cross-match

Although it would be ideal to require blood group identity between donor and recipient, this would disadvantage recipients with rare blood groups out of all proportion to the advantage gained. Blood group compatibility is therefore all that is required, which means that recipients with blood groups A, B and AB can all receive from O donors. Cross-match-positive grafts should be avoided.

The human major histocompatibility complex

Glycoprotein molecules on the surface of all somatic cells act as markers of genetic identity; they allow the immune system to distinguish self from alien cells. When alien cells bearing these markers are transplanted into a host, they trigger an immune response leading to allograft rejection. These molecules were originally detected on leukocytes and are therefore named human leukocyte antigens; they are now universally referred to as HLA antigens. These histocompatibility antigens are genetically controlled by loci on the short arm of chromosome 6 that constitute the major histocompatibility complex. The important antigens in transplantation are the class I antigens, products of the HLA-A, B and C regions, and the class II antigens of the HLA-D region. Foreign class I and class II antigens are capable of stimulating the recipient immune system and triggering lymphocyte sensitization, as described below.

CROSS-MATCHING Testing for preformed antibody is crucial to all forms of transplantation. These antibodies, when present, signify immunological memory of a previous sensitization; if ignored, accelerated rejection will occur. Potential recipients can be screened in advance for the presence of cytotoxic antibodies, and positive results will identify the specificity of the antibodies concerned. The chance of the recipient meeting a donor with cross-reactive antigens can be assessed by comparing the frequency of the antibodies against a panel of common antigens. Forewarned is forearmed, but it is still necessary to perform a direct cross-match against the proposed donor as soon as cells become available. Lymphocytes from the donor are incubated with sera from the recipient in the presence of complement. After incubation the percentage of cell killing (cytolysis) is measured using fluoroscopic microscopy. A positive cross-match is an absolute contraindication to transplantation.

HLA MATCHING HLA matching depends on identifying the degrees of disparity in HLA antigens between donors and potential recipients. For most organ transplants, and particularly for renal allografts, avoiding HLA mismatches both improves the chances of long-term graft survival and avoids unnecessary sensitization. Most laboratories now use molecular biological techniques utilizing the polymerase chain reaction to accurately classify the surface HLA antigens. This has now become a highly reproducible system of classification of the multiple alleles of the HLA antigens. There is still a place for the older serological methods but only to clarify fuzzy results. Matching for DR, where there are only 20 important determinants, can be readily achieved, and evidence suggests that DR matching has a more important influence on allograft survival than matching for the A and B loci.[23,24]

TYPES OF REJECTION

Solid organs are rejected by one or more of three classical mechanisms: instantly in hyperacute rejection; after a week to 10 days in cell-mediated rejection; or slowly, over several months or years, in chronic rejection.

HYPERACUTE REJECTION

Hyperacute rejection occurs in the presence of preformed humoral antibodies to the donor's HLA determinants (the recipient has an immunological memory for some of the donor's antigen specificities), and this will result in the immediate, irreversible destruction of the graft. Hyperacute rejection occurs within a few minutes of revascularization. The preformed antibodies may arise following blood transfusion, as a result of pregnancy (against fetal antigens of paternal origin), or against mismatched determinants of a previous failed transplant. Previous exposure to foreign HLA antigens results in the formation of circulating cytotoxic antibodies in the blood of the potential transplant recipient. Following revascularization of the graft, the recipient's antibodies can become fixed to class I determinants on the vascular endothelium of the donor, resulting

REFERENCES

22. Marshall VC, Jablonski P, Scott DF. In: Morris PJ (ed). Kidney Transplantation, Principles and Practice. 3rd edn. WB Saunders, Philadelphia, 1988
23. Albrechtsen D, Moen T, Thorsby E. Transplant Proc 1983; 15: 1120–1123
24. D'Ardenne AJ, Dunnill MS et al. J Clin Pathol 1986; 39: 144–151

in endothelial cell destruction and activation of the coagulation system. Platelets adhere to the damaged areas, resulting in local intravascular coagulation and then haemorrhage as fibrinogen is rapidly depleted.

Because hyperacute rejection is an irreversible process, it is vital to avoid the reaction by careful preoperative cross-matching against donor cells. A fresh serum sample and serum samples collected from the recipient during the year preceding the transplant should all give a negative reaction when tested with lymphocytes from a prospective donor. In clinical transplantation the risk of hyperacute rejection is a major concern in renal programmes, and it has also been described following cardiac transplantation. The liver, despite expressing HLA-A and B antigens on its endothelium, seems to be much less susceptible to hyperacute rejection.

ACUTE CELL-MEDIATED REJECTION

In all forms of organ transplantation, it is the formation of sensitized lymphoid cells causing acute rejection that poses the greatest threat to the survival of the graft. The initial phase in the process is sensitization (recognition) of donor antigen by the circulating T (thymus-derived) lymphocytes of the recipient. There are two possible means by which this initial sensitization can be achieved. Recipient macrophages may take up antigenic fragments washed out into the circulation following revascularization of the graft. Alternatively, non-sensitized lymphocytes may come into contact with the so-called passenger leukocytes or dendritic cells of the donor, which express class II antigens, in large quantities, on their surface. It is probable that both these mechanisms are involved in antigen presentation.

For transformation of circulating T lymphocytes into activated blast cells to occur, the T lymphocytes also need stimulation by a second signal in the form of a soluble mediator, interleukin-1, which is secreted by the recipient's macrophages. Presence of an accessory signal from the surface of the dendritic cell is also required to fully activate recipient T cells. In the absence of immunosuppression the T lymphoblasts proliferate rapidly and invade the graft.

These activated T cells secrete a number of effector molecules known as lymphokines. Of these, the most important is interleukin-2, which causes clonal expansion of the T-cell population with the generation of cytotoxic T lymphocytes. The cytotoxic cell is able to cause direct cell killing of its target without the involvement of complement. In addition, sensitized T cells can secrete additional factors; for example, macrophage activation factor (also known as interferon-gamma), leukocyte migration inhibition factor and chemotactic factors. These soluble agents probably augment the inflammatory reaction within the graft by involving recipient populations, such as polymorphs and macrophages that are not specifically sensitized to graft antigen.

Acute cell-mediated rejection is characterized by invasion of the graft interstitium by large numbers of proliferating lymphocytes in varying degrees of differentiation. There is always marked inflammatory response but the vascular endothelium is unaffected.

T-lymphocyte sensitization is undoubtedly the main mechanism of graft rejection but stimulation of antibody-secreting B lymphocytes also occurs, and this can result in antibody-mediated rejection, which has a much worse prognosis because it is characterized by prominent vascular damage with fibrinoid necrosis of arterioles. The severity of the rejection response is defined by the Banff international classification (Table 8.1).

Table 8.1 Banff international classification: Banff '97 diagnostic categories for renal allograft biopsies

Grade	Histopathological findings
1	Normal
2	Antibody-mediated rejection (rejection shown to be due at least in part to anti-donor antibody)
2A	Immediate (hyperacute)
2B	Delayed (accelerated acute)
3	Borderline changes: suspicious of acute rejection (this category is used when no intimal arteritis is present but there are foci of mild tubulitis)
4	Acute or active cell-mediated rejection
4ia	Significant interstitial infiltration (25% of parenchyma affected) with foci of moderate tubulitis (more than four mononuclear cells per cross-section)
4ib	Significant interstitial infiltration (> 25% of parenchyma affected) and foci of severe tubulitis (> 10% mononuclear cells per tubular cross-section)
4iia	Mild to moderate intimal arteritis
4iib	Severe intimal arteritis (> 25% of luminal area)
4iii	Transmural arteritis and/or fibrinoid change or necrosis of medial smooth muscle cells and lymphocytic inflammation
5	Chronic sclerosing allograft nephropathy
5i	Mild interstitial fibrosis and tubular atrophy
5ii	Moderate interstitial fibrosis and tubular atrophy
5iii	Severe interstitial fibrosis and tubular atrophy

(From Racussen LC, Solez K et al. Kidney Int 1999; 55: 713–723,[25] with permission from Blackwell Publishing Ltd.[23])

Understanding of the mechanisms of acute rejection and the complex cell–cell interactions involved comes from both animal experimentation and studies on material from human transplants obtained by fine-needle aspiration cytology[26,27] and Tru-cut biopsy.[28] Precise identification of the cells infiltrating the graft has been achieved by the use of monoclonal antibodies able to identify both individual cell types in the white cell series[29] and activation markers such as the interleukin-2 receptor.[30]

CHRONIC REJECTION

In addition to hyperacute rejection caused by cytotoxic antibodies and acute cell-mediated rejection, organ grafts are

REFERENCES

25. Racussen LC, Solez K et al. Kidney Int 1999; 55: 713–723
26. Hayry P, Von Willebrand E et al. Immunol Rev 1984; 77: 85–142
27. Wood RFM, Bolton EM et al. Lancet 1982; ii: 278
28. McWhinnie DL, Thompson JF et al. Transplantation 1986; 42: 352–358
29. Bolton EM, Thompson JF et al. Transplantation 1983; 36: 728–731
30. Robb RJ, Greene WC, Rusk CM. J Exp Med 1984; 160: 1126–1146

also subject to chronic rejection. This can be defined as slow but progressive deterioration in graft function over a prolonged period of months or even years. In many cases chronic rejection is the end result of acute rejection damage with the development of interstitial fibrosis. However, in some cases the process is due to the effects of non-cytotoxic antibodies that bind to antigenic determinants on the vascular endothelium of the graft, stimulating intimal hyperplasia and hence a gradual reduction in the blood supply. A number of cytokines and growth factors play an important role in the pathogenic process that leads to this chronic vasculopathy; among these, tissue growth factor-β is of particular importance, stimulating fibroblastic and myoblastic responses that lead to smooth muscle hyperplasia and subintimal fibrosis. Cyclosporine appears to stimulate tissue growth factor-β.

IMMUNOREGULATORY MECHANISMS

Acute rejection phenomena occur in the early weeks after transplantation, the first 100 days; after that time the risk of rejection recedes and the process appears to switch off. There is no doubt that immunoregulation occurs, although the precise mechanisms are poorly understood. From animal experimentation and in vitro human studies there is evidence that suppressor T cells develop that are capable of subverting the cytotoxic T-cell population.[31] In addition, anti-idiotypic antibodies may form that effectively switch off the reactive sites on the T-cell surface. It has not yet been possible to utilize these suppressor phenomena in any controlled way. Multiple pregnancies (five or more) induce an immunologically privileged status for the mother if and when she needs a transplant. This arises from the repeated injection of paternal HLA antigens from the fetus at each successive pregnancy.

Blood transfusion before transplantation has also been shown to induce a variable degree of immune suppression with a significant improvement in graft survival.[32] The reasons for the transfusion effect have not been defined and the benefit has been outweighed by the risk of transmitting disease.

IMMUNOSUPPRESSION: AGENTS AVAILABLE

ANTI-INFLAMMATORY AGENTS: CORTICOSTEROIDS

Corticosteroids were the first group of drugs to be used for immunosuppression and they remain an important component of many immunosuppressive protocols today. Corticosteroids are the first line of treatment for acute rejection episodes. The use and dosage of steroids has often been abused, and as a result they have been blamed for much of the morbidity associated with clinical transplantation. Despite their proven benefit, the side effects—cushingoid facies, diabetes, hypertension, fragile skin, cataracts and avascular necrosis of bone—are significant, especially with long-term therapy. These complications can be minimized by reducing the dose of steroids. There has always been a considerable interest in withdrawing steroids or avoiding their usage wherever possible.

Mechanism of action

Steroids have both anti-inflammatory and immunosuppressive properties, the two being closely related. Although they have been used clinically for years, their exact mechanism of action is not fully understood. They inhibit the production of T-cell lymphokines such as interleukin-1 and tumour necrosis factor, which are needed to amplify macrophage and lymphocyte responses. Inhibiting interleukin-1 is particularly important because the cytokine provides critical costimulation for interleukin-2 expression by activated T cells. Steroids also have a number of other immunosuppressive effects that are non-specific. They cause lymphopenia secondary to the redistribution of lymphocytes from the vascular compartment back into lymphoid tissue, they inhibit migration of monocytes, and they function as anti-inflammatory agents by blocking various permeability-increasing agents and vasodilators.

Dosage

Treatment is usually started at 2 mg/kg per day, reducing progressively to 0.5 mg/kg per day over the first 10 days. The route of administration or the exact tapering schedule is not important. Acute rejection is usually treated with high-dose intravenous steroids, usually 500 mg/day for 3 days. Steroid dosage is routinely tapered to the lowest possible maintenance dose, often with a view to complete withdrawal. A reasonable alternative to withdrawal is alternate-day steroid treatment.

PURINE ANTAGONISTS

Azathioprine

The first effective immunosuppressive agent was introduced by Calne in 1960[10,11] and shown to prolong survival of human kidney homografts by Murray in 1963.[12]

Mechanism of action

Azathioprine is a purine analogue. It functions as an antiproliferative agent. It is metabolized by the liver to the active drug 6-mercaptopurine, which is subsequently catabolized through the xanthine oxidase pathway. The final metabolites are excreted in the urine. Azathioprine and its metabolites act late in the immune process, affecting the cell cycle by interfering with DNA synthesis and thus suppressing proliferation of activated B and T lymphocytes. Azathioprine also reduces the number of monocytes by arresting the cell cycle of promyelocytes in the bone marrow; it decreases the number of circulating monocytes capable of differentiating into macrophages. Azathioprine is valuable in preventing the onset of acute rejection, but it is not effective in the treatment of acute rejection episodes.

Azathioprine and prednisolone used in combination made solid organ transplantation possible. They remained in continuous use from 1963 until 1984, when they were superseded by the first calcineurin antagonist, cyclosporine. Azathioprine has continued to be used with cyclosporine but is now being replaced by mycophenolate mofetil.

Dosage

Azathioprine is a prodrug. After absorption it is metabolized in the liver to the active drug 6-mercaptopurine. Oral treatment is usually started at between 3 and 5 mg/kg per day and reduced to a maintenance dose of between 1 and 2 mg/kg per day, taken as a single oral tablet. The azathioprine dosage is regulated to maintain the total white cell count between 4000 and

REFERENCES

31. Wang HB, Heacock EH et al. J Immunol 1982; 128: 1382–1385
32. Opelz G, Terasaki PI. Transplantation 1980; 29: 153–158

6000 cells/mm^3. In general, this usually means a maintenance dose of 2.0–3.0 mg/kg per day. Monitoring of drug levels has been shown to have no clinical value.

Adverse effects

The most significant side effect of azathioprine is bone marrow depression. All three haemopoietic cell lines can be affected, leading to leukopenia, thrombocytopenia and anaemia. Bone marrow depression is usually dose-related. Other significant side effects include hepatotoxicity, gastrointestinal disturbances, pancreatitis and alopecia. Azathioprine interacts with allopurinol, resulting in a significant increase in azathioprine toxicity.

Mycophenolate mofetil

Mycophenolate mofetil, despite being discovered by Ellison in 1958, was only approved for use in the prevention of acute rejection after kidney transplantation in May 1995. It has since been incorporated into routine clinical practice in many centres. It is a semisynthetic derivate of mycophenolic acid isolated from the mould *Penicillin glaucum*.

Mode of action

The active immunosuppressive compound mycophenolic acid is a reversible inhibitor of the enzyme inosine monophosphate dehydrogenase, which is a crucial rate-limiting enzyme in the de novo synthesis of purines. This enzyme catalyses the formation of inosine from guanosine nucleotides. Activated lymphocytes have an absolute requirement for de novo synthesis of inosine for clonal expansion. They do not have an alternative pathway. Mycophenolate therefore selectively prevents proliferation of T and B lymphocytes. Although it is an antiproliferative in the same way as azathioprine, it does not have the same bone marrow depressive effect. For these reasons mycophenolate mofetil has largely replaced azathioprine as the antiproliferative agent of choice in immunosuppressive therapy.

Adverse effects

The most significant side effects of mycophenolate mofetil are diarrhoea, gastritis and vomiting. It can also cause clinically important leukopenia.

Dosage

The initial dosage of mycophenolate mofetil should be given within 72 h of transplantation. It is usually administered as 1 g twice a day; 3 g per day is a more effective dosage but leads to a significant increase in side effects.

CALCINEURIN INHIBITORS

Cyclosporine

The action of cyclosporine as an antilymphocyte agent was first described by Jean Borel in 1976,[17] and its application to organ transplantation by Calne in 1977.[18] It was first used in human cadaver transplantation in a small pilot study by Calne in 1978,[19] and its value proved in the Canadian[33] and European[34] multicentre trials reported in 1981 and 1983. The arrival of cyclosporine dramatically altered the field of transplantation. The results after kidney transplantation improved by 30%, and although this had a great impact, the greatest impact was on extrarenal transplants. Graft and patient survival after liver transplantation increased from 30% to 70%. Results for heart, lung and intestinal transplant also improved substantially.

Mechanism of action

Cyclosporine was the first example of an immunosuppressive agent with a specific action ever to be used. It binds with its cytoplasmic receptor protein, cyclophilin, which subsequently inhibits the activity of calcineurin. This impairs the expression of several critical T-cell activation genes, the most important being interleukin-2. As a result, T-cell activation is completely suppressed. The latest formulation, cyclosporine Neoral, is well absorbed, and this has increased the bioavailability of cyclosporine, reducing the intrapatient variation.

Adverse effects

Cyclosporine has a number of non-renal side effects, notably cosmetic complications such as hirsutism and gingival hyperplasia, which may lead to non-compliance. Nephrotoxicity is the most important and troublesome adverse effect of cyclosporine. The nephrotoxicity seen with cyclosporine is complex; the underlying pathogenesis is a powerful vasoconstrictor effect on the afferent arteriole to the glomerulus. This vasoconstriction is transient and reversible to begin with; it is dose-dependent and it causes hypertension and graft dysfunction. Long-term cyclosporine use commonly results in interstitial fibrosis of the renal parenchyma coupled with arteriolar lesions. Cyclosporine may also result in haemolytic uraemic syndrome due to interference with the generation of prostacyclin, which leads to vascular endothelial damage, platelet aggregation, and the formation of thrombi in the microcirculation. Cyclosporine also causes a number of electrolyte abnormalities, the most common being hyperkalaemia, hypomagnesaemia and hyperuricaemia. Cyclosporine also causes neurotoxicity (tremor and hyperaesthesia), disturbances in lipid and glucose metabolism, and a predisposition to infection.

Dosage

The cyclosporine dose is usually given in two divided doses amounting to 7 mg/kg per day. This dose can be reduced over time to maintain a cyclosporine trough level of 100–250 ng/mL.

Tacrolimus (FK506)

Tacrolimus is a calcineurin inhibitor with a similar action to that of cyclosporine. It is a metabolite of the soil fungus *Streptomyces tsukubaensis*, found in Japan. It was in trials in the USA as early as 1983 and released for clinical use, particularly for liver transplantation, in April 1994. It is now widely used in liver, renal and pancreatic transplantation. It is a macrolide lactone structurally related to another new immunosuppressive agent, sirolimus.

Mechanism of action

Tacrolimus, like cyclosporine, acts by binding to immunophilins, ubiquitous and abundant intracellular proteins. Cyclosporine acts by binding cyclophilin whereas tacrolimus acts by binding FK506-binding proteins. This complex of immunophilin plus drug is, in effect, the active agent responsible for the immunosuppressive effect, inhibiting the enzyme calcineurin and preventing the transcription of T4-cell cytokines such as interleukin-2,

REFERENCES

33. Canadian Multi Centre Trial. N Engl J Med 1981; 309; 809–815
34. European Multi Centre Trial. Lancet 1983; 2: 986–9.

interferon-gamma, interleukin-4 and tissue necrosis factor-α. Tacrolimus is approximately 100 times more potent than cyclosporine on a molar basis.

Dosage

Tacrolimus administration should begin within 6–24 h of transplantation. The oral dose is 0.15–0.35 mg/kg per day administered in two divided doses. Once again, the dosage is tailored postoperatively to produce a trough level of between 5 and 10 ng/mL.

Adverse effects

Tacrolimus shares a number of side effects in common with cyclosporine: both cause nephrotoxicity, neurotoxicity, impairment of glucose and lipid metabolism, hypertension, infection and gastrointestinal disturbance. Tacrolimus, however, does not cause hirsutism or gingival hyperplasia. Other common side effects include gastrointestinal upset, diarrhoea and cramps, hypertension, hypercholesterolaemia, hypomagnesaemia and lymphoproliferative disorders.

ANTIPROLIFERATIVE AGENTS: SIROLIMUS (RAPAMYCIN)

Sirolimus is a macrolide antibiotic derived from the fungus *Actinomycetes*, found on Rapanui in the Easter Island group. It has a similar molecular shape to tacrolimus but an entirely different mode of action. It does not affect calcineurin activity; rather, it acts at a step beyond the interaction between the cytokine with its receptor. Even though it binds to cytosolic immunophilin, it does not inhibit calcineurin phosphatase activity because it acts later in the interleukin-2 pathway and does not suppress interleukin-2 production. The sirolimus–immunophilin complex targets two kinases—mammalian targets of rapamycin 1 and 2 (mTOR1 and 2)—that are associated with the cell cycle progression. Inhibition of mTor 1 and 2 by sirolimus blocks lymphocyte activation and the proliferative response of T cells to interleukin-2 by preventing the progression from G1 to S phase of the cell cycle and halting cell division. It is therefore an antiproliferative.

Sirolimus is a powerful immunosuppressive agent in its own right. It is not nephrotoxic and it does not cause hirsutism and gingival hyperplasia. Extensive recent studies have shown that sirolimus allows the withdrawal of cyclosporine after as little as 3 months, with a dramatic improvement in renal function and blood pressure control.[35]

ANTIBODIES

Antithymocyte globulin

Antithymocyte globulin is a potent polyclonal antibody obtained by immunizing animals with human thymocytes. The best antithymocyte globulin is raised by injecting human T cells into rabbits and then separating the sera. It can be used both to prevent rejection and to reverse acute rejection episodes; it acts by destroying circulating T cells. It is more effective than antithymocyte globulin raised in the horse and than the monoclonal antibody OKT3 raised in the mouse. All these agents can cause fever, chills, arthralgia, thrombocytopenia, leukopenia and serum sickness.

Daclizumab and basiliximab

Daclizumab and basiliximab are two IgG_1 isotype monoclonal antibodies that bind to interleukin-2Ra receptor and prevent immune recognition. They are both equally effective in preventing rejection when given during the first 3 months after transplantation. They are used in combination with conventional drugs and have little in the way of side effects.

ALTERNATIVE FORMS OF IMMUNOSUPPRESSION

Radiotherapy

Radiotherapy can be given directly to the graft or to suppress the bone marrow; it has largely been abandoned, but success has been reported with total lymphoid irradiation as a pretransplant preparation for high-risk patients with previous failed grafts who are unable to have dialysis treatment.[36]

Thoracic duct drainage

Thoracic duct drainage to deplete the patient of lymphocytes was one of the techniques employed in the early stages of transplantation, but it has been abandoned now that powerful immunosuppressive drugs have become available.

IMMUNOSUPPRESSIVE PROPHYLAXIS

Immunosuppressive prophylaxis is usually achieved with a combination of cyclosporine, azathioprine and steroids. The dose of cyclosporine is progressively reduced during the first 2 weeks, to achieve maintenance whole blood trough levels of between 100 and 250 ng/mL. Steroid dose is also progressively reduced with a view to withdrawal or alternate day therapy. Tacrolimus is increasingly preferred to cyclosporine because it does not cause hirsutism and gingival overgrowth. Mycophenolate mofetil is often used as an alternative to azathioprine on the grounds that it is less of a bone marrow depressant; the choice is largely dependent on experience and side effects. The common principle is to tail off the dose of all drugs over the first 3 months to minimize the side effects. Where possible, steroids are completely withdrawn, and there is now good evidence that the calcineurin inhibitors should be withdrawn in favour of sirolimus to minimize nephrotoxicity.[35]

DIAGNOSIS AND TREATMENT OF ACUTE REJECTION

Episodes of acute rejection are usually diagnosed indirectly by observing deterioration in graft function. It is important to eliminate other possible causes of change in graft function before diagnosing acute rejection. These would include obstruction, reduced blood supply, infection and, most important of all, drug toxicity. Graft biopsy remains the gold standard for diagnosis of acute rejection.

The first line of treatment is methylprednisolone 500 mg (depending on size) given as an i.v. bolus daily for 3 days. This can be repeated if necessary, provided a response was obtained the first time. In the absence of a response, or when rejection persists, i.v. antithymocyte globulin is given daily for 5–10 days. During treatment with antithymocyte globulin it is essential to monitor

REFERENCES

35. Johnson RWG, Kreiss H, Oberauer R et al. Transplantation 2001; 72: 777–786
36. Najarian JS, Sutherland DER et al. Transplant Proc 1981; 13: 417–424

the lymphocyte count and to give prophylaxis against cytomegalovirus, especially if the donor was positive; cytomegalovirus pneumonia is more often than not fatal in severely immunosuppressed patients.

It is also possible to treat persistent rejection by switching between cyclosporine and tacrolimus and/or by adding mycophenolate mofetil.

LONG-TERM IMMUNOSUPPRESSION

Long-term immunosuppression is the price recipients pay for successful transplantation. The hazards of long-term treatment are drug toxicity, opportunistic infections, and an increased risk of certain malignant tumours.

Of the drug toxicities, nephrotoxicity is the most worrying because there is increasing evidence that this is an important cause of late graft loss in renal allograft recipients and a potent cause of renal failure in recipients of heart, liver and bone marrow grafts. There is an increasing trend to switch from calcineurin inhibitors to sirolimus after 3 months to avoid nephrotoxicity; this exposes the patient to the long-term risk of raised lipoproteins.

OPPORTUNISTIC INFECTION

The risk of opportunistic infections is ever present in immunosuppressed patients, although it diminishes somewhat with time and dose. These infections occur in reasonably predictable time frames.

In the immediate postoperative period, wound infections are relatively rare (less than 0.5%); the most common bacterial infections are usually catheter-related urinary infections. Atelectasis and bacterial pneumonias are fairly frequent, often complicated by herpes simplex and moniliasis.

The most serious opportunistic viral and fungal infections usually commence at around 1 month post-transplant. They are predicated by immunosuppressive dose, treatment of rejection and previous immune status. *Pneumocystis carinii*, cytomegalic inclusion disease, cytomegalovirus, hepatitis B and C, and Epstein–Barr virus are the most common and the most troublesome infections. Nocardia, listeria and tuberculosis are the most common bacterial infections. Aspergillosis and cryptococcosis are the most dangerous fungal problems.

Prophylaxis is to be commended in particular situations. A single dose of a broad spectrum antibiotic at the time of surgery reduces the risk of opportunistic bacterial infection; oral trimethoprim for 3 months eliminates most of the risk of *Pneumocystis carinii*. Intravenous ganciclovir should be given during a course of antibody treatment for rejection because this commonly follows heavy doses of conventional immunosuppression and reduces the patient's defences against cytomegalovirus in particular. Cytomegalovirus viraemia unchecked is commonly fatal; cytomegalovirus can affect all organs of the body but pneumonitis and hepatitis are most common.

OPPORTUNISTIC TUMOURS

The prevalence of tumours increases with time.[37] Skin tumours are the most common; they are often multiple and commonly recur. The tumours may be either basal cell tumours or squamous epitheliomas. They occur on exposed parts of the body and are related to exposure to ultraviolet light. The increased incidence of these tumours is caused by the deposition of azathioprine in the skin and its reaction to ultraviolet light.

Lymphoproliferative disorders caused by exposure to Epstein–Barr virus are among the most challenging; these range from a benign polyclonal process sensitive to reduction in immunosuppressive therapy to aggressive malignant monoclonal extra nodal disease, which is most often fatal.

RENAL TRANSPLANTATION

The waiting lists for renal transplantation in the UK continue to increase at about 2% per annum. This represents a huge drain on national resources for health not only from the cost of long-term dialysis but also as a result of loss of income from people who could be fit and contributing to the economy.

Waiting lists have continued to grow worldwide. The number of patients on dialysis awaiting a renal transplant in the UK has grown from 1592 in the 1970s to 6252 in 2002. This reflects improved availability of renal replacement therapy and the widening of eligibility criteria for acceptance, especially for patients at the extremes of age. Unfortunately, renal transplant activity has remained steady, at around 1700 per year, despite desperate attempts to increase the number of cadaver donors. There has been a continuing slow decline in the number of heart-beating ventilated donors over the last 10 years as a result of a gratifying reduction in the number of deaths from road traffic accidents and better management of intracranial haemorrhage. There is also a shortfall in the number of intensive care beds in which suitable potential donors can be nursed.

In reality there are never going to be enough cadaver donors to meet demand, and therefore it is necessary to look to live kidney donation to bridge the gap between supply and demand. In 2001, living donor transplants represented around 24% of all kidneys transplanted in the UK; this compares unfavourably with 31% in the USA and 40% in Norway. The pressure to increase live donation is only partly due to the shortage; it is also because the long-term results, even from poorly matched grafts, with short ischaemic times are so much better.

LIVE DONOR SELECTION AND WORK-UP

The British Transplantation Society has published clear guidelines on the management of live donation (see http://www.bts.org.uk), which include the recommendation that the donor must be fully informed of all potential complications; these include risk of death (approximately one in 3000 cases); idiosyncratic reactions to anaesthetic and other drugs; general complications of major surgery, such as thromboembolism, intra-abdominal bleeding and abscess formation; wound problems such as haematoma, infection and herniation; chest problems such as pneumothorax, pneumonia and atelectasis; urinary retention or infection; and the possible need for blood transfusion.

Long-term issues need to be explored; these include the possibility of long- or short-term wound pain, the risk of a slight

REFERENCE

37. Sheil AGR, Disney APS, Mathews TH et al. Transplant Proc 1993; 25: 1383–1384

rise in blood pressure, and the possible psychological sequelae of donation, such as anticlimactic depression and the reaction to the graft failing.

Donor selection involves an independent, detailed clinical assessment to exclude transmissible disease and to assess the degree of immunological similarity between donor and recipient. It has to be established that there are two kidneys present and that they are both functioning equally well. The anatomy of the kidneys and their vascular connections need to be fully evaluated, preferably by contrast-enhanced spiral CT scan. Last, the reasons for donation need to be clear and free from any external pressure.

LIVE DONOR NEPHRECTOMY

Live donor nephrectomy is a unique operation in that the surgery is for the benefit of someone else. This places extra responsibility on the surgeon. Most live donor nephrectomies are still carried out as an open procedure through the bed of the 12th rib, an operation—which although it gives good exposure—has a justifiable reputation for postoperative pain and minor chest complications. Increasingly there is a move towards an anterior approach, which can be either trans- or extraperitoneal. This approach is much more acceptable to the patient but the exposure is less satisfactory. Laparoscopic live donor nephrectomy is now widely practised in the USA; it has the advantages of excellent exposure, low blood loss, much less postoperative pain and a very short in-hospital stay. The need to convert to open surgery is low. With increasing expertise it seems probable that this will soon be the standard technique worldwide.

RECIPIENT SELECTION AND PREOPERATIVE PREPARATION

Every patient accepted on to a renal replacement programme should be considered for a renal transplant; there are very few contraindications. Age by itself is not a contraindication provided there are no significant comorbidities; elderly patients do remarkably well with a renal transplant. Elderly patients accepted on to the waiting list should have a life expectancy of at least 2 years after transplantation; their health should be such that neither the operation nor the immunosuppressive therapy will cause premature death or loss of quality of life. Some of these judgements are very subjective and they can be difficult. Although on one hand it would be irresponsible to offer a transplant to someone who has advanced atherosclerosis or recent history of invasive malignant disease, on the other hand patients with incipient left ventricular failure, although a high-risk group, will frequently show an improvement in cardiac function following a successful renal graft.

Transplantation rather than dialysis is the preferred treatment for children with end-stage renal disease as they fail to grow and develop on dialysis. Lack of bladder function is an undoubted problem in a number of children, but kidneys can be successfully transplanted with ureteric drainage into an ileal conduit or into an enhanced bladder with self catheterization.[38]

Severe anomalies of the lower urinary tract are not a contraindication in adults. It may be necessary to remove all or most of the upper urinary tract and establish a resting ileal conduit in preparation for the transplant, a procedure that inflicts considerable hardship because it may cause postural hypotension and anaemia, and require even more severe fluid restriction.

The selection of the most appropriate recipient for a given donor kidney is based on ABO blood group compatibility and HLA matching. Using national and international organ-matching schemes the aim is to avoid mismatches at DR wherever possible and to minimize the number of mismatches at the other loci to no more than two. This should be achievable in at least 60% of cases. Analysis of the European Collaborative Study database demonstrates that these beneficially matched grafts have survival rates in excess of 85% at 1 year, an improvement of more than 10% on all other match grades.[39]

Before proceeding with the transplant a negative cytotoxic cross-match is essential to ensure that the potential recipient does not have circulating antibodies that might precipitate hyperacute rejection.

THE TRANSPLANT OPERATION

The iliac fossa was selected as the site for renal transplantation by the groups in Paris, and later in Boston, who performed the first successful cases in the 1950s. The essential features of the procedure have remained unchanged ever since. The kidney is transplanted extraperitoneally in the iliac fossa; the renal artery is anastomosed to either the internal iliac artery (end to end) or the external iliac artery (end to side) and the renal vein is joined end to side to the external iliac vein. In this position only a short length of ureter is required to reach the bladder.

In mobilizing the iliac vessels it is essential that any lymphatic trunks divided should be carefully ligated to minimize the risk of lymphocyst. The arterial and venous anastomoses are carried out using standard vascular techniques with 5/0 monofilament proline sutures (Fig. 8.3). Many patients in chronic renal failure have low haematocrits and prolonged coagulation times, rendering it unnecessary to employ systemic heparinization during the 25–30 min required to revascularize the graft. Following the release of the clamps the kidney should become pink and firm with immediate urine production. To encourage a diuresis the central venous pressure should be maintained in excess of 10 cm of water, and an infusion of furosemide (frusemide) and mannitol or dopamine will promote an immediate diuresis. The ureter is most commonly implanted through a short submucosal tunnel on the dome or lateral side of the bladder to reduce the risk of reflux and ascending infection in the graft.

Children warrant special consideration; urological disease is the cause of renal failure in 50% of small children. Ureteric reflux, hydronephrosis, megaureter, megacystis, neurogenic bladder and spina bifida are common causes often complicated by long-standing and recurrent infection. Such children require careful investigation prior to transplantation and their parents need expert counselling. Often complete clearance of the infected urinary tract is required with establishment of a resting ileal conduit some months before a transplant can be found. This imposes the special hardship of anuria, hypotension and anaemia on the child, often for a considerable period of time.

Children in renal failure fail to grow and develop normally, and this can make the procedure technically challenging. Children of 20 kg or more can be treated more or less like adults, but below 20 kg the kidney often has to be placed intraperitoneally, especially if it is an adult kidney; this involves an extensive dissection and requires meticulous haemostasis and very careful postoperative fluid and electrolyte control.

REFERENCES

38. MacGregor P, Novick AC et al. J Urol 1986; 135: 686–688
39. Gilks WR, Bradley BA, Gore SM. Lancet 1986; i: 509

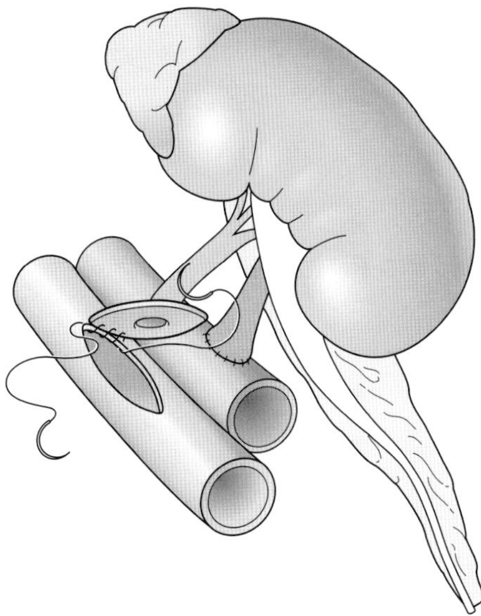

Figure 8.3 The vascular anastomoses in a renal transplant. The renal vein is anastomosed end to side to the external iliac vein. The figure shows the method of anastomosis of the Carrel patch of aorta around the donor renal artery to the recipient's external iliac artery.

POSTOPERATIVE PROBLEMS

Arterial or venous occlusion

Arterial or venous occlusion is a very early complication; the incidence has been reported as high as 10% in some series. Diagnostic features are continuing renal failure and anuria with no evidence of isotope uptake on technetium-99m MAG 3 scan, indicating lack of perfusion. Venous thrombosis is more uncommon (0.9–7.6%); it is often dramatic in presentation, with severe pansuprapubic swelling and haematuria. Sometimes the graft will rupture and haemorrhage may be profuse. Venous thrombosis is usually caused by misalignment of the vein, sometimes by coincidental extraneous compression or by deep vein thrombosis due to a hypercoagulable state.

Graft dysfunction

There are many possible causes of graft dysfunction after transplantation. These include acute tubular necrosis, ureteric obstruction, urinary leak, acute rejection and drug-induced nephrotoxicity. The differential diagnosis can usually be clarified by an ultrasound scan to exclude obstruction and extravasation of urine, blood trough level for cyclosporine or tacrolimus to exclude toxicity, and finally a biopsy to prove rejection. Biopsy can be a hazardous procedure and should not be undertaken lightly; it is, however, the gold standard for diagnosis of rejection. The complications of biopsy include haematuria, perinephric haemorrhage, rupture of the kidney, arteriovenous fistula, blood clot obstruction of the renal pelvis, and accidental damage to surrounding structures.

Urinary leak

Urinary leak can occur in the early postoperative period if the catheter becomes blocked. It is a particular problem in patients with small, contracted bladders. An alternative cause is necrosis of the lower end of the ureter; this is relatively uncommon and tends to present insidiously with suprapubic tenderness and a gradual reduction in urine output 5–10 days after transplantation. In some circumstances it may be possible to reimplant the transplant ureter; however, if necrosis is extensive it will be necessary to use the patient's own ureter or a bladder flap to remedy the situation.

Ureteric stenosis

When ureteric stenosis occurs early it is usually due to a technical error and requires surgical correction. Late-onset ureteric stenosis may be ischaemic and is one of the differential diagnoses in patients with a gradual reduction in renal function. The resulting hydronephrosis is readily detected on ultrasound scanning. The stenosis is frequently localized to the lower end of the ureter. It can sometimes be treated by percutaneous dilatation and stenting. Alternately, surgical reimplantation will be required and is not unduly difficult.

Renal artery stenosis

All large series report late renal artery stenosis, with an incidence ranging from 1.6 to 12%. Classically this is heralded by increasing blood pressure, the presence of a bruit over the graft, and declining function. Surgical correction of renal artery stenosis can be hazardous. A review of 180 cases found that although 76% benefited, there was a 3% mortality rate and a 12% incidence of graft loss.[40] Although good results have been reported following percutaneous transluminal angioplasty, it appears that long-term success is achieved in only a third of cases.[41]

Recurrent disease

Recurrent disease is much under-diagnosed because many patients present in end-stage renal failure, for the first time, too late for a precise histological diagnosis to be made. Patients at particular risk are those with mesangiocapillary type II glomerular nephritis, immunoglobulin A nephropathy, malignant focal glomerulosclerosis[42] and oxalosis. Acceptable graft survival rates can be achieved in patients with oxalosis by ensuring a massive diuresis and using daily dialysis to reduce oxalate load in the immediate postoperative period.[43]

Infection remains one of the major causes of morbidity following transplantation. A wide variety of infections with bacteria, viruses, fungi and protozoa have been reported in transplant recipients.

Diagnosis and treatment of acute rejection

Episodes of acute rejection occur during the first 100 days post transplant. They are usually diagnosed indirectly by observing deterioration in graft function: a rise in serum creatinine, a fall in urine output, or a reduction in uptake of isotope on technetium-99m DTPA or technetium-99m MAG 3 scan. It is important to eliminate other possible causes of change in graft function before diagnosing acute rejection. These would include ureteric obstruction, reduced blood supply, infection, and most important of all drug-induced nephrotoxicity. Graft biopsy remains the gold standard for diagnosis of acute rejection but it is not without hazard.

The first line of treatment is methylprednisolone 500 mg (depending on size) given as an i.v. bolus daily for 3 days. This can

REFERENCES

40. Lohr JW, MacDougall ML et al. Am J Kidney Dis 1986; 7: 363–367
41. Reisfeld D, Matas AJ et al. Transplant Proc 1989; 21: 1955–1956
42. Cameron JS. Transplantation 1982; 34: 237–245
43. Watts RWE, Morgan SH et al. Transplantation 1988; 45: 1143–1145

be repeated if necessary, provided a response was obtained the first time. In the absence of a response, or when rejection persists, i.v. antithymocyte globulin is given daily for 5–10 days. During treatment with antithymocyte globulin it is essential to monitor the lymphocyte count and to give prophylaxis against cytomegalovirus, especially if the donor was positive for cytomegalovirus; cytomegalovirus pneumonia is commonly fatal in severely immunosuppressed patients.

It is also possible to treat persistent rejection by switching between cyclosporine and tacrolimus and/or by adding mycophenolate mofetil.

Results of kidney transplantation

That successful kidney transplantation saves life and improves quality of life is beyond dispute. The question is: for how many and at what price? Even allowing for the high cost of transplantation in the first year, it is still more cost-effective than dialysis and against that benchmark there are significant savings for every year the patient survives beyond the third. The European Collaborative Study has data for more than 100 000 patients receiving renal transplants between 1985 and 2003 (Figs 8.4 and 8.5). These data, which can be examined on the Collaborative Transplant Study website (http://www.ctstransplant.org), report an overall patient survival of 90% at 5 years, rising to 98% for the 6500 fortunate enough to receive a well-matched living donor graft. The overall graft survival for cadaver grafts (90 000) was 85% at 1 year and 70% at 5 years. Noticeably, results for first grafts were significantly better than those for second and subsequent grafts.

All registries have accessible websites (listed at the end of this chapter); they all show that avoiding mismatches for DR antigens gives a 10% advantage in 5-year graft survival and that mismatched live donated grafts survive better than cadaver grafts, however well matched. This is probably a function of avoiding ischaemic injury. Late graft loss is multifactorial in origin. Connolly has shown that there are five key predictive factors: cadaver donor, matching, ischaemia time, relative kidney size and recipient comorbidity.[44] Only about half of the losses at 1 year can be attributed to acute rejection (5%), and only about half of the losses at 5 years can be attributed to chronic rejection. This means that there is room for improvement; unnecessary graft loss must be avoided at all costs.

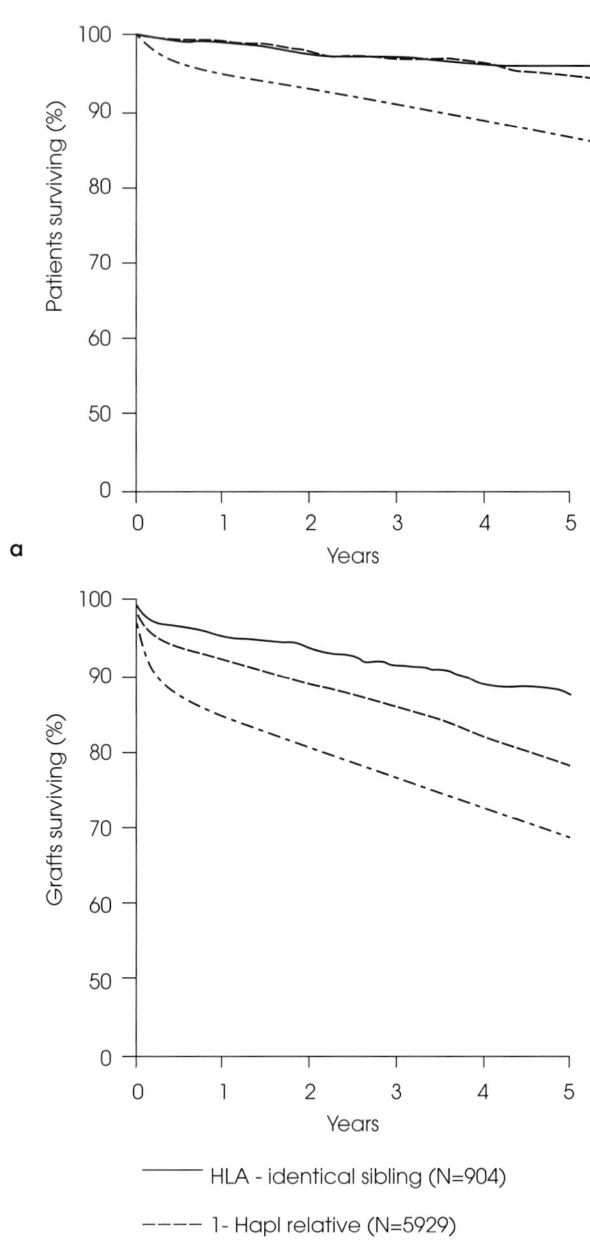

Figure 8.4 Patient (a) and graft (b) survival of more than 100 000 renal transplants reported to the European Collaborative Transplant Study Group between 1985 and 2001. This study confirms the clear advantage of well-matched live related donor transplants. Published with kind permission of Professor Gerhardt Opelz.

CONCLUSIONS

Renal transplantation has become established as the major means of replacement therapy for patients with end-stage renal failure. The indications have widened, with treatment being offered to small children up to patients in their 70s. Transplantation is now associated with better rehabilitation and lower morbidity and mortality rates than either haemodialysis or continuous ambulatory peritoneal dialysis. Despite the economic advantages of kidney grafting, units throughout the world are hampered by a chronic shortage of suitable organs. For donor referral rates to improve, public education programmes will have to be combined with a greater awareness among healthcare professionals of the enormous benefits of successful transplantation.

PANCREATIC TRANSPLANTATION

The syndrome of type 1 insulin-dependent diabetes mellitus includes not only abnormal glucose metabolism but also specific microvascular complications: retinopathy, nephropathy, neuropathy and small vessel peripheral vascular disease. Diabetes mellitus is the leading cause of blindness and chronic renal failure in young adults and a principle cause of amputation and impotence. The discovery of insulin by Banting and Best in 1922 dramatically changed the life expectancy of young diabetic patients; premature death from diabetic ketosis became

REFERENCES

44. Connolly JK, Dyer P, Martin S et al. Transplantation 1996; 61: 709–714

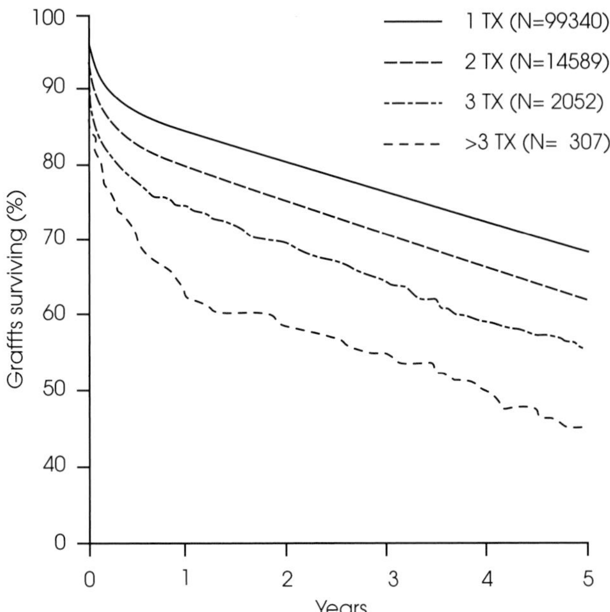

Figure 8.5 Cadaver kidney transplants reported to the European Collaborative Transplant Study Group between 1985 and 2001. Successive renal transplants do progressively less well, particularly after the second. Published with kind permission of Professor Gerhardt Opelz.

preventable.[45] However, by the late 1930s it was clear that this did not resolve the whole syndrome of diabetic disease; patients were still suffering and dying as a result of microangiopathic complications. Diabetic patients were 25 times more prone to blindness, five times more prone to peripheral gangrene and amputation, and 17 times more likely to develop major kidney disease. These major difficulties result in a reduction in life expectation of one-third among diabetic patients; in the USA, insulin-dependent diabetes is now the fifth most common cause of death.[46]

The number of diabetic patients requiring chronic renal replacement therapy continues to increase. In 1976, 6% of dialysis patients in the USA were diabetic; a decade later that figure had risen to 25%.[47] The uraemic diabetic patient presents a formidable clinical management problem because of the ocular, cardiovascular, neurological and psychological complications of diabetes.[48]

The first pancreatic transplantation was performed by Kelly and Lillehei in 1966 in an effort to stabilize the carbohydrate control and to delay or prevent the microangiopathic complications.[49] Since 1966, more than 14 000 pancreatic grafts have been performed worldwide and reported to the International Pancreas Transplant Registry. The rationale behind kidney and pancreas transplantation remains, first and foremost, to resolve the clinical syndrome of diabetes and to improve the patient's quality of life by delaying or preventing the onset of microvascular complications.[50] Increasing evidence suggests that the control of carbohydrate homeostasis has a marked influence on microvascular complications, and that even quite marked diabetic renal damage will improve if optimal carbohydrate control is obtained.[51]

INDICATIONS FOR SIMULTANEOUS PANCREAS–KIDNEY TRANSPLANTATION

Candidates for simultaneous pancreas–kidney transplantation are unstable diabetic patients with impending or frank renal failure (with a creatinine clearance of < 15 mL/min) and with one or more poorly controlled, well-defined secondary complications (such as proliferative diabetic retinopathy or neuropathy), and type 1 diabetic patients on dialysis or with a failing previous renal allograft. At first, only patients with the most advanced complications were considered, but patients with earlier stage disease are now increasingly considered for pancreatic grafting. Careful evaluation, including coronary artery assessment, is needed because of the multiple complications so often encountered in these patients. Investigations usually include electrocardiogram, ultrasound stress electrocardiogram and coronary angiography to assess the extent of coronary artery disease. These are done with increased frequency. Baseline studies of the eyes and of peripheral nerves should also be done.

TECHNICAL SURGICAL CONSIDERATIONS

Pancreatic grafts are obtained from cadaveric donors at the same time as removal of the kidneys and liver. It is usual to avoid dissection of the pancreas prior to perfusion of all the abdominal organs with cold University of Wisconsin fluid, because unnecessary handling may cause graft pancreatitis after reimplantation. Once cooled, liver retrieval is followed by removal of the pancreas, although some groups prefer en bloc liver–pancreas removal with separation on the bench after further cooling. One of the difficulties of segmental or whole-organ pancreatic implantation is the need to provide a drainage system for the exocrine acinar tissue of the graft. The development of an ingenious method of ductal injection with neoprene, a latex polymer glue, by Dubernard was a major factor reawakening interest in pancreatic transplantation.[52] However, this technique resulted in progressive fibrosis and sclerosis of the acinar tissue, leaving a scarred non-functional gland in the long term.

Operative techniques were then developed to drain the pancreas into the bladder on the grounds that inactivated pancreatic enzymes are harmless and, furthermore, monitoring of urinary amylase might prove a predictor of rejection. Neither of these theories proved reliable, and many patients have suffered significant complications due to chemical cystitis and urethritis, dehydration and bicarbonate losses. Enteric drainage is now the preferred procedure, utilizing a duodenal segment from the donor. There are less acute infective complications when the pancreas is drained into the intestine than when drained into the bladder. The pancreas graft is placed intraperitoneally. Unless the coeliac axis and superior mesenteric arteries have been procured on a common aortic cuff, they have to be meticulously reconstructed in ice beforehand using donor common, external and internal iliac arteries as a Y graft. The arterial conduit thus formed is then anastomosed to the external iliac artery of the recipient. In most major centres, systemic venous drainage has

REFERENCES

45. Bliss M. The Discovery of Insulin. Paul Harris, Edinburgh, 1983
46. Carter Center of Emory University. Diabetes Care 1985; 8: 391–406
47. Brunette P. Diabet Nephropath 1985; 4: 103
48. Friedman EA. Diabet Nephropath 1983; 2: 3
49. Kelly W, Lillehei R, Merkle F. Surgery 1967; 61: 827–835
50. Williams PW. Br Med J 1984; 2: 1303
51. The DCCT Research Trial Group. N Engl J Med 1993: 329
52. Dubernard JM, Traeger J, Neyra P. Surgery 1978; 84: 633–639

given way to portal venous drainage: the donor portal vein is anastomosed to the recipient superior mesenteric vein in the root of the small bowel mesentery. The duodenum is anastomosed side to side to jejunum. Ileum can be used, but this tends to cause diarrhoea related to the large volume of exocrine excretion.

POSTOPERATIVE COMPLICATIONS

Postoperative complications include vascular thrombosis, episodes of graft pancreatitis, leaks from the duodenal anastomosis, and infections. These complications are notoriously difficult to diagnose, and high-quality radiology support, particularly CT, is required. Acute rejection is also difficult to diagnose but serum amylase and trypsin levels may be predictive. Fine-needle biopsy can be done but is not without risk. Most grafts are simultaneous with a kidney from the same donor and this is relied on for rejection diagnosis and treatment.

IMPLANTATION OF ISLETS OF LANGERHANS

Ideally the islets of Langerhans, the active organs of insulin release, would be the only cells transferred from donor to recipient, and in small animal models this is a viable proposition. Early attempts at islet transplantation in humans yielded little success;[53] in larger animals and humans the purity of islets and their viability after extraction have until recently been much less satisfactory, and the islet yields have usually been insufficient to control blood sugar. Attempts at cellular microencapsulation of islets within a polyisoprene alginate membrane have been introduced in an effort to reduce the immunological damage.[54] These megaislets, or clusters, can be successfully transferred in animal models without immunological destruction;[55] however, fibrosis around the capsule has proved to be a limiting factor of this technique. The Edmonton group have shown that by repeated infusions of islets over several months they have been able to render patients insulin-free, suggesting that critical mass is an important factor in islet transplantation.[56]

RESULTS OF TRANSPLANTATION

Reports from the international registry show that more than 14 000 pancreatic transplants of all kinds have been performed worldwide; these results can be viewed on the registry website. Results for 5400 simultaneous kidney and enterically drained whole pancreas grafts are broadly similar to those for kidney transplantation alone—patient survival at 1 year is 97% and graft survival 88%—and thus these developing techniques have become increasingly safe. One-year survival after pancreas transplantation alone remains lower (around 60%) than when in combination with the kidney, and this may be attributed to the difficulties in diagnosing acute rejection.[57] Although the clinical syndrome of diabetes mellitus (namely glycosuria, polyuria and polydipsia) is resolved by implantation of a pancreatic graft, the long-term impact on microvascular complications is less certain.[58]

Improvement in nerve conduction studies has been clearly demonstrated with stabilization of the retina, and transplant biopsies of kidney grafts in these same patients have not shown the typical thickening of glomerular basement membrane seen in diabetic nephropathy.

LIVER TRANSPLANTATION

In the 30 years since the first attempts at liver transplantation in humans,[59] this procedure has progressed to become of major benefit to patients with advanced liver disease. Over 4000 liver grafts are performed in Europe alone each year and about 10 000 worldwide, and the development of newer surgical techniques, combined with the introduction of improved immunosuppressive protocols, has led to a significant improvement in overall success rates (see the European Liver Transplant Registry website at http://www.eltr.org).[60]

In the UK there are about 700 liver transplants each year. The number of transplants carried out has remained relatively stable since 1995, but waiting lists have increased, as with those for other organ transplants. New therapies and improved results will most probably increase the demand for liver transplantation from the current level of 12 per million of population per year up to about 20 per million of population per year. The supply of cadaveric donor organs, currently 11.2 per million of population per year, is insufficient to meet this demand. In response to this, new innovations are developing, split liver transplantation (where one organ is divided for two recipients) and live partial liver donation in particular. In countries where there are religious or cultural beliefs that prevent cadaveric donation, liver transplantation is exclusively live related, and excellent results have been achieved in Japan and Korea in particular, with some centres carrying out more than 100 grafts each year. Unfortunately, several live donor deaths have now been reported, and although this approach has been embraced with enthusiasm throughout much of the world, the approach in the UK has been more cautious. An alternative strategy is the use of livers from 'marginal' donors and from non-heart-beating cadaveric donors, and these types of transplant are being carried out cautiously in the most major centres.

CURRENT PATIENT SELECTION

For the most part, patients considered for liver transplantation have developed major hepatic decompensation due to advanced parenchymatous liver disease (Table 8.2). This is most often related to a viral aetiology, most commonly hepatitis C but also hepatitis B. Alcoholic liver disease has also become a major indication, and viral diseases and alcohol account for more than 70% of liver transplants. It is usual to require a significant period of abstinence from alcohol before a patient is accepted on to a transplant list, but there is still a lot of variation between units, particularly in relation to young adults with acute alcoholic liver failure. Some of these patients will have liver diseases complicated by the development of tumours, primarily hepatocellular carcinoma. Although primary hepatocellular carcinoma might appear at first sight to be the most obvious indication for liver

REFERENCES

53. Kendall DM, Robertson RP. Diabetes Metab 1996; 22: 157–163
54. O'Shea GM, Sun AM. Diabetes 1986; 35: 445–446
55. Sun AM, O'Shea GM, Goosen MF. Appl Biochem Biotechnol 1984; 10: 87–99
56. Shapiro AMJ, Lakey JRT, Ryan EA et al. N Engl J Med 2000; 343: 230–238
57. Gruessner A, Sutherland DER. In: Cecka, Terasaki (eds). Clinical Transplants. UCLA Tissue Typing Laboratory, Los Angeles, CA, USA, 1996: 47–67
58. Sollinger HW, Geffner SR. Surg Clin North Am 1994; 74: 1183–1195
59. Starzl TE. Experience in Hepatic Transplantation. WB Saunders, Philadelphia, 1969
60. Levy MF, Goldstein RM et al. Clin Transplant 1993; 14: 161–173

Table 8.2 Adult liver transplant indications in Europe, January 1988 to December 2001

Condition	Percentage of patients
Cirrhosis	59
Virus-related	25
Alcohol-related	18
Primary biliary cirrhosis	8
Cryptogenic	5
Autoimmune	2
Others	1
Cancer	11
Cholestatic diseases	11
Metabolic	6
Acute hepatic failure	9
Others*	4

*Budd–Chiari, benign tumours, polycystic liver disease, and parasitic infections.

Table 8.3 Indications for liver transplantation in children

	Aged 0–2 years (%)	Aged 2–15 years (%)
Cholestasis	74	45
Acute hepatic failure	10	14
Metabolic	9	24
Cirrhosis	3	9
Cancer	2	4

replacement, recurrent cancer is the rule rather than the exception and strict criteria are applied to this patient group. Patients are accepted on to the transplant list if the tumours are small and few, and are a secondary rather than a primary indication for the transplant. Cholangiocarcinoma is now viewed as a contraindication by most transplant groups because results have been disappointing. Acute hepatic failure accounts for about 10% of liver transplants and this relates to drug toxicity, acute hepatitis A or B, or seronegative hepatitis.

CHILDREN

By far the most important indication in children is following a failed correction of biliary atresia. This condition affects one per 8000 live births in western countries,[61] and although in a third of these children satisfactory biliary drainage can be achieved by a Kasai-type procedure,[62] for the most part advanced cirrhosis and decompensation will occur. Such children are best not treated by reintervention but should be urgently considered for hepatic replacement.

Children suffering from primary metabolic disorders or inborn errors of metabolism that do eventually lead to complete liver destruction are also considered for replacement when cirrhosis and portal hypertension develop or if there is a risk of the development of malignancy or systemic metabolic deterioration. Acute liver failure accounts for 10–15% of cases, and this is most commonly due to Wilson's disease and hepatitis A. Hepatoblastoma accounts for the majority of children undergoing liver transplantation for cancer, and chemotherapy is used in conjunction with the transplant (Table 8.3).

SURGICAL TECHNIQUE

Of all the organ transplant procedures currently undertaken, liver transplantation affords the most major technical problems. Not only is the liver a complex biochemical structure with multiple vascular anatomical relationships, but it also seems particularly susceptible to ischaemic damage.

Although up to 60 min of warm ischaemia can be tolerated in some clinical situations, this has rarely been associated with satisfactory function when a period of cold preservation is also required.[63] Therefore meticulous surgical technique in organ retrieval and preservation is required to ensure rapid cooling to below 48°C and, even so, implantation of the liver will normally be required in less than 14 h.

The recipient is prepared for the removal of the diseased liver and subsequent implantation (Fig. 8.6). This complex procedure may be undertaken using venous bypass from the lower inferior vena cava and portal vein to the superior cava to avoid diminished cardiac return during the phase at which the liver is being exchanged. Alternatively, caval preservation techniques can be used to avoid the need for bypass. This is particularly common in paediatric transplantation, where most grafts are partial liver transplants as a result of a split procedure.

POSTOPERATIVE MANAGEMENT

The grafted liver must function immediately, otherwise a consumptive coagulopathy will occur leading to death within 24 h from overwhelming haemorrhage. During this phase, while haemodynamic stability is being re-established, patients are normally ventilated with meticulous monitoring of cardiac output and renal function, and immunosuppression is started to diminish the risk of major hepatic rejection. However, protocols are changing constantly and in some units up to one-third of the patients are extubated as soon as the surgery is finished and hospital stays are reducing rapidly. Gastric and intestinal absorption of the newer forms of calcineurin inhibitor (Neoral cyclosporine and tacrolimus) recovers surprisingly rapidly and it is rare to use intravenous immunosuppressive agents today.

Diagnosis of hepatic rejection has proved difficult compared with that for other organs such as the kidney, and there is a heavy reliance on percutaneous liver biopsy. The patient may develop liver dysfunction because of a combination of reasons that include ischaemia, infection, biliary obstruction or cytomegalovirus infection, and these all need to be excluded before the diagnosis of rejection can be confirmed, usually on liver biopsy. In approximately 5% of patients the graft fails with progressive deterioration in function, and under these circumstances retransplantation may be the only hope of saving the patient.

RESULTS OF LIVER GRAFTING

As in any surgical endeavour, the results of liver transplantation will be largely dependent on the selection criteria. Patients in the

REFERENCES

61. Balistrei WF. J Pediatrics 1985; 106: 171
62. Kasai M. Prog Pediatr Surg 1974; 6: 53–62
63. Shaw BW, Gordon RD et al. Transplant Proc 1985; 17: 26

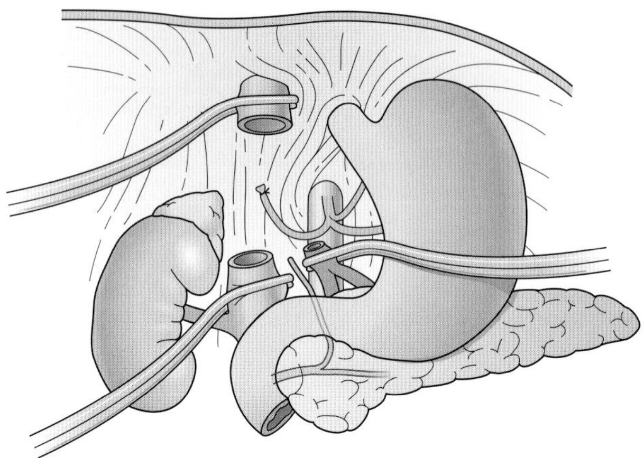

Figure 8.6 Recipient following hepatectomy.

final agonal stages of their disease can often not be offered liver replacement because of the high morbidity and mortality, but almost all adult patients below the age of 70 with terminal liver disease should be considered. Current results from Europe for patients transplanted since 1995 demonstrate an 83% 1-year survival, with 72% still alive and well after 5 years; for children these figures are 82% and 76%, respectively.[64,65]

Late acute and chronic rejection is relatively rare—10-year survival figures approximate to the 5-year survivals—and the long-term outlook for patients is continuing to improve. In the absence of transplantation, these patients' survival is usually measured in months.

REFERENCES

64. European FK506 Liver Study Group. Lancet 1994; 344: 423–428
65. Goldstein RM. Recent Developments in Transplant Medicine. Glerricine, Illinois, 1996

USEFUL WEBSITES

British Transplantation Society (http://www.bts.org.uk)
European Liver Transplant Registry (http://www.eltr.org)
North West Kidney Transplant Audit (http://www.nwkta.org)
UK Transplant Website (http://www.uktransplant.org.uk)
United Network for Organ Sharing (http://www.unos.org)

Principles of plastic surgery and skin tumours

9

David A. Ross, Catharine J. Milroy, Sarah L. Benyon

PRINCIPLES OF PLASTIC SURGERY

INTRODUCTION AND HISTORY

Plastic surgery deals principally with the restoration of structure and function that may be disrupted secondary to a range of causes. These include congenital and developmental abnormalities as well as correcting the impact of trauma or cancer.

This branch of surgery is ancient, and early descriptions date back to at least the sixth century BC. At that time, Susruta described nasal reconstruction using a cheek flap. Reconstruction of the nose was to form the backbone on which plastic surgery as a speciality was developed, culminating in Edward Zeiss coining the term *plastic surgery* to encapsulate the newly developed speciality in 1838.[1] Early nasal reconstruction largely dealt with post-traumatic defects, but with the introduction of anaesthesia extended to reconstruct defects secondary to syphilis and, with migration, to minimize racial stereotyping.

Plastic surgery had a further renaissance during the First World War, when the New Zealander Harold Gilles came to Britain and developed principles of modern plastic surgery.[2] The invention of the parachute just prior to the Second World War meant the survival of young pilots who had sustained horrific injuries by baling out of burning cockpits. Many of the most severely scarred patients were transferred to East Grinstead, where McIndoe further advanced the boundaries of reconstruction.[3] The 'guinea pig club' formed by the patients of McIndoe still meets at East Grinstead.

The scope of modern plastic surgery is extraordinarily varied. It encompasses management from before birth to palliative procedures prior to death that encompass the whole body. Congenital anomalies including cleft lip and palate, hypospadias and hand deformities are all part of plastic surgery. Burns and trauma surgery, particularly of the hand and lower limb, are also included in the remit of the plastic surgeon. An expanding part of plastic surgery includes oncoplastic reconstruction, emphasizing the multidisciplinary nature of contemporary surgical practice.

The application of recent research into anatomy and physiology has resulted in major advances in the speciality. These include the use of microvascular techniques to transfer tissues, sentinel node biopsy in melanoma, and negative-pressure wound care. This chapter describes the principles of plastic surgery and their application to more complex reconstructive problems as well as the diagnosis and management of skin pathology. The first section will discuss basic principles of plastic surgery and cite examples of their application. These techniques have also led to, and developed in tandem with, the evolution of aesthetic surgery.

PRINCIPLES OF SOFT TISSUE RECONSTRUCTION

Simple wounds can be closed by direct approximation and suturing. If an area of tissue has been removed or traumatically lost, skin elasticity and local undermining may permit direct closure. Time-honoured principles dictate how surgical wounds will heal.[4] Skin should never be closed under excessive tension because this will lead to necrosis of skin edge, resulting in infection and wound breakdown. Small defects up to 1.5 cm may be left to heal by second intention. Wound contracture and re-epithelialization across such a wound is speedy and the resultant scar may be minimal. However, for larger defects, scarring and deformity may be avoided only when closure is achieved by resurfacing the wound.

In such a situation, the plastic surgeon is required to assess the defect in terms of site, size, depth, and the involved tissue(s). Furthermore, for three-dimensional defects, such as the lip or pharynx, the defect needs to be considered in terms of cover, support and lining. A graft is any tissue—be it skin, nerve, vessel, bone or cartilage—that is transferred without a blood supply. Its survival therefore becomes dependent on its acquiring a blood supply from a healthy donor bed within a limited period of time. It follows that only limited-volume grafts can be transferred, and that they must be placed into or on to a healthy environment if they are to 'take'. Superficial, large defects may be resurfaced with a split-thickness skin graft. This tissue source is plentiful and commonly used to resurface areas of extensive skin loss. However, it is thin and prone to contraction that may compromise both function and cosmesis if placed on the face or over a joint.

Flaps are defined as tissue transferred with an intact blood supply. At their simplest they consist of local flaps taken from sites adjacent to the defect. Blood supply enters the base of the flap by a random pattern, allowing tissue to be advanced, rotated or transposed. Retaining an independent blood supply facilitates transfer into a potentially unhealthy area where a graft would not take, such as irradiated postmastectomy skin or an open tibial fracture. Axial pattern flaps are fed by an identifiable vessel.[5] This allows flaps to be islanded and rotated over a wide arc. Free flaps

REFERENCES

1. Taylor GI. The twenty-third Sir Harold Gillies memorial lecture. Keeping a head. Br J Plast Surg. 2002; 55: 543–560
2. Gilles H. Principles and Art of Plastic Surgery. Little, Brown, Boston, 1957.
3. McIndoe AH. Bradshaw lecture 1958. Br J Plast Surg 1983; 36: 410–420
4. Gibson T. Br J Plast Surg 1978; 31: 1–2
5. Cormack GC, Lamberty BGH. The Arterial Anatomy of Skin Flaps. 2nd edn. Churchill Livingstone, Edinburgh, 1994: 16–19

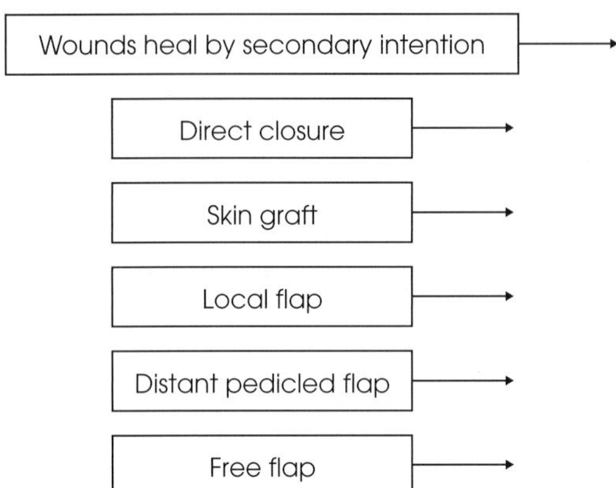

Figure 9.1 The reconstructive ladder.

consist of axial pattern flaps, the vascular pedicle of which has been divided and reanastomosed (usually using microvascular techniques) to vessels at the recipient site. This separation of transferable tissue has been classified as the reconstructive ladder.

RECONSTRUCTIVE LADDER

The above description outlined the concept of a reconstructive ladder (Fig. 9.1) that has evolved to provide the surgeon with various reconstructive options. Several techniques may be available to provide cover in a particular situation. However, technique selection is dependent on several factors, including the patient's health; available surgical experience; microsurgical facilities; and the desired optimum structural, functional and cosmetic outcome. Consequently, a particular reconstructive technique is chosen only after considering the patient's health, nutritional status and fitness for surgery. The chosen method should combine the simplest procedure that provides the optimum functional and aesthetic result with the minimum donor site morbidity and risk to the patient.

SKIN GRAFTS

Skin grafting was first reported in the early 1800s and Reverdin in Paris described use of skin grafts in 1869.[6] Skin grafts may be classified as split skin or full thickness depending on the thickness of dermis transferred. Split-skin grafts heal quickly and reliably, and they can be used to cover large areas of defect. They leave donor sites that re-epithelialize over within 2–3 weeks depending on the thickness of repopulating dermis. Split-thickness grafts are poorly resistant to trauma and tend to contract with time. Full-thickness grafts produce superior-quality wounds and are less prone to contraction. However, they are limited in quantity because the donor site must be closed directly. They are commonly used to resurface defects on the face.

A skin graft consists of epidermis and varying thickness of dermis detached from its blood supply. Vascularity must be quickly acquired from the new bed, and for this reason skin grafts will not survive where the underlying tissue perfusion is inadequate, as in scarred tissues or following radiotherapy. Similarly, graft take will be poor in patients with arteriopathy or severe diabetes. Grafts will not survive on bone denuded of periosteum or on tendon without paratenon. Skin grafts may not survive in the presence of infection, particularly β-haemolytic streptococci.[7]

Skin graft harvest and the donor site

Split-skin grafts can be harvested using a variety of hand knives (Fig. 9.2) or dermatomes. Humby introduced guarded skin graft knives to make harvesting sheets of skin grafts easier, and this was further improved with the introduction of mechanical dermatomes. The most common hand-held skin graft knives are the Watson and Braithwaite modifications of the Humby knife. Electric dermatomes are increasingly used because they facilitate harvesting of uniform-thickness grafts that leave superior donor scars.

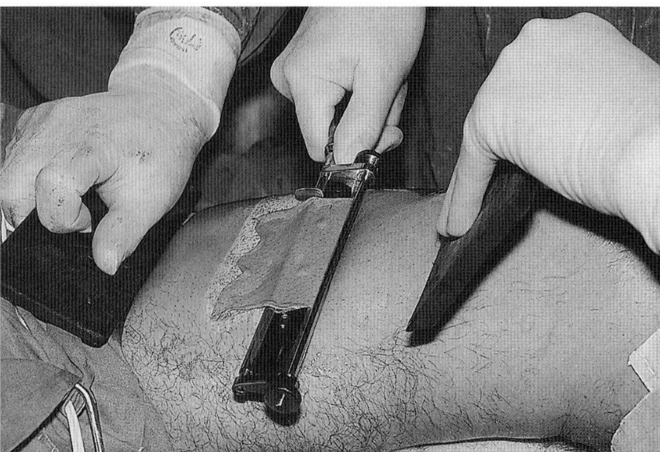

Figure 9.2 A skin graft being taken with a hand knife.

Advances in grafting techniques include meshing sheets of graft to increase the potential area of coverage and allow egress of excess fluid (Fig. 9.3). Other developments have included the improvement of shear-free dressings, such as sponge and staples, as opposed to the traditional proflavine wool tie-over. Research is focusing on artificial graft equivalents to obviate the need for the donor site.

The choice of the donor site depends on the size of the area to be resurfaced and aesthetic considerations of both the recipient and donor site. Following extensive burns, where a large area of skin has to be resurfaced, available donor sites including the scalp and the sole of the foot may be harvested. In general, a site is selected that can be readily concealed, such as the most common donor site of the upper lateral thigh. Elderly skin tends to be thin, and the best donor sites are the lateral thigh or back because the dermis remains thickest. However, donor sites in the elderly are prone to breakdown and prolonged healing difficulties. Efforts to heal resistant sites include further grafting, keratinocyte culture, and reapplication of 1:6 meshed skin to the donor site. Accordingly, for smaller defects in older patients, it is reasonable to avoid using split-skin grafts and to take a full-thickness graft from the upper arm, closing the donor site directly.

Full-thickness skin grafts are harvested using a knife, and the donor site closed directly. The best colour and texture match is obtained if skin graft is taken from a site adjacent to the defect. This is particularly true for full-thickness grafts to the face; common donor sites include pre- and postauricular skin, where the scar can be hidden.

Initially, skin grafts appear pale but they revascularize to a 'blanchable' blush over 3–4 days. A thick split graft taken from the thigh is always a poor colour and texture match for the face, whereas full-thickness postauricular Wolfe grafts provide an

REFERENCES

6. Reverdin JL. Bull Soc Imperiale Chir Paris 1869; 10
7. Medawar PB. J Anat 1944; 78: 157

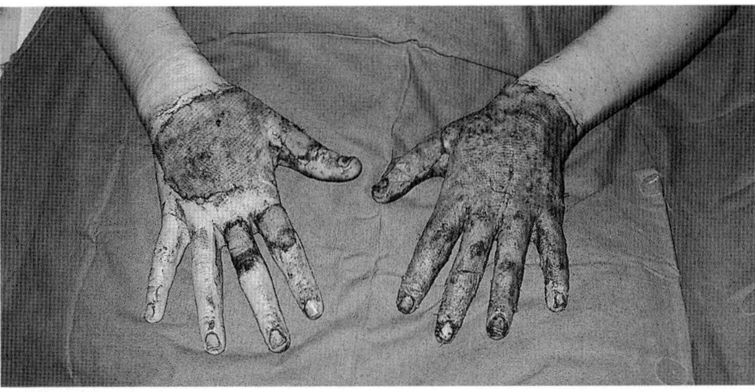

a

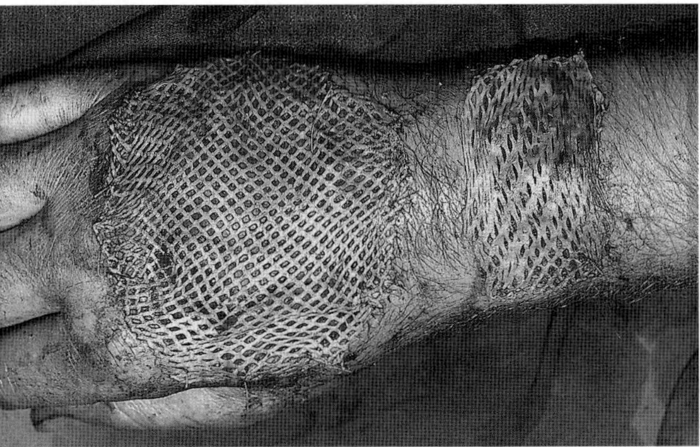

b

Figure 9.3 (**a**) Skin grafts on the dorsum of both hands; (**b**) a meshed skin graft on the dorsum of the hand. Courtesy of Mr A Phipps.

excellent match for the cheek and lower eyelid. The choice of skin graft and donor site therefore depend on aesthetic and functional considerations as well as the size of the area to be covered and the state of the recipient bed.

Skin grafts contract after harvesting (primary contracture) and then again after insetting (secondary contracture). Thin grafts contract more than thick ones, but the mechanisms by which the dermis appears to inhibit the normal wound contractile process are unclear. Thick full-thickness skin grafts die after 3–4 days in storage, whereas thin split-thickness skin grafts may take on a well-vascularized bed up to 14 days after storage.

Meshing and dressing

A graft must be immobile to allow a circulation to become established. Shear forces will prevent take and must be prevented by careful suturing and appropriate dressing. The most common cause of graft failure is build-up of haematoma beneath the skin graft, because this also separates it from the underlying bed. The skin graft can either be held in place with a dressing of sponge or gauze sutured or stapled down to the wound edges, or it can be left exposed. Donor sites heal by epithelialization from pilosebaceous units, and to a lesser extent from sweat glands. Thin skin grafts leave more adnexal structures, allowing faster healing. In a thin split-skin graft, the donor site can be expected to heal in 7–10 days, whereas a thicker graft may take up to 3 weeks. Modern dressing materials promote quicker healing with less discomfort. Alginate dressings were traditionally used, but more recently the raw area has been found to heal more quickly and less painfully if simple adherent dressings such as Mefix are applied directly to the wound.

Skin graft take is a complex process. On a healthy recipient site, the graft rapidly adheres by fibrin formed from extravasated plasma fibrinogen and derives nutrients from the underlying bed. This is known as imbibition.[8] After approximately 48 h, imbibition is superseded by reconnection of blood supply from the bed to vessel remnants within the graft: a process known as vascular inosculation. Full incorporation of the graft requires these processes to occur in parallel with neovascularization.

Imbibition of plasma, drawn up into the capillary bed of the graft, sustains the graft until new capillary in-growth occurs, which is a function of the vascularity and perfusion of the recipient bed. In the first few days after grafting there is great epithelial activity with an increased mitotic rate. The epithelial thickness rapidly increases and desquamation occurs. This process is less florid in full-thickness grafts.[7] Ribonucleic acid content and enzymatic activity also increase after about 4 days, paralleling these epithelial events. The dermal component does not regenerate, and fibroblasts seen in skin graft biopsies are thought to migrate into the graft after the third day. Collagen turnover approaches normal levels at 10–14 days, with 85% being replaced after 5 months—a turnover rate double that of normal skin. Elastin fibres have also regenerated at about 1 month, after initial breakdown. A fine neovasculature connects the graft to capillary buds in the bed by 48 h. This may be by new in-growth of independent vessels or by revascularization of graft vessels.[9] Lymphatic patency is established by the sixth day after grafting. Sensation also returns, with good two-point discrimination as nerves enter the graft from the edge and bed of the recipient site, but full recovery may take months or years.

Meshing of grafts is achieved by passing them through a roller that makes multiple symmetrical perforations. Meshing allows the graft to expand and cover a larger area than would be possible with an unmeshed sheet graft, thus conserving donor site.[10] Expansion of the meshed graft depends on the size of the hole; in large burns a wide mesh is used to facilitate coverage of the largest possible area. Meshing also allows any serum or haematoma to escape through the interstices, reducing graft separation. A major disadvantage of meshed skin grafts is that the final scar appearance is patterned, because the interstices heal by epithelialization alone and contain no dermis. Meshing can be low or high ratio. A 1:1.5 mesh allows fluid drainage but minimizes cosmetic problems; 1:6 meshing produces a very delicate mesh used in large-percentage burns or to over-graft donor sites.[11] This ratio can leave a chequer-board appearance after healing but uses a minimum of skin.

Artificial dermis and cultured epidermis

Intensive effort has been made to find a substitute for autologous skin grafts.[12] This is important, first to reduce donor site problems and second to improve the quality and reliability of grafts. Donor sites are not just cosmetic problems: in situations such as large-percentage burns they simply may not be available.

Both porcine and cadaver skin have long been used as alternatives, but they are temporary and have lost favour due to

REFERENCES

8. Ollier L. Bull Acad Med 1872; 1: 243
9. Converse JM et al. Br J Plast Surg 1975; 28: 274
10. Davison PM, Batchelor AG, Lewis Smith PA. Br J Plast Surg 1986; 39: 462
11. Rees TD, Casson PR. Plast Reconstr Surg 1966; 38: 522
12. Phipps AR, Clarke JA. Br J Plast Surg 1991; 44: 608–611

theoretical problems with disease transmission. Artificial dermis has been developed to address this problem. Collagen constructs can be placed on infection-free vascular beds and allow organized in-growth of host blood vessels. After 2 weeks, sheets of cultured keratinocytes harvested from the tiny areas of host and expanded in vitro can be supported by this newly vascularized bed. The artificial dermis is less robust in resisting infection and requires a more vascular bed than that needed by autogenous skin. The advantage of this technique is that large areas can be grafted without the need for donor sites, and cosmetic results are closer to those of full-thickness grafts rather than thin split-skin grafts.

OTHER TISSUE GRAFTS

Theoretically, any tissue may be grafted to a healthy vascular bed that can supply it with nutrient vessels.[13] Both allografts (same species) and xenografts (different species) have been used but will be rejected by the host immune system within a short space of time.

Bone graft

Bone grafts may be cortical or cancellous. Cortical bone grafts are usually harvested from the iliac crest and should be less than 5 cm if they are to survive. Partial resorption may occur, and long-term bony support in larger defects may require a vascularized bone flap. Cancellous bone can be harvested from the iliac crest but if required in only small amounts, as in hand fractures, can be obtained following osteotomy of Lister's tubercle on the radius.

Nerve graft

Small essential nerves such as the digital nerves are often irredeemably damaged or partially avulsed.[13] Small gaps can be closed with mobilization of the nerve and suture under gentle stretch. Longer gaps must be grafted using less important nerves such as superficial cutaneous nerves of the forearm. Mixed nerve defects such as the median nerve can be bridged by cable grafts. Cable grafting uses several lengths of the same donor nerve sutured in parallel to match the diameter of the nerve. The best source is the sural nerve in the leg. The donor deficit is minimal: a small numb area on the lateral aspect of the foot and several transverse lacerations on the calf. Nerves regenerate after repair at a rate of 1 mm/day, so patients should be warned that postoperative return of function may take many months.

Composite grafts

Composite grafts consist of combinations of tissue types, such as skin and cartilage. Success demands good vascularity and a small defect. Composite grafts harvested from the helical rim of the ear are used to reconstruct alar defects. Another application includes repair of amputated fingertips in young children. The amputated part needs to be in good condition, not crushed, and distal to the nail fold. The part should be preserved as in a potential transplant and wrapped in saline-soaked gauze in a container of ice water. Results of surgery are best in the first few hours after severance, with limited success after 6 h.

FLAPS

DEFINITION AND DEVELOPMENT

In areas of relatively low vascularity, such as bare tendon or bone, a graft will not survive. If tissue is to survive it must bring with it its own blood supply. A flap comprises tissue transferred from one region to another while maintaining a continuous blood supply through a vascular pedicle. This blood supply may consist of small subdermal capillaries, as in *random* pattern, local flaps (Fig. 9.4). Alternatively, larger, more complex *axial* pattern flaps (Fig. 9.4) may be transferred, dependent on an identifiable vascular pedicle.

Composite flaps comprise a combination of tissue types, usually skin muscle and/or bone. They are thus superior to simple grafts in situations where the defect bed is potentially unhealthy due to extensive trauma and bruising, subclinical osteomyelitis or radiotherapy. In addition, replacing the lost tissue of the defect with similar tissue from the donor site allows improved function and cosmesis.

The disadvantage of flaps is that there is often a more significant donor defect than that in skin grafting. Much research in plastic surgery has been aimed towards minimizing donor defects.

The two biggest advances in plastic and reconstructive surgery this past century have been:

- the identification of regional blood supply of skin, and
- the realization that tissue supplied by specific vessels can be disconnected and revascularized elsewhere.

Until the early 1970s, most skin flaps were raised on a random blood supply with no specific artery and vein within the flap.[14] The general rule was that these random pattern flaps should be raised with a length-to-width ratio of 1:1, because longer flaps did not have a reliable circulation, except in the well-vascularized areas of the head and neck. This ratio was largely abandoned with the concept of axial pattern flaps.[15] Anatomists and surgeons had independently described the segmental nature of the blood supply of the skin in the late 1800s, but it was not until 1973 that the distinction between random and axial pattern flaps became appreciated.

All areas of the integument have a segmental blood supply from perforating vessels that enter through the deep fascia, where this is present, from the underlying muscle or intermuscular septum. The understanding of this led to a rapid increase in the discovery of cutaneous axial pattern flaps and composite musculocutaneous, fasciocutaneous and bony composite flaps.[2]

Most early axial pattern flaps were purely cutaneous and had an intact skin bridge. The tube pedicle was the chief tool of reconstructive surgery from its invention, but it is now largely of historical interest only.[16] It was soon apparent that this type of flap could survive isolated on the vessels alone as an island of skin, which made the flap more mobile. The development of microvascular surgery allowed free flaps to be transferred with immediate anastomosis to vessels at the recipient site (Table 9.1).[17]

CLASSIFICATION OF FLAPS

Flaps are defined as tissue brought into an area with its own blood supply, and they can be classified according to their vascular anatomy and the method of transfer or composition. All flaps are

REFERENCES

13. McCarthy J (ed). Plastic Surgery, Vol 1. WB Saunders, London, 1990: 630–697
14. Milton SH. Br J Surg 1970; 57: 502
15. McGregor IA, Morgan G. Br J Plast Surg 1973; 26: 202
16. Gillies HD. NY Med J 1920; 3: 1
17. Hodges PL. Sel Read Plast Surg 1992; 7: 1–31

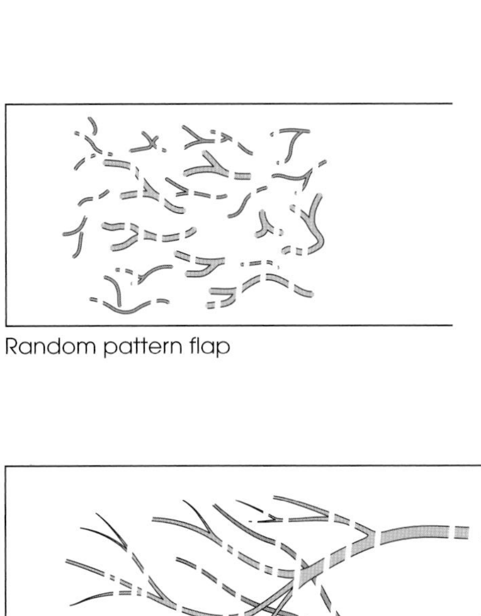

Random pattern flap

Cutaneous axial pedicle

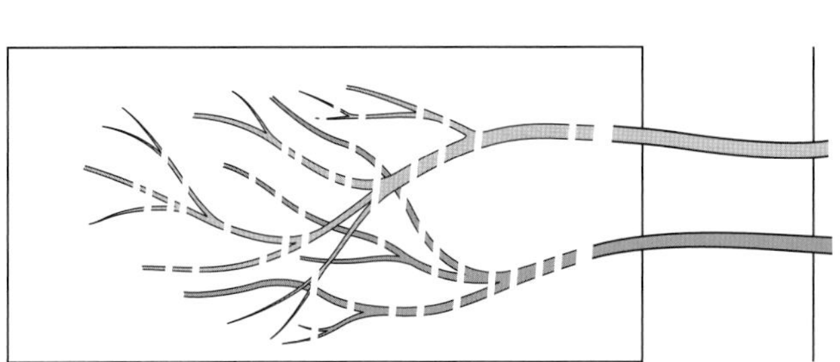

Cutaneous axial island

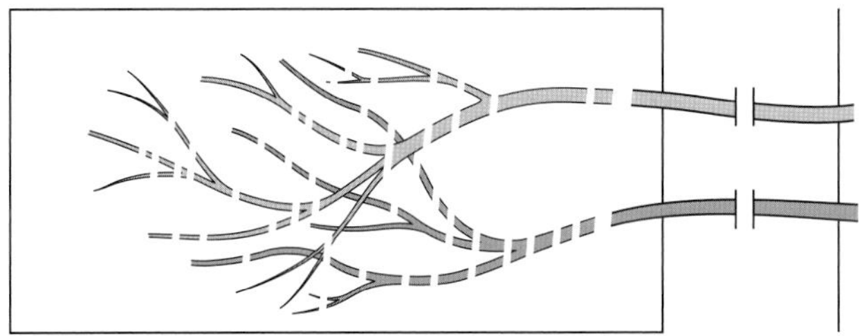

Cutaneous axial free

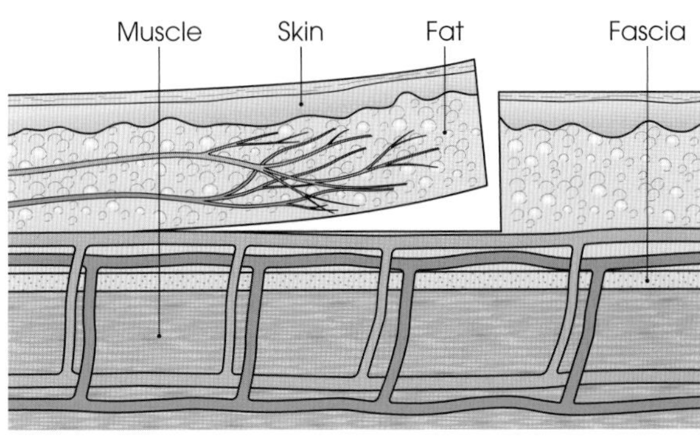

Axial cutaneous

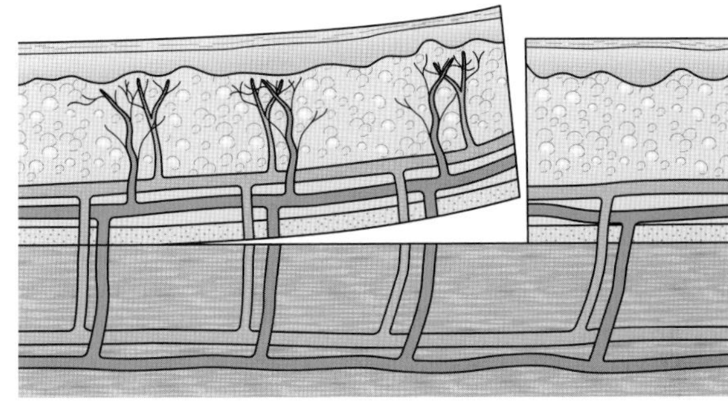

Fasciocutaneous flap

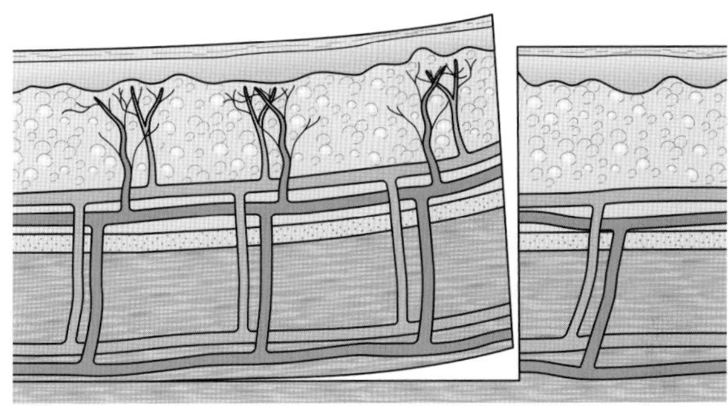

Myocutaneous flap

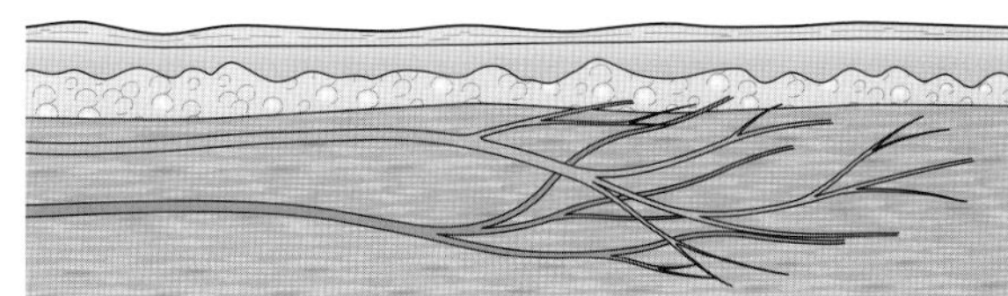

Muscle flap with skin graft

Figure 9.4 Random and axial flaps. Random flaps have a random vascular supply based on the subdermal vascular plexus. Axial flaps have a known vascular supply based on a named artery and vein; this makes them safer and more versatile. Depending on the blood supply to the skin, axial flaps may be raised as skin and fat only; skin, fat and fascia; or skin, fat, fascia and muscle. They may also be fascia or muscle only, which can then be grafted.

random or axial, local or distant, and they can contain any tissue that is capable of transfer, including omentum and bowel. Flaps can be described by their site of origin, shape, method of transfer, blood supply or tissue content. Random pattern flaps are not supplied by a specific artery and are limited in size. Tissues supplied by an identified vessel are known as axial flaps and may be much larger. Axial flaps can be pedicled, islanded, or transferred free with a microvascular anastomosis. Flaps may also contain nerves, tendons or even joints. This allows the surgeon to tailor a flap to suit the requirements of the reconstruction, for example reconstruction of the ramus of the mandible with skin cover and intraoral lining produced by a single flap.

INDICATIONS FOR FLAP RECONSTRUCTION

Flaps are used in situations where grafts will not take, or where the aim is to reconstruct with tissue that is like for like (bone, joint, tendon, nerve, epithelial lining, etc.) and that provides optimal structure, function and cosmesis. Flaps are also used to

Table 9.1 Milestones in the modern evolution of surgical flaps

Date	Surgeon(s)	Milestone(s)
1814	Carpue	Forehead flap rhinoplasty, pedicled random pattern flaps
1818	von Graefe	
Late 19th century, early 20th century	Mutter, Gersuny, Trotter, Volkmann, Deiffenbach, Morax, Syndacker	Random pattern cutaneous flaps
1906	Tansini	Latissimus dorsi muscle flap for breast reconstruction
1907	Syndacker	Platysma flaps
1908	Morax	
1917	Filatov, Ganser, Gillies, Aymard	First tube pedicled flaps, observations of the value of delay
1919	Davis	Observations on pedicled flaps, review of Manchot's work describing vascular territories
1921	Blair	Delay phenomenon in non-pedicled flaps
1936	Salmon	Arterial anatomy of skin flaps (long unrecognized thereafter)
1942	Converse	Median forehead flap
1946	Kazanjian	
1946	Shaw and Payne	Hypogastric flap (tubed)
1950s and 1960s	Conley, DesPrez, Egerton, Wilson, Wookey, Zovikian	Empiric development of head and neck flaps and trunk flaps
1955	Owens	Compound sternomastoid skin flap
1963	Bakamjian	Deltopectoral flap
1963	Goldwyn and colleagues	First experimental free tissue transfer
1963	(In Shanghai, China)	Successfully replanted hand (Chen 1982)
1965	Komatsu and Tamai	First complete thumb replant
1967	Wilson	Arterial anatomy and angiotomes
1967	Cobbett	First toe–thumb transfer
1968	Ger	Muscle flaps rediscovered
1970s	McCraw, Furlow, Vasconez, Mathes, Nahai, Maxwell, Orticochea, Serafin (Atlanta, Georgia, USA)	Muscle and musculocutaneous local and free flaps
1971	Antia and Bush	First English literature reports of human free tissue transfer
1972	McLean and Buncke, Harii and coworkers	
1973	Taylor and Daniel, O'Brien	
1972	McGregor and Jackson	Groin flap
1973	McGregor and Morgan	Formalization of axial and random pattern flaps, arterial anatomical territories and importance of 'dynamic' arterial territories
1973	Behan and Wilson	Angiotomes and 'prop' arteries defined
1976	Radovan	Expanded flaps
1981	Ponten	Fasciocutaneous flaps
1987	Taylor and Palmer	Angiosomes

(After Cormack and Lamberty 1994,[5] and Hodges 1992.[17])

import a blood supply to areas of doubtful viability, such as in the reconstruction of pressure sores or after complex trauma.

Often several flap options may exist for a given defect. The choice of flap will depend on patient factors as well as the surgeon's technical experience and allied support. Donor site morbidity is also an important consideration when planning surgery. The free radial forearm flap is often used for intraoral reconstruction in head and neck cancer, but it can leave an unsightly donor site defect. Other options include the anterior thigh flap, which leaves a more acceptable straight-line donor scar on the thigh.

LOCAL FLAPS

Local flaps lie adjacent to the defect and depend on local tissue laxity to allow donor closure. The flap may be moved into the wound by several methods as described below.

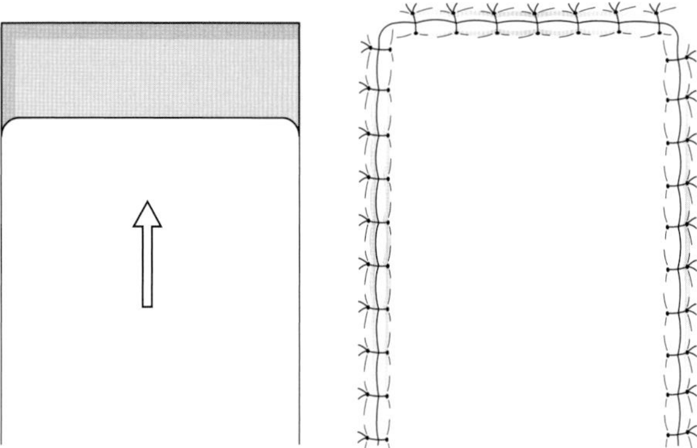

Figure 9.5 An advancement flap.

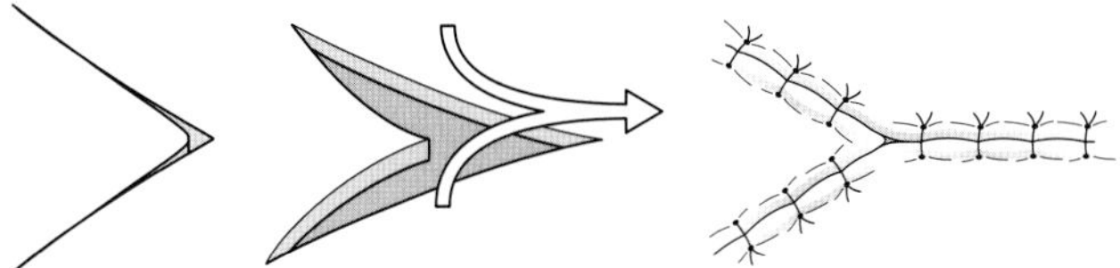

Figure 9.6 A V–Y advancement flap.

Advancement

Advancement (Fig. 9.5) is the simplest type of flap. The skin is undermined and advanced to cover the defect. Direct closure of an elliptical defect is, in effect, the advancement of opposing flaps to allow the skin edges to be primarily sutured.

V–Y flaps

V–Y flaps (Fig. 9.6) are advancement flaps that mobilize skin on a subdermal pedicle containing blood vessels. The skin is mobilized by selective undermining and is retained in its new position by careful suturing to take up the tension. The donor site is directly closed.

Z plasty

Z plasty (Fig. 9.7) is a method of readjusting the length or orientation of a scar to improve aesthetics.

Transposition

A flap of skin is transposed to cover an adjacent defect, leaving a secondary defect (Fig. 9.8). The pivot point of the flap is the base of the flap furthest from the defect and dictates the distance the flap will reach. A Z plasty is a type of transposition flap.

Bilobed

The bilobed flap (Fig. 9.9) is a transposition flap where a secondary, smaller flap is also raised to fill the primary donor defect and the secondary donor defect is directly closed.

Rhomboid

The defect is designed (excised) in a rhomboid shape, and an equivalent rhomboid of adjacent skin is transposed to cover it, such that it is possible to close the secondary defect in the direction of greatest skin laxity (Fig. 9.10). There are four possible geometric flaps for each defect, although only two optimal clinical choices to place the resultant scar in relaxed skin tension lines.[18]

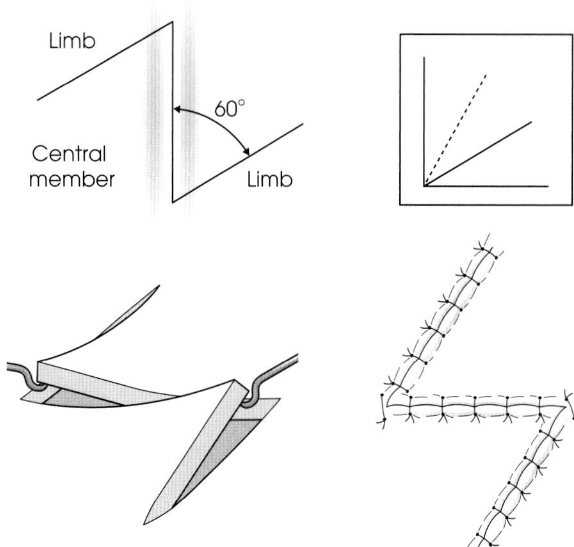

Figure 9.7 A Z plasty for taking the stress off a scar.

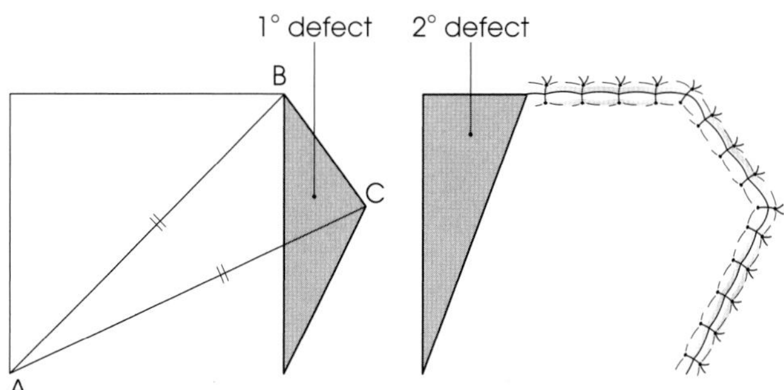

Figure 9.8 A transposition flap.

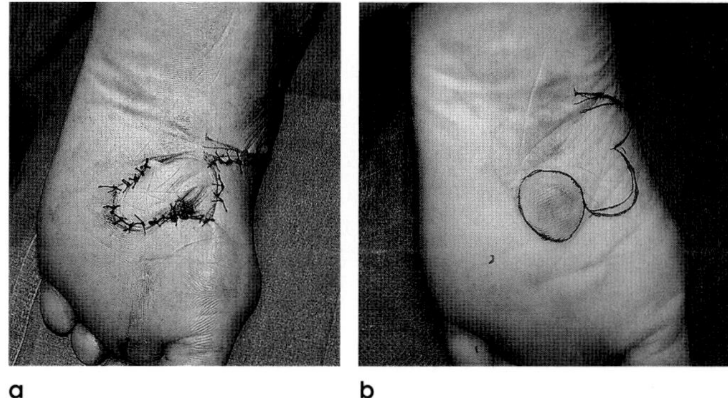

Figure 9.9 A bilobed flap used to resurface a defect on the sole of the foot.

Rotation

A semicircle of skin is rotated to fill an adjacent defect, usually allowing primary closure of the donor defect (Fig. 9.11).[19]

Many flaps combine elements of transposition and rotation. Local skin flaps are particularly useful in the head, face and neck, where there is a greater capillary density in the dermis.

REFERENCES

18. Borges AF. Plast Reconstr Surg 1978; 62: 542–548
19. Pasyk KA et al. Plast Reconstr Surg 1989; 83: 939

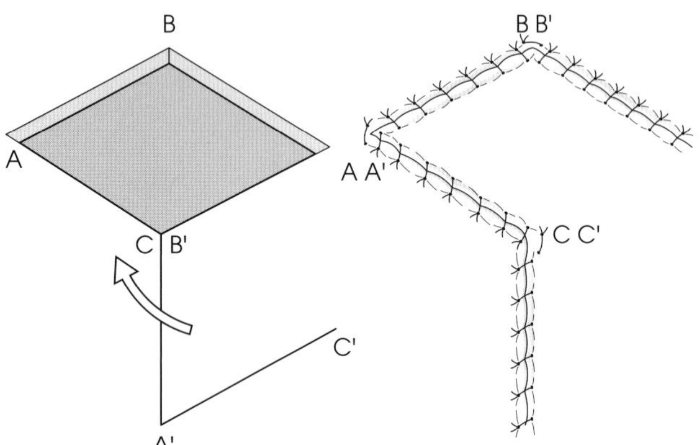

Figure 9.10 A rhomboid flap.

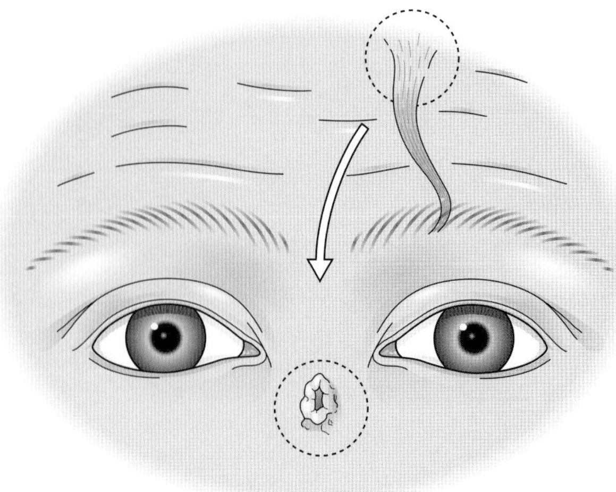

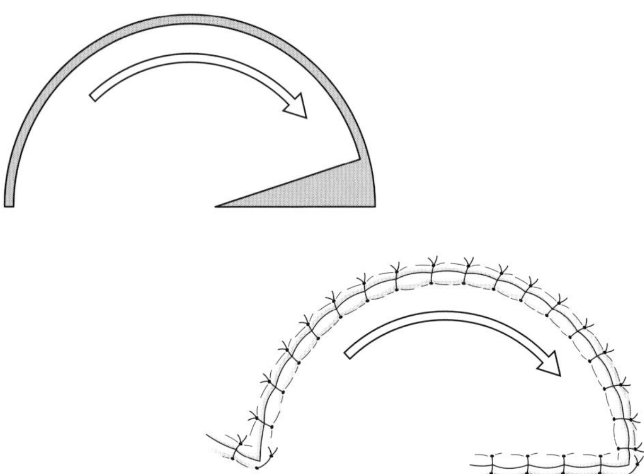

Figure 9.11 A rotation flap.

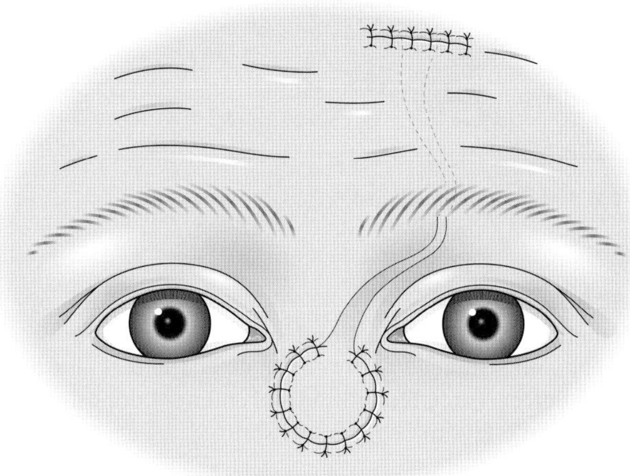

Figure 9.12 An island flap.

DISTANT FLAPS

Distant flaps do not rely on local laxity. They thus have the scope to cover larger defects and also to introduce healthy, well-vascularized tissue into regions that may be damaged by trauma, infection or irradiation, and so contribute to healing.

Pedicled flaps can be islanded, where the skin paddle is entirely isolated except for the vascular pedicle, allowing greater mobility (Fig. 9.12). A *free flap* is a term used to describe transfer of a flap where the pedicle is divided from its origin and anastomosed to a new pedicle at a distant site (Fig. 9.13).

PEDICLED AXIAL PATTERN SKIN FLAPS

Pedicled axial pattern skin flaps (Table 9.2) are based on arteries and accompanying veins that run in the subcutaneous fat, superficial to the deep fascia and parallel to the skin surface. Such end arteries are confined to certain areas of the anatomy, and they are not connected deeply by perforators to the fascial or muscular systems, allowing large mobile skin islands to be raised on them. The territories that they easily perfuse, based on cadaveric injection studies, are termed their *anatomic territories*.

In addition to the arterial territories predicted by cadaveric perfusion studies, each artery has a dynamic territory that it will perfuse through collateral vessels if their perfusion pressure from an alternative source falls. This dynamic territory can be exploited by ligating a neighbouring high-pressure trunk. An example is the forehead flap based on the superficial temporal artery; this can perfuse the territories of the ligated ipsilateral and contralateral supraorbital and supratrochlear arteries as well as the contralateral superficial temporal to provide a much larger flap.

A further potential territory is also available. This is most easily demonstrated by clinical experience and cannot be plotted by knowledge of anatomy alone. The potential territory consists of the area supplied by both the anatomic and dynamic territories, plus a variable area of tissue beyond, perfused by vessels of a random pattern.

PEDICLED AXIAL PATTERN MUSCULOCUTANEOUS FLAPS

Pedicled axial pattern musculocutaneous flaps are composite flaps containing skin, subcutaneous fat, fascia and muscle based on one or more perforating branches to the skin from vessels primarily supplying muscle. Perforating vessels pierce the deep fascia and ramify in the subcutaneous tissues. Musculocutaneous flaps were described in the literature as early as 1906, and isolated descriptions appeared intermittently in the literature. More recently, Ger rediscovered their potential and described the use of muscle flaps with skin grafts to cover difficult lower limb defects and pressure sores.[20]

REFERENCE

20. Ger R. Surgery 1968; 63: 757

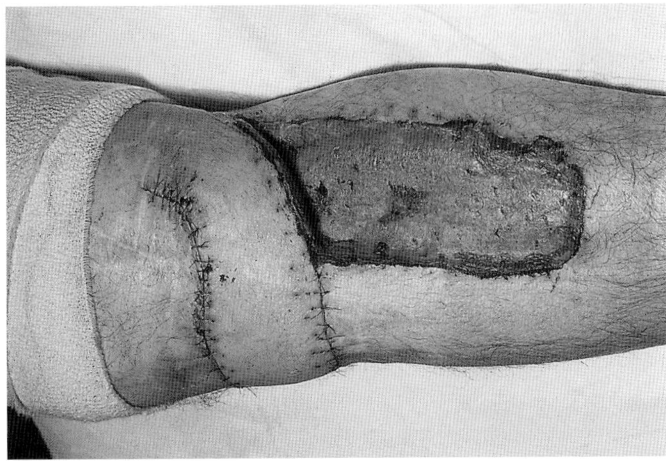

Figure 9.13 A fasciocutaneous flap used to cover a defect of the upper tibia.

Table 9.2 Axial pattern flaps and the vessels on which they are based

Direct cutaneous vessel	Clinical surgical flap
Superficial temporal artery	Forehead flap
Supratrochlear and supraorbital artery	Median forehead flap
Posterior auricular artery	Postauricular flap
Internal thoracic artery (second or third intercostal perforators)	Deltopectoral flap
Superficial circumflex iliac artery	Groin flap
Superficial inferior epigastric artery	Hypogastric flap
Dorsalis pedis artery	Dorsalis pedis flap

The present array of musculocutaneous flaps was mostly described in the 1970s following understanding of the axial flap principle. All or part of the muscle may be detached from its origin, its insertion, or both, and transferred with a paddle of overlying skin as a local, distant or free flap. The blood supply to the muscles of the body varies, making some muscles more suitable than others for use as musculocutaneous or muscle flaps, but there are few, if any, muscles that have not been used in reconstructive surgery.[21]

Increasing anatomical knowledge has allowed selective raising of muscle flaps to leave innervated, perfused muscle bellies behind to minimize donor deficit (e.g. the latissimus dorsi flap) or include them in the flap (e.g. the neurovascular gracilis for facial reanimation surgery). Similarly, combination muscle flaps may be raised together (e.g. the latissimus dorsi with the serratus anterior or the tensor fasciae latae with gluteus medius). Muscle flaps are useful to fill dead space with well-vascularized tissue and to provide the possibility of motor function.

It is important to know whether the muscle is to be raised with skin, and the quantity and mobility of the available skin paddle. Skin can be valuable postoperatively to monitor perfusion of the whole composite flap by its capillary refill, but it is not essential and other flap monitoring (such as laser fluorescence) is increasingly available.

FASCIOCUTANEOUS AND ADIPOFASCIAL PERFORATOR FLAPS

Although the value of taking the deep fascia with a skin flap to improve its blood supply had been suggested in 1920, the role of fascial perforating blood vessels in enhancing the surviving length of skin flaps was not appreciated until 1981.[22] Fascial, adipofascial and fasciocutaneous flaps have less bulk than equivalent musculocutaneous flaps, which is advantageous in certain situations (e.g. inside the mouth or on the dorsum of the hand).

The fasciocutaneous system incorporates vessels passing to the skin along fascial septa, between (rather than through) muscle bellies, to fan out in the deep fascial plexus—predominantly its superficial surface. These plexuses in turn send superficial branches to the skin, thus allowing the fascia to be raised as an adipofascial or fasciocutaneous flap. Initial length-to-breadth ratios of 2.5:1 were achieved in the notoriously difficult area below the knee, dramatically improving choice in the management of both upper and lower limb defects.

MICROVASCULAR SURGERY AND FREE TISSUE TRANSFER (Box 9.1)

An operating microscope has been used in otolaryngology and ophthalmology for decades, but after the pioneering work of Carel, who described triangulation of the vessel ends,[23] and Guthrie in the early 1900s,[24] microvascular and microneural surgery did not resume until the 1960s. Successful replantation of severed limbs and digits were followed in 1969 at East Grinstead by the first elective transfer of a toe to replace an amputated thumb.[25] Improving equipment and techniques coincided with the recognition of axial pattern flaps, and the first successful free skin flap transfer from the groin occurred in 1973.[26]

Initially, free flap transfer was considered a complex and time-consuming procedure, used only where other methods were not available and often occupying a whole day in the operating theatre. Free flaps were felt to be less reliable than conventional flaps, and a great deal of time and ingenuity were put into devices that monitored the flap postoperatively to allow early intervention in case of failure. Increasing experience has demonstrated that microvascular transfer of flaps need take little longer than conventional transfer, and that flap survival is often better than conventional pedicle transfer. Accordingly, free flaps are now routinely used in reconstructive surgery.

Free flap transfers have several advantages over conventional flaps, often making them the procedure of choice in quite simple situations. Microvascular transfer of a flap allows the flap to be exactly tailored to fit the size and position of the defect, without the constraints of a pedicle. It allows a single-stage reconstruction that can dramatically shorten hospital stay, negating the cost of increased operating time. A wide choice of possible donor sites allow the surgeon to use an appropriate flap for a better aesthetic result, often with the minimum donor defect. A free flap may bring in an improved blood supply to an unhealthy or ischaemic

REFERENCES

21. Mathes SJ, Nahai F. Plast Reconstr Surg 1981; 67: 177–187
22. Ponten B. Br J Plast Surg 1981; 34: 215
23. Carel A. Lyon Med 1902; 98: 859
24. Guthrie C. Blood Vessel Surgery and its Application. University of Pittsburgh Press, Pittsburgh, 1912
25. Cobbett JR. J Bone Joint Surg 1969; 51: 677–699
26. Daniel RK, Taylor GI. Plast Reconstr Surg 1973; 52: 111–117

Box 9.1 Commonly used flaps

Cutaneous and fasciocutaneous flaps
- Scalp, forehead
- Temporal fascia
- Supraclavicular
- Deltopectoral
- Scapular, parascapular
- Deltoid
- Axillary
- Lateral arm
- Medial arm
- Radial forearm (Chinese)
- Ulnar forearm
- Groin, hypogastric
- Medial thigh
- Anterior thigh
- Lateral thigh
- Posterior thigh
- Anterior tibial
- Posterior tibial
- Saphenous
- Sural
- Dorsalis pedis
- Sole of foot

Muscle and myocutaneous flaps
- Trapezius
- Pectoralis major
- Pectoralis minor
- Serratus anterior
- Latissimus dorsi
- External oblique
- Internal oblique
- Superior rectus abdominis
- Inferior rectus abdominis
- Superior gluteus maximus
- Inferior gluteus maximus
- Gracilis
- Tensor fasciae latae
- Rectus femoris
- Gastrocnemius

Specialized parts and organs
- Bones
- Rib: alone, with serratus anterior, with latissimus dorsi
- Sternum with pectoralis major
- Humerus with lateral arm
- Scapula with trapezius (spine) or scapular flap (medial border)
- Radius with radial forearm
- Radius with ulnar forearm
- Iliac crest with groin flap
- Fibula with or without skin
- Toe transfers
- Pulp transfers
- Nail bed transfers
- Joint transfers
- Vascularized nerve
- Testes
- Small bowel
- Large bowel
- Omentum

area (e.g. irradiated tissues). Free flaps have a high success rate and can be moved to almost any area of the body.

POSTOPERATIVE CARE

The vascular anastomosis is extremely vulnerable in the first 48 h following surgery and is most susceptible to revision at this time. During this period patients are usually nursed in a high-dependency unit and kept warm, well hydrated and pain-free. These measures are introduced to maintain peripheral perfusion and thus aid flow through the anastomosis into the flap. Observations are made of the urine output, core temperature and blood pressure. Some surgeons use anticoagulants such as dextran or heparin to counter the tendency for platelet aggregation around the anastomosis, but there is little evidence that this improves revision rate.

A healthy free flap should be pink, show normal refilling of the capillaries on digital pressure, have a nominal tissue tension, be at the same temperature as the adjacent tissues, and show normal bleeding in response to a pinprick. Venous failure initially produces a very pink flap with rapid capillary refilling, marked swelling and congestion. The colour will progress to a mottled then purple discoloration indicating immediate surgical exploration of the anastomosis. Experienced flap observation is essential in the first 48 h to ensure early detection and investigation of vascular problems.

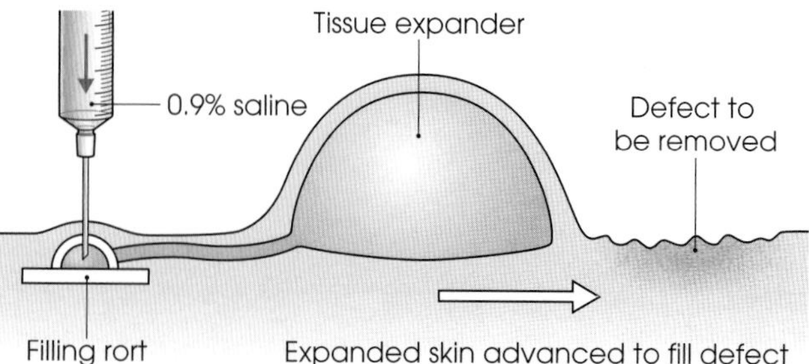

Figure 9.14 The technique of tissue expansion.

TISSUE EXPANSION

Tissue expansion provides adjacent matching skin that has the correct characteristics for that site, such as colour, texture, thickness, hair-bearing (where appropriate) and sensation. There is also no donor site, as with skin grafts or flap repairs. There seem to be few areas of the body that cannot be expanded provided that careful planning and the correct type of expander are used. Tissue expansion has been used to treat traumatic hair loss, male pattern baldness, burns scarring (Fig. 9.14), tattoo removal, port wine stains, giant pigmented naevi and facial reconstruction to date.

Soft tissue expansion was originally described by Dr Charles Neumann in 1957, but first utilized in plastic surgery by Dr Chedomir Radovan in 1976.[27] A silicon bag, similar to a non-inflated balloon, is placed under normal skin adjacent to a defect, scar or area to be excised. This is inflated at weekly intervals by injection of normal saline into a port placed at a distance from the bag but connected to it via a fine-bore tube. The process of inflation stretches the overlying tissue and skin. In this way the skin is expanded, increased in area, and made available for reconstruction (Fig. 9.15). Once sufficient skin has been generated the expander can be removed, the lesion excised, and

REFERENCE

27. Radovan C. Plast Reconstr Surg 1984; 74: 482–492

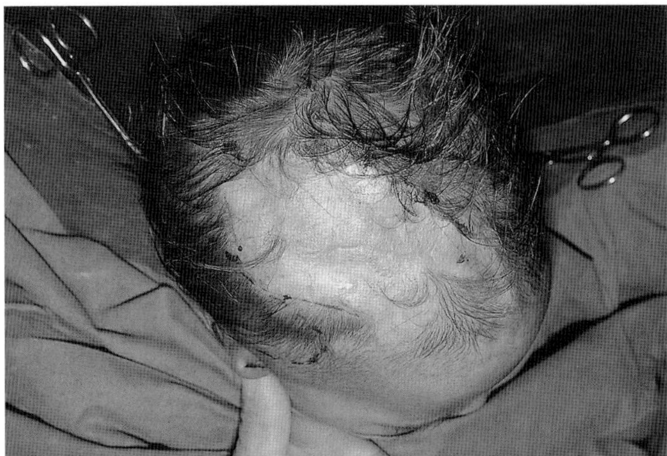

a

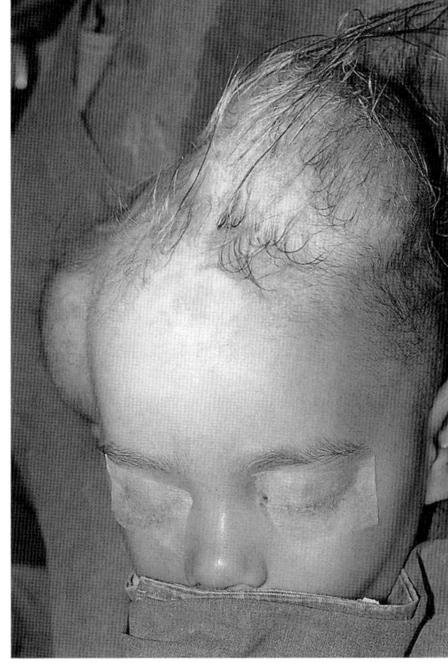

b

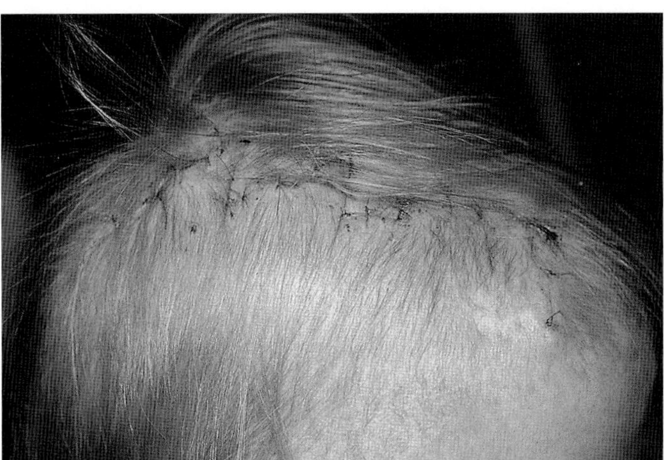

c

Figure 9.15 Tissue expanders used to close a scalp defect caused by a burn: **(a)** scalp defect, **(b)** expanded tissue, **(c)** closed defect.

the resultant defect covered utilizing the excess skin produced by the expander.

Tissue expansion has a number of disadvantages, including the time required: usually 8–20 weeks depending on the site and amount of skin required. During this time the patient has to attend hospital regularly and the process is often very painful, especially for children. The increasingly odd appearance of the expander, particularly on the scalp and limbs, also causes distress to the patients. Adequate preoperative counselling can help to eliminate these concerns for patients. Often the most successful areas for expansion are where the surface is convex with a bony base, as in the scalp or forehead and breast.

Tissue expansion exploits the viscoelastic properties of skin.[28] Mechanical creep is defined as the elongation of skin with a constant load over time. It is demonstrated during intraoperative tissue expansion and skin suturing under tension to facilitate wound closure. Biological creep, however, is the generation of new tissue secondary to a persistent chronic stretching force such as seen in conventional tissue expansion, pregnancy and obesity. The resistance of the skin to a stretching force decreases with time (stress relaxation) and explains why expanded skin, while initially tight, is relaxed by the next clinic appointment.

Expansion is utilized in a number of areas of the body including the scalp, forehead, chest, and upper and lower limbs. Correction of postmastectomy or hypoplastic breasts can be achieved with modified tissue expanders. The cavity is used for permanent insertion of a silicon implant to recreate the breast mound and the expanded skin to provide an envelope for the implant. Expansion is commonly used to replace scars or areas of alopecia on the scalp.[29]

Expanders are available in a variety of different shapes and sizes. Under antibiotic cover, a minimal skin incision is made to insert the expander without bending it, dissecting it usually at the level of the superficial fascia.[30] A subcutaneous pocket is also tunnelled for the injection port at a distance from the expander. A small volume of saline is injected immediately to smooth out the envelope of the expander, the incisions are closed and the wounds left for 3 weeks to heal. Expansion is then begun and repeated at weekly intervals until sufficient skin is ready for advancement.

The amount of expanded skin produced can be estimated by measuring the increase in arc length over the top of the expander. Expansion should continue until there is at least an increase in arc length equal to the width of the defect. Compli-

REFERENCES

28. Wilhelmi BJ, Blackwell SJ, Mancoll JS et al. Ann Plast Surg 41: 215–219
29. Faltaous AA, Yetman RJ. Plast Reconstr Surg 1996; 97: 56–60
30. Matton GE, Tonnard PL, Monstrey SJ et al. Br J Plast Surg 1995; 48: 172–176

cations of tissue expansion include pain, infection, haematoma, rupture, extrusion of the expander or port, and local tissue necrosis.

REGIONAL RECONSTRUCTION

BREAST RECONSTRUCTION

Breast cancer presents women with several significant challenges. In addition to confronting the impact of this diagnosis, patients are often also concerned with effects of surgery—mastectomy in particular. Lumpectomy and radiotherapy may also alter breast shape significantly and may prove equally distressing and abhorrent to the patient. Reconstruction should be discussed with most patients facing mastectomy (ideally as part of the multidisciplinary care of the patient), but should always defer to oncological priorities. Several methods are available and may be offered at the time of mastectomy (immediate reconstruction) or at a later stage (delayed reconstruction).[31] Immediate breast reconstruction is popular in the UK due to reduced costs and overall operating time as well as optimal aesthetics and patient psychology.

Reconstruction of the female breast aims to replace the skin and volume lost due to mastectomy. Techniques may be broadly divided into implant-based methods, which require a prosthesis to provide volume, and autologous techniques that rely on the patient's own tissues to provide both volume and skin. Outdated arguments used to support the notion that delayed reconstructions are superior because they allow the woman to 'mourn' her breast and thus appreciate her reconstructed breast. This is no longer true because immediate techniques, combined with skin-sparing mastectomy, have allowed patients to obtain reconstructions of excellent aesthetic quality.

Implant-based breast reconstruction

Following mastectomy, only a thin layer of skin and subcutaneous fat lies above the chest wall. Prostheses require more substantial soft tissue cover and are usually placed under the pectoralis major muscle. Usually this will demand use of a specific expander prosthesis that can be injected with saline to stretch the overlying muscle over several weeks. Simple implant placement is likely to produce a very obvious result that is only aesthetic in the smaller breast. Women with larger, ptotic breasts will usually require adjustment to the other breast if symmetry of shape is required.

For the larger, ptotic breast, it may be beneficial to provide additional skin and soft tissue cover using the latissimus dorsi muscle.[32] This technique can give excellent symmetry as an immediate technique. However, an expander is required for the larger-breasted woman if used as a delayed technique. The latissimus dorsi flap is raised with the patient in the lateral position, allowing simultaneous mastectomy by the breast surgeon. Incision proceeds through the skin of the back and fatty layer. The muscle is isolated from the distal to proximal to preserve the pedicle entering 10 cm from the apex of the axilla on the underside of the axilla. The pedicle is dissected to ensure that the thoracodorsal artery has not been damaged by lymph node surgery or radiotherapy as it traverses the axilla. The flap may still be raised in these circumstances on the retrograde flow from the arterial branch to the serratus muscle, but this leads to reduced mobility. The nerve is generally divided to prevent twitching of the breast, but this is not mandatory and some surgeons believe leaving it is safer in scarred cases and that muscle volume is preserved. The tendon of latissimus dorsi is attached to the highest point of the anterior axillary fold and is detached to island the muscle so that it can be tunnelled through to the anterior chest. Finally the patient is turned on to her back to allow accurate placement of the implant and shaping of the new breast.

Implant-based reconstructions have several limitations. Implants are medical devices and have a finite lifetime. Modern implants may last two decades or more but are vulnerable to capsular contraction, particularly after radiotherapy. In addition, implants may become infected and require removal.[33]

Autologous reconstruction

Breast reconstruction utilizing the patient's tissues alone has several obvious attractions. It avoids use of a prosthesis and any associated risks. However, these techniques tend to be more technically demanding than implant-based methods and usually require microsurgical skills.

The most established techniques are based on the transverse rectus abdominis myocutaneous (TRAM) flap. This method utilizes the skin and fat below the umbilicus, fed via perforating vessels that penetrate the rectus to reach the overlying skin. These perforators are branches of the deep inferior epigastric artery, which arborizes with the superior epigastric artery. As a consequence, the flap may be raised as a superiorly based pedicled flap or alternatively as a free flap based on the deep inferior epigastric vessels.

These abdominal flaps are considered to give the optimum aesthetic result. However, legitimate concerns exist regarding the time required for surgery (6–8 h) and the potential for injury and long-term damage to the abdominal wall, particularly in the case of pedicled TRAM flaps. Furthermore, free flaps may fail even in the best of hands. Accordingly, surgeons with both experience and specialist training should perform these procedures. Recent advances have led to minimal removal of the rectus muscle, or none at all. Immediate breast reconstruction with a free perforator flap, the deep inferior epigastric perforator (DIEP) flap, is now considered to be the current gold standard (Fig. 9.16).[31]

Free flaps may be extensively moulded and shaped without the danger of venous congestion that is a risk in the pedicled TRAM flap due to the bulky muscle pedicle. The free TRAM flap was originally developed to reduce the need for a muscle pedicle stretched across the chest. The flap is usually plumbed into the internal mammary artery and vein. Previously the thoracodorsal vessels were used, but this risks the arterial supply to the reserve latissimus dorsi should the free flap fail.

If the patient's abdomen is too slim or unsuitable due to previous surgery, other potential autologous donor sites include the superior gluteal artery perforator (S-GAP) flap. This flap consists of skin and fat alone, harvested from the upper aspect of the buttock. It leaves a very good donor site, with minimal trauma; as a result the patients tend to recover quickly. However, the flap is often suitable only for reconstruction of the small to medium breast, and the pedicle is both short and small.[34]

REFERENCES

31. Kroll SS, Baldwin B. Plast Reconstr Surg 1992; 90: 455
32. McCraw JP, Papp C, Edwards A et al. Clin Plastic Surg 1994; 21: 279–288
33. Brody GS. Plast Reconstr Surg 1997; 100: 1314–1321
34. Blondeel PN. Br J Plast Surg 1999; 52: 185–193.

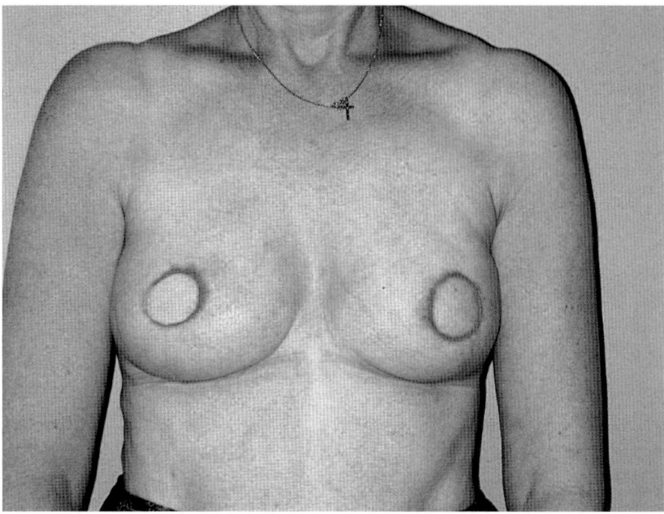
a

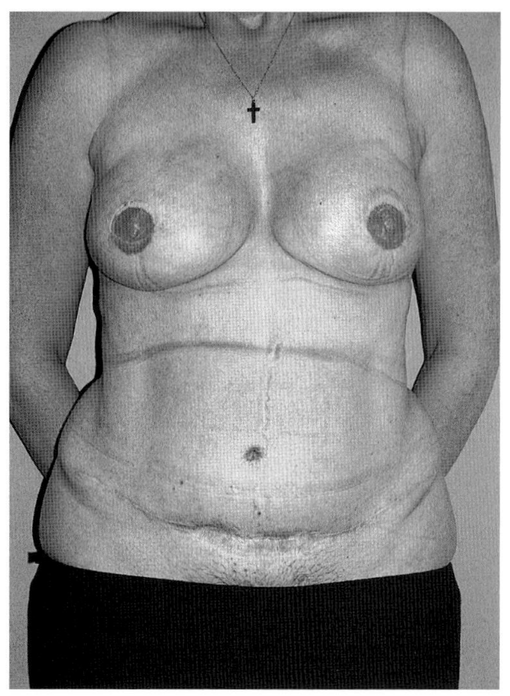
b

Figure 9.16 Breast reconstruction using a DIEP free flap, demonstrating the abdominal scar.

Once reconstruction of the mound has been completed, the nipple and areola may be recreated using a combination of local flaps, such as the modified skate flap. The areola may be obtained using either a full-thickness skin graft from the inner thigh or by using a tattoo. The latter is much less traumatic and can give superb results, although it tends to fade and may need redoing after 2–3 years.

If the patient is seeking symmetry of shape as well as of volume, then it may be necessary to revise the contralateral breast using standard aesthetic techniques to augment, reduce or lift the breast. In this way, excellent aesthetic reconstructions may be achieved.

HEAD AND NECK RECONSTRUCTION

Patients undergoing surgery for head and neck cancer should, ideally, be treated by a multidisciplinary team. Resection of these cancers may compromise important structures and functions, including the airway, eating, vision and speech, as well as having a devastating impact on appearance. Other modalities of treatment are available and should be used where appropriate. In addition, surgical restoration of appearance and function may be further enhanced by application of prosthetics and osseointegrated implants.

Selection of the appropriate method of reconstruction depends on several factors, as described below.

The patient

Patients are usually over 60 years of age and may have other intercurrent illness, including malnutrition, cardiorespiratory disease or diabetes. Furthermore, patients may be referred for surgery following radiotherapy, which may affect the access to vascular pedicles or the availability of local tissues as potential flaps. Percutaneous gastrostomy or nasogastric feeding should be considered if nutritional status is poor and oral feeding is not going to be possible in the postoperative recovery period.

The defect

Assessment of the defect includes consideration of the location and size of the resection and analysis in terms of cover, support and lining. The principles of head and neck reconstruction are to conserve appearance, lip seal and oral continence, swallowing, and speech, as well as to protect the airway and important neurovascular structures. The ultimate aim is to restore physiological and social function.

All surgery in this difficult and crucial area should be planned with a back-up method in the event of failure. The classic example of this is the defensive raising of the pectoralis flap, preserving the pedicle of the deltopectoral flap for use as a salvage procedure should all else fail.

Methods of reconstruction follow the reconstructive ladder, beginning with simple split-thickness skin grafts at one end and proceeding to free tissue transfer at the other. Ascent of this ladder does not always imply a superior result, because in the appropriate circumstances a skin graft may provide the best functional and cosmetic result.

MUCOSAL LESIONS: OROPHARYNX AND ORAL CAVITY

The oropharynx extends from the anterior faucial pillars to the epiglottis and includes the base of the tongue, essential to initiation of the involuntary swallow. Resection within any part of the oropharynx can alter speech or swallowing. Oral cavity includes the anterior tongue and buccal cavity.

Defects following excision of small lesions up to 1.5 cm in diameter may be either closed primarily or left to granulate. For lesions lying on or near the alveolus, this may be made easier if a mandibular rim excision resection has been performed.

Larger defects require flap reconstruction to reconstitute them. Ideally, local oral mucosal flaps should not be used for reconstruction of defects following resection of malignant tumours because they lie within the field of potential malignant change. Local flaps that lie outside the immediate area of mucosa include the nasolabial flap[35] and submental artery flaps.[36] Pedicled flaps include temporalis flap[37] and trapezius flap. The deltopectoral flap is used only as a salvage procedure or when other options are not available. The free radial forearm flap is often the method of choice, providing thin, pliable lining. The pectoralis myocutaneous flap[38] is also commonly used but may introduce too much bulk.

Reconstruction of the tongue base may prove especially problematic because adequate clearance may be gained only at the expense of innervation to the remaining tongue. Resection of large lesions from the tongue base may result in loss of the hypoglossal nerves and usually leads to total or near total glossectomy, producing severe speech and swallowing difficulties. The aim of reconstruction is to fill the defect with bulky tissue using either the latissimus dorsi flap or the pectoralis major flap.[39] The rectus abdominis myocutaneous flap is also of use in this location. The tongue set-back flap has been used to fill in such defects, but the reconstruction relies on local tissue subjected to the same oncogenic stimulus as the original lesion.

Total glossectomy can be complicated by aspiration due to removal of the suprahyoid and extrinsic tongue muscles. This may be ameliorated by laryngoplasty or laryngeal suspension. If aspiration is severe or persists, laryngectomy may be needed to protect the lungs and airway.

LIP RECONSTRUCTION

Wedge excision

Squamous cell carcinoma of the lip is common in smokers and requires excision with a 5-mm margin. An ellipse excision of skin will leave an excess of mucosa. The best cosmetic result is obtained by excision of entire thickness of the lip. Closure results in a simple, unobtrusive vertical scar, but it is essential to carefully appose the edges of orbicularis oris with long-lasting sutures to restore oral competence. Equally important is to exactly match the edge of the vermillion together with the white roll adjacent to it to prevent an obvious step in the scar. Lesions less than one-third of the width of the eyelid can also be excised in this way.

Karapandzic neurovascular flap

Where more than one-third of the width of the lip is lost, then reconstruction is required. This should be sensate and contain muscle to ensure oral competence. The neurovascular fan flap described by Karapandzic transfers skin, muscle and mucosa into the defect by an oral circumference advancement. A degree of microstomia is created because no new tissue is introduced, but this usually stretches. Correct muscle orientation is maintained with preservation of the nerves to the orbicularis.

NASAL RECONSTRUCTION

The nose has very little spare tissue, and direct closure is rarely an option. Small lesions can be excised and skin grafts used. Although these leave obvious scars, small local bilobed flaps are often used, where a flap of tissue is swung 90° into a defect, leaving a donor that is closed with another, smaller flap perpendicular to the first, from an area of greater skin laxity (Fig. 9.17). These flaps are often also poorly cosmetic. This is due to a pin-cushioning effect, with contracture of the scar leading to bulging of the transposed tissue.

The forehead flap has been in use since ancient Indian times. The flap is supplied by the supratrochlear vessels and provides even-toned, well-vascularized facial skin to replace large defects including those of the tip and columella. It can be used in association with cartilage and bone grafts for support and with mucosal grafts for lining.

RECONSTRUCTION OF THE ORAL CAVITY INCLUDING EXTERNAL SKIN COVER

Advanced intraoral carcinomas may infiltrate the cheek and require excision. The reconstructive goals are to provide both lining and cover using thin pliable skin that has an acceptable colour match. In the elderly, cover may be provided by rotating cervical skin up on to the cheek. However, if a large amount of lining has been lost alternative sources will need to be sought. Bipaddled skin flaps with an intermediate de-epithelialized bridge allow use of a single flap to achieve both cover and lining. The pedicled or free latissimus dorsi can be used in this way, as can the rectus abdominis, although both these flaps may prove bulky.

RECONSTRUCTION OF THE ORAL CAVITY INCLUDING BONE

Mandibulectomy produces a dramatic Andy Gump appearance. The physical and psychological hardship for those with such a deformity is immense, and it is further exacerbated by the inability to speak and eat properly. Therefore, where possible, consideration should be given to conserving and/or reconstructing the mandible.

Advances in the knowledge of tumour biology and the way tumours invade the mandible in non-irradiated cases has meant fewer radical bone resections. Tumour control can be achieved by performing rim resections or partial (segmental) resections of the mandible. However, there are still cases where mandibulectomy is required. The aims of mandibular reconstruction are to maintain the dental arch, to allow dental occlusion, and to provide a platform for prosthetic rehabilitation.

The ideal mandibular reconstruction provides bone continuity with adequate alveolar height, good facial cosmesis and arch form, and adequate osseous bulk. There may also be a need for intraoral lining. The reconstruction must be robust enough to enable radiotherapy to be used as part of the treatment regimen. Reconstruction of the mandible requires good bone stock and thin pliable skin for soft tissue cover. No single flap can provide this; the radial forearm flap has thin reliable skin but poor bone stock, whereas the fibula flap has very good bone stock but a relatively unreliable skin paddle. Bone can be supplied by non-vascularized bone grafts such as in titanium trays or reconstruction plates plus bone graft.

Rib grafts harvested with both pectoralis major[40] and latissimus dorsi derive minimal blood supply from the accompanying muscle and are, in effect, also non-vascularized grafts. Vascular-

REFERENCES

35. Gerwitz HS, Eilber FR, Zarem HA. Am J Surg 1978; 136: 508–511
36. Faltaous AA, Yetman RJ. Plast Reconst Surg 1996; 97: 56–60
37. McGregor IA. Br J Plast Surg 1963; 16: 318–335
38. Shemen LJ, Freeman JL, Young S et al. Ear Nose Throat J 1986; 65: 61–72
39. Quillen CG, Sherwin JC, Georgiade NC. Plast Reconst Surg 1978; 62: 113
40. Bell MSG, Barron PT. Ann Plast Surg 1981; 6: 347

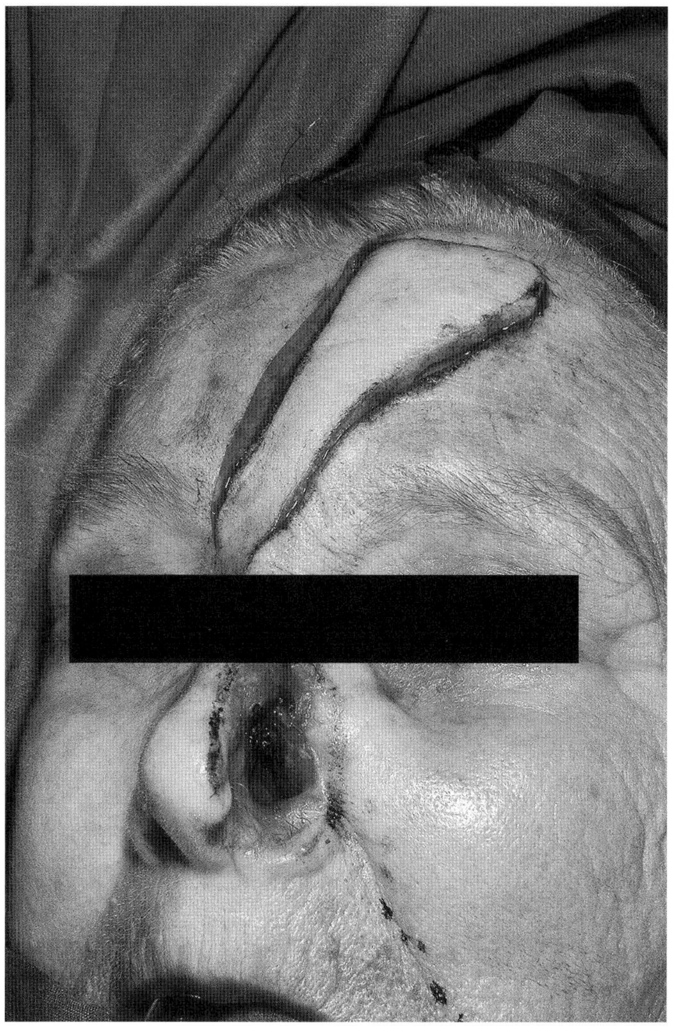

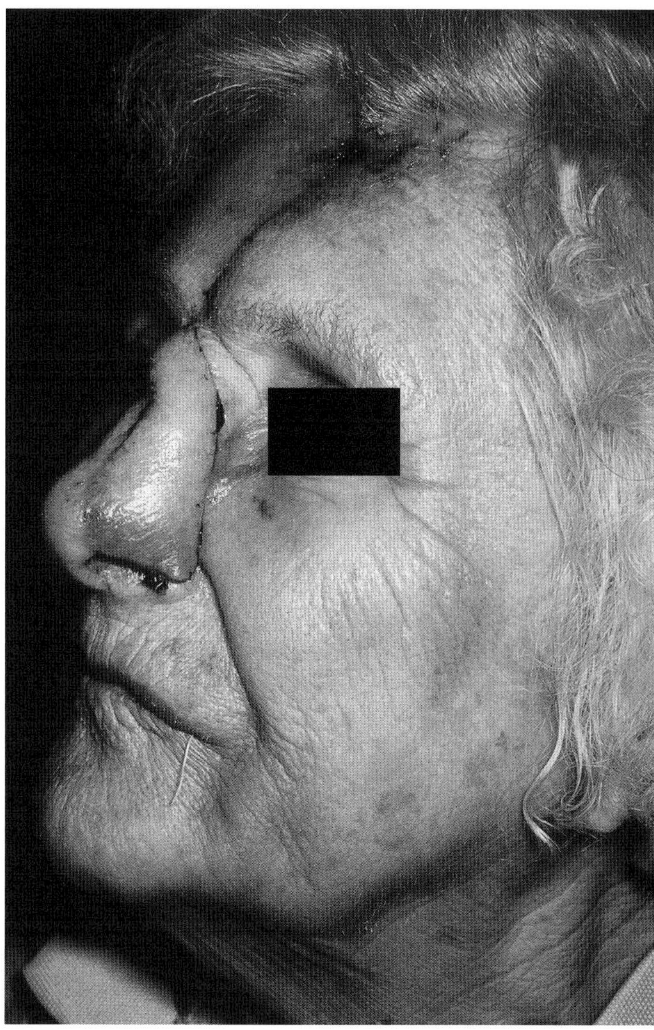

a b

Figure 9.17 A forehead flap to reconstruct alar defect after excision of a basal cell carcinoma.

ized bone flaps include the radial forearm flap,[41] fibula flap,[42] scapula flap,[43] and deep circumflex iliac artery flap.

Vascularized bone is probably the method of choice for mandibular reconstruction. The technique is not so environment-dependent as non-vascularized bone grafting techniques, and it has the ability to incorporate soft tissue for reconstruction within the flap and osseointegrated implants for dental restoration. Defects less than 6 cm in length may be restored using the radial forearm osseofasciocutaneous flap. Defects that are longer than 6 cm in length can be replaced with bone derived from the scapula flap, the deep circumflex iliac artery (DCIA) flap or the fibula flap. Both the DCIA flap and the fibula flap have enough bone stock to enable osseointegration implants to be inserted, whereas the radial forearm flap probably does not.[44]

Radial artery forearm flap (Fig. 9.18)

The radial forearm flap is a fasciocutaneous flap supplied by the radial artery, with perforators travelling in the intermuscular septum to overlying skin and the underlying radius. The latter provide access to vascularized bone.[45]

The radial artery is relatively large and easy to anastamose. The venous drainage of the flap is by either the venae comitantes or the superficial venous system, with some surgeons incorporating the cephalic vein to increase drainage. The radial forearm microvascular free flap provides enough skin to have single, double or triple skin paddles to reconstruct complex three-dimensional defects around the face. The flap can be raised with palmaris longus tendon to act as a sling to support the angle of the mouth following the reconstruction.

The axis of the flap is marked by drawing a line between the palpable brachial pulse in the antecubital fossa and the radial artery pulse at the wrist. The site and size of the skin paddle depends on size of defect, hairiness of skin, length of pedicle required, and superficial venous system. The flap is raised using a tourniquet without exsanguination, to identify necessary veins.

REFERENCES

41. Bhathena A, Karavena NM. Head Neck Surg 1986; 8: 311
42. Hidalgo DA. Plast Reconst Surg 1989; 84: 71
43. Sullivan MJ, Baker SR, Crompton R et al. Arch Otolaryngol Head Neck Surg 1985; 115: 1334
44. David DJ, Tan E, Katsaros J et al. Plast Reconst Surg 1988; 82: 792–801
45. Soutar DS, Shecker LR, Tanner NSB et al. Br J Plast Surg 1983; 36: 1

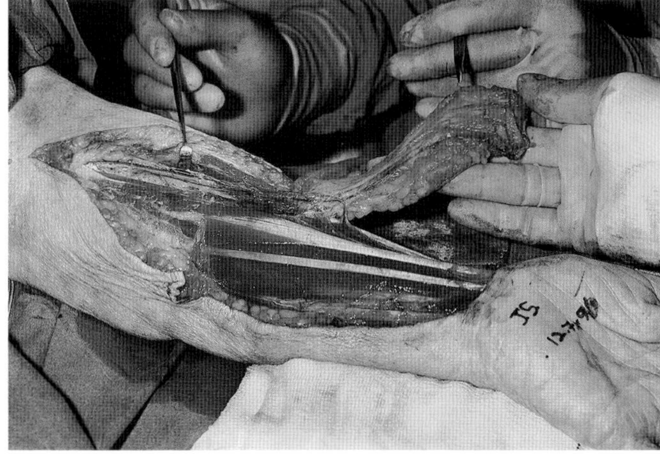

a

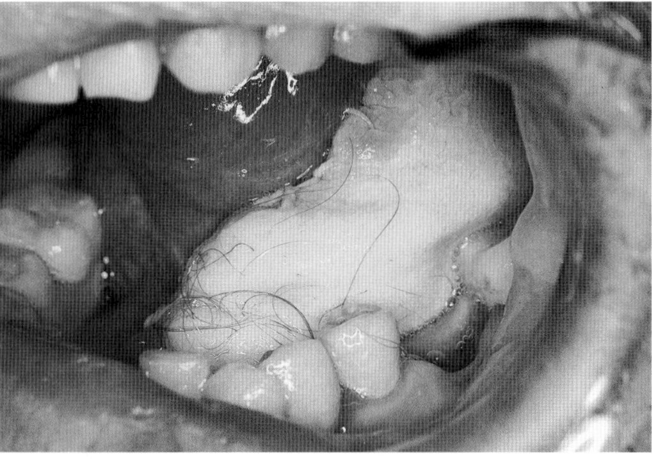

b

Figure 9.18 Radial forearm free flap to reconstruct the side of the tongue and floor of the mouth following excision of a squamous cell carcinoma.

The skin is incised down to and through deep fascia, and raised, preserving the paratenon over the flexor tendons. The dissection proceeds from both ulnar and radial sides to leave the skin paddle attached to the artery and vein alone.

The donor site can be closed with either a split-skin or full-thickness skin graft. If a small paddle is used, the defect can be closed directly by using an ulnar-based rotation flap. When bone is required, the osteotomy should aim to remove an approximately one-third cross-section of radius, with a maximum length of 12 cm. Postoperatively, the patient is placed in a protective above-elbow plaster cast for up to 6 weeks.

When used for intraoral reconstruction, flaps may be innervated using either the medial or lateral antebrachial nerve, usually performing a neurorrhaphy with the ipsilateral lingual nerve. As another variant, if minimal bulk is required the flap may consist of fascia alone and the surface covered with a split-skin graft (although this would not be indicated for intraoral reconstruction).

Fibula flap

The fibula flap is an osseofasciocutaneous flap supplied by the peroneal artery, with septocutaneous and musculocutaneous perforators. The nutrient vessel is a branch of the peroneal entering the shaft in the middle third. The flap provides a large amount of cortical bone up to 25 cm long. It leaves an excellent donor defect, although the distal 5 cm of fibula must be left to maintain ankle stability. The skin paddle can be oriented longitudinally or transversely depending on reconstructive requirements. The bone stock is suitable for osseointegrated implants and can be osteotomized to recreate the mentum.

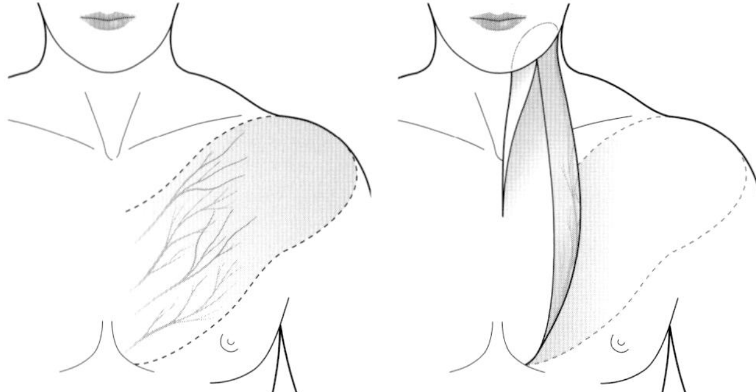

Figure 9.19 Deltopectoral flap.

The peroneal vessels provide a relatively short pedicle, but they remain large throughout their length. As a result, they are suitable for use as recipient vessels if it is necessary to add an additional free flap in series (i.e. radial forearm flap for intraoral lining).

Deep circumflex iliac artery flap

The DCIA flap is supplied by the deep circumflex iliac artery that arises from the external iliac artery, opposite the exit of the deep inferior epigastric artery, just above the inguinal ligament. The major application of this flap is as a source of bone for mandibular reconstruction. It can also provide skin and muscle if required, although vascularity to the skin paddle is not always reliable.

The bone is helpfully shaped for mandibular reconstruction. If a skin paddle is used, it is marked along the iliac crest with approximately two-thirds of its area above the crest and one-third below. The medial end of the skin paddle overlies or is just medial to the anterior superior iliac spine. The donor site is closed carefully in layers to prevent risk of incisional hernia and damage to the lateral cutaneous nerve of the thigh.

Deltopectoral flap

The deltopectoral flap (Fig. 9.19) is a fasciocutaneous flap first described by Bakamjian in 1965.[46] The flap is supplied by the intercostal perforating branches of the internal mammary artery lying at the lateral edge of the sternum between the second to fourth intercostal space. It reaches laterally over the anterior surface of the deltoid, but it can be extended a further 3–5 cm using a delay procedure where the skin is incised but the flap not raised until an enhanced blood supply through the chosen pedicle has been stimulated by the severance of the skin vessels. With an initial delay, the flap can reach as high as the zygomatic arch, but attempts to extend beyond this are likely to result in distal necrosis. Maximal possible flap length is approximately 45 cm.

In centres where microsurgery is available this flap is usually reserved for salvage surgery. However, it remains the flap of

REFERENCE

46. Bakamjian VY. Plast Reconstr Surg 1965; 36: 173

choice where free tissue transfer is contraindicated or where neck skin is involved and requires resurfacing prior to brachytherapy.

The donor site usually requires an SSG and the pedicle is generally divided at 2–3 weeks.

LIMB AND FACE TRANSPLANTATION

Advances in immunosuppression for organ transplants have allowed plastic surgeons to attempt transplantation of allogenic composite flaps. The highly antigenic nature of skin has previously precluded this. In addition, matching must include cosmetic consideration as well as a degree of tissue typing, because it has been found that patients will not accept a limb that does not look similar to their original.

There are a number of difficult ethical problems involved in these transplants. The recommendation is that hand transplants be performed only in bilateral amputees in whom the risk–benefit ratio is best. Face transplantation is still under discussion, and it is likely that, as in hand transplantation, a major hurdle will be the lack of suitable donors.

Lower limb reconstruction

Working party recommendations

Soft tissue cover is absolutely essential if bone healing is to occur. Bone at the fracture site will be lacking healthy periosteum and thus is not able to take a skin graft. Indeed, the vascular supply of the bone is compromised at a time when good nutrition is essential to prevent infection and allow progression of healing. Introduction of soft tissue with an intact blood supply—the flap—is mandatory.

In 1997, a joint working party of the British Orthopaedic Association and the British Association of Plastic Surgeons made recommendations on the management of open tibial fractures.[47] These highlighted the importance of cooperation at an early stage with transfer to specialist centres where appropriate. The recommendations were based on an audit of 1000 consecutive open fractures over a period of 6 years in Edinburgh.

It was noted that 20% of type II, 30% of type IIIA, and 70% of Gustilo type IIIB tibial diaphyseal fractures required flap cover. Guidelines have been set that suggest that to achieve optimal management the case should be discussed ideally at consultant level prior to first surgery, and that initial fixation and debridement should be within 6 h and definitive skin cover attained within the first 5 days, whether that be skin graft, local flap or distant microvascular free flap. Initial debridement involves excision of all devitalized tissue so that a clean, healthy, bleeding edge is achieved for skin, muscle and skin. A 6-L lavage with pulsed pressurized normal saline is recommended. Bony stabilization is the choice of the orthopaedic surgeon, but where external pins are used it is important to stay within the anterolateral aspect of the tibia to avoid compromising future skin flaps.

Compartment syndrome

Compartment syndrome commonly occurs following fractures in the lower leg and is caused by direct crush or reperfusion oedema. It is defined as the increase in pressure within a fascially bounded compartment that threatens muscle and nerve viability by venous obstruction. Tissue pressure can be measured by a needle catheter technique and is normally below 30 mmHg. Compartment release is indicated when the differential pressure (diastolic – compartment pressure) is less than 30 mmHg. More importantly, if clinical suspicion is high due to mechanism of injury or signs such as swelling and pain, then release is a surgical emergency.

Like external fixator pin placement, it is important to perform safe incisions that will not compromise future perforator flaps or level of amputation. The two safe incisions that allow release of all four compartments are the medial incision 2.5 cm posterior to the medial border of the tibia and the anterolateral, 2 cm lateral to the anterior border of the tibia.

Fasciocutaneous rotation and transposition flaps

Fasciocutaneous refers to the composition of local skin and fascia flaps of the leg. These are supplied by several perforators that run in the fascial layer, hence that tissue's inclusion. They are most commonly proximally based because this is considered safer given the general orientation of vessels from proximal to distal, but they can also be distally based. The flap is named *rotation* or *transposition* depending on how the flap is moved across from the donor site to the recipient.

Propeller perforator flaps

Propeller perforator flaps are the ultimate generation of fasciocutaneous flaps. They rely on a single perforator of diameters of around 1–2 mm that can be swivelled 180°, like the blade of a propeller, to introduce healthy tissue into the wound. The skill in performing this flap lies in dissecting the perforator free of attachments that may kink the vessel during this radical swing, while preserving the microscopic venae comitantes that provide venous drainage to the flap.

Gastrocnemius muscle flap

This is a local muscle flap often used to cover defects around the knee, particularly exposed prosthesis. It is a reliable, easily raised flap that is supplied by the proximal vessels entering the heads of the lateral and medial halves of the muscle. Usually only one half is required so that some function is retained. The muscle is raised from distal to proximal and the origin of the muscle divided, leaving the pedicle intact. This islanded muscle flap can then be rotated to cover defects across the anterior knee.

Latissimus dorsi muscle flap

In massively traumatized legs, the area of soft tissue loss is often too great to be covered by a local flap. This is particularly true after degloving type injuries or where large amounts of crushed devitalized tissue require debridement.

The latissimus dorsi flap is probably the largest free flap in the body and is often thought of as the workhorse of free flaps. The thoracodorsal artery is a long, reliable, easily harvested pedicle that can be anastomosed safely out of the zone of trauma. In leg trauma, the latissimus dorsi is normally used as a simple muscle flap because the skin and subcutaneous tissue of the back is thick and inappropriate on the leg. The donor is usually closed directly and a split-skin graft harvested from the thigh to cover the raw muscle when placed in site.

REFERENCE

47. British Orthopaedic Association–British Association of Plastic Surgeons Working Party on the Management of Open Tibial Fractures. Br J Plast Surg 1997; 50: 570–583

Anterolateral thigh flap

This free flap is gaining favour as an exceptionally thin and pliable flap with an excellent donor defect that can be harvested with the patient in the supine position. The flap is supplied by a musculo- or septocutaneous cutaneous perforator from the descending branch of the lateral circumflex femoral artery. The advantages of this flap that consists simply of fascia and skin outweigh the difficulties of the variable anatomy and intricate dissection.

HAND SURGERY: ELECTIVE

Dupuytren's disease

This is a disease with a genetic predisposition thought to have been spread across northern Europe by invading Vikings. The aetiology remains a mystery, but there is thought to be an abnormality of myofibroblasts, possibly responding to growth factors such as transforming growth factor. The result is contraction of bands of abnormal fascia, leading to contraction of fingers and reduced hand function.

Surgery is not curative and is aimed at restoring extension by removing as much of the diseased tissue as is reasonable given the patient's circumstances. In young, fit patients it is desirable to excise as much diseased tissue as possible to reduce recurrence. Dermofasciectomy involves careful dissection of cord of disease while preserving the digital nerves and vessels. Skin may be excised due to involvement or may simply be attenuated, and this may require skin grafting to fingers, although in the palm healing is effective using the open palm technique with regular dressing. In older, less fit patients a fasciotomy, where the cord is simply divided, can be performed under local anaesthetic and will give an immediate if short-term solution.

Carpal tunnel release

The median nerve at the carpal tunnel in the wrist is the most common site of nerve compression in the body. The nerve runs through a tight passage formed by the proximal and distal rows of carpal bones dorsally and the volar intercarpal ligament along with the tendons of the fingers. Conditions causing oedema of synovium can lead to compression of the nerve and frequently the syndrome is seen in pregnancy, thyroid disease, rheumatoid arthritis and diabetes.

The classic symptoms and signs are of paraesthesia in the distribution of the nerve, exacerbated by tapping over the tunnel (Tinel's sign), and worsening of tingling on flexion of the wrists (Phalen's sign). Wasting of the thenar muscles is a late sign that should precipitate urgent action to prevent further permanent nerve damage. Initial treatment is by steroid injection and night-time splinting to prevent the precipitating wrist flexion. Electromyographic studies are often used to establish the diagnosis but are not required prior to surgery if presentation is classic and not responsive to conservative measures.

Rheumatoid disease

Rheumatoid disease is a debilitating autoimmune disease with progressive destruction of the synovium and eventual erosion of bone. Many advances in drug therapy have had a major influence on disease modification. Surgery for rheumatoid disease has an important place, but a multidisciplinary approach is essential and optimization of conservative treatment is ensured prior to undertaking surgery. The basic principle of surgery in rheumatoid disease is to proceed from proximal stabilization to distal procedures. There is little sense in replacing delicate metacarpophalangeal joints where the wrist is unstable and painful, because this will prevent the proper rehabilitation and use of the distal joints.

HAND SURGERY: TRAUMA

Infection

Infection within fascial spaces of the hand can be devastatingly mutilating and potentially limb-threatening. The usual source of entry is from an animal bite or thorn. All such wounds must be thoroughly washed out and foreign bodies excluded. Prophylactic antibiotics covering *Pasteurella multocida* as well as staphylococci and streptococci are indicated for deeply penetrating wounds. Infection within the tendon sheath is relatively common and is indicated by swelling and acute tenderness over the volar aspect of the finger, with inability of the patient to actively flex and exquisite pain on passive flexion. This is a surgical emergency because destruction of the vinculae within the synovial mesentery containing the blood supply to the tendon swiftly follows established infection, and the tendon literally rots inside the sheath.

Treatment is by washout of the sheath, often with 24 h of irrigation. Of particular danger is the fight bite. Contact of the metacarpal heads while in a fist making contact with teeth in the mouth of another person results in implantation of oral flora in the confined joint space and aggressive infection with aerobes (such as staphylococci and streptococci) as well as anaerobes (such as *Eikenella corrodens* and *Bacteroides*). The principles of surgery for hand infections are to debride all non-viable tissue, release compartments under pressure by fasciotomy, elevate the limb, and give appropriate antibiotics. Of prime importance is early intervention with the occupational therapists for splintage and early mobilization with physiotherapists to limit the tendency for the hand to develop function-limiting contractures.

Replantation

All the extremities may be replanted with varying degrees of success. The ideal replant would be a sharp, guillotine injury to a distal part (such as a thumb or penis) in a fit, young non-smoker, where the injury has occurred within 6 h and the part has been transferred wrapped in saline-soaked gauze in a container of ice and water. Even in these circumstances, there may be considerable problems with long-term function, especially that related to sensation.

Relative contraindications to replantation include unfit patients; crushed, contaminated or avulsed parts; and prolonged warm ischaemia time, particularly where muscle bulk is significant. Thus lower limbs are rarely replanted, because the large muscle bulk in these parts generally will result in overwhelming reperfusion injury after even a short time, and usually the mechanism of injury is destructive, resulting in suboptimal nerve repair where extremes of nerve regeneration are already required. A further reason for the rarity of lower limb replantation is the relative success of lower limb prosthesis. Equally, some parts are so valuable and difficult to reconstruct by any other means that they merit heroic attempts to replant. The thumb is a classic example, and replantation is generally attempted even where this requires bone, tendon or vessel grafting, or alternatively segmental reduction. The alternative is significant loss of function of the hand, estimated to be approximately 50% by insurance companies, and the prospect of toe to thumb transfer to restore this function.

Tendon repair

Although repair of extensor tendons is relatively straightforward, the repair of flexor tendons in the hand can be fraught with difficulty. Verdan described zones of tendon injury that correspond to the site of tendon laceration when the fingers are extended rather than to the skin wound. Normally the fingers are in flexion at the time of injury, and the zone of tendon injury lies distal to the skin wound. Verdan's zone II lies between the insertion of the flexor digitorum superficialis tendons distally to the beginning of the A1 pulley on the head of the metacarpal proximally.

For many years, tendon repair in this no mans land zone was so disastrous that most authors recommended leaving the acute injury and attempting only secondary tendon grafting in selected cases. This has changed with improved technique (commonly the modified Kessler core stitch with epitendinous suture), better suture material, and an understanding of the need for accurate splinting and appropriate physiotherapy.

GENITAL RECONSTRUCTION

Lotus petal flaps

These local fasciocutaneous flaps are raised on the plentiful vascular plexus of vessels in the perineum created by the superficial and deep external pudendal vessels anteriorly and the posterior internal pudendal artery that gives rise to the inferior rectal and inferior gluteal vessels.[48] The pattern of potential flaps resembles the petals of the lotus flower. More than one flap may be used in a single reconstruction and donor sites can be closed directly. The flaps are generally used following radical vulvectomy and also to relieve vaginal stenosis.[49]

Gracilis

Although the skin lotus petal flaps have gained popularity, the original vaginal reconstructions were performed using longer sensate muscle flaps. For perineal reconstruction, the gracilis is raised as a proximally based pedicled muscle flap. The major vessel is the ascending branch of the medial circumflex femoral artery. The flap can be rotated to fill tissue defects of the perineum, including ischial pressure sores, and to provide muscle function for the anus.

PENILE RECONSTRUCTION

The penis is complex to reconstruct, and it is usual to attempt lengthening procedures in the first instance in all but the most radical of amputations. Extremely short, sensate stumps can be vastly improved by a combination of suprapubic liposuction, release of superior suspensory ligament, and fat injection into the shaft. There is, nevertheless, a role for complete reconstruction in both oncological reconstruction and gender reassignment.

The grandfather of plastic surgery, Gilles, described the inferiorly based, random-patterned abdominal flap that could be tubed to form a neopenis. This skin is often thick and hairy, and axially patterned flaps tend to be more reliable. The groin flap based on the superficial circumflex iliac artery has thus superseded the abdominal flap. This skin is less hairy, and a hydraulic device can be inserted to simulate the inflation of erection. Urethral reconstruction is more complex, with a high rate of fistula and stricture, and not all patients require this further step.

If the urethra is to be reconstructed, then a good option is the radial forearm free flap, because here the urethra can be formed in one stage. Allen's test should be performed prior to surgery to establish an intact palmar arch and avoid devascularizing the hand by harvest of the radial artery. The distal part of the flap is planned 4 cm proximal to the wrist to help conceal the donor, and a 12 cm × 12 cm area is marked centred on the radial artery and including the cephalic vein. The urethra is tubed from the ulna side of the flap over an 18-Fr catheter, and separated by a de-epithelialized bridge from the radial side that will be used as the body of the penis in a tube around a tube arrangement. The flap is raised suprafascially to include the intramuscular septum containing the skin perforators arising from the vessel. The flap is divided once the phallus is created and transferred to the prepared vessels in the groin, with the medial antecubital nerve being anastomosed to the pudendal nerve for sensation. The donor is repaired using a split-skin graft.

PAEDIATRIC PLASTIC SURGERY

CLEFT LIP AND PALATE (Fig. 9.20)

The Clinical Standards Advisory Group report in 1998 changed the way in which cleft lip and palate patients are treated in Britain. Prior to this, there were numerous low-volume operators around the country with a lack of multidisciplinary input. The report suggested a major reduction in units treating these patients, so that each surgeon now treats a minimum of 50 new patients annually. Cleft lip with or without cleft palate is a separate entity to cleft palate, but both have a genetic predisposition. Inheritance may be chromosomal, such as trisomy 13 (Patau) and 21 (Downs); Mendelian single gene, such as Treacher Collins; or sporadic, associated with developmental abnormalities such as the Pierre Robin sequence, when macroglossia leads to underdevelopment of the palate.

Problems associated with cleft lip and palate include breathing and feeding difficulties, speech impairments, and the cosmetic stigma, which includes tooth, maxilla and nasal development as well as the obvious lip deformity.

HYPOSPADIAS (see Ch. 38)

Hypospadias is characterized by the ventral position of the meatus, with a dorsal hooded foreskin and often an associated ventral curvature of the penis on erection (chordee) related to the short male urethra and deficiency of ventral skin. The aetiology is unclear, but there is a genetic predisposition and there may be a relation to oestrogen exposure during gestation. More proximal hypospadias is associated with abnormalities of the renal tract.

Epispadias is a separate entity both embryologically and in terms of treatment, and may be associated with abnormalities of the anterior abdominal wall. It is said that the ancient Greeks treated hypospadias by amputation of the distal part of the penis and remoulding of the glans with glowing cautery. Modern management centres on one-stage repair in simple distal hypospadias and two-stage repair popularized by Bracka in proximal or recurrent deformity.[50] Treatment is usually started after the age of 3 years because the child is then able to be more compliant but has not been traumatized by school.

REFERENCES

48. Yii NW, Niranjan NS. Br J Plast Surg 1996; 46: 547–554
49. Wee JT, Joseph VT. Plast Reconstr Surg 1989; 83: 701–709
50. Johnson D, Coleman DJ. Br J Plast Surg 1998; 51: 195–201

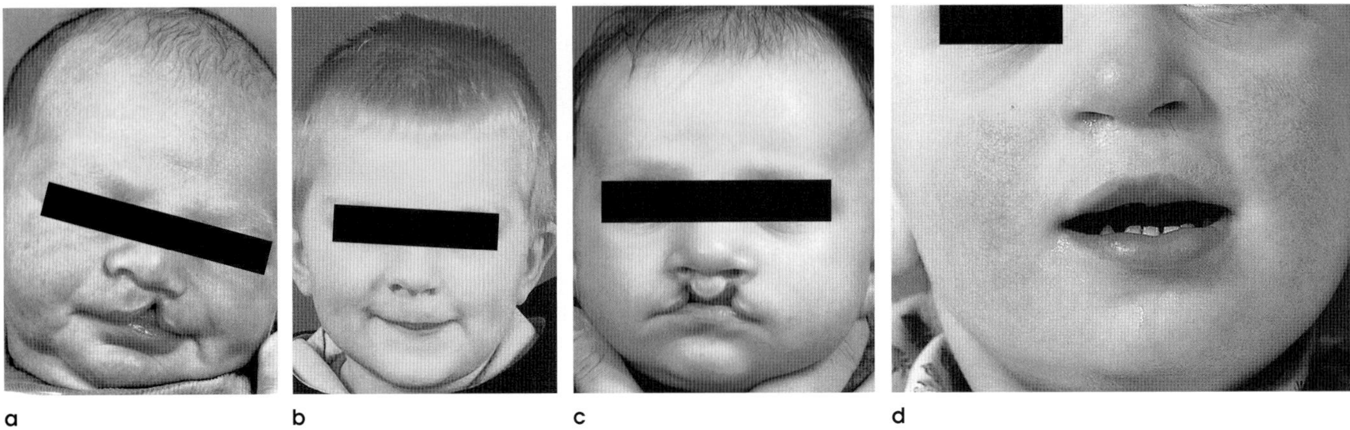

Figure 9.20 Bilateral cleft lip.

CONGENITAL HAND SURGERY

Hand symptoms may be part of a syndrome, and these patients should be screened for other abnormalities, particularly those that might affect the difficulty of performing a general anaesthetic if surgery is to be considered.

Hypoplasia of the thumb is an important functional deformity that has been classified by Blauth. Type I is minimal shortening that requires no action other than reassurance. Types II and III include narrowed first web space, thenar eminence hypoplasia, and metacarpophalangeal joint instability that require some reconstruction. Types IV and V are so rudimentary that index finger pollicization is the best option. This involves shortening the metacarpal and palmar, rotating the head to allow forceful pinch grip. Toe to thumb transfer is possible but pinch grip is more difficult to attain.

CRANIOFACIAL SYNDROMES

This wide-ranging collection of congenital abnormalities causes massive functional disorder and significant disfigurement. A common symptom is craniosynostosis. This is defined as premature fusion of one of the suture lines in the growing skull. Other sutures continue to grow, leading to abnormal elongation of the child's skull. In the case of unilateral lamboidal suture synostosis, this must be distinguished from deformational abnormality caused by positioning the child habitually in one position. Genetic studies have started to unravel the role of growth factors (such as fibroblast growth factor) and their receptors in these disorders, which may aid in management in the future. Treatment involves excision of the affected suture by strip craniectomy. Failure to correct the abnormal growth may lead to impairment of brain development.

Several syndromes include both head and neck, and limb abnormalities. Crouzon's syndrome presents as an infant with midface hypoplasia and exorbitism. If symptoms of syndactyly of the middle digits of hands and feet are also present, then this is termed *Apert's syndrome* and these patients have a higher rate of mental retardation than in Crouzon's (50% as apposed to 5%). Other craniofacial syndromes include facial clefting[51] and metabolic disorders such as Albright syndrome, which is the combination of short neck, low nasal bridge, cataracts and pseudohypoparathyroidism. These patients require multidisciplinary input in major centres, but all medical practitioners should be aware of their potential problems.

FACIAL REANIMATION

Facial palsy may be congenital or acquired as a result of surgical trauma or Bell's palsy. Congenital facial palsy may rarely be bilateral, when it is termed Möbius syndrome. Upper motor neuron lesions present with ipsilateral paralysis, most notably inability to smile on the affected side. Upper face function is preserved due to bilateral innervation.

Reconstruction of these deformities depends on the level and extent of injury as well as the desires of the patient. The gold standard of repair is the two-stage cross-facial nerve graft using interpositional nerve graft (usually sural) from the unaffected side to the paralysed side. Progress of the nerve regeneration is assessed using Tinel's sign that elicits tingling at the extent of the new nerve when tapped proximally. At the second stage, when the nerve has sufficiently regenerated, a free muscle transfer is performed—often pectoralis minor or gracilis. This technique allows restoration of spontaneous expression as well as coordinated synchronized movements of the mouth in 95% of patients and is greatly superior to static fascia lata slings.

EAR RECONSTRUCTION

Ear abnormalities are extremely common and correction of prominent ears is a frequently performed operation to prevent the torment of bullying at school. There are several techniques to reconstruct the usual problem of underdeveloped conchal folding. Posterior skin excision with incision and scoring the cartilage on the anterior aspect reduces the tendency of the cartilage to spring back into the prominent flat shape. There has been a move to reduce the amount of skin excised to lower the incidence of keloid scarring. In addition, many surgeons tend to reduce the amount of anterior dissection to reduce the chance of haematoma or necrosis. Mustarde sutures can be placed to hold the cartilage fold in place.

Reconstruction of absent ears is occasionally necessary due to failure of formation (known as microtia) or loss following trauma. Microtia is thought to result from obliteration of the stapedial artery during embryogenesis. This leads to a form of hemifacial microsomia resulting from first and second branchial arch syndrome. A complete ear can be carved from sixth to ninth

REFERENCE

51. Jones MC. Clin Plast Surg 1993; 20: 599–606

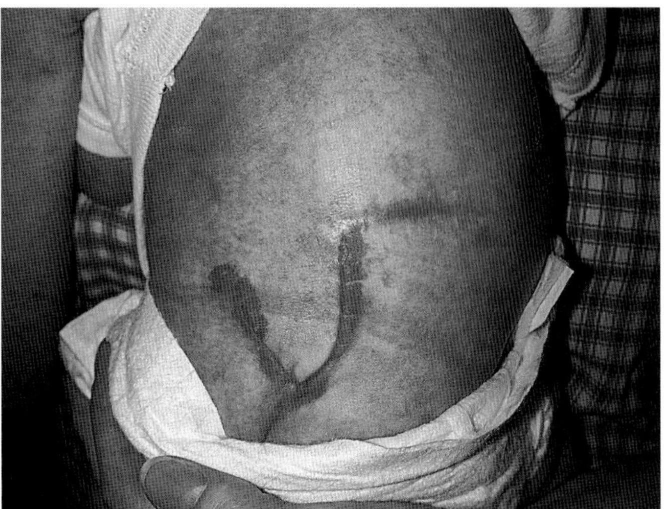

Figure 9.21 A myelomeningocele.

costal cartilage, making use of the vestigial ear parts. This can usually be placed under skin of the scalp, and with further minor procedures can look remarkably realistic. Occasionally the skin envelope is insufficient, necessitating tempoparietal fascial flaps and skin grafts, or alternatively tissue expansion. An alternative to these reconstructions is the Branemark implant together with a realistic prosthesis.

MYELOMENINGOCELE

Myelomeningocele (Fig. 9.21) is seen in one in 1000 live births; it requires the input of neurosurgery to repair cord and meninges and of plastic surgery to repair soft tissue defect. Primary closure may be possible by wide undermining of skin. The undermining may include muscle layers of gluteus and latissimus for extra support. Relaxing incisions laterally have also been used and may be left to granulate or closed using V–Y advancement. Rotation, bilobed and rhomboid flaps have all been used with success.

AESTHETIC SURGERY

BREAST REDUCTION

Breast reduction (Fig. 9.22) is performed within the UK National Health Service under certain guidelines. Patients can be seriously disadvantaged by large, pendulous breasts that may contribute to backache, fungal skin problems and psychosocial embarrassment. Breast reduction involves raising the nipple on a pedicle and transposing it to a higher level on the chest. Skin is excised around the nipple and inferiorly to reduce volume, and the breast is then reshaped and skin sutured. Advances have been made in reducing scarring by use of the Lejour technique of vertical scar resection, and in reducing risk of nipple necrosis by improved understanding of pedicle use. Nevertheless, patients should still be made aware that this is a major surgical procedure.

FACE-LIFT

Patients may gain great psychological benefit from face-lift, but care must be taken to ensure that the patient's goals are realistic and that they do not expect to become a 'different person'. There are many procedures for rhytidectomy but laser, chemical peels, fat injections and botulinum toxin have fairly transient effects, while surgical lifts are more resilient in rejuvenating appearance.

An idea of the effect of a lift is obtained by gentle fingertip traction on the skin in the malar and temporal areas, although the nasolabial fold is never entirely eliminated. Incisions are placed behind the hairline and in the crease anterior to the ear to camouflage them, although care should be taken in excessively coloured hair because this is brittle and tends to break off around the suture line. This may be an indication for endoscopically assisted lifts, and increasingly brow lifts are performed in this manner. Patients must be warned that massive weight loss and smoking are disastrous after face-lift due to the loss of tension and slowed healing, respectively.

Traditionally, surgery has involved subcutaneous dissection with skin flaps advanced from zygomatic cervicofacial and temporal areas with resection of skin. Recently, a more effective

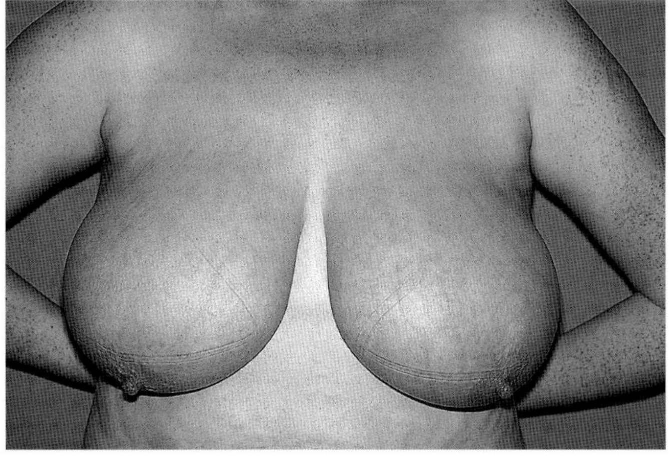

a

b

Figure 9.22 Bilateral breast reduction: (**a**) before and (**b**) after.

technique has been employed to produce a deeper plane of benefit. The platysma of the neck and the superficial musculo-aponeurotic system of the face are included in the flaps and provide increased support to the lift.[37]

BOTULINUM TOXIN

Botulinum toxin is an extremely potent toxin, secreted by *Clostridium* bacteria, that irreversibly blocks acetylcholine receptors in muscle, leading to paralysis. Clinically the effect lasts around 3 months as new receptors are generated. Its action has been exploited for many years in treating facial muscle spasm and in cerebral palsy limbs. More recently, it has found notoriety in cosmetic surgery in treatment of hyperhidrosis and facial wrinkles. Care should be taken when injecting the toxin in the face, and a good knowledge of muscle anatomy is essential to avoid eyelid ptosis.

AUGMENTATION MAMMOPLASTY

Some women have a loss of breast tissue following pregnancy and breast-feeding, while others may have breast asymmetry. The improvement in self confidence produced by augmentation can be gratifying as the patient's body image is restored. The size of implant to be used will largely be determined by the amount of available skin. It is not possible to put a very large implant into a completely flat chest, and conversely a ptotic breast requires a large implant to take up the excess skin.

The implants themselves are made of a pliable silicone envelope containing silicone gel. The skin pocket can be enlarged using an expander, but these usually need to be replaced with a standard implant at a later procedure.

There has been much controversy over the safety of silicone prostheses, and the term *silicone disease* has been introduced to describe the purported detrimental effects of silicone. There is no evidence that silicone disease has any scientific basis, and there is good evidence that silicone bears no association to the incidence of breast cancer or any autoimmune disease.[33] The Chief Medical Officer in the UK has never had any reason to restrict the use of silicone gel implants.

Breast implants can be inserted through a submammary, axillary, circumareolar or transareolar approach. In Great Britain the submammary is most common. Most implants are placed in a subglandular plane, in the layer of loose areolar tissue that separates the breast from the underlying pectoralis muscle, but in thinner patients the submuscular pocket is used. The main complication used to be the development of a firm capsule, but new, textured implant technology has reduced this form of scarring.

Congenital problems may also be treated with augmentation. Hypoplasia or aplasia of the breast in association with hypoplasia or absence of the muscles of the chest wall and brachysyndactyly of the hand (Poland's syndrome) is a rare problem and reason for referral for augmentation or reconstruction. Congenital tubular breasts are more common and are characterized by a constricted breast base and herniation of the areolae to give a Snoopy nose shape. These breasts may also be treated with insertion of breast implants together with resection of excess areolar skin.

FUNCTIONAL ANATOMY OF THE SKIN

The skin is the largest organ of the human body. It is multi-functional and essential to life. Skin is a physical barrier to both dehydration and invasion by infection and toxins. However, skin is also unique in that it provides an important route of interaction with the environment by sensory perception, including fine touch, pain, temperature and vibration.

The skin is an active homeostatic organ controlling body temperature by the regulation of flow through cutaneous capillary beds and by eccrine sweat gland perfusion. It also has a regulatory role in salt and water control. As a closed keratinized surface, it limits body fluid loss and influences temperature control through regulated saline sweat production by the eccrine glands controlled by neuroendocrine mechanisms. Skin also has a hormone function that is essential in vitamin D synthesis: ultraviolet light converts dihydrocholesterol to vitamin D_3, which then undergoes hepatic and renal hydroxylation to potent vitamin D. However, ultraviolet radiation also destroys cutaneous proteins and may injure DNA and lead to tumour formation. Melanocytes produce melanin pigment to provide a degree of protection, while enzyme mechanisms exist to repair genomic damage.

Different areas of the body demonstrate a wide variation in structure and function. The back skin is 10 times thicker than that of the eyelid. Similarly, the hairless skin of the palm, with its profuse ridges and sweat glands, is in sharp contrast to the sebaceous and hairy skin of the scalp. However, skin throughout the body shares the same basic features (Fig. 9.23).

EPIDERMIS

The epidermis is the external aspect of skin and consists of a stratified, keratinized, squamous epithelium. It comprises four distinct layers: the basal cell layer (stratum basale), the prickle cell layer (stratum spinosum), the granular cell layer (stratum granulare), and the keratin layer (stratum corneum). These layers vary in appearance in different areas of the body. The skin

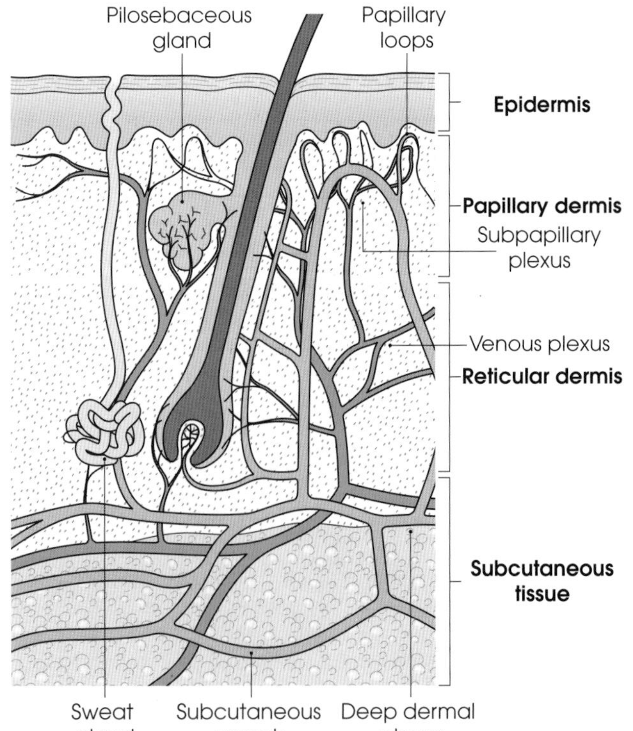

Figure 9.23 Structure of the skin.

appendages (hair follicles, sebaceous glands, sweat glands and nails) are all derived from epidermis and have the potential to reconstitute the skin.

Keratinocytes are the dominant cell type. They develop from basal cells and show a progressive increase in keratin content with loss of their nuclei, so that the most superficial keratin layer itself consists of flat dead cells that are lost through desquamation.

In addition to keratinocytes, the epidermis contains three types of clear cell: melanocytes, Langerhans cells and Merkel cells.

Melanocytes are derived from neuroectoderm, in the basal cell layer of the epidermis, and comprise 10% of the cell population. The number of melanocytes in white and black races is the same, but in darker skin and in freckles more melanin is produced by each cell. Melanocytes supply the surrounding keratinocytes with melanin through their dendritic processes. The pigmented keratinocytes serve to protect the underlying basal cell layer from the effects of ultraviolet radiation.

Langerhans cells are found in the suprabasal layers of the epidermis in similar numbers to melanocytes. Langerhans cells are derived from bone marrow and are related to macrophages. They function in immunosurveillance by processing antigens, either viral or neoplastic, and present them in a form that is recognized by T lymphocytes.

Merkel cells are present in small numbers in the basal layer of the epidermis. They cannot be identified by routine histological staining but can be seen with silver stains. They are thought to be epithelial neuroendocrine cells that act with peripheral nerve endings as slowly adapting mechanoreceptors and are responsible for tactile stereognosis.

HAIR

Adult scalp hair goes through a cycle of growth: anagen, a stage of active growth that lasts 3 years; catagen, a stage of regression lasting 3 weeks; and telogen, a resting period lasting 3 months.

Invagination of the epidermis gives rise to the outer root sheath of the hair follicle that contains the hair bulb. The cells of the hair bulb develop into the inner root sheath and the hair shaft. The outer root sheath is produced by invagination of the epidermis and resembles the superficial epidermis in its upper portion. A sebaceous duct opens into every hair follicle to lubricate and maintain the hair shaft. Each follicle is surrounded by a vascular fibrous tissue sheath into which the erector pili muscle is inserted and allows the hair to stand on end. The outer layer of the hair shaft is a cuticle of overlapping cells originating from a cortex of growing cells that lose their nuclei and keratinize. These in turn surround an inner medulla that is only partially keratinized.

Hair colour is determined by the quantity of melanin produced by melanocytes present in the basal layer of the hair bulb. Curly hair is formed by genetically determined convolutions in the hair follicle. In humans, the hair serves both a decorative and a small protective function. However, follicle cells are of enormous importance as a source of epidermal regeneration following superficial traumatic skin loss, as occurs in dermal burns and at the donor sites of skin grafts.

SEBACEOUS GLANDS

Sebaceous glands secrete a protective coating of mixed lipids known as sebum into the hair follicle via the sebaceous duct. Sebaceous glands are holocrine glands, the secretions of which are formed by disintegration of the cells adjacent to the lumen. In some areas of the body these glands are not associated with hairs, such as on the labia minora, the areola of the breast, and as Montgomery's tubercles around the nipple. The Meibomian glands of the eyelids are modified sebaceous glands.

ECCRINE SWEAT GLANDS

Eccrine glands produce sweat that is similar in composition to plasma; they have a primary heat-regulating function, although sweating also occurs in response to mental stress. Eccrine glands are present in greatest numbers on the soles of the feet and palms of the hands but occur everywhere on the body except the lips, the nail beds, the labia minora, and the glans of the penis.

The secretory part of the gland lies in the lower part of the dermis, at the junction with the subcutaneous fat, and is surrounded by a discontinuous outer layer of myoepithelial cells that aids secretion by contractile activity.

APOCRINE SWEAT GLANDS

Apocrine glands are limited to the axillae, anogenital region and breast. They occur in a modified form in the external auditory meatus as ceruminous glands and in the eyelid as Moll's glands. They become functional at puberty and may have a sexual role. Their basic structure is similar to the eccrine gland, but they lie more superficially in the subcutaneous fat. Gland secretion of cell contents is by formation of a cap of cytoplasm at the apex of the cell that becomes detached.

NAILS

The nail is a tough plate of keratinized cells that originate from the germinal matrix under the nail fold (Fig. 9.24). The distal portion of the germinal matrix is visible as the pale lunula, to which the nail plate is only loosely adherent. Thereafter the nail plate is firmly adherent to the underlying nail bed, so that an injury to the fingertip frequently leaves the nail attached to the bed but avulses it out of the nail fold. Nail bed injuries are common in toddlers exploring closing doors. Minimal damage can be treated conservatively, but permanent nail deformity may

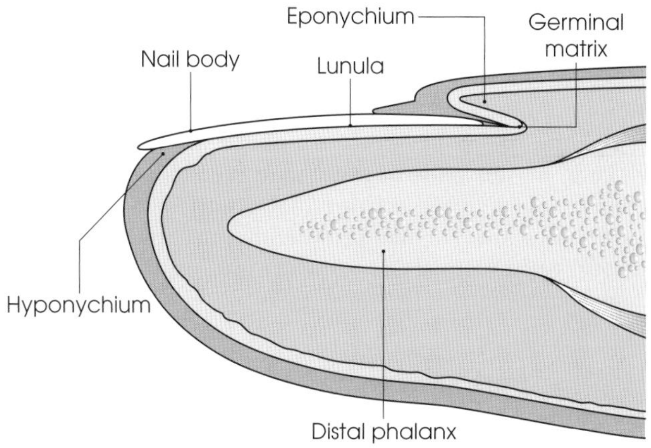

Figure 9.24 The structure of the nail and nail fold.

result without surgical intervention in more severe crush injuries. Nails grow at approximately 0.1 mm a day, although the rate of growth varies with age, site, season, nutrition and disease. Nails support the finger pulp and are important in initiating pinch, especially where small objects are involved.

DERMIS

The dermis is a highly specialized component of skin, and it consists of a collagen and elastic fibre scaffold surrounded by ground substance containing the vascular, neural and cellular elements that support the overlying epidermis. It is divided into two layers: the papillary dermis and the deeper reticular dermis. The papillary dermis is a narrow band lying immediately under the rete ridges of the epidermis, and comprises fine collagen and elastic fibres that are loosely and irregularly arranged. The reticular dermis is responsible for the skin thickness, and the collagen and elastic fibres are organized in thick bundles that lie parallel to the skin surface. These fibres produce the lines of skin cleavage, or relaxed skin tension lines, as demonstrated by Langer.[4]

The primary dermal cell type is the fibroblast, which generates collagen into the ground substance. Collagen turnover is constant and is greater under tension or mechanical stress. Fibroblasts also generate elastin, and these proteins form a matrix embedded in ground substance, which consists of glycosaminoglycans and proteoglycans.

The neural component comprises sensory and autonomic nerves as free nerve endings and special end organs: Pacinian corpuscles detect pressure and vibration, and Meissner's corpuscles and Merkel cell hair discs both appreciate touch sensation.

The vascular network of the dermis comprises a subdermal plexus feeding a more superficial papillary plexus just deep to the epidermis. Veins have a similar arrangement but include a third, mid-dermal plexus. Inflow to the subdermal plexus is from vessels originating beneath the deep fascia and running through the subdermal fat. These vessels pass almost vertically to supply a narrow area of skin, or are angulated longitudinally and in concert with the cutaneous nerves, giving branches to supply a larger skin area. They may be reinforced by anastomoses with branches from other similar vertically oriented subfascial vessels, and may course either through muscles or around them.[5]

The subdermal fatty tissue is a discrete layer of the integument distinct from perineural or perivascular fat, and comprises fat lobules separated by fibrous septa running from the dermis superficially to the deep fascia. Cutaneous nerves and vessels pass in these septa, but the capillary supply to the fat cells lies within each lobule. The epidermis has no blood supply and is nourished by diffusion from the underlying dermis.

Unlike the epidermis, which is replaced by mitosis from the basal layer of the pilosebaceous units, the dermis does not regenerate. Accordingly, scarring may occur following injuries where dermis is lost. This may prove aesthetically and functionally disastrous when dermal loss is extensive, as occurs in full-thickness burn injury.

THE SUBDERMAL INTEGUMENT: FASCIA

The deep fascia consists of two different types. Trunk fascia covers muscle and is relatively distensible. In contrast, limb fascia covers muscle and forms compartments that are relatively inelastic. The deep fascia of the limbs prevents bowstringing of tendons, is continuous with joint capsules, and gives rise to muscular attachments. It therefore has a well-developed blood supply in the form of fascial plexuses that are exploited in the designing of fasciocutaneous flaps for limb reconstruction.

THE MANAGEMENT OF WOUNDS

ACUTE WOUNDS

Acute wounds should not be considered in isolation. It is important to examine the patient carefully to ensure that there are no other injuries in addition to the obvious.

A wound constitutes a break in the epithelial integrity of the skin. Wounds can be classified in a number of ways, for example clean, dirty, infected, partial or full thickness, those with a defined edge or an ill-defined edge, and those with or without skin loss. Surgical wounds can be specifically classified as clean, clean–contaminated, contaminated and dirty. The multiple causes of wounds result in a wide range of clinical presentations and subsequent behaviour. This range in character of wounds renders clinical trials of wound care difficult to design with scientific objectivity and has resulted in a broad range of wound products and clinical therapies. In addition, the explosion in knowledge of the basic science of wound healing has ushered in a range of biological growth factors and chemical wound manipulations that are of dubious clinical benefit. Given the multiple molecular mechanisms involved, it is unlikely that any single successful therapy to accelerate wound healing will be developed.

Optimum wound healing will occur only when the wound is clean, free of infection, and in the presence of adequate nutritional substances. Trauma patients and those post surgery are often in a hypercatabolic state, and therefore have much higher nutritional requirements. Certain systemic illnesses, such as anaemia, diabetes, obesity and cancer, often lead to wound complications and delayed healing. Any deficiencies must be recognized early and corrected as far as possible. Iatrogenic factors, including chemotherapy and radiotherapy, may also retard healing. Failure of wounds to heal may therefore be the result of either systemic or local factors.

SYSTEMIC FACTORS

Nutrition

The nutritional state of the patient may have a major impact in determining the success of the healing process. Malnutrition causes depression of both the immune system and the inflammatory response, increasing the risk of wound infection and delayed healing. A deficiency in protein may inhibit collagen formation and so inhibit the regaining of tensile strength. Sulphur-containing amino acids such as methionine seem to be particularly important, and increasing the intake of this amino acid alone can partially offset the effects of a low protein intake.

There is some evidence that the A, C and E vitamins are particularly important in wound healing. Vitamin A increases epithelial cell turnover. The active form, retinoic acid, acts as a typical steroid hormone and binds to chromatin in the nucleus to increase the synthesis of proteins controlling epithelial cell growth and differentiation. Oral vitamin A therapy stimulates collagen deposition and increases wound tensile strength; topical therapy accelerates wound re-epithelialization. The benefits of vitamin C have been long established and can be summarized as accelerating maturation of fibroblasts contributing to the higher structure of the extracellular matrix, and stimulating angiogenesis. Specifically, vitamin C is a coenzyme for lysine and proline hydroxylase involved in collagen synthesis, and a deficiency leads to inhibition of secretion of collagen fibres by fibroblasts. Of note, dietary loading does not boost supranormal healing. Vitamin E increases the breaking strength of preoperatively irradiated wounds and neutralizes lipid peroxidation, limiting levels of free radicals and thus oxidative tissue damage. Studies differ regarding its effects on collagen synthesis.

Zinc is a ubiquitous component of enzyme systems important to wound-healing physiology. Low zinc levels contribute to reduction in fibroblast and epithelial proliferation, and patients with chronic wounds may benefit from supplementation.

Age

Wound tensile strengths and healing rates decrease with age. This may be a function of reduced metabolic activity and increased susceptibility to insult. However, degradation of the dermal components of skin with resulting loss of elasticity will follow cumulative effects of sun exposure.

Smoking

Nicotine and other components in cigarette smoke act as potent vasoconstrictors. This reduces perfusion and oxygenation to wounds. Smoking is also known to have a negative effect on the immune system, and smokers are more susceptible to wound infection. Carbon monoxide found in cigarette smoke causes carboxyhaemoglobin levels to rise and further decreases the amount of oxyhaemoglobin available to the tissues. Patients should be advised to cease smoking at least 6 weeks before reconstructive procedures. Nicotine substitutes such as gum and patches have a lesser, but still detrimental, effect.

Steroid therapy

High-dose or prolonged courses of steroid therapy may significantly affect wound healing. Corticosteroids inhibit the action of wound macrophages, which are essential to all stages of wound healing, particularly those involved in the demolition and organization phases. Acute inflammation and the handling of bacteria are also impaired. Deficient wound healing and wound infection is more common. Fibroblast function and collagen synthesis are also compromised by steroids, as are myofibroblast-mediated wound contraction and angiogenesis.[52] Non-steroidal anti-inflammatory agents at therapeutic doses have also been shown to significantly reduce collagen synthesis by the prostaglandin pathway, but this is probably not significant in clinical practice.

Chemotherapy and radiotherapy

Chemotherapeutic agents usually decrease fibroblast activity and reduce wound contraction.[53] Accordingly, adjuvant systemic chemotherapy should not commence until at least 2 weeks after surgery. Acute radiation injury is characterized by a vasculitis, intravascular stasis and small-vessel occlusion. In addition, direct irreversible fibroblast damage occurs to also compromise wound healing.

Diabetes mellitus

In diabetes mellitus, polymorphonuclear phagocyte function is impaired, interfering with the acute inflammatory reaction. There is increased incidence of peripheral vascular disease affecting both medium and small vessels, which reduces the blood supply to healing tissues. Diabetic neuropathy reduces sensation to touch and pain, increasing the chance of wound development. Skin ulceration commonly acts as a source of infection. When diabetes is poorly controlled, higher blood and tissue sugar levels encourage bacterial growth.

LOCAL FACTORS

Oxygenation

Fibroblasts are oxygen-sensitive and will not generate collagen synthesis at tissue oxygen tensions of less than 40 mmHg. It has been reported that hyperoxygenation improves collagen synthesis that is directly proportional to the tensile strength of the wound. Hyperbaric oxygenation chambers have been used to improve wound healing, but this is not in general use. Oxygenation also improves host defence mechanisms against microbial infection and may elevate wound re-epithelialization rates. Hypoxia has been reported to be the most common cause of wound infection and failure to heal. Oxygen tension in the healing wound is affected by many variables, including the oxygen fraction in inspired air, the oxygen–haemoglobin saturation dynamics in red cells of adequate number and function, presence of anaemia, and the efficiency of the circulatory system and microcirculation. Any of these mechanisms may be malfunctioning in the susceptible patient.

Denervation

Denervated skin, insensitive to pain, may result in unnoticed wounds that propagate and ulcerate faster and heal more slowly than sensate areas. The classic example of this phenomenon is leprosy.

Presence of infection or a foreign body

The presence of infection or a foreign body will increase the intensity and duration of the inflammatory response. An infected wound stimulates an inflammatory response that is aimed at demolition and bacteriolysis rather than regeneration and repair. Angiogenesis, granulation and epithelialization are impaired by this catabolic response made worse by infection.

Excess mobility

Excess mobility in any tissue will impair healing and prolong the time to full recovery.

Vascular supply

The degree of arterial perfusion and the efficacy of venous drainage play key roles in healing of wounds. In patients with long-standing arterial disease, a trivial injury may give rise to a disproportionate degree of tissue damage, and healing may be delayed or even completely inhibited, resulting in a chronic non-healing ulcer. Impairment of venous drainage will also lead to chronic wounds. Microangiopathy secondary to chronic diabetes may also significantly reduce healing capacity.

REFERENCES

52. Rohrich RJ, Robinson JB. Sel Read Plast Surg 1992; 7: 1–42
53. Rockwell WB, Cohen IK, Erhlich HP. Plast Reconstr Surg 1989; 84: 827–883

Table 9.3 Types of dressing

Dressing type	Use	Example(s)
Dry dressings	Suture lines	Mepore, Steristrips
Film dressings	Suture lines, donor sites	Opsite, Tegaderm
Tulle gras	Skin grafts, surgical wounds	Jelonet
Non-adherent silicone dressing	Skin grafts, second-degree burns, newly granulating wounds, painful wounds	Mepitel
Hydrocolloids	Ulcerated shallow wounds	Granuflex, Duoderm.
Hydrogels	Dry or necrotic wounds, granulating wounds	Intrasite
Alginates	Exudative, open, often deep wounds	Aquacel
Bead dressings	Sloughy, open, often deep wounds	Iodosorb

DRESSING TECHNOLOGY

Over the past 40 years, great advances have been made in understanding the complex processes of wound healing. Different wounds require different dressings. Some simple, closed suture lines require only adhesive paper tape, such as Steristrips, or an absorbent dressing with an adhesive border, such as Mepore. More complex, exuding wounds that are at risk of secondary infection require more extensive management and possibly the use of vacuum dressings. Dressings are now being made to provide the requirements of the ideal wound environment and to include specific epidermal growth factors.

The requirements for the ideal surgical dressing can be summarized as follows.

- Be absorbent and able to remove excess exudate.
- Maintain a moist environment and aid own tissues to debride any necrotic material to allow healing.
- Prevent trauma to underlying healing granulation tissue, particularly during dressing changes.
- Be leak-proof and able to prevent secondary infection, especially when the dressing is soiled or wet.
- Maintain temperature and gaseous exchange.
- Allow pain-free, simple dressing changes.
- Require less frequent dressing changes.
- Be odourless, comfortable and cosmetically acceptable.
- Be cheap.

Much research is undertaken by drug companies each year to improve the quality of dressings available. Furthermore, many problems may stem from lack of knowledge on behalf of medical staff as to the appropriate use of these dressings.

The different types of dressing may be divided into several categories, as shown in Table 9.3.

Dry dressings

Dry dressings are simple absorbent dressings used for post-operative wounds to protect suture lines. They can also be used as a secondary dressing to hydrogel dressings.

Tulle gras dressings

Tulle is a fine cloth named after the French town where it was originally produced, and *gras* is French for grease. The modern Tulle dressing, for example Jelonet, comprises an open-weave fabric with a knotted structure to help maintain its integrity, coated with a soft paraffin mixture to prevent sticking. This is designed to stay on the surface of the wound for 1–3 days, allowing exudates to pass through to an absorbent secondary dressing.

Mepitel is a newer dressing, which consists of fine mesh netting coated in a hydrophobic silicone gel. It does not dry out, is non-adherent, and can be applied, removed and reapplied with minimal discomfort or disturbance to the wound site and healing tissue. It is indicated for use on skin grafts, second-degree burns, and fragile newly granulating wounds. It can be left in place over the wound bed for several days.

Alginates or fibre dressings

Alginates, which include Aquacel, are indicated for use on all types of exuding wounds. They are available as ribbons or strips, suitable for packing large cavity wounds. Most will require a secondary dressing to retain them in the wound. They are constructed from interwoven strands of calcium alginate, mixed in some brands with varying proportions of sodium alginate. On contact with wound exudate the fibres turn to gel, trapping moisture at the wound surface to create a moist environment and making them easy to remove. They are unsuitable for dry or necrotic wounds. Kaltostat is an alginate but unsuitable for use on exudative wounds. It is indicated where haemostasis is required, for example on donor sites and other raw surfaces.

Hydrocolloids

Hydrocolloids are suitable for shallow wounds with a light to medium amount of exudates. They are not suitable for infected wounds. Hydrocolloids consist of a wafer constructed from a thin layer of polyurethane film with an adhesive of varying thickness containing gelatine, pectin and carboxymethylcellulose. The film is impermeable to water and micro-organisms. The wound exudate combines with the ingredients of the adhesive to form a gel, which promotes moist wound healing. Examples of hydrocolloids include Granuflex and Duoderm. They are unsuitable for wounds nearing the stage of epithelialization because they can lead to over-granulation.

Bead dressings

Bead dressings are formed of a paste made up from beads 0.1–0.3 mm in diameter with water and either an ointment base (Iodosorb) or a polyethylene glycol base (Debrisan). The beads are hydrophilic, giving absorbency to the dressing. Movement of the beads in the dressing causes bacteria and necrotic material to be picked up by the dressing. They are indicated for moist, sloughy wounds.

VACUUM-ASSISTED CLOSURE

Vacuum-assisted closure has represented the most significant advance in clinical wound management over the past decade. It

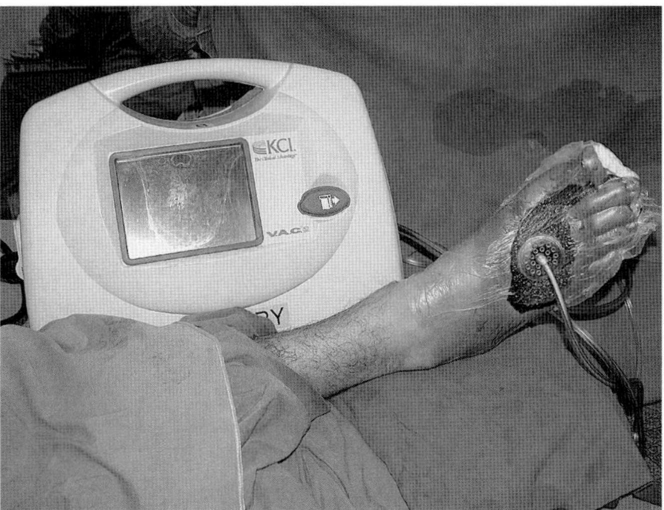

Figure 9.25 The vacuum-assisted closure pump.

was first demonstrated in pigs in 1988 and used on human wounds the following year. The vacuum-assisted closure pump system (Fig. 9.25) delivers a uniform, controlled, subatmospheric pressure to the wound surface. This promotes the removal of exudate, leading to tissue decompression enabling the arterioles in the wound bed to dilate. This in turn improves blood flow and the delivery of oxygen and nutrients to the wound. The improved circulation stimulates angiogenesis and encourages proliferation of granulation tissue that progressively fills the wound.[54] The negative pressure also draws the wound margins closer together. It is also reported that vacuum-assisted closure treatment leads to a significant reduction in bacterial count.

Indications for use include pressure sores, venous leg ulcers, dehisced wounds, surgical wounds and over-meshed skin grafts. Relative and absolute contraindications include patients with bleeding tendencies, patients on anticoagulants, cancer in the wound margins, presence of necrotic tissue, fistulae to organs or body cavities, and untreated osteomyelitis.

The vacuum-assisted closure system consists of the pump or negative-pressure unit, black dressing foam with a drainage tube fixed within the foam, and a semipermeable film-dressing drape. The foam is cut to size to fill the wound cavity, and the tubing is placed either on the foam or inside it. The film dressing is applied over the foam and the drainage tube to make an airtight seal to the surrounding skin. The drainage tube is then connected to the pump via the collection canister, and the pump is switched on. The pressure should be adjusted for patient comfort but is normally around 125 mmHg (range 50–175 mmHg). The programme can be continuous or intermittent. The dressing should be changed every 48 h unless the wound is infected (12 h) or a skin graft (simply remove after 5 days). The system can be switched off for short periods of time to allow a patient to attend to hygiene needs.

PRESSURE SORES

Pressure sores are a significant cause of morbidity, prolonged in-patient stay, and cost to the health service, estimated at £150 million per year in Great Britain. Their aetiology is multifactorial but includes prolonged weight bearing and mechanical shear forces on the soft tissue over bony prominences. This produces a resultant increase in the pressure across small blood vessels, reduced tissue perfusion, and ischaemic necrosis. Sores begin with tissue necrosis near the bony prominence and lead to a cone-shaped area of tissue breakdown with the apex at the skin surface.

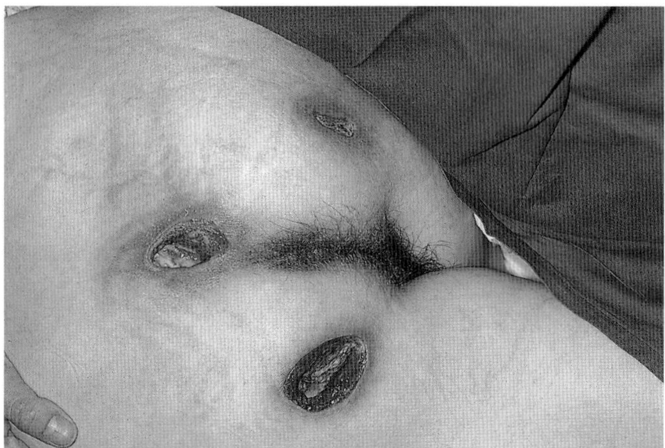

Figure 9.26 Sacral and bilateral ischial pressure sores.

The prevalence of pressure necrosis in the UK hospital population is 7–8%, with the majority occurring in patients over 70 years of age who are often malnourished. Immobility is the primary contributing factor, as well as prolonged periods of bed rest. Pressure sores are also commonly seen in younger patients with neurological injuries or spina bifida. Approximately 80% of paraplegic patients develop a pressure sore. Tissue damage is thought to occur when uninterrupted pressures of greater than 9.3 kPa are sustained,[55] but in healthy sitting people an inverse relationship occurs between tissue pressure and duration of tolerance.[56] Accordingly, the inability to change position puts patients at particular risk. This includes patients undergoing long operative procedures, with implications for patient positioning, especially when there is prolonged iatrogenic hypotension.

Shearing forces are of major importance, initiating tearing of vessels and connective tissue laminae of the subcutaneous fat. This produces subsequent thrombosis and haematoma. Tissue maceration from sweating and incontinence also further reduces tissue integrity.

The most common sites for pressure sores are the sacrum (43%), greater trochanter (12%), heel (11%), lateral malleolus (6%), and ischial tuberosity (5%) (Fig. 9.26). Occipital sores are not uncommon in the bedridden. The American National Pressure Ulcer Advisory Panel classification is the most established classification system in current use.

- Stage 1: non-blanchable erythema of intact skin.
- Stage 2: partial-thickness skin loss involving dermis and epidermis (shallow abrasion wound).
- Stage 3: full-thickness skin loss involving subcutaneous tissue, which may extend down to but not through underlying fascia (deep crater).
- Stage 4: full-thickness skin loss with extensive damage in muscle, bone or joint involvement.

REFERENCES

54. DeFranzo AJ, Argenta LC, Marks MW et al. Plast Reconstr Surg 2001; 108: 1184–1189
55. Kosiak M. Arch Phys Med Rehabil 1961; 42: 19–29
56. Barbanel JC. Prosthet Orthot Int 1991; 15: 225–231

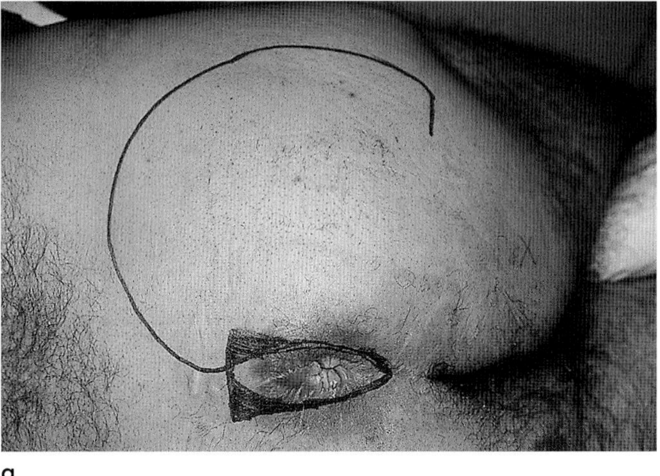
a

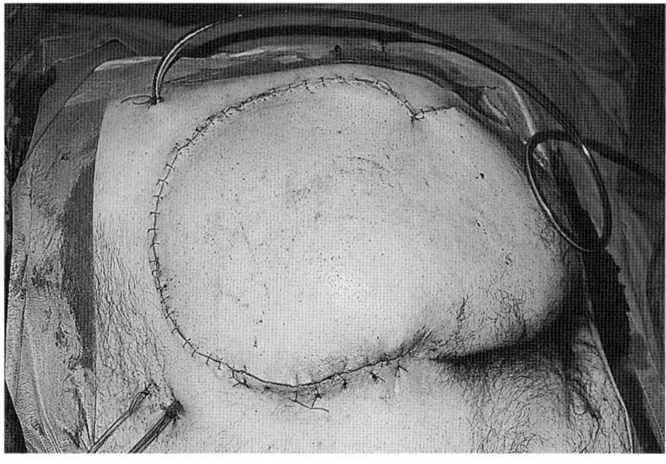
b

Figure 9.27 Gluteal rotation flap for sacral pressure sores: (**a**) before, (**b**) after.

This classification system contradicts a theoretical aetiology of pressure sores, namely that the final common pathway is ischaemic, and that muscle and fat are more poorly tolerant of ischaemia than the fascia or the skin. When pressure sores occur in sites where muscle covers bone, such as the sacrum and trochanters, muscle damage may precede any visible cutaneous signs.

Investigation of cutaneous blood flow with laser Doppler scanning shows reduced cutaneous blood flow over the sacral area compared with the gluteal area, when controlled pressure is applied.[57] An ischaemia–reperfusion injury may also result from continuous small changes in blood flow, and net increases in tissue pressure reduce venous and lymphatic outflow and thus clearance of toxic metabolites. Furthermore, the factors that are known to slow wound healing also contribute to the risk and severity of pressure necrosis.

Repeated laser duplex fluximetry and measurement of serum phosphokinase levels may indicate the onset of pressure necrosis but have yet to replace clinical vigilance.

Prophylactic clinical care is essential. It includes frequent turning (2–4 hourly), skin inspection, massage and toileting. Specially designed aids, mattresses and cushions to even pressure gradients may further reduce risk. A variety of high-cost air-fluidized, alternating air, static air and water mattresses are available and demand evaluation by well-designed clinical trials. Air- and gel-filled cushions are used in wheelchairs to reduce the incidence of ischial sores, where a high body weight to dependent area ratio necessarily occurs.

MANAGEMENT OF PRESSURE SORES

When preventive care fails, management is first conservative and surgical only if required. It is also essential to appreciate the multidisciplinary management of these complex wounds. The surgeon may play only a small role because those of the district nurse, occupational therapist and dietician are of greater importance. The principles are to improve tissue perfusion and oxygenation, correct anaemia and relieve pressure. Wound healing is further optimized by treating infection and providing optimal nutritional support. There is no place for prophylactic antibiotics. There is a need for evaluation of the wide variety of topical dressings, agents from inorganic chemicals to enzymes and growth factors, and the use of hyperbaric oxygen, vacuum-assisted closure pumps, hydrotherapy, ultrasound and electrotherapy. Surgery should not be considered until all correctable indices have been optimized and preventive measures are in place in the ward (i.e. low air-loss mattress) and essential equipment at home.

Surgical options for wound closure include a variety of fascial and composite muscle-containing flaps for each site. Usually the simplest appropriate procedure is selected because these patients may have compromised primary healing, and to appreciate that the procedure may be palliative rather than curative. Large flaps should be used that can be rerotated in case of pressure sore recurrence and that do not preclude the use of other flaps in the area (Fig. 9.27). The cavity produced by the debridement and ostectomy of a pressure sore must be filled by perfused tissue, usually muscle, to introduce a blood supply and encourage healing. It is a misconception that muscle flaps provide padding over a pressure point, because muscle is more vulnerable to ischaemia than the overlying skin. Scars that result from these operations should not be placed over pressure points because they are liable to repeated dehiscence. Where possible, muscle tone and skin sensation should be preserved and the post-operative care of the patient directed towards minimizing the risk of recurrence. Recurrence of pressure necrosis is depressingly common unless aetiological factors can be corrected.

HYPERTROPHIC SCARS AND KELOIDS

A scar is the natural result of the body's attempt to repair an area of epithelial skin loss. There is an enormous individual variation in the degree of scar formation, and it remains unclear as to why some people scar badly and others do not.

Hypertrophic scars and keloids both occur as a result of an exaggerated wound healing response. Hypertrophic scars develop soon after injury. There is excessive deposition of scar tissue, such that the scar is raised above the level of the surrounding skin but does not extend beyond the limits of the original incision. Usually these scars improve with time, although

REFERENCE

57. Schubert V, Fragrell B. Clin Physiol 1989; 9: 535–545

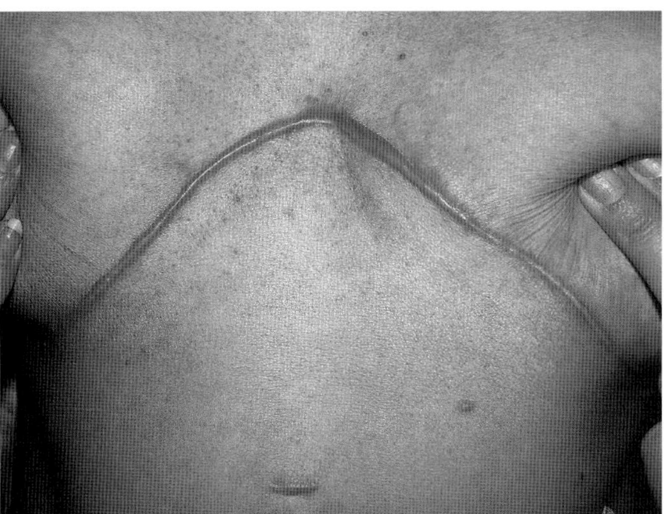

Figure 9.28 A hypertrophic scar.

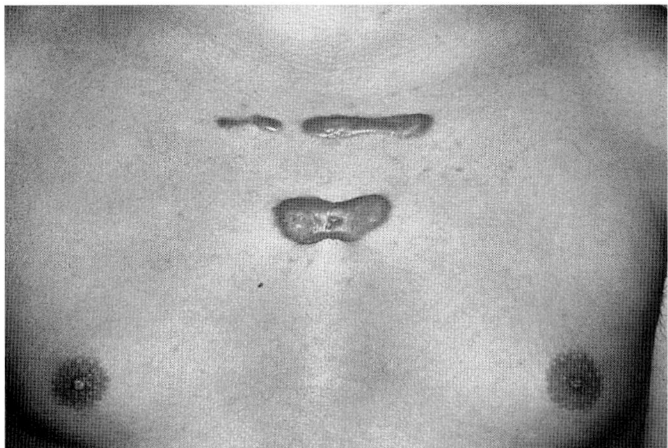

Figure 9.29 A keloid scar.

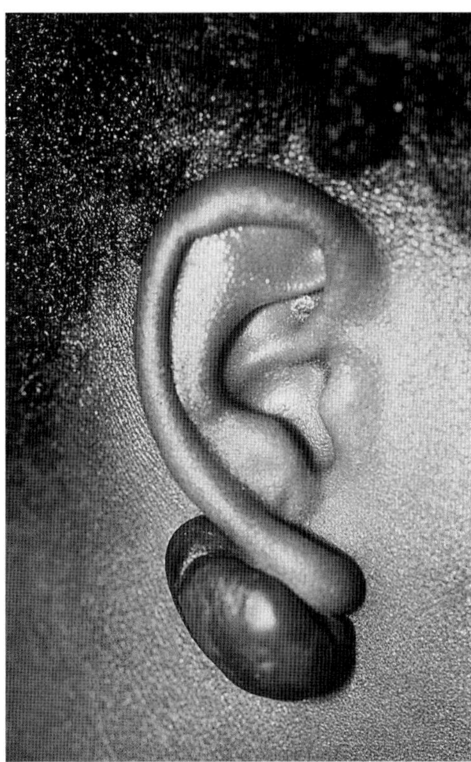

Figure 9.30 A keloid in the ear lobe following piercing.

it may take up to 18 months. In contrast, keloid scars progressively enlarge beyond the limits of the original incision to involve normal skin. They can be grossly elevated, disfiguring lesions that rarely regress spontaneously and are very difficult to treat. They can also prove painful and itchy, particularly in warmer weather. Certain areas of the body are more likely to develop hypertrophic scars or keloid (Figs 9.28 and 9.29), such as the presternal area; the deltoid area, most often following BCG vaccination; and the ear lobe, following piercing (Fig. 9.30).

Keloids were originally described in 2500 BC but were officially named by Alibert in 1806; *cheloide* derives from the Greek *chele*, meaning crab claw, to describe the lateral growth of keloids. Keloids are more common in dark-skinned races, where the incidence has been reported as between 4.5 and 16%. They usually occur in younger patients between the ages of 10 and 30 years. The higher incidence in younger individuals may reflect skin of greater youthful turgor associated with a higher rate of collagen synthesis.

Considerable, and unsuccessful, efforts have been made to elucidate the aetiology of keloids. Significant factors include a genetic predisposition coupled with some form of skin trauma, often minor, such as insect bite or spot. Wounds associated with infection, trauma, burns or tension have a greater incidence of both scar hypertrophy and keloid formation. The predisposition of pigmented races to keloidal scarring has been attributed to abnormal melanocyte physiology, consistent with the observation that areas of low melanocyte density (such as the palms and soles of the feet) have low incidence of abnormal scarring. Keloid formation has been associated with endocrine factors because they frequently occur during puberty or pregnancy and resolve after the menopause. Clinically, the major concern for the individual is the appearance, although they can cause symptoms such as itching and pain.

Under the light microscope, keloid and hypertrophic scars are indistinguishable, each demonstrating dense swirling collagen fibrils and a dense epidermal cell layer containing many fibroblasts and mucinous ground substance. Under the electron microscope, the collagen arrangement of keloid scars can be seen to be more irregular, with a reduction in interfibrillar distance compared with hypertrophic scars. Discrete collagen bundles do not occur; the fibres are haphazardly arranged and not parallel to the epithelial surface as in a normal scar.

Biochemically, there are also differences between the two. Proline hydroxylase activity correlates well with the rate of collagen synthesis, and results have shown its activity is higher in keloids than in hypertrophic and normal scars. Collagenase activity has been shown to be higher in both keloids and hypertrophic scars, indicating that in both total collagen turnover is increased.

MANAGEMENT OF HYPERTROPHIC AND KELOID SCARS (Box 9.2)

Keloids are notoriously difficult to treat, and despite the variety of therapies available the recurrence rates remain high. In contrast, hypertrophic scars respond better to treatment. Treatment options can be divided into non-surgical, surgical and combination therapy. Non-surgical methods can be further subdivided into physical and pharmacological therapy.

Box 9.2 Management options for hypertrophic and keloid scars

Non-surgical

Physical

- Mechanical pressure
- Silicone gel sheeting
- Radiation
- Cryotherapy
- Laser therapy

Chemical

- Intralesional corticosteroids
- Intralesional 5-fluorouracil
- Interferon
- Intralesional bleomycin
- Intralesional verapamil
- Nitric oxide
- Others

Surgical excision

- Intralesional

Combination therapy

- Surgery and pressure
- Surgery and intralesional steroids
- Surgery and radiation

Most hypertrophic scarring is treated conservatively. Hypertrophic scarring resulting from excessive wound tension or infection can be treated effectively with surgical excision combined with postoperative tape or silicone gel sheeting. Where the scar is bridging a flexure, correction of the contracture with techniques such as Z plasty improve both the appearance and mobility of the scar.

Surgery alone for keloid is associated with recurrence rates of between 45 and 100%, although this may be minimized using an intralesional approach. Surgical revision is therefore usually combined with adjuvant radiotherapy, mechanical methods or pharmacological methods. Combining surgery with steroid injections reduces the recurrence rate to less than 50%. Surgery and radiation further reduce recurrence to 10%.

Non-surgical approaches include mechanical pressure and the use of topical silicone gel. Pressure therapy has been used in the management of both hypertrophic scars and keloids since the 1970s and is particularly useful for hypertrophic burn scars. Several studies suggest that uniform, continuous pressure between 24 and 30 mmHg for 24 h a day for up to a year can have beneficial effects. Topical pressure hastens collagen maturation and flattens the scar. Failure occurs principally at sites of mobility where pressure cannot be maintained. Custom-made pressure garments are often worn continuously by postburn patients up to a year or more after injury.

Silicone gel sheeting is now a widely acceptable treatment adopted by many plastic surgeons. Results from randomized controlled trials demonstrate that it is a safe and effective option for both hypertrophic and keloid scars. It has been shown to decrease pain and itching as well as to lead to scar flattening, although the mode of action is unclear. It can be particularly useful in children and those patients who cannot tolerate the pain and discomfort of other methods.

Radiotherapy is usually used in combination with surgery for larger or recurrent resistant keloids. Although it has been used alone, recurrence rates of 50–100% have been noted and monotherapy is not recommended. The potential morbidity and risk of carcinogenesis after radiotherapy has limited its use to scars resistant to surgery, pressure and steroid therapy. The wound should be irradiated 24–48 h after surgery, usually with a single fraction of 8–9 Gy.

Intralesional injection of the steroid triamcinolone remains the first-line therapy for the treatment of small keloid scars (less than 2 cm). The mechanism of action remains unclear, although it is thought to lead to a decrease in normal collagen turnover. Results can often be dramatic, leading to obvious flattening and softening of the lesion. The steroid is injected into the substance of the keloid until it blanches. Injections should be on a regular basis every 4–6 weeks until flattening has occurred. This is often a painful procedure, and children may require a general anaesthetic. Side effects include skin atrophy, hypopigmentation and telangiectasia, and patients should be warned of these risks prior to embarking on a course of treatment. Recurrence rates of 9–50% are reported but are less when corticosteroids are combined with surgery.

New and more innovative therapies have been proposed. Laser therapy, particularly wavelength-specific lasers (YAG and pulsed dye), have been used with variable responses for the treatment of both hypertrophic scars and keloids, but lack of randomized controlled trials and limited follow-up mean that further studies are required. Interferon has been shown to increase collagen breakdown, and studies using intralesional injections of interferon resulted in significant rates of improvement of hypertrophic scars. Additionally, interferon injections were reported to be better than steroid injections at preventing postsurgical recurrence of keloid.

Intralesional 5-fluorouracil, alone as well as in combination with steroids, has been used successfully to treat hypertrophic scars and keloids but, as with other emerging therapies, requires further investigation. The cytotoxic antibiotic bleomycin has also shown good results leading to complete or significant flattening of hypertrophic scars and keloids following injection. Larger-scale prospective studies with appropriate follow-up are needed before these treatments can gain clinical acceptance. Other miscellaneous treatments include topical vitamin E, retinoic acid, colchicine and glycosaminoglycan gel; however, the evidence for these is anecdotal.

EXTRAVASATION INJURIES

An extravasation injury can be defined as the tissue damage caused by leakage of a solution from a vein into the surrounding tissue during intravenous administration. The resultant injury may lead to full-thickness skin loss, skin necrosis, and possible damage to underlying structures such as tendons, nerves and joints. In severe cases, where the vascularity is affected, amputation of the limb may even be necessary. Early identification and prompt, appropriate treatment is essential to reduce morbidity.

Extravasation injuries are a common problem, occurring in 0.1–0.7% of cytotoxic drug administrations. For those patients receiving chemotherapy there is a 4.7% incidence of extravasation. Commonly, agents leading to extravasation injury can be divided into three categories:

1. osmotically active solutions such as parenteral nutrition, calcium, potassium, bicarbonate or solutions of 10% dextrose or higher (extravasation of normal saline and 5% dextrose does not result in long-term tissue damage);

2. chemotherapeutic agents such as cisplatin, vincristine or doxorubicin; and
3. other agents, such as X-ray contrast as well as certain antibiotics and anaesthetic agents.

Certain groups of patients are more at risk of extravasation injury. Cancer patients and the elderly often have fragile skin and friable veins that are difficult to cannulate. Diabetic patients with peripheral neuropathy, intensive care patients, and babies on special care are more susceptible because they are unable to communicate pain easily. Erythema, swelling, blistering and discoloration of the overlying skin may be present. Early, firm induration and pain are indicative of changes that may lead to ulceration.

Common locations for cannulae resulting in injuries are dorsum of hand, forearm, cubital fossa, and dorsum of the foot, where there is little soft tissue coverage. Extravasation is usually the result of leakage around the original puncture site. When the flow of blood proximal and distal to the cannula becomes occluded, there is a rise in intraluminal pressure leading to leakage of fluid from the puncture site. If the infused fluid is acidic, this may cause phlebitis leading to vasoconstriction and impaired blood flow.

The damage caused varies in extent according to the nature and amount of drug infused. Many cytotoxic medications are also vesicants, and in addition to causing immediate injury may bind to tissue DNA. The drug can then be released slowly over a period of time, resulting in a gradual increase in ulcer size. Doxorubicin has been shown to remain in tissues for 5 months after extravasation, presenting late with extensive tissue destruction. Calcium and potassium infusions, in addition to their acidity and hypertonicity, may cause direct cellular damage by protein precipitation.

Several methods exist to treat extravasation injuries, all sharing similar aims to wash the agent out as soon as possible to prevent progression to tissue necrosis and ulceration.[58] The mainstay of treatment remains flushing the area with large volumes of saline to remove the extravasated material and liposuction to aspirate extravasated material. Hyaluronidase is an enzyme that breaks down hyaluronic acid and therefore reduces the viscosity of the connective tissue matrix to facilitate absorption and dispersal. It is injected locally as soon as possible and has been shown to help reduce damage from vinca alkaloids, calcium, potassium and dextrose. The use of ice and topical steroids has been suggested to minimize inflammation, although in many cases this is not a feature.

Patients referred late often already have well-demarcated areas of necrosis. These areas should be debrided extensively to create a healthy bed for flap or graft repair. Preventive measures should be adopted to minimize the number of extravasation injuries and include the use of a large central vein for administration, hypervigilance among specialist nursing staff, a clear treatment protocol, and early discussion with a plastic surgeon.

PROTOCOL FOR ACUTE MANAGEMENT OF EXTRAVASATION INJURIES

1. Stop the infusion immediately and remove 3–5 mL of blood back from the cannula.
2. Remove the cannula and mark out the area of extravasation. Apply ice or cold pack.
3. Infiltrate the area with 1500 units of hyaluronidase in 5 mL of 1% lidocaine (lignocaine).
4. Make several stab incisions around the area and flush using a syringe with a large volume of normal saline (500 mL). The saline should be injected through each incision in turn.
5. Elevate the area to minimize swelling and reapply the ice pack. Encourage movement.
6. Hydrocortisone cream can be applied topically twice daily if erythema is present.
7. Careful observation for pain, induration and necrosis for several days.
8. The patient's condition should be reviewed by a plastic surgeon.

BENIGN AND MALIGNANT SKIN TUMOURS

As noted earlier, skin is composed of many cell types. Benign and malignant tumours can arise from each of these cell types. Furthermore, some of the malignant lesions may prove to be very aggressive and associated with early metastasis and death. Accordingly, prevention and early diagnosis are important. Skin lesions may present in a variety of shapes, textures and colours. The same skin tumour may have a very different presentation in different individuals, or in different body sites of the same individual. It is therefore important to have a common language and set of descriptive terms applied to these lesions, both to facilitate communication between clinicians and to reduce confusion and anxiety for the patient. For brief definitions of common terms see Table 9.4.

NON-PIGMENTED LESIONS (BENIGN)

EPIDERMAL CYSTS

Epidermal cysts and trichilemmal cysts are also referred to as sebaceous cysts (Figs 9.31 and 9.32). Neither, however, is derived from sebaceous glands, and although they are clinically indistinguishable they can be separated histologically. Cysts are usually solitary and may occur at any age and at almost any site; they are most common, however, on the face, trunk, neck, extremities and scalp. They are thought to arise from hair follicles. Multiple cysts occur in Gardner's syndrome in association with intestinal polyposis, desmoid tumours and osteomas.[59]

An identical cyst occurs from traumatic implantation of epidermis, known as an implantation or inclusion dermoid cyst. Milia are also similar and present as small, white, superficial spots that can occur in large numbers on the face as an almost normal feature of newborn babies. Like epidermal cysts, they are derived from hair follicles. Epidermal cysts can be of almost any size and present as a round, smooth, firm to soft swelling that is attached to the skin. A punctum is normally present near the apex of the cyst, which may exhibit a plastic deformation that helps to distinguish it from a lipoma. Cysts can become infected, with subsequent discharge of foul-smelling, cheesy, keratinous debris contents. Treatment is by excision, although recurrence is possible if cyst lining is left behind. These lesions often arise on visible sites and can be extracted piecemeal through a 3-mm punch biopsy excision opening.

REFERENCES

58. Gault DT. Br J Plast Surg 1993; 46: 91–96
59. Lever WF, Schaumberg-Lever G. Histopathology of the Skin. JB Lippincott, Philadelphia, 1990: 670

Table 9.4 Skin lesion terminology

Term	Definition
Cyst	A tumour that contains fluid.
Hamartoma	An overgrowth of one or more cell types that are normal constituents of the organ in which they arise. The commonest examples are haemangiomas, lymphangiomas (see Ch. 10) and neurofibromas.
Macule	A flat, impalpable lesion (e.g. a port wine stain).
Naevus	A lesion present from birth, composed of mature structures normally found in the skin but present in excess or in an abnormal disposition. This type of lesion is also referred to as a hamartoma. The term naevus is also used to describe lesions comprising naevus cells, as in melanocytic or pigmented naevi.
Papilloma	A benign overgrowth of epithelial tissue.
Papule	A small, elevated lesion.
Plaque	An elevated area, usually larger than 2 cm across.
Pustule	A raised lesion that contains pus.
Tumour	Literally, a swelling. Commonly but inaccurately used to mean a malignant swelling.
Ulcer	An area of dissolution of an epithelial surface.
Vesicle	A small blister.

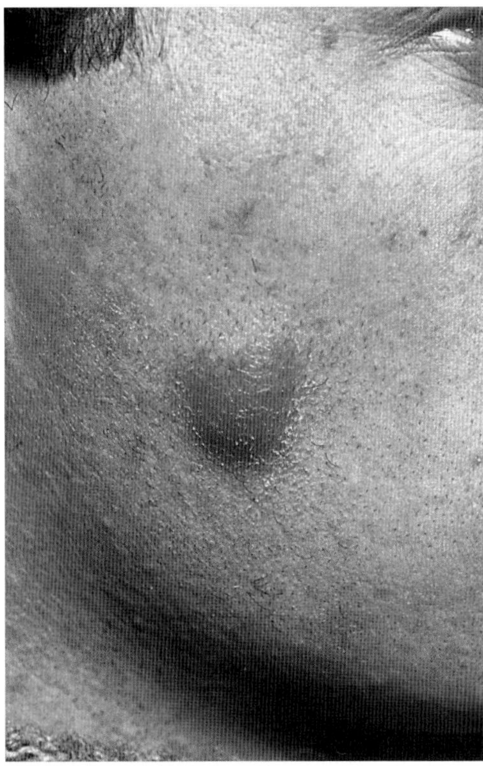

Figure 9.31 An epidermal cyst.

The proliferating trichilemmal cyst or tumour is usually solitary and, like the trichilemmal cyst, mainly occurs on the scalp. The tumour may reach a very large size and ulcerate, when it is called a Pott's peculiar tumour (Fig. 9.33), and may resemble a squamous carcinoma both clinically and histologically. The tumour nearly always behaves in a benign manner, although it can recur after excision.

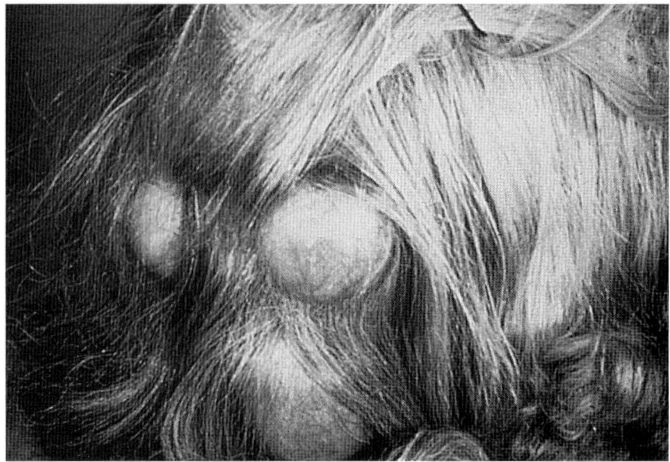

Figure 9.32 Multiple epidermal or trichilemmal cysts.

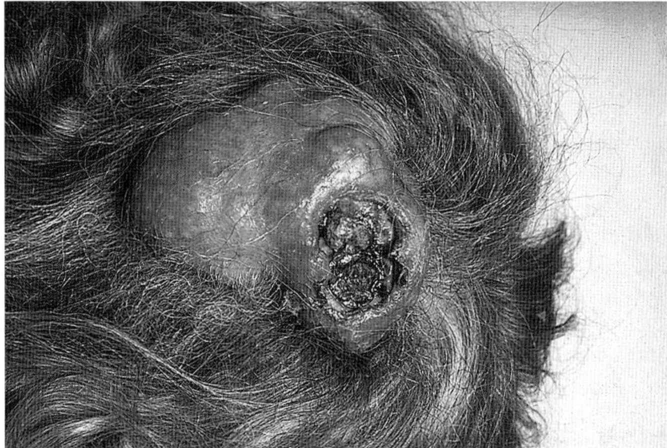

Figure 9.33 A Pott's peculiar tumour.

DERMOID CYSTS

Dermoid cysts are congenital subcutaneous cysts and are the result of the developmental inclusion of epidermis along lines of fusion. The cyst is lined by stratified squamous epithelium but, unlike the epidermal cyst, the wall also contains functioning epidermal appendages such as hair follicles, sweat glands and sebaceous glands. Common sites are the lateral and medial ends of the eyebrow, known as external and internal angular dermoid cysts (Fig. 9.34); the midline of the nose; sublingually; and the midline of the neck, perineum and sacrum.

Treatment consists of complete excision, but great care must be taken to establish the extent of the cyst prior to surgery. An external angular dermoid frequently creates a bony depression and rarely penetrates down to the dura. A nasal dermoid may present as a deceptively small superficial pit that is the only visible part of an extensive cyst that passes between the nasal bones towards the sphenoid sinus in a dumb-bell fashion. Skull radiographs and a CT scan may be indicated. Surgery needs appropriate planning, with specialist neurosurgical involvement if indicated. These are not cysts that should be excised by an inexperienced surgeon under local anaesthetic.

HAIR FOLLICLE TUMOURS

Trichofolliculomas and trichoepitheliomas present as firm, pink nodules, usually on the head and neck in early adult life. They are

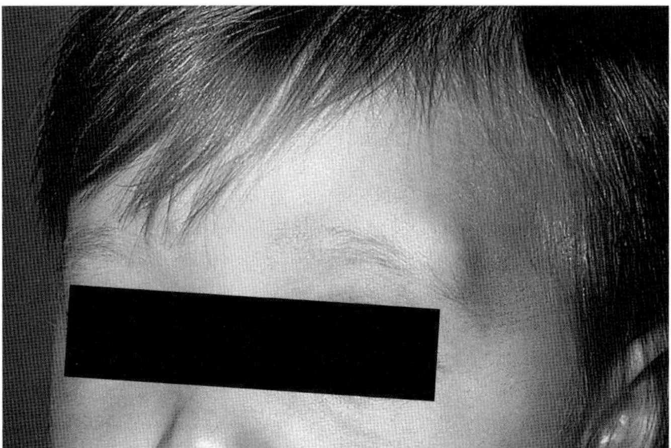

Figure 9.34 An external angular dermoid cyst.

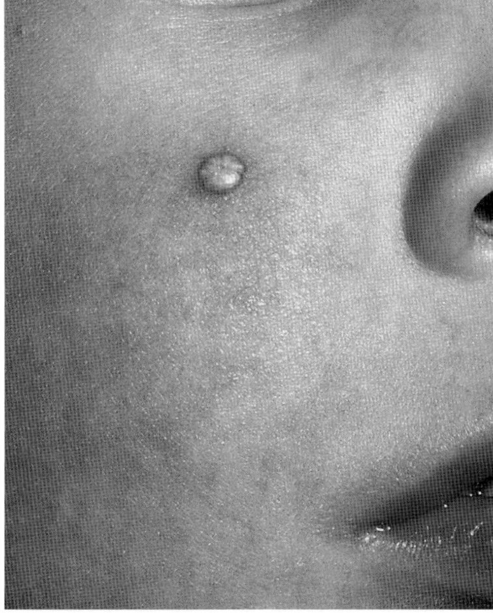

Figure 9.35 A pilomatrixoma.

slow-growing and benign but may require excision to allow histological differentiation from basal cell carcinoma. They are histologically derived from hair follicles, and trichofolliculomas produce hairs growing from a central depression.

Solitary trichilemmomas present in middle life and are pinky brown papules that may also be mistaken for basal cell carcinomas. They can resemble warts and similarly may be found on the lips and tongue. Cowden's disease is an autosomal dominant syndrome with multiple trichilemmomas associated with fibrous hamartomas and visceral malignancies.

Pilomatrixoma is also known as calcifying epithelioma of Malherbe due to the white granular calcification visible superficially on the reddish nodules (Fig. 9.35). Invasive growth has been reported, but simple excision is the treatment of choice.

SEBACEOUS TUMOURS

Sebaceous adenomas are rare, solitary, smooth, firm tumours often found on the face and scalp in middle age and measuring less than 1 cm in diameter. Multiple sebaceous adenomas have been described in association with the Muir–Torre syndrome, in which visceral malignancies are associated with sebaceous lesions and sometimes keratoacanthomas.

Generally of elderly men, senile sebaceous hyperplasia is a fairly common lesion occurring on the forehead or cheeks as solitary or multiple soft yellowish papules, often with a central depression. Like most of these lesions, it may be confused with basal cell carcinoma.

Naevus sebaceus of Jadassohn is not a true sebaceous tumour but an organoid naevus that involves more than adnexa. The scalp is the most common site, and the lesion presents at birth as a yellowish papillomatous hairless area. At puberty, hyperplasia of sebaceous glands gives rise to a soft warty lesion. A significant number go on to develop tumours within the naevus that are generally benign, but patients are often referred for removal of these lesions due to their potential to lead to basal cell carcinoma.[60] Epidemiological studies suggest that development of basal cell carcinoma is more rare than previously described, and excision should be on cosmetic grounds.

RHINOPHYMA

Rhinophyma (Fig. 9.36) is an overgrowth of the sebaceous glands of the nose, leading to abnormal thickening of the skin. Nasal cartilages and bone are spared. Men are mainly affected in middle life. It is probably a form of acne rosacea, and no association with alcohol has been established.[61] Malignant transformation into both squamous and basal cell carcinoma has been reported but is unusual.

The most common and effective treatment is surgical planing of the nose until the base of the sebaceous glands is reached, from which re-epithelialization can occur. This is usually achieved with a scalpel or skin graft knife, but laser and electrocautery have also been used. The surface is generally left raw with a light dressing to re-epithelialize, but the first layer of the nose can be removed as a skin graft to resurface any inadvertent full-thickness defects.

SEBACEOUS CARCINOMA

Sebaceous carcinoma is a rare malignant tumour arising from cutaneous sebaceous glands. It chiefly occurs in the fifth and sixth decades, with women affected more often than men. It develops on the eyelids, where it has its origin from Meibomian glands, but also arises elsewhere on the head and neck. It presents as a nodule, with a red-yellow discoloration, which increases in size and may ulcerate. Histologically, the tumour consists of lobules of undifferentiated cells in the dermis; some of the cells have foamy cytoplasm, suggesting a sebaceous origin. Pagetoid spread of the tumour cells in the epidermis occurs in the eyelid tumours. Stains for fat are positive, confirming the diagnosis. Treatment is by local excision.

SWEAT GLAND TUMOURS

Eccrine poroma is a common, benign, red-pink, sessile or pedunculated nodule usually found on the plantar surface of the feet or the palms of the hands in adults. They can be confused clinically with granuloma pyogenicum or amelanotic malignant melanoma.

Eccrine spiradenoma is a solitary and often painful tumour that may be mistaken for a glomus tumour. It occurs as a subcutaneous, firm nodule anywhere on the body in young adults. Malignant transformation has been reported in all these

REFERENCES

60. Mehregan AH, Pinkus H. Arch Dermatol 1965; 91: 574
61. Acker DW, Helwig EB. Arch Dermatol 1967; 95: 250–254

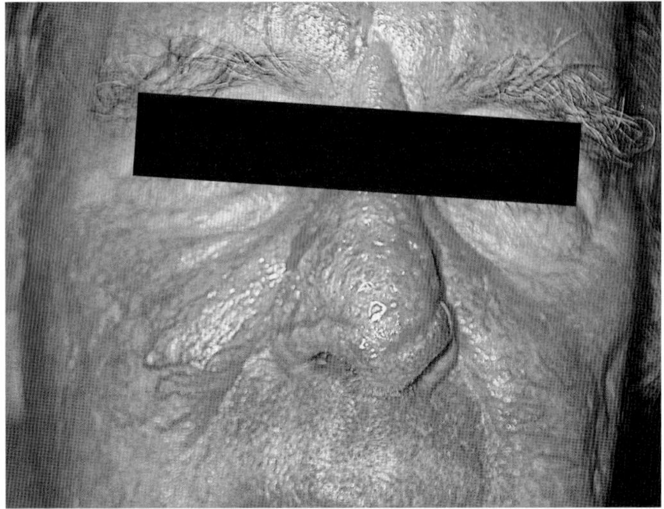

a

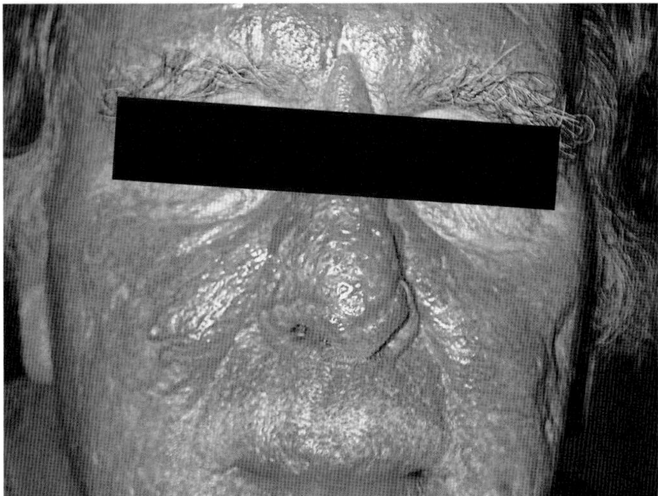

b

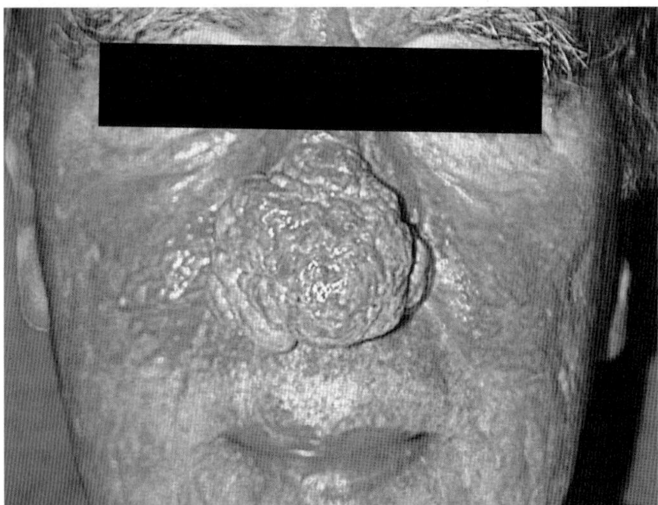

c

Figure 9.36 A rhinophyma.

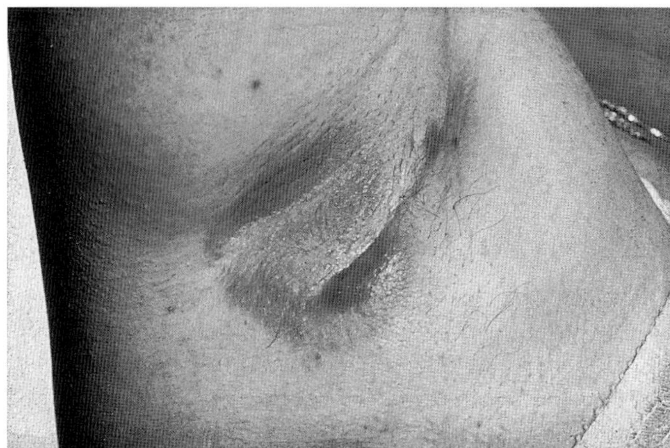

Figure 9.37 Hidradenitis suppurativa.

types of tumour, but it is extremely rare and treatment is by complete simple excision.

Syringomas are usually multiple, tiny, yellowish papules around the lower eyelids and cheeks of women. They appear at puberty or in later life. They are rarely associated with cicatricial alopecia when they are present on the scalp in large numbers.

Cylindromas occur as either solitary or multiple smooth, pink nodules on the head and scalp. Multiple tumours are inherited as a genetic dominant and may form coalescing clusters on the scalp, the so-called 'turban tumour'. They arise in adult life and grow slowly. These tumours are associated with multiple trichoepitheliomas that have the same pattern of inheritance.

Tumours derived from apocrine cells are rare. The apocrine hidrocystoma or cystadenoma occurs on the face of adults as a small cystic nodule with a bluish hue that can cause confusion with a blue naevus or melanoma. Syringocystadenoma papilliferum is usually present at birth or arises in early childhood. It consists of one or several verrucous nodules in a linear arrangement on the scalp or face. The tumour may arise at puberty in a pre-existing naevus sebaceous of Jadassohn.

INFECTION AND SKIN LESIONS

Hidradenitis suppurativa (Fig. 9.37), acne conglobata and perifollicular capitis are chronic and recurrent deep-seated cutaneous infections of the skin. Staphylococcal, streptococcal and anaerobic bacteria have been isolated from the affected area, but some abcesses are sterile and the exact aetiology is unknown. Recurrent infection in a susceptible individual may lead to scarring and propagation of the disease. It has been suggested that these conditions are the result of an antigen–antibody reaction with blockage of follicular secretions and subsequent abscess formation. Hidradenitis affects the axillae and the perineum and occurs most frequently in overweight women; acne conglobata affects the back, buttocks and chest, and occurs in either sex; perifolliculitis capitis affects the scalp. The severity of the disease varies from the occasional well-localized abscess that responds to incision and antibiotics to widespread watering can sinuses that require radical excision and skin grafting or local flaps. Hyperhidradentis or excessive sweating can be treated by botulinum toxin.

Necrotizing fasciitis

Necrotizing fasciitis is a potentially fatal synergistic infection of the subdermal layers of the skin. A prior history of skin injury or

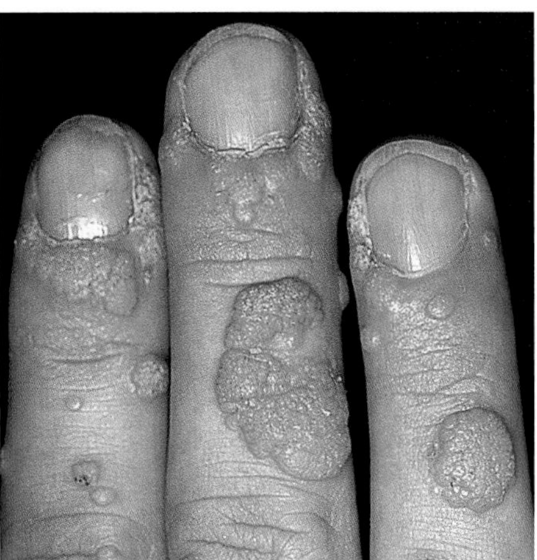

Figure 9.38 Warts on the hand. From Habif 2003,[62] with permission.

surgery may be present. Micro-organisms lead to endarteritis of the fascia, which in turn affects blood supply to the overlying skin and extensive necrosis. The initial virulence of the infection may be missed, however, and a high index of suspicion is necessary to allow early diagnosis and aggressive treatment. Subtle signs of cellulitis associated with systemic illness should raise the possibility of necrotizing fasciitis, particularly in susceptible individuals such as immunocompromised and diabetic patients. It is also described in infants following chickenpox. Fournier's gangrene is simply an eponymous name for necrotizing fasciitis of the perineal area. Skin will initially appear normal but becomes erythematous and shiny, progressing to blistering and crepitus associated with gas on X-ray.

Treatment includes resuscitation with high-dose, broad-spectrum antibiotics and extensive debridement. Patients usually require several further visits to theatre to ensure that all non-viable tissue has been removed. The vacuum-assisted closure pump has a particular role to play here in aiding debridement and encouraging granulation. Once the wound is stable and free of gross infection, it can be resurfaced using split-skin graft.

Viral warts (verruca vulgaris)

Warts are the result of infection of the squamous epithelium of the skin by human papillomavirus. Most common are human papillomavirus 1, 2 and 4 causing hand warts (Fig. 9.38). They present as small, hyperkeratotic, papillomatous lesions, frequently multiple and occurring in groups.

Cell-mediated immunity is thought to be responsible for the spontaneous regression that occurs after a period of time, and this unpredictability can make analysis of treatment difficult. Topical applications of keratolytics such as salicylic acid or cytotoxics such as podophyllin are often effective, as is cryotherapy. More resistant warts can usually be eradicated by curettage and diathermy, and increasingly laser therapy is used to this end. In immunosuppressed and elderly patients there is evidence that viral warts can undergo malignant transformation to squamous cell carcinoma.

Condylomata acuminata are sexually transmitted warts occurring in the anogenital region. They can reach a large size, presenting as cauliflower-like masses. Human papillomavirus 6 and 11 have been isolated in these lesions. In women, similar human papillomavirus 16 and 18 wart viruses are strongly associated with cervical dysplasia and neoplasia.

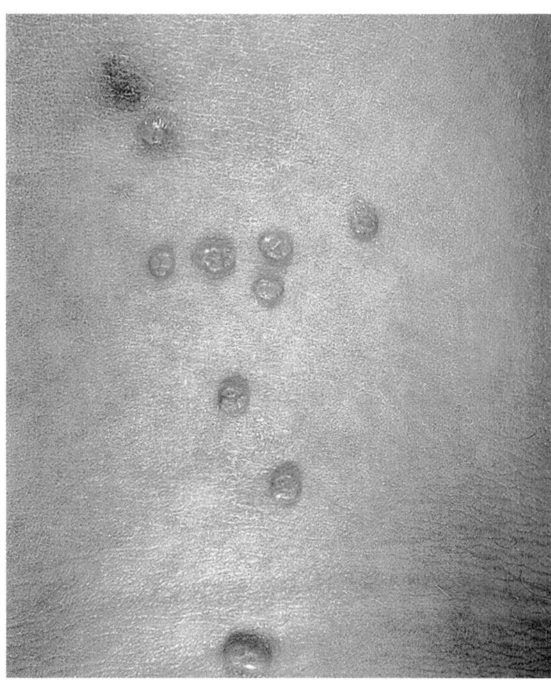

Figure 9.39 Molluscum contagiosum. From Habif 2003,[62] with permission.

Molluscum contagiosum are wart-like lesions caused by poxvirus (Fig. 9.39). They are common in young children and occur on the face and trunk as a result of direct contact. Clinically the lesions are smooth, pale, firm nodules about 2–5 mm in diameter, with a central depression.

HAMARTOMA

Hamartomas are not true tumours but represent an overgrowth of one or more cell types that are normal constituents, but arranged in an irregular fashion, of the organ in which they arise. The most common examples are haemangiomas, lymphangiomas, lipomas and neurofibromas.

Haemangioma

Pyogenic granulomas are small, benign, haemorrhagic, friable nodules that may be sessile or pedunculated and usually measure less than 1 cm across (Fig. 9.40). There is often a preceding history of injury. They are common in small children and may resolve spontaneously, although more often require curettage with diathermy of the base if they persist. Specimens should be sent for histology, particularly in the older patient, to exclude a malignant haemangioendothelioma or an amelanotic melanoma.

Strawberry naevus is a form of haemangioma appearing particularly on the head and neck spontaneously soon after birth (Fig. 9.41). These lesions often start as a small, pinkish, 'herald' patch but then grow rapidly, occasionally to an alarming size, in the first year of life. The majority of lesions arise on the head and neck. Approximately 70% will involute within 7 years, and therefore surgery is not indicated unless there are complications. These include bleeding, ulceration, infection and obstruction.

REFERENCE

62. Habif T. Clinical Dermatology. 4th edn. Mosby, London, 2003.

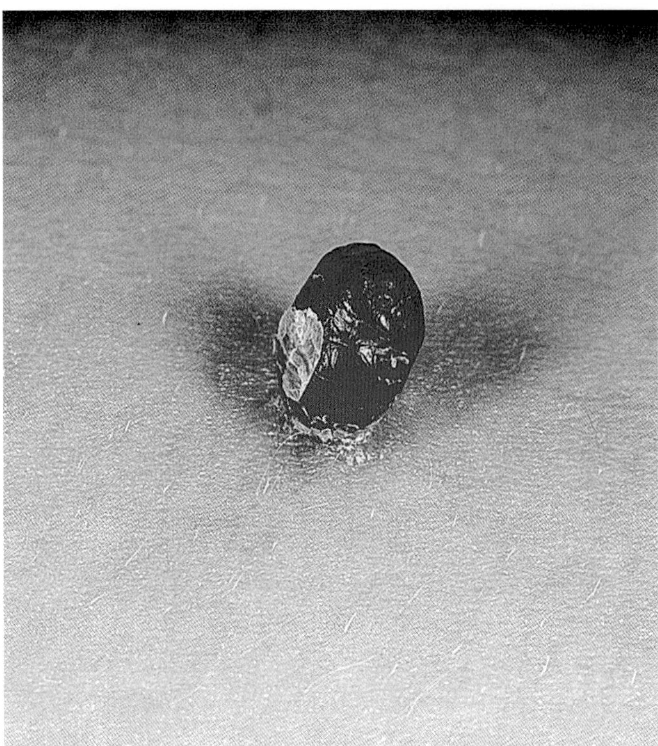

Figure 9.40 A pyogenic granuloma. From Habif 2003,[62] with permission.

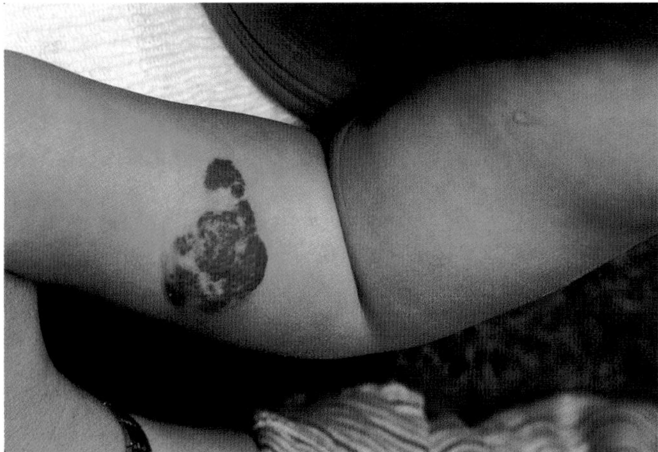

Figure 9.41 A strawberry naevus.

Rarely, platelets may be trapped in large lesions, producing a thrombocytopenia. Obstructive problems may arise from intraoral lesions or those near the visual axis (obstructive amblyopia). Treatments include systemic and intralesional steroids, surgery and interventional radiology. Large or complex lesions are best managed using a multidisciplinary approach.

It is important to distinguish haemangiomas from vascular malformations because the prognosis and management are very different. Vascular malformations are usually present at birth and grow in size with the child. They do not regress and may result in significant deformity and morbidity.

Lymphangioma

Like haemangiomas, lymphangiomas consist of abnormal vessels producing cystic spaces of variable size, lined with a single layer of endothelium. The majority are present at birth and grow with the child.

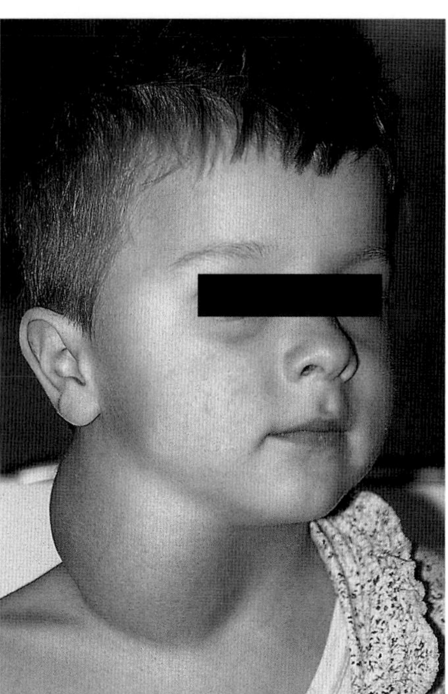

Figure 9.42 A cystic hygroma.

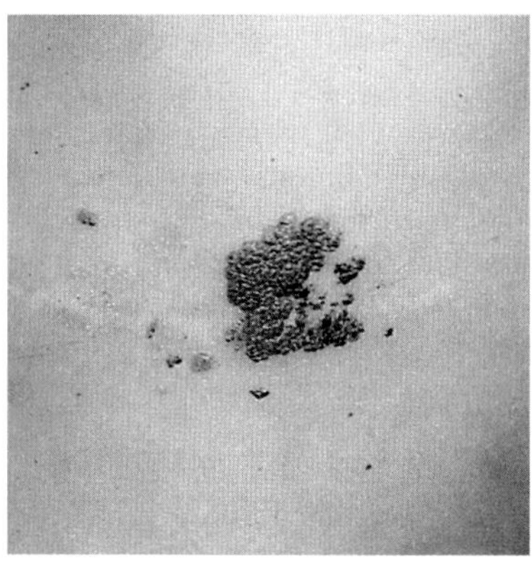

Figure 9.43 Lymphangioma circumscriptum.

The classification of lymphangiomas is complex. The clinical varieties are:

- cystic (cystic hygroma),
- solid,
- mixed vascular and lymphatic hamartoma (lymphohaemangioma), and
- cutaneous (lymphangioma circumscriptum).

Cystic hygroma presents at birth as a soft, fluctuant swelling in the supraclavicular area, which brilliantly transilluminates (Fig. 9.42). The overlying skin is normal. Regression of loculated areas is the rule by the time the child is 4 years old, and generally surgery is avoided until then. Excision is potentially mutilating and should be undertaken only by specialists.

Solid or diffuse lymphangiomas and lymphohaemangiomas occur throughout the body and may be associated with local tissue overgrowth. The diffuse nature of the lesion makes complete surgical excision difficult, and local recurrence and regrowth are common.

Cutaneous lymphangioma presents as small multiple vesicles of skin and mucosa (Fig. 9.43). They may be present at birth but usually develop in childhood. Point diathermy may be used to

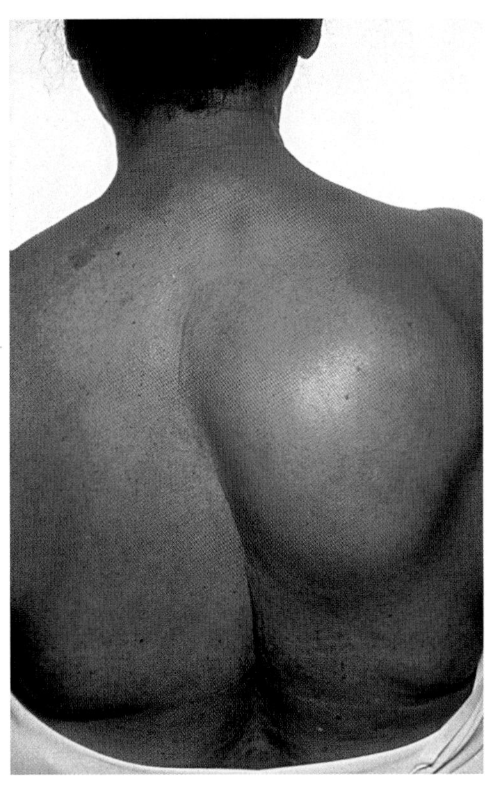

Figure 9.44 A lipoma.

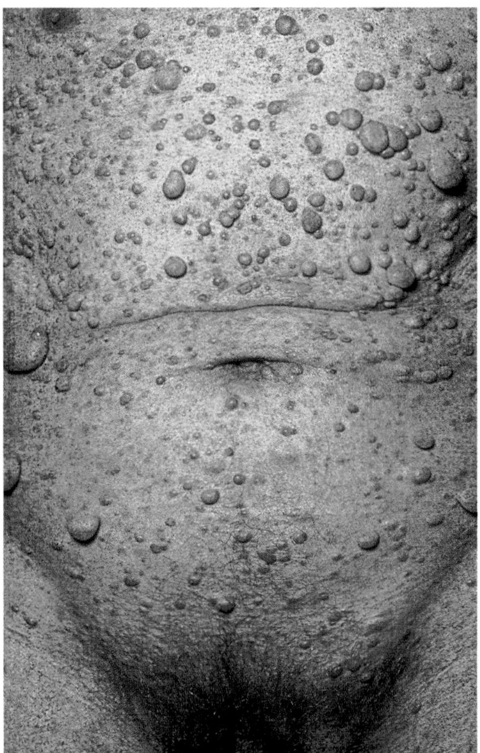

Figure 9.45 Multiple neurofibromas (von Recklinghausen's disease).

control symptoms such as bleeding. Excision may be necessary in recurrent painful infection but can be difficult due to the extent of the lesion, which consists of interconnecting reservoirs of fluid that reconstitute after incomplete excision.

Lipoma and liposarcoma

Lipomas are tumours of fat cells that commonly arise in the subcutaneous layer of skin, particularly on the trunk (Fig. 9.44). They are soft to firm and usually lobular. They are distinguished from sebaceous cysts by their mobility and lack of punctum. Multiple lipomas occur in Dercum's disease.[63] Angiolipomas have a prominent vascular component and may become painful in puberty. Superficial lipomas can be excised through small remote incisions or by liposuction,[64] although the latter carries an increased risk of recurrence. Submuscular lipomas feel more diffuse on examination and require penetration of the muscular plane prior to extraction.

Liposarcomas arise de novo, not from pre-existing lipomas, and are usually large, occur in an older age group, and tend to arise in submuscular or subfascial lesions.

Neurofibroma

Neurofibromas are benign tumours arising from peripheral nerve elements. Multiple tumours are seen in von Recklinghausen's disease, characterized by café-au-lait spots on the skin (Fig. 9.45).[65] Other associated features include scoliosis, intracranial anomalies and mental retardation. The disease is autosomally dominant in those with a family history.

Patients often require removal of multiple small lesions under local anaesthetic. Larger lesions require careful imaging and multidisciplinary assessment prior to surgery, because resection and reconstruction may be complex and associated with considerable blood loss. Malignant transformation of neurofibromas is rare but has poor prognosis.

DERMATOFIBROMA

Dermatofibromas, or fibrous histiocytomas, are small, firm, subcutaneous nodules frequently found on the legs of young to middle-aged women (Fig. 9.46). They usually appear pigmented or light brown and can be confused with melanoma. There is often a past history of minor trauma or insect bite, and this led to a belief that these were not true tumours but reactive. They are likely to originate from dermal fibroblasts.[66]

XANTHOMA AND XANTHELASMATA

Xanthomata are formed by collections of lipid-laden macrophages that occur in the dermis or around tendons and have a yellowish colour. They occur typically in patients with primary or secondary hyperlipidaemic states. Xanthelasmata are yellow plaques on the eyelids. These are associated with elevated lipid levels in only one-third of patients. Treatment is by excision, which is easily performed under local anaesthetic. Juvenile xanthogranuloma presents in early infancy as a small, solitary, yellowish red nodule (often on the face), which can also be excised simply.

SEBORRHOEIC KERATOSIS

Also known as basal cell papilloma or seborrhoeic warts, seborrhoeic keratoses are very common skin plaques found over the torso in later life (Fig. 9.47). They present as greasy lesions that have a characteristic stuck on appearance. They can be

REFERENCES

63. Blomstrand R, Juhlin L. Acta Dermatol Venereol 1971; 51: 243–250
64. Illouz Y-G. Body Sculpturing Lipoplasty. Churchill Livingstone, Edinburgh, 1989: 373
65. Griffith BH, McKinney P. Plast Reconstr Surg 1972; 49: 647–653
66. Cerio R, Spaull J et al. Br J Dermatol 1989; 120: 197–206

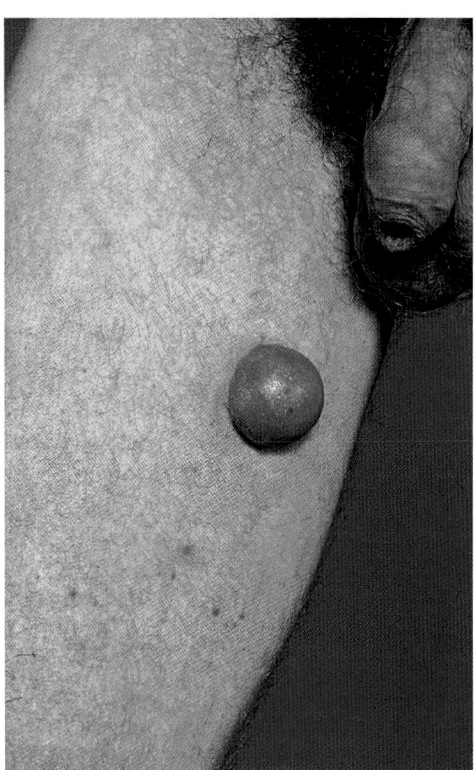

Figure 9.46 A dermatofibroma.

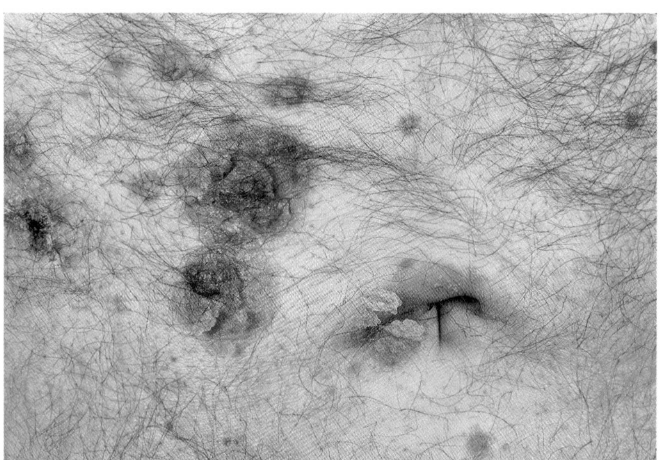

Figure 9.47 A seborrhoeic keratosis.

variably pigmented, from light brown to black, but are rarely mistaken for melanoma due to the surface texture, which ranges from velvety to warty. Multiple seborrhoeic keratoses have rarely been associated with internal malignancy (the Leser–Trélat sign).

KERATOACANTHOMAS

Keratoacanthomas are rapidly growing skin tumours that can be mistaken, both clinically and histologically, for well-differentiated squamous cell carcinoma. They develop over 6 weeks as a dome-shaped lesion, measuring up to 2.5 cm in diameter, with a central keratin-filled crater on sun-exposed parts of the body (Fig. 9.48). They involute in approximately 6 months if untreated, leaving only a depressed scar behind. When there is deviation from the classic timing and appearance, an excision biopsy is essential to exclude squamous cell carcinoma, because the histological diagnosis depends more on the architecture than on the cytological features. Sometimes it may not be possible to distinguish keratoacanthomas from well-differentiated squamous carcinomas, and in the elderly patient they should be regarded with great suspicion and excised completely with an adequate margin.

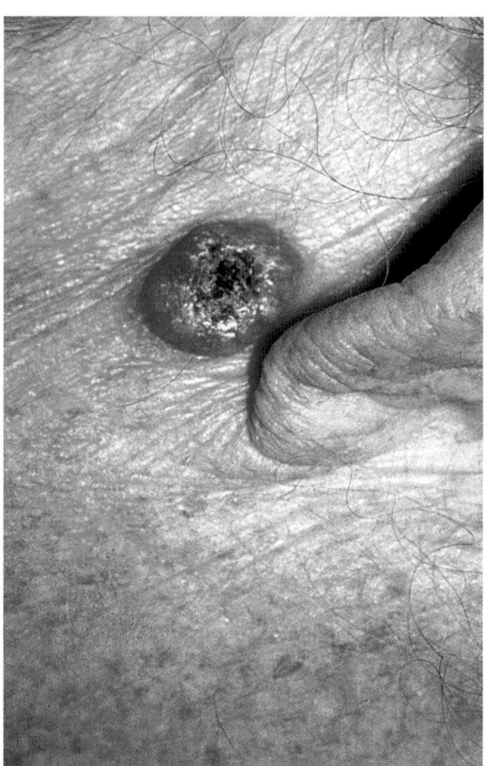

Figure 9.48 A keratoacanthoma.

NON-PIGMENTED LESIONS (PREMALIGNANT)

ACTINIC KERATOSIS

Also known as solar or senile keratosis, these erythematous scaly plaques are often multiple and represent in situ squamous cell carcinomata. They occur on the sun-exposed sites of the face and dorsum of the hands of elderly people. If left untreated, 25% will progress to an invasive squamous carcinoma after a number of years. Cryotherapy or topical application of the cytotoxic agent 5-fluorouracil are effective treatments, and have the advantage of being quick and simple as well as suitable for repeated treatment courses for new multiple lesions. Lesions that persist after several applications, however, should be surgically excised. It has been suggested that retinoic acid, used for treating acne, may also be of benefit in reversing the damaging effects of sunlight, but this is probably only a temporary effect.

BOWEN'S DISEASE

Bowen's disease (Fig. 9.49a) is an intraepidermal carcinoma. It presents as a single, red-brown, irregular plaque that may be ulcerated or crusty. Bowen's disease of the glans penis is called erythroplasia of Queyrat (Fig. 9.49b).[67] There may be an asso-

• REFERENCE •

67. Andersen SL, Nielsen A et al. Arch Dermatol 1973; 108: 367–370

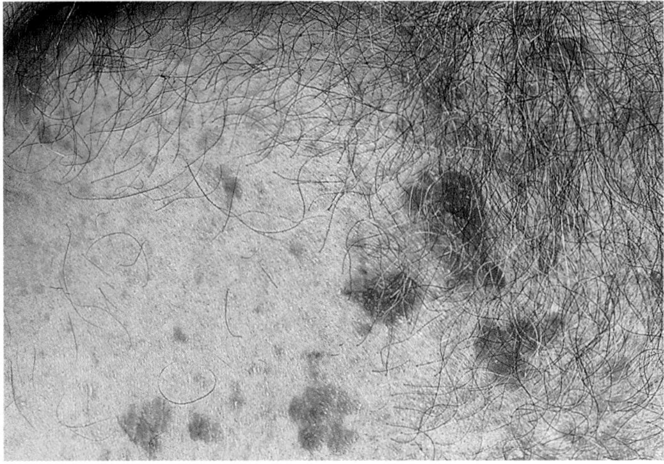

a

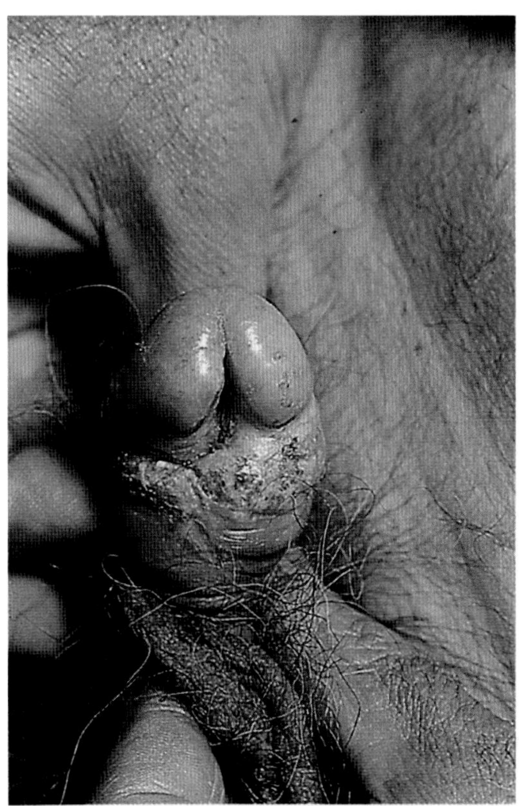

b

Figure 9.49 (**a**) Bowen's disease and (**b**) erythroplasia of Queyrat.

ciation between Bowen's disease and the development of an internal malignancy, usually 5–7 years later, particularly if it occurs in an area that has never been exposed to the sun. A small percentage progress to invasive squamous cell carcinoma. Treatment is by excision with at least a 0.5 cm margin.

LEUKOPLAKIA

Leukoplakia is a clinical description of a white patch that occurs on the vermilion border of the lips, the oral mucosa or the vulva, and that will not rub off and is not due to any other specific disease entity (e.g. lichen planus or *Candida albicans* infection). It is the visible end result of thickening and maceration of the keratinized squamous epithelium of the mucosa. Eighty per cent of cases are benign and are caused by external irritation, such as dentures. The remaining 20% show varying degrees of dysplastic change, and 3% of these already have invasive carcinoma. This occurs more frequently in leukoplakia of the floor of the mouth (68%) than in the buccal mucosa (4%). Because it is impossible to detect the development of carcinoma by clinical examination, it is necessary to biopsy any area of leukoplakia that persists for more than a few weeks after the suspected cause has been removed.

The term erythroplakia describes red patches on the oral mucosa, with or without leukoplakia, that always demonstrate in situ or invasive carcinoma.

NON-PIGMENTED LESIONS (MALIGNANT)

BASAL CELL CARCINOMA

Basal cell carcinomas are also known as rodent ulcer. This is a response to the relatively benign nature of the tumour in the majority of cases. Basal cell carcinoma is the most common skin malignancy and usually occurs on hair-bearing skin of elderly people, most commonly on sun-exposed areas and particularly around the eye. The majority can be treated simply with local excision with narrow margins. Occasionally these tumours are traps for the unwary, however, and local recurrence can result in increasingly aggressive behaviour resulting in destruction of features. Excessive sun exposure, particularly to ultraviolet light in the UVB range, predisposes to their development. There is also an increased incidence in patients with xeroderma pigmentosum and radiotherapy scars. Several different clinical types are recognized, as described below.

Nodular or noduloulcerative

Nodular or noduloulcerative (Fig. 9.50) is the most common type. It usually has a clearly defined margin, and these tumours are easy to remove completely. As it enlarges, central ulceration may occur. The nodule is associated with surface telangiectasia and a rolled edge that can often be more clearly observed using the stretch test, where the skin on either side of the tumour is stretched taught to highlight the characteristic edge. Occasionally these basal cell carcinomas may be pigmented due to melanin deposition (Fig. 9.51) and can cause confusion with malignant melanoma.

Infiltrative

Infiltrative tumours (Fig. 9.52) include morpheic or sclerosing. The tumour is flat or even depressed, with a poorly defined edge, and skin ulceration occurs late. The lack of a clearly defined border and the infiltrative nature often results in incomplete excision. These tumours are dangerous, particularly in the deep planes of the face such as the nasolabial fold and inner canthus, where incomplete excision is common and deep extension difficult to control.

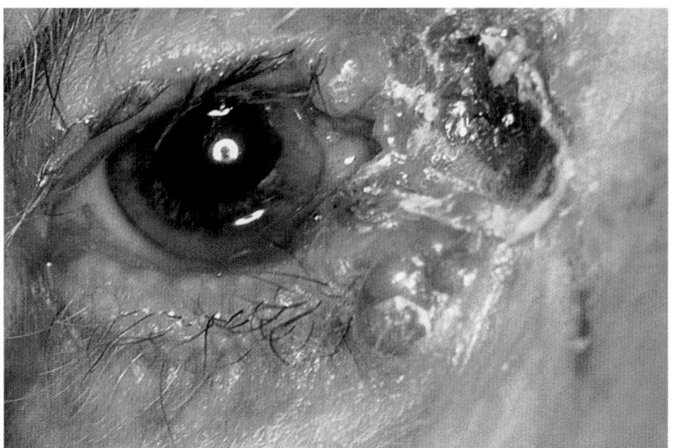

Figure 9.50 A noduloulcerative basal cell carcinoma.

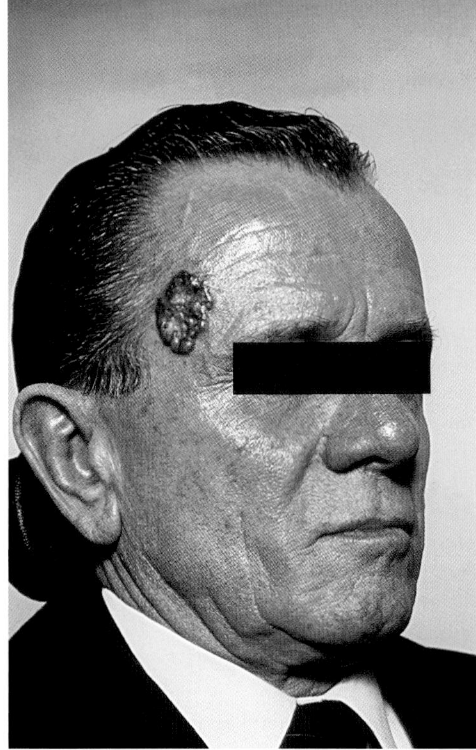

Figure 9.51 A pigmented basal cell carcinoma.

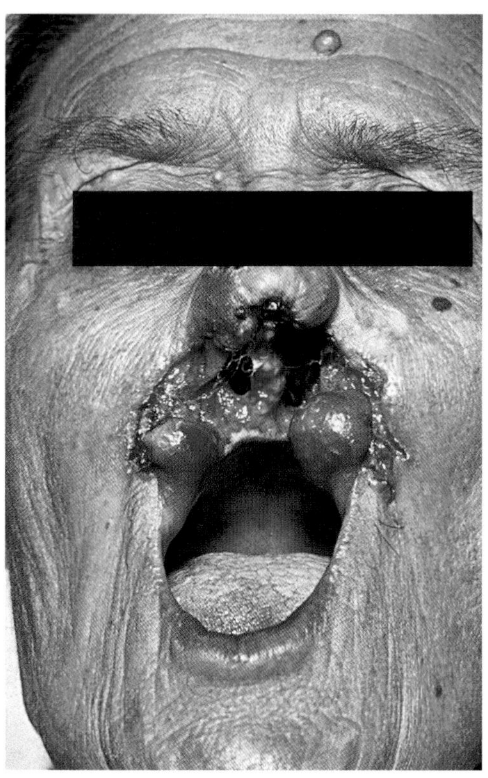

Figure 9.52 An infiltrative basal cell carcinoma that has completely destroyed the nose.

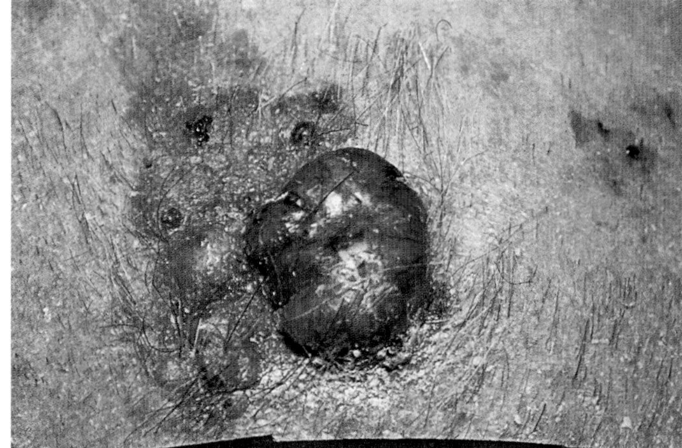

Figure 9.53 A naevoid basal cell epithelioma (Gorlin's syndrome).

Micronodular

Micronodular tumours resemble nodular basal cell carcinoma, but histologically they are arranged in small groups that can make the margin difficult to ascertain and thus lead to higher rates of incomplete excision and potential recurrence.

Superficial

Superficial basal cell carcinomas occur on the trunk and present as reddened scaly patches that increase in size. They should not be confused with Bowen's disease. A subtype includes cicatricial (field fire, bush fire). This presents as multiple, superficial, erythematous lesions interspersed with pale atrophic 'burnt out' areas.

Multiple basal cell carcinomas can occur both in susceptible individuals with sun-damaged skin and as an inherited condition. The naevoid basal cell epithelioma syndrome, or Gorlin's syndrome (Fig. 9.53), is autosomal dominant and presents in early adult life with multiple basal cell carcinomas, keratocysts of the jaw, skeletal abnormalities and palmar and plantar pits.[68]

Microscopically, basal cell carcinomas have several patterns, but all consist of nests and islands of basaloid cells in the dermis, similar to those seen in the basal layer of the epidermis. There is peripheral palisading in the nests of cells, and there is a high mitotic rate. The epidermis is frequently ulcerated. Areas of squamous differentiation may be seen, but the tumour has the overall architecture and behaviour of a basal cell carcinoma.

Basal cell carcinomas are only locally invasive, although they can be horrifyingly destructive due to their location. Metastasis has been reported but is extremely rare. Treatment is by local

REFERENCE

68. Gorlin RJ, Sedano HO. Birth Defects 1971; 8: 140–148

excision. For discrete nodular tumours the usual excision margin is 3 mm, but poorly defined or indurated tumours require a wider margin of excision, especially at the inner canthus of the eye, the nasolabial fold, the nasal floor and the ear. Adequate clearance is important in basal cell carcinoma because it becomes increasingly difficult to eradicate the tumours when hampered by scarring and recurrence causing increasingly destructive tissue damage. Recurrent lesions require wider resection and have a significantly higher recurrence rate themselves. Overall, the incomplete excision rate of these tumours is around 10%. A decision to re-excise depends on the histological nature of the tumour and the circumstances of the patient. In young patients with infiltrative basal cell carcinoma complete excision should be obtained, but in frail elderly patients with superficial or nodular lesions then a policy of watchful waiting can be employed because only 30% of basal cell carcinomas actually recur after incomplete excision. It is thought that this may be due to the inflammatory response of healing following the initial excision destroying a minimal residual load of malignant cells.

Excellent results can also be obtained with radiotherapy, although there is no histological guide to type or margin of excision and cosmetic results are said to be inferior to surgery. Mohs surgery is chemosurgery with frequent histological assessment of margins, which gives improved rates of incomplete excision. This technique is expensive and time-consuming but may be appropriate in re-recurrent tumours in cosmetically sensitive areas. The choice of technique is dependent on the site and extent of the lesion and the experience of the surgeon.

SQUAMOUS CELL CARCINOMAS

Squamous cell carcinomas (Fig. 9.54) are the second most common cutaneous malignancy. They are also known as epidermoid carcinoma. They arise from the keratinizing cell layer of the epidermis. They may develop in a pre-existing actinic keratosis or in an area of Bowen's disease, or they may arise de novo. Immunosuppressed patients may develop multiple squamous cell carcinomas. This may be related to reduced immunosurveillance or predisposition to viral infection. The principal aetiological factors are sun exposure, radiation, certain chemicals, chronic sinuses, and chronic cutaneous ulceration such as in Marjolin's ulcer (squamous carcinoma in chronic venous ulcers) and long-standing unhealed burn wounds.

Squamous cell carcinomas present as enlarging keratotic nodules with a heaped up border. Central ulceration occurs as the tumour enlarges. A well-differentiated lesion may present as a keratin horn. Suspicious lesions should be biopsied, because squamous cell carcinomas are commonly mistaken for keratoacanthoma, basal cell carcinoma, amelanotic melanoma and adnexal tumours.[69]

Microscopically there are long, irregular tongues of dysplastic-looking squamous epithelium arising from the epidermis or ulcer base that extend into the deep dermis and subcutaneous fat in a haphazard fashion. The adjacent epidermis usually shows evidence of intraepidermal carcinoma. The tumour may be well differentiated with keratin production, moderately differentiated or poorly differentiated, where the spindle cell morphology has to be differentiated from melanoma, atypical fibroxanthoma and cylindroma.

Untreated squamous carcinomas are locally destructive and may metastasize to local lymph nodes. Treatment is as for basal cell carcinoma, although a wider excision margin of 1 cm is usual because the local recurrence rate for squamous cell carcinoma is twice that of basal cell carcinoma. Metastasis to regional nodes occurs in 5–10%, but is very low in those tumours arising in sun-damaged skin (0.5%) and highest in tumours that arise in mucosal surfaces, irradiated areas, and the edges of ulcers and sinuses (20%). Regional node spread is treated by surgical block dissection, radiotherapy, or both. This reduces local recurrence and long-term mortality. Trials of sentinel node biopsy for squamous cell carcinoma are currently ongoing.

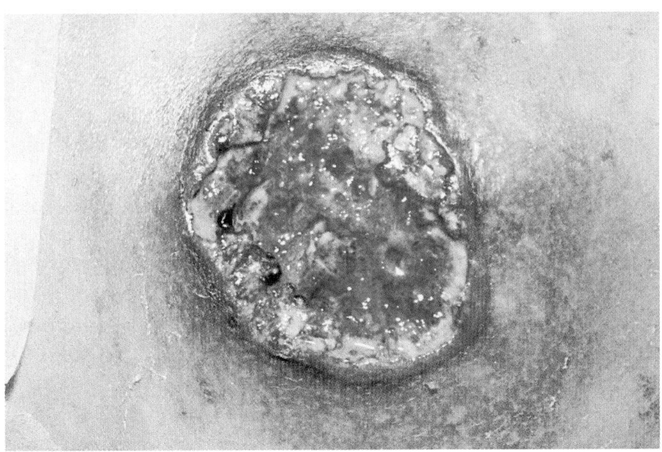

Figure 9.54 A squamous cell carcinoma.

CUTANEOUS MALIGNANT LYMPHOMA

The skin may be infiltrated by leukaemic cells and by malignant lymphocytes early in non-Hodgkin's lymphoma. Five per cent of B-cell lymphomas arise in the skin. Skin involvement presents as a smooth plaque of variable colour that slowly enlarges. Histologically there is lymphoid infiltrate, and immunohistochemistry confirms the presence of B cells producing immunoglobulin with only one of the light chains, kappa or lambda (light-chain restriction). T-cell lymphomas include specific types with skin involvement. Mycosis fungoides presents as areas of localized eczema and Sezary syndrome presents as generalized exfoliative erythroderma.

Involvement of the skin by Hodgkin's disease usually occurs late in the course of the illness and presents as a plaque, nodule or ulcer. Microscopically there is a heavy lymphoid infiltrate and occasional Reed–Sternberg cells are seen.

Surgical biopsy is required to make a diagnosis, but treatment is by radiation and cytotoxic chemotherapy.

CUTANEOUS METASTASIS

The most common primary sites are the bronchus or oesophagus in men and the breast or ovaries in women. Metastases occur in all areas of the skin, but the chest wall is the most common site, especially when the primary is a carcinoma of the breast. Sister Joseph's nodule is an umbilical metastasis usually from ovarian carcinoma. These metastases are generally a late sign and indicate poor prognosis.

MERKEL CELL CARCINOMA

This rare but highly aggressive tumour is believed to be derived from the Merkel cell population, which are primitive neuro-

• REFERENCE •

69. Paletta FX. Clin Plast Surg 1980; 7: 313–336

endocrine cells in the skin. The tumour presents in the elderly as a firm, painless nodule. The overlying epidermis may be violaceous.

Histologically the lesion is quite distinctive, and it consists of an ill-defined dermal nodule made up of cords and trabeculae of medium-sized cells with very little cytoplasm and with a high mitotic and apoptotic rate. Foci of squamous or eccrine differentiation may also be present. The diagnosis is one of exclusion, with malignant lymphoma and metastatic small cell carcinoma being the two conditions that require differentiation. Immunohistochemistry is very helpful in excluding a lymphoma, but a metastatic small cell carcinoma often needs to be excluded clinically.

The prognosis is poor, with a local recurrence developing in 36% and metastasis in 28%. Approximately half of patients are dead within 2 years.

PAGET'S DISEASE

Mammary and extramammary Paget's disease are two distinct entities in which the epidermis is infiltrated by adenocarcinoma cells. Paget's disease of the breast is discussed in Ch. 23.

Extramammary Paget's disease occurs in the genital and perianal region, predominantly in women. It has also been described in the axilla, and therefore occurs where apocrine glands are situated. It can occur in association with a mucin-secreting carcinoma of the rectum or endocervix. In the majority of cases, unlike the disease in the breast, an underlying carcinoma is not found.

Clinically it presents as an eczematous, red, velvety area, with oozing and crusting. It is intensely pruritic. Malignant melanoma has to be excluded, and this can be achieved by performing an S100 stain, which is positive only in melanoma.

Treatment is by surgical excision, but local recurrence is common because the margins of the tumour are very difficult to define and Paget's disease is often multifocal. The prognosis is good when Paget's disease is not associated with a tumour, but poor when it is.

PIGMENTED LESIONS (BENIGN)

FRECKLES

Freckles are lightly pigmented macules that are related to exposure to sunlight and are more common in individuals with red hair and blue eyes. Histologically the freckle is simply related to a localized increase in pigmentation, and the architecture of the epidermis is normal with no increase in numbers of melanocytes.

SOLAR LENTIGO

Solar lentigo are benign pigmented macules that occur in the sun-damaged skin of the elderly and are therefore common on the face and dorsum of the hands. They vary in size but can reach 1–2 cm in diameter and may coalesce. Microscopically there is solar damage to collagen, hyperkeratosis, and an increase in melanocytes and pigment along the basal layer. There is, however, no cellular atypia.

NAEVI

Evolution of naevi

Histologically, melanocytic naevi are proliferative collections of melanocytes, which in normal skin are scattered along the basal layer of the epidermis between the keratinocyte population. Melanocytic naevi can be congenital, but most are acquired. Acquired naevi first appear in childhood and adolescence, mature through middle age, and decrease in number thereafter. Many naevi pass through recognizable stages, starting flat in childhood and eventually becoming intradermal in late adult life. Clinically, flat naevi tend to be a lentigo or a junctional naevus. Slightly elevated naevi tend to be compound, and papular or papillomatous naevi are usually intradermal. The normal evolution of naevi is important in the context of understanding lesions suspicious of malignant melanoma. It is important to note that evidence of pre-existing naevi is present in only 20% of malignant melanomas.[70] The majority of melanomas arise in previously normal skin.

Lentigo simplex

Lentigo simplex macules (Fig. 9.55a) are often jet black and usually less than 5 mm in diameter. They occur in infancy and early childhood. Histologically there is a proliferation of melanocytes along the basal layer in a linear fashion, and the colour is produced by abundant melanin pigment. The association of multiple lentigo around buccal mucosa is seen in Peutz–Jeghers syndrome, which is an inherited autosomal dominant condition. The patients also have multiple hamartomatous polyps throughout the gastrointestinal tract.

Junctional naevi

Junctional naevi (Fig. 9.55b) is the stage after lentigo simplex in the development of naevi. These are still flat but tend to be larger and a lighter homogenous brown-black in colour. Histologically, numerous melanocytes now form clusters or nests of cells in the basal layer. New melanocytic lesions in adults with abundant junctional activity should be carefully studied by the pathologist to rule out malignancy.

Compound naevi

Naevi mature in adolescence and can become raised and papular (Fig. 9.55c). Histologically, cells start dropping down into the dermis and the naevus may become even more pale.

Intradermal naevi

By the end of the third decade, most naevi are of the intradermal type (Fig. 9.55d) and appear as flesh-coloured papules with little pigment. Clinically they are common as the occasional pigmented, hairy mole on the face of the middle-aged. Histologically all the melanocytic nests are confined to the dermis.

Other naevi of note

Spitz naevus (juvenile melanoma)

Spitz naevi are a variant of benign melanocytic lesions and have distinctive clinical and histological features; their recognition is important because they can be mistaken histologically for a malignant melanoma. They usually occur in children and young adults under 30 years of age. Spitz naevi can occur in any area of the body and present as a single, pink, dome-shaped nodule less than 1 cm in diameter.[71]

REFERENCES

70. English DR, Armstrong BK. Br Med J Clin Res 1988; 296: 1285–1288
71. Weedon D, Little JH. Cancer 1977; 40: 217–225

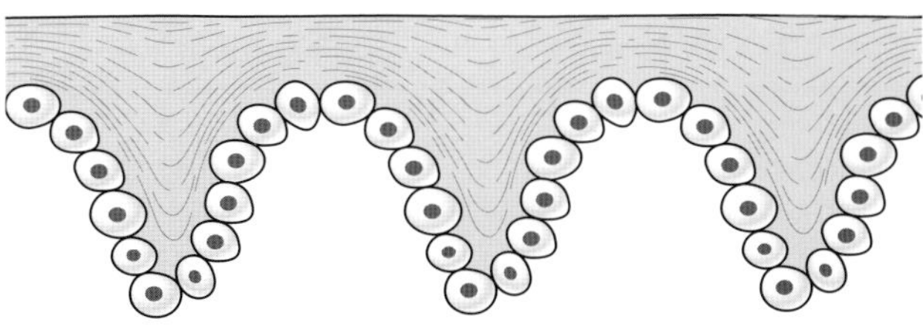
a

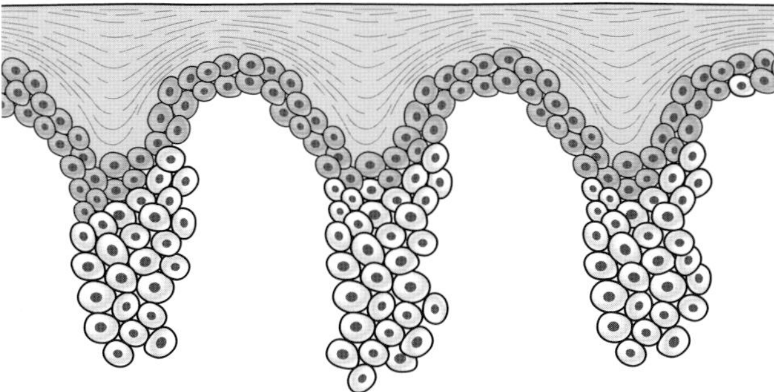
b

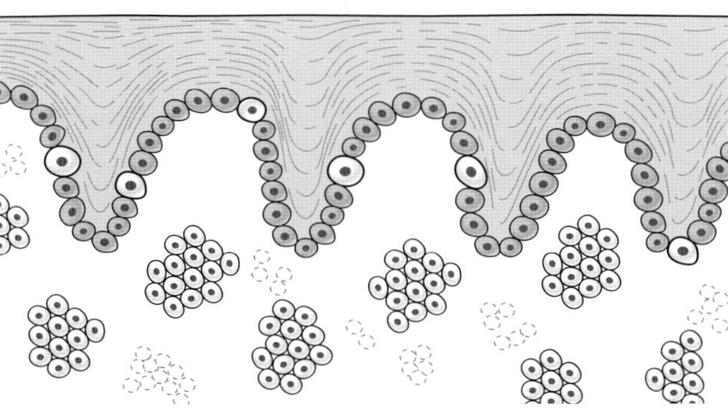
c

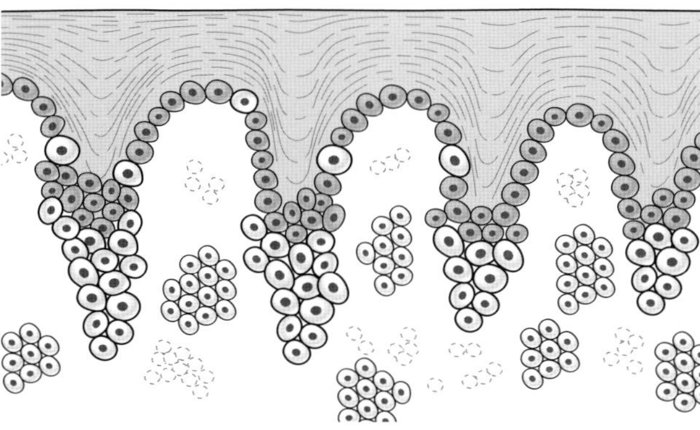
d

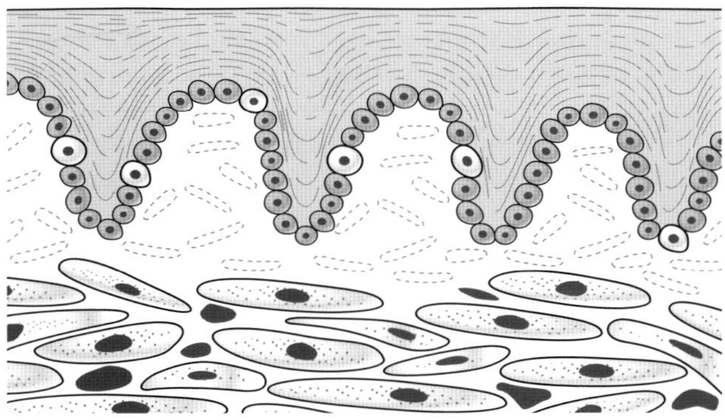
e

Figure 9.55 Naevi: (**a**) simple, (**b**) junctional, (**c**) compound, (**d**) intradermal and (**e**) blue.

Histologically, one of the most important features is the symmetry of the lesion on low-power examination. The melanocytic cells lie in an oedematous and vascular stroma. The overlying epidermis usually exhibits hyperplasia. Pigment deposition is not prominent. The most important differential diagnosis is that of malignant melanoma, and this is a particular problem in the naevi that do not show the classic features. Worrying histological features include marked nuclear atypia, lack of maturation at the deep aspect of the naevus, atypical mitoses, and lack of symmetry on low-power examination. Spitz naevi are benign, needing only local excision, often as an excision biopsy to exclude melanoma.

Halo naevi

Halo naevi are benign pigmented naevi surrounded by an area of depigmentation. They may be solitary or multiple, and the halo represents destruction of melanocytes by invading lymphoid cells. The reasons for this are not known, but the mechanism appears to be that the naevus cells produce an antigen that stimulates an antibody in the surrounding lymphocytes.[72] The area of depigmentation may persist for years, but repigmentation occurs in almost all cases. No treatment is required unless there are other features of the mole that suggest malignant change, such as depigmentation and regression, and that may also occur around a malignant melanoma.

Blue naevi

Blue naevi (Fig. 9.55e) are benign melanocytic lesions that are recognized clinically by their slate-blue colour. Less than 1% undergo malignant transformation. There are two types. The common blue naevus occurs relatively frequently and the classic patient is a woman in her thirties. They are seen most often on the face and dorsum of the hands. Macroscopically they are dome-shaped, blue-black lesions measuring up to 1 cm. The cellular blue naevus is uncommon. More than half are located in the sacrococcygeal area and buttocks. Clinically they present as painful and sometimes ulcerated blue-black lesions 2 cm or more in size. Histologically they comprise a dermal cellular population, heavy with melanin pigment and extending occasionally into subcutaneous fat.

Congenital naevi

Congenital melanocytic naevi are present at birth and may be hairy. They grow in proportion to the child. *Giant pigmented naevi*, which may be called giant hairy naevi or bathing trunk naevi, have no agreed definition, but the term should probably be reserved for naevi that are at least 20 cm in diameter or 1% of the total surface area of skin.[73] Giant naevi of the neck or scalp may be associated with intracranial involvement, which can present with epilepsy. Histologically they can be compound or intra-

REFERENCES

72. Lever WF, Schaumberg-Lever G. Histopathology of the Skin. JB Lippincott, Philadelphia, 1990: 764
73. Kopf AW, Bart RS et al. J Am Acad Dermatol 1979; 1: 123–130

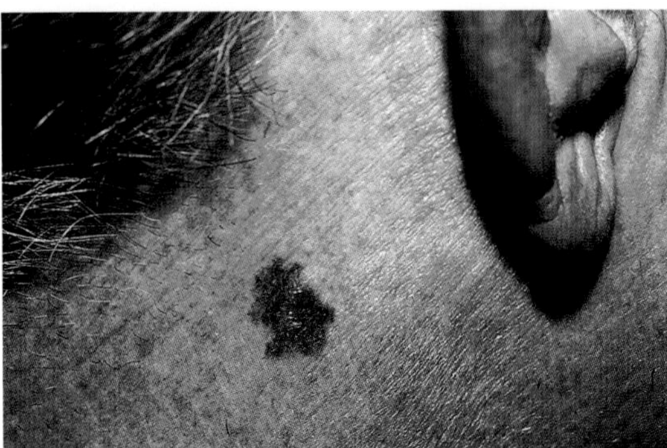

Figure 9.56 A Hutchinson's freckle (lentigo maligna). From Habif 2003,[62] with permission.

dermal, similar to the acquired naevi, but there are subtle histological differences. Malignant melanoma may develop in these large pigmented naevi, mostly before the age of 15 years, and carries a particularly poor prognosis. The lifetime risk for developing malignant melanoma in these patients has been variously estimated at between 1 and 42%, but it is probably nearer to 8%.

Treatment of giant naevi is very difficult. Shaving the naevus and laser treatment in the first few weeks of life rarely works in the occasions where melanocytes are superficial. In the majority the naevus is predominantly intradermal, superficial treatments are ineffective, and recurrence inevitable. Total excision and skin grafting produces a very poor cosmetic result, with some pigment recurring in both the graft and the donor sites; it is also a painful and protracted procedure for the child. Tissue expansion and serial excisions are extremely useful in these naevi, but again may need multiple procedures.

PIGMENTED LESIONS (PREMALIGNANT)

LENTIGO MALIGNA (HUTCHINSON'S MELANOTIC FRECKLE)

Lentigo maligna presents as a flat, pigmented, brown to black freckle with an irregular outline, which gradually enlarges over the years (Fig. 9.56). Atypical melanocytes proliferate along the dermoepidermal junction, but there is no dermal invasion and the lesion represents the carcinoma in situ stage of malignant melanoma.

After 10–30 years, the lentigo maligna transforms into a malignant melanoma, detected clinically by the development of a black or tan nodule within the flat lesion, and histologically by the spread of the atypical melanocytic cells from the dermoepidermal junction into the dermis.

DYSPLASTIC NAEVUS SYNDROME (B–K MOLE SYNDROME, FAMM SYNDROME)

Dysplastic naevi are melanocytic lesions with distinctive clinical and histopathological features, and the use of the term should be restricted to naevi with both of these components.[74]

There is controversy over the relationship of dysplastic naevi, family history and melanoma. There is certainly a markedly increased risk of developing malignant melanoma in those patients who have dysplastic naevi and a family history of melanoma, although there is no proved increased risk of melanoma in patients with solitary dysplastic naevi without a family history. The naevi tend to occur on the trunk; have an irregular, ill-defined border; are usually greater than 5 mm in diameter; and have a variegated colour of tan through to dark brown on a pink background. Surrounding erythema is common.

The lifetime risk for the development of melanoma from dysplastic naevi is in the order of 20% in patients with no family history of melanoma. In the familial syndrome, where at least two members have had a malignant melanoma, the actuarial lifetime risk of developing melanoma for a family member who has cutaneous dysplastic naevi is close to 100%. The majority of dysplastic naevi do not undergo malignant transformation; environmental factors such as sunlight may be important in their natural history. Patients with dysplastic naevi should be examined carefully, over the whole of the body surface, and a family history obtained. Whole-body photographs have been used to quantify changes in individual moles and to detect new lesions.

Box 9.3 Risk factors for developing melanoma

Moderate risk
- Previous melanoma
- Many moles or unusual, atypical moles
- Fair skin, blonde hair, blue eyes; patients who sunburn easily, do not tan, or tan only with difficulty
- A history of severe sunburn either as children or teenagers

High risk
- Strong family history of melanoma
- Giant pigmented hairy naevi

PIGMENTED LESIONS (MALIGNANT)

CUTANEOUS MELANOMA

In 1857, William Norris, a Stourbridge GP, published the first formal treatise on melanoma. He noted the disease to be rare but to occur in individuals with moles and fair skin. Furthermore, Norris postulated that melanoma might have a hereditary element and be associated with the presence of other cancers (Box 9.3). He advised that surgery provided the only effective treatment and recognized that neither medicine nor surgery would be of benefit once the disease had spread.

Over the past 50 years, Norris's observations have held, but the incidence of melanoma has dramatically increased, almost doubling each decade, to grow at a rate faster than any other cancer. The causes for this are varied, but are largely ascribed to the excessive exposure of fair-skinned individuals to sunlight and, in particular, ultraviolet radiation. In the UK, melanoma affects approximately eight in 100 000 of the population and will result in the death of over 1200 people each year. Studies have shown a correlation between the incidence of hours of sunshine and the incidence of the disease. What is also evident is that exposure in childhood and sunburn may be associated with development of melanoma in later life—hence the importance of good sun protection for children and adolescents.

Between 40 and 70% of melanomas are associated with a pre-existing mole. Most people have moles that increase in number

REFERENCE

74. Clark WH Jr, Reimer RR et al Arch Dermatol 1978; 114: 732–738

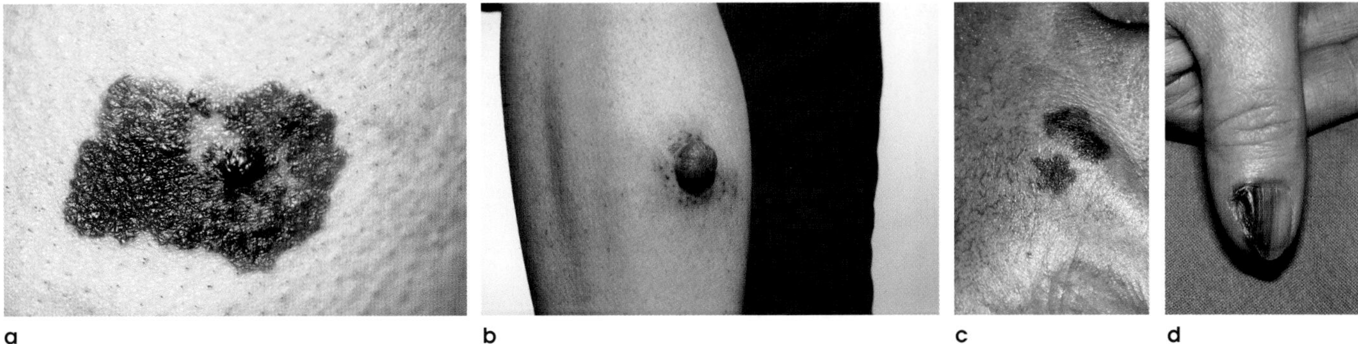

Figure 9.57 (**a**) A superficial spreading melanoma, (**b**) a nodular malignant melanoma, (**c**) a lentigo maligna melanoma, and (**d**) an acral lentiginous melanoma.

with age and sun exposure. The vast majority of these are quite normal and will remain so; accordingly there is no role for prophylactic excision of otherwise normal naevi. However, to make an early diagnosis it is important to identify, through health education and screening, those people most at risk of developing melanoma.

Early diagnosis can be achieved by self-screening and opportunistic screening by the GP and other clinicians. It is important to ensure rapid referral of suspicious lesions to a surgeon or dermatologist with a recognized interest in pigmented lesions or melanoma. Pigmented lesion clinics are also beneficial because they combine specialist input with early diagnosis and biopsy facilities.

Identification of change in otherwise normal naevi or any new lesions can be helped using the ABCD rule and should be taught to susceptible patients. Changes indicative of suspicious lesions or malignant change in moles include the following.

- A: asymmetry.
- B: border. Benign naevi tend to have a relatively symmetrical border, whereas malignant lesions tend to be uneven with scalloped or notched edges.
- C: colour. Benign lesions tend to be uniform in colour, whereas malignant lesions tend to be variegated.
- D: diameter. Lesions larger than 6 mm are more likely to be malignant, particularly if accompanied by changes in the above categories.

Additional minor signs include itching and bleeding.

Morphologically, four types of tumour are recognized.

Superficial spreading melanoma

Superficial spreading melanoma (Fig. 9.57a) accounts for approximately 70% of all tumours.[75] It may develop from a pre-existing mole, initially as a flat lesion with irregular borders and variable pigmentation. Tumour cells initially grow outwardly in a horizontal plane above the basement membrane. This lateral spread of cells is termed the *radial growth phase*. Over a period of months, areas within the tumour may become more nodular as the tumour begins to penetrate the basement membrane. This constitutes the *vertical growth phase*, when the tumour becomes invasive and liable to metastasize.

Nodular melanomas

Nodular melanomas (Fig. 9.57b) are the second most common type of lesion and account for approximately 25% of cases. These can arise de novo and usually present with a shorter history. They are more protuberant and symmetric in shape than superficial spreading melanomas. Of most importance, they are characterized by direct vertical growth phase and are clinically aggressive.

Lentigo melanoma

Lentigo melanomas (Fig. 9.57c) account for approximately 4% of all tumours and are the only type of melanoma to display an overt dose–response relationship with sun exposure. These tumours arise on exposed areas over a period of many years, usually on the face. There is usually a premalignant phase consisting of a large pigmented patch, known as a lentigo maligna, which resembles a large freckle. Over a period of years, a lentigo may develop areas of increased pigmentation representing radial growth phase tumour. In time, these areas progress to an invasive vertical growth pattern, at which point the tumour will be of similar metastatic potential to other melanoma types of similar thickness.

Acral lentiginous melanomas

The final group consists of the acral lentiginous melanomas (Fig. 9.57d). These are rare among fair-skinned individuals, accounting for approximately only 1% of tumours. However, this is the most common form of tumour seen in Afro-Caribbean or East Asian patients. This subtype includes subungual lesions and those found on the palms or soles of the feet. Due to their relative rarity, they tend to present at a more advanced stage and are thus associated with a worse prognosis.

Suspicious naevi should undergo excision biopsy with a 2-mm margin. Incision and shave biopsies may prevent accurate histological assessment and should not be used other than for very large lesions. The key histopathological prognostic observations of a melanoma include the tumour (Breslow) thickness (Fig. 9.58), lymphocytic invasion of the tumour (Fig. 9.59), and the presence of ulceration.

Once the diagnosis is confirmed, the patient usually requires a wider excision. Randomized studies suggest 1 cm per mm thickness of tumour, up to 2 mm thick. Several studies have attested to the efficacy of narrow margins for thin (less than 2 mm) lesions.[76] However, little mature randomized data exist for the management of thick (greater than 2 mm) tumours. The British Association of Plastic Surgeons, in conjunction with the

REFERENCES

75. Langley RGB, Fitzpatrick TB, Sober AJ. Cutaneous Melanoma. Quality Medical Publishing, St Louis, 1998: 81–102
76. Lens MB, Dawes M, Goodacre T et al. Arch Surg 2002, 137: 1101–1105

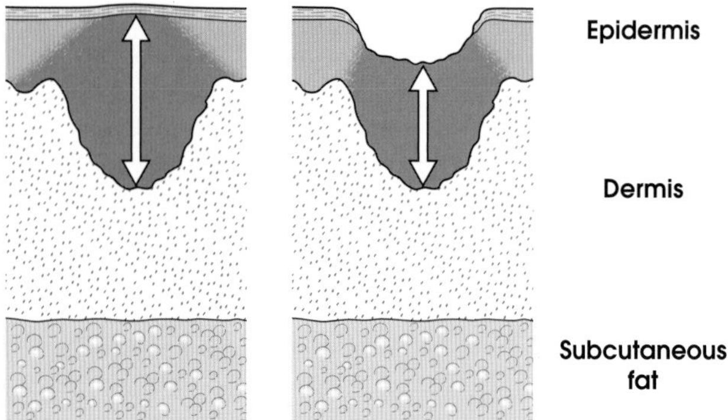

Figure 9.58 Breslow's thickness of malignant melanoma.

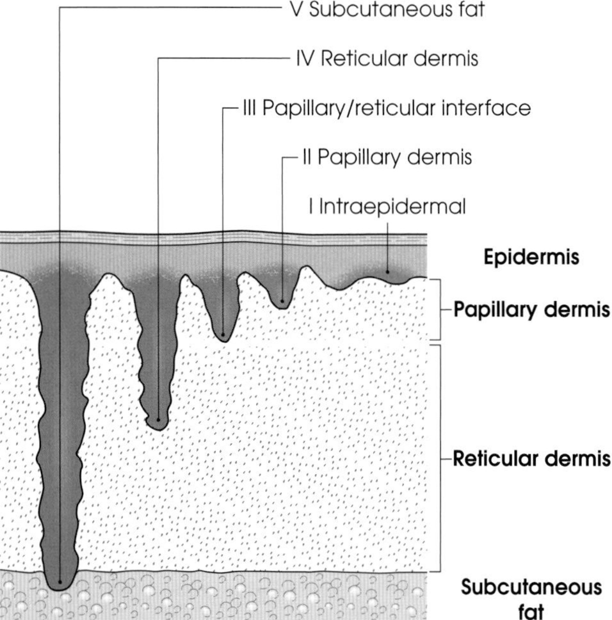

Figure 9.59 Clark's level of melanoma invasion.

Melanoma Study Group, presented early data to suggest that narrow excision margins will not suffice for tumours in excess of 2 mm thick. This study randomized tumours greater than 2 mm thick to 1-cm versus 3-cm excision margins and found a significant increase in local recurrence for those treated with a narrow margin.

Usually the excision defect can be primarily closed, or covered with a skin graft or local flap. Patients should undergo a baseline chest X-ray or CT scan, although bone scans are of little proved benefit at this stage.

Disease progression

Melanomas metastasize via a number of routes, but initially and principally via the lymphatics. Almost 70% of tumours will spread via the regional nodes, although controversy still surrounds their optimum management. Of significance, occult micrometastases are noted in about 20% of regional nodes at the time of primary presentation. A major, as yet unanswered, question is whether they should be removed at the same time as the primary tumour (elective node dissection). Randomized controlled studies have not shown this to improve patient survival, and it may subject patients only to unnecessary surgery and morbidity.[77] In the UK, we have tended to offer a watch and wait policy, whereby removal of the primary melanoma is followed by regular review to detect evidence of recurrent nodal disease, performing a therapeutic node dissection in the presence of palpable disease. However, retrospective data suggest that elective node dissection may be of benefit, particularly for intermediate thickness tumours (1.5–3 mm).

Table 9.5 Tumour thickness and clinical prognosis of malignant melanoma

Tumour thickness (mm)	Survival at 10 years (%)
< 0.75	98
0.75–1.5	91
> 3	55

In 1992, Morton and coworkers elaborated on earlier work by Cabanas to postulate that areas of skin drain to specific lymph nodes within a nodal basin that may be predictive of its tumour status.[78] The sentinel node is defined as the first node to which a tumour drains, and may be identified with lymphoscintigraphy. Sentinel node biopsy has been proposed to settle the controversy between elective node dissection and TLND by allowing objective selection of patients for lymphadenectomy, and the first major trial to assess the predictive value of sentinel node status has now closed. Presently, if micrometastases are present, the patient can be offered formal lymph node clearance. Patients with a negative biopsy can be reassured and followed up routinely.

The introduction of sentinel node biopsy has made several important contributions to the management of primary melanoma, and it has now become the standard of care in most major cancer centres worldwide. Presence of micrometastases are recognized to be the most powerful prognostic factor identified to date, including primary tumour thickness (see Table 9.5). Furthermore, the volume of micrometastases may be correlated with outcome. Use of this technique allows accurate staging, and therefore accurate stratification of patients for clinical trials. Finally, experience with this technique has revealed that skin tumours do not follow predictable routes of lymphatic spread; 25% of upper back melanomas drain initially to nodes in the triangular space.

Present indications for sentinel node biopsy include melanomas over 1 mm thick or thinner tumours with ulceration or histological regression. The role of sentinel node biopsy in tumours greater than 4 mm is controversial. The risk of haematogenous spread is greater in this group of patients, and therefore selective lymphadenectomy is less likely to provide disease control. Usually more than one sentinel node is found in each basin. Furthermore, torso lesions may have sentinel nodes in more than one basin. As a result, patients usually undergo preoperative lymphoscintigraphy using a technetium-labelled tracer to identify the route of drainage as well as the number and site of sentinel nodes. Immediately preoperatively, patent blue dye is injected intradermally around the tumour. This allows

REFERENCES

77. Ross DA, Ross MI. Melanoma, Critical Debates. Blackwell, London, 2002: 133–149
78. Morton DDL, Wen D-R, Wong JH et al. Arch Surg 1992; 127: 392–399

further intraoperative detection of afferent lymphatics and staining of the sentinel node itself. Handheld gamma probes have further refined detection of the sentinel node, improving detection rates to almost 100%.

Sentinel node biopsy makes considerable demand of the pathologist. Serial sections are essential to identify micrometastases. Histologically negative nodes may still prove positive for micrometastases using immunohistochemistry with S100 or HMB45. Tyrosinase mRNA can also identify histologically occult micrometastases using PCR, although its clinical significance is still under evaluation.

Once the disease has spread, surgery still has a role in resecting isolated skin metastases or visceral metastases localized to one lobe of the liver, lung, or even the brain. Isolated limb perfusion with high-dose chemotherapy provides good local control of extensive limb disease but does not affect outcome. The CO_2 laser may also be beneficial in treating multiple skin metastases.

Chemotherapy and immunotherapy

Melanoma has proved to be resistant to most forms of chemotherapy. The standard, dacarbazine, produces a 3–5% complete response rate, which may be marginally increased with combination regimens. Considerable interest has centred on the role of interferon, initially thought to produce a 10% increase in survival. Unfortunately this initial optimism was not supported in later studies,[79] and further investigation is required. Other avenues of research include the study of tumour vaccines. Melanomas are known to produce specific antibodies, and much interest centres on their potential use as tumour vaccines. Radiotherapy has been under-utilized but has a recognized role in palliation of recurrent skin and cerebral metastases.

Prevention

Prevention remains one of the major areas whereby all clinicians can contribute to reducing the impact of this condition. Opportunistic screening provides an excellent opportunity to advise patients on good sun care (see Box 9.4).

SOFT TISSUE SARCOMAS

Sarcomas are rare, malignant tumours arising from or differentiating towards a tissue of mesenchymal origin, and they can arise anywhere in the body.[80] Numerous histological variants of these tumours exist; they have a range of biological behaviour from indolent growth and local recurrence to rapid growth, invasion and dissemination. Treatment may be difficult, and generally these tumours should be referred to specialist units. Multidisciplinary teams are the ideal for management and aim to preserve skin where possible and to spare limbs. Surgical excision is the first line of treatment, followed by adjuvant radiotherapy. Enneking staging is helpful in managing these tumours, but the overall prognosis is 50% survival at 5 years.

The clinical picture is an essential component of the eventual diagnosis, because many of these tumours display age, site and gender predominance: cutaneous angiosarcomas occur in the elderly, liposarcomas and malignant histiocytomas are tumours of adults, embryonal rhabdomyosarcoma is a tumour of children. Synovial sarcoma is commonly a tumour of the lower limb in young adult males, whereas epithelioid sarcoma occurs in the upper limb in the same patient group.

The speed of growth and the plane or depth of origin of the tumours also give important clues to the diagnosis. Deeper tumours tend to be more aggressive than superficial ones such as dermatofibrosarcoma protuberans and fibrosarcoma. Care must be taken, however, because both angiosarcomas and epithelioid sarcomas are both superficial and highly malignant.[81] A few important examples are discussed here.

Box 9.4 Prevention of malignant melanoma

- Physical protection, i.e. shade and avoidance of direct sunlight within 2 h either side of the solar noon.
- High-protection fabrics, long-sleeved shirts and hats.
- Sunscreens and creams should be used as an adjunct to the use of physical protection, with a minimal sun protection factor of 15 plus. It should be remembered that sunscreens act as filters, and that sun damage continues despite their use.
- Patients should be given advice regarding the potential risk of sunbeds and tanning lamps.
- Prevention and protection of children is essential because sun exposure in this age group is grossly related to the development of moles. Furthermore, as noted in the text, the presence of multiple naevi is a strong risk factor for melanoma.

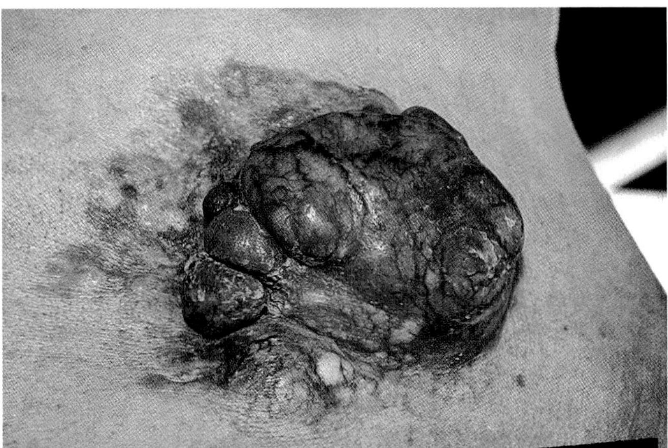

Figure 9.60 A dermatofibrosarcoma protuberans.

Dermatofibrosarcoma protuberans

Dermatofibrosarcoma protuberans (Fig. 9.60) is commonly encountered as a firm, dermal, multinodular, plaque-like growth. The tumour is non-tender, with a dark hue. Dermatofibrosarcoma protuberans is infiltrative and recurs if not widely excised. Aggressive sarcomatous change and metastasis follow multiple recurrences, thus the tumour demands careful diagnosis and wide local excision on the first occasion.[82]

Malignant peripheral nerve sheath tumours

The sarcomas of nerve and nerve sheath are classified as the malignant peripheral nerve sheath tumours. Schwann cell differentiation is the most common pattern.[83] Although malignant peripheral nerve sheath tumours occur in normal patients, they are common in patients with neurofibromatosis,

REFERENCES

79. Kirkwood JM. Surg Clin North Am 2003; 83: 283–322
80. Fisher C. Br J Plast Surg 1996; 49: 27–33
81. Girard C, Johnson WC et al. Cancer 1970; 26: 868–883
82. Kahn LB, Saxe N et al. Arch Dermatol 1978; 114: 599–601
83. Ricardi V. N Engl J Med 1981; 305: 1617–1626

who have a 4% incidence of malignant change in their numerous neurofibromas. The outcome of these tumours is difficult to predict, although those with neurofibromatosis tend to have a worse prognosis.

Epithelioid sarcoma

Epithelioid sarcoma presents as an ulcerating nodule on the upper limb. The tumours are slow-growing, painless, intradermal or subcutaneous nodules that are often multiple. The diagnosis is almost always made histologically (aided by cytokeratin immunostaining) rather than clinically, which results in the primary excision margins often being inadequate. The tumour spreads insidiously along tendons, nerves and fascial planes, and early nodal involvement is common. Treatment is by early wide excision, which frequently necessitates amputation. The local recurrence rate even after adequate surgery is approximately 75%; metastases develop in approximately 30–50%.

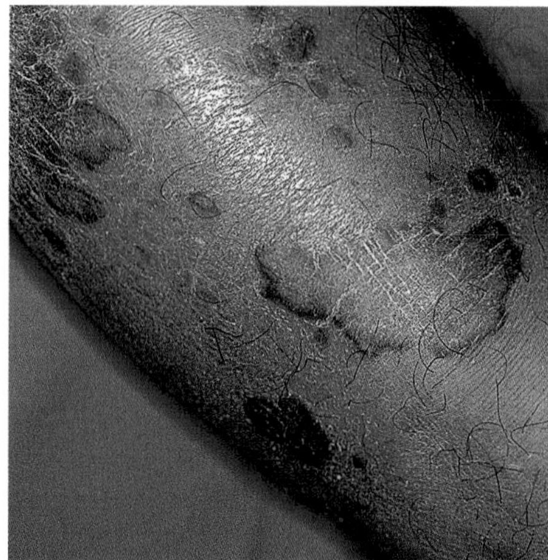

Figure 9.61 Kaposi's sarcoma. From Habif 2003,[62] with permission.

Kaposi's sarcoma

This sarcoma (Fig. 9.61) was described by Kaposi in 1872 as a painless, red or brown nodule, later ulcerating, usually on the leg or foot of elderly male patients. In 10% the viscera are involved; the gastrointestinal tract, liver and lungs are most often affected. More recently, Kaposi's sarcoma has been considered a major indicator of AIDS, heralding the conversion of the latency of the virus to the actual syndrome. These lesions are often smaller but more widely distributed than those of the classical form, and they often involve the mucous membranes.[84]

Angiosarcoma

Angiosarcoma is one of the most aggressive of the sarcomas.[85] The clinical diagnosis is usually delayed because presentation is variable in an elderly, frail population. Lesions appear as bruises, cellulitis or friable haemorrhagic plaques. Extensive local excision is necessary to eradicate the lesion.

Stewart–Treves syndrome describes lymphangiosarcoma that may develop in limbs with chronic lymphoedema, for example in the arm following axillary treatment for breast carcinoma.[86]

REFERENCES

84. Ziegler JL, Templeton AC et al. Semin Oncol 1984; 11: 47–52
85. Girard C, Johnson WC et al. Cancer 1970; 26: 868–883
86. Stewart FW, Treves N. Cancer 1948; 1: 64–81

The arteries

10

Peter R. Taylor, John A. Murie, Matthew M. Thompson, Julian Scott

INTRODUCTION

Atherosclerosis is responsible for nearly 90% of arterial disease in the western world.[1] The prevalence of atherosclerosis in Africa, the Indian subcontinent, and the Far East is much lower,[2] while arteritis, although still relatively rare, is more common in India and the Far East.[3] Vasospastic diseases, which are accentuated by a cold climate, appear to be increasing in incidence,[4] but syphilitic arteritis has almost disappeared.

The prevalence of arterial injury has risen proportionally with the increase in road traffic accidents,[5] operative surgery and interventional procedures, but armed insurrection and wars[6] are still responsible for sudden surges in the frequency of serious vascular injury. In the USA, there has been a steady increase in the number of vascular injuries in civilians caused by knife and gunshot wounds.[7] This type of trauma remains relatively rare in Europe, but its incidence is slowly increasing.

True arterial tumours are extremely rare, but AIDS has led to an epidemic of Kaposi's sarcoma (although there is dispute as to whether this is a true tumour).[8] The majority of angiomata are hereditary malformations and should therefore be classified as hamartomas.

Aneurysmal disease of arteries appears to be increasing,[9] but the incidence of arterial emboli appears to be falling in parallel with a decline in rheumatic heart disease.[10] This may also be related to the increased prescribing of warfarin to patients in atrial fibrillation.[11]

Heredity, diet, and racial and environmental factors all influence the prevalence of arterial disease, and fluctuations in these factors in various parts of the world are probably responsible for the differing proportions of arterial pathology that are found in individual countries.

The symptoms caused by arterial disease are dependent on the vessels that are affected, but there are many pathophysiological outcomes, symptoms and signs that are common to all arterial diseases. These are discussed first, before the individual pathological processes are described in detail in the subsequent sections.

PATHOPHYSIOLOGY OF ARTERIAL DISEASE

Disease in the arterial wall can lead to narrowing or dilatation of the vessel lumen; both outcomes can result from the same pathological process (e.g. atheroma) and can even develop simultaneously at different sites in the same individual. Three main territories are affected:

- cardiac,
- cerebrovascular, and
- aorta and limbs.

Visceral and mesenteric involvement is less common, and atherosclerotic disease of the upper limb is very rare.

ARTERIAL STENOSIS

A reduction in the cross-sectional area of the arterial lumen has little consequence at first, because flow is governed by Poiseuilles's law, which states that flow is proportional to the radius of the vessel to the power four and inversely proportional to the length of the vessel and the viscosity of the blood. Therefore the radius of the vessel wall has to be considerably reduced before there is any reduction in flow.

Blood flow in normal arteries is smooth and laminar, but wall abnormalities set up eddy currents and these alter shear forces, which accentuate arterial damage. A haemodynamically significant stenosis, causing appreciable changes in pressure and flow, does not occur until the cross-sectional area has been decreased by 75% (equivalent to a diameter reduction of at least 50%).[12] Stenoses of this magnitude do not allow an increase in blood flow when distal vasodilatation is caused by increased demand, and the tissues supplied by the artery are therefore deprived of oxygen. An oxygen debt then develops, leading to anaerobic metabolism and accumulation of unwanted metabolites. This process results in symptoms of **intermittent claudication** in the lower limbs.

The exact mechanism for the development of the pain of claudication remains obscure but may be related to anoxia, acidosis, and the accumulation of metabolites. The pain may be the result of 'defective terminal circulation interfering with the insulation of nerve fibres permitting the overflow of efferent sympathetic stimuli to neighbouring sensory fibres'.[13] Claudication was thought to be caused by accumulation of substance P within the muscles.[14] Little new has been added to these theories in recent years.

REFERENCES

1. Robertson WB. Pathol Microbiol 1967; 30: 810
2. McGill HC. Lab Invest 1968; 18: 465
3. Tejada C, Strong JP et al. Lab Invest 1968; 18: 509
4. Olsen N, Nielsen SL. Scand J Clin Lab Invest 1978; 37: 761
5. Trunkey DD. Sci Am 1983; 249: 28
6. Rich NM, Baugh JH, Hughes CW. J Trauma 1970; 10: 359
7. Rich NM. In: Bongard FS, Wilson SE, Perry MO (eds). Vascular Injuries in Surgical Practice. Prentice Hall, London, 1991: 1–31
8. Durack DT. N Engl J Med 1981; 305: 1465
9. Collin J. Br J Surg 1987; 74: 332
10. Abbott WM, Maloney RD et al. Am Surg 1982; 143: 460
11. Petersen P et al. Lancet 1989; 1: 175
12. Sumner DS. In: Rutherford RB (ed). Vascular Surgery. 4th edn. WB Saunders, London, 1995: 18–25
13. Cohen S. Postgrad Med J 1946; 22: 1
14. Lewis T, Pickering GW, Rothschild P. Heart 1929; 15: 359

Intermittent claudication is a cramp-like pain caused by muscle ischaemia. Claudication pain is experienced in the muscles of the thigh and buttock if there is a stenosis or occlusion of the aorta or the iliac vessels, and in men this may be associated with impotence. Claudication pain is most commonly felt in the large muscles of the posterior calf, where it is often the result of a stenosis or occlusion of the superficial femoral artery at the adductor hiatus. Occasionally it affects the muscles of the upper limb, and very rarely the small muscles of the foot. Claudication pain can occur in the jaw muscles of patients with Takayasu's disease.

Claudication pain increases with exercise and is relieved completely by rest. The distance at which the pain develops (the claudication distance) may vary from day to day, often depending on the ambient temperature. This distance shortens if the disease extends or the vessel occludes. It is usually worse on walking up hills and better when walking on the level or downhill. Claudication pain can be categorized into a series of grades depending on the severity of the symptoms,[15] but the distance to the onset of the pain and the maximum distance that can be achieved by the patient is simpler to comprehend and can be objectively measured on a treadmill.

Stenosis of the extracranial vessels is most commonly found at the junction of the common, internal and external carotid arteries. Stenotic disease of one carotid bifurcation rarely produces symptoms as the result of reduced blood flow. Symptoms may occur, however, if there is a severe stenosis or a total occlusion of the opposite carotid, or if the circle of Willis is incomplete. Symptoms from a unilateral stenosis are invariably the result of platelet emboli breaking loose from the diseased arterial wall, causing transient ischaemic attacks that recover within 24 h, episodes of fleeting blindness usually lasting a few minutes (called amaurosis fugax), or completed strokes where the neurological deficit lasts longer than 24 h. Stenoses in the vertebrobasilar system may give rise to loss of consciousness and vertigo on sudden changes of posture or after rapid neck movements. Occasionally, severe carotid stenosis may follow neck irradiation for lymphomas or carcinoma of the thyroid gland or larynx.

A severe stenosis of one renal artery was shown experimentally by Goldblatt and colleagues to promote the release of renin.[16] Renin acts on angiotensinogen, a plasma globulin proenzyme, to produce angiotensin, which acts directly on the arterial wall to cause generalized arteriolar contraction and hypertension. Renal artery stenosis is an important treatable cause of hypertension and can also cause chronic renal failure. Stenoses of the coeliac and mesenteric vessels can produce severe abdominal pain after meals. This is called **intestinal angina**, and must be differentiated from other more common causes of severe indigestion. Patients usually stop eating to avoid the pain and may rapidly lose weight. They literally have a fear of food. Arterial impotence is the result of an inability to increase blood flow through the helicine arteries of the penis. Arterial influx must exceed venous drainage to produce and maintain tumescence (see Ch. 38).

ACUTE ARTERIAL OCCLUSION

Stenotic disease of the arterial wall may progress until the lumen is completely obliterated, but this usually follows an acute thrombosis. Atheromatous plaque within the arterial wall may fissure and rupture, allowing blood to enter the plaque and red cells and fibrin to accumulate within the arterial wall.[17] This occludes the lumen and usually results in propagated thrombosis extending as far as the next major collateral branch and occasionally beyond. Acute arterial occlusions may also be produced by emboli, thrombosis of an aneurysm, arterial dissection, external compression, ligation or injury. Rarely, massive trauma may disrupt the artery, but more commonly intimal tears can result from fractures of bones adjacent to arteries, particularly the brachial artery in supracondylar fractures of the humerus in children and the popliteal artery in fractures around the knee caused by hyperextension injuries in adults (Fig. 10.1).

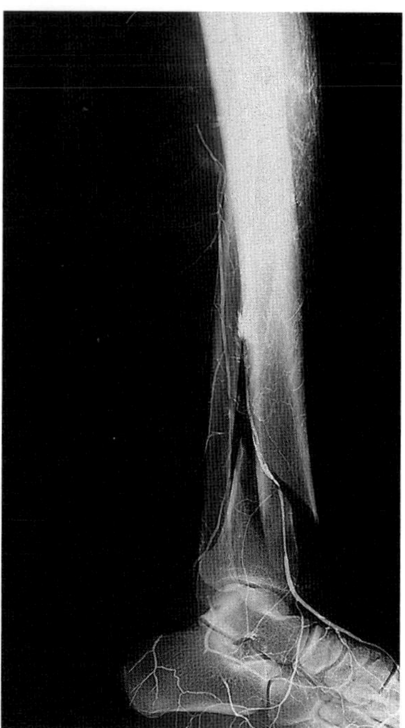

Figure 10.1 Fractured tibia causing disruption of tibial vessels.

Both the speed of the occlusion and the available collateral circulation determine the subsequent symptoms. When the occlusion is gradual and the collaterals good, the symptoms may be minimal, but if the occlusion is sudden and the collateral circulation poor, then symptoms of acute ischaemia and tissue infarction rapidly develop.

Coronary arteries

An acute occlusion of one of the coronary vessels can be symptomless but frequently produces a myocardial infarct, a cardiac arrhythmia or cardiac arrest (see Ch. 22).

Aorta, and iliac and lower limb arteries

Acute occlusion of the aorta and iliac vessels is rare but may occur if an aneurysm thromboses, or if acute thrombosis supervenes on atheromatous disease. A saddle embolus may lodge at the aortic bifurcation and occlude both iliac arteries. When an acute aortic occlusion occurs the patient first complains of sudden severe pain in both lower limbs, which are noted to be pale and cold. The pallor may persist, but if the surroundings are warm the pallor is soon replaced by cyanosis, which can spread to the level of the

REFERENCES

15. Fontaine R, Kieny R et al. J Cardiovasc Surg 1964; 4: 463
16. Goldblatt H, Lynch J et al. J Exp Med 1934; 59: 347
17. Davis MJ, Thomas AC. Br Heart J 1985; 53: 363

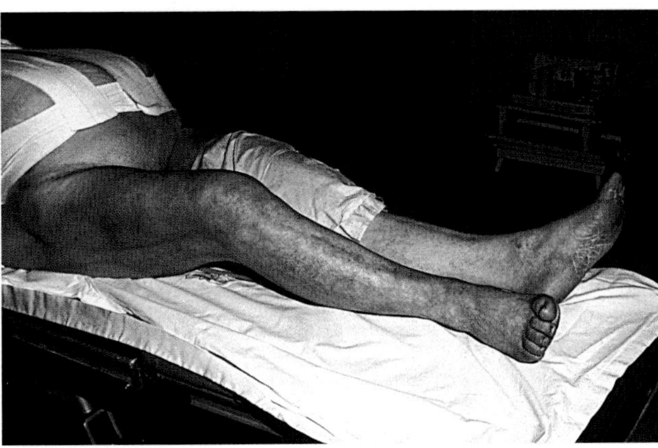

Figure 10.2 Right leg with acute ischaemia, showing mottling and marble-like appearance.

umbilicus. White patches called Bier spots[18] appear among the blue or purple background after several hours, and these then coalesce to produce a mottled appearance. Streaking by pigment-stained venules completes the similarity to marble (Fig. 10.2). This state may take some days to develop and is reversible in its early stages. Blood blisters indicate cutaneous damage, and these easily brush off to leave superficial oozing ulcers. The limbs continue to cool centripetally and may later become oedematous.

Pain is often severe and of a bursting nature, although it may occasionally be mild, amounting only to numbness and paraesthesia. When the blood supply is restored after some delay, neuritic pain may persist, with hypersensitivity to both painful and thermal stimuli. Nerve and muscle function rapidly cease if ischaemia persists, with nerve conduction disappearing between 15 and 30 min and permanent muscle damage developing within a few hours. The limbs may become anaesthetic at the same time, and this anaesthesia has a stocking-type distribution.

Although skin tolerates periods of ischaemia up to 48 h reasonably well, recovery in nerve and muscle is much more variable and is usually incomplete. The muscles of the anterior compartment of the lower leg are invariably the most severely affected, with the extensor hallucis longus muscle often the last to recover. The muscles of the plantar compartment recover poorly, if at all, and the skin of the sole may remain anaesthetic even after the rest of the leg has returned to normal. Human striated muscle virtually never regenerates after a period of severe ischaemia; it is replaced by fibrous tissue that causes severe contracture.[19]

At an advanced stage of acute ischaemia, revascularization of the limb is hazardous because toxic metabolites, myoglobin, and large quantities of potassium[20] may be released into the circulation, causing sudden death from cardiac arrhythmia, renal failure, respiratory distress syndrome or general toxaemia. A history of ischaemia extending beyond 24 h, associated with anaesthesia, muscle tenderness and swelling, should alert the clinician to this risk, and any attempt at revascularization must then be carefully considered and accompanied by the judicious use of extensive fasciotomies. Amputation may be safer in these circumstances.

An identical picture can be produced in a single limb by an embolus or thrombosis of the superficial femoral and profunda femoris bifurcation.[21] Acute occlusions below this point rarely cause such a florid picture because of the better collateral channels that are available. An acute thrombosis of a popliteal aneurysm, when the crural vessels have already been occluded by distal emboli, is an exception to this rule, and is an important cause of severe acute ischaemia of the calf and foot. A combination of an acute proximal thrombosis with prior disease of the crural or popliteal vessels from any cause also produces acute ischaemic changes.

Extracranial vessels

An acute occlusion of either the common or internal carotid artery may be well tolerated because an adequate circle of Willis is capable of supplying the opposite hemisphere from a patent vertebral or contralateral carotid artery.[22] A carotid occlusion usually results in cerebral infarction and a major stroke if the circle of Willis is congenitally incomplete or diseased, or if there are additional stenoses or occlusions in the other extracranial vessels (Fig. 10.3). This presents as a sudden onset of monoplegia or hemiplegia, which may be accompanied by dysphasia, dysarthria, visual disturbance, cognitive loss and emotional lability. Recovery depends on the size of the initial infarct and the adequacy of the collateral circulation. Cerebral infarcts can also follow occlusions of the brachiocephalic trunk and the vertebrobasilar vessels, but most strokes that are not the result of a carotid occlusion are caused by small vessel disease, an intracerebral haemorrhage, or a thrombosis or an embolism of the intracerebral vessels.

Upper limb arteries

Thrombosis or embolism can cause sudden occlusions of the subclavian, axillary or brachial arteries. Occasionally, occlusion of an aneurysm related to a cervical rib or from an arteritis in the vessel wall may be responsible. Atherosclerotic occlusions of the upper limb are uncommon, but they can give rise to ischaemic pain on exercise, subclavian steal syndrome, and even acute ischaemia of the upper limb.

The subclavian steal syndrome occurs when a block in the first part of the subclavian artery leads to the stealing of blood from the circle of Willis by retrograde flow down the vertebral artery, which acts as a collateral to the arm during muscular exercise (Fig. 10.4).[23] This is a rare disorder that produces multiple symptoms during arm exercise, including visual disturbance, vertigo, ataxia, syncope, motor and sensory deficits, dysarthria and dysphasia. Some still doubt the existence of the syndrome.

Acute ischaemia of the upper limb is identical in presentation and appearance to that of the lower limb.

Visceral vessels

The three anterior abdominal aortic branches—the coeliac, and the superior and inferior mesenteric vessels—may all occlude acutely as a result of thrombosis, embolism, a dissecting aneurysm or vasculitis. There is normally a good collateral circulation between all three visceral arteries, and patients may remain symptomless despite occlusions of all three major vessels. An

REFERENCES

18. Lewis T. Vascular Disorders of the Limbs. Macmillan, London, 1944
19. Von Volkman R, Von Pitha, Bilroth H (eds). In: Handbuch der Allgemeinen und Specielsen Chirurgie, Vol 2. Stuttgart, 1872
20. Haimovici H. Contemp Surg 1980; 17: 33
21. Blaisdell WF, Steele M, Allen RE. Surgery 1978; 84: 222
22. Fields WS, Bruetman ME, Weibel J. Monographs in the Surgical Sciences. Williams & Wilkins, Baltimore, 1965
23. (Editorial). N Engl J Med 1961; 265: 912

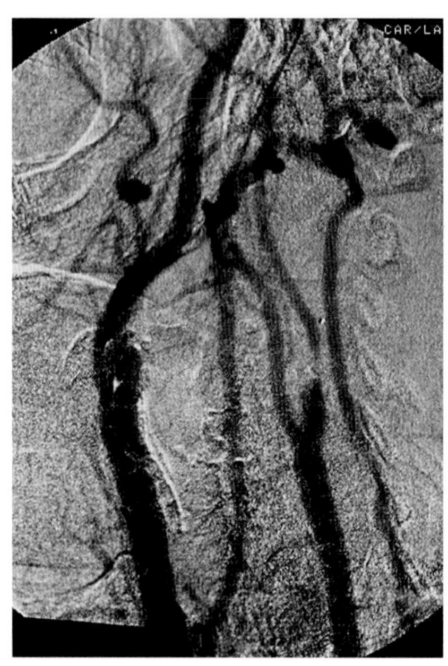

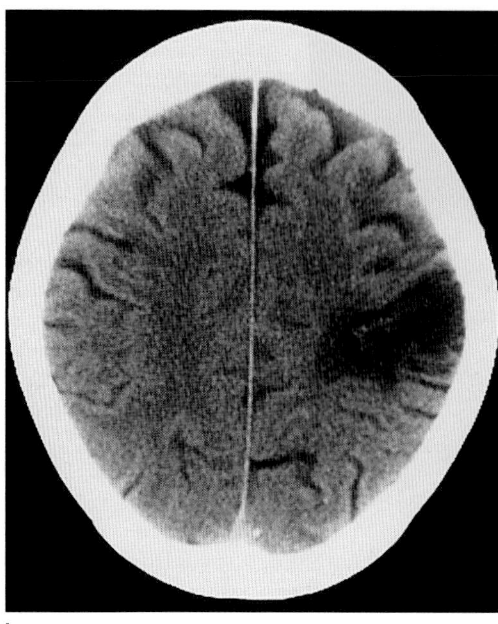

a b

Figure 10.3 An intravenous digital subtraction angiogram showing a stenosed carotid artery. This resulted in the cerebral infarct shown on the CT scan of the brain (**b**).

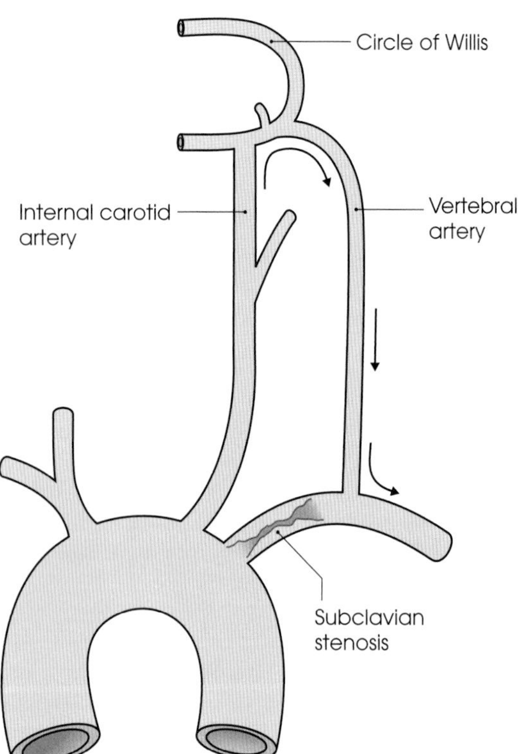

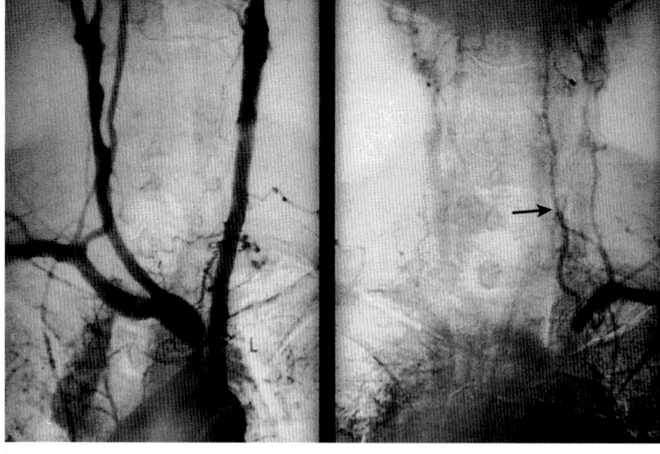

Figure 10.4 The subclavian steal syndrome: (**a**) diagrammatic representation of flow and (**b**) intravenous digital subtraction angiography showing occlusion of the left subclavian artery with (**c**) late filling of this vessel by retrograde flow down the vertebral artery (arrow).

acute embolus or thrombosis lodging at the origin of the superior mesenteric artery usually produces a mesenteric infarct, because this is an end artery. Patients with mesenteric infarction complain of persistent, severe and generalized abdominal pain. The severity of the pain is often matched by a paucity of physical signs. Patients rapidly become toxic and shocked, and die from the consequences of septic shock if left untreated.

The infarcted bowel is at first pale, but then becomes oedematous and suffused, before rapidly discolouring and turning dark blue as the stagnant blood becomes deoxygenated and the anaerobic putrefactive organisms begin to multiply. Initially the mucosa ulcerates, but as the ischaemia progresses it necroses and separates. The serosal surface becomes dull and eventually black with the cessation of peristaltic movement. No pulsation can be felt in the mesenteric blood vessels.

Miscellaneous arteries

The arterial supply of the kidneys, spleen and liver can also become acutely occluded. Splenic infarcts are commonly associated with sickle cell anaemia or hypersplenism and can result in splenic atrophy, which is often referred to as an autosplenectomy. The liver, like the lungs, receives a dual blood supply and therefore rarely infarcts, even when the hepatic artery is accidentally or deliberately ligated or embolized to treat metastatic tumours (Ch. 29).

GANGRENE

Gangrene is irreversible tissue necrosis, often associated with putrefaction, and is usually caused by an acute occlusion of the blood supply to an organ or extremity. Gangrene occurs most commonly in the lower limb, but the upper limb and intestine may also be affected. It has two forms—wet and dry—but gradations occur, from the waterlogged gangrene of rapidly extending infection to the mummification of gradual arterial occlusion.

Wet gangrene follows an acute arterial occlusion that is left untreated, particularly if the limb is oedematous or has defective venous drainage. Wet gangrene occurs if the arterial occlusion is sufficiently sudden to prevent the loss by evaporation of the normal tissue fluid. Micro-organisms secondarily invade the dead tissue, which provides an excellent medium for bacterial growth. Wet arterial gangrene has to be differentiated from infected clostridial or non-clostridial gas gangrene (see Ch. 4). Antibiotics often fail to prevent infection because the drugs cannot reach the ischaemic tissues. They may, however, be useful in preventing the spread of organisms to healthy tissues and in encouraging demarcation. Wet gangrene has a dusky appearance, often intermingled with the erythema of inflammation, which has an ill-defined and spreading edge (Fig. 10.5). The skin may blister, and the digits soon become insensitive and immobile because of ischaemic changes in the nerves and muscles of the limb. Gas bubbles may form within the tissues, causing crepitus (surgical emphysema); if left untreated the limb gives off a characteristic putrefying stench.

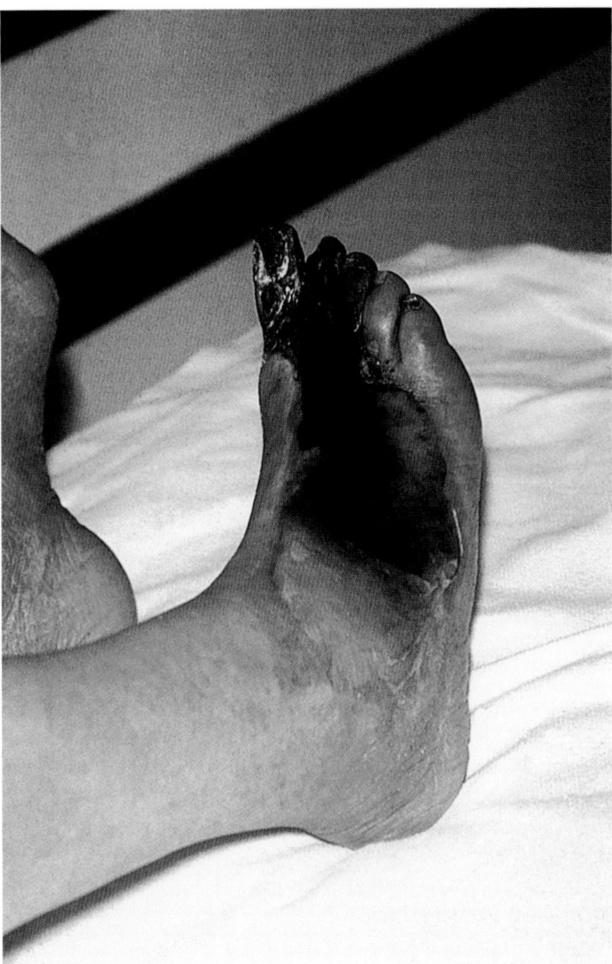

Figure 10.5 A limb with an area of wet gangrene.

CHRONIC OCCLUSION

When a severe arterial stenosis pre-dates an acute arterial occlusion, pre-existing collateral channels usually ensure that the symptoms of acute ischaemia and wet gangrene do not develop. In some instances where there are very good collateral pathways, patients may even remain free of symptoms, and should gangrene occur the changes are often minimal. In many instances the eventual occlusion leads to a sudden but rapid deterioration in symptoms, which then usually improve as collateral channels open up in response to the new ischaemic stimulus.

Acute on chronic occlusions invariably develop on top of pre-existing disease of the arterial wall, and atherosclerosis or arteritis is usually responsible. Rupture of an atheromatous plaque with resultant intraplaque haemorrhage is still the most common cause of the final arterial thrombotic occlusion,[23] but gradual thickening of the subintimal layer with platelet deposition may also account for some of the more chronic occlusions. Rupture of an atheromatous plaque may shower emboli into the distal circulation, causing occlusion of the digital arteries. This gives rise to the blue toe syndrome, or if the upper limb is affected, the blue finger syndrome.[24] When the emboli are more extensive and produce widespread ischaemic areas, the changes are often called **trash foot**.

Aorto-iliac and lower limb vessels

A chronic aorto-iliac occlusion often presents with new or deteriorating claudication, which is usually experienced in both thighs and buttocks as well as in the lower leg and calf. Erectile impotence and muscle wasting are additional features of Leriche's syndrome.[25] A single common iliac occlusion may cause unilateral buttock claudication, while an external iliac occlusion usually produces unilateral thigh claudication. An acute or chronic aorto-iliac occlusion almost never causes rest pain or dry gangrene of the feet, unless there are additional stenoses or occlusions of the distal vessels. The external iliac and the common femoral arteries may also become chronically occluded, and the profunda femoris artery is often narrowed or occluded at its origin, although this vessel is usually disease-free in some part of its course.[26]

The most common site of stenosis in the lower limb is in the superficial femoral artery as it passes through the adductor canal.[27] This artery may later occlude, while the popliteal artery, particularly in its lower third, is often comparatively disease-free (Fig. 10.6). Individual crural vessels, the pedal arches, and the metatarsal and digital arteries may all become chronically

REFERENCES

24. Karmody AM, Powers SR et al. Arch Surg 1976; 111: 1263–1268
25. Leriche R. Presse Med 1940; 48: 601
26. Dibble JH. The Pathology of Limb Ischaemia. Oliver and Boyd, Edinburgh, 1966
27. Beales JSM, Adcock FA et al. Br J Radiol 1971; 44: 854

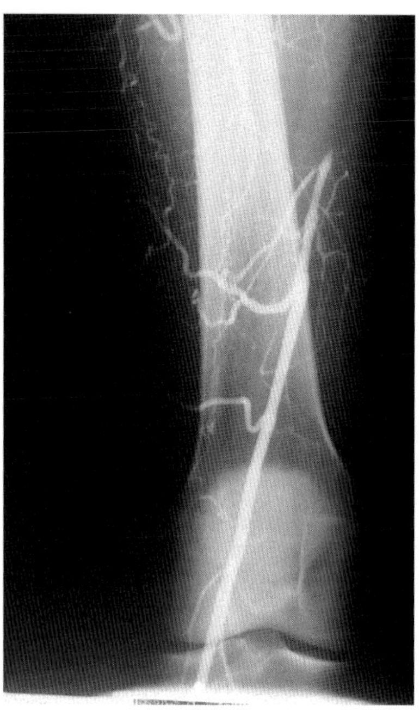

Figure 10.6 An aortogram showing an occluded superficial femoral artery on the right with a relatively spared popliteal artery.

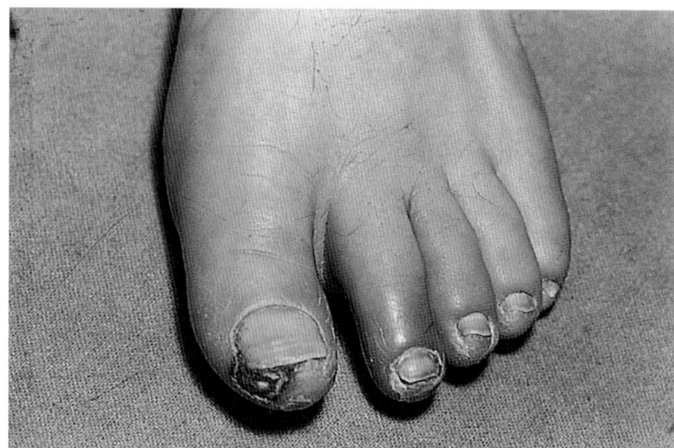

Figure 10.7 An ischaemic nail fold.

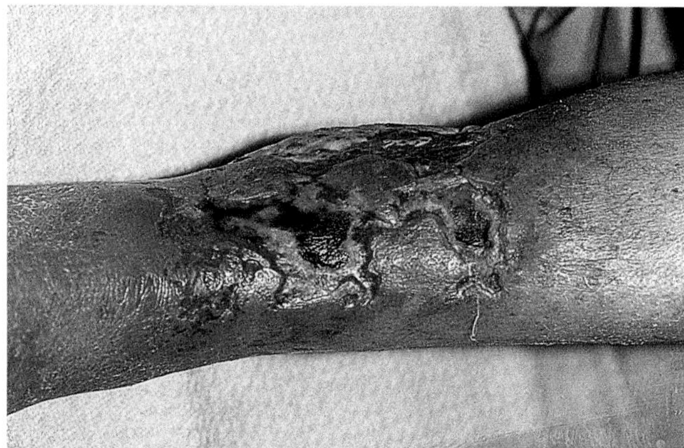

Figure 10.8 An ischaemic ulcer.

occluded as the result of mural disease. The more distal the occlusion, the less the prospect of collateral pathways and the greater the likelihood of ischaemic rest pain, ulceration and gangrene. Diabetic patients commonly have disease of multiple segments, which often affects the arteries distal to the popliteal trifurcation.

Critical limb ischaemia

Critical limb ischaemia has been defined as rest pain, ulceration or gangrene associated with a Doppler pressure at the ankle of less than 50 mmHg, or at the toe of 30 mmHg, in patients who are not diabetic. Tissue necrosis will almost inevitably ensue in limbs with critical ischaemia if the circulation cannot be improved.

Rest pain

Rest pain is usually experienced in the dorsum of the foot and the toes, being worse at night. The pain is dull and severe, and it usually requires opiate analgesia for symptomatic relief. The patient wakes up with a painful cold foot, which is relieved by hanging the foot over the side of the bed or by walking around. Placing the leg in a dependent position allows gravity to improve the blood flow, and exercise also increases the blood flow to the limb. Patients may even take to sleeping in a chair to avoid the pain associated with elevation of the legs. The pain comes on at night because of the reduction in cardiac output that accompanies sleep, with a decrease in blood pressure and an increase in peripheral vasodilatation. Although the exact mechanism of rest pain remains obscure, a reduced blood supply to peripheral nerves and an accumulation of metabolites have both been implicated.

Dry gangrene

Nutritional changes vary in extent from dry necrosis of the skin of the fingertips or toes, which can occur in Raynaud's disease or scleroderma, to gangrene of one or more limbs. Sometimes the first sign of arterial insufficiency is a nail fold infection in, for example, a patient with thromboangiitis obliterans (Fig. 10.7). Ulceration of the legs that fails to heal (Fig. 10.8) or tiny fissures in the skin of the feet may be early signs of incipient gangrene.

Dry gangrene develops from the gradual interruption of the blood supply of tissues free from oedema, liberally drained by open veins, exposed to evaporation and remaining uninfected. An area of skin, often at the tip of a digit or at a point of contact between two adjacent toes, becomes dark and blackens. This area is often small at first but may then extend for a varying distance. Sensation is lost, and the gangrenous part becomes shrunken and wrinkled. This process of tissue death extends until a level is reached where an adequate blood supply remains. The vessels at this level dilate, and signs of mild inflammation arise to produce a barrier of granulation tissue—the line of demarcation between living and dead tissue (Fig. 10.9).

When the process is allowed to proceed uninterrupted, the gangrenous extremity separates, and as the superficial tissues are dried by evaporation to a more proximal level than the deep tissues, the resultant stump is conical with an apex of exposed bone, which may later separate as a sequestrum before being covered by epithelium. It is rarely possible or practical to await this process of autoamputation when gangrene extends into the forefoot or above the level of the heel (Fig. 10.10), and surgical ablation is invariably required to relieve pain and provide a functional myoplastic stump (see p. 264).

Extracranial vessels

Chronic occlusion of the common carotid, external and internal carotid vessels is the normal progression of severe stenosis in these vessels. The vertebral and basilar arteries may also occlude,

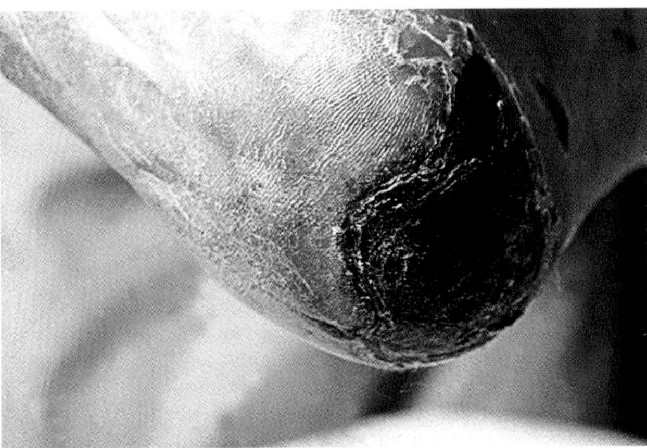

Figure 10.9 A clear line of demarcation between living and dead tissue.

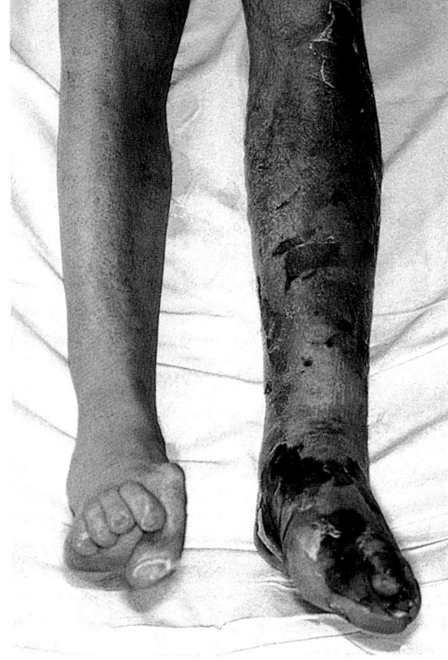

Figure 10.10 Extensive gangrene involving the foot and lower leg. The heel could not have been preserved even if the limb had been successfully revascularized.

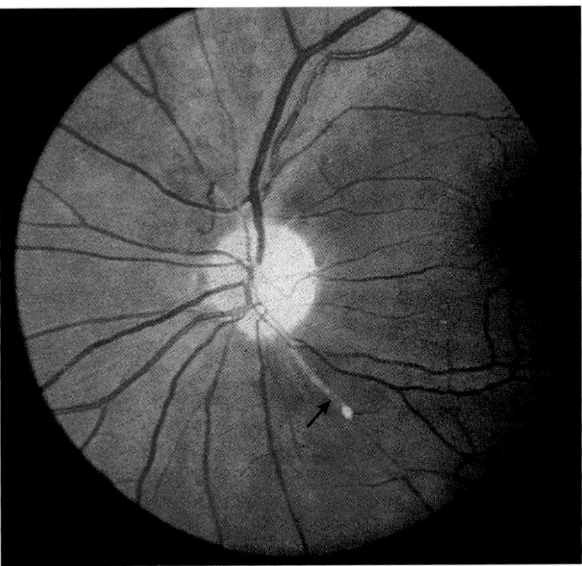

Figure 10.11 A cholesterol embolus occluding a branch of the retinal artery.

as may the main brachiocephalic or innominate trunk. Chronic occlusions of individual vessels may be symptomless in the presence of a well-formed circle of Willis, or may be associated with transient ischaemic attacks, progressive dementia, blindness and cerebral infarction.[28]

Transient ischaemic attacks are reversible episodes of focal cerebral malfunction, which recover within 24 h.[29] The majority of these abate within a few minutes or a couple of hours, although minor neurological signs may persist for longer. The majority of transient ischaemic attacks are the result of platelet clumps breaking off from ulcerated plaques in the extracerebral vessels and embolizing into the cerebral or retinal vessels, where they lodge temporarily, occluding the blood supply, before subsequently breaking up.[30,31] Transient ischaemic attacks can occur in patients with occluded cerebral vessels, and it is still debatable whether these are the result of platelet emboli arising from the proximal end of an occluded vessel, or whether they represent true cerebral hypoperfusion as the result of critically reduced blood flow.[32] Cerebral hypoperfusion certainly does exist,[33] while the former hypothesis remains speculative. Hypoperfusional transient ischaemic attacks tend to follow exertion or vasodilatation and may occur many times a day. They usually affect patients with one or more occluded extracranial vessels (i.e. both carotids and one vertebral).

Many extracerebral arterial occlusions cause cerebral infarction, which produces an area of hyperaemic congested brain that rapidly becomes oedematous. The oedema may spread into the surrounding normal brain, causing raised intracranial pressure, tentorial herniation, and eventually coning of the brain stem. The infarct then becomes softened and pulpy, containing a white emulsion consisting of fatty globules, the remains of cells and fibres, containing many phagocytes. Later the infarct may liquefy and even calcify before being replaced by scar tissue, although a central cystic area can persist.

A platelet or cholesterol embolus arising from disease in the wall of the aorta, the brachiocephalic artery or the carotid vessels may cause transient monocular blindness (amaurosis fugax), or permanent loss of vision if the retinal artery or one of its major branches remains occluded. Fundoscopy may show emboli within the retinal vessels (Fig. 10.11) or may show pale areas of retinal infarction (Fig. 10.12). Areas of visual field may be lost.

Progressive dementia is a rare but important consequence of chronic occlusive and embolic disease of the extracranial and intracerebral vessels. It is less common than other forms of dementia such as Alzheimer's disease but must be considered in all patients presenting with presenile dementia. Loss of the superficial temporal or carotid pulse, poor pulsation seen in the retinal vessels, extracranial or postorbital bruits, and evidence of ischaemic vascular disease elsewhere should all alert the clinician to the possibility of a vascular cause for dementia.

REFERENCES

28. Mitchell JRA, Schwartz CJ. Arterial Disease. Blackwell, Oxford, 1965
29. Fisher CM. Neurol Psychiatry 1951; 65: 356
30. Harrison MGH, Marshall J. Br Med J 1975; 1: 616
31. Hollenhorst RW. JAMA 1961; 178: 23
32. Barnett HJM, Peerless SJ, Kaufman JCE. Stroke 1978; 9: 448
33. Gibbs JM, Wise RJS et al. Lancet 1984; i: 310

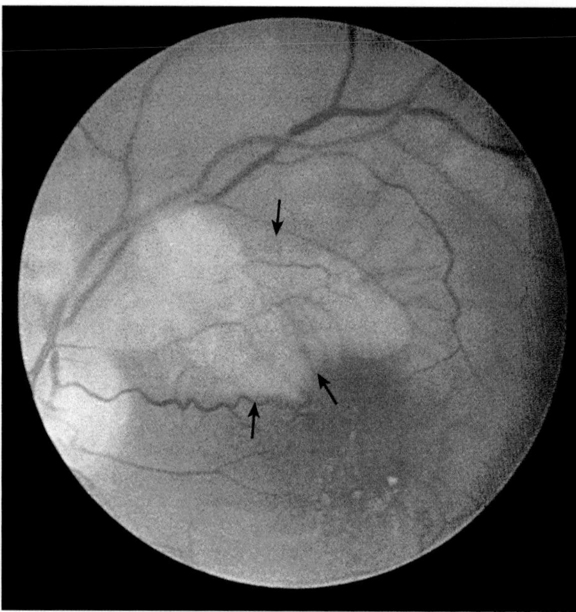

Figure 10.12 A retinal infarct.

Visceral vessels

Chronic occlusions of one of the visceral vessels may, like a severe stenosis, pass unnoticed providing the other major vessels are free of disease. An acute occlusion of the superior mesenteric artery usually causes mesenteric infarction because collateral channels may not be able to dilate sufficiently swiftly.

Symptoms of intestinal angina and mesenteric infarction invariably follow a major visceral occlusion if there is stenotic or occlusive disease in the other two vessels.[34] A poor marginal artery in association with a chronic reduction in mesenteric blood flow can lead to ischaemic colitis, which presents with persistent and sometimes blood-stained diarrhoea, abdominal pain and weight loss (see Ch. 28).

Chronic stenosis of a single renal artery causes hypertension and a decrease in renal size. Bilateral stenoses also result in hypertension, a decrease in renal size, and eventually a progressive deterioration in renal function, which finally results in renal failure.

CLINICAL HISTORY OF ARTERIAL DISEASE

The name, sex and age of the patient, together with his or her occupation, are essential. The initial symptoms, the time of their first presentation, and any subsequent change must be documented. For example, if the complaint is of intermittent claudication of the lower limb, the time of onset, the site of the pain, the exact distance at which it develops, the maximum walking distance, and the time taken for the pain to pass off must be determined. In addition, the progression and regression of symptoms from their first presentation should be carefully noted.

Direct questioning must exclude rest pain, and evidence of vascular disease in other territories must be carefully sought in all patients presenting with symptoms of an arterial nature. The effect of the symptoms on the patient's daily life, work and hobbies must also be assessed from the history, and all patients with vascular symptoms must be closely questioned on their tobacco habits. A family history of vascular disease may be important in aneurysms and vasospastic disorders, and the patient's occupation may provide useful information. For example, regular usage of vibrating tools may induce vasospasticity in the digital vessels. A history of significant trauma, however long ago, must not be overlooked; neither should a history of frostbite. A detailed history of drug intake and allergy may be important, and the patient's previous and present general health may also provide useful information. A past history of rheumatic fever, atrial fibrillation, diabetes, syphilis, rheumatoid arthritis and ergot intake may also provide important clues to the diagnosis of the underlying arterial disorder.

PHYSICAL SIGNS OF ARTERIAL DISEASE

Many of the physical signs associated with arterial disease have already been discussed in the description of the pathophysiology of arterial disease, but they are summarized here. The lower limbs are used as examples of the physical signs associated with peripheral arterial disease.

The temperature of the limb should be assessed and compared with the opposite side. Relative coolness indicates a significant reduction in blood flow, while frigidity follows an acute occlusion with poor collaterals.

Colour changes in the skin range from pallor, through normal skin colour, to cyanosis and rubor. These changes may remain constant, vary with position, or undergo cyclical changes in vasospastic disease. Intense pallor is usually seen in the early stages of an acute arterial obstruction with poor collaterals. At a later stage, the limb becomes cyanotic before gangrene develops. Chronic ischaemia is often associated with cyanosis and rubor, as accumulated metabolites attempt to stimulate capillary vasodilatation, but the poor blood flow results in desaturation of the stagnant blood. Buerger's test exploits the response of ischaemic tissues to elevation. Buerger's angle of circulatory insufficiency is the angle at which a limb is held to produce pallor.[35] This test is very inaccurate but can be used to compare a normal and an abnormal limb if both limbs are elevated to 60° for 2 min.[36] Pallor is then obvious on the sole of the ischaemic foot. The time taken for each limb to become pallid is observed. The veins in the elevated ischaemic limb may become empty, causing venous guttering, and if the legs are then placed in a dependent position, the ischaemic limb shows a delayed but pronounced hyperaemic response.

Evidence of early ischaemic change is seen in rapidly growing tissues. The nails become brittle and short, and hair growth is said to be poor, although it is often difficult to detect marked differences in hair growth between normal and abnormal limbs.

In advanced chronic ischaemia, cracks may develop over the heel (Fig. 10.13); the pulp spaces may become infected and ulceration may appear over the pressure points and between the toes. Eventually frank gangrene is seen in the distal tissues (Figs 10.7–10.10 and 10.14).

In acute ischaemia, the leg is pallid and rapidly becomes swollen over the muscle compartment. Later the muscles become

REFERENCES

34. Dick AP, Graff R et al. Gut 1967; 8: 206
35. Buerger L. Circulatory Disturbances of the Extremities. WB Saunders, Philadelphia, 1924
36. Insall RL, Davies RJ, Prout WG. J R Soc Med 1989; 82: 729

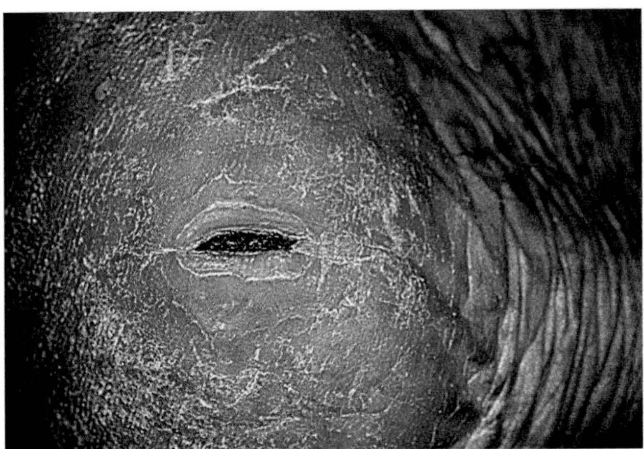

Figure 10.13 An ischaemic crack over the heel.

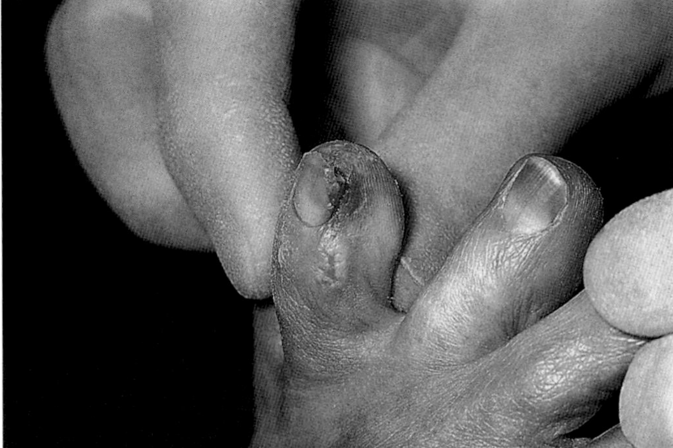

Figure 10.14 Ischaemic ulceration appearing between the toes.

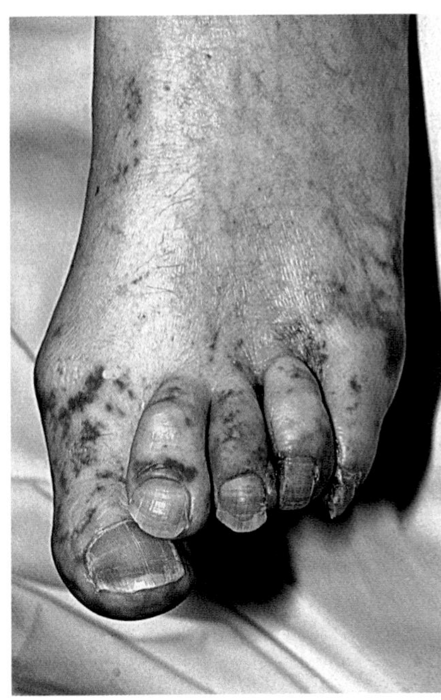

Figure 10.15 The appearance produced by showers of platelet emboli lodging in the capillaries of the feet.

tender as neuromuscular weakness and finally paralysis develop. This is associated with loss of sensation in the skin to light touch and pain. Such a neurosensory deficit indicates severe ischaemia.

The presence and extent of any gangrene should be carefully inspected and recorded, and the existence of a clear line of demarcation noted (Figs 10.9 and 10.10). Ischaemic ulceration can occur anywhere on the toes, foot, or around the ankle. Ischaemic ulcers do not have any distinguishing signs. They have sloping terraced edges. They are not surrounded by lipodermatosclerosis but usually have a slough-covered surface and poor pale granulation tissue in their base. Multiple showers of tiny emboli have the characteristic features already described (Fig. 10.15). Their appearance should lead to a careful search for a proximal aneurysm or an ulcerated plaque.

Absence of arterial pulsation indicates arterial occlusion, which may be assumed to lie below the lowest palpable and above the highest impalpable pulse. Large collateral vessels may maintain a reduced distal pulse even when the main artery is occluded. In the lower limbs the aortic, both femoral, popliteal, posterior tibial and dorsalis pedis pulses must be palpated and recorded as present, diminished, absent or enlarged. Although a complicated grading system has been proposed to gauge pulse volume,[37] the use of these four simple descriptions is probably more valuable. It is important to remember that anatomical variations can exist: the dorsalis pedis is absent from its normal position in 14% of the population, and the peroneal artery replaces the posterior tibial artery in 5%.[38] The astute clinician will also feel for the peroneal trunk as it lies in front of the lateral malleolus.

A true expansile pulsation must be distinguished from transmitted pulsation, and the upper and lower extent of any aneurysm must be determined. When an aneurysm is found, all other aneurysmal sites must be carefully palpated to exclude the presence of multiple aneurysms. An aneurysm in the popliteal fossa is easily missed by the conventional method of palpation. It may be better felt if the knee is hyperextended by one hand, pushing the artery on to the flexed fingers of the other hand.

All the arteries that supply the lower limbs must be carefully auscultated to detect bruits or machinery murmurs. It is important to listen over the aorta, the iliac vessels, the common femoral arteries and the superficial femoral artery in the adductor canal, and the popliteal artery because these are the common sites of arterial stenoses.

In patients suspected of having vascular disease, all the other major vessels must be examined by palpation and auscultation. The superficial temporal artery pulse should be felt in front of the external auditory meatus, and middle cerebral bruits may be heard through the closed upper eyelid. Carotid pulsation and carotid bruits may be felt and auscultated at the anterior border of the sternomastoid behind and below the angle of the jaw. Subclavian and vertebral bruits are listened for in the supraclavicular fossa. All bruits heard over the vessels of the head and neck can be transmitted from cardiac murmurs, and it is therefore important to auscultate over the precordium to exclude this possibility. In the upper limb the brachial, radial and ulnar pulses should be palpated and the blood pressure taken in both antecubital fossae. The presence of a cardiac irregularity is noted

REFERENCES

37. Adachi B. Das Arteriensystem. Arf Maruzen, I Paner, Kyoto, 1920
38. Ludbrook J, Clark AM, McKenzie JK. Br Med J 1962; 1: 1724

when the pulses are examined, and any abnormality of the jugular venous pressure must also be recorded.

The heart and lungs must be fully examined because abnormal findings may support a particular diagnosis and influence management. A general examination of the patient should enable anaemia, polycythaemia, xanthomata, xanthelasmata, arcus senilis, and other major pathology to be detected (Fig. 10.16).

A full neurological examination including fundoscopy must be carried out if the patient complains of transient ischaemic attacks, amaurosis fugax, vertebrobasilar insufficiency or completed strokes. It is also essential if a cervical bruit is found on routine examination.

There are few physical signs of chronic mesenteric ischaemia apart from the doubtful relevance of an abdominal bruit. Even when an acute mesenteric infarct develops, there may be little in the way of physical signs, the patient complaining of severe abdominal pain out of proportion to the findings on clinical examination. Patients subsequently develop signs of acute peritonitis with generalized tenderness, rebound tenderness, guarding, rigidity and absent bowel sounds. Eventually, abdominal distension and septic shock supervene (see Ch. 25).

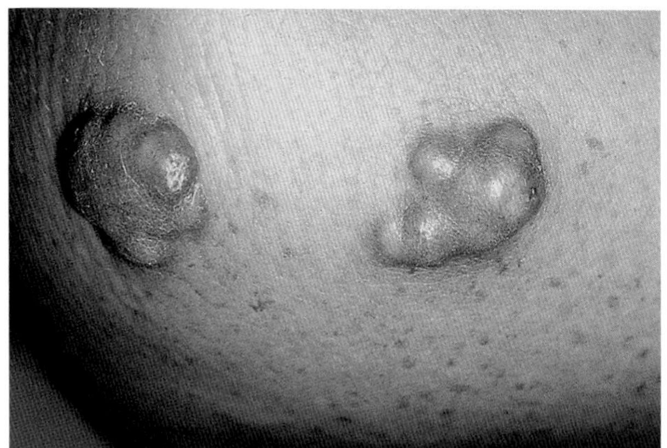
a

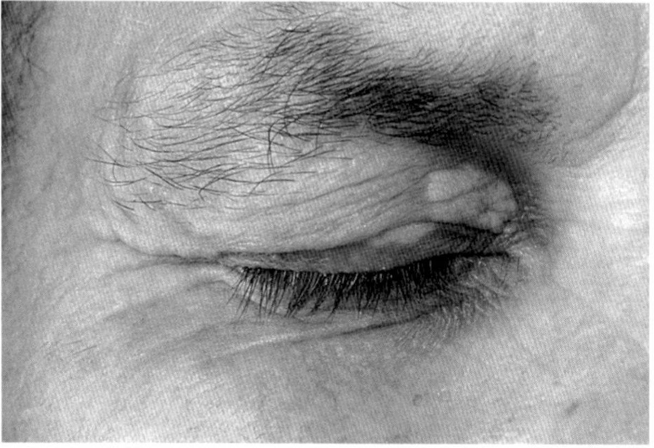
b

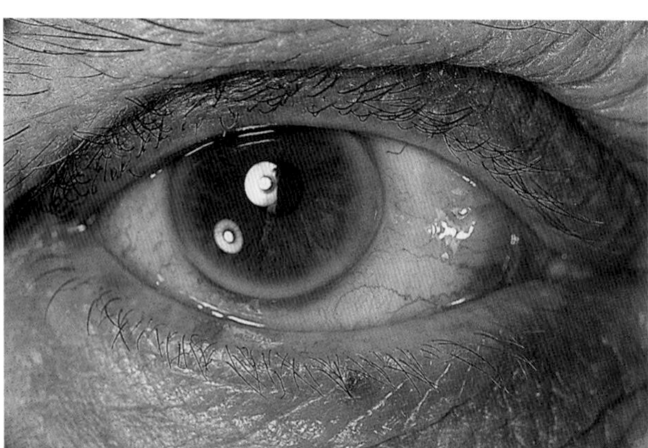
c

Figure 10.16 Examples of (a) xanthomata, (b) xanthelasmata and (c) arcus senilis.

Machinery murmurs may be heard over arteriovenous fistulae or over their major feeding vessels. The neck veins may be elevated if a fistula is causing cardiac embarrassment, and a left ventricular heave may be detected on palpation of the precordium. An indication of the amount of the circulatory embarrassment produced by arteriovenous fistulae within the limbs can be obtained by Branham's test.[39,40] In this test, the pulse rate is recorded for 1 min before a pneumatic tourniquet is placed around the root of the affected limb and inflated above systolic pressure to occlude arterial inflow before the pulse rate is retaken. A marked fall in the pulse rate indicates a large left-to-right shunt and potential cardiac embarrassment. Occasionally an abdominal aortic aneurysm may rupture into the inferior vena cava. The classical signs are lower limb oedema and cyanosis, a machinery murmur on abdominal auscultation, and marked elevation of the jugular venous pressure.

Patients with vasospastic disease may have their symptoms provoked by exposure to cold. The integrity of the palmar arch can be assessed by Allen's test.[41] In this test, digital compression is applied over the ulnar and radial arteries at the wrist, while the patient is instructed to make a fist repeatedly to empty the capillary circulation of the hand. Partial or complete palmar flushing is seen when the pressure over one of the vessels is released. The continuity of the palmar arch and its dependent vessels of supply can be deduced if this test is repeated for the other feeding vessel.

Thoracic outlet syndrome may cause occlusion of the subclavian artery. This syndrome is most commonly associated with a cervical rib but can be caused by a tight band, bony exostoses or hypertrophied muscle. The radial pulse, which is palpable when the arm is at rest by the side, will fade or disappear when the arm is abducted and externally rotated to 90°, and exercise of the hand in this position rapidly causes ischaemic pain associated with pallor. This test is not specific and can be positive in normal individuals.

Popliteal entrapment syndrome occurs when the popliteal artery passes beneath the medial head of gastrocnemius. Normal pedal pulses are present at rest but become impalpable on plantar flexion of the ankle against resistance.

INVESTIGATION OF VASCULAR DISEASE

BLOOD AND URINE TESTS

All patients with vascular disease should have a full blood count, which includes the haemoglobin, packed cell volume, differential white blood cell count and platelet estimation, and a blood film where necessary. The absolute leukocyte count in peripheral blood relates to the prevalence of cardiovascular disease,[42] which

REFERENCES

39. Branham HH. J Surg 1890; 3: 250
40. Nicoladoni C. Arch Klin Chir 1875; 18: 252
41. Allen EV. Am J Med Sci 1929; 178: 237
42. Dormandy JA, Murray GD. Eur J Vasc Surg 1991; 5: 131–133

may in part be from the effect of smoking. A fall in the leukocyte count is accompanied by a reduction in deaths from heart disease, which was independent of other cardiovascular risk factors.[43] Polycythaemia is an important cause of peripheral vascular symptoms, and anaemia may make symptoms of ischaemia worse. Leukaemia and thrombocythaemia can lead to thrombosis of the microcirculation.

The erythrocyte sedimentation rate or blood viscosity and C-reactive protein are elevated in autoimmune conditions such as collagen diseases, including rheumatoid arteritis, and other disorders such as Buerger's disease or inflammatory aneurysms. The urea, electrolytes and creatinine assess renal function and may be abnormal if patients have been on long-term diuretic treatment.

Elevated serum cholesterol and fasting triglyceride concentrations are important risk factors, which can be treated with dietary and pharmacological manipulation to prevent rapid progression of atherosclerotic disease. Family screening and counselling can be performed in patients with inherited hyperlipidaemias.

The urine should be tested for sugar and a random blood glucose measured to exclude diabetes. A glycosylated haemoglobin and a glucose tolerance test are indicated if the screening tests are equivocal or if diabetes is suspected. Serum autoantibodies may be raised in the collagen diseases, and blood should be screened for antinuclear factor, anti-DNA, Rose–Waaler and latex agglutination, antinuclear cytoplasmic antibody, immunoglobulins and complement (C3, C4) in patients suspected of having a vasculitis or an inflammatory arteritis.

A coagulation screen comprising the prothrombin time, the activated partial thromboplastin time, and the thrombin time may be helpful, particularly in patients with liver disease and in those having major surgery (see Ch. 3). The clotting time provides a global measure of coagulation. Young patients who present with arterial occlusion, and patients who thrombose bypass grafts for no technical reason, should have a thrombophilia screen that includes protein C and S estimation, antithrombin III levels and antiphospholipid antibodies (see Ch. 3). Activated protein C should also now be measured because this is the most common form of thrombophilia. Raised levels of homocysteine have also been shown to be an important risk factor for thrombosis.[44] Other tests—such as platelet aggregation tests, thrombomodulin assay, and the thromboelastograph—have not yet found their way into the routine assessment of arterial disorders (see Ch. 3).

CARDIORESPIRATORY INVESTIGATIONS

A chest radiograph and an electrocardiogram are essential in patients with atheromatous peripheral vascular disease. The chest radiograph allows an assessment of cardiac size and chamber dilatation to be made, and detects significant pulmonary pathology such as carcinoma of the bronchus, which is an important concomitant condition in heavy smokers with severe atherosclerosis. Peak expiratory flow rate is a useful test of respiratory function, and spirometry and arterial blood gases may be measured in some patients with asthma or chronic obstructive airways disease. Spirometry and the partial pressure of carbon dioxide (P_aCO_2) unfortunately appear to be of variable predictive value, and a careful history and physical examination are still the most important predictors of pulmonary complications.[45]

The electrocardiograph diagnoses arrhythmias and may also provide evidence of myocardial ischaemia. An exercise electrocardiograph may uncover ischaemic changes that are not present at rest. An echocardiogram is useful in determining left ventricular function and confirming the diagnosis of cardiac valvular disease. Transthoracic echocardiography will rarely image the atrial appendage, and in cases of suspected intracardiac thrombus the transoesophageal route is more sensitive. It can also assess abnormalities of the heart and great vessels.[46] Echocardiography before and after dobutamine may detect abnormalities of wall motion secondary to reversible coronary ischaemia. Thallium scanning before and after vasodilatation with dipyridamole also defines areas of cardiac ischaemia. Thallium is taken up into healthy myocardium, but infarction produces cold spots. A cold spot, which appears after dipyridamole, suggests an area of reversible ischaemia. Dobutamine stress echocardiography and thallium scanning are equivalent tests, and the choice is dependent on local availability. Coronary catheterization and angiography may be necessary in patients with severe angina and in those who have positive stress tests. Positron emission tomography is a research tool, which is very good at assessing cardiac ischaemia but is very expensive and only available at a limited number of hospitals.

In patients with suspected renovascular disease, ultrasound examination can determine the size of the kidney and the presence of renal artery stenosis. This should be confirmed by gadolinium-enhanced magnetic resonance angiography.

Intravenous pyelography and barium contrast studies may be helpful in assessing patients suspected of renal vascular disease or mesenteric occlusions. Small ischaemic kidneys may be seen on the renogram phase of the pyelogram, with delay in the appearance of contrast, which often appears to be very concentrated. Reduced function can be confirmed by an isotopic renogram.[47] Thumb-printing or ischaemic strictures may occasionally be seen in patients with ischaemic colitis (see Ch. 28), but at present there are no satisfactory tests for detecting intestinal ischaemia other than arteriography, and even then the anatomical appearances do not always relate to the pathophysiology of the condition.

SPECIFIC VASCULAR INVESTIGATIONS

Doppler ultrasound pressure measurement

Ultrasound probes emit and receive continuous high-frequency sound waves through two crystals. When the emitted sound strikes a moving object, such as the red cell, it is reflected back. This is detected by the probe as an increase or decrease in frequency, depending on the direction of movement of the object. This is known as the Doppler shift or Doppler effect. This Doppler shift is perceived as a change in the pitch of a siren or train whistle as an ambulance or train passes an observer. The increase in frequency is proportional to the velocity of the moving particle. This increased frequency is detected audibly as an increase in pitch, and can be recorded and quantified by its spectral wave form.[48] The peak of the spectral trace is related to the highest velocity in the lumen—usually found in the centre of the vessel.

REFERENCES

43. Grimm RH Jr., Neaton JD, Ludwig W. JAMA 1985; 254: 1932–1937
44. Macy PA. Clin Lab Sci 2001; 14: 272
45. Smetana GW. N Engl J Med 1999; 340: 937–944
46. Lagattolla NR, Burnand KG, Stewart A. Br J Surg 1995; 82: 16651
47. Maxwell MH, Lupu AN, Taplin EV. J Urol 1968; 100: 376
48. Strandness DE. Cardiovasc Surg 1970; 11: 192

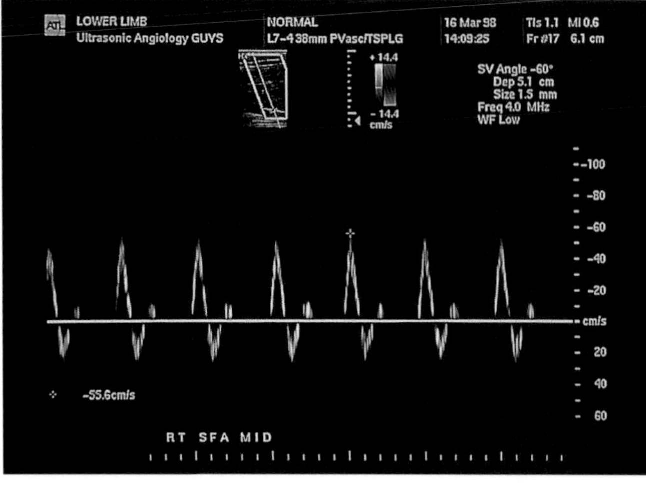

a

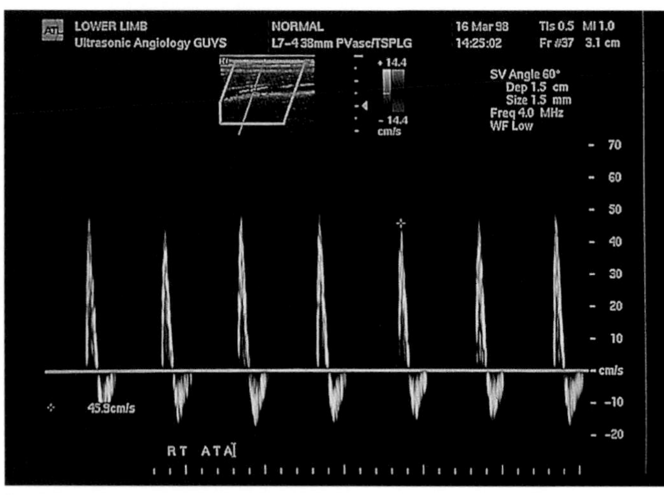

b

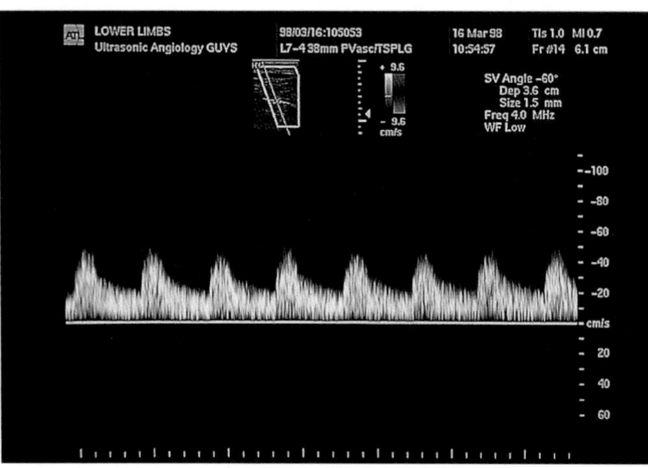

c

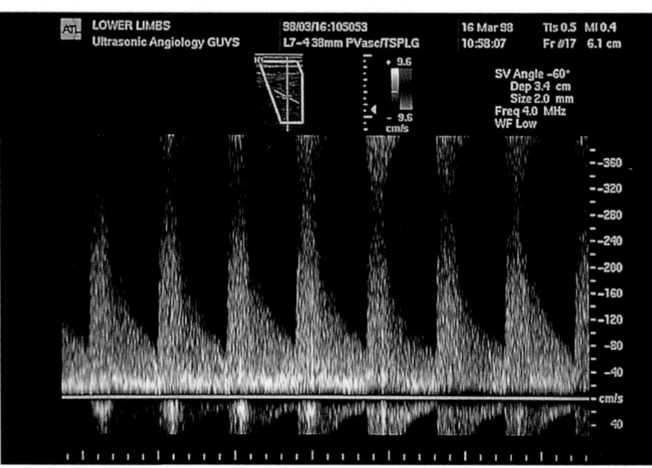

d

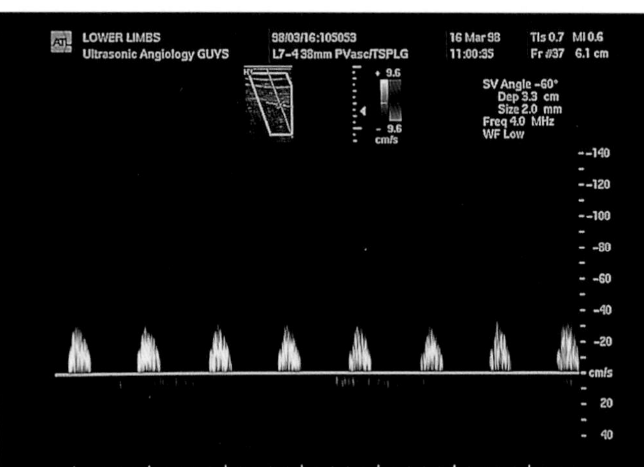

e

Figure 10.17 (a) Normal triphasic waveform: forward systolic flow with sharp well-defined peak, reversed flow component in diastole, and small forward flow due to elastic recoil of arteries consistent with normal flow in high-resistance peripheral arteries. (b) Biphasic waveform: forward systolic flow with reversed flow in diastole, without the third phase of forward flow. (c) Monophasic waveform with continuous forward diastolic flow, which shows spectral broadening compared with (a), consistent with low-resistance flow (e.g. internal carotid artery or renal artery). (d) Very high-velocity with spectral broadening, consistent with a significant stenosis. (e) Monophasic damped low-velocity waveform with no diastolic flow, consistent with waveforms found distal to an occlusion, or in a vessel with very low flow.

When the lumen is narrowed, the velocity must increase to maintain flow, and this is reflected by an increase in the spectral wave form. The stenosis produces local turbulence with a wide variation in velocities at any one point, and this causes a spectral broadening. The normal wave form is triphasic, with a sharp upstroke related to acceleration, a downstroke from deceleration (reversal of flow), and a small component representing forward flow. The wave form distal to a stenosis may become bi- or uniphasic (Fig. 10.17).

The Doppler probe should be held at 45–60° to the skin overlying the vessel, and an acoustic gel used to obliterate air from the interface to ensure good coupling. The probe can be used in combination with a sphygmomanometer cuff to measure the pressure in peripheral arteries,[49] which is very useful if the

REFERENCE

49. Yao JST, Hobbs JT, Irvine WT. Br J Surg 1969; 56: 676

pulse is impalpable or weak. When the cuff of the sphygmomanometer is inflated above the systolic pressure, the lumen of the vessel is occluded by the external compressive force, blood flow ceases, and the sound disappears. As the tourniquet is released flow and sound return, and this pressure is recorded. By comparing the pressure in the dorsalis pedis, peroneal and posterior tibial arteries at the ankle with the normal brachial systolic pressure measured by the same technique, a Doppler index is obtained (the ankle:brachial pressure index). In normal vessels this index is close to unity.[49] In moderate occlusive disease the index is between 0.5 and 0.9, and in severe disease with rest pain or gangrene it is less than 0.4. Absolute pressures may give a more accurate picture. The pressure is normally above 50 mmHg in at least one ankle vessel in moderate disease, and below this level in all vessels if the limb is critically ischaemic.[50] This index is usually reproducible and can be used to follow patients over time and assess the results of revascularization procedures.

Doppler pressures are incongruously high in patients with heavily calcified peripheral vessels because these arteries resist compression by the tourniquet and the Doppler signal persists. For this reason, pressure measurements in patients with diabetes and/or renal failure are unreliable.[51] Pulses below 75–85 mmHg are usually impalpable, therefore the combination of an impalpable pulse with a high Doppler pressure (greater than 120 mmHg) is diagnostic of incompressible arteries.

A treadmill with adjustable speed and gradient provides an objective and reproducible assessment of the claudication distance.[52] It may help to differentiate pain on walking caused by arterial disease from other causes such as spinal claudication. A fall in Doppler pressure of more than 15 mmHg after exercise (3 min of walking at 4 km/h on a 10° slope) can identify patients with stenotic arterial disease.[53] The routine use of exercise testing, however, adds little to the information given by the resting ankle brachial pressure index.

A number of methods have been used to assess the sonogram waveform in greater detail in an attempt to separate the relative importance of proximal and distal stenoses and occlusions, when both problems coexist in the same patient. None of these measurements, however, has shown a perfect correlation with the findings of biplanar arteriography, and they have not found their way into routine vascular surgical practice.[54]

In some patients with severe critical ischaemia, the Doppler probe may not be sensitive enough to detect flow at the ankle. The signal can be augmented by inflating a pneumatic cuff around the calf, a technique called pulse-generated run-off. This may detect patent distal arteries, which are not detected on Doppler examination or on arteriography.[55] This technique has been largely superseded by the rapid advances in intra-arterial digital subtraction angiography and associated software developments. Handheld Doppler assessment of the tibial vessels in the dependent leg position will often detect flow if the vessels are patent, and is therefore a useful adjunct in determining suitability for femorodistal grafting.

Doppler mapping

This technique of individual insonation of the digital vessels has been used to assess vasospastic disease in the hand. The more severe the vasospasm, the fewer the number and lengths of vessel that can be insonated.

B-mode ultrasound imaging

The simple Doppler probe uses continuous wave ultrasound signals, which cannot give anatomical information. Pulsed ultrasound probes send out short bursts of ultrasound waves; this allows the depth to be calculated by noting the time for the signal to return to the transducer. A two-dimensional image is built up based on the reflection of ultrasound waves from changes in tissue density. The greyscale is related to the strength of the returning signal. The signal is very strong and is represented as white if all the sound waves are returned to the probe. When no signal is detected the area is black. Intermediate signal strength is depicted as varying shades of grey. Abdominal B-mode ultrasound scanning[56] is an excellent technique for identifying and measuring the dimensions of infrarenal abdominal aortic aneurysms. The most accurate measurement is the anteroposterior diameter. Difficulties may arise when there is a poor acoustic window, often present in obese patients, and in those with a large amount of bowel gas.

Ultrasound can be used as a screening technique for abdominal aortic aneurysms in men aged 65–80 years. A randomized controlled study showed that screening significantly decreased the incidence of rupture and mortality when compared with an unscreened control group.[57]

Duplex ultrasound scanning

The combination of pulsed Doppler and B-mode imaging is known as duplex imaging. The direction of flow is depicted by a change in colour (colour flow imaging), with flow directed towards the probe seen as one colour and flow away as another (usually red and blue). The velocity of flow can also be encoded in colour, making areas of high velocity readily identifiable. The addition of colour renders the vessel and areas of disease easier to visualize, and therefore decreases the time taken to perform the study. This makes duplex scanning of the peripheral arteries a viable alternative to contrast radiology. Power Doppler detects the amplitude of the signal and therefore encodes for velocity of flow but not for direction. It is particularly useful for determining the presence of flow before an impending occlusion. It has the disadvantage that it increases the number of artefacts. There are now a number of ultrasound contrast agents that enhance the acoustic backscatter from moving blood and may improve its definition.[58] Duplex scanning has become established as the first investigation for many patients with arterial disease. Its value in assessing carotid stenoses is well established.[59] The excellent images now obtained have been used to characterize the morphology of atheromatous plaques at the carotid bifurcation.[58]

Duplex can also be used to measure stenoses in native limb arteries and in arterial bypass grafts.[60] Localized changes in peak systolic velocity with a ratio greater than 2 suggest that the stenosis

REFERENCES

50. Jamieson CW. Br J Surg 1982; 69 (Suppl 2): 52
51. Quin RO, Evans DH, Bell PRF. J Cardiovasc Surg 1975; 16: 586
52. Clyne CAC, Tripolitis A, Jamieson CW. Surg Gynecol Obstet 1979; 149: 727
53. Laing SP. Br Med J 1980; 1: 13
54. Campbell WB, Cole SLA et al. Br J Surg 1984; 71: 302
55. Beard J et al. Br J Surg 1988; 75: 761–763
56. Leopold GR. Radiology 1970; 96: 9
57. Scott RAP et al. Br J Surg 1995; 82: 1066
58. Strandness DE. In: Greenhalgh RM (ed). Vascular Imaging for Surgeons. WB Saunders, London, 1995: 41–50
59. Nicholls SC, Phillips DJ et al. J Vasc Surg 1985; 2: 375
60. Bandyk D et al. J Vasc Surg 1989; 9: 286

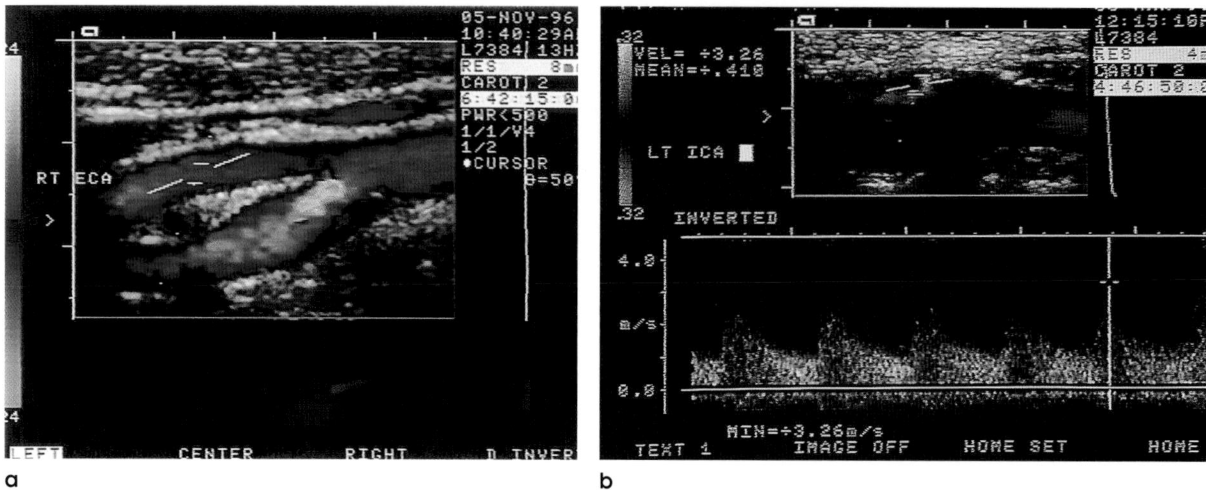

a b

Figure 10.18 Doppler scans indicative of (a) normal carotid arteries and (b) a tight stenosis.

is haemodynamically significant, i.e. equivalent to a 75% reduction in cross-sectional area or 50% diameter reduction (Fig. 10.18). The identification of grafts with significant stenoses is important because remedial measures may maintain graft patency.[61] Although the circumstantial evidence is strong for the efficacy of graft surveillance programmes using duplex, no randomized controlled study has yet been published. Duplex scanning has also been used to guide and monitor percutaneous transluminal angioplasty of lower limb arteries.

Intravascular ultrasound

An ultrasound catheter is inserted into the lumen of the vessel over a guide wire, and a series of cross-sectional scans are recorded as it is pulled back.[62] These scans can be combined to produce a three-dimensional image of the inside of the artery, which can be rotated to view all aspects. This technique has been widely used following balloon angioplasty and after the placement of stents and stent grafts; however, there is no good evidence to support its routine use.

Contrast arteriography

Non-invasive tests are now able to diagnose the extent of arterial disease with considerable accuracy. The role of diagnostic contrast arteriography has therefore diminished. Some clinicians use non-invasive tests such as Doppler and duplex alone to assess the vessels before intervention. The majority of surgeons and radiologists still, however, use contrast radiography to visualize arterial stenoses or occlusions before treatment. There are a number of different techniques for obtaining arteriograms, and these are now described with an account of their relative advantages and disadvantages, and indications and contra-indications.

Direct needle puncture

Direct needle puncture was first described by Dos Santos and coworkers in 1929.[63] A hollow needle is inserted directly into the arterial lumen upstream of the area of interest. A bolus of radiopaque contrast medium is injected directly into the lumen of the vessel, and a rapid series of radiographs is taken of the vessels downstream of the injection site. Any direct puncture into an artery carries the risk of local damage, wall dissection, haemorrhage, false aneurysm formation, thrombosis and embolism.[64] Any injection of contrast can produce allergic and anaphylactic reactions, but this risk is reduced by using an iso-osmolar contrast medium.[65] Translumbar aortography is now rarely used. Although useful in the operating theatre, direct arterial puncture has been superseded by the Seldinger technique.

Seldinger retrograde arteriography

The Seldinger technique uses a small plastic cannula, which is inserted into the artery over a flexible guide wire placed in the vessel through a hollow needle.[66] This allows a catheter to be passed both retrogradely into a proximal vessel and antegradely into a distal vessel. The femoral artery is the most commonly used access site.

The advent of guidable and steerable catheters[67] has permitted retrograde insertion of these catheters into the root of the aorta. Views of the aortic arch and great vessels can be obtained from an unselective arch injection.

Selective studies can be performed when a catheter is inserted into the origins or even passed up the individual great vessels for more detailed images. Selective carotid angiograms can provide information about the circle of Willis, but the risk of stroke is higher than for arch injections.[68]

Retrograde insertion to the level of the renal arteries allows an assessment to be made of renal artery stenoses in hypertensive patients with peripheral vascular disease. A catheter inserted to this level also produces good views of the infrarenal aorta and the iliac, femoral and popliteal arteries. It is conventional to pass the catheter up the normal femoral artery or least diseased side. Retrograde insertion to the level of the iliac vessel can be

REFERENCES

61. Ramaswami G et al. Eur J Vasc Surg 1994; 8: 214
62. Gerritsen GP et al. J Vasc Surg 1993; 18: 31
63. Dos Santos R, Lamas AC, Caldas JP. Arteriographie des Membres et de L'Aorte Abdominale. Masson, Paris, 1931
64. McAffee JG. Radiology 1957; 68: 825
65. Alment T, Aspelin P, Levin B. Invest Radiol 1975; 10: 519
66. Seldinger SI. Acta Radiol 1953; 39: 368
67. Neiman HL, Brand TD, Greenberg M. Arch Surg 1981; 116: 821
68. Hankey GJ, Warlow CP, Sellar RJ. Stroke 1990; 21: 209

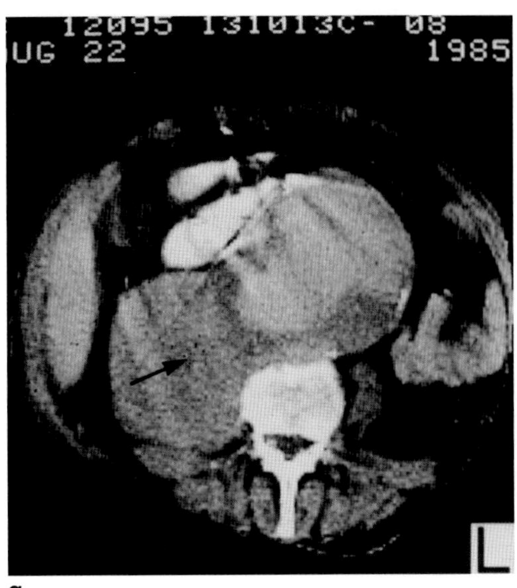

a

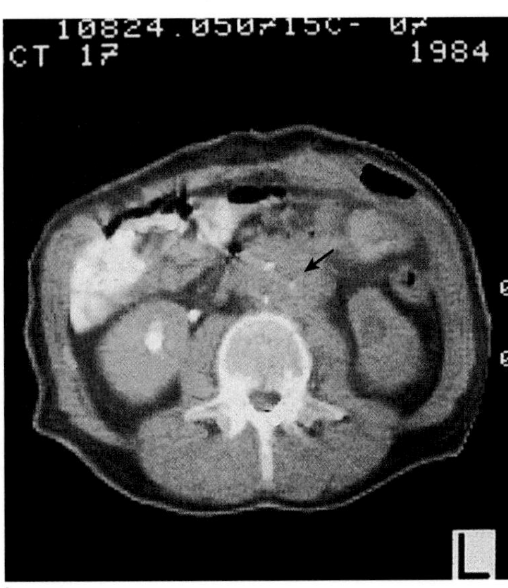

b

Figure 10.19 (a) A CT scan showing a controlled rupture of an aortic aneurysm (arrowed). (b) A CT scan showing the features of an inflammatory aneurysm; a soft tissue mass outside the wall is seen (arrowed).

performed by insertion of the catheter into the ipsilateral femoral artery when proximal disease is not suspected and no views of the other leg are required. The contrast medium then passes down the single limb, giving good views of the distal vasculature in the leg and the foot.

Antegrade femoral puncture is occasionally required for diagnostic purposes and is useful when angioplasty of distal stenoses is being contemplated, especially if these cannot be reached via the iliac bifurcation from puncture of the contralateral femoral artery or the arm.

It is possible to damage the vessel wall by the Seldinger technique, but general anaesthesia is avoided. There is still a risk of contrast allergy, and the contrast load can cause a deterioration of renal function or cardiac failure.

Digital subtraction arteriography

Digital subtraction arteriography has now become the preferred radiological method for imaging arteries and can be performed with contrast injected into either the veins or the arteries. Images are taken of the field of interest and these are digitized. Contrast medium is then injected into the circulation and further views taken. The control images can be subtracted from those taken after contrast, giving high-quality images of the arteries.[69] The patient must not move, and poor images are obtained if involuntary movement takes place, particularly in the abdomen, when bowel peristalsis can cause gas artefacts. If intravenous contrast is used, this passes through the right heart and pulmonary circulation before reaching the left heart and the peripheral arteries. The patient must have good cardiac function because a large volume of contrast medium has to be used in intravenous studies. The technique is contraindicated in patients with poor cardiac output and also in patients with renal failure.[70]

In patients with renal impairment, a variety of techniques have been used to minimize the nephrotoxic effects of the contrast. More recently, the prophylactic oral administration of acetylcysteine combined with hydration has been claimed to protect the kidneys following conventional angiography.[71] Carbon dioxide angiography has been used as an alternative in patients with renal impairment, cardiac failure, and previous allergic reactions to contrast agents. It is well tolerated and can be used as a sole agent in 88% of cases.[72] It is, however, contraindicated in the assessment of the cerebrovascular system.[73] The hazards of direct arterial puncture are avoided by the intravenous technique, although of course those of contrast sensitivity remain.

The advantages of seeing the vessels without background interference from bone, together with the low volume of contrast that is required for intra-arterial injection, have established digital subtraction angiography as the technique of choice.

Both intravenous and intra-arterial digital angiography are particularly useful for imaging the carotid vessels, the aortic arch, and the thoracic and abdominal aorta.[74] Other arteries that require intra-arterial delivery of contrast are the intracerebral vessels, the renal and visceral arteries, and the coronary vessels.

Abdominal grey-scale ultrasound scanning and CT scanning are excellent methods of imaging and sizing aortic aneurysms; CT is particularly useful in determining the extent of the aneurysm, the possibility of a controlled rupture (Fig. 10.19a),[75] or the presence of periaortic fibrosis (Fig. 10.19b).[76] The development of spiral CT scanning allows rapid acquisition of data as the patient is moved continuously through the scanner. This has provided much thinner slices, which can be reconstructed in three dimensions, giving better identification of the relationship of the neck of an abdominal aortic aneurysm to the renal and visceral vessels.[77] The latest CT scanners use multiple detectors (multislice scanners), which markedly decrease the time taken to scan, improving the quality and sensitivity of the images.

Magnetic resonance imaging provides a non-invasive method of assessing aortic aneurysms and has the ability to image vessels in the coronal plane. One disadvantage of MRI is that turbulence

REFERENCES

69. Chilcote WA, Modie MT et al. Radiology 1981; 139: 287
70. Dawson P. Clin Radiol 1988; 39: 474
71. Tepel M, van der Giet M, Schwarzfeld C et al. N Engl J Med 2000; 343: 210–212
72. Kessel DO, Robertson I, Patel J et al. Cardiovasc Intervent Radiol 2002; 25: 476–483
73. Wilson AJ, Boxer MM. Invest Radiol 2002; 37: 542–551
74. Buonocore E, Meany TF et al. Radiology 1981; 139: 281
75. Senepati A, Hurst AE et al. J Cardiovasc Surg 1986; 27: 719
76. Baskerville PA, Blakeney CG et al. Br J Surg 1983; 70: 381
77. Rubin GD, Dake MD et al. Radiology 1993; 186: 147

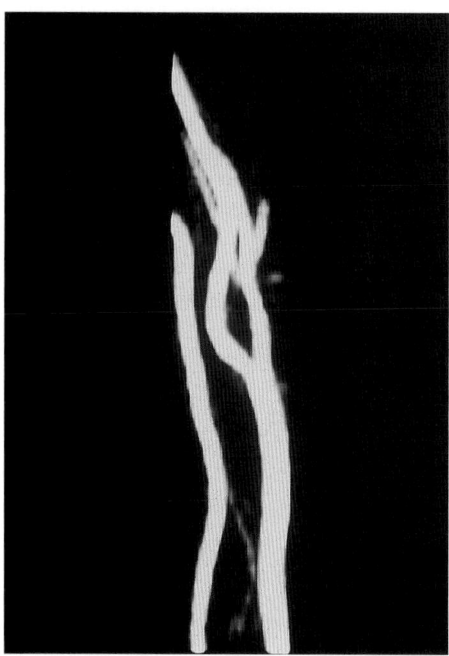

Figure 10.20 Magnetic resonance angiography of the left carotid vessels.

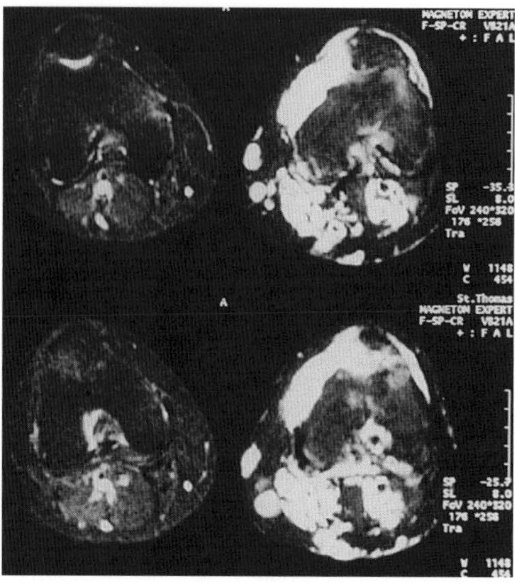

Figure 10.21 An MRI scan of a congenital vascular anomaly.

can result in signal loss, but this can be overcome by the infusion of gadolinium, which provides good images of arterial pathology.[78] An angiogram can be obtained from the acquisition of magnetic data (magnetic resonance angiography, Fig. 10.20).[79] This technique may at some stage abolish the need for contrast arteriography.

Computerized tomography, MRI and ultrasound scanning may be used to investigate aneurysms at other sites, and CT and MRI can determine the extent of a congenital vascular anomaly (Fig. 10.21).[80] Magnetic resonance and CT scans of the brain delineate areas of infarction and generalized cerebral atrophy.[81]

Cerebral vascular disease

Patients with cerebral vascular disease may require CT and MRI scans of the brain to exclude other pathology such as a space-occupying lesion. Positron emission tomography of the brain,[82] or xenon clearance with and without inhalation of carbon dioxide,[83] provides an estimation of the cerebral vascular reserve where cerebral hypoperfusion is suspected, although these tests are largely research tools at present. Middle cerebral Doppler velocity before and after inhalation of carbon dioxide is a less expensive alternative.[84]

Renal vascular disease

Ultrasound has become the first-line investigation for renal disease. Not only can it detect abnormalities in morphology, but with the addition of pulse Doppler, colour Doppler, power Doppler and ultrasound contrast agents, the renal vasculature can now be assessed.[85] Spiral CT angiography with three-dimensional reconstruction can provide excellent images of the renal arteries (Fig. 10.22),[86] as can magnetic resonance angiography.[87] Intra-arterial digital subtraction angiography still remains the best form of imaging.[88]

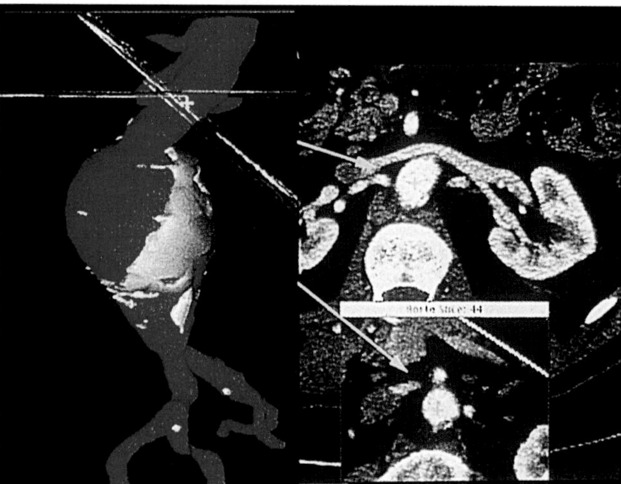

Figure 10.22 Spiral CT angiography with three-dimensional reconstruction to show renal arteries.

Gastrointestinal tract blood vessels

Duplex Doppler assessment of the visceral arteries should be undertaken in starved patients. The coeliac axis and the superior mesenteric arteries can be visualized, but only the proximal part of the inferior mesenteric artery can be seen. Intra-arterial digital subtraction arteriography remains the best method of detecting disease in the visceral arteries, but the anatomical appearances do not always relate to the extent of the bowel ischaemia.

REFERENCES

78. Prince MR. Radiology 1994; 191: 155
79. Anderson CM, Edelman RR, Turski PA (eds). Clinical Magnetic Resonance Angiography. Raven Press, New York, 1993
80. Avigdor M, Saks FFR et al. Radiology 1995; 194: 908
81. Bradshaw JR, Thompson JLG, Campbell MJ. Br Med J 1983; 286: 277
82. Wise RJS, Bernandi S et al. Brain 1983; 106: 197
83. Norving B, Nilssons B, Risberg J. Stroke 1982; 13: 155
84. Bishop CCR, Powell S et al. Stroke 1986; 17: 913
85. Scoutt LM, Taylor KJW. In: Taylor KJW, Burns PN, Wells PNT (eds). Clinical Applications of Doppler Ultrasound. Raven Press, New York, 1995: 155-178
86. Rubin GD, Dake MD et al. Radiology 1994; 190: 181
87. Debatin SF, Spritzer CE et al. Am J Roentgenol 1991; 157: 981
88. Kim D, Porter DH et al. Angiology 1991; 42: 345

OTHER TECHNIQUES

Plethysmography by a variety of different techniques and isotopic clearance studies[89] have been used to measure regional blood flow, but are still largely research tools and have not found a definite place in clinical diagnosis.

A transcutaneous oxygen electrode can be used to determine the flux of oxygen across the skin; this is dependent on blood flow and oxygenation of arterial blood. Absolute oxygen levels, arm:leg ratios, and the percentage of oxygen fall on exercise have been used to assess patients with claudication or critical leg ischaemia,[90] and transcutaneous oxygen readings have been used by some to decide on the level of amputation.[91]

Intravenous guanethidine retained in the limb by a sphygmomanometer cuff may abolish vasospasm; this test, in combination with local anaesthetic symptomatic ganglion block, may be used to confirm the diagnosis of vasospastic disease and assess the likely effect of treatment.

CONGENITAL ARTERIAL DISORDERS

ARTERIOVENOUS FISTULAE

Arteriovenous fistulae are found in many tissues at many sites but are most commonly found in the head, the neck, and the extremities.[92] Congenital arteriovenous fistulae may be localized or diffuse, and may be between large or small vessels. They may on occasions form arteriovenous aneurysms. Congenital fistulae are uncommon, and their incidence is probably less than 1 per million live births.[93] Although they are present from birth, they often increase in size during puberty or pregnancy.

Localized fistulae (cirsoid aneurysms)

These commonly arise in the head and neck, often appearing in the scalp from the superficial temporal vessels, but are also found in the limbs. They appear as a soft warm pulsatile swelling, which is often covered by dilated cutaneous vessels in the overlying skin or mucous membrane (Fig. 10.23). Patients often complain because the lesion is unsightly; it may enlarge, and as it does so it can cause aching pain. The overlying mucous membrane or skin may ulcerate, and this can give rise to repeated and frightening haemorrhages. Platelets are occasionally sequestrated by these anomalies, but heart failure is an unusual complication. The small arteries, veins, and even the capillaries are dilated and produce a swelling that is like a bag of pulsating worms. There is often a palpable thrill over the swelling, and a machinery murmur can be heard on auscultation. Pressure over the main feeding vessel that abolishes the pulsation may cause a bradycardia if the fistula is large (Branham's test).

Selective arteriography (Fig. 10.24), magnetic resonance angiography and CT scanning establish the extent and connections of a cirsoid aneurysm, which can easily be distinguished from a pure venous angioma by its physical signs. A highly vascular secondary deposit (e.g. a thyroid carcinoma) must be considered in the differential diagnosis of a pulsatile mass of late onset, and an acquired traumatic arteriovenous fistula must also be differentiated from the congenital variety.

When a cirsoid aneurysm develops during pregnancy it should be treated expectantly, as should all small localized fistulae that are not enlarging or causing symptoms. Lesions that enlarge in pregnancy commonly regress after delivery.[94] If they are expanding or producing symptoms, the risks of treatment have to be weighed against the improvement that can be expected and the final cosmetic result that can be achieved in each individual patient.

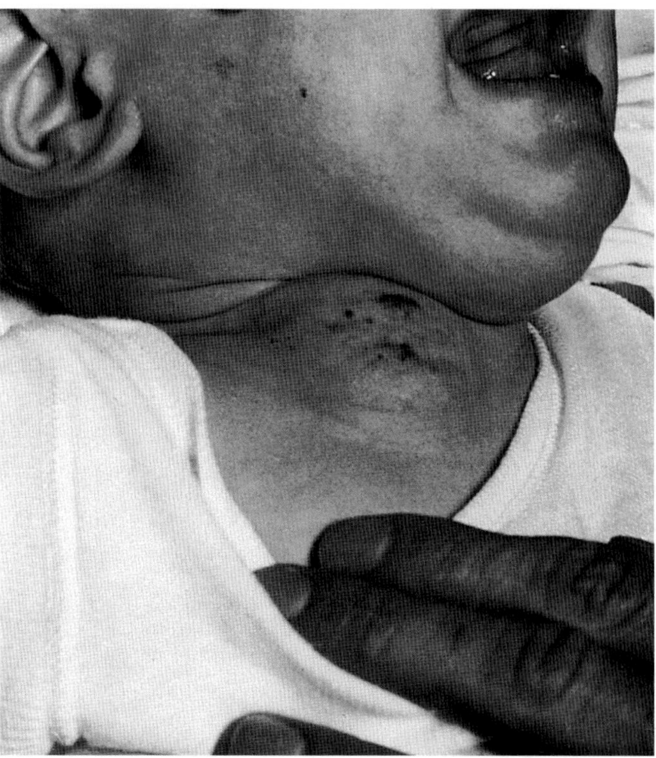

Figure 10.23 An arteriovenous malformation presenting as a localized pulsatile swelling. Dilated vessels can be seen in the overlying skin.

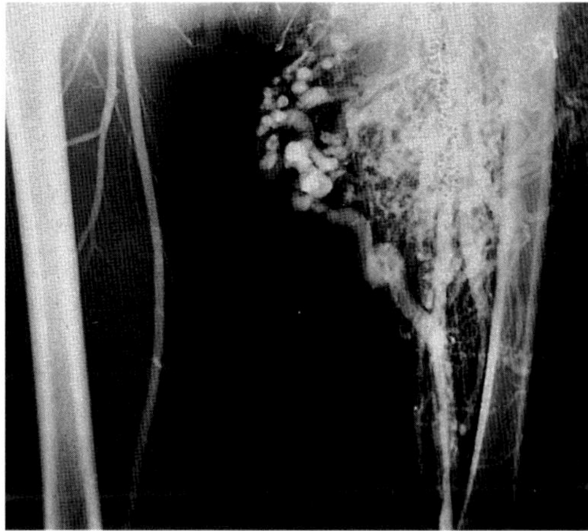

Figure 10.24 An arteriogram showing massive venous filling from an arteriovenous fistula.

Treatment can be by therapeutic embolization[95] or by occlusion of the feeding vessel combined with excision of the

REFERENCES

89. Gutajar CL, Brown NJG, Marston A. Br J Surg 1971; 58: 532
90. Franzeck HK, Talke P et al. Am Surg 1984; 147: 510
91. Mustapha NM, Redhead RG, Jain SK. Surg Gynecol Obstet 1983; 156: 282
92. Szilagyi DE, Elliott JP et al. Surgery 1965; 57: 61
93. Mulliken JB, Young AE. Vascular Birthmarks. WB Saunders, Philadelphia, 1978
94. Fontaine R. Lyon Chir 1967; 62: 3332
95. Stanley RJ, Cubillo E. Radiology 1975; 115: 609

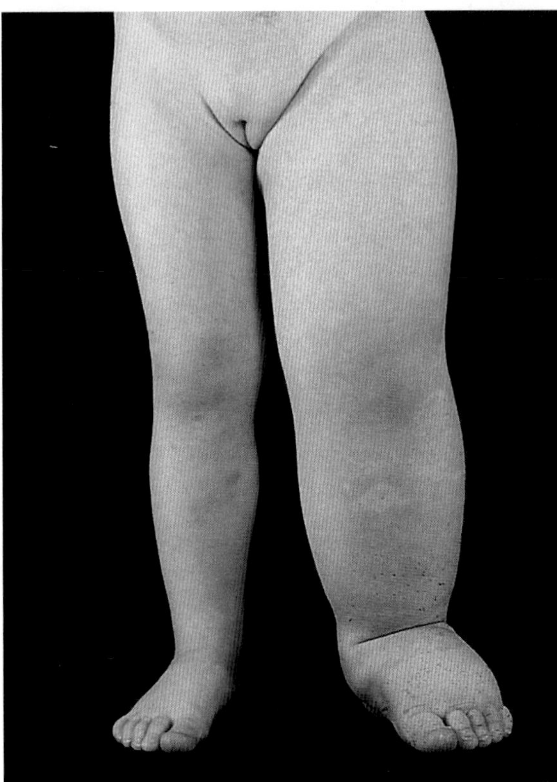

Figure 10.25 A limb with Parkes Weber syndrome.

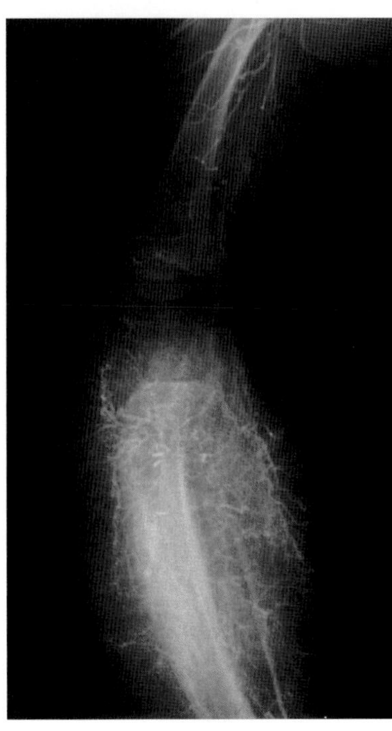

Figure 10.26 An arteriogram of a limb with multiple arteriovenous fistulae. Many abnormal vascular channels are seen with early filling of the veins.

mass.[96] The risks of inadvertent cerebral embolization during therapeutic embolization of arteriovenous fistulae in the head and neck mean that this treatment must be carried out by a very experienced radiologist using great care,[97] and many anomalies in this situation are best treated by surgical excision.

In the limbs, the risk of inadvertent misplaced embolism is less but digital gangrene is not unknown. Blood clot, Gelfoam, skeletal muscle, lead shot, alginates and tungsten coils have all been used to occlude feeding vessels, with varying success. Improvements are often temporary, and repeated embolization may be required at regular intervals.[98] Simple ligation of some feeding vessels is always ineffective, and this abolishes a potentially useful site of access for future therapeutic embolization. Any attempt at surgical obliteration of the feeding vessels must, if possible, be followed by an immediate attempt to excise the whole abnormality.

Multiple arteriovenous fistulae (Parkes Weber syndrome)

Multiple arteriovenous fistulae[99] usually present with an overall increase in the size of a limb, which is the common site of occurrence. The limb is often deformed, covered with dilated veins, and may later develop severe lipodermatosclerosis and intractable ulceration (Fig. 10.25). Usually multiple arteriovenous fistulae eventually cause high-output cardiac failure[100] and may occasionally cause severe thrombocytopenia.[101] The limb is usually hot, and is increased in width as well as length with an overgrowth of bone. Bruits and thrills may be audible or palpable, but they are not always present. A tourniquet inflated around the root of the limb usually causes slowing of the pulse.

The condition needs to be distinguished from Klippel–Trenaunay syndrome, where there is bony and soft tissue overgrowth associated with a venous malformation, primitive varicose veins and a capillary naevus, but no arteriovenous fistulae are present (see Ch. 11). Local gigantism and lymphoedema (see Ch. 12) must also be considered in the differential diagnosis.[102]

The increase in cutaneous temperature and local blood flow can be confirmed by thermography or plethysmography; arteriography shows the characteristic appearance of rapid blushing through the abnormal communications with early arrival of the dye in the veins (Fig. 10.26). It is often impossible to visualize individual fistulae unless they are very large. In early life the condition is probably best treated expectantly, unless severe deformity or evidence of cardiac overload develops. It is usually impossible to embolize or excise all the fistulae, but if they are derived from a single peripheral artery, embolism may be attempted.

Where microfistulae are present throughout a limb, an attempt can be made to inject microspheres of a known diameter into the feeding vessels, in the hope that these will preferentially enter and occlude large numbers of fistulae because of their increased blood flow.[103] This technique may be repeated on many occasions but does carry the risk of causing distal ischaemia, and it has not proved very effective in the long term.

It is occasionally worthwhile inserting orthopaedic staples across the epiphysis of the limb in an attempt to slow down bone growth.[104] If this fails, a shoe raise for the heel of the opposite foot may level the stance and prevent pelvic tilting. Graduated elastic stockings reduce superficial venous hypertension, compress

REFERENCES

96. Biller HF, Krepski YP, Som PM. Otolaryngol Head Neck Surg 1982; 90: 37
97. Castaenda-Zuniga WR, Tadavarthy SM et al. Radiology 1981; 141: 238
98. Barth KH, Stranberg JD, White RI. Invest Radiol 1977; 12: 273
99. Parkes Weber F. Br J Dermatol 1907; 19: 231
100. Reid MR. Bull Johns Hopkins Hosp 1920; 31: 43
101. Kasabach HH, Merritt KK. Am J Dis Child 1940; 59: 1063
102. Robertson DJ. Ann R Coll Surg Engl 1956; 18: 73
103. Berenstein AM, Kricheff I. Radiology 1979; 132: 631
104. Blount WP, Clarke GR. J Bone Joint Surg 1949; 319: 464

dilated surface veins, and may prevent or delay the development of lipodermatosclerosis and ulceration.

After childhood, an attempt may be made to ligate all the branches of the feeding artery under tourniquet control. This process of deafferentation, or skeletonization,[105,106] is an effective method of treating fistulae derived from a single artery and allows the main sites of communication to be ablated. It too carries the risk of producing distal ischaemia and is followed by a high incidence of recurrence. It may therefore be preferable to carry out repeated selective embolization of the main sites of fistulation. This treatment is usually required at regular intervals throughout life as new fistulae are constantly developing. The cardiac output must also be regularly monitored.

Ablation of the affected part is the final option if pain, deformity or cardiac failure become serious problems. This may require radical amputation of abnormal limbs, with the prospect of poor mobility. This option should be reserved for severe complications when all other methods of treatment have failed. There are a number of other syndromes where congenital arterio-venous fistulae extend throughout the brain, the liver or the intestine.[107,108] These can cause compression of surrounding tissues, recurrent haemorrhage, congestive cardiac failure or platelet consumption. The same principles apply to their management as those already discussed; unfortunately, other congenital malformations commonly coexist.

VASCULAR MALFORMATIONS

Most malformations display arterial, venous and lymphatic elements in some part of their structure. Those malformations that are predominantly venous or lymphatic are discussed in Chapters 11 and 12, but all other vascular malformations are discussed here.

Vascular malformations have in the past been called angiomas, to which the prefixes haem-, lymph-, capillary or cavernous are then applied. The term *angioma* is, however, a misnomer, because the lesion is not a true tumour of blood vessels but a malformation or hamartoma. These malformations are thought to develop as an abnormal proliferation of the embryonic vascular network. It has been suggested that angiogenic[109] and hormonal factors may be responsible for their development, which might explain why they are found more commonly in the female sex. All angiomata may ulcerate and induce hyperkeratosis in the overlying stratum corneum. They rarely, if ever, undergo malignant change.

CAPILLARY MALFORMATIONS

These lesions account for two-thirds of all vascular malformations and include naevi, port wine stains, telangiectasis and spider naevi. Their incidence is between 1 and 2.6%.[110] Half occur as a single lesion, and 20% of affected infants have more than one malformation.

Cutaneous naevi

Naevus flammeus neonatorum (salmon patch)

This is a pink or red network of small capillaries without much cellular proliferation, radiating from a central punctum, which is formed by an artery in the subcutis that supplies the tumour. It can occur anywhere on the skin surface but most commonly arises on the face; it appears as a salmon-coloured patch that lies flush with the skin surface unless there is an overlying cutaneous proliferation (Fig. 10.27). Naevi may be multiple and their size can vary enormously, but they are usually unilateral and rarely transgress the median plane. They can arise on mucous membranes and in the central nervous system, where they occasionally appear as small red spongy tumours embedded in the walls of cysts.

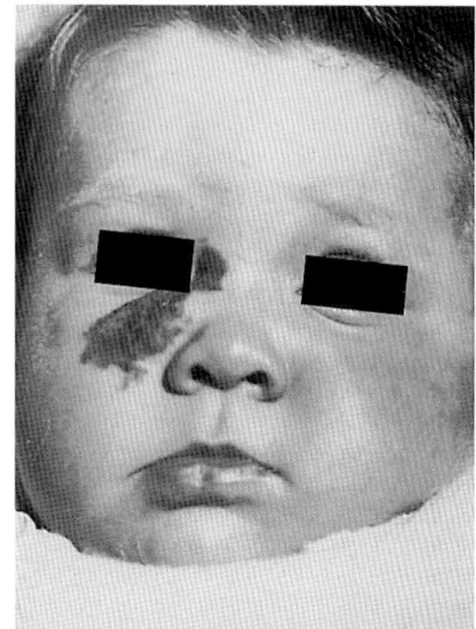

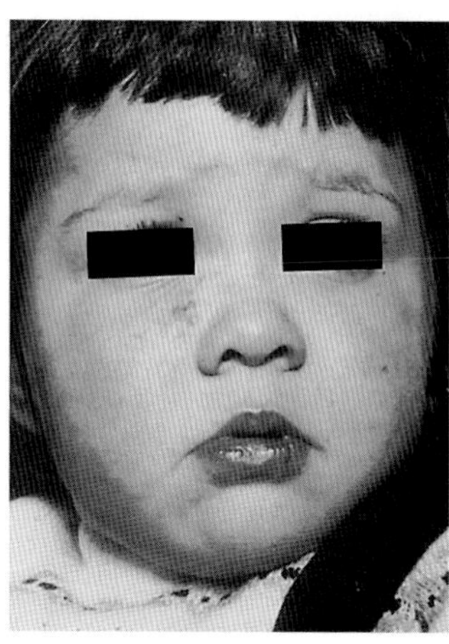

a b

Figure 10.27 A cutaneous naevus on the face (a) and its spontaneous resolution over time (b).

Strawberry patch

Strawberry patch is another descriptive term given to certain naevi that appear bright red, lobulated, and raised above the surface. This naevus often develops external extensions that separate from the tumour at first but later fuse with the main haemangioma; this variety commonly ulcerates.

Telangiectasis

Telangiectasis is simply a dilatation of normal capillaries rather than a vascular malformation. They arise after skin irradiation, and certain syndromes are recognized where multiple telangiectases are associated with gastrointestinal haemorrhage, epistaxis, haematuria, and even intracerebral haemorrhage.[111]

Spider naevus (naevus araneus)

Spider naevus is a form of telangiectasis that occurs over the upper torso, head and neck in adults, often in association with liver insufficiency or pregnancy.[112] The presence of more than five spider naevi is regarded as pathological (see Ch. 29).

Hereditary haemorrhagic telangiectasia (Rendu–Osler–Weber syndrome)

Hereditary haemorrhagic telangiectasia[111–113] is inherited as a Mendelian dominant, with incomplete penetrance. It is a rare disease, with an incidence of one or two per 100 000. Tiny capillary haemangiomas scattered over mucous membranes and sometimes the skin may give rise to overt and occult haemorrhage

REFERENCES

105. Malan E, Puglionise A. J Cardiovasc Surg 1965; 6: 255
106. Cotton LT, Sykes BJ. Proc R Soc Med 1969; 62: 245
107. Sturec WA. Trans Clin Soc Lond 1879; 12: 162
108. Parkes Weber F. Proc R Soc Med 1929; 22: 431
109. Folkman J, Haundschild C. Nature 1980; 288: 551
110. Pratt AG. Arch Dermatol 1967; 67: 302
111. Rendu M. Bull Soc Med Hop Paris 1896; 13: 731
112. Barter RH, Letterman ES, Schurter M. Surg Gynecol Obstet 1963; 87: 628
113. Osler W. Bull Johns Hopkins Hosp 1901; 12: 333

presenting as haematemesis, haematuria, melaena or iron deficiency anaemia.

Campbell de Morgan's spot

Campbell de Morgan's spot is a uniformly red capillary naevus that is usually 2–3 mm in diameter. It often develops on the trunk in middle age. It is of no clinical significance.

Port wine stain (naevus vinosus)

Port wine stain is a purple-blue naevus of skin that commonly arises on the face and may involve the lips and mucous membrane of the mouth. These naevi also arise on the limbs in association with Klippel–Trenaunay syndrome (see Ch. 11).

Clinical features

All vascular naevi appear to contain blood vessels and empty on compression, although often incompletely. A glass slide can be used to demonstrate the sign of emptying. Doubts about the diagnosis can be clarified by biopsy.

Management

The presence of other conditions, such as the Klippel–Trenaunay syndrome and Rendu–Osler–Weber syndrome, must be considered. The majority of capillary naevi do not require treatment unless they are causing symptoms. Camouflage paint produces acceptable cosmesis in many instances.[114] Carbon dioxide snow (cryotherapy)[115] and laser photocoagulation[116] have been used to destroy capillary naevi and are effective methods of treatment, although time-consuming and expensive. The red-blue discoloration of the naevus is often exchanged for white scar tissue unless these treatments are carefully applied. Radiotherapy, electrolysis, thermocautery, sclerotherapy, surgical excision and skin grafting have also been used, with variable success. Tattooing has been tried, but camouflage paints are usually preferable. Corticosteroids may reduce the size of large angiomas and restore platelet counts to normal.[117]

CAVERNOUS HAEMANGIOMA (STRAWBERRY PATCH)

Cavernous haemangioma occurs in the subcutaneous tissue of the skin or beneath mucous membranes, and becomes apparent as a bluish, slightly elevated patch a few weeks after birth. Cavernous haemangiomata can also arise in the liver and other internal organs. They consist of dilated blood spaces with thin walls supported by a tenuous stroma.

Sixty per cent of these malformations undergo spontaneous resolution by the age of 3, and some may then organize and calcify. The overlying skin may occasionally break down and ulcerate (Fig. 10.28). These haemangiomata may also occasionally cause thrombocytopenia and cutaneous bleeding.

When spontaneous resolution does not occur, the malformation usually requires excision and some form of plastic repair if treatment is justified on cosmetic grounds. Repeated diathermy coagulation and cryotherapy have also been tried, but the recurrence rate is high.[118]

MIXED NAEVI

Mixed naevi have a combination of capillary and cavernous elements, often with diffuse endothelial proliferation compressing the dilated capillary channels. These naevi also have a high incidence of spontaneous regression, but they may occasionally ulcerate and become infected. Excision with reconstruction or radiotherapy are the two main techniques that have been used in treatment.[119] The complications that can follow radiotherapy favour surgical excision where this is possible.

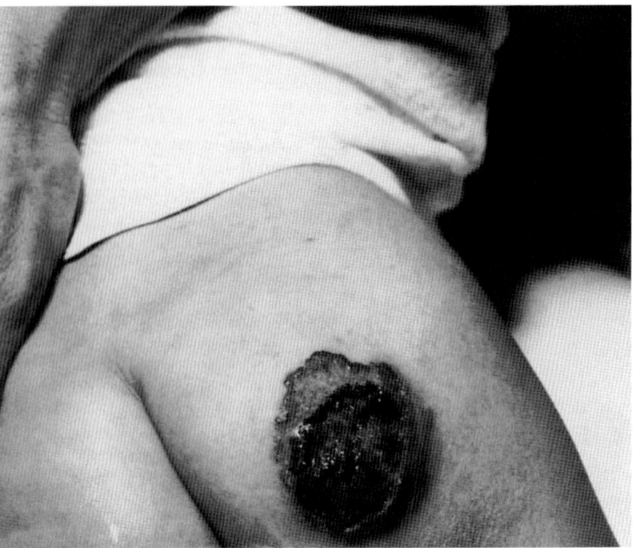

Figure 10.28 Ulceration over a cavernous haemangioma.

CYSTIC DISEASE OF THE ARTERIAL WALL

Although this condition is grouped with congenital disorders of the arteries, it is debatable if it is truly congenital. The diagnosis is usually made when the vessel occludes, which is almost always in early adult life.[120] Claudication or acute ischaemia developing in a young adult suggest the possibility of an arterial cyst, but it must be differentiated from an entrapment syndrome, an embolus, or premature atherosclerosis. The cyst is filled with mucopolysaccharide and forms in the layers of the arterial wall; it has a similar structure to a ganglion. Cysts are most commonly reported to occur in the popliteal artery. The diagnosis is by arteriography and duplex ultrasound or CT scanning of the popliteal fossa.

Treatment is by deroofing or excising the cyst if possible and extracting distal thrombosis, if this is present, with a Fogarty balloon catheter.[121] The abnormal vessel wall must be resected and replaced by a vein graft or prosthetic material if deroofing is impossible. Excision of the cyst with a primary end-to-end arterial anastomosis is rarely possible.[122]

CONGENITAL ENTRAPMENT SYNDROMES

The most common sites of arterial entrapment are at the thoracic outlet, often by a cervical rib, and in the popliteal fossa by an abnormal attachment of the popliteus or gastrocnemius muscles. Other rarer causes of entrapment include the anterior tibial syndrome, vertebral artery compression, and coeliac axis compression.

REFERENCES

114. Cosman B. Lasers Surg Med 1980; 1: 133
115. Blaisdell JH. N Engl J Med 1936; 215: 485
116. Adams SJ, Swain CP et al. Br J Dermatol 1987; 117: 487
117. Brown SH, Neerhout RC, Fonkalsrud EW. Surgery 1972; 71: 168
118. Matthews DN. Plast Reconstr Surg 1968; 41: 528
119. Webber TR, West KW, Cohen M. J Vasc Surg 1984; 1: 423
120. Bliss BP. Am Heart J 1964; 68: 838
121. Lewis GJT, Douglas DM et al. Br Med J 1967; 3: 411
122. Tracey GD, Ludbrook J, Rundle FF. J Vasc Surg 1969; 3: 10

Thoracic outlet syndrome

A cervical rib can definitely compress, occlude, and damage the subclavian artery, but a fibrous band situated in the position of a cervical rib or muscular hypertrophy is a more contentious cause of compression at the thoracic outlet. Because the diagnosis is difficult to refute—or for that matter to prove—many patients in certain parts of the world have undergone thoracic outlet decompression on fairly nebulous grounds, often perhaps for disease in the cervical spine.

Cervical rib

This occurs in 0.4% of the population, with 70% having bilateral cervical ribs,[123] but it is symptomatic in approximately 60%. Of the patients with symptoms, neurological manifestations of cervical rib outweigh vascular complications by approximately 20 to 1. A cervical rib was first resected by Coote in London in 1861,[124] some 40 years before Bramwell suggested that a normal first rib could compress the brachial plexus.[125]

Patients with symptomatic cervical ribs complain of cramping pain in the arm and hand, which may become pallid, cyanosed or oedematous during use. Paraesthesiae, weakness and numbness commonly coexist as a result of compression of the T1 nerve root, but vascular symptoms do occasionally occur in isolation. A cervical rib can cause secondary vasospasm, which may progress to fingertip necrosis and even digital gangrene. Emboli from a subclavian false aneurysm are usually the cause of patchy necrosis and gangrene of the hand and digits. Acute thrombosis of the subclavian artery is unusual but can cause extensive ischaemia of the upper limb. Patients occasionally present because they have noticed a mass or pulsation in the neck. Obstruction to the venous return from the arm may also occur in isolation or in association with neuritic or vascular symptoms. Venous symptoms consist of engorgement, oedema, cyanosis, and discomfort during exercise, but the first sign is often an acute axillary venous thrombosis (see Ch. 11).

The signs of a cervical rib fall into four distinct categories: local signs from the rib and artery; signs of venous obstruction or occlusion; neurological signs in the upper limb; and least common but most serious, signs of arterial spasm or ischaemia, usually affecting the fingers and hand. In a thin person, it may be possible to observe and palpate a bony swelling in the supraclavicular fossa above the clavicle (Fig. 10.29). The subclavian pulse may be palpable above the bony mass, or it may simply appear more prominent. A truly expansile pulsation usually signifies a traumatic false aneurysm. This is uncommon and must be carefully distinguished from a 'prominent' pulsation. A bruit may be heard over the artery in the supraclavicular fossa, and this may vary in differing degrees of abduction of the arm. Signs of venous obstruction are most obvious during periods of increased flow, such as exercise. The subcutaneous veins of the arm become distended and may remain so even during arm elevation. The hand and arm may be cyanosed, and there may be mild swelling that is apparent as pitting oedema on the dorsum of the hand. These signs all become more obvious if the axillary vein thromboses, when collateral veins develop in the skin over the anterior shoulder and the scapula (see Ch. 11). The neurological signs are the result of T1 root compression as this loops over the cervical rib. There is weakness and wasting of the small muscles of the hand, and anaesthesia over the T1 and occasionally C8 dermatomes.

The radial and ulnar pulses are usually present and of normal volume, but they may be reduced in amplitude or obliterated in

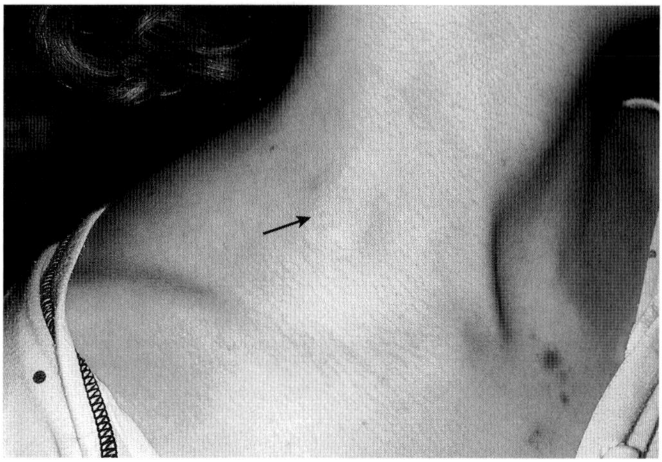

Figure 10.29 A visible cervical rib (arrowed) causing a swelling above the clavicle.

certain positions of the shoulder joint. These positions include the position of attention, with the shoulder pressed down; when the shoulder is braced backwards; when the shoulder is abducted against resistance; when it is abducted or adducted and extended backwards; and when the neck is hyperextended.[126] Unfortunately, all these manoeuvres can reduce the pulse of a normal individual, and little reliance can be placed on these signs.[127] The vascular symptoms and signs of a cervical rib are almost always unilateral, but they tend to progress after they have developed; areas of necrosis, patchy gangrene, and eventually more extensive gangrene can appear if the arterial compression is left untreated (Fig. 10.30). An acute thrombosis of the subclavian artery leads to massive ischaemia of the upper limb, but this is unusual because of the excellent potential for a collateral circulation.

Mechanism of symptoms

A number of mechanisms for the symptoms of cervical rib or thoracic outlet compression have been postulated. It has been suggested that the artery is compressed between the rib and the scalenus anterior,[128] between the rib and the clavicle (costoclavicular compression),[129] between a band arising from the rib and the clavicle, between the two heads of scalenus medius, or between the converging heads of the median nerve.[130]

The thoracic outlet syndrome may follow fracture of the clavicle, which causes distortion. It may also be caused by fibrous bands coming off a large transverse process of the seventh cervical vertebra, or by a rudimentary cervical rib. Hypertrophy of the scalene muscles, which may be found in bodybuilders, champion swimmers or gymnasts, can also cause compression. An abnormality of the first rib, caused by a congenital enlargement, a fracture or a tumour, is a rare cause of symptoms.[131] The axillary vein may occasionally be compressed by the phrenic nerve or by an accessory pectoral muscle.[132]

REFERENCES

123. Young HA, Hardy DG. Br J Hosp Med 1983; 1: 487
124. Coote H. Lancet 1861; i: 360
125. Bramwell F. Rev Neurol Psychiatry 1903; 1: 236
126. Adson AW, Coffey JR. Ann Surg 1927; 69: 203
127. Warrens AN, Heaton JM. Ann R Coll Surg Engl 1987; 69: 203
128. Murphy JB. Surg Gynecol Obstet 1906; 3: 574
129. Telford ED, Mottershead S. Br Med J 1947; 1: 325
130. Todd TW. J Anat Physiol 1911; 45: 293
131. Coote H. Med Times Gaz 1861; 2: 108
132. Boontje AH. Br J Surg 1979; 66: 331

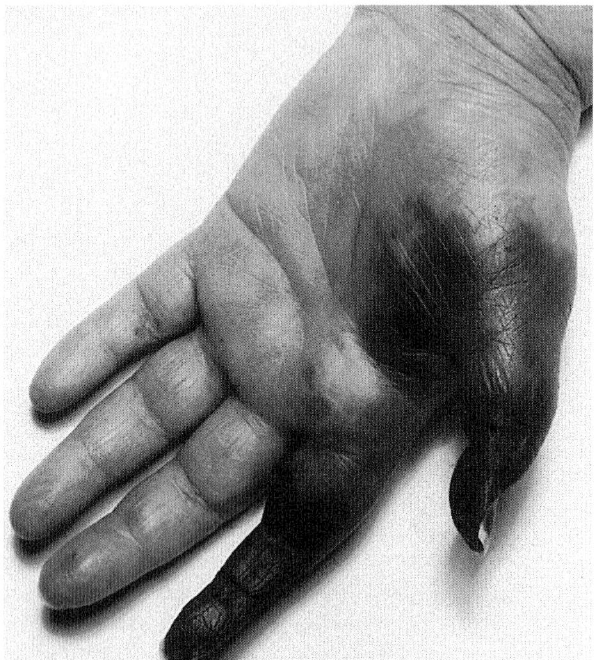

Figure 10.30 A gangrenous hand caused by a thrombosed subclavian artery.

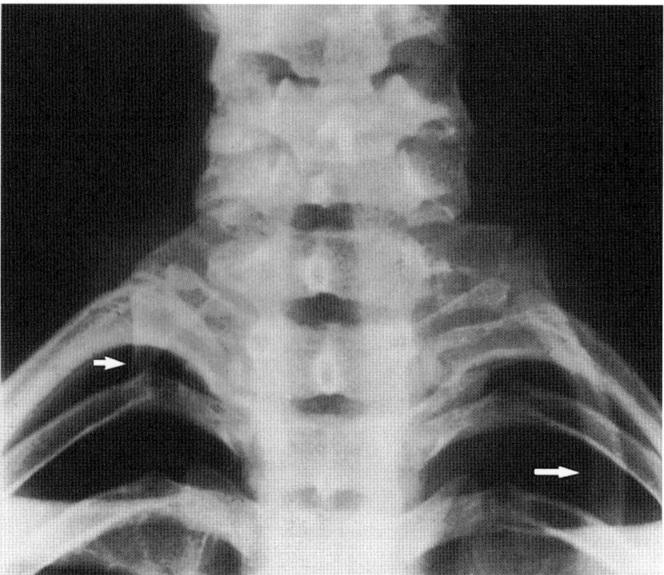

Figure 10.31 A plain radiograph of the thoracic inlet showing cervical ribs (arrowed).

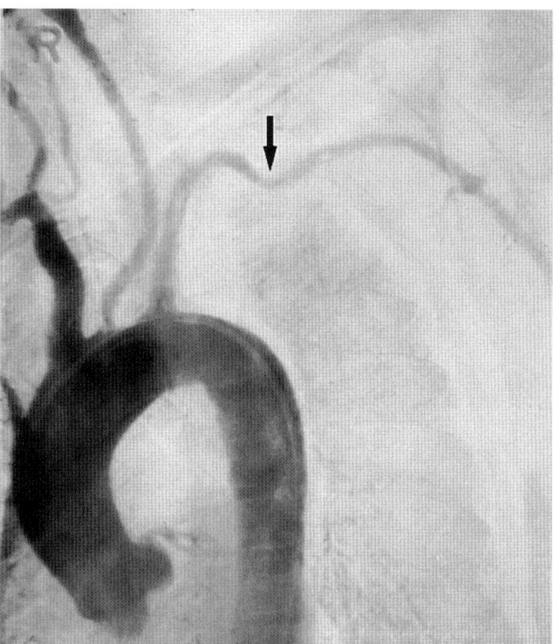

Figure 10.32 An arch aortogram showing a kink in the subclavian artery caused by a fascial band.

The thoracic outlet syndrome is a condition that is often overdiagnosed, and the neurological symptoms must be carefully differentiated from those of cervical spondylosis, cervical disc protrusions, and spinal cord tumours. Syringomyelia, a Pancoast's tumour, osteoarthritis of the shoulder, supraspinatus tendonitis, ulnar neuritis and carpal tunnel syndrome are other conditions that can cause similar symptoms. Impaired conduction velocity down the ulnar nerve on electromyography may help to confirm the diagnosis,[133] but this is not always present and is not essential for diagnosis. Venous symptoms must be differentiated from an axillary vein thrombosis. The arterial symptoms of a cervical rib must be differentiated from atherosclerotic disease of the subclavian artery, Takayasu's disease, Buerger's disease, and both primary and secondary vasospastic disorders. The presence of a cervical rib or a large transverse process of the seventh cervical vertebra on plain radiographs of the thoracic inlet (Fig. 10.31) provides some support for the diagnosis, and at the same time radiographs of the cervical spine and shoulder should be obtained to exclude some of the other conditions from which the outlet syndrome must be differentiated. Duplex scanning should be performed with the arm in the position that promotes the patients' symptoms. Axillary phlebograms and arteriograms with the arms in different degrees of abduction may show a marked kink in the artery or vein (Fig. 10.32), and this also provides support for the diagnosis.[134] At a later stage, these investigations may show evidence of a thrombosis in the axillary vein or artery, and sometimes signs of multiple emboli within the small vessels of the hand. Occasionally a localized aneurysm related to the rib is demonstrated (Fig. 10.33).

Management of thoracic outlet syndrome

The final decision to decompress the thoracic outlet is a clinical one if all investigations remain inconclusive. When the diagnosis remains in doubt, it is better to err towards caution and try to improve posture and strengthen the trapezius muscle with a course of exercises, reserving decompression for persistent or deteriorating symptoms. Patients must be warned that decompression does not always relieve symptoms, and can cause the complications of Horner's syndrome or brachial neuritis. A neurologist's opinion is always helpful to rule out other causes of symptoms that the surgeon may have overlooked.

REFERENCES

133. Urshel HC, Paulson DL, McNamara JJ. Ann Surg 1968; 6: 1
134. Lang EK. Radiology 1965; 84: 296

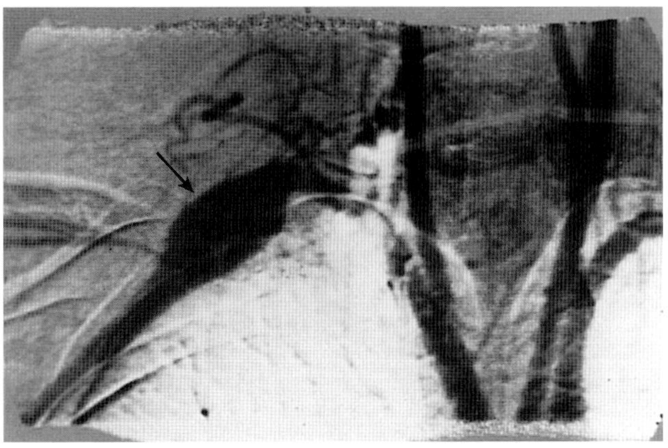

Figure 10.33 A digital subtraction angiogram showing a subclavian aneurysm caused by a cervical rib.

Decompression of the thoracic outlet: resection of a cervical rib

The operation can be performed through a supraclavicular approach. The clavicular fibres of sternomastoid and the omohyoid muscle are divided (Fig. 10.34). The scalene fat pad is dissected off the scalenus anterior, and the phrenic nerve is retracted off this muscle before it is divided. The subclavian artery, which lies directly behind the muscle, is dissected free from its sheath and is retracted upwards or downwards before the pleurocervical fascia (Sibson's fascia) is divided. The pleura is exposed and reflected off the inner surface of the first rib. A cervical rib is then felt as a bony spur directed towards the inner surface of the first rib. The T1 nerve root is located, passing up over the neck of the first rib and looping over the cervical rib as it passes laterally to form the brachial plexus (Fig. 10.34). A cervical rib often passes between the nerve trunks of the brachial plexus as it is traced upwards and backwards towards its articulation with the transverse process and body of the seventh cervical vertebra. The rib is removed by bone nibblers as close to the vertebral articulation as possible.

When a subclavian aneurysm is present, its limits must be defined and the vessel isolated, before it is cross-clamped and the aneurysm resected. It is extremely unusual for there to be enough arterial length to allow an end-to-end anastomosis to be made, and the resected aneurysm is normally replaced by a segment of reversed long saphenous vein or a prosthetic graft. Embolectomy, thrombectomy, thrombolysis, and occasionally bypass surgery are required for ischaemic complications, when the results are much more unpredictable.

The thoracic outlet can be decompressed through a transaxillary approach.[135] Specially designed rib-cutting shears were developed along with a T1 nerve retractor. This allows full decompression of the space from the costochondral junction to the neck of the first rib (Fig. 10.35). This approach does not allow cervical ribs to be seen but is favoured by Roos for patients with thoracic outlet syndromes who do not have cervical ribs. The first rib can also be resected from above using a supra- and infraclavicular approach. The results of surgery are good in patients with a true outlet syndrome,[136] but ribs can re-form if the periosteum is left intact. Complications include pneumothorax, intercostobrachial and supraclavicular paraesthesia, Horner's syndrome, and damage to the brachial plexus and subclavian artery. Patients can die from major vascular injuries, and the hand may have to be amputated if ischaemia cannot be reversed.

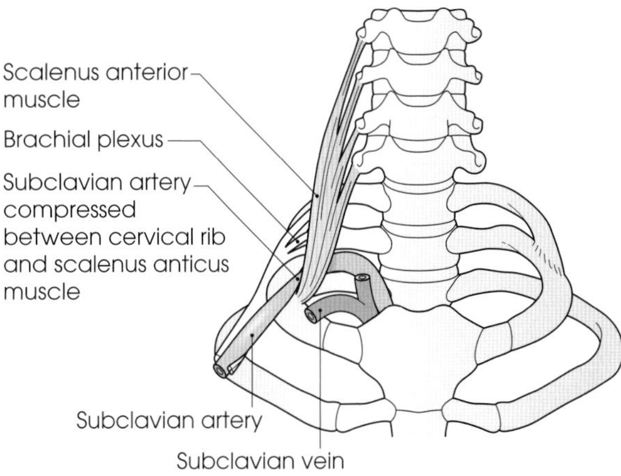

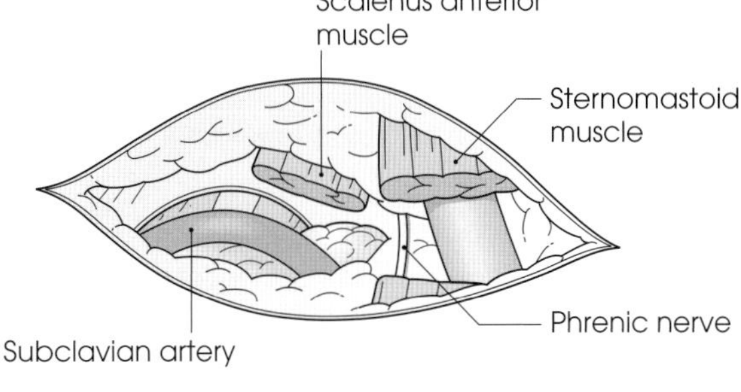

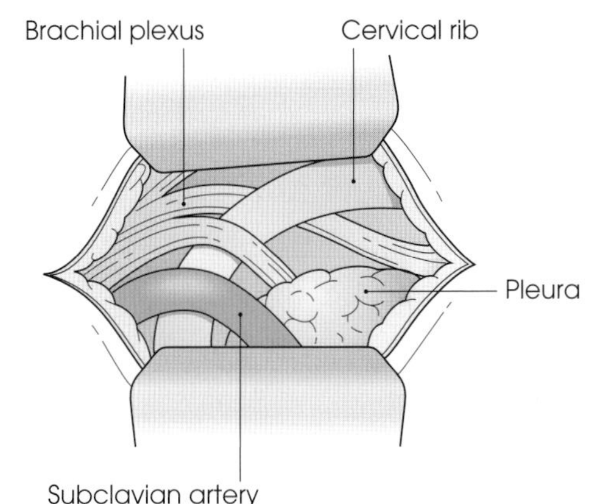

Figure 10.34 Resection of a cervical rib.

Popliteal entrapment

The popliteal artery may pass medially around the anatomically normal medial head of the gastrocnemius muscle, or it may pass beneath an aberrant band arising from any of the muscles in the popliteal fossa (Fig. 10.36).[137] A number of other variations have been described but all are rare. Contraction of the fibres of these muscles can occlude the artery and cut off the blood supply to the calf, causing claudication. Eventually the repeated occlusion or the constant trauma of muscle contraction can damage the arterial wall and result in intimal thickening, plaque formation, fibrosis and thrombosis. This often occurs after a particularly violent episode of exercise.

REFERENCES

135. Roos DB. Surgery 1982; 92: 1077
136. Lepanto M, Lindgren K-A et al. Br J Surg 1989; 76: 1255
137. Insua JA, Young JR, Humphries AW. Arch Surg 1970; 101: 771

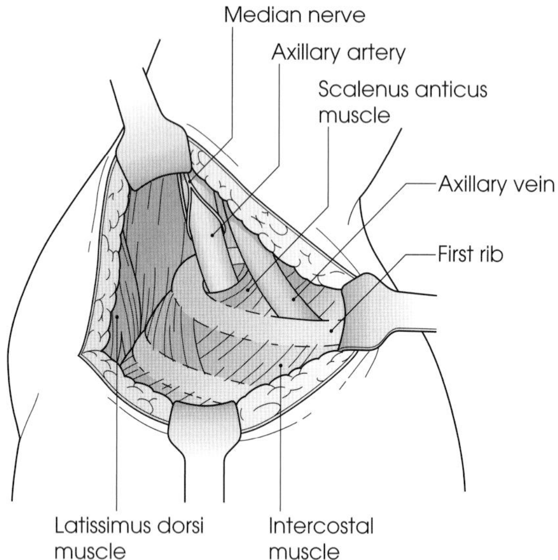

Figure 10.35 The axillary approach used to resect the first rib.

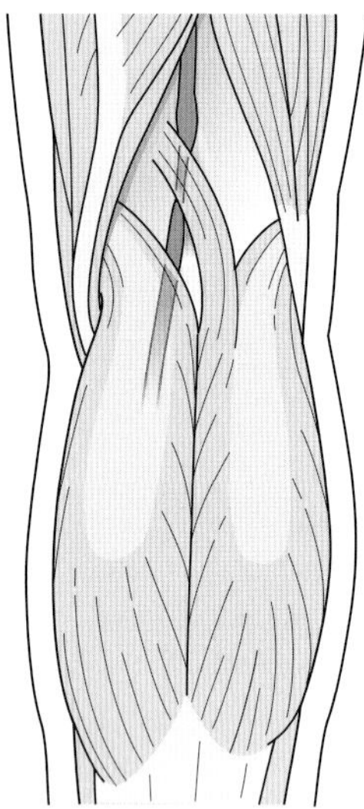

Figure 10.36 Popliteal entrapment by a third head of the gastrocnemius muscle.

The condition should be suspected in a young and often physically fit man who complains of claudication on exercise. Contraction of the calf muscles against resistance often causes the foot pulses to disappear. Popliteal entrapment must be differentiated from popliteal cystic disease, premature atherosclerosis, arteritis, chronic compartment syndrome and embolism.

Duplex scanning at rest and during muscle contraction may confirm cessation of blood flow. Arteriography often shows a medial deviation in the artery as it crosses the popliteal fossa, and CT or MRI scan at knee level shows muscle passing either side of the vessel.[138] Magnetic resonance scanning also provides very good images of this anomaly.

Division of the muscle belly is all that is required if the vessel has not occluded, but thrombectomy and replacement of the damaged vessel is necessary if thrombosis has occurred. Muscle division is curative, but if the vessel has thrombosed the end result is less predictable.[139] The opposite popliteal fossa must be carefully examined; muscle division should be undertaken prophylactically if there are signs of compression.

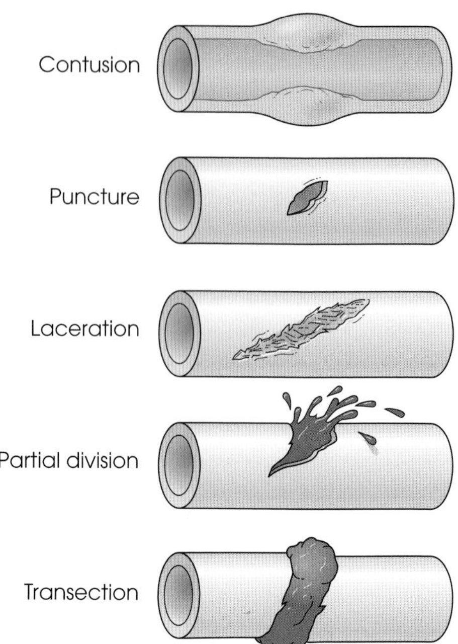

Figure 10.37 The different types of arterial injury.

ARTERIAL INJURY

Arterial injuries may be either open or closed and can be caused by direct damage from a missile, a stabbing weapon, or a piece of shrapnel; alternatively, they may be caused indirectly by a bony injury that secondarily impinges on or lacerates the vessel wall.[140] A significant proportion of all arterial injuries are now the result of medical, surgical or radiological intervention, and these iatrogenic injuries are increasing every year.[141] Arteries may also be damaged by extremes of temperature and inadvertent injections of noxious agents.

The injured artery may be contused, punctured, lacerated or partially divided; the intima may be damaged, or the vessel may be completely divided with separation of the ends (Fig. 10.37). These injuries result in haemorrhage, spasm, occlusion, thrombosis, dissection, or the development of false aneurysms and arteriovenous fistulae.

ARTERIAL HAEMORRHAGE

Arterial haemorrhage may be primary, secondary or reactionary, and can be either concealed or revealed, depending on whether the injury is open or closed. Most lacerations or missile injuries that partially or completely sever an artery result in a visible haemorrhage that is bright red and pulsatile. Both sharp arterial transections and crushing tearing injuries of the vessels cause arterial spasm; this, combined with the hypotension caused by blood loss and rapid platelet deposition, quickly leads to a reduction in or cessation of bleeding. Bleeding may be prolonged if there is a lateral tear in the artery or if the laceration is held

REFERENCES

138. Muller N, Morris DC, Nichols DM. Radiology 1984; 151: 157
139. Barabas AP, Macfarlane R. Br J Hosp Med 1985; 1: 304
140. Makin GS, Howard JM, Green RL. Surgery 1966; 59: 203
141. McMillan I, Murie JA. Br J Surg 1984; 71: 832

open. When the blood pressure recovers, muscle spasm may wear off and platelet thrombi are expelled, resulting in a reactionary haemorrhage. A secondary haemorrhage can occur if infection erodes the arterial wall; this is usually between 7 and 10 days after the initial injury.

Arteries may also be torn or damaged and bleed internally. The profunda femoris or one of its perforating arteries, for example, is commonly torn by a fracture of the shaft of the femur, producing a massive haematoma in the thigh without overt signs of haemorrhage (see Ch. 55). Concealed bleeding may occasionally cause a rise in the intercompartmental pressure that occludes arterial inflow and leads to ischaemic necrosis.

The first-aid management of arterial haemorrhage is to apply external pressure directly over the bleeding point—or at one of the well-recognized compression points along the proximal course of the damaged artery where it crosses a bony prominence—to produce occlusion. A tourniquet should only be used if haemorrhage cannot be controlled by pressure, and then its application must be carefully monitored because the risk of distal ischaemia and metabolic derangement following release is considerable. The application of a tourniquet in theatre may on occasion make the subsequent exploration and arterial reconstruction much easier. Artery forceps (haemostats) should not be used in the accident and emergency department to control bleeding arteries in the depths of wounds unless patients are in extremis and arteries that are bleeding cannot be controlled by the measures described above.

Local pressure followed by resuscitation should normally proceed to rapid exploration under general anaesthesia. There is no place for arteriography or other investigations if arterial haemorrhage is massive, but an appropriate quantity of blood must be sent for cross-matching before the patient is taken to theatre. Plain radiographs and arteriography can be obtained if the patient is stable and there is no overt external bleeding. This will confirm the sites of injury and detect bony damage and foreign body fragments such as shrapnel.

At operation, after proximal and distal control of the bleeding vessel has been achieved, the artery is repaired, extending the skin wound as necessary. Few arteries should be ligated if they can be repaired, although individual vessels in the forearm and calf can usually be tied off with safety. Once a suitable length of normal artery has been exposed above and below the site of the injury, the patient should be given systemic heparin (5000 units, with smaller doses in children) before arterial occluding clamps are applied on either side of the injured segment.

When the extent of the arterial damage is not apparent from external inspection, or when it is suspected that a distal vessel is occluded by thrombus arteriography should be carried out on the operating table using a fine needle or catheter inserted directly into the vessel, with films wrapped in sterile towels placed beneath the injured part. Alternatively, a C arm with digital subtraction facilities can be used, providing the patient is on a radiotranslucent table. The artery should be opened and the lumen inspected if there is any evidence of intimal damage or distal propagation of thrombus shown on the arteriogram. The damaged portion of the vessel must be resected and a Fogarty catheter passed distally to remove propagated thrombus. A completion arteriogram should be obtained to ensure that all the distal thrombus has been removed after a repair of the artery has been effected.

Arterial repair may be by simple suture, lateral continuous suture, patch repair, end-to-end anastomosis or interposition grafting (Fig. 10.38). The type of injury determines the type of repair. A small puncture wound commonly occurring after radiological or cardiac catheterization can usually be closed by one or two simple sutures placed in the axis of the vessel to avoid narrowing. A linear laceration or a small branch avulsed from the side of the vessel can usually be closed by a single continuous suture, provided that arterial wall has not been lost, and provided that the lumen will not be narrowed by this type of repair. A patch should be inserted to repair any defect where there is a risk of stenosis. Vein is usually the material of choice for the patch, but prosthetic material (Dacron or polytetrafluoroethylene) can be used when a suitably thick-walled vein is not available, providing there is no risk of infection.

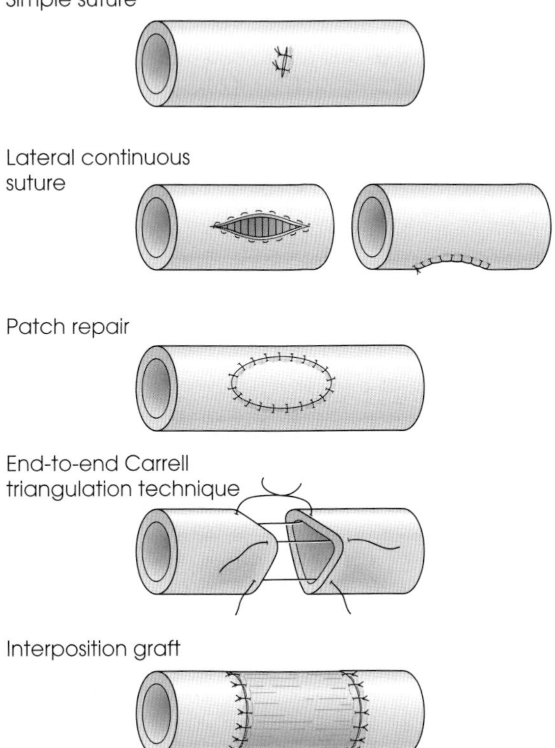

Figure 10.38 Methods of repairing arterial injuries.

Occasionally it is possible to mobilize a sufficient length of artery to excise the damaged arterial wall and carry out an end-to-end anastomosis. This is possible when the vessel has been neatly transected, but should not be attempted if the anastomosis has to be made under tension, or if a damaged segment of vessel must be retained to allow a satisfactory anastomosis to be made. An end-to-end anastomosis may be made using a double-ended suture or by the triangulation method of Carrel (Fig. 10.38).[142]

An interposition graft of vein or prosthetic material should be used to replace any segment of severely damaged vessel if excision and end-to-end anastomosis are not possible (Fig. 10.38). Long saphenous vein is usually the material that is chosen for this purpose in patients with arterial damage in the limbs, but this vein must not be taken from a limb with a concomitant venous injury, because this may sacrifice an important collateral.[143] The

REFERENCES

142. Carrel A. Lyon Med 1902; 98: 859
143. Barros D'Sa A. Ann R Coll Surg Engl 1982; 64: 37

long or short saphenous vein of the contralateral undamaged limb or the cephalic vein is used instead. The internal and external jugular veins and the brachial veins provide useful alternatives if arteries of the calibre of the iliac, carotid or subclavian arteries have been damaged.[144] Alternatively the cephalic or saphenous veins can be fashioned into a larger calibre panel composite or compilation graft.[145] Prosthetic materials can be used to replace major vessels if vein is unavailable or unsuitable, but should not be used in contaminated wounds because of the dangers of graft infection. An indwelling shunt of the Javid or Pruitt type can be used to maintain the arterial inflow and venous outflow while other injuries are being repaired.[146] Many now prefer to perform the vascular repairs first and stabilize bones or repair nerves and soft tissue later.[147] The internal iliac artery can be used as a free graft if the arterial injury is within the abdomen.

ARTERIAL SPASM

It is now recognized that post-traumatic arterial spasm is a dangerous diagnosis to make, because it is often associated with intimal damage and intraluminal thrombosis, which can be excluded only by arteriography or exploration. Traumatic spasm certainly does occur, but should be diagnosed only in retrospect after arteriography has shown typical appearances or arteriotomy fails to demonstrate intimal damage.

Arterial spasm is often the only visible sign of a severe arterial injury, with wall contusion and intimal damage underlying the area of spasm.[148] Urgent arteriography should be carried out when a patient presents with a cold extremity following a direct or crushing injury, especially if this is associated with a bone fracture such as supracondylar fracture of the humerus (see Ch. 53), and the distal pulses are impalpable or cannot be detected with a Doppler ultrasound probe. Surgical exploration is indicated if the artery is locally stenosed or occluded on arteriogram. When the vessel has been exposed and the haemorrhage controlled, areas of arterial contusion or persistent spasm should be investigated by intraoperative arteriography, or alternatively the luminal surface can be directly inspected through an appropriately sited arteriotomy.

Intramuscular or intraluminal injections of papaverine and careful division of the adventitia may alleviate the stenosis;[149] the arteriogram confirms smooth spasm of the wall. This can be confirmed by repeating the arteriography. Persistent spasm is an indication for inspection of the luminal surface. Damaged arterial wall is dealt with by the methods described earlier.

ARTERIAL OCCLUSION

Arterial occlusion follows severe wall contusion with mural thrombus or intimal tears, and also occurs when the vessel has been completely transected. The symptoms and signs are those of arterial haemorrhage combined with evidence of an acute arterial occlusion. Occasionally, arterial occlusion may be difficult to diagnose, particularly when the patient has sustained a fracture. The absence of a distal pulse may be explained by a raised compartment pressure, and the presence of distal arterial Doppler signals may provide false reassurance.

The common sites of arterial damage in combination with fractures include the superficial femoral artery in fractures of the femur, the popliteal artery in injuries of the knee (particularly posterior dislocation), and the brachial artery in supracondylar fractures of the humerus. Rarely, the axillary artery can be damaged by a fractured clavicle and the brachial artery by fractures of the humerus. A high index of suspicion must be maintained in these circumstances, and arteriography is indicated if there is any doubt. Arteriography is helpful to determine the upper limit of the occlusion, but rarely shows the distal arterial tree because the collateral pathways have not yet had time to develop. When an occluded artery is exposed, it appears swollen, discoloured and solid, and is either not pulsatile or feebly pulsatile. The vessel lumen is explored through an arteriotomy, which is begun above the damaged segment and extended through the injured portion of the vessel. Distal thrombus is removed by a Fogarty catheter before the damaged artery is repaired or excised. When the vessel has been completely divided, the two ends of the transected artery are mobilized and occluded by clamps before continuity is restored by end-to-end anastomosis or interposition grafting.

Limbs that have sustained acute arterial occlusions should have early and adequate fasciotomies made to prevent massive rises in compartment pressure[150] when the period of acute ischaemia has been considerable (more than 3 or 4 h), or when there has been any associated venous injury. Distal pulses must be monitored postoperatively by regular clinical examination, supplemented if necessary by Doppler ultrasound pressure measurement. Disappearance of pulsation is an indication for re-exploration of the vessel. Patients should be given systemic antibiotics to try to prevent secondary infection. Tissues that are not viable must be excised, but it is important to achieve soft tissue cover of all arterial suture lines.

ARTERIAL DISSECTION

Arterial dissection is the consequence of an intimal tear with arterial blood entering the media, and it becomes apparent when the vessel occludes. The dissection rarely extends for any great distance down the vessel because the media is normal and not weakened from cystic median necrosis. Arteriography usually shows a smoothly narrowed vessel with contrast outlining the origin of the dissection. The damaged segment of artery must be excised and replaced.

TRAUMATIC OR FALSE ANEURYSM (PULSATING HAEMATOMA)

A laceration through part of an arterial wall results in a local haematoma that may eventually be contained by the surrounding normal tissues. Fibrous tissue develops around this haematoma; this then contracts to give a false sac containing thrombus, which remains in continuity with the vessel lumen. Continued arterial pulsation erodes the wall of a false aneurysm, increasing the cavity in the haematoma.[151]

There is often a history of considerable primary haemorrhage from a small wound, and there may be signs of marked swelling and local oedema. Distal pulsation is usually maintained, but a local bruit may precede the appearance of the expansile

REFERENCES

144. Thompson BW, Read RC, Casali RE. Am J Surg 1975; 130: 733
145. Livingston RH, Wilson RI. Br Med J 1975; 1: 667
146. Radonic V, Baric D, Petricevic A et al. Br J Surg 1995; 82: 777
147. Kinmonth JB. Br Med J 1952; 1: 59
148. Barros D'Sa A. Vasa-Suppl 1991; 33: 66
149. Patman RD, Thompson JE. Arch Surg 1970; 101: 663
150. Patterson-Ross J. Br Med J 1946; 1: 1
151. Hajarizadeh H, La Rosa CR. J Vasc Surg 1995; 22: 425

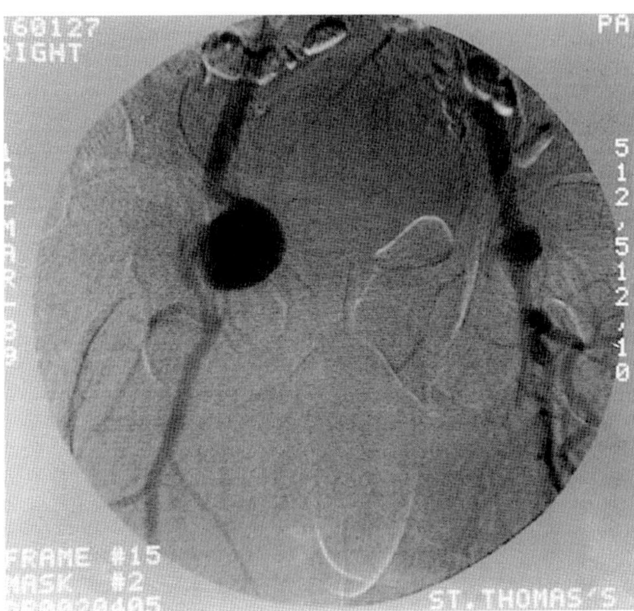

Figure 10.39 A digital subtraction arteriogram showing a false aneurysm.

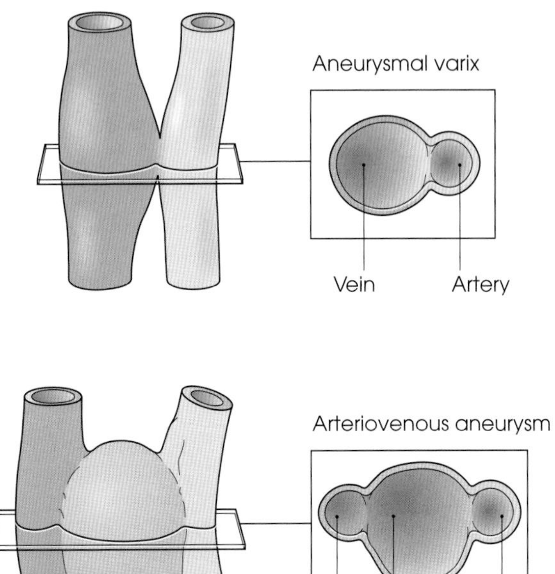

Figure 10.40 Different types of arteriovenous fistula.

pulsation. Surrounding structures are compressed as the aneurysm expands, and limb oedema, deep vein thrombosis, and nerve damage causing pain may all complicate its development. It is extremely rare for the artery to occlude, however, and treatment rarely needs to be urgent unless there is danger of skin necrosis or sepsis developing over the sac. At first it may be difficult to decide whether there is just a local haematoma lying over the vessel with transmitted pulsation. Re-examination over a period of days invariably dispels doubt, but a colour duplex scan usually confirms the presence of a false aneurysm.

It may be possible to occlude the site of the leak using the duplex scanner probe to provide precise pressure if it is found early and the defect is small.[152] This technique has been superseded by direct thrombin injection, which is associated with a 94–98% occlusion rate of the false femoral aneurysms.[153] This technique causes less pain and is even effective in patients on anticoagulation. Digital or conventional arteriography[154] usually confirms the presence and exact location of a false aneurysm (Fig. 10.39), which can be repaired electively when compression fails. Arteriography also demonstrates the state of the distal arterial tree. When the vessels proximal and distal to the aneurysm have been displayed and controlled, the sac is opened and the arterial defect is closed. When all the vessels entering the false sac cannot be easily controlled before it is opened, troublesome back-bleeding can be prevented by inserting Fogarty catheters into the relevant branches and inflating the balloons until the bleeding ceases. Closure with simple sutures often suffices if the defect is small, but if it is large, a patch or interposition graft may be required.

There is almost no place today for arterial ligation in the treatment of false aneurysm, unless access to the sac is extremely difficult. The results of surgical repair are very good; providing the false aneurysm is tackled before it becomes too large or complications have developed, repairs carry a low morbidity and mortality[155] and can normally be carried out without compromising arterial patency. The development of covered stents allows false aneurysms to be easily obliterated, and is the method of choice if the patient is old and unfit and if the aneurysm is in an inaccessible site.[156] The undistended stent is inserted over a guide wire, positioned across the neck of the false sac, and expanded to occlude the opening.

TRAUMATIC ARTERIOVENOUS FISTULA

Traumatic arteriovenous fistula usually develops when there is a simultaneous partial laceration of a vein and artery lying in close apposition, with both vessels opening into a common haematoma cavity (an arteriovenous aneurysm). Occasionally the vessels communicate directly, with complete or partial redirection of arterial blood into the vein (an aneurysmal varix). Sometimes a second injury of the arterial wall may produce a false aneurysm in the artery in addition to the arteriovenous aneurysm, and rarely the proximal end of the divided artery appears to join the distal end of the divided vein (Fig. 10.40).

Arteriovenous fistulae do not form immediately after wounding, usually taking some days to develop. The patient may notice a thrill or even become aware of a buzzing noise if the fistula is situated in the head or neck. Fistulae usually follow an open wound but may also follow a closed injury, which may be trivial; they can occasionally occur after mass ligation of an artery and its adjoining vein.[157] A traumatic fistula may develop between two insignificant peripheral vessels or may involve vessels as large as the aorta and inferior vena cava. Many are now caused by

REFERENCES

152. Olsen DM et al. J Vasc Surg 2002; 36: 779–782
153. Mohler ER III, Mitchell ME, Carpenter JP et al. Vasc Med 2001; 6; 241–244
154. McMillan I, Murie JA. Br J Surg 1984; 71: 832
155. Elkin DC, Shumacker HB. Surgery in World War II, Vascular Surgery. Government Print Office, Washington, 1955
156. Parodi JC. J Vasc Surg 1995; 21: 549
157. Holman E. Arteriovenous Aneurysm. Macmillan, New York, 1937

needles or catheters inserted by cardiologists or radiologists as part of investigation or treatment.

The symptoms and signs are initially similar to those of a traumatic aneurysm, although the swelling is often less and a thrill or bruit predominates. Later the adjoining veins around the fistula dilate and may form a plexiform pulsating mass. A machinery murmur is heard loudest over the fistula, but it is usually transmitted for some distance in all directions. The murmur is usually loudest in systole and can be abolished by direct pressure over the fistula. When the fistula is large, it may at first cause a fall in both the systolic and diastolic pressure, an increase in heart rate, and raised venous pressure both proximal and distal to the fistula.[157] The cardiac output increases as a result of the increased venous return, and the venous oxygen content also rises. The arterial blood flow beyond the fistula is reduced, and rarely this may cause gangrene. As the patient acclimatizes to the fistula, the circulating blood volume increases, both the systolic and diastolic pressure rise, and the pulse rate returns to normal. The adjoining vessels continue to enlarge if the fistula is not repaired at this stage and may even develop atherosclerosis and phlebosclerosis. The heart then begins to dilate and may eventually fail. When the fistula is situated in a limb, this may hypertrophy and lengthen,[157] and the chronic venous hypertension may lead to lipodermatosclerosis and venous ulceration. Most of these effects are reversed when the fistula is closed. Bacterial endocarditis is a rare but potentially lethal complication.[158]

Confirmation of the effect

Confirmation of the effect of the fistula on cardiac output is demonstrated by the bradycardic reaction of Branham.[39,40] The pulse rate is recorded for a minute before the fistula is occluded. It is then measured for a further minute, and a marked fall in pulse rate in the second period is indicative of a sizeable left-to-right shunt with cardiac compensation. The fistula can be safely treated by ligation if the distal vessels still pulsate when the fistula is occluded (the Henle–Coenen sign),[159,160] but in practice surgical correction should always aim to separate the vessels and close the defect.

Before operation, arteriography should be obtained to delineate the site of the fistula and confirm the presence of a normal distal arterial tree (Fig. 10.41). It is occasionally helpful to measure the cardiac output and pulmonary oxygen saturation. A small fistula, which can be held occluded by pressure from a duplex probe, may occasionally close spontaneously.[161] If this fails, the choice lies between inserting a covered stent over the defect[156] or direct operative closure. A large fistula in an unfit patient is ideal for stenting, whereas a small peripheral fistula in a fit young patient should be corrected by operation. At operation the artery and the vein should be controlled above and below the point of connection; after systemic heparin has been given, the vessel can be occluded by clamps and separated. The defect in both the artery and the vein should be directly closed if possible. Occasionally, in for instance a large aortocaval fistula, it may be difficult to obtain direct access to the fistula; under these circumstances it may be preferable to open the artery and close the fistula from within the lumen.[162] A covered stent placed over the defect is then an attractive alternative. The draining veins should not be ligated if possible because symptoms of defective venous drainage may develop in the future. Closure of the fistula almost instantly cures cardiac failure, which may have needed intensive treatment before the operation.

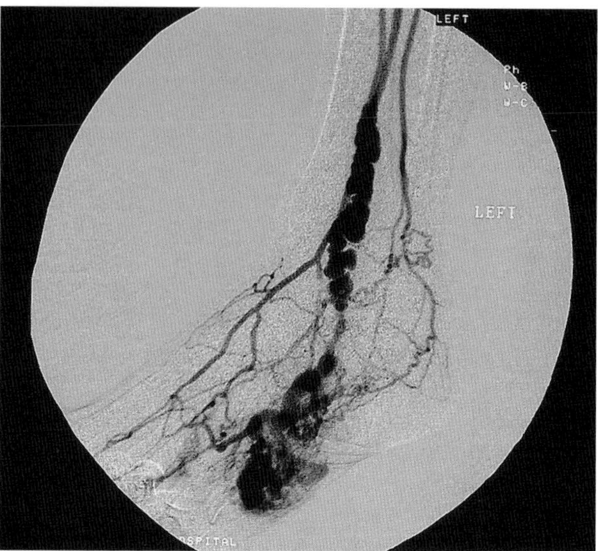

Figure 10.41 An angiogram showing an arteriovenous fistula.

IATROGENIC ARTERIAL INJURIES

Ligation

In any operation, sudden life-threatening haemorrhage may require rapid surgical control, and the application of haemostatic artery forceps and ligatures forms part of all operations. There are no undesirable consequences providing the tissues supplied by the occluded vessels have an alternative means of blood supply or are being removed as part of the operation, but from time to time a major vessel is inadvertently ligated. This must be recognized immediately and appropriate steps taken to restore blood flow. This may simply entail removal of the ligature, but if the arterial wall has been devitalized by its application the damaged vessel must be resected. The principles of vascular repair of an injured artery have already been described. There is almost never a good reason for not restoring arterial inflow and relying instead on collateral pathways to develop.

External compression from plasters, bandages and splints

Plasters, bandages and splints may produce arterial occlusion in a number of ways. First, the edge of the splint or plaster cast may compress an area of skin and occlude the underlying vessels. Second, the plaster or bandage is applied too tightly, occluding the veins, causing oedema and raising the tension beneath the external occlusion until the arteries eventually become obstructed. Third, the patient may keep the leg in a dependent position and so develop oedema of the limb, which will compromise the blood supply if the external compression is non-compliant. Finally, the patient may develop heart failure or stop taking diuretic tablets for heart failure and so develop lower limb oedema, with disastrous consequences.

REFERENCES

158. Reinhoff WH, Hamman L. Ann Surg 1935; 102: 905
159. Henle AR. Zentralbl Chir 1914; 41: 92
160. Coenen H. Zentralbl Chir 1913; 40: 191
161. Feld R, Patton GMN, Carabasi A. J Vasc Surg 1992; 16: 832
162. McClelland RM, Canizaro PC, Shires GT. Major Probl Clin Surg 1971; 3: 146

This complication should be entirely preventable if the digits of all limbs encased in plasters or tight dressings are regularly inspected and by responding to all complaints of excessive pain by releasing dressings, splitting plasters, and inspecting encased limbs. Cold digits and absent distal pulsation are late signs.

Iatrogenic arterial puncture damage

Radiologists and cardiologists are regularly required to perform arterial punctures for contrast arteriography and cardiac investigation, and doctors of all specialities sample arterial blood for gas and pH analysis. Any arterial puncture carries the risks already described of dissection, haemorrhage, thrombosis, false aneurysm and arteriovenous fistula formation. These risks must be recognized, and are minimized by careful technique and adequate external pressure applied for an appropriate period (2–5 min) over all arterial puncture sites. Punctures into the external iliac artery above the inguinal ligament or into the profunda femoris artery are more difficult to control. Careful monitoring should detect developing complications, which can be rapidly corrected by the appropriate surgical manoeuvres.

Intra-arterial injection of drugs and chemicals

A number of compounds, given intravenously with complete safety, have disastrous consequences if injected into an artery. Short-acting barbiturates for anaesthesia,[163] sodium tetradecyl sulphate as a vein sclerosant,[164] and quinine given for malaria are examples of drugs that can be safely injected into veins but severely damage arteries. Drug abusers may inadvertently self-administer barbiturates or benzodiazepines into arteries, with disastrous consequences.[165] Because arteries often lie in close proximity to veins, these complications are well recognized. They may be prevented if bright red pulsatile blood is noted to enter the barrel of the syringe; even when the injection has begun, disaster may still be averted if further injection is immediately abandoned when the patient complains of severe limb pain.[164]

The limb may be lost from gangrene or severely compromised by the development of a Volkmann's contracture if a toxic compound is inadvertently injected into a peripheral artery before it is recognized. Limbs that recover may later develop Raynaud's phenomenon.

In many patients who receive an inadvertent arterial injection there is a congenital arterial anomaly. In 10% there is a high bifurcation of the brachial artery, with the ulnar artery passing superficial to the common flexor origin and so presenting more readily to the needle. The antecubital fossa should not be used for thiopentone injections, and a pause should always be made after a small quantity of barbiturate has been injected to discover if this is painful. The vessel thromboses because of acute intimal damage, perhaps as a result of the release of noradrenaline or the high pH of thiopentone, and the thrombosis rapidly extends into all the major tributaries. The moment this disaster is recognized, the syringe should be removed from the needle and an injection of heparin given through the same needle. An intravenous infusion of dextran may be started, and the patient should be continued on systemic anticoagulants.[164] Alternatively, a prostacyclin infusion may be tried. A stellate ganglion block, a lumbar sympathectomy, or a local periarterial sympathetic block may abolish arterial spasm, while external cooling may help to prevent tissue loss. Urgent arteriography may indicate the need for thrombectomy if these measures fail to improve the circulation, although the results of this desperate surgery are often poor. A significant proportion of these injuries end in amputation and litigation.[166]

Ergot poisoning

Ergot poisoning is rare but is discussed in more detail under *Ergotism* (p. 258).

ENVIRONMENTAL ARTERIAL INJURY

Frostbite

Frostbite affects high-altitude mountaineers and those who are exposed in cold climates without adequate protection. The dangers of cold weather and suggestions for withstanding its effects are recorded in ancient Aryan and Assyrian texts. Hippocrates and Galen also recognized the signs of cold injury[167] and suggested methods to protect against its development. Xenophon recorded that during the retreat of the Greek soldiers from Persia 'they left behind soldiers who had lost their eyesight because of snow blindness and also those whose toes rotted off because of the cold'.[168] He suggested that it was beneficial to keep moving and to take sandals off at night. He noted that 'the straps cut into the feet' of those who went to sleep wearing their sandals. Matters were made worse when new uncured leather was used to make replacements for sandals that had worn out. Larrey, Napoleon's surgeon in the Polish campaign, provided a classical description of the ravages of frostbite,[169] and cold injury still caused many casualties in the Second World War despite the improvements in protective clothing; it proved a particular hazard in high-altitude aerial combat.[170] Even in the Falklands conflict, cold injury proved a major problem.[171] There is a strong association between the extent of the ischaemia and the outcome of each finger and toe.[172]

Response to freezing

The first signs of cold injury appear in the extremities at tissue temperatures of 15°C.[173] The fingers and toes redden because of a relative oxygen surplus: oxygen consumption is less than demand. At 10°C the skin is red and hypersensitive, and digital movements become clumsy. Below 10°C the skin becomes pink and painful; at lower temperatures the vessels become permanently contracted and the tissues appear cold and white (Stray's sign).[174] At 2.5°C ice crystals form in the tissues, which become anaesthetic and immobile, sometimes with scattered areas of cyanosis. Even at this stage, recovery can occur because cells have the capacity to supercool beyond their freezing point without solidifying. Tissue destruction occurs between −4 and −10°C, and true freezing may not develop until a temperature of −20°C is reached.

REFERENCES

163. Kinmonth JB, Shepherd RC. Br Med J 1959; 2: 914
164. MacGowan WAL, Holland PDJ et al. Br J Surg 1972; 59: 103
165. Wright CB, Lamoy RE, Hobson RW. Surgery 1976; 79: 425
166. Macgowan WAL. J R Soc Med 1985; 78: 136
167. Schechter DC, Sarot IA. Surgery 1968; 63: 527
168. Xenophon. Anabasis, Vol IV. Bristol Classic Press, Bristo, 1981
169. Dunning MWF. Br J Surg 1964; 51: 883
170. Simeone FA. Arch Surg 1960; 80: 396
171. Oakley EH. Ergonomics 1984; 27: 631
172. Cauchy E, Chetaille E, Marchand V et al. Wilderness Environ Med 2001; 12: 248–255
173. Meryman HT. Physiol Rev 1957; 37: 233
174. Stray L. Publ Norw Acad Sci 1943: 3

When water is transformed to ice the osmolality of the extracellular space increases, leading to diffusion of water from the intracellular space. Protein denaturation, pH changes, cellular dehydration, rupture of cell membranes, and destruction of cellular enzymes are all caused by freezing. Long periods of oxygen lack at this temperature are well tolerated because the cellular metabolism becomes suspended. The cold, which is amplified by wind chill, stimulates the autonomic nervous system, causing vasoconstriction. The slowing of the blood flow leads to haemoconcentration, increasing viscosity, causing capillary sludging and further reducing the blood supply of the frozen part. Eventually thrombosis leads to ischaemia and gangrene. Initially there is discomfort and local blanching, but this usually disappears as sensation is lost. Numbness and tingling give way to a wooden feeling. The affected person is often unaware of the blanching, which is most common on the ear and face, and an appreciation of the potential risks by colleagues may be valuable.

Recovery

Pain and swelling are common as the tissues rewarm. Arteriolar spasm relaxes and the capillaries dilate, allowing plasma to circulate. Blisters develop as fluid leaks out of damaged capillaries, and the skin changes to a dull red colour as cellular metabolism restarts. Diagnosis is rarely difficult. A Doppler probe may be used to assess the patency of the small vessels.

Prophylaxis

Prophylaxis is always preferable to treating the established condition, which is essentially incurable. Many factors have been implicated in the development of frostbite, including poor physical fitness, excessive alcohol intake, smoking, and the use of tight-fitting and wet clothes, as well as the presence of pre-existing vascular disease. In wartime, cold exposure often cannot be avoided, and great care must then be taken of both hands and feet. Insulated boots and gloves are now standard issue in arctic conditions, and tight shoes and straps must be avoided. Warm hats with ear flaps are also valuable. Depression, misery, and lack of exertion all encourage frostbite, and a positive attitude and enforced exercise may delay its development.

Treatment

There is disagreement over whether rewarming should be slow or rapid,[175] but frozen extremities should probably be left exposed in a cool moist environment or gently heated in warm water at a temperature not exceeding 60°C. Rapid rewarming in a whirlpool bath at 37–40°C now appears to be the most popular method of treatment.[175] The whole body should be gently warmed before the extremity is heated. Blisters should be left alone unless they reach massive proportions, when their contents may be aspirated through a sterile needle.

Topical applications of Flamazine or other antibiotics may prevent secondary infection if the skin separates, and systemic antibiotics are given for established infection. Thrombosis may be reversed by full doses of heparin administered by the intravenous or subcutaneous routes, although the evidence for its effectiveness is fairly weak.[176] Dextran may improve tissue survival by preventing capillary sludging[176] but carries an increased risk of bleeding, especially if used in combination with heparin. The place of sympathectomy is disputed, but it is probably beneficial,[177–179] and temporary stellate ganglion or brachial plexus block has never been tested in a controlled trial. Phenoxybenzamine, pentoxifylline (400 mg t.d.s. for 2–6 weeks) and hyperbaric oxygen have also been advocated on an anecdotal basis.[180] Good results have also been achieved using a topical thromboxane inhibitor (*Aloe vera*) in combination with aspirin used as a systemic antiprostaglandin, but this regimen was assessed in a consecutive series of patients without a control group.[181] Preliminary reports suggest that thrombolysis may be helpful,[182] but treatment with a prostaglandin analogue (iloprost) may be preferable.[183]

Local amputations of necrotic digits should be carried out when a clear line of demarcation has developed, although sometimes pain or the onset of infection may necessitate an earlier intervention. Amputation should be delayed as long as possible—between 30 and 90 days after freezing appears to be ideal. Fasciotomies may be required if there is evidence of a compartment syndrome. Split-skin grafts may be used to provide skin cover, but more complex reconstructions using plastic surgical techniques may be required to retain digit length and provide a functional hand (see Ch. 9).

When recovery is underway, active movements should be encouraged by a physiotherapist. Severe cold must always be avoided after an episode of frostbite, because of increased susceptibility to further damage and an often exaggerated response of the affected limbs to cold and heat. Causalgia and Raynaud's syndrome are late complications that can follow severe frostbite. Hyperhidrosis may also be a problem during recovery. It is often difficult to judge the extent of the final tissue loss at an early stage, but a knowledge of the conditions and the length of the exposure may allow a sensible estimation to be made.[184]

IMMERSION FOOT (TRENCH FOOT, SHELTER FOOT)

These conditions have long been familiar to mariners. Shannon, marooned in the Arctic for 7 days in 1832, lost 30 of his company of 49 men from trench foot, and Shackleton and his comrades were also affected by it on their passages from Elephant Island to South Georgia. Some of the British marines and paratroopers in the Falkland Islands campaign fell victims to trench foot,[185] and more recently it has been highlighted as a problem for the homeless.[186] It is often seen in survivors of shipwrecks in cold waters, and in those who sleep outside in cold and wet environments wearing tight, constricting footwear. Because the sea freezes at −1.9°C and the tissues freeze only at −2.5°C, exposure to unfrozen sea is not capable of freezing tissues, but the wet increases the conduction of cold and heat losses, preventing the supercooling that protects against frostbite.[187] In addition, injury

REFERENCES

175. Mills WJ. Out in the Cold. EM Books, New York, 1979
176. Mundth ED. In: Viereck (ed.). Proceedings of the Symposia on Arctic Medicine and Biology in Frostbite. Arctic Aero Medical Laboratory, Fort Wainwright, 1964
177. Isaacson NH, Harrel JB. Surgery 1953; 33: 810
178. Schumaker HB, Kilman JW. Arch Surg 1964; 89: 575
179. Taylor MS. Mil Med 1999; 164: 566–567
180. Hayes DW Jr, Mandracchia VJ, Considine C et al. Clin Podiatr Med Surg 2000; 17: 715–722
181. McCauley RC, Hing DN et al. J Trauma 1983; 23: 143
182. Skolnick AA. JAMA 1992; 267: 2008
183. Groechenig E. Lancet 1994; 34: 1152
184. Knize DM, Weatherley-White RCA et al. J Trauma 1969; 9: 749
185. Marsh AR. J R Soc Med 1983; 76: 972
186. Wrenn K. Arch Int Med 1991; 151: 785
187. White JC, Scoville WB. N Engl J Med 1945; 232: 415

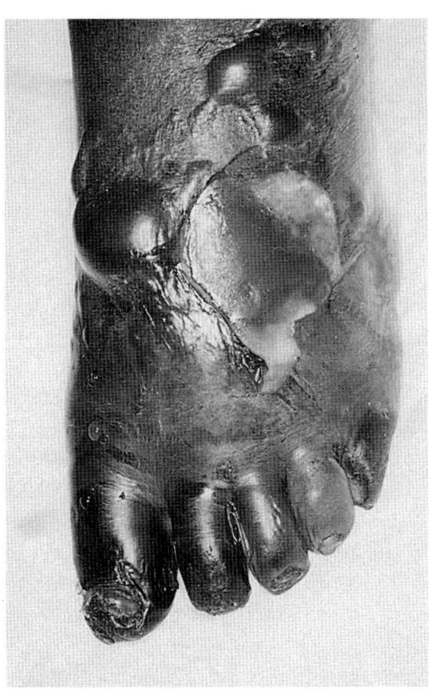

Figure 10.42 A trench foot.

by water absorption in the stratum corneum of the skin of the feet is thought to be important. The extremities become numb during the period of exposure, and victims feel as though they are walking on cotton wool. Pain is unusual but cramp may occur; after a few days the feet swell, producing a feeling of constriction in shod feet. The skin at this stage turns red, then pale, then yellow, blue, and eventually black (Fig. 10.42).

When the limbs are removed from this environment and released from their constraining footwear, they at first remain cold, swollen, discoloured, numb and powerless. The pedal pulses are usually impalpable and gangrene may develop. When this does not occur, the limb usually becomes hyperaemic and swollen, and this is accompanied by pain and paraesthesia. The small muscles of the affected feet and hands become weak and wasted. The skin blisters and may ulcerate. Even at this stage, which often lasts 6–10 weeks, gangrene may still develop. The normal temperature gradient is often lost, with the affected skin feeling warm or warmer than the skin of the groins and axillae. The extremities usually redden with dependence and blanch with elevation. Shooting pains are common, occurring at night and brought on by warmth, dependence, exercise or cold. Glove and stocking anaesthesia may develop in the affected skin, but often has a variable and irregular upper limit. Hair may fall out and nails may be shed, and patients often feel unwell with a low fever, weight loss and tachycardia. Eventually most limbs recover completely, but patients with severe initial damage may develop hyperaesthetic, smooth, shining, hairless skin; pigmentation; telangiectases; hypersensitivity to extremes of temperature; and wasted and pointed digits with stiff joints.[188]

Treatment

When first seen or rescued, the patient should have their boots and clothes cut away and should then be gently warmed while the extremities are protected from heat, although not over-cooled.[189] The patient should be placed in a draught from an open window or an electric fan, but the skin should be kept dry. The value of sympathectomy at an early stage is disputed.[28,190] Ice packs may provide symptomatic relief during the hyperaemic phase, and patients should be kept in bed until the swelling has disappeared and walking is painless. Smoking is prohibited, and sympathectomy may be valuable during recovery if vasospasm is a problem. Prostaglandin infusions may also be beneficial.[183] Local amputation may be required at this stage to remove necrotic digits. It is best to delay amputation as long as possible to avoid unnecessarily excising potentially recoverable tissue.

ATHEROSCLEROSIS

Atherosclerosis is a focal intimal accumulation consisting of lipids and fibrous tissue (collagen and elastin) associated with smooth muscle proliferation, found mainly in large and medium-sized arteries.[28] It develops as a plaque or series of plaques beneath the endothelium, called atheroma from the Greek word meaning gruel or porridge.

PATHOLOGY

The fatty streak is the earliest change: it has been seen in the large and medium-sized arteries of both children and adults.[28] It is simply a collection of lipid, usually forming as a longitudinal streak beneath the aortic endothelium. It is not known if this streak is capable of regressing or extending to form the more advanced gelatinous plaque. The latter is thought to develop into the fully mature fibrolipid plaque, which has a cholesterol lipid–rich base covered by a fibrous cap, surrounded by proliferating smooth muscle cells.

Lipids are first seen in the vessel wall within macrophages, which then coalesce before becoming surrounded by smooth muscle cells. These macrophages have been shown to originate from blood monocytes.[190] The accumulation of lipid in the arterial wall may disrupt the overlying endothelium, exposing the subendothelial tissues. This encourages platelet adherence, with the release of thromboxane, which further stimulates the accumulation of platelets, and the release of platelet-derived growth factor, which may be responsible for the smooth muscle proliferation.[191] The initial problem is thought to be endothelial dysfunction caused by biochemical and haemodynamic stresses. Oxidation of low-density lipoprotein cholesterol stimulates leukocyte adhesion and the production of the monocyte chemoattractant protein.[192]

The mature plaque accumulating in the arterial wall narrows the vessel lumen and prevents blood flow from increasing during periods of maximum demand. Plaques that erode through the endothelial lining present a roughened, ulcerated surface that is highly thrombogenic. Platelets adhere to these ulcers and accumulate, projecting into the lumen. Platelet accumulation produces a further reduction in blood flow and encourages thrombosis. Large clumps of platelets and even cholesterol break off and embolize distally to obstruct the peripheral circulation and produce small infarcts.

REFERENCES

188. Ungley CC, Blackwood W. Lancet 194; ii: 447
189. Learmonth JR, Wingley CC. Proc R Soc Med 1943; 36: 515
190. Gerrity RG. Am J Pathol 1981; 103: 191
191. Harker LA, Ross R, Glomset J. Ann NY Acad Sci 1976; 275: 321
192. Ross R. Nature 1993; 330: 1431

Mature plaques may fissure and rupture, allowing blood to track into the wall, resulting in rapid swelling of the plaque, which then occludes the vessel and leads to distal thrombosis.[193] Some plaques appear to weaken the vessel wall, allowing aneurysms to develop,[194] while dystrophic calcification can occur in atheroma at any site. Whether atheroma is really responsible for aneurysm development is still open to dispute, because proteolytic degeneration and remodelling appear to be more important (see p. 242–243).

The cause of atheroma is still not known, but a number of theories have been put forward in an effort to explain its development. In view of the lipid nature of the plaque, it was originally proposed that cholesterol, cholesterol esters and other triglycerides were absorbed through the endothelium, where they accumulated within the intima.[195] An active transport mechanism for lipid absorption has been postulated, because this process takes place across a concentration gradient.[196] Because cholesterol and triglycerides are almost insoluble in aqueous solutions, they are transported in the blood in water-soluble molecules called lipoproteins.

Epidemiological studies have shown that elevated lipoprotein concentrations in the blood, especially of the low-density lipoproteins, are associated with an increased risk of atherosclerotic disease.[197] Lipoproteins can be subdivided into five classes by their density characteristics on ultracentrifugation.[198] These five classes are chylomicrons, very low-density lipoproteins, low-density lipoproteins, intermediate-density lipoproteins, and high-density lipoproteins. The plasma cholesterol concentration correlates with the level of low-density lipoproteins in the blood,[199] and the plasma triglyceride level is reflected by the chylomicrons and very low-density lipoprotein concentration. High-density lipoproteins vary independently of cholesterol and triglycerides, and high levels of these compounds appear to be beneficial because they prevent low-density lipoproteins from entering the vessel wall.[200]

Experimental animals fed a diet high in cholesterol and animal fat develop similar lesions to human atheroma.[201] In these models, mucopolysaccharide accumulates within the intima before lipid deposition occurs, suggesting that the high levels of cholesterol and low-density lipoprotein may cause chemical damage to the endothelium and stimulate atheroma formation. Human endothelial cells grown in tissue culture have been shown to have a surface receptor that is capable of recognizing and binding low-density lipoproteins, which are then absorbed and transported to the lysozymes, where hydrolysis occurs.[202] The cholesterol ester core of low-density lipoprotein is hydrolysed to release free cholesterol and fatty acids into the cell cytoplasm.

The absorption of lipid does not explain the focal nature of atheromatous disease; Rokitansky[203] and Duguid[204] suggested that mural thrombi are encrusted by endothelium and incorporated into the vessel wall at many sites in the arterial tree. These intimal thrombi were then thought to be replaced with lipid to form atheromatous plaque. Evidence of widespread intravascular thrombosis has, however, never been confirmed. Traumatic intimal damage may lead to platelet adherence with release of mitogens into the vessel wall, which stimulate smooth muscle cell proliferation.[205] These smooth muscle cells may migrate into the intima and metaplase to form cells that are thought to encourage the deposition of lipid. Mechanical damage from shear stress, hypertension, arterial bending and muscle or tendon trauma, and chemical damage from hyperlipidaemia, adrenaline and nicotine, have all been implicated as causes of intimal damage.[206] There is little firm evidence that structural intimal damage occurs, but endothelial permeability may be increased, and this may allow fibrinogen and lipoproteins to enter the vessel wall.

The recognition that atheroma occurs near bifurcations and that blood flow is not uniform throughout the arterial tree has led to the investigation of mechanical factors as aetiological agents in atherogenesis. It was originally thought that high shear stresses—which are a function of the velocity of blood flow, the viscosity of blood, and the radius of the vessel wall—might disrupt the endothelium.[207] Experimental studies in animal models fed atherogenic diets, however, showed that plaques developed in segments of low shear stress, such as the iliac artery ostia, and similar sites are affected in humans.[208] It seems possible that low levels of shear stress reduce the transport of atherogenic-promoting substances away from the wall and encourage their accumulation in or on the vessel wall.[209] Low shear stress may also interfere with endothelial metabolism.

Atheroma depositing in the carotid bifurcation, a common site for the disease, may be influenced by the flow patterns of blood passing through the carotid sinus, which by its bulbous shape encourages flow separation.[210] This is responsible for a low shear velocity along the posterior wall, with a reversal of axial flow and the development of vortical patterns in the formed elements of the blood. This again allows particles to have a longer time in contact with the endothelium, increasing the chance of adhesion and absorption. The development of early plaques may also encourage turbulence, seen as random patterns in the passage of blood particles, which may stimulate or encourage further deposition on the wall.

Atheroma is found only in the pulmonary arteries of patients with pulmonary hypertension and in vessels above a coarctation, which have a raised blood pressure, implying that raised blood pressure may encourage atherogenesis. There is, however, no

REFERENCES

193. Davies MJ, Thomas AC. Br Heart J 1985; 53: 363
194. Greenhalgh RM, Laing S, Taylor GW. J Cardiovasc Surg 1981; 21: 559
195. Virchow R. Phlogose und Thrombose Im Gefass-system. Gesammelte Abhandlungen zur Wissenschaftlichen Medizin. Meidinger, Frankfurt, 1856
196. Dayton S, Hashimoto S. Circ Res 1966; 19: 1041
197. Miller GJ, Miller NE. Lancet 1975; i: 16
198. Lewis B. The Lipoproteins of Plasma in the Hyperlipidaemias: Clinical and Laboratory Practice. Blackwell, Oxford, 1976
199. Brown MS, Faust JR, Goldstein JL. J Clin Invest 1975; 55: 783
200. Carew TE, Koschinsky T et al. Lancet 1976; i: 1315
201. Anitschkow NN. In: Cowdry EV (ed). Experimental Atherosclerosis in Animals—a Summary of the Problem. Macmillan, New York, 1933
202. Brown MS, Ho YK, Goldstein JL. Ann NY Acad Sci 1976; 275: 224
203. Rokitansky C. Handbuch der Pathologischen Anatomie, Vol 2. Bradmuller & Seidel, Vienna, 1844
204. Duguid JB. J Pathol Bacteriol 1946; 58: 207
205. Ross R, Glomset JA. N Engl J Med 1976; 295: 369
206. Woolf N. Pathology of Atherosclerosis. Butterworths, London, 1982
207. Reidy MA, Bowyer DE. Atherosclerosis 1977; 26: 181
208. Zarins CK, Trylor KE, Lundell MI. Proceedings of Specialist Workshop in the Role of Fluid Mechanics in Atherosclerosis. 1978
209. Caro C, Fitzgerald JM, Schroter RC. Nature 1969; 223: 1159
210. Zarins CK, Giddens DP, Bharadvaj BK. Circ Res 1983; 53: 502

evidence of increased coronary artery disease in patients with mild or moderate hypertension.[211] Cigarette smoking, obesity, lack of physical exercise, anxiety and personality disorders, diabetes, renal failure and dietary fat intake have all been incriminated as risk factors in the development of atherogenesis, and there are others—including the hardness of the drinking water, diminished thyroid function, and various forms of hyperlipidaemia—that may also play a part. It is possible that reduced production of nitric oxide may also be implicated in the genesis of atheroma. The aetiology of this complex disease appears to be multifactorial.

CLINICAL FEATURES AND TREATMENT

Obliterative atherosclerosis produces symptoms as the result of a reduced blood supply to the tissues in the distribution of the arteries affected by the disease. It is a generalized disease, and simultaneous symptoms can occur in several different sites. Most of the presentations have already been discussed, but the symptoms, signs, investigation and treatment of stenosing atherosclerosis will now be summarized for each commonly affected vessel.

INTRACRANIAL ATHEROSCLEROSIS

Originally, atherosclerosis was thought to often affect the intracerebral vessels, where it was held to be the major cause of cerebral thrombosis and cerebral infarction. In the 1950s, however, it was recognized that atherosclerotic plaques were commonly present in the carotid bifurcations of patients dying of stroke,[212] and subsequent post-mortem surveys confirmed that the carotid bifurcation was the site of predilection for atheroma in the arteries of the head and neck.[28] The pendulum has, however, swung too far, and it seems to have been forgotten that atherosclerosis can and does involve the intracranial carotid arteries, the basilar artery, and all the cerebral arteries, including those that make up the circle of Willis. Patients with disease in the intracranial vessels can present with transient ischaemic attacks, strokes and progressive dementia. These symptoms have to be differentiated from those of extracranial atherosclerosis, which causes reduced cerebral perfusion and acts as a source of platelet emboli.

Other conditions that need to be considered in the differential diagnosis of stroke and transient ischaemic attacks include cerebral tumours, cerebral haemorrhage, hypertensive encephalopathy, migraine, demyelinating disease, cardiac arrhythmias, sickle cell disease, systemic lupus erythematosus, polycythaemia and Alzheimer's disease, which may all have similar neurological presentations. Referral to a neurologist and investigation with CT or magnetic resonance scanning may be necessary to exclude these disorders.[213] Patients with transient ischaemic attacks, or progressive dementia with a carotid or cerebral bruit, should have a duplex Doppler assessment of the extracranial vessels supplemented by intravenous digital subtraction angiography or magnetic resonance angiography.[214,215] Intra-arterial arteriography is necessary to confirm a diagnosis of intracerebral atherosclerosis with certainty, but it carries the risk of precipitating a stroke. There is no surgical procedure that is capable of curing diffuse intracerebral disease that has caused dementia, or localized disease that has resulted in cerebral infarction. Aspirin and dipyridamole may reduce platelet embolization[216] but do not improve cerebral perfusion. Extracranial–intracranial bypass has been shown to improve cerebral perfusion, although there is no evidence that it extends life.[217,218]

INTERNAL CAROTID ARTERY ATHEROSCLEROSIS

Atheroma in the carotid arteries is usually localized to the carotid bifurcation.[28,206] Unfortunately, the majority of patients still present for the first time with completed strokes. Many patients, however, have transient ischaemic attacks, which are usually hemispheric, affecting the contralateral limbs, or they develop amaurosis fugax in the ipsilateral eye.[219] These symptoms are usually the result of repeated microemboli derived from carotid plaque, consisting of either platelet aggregates or cholesterol intraplaque debris after ulceration of the plaque. True cerebral hypoperfusion is rare unless extensive stenoses or occlusions are present in the other cerebral vessels, or there is a poorly formed circle of Willis.[220]

The superficial temporal pulse is impalpable if the common carotid artery is occluded. A bruit is heard in 80% of patients with some degree of carotid stenosis, although bruits are often not heard in patients with severe stenoses. Bruits may also be picked up on routine examination of symptomless patients. A neurological examination may confirm evidence of an upper motor neurone lesion if cerebral infarction has occurred. Retinal examination may disclose evidence of cholesterol emboli or retinal infarction (Figs 10.11 and 10.12).

Migraine, epilepsy and Stokes–Adams attacks must be differentiated from transient ischaemic attacks, and another source of emboli must also be considered. The heart and the aortic arch are the two most common alternative sources of emboli, and transoesophageal echocardiography may be useful if a cardiac cause is suspected. Some patients have a patent foramen ovale, which may allow paradoxical emboli from the systemic venous circulation to enter the cerebral circulation. Space-occupying cerebral lesions, intracerebral arterial disease, and hypertensive encephalopathy may also present with similar symptoms. Takayasu's disease, fibromuscular hyperplasia, carotid aneurysms and carotid kinking are other rare causes of transient ischaemic attacks.

Most patients with transient ischaemic attacks, without evidence of a cardiac cause, should have the carotid bifurcation imaged by duplex ultrasound scanning; vessels proximal to the bifurcation may be assessed by intravenous digital subtraction angiography.[215] Intravenous or intra-arterial digital subtraction angiography (possibly with selective injection of the individual extracranial vessels) should be considered if duplex scanning is equivocal or if the duplex and intravenous angiogram produce conflicting results. Conventional intra-arterial arteriography has about a 2% risk of stroke,[221] and even digital subtraction techniques are not free from major complications. There has

REFERENCES

211. MRC Working Party. Br Med J 1988; 296: 1565
212. Fisher CM. Arch Neurol Psychiatry 1957; 72: 187
213. Oxfordshire Community Stroke Project. Br Med J 1983; 287: 713
214. Turnipseed WD, Sakett JF et al. Arch Surg 1981; 116: 470
215. Horrocks M. Br J Med 1986; 2: 53
216. Canadian Cooperative Study Group. N Engl J Med 1978; 299: 53
217. EC/IC Bypass Study Group. N Engl J Med 1985; 313: 1191
218. Bishop CCR, Burnand KG et al. Br J Surg 1987; 74: 802
219. Ross Russell RW. Lancet 1961; ii: 422
220. Fields MS, Bruetman ME, Weibel J. Collateral Circulation of the Brain. Williams & Wilkins, New York, 1965
221. Leow K, Murie JA. Br J Surg 1988; 75: 428

therefore been a trend in recent years to rely on ultrasonographic evidence alone if a satisfactory duplex scan is obtained by an experienced operator. The introduction of magnetic resonance angiography may avoid these complications and provide satisfactory images. Many still favour a combination of duplex scanning and intravenous digital subtraction angiography.

Patients with carotid territory transient ischaemic attacks or amaurosis fugax related to an internal carotid artery found to have a significant stenosis of 70% or more (by diameter) should be offered carotid endarterectomy.[222,223] Surgery should take place as soon after diagnosis as practically possible, because the benefits are reduced if there is a delay of more than 6 months from the onset of symptoms. Patients with lesser degrees of stenosis should be treated with antiplatelet agents and only operated on if their medication fails to arrest symptoms.

It has been suggested that certain features of the atheromatous plaque, other than the degree of stenosis, may render it particularly liable to cause embolism. Duplex scanning may indicate plaque friability and identify those at particular risk of stroke.[224] Patients with an occluded carotid artery can usually be treated conservatively. In the rare instance of continuing symptoms from proved hypoperfusion, extracranial–intracranial bypass may relieve symptoms.[218] Percutaneous transluminal balloon angioplasty of carotid stenosis has been carried out successfully in many centres, but its place in the overall management of carotid disease is not yet clear.[225] Carotid angioplasty with or without stenting should be carried out only within the confines of a clinical trial at present. Better results appear to be achieved by carotid stenting used in association with a cerebral protection device, and trials are under way to compare this treatment with carotid endarterectomy.

Carotid endarterectomy

The carotid artery is approached through an incision along the anterior border of the sternomastoid. The internal jugular vein is mobilized posteriorly after the common facial vein has been ligated and divided (Fig. 10.43a, b). The common, internal and external carotid arteries are then dissected free, taking care to preserve and protect the vagus and the hypoglossal nerves. The carotid sinus nerve is blocked with local anaesthetic to prevent excessive variations in blood pressure, which may occur during dissection. When the upper and lower limits of the diseased arterial segment have been defined, systemic heparin is given and the vessels are clamped. An arteriotomy in the common carotid artery is continued cephalad through the narrowed internal carotid ostium and as far as normal vessel. When an intraluminal shunt of the Javid or Pruitt type[226,227] is to be used, it is inserted at this stage to allow continuation of cerebral perfusion via the operated internal carotid vessel (Fig. 10.43b). The plane between the plaque and the residual arterial wall is developed and the full extent of the plaque is removed, taking care to avoid leaving residual disease or an intimal flap at the upper end of the endarterectomy. When a smooth intraluminal surface has been achieved, the arteriotomy is closed with a continuous monofilament suture. Before completion of the suture line, arterial clamps are reapplied and the shunt removed.

The use of a patch of vein or prosthetic material to prevent narrowing of the lumen during closure of the arteriotomy is widely advocated.[228] This technique is particularly attractive for vessels of narrow calibre, especially in women, when it may prevent late restenosis. When a vein patch is used, saphenous vein should be taken from the upper end near the saphenofemoral

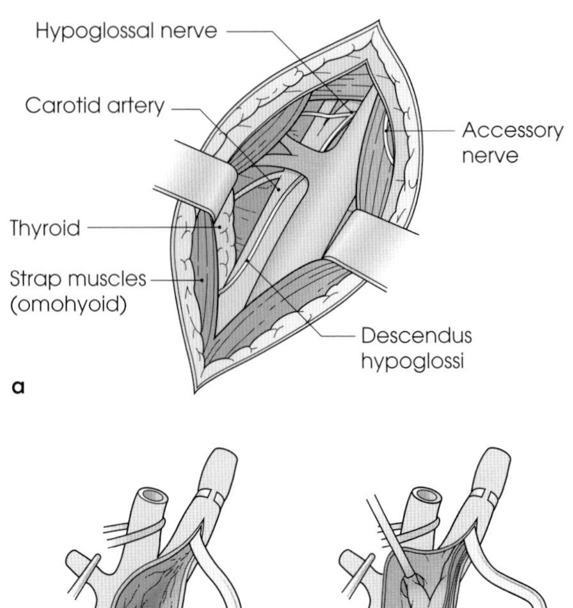

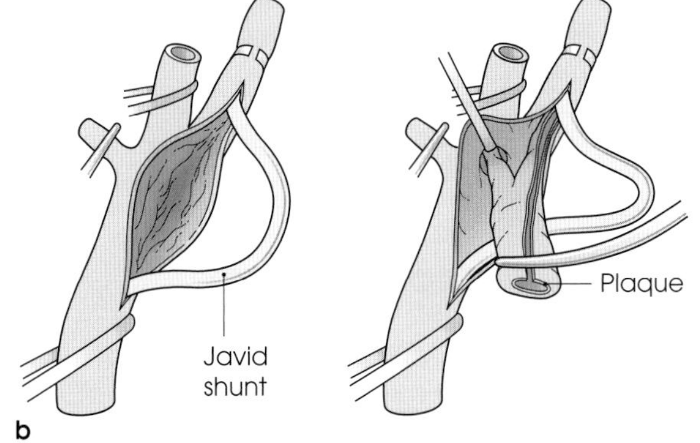

Figure 10.43 Carotid endarterectomy.

junction, because the lower part of the vein is prone to rupture.[229] Dacron patches are usually more practical but infection can be a hazard.

The number of surgeons who never use a shunt during this operation has dwindled. Most either shunt routinely or selectively, although the basis of selection for shunting varies. A shunt should be used if there is severe contralateral disease or a low pressure in the carotid after it has been clamped (a stump pressure of below 50 mmHg).[230] The operation can be carried out under local anaesthesia,[231] and a shunt inserted if the patient starts to develop ischaemic symptoms or signs.

The debate about local versus general anaethesia is being tested in the General Anaesthetic Versus Local Anaesthetic for Carotid Surgery (GALA) trial. A variety of intraoperative tools have been used to monitor the patient during surgery; none have

REFERENCES

222. European Carotid Surgery Trialists' Collaborative Group. Lancet 1991; 337: 1235
223. North American Symptomatic Carotid Endarterectomy Trial Collaborators. N Engl J Med 1991; 325: 445
224. European Carotid Plaque Study Group. Eur J Vasc Surg 1995; 10: 23
225. McGuinness C, Burnand KG. Br J Surg 1996; 83: 1171
226. Javid H, Julian OC et al. World J Surg 1979; 3: 167
227. Pruitt C. Contemp Surg 1983; 23: 1
228. Eikelboom BC, Ackerstaff RGA et al. J Vasc Surg 1988; 7: 240
229. John TG, Bradbury AW, Ruckley CV. Br J Surg 1993; 80: 852
230. Hays RJ, Levinson SA, Wylie EJ. Surgery 1972; 72: 953
231. Connolly JE, Kwaan JHM, Stemmer EA. Ann Surg 1977; 186: 334

gained universal acceptance. Electroencephalography can be used to monitor cerebral function during general anaesthesia.[232] The introduction of transcranial Doppler ultrasonography to monitor flow in the middle cerebral artery throughout may indicate the need to insert a shunt if the signal disappears. When the vessel is clamped, light-reflective cerebral oximetry may also be used to assess cerebral perfusion. In this technique, near infrared light is transmitted to the brain through the scalp, and spectroscopy is performed on the reflected wave. A marked reduction of cerebral oxygenation indicates the need for a shunt.[233] Although the initial research evidence supported its use, it has not gained wide acceptance as a valid intraoperative tool. Intraoperative angioscopy[234] allows the endarterectomy to be inspected, but these types of device have subsequently been withdrawn.

Patients with fibromuscular hyperplasia, recognized by the string of beads appearance on angiography (Fig. 10.44),[235] are best treated by angioplasty with or without stenting.[236] Kinked carotid arteries are best left untouched, unless patients are having severe recurrent transient ischaemic attacks for which no other cause is evident.[237] Operative correction is by division, resection and reanastomosis of the artery.

Results

Two major prospective randomized trials have confirmed the value of carotid endarterectomy in patients with symptoms.[222,223] Patients with carotid territory transient ischaemic attacks,

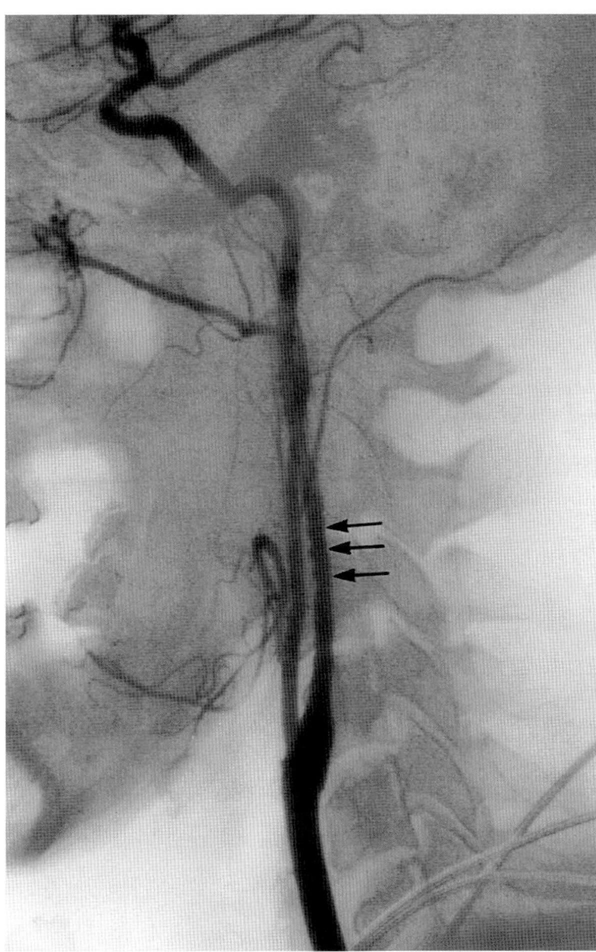

Figure 10.44 An arteriogram showing the appearances of fibromuscular hyperplasia of the carotid artery.

amaurosis fugax or a mild stroke, with a 70% or greater (diameter) stenosis, should be offered carotid endarterectomy. Those with a stenosis of less than 70% are less likely to benefit from surgery, although the trials of this subgroup are still continuing. Patients with ulcerated plaques who are continuing to have symptoms on antiplatelet agents should also be offered surgery, although there are no studies to support this. The degree of benefit for those in whom operation is indicated is substantial: a sixfold reduction in stroke at 3 years compared with best medical management.[222] It should not be forgotten, however, that good surgical results depend on good operative technique. Carotid endarterectomy has a mortality of 1–2% in experienced hands, with a stroke risk of 1–2%,[238,239] but these figures are doubled if less experienced surgeons operate.[240]

There is little justification for operating on patients who have progressing or completed strokes. The indications for operation in those with a symptomless carotid stenosis are not yet clear. Two multicentre randomized studies, the Asymptomatic Carotid Atherosclerosis Study (ACAS)[241] and its European counterpart, the Asymptomatic Carotid Surgery Trial (ACST),[242] have reported. They indicate that in certain well-defined circumstances, a tight stenotic lesion merits surgical correction. The symptomatic trials demonstrate that four carotid endarterectomies are required to prevent one stroke per year, while the symptomless studies suggest that nearly 20 operations are needed in symptomless patients to prevent one stroke every 5 years.

A number of patients develop recurrent stenosis of the endarterectomized vessel. In the early months this is usually the result of myointimal hyperplasia, and is often symptomless unless it is severe and bilateral. The role of aspirin and patching in preventing the complication has not yet been established.[243] After several years atheroma can recur and may give rise to new symptoms. Reoperations are difficult; however, 5-year freedom from stroke rates of 92% have been reported.[244] A higher rate of cranial nerve injury is reported, and carotid stenting has been advocated in this setting.[245] The restenotic lesion can be resected and replaced with vein or polytetrafluoroethylene.[246]

VERTEBROBASILAR ATHEROSCLEROSIS

Patients with vertebrobasilar insufficiency usually present with vertigo, faintness, giddiness or loss of consciousness, which is often brought on by changes in posture. Cerebellar symptoms

REFERENCES

232. Callow AD. Am J Surg 1980; 140: 181
233. Williams IM, Picton A et al. Br J Surg 1994; 81: 1291
234. Lennard N, Smith JL et al. Eur J Vasc Endovasc Surg 1999; 17: 234–240
235. Wylie EJ, Binkley FM, Palubinskas AJ. Am J Surg 1966; 112: 149
236. Morris GC, Carson WP et al. Surgery 1971; 69: 498
237. Riser MM, Geraud J, Ducoudray J. Rev Neurol 1951; 85: 145
238. Browse NL, Ross-Russell RW. Br J Surg 1984; 71: 53
239. Hertzer N. J Vasc Surg 1988; 7: 610
240. Cafferata HT, Gainey MD. J Cardiovasc Surg 1986; 27: 557
241. Executive Committee for the Asymptomatic Carotid Atherosclerosis Study JAMA 1995; 273: 1421
242. Warlow C. Lancet 1995; 345: 1254
243. Hertzer NR, Bevan EG et al. Ann Surg 1987; 206: 628
244. O'Hara PJ et al. J Vasc Surg 2001; 34: 5–12
245. AbuRahma AF, Bates MC et al. J Endovasc Ther 2002; 9: 566–572
246. Lattimer C, Burnand KG. Br J Surg 1997; 84: 1206

and occipital visual disturbances can also occur. There is a considerable overlap between the symptoms of carotid and basilar ischaemia, and differentiation may be difficult. There may be few signs, although a bruit may be audible over the course of the vertebral artery, and nystagmus may be present. Vertebrobasilar insufficiency must be differentiated from cervical spondylosis, migraine, and other conditions that cause brain stem compression or infiltration.

Many patients with mild symptoms can be treated by advice to avoid rapid changes in posture, and prescription of antihistamines to prevent vertigo and nausea. Operative endarterectomy of the lower end of the vertebral artery has been performed for disabling symptoms associated with a localized stenosis,[247] and more radical bypasses have been suggested for relief of symptoms. These procedures have not been tested in good controlled clinical trials, and their value has therefore not been established.

AORTIC ARCH, INNOMINATE AND COMMON CAROTID ATHEROSCLEROSIS

These vessels are much less commonly affected by atheroma than the carotid bifurcation or the vertebrobasilar arteries, and they are therefore a rarer source of ischaemic attacks and stroke. Takayasu's disease does, however, cause significant stenoses in these vessels. Surgical treatment is rarely indicated unless symptoms are the result of hypoperfusion or persist despite antiplatelet treatment. Often carotid–carotid bypass in the neck or another extra-anatomical bypass is possible, with a lower mortality than major thoracocervical procedures.[248, 248a]

Subclavian, axillary and brachial atherosclerosis and the subclavian steal syndrome

Atherosclerosis rarely produces symptoms in the vessels supplying the upper limbs. This is principally because the collateral pathways are so extensive that ischaemic symptoms do not develop, but atheroma also affects these vessels less frequently. Upper limb claudication and digital gangrene can occur, and if the occlusion or stenosis is in the proximal part of the subclavian artery patients may experience vertebrobasilar symptoms when they exercise the affected limb.[249] This is the result of a reversal of flow in the vertebral artery on the side of the stenosis, which acts as a collateral to supply blood to the ischaemic arm, stealing blood from the circle of Willis and cerebral vessels (Fig. 10.4a). Many doubt the existence of this syndrome, which is often associated with carotid stenoses. The finding of diminished pulses at the wrist or a reduced blood pressure in the affected arm supports the diagnosis if the patient gives a good history of arm claudication, or symptoms consistent with a subclavian steal. Other causes of subclavian obstruction include arteritis, embolism and cervical ribs. Some patients who have had coronary artery bypass using the left internal mammary artery complain of angina on using their left arm. They usually have a tight stenosis or occlusion of the origin of the left subclavian artery, so that the arm steals blood from the coronary circulation during exercise—the so-called 'coronary–subclavian steal syndrome'.[250]

Duplex ultrasound scanning showing reversed flow in the vertebral artery, which is enhanced by exercise, provides confirmation of the diagnosis.[251] Many symptomless patients may, however, have reversed flow in the vertebral artery, and intervention is not required in these patients.[252] Arteriography, by catheter or intravenous digital subtraction, should be used to confirm the diagnosis before reconstruction is contemplated.

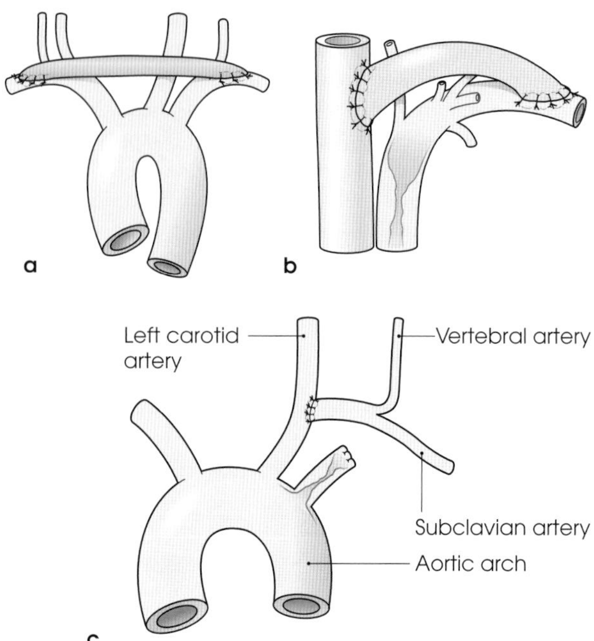

Figure 10.45 (**a**) Subclavian–subclavian bypass, (**b**) carotid–subclavian bypass, and (**c**) subclavian–carotid anastomosis.

Reconstruction of the subclavian artery can be by subclavian–subclavian bypass (Fig. 10.45a), by carotid–subclavian bypass, or by carotid–axillary bypass[253] using vein or prosthetic material (Fig. 10.45b). Many surgeons prefer division of the subclavian artery with end-to-side anastomosis of the vessel to the carotid artery (Fig. 10.45c). One study comparing transposition with bypass showed improved patency in patients treated by transposition.[254] Angioplasty with or without stent insertion is often selected as best first-line treatment for subclavian stenoses. There have not been any controlled trials comparing these treatments with surgical bypass. A long vein bypass must be taken from a healthy artery above an occlusion of the axillary or brachial artery to an unaffected segment beyond, tunnelling the bypass through the thoracic outlet. These bypasses are often difficult to perform and tend to occlude early, perhaps because of kinking during shoulder movement.

EXTERNAL CAROTID ATHEROSCLEROSIS

A stenosis of the origin of the external carotid artery is usually treated at the same time as bifurcation disease. External carotid

REFERENCES

247. Edwards WH, Mulherin JL. Surgery 1980; 87: 20
248. Thevenet A. Med Hyg 1980; 38: 4154
248a. Modarai B, Burnand KG. Br J Surg 2004; 91: 1453
249. Reivich MH, Helling HE et al. N Engl J Med 1961; 265: 878
250. Bryan FC, Allen RC, Lumsden AB. Ann Vasc Surg 1995; 9: 115–122
251. Berguer R, Higgins R, Nelson R. N Engl J Med 1980; 302: 1349
252. Thomassen L, Aarli JA. Acta Neurol Scand 1994; 90: 241–244
253. Jacobsen JH, Mozersky DJ et al. Arch Surg 1983; 166: 24
254. Kretschmer G, Teleky B, Marosi L. J Cardiovasc Surg 1991; 32: 334
255. Jackson BB. Am J Surg 1967; 113: 375

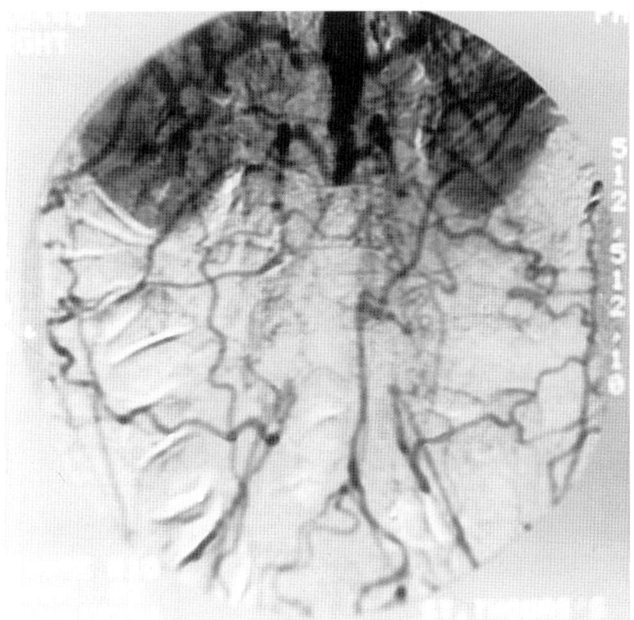

Figure 10.46 An intravenous digital subtraction arteriogram demonstrating an aortoiliac occlusion.

endarterectomy is justified only as an isolated procedure if the patient develops eye symptoms on the side of an internal carotid occlusion,[255] when there is an associated tight external carotid stenosis. External carotid endarterectomy can also be performed as a prelude to extracranial–intracranial bypass.

ATHEROSCLEROSIS OF THE THORACIC AORTA

Although atheroma is quite commonly found in this vessel, it rarely causes a stenosis or occlusion, and only produces symptoms if embolism or aneurysmal dilatation occurs. The former may occur during radiological manipulation of wires around the arch. The thoracic aorta is probably the main source of emboli during coronary artery bypass grafting, when the aorta is cross-clamped.

ATHEROSCLEROSIS OF THE ABDOMINAL AORTA, THE RENAL ARTERIES AND THE ILIAC VESSELS

The abdominal aorta and iliac bifurcations are common sites for atheroma to develop, and the trunks of the aorta and iliac vessels are often affected by more diffuse disease, which may extend into the renal arteries. In some patients the disease appears to be localized to the aortoiliac segment, while others have much more diffuse disease involving all the vessels of the lower limb.[28]

Rest pain or gangrene does not usually occur if the atheroma is confined to the aorta and iliac vessels, because the collateral circulation is normally adequate (Fig. 10.46); even if these vessels are totally occluded, patients complain only of intermittent claudication providing the other vessels in the limb are not occluded or stenosed. Patients with aortoiliac disease usually develop buttock and thigh claudication and may lose the ability to achieve penile erection, a syndrome that Leriche and Morel felt was the result of a hypoplastic aorta.[256] When severe distal disease is already present, rest pain and gangrene usually supervene when the aortoiliac segment occludes. Patients occasionally present with symptoms of distal emboli in their feet (Fig. 10.15).

It is important to differentiate aortic claudication from disease of the spinal cord (see Ch. 48).[257] Absent or weak femoral pulses are always present in patients with severe aortoiliac disease, and appropriately sited bruits may be heard over critical stenoses.

There is often only a marginal reduction in the resting Doppler pressure index, but this is invariably accentuated by exercise. The Doppler waveform of the femoral pulse may show characteristic features and help to determine the major site of disease.[258] Intravenous digital subtraction arteriography or intra-arterial contrast aortography confirms the diagnosis and displays the distal arterial tree (Fig. 10.46). Duplex ultrasound may now provide enough information, although bowel gas may make aortoiliac visualization difficult unless special measures are taken. A reasonable period should be allowed from the onset of symptoms for collaterals to develop as symptoms may improve; all patients with claudication should be encouraged to stop smoking. Intervention is clearly indicated in patients with rest pain or early gangrene, and may be requested by patients if the claudication pain is interfering with their work or hobbies. This is a reasonable request and should be acceded to, providing the patients are otherwise fit and well.

Reconstruction for atherosclerosis of the aortoiliac segment

Single stenoses of the iliac vessels can be treated very adequately with balloon angioplasty (percutaneous transluminal angioplasty) with good long-term results.[259] More extensive stenoses or occlusions may also be treated by balloon angioplasty, although extensive or recurrent lesions usually require endovascular stenting.[260] Angioplasty is much simpler than surgery, having a lower morbidity and mortality, and a much shorter hospital stay. The long-term patency following dilatation of the iliac vessels is in excess of 80%, making aortoiliac endarterectomy a rare operation, because the majority of the lesions previously treated by endarterectomy can now be satisfactorily treated by angioplasty, followed by placement of an intraluminal stent if there is residual narrowing or dissection. Long occlusions are best treated by primary stenting.[261] The number of angioplasties performed has increased enormously,[262] and surgery tends to be reserved for failed passage of the guide wire (Fig. 10.47). Intraluminal stents are made of strong flexible metal or nitrinol, and are inserted over the guide wire before being expanded across the stenosis or occlusion by balloon dilatation (Fig. 10.48). Short aortic occlusions and bilateral common iliac artery occlusions can also be treated by stenting, with good results. The place of localized aortoiliac endarterectomy using closed Volmar ring strippers or a Moll ring cutter is debatable and has not been evaluated in controlled clinical trials.

A bifurcated Dacron bypass graft is the best means of improving the blood supply to the lower limbs if the disease is more extensive. This is the operation of choice where the whole

REFERENCES

256. Leriche R, Morel A. Ann Surg 1948; 127: 193
257. Snyder EN, Mulfinger GL, Lambret RW. Am J Surg 1975; 130: 172
258. Woodcock JP, Gosling RG, Fitzgerald DE. Br J Surg 1972; 59: 226
259. van Andel GJ, van Erp WFM. Radiology 1985; 156: 321
260. Gunther RW, Vorwerk D. AJR Am J Roentgenol 1991; 156: 389
261. Palmaz JC, Garcia OJ et al. Radiology 1990; 174: 969
262. Pell JP, Whyman MR, Ruckley CV. Br J Surg 1994; 81: 832

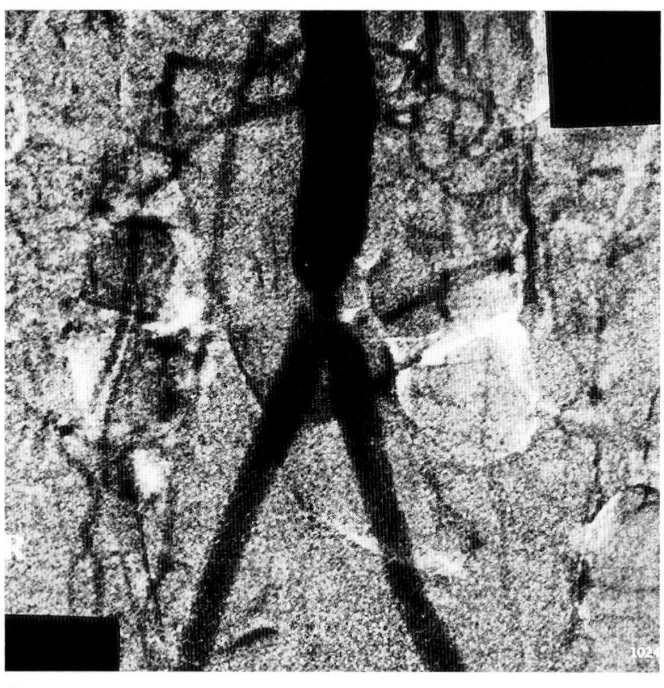

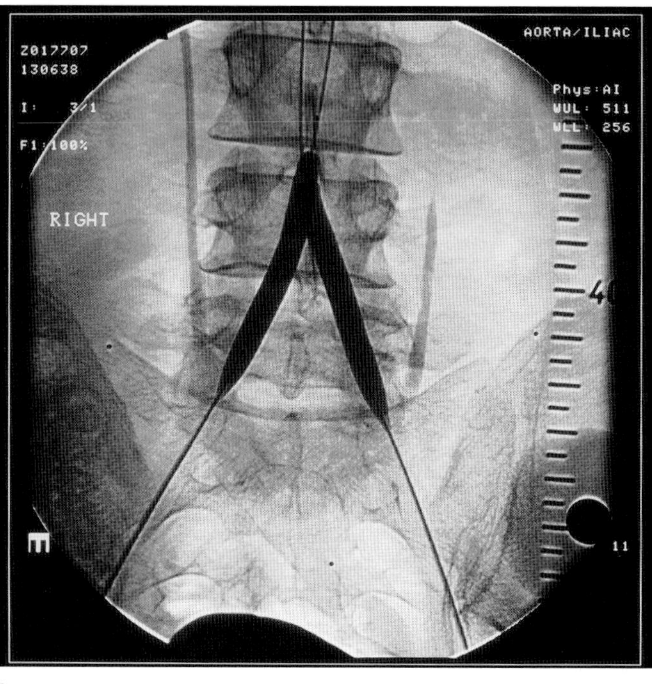

a b

Figure 10.47 (a) Distal aortic stenosis; (b) treatment by the kissing balloon technique.

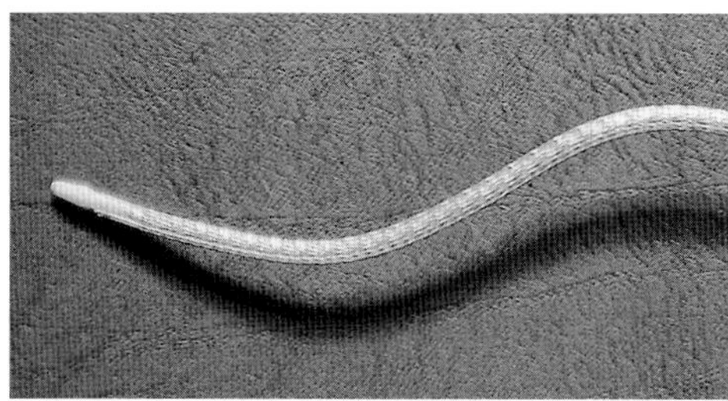

a

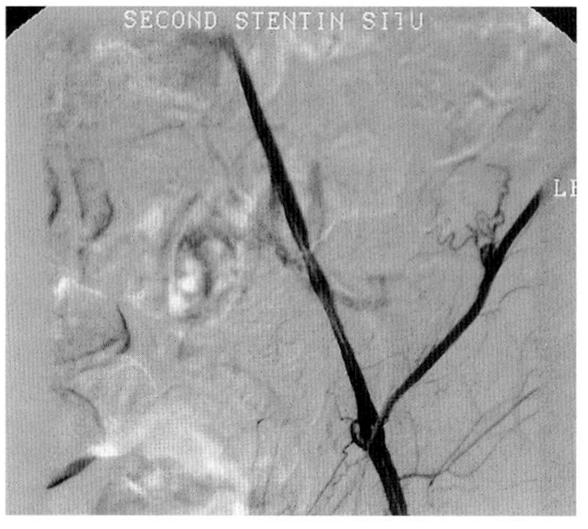

b

Figure 10.48 Stent grafts in iliac arteries: (a) an undistended wall stent and (b) arteriogram of an expanded wall stent.

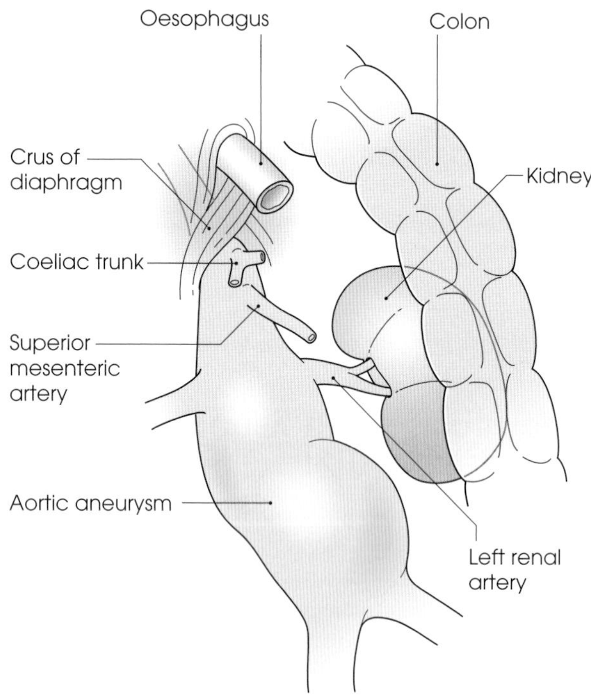

Figure 10.49 Retroperitoneal approach to aorta.

aorta and iliac system is occluded up to the renal arteries.[263] The trunk of the prosthesis can be sewn end-to-end to the divided aorta, suturing off the distal aortic lumen, or end-to-side on to the anterior surface of the aorta. Debate continues as to which of these two options is preferable.[264] Whatever technique is used, the graft should be sutured to the most normal piece of aorta, which is usually at or just below the renal arteries.

Surgeons differ in their approach to the abdominal aorta (Fig. 10.49), some using long transverse abdominal incisions, others choosing long midline incisions, while oblique incisions with an extraperitoneal approach extending behind or through the pleural cavity may be used, especially if the suprarenal aorta is to be exposed. More recently, there have been several reports

REFERENCES

263. Szilagyi DE, Smith RF, Whitney DG. Arch Surg 1964; 89: 827
264. Brewster DC, Darling RC. Surgery 1978; 84: 739

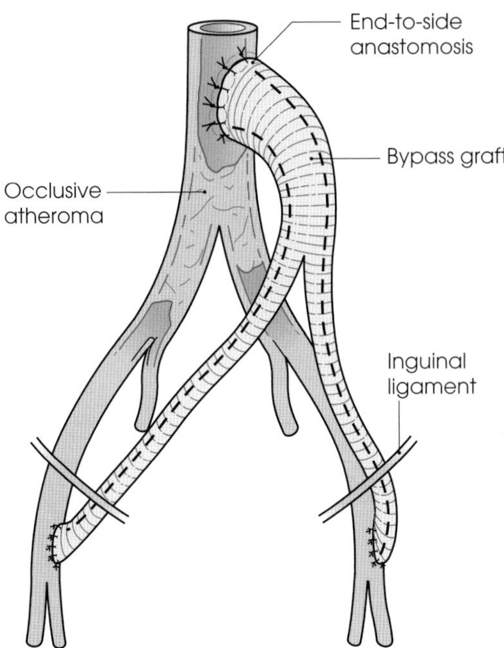

Figure 10.50 An aortofemoral bypass in place.

of total or hand-assisted laparoscopic aortofemoral grafting. This technique is in its early stage of development and requires very specific advanced laparoscopic skills. When an open transperitoneal approach is used, the small intestine can be packed away inside the abdomen or exteriorized in a plastic bag. The aorta is reached by mobilizing the fourth part of the duodenum to the right and dividing the posterior peritoneum vertically over the front of the aorta. The periaortic fat and lymph glands must also be divided to expose the anterior surface of the aorta. The whole procedure is facilitated by a large self-retaining retractor such as the Buckwalter or the Omnitract, both of which fix to the operating table.

A short segment of undiseased subrenal aorta is mobilized and 5000 units of heparin is administered. The aorta is clamped proximally and distally. Depending on the type of the proximal anastomosis (end to end or end to side), the aorta is either transected or a longitudinal arteriotomy made in the anterior wall. In the latter, there may be back-bleeding from lumbar vessels, which must be controlled. A bifurcated Dacron or polytetrafluoroethylene graft is cut to length with a short body. It is anastomosed using a monofilament suture and the clamps released. The distal limbs of a bifurcated graft can be passed down in a retroperitoneal tunnel behind the inguinal ligament. It is best to identify the inferior epigastric vein, which passes over the anterior aspect of the terminal portion of the external iliac artery. Damage to this vein can result in torrential bleeding, which can be difficult to control. The distal anastomosis is performed end to side to the common, superficial or profunda femoris vessels (Fig. 10.50). The common femoral and profunda femoris arteries may require a localized endarterectomy. This anastomosis should extend into an undiseased portion of the profunda artery if the superficial femoral artery is occluded, and some surgeons routinely bypass to the profunda.[265]

When the aortic occlusion extends up to the renal artery orifices, the segment of aorta immediately beneath these vessels is dissected free. A vertical incision is made in the prepared segment of vessel before clamps are applied, and the surgeon's thumb is pressed back on the pulsating portion of the vessel at the level of the renal arteries, and gently but firmly squeezed down to extrude the thrombus from the arteriotomy by compressing it like toothpaste between the thumb and the vertebral column. The atherothrombotic plug is expelled from the vessel and is followed by a rapid gush of blood. Bleeding is controlled by finger pressure, while a clamp is applied across the aorta between the arteriotomy and the renal arteries.[266] The graft limbs are usually tunnelled retroperitoneally and anastomosed end to side to the common or profunda femoris arteries, which are exposed through oblique or vertical groin incisions.

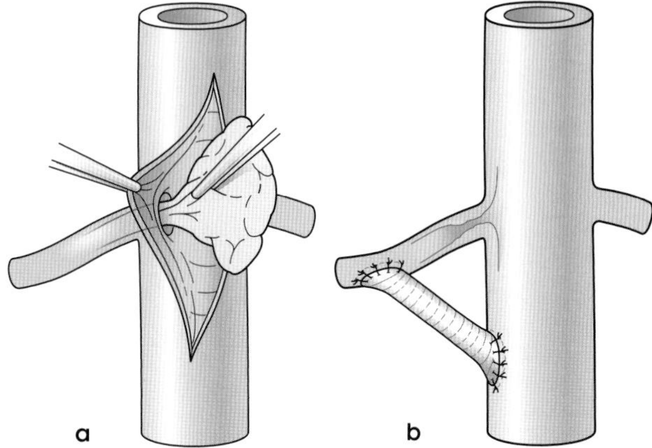

Figure 10.51 Techniques for revascularizing the renal arteries.

The suprarenal aorta and the renal arteries may be dissected out if there is extensive atheroma extending into and narrowing the renal vessels. An extensive endarterectomy of this whole segment can then be carried out through an appropriately sited arteriotomy.[267] It is rarely necessary to begin the bypass above the renal vessels. Side grafts of vein or prosthetic material can be taken off the main stem to revascularize the renal arteries if necessary (Fig. 10.51). On most occasions, it is better to ignore mild or moderate concomitant stenotic disease of the renal vessels and simply treat hypertension with drugs, because there is little evidence that renal revascularization cures hypertension, although it may prevent renal failure.

Disease in a single external iliac artery can be treated by endarterectomy by iliofemoral or aortofemoral bypass, or by femorofemoral cross-over grafts (Fig. 10.52), providing the vessels of the opposite limb are undiseased. There are advantages and disadvantages to each of these procedures, but they have largely been eclipsed by the development of angioplasty and stenting (see earlier text). External iliac endarterectomy may be performed with Volmar strippers from below, taking great care to avoid leaving loose distal plaque. Patches of vein or Dacron must be used to close the arteriotomies if there is any risk of narrowing. The vertical incision made over the femoral artery can be extended up over the abdomen as an alternative means of exposing the iliac vessels. This gives excellent access to the whole of the external iliac artery, but the inguinal ligament has to be divided and resutured. This increases the risk of a subsequent prevascular hernia. An oblique muscle-cutting extraperitoneal approach can be used to bypass this segment with an externally

REFERENCES

265. Malone JM, Goldstone J, Moore WS. Ann Surg 1978; 188: 817
266. Starrett RW, Stoney RJ. Surgery 1974; 76: 890

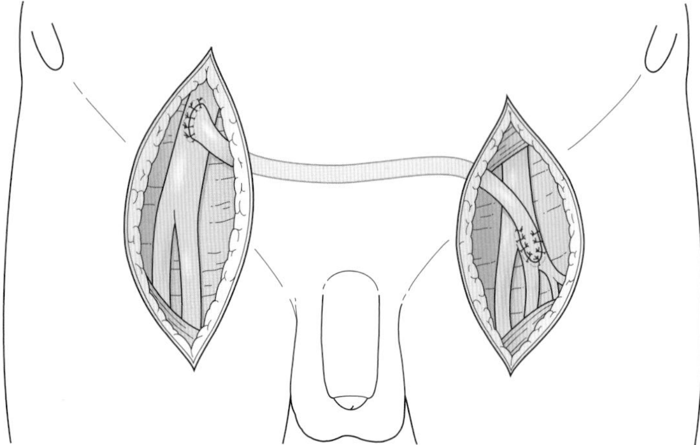

Figure 10.52 Technique for dealing with a single iliac artery occlusion: femorofemoral bypass.

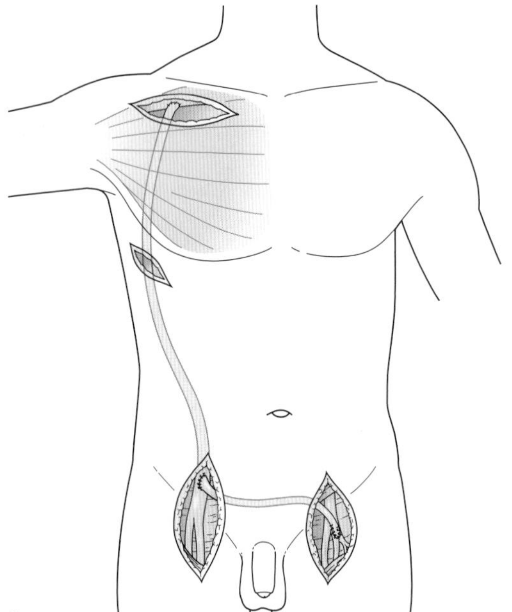

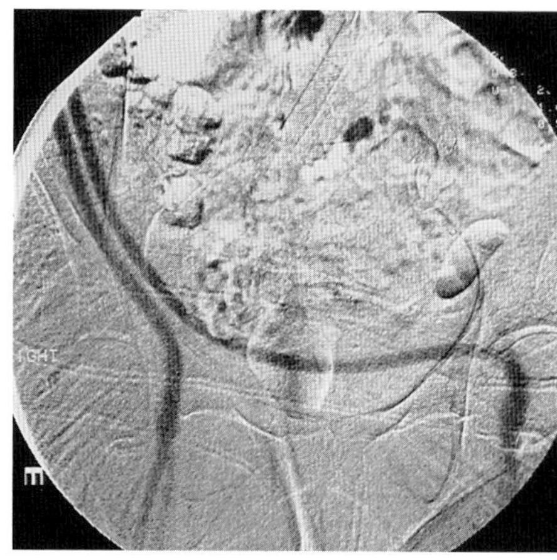

Figure 10.53 (a) The technique for performing an axillobifemoral graft. (b) an arteriogram showing a successful axillobifemoral bypass.

supported Dacron or polytetrafluoroethylene anastomosed end-to-side above and below the diseased segment, the prosthesis being blindly tunnelled retroperitoneally beneath the inguinal ligament.

In a cross-over femorofemoral graft, the external iliac or femoral vessels of the normal side are exposed and a tunnel is made in the subcutaneous fat above the pubis, although some make the tunnel behind the rectus abdominis muscles.[268] A tube of externally supported Dacron, polytetrafluoroethylene, or (if infection is considered a risk) a reversed saphenous vein is sutured end to side to the donor vessels and to the common femoral or profunda femoris artery of the opposite side, below the level of the obstruction. In old or unfit patients, an axillobifemoral graft may be used to bypass an occluded aorta.[269] A bifurcated Dacron or polytetrafluoroethylene graft is tunnelled subcutaneously and anastomosed end to side to the axillary and femoral arteries (Fig. 10.53).

The graft may be strengthened by an external support[270] to prevent occlusion during flexure. The axillary artery is approached by splitting the pectoralis major muscle below the clavicle and dividing pectoralis minor. The graft is anastomosed to the inferior surface of the axillary artery; this is simply achieved by clamping the artery and rotating the vessel forwards by 60–90°. One randomized clinical trial has confirmed significant improvement in graft patency with a flow splitter Y configuration compared with the conventional 90° arm.[271] The graft is tunnelled subcutaneously and anastomosed end to side to the femoral vessels exposed through two groin incisions.

Results of reconstruction of the aortoiliac segment

Aortoiliac and aortofemoral Dacron grafts have a 90–95% 5-year patency, providing there is a good distal arterial tree.[264,272] The patency of endarterectomy is probably not quite as good.[264,273]

REFERENCES

267. Stoney PJ. In: Rutherford RB (ed). Vascular Surgery. WB Saunders, Philadelphia, 1968
268. Tyson RR, Reichel FA. Surgery 1972; 72: 401
269. Mannick JA, Nabseth DC. N Engl J Med 1968; 278: 461
270. Kenny DA, Sauvage LR et al. Surgery 1982; 931: 946
271. Wittens CH, van Houtte HJ, van Urk H. Eur J Vasc Surg 1992; 6: 115–123
272. Taylor GW, Calo AR. Br Med J 1962; 1: 507
273. Cockett FB, Maurice BA. Br Med J 1963; 40: 153

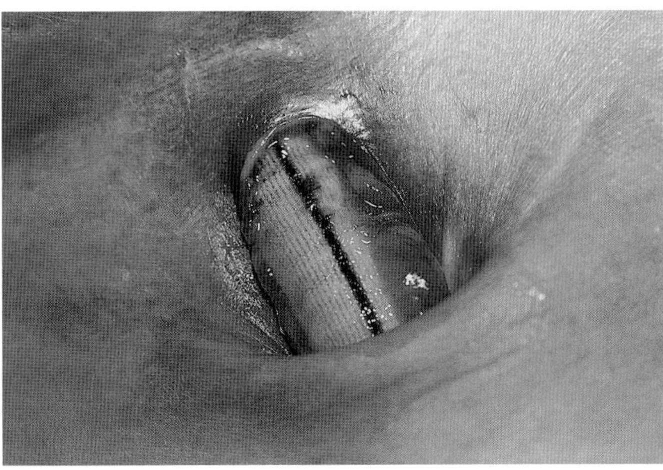

Figure 10.54 An infected limb of dacron bypass graft in the groin.

Cross-over bypass grafts have a 5-year patency of between 70 and 80%,[274,275] and axillofemoral grafts have a lower patency of about 60–70%.[276] Angioplasty of single iliac stenoses has a 7-year patency of 90%,[259] and the results of stenting may improve the results of dilating longer stenoses and occlusions.

Complications

Aortic operations have an operative mortality of between 2 and 5%.[264,277] Patients die from chest infection, myocardial infarction and pulmonary embolism. Careful preoperative cardiac assessment, combined with fastidious intraoperative monitoring to reduce cardiac work to a minimum, may further reduce mortality. Graft infection (Fig. 10.54) and aortograft–enteric fistulae are the major postoperative disasters, which usually necessitate graft removal and an extra-anatomical reconstruction using axillo-bifemoral grafts[278] or tunnelling a bypass through the obturator foramen. More recently, composite vein grafts using the common femoral veins of both lower limbs have been used to replace the aorta.[279] Graft infection and graft–enteric fistulae have a high mortality, of around 50%.[280] Other late problems include false aneurysm formation[281] and graft thrombosis; these require reanastomosis, extra-anatomical bypass, graft thrombectomy, and procedures to improve the outflow of the graft.

ATHEROSCLEROSIS OF THE FEMOROPOPLITEAL, PROFUNDA FEMORIS AND CRURAL ARTERIES

The most common site of atheromatous plaque is in the superficial femoral artery as it passes through the adductor canal. Patients complain of intermittent claudication if this vessel is severely stenosed or occluded, providing that the aortoiliac and crural vessels are not also diseased. Rest pain and gangrene are liable to ensue when there are additional occlusions in other arteries. Diffuse atheroma can involve the whole of the superficial femoral artery, and occlusions up to the origin of the profunda femoris are common.

The profunda femoris artery is often relatively disease-free, although posterior plaque in the common femoral artery extending into the profunda origin may narrow or occlude its proximal portion. There are, however, many exceptions to this adage, and on occasion disease may spread for a considerable distance down the profunda femoris artery and even involve its muscular branches. Combined occlusions in the profunda and superficial femoral arteries are more likely to cause rest pain and gangrene.

The infragenicular segment of the popliteal artery is another site that is often spared from significant disease, but there are also many exceptions to this observation, and the entire popliteal artery and trifurcation, including the origins of the crural vessels, are often occluded. This situation is invariably associated with severe claudication, rest pain or gangrene.

It is now recognized that atherosclerosis can cause stenoses and occlusions of all the crural vessels, and even involve the dorsalis pedis artery and the plantar vessels of the foot.[282] A widely patent plantar arch may affect the outcome of bypasses to the crural vessels, although this observation is still disputed.[283]

Atheromatous disease in the vessels of the lower limb may lead to embolism and thrombosis, which may in turn cause occlusions of the digital vessels. Peripheral arterial revascularization should rarely be attempted if there is extensive gangrene spreading on to the forefoot (Fig. 10.10), especially if the heel cannot be preserved by a conservative amputation. Reconstruction is also rarely justified to allow a major amputation to be performed at a lower level (e.g. below rather than above the knee), although there are occasional exceptions to this rule. The absolute indication for peripheral reconstruction (below the groin) of the arteries of the lower limb is rest pain or early gangrene (critical ischaemia), providing that there is a suitable conduit and vessel in the distal part of the limb that is capable of accepting a bypass.

Investigation

Attempts were originally made to define critical limb ischaemia according to the ankle systolic pressure. Further evidence showed that arbitrary blood pressure measurements are of little clinical relevance,[284] and no definition of chronic limb ischaemia can predict which patients with diabetes will require amputation.[285]

The suitability of a vessel in the distal part of the limb to accept a bypass is usually determined by arteriography, but Doppler mapping, Doppler scanning and intraoperative arteriography have also been used to assess the run-off. The technique of pulse-generated Doppler run-off was first described in 1986,[286] and is probably better at detecting vessels communicating with the pedal arch than arteriography, although dependent Doppler has been found to be equally effective.[287] Digital subtraction angiography with multiple exposures provides detailed views of all the vessels below the knee. It is important to assess the amount of disease in the aortoiliac segment because the inflow influences the patency of a distal bypass. Intra-arterial pressure measurements at rest and after administration of papaverine provide

REFERENCES

274. Helsby R, Moosa AR. Br J Surg 1975; 62: 596
275. Dick LS, Brief DR et al. Arch Surg 1980; 115: 1359
276. Burrell MJ, Wheeler JR et al. Ann Surg 1982; 195: 6796
277. Jamieson CW. Surgical Management of Vascular Disease. Heinemann, London, 1982
278. Trout HH, Kozloff L, Giordano JM. Ann Surg 1984; 199: 669
279. Van-Det RJ, Brands LC. Surgery 1981; 89: 543
280. Perdue GD, Smith RB et al. Surgery 1980; 192: 237
281. Benhamou DE, Kieffer E et al. J Cardiovasc Surg 1984; 25: 118
282. Aston N, Lea Thomas M, Burnand KG. Eur J Surg 1992; 6: 73
283. Ascer E, Veith FJ et al. J Vasc Surg 1984; 1: 817
284. Thompson MM, Sayer RD. Eur J Vasc Surg 1993; 7: 420
285. Tyrell MR, Wolfe JHN. Br J Surg 1993; 80: 177
286. Beard JD, Lee RE et al. J Vasc Surg 1986; 4: 588
287. Currie IC, Baird RN, Lamont PM. Br J Surg 1994; 81: 1448

functional information about the inflow but are rarely used clinically. Duplex scanning, assessing the peak systolic velocity above and below a stenosis, may be a better method of assessing haemodynamically significant stenoses than simply feeling the femoral pulse.[288]

Management

Conservative measures

Arterial reconstruction is not essential in patients presenting with claudication, and a period of conservative management is almost always indicated before surgery is considered. Patients should always be advised to stop smoking and to try to walk through the pain to encourage the development of collateral vessels.[289] Any polycythaemia or anaemia should be corrected, and coincidental diabetes should be treated. β-Blockers should be discontinued because these may cause a diminution of the claudication distance, although the value of this is debated.[290] The serum cholesterol and triglycerides should be lowered by a statin or a fibrate. Any cardiac irregularities should be treated or controlled if possible.

Vasodilating drugs are of little value, and any improvement achieved in the claudication distance is almost always marginal. On theoretical grounds, it is unlikely that these drugs can improve much on nature, because ischaemic tissue is the most powerful vasodilatory stimulus that is known. Therapeutic haemodilution has proved equally ineffective, and many other drugs, including haemorheological agents, antiplatelet drugs, fibrinolytic stimulants and anticoagulants, have also been tried without success.[291] Cilostazol, which is a type III phosphodiesterase inhibitor, has been shown in eight prospective, randomized, double-blind, placebo-controlled trials to improve walking distance and quality of life measures in patients with claudication.[292] Supervised exercise training programmes have also been shown to be as effective as angioplasty in improving the claudication distance.[293] Further controlled trials to evaluate exercise training against angioplasty are underway.

Indications for revascularization and selection of the procedure

Angioplasty and operations for claudication may be considered when symptoms are seriously interfering with the patient's occupation or enjoyment of life, providing that the symptoms have been present for 6 months or more, so that there has been time for collaterals to develop and maximum spontaneous improvement to occur. Patients should also have given up smoking and be reasonably fit. These rules may perhaps be relaxed a little where clinical features such as weak distal pulses with midthigh arterial bruits and reduced postexercise Doppler ankle systolic pressures suggest that a stenosis might be suitable for angioplasty.[294] The long-term outcome remains poor if patients continue to smoke. Colour duplex scanning may also be very helpful in selecting suitable patients for angioplasty,[295] but arteriography is still usually required to get a detailed picture of the distal arterial tree.

Patients with rest pain or digital ischaemia rarely have isolated superficial femoral occlusions. They usually have associated aortoiliac disease, a diseased profunda femoris artery, crural vessel obstruction, or distal occlusions within the pedal vessels. Lumbar sympathectomy may help patients with mild rest pain, although it is probably most effective in treating symptoms of coldness, numbness and tingling. Sympathectomy may aid the healing of superficial ulcers as it increases skin blood flow, but it is ineffective once there is frank gangrene. It is doubtful if sympathectomy ever saves a threatened limb from amputation. Phenol ablation of the sympathetic chain by percutaneous injection is now the preferred technique.

An associated stenosis of the aortoiliac segment may require angioplasty, stenting, endarterectomy, or bypass in combination with a femoropopliteal bypass.[296] The saphenous vein should be assessed preoperatively with either saphenous phlebography[297] or colour duplex scanning,[298] which has the advantage that the site of branches can be marked on the skin. Prosthetic material may be used to bypass occlusions in the limb vessels in patients with arterial ischaemia if the saphenous vein is unsuitable or has been previously removed. Prosthetic grafts are more prone to occlude than vein.[299] Improved results have been reported when a cuff of vein is interposed between the distal end of the graft and the recipient arteries at or below the level of the infrapopliteal artery.[300–302] The short saphenous vein, the cephalic and basilic veins,[303,304] and even the femoral vein have been used as an alternative to prosthetics.[305] Long endarterectomies of the superficial femoral artery are also possible.[273]

Amputation is the final option for both acute and chronic ischaemia of the lower extremities if revascularization procedures are impossible or ineffective. There is some evidence that the number of patients coming to amputation is decreasing as attempts at revascularization increase.[306]

Femoropopliteal vein bypass grafting

The popliteal artery is explored first if the distal run-off is questionable, otherwise the long saphenous vein is dissected out, either through a long incision placed over the vein or through a series of short incisions. The vein is either reversed or anastomosed in situ. The tributaries of the long saphenous vein are ligated and divided for an appropriate distance to allow the vein to be used as a reversed bypass graft. Alternatively, it can be

REFERENCES

288. Legemate DA, Teeuwen C, Eikelboom BC. Br J Surg 1991; 78: 1003
289. Larsen DA, Lassen NA. Lancet 1966; ii: 1093
290. Radack K, Deck C. Arch Intern Med 1991; 151: 1769
291. Ruckley CV. Br Med J 1986; 292: 970
292. Thompson PD, Zimet R, Forbes WP et al. Am J Cardiol 2002; 90: 1314–1319
293. Creasy TS, McMillan PJ, Fletcher EWL. Eur J Vasc Surg 1990; 4: 135
294. Nicholson ML, Byrne RL, Callum KG. Eur J Vasc Surg 1993; 7: 59
295. London NJM, Nydahl S. In: Greenhalgh RM (ed). Vascular Imaging for Surgeons. WB Saunders, London, 1995: 321
296. Wake P, Mansfield AO. Br J Hosp Med 1980; 120: 129
297. Senapati A, Burnand KG et al. Ann R Coll Surg Engl 1985; 72: 183
298. Davies AH, Magee TR. Eur J Vasc Surg 1991; 5: 633
299. Szilagyi DE. J Cardiovasc Surg 1982; 23: 183
300. Miller JH, Foreman RK. Aust NZ J Surg 1984; 54: 283
301. Taylor RS, McFarland RJ, Cox MI. Eur J Vasc Surg 1987; 1: 335
302. Tyrell MR, Wolfe JHN. Br J Surg 1991; 78: 1016
303. Campbell DR, Hoar CS, Gibbons GW. Ann Surg 1979; 190: 740
304. Harris RW, Andros G et al. Ann Surg 1984; 200: 785
305. Schulman ML, Badhey MR. Arch Surg 1981; 116: 1141
306. (Anonymous). Department of Health and Social Security and Office of Population Censuses and Surveys Hospital Inpatient Enquiry (1974–1984). HMSO, London

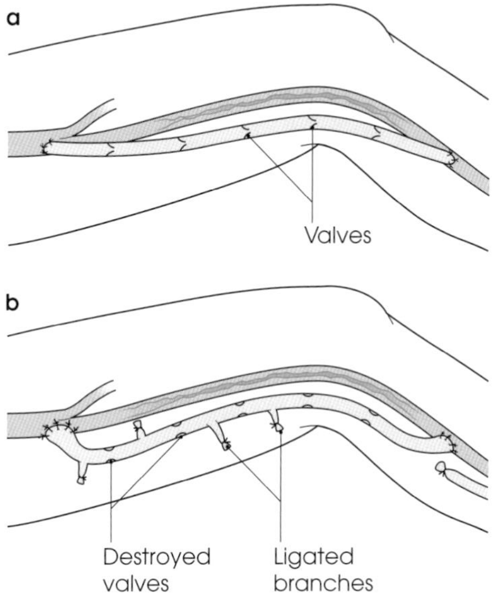

Figure 10.55 The techniques of femoropopliteal vein bypass grafting: (a) reversed and (b) in situ.

left in situ if this is the preferred operation, when the tributaries are ligated or clipped in continuity. The common femoral, profunda femoris and superficial femoral artery are dissected free and isolated through the upper end of the incision used to mobilize the vein. The upper end of the reversed vein is normally anastomosed to the common femoral artery, and the lower end is anastomosed to the popliteal artery, either above or below the knee depending on the condition of the vessel (Fig. 10.55). The vein can be placed subcutaneously or tunnelled through the adductor muscles to the popliteal fossa.

The popliteal artery is either dissected out above the knee, if this segment of artery is patent and relatively free of disease, or alternatively the infrageniculate portion of the vessel, which is often less severely diseased, is dissected free from its accompanying veins. The suprageniculate popliteal artery is approached by mobilizing the sartorius along either its anterior or posterior border. The infrageniculate popliteal artery is found by incising the deep fascia longitudinally just behind the posteromedial border of the tibia, taking care to avoid the saphenous nerve. The space between the medial head of the gastrocnemius and the tibia is then opened and retracted using an asymmetric Browse retractor. A new passage is made using a special tunnelling instrument if the reversed vein is to be used. Several techniques have been described:

- passing from the popliteal fossa, through the adductor magnus and the subsartorial canal, up into the femoral triangle; and
- by simultaneously creating a tunnel behind the medial head of gastrocnemius into the above-knee popliteal space.

The graft can then be tunnelled subfascially to the common femoral artery. The carefully prepared vein is then positioned in this channel, and end-to-side anastomoses are made to the common femoral artery in the groin and the chosen segment of the popliteal artery behind the knee.

In situ grafting, which is the method of choice in crural and pedal anastomoses, leaves the long saphenous vein in its anatomical position.[307] After the major tributaries have been ligated, the upper end is freed, mobilized and detached from the femoral vein, which is over-sewn using a monofilament suture. The cusps of the most proximal saphenous valve are excised under direct vision. The vein is then anastomosed end to side to

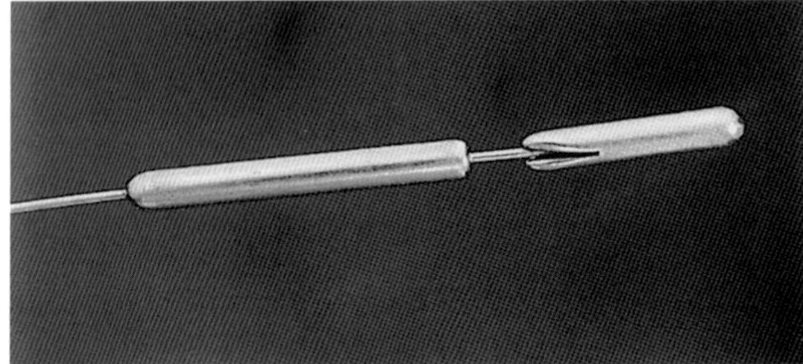

Figure 10.56 Hall's valvulotome used for excising the saphenous valves during in situ vein bypass grafting.

the femoral artery. It is important to position the proximal vein over the femoral artery prior to any arteriotomy. In the case of severe common femoral artery disease, a localized endarterectomy should be undertaken and closed with a patch before the graft is anastomosed to the patch. After the arterial clamps have been released, blood is allowed to distend the upper end of the vein as far as the first competent valve.

A valvulotome is then passed up the vein through its divided lower end to the upper anastomosis, and this is then gently withdrawn, engaging the valves one by one before being gently pulled through them. This avulses the cusps and renders each valve incompetent. A number of different valvulotomes have been devised for this operation; the Hall's strippers (Fig. 10.56), Cartier's, and Leather and Karmody's instruments are still popular.[307,308] The one-size disposable Le Maitre valvulotome is simple to use and expands to the size of the vein as it is withdrawn. A good flow of arterial blood should be obtained from the cut end of the divided vein when the valvulotome is delivered from the distal venotomy. The valvulotome should be inserted and pulled down a second time if the flow remains poor. Small-diameter valvulotomes may be followed by progressively larger instruments, although care must be taken not to damage the intima by inserting oversized valvulotomes. Persistently poor blood flow from the divided distal vessel suggests the presence of a large unligated tributary, and further examination of the vein by on-table angiography or angioscopy may confirm its presence. Alternatively, the valves can be disrupted under direct vision using the angioscope if this is available. When a good flow has been achieved, the distal anastomosis is performed.

Alternatives

A prosthetic graft can be used if the vein is known to have been stripped out in the past, is judged to be inadequate on preoperative saphenography or duplex scanning, or is found to be poor or absent at operation. Alternatively, a composite graft can be made from arm veins, the short saphenous vein, or a segment of undamaged long saphenous vein.[309] The long saphenous vein from the opposite limb may be used if this is of adequate quality. Prosthetic grafts can be of Dacron, which may be externally supported;[271] polytetrafluoroethylene;[310] or glutaraldehyde-tanned human or animal umbilical veins, which have to be externally

REFERENCES

307. Leather RP, Powers SR, Karmody AM. Surgery 1979; 86: 453
308. Hall KV. Surgery 1962; 51: 492
309. Edwards WS, Gerety E et al. Surgery 1976; 80: 722
310. Veith FJ, Moss CM et al. JAMA 1978; 240: 1867

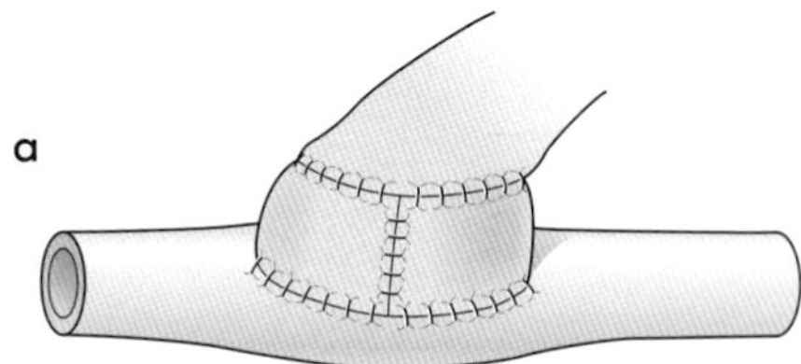

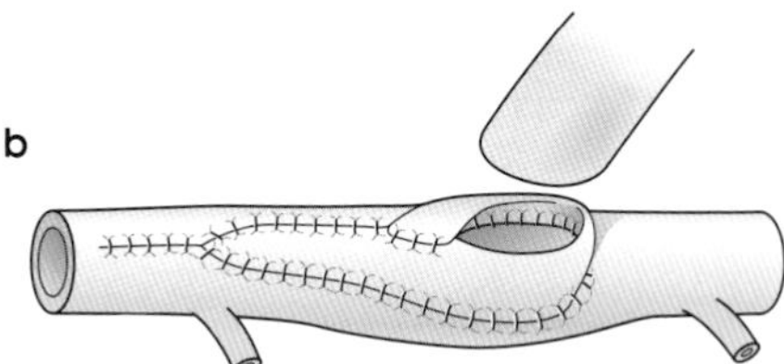

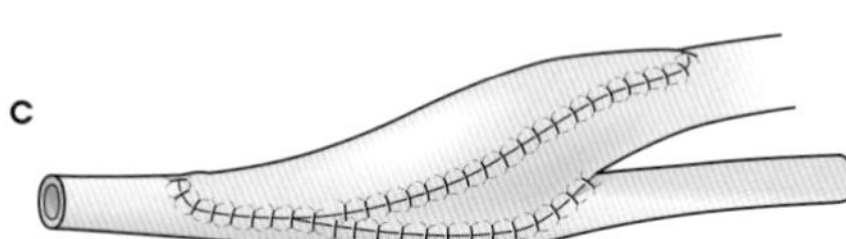

Figure 10.57 (a) Miller cuff, (b) St Mary's boot and (c) Taylor patch.

supported to prevent aneurysm formation.[311] The anastomosis between the prosthetic and lower vessel may be made via a Miller cuff,[300] a Taylor patch,[301] or a St Mary's boot (Fig. 10.57).[302]

A long endarterectomy can be performed using a Volmar's ring stripper to core out the atheroma.[273] This may also be carried out through a long open incision into the artery, but a vein graft is then usually required to prevent stenosis during closure. After endarterectomy, the luminal surface should be inspected by arteriography or with an angioscope[312] to ensure that it is smooth. The rough luminal surface can be lined by a smooth prosthesis.

Angioplasty now provides a credible alternative to vein bypass grafting, and the use of the subintimal route and stenting may continue to improve results.[313] Patients considered for femoropopliteal angioplasty should also be considered appropriate for surgical bypass, which may be urgently required if complications develop.

Femorocrural and pedal grafts

Ipsilateral long saphenous vein, preferably using the in situ technique, is again the material of choice for bypasses to the posterior tibial proximal or mid-third calf peroneal and dorsalis pedis arteries. Grafts to the anterior tibial artery are best performed via a lateral route; this avoids a subcutaneous tunnel over the anterior aspect of the tibia. Distal third peroneal grafts are again best approached from the lateral route. In the case of composite vein grafts, it is important to place the tunnelling incisions at the sites of the end-to-end anastomoses. This facilitates the occasional haemostatic suture!

Prosthetic bypasses to these small vessels are much less satisfactory, but improved results have been reported using vein cuffs,[300] patches[301] or boots[302] via which the polytetrafluoroethylene grafts are anastomosed to the distal vessels. The anterior and posterior tibial arteries and the peroneal vessels can all be easily exposed in the lower part of the calf. The posterior tibial artery passes down behind the soleal arch and lies on the muscles on the posterior surface of the tibia, almost directly beneath the long saphenous vein. The anterior tibial artery lies deep in the anterior compartment almost on the interosseous membrane, and continues down as the dorsalis pedis artery over the front of the ankle between the tendons of the anterior compartment. The peroneal artery lies deep to the fibula, and can be easily reached by resecting the middle third of this bone, or with more difficulty by burrowing across the posterior compartment of the calf from the medial side.

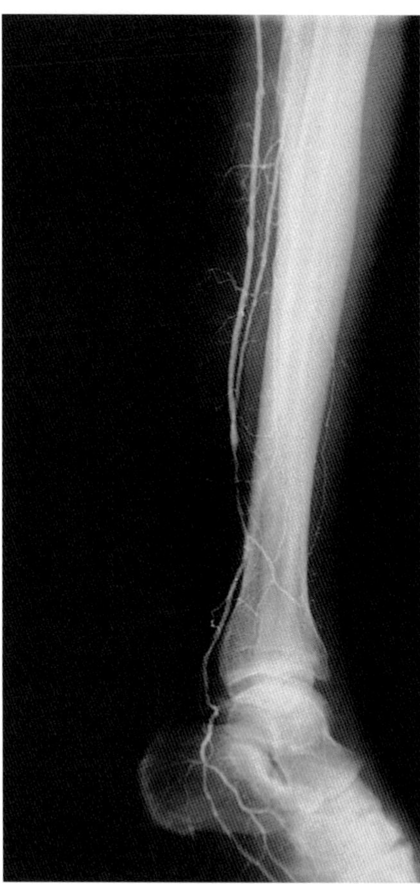

Figure 10.58 An operative arteriogram showing a femoro-posterior tibial vein graft.

The technique for femorodistal or crural bypass is otherwise identical to femoropopliteal grafting, although postoperative on-table arteriography and/or intraoperative Doppler flow or peripheral resistance measurements before and after papaverine are required to ensure a technically satisfactory graft (Fig. 10.58). Many surgeons use (× 2.5) magnifying loops to allow them to place their sutures with greater accuracy, because of the small size of the vessels. When the distal run-off is poor, anastomosis to more than one crural vessel may improve graft patency,[309] and some surgeons have made a common ostium arteriovenous anastomosis at the distal end to prevent grafts occluding by decreasing the peripheral resistance,[311] although at present there is no evidence that this improves patency.[314]

Angioplasty

Transluminal balloon dilatation of the distal vessels is effective for stenotic lesions; it has proved less successful in occlusive disease,[315] although some good results have been obtained with

REFERENCES

311. Dardik H, Dardik I. Ann Surg 1976; 183: 252
312. Itoh T, Hori M. Surgery 1983; 93: 391
313. Varty IC, Nydahl P, Butterworth P. Br J Surg 1996; 83: 953
314. Harris PL, Campbell H. Br J Surg 1983; 70: 377
315. Gruntzig A. Lancet 1978; i: 263

low-profile catheters and steerable guide wires.[316] A guide wire is passed through the stenosis or occlusion under radiographic control, and coaxial plastic balloon catheters are distended within the diseased segment to dilate the stenosis. It is not fully understood how the compressed atheroma disappears, but it is split by the dilating process into a number of longitudinal fissures. The vessel itself is also dilated. The procedure may be repeated regularly, but it can cause vessel rupture, dissection and thrombosis, especially in inexperienced hands. It is more effective in the aortoiliac segment than in the distal vasculature, and is better for treating stenotic than occlusive disease, although this tenet is being challenged by use of the subintimal technique and greater application of stents.

Profundaplasty

Profundaplasty,[317] which is widening of the profunda orifice, or the modification of extended deep femoral angioplasty[318] are now rarely considered to be effective on their own, and are usually combined with an aortic graft or some form of femoropopliteal or distal bypass.

COMBINATION DISEASE (AORTOILIAC AND FEMOROCRURAL DISEASE)

There is a small group of patients in whom an aortoiliac occlusion exists in association with severe profunda disease and a superficial femoral occlusion, where adequate outflow from an aortic graft can be achieved only by a synchronously performed aortic procedure and femoropopliteal bypass. In a number of patients, it is difficult to determine whether apparently mild aortic disease will reduce the patency of a femorodistal bypass. A proximal bypass should take precedence; angiography can be performed in cases of doubt and may be carried out in theatre at the time of the distal bypass. Many of these patients can be treated by preoperative or intraoperative iliac angioplasty and stenting combined with a distal vein bypass graft.

POSTOPERATIVE CARE

Fibrous strictures develop in between 20 and 30% of vein grafts in the first 12 months after operation.[319] For this reason vein graft surveillance programmes have been advocated, although conflicting results have questioned their value.[320] Colour duplex scanning is probably the most cost-effective technique, and at-risk grafts should be imaged and potentially treated at the time of intra-arterial digital subtraction angiography. These stenoses do not appear to be usually related to vascular clamp sites, tributaries, or residual valve cusps.[321] A trial of in situ versus reversed femoropopliteal vein grafts showed no difference in the short term, or longer term results up to 6 years.[322] The main advantage of the in situ technique is that the smaller lower end of the vein more closely matches the distal artery, and most surgeons choose this technique for anastomoses to the crural vessels. After 12 months, progression of proximal and distal atherosclerosis accounts for the majority of stenoses identified within a graft surveillance programme.

Results

Femoropopliteal bypass grafts performed for intermittent claudication have a cumulative patency of between 60 and 80% at 5 years and 30–40% at 10 years.[323] Prosthetics, endarterectomies and angioplasties have not achieved the same patency to date, being between 20 and 30% worse than vein.[324] Graft patency is even worse in patients with digital gangrene and critical ischaemia, and is significantly reduced in single crural vessel bypasses when compared with popliteal bypasses.[325] Graft failure does not always equate with limb loss, which must remain the final arbiter in determining graft success. Regular graft surveillance followed by intervention with angioplasty or further surgery appears to have improved (secondary) graft patency to 80% at 5 years,[326] although as stated this is still debated.

ISCHAEMIA OF THE GASTROINTESTINAL TRACT

The coeliac axis, and superior and inferior mesenteric arteries, with branches from the internal iliac artery supply the whole of the gastrointestinal tract with blood. Because of the many connections between the branches of these arteries, single or even multiple occlusions within the main vessels are often well tolerated, providing they are of gradual onset. Only an acute occlusion of the superior mesenteric artery is usually capable of producing small bowel infarction.

Atherosclerotic aortic disease may gradually narrow the orifices of all the visceral vessels, and may on occasion cause an acute thrombosis. Emboli can impact within the visceral arteries, and this aetiology accounts for at least 25% of all acute mesenteric occlusions.[327] Mesenteric venous thrombosis is another important cause of acute mesenteric ischaemia,[327] and low cardiac output can cause bowel ischaemia without there being any occlusions of the mesenteric vessels.[328] It has been reported that the coeliac artery can be compressed by the median arcuate ligament of the diaphragm, causing the coeliac axis compression syndrome, although some doubt its existence.[329] Chronic mesenteric ischaemia is almost invariably caused by atherosclerotic disease involving the aorta or the trunks of the major visceral vessels, although Buerger's disease, other forms of vasculitis, aortic dissection, fibromuscular hyperplasia and external compression are occasionally responsible.

CLINICAL FEATURES

Acute mesenteric ischaemia is described in Chapter 27. Chronic mesenteric ischaemia usually presents with severe postprandial pain that develops soon after food is taken and lasts for several hours. This pain, which has been called intestinal angina, is usually felt in the epigastrium. There is often a genuine fear of food because of the pain that it will produce. Weight loss is usually

REFERENCES

316. Schwarten DE, Cutcliff WB. Radiology 1988; 169: 71
317. Martin P, Bouhoutsos J. Br J Surg 1977; 64: 194
318. Berguer R, Cotton L, Sabri S. Br Med J 1973; 1: 469
319. Grigg MJ, Nicolaides AN, Wolfe JHN. Br J Surg 1988; 75: 737
320. Harris PL. Br J Surg 1992; 79: 97
321. Moody AP, Edwards PR, Harris PL. Eur J Vasc Surg 1992; 6: 509
322. Moody AP, Edwards PR, Harris PL. Br J Surg 1992; 79: 750
323. DeWeese JA, Robb CG. Surgery 1977; 82: 775
324. Bergan JJ, Veith FJ et al. Surgery 1982; 92: 921
325. Harris PL, Cave-Bingley DJ, McSweeney L. Br J Surg 1985; 72: 317
326. Moody P, Gould DA, Harris PL. Eur J Vasc Surg 1990; 4: 1117
327. Jackson BB. Occlusion of the Superior Mesenteric Artery. Thomas, Springfield, 1963
328. Britt LG, Cheek RC. Ann Surg 1969; 169: 704
329. (Anonymous). Br Med J 1970; 1: 317

marked, and if the inferior mesenteric artery is occluded, diarrhoea and rectal bleeding predominate. An abdominal bruit is the only physical sign that may be present; this is heard in 75% of patients with this condition.[330] It is not diagnostic, and other much more common causes of chronic abdominal pain must be excluded by endoscopy, ultrasound, and endoscopic retrograde cholangiopancreatography. The differential diagnosis includes peptic ulcer disease, chronic cholecystitis, chronic pancreatitis, irritable bowel syndrome, and obscure slow-growing intra-abdominal tumours (see Ch. 25).

INVESTIGATIONS

Duplex scanning of the visceral arteries can be performed before and after a standard meal, but the investigation of choice remains an intra-arterial digital subtraction angiography. Lateral aortography may show a stenosis or occlusion of one or more of the major vessels (Fig. 10.59).[331] It is important at the time of diagnostic angiography not to cannulate a stenosed coeliac axis or superior mesenteric artery, because this may precipitate acute thrombosis and severe visceral ischaemia. Thumb-printing or pseudopolyposis of the colonic mucosa may be seen in patients with ischaemic colitis on barium enema. Gastroduodenal biopsy may demonstrate the features of ischaemia on histological examination. Evidence of malabsorption may be provided by a Schilling test, a D-xylose test, faecal fat estimation or chromium-labelled albumin. The diagnosis rests on a high index of suspicion combined with appropriate arteriographic findings.

TREATMENT

Once the diagnosis has been made, patients should be considered for balloon angioplasty with or without stenting, or surgery. The results are similar, with mortality rates ranging between 2 and 10%; however, balloon angioplasty for revascularization is associated with a higher rate of restenosis. If the superior mesenteric artery is narrowed, there are a number of surgical options including revascularization; a vein bypass graft from the aorta;[332] endarterectomy,[333] which is technically difficult; or a side-to-side anastomosis between the ileocolic and right common iliac arteries.[334] Depending on the state of the infrarenal aorta and the general habitus of the patient, an externally supported bifurcated Dacron graft can be anastomosed to either the supracoeliac or infrarenal aorta and the superior mesenteric artery and the hepatic artery. The grafts are tunnelled behind the pancreas and usually lie in a reasonable position, which contrasts with vein grafts that often kink. Operative treatment carries a considerable risk (10% mortality at least), but can produce good results in selected patients, with 90% or more being symptom-free after surgery.[333]

A reduction in blood flow to the colon often preferentially damages the mucosa, causing mucosal sloughing. A similar picture may be seen with clostridial infection. Patients with full-thickness gangrene of the small or large bowel require resection, but patients at an earlier stage of ischaemic colitis may be best treated at first with intravenous fluids and broad-spectrum antibiotics.[335]

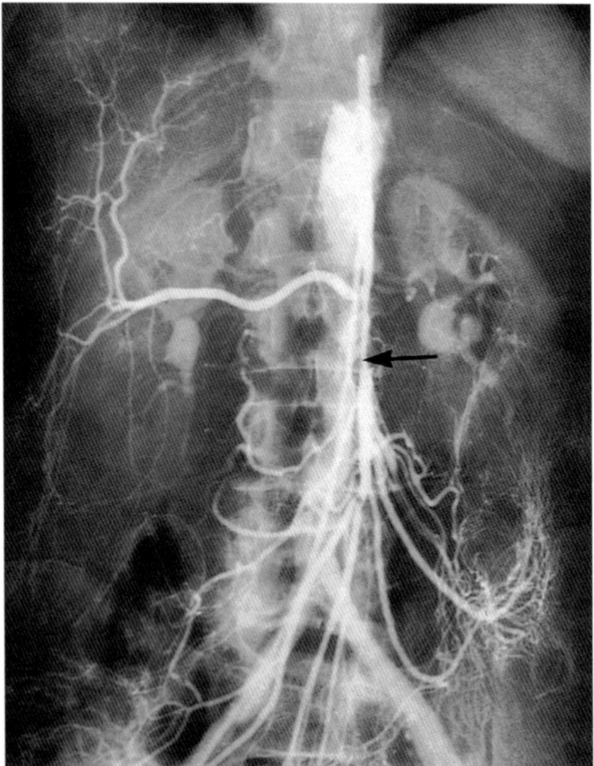

Figure 10.59 An aortogram showing narrowing of the superior mesenteric artery near its origin and occlusion of the inferior mesenteric artery.

RENOVASCULAR HYPERTENSION

RENAL ARTERY STENOSIS

Renovascular disease is present in 6.8% of Americans over the age of 65. It is associated with low levels of high-density lipoprotein, a low cholesterol, and hypertension.[336] Renal artery stenosis is a well-recognized cause of hypertension, but more recently it has also been demonstrated to be an important cause of renal failure. Hypertension is a condition in which there is permanent elevation of both the systolic and diastolic pressure; if the diastolic pressure is persistently above 95 or 100 mmHg, some form of treatment is required. In most patients with hypertension, no cause is found and the hypertension is therefore called essential. A number of causes for hypertension are, however, recognized including Cushing's syndrome, Conn's syndrome (see Ch. 34), phaeochromocytomas (see Ch. 34), coarctation of the aorta (see Ch. 22), and renovascular disease. Renovascular hypertension and renal failure are discussed here.

Pathophysiology

Hypertension

Goldblatt and colleagues showed that partial compression of one renal artery by a clamp produced experimental hypertension.[337] This effect persisted when the kidney was transplanted to another site, indicating that it was independent of any nervous

REFERENCES

330. Stoney RJ, Wylie EJ. Ann Surg 1966; 164: 174
331. Dick AP, Graff R et al. Gut 1967; 8: 206
332. Mikkelsen WP. Am J Surg 1957; 94: 262
333. Stoney RJ, Ehrenfeld WK, Wylie EJ. Ann Surg 1977; 186: 468
334. Mavor GE, Lyall AD et al. Br J Surg 1962; 50: 219
335. Marcuson RW. Br J Hosp Med 1974; 203
336. Hansen KJ, Edwards MS, Craven TE et al. J Vasc Surg 2002; 36: 443–451
337. Goldblatt H, Lynch et al. J Exp Med 1934; 59: 347

mechanism. The experimental hypertension was abolished by the removal of the clamped kidney. This renovascular hypertension was later shown to be caused by release of renin from the juxtaglomerular apparatus into the renal venous blood. The renin converts angiotensinogen, a circulating protein, into the pressor angiotensin I, which is itself rapidly converted to the even more potent angiotensin II.[338] When this substance is infused into a peripheral vein, it produces a substantial rise in both the systolic and diastolic pressure. Hypertension in between 2 and 7% of all patients with the condition has a renovascular cause,[339] although some have suggested that this figure is an overestimate.[340] After the age of 50, identification of renovascular disease is probably unnecessary unless the hypertension is severe and uncontrollable by drugs.

Renal failure

Acute renal failure can be caused by atherosclerotic renovascular disease, and is often precipitated by the use of angiotensin-converting enzyme inhibitors, non-steroidal drugs and aminoglycosides. In a prospective study, angiography performed when there was evidence of atherosclerotic disease elsewhere showed that in 14% the renal failure was the result of atherosclerotic renal vascular disease.[341] A prospective study has shown that 5% of patients presenting with a greater than 60% stenosis of the renal artery progressed to arterial occlusion within 1 year and 11% at 2 years.[342] This study also showed that progression from less than 60% stenosis to greater than 60% stenosis or occlusion occurred in 23% at 1 year and in 42% at 2 years. Another prospective duplex study has shown that 19% of patients with greater than 60% stenosis of the renal artery lose 1 cm or more in length of the kidney in the next 12 months. No change in renal dimensions was found if the stenosis was less than 60%.[343] Acute occlusion of the renal artery can lead to death of the kidney. The pathological events occurring in gradual occlusion are more complex and are still not fully understood. A severe stenosis of 80–85% will cause a reduction in flow below the critical perfusion pressure.[344] Eventually there is loss of renal parenchyma, resulting in a decrease in renal length and the onset of renal failure.

Aetiology

Hypertension

Atherosclerotic disease accounts for approximately two-thirds of all cases of renovascular hypertension, and fibromuscular hyperplasia accounts for most of the rest. Polycystic kidneys, pyelonephritis and hydronephrosis are other conditions that can cause renal hypertension, and vascular malformation, aortic dissections, various forms of arteritis, and emboli are rare causes of renovascular hypertension.

Flash pulmonary oedema

Patients who have a severe stenosis of a single kidney or who have bilateral tight stenoses may present with a sudden onset of severe pulmonary oedema.[345] These patients usually have atherosclerosis, although it has been described in renal transplant patients who have proximal iliac disease. All patients have normal cardiac function.

Diagnosis and investigation

The diagnosis of renovascular hypertension must be suspected in young males if there is a relatively sudden onset of symptoms (headaches, giddiness, epistaxis, visual disturbances or dyspnoea), especially if there is evidence of an abdominal bruit or if casts of red and white cells are found within the urine. A family history of arterial disease, an early age at onset, and drug resistance are other pointers to a possible renal cause. Patients presenting with chronic renal failure who have atheromatous disease elsewhere should be suspected of having a renal artery stenosis.

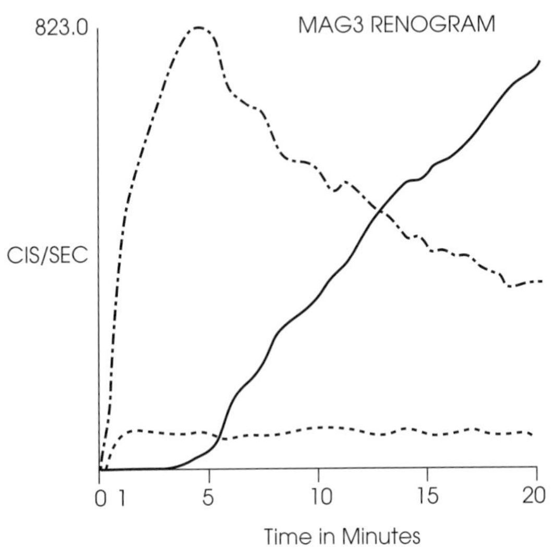

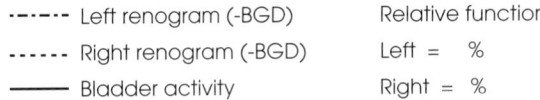

Figure 10.60 An isotope renogram showing delayed uptake and secretion characteristic of ischaemia.

An ultrasound scan may reveal loss of renal length and thinning of the renal cortex in patients with renal failure. Duplex ultrasound scanning can be used to detect renal artery stenosis by finding a peak systolic velocity of greater than 200 cm/s within the renal arteries, although the renal artery can be difficult to visualize.[346] The use of a renal resistance index (80 or higher) has been used to identify patients at greater risk of renal deterioration.[347] An intravenous pyelogram may confirm renal disease. The nephrogram is delayed and the contrast appears to be more concentrated in a smaller kidney if it is ischaemic.

The serum creatinine is often raised and the creatinine clearance is reduced. Isotope renography shows an ischaemic pattern with delayed uptake and secretion (Fig. 10.60). Isotope renography before and after the administration of captopril is a sensitive technique for displaying renal artery stenosis. Selective ureteric catheterization should confirm a low sodium excretion on the side of the stenosis, and selective venous catheterization should demonstrate elevation of renin in the appropriate renal

REFERENCES

338. Lentz KE, Skeggs LT et al. J Exp Med 1956; 103: 183
339. Dean RH, Kieffer RW et al. Arch Surg 1981; 116: 1408
340. Tucher RM, Labarthe DR. Mayo Clin Proc 1977; 52: 549
341. Scoble JE et al. Clin Nephrol 1989; 31: 119
342. Zierler RE et al. J Vasc Surg 1994; 19: 250
343. Guzman RP et al. Hypertension 1994; 23: 346
344. May AG et al. Surgery 1963; 53: 513
345. Pickering TG, Herman L, Devereux RB et al. Lancet 1988; 2: 551–552
346. Hoffman U et al. Kidney Int 1991; 39: 1232
347. Radermacher J, Ellis S, Haller H. Hypertension 2002; 39: 699–703

vein.[348] A renal vein renin ratio of 1.5 is highly suggestive of the diagnosis,[349] but before this is measured all antihypertensive treatment must be stopped. False positive and negative results do occur, but this investigation is the most sensitive diagnostic test and can be repeated if necessary. Arteriography by digital subtraction or by selective catheterization[350] confirms the renal artery stenosis.

Management

Many patients who are elderly and have well-preserved renal function are best treated by antihypertensive medication. Surgery is contraindicated in elderly patients with extensive bilateral disease who have serious concomitant pathology.[351] In the young or middle-aged, an attempt should be made to treat a symptomatic vascular stenosis. Percutaneous transluminal angioplasty is a simple manoeuvre that is particularly effective in treating isolated short stenoses in the main trunk of the renal artery, especially in patients with fibromuscular hyperplasia.[352] An endovascular stent can be inserted if this technique fails or if the stenosis is mainly at the ostium of the renal artery. Although early results have been encouraging, long-term follow-up studies are necessary to compare stenting with the proven benefit of surgery.[353]

Aortorenal vein bypass is probably the open surgical treatment of choice (Fig. 10.51b). Saphenous vein, hypogastric artery and synthetic material have all been used for this purpose.[354] A bypass from the splenic or hepatic arteries is a useful alternative when the aorta is severely diseased but does not require replacement. The San Francisco surgeons have championed extensive aortorenal endarterectomy[354] in patients with severe aortorenal atheroma, and this approach is very useful if there is extensive coexistent aortic disease above the renal arteries extending into the superior mesenteric or coeliac arteries (Fig. 10.61).

The kidney should be cooled and removed if the stenosis extends into its hilum, particularly in patients with fibromuscular hyperplasia.[355] Careful surgical repair can then be performed on the bench using vein grafts to widen the renal branches before the kidney is reimplanted, usually on to the internal iliac artery and common iliac vein. The ureter is then reimplanted into the bladder. Nephrectomy is indicated if the kidney function is poor and there is little remaining cortex, providing that the function of the other kidney is normal. It is also indicated if reconstruction is considered impossible or dangerous.

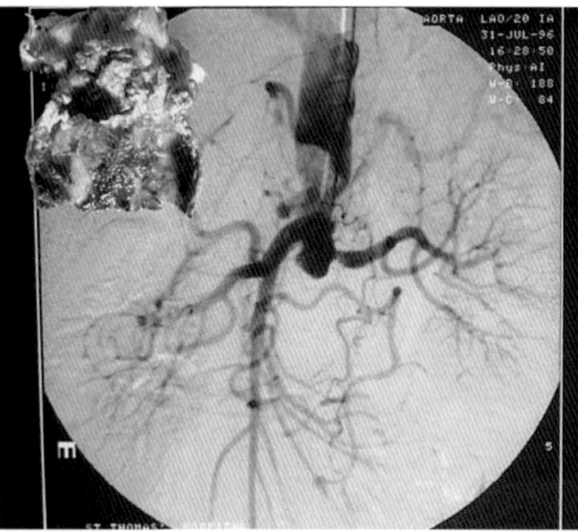

Figure 10.61 Angiogram showing suprarenal plaque. The excised plaque is shown top left.

Results

Transluminal angioplasty has an early success of about 90% in patients with fibromuscular hyperplasia, but it is usually poorly maintained, with nearly half the patients requiring a further dilatation within 2 or 3 years.[356] This treatment is less successful in atherosclerotic disease, and a randomized trial has shown that restenosis in ostial disease is significantly reduced by stenting.[357] Surgical bypass is also effective in lowering the blood pressure to normal in 90% of patients with fibromuscular hyperplasia but is less effective in atherosclerotic disease, producing an improvement in blood pressure control in about 50–60% without preserving renal function.[354] Patients with flash pulmonary oedema can be cured with intervention, and this condition is thought to be an absolute indication for treatment.[345] The results of intervention for hypertension in older patients are poor, with three randomized trials showing no benefit of angioplasty over best medical therapy. A 2003 meta-analysis of randomized controlled trials of balloon angioplasty versus best medical therapy for hypertensive patients with atherosclerotic renal artery disease concluded that it should be reserved for patients with poorly controlled hypertension.[358] Patients who have intervention for renal dysfunction may benefit, but level-one evidence is lacking. Trials are under way to determine the place of intervention for patients with renal dysfunction secondary to atherosclerosis.

DIABETIC ISCHAEMIA

Diabetes is a common disease that affects approximately 5% of the population. The Framingham study showed that diabetic patients were three to four times more likely to have intermittent claudication than those without diabetes.[359] This was true of both insulin-dependent diabetes and maturity-onset diabetes, and was also related to smoking. The natural history of peripheral vascular disease is worse in diabetic patients, with an increase in both mortality and limb loss.[360] This may be related to abnormalities in serum lipids and lipoproteins, to an increase in platelet aggregation, and to a prothrombotic tendency.

Diabetes can affect the foot because of three inter-related factors: neuropathy, infection and ischaemia. The neuropathy can affect both somatic and autonomic nerves. Absence of pain allows mechanical damage to the foot from tight shoes, penetrating injuries and nail cutting to pass unnoticed. Loss of temperature sensation can result in similar thermal injuries from bathing in hot water and keeping the feet too close to a hot water

REFERENCES

348. Kaufman JJ, Lupu AN et al. J Urol 1970; 103: 702
349. Dean RH, Foster JH. Surgery 1973; 74: 926
350. Gomes AS, Pais SO, Barbaric ZL. Am J Radiol 1983; 140: 779
351. Hallet JW, Fowl R, O'Brien PC. J Vasc Surg 1987; 5: 622
352. Gruntzig A, Vetter W et al. Lancet 1978; i: 801
353. Raynaud AC et al. J Vasc Interv Radiol 1994; 5: 849
354. Dean RH, Krueger TC et al. J Vasc Surg 1984; 1: 234
355. Belzer FO, Salvatierra O. Ann Surg 1975; 182: 456
356. Ramsay LE, Waller PC. Br Med J 1990; 300: 569
357. van de Ven PJG, Kaatee R, Beutler JJ et al. Lancet 1999; 353: 282–286
358. Nordmann AJ, Woo K et al. Am J Med 2003; 114: 44–50
359. Garcia C et al. Diabetes 1980; 29: 105
360. Shadt DC et al. JAMA 1961; 175: 937

bottle, fire or radiator. Damage to motor fibres causes wasting and weakness of the intrinsic muscles of the feet, resulting in a cavus deformity, claw toes, abnormal weight distribution, and callus formation. Degeneration of the sudomotor axons results in loss of sweating, causing dry skin, cracks, fissures and ulceration. Neuropathic ulceration results from the alteration of weight distribution, which produces callosities and subkeratotic haematomas. This causes tissue necrosis below the callus, which may ulcerate and encourage infection. Neuropathic ulcers are painless, surrounded by callus, usually circular, and punched out. They may be very deep, extending to the bone. They usually develop beneath the metatarsal heads and the tips of the toes, but may also occur over the dorsal interphalangeal joints of clawed toes and over both malleoli where they rub against footwear. Pedal pulses are usually easily palpable.

Infection in diabetic patients occurs because of an impaired immune response. The polymorph leukocyte has a reduced activity, particularly against *Staphylococcus aureus* and *Escherichia coli*.[361] Wound healing is also impaired, which makes minor injuries slow to heal. Non-clostridial gas-forming organisms quite commonly invade diabetic feet and produce gas in the tissues. Crepitus is present and a characteristic putrefying stench is apparent. Plain radiographs show the free gas in the tissues. Ischaemia is the result of both large and small vessel disease, although the importance of the latter may have been over-emphasized. Large vessel atherosclerosis presents at an earlier age, and is more severe in diabetic patients compared with non-diabetic controls. The proximal vessels are usually spared, with the majority of the disease affecting the arteries below the knee. Occlusions are more likely to occur at multiple levels and to be bilateral. The blood flow through diabetic feet is often greater than in equivalent atherosclerotic patients without diabetes;[362] this may be the result of arteriovenous shunting. The basement membrane of the capillaries is thickened and more permeable, although the significance of this is disputed. Crural arterial occlusion is the most important cause of digital and pedal gangrene, although secondary infection is quite common. The ulceration associated with ischaemia has no surrounding callus, and frequently affects the first and fifth metatarsal heads and the toes. There is usually a preceding history of intermittent claudication and rest pain.

A full blood count, blood glucose, and blood glycosylated haemoglobin should be obtained. Swabs should be taken from the ulcers for bacterial culture and sensitivity to antibiotics. Plain radiograph of the foot may confirm osteomyelitis or septic arthritis, although evidence of bone destruction is often late. Calcification of the digital vessels and the presence of gas in the tissues may also be shown. Doppler pressures are usually misleading because calcification in the walls of the crural arteries prevents their compression by the sphygmomanometer cuff. Duplex examination may identify arterial occlusions and stenoses but may also be hampered by calcification in the vessels. Intra-arterial digital subtraction angiography should be performed whenever ischaemia is suspected. Magnetic resonance imaging scans are good at detecting early osteomyelitis and abscesses in the foot.

The diabetic foot is best managed by a team consisting of a diabetic physician, a vascular surgeon, an orthopaedic surgeon, a diabetic nurse, a chiropodist, a physiotherapist, an orthotist and a limb fitter. All diabetic patients, especially those with claudication or neuropathy, should be encouraged to inspect their feet every night; a mirror is useful to examine the sole of the foot. Progression of early skin damage may be avoided by bed rest and antibiotics.

Established neuropathic ulceration is treated by removing the callus, eradicating infection, and reducing weight-bearing forces. All patients should be prescribed broad-spectrum antibiotics until healing is complete. Infections are usually caused by a number of different bacterial species including Gram-positive, Gram-negative, enteric and anaerobic organisms. The most common are staphylococci, enterococci, enterobacteria, and anaerobes such as *Peptostreptococcus* and *Bacteroides*.[363] The patient should be admitted to hospital for bed rest and limb elevation if cellulitis is present. Blood cultures should be performed before intravenous antibiotic therapy is begun. An insulin infusion and sliding scale may be required to control the blood glucose. Any associated cardiac failure should be treated. When healing has been achieved, patients should be advised on footwear, chiropody, smoking, obesity and diabetic control. Surgical debridement of dead tissue and infected bone should be performed and all pockets of pus should be drained.

Distal atherosclerotic arterial disease should be treated by angioplasty or bypass surgery. The distal nature of the disease in diabetic patients means that the superficial femoral and the popliteal arteries can be used as the donor vessel.[364] Bypasses are usually made to the crural arteries near the ankle. Sympathectomy is usually ineffective in diabetic patients who are already autosympathectomized, and the results of prostaglandin infusion are also poor. Trophic ulcers of the sole of the foot may heal if the limb is enclosed in a below-knee plaster with a rocker.[365] Alternative therapies include the use of suction devices and the use of free flaps. Recurrence may be prevented by excising the metatarsal heads.[366]

In every ischaemic diabetic foot it is important to determine the extent of the ischaemia, neuropathy and infection before deciding on the best method of treatment. A gangrenous digit in a warm foot with impaired proprioception and deep pain but normal foot pulses can be treated by digital, transmetatarsal or ray amputation with a reasonable chance of success.[366] A cold foot with absent pulses must be investigated by arteriography with a view to simultaneous reconstruction and amputation if possible.

ARTERIAL DILATATION

Generalized dilatation of the whole arterial tree is known as arteriomegaly. A vessel that has increased in size to less than twice its normal diameter is said to be ectatic. An arterial aneurysm is defined as a localized or segmental pathological dilatation to more than twice the diameter of the normal vessel. Arteriomegaly is an ill-understood condition in which many vessels become dilated. Patients with this condition are liable to develop multiple aneurysms.[367] Multiple aneurysms and arteriomegaly, which are

REFERENCES

361. Rayfield EJ et al. Am J Med 1982; 72: 439
362. Rayman G et al. Br Med J 1986; 292: 87
363. Wheat LJ et al. Arch Intern Med 1987; 4: 475
364. Veith FJ et al. Surgery 1981; 90: 980
365. Pollard JP, Le Quesne LP. Br Med J 1983; 286: 436
366. Singer A. Arch Surg 1976; 111: 964
367. Lea Thomas M. Br J Surg 1971; 58: 690

endemic in certain strains of mice, were thought to be associated with copper deficiency,[368] but this has not been confirmed. Proteolytic degeneration and remodelling are now thought to be important in the aetiology, and the role of atheroma as a causative agent is disputed.

ANEURYSMS

Aneurysms are classified into true and false, depending on the involvement of the arterial wall in the aneurysmal process. In true aneurysms the dilatation involves all layers of the arterial wall. In false aneurysms the wall of the vessel has been breached, and the aneurysmal sac is made up of surrounding structures that have been compressed by the escaping blood. A false aneurysm usually starts as a pulsating haematoma. The blood that escapes from a partially divided artery normally thromboses, but eventually the pulsation beating through the defect in the wall may excavate a cavity in the haematoma. The surrounding tissues are eroded by the continuing pulsation as the aneurysm expands.

Sometimes a nearby artery and vein are damaged by the same injury, with both vessels opening into the one haematoma cavity. The same process of haematoma cavitation can then occur, with the aneurysmal sac communicating with both the artery and vein to give an arteriovenous aneurysm. This type of aneurysm is also found as a developmental abnormality. If the arterial flow is directly diverted into the vein, this distends and becomes an aneurysmal varix. The femoral arteries are the most common site for false aneurysms, which are often iatrogenic. These may be treated surgically, by ultrasound-guided compression, or by thrombin injection if large or symptomatic.[369]

True aneurysms are subdivided into fusiform (spindle-shaped enlargement of the whole luminal circumference) or saccular (when only a small segment of arterial wall balloons outwards as a rounded bulbous mass). The aetiology of non-specific aneurysms remains largely undefined but has a substantial genetic component. Histologically, mature aneurysms are characterized by a loss of elastin and smooth muscle cells from the arterial media and a compensatory increase in adventitial collagen. The main pathological processes involved in aneurysm expansion are widespread inflammation throughout the vessel wall, proteolytic degradation, and remodelling of the extracellular matrix.[370]

Atherosclerosis was considered to be the most common cause of true aneurysms, but the reason that dilatation developed in some, while stenosing disease occurred in the majority, remains obscure. It has been suggested that the lipoprotein profile may differ,[371] or that the amounts of elastin in the wall may influence development.[372] The causative role for atherosclerosis in aneurysmal disease is disputed. A genetic or familial predisposition has also been established.[373] Syphilis is an unusual cause of aneurysms today, but used to produce mainly saccular aneurysms occurring in any vessel. Marfan's and Ehlers–Danlos syndromes, and pseudoxanthoma elasticum are rare collagen diseases associated with the development of saccular or dissecting aneurysms. Congenital aneurysms found on the circle of Willis are called berry aneurysms; it is not known how or why they develop. Aortic dissections should not be classified as aneurysms (see Ch. 22). Mycotic aneurysms develop when a vegetative endocarditis or an infected embolus lodges in the systemic circulation. This usually occurs at a bifurcation, allowing the contained organisms to proliferate and weaken the arterial wall.

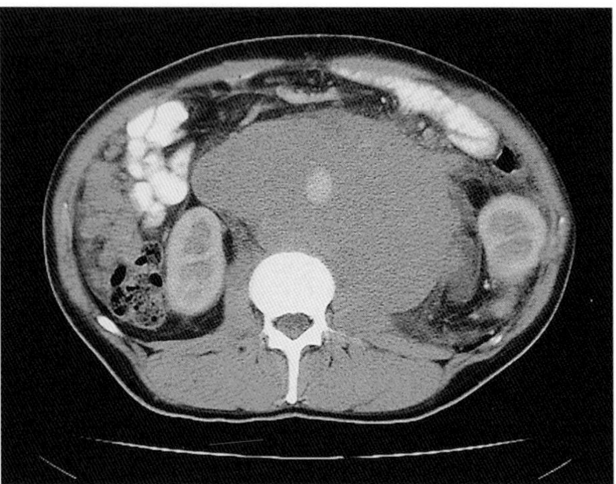

Figure 10.62 Aorta surrounded by a mass of lymphomatous lymph nodes.

CLINICAL FEATURES

Arteriomegaly is usually symptomless until aneurysmal dilatation occurs at specific sites. Aneurysms often cause no symptoms, but the abnormally large pulsation may occasionally be noticed by the patient or found by a doctor during routine examination. Aneurysms may compress and erode surrounding structures (including nerves, intestine and bone) and they may rupture, causing haemorrhage into serous cavities, into hollow viscera, or on to the skin surface. Intraluminal thrombus may embolize distally, and rarely the whole aneurysm may thrombose. The expansile pulse of an aneurysmal artery must be differentiated from the transmitted pulse of a mass overlying a vessel. An expansile pulse expands in two planes, while a transmitted pulse is felt only in one. Occasionally a highly vascular tumour may prove difficult to differentiate from an aneurysm. Also, a mass of retroperitoneal nodes plastered around the aorta may feel like an aneurysm (Fig. 10.62). Aneurysms are most frequently found in the abdominal aorta, the iliac vessels, and the femoral and popliteal arteries. A very tortuous artery may also be mistaken for an aneurysm.

MANAGEMENT

Modern techniques have rendered obsolete the proximal ligation of Hunter above a popliteal aneurysm,[374] the distal ligation of Bradsor for an innominate aneurysm,[375] and a combination of proximal and distal ligation without reconstruction. Endo-

REFERENCES

368. Andrews EJ, White WJ, Bullock LP. Am J Pathol 1975; 78: 199
369. Weinmann EE, Chayen D et al. Eur J Vasc Endovasc Surg 2002; 23: 68–72
370. Wills A, Thompson MM, Crowther M et al. Eur J Vasc Endovasc Surg 1996; 12: 391
371. De Palma RG. In: Bergan JJ, Yao JST (eds). Aneurysms, Diagnosis and Treatment. Grune & Stratton, New York, 1982
372. Powell JT, Campa J et al. Br J Surg 1985; 72: 401
373. Clifton MA. Br J Surg 1977; 64: 765
374. Hunter JA. In: Palmer JF (ed). The Works of John Hunter. Longman, London, 1837: 601
375. Deschamps F. In: Observations on Aneurysm. Sydenham Society, London, 1844

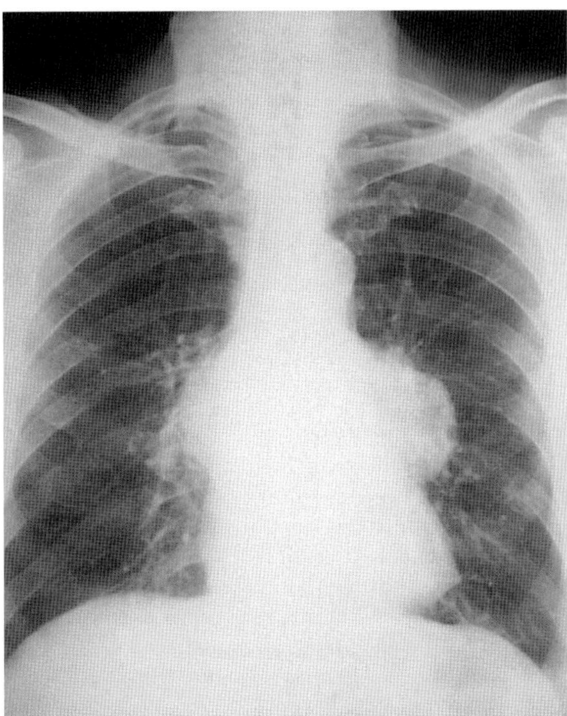

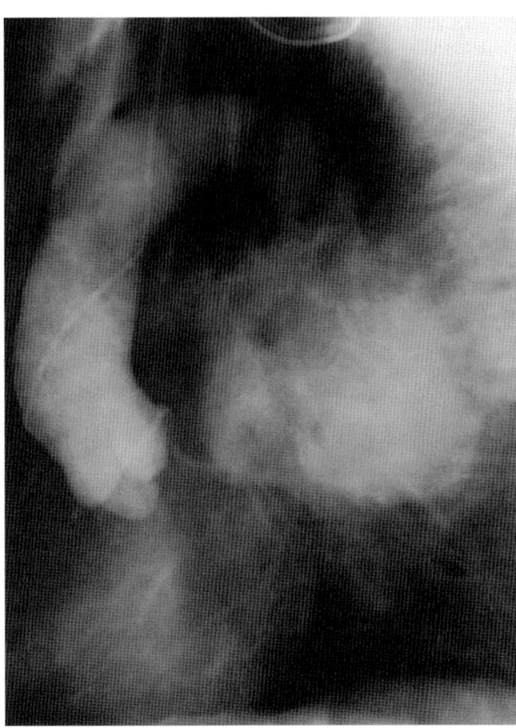

a b

Figure 10.63 A chest radiograph (**a**) showing a soft tissue mass that was subsequently shown to be a thoracic aneurysm on arteriography (**b**).

aneurysmorrhaphy,[376] which consists of closure of a saccular aneurysm from within the neck, is also now rarely practised, and wrapping[377] and intra-aneurysmal wiring[378] have all given way to the technique of resection and reconstruction. There is considerable interest in the use of endovascular stented grafts for lining and treating aneurysms, particularly in the thoracic and abdominal aorta. The long-term results of endovascular repair are not yet available, but controlled trials of this new treatment against standard operation are being conducted.[379]

ANEURYSMS OF INDIVIDUAL VESSELS

Thoracic aorta

Thoracic aneurysms are much less common than abdominal aortic aneurysms.[380] A true aneurysm of the thoracic aorta needs to be differentiated from an unfolded aorta, an aortic dissection, and occasionally a mediastinal tumour, especially if it presents a shadow on a chest radiograph (Fig. 10.63). Computerized tomography scanning, MRI and trans-oesophageal ultrasound may establish that a true dilatation of the aorta is present and exclude the double lumen seen in a dissecting aneurysm (see Ch. 22). Thoracic aneurysms may also present with back pain from bone erosion, and dysphagia and stridor as the result of compression of the oesophagus and trachea, respectively. They may also occasionally rupture, causing severe shortness of breath and shock.

The risks involved in treating thoracic aneurysms have been highlighted in the audit of cardiothoracic centres in the UK, which showed a 28% mortality rate for surgery on the descending thoracic aorta.[381] Natural history data have, however, shown that aneurysms greater than 7 cm in diameter have a risk of rupture, which is 14 times greater than that of those measuring 5 cm or less.[382]

Symptomless thoracic aneurysms in elderly patients are probably better left alone, but a large expanding or symptomatic aneurysm in a young fit patient should be resected if possible. The risk of producing a paraplegia by interrupting the blood supply of the spinal cord, which is provided by the arteries of Adamkiewicz, may be reduced by reimplanting these vessels if they have been accurately located preoperatively.[383] Patients with ruptured thoracic aneurysms rarely reach the operating room.

In an elective case the upper and lower limits of the aneurysm are controlled, and a Dacron prosthesis is inserted end to end with the normal artery above and below the dilatation. Major side branches are reimplanted. The inlay technique described by Crawford (Fig. 10.64)[380] has replaced the side branch technique described by De Bakey (Fig. 10.65).[384]

Endovascular stent grafts have been used with increasing success in treating localized thoracic aneurysms.[385,386] A stent graft is inserted via the femoral arteries through the aneurysm, and anchored in normal aorta both proximally and distally to exclude the aneurysm from the circulation. The reported mortality of endovascular thoracic aneurysm repair (5%) is

REFERENCES

376. Matas R. Ann Surg 1903; 37: 161
377. Benson EA. Ann R Coll Surg Engl 1977; 59: 65
378. Power DA, Colt GH. Lancet 1903; ii: 808
379. Yusuf SW, Hopkinson BR. In: Greenhalgh RM, Fowkes FGR (eds). Trials and Tribulations of Vascular Surgery. WB Saunders, London, 1996: 193–202
380. Crawford ES. Ann Surg 1974; 179: 763
381. Keogh BE, Kinsman R. National Adult Cardiac Database Npost 1998 Concord Services, London, 1999
382. Coady MA, Rizzo JA, Hammond GL et al. Ann Thorac Surg 1999; 67: 1922–1926
383. Connolly JE, Zuber WF et al. Ann Surg 1970; 172: 909
384. De Bakey ME, Crawford ES et al. Ann Surg 1965; 162: 650
385. Semba CP, Dake MD. In: Chuter TAM, Donayre CE, White RA (eds). Endovascular Prostheses. Little Brown, Boston, 1995
386. Taylor PR, Gaines PA, McGuinness CL et al. Eur J Vasc Endovasc Surg 2001; 22: 70

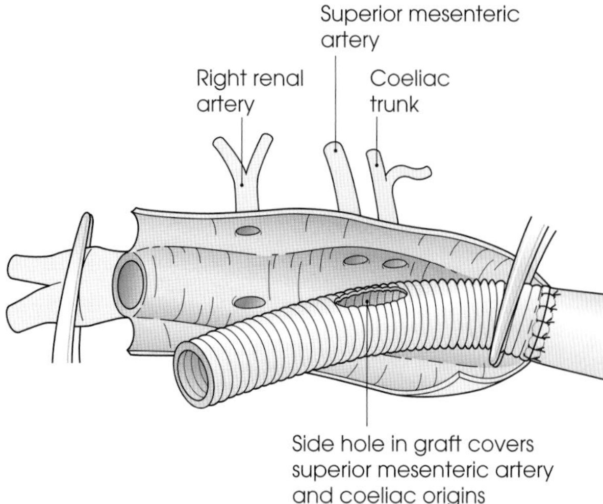

Figure 10.64 The Crawford technique for repairing thoracoabdominal aneurysms.

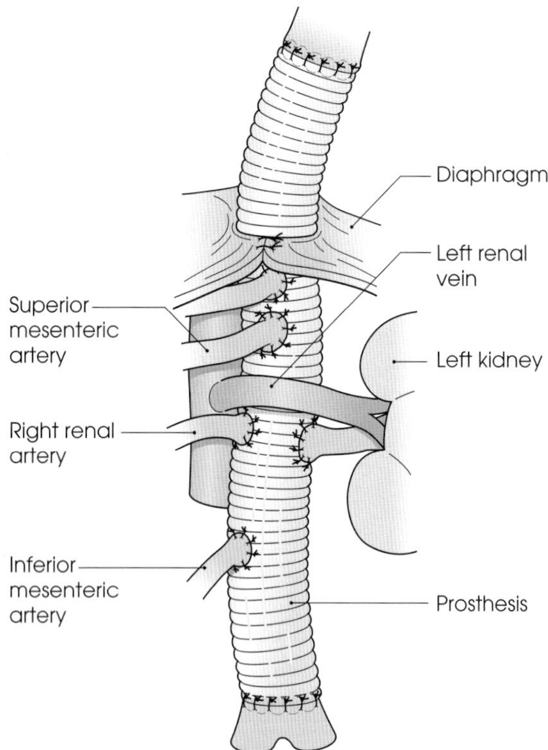

Figure 10.65 The De Bakey technique for repairing thoracoabdominal aneurysms. Each artery is anastomosed to a Dacron side branch sutured on to the main graft.

considerably less than that of conventional surgery, and endovascular procedures are likely to become the treatment of choice for thoracic aneurysms. Endovascular prostheses do suffer from stent fractures and graft displacement, which may allow blood to perfuse the aneurysm sac (an endoleak), causing continued aneurysm expansion.[387] The initial reduction in mortality from endovascular surgery seems to outweigh any potential long-term considerations of durability in the thoracic aorta. This may not be the case in abdominal aneurysms (see below).

Table 10.1 Results of surgical treatment of thoracoabdominal aortic aneurysms

Extent	No. of patients	Deaths (%)	Paraplegia (%)	Haemodialysis (%)
I	270	23 (9)	38 (14)	20 (7)
II	353	36 (10)	102 (29)	34 (10)
III	285	25 (9)	16 (6)	28 (10)
IV	285	19 (7)	10 (4)	24 (8)
Total	1193	103 (9)	166 (14)	106 (9)

Thoracoabdominal aneurysms

There are four types of thoracoabdominal aneurysm; these are shown in Fig. 10.66. Type II is the most extensive and treatment has the highest risk in this category. Thoracoabdominal aneurysms should be operated on only if the patient is fit and there is evidence of continued expansion. The Crawford technique of clamp and go has mostly been replaced by the more controlled conditions provided by atriofemoral bypass. The inlay technique of Crawford is, however, still favoured. His results are shown in Table 10.1.

The risk of paraplegia remains high. Some surgeons use continuous drainage of cerebrospinal fluid to increase the spinal cord perfusion pressure during aortic cross-clamping. This may reduce the risk of paraplegia. A randomized study has shown a significant reduction in spinal cord problems if cerebrospinal fluid drainage is performed.[388] Some advocate the use of motor evoked potentials to identify patients at risk of paraplegia who would benefit from intercostal reimplantation.[389] Others routinely implant intercostal vessels in the region of T8 to L2.[390] The risk of paraplegia remains high at 10–20% even in expert hands, and there is considerable mortality (10–50%). Renal failure is also a common complication following surgical repair of thoracoabdominal aneurysms, and is predictive of a poor long-term outcome.[391] The use of sequential clamping with partial left heart bypass may improve outcome,[392] but the role of selective visceral and renal perfusion remains controversial.[393]

Abdominal aortic aneurysms

The abdominal aorta is the most frequent site of aneurysms, and abdominal aortic aneurysms are found in 2% of all post-mortems.[394] The incidence of abdominal aortic aneurysm appears to be genuinely increasing in a number of countries, and in some the condition appears to be reaching epidemic proportions.[395] The dilatation usually begins below the renal

REFERENCES

387. Veith FJ et al. J Vasc Surg 2002; 35: 1029
388. Coselli JS, LeMaire SA, Koksoy C et al. J Vasc Surg 2002: 35: 631
389. Jacobs MJ, de Mol BA, Elenbaas T et al. J Vasc Surg 2002; 35: 30
390. Safi HJ, Miller CC, Carr C et al. J Vasc Surg 1998; 27: 58
391. Svensson LG et al. J Vasc Surg 1989; 10: 230
392. Safi HJ, Hess KR, Randel M et al. J Vasc Surg 1996; 23: 223
393. Safi HJ, Miller CC, Yawn DH et al. J Vasc Surg 1998; 27: 145
394. Turk KAD. Proc R Soc Med 1965; 58: 869
395. Collin J. Br J Hosp Med 1988; 64: 67

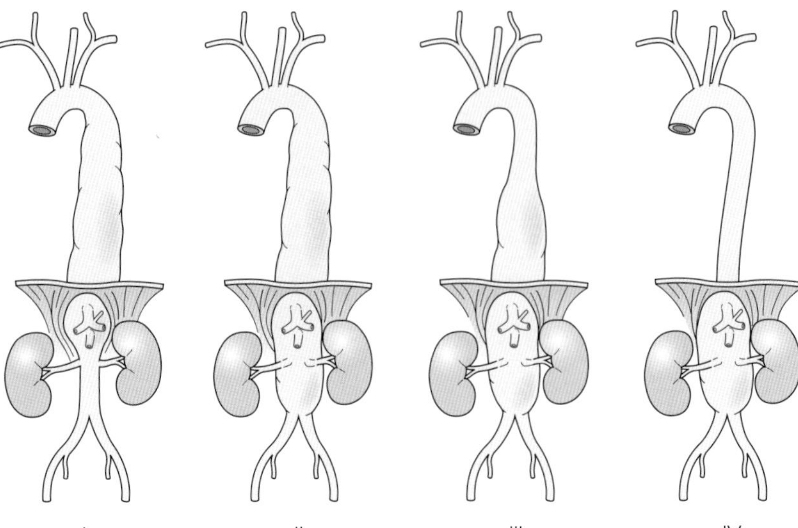

Figure 10.66 The Crawford classification of thoracoabdominal aneurysms.

arteries and extends to the aortic bifurcation or below. Aortic aneurysms are often associated with aneurysms of the iliac, femoral and popliteal arteries, especially when they occur in patients with generalized arteriomegaly. Only 1–2% of abdominal aneurysms are associated with aneurysmal dilatation extending above the renal arteries (see earlier). The incidence of abdominal aneurysm appears to be greatest in elderly (above the age of 60) male hypertensive individuals who smoke. Abdominal aortic aneurysms cause approximately 8000 deaths annually in the UK. The majority of deaths are caused by aneurysm rupture in patients with previously undetected, symptomless aneurysms. Fifty per cent of deaths attributable to ruptured abdominal aortic aneurysms occur at home, and of the remaining half who reach hospital, less than half survive.[396]

Aortic aneurysms are often found on routine medical examination when a central abdominal pulsatile mass is discovered during abdominal palpation. They also cause severe abdominal pain and shock when they rupture; many patients develop symptoms of chronic back pain as the result of pressure on the lumbar vertebrae, which may be eroded. Thrombosis, distal embolization, and rupture into the intestine or vena cava are rare complications.

Community-based screening has been suggested as a mechanism to reduce death from ruptured abdominal aneurysms, by identifying symptomless patients before rupture occurs. Screening programmes target men over 65 years of age and determine the diameter of the aorta using portable B mode ultrasound. Aneurysm screening identifies abdominal aortic aneurysms (most relatively small) in 5% of the elderly male population, who may then be treated appropriately. Patients with small aneurysms (less than 5.5 cm) are followed with serial ultrasound scans, while patients with larger aneurysms may be considered for surgery. The benefit of community-based screening for abdominal aortic aneurysm has been established by a randomized clinical trial that demonstrated a 53% reduction in aneurysm-related death in the screened group.[397]

Patients who present electively must be fully examined to determine their general fitness for surgery and the state of their distal vasculature. Patients with comorbid medical pathology should be made as fit as possible prior to surgery. There is evidence that preoperative β-blockade reduces cardiac death and myocardial infarction in the perioperative period.[398] Aortic dilatation may be confirmed by plain radiograph (Fig. 10.67), ultrasound scanning (Fig. 10.68) or CT scanning (Fig. 10.69). Magnetic resonance imaging can also be used in the identification of an inflammatory aneurysm.[399] All these scans allow a more accurate assessment of the width and extent of the aneurysm. Ultrasound is the least expensive, but spiral CT gives a more

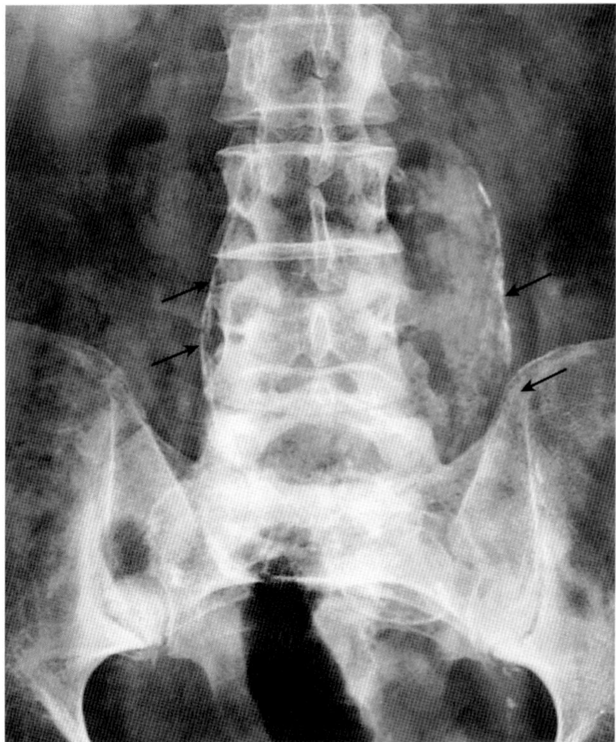

Figure 10.67 A plain abdominal radiograph of an abdominal aortic aneurysm, showing calcification in the wall and a soft tissue mass.

REFERENCES

396. Thompson MM, Bell PR. Br Med J 2002; 320: 1193
397. Ashton HA, Buxton MJ et al. Lancet 2002; 360: 1531
398. Poldermans D et al. N Engl J Med 1999; 341: 1789
399. Tennant WG, Hartnell GG, Baird RN et al. J Vasc Surg 1993; 17: 703–709

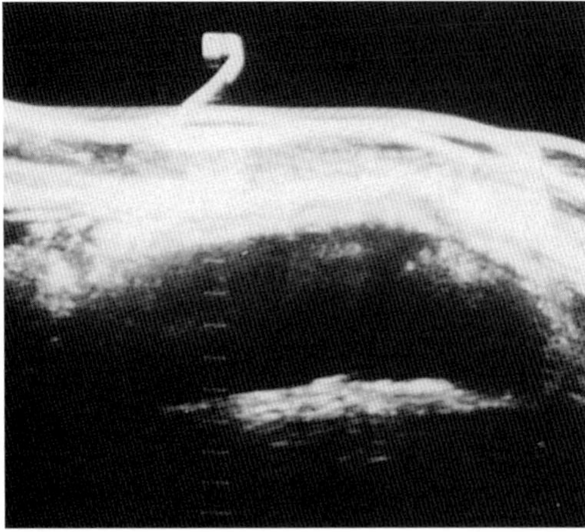

a

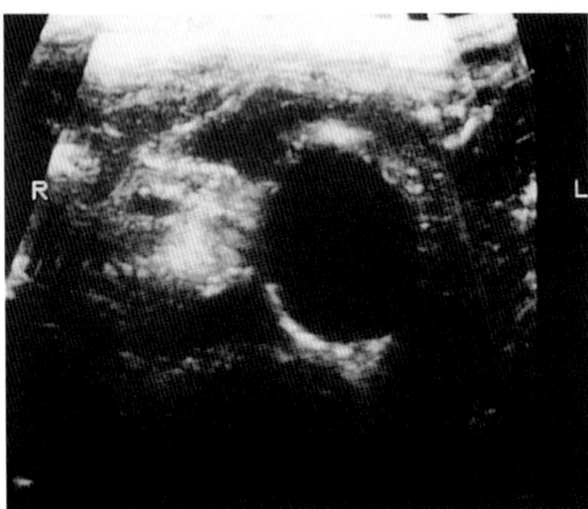

b

Figure 10.68 An ultrasound scan of an abdominal aortic aneurysm: (a) longitudinal and (b) transverse.

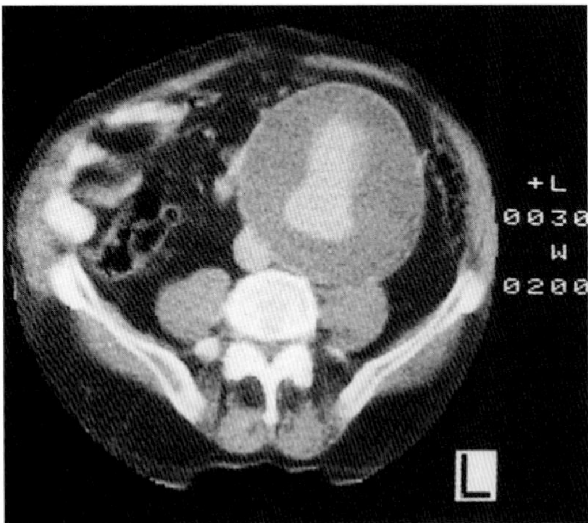

Figure 10.69 A CT scan showing a large aortic aneurysm.

accurate size estimation and has the advantage that the renal arteries and periaortic structures can usually be clearly seen. Arteriography is obtained if involvement of the renal arteries is suspected, or the state of the distal vascular tree is in doubt (Fig. 10.70).[400]

An elevated erythrocyte sedimentation rate and/or C-reactive protein should arouse suspicion of inflammatory change,[401] which can be confirmed by CT or MRI scan (see Fig. 10.19).[402]

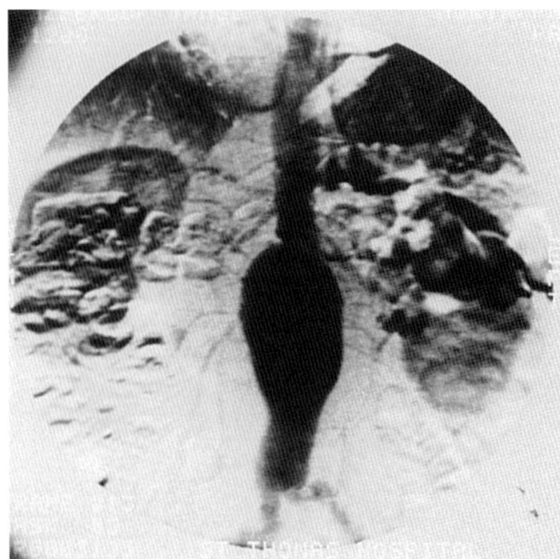

Figure 10.70 A digital subtraction arteriogram showing the extent of an abdominal aneurysm.

The aetiology of inflammatory aneurysms (periaortic fibrosis) is not known, but surgery is invariably difficult because of varying degrees of retroperitoneal fibrosis, occasionally because of involvement of the renal vein at the neck, and difficult access to the iliac vessels. There are a number of anecdotal reports on steroid therapy to reduced the size of the inflammatory mass.[403] There is an association between an inflammatory aneurysm and retroperitoneal fibrosis. The ureters may have to be lysed at the time of aneurysm surgery, although insertion of lighted double-J stents can also be used to ensure patency of the ureter and identification at the time of surgery.[403]

Ruptured and symptomatic abdominal aortic aneurysms require emergency or urgent surgical repair, unless this is prohibited by coexistent pathology. The decision to repair a symptomless abdominal aortic aneurysm must be made on an individual basis, because the risks of operation must be balanced against the risk of death from ruptured aneurysm. The main factors in this equation are the maximum size of the aneurysm and the general health of the patient. The risk of aneurysm rupture is related to the maximum aortic diameter. Exact rupture rates are difficult to estimate, but pooling of available data and information from a prospective study suggest that the annual rupture rate starts to increase exponentially above aneurysm diameters of 5.5 cm.[404] The decision to repair abdominal aortic aneurysms less than 5.5 cm is still controversial. Two multicentre trials have reported the results of randomization between early surgery and ultrasound surveillance in patients with aneurysms 4.0–5.5 cm in diameter.[404,405] These studies failed to show any advantage for early surgery, although most patients in the observation arm eventually had aneurysm repairs.

REFERENCES

400. Brewster DC, Retana A et al. N Engl J Med 1975; 292: 822
401. Walker DI, Bloor K et al. Br J Surg 1972; 59: 609
402. Baskerville PA, Blakeney CG et al. Br J Surg 1983; 70: 381
403. Bainbridge ET, Woodward DAK. J Cardiovasc Surg 1982; 23: 365
404. Lederle FA, Wilson SE et al. N Engl J Med 2002; 346: 1437
405. UK small Aneurysm Trial Participants. Lancet 1998; 352: 1649

Patients who are found to have a 6-cm diameter aneurysm should be offered surgical repair, providing they are reasonably fit and can be expected to survive the operation. The risk of smaller aneurysms rupturing is much less. Aneurysms that are greater than 7 or 8 cm are very liable to rupture, and such patients should be offered early operations.[406] The growth rate of aneurysms is unpredictable but may be monitored by serial ultrasound examinations.[407]

Elective aortic aneurysm repair

The aorta is approached as described on p. 230/231. The neck of the aneurysm is defined and controlled, and the iliac arteries are dissected free. After heparin has been given and clamps have been applied, a tube graft is inlayed into the aorta if the iliac arteries are not severely diseased. The lumbar arteries and inferior mesenteric artery are sewn off if they bleed. Aortoiliac or femoral bypass is required if the iliac arteries are aneurysmal or occluded. At least one internal iliac artery must be revascularized to avoid colonic or buttock ischaemia. The inferior mesenteric artery can be reimplanted if colon ischaemia is apparent.

The mortality for elective aortic aneurysm repair should be between 5 and 8%,[408–410] and a 2–4% mortality has been achieved in some selected series.[411–414] In the immediate postoperative period, myocardial ischaemia is responsible for the majority of deaths. Other common early complications include respiratory and renal failure, bleeding, and prolonged ileus. In the longer term, graft infection may lead to septicaemia, sinus formation or aortic graft–enteric fistula, which requires removal of the graft and restoration of the distal blood flow by an axillobifemoral graft or venous composite graft.[415] This complication should be suspected in patients presenting with an upper gastrointestinal bleed who have previously had an aortic aneurysm repair. Prophylactic antibiotics and careful wrapping of the graft by the aneurysm sac or omentum may reduce the incidence of this complication. Early graft occlusions are rare in patients with aneurysms.

False aneurysms usually develop at groin anastomoses and require reoperation, excision of the false sac, and reanastomosis.[416] This complication usually develops several years after the initial operation. Myocardial infarction, deep vein thrombosis, pulmonary embolism, chest infection, stroke and multisystem organ failure are all recognized complications.

Endovascularly placed stent grafts

The first endovascular repair of an abdominal aortic aneurysm was performed in the early 1990s,[417] but the technique has become widespread in the past 5 years. Endovascular aneurysm repair relies on the endoluminal placement of a covered endoprosthesis to exclude the aneurysm sac from the circulation, facilitating aneurysm thrombosis, and thus reducing the risk of aneurysm rupture.

Endovascular aneurysm repair is not feasible in all infrarenal aneurysms because of morphological constraints. To ensure adequate fixation of the proximal endograft, there is an obligatory requirement for a length of normal aorta immediately distal to the renal arteries. In addition, favourable proximal neck morphology must be present. This means that there must be minimal angulation, absence of thrombus, and a parallel-sided neck (not cone-shaped). The neck should have a diameter of less than 32 mm and there should be suitable iliac landing sites. These should not be aneurysmal and the iliac tortuosity should not be excessive. Adequate access must be available through the iliac system. Only half of all abdominal aneurysms can be treated by endovascular techniques.[419]

The advantages of endovascular aneurysm repair are related to avoiding the abdominal incision, and the need for aortic clamping. Comparative studies have demonstrated that endovascular aneurysm repair causes less derangement of the heart, lungs and gastrointestinal tract than conventional surgery, and reduces the need for organ support, transfusion and analgesia.[420] Endovascular repair may be utilized in situations where standard open surgery is difficult. Ninety-five per cent of patients selected for endovascular aneurysm repair have a successful procedure without the need for revisional open surgery, and the early mortality rate may be as low as 1–2%.[421]

The long-term durability of these procedures remains a problem, however, and there are specific, procedure-related complications of stent migration, endoleak and device failure, all of which can cause late aneurysm rupture. There is as yet no fully reliable long-term follow-up. Registry data suggest that the annual incidence of endoleak may be as high as 10%, and the late aneurysm rupture rate is 1%.[422] This is worrying because most aneurysms treated by endovascular repair are small, and the rupture rate of aneurysms below 5.5 cm diameter is 1% per year. The Endovascular Aneurysm Repair (EVAR) trials in the UK are randomizing medically fit patients to conventional or endovascular surgery (EVAR 1), and unfit patients to endovascular surgery or best medical therapy (EVAR 2). Endovascular repair may at present be recommended in high-risk patients, or in those with contra-indications to conventional surgery. Patients with a long life expectancy and medically fit for conventional surgery may be better served by a definitive open procedure.

Measurement of the length and the diameter of the neck of the aortic aneurysm is extremely important, because each graft must fit perfectly and is therefore usually slightly oversized. The diameter is measured by spiral CT scan, and the length by performing angiography with a catheter marked at 1-cm intervals (Fig. 10.71).

The endovascular graft consists of a vascular prosthesis supported by metallic stents, compressed inside a sheath (Fig. 10.71). The device is usually deployed via bilateral femoral arteriotomies, although aorto-uniiliac prostheses can be used (Fig. 10.72).[418] Straight grafts are no longer used because of the high incidence of endoleak.

A bifurcated prosthesis is inserted into the aorta via the femoral arteries. The graft is assembled within the aneurysm sac using a main body and a contralateral iliac limb. Aneurysms

REFERENCES

406. Darling RC. Am J Surg 1970; 179: 397
407. Bernstein EF, Dilley RB et al. Surgery 1976; 80: 765
408. Fielding JWL, Black J et al. Br Med J 1981; 283: 355
409. Berridge D, Chamberlain J et al. Br J Surg 1995; 82: 906
410. Kazmers A, Jacob L et al. J Vasc Surg 1996; 23: 191
411. Soreide O, Lillestol J et al. Surgery 1982; 91: 188
412. Campbell WB, Collin J, Morris PJ. Ann R Coll Surg Engl 1986; 68: 275
413. Whittemore AD, Clowes AW et al. Ann Surg 1980; 192: 414
414. Mutirangura P, Stonebridge PA et al. Br J Surg 1989; 76: 1251
415. O'Brien T, Collin J. Br J Surg 1992; 79: 1262
416. Szilagyi DE, Smith RF et al. Surgery 1975; 78: 800
417. Parodi JC, Palmaz JC, Barone HD. Ann Vasc Surg 1991; 5: 491
418. Ingle H, Fishwick G et al. J Endovasc 2002; 9: 481

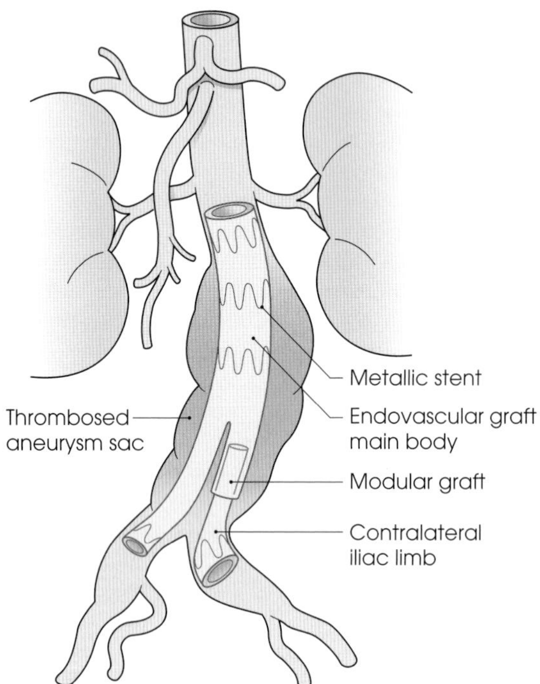

Figure 10.71 An endovascular modular stent graft placed in an abdominal aortic aneurysm.

that are excluded from the circulation usually decrease in size, and patients with significant endo-luminal leaks have sacs that continue to expand and remain at continued risk of rupture.[423]

Ruptured abdominal aortic aneurysm

Patients with ruptured abdominal aneurysms present as emergencies with severe abdominal pain and shock. The pain commonly radiates to the back, and patients often collapse with the onset of pain. The finding of a tender pulsatile central mass on examination of the abdomen clinches the diagnosis, but hypotension may render the mass impalpable, and signs of hypovolaemia may predominate. Mesenteric thrombosis, myocardial infarction, acute pancreatitis, perforated peptic ulcer, ureteric calculus and mesenteric volvulus are other diagnoses that must be considered. Dilatation of the femoral or popliteal arteries corroborates the diagnosis. Abdominal radiographs may show calcification in the wall of the aneurysm, and the psoas shadow may be lost.

Computerized tomography scanning may confirm a localized haematoma in patients with pain and no signs of shock (Fig. 10.19a), but this investigation may be falsely negative and is only indicated if the patient is in a stable condition.[424] An electrocardiogram and chest radiograph may be helpful as part of the initial assessment, but urgent surgery should not be delayed by over-investigation, and once the diagnosis has been made the aim should be to get the patient to theatre as quickly as possible.

Ten or 12 units of blood should be urgently cross-matched, but grouped uncross-matched blood can be given before cross-matched blood is available. It is unwise to resuscitate the patient over-vigorously until the aorta has been cross-clamped, because a reactionary haemorrhage may prove fatal as the blood pressure rises. Patients with severe hypotension and hypovolaemia must, however, receive blood or plasma expanders to produce a recordable blood pressure. A urinary catheter and a number of intravenous lines should be inserted, one of which should be a central line. The patient should have a crash induction of anaesthesia in theatre, having already been prepared and draped, with the surgeon poised to open the abdomen the moment that anaesthesia is established. A cell salvage device is a useful adjunct.

The abdomen is swiftly entered through a long midline incision, the diagnosis is confirmed, and the aneurysm neck is rapidly controlled by the application of a clamp. Many different approaches have been described to isolate the neck of the aneurysm in order to apply the clamp; using two suckers, a direct approach through the haematoma after exteriorizing the bowel is usually straightforward. The haematoma often facilitates the dissection. If difficulties arise with severe, uncontrolled bleeding, a clamp may be applied to the suprarenal aorta below the diaphragm for a short period, or alternatively an occluder can be used to compress the supracoeliac aorta at the same level. A large Foley catheter on an introducer can also be inserted through the rupture, and the balloon blown up in the upper aorta to control haemorrhage.[425] It is even possible to insert a Fogarty catheter into the aorta above the aneurysm via a cut-down in a peripheral artery before the aneurysm is opened.[426] The right colon and duodenum can be mobilized to the left if access to the neck of the aneurysm is difficult. The aorta is then approached from the right side, avoiding the haematoma. Once the haemorrhage has been controlled, vigorous resuscitation restores blood volume, blood pressure and urine output, which may be further stimulated by mannitol, diuretics and dopamine, although there is little evidence that these urinary stimulants have any effect other than to please the surgeon and anaesthetist!

Repair of a leaking aneurysm then proceeds using identical techniques to those employed for elective repair (Fig. 10.73). Occasionally the neck of the aneurysm is so poor that sutures cut out. In this situation the anastomosis can be buttressed with a Teflon® strip or pledglets. Under exceptional circumstances the aorta can be closed off with a suture, balloon, or even an orthopaedic staple, before an axillobifemoral graft is used to restore blood flow to the legs.[427]

Results

Many patients with aortic aneurysms that rupture fail to reach hospital,[428] when sudden death is often ascribed to other causes, but of those reaching hospital, the mortality rate should be less than 50%. A 32% mortality rate has been achieved.[429] Death is commonly the result of renal failure, uncontrolled bleeding, myocardial infarction, and respiratory and multisystem organ failure. Some encouraging results have been reported using endoluminal repair for ruptured abdominal aortic aneurysms;

REFERENCES

419. Schumacher H, Allenberg JR, Eckstein HH. Br J Surg 1996; 83: 949
420. Boyle JR, Goodall S et al. J Endovasc Ther 2000; 7: 359
421. Vallabhaneni SR, Harris PL. Eur J Radiol 2001; 39: 34
422. Harris PL, Vallabhaneni SR et al. J Vasc Surg 2000; 32: 739
423. Parodi JC. J Vasc Surg 1995; 21: 549
424. Senapati A, Hurst PAE et al. J Cardiovasc Surg 1986; 27: 719
425. Wyatt AP. Ann R Coll Surg Engl 1976; 58: 52
426. Hyde GL, Sullivan DM. Surg Gynecol Obstet 1982; 154: 197
427. Berguer R, Scheider J, Wilner HI. Surgery 1978; 83: 425
428. Armour RH. Br Med J 1977; ii: 1055
429. Jenkins AM, Ruckley CV, Nolan B. Br J Surg 1986; 73: 395
430. Hinchliffe RJ, Yusuf SW, Macierewicz JA et al. Eur J Vasc Endovasc Surg 2001; 22: 528

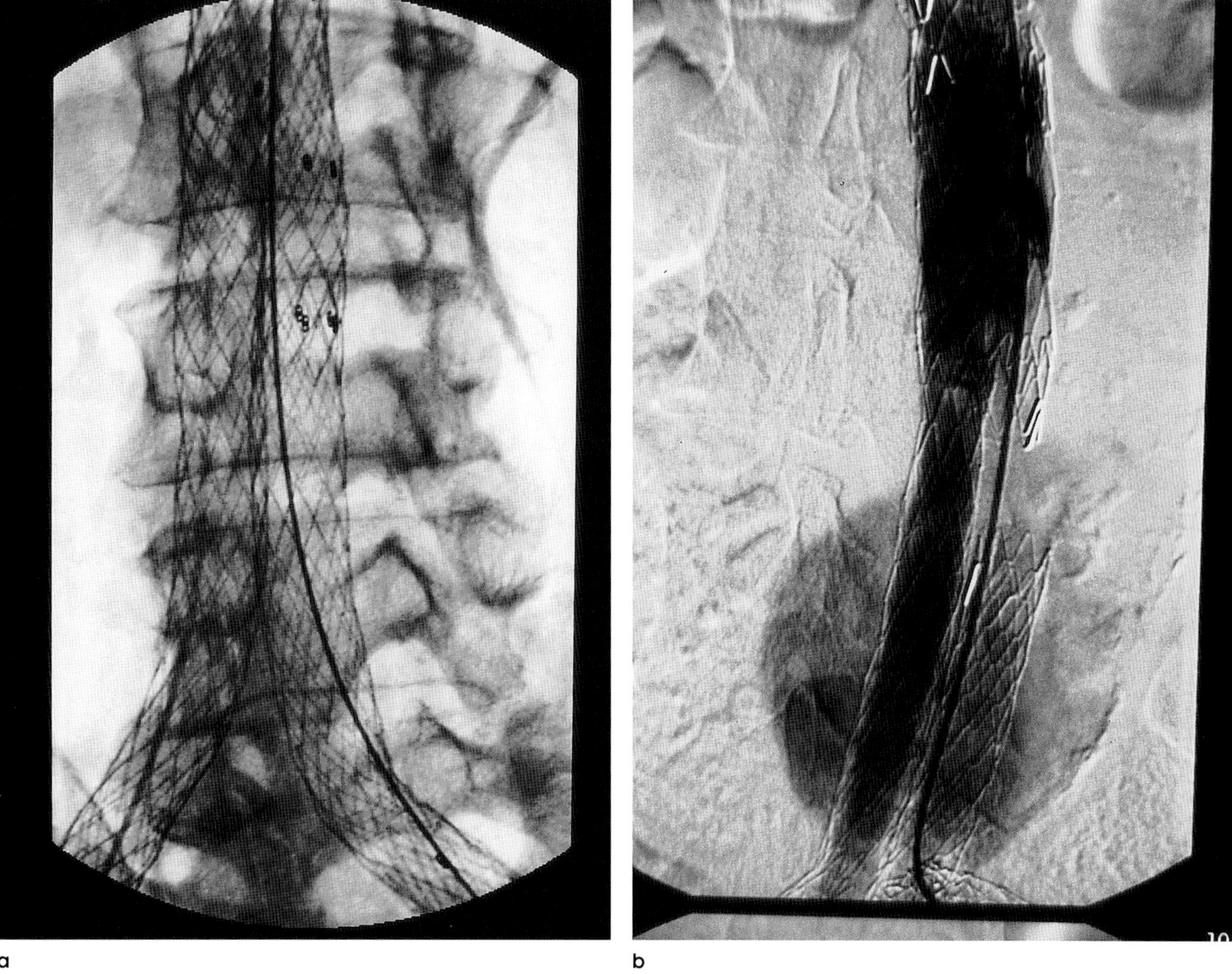

a b

Figure 10.72 (a) Aortic stent graft; (b) dislocation of an isolated iliac limb causing a type III endoleak.

however, the numbers are small and the cases are probably highly selected.[430] Large randomized trials need to be conducted to assess the role of endoluminal repair for ruptured abdominal aortic aneurysms.

Complications of surgery

Graft infections may lead to septicaemia, sinus formation, or aortic graft–enteric fistula, which requires removal of the graft and restoration of the distal blood flow by an axillobifemoral or composite vein graft.[415,431] This should be suspected in patients presenting with an upper gastrointestinal bleed who have previously had an aortic aneurysm repair. Prophylactic antibiotics and careful wrapping of the graft by the aneurysm sac or omentum may reduce the incidence of this complication. Early graft occlusions are rare in patients with aneurysms. Mesenteric ischaemia may be treated by reimplantation of the inferior mesenteric artery, but when established requires bowel resection (see Chapter 27).

False aneurysms usually develop after groin anastomoses, and require reoperation, excision of the false sac, and reanastomosis.[416] This complication usually develops several years after the initial operation. Myocardial infarction, deep vein thrombosis, pulmonary embolism, chest infection, stroke and multisystem organ failure are all recognized complications following emergency surgery on aneurysms.

Femoral artery aneurysms

Aneurysms of the femoral artery are usually part of a generalized arterial dilatation, although isolated aneurysms of the common femoral vessels are recognized.[432] The majority are symptomless; they rarely rupture but they may be a source of distal emboli and they occasionally thrombose. A pulsatile swelling in the femoral triangle must be differentiated from other masses in this region. Confirmation of an expansile mass makes other diagnoses unlikely. Repair is by insertion of a prosthetic graft or reversed saphenous vein (although this is rarely of sufficient size) between

REFERENCES

419. Schumacher H, Allenberg JR, Eckstein HH. Br J Surg 1996; 83: 949
420. Boyle JR, Goodall S et al. J Endovasc Ther 2000; 7: 359
421. Vallabhaneni SR, Harris PL. Eur J Radiol 2001; 39: 34
422. Harris PL, Vallabhaneni SR et al. J Vasc Surg 2000; 32: 739
431. Hannon RJ, Wolfe JH, Mansfied AO. Br J Surg 1996; 83: 654
432. Cutler BS, Darling RC. Surgery 1973; 74: 764

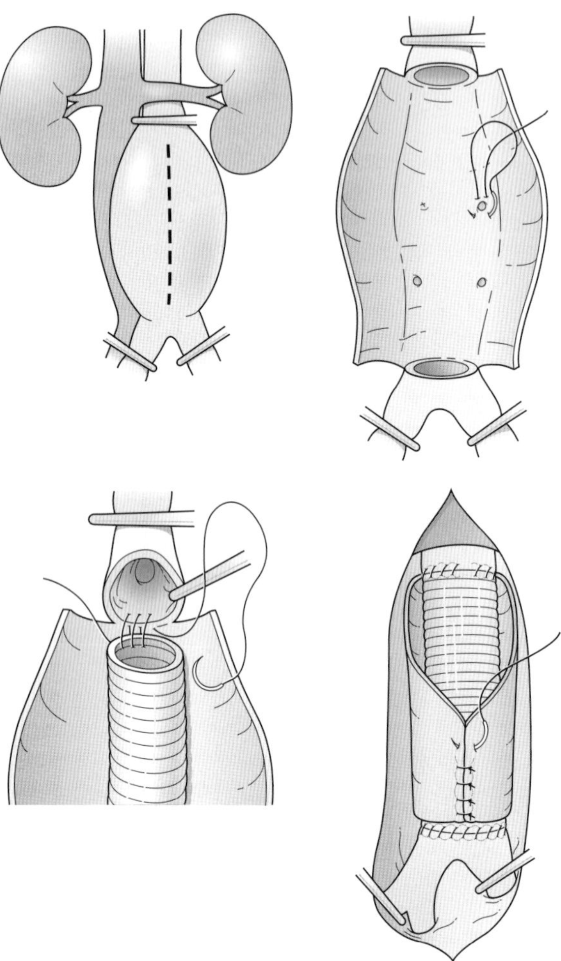

Figure 10.73 The technique for repairing an abdominal aortic aneurysm.

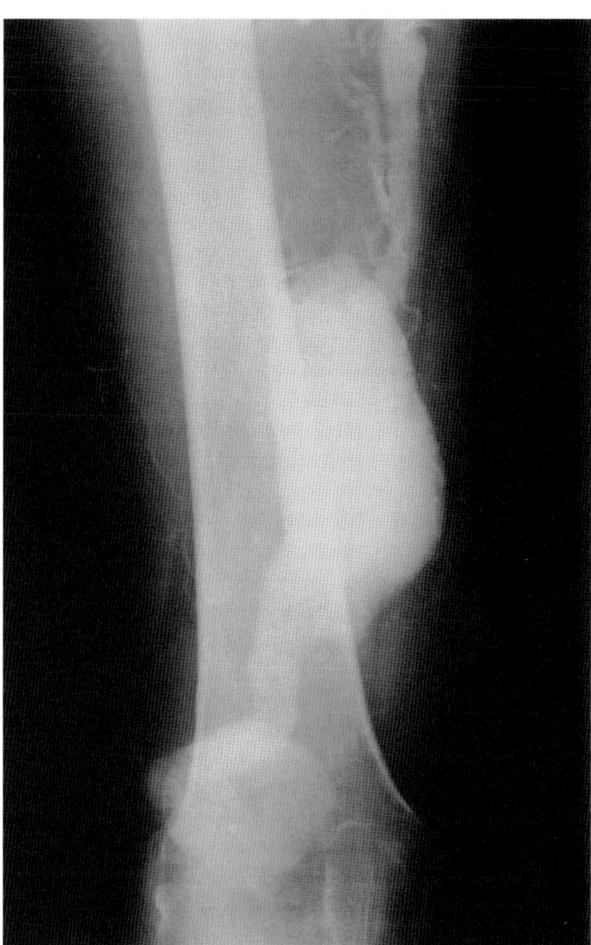

Figure 10.74 An arteriogram showing a popliteal aneurysm.

the external iliac artery and the superficial femoral artery, incorporating the profunda artery orifice if possible in the distal anastomosis. The profunda artery may be separately anastomosed to the graft if it cannot be retained on the lower patch. Aneurysms of the profunda femoris artery are rare but do occur.[433] They can usually be safely ligated but can be resected and replaced if necessary.

Popliteal artery aneurysms

The popliteal artery is the second most common site of aneurysms, accounting for 70% of all peripheral aneurysms.[434] Popliteal aneurysms occasionally present as large pulsatile masses noticed by the patient or physician, but are much more commonly diagnosed when the patient presents with peripheral ischaemia from embolization of contained thrombus or when the aneurysm itself thromboses. Popliteal artery aneurysms are often part of arteriomegaly with multiple sites of aneurysmal dilatation. The diagnosis can be confirmed by arteriography, ultrasound or CT scan (Fig. 10.74),[435] and femoral arteriography or duplex scanning is also helpful to assess the patency of the crural vessels.

A symptomatic popliteal aneurysm should be treated by vein bypass with either resection, or proximal and distal ligation of the aneurysm, and replacement by a vein bypass graft (Fig. 10.75) to avoid the considerable risk of gangrene and limb loss.[436] It is important to open the sac and ligate all the geniculate branches to avoid continued aneurysmal dilatation. The approach is otherwise similar to a femoropopliteal vein bypass graft. In an acutely ischaemic limb, infusions of streptokinase or tissue plasminogen activator should be given to lyse the thrombus before the aneurysm is repaired.[437] Alternatively, the thrombus may be retrieved at operation and the run-off lysed intraoperatively.

There is still debate over the management of symptomless popliteal aneurysms. Some suggest that all should be repaired to prevent the disastrous consequences of thrombosis,[438] while others argue that surgery carries risks that may outweigh the natural history of the disease, and recommend conservative management until thrombosis occurs.[439] A consensus approach recommends repair of popliteal aneurysms that exceed 2.5 cm in diameter, especially if they contain a large amount of thrombus.

Innominate and extracranial carotid arteries

Many so-called ‘aneurysms’ in these sites are produced by tortuous, kinked and atherosclerotic vessels. These are called student’s aneurysms. True aneurysms do rarely occur and may

REFERENCES

433. Symes JM, Eadie DG. J Cardiovasc Surg 1973; 14: 220
434. Linton RR. Surgery 1949; 26: 41
435. Davis RP, Neiman ML et al. Arch Surg 1977; 112: 55
436. Graham AR, Lord RSA et al. Aust NZ J Surg 1983; 53: 99
437. Ramesh S, Michaels JA, Galland RB. Br J Surg 1993; 80: 1531
438. Halliday AW et al. Ann R Coll Surg Engl 1991; 73: 771
439. Hands LJ, Collin J. Br J Surg 1991; 78: 996

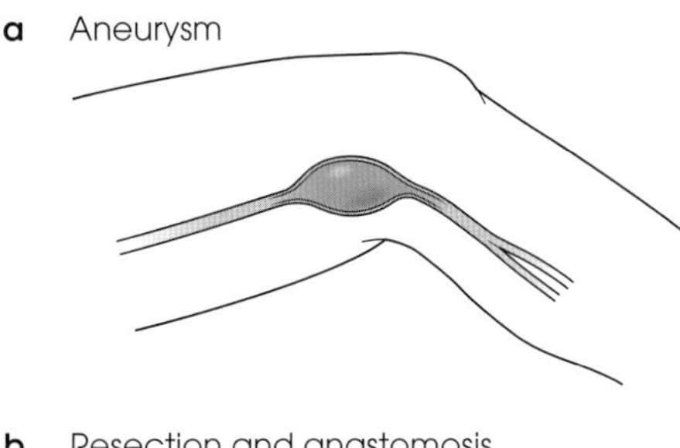

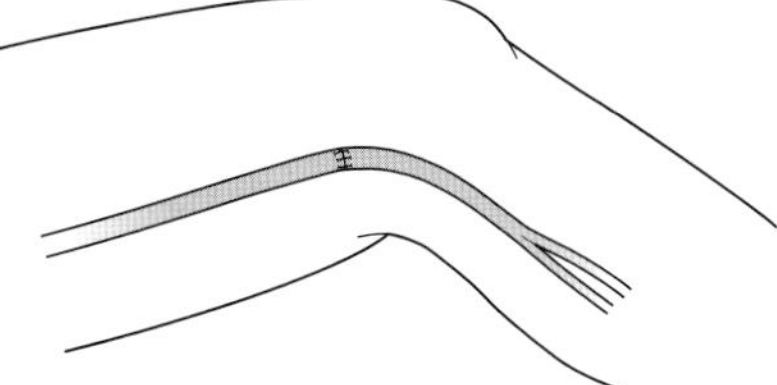

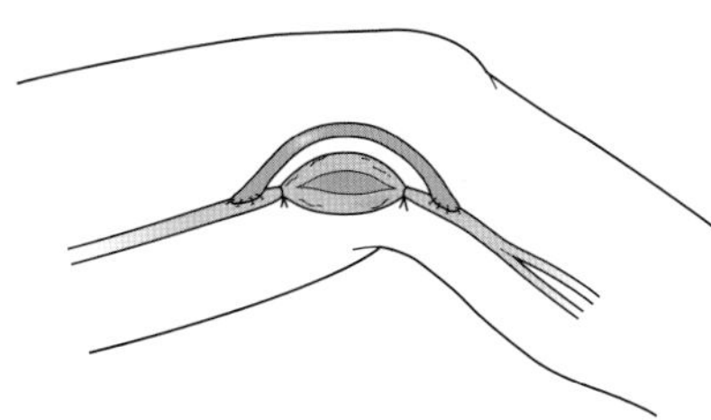

Figure 10.75 The techniques used to repair a popliteal aneurysm.

require resection and replacement, especially if they are a source of emboli.

Subclavian and axillary arteries

Subclavian aneurysms used to develop in dock labourers and coal heavers, but mechanization has almost abolished this particular occupational hazard; aneurysms of these vessels are now usually found in relation to a cervical rib as a poststenotic dilatation. The use of stent grafts should be avoided because they are likely to undergo structural failure due to the repeated entrapment between the first rib and clavicle. Axillary aneurysms used to occur in patients using crutches but are rarely seen today.

Radial arteries

Radial artery aneurysms are usually traumatic or iatrogenic false aneurysms, and are most commonly seen after insertion of radial artery catheters. They can be treated by proximal and distal ligation if the Allen's test (page 202) is normal, or the artery can be reconstructed using vein if the vascularity of the hand is in doubt.

Splenic, hepatic, mesenteric and renal artery

Aneurysm of the splenic artery is the second most common intra-abdominal aneurysm (0.01–0.08%), affecting women four times as commonly as men, principally during the childbearing years.[440] They are normally symptomless unless they rupture. This is the only important complication and it occurs in a quarter of all cases. Rupture is most likely in the third trimester of pregnancy. Portal hypertension and pancreatitis are both thought to predispose to splenic aneurysm formation. The chance finding of a ring of calcification in the epigastrium or left hypochondrium on a plain abdominal radiograph (Fig. 10.76) may allow the diagnosis to be made before rupture. Operation is indicated for aneurysms greater than 3 cm in diameter and in pregnant patients.[441] Aneurysms can be excised and the artery reconstituted by end-to-end anastomosis or an interposition graft. If reconstruction is difficult or impossible, ligation on either side of the aneurysm does not always presage splenectomy. Splenic artery aneurysms have also been induced to thrombose by percutaneous embolization.[442]

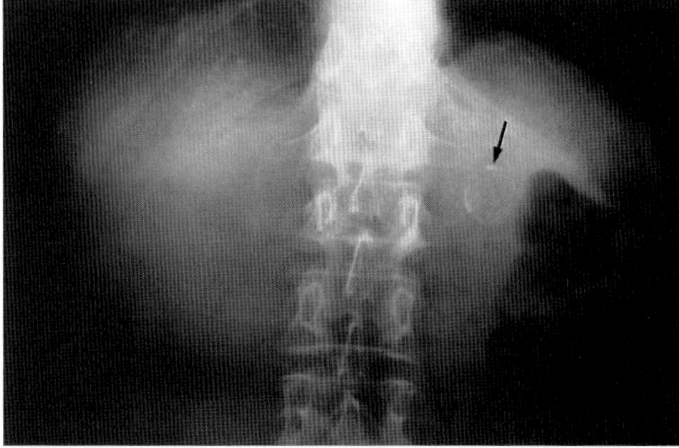
a

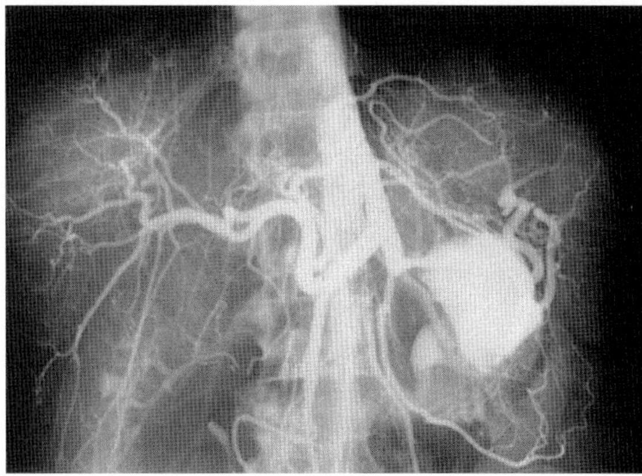
b

Figure 10.76 (a) A ring of calcification in the wall of a splenic artery aneurysm. (b) An arteriogram of a splenic artery aneurysm.

Hepatic artery aneurysms, which are one-third as common as splenic aneurysms, commonly present when they rupture into the biliary system or the peritoneal cavity. Intrabiliary rupture produces abdominal pain, gastrointestinal bleeding and jaundice. Excision of the aneurysm and, if possible, reconstruction of the artery by a vein graft are required for large extrahepatic aneurysms, although aberrant anatomy or good collaterals may make reconstruction unnecessary.[443] Intrahepatic and extrahepatic saccular aneurysms are best treated by therapeutic embolization.[444]

Coeliac (Fig. 10.77) and mesenteric artery aneurysms usually present with non-specific abdominal pain, which may or may not

REFERENCES

440. Stanley JC, Fry WJ. Surgery 1974; 76: 898
441. Trastek VF, Bairolero PC et al. Surgery 1982; 91: 694
442. Probst P, Castaneda-Zuniga WR et al. Diagn Radiol 1978; 128: 619
443. Dwight RW, Ratcliffe JW. Surgery 1952; 31: 915
444. Kadir S, Athanasoulis CA et al. Radiology 1980; 134: 335

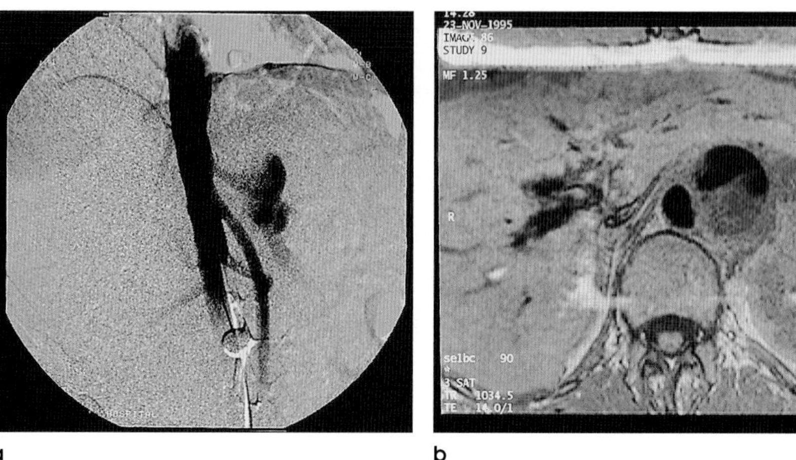

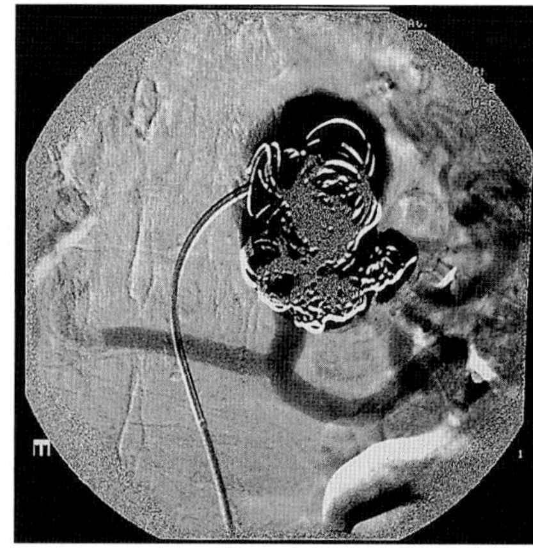

a b c

Figure 10.77 Coeliac artery aneurysm: (a) arteriogram, (b) MRI scan, and (c) with coils inserted.

be associated with a mobile pulsatile mass. They are often mycotic and may be related to pancreatitis, biliary sepsis and intravenous drug abuse. Surgical resection and reconstruction are required, but the collateral circulation is often good enough to maintain viability if the aneurysm is ligated.[445] More recently, these aneurysms have been treated by therapeutic embolization. Renal artery aneurysms are rare, and are often associated with hypertension. They are usually saccular and found at the bifurcation of the renal arteries. They are commonly the result of medial necrosis, but atherosclerosis and fibromuscular hyperplasia may also be causative factors. Rupture is unusual but can occur in pregnancy. These aneurysms normally present as a chance finding during the investigation of hypertension. They can usually be safely ignored, but occasionally large aneurysms require excision, cold perfusion, bench surgery, and reimplantation of the kidney into the pelvis.

Aneurysms of the intracerebral arteries are discussed in Chapter 15.

ARTERIAL EMBOLISM AND ACUTE THROMBOTIC ISCHAEMIA

An embolus is the passage of matter from one part of the circulation to another through a vascular lumen. The common site of origin of arterial emboli is the myocardium, the most frequent cause being thrombus in the atrial appendage secondary to atrial fibrillation.[446]

Mural thrombus on a myocardial infarct is another important source of embolism. Endocarditis on a rheumatic heart valve is rare, but acute bacterial endocarditis after intravenous drug abuse with unsterile needles is an important source of peripheral emboli. Occasionally, emboli may derive from prosthetic cardiac valves. Small emboli may also originate from mural arterial disease anywhere within the vascular tree—so-called 'artery-to-artery' emboli. Thrombus within an aneurysm may become dislodged, as may platelet aggregates or cholesterol debris from the surface of an atherosclerotic plaque. The former, like cardiac emboli, may occlude major vessels, while the latter usually produce small distal infarcts or temporary ischaemia (e.g. the blue toe syndrome). Cholesterol emboli are now a well-recognized complication of balloon angioplasty and endovascular stenting. Tumour emboli and paradoxical emboli are rare causes of arterial embolization. Tumour emboli are almost always microscopic, but large macroscopic tumour emboli may occasionally be encountered and left atrial myxoma is a well-recognized but rare source of peripheral embolism.[447] Paradoxical embolism occurs when a venous embolism, derived from a deep vein thrombosis, passes into the systemic arterial circulation via a large congenital communication between the right and left heart circulation.[448] Very rarely, a bullet may pass through the arterial circulation,[449] and other foreign bodies, such as intravenous catheters or disrupted prosthetic cardiac valves, may also embolize.

Emboli usually lodge at the bifurcation of the aorta or in the femoral, popliteal, brachial or carotid arteries; they may also lodge in branches of the aorta. The effects of embolism depend on the site of obstruction, the level of occlusion, the potential for collateral formation, and the speed of collateral development. Small emboli of platelet aggregates or cholesterol debris arising from the arch of the aorta and extracranial vessels are the most frequent cause of amaurosis fugax and transient ischaemic attacks (see pages 199–225). In the upper limb, small peripheral emboli may arise from a subclavian aneurysm complicating a cervical rib (see page 213). These may cause distal vasospasm and secondary Raynaud's syndrome, or even small areas of digital gangrene in the tips of the fingers. Distal emboli may also affect the lower limbs; they may arise from aortic atherosclerosis and aortic, femoral and popliteal aneurysms. These cause vasospasm and occlusion of the distal vessels, leading to claudication, rest pain, and eventually frank gangrene. Cutaneous gangrene secondary to small peripheral emboli has a characteristic appearance, with showers of dark spots appearing at multiple sites in the foot (Fig. 10.15). This appearance is almost pathognomonic of peripheral emboli but must be differentiated from polycythaemia or a platelet abnormality.

An embolus of vegetations arising on a heart valve with bacterial endocarditis may lodge at an arterial bifurcation, where it can erode the arterial wall and produce a mycotic aneurysm.

REFERENCES

445. Deterling RA. J Cardiovasc Surg 1971; 12: 309
446. Baxter-Smith D, Ashton F, Slaney G. J Cardiovasc Surg 1988; 28: 453
447. Mercier AL, Suggon MG et al. Am J Cardiol 1978; 41: 437
448. Thompson T, Evans W. Q J Med 1930; 23: 135
449. Cooper FW, Harris MH, Kahn JW. Ann Surg 1948; 127: 1

The incidence of this complication has declined with the reduced incidence of bacterial endocarditis and the advent of effective antibiotics. Air embolism is a rare condition that may cause cerebral infarction and cardiac arrest. Fat embolism may complicate the recovery of patients with multiple fractures (see Ch. 52). The fat globules that enter the circulation usually impact in the brain and lungs, causing hypoxia and confusion. It is not appropriate to discuss amniotic emboli here because they are almost exclusively a gynaecological problem.

CLINICAL FEATURES

Large emboli present with symptoms of acute arterial occlusion beyond the point of obstruction. Embolism is no longer the most common cause of acute lower limb ischaemia in western nations; that distinction now belongs to acute thrombosis on pre-existing atheroma.[450] It is often difficult to distinguish between the two pathologies on clinical grounds. When there is a potential embolic source and there is no history of claudication or other evidence of significant atherosclerosis, an embolism is the most likely cause. Most patients, however, present a diagnostic challenge, with some blurring of the classical picture. It is then helpful to obtain an angiogram, which is preferable to blind exploration. It not only assists diagnosis, but also provides access for thrombolysis. Pain, pallor, and paralysis with muscle tenderness and a greater than six hour history indicate the heed for urgent revascularisation.

Other causes of acute arterial occlusion that must be considered include an aortic dissection and a thrombosed aneurysm, the latter especially at the popliteal site. Acute traumatic occlusions and occlusions secondary to arteritis rarely cause diagnostic difficulty. Acute occlusions can also be caused by arterial entrapment and congenital abnormalities of the arterial wall, such as cysts.

INVESTIGATIONS

Angiography usually shows an occlusion with a sharp cut-off at the upper end (Fig. 10.78), and there may be evidence of occlusion in other vessels, suggesting fragmentation or multiple emboli. Collaterals are usually poor unless there is coexisting atherosclerosis, when even angiography may fail to distinguish the two conditions. An electrocardiogram and chest radiograph—along with a full blood count, and urea and electrolyte estimation—should be obtained before operation. Transoesophageal echocardiography is the best way of demonstrating residual thrombus within the heart. It also delineates valvular disease and anatomical abnormalities such as a patent ductus or an atrial septal defect.[451] This investigation is obtained after the embolus has been treated, when it will influence the strategy for preventing recurrent emboli.

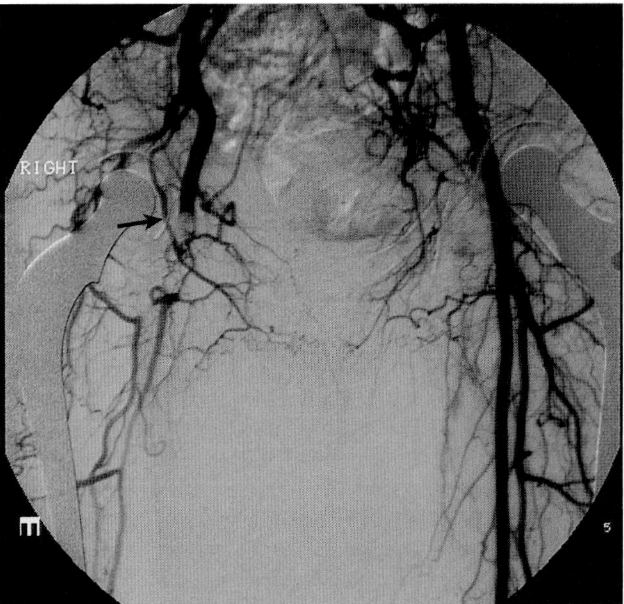

Figure 10.78 An arteriogram showing an occlusion of the right femoral artery with a sharp cut-off indicative of an embolic occlusion.

MANAGEMENT

In a few patients the embolus passes into a small peripheral vessel and disintegrates, causing minimal symptoms that quickly resolve. Under these circumstances it is only necessary to determine the source of embolus and prevent recurrence, usually by anticoagulation. In the majority of patients, persistence of acute ischaemia demands more active management by operative embolectomy or catheter-directed intra-arterial thrombolysis. It is wise to commence full anticoagulation with intravenous heparin once acute ischaemia has been diagnosed. This measure is essential to prevent thrombus propagation in the relatively static columns of blood distal and proximal to the site of arterial occlusion. Surgeons should also remember not to devote all their attention to the peripheral problem; patients with emboli are systemically unwell, usually from a cardiac cause. It is the central, not the peripheral, problem that mainly accounts for the mortality rate of up to 30% that is associated with major arterial embolism to the lower limbs,[452] and it is wise to involve a physician or cardiologist at an early stage of management.

Surgical embolectomy

The operation may be performed under local, regional or general anaesthesia, depending on the patient's fitness. When local anaesthetic is used, an anaesthetist should be present throughout the proceedings to monitor the patient. Both common femoral arteries are exposed through vertical or oblique groin incisions and controlled if a saddle embolus has lodged at the aortic bifurcation. The deep and superficial femoral arteries are also exposed and encircled with slings. An arteriotomy is made without the application of clamps if no pulsation is felt in the vessels. Thrombus may be encountered in the lumen, or there may be a small amount of back-bleeding from collaterals. This is easily controlled by temporary application of clamps or by traction on the slings. A Fogarty balloon catheter[453] of Fr gauge 4 or 5 is passed up from both groins into the abdominal aorta. The balloon is inflated and the catheter withdrawn (Fig. 10.79a). This should extrude the embolus from the arteriotomy and establish down-flow. A Fr gauge 3 or 4 catheter is then used to clear any fragmented embolus or propagated thrombus from the distal femoral vessels (Fig. 10.79b). When the distal vessels have

REFERENCES

450. Mills JL, Porter JM. Ann Vasc Surg 1991; 5: 96
451. Lagattolla N, Burnand KG, Stewart A. Br J Surg 1995; 82: 1651
452. Murie JA, Mathieson M. J Cardiovasc Surg 1987; 28: 516
453. Fogarty TJ, Cranley JJ et al. Surg Gynecol Obstet 1963; 116: 241

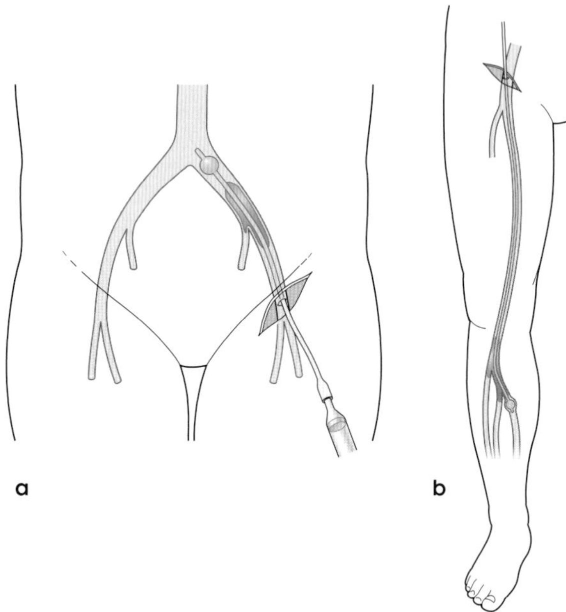

Figure 10.79 The technique of embolectomy.

been cleared there should be adequate backflow. A perioperative angiogram should be obtained at this point to ensure that all distal emboli have been removed. Anticoagulation may have to be continued long term, depending on the cause of the embolism; in such circumstances warfarin is substituted for heparin.

Variations

The aorta may have to be explored if satisfactory inflow cannot be established. When the catheter will not pass proximally with ease, the probable cause is atherosclerosis; if it passes easily but no blood flow is obtained on withdrawal, the probability of aortoiliac dissection should be considered.

Poor backflow despite the easy passage of the catheter distally to the ankle may indicate residual thrombus in the tibial vessels. This can be confirmed by perioperative angiography. Further passage of the catheter may complete the removal of distal emboli or thrombus. If not, the tibial vessels may be individually swept by a small Fogarty catheter inserted via an arteriotomy in the infrageniculate popliteal artery. Perioperative thrombolysis via the common femoral arteriotomy is another option. This is performed by injecting a lytic solution into the vessels and allowing a suitable time for clot dissolution. Although early reports of the use of streptokinase were disappointing, more recent studies using streptokinase (100 000 units in 100 mL of normal saline infused over 30 min) or urokinase have been more encouraging.[454] Tissue plasminogen activator may also be effective.[455]

The popliteal artery may have to be explored if poor backflow is still obtained or the operative arteriogram shows that there is residual thrombus within the crural vessels. Further passage of balloon catheters into the crural arteries should enable complete removal of distal emboli, but occasionally these vessels need to be exposed at the ankle. Arteriotomies in the popliteal artery and distal vessels need to be carefully closed with vein patches.

Thrombosis in the microcirculation is likely if adequate revascularization is not achieved despite good inflow to the groin and clear distal vessels. This may result in limb loss. Occlusive atheromatous disease is present if the Fogarty catheter will not pass to the ankle; in this situation a bypass graft, from the common femoral to the popliteal artery or crural vessel, may save the limb. An operative arteriogram may indicate potential target vessels. Emboli can also be removed from the femoral, popliteal and brachial bifurcations using the same techniques, and mesenteric emboli can also be removed by balloon catheter (see Ch. 27).

Thrombolysis

Streptokinase, urokinase and tissue plasminogen activator can be infused directly into an embolus or thrombus developing at a site of pre-existing atheroma via a small-calibre catheter inserted percutaneously.[456] The most common route is via the common femoral artery in the groin, the catheter being advanced distally if the occlusion is in the leg vessels, or proximally over the aortic bifurcation to the contralateral side if the iliac vessels are occluded. Fibrinolysis is also now used to remove emboli, but it is particularly useful for acute on chronic ischaemia secondary to thrombosis. In either case, it can be used only if the state of the limb allows, i.e. if sensation and motor power have not been lost. If, on the other hand, the neurological deficit is marked, operation should be undertaken, because there is inadequate time for lysis to be effective before irreversible ischaemic change occurs. Other contraindications to lysis include conditions with a risk of haemorrhage, a stroke within the preceding 2 months, and major surgery within the preceding few days. Many dosage and time regimens have been described, and time to lysis can be reduced by using a spray catheter and injector programmed to deliver the lytic solution in pulses, the so-called 'pulse spray' technique.[457] Using such modern systems, a mean time to lysis of less than an hour has been achieved in some cases but, because lysis cannot be guaranteed, surgery will still be preferable if the situation is critical. Lysis of iliac thrombus can be dangerous, because it can cause major problems if it migrates into the distal limb vessels.

It should be appreciated that the technique of intra-arterial thrombolysis is evolving, and no established technique has yet been developed. Angiographic patency can be achieved in up to 90% of selected cases, but the clinical results are not as good because a fair proportion of arteries reocclude.[458] Although the delivery of the lytic agent directly into the embolus or thrombus aims to prevent widespread systemic lysis, the technique is nevertheless associated with significant bleeding complications, and its use should be restricted to vascular surgical units with experienced interventional radiological and surgical staff. A controlled trial in patients with subacute peripheral ischaemia showed that thrombolytic therapy produced fewer complications and had a lower mortality than immediate surgical revascularization. The limb salvage rate was similar in the two groups.[459]

REFERENCES

454. Beard JD, Nyamekye I et al. Br J Surg 1993; 80: 21
455. Ad Hoc Committee on Clinical Research. J Vasc Surg 1992; 15: 886
456. Braithwaite BD, Earnshaw JJ. Br J Surg 1994; 81: 1705
457. Yusuf SW, Whitaker SC et al. Eur J Vasc Endovasc Surg 1995; 10: 136
458. Andaz S, Shields DA, Scurr JH et al. Eur J Vasc Surg 1993; 7: 595
459. Ouriel K, Shortell CK, DeWeese JA. J Vasc Surg 1994; 19: 1021
460. Blaisdell FW, Steele M, Allen RE. Surgery 1978; 84: 822

Complications and results of surgery

The mortality associated with surgical embolectomy remains depressingly high at between 10 and 20%.[452,460] This is largely the result of the poor general condition of the patients, especially those with emboli arising from mural thrombus on a myocardial infarct. A significant proportion of patients who present after a prolonged period of acute ischaemia develop severe metabolic problems after revascularization. This is usually the result of large amounts of potassium, myoglobin, and other toxic metabolites being released back into the systemic circulation following the restoration of the blood supply.[461] Cardiac arrest and renal failure may ensue. Glucose and insulin, mannitol and haemodialysis may be helpful in reducing some of these complications.[462] Restoration of blood flow may also cause compartment syndromes; fasciotomies should be performed if this complication is considered probable and are essential if it occurs. Ischaemic contractures (e.g. Volkmann's) may develop if there is a delay in restoring the blood supply in the face of severe ischaemia. Amputation may be necessary if the limb remains ischaemic after all reasonable attempts at revascularization. Delayed embolectomy can be carried out successfully up to a few weeks after the acute event, providing irreversible ischaemia has not developed and the embolus has not become too adherent to the arterial wall.[463]

ARTERIAL VASOSPASM (VASOMOTOR DISEASE)

Arterial spasm may be either a primary vasomotor malfunction or may be secondary to another pathological process affecting the vessel wall. A number of primary vasomotor disturbances are recognized by the appearances they produce, but their aetiology still remains largely conjectural. These disorders include Raynaud's disease, acrocyanosis, erythrocyanosis frigida and erythromelalgia. The vasospasm of the first three conditions is precipitated by cold, while arterial vasodilatation in erythromelalgia appears to be related to venous congestion, warmth or pressure.[464] The primary vasospastic disorders cause considerable misery in cold climates, where numb and painful digits may progress to ulceration and even frank necrosis and gangrene during winter months (Fig. 10.80).

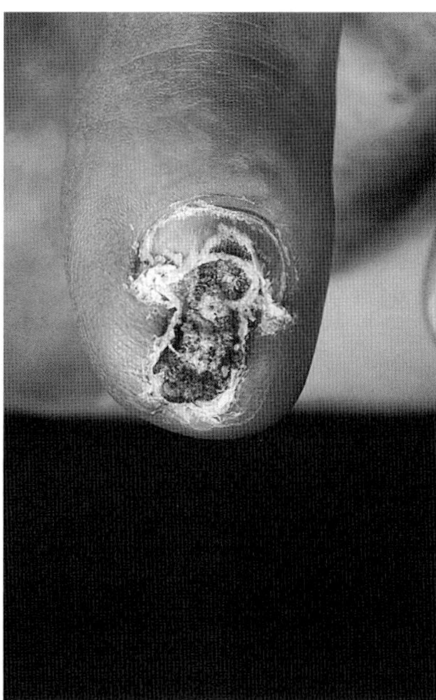

Figure 10.80 Raynaud's disease with necrosis of fingertips.

Vasomotor changes can follow division of peripheral nerves and are common after poliomyelitis. Paralysed limbs may become cold, oedematous and cyanotic. Sympathectomy is beneficial if severe chilblains or cutaneous necrosis develops.[465] Collagen diseases, repeated trauma, nerve damage, obliterative vascular disease, vessel entrapment syndromes, and certain drugs and poisons may all cause secondary vasospasm and must be differentiated from a primary disorder.[466] Collagen diseases, in particular, give rise to severe vasospasm in the small arteries of the hand, foot, toes and fingers, with a greater incidence of digital necrosis and gangrene than is found in the primary vasospastic disorders.

Arterial spasm may complicate intraluminal thrombosis or embolism, and is also an important cause of morbidity after inadvertent intra-arterial injection of noxious substances including thiopentone, other barbiturates, venous sclerosants, quinine and hypertonic solutions. Spasm also occurs after poisoning by arsenic, heavy metals and ergot.

RAYNAUD'S PHENOMENON (OR SYNDROME) AND RAYNAUD'S DISEASE

Maurice Raynaud published his thesis on local asphyxia and gangrene of the extremities in 1862.[467] He described a set of symptoms in a series of patients, and this collection of symptoms came to be called Raynaud's disease. In 1946, Lewis suggested that the term *Raynaud's disease* should be reserved for those patients with typical symptoms of intermittent digital vasospasm in whom no cause could be found,[468] while *Raynaud's phenomenon* or *syndrome* should be applied to patients with an established cause.[469] It has been suggested that most patients thought to have primary Raynaud's disease actually have some autoimmune abnormality, and the term may become obsolete as new causes for the phenomenon are established. The episodic digital ischaemia is provoked by emotion, trauma, hormones and drugs, in addition to the normal cold trigger.

Raynaud described three classic phases: local syncope or blanching of the digits from digital arterial spasm; local asphyxia or cyanosis, when the fingers become swollen, blue and painful from stagnant anoxia; and recovery or reactive hyperaemia, when the fingers become red and tingling as the accumulation of metabolites causes vasodilatation. These attacks are episodic, and can occur in either the fingers or toes in response to cold or emotional stimuli. Many attacks do not pass through all the colour changes described here, with either blanching or cyanosis predominating and the hyperaemic phase often being dimly

REFERENCES

461. Haimovichi H. Surgery 1979; 85: 461
462. London PS. J Hosp Med 1968; 1: 312
463. Ammann J, Seiler H, Vogt B. Br J Surg 1976; 63: 73–76
464. Lewis T. Clin Sci 1933; 211: 175
465. Kinmonth JB, Rob CG, Simeone FA. Vascular Surgery. Arnold, London, 1962
466. Rivers SP, Porter JM. In: Bergan JJ (ed). Arterial Surgery. Churchill Livingstone, Edinburgh, 1984
467. Raynaud M. On Local Asphyxia and Symmetrical Gangrene of the Extremities. New Sydenham Society, London, 1888
468. Lewis T. Vascular Disorders of the Limbs. Macmillan, London, 1946
469. Allen EV, Brown GE. Am J Med Sci 1932; 183: 187

Box 10.1 Diseases associated with Raynaud's colour changes

Connective tissue disorders
- Systemic sclerosis (scleroderma)
- Systemic lupus erythematosus
- Polyarteritis nodosa
- Rheumatoid arthritis
- Sjögren's syndrome

Arterial disease
- Atherosclerosis
- Buerger's disease (thromboangiitis obliterans)
- Embolism from cervical rib

Trauma
- Vibration-induced white finger
- Sequel to frostbite

Blood disorders
- Cold agglutinins
- Cryoglobulinaemia
- Hyperviscosity (polycythaemia)

Drugs
- Oral contraceptives
- β-Blockers

perceived. The spectrum of attacks ranges from mild episodic pallor and paraesthesiae to constant pain, ulceration and frank necrosis (Fig. 10.80). Box 10.1 lists some of the many diseases that have been associated with Raynaud's colour changes.

Pathophysiology

Fixed obstruction of the small vessels may predispose to Raynaud's phenomenon without any increase in vasomotor activity, as a normal response to a cold challenge may cause temporary closure of the already diseased small vessels; a proximal occlusion may produce a similar effect by reducing the distal pressure and flow. In patients with normal vessels, there is evidence that there is some fault in the α-receptors of the vascular smooth muscle.[470] This local fault must be an abnormality either of smooth muscle contraction or of arterial wall elasticity. Much work has centred on associated haemorheological faults; hyperviscosity, platelet dysfunction, hyperfibrinogenaemia, cold agglutinins and cryoglobulins have all been incriminated as a cause of vasospasm in some patients.

Clinical features

Between 60 and 90% of all sufferers from Raynaud's phenomenon are women. The majority are teenagers or young adults at onset.[471] The prevalence of this condition is said to range from 5 to 20%,[472] but the criteria accepted for diagnosis are fairly non-specific and are influenced by the ambient temperature. Environmental factors obviously affect the prevalence of the condition, with half of the food-processing employees exposed to intermittent hot and cold conditions being affected,[473] and a similar proportion of those who constantly use vibrating tools.[474] The diagnosis is usually made from the clinical history of the attacks, but some use digital plethysmography and cold provocation tests as a means of confirmation.[475] Doppler mapping after cold stimulation may be a useful method of quantifying the severity of attacks.[476] Unilateral disease suggests a local organic cause such as a thoracic outlet syndrome or disease of the arterial wall, but unilateral vasospasm is also recognized.

The fingers of patients with Raynaud's syndrome often appear red or reddish blue between attacks; the skin is usually dry and the nails brittle. Trophic changes develop in the finger pulps in more advanced cases, with chronic paronychia, ulceration and gangrene (Fig. 10.80). The wrist pulses are normally present; their absence suggests that the Raynaud's syndrome is secondary to disease of the large vessels. The neck must be examined to exclude cervical ribs, aneurysms and bruits (see page 213). Digital pulses may be insonated with Doppler ultrasound and the pattern of occlusion after cold provocation can be recorded.[477] Arteriography is indicated if proximal atherosclerosis or digital occlusions are suspected. Plethysmography reveals low flow, and thermography shows a temperature gradient developing between the hand and the fingers during body cooling and rewarming. Raynaud's phenomenon must be distinguished from acrocyanosis and other vasospastic disorders, including the normal cold response. Once a diagnosis of Raynaud's phenomenon is made, a battery of tests is indicated to exclude a possible cause. A full blood count and measurements of urea and electrolytes, erythrocyte sedimentation rate, cryoglobulins, antinuclear factor, rheumatoid antibodies, and antimitochondrial and antithyroid antibodies should all be obtained.[478] When there is a history of dysphagia, a barium swallow may confirm the disordered peristalsis that is found in patients with scleroderma.

Management

Patients must be advised to keep warm and to avoid going out in ice and snow without gloves. Some may be able to move to a warm climate, and if this opportunity is available it should be taken. Cigarette smoking should be abandoned, and β-blockers and ergot-containing drugs should be avoided. Heated gloves may be helpful in reducing the number of attacks in winter.[479]

Numerous vasodilatory drugs such as inositol nicotinate, thymoxamine and naftidrofuryl oxalate have been tried and may help some patients.[480] Reserpine in a dose of 0.25 or 0.5 mg has a proved effect,[481] but it can cause depression and other unpleasant side effects. It, like guanethidine, can be used intravenously; reserpine has also been given intra-arterially.[479] Methyldopa and prazosin have also been used with some success,[482] and calcium-blocking agents such as nifedipine have gained in popularity.[483] The serotonin antagonist ketanserin has also been used to treat

REFERENCES

470. Jamieson GG, Ludbrook J, Wilson A. Circulation 1971; 44: 254
471. Olsen N, Nielsen SC. Scand J Clin Lab Invest 1978; 37: 761
472. Heslop J, Coggon D, Acheson ED. J R Coll Gen Pract 1983; 33: 95
473. Mackiewisz A, Piskortz A. J Cardiovasc Surg 1977; 18: 151
474. Taylor W. The Vibration Syndrome. Academic Press, London, 1974
475. Rosch J, Porter JM, Gralion BJ. Circulation 1977; 55: 807
476. Krakenbuhl B, Nielsen SL, Lassen NA. Scand J Clin Lab Invest 1977; 37: 71
477. Yao JST, Gourmos G et al. Surg Gynecol Obstet 1972; 135: 373
478. Porter JM, Rivers SP et al. Am J Surg 1981; 142: 183
479. Kempson GE, Coggon D, Acheson ED. Br Med J 1983; 286: 268
480. Coffman JD. N Engl J Med 1979; 300: 713
481. Krakenbuhl B, Nielsen SL, Lassen NA. Scand J Clin Lab Invest 1977; 37: 71
482. Varadi DP, Lawrence AM. Arch Intern Med 1969; 124: 13
483. Kahan A, Weber S et al. Ann Intern Med 1980; 94: 546

Raynaud's disease.[484] Prostacyclin and prostaglandin E_1, orally or by intravenous infusion, have been used to good effect, especially in patients with digital gangrene.[485] Repeated plasmapheresis has helped some severely affected patients,[486] but its place in management of this condition is not fully established. The anabolic steroid stanozolol, which enhances fibrinolysis, reduced the severity and frequency of attacks in some patients but its value is unpredictable.[487] Oxypentifylline, another agent that reduces blood viscosity, may also be helpful,[488] and transdermal glyceryl trinitrate and prostaglandin analogues have been found to be of some benefit.[489]

Many patients with Raynaud's disease can achieve a satisfactory quality of life with minimal symptoms by cold avoidance, tobacco abstinence, using warm or heated gloves in the winter months, and taking vasodilatory drugs during severe attacks. A few, however, develop severe irreversible ischaemia of the digits and require more drastic measures. Regular prostacyclin or prostaglandin analogue infusions at 4–8-weekly intervals may tide some patients through severe winters, and others should be considered for cervical sympathectomy.[490] This operation usually produces a dramatic early benefit, but this is invariably short-lived and after a year or two there is usually only a marginal improvement. Developments in minimally invasive therapy have established the endoscopic transthoracic approach for cervical sympathectomy.

Prognosis

Raynaud's phenomenon is an incurable disorder that may be alleviated by a number of treatments, as outlined here. Severe ischaemia of the fingertips may have to be treated by amputation in a small proportion of patients (usually those with collagen diseases such as scleroderma, which invariably have a more severe course).

Those with occupational Raynaud's phenomenon should be encouraged to change jobs. In the first edition of this book, Aird emphasized the importance of vibration-induced white finger (occupational Raynaud's phenomenon) in cold riveters, and suggested that Sorbo pads in the gloves or on the handles of machines might help, together with a change to soft riveting every few months.

ACROCYANOSIS

Acrocyanosis is a generalized cyanosis of the hands, which follows exposure to cold and principally affects women. It is bilateral and symmetrical; although its intensity may vary, it is often associated with sluggish and awkward finger movements and a loss of sensation. As the attacks subside, the hands become warm, red, swollen and painful. Between attacks the hands remain cold and the palms feel sweaty.

In contrast to the digital artery spasm found in Raynaud's disease, the spasm of acrocyanosis occurs in the smaller arteries and arterioles, thus slowing the circulation through the capillary bed.[491] The stagnant anoxia that develops encourages the accumulation of metabolites that cause the capillaries to dilate, increasing stagnation and producing the typical cold, blue, cyanotic appearance. Cold avoidance is the mainstay of treatment, and the benefits of vasodilators and sympathectomy are usually marginal.

ERYTHROCYANOSIS FRIGIDA

This disorder, sometimes known as Bazin's disease,[465] affects healthy young women of stout build, with fat and often hairless legs. As in acrocyanosis, the capillaries dilate while the arterioles remain constricted. In cold weather, the legs develop dusky reddish purple blotches in the skin of the calf just above the ankles, and in severe cases the skin of the lower half of the leg is purple. The affected area blanches with pressure and is tender to friction, warmth and touch. Induration and nodularity are often palpable within the subcutaneous fat, and the skin overlying these chilblains often feels cold to the touch. These areas may ulcerate, and they then have to be differentiated from other types of cutaneous leg ulcers (see Chapter 11). In severe, long-standing cases the whole limb develops a solid and persistent oedema. Histology of the nodules shows areas of fat necrosis with occasional giant cells, which is why the condition was originally thought of as a form of cutaneous tuberculosis.[492]

Yet again, patients should be advised to protect themselves from the cold. Vasodilators and sympathectomy may be helpful in healing chilblains in the most severely affected cases. Weight loss is also advised.

ERYTHROMELALGIA

This condition is characterized by redness of the extremities, which is often associated with burning pain.[493] The erythema and pain are accentuated by dependence, and even by the pressure of bed coverings or shoes. The pain may be eased by elevating and cooling the limbs. Erythromelalgia is a rare disorder that affects women more than men, and it is usually worse in the summer months. The cause appears to be related to an inappropriate release of vasodilator substances, which dilate the capillaries and stimulate pain endings. Serotonin accumulation within the tissues may be responsible for the condition. Little has been added to this hypothesis in 20 years.

Erythromelalgia must be differentiated from polycythaemia, pernicious anaemia, Buerger's disease, gout, systemic lupus erythematosus, rheumatoid arthritis, venous insufficiency and peripheral neuritis. It may not be a distinct disorder. Treatment is empirical. Cooling may be helpful but is often unpredictable. Lumbar sympathectomy has helped some patients but in others the condition has been made worse,[465] and a local anaesthetic injection that allows the effect of sympathectomy to be evaluated should be tried first. Many patients are best treated by reassurance, combined with analgesic and psychotropic drugs where necessary. Aspirin, ergotamine and methysergide have also been used to treat the condition,[494] and the serotonin blocker ketanserin may also be worth trying. Nerve section has been used to relieve pain in patients with severe symptoms.

LIVEDO RETICULARIS

Livedo reticularis is another rare vasospastic disorder in which cyanotic blotchy mottling of the skin, especially of the lower

REFERENCES

484. Stranden E, Roald OK, Krohg K. Br Med J 1982; 285: 1069
485. Pardy BJ, Lewis JD, Eastcott HHG. Surgery 1980; 88: 826
486. Talpos G, White JM et al. Lancet 1978; i: 416
487. Jarrett PEM, Morland M, Browse NL. Br Med J 1978; 2: 523
488. Roath S. Br Med J 1986; 293: 88
489. Franks AG. Lancet 1982; i: 76
490. Baddeley RM. Br J Surg 1965; 52: 426
491. Stern ES. Br J Dermatol 1937; 49: 100
492. McGovern T, Wright IS. Am Heart J 1941; 22: 583
493. Weir Mitchell SW. Am J Med Sci 1878; 76: 2
494. Catchpole BN. Lancet 1964; i: 909

extremity, develops the appearance of an irregular network. This change has been linked to systemic lupus erythematosus and the anticardiolipin antibody.[495] The cutaneous changes are produced by spasm of the arterioles and dilatation of the capillaries and venules, causing local stagnation. The meshwork appearance may be the result of the anatomy of the cutaneous circulation, with the pale areas representing the sites of arterial inflow and the cyanotic lacework the sluggish peripheral capillaries and venules. Histological examination of the arterioles shows proliferation of the intima, with a perivascular infiltration of inflammatory cells. Apart from its bizarre appearances, the major reason for seeking advice is the development of cutaneous ulceration, which is often indolent and resistant to treatment.

Patients should be advised to avoid cold, and occasionally lumbar sympathectomy or prostaglandin infusions may help to heal ulceration.

ERGOTISM

A diet of rye contaminated by *Claviceps purpurea* causes dry gangrene of the extremities if ingested for long periods.[496] Chronic migraine sufferers may also overdose with ergotamine tartrate. There is a rapid response to withdrawal of the drug, providing gangrene has not become established. The chronic intake of ergot produces spasm of the small vessels and eventually intimal proliferation. Captopril, which inhibits angiotensin conversion, may be of specific benefit in reversing ergotamine-induced ischaemia.[497]

HYPERHIDROSIS

Hyperhidrosis is excessive sweating, which is unrelated to heat but often stimulated by anxiety. It affects the palms of the hands and the soles of the feet, although the whole body, especially the axillae and groins, may be involved. It is debatable whether hyperhidrosis is a true vasomotor abnormality, but Aird (in the 1st edition) classified it as such. It is no longer true to say that it is more common in men than in women: the reverse is true.[498] It is a social stigma that discourages physical contact. It also interferes with writing, and although ledgers are now a thing of the past, Uriah Heep is the archetypical hyperhidrosis patient. The feet may also be affected, but are rarely considered as important as the hands. The axillae are another common site for hyperhidrosis, leaving unsightly damp patches on the armpits of shirts, blouses and dresses.

Hyperhidrosis erythematosus traumatica is a rare occupational form of the condition in which excessive sweating occurs in skin that is in contact with a vibrating surface, especially a capstan lathe.[499] Symptoms disappear when the stimulus is removed. Hyperhidrosis can also occur on the face of patients with syringomyelia and in those with Frey's syndrome. The cause of the condition is not known, but thyrotoxicosis must always be excluded.[500]

Treatment

Regular painting with aluminium hexachloride solution or repeated subcutaneous botulinum toxin injections may reduce axillary hyperhidrosis,[501] but many patients request a permanent cure. Good results are obtained by excising the hair-bearing area of the axillary skin, and this is the treatment of choice for axillary hyperhidrosis.[502] Cervical sympathectomy is an effective way of abolishing excessive palmar sweating, and lumbar sympathectomy alleviates its plantar counterpart.[503] Cervical sympathectomy may be performed by the cervical,[504] transaxillary[505] or thoracoscopic route,[506] depending on surgical preference. Total sympathectomy may produce debilitating postural hypotension, and in addition excessive sweating around the midriff may be annoying.[507] This procedure is, if possible, best avoided. Cervical or thoracoscopic sympathectomy provides excellent and long-lasting relief of symptoms; however, the patient should be aware of the potential complications of pneumo- or haemothorax, Horner's syndrome, compensatory sweating and gustatory sweating.[508]

THE VASCULITIDES

The vasculitides are a group of diseases in which inflammatory cells (principally lymphocytes, plasma cells and histiocytes) invade the arterial wall, causing swelling and obstruction. A number of different patterns are seen, with varying outcomes.

THROMBOANGIITIS OBLITERANS (BUERGER'S DISEASE)

This disease, originally called endarteritis by von Winiwarter,[509] almost exclusively affects young men in their twenties or thirties who are tobacco addicts. Although it was first described in the American Jewish population,[510] it is now recognized in all races and appears to be particularly common in Arab, Indian and Chinese people.[511] Some have cast doubt on the existence of the condition, regarding it as a variant of accelerated atherosclerosis, but most regard it as a separate disorder.

Pathology

The distal (medium-sized) arteries of the lower limb become progressively obliterated, and these changes are also found in similar-sized arteries in the upper limb. Histology of the vessels shows a transmural round cell infiltration, which is associated with intimal proliferation. Luminal thrombosis is common. The accompanying veins and nerves may also become involved in the inflammatory process, and recurrent superficial venous thrombosis is quite common. Collagen is laid down around the vessels, encasing them in a thick fibrous coat. The vasculitis may rarely involve the intra-abdominal vessels, including the mesenteric and renal arteries, and may even occasionally affect the cerebral and coronary vessels.

REFERENCES

485. Pardy BJ, Lewis JD, Eastcott HHG. Surgery 1980; 88: 826
486. Talpos G, White JM et al. Lancet 1978; i: 416
496. Merhoff GC, Porter JM. Ann Surg 1974; 180: 773
497. Zimran A, Ofek B, Herschko C. Br Med J 1984; 288: 364
498. Ellis J. J R Coll Med 1982; 75: 555
499. Davies J. Br J Ind Med 1951; 8: 95
500. Ellis H. Br J Hosp Med 1972; 1: 641
501. Scholes KT, Crow KD et al. Br Med J 1978; 2: 84
502. Ellis H. Am J Surg 1976; 45: 546
503. Gillespie JA. Br J Hosp Med 1975; 418
504. Telford ED. Br J Surg 1935; 23: 448
505. Atkins HJB. Lancet 1949; ii: 1152
506. Hederman WP. In: Greenhalgh RM (ed). Vascular and Endovascular Surgical Techniques. WB Saunders, London, 1994: 281–284
507. White JC, Smitchwick RH. The Autonomic Nervous System. Kimpton, London, 1946
508. Greenhalgh RM, Rosengarten DS, Martin P. Br Med J 1971; 1: 332
509. von Winiwarter F. Arch Klin Chir 1879; 23: 203
510. Buerger L. Am J Med Sci 1908; 136: 567
511. Goodman RM, Ewan B et al. Am J Med 1965; 39: 601

Clinical features

Patients usually present with chronic paronychias, poorly healing ulcers, or digital gangrene. These symptoms may have been preceded by a history of claudication. Superficial and deep vein thrombosis may be the first manifestation of Buerger's disease in a few patients, and erythema nodosum is occasionally one of the presenting complaints. In the lower limbs the popliteal pulse is usually preserved, but the pedal pulses are often missing. The thickened vessels may themselves be palpable and tender. Buerger's disease must be differentiated from early-onset atherosclerosis, diabetic arterial disease, thrombocythaemia, polycythaemia, recurrent embolism from the heart or an aneurysm, thrombophlebitis migrans, rheumatoid arteritis, homocysteinaemia and Behçet's disease. Arteriography shows a characteristic pattern of normal proximal vessels and distal occlusions with many corkscrew collaterals (Fig. 10.81).[512] Biopsy of an occluded vessel may provide histological confirmation of the diagnosis,[513] but can risk making the ischaemia worse and may heal poorly. Circulating antibodies to collagen are present in the blood of 45% of patients with Buerger's disease, who often test positive for human leukocyte antigen B5.[514]

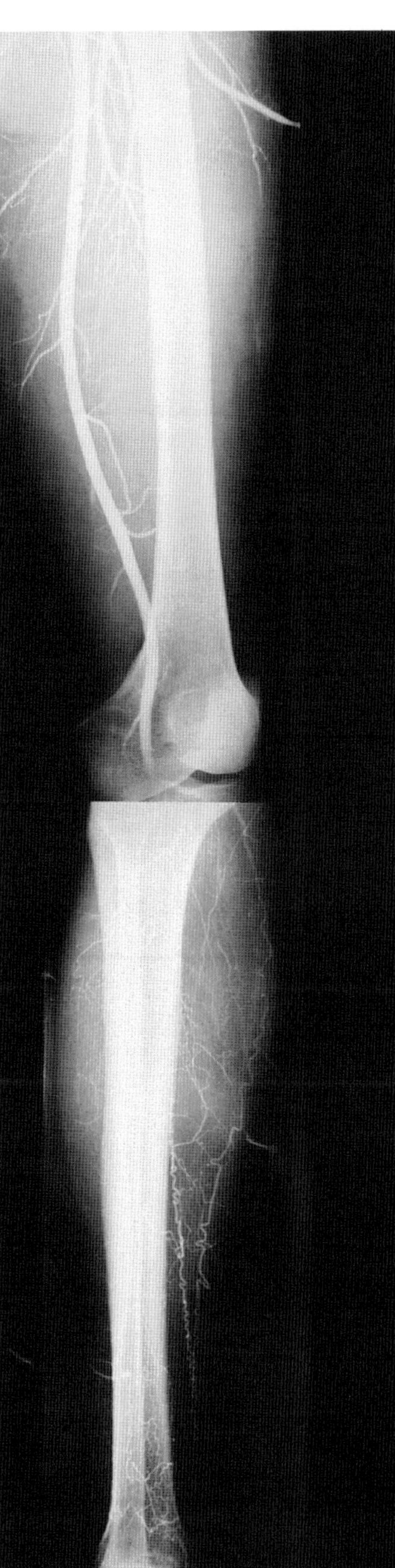

Figure 10.81 An arteriogram showing the typical features of Buerger's disease. The proximal arteries are normal. Multiple peripheral arterial occlusions are bypassed by corkscrew collaterals.

Management

Patients must be encouraged, bullied or cajoled to stop smoking. The risks of ignoring this advice must be clearly explained.[515] Progressive ischaemia leads first to digital and then more major amputations of all limbs. Sympathectomy often relieves rest pain and allows nail fold infection and small incipient patches of gangrene to heal.[516] It is particularly valuable in Buerger's disease, perhaps because there is an important element of arterial spasm in the affected vessels. Surgical rather than chemical sympathectomy is often preferred to ensure complete and permanent nerve section.

Lumbar sympathectomy

The lumbar sympathetic chain is approached through a transverse incision at the level of the umbilicus on the side to be denervated. The oblique muscles of the abdominal wall are split or divided in the line of the incision until the peritoneum is exposed. This is freed off the deep surface of the transversus abdominis muscle by blunt dissection, and retracted medially to allow the retroperitoneal space to be entered. The front of the psoas is displayed, and the groove between the medial border of psoas, the lumbar vertebrae, and the aorta on the left or the vena cava on the right is defined. The lumbar sympathetic chain can usually be palpated as a firm cord, punctuated by a number of swellings lying in the fibrofatty tissue of this groove on the front of the vertebrae. The chain is defined and picked up with a nerve hook, before it is dissected down to the pelvic brim and up to the crura of the diaphragm. All the rami that join the ganglia are divided. The first, second and third lumbar ganglia are resected. The wound is closed in layers with suction drainage.

Alternative treatments and progress

Apart from sympathectomy, there is little that avoids digital ablation, which is reserved for dead and devitalized tissue or bone. Bypass surgery is often impossible and fruitless, although it

REFERENCES

512. Szylagyi DE, Derusso FJ, Elliot JP. Arch Surg 1964; 88: 824
513. McKusick VA, Harris WS et al. JAMA 1962; 181: 5
514. McLoughlin G, Helsby R et al. Br Med J 1976; ii: 1165
515. Hill GL. Br J Surg 1974; 61: 476
516. Kunlin J, Lengua F et al. J Cardiovasc Surg 1973; 1: 21

can be successful.[517] Antibiotics, foot care, prostaglandins[518] and analgesics may all be tried in an attempt to tide patients over periods of acute ischaemia until collaterals develop. Many patients who cannot abandon smoking end up with one or more major amputations.

TAKAYASU'S DISEASE (PULSELESS DISEASE)

In 1908, Takayasu reported that young Japanese women developed a disease in which they lost pulses in one or more branches of the aortic arch.[519] It is now recognized that this disease occurs in occidental as well as east Asian people, and in men as well as women.[520] Many patients seen in the West have a Turkish and Middle Eastern ancestry. The symptoms depend on which vessel is affected, but disease in the carotid and subclavian arteries can cause transient ischaemic attacks, blindness, stroke or arm claudication, and ischaemia. Aortic disease must be differentiated from coarctation and produces similar symptoms. The aortic arch and its branches, the descending, thoracic and abdominal aorta, can all be affected. The arteritis gives rise to local pain, and is often accompanied by pyrexia, malaise, and an elevated sedimentation rate in the acute stage. Arteriography demonstrates a smooth, tapering stenosis (Fig. 10.82) or total occlusion. This disease can also give rise to aneurysm formation.

Surgical bypass to normal vessels beyond the limits of the disease is required for ischaemic symptoms, and has rewarding results.[521] The disease tends to burn itself out with time, and the place of steroids in reducing inflammation remains unproved. The same is true of azathioprine and cyclosporine. Five-year survival from the time of diagnosis ranges from 60 to 80%.[522,523]

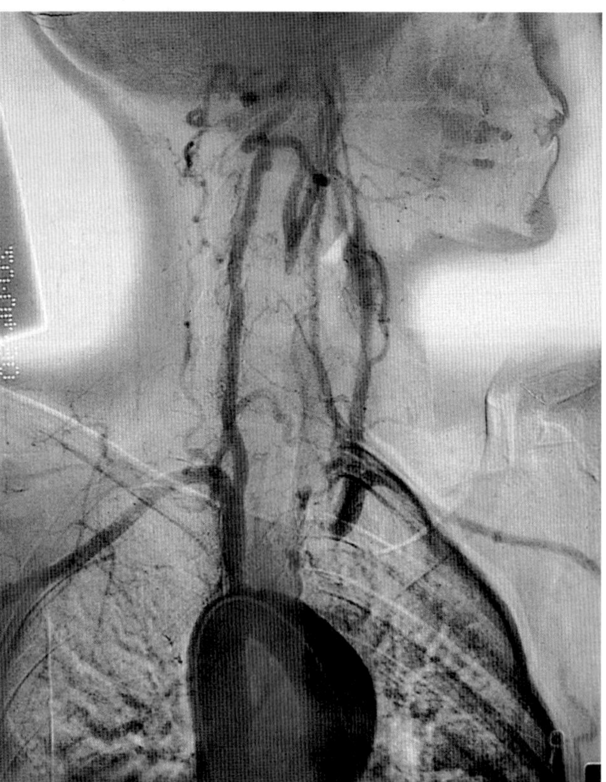

Figure 10.82 An arch arteriogram showing changes consistent with Takayasu's disease. The right and left common carotid arteries are occluded as is the left subclavian artery.

TEMPORAL ARTERITIS

This condition, first described by Jonathan Hutchinson in 1889,[524] is usually seen after the age of 60, and is twice as common in women as in men. The arteritis usually starts with malaise, fever and myalgia, which often persist for several months. A fronto-parietal headache then develops, and the skin over the affected area is tender to touch and sometimes red. The superficial temporal artery may be visible, thickened and tender, with absent pulsation. Visual loss occurs in between one-third and one-half of all cases; if this is left untreated it becomes permanent.[525] Retinoscopy is initially normal, but at a later stage ischaemic papillopathy develops and there may be evidence of occlusion of the central retinal artery or its branches. Ophthalmoplegia also occurs. There may be an associated arteritis in the peripheral vessels, causing, for example, brachial artery occlusion.

The diagnosis is usually made by taking a segment of the superficial temporal artery for biopsy under local anaesthetic, through an incision placed directly over the vessel. Histology shows a florid intimal thickening; a round cell infiltration through all coats of the arterial wall, which is associated with destruction of the internal elastic lamina; and the presence of a few giant cells. Treatment is by systemic steroids, which should begin immediately in large doses (60 mg of prednisone a day) but can then be reduced at a later stage.[526] Steroids reduce the incidence of blindness. Some 40% of biopsies do not show any of the characteristic histological features; if the diagnosis is strongly suspected on clinical grounds, treatment with steroids should be started without delay. Azathioprine may also be used to treat patients with this condition and has an important steroid-sparing role.[527]

VASCULAR TUMOURS

Angiomas have been discussed and are properly considered as malformations (hamartomas) rather than as benign tumours.

GLOMUS TUMOUR (ANGIOMYONEUROMA, GLOMANGIOMA)

This is the only true benign tumour of blood vessels. It is a small painful tumour originally described by Wood in 1829.[528] The glomus tumour lies in the skin but may grow into the deeper layers, although its greatest diameter is seldom more than a few millimetres. It usually has a well-marked capsule, especially on the deep surface of the tumour. Histologically the tumour consists of a tangled mass of blood vessels lined by a layer of flattened or swollen endothelial cells on a supporting fibrous

REFERENCES

517. Shionoya S, Ban I et al. Br J Surg 1976; 63: 841
518. Szczeklik A, Cryglewski RJ et al. Thromb Res 1980; 191: 1–15
519. Takayasu M. Acta Soc Ophthalmol 1908; 12: 554
520. Schire V, Asherton RA. Q J Med 1964; 33: 439
521. Fraga A, Mintz G et al. Arthritis Rheum 1976; 15: 617
522. Ishikawa IC. Circulation 1970; 57: 27
523. Urban-Waern A, Anderson P, Hemmingsson A. Angiology 1983; 17: 311
524. Hutchinson J. Arch Surg (Lond) 1889; 1: 323
525. Graham E, Holland A et al. Br Med J 198; 282: 269
526. Hunder GG, Sheps SG et al. Ann Intern Med 1975; 82: 613
527. Desilva M, Hazelman BL. Ann Rheum Dis 1986; 445: 136
528. Wood W. Trans Med Chir Soc Edinb 1829; 3: 317

stroma, surrounded by epithelial cells and smooth muscle fibres, the latter being well differentiated or taking the form of muscle fibrils within the epithelial cells. The epithelioid glomus cells, which have well-defined outlines, have short contractile fibrils within their cytoplasm; the glomus cells often lie both inside and outside the muscular layer of the vessel wall and are mixed up with myelinated and non-myelinated nerve fibres. The haemangiopericytoma first described by Stout and Murray[529] is a similar type of tumour but is not as painful or as vascular. The cutaneous myoma arising from the erector pili may also occasionally be mistaken for a glomus tumour.

Clinical features

Glomus tumours usually occur in the extremities; two-thirds are in the upper limb but some arise on the trunk. Half develop in the digits, one-third in a subungual position. Tumours tend to develop on the fingers and toes in women, while in men they are usually more centrally placed. The peak incidence is in the twenties. Less than 2% are painless.

Most tumours give rise to exquisite pain, which is burning, throbbing or bursting in nature, occurring in paroxysms that are brought on by pressure, heat or cold, although the pain can arise spontaneously. Relief is often sought by the application of heat or cold, and a bandage or glove is occasionally worn for protection. The pain may be localized or so diffuse that the tiny trigger spot cannot be located. The nail is often left uncut by the patient if the tumour is subungual; sudden unexpected trauma can cause fainting. Occasionally relief is obtained by gentle pressure to empty the tumour, rendering it colourless and painless for several hours. The pain is so disproportionate to the size of the tumour that a psychoneurosis may be suspected.

The pain may be precisely located by stroking the affected area with a pinhead. The pain pathways are not clearly understood because pain is not abolished by blocking both the sympathetic and somatic nerves. The affected extremity may occasionally become flushed and warm, or pallid, cold and sweaty. Most tumours are blue or purplish in colour; few are red. The colour may change with alteration in the position of the limb or compression of the feeding and draining vessels. The colour of a subungual tumour does not show through the nail, making it difficult to detect, and many of the superficial cutaneous tumours are impalpable and invisible because the overlying skin is often thick and wrinkled. The nail overlying a subungual tumour is often thickened, unduly convex, and longitudinally striated from retarded growth. The bone of the underlying phalanx may be eroded, excavated or rarefied, and the affected extremity is usually warmer than its fellow of the opposite side. During an attack of pain the whole extremity may become cool and sweaty, and a unilateral Horner's syndrome may even develop.

Treatment is by surgical excision. A wide margin of tissue must be taken around the possible site of an invisible, impalpable tumour to ensure its satisfactory removal.[530]

ANGIOSARCOMA

This tumour affects young men and women, and usually develops in the skin and soft tissues of the extremities. Rapid growth produces a bulky, painful, hot tumour, which is liable to bleed. A special variety affects the nasal cavity. Death is usually the result of lung metastases. Although angiosarcomas are radiosensitive and respond to chemotherapy, radical amputation is still advised.

A number of subtypes are recognized.

- A haemangioendothelioma arises in bone and may also affect the spleen.[531]
- Angiosarcomas may occasionally develop in a long-standing developmental angioma. This is a rare condition but should be considered if a long-standing angioma suddenly increases in size or becomes painful. Surgical excision for biopsy is then indicated.
- Angiosarcomas can arise in the liver, causing massive hepatic enlargement and ascites.[532] These tumours occur in children and young adults, and must be differentiated from other liver tumours, such as hepatoblastomas (see Ch. 29). The prognosis is poor.
- Angiosarcomas can arise in chronically lymphoedematous limbs, although lymphangiosarcoma is the more usual lesion (see Ch. 12).[533]

KAPOSI'S MULTIPLE HAEMANGIOSARCOMA[534]

The incidence of this 'tumour' has increased dramatically with the advent of AIDS.[535] Until the 1980s, this was a rare tumour predominantly affecting young Mediterranean men between their teens and forties.[536] It was also reported to be common in Bantu people and in other African nationalities.[537]

It usually starts in the skin of the lower extremity or the penis. A bluish red, well-demarcated macule appears first and grows. Other macules then appear close by and these enlarge to fuse with the first macule, becoming elevated as they grow (Fig. 9.61). The other lower limb is often affected at the same time, and the lesion spreads up the leg and on to the lower part of the trunk. The nodules are painless, apart from those on the penis or the soles of the feet. Spread is usually by the bloodstream to the liver and lungs. This diagnosis should be suspected in all homosexual or haemophiliac patients who develop suggestive skin lesions. The diagnosis is confirmed by biopsy and by testing the blood for antibodies to HIV.[538] Histologically, the blood spaces within the tumour are surrounded by anaplastic fibroblasts with nuclear atypia and multiple mitotic patterns.

Patients should be on appropriate antiretroviral medication, and treatment of the tumour is by a combination of cytotoxic chemotherapeutic agents and superficial irradiation.[539] In some patients a good initial response is obtained, but eventually all tumours recur and death is inevitable.

CAROTID BODY TUMOURS (CHEMODECTOMAS)

The carotid body is situated at the carotid bifurcation, and contains numerous sinusoidal capillaries that allow the blood to come in close contact with the glomus cells that form its main structure. These cells are thought to originate from para-ganglionic cells derived from neural crest. They are richly

REFERENCES

529. Stout AP, Murray MR. Ann Surg 1942; 116: 26
530. Strahan J, Bailie HWC. Br J Surg 1972; 59: 91
531. Stout AP. Ann Surg 1943; 118: 445
532. Pollard S, Millward-Sadier GH. J Clin Pathol 1974; 27: 214
533. Stewart FW, Treves N. Cancer 1948; 1: 64
534. Kaposi M. Arch Dermatol Syp 1872; 4: 265
535. Sonnabend J, Wilkins SS, Purtilo T. JAMA 1983; 249: 2370
536. McCarthy WD, Pack GT. Surg Gynecol Obstet 1950; 91: 465
537. Rothman S. Arch Dermatol 1962; 85: 311
538. Pinching A. J Clin Exp Immunol 1984; 56: 1
539. Volberding P. Semin Oncol 1984; 11: 60

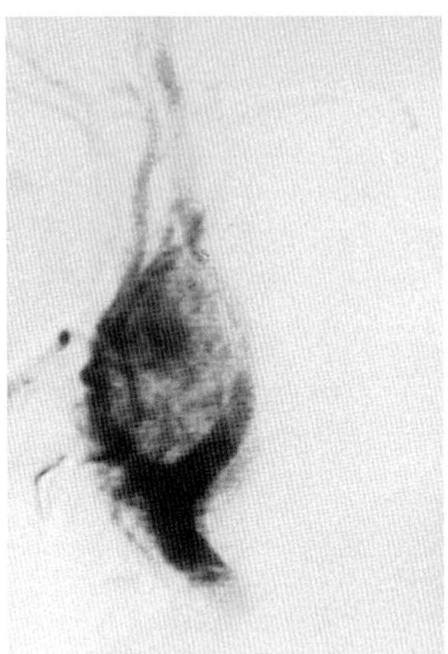

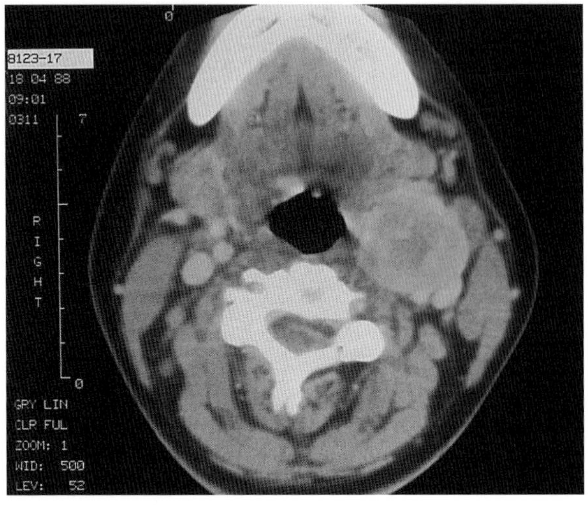

a b

Figure 10.83 (a) A carotid body tumour causing splaying of the carotid bifurcation; the vascularity of the tumour can be seen. (b) Computerized tomography scan of the neck also shows the tumour.

supplied by afferent nerve endings (chemoreceptors) and are sensitive to changes in the oxygen, carbon dioxide content, and pH of the perfusing blood. They stimulate the cardiovascular and respiratory centres to alter the heart rate and sympathetic tone to maintain homeostasis. Chemoreceptors are also found in the aortic arch, the internal jugular vein, the middle ear, the ganglion nodosum of the vagus nerve, and the retroperitoneum around the abdominal aorta in the organ of Zuckerkandl.

Pathology

Tumours of the carotid body are rare but well recognized. Just over 200 cases had been reported by 1943,[540] and 546 by 1960;[541] chemodectomas at other sites are rarer still. These tumours have an equal sex distribution and occur over a wide age range, with a median in the fifth decade. They can be familial, and a third of the familial tumours are reported to be bilateral. Ten per cent of non-familial tumours are bilateral.[542] Chronic hypoxia is thought to be a causal factor, and there is a high incidence of carotid body tumours in Peru and Mexico City.[543]

Chemodectomas are ovoid tumours arising in the carotid bifurcation, distorting and encasing the carotid vessels. Hutchinson called them 'potato tumours' because he thought a potato could be likened to their macroscopic appearance on transection, but they usually appear more reddish brown and are highly vascular, making them easily compressible. The tumour cells are polygonal or spindle-shaped, and the neoplastic cell masses are enclosed in a box-like framework of fine connective tissue with an extensive sinusoidal blood supply. The microscopic appearances are unhelpful in predicting malignant behaviour; local invasion and lymphatic or blood-borne metastases occur in between 2.5 and 50% of cases,[544] although some regard all these (or carotid body) tumours as malign.[545] Left untreated, about 5–10% develop metastases within 10 years.

Clinical features

Patients present with solitary or bilateral lumps just in front of and deep to the anterior border of the sternomastoid muscle. The mass is closely related to the carotid pulse, usually at the level of the hyoid bone. The carotid pulse is transmitted by the tumour, but on occasions the tumour is so vascular that it appears to be truly expansile. The tumour may decrease in size with compression, and in 20% there is a thrill or an audible bruit over a highly vascular tumour.[546] The mass can be shown to move laterally but not vertically, and this movement displaces the carotid pulse. A carotid body tumour must be differentiated from a branchial cyst, a neurofibroma, and an enlarged lymph node. A third are incorrectly diagnosed on clinical examination. Further dissection should be abandoned without a biopsy being taken if a tumour is found unexpectedly at operation. Re-exploration can then be carried out by an experienced vascular surgeon after appropriate investigation.

Investigations

Duplex ultrasonography is almost always diagnostic.[547] Carotid arteriography by intravenous digital subtraction arteriography[548] shows a splayed carotid bifurcation containing a highly vascular tumour (Fig. 10.83a). Computerized tomography scans may be helpful in assessing tumour size (Fig. 10.83b), and magnetic resonance angiography also provides detailed images.

Management

Carotid body tumours enlarge slowly but inexorably if left untreated and may eventually obstruct the carotid vessels. There is a greater risk of malignancy as their size increases, and the larger the tumour the more difficult the operation. The carotid bifurcation is exposed as for a carotid endarterectomy. The vessels are isolated above and below the tumour and taped. The tumour is then dissected off the vessels in the subadventitial plane,[549] using careful sharp dissection and meticulous haemostasis, with under-running of large branches and diathermy of the smaller feeding vessels. There is usually a plane of cleavage along the posterior border of the internal carotid artery. The external carotid artery can be ligated and divided if necessary to provide

REFERENCES

540. Kinmonth JB, Lockhart KT. St Thomas' Gaz 1943; 41: 4
541. Dallachy R, Simpson IC. J Laryngol Otol 1960; 74: 217
542. Rush BF. Ann Surg 1963; 157: 633
543. Farr HW. Cancer J Clin 1980; 30: 260
544. Harrington SW, Clagett OT, Dockerty MB. Ann Surg 1941; 114: 820
545. Dent TL, Thompson NW, Fry WY. Surgery 1976; 80: 365
546. Wilson R. Surgery 1966; 59: 483
547. Dickinson PH, Griffin SM et al. Br J Surg 1986; 72: 14
548. McPherson GAD, Halliday AW, Mansfield AO. Br J Surg 1989; 76: 33
549. Gordon-Taylor G. Br J Surg 1940; 28: 163

better access. A shunt and interposition vein graft can be used if the internal carotid artery has to be sacrificed during removal of the tumour.[550]

Results and complications

Surgical treatment is the method of choice in patients under the age of 50, but in older patients a watch policy may be adopted. The small risk of hemiplegia (1–2%) and the greater risk of nerve palsy, which varies between 12 and 40%, must be explained to the patient before operation; some will then decline surgery.[548] Radiotherapy has been shown to be effective, and this may be used as the treatment of choice in elderly, high-risk patients. It may also be employed to treat patients with residual tumour or local recurrence. Preoperative embolization has been advocated to reduce the size and vascularity of large tumours, but few use this technique.[551] The mortality rate of the operation has declined considerably in recent years and should be in the order of 1–2%.[546–548,552]

GLOMUS JUGULARE TUMOUR

This is a rare tumour arising in the jugular bulb, presenting as a lump situated between the posterior border of the mandibular and the mastoid processes.[553] Apart from noticing the mass, patients may complain of buzzing in the head. This tumour may easily be mistaken for a carotid body tumour (it is usually too high) or a parotid neoplasm (it is usually too deep). Glomus jugulare tumours may arise in the vagus, glossopharyngeal or hypoglossal nerves, and can extend up into the middle ear or into the cranial cavity. Excision may be followed by palsies of the 10th, 11th and 12th nerves. Radiotherapy is an alternative method of treatment but associated with a high recurrence rate.

MISCELLANEOUS CONDITIONS

RADIATION ARTERITIS

Radiation arteritis follows high doses of irradiation applied near major arteries. The carotid and iliac arteries are often affected, because irradiation to the neck and pelvis is the usual treatment for cervical lymphomas and pelvic tumours.[554] Damage to the vasa vasorum leads to intimal thickening, to transmural fibrosis, and eventually to arterial occlusion. Occluded segments can be treated by bypass to healthy vessels.

AINHUM (DACTYLOLYSIS SPONTANEA)

Ainhum is a rare condition affecting black races.[555] Digital gangrene develops in a single digit, usually the fifth toe, which mummifies and either separates or is amputated. The aetiology of this condition is obscure, but it appears to be self-limiting. A local vasculitis is suspected.

CAROTID SINUS SYNDROME

The baroreceptors of the carotid sinus normally maintain a constant blood pressure by means of reflex changes in the heart and peripheral blood vessels.[556] Pathological instability or hypersensitivity of the carotid sinus may cause episodes of bradycardia or asystole, transient falls in blood pressure, or syncopal attacks. These attacks may be initiated by sudden turning of the head or follow undue pressure on the neck. Attacks can be reproduced by pressure over the sinus and, if troublesome, may be abolished by sectioning the carotid sinus nerve.[557]

LEIOMYOMAS AND LEIOMYOSARCOMAS

Leiomyomas and leiomyosarcomas are extremely rare in arteries. They are much more common in veins (see Chapter 11).

AMPUTATION

Successful revascularization procedures in the lower limb may allow limited digital or transmetatarsal amputations, which inevitably fail if the blood supply of the foot cannot be improved. Every effort should be made to obtain a successful below-knee amputation in patients in whom reconstruction is impossible, and through-knee and above-knee amputation should be regarded as inferior options to be avoided whenever possible. There are a few exceptions, for example when the patient has severe arthritis of the knee or a marked fixed flexion deformity, or when the limb to be amputated is paralysed from a stroke so that a prosthesis is unlikely to be used.

THE IDEAL STUMP

This should heal by first intention; the scar should not have to transmit pressure and should be freely mobile; the soft tissue should not be redundant, but should fit snugly over a well-rounded bone end; and the stump should be conical in shape and free from pain. The joints above the stump should be fully mobile.

AFTER TREATMENT

The stump should be inspected at 5–7 days if the postoperative course is uncomplicated, but the dressings may be taken down earlier if infection or poor healing is suspected. Patients should start to carry out exercises to strengthen the upper limb muscles as soon as possible; these should ideally begin before surgery. The amputation stump can be mobilized and strengthened by exercises from 24 to 48 h after operation, but weight-bearing should not start until 5 or 6 days have passed, and the fashion of immediate application of a temporary prosthesis in theatre with very early weight-bearing has now been largely abandoned. If the stump is satisfactory by 5 or 6 days, then the pneumatic postamputation mobility aid (Fig. 10.84)[558] can be applied to the stump to allow relatively early mobilization. This apparatus consists of an inflatable bag inside a metal frame that is attached to a pylon. The pneumatic bag is inflated to act as a socket, and this allows early walking practice without the necessity for casting a formal socket. Less emphasis is now placed on bandaging, and more on the early use of the pneumatic mobility aid. Early measurement and assessment of the stump by a prosthetist allows prompt fitting of the definitive limb. The development of lightweight (carbon-fibre) modular prostheses[559] has reduced production time and increased mobility.

REFERENCES

550. Javid H, Chawla SK et al. Arch Surg 1976; 111: 344
551. Vanasperen DC, Boer FRS et al. Br J Surg 1981; 68: 433
552. Browse NL. Br Med J 1982; 284: 1507
553. Glenner GG, Grimley PM. In: Hymes V (ed.). Atlas of Tumour Pathology. Armed Forces Institute of Pathology, Washington, 1974
554. Lawson JA. J Cardiovasc Surg 1985; 26: 151
555. Hircherson DC. Ann Surg 1950; 132: 312
556. Waller A. Proc R Soc Med 1862; 11: 302
557. Eascott HHG. Arterial Surgery. Pitman, London, 1969
558. Little JM, Gosling L, Weeks A. Med J Aust 1972; 1: 1300
559. Foorte J, Lawrence RB, Davies RM. Int Rehabil Med 1984; 6: 72

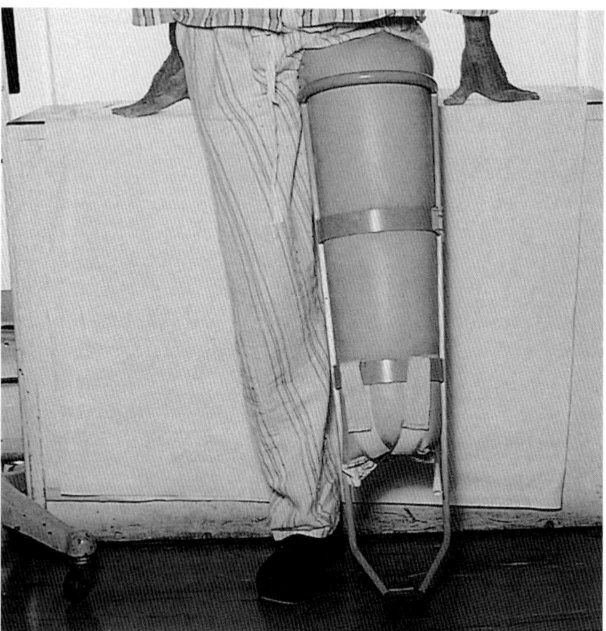

Figure 10.84 The pneumatic postamputation mobility aid.

COMPLICATIONS

Haematoma formation

Haematoma formation can be avoided by careful haemostasis and the provision of adequate drainage. Should it occur, formal evacuation is sometimes required.

Infection

Infection cannot be completely avoided, especially if there is infected gangrene in the amputated tissues. Avoidance of haematomas is important. A swab should be taken if possible 2 or more days prior to operation so that appropriate antibiotics can be given. Penicillin and metronidazole are effective against clostridia and other anaerobes. Formal drainage is occasionally required, and healing often then takes place by secondary intention. Prophylactic antibiotics should always be given for amputations.

Ischaemic necrosis

Ischaemic necrosis is the most common complication after amputations performed for ischaemia and is often the result of poor technique. Haematomas, suturing under tension, and incorrect selection of the level of amputation with persisting ischaemia of the skin flaps are usually responsible.

Osteomyelitis

Osteomyelitis has been relatively unusual since the advent of antibiotics. If it occurs, it may necessitate reamputation at a higher level.

Spurs and osteophytes

Spurs and osteophytes require treatment, which usually consists of revision of the amputation to a higher level, only if they cause pain.

Ulceration of the stump

Ulceration of the stump can be the result of infection and ischaemia, or pressure and friction from the prosthesis. This usually requires refashioning of the stump or recasting the socket.

An adherent or uncomfortable scar may require refashioning.

Stump neuroma

Stump neuroma is usually the result of a failure to cut back the nerves far enough. A thick bulbous neuroma forms on the transected nerve; this is exquisitely painful when compressed by a prosthesis. Shooting pain is produced by localized pressure. Local anaesthetic infiltration usually abolishes the pain and confirms the diagnosis. The pain may also be helped by repeated percussion or application of a mechanical vibrator.[560] Transcutaneous electrical nerve stimulation may also prove effective (see Ch. 5). The definitive treatment is to section the nerve at a higher level, but the neuroma may still recur.

Phantom limb

Pain is a curious phenomenon and is experienced by most amputees to some extent.[561] In some, the painful sensation derived from a non-existent limb becomes unbearable and disrupts their life, making treatment imperative. Antidepressant tablets, tranquillizers, hypnotherapy and acupuncture have all been tried with some success, but carbamazepine and nerve division appear to be of greater value.

The phantom limb pain is thought to be caused by persistence of the sensory cortex, and is often most severe in the fingers and toes, which have the largest cortical representation. In most cases it quickly fades, but may persist as 'telescoping', with the feeling that the foot is attached to the thigh, or the hand to the upper arm when the patient goes to scratch the non-existent digit. It is a strange fact that if several fingers are amputated, only the first is affected by phantom feelings, and if multiple amputations are required, only the first ever causes a phantom.

Local and repeated percussion with a patella hammer over a painful spot may occasionally alleviate a painful phantom. Prior insertion of epidural anaesthesia often avoids the subsequent development of phantom limb,[562] although this has been disputed. Gabapentin is also being used in this condition, with some good results.

Causalgia

Causalgia is an intractable burning type of pain thought to result from sympathetic fibres growing down systemic nerves. It is often associated with a smooth, red, shiny skin. Guanethidine blocks or sympathectomy may bring relief.[563]

Jactitation

Jactitation, an unexplained sudden jumping of the leg, may result from a neuroma or from a psychogenic cause.

Aneurysms and arteriovenous fistulae

These are rare complications that may occasionally require treatment.

REFERENCES

560. Richie Russell WMR. Med J 1949; 1: 1024
561. Weir-Mitchell S. Injuries of Nerves and Their Consequences. Lippincott, Philadelphia, 1872
562. Bachs S, Noreng M, Tjellden N. Pain 1988; 33: 297
563. Glynn CJ, Basedow RW, Walsh JA. Br J Anaesth 1981; 53: 1297

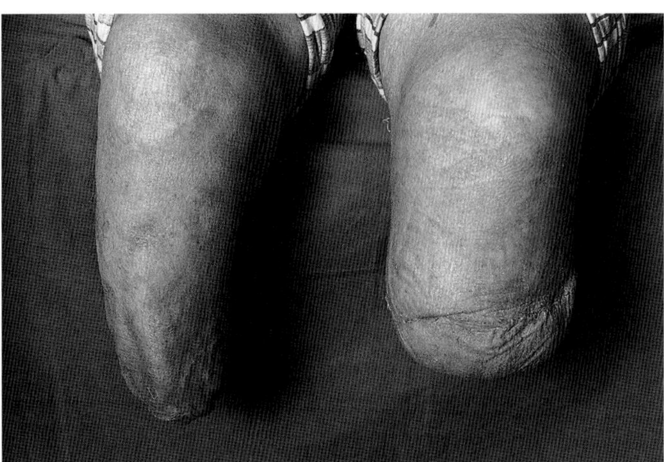

Figure 10.85 A poor below-knee stump caused by muscle retraction on the right leg, and a good stump on the left leg.

Fixed flexion deformity

Fixed flexion deformity develops if patients with rest pain or gangrene are left in severe pain for some time before coming to amputation. The hip and knee are flexed in an effort to provide relief; if this position is maintained for long periods, contractures can develop. This complication is best avoided by regular active movements. Physiotherapy may help, or manipulation under anaesthesia may be necessary, and even this fails when the contracture is long-standing. Amputation at a higher level is then required.

Muscle herniation

Muscle herniation can occur when the muscles slip off the bone, leaving it uncovered. The shape of the stump is ruined, and it may no longer fit its socket (Fig. 10.85). Refashioning is required.

Non-union

Non-union may occur between the patella and the end of the femur after a Stokes–Gritti amputation.[564] The stump should be refashioned to an above-knee amputation if this happens.

Disruption of the amputation stump

Disruption of the amputation stump following falls is a major problem that often requires refashioning to a higher level.

GUILLOTINE AMPUTATION

This method of amputation is used when healing cannot be guaranteed in the presence of severe tissue trauma or infection. It aims to remove all the dead and potentially dangerous tissue. Flaps are raised and the tissues are divided down the bone, which is then transected. The flaps are left open, with the end of the stump being covered by sterile dressings. The operation can be performed in a field hospital during wartime, allowing definitive surgery to be carried out in a more formal setting 3–5 days later, when further excision of any necrotic tissue is undertaken before the flaps are sutured.

AMPUTATIONS AT SPECIFIC SITES

The toes

Toe amputations are carried out through racket-shaped incisions, with the bone being divided through the shaft of the phalanx or through the neck of the underlying metatarsal bone.

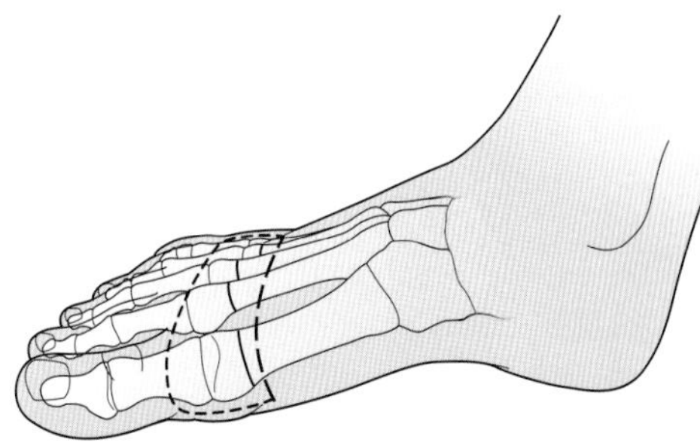

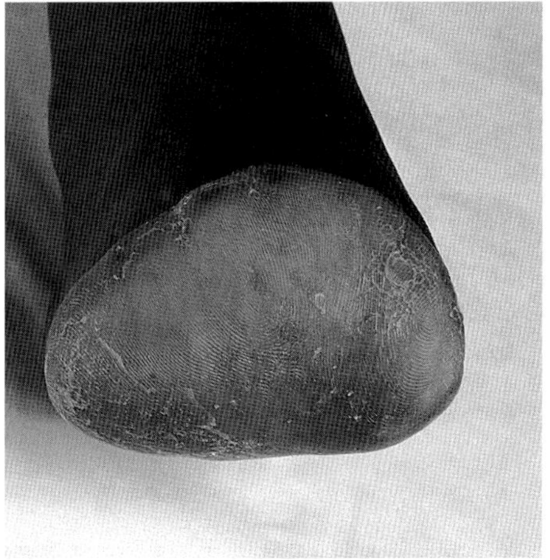

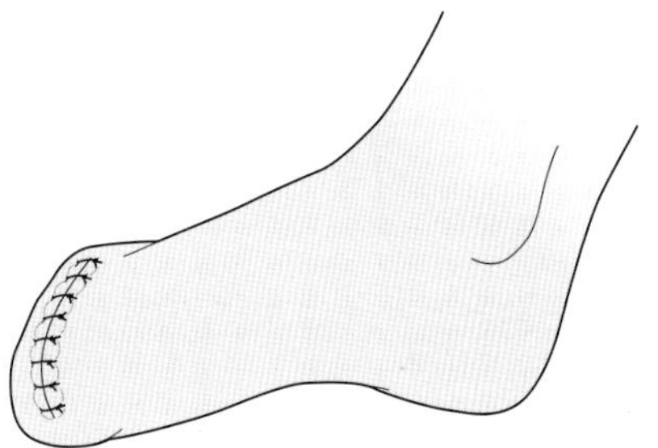

Figure 10.86 The transmetatarsal amputation.

Amputations of the first toe should include excision of the associated sesamoid bone. Although it is tempting to amputate through a joint, this leaves avascular cartilage beneath, which may cause poor healing. The dorsal and ventral tendons are divided at the same level as the bone, and the digital vessels are ligated. Most digital amputation sites with a reasonable blood supply will heal in 2–3 months. Individual toes cannot be successfully amputated for ischaemia unless the blood supply has been improved. Infective diabetic gangrene of individual toes responds well to digital amputation in the presence of a good blood supply.

The foot

A transmetatarsal amputation can be used in diabetic patients who have gangrene of the forefoot, or in patients with many toes that remain irreversibly ischaemic after a successful revascularization. The patient is provided with a good stump, and walking is usually excellent. The only prosthesis that is required is a shoe-filler.

The amputation is made at the level of the metatarsal necks; a long plantar flap is used to close the defect because this skin has

REFERENCES

564. Martin P, Wickham J. Lancet 1962; ii: 16

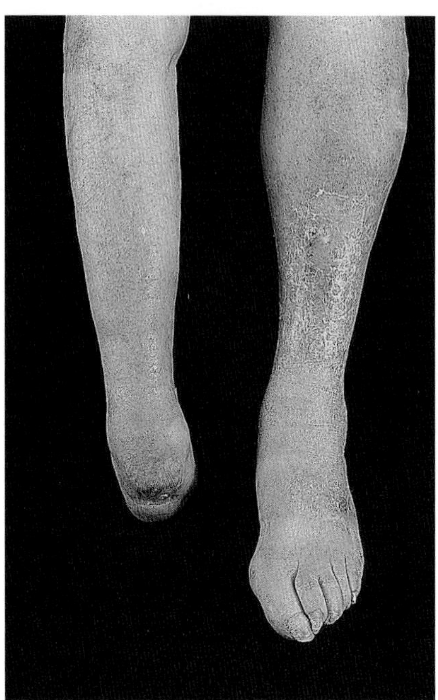

Figure 10.87 Chopart's amputation of the right foot.

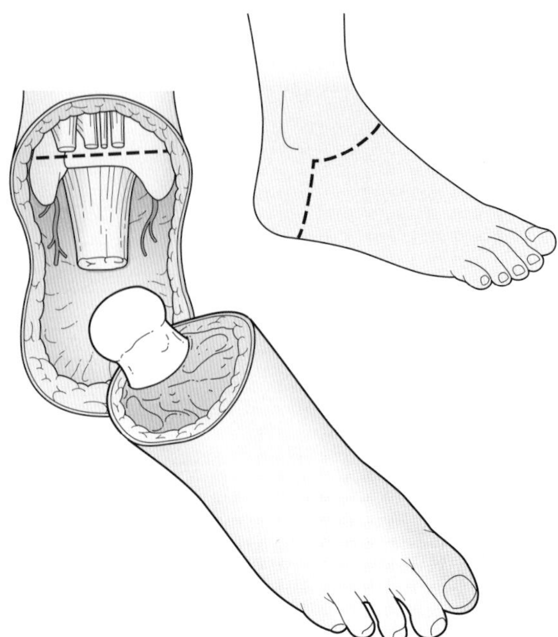

Figure 10.89 The technique of Syme's amputation.

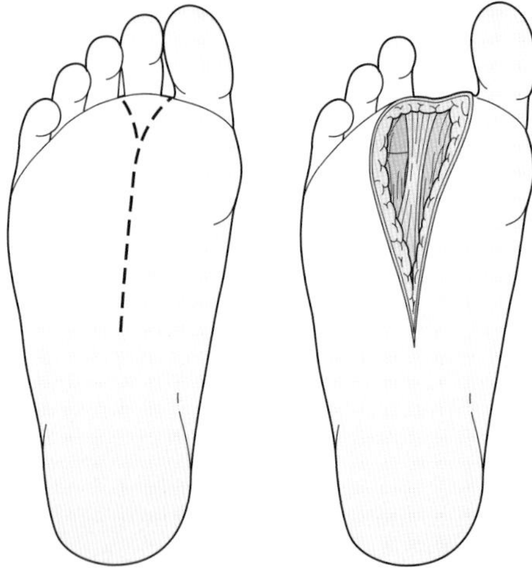

Figure 10.88 A ray amputation for diabetic gangrene.

the best blood supply (Fig. 10.86). The bones may be individually divided by a vibrating saw or a Gigli saw. Suturing the flap should be avoided, especially in those patients with poor skin. Chopart's and Lisfranc's amputations,[565,566] which are made through the tarsal bones, are rarely performed because the heel tends to develop equinovarus with inversion, restricting subsequent mobility. Nevertheless, some patients have maintained good mobility for many years on this type of stump, and they are slowly coming back into fashion (Fig. 10.87).

Individual rays consisting of one or more toes with their related metatarsal from the medial, lateral or central part of the forefoot can be excised. This amputation is useful in diabetic gangrene when infection spreads back along the line of the toe and its metatarsal. It heals up well by secondary intention (Fig. 10.88).

The heel (Syme's amputation)

Syme's amputation[567] is still popular with some orthopaedic surgeons but is rarely performed for ischaemia, and is not favoured by the limb-fitters. Although it is classed as an end-bearing stump, few such stumps continue to weight-bear, and any prosthesis used does not have enough room for ankle or sole springs. Most prosthetists feel the patient is better served by a good below-knee amputation. The prosthesis required is ugly, and the operation is technically difficult and requires considerable expertise before success is consistently achieved. Patients can, however, walk without a prosthesis while at home, having the advantage of what the Germans call *earth feeling*.

In the classical Syme's amputation, the bones are divided just above the ankle, with the malleoli being sawn off and a bulky heel fashioned over the divided bone. The details of the operation can be found in textbooks of operative surgery.[568] The approach has been modified to divide the bone slightly higher (2 cm above the joint space), and Fig. 10.89 shows the skin incision and the general technique with the modification. The incision joins the two malleoli anteriorly and drops vertically down to encircle the heel just in front of its prominence. A third of Syme's amputations are subsequently revised to a higher level because of poor healing, ulceration or poor function.[569]

Below-knee amputation

This is the level of amputation that most surgeons try to achieve in patients who require a major amputation for severe ischaemia of the lower limb. It has been shown that 80% of patients with

REFERENCES

565. Chopart F, Desault PJ. Traite des Maladies Chirurgicales et des Operations qui Leur Conviennent. Vulier, Paris, 1795
566. Lisfranc J. Nouvelle Method Operatoire Pour L'Amputation Partielle du Pied: Son Articulation Tarso-metafarsienne: Methode Precedes des Nombreuses Modifications qu'a Susbies Cette de Chopart. Gambon, Paris, 1815
567. Syme J. Mon J Med Sci 1843; 3: 93
568. Fiddian NJ. Amputations in General Surgical Operations. Churchill Livingstone, London, 1987: 416
569. Aird I. A Companion in Surgical Studies. E & S Livingstone, Edinburgh, 1958

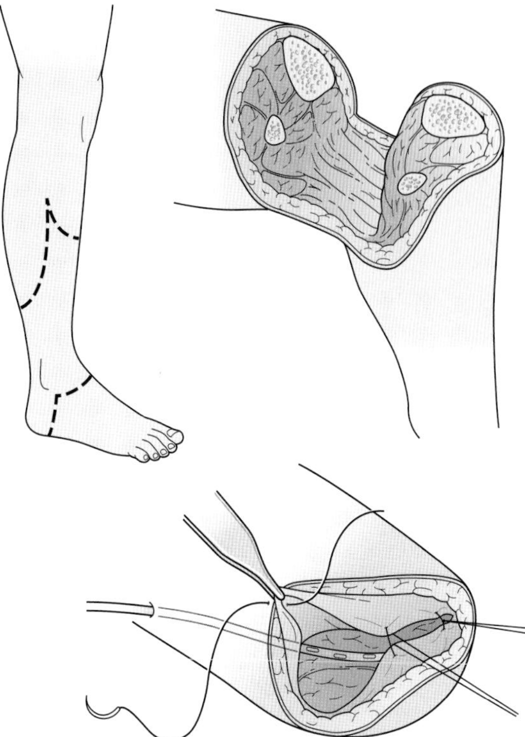

Figure 10.90 The Burgess technique of below-knee amputation utilising a long posterior flap.

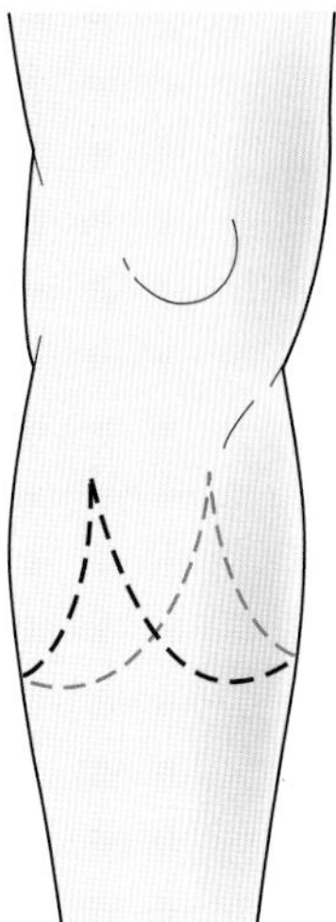

Figure 10.91 The technique of below-knee amputation using a skew flap (Robinson).

ischaemic gangrene can have a successful amputation at this level.[570] There is some evidence that failed arterial reconstruction leads to a high level of amputation, although more recent work seems to refute this.[571]

A number of tests, including Doppler ankle pressures, oximetry, isotope clearance, arteriography, thermography and plethysmography, have been used in an effort to determine the likely success of amputation at this level. The proponents of oximetry and thermography make reasonable claims for their value, but they are not in standard clinical practice around the world, and sound clinical judgement combined with inspection of flap bleeding is probably the best guide to success.[572] Although this was stated over 20 years ago, it is probably still true.

The two methods that are commonly used to perform this operation are the long posterior flap of Burgess[573] and the skew flap of Kingsley Robinson and coworkers.[574] Early studies suggested that healing might be better with a skew-flap operation, but when the two techniques were evaluated in a controlled clinical trial there was little difference in the healing rate.[575] A subsequent study also showed no difference in the healing rate, but did show earlier limb-fitting and mobilization with skew flaps;[576] this was thought to be because it is easier to get a nicely rounded stump with the skew-flap operation.

Several techniques have been described. The rule of three is based on the circumference of the calf a hand's breadth from the tibial tubercle. The circumference is divided into thirds. Two-thirds represent the proximal bone section, and the remaining third the posterior myoplastic flap. Alternatively, the incision extends from the medial border of the tibia horizontally across the front of the leg to the lateral border of the leg, approximately 15 cm below the tibial tuberosity. Another method of arriving at the correct level of amputation is to measure 1 inch below the tibial tubercle for every foot of the patient's height (i.e. 5 inches for a 5-foot individual and 6 inches for a 6-foot individual). This leaves a reasonable stump to fit in a prosthesis without leaving it too long, which can make subsequent limb-fitting difficult. The incision then extends vertically down the leg on either side, and joins across the calf just above the origin of the Achilles tendon (Fig. 10.90). The posterior flap can be trimmed later when the muscles are thinned.

Details of the operative technique can be found in textbooks of operative surgery.[577] The important points are that the end of the tibia must be carefully bevelled and filed smooth. The soleus is removed to prevent persistent muscle ischaemia and to reduce the size of the musculocutaneous flap. The skin is carefully approximated with very gentle non-absorbable sutures or a subcuticular suture. The patient can be mobilized on a postamputation mobility aid at 7–10 days. It is important that the patient's bed is fitted with a monkey ladder and/or pole and triceps springs. All these aids are useful in maintaining mobility and upper body strength. In the skew-flap procedure, the skin flaps are raised as shown in Fig. 10.91, and the final suture line runs obliquely anteroposteriorly. Otherwise the technique is similar to the Burgess operation.

Through-knee amputation

Equal lateral flaps are normally used for this amputation, which is not popular in ischaemic disease because it heals poorly. Even if primary healing is obtained, it leaves a large bulbous stump, which makes it difficult to fit a prosthesis. It has the advantage that it is quick to perform and relatively atraumatic. The stump is end-bearing.

REFERENCES

570. McCollum PT, Spence VA, Walker WA. Br J Surg 1988; 75: 1193
571. Cook TA, Davies AH, Horrocks M et al. Eur J Vasc Surg 1992; 6: 599
572. Browse NL. Scand Clin Lab Invest 1973; 128 (Suppl): 249
573. Burgess EM. Clin Orthop 1967; 37: 17
574. Robinson KP, Hoile R, Coddington T. Br J Surg 1982; 69: 554
575. Ruckley CV, Prescott RJ. In: Greenhalgh RM (ed). Limb Salvage and Amputation for Vascular Disease. WB Saunders, London, 1988
576. Reynolds J, Callum KG. Br J Surg 1991; 78: 370
577. McCollum CN. In: Greenhalgh RM (ed.). Vascular Surgical Techniques. WB Saunders, London, 1989: 340

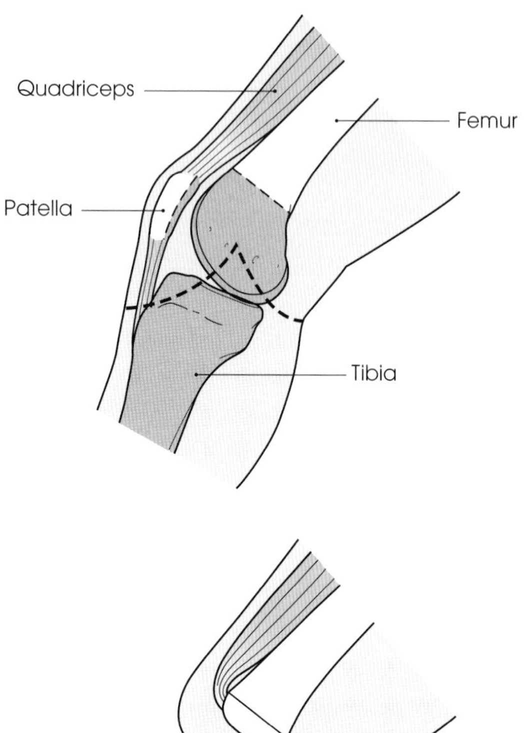

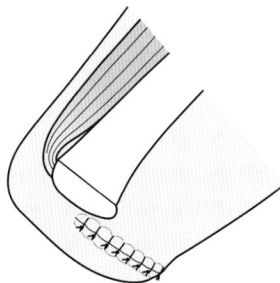

Figure 10.92 The technique of Gritti–Stokes amputation.

Supracondylar (Gritti–Stokes) amputation

Supracondylar amputation[578] leaves a longer stump than the standard above-knee amputation, which may be an advantage in a bilateral amputee who wishes to change position in bed or on a chair when a prosthesis is not being worn. Because of the length of the stump, it is difficult to fit an internal knee mechanism in the prosthesis, and this has made this amputation unpopular with prosthetists.

The skin flaps are shown in Fig. 10.92. The knee joint is entered by deepening the anterior incision through the patella tendon and the joint capsule, before the knee is disarticulated by dividing the capsule above the meniscus and sectioning the cruciate ligaments. The vessels that are found behind the bone are ligated and divided. The nerves are pulled down and transected. The anterior flap and patella are turned upwards, and the femur is divided immediately above the condyles before the articular surface of the patella is removed with a saw. The patella is then wired to the end of the femur or carefully fixed with non-absorbable sutures. There is less tendency for the patella to dislocate off the femur if the transected femur is angled slightly backwards.[579] There is some evidence that mobility with a prothesis is better after a Gritti–Stokes than after an above-knee amputation.

Above-knee amputation

In this amputation, equal anterior and posterior semicircular flaps are cut with their upper limit at the level of the bone section, which is ideally 25–30 cm below the tip of the greater trochanter. Enough room must be left for a knee mechanism to fit beneath the stump (usually 12 cm up from the knee joint). The divided vasti and quadriceps must be sutured over the end of the conically bevelled bone to provide a well-shaped myoplastic stump. The muscles may be sutured to the bone end (a myodesis),[580] but this refinement is almost certainly unnecessary. There is some evidence that suturing the adductor longus tendon to the lateral aspect of the femur maintains the femoral line in a varus position, which is thought to aid postoperative mobilization.

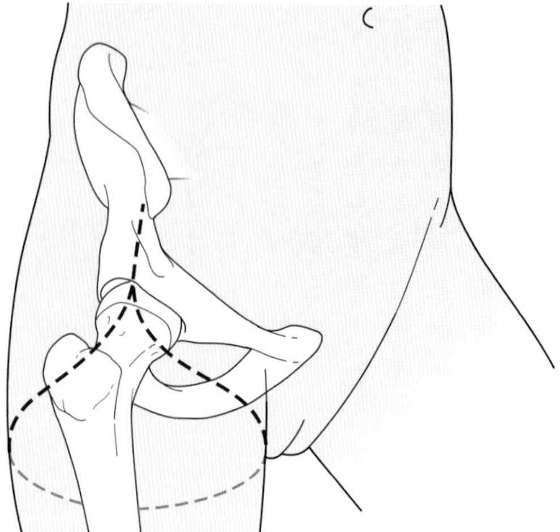

Figure 10.93 The technique of hip disarticulation.

Disarticulation of the hip

Disarticulation of the hip[581] is hardly ever required for vascular disease and is mainly performed to eradicate soft tissue and bony tumours in the upper thigh (see Ch. 42). A long posterior flap is used to cover the defect (Fig. 10.93). The femoral vessels are carefully ligated, the capsule of the joint is divided, and the head of the femur is dislocated forwards before the round ligament is divided. The obturator and gluteal vessels are then ligated and divided, and the sciatic nerve is cut back. The procedure is best done in conjunction with an orthopaedic surgeon.

Hindquarter amputation

Hindquarter amputation was devised to treat bony and soft tissue tumours in the pelvic bones, the upper femur, and the soft tissues of the upper thigh and buttock (see Ch. 42). It has also been used for severe traumatic injuries in this region causing unreconstructable damage to the blood supply. It was first performed in 1891 by Billroth, whose patient did not survive,[582] and later by Girard, whose patient lived.[583] Gordon-Taylor[584] popularized the operation in the UK and was its chief exponent, but it is relatively rarely performed today (at present).

Amputations of the fingers

See Chapter 47.

REFERENCES

578. Gritti R. Ann Univ Med (Milano) 1857; 161: 5
579. Doran J, Hopkinson BR, Makin GS. Br J Surg 1978; 65: 135
580. Robinson KP. Br J Hosp Med 1976; 629: 631
581. Boyd HB. Surg Gynecol Obstet 1947; 84: 346
582. Gordon-Taylor G, Wiles P. Br J Surg 1935; 22: 695
583. Girard C. Congr Fr Chir 1895; 9: 823
584. Gordon-Taylor G, Wiles P. Br J Surg 1935; 22: 671

Amputations in the upper limbs

These can be made through the forearm or arm above the elbow. A stump of 15 cm from the tip of the olecranon is ideal, and above the elbow 19 cm from the acromion to the cut end of humerus is preferred. These stumps should not be less than 10 and 7.5 cm, respectively. Amputations through the arm are occasionally required for ischaemia, but the majority are required for trauma, vascular malformation, infection or tumours. The shoulder joint may be disarticulated, and a forequarter amputation is occasionally required for malignancy.

OTHER INDICATIONS FOR AMPUTATION

Between 80 and 90% of all amputations are carried out for ischaemic arterial disease, including Buerger's disease, diabetic vasculitis, emboli and trauma. Rare indications include arterio-venous fistulae, gas gangrene, septic arthritis, osteomyelitis (now rare), intractable venous ulceration, congenital deformities, malignancy and painful paralysed limbs.

The veins

11

Kevin G. Burnand, Andrew W. Bradbury, Rachel C. Sam

INTRODUCTION

The veins of the lower limb, including those of the pelvis and abdomen, are much more commonly the subject of disease and disorder than are the veins of the head and neck, the upper limb, and the thorax. This may relate to the special demands placed on the veins in the lower half of the body: to continue to function and overcome the influence of gravity that has resulted from the adoption of the erect stance.

The presence of large saccular veins within the powerful posterior muscles of the calf provides an accessory pumping mechanism or peripheral heart capable of augmenting venous return against the hydrostatic gradient. The calf pump, in combination with the less efficient foot and buttock pumps, forces blood out of the lower extremities during exercise.[1] Closure of the valves in the deep and communicating veins prevents reflux and avoids the transmission of high pressure into the superficial venous bed during exercise. This mechanism prevents the development of high superficial venous pressures, which can over-distend the subcutaneous veins and interfere with capillary flow and exchange. Chronic disorders of the veins of the lower extremities are usually the result of valve malfunction, which interferes with the action of the calf muscle pump. Veins provide the capacitance required for changing circulatory filling because of their ability to distend and empty rapidly without altering their resistance to flow.[2] Veins can undergo large changes in volume with little change in transmural pressure. The venous system must accommodate enormous variations in the rates of flow at different sites in the body. Thrombus formation is a major problem throughout the venous system, and this risk is exacerbated by low blood flow.

ANATOMY AND EMBRYOLOGY

The veins develop from an intercommunicating network of blood islands that coalesce and differentiate into a number of dominant pathways as flow becomes established.[3] Not surprisingly, this complex process fails on occasions and congenital venous anomalies are quite common. The major veins of the lower limb, abdomen and thorax develop from pairs of anterior, posterior, superior and subcardinal veins. These vessels interconnect in a complex manner, and the iliac veins, the inferior and superior venae cavae, and the azygos veins are formed by the development of dominant flow pathways through certain sectors of this network (Fig. 11.1). Normally the right common cardinal vein, which is formed by the coalescence of the anterior and posterior cardinal veins behind the heart, achieves dominance. Paired venae cavae, multiple cross-connecting vessels, total agenesis, and a retroaortic left renal vein can all occur when this fails to occur.[3–5] In the limbs, a failure of regression of the original axial veins results in a persistent lateral vein, which may be associated with agenesis of all or part of the main venous channels.[6] Most venous anomalies can be classified as aplasias, hypoplasias, reduplications, or persistence of vestigial vessels. Agenesis of venous valves and structural defects in the composition of the vein wall can also occur.

The superficial venous system of the lower limb is made up of the long and short saphenous veins and their tributaries. These veins interconnect at many points. The deep system consists of paired calf veins, which accompany each named artery before joining the popliteal vein (which may itself be duplex). The femoral vein is formed when the popliteal vein passes through the adductor canal and receives the profunda femoris vein in the upper thigh. This in turn becomes the external iliac vein as it passes behind the inguinal ligament. It joins with the internal iliac vein in the pelvis to become the common iliac vein, which merges with its opposite counterpart to form the inferior vena cava. This ascends on the right of the aorta to enter the lower part of the right atrium after passing behind the liver. The superficial and deep systems of the limb connect at various points through communicating veins, which include the saphenofemoral and saphenopopliteal junctions and the perforating or communicating veins of the calf.

APLASIA AND HYPOPLASIA

Agenesis may be extensive or localized with a 'membrane' crossing the lumen.[7] Reduplication is also common but is of little clinical significance.

CONGENITAL ABNORMALITIES

VENOUS ANGIOMAS

Venous angiomas are a confluent mass of anomalous veins, which vary from small localized collections of abnormal surface veins to an extensive network that can extend deeply into the soft tissues, bones and joints.[8] Most angiomas are first noticed as a variable

REFERENCES

1. Ludbrook J. Aspects of Venous Function in the Lower Limbs. Thomas, Illinois, 1966
2. Shepherd JT, Vanhoutte PM. Veins and their Control. Saunders, Philadelphia, 1975
3. Langman J. Medical Embryology. 4th edn. Williams & Wilkins, Baltimore, 1981
4. Hirsch DM, Chan K. JAMA 1963; 185: 729
5. May R, Nissl R. In: May R (ed). Surgery of the Veins of the Leg and Pelvis. Thieme, Stuttgart, 1979
6. Servelle M, Babillot J. Phlebologie 1980; 33: 31
7. Sen PK, Kinare SG et al. J Cardiovasc Surg 1987; 8: 344
8. Arland R. Phlebologie 1980; 33: 547

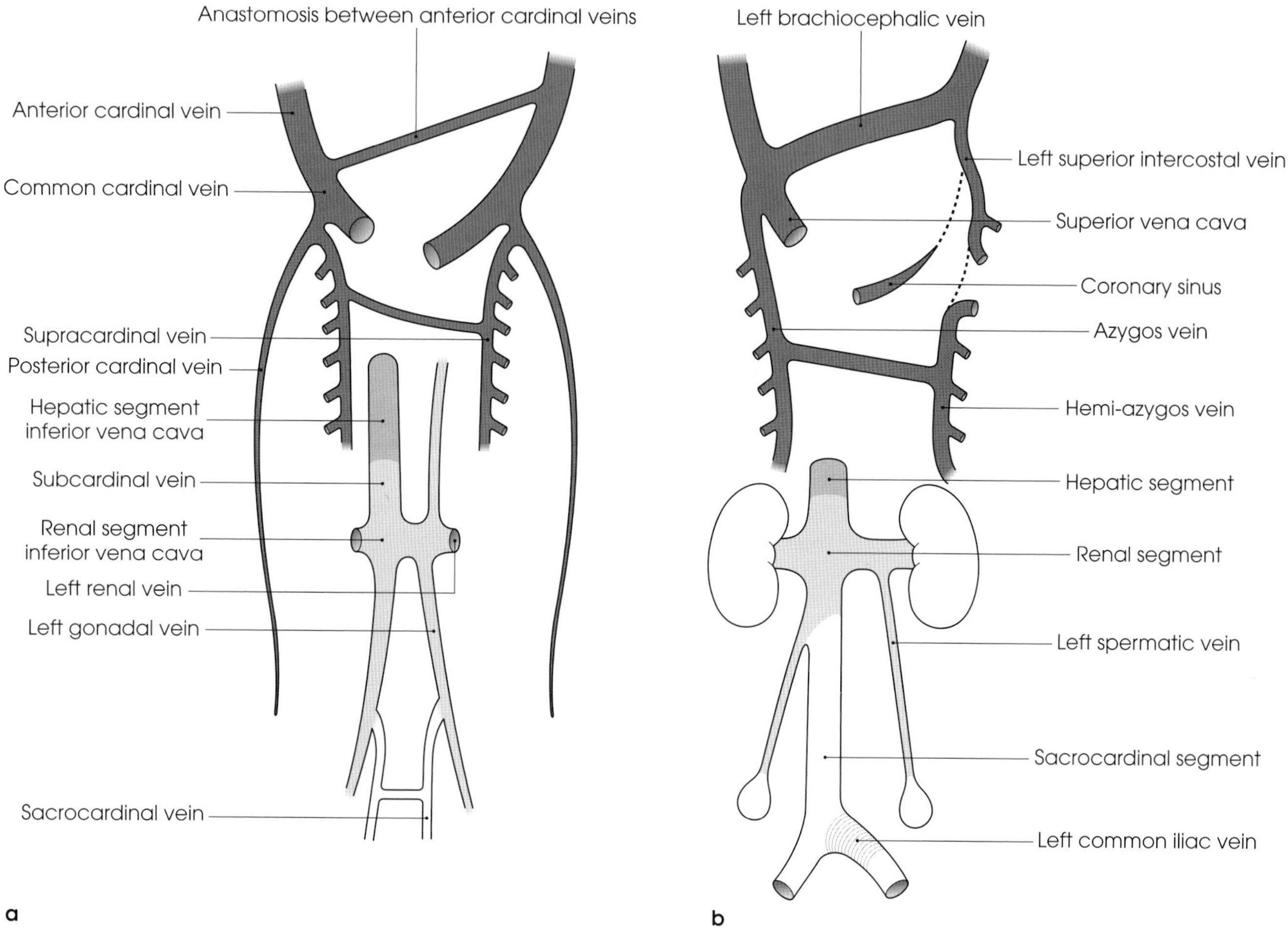

Anastomosis between anterior cardinal veins
Anterior cardinal vein
Common cardinal vein
Supracardinal vein
Posterior cardinal vein
Hepatic segment inferior vena cava
Subcardinal vein
Renal segment inferior vena cava
Left renal vein
Left gonadal vein
Sacrocardinal vein
a

Left brachiocephalic vein
Left superior intercostal vein
Superior vena cava
Coronary sinus
Azygos vein
Hemi-azygos vein
Hepatic segment
Renal segment
Left spermatic vein
Sacrocardinal segment
Left common iliac vein
b

Figure 11.1 Development of the venous pathways from the lower limb: (**a**) embryonic veins, and (**b**) final appearance showing deviation from originals.

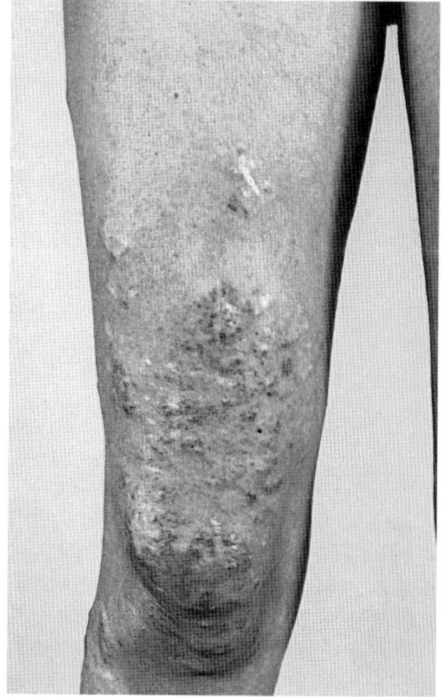

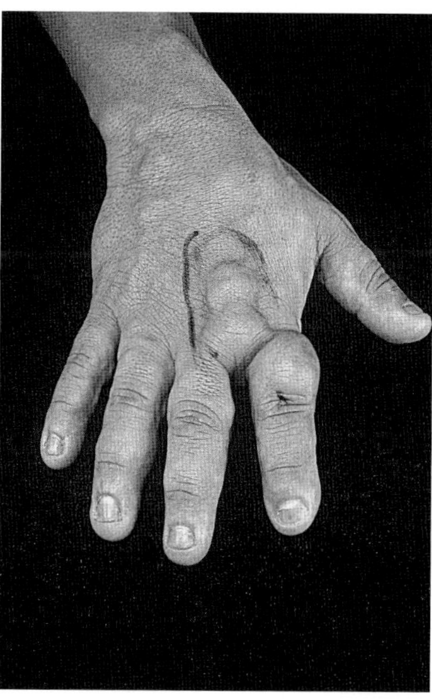

Figure 11.2 Venous angioma: (**a**) on the leg, and (**b**) on the hand.

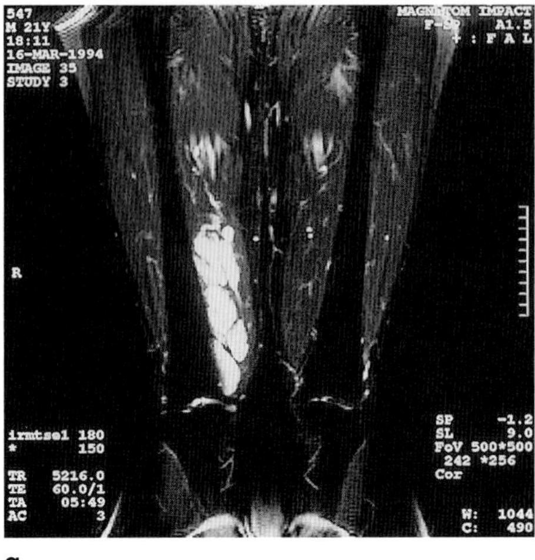

a

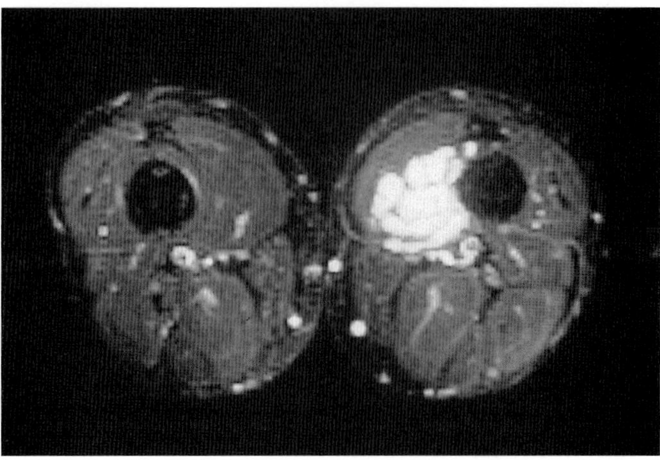

b

Figure 11.3 Venous angioma shown by MRI scan using STIR sequence: (**a**) transverse cut, and (**b**) vertical cut.

swelling, often situated beneath a cluster of dilated cutaneous veins or seen as bluish 'tumour' (Fig. 11.2). Deep angiomas may not cause a swelling and present with local pain or with episodes of haemorrhage or thrombosis. Angiomatous swellings are compressible and collapse when raised above the level of the heart. Venous angiomas must be differentiated from capillary haemangiomata, multiple arteriovenous fistulae, and lymphangiomata (see Ch. 10 and Ch. 12). Occasionally a venous angioma may be mistaken for a soft tissue sarcoma or an abscess if it is complicated by thrombosis or haemorrhage. The extent and nature of the angioma can be determined by CT scanning of the limb after contrast, but a short T1 time inversion recovery (STIR) sequence of magnetic resonance provides even better information (Fig. 11.3).[9]

Venous angiomas are often difficult to excise completely, yet this remains the best form of treatment.[10] Sclerotherapy may be beneficial but embolization is ineffective. The extent of the lesion determines the prospect of surgical success. Tissue defects left after excision can be covered by split-skin grafts, pedicle flaps, or even vascularized free flaps.[11]

Partial removal with over-sewing of residual angiomatous tissue usually produces an improvement, even in more extensive lesions. It is, however, vital to avoid damaging nerves or major arteries, and it is often preferable to leave some of the angioma and carry out a further excision on a later occasion than to produce unnecessary complications by an overambitious initial operation. Excision of angiomas from limbs is easier if the limb is exsanguinated and the operation is performed after a tourniquet has been applied.

VALVE ABNORMALITIES

Total venous valvular agenesis is extremely rare, with fewer than 50 cases having been reported.[12] The edges of the valve cusps may be floppy, which leads to inversion and venous reflux. These floppy valves can be tightened using a variety of open and closed techniques. A brachial valve may be transplanted into the femoral or popliteal veins but the benefits of these operations are still debated.[13]

KLIPPEL–TRENAUNAY SYNDROME

This syndrome was first described by Klippel and Trenaunay in 1900[14] and consists of the combination of a cutaneous naevus, varicose veins, and bone and soft tissue deformity affecting one or more limbs. The condition must be differentiated from Parkes–Weber syndrome, in which there are multiple arteriovenous fistulae that also cause limb hypertrophy. The Klippel–Trenaunay syndrome is a diffuse mesodermal abnormality often associated with lymphatic and other congenital abnormalities. The naevus, limb hypertrophy, and visible veins are present at birth or develop in childhood. The naevus is variable in extent, usually pale purple, affecting part or all of the limb and extending on to the trunk in many instances. It characteristically has a metameric distribution (Fig. 11.4). The varicose veins are often extensive and are usually situated over the lateral surface of the limb, where they connect with a persistent primitive lateral limb vein that has failed to regress (Fig. 11.4).[14] Approximately a quarter of the

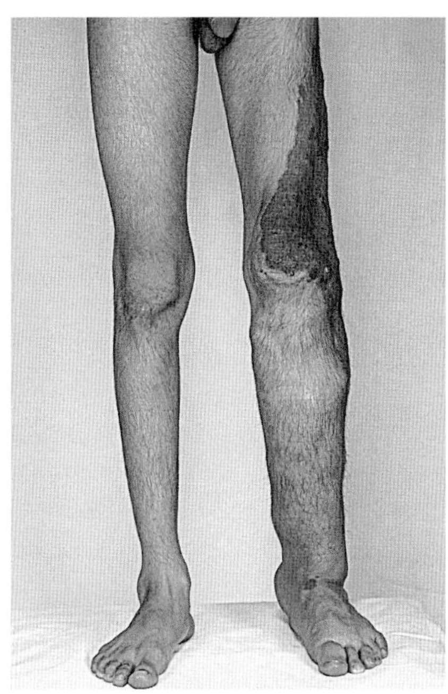

Figure 11.4 Klippel–Trenaunay syndrome.

REFERENCES

9. Sacks AM, Paterson FC, Irvine A et al. Radiology 1995; 194: 908–911
10. Christenson JT, Gunterberg B. Br J Surg 1985; 7: 748
11. Multiken JB, Young AE. Vascular Birthmarks. Saunders, Philadelphia, 1989
12. Lodin A, Lindvall N, Gentele H. Acta Chir Scand 1958; 116: 256
13. Perrin M, Calvignac JL, Hiltbrand B et al. Phlebology 1995; Suppl 1: 968
14. Klippel M, Trenaunay P. Arch Gen Med (Paris) 1900; 185: 641

patients who have the syndrome have pelvic venous anomalies that may give rise to rectal bleeding or haematuria.[15] Aplasia of the deep veins is present in 5 or 10% of patients, and poor venous drainage, soft tissue hypertrophy, and lymphatic obliteration cause limb swelling and ankle oedema.[16,17]

There is an increased incidence of deep vein thrombosis and pulmonary embolism in patients with the Klippel–Trenaunay syndrome, and there may be an associated activated protein C resistance. Lipodermatosclerosis and ulceration can develop. Bone hypertrophy and limb lengthening may lead to an abnormal gait, which in turn may cause joint problems and lumbar backache.[17,18] Other congenital abnormalities, which include spina bifida and syndactyly, may also be present. Klippel–Trenaunay syndrome can usually be distinguished from Parkes–Weber syndrome on clinical examination, but if this proves difficult blood flow estimation and arteriography are diagnostic.[15] Deep venous agenesis must be excluded by duplex scanning or phlebography before any surgery is undertaken on the superficial veins.

Elastic support stockings, which relieve aching and swelling, may prevent the development of lipodermatosclerosis and ulceration. Surgical eradication of the superficial veins should be advised only if the deep veins are normal and the symptoms are not relieved by stockings. Sites of superficial to deep communication should be disconnected and surface varices can be stripped out or avulsed,[15] but some recurrence is inevitable. The naevus may be disguised by camouflage cream or laser photocoagulation.

Local amputations may be required for gigantism of the toes and forefoot. Excessive limb growth may be controlled by epiphyseal stapling or epiphysiolysis,[19] but a heel raise for the opposite limb may be all that is required.

POPLITEAL VEIN ENTRAPMENT

Popliteal vein entrapment is similar to popliteal arterial entrapment (see Ch. 10). Patients present with intermittent swelling and discomfort that comes on during exercise, or they develop a deep venous thrombosis.[20] When the condition is diagnosed before thrombosis has occurred, the entrapment can be treated by dividing the abnormal muscle, which is usually one head of the gastrocnemius.

THORACIC INLET SYNDROME

The axillary vein may be compressed at its entry through the thoracic inlet, in a similar manner to the subclavian artery and the T1 nerve root (see Ch. 10).[21] Obstruction to the venous return is the most common cause of an axillary vein thrombosis. Resection of a cervical or the first rib may prevent thrombosis and relieve symptoms. This may be carried out through an axillary approach or through combined supra- and infraclavicular incisions.

CYSTIC DEGENERATION OF THE VEIN WALL

Cystic degeneration of the vein wall has similarities to cystic change in the arterial wall (see Ch. 10). The cysts contain a transparent gelatinous material that is identical to the contents of a ganglion.[22] Patients present with a mass related to the vein or with signs of venous obstruction and thrombosis. The cyst may be visible on CT scanning or duplex ultrasound imaging as a smooth swelling compressing the vessel lumen. The cyst may be deroofed and the contents expelled or the affected segment of vein can be resected and replaced with a short vein graft.[23,24]

Table 11.1 Incidence of combined arterial and venous injuries in the Vietnam War

Artery injured	Number of arterial injuries	Number of concomitant venous injuries (%)
Axillary	59	20 (33.8)
Brachial	283	54 (19.0)
Iliac	26	11 (42.3)
Common femoral	46	17 (36.9)
Superficial femoral	305	139 (45.5)
Popliteal	217	116 (53.5)
Total	936	357 (37.9)

(From Rich et al. 1970.)

VENOUS INJURY

Any injury to soft tissue or bone is associated with some damage to small and medium-sized veins, but haemorrhage or occlusion of these vessels can usually be safely ignored. When a haematoma develops, it may occasionally require drainage. When similar-sized veins are damaged during operations they can be safely ligated, but injuries to the large axial veins of the limbs, pelvis and abdomen cannot be ignored, nor can these vessels be safely ligated because this results in acute or chronic venous obstruction.

Many major venous injuries unfortunately still pass unnoticed and only come to light when the post-thrombotic syndrome develops some years later. It is therefore impossible to provide an accurate figure for the incidence of major venous injury, although a number of large series of vascular injuries during war or civil unrest have been reported.[25–29] These reports have shown that when a patient has an arterial injury (see Ch. 10) a concomitant venous injury is common (Table 11.1). The risk of

REFERENCES

15. Baskerville PA, Ackroyd JS et al. Br J Surg 1985; 72: 232
16. Young AE. Birth Defects Orig Artic Ser 1978; 14: 289
17. Van Der Molen H. R Soc Fr Phleb 1968; 2: 187
18. Vollmar J, Vogt K. Chirurgie 1976; 47: 205
19. Blount WP, Clark GR. J Bone Joint Surg 1949; 31A
20. Rich NM, Hughes CW. Am J Surg 1967; 113: 696
21. McLeer RS, Kesterson JE et al. Ann Surg 1951; 133: 588
22. Mentha C. Presse Med 1963; 71: 2205
23. Browse NL, Burnand KG, Lea Thomas M. Diseases of the Veins. Arnold, London, 1988
24. Fyfe NCM, Sillocks PB, Browse NL. J Cardiovasc Surg 1980; 21: 703
25. De Bakey ME, Simeone FA. Ann Surg 1946; 123: 534
26. Hughes CW. Surg Gynecol Obstet 1954; 99: 91
27. Rich NM. J Cardiovasc Surg 1970; 11: 368
28. Livingstone RH, Wilson R. Br Med J 1975; 1: 667
29. Schramek A, Hashmonai M. Br J Surg 1977; 64: 644
30. Rich NM, Baugh JH, Hughes CWJ. J Trauma 1970; 10: 359

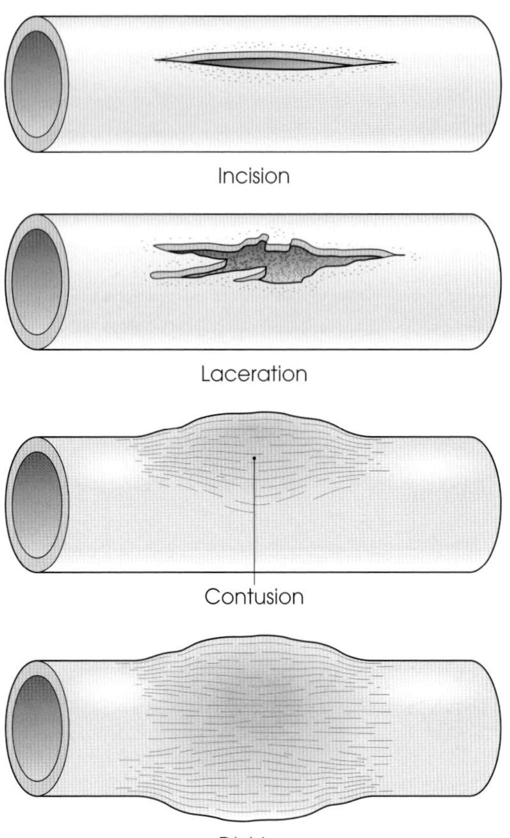

Figure 11.5 Types of venous injury. (From Browse et al. Diseases of the Veins Pathology, Diagnosis and Treatment, 1988. Reproduced by permission of Hodder Arnold.[23])

major venous injury in civilian life has increased in recent years.[31–34]

METHOD AND TYPE OF INJURY

Veins may be injured in one of five ways: they can be incised, lacerated (torn), contused, stretched or divided (Fig. 11.5). A number of external forces are responsible for these injuries. These include stab wounds, bullet wounds and bomb fragments (shrapnel), which can produce incisions, lacerations, contusions or transections of the vein wall. Blows or crushing injuries that fail to disrupt the vein wall produce contusions or intimal damage, both of which may lead to secondary thrombosis. Veins lying close to fractures or dislocations may be overstretched, disrupting one or more layers of the vein wall and predisposing to thrombosis.

Iatrogenic venous injuries are an important cause of vein damage.[33] Large veins can be inadvertently damaged at operation, especially during difficult arterial surgery (e.g. abdominal aneurysms). Veins can also be damaged by direct puncture when a catheter or needle is inserted for monitoring or nutrition and during cardiac or radiological investigations. Toxic substances injected into the veins in error may also cause intimal damage and thrombosis.[35]

SYMPTOMS, SIGNS AND INVESTIGATIONS

A venous injury produces either concealed or revealed haemorrhage. The latter is seen as dark blood that wells up out of the wound. Concealed blood loss may only be suspected when hypovolaemic shock develops. There may also be signs of venous obstruction in the affected part, indicated by the presence of cyanosis and oedema. Investigations are irrelevant if the patient is actively bleeding, and adequate resuscitation should be followed by operation and venous repair. Duplex scanning and phlebography may be helpful when late signs of venous obstruction or thrombosis develop.

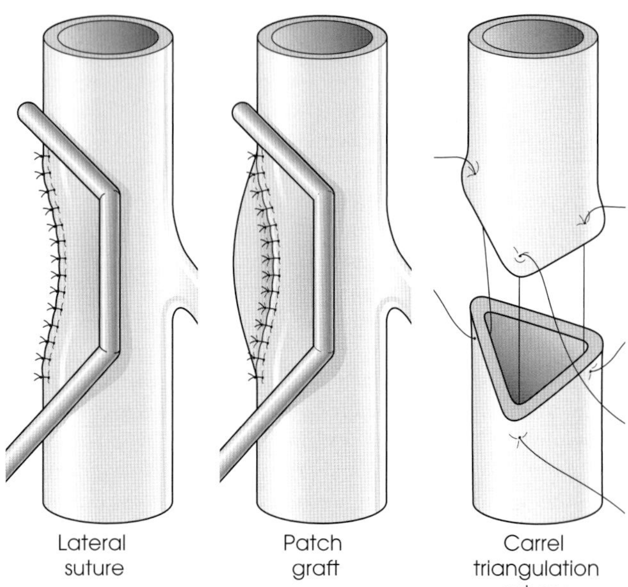

Figure 11.6 Methods of repairing venous injury. (From Browse et al. Diseases of the Veins Pathology, Diagnosis and Treatment, 1988. Reproduced by permission of Hodder Arnold.[23])

MANAGEMENT

Pressure and elevation are effective first aid treatment, but the patient should be quickly transferred to hospital, where resuscitation and cross-matching of blood should be followed by operative exploration of the wound under general anaesthesia. Skin wounds are extended to visualize the bleeding point or points, and suction helps to display the anatomy. Haemorrhage from a large vein can usually be controlled by finger pressure on either side of the laceration, which allows the vein wall to be dissected out and inspected. Fogarty catheters can be inserted through the venous defect if control cannot be achieved by pressure, and balloon inflation helps to control blood loss.

Once the vein has been dissected free, a small laceration can be closed by a simple or continuous suture while a more complicated venous injury may require repair by a vein patch or an interposition graft (Fig. 11.6).[32] Heparin should be given unless a coagulopathy is present. Once the bleeding has been controlled, the wound must be inspected to exclude any associated injuries to other important structures such as accompanying arteries and nerves. The continuity of major veins should be restored at an early stage, before other structures are repaired. This is especially important if an associated artery

REFERENCES

31. Gaspar MR, Treiman RL. Am J Surg 1960; 100: 171
32. Drapanas T, Hewitt RL et al. Ann Surg 1970; 172: 351
33. Vollmar J. In: May R (ed). Surgery of the Veins of the Leg and Pelvis. Thieme, Stuttgart, 1979
34. Nypaver TJ, Schuler JJ, McDonnell P et al. Vasc Surg 1992; 16: 762
35. MacGowan WAL, Holland PDJ et al. Br J Surg 1972; 59: 103

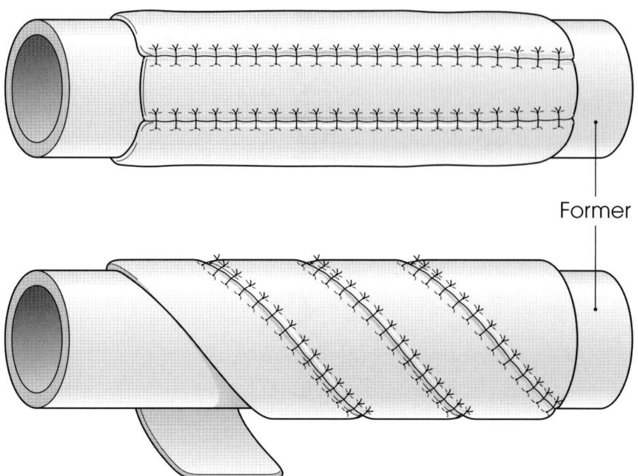

Figure 11.7 Methods of producing a composite venous graft. (From Browse et al. Diseases of the Veins Pathology, Diagnosis and Treatment, 1988. Reproduced by permission of Hodder Arnold.[23])

is also damaged. Autogenous vein is the material of choice for venous reconstruction, but this should not be taken from the injured extremity because all veins may act as useful collaterals should the graft fail. When a segment of vein wall has been lost, a vein patch must be used to prevent narrowing (Fig. 11.6).[33,36] An interposition vein graft may be made up as a composite to provide the desired diameter to replace a damaged or transected vessel. The long and short saphenous, the cephalic, the brachial and the internal jugular veins can all be used for this purpose. These veins can be split open and sewn spirally[37] or joined as a series of panels[38] to produce a graft of appropriate diameter (Fig. 11.7).

Heparin should normally be administered for several days after a vein repair, although its value in preventing thrombosis has been questioned.[39] A flow-enhancing distal arteriovenous fistula or pneumatic compression leggings may also reduce the risk of a perioperative or postoperative thrombosis.[40,41] Fasciotomies should be performed if there has been extensive venous damage or associated arterial damage. The damaged vein should not be left exposed but an effort must be made to cover it with viable muscle. Blood loss from large veins can be prevented by isolating the injury with an intraluminal shunt,[42] which also provides an ideal environment for venous repair (Fig. 11.8). Patients who sustain blunt trauma to the abdomen and pelvis with associated pelvic fractures may have significant venous injury. Blind exploration of the patient can cause death from uncontrollable haemorrhage. The absence of continuing bleeding after initial resuscitation is an indication to adopt a conservative approach.

RESULTS

The simultaneous repair of damaged veins and arteries has been shown to increase the prospects of limb survival.[28] The long-term patency rates of vein repair have not been well documented but between 30 and 70% of repairs appear to be successful.[37]

COMPLICATIONS

Major venous injuries may be complicated by the development of arteriovenous fistulae, air embolism, deep vein thrombosis, pulmonary embolism, post-thrombotic limb, secondary infection and haemorrhage.[33,36]

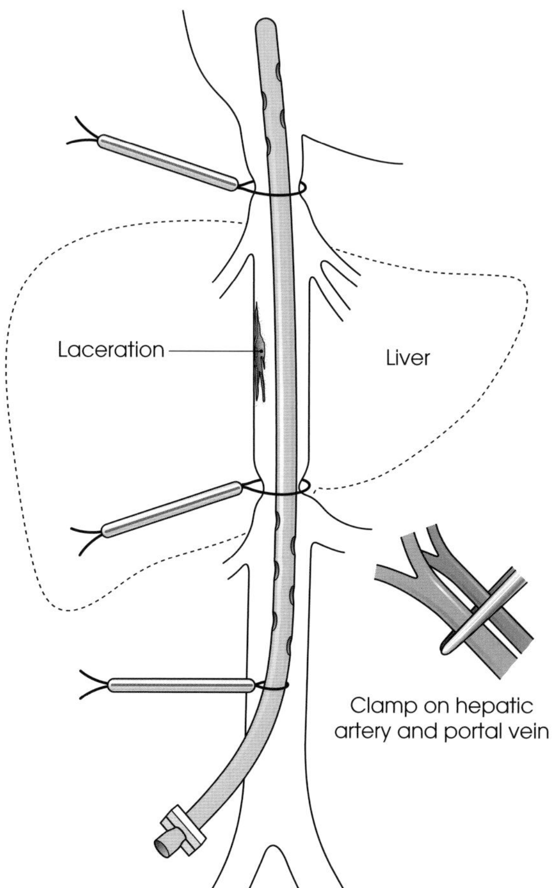

Figure 11.8 Insertion of an intraluminal shunt, which allows venous repair to be carried out in a bloodless field.

VARICOSE VEINS

A varicose vein is a vein that is tortuous and dilated, and varicose veins are invariably associated with valvular incompetence. The prevalence of this condition in Europe and the USA has been shown by a number of large surveys to be about 2%, with a slightly higher incidence in women than in men; this incidence increases with age.[43–46]

REFERENCES

36. Rich NM, Hughes GW, Baugh JH. Ann Surg 1970; 171: 724
37. Hobson RW, Yeager RA et al. Am J Surg 1983; 146: 220
38. O'Reilly NJH, Hood JM et al. Br J Surg 1980; 67: 337
39. Hobson RW, Groom RD, Rich NM. Ann Surg 1973; 178: 773
40. Hobson RW, Lee BC et al. Surg Gynecol Obstet 1984; 159: 284
41. Bryant ME, Lazenby WD, Howard JM. Arch Surg 1958; 76: 289
42. Matto KL. Surgery 1982; 91: 497
43. Borschberg E. The Prevalence of Varicose Veins of the Lower Extremity. Karger, Basel, 1967
44. Widmer LK. Peripheral Venous Disorders. Prevalence and Socio-medical Importance. Hans Huber, Berne, 1978
45. US Department of Health Education and Welfare. National Health Survey 1935–1936. US Department of Health Education and Welfare, Washington, 1938
46. Callum M. Br J Surg 1994; 81: 167

PATHOLOGY

Varicose veins may be defined as primary if the cause is not known, or they may be secondary to other conditions, which include post-thrombotic damage, pregnancy, pelvic tumours, and congenital disorders such as the Klippel–Trenaunay syndrome.

The influence of heredity on the development of varicose veins has been clearly demonstrated,[46–48] but the role of valvular damage versus a wall defect is still debated.[49,50] There is anatomical evidence that venous dilatation occurs below rather than above valves.[51] The collagen and mucopolysaccharide content of the vein wall is abnormal in patients with established varicosities and in their relatives before varicose veins have developed.[52] These findings are in favour of an inherited abnormality of the vein wall, causing secondary valvular incompetence.[50] Congenital valvular agenesis is an extremely rare but well-documented cause of varicose veins.[53] In situ vein bypass grafts in which all the valves have been deliberately destroyed do not, however, become varicose or aneurysmal. Varicose veins affect only humans, suggesting that the erect stance is important. Hormonal and haemodynamic factors may encourage varicosis. The concept that all varicose veins are secondary to incompetence of the communicating veins is no longer tenable.

Other factors that have been thought to predispose to varicose veins include age, female gender, parity,[54] occupations that involve prolonged standing[55] and tight clothing especially around the waist.[56] It has even been suggested that varicosities are the result of faulty bowel habit causing faecal masses to interfere with the venous return from the lower limb.[57] The sedentary position for defecation adopted by western societies does not appear to be important![46]

Histological studies of varicose veins have shown that there is a considerable increase in the fibrous tissue within the vein wall, which breaks up the smooth muscle and extends into all coats of the vein wall.[50] The valve sinuses are at first overstretched, causing the valves to atrophy. Varicosities usually occur in the tributaries of the saphenous vein rather than in the main trunks, although the saphenous veins can occasionally develop some abnormal sacculation.[51]

SYMPTOMS

Most patients with varicose veins do not seek medical advice. Unsightliness or disfigurement of the legs is one of the main reasons why patients with varicose veins, particularly women, present for treatment. Varicose veins can also cause discomfort, which is characteristically an ache felt in or over the veins, usually worse after prolonged standing or at the end of the day. The pain does not appear to be related to the size of the varicosities.[23] Pain and tenderness of the varicosities can be a prominent feature in women just before and during their period. Night cramps, ankle swelling, itching and restless legs are other common complaints.

The relationship between venous symptoms and the presence of venous reflux has not been confirmed. Varicose veins have an increased tendency to develop superficial thrombophlebitis, and they occasionally rupture spontaneously and bleed dramatically. Varicose veins are also associated with lipodermatosclerosis (pigmentation, induration and inflammation in the calf skin), which can be complicated by venous ulceration. Because varicose veins can develop in a post-thrombotic limb, it is important to try to exclude this on the history. Previous fractures of the limbs, major surgery, or a swollen leg in pregnancy are all indicators.

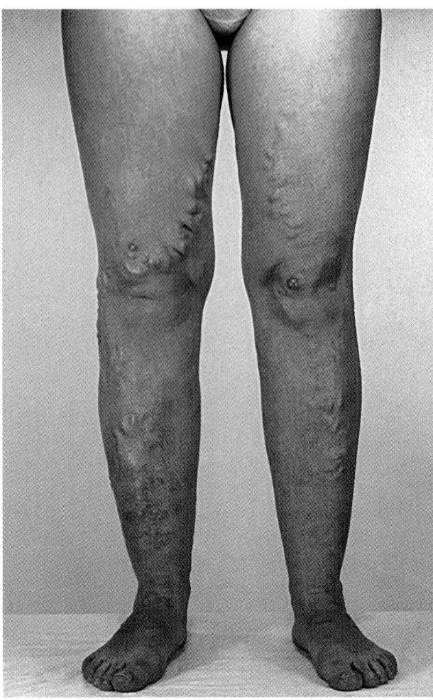

Figure 11.9 Long saphenous varicosities.

EXAMINATION

The patient should be examined standing on a low stool or platform in a well-lit and warm room with the lower limbs fully exposed from the groin to the toes. The distribution of all the major subcutaneous varicosities on both aspects of the limb should be carefully recorded on outline diagrams of the leg.[58] An attempt should be made to determine which major tributaries have become varicose, and any unusual channels should also be recorded. Careful inspection may reveal a saphena varix (Fig. 11.9) or a dilated short saphenous termination. The presence of an ankle flare, indicative of venous hypertension, or dilated calf blow-outs is suggestive of incompetent calf communicating veins (Fig. 11.10).[59] Any skin change around the ankle, especially lipodermatosclerosis, ulceration and eczema, indicates the possibility of post-thrombotic damage, which is further supported by findings of dilated veins over the groin or abdomen.

Some varicose veins are more easily felt than seen, and it is advisable to run a hand lightly over the course of both the long and the short saphenous territories.[23] Ankle oedema and a temperature difference between the limbs may also be detected by this type of palpation, which will often pick up thickening in the gaiter skin (which may be the first sign of lipodermato-

REFERENCES

47. Virchow R. Cellular Pathology. Churchill, London, 1860
48. Gundersen J, Hauge M. Angiology 1969; 20: 346
49. Ludbrook J. Lancet 1963; ii: 1289
50. Rose SS, Ahmed A. J Cardiovasc Surg 1986; 27: 534
51. Cotton L. Br J Surg 1961; 48: 589
52. Svejcar J, Prerovsky I et al. Clin Sci 1963; 24: 325
53. Lindvall N, Lodin A. Acta Chir Scand 1962; 124: 310
54. Foote RR. Varicose Veins. Butterworths, London, 1954
55. Lake M, Pratt GH, Wright IS. JAMA 1942; 119: 696
56. Mekky S, Schilling RSF, Walford J. Br Med J 1969; 2: 591
57. Burkitt DP. Br Med J 1972; 2: 556
58. Dodd HJ, Cockett FB. The Pathology and Surgery of the Veins of the Lower Limb. Churchill Livingstone, Edinburgh, 1976
59. Cockett FB. Br Med J 1953; 2: 1399

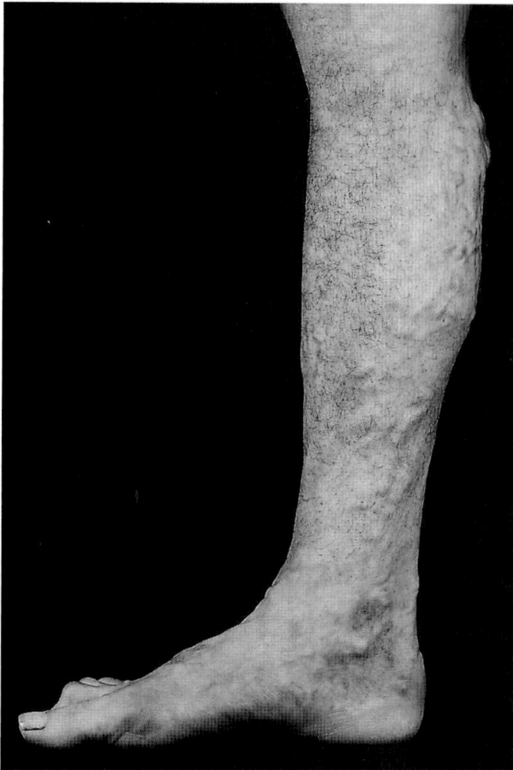

Figure 11.10 An ankle flare indicative of venous hypertension and incompetent calf communicating veins.

sclerosis). A cough impulse should be examined for over the saphenofemoral junction and over any large varices further down the limb.[18,60] If a thrill is present, the upper valves of the long saphenous vein must be incompetent. Valvular incompetence can also be assessed by percussing over a varix and finding an impulse passing up and down a dilated and valveless vein. Although it has been suggested that palpation over the medial calf may detect fascial defects where incompetent communicating veins pierce the deep fascia,[61] this test has been shown to be hopelessly inaccurate.[62] The use of a sliding finger to control reflux through incompetent perforating veins has been championed by some,[63] but others have found this test to be equally ineffective for localizing the communicating veins. An arteriovenous fistula is suspected if a murmur is heard over a localized collection of varices.

TOURNIQUET TESTS

The Brodie–Trendelenburg test[64,65] consists of the application of a single tourniquet around the upper thigh after all the surface veins have been emptied by elevation of the limb and gentle massage.[23,54,58] Long saphenous incompetence is confirmed if the varicosities remain empty when the patient stands erect (Fig. 11.11). The varicosities should rapidly refill from above downwards when the tourniquet is released. When the varices are not controlled by the thigh tourniquet, the test should be repeated with the tourniquet placed just above the knee. Control at this level indicates the presence of an incompetent midthigh perforating vein. Control of the varices by a below the knee tourniquet is indicative of short saphenous incompetence. Multiple tourniquets applied at intervals along the leg have been used to try to determine the position of incompetent calf communicating veins, but these tests are extremely difficult to

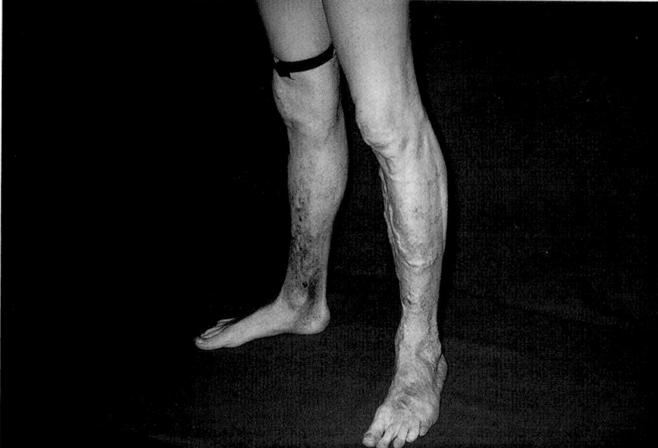

a

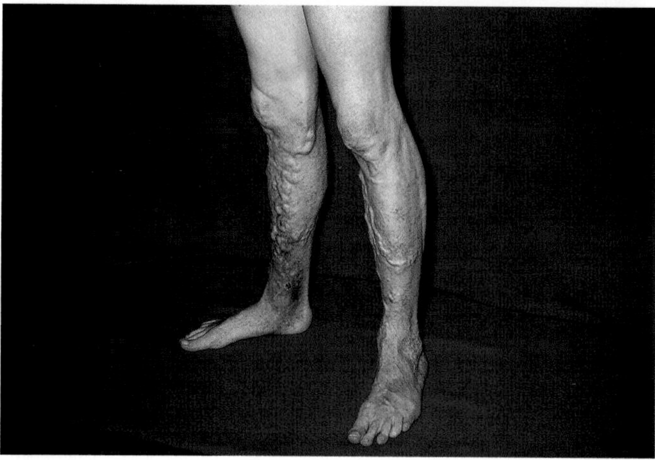

b

Figure 11.11 The Brodie–Trendelenburg tourniquet test: **(a)** the varicose tributaries of the long saphenous vein are kept empty by the tourniquet and **(b)** fill on release.

interpret. In the Perthes walking test,[66] a single tourniquet is applied around the thigh or knee and the patient asked to heel-raise or walk. The patient has normal calf communicating veins and deep veins if the surface veins empty. This test is useful in providing an overall assessment of the competence of the deep and communicating veins.

DIAGNOSIS

The majority of varicose veins can be assessed from the history and a careful clinical examination supplemented by the tourniquet tests,[23,54,58] but in many patients the history or physical signs indicate that varicose veins are not responsible for the patient's symptoms and that additional tests are required to exclude disorders of the hips, knees, spine, peripheral vessels

REFERENCES

60. Chevrier L. Arch Gen Chir 1908; 2: 44
61. Fegan WG. Varicose Veins: Compression Sclerotherapy. Heinemann, London, 1967
62. O'Donnell TF, Burnand KG et al. Arch Surg 1977; 112: 31
63. Hobbs J. Arch Surg 1974; 109: 793
64. Brodie B. Lectures Illustrative of Various Subjects in Pathology and Surgery. Longmans, London, 1846
65. Trendelenburg F. Klin Chir 1891; 7: 195
66. Perthes G. Dtsch Med Wochenschr 1895; 21: 253

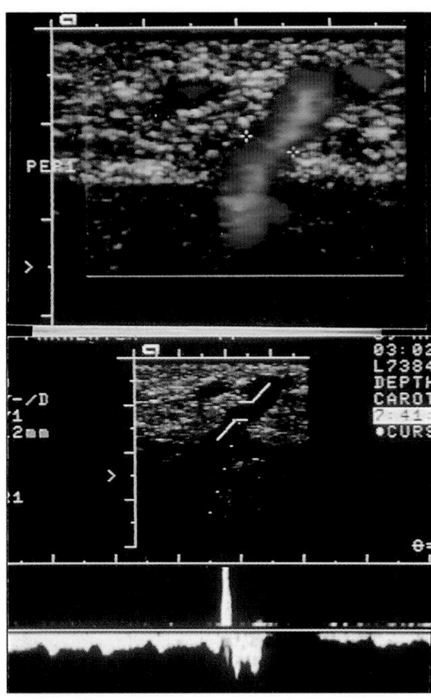

Figure 11.12 Duplex scan showing incompetent calf communicating veins.

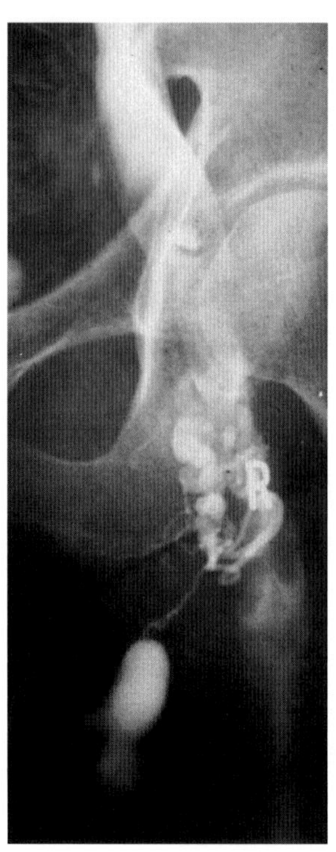

a

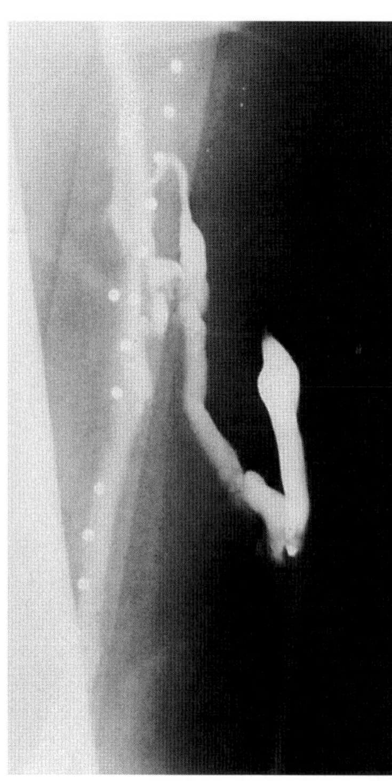

b

Figure 11.13 Varicograms showing (**a**) groin recurrences and (**b**) an incompetent Hunterian communicating vein connecting to previously ligated long saphenous vein.

or nervous system. The varicose veins that are present may be secondary to another cause, or it may not be possible to determine the extent and connections of the varicosities from the clinical examination. Further investigations are then necessary.

Doppler ultrasound testing of venous reflux in the long saphenous, short saphenous,[67] and calf communicating veins[68] is a simple investigation available in the clinic. It is valuable in confirming long saphenous reflux but cannot locate short saphenous incompetence or incompetent calf communicating veins with any accuracy.[62] The presence of a bidirectional signal on calf compression (forward and backward flow) or retrograde flow on tourniquet release or calf compression indicates incompetence of the long saphenous main trunk. Duplex ultrasound, which determines the presence of retrograde flow in a defined vein, has revolutionized the assessment of long and short saphenous incompetence in patients for whose conditions clinical examination or simple Doppler[69] fails to establish a clear diagnosis. Duplex may also be valuable in determining valvular incompetence in the communicating (Fig. 11.12) and deep veins, although it is not completely accurate in detecting post-thrombotic changes in the deep veins, where phlebography still has a place.[70] Bipedal ascending phlebography consists of injecting non-ionic contrast media into foot veins, with ankle tourniquets to direct the contrast into the deep system. This is still the most accurate method of detecting post-thrombotic damage.[71] Direct injection of contrast media into surface veins (varicography) outlines the extent and connections of varicosities and is particularly useful if the clinical tests and duplex are equivocal, or if the patient has had previous operations for varicose veins (Fig. 11.13).[72–74]

MANAGEMENT

When patients with varicose veins have been fully assessed, they should be placed in one of several categories.

- Definite long or short saphenous varicosities with a single saphenous vein incompetence or a combination of both long and short saphenous incompetence, which is often more difficult to diagnose and may require Doppler, duplex or varicography to confirm the diagnosis.
- A combination of saphenous incompetence and incompetence of communicating veins in the calf or thigh.
- Isolated calf communicating vein incompetence (rare).
- Minor tributary vein incompetence without evidence of saphenous or communicating vein incompetence.

The venous system requires a more detailed evaluation if there is suspicion of post-thrombotic damage or when the skin changes associated with venous hypertension are present in the gaiter region of the calf.

TREATMENT

Patients with minor cosmetic varicosities or visible veins can be treated by reassurance or elastic support stockings. Patients with clear evidence of long or short saphenous incompetence or with a combination of the two, almost always associated with branch vein varicosities, should have the saphenofemoral or sapheno-

REFERENCES

67. Hoare MC, Royle JP. Aust NZ J Surg 1984; 54: 49
68. Miner SS, Foote AV. Br J Surg 1974; 61: 653
69. Coleridge-Smith PD, Scurr JH. Curr Pract Surg 1995; 7: 182
70. De Maeseneer MG et al. Cardiovasc Surg 1993; 1: 686
71. Baker S, Burnand KG, Sommerville KM et al. Lancet 1993; 341: 400
72. Corbett CR, McIrvine AJ et al. Ann R Coll Surg Engl 1984; 66: 412
73. Bradbury AW, Stonebridge PA, Callum MJ et al. Br J Surg 1994; 81: 373
74. Bradbury AW, Stonebridge PA, Ruckley CV. Br J Surg 1993; 80: 849

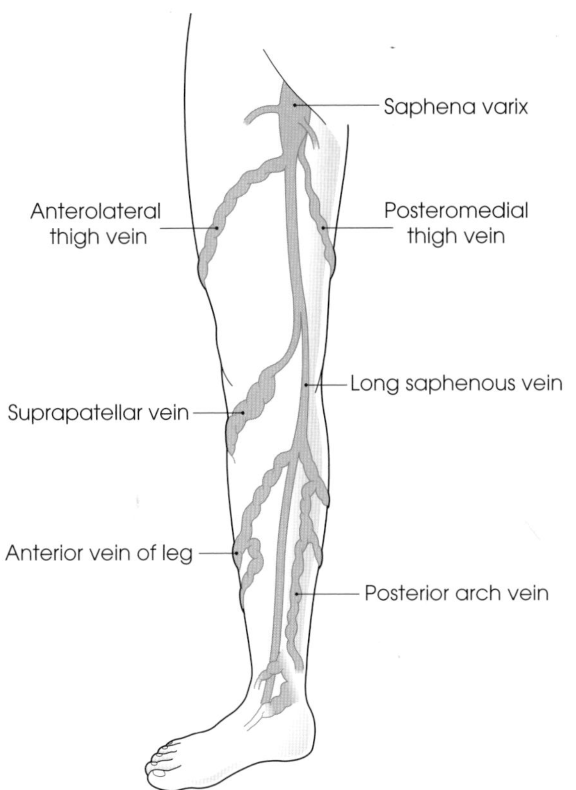

Figure 11.14 The major tributaries that join the long saphenous vein in its course up the leg.

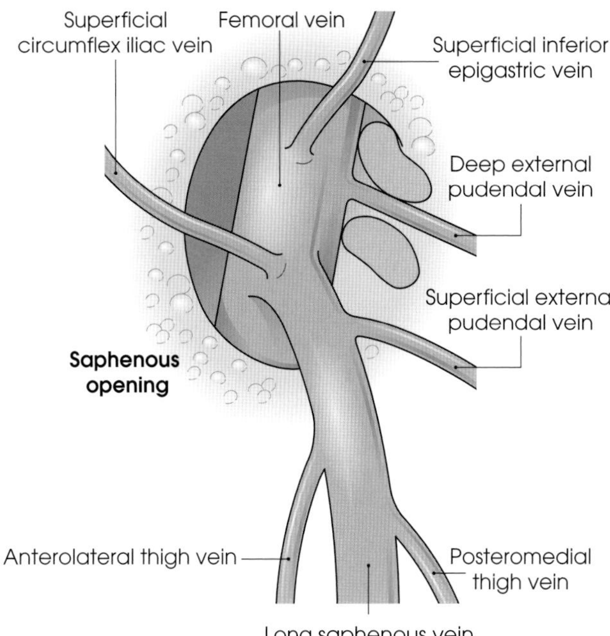

Figure 11.15 The tributaries that enter the long saphenous vein near its termination.

popliteal junction surgically ligated if their symptoms justify intervention. This should be combined with stripping of the incompetent long saphenous vein to the knee, or the incompetent short saphenous vein to the ankle, and avulsion of all the varicose tributaries. These operations have been shown by Hobbs to have a lower incidence of recurrence than sclerotherapy when major saphenous incompetence is present.[75]

The saphenous veins must be disconnected flush with the femoral and popliteal veins, and all the tributaries near their termination must be ligated and divided to prevent recurrence.[23,54,58,59] The value of vein stripping has been confirmed by clinical trials.[76–78] It prevents the possibility of reconnection and removes some of the communicating veins as well as disconnecting the venous tributaries from the main channels (Fig. 11.14).

The saphenofemoral junction is approached with the patient lying flat with legs abducted and elevated. An oblique incision is made 2 cm below and lateral to the pubic tubercle, and the long saphenous vein is found by blunt dissection as it passes up through the subcutaneous fat. It is traced to its termination with the femoral vein as it dips down through the cribriform fascia and fossa ovale. The superficial inferior epigastric vein, the superficial external and deep external pudendal veins, and the superficial external iliac veins usually join the long saphenous vein near its termination (Fig. 11.15). These tributaries must be carefully ligated and divided. When the saphenofemoral junction has been defined, the vein is divided and ligated before a flexible intraluminal stripper is passed down the vein to knee level or just below. The stripper is recovered through a small incision placed over its tip, and the vein is avulsed by steady downwards traction on the distal end. An additional stripper may be passed up from a separate incision made over the vein near the knee or at the ankle (Fig. 11.16) if the stripper will not pass down the vein. Pin stripping, developed by Oesch,[79] invaginates the vein and may reduce the postoperative bleeding but this has not been confirmed by controlled trials.[80,81] Laser or thermal destruction of the long saphenous vein has been introduced, but these techniques require good controlled trials to establish their efficacy.

The short saphenous vein is approached with the patient lying prone. An incision is made at the ankle and the vein is dissected off the sural nerve. The vein is ligated and the stripper is inserted through a venotomy and passed up towards the knee, where it can be felt to 'kick' and pass deeply at the level of the saphenopopliteal junction. The short saphenous termination is more accurately located by on-table phlebography or by preoperative duplex scanning or varicography.[82,83] An appropriately sited transverse incision is then made over the saphenopopliteal junction, and the short saphenous vein containing the stripper is located lying beneath the deep fascia (Fig. 11.17) before being traced to its T-junction with the popliteal vein. The short saphenous vein is then disconnected, its stump is ligated, and the distal vein is stripped out. Many surgeons simply ligate the short saphenous vein without stripping it, but the recurrence rate of this approach is considerable.

Branch varicosities are avulsed through multiple minute incisions placed directly over the varicosities at appropriate

REFERENCES

75. Hobbs JT. Br J Surg 1968; 55: 777
76. Sarin S, Scurr JH, Coleridge-Smith PD. Br J Surg 1992; 79: 889
77. Bergan J. J Cardiovasc Surg 1993; 1: 624
78. Woodyer AB, Dormandy JA. Phlebology 1996; 1: 221
79. Oesch A. Phlebology 1993; 4: 171
80. Coleridge-Smith PD, Butler CM, Sommerville KM et al. Phlebology 1995; 1: 493
81. Tyrell MR, Rocker N, Maisey N et al. Phlebology 1995; 1: 451
82. Hobbs JT. Br Med J 1980; 2: 1528
83. Burnand KG. Phlebologie 1983; 1: 269

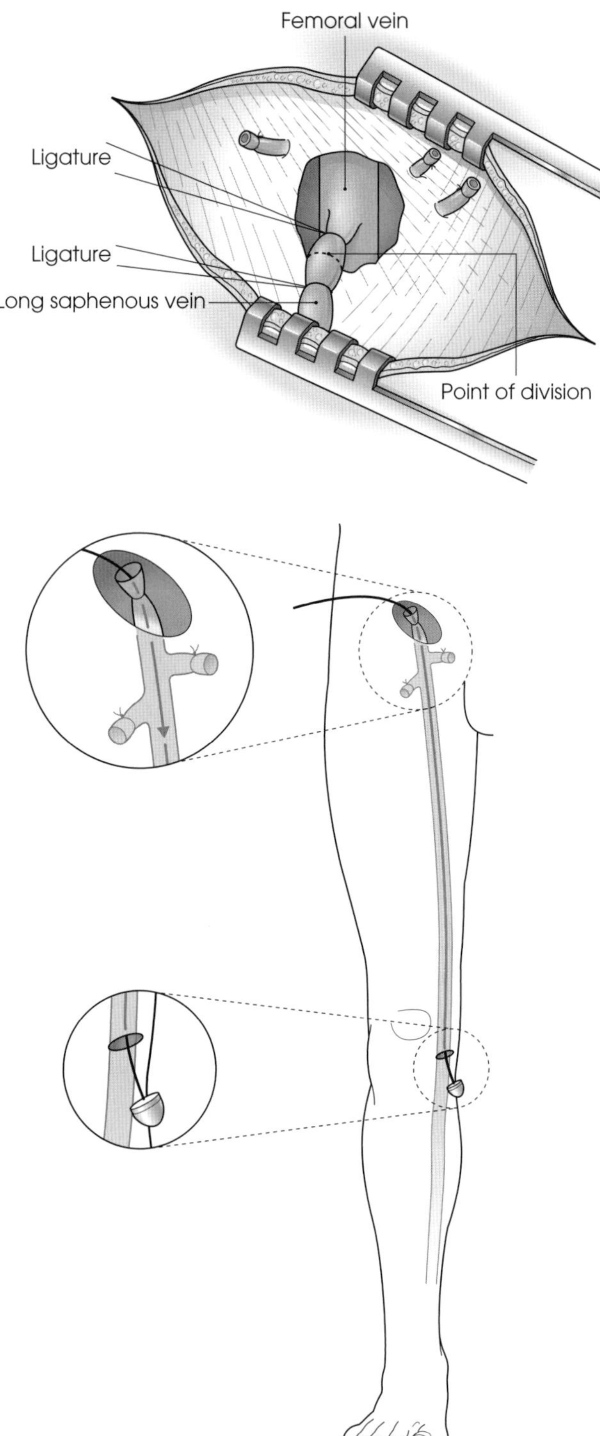

Figure 11.16 High saphenous ligation and stripping of the long saphenous vein.

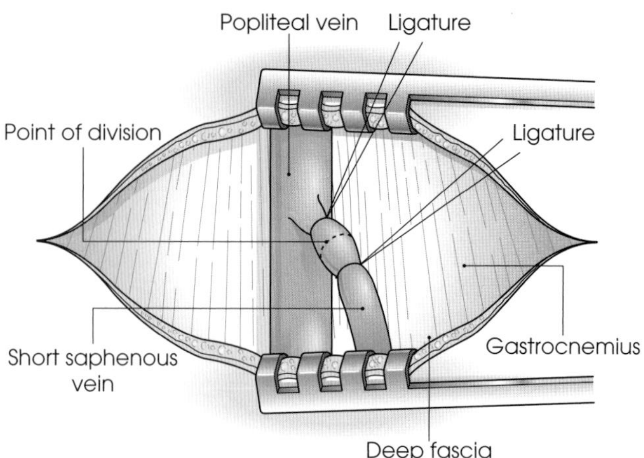

Figure 11.17 The popliteal dissection for short saphenous incompetence.

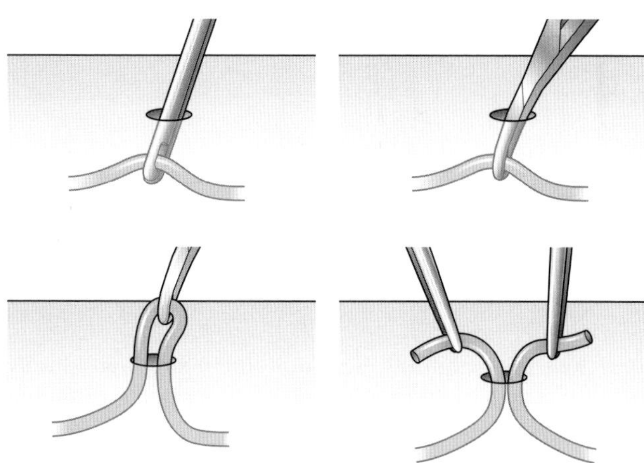

Figure 11.18 Avulsion of varicose tributaries.

intervals of about 5–10 cm (Fig. 11.18).[84] The veins are teased out using specially designed hooks or mosquito forceps, and the whole process may be easier and relatively bloodless if a tourniquet is used to exsanguinate the limb. Incompetent communicating veins are ligated through short incisions placed in Langer's lines if they can be located preoperatively. A minimally invasive approach has been developed using a specially designed telescope inserted beneath the deep fascia through a small incision in the upper calf.[85,86] The incompetent calf communicating veins are ligated and divided through the endoscope (Fig. 11.19). The major advantage of this operation is that in patients with established lipodermatosclerosis an incision through the affected area can be avoided. A recent trial failed to show that this technique was of any value in healing ulcers or preventing their recurrences.

Patients with minor branch varicosities who demand treatment, or patients who develop tributary recurrences after correctly performed saphenous surgery, are best treated by injection sclerotherapy. There are still some who will treat all varicosities by this technique. Introduced originally by Tavel,[87] and popularized by Tournay in France[88] and Fegan in Ireland,[89] sclerotherapy has been shown to be an effective method of eradicating varicose veins providing that major saphenous incompetence is not present or has been eradicated.[75] Sodium tetradecyl sulphate 1%, a detergent, is a popular sclerosant,

REFERENCES

84. Rivlin S. Br J Surg 1975; 62: 413
85. Gloviczki MD, Robert A, Camria MD et al. J Vasc Surg 1996; 23: 517
86. Hauer G, Borkun J, Wigger I et al. Surg Endosc 1988; 2: 5
87. Tavel E. Dtsch Z Chir 1912; 116: 735
88. Tournay R. Bull Med Paris 1931; 45: 73
89. Fegan WG. Lancet 1963; ii: 109

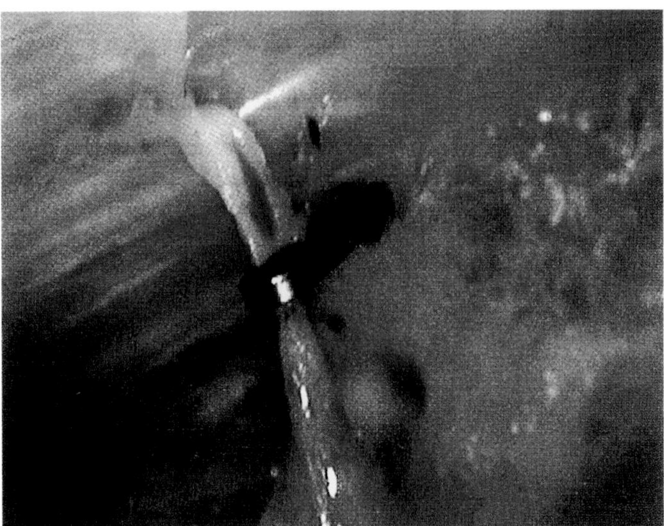

Figure 11.19 Ligated incompetent calf communicating veins (viewed through an endoscope). Subfascial endoscopic perforator surgery (SEPS): ligation of incompetent perforator.

although polidocanol and foam sclerosants are becoming more popular. Empty veins are injected, and are compressed and bandaged for a period of 3–6 weeks. Injections can be repeated on many occasions until all the varices have been eradicated. Extravasation of sclerosant and inadvertent intra-arterial injections[90] are disasters that can be avoided by careful technique. Skin pigmentation and telangiectatic matting are unwanted side effects. Sclerotherapy using duplex scanning to define the venous anatomy and confirm obliteration may improve results. It is not known if this approach is cost-effective. Foam sclerosants have been claimed to be made effective but this substance also requires further evaluation.

RESULTS

Varicosities can always develop in superficial veins that were not treated initially because at the time they were not affected. Despite this, good results have been reported for both surgery[84] and sclerotherapy,[89] although there are no series that have been subjected to independent scrutiny. About two-thirds of patients never demand further treatment, although a third of these develop some new veins.

RECURRENCES

Patients should be warned that varicose veins can always recur. Inadequate or incorrect surgery requires reoperation. This surgery is difficult and has a greater risk of complications.[23,58] Groin recurrences are most common, and after their presence has been confirmed by duplex scan or varicography the saphenofemoral junction should be approached over the front of the femoral artery. The stump of the long saphenous vein is ligated, and any tributaries entering this segment of the femoral vein are disconnected. Popliteal fossa recurrences are even more difficult to treat and can be approached through a lazy S incision, dividing all veins entering the popliteal vein.

VENOUS LIPODERMATOSCLEROSIS

Skin changes develop in the gaiter skin around the ankle of some patients with primary varicose veins and also develop some years after a deep vein thrombosis. The skin and subcutaneous tissues become pigmented, indurated, tender and inflamed (Fig. 11.20).[23,58] The skin pigment is from both melanin and haemosiderin. Lipodermatosclerosis is invariably associated with incompetence of the ankle communicating veins and dilated capillaries beneath the malleolus (an ankle flare).[59] When these changes are present they commonly precede the development of venous ulceration (Fig. 11.12).

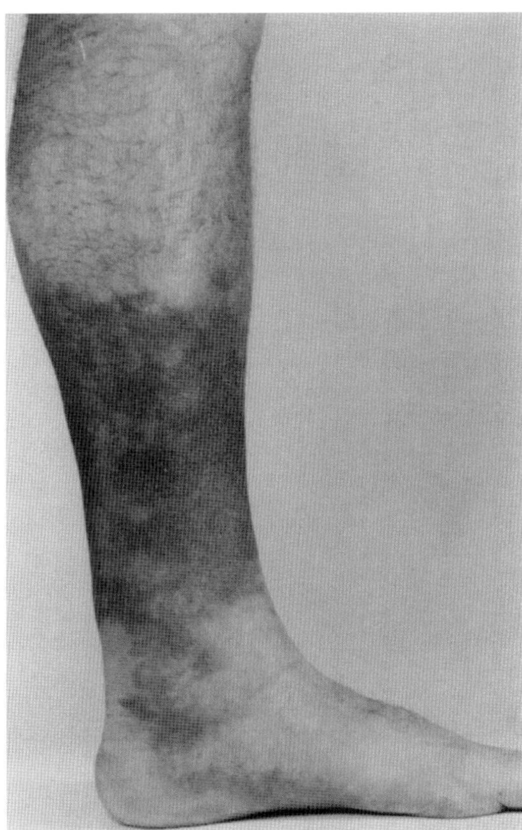

Figure 11.20 The changes of lipodermatosclerosis.

VENOUS ULCERATION

An ulcer is the dissolution of an epithelial surface. It can develop spontaneously, but often a minor injury breaks the continuity of skin already damaged by lipodermatosclerosis. The factors involved in the genesis of ulcers include a high venous pressure, pericapillary fibrin deposition, white cell activation, and trapping and increased production of free radicals.[91–95] The exact mechanism responsible for the skin breakdown is still not known.

REFERENCES

90. MacGowan WAL. J R Soc Med 1985; 78: 136
91. Burnand KG, Whimster I, Clemenson G et al. Br J Surg 1981; 68: 297
92. Browse NL, Burnand KG. Lancet 1982; 2: 243
93. Burnand KG, Whimster I, Naidoo A et al. Br Med J 1982; 285: 1071
94. Thomas PRS, Nash GB, Dormandy JA. Br Med J 1988; 296: 1693
95. Coleridge-Smith PD, Thomas P, Scurr JH et al. Br Med J 1988; 296: 1726

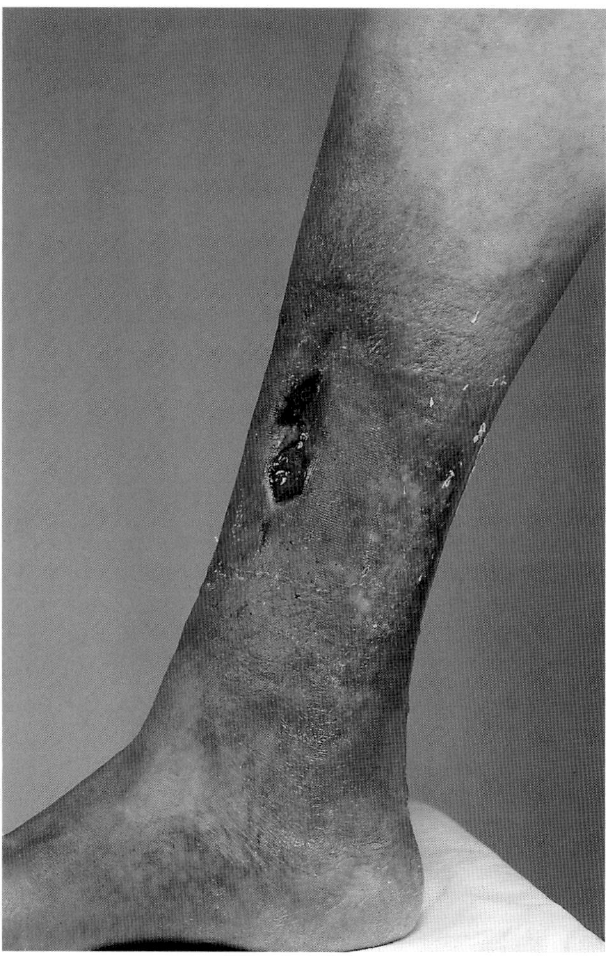

Figure 11.21 A venous ulcer.

A number of surveys have shown that the prevalence of venous ulceration is around 0.3%,[96,97] although this may represent an underestimate.[98,99] Between a half and a third of venous ulcers occur in limbs that have sustained a previous deep vein thrombosis (post-thrombotic ulcers), but the rest are associated with superficial venous incompetence (varicose ulcers).

Venous ulcers are terraced simple ulcers with gently sloping edges (Fig. 11.21). The granulations in their base vary with the state of healing of the ulcer. They appear red and velvety if the ulcer is uninfected and healing well, white and fibrous if it is long-standing and stationary, and yellow and offensive if it is infected and enlarging. Venous ulcers invariably occur within an area of lipodermatosclerosis in the gaiter skin, but they are not always associated with visible varicose veins. The nature of the venous incompetence must be carefully determined by clinical examination and special investigations. Venous ulcers must be differentiated from other types of ulcer (Fig. 11.22), including ischaemic ulcers, traumatic ulcers, vasculitic ulcers (e.g. rheumatoid or scleroderma), and neoplastic ulcers (basal cell or squamous cell carcinomas). Other rare causes of leg ulceration include neuropathic damage (e.g. diabetes), syphilis, tuberculosis, pyoderma gangrenosum, necrobiosis lipoidica, arteriovenous fistulae, blood dyscrasias and artefactual damage.[23,58]

The peripheral pulses must always be palpated, and if they cannot be felt Doppler pressures must be measured. A full blood count and erythrocyte sedimentation rate is obtained. Autoantibodies should be measured if there is any suspicion of vasculitis or rheumatoid arthritis. Serological tests should be performed for syphilis if the cause of the ulcer remains obscure. The urine and blood should be tested for sugar, and if there are any signs of neuropathy (e.g. loss of deep pain and proprioception) an electromyogram may be helpful. When an ulcer fails to heal, a biopsy must be taken, and this should be done at once if there is any suspicion of malignancy (elevated and overhanging edge), which can develop in a long-standing venous ulcer (Marjolin's ulcer).[100]

MANAGEMENT

Most ulcers that are considered on initial assessment to be venous are treated conservatively at first. Occlusive dressings are applied to the ulcer and covered by compression bandages or stockings worn from the foot to the knee. Many different types of dressing and bandage have been used. Provision of adequate compression over the calf pump is probably more important than the type of dressing; however, a number of studies have compared the efficacy of different dressings and compression regimens in promoting ulcer healing.[101,102]

Dry, non-adherent dressings or paste bandages, both covered by elasticated bandages, are the most popular methods of achieving compression (Fig. 11.23). The ulcer is gently cleaned once a week, and the dressing and bandages are carefully reapplied. More frequent changes of dressings and bandages may be required if there is copious exudate from the ulcer. The area of ulceration should be measured at each attendance and, providing the ulcer is closing, conservative treatment may be continued. Between 50 and 70% of ulcers are healed at 3 months and 80–90% by 12 months.

In-patient management is indicated if the ulcer remains static or if it enlarges. This consists of excising the ulcer base back to healthy tissue and applying pinch grafts[103] or mesh grafts to the defect.[104] There is no evidence that antibiotics, antiseptics or local applications speed ulcer healing.

When the ulcer has healed, the patient should be investigated by duplex Doppler, venous pressure measurements (or an equivalent test of calf pump function), and phlebography. The underlying venous abnormality should then be corrected if possible. Saphenous surgery is successful in preventing reulceration in patients with normal deep veins but has not proved effective in post-thrombotic limbs. The relative value of saphenous and communicating vein surgery is disputed and awaits further clinical trials.[105] Graduated elastic support stockings, stimulation of fibrinolysis, and reduction of viscosity by

REFERENCES

96. Callum MJ, Ruckley CV, Harper DR et al. Br Med J 1985; 290: 1855
97. Edwards AT, MChir Thesis 1997, University of Wales
98. Nelzen O, Bergqvist D, Lindhagen A. Br J Surg 1996; 83: 255
99. Baker SR, Stacey MC, Jopp-McKay AG et al. Br J Surg 1991; 78: 864
100. Marjolin JN. Ulcere Diet de Med Practique. 2nd edn. Paris, 1846
101. Burnand KG, Northeast ADR et al. Br J Surg 1989; 76: 1332
102. Blair SD, Wright DDI et al. Br Med J 1988; 297: 1159
103. Poskitt KR, James AJ et al. Br Med J 1987; 294: 674
104. Chilvers AS, Freeman GK. Lancet 1969; ii: 1087
105. Burnand KG, O'Donnell TF et al. Lancet 1976; 1: 936

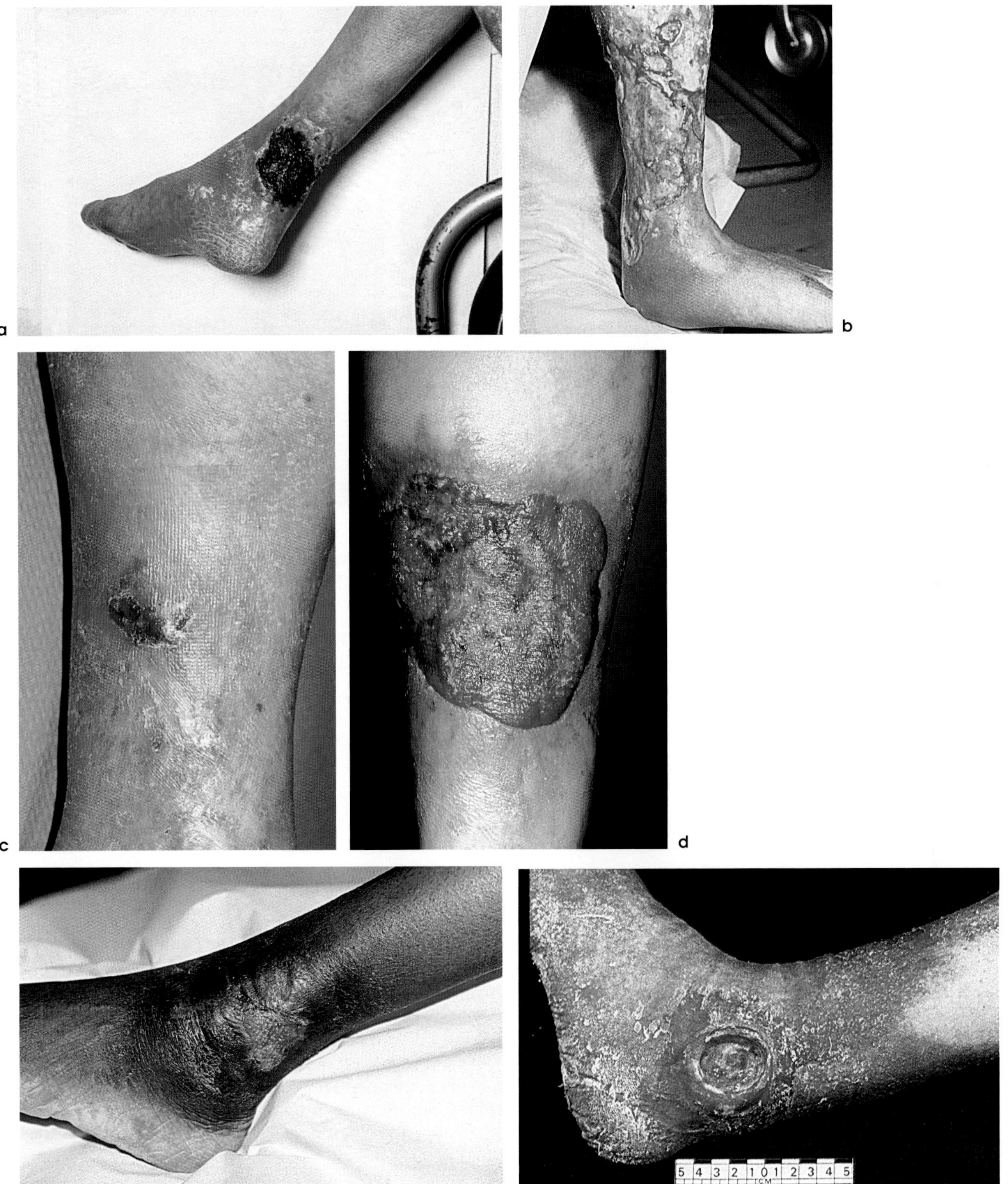

Figure 11.22 Examples of non-venous ulcers: (**a**) ischaemic, (**b**) rheumatoid, (**c**) basal cell carcinoma, (**d**) and (**e**) squamous cell carcinoma, (**f**) spina bifida. *Continued.*

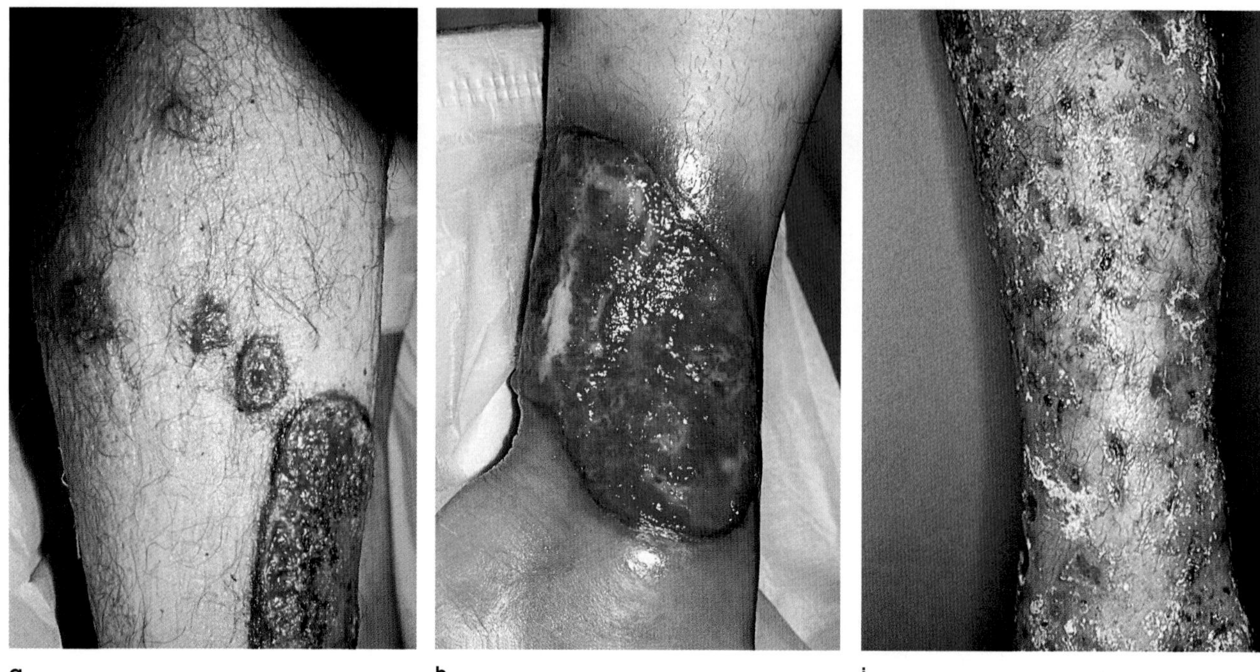

g h i

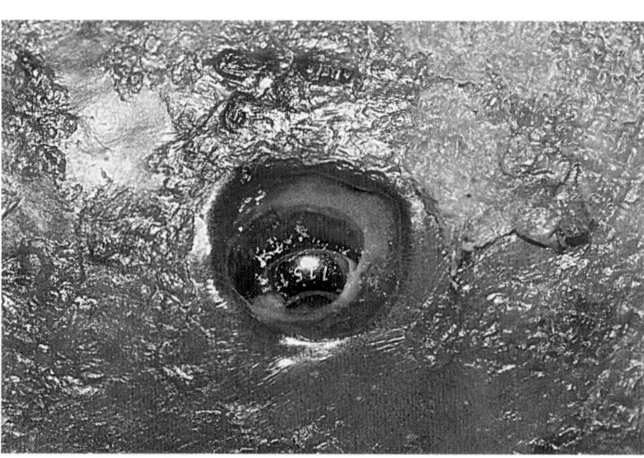

j

Figure 11.22, *cont'd* Examples of non-venous ulcers: (**g**) pyoderma gangrenosum, (**h**) sickle, (**i**) self-inflicted, (**j**) ulceration in AIDS, and (**k**) a foreign body orthopaedic screw causing ulceration.

drugs,[106] venous reconstruction[107] and valvular transplantation[108] have all been used in post-thrombotic limbs in an attempt to prevent reulceration (Fig. 11.24).[23] No good prospective trials have yet been published. Permanent elastic hosiery should be prescribed for all those who have had a venous ulcer, and patients should be warned to take care of their legs because there is always the possibility of reulceration, especially after minor trauma.[109]

DEEP VEIN THROMBOSIS

A thrombosis is a semisolid mass, formed from blood constituents, which develops within the bloodstream. Venous thrombosis is a common condition that can arise in the deep and superficial veins of the lower limb and in the veins of the pelvis. It may also occur in the veins of the upper limb in association with thoracic inlet syndrome or iatrogenic trauma.

INCIDENCE AND PREVALENCE

Ninety-eight per cent of all venous thrombi arise in the deep veins of the legs and pelvis, and 2% develop at other sites.[110] The true incidence of venous thrombosis in the general population is not known, although clinical and phlebographic studies in patients from a defined population presenting with symptoms suggest that the incidence is approximately 0.5%.[111] Nearly a third of all patients over the age of 40 undergoing major surgical operations develop a deep vein thrombosis if no prophylaxis is used.[112] After major hip surgery, the incidence of thrombosis rises to 60%,[113] and after major gynaecological surgery it occurs in 20–30% without any form of prophylaxis.[114] Deep vein thrombosis is not confined to surgical patients, and the incidence in medical

REFERENCES

106. Burnand KG, Pattison M, Browse NL. In: Davidson JF, Bachman F et al (eds). Progress in Fibrinolysis, Vol 6. Churchill Livingstone, Edinburgh, 1983
107. Bergan JJ, Yao JST et al. J Vasc Surg 1986; 3: 174
108. Taheri SA, Lazar L et al. Surgery 1982; 91: 28
109. Browse NL. Br Med J 1983; 286: 1920
110. Gibbs NM. Br J Surg 1957; 191: 15
111. Bergqvist D, Lindblad N. Br J Surg 1985; 72: 105
112. Carr K, Nicolaides VV et al. Lancet 1972; i: 540
113. Hull R, Hirsch J et al. Thromb Res 1979; 15: 227
114. Clark-Pearson DL, Synan IS et al. Obst Gynaecol 1984; 63: 92

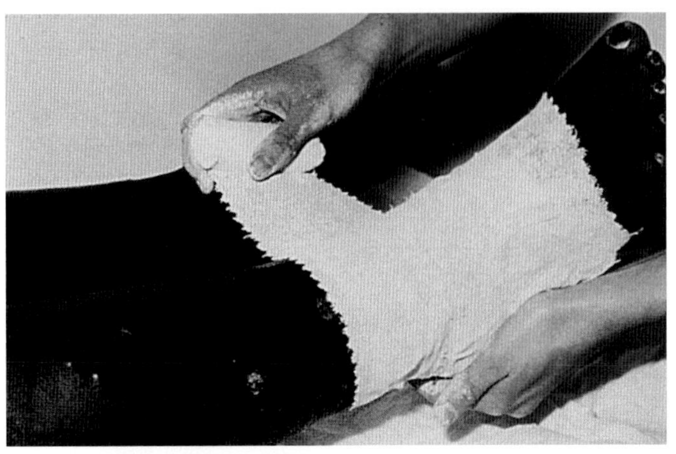

a

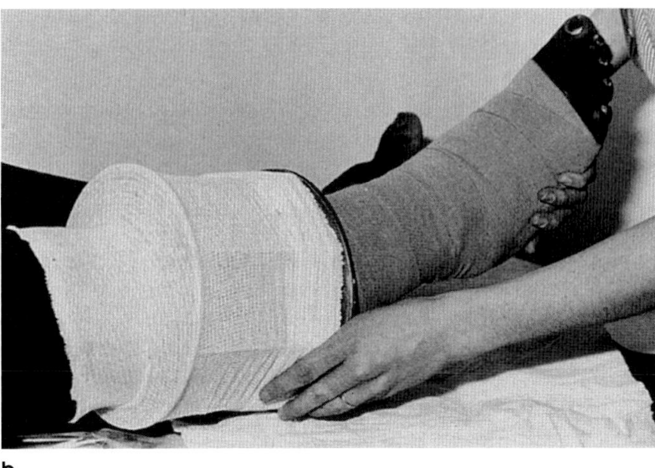

b

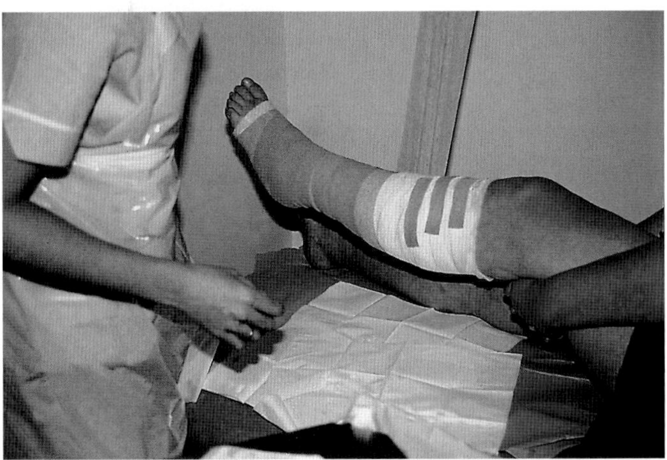

c

Figure 11.23 A paste bandage being applied to an ulcerated limb (**a,b**) and application of a four-layer bandage (**c**).

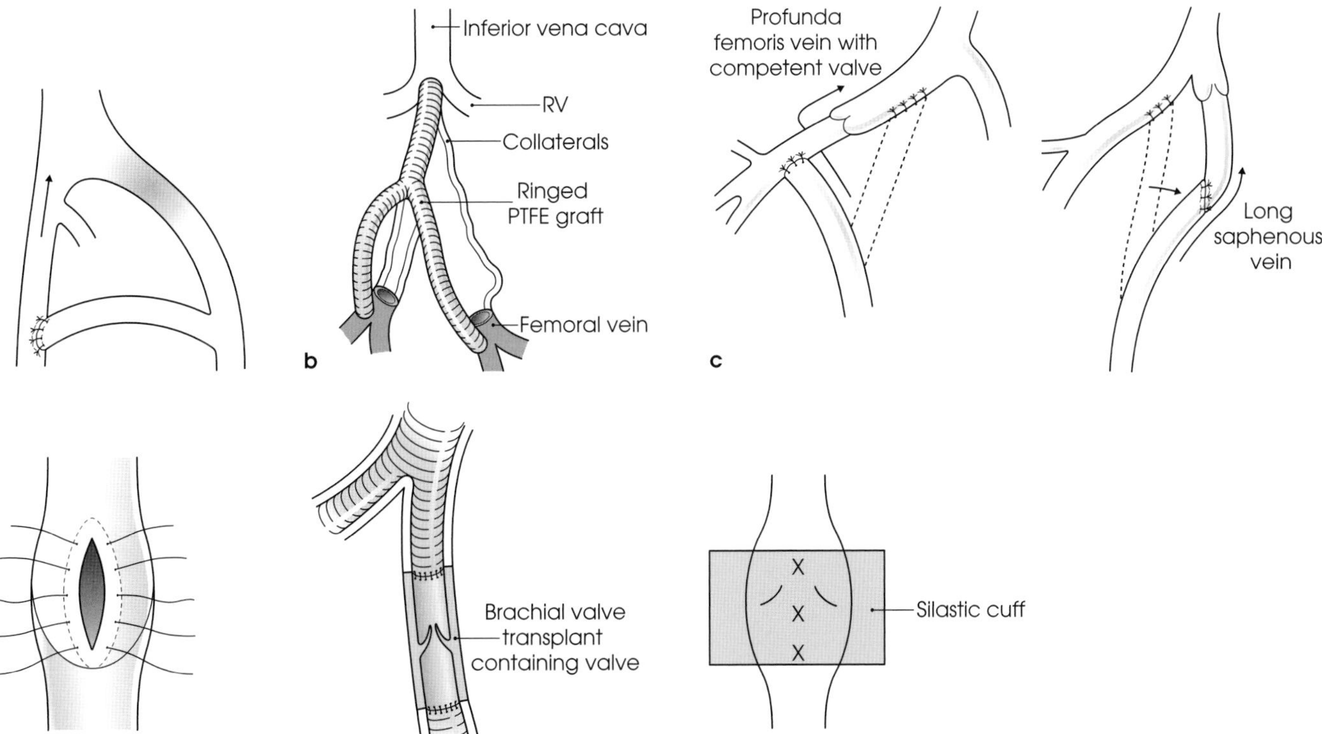

Figure 11.24 Techniques that have been used to bypass obstructed deep veins or restore valvular competence: (**a**) Palma, (**b**) Dale, (**c**) Kistner, (**d**) Jones, (**e**) Taheri and (**f**) Lane.

patients after myocardial infarction and cerebrovascular accidents is 20%.[115] The incidence of deep vein thrombosis in patients under the age of 40 having major surgery was less than 5%, but in patients over the age of 80 it was much greater. Prophylactic measures have now reduced the incidence of deep vein thrombosis in hospitals.

AETIOLOGY

Thrombosis develops from an interaction between the vessel wall, the platelets, and the coagulation system. In 1856, Virchow proposed the triad of stasis, vein wall damage, and increased coagulation of blood, which he felt was responsible for the development of deep vein thrombosis.[47] Alterations in the coagulation system, which include congenital deficiencies or acquired abnormalities, increase the risk of venous thrombosis. The importance of antithrombin, the lupus anticoagulant, heparin cofactor, protein C, protein S and activated protein C resistance is now recognized.[116,117] Subtle changes in the structure and function of the endothelium may encourage white cells and platelets to adhere to the wall and thrombus to accumulate.[118] The initial thrombus is encouraged to propagate if stasis or hypercoagulability coexist. Increasing age, pregnancy, coexisting malignancy, a past history of venous thrombosis or pulmonary embolism, obesity, administration of oestrogens, and varicose veins are all associated with an increased risk of deep vein thrombosis.[119] The risk factors for deep vein thrombosis are summarized in Box 11.1.

Prolonged sitting on international airline flights and immobility on the operating table may predispose to thrombosis.

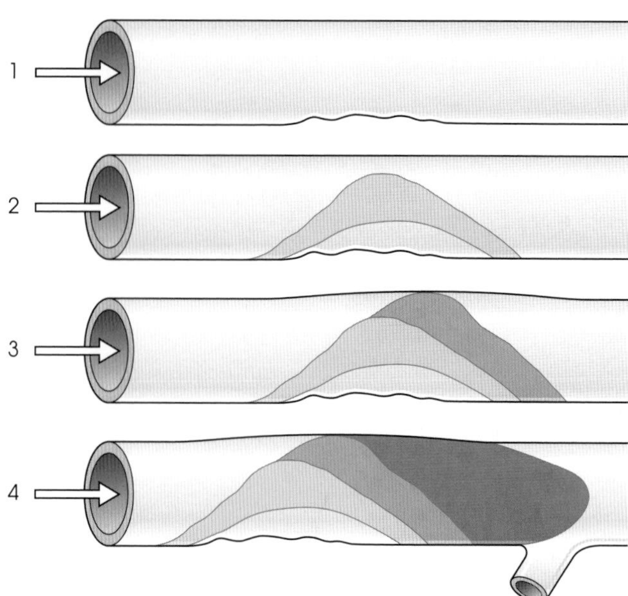

Figure 11.25 Stages in the development of a venous thrombosis. **(a)** The initial platelet cluster adheres to the vein wall as a grey amorphous thickening. **(b)** Laminated coralline thrombus develops on the surface of the platelet cluster, with alternative layers of fibrin and red cells trapped between layers of fibrin and platelets (the lines of Zahn). **(c)** As the thrombus grows across the flowing blood, it bends in the direction of the blood flow, making the lines of Zahn oblique. **(d)** When the vein is totally occluded, non-adherent, jelly-like propagated thrombus spreads up the vessel as far as the next major tributary; this thrombus is dark red and consists only of fibrin and red cells.

PATHOLOGY

Initially, platelets adhere to the endothelial surface and form a grey amorphous cluster. More platelets then adhere, with fibrin and red cells becoming deposited between the layers of platelets, giving the laminated appearance known as the lines of Zahn (Fig. 11.25). The coralline (coral-like) thrombus extends into the bloodstream, becoming bent in the direction of flow.[120] The flow past the thrombus decreases and eventually ceases with the rapid extension of red, jelly-like propagated thrombus, consisting of a fibrin and red cell meshwork extending up the vein as far as the next tributary.[121,122] The thrombus can continue to extend up the vein if the orifice of the tributary becomes occluded, and it may reach several feet in length. At this stage, the thrombus that is loosely attached or lying free becomes easily detached, increasing the risk of pulmonary embolism. Thrombus that becomes tightly adherent to the wall contracts and organizes, producing valve destruction and luminal occlusion, responsible for the eventual development of the post-thrombotic limb. This process usually starts in the valve cusps of the soleal sinusoids (Fig. 11.26), although thrombosis may originate in the profunda femoris, common femoral, internal iliac, and even the renal veins.

Box 11.1 Risk factors for deep vein thrombosis

- Increasing age
- Gender
- Season
- Race
- Type of operation
- Type of anaesthetic
- Length of operation
- Pregnancy and puerperium
- General injury
- Local injury
- Immobilization
- Bed rest
- Malignancy
- Previous venous thrombosis
- Varicose veins
- Obesity
- Cardiac failure
- Myocardial infarction
- Arterial ischaemia
- Contraceptive pill
- Intravenous saline (haemodilution)
- Haemostatic drugs
- Other drugs
- Vasculitis (Buerger's disease, Behçet's syndrome)
- Congenital venous abnormalities (Klippel–Trenaunay syndrome)

REFERENCES

115. Nicolaides AM, Kakkar VV et al. Br Med J 1971; 1: 132
116. Melissari E, Bonte G, Lindo VS et al. Blood Coagul Fibrinolysis 1992; 3: 749
117. Weston-Smith S, Revell P, Savidge GF. Br J Hosp Med 1989; 41: 368
118. Stewart GR, Ritchie WGM, Lynch PE. Am J Pathol 1974; 74: 507–532
119. Nicolaides AN, Gordon-Smith I. In: Nicolaides AN (ed). Thromboembolism. MTP, Lancaster, 1975
120. Aschoff L. Beitr Pathol Anat 1912; 52: 207
121. Sevitt S. J Clin Pathol 1974; 27: 517
122. Hadfield C. J R Coll Surg Engl 1950; 6: 219

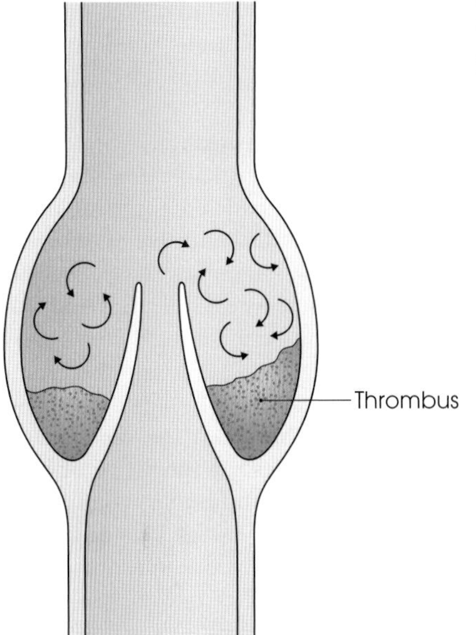

Figure 11.26 Thrombus developing in a valve pocket.

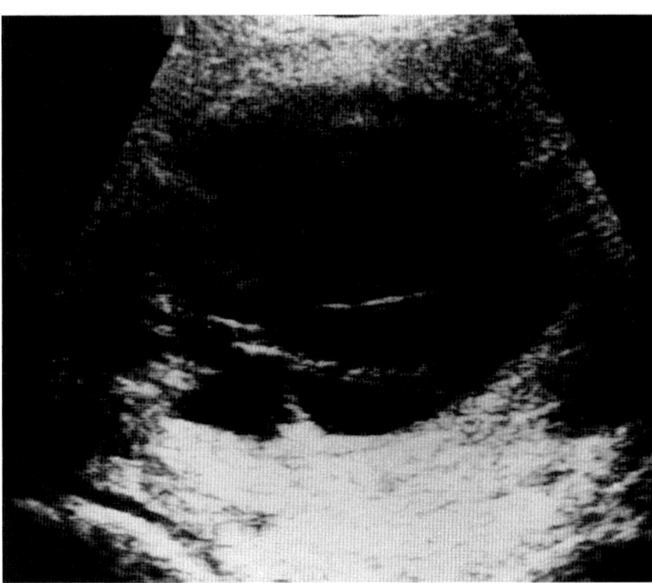

Figure 11.28 An ultrasound of a ruptured Baker's cyst.

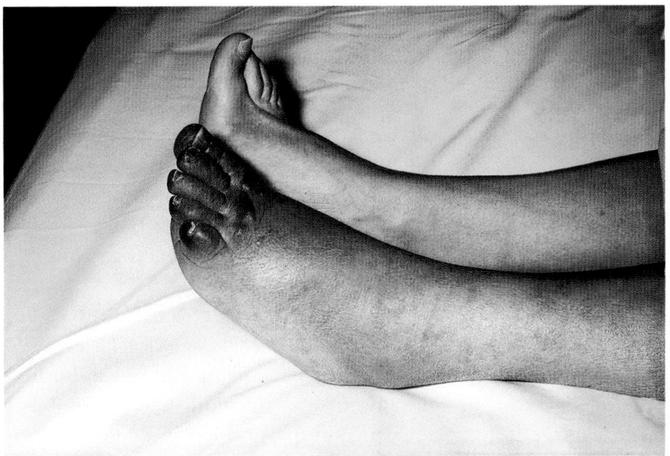

Figure 11.27 Leg with venous gangrene of the toes.

Box 11.2 Differential diagnosis for deep vein thrombosis

- Torn gastrocnemius muscle
- Ruptured Baker's cyst
- Calf haematoma
- Lymphoedema with cellulitis
- Acute arterial ischaemia
- Extrinsic obstruction of veins and lymphatics in pelvis
- Pathological fracture of femur
- Superficial thrombophlebitis
- Acute arthritis of the knee
- Haemarthrosis of the knee
- Torn meniscus
- Achilles tendonitis
- Oedema from congestive cardiac failure of the nephrotic syndrome
- Rapidly growing sarcoma
- Myositis ossificans
- Münchhausen's syndrome

CLINICAL FEATURES

The symptoms of deep vein thrombosis include limb swelling, calf pain, tenderness, and a low-grade pyrexia. Even with extensive deep vein thrombosis, symptoms may not be experienced; a pulmonary embolism or the subsequent development of a post-thrombotic limb may be the only indication of a previous venous thrombosis.[123] Occasionally, patients with a severe iliofemoral thrombosis present with a very swollen white oedematous limb (phlegmasia alba dolens). More commonly, a massive proximal thrombosis causes a blue leg (phlegmasia cerulea dolens), and this may eventually progress to true venous gangrene in a few patients (Fig. 11.27). Confirmation of swelling, tenderness over the deep veins, ankle oedema (especially if it is unilateral), and dilated superficial veins support the diagnosis. Homan's dorsiflexion test is inaccurate and should be abandoned. Clinical signs are often unreliable and special tests are essential to confirm the diagnosis. Only half of the patients with deep vein thrombosis present with clinical signs, and 30–50% of patients with an indicative history and physical signs have normal deep veins on phlebography.[124] A ruptured Baker's cyst (Fig. 11.28), cellulitis, lymphoedema, torn calf muscles, and calf haematomas can all mimic the signs of deep vein thrombosis. The full differential diagnosis is given in Box 11.2.

INVESTIGATIONS

Bipedal ascending contrast phlebography outlines the thrombus with a high degree of accuracy (Fig. 11.29), but venous imaging using B-mode ultrasound is now the most common method of diagnosis.[125] It is less accurate than phlebography in the diagnosis of calf thrombosis but has become the investigation of first choice. Thrombus may be imaged or assumed if the vein cannot be compressed (Fig. 11.30). If this test is negative, follow-up investigation should be undertaken, using phlebography in patients in whom there is a high suspicion of deep vein thrombosis or a repeat ultrasound in 2–3 days in those in whom

REFERENCES

123. Jeffrey BC, Immelman EJ, Banatar SR. S Afr Med J 1957: 643
124. Kakkar VV. Arch Surg 1972; 104: 152
125. Sullivan ED, Peter DJ, Cranley JJ. J Vasc Surg 1984; 1: 465

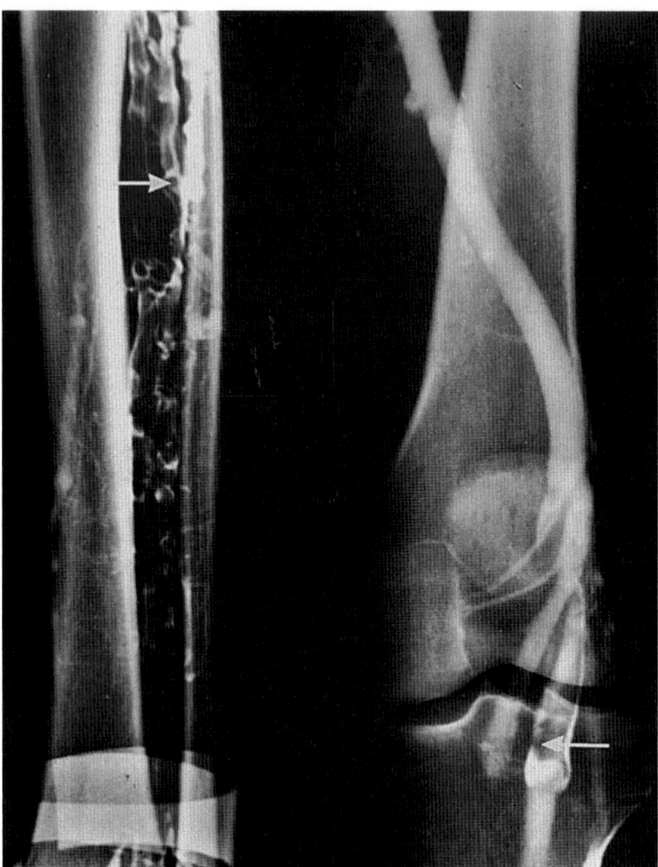

Figure 11.29 Phlebogram showing deep vein thrombosis.

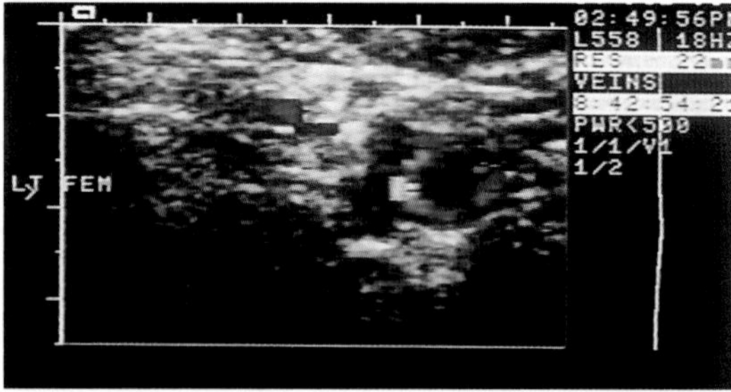

Figure 11.30 Duplex scan showing thrombus surrounded by flow.

there is a low suspicion.[126] D-Dimer, which detects breakdown products of thrombus, is a useful negative predictor of thrombosis and can be used to screen patients who do not need a duplex scan.

Plethysmography, which detects a reduced venous capacitance and reduced venous outflow, may be used as a screening test, but its accuracy for non-occlusive calf thrombi is poor.[127] Thermography has also been used to screen for thrombosis, but its specificity is poor[128] and the equipment is expensive to purchase. The radioactive iodine-125 fibrinogen uptake test was a valuable research tool but has been withdrawn because of the risk of AIDS.[129]

PREVENTION

Much attention is being paid to deep vein thrombosis prophylaxis in the postoperative period. Patients can be classified into high risk (elderly, previous thrombosis, malignancy, extensive pelvic surgery), medium risk (most major operations), and low risk (young and minor surgery).[130] The methods employed fall conveniently into mechanical methods of prophylaxis and antithrombotic methods.

Graduated compression stockings provide a simple and economical form of prophylaxis that is suitable for low- and medium-risk patients. Intermittent pneumatic compression using either single or multichamber devices is also effective in reducing the incidence of deep vein thrombosis. Pneumatic devices can be combined with graduated elastic compression stockings and this appears to be synergistic.[131] Electrical stimulation is now rarely used.

Full-scale anticoagulation increases the risk of postoperative bleeding, and subcutaneous heparin has been the most widely studied method of prophylaxis. It reduces the incidence of both postoperative venous thrombosis and pulmonary embolism, albeit at the expense of a small increased risk of bleeding. Low-molecular-weight heparin fragments are effective in reducing the incidence of deep vein thrombosis, and they may be associated with a reduced incidence of bleeding complications. A lower dose given once a day seems to provide adequate prophylaxis even in patients having hip replacements, and the reduced frequency of administration and increased efficacy have made this the most popular form of prophylaxis.[132–134]

Antiplatelet agents are of low efficacy.[135] Even with 'ideal' prophylaxis, between 5 and 20% of all patients still develop a deep vein thrombosis and up to 0.2% still have a fatal pulmonary embolism.[136] Patients remain at risk even after they have been discharged home, and prophylactic measures should ideally be continued for several weeks. Newer agents such as the pentosaccharides and antithrombosis may also be efficacious.

TREATMENT OF ESTABLISHED DEEP VEIN THROMBOSIS

The presence and extent of the thrombosis should be established by duplex scan or phlebography.[137] Established thrombosis requires urgent anticoagulant therapy, and low-molecular-weight heparin is usually given via the subcutaneous route.[138,139]

Warfarin therapy may be begun after 24 or 48 h. Several flexible dose schedules for warfarin therapy have been devised, and if a 10-mg loading dose is given on the first day, followed by 5 mg on the second, third and fourth days, the majority of patients will fall within the therapeutic range of the international

REFERENCES

126. Hyman JH, O'Sullivan E, Thomas E. Br J Surg 1973; 60: 52
127. Negus D, Pinto DJ et al. Br J Surg 1968; 55: 835
128. Barnes RW, Collicott PE et al. Surgery 1972; 72: 971
129. Cooke ED, Pitcher MP. Br J Surg 1974; 61: 971
130. Browse NL. Ann R Coll Surg 1977; 59: 138
131. Scurr RH, Coleridge Smith PD, Hasty JH. Surgery 1987; 5: 816
132. Lassen MR, Borris LC, Christiansen HM et al. Semin Thromb Hemost 1991; 17 (Suppl 3): 284
133. Nurmohamed MT, Rosendaal FR, Büller H et al. Lancet 1992; 340: 152
134. Leizorovicz A, Haugh MC, Chapuis FR et al. Br Med J 1992; 305: 913
135. Nicolaides AN, Arcelus J, Belcaro G et al. Int Angiol 1992; 11: 151
136. Willie-Jorgensen P, Fischer A et al. Br J Surg 1985; 72: 574
137. Ramsay LE. Br Med J 1983; 286: 698
138. Bentley PG, Kakkar VV et al. Thromb Res 1980; 18: 177–187
139. Walker MG, Shaw JW et al. Br Med J 1987; 294: 1189

normalized ratio, as long as the sample has been collected less than 12 h after stopping the heparin infusion.

Patients receiving antibiotics or other drugs known to interfere with the vitamin K:warfarin balance require smaller loading and maintenance doses. Warfarin treatment is normally maintained for 3–6 months, and there is clear evidence that its early cessation leads to an increased risk of rethrombosis.[140] In some patients with coagulation abnormalities, such as antithrombin deficiency or recurrent venous thrombosis, it may be necessary to give warfarin indefinitely. The dosage of warfarin is maintained by weekly or twice-weekly international normalized ratio estimations.

The fibrinolytic agents streptokinase, urokinase, and tissue plasminogen activator may be used selectively if patients are shown to have an extensive fresh venous thrombosis. The use of high doses of thrombolytic treatment delivered directly into the thrombus is being studied. The role of surgical thrombectomy has never been clearly established. In the acutely ischaemic limb with phlegmasia cerulea dolens as the result of an iliofemoral thrombus, surgical thrombectomy or lysis is indicated and may prevent limb loss.[141] After the femoral vein or veins have been exposed and snared, Fogarty catheters are passed in an antegrade and, if possible, in a retrograde direction to remove thrombus. An arteriovenous shunt made beyond the venotomy may help to prevent rethrombosis[142] and full anticoagulation is required postoperatively. Thrombectomy has no place in the management of early distal venous thrombosis or in thrombus that is more than 5 days old. All thromboses are associated with intimal and valvular damage, and although thrombus can be removed the valves may still be permanently destroyed.[143,144]

The risk of pulmonary embolism increases if extensive loose venous thrombus is present, and under these circumstances venous interruption must be considered, especially if the patient has had a small herald embolus.[145] The insertion of transvenous filters to prevent venous emboli reaching the lung is clearly established although rarely necessary. The Mobin–Uddin filter was the first effective transvenous filter, but the high incidence of thrombosis that it caused led to the development of the Greenfield–Kimray filter (Fig. 11.31a), and there are now many other filters that can be inserted percutaneously (Fig. 11.31b, c). The Greenfield–Kimray filter is positioned into the vena cava via the internal jugular vein. The filter, which is shaped like a shuttlecock, is held closed within a special introducing catheter. This catheter is inserted percutaneously and is passed through the right atrium until the tip of the catheter comes to lie within the vena cava beneath the renal veins. Correct positioning of the filter is confirmed by contrast radiography before it is ejected. As the filter springs out, the little barbed feet hook into the vein wall and prevent it from becoming dislodged. The principal indication for inserting an inferior vena cava filter remains recurrent pulmonary embolism in patients who have received or are receiving full and adequate anticoagulation. Filters are also inserted into patients who cannot be given anticoagulants because of the risk of haemorrhage,[146,147] for example from a peptic ulcer.

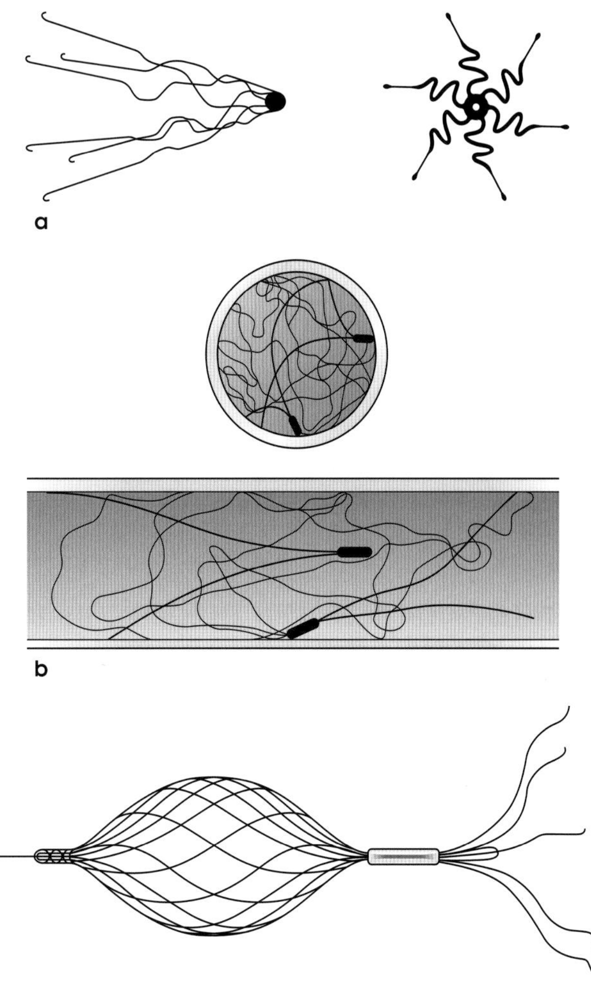

Figure 11.31 Types of filter for interruption of inferior vena cava: **(a)** the Greenfield filter, **(b)** bird's nest, and **(c)** Günther.

COMPLICATIONS AND RECURRENCES

All patients who have had one deep vein thrombosis have an increased risk of developing another. Some patients develop recurrent spontaneous venous thromboses, and these patients should be tested for activated protein C resistance, antithrombin and protein C deficiencies, anticardiolipin antibodies, and protein S deficiency (thrombophilia). These tests need to be performed when the patient is not on any form of anticoagulation that interferes with their accuracy.[23] Patients should also be screened for an occult neoplasm. Long-term anticoagulation is advisable in patients who develop recurrent venous thrombosis or who have a thrombophilia. Many patients with recurrent, apparently idiopathic thromboses are later found to have an occult malignancy.[148,149]

REFERENCES

140. Lagerstedt CI, Olsson CG et al. Lancet 1985; ii: 518
141. Mahorner H, Castleberry JW, Coleman WC. Ann Surg 1957; 146: 510
142. Eklof B, Linarsson E, Plate G. In: Bergan JJ, Yao JST (eds). Surgery of the Veins. Grune & Stratton, Orlando, 1985
143. Edwards AE, Edwards JE. Surg Gynecol Obstet 1937; 65: 310
144. Plate G, Einarsson E et al. Vasc Surg 1984; 1: 867
145. Browse NL, Lea Thomas M et al. Br Med J 1969; 3: 382
146. Greenfield LJ, Zocco J et al. Ann Surg 1977; 185: 692
147. Scurr JH, Jarrett P, Wastell C. Ann R Coll Surg 1983; 65: 233
148. Sproul EE. Am J Cancer 1938; 34: 566
149. Lagattolla NRF, Burnand KG, Irvine A et al. Ann R Coll Surg 1996; 78: 336

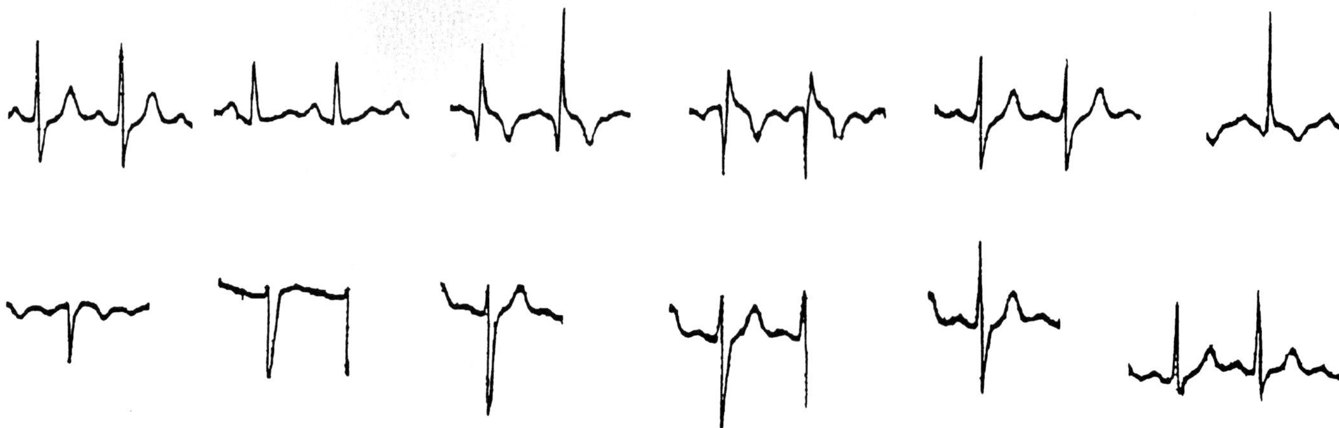

Figure 11.32 An electrocardiogram showing the classical changes associated with a moderately severe pulmonary embolism.

RELATIONSHIP OF DEEP VEIN THROMBOSIS TO PULMONARY EMBOLISM

The majority of pulmonary emboli arise from venous thromboses developing within the lower limbs or pelvis. Most clinically significant pulmonary emboli arise from the femoral, iliac and pelvic veins. Venous thromboses in the calf veins seldom give rise to large pulmonary emboli until they propagate into the proximal veins.[110] There is good circumstantial evidence to suggest that reducing the incidence of deep vein thrombosis in the lower leg reduces the incidence of propagated thrombus in the proximal axial veins, and as a consequence the incidence of pulmonary embolism is reduced.[150]

POST-THROMBOTIC LIMB

VENOUS GANGRENE

Venous gangrene is a rare complication of massive iliofemoral thrombosis. The gangrene is usually limited to the feet, and its symmetry (Fig. 11.27) distinguishes the condition from arterial ischaemia. It is treated by lysis or thrombectomy (see earlier).

PULMONARY HYPERTENSION

Pulmonary hypertension is caused by recurrent pulmonary emboli, which progressively obstruct the pulmonary vasculature. The emboli are often small and the onset of pulmonary hypertension is insidious. Pulmonary artery pressures are high. Medical treatment is generally unsuccessful, but surgical interruption of the inferior vena cava is indicated if further defects develop on lung scanning despite adequate anticoagulation. Pulmonary thromboembolectectomy and lung transplantation are reserved for those who are severely disabled.

PARADOXICAL EMBOLISM

A patent foramen ovale, a patent ductus arteriosus, or a ventricular septal defect allows a paradoxical embolism to occur; an embolus arising in the venous circulation enters the arterial circulation, producing an arterial occlusion. This rare complication should be suspected in any patient with a cardiac murmur who has a swollen leg and develops an acute arterial obstruction. The embolus must be removed, the venous thrombosis treated, and the cardiac defect closed.

PULMONARY EMBOLISM

Pulmonary emboli invariably originate from thrombi in deep veins of the lower limbs or pelvis. The symptoms of a pulmonary embolism include acute pleuritic pain, dyspnoea, haemoptysis and sudden death. Many patients remain symptom-free and the diagnosis is made only by special tests or inferred from the subsequent development of pulmonary hypertension (see earlier). The symptoms and signs of a deep vein thrombosis may predominate, but the presence of cyanosis, raised neck veins, a pleural rub, and a fixed split-second heart sound are all indicative of a pulmonary embolism.

The diagnosis of pulmonary embolism is supported by oligaemia; wedge-shaped areas of consolidation and enlarged hilar shadows on chest radiograph; an S wave in lead 1, a Q wave in lead 3, and inverted T waves over the right chest on electrocardiogram (Fig. 11.32); and hypoxia combined with hypocarbia in the arterial blood. Ventilation perfusion scanning provides useful confirmation (Fig. 11.33), but spiral CT scanning or pulmonary angiography (Fig. 11.34) can confirm the embolism if the scan is equivocal.

It is wrong to consider all emboli together because the size, significance and outcome of a pulmonary embolism are so variable. Miller suggests that pulmonary embolic can be classified into one of four main groups:[151]

- acute minor,
- acute massive,
- subacute massive, and
- chronic (pulmonary hypertension).

In patients with a minor embolism, anticoagulation using heparin and warfarin is appropriate providing that the source of the embolism is confirmed and further embolism is prevented. Acute massive pulmonary embolism is associated with significant pulmonary artery occlusion and marked outflow obstruction, indicated by a significant rise in the pulmonary artery pressure.

REFERENCES

150. Gaylan JE, Alpert JS. Prog Cardiovasc Dis 1975; 17: 259
151. Miller G. In: Browse NL, Burnand KG, Lea Thomas M (eds). Diseases of the Veins. Arnold, London, 1988

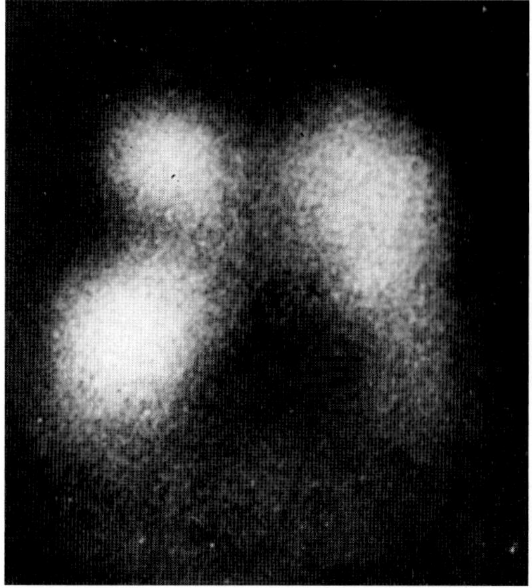

a

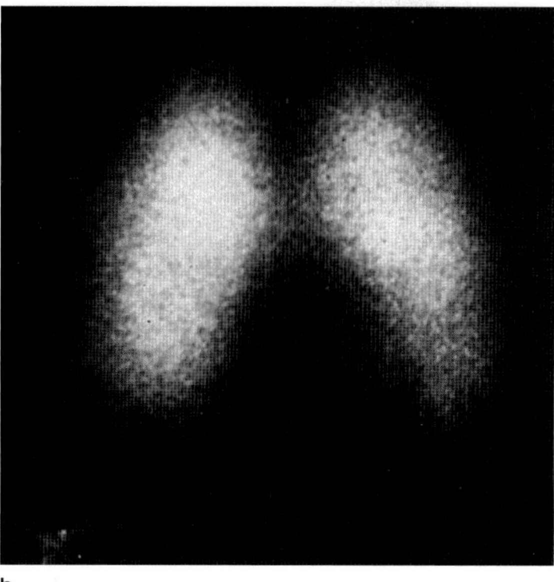

b

Figure 11.33 A ventilation perfusion lung scan showing unmatched perfusion defects indicative of a pulmonary embolism.

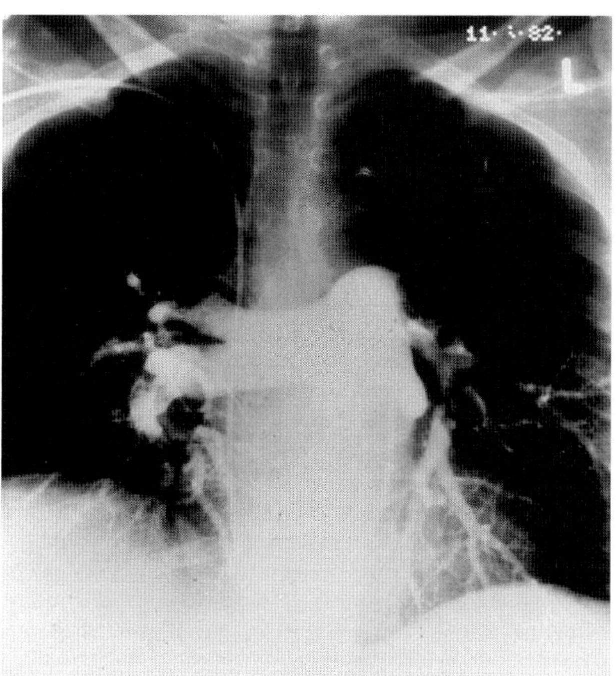

Figure 11.34 A pulmonary angiogram showing multiple filling defects from repeated emboli.

Emergency embolectomy can save the patient's life in these circumstances.[152,153] With smaller emboli, anticoagulation or fibrinolytic treatment may be effective.

After all types of pulmonary embolism the following outcomes are possible.[23,150] Ten per cent of patients die within the first hour, before the diagnosis can be confirmed; of the 90% or so who survive the initial insult, the diagnosis is confirmed only in one-third. When the diagnosis is confirmed and appropriate treatment instituted, the mortality is still 15%. Treatment is not instituted in patients in whom the diagnosis cannot be confirmed, and in these patients the mortality is even greater, with more than half dying.

Up to 70% of those patients presenting with the clinical features of a pulmonary embolism have normal pulmonary arteriograms. Spiral CT angiography has improved the diagnostic accuracy of standard contrast studies.

When the patient has survived the initial pulmonary embolus, duplex Doppler scans must be obtained to assess the presence and extent of any residual thrombus within the deep veins of the lower limbs. Unfortunately, the detection rate of these studies is disappointing, with thrombus confirmed in between 20 and 30%. Recurrent embolism in the presence of adequate anticoagulation is the best indication for interrupting the inferior vena cava (see p. 289).

SUPERFICIAL THROMBOPHLEBITIS

Thrombosis may affect the superficial veins. Varicose veins are the most common predisposing cause,[154] but trauma, chemical irritation and local sepsis may also play a part.[155] Patients present with a painful, hard, hot and reddened subcutaneous cord. Surgical treatment is rarely indicated, unless the upper end of the long saphenous vein is involved, when ligation should be considered to prevent propagation.

The majority of patients are treated by anti-inflammatory agents and external elastic support. The condition is usually self-limiting, but recurrences indicate the possibility of thrombophlebitis migrans, often associated with an underlying carcinoma.[156] Many patients with superficial thrombophlebitis have a coexistent deep vein thrombosis.

REFERENCES

152. Trendelenburg F. Arch Klin Chir 1908; 86: 686
153. Clarke DB, Abrahams LD. Lancet 1972; i: 767
154. Edwards EA. Surg Gynecol Obstet 1938; 66: 236
155. Woodhouse C. J R Ann R Coll Surg Engl 1980; 62: 364
156. Edwards EA. N Engl J Med 1949; 240: 1031

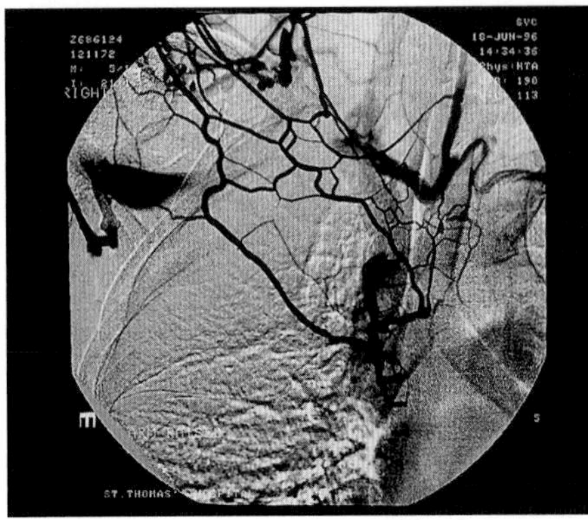

a

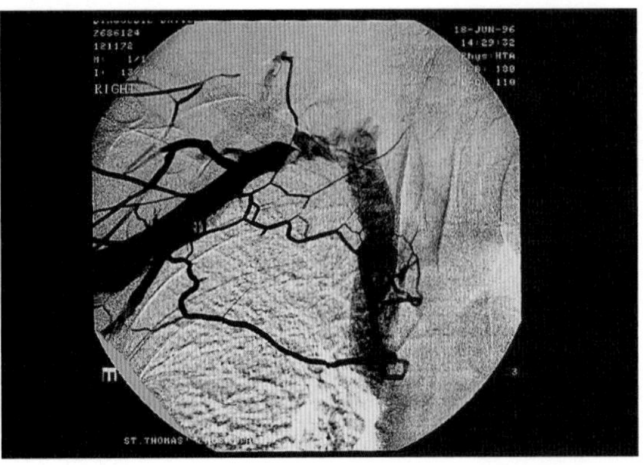

b

Figure 11.35 Axillary phlebograms showing axillary vein thrombosis **(a)** before lysis and **(b)** post lysis.

AXILLARY OR SUBCLAVIAN VEIN THROMBOSIS

This condition was originally described by Sir James Paget in 1875[157] and independently by Von Schrotter in 1884.[158] It is responsible for 1–2% of all venous thromboses and may be idiopathic or secondary to a recognized cause.

Thrombosis is more common on the right, often developing after excessive or unusual exercise, and therefore has been nicknamed 'effort thrombosis'.[159] It often occurs in patients with cervical ribs or thoracic inlet obstruction (see Ch. 10) and may be the cause of all axillary vein thromboses,[160] although the aetiology is probably multifactorial.[161,162] Thrombosis commonly follows the insertion of catheters into the subclavian vein (central vein lines, Swan–Ganz catheters, or venous access for chemotherapy).

Most patients are men between 35 and 45 years of age who present with discomfort and swelling in their dominant arm 24 h or so after an episode of excessive or unusual exercise. The hand and forearm feel cool and are swollen and blue. The finger movements are often diminished. There is usually pitting oedema on the dorsum of the hand, and the subcutaneous veins are distended, with collateral veins later enlarging and becoming visible over the shoulder and chest. A tender cord can sometimes be felt along the course of the axillary vein. In the early stages arterial ischaemia may be suspected, and similar symptoms may be produced by external compression of the vein by a Pancoast tumour or secondary malignant lymph glands.

A chest radiograph and a CT scan of the lungs may be helpful in excluding the above conditions, but brachial phlebography is required to confirm the diagnosis and to provide the necessary information for the proper management of the condition (Fig. 11.35).[163] Duplex scanning is now an alternative means of diagnosis, but the therapeutic infusion of fibrinolytic drugs requires venous access.

Many patients present days or weeks after the onset of symptoms, when active management has no part to play. When patients are seen at an early stage, treatment by chemical thrombolysis (streptokinase or urokinase) or thrombectomy followed by surgical decompression of the thoracic inlet may reduce late sequelae (see Ch. 10).[164,165] Angioplasty and stent placements are contraindicated. The occluded segment can be bypassed if incapacitating late symptoms of discomfort and oedema of the arm develop. The internal jugular vein appears to be the best conduit.[165] Anticoagulants are usually given for 3 months to prevent propagation of thrombus and the faint possibility of pulmonary embolism. Most untreated patients develop good collateral pathways, and after a few months become symptom-free.[160]

SUPERIOR VENA CAVAL THROMBOSIS

Thrombosis of the superior vena cava is usually an acute event and is often associated with a rapidly enlarging carcinoma of the bronchus, although it may also be caused by other neoplasms such as thymomas, lymphomas, and carcinoma of the thyroid.[23] A more chronic obstruction of the superior vena cava may develop in patients with a retrosternal goitre, in benign or slow-growing mediastinal tumours, and in patients with constrictive pericarditis or mediastinal fibrosis. Acute thrombosis most commonly follows intravenous cannulation of the internal jugular and subclavian veins for intravenous feeding, in which hyperosmolar solutions are usually infused.[155]

Patients present with swelling of the neck and face, accompanied by shortness of breath. Rare symptoms include tinnitus headache, epistaxis, a non-productive cough, and dysphagia. On examination the head and neck are suffused and cyanosed, with obviously distended neck veins that do not collapse on elevation or with respiration.[23]

A chest radiograph often shows a bronchogenic or mediastinal tumour, and CT scanning may be helpful in defining the extent of the neoplasm. Bilateral brachial vein injections of contrast determine the extent of the occlusion, but a tissue diagnosis should be obtained before treatment is begun.

Radiotherapy produces a rapid improvement in symptoms by shrinking bronchogenic and other rapidly growing neoplasms, but this improvement is always temporary unless the patient

REFERENCES

157. Paget J. Clinical Lectures and Essays. Longman's Green, London, 1875
158. Von Schrotter L. In: Nothnagel CNH (ed). Handbuch der Pathologie und Therapie. Holder, Vienna, 1884
159. Kleinsasser LJ. Arch Surg 1949; 59: 258
160. Adams JT, McEvoy RK, De Weese JA. Arch Surg 1965; 91: 29
161. Tilney NL, Griffith HJG, Edwards EA. Arch Surg 1970; 101: 792
162. Sundquist SB, Hedner U et al. Br Med J 1981; 283: 265
163. Stevenson IM, Parry EW. J Cardiovasc Surg 1975; 16: 580
164. Dunant JH. Int Angiol 1984; 3: 157
165. Witte LC, Smith AC. Arch Surg 1966; 93: 664

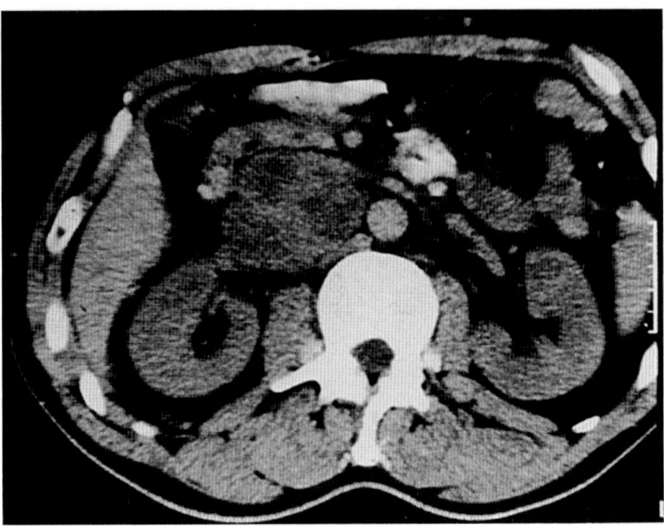

Figure 11.36 A CT scan of the abdomen, showing a leiomyosarcoma of the inferior vena cava.

dies of another cause before symptoms recur. Individual cases of caval bypass have been reported using vein or synthetic graft anastomosed to the right atrium.[166] Thrombolysis, angioplasty and stenting are now the treatment of choice, especially if the condition is a complication of intravenous feeding.

VENOUS TUMOURS

Leiomyomas, which are usually low-grade leiomyosarcomas, are rare tumours arising in the vein wall; the inferior vena cava is the most common site of occurrence.[167] They present with symptoms and signs of venous obstruction, and a mass may be palpable. The extent of the tumour is determined by phlebography and CT scanning (Fig. 11.36). The tumour is resected if possible and the vein bypassed or reconstructed.[166] These tumours often recur locally and the eventual prognosis is poor, although the patients may live for many years.

REFERENCES

166. Skinner DB, Saltzman EW, Scannell JC. J Thorac Cardiovasc Surg 1976; 53: 549
167. Kieffer E, Berrod JL, Chomettor G. In: Bergan JJ, Yao JST (eds). Surgery of the Veins. Grune & Stratton, Orlando, 1995

Disease of the lymphatics

12

Catharine L. McGuinness, Kevin G. Burnand

INTRODUCTION

Lymphoedema is defined as the excessive accumulation of tissue fluid that results from impaired lymphatic drainage, and the term *lymphoedema* should be confined to describing oedema in patients in whom a lymphatic abnormality has been confirmed. Lymphoedema principally involves the legs (80%), although the arms, genitalia and face can also be affected. In the majority of cases of lymphoedema a cause can be identified, and therefore by definition the lymphoedema is secondary. The recent rapid improvements in genetic technology and human genome mapping have resulted in major advances in the understanding of the process of lymphatic development, and subsequently the mechanisms involved in some types of primary lymphoedema have been identified.

MECHANICAL FUNCTION OF THE LYMPHATIC SYSTEM

The first major mechanical function of the lymphatic system is to clear the interstitial space of large molecules and excess fluid; the second is to return lymphocytes from the lymph back into the bloodstream. Starling's original hypothesis,[1] which proposed that there was no protein transport across the capillary endothelium, was modified by Pappenheimer and Soto-Riviera,[2] who demonstrated that the rate of capillary filtration is a function of hydrodynamic and colloid osmotic pressures, and is directly proportional to their difference. Four factors govern this exchange: the capillary blood pressure (hydrostatic pressure), the oncotic (osmotic) pressure of plasma proteins in the blood, the interstitial pressure (hydrostatic pressure), and the oncotic (osmotic) pressure of proteins in the interstitial fluid. The interstitial space has a negative pressure and this, combined with the hydrostatic pressure of the capillaries, encourages fluid to escape from the intravascular compartment despite the intravascular oncotic pressure. The intraluminal pressure of the lymphatics is similar to that of the interstitial fluid, therefore the terminal lymphatics must actively absorb protein through their pores, but the mechanism by which this is achieved is not known.

The protein content of blood and lymph are different, and there is always relatively more albumin than globulin in lymph.[3] Between 50 and 80% of the intravascular protein is returned to the bloodstream every day via the thoracic duct (Fig. 12.1). Even when the lymph flow is reduced, some 40% of the intravascular plasma proteins pass through the thoracic duct in 24 h.[4] This vast flux of protein can occur only in a fully functional lymphatic system. In addition to the accumulation of interstitial fluid as a consequence of impaired clearance, lymphoedema also involves decreased transport of autologous and foreign proteins. The parenchymal and immune cells secrete cytokines that may be responsible for the fibroblastic and epithelial proliferation that cause the sclerotic changes of the skin and subcutaneous tissues seen in long-standing lymphoedema.

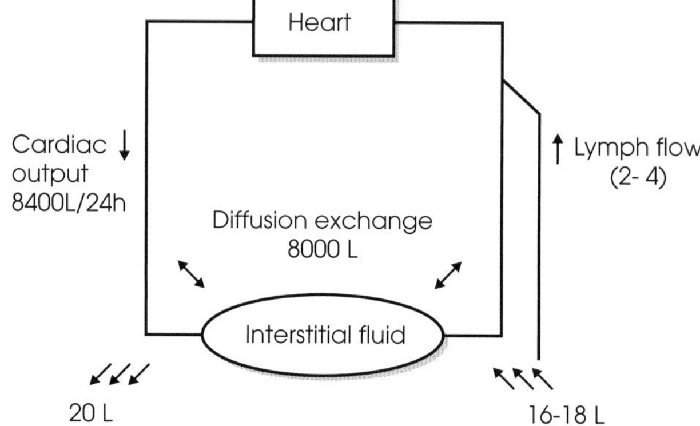

	Filtrate	Absorbate	Lymph
Fluid	20 L	16-18 L	2-4 L
Protein	80-200g	0-5g	75-195g

Figure 12.1 The interstitial circulation: the volumes of fluid taking part in exchange.

LYMPH FLOW

Lymph flow depends mainly on the intrinsic contractility of the lymphatic vessels and extrinsic factors. This is a potent force in the propulsion of lymph in the resting leg but may be assisted during exercise by other extrinsic factors. These include muscular activity, thoracic and abdominal pressure changes, and even perhaps the pulsation of local blood vessels.[5]

REFERENCES

1. Starling EH. J Physiol (Lond) 1896; 19: 312
2. Pappenheimer JR, Soto-Riviera A. Am J Physiol 1948; 152: 471
3. Wooley G, Courtice FC. Aust J Exp Biol Med Sci 1962; 40: 121
4. Yoffey JM, Courtice FC. Lymphatics, Lymph and the Lymphomyeloid Complex. Academic Press, London, 1970
5. Parsons RJ, McMaster PD. J Exp Med 1938; 68: 353

Lymph flow is sluggish at rest, and under these circumstances lymph nodes may produce a significant resistance to flow. The role of a lymph node is to act as a filter, which results in a reduction in flow as the lymphatic drainage is interrupted at each lymph node.

CLASSIFICATION AND SUBDIVISIONS

Lymphoedema can be divided into primary and secondary, the latter being much more common. Secondary lymphoedema occurs as a result of disruption to the lymphatic system. Primary or 'idiopathic' lymphoedema is much rarer, although the exact incidence is unknown because mildly affected individuals may never seek a medical opinion and there is a dearth of population-based studies using objective confirmatory tests.

PRIMARY LYMPHOEDEMA

Although the incidence of primary lymphoedema remains poorly documented, the frequency at birth of those who will develop primary lymphoedema is thought to be 1:6000, with a male to female ratio of 1:3.[6]

CLASSIFICATION OF PRIMARY LYMPHOEDEMA

Subdivisions of primary lymphoedema have been made on the basis of anatomical abnormalities found during lymphangiographic studies.[7]

First, the lymphatic channels may be absent (aplastic) or hypoplastic with few vessels petering out proximally. Second, there may be an excessive number of abnormally functioning lymphatics (numerical hyperplasia),[8] or third, there may be dilated ectatic vessels (megalymphatics), which are often associated with lymphatic fluid collections or leaks such as chylothorax, chylous ascites and lymphatic reflux. Last, the lymphatics may be obstructed secondary to a primary fibrotic reaction in the more proximal lymph nodes (Boxes 12.1 and 12.2).[9]

Although the definitive diagnosis is made by lymphangiography, the clinical presentation of the patient often identifies a particular subtype of the disease. For example, a capillary naevus on the trunk associated with lymph vesicles suggests the presence of megalymphatics, and patients with this condition often have symptoms related to chylous fistulae in the abdominal or thoracic cavity. Patients with lymphoedema affecting the whole of one leg, including the thigh and buttock, are likely to have pelvic obstruction, whereas patients with mild ankle and foot oedema are much more likely to be women with distal obliteration of the lymphatics below the groins.

AETIOLOGY OF PRIMARY LYMPHOEDEMA

By definition, the cause of primary lymphoedema is not known, but it is now apparent that genetic predisposition is an obvious factor in its development. Thirty per cent of patients with primary lymphoedema have a family history of swollen legs, which suggests that a genetic defect may be important.

In a small number of babies who have lymphoedema present at birth, the affected limb has 'aplasia' or complete absence of lymphatic vessels (Milroy's disease). Milroy reported a large family in North America with a dominantly inherited congenital lymphoedema and concluded that there was a genetic cause.[10] Genetic studies performed in North America and the UK on similarly affected families mapped the condition to a region of chromosome 5q (5q34–q35). This region contains the gene for vascular endothelial growth factor receptor-3 (*VEGFR3*), which encodes for a receptor tyrosine kinase that is specific for lymphatic vessels. It appears that defective *VEGFR3* signalling is the cause of the congenital hereditary lymphoedema linked to 5q34–q35.[11]

Meig's disease is a much more common form of primary lymphoedema in which the swelling develops around the teenage years. Studies have shown that there is a one-in-three risk of inheriting the condition, and females are three times more likely to be affected than males. As yet, the genetic abnormality responsible is undiscovered.

Box 12.1 Differential diagnosis of lymphoedema

- Systemic disorders
- Cardiac failure
- Renal failure
- Hepatic cirrhosis
- Hypoproteinaemia
- Allergic disorders
- Hereditary angioedema
- Idiopathic cyclic oedema
- Venous disorders
- Post-thrombotic syndrome
- Iliac venous (obstructive) disease
- Extrinsic pressure (e.g. by tumour, pregnancy or retroperitoneal fibrosis)
- Klippel–Trenaunay syndrome
- Miscellaneous disorders
- Arteriovenous malformations
- Lipoedema/lipodystrophy
- Disuse and factitious oedema
- Gigantism

Box 12.2 Kinmonth classification of patients with lymphoedema

- *Hypoplasia or aplasia, distal*: the lymph vessels are small and few (fewer than five vessels shown in the thigh) or obliterated.
- *Hypoplasia, proximal*: lymph vessels and nodes are small and few in the groin and pelvis; vessels in the limbs distal to the site of hypoplasia are numerous and dilated (i.e. obstructed and distended).
- *Hypoplasia, distal and proximal*: a combination of the two previous conditions; vessels and nodes are small and few in limb and pelvis.
- *Hyperplasia*: numerous lymphatics are seen in both limbs, with many large nodes in the groin and trunk, and a non-filling or distorted thoracic duct. Megalymphatics, many large, tortuous, varicose lymphatics in limbs and trunk, with diffuse scattered nodes often numerous and almost always unilateral.

REFERENCES

6. Dale RF. J Med Genet 1985; 22: 274–278
7. Kinmonth JB. Clin Sci 1952; 11: 13
8. Kinmonth JB. Lymphatics, Surgery, Lymphography and Diseases of the Chyle and Lymph System. 2nd edn. Edward Arnold, London, 1982
9. Wolfe JHN. Ann R Coll Surg 1984; 66: 251–257
10. Pfleger L, Kaindl F et al. In: Collette JM (ed). New Trends in Basic Lymphology. Birkhauser Verlag, Basel, 1967
11. Irrthum A, Karkkainen MJ, Devriendt K et al. Am J Hum Genet 2000; 67: 295–301

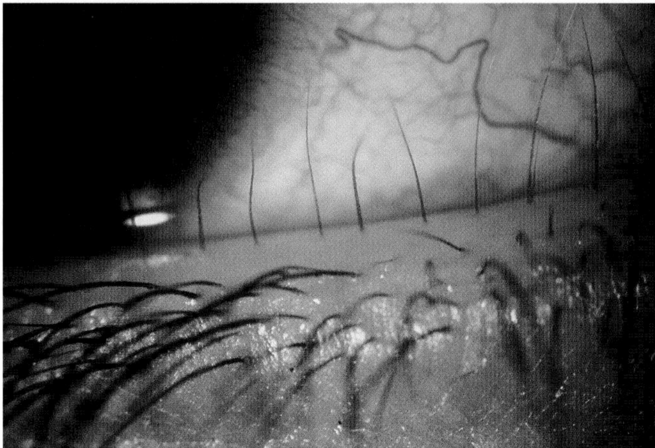

Figure 12.2 Distichiasis.

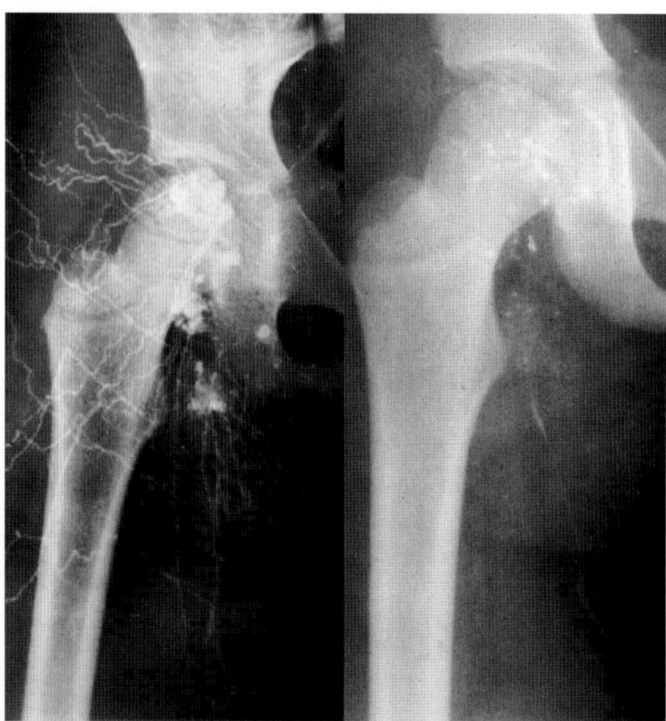

Figure 12.3 The lymphogram on the left shows pelvic obliteration of lymphatics and collaterals, but 9 months later (right) the distal pathways have also been obliterated.

Hereditary lymphoedema–distichiasis is a rare autosomal dominant disorder that presents with primary limb lymphoedema of variable age onset and distichiasis (extra aberrant growth of eyelashes from the Meibomian gland, often appearing as a second set of eyelashes; Fig. 12.2). Other eye findings may include ptosis, congenital cataracts, exotropia, congenital ectropion and photophobia. Genetic studies on families attending Moorfield's, St George's and St Thomas' hospitals in the UK revealed that this rare condition was mapped to the q24 position on chromosome 16. This area was subsequently identified as the *FOXC2* gene.[12,13] Mutations have now been reported in this transcription factor gene, and many other clinical findings including varicose veins, cleft palate, spinal extradural cysts and congenital heart disease have now been associated with lymphoedema–distichiasis. Imaging of the lymphatics in persons with lymphoedema–distichiasis has revealed normal or increased numbers of lymphatic vessels, in contrast with hypoplasia or aplasia seen in other forms of primary lymphoedema.

Yet another gene of interest is the *Prox1* gene, which is expressed by the subpopulation of endothelial cells that form the lymphatic vessels. In *Prox1* nullizygous animal embryos the lymphatics fail to develop but vasculogenesis and angiogenesis continue normally. This suggests that *Prox1* is a crucial specific regulator of lymphangiogenesis.[14]

Lymphoedema is associated with many other syndromes in which chromosome abnormality is the cause, including Pierre–Robin (skeletal abnormalities and micrognathia), Noonan's,[15,16] yellow nail (yellow discolouration of the nails, pleural effusion and primary lymphoedema), Down's, Aagenaes[17] (cholestasis and lymphoedema) and autosomal dominant microcephaly–lymphoedema–chorioretinal dysplasia syndrome.[18] A lymphoedema-critical region in the X chromosome has now been identified in Turner's syndrome.

Some degree of inheritance can be shown in one-third of patients with lymphoedema, but how or why the lymphatic vessels are malfunctioning in some patients is unknown. Even finding the absence or abnormality of lymphatics makes it difficult to explain the late onset of signs in the majority of patients with primary lymphoedema, the most common age of onset being between 10 and 25 years of age.

It is possible that in the presence of a primary abnormality there is continuing damage to any existing lymphatic vessels or lymph nodes by the constituents of lymph. Lymph may contain large amounts of fibrinogen, which may coagulate within the vessels or nodes in conditions of low flow. This may result in the 'die-back' or damage of previously functioning distal lymphatic vessels (Fig. 12.3) or the disappearance of lymphangioles resulting in hypoplasia. Anticoagulation has been reported to result in improvement in patients with lymphoedema, suggesting that the hypothesis that hypercoagulability of lymph is harmful may be correct. Benzopyrones are a group of drugs that increase proteolysis by macrophages and have been reported to reduce lymphoedema clinically. The pathophysiological causes of hyperplastic or dilated megalymphatics have, however, still not been elucidated.

The initial cause of lymphatic failure in many cases of primary lymphoedema remains an enigma. Theoretically the condition can be caused by abnormalities in lymph formation or lymph clearance. Venous obstruction increases the capillary filtration by causing a persistent elevation in venous pressure. This in turn increases lymph formation. Despite the undoubted effect of venous disease on an inadequate lymphatic system, the hypothesis that lymphoedema develops secondary to venous disease remains to be confirmed.

REFERENCES

12. Fang J, Dagenais SL, Erickson RP et al. Am J Hum Genet 2000; 67: 1382–1388
13. Bell R, Brice G, Child AH et al. Hum Genet 2001; 108: 546–551
14. Petrova TV, Makinen T, Makela TP et al. EMBO J 2002; 21: 4593–4599
15. Ho WL, Wang JK, Li YW. Pediatr Radiol 2003; 33: 200–202
16. Lanning P, Simila S, Suramo I et al. Pediatr Radiol 1978; 7: 106–109
17. Bull LN, Roche E, Song EJ et al. Am J Hum Genet 2000; 67: 994–999
18. Simonell F, Testa F, Nesti A et al. J Pediatr Ophthalmol Strabismus 2002; 39: 288–292

Lymphoedema is usually caused by an abnormal clearance of lymph, which may occur at the lymphatic capillary bed. The collecting vessels have been found to be abnormal on histological examination.[19] Sometimes biopsies reveal evidence of peri-lymphangitis and endolymphangitis proliferans, although others show lymphangiectasia (a dilated lymphangiole with atrophy of its wall). Almost all adults with primary lymphoedema have evidence of abnormal or occluded lymph vessels in their feet. Total aplasia of the lymph trunks is extremely rare, except in Milroy's disease, which in itself is a rare condition (3% of primary lymphoedema). In a few patients there is a radiologically demonstrable abnormality of the thoracic duct that may interfere with lymph flow, and these patients tend to have increased numbers of distal lymphatics. In 1948, Mowlem suggested that abnormalities in the lymph node are the cause of primary lymphoedema, but this suggestion was not re-examined for many years.[20] Extensive nodal fibrosis has been found in some patients with primary lymphoedema and it has been suggested that this may be the cause, rather than the result, of the condition. The reason for this fibrosis remains obscure and it particularly occurs in those with complete limb swelling (Fig. 12.4).

The fact that many girls develop lymphoedema around the age of puberty has led to conjecture that increased lymphatic return, secondary to fluid retention caused by an increase in reproductive hormones, might play a part in precipitating lymphoedema.

SECONDARY LYMPHOEDEMA

All patients presenting with lymphoedema must have a possible cause excluded by careful examination and special tests where necessary.

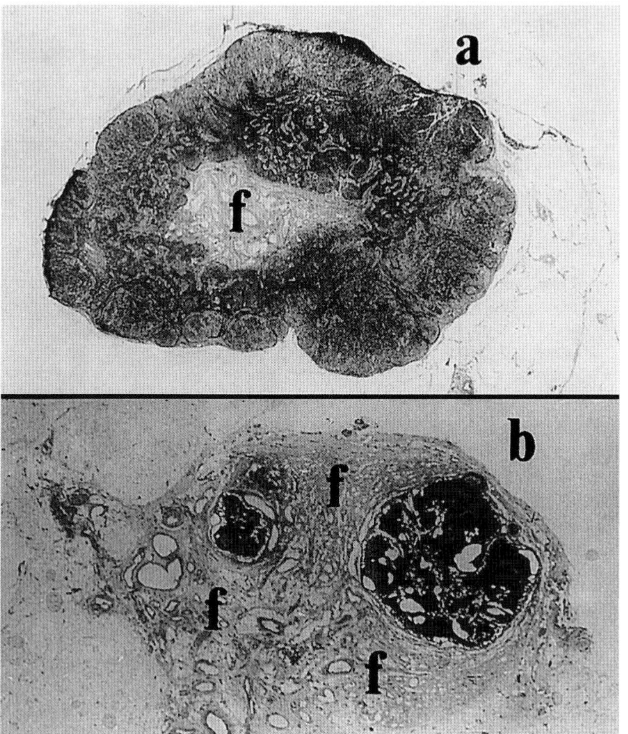

Figure 12.4 (a) Normal lymph node with central fibrosis (f) and (b) fibrotic lymph node from a patient with primary lymphoedema.

Secondary lymphoedema in Europe and North America is usually the result of surgical excision and radiotherapy of local lymph nodes to treat malignant spread, but on a global scale infection is of much greater importance.

FILARIASIS

The most important cause of lymphoedema worldwide is this helminthic infection. There are three filarial worms which cause lymphatic filariasis: *Wuchereria bancrofti*, *Brugia malayi* and, least often, *Brugia timori*. Infection results from a bite from an infected arthropod. The larvae mature into adult worms within the human host, and the female produces microfilariae that are then transmitted to other biting insects, thus completing the life cycle. Approximately 80 million people in 76 countries are infected with filarial parasites.[21] *Wuchereria bancrofti* accounts for about 90% of infections and *Brugia malayi* for most of the remaining cases. About two-thirds of infected people live in China, India and Indonesia. Filariasis causes lymphoedema because the worms enter the lymphatics and produce a fibrotic inflammatory reaction, particularly in the lymph nodes. The severe swelling (usually of the lower limbs) that results is called elephantiasis.[22]

The diagnosis is confirmed by finding microfilariae, which enter the blood in large numbers at night. A strongly positive complement fixation test suggests active or past filariasis.

Treatment with diethylcarbamazine destroys the filariae but cannot reverse established lymphoedema, although progression of the disease may be slowed or prevented. Established lymphoedema is treated by the same methods as those used to treat primary lymphoedema.

NON-FILARIAL ELEPHANTIASIS

Podoconiosis is a form of endemic non-filarial elephantiasis, which Price reported in certain parts of East Africa and Ethiopia where filariasis does not exist.[23] He showed that elephantiasis was associated with areas where the soil was rich in silica. These silica particles, which became surrounded by dense fibrotic reaction, could be seen in the inguinal lymph nodes of the barefoot tribesmen. The condition is therefore thought to be the result of an obstructive lymphopathy caused by aluminosilicate and silica absorbed from soil through the soles of the feet.

MALIGNANCY

Any malignant process that spreads to the lymph nodes can cause secondary lymphoedema,[24] but it is more common after surgical resection or radiotherapy to treat nodal deposits of tumour. Hodgkin's disease and the non-Hodgkin's lymphomas occasionally present with lymphoedema, which may also complicate malignant melanomas and testicular seminomas (Fig. 12.5). The mass effect of large tumours can also obstruct lymph flow.

REFERENCES

19. Casley-Smith JR. In: Zweitach BW (ed). The Inflammatory Process. Academic Press, New York, 1973
20. Mowlem R. Br J Plast Surg 1948; 1: 48
21. Ngwira BM, Jabu CH, Kanyongoloka H et al. Ann Trop Med Parasitol. 2002; 96: 137–144
22. Molyneux DH, Taylor MJ. Curr Opin Infect Dis 2001; 14: 155–159
23. Price EW. Trans R Soc Trop Med Hyg 1972; 66: 150
24. Mogulkoc N, Onal B, Okyay N et al. Eur Respir J 1999; 13: 1489–1491

SURGICAL BLOCK DISSECTION AND RADIOTHERAPY

Block dissections are usually carried out to treat malignancies affecting lymph nodes, although in many cases they form part of a staging or prophylactic procedure. The carcinomas commonly treated by block dissections are those of the breast and uterus, although malignant melanoma and testicular tumours are also often treated by block dissection or irradiation.

The incidence of secondary lymphoedema following surgical excision of pelvic and inguinal lymph nodes varies considerably. The main determining factors are the primary pathology and whether adjuvant radiotherapy was given. The incidence of lymphoedema following iliac and inguinal lymphadenectomy for vulval and penile carcinoma is 15%,[25–29] but following inguinal lymphadenectomy for cutaneous carcinoma it may be as high as 55%.[30] Surgical interruption of inguinal lymphatics most commonly occurs after varicose vein surgery, especially following redo groin incisions (Ch. 11). The incidence of lymphoedema following this type of surgery is reported to be in the range of 0.5%.[31] Secondary lymphoedema of the upper arm usually follows an axillary clearance with or without adjuvant radiotherapy for breast cancer.[32] The incidence varies between 2.7 and 7.6%, depending on the level of axillary clearance.[33,34] As the lymphatics have excellent regenerative properties, lymphoedema becomes more likely if the lymphatic extirpation is associated with infection or irradiation. The subsequent block of fibrous tissue cannot be transgressed by the new lymphatic pathways and lymphoedema ensues. In a number of patients an associated venous occlusion may increase the lymphatic load and tip the balance towards clinical oedema. It is hoped that the introduction of sentinel node biopsies in these conditions (see Ch. 23) may reduce the incidence of limb swelling caused by unnecessary block dissections.

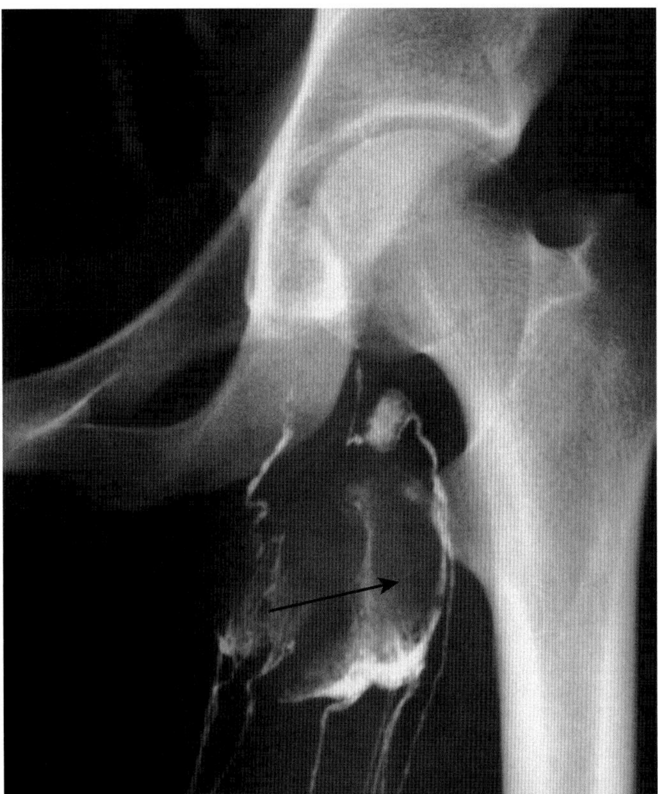

Figure 12.5 Second dep. Top malignant melanoma blocking an inguinal lymph node.

Radiotherapy was a common cause of secondary lymphoedema of the upper limb in patients with breast carcinoma in the 1970s and 1980s, especially when given after an axillary clearance. The combination of radiotherapy and surgery carries a higher risk of lymphoedema than either treatment in isolation. Radiotherapy results in nodal fibrosis, which causes obstruction of the lymphatic vessels. Recurrent tumour in an irradiated field may also be responsible for lymphoedema developing some years after treatment of the primary disease.

TRAUMA

Severe trauma occasionally causes tissue loss that includes lymph nodes or lymphatic channels. This is particularly common after severe degloving injuries.

CHRONIC INFECTION AND CHRONIC INFLAMMATION

Although tuberculosis has often been cited as a cause of lymphoedema,[35] it is uncommon today. Severe rheumatoid disease,[36] psoriatic arthritis,[37] chronic eczema and allergic dermatitis[38,39] are all recognized causes of lymphoedema from the chronic stimulation of the lymph nodes that results in fibrosis and mild obstruction to the lymphatic drainage.

ACUTE INFECTION

Severe cellulitis can occasionally damage the local subcutaneous lymphatics and cause mild lymphoedema. Patients suffering from subclinical primary lymphoedema may also develop a secondary cellulitis and the two presentations can be difficult to distinguish.

SELF-INDUCED OR ARTEFACTUAL LYMPHOEDEMA

This quite common form of Munchausen's syndrome is produced by repeated tight application of a tourniquet around a limb to produce lymphoedema artefacta (Fig. 12.6). Total disuse of a limb can also cause swelling. This form of self-induced

REFERENCES

25. Petereit DG, Mehta MP, Buchler DA et al. Int J Radiat Oncol Biol Phys 1993; 27: 963–967
26. Ornellas AA, Seixas AL, De Moraes JR. J Urol 1991; 146: 330–332
27. Lin JY, Du Beshter B, Angel C et al. Gynecol Oncol 1992; 47: 80–86
28. Ravi R. Jpn J Clin Oncol 1993; 23: 53–58
29. Cavanagh D, Fiorica JV et al. Am J Obstet Gynecol 1990; 163: 1007–1015
30. James JH. Scand J Plast Reconstr Surg 1982; 16: 167–171
31. Ouvry PA, Guenneguez H. Phlebology 1993; 46: 563–568
32. Sparaco A, Fentiman IS. Int J Clin Pract 2002; 56: 107–110
33. Siegel BM, Mayzel KA, Love SM. Arch Surg 1990; 125: 1144–1147
34. Hoe AL, Iven D, Royle GI et al. Br J Surg 1992; 79: 261–263
35. Ramesh V, Ramesh V. Genitourin Med 1997; 73: 226–227
36. Schmit P, Prieur AM, Brunelle F. Pediatr Radiol 1999; 29: 364–366
37. Bohm M, Riemann B, Luger TA et al. Br J Dermatol 2000; 143: 1297–1301
38. Gach JE, King CM. Acta Derm Venereol 2001; 81: 437–438
39. Fitzgerald DA. Contact Derm 1994; 30: 310

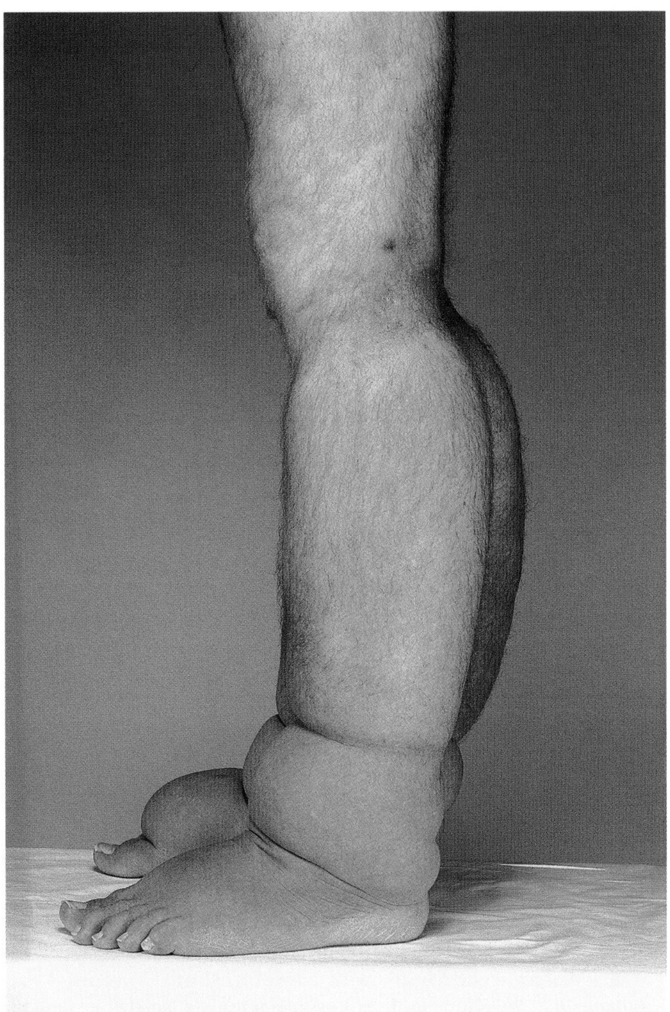

Figure 12.6 Artefactual lymphoedema caused by a tourniquet, producing indentation.

lymphoedema should be suspected if passive movement of the limb is not possible. Lymphograms are usually normal or only mildly unusual. The cause should be suspected if there is a sharp cut-off to the lymphoedema demarcated by a dent caused by application of the tourniquet. Patients should be referred for psychiatric advice, although this is often not of much help.

DIFFERENTIAL DIAGNOSIS

All possible causes of tissue oedema must be considered before a diagnosis of lymphoedema is made. The most common causes of oedema rarely represent a diagnostic problem (Box 12.3).

Cardiac oedema should be apparent from examination of the central venous pressure, heart and lungs, while the oedema of chronic renal failure and hypoproteinaemia from malnutrition, malabsorption or hepatic cirrhosis should be diagnosed from the initial blood investigations.

Allergic disorders must also be considered, but they can usually be diagnosed from the history. Hereditary angioedema, from a deficiency in the complement system regulation, is inherited as an autosomal dominant. It presents with attacks of swelling of the face and extremities that subsequently resolve. The oedema is sometimes associated with erythema.

Box 12.3 The Browse-Stewart classification of patients with lymphoedema

Secondary lymphoedema

All forms of lymphoedema caused by disease not originating in the lymph-conducting elements of the vessels and nodes.

Primary lymphoedema

Lymphoedema caused by abnormalities or disease originating in the lymphatics or the lymph-conducting elements of the lymph nodes.

Congenital

- Congenital aplasia or hypoplasia of peripheral lymphatic (lymphatic abnormality and/or oedema present at or appearing within 2 years of birth).
- Congenital abnormalities of the abdominal or thoracic lymph trunks.
- Congenital valvular incompetence. This is always associated with megalymphatics and often with chylous reflux.

Acquired

Intraluminal or intramural lymphangio-obstructive oedema

- *Distal*: acquired obliteration of the distal limb lymphatics, of unknown cause.
- *Proximal*: acquired obliteration of the lymphatics in the proximal part of the limb, usually associated with distal dilatation, of unknown cause.
- *Combined*: acquired obliteration of all the lymphatics of the limb.

Obstruction by the lymph nodes

Obliteration of the lymph-conducting pathways through the node by hilar fibrosis. This may cause the changes classified above as lymphangio-obstructive oedema. These two conditions often coexist, and acquired valvular incompetence may follow any form of obstruction.

Idiopathic cyclic oedema, which commonly occurs in young women during their childbearing years, can be mistaken for mild bilateral distal lymphoedema, and this condition has been shown to be exacerbated by diuretics.[40] The cyclical nature of the swelling, which usually occurs in the week before menses, should also alert the clinician to this diagnosis. The lymphatics are entirely normal, and patients may be helped by remedies designed to help premenstrual syndrome.[41]

The most common cause of unilateral ankle oedema is long-standing venous disease. The diagnosis is often suggested by the presence of abnormal cutaneous veins, ankle flares or lipodermatosclerosis in the ankle skin. These changes may not, however, be present in limbs with iliac vein compression syndrome, or in patients with an inferior vena caval occlusion. A lower limb duplex scan and a venogram should establish the diagnosis if doubt exists. Unless there is a failure of the lymphatic system, venous occlusion cannot cause lymphoedema. Subclinical lymphoedema may occasionally become apparent as a result of venous thrombosis. Under these circumstances, poorly functioning lymphatics that were able to drain the interstitial space cannot cope with the extra fluid and protein forced out of the capillary bed.

REFERENCES

40. MacGregor GA, Markandu ND, Roulston JE et al. Lancet 1979; i: 397–400
41. Streeten DPH, Dalakos DG et al. Clin Sci Mol Med 1973; 45: 347

Klippel–Trenaunay syndrome, in which congenital varicose veins are associated with bony and soft tissue deformity, elongation of the limb, capillary naevi, and often an abnormal deep venous system, may also cause limb oedema. Some patients with this syndrome have an associated primary abnormality of their lymphatics: 55% in one report (see Ch. 11).[42]

Malignant disease may also cause unilateral oedema, and because the lymphatic obstruction is frequently deep in the pelvis the clinical diagnosis is easily missed. Pelvic ultrasound or CT scanning can usually detect enlarged pelvic lymph nodes with a reasonable degree of accuracy.

Disuse or hysterical oedema is produced by voluntary or involuntary immobility. This condition may develop in patients with long-standing paralysis from causes such as poliomyelitis, but it may also occur in patients with psychological disturbances.

There remain a few obscure causes of leg swelling that must be differentiated from lymphoedema. In lipodystrophy or lipoedema there is excessive deposition of fat in the legs. In some patients there is a family history, suggesting that there may be a genetic cause. Almost all patients with this condition are female and some have generalized gross obesity (Fig. 12.7). In others, the subcutaneous fat deposition is confined to the lower half of the body or the legs alone. Most patients complain of pain and report that their ankles have always been 'heavy'. Their 'swollen' limbs do not 'pit' and an isotope lymphogram is normal. Erythrocyanosis frigida is a relatively common condition in young, often heavily built women, in whom the skin is cold to the touch and has reddish blue blotchy areas of discolouration owing to sluggish cutaneous circulation. The condition is almost always bilateral and the ankles are thickened, but the feet are not usually swollen. There is an overlap of this condition with lipodystrophy.

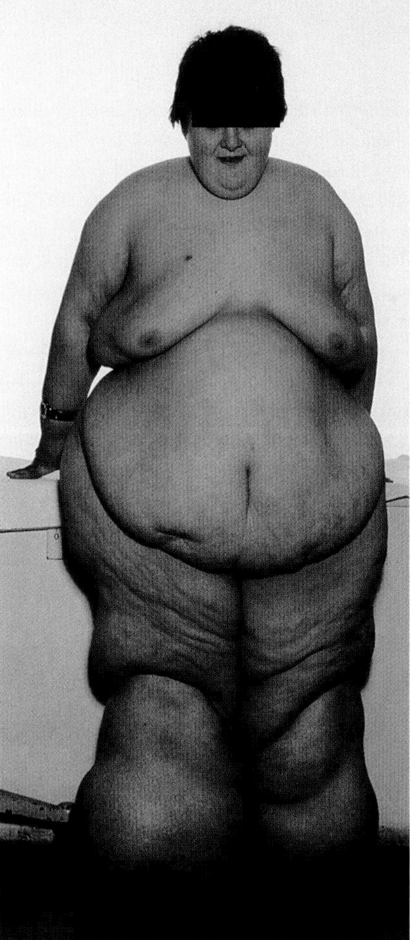

Figure 12.7 Gross obesity should not be confused with lymphoedema.

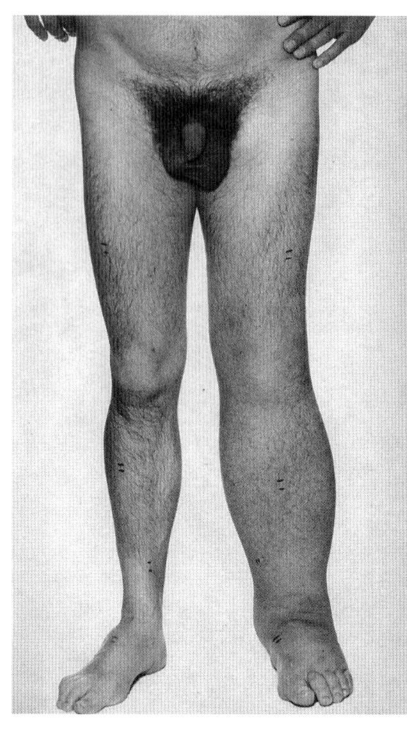

Figure 12.8 Primary lymphoedema. The clinical diagnosis in this patient is evident, but lymphography may be useful for confirmation and in considering treatment.

True gigantism of a limb is rare. It may be associated with varying degrees of hypertrophy of the subcutaneous tissue, but the skin texture, the blood supply and lymph drainage are all normal. Patients with multiple arteriovenous fistulae (the Parkes–Weber syndrome) also develop limb swelling and lengthening. The limb feels hot and machinery murmurs may be heard (see Ch. 10).

CLINICAL PRESENTATION

The majority of patients present with swelling of one or both lower limbs, but the lower abdomen, the genital region, one or both upper limbs, and (rarely) the face or chest can be lymphoedematous. In the legs, swelling usually develops around the ankle and on the dorsum of the foot, and spreads proximally (Fig. 12.8). In most patients the oedema does not spread above the knee, but severe oedema of the whole limb including the buttock suggests a proximal nodal lymphatic block (see Fig. 12.13). Patients with proximal lymphatic occlusions may, however, have no oedema of the ankle or foot. A detailed past and family history should exclude secondary causes of lymphoedema and should suggest a genetic cause of the primary condition.

Because lymphatic oedema results in a fibrotic reaction in the subcutaneous tissues, it is more resistant to pitting than 'acute' oedema associated with cardiac failure or hypoproteinaemia. Prolonged digital pressure will always produce a pit. If pitting cannot be demonstrated the diagnosis of lymphoedema is unlikely and another cause for the swelling should be sought.

REFERENCES

42. Baskerville PA, Ackroyd JS et al. Br J Surg 1985; 72: 232

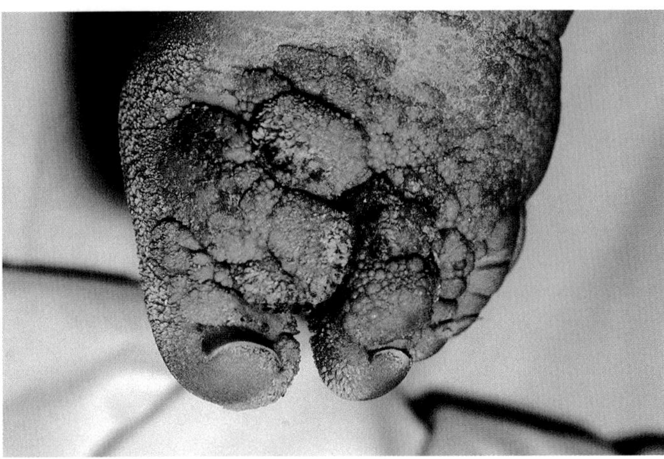

Figure 12.9 Warty excrescences on toes: the typical skin changes associated with lymphoedema.

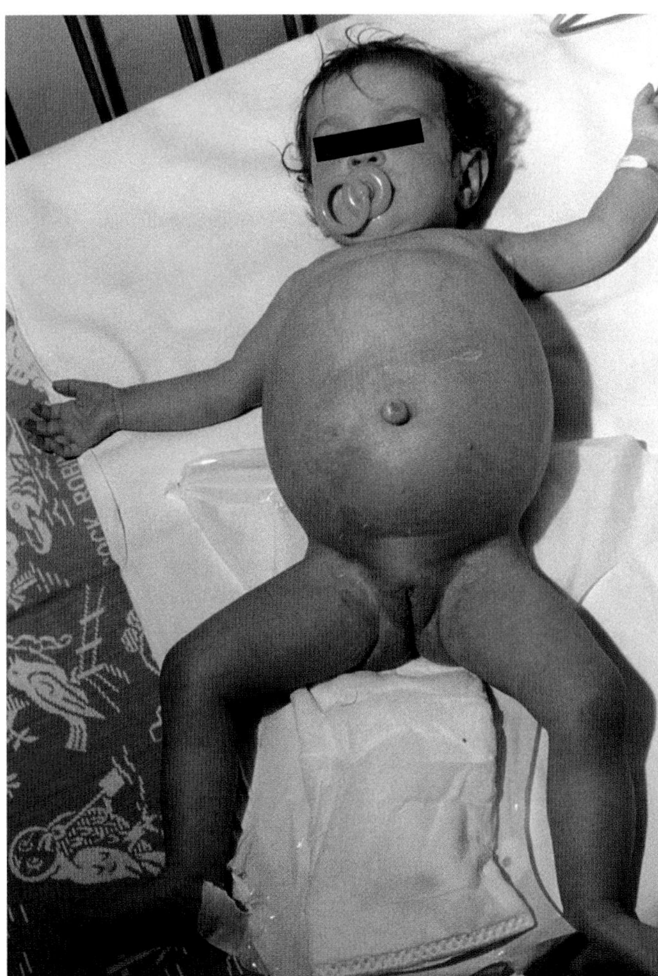

Figure 12.10 Chylous ascites.

The onset of the lymphoedema is usually insidious, but the majority of patients report that the swelling decreases during sleep and is maximal at the end of the day. The patient may attribute the onset of the swelling to a minor infection, insect bite or a mild injury, such as a twisted ankle. It is quite conceivable that such an episode did, indeed, produce the lymphatic overload that initiated the irreversible process of lymph accumulation in a patient with already inadequate or damaged lymphatics.

The onset can occasionally be sudden, and progression rapid. This is often associated with cellulitis, which can be both a cause and a result of the lymphoedema. Patients with sudden severe swelling usually have a proximal lymphatic occlusion and may have an underlying cause for this. Patients with malignant obstruction of both the veins and lymphatics often develop a severe oedema of rapid onset that can cause intractable pain, which may be very difficult to alleviate. As the condition progresses, a few patients develop marked cutaneous thickening and skin excrescences, which can progress to lymphatic warts (condylomata) and often multiple coarse papillae over their toes (Fig. 12.9). The skin of the lower leg becomes thickened and pigmented. Other patients are troubled by repeated attacks of infection. The infecting agent often enters through the hyperkeratotic skin or through cracks in the interdigital clefts that occur in athlete's foot.

The inguinal nodes may be enlarged, particularly in patients with a proximal pelvic lymphatic obstruction. Occasionally patients develop numerous vesicles in the skin that may leak clear lymph or, occasionally, chyle. The presence of small lymph vesicles or blisters and a cutaneous capillary naevus is suggestive of a megalymphatic problem. Vesicles usually arise over the upper thighs or on the external genitalia, and they may also act as a portal of entry for bacteria. A few patients have chylometrorrhoea, chyluria, chylous ascites or chylothorax: all features of megalymphatics and associated lymphatic fistulae. Other associated congenital abnormalities may be present, including yellow nails, distichiasis (two layers of eyelashes) and cardiac anomalies. Other rare conditions include Pierre–Robin, Noonan's and Turner's syndrome.

Lymphoedema of the male genitalia is embarrassing, uncomfortable, and interferes with urination and sexual relationships. Leaking vesicles and recurrent attacks of cellulitis often complicate the condition. Women with genital oedema usually have fewer problems but massive labial swelling can occur.

Lymph leakage into the abdominal and pleural cavities causes chylous ascites (Fig. 12.10) and pleural effusions, respectively. Patients present with abdominal distension or dyspnoea. These problems are usually the result of leakage from refluxing megalymphatics. Chyluria (leak into the bladder or ureters) and chylous leakage from the vagina (chylometrorrhoea) are rare complications. Chylous leak into the bowel can result in a protein-losing enteropathy and severe weight loss. The chylous leakage from the serosal surface of the bowel may increase the ascites.

Lymphoedema may occasionally affect the upper limb, including the fingers, and unilateral pectoral swelling can also occur. Oedema of the face usually presents as swelling of the eyelids, which are the most lax tissues in this region.

Patients with lymphoedema usually seek advice because they want to know the cause of the swelling, which can cause major cosmetic embarrassment but is more often only a nuisance. Severe swelling may make it impossible to buy shoes or trousers, and an enormously heavy limb may reduce mobility. Recurrent attacks of cellulitis may also be a major problem, causing the patient to lose time off school or work. Severe attacks may require admission to hospital for intravenous antibiotics and may even be life-threatening.

Several tumours are known to be associated with lymphoedema. Lymphangiosarcoma (Stewart–Treves syndrome) is an extremely rare but highly lethal complication of chronic lymph-

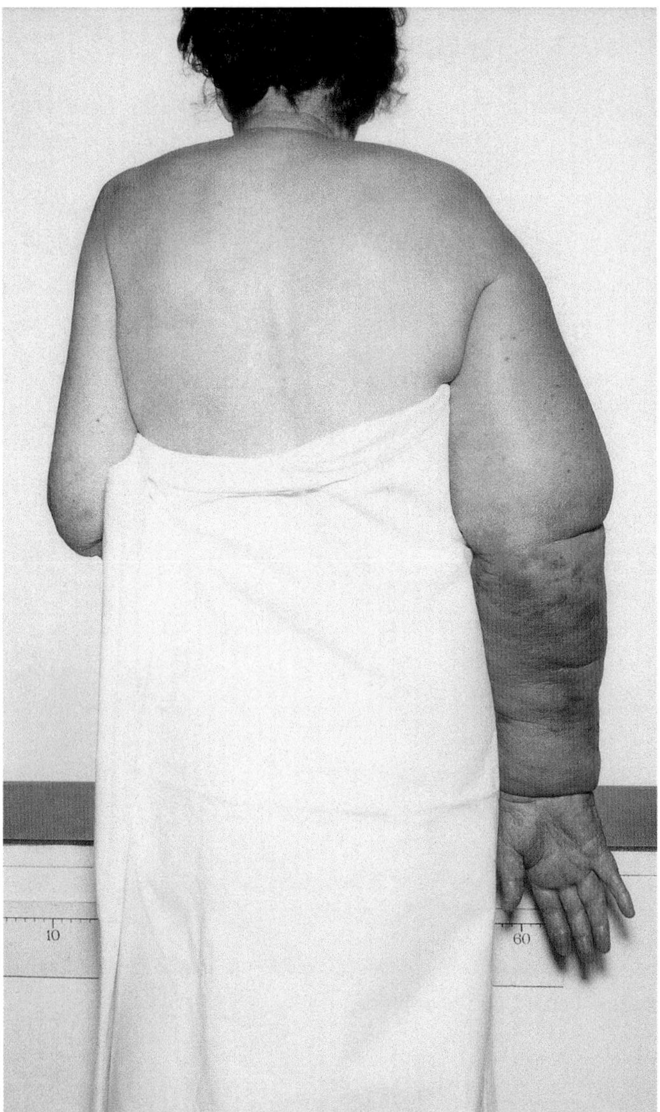

Figure 12.11 Lymphangiosarcoma (Stewart–Treves syndrome).

oedema (Fig. 12.11).[43,44] Lymphangiosarcoma rarely develops in limbs following long-standing primary lymphoedema, and more often develops in patients with secondary lymphoedema. Treatment of postmastectomy lymphangiosarcoma is still unsatisfactory. Early recognition and radical ablative surgery seem to provide the best chance for survival. Squamous cell carcinoma,[45] cutaneous plasmacytoma,[46] angiosarcoma and Kaposi's sarcoma[47–49] have all been reported in lymphoedematous limbs.

EXAMINATION

Apart from confirming the presence of pitting, physical examination excludes other causes of limb swelling and reveals any associated abnormalities. Examination of the feet may confirm the presence of 'square toes', which result from footwear preventing toe expansion. It is important to inspect the web spaces between the toes for athlete's foot, which is especially common in lymphoedematous limbs and is an important portal of entry for bacteria that cause recurrent cellulitis. Yellow nail syndrome is occasionally associated with lymphoedema, as is distichiasis (two layers of eyelashes). Occasionally other skeletal abnormalities are present, and congenital cardiac anomalies are found also in patients with lymphatic hyperplasia.

The volume of the limb must be assessed to allow the results of therapy to be evaluated. The length of the limbs should also be recorded and the presence of any abnormal veins should be noted. The abdomen and chest should be carefully examined for ascites or effusions. The groins, axillae and neck should be palpated for pathologically enlarged lymph nodes. Rectal and vaginal examinations are indicated if a pelvic malignancy is suspected.

DIAGNOSIS

The history and physical examination should indicate whether the patient has primary or secondary lymphoedema, but unequivocal confirmation of the diagnosis is desirable. Other investigations are necessary if the swelling is not considered to be the result of lymphoedema.

An absence of venous stigmata makes the diagnosis of lymphoedema very likely if the appearances are typical. Isotope lymphography[50] should, however, always be performed to confirm the diagnosis and to determine whether a proximal block is present that requires further assessment with a view to bypass surgery. Isotope lymphography is also the investigation of first choice if the diagnosis is in doubt. Rhenium and antimony sulphide microcolloids labelled with technetium-99m, when injected into a web space, are taken up by the lymphatic system and pass up through the lymphatics to be concentrated in the proximal nodes. The percentage of uptake can therefore be measured and, although normal values should be ascertained by each laboratory, an ilioinguinal colloid uptake of less than 0.3% at 30 min after the injection into the toe web spaces is probably diagnostic of lymphoedema.[51] An abnormally rapid clearance occurs in patients with venous oedema, resulting in early ilioinguinal lymph node uptake (Fig. 12.12).

Other methods for interpreting lymphoscintigrams are the Kleinhans transport index, where a score of less than 10 is considered diagnostic, and time–activity curve analysis of different limb segments.[52] Lymphoscintigraphy is minimally invasive and moderately reliable in diagnosing lymphoedema but does not discern between the various subgroups of primary lymphoedema and between primary and secondary lymph-

REFERENCES

43. Aygit AC, Yildirim AM, Dervisoglu S. J Hand Surg (Br) 1999; 24: 135–137
44. Stewart FW, Treves N. Cancer 1948; 1: 64–81
45. Lister RK, Black MM, Calonje E et al. Br J Dermatol 1997; 136: 384–387
46. Corazza M, Lombardi A, Strumia R et al. Eur J Dermatol 2002; 12: 191–193
47. Azurdia RM, Guerin DM, Verbov JL. Clin Exp Dermatol 1999; 24: 270–272
48. Atillasoy ES, Santoro A, Weinberg JM. J Eur Acad Dermatol Venereol 2001; 15: 364–365
49. Schwartz RA, Cohen JB, Watson RA et al. Br J Dermatol 2000; 142: 153–156
50. Burnand KG, McGuinness CL, Lagattolla NR et al. Br J Surg 2002; 89: 74–78
51. Stewart G, Gaunt JI et al. Br J Surg 1985; 72: 906
52. Kleinhans E, Baumeister RGH, Hahn D et al. Eur J Nucl Med 1985; 10: 349–352

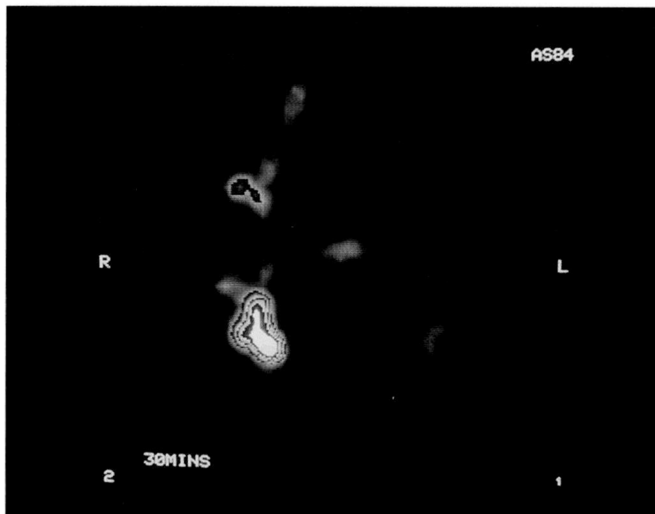

Figure 12.12 A lymphoscintigram with technetium-labelled rhenium sulphur colloid. Inguinal lymph nodes are taking up isotope on the right but there is no uptake on the left, indicating poor distal lymphatic function.

oedema.[53] Both false positive and false negative scans occur. False positive scans are common when there is a proximal block associated with normal distal lymphatics or when nodal uptake is normal and the region of interest continues to accumulate isotope. False negatives occur when the isotope is incorrectly injected.

Formal contrast lymphography using an oily contrast medium (Lipiodol) is now reserved for equivocal results from the isotope lymphography, especially if a proximal lymphatic block is suspected and where bypass is being considered. It is also very valuable if reflux is suspected, and the site and extent need to be carefully determined before treatment is undertaken. Patent blue green violet is injected between the web spaces before an incision through the skin on the dorsum of the foot defines a lymphatic and allows direct cannulation using an operating microscope. Immediate and delayed radiographs define the lymphatic anatomy with precision (Fig. 12.13).

TREATMENT

Ninety per cent of all patients with primary or secondary lymphoedema respond to active conservative management. Patients are often given pessimistic, nihilistic advice and feel frustrated and impotent in the face of an incurable condition. Interstitial fluid can be compressed out of the subcutaneous tissues by the regular use of an intermittent pneumatic compression device (Flowtron, LymphaPress),[54] which is then maintained by adequate elastic stockings (40 mmHg compression or more). Adoption of these measures often produces good results.[55,56] Potential portals of entry of infection must be rigorously eradicated and cellulitis treated immediately with systemic antibiotics.

Many private clinics now specialize in a combination of regular massage (manual lymphatic drainage), pneumatic compression and tight bandaging to bring the swelling under control. This is followed by application of tight, correctly fitted compression hosiery. Patients should also be advised to lose weight and elevate the leg whenever possible. Regular exercise is also advocated. There are, however, disappointingly few trials that confirm the benefits of these measures and rely on compression hosiery to maintain any benefits produced.

Benzopyrones statistically reduce the size of lymphoedematous limbs but the reduction achieved is small.[57,58] They act through enhancing macrophage activity and the best results are usually achieved in combination with physiotherapy.[59]

Diuretics are inadvisable because fluid depletion throughout the body eventually results in only a marginal reduction in the size of the oedematous limb.

OPERATIONS

Surgery should be considered only for a small group of patients.

- In 2 or 3% it is possible to improve lymphatic drainage with an operation designed to bypass the lymphatic occlusion.
- In a huge limb that has become functionally impaired bulky tissue can be removed, especially when conservative treatment has failed.
- Patients with megalymphatics and lymphatic fistulae can be treated effectively by the judicious use of lymphatic ligation.[8]
- Cosmetic surgery for lymphoedema is not indicated because patients will be disappointed with the results.

Debulking operations

Many operations attempt to improve the lymphatic drainage of the subcutaneous tissues while reducing the bulk of the leg. Kondoleon hoped that by cutting windows in the deep fascia some lymph would drain into the deep compartment.[60] Sistrunk modified this operation with the same aim.[61]

Homans's operation[62] (first described by Auchincloss[63]) is moderately successful but leaves large scars on the leg (Fig. 12.14). Providing the skin is healthy, flaps are raised and a segment of subcutaneous tissue is removed. The anterior and posterior skin flaps are then sutured together to lie snugly on the deep fascia, once a gusset has been removed to avoid redundant skin. The first operation is usually performed on the medial side of the leg, and sometimes a second operation is required on the lateral side. The circumference of the limb is usually reduced by about a third for each operation and the surgery can be repeated.

Thompson and Wee tried to combine tissue excision with an improvement in lymphatic drainage.[64] They hoped that by burying a dermal flap, lymph would pass through skin lymphatics into the deep fascial compartment. The results are no better than

REFERENCES

53. Cambria RA, Gloviczki P, Naessens JM et al. J Vasc Surg 1993; 18: 773–782
54. Zelikovski A, Monoach M et al. Lymphology 1980; 13: 68
55. Casley-Smith JR, Casley-Smith JR. Australas J Dermatol 1992; 33: 69–74
56. Pecking A. Bull Cancer 1991; 78: 373–377
57. Casley-Smith JR, Wang CT, Casley-Smith JR et al. Br Med J 1993; 307: 1037–1041
58. Casley-Smith JR, Morgan RG, Piller NB. N Engl J Med 1993; 329: 1158–1163
59. Casley-Smith JR, Casley-Smith JR, Cluzan RV. Progress in Lymphology XIII. Elsevier, Amsterdam, 1992: 537–538
60. Kondoleon E. Munch Med Wochenschr 1912; 59: 525
61. Sistrunk WE. JAMA 1918; 71: 800
62. Homans J. N Engl J Med 1936; 215: 1099
63. Auchincloss H. Puerto Rico J Pub Health Trop Med 1930; 6: 149
64. Thompson N, Wee JTK. Chir Plast (Berl) 1980; 5: 147

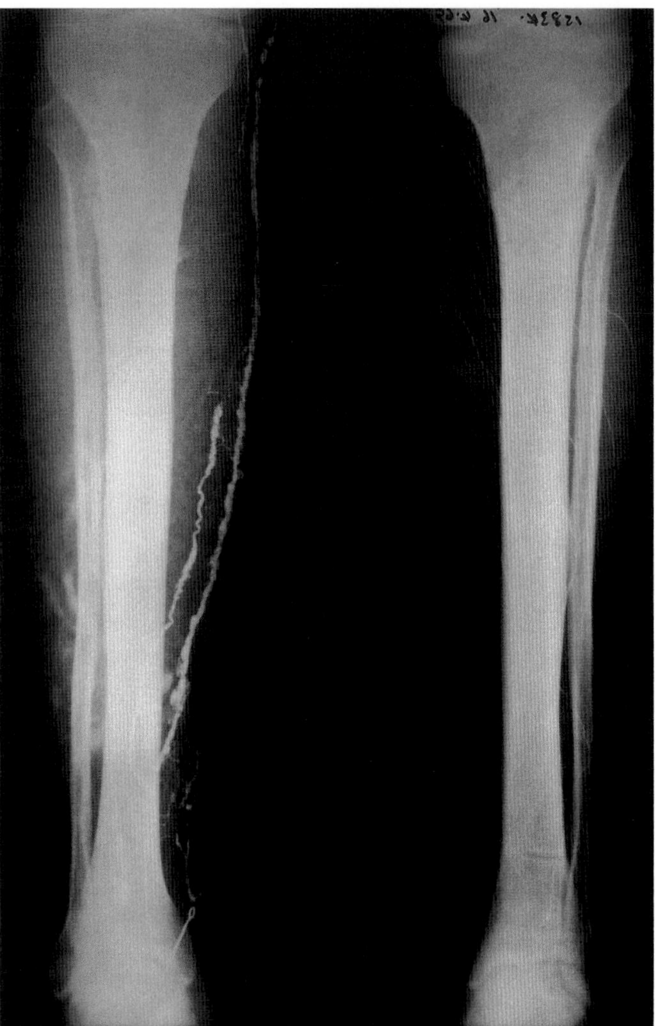

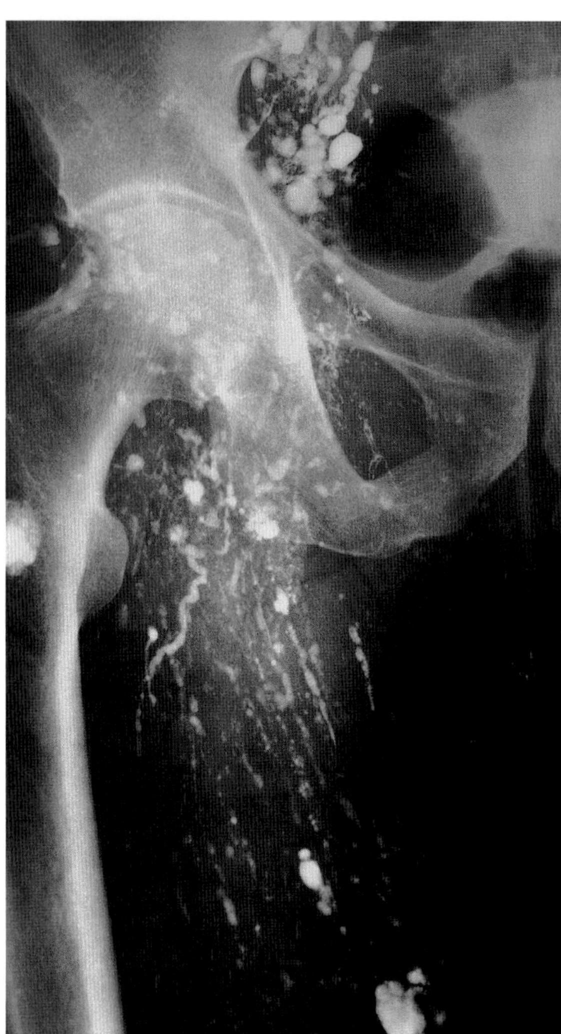

Figure 12.13 A contrast lymphogram showing obstructed lymphatics in the right iliac region causing dilation of all the lymphatic channels in the limb.

Homans's operation and the complications are greater. There is no sign of the buried dermal flap if the operation has to be revised. Pilonidal sinuses in the buried flap provide additional complications and this procedure has now largely been abandoned.

A Charles procedure is indicated if the skin has become grossly thickened and involved in the lymphoedematous process.[65] It is also the best way of treating massive swelling. All the skin and subcutaneous fat are excised between the ankle and knee before split-skin grafts are placed on the denuded deep fascia (Fig. 12.15). Care must be taken to shape flaps at the upper end to avoid a pantaloon effect and to keep the mature skin over both joints to ensure mobility.

Some patients who, after a Charles procedure, develop gross keratotic and warty excrescences protruding from a deeply fissured surface benefit by having these keratoses shaved down.

Lymph drainage operations

Many different procedures have been tried in an attempt to drain lymph from an affected leg but most have failed. The insertion of silk threads was introduced by Handley in the hope that lymph would drain along them.[66] This does not work and has been abandoned. Two operations that are moderately successful are the mesenteric bridge procedure and lymphovenous anastomosis.

Lymphovenous fistulae

Lymphonodal to venous anastomosis was originally attempted by Nielbowicz and Olszewski,[67] but the results were disappointing in patients with primary lymphoedema. Direct lymphovenous anastomosis may be more effective in patients with secondary lymphoedema than in patients with primary lymphoedema.[68] Nevertheless, there are several advocates of this painstaking technique in which lymphatics are dissected out with the operating microscope and anastomosed to nearby veins. Good results are claimed but they are masked by the concomitant use

REFERENCES

65. Charles RH. In: Latham A, English TC (eds). Elephantiasis Scrotii, a System of Treatment, Vol 111. J & A Churchill, London, 1912
66. Handley WS. Lancet 1908; i: 783
67. Nielbowicz J, Olszewski W. Minerva Cardioangiol 1967; 15: 254–256
68. O'Brien B. Microvascular Reconstructive Surgery. Churchill Livingstone, Edinburgh, 1977

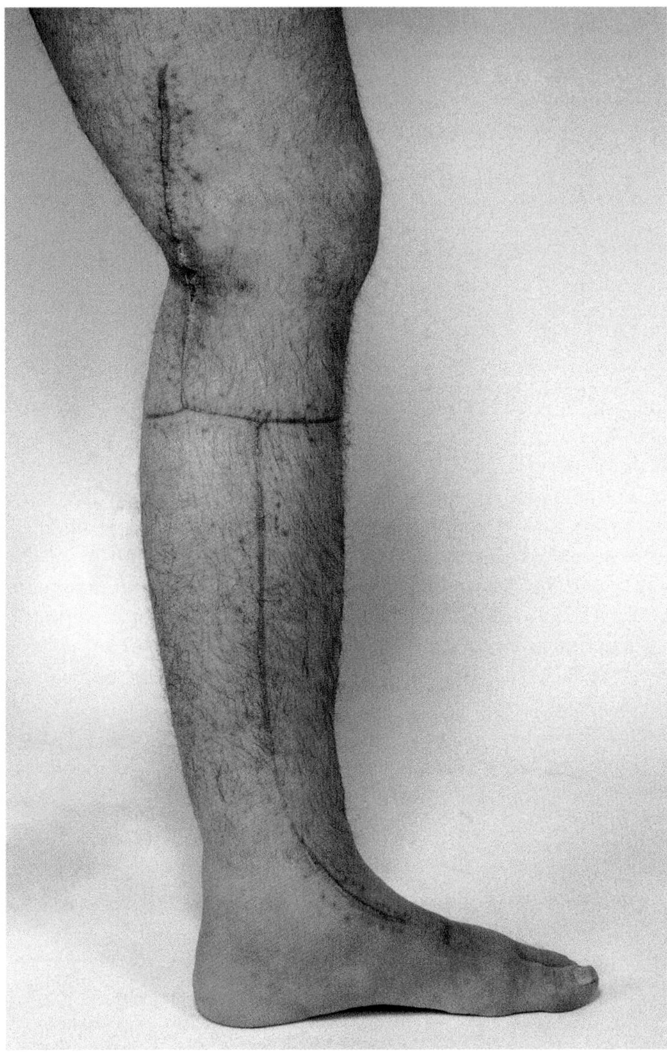

Figure 12.14 Scars of Homans's operation.

of improved conservative management and additional excisional procedures. In many countries initial enthusiasm has given way to eventual disillusionment.

Bridging operations

Many bridging operations have failed because lymphatic communication was not achieved. The omentum does not have sufficient lymphatics to be of value, but the introduction of the enteromesenteric bridge, developed by Kinmonth, may be successful in a small group of patients. The rich submucosal lymphatics of the ileum are utilized by isolating and opening up a pedicle of small bowel. The bowel is opened along its antimesenteric border and the mucosa is then stripped off to expose the rich lymphatic submucosal plexus, which is brought into direct apposition with a bivalved lymph node or group of nodes in the iliac or inguinal region (Fig. 12.16). Because lymphatics have considerable powers of regeneration, a 'low-resistance' connection soon develops between the lymph nodes of the lymphoedematous leg and the enteromesenteric pedicle. Providing the main lymphatic drainage is patent at the level of the cisterna chyli, or more proximally in the thoracic duct, good results can be obtained in just over half the patients in whom it is attempted.[69,70] It is, however, a relatively major operation and carries the potential risk of small bowel obstruction from strangulation around the mesenteric pedicle. Previous radiation is usually a contraindication and it is not effective when a long-standing proximal obstruction has caused distal lymphatic obliteration.

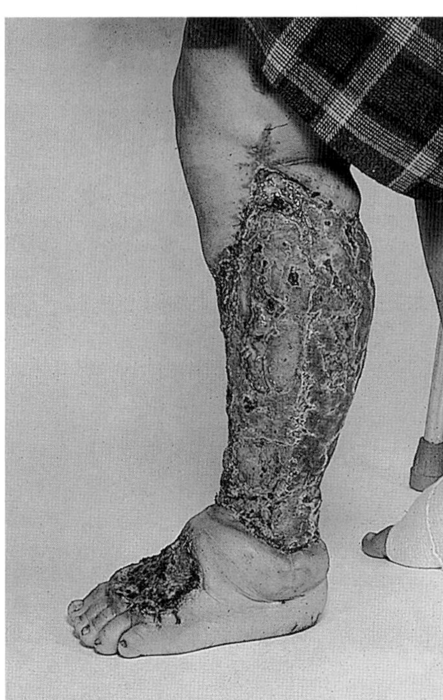

Figure 12.15 A successful Charles reduction.

Summary of surgical operations for lymphoedema

There is no surgical procedure that returns a severely lymphoedematous limb to total normality. Patients should be referred to a specialist centre, where appropriate investigations and careful assessment based on experience offer the optimum management.

The published results of the different procedures described in this chapter are summarized in Table 12.1. These results must be accepted with caution because none were subjected to independent scrutiny and most are only categorized into good, moderate and poor.

CHYLOUS REFLUX

Chylous reflux occurs when there is massive lymphatic ectasia with valvular incompetence. Leakage of chyle from vesicles, chyluria and chylous ascites are common (Fig. 12.10). Lymph-angiography with contrast may determine the site of leakage and allow ligation or excisional operations to be carried out. Chylous ascites may also be treated by peritoneovenous shunts, but these often block and need to be replaced. Chylothorax is well treated by pleurectomy.

PROGNOSIS

The clinical pattern of the disease appears to be determined early in its natural history. Although girth of an affected limb can

REFERENCES

69. Kinmonth JB, Hurst PAE et al. Br J Surg 1978; 65: 829
70. Hurst PAE, Stewart G et al. Br J Surg 1985; 72: 272–274

Table 12.1 Results of surgical procedures for primary and secondary lymphoedema

Procedure	No. of patients	Outcome
Charles	34 with primary and filarial lymphoedema	Good functional results and 88% graft take
Modified Thompson's	74	Good, 21.6%; moderate, 60.8%; and poor, 17%
Lymphovenous anastomosis	91 with secondary lower limb lymphoedema	Good, 72%; moderate, 15%; and poor, 4%
Enteromesenteric bridge	8 primary lower limb	75% showed improvement
Microlymphatic anastomosis	79	Good results in 30%, fair results in 53%

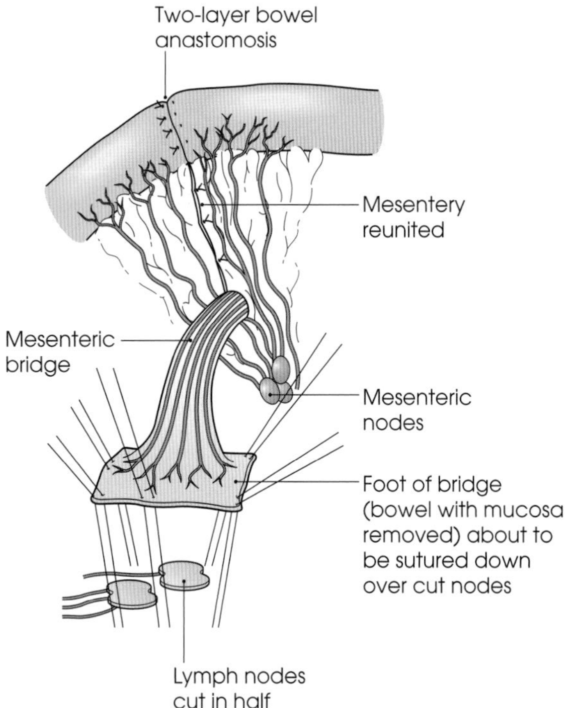

Figure 12.16 A representation of the ileal mesenteric bridging operation (with thanks to Mr P.A. Hurst).

increase, it is unusual for the oedema to spread up the leg if only the lower leg has been involved for more than 5 years. When oedema develops in the opposite leg it is usually less severe.

The majority of patients with primary lymphoedema have obliterated distal lymphatics (90%). This process predominantly affects the distal lymphatics of ovulating women, and it can be contained by a pneumatic compression device and adequate compression stockings. The less common pelvic lymphatic obstruction may be amenable to a lymph drainage procedure because the distal lymphatics often remain patent. As time passes, these distal lymphatics obliterate so that the opportunity for successful surgery is lost.[71]

Lymphoedema may also affect the eyelids and the genitalia, where excisional operations may be beneficial.

REFERENCE

71. Fyfe NCM, Wolfe JHN, Kinmonth JB. Lymphology 1982; 15: 66–69

The face, mouth, tongue and jaws: the maxillofacial region

13

Peter Ward Booth, Mike Corrigan, Mark McGurk

INTRODUCTION

Knowledge of the anatomy and function of the face, neck, mouth and jaws is extremely important if the outcomes of treatment are to be improved in patients with maxillofacial problems.

CRANIOMAXILLOFACIAL DEFORMITY

Many acquired conditions as well as congenital and developmental deformities of the craniofacial skeleton are now treated using the principles and techniques of craniofacial surgery (Box 13.1). The congenital and developmental conditions described in this chapter require a team of maxillofacial surgeons, neurosurgeons, plastic surgeons, psychologists, ophthalmologists, speech and language therapists, orthodontists, audiologists and geneticists to assess and treat affected children. A nurse coordinator is also an important member of the team.

Although the diagnosis of facial deformity may be obvious, categorizing the deformity can be extremely difficult, as the deformity rarely fits neatly into one pigeon-hole. It is possible to create a broad classification.

It is important to understand some important features of facial deformity.

- The face is attached to the skull base. Thus deformity of the cranium may also be seen as a facial deformity; indeed, this may be more obvious than the skull deformity.
- The skin drapes over the bony skeleton, and so most (but not all!) facial deformities are caused by bone abnormalities (Fig. 13.1). Soft tissue anomalies rarely occur alone. When soft tissue anomalies do occur, there are commonly secondary skeletal abnormalities.
- Most facial deformities are caused by errors in the growth process, often beginning in utero.
- The pubertal growth spurt usually exaggerates any deformity.

Box 13.1 The scope of craniomaxillofacial surgery

Congenital and developmental deformities
- Craniosynostosis
- Craniofacial clefts
- Craniofacial cephaloceles
- Orthognathic deformities

Acquired conditions
- Craniomaxillofacial trauma
- Tumour access

Deformities can be broadly subdivided into
- craniofacial anomalies,
- clefting anomalies, and
- dentofacial anomalies.

There is often a crossover into other categories, for example most children with cleft lips and palates have a broad skull and a degree of hypertelorism (their eyes are too far apart).

Some facial deformities have other associated systemic genetic abnormalities and traits. For example, some patients with a cleft palate have a generic abnormality at chromosome 22q.11; this is the so-called velocardio facial syndrome, which is associated with cardiac and personality abnormalities. In Apert's syndrome, there is premature fusion of the cranial sutures and also syndactyly.

CRANIOFACIAL SYNDROMES

Many facial anomalies also have a cranial element, but pure craniofacial deformities are rare. Crouzon's syndrome, which is one of the more common syndromes, has an incidence of 1 in 25/100 000 live births. It lies within the largest group of craniofacial deformities, the craniosynostoses, in which the underlying problem is premature fusion of one or more of the cranial sutures. This causes raised intracranial pressure and deformities of the head shape. The cranium is subject to normal moulding deformities, which are self-correcting. A true craniosynostosis will distort the shape of the skull as the brain attempts to grow against the fused sutures. The deformity worsens as the brain grows. The condition causes a broad tall head if symmetrical, or a rotated asymmetrical shape, so-called plagiocephaly, if a lateral fusion has occurred. Hypertelorism (increased width between the eye sockets) is often a feature, and as growth continues the failure of the skull base to grow forwards causes the maxilla to be held back. This makes the eyes seem proptosed and the face to have a 'dished in' appearance (Fig. 13.2).

In the early years, the increased intracranial pressure may lead to brain damage, and in severe cases blindness. Later in life, the characteristic facial appearance may interfere with the airway and ability to masticate. The maxilla is so far back that this reduces the airway and can cause severe dental malocclusion, with an apparent prominence of the mandible (which has grown normally). The retrusive maxilla may also cause severe proptosis.

The timing of surgery is dependent on the severity of the deformity. The facial surgery is normally straightforward, but the neurosurgical management, especially in very young children, is complex and difficult. The treatment of these craniofacial deformities is concentrated in five or six supraregional centres in the UK. Only a brief account is indicated, because this is very rare surgery.

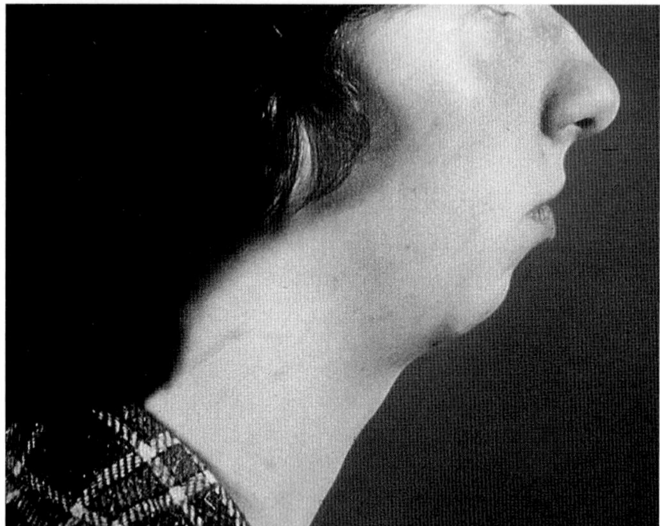

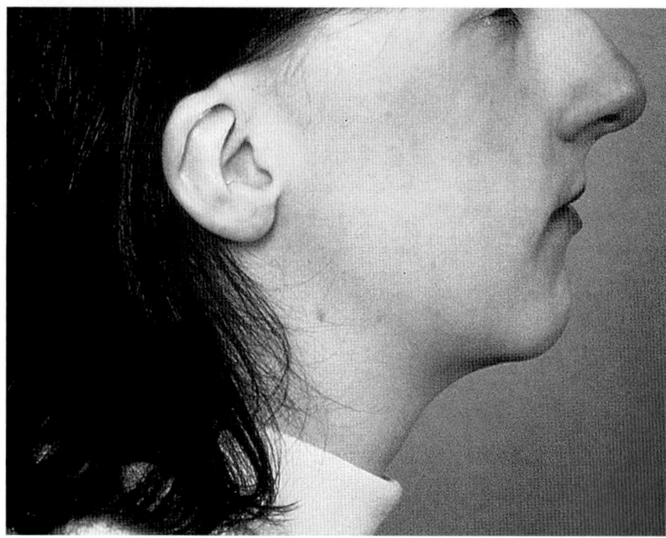

Figure 13.1 Example of a facial deformity: this patient's short lower jaw is a skeletal problem (a) corrected by bone surgery (b).

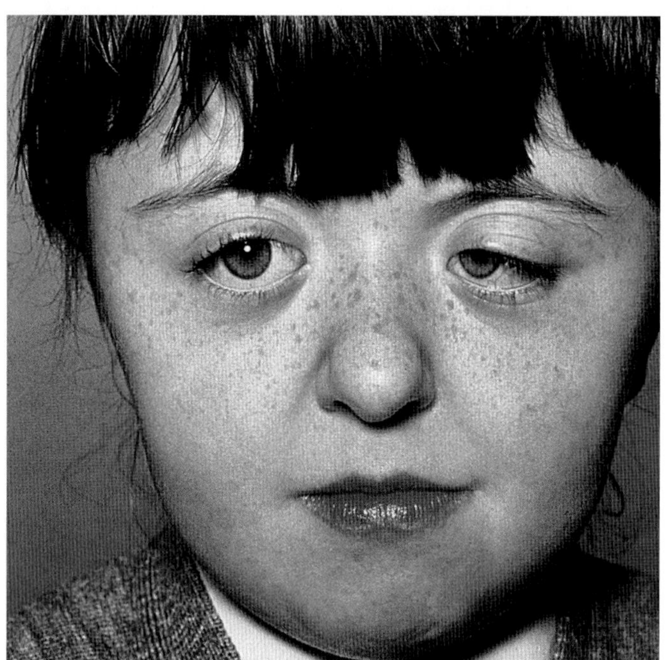

Figure 13.2 An example of Apert's syndrome, caused by premature fusion of cranial sutures. Notice the hypertelorism and hypoplastic maxilla caused by lack of forward growth of the skull base.

Surgery is directed at releasing the synostosis in the hope that this produces a normal-shaped head, reduces the possibility of raised intracranial pressure, and allows normal anterior–posterior skull base growth. Surgery to the face at a high Le Fort III level (see Fig. 13.13) is undertaken to advance the retrusive maxilla if this fails or if the child presents late. Cranial surgery may also be needed at this stage. These principles can be applied to the wide spectrum of syndromes and to idiopathic cranial facial anomalies.

Once the bones have been mobilized by osteotomies, they are stablized with small bone plates (often resorbable in children). Bone grafts may be required to cover large defects. Osteogenic distraction may also have a useful role. The bones are separated by osteotomy cuts before waiting a week for the healing callus to form. Traction is then applied across the callus. This avoids the need for bone grafts, and more importantly slowly expands the soft tissue envelope, which it is hoped leads to greater stability. It is a simple and attractive option when large skeletal movements are required.

CRANIOFACIAL CLEFTS

Craniofacial clefts can be defined as areas of partial or complete failure of development of one or more tissues. They are classified as true or pseudoclefts. True facial clefts are the result of failure of the facial processes to fuse, whereas pseudoclefts arise from faulty differentiation of tissues after the fusion of the processes has occurred normally.

Clefts can be further classified according to the region affected: craniofacial, cranial or facial. Tessier proposed a classification relating the site of the cleft to the orbits.[1] This system has been widely adopted. The management of clefts of the lip and palate (facial cleft 2), hemifacial microsomia (facial clefts 6 and 7), and Treacher Collins syndrome (facial clefts 6, 7 and 8) is important.

Figure 13.3 illustrates the wide number of clefting defects that can present. An important feature of clefting defects is that although there may appear to be defects in bone, muscle and skin (in any combination), the basic structures are essentially all present, albeit misaligned. Surgery should therefore be primarily concerned with realigning, not adding or removing, tissues.

One of the major problems associated with clefting defects is that the defect occurs in utero. As a result, the pull of unopposed muscles either side of the cleft distorts the tissues. This is particularly seen in patients with cleft lips and palates, in whom the nose is deviated and broadened, because the circumoral muscles have been misaligned during the uterine growth period. It is why the operations should be directed at correcting not only the cutaneous and mucosal deficiency, but also redirecting the muscles into the correct position to mitigate the distortion caused in utero. The deformity is not so severe at birth if the skin and mucosa are intact and there is only a bony defect (as seen in Treacher Collins syndrome). Once facial growth begins,

REFERENCE

1. Tessier PJ. Maxillofac Surg 1976; 4: 69

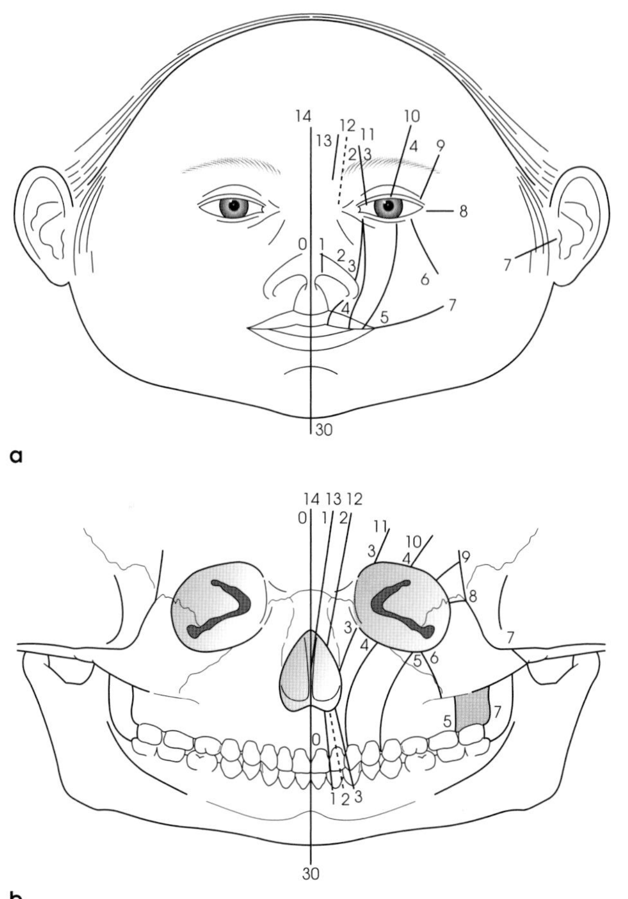

Figure 13.3 Facial clefting. (After Tessier PJ. Maxillofac Surg 1976; 4: 69, with permission from The European Association for Cranio-Maxillofacial Surgery.)

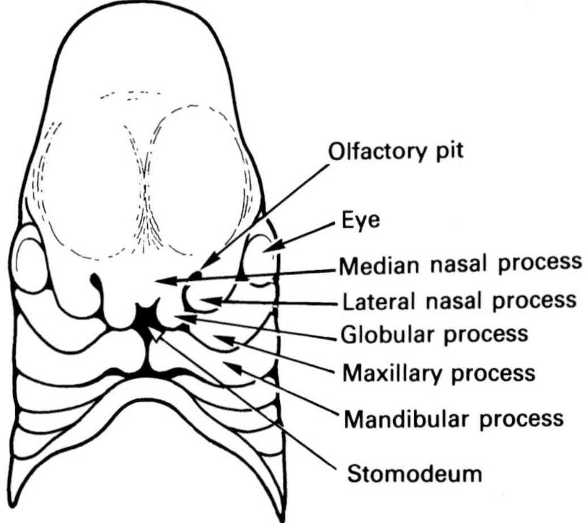

Figure 13.4 Head of embryo at 6 weeks' gestation.

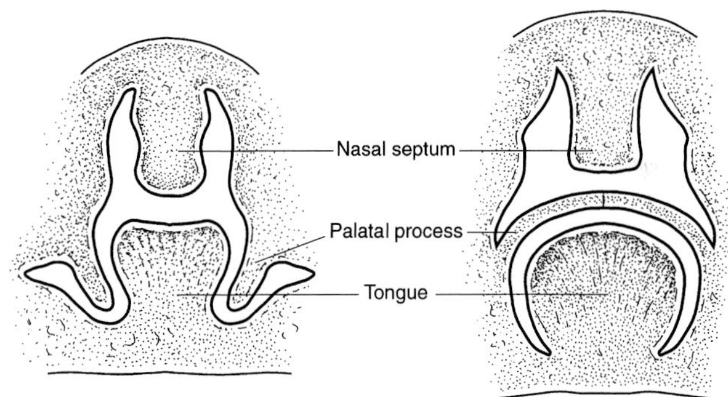

Figure 13.5 Development of the palate at 7 weeks' gestation.

particularly during the pubertal growth spurt, the deficiency of the bony skeleton becomes more obvious.

CLEFTS OF THE LIP AND PALATE

A knowledge of the embryology of the head is essential for understanding the development and management of clefts of the lip and palate.

Embryology

The cleft lip deformity becomes established in the first 6–8 weeks of pregnancy, and is usually considered to be caused by failure of fusion of the maxillary and median nasal processes (Fig. 13.4).[2] It may also be caused by incomplete mesodermal in-growth into these processes, with subsequent breakdown of epitheliuim.[3]

The median nasal processes grow more rapidly than the lateral processes and approach each other in the midline. They fuse to give rise to the central part of the lip (the philtrum), the alveolus, and the palate in front of the incisive foramen.

The extent of the deficiency in mesodermal migration determines the degree of clefting. This varies from a notch in the vermilion (an incomplete cleft) to a fissure extending through the lip to the nostril and involving the alveolus and anterior palate. The nostril is deformed and the columella is deflected to the opposite side. In bilateral cleft lip, the central portion of the alveolus is covered anteriorly by the skin of the columella and philtrum, and hangs from the tip of the nasal septum. Teeth that should develop at the site of the cleft are often deformed, unerupted, or absent altogether.

A palatal cleft is the result of failure of fusion of the palatal shelves of the maxillary processes. These shelves are initially separated by the tongue, which descends by the eighth week of pregnancy, allowing the shelves to fuse (Fig. 13.5). This starts anteriorly and is followed by the development of centres of ossification, which form the hard palate. Differentiation into the muscles of the soft palate occurs posteriorly from mesoderm that has migrated from the pharyngeal wall. The extent of the cleft may range from complete, extending bilaterally on either side of the premaxilla, to a simple bifid uvula. Submucosal clefts are probably the result of failure of mesodermal migration, and consist of notching of the hard palate, a bifid uvula, and diastasis of the palatal muscles.

Aetiology

The aetiology of cleft lip is multifactorial, involving both genetic and intrauterine factors. The mode of inheritance is not clear, but it is likely to be polygenic.[4] Cleft palate alone is genetically and embryologically distinct, being inherited as a simple dominant

REFERENCES

2. Berkovitz BKB, Holland GR, Moxham BJ. Colour Atlas and Textbook of Oral Anatomy. Wolfe Medical, London, 1978
3. Veau V, Politzer J. Ann Anat Pathol 1936; 12: 275
4. Fogh-Andersen P. Inheritance of Harelip and Cleft Palate. Nyt Nordisk Forlag, Arnold Busck, Copenhagen, 1942

with variable penetrance.[5] When unaffected parents have a child with a cleft lip, there is a 5% risk of a subsequent child having cleft lip and palate, rising to 9% if there are two affected siblings. The risk is three times greater than normal if one parent and one child are affected.[6] Although heredity is the most important aetiological factor in typical cleft deformities, drugs such as thalidomide and cytotoxic agents have been incriminated in the formation of facial clefts.[7] Many cases are associated with anomalies or syndromes affecting other parts of the body, with a frequency varying from 10 to 50%.[8]

Clefts of the lip are among the most common birth defects, occurring in about one in 750 live births in the UK and affecting male babies more frequently than female ones.[9] Clefts of the palate are, however, rarer, occurring in about one in 2000 live births and affecting female babies more often than male ones.[10] In about half of the cases, clefts of the lip and palate occur together.

Classification

Several methods of classification have evolved since that of Veau,[11] and most are based on the system recommended by Kernahan & Stark.[12] Clefts of the lip and palate are classified in Box 13.2. Cleft lip may be incomplete or complete, with or without involvement of the alveolus. It may occur unilaterally (70% on the left side), bilaterally (25%) or, rarely, in the midline. Clefts of the palate alone (32%) involve the soft palate and the posterior third of the hard palate. They may be complete, incomplete or submucous. Clefts of the soft and hard palate involving the alveolus and associated with cleft lip (52%) may be unilateral or bilateral.[12] About 85% of bilateral cleft lips and 70% of unilateral cleft lips are associated with a cleft palate.[13]

Diagnosis

Traditionally, the diagnosis was made at birth and came as a great shock to both parents and doctors. Most cleft lips can now be detected in utero using ultrasound diagnostic imaging. The cleft lip can usually be diagnosed after about 24 weeks of gestation. This gives the family much more time to come to terms with the defect, and provides an opportunity for support teams to talk to the family about the condition. It is, however, very difficult, if not impossible, to diagnose an isolated cleft palate in utero. This is important because children with an isolated cleft palate have a higher incidence of associated defects, for example, cardiac anomalies.

Facial deformity arising in association with cleft lip and palate causes special problems. The condition requires observation and often surgery throughout the growth period. The condition is not simply a problem of aesthetics, because the patient with the cleft lip and palate can have a variety of functional problems. One of the most important complications of a cleft lip and palate is the inability of the palate to work properly, giving rise to speech difficulties. The poor function of the palatal muscles also interferes with Eustachian tube opening, giving rise to middle ear problems and causing hearing difficulties. It is important to define the extent of the condition. The clefting defect is more complex if there is a bilateral cleft lip and a cleft palate rather than a unilateral incomplete cleft. The problem is compounded by other problems, such as systemic disease and learning difficulties.

An important aspect of the surgical management is the documentation of the cleft with appropriate photographs and casts. These will act as a reference point for later audit of the outcome of treatment.

Box 13.2 Classification of clefts of the lip and palate

Cleft lip
- Unilateral, bilateral or median
- Complete or incomplete

Cleft palate
- Unilateral, bilateral or midline
- Complete, submucous or incomplete (soft palate)

Treatment

The fundamental principles in the management of craniofacial clefts are to achieve a functional and anatomical repair of the bony and soft tissue defects of the lip and palate to promote normal speech, hearing, growth, and social integration.

Surgical management is full of controversy, primarily because of the difficulty of auditing outcome. Measuring 'good' aesthetic results is very subjective; even measuring facial growth, dental development, and speech is not precise. Patients must be followed up for many years, because growth changes the outcome. Every operation on the growing face adversely affects growth, and procedures should be kept to a minimum (Figs 13.6 and 13.7).

Pre-surgical measures

Sometimes intraoral or extraoral appliances are employed to approximate the palatal cleft segments into a symmetrical arch form, so as to facilitate cleft lip and palate repair.[14]

Cleft lip and palate repair

It is normal practice to close the lip defect at about 3 months, and the cleft palate at about 9 months. Many surgeons, however, combine lip closure with closure of the soft palate. This not only encourages normal function of the soft palate but also helps to close any defect in the hard palate. It is important that surgical interventions are kept to a minimum, and each surgical procedure must be carried out with meticulous care. It is surprising that despite the many publications on the management of cleft lip and palate, it is only very recently that reconstructing and realigning

REFERENCES

5. Roberts JAF. Multifactorial inheritance and human disease. In: Steinberg AG, Bern AG (eds). Advances in Medical Genetics. Grune & Stratton, New York, 1964
6. Fogh-Andersen P. In: Edwards M, Watson ACH (eds). Advances in the Management of Cleft Palate. Churchill Livingstone, Edinburgh, 1980: 43
7. Poswillo D. Oral Surg 1973; 35: 302
8. Gorlin RJ, Pindborg JJ, Cohen MM. Syndromes of the Head and Neck. 2nd edn. McGraw Hill, New York, 1976: 137
9. Drillien CM, Ingram TTS, Walkinson EM. The Causes and Natural History of Cleft Lip and Palate. E & S Livingstone, Edinburgh, 1966
10. Wilson MEA. Br J Plast Surg 1972; 25: 224
11. Veau V. Division Palatine. Masson, Paris, 1931
12. Kernahan DA, Stark RB. Plast Reconstr Surg 1958; 22: 435
13. Reidy JP. Br J Plast Surg 1960; 12: 215
14. Jackson IT, Vandevord JE et al. Br J Plast Surg 1976; 29: 295

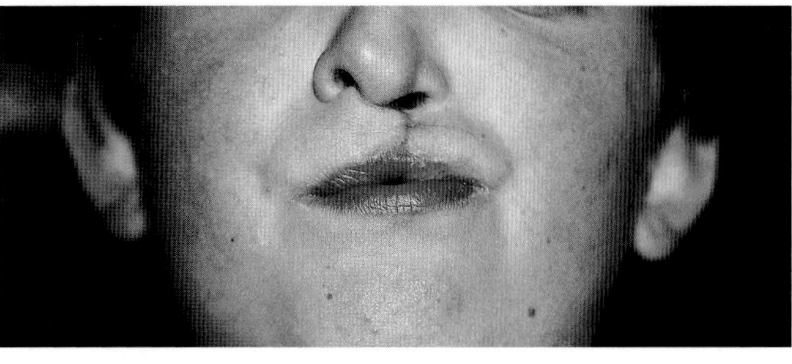

a

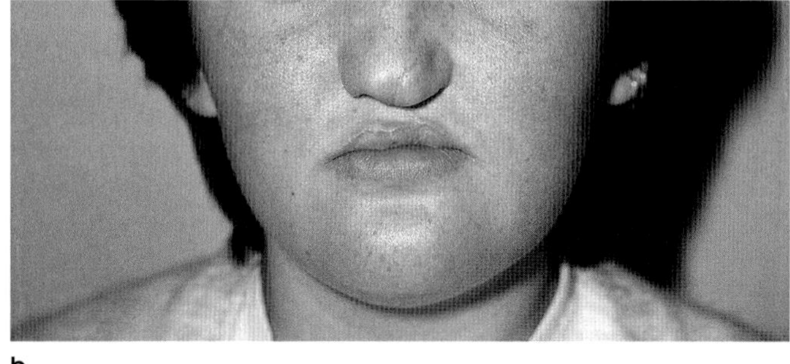

b

Figure 13.6 Two examples of a poor outcome. Panel (a) clearly shows no muscle repair or realignment; as a result, the base of the nose has been pulled further laterally, distorting the alar cartilage. Panel (b) shows a prominent and unnecessary scar on the dome of the distorted nose. The maxilla in both cases is retrusive. Both these cases came from a high-volume surgeon.

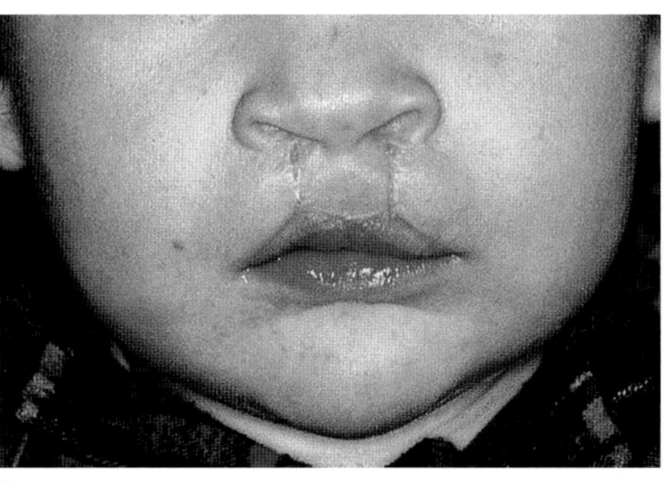

a

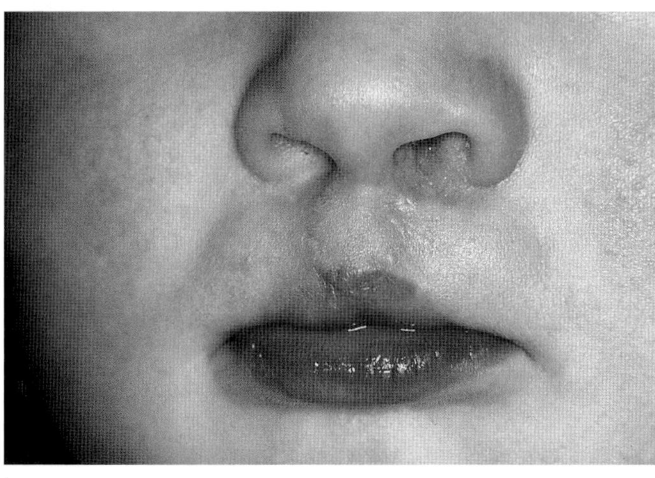

b

Figure 13.7 Both these similar bilateral clefts were treated by the same surgeon. The patient in (a) was treated by traditional methods, but (b) used a careful muscle realignment; notice the narrow well-shaped nose and good lip projection. (Courtesy of Professor Hemprich.)

the muscles around the nose and lip has become an important aspect of closure. Careful muscular reconstruction clearly benefits not only the function of the palate but also the shape of the nose and the function of the lip (see Figs 13.6 and 13.7).[15]

Many techniques have been described for cleft lip repair. The advancement–rotation method of Millard (1957)[16] is the most popular at present (Fig. 13.8). This technique involves equalizing the heights of the lip on either side of the cleft by rotation of the medial edge of the cleft down to its normal position. The lateral edge of the cleft across is then advanced to meet the medial edge. In this way, a symmetrical cupid's bow is created. The technique requires careful measurement to develop medial, lateral and central flaps. The medial flap is rotated down, thereby opening a gap into which the lateral flap is advanced. The central flap is used to lengthen the shortened columella.

In bilateral cleft lips, setting back the premaxilla causes retardation of forward maxillary growth; Millard's technique for closure of the bilateral cleft lip is therefore performed in two stages. Initially, the muscle layer is brought behind the prolabium and in front of the premaxilla. At the second stage, the lip is freed from the septum, the columella is lengthened, and the tip of the nose is raised.

Delaire in 1975 invented the concept of a functional repair.[17] The objective was to facilitate normal growth, thus avoiding the development of compensatory secondary deformities and

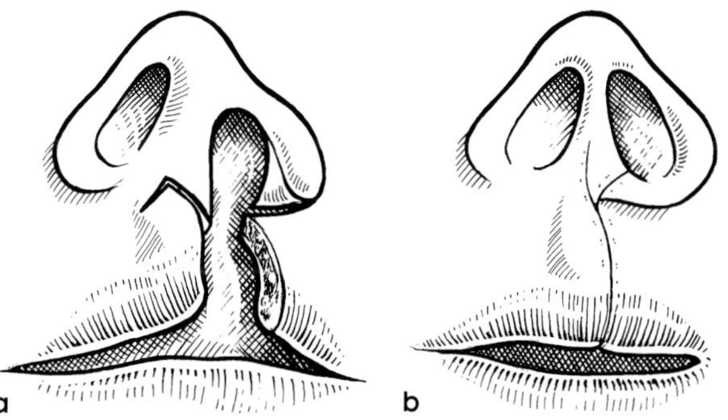

Figure 13.8 (a) Inset of the flaps of rotation-advancement technique of cleft lip repair. (b) The completed unilateral cleft lip repair by the rotation-advancement method.

REFERENCES

15. Markus AF, Smith WP, Delaire J. Br J Oral Maxillofac Surg 1993; 31: 281
16. Millard DR. Cleft Craft. Little Brown, Boston, 1976
17. Markus AF, Delaire J. Br J Oral Maxillofac Surg 1993; 31: 281

the need for their later correction. Functional repair involves repositioning of displaced nasal skin on the lip back into the nostril, anatomical reconstruction of the nasolabial musculature, and correct positioning of distorted neighbouring soft tissues.

Cleft palate repair (Fig. 13.7)

The muscles of the soft palate are oriented anteroposteriorly rather than transversely, and inserted into the posterior edge of the hard palate and along the medial edge of the cleft. The correct repositioning of the soft palate muscles is essential to avoid nasal escape of air during speech. The hard and soft palate repair can be undertaken at the same time or as a two-stage procedure. There are a number of techniques available for repairing palatal clefts. In the one-stage procedure of Von Langenbeck,[18] long mucoperiosteal flaps are first raised in the hard palate by making medial incisions along the cleft margins and lateral incisions close to the gingival margins (Fig. 13.9). The latter are extended posteriorly on to the anterior pillar of the fauces and may be joined with medial incisions anteriorly (Veau flaps).[11] The muscles of the soft palate are then detached from their abnormal insertions, and the flaps that have been raised on either side are transposed medially before closure is achieved in three layers: nasal mucosa, muscular, and oral mucosa. Delaire has emphasized the importance of a precise anatomical and functional repair of clefts of the soft palate (functional palatoplasty).[15] This involves radical mobilization and repositioning of the muscles of the soft palate and closure of the nasal and oral mucosal layers.

In the two-stage procedure, after the initial repair of the soft palate, growth brings the palatal segments closer together, reducing the width of the defect. This makes the subsequent repair of the hard palate easier and more successful.

An alveolar cleft associated with a cleft lip should be closed at the same time as the lip is repaired, otherwise a troublesome oronasal fistula results. The nasal floor may be closed in one layer by elevating the septal mucoperichondrium and suturing to the mucoperiosteum of the lateral wall of the nose. The second oral layer may be obtained from the labial mucosa.[19,20]

Speech

Normal speech can be expected in about three-quarters of the children who have had cleft palates repaired. Correct phonation depends on the ability of the soft palate to complete a sphincter between the lateral and posterior walls of the oronasal pharynx. This can be objectively assessed using cinefluoroscopy and endoscopic examination, enabling selection of the most appropriate procedure for the correction of velopharyngeal incompetence, should this persist following cleft palate repair.[21]

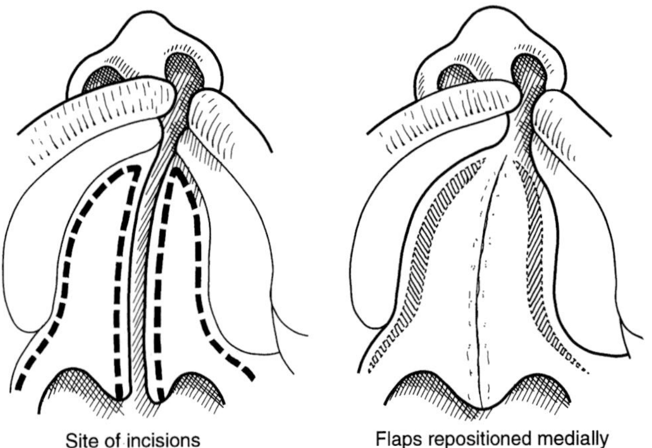

Figure 13.9 The use of Veau flaps for repair of the cleft palate.

Hearing

Many children with cleft palates become deaf from recurrent middle ear infection. This may be the result of drainage problems along the Eustachian canal associated with abnormalities of the tensor palati muscles.[22] Treatment of the ear infections must be prompt and effective, as loss of hearing has additional deleterious effects on the development of speech.

Secondary procedures

Throughout the formative years, an orthodontist must monitor the growth and development of the jaws. Teeth are often congenitally absent, deformed, or displaced at the site of the cleft. Maintenance of oral hygiene and preservation of the secondary dentition are important measures that encourage oral rehabilitation. To achieve this, the alveolar bone cleft must be repaired. Closure in the baby, using bone grafts, leads to a failure of midface and alveolar growth. The closure of the cleft by a bone graft is therefore done as late as possible. The aim of the graft is to allow the teeth to erupt as normally as possible and not into the cleft fistula. Creating a normal alveolus also improves the shape of the nose and provides an intact maxilla. Importantly for the patient, it also closes a very unpleasant oral nasal fistula. The operation is usually carried out after the transverse growth is nearly complete. In practical terms, this is at about the age of 8, when the canine tooth is two-thirds formed, because this is a non-vascularized free bone graft. It is important to obtain good closure of the nasal and muscosal layers at the same time as the alveolus is nearly complete.

HEMIFACIAL MICROSOMIA (FACIAL CLEFTS 6 AND 7, FIRST AND SECOND BRANCHIAL ARCH SYNDROME, OTOMANDIBULAR DYSOSTOSIS, CRANIOFACIAL MICROSOMIA)

This defect was originally believed to be the result of bleeding from the stapedial arterial system during early embryonic development.[23] The clinical features consist of inferior displacement of the lateral canthus, a prominent and inferiorly displaced ear, midfacial flattening (zygomatic hypoplasia), deviation of the chin, a hypoplastic mandible, upwards tilting of the occlusal plane, nasal deviation, facial paresis, upper eyelid colobomas (V-shaped defects), and occasionally cleft lip and palate.[24] When syndactyly, fusion of fingers and toes, is also present, the condition is termed Goldenhar's syndrome. The deformity is essentially unilateral, although in up to a third of cases the features may be bilateral.

The treatment varies according to the severity of the deformity. Some deformities, such as skin tags and macrostomia, are treated during early childhood, whereas the treatment of the bony

REFERENCES

18. Watson ACH. Advances in Management of Cleft Palate. Churchill Livingstone, Edinburgh, 1980
19. Muir FK. Br J Plast Surg 1966; 29: 30
20. Burian F. The Plastic Surgery Atlas. Macmillan, New York, 1978
21. Moore FT. Br J Plast Surg 1960; 47: 424
22. Bluestone C. Ann Otol Rhinol Laryngol 1971; 80: 1
23. Poswillo DE. Oral Surg 1973; 35: 302
24. Poole MD. World J Surg 1989; 13: 396

deformity is delayed until growth can be assessed. Some believe in delaying treatment of the mandibular hypoplasia until growth has ceased, when the deformity can be fully corrected in a single stage.

TREACHER COLLINS SYNDROME (FACIAL CLEFTS 6, 7 AND 8)

Also known as mandibulofacial dysostosis, this is an autosomal dominant disorder. The syndrome produces a symmetrical deformity of varying severity. The clinical features consist of anti-mongoloid palpebral fissures; a lower eyelid coloboma; absence of the medial half of the lower eyelashes; hypoplasia of the external and middle ears, zygoma and mandible; a V-shaped patch of hair extending on to the cheeks; a parrot beak-shaped nose; dental crowding; and an anterior open bite with malocclusion.[25] Treatment of this condition requires correction of both the mid and lower facial deformities.

ORTHOGNATHIC DEFORMITIES

Orthognathic surgery involves repositioning parts of the facial skeleton to correct facial deformity. In addition to improving the facial appearance, functional improvements can be expected in the temporomandibular joint function and dental occlusion.

CLINICAL EVALUATION

Clinical assessment is the most important technique for evaluating facial deformity. Facial symmetry is the single most important feature of a pleasing facial appearance.[26] Palpation from behind the patient allows assessment of retrusion of the supraorbital and infraorbital margins, the zygomatic prominences, and paranasal areas.

The facial profile must be assessed. The profile of the nose, lips and chin should take the shape of a cupid's bow. This is influenced by the relationship of the maxilla to the mandible and the inclination of their incisor teeth. The inclination of the teeth often compensates for the underlying skeletal deformity. Normally, the upper incisor teeth are 1–2 mm in front of the lower ones. The teeth may, however, be proclined, retroclined, or even reversed, with the lower teeth occluding in front of the upper ones. Normally, only about 1–2 mm of the crowns of the upper incisor teeth show beneath the upper lip at rest, whereas about two-thirds of the crowns are visible on smiling.

RADIOLOGICAL EVALUATION

The average lengths, proportions and angles of various parts of the skull have been ascertained by analysing standardized cephalometric radiographs from a large population. Quantitative comparisons of measurements can be made between these 'norms' and individual cases to identify the areas of deformity and grade their severity.

TREATMENT PLANNING

The objective of treatment is to achieve an optimal appearance and accurate dental occlusion. Treatment usually begins with a prolonged course of orthodontics to align and correct the angulation of the teeth and to coordinate the dental arches into compatible shapes. Osteotomies are made in the maxilla and mandible to shift them appropriately to correct the facial deformity.

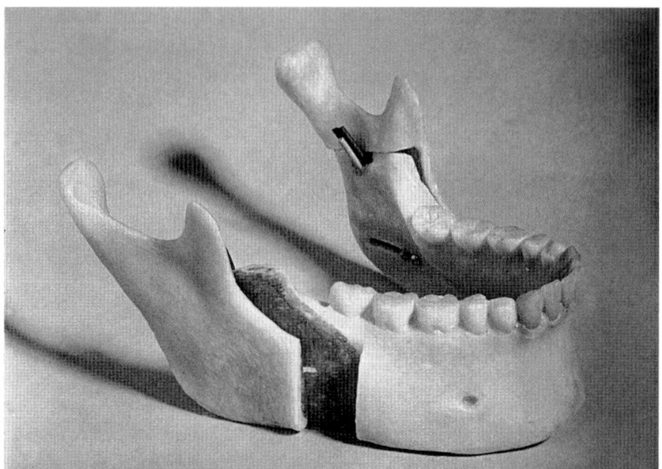

Figure 13.10 A sagittal split mandibular osteotomy.

MAXILLARY OSTEOTOMIES

The Le Fort I osteotomy is the most commonly performed maxillary procedure. It allows correction of both anteroposterior and vertical facial disproportions, namely midfacial retrusion, as well as long or short faces. The Le Fort II and III maxillary osteotomies are mainly used to advance different areas of the midface. Segmental osteotomies of the maxilla allow the correction of more localized deformities.

MANDIBULAR OSTEOTOMIES

Osteotomies can be performed on the mandible at various sites. The ramus is the site most commonly chosen for both advancement and setback procedures, the sagittal split osteotomy being the most commonly used (Fig. 13.10).[27–29] Other advancement procedures of the mandible include the vertical subsigmoid and inverted L osteotomies, both of which require interposition bone grafts.

GENIOPLASTIES

These procedures enable correction of deficient or excessive chin projection and lower anterior dental height discrepancies. An osteotomy is made in the anterior part of the mandible below the teeth and repositioned.

MAXILLOFACIAL TRAUMA

In the UK, the commonest cause of facial trauma is direct interpersonal violence. Road traffic accidents and sporting injuries are also a major aetiological factor, and falls, which have many causes, including simple syncope, are another large group.[30] The number of industrial accidents is reducing as heavy

REFERENCES

25. Argenta SC, Iacobucci JJ. World J Surg 1989; 13: 401
26. Epker BN, Fish LC. Dentofacial deformities—integrated orthodontic and surgical correction, Vols 1 and 2. Mosby, St Louis, 1986
27. Obwegeser H. Oral Surg 1957; 10: 677, 787, 899
28. Dal Pont G. J Oral Surg Anesth Hosp Dent Serv 1961; 19: 42
29. Hunsuck EE. J Oral Surg 1968; 26: 249
30. Hussain K, Wijetunge DB, Grubnic S et al. J Trauma 1994; 1: 106

industry becomes safer. In the interpersonal violence group, men who are either unemployed or undertake unskilled work form the largest group. Most are intoxicated at the time of injury. Sadly, the level of violence and the severity of injury appear to be increasing, as is the number of patients seeking treatment (Fig. 13.11)[6,7]

As craniomaxillofacial trauma is often associated with other injuries, a full assessment must be made of the whole patient. Advanced Trauma Life Support® (ATLS®) is discussed in detail in Chapter 7.[31] Maxillofacial trauma may compromise the airway and circulation, and cervical and head injuries are often associated.

Conscious patients with facial fractures are usually able to guard their airway by sitting up and leaning forwards.[32] This is not possible in unconscious patients. Multiple dental fractures and fractured dental restorations are liable to be inhaled and obstruct the airway when associated with a posteriorly displaced Le Fort maxillary fracture. They need to be removed with the aid of a good light and a suction catheter. The soft palate may lie against the pharyngeal walls and base of the tongue, obstructing the airway. This may be prevented by the insertion of an oropharyngeal or nasopharyngeal airway, an endotracheal tube, or immediate manual disimpaction of the maxilla. Occasionally, midfacial fractures may be associated with torrential nasopharyngeal haemorrhage, preventing endotracheal intubation, and postnasal packing and/or cricothyrotomy may then be necessary as an emergency procedure.

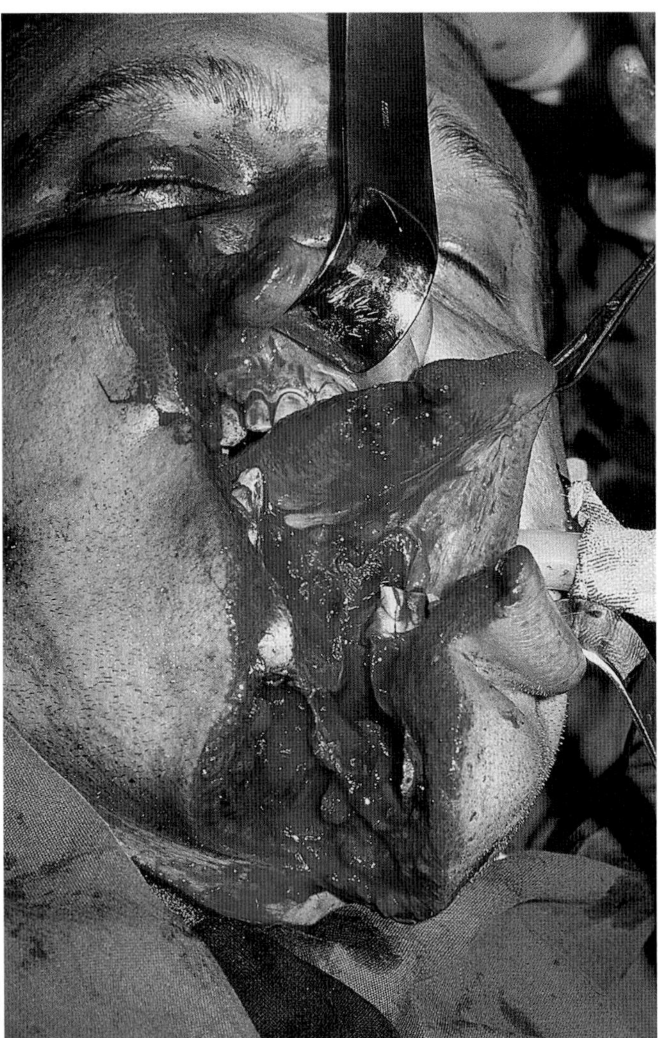

Figure 13.11 An industrial accident from a cutting disc.

The airway may also be compromised after some types of mandibular fracture. In bilateral parasymphyseal mandibular fractures, the central fragment is displaced posteriorly by the pull of the genioglossus muscles, allowing the tongue to fall back against the posterior pharyngeal wall, occluding the airway. Insertion of an oropharyngeal or nasopharyngeal airway relieves the obstruction. A large suture can be placed through the tongue to allow forward traction if these are not available.

Haemorrhage resulting from midfacial fractures is not normally prolonged, but persistent haemorrhage can usually be controlled by anterior and posterior nasal packing. If packing fails, carotid angiography may be indicated to identify bleeding vessels prior to ligation, for example the anterior ethmoidal or external carotid arteries. Therapeutic embolization is an alternative.

EXAMINATION

The examination begins with an inspection of the cranium; this may reveal the presence of haematomas and lacerations, suggesting an associated intracranial injury. Concomitant orbital injuries may also be present.

Orbital examination

It is important to undertake a basic ocular examination (visual acuity, pupillary size and reactivity, and depth of the anterior chamber) of the traumatized eye, even when the lids are closed by swelling. Infraorbital nerve hypoaesthesia is usually associated with fractures of the infraorbital canal along the floor of the orbit. It can also be caused by direct blunt injury of the infraorbital nerve where it emerges from the infraorbital foramen. The presence of diplopia is important, and this should always be tested. It may simply be the result of oedema and should be allowed to settle for a few days before investigations are requested. Surgical emphysema is indicative of an orbital fracture involving one or more of the paranasal air sinuses.

Fractures of the orbital walls are inevitable with nasoethmoidal, zygomatic, and Le Fort complex fractures. An isolated 'blow-out' fracture of the orbital wall can result from direct impact. Prolapse of periorbital fat and/or extraocular muscles through the defect may produce enophthalmos, and restriction of ocular movement can cause diplopia (see Fig. 13.12).

Nasal and nasoethmoidal examination

The nasoethmoidal complex extends from the dorsum of the nose and the cribriform plate above to the palate below, and from the lateral nasal and medial orbital walls on one side to those on the other side.

The clinical features associated with nasal fractures are contusion, epistaxis, and nasal deformity. The nose may be displaced laterally or posteriorly. Powerful frontal blows displace the nasal structures posteriorly into the space between the medial orbital walls, producing nasoethmoidal fractures. Additional signs

REFERENCES

31. Committee on Trauma, American College of Surgeons. Advanced Trauma Life Support® Student Manual. American College of Surgeons, Chicago, 1989
32. Rowe NL, Williams JL (eds). Maxillofacial Injuries. Churchill Livingstone, Edinburgh, 1985

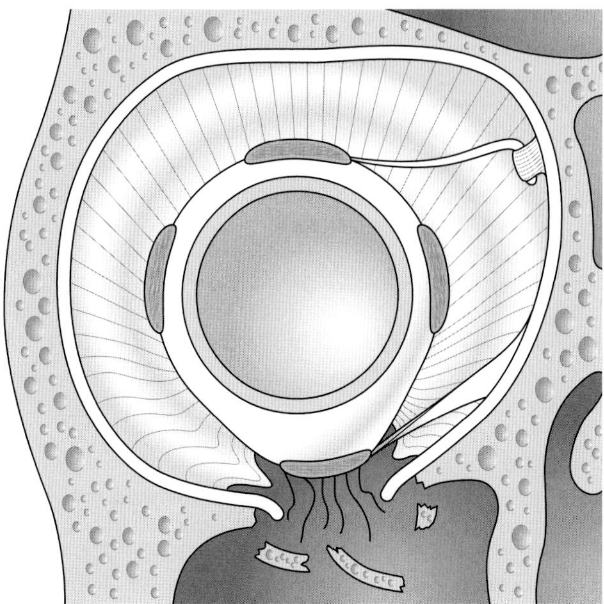

Figure 13.12 In fractures, soft tissue may be incarcerated in fracture segments and, by virtue of this incarceration, the full extraocular motion of the extraocular muscles may be impaired. Release of the soft tissue releases this incarceration and conceptually replaces the soft tissue in a position where correct healing is most likely. (From Ward Booth et al. 1999.[33])

of nasoethmoidal fractures are a laceration over the root of the nose, telecanthus, an upturned nasal tip, a stretched columella, and cerebral spinal fluid rhinorrhoea.

Zygomatic examination

Although zygomatic fractures may involve only part of the bone, for example its arch, adjacent bones—such as the frontal process of the maxilla, the zygomatic process of the temporal bone, and the floor and lateral walls of the orbit—are also often damaged. These fractures are therefore known as zygomatic complex fractures. The associated clinical signs are tenderness and 'stepping' of the infraorbital margin and the zygomaticofrontal suture. Midfacial flattening and trismus are also sometimes found in conjunction with orbital fractures.

Maxillary examination

Fractures of the maxilla are the result of considerable force and are often associated with craniocerebral injury (see Ch. 7). The maxilla offers a high resistance against forces directed upwards but relatively little resistance if the impact is directed horizontally. Fractures may occur at three levels, Le Fort I, II and III, and may be unilateral or bilateral (Fig. 13.13). The palate may also be fractured in the midline.

The Le Fort I fracture passes from the lower end of the pyriform fossa backwards, across the maxilla above the roots of the teeth to the pterygomaxillary fissure. The fracture also extends from the piriform fossa along the lateral walls of the nose and nasal septum at the same level. The Le Fort I segment therefore consists of the teeth, their supporting alveolar bone, and the hard palate.

The Le Fort II fracture is pyramidal in shape, passing from the dorsum of the nose backwards across the medial walls of the orbit (posterior to the nasolacrimal apparatus) to the inferior orbital margins and medial to the infraorbital foramina. It then continues across the maxilla, below the bodies of the zygomatic bones and above the roots of the maxillary teeth, to the pterygomaxillary fissure.

Le Fort III fractures are the most severe of all facial fractures, and are the result of disjunction of the midfacial skeleton from the anterior cranial base. The fracture line passes from the dorsum of the nose and cribriform plate, along the medial walls

REFERENCES

33. Ward Booth P, Schendel SA, Hausamen J.-E. (eds). Maxillofacial Surgery. Churchill Livingstone, Edinburgh, 1999

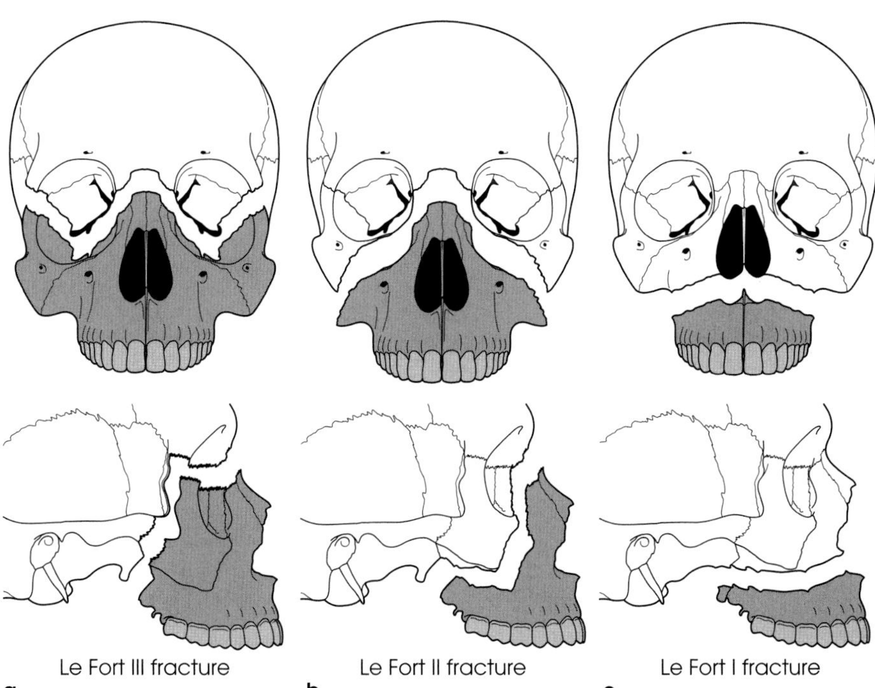

Figure 13.13 The Le Fort fracture lines: (**a**) Le Fort III, (**b**) Le Fort II, and (**c**) Le Fort I. (From Ward Booth et al. 1999.[33])

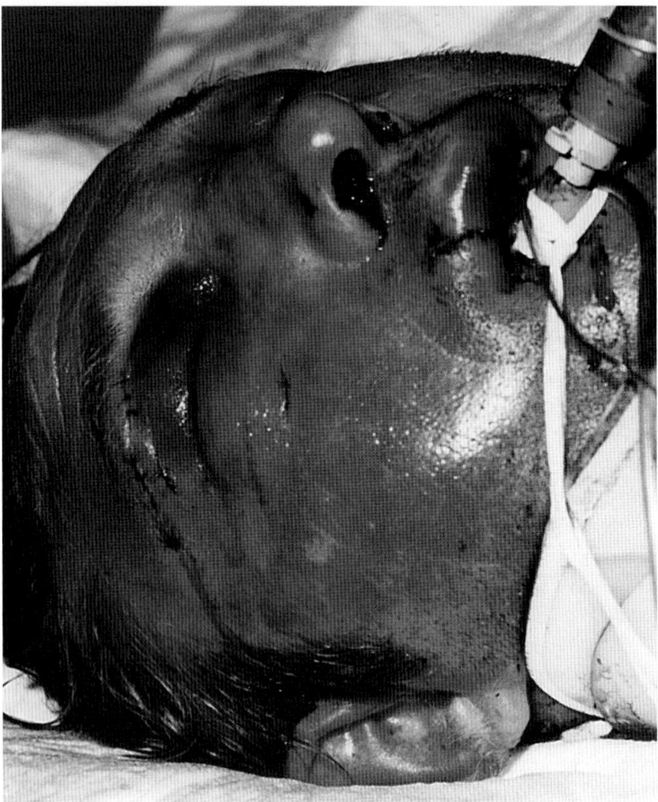

Figure 13.14 Facial bone fractures in polytrauma patients involved in traffic accidents: mandible (61.0%), maxilla (46.3%), zygoma (26.8%) and nasal bone (19.5%). (After Ward Booth et al. 1999.[33])

of the orbit, to the inferior orbital fissure. It then continues up across the lateral walls of the orbits to the zygomaticofrontal sutures. The zygomatic arches are also fractured.

The clinical symptoms and signs vary according to the level of fracture. Dental malocclusion is associated with displaced fractures at any level. Le Fort II and III fractures cause the features of orbital wall and nasoethmoidal fractures. The symptoms and signs of Le Fort III maxillary fractures are fairly characteristic and include panda or raccoon appearance (bilateral black eyes), gross midfacial swelling, bilateral epistaxis, cerebrospinal fluid rhinorrhoea, and dental malocclusion (Fig. 13.14). The face swells like a balloon because the tissues offer little resistance to oedema formation in the absence of a deep fascial layer. The clinical diagnosis of a Le Fort fracture is confirmed by mobility of the fractured segment (Fig. 13.15).

Mandibular examination

The symptoms and signs of a fractured mandible include pain and swelling over the fracture site as well as trismus and malocclusion. Displaced fractures of the body of the mandible may produce hypoaesthesia of the lower lip. The relative incidence of fractures of the mandible at various sites is shown in Fig. 13.16.

INVESTIGATIONS

Radiology is necessary to diagnose facial fractures with certainty and assess their severity. 158 and 308 occipitomental plain radiographs are useful to diagnose maxillary, zygomatic and orbital fractures (Fig. 13.17). They may show the classical 'hanging drop' sign in the maxillary antrum, which is indicative of an orbital floor injury. High-resolution cross-sectional CT and MRI are invaluable for demonstrating midfacial fractures and herniation of orbital soft tissues.

An orthopantomograph and a posteroanterior plain mandibular radiograph show the vast majority of fractures of the mandible in two planes (Fig. 13.18). Mandibular fractures do not normally pose a diagnostic problem, but condylar fractures are easily overlooked. Preauricular tenderness, especially if accompanied by a laceration on the point of the chin, demands a careful radiological evaluation of the condyle.

MANAGEMENT OF MAXILLOFACIAL TRAUMA

It should always be remembered that hard and soft tissue injuries commonly occur together.

Primary care

On arrival at the accident and emergency department, facial trauma must be managed in a logical way using the ATLS® triage process, which is discussed in Chapter 7. There are special problems associated with the early management of facial trauma.

Bleeding

Facial injuries are commonly associated with bleeding, marked bruising, and oedema, which can adversely affect the airways. The combination of brisk bleeding, swelling, and possible head injury and/or alcohol intoxication puts patients at great risk.

The management of profuse bleeding can be exceptionally difficult. Bleeding arising from skin or mucosal vessels is readily staunched. Bleeding from the scalp can be more troublesome. Rarely, the facial or superficial temporal arteries are divided and require ligation. Penetrating injuries, particularly by a knife or glass shards, may damage the deeper vessels of the face and neck. Venous damage is particularly deceptive, because the bleeding may be intermittent yet profuse. Involvement of the major vessels requires temporary tamponade and urgent exploration via an open approach (see Ch. 10).

Profuse haemorrhage from the lingual arteries can obstruct the airway, which should be secured by nasal intubation. The wound can then be explored and the bleeding controlled. Haemorrhage can also occur from the maxillary artery, in the temporal fossa, in association with maxillary fractures. Access to the bleeding point is difficult, and ligation of the external carotid artery is slow and often ineffective because of cross-circulation from other vessels. The bleeding is usually profuse from the nose, and posterior and anterior nasal packs should be applied. In some cases, packs are ineffective and immediate stabilization of the maxillary fracture is required. Packing through the posterior maxillary wall has been advocated in certain circumstances.

Airway

Facial swelling can look dramatic, (see Fig. 13.14) but it is generally confined to the superficial tissues and rarely extends into the oropharynx. In the majority of instances, it is not the swelling that compromises the airway but the associated oral or nasal bleeding.[34,35]

REFERENCES

34. Brickley MR. The circumstances and aetiology of urban violence. MScD thesis, University of Wales
35. Telfer M, Jones GM, Sheperd JP. Br J Oral Maxillofac Surg 1991; 29: 250–255

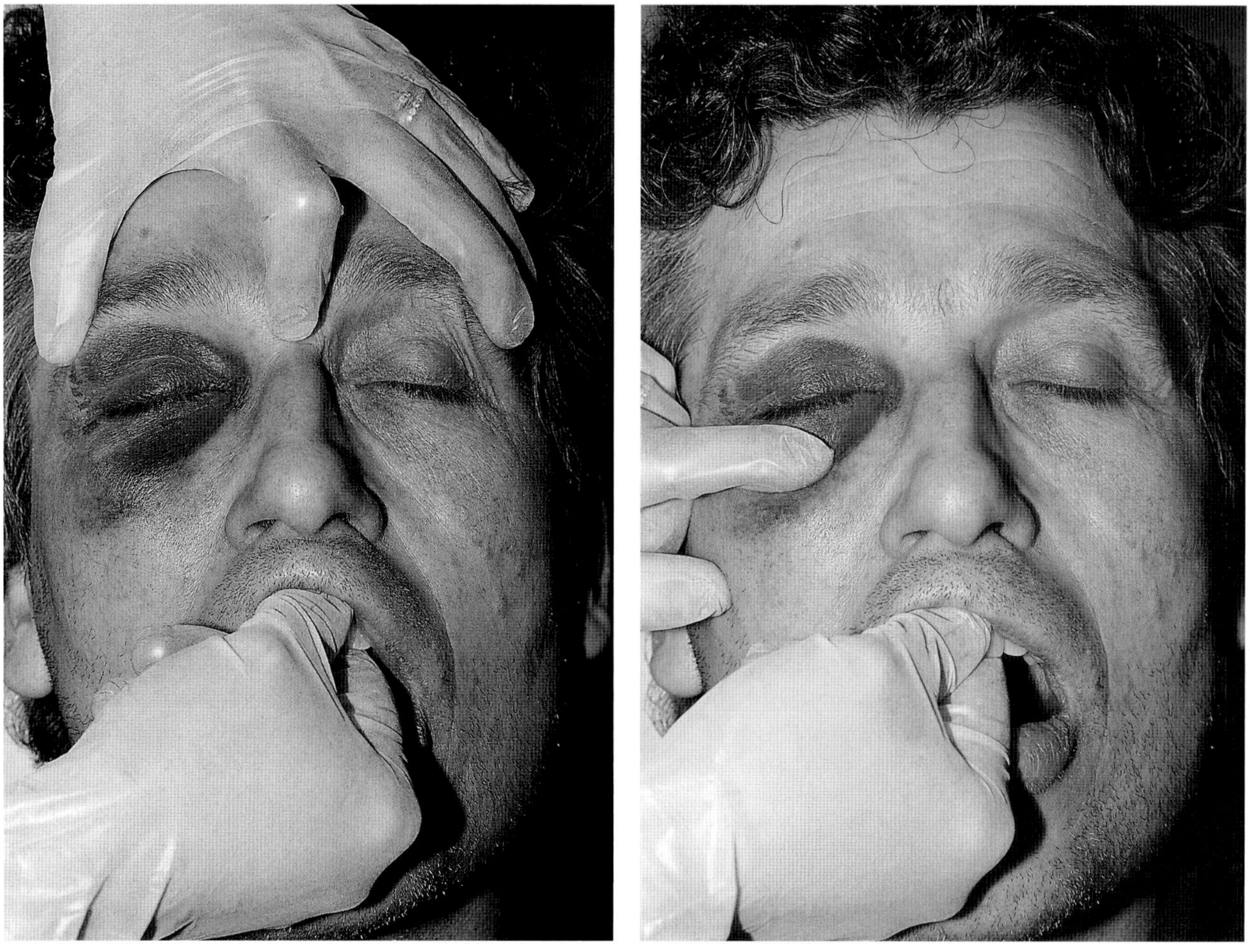

a

b

Figure 13.15 Polytrauma patients have various other injuries; the commonest concomitant ones associated with facial fractures are shown. (From Ward Booth et al. 1999.[33])

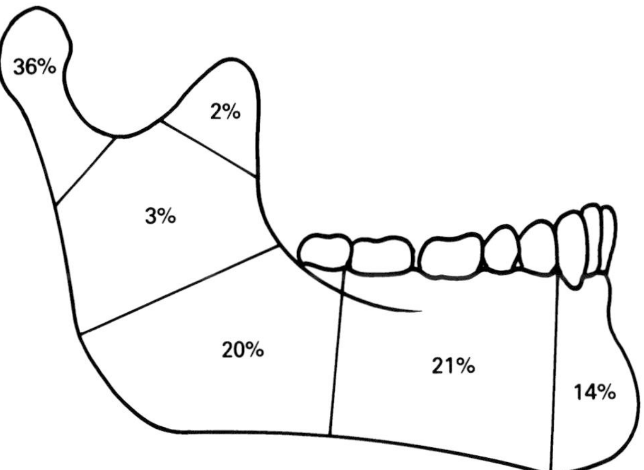

Figure 13.16 The incidence of fractures occurring at various sites of the mandible.

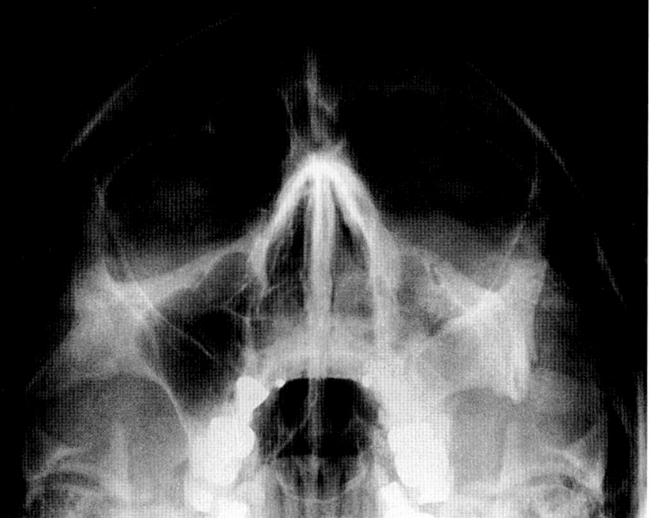

Figure 13.17 A 15° occipitomental radiograph showing a zygomatic complex fracture.

Oedema of the mucosa, coupled with possible disruption of the cartilaginous skeleton, may give rise to significant airway embarrassment if the trachea or larynx is damaged. Protection of the airway is essential if there is an associated head or chest injury.

Nerve damage

The early identification of nerve damage, especially of the facial nerve, is critical to a good outcome. It can be difficult to make a formal assessment, because of severe facial swelling and the common association with either a head injury or intoxication. Knowledge of the facial anatomy of the nerve and the parotid duct is helpful when examining facial wounds.

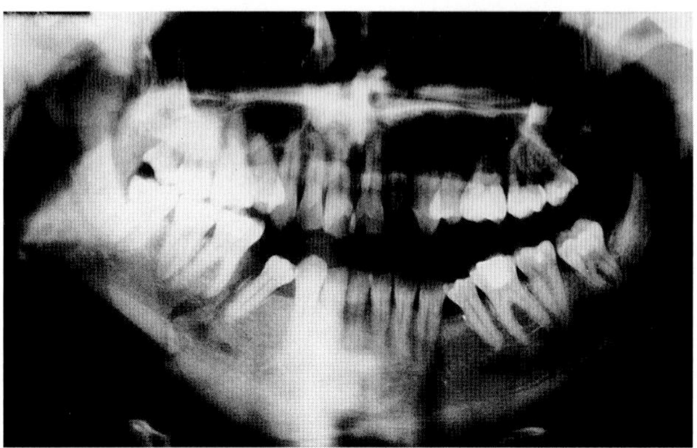

Figure 13.18 An orthopantomograph view showing mandibular fractures.

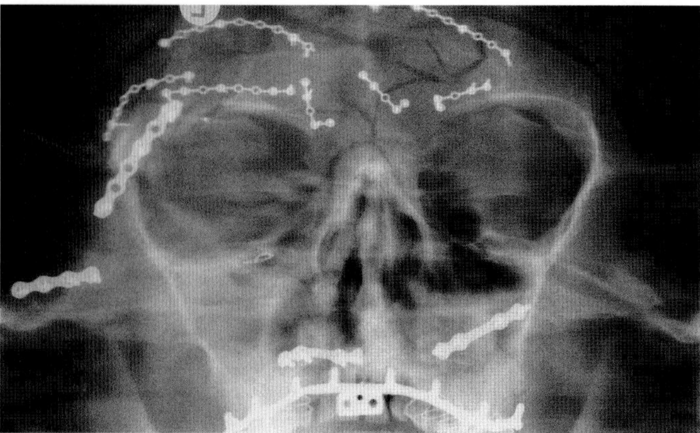

Figure 13.19 Small plates placed through carefully designed access surgery improve the quality of the reduction, create better postoperative aesthetics and function, and allow shorter hospital stays.

Other injuries

Associated injuries affect the timing of the treatment of maxillofacial injuries.

Principles of treatment

The principles of treatment that are common to all fractures are reduction, fixation, and restoration of function. Rigid intermaxillary fixation is no longer a requirement. The modern approach is to expose the fracture, followed by reduction and fixation with stable microplates. There is now no place for heavy-compression plating systems. Reconstruction plates may be needed as a temporary measure if there is bone loss or gross comminution. The use of resorbable plates as opposed to traditional titanium plates may have a limited role in fracture of the upper face and cranium.

Surgical access has developed, almost as an art, to avoid unnecessary skin incisions. Scars are now rarely placed on the visible skin surfaces. Access is gained whenever possible through the oral cavity using long mucosal incisions, which have minimal morbidity. Most fractures of the mandible and lower facial skeleton can be exposed to rough oral incisions. Access to the periorbital area is made through an incision in the lower conjunctiva, which may be extended through the lateral canthus. Coronal incisions made high in the hairline allow access to the upper and midface. The only fractures where open access requires significant visible skin incisions are those of the mandibular condylar neck. To undertake secondary rhinoplasty using the open approach, a small V incision in the columella is created, which has been described as visible only to dogs and lovers!

Timing of surgery

'As soon as possible' is still a reliable maxim. Postinjury swelling makes the correct placement of incisions difficult, and most surgeons like to await the reduction of swelling, or ideally operate before the swelling has developed. Other factors, such as concurrent head or chest injuries, or alcohol intoxication, may prevent early intervention.

Complex facial fractures are very time-consuming to treat, requiring meticulous reduction and fixation, often with a large number of plates (Fig. 13.19). A nasotracheal airway is preferred because of the requirement to restore the dentition and occlusion. Tracheal intubation through a badly traumatized midface is never easy. Occasionally, an elective tracheostomy is indicated. It is accepted practice to use nasal intubation even in patients with midface fractures, despite older literature highlighting the risk of introducing infection or passing the tube itself through the cribriform plate. The risk of infection is not significant, and an experienced anaesthetist would not expect to pass the tube through the cribriform plate. Perioperative antibiotics are routinely prescribed.

Treatment

It is no longer common practice to wire the teeth together, either temporarily or for a fixed period, because of the routine availability of miniplate osteosynthesis systems. It is certainly not necessary to wire the teeth in the postoperative period in the vast majority of patients with facial fractures. This has significantly improved their safety and comfort.

The aim of open reduction and fixation is to return the patient to normal form and function. Function means preserving motor and sensory nerve function, correcting the ocular position and movements, restoring the nasal and oral airway, and restoring normal dental occlusion.

The underlying principle of the modern management of maxillofacial trauma, based on extensive outcome reviews,[8,9] is open reduction and fixation with small-plate osteosynthesis. When large orthopaedic and compression plates were used in the past, plate fixation had a poor reputation. Champy and others demonstrated that the unique healing properties, biomechanical loads, and aesthetics of the facial skeleton require only small, non-compressive plates located with monocortical screws. In the mandible, 2.0 mm-thick plates are used, with 1.5-mm or 1-mm plates used elsewhere. In most countries, the plates are made of titanium and are only removed if they become infected or palpable (10%). The role of absorbable plates and screws has not yet been established. Biomechanically, they do not perform as well as metal. The resorption is slow, and the fragments may be retained in the lymphatic system indefinitely.

The key to open reduction is good surgical access. Any associated facial lacerations can be used, but if the skin is intact transmucosal incisions should be used wherever possible. In the upper facial skeleton, a high coronal incision affords access to the frontal bone, zygoma, and upper nasal skeleton. For isolated zygomatic and orbital floor fractures, an extended inferior transconjunctival incision is ideal. Upper blepharoplasty incisions may also be used.

A logic approach is required for the reduction of panfacial fractures, starting from the most posterior aspect (the base of the zygomatic arch and the mandibular condyles) and working forwards.

ORBITAL FRACTURES

The aim of treatment is to restore orbital wall continuity and volume. Herniated periorbital soft tissue is replaced within the orbital cavity (see Fig. 13.12), and the defect is reconstructed with bone graft or an alloplastic material. Access may be obtained through the conjunctiva or an incision through the eyelid.

NASAL FRACTURES

Nasal fractures are the most common type of facial fracture (44%). They are often inadequately treated, leaving a facial deformity and a compromised nasal airway.[36] The 'open book' and laterally displaced types of nasal fracture are usually treated by closed reduction. Care should be taken to ensure that the septum is in the midline to avoid the risk of late nasal deformity. Nasal fractures must be carefully splinted postoperatively. Displaced naso-ethmoidal fractures are treated by internal fixation and reconstruction of the orbital walls.

ZYGOMATIC FRACTURES

Non-displaced fractures do not require surgery. Simple displaced fractures are the result of low-impact trauma and are usually adequately treated by one of a number of closed reduction techniques, the most common being that of Gillies' temporal reduction (Fig. 13.20). Grossly displaced and comminuted zygomatic complex fractures result from high-impact trauma and require anatomical open reduction and internal fixation with miniplates.

Residual midfacial flattening, neurapraxia of the infraorbital nerve, and trismus are complications of poorly treated zygomatic complex fractures. Diplopia and enophthalmos may persist after the treatment of orbital fractures.

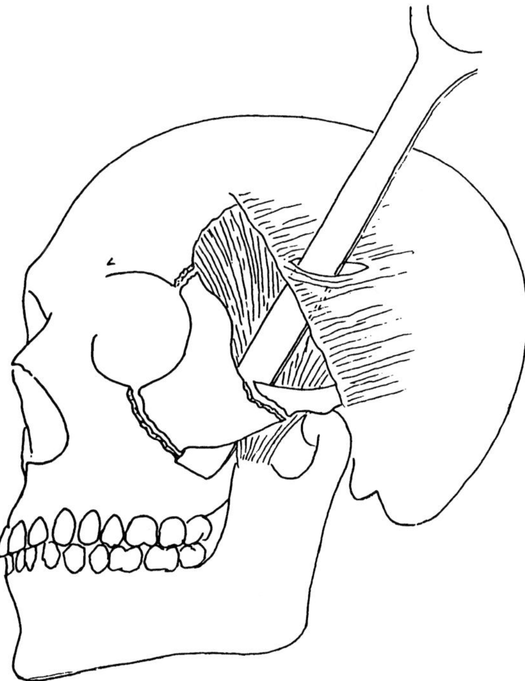

Figure 13.20 The Gillies temporal approach for reduction of a zygomatic complex fracture.

MAXILLARY FRACTURES

Undisplaced fractures are treated conservatively. Displaced fractures are now normally realigned by open reduction and internal fixation using miniplates, although occasionally the traditional method of closed reduction and external fixation is still used. The mandible is used to align the maxilla using the dentition or dentures as a guide. If the mandible is fractured, its continuity should be restored first. Once correct jaw alignment is achieved, repositioning and immobilization of adjacent bone fragments is undertaken.

The complications of maxillary fractures include suboptimal restoration of the contour of the midface, altered dental occlusion, and infraorbital paraesthesia. Malunion is rare.

MANDIBULAR FRACTURES

The mandibular condyle is unusual in two ways: it acts as a growth centre and, in children with condylar injuries, a quarter develop some degree of mandibular growth retardation. This may produce secondary facial deformity. Fractures of the condyle heal spontaneously without immobilization of the jaw. The condyle may fuse with the temporal bone in children below 10 years of age. This can have disastrous consequences for facial growth, and all condylar fractures in children should be mobilized early to avoid this complication.

Fractures of the condyle are usually extracapsular, and the majority are treated conservatively, especially in children. Providing that dental occlusion is not affected, the jaw must be rested by giving a soft diet and administering appropriate analgesia. The jaw may be immobilized by means of mandibulo-maxillary wire, or preferably by elastic fixation, for a period of about 3 weeks, if malocclusion is present. When the head of the condyle is dislocated medially from the glenoid fossa by the pull of the lateral pterygoid muscle, open reduction and internal fixation is indicated, especially when the displacement is such that it interferes with dental occlusion. It is also indicated when both condyles are fractured and displaced, leading to a reduction in the height of the ramus and gagging of the mandible on the molar teeth. This is especially true if the maxilla is also displaced and therefore reliant on the mandible to establish the correct jaw alignment.

Fractures of the angle and body of the mandible are usually caused by a direct blow over the affected area or an indirect force transmitted from a blow over the contralateral parasymphyseal area of the bone. Undisplaced angular fractures, without mobility or dental malocclusion, are treated conservatively with rest, a soft diet, and analgesia. Reduction and immobilization of the fracture by miniplates is indicated if the fracture site is mobile, or dental occlusion is affected.

Complications arising from the treatment of mandibular fractures are surprisingly uncommon but include infection, malocclusion, trismus, delayed union, non-union, and growth reduction in children.

PANFACIAL (MULTIPLE) FRACTURES

The management of multiple facial fractures is the same as that of fractures of the individual bones. These are normally caused by high-velocity injuries and consist of comminuted fractures of

REFERENCES

36. Stell PM. Clin Otolaryngol 1980; 5: 362

the orbital, nasoethmoidal, zygomatic and maxillary complexes, as well as of the mandible. They are difficult to treat. Excellent results can be achieved with careful preservation of the multiple fractured bony fragments and their anatomical open reduction and internal fixation.

INFECTIONS OF THE MOUTH

BACTERIAL INFECTION

Dental caries is the most common bacterial disease in the head and neck, and results from acid demineralization of first enamel and then the dentine of the crowns of teeth; this process can be arrested in the early stages. Decay results in destruction of the tooth and infection of the pulp, which in turn leads to necrosis and death of the tooth. Infection may then extend along the root canal to the periapical tissues within the alveolar bone.

Dento-alveolar abscess

These may form as a result of an acute infection at the apex of a tooth and the discharge of pus into the mouth via a sinus on the alveolus. It may rarely spread to cause a facial abscess. Involvement of the submandibular lymph nodes, especially in children, may cause large swellings and abscess formation.

A periapical abscess requires drainage and elimination of the source of infection. A minor infection can be alleviated by root canal therapy, which may be performed in conjunction with open drainage of the abscess. Alternatively, tooth extraction provides drainage and removes the cause.

The infection from a periapical abscess penetrates the adjacent bony cortex, and if left untreated tracks beneath the periosteum to discharge into the mouth. This is usually accompanied by significant pain relief. Most abscesses point into the oral cavity. An infection can drain into the submandibular space via the posterior aspect of the mandible, where the mylohyoid attachment becomes superficial and the apices of the teeth project below it. Infection beneath a wisdom tooth may spread into a variety of spaces and can present unexpectedly as a parapharyngeal or submasseteric abscess. Retromolar infections can be distinguished from a tonsillar quinsy because they invariably cause trismus.

Soft tissue infections

Soft tissue infection of dental origin may be acute or chronic. Acute infection may take the form of an abscess, which in most instances presents as a submandibular swelling or periorbital oedema if the maxillary teeth are involved. The majority of such infections can be easily treated by drainage, antibiotics, and removal of the source of the infection. Occasionally, a virulent bacterium such as the β-haemolytic streptococcus can cause a spreading 'cellulitis', which in its severe form may result in Ludwig's angina. It is important with cervicofacial infections to exclude predisposing conditions such as diabetes mellitus and immunosuppression.

Patients are unwell, with systemic symptoms such as fever and malaise. Spreading infection can cause a compromised airway, preceded by an elevated tongue and difficulty in swallowing. The presence of trismus makes intraoral examination difficult, but an orthopantomograph helps to identify carious teeth. The infection can spread to involve the sublingual space anteriorly, and the superficial pterygoid, deep temporal, and parapharyngeal spaces posteriorly.

All patients, except those with limited submandibular swellings, should be admitted to hospital, given intravenous antibiotics, and rehydrated if necessary. The abscess is then incised and drained. Intubation may be very difficult, and a tracheostomy may occasionally be required. After an incision has been made over the swelling, Hilton's method of blunt dissection is used to avoid damage to the mandibular branch of the facial nerve. The fibrous septa in the abscess cavity are broken down digitally.

Ludwig's angina

This condition causes bilateral infection of the submandibular, sublingual and submental spaces. It usually arises from dental sepsis in a mandibular molar tooth. The infection may spread rapidly along the deep cervical and parapharyngeal fascial planes to produce supraglottic oedema and airway obstruction. Dyspnoea, dysphagia and dysphonia are sinister symptoms of impending airway obstruction. Patient exhaustion and complete airway obstruction can quickly supervene.

This condition is a surgical emergency. The first priority in severe cases is to secure the airway by endotracheal intubation or tracheostomy. Intravenous antibiotics are commenced. The submandibular, sublingual and submental spaces are then drained before the cause is removed (e.g. a carious tooth).

VIRAL INFECTIONS

Herpetic stomatitis

The primary infection usually occurs in childhood and may be accompanied by a severe systemic upset. The herpes type I virus is the common cause of infection, but the type II virus, which is normally associated with genital disease, has become an increasing cause of herpetic stomatitis. Multiple small painful ulcers are preceded by vesicles affecting any part of the oral mucosa but mostly on the gingivae, hard palate, and tongue, with accompanying cervical lymphadenopathy. Recovery may take a week or more. Topically applied antiviral agents such as acyclovir can be used to treat severe cases[37] but are not very effective once the infection is established.

Herpes labialis

About one-third of the population who have had primary herpes are subject to recurrent herpetic lesions affecting the lips. The virus persists in a latent form in the trigeminal ganglia, and is reactivated by local or systemic factors such as fever or over-exposure of the lips to sunshine, cold, or local trauma. The first sign is swelling of the lip before a crop of vesicles develop that burst and form the familiar cold sore. Treatment with acyclovir is effective if begun early[37] and is indicated in the immunocompromised.

Hand, foot and mouth disease (caused by strains of the Coxsackie A virus)

This is an acute but mild viral infection. It often produces minor epidemics in children and is characterized by painful oral ulceration with a rash on the hands and feet.[38] There is no specific treatment.

REFERENCES

37. Jaffe EC, Lehner T. Br Dent J 1968; 125: 392
38. Cawson RA, McSwiggan DA. Oral Surg 1969; 217: 451

Herpes zoster of the trigeminal nerve (shingles)

This condition is more common in the elderly or the immunologically compromised, and is accompanied by prodromal pain and a vesicular rash in the distribution of one or more divisions of the nerve.[39] The trigeminal nerve is affected in 15% of cases. Involvement of the ophthalmic division may lead to corneal ulceration. In a few cases, the facial nerve is the focus of the viral infection, resulting in intense pain over the mastoid, followed by vesicles developing on both the soft palate and external auditory meatus in conjunction with a facial palsy (Ramsay Hunt syndrome). Herpes zoster responds to topical application of acyclovir. Antibiotic creams are useful to prevent secondary infection of skin lesions, and analgesics are usually required. Post-herpetic neuralgia is an uncommon but troublesome complication in the elderly and responds poorly to treatment.

Human immunodeficiency virus

This virus can cause oral ulceration, Kaposi's sarcoma, candidiasis, and hairy leukoplakia in the mouth; only Kaposi's sarcoma is pathognomonic of the virus.[40]

FUNGAL INFECTIONS

Candidiasis

The single-celled yeast organism *Candida albicans* is a commensal in humans. Infection occurs in patients whose resistance is diminished, or where local factors such as chronic trauma, or maceration from dentures, encourage establishment of the infection.

Acute infection (thrush)

Acute infection is characterized by creamy white patches that can be rubbed off. They are produced by proliferation of the invaded epithelium. Acute infection complicates malnutrition, postoperative debility, antibiotic therapy, and immunosuppressive treatment.[41] Antifungal agents such as nystatin or amphotericin B should be prescribed, and antibiotics should be withdrawn if possible.

Chronic infection

Chronic infection is associated with ill-fitting dentures, where the underlying mucosa becomes red and oedematous. The infection is often associated with angular cheilitis, in which the epithelium at the angle of the mouth is broken down, inflamed and crusted.[42] Persistent white hyperplastic plaques, indistinguishable from leukoplakia, may also be found on the buccal mucosa, tongue, and occasionally the palate. The diagnosis can be made with certainty only by biopsy. Antifungal agents have variable success rates in the treatment of established chronic infection.[43] Dentures should be kept scrupulously clean and constructed to support the lips to eliminate the skin folds at the corners of the mouth. Thick white patches sometimes need to be removed by surgical excision.

Actinomycosis

Actinomycosis is a chronic suppurative infection of the cervicofacial region caused by *Actinomyces israelii* (see Ch. 4). It is characterized by widespread fibrosis and multiple skin sinuses. The matted colonies form into 'sulphur granules' and are discharged in the pus. Penicillin or tetracycline should be given for several weeks and will eventually produce complete resolution.[44] The condition is uncommon in the head and neck.

FUSOSPIROCHAETAL INFECTIONS

Acute ulcerative gingivitis (Vincent's gingivitis, trench mouth)

This is an acute ulcerative infection of the gingivae from synergistic infection by the spirochaete *Borrelia vincentii* and the spindle-shaped bacterium *Fusobacterium nucleatum*. Predisposing factors (apart from a neglected mouth) are stress, anxiety, smoking, and upper respiratory tract infections. The term 'trench mouth' was coined in the First World War. The main symptoms are painful bleeding gums and marked halitosis. Treatment is with penicillin and improved oral hygiene. The condition is uncommon today.

Cancrum oris (noma, phagedaena)

This disease occurs mainly in tropical countries. It commences as an acute ulcerative gingivitis and progresses to necrosis of the soft tissues overlying the jaws. It affects debilitated children and seriously ill adults suffering from malnutrition. The ulceration and necrosis are progressive, affecting the lips, cheek and tongue, and exposing large areas of alveolar bone. A fatal outcome from exhaustion and bronchopneumonia occurs in 90% of untreated cases.[45] Treatment is with penicillin and metronidazole combined with correction of the nutritional deficiency. Treatment must also be given for underlying diseases such as anaemia from hookworm infestation and malaria. The ulceration heals by fibrosis, causing contractions, extra-articular ankylosis, and severe disfigurement.

Tuberculosis and syphilis (see Ch. 4)

These conditions are relatively uncommon in the western population today, especially as a cause of oral ulceration. The primary tuberculosis complex is rare and presents as an indolent painless ulcer associated with marked regional lymphadenopathy. Primary syphilitic ulcers (chancres) are also painless, with a raised indurated edge. The regional lymph nodes are often enlarged (bubos), but serological tests are often negative. The second stage (6–8 weeks) is associated with a mild febrile illness, lymphadenopathy, skin rashes, and flat greyish oral ulcers, enlarging in a snail track manner. Tertiary syphilis presents several years later and classically affects the hard palate.[46]

ORAL ULCERATION

Persistent oral ulceration that cannot be identified must be regarded as neoplastic and biopsied to establish a diagnosis.

TRAUMATIC ULCERATION

Traumatic ulceration is relatively common but seldom serious. The ulcers often occur in the buccal mucosa of the cheeks, either at the level of dental occlusion or adjacent to a misaligned or sharp-edged tooth. Ulcers can also arise on the lateral margins

REFERENCES

39. Hudson CD, Vickers RA. Oral Surg 1971; 31: 494
40. Lozada F, Silverman S et al. Oral Surg 1983; 56: 491
41. Lehner T. Dent Pract 1967; 17: 209
42. Holbrook WP, Rodgers GD. Oral Surg 1980; 49: 122
43. Cawson RA. Oral Surg Oral Med Oral Pathol 1966; 22: 53
44. Bramley P, Orton HS. Br Dent J 1960; 109: 235
45. Emslie RD. Dent Pract 1963; 13: 481
46. Meyer I, Shklar G. Oral Surg 1967; 23: 45

of the tongue, where they may be mistaken for a carcinoma, or on the buccal or lingual sulci from ill-fitting dentures. Removal of the source of irritation effects a cure within a few days, but if the ulcer persists it should be biopsied.

APHTHOUS ULCERATION

Aphthous ulceration is the most common disorder affecting the oral mucous membrane.[47] Three forms exist: minor, which occurs in crops of two or three ulcers that resolve within 10 days; major, large, deep and persistent ulcers that take a number of weeks to resolve, leaving scars; and a herpetiform type that presents with multiple tiny ulcers. The minor form is most common. Suggested aetiological factors include infection, trauma, hormonal imbalance, immunological mechanisms, and gastrointestinal disease.[48] Some patients may have low serum iron, folic acid, or vitamin B_{12} levels.[49]

The condition begins in childhood, seems to affect patients with mouths that are well cared for, and is rarely seen in the elderly edentulous patient. Minor aphthous ulcers vary in size, number and frequency. They characteristically occur on the non-keratinized mucosa and last for 3–7 days. They are round or oval, with a shallow grey–yellow slough covered base and surrounding erythema. There is no totally effective treatment, but topical antiseptics and anaesthetics may be tried and some patients find relief from locally applied corticosteroid preparations.[50] Large ulcers may be several centimetres in diameter and persist for up to 3 months, resembling a carcinoma. When there is doubt, they should be biopsied.

Association with gastrointestinal disorders

Many of the disorders affecting the lower gastrointestinal tract also have oral manifestations. Patients with Crohn's disease have a characteristic cobblestone appearance of the oral mucosa, and may suffer from mouth ulcers and granulomatous enlargement of the lips. Ulcerative colitis is associated with severe oral aphthous ulceration, and coeliac disease with recurrent ulcers of the herpetiform variety.

BEHÇET'S SYNDROME

This condition is a rare, autoimmune disease characterized by oral ulceration (indistinguishable from aphthae), anterior uveitis, and genital ulceration. Young males are mainly affected. Non-suppurative arthritis occurs in one-third of cases. Treatment is symptomatic, and systemic steroids are necessary in the acute condition.[51]

AGRANULOCYTOSIS AND NEUTROPENIA

Any condition that interferes with cell proliferation can cause early symptoms or signs within the mouth. Oral ulceration may be the presenting feature of blood dyscrasias from cytotoxic drugs or bone marrow disease. The ulceration may progress to extensive necrotic lesions. Treatment should be directed at the underlying disease.[52]

VESICULOBULLOUS LESIONS

Many dermatological conditions affect the oral mucosa. Vesiculobullous diseases often present with oral ulceration.

Epidermolysis bullosa is a rare inherited disorder. Intra-epithelial bullae form in response to minor trauma.[53] A severe dystrophic form affecting the skin causes scarring and is sometimes fatal. There is no effective treatment.

Pemphigus is a progressive disease also characterized by intra-epithelial bullae of the skin and mucous membranes. The epithelium may be rubbed off by light finger pressure, Nikolsky's sign.[54] Benign mucous membrane pemphigoid, in contrast, consists of subepithelial bullae and results in scar formation. Immunosuppressive drugs may produce remission.

Erythema multiforme (Stevens–Johnson syndrome) is a rare but serious ulcerative condition of immune origin.[55] Drug allergy is known to produce it, especially to sulphonamides and barbiturates, as well as certain infections, such as mycoplasma pneumonia, but often no cause can be found. Teenagers and young adults are predominantly affected. Oral ulceration can be diffuse, with target lesions and extensive crusting of the lips at the mucocutaneous junction. Attacks may last up to 3–4 weeks, and there may be associated conjunctivitis, tracheitis and dysphagia.[56] Corticosteroids, supportive treatment, and antibiotics are given in severe cases.

WHITE PATCHES IN THE ORAL CAVITY

White patches commonly arise on the oral mucosa. It is estimated that they are present in 2% of the population; although the majority of cases are inconsequential, approximately 2% are epithelial dysplasia. *Leukoplakia* is a term used to describe a white patch or plaque that cannot be characterized clinically or pathologically as any other condition (Fig. 13.21). This definition does not imply any specific histological changes.[57] White patches have three main histological features: abnormal keratinization, hyper- or hypoplasia of the epithelium, and disordered maturation (dysplasia). Dysplasia is the only significant histological guide to the possibility of malignant change.

FRICTIONAL KERATOSIS

Frictional keratosis is caused by abrasion of the mucosa by irritants such as sharp teeth, ill-fitting dentures, and cheek-biting. Removal of the cause effects a cure within a few days.

SMOKER'S KERATOSIS

This characteristically occurs on the palate of heavy smokers. There is a pale white thickening of the mucosa and multiple small red swellings that mark the ducts of the minor mucous glands. It is not considered to be premalignant and disappears if the patient stops smoking.

LICHEN PLANUS

Lichen planus is the most common cause of persistent white patches in the mouth. The patches are often striated, forming a lace-like pattern, but can also be papular and confluent,

REFERENCES

47. Gayford JJ, Haskell R. Clinical Oral Medicine. 2nd edn. John Wright, Bristol, 1979: 1
48. Williams BD, Lehner T. Br Med J 1977; 1: 1387
49. Wray D, Ferguson MM et al. Br Med J 1975; 2: 490
50. MacPhee IT, Sircus W, Farmer ED. Br Med J 1968; 2: 147
51. Lehner T. Gut 1977; 18: 491
52. Scully C, MacFadyen E, Campbell A. Br J Oral Surg 1982; 20: 96
53. Winstock D. Br J Dermatol 1962; 74: 431
54. Firkin BG, Whitworth JA (eds). Dictionary of Medical Eponyms. Parthenon, Lancashire, 1987: 374
55. Ashby DW, Lazar T. Lancet 1951; i: 1091
56. Lozada F, Silverman S. Oral Surg 1987; 36: 628
57. Eveson JW. Cancer Surv 1983; 3: 405

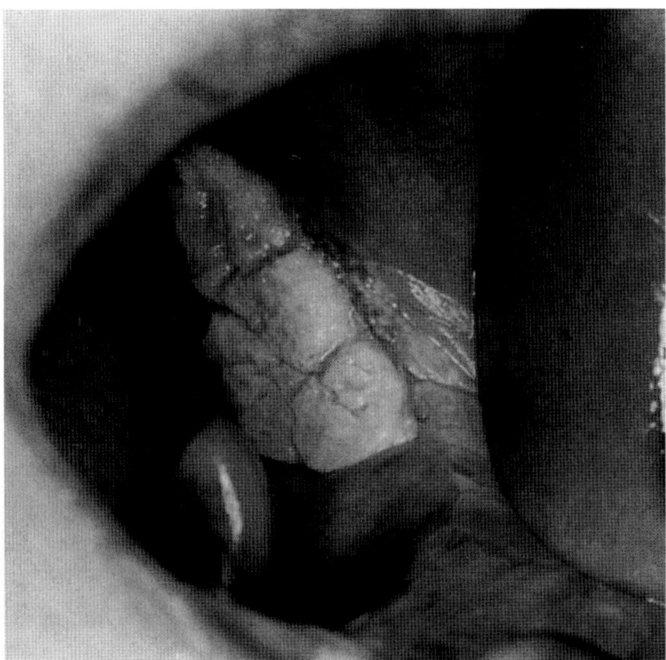

Figure 13.21 Leukoplakia of the buccal mucosa.

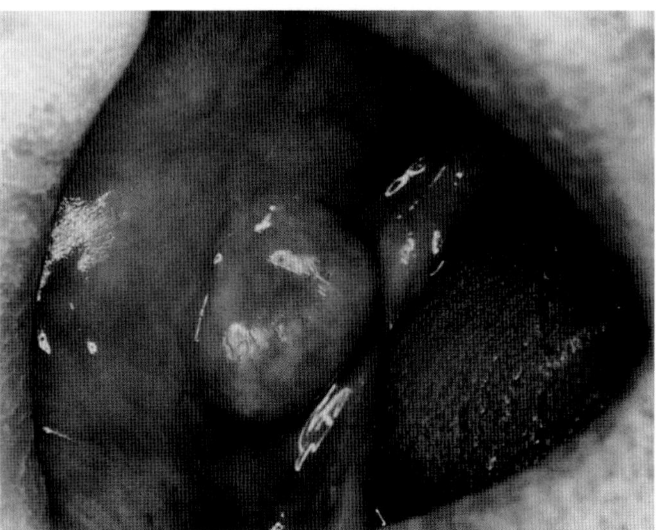

Figure 13.22 A fibroepithelial polyp of the buccal mucosa.

especially on the tongue. They are often bilateral, affecting the cheek mucosa, and can be erosive and painful. Some patients may also have itchy skin papules on the flexor surfaces of their limbs. The condition is often associated with anxiety or stress. The oral lesions can be improved by removing any irritating factors or trauma, and the erosive lesions should be treated by the local application of corticosteroids.

TRANSIENT WHITE PATCHES

Other common causes of white patches are candida, infection, and chemical burns, for example prolonged mucosal contact with aspirin. Small submucosal sebaceous glands (Fordyce spots) can also give the appearance of a white patch. Familial thickening of the mucosa occurs in patients with a white sponge naevus. Syphilitic leukoplakia is now only of historical interest.

GRANULOMATOUS SWELLINGS IN THE MOUTH

These are frequently the result of chronic inflammatory hyperplasia caused by recurrent minor injury or infection, and are the most common cause of localized swellings in the mouth. When they arise from the gingivae, the term *epulis* (on the gum) is used.

PYOGENIC GRANULOMA

Pyogenic granulomas are caused by overproduction of granulation tissue in response to chronic infection or foreign bodies. They may be associated with chronic sinuses, infected tooth sockets, and gingival infection. Minimal provocation is required for their induction in pregnancy (pregnancy epulis).[58] They should be excised, and any local cause should be treated.[59]

FIBROEPITHELIAL POLYP

These swellings arise as the result of hyperplasia of the subepithelial tissue and are covered by stratified squamous epithelium.[60] They are caused by chronic irritation on the insides of the cheeks (occlusal trauma; Fig. 13.22) or at the periphery of ill-fitting dentures. They are smooth pink swellings that are sessile or pedunculated and regress when the local irritant is removed. Occasionally, an enlarged parotid papilla pouting from the cheek can be confused with a polyp. Phenytoin and cyclosporine A can stimulate an exuberant fibrous response to gingival inflammation, producing gingival hyperplasia. This is managed by improving oral hygiene and gingival trimming.

UNCOMMON GRANULOMATOUS CONDITIONS

Peripheral giant cell granuloma

These giant cell granulomas arise only anterior to the first molar teeth and are related to the process of deciduous tooth resorption. During removal, the underlying bone should be curetted to prevent recurrence.[61]

Malignant granuloma

Two distinct conditions exist: Wegener's granuloma and midline lethal granuloma. They have a similar mode of presentation, which normally consists of granulomatous inflammation in the nose and central maxilla. Wegener's granulomatosis is a vasculitis that also affects the kidneys and lungs,[62] and it is often fatal.[63] Midline lethal granuloma is a T-cell lymphoma, but the histological features may not be typical. In a third of cases, the diagnosis is made on the clinical features alone. Treatment for the former disease includes steroids and cytotoxic drugs; the latter is treated by radiotherapy.

REFERENCES

58. Angelopoulos AP. J Oral Surg 1971; 29: 840
59. Bhaskar SN, Jacoway JR. J Oral Surg 1966; 24: 391
60. Barker DS, Lucas RB. Br J Oral Surg 1967; 5: 86
61. Killey HC, Kay LW. J Int Coll Surg 1965; 44: 262
62. Fauci AS, Haynes BF, Katz P et al. Ann Intern Med 1983; 98: 76
63. Butler DJ, Thompson H. Br J Oral Surg 1972; 9: 208

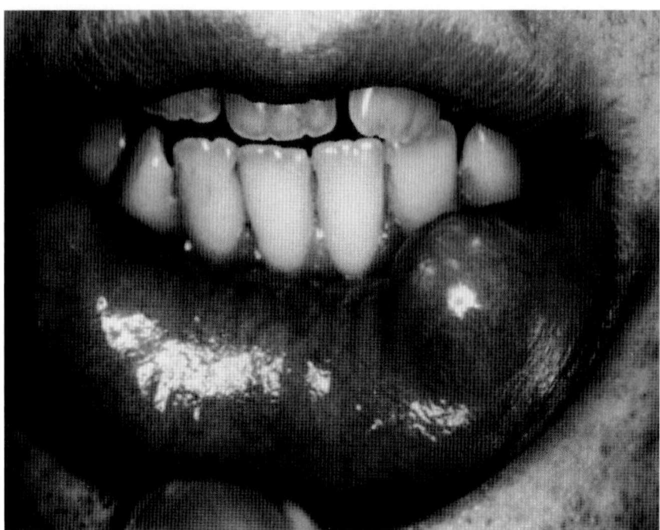

Figure 13.23 A mucocele of the lip.

CYSTS OF THE MOUTH

MUCOCELES

Mucoceles probably arise from trauma to the ducts of minor salivary glands and are found particularly on the lip.[64] They are in reality mucus extravasation cysts, as the histological appearances suggest that the duct has been torn, allowing escape of mucus into the tissues.[65] They are superficial, bluish in colour, and may fluctuate in size, reaching 1–2 cm in diameter (Fig. 13.23). They should be excised with an ellipse of overlying mucosa, but the cyst wall is thin and fragile, and unless care is taken they are easily ruptured at operation. Recurrence is common. Mucoceles may also be treated by cryosurgery.[66]

RANULA

This term *ranula* ('like the belly of a frog') is used to describe a salivary extravasation cyst that develops in the floor of the mouth. It is larger than a mucocele, because of the loose, areola-filled spaces in the floor of the mouth into which it extends. It arises from the sublingual gland.[67] Ranulas develop on one side of the floor of the mouth, and slowly enlarge to form a bluish, dome-shaped, fluctuant swelling beneath the sublingual mucosa (Fig. 13.24). They may extend between the muscle layers, and present as a submental swelling or a plunging ranula if the myelohyoid diaphragm is penetrated. These cysts have very thin walls and are easily ruptured. This is a cause of recurrence unless the sublingual gland is removed.[68] Care must be taken not to damage the submandibular duct or the lingual nerve at the time of excision. Surgery is technically demanding, and recurrence is common in inexperienced hands.

OTHER MIDLINE CYSTS

Sublingual dermoid cysts are uncommon. They originate from the embryonic branchial arches. They are thick-walled, lined with squamous cell epithelium, and present as pink doughy swellings that may elevate the tongue. They may extend almost to the hyoid bone before the patient presents. Large cysts, or those that are adherent because of infection, are more easily approached from the neck (see Ch. 16).[69]

Thyroglossal cysts rarely present in the mouth and occur more frequently in the hyoid area (see Ch. 16).

Lipomas, neuromas, and other benign tumours may also present as a mass in the floor of the mouth.

BENIGN TUMOURS OF THE ORAL CAVITY

SQUAMOUS CELL PAPILLOMA

These small tumours arise from the epithelium and occur mainly on the palate, fauces and gingivae in children and young adults. They are of viral origin, and their surface is covered in white, finger-like processes or has a pink, cauliflower-like appearance if the keratin is lost. They have no malignant potential. Most are excised.

LIPOMAS

Intraoral lipomas are rare but may occur in the floor of the mouth or in the cheeks as slow-growing, soft, lobulated, fatty swellings.[70]

HAEMANGIOMA AND LYMPHANGIOMA

More than half of these angiomas occur in the head and neck, and can present problems with respect to airway management, disturbed growth, and haemorrhage.

GRANULAR CELL MYOBLASTOMA

This uncommon benign tumour usually occurs in the tongue and affects adults in middle age. The tumour presents as a small rounded swelling in or beneath the mucosa.[71] It does not recur if it is adequately excised.

NEURAL TUMOURS

These are occasionally seen in the oral cavity as small painless nodules, although a central neurilemmoma or Schwannoma can develop in the mandible in the inferior dental nerve. Von Recklinghausen's neurofibromatosis (see Ch. 43) can involve the face and mouth, often extensively. The plexiform variety of neurofibroma infiltrates the facial tissues, producing pendulous masses; it can involve the underlying bone, causing deformity and interfering with tooth eruption.[72] Surgery is undertaken for cosmetic and functional reasons (see Ch. 43).

MALIGNANT AND PREMALIGNANT TUMOURS OF THE ORAL CAVITY

Squamous cell carcinoma is the principal cancer of the upper alimentary tract. Much like its counterpart in the lung, it is an aggressive tumour, and the untreated patient has a life expectancy of approximately 18 months from the time of

REFERENCES

64. Cohen L. Oral Surg 1965; 19: 365
65. Harrison JD. Oral Surg 1975; 39: 268
66. Leopard P J. Br J Oral Surg 1972; 13: 128
67. Roediger WEW, Lloyd P, Lawson HH. Br J Surg 1973; 60: 720
68. Parekh D, Stewart M, Joseph C et al. Brit J Surg 1987; 74:307
69. Seward GR. Br J Oral Surg 1965; 3: 36
70. Greer RO, Goldman HM. Oral Surg 1974; 38: 43
71. Cawson RA, Eveson JW. Oral Pathology and Diagnosis. Heinemann, London, 1987: 10–18
72. O'Driscoll PM. Br J Oral Surg 1965; 3: 22

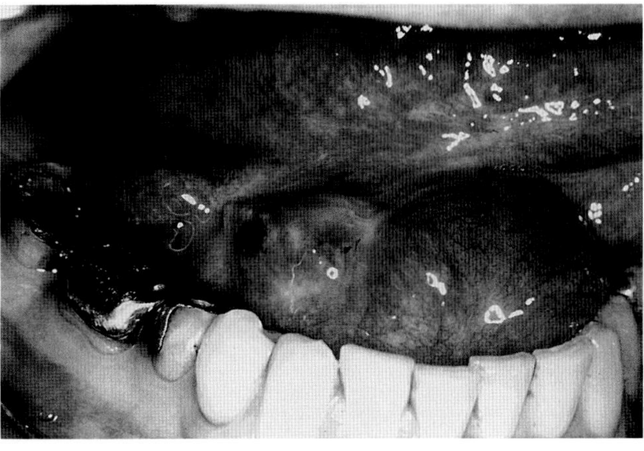
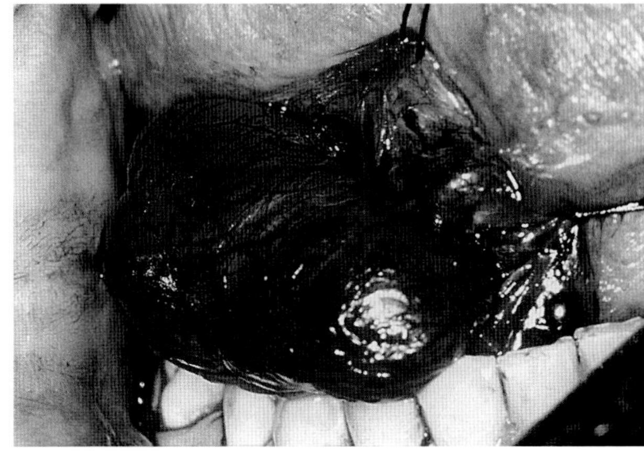

a b

Figure 13.24 Extravasation cyst in the floor of the mouth (ranula).

diagnosis. Disease of the upper alimentary tract has an incidence of 2–3 per 100 000 of the UK population per annum, but poses a much larger health problem in developing countries, where it represents the third most common cancer.[73] Between 70 and 80% of patients with stage 1 or 2 tumours, and half of those with stage 3 disease, can be cured. In contrast, only 25–30% with stage 4 disease are curable.[74] Unfortunately, over two-thirds of patients present with late-stage disease.

PREMALIGNANT CONDITIONS

Leukoplakia is a diagnosis established by exclusion of other known causes of oral white patches. Only a small proportion (2–4%) of leukoplakias series to malignancy.[75] They do so through a series of identifiable stages, much like dysplasia of the cervix. Some areas become red and speckled—erythroplakias; half of these progress to cancer. Patches on the lateral border of the tongue or floor of the mouth also have a risk of malignant change. The risk of malignant change increases with age, the duration of the lesion, the site, the patient's smoking and drinking habits, and the degree of dysplasia.

Submucous fibrosis is peculiar to people of Asian descent[76] and is related to pan and betel nut chewing. The ingredients of pan (betel nut, slake lime, and tobacco) cause a dense submucous fibrosis that carries a small risk of neoplastic change (4% over 15 years).

Lichen planus

Lichen planus is an autoimmune disorder (see Ch. 17). At the extreme end of the disease spectrum is an atrophic and erosive form of lichen planus, and a small percentage of these (0.3%) can convert to squamous cell carcinoma.

Sideropenic dysphagia

There is a significant association between cancer of the mouth and cervical oesophagus, and sideropenic dysphagia (Paterson–Kelly syndrome).[77]

AETIOLOGICAL FACTORS IN ORAL MALIGNANCY

A range of factors, including syphilis, candidal infection, papilloma virus, and repeated trauma, are reported to induce oral cancer but definitive evidence is lacking. Epstein–Barr virus has an association with nasopharyngeal carcinoma,[78] and women with iron deficiency anaemia and oesophageal stricture are at risk of hypopharyngeal cancer in Plummer–Vinson syndrome (see Ch. 20). The immune suppression required after organ transplantation (see Ch. 8) is associated with skin rather than mucosal squamous cell carcinoma, and AIDS is not associated with oral squamous cell cancer. Excessive exposure to sunlight is associated with lip cancer.[79] The two overriding aetiological factors are excessive smoking and alcohol consumption, and their effects are synergistic. The odds ratio over normal is 15 for combined consumption and only 3–5 for single-agent use.[80]

Retinoids may help to stabilize the epithelium, but the evidence of their efficacy in preventing oral cancer is as yet unsubstantiated.

CLINICAL PRESENTATION

A delay of more than 3 months occurs from the onset of symptoms to diagnosis in about a third of cases. The patient is responsible for the delay in the majority of cases, but the remainder (approximately 20%) relate to medical personnel.[81]

The median age at presentation is 61 years, and men are more commonly affected than women. Tumours usually arise in the salivary gutters of the mouth (Fig. 13.25), and the four most common symptoms are ulcer, swelling, neck lump, and pain. A history of pain radiating to the ear is an ominous symptom and demands careful evaluation. Pain and nerve involvement suggest invasion of the skull base. Posterior invasion causes trismus and

REFERENCES

73. Johnson NW. In: Johnson NW (ed). Risk Markers for Oral Diseases, Vol 2. Oral Cancer. Cambridge University Press, Cambridge, 1991: 3
74. Franceshi D, Gupta R, Spiro RH et al. Am J Surg 1993; 166: 360–365
75. Harris M. In: Johnson NW (ed). Risk Markers for Oral Diseases, Vol 2. Oral Cancer. Cambridge University Press, Cambridge, 1991: 157
76. McGurk M, Craig GT. Br J Oral Maxillofac Surg 1984; 22: 56
77. Larsson LG, Sandstrom A, Westling P. Cancer Res 1975; 35: 3308
78. Yip TTC, Ngan RKC et al. Cancer 1994, 74: 2414
79. Jorgensen K, Elbrand O, Anderson AP. Acta Radiol Oncol Radiat Phys Biol 1973; 12: 177
80. Binnie WH. In: Johnson NW (ed). Risk Markers for Oral Diseases, Vol 2. Oral Cancer. Cambridge University Press, Cambridge, 1991: 64
81. Kowalski LP, Franco EL et al. Oral Oncol Eur J Cancer 1994; 30B: 267

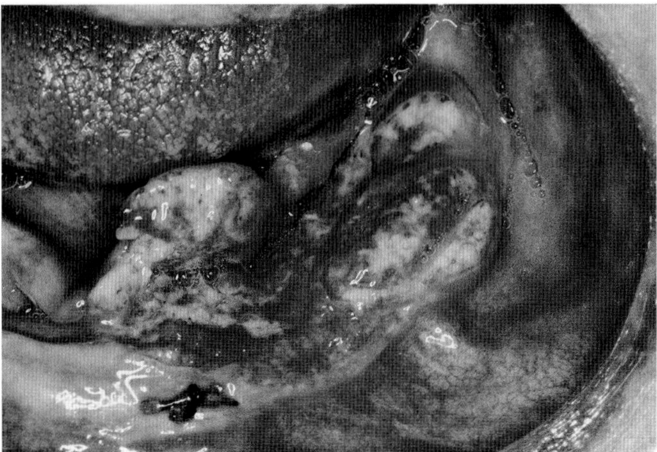

Figure 13.25 Typical oral cancer, a common site: the floor of the mouth, large ulcer, raised rolled edges, with adjacent abnormal mucosa showing speckled leukoplakia.

superior invasion proptosis, dystopia and diplopia. Epiphora and unilateral epistaxis are other rarer presenting symptoms.

Tumours normally metastasize to cervical lymph nodes, with systemic dissemination occurring in only 10% of cases if the primary cancer can be controlled. A palpable lymph node is present in 20% of cases when they are first seen, and in a further 10% it is the only sign at diagnosis.[82] The latter mode of presentation can lead to mismanagement, as open biopsy of the node may reduce survival by 30% by ensuring local dissemination of the tumour. The first step should be a careful evaluation of the upper alimentary tract, the nasal passages, and the larynx, which will normally reveal the primary tumour (see Ch. 20). Approximately 5% of patients have a second synchronous tumour at presentation, and a further 10% develop a metachronous tumour within 6 months.[83] There is a 2% cumulative risk of developing a second primary cancer per year of life.

INVESTIGATION

An incisional biopsy confirms the diagnosis. This should cross the advancing edge of the tumour and include a small sample of clinically normal tissue as well as the obviously abnormal tissue. When biopsying premalignant lesions, skill and judgement are required to take the biopsy from the most aggressive part of the tumor. The sample should be handled carefully to avoid crush artefacts. Multiple biopsies may be necessary in doubtful lesions to minimize the risk of sampling errors giving a false negative result.

Triple endoscopy (nasal, oesophageal and laryngeal–tracheal) may be useful to exclude multiple synchronous primaries in the aerodigestive tract. Computerized tomography and MRI of the face, mouth and neck help to exclude second primary tumours, and provide information on both the extent of the cancer and the invasion of surrounding structures by the tumour (Fig. 13.26). Invasion of bone is better imaged using MRI. Ultrasound, often with ultrasound-guided fine-needle aspiration, as well as CT and MRI, is used to evaluate the neck for the presence of nodes, but no single technique, including clinical examination, is conclusive.

The tumour, node, metastasis (TNM) staging is governed by both the size and the involvement of local structures, therefore the criteria vary through the upper aerodigestive tract.[84] A simplified description is shown in Box 13.3.

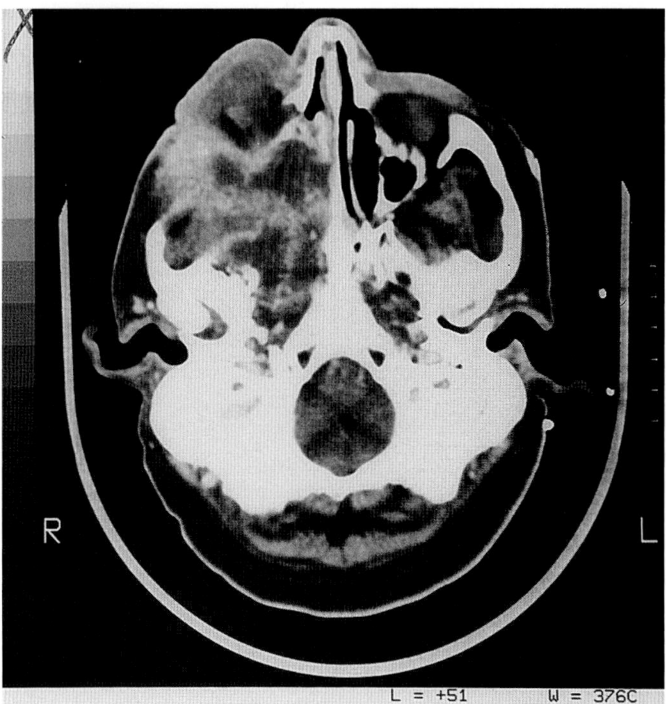

Figure 13.26 A very large, neglected antral tumour, which had recently produced symptoms.

Box 13.3 Simplified staging criteria

- Stage 1: T1, N0, M0
- Stage 2: T2, N0, M0
- Stage 3: T3, N0, M0; T1–3, N1, M0
- Stage 4: T4, N0, M0; T1–4, N1–3, M0–1

Tumour
- T1: 0–2 cm
- T2: 2–4 cm
- T3: 4–6 cm
- T4: > 6 cm

T staging is not strictly based on size but also takes account of invasion of anatomical structures and varies with position in the aerodigestive tract.

Node
- N0: no cervical node involvement
- N1: single ipsilateral node < 3 cm
- N2:
  a Single ipsilateral node > 3 and < 6 cm
  b Multiple ipsilateral nodes < 6 cm
  c Bilateral contralateral nodes < 6 cm
- N3: > 6 cm

Metastasis
- M0: no distant metastasis
- M1: distant metastasis

REFERENCES

82. Lefebvre JL, Coche-Dequeant B et al. Am J Surg 1990; 160: 443
83. Pamosetti E, Luboinski B, Mamelle G et al. Laryngoscope 1989; 99: 1267
84. Urken ML, Buchbinder D, Weinberg H et al. Laryngoscope 1991; 101: 935–950

MANAGEMENT

Squamous cell carcinomas of the oral cavity, including the tongue, cheek, and floor of the mouth, are treated in a similar manner and are therefore considered as one entity.

An essential part of the treatment is a joint clinic that brings together all the clinicians who may contribute to the longitudinal care of the patient. The team should include a maxillofacial surgeon, an oncologist, a pathologist, and a radiologist. In addition, a restorative dental surgeon may be useful because of the state of the dentition and the requirement for pre- and post-treatment oral care. Oncology specialist nurses help patients come to terms with their disease, and their support should continue into the postoperative period.

The immediate postoperative problems should be considered at an early stage. Many patients have feeding difficulties, either from the surgery or from mucositis induced by radiotherapy. Good nutrition is extremely important in the perioperative period, and the use of an elective percutaneous gastrostomy should be considered. A convenient time to place this is during any triple endoscopy or examination under anaesthesia.

TREATMENT

The debate over whether radiation or surgery is the more effective in treatment has now been largely resolved.[85] Unequivocal indications for surgery are failed radiotherapy, bone invasion, and cervical metastasis. Small stage 1 and 2 tumours are equally well treated by radiotherapy or surgery, and the choice depends on the preference of the clinician. Small tumours arising in the anterior two-thirds of the tongue can be treated by local implantation of radioactive needles (caesium wire, 5–7 days) under general anaesthesia[86] or can equally well be excised, as the morbidity is low compared with a course of external beam radiotherapy. Large tumours, stage 3 and 4, or those with cervical metastasis respond best to surgery followed by adjuvant radiotherapy. The role of chemotherapy to treat the primary tumour is limited, with an estimated maximum improvement in survival of 0–6%.[87] The role of chemotherapy as an adjuvant to surgery or radiotherapy is being explored.

The single most important prognostic indicator of survival is cervical node metastasis, which halves survival.[88] The prognosis is also reduced if the capsule of the tumour has been breached, the chance of which increases with increasing size of the tumour and the number of metastatic lymph nodes. Adjuvant radiotherapy is advocated if more than two metastatic nodes are present in a specimen. Open node biopsy should not be carried out without continuing to perform a neck dissection. Radiotherapy should be avoided if there is bone involvement or the tumour is very large.

Surgery

The three roles of surgery are management of the primary site, management of node spread, and reconstruction.

Primary site

The aim is to excise the tumour with a 5-mm or greater microscopic margin of normal tumour-free tissue. Microscopic evidence of positive or 'close' margins (tumour within 2 or 3 mm of the resection margin) leads to an unacceptably high recurrence rate. Some squamous cell carcinomas and most adenoid cystic carcinomas of salivary glands spread along the perineurium. Most surgeons attempt a clearance of at least 1 cm (preferably 2 cm) beyond the margin of the visible tumour, because this can allow skip lesions, with lengths of normal unaffected nerve separating islands of tumour cells. There is inevitable shrinkage of the specimen during fixation, and this may confuse histological interpretation.

Non-irradiated periosteum can act as a barrier to tumour spread, and invasion of the mandible is more likely to occur through the alveolus than through the medial or lateral cortices. Magnetic resonance imaging is more useful than CT in demonstrating bone involvement preoperatively, but if doubt exists it is prudent to err on the side of caution and resect bone. The resection must then take account of the rapidity with which the tumour can spread within the medullary cavity.

When the maxilla is involved, it is usual to resect the bone en bloc with the specimen, leaving tumour-free bony resection margins behind. In the mandible, it is possible to carry out either partial-thickness or rim resections, the morbidity of which is much less than with a full-thickness bone resection. Although radiological examinations (MRI, CT, plain films, and bone scans) are helpful in demonstrating bone invasion preoperatively, direct inspection by periosteal stripping is probably the most successful way of determining bone involvement. Tumours are complex three-dimensional shapes, and clear resection margins must be achieved in all planes, particularly the deep surfaces.

Neck

Surgery has a dual role: to resect metastatic disease and to 'stage' the neck. Tumour spread in the neck is unpredictable, and skip deposits down the cervical lymphatic chain are common. Spread beyond the neck is very rare. Most tumours spread only to one side of the neck, except for midline tumours and carcinomas of the posterior maxilla that can spread to the retropharyngeal nodes.

For many years, the standard management of metastatic lymph nodes was by a radical neck dissection. This consisted of removal of all lymph nodes at all levels of the neck (see Box 13.4).

During the radical neck dissection, the structures adjacent to the lymph nodes were also removed to ensure that a 'safe' margin of tissue was removed. The structures removed included the sternocleidomastoid muscle, the accessory nerve, and the internal jugular vein. The removal of these structures has important functional and aesthetic significance, giving rise to poor cosmetic appearance, shoulder girdle dysfunction, and, particularly after bilateral dissections, reduced venous outflow from the head and neck region, resulting in widespread oedema including cerebral oedema.

Despite this radical approach, many lymph nodes are excised with minimal clearance; however, despite the close resection margins, recurrence in the neck is rare. As a consequence, it is now common to undertake a functional or modified dissection of the neck, unless there is evidence before or at operation of extranodal extension which involves adjacent structures. Three types of modified neck dissection exist (see Box 13.5).

REFERENCES

85. Renehan A, Gleave EN et al. Br J Surg 1996; 83: 1750
86. McGurk M, Williams RG, Calman FMB. In: de Burgh Norman JE, McGurk M (eds). Color Atlas and Text of the Salivary Glands. Diseases, Disorders and Surgery. Mosby-Wolfe, London, 1995: 181
87. Spiro RH, Armstrong J et al. Arch Otolaryngol Head Neck Surg 1989; 115: 316
88. McGurk M, Hussain K. Ann R Coll Surg Engl 1997; 79: 198–202

Box 13.4 Lymph nodes at different levels of the neck

- Level I: submandibular triangle
- Level II: upper jugular nodes
- Level III: middle jugular nodes
- Level IV: lower jugular nodes
- Level V: posterior nodes

Box 13.5 Types of modified neck dissection

- Type I: radical but with preservation of accessory nerve
- Type II: with addition preservation of internal jugular vein
- Type III: with additional preservation of sternomastoid muscle

Radical dissection is still considered when there are multiple nodes at multiple levels; there is evidence of extracapsular spread preoperatively; or if intraoperatively extracapsular spread is evident, at which point the functional approach is converted to a radical one. Postoperative radiotherapy is usually given if there are multiple nodes at multiple levels or evidence of extracapsular spread.

It is not possible with certainty to stage the nodal neck disease preoperatively, and the initial TNM staging is modified after surgery in the light of the histological findings. Clinical examination, CT and MRI all have approximately 15% false negatives. Ultrasound-guided fine-needle aspiration,[4] carried out by an expert, is regarded as the most accurate method currently available. Newer techniques, including positron emission tomography scanning, have yet to prove their worth for preoperative staging.

Reconstruction

Urken was probably one of the earliest to document that reconstruction was not just about filling a defect created by ablative surgery.[84] Clearly, filling the defect is important, but if the patient's quality of life is to return to acceptable levels, then the surgery has to be taken beyond reconstruction to rehabilitation. The survival rates for oral cancer have only marginally improved, but great strides have been achieved in rehabilitation.

The mouth and jaws can be divided into functional units: mandible, floor of mouth and tongue, and palate (soft and hard palate). Each has different functions and hence demands (Fig. 13.27).

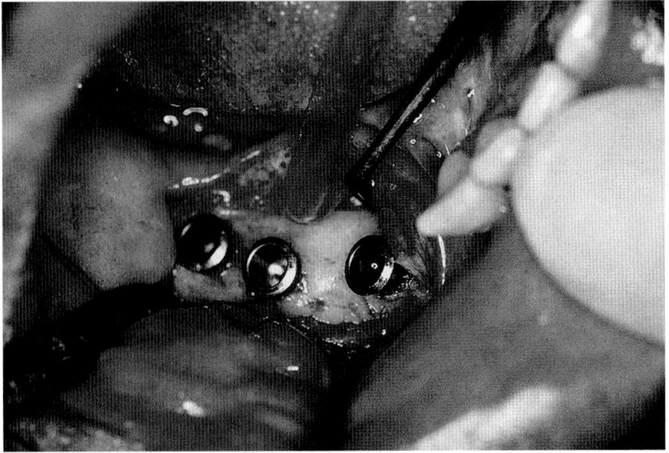

Figure 13.27 Dental implants into bone grafts, again improve the quality of the rehabilitation.

Different methods of reconstruction

MANDIBLE The mandible is crucial in maintaining the facial shape. It also supports the lips and musculature, maintaining oral competence. Its projection supports the muscles of the floor of the mouth, helping to maintain swallowing and the oropharyngeal airway. It also has a central role in mastication by supporting the dentition, either natural or prosthetic.

It is difficult to reconstruct the mandible. Attempts have been made to either avoid mandibular resections or to use simple replacements such as reconstruction plates. The former runs the risk of incomplete tumour ablation or subsequent fractures of the small remnant of mandible, while the latter has proved disastrous, failing on all counts of rehabilitation and usually fracturing or becoming exposed through the skin or mucosa.

Free composite tissue transfers achieve the most successful reconstructions. The osseocutaneous radial forearm flap has low donor-site morbidity (occasional fracture of the residual radius occurs) but provides small bone stock. Larger bone stock is provided by the iliac crest, but the morbidity at the donor site is high. Fibula free grafts lie somewhere in between the two. The choice of donor site depends on the size of the defect and the potential to replace the dentition with osseointegrated dental implants. Although the primary reconstruction is undertaken at the time of ablation, the placement of implants is usually undertaken later. Subsequent soft tissue manipulation or grafting is usually required to develop the appropriate mucosal attachment necessary for implants.

FLOOR OF MOUTH AND TONGUE In contrast to the rigidity of the mandible, the tongue is highly muscular and in constant motion to fulfil its function in speech and deglutition. Attempts at introducing innervated tissue to replace it are still in development. The aim of reconstruction is to maximize existing movements, because it is exceptionally rare for the whole tongue to require resection. Flaps must therefore be thin and mobile, and the radial forearm is excellent for reconstruction. The fascia alone may be used to cover small defects. Larger defects can be closed by thin muscular flaps such as rectus abdominis muscle, which unlike skin has the advantage of allowing mucosalization.

HARD AND SOFT PALATE The hard and soft palate are rarer sites for malignancy but potentially a devastating area to ablate. It is always involved in maxillary sinus surgery, and whether the lesion arises primarily on the oral aspect of the palate or in the sinus, the surgical defect creates a communication into the maxillary sinus and may involve the soft palate. There is some controversy over the use of obturators over free tissue transfer to reconstruct the defect caused by the surgery. No one method is suitable for all circumstances.

LIPS Primary closure following resection is usually possible if less than half of the lip length has been resected. The key to a successful primary repair is to ensure correct approximation and alignment of the orbicularis oris muscle and the vermilion border. Loss of lip height, notching, and an incompetent sphincter may result if the lip is not properly repaired. Primary closure can still be carried out where the loss extends to half of the lip, but some degree of microstomia will result. Flap repair is

Table 13.1 The proportion of benign and malignant salivary gland neoplasms by site

	Malignant (%)	Benign (%)
Parotid	20	80
Submandibular	50	50
Minor salivary glands	60	40

required when more than half of the lip, or the commissure, has been resected.

MINOR SALIVARY GLAND TUMOURS OF THE ORAL CAVITY

Although the management of these tumours is similar to that of major salivary gland tumours (see Ch. 14), there are subtle differences.

General characteristics

Benign and malignant tumours arise in the submandibular and minor salivary glands with about the same frequency, and together represent approximately 30% of salivary neoplasms. The rest originate in the parotid gland (see Ch. 14). About 60% present as an apparently benign lump, because salivary gland cancers are often slow-growing.[85] The risk of encountering a malignant salivary gland tumour increases depending on the site of origin (Table 13.1), being greater in the parotid than in the submandibular gland, and being even more likely in the minor salivary glands.

The histological classification of salivary gland cancers is unwieldy (see Ch. 14) and adds little to the surgical management, which is simply governed by tumour stage (notably the size of the lump) and the clinical grade of the tumour. Salivary gland cancers can be broadly divided into three prognostic groups. The histological subtypes that are high-grade include malignant pleomorphic carcinoma, squamous cell carcinoma, and anaplastic carcinoma. Low-grade tumours are mucoepidermoid carcinomas (although 20% of these are high grade) and acinic cell carcinomas. An intermediate group consists of adenoid cystic carcinomas and adenocarcinomas. The relative incidence of the different histological types is similar in the mouth and parotid gland, but the submandibular gland has a higher proportion of adenoid cystic carcinomas (Table 13.2).[86] Wide local excision of the submandibular triangle, with some form of selective neck dissection, ensures survival rates comparable with those achieved in the parotid and the mouth.[87]

Clinical presentations

The majority of oral salivary gland neoplasms present as a smooth lobulated mass that often has a blue appearance. Benign tumours present at a median age of 48 years, about a decade earlier than malignant tumours. A delay in presentation of 2–3 years is a feature of these slow-growing tumours. Malignancy is suspected when an indurated lump is fixed to the overlying mucosa (Table 13.3). Perineurial invasion is a feature of adenoid cystic carcinoma, as is pain, although this symptom is still uncommon (10–20% of cases), as is cervical lymph node metastasis.[86]

The definitive diagnosis is established by open biopsy prior to surgery in the majority of instances. Where this is not possible, fine-needle aspiration cytology correctly identifies over 90% of malignant tumours.[88] Surgery is the treatment of choice for both benign and malignant salivary neoplasms.

Pleomorphic adenoma

Pleomorphic adenomas can be removed with a thin margin of normal tissue.[89] The subperiosteal plane (the surgeon's friend) should be used for dissection whenever possible, as most will be at the junction of the hard and soft palate.

Carcinoma

Minor salivary gland cancers are minor in name only.[90] Small malignant lesions (T1) can be treated adequately by wide local excision, but with increasing size the management is similar to that for squamous cell carcinoma at this site, namely an in-continuity local and selective neck resection.

Several studies have demonstrated that both local control and improved survival are achieved with adjuvant radiotherapy, and it is advocated particularly in large or high-grade cancers. The prognosis for minor salivary gland cancers in the oral cavity is similar to that expected for major salivary gland cancer: 75%, 62% and 56% at 5, 10 and 15 years, respectively.[91]

Mucosal malignant melanoma

This tumour is uncommon in the face and oral cavity, and represents only 1–2% of all malignant melanomas (see Ch. 9). Slightly more than half occur in the nose and paranasal sinuses; the remainder arise in the mouth and oropharynx. The mean age of presentation is in the fifth decade, and most have an insidious onset. Symptoms include nasal obstruction, discharge and bleeding if the primary tumour is in the nose. It usually present as a mass if it arises in the oral cavity. Delay in presentation is usual, but the disease is often confined to the primary site and cervical lymph node metastasis is uncommon at presentation.

Local resection has been the traditional approach to treatment, but it is difficult to ensure that the surgical margins are adequate because of diffuse submucosal lymphatic permeation. Local control is associated with prolonged survival if the tumour is small and resectable. Malignant melanoma may also occasionally be responsive to radiation therapy,[92] but immuno- and chemotherapy have no established place in its management (see Ch. 9).

The prognosis is poor, with only 10–40% of patients surviving 5 years.[93]

SARCOMA

Sarcoma of the head and neck is another relatively uncommon tumour, constituting about 15% of all sarcomas but fewer than 1% of malignant tumours in the head and neck. The response to treatment can be affected by the site, grade, and the age of the host (e.g. adult or child). The majority of tumours occur in

REFERENCES

89. McGurk M, Renehan A, Gleave EN et al. Br J Surg 1996; 83: 1747
90. de Burgh Norman JE. In: de Burgh Norman JE, McGurk M (eds). Colour Atlas and Textbook of the Salivary Glands. Diseases, Disorders and Surgery. Mosby-Wolfe, London, 1995: 197
91. Spiro RH, Thater HT et al. Am J Surg 1991; 162: 330
92. Sause WT, Cooper JS et al. Int J Radiat Oncol Biol Phys 1991; 20:429
93. Stern SJ, Guillamondegui OM. Head Neck 1991; 13: 22

Table 13.2 Relative proportion of the seven main histological cancers by site in a review of 670 minor, 585 submandibular, and 2150 parotid cancers[85]

	Tumour site (%)		
Carcinoma	Minor salivary glands	Parotid	Submandibular
Mucoepidermoid	41	31	22
Adenoid cystic	27	13	41
Adenocarcinoma	19	14	9
Malignant pleomorphic	5	13	12
Acinic cell	3	12	2
Squamous cell	3	6	7
Anaplastic	2	10	7

Table 13.3 Distribution of benign and malignant minor salivary gland tumours by site in a review of 3079 reported cases[85]

	Tumour (%)	
Site	Benign	Malignant
Palate	50	50
Floor of mouth	12	88
Retromolar	9	91
Lip	54	46
Tongue	9	91
Cheek	41	59

adults, with a median age at presentation of 45 years, most arising in soft tissue (80%) rather than bone (20%). The common presenting symptoms include a mass, pain, and skin involvement.

A wide range of histological types exist depending on the mesodermal site of origin. The prognosis is related principally to the grade and tumour size; histological type is less influential, although some, such as rhabdomyosarcoma, have a greater proportion of high-grade neoplasms. The prognosis for patients with high-grade lesions is less than 40% at 5 and 10 years, compared with approximately 80% for low-grade sarcomas.[94] The pattern of failure is usually local recurrence, normally within 2 years, with or without distant metastasis.

Wide surgical excision remains the best treatment. Prophylactic neck dissections, except for access purposes, are not advocated. Multivariate analysis of prognostic factors has shown that local recurrence is largely a function of the adequacy of excision.[95] Microscopic extension of the tumour makes this difficult to achieve in half the cases, but adjuvant radiotherapy has proved effective in reducing local recurrence.[95]

LYMPHORETICULAR NEOPLASMS

This group of tumours usually present in the head and neck region as a cervical lymphadenopathy (see Ch. 34). Multiple myelomatosis may affect the jaws: deposits cause pain and swelling, and even pathological fracture. The osteolytic lesions, which are also common in the skull bones, need to be distinguished from other causes of radiolucency. A raised sedimentation rate and Bence Jones proteinuria support a diagnosis of myeloma.

Burkitt's tumour

This is a tumour of lymphoid tissue occurring in children in tropical Africa and Brazil.[96] It is thought to follow infection with the Epstein–Barr virus.[97] The jaws are initially affected, with rapidly enlarging swellings destroying bone, often at several sites (Fig. 13.28). Later, deposits appear in all the abdominal organs. Treatment is by cytotoxic drug regimens, which may provide rapid remission, but the overall mortality remains high. Remission for more than 2 years is associated with a survival rate of 50%.[98]

Lymphoma

Non-Hodgkin's lymphomas (see Ch. 34) can present in the oral cavity as isolated extralymphatic deposits, but more commonly present as cervical lymphadenopathy or enlargement of Waldeyer's ring. Patients with Sjögren's syndrome can develop mucosa-associated lymphoid tissue (MALT) lymphomas, which normally present as a discrete parotid mass.[99]

Leukaemia

Oral manifestations of acute leukaemia are seen in half the patients with this disease and may be its primary presentation. Mucosal pallor, gingival bleeding, or purpura is the first sign, followed by gingival swelling, which may progress to ulceration. Necrotic ulcers and osteolytic lesions may also develop.[100]

Secondary neoplasms

Metastases from primary tumours elsewhere in the body occasionally occur in the mouth. Spread is via the bloodstream from sites such as the bronchus, breast, kidney, prostate and

REFERENCES

94. Mandard AM, Petiot JF. Cancer 1989; 63: 1437
95. Elias AD, Antman KH. Semin Oncol 1989; 16: 305
96. Burkitt DJ. Dent Res 1966; 45: 554
97. Klein G. N Engl J Med 1975; 293: 1353
98. Ziegler JL, MacGrath IT, Olweny CLM. Lancet 1979; ii: 936
99. Isaacson PG. In: de Burgh Norman JE, McGurk M (eds). Color Atlas and Text of the Salivary Glands. Diseases, Disorders and Surgery. Mosby-Wolfe, London, 1995: 289
100. Pollock A. Br Dent J 1977; 142: 369

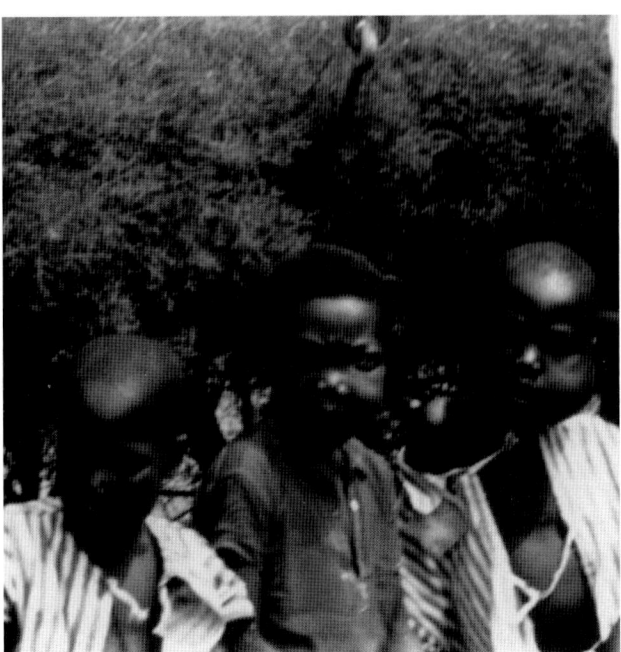

Figure 13.28 Burkitt's lymphoma.

thyroid. The deposits develop as rapidly proliferating masses within the gingival tissues, or they may present as osteolytic lesions in the jaws. Pain, anaesthesia, or even pathological fracture can occur. The underlying disease should be treated if possible and the local metastasis can be excised or irradiated.[88]

THE TONGUE

CONGENITAL ABNORMALITIES

Bifid tongue

Bifid tongue may occur as an isolated phenomenon or can be associated with chromosomal syndromes. It sometimes occurs in the Pierre Robin syndrome and may be associated with a medial cleft of the lower lip. It is a constant feature in the orofacial–digital syndrome.[101]

Fissured tongue

In this condition, the dorsum of the tongue is crossed by irregular 3–4 mm-deep fissures running longitudinally or diagonally. The mucosa is covered with normal papillae, and the only significance of the condition is that some patients complain of soreness from inflammation at the base of the fissures. Antifungal agents may then be beneficial.

Tongue tie (ankyloglossia)

This condition is the result of varying degrees of shortness of the lingual fraenum, which in the most extreme case attaches the tip of the tongue to the mucosa behind the lower incisor teeth. Children with tongue tie cannot protrude the tongue, but treatment is only indicated if the tongue's contribution to controlling food and oral hygiene is compromised. Ankyloglossia rarely, if ever, affects speech.

Fraenectomy is carried out by excising the fraenum from its attachments, allowing the tip of the tongue to be pulled away from the floor of the mouth.[102] The resulting defect, which runs from behind the incisor teeth between the submandibular duct orifices and along the ventral surface of the tongue, should be carefully sutured to prevent scarring.

GEOGRAPHICAL TONGUE (ERYTHEMA MIGRANS LINGUAE)

This common condition is characterized by smooth red patches that appear to migrate across the dorsum of the tongue like fairy rings. The scalloped edge is well defined by mild hyperkeratinization of the unaffected mucosa.[103] Histologically, there is thinning of the epithelium, for which there is no explanation. The patient should be reassured that the appearance is of no significance and can be ignored.

MEDIAN RHOMBOID GLOSSITIS

This reddish, diamond-shaped patch arises in the midline of the dorsum of the tongue anterior to the circumvallate papillae. It is seen only in adults, and its cause is unknown, although it was once thought to be the result of persistence of the tuberculum impar. Histologically, there is depapillation with acanthosis, irregular hyperplasia, and chronic inflammatory infiltration. It is not premalignant. There are no symptoms and the patient should be reassured.[104]

BLACK HAIRY TONGUE

Black hairy tongue is the result of overgrowth of the filiform papillae, which form a thick, brownish-black, hairy mat on the dorsum of the tongue.[105] The discoloration is from pigment-producing organisms or fungi. The cause is unknown, although heavy smoking, sucking antiseptics, and antibiotics have been blamed. The patient should be reassured that the condition is not dangerous and advised to scrape or brush the tongue to remove the overgrowth.

GLOSSITIS

This is a term used to describe a red, smooth (depapillated) and sore tongue. It occurs in iron deficiency, pernicious anaemia, and other vitamin B group deficiencies, which are now rarely seen. It may also be caused by candida infection.[106]

SORE TONGUE

There are usually no abnormal appearances, and once haematological abnormalities have been excluded, the cause is usually ascribed to psychogenic disorders.[107] It occurs principally in postmenopausal females, and hormonal changes are known to induce mucosal atrophy.

MACROGLOSSIA

Enlargement of the tongue occurs in acromegaly and sometimes neurofibromatosis. The tongue may also be enlarged when it

REFERENCES

101. Gorlin RJ, Pindborg JJ, Cohen MM. Syndromes of the Head and Neck. 2nd edn. McGraw Hill, New York, 1976: 32, 91
102. Killey HC, Seward GR, Kay LW. An Outline of Oral Surgery, Part 1. John Wright, Bristol, 1975: 65
103. Hume WJ. J Dent 1975; 3: 25
104. Baughman RA. Oral Surg 1971; 31: 56
105. Neville BW, Damm DD, Allen CM et al. In: Neville BW, Damm DD, Allen CM et al (eds). Oral and Maxillofacial Pathology. WB Saunders, Philadelphia, 1995: 12
106. Jensen H, Kjerulf K, Hjorting-Hansen E. Acta Med Scand 1965; 178: 651
107. Lamey P-J, Lamb AB. Br Med J 1988; 296: 1243

contains a vascular malformation such as a haemangioma, lymphangioma, or more often a mixture of the two. The growth of these angiomas can have a secondary effect on the size of the mandible.[108] The tongue may also contain an angioma in patients with the Sturge–Weber syndrome.

Macroglossia can develop in a quarter or more of patients with primary amyloidosis.[109] Macroglossia also occurs in the mucolipidoses (especially Hurler's syndrome), in the mucopolysaccharidoses, and in other genetic syndromes.[110] Hemihypertrophy of the face is associated with diffuse or unilateral macroglossia, which may be associated with hypertrophy of the fungiform papillae. Macroglossia is also a major component of the Beckwith–Wiedeman syndrome.[111] The apparent enlargement of the tongue in the Pierre Robin syndrome and some muscular dystrophies is caused by glossoptosis.

The enlarged tongue may have its size reduced by wedge resection of the anterior two-thirds to treat some of these conditions.[112]

INFECTION OF THE JAWS

The most common dental infection is caries, and it may go on to produce dentoalveolar and soft tissue infection.

ACUTE OSTEOMYELITIS

This condition is still encountered but, in view of the large number of dental infections that arise from within the medullary bone, it has a surprisingly low incidence. The virulence of the organism and a reduced host response from immunosuppression play a part in its development. It causes intense pain, fever and, if the mandible is involved, paraesthesia of the inferior dental nerve. After 5–10 days, pus starts to discharge and the teeth loosen.

Treatment is by a combination of antibiotics and debridement.[113] Early disease may be aborted by intravenous penicillin or clindamycin until the systemic symptoms improve, when oral antibodies can commence. It is important to culture the organism whenever possible and determine antibacterial sensitivities. Some patients progress to a subacute or chronic form. Sequestration, decortication, or even bone resection may be required to eradicate the infection if fistulae develop or the purulent discharge persists.

Infantile osteomyelitis is an uncommon but serious condition that carried a significant mortality before the introduction of antibiotics. The infection is disseminated through the bloodstream and targets highly vascularized bone, for example the maxilla or temporomandibular joints. The destruction and scarring that result can have a deleterious effect on growth. The condition usually presents in the first few weeks of life with local periorbital cellulitis and systemic malaise, fever and pyrexia. The organism is usually a staphylococcus and intravenous penicillin is the treatment of choice, together with simple drainage where necessary.

CHRONIC OSTEOMYELITIS

The mandible may respond to chronic irritation by forming focal condensations of sclerotic bone in young adults.[114] The source of the irritation is usually a chronically infected tooth. Garré's sclerosing osteomyelitis is a proliferative response to irritation in the periosteum of the jaw that leads to thickening of the membrane and cortical proliferation of bone.[115] The condition primarily affects children and young adults, and reflects the growth and proliferative potential of bone at this age.

Initially, the condition is painless with dark ebony-like bone exposed in the floor of the mouth. Later, it becomes painful as secondary infection develops. Long courses of tetracycline may improve the symptoms, but the mucosal defect seldom heals. Minor surgical debridement with primary mucosal closure may be successful in localized disease and is worth trying. In advanced cases, new vascularized tissue is required to facilitate healing. This may be achieved by surgical excision and reconstruction with a vascularized bone graft.

Box 13.6 Classification of cysts of the jaws

Odontogenic cysts

Inflammatory
- Apical
- Lateral periodontal
- Residual

Developmental
- Dentigerous
- Primordial
- Keratocyst
- Calcifying odontogenic

Non-odontogenic cysts

Epitheliated
- Globulomaxillary
- Median palatine
- Nasopalatine

Non-epitheliated
- Aneurysmal
- Solitary bone
- Stafne's bone cavity

CYSTS OF THE JAWS

Cysts are a frequent occurrence in the jaws because epithelial remnants persist in the bone after tooth formation: odontogenic cysts (Box 13.6). Other cysts develop from epithelial residues at the lines of fusion of embryonic processes, so-called fissural cysts. For an understanding of the origin of the odontogenic cysts and also the rarer odontogenic tumours of the jaws, a brief description of tooth development is necessary.[116]

REFERENCES

108. Gupta OP. Arch Otolaryngol 1971; 93: 378
109. Keith DA. Br J Oral Surg 1972; 10: 107
110. Neville BW, Damm DD, Allen CM et al. In: Neville BW, Damm DD, Allen CM et al (eds). Oral and Maxillofacial Pathology. WB Saunders, Philadelphia, 1995: 8
111. Gorlin RJ, Pindborg JJ. Syndromes of the Head and Neck. McGraw Hill, New York, 1976: 42
112. Hendrick JW, Antonio S. Surgery 1956; 39: 674
113. Adekeye EO, Cornash J. Br J Oral Maxillofac Surg 1985; 23: 24
114. Eversole LR, Stone CE, Strub D. Oral Surg Oral Med Oral Path 1984; 58: 456
115. Felsberg GJ, Gore RL, Schweitzer ME. Oral Surg Oral Med Oral Path 1990; 70: 117
116. Osborn JW, Tencate AR. Advanced Dental Histology. 3rd edn. John Wright, Bristol, 1977

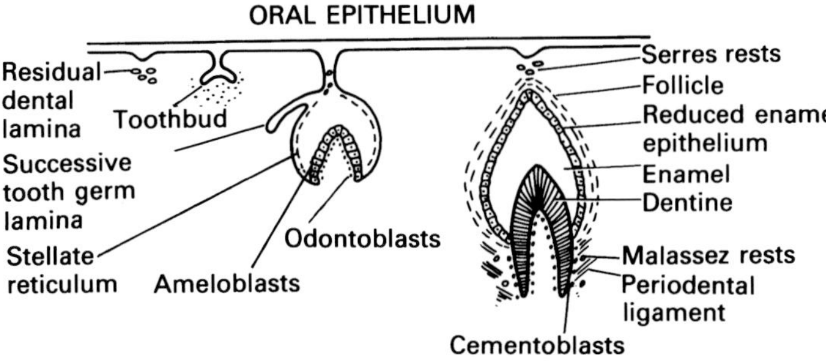

Figure 13.29 The stages of tooth development and the origin of various cell remnants.

At about the sixth week of fetal life, a band of proliferating oral epithelium called the dental lamina protrudes into the underlying mesoderm along the tooth-bearing region of each jaw. Small clumps of mesenchymal cells form in regions that correspond to those of the subsequent tooth germs and become surrounded by stalks of proliferating epithelium, thus establishing the tooth buds. The cap of epithelium, now known as the enamel organ, remains joined to the oral epithelium by a chord of cells, but like the dental lamina between the tooth buds, this eventually breaks down and disappears. Residual epithelium may remain as cell rests (Fig. 13.29).

The enamel organ undergoes differentiation: cells on the inner aspect become cuboidal, there are central star-shaped cells, and somewhat flatter cells form the outer enamel epithelium. The condensation of mesenchymal cells known as the dental papilla is continuous with a layer of connective tissue surrounding the enamel organ called the dental follicle, and eventually this forms the periodontal membrane. The cells immediately adjacent to the enamel epithelium differentiate into a single layer of odontoblasts, which form the dentine. Once this process begins, the cells of the enamel epithelium start laying down enamel and are then known as ameloblasts.

When the crown of the tooth has been formed, the rim of epithelium around its base proliferates downwards as the sheath of Hertwig, inducing cells to form the dentine of the root. The coronal part of the sheath breaks up, and cementoblasts differentiate from the follicular tissue around the root of the tooth and lay down cementum on the root surface, incorporating collagen fibres that make up the periodontal ligament. Residual epithelium remains in this membrane throughout life as the cell rests of Malassez.

ODONTOGENIC CYSTS

Inflammatory cysts

Apical or residual cysts

Apical cysts occur most frequently (55%), and are the result of dental infection stimulating the epithelial remnants to coalesce. They are usually symptomless but may present with acute pain if they become secondarily infected.[117] Radiologically, they appear as well-defined unilocular radiolucencies (Fig. 13.32). Multilocular cysts or those that erode teeth suggest that a more aggressive pathological process is responsible. Small cysts (< 1 cm in diameter) often resolve after root canal therapy or extraction of the tooth, but occasionally may persist. Large cysts require enucleation and, if very large, may warrant marsupialization.

Lateral periodontal cyst

Lateral periodontal cysts are uncommon and have the same aetiology and pathogenesis as apical cysts. Their treatment is the same.

Developmental cysts

Follicular or dentigerous cyst

Follicular or dentigerous cysts are relatively common, and are the result of a cystic degeneration within the follicle around the crown of the tooth. They present as a slowly enlarging, painless swelling and are seen as a unilocular radiolucency related to the crown of a tooth.

Primordial keratocyst

Primordial keratocysts arise from degeneration of the dental stellate reticulum before the tooth forms. They are usually symptomless and present late as painless swellings of the jaw. The mandible is primarily involved at either its angle, the body, or ramus. They are capable of aggressive behaviour and must be correctly diagnosed preoperatively if recurrence is to be avoided. Diagnosis is possible because the aspirated cystic fluid is characterized by a soluble protein content of < 3.5 g/dL. Smaller unilocular cysts are treated by simple enucleation, but this technique is not effective for large multilocular lesions, and a recurrence rate as high as 60% is reported.

Other odontogenic cysts

Calcifying epithelial odontogenic cysts are very rare; one type is a simple cyst, the other a neoplasm. They present as painless swelling of the anterior parts of the jaws, and radiographs demonstrate calcification within the cyst. The simple cysts are treated by enucleation, the others usually by local marginal resection.

Epstein's pearls (Bohn's nodules)

These are gingival cysts, common in the newborn, which tend to rupture spontaneously or involute and are rarely seen after 3 months of age. They form small white nodules 2–3 mm in diameter and are found on the crest of the maxillary and mandibular ridges, and in the midline of the palate. Those arising along the midpalatal raphe develop from epithelial inclusions in the line of fusion of the palatal processes.[118] No treatment is required.

NON-ODONTOGENIC CYSTS (NON-EPITHELIAL CYSTS)

The non-odontogenic cysts are classified according to the lining of the cyst wall. Fissural cysts are lined by epithelium, whereas aneurysmal and solitary bone cysts are lined only by connective tissue.

Aneurysmal bone cysts are rare. Their cause is unknown, and they also affect the axial skeleton (usually the vertebrae and long bones of middle-aged adults). In the jaws, the mandible is affected more frequently than the maxilla, and there is a predilection for the posterior regions of the jaws. Clinically, they present as painful firm swellings with displacement of the associated teeth. Despite their name, they are not pulsatile nor

REFERENCES

117. Killey HC, Kay LW, Seward GR. In: Killey HC, Kay LW, Seward GR (eds). Benign Cystic Lesions of the Jaws, their Diagnosis and Treatment. Churchill Livingstone, Edinburgh, 1977: 75
118. Shear M. Cysts of the Oral Regions. 2nd edn. John Wright, Bristol, 1983: 35

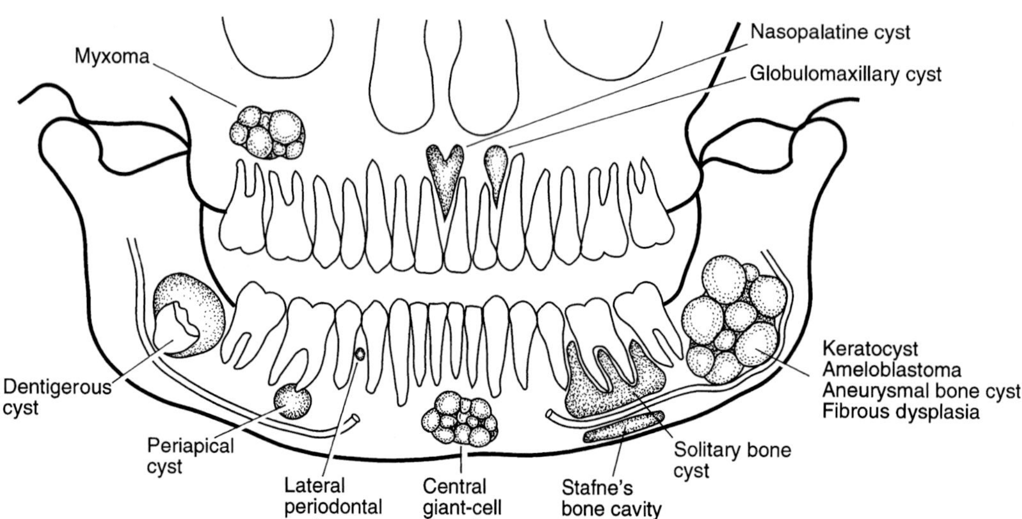

Figure 13.30 Radiolucent lesions of the jaws and their sites of predilection.

are they associated with a bruit. They may present radiologically as unilocular or multilocular radiolucencies (Fig. 13.30). They are treated by curettage and have a recurrence rate of about 25%.

Solitary bone cysts are idiopathic and tend to occur at a younger age (10–20 years) than with aneurysmal bone cysts. They are usually diagnosed as an incidental radiographic finding but can present with swelling and pain. They have a similar distribution in the jaws to aneurysmal bone cysts, and radiographically appear as scalloped radiolucencies above the level of the inferior dental canal (Fig. 13.30). They contain straw-coloured liquid and are treated by curettage.

Stafne's bone cavities are not cysts of the jaws but simply depressions on the lingual aspect of the mandible produced by the submandibular salivary gland. Radiographic images depict the depression as a well-circumscribed unilocular radiolucency below the level of the inferior dental canal (Fig. 13.30).

Non-odontogenic (fissural) cysts

All four fissural cysts occur infrequently and can be surgically enucleated.

Nasopalatine cysts are the most common type of fissural cyst, occurring in about 1% of the population. They develop from epithelium trapped between the median nasal and palatal processes, and are located between or above the roots of the maxillary central incisor teeth (Fig. 13.30).

Globulomaxillary cysts develop from epithelium trapped between the median nasal and maxillary processes, and therefore present as discrete radiolucencies between the maxillary lateral incisor and canine teeth (Fig. 13.30). They are usually an incidental radiographic finding, but when infected are acutely painful.

Median palatal cysts develop from epithelium trapped between the palatal processes and usually present as painless swellings in the affected area.

Median mandibular cysts develop from epithelium trapped between the mandibular processes.

OSTEODYSTROPHIES

The diseases of bone included under this heading are neither inflammatory nor neoplastic but are genetic, metabolic, or of unknown cause.

GENETIC BONE DISEASES

Osteogenesis imperfecta

This is a hereditary disorder in which the bones are poorly formed and fragile. The underlying defect is one of collagen synthesis: although cartilaginous growth is normal, cortical plates of compact bone are not formed.[119]

Cleidocranial dysostosis

Cleidocranial dysostosis is a rare familial disorder in which anodontia and delayed eruption of teeth are accompanied by defective formation of the clavicles, delayed closure of fontanelles, and maxillary hypoplasia.[120]

METABOLIC BONE DISEASES

Rickets

Disorders of calcium and phosphorus metabolism caused by deficiency of vitamin D, in rickets or chronic renal disease, result in defects in the development of bone but rarely of the teeth. Eruption of the teeth may be delayed, and hypocalcification of dentine occurs only in severe cases.[121] A diagnosis is made on clinical and radiological examination, and is confirmed by finding low serum levels of calcium and phosphorus with a raised alkaline phosphatase.

Hyperparathyroidism

The jaws are commonly affected by the giant cell 'tumours' (brown tumours) that occur in hyperparathyroidism.[122] This condition should always be considered, in the older female patient, when a giant cell granuloma of the jaw is diagnosed histologically or if there is a recurrence after adequate excision. Granulomas can develop in either jaw, causing radiolucent cyst-like swellings of the bone and loosening of the teeth. Successful treatment of the hyperparathyroidism causes the osteolytic lesions to regress.

REFERENCES

119. Lewis NA et al. Oral Surg 1958; 11: 289
120. Gorlin RJ, Pindborg JJ. Syndromes of the Head and Neck. McGraw-Hill, New York, 1976
121. Cawson RA. Brit Dent J 1964; 117: 141

Central giant cell granuloma

Central giant cell granulomas are idiopathic lesions of the jaw bones that occur most commonly in young adults and females. They present clinically with swelling and tooth displacement. The anterior parts of the jaws, and particularly the mandible, are the most commonly affected sites. Radiologically, these granulomas have a unilocular appearance. The diagnosis is established by means of an incisional biopsy. A small proportion of giant cell granulomas are associated with secondary hyperparathyroidism. Histologically, they consist of focal collections of giant cells, and they need to be distinguished from other intraosseous giant cell lesions such as osteoclastomas and aneurysmal bone cysts. The treatment usually consists of enucleation, although a favourable response to calcitonin has also been described.[123] Those cases caused by hyperparathyroidism respond to treatment of the underlying condition (see Ch. 15).

Scurvy

Deficiency of vitamin C (ascorbic acid) is normally the result of gross dietary deprivation. It may occur subclinically in elderly people whose diets do not include fresh fruit.[124] It results in the defective formation of collagen and osteoid tissue.

Swollen oedematous and bleeding gums occur in patients with poor oral hygiene. There is a haemorrhagic tendency from increased capillary fragility. The Hess capillary fragility test produces capillary rupture, and areas of ecchymosis are common both intraorally and on the skin. Patients with these symptoms may have leukaemia, which must be excluded.

BONE DISEASE OF UNKNOWN CAUSE

Paget's disease (osteitis deformans)

The aetiology of Paget's disease (see Ch. 41) is unknown. It affects patients past middle age and occurs in 3% of patients over 40 years old. The incidence rises in the seventh decade to 70% in men and 30% in women.[125] The most frequently involved bones are the pelvis, femora, vertebrae and skull, when the jaws may also be affected.

There is a rapid, irregular and exaggerated resorption and replacement of bone, causing thickening, swelling, and increased vascularity, often with severe, intractable pain. Serum calcium and phosphorus levels are normal, but the alkaline phosphatase level is raised. When the skull is affected, it slowly enlarges, as do the jaws; the maxilla more frequently than the mandible, necessitating frequent adjustments to dentures.[126] The teeth may become displaced and are affected by hypercementosis, which fuses them to the bone, complicating extractions. In the osteolytic phase of the disease, oral surgery can be complicated by severe haemorrhage, and in sclerotic disease, surgery may be followed by chronic osteomyelitis.

The main radiological changes are irregular patches of sclerosis and radiolucency (cotton-wool appearance), enlargement of the bone, and hypercementosis of the roots of the teeth.[127] When the jaws alone are affected, general treatment to suppress bone metabolism is not required.

Fibrous dysplasia

Fibrous dysplasia may be monostotic or polyostotic; the latter can be further classified as Jaffe's disease and Albright's syndrome.[128]

Albright's syndrome has an insidious onset between 10 and 20 years of age with skeletal, cutaneous and endocrine manifestations. The skeletal involvement tends to be unilateral and affects the cranium (50%), mandible (30%), and long bones. Bone pain is the most common presenting symptom. Involvement of the facial bones can cause significant disfigurement. Café-au-lait spots are a feature, and there are endocrine abnormalities of the pituitary, thyroid and parathyroid glands. Sexual precocity occurs in female patients.

Jaffe's variety of polyostotic dysplasia has a more restricted bony involvement than that of Albright's syndrome. Café-au-lait spots are also present but endocrine abnormalities do not occur.

In the monostotic variety, single bones are affected. It presents as a slowly progressive facial deformity with displacement of teeth and visual disturbance from orbital wall and optic canal involvement.

A familial form of fibrous dysplasia called cherubism causes bilateral deformity. When the maxilla is affected, there is subperiosteal deposition of bone on to the floor of the orbits, displacing the eyes upwards and exposing the sclerae, producing the appearance of a cherub. The condition stabilizes at about 7 years of age, when the deformity can be corrected.

TUMOURS OF THE JAWS

Primary tumours of bone can arise in the jaws or invade the jaws from adjacent structures. Metastases also occur. Tumours can also arise from odontogenic tissue (Box 13.7). This tissue, which is responsible for the highly complex process of tooth formation, can be the origin of true neoplasms, malformations of dental tissues known as odontomes, or mixtures of both of these.

Both primary and odontogenic tumours are uncommon. The most common cause of a jaw tumour is local invasion from adjacent epithelium.

ODONTOGENIC TUMOURS

Ameloblastoma

The most common odontogenic tumour is the ameloblastoma, with an annual incidence of one per 10^6 in the UK population, thus most of these odontogenic tumours are little more than curiosities. They are generally low-grade tumours. Ameloblastoma is so called because the cells have histological similarity to ameloblasts. It is virtually restricted to the jaws and is locally invasive.[129] Various histological patterns are seen, some closely resembling the enamel organ. Cyst formation is common and occurs as microcysts in a predominantly solid tumour or as large unilocular cysts, often indistinguishable from non-neoplastic cysts.[130] Most tumours develop in middle age, predominantly in the mandible, and usually in the molar region or ascending ramus. They present as symptomless, slow-growing swellings, sometimes attaining a large size if left untreated. Radiologically,

REFERENCES

122. Silverman S Jr, Ware WH, Gillooly C Jr. Oral Surg 1968; 26: 184
123. Harris M. Br J Oral Maxillofac Surg 1993; 31: 89
124. Tillman HT. Oral Surg 1961; 14: 877
125. Collins DH. Lancet 1956; ii: 51
126. Smith BJ, Eveson JW. J Oral Pathol 1981; 10: 233
127. Beeching B. Interpreting Dental Radiographs. Update Books, London, 1981: 137
128. Neville BW, Damm DD, Allen CM et al. In: Neville BW, Damm DD, Allen CM et al (eds). Oral and Maxillofacial Pathology. WB Saunders, Philadelphia, 1995: 460
129. Small IA, Waldron CA. Oral Surg 1955; 8: 281
130. Robinson L, Martinez MG. Cancer 1977; 40: 227

Box 13.7 Classification of primary odontogenic neoplasms of the jaw bones

Epithelial (ectodermal) origin
- Ameloblastoma
- Calcifying epithelial odontogenic tumour
- Adenomatoid tumour
- Ameloblastic odontoma
- Ameloblastic fibroma
- Ameloblastic fibro-odontoma
- Ameloblastic fibrosarcoma

Connective tissue (mesodermal) origin
- Cementoblastoma
- Myxoma

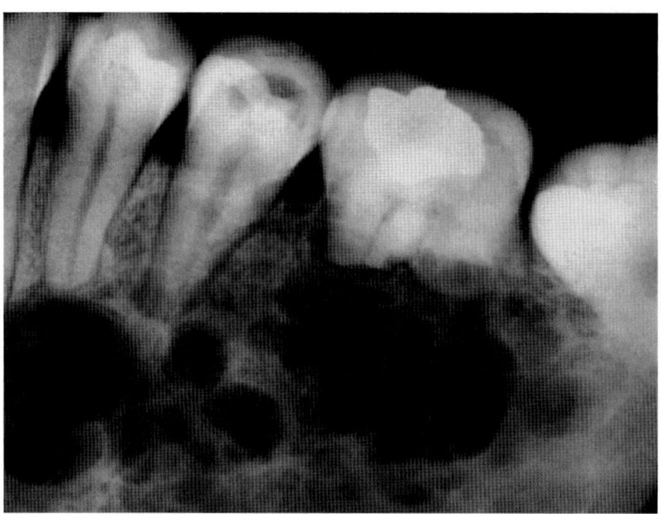

Figure 13.31 The multilocular appearance of an ameloblastoma.

there is a well-defined radiolucent area that is characteristically multilocular with small daughter cysts on the periphery (Fig. 13.31).

Treatment

The ameloblastoma tends to penetrate medullary spaces, and thus should be removed with a margin of up to 1 cm of cancellous bone. A subperiosteal excision can usually be carried out with a small chance of recurrence. Some cases require a full-thickness excision of the affected part of the jaw and restoration with a bone graft.

Follow-up should be indefinite, as recurrences may occur up to 20 years or more later.[131]

Cementoma

These tumours are characterized by continuing proliferation of cementum.[132]

Benign cementoblastoma mainly develops in young adults as an irregular or rounded mass of cementum attached to the root of a mandibular molar or premolar tooth.

Cementifying fibroma is a mass of connective tissue that forms within the jaw, containing nodules of cementum-like material. It occurs in the molar region in middle-aged patients.

In gigantiform cementoma, several tumours may coalesce and grow until there is enlargement of the jaw. Radiographically, the tumours appear as lobulated radiopaque masses with a radiolucent border.

Myxoma

This tumour is seen only in the jaws and is regarded as being of odontogenic origin. It is a different entity from the myxomatous change that occurs in other tumours. These tumours consist of spindle-shaped cells, scantily distributed in a mucoid intercellular material showing a resemblance to dental mesenchyme. Young people are mainly affected and present with a slow-growing, painless swelling of the jaw.[133]

Radiologically, a finely trabeculated 'soap bubble' radiolucency is seen expanding the bone. The tumour is infiltrative, and recurrence after excision is common.

Odontomes

This term is now used for malformations of dental tissue of developmental origin. These 'tumours' are really hamartomas in that the enamel, dentine, pulp and cementum are found in relationship to one another.

BENIGN NON-ODONTOGENIC TUMOURS OF THE JAW

Fibroma

This rare tumour may arise in the bone or beneath the periosteum. Histologically, it consists of fibroblasts and bundles of collagen fibres in a whorled arrangement. Fibromas present as a slow-growing, round mass on the surface of the jaw or, if endosteal, will eventually expand the bone. They may invade the antrum and become quite large before symptoms occur.[134]

Ossifying fibroma

This uncommon tumour usually arises in children's mandibles and presents as a slow-growing, painless swelling. Radiologically, it appears as a well-defined radiolucent area with speckled opacities throughout; these are small areas of calcification that are seen in the cellular fibrous tissue.[135] Local surgical excision is indicated.

Chondroma

Chondroma rarely occurs in the jaws. The tumour presents as a rounded hard mass that may cause asymmetry of the mandible or a radiolucent expansion of either jaw.[136] Sarcomatous change can occur, and wide excision is necessary.

Osteoma

Compact or cancellous osteomas are occasionally seen in either jaw, but localized overgrowths known as exostoses are more common, especially in the maxilla.

Torus palatinus

Torus palatinus is an exostosis peculiar to the palate, and develops in early adult life as a smooth, rounded, symmetrical swelling in the midline of the hard palate (Fig. 13.32).[137] It need only be removed if it interferes with a denture.

REFERENCES

131. Gardner DG, Pecak AM. Cancer 1980; 46: 2514
132. Pindborg JJ, Kramer IR. Histological Typing of Odontogenic Tumours. World Health Organization, Geneva, 1971: 31
133. Killey HC, Kay LW. Br J Oral Surg 1964; 2: 124
134. Wesley RK, Wysocki GP, Mintz SM. Oral Surg 1975; 40: 235
135. Langdon JD, Rapidis AD, Patel MF. Br J Oral Surg 1976; 14: 1
136. MacGregor AB. Br Dent J 1952; 94: 39
137. Kolas S, Walperin V et al. Oral Surg 1953; 6: 1134

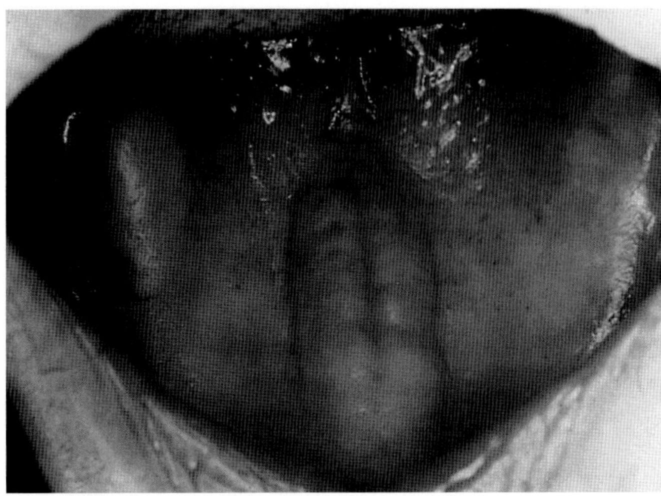

Figure 13.32 Torus palatinus.

Torus mandibularis

Torus mandibularis is a similar exostosis found bilaterally on the lingual side of the mandible in the premolar region. It need not be removed.

Juvenile angiofibroma

This neoplasm occurs primarily in males and is characterized by aggressive local growth. It arises from the pterygopalatine area and is particularly vascular. It extends as finger-like protrusions into local structures, especially the nose, pterygomaxillary fissure, maxillary antrum, ethmoid, and sphenoidal sinus. Occasionally, it extends through foramina in the skull base to enter the cranial cavity. It usually presents as a nasal mass accompanied by frightening epistaxis.

Almost all tumours occur in males between 10 and 20 years of age, and they are known for spontaneous regression.[138] The predominance in adolescent males suggests an endocrine origin. Numerous ways have been found to manage these tumours, including cryotherapy, embolization, sclerotherapy, chemotherapy, and surgical excision.[139] Operative excision is preferred and is successful in 80–100%.[140] Radiotherapy has been used in difficult cases.

MALIGNANT TUMOURS OF THE JAW

Osteogenic sarcoma

Osteogenic sarcoma is a highly malignant tumour (see Ch. 42) that rarely develops in the jaws. It usually affects young adults but may occur in the elderly after irradiation.[141] The tumour is osteoproliferative with osteoblasts, fibroblasts, or cartilage cells seen on histological examination. The presence of osteoid is diagnostic.

The tumour forms a rapidly growing swelling that may be painful. Radiographs show resorption of normal bone with expansion and occasional radiopacities from bone formation throughout the tumour. Metastasis may already be present in the lungs at the time of diagnosis. Treatment is the same as that for other soft tissue sarcomas (see Ch. 42).

Secondary neoplasms in the jaws

Metastatic deposits in the jaws usually arise from primary growths in the bronchus, breast, liver, thyroid or kidney. Deposits tend to occur at the lingula (mandibular foramen) or the mental foramen. The jaws are occasionally the site of the first apparent metastasis, but a skeletal survey often shows widespread symptomless secondaries elsewhere.[142]

Common symptoms are pain and swelling of the gingival tissue overlying the bone. Anaesthesia of the lip is often present as the result of sensory nerve involvement at an early stage. Biopsy confirms the diagnosis. Treatment is palliative, and symptoms may be relieved by local excision or by radiotherapy.[143]

Carcinoma of the maxilla

Carcinoma affecting the upper alveolus or palate is a consequence of oral cancer. Tumours at these sites present as a swelling or oral ulceration. The treatment is usually surgical excision of part or the whole of the maxilla, depending on the site and the extent and type of tumour. A neck dissection is not normally indicated, but otherwise the same principles apply as in other tumours of the mouth.

Squamous cell carcinoma of the maxillary antrum is a separate entity. It is the most common malignant tumour of the maxilla (63%) and arises from the mucosal lining of the paranasal sinuses. Adenocarcinoma accounts for a further 16%, and various sarcomas, reticuloses, and salivary gland tumours are occasionally seen.[144] Adenocarcinoma has a predilection for the ethmoid air cells; wood dust has been confirmed as one aetiological factor.[145]

Squamous cell carcinoma of the maxillary antrum has a high mortality (60%) because the tumour is usually advanced when first diagnosed. Lymph node involvement, present in less than 10% of patients at presentation, is a contraindication to aggressive curative surgery.[146,147]

This tumour arises in the hidden bony compartment of the maxilla, accounting for its late presentation. Pain, swelling, and nasal obstruction are the common initial symptoms. Proptosis develops if there is invasion of the orbit superiorly. Anterior invasion is associated with infraorbital nerve paraesthesia, and medial invasion causes nasal obstruction. The disease is advanced and has a poor prognosis if the pterygoid plates and muscles are involved, with accompanying trismus.

Computerized tomography is essential for estimating the size and extent of the tumour. Recent advances that allow accurate superimposition of positron emission tomography images on CT or MRI scans have improved the clinician's appreciation of tumour extent.[148] Biopsy may be carried out via a Caldwell–Luc approach but is best done via the intranasal route, as the lateral wall of the nose is always removed in the subsequent operation.

REFERENCES

138. Cummings BJ. In: Harris DFN (ed). Dilemmas in Otolaryngology. Churchill Livingstone, Edinburgh, 1988: 223
139. Fitzpatrick PJ, Briant TD, Berman JM. Arch Otolaryngol 1980; 106: 234
140. Witt TR, Shah JP, Sternberg SS. Am J Surg 1983; 146: 212
141. Garrington GE, Scofield HH et al. Cancer 1967; 20: 377
142. Hatziotis JC, Constantinidou H, Papanayotou PH. Oral Surg 1973; 36: 544
143. Henk JM, Langdon JD. Malignant Tumours of the Oral Cavity. Edward Arnold, London, 1985: 211
144. Lewis JS, Castro EB. J Laryngol Otol 1972; 86: 255
145. Hadfield EH. Ann Coll Surg Engl 1970; 46: 301
146. Stell PM. Proc R Soc Med 1975; 68: 83
147. Harrison PF. Laryngol Otol 1976; 90: 69
148. Wong WL, Hussain K et al. Am J Surg 1996; 172: 628

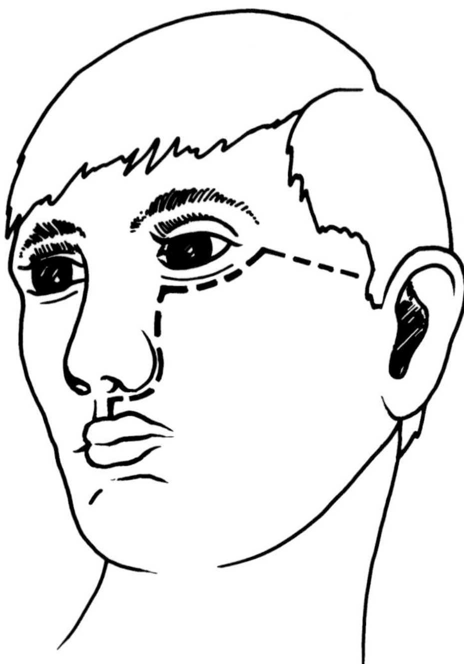

Figure 13.33 The Weber–Fergusson approach for a maxillectomy.

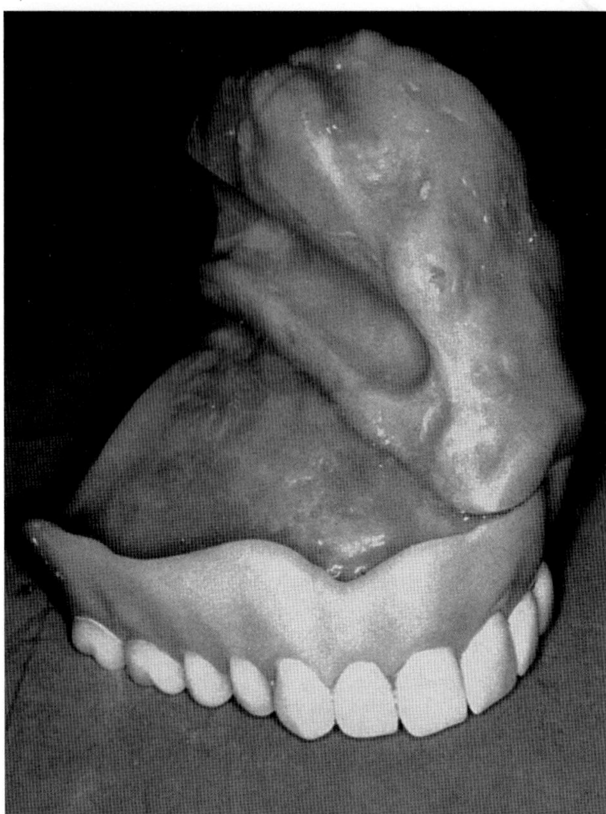

Figure 13.34 A hollow box obturator attached to an upper denture.

Treatment

The prognosis for this condition is relatively poor: 6 out of 10 patients are incurable because of advanced disease. Surgery is disfiguring, especially when it involves maxillectomy with enucleation of the eye, although a dental obturator maintains good function. Surgical resection with adjuvant radiotherapy gives the best prospect of cure.[149] Chemotherapy and radiotherapy have been used, with surgery reserved as a debulking procedure,[150] but this has not yet received widespread acceptance.

MAXILLECTOMY Maxillectomy is a difficult operation to perform, as there are no fascial planes to follow and the tumour frequently extends to the posterior maxillary wall and into the pterygoid area. A temporary tarsorrhaphy should be performed first. The Weber–Fergusson skin incision is most commonly employed (Fig. 13.33).[151] This begins in the midline of the upper lip, skirts the ala margin, and runs upwards along the lateral border of the nose to the medial canthus. The incision is continued laterally about 5 mm below the lower lid to end over the zygoma. A cheek flap is then elevated in a supraperiosteal plane by incising the mucosa along the buccal sulcus. The alveolus and palate are split in the midline, and the nasal process of the maxilla is divided. The orbital contents may be preserved if the orbital floor is not involved. The antral wall can then be entered just below the orbital rim. The ethmoids are sectioned below the ethmoidal arteries if the eye is not to be preserved, and the bone cut continued inferiorly across the orbital floor to meet the inferior orbital fissure.

The malar process is divided or, if this bone is also to be removed, the zygomatic arch and frontal process of the maxilla must be separated by division of the frontozygomatic suture down through the lateral orbital wall to the inferior orbital fissure.

The ramus or coronoid process of the mandible can be resected to give free access to the infratemporal fossa and pterygoid plates if the tumour has breached the posterior maxillary wall. The latter are separated from their attachment to the base of the skull. The soft palate is now divided as dictated by the tumour extension before the maxilla is mobilized. Much of the final dissection in the nasopharynx has to be done blind.

After the antrum has been removed, it is essential to support the cheek. Traditionally, the raw surface of the cheek flap is skin-grafted to prevent scarring, and the cavity packed by a previously constructed base plate or denture and held in place by wire.[153] Frontal wiring should be employed to retain the prosthesis if the zygoma and orbital rim have been removed.

The definitive obturator, usually soft-lined and of hollow box construction, may be fitted when healing has been completed, and in most cases overcomes major disfigurement (Fig. 13.34). Primary reconstruction with microvascular flaps and dental implants is now an alternative. This helps to improve the stability of the eye prosthesis.

REFERENCES

149. Ketcham AS, Van Buren JM. Tumours of the paranasal sinuses: a therapeutic challenge. Am J Surg 1985; 150: 406
150. Sakai S, Hohki A, Fuchilate H et al. Cancer 1983; 52: 1360
151. Stell PM, Maran AGD. Head and Neck Surgery. 2nd edn. Heinemann, London, 1978: 270
152. Harrison DFN. In: Dudley H, Carter D (eds). Rob and Smith's Operative Surgery, Nose and Throat. 4th edn. Butterworths, London, 1978: 145
153. Rayne J. In: Norman J, Bramley PA (eds). Textbook and Colour Atlas of Temporomandibular Joint Diseases, Disorders and Surgery. Wolfe Medical, London, 1990: 151

THE TEMPEROMANDIBULAR JOINT

The initial movement on opening the jaw is rotational between the condyle and meniscus, then the meniscus glides down the slope of the articular eminence. Maximal opening is again a rotational movement.[153]

DISLOCATION OF THE JAW

Dislocation of the mandible can be acute or chronic. The mandibular condyle can be displaced superiorly, posteriorly or anteriorly; the last of these is the most common when associated with a fracture. The condyle can also be displaced laterally or, more commonly, medially, as this is the direction of muscle pull. Acute dislocation is relatively common and may be the result of trauma or excessive mouth opening. It can also occur in patients with psychiatric disorders. In chronic disease, lax ligaments predispose to recurrent dislocation. Long-standing dislocation is often overlooked, especially in a withdrawn psychiatric or geriatric patient.

Condylar dislocation normally occurs on one side and results in the chin deviating to the opposite side with an inability to close the mouth (Fig. 13.35). A preauricular depression and radiological evidence of an empty glenoid fossa confirm the diagnosis. The acute dislocation is painful, and the masticatory muscles soon go into spasm. Simple reduction may prove impossible unless undertaken immediately; muscle relaxants and intravenous diazepam (Valium) are usually required. Reduction is accomplished by applying downward pressure in the molar region, with thumbs well protected by padding, and at the same time elevating the chin point with the fingers.

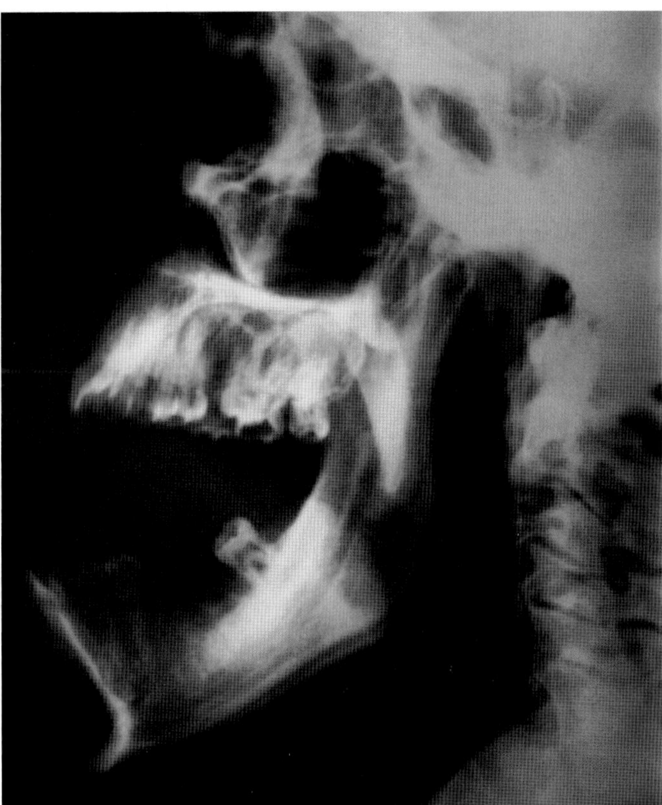

Figure 13.35 A lateral skull radiograph showing bilateral dislocation of the temporomandibular joints.

Recurrent dislocation is a distressing condition, each episode being accompanied by pain and requiring reduction. The restraining capsule around the joint can be tightened with sclerosing agents or surgery. Alternatively, the articulating eminence can be removed to allow the condyle to move freely over the surface, or conversely augmented with bone grafts to block the passage of the condyle. All these surgical procedures induce a degree of local fibrosis, which contributes to limitation in joint movement. A long-standing dislocation can be difficult to reduce, and coronoidectomy may be required to release the powerful temporalis muscle.

TRISMUS

Trismus is a functional inability to open the mouth, and is a symptom rather than a disorder in its own right. The most frequent cause is temporomandibular joint dysfunction, and it may also follow an inferior dental nerve block from trauma or haematoma in the medial pterygoid muscle. Direct invasion of muscles by a carcinoma is another unremitting cause of trismus. Disorders of the central nervous system in which trismus is an incidental feature include tetanus, motor neurone disease, dyskinesia produced by phenothiazine drugs, and hysteria. Symptoms regress with the treatment of the underlying condition.

ANKYLOSIS

Permanent limitation of movement of the jaw may be caused by fibrous, bony ankylosis or mechanical obstruction of mandibular movement. There may be an associated deficiency in mandibular growth if it occurs in childhood. The majority of patients have surprisingly little difficulty in taking an adequate diet.

Ankylosis is an uncommon condition in developed countries. The majority of cases follow injury or occasionally infection in children under 10 years of age.

Unilateral ankylosis causes deviation of the mandible to the affected side. In children, bilateral ankylosis results in a 'bird face', with a tiny, retruded mandible and compensatory growth of the alveolar bone around the teeth in an attempt to maintain dental occlusion.

Management

In children, it is important to re-establish mandibular mobility and function; facial aesthetics are of secondary concern as they maintain a potential for growth. Reconstructive procedures are delayed until the teenage years. In adults, once the ankylosis has been convincingly eradicated (recurrence is common), reconstruction of the mandible is undertaken. In long-standing ankylosis, it is necessary to remove both the coronoid processes to release the vice-like grip of the fibrotic temporalis muscles. Once the segment of ankylosed bone is removed from around the condyle, a strip of temporalis muscle is rotated inferiorly to line the glenoid area, and an interpositional graft is used to replace the condylar segment to maintain the vertical height of the ramus. Early mobilization of the joint is encouraged to avoid reankylosis.

TEMPOROMANDIBULAR JOINT DYSFUNCTION

This troublesome condition is characterized by one or more of the symptoms of pain, clicking, and limited jaw opening. The cause of this disorder is still poorly understood, but it appears to be caused by abnormalities of the tripartite joint structure. There is a strong psychological component in many patients, who often exhibit neuroticism, anxiety and depression. It is usually a self-limiting condition, and the vast majority of patients spontaneously improve within a few months.[154] The underlying mechanism is probably related to overloading of the joint or abnormal joint use. Surgery should be limited to arthroscopy and lavage unless identified pathology is present.

ARTHRITIS OF THE TEMPOROMANDIBULAR JOINT

Rheumatoid arthritis

The temporomandibular joint is never involved alone: patients usually seek treatment for other affected joints. Surgical intervention is rarely required in adults, but in Still's disease the childhood condyle may lose its growth potential, leading to a bird face.

Osteoarthritis

Although the mandibular joint is not weight-bearing, degenerative changes are occasionally seen.[155] The condition is self-limiting.

Suppurative arthritis

Suppurative arthritis is rare, as most infections are now promptly treated with antibiotics. The joint is swollen and painful, with marked trismus. Destruction of bone may lead to ankylosis if left untreated. Treatment is by antibiotics combined with bone and joint debridement.

REFERENCES

154. Toller PA. Scientific Foundation in Dentistry. Heinemann, London, 1974: 596
155. Ogus H. Br J Oral Surg 1979; 17: 17

Diseases of the salivary glands

14

Michael Gleeson, Victoria M. M. Ward

INTRODUCTION

Salivary tissue is found in large, localized aggregates as the parotid, submandibular and sublingual glands, and as solitary, isolated mucosal or minor glands that are liberally distributed throughout the mouth and pharynx. The diseases described in this chapter can affect salivary tissue in both the major and the minor glands. However, for the most part, it is the management of major gland disease processes, particularly tumours, that attracts most surgical attention.

The quality, quantity and constituents of saliva vary according to the site of its production and the circumstances of its generation. The parotids produce serous saliva while the submandibular and sublingual glands produce a more mucoid secretion. Saliva stimulated in response to the sight and smell of food, or in the process of mastication, differs from that secreted at other times. About 1.5 L of saliva is produced every day. Saliva contributes to preparation of food for swallowing, initiates carbohydrate digestion, and helps maintain oral and dental health. Disorders that disturb its production affect these functions.

In the sections that follow, the management of focal and generalized salivary gland swelling is considered. Some of these conditions are associated with functional changes while others are not. Conditions that cause decreased or abnormal salivary secretion are discussed, and guidelines for the management of trauma to the salivary glands are detailed.

SALIVARY GLAND SWELLING

Swellings of the salivary glands can be either localized or generalized, and can be caused by a number of pathological processes that range from inflammation to infiltration and neoplasia.

INFLAMMATORY AND INFILTRATIVE DISORDERS

Acute viral sialadenitis

Better known as mumps, acute viral sialadenitis is caused by the paramyxovirus. An infection spread by droplets, it has an incubation period of 18–21 days. It affects children mainly, although presentation in adult life is not uncommon. Immunization against the mumps virus is available and administered to most children in the first year of life. As a consequence of the immunization programmes throughout the world, mumps is now relatively rare and clinicians may fail to consider it in their differential diagnosis of acute salivary gland enlargement.

Clinical features

After a prodromal period of malaise and anorexia, tense, tender swelling of one or both parotid glands develops, accompanied by fever. The submandibular glands may also be affected. After puberty, 20% of men with mumps develop orchitis, but sterility seldom results.

Investigation and treatment

Mumps can be distinguished from other forms of acute parotitis by the absence of a neutrophil leukocytosis in the blood, and the diagnosis can be confirmed by serological tests. Mumps is normally a self-limiting disease, requiring little more than sympathetic supportive care. However, complications in severe cases can include aseptic meningitis, sterility and permanent unilateral sensorineural deafness.

Acute suppurative sialadenitis

Acute suppurative sialadenitis affecting the parotid glands was a common postoperative complication during the early part of the past century. Preoperative dehydration, oral sepsis and generalized septicaemia predisposed to the development of this condition. Nowadays, the single most important factor in its genesis is reduced salivary flow, perhaps the consequence of Sjögren's syndrome, radiation damage, and tricyclic or phenothiazine drug treatment.

Clinical features

Most patients with acute parotitis are middle-aged or older. Women are more often affected than men. The parotid is swollen, tense, extremely tender, and hot, and the overlying skin is inflamed. There may be a regional lymphadenopathy. The parotid papilla is often hyperaemic and sometimes oedematous. Pus can sometimes be milked from the duct by massaging the patient's cheek (Fig. 14.1). Later on, areas of the gland may become fluctuant as an abscess forms, and occasionally facial weakness may develop.

Acute suppurative sialadenitis of the submandibular gland is usually caused by duct obstruction by stones: sialolithiasis. Patients with this condition develop a brawny swelling in their submandibular triangle, and pus often exudes from Wharton's duct.

Staphylococcus aureus is the most commonly isolated organism but anaerobes may also be grown.

Investigation and treatment

In the acute phase, pus from the gland should be sent for culture and sensitivity tests. Treatment is best started with flucloxacillin 500 mg q.i.d. i.v. and metronidazole 500 mg t.i.d. i.v. Adequate hydration must be maintained with intravenous fluids if necessary. Surgical intervention, other than to remove a stone impacted at the orifice of the duct, is seldom required but sometimes drainage of an abscess becomes necessary. When the infection has settled, a sialogram will show the presence of any stones that may require surgical removal at a later date.

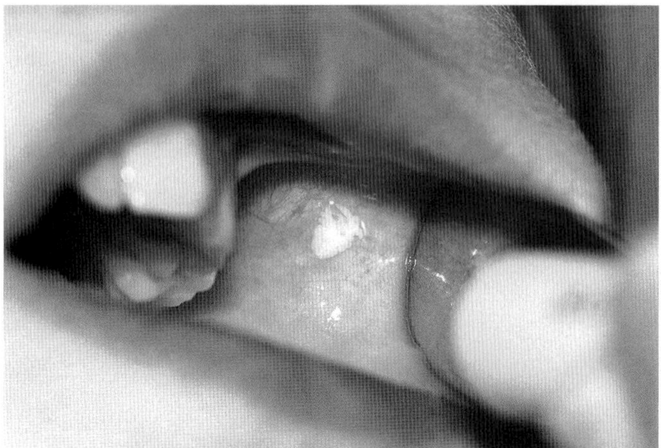

Figure 14.1 Pus has been milked from the parotid duct in this case of acute sialadenitis.

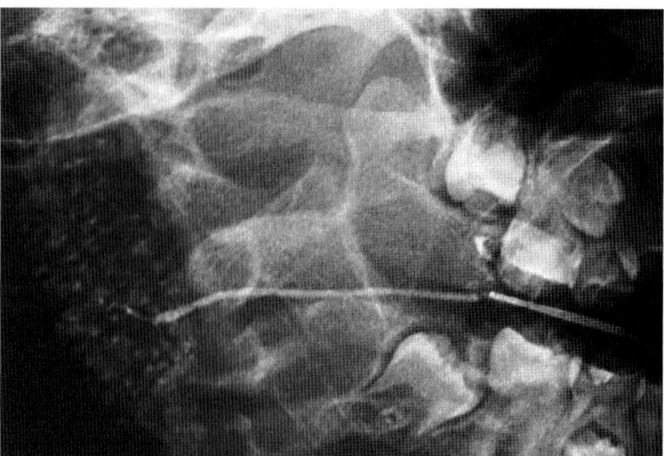

Figure 14.2 Sialogram showing widespread punctate sialectasis in a patient with chronic sialadenitis.

Chronic recurrent sialadenitis

Chronic sialadenitis is more common in the submandibular gland than in the other glands. Obstruction of the duct by stones or mucous plugs is probably the major cause. In a small subset of patients, disease is restricted to the parotid glands, where it is often bilateral and not the result of calculus obstruction. Both adults and children may be affected. In adults, chronic parotitis usually runs a steadily progressive course with shorter intervals between acute attacks, but in children it often regresses spontaneously during adolescence.

Investigation and treatment

Sialography remains the most popular and best method of assessment of ductal inflammatory and degenerative disease, despite the more sophisticated imaging techniques available. Focal or diffuse ductal strictures and ectasia are easily demonstrated. In severe cases, destruction of the gland parenchyma gives rise to the classic appearance of punctate sialectasis (Fig. 14.2). However, its use is limited by the fact that space-occupying lesions are neither reliably detected nor localized. Sialography should be restricted therefore to patients with recurrent parotid or submandibular swelling in which no discrete mass, other than a calculus, can be palpated.

Antibiotic therapy is the only appropriate treatment for acute episodes, but eventually even this becomes ineffective as bacterial resistance develops. Resection of the gland is necessary for these patients. Dissection of salivary glands affected by chronic sialadenitis can be difficult, because recurrent inflammatory episodes cause dense adhesions to form between the salivary tissue and adjacent structures. Furthermore, in chronic parotitis it is insufficient merely to remove the superficial lobe; a total conservative parotidectomy is required. All parotid tissue must be resected, while preserving every element of the facial nerve. This form of parotid surgery should be reserved for surgeons with special expertise, because it can be extremely testing. Iatrogenic deficits of facial, lingual and hypoglossal nerve function are easily acquired during surgery, and patients should be forewarned about these potential complications.

Sialolithiasis: salivary gland calculi

Sialolithiasis affects 12 per 1000 of the adult population. Calculi may develop in both the submandibular and the parotid glands, but the majority arise in the former. Sialolithiasis is seen most commonly in the fourth and fifth decades of life and is more common in men. There are a number of predisposing conditions, such as reduced salivary flow rates, duct obstruction and dehydration.

Clinical features

Stones may be asymptomatic if in the body of the gland but become symptomatic when lodged in the duct. Patients with sialolithiasis complain of pain and swelling in the affected gland at mealtimes, when the surge of salivary secretion is dammed up behind the obstruction. They are also subject to recurrent infection.

Investigation and treatment

Plain radiographs of the gland usually confirm the presence of calculi, although only about 40% of parotid calculi and 20% of submandibular calculi are radiolucent. In these cases, sialography can locate the site of obstruction.

Calculi should be removed if large enough to cause obstructive symptoms or if they have led to painful sialadenitis. Fragmentation of the stone by lithotripsy is gaining popularity, but a simple ductotomy may allow some stones to be expelled spontaneously. Others can be extracted using a steerable catheter. Surgical resection of the whole gland is the only possible treatment for giant stones (Fig. 14.3).

Sjögren's syndrome

The term *Sjögren's syndrome* describes the combination of dry eyes and dry mouth caused by an autoimmune lymphocytic infiltrate that causes destruction of glandular tissue. When rheumatoid arthritis or another connective tissue disorder is associated, the condition is called secondary Sjögren's syndrome. Primary Sjögren's syndrome comprises dry mouth and eyes without an associated connective tissue disease. It is usually more severe than secondary Sjögren's syndrome, affects other exocrine glands, and is often complicated by the development of lymphoma. There is a strong association with HLA DR3 in the case of primary Sjögren's syndrome and with HLA DR4 in secondary Sjögren's syndrome.

Clinical features

Sjögren's syndrome[1] is seen principally in the middle-aged, and in women much more often than in men. There is another smaller

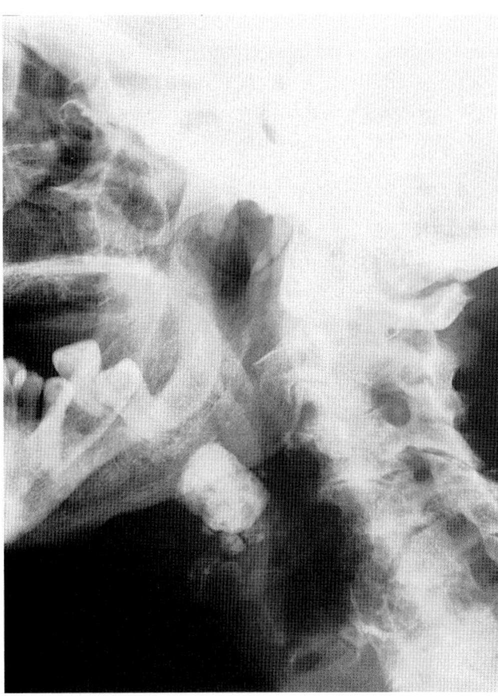

Figure 14.3 A giant stone in the body of the submandibular gland is evident on this lateral neck X-ray; the patient had sustained numerous infective episodes. Operative specimen; the calculus can be seen to occupy the majority of the gland.

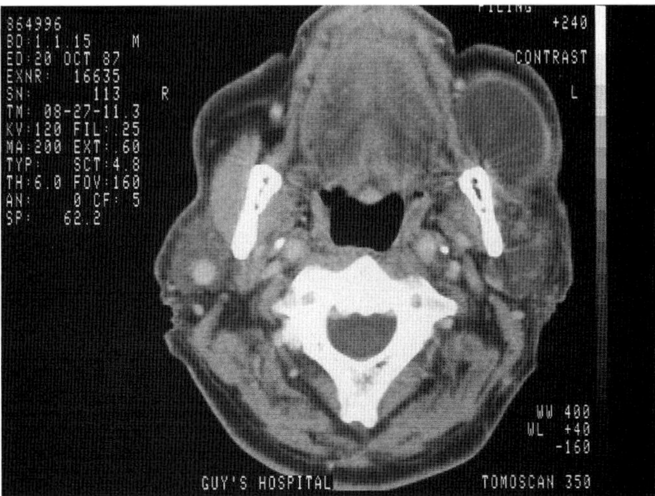

Figure 14.4 An MRI scan of the parotid glands of a patient with HIV infection. Cystic lesions characteristic of this condition are seen.

peak of incidence at the age of approximately 30 years. Unless complete xerostomia develops and the patient has parchment-dry mucosa, it is often difficult to perceive reduced salivary flow by mere clinical inspection. The dorsum of the tongue typically becomes lobulated, and frequently the oral mucosa is red and sore as a result of infection by *Candida albicans* secondary to the reduced salivary flow. Angular stomatitis may also result from the same infection.

Investigation and treatment

Investigations that aid diagnosis include sialography, which may show punctate sialectasis. Schirmer's test may demonstrate a reduction of lacrimal flow and there may be raised serum autoantibody titres (antinuclear and rheumatoid factor). Labial gland biopsy characteristically demonstrates periductal lymphocytic infiltrates.

Treatment is largely palliative and involves the prescription of artificial tears and saliva. Patients with Sjögren's syndrome should undergo regular dental and ophthalmological assessment because they are highly susceptible to dental caries and corneal damage. These patients should be kept under intermittent clinical review because lymphoma develops in 2%.

HIV-associated salivary gland disease

Salivary gland disease is often associated with HIV disease and is similar to Sjögren's disease.[2]

Clinical features

The disease is characterized by a painless, cystic swelling of the gland that is bilateral in 80% of cases. The patients usually have a variable degree of xerostomia. This particular manifestation is common in children with HIV disease. Parotid involvement is more frequent than that of the other major glands and is often seen in conjunction with the lymphadenopathy syndrome of HIV disease.

Investigation and treatment

The diagnosis should be considered in all patients where risk factors for HIV exist. Where the diagnosis has already been established, fine-needle aspiration cytology may be helpful in excluding lymphoma. If the diagnosis remains in doubt, MRI will show the characteristic multicentric cystic nature of the salivary gland disease (Fig. 14.4).

There is no specific treatment. Management is centred on symptom control. Good oral hygiene should be advised, and where cysts exist repeat aspiration may be performed. Superficial parotidectomy may become necessary if the diagnosis is in doubt, for cosmetic reasons and for those patients where the cysts reform despite aspiration.

Sialosis

Sialosis is an uncommon type of non-inflammatory swelling that often develops in the parotid glands. It is associated with a variety of systemic diseases but sometimes affects those without such diseases. Its pathogenesis remains uncertain.

Clinical features

Patients are usually in their late middle age. Diseases that may be associated include diabetes mellitus, any endocrine disorder, or alcoholism. Sialosis can also be induced by agents such as sympathomimetic drugs in long-term use for asthma and some of the older antihypertensive drugs, particularly guanethidine. In a significant number of patients no underlying disorder can be found.

REFERENCES

1. Cawson RA, Gleeson MJ, Eveson JW. In: Cawson RA, Gleeson MJ, Eveson JW (eds). Pathology and Surgery of the Salivary Glands. Isis Medical Media, Oxford, 1997: 49–55
2. Finfer MD, Schinella RA, Rothstein SG et al. Arch Otolaryngol Head Neck Surg 1988; 114: 1290–1294

Investigation and treatment

Diagnosis depends largely on the clinical features and medical history, but absolute confirmation depends on aspiration cytology or biopsy. Treatment for sialosis is unsatisfactory. Endocrine-associated sialosis is usually persistent even when control of the underlying disease is achieved. Drug-associated sialosis may regress when the drug responsible for the condition is withdrawn.

Sarcoidosis

This multisystem disease often affects salivary tissue but this is rarely the first sign.

Clinical features

Parotid gland involvement is well recognized but swelling of the gland develops in only 10% of cases. The most severe type of parotid involvement is seen in Heerfordt's syndrome, which comprises parotid swelling, anterior uveitis, facial palsy and fever. Xerostomia may result.

Investigation and treatment

Diagnosis of sarcoidosis can be difficult because there is no single pathognomonic feature and no test is reliably confirmatory. The Kveim test has been discarded because it involved the use of human splenic tissue. Raised angiotensin converting enzyme levels are helpful but not diagnostic. Diagnosis can be made only on the basis of clinical and radiographic findings together with laboratory tests. Histological confirmation of granuloma formation is mandatory. If the chest radiograph changes are compatible with sarcoidosis, demonstration of granuloma formation is frequently possible by biopsy of labial salivary glands.

Acute cases are generally self-limiting, and spontaneous resolution can be expected in about 50% of cases. The main treatment for patients with significant respiratory impairment, hypercalcaemia, uveitis or other serious complications is corticosteroids, particularly prednisolone, usually in a course of about 6 weeks. Symptomatic control of xerostomia with synthetic saliva may be helpful.

TRAUMATIC DISORDERS

Parotid gland

Trauma to the parotid gland may happen as a result of facial laceration or iatrogenic damage during surgery. In either situation the facial nerve may also be damaged, either in its entirety or in part. Surgery to repair or graft the nerve may be necessary, and any injury to the parotid gland where nerve damage is suspected should be explored as soon as possible through a parotidectomy incision. Most salivary fistulae close spontaneously within a few weeks. More persistent fistulae require surgical treatment, either by repair or by reimplantation of the duct. In some it becomes necessary to remove the whole gland.

SALIVARY GLAND TUMOURS

Fewer than 3% of all neoplasms originate in salivary glands, and at least 75% of these tumours are benign. In England and Wales in 1985, the registration rate of malignant salivary tumours developing in major glands was 1.2 per 100 000 of the population.[3] Malignant salivary tumours are certainly uncommon. The peak incidence of malignant salivary neoplasms is in the sixth and seventh decades of life for both men and women. In the major series, salivary tumours have been found to be slightly more common in females than in males. Only previous radiation has been shown convincingly to have any significant influence on the development of salivary gland neoplasms. The survivors of the Hiroshima atomic bomb experienced an increased incidence of both benign and malignant salivary gland tumours. The incidence of benign tumours was 2.6 times higher than that of a similar non-exposed population, while that of malignant tumours was 10 times greater.[4,5]

General considerations

From a clinical standpoint, it is unfortunate that the vast majority of malignant salivary tumours have no features that distinguish them from benign tumours at presentation. Figure 14.5 is a useful clinical algorithm for the investigation and management of salivary gland masses in general. Regrettably, the diagnosis of many malignant tumours is made after an operation designed to control benign disease, an operation that was probably not as radical as might have seemed prudent in retrospect. Pain, rapid growth pattern, progressive facial weakness, lymphadenopathy and ulceration are features of advanced and possibly, but not always, incurable malignancy. To make matters worse, even the most commonly encountered and benign salivary tumour, pleomorphic adenoma, can pose considerable management problems as it recurs locally if inadequately resected, ruptured or biopsied. If untreated it also has the potential to undergo malignant change.

Perhaps the feature that makes many malignant salivary gland tumours stand apart from neoplasms in other organs is that their natural history is usually measured in decades rather than in years. The slow growth pattern of these tumours may lull the patient into a false sense of security but does not lessen their malignant nature. Despite treatment, these tumours recur or return as metastatic disease many years later, inflicting considerable morbidity and mortality. The World Health Organization classification of salivary gland tumours recognizes their full malignant potential (Table 14.1).

Investigation

Fine-needle aspiration cytology

Preoperative diagnosis of tumours can often be made by fine-needle aspiration cytology. It should be possible to differentiate malignant from benign salivary gland tumours with over 90% accuracy, and the technique avoids the risk of seeding tumour cells that is associated with open biopsy.[6,7] The only potential drawback is that not all cytologists have the opportunity to develop their diagnostic skills in salivary gland disease. Nevertheless, it can be extremely useful and warns surgeons and their patients of an unexpected malignant tumour.

Imaging

Computerized tomography and magnetic resonance images are often acquired in the management of patients with salivary gland masses. Neither imaging modality can predict the nature of a

REFERENCES

3. Office for National Statistics. OPSC Cancer Statistics: Registrations, Series MB1, No. 18. HMSO, London, 1985
4. Takeichi N, Hirose F, Yamamoto H et al. Cancer 1983; 52: 377–385
5. Shore-Freedman E, Abrahams C, Recant W et al. Cancer 1983, 51: 2159–2163
6. Eneroth CM, Franzen S, Zajicek J. Acta Otolaryngol Suppl 1967; 244: 168–171
7. Sismanis A, Merriam JM, Kline TS et al. Head Neck Surg 1981; 3: 482–489

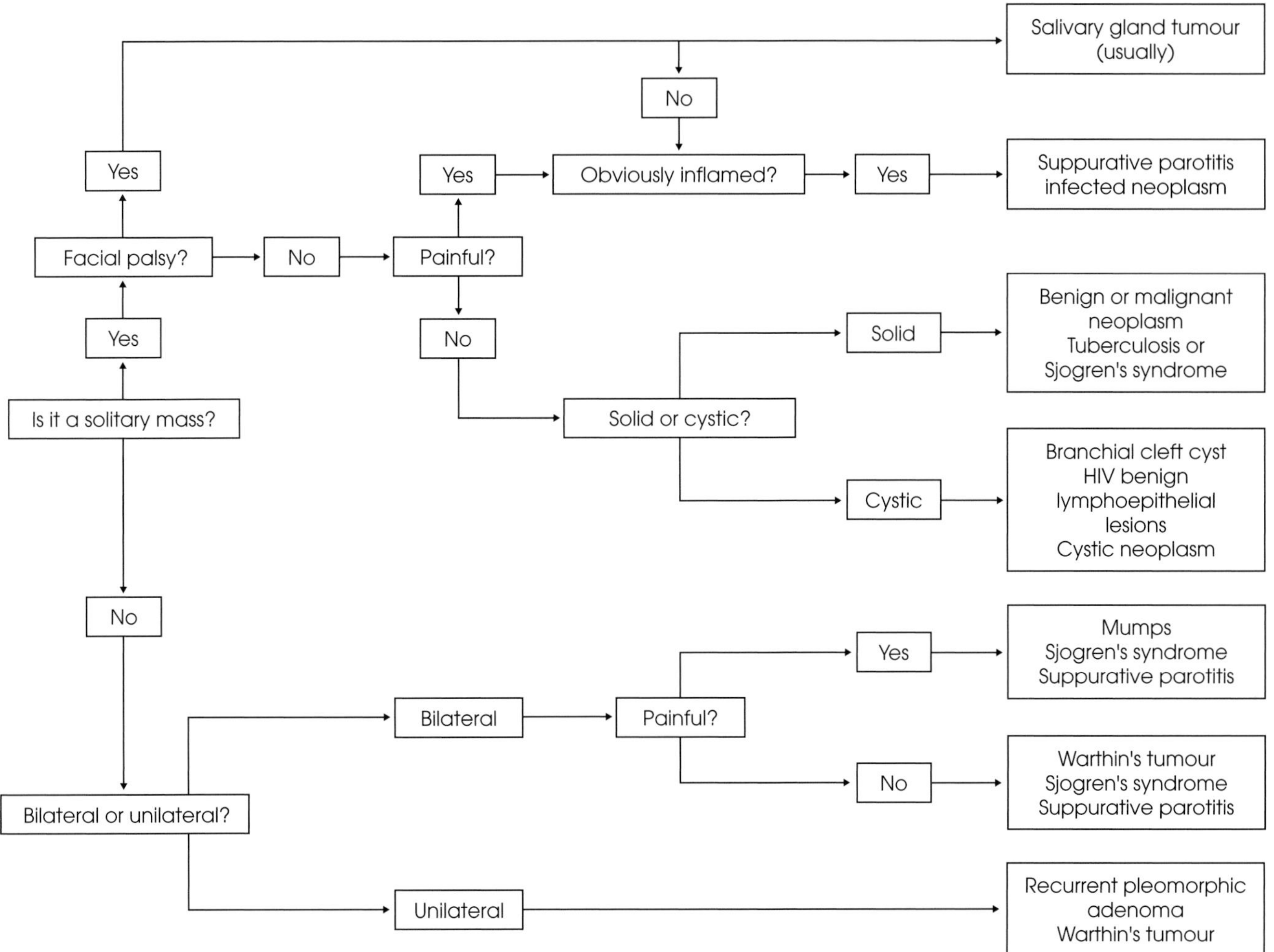

Figure 14.5 Clinical algorithm for the investigation and management of salivary gland masses.

tumour accurately, and for the majority of patients imaging adds little to their management other than cost. Those cases in which it can be helpful include the following:

- Tumours confined to the deep lobe of the parotid gland, where the full extent and relationships of the tumour can be seen (Fig. 14.6).
- Tumours with involvement of both the deep and the superficial lobes of the parotid gland (dumb-bell tumours) in which the integrity of the facial nerve is at increased risk.
- Tumours presenting with facial weakness, other neural deficit, or indication of malignancy where it is difficult to assess the extent of disease by clinical examination only.
- Congenital parotid masses, some of which may be vascular.
- Recurrent disease, because it is often multifocal and extremely difficult to define (Fig. 14.7).

In the sections that follow, features of specific salivary gland neoplasms are discussed to give guidelines about clinical management and likely outcomes.

BENIGN SALIVARY GLAND TUMOURS

Pleomorphic adenoma

As the most common tumour to develop in the parotid gland, pleomorphic adenoma accounts for 80% of all benign parotid tumours. It is also the most common tumour of the submandibular and minor salivary glands. Pleomorphic adenomas may develop at almost any age from childhood to senescence. The mean age at presentation in most series is 46 years. Overall there is a slight female predominance.

Clinical features

The great majority of pleomorphic adenomas are found in the parotid glands, where they form slow-growing, usually painless, firm swellings that are not attached to the overlying skin. Any impairment of facial nerve function, pain or ulceration of the overlying skin strongly suggests malignant disease. Eighty per cent of parotid pleomorphic adenomas are within the superficial lobe, and 20% arise either within the deep lobe or involve it by direct growth from the superficial lobe. Deep lobe tumours usually present as a parapharyngeal mass, displacing the soft palate and tonsil medially. Difficulty in swallowing is unusual, and most deep lobe tumours are incidental findings at consultations for other complaints. These tumours have frequently reached a very large size by this time.

As for the other salivary glands, 11% of all pleomorphic adenomas are found in the submandibular glands and a similar proportion is found in minor salivary glands. In the minor glands, the majority are found in the palate; the next most common sites are the lips and the cheeks. These adenomas may also occasionally be found in other sites, such as the tongue, retromolar trigone, pharynx or tonsil. Occasionally, pleomorphic

Table 14.1 World Health Organization classification of salivary gland tumours

WHO class	Tumour	ICD-O* morphology code
1	**Adenoma**	–
1.1	Pleomorphic adenoma	8940/0
1.2	Myoepithelioma	8982/0
1.3	Basal cell adenoma	8147/0
1.4	Warthin tumour (adenolymphoma)	8561/0
1.5	Oncocytoma (oncocytic adenoma)	8290/0
1.6	Canalicular adenoma	–
1.7	Sebaceous adenoma	8410/0
1.8	Ductal papilloma	8503/0
1.8.1	Inverted ductal papilloma	–
1.8.2	Intraductal papilloma	8503/0
1.8.3	Sialadenoma papilliferum	–
1.9	Cystadenoma	8440/0
1.9.1	Papillary cystadenoma	8450/0
1.9.2	Mucinous cystadenoma	8470/0
2	**Carcinoma**	–
2.1	Acinar cell carcinoma	8550/3
2.2	Mucoepidermoid carcinoma	8430/3
2.3	Adenoid cystic carcinoma	8200/3
2.4	Polymorphous low-grade adenocarcinoma (terminal duct adenocarcinoma)	8525/3
2.5	Epithelial–myoepithelial carcinoma	8562/3
2.6	Basal cell adenocarcinoma	8147/3
2.7	Sebaceous carcinoma	8410/3
2.8	Papillary cystadenocarcinoma	8450/3
2.9	Mucinous adenocarcinoma	8480/3
2.10	Oncocytic carcinoma	8290/3
2.11	Salivary duct carcinoma	–
2.12	Adenocarcinoma	8140/3
2.13	Malignant myoepithelioma (myoepithelial carcinoma)	8982/3
2.14	Carcinoma in pleomorphic adenoma (malignant mixed tumour)	8941/3
2.15	Squamous cell carcinoma	8070/3
2.16	Small cell carcinoma	8041/3
2.17	Undifferentiated carcinoma	8020/3
2.18	Other carcinomas	–
3	**Non-epithelial tumours**	–
3.1	Angiomas	–
3.2	Lipomas	–
3.3	Neural tumours	–
3.4	Other benign mesenchymal tumours	–
3.5	Sarcomas	–
4	**Malignant lymphomas**	–
5	**Secondary tumours**	–
6	**Unclassified tumours**	–
7	**Tumour-like lesions**	–
7.1	Sialadenosis	71000
7.2	Oncocytosis	73050
7.3	Necrotizing sialometaplasia (salivary gland infarction)	73220
7.4	Benign lymphoepithelial lesion	72240
7.5	Salivary gland cysts	33400
7.6	Chronic sclerosing sialadenitis of submandibular gland (Kuttner tumour)	45000
7.7	Cystic lymphoid hyperplasia in AIDS	–

*International Classification of Diseases for Oncology.

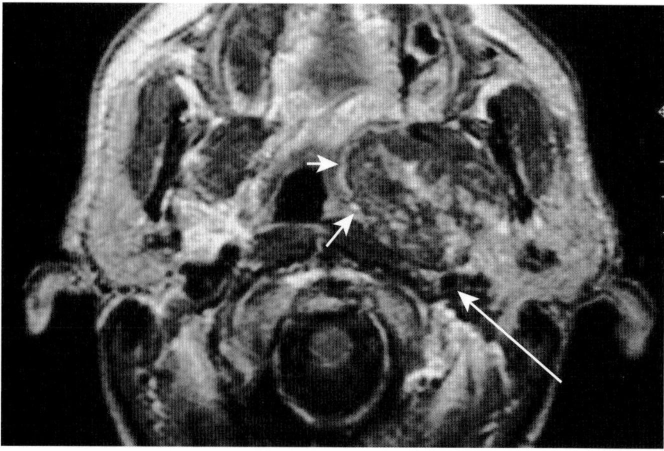

Figure 14.6 An MRI scan of a deep lobe parotid tumour (arrowheads). The tumour is in continuity with the remaining parotid tissue and the internal carotid artery lies immediately posterior to it (arrowed).

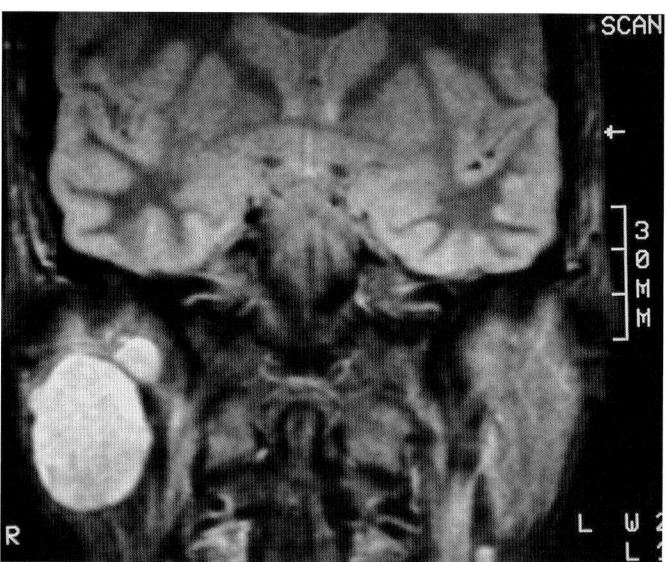

Figure 14.7 An MRI scan of a recurrent pleomorphic adenoma. It can be seen that the mass that was easily palpable in the patient's neck was, in fact, two recurrences. Many other recurrences were found at exploration.

adenomas are found in the nasal cavity, trachea, bronchi, the middle ear, external auditory meatus and lacrimal glands. The clinical features of pleomorphic adenomas in the other major or minor salivary glands do not differ significantly from those of pleomorphic adenomas in the parotids.

Investigation and treatment

Fine-needle aspiration cytology usually confirms the clinical diagnosis, and MRI scans should be obtained in selected cases as outlined earlier. In the parotid gland the treatment of choice is surgical excision ensuring that the tumour is contained and removed with a cuff of normal salivary tissue around it. This reduces the risk of damage to the capsule and spillage of tumour. Because most tumours are contained in the superficial lobe, a lateral or superficial parotidectomy is required. The importance of the capsule is a subject of considerable controversy. It may be complete or incomplete and in any tumour can be extremely variable; thick and fibrous in one part while completely absent in other places.[8]

The degree of encapsulation and the ability of these tumours to extend through the capsule are of practical importance in their surgical management. In the past, some surgeons enucleated these tumours and subsequent recurrence was commonplace. Nowadays, some surgeons perform a variation of enucleation that they call an extracapsular dissection.[9] This operation is performed using a microscope or with loupes. It is claimed to be as effective as superficial parotidectomy for the control of benign disease. It would certainly provide suboptimal treatment in the case of a malignant tumour, where excision with a cuff of normal tissue around the tumour offers the best chance of cure. Removing the tumour with a good margin of healthy tissue limits the risk of rupture, tumour spillage, contamination, and seeding of the wound regardless of whether the tumour is benign or malignant. It is worth remembering that tumour spillage definitely increases the risk of recurrence of pleomorphic adenoma, and revision surgery to remove recurrence is associated with an increased incidence of facial nerve damage.[10]

Recurrent pleomorphic adenoma

The precise incidence of recurrence following primary surgery for pleomorphic adenoma is not known and depends, to some extent, on the technique used to remove the primary tumour. Recurrence can develop 15–20 years after seemingly uneventful surgery, and it is this fact that many ignore when reporting their operative results. When recurrence develops, both surgeon and patient are confronted with a formidable problem because the disease is often multifocal and the facial nerve can be encased in scar tissue, making it impossible to find without inflicting damage. Further recurrence has been reported to develop in up to 40% of patients, and malignant change takes place in about 10%. Surgical resection followed by radiotherapy in those with diffuse disease is widely advocated.[11–13] Because the risk of facial nerve damage at reoperation is considerable, this surgery should be undertaken only by those capable of reconstructing the nerve if it is damaged or needs to be resected.

Warthin's tumour

Warthin's tumour accounts for 14% of all salivary gland neoplasms and is the second most common tumour to develop. It is sometimes referred to as adenolymphoma, but this term is misleading, implying malignancy in a benign lesion.

Clinical features

Warthin's tumour is almost always found in the parotid glands. These tumours can develop at any age but are more common in the elderly, and most patients are smokers.[14] The typical growth pattern is slow, and they present as painless swellings usually at the lower pole of the parotid gland. Pain may be a significant feature in a few, being described as earache. Warthin's tumours appear capable of giving rise to a greater variety of symptoms than other benign tumours, and the complaints of pain and of sudden increase in size of the mass, presumably as a result of cystic expansion, may falsely suggest malignancy.[15] Carcinomatous change in Warthin's tumours is exceedingly rare. Small foci of incipient tumour formation may also be found in the surrounding parotid tissue. Such multiple foci almost certainly account for the rare recurrences that have been reported. However, the infrequency of such reports suggests that small Warthin's tumours may spontaneously abort.

Investigation and treatment

Excision (superficial or total conservative parotidectomy) is curative, and there is a view that careful enucleation of these well-demarcated tumours is sufficient if a confident diagnosis has been made on fine-needle biopsy.[16–18]

MALIGNANT SALIVARY GLAND TUMOURS

Adenoid cystic carcinoma

Adenoid cystic carcinoma is the most common malignant salivary neoplasm. As with the other tumours, its distribution varies between sites. It is far more common in the submandibular, sublingual and minor glands, where it constitutes 16%, 28% and 13% of all neoplasms in these glands, respectively. However, in the parotid gland only 2% of tumours are of this type.

Clinical features

Adenoid cystic carcinoma usually presents as a mass or a submucosal swelling that can be either painless or painful. It rarely ulcerates. Facial palsy develops in up to 20% of parotid tumours, and palpable lymph node involvement or direct invasion of adjacent tissues is found in 15%.

Adenoid cystic carcinoma grows slowly and insidiously, with a characteristic propensity for perineural infiltration, and spread along the Haversian systems and neural canals of bones. Widespread infiltration by this route is often achieved with little apparent bone erosion. This pattern is reflected in the local recurrence and cumulative mortality rates for this tumour, namely 5-year survival of 62%, 10-year survival of 39%, 15-year survival of 26%, and 20-year survival of 21%. Nodal involvement is normally the result of direct growth of tumour rather than by lymphatic spread. Metastases develop late in the disease and are usually pulmonary. Local recurrence is extremely common and appears in at least 50% of patients. Even multiple local recurrences or distant metastases are compatible with prolonged survival. While 33% of patients die within 1 year of the recognition of their metastatic disease, 20% of those with pulmonary secondaries survive with this increased tumour load for longer than 5 years.[19–21]

REFERENCES

8. Webb AJ, Eveson JW. Clin Otolaryngol 2001; 26: 134–142
9. Maynard JD. Br J Surg 1988; 75: 305–308
10. McGurk M, Reneham A, Gleave EN et al. Br J Surg 1996; 172: 710–714
11. Yugueros P, Goellner JR, Petty PM et al. Ann Plast Surg 1998; 40: 573–576
12. Phillips PP, Olsen KD. Ann Otol Rhinol Laryngol 1995; 104: 100–104
13. Leverstein H, Tiwari RM, Snow GB et al. Eur Arch Otorhinolaryngol 1997; 254: 313–317
14. Xu GY, Liu XB, Li ZL et al. Br J Oral Maxillofac Surg 1998; 36: 183–185
15. Eveson JW, Cawson RA. Oral Surg Oral Med Oral Pathol 1986; 61: 256–262
16. Raymond MR, Yoo JH, Heathcote JG et al. J Otolaryngol 2002; 31: 263–270
17. Lewis DR, Webb AJ, Lott MF et al. Br J Surg 1999; 86: 1275–1279
18. Yu GY, Ma DQ, Liu XB et al. Br J Oral Maxillofac Surg 1998; 36: 186–189
19. Spiro RH, Huvos AG, Strong EW. Am J Surg 1974; 128: 512–520
20. Hamper K, Lazar F, Dietel M et al. J Oral Pathol Med 1990; 19: 101–107
21. Shannon Allen M, Marsh WL. Cancer 1976; 38: 2017–2021

Investigation and treatment

Fine-needle aspiration cytology is usually very accurate and MRI should be obtained in every case. This tumour should be excised as widely as possible and postoperative radiotherapy given to improve local control. For a parotid tumour this surgery implies total parotidectomy. The facial nerve is conserved only if there is no evidence of invasion by tumour. Subtotal petrosectomy has been advocated for patients with clinical evidence of facial nerve invasion. It is essential to appreciate that this tumour spreads along the perineurium in both peripheral and central directions. Great care must be taken to excise the neural spread of tumour in both directions. Part of the mandible, the maxillary tuberosity, and the contents of the infratemporal fossa must also be resected in some of these patients. Radical neck dissection is indicated only for those patients with obvious nodal disease or those in whom a large soft tissue cuff must be removed. The treatment plan must take full account of the patient's age, general health and attitude to their illness; the realistic extent of microscopic disease; and the likely benefit that the patient might derive from mutilating surgery.

Submandibular disease is best managed by en bloc resection of the gland encompassing the lingual, hypoglossal and marginal mandibular nerves, together with a suprahyoid nodal clearance. Palatal tumours require wide local resection to include the floor of the maxillary sinus at least. Recurrent tumour is best dealt with by surgery followed by radiotherapy if possible. Advanced and incurable disease is sometimes palliated by radiotherapy that makes salvage surgery feasible for a few.

Mucoepidermoid carcinoma

Mucoepidermoid carcinoma is the most common malignant salivary gland tumour to arise in childhood. The parotid and minor glands of the palate are the most frequently affected sites. Mucoepidermoid carcinoma is composed of two distinct cell types: epidermoid cells and mucous cells. Both cell types may show varying degrees of differentiation. Increased mitotic activity is not necessarily seen, even in high-grade tumours – a feature partially responsible for the unpredictable nature of this particular neoplasm.[22]

Clinical features

Mucoepidermoid carcinomas grow slowly and recur locally. Lymph node metastases develop in up to 30% of patients and are present at presentation in 15%. Metastases to the lungs, bones and brain develop in approximately 15%. It has been claimed that recurrence and survival rates are strongly influenced by the histological grading of the tumour and its size at presentation. Low-grade tumours are said to be compatible with an 80% 15-year survival rate, while a similar measure for high-grade tumours is reported to be only 33%.[23,24]

Investigation and treatment

Fine-needle aspiration cytology often indicates the diagnosis, and MRI should be obtained in all cases suggested by fine-needle aspiration cytology. Low-grade tumours should be managed by local resection and prolonged follow-up. High-grade lesions require more radical resection with adjunctive radiotherapy. If local recurrence occurs it is likely to appear within 12 months of the primary procedure.

Carcinoma in pleomorphic adenoma

Carcinoma in pleomorphic adenoma is a rare entity. Almost all are adenocarcinomas or undifferentiated carcinomas and are clearly seen to arise close to, or within, a pleomorphic adenoma. The majority of these carcinomas have been found to develop in recurrences.[25]

Clinical features

Rapid growth of a pleomorphic adenoma, the development of facial palsy, or the onset of pain all suggest malignant change. It is an aggressive disease with reported 5-year survival rates of 50%. All patients die if the carcinoma extends more than 8 mm beyond the residual benign tumour or has invaded bone. Perhaps this is a pessimistic assessment of this disease, because many more may have been missed due to the limitations of processing large pleomorphic tumours.

Investigation and treatment

Radical local resection and radiotherapy offer the best chance of control.

Acinic cell carcinoma

Acinic cell carcinoma accounts for 2.5% of all salivary gland tumours and predominantly affects the parotid gland. A very small proportion may be bilateral. This tumour exerts a mortality many years after other salivary neoplasms would have been considered cured. Survival rates of 85%, 65% and 50% for 5, 10 and 15 years, respectively, have been reported. A number of histological variants have been described but no histological features or grading scheme appears to correlate with poor prognosis.[26]

Clinical features

As with adenoid cystic carcinoma, this tumour is very slow-growing. Local recurrence or the development of metastases after a prolonged disease-free interval is common.

Investigation and treatment

Fine-needle aspiration cytology often indicates the diagnosis, and MRI should be obtained in all cases suggested by fine-needle aspiration cytology. The management of this carcinoma is excision of the gland with conservation of all uninvolved nerves. Because nodal disease is uncommon and develops in no more than 10% of patients, elective neck dissection is not indicated.

Adenocarcinoma

Adenocarcinoma accounts for 2.5% of parotid tumours and a much higher percentage of tumours in other glands. A wide spectrum of adenocarcinomas is recognized. The grade of the neoplasm is judged by mitotic rate, cellular pleomorphism and stromal invasion. High-grade tumours tend to present with locally advanced disease, often with nodal involvement, and are reported to have significantly poorer prognosis.[27] A subset of adeno-

REFERENCES

22. Batsakis JG, Luna MA, El-Naggar A. Ann Otol Rhinol Laryngol 1990; 99: 1007–1009
23. Spiro RH, Huvos AG, Berk R et al. Am J Surg 1978; 136: 461–468
24. Evans HL. Am J Clin Pathol 1984; 81: 696–701
25. Batsakis JG. Ann Otol Rhinol Laryngol 1982; 91: 342–343
26. Batsakis JG, Chin EK, Weimert TA et al. J Laryngol Otol 1979; 93: 325–340
27. Spiro RH, Huvos AG, Strong EW. Am J Surg 1982; 144: 423–431

carcinoma, the polymorphous low-grade adenocarcinoma, affects the minor salivary glands, particularly those of the palate. It has aggressive histological features, such as perineural and perivascular invasion, that are misleading. This type of adenocarcinoma rarely metastasizes but tends to recur locally.[28]

Clinical features

Most adenocarcinomas present as masses, half of which are fixed. Some are painful and a few will have produced a facial palsy. One in five patients has nodal disease at presentation, and a further 10% develop it later. Failure to control disease is usually manifest as local or regional recurrence, but distant metastasis, usually to the lungs, is also common.

Investigation and treatment

Fine-needle aspiration cytology is extremely useful for this neoplasm, and MRI should be obtained in all cases. The clinical management of this tumour is determined by the histological grade and the circumstances of the patient. It would be inappropriate to manage an elderly patient with a high-grade tumour with anything other than a palliative procedure, whereas an identical tumour in a younger patient ought to be treated aggressively. Surgical treatment should be planned to provide a generous cuff of healthy tissue around the tumour. Because nodal disease is present in 20% of patients at presentation and a further 10% go on to develop it, the need for a radical neck dissection should be considered in all cases.

Lymphoma

Primary lymphomas of salivary glands are rare. The origin of salivary gland lymphomas has frequently been assumed to be from mucosa-associated lymphoid tissue and many probably are. However, others develop in intra- or juxtaglandular nodes. The vast majority are non-Hodgkin's lymphomas, and 90% are well differentiated with the remainder being poorly differentiated. The incidence of salivary gland lymphomas in association with HIV infection appears to be high.

Clinical features

Most salivary gland lymphomas develop in the parotid gland as firm swellings that in the majority of cases are painless. There is sometimes fixation to deep or superficial tissues. Facial palsy is most uncommon. The prognosis of primary salivary gland lymphomas appears to be better than that of nodal lymphomas.[29]

Investigation and treatment

The first essential is precise histological categorization, followed by staging to determine whether the tumour is a primary salivary gland tumour or, if not, the extent of the disease. If it can be established that the lymphoma is limited to a salivary gland, parotidectomy followed by radiotherapy is an acceptable option, although rarely indicated because the disease is usually more advanced. Total conservative parotidectomy in this condition, preserving every branch of the facial nerve, is extremely difficult. In almost all cases the treatment and prognosis will be determined by the stage and histological subtype of the lymphoma, and treatment should be according to accepted protocols.

SALIVARY GLAND SURGERY

Parotid gland

Removal of the lateral part of the parotid gland (superficial parotidectomy) is adequate treatment for the majority of tumours. Those arising within or involving the deep lobe demand a total conservative parotidectomy in which all, or almost all, parotid tissue is removed, leaving the facial nerve intact. This is also the operation of choice for the control of recurrent sialadenitis. Total parotidectomy, removal of the entire parotid gland and facial nerve, is indicated for malignant tumours that have infiltrated the facial nerve. Enucleation or extracapsular dissection is acceptable in those rare situations when the tumour is hanging off the inferior pole of the parotid gland. Poor general health is the only valid contraindication to surgery on this gland.

Informed consent

Prior to superficial or total conservative parotidectomy the patient should be warned about the following serious or frequent complications.

Facial weakness

The risk of temporary or permanent facial weakness must be carefully explained, because it has a very significant impact on quality of life. The risk of facial nerve damage is related to the extent of the disease, the type of resection, and the experience of the surgeon. Neuropraxia usually recovers within 4–6 weeks. More severe injuries cause some degree of degeneration, and recovery may never be complete and may take 6–12 months or even longer to take place.

Facial anaesthesia

Anaesthesia in the distribution of the greater auricular nerve, over the angle of the mandible and inferior two-thirds of the pinna, is unavoidable. Most patients learn to accept this deficit and few are severely troubled by it.

Cosmetic defects

The cosmetic appearance of the incision rarely causes concern. Loss of bulk behind the ramus of the mandible may result in a mildly unsightly dent in the normal outline of the jaw.

Frey's syndrome

Gustatory sweating or flushing (Frey's syndrome) is a socially embarrassing complication of parotidectomy. Following surgery it develops in nearly all patients to some degree. The frequency of this complication is sufficient to warrant preoperative explanation, together with the reassurance that it is rarely significantly disconcerting and usually amenable to the simple preventive measures, for example the application of an antiperspirant or local, subdermal injections of botulinum toxin.

Operative procedure: superficial and total conservative parotidectomy

The fundamental principle of parotidectomy is exposure of the facial nerve then removal of the gland and diseased tissue from around it. The surgeon should be aware that the branching pattern of the facial nerve can be quite varied and that the nerve may have been displaced from its normal position by tumour. Identification of the facial nerve and safe manipulation of the tissues around it can be significantly aided by the use of a facial nerve monitor.

REFERENCES

28. Evans HL, Batsakis JG. Cancer 1984; 53: 935–942
29. Gleeson MJ, Bennett MH, Cawson RA. Cancer 1986; 58: 699–704

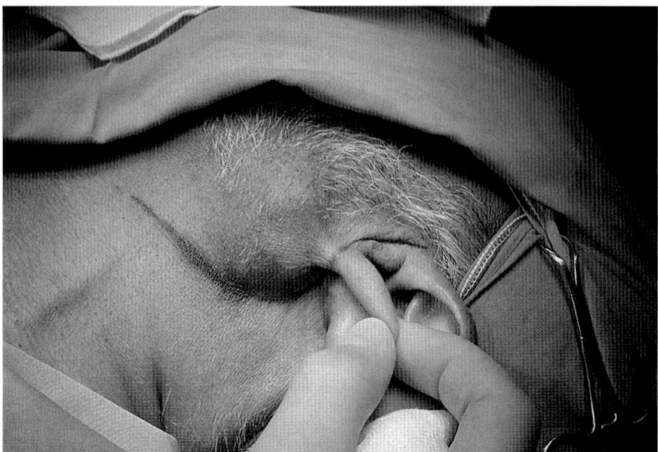

Figure 14.8 The 'lazy S' incision has been marked out on the patient. The outline of the tumour is very clearly seen.

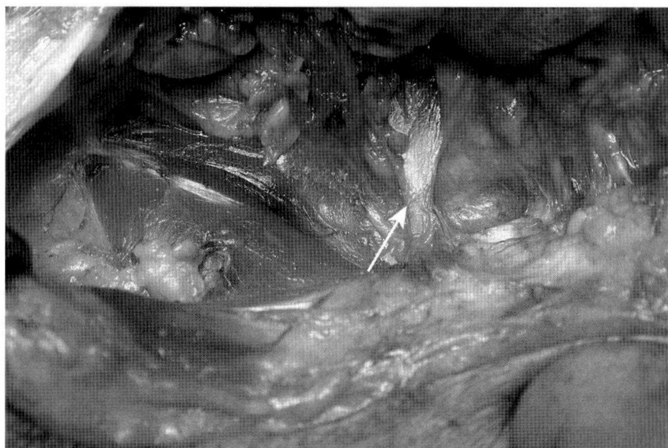

Figure 14.10 The main trunk of the facial nerve has been identified just anterior to the posterior belly of the digastric muscle (arrowed).

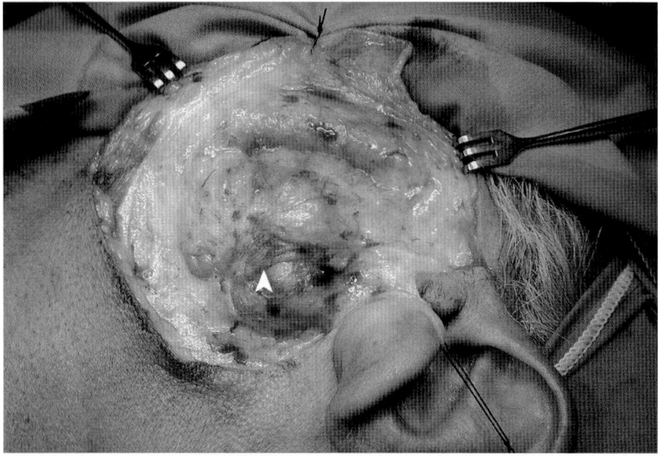

Figure 14.9 Flaps have been raised and the greater auricular nerve can be seen coursing over the parotid fascia (arrowed).

Most tumours can be removed through a 'lazy S' incision (Fig. 14.8) but, in some, extension of the incision into the hairline aids exposure. Infiltration of the area with 1:200 000 adrenaline (epinephrine) reduces haemorrhage and makes identification of the facial nerve slightly easier. Skin flaps are raised that contain the subcutaneous tissue lateral to the parotid fascia (Fig. 14.9). The parotid is then mobilized from the cartilage of the external auditory canal and adjacent muscles, the sternocleidomastoid and digastric muscles. In this process it is necessary to section the greater auricular nerve.

The facial nerve trunk is then identified. A number of anatomical landmarks facilitate this part of the operation:

- The inferior portion of the cartilaginous external auditory canal; the facial nerve lies 1 cm deep and inferior to its tip.
- The groove between the cartilaginous and bony external auditory meatus. The facial nerve lies immediately deep and inferior to this at its point of exit from the skull. This groove is very easy to feel.
- The anterior border of the posterior belly of the digastric muscle. The facial nerve leaves the skull immediately anterior to the attachment of this muscle. The facial nerve can be exposed by careful dissection in the area immediately anterior to the posterior belly of the digastric in the region of the mastoid process (Fig. 14.10).

In some cases, for example recurrence surgery, it is neither possible nor wise to expose the facial nerve trunk at the skull base at the outset of the operation. In these cases it is better to locate and identify one of the major branches and dissect centrally or peripherally from there. The mandibular branch can be found at the angle of the mandible, as it lies superficial to the facial vessels. The cervical branch of the nerve can be located at the point where it pierces the deep fascia, below the body of the mandible. The zygomatic and temporal branches of the upper trunk cross the zygomatic arch anterior to, and within 1–2 cm of, the superficial temporal artery.

In summary, there are a variety of landmarks that can be used to aid identification of the facial nerve and its branches. With experience the surgeon learns how and when to use this information. The routine use of facial nerve monitoring for parotid surgery also helps in this process and cannot be recommended too strongly. Not only does it predict the impending proximity of the facial nerve trunk, but it also helps minimize trauma to its finer branches that can be irrevocably damaged all too easily.

After identification of the nerve, the superficial lobe of the parotid gland and tumour are then dissected off its main divisions and branches. By this means the superficial lobe of the gland is separated from the deeper tissues (Fig. 14.11). If a tumour ruptures, the spillage should be contained and the tissues immediately deep to it removed.

Haemostasis is then achieved and the wound closed in two layers. Either active or passive drains should be used. Great care should be exercised when placing vacuum drains, particularly if there are sections of unsupported facial nerve within the field, because drains can cause inadvertent neuropraxia.

Occasionally it is necessary to remove the deep lobe of the gland for chronic infection or a tumour within it. For the control of chronic sialadenitis, the segments of parotid tissue deep to and in between the branches of the facial nerve must be removed. This can be performed in a piecemeal fashion. In the case of a tumour within the deep lobe, the facial nerve must be mobilized with great care. In the first instance it is best to develop a plane deep to the main trunk. The remaining peripheral mobilization can be facilitated by gentle elevation of the trunk with a nerve hook. A piecemeal approach is not appropriate in these circumstances, and the tumour must be removed with as much

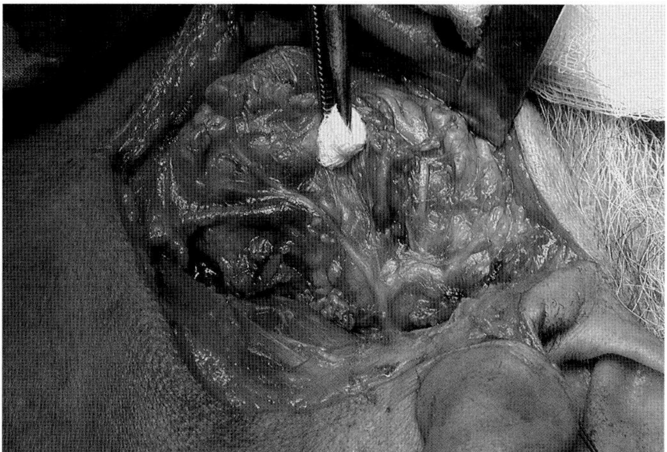

Figure 14.11 The completed dissection; some parotid tissue is still present peripherally but its removal was unnecessary.

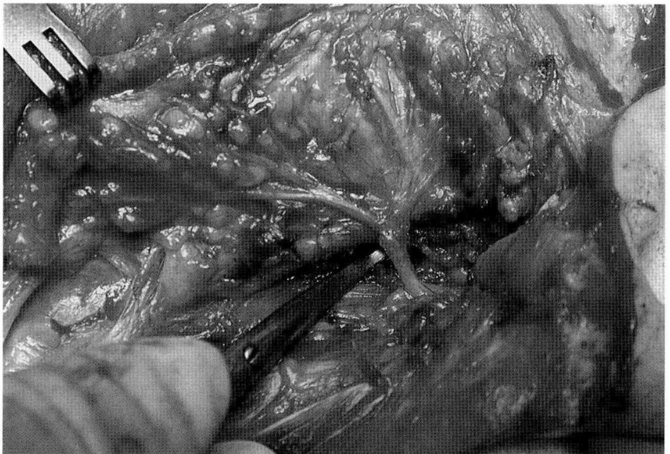

Figure 14.12 A total conservative parotidectomy has been undertaken in this patient to remove a tumour that had an extension deep to the main trunk of the facial nerve. The main trunk has been completely mobilized.

normal parotid tissue as possible, although that it is usually very scant (Fig. 14.12). Access to the tumour can be improved by sectioning the digastric muscle and by counterpressure applied to the tumour by an assistant with their index finger in the patient's oropharynx.

Submandibular gland

Removal of the submandibular gland is indicated for neoplasms or intractable infection.

Informed consent

Before resection of the submandibular salivary gland the patient should be warned about the following serious or frequent complications.

Damage to the marginal branch of the facial nerve

This may result in either a temporary or permanent weakness of the angle of the mouth that will be most noticeable on smiling and puckering the lips. In cases of malignant disease involving or abutting this nerve it may be necessary to resect it together with the gland, and the neural deficit is then unavoidable.

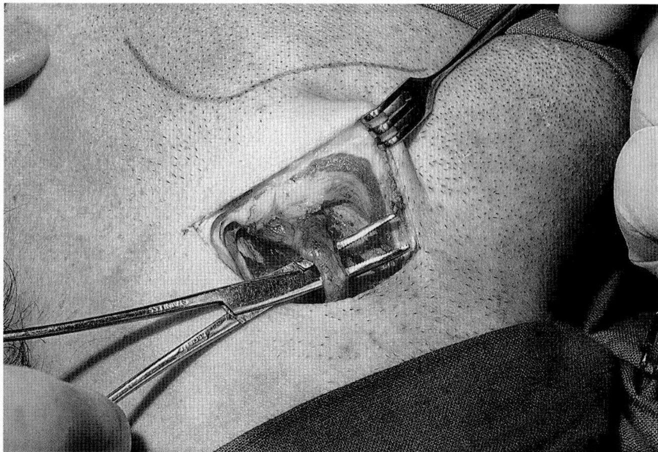

Figure 14.13 Skin flaps have been raised and the facial vessels mobilized prior to ligation.

Lingual and hypoglossal nerve damage

Neuropraxia of the lingual and hypoglossal nerves is unusual but possible, especially in those patients who have sustained numerous infective episodes. In these cases the gland is likely to be densely tethered to adjacent structures that become more difficult to identify and preserve. Planned resection of these nerves is necessary in locally advanced malignant disease and will result in hemianaesthesia of the anterior two-thirds of the tongue and limitation of tongue movements. A sensory deficit in the presence of malignant disease is usually tolerated well by the patient, but is a common source of litigation in those with benign or inflammatory pathology. Motor dysfunction of the tongue initially impairs articulation and mastication, but the patient rapidly compensates. Ultimately the tongue muscles waste on that side but without further symptomatic deterioration.

Cosmetic defects

The patient should be reassured that a properly placed skin incision is unlikely to leave a cosmetically unsightly scar.

Operative procedure: submandibular gland resection

The incision is made in or parallel to a natural skin crease approximately 2.5 cm below the lower border of the mandible and extending for approximately 10 cm anterior to sternomastoid muscle. It is deepened through the platysma muscle and flaps developed in the fascial plane immediately beneath it. Care must be taken in development of the superior flap as the marginal mandibular branch of the facial nerve runs in the same tissue plane. This nerve enters the neck 1 cm in front of the angle of the mandible, then loops over the facial artery and vein 2 cm below the lower border of the body of the mandible before sweeping superiorly to the angle of the mouth. The mandibular branch of the facial nerve can be protected from inadvertent damage by one of two manoeuvres. In the first, the facial vessels are transected at a low level on the surface of the submandibular gland and reflected superiorly (Fig. 14.13). The nerve, which lies lateral to the facial vessels, can thereby be lifted out of the operative field. Alternatively, the capsule of the gland can be opened at the level of the hyoid bone and dissection continued beneath it. The elevated capsule protects the nerve in a similar fashion to the first technique. Occasionally it is very difficult to identify the mandibular branch, and in these cases a nerve stimulator or monitor with sensing electrodes inserted into the orbicularis oris is helpful.

The superficial part of the gland is mobilized by either blunt or sharp dissection and retracted posteriorly to expose the deep portion that lies on the hyoglossus muscle and is partly covered by the mylohyoid muscle. Retraction of the mylohyoid anteriorly, together with posterolateral traction on the gland, brings the lingual nerve, duct and more proximal part of the facial artery into the operative field. The lingual nerve appears as a ribbon-like band loosely attached to the body of the gland by a few fibres: the parasympathetic secretomotor supply. Section of these fibres releases the nerve from the gland and permits it to assume a more superior relation. At this stage the hypoglossal nerve may be seen inferior and parallel to the lingual nerve but is sometimes partially covered by the posterior belly of the digastric muscle. The proximal part of the facial artery is usually ligated at this point. The gland is then further mobilized from the hyoglossus muscle and about its duct so that this may be ligated and transected as far anterior as possible. A small vacuum drain is inserted and brought out through the skin posteriorly. The wound is closed in two layers.

Skull and brain

15

Peter Bullock, Aabir Chakraborty

INTRODUCTION

Neurosurgery has advanced over the past decade largely as the result of developments in neuroradiology and neuroanaesthesia. This has led to expectations of improved outcome. An optimum outcome is still dependent on a clear history and a detailed examination being undertaken rather than relying solely on modern diagnostic technology. This chapter aims to review the presentation and management of the most frequently encountered neurosurgical conditions (Box 15.1).

Box 15.1 Common cranial neurosurgical conditions

Trauma
- Acute extradural haematoma
- Acute or chronic subdural haematoma
- Diffuse axonal injury and cerebral contusions
- Depressed skull fractures or complex fractures

Neoplastic
- Benign: meningioma, acoustic neuroma, pituitary adenoma
- Primary malignant: glioma (grades I–IV)
- Secondary malignant: lung, breast, gastrointestinal tract, melanoma

Vascular
- Aneurysmal subarachnoid haemorrhage
- Arteriovenous malformations
- Primary intracerebral haemorrhage

Infection
- Cerebral abscess
- Subdural empyema
- Meningitis

Hydrocephalus
- Congenital
- Acquired
- Communicating
- Obstructive

Functional
- Treatment of trigeminal neuralgia
- Epilepsy

ANATOMY AND PHYSIOLOGY[1]

The brain is protected by the cranial vault and is surrounded by the meninges, which form folds to separate the different compartments.

The brain is divided into two compartments (Fig. 15.1).

1. The supratentorial compartment comprises the two cerebral hemispheres, separated by the longitudinal fissure and

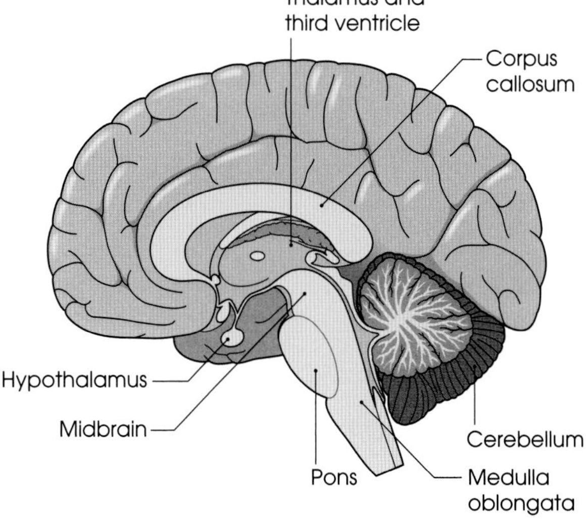

Figure 15.1 Anatomy of the brain.

   interconnected by the corpus callosum. The paired hemispheres encase the lateral and third ventricles, and merge with the diencephalon, the deep grey matter that includes the thalamus and the hypothalamus.
2. The infratentorial compartment comprises the cerebellum and brain stem, which continues down to the spinal cord.

The ventricles are a series of fluid-filled cavities within the brain that are in communication with the subarachnoid space, a thin layer of fluid over the surface of the brain.

The blood supply to the brain is from the internal carotid and vertebral arteries; these communicate with each other through the circle of Willis, which lies on the skull base under the centre of the cerebral hemispheres.

MICROSCOPIC ARRANGEMENT

The brain comprises neurons, neuroglia and microglia. The neuroglia act as support for the neurons. The three common cells of the neuroglia are the astrocyte, which is involved in providing physical and biochemical support for the neurons; the oligodendrocyte, involved in myelin production; and the ependymal cells that line the cerebrospinal fluid pathways. The microglia act as the monocyte–phagocyte system within the central nervous system.

Intrinsic brain tumours usually arise from astrocytes (astrocytomas), oligodendrocytes (oligodendrogliomas), and the

• REFERENCE •

1. Sinnatamby CS (ed). Last's Anatomy: Regional and Applied. 10th edn. Harcourt, Edinburgh, 1999

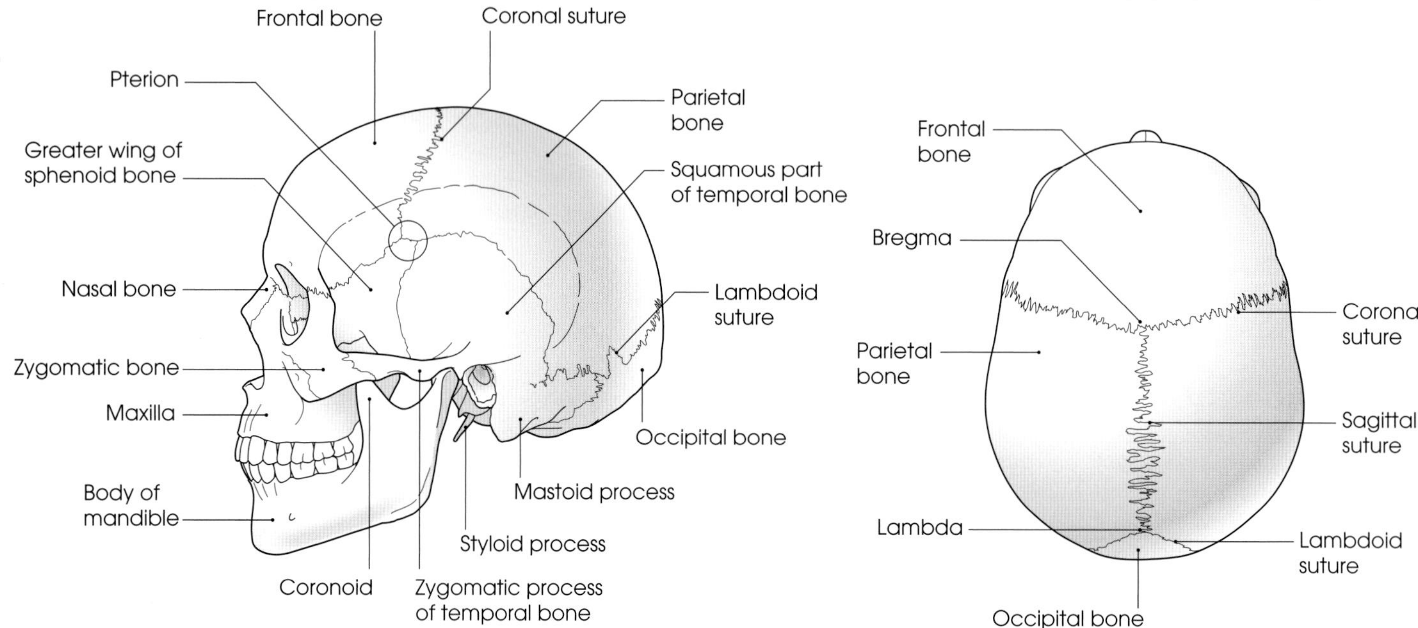

Figure 15.2 The bones of the skull and its sutures.

ependymal lining (ependymomas). This group of intrinsic brain tumours is collectively known as gliomas.[2]

THE SKULL

The skull (Fig. 15.2) is divided into the cranium and the facial skeleton. The cranium is divided into the vault (calvarium) and the skull base. The vault is formed by a number of individual bones that fuse after birth. This allows overlap of the bones during labour, facilitating delivery. Brain growth, and therefore increase in head circumference, is most marked in the first 6 months of life. It is unusual for premature fusion of one or more of the skull vault bones, known as craniosynostosis, to restrict brain growth, but it can lead to marked asymmetry of the skull.[3] It is therefore useful to recognize even single-suture craniosynostosis at an early stage so that any correction can be more effective. The complexity of the surgery required depends on the number of sutures involved. The procedures range from the excision of a single vault suture in sagittal craniosynostosis to complex staged craniofacial reconstructions undertaken by a multidisciplinary team for Crouzon's and Apert's syndromes.

Tumours of the vault are often benign. The most common types are osteomas and haemangiomas. Metastases can involve the skull in patients with advanced malignancy. Primary malignant tumours (e.g. osteogenic sarcoma) of the vault are very rare.

The inside of the skull base is divided into the anterior, middle and posterior cranial fossae. The anterior and middle cranial fossae have an irregular and undulating surface. In head injuries the brain may impact against these bony surfaces and this may lead to contusions of the inferior surfaces of the frontal and temporal lobes in typical coup and contrecoup fashion.

THE MENINGES[1]

The meninges are membranes that line the skull, and enclose and support the brain (Figs 15.3 and 15.4). There are three layers of meninges: the dura mater, the arachnoid mater, and the pia mater.

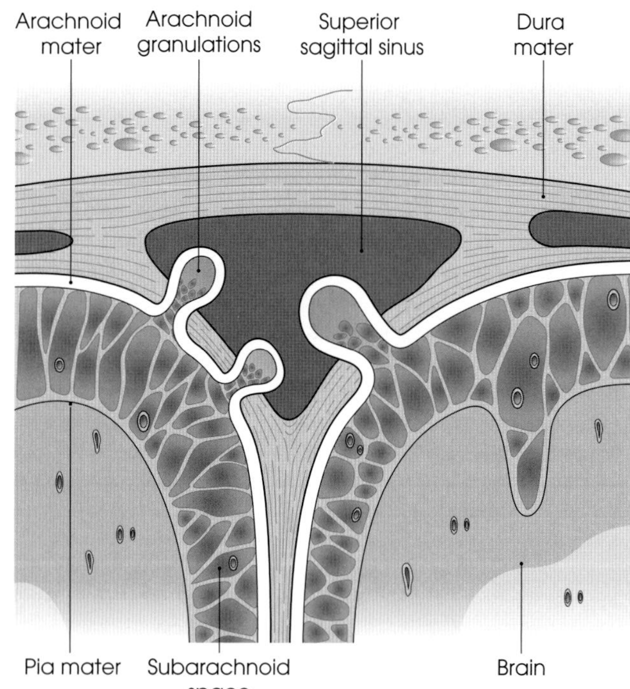

Figure 15.3 The relationship of the major venous sinuses with the dural folds.

REFERENCES

2. Youmans JR (ed). Neurological Surgery. 4th edn. Elsevier Science, Philadelphia, 1997
3. McLone DG, Reigel DH, Marlin AE (eds). Paediatric Neurosurgery: Surgery of the Developing Nervous System. 4th edn. Saunders, Philadelphia, 2000

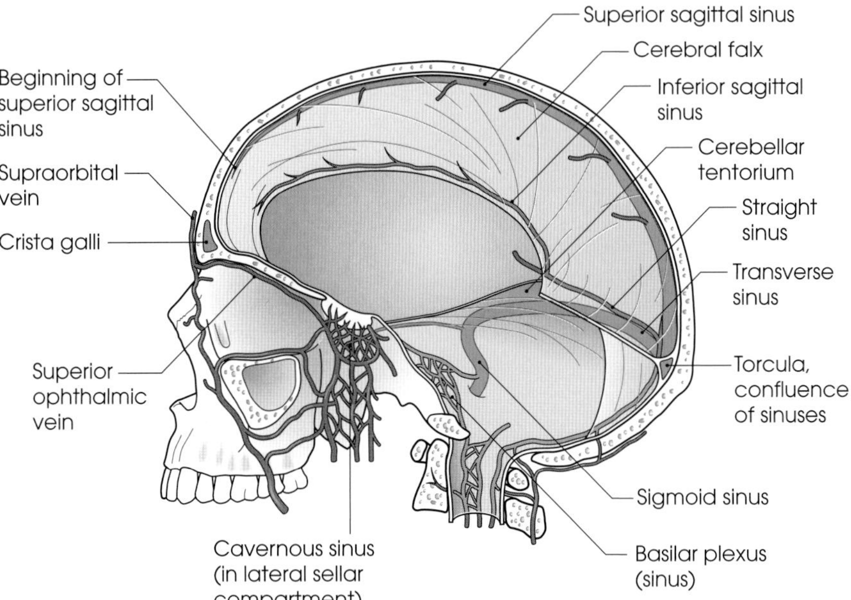

Figure 15.4 The scalp, calvaria (skull cap) and meninges: anterior view of the coronal section. Observe the layers of the scalp. The skin is bound tightly to the epicranial aponeurosis (aponeurosis epicranialis), which moves freely over the pericranium and skull because of the intervening loose connective tissue. The aponeurosis is the flat intermediate tendon of the occipitofrontalis muscle.

The dura mater

The dura mater is the fibrous outer layer of the meninges. This layer forms two major dural folds that support the brain. The midline falx cerebri separates the two cerebral hemispheres. The major superficial venous sinuses are formed between the layers of the dura mater. The falx cerebri carries the superior sagittal and inferior sagittal sinuses. The tentorium cerebelli is the other major dural fold that separates the cerebral hemispheres from the cerebellum. It is tent-shaped and projects from the margin of the transverse sinuses and superior petrosal sinuses up to the posterior clinoid processes. The tentorium cerebelli therefore divides the supratentorial and infratentorial compartments. The brain stem traverses the tentorial hiatus.

Brain shift and herniation is seen with expanding space-occupying lesions. This is most dramatically illustrated by a rapidly expanding extradural haematoma. Typically this haematoma occurs in the middle fossa and causes lateral shift of the hemisphere. The medial aspect of the temporal lobe (uncus) then compresses the midbrain and third cranial nerve. Clinically this is manifest by a decreasing conscious level, an ipsilateral dilated pupil, and a contralateral hemiparesis. In some patients with uncal herniation the posterior cerebral artery may also be compressed, giving rise to infarction of the occipital lobe.

Arachnoid mater and pia mater

The arachnoid mater is a fine membrane that is closely applied to the inner layer of dura mater and is separated from the surface of the brain by a thin layer of cerebrospinal fluid. This subarachnoid space also contains the major cerebral arteries. The basal cisterns are large subarachnoid spaces at the base of the brain. These are the sites where blood is most evident following a subarachnoid haemorrhage. Meningiomas are usually benign tumours that are thought to arise from cells in the arachnoid mater. The pia mater is a delicate membrane that invests both the brain and the spinal cord.

BLOOD–BRAIN BARRIER[4]

The blood–brain barrier is a physiological barrier formed by the tight junctions of the capillary endothelial cells. These tight circumferential junctions between endothelial cells in cerebral vessels restrict permeability, and this property distinguishes them from extracerebral capillaries. The tight junctions provide an anatomical barrier as well as high electrical impedance that restricts the passage of polar solutes (molecules with charged particles). Lipid-soluble molecules can still pass freely, but amino acids and sugars require specific carrier-mediated mechanisms. Mitochondria are found in three times the density in cerebral endothelial cells than in extracerebral vessels. This reflects the high-energy demands required to maintain these selective transport mechanisms. Pinocytic vesicles provide another form of passage in extracerebral vessels but are virtually absent in the cerebral capillaries. This probably explains the relative exclusion of plasma proteins from the cerebrospinal fluid.

The intact barrier limits the delivery of antibiotics and chemotherapeutic agents to the brain. The barrier is, however, breached in a range of pathological processes: where there is damage to the capillary bed, as seen in head injuries, or there is proliferation of new vessels with increased vascular permeability, as occurs with malignant brain tumours.

BLOOD SUPPLY[1]

Arterial supply

The internal carotid artery enters the skull vault from the carotid canal. It has a tortuous course through the petrous temporal bone and cavernous sinus. The supraclinoid portion bifurcates into the anterior cerebral artery and the middle cerebral artery. The vertebral artery joins its counterpart to form the basilar artery in the posterior fossa. The basilar artery bifurcates to form the posterior cerebral arteries that complete the posterior circle of Willis (Fig. 15.5). The circle of Willis is an anastamotic arrangement that maintains cross-flow after occlusion of one or more of the four parent vessels. Cerebral artery aneurysms most frequently arise at the junctions of the circle of Willis.

REFERENCE

4. Carpenter R. Neurophysiology. 4th edn. Arnold, London, 2002

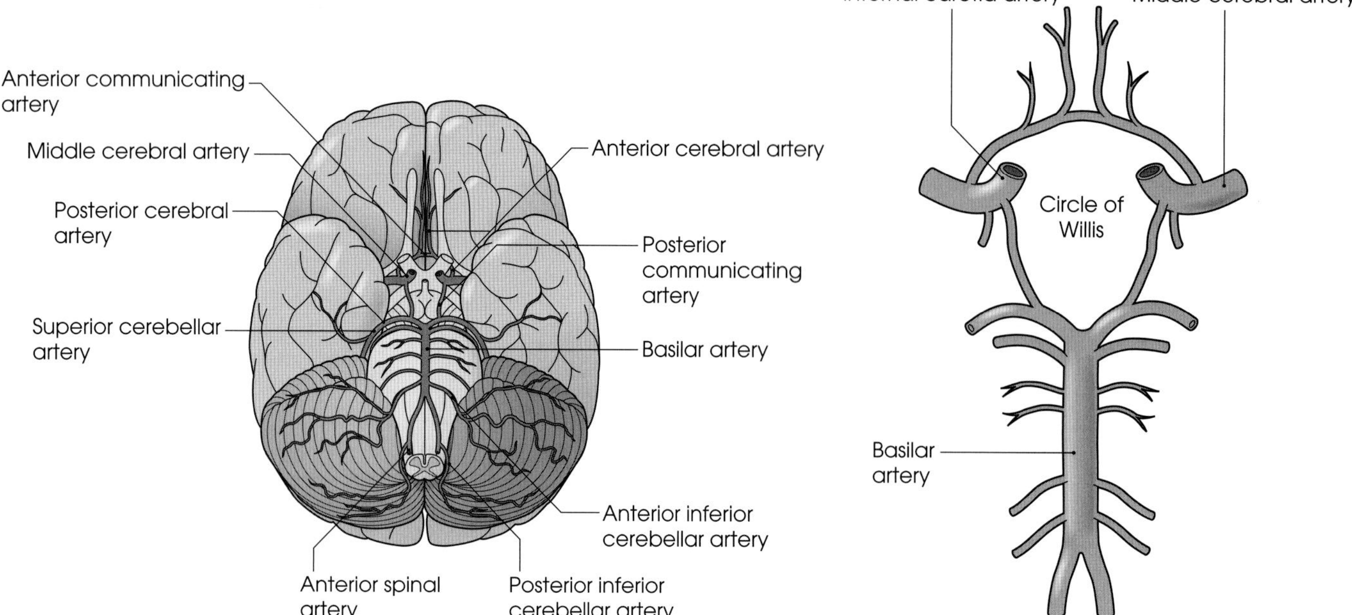

Figure 15.5 The circle of Willis: anastomotic arrangement between anterior and posterior communicating arteries.

Venous drainage

The cerebral veins are divided into a superficial group that drain the cortical surfaces, and a deep group that drain the deep white and grey matter. The deep venous channels course through the walls of the ventricles and basal cisterns to drain into the internal cerebral and basal veins via the lateral sinus into the internal jugular vein (Fig. 15.3). There are also connections between the intracranial and extracranial veins. These include the superior and inferior ophthalmic veins. It is important to recognize that periorbital cellulitis can lead to intracranial venous sinus thrombosis via these vessels. In addition, mastoiditis can give rise to thrombosis of the lateral sinus.

CEREBROSPINAL FLUID[1]

Cerebrospinal fluid is clear, water-like fluid that is largely produced by the choroid plexus. This is a continuous process, and approximately 500 mL are produced and absorbed in a day. The choroid plexus is in the third, lateral and fourth ventricles. Cerebrospinal fluid normally flows from the lateral ventricles via the foramen of Monro into the third ventricle (Fig. 15.6). It then passes through the aqueduct of Sylvius into the fourth ventricle and out via the foramina of Luschka and Magendie into the subarachnoid space over both cerebral hemispheres. The cerebrospinal fluid is absorbed by arachnoid villi that invaginate the superior sagittal sinus. The arachnoid granulations contain specialized cells that absorb cerebrospinal fluid and redistribute it to the venous system. In the normal state, cerebrospinal fluid passes freely between the cranial and spinal compartments.

Any obstruction to the cerebrospinal fluid pathways leads to hydrocephalus.[5] The typical obstructions seen in childhood are the result of congenital narrowing of the pathways (e.g. aqueduct stenosis). In adults, obstruction is more commonly from tumours and haemorrhage. A failure of absorption at the arachnoid granulations can be seen at any age. The arachnoid granulations can be occluded by meningitis, e.g. infection, and subarachnoid haemorrhage. This is described as a communicating hydrocephalus where the ventricles are in communication with the subarachnoid space. Thus any rise in intracranial pressure seen with a communicating hydrocephalus is distributed throughout the length of the craniospinal axis. This is of practical importance because it is safe to undertake a lumbar puncture in these circumstances. Box 15.2 shows the common causes of hydrocephalus.

Treatment of hydrocephalus involves diversion of cerebrspinal fluid to areas where the cerebrospinal fluid can be absorbed or by removal of the obstruction causing the blockage (usually a tumour).[5] The most common method of diversion is by inserting a ventriculoperitoneal shunt, although ventriculoatrial, lumbo-peritoneal and ventriculopleural shunts can also be used occasionally.

Third ventriculostomy is frequently used to treat obstructive hydrocephalus. An endoscope is inserted into the frontal horn of the lateral ventricle and then into the third ventricle via the foramen of Monro. A new pathway is opened through the floor of the third ventricle into the basal cisterns, thus bypassing the blockage.

VISUAL PATHWAYS[1]

The visual pathways pass from the eye via the optic nerves, tracts and radiations to the occipital lobes. The suprasellar area has a high incidence of tumours, and knowledge of the visual fields is essential for localizing these lesions. Bedside testing of the visual fields should be routine in any patient with a suspected pituitary lesion.

The ocular motor pathways have a complex integrated arrangement that is essential for normal ocular movements and balance. Assessment of the pupils and the presence of any ptosis or proptosis precedes testing of eye movements. Double vision is often caused by raised intracranial pressure consequent on a sixth nerve palsy. This is a non-localizing sign that can be bilateral.

• REFERENCE •

5. Arriada N, Sotelo J. Surg Neurol 2002; 58: 377

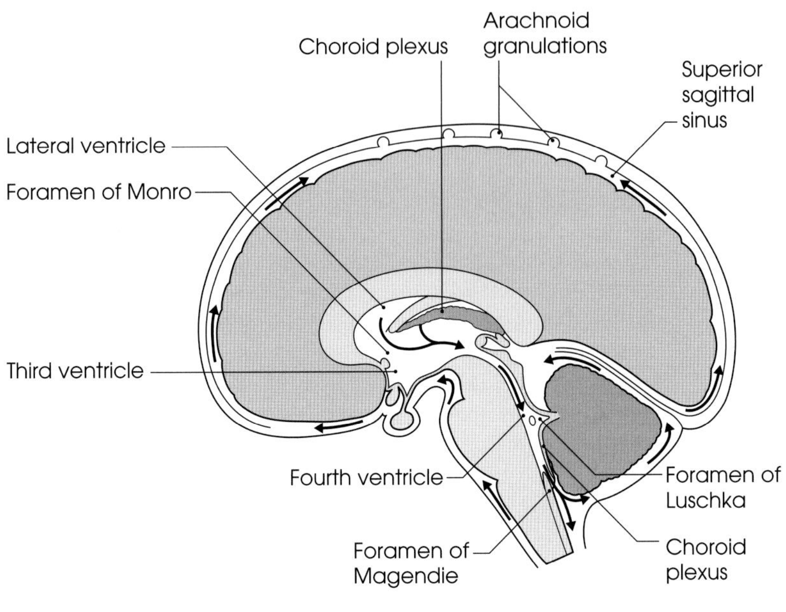

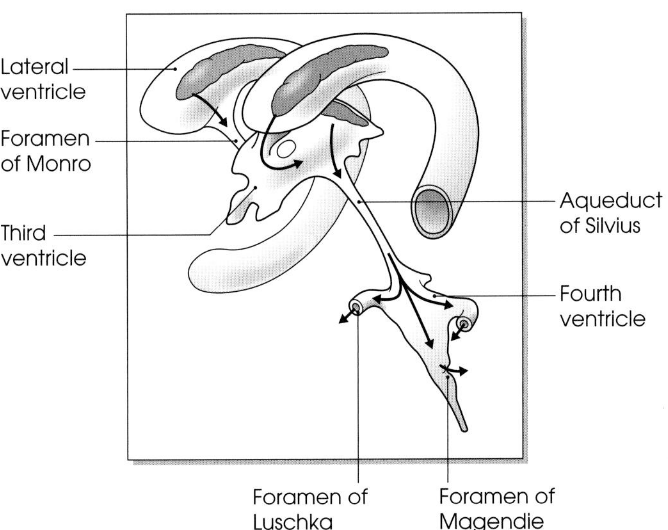

Figure 15.6 Midline sagittal section of the brain, showing the direction of cerebrospinal fluid flow. Cerebrospinal fluid is produced from the choroid plexus of the third and lateral ventricles. It passes through the foramen of Monro into the fourth ventricle. It then circulates over the surface of the brain and spinal cord through the median aperture in the fourth ventricle, called the foramen of Magendie, and the lateral apertures, called the foramina of Luschka. Absorption of cerebrospinal fluid occurs at the arachnoid granulations that are located along the superior sagittal sinus.

Box 15.2 Common causes of hydrocephalus

Loss of normal circulation (obstructive)
- Congenital: aqueduct stenosis, Chiari malformation, Dandy–Walker malformation
- Space-occupying lesions (e.g. tumour, haemorrhage, infection): posterior fossa, intraventricular

Underdrainage (communicating)
- Post meningitis
- Post traumatic
- Past subarachnoid haemorrhage
- Normal pressure hydrocephalus
- Intraventricular haemorrhage

Overproduction (rare)
- Choroid plexus papilloma

Figure 15.8 summarizes the visual pathways and the effects of lesions.

INTRACRANIAL PRESSURE REGULATION[4]

Monro–Kellie doctrine

The skull vault is a rigid box that has a constant volume of approximately 1700 mL in the adult. Its contents are brain (80%), cerebrospinal fluid (10%), and venous and arterial blood (10%). Compliance within the cranial cavity is usually high, and a slow growing tumour can reach a considerable size with little change in the intracranial pressure (Fig. 15.7). The modified Monro–Kellie doctrine explains the compensatory mechanisms that occur with a more rapidly expanding intracranial mass, such as a haematoma, abscess or malignant tumour. The intracranial volume is fixed, so there is a reciprocal decrease in the volume of venous blood and cerebrospinal fluid. Once these compensatory mechanisms are exhausted, then the intracranial pressure rises exponentially compared with any increase in the volume of the mass. This is the basis of the Monro–Kellie doctrine and explains the rapid rise in intracranial pressure and the deterioration in conscious level sometimes seen in neurosurgical patients.

CEREBRAL BLOOD FLOW[4]

Normal cerebral blood flow is high in order to maintain the metabolic demands of the brain. Blood flow averages 55 mL per 100 g of brain tissue per minute. Grey matter has higher metabolic demands and often averages 75 mL per 100 g. The natural ability to maintain cerebral blood flow over a range of blood pressures is termed *autoregulation.* This is usually effective within a range of mean arterial pressures of 50 and 160 mmHg.

Carbon dioxide tensions also influence cerebral blood flow. Hyperventilation leads to vasoconstriction and decreases cerebral blood volume. This manoeuvre is sometimes employed to reduce intracranial pressure. In contrast, vasodilatation and rises in intracranial pressure are seen with graded increases in carbon dioxide.

The cerebral perfusion pressure is the most significant factor that determines cerebral blood flow. It is routinely calculated in patients monitored in intensive care units. Cerebral perfusion pressure is defined as the mean arterial pressure minus the intracranial pressure. Thus with increasing intracranial pressure there may be a fall in cerebral perfusion pressure. At this point, measures may be taken to either lower the intracranial pressure or to raise the blood pressure. Normal intracranial pressure is 10–15 mmHg. The optimum cerebral perfusion pressure value is 80 mmHg. In brain death the intracranial pressure has reached a level where there is no cerebral perfusion, and a cerebral angiogram demonstrates the absence of intracerebral flow.

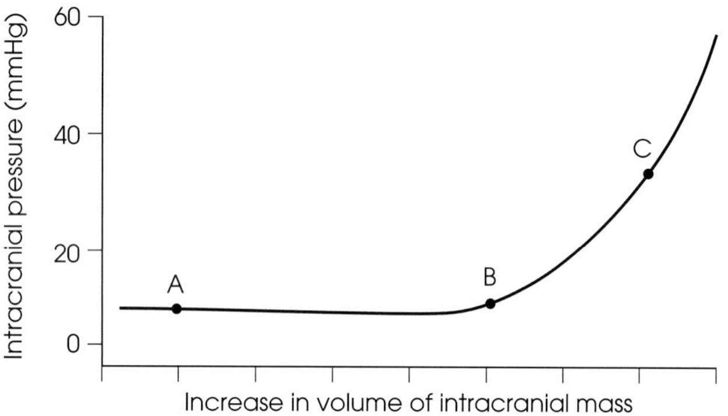

Figure 15.7 Development of intracranial hypertension: the pressure–volume curve. **A.** The intracranial mass (e.g. haematoma) begins to expand but intracranial pressure (ICP) does not increase because of displacement of cerebrospinal fluid and venous blood. **B.** The intracranial pressure is still normal but 'compensatory' mechanisms are exhausted. **C.** Any further increase in volume of the intracranial mass causes a marked increase in intracranial pressure.

CLINICAL PRESENTATION[6]

In general, space-occupying lesions in the brain have one or a combination of three main clinical presentations: headaches and drowsiness caused by raised intracranial pressure, focal neurological signs such as hemiparesis, and fits that may be focal or generalized. This combination of symptoms and signs is common to any space-occupying lesion such as tumour, brain abscess or haematoma. Time should be spent interviewing friends and family, because many patients with neurosurgical conditions are unable to give a detailed history themselves. Witnesses of road traffic accidents or falls often provide useful information not available from the unconscious patient. The patient may have complained of chest pain or suffered a fit before the fall.

Subarachnoid haemorrhage is one of the conditions that can be diagnosed on the history alone. The typical history is of a middle-aged individual, often a smoker, collapsing with the sudden onset of the worst headache of his or her life. The working diagnosis is a ruptured cerebral artery aneurysm (a berry aneurysm on the circle of Willis). A vascular malformation needs to be ruled out by angiography, but other rare causes of a spontaneous intracranial haemorrhage—such as vasculitis from cocaine abuse—can be excluded only by a careful history. The history enables the likely pathology to be identified and the examination localizes the region of the nervous system involved.

REFERENCE

6. Patten JP. Neurological Differential Diagnosis. 2nd edn. Springer-Verlag, Berlin, 1995

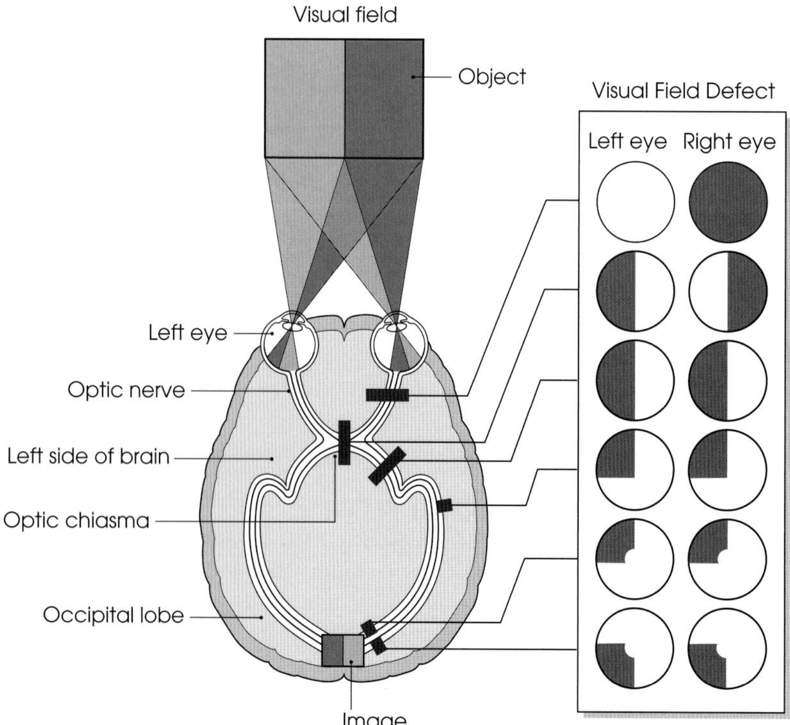

Figure 15.8 The optic pathway and visual disturbances created by specific lesions.

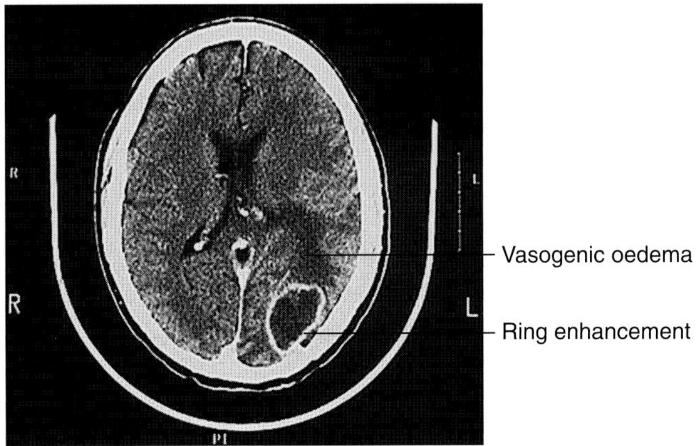

Figure 15.9 A contrast-enhanced CT scan showing a ring-enhancing lesion. A differential diagnosis would include tumour (primary or secondary) or infection. Careful history will give clues as to the aetiology. Note the vasogenic oedema and the asymmetry of the posterior horns of the lateral ventricles.

Table 15.1 The Glasgow coma score

Factor	Score
Best verbal response	
Orientated	5
Not orientated	4
Inappropriate words	3
Incomprehensible sounds	2
No response	1
Eye opening	
Spontaneously	4
To speech	3
To pain	2
No response	1
Best motor response	
Obeys commands	6
Localizes pain	5
Withdraws to pain	4
Flexion (abnormal) to pain	3
Extension to pain	2
No response	1

A working clinical diagnosis can be made in the majority of patients, and imaging then confirms the clinical findings. In a small group of patients the nature of the space-occupying lesion may not be evident; CT and MRI scans may simply demonstrate a ring-enhancing lesion, when the differential diagnosis can be wide, including opportunistic infections or lymphoma. A biopsy is required to provide a definite diagnosis in these patients, who are often immunosuppressed after organ transplant or have AIDS. Figure 15.9 shows the image for differential diagnosis of a ring-enhancing lesion.

THE GLASGOW COMA SCORE[7]

The Glasgow coma score is a practical scoring system of a patient's conscious level whatever the pathology. It enables a wide range of staff to reliably score the conscious level over an extended period of time. Teasdale and Jennett initially introduced this score in 1974 for the management of patients with head injuries in Glasgow. It is now used throughout the world for the assessment of neurosurgical patients whatever the underlying condition.

Three features are independently observed: eye opening, motor response and verbal performance. Table 15.1 summarizes the components of the score. It is the best response for each activity that is recorded. An overall score that ranges from 3 to 15 can be obtained by adding each individual activity. A score of 8 or less is generally accepted as a definition of coma. Patients in coma are routinely intubated and ventilated to protect their airway. An obstructed airway is the commonest cause of deterioration in patients with head injury.

TUMOURS[6]

Patients with brain tumours present with symptoms and signs of raised intracranial pressure, such as increasing headache, focal signs such as hemiparesis, or fits. The most common presentation of brain tumours is with a focal neurological deficit, usually a weakness of an arm and leg. Increasing headache is present in about half of patients with brain tumours at the time of diagnosis. The actual combination of symptoms and signs is dependent on the location and rate of growth of the tumour. Typically a rapidly growing, intrinsic, malignant glioma will present with both raised intracranial pressure and focal weakness. Fits are the presenting symptom in approximately one-third of patients with brain tumours.

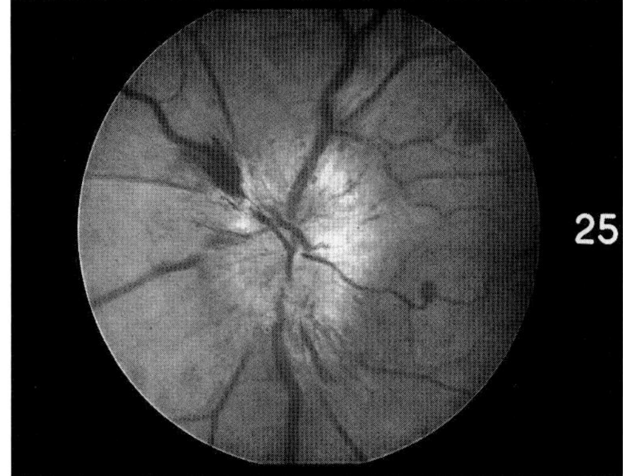

Figure 15.10 Papilloedema. Note the blurring of the optic disc.

Symptoms and signs of raised intracranial pressure

Headache, vomiting and drowsiness are the cardinal features of raised intracranial pressure. The headache is typically progressive and is often worse when lying down. It may wake the patient and be accompanied by vomiting that is not preceded by nausea. The headache is not usually localized to any one side and is usually severe and progressive. Younger patients with raised intracranial pressure are more likely to have papilloedema (Fig. 15.10). The absence of papilloedema is no guarantee that the pressure is normal. Fundoscopy should be performed on all patients with headache. The increasing frequency and severity of the headache reflects loss of intracranial compliance. Increasing brain shift and distortion lead to alterations in the conscious level. Lethargy and somnolence may be present by the time the diagnosis of a brain tumour is made. Drowsiness is a sign of raised intracranial pressure, and if untreated can progress to coma. Cushing's triad refers to bradycardia, hypertension and respiratory irregularities

• REFERENCE •
7. Teasdale G, Jennett B. Lancet 1974; 2: 81

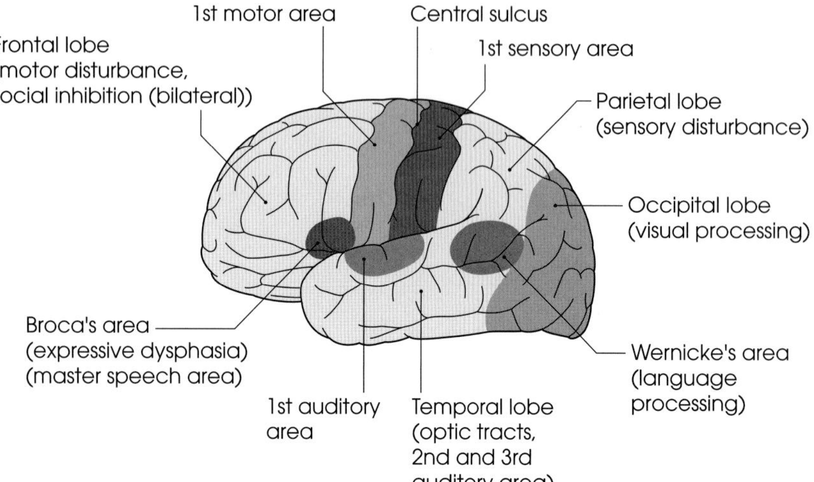

Figure 15.11 The functional localization of the cerebral hemispheres.

in coma. These are agonal events and reflect compression of the brain stem at the foramen magnum (coning) that can lead to brain death.

Focal neurological signs

Focal signs enable the site of the tumour to be localized. In a right-handed patient who presents with dysphasia and hemiparesis, the tumour is usually situated in the dominant temporal lobe. Dysphasia is often mistaken for confusion. Changes in personality and mentation are especially common in frontal lobe tumours. Tumours in the parietal lobe present with contralateral hemiparesis and sensory neglect. Occipital lobe tumours may cause a homonymous hemianopia. Cerebellar tumours present with ataxia and nystagmus. Figure 15.11 summarizes the correlation between common symptoms and focal signs and the site of the tumour.

Cranial nerve palsies are more commonly seen with tumours of the skull base. Unilateral deafness is a presenting feature of an acoustic neuroma and may be the only symptom for many years. Visual loss is seen with suprasellar extension of pituitary tumours and compression of the optic chiasm. Clinical features of pituitary tumours vary with the size of the tumour and whether it is secreting abnormally high levels of pituitary hormones. Secreting tumours produce a range of endocrine syndromes and tend to be diagnosed earlier than non-functioning pituitary tumours. The characteristic syndrome of acromegaly is from excessive growth hormone release. Cushing's disease is caused by central hypersecretion of adrenocorticotrophic hormone. Amenorrhoea and or galactorrhoea are seen with prolactinomas. Non-functioning adenomas are often macroadenomas by the time the diagnosis is made. They are associated with hypopituitarism and chiasmal compression causing bitemporal hemianopia. Patients may describe pain behind the eye, with diplopia or facial numbness if there is invasion of the cavernous sinus.

Epilepsy

Fits are a common presenting symptom, particularly in patients with low-grade tumours. Focal fits are witnessed in half of this patient group. A focal fit provides valuable clinical information on the likely site of the underlying tumour. Tumours involving the frontal and temporal cortex are particularly associated with both focal and generalized epilepsy.

NEUROVASCULAR DISEASE[6]

Subarachnoid haemorrhage

The most common cause of spontaneous subarachnoid haemorrhage is the rupture of a berry aneurysm at a junction of the circle of Willis (Fig. 15.5).[8] It is a devastating illness and many patients die before reaching hospital. A third of those affected are left disabled and a third go on to make a good recovery. Rebleeding and vasospasm are the major cause of morbidity and mortality in patients surviving the first bleed.

The classical history of a sudden onset of a severe headache is characterized by the headache being at its maximum within seconds or minutes. Patients often report that they feel they have been hit over the head. The subarachnoid blood fills the basal cisterns and leads to a chemical meningitis. Patients suffer intense headache, neck stiffness and photophobia. Focal neurological signs such as hemiparesis can often occur with middle cerebral artery aneurysms. Predisposing factors include smoking and hypertension. A family history is noted in less than 5% of patients. Congenital disorders such as polycystic kidney disease and coarctation of the aorta need to be excluded. Aneurysms can also present because of their local mass effect prior to rupture.

Arteriovenous malformations

Arteriovenous malformations are developmental anomalies that allow blood to pass directly from arteries into veins because the embryonic capillary bed fails to develop.[9] They can be classified by their size, the number of feeding vessels, and whether the venous drainage is superficial or deep. Their location is also important. They can be deep, superficial, or in an eloquent area, and there are frequently associated vascular abnormalities. High flows generate an increased incidence of aneurysms on the arterial feeding vessels, and on the venous side varices and stenosis can occur.

Arteriovenous malformations have a variety of clinical presentations, with intracranial haemorrhage being the most common. The haemorrhage is usually intraparenchymal, but rupture into the ventricles and subarachnoid space is common.

REFERENCES

8. van Gijn J, Rinkel GJ. Brain 2001; 124: 249
9. Fleetwood IG, Steinberg GK. Lancet 2002; 359: 863

The majority of patients survive the ictus and, unlike an aneurysmal bleed, the risk of rebleeding or vasospasm is much reduced. Fits are a frequent presentation, and these may be focal or generalized without signs of haemorrhage. Headaches are not infrequent and can be mistaken for migraine. They may be unilateral or generalized. Progressive neurological deficit developing over a long period can also result from ischaemia caused by a chronic steal syndrome.

INFECTION[2]

Intracranial abscess and subdural empyema are usually secondary to untreated sepsis in the frontal sinus or middle ear.[10] Intracranial abscess is rarely seen after head injuries because of the early aggressive debridement of open head injuries and the increasing use of prophylactic antibiotics. Advances in the care of patients with congenital cardiac and pulmonary conditions have also reduced the frequency of metastatic brain abscess. Immunosuppressed patients with HIV–AIDS or following transplants are at risk of a wider range of opportunistic organisms (see Ch. 4).

Brain abscess

Patients with a brain abscess present with a combination of raised intracranial pressure, hemiparesis and fits. *Streptoccocus milleri* is most commonly the only organism isolated from a brain abscess secondary to a frontal sinus infection. A mixed growth is more often seen in a brain abscess arising from a middle ear infection. Thus *Streptococcus*, *Staphylococcus*, coliforms and *Haemophilus* can be identified in a temporal lobe or cerebellar abscess. Pyrexia is not a major feature of a brain abscess because it is usually well encapsulated. Inflammatory markers such as erythrocyte sedimentation rate and C-reactive protein may be normal.

Subdural empyema

Infection in the subdural space over the cerebral hemisphere is less common but more serious. It is usually secondary to infection of the ear or frontal sinus (see Ch. 19). The infection is progressive and rapidly involves the whole surface of a hemisphere. A reduced level of consciousness follows headache with rapidly progressive focal neurological signs and meningism. The pus spreads widely over the cortical surface, causing thrombosis of the cortical veins. Infarction and swelling of the brain follow. Seizures are almost invariable.

Meningitis

Cerebrospinal fluid may leak from the nose or ear after a head injury associated with a fracture of the floor of the anterior or middle fossae. This cerebrospinal fluid rhinorrhoea or otorrhoea can lead to meningitis. Prompt treatment with antibiotics should be instituted once a diagnosis of meningitis is made. The site of the cerebrospinal fluid leak can be repaired later, once the infection has been cleared.

FUNCTIONAL NEUROSURGERY[6]

Trigeminal neuralgia

The trigeminal nerve provides sensation to the face. Trigeminal neuralgia is characterized by severe shooting pains in the distribution of the trigeminal nerve. There are often precipitating events that initiate an attack, such as eating, brushing teeth, combing hair, or even walking in a cold wind. Patients cannot eat because chewing triggers the pain. They commonly lose weight in severe attacks. The intractable pain can lead to suicide.

The cause of primary trigeminal neuralgia is thought to be a vascular loop compressing the nerve root entry zone. Secondary trigeminal neuralgia results from distortion of the trigeminal nerve in the cerebellopontine angle by tumours, cysts and aneurysms. It may also be a feature of multiple sclerosis. The neurological examination of a patient with primary trigeminal neuralgia is usually normal. Brain MRI is undertaken to exclude secondary causes of trigeminal neuralgia.

Epilepsy[6]

For the convenience of classification, epilepsy can be divided into localized and non-localized attacks. Further subdivision into idiopathic and symptomatic is more useful. More than 65% of all patients with epilepsy achieve good control with medical therapy. Patients with generalized idiopathic epilepsy respond to medical therapies more consistently. Patients with intractable complex partial seizures require assessment by a multidisciplinary team.

Standard preoperative evaluations include video-electroencephalogram telemetry, neuropsychological testing, intracarotid sodium amytal (Wada test), and neuroimaging studies. All these tests are designed to help localize the seizure focus. Electrophysiological cortical mapping and studies of the sulci and gyri on MRI play a role in directing any operative approach. Patients may be considered for focal resection to stop the fits, or hemispherectomy in refractory epilepsy and hemiplegia. Temporal lobectomy represents the largest subgroup of cortical resection in the treatment of complex partial seizures. Corpus callosotomy is undertaken when no focus has been identified and aims to alleviate the intensity and severity of the fits.

Movement disorder surgery

Deep brain stimulation and small discrete thermocoagulation lesions of the basal ganglia have been shown to effectively control symptoms in patients with advanced Parkinson's disease, dystonia and essential tremor, as well as conferring improved quality of life and a reduction in drug dosage. Tissue transplantation of adrenal tissue to the brain has brought modest benefits and remains an experimental option for Parkinson's disease.

INVESTIGATIONS

Investigations that are routinely employed in the preoperative assessment of neurosurgical patients include urea and electrolytes, because disturbances of fluid and salt balance are common in patients with intracranial pathology. Clotting studies are performed to reduce the risk of complications from bleeding. Rarely, tumour markers are detected for pineal tumours and are useful in the diagnosis of functioning pituitary tumours. Patients presenting with a solitary brain tumour need a general assessment to exclude metastatic disease. Computerized tomography of the thorax, ultrasound of the abdomen, and mammography should be considered to exclude primary tumours of the lung, breast, kidney and gastrointestinal tract. A lumbar puncture is useful in suspected cases of subarachnoid haemorrhage. Cytology and the identification of tumour markers can also be helpful in patients with leptomeningeal tumour spread. It is important that lumbar

• REFERENCE •

10. Rushing EJ, Burns DK. Neuroimaging Clin North Am 2001; 11: vii

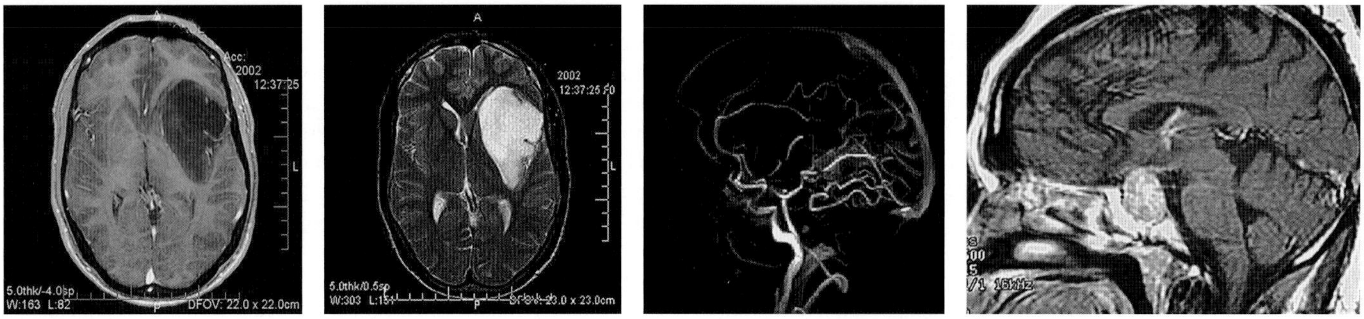

Figure 15.12 Magnetic resonance imaging and its applications to the brain. (**a**) T1-weighted and (**b**) T2-weighted MRI scans of the same patient. This demonstrates how the T1-weighted image gives excellent anatomical detail whereas the T2-weighted image gives more pathological detail. (**c**) Sagittal magnetic resonance venogram showing the major veins in the brain. (**d**) Midsagittal, contrast-enhanced, T1-weighted MRI scan showing a pituitary space-occupying lesion.

puncture is undertaken only in patients with communicating hydrocephalus and not in patients with raised intracranial pressure and focal signs.

SKULL X-RAY[11]

Plain skull X-rays are not routine investigations since CT and MRI have become more widely available. Skull X-rays still have a role in the management of mild to moderate head injuries. In this situation the presence of a skull fracture should alert the clinician to the increased likelihood of an underlying intracranial haematoma. Ninety per cent of patients with an acute extradural haematoma and 66% of patients with an acute subdural haematoma will have a linear skull fracture.

Skull X-rays are also indicated in patients with shunt dysfunction to ensure that there is no disconnection of the shunt tubing.

COMPUTERIZED TOMOGRAPHY[11]

In neurological emergencies, CT scanning is the investigation of choice, and it is often the primary investigation in many patients with a neurological complaint. It is widely available and the images can be electronically transmitted to the regional neurosurgical unit. The presence of extradural and subdural haematomas can be rapidly demonstrated. In the detection of brain tumours CT scan reliably detects over 95% of brain tumours, but very small tumours can be overlooked. The use of contrast enhancement is also essential to distinguish isodense lesions such as meningiomas from the surrounding brain. Faster multislice CT scanners are now widely available and allow three-dimensional reconstruction. The images can be adjusted to highlight bone or brain parenchyma. In addition, fine multislice imaging with contrast allows detailed imaging of vascular structures such as aneurysms. Computerized tomography scans are better tolerated than MRI, but because the radiation dose is considerably higher serial imaging should be avoided, particularly in children.

MAGNETIC RESONANCE IMAGING[11]

This is the preferred imaging technique for the initial evaluation and follow-up of brain tumours. The limiting factors are accessibility, time constraints, and tolerance of the procedure. MRI is more sensitive and has superior resolution when compared to CT and will detect smaller tumours. As with CT scan, the administration of contrast agents greatly increases the sensitivity of the study. Magnetic resonance imaging provides more detailed anatomy that can be viewed in multiple planes. However, it is not generally useful in the context of acute trauma.

The principles of MRI need to be appreciated to reduce the risk to the patient. The patient is placed in a strong magnetic field. Thus it is important that the patient has no cardiac pacemaker and no intracranial aneurysm clips. In the case of an anaesthetized patient, the anaesthetic equipment has to be specially modified. The strong magnetic field causes the protons in the water content of the body to align, and then a radiofrequency pulse is introduced that causes the spinning protons to move out of alignment. Once the radiofrequency excitation stops, the protons return to their resting state and give off a small amount of radiofrequency energy. Surface coils within the scanner detect this signal. T1-weighted images provide better anatomical detail, while T2 images are more sensitive to the water content. The intermediate or proton density images provide improved contrast between lesions and cerebrospinal fluid. Fluid-attenuated inversion recovery is a pulse sequence that abolishes the cerebrospinal fluid signal, enabling pathology adjacent to the cerebrospinal fluid to be seen more clearly. Advanced MRI can provide information on diffusion and perfusion in different regions of the brain. Magnetic resonance spectroscopy also provides information on regional and tumour metabolism. Figure 15.12 shows some common applications of MRI scanning in neurosurgery.

ANGIOGRAPHY[11]

The role of cerebral angiography has changed with the increasing demand for interventional procedures. Diagnostic angiography for a suspected aneurysm is now more often followed by an endovascular procedure such as coiling rather than an open operation and clipping of the aneurysm. Interventional neuroradiologists undertake a wide variety of procedures, including coiling of aneurysms in patients who have had a subarachnoid haemorrhage, and with the development of microcatheters, superselective embolization of arteriovenous malformations is routine. Both CT and MRI angiography have improved and taken the place of many of the previous indications for conventional angiography.

REFERENCE

11. Osbourn AG. Diagnostic Neuroradiology. Mosby, St Louis, 1993

ULTRASOUND[11]

Ultrasound is a valuable imaging tool in the first year of life when the anterior fontanelle is open. It allows a detailed review of the subdural space and ventricular system. In adults, Doppler studies are routinely used in the assessment of the carotid arteries (see Ch. 10). Ultrasound can also be used intraoperatively to localize superficial brain tumours.

FUNCTIONAL MAGNETIC RESONANCE IMAGING[11]

Functional MRI is used to measure small metabolic changes in active parts of the brain. This can be used to map those parts of the brain that handle critical functions such as speech, vision and movement. Brain mapping is undertaken by advanced MRI techniques such as echo planar imaging. Images are captured in less than 100 ms. Serial images provide information on changes in local blood flow after stimulation. This has clinical applications, for instance it can localize the motor strip prior to surgery for tumours in the region. During a functional MRI study the patient performs a particular task while the imaging is taking place. The metabolism in the area of the brain responsible for that task will increase, and the signal in the magnetic resonance image will change. By performing specific tasks that correspond to different functions, it is possible to locate the area in the brain that governs that function. The patient with an intrinsic parietal tumour will be asked to tap the index finger against the thumb to highlight the contralateral motor strip and determine its relationship to the tumour.

POSITRON EMISSION TOMOGRAPHY[11]

Positron emission tomography is a nuclear imaging technique that uses small amounts of radioactive isotopes (radionuclides) to measure cellular and tissue metabolism. Radionuclides are absorbed by healthy tissue at a different rate from pathological tissue. Positron emission tomography scans therefore provide a dynamic map of the metabolism of the brain. This can be coregistered with CT or MRI for planning surgery. The most commonly used positron-emitting isotope is fluorine-18 fluorodeoxyglucose. This is taken up into brain cells and tumour cells in a similar proportion to glucose uptake. The rate of uptake reflects the local metabolic rate. Low-grade glial tumours can be identified by their low uptake of fluorine-18 fluorodeoxyglucose. Its overall use is limited by its high cost, restricted availability, and poor spatial resolution compared with MRI or CT.

IMAGE-GUIDED STEREOTACTIC SURGERY[2]

This new technology gives surgeons the ability to navigate complex anatomy and remove deep-seated tumours.[12] By anticipating and avoiding important structures, blood vessels and functional areas, neurosurgeons can perform safer and more aggressive resection of tumours. This is a rapidly developing field with new innovations being regularly introduced. The aim is to accurately localize a lesion using minimum access and to prevent damage to surrounding structures. This can be achieved by a number of approaches.

Framed stereotactic methods

This is a method of targeting using a fixed head frame. The patient is fitted with the stereotactic frame under local or general anaesthetic. An MRI or CT scan is performed that incorporates the frame, allowing the target to be precisely localized in space. The position of the lesion relative to the frame is then measured, and the computer then calculates the X, Y and Z stereotactic coordinates directly. Lesions can be biopsied safely and rapidly with an accuracy of 2 mm. Stereotaxy also enables the accurate placement of deep electrodes to record or stimulate thalamic nuclei to treat movement disorders.

Frameless stereotaxy

The equipment complements a surgeon's visualization before and during surgery by taking image data from a CT scan or MRI and transforming it into three dimensions. The frameless systems use bony landmarks and skin markers to register the patient's skull in relation to deeper structures. A preoperative CT or MRI scan is performed on the patient with multiple small markers on the head. In theatre, a camera situated above the operating table registers the surface markers. This information is then transferred to the workstation and superimposed on to the preoperative scan using the markers as reference points. Optical sensors can then track instruments and relate them to the target area. This allows real-time localization based on the preoperative scan, but it does not compensate for potential shift of intracranial structures during the operation.

Intraoperative magnetic resonance imaging[2]

Intracranial navigation using a low-field intraoperative MRI allows the surgeon to reassess anatomical relationships in near real time. Neuronavigation provides intraoperative orientation to the surgeon, helps in planning a precise surgical approach to the targeted lesion, and defines the surrounding neurovascular structures. Co-registration of the functional data provided by functional MRI with neuronavigation helps to define the eloquent areas of the brain during surgery. An intraoperative MRI enables radical resection of the lesions and provides updates with intraoperative images to compensate for brain shift.

DIFFERENTIAL DIAGNOSIS[2]

TRAUMA[2]

Patients with head injuries are usually first seen in accident and emergency departments.[13,14] The diagnosis is straightforward in the majority. Doubt about the diagnosis can occur in a confused or unconscious patient where there is no clear history. Drug and alcohol abuse are increasing and can lead to diagnostic difficulties in the young, as can cerebrovascular accidents or fits in the elderly. Each of these conditions can also result in a head injury. The history from a friend or the family can be crucial. Information from ambulance personnel or police should be actively sought. Primary and secondary surveys are essential to rule out injuries elsewhere. At least a third of patients rendered unconscious from serious head injuries have injuries at other sites that can be overlooked. In adults, hypotension is rarely caused by

REFERENCES

12. Gildenberg PL, Woo SY. Stereotact Funct Neurosurg 2000; 75: 147
13. Molyneux A, Kerr R, Stratton I. Lancet 2002; 360: 1267
13. The Brain Trauma Foundation et al. J Neurotrauma 2000; 17: 457
14. Brain Trauma Foundation. Guidelines for the Prehospital Management of Traumatic Brain Injury. BTF, New York, 2000

a head injury and a ruptured spleen or liver need to be ruled out in such cases.

TUMOUR[2]

There is no single symptom or sign for diagnosing a cerebral tumour. A brain abscess can have a similar clinical presentation to a fast-growing malignant tumour. Both CT and/or MRI are essential to characterize whether a space-occupying lesion is a tumour and whether it is malignant or benign. In patients found to have a ring-enhancing brain lesion the differential diagnosis can be quite wide. A biopsy is usually indicated to provide a histological diagnosis. Without a biopsy a benign process can be overlooked (Fig. 15.8). A middle-aged woman treated for breast cancer presented with a fit and was discovered to have a solitary ring-enhancing brain lesion. It proved to be an abscess from a tooth infection rather than a metastasis.

It is increasingly common for patients to be referred with incidental findings. Meningiomas are a frequent finding with increasing age.[15,16] These tumours are often symptomless and found in elderly women. They do not all need surgery and often can be simply reviewed annually with follow-up scans. A middle-aged woman being investigated for tinnitus had a small convexity meningioma uncovered on scanning. It was not responsible for the tinnitus but she was referred for surgery. In these cases the natural history of the condition must be weighed against the risks of surgery. In some patients it can be difficult to determine whether the tumour is symptomatic, and a multidisciplinary team is helpful to provide sensible advice to the patient. An elderly patient may have an incidental meningioma discovered without any mass effect while being investigated for a transient ischaemic attack. In this case, carotid Doppler studies and an echocardiogram are more likely to provide the answer.

Computerized tomography brain scans (Fig. 15.8) show space-occupying lesions, both of which are causing midline shift from vasogenic oedema, and they enhance with contrast. The differential diagnosis includes a metastasis, a malignant glioma, and a cerebral abscess. The history, examination and investigations may help to narrow down the differential diagnosis, but the only certain way to make an accurate diagnosis is to take a biopsy.

A wide differential diagnosis is possible with sellar and suprasellar lesions. Pituitary adenomas are the most common pathology seen in this area (Fig. 15.12d) however other pathologies such as craniopharyngioma, sarcoid, metastasis and tuberculosis to name a few are also seen.

VASCULAR LESIONS[6]

The range of potential diagnoses is based on a detailed history and examination.[8] The history provides a likely pathology, for example sudden collapse with headache is likely to be the result of a brain haemorrhage. The neurological examination should allow the site of the haemorrhage to be localized. There are multiple causes for headache. The surgically important diagnosis is a subarachnoid haemorrhage. The first investigation is a CT scan, which will confirm 90% of subarachnoid haemorrhages. There is a small group of patients who have had a very small bleed that is not detectable on the CT scan. If there are no contra-indications a lumbar puncture should be performed. A normal lumbar puncture and CT scan effectively rule out a subarachnoid haemorrhage. Box 15.3 shows the range of diagnoses that present with a sudden-onset severe headache. This still leaves a wide differential diagnosis, and the priority is to exclude a structural abnormality. Ruptured cerebral aneurysms give rise to classical presentation of sudden onset of severe headaches with vomiting. An early CT brain scan will demonstrate blood in the basal cisterns, confirm the diagnosis of subarachnoid haemorrhage, and rule out a bleed from a tumour. When there are multiple aneurysms, an early CT scan may also identify the responsible aneurysm from the pattern of haemorrhage.

Box 15.3 Causes of sudden-onset severe headache

- Subarachnoid haemorrhage
- Venous sinus thrombosis
- Temporal arteritis
- Acute hypertension
- Arterial dissection
- Migraine
- Cluster headache
- Hydrocephalus
- Pituitary apoplexy
- Infection (cranial and non-cranial)
- Referred neck pain
- Benign exertional headache
- Post traumatic
- Temporal arteritis

Sudden onset of headache may be caused by a range of conditions (Box 15.3). How far should a severe headache be investigated in the absence of physical signs? Any neck stiffness or photophobia may have passed. The clinical management is therefore based entirely on the history. A conventional angiogram is required to fully exclude an underlying aneurysm. This is not without risk and therefore is not undertaken unless the history is strongly suggestive of a haemorrhage. Magnetic resonance angiography carries no risk but may miss a small aneurysm (less than 5 mm). An arteriovenous malformation will be excluded by conventional angiography. In other patients, vasculitis secondary to cocaine abuse may be responsible for the haemorrhage. In the absence of a good history the underlying cause of the haemorrhage could be overlooked. Magnetic resonance imaging is useful in the case of a negative angiogram; it may reveal a cavernous angioma not seen on conventional angiography.

DEMENTIA[6]

Dementia is common however there are a only a few conditions such as normal pressure hydrocephalus or a frontal tumour that with surgery allow the dementia to be reversed. The history is the most valuable element in a patient's assessment, and this may not be straightforward. A patient with a frontal tumour may also have Alzheimer's. This produces a progressive dementia associated with motor difficulties. A patient with dementia may have both communicating hydrocephalus and multi-infarct dementia. Magnetic resonance imaging cannot determine which is responsible and whether any intervention will be beneficial.

INFECTION[2]

The number of immunosuppressed patients is increasing with the increase in transplants and AIDS. Both groups of patients are

REFERENCES

15. DeAngelis LM. N Engl J Med 2001; 344: 114
16. Behin A, Hoang-Xuan K, Carpentier AF et al. Lancet 2003; 361: 323

at risk of a wide range of opportunistic organisms that can cause both systemic and brain infections.[10] Biopsy and aspiration may be the only method of establishing the organism responsible.

TRAUMA[17]

INTRODUCTION

Every year in the UK, one million patients attend accident and emergency departments with a head injury. The majority are cared for outside neurosurgical units. Guidelines have been developed to make it easier to recognize those patients with minor or moderate head injuries who need referral because of the risk of developing intracranial complications such as bleeding and infection. All patients with severe head injuries should be urgently referred for a neurosurgical opinion. Early recognition and treatment of severe head injuries reduce morbidity and mortality. The commonest causes of severe head injuries are road traffic accidents, falls, sporting accidents, assault, and accidents at home or at work. Alcohol and drug abuse are contributory factors in many severe head injuries.[18]

INJURIES TO THE SCALP[2]

There is a potential large space beneath the scalp (subaponeurotic space) that can be involved in trauma. The condition of patients with any form of scalp lacerations should be taken seriously. The scalp laceration should be fully debrided before being closed under local anaesthetic. A simple puncture wound may harbour a deeper penetrating injury. An X-ray or CT scan excludes an underlying skull fracture.

Cephalohaematoma

Cephalohaematoma (subpericranial haematoma) occurs as a result of a scalp injury in young infants. The haematoma is closely demarcated by the attachment of the pericranium at the suture lines. The edge of the haematoma can be mistaken for a fracture line. The haematoma is normally left to resorb, but the infant's haemoglobin should be monitored. The haematoma should not be aspirated because of the risk of infection.

Subaponeurotic haematoma

Subaponeurotic haematomas can follow a head injury at any age. After a few days they form large fluctuant swellings, often extending from the frontal region to the occiput. They occupy the space between the galea and the pericranium. Once again, these haematomas should not be aspirated and are best left to spontaneously resorb.

INJURIES TO THE SKULL

Fractures of the skull vault may be linear, comminuted or depressed. The detection of skull fractures is important because they indicate an increased risk of an intracranial haematoma. A linear fracture is seen in 90% of adult patients with extradural haematomas. Patients with skull fractures should all have a CT brain scan to exclude any underlying intracranial pathology.

Skull fractures may be simple or compound. Compound depressed fractures of the vault have a significant risk of causing intracranial infection. Fractures of the skull base are also often compound because they can open into the pharynx, nose, ear or sinuses. The diagnosis of a base of skull fracture is usually made on the clinical findings. Bilateral black eyes (panda sign) occur in fractures of the anterior fossa, and bruising over the mastoid process (Battle's sign) is seen with a fracture of the petrous bone.

Fractures of the skull base are often associated with cerebrospinal fluid rhinorrhoea or otorrhoea as well as cranial nerve palsies. These injuries also increase the risk of meningitis or abscess formation. Patients with cerebrospinal fluid rhinorrhoea should be advised not to blow their nose because there is a risk of forcing air inside the head (pneumocephalus). This can cause a severe headache and increases the risk of infection.

BRAIN INJURIES[2]

The pathological sequelae of injuries to the brain can be subdivided into effects caused by the initial impact and those arising from secondary complications.[13,14]

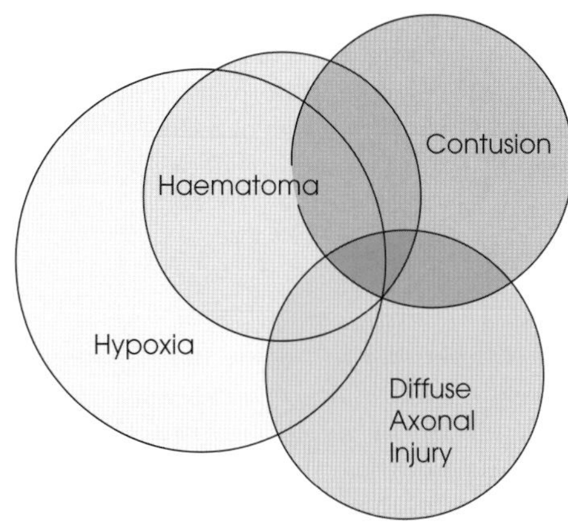

Figure 15.13 Causes of brain damage after severe head injury.

Primary injury[2]

The damage caused by the initial impact can be seen when a head strikes a surface such as a windscreen at high speed. The frontal and temporal regions of the brain impact on the inside of the skull, leading to local contusions. A contrecoup injury of the occipital pole may also occur. Such a pure anteroposterior movement is exceptional, and there is more often major rotational force leading to widespread damage by shearing of the white matter tracts. Thus acceleration and deceleration forces result in local cortical contusions at the site of impact as well as a more diffuse axonal injury. The significance of cortical contusions is that they can enlarge, coalesce, and produce significant mass effect, which is called a delayed traumatic intracerebral haematoma.

Diffuse axonal injury indicates widespread microscopic damage to the white matter tracts and usually reflects a high-speed deceleration injury. A CT brain scan soon after injury may be normal in a patient who is deeply comatose from diffuse axonal injury. Diffuse axonal injury is part of a spectrum, and in its most severe form patients never recover from deep coma, while in others it leaves long-term difficulties with memory and behaviour.

REFERENCES

17. Working Party on the Management of Patients with Head Injuries. Report of the Working Party on the Management of Patients with Head Injuries. Royal College of Surgeons of England, London, 1999
18. McEvoy AW, Kitchen ND, Thomas DG. Br Med J 2000; 320: 1322

Secondary injury[2]

Traumatic brain injury is the most common cause of death and disability in young adults. Early identification of severe traumatic brain injury with proper management along accepted guidelines can minimize the risk of secondary brain injury from hypoxia and hypotension, and improve the overall outcome. Respiratory obstruction and hypotension are common reasons for deterioration in patients with head injury. All patients with severe head injuries require early intubation and ventilation to prevent hypoxia and hypercarbia.[19,20] Hypoxia and hypercarbia promote anaerobic metabolism, which leads to a localized acidosis, and this subsequently leads to neuronal death as a secondary effect. Almost a third of patients with severe head injuries have additional injuries such as a ruptured viscus or an associated spinal injury. The more severe the head injury, the more likely is there to be other systemic injuries (see Ch. 7). Treatment is directed principally at preventing secondary brain damage (keeping the patient well oxygenated and normotensive) and at obtaining early identification of any intracranial haematoma. Fits also aggravate the primary damage and need to be rapidly controlled (Fig. 15.15).

ASSESSMENT[17]

Head injuries are classified by their severity as well as by the mechanism of injury. It is never safe to assume that a patient's impaired conscious level is the result of alcohol or drugs. Guidelines have been developed to identify patients at risk of intracranial complications, and the indications for skull radiographs are being replaced by the need for an early CT scan.

Mild head injuries

The majority of patients with head injuries seen in accident and emergency departments have suffered a mild injury with a Glasgow coma score between 13 and 15. Those patients who are fully alert with a normal skull radiograph can be sent home with a head injury card. It is important that they are discharged to the care of a responsible adult who has written instructions to return if there is any deterioration in the patient's condition. Patient should not be discharged if they have severe headache or drowsiness. Follow-up in the department or by the general practitioner should be arranged.

Moderate head injuries

Patients with coma scores of 9–12 are all admitted for observation because of a moderate risk of an intracranial haematoma. Early CT brain scans can reduce the morbidity and mortality from intracranial haematomas. In hospitals where CT scanning is not available there may still be a role for plain skull radiographs. A normal skull X-ray can help in the management of both minor and major head injuries. Identification of a skull fracture remains important because, despite the patient appearing well when first seen, it increases the possibility of an intracranial haematoma. A skull radiograph may also reveal an unsuspected depressed skull fracture.

Severe head injuries and multiple trauma[17,21]

Severe head injuries are defined as those with a Glasgow coma score of 8 or less. The priorities for all clinicians involved in the early resuscitation of an injured patient are the same regardless of specialty (see Ch. 7). In addition, the more severe the head injury, the more likely there is to be an associated systemic injury. One-third of head-injured patients in coma have a major injury elsewhere in the body. Rapid assessment and management take place along the lines recommended by the Advanced Trauma Life Support® system. Thus the airway, breathing and circulation are given the first priority to prevent hypoxia, hypercarbia and hypotension, all of which exacerbate secondary head injury. Immobilization of the neck is important until a cervical spine injury has been excluded (see Ch. 56).

Airway

The patient should have no respiratory obstruction. Sometimes a cricothyroidotomy may be required to establish an airway. At the same time, the patient should have his or her cervical spine immobilized using a hard collar, sandbags around the head, and strapping. The patient should be on a spinal board.

Breathing

The patient should be intubated and adequately ventilated to prevent hypoxia and hypercarbia and also to prevent aspiration of gastric contents. Inadequate ventilation may be the result of an underlying lung problem such as a pneumothorax, which should be treated at this stage.

Circulation

The patient needs to be haemodynamically stable with adequate intravenous access.[19] A source of bleeding must be sought and controlled in a patient who shows evidence of haemodynamic instability. Common sites include the chest, abdomen, retroperitoneum and long bones. Hypotension in an adult with a head injury is almost always caused by an extracranial injury.

Disability

The first neurological examination is aimed at diagnosing potentially life-threatening conditions that require urgent treatment. This should be performed before any sedation or paralysing agents are given if the patient is to be intubated or ventilated. The Glasgow coma score is assessed, as are the pupil responses. Subsequent assessments are performed to monitor progress. The neurological examination may improve after the patient has been resuscitated.

All patients with a depressed conscious level require a CT brain scan. Almost half of severely head-injured patients harbour a significant intracranial haematoma and require urgent transfer to a neurosurgical service. The most important indicator of an intracranial haematoma and the need for neurosurgical consultation is a decreasing conscious level. A patient unconscious from the time of the accident, and with equal pupils and no other lateralizing signs, is likely to have a diffuse head injury without any significant intracranial haematoma. They still require an urgent CT scan.

Exposure

The patient is fully exposed to rule out any other injuries that have been missed. The patient is also warmed at this stage.

REFERENCE

19. The Brain Trauma Foundation et al. J Neurotrauma 2000; 17: 471
20. Teasdale GM, Graham DI. Neurosurgery 1998; 43: 723
21. Committee on Trauma of the American College of Surgeons. Advanced Trauma Life Support for Doctors: Student Manual. 7th edn. American College of Surgeons, Chicago, 2001

X-rays

X-rays of the cervical spine, chest and pelvis are taken in all patients following major trauma.

Secondary survey

The whole scalp should be examined for abrasions and deep lacerations. There is a high incidence of cervical spine injuries in patients with head injuries. It is important to remember to exclude a neck injury in any patient with a facial or head injury. Children in particular can have significant spinal cord damage without bony injury. In patients with unexplained hypotension a spinal cord injury must be ruled out. Depending on the forces involved, a patient with one level of spinal injury must be fully examined to exclude a second spinal injury. The more severe the primary head injury, the more likely there are to be other systemic injuries.

TRANSFER TO A NEUROSURGICAL CENTRE[17]

A telephone consultation and an image link usually precede transfer of a patient to a neurosurgical centre. The patient should be fully stabilized before transfer. All patients with a Glasgow coma score of 10 or less, and those at risk of airway compromise, require endotracheal intubation before transfer. Bladder catheterization is also helpful. The personnel accompanying the patient must be familiar with the equipment and working environment of the transfer vehicle, and must be able to monitor the patient's condition accurately and perform any necessary procedures in the ambulance. It is also vital to ensure that all the documents and radiographs are sent with the patient. Interhospital transfers can be hazardous and must be planned carefully.

MANAGEMENT OF INTRACRANIAL HAEMATOMAS

Acute extradural haematoma[2,22] (Fig. 15.14)

Prompt evacuation of acute extradural haematoma is associated with an excellent outcome because there is often no underlying primary brain injury. It is therefore vital to diagnose the condition early.

Clinical presentation

Frequently the initial injury is not severe, and the patient may have been knocked down but not out. The impact is frequently to the temporal region, where the relatively thin skull is fractured over the middle meningeal artery. The fracture tears the meningeal artery, which bleeds into the extradural space. Patients complain of increasing headache. Vomiting and drowsiness follow. The patient readily falls asleep and is difficult to rouse. Lateralizing signs develop with an ipsilateral dilated pupil and a contralateral hemiparesis. Finally there is coma with bilaterally fixed dilated pupils, terminating in a respiratory arrest. The majority of patients progressively deteriorate from the time of the injury. The well-known lucid interval of an extradural haematoma is the exception. It is important not to wait until the patient is in coma before making the diagnosis. The outcome is directly related to the patient's conscious level before surgery. The mortality is close to zero for those with a coma score of 9 or above at the time of diagnosis.

Treatment

Extradural haematomas are ideally evacuated by a trained neurosurgeon. A craniotomy is rapidly undertaken with a power drill, and the haematoma evacuated before the bleeding meningeal vessel is secured. Other surgical personnel may undertake this procedure in an emergency if a neurosurgeon is not on site. An exploratory operation may need to be undertaken if the patient is rapidly deteriorating. Exploratory burr holes are indicated on the same side of the skull fracture or of the pupil that first dilates. Such a procedure should be undertaken only after neurosurgical consultation. The aim is to identify and evacuate the haematoma and to reduce the intracranial pressure. Mannitol, an osmotic diuretic, is given in a dose of 0.5 g per kg of body weight in adults as a single intravenous bolus over 15 min to 'buy time' on the way to theatre or during transfer.[23] Any patient who has been given mannitol should be catheterized.

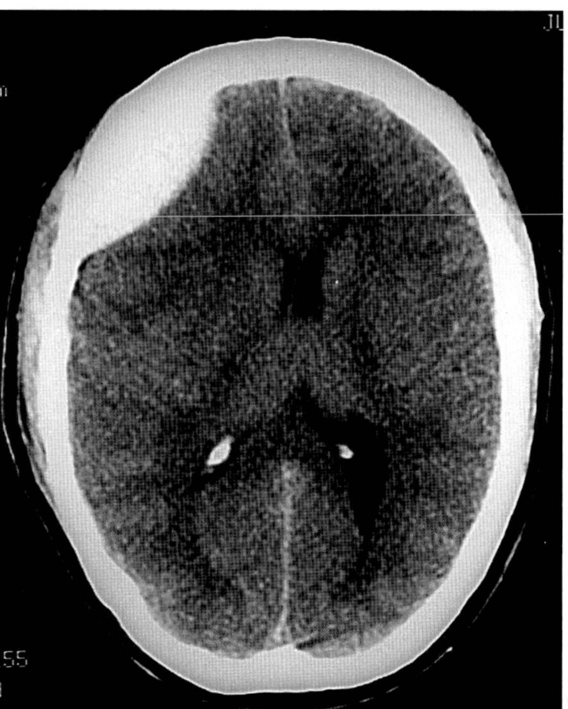

Figure 15.14 CT scan appearance of an extradural haematoma – typically a biconvex high density mass lesion causing midline shift.

Acute subdural haematoma[2,22] (Fig. 15.16)

Clinical presentation

Acute subdural haematomas usually result from high-speed injuries and are more frequent than extradural haematomas. These patients frequently have systemic injuries. The brain injury carries a high mortality and morbidity. Patients are often unconscious with lateralizing signs from the time of the accident. There is major damage to the hemisphere that is swollen. The surface of the brain is torn, and blood extends widely over the surface of the hemisphere (Fig. 15.15). The priorities are to evacuate the haematoma and then control the brain swelling.

REFERENCES

22. Schmidek HH, Sweet WH (eds). Operative Neurosurgical Techniques. 4th edn. Saunders, Philadelphia, 2000
23. Schrot RJ, Muizelaar JP. Lancet 2002; 359: 1633

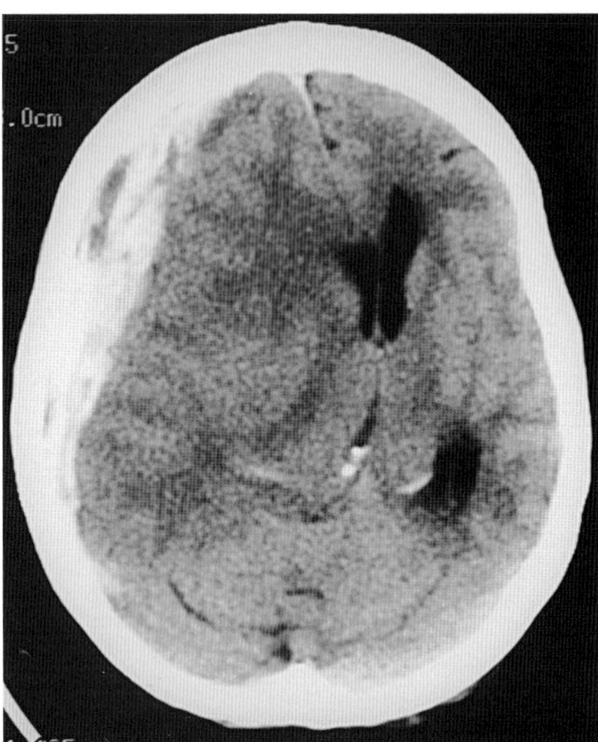

Figure 15.15 A CT scan appearance of a typical subdural haematoma, which follows the surface of the brain.

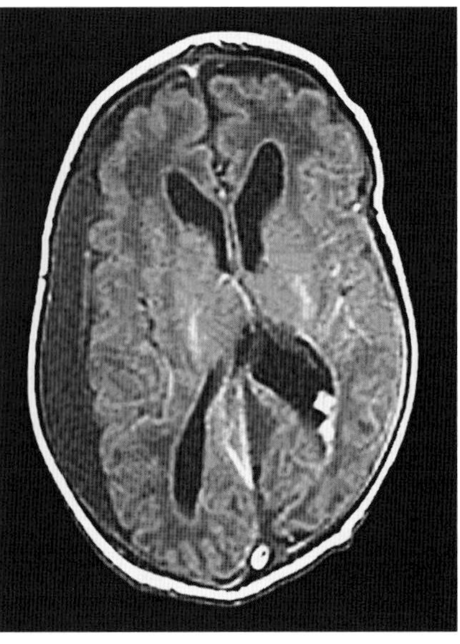

Figure 15.16 A CT scan appearance of a typical acute subdural haematoma, which follows the brain. Note the massive midline shift.

Treatment

Early evacuation reduces morbidity and mortality; however, the overall outcome is considerably worse than with an extradural haematoma. The mortality rate varies between 30 and 45%, the same number being significantly disabled, and 30% making only a moderate recovery.

Chronic subdural haematoma[2,22]

Chronic subdural haematomas have their peak incidence in the elderly.[24,25] They are often triggered by minor trauma. The atrophied brain is mobile, and as a result this puts the surface bridging veins at risk of stretching and rupturing from modest injury. Epileptic patients, alcoholic patients, and patients on anticoagulants have an increased incidence. Patients may not become symptomatic for many days or weeks after an otherwise minor head injury. Progressive symptoms of headache, failing intellect, hemiparesis, and a fluctuating conscious level are common. These subdural collections are often liquid by the time of diagnosis and can be drained by burr holes under local anaesthetic. The results of treatment of chronic subdural haematoma are generally good despite the advanced age of many of the patients. Up to 90% recover their premorbid function (Fig. 15.16).

SURGICAL PROCEDURES

Figure 15.17 shows the instruments commonly used for performing a burr hole and craniotomy.

Procedure for making a burr hole[2,22]

Burr holes are sited in the standard positions (Fig. 15.18).

1. Clean, shave, prepare and mark the area where the burr hole is to be made, also marking the major venous sinuses to prevent inadvertent injury.
2. Infiltrate with local anaesthetic.
3. Make a short incision down to the bone.
4. Insert self-retaining retractors and dissect the periosteum off the bone.
5. Using the perforator drill bit on the Hudson brace, drill into the bone until rocking is felt. This indicates that the perforator has pierced the inner table.
6. Use the burr drill bit to widen the hole. Never press down into the hole.
7. Use the sucker to evacuate the immediately visible haematoma.
8. If no blood is found, open the dura with a tenotome and sharp hook to decompress the subdural compartment.

Procedure for performing a trauma craniotomy[2,22]

Blood must be cross-matched for the patient and must be in theatre for a child. The most common trauma craniotomy is made using a question mark skin incision to give access to the frontal, parietal and temporal lobes (Fig. 15.19).

1. Clean, shave, prepare and mark the area where the burr hole is to be made, also marking the major sinuses to prevent inadvertent injury. Infiltrate with local anaesthetic if there is time.
2. Make the temporal burr hole as described above. This should be performed as quickly as possible to decompress the underlying haematoma.
3. Using the skin knife, the incision should be extended along the marks made. Cut through the skin, subcutaneous tissue and galea. Haemostasis can be achieved by applying clips to the flap.
4. Develop the plane between the galea and the temporalis muscle and pin the flap back out of the way.
5. Using a periosteal elevator and cutting diathermy, mark out the outline of the bone flap. The temporalis muscle should retain its pedicle inferiorly.
6. Make two or three further burr holes in the appropriate positions. Avoid making holes over the venous sinuses.

REFERENCES

24. Maurice-Williams RS. Lancet 2001; 357: 1308
25. Maurice-Williams RS. Br J Neurosurg 1999; 13: 547

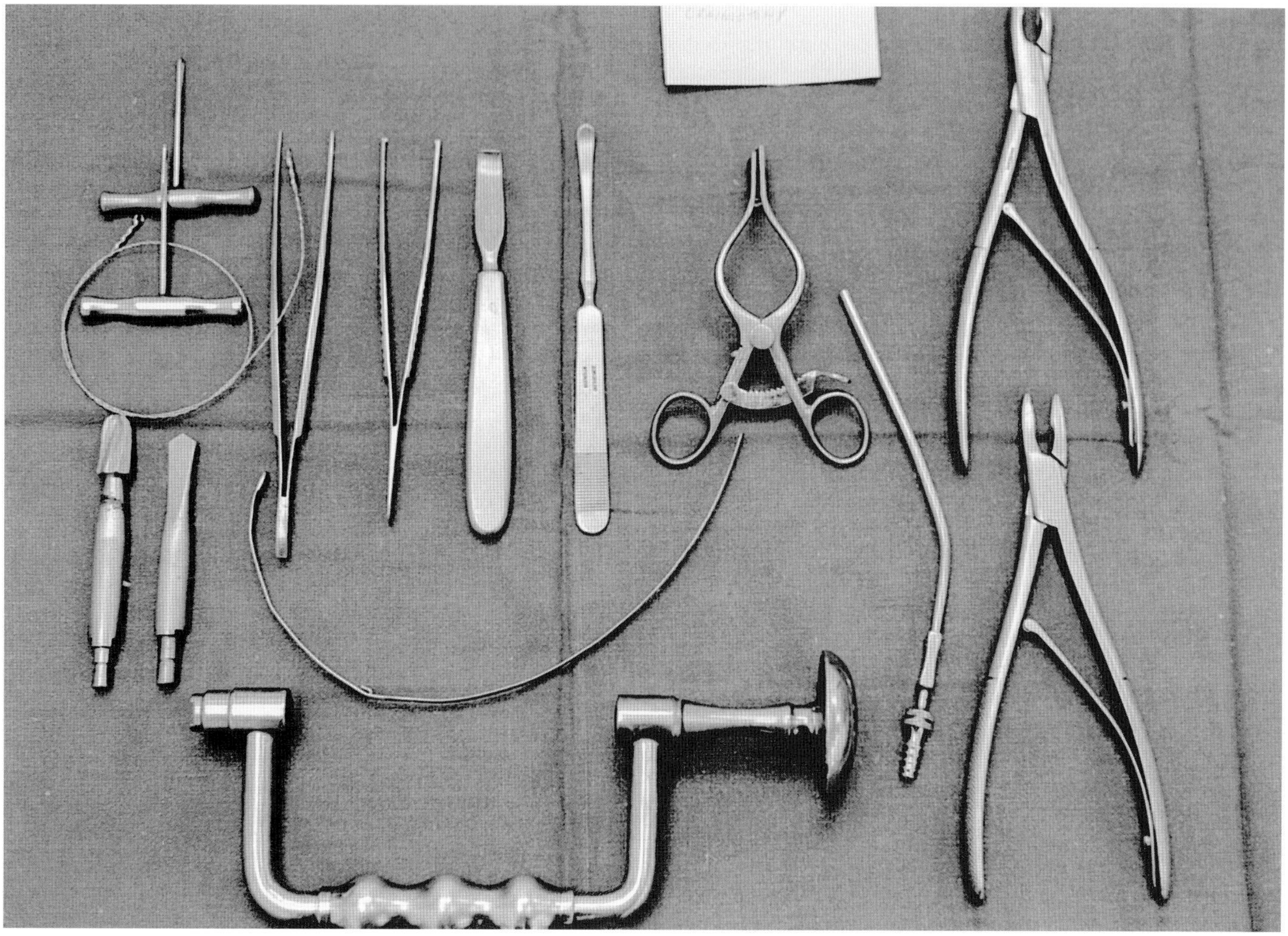

Figure 15.17 Tools required for a burr hole. Gigli saw, Periosteal elevator, Retractor, Bone nibblers, Burr, Perforator, Hudson brace and sucker.

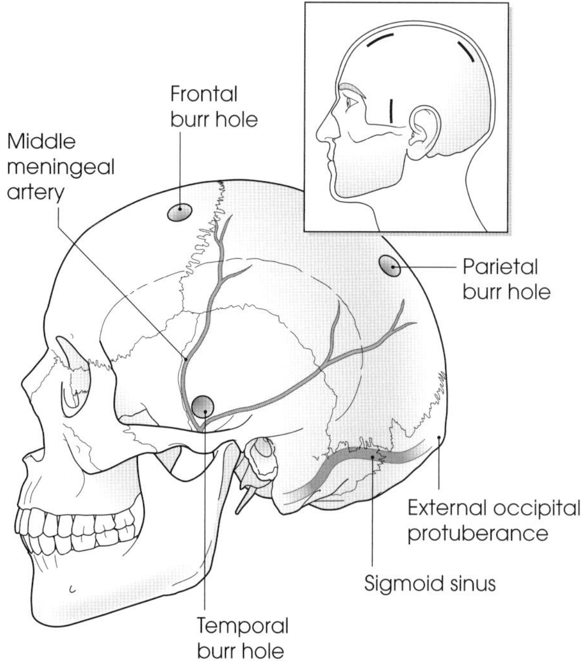

Figure 15.18 Cranial landmarks, standard positions of exploratory burr holes.

7. The burr holes can be connected up using a Gigli saw. This instrument has a guide that strips the dura and also protects the underlying surface. The Gigli saw acts like a cheese cutter.
8. The bone flap with the overlying temporalis muscle should be carefully retracted back to expose the extradural haematoma.
9. In the first instance, even if it is dark and bulging, the dura should only be opened with a small incision to release any subdural blood and prevent excessive brain herniation.

MANAGEMENT OF THE PATIENT WITH A SEVERE HEAD INJURY IN THE INTENSIVE CARE UNIT[2]

Intracranial pressure monitoring

The current management of patients with brain injury but who do not have intracranial haematomas includes sedation and controlled hyperventilation to reduce the swelling and maintain optimum cerebral perfusion. The neurological examination is restricted to monitoring the pupil responses, where changes are seen only after major rises in intracranial pressure. Intracranial pressure monitoring is therefore of value and provides a means of calculating cerebral perfusion, as well as detecting early rises in intracranial pressure caused by brain swelling, or the formation of an intracranial haematoma.

Cerebral perfusion pressure

The maintenance of an adequate cerebral perfusion pressure is considered to be one of the fundamental aims in the management of patients with severe head injuries. It is calculated by subtracting the intracranial pressure from the mean arterial blood pressure. The optimum range is 60–80 mmHg.

Methods for reducing intracranial pressure

Most centres have written protocols on the stepwise introduction of therapeutic measures to control a rising intracranial pressure. Although the medical management of raised intracranial pressure forms an important part of the treatment of the head-injured patient, it must be remembered that surgical evacuation of an intracranial haematoma provides the most effective means of controlling raised pressure. A repeat CT scan should be considered in ventilated patients with an unexplained rise in intracranial pressure to exclude a delayed haematoma.

Hyperventilation remains the primary method by which raised intracranial pressure is controlled. In patients with severe head injuries, the brain swells in the fixed space of the skull and displaces the cerebrospinal fluid. The brain swelling also reduces the venous space, and if hypercapnia occurs it leads to further rises in intracranial pressure from cerebral vasodilatation. Even mild hypercapnia can cause a marked rise in intracranial pressure. Controlled hyperventilation aims to reduce the partial pressure of arterial carbon dioxide to between 3.5 and 4.5 kPa. Reducing the levels below pCO_2 3.5 kPa results in vasoconstriction, and this causes further ischaemic damage to areas adjacent to the injury. The patient's position in bed is also important, and the simple manoeuvre of elevating the head and upper body to 30° maximizes the cerebral venous return and lowers the intracranial pressure. Intravenous mannitol given in regular small doses can be effective (0.2 g/kg) in the absence of a raised osmolality and may be continued for several days. In a single larger dose (0.5 g/kg), it can reduce intracranial pressure rapidly when there is evidence of imminent cerebral herniation despite adequate hyperventilation. Induction of moderate hypothermia and barbiturate coma are other techniques occasionally used to control raised intracranial pressure.

COMPLICATIONS OF HEAD INJURIES[2]

Basal skull fracture

Cerebrospinal fluid leak (otorrhoea and rhinorrhoea), pneumocephalus and meningitis are potential complications of a base of skull fracture. Treatment is usually conservative, although repairs may be required if the leak persists or infective complications develop. Antibiotics should not be given while the cerebrospinal fluid leak is present, unless the patient becomes septic.

Anosmia can occur following a base of skull fracture as a consequence olfactory nerve damage.

Post-traumatic epilepsy

The overall risk of late epilepsy after head injury is approximately 5%. The three most significant factors that increase the likelihood of late epilepsy after a head injury are an early seizure, an intracranial haematoma, or a depressed fracture. When none of these factors is present the incidence is only 1%. Early seizures occur more frequently in patients with contusions, acute subdural haematomas, and penetrating injuries. Early seizures increase the risk of late epilepsy. Three-quarters of patients developing late epilepsy suffer their first fit within 1 year of the injury. After a depressed fracture the overall risk of late epilepsy is 15%, but this is increased by the presence of a dural tear, focal signs, post-traumatic amnesia over 24 h, or early epilepsy. The risk of late epilepsy is not influenced by whether the bone fragments are elevated or not.

Prophylactic anticonvulsants remain controversial but are not given routinely in head-injured patients because trials have not shown convincingly that they reduce either the incidence of early seizures or the prevention of late epilepsy. Prophylaxis is of benefit in patients with penetrating injuries or those patients who have suffered an infective complication, where the risk of developing seizures is high.[26]

Caroticocavernous sinus fistula

Carotid cavernous fistulas are abnormal communications between the carotid artery and the cavernous sinus. A traumatic fistula may result from a fracture of the floor of the middle cranial fossa tearing the wall of the carotid artery at its entry to the cavernous sinus. A high-flow fistula leads to considerable back-pressure in the orbital draining vessels. This causes marked proptosis and hyperaemia of the eye. The patient usually complains of the noise from the fistula, and a bruit can be heard over the eye. The proptosis is pulsatile. The dangers of this fistula are loss of vision, ophthalmoplegia, and the risk of a catastrophic nasal haemorrhage. Treatment is by occlusion of the fistula using endovascular techniques. A variety of agents have been used to occlude the fistula, including balloons, glue and coils.

Stab wounds and other penetrating injuries may also result in a direct fistula. Patients who suffer a stab injury to the head should undergo cerebral angiography to exclude a fistula.

TREATMENT AND OUTCOME

The range and complexity of neurosurgical procedures has increased over the past decade. Most brain surgery carries considerable benefits as well as a small risk of serious complications that still involve a risk to life and limb. Patients and their families now regularly demand a fuller understanding of the surgeon's goals as well as the setbacks they could face. It is therefore important that sufficient time is given to answer these questions. In general, a fully informed patient is more likely to be a surgeon's ally. It is also worth emphasizing that outcome from any intervention cannot just be considered in terms of morbidity and mortality, but that the quality of outcome is also important. These broader dimensions are difficult to measure and include functional ability, pain and well-being, which are inevitably based on subjective feelings and different cultural attitudes.

SURGERY[22]

Major operations on the skull and brain are usually performed with controlled anaesthesia. The ability to undertake microsurgery has been enhanced by three-dimensional visualization before and during operations as well as more advanced operating microscopes. Optimum surgical corridors can be planned more accurately, and this can improve outcome. Many lesions are deep within the brain, so navigation to the target is routinely

REFERENCE

26. Chang BS, Lowenstein DH. Neurology 2003; 60: 10

incorporated. Various approaches are used to enter various parts of the cranial vault.

SPECIFIC DISEASES[2]

Outcome in head trauma

The outcome for patients with head injuries usually depends on the severity of the initial impact. The quality of outcome after mild or moderate head injury depends not only on the kind of injury but also on the kind of brain. It has been shown that a previous head injury delays the recovery rate after a mild or moderate head injury. It is clear that for many patients the long-term outcome is determined primarily by their intellectual and behavioural disabilities rather than by any physical impairment.

In severe head injuries the recognized risk factors conferring a poor prognosis include age, and motor and pupil response. Older patients have a higher mortality rate, with a predisposition to both intracerebral and subdural haematoma. The motor response has independent prognostic significance at any age. The poorer the motor response, the poorer is the outcome. The loss of pupil reactions is an ominous sign and reflects brain stem compression with evidence of herniation. The majority of patients with fixed and unreactive pupils after a severe head injury do not survive.

Tumour

The surgical management of brain tumours ranges from craniotomy and complete excision of surface tumours such as meningiomas to the stereotactic biopsy of a deeply seated malignant tumour of the brain stem.[15,16,27,28] The surgical management of malignant brain tumours includes tumour biopsy and debulking procedures to improve the quality and length of survival, and provides the best platform for adjunctive radiotherapy and chemotherapy.

The advances in both imaging and intraoperative technology enable a very accurate biopsy to be taken of a tumour in any site with very low morbidity and mortality. Sophisticated planning of approaches to tumours is possible with three-dimensional reconstruction of both CT and magnetic resonance images, which is particularly valuable for tumours around the base of the skull. Intraoperative localization by frameless stereotaxy or ultrasound is now routinely available, as is endoscopy for intraventricular tumours. Intraoperative monitoring of the facial and auditory cranial nerves ensures identification and preservation of function. Electrocorticography and functional mapping can be of value in tumours that are adjacent to the motor strip.

The craniotomy can be undertaken under local anaesthetic for tumours in eloquent regions, for example temporal lobe tumours to preserve speech function. Removal of deeply sited thalamic tumours by ultrasonic aspirators and lasers can be improved by overlapping the computer-generated image of the tumour on to the microscope image to ensure that the full extent of the tumour has been reached. Robotic surgery is also being developed. Virtual reality is being explored for training purposes, allowing the neurosurgeon to rehearse different approaches to the same region and identify various anatomical structures en route.

In most cases a biopsy is recommended as a minimum to establish the diagnosis once a solitary space-occupying lesion has been demonstrated. Surgery can be graded by the extent of tumour removal. Generally, complete excision has a better long-term outcome than subtotal resection or incomplete removal. Patients with a suspected malignant tumour who do not undergo biopsy and are treated on the MRI or CT appearance run the risk of a more benign process, such as an abscess or a benign tumour, being overlooked.

Chemotherapy has a primary role in some rare brain tumours. Cisplatin and its derivatives are successful in the treatment of intracranial germ cell tumours, but most of the common malignant brain tumours are relatively unresponsive to chemotherapy. The nitrosoureas are of benefit in a third of patients with malignant gliomas because they are fat-soluble and cross the blood–brain barrier without difficulty.[29]

Radiation therapy is commonly used in the treatment of malignant brain tumours.[30] It usually takes the form of external beam irradiation that can be delivered focally or to the whole brain. A number of advances in the delivery of radiotherapy have improved both its efficacy and its safety. Radiosurgery, or the Gamma Knife, is the single delivery of a finely focused beam to a small volume. The dose by any form of radiation therapy is limited by the tolerance of the surrounding brain. Recurrent tumours may be treated with stereotactic focal irradiation (Linac or Gamma Knife) or by brachytherapy, which is the implantation of a local radiation source.[31] The side effects from radiation include early hair loss, and in later years the possibility of hypopituitarism and radiation necrosis. Radiation necrosis can often be distinguished from recurrent tumour by positron emission tomography. An additional late risk from radiation therapy is the development of a second malignancy.

Meningiomas[32] (Fig. 15.19)

Meningiomas are generally regarded as having a good prognosis. They can occur anywhere on the inner surface of the skull from the base to the convexity. They are found twice as often in women and usually in later life. The mainstay of treatment is surgical removal. Complete excision can, however, still be a challenge when the tumour has encircled vital structures such as the carotid artery or invaded the sagittal sinus. Radiotherapy may be recommended for patients with residual tumour or for those patients with an aggressive histological variant. Not every patient requires an operation. In more and more patients, symptomless tumours are being uncovered on imaging. A period of observation for these patients is often recommended.

Gliomas[2,32] (Fig. 15.20)

Low grade gliomas

Most histologically benign forms of astrocytoma occur in childhood.[33] The cerebellar pilocytic form usually presents with ataxia and headaches, and is potentially the most curable with surgery alone. Other forms of low-grade astrocytomas include the optic nerve gliomas. This group may be associated with neurofibromatosis and have a more indolent course. The diffuse low-grade astrocytoma and mixed oligoastrocytoma are more

REFERENCES

27. Ewend MG, Carey LA, Morris DE et al. Curr Treat Options Oncol 2001; 2: 537
28. Dunn IF, Black PM. Neurosurgery 2003; 52: 1411
29. Batchelor T. Lancet 2000; 355: 1115
30. Laperriere N, Zuraw L, Cairncross G. Radiother Oncol 2002; 64: 259
31. Sansur CA et al. Stereotact Funct Neurosurg 2000; 74: 37
32. Fuller GN, Goodman JC. Practical Review of Neuropathology. Lippincott, Williams & Wilkins, Philadelphia, 2001
33. Stieber VW. Curr Treat Options Oncol 2001; 2: 495

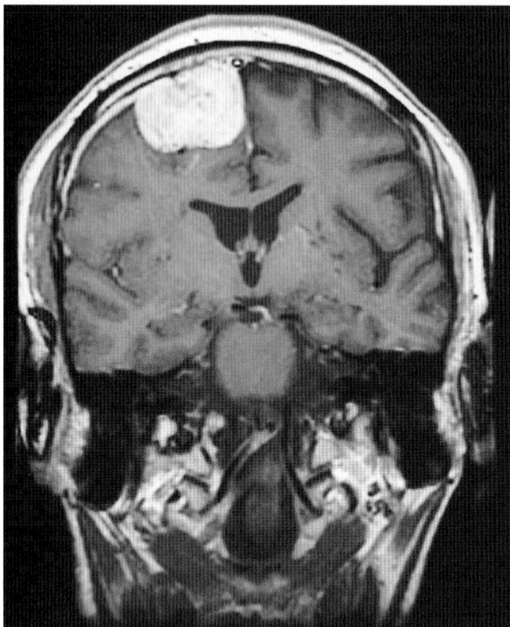

Figure 15.19 MRI scan of a right parasagittal meningioma.

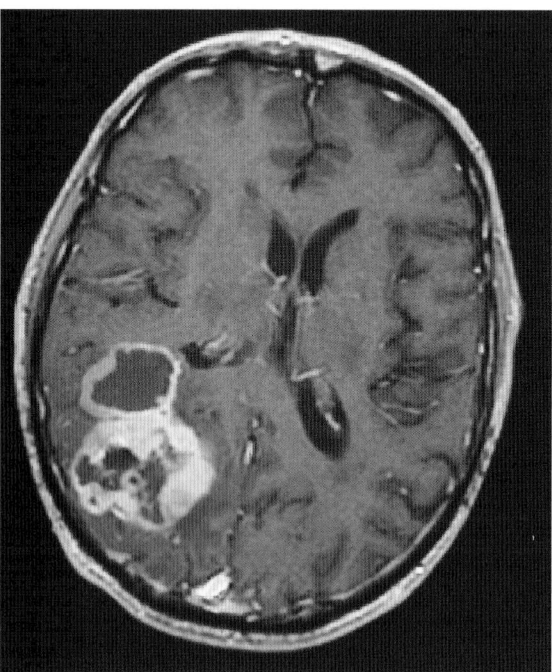

Figure 15.20 A parieto-occipital high grade glioma.

common in young adults and typically arise in the frontal lobe. Seizures are the most common presenting symptom. It is important to note that many low-grade gliomas transform into malignant gliomas with time. The median survival is between 7 and 12 years.

HIGH GRADE GLIOMAS

High-grade gliomas should be maximally debulked and then irradiated.[28] Surgical procedures are generally graded by the extent of tumour removal: from complete, to subtotal, to incomplete, to biopsy only. For gliomas the extent of tumour resection is largely related to the site of the tumour. Deep lesions in the brain stem or thalamus may be managed by biopsy alone. Unfortunately, management of malignant gliomas generally remains palliative, with a median survival of approximately 18 months even with a combination of surgery and radical radiotherapy. Younger patients have a slightly better prognosis.

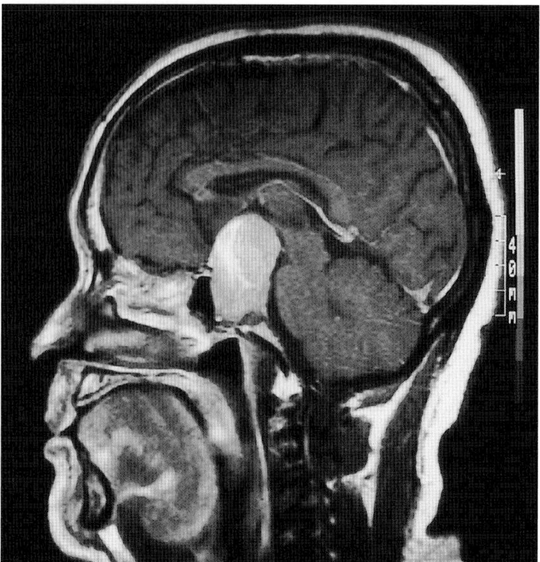

Figure 15.21 Mid sagittal MRI showing a pituitary macroadenoma.

Pituitary tumours[2,32] (Fig. 15.21)

The best outcome for patients with pituitary tumours is achieved by a multidisciplinary team of an endocrinologist, neurosurgeon and radiotherapist.[34] Patients require the minimum of a full endocrine and visual assessment with detailed MRI. Simple observation may be indicated for patients with small tumours that are not producing significant endocrine disturbance. Prolactinomas are best treated medically with a dopamine agonist such as cabergoline in the first instance, and the tumour is monitored in the first 6 months to see if it is shrinking. Surgical therapy remains the treatment of choice for all other pituitary tumours. The trans-sphenoidal route is the best approach for the majority of pituitary tumours, with craniotomy being infrequently undertaken. The recognized complications of the trans-sphenoidal route include a cerebrospinal fluid leak, bleeding, infection, and leaving the patient with hypopituitarism. Acromegaly and Cushing's disease can be cured by surgery. Radiotherapy is used to treat residual or recurrent tumour. External beam or focal stereotactic radiotherapy can be employed. Long-term endocrine follow-up is essential.

Acoustic neuromas[2,32]

Acoustic neuromas are slow-growing nerve sheath tumours that fill the cerebellopontine angle. Most tumours are unilateral, and when bilateral are associated with neurofibromatosis type 2. Presenting symptoms and signs include deafness, ataxia and tinnitus. Small tumours may be treated with stereotactic radiosurgery or kept under review and managed conservatively.[35,36]

REFERENCES

34. Arafah BM, Nasrallah MP. Endocr Relat Cancer 2001; 8: 287
35. Battista RA, Wiet RJ. Am J Otol 2000; 21: 371
36. Wright A, Bradford R. Br Med J 1995; 311: 1141

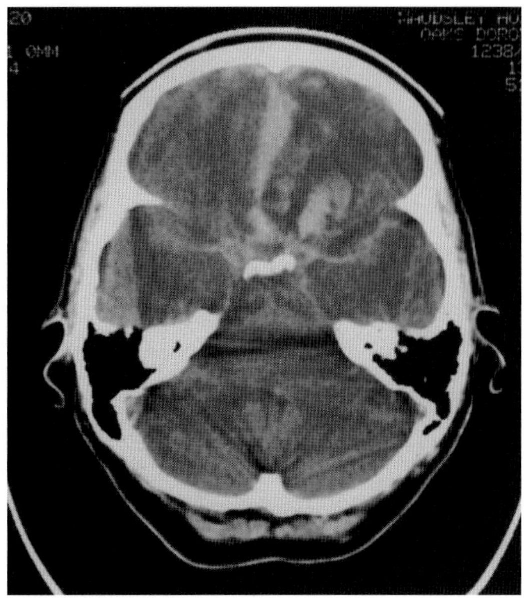

Figure 15.22 CT scan showing subarachnoid haemorrhage possibly from a ruptured anterior communicating artery aneursym.

Larger tumours require surgery, often using the translabyrinthine approach. The size of the tumour is directly related to the likely outcome, with tumours more than 4 cm having an increased risk of a facial nerve palsy. Complete excision should be seen as curative.

Subarachnoid and intracerebral haemorrhage[2]

(Fig. 15.22)

The traditional approach over the past 30 years has involved a craniotomy and direct clipping of the neck of the aneurysm to prevent rebleeding.[8,37] The rapid development of the endovascular technique now provides a useful alternative. This involves packing small, soft, platinum coils into the aneurysm sac that excludes it from the circulation. Only aneurysms that have a relatively narrow neck are amenable to this technique, which is generally undertaken by an interventional neuroradiologist. The International Subarachnoid Aneurysm Trial has shown that the overall outcome with coiling of small anterior circulation aneurysms can be better than with open surgery.[38]

The majority of aneurysms treated are those that have ruptured. In treating symptomless unruptured aneurysms, the risks of haemorrhage must be balanced against the risks of intervention. The risk of rupture increases with size, and the current consensus is that an aneurysm of more than 1 cm in diameter carries a significant risk if left untreated.

The outcome from subarachnoid haemorrhage is often dependent on the clinical condition of the patient at the time of presentation. In addition, the patient's age and volume of blood on the CT scan can influence the outcome. There are several grading systems used to classify all of these factors that in turn reflect the extent of the initial brain damage. A good grade reflects an alert patient who is free of any neurological deficit. A patient in poor grade may remain in coma from the initial ictus. Some patients may die before reaching hospital. The overall outcome can be disappointing, with many successfully treated patients unable to return to their former work because of problems with memory and concentration. A grading system is shown in Table 15.3.

Table 15.3 The World Federation of Neurological Surgeons (WFNS) grading of subarachnoid haemorrhage

WFNS grade	Glasgow coma score	Focal neurological deficit
I	15	Absent
II	13–14	Absent
III	13–14	Present
IV	7–12	Present or absent
V	3–6	Present or absent

Intracerebral haemorrhage is the commonest presentation of cerebral arteriovenous malformations. Fits may be present for years before the haemorrhage, but the majority of the morbidity and mortality is related to the haemorrhage. Cerebral arteriovenous malformations are about one-tenth as common as aneurysms. Treatments include surgical excision, endovascular occlusion and radiotherapy. The management therefore needs a multidisciplinary team. All symptomatic patients should be offered definitive treatment, while symptomless patients should be reviewed and the individual risks and benefits of any treatment option considered.

Infection[2]

Brain abscess

A bacterial brain abscess should be treated by drainage or excision followed by intravenous antibiotics. A generous craniotomy and wash out is the most effective treatment for subdural empyema, followed by prolonged intravenous antibiotics and anticonvulsants. Improved outcome is related to early diagnosis, more accurate localization, and more potent antibiotics. The main prognostic factor remains the neurological condition at the time of diagnosis, as is true for a wide range of intracranial pathologies. Patients in coma at the time of diagnosis are less likely to survive. Prophylactic anticonvulsants are recommended for all patients because of the high risk of fits.

Functional surgery

Trigeminal neuralgia

Trigeminal neuralgia is a severe facial pain that can be rapidly diagnosed and effectively treated. It is thought to occur as a result of vascular compression of the trigeminal nerve at its origin from the brain stem. Medical treatment with carbamazepine or gabapentin is often the first choice. Surgery is recommended in patients who still have pain on maximum therapy. The surgical options range from partial destruction of the nerve by selective thermocoagulation of the retrogasserian region via the foramen ovale to microvascular decompression via a direct posterior fossa exposure. This technique is successful in the majority of patients when a vascular loop is identified. Other treatments include stereotactic radiosurgery (Gamma Knife).

REFERENCES

37. Lawton MT, Spetzler RF. Neurosurg Clin North Am 1998; 9: 725
38. Molyneux A et al. Lancet 2002; 360: 1267

Epilepsy

Many patients with intractable epilepsy can be helped by surgery to reduce the number of fits. Temporal lobectomy provides good seizure control for 60–80% of individuals who previously suffered intractable fits. A good outcome correlates closely with uncovering specific pathology.

There are very few studies that have addressed the quality of life in patients after epilepsy surgery. Measures of surgical outcome are often very basic and do not look at psychosocial factors. Broader outcome measures incorporating all dimensions of day-to-day living are difficult to measure and therefore not frequently included. Surgery for epilepsy cannot necessarily reverse the other disabilities that these patients may suffer, such as intellectual impairment, social difficulties, or psychiatric disorders.

The neck

16

Anthony E. Young

INTRODUCTION

The clinical problem most often encountered in the neck by surgeons is a swelling. The diagnosis of such swellings is one of the classical exercises in clinical expertise. It requires not only knowledge of the anatomy of the neck, but also the skills of focused history-taking and careful examination; these two alone will yield a diagnosis in the majority of cases.

A swelling in the neck may be of a type common elsewhere in the body, such as a sebaceous cyst or lipoma; if the swelling is lymphadenopathy it may reflect systemic disease, but the majority of lumps that present in the neck are, or reflect, specific local disease (Fig. 16.1). The causes of such swellings are reviewed in this chapter, but the details of specific disease may be described in other chapters.

CAUSES OF A SWELLING IN THE NECK

The specific causes are summarized in Box 16.1.

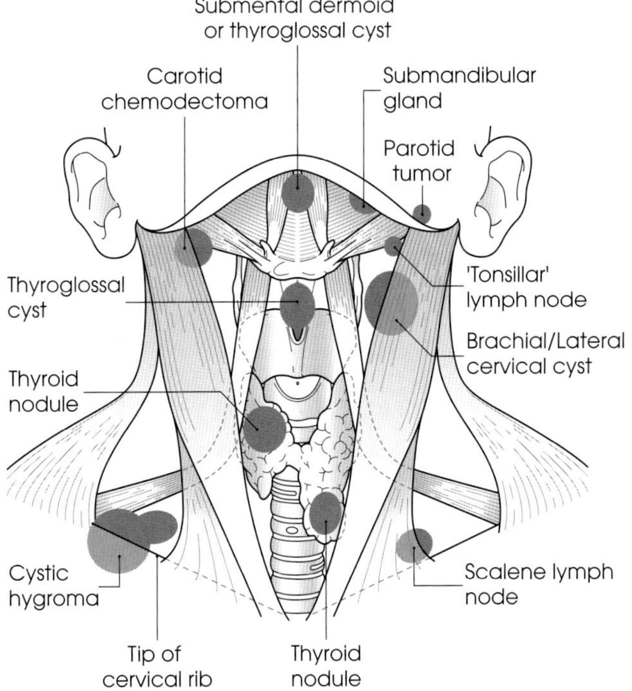

Figure 16.1 Anatomical location of the most common swellings in the neck.

THYROGLOSSAL TRACT

The thyroglossal tract is the remnant that marks developmental descent of the thyroid gland. The thyroid appears as a midline diverticulum at the fourth week of development, and promptly descends ventrally to the pharynx between the developing second branchial arch (Fig. 16.2). The duct formed during descent becomes solid and then normally involutes. Various clinical results are obtained if this process is not smooth:

- Persistence of the origin of the tract may remain as a midline dimple at the junction of the filiform and valate papillae of the tongue: the foramen caecum.
- The tract itself may persist whole as a thyroglossal duct or in part as a thyroglossal cyst.
- Solid thyroid tissue may persist and develop at any stage along the tract, in particular as a lingual thyroid, as tissue in the wall of the patent duct or cyst, or most commonly as a pyramidal lobe of a normal thyroid (see *Lingual thyroid* section of Ch. 17.

Thyroglossal cyst

Thyroglossal cysts may appear in association with patent or closed thyroglossal ducts. Some 40% present during the first decade of life, the remainder at any time; these cysts even appear in octogenarians. Only rarely is a thyroglossal cyst noted at birth. The incidence is approximately equal in males and females. Both

Box 16.1 Causes of a swelling in the neck

Congenital abnormalities
- Thyroglossal tract abnormalities
- Branchial (lateral cervical) cysts
- Cystic hygroma
- Cervical rib

Tumours
- Thyroid tumours (see Ch. 17)
- Salivary gland tumours (see Ch. 14)
- Sarcoma, lipoma, neuroma, fibroma etc.
- Chemodectoma

Lymph node enlargements
See Box 16.2.

Benign enlargements of glands
- Salivary gland (see Ch. 14)
- Thyroid gland (see Ch. 17)

Diverticula
- Laryngocele (see Ch. 19)
- Pharyngeal pouch (see Ch. 19)

Traumatic
- Sternomastoid 'tumour'

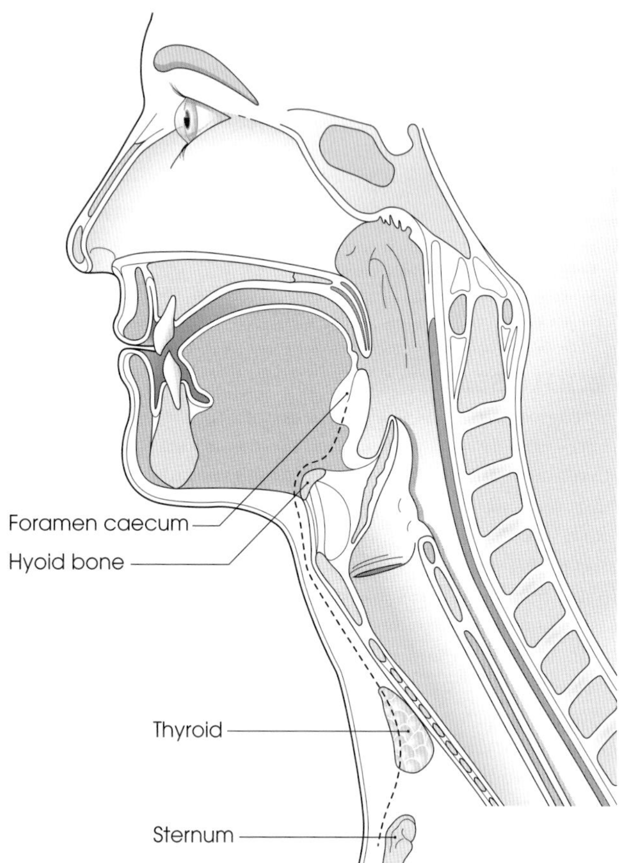

Figure 16.2 The thyroglossal tract. Thyroglossal cysts are usually located between the hyoid and the pyramidal lobe, but can occur anywhere from the foramen caecum to the sternum.

variants are smooth, rounded, unattached to the strap muscles, and typically in the midline, although a quarter may be a little to the right or the left (Fig. 16.3). Very occasionally a cyst is found as far out as the lateral tip of the hyoid. The cysts are usually just above or just below the hyoid, attached to a remnant of the thyroglossal tract. Thus a cyst may rise on protrusion of the tongue and during deglutition. Elevation on protrusion of the tongue differentiates a thyroglossal cyst from a nodule in the thyroid isthmus or pyramidal lobe. Thyroglossal cysts rarely transilluminate.

Thyroglossal cysts are the most common midline neck tumour of infancy, and may be confused with epidermoid cysts, dermoid cysts, enlarged lymph nodes, subhyoid bursae, and pyramidal lobe thyroid nodules. The cysts are lined by stratified squamous epithelium or ciliated pseudostratified columnar epithelium. There may be thyroid or lymphoid tissue in the wall, and any of these elements may undergo malignant change. Indeed, it has been asserted that the thyroid tissue is usually dysplastic and thus particularly at risk of malignant change. Malignancies are most commonly of thyroid papillary type,[1] but there is no evidence that the disease is multicentric, and it is not necessary to excise the thyroid as well as the thyroglossal tumour.

Thyroglossal fistula (sinus)

A thyroglossal fistula is almost invariably an acquired lesion. It originates following rupture or incision of a thyroglossal cyst. The external opening is usually directed cranially and overlaid by a crescent-shaped fold of stretched skin. There is intermittent

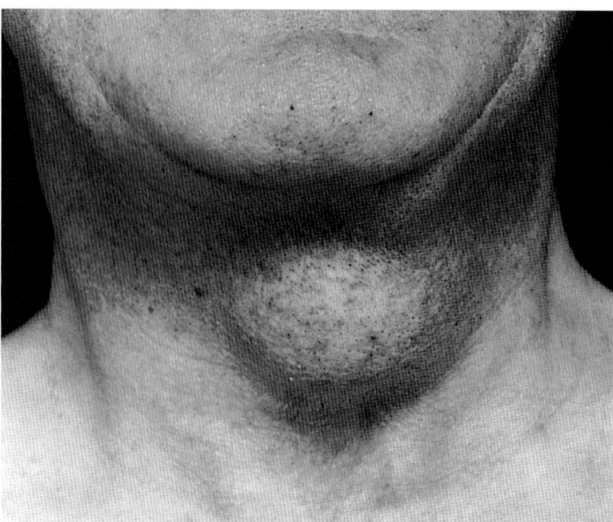

Figure 16.3 A large thyroglossal cyst located just below the hyoid.

seropurulent discharge. It is difficult, either surgically or with dyes, to show any communication between the orifice and the foramen caecum of the tongue, and these fistulae are more appropriately classified as sinuses because they do not connect two epithelial surfaces.

Treatment of thyroglossal cyst and fistula

Where part of or all the thyroglossal duct is patent, the treatment of choice for both cyst and sinus is Sistrunk's operation. A patent track may be injected with dye before the operation is begun. The cyst or sinus is then mobilized via a transverse incision made over it. The track is followed up between the infrahyoid muscles to the level of the hyoid bone. Its relationship to this bone is complex, and the only sure way of ablating the track is to excise the central portion of the hyoid bone. The track is then followed upwards and backwards to the base of the tongue. Usually in this part of its course, the track is incomplete and represented only by isolated fragments of epithelial tissue. A blind dissection must therefore be done in the midline between the geniohyoids and genioglossae. This suprahyoid part of the operation may be omitted where the cyst is infrahyoid and no proximal track can be demonstrated. It may be employed, however, with suprahyoid cysts and should ideally be taken to the foramen caecum. Failure to excise the central portion of the hyoid bone is associated with a high incidence of recurrence.[2] Excision of the hyoid is not attended by any disability, and is not associated with osteomyelitis when performed in the presence of sepsis.

BRANCHIAL (LATERAL CERVICAL) CYST

The second most common congenital swelling in the neck is the so-called branchial cyst. This name presupposes an origin from embryonic branchial cleft tissue remnants. This view is encouraged by the fact that when such cysts become infected they discharge through the skin, and the sinus that may subsequently develop is at the anterior border of the sternomastoid muscle at

REFERENCES

1. Saharin PC. Br J Surg 1975; 62: 689–691
2. Pollock WF, Stevenson EO. J Surg 1966; 112: 225–231

a similar site to the external opening of a true branchial fistula (see below). Further evidence of a branchial cleft origin is supported by the very occasional tract that is discovered running from the deep surface of these lesions towards the pharynx. By contrast, it has been noted that almost all branchial cysts have lymphoid tissue in their walls and may thus represent merely cystic degeneration in cervical lymphatic tissue. Linking these two disparate hypotheses is the notion that trapped embryological remnants, or acquired additional epithelial tissue originating from the tonsil, may stimulate this degeneration.[3] The cysts themselves are lined by heterotopic squamous epithelium. The debate is arcane and of little practical value except that it supports the view that these cysts should be defined as *lateral cervical cysts* rather than *branchial cysts*, and that at operation 'what you see is what you get'; thus there is no requirement to dissect out a hypothetical deep tract leading to the pharynx.

Most lateral cervical cysts present in the third decade. There is no dominant side or predilection for either sex. Patients complain of an enlarging lump, usually presenting from behind the junction of the upper and middle thirds of the sternomastoid muscle, although it may present anywhere behind or just in front of the upper sternomastoid (Fig. 16.4). There may be pain and even frank infection, which is usually responsive to antibiotics. Established or recurrent infection can lead to the development of a brawny or fibrotic mass with fixity to surrounding structures. The diagnosis is primarily clinical, but if there is doubt or if excision is not planned, a fine-needle aspiration biopsy must be done to exclude the differential diagnosis of a cystic cervical metastasis.[4] A true lateral cervical cyst yields an opalescent fluid containing cholesterol crystals or frank pus.

Once diagnosed, the lateral cervical cyst should be treated by surgical excision. This must be preceded by a course of antibiotics if there is infection. The cyst that has never been infected can be readily excised through an oblique skin-crease incision and a plane developed outside the cyst. The previously infected cyst will, however, be fixed wholly or in part to surrounding structures, including the jugular vein, and excision may be difficult. Care must be taken to excise the whole of the cyst; failure to do so risks recurrence or the development of a chronic, discharging sinus in the wound. There is no need to search for a tract leading to the pharynx from the deep surface.

BRANCHIAL FISTULAE AND SINUSES

The term *branchial* is derived from the Greek word for a gill. At 5 weeks, the human embryo exhibits four branchial clefts externally and five matched pharyngeal pouches internally.[5]

The first pair form the middle ear and Eustachian tube. Anomalies of the first cleft may appear as a sinus posterior or anterior to the external ear, and are rarely appreciated until they become infected, usually in a young adult (Fig. 16.5). These sinuses extend deeply and may be difficult to eradicate surgically. If the surgeon is tempted to operate on a recurrent sinus anterior to the meatus, it should be remembered that the deeply extending track will pass close to the facial nerve, which is therefore at risk.

Second cleft anomalies are uncommon. True fistulae may be bilateral; their anterior openings are in the line of the anterior border of the sternomastoid muscle. From this opening the fistula passes deeply between the stylohyoid muscles and the posterior belly of digastric, anterior to the hypoglossal nerve, through the bifurcation of the internal and external carotid arteries, and enters the pharynx in the tonsillar fossa.[6]

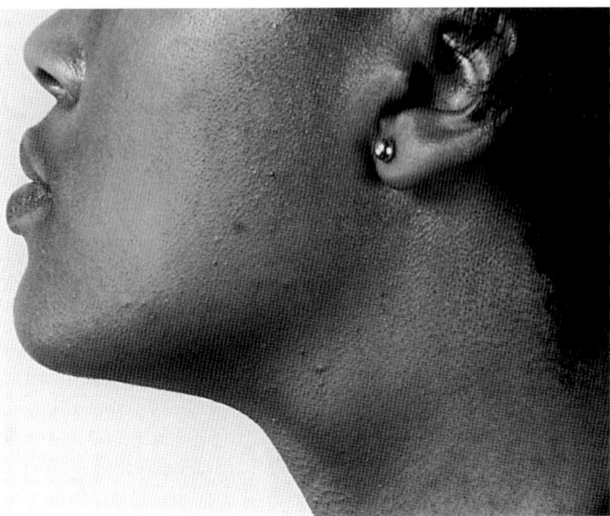

Figure 16.4 A branchial cyst emerging anteriorly to the upper third of the sternomastoid.

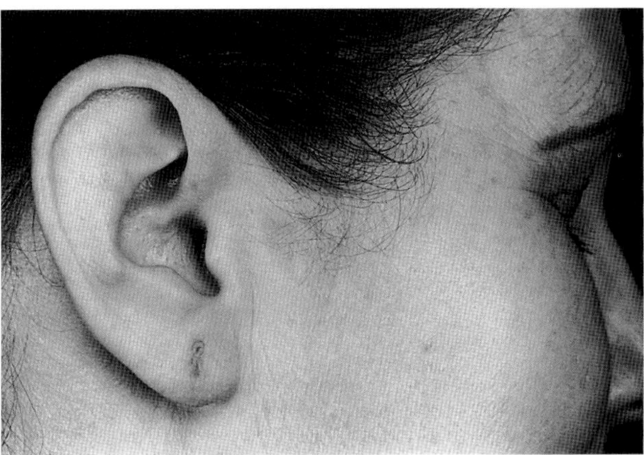

Figure 16.5 A large, quiescent preauricular sinus.

CYSTIC HYGROMA

Cystic hygroma is an old but widely used term describing a congenital, cystic, lymphatic malformation at the root of the neck. Cystic hygromas probably represent a developmental anomaly during the coalescence of primitive lymph elements into the adult pattern. The malformation consists of thin-walled, single or multiple interconnecting or separate cysts that insinuate themselves widely into the tissues at the root of the neck; 50–65% are present at birth and if very large may even obstruct delivery. After delivery large cysts may obstruct respiration and swallowing.[7] Presentation is occasionally delayed until adulthood.

The diagnosis is usually made by clinical examination of these transilluminable thin-walled cysts, but a chest radiograph is

REFERENCES

3. Golledge J, Ellis H. J Laryngol Otol 1994; 108: 653–659
4. Sheahan P et al. Otolaryngol Head Neck Surg 2002; 127: 294–298
5. Wendell Todd N. Surg Clin North Am 1993; 73: 599–610
6. Parke WW, Settles HE. Clin Anat 1991; 4: 285
7. Bill AH, Sumner DS. Surg Gynecol Obstet 1965; 120: 79–86

important to map their caudal extents, and CT or MRI may be helpful if they are complex. The injection of sclerosant after aspiration may be effective treatment, but in general excision is necessary and this should preferably be performed as a one-stage procedure.

CERVICAL RIB

About 1% of the population have a supernumerary rib arising from the lowest cervical vertebra. It is bilateral in 80%. The rib is an incomplete stub, and its anterior portion can be felt as a fixed, hard swelling in the supraclavicular fossa, where it may mimic metastatic disease. Cervical ribs themselves rarely cause symptoms, although occasionally symptoms of thoracic outlet syndrome may be produced due to disturbance of the adjacent brachial plexus or subclavian vessels. These do not pass over the rib, however, and other causes of thoracic outlet syndrome should be sought before the symptoms are attributed to cervical rib.

The rib is readily identified on simple radiography. Resection of cervical ribs is indicated only in the rare circumstances of their being confidently shown to be the cause of thoracic outlet syndrome. Anterior, posterior and transaxillary routes have been described,[8] but the standard approach is a supraclavicular collar incision with exposure of the upper and mid trunks of the brachial plexus, before excision of the rib as far back as is necessary to relieve pressure on nerves or vessels.[9]

TUMOURS IN THE NECK

THYROID

Thyroid disease, whether solitary nodules or multinodular goitre, often presents as the finding of a nodule in the neck. A nodule located in the upper pole of the thyroid may be felt surprisingly high in the neck. Nevertheless, in all cases the thyroid nodule will move on swallowing; its relationship to the thyroid may be confirmed on ultrasound scanning, and its nature initially investigated with a fine-needle aspiration biopsy (see Ch. 17).

SALIVARY GLAND

Salivary gland tumours and benign swellings are common causes of a swelling in the neck. The uninitiated will often misdiagnose a tumour in the tail of the parotid as a cervical node (Fig. 16.6), but the history distinguishes benign whole-gland swellings, such as sialectasis and Sjögren's syndrome, while fine-needle biopsy can reliably diagnose tumours without risk of seeding the disease into the needle track (see Ch. 14).

CHEMODECTOMA (CAROTID BODY TUMOUR)

Chemodectomas are tumours of the paraganglion cells of the carotid body located at the bifurcation of the common carotid artery (see Ch. 10). These tumours are usually benign but locally invasive. Between 5 and 10% are malignant and have potential to metastasize to local lymph nodes. They may be bilateral and may also be familial.[10] Patients with chemodectomas may have other head and neck paraganglionic tumours, including vagal and glomus jugulare tumours.

The tumour presents as a slow-growing, often painful, pulsatile mass at the angle of the jaw; if untreated it spreads cranially to the base of the skull as well as forwards to become a more pronounced tumour in the neck. Investigation is initially by Doppler ultrasound to confirm the diagnosis, and then by angiography. If there is doubt about the extent of the tumour, a CT or MRI scan may be helpful and cytology, although difficult to interpret, may clinch the diagnosis.

REFERENCES

8. Fulford PE et al. Cardiovasc Surg 2001; 9: 620–624
9. Sharrard WJW. In: Paediatric Orthopedics and Fractures. Blackwell, Oxford, 1993: 915
10. Gardner G et al. Am J Surg 1996; 172: 196–199

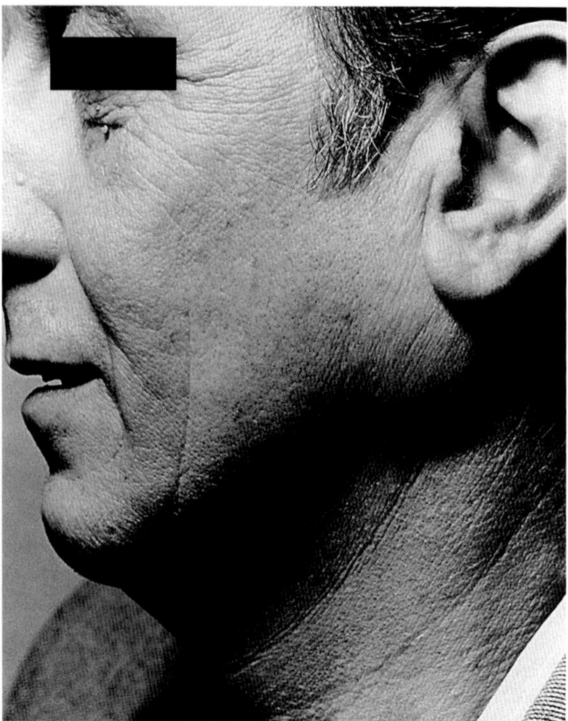
a

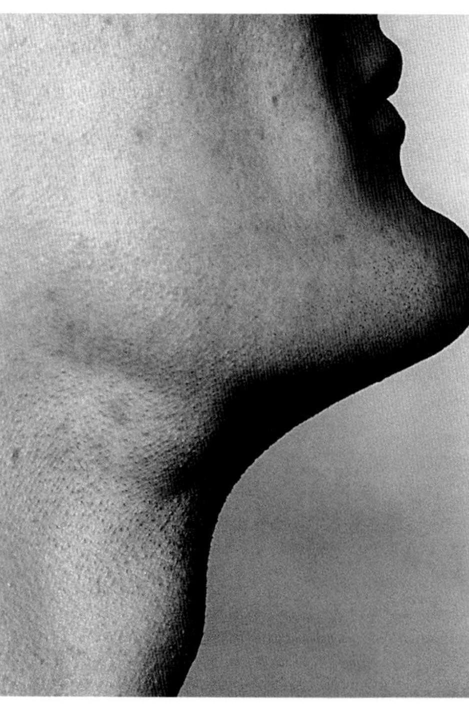
b

Figure 16.6 (**a**) A pleomorphic adenoma in the tail of the parotid. (**b**) Enlargement of a submandibular gland obstructed by a stone.

The preferred management is by surgery, but it should be remembered that there is only endothelium between the tumour and the lumen of the carotid artery. Surgery should be undertaken only when the necessary vascular surgical skills are available, remembering that postoperative neurological deficit can complicate the resection even of small tumours.[11] If the tumour is large but resectable, surgery of these highly vascular tumours may be made more straightforward by preoperative embolization.[12] This is, however, a potentially dangerous addition to the management. Wax and Briant have described the use of the ultrasonic surgical dissector to facilitate removal of these tumours.[13]

Excellent results have been achieved with radiotherapy instead of surgery in patients who are unfit for surgery or who have large tumours. There are a number of reports of excellent long-term follow-ups without progression of disease in these patients.[14]

CERVICAL LYMPHADENOPATHY

Cervical lymph nodes may be enlarged by inflammatory changes or by primary or metastatic malignancy (see Box 16.2).

The most common cause of a swelling in the neck is cervical lymphadenopathy, and the causes are usually benign. Although only one node may be visible or palpable, other adjacent nodes are often enlarged, and the extent of the lymphadenopathy is best assessed by ultrasound, which may also suggest a diagnosis based on sonographic detail.[15] One-third of the lymph nodes in the body are situated in the head and neck region, and an understanding of the possible causes of cervical lymphadenopathy requires a knowledge of their anatomy (Fig. 16.7). The habit of naming particular groups of cervical nodes might imply that there are anatomically discrete groups of such nodes. In fact, these names are largely a conventional way of subdividing an extensive interconnecting network of nodes and do not imply anatomical separateness. The surgeon must understand the pattern of lymph drainage in the head and neck if the correct investigations are to be undertaken in a patient with metastatic disease in lymph nodes (Figs 16.8–16.10).

Box 16.2 Causes of cervical lymphadenopathy

Primary malignancy
- Lymphoma: Hodgkin's and non-Hodgkin's
- Leukaemia, especially chronic lymphatic leukaemia

Metastatic malignancy
- Skin: melanoma, squamous cell carcinoma
- Nasopharynx: nose, sinuses, pharynx, larynx
- Mouth: oral cavity, tongue, lips
- Oesophagus
- Thyroid
- Infraclavicular: lung, bronchus, gastrointestinal tract, seminoma, breast, cervix
- Occult primary

Lymphadenitis
- Non-specific: sore throat, tonsillitis, idiopathic histiocytic necrotizing lymphadenitis, infected scalp.
- Specific: infectious mononucleosis, HIV/AIDS, toxoplasmosis, cat scratch fever.
- Granulomatous: tuberculosis, sarcoidosis, fungal.
- Other: Rosai–Dorfman disease, Castleman's disease, angioimmunoblastic lymphadenopathy.

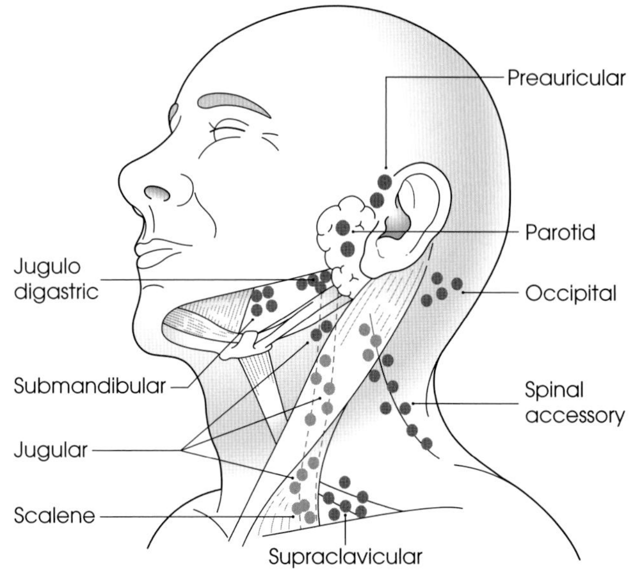

(a)

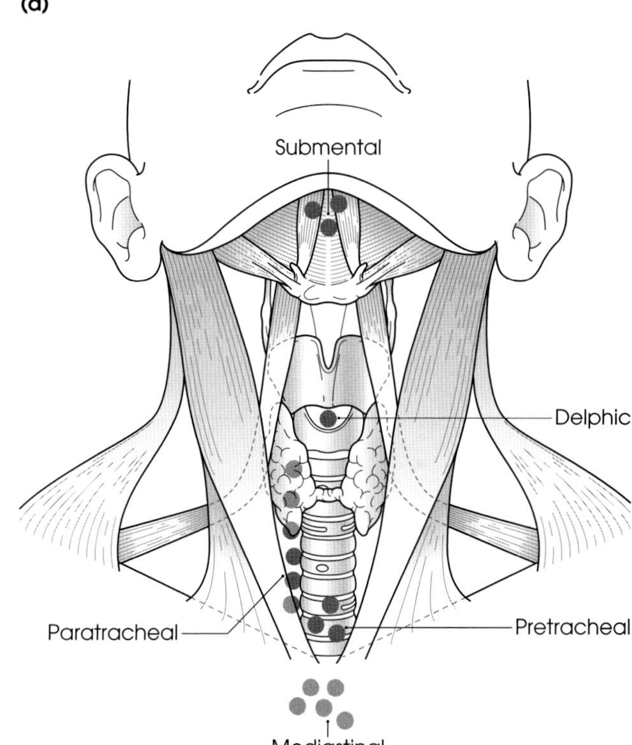

(b)

Figure 16.7 Lateral view (**a**) and anterior view (**b**) of the neck to show typical grouping of lymph nodes.

REFERENCES

11. Westerbrand A et al. J Vasc Surg 1998; 28: 84–92
12. Fruhwith J et al. Eur J Surg Oncol 1996; 22: 88–92
13. Wax MK, Briant TD. Otolaryngol Head Neck Surg 1994; 114: 678
14. Schild SE et al. Mayo Clin Proc 1992; 67: 537–540
15. Ahuja A, Ying M. Clin Radiol 2003; 58: 359–366

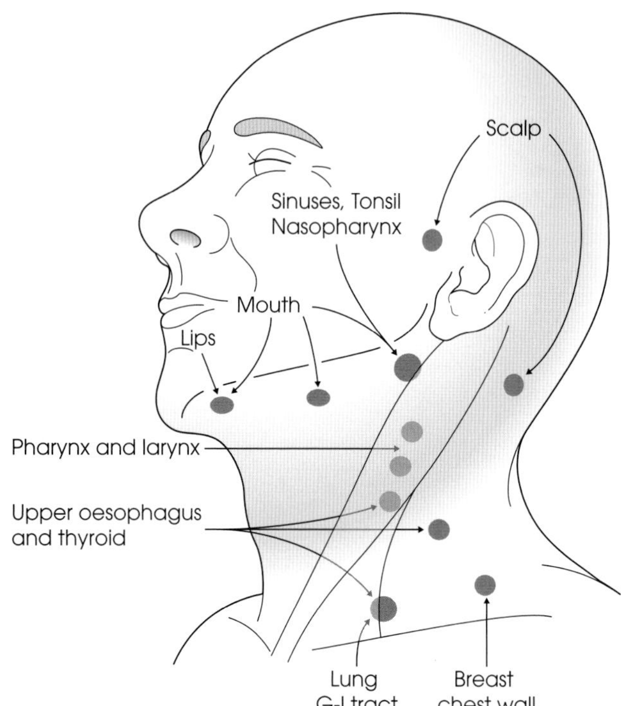

Figure 16.8 Typical lymph drainage pattern towards cervical lymph nodes. These patterns are not exclusive: there are extensive interconnections of lymphatic pathways in the neck.

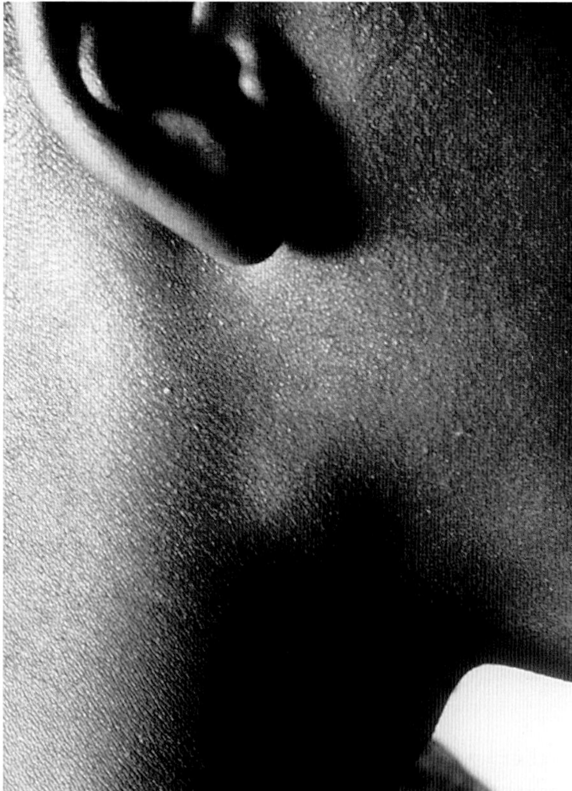

Figure 16.9 A jugulodigastric node enlarged by tonsillitis.

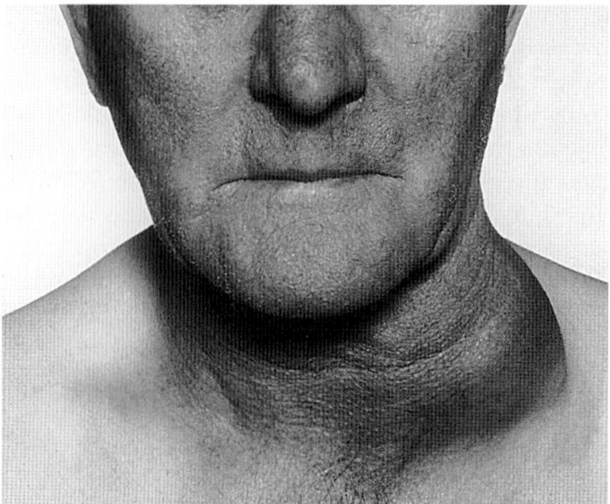

Figure 16.10 A mass of indurated nodes in the root of the neck with reddening of the overlying skin. The differential diagnosis lies between inflammatory lymphadenitis, including tuberculosis, and metastatic nodes. In this patient the nodes were metastatic and the presenting feature of a carcinoma of the bronchus.

IDENTIFYING THE CAUSE OF CERVICAL LYMPHADENOPATHY

Careful clinical history-taking and examination yield a diagnosis in the majority of cases. Particular note should be taken of ear, nose and throat symptoms, weight loss, fever, rashes or night sweats. Pain in lymph nodes after drinking alcohol is said to be a symptom of lymphoma, but has been recorded in other non-malignant causes of lymphadenopathy. The social history should include enquiry about risk factors for human immunodeficiency virus infection, foreign travel, and contact with animals. Examination should include the scalp (to exclude hidden melanoma), the tongue, lips and tonsils, and the thyroid gland. A more general examination should seek evidence of distant malignant disease or hepatosplenomegaly.

The first step in investigation is the taking of a fine-needle aspiration biopsy. A review by Donahue and colleagues showed that most studies of fine-needle biopsy show a false negative rate of around 1–10% and a false positive rate of 0–3%.[16] If the samples are taken by an experienced clinician who can reduce the number of smears that are inadequate for diagnosis, and if the cytologist has appropriate experience, then in almost all patients useful information may be gleaned. An exact diagnosis is not always crucial. The questions particularly to be answered are:

- Is it malignant?
- If so, is it a squamous cell malignancy?
- Is it inflammatory?
- If so, is it tuberculous?

An excision biopsy of a cervical lymph node should never be undertaken without a preliminary fine-needle biopsy. This is particularly important in cases of squamous malignancy and tuberculosis. An open lymph node excision biopsy in squamous malignancy may spoil the field for subsequent block dissection of the neck and, indeed, even reduce the potential of that operation to cure the patient.[17] If squamous metastatic disease is detected

REFERENCES

16. Donahue BJ, Cruickshank JC, Bisop JW. Ear Nose Throat J 1995; 74: 483–486
17. McGuirt WF, McCabe WF. Laryngoscope 1978; 88: 594

on fine-needle aspiration biopsy, there should be prompt referral to an ear, nose and throat surgeon for a full assessment, which will usually include panendoscopy. If this does not disclose a primary tumour, random biopsies from multiple sites are sometimes necessary, although it is very rare to discover the primary site from such blind biopsies. Chest radiographs and sputum cytology should also be obtained. The subsequent management of head and neck squamous cancers where the primary site is discovered is discussed in the relevant chapters elsewhere. Sometimes, however, no primary site is discovered (see next section, *Cervical lymph node metastases from an occult primary*). Immunohistochemical techniques are improving and even lymphomas may now be dignosed confidently from fine-needle aspirates,[18] although in general an open excision biopsy will be required if the cytology diagnoses lymphoma.

If fine-needle biopsy of a node in the supraclavicular fossa discloses adenocarcinoma, a search for a gastric, pancreatic or other abdominal malignancy is begun. Such marker nodes are usually found on the left and referred to as Virchow's nodes, but they may also be found on the right. A previously treated breast cancer is also sometimes found to be the cause of isolated adenocarcinomatous metastatic nodes in the neck.

Mobile metastatic nodes of squamous malignancies are, in general, treated by block dissection of the nodes in conjunction with treatment of the primary tumour. Radiotherapy may be added. Where the cervical node or nodes are fixed at presentation, the prognosis is grave regardless of the site of the primary tumour. The most common patients presenting with fixed nodes are those without a demonstrable primary tumour, a third of whom present in this way.

CERVICAL LYMPH NODE METASTASES FROM AN OCCULT PRIMARY

In a 12-year study from the Sloan-Kettering Cancer Center, reported in 1983, it was noted that in 6% of all cases of head and neck malignancy no primary malignancy was apparent, and in 60% of these cases the tumour was squamous.[19] All patients were treated with radical neck dissection or with radiotherapy. Interestingly, half were alive 5 years later—a much better result than would have been predicted from identified primary squamous carcinomas in the neck. In only 15% was the site of the primary tumour ever discovered from its later appearance and detection at follow-up.

In the 1940s and 1950s, tumours where no primary was found were considered to be the result of malignancy arising in squamous inclusions in cervical lymph nodes, the so-called branchogenic carcinomas. In the 1960s and 1970s, this concept was largely abandoned, but the issue remains unresolved. The proposed treatment policy for such patients is one of a basic search for a primary tumour, as outlined earlier in this chapter, followed by radical neck dissection, because failure to offer radical treatment is followed by a high incidence of uncontrolled local recurrence. Radiotherapy is advised if more than one lymph node is involved or if there is extracapsular spread. Radiotherapy achieves better results if given to both sides of the neck and the whole of the pharyngolaryngeal mucosa.[20]

SPECIFIC INFECTIONS

Infectious mononucleosis (Epstein–Barr virus infection)

This viral infection, a consequence of infection with the Epstein–Barr herpes virus, begins as a prodromal systemic illness with fever, malaise, a headache, and sometimes abdominal pain. The patient then typically develops pharyngitis or exudative tonsillitis and sometimes a rash, particularly if penicillin is prescribed. The lymphadenopathy that appears after the prodrome is predominantly cervical. Although the nodes may be substantially enlarged, the enlargement is always of multiple nodes and the distribution is symmetrical. The great majority of patients are adolescents, teenagers or young adults, and the diagnosis is readily confirmed by the appearance of atypical mononuclear cells in the blood film, associated with a positive serological test. The lymphadenopathy often persists for several months, and is associated with hepatosplenomegaly in 10–20% of patients. There is almost never an indication to biopsy a node to establish the diagnosis. There are reports of emergency tonsillectomy being required for life-threatening upper airway obstruction occurring during the pharyngitic phase of this illness,[21] but this is an exceptionally rare event.

Toxoplasmosis

Toxoplasmosis is a consequence of infection with the parasite *Toxoplasma gondii*; it may occur congenitally as a consequence of infection *in utero*, or be acquired. Lymphadenopathy is only a feature of the acquired disease. The neck is the most common site of lymphadenopathy and usually only a few nodes are enlarged, hence the presentation of these patients to surgeons. The nodes are usually tender for the first 1–2 weeks after their appearance, but after that are painless and may persist for many months; they never suppurate. There are usually few if any concomitant symptoms with the lymphadenopathy; sometimes there is slight fever and malaise. Fine-needle biopsy of the nodes shows non-specific changes. The blood may show slight leukopenia with some atypical lymphocytes, but these are not diagnostic. Specific IgG antibodies appear 2 weeks after the onset of the illness, but are a poor guide to diagnosis because there is a high prevalence in the normal population. Seropositivity rates are normally quoted for a population of fertile women: the rate is 72% in Paris and 21% in London, probably reflecting dietary differences. Toxoplasmosis is seen as an opportunistic infection in AIDS patients, and in these patients specific antibody levels may be low. The node enlarged because of toxoplasmosis is thus difficult to diagnose with certainty. If the patient is well no specific treatment is required, but if the patient is unwell a 1–2-month course of spiramycin is indicated.[22]

Cat scratch fever

Lymphadenopathy is the most common presenting feature of cat scratch disease. The infecting bacillus, *Bartonella henselae*, enters through a scratch from a cat, usually a kitten, and causes the development of a local inflamed papule 3–10 days later; 1–7 weeks afterwards there is enlargement of the regional lymph nodes. These are initially painful, may suppurate, and may persist for up to 4 months in association with vague systemic symptoms

REFERENCES

18. Nasuti JF et al. Diagn Cytopathol 2001; 25: 351–355
19. Spiro RH, DeRose G, Strong EW. Am J Surg 1983; 146: 441–446
20. Grau C et al. Radiother Oncol 2000; 55: 121–129
21. Stevenson DS, Webster G, Stewart IA. J Laryngol Otol 1992; 106: 989–991
22. Courvieur J, Thulliez P. In: Oxford Textbook of Medicine. 3rd edn. Oxford University Press, Oxford, 1996: 865–869

in 30% of patients. Traditionally, the diagnosis is made by aspiration of a node and the microscopic demonstration of the bacillus by Warthin–Starry silver stain. A polymerase chain reaction test is now available to detect *B. henselae* DNA in lymph nodes, but is only diagnostic in the first 6 weeks of the lymphadenopathy;[23] a serological IgG test is also available. Usually no treatment is needed, although large pus-filled nodes may need to be aspirated, and antimicrobial therapy is occasionally needed for systemic symptoms.[24]

GRANULOMATOUS LYMPHADENITIS

Sarcoidosis

Thirty per cent of patients with sarcoidosis have palpable cervical nodes, and in 75% of all patients with sarcoidosis, scalene node biopsy discloses the diagnosis even when the nodes are impalpable. However, in white patients sarcoidosis only presents as a cervical lymphadenopathy in 3%, because the disease is usually predominantly mediastinal; by contrast, nodal disease is the presenting feature in 17% of Asians and 34% of blacks. The nodes are discrete, painless, rubbery, and similar in feel to the nodes encountered in Hodgkin's disease. They do not suppurate. The diagnosis is by fine-needle or open biopsy backed up by a significant elevation of serum angiotensin I-12-converting enzyme or the Kveim skin test.[25]

Tuberculosis in cervical lymph nodes

Tuberculosis may involve cervical nodes by lymphatic or haematogenous spread. Historically, the most common situation is for the organism to enter through the tonsillar bed as a consequence of drinking infected milk, and this pharyngeal point of entry leads to jugulodigastric node enlargement as part of the primary complex. More common in developed countries is the appearance of tuberculous lymphadenitis low in the neck, secondary to pulmonary tuberculosis; in this instance infection is noted primarily in the supraclavicular nodes, the lower jugular nodes, or posterior triangle nodes. In these patients radiology of the chest may disclose a mediastinal lymphadenopathy. Although tuberculous lymphadenitis is now uncommon in western countries, it is nevertheless seen in immigrants from other countries (especially those of the Indian subcontinent, where tuberculosis is still endemic), and is also commonly encountered in the socially disadvantaged and malnourished and in immunocompromised patients, especially those with HIV/AIDS.

In developing countries tuberculosis remains extremely common, and is the most common cause of cervical lymphadenopathy.[26]

Tuberculosis notifications in England and Wales show that there is a racial difference in the form of presentation of extrapulmonary tuberculosis. In whites, 37% present with cervical node involvement, whereas the figure for those originating from the Indian subcontinent is 52%.

Despite the relative infrequency of cervical tuberculosis in developed countries, it should always remain in the differential diagnosis of cervical lymphadenopathy because less than 50% will have any systemic symptoms, and the enlarged or suppurating neck nodes may be the only marker of the disease.

In the early stages of tuberculous lymphadenitis the nodes enlarge but remain discrete. With progression of the disease the nodes caseate and coalesce; if the process proceeds slowly then there is gross surrounding fibrosis. Eventually marked, dense induration is noted, mimicking malignancy. Progressive caseation leads to coalescence of caseous foci into a deep abscess, with softening of the node mass. If the nodes are deep-seated, the pus penetrates the deep fascia and forms a fluctuant cold abscess under the skin. This is the famous but now rarely seen collar stud abscess. Whenever tuberculous infection appears under the skin it causes a dusky cold induration of that skin, and eventually discharges through the skin with the development of a chronic sinus. Secondary infection can now occur. Chronic tuberculosis in the skin produces the changes identified as scrofula.

Management

Once tuberculosis has been suspected it is readily diagnosed by fine-needle aspiration biopsy cytology; this will show caseous changes and/or epithelioid cells in 85%,[27] but acid-fast bacilli will be seen in the cytological preparation in only 50%. Pus should therefore be aspirated for culture. Aspiration is not only crucial in providing material for determining antibiotic sensitivities, but is also therapeutic when combined with drug therapy. Ultrasound or radiographic imaging is not useful in confirming a diagnosis of tuberculosis, but may help to map abscesses and guide aspiration. A positive or suspicious fine-needle aspiration biopsy coupled with a strongly positive purified protein derivative or Heaf skin test is sufficient diagnosis to allow initiation of treatment without the need for open biopsy. It should, however, be remembered that immunocompromised patients may have an anergic response to skin testing; these and other patients where the diagnosis is uncertain may still need diagnostic excision of a node for histology and culture.

The role of surgery in the treatment of tuberculous lymphadenitis is very limited; it should be avoided, if possible, because of the risk of development of chronic sinuses at the site of biopsy or drainage. It should be considered only if there is a persistent large mass or a sinus after a full course of medical treatment. Surgery should take the form of extirpation of the tuberculous mass as if it were a low-grade malignancy. The procedure is technically difficult, and surrounding structures are at considerable risk. If sinuses or ulcers have developed then surgery combined with medical therapy helps to obtain a cosmetically acceptable scar.[28]

ATYPICAL MYCOBACTERIAL INFECTION

Several other mycobacteria can cause cervical lymphadenitis, mostly *Mycobacterium avium* or *M. intracellulare*, and the infections occur almost exclusively in children and the immunocompromised, especially those who have had contact with birds. The patients tend to present with nodes higher in the neck than is found in tuberculous patients; the lymphadenopathy is more often unilateral, and there is usually no concomitant systemic illness. This form of lymphadenitis often shows minimal response to drug therapy,[29] and surgical treatment, ideally with node excision, should be undertaken.[30]

REFERENCES

23. Margolis B et al. Arch Pathol Lab Med 2003; 127: 706–710
24. Margileth AM. Pediatr Infect Dis J 1992; 11: 474
25. Studdy PR. In: Oxford Textbook of Medicine. 3rd edn. Oxford University Press, Oxford, 1996.
26. Watters AK. Br J Surg 1997; 84: 8–14
27. Dasgupta A et al. J Indian Med Assoc 1994; 92: 44–46
28. Subramanyam M. Br J Surg 1993; 80: 1547–1548
29. Bailey WC. Chest 1983; 84: 625
30. Tunkel DE, Romaneschi KB. Laryngoscope 1995; 105: 1024–1028

HIV/AIDS AND CERVICAL LYMPHADENOPATHY

Cervical lymphadenopathy is often encountered in patients with HIV infection and in those with AIDS. Persistent generalized lymphadenopathy is a feature of the pre-AIDS state. In these patients, as well as in patients with established AIDS, the clinical decision to be made is whether the appearance of enlarged cervical nodes is part of the lymphadenopathy associated with the disease itself, or whether it signals the appearance of an associated lymphoma, tuberculosis, or other opportunistic infection in an immunocompromised patient. Fine-needle aspiration biopsy is indicated in an attempt to resolve this issue, especially if there is asymmetrical primarily cervical lymphadenopathy. The results of this will indicate the small number of patients in whom biopsy excision is justified. Widespread open excision biopsy of enlarged lymph nodes in these patients is rarely justified. In an analysis of studies of unselected biopsy for persistent, generalized lymphadenopathy in HIV-positive patients, the management was only shown to be altered in 3% of patients as a consequence of the histological findings.[31]

KIKUCHI–FUJIMOTO DISEASE

Kikuchi–Fujimoto disease (necrotizing histiocytic lymphadenitis) is a disease of unknown aetiology predominantly affecting young women, especially those of east Asian ethnicity, between the ages of 20 and 30. Usually it presents as posterior cervical lymphadenopathy. It may be associated with a flu-like prodrome and a relapsing course. Although C-reactive protein levels and the erythrocyte sedimentation rate may be raised and the white cell count low, there is no means to confirm the diagnosis other than by seeing the complex but typical histological changes in an excision biopsy of the involved node. The lymphadenopathy normally resolves without treatment within 6 months.[32]

STERNOMASTOID TUMOUR

Sternomastoid tumours appear 1–2 weeks after birth, usually following a complicated or breech birth. The tumour is unilateral, usually occupies the lower half of the muscle, and occupies both heads. At the outset it is in fact an interfascicular haematoma of the sternomastoid with associated muscle degeneration. It is at first tender and often associated with torticollis. If sternomastoid tumour is diagnosed early the optimal treatment is conservative, with active stimulation and passive stretching; during this regimen the tumour normally disappears over the first 4–6 months of life. Only those cases that are noted late and are unresponsive to conservative treatment require surgery.[33] If the condition is not treated a permanent wry neck deformity may begin to develop at about 4 years of age.

SURGERY OF CERVICAL LYMPH NODES

LYMPH NODE BIOPSY

Excision of a cervical node for biopsy is necessary if fine-needle biopsy has failed to produce a diagnosis where it is clinically necessary to achieve one. It is also important if the proposed diagnosis is lymphoma, in which instance a whole node is required for detailed histology and marker studies. The most discrete, mobile, superficial yet clearly abnormal gland should be chosen for excision. Biopsy under local anaesthetic is feasible, but general anaesthetic is often preferred because the surgery may prove more difficult than it appears at first sight.

Damage to the spinal accessory nerve is a particular risk during biopsies in the posterior triangle. The nerve is intimately related to the posterior triangle nodes, is only 2 mm in diameter, and is surprisingly superficial. Damage leads to pain in the shoulder and arm, paralysis of the trapezius muscle, winging of the scapula, and frequently also to litigation. If the injury is recognized the patient should be promptly referred for neurolysis or nerve grafting.[34,35]

An inexperienced surgeon should not be allowed to undertake an unsupervised biopsy of posterior neck nodes without being apprised of the anatomical dangers.

BLOCK DISSECTION OF THE NECK

The classical block dissection of the neck for clearance of the cervical lymph nodes has remained unchanged for most of the past century, and it remains the standard operation for extensive nodal disease from squamous carcinoma, malignant melanoma, and patients with extensive medullary carcinoma of the thyroid. The classical procedure removes the sternomastoid muscle, the jugular vein and the accessory nerve (Fig. 16.11), leaving a considerable cosmetic and functional deficit. Therefore in many situations more limited operations are now undertaken, a stance reinforced by the widespread use of high-quality, effective adjuvant radiotherapy. Differentiated thyroid cancer has always been managed effectively with limited block dissection,[36] and it is only in medullary or very advanced papillary or follicular tumours that radical procedures are undertaken (see Ch. 17). It has been proposed that, for node-negative and early node-positive oral and oropharyngeal carcinoma, a supraomohyoid dissection will suffice, and that for hypopharyngeal and pharyngeal tumours a lateral neck dissection is sufficient.[37]

RADICAL NECK DISSECTION

The purpose of the standard, full radical neck dissection is the clearance of all lymphatic tissue from the mandible above to the clavicle below, and from the midline to the anterior border of the trapezius muscle laterally. Normally, only unilateral block dissection is undertaken, but with the introduction of modified operations, particularly those sparing the jugular vein, bilateral dissections are sometimes feasible.

Many incisions are in use (Fig. 16.12). The McFee incision consists of two horizontal limbs, one below the mandible and the other above the clavicle, and is particularly used if the patient has been previously irradiated. The standard Y incision comprises a horizontal component that extends from the mastoid to the hyoid bone and then up to the point of the chin. The vertical component commences in the centre of the horizontal incision and descends vertically in a 'lazy S' shape to the clavicle.

REFERENCES

31. Godley MJ. Br J Surg 1986; 73: 170–171
32. Lin HC et al. Otolaryngol Head Neck Surg 2003; 128: 650–653
33. Cheng JC, Au AW. J Paediatr Orthop 1994; 14: 802–808
34. Williams WW et al. Ann R Coll Surg Engl 1996; 78: 521–525
35. London J, London NJ, Kay SP. Ann R Coll Surg Engl 1996; 78: 146–150
36. Orsenigo E et al. Eur J Surg Oncol 1997; 23: 286–288
37. Shah JP, Andersen PE. Ann Surg Oncol 1994; 1: 521–532

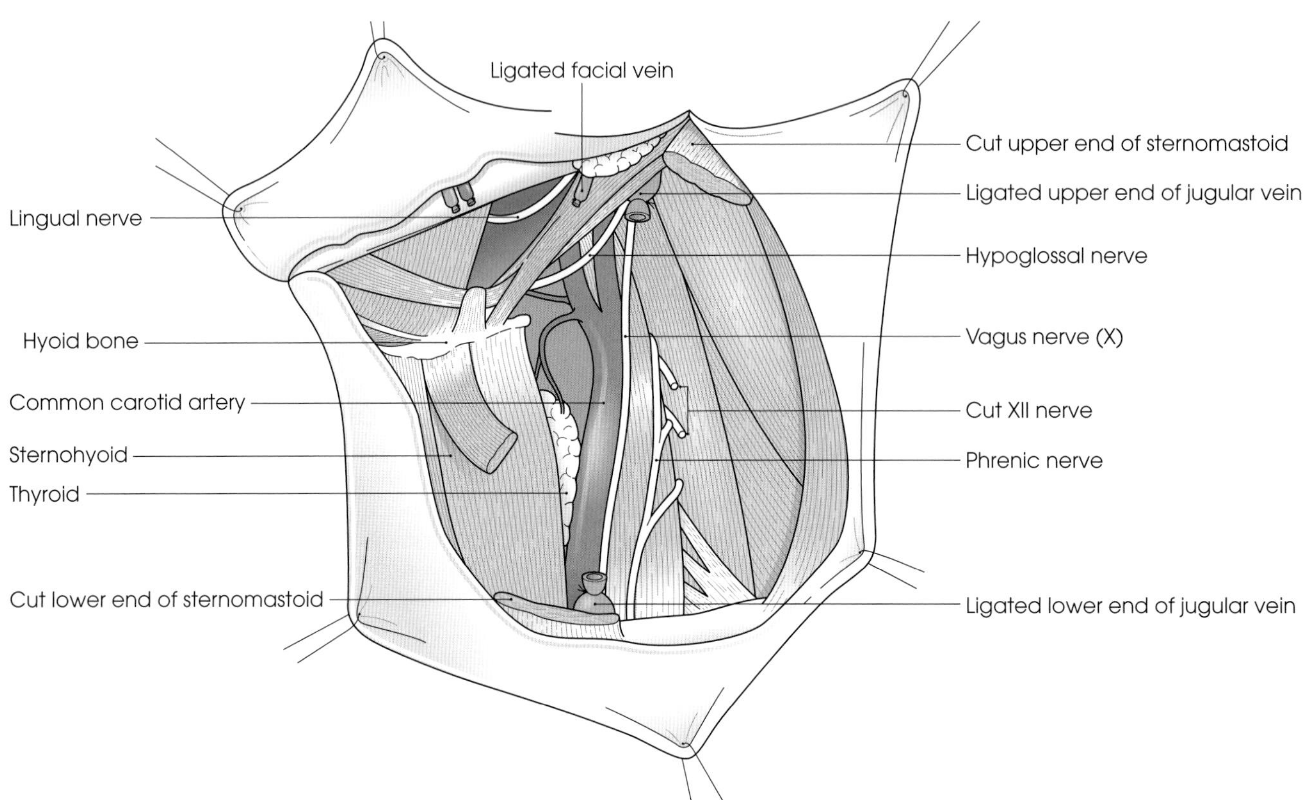

Figure 16.11 Anatomical structures exposed at the end of a radical block dissection of the neck. Note the cut ends of the excised sternomastoid, accessory nerve and jugular vein.

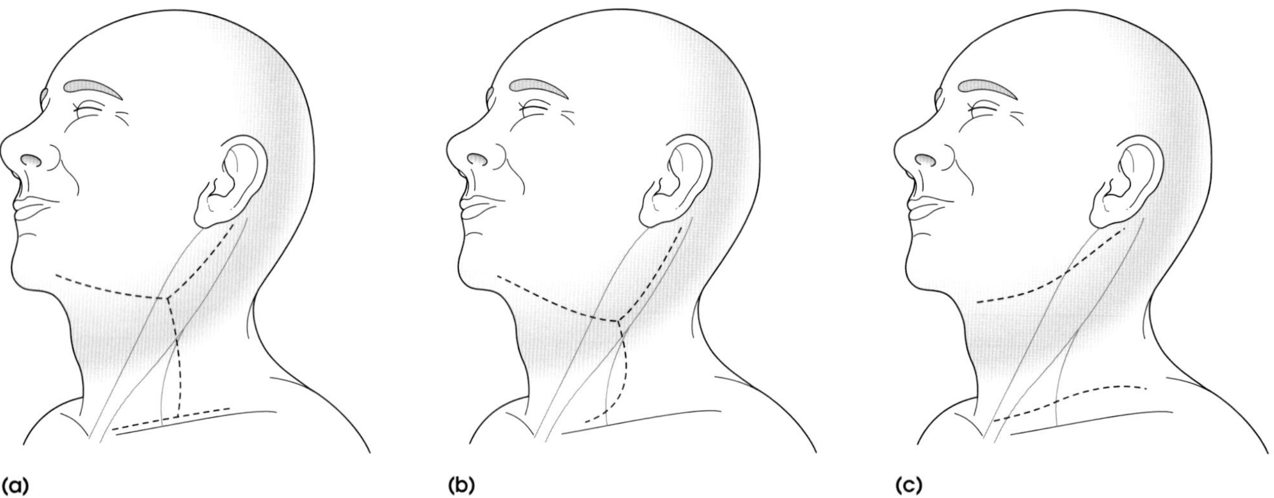

Figure 16.12 Examples of incisions used for block dissection of the neck: (**a**) 'wine glass', (**b**) standard Y incision, and (**c**) McFee.

Skin flaps are raised together with the platysma, taking care to protect the mandibular branch of the facial nerve under the upper skin flap. The lower limit of the dissection is extended, and the distal end of the sternomastoid muscle is divided. Next the internal jugular vein is exposed and divided. The divided upper end of the vein, together with the lymphatic and connective tissues surrounding it, is lifted away from the common carotid artery and the vagus nerve. This block of mobilized tissues is now gently separated from the prevertebral fascia, sparing the phrenic nerve on the anterior surface of scalenus anterior. During the mobilization the transverse cervical artery and vein are divided and ligated. The anterior border of the trapezius is defined and the posterior triangle is cleared, dividing the accessory nerve centrally and distally to the mobilized block of lymphatic tissue. The dissection is continued upwards beside the common carotid artery to its bifurcation. The cranial end of sternomastoid is then separated from the mastoid process; the internal jugular vein is exposed, ligated and divided.

The dissection continues forwards, ligating the posterior facial vein and usually dividing the tail of the parotid gland. The hypoglossal nerve is traced forwards to the submandibular triangle and spared. The upper border of the submandibular gland is freed by dividing and ligating the facial vessels. The lingual nerve is identified and separated from the submandibular duct, which can then be divided. The gland is delivered after the facial artery has again been divided on its posterior border. If the tumour is situated in the anterior portion of the oral cavity the submental triangle should also be included in the dissection.

If the skin flaps are involved, irradiated or unhealthy, extra tissue may have to be brought in to close the wound of a block dissection of the neck. This can be a free graft, skin flaps or free tissue transfer with microanastomosis (see Ch. 9).

The thyroid gland

17

David M. Scott-Coombes, Anthony E. Young

INTRODUCTION

The thyroid gland develops from the endodermal lining of the pharynx in the floor of the mouth. In 10% of adults, the embryological scar is visible as the foramen caecum, a pit in the midline at the junction of the anterior two-thirds and posterior one-third of the tongue. The gland descends along the thyroglossal duct to rest anterior to the trachea. The upper poles of the gland are invaded by neural crest cells derived from the ultimobranchial body and fourth pharyngeal pouch, which develop into the parafollicular C cells.

The principle function of the thyroid gland is to synthesize the hormones tetraiodothyronine (thyroxine) and tri-iodothyronine (Fig. 17.1). Dietary iodide is trapped by the thyrocyte and oxidized by the enzyme thyroid peroxidase to iodine. Thyroglobulin, a tyrosine-rich protein at the apex of the thyrocyte, becomes iodinated. Linkage of iodide to tyrosine residues results in the formation of monoiodotyrosine and di-iodotyrosine. Coupling reactions between the iodinated tyrosine residues produce tri-iodothyronine and thyroxine, which are secreted into the systemic circulation.

The main physiological stimulator of the thyroid gland is thyrotropin secreted from the anterior pituitary gland. The production of thyrotropin is stimulated by thyrotropin-releasing hormone from the hypothalamus, and suppressed by the thyroid hormones, in particular tri-iodothyronine. The C cells of the thyroid gland secrete calcitonin. While it inhibits bone resorption, the physiological role of this hormone is not fully understood.

DIAGNOSIS OF THYROID DISEASE

GENERAL CONSIDERATIONS

Patients with thyroid pathology present in two ways: endocrine dysfunction (thyrotoxicosis or myxoedema) or goitre.

DIFFERENTIAL DIAGNOSIS

Goitre is a term used to describe any enlargement of the thyroid gland. Goitres may be solitary (unilateral) or diffuse (bilateral), and diffuse goitres have either a smooth or a nodular surface. Knowledge of the thyroid status from history, examination, and thyroid function tests, coupled with the clinical impression of the type of goitre, permits the surgeon to develop a differential diagnosis (Table 17.1).

CONGENITAL ABNORMALITIES

THYROGLOSSAL DUCT ABNORMALITIES

See Chapter 16, *The neck*.

LINGUAL THYROID

Lingual thyroid is a very rare developmental abnormality characterized by non-descent of all or part of the embryonic thyroid. In 70% of cases it constitutes the entirety of thyroid

REFERENCES

1. Clark OH. Endocrine Surgery. CV Mosby, St Louis, 1985

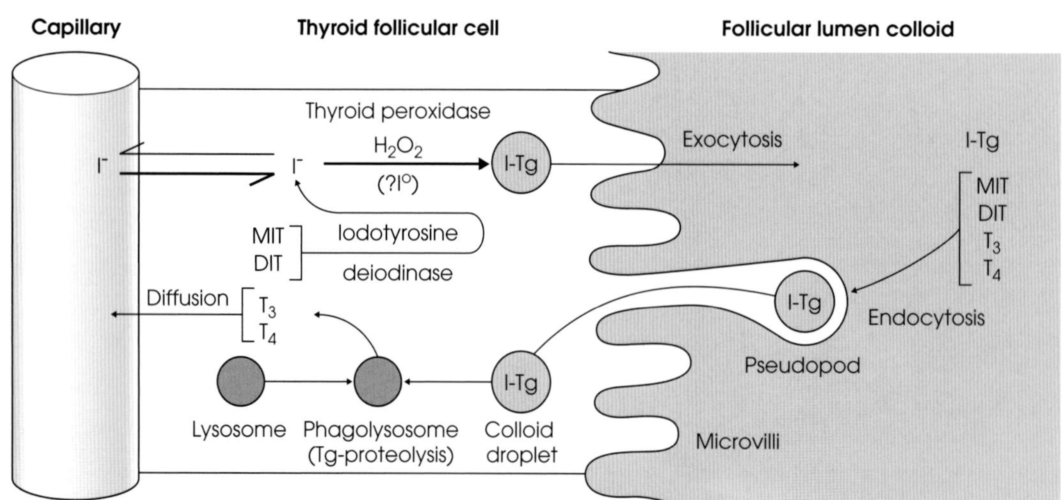

Figure 17.1 Pathways of thyroid hormone synthesis. Tg, thyroglobulin; MIT, monoiodotyrosine; DIT, di-iodotyrosine; T_3, tri-iodothyronine; T_4, tetraiodothyronine (thyroxine). (Reproduced from Clark OH. Endocrine surgery. CU Mosby, St Louis, 1985, with permission.[1])

Table 17.1 Differential diagnosis of a goitre

Thyroid hormonal status	Type of goitre		
	Solitary	Diffuse smooth	Diffuse nodular
Euthyroid	Dominant nodule in multinodular goitre Adenoma Cancer	Simple physiological goitre Endemic goitre Lymphoma	Multinodular goitre
Thyrotoxic	Toxic adenoma	Graves' disease	Plummer's syndrome
Myxoedematous		Hashimoto's	Hashimoto's

tissue. It may either be symptomless or suffer from any of the diseases to which the thyroid is liable. One-third of patients develop hypothyroidism. Examination reveals a smooth, hypervascular, reddish brown, mucosal-covered projection at the back of the tongue, often only clearly visible by laryngoscopy. Most presenting patients are young women, where enlargement is due to the physiological hyperplasia of pregnancy or to the development of an adenoma.[2] Rarely it may cause dysphagia, dysphonia or airways obstruction, and it may bleed. Lingual thyroid carcinoma is exceptionally rare.[3]

A technetium isotope scan is essential to confirm the diagnosis, but more importantly to establish the presence or absence of other thyroid tissue.[4] An asymptomatic lingual thyroid that is stationary in size is left alone. Hypertrophy may be limited by therapeutic doses of thyroxine, by antithyroid drugs, or by radioiodine. Excision may be necessary, particularly if malignant disease has occurred. Removal is undertaken via a transoral approach, bisecting the tongue longitudinally to access the tumour.

OTHER ECTOPIC THYROID TISSUE

Thyroid tissue is sometimes identified as discrete nodules physically separate from the thyroid, but immediately adjacent to it. These sequestered thyroid nodules may be mistaken for parathyroid glands.[5] Thyroid tissue may also occur in the mediastinum as far distal as the pericardium, and within the wall of the trachea or larynx, oropharynx and oesophagus.

Historically, thyroid in lymph node areas deep to the sternomastoid muscle was believed to arise as ectopic thyroid tissue derived from the ultimobranchial body; this was the 'lateral aberrant thyroid'. It is now known that these lesions are lymph node metastases from differentiated intrathyroid cancers.

BENIGN GOITRE

PATHOLOGY

Non-toxic goitre is the commonest form of thyroid abnormality. It may be either endemic or sporadic. The trigger for the development of goitre is a failure to meet the physiological demands for thyroxine, either due to increased demands or because of impaired production of thyroxine leading to fluctuating levels of thyrotropin, which drives the hyperplasia. Initially the goitre is diffuse and smooth, but the end-stage of thyroid hyperplasia is multinodular goitre. The mechanism of this transformation remains difficult to define. As time passes some follicles rupture, producing inflammatory changes, or they outrun their blood supply, producing infarction, haemorrhage, fibrosis, calcification and cyst formation. The overall effect of these changes is to produce a gland studded with nodules of varying size, maturity, activity and physical structure. These nodules are typically non-functioning, but sometimes they may secrete thyroxine, autonomously of thyrotropin.

PHYSIOLOGICAL GOITRE

Physiological goitre is secondary to demands for thyroxine, as in puberty, pregnancy and lactation.

IODINE-DEFICIENCY GOITRE

Seven per cent of the world population suffers from clinically apparent goitre,[6] with prevalences ranging from almost zero in Japan, South Africa and the USA, to 80% in parts of the Andes, Zaire and New Guinea. Although iodine has been introduced into salt, food or water, endemic goitre remains a common problem. Worldwide differences in the prevalence of iodine-deficiency goitre are not entirely attributable to iodine intake. Familial and racial traits of dyshormonogenesis and the intake of goitrogenic foods are also considered to play a role.

Dyshormonogenesis

The enzymes responsible for thyroxine synthesis may be partially or completely deficient.[6] Such defects are familial. With a severe inborn error of thyroid metabolism, thyrotropin levels are very high and the infant gland becomes diffusely enlarged. More typically the underproduction of thyroxine is less severe and may be intermittent.

Severe defects tend to cretinism, but less severely affected individuals develop an enlarging goitre, usually from childhood. Peroxidase deficiency may be associated with deafness as well as goitre (Pendred's syndrome).[7] Treatment is the same for each specific enzymatic defect, namely thyroxine replacement.

REFERENCES

2. Montgomery ML. West J Surg Gynecol Obstet 1935; 43: 661–669
3. Massine RE et al. Thyroid 2001; 11: 1191–1196
4. Aktolun C, Demir H et al. Clin Nucl Med 2001; 26: 933–935
5. Sackett WR, Reeve TS et al. J Am Coll Surg 2002; 195: 635–640
6. Kelly FC, Snedden WW. Bull World Health Organ 1958; 18: 5–173
7. Fraser GR, Morgans ME, Troller WR. Q J Med 1960; 53: 279–295

Goitrogens

Goitrogens are substances that impair thyroxine synthesis, and the resultant increase in thyrotropin secretion causes hypertrophy. These substances may be grouped as follows:

- Drugs that interfere with thyroxine synthesis: propylthiouracil, carbimazole, perchlorate, thiocyanate, iodides (as in seaweed tablets or in amiodarone), resorcinol, sulphonamides, cobalt and aminoglutethimide.
- Dietary agents.

Dietary agents have an ill-understood role. Excess intake of halogens such as chloride or fluoride displaces iodine; high levels of calcium in drinking water from limestone areas appear to influence the incidence of goitre where there is coexisting iodine deficiency. Pollution of drinking water by *Escherichia coli* is also implicated.[8] Cassava and soya beans, members of the *Brassica* genus of vegetables, contain goitrogens,[9] but there is no evidence of a clinically significant effect in humans.

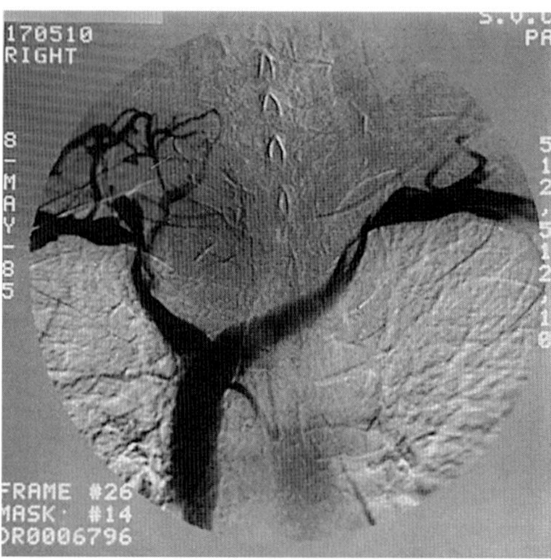

Figure 17.2 Digital subtraction angiogram showing compression of the great veins by a retrosternal multinodular goitre.

Radiation

Low doses of radiation (2–15 Gy), at one time used predominantly in the USA to treat a variety of benign head and neck diseases of childhood, have been implicated not only in the later development of cancer but also in a 20% incidence of nodular goitre 10–30 years later.[10]

THYROIDITIS

Clinical presentation

Patients present for one or more of the following reasons:

- cosmetic appearance;
- discomfort;
- tracheal compression;
- oesophageal compression;
- retrosternal extension;
- anxiety about malignancy;
- development of hyperthyroidism; or
- hoarseness.

Whether a goitre is cosmetically acceptable depends on the patient's personality and cultural background. Discomfort may arise either acutely, secondary to haemorrhage into a nodule, or episodically, during neck movements or swallowing. Tracheal compression is insidious in its onset. Persisting minor cough is an early sign, and stridor develops late. Oesophageal compression is unusual without retrosternal extension. Food may occasionally stick, but if there is persistent dysphagia other causes should be sought before the cause is attributed to the goitre.

Most goitres enlarge harmlessly forwards from the neck, but 10% will plunge into the chest. Extension is generally into the anterior mediastinum, but a posteriorly situated nodule may descend behind the oesophagus. Once in the confines of the bony thorax, compressive symptoms are more common and the great veins may be obstructed (Fig. 17.2). Rarely the whole of the goitre is confined within the thorax.

Many multinodular goitres present as a single nodule (the dominant nodule of a multinodular goitre), raising the possibility of a thyroid malignancy. Fine-needle aspiration biopsy should therefore be performed.

Hyperthyroidism occurs in a small number of long-standing nodular goitres due to the development of one or more autonomous hyperfunctioning nodules; this is Plummer's syndrome (discussed later in this chapter).

Voice changes (hoarseness) may be produced by distortion of the larynx by the goitre or by recurrent laryngeal nerve palsy. The latter should be taken as a warning of the possibility of thyroid malignancy.

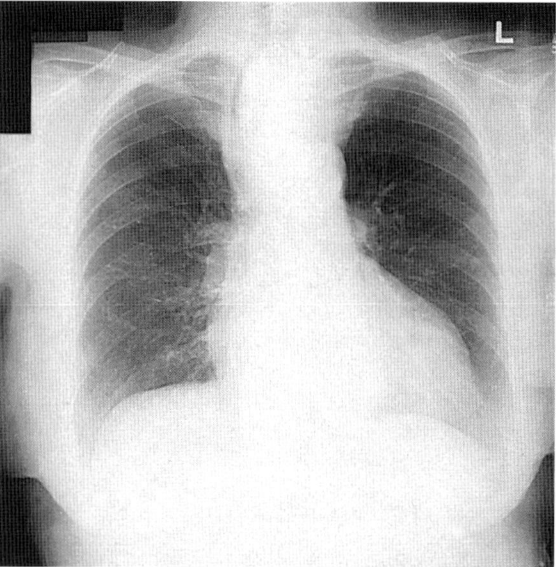

Figure 17.3 Chest radiograph showing a retrosternal goitre. Note the trachea narrowed and displaced to the right.

Investigation

Thyrotropin, thyroxine and tri-iodothyronine should be assessed in all patients. If there is any suspicion of thyroiditis, autoantibodies should be assayed. All clinically dominant nodules should undergo fine-needle aspiration biopsy. Either ultrasound or technetium scintigraphy will distinguish a solitary nodule from a multinodular goitre, although isotope scans are better for retrosternal goitres. An abnormal chest X-ray is often the first indication of a retrosternal goitre (Fig. 17.3). If tracheal compression is suspected, cross-sectional imaging (CT or MRI) provides views of the airway (Fig. 17.4). When there is anxiety about malignancy, cross-sectional imaging may show that the gland capsule has been transgressed, but iodine-containing

REFERENCES

8. Carbon JA, Hung L, Jones D. Fed Proc 1965; 24: 486
9. McCarrison RM. Chir Tr 1906; 89: 437
10. Greenspan FS. JAMA 1976; 237: 2089–2091

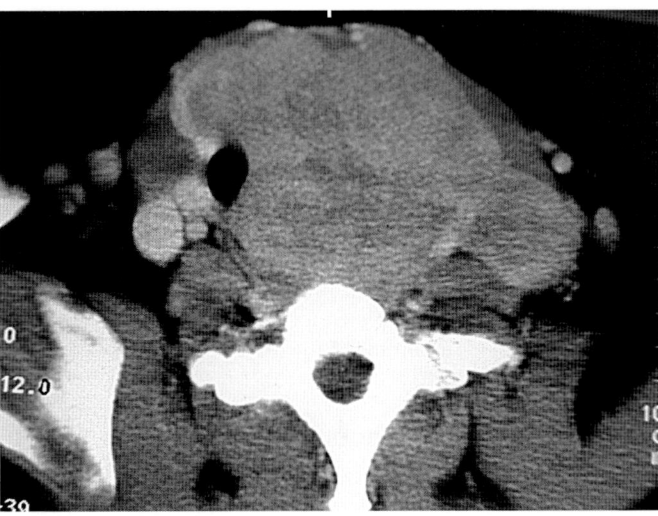

Figure 17.4 A CT scan of the neck, demonstrating enlargement of the lobe of the thyroid gland with compression of the trachea.

contrast should be avoided because it may delay subsequent radioiodine therapy. Dysphagia should always be investigated by contrast studies before it is confidently ascribed to pressure from the thyroid.

Treatment

Medical

Endemic goitre may be partly prevented and treated by ensuring a daily iodine intake of 150–300 mg. Older patients with developed multinodular goitre should not, however, be given iodine therapy because thyrotoxicosis may be induced (the Jod-Basedow effect). Goitrogens should be excluded from the diet.

Thyroxine has been widely used in the treatment of multinodular goitre because of the presumed role of a raised thyrotropin level in its genesis. Some 70% of smooth dyshormogenic goitres in young people may regress with suppressive doses of thyroxine,[11] but there is little convincing published evidence that thyroxine will significantly affect the size of an established nodular goitre.

Surgery

The indications for surgery are:

- suspicion of malignancy;
- tracheal compression;
- oesophageal compression;
- true retrosternal goitre; and
- cosmesis.

The management of the potentially malignant nodule is described later in this chapter. Any tracheal narrowing by a multinodular goitre should be regarded as an indication for surgery. If there is already stridor, surgery should be undertaken urgently.

If all risk of recurrence is to be avoided, the correct procedure is a total thyroidectomy by an experienced thyroid surgeon. Lesser surgery reduces the risks of recurrent laryngeal nerve injury and hypoparathyroidism, but greatly increases the risk of recurrent goitre and the associated increased risks of reoperative thyroid surgery.[12] Postoperatively, the patient should be started on a replacement dose of thyroxine.

Surgery is normally indicated for true retrosternal goitre because these patients are particularly at risk of compressive symptoms, and because continued growth of the goitre may be difficult to assess. Furthermore, the hazards of surgery increase proportionately with the size of the goitre. Even large retrosternal goitres can be safely extracted via the cervical incision as they derive their blood supply from normal thyroid vessels in the neck.[13] However, if the nodules are very large they may need to be removed piecemeal.[14] If there is definite malignant change with fixity of the goitre in the chest an upper midline sternotomy may be necessary.

In some elderly patients with asymptomatic retrosternal goitres that are shown on sequential imaging to be enlarging very slowly or not at all, a policy of continuing observation may be safer than surgery.

TUMOURS OF THE THYROID GLAND

In all, 3–5% of the population have a clinically palpable thyroid nodule,[15] at autopsy 50% of adults are found to have a thyroid nodule,[16] and 30% of all adults can be shown by ultrasound to harbour a nodule.[17] The incidence is substantially higher in areas of iodine deficiency and endemic goitre. By contrast, the incidence of true thyroid cancer is low: around four per 100 000 per year.[18] Therein lies the clinical problem. The palpable nodule is the end-point of many different pathological processes, benign and malignant. Distinction between these simply by clinical examination is often impossible, and referral to specialists is both appropriate and common. The death rate from thyroid cancer (six per million per year) is low, but this reflects not just the relative indolence of some thyroid cancers but also the success of treatment. For this reason, the proper assessment of thyroid nodules and the vigorous treatment of thyroid cancer are fully justified.

Thyroid tumours may be classified as shown in Box 17.1.

BENIGN THYROID TUMOURS

Almost all benign thyroid tumours are follicular adenomas. They are encapsulated and usually 2–4 cm in diameter at presentation. They are clinically and cytologically indistinguishable from follicular carcinomas, and all follicular lesions should be excised. The final diagnosis is made on histology, because the distinction between these lesions is based on the presence of vascular or capsular invasion.

The follicular adenoma encompasses many categories, such as embryonal, fetal, simple, colloid, macrofollicular and microfollicular adenomas. Embryonal adenomas are at one end of the spectrum, having rudimentary acini and no colloid, whereas the colloid adenomas at the other end are bulging with colloid. A difficult category to assess is the Hürthle cell adenoma (Askanazy

REFERENCES

11. Astwood EB, Cassidy CE, Amback GD. JAMA 1960; 174: 459–464
12. Reeve TS, Delbridge L et al. Ann Surg 1987; 206: 782–786
13. Lahey FH. Surg Clin North Am 1945; 25: 609–618
14. Allo MD, Thompson NW. Surgery 1983; 94: 969–977
15. Wang C, Crapo LM. Endocrinol Metab Clin North Am 1997; 26: 189–218
16. Mortensen JD, Woolner LB et al. J Clin Endocrinol 1955; 15: 1270
17. Brander A, Viikinkoski P et al. Radiology 1991; 181: 683–687
18. Thompson NW, Kiskiyama RH, Harknen JK. Curr Probl Surg 1978; 15: 1–67

Box 17.1 Classification of thyroid tumours

Benign
- Follicular adenoma
- Teratoma

Malignant
- Differentiated carcinoma
  - Papillary
  - Mixed papillary–follicular
  - Follicular
  - Medullary
- Undifferentiated (anaplastic)
- Lymphoma
- Miscellaneous
- Squamous
- Sarcoma
- Teratoma
- Plasmacytoma
- Metastatic

cell tumour, oncocytoma, or oxyphil tumour). They may be particularly difficult to differentiate from malignant tumours, and it is claimed that some will develop metastases. Nevertheless, in general these tumours may be regarded as benign and lobectomy is adequate treatment.[19]

Thyroid cysts

True cysts (i.e. those with a completely smooth wall) are very rare. The majority identified by ultrasound are composite lesions representing colloid degeneration, necrosis or haemorrhage in benign or malignant tumours. The cyst should undergo fine-needle aspiration biopsy, but negative fluid cytology does not exclude a neoplasm. Fine-needle aspiration biopsy should be repeated if a residual nodule can be palpated following aspiration. It is reasonable to aspirate the cyst up to three times before recommending excision. One-third of malignant thyroid cysts have false-negative cytology.[20]

Toxic adenomas

See *Hyperthyroidism* section, p. 398.)

MALIGNANT THYROID NEOPLASMS

Aetiology of thyroid neoplasia

Thyroid neoplasia can occur in any part of the thyroid or in ectopic thyroid tissue. While there is no difference in the prevalence of thyroid cancer between geographic areas of differing iodine intake, the different types of malignancy vary in their distribution. In areas of relatively high iodine intake there is a predominance of papillary thyroid cancer (80%), whereas in iodine-deficient regions there is a greater proportion of follicular (50%) and anaplastic tumours. Iodine is known to have a growth-inhibiting effect on the thyrocyte. Growth factors, thyrotropin and other hormones (i.e. oestrogen) increase thyrocyte growth. Neoplasia may result from mutations of growth-factor receptors and deregulation of tumour-suppressor genes.[21] The sequence of genetic and hormonal events involved in the induction of differentiated thyroid malignancy is complex and incompletely understood.[22] But we do know that most differentiated thyroid cancers need thyrotropin for continued growth while undifferentiated and medullary cancers do not.

Ionizing radiation exposure and family history are two recognized aetiological factors. The small doses of radiation once administered to the neck of children for the management of various minor childhood ailments is now known to be a potent carcinogen, with a risk of malignancy in a palpable nodule as high as 50%.[23] Larger doses of radiation administered in the treatment of, for example, Hodgkin's disease may also lead to thyroid cancer after a latent period of 6–35 years.[24] The nuclear accident in Chernobyl has been succeeded by an epidemic of aggressive childhood papillary cancer in nearby parts of the Ukraine.[25] The use of iodine-131 for the treatment of thyrotoxicosis has not been shown to lead to an increase in thyroid malignancy.

A family history of multiple endocrine neoplasia type 2 is a risk factor in medullary carcinoma of the thyroid. Papillary carcinoma may rarely be familial.[26]

Assessment of thyroid nodules

Palpation cannot exclude thyroid cancer. Hardness, fixity to surrounding structures, or the presence of one or more palpable nodes is very suspicious. Recurrent laryngeal nerve palsy or persisting pain and dysphagia may also be indicators of malignancy. Concomitant thyrotoxicosis makes malignancy less likely but does not exclude it.

Fine-needle aspiration biopsy is the best way of assessing the chance of malignancy in a thyroid nodule.[27] Technetium-99m scintiscanning and/or neck ultrasound demonstrate whether an apparently solitary nodule is in fact part of a multinodular goitre, and fine-needle aspiration biopsy should be directed to the clinically dominant nodule. Excision of the thyroid nodule can then be avoided if the cytopathology is unequivocally benign. However, surgery is indicated on patients with pressure symptoms or cosmetic anxieties. Core biopsies are considered unsafe for the assessment of all but very large thyroid nodules.

Fine-needle aspiration biopsy

Fine-needle aspiration biopsy is acceptable to the patient, requires no anaesthesia, is safe, and can be repeated, and the processing of the sample is quick, easy and cheap. In the standard technique of fine-needle aspiration biopsy, a 22-gauge needle attached to a syringe is passed through the lesion four to eight times in different directions without withdrawing the needle from the cutaneous entry site. Obtaining adequate specimens and making satisfactory slides is not difficult but requires experience.[28] Difficulties in interpretation are encountered, and rebiopsy may be necessary. In experienced hands, cytological assessment allows a confident diagnosis of benign colloid,

REFERENCES

19. Bondeson L, Bondeson AG et al. Am Surg 1981; 194: 677–680
20. Cusick EL, McIntosh CA et al. Br J Surg 1988; 75: 984–987
21. Goretzki PE, Dotzenrath C et al. Arch Surg 1999; 384: 1–8
22. Wynford-Thomas D. In: Wheeler MH, Lazarus JH (eds). Diseases of the Thyroid. Chapman & Hall, London, 1994
23. Favus MJ, Schnieder AB et al. N Engl J Med 1976; 294: 1019–1025
24. Naunkeim KS, Kaplan EL. Surgery of the Thyroid and Parathyroid Glands. Churchill Livingstone, Edinburgh, 1983: 51–62
25. Williams D. Nature 1994; 371: 556
26. Ozaki O et al. World J Surg 1988; 12: 565–571
27. Carpi A, Ferrari E et al. J Clin Oncol 1996; 14: 1704–1712
28. Abele JS, Miller TR. Endocrine Surgery of the Thyroid and Parathyroid Glands. CV Mosby, St Louis, 1985: 293–366

involutional nodules, papillary, medullary and anaplastic carcinoma, but cannot differentiate between follicular adenoma and follicular carcinoma.

In the literature the false-positive rate for malignancy is less than 2% and false-negative rate around 5%,[29] but the false-negative rates may be as high as 30% for large and partly cystic nodules.[30] If after biopsy any doubt remains about the benignity of the thyroid swelling, it should be excised surgically. A management plan for thyroid nodules is shown in Fig. 17.5.

MANAGEMENT OF DIFFERENTIATED THYROID CANCER

Differentiated thyroid cancer accounts for 80% of thyroid neoplasms and encompasses two major groups: papillary and follicular cancer. Papillary and follicular thyroid cancers are biologically different tumours. Papillary is multifocal, unencapsulated, invades lymphatics, and spreads to lymph nodes. Follicular cancer is solitary, encapsulated, invades veins, and spreads to bones. Between 70 and 80% of differentiated thyroid cancers are papillary and 20–30% follicular.

Papillary and mixed tumours

Pathology

Papillary thyroid carcinomas have a 4:1 predominance in women and tend to present in the young and middle-aged. There are a number of pathological variants. The commonest morphology is that of abundant papillary structures, but the follicular variants are composed almost entirely of follicular structures, and distinction from a follicular neoplasm by fine-needle aspiration biopsy can be difficult. Micropapillary carcinomas (less than 10 mm in diameter) are usually clinically silent and frequently an incidental finding in glands excised for other reasons. The diffuse sclerosing and tall cell variants are both aggressive tumours that predominate in young and elderly patients, respectively.

These tumours tend to be small at presentation (50% less than 2 cm in diameter) and have a propensity for multicentricity (30–50%) and early lymph node metastasis. Psammoma bodies (calcific concretions) are a classical finding in papillary cancer and correlate with lymph node metastasis. There is no single discriminating factor that determines prognosis. Factors that implicate a worse prognosis include age and sex (over 50 years for women, over 40 years for men), tumour size (greater than 40 mm), and the presence of local invasion.[31]

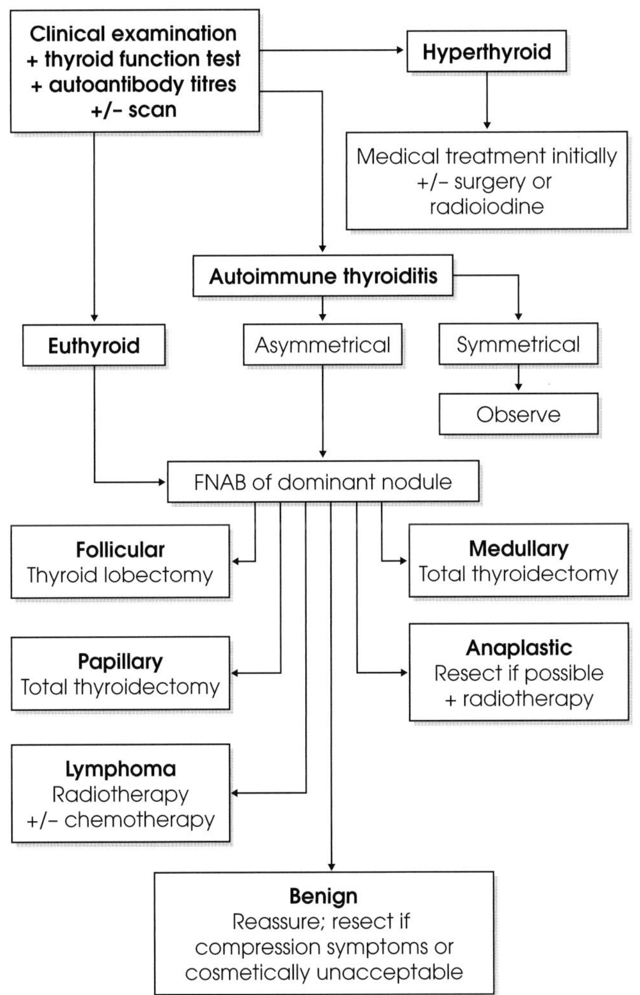

Figure 17.5 Management plan for a thyroid nodule. FNAB, fine-needle aspiration biopsy.

Treatment

Papillary thyroid cancer includes a wide spectrum of tumours, from those for which the clinical significance is unclear to those that are lethal, and so controversy exists about the best management of this disease, particularly for those in a low-risk group. Unfortunately, no randomized studies exist that compare radical with conservative thyroid resection. Analyses do, however, show that patients at high and low risk can be separated.[32] The surgical options are either a total thyroidectomy, with or without a lymph node dissection, or a total thyroid lobectomy (including the isthmus). Consensus exists for the following:

- The minimal resection is a total thyroid lobectomy with isthmusectomy.
- Microcarcinoma without capsular invasion and without enlarged metastatic lymph nodes is adequately treated by lobectomy and isthmusectomy.
- Total thyroidectomy is indicated in patients with local invasion or distant metastases, in those with a previous history of head and neck radiotherapy, and in those younger than 18 years because these tumours behave aggressively in children.[33]

Multicentricity is frequently cited as an indication for total thyroidectomy for all papillary cancers.[34] Others have observed that when a small (less than 2 cm) solitary papillary cancer is treated by lobectomy and suppression of thyrotropin (by the administration of thyroxine), the incidence of recurrence in the opposite lobe is very low and the mortality rate just as low compared with total thyroidectomy.[35] Others advocate a total thyroidectomy followed by radioiodine ablation to reduce local recurrence rates.[36]

Total thyroidectomy has the benefits of permitting iodine-131 ablation and increasing the sensitivity of thyroglobulin surveil-

REFERENCES

29. Gharib H. Mayo Clin Proc 1994; 69: 44–49
30. Kohler F, Kohler H. In: Romer H-D, Clark OH (eds). Thyroid Tumours. Karger, Basel, 1988
31. Mazzaferi EL, Jhiang SM. Am J Med 1994; 97: 418–428
32. Mazzaferri EL, Young RL. Am J Med 1981; 70: 511–518
33. Harrach HR, Williams ED. Br J Cancer 1995; 72: 777–783
34. Clark OH. Am Surg 1982; 196: 361–370
35. Rossi RL, Cady B et al. World J Surg 1986; 10: 612–622
36. DeGroot LJ, Kaplan EL et al. World J Surg 1994; 18: 123–130

lance. The arguments against a total thyroidectomy, and even more against central node dissection, are the higher risks of hypoparathyroidism and recurrent laryngeal nerve injury. One could conclude that in low-risk patients the extent of surgery should be determined by the experience of the surgeon. The optimal solution involves limiting thyroid surgery to a smaller number of surgeons with greater experience.[37] Radioactive iodine is indicated in most patients with distant metastatic disease and in those with locally invasive neck disease.[32]

Further controversy surrounds the necessity for adjuvant lymph node dissection.[38] The current consensus is that lymph node dissections are indicated in patients with clinical or macroscopic lymph node metastases.[39] The lymphatic drainage of the neck is functionally separated into central and lateral compartments. The central area (prelaryngeal, pretracheal and paratracheo-oesophageal) is the primary zone of lymphatic drainage, whereas the lateral area (internal jugular and posterior triangles) is a secondary zone. Because metastatic cancer in lymph nodes rarely escapes the confines of the nodes, traditional forms of radical block dissection sacrificing the jugular vein, sternomastoid muscle and nerves are almost never indicated, and a modified block dissection spares these structures and is appropriate. It can be performed through the extended thyroidectomy incision, sometimes supplemented by another higher, parallel, skin-crease incision on the affected side. The dissection need not be carried above the hyoid, but needs to extend distally into the upper mediastinum, especially along the tracheo-oesophageal groove.

Follicular carcinoma

Pathology

There are three categories of follicular neoplasm:

1. Follicular tumours without invasion of the capsule or blood vessels, which may be considered benign (follicular adenoma).
2. Follicular tumours with papillary differentiation, which are regarded as variants of papillary cancer and treated as such (follicular variant of papillary thyroid carcinoma).
3. Invasive, purely follicular carcinoma.

Follicular carcinoma typically occurs in patients over 50 years, involves the cervical lymph nodes in only 6%, and is prone to distant metastases when angioinvasive.

For a minority of tumours, distinction between benign and malignant on histology may be very difficult because the signs of invasion may be minimal. Such tumours are frequently described as minimally invasive and treated as benign.

Treatment

The proper treatment of invasive follicular carcinoma is total thyroidectomy followed by radioiodine therapy. When regional nodes are involved they should be excised by modified block dissection. All patients must receive lifelong suppressive thyroxine therapy.

Where a follicular neoplasm has been diagnosed on fine-needle aspiration biopsy, a total thyroid lobectomy is done and paraffin-section histology awaited, because frozen-section diagnosis is unreliable. If follicular carcinoma is diagnosed, the residual lobe can be removed at a second operation, followed by radioiodine ablation.

Adjunctive therapy for thyroid carcinoma

Radioiodine therapy

Radioiodine therapy will only be effective after a total thyroidectomy. If only one lobe has been removed at operation, the second may occasionally be ablated with radioiodine rather than a second operation. Following operation, patients are rendered euthyroid with tri-iodothyronine 60–100 μg/day until recovery from operation is complete. The tri-iodothyronine is then discontinued 2 weeks before the planned time for radioiodine therapy. The resultant hypothyroidism stimulates maximal thyrotropin secretion, encouraging uptake of the isotope by any residual functioning thyroid tissue. Because the period of hypothyroidism following tri-iodothyronine withdrawal is unpleasant for patients, the current trend is to increase radioiodine uptake by giving synthetic thyrotropin. There is debate over whether to perform a preablation scintiscan or to proceed directly to a therapeutic dose (30–150 mCi).[39] If multiple avid metastases are demonstrated, a further higher dose up to 200 mCi is sometimes given. Where uptake has been demonstrated, the process may be repeated to a total dose of 800–1000 mCi (Fig. 17.6). Although no randomized study exists, treatment with radioiodine reduces the risk of both recurrence and death.[40]

External radiotherapy

In differentiated cancer, external radiotherapy is primarily of value where there is residual metastatic disease after radioiodine therapy, where there is no uptake of radioiodine by metastases that can be imaged by alternative means, or where there is a large unresectable primary tumour.

Follow-up

Patients should be examined in a multidisciplinary clinic for clinical signs of local recurrence. The use of thyroxine postoperatively in all patients significantly reduces recurrence and

REFERENCES

37. Sosa JA, Bowman HM et al. Ann Surg 1998; 228: 320–323
38. Simon D, Goretzki PE et al. World J Surg 1996; 20: 860–866
39. Mazzaferri EL, Kloos RT. J Clin Endocrinol Metab 2001; 86: 1447–1463
40. Sherman SI. Lancet 2003; 361: 501–511

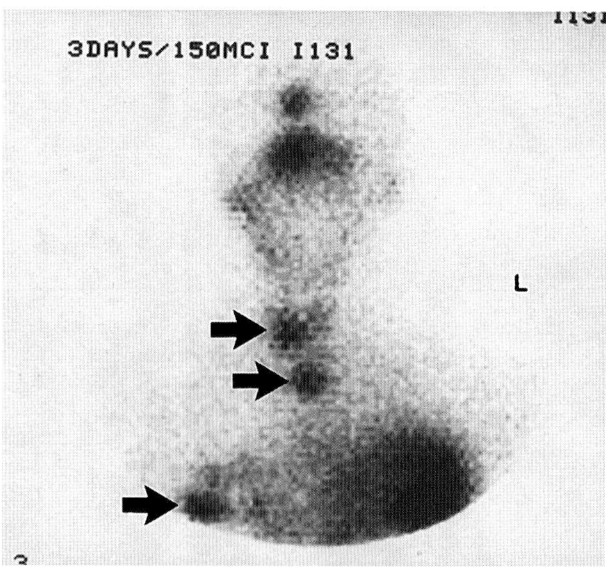

Figure 17.6 Radioiodine scan showing metastatic follicular thyroid carcinoma in the neck and lungs (arrows).

improves survival.[41] The dose of thyroxine to achieve thyrotropin suppression without toxicity usually lies between 175 and 300 µg/day. Thyroid function tests should be monitored to confirm thyrotropin suppression. Thyroglobulin is only produced by functioning thyroid tissue, and its presence in the serum after total thyroidectomy or ablation suggests recurrent disease. It can be used as a guide for the need for further radioiodine therapy, and it should probably be assayed 6-monthly.[42,43]

Prognosis

The prognosis of differentiated thyroid cancer, even when metastases are present at the time of discovery, is excellent (Fig. 17.7). Prognosis is particularly favourable in patients between the ages of 20 and 50 years. Although differentiated thyroid carcinoma is uncommon in children, the rates of recurrence are higher and prognosis less good.

MEDULLARY THYROID CANCER

Medullary thyroid cancer is cancer of the parafollicular cells (C cells), which produce calcitonin, a useful tumour marker. It accounts for 5–8% of all thyroid neoplasms, and it occurs in several distinct clinical contexts:

- sporadic (75%);
- familial, in association with multiple endocrine neoplasia type 2; and
- familial, without other stigmata of multiple endocrine neoplasia.

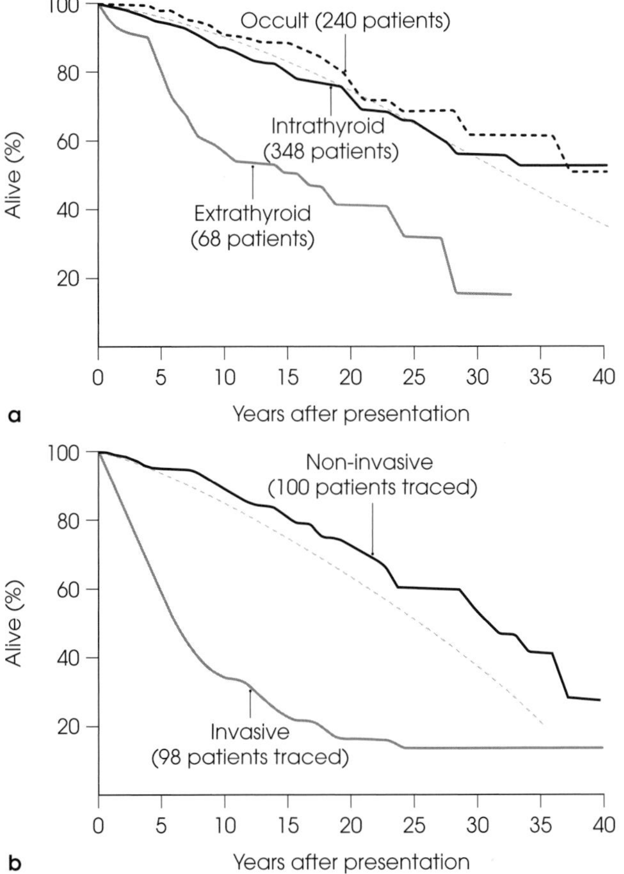

Figure 17.7 Survival after treatment of (**a**) papillary and (**b**) follicular thyroid carcinoma. Broken lines show the survival of a normal population. (From Woolner et al 1968,[44] with permission.)

Clinical features

Most sporadic cases present in patients over the age of 40 years with a goitre, and 25% of patients have palpable lymph node metastases. Sporadic medullary thyroid cancer is usually solitary and unilateral, whereas hereditary forms are bilateral and multicentric. They occur in the middle to upper third of the gland, where the C cells are most numerous. In the familial form of the disease, C-cell hyperplasia is present prior to invasive tumour development. Those with multiple endocrine neoplasia type 2a may also have clinical signs of phaeochromocytoma (40%) and/or hyperparathyroidism (20%). In multiple endocrine neoplasia type 2b, patients will additionally display multiple mucosal neuromas, especially of the lips and tongue, and a marfanoid habitus.

Genetics

Multiple endocrine neoplasia type 2 has an autosomal dominant inheritance. The precise genetic defect has been localized to mutations in the *RET* proto-oncogene on chromosome 10. In multiple endocrine neoplasia type 2a most mutations occur at codon 634, whereas codon 618 is usually implicated in familial medullary thyroid carcinoma and codon 918 in type 2b. The availability of accurate, cost-effective genetic screening has enabled earlier surgery in affected children, resulting in detection of early disease and a significant prospect of surgical cure.[44] Where present, these mutations carry a 100% risk of developing medullary carcinoma, and 'prophylactic' thyroidectomy should be undertaken around the age of 5 years for multiple endocrine neoplasia type 2a and in the first year of life for type 2b.[45]

Investigation

When medullary thyroid cancer is suspected on fine-needle aspiration biopsy or from the clinical history, or if there is bilateral upper polar calcification or concurrent signs of phaeochromocytoma or hypercalcaemia, then calcitonin should be measured. If calcitonin is raised, a coexisting phaeochromocytoma must be excluded. Medullary thyroid cancer produces not only calcitonin but also other substances, including serotonin, prostaglandin, 5-hydroxyindoleacetic acid, carcinoembryonic antigen, histaminase, adrenocorticotrophic hormone and prolactin. These can be used to assess the presence, extent and recurrence of the disease. Usually only calcitonin and carcinoembryonic antigen are assayed.

Genetic screening should be performed on all patients diagnosed with medullary thyroid carcinoma. If a familial trait is identified, then formal family-tree analysis and reporting to the national multiple endocrine neoplasia database is appropriate.

Treatment

Medullary thyroid cancer is more aggressive than differentiated thyroid cancer; 50% of cases have involved nodes at operation

REFERENCES

41. Pujol P, Daures J-P et al. J Clin Endocrinol Metab 1996; 81: 4318–4323
42. Ericsson UB, Tegler L et al. Acta Chir Scand 1984; 150: 367–375
43. Ashcroft MW, Van Herle AJ. Am J Med 1981; 71: 806
44. Woolner LB et al. In: Young S, Ingman IR (eds). ICRF Symposium on Thyroid Neoplasia. Academic Press, London, 1968
45. O'Riordain D, O'Brian T et al. Surgery 1994; 116: 1017–1023

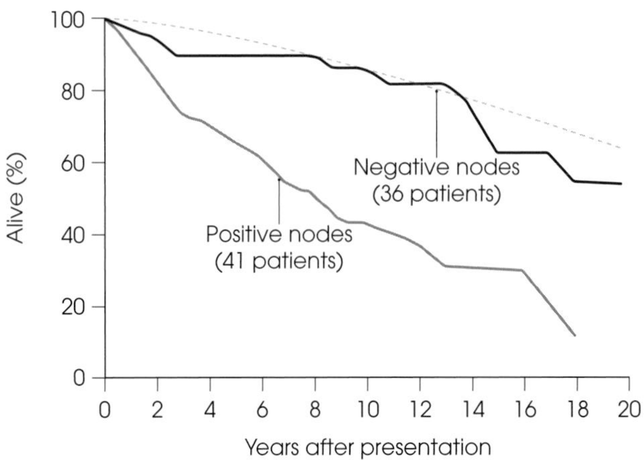

Figure 17.8 Survival after treatment of medullary thyroid carcinoma. (From Woolner et al 1968,[44] with permission.)

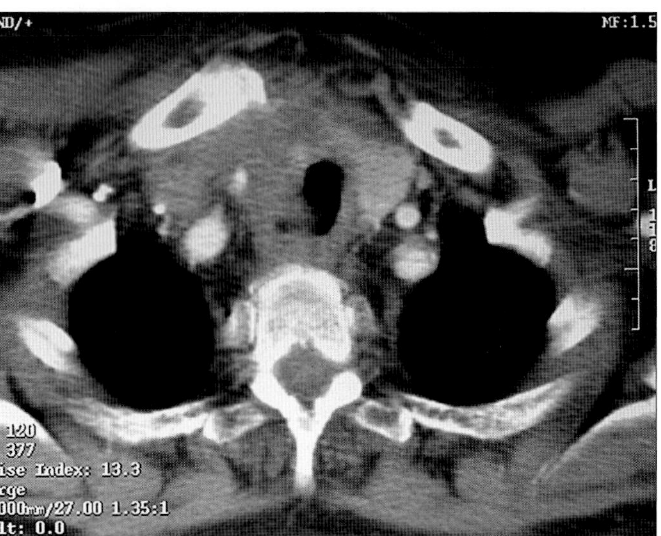

Figure 17.9 A CT scan of the neck, demonstrating anaplastic carcinoma of the right lobe of the thyroid gland with tracheal invasion.

even where the primary lesion is tiny. The mainstay of treatment is radical surgery. The addition of node dissection to thyroidectomy has been shown to improve the 10-year prognosis from 43 to 67%.[46] Prognosis is shown in Fig. 17.8.

The diagnosis of medullary thyroid cancer should be established preoperatively by fine-needle aspiration biopsy. Total thyroidectomy should be performed, as well as ipsilateral resection of all lymphatic tissue from the thyroid cartilage to the upper mediastinum, including the thymus, and laterally to the outer border of the sternomastoid. Bilateral neck dissection should be performed if there is multicentric or familial disease. If a preoperative diagnosis was not made, or if thyroidectomy was performed in a familial case with impalpable disease, later neck dissection is only indicated if calcitonin levels do not fall to normal or near-normal levels postoperatively, or if frozen-section analysis of a node shows metastatic deposits. Radioiodine, external radiotherapy and chemotherapy have no role in the management of the primary disease.

Postoperatively, patients must be followed by sequential calcitonin assays. A raised postoperative calcitonin level strongly suggests recurrent or persistent disease. Other causes for elevated calcitonin include other malignancies, renal failure and pregnancy. After total thyroidectomy and node resection, the serum calcitonin should be immeasurably low. Many surgeons dealing with this condition are, however, familiar with the scenario of a low but stable calcitonin level that does not seem to be associated with progressing disease,[47] but others favour extensive investigation and aggressive reoperative strategies for such patients. Recurrent disease may be imaged with neck ultrasound, technetium-99m 111-dimercaptosuccinic acid (DMSA), octreotide, or positron emission tomography isotope scans. There is no evidence that reoperation in the presence of a persistently raised calcitonin level but without palpable or imaged disease is beneficial.

Metastatic medullary thyroid cancer may be troublesome because of local recurrent disease or diarrhoea. Debulking of metastases or therapy by external radiotherapy[47] or chemotherapy is occasionally feasible.

ANAPLASTIC THYROID CANCER

Anaplastic malignancies of the thyroid are the worst of all thyroid malignancies and one of the most aggressive of all human neoplasms. Death occurs within a year of diagnosis in 90% of patients. They account for 3–30% of all thyroid neoplasms depending on the geographic area, and are commonest in areas of endemic goitre. The tumour is almost entirely confined to elderly patients, in whom it presents late, probably having begun as an unrecognized or ignored differentiated tumour of papillary or follicular type. Such tumours often histologically coexist with anaplastic cancer. This favours a more aggressive approach to the management of differentiated carcinoma in an attempt to avoid dedifferentiation into anaplastic disease.

At presentation the patient usually has a fixed mass in the centre of the neck, surrounding the trachea and infiltrating local structures with great tenacity; even the carotid arteries and the lumen of the trachea are not excluded from invasion (Fig. 17.9). Stridor from tracheal invasion, dysphagia from oesophageal involvement, and recurrent nerve palsy and pain are all common.

Management

Biopsy is essential to distinguish between lymphoma and anaplastic cancer. This distinction is not always possible on fine-needle aspiration biopsy, and open or core biopsy may be necessary. When undifferentiated and differentiated cancers are found to coexist, the prognosis is no better than when the tumour is solely undifferentiated.

Curative surgery is almost never feasible.[48] Traditionally, debulking surgery is attempted when feasible, but in fewer than half the patients is the limited objective of freeing the trachea and oesophagus from encroachment achievable.[49] Indeed, the sole result may be to allow tumour to fungate through the wound. Super-radical surgery has been advocated, but is not generally

REFERENCES

46. Johnston LB, Chew SL et al. Clin Endocrinol 2000; 52: 127–136
47. Van Heerden JA, Hay ID. In: Wheeler MH, Lazarus JH (eds). Diseases of the Thyroid. Chapman & Hall, London, 1994: 400–401
48. Jereb B, Stjernsward J, Lowhagen T. Cancer 1975; 35: 1293–1295
49. McIver B, Hay ID et al. Surgery 2001; 130: 1028–1034

accepted as useful.[50] Preoperative radiotherapy has not been found to shrink the tumour sufficiently to allow radical surgery. Some have advocated following surgery by radiotherapy and chemotherapy,[51] but most older patients cannot tolerate this triple insult, and such aggressive intent should be restricted to the rare younger patient presenting with this disease. For the majority of patients, biopsy followed by attempted palliation with radiotherapy is all that is indicated.

LYMPHOMA OF THE THYROID

Lymphoma may involve the thyroid primarily or secondarily. Primary lymphoma must be distinguished from small cell anaplastic cancer. There is sometimes a history of coexisting lymphocytic thyroiditis, and histological changes of Hashimoto's thyroiditis are found in 36% of resected lymphomas of the thyroid. The lymphoma is typically of the B-cell type, and many arise from mucosa-associated lymphatic tissue.[52] Patients present with a rapidly expanding goitre associated with compression symptoms. The role of surgery is confined to surgical biopsy when fine-needle aspiration biopsy fails to yield a diagnosis, and possibly a thyroidectomy for lymphoma localized to the thyroid gland.[53] There is no evidence that surgery improves the prognosis of patients presenting with extrathyroid disease. Following a confident biopsy result, patients should be treated by a combination of radiotherapy and chemotherapy. Recurrent or distant metastatic disease is treated by chemotherapy.

The 5-year survival rate is 86% when the disease is confined at presentation to the thyroid, but only 38% where soft tissue or nodal involvement is present.[54] Prognosis is also critically related to the grade of the tumour: low-grade and intermediate-grade tumours have a 5-year survival rate of around 80%, whereas for high-grade lesions it is less than 20%.[51]

SQUAMOUS CARCINOMA

Squamous carcinoma is very rare and should be distinguished from squamous metaplasia in papillary carcinoma. True squamous carcinoma arises in embryonal remnants and may coexist with adenocarcinoma. Squamous carcinoma of the thyroid is an extremely aggressive, essentially untreatable malignancy.[55]

TERATOMA

Teratomas are tumours that contain tissue from all three germ layers. They are benign in children but usually malignant when encountered in adults, in which context they are very aggressive and prognosis is usually survival for less than 1 year.[56]

HYPERTHYROIDISM

Three diseases account for 95% of causes of thyrotoxicosis: Graves' disease (80%), toxic multinodular goitre (15%), and toxic adenoma (5%). Other causes of thyrotoxicosis are listed in Box 17.2. The clinical features of thyrotoxicosis are broadly similar for all causes, and the principle symptoms are listed in Table 17.2. Elevated thyroid hormones and suppression of thyrotropin confirm the diagnosis. Autoantibodies are elevated in patients with Graves' disease. A thyroid scintiscan differentiates Graves' disease from toxic nodular goitre or a hyperfunctioning adenoma (Fig. 17.10). A quantitative measure of the uptake of the isotope will also indicate the severity of the disease.

Box 17.2 Causes of hyperthyroidism

- Diffuse toxic goitre (Graves' disease)
- Hyperfunctioning adenoma
- Toxic multinodular goitre (Plummer's syndrome)
- Overdose of thyroxine (iatrogenic or factitious)
- Subacute or acute thyroiditis
- Thyroid-stimulating hormone-secreting tumours (choriocarcinoma, hydatidiform mole, embryonal testicular cancer)
- Functioning thyroid carcinoma
- Over-treatment of nodular goitre with iodine (Jod–Basedow effect)
- During iodine-131 therapy
- Struma ovarii

GRAVES' DISEASE

Pathology

In this autoimmune condition IgG immunoglobulins are raised against thyrotropin receptors. These immunoglobulins mimic thyrotropin to stimulate the production of thyroid hormones. The aetiology remains unclear, but patients of HLA Dw3 seem particularly at risk, implying a genetic predisposition. Unique to Graves' disease is the involvement of the eyes. Lymphocytes are directed against an undetermined antigen and infiltrate the orbital tissues.

Clinical features

Graves' disease is predominantly a disease of women (female:male, 10:1), among whom the incidence is 20 per 1000. The peak incidence is at 20–40 years, but any age from birth to death may be affected. Clinically, patients have the typical features of thyrotoxicosis with a predominance of central nervous system symptoms. Most are the result of excessive circulating thyroxine, but exophthalmos, pretibial myxoedema and thyroid acropachy have a different causation. The thyroid is uniformly enlarged, smooth and firm. It is rarely very large but is frequently hypervascular; a thrill may be palpable and a strong bruit audible.

A total of 75% of cases have associated eye disease, but only 2–3% develop severe exophthalmos.[57] The typical appearances of exophthalmos are a combination of proptosis, lid retraction due to a direct effect of thyroxine on the muscles, conjunctival oedema and redness, and oedema of the eyelids. In severe cases there is ophthalmoplegia following paralysis of the voluntary eye muscles. This may cause squint. Finally, optic nerve damage and loss of vision may occur.

Treatment

All patients with Graves' disease must be treated, otherwise 25% will die and 50% will be left incapacitated to some degree. There

REFERENCES

50. Djalilian M, Beahrs OH et al. Am J Surg 1974; 128: 500–504
51. Nilsson O, Lindeberg J et al. World J Surg 1998; 22: 725–730
52. Derringer GA, Thompson LDR et al. Am J Surg Pathol 2000; 24: 623–639
53. Pasieka JL. World J Surg 2000; 24: 966–970
54. Devine RM, Edis AJ, Banks PM. World J Surg 1981; 5: 33–38
55. Harada T, Shimaoka K, Yakumaru K et al. J Surg Oncol 1982; 19: 36–43
56. Kimler SC, Mulh WF. Cancer 1978; 42: 311–317
57. Hamilton RD, Mayberry WE, McConahey WM et al. Mayo Clin Proc 1967; 42: 812–813

Table 17.2 Clinical features of hyperthyroidism

General	Cardiovascular system	Neuromuscular	Gastrointestinal	Skin	Reproductive	Eyes	Bone
Weight loss Increased appetite Fatigue Sweating Heat intolerance	Palpitations Angina Sinus tachycardia or atrial fibrillation Cardiac failure Vasodilatation	Tremor Emotional lability, psychosis Proximal myopathy Myasthenia gravis Choreoathetosis	Vomiting Diarrhoea Steatorrhoea	Increased pigmentation Thyroid acropachy* Spider naevi Palmar erythema Pretibial myxoedema* Onycholysis	Oligomenorrhoea Gynaecomastia Reduced libido	Lid lag Proptosis* Ophthalmoplegia* Chemosis and corneal ulceration*	Osteoporosis

*Only noted in Graves' disease.

Table 17.3 Advantages and disadvantages of definitive therapy for Graves' disease

Surgery		Radioiodine	
Advantages	**Disadvantages**	**Advantages**	**Disadvantages**
Immediate control Possibility of avoiding thyroxine	Risks of surgery recurrent laryngeal nerve injury Hypoparathyroidism Cost and inpatient stay Scar	Outpatient therapy Avoids risks of surgery Avoids scar	Unknown long-term side effects of iodine-131 Short-term social restrictions Inevitable hypothyroidism Takes longer to become euthyroid Worsens eye disease?

are three forms of treatment: antithyroid drugs, radioiodine and surgery. No one form of treatment is optimal, and the timing and choice of treatment must be carefully matched to the patient's disease, social circumstances and wishes. All treatment must therefore be preceded by full discussion of the benefits and complications of each form of treatment. The Royal College of Physicians of London has produced a consensus statement for good practice in the management of hyperthyroidism.[58]

Medical therapy

The first-line treatment for Graves' disease is medical therapy using drugs that block the synthesis of thyroxine. The thionamides (propylthiouracil, methimazole and carbimazole) inhibit thyroid peroxidase. In addition, antithyroid drugs have direct effects on the autoimmune process, leading to a reduction in thyroid autoantibodies. Thyrotoxicosis can usually be controlled within 10–14 days, but it may take 2 months. Some clinicians give a higher dose of carbimazole to maximize its immunosuppressive properties in conjunction with thyroxine to maintain a euthyroid state (the 'block and replace' regimen).

Patients are maintained on antithyroid drugs for a limited time once a euthyroid status has been established. This cannot be indefinite owing to the rare (0.4%) but serious complication of agranulocytosis. Patients must be warned about the risk and advised to seek urgent medical advice if they develop a sore throat, which usually heralds this complication. There is no agreement as to the optimal duration of the first course of treatment. Practices range from 3 to 18 months, after which up to 50% of patients will stay in remission, although quoted figures range from 15 to 80%.[59] Remission is most likely to occur where the goitre is small, the thyrotoxicosis mild, and where there is a rapid response to the treatment by the shrinkage of the gland.

When a patient relapses into a thyrotoxic state, definitive therapy by means of either surgery or radioiodine is indicated. Antithyroid medication is recommenced in preparation for definitive treatment.

Definitive therapy

The principle of definitive therapy is to destroy sufficient thyroid tissue to prevent the excess secretion of thyroxine. The choice between radioiodine and surgery is influenced by the patient's age, the size of the goitre, the degree of hyperthyroidism, and the presence of ophthalmopathy, as well as the patient's choice and the availability of surgical expertise. The main advantages and disadvantages are shown in Table 17.3.

Radioiodine therapy

Radioiodine as iodine-131 is given as a single oral dose, and exerts its action by direct radiation damage to the replicative mechanisms of the follicular cells. A response is generally achieved in 6–10 weeks, and control of hyperthyroidism by drugs will be necessary in the interim. If no control is achieved at 4 months, further radioiodine is given.

The benefits of radioiodine therapy are its simplicity, its cheapness, and its short-term safety. The risks in theory include the possible induction of thyroid and other malignancies, especially leukaemia, and the induction of genetic abnormalities in future children. While these risks appear to be very small,[60,61]

REFERENCES

58. Vanderpump MPJ, Ahlquist JA et al. Br Med J 1996; 313: 39–544
59. Franklyn JA. Baillières Clin Endocrinol Metab 1997; 11: 561–571
60. Stoffer SS, Hamburger JI. J Nucl Med 1970; 17: 146–149
61. Hall P, Berg G, Bjelkengren G et al. Int J Cancer 1992; 50: 886–890

there is insecurity about the delayed effects of radiation. The major drawback is the high incidence of late hypothyroidism and the unpredictability of its time of onset. In the first 3 years this ranges from 10 to 40%.[62] Thereafter there is a 3% per annum increment. It is the treatment of choice for those with recurrent thyrotoxicosis following surgery because reoperation carries greater risks.

A significant disadvantage of radioiodine therapy is the short-term social restrictions following therapy. Patients must not be pregnant at the time of therapy and should avoid pregnancy for at least 4 months. In addition, patients must avoid non-essential close personal contact with children for as long as 4 weeks,[63] a significant restriction on a predominantly young female patient population.

Radioiodine therapy carries a small, but definite, risk of progression of Graves' ophthalmopathy.[64] At-risk patients treated with radioiodine should receive concomitant steroid therapy.

Surgery

Thyroidectomy brings about a rapid cure for hyperthyroidism and is indicated for the following groups:

- severe ophthalmopathy;
- ongoing or planned pregnancy;
- large or nodular goitres; and
- patients who refuse radiation therapy.

It is also preferable for those in whom follow-up or compliance with medical treatment is uncertain, owing to the lower incidence of hypothyroidism in surgically treated patients and the fact that the majority of postoperative hypothyroidism declares itself within 1 year of operation.[63]

Preparation for surgery

The patient should be biochemically euthyroid when operated on. The addition of beta blockers (when not contraindicated) may be considered. Some surgeons use iodine as potassium iodide or Lugol's iodine 7–10 days preoperatively to reduce thyroid vascularity.[65]

Operation

The goals of surgery are to minimize recurrence of thyrotoxicosis, minimize morbidity, and render the patient euthyroid without the need for thyroxine supplementation. The risks of operation are the normal risks of thyroidectomy, to which is added the risk of fulminating hyperthyroidism after operation if a preoperative euthyroid has not been achieved. The technical difficulties of thyroidectomy for Graves' disease should never be underestimated. Even in the fully controlled patient, the gland often remains very vascular and difficult to handle, especially in the young patient. This surgery should be restricted to those surgeons who are experienced and have a documented low rate of postoperative complications.

The conventional operation is bilateral subtotal thyroidectomy, but a hemithyroidectomy and contralateral subtotal lobectomy is another option.[66] The weight of the thyroid remnant(s) left to attain postoperative euthyroidism is difficult to judge, both in theory and practically at the time of operation. A total remnant weight between 4 and 10 g is reasonable.[67,68] A minority of surgeons routinely perform a total thyroidectomy, accepting the inevitability of hypothyroidism as the price of abolishing any risk of recurrence.

Results of surgery

The recurrence rate after subtotal thyroidectomy is about 5% at 5 years, and some recurrences occur after that, especially in areas of high iodine intake.[69] Recurrence is treated with radioiodine, because further surgery carries an unacceptable risk of complications.

Postoperative hypothyroidism develops in between 9%[70] and 49%[71] of patients. The incidence is higher with small remnants, pronounced lymphocytic infiltration of the gland, raised thyroid autoantibody titres, and low iodine intake. The reported incidence of hypothyroidism depends on its definition. Many patients have a raised thyrotropin and a marginally low thyroxine in the first few months after surgery, but many of these will remain clinically euthyroid and the thyroid function reverts to normal after 6–12 months.[67] Such patients need not take replacement thyroxine but need regular careful review. Definite clinical hypothyroidism requires lifelong replacement therapy with thyroxine. Although 90% of incidences of continuing postoperative hypothyroidism will declare themselves in the first year, there is a 1–2% addition to this total in each of the following years, and follow-up should be lifelong.

Eyes

In the majority of cases, there will be regression or arrested progression of exophthalmos after successful management of the thyroid gland in Graves' disease. Progressive eye disease will, however, occur in 3–10%,[71] and may require high-dose steroids, immunosuppression, or even surgical orbital decompression.[72]

THYROTOXICOSIS IN CHILDHOOD

Medical control of thyrotoxicosis in childhood may be difficult and more complicated than it is in the adult, but should always be the first line of treatment. When control cannot be achieved or maintained, the tendency in the past has been to prefer surgical treatment,[73] but there is now enough long-term experience with radioiodine treatment to confirm that it is safe in this age group.[74] Surgery may be preferred by children and adolescents who do not wish to take antithyroid drugs, and is indicated in children with a large goitre, particularly if retrosternal.

THYROTOXICOSIS IN PREGNANCY

The prevalence of thyrotoxicosis in pregnancy is 0.05%.[75] The diagnosis is difficult, because more than 50% of pregnant women

REFERENCES

62. Nofal MM et al. JAMA 1966; 197: 608
63. Lazarus JH. J R Coll Physicians Lond 1995; 29: 464–469
64. Bonnema SJ et al. Eur J Endocrinol 2002; 147: 1–11
65. Marigold JH, Morgan AK et al. Br J Surg 1985; 72: 45–47
66. Andaker L et al. World J Surg 1992; 16: 765–769
67. Michie W, Pegg CAS, Bewsher PD. Br Med J 1972; 1: 13–17
68. Cusick EL, Krukowski ZH, Matheson NA. Br J Surg 1988; 74: 780–783
69. Kalk WJ, Kantor S, Durback D. Lancet 1978; i: 291–294
70. Caswell HT, Maier WP. Surg Gynecol Obstet 1972; 134: 218–220
71. Michie W. Br J Surg 1975; 62: 673–682
72. Fells P. In: Lynn J, Bloom SR (eds). Surgical Endocrinology. Butterworth Heinemann, Oxford, 1993: 312–323
73. Soreide J-A, van Heerden JA et al. World J Surg 1996; 20: 794–800
74. Hamburger JI. J Clin Endocrinol Metab 1985; 60: 1019
75. Drury MI. J R Soc Med 1986; 79: 317–318

have a goitre and the signs of pregnancy can mimic thyrotoxicosis. If the diagnosis is made during pregnancy, cautious treatment with the lowest effective dose of carbimazole, methimazole or propylthiouracil is indicated,[76] and beta blockers should be used with caution. The use of radioiodine for investigation or treatment is absolutely contraindicated, because it crosses the placenta and destroys the fetal thyroid. When medical control fails, surgery may be necessary and is best planned towards the end of the second trimester. Preoperative preparation with iodides is not permitted.

PLUMMER'S SYNDROME (TOXIC MULTINODULAR GOITRE)

This condition, also termed *secondary thyrotoxicosis*, is caused by an autonomous overproduction of thyroxine by nodules in a longstanding goitre. Patients are therefore older (over 40 years) and have a preceding history of goitre. The resultant hyperthyroidism predominantly affects the cardiovascular system and is not associated with exophthalmos, myopathy, or the serological changes seen in Graves' disease. The explanation for how previously non-functioning colloid nodules develop into overfunctioning units remains unclear, but is likely to involve mutations of growth factor receptors.

Treatment

The choice rests between surgery and radioiodine. The use of antithyroid drugs is restricted to control prior to definitive therapy. Subtotal thyroidectomy is indicated in patients with a large goitre and compressive symptoms, particularly with retrosternal extension. Those with mild hyperthyroidism in small multinodular glands can be successfully treated with radioiodine. There is a high incidence of hypothyroidism after surgery: 70% at 2 years in the Mayo Clinic series.[77]

TOXIC ADENOMA

Toxic adenoma is a hyperfunctioning follicular adenoma; nine out of 10 cases are in females and they can occur at any age. Some 54% present because of a nodule, 37% because of thyrotoxicosis;[78] 90–96% of such adenomas are benign.[79] The autonomous overproduction of thyroxine or tri-iodothyronine suppresses thyrotropin. Diagnosis is easily made with a technetium scintiscan (Fig. 17.10), which shows uptake of the isotope solely in the nodule; the remainder of the gland is not imaged. This favours treatment by radioiodine, which is selectively taken up by the adenoma; the suppressed normal thyroid tissue is usually protected from destruction. However, a neoplasm could go undiagnosed and posttherapy hypothyroidism can occur. A thyroid lobectomy is an equally effective alternative, has the advantage of providing a histological diagnosis, and should always be undertaken for larger lesions (over 4 cm).

HYPOTHYROIDISM

Hypothyroidism exists when there is inadequate thyroid hormone action on the peripheral tissues. This can occur by reduced production of hormone by the gland (primary hypothyroidism), failure of thyroid-stimulating hormone production (secondary hypothyroidism), failure of production of thyroid-stimulating hormone-releasing hormone (tertiary hypothyroidism), or resistance of the peripheral tissues to thyroxine. The causes of hypothyroidism are outlined in Box 17.3. The end results of all these processes are the same, and may be symptomatic (myxoedema) or asymptomatic.

Box 17.3 Causes of hypothyroidism

Primary hypothyroidism

- Hashimoto's thyroiditis
- Radioactive iodine therapy for Graves' disease
- Thyroidectomy
- Antithyroid drug therapy for Graves' disease
- Excessive iodide intake
- Subacute thyroiditis
- Miscellaneous rare causes
- Iodide deficiency
- Goitrogens
- Inborn errors of thyroid metabolism

Secondary hypothyroidism

- Ablative therapy for pituitary adenoma
- Chromophobe pituitary adenoma
- Other causes of pituitary destruction
- Tertiary hypothyroidism
- Peripheral resistance to thyroxine

CLINICAL SYMPTOMS

The hypothyroid infant (cretin) is somnolent, feeds poorly, fails to thrive, and is constipated. The tongue is large, the face puffy, the abdomen protuberant, and umbilical hernias are common. Onset of hypothyroidism in childhood leads to growth failure and slowing of sexual, physical and intellectual development. In adults the onset of hypothyroidism is usually insidious and subtle, and unnoticed by patient and relatives. There is weight gain, coldness, thickening and dryness of the skin, facial puffiness and pallor, dry brittle scanty hair, and hoarseness. Sometimes there is anorexia, deafness, dyspnoea or palpitations. In almost all patients there is noticeable slowing of the intellect.

Once suspected, myxoedema is readily diagnosed if thyrotropin is raised, but thyrotropin will be low in secondary and tertiary myxoedema. Free thyroxine and tri-iodothyronine are low in established myxoedema.

Treatment is ideally by synthetic thyroxine. It has a predictable biological activity and long half-life (1 week), and is palatable and cheap. In elderly patients and those with coronary atherosclerosis, thyroxine therapy must be introduced with extreme care if angina is to be avoided. It is usual to start with one-tenth to one-fifth of the full replacement dose and increase gradually to the full dose over 2 months.[80]

SICK EUTHYROIDISM

Any severe illness may cause a low plasma total thyroxine concentration. Thyrotropin levels are usually normal or slightly high. Triiodothyronine levels may be low. Assessment of thyroid function is best deferred until the patient has recovered from the illness.

REFERENCES

76. de Swiet M, Lynn J. In: Surgical Endocrinology. Butterworth Heinemann, Oxford, 1993: 85–86
77. Mensen MD, Gharib H et al. World J Surg 1986; 10: 673–680
78. Bransom CJ, Talbot CH et al. Br J Surg 1979; 66: 590–595
79. Johnson IDA. Br J Surg 1975; 62: 765–768
80. Rapoport B. Endocrine Surgery of the Thyroid and Parathyroid Gland. CV Mosby, St Louis, 1985: 144–17

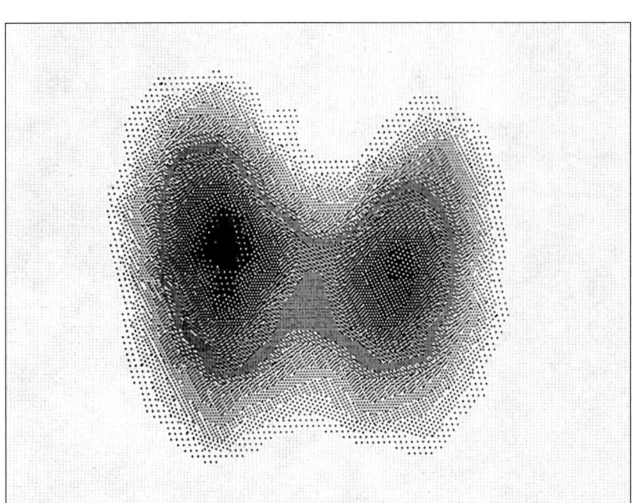

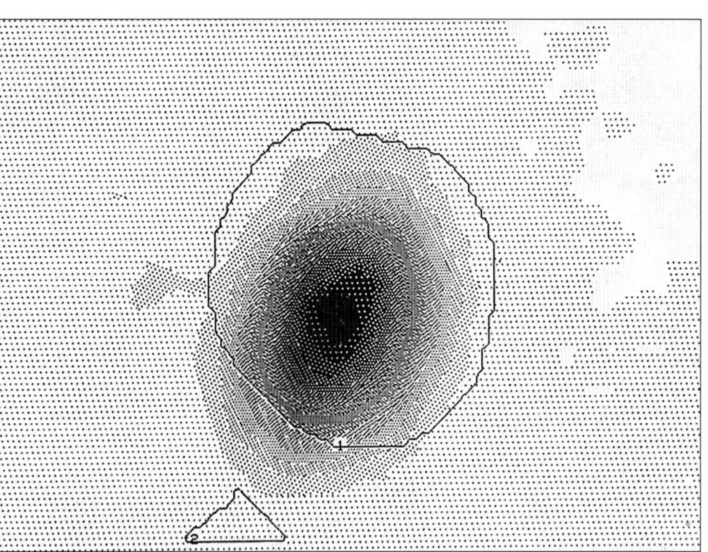

Figure 17.10 Technetium isotope scans. (**a**) Graves' disease. Uptake of the isotope was 5.3%; normal is 0.7–3% at 20 min. (**b**) Functioning thyroid adenoma. The triangle marks the sternal notch. Uptake was 5.16%. The right lobe is not imaged as it is suppressed by the hyperfunctioning left lobe.

Table 17.4 Classification of thyroiditis

Type	Name	Haplotype	Aetiology	Autoimmune
Acute suppurative	–	–	Infection	No
Subacute (transient)				
Granulomatous				Possible in part
Lymphocytic	De Quervain's*	HLA Bw35	Viral and genetic predisposition	
Sporadic	'Silent' or painless	HLA DR3	Unknown	Possibly
Postpartum	Postpartum	HLA DR3, DR5	Thyroid stimulation in pregnancy	Probably
Chronic lymphocytic				
Non-goitrous	Atrophic	HLA DR3	Surface expression of antigens *and* organ-specific defect in suppressor T cells *leads to* autodestructive antibody production	Definitely
Goitrous	Hashimoto's†	HLA DR5, B8, Dw3		
Chronic fibrous	Riedel's‡	–	Systemic fibrosis of unknown origin	Possible

*Fritz de Quervain (1868–1940) became reader to Kocher in Bern and succeeded him as Professor of Surgery. He described the thyroiditis that bears his name in 1902.
†Hakura Hashimoto (1881–1934), a Japanese surgeon, described thyroiditis in 1912, and in 1956 it was found to be autoimmune.
‡Bernhard Riedel (1846–1916), Professor of Surgery at Jena, described thyroiditis in 1896.

THYROIDITIS

Inflammatory changes in the thyroid are common and may or may not be associated with a change in the function of the gland. Their categorization is confused by ignorance of their aetiology, but from a clinical point of view the traditional groupings of acute, subacute, Hashimoto's and Riedel's thyroiditis are adequate (Table 17.4). However, because there are several definite clinical variants among patients previously categorized as Hashimoto's thyroiditis, the term *autoimmune thyroiditis* is now more appropriate.

ACUTE SUPPURATIVE THYROIDITIS

This condition, now rarely encountered, is secondary to haematogenous or local spread of bacterial, fungal or parasitic infection from elsewhere in the body. Typically, *Staphylococcus aureus*, haemolytic streptococci and *Streptococcus pneumoniae* are responsible. The goitrous gland is more vulnerable than the normal one.

The clinical features are those of acute infection: pain in the thyroid radiating to the ear, occiput or jaw, and worsened by movement or swallowing; and fever, tachycardia, and local oedema that may involve the larynx, trachea or oesophagus. The diagnosis is clinical. Identification of the organism may require needle aspiration and culture. Treatment is by the appropriate antibiotic, but occasionally open drainage or thyroidectomy is indicated.[81]

SUBACUTE (TRANSIENT) THYROIDITIS

Granulomatous thyroiditis (de Quervain's)

This is a self-limiting inflammation of the gland, pathologically characterized by localized destruction of thyroid follicular epithelium with giant cell formation and a mixed inflammatory

REFERENCES

81. Hashimoto H. Arch Klin Chir 1912; 97: 219–248

response. The aetiology is probably primarily viral; mumps, measles, influenza, Epstein–Barr, coxsackie and adenoviruses have all been implicated. Thyroid symptoms are usually preceded by a sore throat and an upper respiratory tract infection. The gland then becomes tender and enlarged, usually bilaterally. The patient feels unwell, has a low-grade fever and sometimes an associated myalgia. In 50% of patients, there may be transient signs of mild hyperthyroidism due to release of stored thyroxine by destruction of the thyroid parenchyma. Over ensuing weeks or months, the gland shrinks. Thyroid function tests return to normal, but a quarter of patients become mildly hypothyroid.

Investigation shows a raised erythrocyte sedimentation rate, usually above 50 mm/h. The hyperthyroidism can be distinguished from Graves' disease by the low uptake of isotope on scintiscanning. Biopsy is not necessary. Non-steroidal anti-inflammatory drugs ease the discomfort in the acute stage, and steroid therapy is very occasionally necessary. Antithyroid drugs are of no value in the hyperthyroid stage, but beta blockers may produce symptomatic relief.[82] The disease may run an erratic course, with recurrence of symptoms when recovery seems under way.

Lymphocytic 'silent' thyroiditis

Sporadic

Patients may be asymptomatic or present at any age with mild hyperthyroidism. The thyroid is moderately enlarged but painless and non-tender, and there is no elevation of markers of inflammation. Tri-iodothyronine and thyroxine are initially raised and thyrotropin suppressed. Radioiodine uptake is decreased. The hyperthyroid phase lasts for 1–12 months, followed by a transient myxoedema (possibly due to follicular depletion). The patient becomes euthyroid after the recuperative phase, but there is a recurrence rate of 10–15%.[83] Usually there is no need for therapy, but beta blockers may be indicated in severe cases.

Postpartum

This autoimmune thyroiditis occurs in about 5% of postpartum women, several weeks after delivery.[84] In many ways it is identical to the sporadic form, but the recuperative phase is often incomplete, leading to persistent myxoedema. It has been postulated that this disorder could be responsible for postpartum depression.

CHRONIC LYMPHOCYTIC THYROIDITIS

Autoimmune lymphocytic thyroiditis affects predominantly women (10-fold) in the 30–60-year age range. It is characterized by a lymphoid and plasma cell infiltration. There are two clinical subtypes: goitrous (Hashimoto's) and atrophic.

Hashimoto's thyroiditis

Pathology

Over 90% of cases of hypothyroidism are secondary to this condition. The aetiology is autoimmune, and 95% of patients have circulating autoantibodies to thyroglobulin and thyroid microsomes (now known to be the enzyme thyroid peroxidase). The predominance of HLA antigens DR5, B8, and Dw3 suggests that genetic factors are important. The pathophysiology is believed to be due to aberrant expression of MHC class 2 molecules on the thyrocytes, permitting autoantigen presentation to T-helper cells inducing B-lymphocytes to secrete autoantibodies. In addition, there may be defects in the suppressor T-cell function. The consequences of this autoimmune process are that of cell-mediated cytotoxicity and complement fixation leading to cellular destruction. Histologically, there is infiltration by lymphoid cells organized in clumps or germinal centres and associated with hyperplasia, fibrosis and increased oxyphil (Askanazy) cells.

Clinical features

Patients insidiously develop myxoedema in the presence of a goitre. Hypothyroidism is more pronounced in the elderly. The goitre is usually moderate but sometimes gross. The enlargement is painless and the symptoms are due only to pressure. The goitre is rubbery and may be solitary or diffuse, smooth or nodular. The diagnosis is primarily by autoantibody titre estimations. Fine-needle aspiration biopsy should always be undertaken to exclude coexisting malignant disease if the goitre is asymmetrical.

Treatment

Thyroxine is always given if the patient is hypothyroid. With progression of the disease the goitre shrinks. Surgery is only indicated where the goitre presents with compressive or aesthetic complications, or where malignancy is suspected on clinical, histological or cytological grounds.[85]

Hashimoto's and neoplasia

A prospective study of 829 patients with Hashimoto's followed for 8 years and compared with 829 controls with colloid goitre showed a sevenfold increase of malignant lymphoma in the Hashimoto patients.[86] Nevertheless, only a tiny fraction of a per cent of patients with Hashimoto's progress to thyroid lymphoma. There is also a marginally increased link of differentiated carcinoma.

Atrophic thyroiditis

In this group of patients, the thyroid undergoes follicular destruction or atrophy with fibrosis and a lesser degree of lymphocytic infiltration. Autoantibodies are measurable in only 55% of patients. It is believed that thyrotropin receptor-blocking antibodies have the prevailing action.[83] Clinically, patients develop myxoedema without goitre and the treatment is medical.

Riedel's thyroiditis

This very rare process is one of dense fibrosis of all or part of the gland with invasion of adjacent tissues. It is probably related to other idiopathic fibroses (retroperitoneal, mediastinal, retro-orbital and sclerosing cholangitis). Patients present with compressive symptoms and occasionally a mass, which may be painful. Clinically, the thyroid is non-tender and stony-hard, and the diagnostic difficulty lies in excluding malignancy. Fine-needle aspiration biopsy yields an acellular specimen, and open biopsy is often required. Anecdotal reports suggest that steroids may be of value, but there are no controlled trials.[87] Debulking surgery may be necessary to release the trachea or oesophagus, but the obli-

REFERENCES

82. Volpe R. The Thyroid. Harpers & Row, Hagerstown, 1978: 986–994
83. Dussault JH, Rousseau F. Endocrinol Metab Clin North Am 1987; 16: 417–429
84. Amino N, Mori H et al. N Engl J Med 1982; 306: 849–852
85. Thomas CG, Rotledge RG. Am Surg 1981; 193: 769–776
86. Holm LE, Blomgrem H, Lowhagen T. N Engl J Med 1985; 312: 601–604
87. Vaidya B, Harris PE et al. Postgrad Med J 1997; 73: 817–819

teration of normal tissue planes renders the dissection difficult and hazardous.

THYROIDECTOMY

Thyroid function tests should document that the patient is euthyroid. Indirect laryngoscopy is undertaken to document the preoperative vocal cord function in patients with voice change or previous thyroid change. An anaesthetic opinion should be sought regarding fitness for general anaesthesia, and particularly to anticipate difficulty of intubation. Where the patient is really unsuitable for general anaesthesia, regional anaesthesia is sometimes feasible.[88] The patient should be asked for consent after explicit discussion of the risks of permanent injury to the recurrent laryngeal nerve and parathyroid glands, and the possibility of lifelong thyroxine therapy. For benign disease, the rate of permanent nerve injury should be no greater than 1–2%.

A standard symmetrical skin-crease collar incision is undertaken about one fingerbreadth superior to the suprasternal notch. For small goitres the midline raphe of the straps is incised, whereas division of the straps muscles in the presence of a large goitre improves access without functional loss.[89] The sternothyroid and sternothyroid muscles are separated from the thyroid capsule and reflected laterally.

Prior to any resection, a careful search is made for the parathyroids, and the full course of the recurrent laryngeal nerve in the neck is identified.

RESECTION

After identification of the key structures, the resection can begin with the dissection, ligation and division of the superior thyroid vessels, avoiding injury to the external branch of the superior laryngeal nerve. The nerve is small and flattened, and usually passes just medial to the superior thyroid artery lying on the inferior pharyngeal constrictor. However, in 20% it may be intimately involved with the superior thyroid artery, sometimes winding around it.[90] Mobilization of the superior pole facilitates the dissection of the recurrent laryngeal nerve. The surgeon who is not constantly anxious about the possibility of damaging the recurrent laryngeal nerve should not be performing thyroid surgery. The nerve should be routinely exposed throughout its journey in the neck up to the point it enters the larynx under the ligament of Berry. During its exposure the individual branches of the inferior thyroid artery are dissected and divided using a variety of ligatures, clips or the harmonic scalpel. Care must be taken not to exert undue traction on the thyroid gland as the nerve may be injured at the point it enters the larynx. The inferior thyroid veins are divided and the thyroid gland sharply dissected off the trachea. Attention is then directed to resecting the pyramidal lobe. Failure to do this can result in an unsightly midline swelling in the postoperative period.

Rarely (less than 1%), the right laryngeal nerve is non-recurrent, arising directly from the cervical vagus to run transversely, reaching the thyroid at any point from the superior to the inferior pole.[91] It is most at risk when it is adherent to the inferior thyroid artery, and may thus be included in a ligature passed around that artery. Its occurrence is thought to be due to failure of the fourth arch vessel to develop.

The extent of thyroid resection is dictated by the pathology and the individual surgeon's practice. A total thyroid lobectomy is the minimal operation for lesions where malignancy is suspected. There is no place for 'shelling out' a lesion, aside from the occasions when a patient has a solitary nodule in the isthmus, when an isthmusectomy is permissible. When a subtotal resection is performed (e.g. Graves' disease) a remnant between 5 and 10 mg should be left behind.

At the conclusion of the operation, the patient is tilted head down, and the anaesthetist performs a Valsalva manoeuvre on the patient in an attempt to identify any venous haemorrhage. It is prudent to place a vacuum drain in the wound, although it has been claimed that this is not necessary.[92] Thyroidectomy wound closure produces an excellent cosmetic result regardless of the method chosen. Local infiltration of the wound with local anaesthetic is helpful, but care must be taken that the anaesthetic does not track down to the recurrent laryngeal nerve to produce temporary vocal cord paralysis. Immediate postoperative assessment of vocal cord movement by the anaesthetist using the laryngoscope is unreliable and unnecessary.

POSTOPERATIVE CARE

The serum calcium should be measured on the first postoperative day for patients undergoing a bilateral dissection. Most patients are fit for discharge 48 h after surgery.

COMPLICATIONS OF THYROIDECTOMY

Haemorrhage

If haemorrhage occurs it does so within a few hours of operation, and may quickly give rise to asphyxia. The danger is normally not directly from the haematoma itself, but the secondary laryngeal oedema that can occur even in the presence of quite small amounts of blood in the neck. The condition is recognized by deterioration in the patient's condition, and by a crowing respiration not dissimilar to that of recurrent laryngeal paralysis. When haemorrhage or marked laryngeal oedema occurs, the patient should be promptly reintubated and the neck wound reopened. It is unusual to find a specific bleeding point and not all the haematoma can be evacuated, because it tends to suffuse all the layers of the neck. After re-exploration the wound should be resutured with generous drainage; prophylactic antibiotics should be given.

Wound complications

Sepsis

Sepsis is uncommon in thyroid surgery, and prophylactic antibiotics are not normally indicated. When sepsis does develop, it may be in the form of cellulitis or an infected haematoma. Both may present within days of surgery and discharge through the wound.

Oedema of the wound

Oedema of the wound flaps is common, and may persist for weeks after operation, particularly in the upper flap.

REFERENCES

88. Saxe AW, Brown E, Hamburger SW. Surgery 1988; 103: 415–420
89. Jaffe V, Young AE. Ann R Coll Surg Engl 1993; 75: 118
90. Moosman DA, De Weese MS. Surg Gynecol Obstet 1968; 122: 1011–1016
91. Stewart GR, Mountain JG, Colcock BP. Br J Surg 1972; 59: 379–381
92. Kristoffersson A, Sandzen B, Jarhult J. Br J Surg 1986; 73: 121–122

Hypertrophic scarring

Although most thyroidectomy wounds will heal with almost invisible scars, some will become hypertrophic, especially in their centre. Local steroid application will sometimes be of benefit. In known keloid formers, an approach to the thyroid through bilateral submammary excisions has been proposed.[93]

Respiratory obstruction

Respiratory obstruction[94] after thyroidectomy may be due to oedema of the laryngeal mucosa, clot formation deep to the strap muscles, bilateral recurrent laryngeal nerve paralysis, mediastinal emphysema with extrapleural pneumothorax, or collapse of a trachea the cartilage of which has been made soft by long-standing compression by a goitre. This last factor is known as tracheomalacia; it is very rare.

Whenever there is progressing airways obstruction after thyroidectomy, as evidenced by stridor, prompt reintubation is indicated. Unless a definite cause of the obstruction is known, subsequent extubation should be in the presence of an ear, nose and throat specialist equipped to assess the airway endoscopically.

Nerve damage

The recurrent and superior laryngeal nerves are at risk, and in extensive thyroid surgery the vagus and the sympathetic trunks are also at risk. Close attention must be paid to the patient in the immediate postoperative period, and any doubts about the adequacy of the airway reported immediately to the anaesthetist and surgeon.

Recurrent laryngeal nerve damage may be unilateral or bilateral, partial or complete. With partial paralysis the cord lies in the midline, whereas the cord lies in the cadaveric position with complete laryngeal paralysis. The consequences of nerve injury range from hoarseness of the voice with mild dyspnoea to severe dyspnoea and stridor. Resuture of the nerves is not generally beneficial either immediately or later,[95] although there have been claims that accurate resuture will improve phonation.[96] If recurrent laryngeal nerve palsy is suspected at any time, an ear, nose and throat surgeon should document it using fibre-optic laryngoscopy. Most cases will recover spontaneously and reoperation is not indicated.

The external motor branch of the superior laryngeal nerve supplies the cricothyroid muscle. Its internal branch transmits supraglottic sensory information. Nerve damage causes a variable huskiness and weakness of the voice, and a decrease in volume, range and pitch that may be of crucial importance to public speakers and to singers. Damage can also lead to a permanent postdeglutition cough with occasional choking.

Hypocalcaemia

Calcium levels may fall after thyroidectomy for two reasons: metabolic and anatomical.

Metabolic

Mild hypocalcaemia is occasionally observed even in unilateral thyroidectomy, but the fall is rarely to below 2.0 mmol/L and almost never symptomatic. The cause is not understood, but the release of calcitonin during manipulation, the reversal of thyrotoxic osteodystrophy, and a reduction of renal tubular reabsorption of calcium without a change in parathormone or calcitonin levels have been proposed.[97,98]

Anatomical

Hypoparathyroidism and hypocalcaemia result from bruising or removal of parathyroid tissue. Careful identification and preservation of the parathyroids during thyroidectomy remain the most appropriate prophylaxis. When recognized during thyroidectomy, inadvertently excised parathyroid glands should be diced and autotransplanted into pockets in the sternomastoid muscle, where they may revascularize and function.

Mildly symptomatic hypocalcaemia need not normally be treated if the calcium is over 2.0 mmol/L. If it fails to resolve, or if the calcium continues to fall, treatment with oral calcium supplements or 10% calcium gluconate given slowly via a central vein may be necessary. If hypocalcaemia persists, treatment with synthetic vitamin D and oral calcium will be necessary. A return of parathyroid function may take 3–6 months.

Pneumothorax

Pneumothorax is uncommon, except during extraction of retrosternal goitres.

Air embolism

Air embolism is also rare, but may be produced if a large vein in the neck is opened when the patient is in the head-up position.

Thyroid crisis

This rare complication only occurs when the thyrotoxic patient is operated on without adequate preliminary preparation. It occurs soon after operation, and takes the form of fulminating thyrotoxicosis with hyperpyrexia, arrhythmias and cardiac failure. It is treated by large doses of carbimazole (60–120 mg) or propylthiouracil (600–1200 mg) followed by Lugol's iodine. The cardiac effects are blocked with propranolol; digoxin may also be necessary. Dexamethasone reduces the conversion of thyroxine to bi-iodothyronine peripherally, and hyperpyrexia is treated by largactil and cooling. Extreme cases may require plasmapheresis or even exchange transfusion.

Recurrent hyperthyroidism

Recurrent hyperthyroidism may occur after thyroidectomy for thyrotoxicosis and is discussed in the *Thyrotoxicosis* sections of this chapter (p. 397).

Hypothyroidism

All patients treated by total thyroidectomy will develop hypothyroidism, but only a small percentage of those treated by bilateral subtotal thyroidectomy will develop thyroid insufficiency unless the underlying disease is thyrotoxicosis, in which case the incidence is much higher and is discussed in the *Thyrotoxicosis* sections. Because a small number of those undergoing lobectomy as treatment for a nodule may fail to remain euthyroid after operation, all lobectomy patients should have their thyrotropin measured at follow-up.

REFERENCES

93. Aghaji MAC. Br J Surg 1988; 75: 1034
94. Wade JSH. Ann R Coll Surg Engl 1980; 62: 15–24
95. Gordon JH, McCabe BF. Laryngoscope 1968; 78: 236–239
96. Ezaki H, Ushio H et al. World J Surg 1982; 6: 342–346
97. Percival RC, Hargreaves AW, Karis JA. Acta Endocrinol (Copenh) 1985; 220–226
98. Michie W, Duncan T et al. Lancet 1976; i: 508–514

The parathyroid glands

18

Paul R. Maddox, Radu Mihai

INTRODUCTION

It was only just over 100 years ago that Sandstrom first described the appearance of the human parathyroid glands.[1] The first operation for hyperparathyroidism was carried out by Mandl in 1926,[2] but the physiology of the parathyroids was not fully understood until the 1940s. The cloning of the calcium receptor in 1993 boosted the interest in basic laboratory research about parathyroid function. In recent years, the advent of accurate imaging techniques has allowed the development of new surgical techniques, such as minimally invasive neck surgery, for patients with hyperparathyroidism.

EMBRYOLOGY AND CLINICAL ANATOMY

The parathyroid glands form during the fifth week of embryological development from the endoderm of the dorsal wings of pharyngeal pouches III and IV, with the probable involvement of placodal ectoderm. This ectodermal component allows an appreciation of how the parathyroid glands can be accommodated within the amine precursor uptake and decarboxylation system. Pouch III (ventral wing) gives origin to the thymus, the relative caudal descent of which also involves the parathyroid III, so that parathyroid III comes to lie below parathyroid IV (Fig. 18.1).

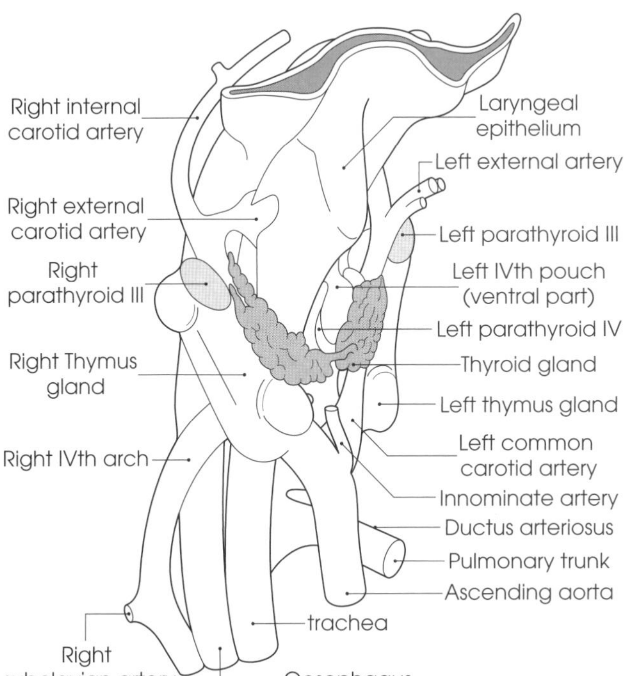

Figure 18.1 The pharyngeal and laryngeal regions and associated pharyngeal derivatives of a human embryo of around 16.8 mm.

During separation of the parathyroid 'buds' from the endoderm microscopic fragmentation is observed, and the development of such fragments might account for accessory parathyroid glands within the thymus.

In a consecutive series of 428 necropsies, Gilmour was the first to report the variability of gland number: four glands were present in 87%, while 0.2% had only two glands, 6.1% had only three glands, 6% had five glands, and 0.5% had six glands.[3] He acknowledged that all glands might not have been found. A more recent autopsy study suggested that a fourth gland was absent in only 3% of patients, and supernumerary glands were found in 13%, most often in the thymus.[4] Symmetry can be expected in 80% of patients. These figures should be borne in mind as the surgeon struggles to find four glands during bilateral neck exploration. The presence of detectable plasma levels of parathyroid hormone (PTH) after total parathyroidectomy in patients with renal failure[5] also suggests that additional or ectopic parathyroid tissue might exist more frequently than previously believed.

The commonest positions are for the superior gland to be found just above the intersection of the recurrent laryngeal nerve and the inferior thyroid artery, and for the inferior gland to be sited caudally at the lower pole of the thyroid, in the thymus or the thyrothymic ligament. The 'lower' glands sometimes appear higher in the neck because of failure of descent during development. The relative frequency with which the glands are found in different sites is illustrated in Fig. 18.2. Most 'failed' cervical explorations by experienced endocrine surgeons will eventually prove to have mediastinal adenomas.

PRIMARY HYPERPARATHYROIDISM

Primary hyperparathyroidism is the spontaneous occurrence of excess production of PTH, causing hypercalcaemia. In most patients the cause is a single parathyroid adenoma, but up to 15% of patients have multiple gland hyperplasia; carcinoma of the parathyroid is very rare (1%). A very small number of patients will have two parathyroid adenomata.

REFERENCES

1. Sandstrom I. Upsala Lakarforenings Forth 1880; 15: 441
2. Mandl F. Arch Klin Chir 1926; 143: 245
3. Gilmour JR. J Pathol Bacteriol 1938; 46: 133
4. Akerström G, Malmaeus J, Bergstrom R. Surgery 1984; 95: 14

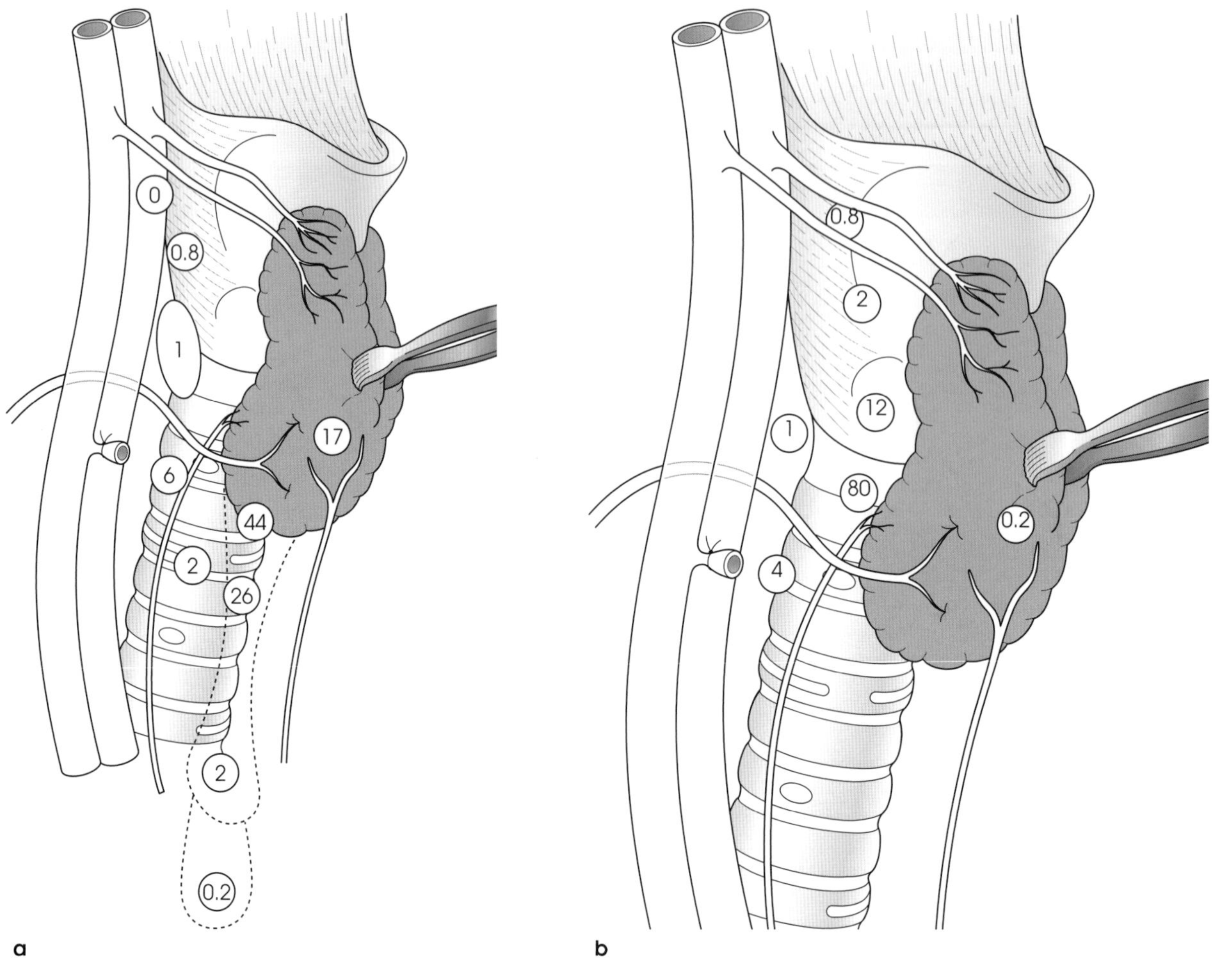

Figure 18.2 The relative frequency of location of (**a**) the lower parathyroid glands and (**b**) the upper parathyroid glands. (After Akerström et al Surgery. 1984; 95: 14–21, with permission.[4])

BASIC SCIENCE SUMMARY

CALCIUM

Calcium is a critically important cation for cell membrane stability, nerve conduction, muscle contraction, enzyme and hormone activation, blood coagulation, and bone mineral deposition. All but 1% is found within the skeleton, and plasma concentrations remain remarkably constant. Some 40% of circulating calcium is bound to proteins (80–90% to albumin and 10–15% to globulins), 10% is complexed (e.g. to phosphate, lactate, and bicarbonate), and 50% is ionized.

Calcium is the main modulator of parathyroid secretion. Hypercalcaemia inhibits PTH secretion and hypocalcaemia stimulates PTH secretion.

CALCIUM-SENSING RECEPTOR

The calcium-sensing receptor (CaR) is expressed on the plasma membrane of parathyroid cells,[6] and enables them to detect and respond to minute changes in extracellular calcium levels. Inactivating mutations of the CaR cause autosomal dominant hypercalcaemic disorders: familial hypocalciuric hypercalcaemia and neonatal severe hyperparathyroidism. No such mutations have been identified in parathyroid adenomas,[7] but CaR expression appears to be substantially reduced in parathyroid adenomas,[8] explaining the impaired control of PTH secretion by extracellular calcium. In addition to the CaR, a member of the low-density lipoprotein receptor superfamily was reported to be another putative calcium sensor protein on parathyroid cells[9] with reduced expression in primary hyperparathyroidism.[10]

PHOSPHATE

Phosphate is contained mainly within the skeleton (85%) and within intracellular pools. Fifteen per cent of serum phosphate is bound to proteins, and the rest is ionized or complexed with cations. It is predominantly excreted by the kidneys and variations in plasma concentrations directly affect the concentration of serum calcium. Increased plasma levels of phosphates have a direct stimulatory effect on parathyroid glands and represent a pathogenic mechanism of secondary hyperparathyroidism in patients with renal failure.

REFERENCES

5. Nicholson ML, Feehally J. Brit J Surg 1995; 82: 1427
6. Brown EM, Gamba G et al. Nature 1993; 366: 575
7. Hosokawa Y, Pollak MR et al. J Clin Endocrinol Metab 1995; 80: 3107
8. Kifor O, Moore FD et al. J Clin Endocrinol Metab 1996; 81: 1598
9. Saito A, Pietromonaco S et al. Proc Natl Acad Sci USA 1994; 91: 9725
10. Juhlin C, Klareskog L et al. Endocrinology 1988; 122: 2999

PARATHYROID HORMONE

An 84-amino acid peptide, PTH has a short half-life (minutes) in the circulation before it is broken down into an amino-terminal fragment (amino acids 1–34) and a carboxy-terminal fragment. Only the 1–34 fragment retains biological activity. A raised or detectable (i.e. inappropriately inhibited) PTH level in the face of hypercalcaemia is usually diagnostic of hyperparathyroidism. Modern assays measure the intact hormone by radioimmunoassays or by chemiluminescent immunoassay.[11]

Receptors for PTH are widely distributed in cells other than the traditional renal and bone target cells; other cells include fibroblasts, chondrocytes, vascular smooth muscle cells, fat cells, and placental trophoblasts. Interaction of PTH with specific receptors on the proximal and distal renal tubular cells leads to increased excretion of phosphate, sodium, potassium and bicarbonate, and a decreased excretion of magnesium and hydrogen ions. Although the physiological effect of PTH is to reduce renal excretion of calcium, in primary hyperparathyroidism this effect is overwhelmed and hypercalcaemia-induced hypercalciuria occurs. The intracellular signalling for these effects relies on intracellular cyclic AMP, the increased urinary secretion of which is a biochemical marker of primary hyperparathyroidism.

Osteoclast-mediated bone reabsorption is stimulated by PTH, resulting in increased alkaline phosphatase activity and increased urinary excretion of hydroxyproline from increased breakdown of bone matrix.

Several of these PTH-induced effects may be used to refine the diagnosis of hyperparathyroidism:

- hypophosphataemia;
- hyperchloraemia;
- increased chloride:phosphate ratio;
- hypercalciuria;
- increased serum alkaline phosphatase;
- increased urinary excretion of cyclic AMP; and
- increased urinary excretion of hydroxyproline.

VITAMIN D

Vitamin D is represented by two sterols, ergosterol in plants and dihydrocholesterol in the skin, which are converted on exposure to ultraviolet light to vitamin D_2 and D_3, respectively. These forms are absorbed from the small intestine. Vitamin D_3 becomes protein-bound and is 25-hydroxylated in the liver before a second hydroxylation occurs in the kidney (under PTH stimulatory control) to produce 1,25-dihydroxycholecalciferol, a very potent form of vitamin D.

Active vitamin D_3 is an important regulator of parathyroid cell growth and inhibits *PTH* gene transcription. It is assumed that impaired effects of vitamin D_3 may contribute to the enhanced secretion and proliferation seen in primary hyperparathyroidism.

CLINICAL FEATURES

SYMPTOMATIC HYPERPARATHYROIDISM

It is not understood why the similar levels of biochemical abnormality can be associated with renal disease, bone disease, or a combination of the two. Relatively mild elevations in serum calcium can produce severe systemic effects in some patients and no symptoms in others.

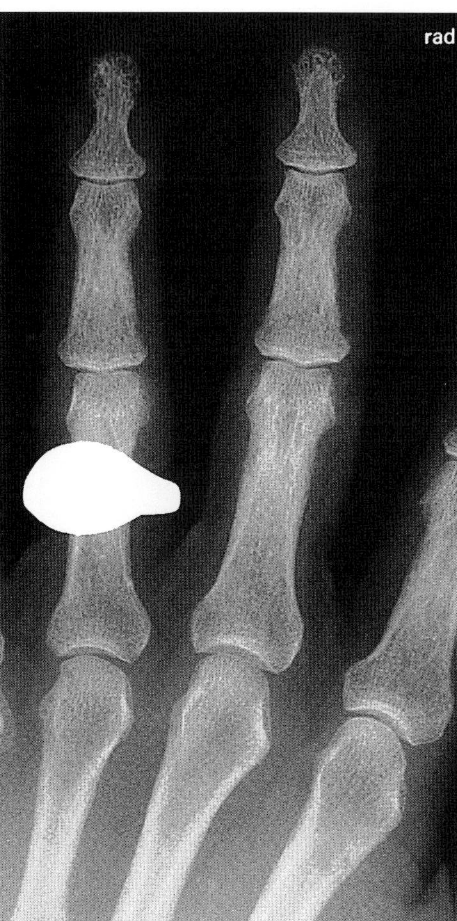

Figure 18.3 Magnified view of the middle and ring fingers of a young man with hyperparathyroidism, showing erosion of the terminal tufts of the distal phalanx and subperiosteal erosion, especially on the radial side (rad) of the proximal phalanges.

Bone disease

Bone disease in its florid form is called *osteitis fibrosa cystica* and is now rarely seen. The earliest changes are seen on X-rays of the hands, where subperiosteal erosions can be detected in the phalanges (especially the radial aspect of the middle phalanges) and terminal tufts (Fig. 18.3). The skull demonstrates a mottled appearance with lucent cystic areas ('pepper pot skull' in its most florid form; Fig. 18.4), and any bone may demonstrate cystic lesions due to osteoclastomas or 'brown' tumours. These lesions produce skeletal pain and may lead to pathological fractures. Subtle bone changes are rarely detected on skeletal surveys, and there is little justification for a skeletal survey to aid diagnosis of hyperparathyroidism unless there are specific symptoms.

Dual-energy X-ray absoptiometry (DEXA) scanning is now widely used to evaluate bone mass. There are region-specific differences in bone mass, with low values in areas with cortical bone (e.g. radius) and normal or high values in vertebrae and iliac crest (trabecular bone). In many patients there is an initial rapid loss in bone mass, followed by a period of stable disease with little progression at the time of diagnosis of primary hyperparathyroidism. Parathyroidectomy induces an increase in bone density of up to 20%, and the increased risk for fractures returns to normal after 1 year.

REFERENCES

11. Farndon JR, Geraghty JM et al. World J Surg 1987; 11: 252

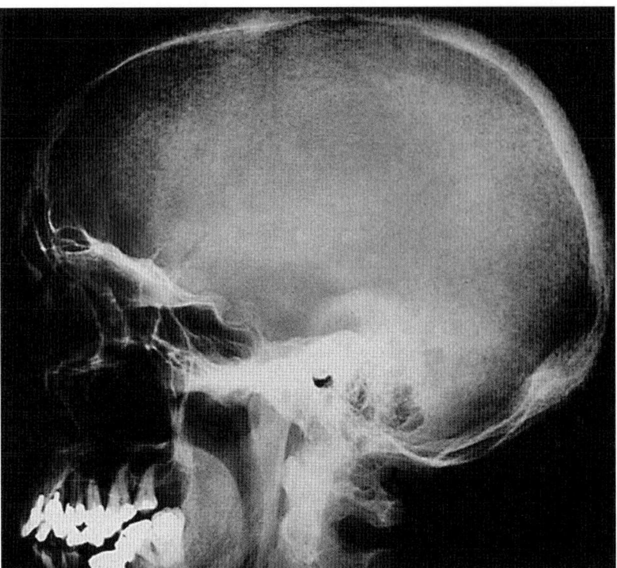

Figure 18.4 Skull X-ray of the patient shown in Fig. 18.3, demonstrating a classical 'pepper pot' skull.

Renal disease

Renal disease usually presents as a result of stone production or nephrocalcinosis, with the patient complaining of polyuria, polydypsia, ureteric colic, renal pain, haematuria, and symptoms of renal tract infections. The degree of hypercalcaemia is often not severe. A beneficial surgical outcome is more difficult to achieve in this setting, and some postulate that this early presentation with a mild biochemical abnormality and hyperplastic glands might be the precursor of more severe adenomatous disease.[12]

Hypertension

Hypertension is present in many patients with primary hyperparathyroidism. A parathyroid hypertensive factor has been purified from plasma of spontaneously hypertensive rats. Its levels in patients with primary hyperparathyroidism have been found to correlate with hypertension, and also to fall after parathyroidectomy in parallel with normalization of blood pressure.

Left ventricular hypertrophy has a high prevalence in patients with primary hyperparathyroidism, and responds within 6 months after parathyroidectomy.[13] In many patients, however, concretion of hypercalcaemia has little or no effect on coexisting hypertension.

Gastrointestinal symptoms

Gastrointestinal symptoms may be related to peptic ulcer disease, constipation, pancreatitis or gallstones, all of which may be linked to hyperparathyroidism. However, these are all common conditions, and in most patients the association may be by pure chance. Nevertheless, in some situations the link is quite definite; for example, peptic ulcer due to hypergastrinaemia from a gastrinoma associated with parathyroid hyperplasia or adenomas as part of the multiple endocrine neoplasia type I syndrome.

Psychiatric and neuromuscular symptoms

Vague psychiatric and neuromuscular symptoms are recognized in 30% of patients diagnosed with hyperparathyroidism. These symptoms can be reversed after parathyroidectomy, but their severity is not related to the degree of hypercalcaemia.

Increased risk of premature death

A population-based cohort study with 14 years' follow-up has demonstrated that, among persons aged 70 years or less at the time of detection of the hypercalcaemia, survival was lower in the hypercalcaemic group than in a normocalcaemic age- and sex-matched control group.[14] A further study revealed an increased risk of premature death even after treatment for hyperparathyroidism, but with better survival for patients who underwent parathyroidectomy at an early stage of disease.[15] The additional mortality was mainly due to cardiovascular disease.

'ASYMPTOMATIC' HYPERPARATHYROIDISM

The advent of multichannel biochemical analysers has led to identification of an increasing number of patients with hypercalcaemia who have minimal or no symptoms. The definition of 'asymptomatic' can be very difficult: what might be attributable to old age in an 80-year-old would be unacceptable to most 40-year-olds. Symptoms can develop so insidiously over months or years that they are often ascribed to ageing. It is often only after restoration of biochemical normality that the true cause of the symptoms is appreciated.

The changing presentation of primary hyperparathyroidism is exemplified by three different studies. Haff and his colleagues in 1970 reported an incidence of hyperparathyroidism of one in 2000 of the population.[16] More recently, in a hospital population the incidence was found to be as high as one in 680. In the UK, hyperparathyroidism presents in about one in 4000, the majority of these patients being 'asymptomatic'.[17]

NORMOCALCAEMIC HYPERPARATHYROIDISM

Normocalcaemic hyperparathyroidism is defined as normal total serum calcium in the presence of symptoms or complications attributable to primary hyperparathyroidism. Factors known to decrease calcium levels (such as decreased serum albumin, vitamin D deficiency, severe pancreatitis, increased phosphate intake, and hypomagnesaemia) should be eliminated during the diagnostic work-up.

Most such patients present with a renal calculus, and most have hypercalciuria.[18] Cases present a diagnostic challenge to differentiate from idiopathic hypercalciuria (assumed to be due to increased intestinal absorption or renal calcium leak). A failure to distinguish these two possibilities may lead to inappropriate neck exploration in patients with idiopathic hypercalciuria, or to an overlooked diagnosis in those with primary hyperparathyroidism. A diagnosis is supported by a trial of thiazide diuretics, which induces overt hypercalcaemia in patients with primary hyperparathyroidism.

REFERENCES

12. Akerstrom G, Bergstrom R et al. World J Surg 1986; 10: 696
13. Piovesan A, Molineri N, Casasso F et al. Clin Endocrinol (Oxf) 1999; 50: 321–328
14. Palmer M, Adami HO, Bergstrom R et al. Lancet 1987; 1: 59–62
15. Hedback G, Oden A, Tissel LA. Surgery 1995; 117: 134–139
16. Haff RC, Black WC, Ballinger WF. Ann Surg 1970; 171: 85
17. Mundy GR, Cove DH et al. Lancet 1980; i: 1317
18. Monchik JM. Surgery 1995; 118: 17–23

HYPERCALCAEMIC CRISIS

Hypercalcaemia may present as a metabolic emergency, and in this context the severity of clinical manifestations often correlates with the degree of hypercalcaemia. Neuromuscular, renal and gastrointestinal manifestations are influenced by the speed of onset of hypercalcaemia and by intercurrent medical conditions.

Marked dehydration due to anorexia, nausea or vomiting leads to more severe hypercalcaemia. Weakness and lethargy lead to immobilization, which accentuates bone resorption. Confusion, significant cognitive impairment and even coma are possible. If untreated, the condition will proceed to oliguric renal failure, cardiac arrhythmia and death.

Hypercalcaemia associated with malignancy is the most common cause of severe hypercalcaemia.

Acute primary hyperparathyroidism is more frequent in patients with long-standing hypercalcaemia, radiographic evidence of bone disease, and a history of nephrolithiasis.

Sarcoidosis, milk-alkali syndrome, and adrenal insufficiency are very rare causes of hypercalcaemic crisis.

FAMILIAL HYPERPARATHYROIDISM

Multiple endocrine neoplasia

An association of parathyroid hyperplasia with pancreatic islet cell and pituitary tumours occurs in multiple endocrine neoplasia type I. In such patients, adrenocortical, thyroid and carcinoid tumours may also be associated. Ninety per cent of patients with multiple endocrine neoplasia type I syndrome have parathyroid hyperplasia with less pronounced hypercalcaemia, but present at an earlier age than the non-familial or sporadic variant.

The association of medullary thyroid carcinoma, phaeochromocytoma and hyperparathyroidism constitutes the multiple endocrine neoplasia type II syndrome. Some 20–60% of patients with this syndrome have parathyroid hyperplasia, but the parathyroid disease is usually mild and insignificant compared with the effects produced by the other tumours. There is no value in screening for these familial syndromes by measurement of other hormonal products in a population of patients undergoing surgery for apparently 'uncomplicated' primary hyperparathyroidism, unless there is a positive family history or suggestive symptoms.[11]

Familial isolated hyperparathyroidism

Familial isolated hyperparathyroidism is a rare syndrome inherited as an autosomal dominant disorder. This syndrome has an increased risk of malignant parathyroid transformation,[19] and may be associated with jaw tumours.

DIAGNOSIS

Simple investigations can suggest the diagnosis—the ionized calcium, serum phosphate and serum chloride (as the chloride:phosphate ratio)—but PTH measurement is crucial to clinch the diagnosis.

The daily excretion of calcium in the urine is a valuable assessment. Excess urinary calcium can support the diagnosis of primary hyperparathyroidism but, more importantly, loss of less than 2 mmol of calcium per day must alert the clinician to the diagnosis of familial hypercalcaemic hypocalciuria. This autosomal dominant condition may mimic primary hyperparathyroidism very closely, with normal PTH levels that are judged to be inappropriate in the face of hypercalcaemia. A repeat urinary calcium determination, enquiry into family history, and measurement of the serum calcium in first-degree siblings (because it is inherited as an autosomal dominant disease) will confirm the correct diagnosis and save the patient an unnecessary neck exploration.

DIFFERENTIAL DIAGNOSIS OF HYPERCALCAEMIA

More than 80% of patients with persistent hypercalcaemia will have either primary hyperparathyroidism or malignancy and, in general, the history and physical examination can often provide pointers to the correct diagnosis without recourse to complex or expensive investigations.

Causes of hypercalcaemia can be divided into two groups:

- *PTH-mediated*: primary hyperparathyroidism, tertiary hyperparathyroidism, familial hypocalciuric hypercalcaemia; treatment with thiazide diuretics and lithium.
- *Non-PTH-mediated*: malignancy (multiple myeloma; skeletal metastasis from breast, prostate, renal and thyroid cancer), Paget's disease, thyrotoxicosis, granulomatosis (sarcoidosis), excess intake of vitamin D and/or calcium, and adrenocortical insufficiency.

The inter-relationships between malignancy and hyperparathyroidism are complex. Most tumours associated with hypercalcaemia produce PTH-related peptide. Although their coding genes and chemical structure differ, PTH and PTH-related peptide act on the same receptor.[20] Furthermore, primary hyperparathyroidism and breast cancer, for example, occur so frequently in the population that the two diseases can often be present in the same patient. Those with hyperparathyroidism have earlier-stage breast disease, whereas in 97% of those with hypercalcaemia of malignancy there is advanced disease.

DIAGNOSTIC PROCEDURES

LOCALIZATION TECHNIQUES

Most surgeons agree that localization procedures are not justified before bilateral neck exploration for primary hyperparathyroidism. In the past several years, the growing interest in minimally invasive parathyroid surgery has relied on the development of modern localization techniques that allow exploration of only one side of the neck.

Scintigraphy using technetium-99m sestamibi has become the initial investigation of choice.[21] This completely replaced the previous scans using thallium–technetium or thallium–iodine isotopes (Fig. 18.5). Sestamibi accumulates in the mitochondria of parathyroid cells in a manner similar to that described for thallium, but its emission spectrum enhances the sensitivity for both smaller and deeper lesions. In addition, sestamibi permits single-photon emission computerized tomography (SPECT) imaging, with a three-dimensional data display and markedly

REFERENCES

19. Wassif WS, Moniz CF, Friedman E et al. J Clin Endocrinol Metab 1993; 77: 1485–1489
20. Brown EM, Segre GV, Goldring SR. Baillières Clin Endocrinol Metab 1996; 123–161
21. Mitchell BK, Kinder BK et al. J Clin Endocrinol Metab 1995; 80: 7

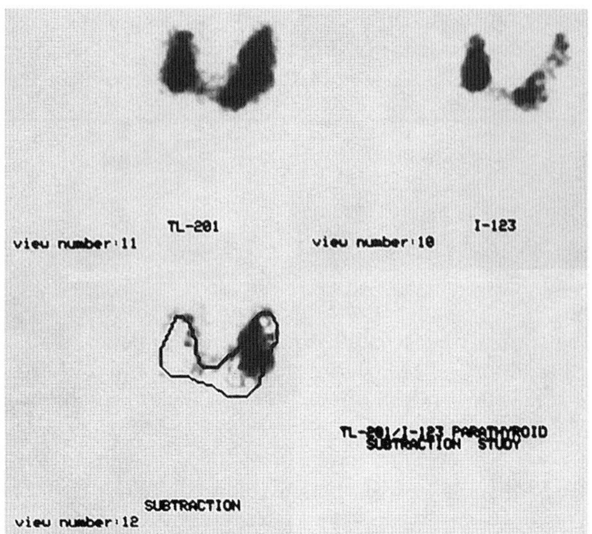

Figure 18.5 A thallium–iodine subtraction scan. Top left, thallium image; top right, iodine image. There is a suggestion of a filling defect consistent with poor uptake in a parathyroid nodule compressing the left lobe of the thyroid. Subtraction of the images (bottom left) reveals excess thallium uptake confined solely within a large parathyroid adenoma behind the left thyroid lobe.

improved spatial resolution. A combination of sestamibi scanning with ultrasound is the preferred approach in most centres performing 'focused' explorations, because it offers 96% sensitivity for the localization of abnormal parathyroid glands.[22] It may also be useful for identifying ectopic parathyroid adenomas (Fig. 18.6).

Ultrasonography alone has an accuracy of 76%, a sensitivity of 82%, and a positive predictive value of 81%.

Computerized tomography provides acceptable results (accuracy 76%, sensitivity 57%, and positive predictive value 80%), but is less accurate than MRI. Both techniques can be considered following failed initial neck exploration as a method to identify ectopic glands. They are not indicated before the first neck exploration.

A preoperative infusion of methylene blue stains adenomas and hyperplastic glands a deep blue colour at surgery. Although perhaps unnecessary for the straightforward case, this is a valuable asset for a difficult cervical exploration. The timing of the infusion is crucial to its success, and hypersensitivity to the dye is occasionally encountered.

Ultrasound-guided fine-needle aspiration biopsy for cytology can be used for assessment of suspected lesion by measuring PTH concentration in the needle aspirate, but this approach has very limited application.

In earlier years, arteriography and selective venous catheterization with sampling for PTH assay (Fig. 18.7) were localization procedures that gave reasonable results, but are rather obsolete in modern practice except in the context of reoperation for persistent or recurrent hyperparathyroidism.

QUICK PTH ASSAY

Rapid immunoradiometric and immunochemiluminometric assays have been developed that can provide results for intact PTH concentrations within 10–20 min. This technique can be used intraoperatively to confirm removal of all overactive parathyroid tissue. Because the half-life of circulating intact PTH is 3–4 min, a decline by 50% or more at 5–10 minutes after excision of an enlarged gland provides evidence of a complete procedure (Fig. 18.8).[24]

This technique is reserved for patients treated by focused neck exploration based on localization scans. There are acknowledged pitfalls with the interpretation of this test, such as uncertainty whether the basal level should be considered as that before the operation or the level just before excising the parathyroid adenoma (because surgical manipulation of the neck can potentially induce a rise in PTH level). A 10% failure rate for this test has been quoted.

A similar method has been proposed for lateralization of parathyroid adenomas by PTH estimation in left versus right internal jugular veins at the beginning of surgery.[25]

PATHOLOGY

ADENOMA

Chief cells, oxyphil cells and water-clear cells are present in differing proportions in parathyroid adenomas. An acinar pattern can be observed in some tumours. The presence of a rim of compressed normal tissue supports the diagnosis of an adenoma. Their weight ranges from 70 mg to 20 g.

DOUBLE ADENOMAS

Double adenomas are considered a distinct entity. Patients with persistent or recurrent primary hyperparathyroidism caused by missed or unrecognized double adenomas are older, nephrolithiasis is less common, while muscle weakness, neuropsychiatric disorders, constipation, and weight loss are more severe than in patients with persistent or recurrent primary hyperparathyroidism caused by hyperplasia.[26]

HYPERPLASIA

The aetiology of primary parathyroid hyperplasia is not understood. It can occur alone or in association with certain familial endocrinopathies as part of multiple endocrine neoplasia syndromes. Intraoperative assessment is not always easy, even with the help of frozen sections and a skilled pathologist, because the hyperplastic glands may be of different sizes and only one may appear enlarged, mimicking an adenoma.

CARCINOMA

Carcinomas of the parathyroids occur in less than 1% of cases.

ECTOPIC PARATHYROID HORMONE SECRETION

Ectopic PTH secretion is extremely rare, quoted only as case reports of small cell lung cancer and ovarian carcinoma, where DNA rearrangement and amplification in the regulatory region of one *PTH* gene allele have been demonstrated.

REFERENCES

22. Arici C, Cheah K, Ituarte PHD et al. Surgery 2001; 129: 720–729
23. Tibblin SA, Bergenfeltz AOJ. In: Clark OH, Duh QY (eds). Textbook of Endocrine Surgery. WB Saunders, Philadelphia, 1997: 367
24. Irvin GL, Dembrow VD, Prudohomme DL. Am J Surg 1991; 162: 299–302
25. Taylor J, Fraser W, Banaszkiewicz P et al. Br J Surg 1995; 82: 1428–1429
26. Tezelman S, Shen W et al. Surgery 1995; 118: 1115

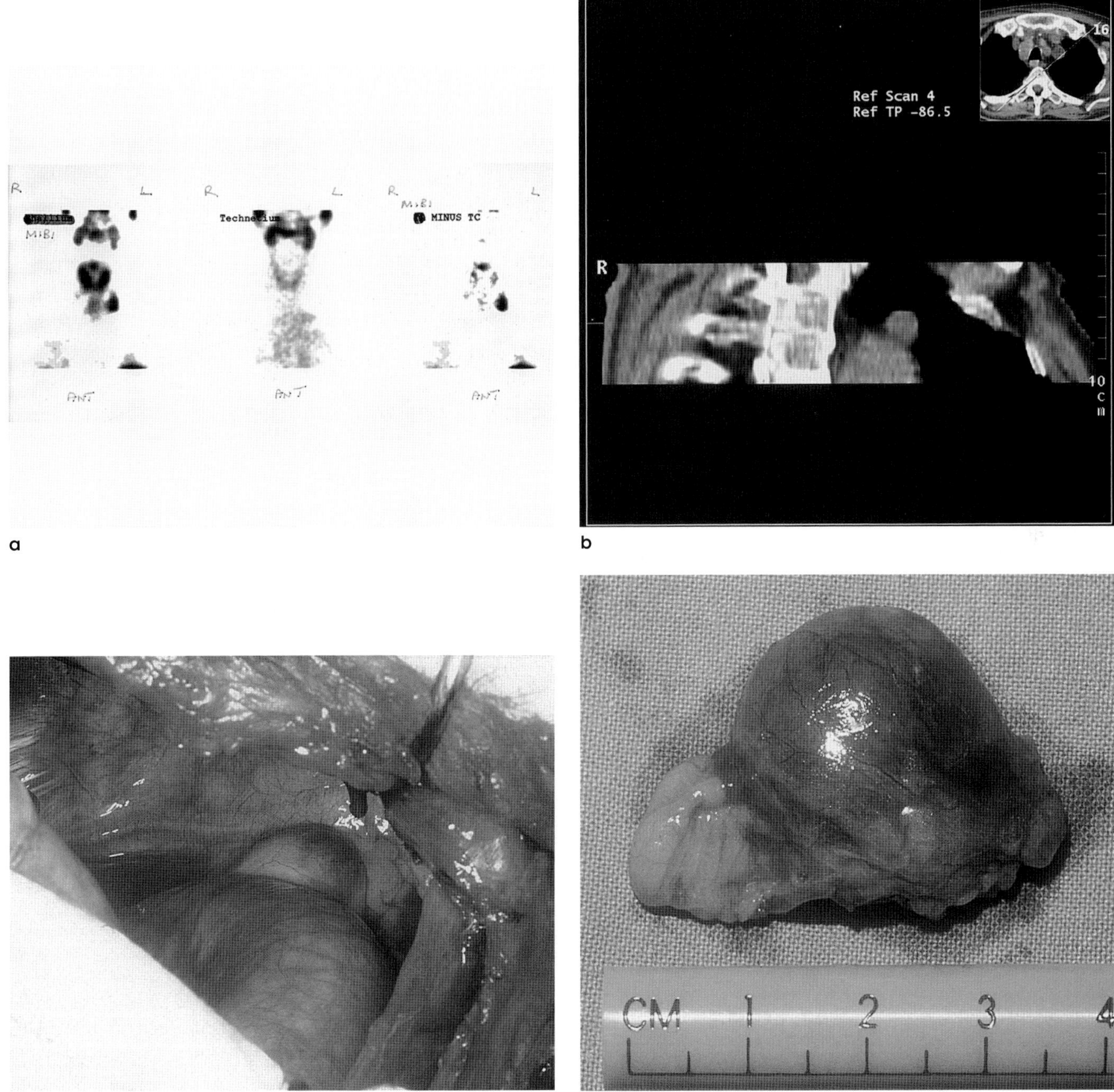

Figure 18.6 Localization techniques for an ectopic parathyroid adenoma. Following a negative cervical exploration, an ectopic intrathoracic fifth parathyroid gland adenoma was identified with sestamibi scanning (**a**) and reconstruction images of CT thorax (**b**). This middle mediastinal tumour can be seen perched on the aortic arch, nestled close to the junction with the left subclavian artery. It was excised through a left fifth rib thoracotomy (**c**) by Mr P. R. Moddox and Mr C. Forrester-Wood, consultant thoracic surgeon, Bristol Royal Infirmary. Note the glistening capsule (**d**).

NEONATAL HYPERPARATHYROIDISM

Neonatal hyperparathyroidism is a genetically transmitted autosomal dominant disease characterized by life-threatening severe hypercalcaemia, and intense parathyroid hyperplasia and hypercellularity. The disease is due to a mutation in the calcium receptor gene, which induces chief cell hyperplasia leading to severe hypercalcaemia, which is fatal if not recognized and treated early. Patients appear to be homozygous for CaR mutations that determine familial benign hypocalciuric hypercalcaemia in heterozygotes.[27] Near-total parathyroidectomy controls the disease.

REFERENCES

27. Pearce SHS, Brown EM. J Clin Endocrinol Metab 1996; 81: 1309

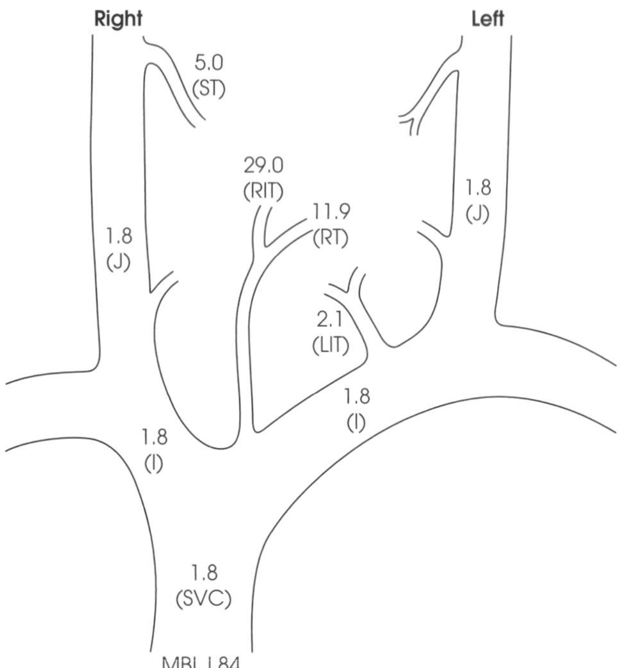

Figure 18.7 Results of selective venous sampling for PTH estimation in a patient with a parathyroid adenoma in the right lower position. The mean blood level of mainstream and vena caval samples represents a background reading of 1.84. The selective samples from the right inferior thyroid (RIT) vein demonstrate a marked gradient consistent with an adenoma in this position. ST, superior thyroid vein; J, jugular vein; LIT, left inferior thyroid vein; I, innominate vein; SVC, superior vena cava; MBL, mean blood level.

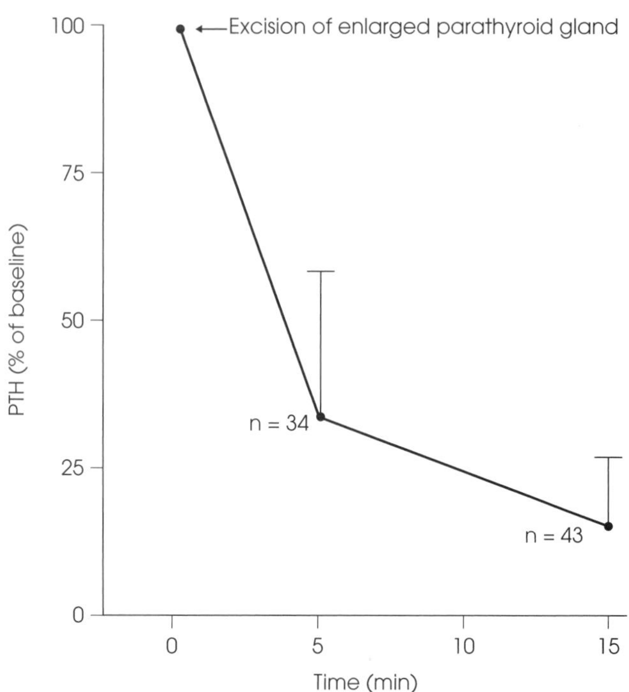

Figure 18.8 Monitoring PTH during parathyroidectomy. Decline of intact PTH after excision of one enlarged parathyroid gland in 43 patients with parathyroid adenoma. Results shown as a percentage of baseline value and means. (After Tibblin SA, Bergenfeltz AOJ. Surgical approach to primary hyperparathyroidism. In Clark OH, Duh QY (eds). Textbook of Endocrine Surgery. WB Saunders, 1997, with permission.[23])

NATURAL HISTORY

Because primary hyperparathyroidism is encountered in up to 1% of the adult population over 60 years of age, it is important to decide which patients need treatment. Several prospective studies followed patients with asymptomatic mild primary hyperparathyroidism for 10 years, and found that 25–33% of patients had progression of their disease.[28] In most patients primary hyperparathryoidism progresses slowly if at all, yet may be associated with subclinical symptoms and premature death. These factors create controversy regarding the indications for surgery.

The National Institutes of Health Consensus Development Conference concluded in 1990 that in asymptomatic patients surgery should be offered to all patients with severe hypercalcaemia (greater than 3 mmol/L) and to those with mild hypercalcaemia (2.8–3 mmol/L) if one of the following criteria were fulfilled: age below 50 years; urinary calcium excretion greater than 400 mg/24 h; bone mass two standard deviations below that of age- and sex-matched controls; and creatinine clearance reduced by at least 30%.[29] Patients who do not undergo surgery should be re-evaluated clinically and biochemically at 12 months' interval and should have a repeat bone-density scan. Since that widely quoted consensus statement, knowledge of the dangers of untreated hyperparathyroidism have become more widely appreciated, and surgery is now more often recommended, especially in those under the age of 60.[30]

TREATMENT

The only curative treatment is surgical excision of the abnormal parathyroid gland(s). The majority of patients proceed to surgery in a planned manner. Surgeons have a responsibility to counsel patients about possible morbidity, for example, persistent hypercalcaemia due to failure to recognize and/or remove all abnormal glands, the possibility of ectopic glands, recurrent laryngeal nerve injury, and hypocalcaemia. Complications are rare and most patients are hospitalized for only 1–2 days.

British Association of Endocrine Surgeons guidelines recommend that all patients are fully informed of potential complications, and should routinely be given an information sheet before being asked to provide informed consent.

HYPERCALCAEMIC CRISIS

Intensive medical treatment will be required before surgical intervention. Intravenous fluids correct dehydration and restore diuresis, facilitating the renal excretion of calcium.

REFERENCES

28. Silverberg SJ, Shane E, Jacobs TP et al. New Engl J Med 1999; 341: 1249–1255
29. NIH Consensus Development Conference Statement. J Bone Miner Res 1991; 6: 9–13
30. Roche NA, Young AE. Br J Surg 2001; 87: 1640–1649

Antiresorptive drugs (bisphosphonates) have become one of the mainstays of therapy for severe hypercalcaemia and intravenous pamidronate is very effective.

Calcitonin has the advantage of a very rapid onset of action (within minutes), but is indicated in only the first 24–48 h of treatment of acute severe hypercalcaemia, in conjunction with more potent but slower-acting therapies (i.e. bisphosphonates).

Intravenous phosphate solution should not be used because of the risk of precipitation of calcium salts.

MEDICAL TREATMENT

All patients diagnosed with primary hyperparathyroidism should be advised to avoid prolonged bed rest or dehydration, and to ask medical advice if persistent vomiting or diarrhoea develop (because these can trigger a hypercalcaemic crisis). A moderate dietary calcium intake is advisable, because low intake further stimulates the parathyroids and high intake accentuates hypercalcaemia.

No satisfactory medical therapy exists for the treatment of primary hyperparathyroidism. Calcitonin and bisphosphonates do not give good long-term control. The somatostatin analogue octreotide has no role in the management of primary hyperparathyroidism. Hormone replacement therapy in postmenopausal women may partly offset the effects of hyperparathyroidism on the bones.

Calcium-sensing receptor agonists

The cloning of the CaR has triggered efforts to develop drugs that could increase the affinity of CaR for extracellular calcium, and thereby potentially correct the biochemical abnormalities in primary hyperparathyroidism. One such compound is NPS R-568, an allosteric modulator of the CaR, which potentiates the effects of cation agonists on CaR.[31]

SURGICAL STRATEGY FOR BILATERAL NECK EXPLORATION IN PRIMARY HYPERPARATHYROIDISM

Once the biochemical diagnosis is confirmed there is no need to proceed to localization procedures if bilateral neck exploration is anticipated. A curved collar incision is made about 2 cm above the suprasternal notch, and this is deepened through platysma before superior and inferior flaps are mobilized, elevating the skin to the level of the thyroid prominence superiorly and the suprasternal notch inferiorly. The strap muscles are separated in the midline and elevated from the underlying thyroid.

There may be a need to divide the middle thyroid vein or the inferior thyroid veins to allow adequate mobilization of the thyroid.

The thyroid lobe is then gently retracted towards the midline, sweeping areolar tissue away, beginning in those areas where the glands are most likely to be found: just above the inferior thyroid artery and around the lower thyroid pole. The carotid sheath is the lateral boundary, and the trachea and oesophagus the medial boundary; the prevertebral muscles and fascia lie posteriorly.

The recurrent laryngeal nerve must always be identified and protected. Its feeding vessel is very small and usually easily seen within its substance ('toothpaste sign'). Undue dissection or palpation near or directly on the nerve is liable to cause intraneural haematoma, which may interfere with nerve function. The nerve is sometimes closely applied to an abnormal parathyroid and must be carefully dissected free. Diathermy should not be used in the vicinity of the nerve.

The vessels supplying a normal gland can be seen coursing into its substance, and care must be taken not to devascularize these structures unwittingly. If a biopsy is taken, it should be a sliver from the distal pole of the gland away from the feeding vessels.

All four glands should be visualized before a policy of resection and biopsy is decided. If there appears to be one large adenoma and three apparently normal glands, then excision of the adenoma is all that is required. Care should be taken to avoid rupture of the capsule of the adenoma, because any spilt cells may seed and lead to later recurrence.

The difficult cervical exploration

If a parathyroid adenoma is not found in any of the usual positions, a step-by-step systematic search is needed. Useful tips for such a dissection have recently been formulated:[32]

1. The majority of parathyroid glands are located within a 1–2-cm circle around the intersection of the inferior thyroid artery and the recurrent laryngeal nerve.
2. Rule of symmetry: it can be assumed that the glands on one side are located similarly to the ones on the other side.
3. The upper gland can be displaced posteriorly and caudally to lie beside the oesophagus, just in front of the vertebral column.
4. The lower gland can be either below the lower pole of the thyroid in the thyrothymic ligament or thymus itself, or in the carotid sheath.
5. According to embryology, the lower parathyroid gland may be high up in the neck, above the upper thyroid pole and medial to the carotid sheath, as high as the submandibular gland.
6. Less than 1% of glands are truly intrathyroid.

The exploration must be carried superiorly as far as possible, and certainly above the upper thyroid pole, behind the pharynx and oesophagus; a full exploration and excision of the thymic upper poles should be performed, opening the carotid sheath and exploring the lower thyroid poles. Intrathyroidal adenomas may be detected by intraoperative ultrasonography. In any event, a careful description with a map should be kept, with the location of all glands, with a notation whether biopsy was proven or not, and the presence of identifying landmarks (e.g. non-absorbable sutures or silver clips that might mark retained glands or biopsy sites). If an adenoma is not found, normal glands should not be removed.

Unilateral exploration in primary hyperparathyroidism

The advantage and cost-effectiveness of preoperative localization and unilateral neck exploration in primary hyperparathyroidism are becoming less controversial issues. Some say that preoperative localization of a solitary parathyroid adenoma (eventually coupled with confirmation of excision of all hyperfunctional tissue by quick PTH assay) may optimize operative time with unilateral neck exploration.[33] Others report unacceptably high surgical failure rates for unilateral neck exploration guided by

REFERENCES

31. Hammerland LG, Garrett JE, Hung BCP et al. Molec Pharmacol 1998; 53: 1083–1088
32. Rothmund M. Br J Surg 1999; 86: 725–726
33. Wei JP, Burke GJ. Am J Surg 1995; 170: 488

localizing studies compared with a bilateral neck exploration by an experienced endocrine surgeon.[34]

One alternative approach to such surgical strategy is based on radioguided parathyroid exploration. Following sestamibi scan, patients undergo unilateral neck exploration guided by a hand-held gamma probe, which is also used to measure ex vivo the radioactivity of the excised tissues. The technique was successful in 97% of cases in a first series of 52 patients.[35] It is not a widely used technique.

Minimally invasive surgery

In recent years, alternative approaches to parathyroid surgery have been reported, but are yet to demonstrate their advantage over the traditional technique.

Video-assisted parathyroidectomy by a lateral approach

Henry and colleagues in Marseille have implemented VAPLA.[36] It is indicated only for patients with a small single adenoma clearly localized by a combination of sestamibi and ultrasound scanning. Patients with ipsilateral previous neck surgery, associated nodular goitre, or suspicion of multiglandular disease are not eligible.

Minimally invasive video-assisted parathyroidectomy

The MIVAP procedure is performed as described originally by Miccoli and coworkers in Pisa.[37] The procedure is carried out through a 15-mm incision at the suprasternal notch; the blunt dissection of the thyroid lobe continues under direct vision from a 30° 5-mm endoscope, and small instruments (2 mm) are used for further dissection. A randomized study involving 38 patients has shown that, compared with conventional parathyroidectomy, MIVAP is associated with a shorter operative time, a better cosmetic result, and a less painful recovery.[38]

Endoscopic parathyroidectomy

Endoscopic parathyroidectomy was first described by Gagner in 1996. It is carried out under a steady gas flow not exceeding 8 mmHg of pressure, using a 5-mm endoscope introduced through a central trocar and two or three additional ports.

Bilateral oblique approach

A new bilateral oblique approach has been described, avoiding infrahyoid dissection, enabling exploration of unusual locations of parathyroid glands (e.g. retro-oesophageal space, jugulo-carotid sheath, and thymus), and being without any additional morbidity in a large series of 600 patients.[39]

TREATMENT OF PARATHYROID HYPERPLASIA IN PRIMARY HYPERPARATHYROIDISM

Hyperplasia can occur with or without adenomas of the parathyroid glands. Excision of the enlarged glands, leaving normal-sized glands intact, is adopted by some surgeons,[40] whereas others recommend that three and a half glands are excised.[41] Recent data in favour of conservative surgery (i.e. resecting the grossly enlarged glands without biopsying the macroscopically normal glands) are reported in a series of 300 patients with primary hyperparathyroidism who presented with multiple gland enlargement in seemingly sporadic cases.[42] When followed-up for an average of 90 months, 90% were normocalcaemic, 5% hypocalcaemic and 5% hypercalcaemic, suggesting that conservative surgery is an acceptable treatment for such patients.

Persistent or recurrent disease can be a problem with subtotal resections; it is encountered in 88% of those having up to two and a half glands resected and 33% of those with three to three and a half glands resected.

MANAGEMENT OF 'ASYMPTOMATIC' HYPERPARATHYROIDISM

There is an ongoing debate related to the question, 'Does mild, symptomless hyperparathyroidism require surgery?' Some advocate parathyroidectomy for all patients with symptomless mild primary hyperparathyroidism,[43] because:

1. Subtle physical and psychological changes are appreciated only on restoration of biochemical normality.
2. There is a risk of developing renal failure in the long term.
3. There is a risk of bone loss: this is especially important in elderly women.
4. Hypercalcaemia may contribute to confusion in the elderly.
5. There is a risk of hypercalcaemic crisis in the elderly, especially if there is intercurrent illness producing dehydration.
6. The incidence and mortality from cardiovascular disease may be increased.
7. The expense and distress of intensive medical follow-up outweigh the cost of an operation.

Not all these conclusions are very firm. For example, in the short term (about 4 years), there is no sign of deterioration in plasma creatinine when age-matched unoperated controls were compared with those who had undergone parathyroidectomy. Furthermore, clodronate sodium can be used for primary hyperparathyroidism patients in whom suppression of bone disease is desirable before surgery or when surgery is contraindicated.[44]

CLINICAL OUTCOMES

Armed with a full knowledge of parathyroid anatomy and embryology, a competent surgeon can successfully identify and remove abnormal parathyroid tissue in 95% of patients.[45] This standard has been adopted by the British Association of Endocrine Surgeons in the current *Guidelines for Surgical Management of Endocrine Disease.*[46] In some centres of excellence,

REFERENCES

34. Zmora O, Schachter PP et al. Surgery 1995; 118: 932
35. McGreal G, Winter DC, Sookhai P et al. Ann Surg Oncol 2001; 8: 856–860
36. Henry JF, Iacobone M, Mirallie E et al. Surgery 2001; 130: 999–1004
37. Miccoli P, Bendinelli C, Vignali E et al. Surgery 1998; 124: 1077–1080
38. Miccoli P, Bendinelli C, Berti P et al. Surgery 1999; 126: 1117–1122
39. Chaffanjon PCJ, Brichon PY, Sarrazin R. Ann Surg 2000; 231: 25–30
40. Thompson NW, Sandelin K. Acta Chir Aust 1994; 26: 44–47
41. Grant CS, Weaver A. Acta Chir Aust 1994; 26: 41–44
42. Proye C, Carnaille B, Quievreux JL et al. World J Surg 1998; 22: 526–529
43. Stevenson JC, Lynn JA. Br Med J 1988; 296: 1017
44. Douglas DL, Kamis JA et al. Br Med J 1983; 286: 587
45. Thompson NW, Eckhauser FE, Harness JK. Surgery 1982; 92: 814
46. British Association of Endocrine Surgeons. Guidelines for Surgical Management of Endocrine Disease and Training Requirements for Endocrine Surgery. 2nd edn, 2004 BAES Royal College of Surgeon of England. www.baes.info.

the outcome of bilateral exploration has been reported to be 100%.[47] However, such results can be difficult to achieve, even by trained endocrine surgeons, in standard practice.[48]

The presence of four normal glands may mean the wrong diagnosis, because a fifth ectopic and abnormal gland is rare. Familial hypocalciuric hypercalcaemia is one of the commonest confounding diagnoses. Most important is an awareness of the frequency and usual location of ectopic adenomas. The identification of all glands is of importance, because the search for a specific missing gland can then proceed logically based on anatomical and embryological knowledge.

COMPLICATIONS

RECURRENT AND PERSISTENT HYPERPARATHYROIDISM

Persistent hyperparathyroidism is the commonest cause of postoperative hypercalcaemia. It is defined as continued hypercalcaemia in the immediate postoperative period or occurring within 1 year of surgery.

Recurrent hyperparathyroidism is defined as hypercalcaemia occurring after parathyroidectomy when the following criteria have been met:

- identification and biopsy proof of all four parathyroids at the initial operation;
- complete removal of all abnormal tissue;
- a normocalcaemic phase of at least 1 year; and
- abnormal tissue uncovered at re-exploration at a site of a previously normal gland.

True recurrent disease might account for 1% of recurrent hypercalcaemia.

If persistent disease is suspected, the diagnosis of primary hyperparathyroidism must be confirmed. Localization tests are not indicated if the patient's general condition would not withstand re-exploration and its associated morbidity. Similarly, if the patient was asymptomatic this may also allow a conservative approach, especially if it could be shown that kidneys, bones and eyes were not being damaged overtly by the disease.

If a decision is made to offer re-exploration, then a full battery of localization tests is indicated, with imaging directed to areas where a gland was not formally identified and specifically looking for an ectopic mediastinal tumour (Fig. 18.6).

However, the initial surgical failure is nearly always the result of an inadequate neck exploration. This may be due to a joint error between the surgeon and pathologist; for example, failure to recognize familial hyperparathyroidism or multiple endocrine neoplasia syndromes.[49] If the lower glands were not found at the first exploration then thymus is the usual site, but the lower pole of the thyroid occasionally harbours a parathyroid adenoma. Ultrasound may detect such tumours, but often incision of the thyroid lobe or lobectomy is required.

There is an increased morbidity with second neck exploration for recurrent or persistent hyperparathyroidism: 6% temporary recurrent nerve neurapraxia, 4% permanent unilateral cord paralysis, and 13% hypoparathyroidism.[50] In view of these likely problems, the surgery should not be undertaken by the occasional parathyroid surgeon.

HYPOPARATHYROIDISM

The rapid onset of hypoparathyroidism can cause hypocalcaemia, with consequent paraesthesia, muscle spasm (i.e. tetany), and seizures.

Injury or removal of normal parathyroid glands during neck surgery is the most common cause of hypoparathyroidism. An operative strategy of parathyroid exploration, which includes an aggressive biopsy policy, will lead to a higher incidence of temporary hypocalcaemia without necessarily improving the overall success of the surgery.[51] Currently, there is a tendency to avoid biopsy of normal glands by using intraoperative PTH monitoring (see previous section) as a proof of complete excision of all abnormal parathyroid tissue, although pitfalls with the interpretation of this test have been reported.

It is essential to monitor calcium levels in the postoperative period, and it is advisable to counsel patients that a period of hypocalcaemia (normally temporary) may follow parathyroid surgery. This may relieve anxiety over any symptoms of hypocalcaemia that might develop. The biochemical threshold at which symptoms develop is variable and unpredictable.

The requirement for an intravenous bolus or infusions of calcium is rare, but can be needed for those elderly patients with severe bone disease ('hungry bones'). Use of intravenous 10% calcium gluconate can cause severe phlebitis if undiluted and tissue damage if there is extravasation. Mild hypocalcaemia can be managed with oral replacement synthetic vitamin D and regular outpatient checks of serum calcium.

PARATHYROID CARCINOMA

The incidence of parathyroid carcinoma is very low. It accounts for about 1% of all patients with primary hyperparathyroidism, with an equal male:female incidence at a mean age of 50 years.

Data from the first prospectively accrued series of 286 patients with parathyroid carcinomas treated in the USA between 1985 and 1995 have been reported.[52] There were no clinical or biochemical markers to allow the preoperative recognition of patients with carcinoma. Furthermore, even in centres with experienced endocrine surgeons, up to 86% of cases have not been appreciated initially by the surgeons, and carcinoma was often confirmed only when the patient subsequently developed local recurrence or metastases. Tumours were rather large (median tumour size 3.3 cm), and lymph node metastasis was identified in 16 of the 105 cases when lymph node status was evaluated at the time of the initial operation.

The classic pathological features include the presence of fibrous bands, stromal and intracytoplasmic fat content, mitotic figures, and nuclear characteristics, which have all been used to help distinguish carcinoma from hyperplasia and adenoma, but the diagnosis usually hinges on the presence of vascular and capsular invasion (Fig. 18.9). Mitotic activity constitutes a prognostic risk factor but is of limited diagnostic significance.

REFERENCES

47. Miura D, Wada N, Arici C et al. World J Surg 2002; 26: 926–930
48. Scott-Coombes D. Br J Surg 2001; 88: 1274
49. Clarke OH, Way LW, Hunt TK. Ann Surg 1976; 184: 391
50. Grant CS, Van Heerden JA et al. World J Surg 1986; 10: 555
51. Kaplan EL, Bartlett S et al. Surgery 1982; 92: 827
52. Hundahl SA, Fleming ID, Fremgen AM et al. Cancer 1999; 86: 538–544

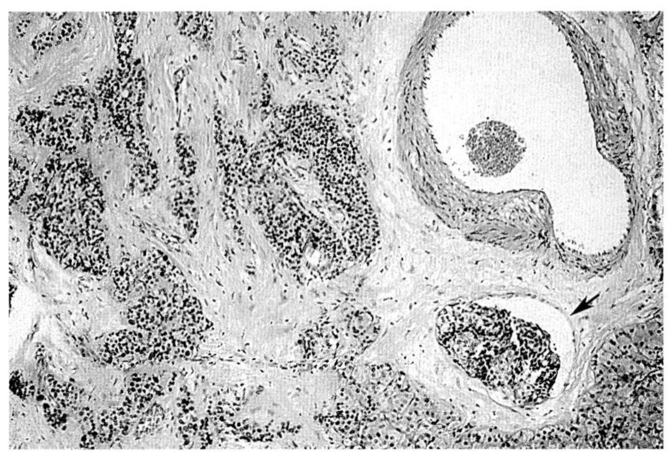

a

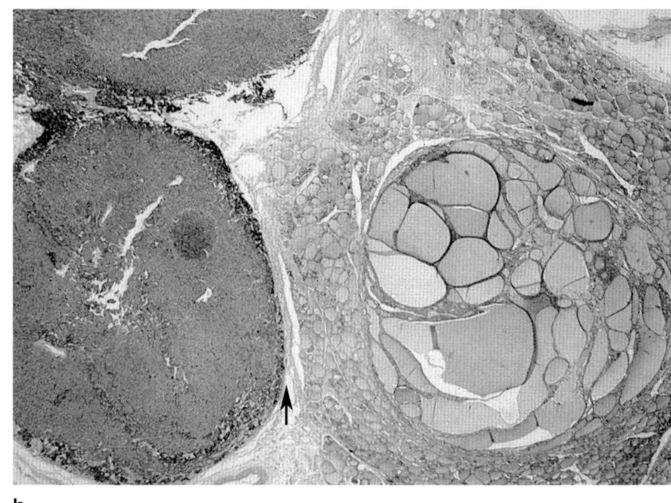

b

Figure 18.9 Pathological features of parathyroid carcinoma: typical broad fibrous septa between clusters of tumour cells, with invasion of blood vessel, depicted above (see arrow) and invasion of capsule and adjoining thyroid gland below. (Courtesy of Dr E. Sheffield, consultant pathologist, Bristol Royal Infirmary.)

Parathyroid carcinoma has a low malignant potential. It tends to recur locally, and metastases occur late in the course of the disease, commonly in cervical nodes (30%), lung (40%), and liver (10%). Most metastases are functional and generate severe hypercalcaemia.

If the condition is recognized preoperatively or at operation, en bloc resections offer the best results, with central compartment dissection when there is evidence of regional node metastases.

Recurrence in the neck or lungs can often be treated by further surgery with en bloc radical dissections, mediastinal lymph node clearance, and limited pulmonary resections.[53] This surgery is rarely curative but palliation is obtained by reducing hypercalcaemia. Radiotherapy is of little use. Attempts to control tumour burden with chemotherapy have been disappointing.

Mithramycin is a potent hypocalcaemic agent that is often effective for many months. Symptomatic relief has been obtained by using disodium clodronate. Treatment of one patient with hypercalcaemia secondary to parathyroid carcinoma with the calcium receptor agonist over 2 years produced no adverse clinical effects, and the drug appeared effective in long-term control of hypercalcaemia.[54]

The outlook is variable and, as with many endocrine tumours, some patients survive for many years with known metastatic disease.

SECONDARY AND TERTIARY HYPERPARATHYROIDISM

Secondary parathyroid hyperplasia occurs in response to a biochemical stimulus. The commonest situation is the hyperphosphataemia, relative hypocalcaemia, and disordered vitamin D metabolism associated with chronic renal failure. The duration of the renal failure and the length of dialysis contribute to the severity of the disease.

Secondary hyperparathyroidism can evolve into an autonomous condition that is not reversed if renal function is restored to normal (i.e. after renal transplantation). This is called tertiary hyperparathyroidism. In such patients hypercalcaemia develops as in primary disease, and a dominant adenoma or adenomas will be found within hyperplastic glands.

The frequency and severity of symptoms of secondary and tertiary hyperparathyroidism are highly variable.

BONE DISEASE

Patients develop osteitis fibrosa cystica or, less frequently, osteomalacia, which may eventually lead to skeletal deformities or fractures. Bone pain occurs primarily in the thoracolumbar spine and lower extremity.

SOFT TISSUE CALCIFICATION

This complication appears in up to 60% of those who have been dialysis-dependent for more than 5 years. Calcification may involve soft tissues, blood vessels, kidneys (nephrocalcinosis), lungs, heart and skin, and can cause pain, organ dysfunction and cosmetic deformities. The majority of such patients benefit from parathyroidectomy.

CALCIPHYLAXIS

Calciphylaxis is a rare condition associated with high PTH values and an increased serum calcium × phosphate product. Patients present with severe calf pain and tenderness due to extensive, non-ulcerating, large, hard and tender subcutaneous plaques in the calves. Involvement of the distal fingers and toes is characteristic. Calcium deposition can be confirmed radiologically and by bone scanning.

PRURITUS

Pruritus is a disabling symptom that affects up to 90% of patients on dialysis. Parathyroidectomy appears to reduce pruritus in both short-term and long-term follow-up.

REFERENCES

53. Fujimoto Y, Obara T. Surg Clin North Am 1987; 67: 343
54. Collins MT, Skarulis MC, Bilezikian JP et al. J Clin Endocrinol Metab 1998; 83: 1083–1088

CARDIOTOXICITY OF PARATHYROID HORMONE

In a 5-year longitudinal echocardiographic study including patients dependent on haemodialysis, one of the best clinical predictors for the presence of left ventricular hypertrophy was raised PTH.

If, despite medical measures to control serum calcium and phosphate levels and the use of a variety of vitamin D sterols, tertiary hyperparathyroidism responds transiently or not at all, parathyroidectomy is necessary. The criteria indicating the need for surgical intervention are not clearly defined.

SURGICAL STRATEGIES

After standard transverse neck incision, all four glands are located and resected parathyroid tissue confirmed by frozen section. Transcervical thymectomy should be routine, aiming to remove supranumerary glands or embryonic rests. If all four glands are not found in the classical locations, the retro-oesophageal space, superior thyroid pedicles, and areas along the carotid sheath should be explored. If, despite rigorous search, all four glands are not identified, the operation should be concluded. Median sternotomy is not performed as part of the initial operation.

Subtotal parathyroidectomy

Subtotal parathyroidectomy involves resection of three glands, leaving approximately 50 mg of viable tissue in situ. If permanent dialysis is anticipated, the remnant should be small (due to long-term hypertrophy of the remnant), whereas it should be larger if renal transplant is likely (to avoid subsequent hypoparathyroidism). The disadvantage of this approach is that a second cervical exploration would be needed if persistent or recurrent hyperparathyroidism occurs.

Total parathyroidectomy plus autotransplantation

Total parathyroidectomy plus autotransplantation was introduced around 1975 by Wells, and in some centres is still the preferred procedure. The gland that macroscopically looks most normal, and on frozen sections shows predominantly diffuse hyperplasia (and not nodular hyperplasia), is selected for autografting and diced fragments inserted into adjacent intramuscular pockets in the forearm. Some fragments can be cryopreserved. Primary graft failure is rare. Advantages with this technique are:

- Parathyroid mass can be reduced effectively with immediate biochemical benefit.
- Graft-dependent recurrent disease can be treated by graft reduction under local anaesthetic, obviating the need for re-exploration of the neck.
- Graft function can be closely monitored by measuring PTH directly in antecubital veins that drain directly from the graft site.

When autotransplantation is undertaken, all four parathyroid glands are removed from the neck. The gland selected for autotransplantation is usually the smallest, without nodule formation, and showing diffuse hyperplasia on frozen section.

Total parathyroidectomy alone

Total parathyroidectomy alone may now be preferred, and in a series appears to be a safe and effective option with all patients having symptomatic and biochemical improvement. If followed up for several years, most patients are found to have detectable levels of PTH, suggesting that total parathyroidectomy was not 'complete' and that residual parathyroid cells or parathyroid cell rests become activated under the continued biochemical stimulus of chronic renal failure.

SUMMARY

Although major insights into the management and pathophysiology of primary hyperparathyroidism have been gained since Mandl performed the first parathyroidectomy in 1924, primary hyperparathyroidism remains an area with many unsolved questions. Genetic alterations and molecular pathways involved in parathyroid gland physiology and pathology, and the relationship between abnormal parathyroid cell growth and hormone secretion in primary hyperparathyroidism, are not yet integrated into a simple model. The appropriate aggressiveness of treatment for patients with mild symptomatic disease is still not agreed. There is continued controversy concerning the advantages of bilateral exploration versus unilateral neck dissection in patients with positive imaging of one parathyroid adenoma. However, when parathyroid surgery is performed by fully trained, competent endocrine surgeons a very high success rate (with an acceptable low morbidity) can be attained.

Ear, nose and throat

19

Sean Carrie

THE EAR

SURGICAL ANATOMY

The ear may be divided into:

- an external portion, comprising the pinna and external auditory meatus;
- the middle ear cleft, composed of the middle ear, the Eustachian tube, and the mastoid air cells; and
- the inner ear, or labyrinth, comprising the cochlea and vestibular labyrinth supplied by the VIII (vestibulocochlear or auditory) nerve.

In the adult, the external ear canal is approximately 3 cm in length and is slightly curved. Thus, to view the tympanic membrane that divides it from the middle ear, the canal must be straightened by gently retracting the pinna upwards and backwards. The tympanic membrane is divided into a small upper portion, the pars flaccida, so called because it lacks much fibrous support, and a lower portion, the pars tensa, which is responsive to sound and appears relatively transparent, exhibiting a light reflex on otoscopic examination (Fig. 19.1). The malleus handle can be seen embedded in the drum and, with the stapes and incus, forms the ossicular chain. Sounds transmitted through the ossicular chain result in movement of the perilymphatic fluids that stimulate the hair cells of the cochlea.

The middle ear lies in close proximity to important structures that may be involved by infection. The temporal lobe in the middle cranial fossa lies superiorly and is only separated from the middle ear by a thin bony plate, the tegmen tympani. Posteriorly, the mastoid air cells are adjacent to the cerebellum in the posterior cranial fossa and lateral (sigmoid) sinus. Medially, the lateral semicircular canal allows access to the inner ear, and the facial nerve passes through the middle ear from the internal auditory meatus to the stylomastoid foramen. The Eustachian tube connects the middle ear to the nasopharynx, and is important in keeping pressure equal between the two. It is relatively short and horizontal in infancy, but during childhood becomes elongated with a more downward angulation.

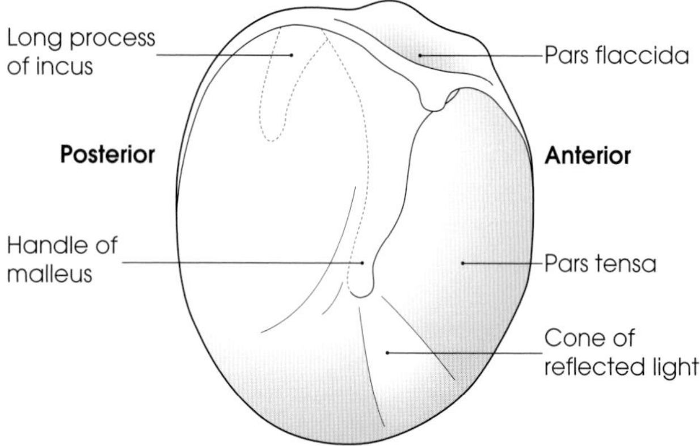

Figure 19.1 The right eardrum.

The cochlea is a spiral structure of two and a half turns, containing perilymph and endolymph partitioned by membranes. Sound vibrations are transmitted in the perilymph compartment, vibrating the basilar membrane and thus stimulating the hair cells that generate neural impulses along the cochlear division of the VIII nerve. The organs of balance are contained in the bony labyrinth. The vestibulocochlear nerve runs into the internal auditory canal, where it is joined by the facial nerve crossing the cerebellopontine angle to the brain stem.

CLINICAL EXAMINATION

The five main symptoms of ear disease are earache, deafness, discharge, tinnitus and vertigo. In a full otological examination, examination of the external ear and eardrum may be performed with an otoscope, an aural speculum, and a headlight or microscope, or with a rigid endoscope. Tuning fork and free-field speech testing give some indication of hearing loss. The audiogram can quantify a hearing loss and indicate whether it is sensorineural, secondary to lesions in the inner ear or central connections, or conductive, as a result of lesions of the outer or middle ears. Tympanometry is mainly used to demonstrate mobility of the drum, and thus the presence of fluid in the middle ear. Other auditory tests include speech audiometry, evoked response audiometry, and otoacoustic emissions. Caloric testing and electronystagmography assess the vestibular system. Electroneuronography is used in the assessment of facial nerve function. High-resolution CT scanning and MRI are both useful in the investigation of ear pathology.

TRAUMA AND FOREIGN BODIES

The pinna may suffer lacerations, avulsion, thermal injury and blunt injury, causing a haematoma. The haematoma forms between the perichondrium and the pinna cartilage, depriving the cartilage of its blood supply and resulting in cosmetic deformity: a ‘cauliflower ear’. The haematoma should be drained under antibiotic cover through an incision on the medial aspect of the pinna. A through-and-through mattress suture tied over a bolster prevents a recurrent haematoma.

The external meatus may also be injured; inserted foreign bodies require careful removal to avoid perforation of the eardrum. In addition to penetrating injuries, the middle ear may be injured by severe barotrauma (e.g. from bomb blasts) or overzealous ear-syringing. Perforation of the eardrum, ossicular disruption, haemotympanum and/or a perilymph fistula may result in, and are characterized by, varying degrees of hearing loss, tinnitus and vertigo. Traumatic perforations usually heal

Table 19.1 Differentiation between furunculosis and acute mastoiditis

	Furunculosis	Mastoiditis
Postauricular tenderness	Diffuse	Maximal over mastoid antrum
Displacement of pinna	Forwards	Forwards and downwards
Enlarged lymph nodes	Present	Absent
Pressure on tragus, moving pinna	Pain	No pain
Computerized tomography	Mastoid air cells clear	Mastoid air cells opacified
Examination of eardrum	If visible normal, usually hidden by swelling of canal	Before perforation, red and bulging

spontaneously, and the external auditory canal should be protected from water until this happens.

Wax may become impacted in the external canal, but the hearing loss is generally small unless there is complete obstruction. If the wax is hard, sodium bicarbonate drops may be used for a couple of weeks to soften it sufficiently to allow syringing or removal under direct vision. Syringing is contraindicated immediately after injury to the ear, or when there is a history of tympanic perforation.

Skull fractures involving the temporal bone may result in a temporary or permanent hearing loss. These fractures may be longitudinal or transverse, or a combination of the two. Facial nerve paralysis is more often associated with transverse fractures, as are vertigo and cerebrospinal fluid leaks.[1,2] Bruising over the mastoid bone (Battle's sign), blood in the external ear, and a cerebrospinal fluid otorrhoea or rhinorrhoea (into the nose via the Eustachian tube) strongly suggest a temporal bone fracture; CT imaging is necessary and audiological, vestibular and facial nerve function should be assessed. The role of systemic steroids and surgical exploration is uncertain.

INFECTION

Otitis externa

Otitis externa is a non-specific inflammation of the external auditory canal, with swelling, discharge and retained debris. The inflammation may spread to involve the pinna, and is often associated with discomfort and itching. Frequent aural toilet with microsuction, topical antibiotic or steroid sprays, or packing with gauze or a wick soaked in a topical agent (such as aluminium acetate solution) are more effective than oral antibiotics. The patient is advised to keep irritants and water away from the ear.

A much more severe form, malignant otitis externa, can occur in patients with diabetes or the immunocompromised; this can produce significant skull base destruction and cranial nerve palsies. Prolonged courses of high-dose antibiotics, such as ciprofloxacin, to treat pseudomonas are required.[3] Radical surgical debridement is occasionally necessary.

Localized infection of a hair follicle, usually with *Staphylococcus*, produces a furuncle that causes severe pain. This may require incision and drainage. An infiltrating squamous cell carcinoma, although very rare, should be considered as a differential diagnosis, particularly in an individual with a history of chronic otitis media.

Features that distinguish furunculosis from acute mastoiditis are summarized in Table 19.1.

Acute otitis media

Acute otitis media is a common condition, especially in childhood. Severe otalgia followed by otorrhoea when the drum perforates is the classical picture. Prior to that, the drum will be red and bulging. In the young child there may be systemic upset masking the otological symptoms. Treatment is generally supportive and antibiotics are not routinely required. Some surgeons advocate myringotomy if perforation has not already occurred.[4]

Chronic suppurative otitis media

Once the acute phase has settled, the perforation usually heals spontaneously; occasionally a more chronic infection develops. This may be associated with cholesteatoma. The exact cause of cholesteatoma is unknown, but is related to a collection of keratinizing squamous epithelium in the middle ear, possibly in a retraction pocket in the tympanic membrane, which gradually erodes into the middle ear and adjacent structures. Cholesteatoma must be suspected if examination of the eardrum reveals a perforation or pocket full of white debris in the attic. By contrast, perforations in the pars tensa are usually 'safe'. The hearing loss is conductive, although it may be less than expected because of conduction of sound through the cholesteatoma. 'Safe' chronic suppurative otitis media may often be managed medically, although a myringoplasty to repair the eardrum may be performed to improve hearing loss or prevent ear infections. Cholesteatoma requires exploration of the middle ear and mastoid with regular follow-up.

Chronic serous otitis media

Following acute otitis media, a serous effusion or 'glue ear' may persist within the middle ear cavity, especially in younger children. Myringotomy and grommet insertion are performed to improve hearing loss and developmental delay (Fig. 19.2). A persistent unilateral middle ear effusion in an adult requires further investigation to exclude a nasopharyngeal tumour.

Complications of otitis media

In the acute phase, if there is any suggestion of mastoid tenderness or swelling, or excessive malaise, headache or drowsiness, the local and intracranial complications of acute otitis media must be considered, because middle ear infection is one of the

REFERENCES

1. Aguilar EA, Yeakley JW, Ghorayer M et al. Head Neck Surg 1987; 9: 162
2. Avrahami E, Chen Z, Solomon A. Neuroradiology 1988; 30: 166
3. Brody T, Prasak ML. Am J Otol 1991; 12: 477
4. Mori Y, Iwasaki S, Kurota IC et al. J Otolaryngol Soc Jap 1992; 95: 48–64

Table 19.2 Intracranial complications of otitis media

Condition	Clinical features
Meningitis	Neck stiffness, photophobia, positive Kernig's sign
Lateral sinus thrombosis	Headache, rigors, spiking temperature, papilloedema, positive blood culture
Extradural abscess	Headache, early meningism
Temporal lobe abscess	
Initial	Chills, rigors, meningism, nausea, vomiting, headaches, psychological changes, tachycardia
Latent (may last for weeks)	Malaise, epileptiform attacks, neurological signs, temperature and periodic slowing of the pulse
Manifest with raised intracranial pressure	Papilloedema, cranial neuropathies III–VII, nominal aphasia, central hearing disorders, acoustic hallucinations, visual disturbance (e.g. homonymous hemianopia), contralateral paralysis
Terminal	Increasing headache, vomiting, stupor, coma, bradycardia, Cheyne–Stokes respiration
Cerebellar abscess	Headache, ataxia, cerebellar signs (e.g. rhombergism, dysdiadochokinesia)
Otitic intracranial hypertension	Headache, papilloedema, VI nerve palsy

commonest sources of a brain abscess, particularly in the temporal lobe but also in the cerebellum (Table 19.2).[5]

Acute mastoiditis is now relatively uncommon in the West. It affects children more often than adults, and is due to extension of infection from the middle ear cleft into the pneumatized mastoid. From there it may spread to adjacent structures, notably the intracranial cavity. In addition to the clinical signs of the otitis, there is significant pain and swelling over the bone, which displaces the pinna forwards and downwards (Fig. 19.3). The clinical presentation may be less obvious if the patient has partially responded to oral antibiotics (i.e. 'masked mastoiditis'). Computerized tomography is the imaging modality of choice because it can demonstrate intracranial involvement. However, a normal CT scan does not exclude intracranial suppuration.

Acute mastoiditis responds to high-dose, parenteral, broad-spectrum antibiotics if treated promptly; if there is incomplete resolution or progression mastoid exploration is required. Other clinical symptoms and signs of intracranial extension may indicate the need for an early neurosurgical opinion and intervention combined with mastoid exploration.

SUDDEN DEAFNESS

The majority of cases of sudden deafness are conductive, caused by occlusion of the external auditory meatus (wet wax or impacted wax on the drum) or due to middle ear effusion. Tuning fork tests highlight the conductive nature of the lesion. Sudden sensorineural deafness is most frequently idiopathic, and probably related to a viral infection or vascular accident. Treatment with steroids and vasodilators is controversial. Rarely an acoustic neuroma may present with a sudden hearing loss.

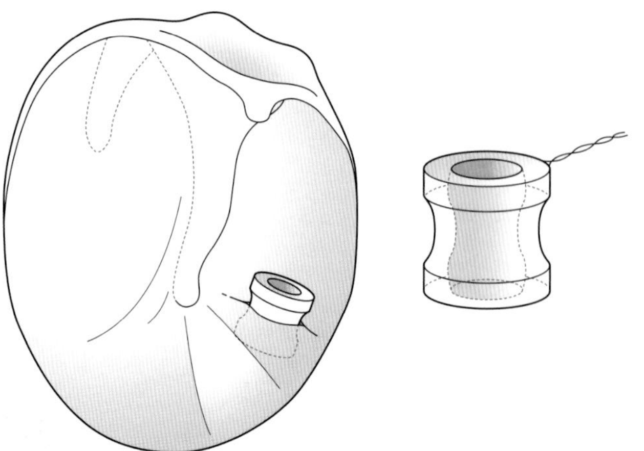

Figure 19.2 Position of myringotomy in anterior tympanic membrane and grommet in situ.

HEARING AIDS

Digital processing technology is now widely available in standard hearing aids, with a concomitant improvement in the quality of the output signal for the user. Other new developments include the osseointegrated bone-anchored hearing aid for selected cases of conductive hearing loss, and cochlear implantation for those with a profound sensorineural hearing loss.

REFERENCES

5. Kului A, Ozatik N, Topou I. Acta Neurochurgica 1990; 107: 140

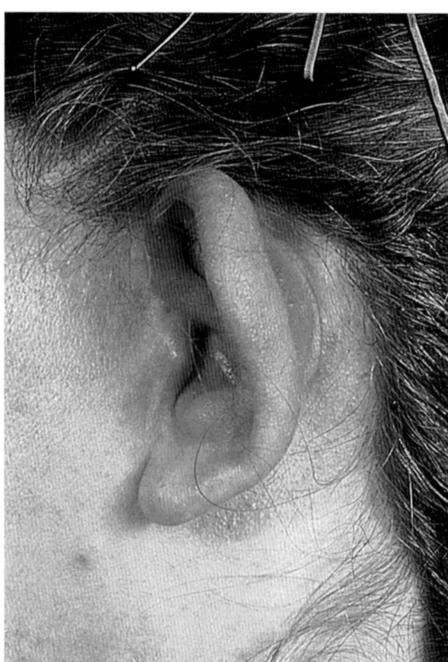

Figure 19.3 Acute mastoiditis associated with acute otitis media pushing pinna forwards.

ACUTE VERTIGO

Vertigo can be defined as the inappropriate sensation of motion. Acute vertiginous symptoms most commonly follow an episode of vestibular failure, possibly viral in origin, when no hearing loss occurs. The vertigo is rotational and associated with nausea and vomiting. Other peripheral causes of vertigo include Ménière's disease (associated fluctuant hearing loss, episodic tinnitus, and a feeling of fullness in the affected ear), chronic suppurative otitis media, and benign paroxysmal positional vertigo, a condition of undetermined aetiology where the vertigo is associated with positional changes only. In the acute phase, treatment is with labyrinthine sedatives, of which buccal prochlorperazine is the most useful. A careful explanation, avoidance of long-term sedatives, and rehabilitative labyrinthine exercises underpin management of patients with chronic symptoms.

When the vertigo is progressive and unrelenting, a central lesion (e.g. cerebral tumour or demyelination) must be considered.

FACIAL NERVE PARALYSIS

The facial nerve has a complex path through the middle ear, within a bony canal and mastoid cells to emerge in the neck through the stylomastoid foramen deep to the tip of the mastoid. It then divides into a number of branches within the parotid gland to supply the muscles of facial expression. A lower motor neuron paralysis may result from damage at any point in its course, conveniently divided into intracranial, intratemporal and extratemporal (Table 19.3). A careful history with ear, nose and throat and neurological examination usually determines a likely cause. Displacement of the tonsil or lateral pharyngeal wall due to a mass in the deep lobe of the parotid should be sought. Appropriate audiometry, electroneuronography, CT and MRI should be requested.

Bell's palsy, an idiopathic lower motor neuron paralysis, is a diagnosis of exclusion. In the majority (85%) of cases, recovery is complete and spontaneous, so the relative value of steroids, vasodilators and surgical decompression is difficult to determine. In common with all facial palsies, protection of the cornea is most important, because without a blink reflex the cornea may ulcerate. Corneal protection is achieved by a lateral tarsorrhaphy, either temporary or permanent, combined with lubricants and artificial tears.

In addition to the treatment of an established cause for the facial palsy—for example parotidectomy for a malignant tumour or removal of an acoustic neuroma—the entire course of the facial nerve is accessible for repair where appropriate. This may include an end-to-end repair or the interposition of a nerve graft.

Table 19.3 Causes of facial nerve paralysis

Intracranial
- Cerebrovascular accident
- Acoustic neuroma
- Meningitis (rarely)

Intratemporal
- Acute and chronic otitis media
- Trauma: surgical or accidental (e.g. skull base fracture)
- Herpes zoster (Ramsay Hunt syndrome)
- Idiopathic (Bell's palsy)
- Tumours (rarely): glomus, paraganglioma; squamous cell carcinoma of external or middle ear; metastases (e.g. breast)

Extratemporal
- Parotid malignancy
- Trauma: surgical or accidental (e.g. facial lacerations)

TUMOURS

Fortunately, malignant tumours of the ear are very rare, but several benign growths may have serious consequences because of their site of origin. An acoustic neuroma (vestibular schwannoma) may arise from the vestibular nerve within the internal auditory canal, expansion of which causes unilateral hearing loss and tinnitus. Other cranial nerve palsies, raised intracranial pressure, and compression of the brain stem ultimately ensue. Magnetic resonance imaging is the most reliable diagnostic technique (Fig. 19.4).

Another benign lesion that is also best demonstrated by MRI is the glomus tumour arising from paraganglionic tissue. This can be found in a number of sites in the head and neck, including the middle ear (glomus tympanicum) and jugular bulb (glomus jugulare). It characteristically produces pulsatile tinnitus, hearing loss, and ultimately cranial nerve palsies (VII, IX, X, XI, and XII). The size of the lesion and age of the patient determine whether treatment is by surgery, radiotherapy, or a combination of both.

THE NOSE

SURGICAL ANATOMY

The nasal cavities begin anteriorly at the nasal vestibule and end posteriorly at the choanae, where the nasopharynx begins. The nasal septum is cartilaginous anteriorly and posteriorly is made up of the perpendicular plate of the ethmoid and vomer (Fig. 19.5). The lateral wall of the nose has three (or sometimes four) turbinates covering meatuses into which the sinuses drain. The anterior ethmoids, and maxillary and frontal sinuses drain into the middle meatus (the ostiomeatal complex), the posterior ethmoids into the superior meatus, and the sphenoid into the

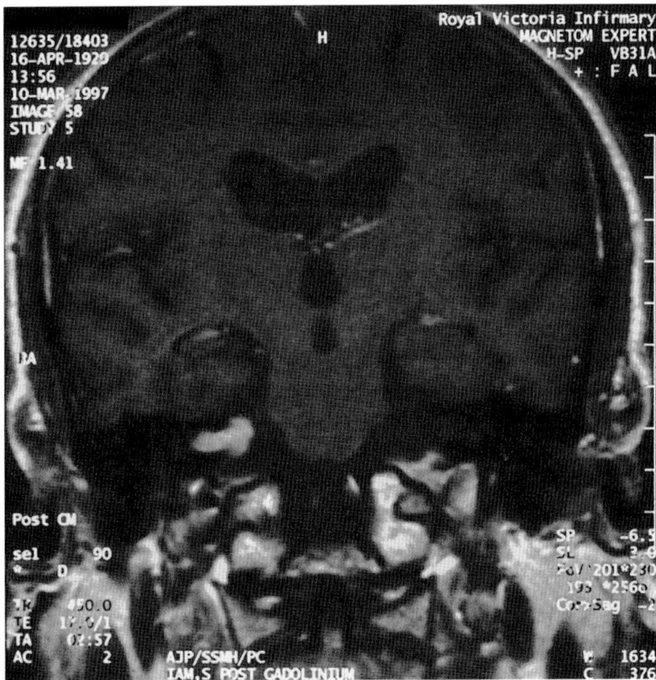

Figure 19.4 Coronal gadolinium-enhanced T_1 MRI scan of acoustic neuroma.

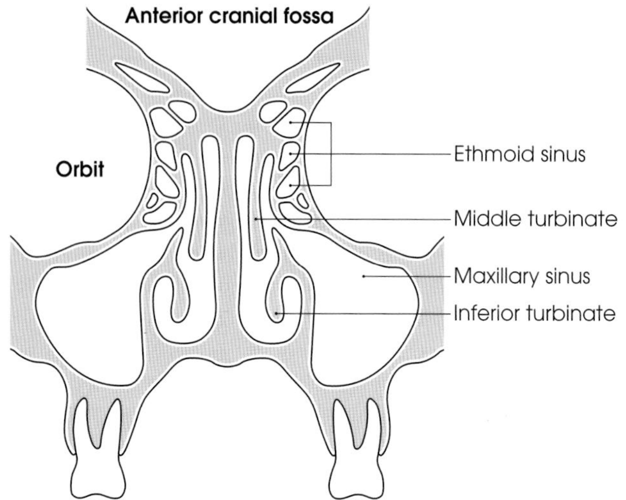

Figure 19.5 Coronal section through nasal cavity.

sphenoethmoidal recess above the posterior choana. The nasolacrimal duct drains into the inferior meatus.

Most of the nasal mucosa is respiratory ciliated epithelium, except superiorly in the roof, where olfactory epithelium lies. The cilia waft mucus produced by seromucinous glands and goblet cells from the sinuses and nasal cavity, via the nasopharynx, into the oropharynx, whence it is swallowed. The sinuses drain by predetermined pathways into the nose through clefts that are vulnerable to obstruction, leading to secondary bacterial infection. The close proximity of the sinuses to the orbit and anterior cranial cavity renders the latter structures at risk of involvement in severe acute infection and, less commonly, from the spread of sinonasal malignancy.

INVESTIGATION

The nose can be examined with a headlight and nasal speculum, a fibre-optic speculum, and rigid or flexible endoscopes. Examination is assisted by the use of local anaesthetics and vasoconstrictors, for example cocaine, lidocaine (lignocaine), and adrenaline (epinephrine). Computerized tomography scanning is preferred for its optimal demonstration of the anatomy and pathology;[6] CT may be combined with MRI in the imaging of neoplasia.[7,8] Other investigations include tests for allergy, airway patency, mucociliary clearance and immune function, and olfactory acuity.

RHINOSINUSITIS

Rhinosinusitis may be broadly defined as inflammation of the nose and sinuses characterized by one or more of the following symptoms: nasal congestion, rhinorrhoea, sneezing, itching and hyposmia. Table 19.4 lists a classification of aetiologies.

Infectious rhinosinusitis covers a range of acute and chronic infections: viral, bacterial and fungal. Acute rhinosinusitis usually resolves spontaneously or with a short course of oral antibiotics, but may be seen in hospital practice when a serious complication occurs. Involvement of the orbit and/or intracranial cavity constitutes a medical emergency (Fig. 19.6, Table 19.5). In the orbit, vision may be lost and rarely recovers. The intracranial complications can be life-threatening, requiring neurosurgical intervention (Fig. 19.7).[10]

In addition to the usual symptoms of nasal obstruction, purulent discharge, facial pain or headache, and pyrexia, there

Table 19.4 Classification of rhinosinusitis

Allergic • Seasonal • Perennial **Non-allergic: infectious** • Acute • Chronic **Non-allergic: non-infectious** • Idiopathic • Occupational **Non-allergic rhinitis with eosinophilia (NARES)** • Hormonal • Drug-induced • Irritants • Food • Emotional • Atrophic **Differential diagnosis** ***Polyps***	***Mechanical factors*** • Deviated septum • Hypertrophic turbinates • Adenoidal hypertrophy • Anatomical variants in the ostiomeatal complex • Foreign bodies • Choanal atresia ***Tumours*** • Benign • Malignant ***Granulomas*** • Wegener's granulomatosis • Sarcoid • Infective: tuberculosis • Leprosy • Malignant: midline destructive granuloma (T-cell lymphoma) ***Cerebrospinal rhinorrhoea***

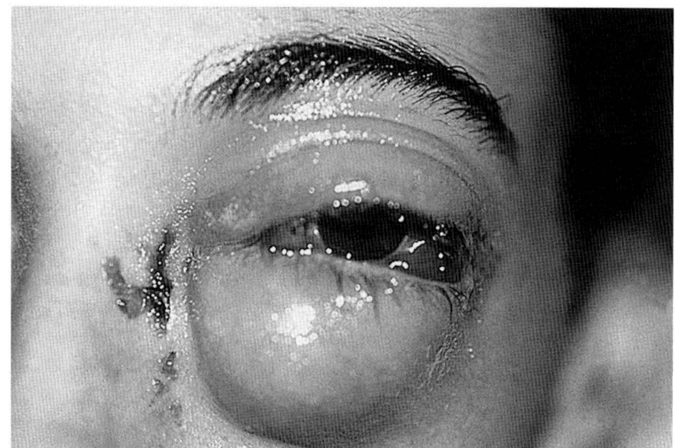

Figure 19.6 Acute orbital cellulitis with intraperiosteal abscess associated with acute pansinusitis.

may be significant swelling around the eye, with proptosis, limitation of eye movement, and visual loss depending on the degree of orbital involvement. It is mandatory that the eye be adequately examined and kept under review irrespective of the associated discomfort. Ideally, an ophthalmologist's opinion should be sought. Symptoms of intracranial involvement, such as headache and malaise, may be obscured by sinusitis. However, signs of meningism, raised intracranial pressure, focal

REFERENCES

6. Zinreich SJ, Kennedy DW, Rosenbaum AE et al. J Radiol 1987; 163: 769
7. Lund VJ, Howard DJ, Lloyd GAS et al. Head Neck Surg 1989; 11: 279
8. Lund VJ, Lloyd GAS, Howard DJ et al. Laryngoscope 1996; 106: 553
9. Mackay IS, Bull TR (eds). Scott-Brown's Otolaryngology: Rhinology. Butterworth-Heinemann, Oxford, 1997
10. Clayman GL, Adams GL, Paugh DR et al. Laryngoscope 1991; 101: 234

Table 19.5 Complications of rhinosinusitis

Acute

Local

Orbital
- Preseptal cellulitis
- Orbital cellulitis without abscess
- Orbital cellulitis with sub- or extraperiosteal abscess
- Orbital cellulitis with intraperiosteal abscess
- Cavernous sinus thrombosis

Intracranial
- Abscess: extradural, subdural, intracerebral
- Meningitis
- Encephalitis
- Cavernous or sagittal sinus thrombosis

Bony
- Osteitis or osteomyelitis (Pott's puffy tumour)

Dental

Distant
- Toxic shock syndrome

Chronic
Mucocele or pyocele

Associated diseases
- Otitis media, adenotonsillitis, bronchiectasis

neurological signs, and drowsiness should alert the physician to this possibility.

High-dose, broad-spectrum, parenteral antibiotics covering likely aerobes and anaerobes should be commenced immediately, and intranasal vasoconstrictor drops may be used. A CT scan will confirm the sinusitis and define the complications. Time should not be lost, however, if the orbit is involved and vision is clearly failing; under these circumstances drainage of the sinuses should be undertaken immediately.[11]

INJURY

The nose is frequently subject to injury, either as a circumscribed injury or as part of a more severe midfacial injury as in a road traffic accident. Fractures may be linear or severely comminuted 'smash' fractures involving frontal and lacrimal bones, orbital rim and ethmoid, including the cribriform plate.[12] The latter may produce a leak of cerebrospinal fluid and/or loss of the sense of smell. Radiographs of the nasal bones are frequently unhelpful. Oedema of the overlying tissues usually obscures the deformity unless the patient is seen within 1–2 h of the injury, so the majority of patients are referred to an ear, nose and throat surgeon for manipulation under anaesthesia, ideally within 10 days. If a septal haematoma is suspected, however, this should be immediately drained under antibiotic cover to avoid necrosis of septal cartilage and cosmetic deformity.

FOREIGN BODIES

There is often a unilateral, foul-smelling, purulent discharge that, together with mucosal swelling, may obscure any view; a radiograph will help only if the object is radiopaque. If the history is strong enough, the patient should be referred for an ear, nose and throat opinion and examination under general anaesthetic.

EPISTAXIS

Nosebleeds can result from a wide range of local and systemic conditions, of which trauma is the most common (Table 19.6). Bleeding from Little's area on the anterior nasal septum is often post-traumatic. Epistaxis can range from occasional slight spotting to torrential life-threatening haemorrhage, and the severity obviously dictates management. Many minor bleeds stop with simple pressure, with or without intranasal instillation of local anaesthetic or vasoconstrictor and cauterization of an obvious bleeding spot. More severe bleeds necessitate general resuscitation. If bleeding is too profuse to adequately examine the nose, a sponge nasal pack should be inserted into the nostril. Alternatively, gauze impregnated in bismuth and iodoform paraffin paste (BIPP) can be used. If layered carefully, 2 m of gauze can be inserted in each nostril. If bleeding continues despite this, a postnasal pack may be required. In either case,

REFERENCES

11. Lund VJ. In: Mackay IS, Bull TR (eds). Scott-Brown's Otolaryngology: Rhinology, Vol 4. Butterworth-Heinemann, Oxford, 1997: 1–11
12. Starkhammar H, Olofsson J. Clin Otolaryngol 1982; 7: 405

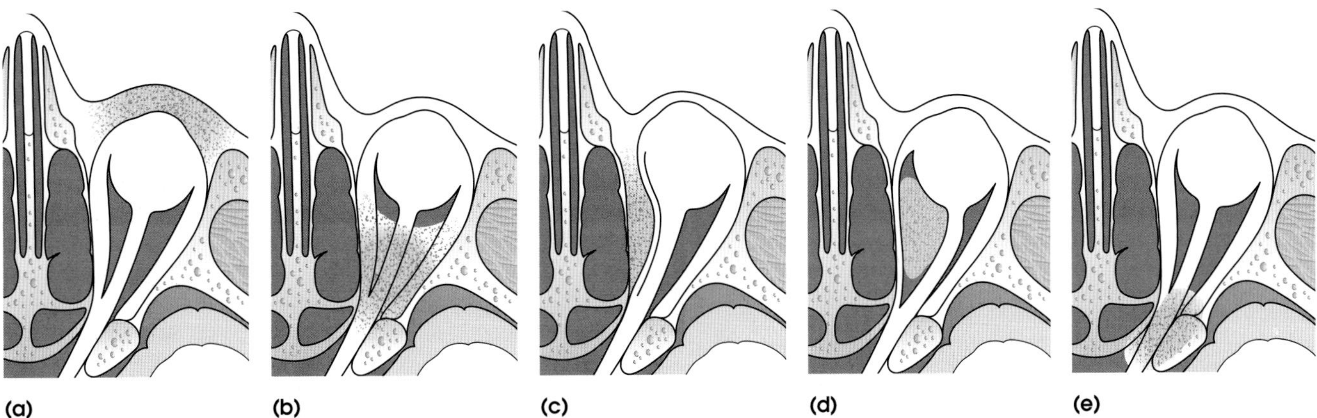

Figure 19.7 Spectrum of orbital complications associated with acute sinusitis: (**a**) preseptal inflammation; (**b**) orbital cellulitis; (**c**) orbital cellulitis with subperiosteal (extraperiosteal) abscess; (**d**) orbital cellulitis with intraperiosteal abscess; and (**e**) cavernous sinus thrombosis. (After Mackay IS, Bull TR (eds). Scott-Brown's Otolaryngology: Rhinology. Oxford: Butterworth-Heinemann, 1997, with permission.[9])

Table 19.6 Causes of epistaxis

Local	***Coagulation disorders***
Idiopathic	*Congenital*
Trauma	• Haemophilia
• Self-inflicted	• Christmas disease
• Facial fractures	• Von Willebrand's
• Iatrogenic: surgery	*Acquired*
• Septal deviation	• Renal and liver failure
• Foreign bodies	• Massive transfusion
• Septal perforation	• Vitamin deficiency
Inflammatory	• Anticoagulants
• Atrophic rhinitis	• Myelosuppressive drugs
Infectious	***Haemopoietic***
Tumours	• Leukaemia
• Benign (e.g. angiofibroma)	• Aplastic anaemia
• Malignant	• Lymphoma
	• Widespread metastases
General	***Hereditary haemorrhagic telangiectasia***
Atherosclerosis	*Endocrine*
Bleeding dyscrasia	• Vicarious menstruation
	• Pregnancy

the patient must be admitted for observation and placed on antibiotics. Occasionally, packing under general anaesthesia and arterial ligation or embolization may be required.

NASAL POLYPS

Nasal polyps are pedunculated masses composed of oedematous mucosa arising within the clefts of the lateral wall of the nose and sinuses (Fig. 19.8). They may occur in association with cystic fibrosis (25% in children,[13] 45% in adults[14]), asthma,[15] and as part of aspirin idiosyncrasy.[16] Complete cure is unusual, but symptomatic relief can be achieved by a combination of steroids (intranasal and parenteral) and surgical removal.[17]

CHRONIC RHINOSINUSITIS

Chronic rhinosinusitis is deemed to exist after symptoms have persisted for more than 12 weeks.[18] Patients may improve with intensive medication, for example long-term oral antibiotics and intranasal steroids, but surgery is frequently required. A more conservative approach has prevailed in recent years, complemented by the improved visualization afforded by CT scanning and by the rigid endoscope. The term *functional endoscopic sinus surgery* has been applied to precise endoscopic surgery dictated by the pathology.[19]

TUMOURS

Sinonasal neoplasia is relatively rare but should be suspected when symptoms persist, particularly if they are unilateral. Patients often present with advanced disease, and oncological treatment is frequently compromised by the close proximity of the orbit and intracranial cavity. Although squamous cell carcinoma is the commonest tumour encountered, this region offers the greatest histological diversity in the body. Specialized histology and imaging (contrast-enhanced CT and MRI) are necessary to determine the diagnosis and extent. Depending on histology, therapy consists of surgery and/or radiotherapy with occasional additional chemotherapy. A number of surgical approaches are available. For any tumour that has transgressed the anterior skull base, a craniofacial resection offers the best chance of cure. For lesions of the nasal cavity and maxillary sinus, a lateral rhinotomy, midfacial degloving approach, and maxillectomies of varying extent may be chosen. Prostheses for both the maxilla and orbit may be required.

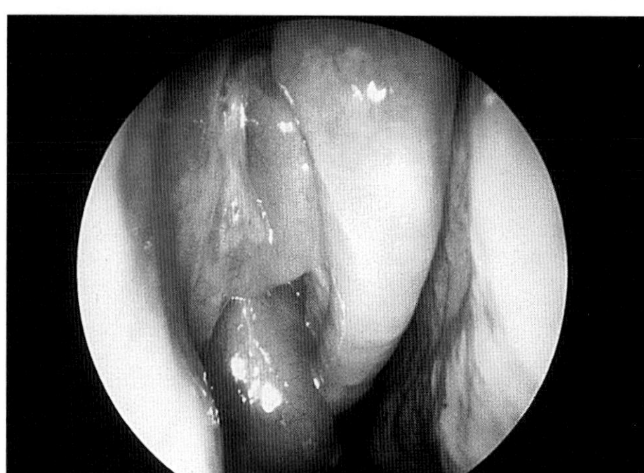

Figure 19.8 Endoscopic view of nasal polyps in right middle meatus.

NASOPHARYNX

SURGICAL ANATOMY

The nasopharynx or postnasal space is situated with the posterior choana anteriorly and the soft palate inferiorly. Superiorly it is related to the skull base and posteriorly to the vertebral bodies. The cartilaginous pharyngeal Eustachian tube enters the space superolaterally. The adenoids are found on the posterior pharyngeal wall. Examination of the postnasal space can be achieved by retrograde mirror examination from the mouth, or using either a flexible or rigid endoscope.

ADENOIDECTOMY

Adenoidectomy is still one of the most frequently performed operations in paediatric practice. Indications for surgery include nasal blockage, especially when associated with a sleep apnoea syndrome, and otitis media with effusion (glue ear).[20,21] Adenoids are curetted from the posterior pharyngeal wall using an adenotome. Adenoidectomy is contraindicated in children with cleft palate abnormalities because a speech defect, rhinolalia aperta, may result.[22]

REFERENCES

13. Stern RC, Boat TF, Wood RE. Am J Dis Child 1982; 136: 1067
14. DiSant'Agnese PA, David PB. Am J Med 1979; 66: 121
15. Drake-Lee AB, Lowe D, Swanston A et al. J Laryngol Otol 1984; 98: 783
16. Spector SL, Wangaard CH, Farr RS. J Allergy Clin Immunol 1979; 64: 500
17. Lund VJ. Br Med J 1995; 331: 1411
18. Kennedy D, Stammberger H, Lund VJ. Ann Otol Rhinol Laryngol 1995; (Suppl 167)
19. Kennedy DW, Zinreich SJ, Rosenbaum AE et al Archiv Oto-Rhino-Laryngol 1985; 111: 576
20. Bluestone CD, Cantekin EI, Berry QC. Laryngoscope 1975; 85: 113
21. Merck W. HNO (Berlin) 1974; 22: 198
22. Goode RL, Ross J. Arch Otolaryngol 1972; 96: 223

NASOPHARYNGEAL CARCINOMA

Nasopharyngeal carcinoma generally accounts for only 4% of head and neck tumours, but in China it accounts for 21% of all malignant neoplasms.[23] Many aetiological factors have been suggested, including a genetic basis (Cantonese Chinese) and the Epstein–Barr virus.

Nasopharyngeal carcinoma most frequently presents in the fourth decade, is more common in men, and is frequently poorly differentiated.

The most common presentations are nasal blockage with a sanguinous rhinorrhoea, sometimes frank epistaxis, a conductive hearing loss due to fluid in the middle ear, and cervical lymph node enlargement. Pain, usually perceived in the ear as a referred otalgia, and cranial nerve neuropathies may occur.

The postnasal space must be carefully examined under general anaesthetic and even if no tumour is visible, endoscopic guided biopsies must be taken in any adult with persistent unilateral fluid in the middle ear. Computerized tomography and MRI scanning will optimally delineate the tumour and act as an aid for planning radiotherapy.

Radiotherapy is the primary modality of treatment, although increasingly data suggest improved results with combined platinum-based chemoradiotherapy.[24] The field must include the cervical nodes, even if they are clinically free of disease. The best 5-year survival rates for tumours confined to the nasopharynx is in the region of 90%, falling to less than 60% in tumours that have spread laterally from the nasopharynx. The presence of lymphatic metastases reduces these figures, although not greatly.[25]

Other tumours may arise or present in the nasopharynx, including neurilemmoma, chordoma, lymphoma, plasmacytoma and rhabdomyosarcoma. Juvenile angiofibroma, a hamartomatous lesion occurring exclusively in young males, arises in the region of the sphenopalatine foramen and extends from the nasal cavity into the nasopharynx, where it presents as a unilateral polyp. Biopsies should never be undertaken because the angiofibroma is highly vascular in nature, but a definitive diagnosis may be made with the pathognomonic features seen on CT scanning and MRI.[26]

THE TONGUE AND OROPHARYNX

SURGICAL ANATOMY

From an embryological perspective, the tongue is divided into an anterior two-thirds (anterior to the vallate papillae) and a posterior third. The interlacing muscle fibres of the tongue form an easy pathway for tumour spread through the tongue substance and early dissemination to the cervical lymph nodes, which may be bilateral and involve the upper and lower cervical nodes.

The oropharynx stretches from the soft palate to the pharyngoepiglottic fold. Anterolaterally are the faucial pillars (anterior pillar, the palatoglossus muscle; posterior pillar, the palatopharyngeus muscle) that guard the palatine tonsils. Anteroinferiorly is the posterior third of the tongue, bounded anteriorly by the sulcus terminalis and inferiorly by the lingual tonsil. The lymphoid drainage of this region is often to both deep cervical chains, with the tonsil specifically draining to the jugulodigastric node. The palatine tonsils atrophy in the adult.

THE TONSILS

Acute tonsillitis is characterized by a severe sore throat that usually produces difficulty in swallowing and may be associated with pyrexia, general malaise and earache. Tonsillar enlargement, both unilateral and bilateral, may occur when neoplasia affects the lymphoid tissue (e.g. leukaemia and lymphoma). Diagnosis may be assisted by a throat swab, full blood count and differential, and a Paul–Bunnell test. Tonsillitis is usually streptococcal in origin and therefore should be treated with penicillin.

Simple tonsillar hypertrophy is not necessarily pathological and its presence is not an indication for tonsillectomy. Tonsillectomy is indicated if there is respiratory obstruction, sleep apnoea, recurrent attacks of acute follicular tonsillitis, or more than one episode of peritonsillar abscess.

Primary postoperative bleeding from the tonsillar bed occurs immediately after surgery, and re-exploration is then frequently necessary, especially in a child. Secondary haemorrhage occurs in approximately 1% of patients, usually between the fifth and eighth day postoperatively, and is due to infection. Operative intervention is usually not indicated; simple supportive measures and parenteral antibiotic therapy suffice.

FOREIGN BODIES

The most common foreign body found in the oropharynx is a fishbone embedded in the palatine or lingual tonsil. Careful inspection after the application of good local anaesthesia reveals the offending bone. Direct removal using Tilley's forceps is feasible for a bone stuck in the tonsil, but endoscopic assistance is usually required for those in the lingual tonsil or tongue base. Because fishbones are frequently radiolucent, plain radiographs are of limited value.

PHARYNGEAL ABSCESSES

The quinsy, or peritonsillar abscess, follows an acute tonsillar infection in which pus collects in the peritonsillar space. It presents with pain and excessive salivation, and the speech is thick and muffled. The abscess tends to point in the soft palate (Figs 19.9 and 19.10). Drainage is achieved under a local anaesthetic by lancing the abscess through the mouth using a guarded no. 11 blade. The symptomatic relief of pain is nearly always instantaneous.

White concretions protruding from the tonsillar clefts, known as tonsilloliths, result from the collections of squamous epithelium in the crypts and are not associated with any symptoms or pathology.

The retropharyngeal nodes, which normally regress by the age of 7 years, may on occasion be associated with suppuration and abscess formation, resulting in airway obstruction (Figs 19.9 and 19.10). Computerized tomography imaging clearly identifies the site and extent of the abscess, which may extend into the thorax. Parapharyngeal abscesses present in the lateral pharyngeal space, which is bounded superiorly by the sphenoid and ends as the tip of an inverted cone at the level of the hyoid; laterally is the superficial layer of the deep fascia and medially the deep layer of the deep investing cervical fascia, posteriorly the carotid sheath

REFERENCES

23. Buell PJ. Cancer 1965; 19: 459
24. Al Sarraf M, LeBlanc M, Giri PGS et al. J Clin Oncol 1998; 16: 1310
25. Watkinson JC, Gaze MN, Wilson JA. Stell and Maran's Head and Neck Surgery. 4th edn. Butterworth-Heinemann, Oxford, 2000
26. Fagan JJ, Snyderman CH, Carral RJ et al. Head Neck 1997; 19: 391

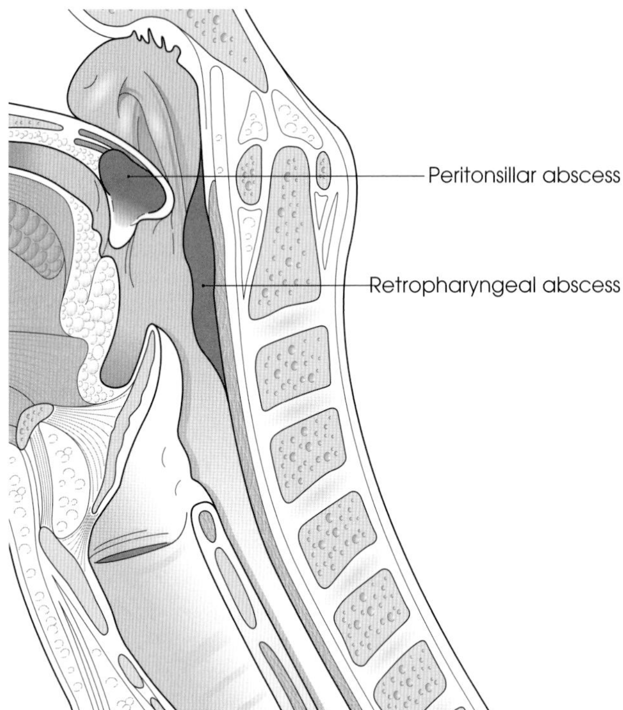

Figure 19.9 The pharynx and larynx: midsagittal section.

and the cranial nerves IX–XII (Fig. 19.10). Pus in this space may have arisen in the peritonsillar space or may have followed pharyngeal trauma, either from a foreign body or during endoscopy. Drainage should be performed externally using an incision along the anterior border of the sternomastoid and the carotid sheath retracted laterally. A corrugated or tube drain should be used without suction. Parenteral antibiotics, providing cover for anaerobic organisms, should be administered. A tracheostomy may be required if there is airway compromise.

CARCINOMA OF THE TONGUE

The predominant tumour of the tongue is squamous cell carcinoma, most of which are well differentiated. This is a disease of middle-aged or elderly patients, and usually presents as a painless lesion. Tobacco and, probably to a greater extent, alcohol are important aetiological factors. Approximately 50% of tumours arise on the anterior two-thirds of the tongue, of which 85% occur on the lateral border. Macroscopically the lesions may appear exophytic or ulcerative and infiltrative. However, the apparent size as judged by the mucosal lesion is deceptive, and one should always assume that a further 2 cm of peripheral tissue may be infiltrated by disease. Palpation gives an indication of extent, and this evaluation is best done under general anaesthetic, when a deep biopsy can be taken. Modern imaging with high-resolution CT and gadolinium-enhanced MRI is useful to assess tumour extent.

If a tongue lesion is detected at an early stage, local excision (sometimes using a CO_2 laser)[27] or radiotherapy (interstitial or external beam)[28] may be appropriate. As already indicated, however, it is easy to underestimate the local extent of these tumours, and hemiglossectomy is appropriate. Even in the absence of palpable nodes, this will be combined with some form of neck dissection to provide staging. Postoperative radiotherapy should follow where any doubt still exists about the margins.

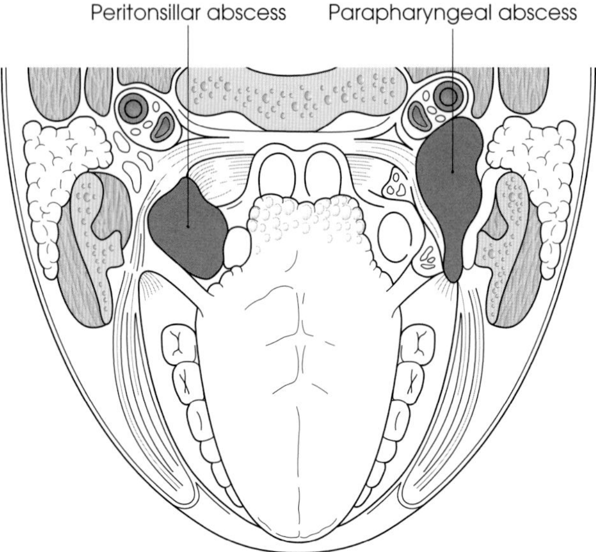

Figure 19.10 Position of pharyngeal abscess.

These procedures may be performed without splitting the mandible, and a range of myocutaneous and free flaps are available for reconstruction.[29] Total glossectomy is rarely performed; the associated morbidity and loss of function is such that, in general, both patients and surgeons decline the procedure.

OROPHARYNGEAL NEOPLASIA

Seventy per cent of oropharyngeal neoplasms are carcinomas, 25% lymphomas, and 5% miscellaneous tumours, including minor salivary gland tumours arising from the glandular epithelium in the oropharynx.[30] Of the squamous carcinomas, half present in the tonsil and half in the posterior third of the tongue, usually with ulceration. Referred otalgia via the glossopharyngeal nerve, dysphagia and a sore throat are common features in the history; some patients notice an ulcer on the tonsil, and in 25% a node in the neck is the presenting feature. In an adult, unilateral tonsillar enlargement that is not ulcerated must be considered a lymphoma until proven otherwise. Examination of the oropharynx must include mirror examination of the posterior third of the tongue and the lingual tonsil, and a thorough manual palpation of this area. Tissue diagnosis is obtained by excision tonsillectomy or deep biopsy.

The choice of treatment between primary radiotherapy and surgery is often difficult.[31] If there is no clinical lymph node involvement, radiotherapy is used as the primary treatment, with salvage surgery held in reserve for any recurrent or residual tumour. When there is lymph node or bony involvement, a combination of surgery and radiotherapy should be considered from the outset. Surgery should include a radical neck dissection

REFERENCES

27. Panje WR, Scher N, Karnell M. Arch Otolaryngol Head Neck Surg 1989; 115: 681
28. Mendenhall WM, Parsons JT, Stringer SP et al. Head Neck 1989; 11: 129
29. Conley J, Sachs ME, Parke RB. Otolaryngol Head Neck Surg 1992: 90: 58
30. Rhys Evans P. In: Hibbert J (ed). Scott-Brown's Otolaryngology, Vol 5. Butterworth, London, 1997
31. Jones AS, Beasely N, Houghton DJ et al. Clin Otolaryngol 1998; 23: 172–176

to remove palpable nodes or a selective neck dissection in cases where the neck is clinically clear of metastases. The surgical objective of a composite en bloc resection of the primary tumour site, allowing a 5–10-mm margin, is achieved and often requires partial glossectomy and partial mandibulectomy. Reconstruction following this radical procedure, often termed a 'commando operation', requires new internal lining for the pharynx, which will allow tongue mobility. Reconstruction can be by a musculocutaneous flap based on the pectoralis major, or preferably a free flap taken from the forearm.[32] If reconstruction of the mandible is needed, then an en bloc resection of the inner plate of the radius can be taken and inserted along with the flap between the two ends of the mandible; because this is a vascularized autologous graft it offers the best chance of success.[33] The effects of not reconstructing the mandible are predominantly cosmetic, in that although mastication is not unduly impaired there is difficulty with speech; the reconstruction should be designed to produce as mobile a tongue tip as possible.

Care must be taken not to misdiagnose deep parotid tumours presenting as a mass in the lateral oropharyngeal wall. A biopsy in such cases is contraindicated because it tends to seed the tumour into the pharynx.

OBSTRUCTIVE SLEEP APNOEA AND SNORING

Snoring is the noise associated with vibration of the pharyngeal soft tissues during sleep. Obstructive sleep apnoea syndrome is apnoea related to airways collapse, resulting in hypoxia. In the long term this may lead to pulmonary hypertension and cor pulmonale. Obstructive sleep apnoea syndrome is characterized by snoring, daytime somnolence and lethargy. A sleep study including monitoring of an overnight ECG, oxygen saturation, and chest wall and abdominal movements will determine whether sleep apnoea is present. Management involves weight loss, smoking cessation, and reduced alcohol consumption. Home continuous positive pressure airways (CPAP) ventilation is an effective treatment for sleep apnoea syndrome. Surgery is reserved for simple snoring and mild sleep apnoea. Treatment options include uvulopalatopharyngoplasty (UVPPP) and laser palatal surgery, both of which stiffen the soft palate. Tongue base collapse may be corrected by mandibular splints. Tracheostomy is understandably reserved for the most severe cases.

THE HYPOPHARYNX

SURGICAL ANATOMY

Anteriorly the hypopharynx descends from the pharyngoepiglottic fold to the level of the cricopharyngeus and cricoid cartilage. It may be conveniently divided into three separate anatomical areas:

1. The posterior pharyngeal wall extends from the level of the pharyngoepiglottic fold as far as the oesophageal opening.
2. The pyriform sinus or fossa lies below the pharyngoepiglottic fold, and is bounded laterally by the mucosa covering the inner aspect of the thyroid cartilage and medially by the back of the aryepiglottic fold. Inferiorly it extends down to the oesophageal opening and posteriorly it opens into the hypopharynx proper.
3. The postcricoid region extends from the level of the arytenoid cartilages above to the lower edge of the cricoid cartilage below.

CLINICAL FEATURES

The primary symptom of any hypopharyngeal disorder is dysphagia, often associated with pain. The pain is classically referred to the ear, being conducted through the internal branch of the superior laryngeal nerve and the auricular branch of the vagus. It is important to distinguish these symptoms from the globus sensation characterized by the 'feeling of a lump in the throat', often worse when swallowing saliva. There is often a strong functional element to globus, although acid reflux into the pharynx may be associated with it in some cases. In all disorders of swallowing, indirect mirror examination of the larynx and pharynx and flexible endoscopy, followed if necessary by video fluoroscopy swallow and often direct endoscopy under general anaesthesia, are necessary. Lesions may be missed when examination of the hypopharynx is made by a flexible endoscope, because the redundant mucosa closes around the endoscope and restricts the view.

FOREIGN BODIES

Hypopharyngeal foreign bodies, often a meat bolus, are usually found at or just above the cricopharyngeal sphincter. They impact on the sphincter and produce acute dysphagia (which is commonly complete), pain, and sometimes voice change. The history of ingestion is usually clear. Plain lateral radiographs of the cervical spine demonstrate radiopaque foreign bodies anterior to the body of the C6 vertebra. An air shadow may be seen in the upper oesophagus, which is normally closed. In cases where there has been penetration of the foreign body through the pharyngeal wall, surgical emphysema occurs, with its characteristic radiological features. If there is any doubt about the diagnosis a rigid endoscopy is performed. If the mucosa has been perforated either by the foreign body itself or during instrumentation, a nasogastric tube should be passed and the patient kept on nil by mouth and given parenteral broad-spectrum antibiotics. One must be alert clinically to the subsequent development of a mediastinal abscess and also, in the older patient, to the possibility that a malignant stricture may underlie the symptoms.

PHARYNGEAL PALSIES

Neurological disorders such as cerebrovascular disease or motor neuron disease may involve the pharynx, resulting in dysphagia and aspiration. The management of this condition is difficult, and should be multidisciplinary with involvement of swallowing therapy. A cricopharyngeal myotomy may produce relief of symptoms. Protection of the airway with a tracheostomy may have to be considered.

PHARYNGEAL WEB

A pharyngeal web, which usually develops in the postcricoid area of middle-aged women, presents with dysphagia and with symptoms of an iron-deficiency anaemia (Paterson–Brown Kelly or Plummer–Vinson syndrome). Care should be taken to examine the patient for koilonychia, angular cheilitis and glossitis, along with splenomegaly. Following a barium swallow all patients with webs should have a rigid oesophagoscopy, both

REFERENCES

32. Panje WR. Otolaryngol Clin 1984; 17: 401
33. McGregor IA, McGregor FM. Cancer of the Face and Mouth. Churchill Livingstone, Edinburgh, 1986

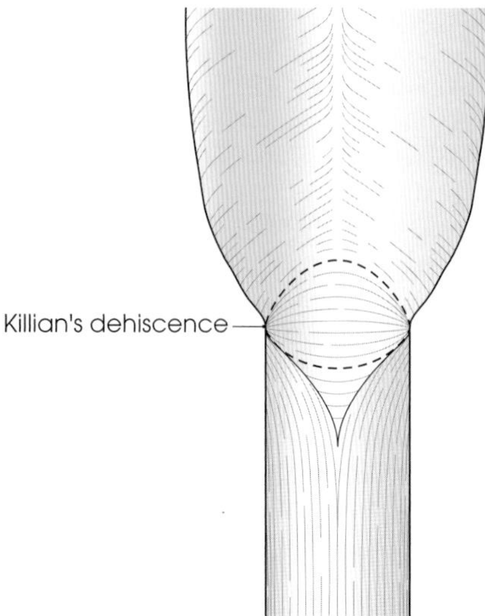

Figure 19.11 Posterior view of pharyngo-oesophageal junction.

to rule out an associated neoplasm and as a treatment to break down the web and relieve dysphagia. Close follow-up is required in all patients because the incidence of postcricoid carcinoma is significant.

PHARYNGEAL POUCH

Pharyngeal pouches are most commonly seen in the elderly, and present with dysphagia associated with regurgitation of undigested foods and consequent weight loss. Pulmonary overspill is a problem, and on occasions hoarseness and chest infections may be the only presenting symptoms. Neoplasia has been reported in less than 1% of pouches.[34] Rarely, a pouch full of fluid may be palpable externally in the neck, producing a squelching sound.

The aetiology of pharyngeal pouches is not known, but pressure studies suggest that there is neuromuscular incoordination resulting in high intraluminal pressure in the pharynx, leading to herniation of the mucosa through its muscular coat. The weakest point is Killian's dehiscence between the thyropharyngeal and cricopharyngeal muscles that make up the inferior constrictor (Fig. 19.11). Barium swallow examination is usually diagnostic (Fig. 19.12). Although pharyngeal pouches may be approached externally, increasingly the treatment of choice is endoscopic stapling.[35]

HYPOPHARYNGEAL NEOPLASIA

Malignancies in this region are almost invariably squamous carcinomas, and the management of patients with these tumours depends on accurate localization of the neoplasm. Assessment requires a thorough clinical examination, barium swallow, and rigid endoscopy of the pharynx and oesophagus. Hypopharyngeal tumours may be missed by flexible gastroscopy.[36] The presence of cervical lymphadenopathy and an assessment of any fixity may also influence the method of treatment. Patients with hypopharyngeal tumours tend to lose weight, and therefore preoperative nutritional support may be valuable.

It is important to recognize at the outset that approximately 25% of hypopharyngeal carcinomas are incurable at presentation. In such cases surgical excision or radiotherapy provides little or no palliation, increases the morbidity of the condition, and does not influence survival.[37] Although each case must be individually assessed, tumours that have spread outside the pharynx, and those associated with bilateral fixed nodes greater than 3 cm in diameter may be considered to be in this category.[38]

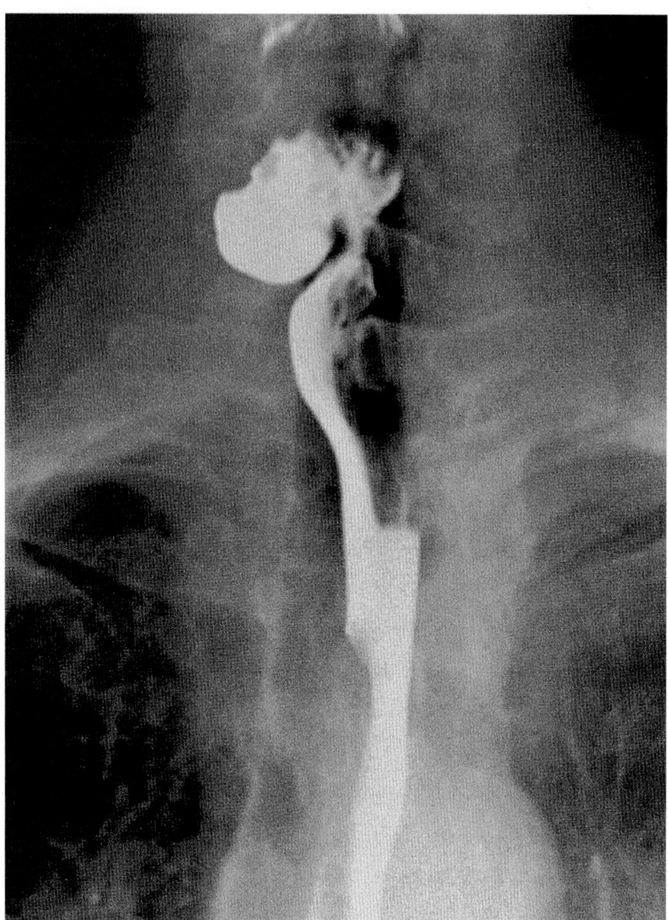

Figure 19.12 Barium swallow of pharyngeal pouch.

Those tumours suitable for primary radiotherapy include vertical tumour length less than 5 cm, mobile vocal folds, and a node-negative neck.[25]

When the tumour is confined to the lateral aspect of the pyriform fossa, a partial pharyngectomy with conservation of the posterior pharyngeal wall and the contralateral pyriform fossa may allow a primary closure.[39] If there is any doubt that a stenosis will result, a vascularized graft should be used to close the defect. If only the posterior pharyngeal wall is involved excision and grafting may suffice. The mainstay of surgical treatment for most hypopharyngeal tumours is total pharyngolaryngectomy and some form of visceral repair. Larger tumours involving the cervical oesophagus will require an oesophagectomy too. In cases where lymph node metastases are present, a contiguous

REFERENCES

34. Huang B, Unni KK, Payne WA. Ann Thor Surg 1984; 38: 207–210
35. Siddiq MA, Sood S, Strachan D. Postgrad Med J 2001; 77: 506–511
36. Fenton JE, Hone S, Gormley P et al. Br Med J 1995; 311: 623
37. Stell PM, Swift AC. In: Kerr AG (ed). Scott-Brown's Otolaryngology. Butterworth, London, 1988
38. Harrison DFN, Thompson AE. Head Neck Surg 1986; 8: 418
39. Ogura JH, Mallen RW. Cancer of the Head and Neck. Appleton-Century-Crofts, St Louis, 1967

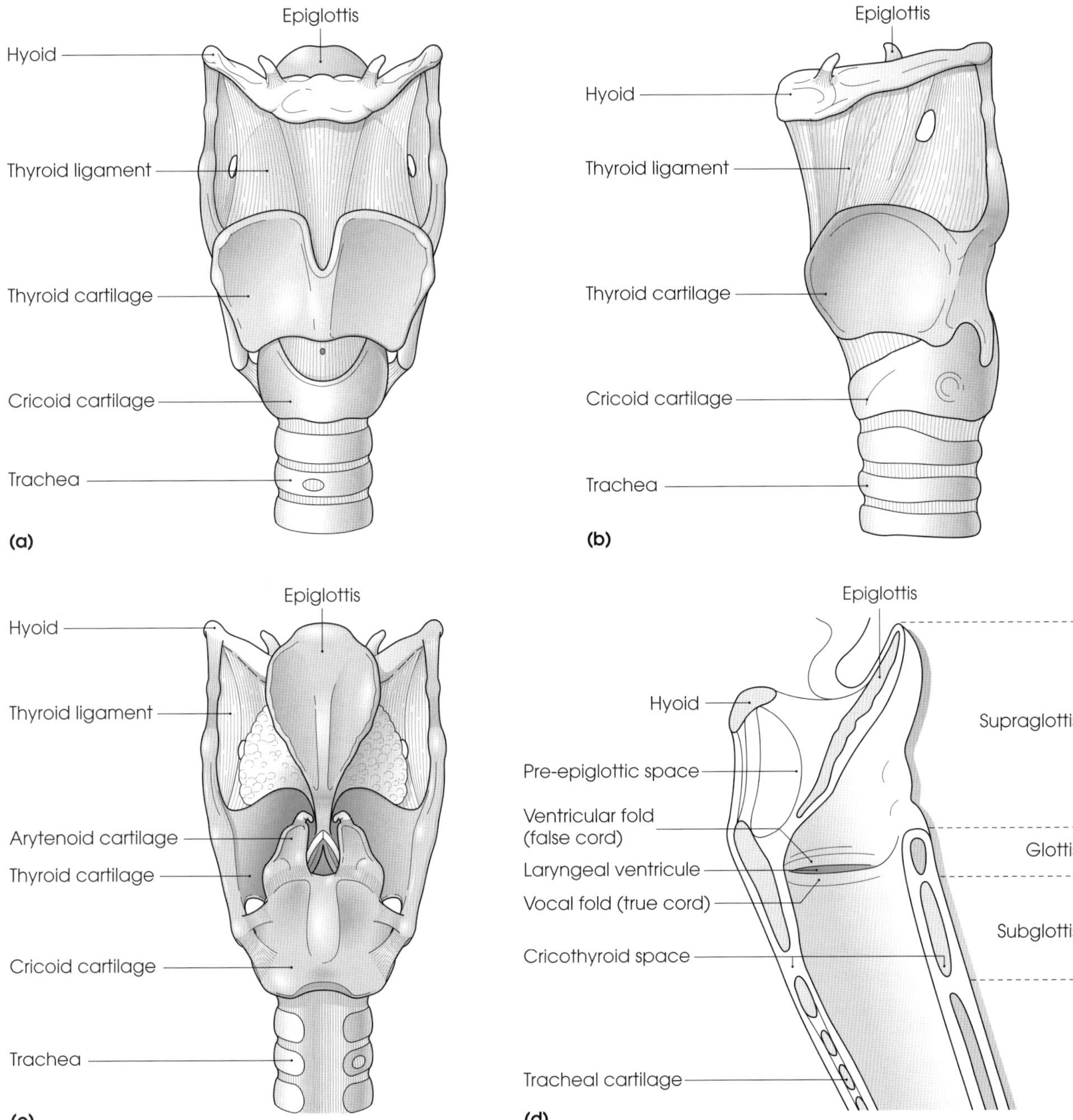

Figure 19.13 The anatomy of the larynx: (**a**) anterior, (**b**) lateral, and (**c**) posterior views; (**d**) sagittal section.

block dissection is indicated. A selective neck dissection may be performed on a node-negative neck. A free jejunal graft is the method of choice for pharyngeal reconstruction.[40] The alternatives include stomach pull-up, colon transplant, and skin flaps that may be either pedicled[41] or free, utilizing a microvascular anastomosis.

THE LARYNX

SURGICAL ANATOMY

The larynx, trachea and bronchi develop embryologically from the foregut in the form of an outpouching.[42] Functionally the larynx is primarily a protective sphincter for the lungs, and only later phylogenetic development results in phonation. The larynx lies in the neck in front of the third to sixth cervical vertebrae. The laryngeal framework or skeleton consists of the hyoid bone, and the thyroid, cricoid, epiglottic and arytenoid cartilages; all these may be seen on a lateral radiograph of the cervical spine. The larynx lies in the hypopharynx, and inferiorly is in continuity with the trachea. It extends superiorly from the free edge of the epiglottis and aryepiglottic folds to the cricoid cartilage inferiorly, and includes the false vocal folds and the true vocal cords (Fig. 19.13).

REFERENCES

40. Shah J. In: Head and Neck Surgery. 2nd edn. Mosby-Wolfe, London, 1996: 235–265
41. Ayshford CA, Walsh RM, Watkinson JC. J Laryngol 113: 145–148
42. Langman J. Medical Embryology. 4th edn. Williams & Wilkins, Baltimore, 1985

The extrinsic muscles of the larynx can broadly be divided into elevators of the larynx—namely the thyrohyoid, stylopharyngeus, palatopharyngeus, mylohyoid, geniohyoid and stylohyoid muscles—and depressors consisting of the sternohyoid, sternothyroid and omohyoid muscles. Such movement is important in deglutition, because elevation and tilting of the larynx allow airway protection by apposing the epiglottis to the aryepiglottic folds, so encouraging the food bolus to pass into the lateral food channels.

The intrinsic muscles may be divided into abductors and adductors of the vocal cords. The posterior cricoarytenoid is the sole abductor of the vocal cord; it arises from the posterior aspect of the cricoid lamina and is inserted into the back of the muscular process of the arytenoids.

The adductors of the larynx are the lateral cricoarytenoid and the transverse and oblique arytenoids. These are supported by the tensors of the vocal cord, the thyroarytenoid (the vocalis), and the cricothyroid muscles. The aryepiglottis and thyroepiglotticus are the muscles that protect the vocal tract during deglutition.

The nerve supply to the larynx is contained in the vagus. The superior laryngeal branch divides into the internal and external laryngeal nerves. The internal branch pierces the cricothyroid membrane above the superior laryngeal artery, and provides sensory input to the larynx above the cords, in addition to having a parasympathetic secretor motor function. The smaller external branch continues down into the inferior constrictor, entering the cricothyroid muscle and acting as its motor nerve. Contraction of the cricothyroid increases the distance between the vocal process of the arytenoid and the thyroid notch, thus increasing the tension of the vocal cord. The recurrent laryngeal nerve on the left leaves the vagus as it crosses the aorta, passing under the arch and the ligamentum arteriosum before ascending again in the groove between the oesophagus and trachea. On the right, the nerve originates from the vagus as it crosses the subclavian artery, passing under the artery to ascend in the tracheo-oesophageal groove. At the lower border of the cricopharyngeus, both nerves pass deeply with the laryngeal branches of the inferior thyroid artery to enter the larynx. The recurrent laryngeal nerve is the motor supply of all muscles of the larynx, with the exception of the cricothyroid.

Stridor is noisy breathing produced by narrowing of the laryngeal airway, has a musical quality, and may be produced on both inspiration and expiration. The common underlying causes are outlined in Table 19.7. In infancy the larynx is proportionally smaller than the adult larynx, and thus small changes in its dimensions may lead to significant reduction in the airway.[43]

Table 19.7 Conditions producing stridor

Lumen	Impacted foreign body
Mural	
Congenital	Laryngeal web Laryngomalacia Subglottic stenosis
Acquired	
Inflammatory	Angioneurotic oedema Granulomas (e.g. Wegener's, sarcoid)
Traumatic/iatrogenic	Post-tracheostomy Postirradiation
Infective	Laryngotracheobronchitis Epiglottitis
Neoplasia	Laryngeal papillomas Malignancy
Extramural	
Traumatic/iatrogenic	Thyroidectomy
Neoplasia	Bronchus, oesophagus, thyroid lymphadenopathy
Neurological	Lower motor neuron disease

CLINICAL EXAMINATION OF THE LARYNX AND ITS FUNCTION

Visualization of the larynx can be by indirect examination with a mirror, direct examination with a rigid endoscope, or more commonly by flexible endoscopy. Stroboscopy provides information about the mucosal wave in the vocal fold mucosal wave. Under general anaesthesia, direct laryngoscopy allows excellent visualization of the larynx. This may be refined using the operating microscope, a technique known as microlaryngoscopy.

ACUTE LARYNGITIS

Acute laryngitis is a complication of the common cold, and is caused by an adenovirus or influenza virus. The condition is self-limiting, and the symptoms consist of hoarseness and paroxysmal cough with sore throat. Resting the voice, abstinence from cigarettes, and soluble aspirin gargles normally control the symptoms.

CHRONIC LARYNGITIS

Hoarseness is usually of insidious onset and may be associated with a discrete attack of laryngitis. Sufferers are most frequently smokers, and there is usually very little accompanying pain. Examination may reveal leukoplakia of the vocal cords, which on histological examination can display a spectrum of epithelial change from simple hyperplasia, with or without cellular atypia, to carcinoma in situ.[44] The term *leukoplakia* thus only indicates the naked-eye appearances of the larynx and not a histological diagnosis.

The most important treatment for chronic laryngitis is removal of the contributory factors, such as tobacco and alcohol. However, because of its chronic nature the epithelial changes may become irreversible, and the condition will respond only to removal of the mucosa using a microlaryngoscopy technique.[45] If the presence of a carcinoma in situ is confirmed on subsequent histology, careful follow-up and review microlaryngoscopy 3 months later are necessary.[44]

VOCAL POLYPS AND NODULES

As a result of poor or excessive voice usage, the vocal cords may develop nodules or become oedematous and develop polyps. Nodules are seen more frequently in children and women, while polyps are more common in adult men. Smoking tends to accentuate any vocal cord trauma. Nodules are usually found at the anterior end of the cord about a third of the way from the

REFERENCES

43. Batch AJB. J Laryngol 1988; 99: 783
44. Helquist H, Lundgren J, Oloffson J. Clin Otolaryngol 1982; 7: 11
45. Kleinsasser O. Microlaryngoscopy and Endolaryngeal Surgery. Saunders, Philadelphia, 1976

anterior commissure. Such lesions can resolve in the acute phase if the voice is rested and re-educated,[46] but larger lesions will require precise surgical removal.

Vocal cord polyps can occur anywhere along the vocal cord, but are frequently seen close to the anterior commissure. Surgery for polyps and nodules may permanently damage or alter the patient's voice, particularly when the lesion is at the anterior commissure because there is a danger that an anterior web may form after surgery.[47]

LARYNGOCELE

When the laryngeal saccule is expanded with air it is termed a *laryngocele*. Any activity that increases intraglottic pressure, such as straining or blowing wind instruments, may cause laryngoceles. These may spread superiorly and present in the false cord (internal laryngocele) or may pass through the thyrohyoid membrane and present as a lump in the neck. Internal laryngoceles can be decompressed through the false cords, but external laryngoceles must be approached through the neck, with the dissection and excision taken as close to their origins as possible.[48]

LARYNGEAL PARALYSIS

Superior laryngeal nerve palsy

Lesions of this nerve are often not recognized clinically unless patients use their voice professionally. A cricothyroid muscle palsy results in a loss of adduction and tension, causing a slightly bowed cord and an asymmetrical larynx (Fig. 19.14b). Compensation usually occurs over time.[49]

Recurrent laryngeal nerve palsy

A unilateral recurrent laryngeal nerve palsy rarely produces inspiratory problems, but because the cords tend to lie in the paramedian position the voice is often seriously compromised, being very breathy and hoarse. As compensation occurs the contralateral vocal cord crosses the midline, probably due to activity of the intra-arytenoid muscle, and the voice disability is reduced (Fig. 19.14c).[50]

The aetiological factors known to cause recurrent laryngeal nerve palsy include injury, surgery (thyroidectomy or thoracic surgery), neoplasm (bronchial and thyroid carcinomas), neurological lesions, infections and inflammations; 40% of cases are idiopathic.[25]

The management of a cord palsy depends on defining the underlying pathology. A significant proportion of idiopathic palsies recover spontaneously, and speech therapy may aid compensation by increasing glottic closure on phonation.[51] In palsies of malignant origin (e.g. carcinoma of the lung), or if at least 9 months have elapsed following surgical damage at thyroidectomy, measures should be taken to obtain glottic closure. Vocal cord injection by Teflon® or collagen can be performed using microlaryngoscopy.[52] The injection is made into the cord just lateral to the vocalis muscle. More recently thyroplasty, the use of a silastic shim, has proved a popular alternative. This is placed through a window in the thyroid cartilage via a small external incision that allows accurate medialization of the cord.[53]

Bilateral recurrent nerve palsy

Damage to the recurrent laryngeal nerve during thyroidectomy is the most common cause of this problem. In the acute phase, often on awaking from the anaesthetic, the patient has a good voice but significant inspiratory stridor. Reintubation is appropriate at this stage, followed by formal appraisal by an ear, nose and throat surgeon. At this time, if the diagnosis is confirmed, laser arytenoidectomy or even tracheostomy may be required (Fig. 19.14d).

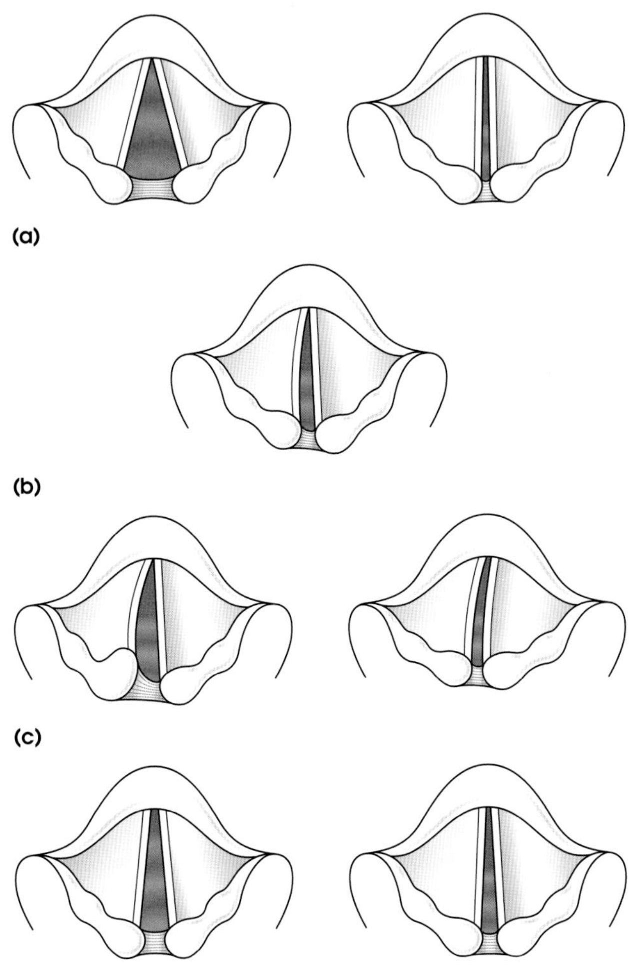

Figure 19.14 (**a**) The normal larynx in abduction (left) and adduction (right). (**b**) Unilateral superior laryngeal nerve palsy in adduction. (**c**) Unilateral recurrent laryngeal nerve palsy: adduction in acute palsy (left) and after compensation (right). (**d**) Bilateral recurrent laryngeal nerve palsy in abduction (left) and adduction (right).

LARYNGEAL TRAUMA

Blunt injuries

Fortunately, the larynx is protected from most injuries by the anterior position of the mandible, which on flexion of the head

REFERENCES

46. Boone H. The Voice and Voice Therapy. 3rd edn. Prentice Hall, New York, 1981
47. Monday LA, Cornut G et al Ann Otol Rhinol Laryngol 1983; 92: 124
48. Stell PM, Maran AGD. J Laryngol 1975; 89: 915
49. Howard DH, Lund VJ. Br Med Bull 1986; 42: 234
50. Dedo H, Urrea RD, Lawson L. Ann Otol Rhinol Laryngol 1973; 82: 661
51. Howard DH. In: Hibbert J (ed). Scott-Brown's Otolaryngology, Vol 5. Butterworth, London, 1997
52. Montgomery WW. Ann Otol 1979; 88: 647
53. Isshiki N. Folia Phoniatrica 1980; 32: 119–154

absorbs most traumatic forces. Thus mandibular fractures are significantly more common than laryngeal fractures. If the larynx is damaged by blunt injury, the cartilage may be crushed against the cervical spine. Surprisingly, symptoms may not develop immediately, stridor appearing only as laryngeal oedema accumulates. When the oesophagus or hypopharynx is damaged surgical emphysema results. Early tracheostomy is required if there is any question of airway obstruction. The anaesthetist should be warned that intubation may be difficult and that tracheostomy, using local anaesthesia, may be necessary. Reconstruction of the larynx demands preservation of as much laryngeal cartilage as possible, and the fixation of the laryngeal skeleton around a solid stent kept in place by stainless steel sutures. Problems may arise if there has been dislocation and rupture of the epiglottis or tearing of the anterior commissure; this can be reconstructed by a keel repair.[54]

Sharp injuries

Stab injuries and self-inflicted knife wounds should be treated by protection of the airway while the haemorrhage is controlled. Induction of anaesthesia in such cases often results in loss of post-traumatic spasm, causing a brisk haemorrhage and loss of the airway.

FOREIGN BODY IN THE LARYNX

The glottis protects the airway by initiating a marked cough reflex, but occasionally a foreign body, often food, still manages to become impacted in the larynx and this may prove fatal. The victim suddenly collapses, perhaps clutching the throat, and quickly becomes cyanosed. Treatment must be immediate. The victim is grasped from behind with the operator's fist placed just below the sternum, and jerked with a strong upward thrust with the intention that the air displaced from the lungs will pop the offending bolus from the larynx (Heimlich's manoeuvre).[55] An alternative, if time and facilities are available, is a cricothyroidotomy.

TUMOURS OF THE LARYNX

Malignant

The great majority of malignant laryngeal tumours are squamous carcinomas developing from the squamous epithelial lining of the vocal cord or from respiratory-type epithelium that has undergone squamous metaplastic change. It often presents early with hoarseness, and a high cure rate is possible.

The annual incidence of laryngeal cancer in the UK is four in 100 000 of the population, which is considerably less than that found in Brazil and the USA (more than 10 per 100 000 of the population), but more than in Japan or Sweden (fewer than three per 100 000). It represents about 1% of all malignancies in the UK. There is usually a long history of cigarette smoking, often combined with alcohol abuse. Men (aged 60–70 years) are affected significantly more frequently than women, in a ratio of 6:1. Hoarseness is the symptom most usually associated with laryngeal cancer; it is always continuous and often progressive. Stridor and dyspnoea are late features.

Examination by indirect laryngoscopy usually reveals the tumour clearly, but a microlaryngoscopy should always be performed and biopsies taken. General anaesthesia in patients with laryngeal cancer may be hazardous, and the anaesthetist should be forewarned to expect a difficult intubation. In some cases an initial tracheostomy must be performed, but this procedure is not without its own problems because airway obstruction may occur when the patient is placed in the supine position, and the tracheostomy must be placed below the tumour's inferior limit.

Inspection of the hypopharynx, upper oesophagus, and trachea must be routine when the larynx is examined under anaesthesia. Biopsies are taken for histology.

Examination of the neck may identify the spread of the tumour in the form of a mass adjacent and fixed to the laryngeal skeleton or as lymph node metastases. Incisional biopsy of the cervical lymphadenopathy associated with clinical laryngeal neoplasia should be avoided, although fine-needle aspiration is useful. Both CT and MRI determine the size and extent of larger laryngeal lesions. Imaging in smaller lesions is not usually required where tumour volume is low and neck metastases are unusual. Staging is performed using the International Union Against Cancer classification based on site, extent and fixation of the lesion. Distant metastases are uncommon, although a synchronous second primary squamous carcinoma in the head and neck occurs in 10% of patients.[37]

Management of laryngeal cancer

Curative treatment usually involves radiotherapy, surgery, or a combination of the two. Chemotherapy in the form of radiosensitizers may be used, but there is no evidence to suggest that preoperative cytotoxic agents either increase survival or decrease morbidity. The aim of a curative treatment must include the preservation of as much normal function as possible. With carcinomas of the larynx this precept is of paramount importance, and this is why radiotherapy is the primary form of treatment in most early lesions (T1 and T2). By contrast, primary surgery is indicated for carcinoma in situ because local excision in the form of vocal cord stripping may be effective. The CO_2 laser may also be used with good effect for this purpose and for the earliest T1 lesions that do not involve the anterior commissure. More extensive surgery should be selected for larger tumours (most T3 and T4 tumours), especially those associated with cervical lymphadenopathy, and for non-squamous carcinomas including adenocarcinomas, chemodectomas and chondrosarcomas, where radiotherapy is less satisfactory or is ineffective.

Following radical radiotherapy, salvage surgery is indicated if the tumour is still present or if it recurs. Although total laryngectomy is by far the most common definitive surgical operation for laryngeal cancer, a range of partial and subtotal laryngectomies is sometimes indicated.[56,57] Five-year survival rates for T1 tumours of the vocal cords exceed 95%. Larger lesions have reduced survival rates, with T3 lesions having corresponding survival rates of 40–70% depending on tumour bulk and treatment modality.[58] Surgical voice restoration following total laryngectomy is now the norm. Surgically created tracheo-oesophageal fistulas are fitted with a one-way valve. Air forced from the lungs through the valve, when the patient occludes the

REFERENCES

54. McNaught RD. Laryngoscope 1950; 60: 264
55. Heimlich HJ. JAMA 1975; 234: 398
56. Stell PM. In: Harrison DFN (ed). Dilemmas in Otorhinolaryngology. Churchill Livingstone, Edinburgh, 1988
57. Robin PE, Olofsson J. In: Hibbert J (ed). Scott-Brown's Otolaryngology, Vol 5. Butterworth, London, 1997
58. Jones AS, Cook JA, Phillips DE et al. Clin Otolaryngol 1992; 17: 433–436

Table 19.8 Indications for tracheostomy

- Emergency: acute upper airway obstruction
- Foreign body
- Infection, inflammation
- Haemorrhage into upper airway
- Elective: protection of the airway when laryngeal and cough reflexes are suppressed.
- Coma
- Neurological disease
- Prolonged ventilation
- Bronchiolar toilet
- To decrease dead space

tracheostome, vibrates the pharynx and proximal oesophagus, producing speech.[59,60]

TRACHEOSTOMY

Tracheostomy may be an emergency or elective procedure. The commonest indications are respiratory and ventilation failure, usually associated with retained bronchial secretions and upper airway obstruction (Table 19.8). It is always important to remember the old surgical rule: 'do a tracheostomy when you think about it; don't wait until it becomes an emergency'.

Surgical technique

Tracheostomy is best performed under general anaesthesia in an operating theatre. The inexperienced surgeon should not be persuaded into performing the operation in an intensive care unit or ward except as a dire emergency; little advantage is gained and complications are more difficult to cope with.

A horizontal skin incision is marked on the skin, midway between the lower edge of the thyroid cartilage (cricoid ring) and the suprasternal notch. In the emergency situation a vertical midline incision may be used, but the surgeon must take care not to veer laterally from the trachea (Fig. 19.15). At all times the surgeon should check the position of the trachea by manual palpation, and thus avoid dissection into the paratracheal space. The thyroid isthmus is divided between clamps and ligated with transfixion sutures. On occasions it may be retracted upwards or downwards. The cricoid ring is identified and retracted upwards by means of a cricoid hook. In children, a vertical incision is made in the second and third tracheal rings; no cartilage is removed. In the adult, a square window is excised between the second and fourth rings, large enough to accept the tracheostomy tube: 30–34 Fg in women, 32–38 Fg in men. At this stage, the anaesthetist should be asked to remove the orotracheal tube slowly from the mouth, and when its distal end moves past the tracheostomy the anaesthetist pauses while the tracheostomy tube, with its obturator inside, is inserted. Haemostasis is achieved, and the tracheostomy tube is securely fastened by means of tapes around the neck tied with the head in flexion. As an additional precaution the flange of the tube may be sewn to the skin by a heavy suture, which can be removed at the first change of tube. The skin incision should only be loosely sutured to avoid surgical emphysema.

Percutaneous tracheostomy has become increasingly popular in the past decade. There are several different techniques available commercially, but most involve the use of a guide wire and dilators to create a tracheostome. Complications include the possibility of false passage and puncture through the side or back wall of the trachea.[62] Risks are minimized by performing simultaneous endoscopic monitoring of the tracheal lumen. The percutaneous technique should be avoided in patients with potential airway obstruction.

Table 19.9 Complications of tracheostomy

Early complications	Late complications
Haemorrhage	Difficult decannulation
Accidental extubation	Tracheocutaneous fistula
Tracheal and paratracheal trauma	Tracheo-oesophageal fistula
Tube lumen obstruction	Tracheoinnominate artery
Subcutaneous emphysema	Haemorrhage
Pneumothorax	Tracheal stenosis
Infection	
Swallowing dysfunction	
Apnoea/death	

Postoperative management

Because the ability to cough is lost, the patient is unable to clear secretions from the tracheobronchial tree; frequent suction is therefore necessary. There is usually no need to change the tracheostomy tube in the first 48 h and, indeed, to change a tube during this period can be positively dangerous because the track has not organized, making replacement of the tube difficult. Crusting frequently occurs as cold dry air thickens the tracheobronchial secretions, and therefore humidified air should be administered either by means of a commercial humidifier or by a regular droplet infusion into the tracheostomy tube. More serious complications can occur in the immediate postoperative period or some time later (Table 19.9).

Tracheostomy tubes

Non-metal

Silastic is the material most frequently used for tracheostomy tubes (Fig. 19.14a). These tubes may be cuffed or uncuffed, and low-pressure cuffs that produce less tracheal pressure are now available.[63] The obturator from the tracheostomy tube should be kept by the patient in case emergency re-intubation is necessary.

Metal tubes

Silver tubes are used for long-term tracheostomy patients. They have an outer and an inner tube, which allows cleaning of the inner tube while maintaining the airway. The inner tube is designed to be slightly longer than the outer tube, thus allowing secretions to be collected on removal of the tube. A third tube, which is placed inside the other two, is fitted with a small flap valve and allows phonation.

REFERENCES

59. Singer MI, Blom ED. Ann Otol 1986; 89: 529
60. Hilgers FJM, Balm AJM. Clin Otol 1993; 18: 517–523
61. Howard DJ. In: MacGregor IA, Howard DJ (eds). Rob and Smith's Operative Surgery. Head and Neck, Part 1. Butterworth, Oxford, 1992
62. Wang MB, Berke GS, Ward PH et al. Ann Otol Rhinol Laryngol 1992; 102: 157–162
63. Sawada Y, Kozima Y, Fonkalsrud E. W Surg Gynecol Obstet 1982; 154: 648

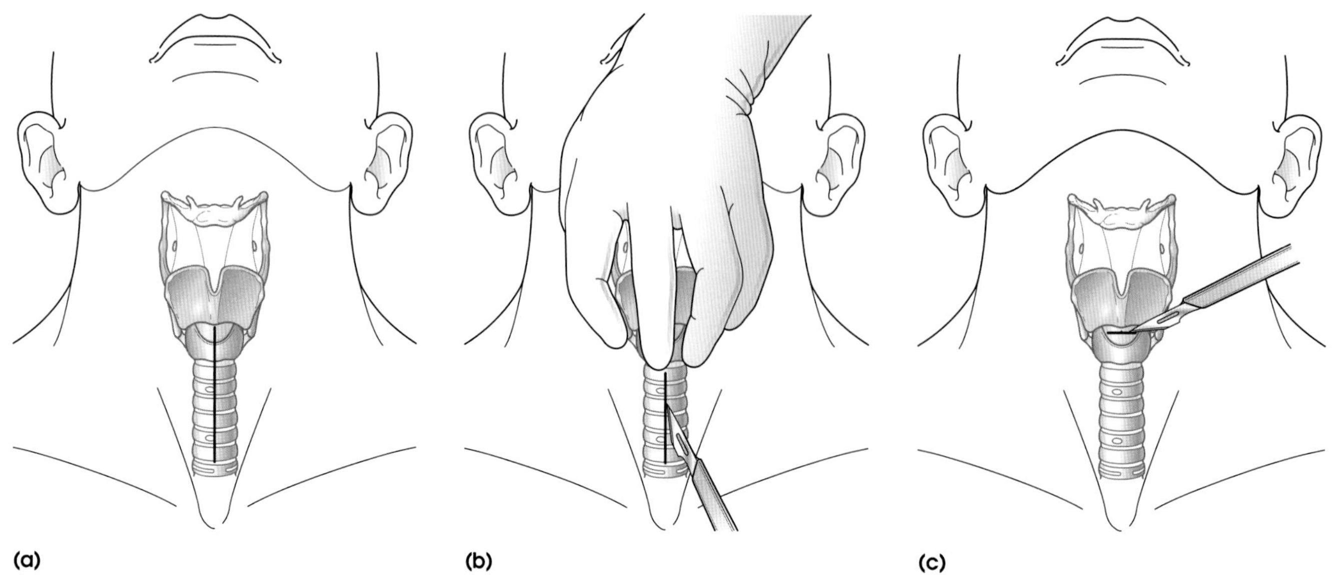

Figure 19.15 (**a**) The position of skin incision in relation to laryngeal landmarks for emergency tracheostomy. (**b**) The position of vertical incision at the level of the second to fourth tracheal rings. (**c**) The position of incision for a cricothyroidotomy (laryngotomy). (After Howard DJ, Emergency and elective airway procedures. In: MacGregor IA, Howard BJ (eds). Rab and Smiths's Operative Surgery. Head and Neck Part I. Oxford: Butterworth-Heinemann, 1992, with permission.[61])

LARYNGOTOMY OR CRICOTHYROTOMY

Emergency entry to the airway in the absence of a previously positioned endotracheal tube is best achieved via the cricothyroid membrane. The thyroid cartilage is steadied and slightly rotated upwards before a scalpel blade is used to make a vertical incision down to and through the cricothyroid membrane. A pair of artery forceps may be inserted to widen the aperture so that a small endotracheal tube may be inserted. Once the airway has been secured, a formal endotracheal intubation or tracheostomy is performed.

MINITRACHEOSTOMY

In cases where tracheobronchial toilet alone is needed, the minitracheostomy is a useful technique. A cricothyrotomy is performed and a small-gauge cannula is railroaded over a flexible introducer. Care should be taken to ensure that the cannula tip has not passed the carina.[64] This technique is not suitable for ventilation except in the very short term.[65]

ACKNOWLEDGEMENT

To the authors of this chapter in previous editions – much of the original work is unchanged.

REFERENCES

64. McGill J, Clinton JE, Ruiz E. Ann Emerg Med 1982; 113: 61
65. Mathews HR, Hopkinson RB. Br J Surg 1982; 71: 147

The oesophagus

20

John Bancewicz, William J. Owen

CONGENITAL OESOPHAGEAL DISORDERS

Oesophageal atresia and tracheo-oesophageal fistula are discussed in Chapter 40.

Dysphagia lusoria is caused by an anomalous subclavian artery or double aortic arch crossing the oesophagus. The aberrant artery can be divided with relief of symptoms.

INJURY

Damage to the oesophagus may arise in various ways, ranging from missile injuries and instrumental injury to damage by drugs or ingested corrosives.

SPONTANEOUS RUPTURE

So-called spontaneous rupture of the oesophagus has been reported many times since Boerhaave of Leiden first reported the case of Baron Wassenaar, Grand Admiral of the Dutch Fleet, a notorious glutton who had cultivated the Roman habit of autoemesis, when, exercising this habit after a meal, he sustained a fatal perforation of the oesophagus just above the diaphragm.[1] Most cases still occur in similar, if less extreme, circumstances. The typical history is that severe pain in the chest or upper abdomen occurs suddenly after an episode of vomiting. This is followed rapidly by cardiovascular collapse as the result of a chemical mediastinitis. When the pain is predominantly in the upper abdomen there is often some degree of abdominal rigidity as well, which may suggest gastroduodenal perforation. Otherwise the condition is most likely to be confused with myocardial infarction or dissecting aneurysm. The tear is usually on the left posterior aspect of the oesophagus just above the cardia. Occasional cases of intra-abdominal rupture have been recorded.

In typical cases subcutaneous emphysema of the neck and upper chest appears, but this is not always marked and may be absent. A chest X-ray usually reveals mediastinal gas or a pleural effusion (Fig. 20.1), but a normal X-ray does not exclude rupture. A contrast swallow (Fig. 20.2) should always be obtained as quickly as possible if the diagnosis is suspected. A delay in making the diagnosis is the greatest single factor contributing to a poor prognosis.

Primary repair is the treatment of choice and should be carried out within a few hours of the rupture. The mortality can be as low as 10%,[2] but may be four or five times this level if the diagnosis is delayed.[3]

PENETRATING INJURY

Penetrating injuries of the oesophagus are uncommon, even in war, as other intrathoracic organs present a much larger target (see Ch. 7). Bullets and knives are the usual implements, but chest drains may occasionally be responsible.[4] By far the largest experience in modern times is reported in the American and South African literature.[5,6] The management is obviously affected by the presence of injury to other organs (see Ch. 7). In the case of missile injuries, especially with high-velocity missiles, there may be a considerable amount of shock-wave damage to surrounding tissues that is not apparent on gross inspection. In such circumstances generous resection may be the only option available. Continuity may be restored by oesophagogastric anastomosis. More complex reconstructions, for example by colonic interposition, should not be attempted in emergency cases.

INSTRUMENTAL PERFORATION

Instrumentation of the upper gastrointestinal tract is the commonest cause of perforation of the oesophagus. The old rigid oesophagoscope could perforate the oesophagus in its upper part, especially in a patient with prominent osteophytes in the

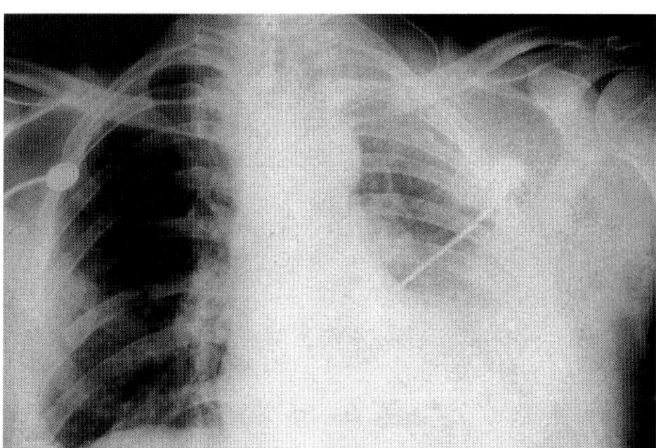

Figure 20.1 Pleural effusion following oesophageal perforation.

REFERENCES

1. Boerhaave H. Atroces, Nec Descripti Primus. Morbi Historia. Secundem Artes Legis Conscripta. Lugdini Batavorum Boutesteniana, Medici, 1724
2. Jones WG II, Ginsberg RJ. Esophageal perforation: a continuing challenge. Ann Thorac Surg 1992; 53: 534–543
3. Reeder LB, DeFilippi VJ, Ferguson MK. Current results of therapy for esophageal perforation. Am J Surg 1995; 169: 615–617
4. Clifford PC. An unusual oesophageal perforation during intercostal drainage for empyema. Br J Surg 1980; 67: 451–452
5. Asensio JA, Chahwan S, Forno W et al. J Trauma. 2001; 50: 289–296
6. Degiannis E, Benn CA, Leandros E et al. Surgery 2000; 128: 54–58

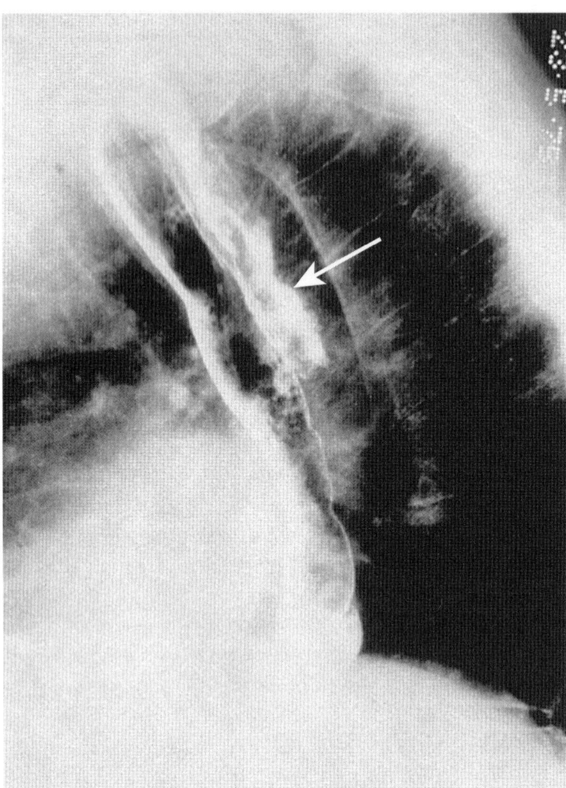

Figure 20.2 Oesophageal perforation (arrow).

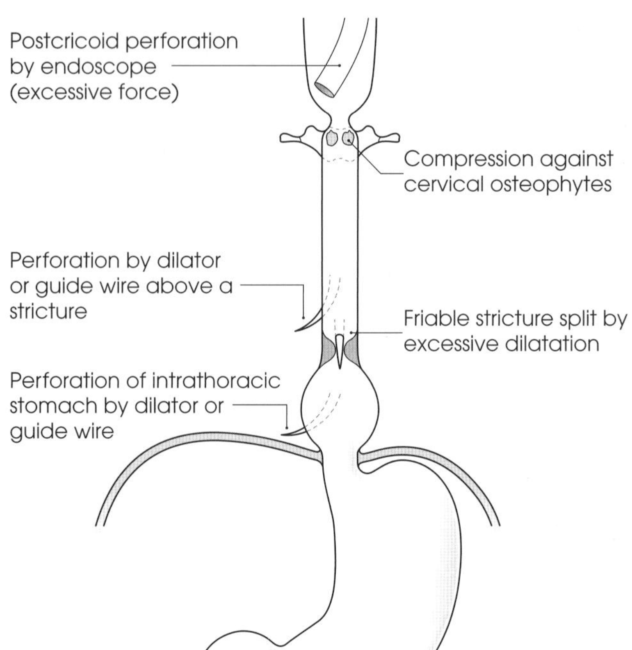

Figure 20.3 Mechanisms responsible for instrumental perforation of the oesophagus.

cervical spine (Fig. 20.3). This is much less common with a modern flexible endoscope, but it is possible to perforate the pharynx above cricopharyngeus, especially in elderly patients whose tissues are friable. The thoracic or occasionally the abdominal oesophagus is more commonly injured during dilatation of strictures or pneumatic dilatation for achalasia. Passage of dilators over a guide wire is normally safe, but only if the wire is correctly placed and its position does not change during instrumentation.

Endo-oesophageal intubation for carcinoma may split a friable growth, but the leak is usually sealed by the stent. It is now well recognized that dilatation of a tumour is potentially dangerous and this should be kept to a minimum.

FOREIGN BODY PERFORATION

Foreign bodies of many sorts, including pins, dentures and other implements, can be retrieved safely from the oesophagus. Perforation may, however, occur during their removal and a foreign body that has been left in situ for several days may erode through the oesophageal wall.

PATHOLOGICAL PERFORATION

Pathological perforation of the oesophagus is unusual, but peptic ulcers and neoplasms may cause free perforation into the mediastinum or pleural cavity. Erosion into the aorta or even the ventricle may occur, with rapidly fatal results.[7] Carcinomas, of course, more commonly cause tracheo-oesophageal fistulas, which are discussed separately (see *Carcinoma of the oesophagus* section, p. 449).

MEDIASTINITIS

Following oesophageal perforation the loose areolar tissues of the posterior mediastinum allow rapid spread of gastrointestinal contents. Mediastinitis is a very dangerous condition that produces marked systemic disturbance and cardiovascular collapse. Cardiac dysrhythmias are common.

The clinical signs of mediastinitis are those of severe systemic sepsis, but there is usually a more marked tachycardia than the patient's condition would appear to indicate. Atrial fibrillation is the commonest dysrhythmia and may seriously interfere with cardiac output in an already compromised patient. There are few specific clinical signs, but a mediastinal 'crunch' may be heard on auscultation if gas is present around the pericardium. The crunching, which sounds like footsteps in soft snow, occurs in synchrony with the heart sounds.

DIAGNOSIS

Awareness of the possibility of perforation is the most important aspect of diagnosis. Any upset or pain following oesophageal instrumentation should raise the suspicion of perforation. Severe chest or abdominal pain following an episode of vomiting is likewise suggestive of perforation.

Investigation has two purposes: first, to demonstrate the perforation, and second, to look for other oesophageal pathology that may influence treatment. A chest X-ray may show subcutaneous gas, mediastinal gas, a pleural effusion or a pneumothorax, depending on the site and size of the perforation and whether it communicates with the pleural cavity. A contrast swallow is almost always required to provide firm proof of the diagnosis, to demonstrate the extent of the problem, and to provide good anatomical definition of the injured oesophagus that may aid rational management. For this purpose barium is preferred to water-soluble contrast media, which produce indifferent pictures. Contrary to popular opinion, barium is not harmful in such

REFERENCES

7. Ming SC. In: Atlas of Tumor Pathology, Series 2, Fascicle 7. Armed Forces Institute of Pathology, Washington, 1973

circumstances provided that it is used in moderation.[8] If a water-soluble contrast medium is used it should be a non-ionic preparation that, unlike Gastrografin, is not harmful to the respiratory tree when aspirated.

Occasionally, careful endoscopy is required in the presence of an established perforation to give additional anatomical or pathological information.

TREATMENT OF OESOPHAGEAL PERFORATION

There is still controversy and even confusion about the best management of oesophageal perforation. The factors that determine the outcome are the size of the perforation, the degree of contamination (the septic load), cardiovascular collapse, communication with the pleural cavity, the general condition and previous health of the patient, the presence of other oesophageal pathology, and the interval between perforation and treatment. Delayed diagnosis is the commonest reason for a poor outcome, and failure to think of the possibility of oesophageal rupture is the main reason for diagnostic error. Paradoxically, the outlook is better in those who are not diagnosed for 48 h or more.[9] This is presumably the self-selection of those with the capacity for survival.

Recommended forms of management range from conservative treatment with intravenous fluids and antibiotics to total oesophagectomy. The range of options is given below.

- Antibiotics and intravenous fluids combined with restriction of oral intake.
- As above, plus pleural drainage using a percutaneous drain or thoracotomy.
- Primary repair.
- Exclusion of the oesophagus and drainage of the chest (Fig. 20.4).
- Oesophageal resection with immediate or delayed reconstruction.

Good results have been claimed for all these methods, but not all are applicable in every situation. Conservative treatment is appropriate for small perforations that are diagnosed promptly, have a small septic load (e.g. following instrumental perforation in a starved patient), and do not produce severe systemic disturbance, particularly if the perforation is confined to the mediastinum. Occasionally perforation will not be diagnosed until several days after the event, when nothing more than drainage of an empyema is feasible, but this is rare.

A reasonably safe general rule is that the worse the systemic effect of the perforation, the greater is the need for a surgical solution. Simple closure of the perforation is an effective form of management provided that it is performed within 12 h and, ideally, sooner. Repair may be impossible if the diagnosis is delayed, because of the condition of the tissues and the problem of wound healing in the presence of sepsis.

When repair is attempted it should be remembered that the defect in the mucosa is often longer than the defect in the muscle. The first stage, therefore, is to incise the muscle layer so that the edges of the mucosa can be clearly seen and sutured, preferably in layers. The repair may be strengthened by applying a flap of intercostal muscle, diaphragm,[10] or the adjacent fundus of the stomach.[11] Only normal oesophageal tissue should be closed, otherwise resection should be considered.

Treatment by exclusion and drainage (Fig. 20.4) has been advocated for perforations that are diagnosed late and associated with heavy contamination.[12] Many other ingenious methods for exclusion and drainage have been reported using a variety of tubes. The object is always the same, namely to drain the chest and divert salivary and gastric secretion away from the perforation. A difficult perforation should be preferentially repaired by closing the oesophagus around a T tube and draining the mediastinum. Subtotal oesophagectomy with construction of a cervical oesophagostomy and a gastrostomy is the ultimate treatment for the extreme situation. Continuity can then be restored several months later, usually by substernal transposition of the stomach.

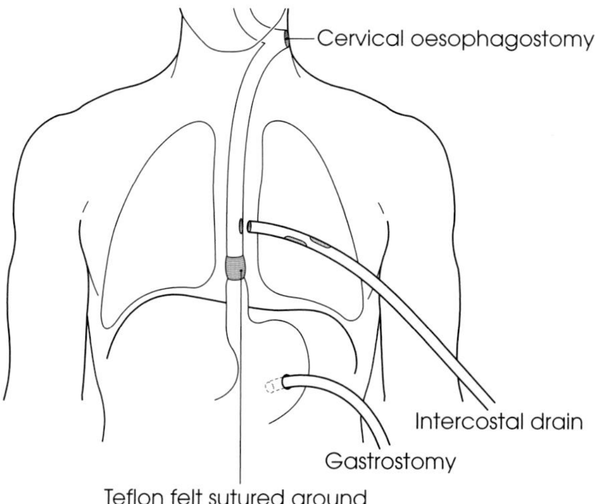

Figure 20.4 Exclusion of the oesophagus for perforation.

MALLORY–WEISS SYNDROME

Mucosal tears at the cardia are quite common during prolonged or violent vomiting.[13] They present with haematemesis, usually of a modest degree. Endoscopy reveals a short longitudinal tear in the mucosa usually just distal to the cardia, or in the lower oesophagus just above the cardia. Some patients may develop chest pain, which raises the suspicion of complete rupture. Occasionally the bleeding may be so severe as to require surgical exploration (by laparotomy) and over-sewing, but this is rare. Endoscopic injection or clipping is now the treatment of choice for dealing with severe bleeding.[14]

REMOVAL OF FOREIGN BODIES

Impacted foreign bodies, ranging from fishbone to false teeth, may present a considerable challenge to remove. There is no place for conservative management—at least not for more than a few hours. Fishbone and coins are not usually difficult to remove, but open safety pins and dentures may tax the skills of even the most experienced endoscopist. In general, the fibre-optic gastroscope is the best tool and an over-tube is useful (Fig. 20.5). Most foreign bodies can be removed with simple grasping

REFERENCES

8. Foley MJ, Ghahremani GG, Rogers LF. Radiology 1982; 144: 231–237
9. Banks JG, Bancewicz J. Br J Surg 1981; 68: 580–584
10. Westaby S. Br J Surg 1980; 67: 801–803
11. Thal AP. Ann Surg 1969; 168: 542–550
12. Urschel HC Jr, Razzuk MA, Wood RE et al. Ann Surg 1974; 179: 587–591
13. Mallory GK, Weiss S. Am J Med Sci 1929; 178: 506–515
14. Huang SP, Wang HP, Lee YC et al. Gastrointest Endosc 2002; 55: 842–846

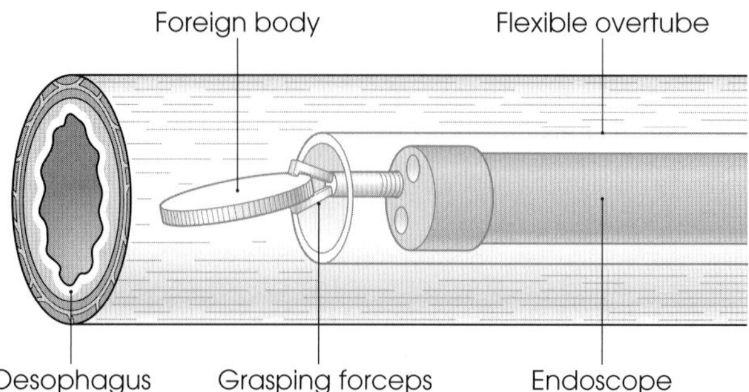

Figure 20.5 Removal of foreign body from the oesophagus using an over-tube and video-endoscope.

forceps, but dentures may need to be broken into small pieces with a cutter that can only be passed down a rigid endoscope. The classic problem is that of the open safety pin; the solution was elegantly discussed by Chevalier Jackson.[15] If the point is downwards, the pin may be held by forceps while the oesophagoscope (or over-tube) is advanced over the pin. If the point faces upwards, the pin can sometimes be pushed into the stomach and then drawn into the tube or endoscope. Alternatively, it may be turned in the oesophagus. This has to be done with a rigid endoscope and grasping forceps. In this manoeuvre the spring of the pin is grasped and moved to one side of the oesophagus. Continued lateral pressure is applied to widen the lumen and the instruments are carefully withdrawn.

CORROSIVE INJURY

Ingested corrosives are highly damaging to the upper gastrointestinal tract. The most commonly taken are caustic soda (lye) or sulphuric acid from car batteries in attempted suicide.[16] Bleach may be drunk by young children. All these agents can cause extensive damage to the pharynx, larynx, oesophagus and stomach. Usually the pharynx is relatively spared because of the short contact time, but oedema of the laryngopharynx may produce respiratory difficulty.

The oesophagus takes the brunt of the injury, especially with caustic soda, and it may even perforate at a very early stage. More often there is severe mucosal and submucosal injury that later gives rise to strictures. The stomach is relatively protected because its contents dilute whatever has been swallowed. Gastric acid will also neutralize at least some of any ingested alkali. Despite this, injury to the stomach may occur with perforation within a few hours or up to 3 weeks after the injury. Later on, part or all of the stomach may contract if the injury has been severe.

The management of caustic injuries has been well reviewed by Bremner and Wright.[17] Early endoscopy within a few hours of injury is the key. A fine video-endoscope is passed by an experienced operator to inspect the whole of the oesophagus and stomach if possible. Complete endoscopy should not be attempted if there is a severe necrotizing lesion, and air insufflation is kept to a minimum. Patients with minor injuries may be discharged early. Those with severe mucosal damage should be treated with steroids for 3 weeks and then begin a programme of regular oesophageal dilatation.

Early resection should be undertaken if full-thickness oesophageal necrosis is suspected.

DRUG-INDUCED INJURY

Medication may injure the oesophagus, both by direct irritation and by its pharmacological effects. Many tablets and capsules lie in the oesophagus for long periods, especially if swallowed in the recumbent position without an adequate drink.[18] Release of irritant constituents in the oesophagus may then cause local damage, giving rise to pain, dysphagia and even stricture formation.[19]

Smooth muscle relaxants may induce gastro-oesophageal reflux and hence injure the oesophagus. They may also reduce the effectiveness of peristalsis and increase the risk of direct mucosal injury. For these reasons a full drug history must be taken from all patients with oesophageal symptoms, especially elderly patients.

RADIATION INJURY

Radiotherapy for cancers of the oesophagus itself and the lung or the breast may produce oesophageal damage. Usually the injury is slight, but considerable dysphagia and odynophagia (painful swallowing) can occur. Inspection of the oesophagus usually reveals very little in the way of gross mucosal injury. Treatment is essentially supportive until the injury has subsided.

By contrast, radiation-induced strictures following treatment of oesophageal cancer may be troublesome.[20] They are often resistant to dilatation, may conceal a local recurrence,[21] and may require resection if the patient's condition will permit. Resection, however, may be a technical challenge because of extensive radiation fibrosis.

NASOGASTRIC INTUBATION

Prolonged nasogastric intubation may occasionally cause an oesophageal stricture. Whether this happens in a normal oesophagus is open to debate.[22] Most of those afflicted have pre-existing reflux disease and intubation simply aggravates matters. The upper oesophageal sphincter may also be rendered incompetent by intubation. This may increase the risk of aspiration pneumonia.

DISORDERS OF THE PHARYNGO-OESOPHAGEAL JUNCTION

There are several conditions that may affect the pharyngo-oesophageal junction and cause dysphagia. Tumours and webs will not be mentioned here as they are discussed in Chapter 19. In practice, dysphagia arising from disorders of the upper oesophagus is often misdiagnosed and may be wrongly labelled as hysterical dysphagia. True psychogenic dysphagia is extremely rare and usually presents as obvious delusions about the act of swallowing.

REFERENCES

15. Jackson C. Ann Otol Rhinol Laryngol 1924; 33: 1009–1179
16. Paul ATS. Surgery (Oxford) 1987; 49: 1156–1159
17. Bremner CE, Wright NC. In: Hennessy TPJ, Cuschieri A (eds). Surgery of the Oesophagus. Baillière Tindall, London, 1992
18. Channer K, Virjee J. Br Med J 1982; 285: 1702
19. Heller SR, Fellows IW, Ogilvie AL et al. Br Med J 1982; 285: 167–168
20. Hennessy TP. Br J Surg 1988; 75: 193–194
21. Xian Zhi Gu. In: Huang GJ, K'ai WY (eds). Carcinoma of the Esophagus and Gastric Cardia. Springer Verlag, Berlin, 1984: 257–274
22. Banfield WJ, Hurwitz AL. Arch Intern Med 1974; 134: 1083–1086

FUNCTIONAL DISORDERS

Three types of problem may be encountered:

1. Diminished pharyngeal propulsion.
2. Relaxation anomalies.
3. Incoordination.

Diminished pharyngeal propulsion

Diminished pharyngeal propulsion is essentially a neurological problem. Motor neuron disease and myaesthenia gravis are the best known conditions that produce swallowing difficulty by reducing the power of pharyngeal propulsion. Oculopharyngeal muscular dystrophy is an inherited condition that is mainly confined to French Canadians.[23]

Cerebrovascular accidents may also interfere with pharyngeal power if the ninth, 10th or 12th cranial nerves are involved, but in addition there is usually a severe disturbance of coordination of the act of swallowing.

Treatment is that of the underlying condition. Cricopharyngeal myotomy has a small part to play in palliative management.[24] Provided that some pharyngeal power is preserved, myotomy reduces the resistance of the upper sphincter and may improve swallowing.

Relaxation anomalies

Relaxation anomalies are uncommon and masquerade under a variety of unsatisfactory names, such as cricopharyngeal bar and upper oesophageal achalasia.[24,25] Little is known of their nature, but Cruse and colleagues have described chronic inflammatory changes in the cricopharyngeus muscle in a small number of patients.[26] This seems to produce stiffening of the muscle, which cannot open up to allow food to pass. Cine or video barium studies are the most helpful form of investigation. The commonest finding is a prominent indentation posteriorly at the level of the cricopharyngeus (Fig. 20.6). Endoscopy is essential to exclude a post-cricoid carcinoma. Sometimes the resistance is so severe that it can actually be felt with an endoscope or a dilator.

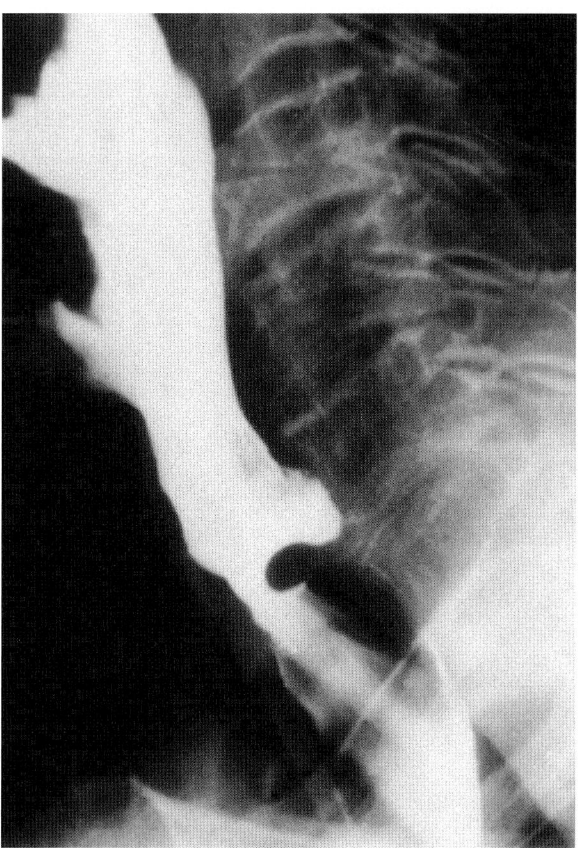

Figure 20.6 Cricopharyngeal bar.

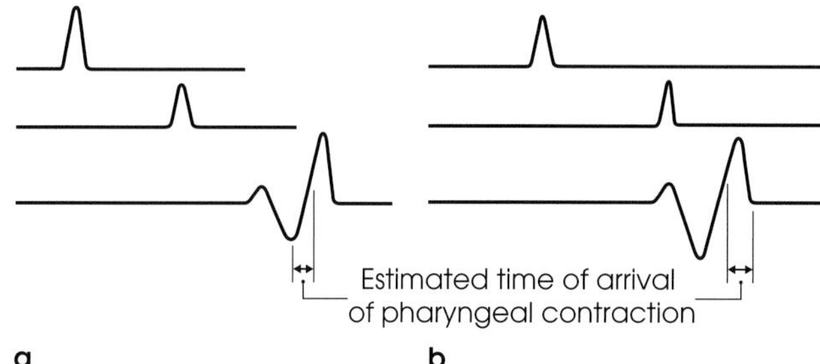

Figure 20.7 Cricopharyngeal incoordination. (**a**) Coordinate response; (**b**) incoordinate response.

Cricopharyngeal myotomy is usually very successful in the management of these conditions.[25–27]

Incoordination

Normally the upper oesophageal sphincter relaxes in time with the arriving pharyngeal contraction to allow food to enter the upper oesophagus. Dysphagia may occur if this response is disturbed (Fig. 20.7). Gross incoordination in swallowing is common following strokes and may occur in other neurological conditions.

Treatment is again directed at the underlying condition, and a speech therapist may be able to help. In severe cases a feeding gastrostomy or jejunostomy is usually required.

PHARYNGEAL (ZENKER'S) DIVERTICULUM[28]

A pharyngeal diverticulum is an out-pouching of mucosa first observed by Ludlow in 1767.[29] It protrudes from the back of the pharynx through Killian–Jamieson's dehiscence just above the cricopharyngeus muscle (Fig. 20.8). Large diverticula may extend into the mediastinum, reaching as low as the arch of the aorta. The reason why diverticula occur has been the subject of speculation for many years. Most agree that they are likely to be the result of a chronic functional obstruction at the upper sphincter.[30] Establishing this as fact, however, has been impossible. Some report a high incidence of cricopharyngeal incoordination,[31] while others deny this.[32] The most convincing

REFERENCES

23. Duranceau AC, Beauchamp G, Jamieson GG et al. Surg Clin North Am 1983; 63: 825–832
24. Duranceau AC, Jamieson GG, Beauchamp G. Surg Clin North Am 1983; 63: 833–839
25. Belsey R. Thorac Cardiovasc Surg 1966; 52: 164–188
26. Cruse JP, Edwards DA, Smith JF et al. Histopathology 1979; 3: 223–232
27. Blakeley WR, Garety EJ, Smith DE. Arch Surg 1968; 96: 745–762
28. Zenker FA, Ziemssen H. In: Zeimssen H (ed). Handbuch des Speciellen Pathologie und Therapie, Vol 7 (Suppl). FCW Vogel, Leipzig, 1877: 1–208
29. Ludlow A. Med Obs Inq 1767; 3: 85–97
30. Payne WS, King RM. Surg Clin North Am 1983; 63: 815–824
31. Ellis FH Jr, Schlegel JF, Lynch VP et al. Ann Surg 1969; 170: 340–349
32. Knuff TE, Benjamin SB, Castell DO. Gastroenterology 1982; 82: 734–736

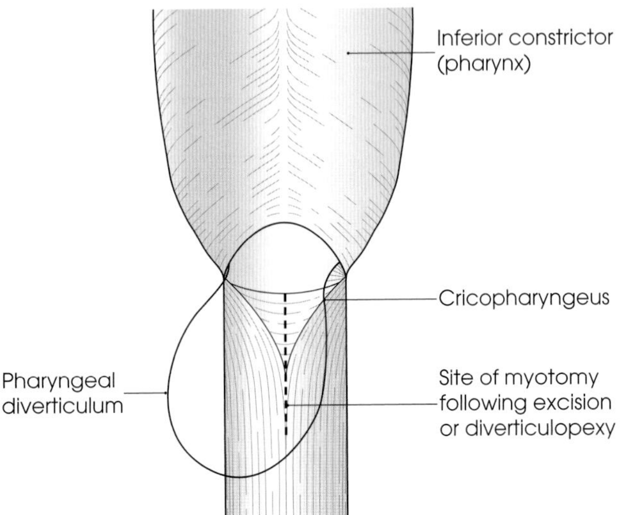

Figure 20.8 Pharyngeal diverticulum presents posteriorly and (usually) to the left.

explanation is that there may be an inflammatory degeneration in the cricopharyngeus muscle with a change in its elastic and contraction properties, i.e. similar to the relaxation anomalies mentioned earlier.[33,34] Diverticula may also be associated with severe symptoms even when they are small.

There are two classic problems in diagnosis. First, a diverticulum can be ruptured during injudicious endoscopy,[35] and second, carcinomas may arise within the diverticulum itself, although this is really quite rare.[36] A barium swallow should be obtained before endoscopy if a pharyngeal diverticulum is suspected.

The classic treatment is excision combined with a crico-pharyngeal myotomy. Small diverticula may be left and treated by myotomy alone. Belsey has suggested that large diverticula may be dealt with by myotomy and diverticulopexy so that the inverted pouch does not fill with food.[25] Dohlman and Mattsson described an endoscopic procedure in which the septum between the diverticulum and the oesophagus is divided by diathermy.[37] The modern version of this is to use a laparoscopic linear cutter staple gun inserted via a short bivalved pharyngoscope.[38,39] It is common to have slight residual dysphagia with this method, but it is a simple procedure with minimal complications.

GASTRO-OESOPHAGEAL REFLUX

AETIOLOGY

An association between sliding hiatus hernia, gastro-oesophageal reflux and symptoms was first described by Allison in 1951,[40] but it is now known that the presence or absence of a hiatus hernia is not the only determinant of reflux. The competence of the gastro-oesophageal junction depends on a combination of normal anatomy, the pressure and length of the lower oesophageal sphincter, particularly the intra-abdominal length,[41] and the occurrence of transient relaxations of the lower oesophageal sphincter.[42] It is important to distinguish *physiological reflux* that occurs mainly after meals from *pathological reflux*, often referred to as *gastro-oesophageal reflux disease*, that causes symptoms. Duodenogastric reflux, occurring especially after gastric resection, may promote reflux of alkaline duodenal contents into the oesophagus. Gastric outlet obstruction may raise intragastric pressure and encourage acid to reflux into the oesophagus.

CLINICAL FEATURES

Reflux symptoms are remarkably common in westernized countries, occurring in up to a quarter of individuals in the community.[43] The typical epigastric and retrosternal burning pains of reflux are well recognized. There are other modes of presentation that may give rise to difficulty in diagnosis and these are therefore enumerated.

1. Anginal-type chest pain, as some patients have reflux symptoms that are strongly related to exercise. The diagnosis may be made by pH monitoring while they exercise on a treadmill.[44] Up to one-third of patients admitted to hospital with suspected cardiac pain have been found to have an oesophageal problem, but it must be emphasized that there are many potential causes of chest pain in patients with angiographically normal coronary arteries.[45] The association between chest pain and reflux needs to be checked carefully in individual patients.
2. Painful swallowing (odynophagia) that is experienced particularly when swallowing hot beverages, citrus drinks or spirits.
3. The reflux of food, which is often confused with vomiting. The clue is that reflux is effortless and provoked by bending or lying down, whereas vomiting involves a powerful contraction of the abdominal wall muscles.
4. Pulmonary aspiration may result in nocturnal coughing, early morning hoarseness, and a clinical picture akin to asthma. The association between respiratory symptoms and nocturnal acid reflux can be documented with pH monitoring, but there is still controversy about the nature of the association and its relevance to treatment.[46,47]

REFERENCES

33. Lerut T, Guelinckz P, Dom R et al. In: Siewert JR, Holscher AH (eds). Diseases of the Esophagus. Springer-Verlag, Berlin, 1988: 1018
34. Lerut T, van Raemdonck D, Guelinckz P et al. In: Little AG, Ferguson MK, Skinner DB (eds). Diseases of the Esophagus, Vol 2. Futura, New York, 1990, 313–323
35. Triggiani E, Belsey R. Thorax 1977; 32: 241–249
36. Wychulis AR, Gunnlaugsson GH, Clagett OT. Surgery 1969; 66: 976–979
37. Dohlman G, Mattsson O. Arch Otolaryngol 1960; 71: 744–752
38. Collard JM, Otte JB, Kestens PJ. Ann Thorac Surg 1993; 56: 573–576
39. Sommer KD, Ahrens KH, Reichenbach M et al. Laryngorhinootologie 2001; 80: 470–477
40. Allison PR. Surg Gynecol Obstet 1951; 92: 419–431
41. DeMeester TR, Wernly JA, Bryant GH et al. Am J Surg 1979; 137: 39–46
42. Dodds WJ, Dent J, Hogan WJ et al. N Engl J Med 1982; 307: 1547–1552
43. Jones RH, Lydeard SE, Hobbs FD et al. Gut 1990; 31: 401–405
44. Schofield PM, Bennett DH, Whorwell PJ et al. Br Med J 1987; 294: 1459–1461
45. Cook RA, Anggiansah A, Smeeton NC et al. Br Heart J 1994; 72: 231–236
46. Pellegrini CA, DeMeester TR, Johnson LF et al. Surgery 1979; 86: 110–119
47. Field SK. Can Respir J 2000; 7: 167–176

DIAGNOSIS

No test is infallible, but a carefully taken history is essential. Odynophagia is a good pointer towards reflux. The effects of posture on symptoms, the beneficial effects of antacids, and the acidic taste of refluxed material into the mouth are also helpful indicators.

Radiology

A routine barium swallow is not a particularly accurate test for reflux, and it cannot be recommended for this purpose.[48] Barium radiology can, however, be a sensitive and accurate test for reflux if there is strict quality control and a standard protocol is followed.[49] This ideal is not often attained in practice. Barium radiology can also give useful anatomical information about the presence of a pharyngeal pouch, stricture or hiatus hernia.

Endoscopy

In routine clinical practice endoscopy is the most frequent investigation for suspected reflux. The earliest sign of reflux oesophagitis is the presence of small, discrete, linear erosions extending up from the squamocolumnar junction. Later, these erosions become confluent and involve the entire circumference of the oesophagus. Stricture or frank ulceration represents a more advanced stage of oesophagitis. Mucosal hyperaemia is not a reliable sign of reflux, and it should be remembered that endoscopy is normal in at least half of the patients with proven gastro-oesophageal reflux. Mucosal biopsies taken with a suction biopsy capsule 5 cm above the gastro-oesophageal junction may show the characteristic hyperplasia of the basal zone and elongation of the papillae.[50] However, standard pinch biopsies are too small to be accurate, and even a normal suction biopsy does not rule out the disease because biopsies are normal in approximately 20% of those with reflux.

Oesophageal pH recording

In 1969, Spencer introduced pH monitoring of the oesophagus.[51] Ambulatory 24-h recording of oesophageal pH is now generally accepted as the most accurate method for diagnosing reflux. It is, however, an uncomfortable and relatively expensive investigation that is used only in cases in which resolution of diagnostic doubt is important, for example before performing surgery for reflux. The pH probe is positioned 5 cm above the lower oesophageal sphincter and connected to a recorder. Patients are then told to resume their daily activities but to avoid acidic drinks; they are asked to keep a diary of symptoms and events for the duration of the test. The results are expressed as the number and duration of reflux episodes over 24 h. An abnormal result is indicated by a pH of less than 4 for more than 3% of the time, when patients are supine, and for more than 8% of the time when they are erect.[52] The DeMeester scoring system incorporates supine and erect reflux, the total number of reflux episodes, the duration of the longest episode, and the number of episodes lasting more than 5 min. It can be calculated automatically by most modern computerized recording systems and is useful in clinical practice.

Bernstein test

The Bernstein acid perfusion test is useful in confirming that the pain described by a patient arises from the oesophagus. Hydrochloric acid (0.1 mol/L) is perfused at the rate of 6 mL/min into the oesophagus through a tube, the tip of which is positioned 5 cm above the gastro-oesophageal junction. The response to acid is compared with that to saline, which is used as a control solution. Acid perfusion reproduces the symptoms of oesophagitis in approximately 70% of those with reflux.

Oesophageal manometry

Oesophageal manometry plays only a minor role in the routine evaluation of reflux, although of course it is the investigation of choice in the assessment of motility disturbances. Much has been made of the importance of preoperative motility assessment to allow 'tailoring' of antireflux operations, but this concept has not been supported by recent studies (see *Tailored antireflux surgery*, p. 441).

COMPLICATIONS

Oesophageal stricture

Strictures occur in approximately 10% of patients with gastro-oesophageal reflux and their frequency increases with age. With modern high-resolution video-endoscopy the gross appearances of benign and malignant strictures can be distinguished quite reliably, but it is always best to be sceptical and take generous biopsies. A short history of progressive or total dysphagia favours the latter. It is important to stress that negative biopsies do not necessarily exclude malignancy, and suspicious gross appearances should trigger further investigation. The inflammation may be mucosal or transmural, and a particularly tight stricture may develop after prolonged nasogastric aspiration in association with reflux, which may be resistant to dilatation therapy. Rarer causes that must be considered in a differential diagnosis of benign stricture include caustic strictures following ingestion of certain tablets (such as some potassium preparations, tetracycline, or non-steroidal anti-inflammatory drugs), radiotherapy, fungal infections, tuberculosis, Crohn's disease and anastomotic strictures.

Most reflux-induced strictures are effectively treated by dilatation and a proton pump inhibitor. Recurrence is relatively uncommon and is often a sign that the patient is on an inadequate dose of drugs or that the diagnosis is not correct. A variety of dilators are available, such as the Celestin or Savary–Gillard bougies that are introduced over a metal guide wire. Balloon dilators that can be passed down the biopsy channel of an endoscope have improved in recent years and are probably now the instrument of first choice. The risk of perforation is less than half a per cent.

Antireflux surgery should be considered in young patients and in those with a recurring stricture needing frequent dilatation. When oesophageal shortening is a problem, a Collis gastroplasty as an oesophageal lengthening procedure can be combined with a Nissen fundoplication with good results.[53] The rare undilatable stricture with transmural fibrosis may require resection.

REFERENCES

48. Richter JE, Castell DO. Ann Intern Med 1982; 97: 93–103
49. Sellar RJ, De Caestecker JS, Heading RC. Clin Radiol 1987; 38: 303–307
50. Ismail-Beigi F, Horton PF, Pope CE. Gastroenterology 1970; 58: 163–174
51. Spencer J. Br J Surg 1969; 56: 912–914
52. Richter JE, Bradley LA, DeMeester TR et al. Dig Dis Sci 1992; 37: 849–856
53. Henderson RD, Marryatt GV. Ann Thorac Surg 1985; 39: 74–79

BARRETT'S OESOPHAGUS

In 1950, Barrett described the presence of a gastric-lined oesophagus, which is now recognized as a metaplastic response to reflux.[54] A Barrett's oesophagus can be recognized endoscopically. The lower oesophagus is covered with a pink, velvety, gastric type of epithelium extending up from the gastro-oesophageal junction. In so-called classic Barrett's the squamocolumnar junction is at least 3 cm above the gastro-oesophageal junction. A study by Singh and coworkers compared patients with Barrett's with patients with uncomplicated reflux, and found a significant reduction in the lower oesophageal sphincter pressure and an increase in the acid exposure in the Barrett's group when compared with the uncomplicated patients.[55] Furthermore, they found that the length of the Barrett's oesophagus bore a direct correlation to the degree of acid exposure. A study using a bile probe (Bilitec™ 2000) found increased bile reflux into the oesophagus in Barrett's patients as compared with patients with uncomplicated reflux.[56] Barrett's oesophagus is seen in about 10% of patients undergoing endoscopy for the assessment of reflux, and carries with it an approximately 30-fold increased risk of developing an adenocarcinoma of the oesophagus. This tumour may be multifocal and may be preceded by the development of high-grade dysplasia. It is now recognized that the original definition of a classic Barrett's oesophagus in the literature was arbitrary, and the concept of *short segment Barrett's*[57] is now accepted. The increased risk of malignancy seems to be associated with the histological finding of intestinal metaplasia and increases with increasing length of the columnar-lined segment. Even now, the natural history of classic and short segment Barrett's remains controversial,[58] and the confusion is further complicated by the recognition of intestinal metaplasia at the oesophagogastric junction. The need for regular screening endoscopy in Barrett's oesophagus also remains contentious. Most authorities currently advocate screening endoscopy at intervals of 2–3 years. The discovery of dysplasia on biopsy is an indication for more frequent endoscopic surveillance. The management of high-grade dysplasia is also controversial. Some advocate continued surveillance until an early adenocarcinoma is detected,[59] while others recommend oesophagectomy because of the failure to differentiate high-grade dysplasia from adenocarcinoma. Certainly, close liaison between the surgeons and pathologists is essential in such cases.[60]

Barrett's oesophagus may present as a benign stricture at the squamocolumnar junction and may be situated high in the oesophagus (Fig. 20.9). It may also be associated with deep penetrating ulcers involving the gastric-lined oesophagus, which may bleed and, rarely, perforate. There are reports of regression of the columnar-lined oesophagus after antireflux surgery, but most would regard a Barrett's oesophagus as a late and irreversible change that does not regress after surgical or medical treatment. Treatment is tailored to the attendant problems: dilatation for strictures, antireflux surgery if symptoms demand, surveillance for dysplasia, and resection for carcinoma.

HAEMORRHAGE

Haemorrhage is an uncommon complication of reflux, although severe haemorrhage can occur from a Barrett's ulcer. Occasionally patients with oesophagitis are found to be anaemic, but other more common causes of gastrointestinal bleeding should be excluded before ascribing the anaemia to the oesophagus (see Ch. 26).

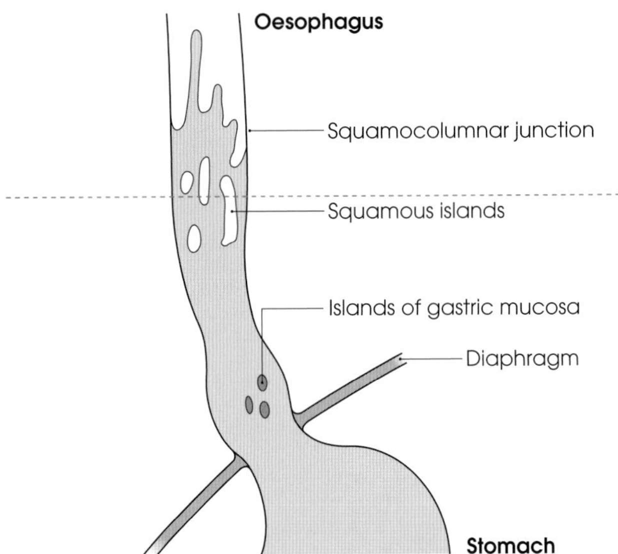

Figure 20.9 Barrett's oesophagus showing replacement of the lower oesophagus with gastric-type mucosa (exceeding 3 cm) and showing islands of squamous epithelium in the columnar-lined segment.

TREATMENT OF UNCOMPLICATED GASTROINTESTINAL REFLUX

MEDICAL

Most patients with gastro-oesophageal reflux respond well to medical therapy. Proton pump inhibitors are so effective that it can be difficult to persuade patients to make sensible lifestyle changes, such as losing weight, stopping smoking, or avoidance of excessive alcohol. However, sensible lifestyle change should be encouraged. The classic manoeuvre of elevation of the head of the bed can significantly reduce nocturnal acid reflux,[61] but if this is uncomfortable serious consideration should be given to surgical treatment. There is still a place for simple antacids, antacid–alginate preparations and H_2 blockers, but the mainstay of treatment is usually a proton pump inhibitor that can be expected to achieve symptom relief in up to 95% of patients with appropriate dose escalation.[62,63]

REFERENCES

54. Barrett NR. Br J Surg 1950; 38: 175–182
55. Singh P, Taylor H, Colin-Jones DG. Am J Gastroenterol 1994; 89: 349–356
56. Vaezi MF, Lacamera RG, Richter JE. Am J Physiol 1994; 267: G1050–G1057
57. Spechler SJ, Zeroogian JM, Anatoniolo DA et al. Lancet 1994; 344: 1533–1536
58. Nandurkar S, Talley NJ. Am J Gastroenterol 1999; 94: 30–40
59. Levine DS, Haggitt RC, Blount PL et al. Gastroenterology 1993; 105: 40–50
60. Peters JH, Clark GW, Ireland AP et al. J Thorac Cardiovasc Surg 1994; 108: 813–822
61. Johnson LF, DeMeester TR. Dig Dis Sci 1981; 8: 673–680
62. Hallerback B, Une P, Carling L et al. Gastroenterology 1994; 107: 1305–1311
63. Klinkenberg Knol EC, Festen HP, Jansen JB et al. Ann Intern Med 1994; 121: 161–167

SURGICAL

Surgical procedures to control reflux may be used as an alternative to long-term medication in patients whose symptoms are not well controlled by drugs or who prefer a surgical option after careful discussion of the risks and possible benefits. When regurgitation is the dominant symptom it often responds rather poorly to medication, and surgery is a good option in such cases.[64]

Nissen fundoplication

The early attempts at correction of reflux concentrated on reducing the hiatus hernia and carrying out a crural repair,[40] but the most popular operation is now a Nissen fundoplication. It is not known exactly how this operation prevents reflux. The traditional view is that it improves the lower oesophageal sphincter tone and increases the length of the intra-abdominal oesophagus.[65] Lower oesophageal sphincter pressure certainly increases in most of those who have successful control of reflux, but there is a sizeable group of patients in whom the pressure actually falls but who are still cured of reflux.[66] Furthermore, there is often no increase in the length of the intra-abdominal oesophagus. It may well be that fundoplication acts largely as a flap valve. The wrap may also prevent distraction and weakening of the lower oesophageal sphincter when the intragastric pressure increases and threatens to produce reflux.[67]

The concept of the 'floppy' Nissen fundoplication is important and was first described by Donahue and colleagues.[65] The lower oesophagus is mobilized via the abdominal route. The greater curvature is then mobilized by division of the short gastric vessels, and the mobilized fundus is wrapped around the lower oesophagus (Fig. 20.10). The tightness of the wrap depends in part on the extent of gastric mobilization, but also on the placement of sutures used to secure the wrap. The essential feature of the operation is to produce a loose fundoplication using a fully mobilized fundus. This allows a short 1–2-cm wrap to be constructed around a 50-FG oesophageal bougie placed within the oesophagus. The looseness of the fundoplication is confirmed by the easy passage of a finger, or instrument of similar calibre, within the wrap. The lower suture picks up the oesophagogastric junction to prevent slippage, and a posterior crural repair is added to stop upward displacement of the fundoplication. This procedure has approximately a 90% chance of success;[68] the incidence of the 'gas bloat syndrome' is markedly reduced by keeping the wrap loose and short so that the patient maintains some ability to belch.[65] Dysphagia in the immediate postoperative period is common, but is usually mild. Long-term dysphagia occurs in approximately 5% of patients, but again is usually mild. Its occurrence is minimized by the use of the 50-FG bougie. Recurrent reflux is seen in about 5–10% and may be from disruption or slippage of the fundoplication.

Most Nissen fundoplications are now done through a laparoscopic approach. This has significantly improved the acceptability of the procedure, but it is essential to pay attention to the minutiae of technique. During the early experience of laparoscopic fundoplication, a number of authors reported large paraoesophageal hernias occurring in the early postoperative period, sometimes associated with perforation, or even gangrene of the stomach. Because of this, it is recommended that meticulous crural repair be done as a routine.

Partial fundoplication

An alternative approach is some form of partial fundoplication, in which the fundus covers approximately 270° of the circumference of the oesophagus. Lesser degrees of fundoplication tend not to be so effective in controlling reflux. There are many different descriptions of partial fundoplication, but the Toupet posterior fundoplication is probably the most popular. As a generalization, partial fundoplication gives rise to less gas bloat and dysphagia, but is more prone to recurrent reflux. This generalization seems to hold true in many series, but there are significant exceptions and there are also large series with excellent reflux control.[69] Partial fundoplication is probably somewhat more demanding technically, but it should be stressed that all reflux surgery is inherently prone to variation, and the minutiae of technique can make a big difference to outcome, whatever type of fundoplication is done.

Tailored antireflux surgery

It has been suggested that patients with abnormal oesophageal motility are more likely to develop dysphagia if they have a full 360° fundoplication rather than a partial fundoplication.[70] This led to the concept of the tailored fundoplication, in which patients with normal motility are offered a Nissen fundoplication and those with abnormal motility are offered a partial fundoplication. The idea has a certain logic to it, but several recent studies have shown that severe motility disturbance detected by manometry does not indicate a high risk of dysphagia.[71,72]

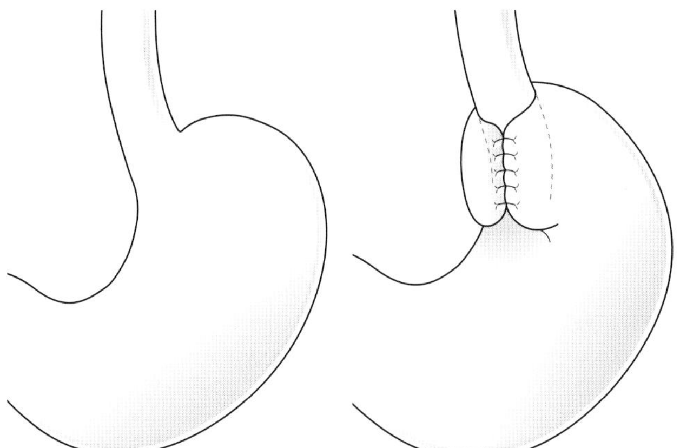

Figure 20.10 Nissen (complete) fundoplication.

REFERENCES

64. Lundell L. Baillières Best Pract Res Clin Gastroenterol 2000; 14: 793–810
65. Donahue PE, Samelson S, Nyhus LM et al. Arch Surg 1985; 120: 663–668
66. Bancewicz J, Mughal MM, Marples M. Br J Surg 1987; 74: 162–164
67. Jamieson GG. Br J Surg 1987; 74: 155–156
68. DeMeester TR, Bonavina L, Albertucci M. Ann Surg 1986; 204: 9–20
69. Zugel N, Jung C, Bruer C et al. Langenbecks Arch Surg 2002; 386: 494–498
70. Kauer WK, Peters JH, DeMeester TR et al. J Thorac Cardiovasc Surg 1995; 110: 141–146
71. Heading RC. Gut 2002; 50: 592–593
72. Booth M, Stratford J, Dehn TC. Dis Esophagus 2002; 15: 57–60

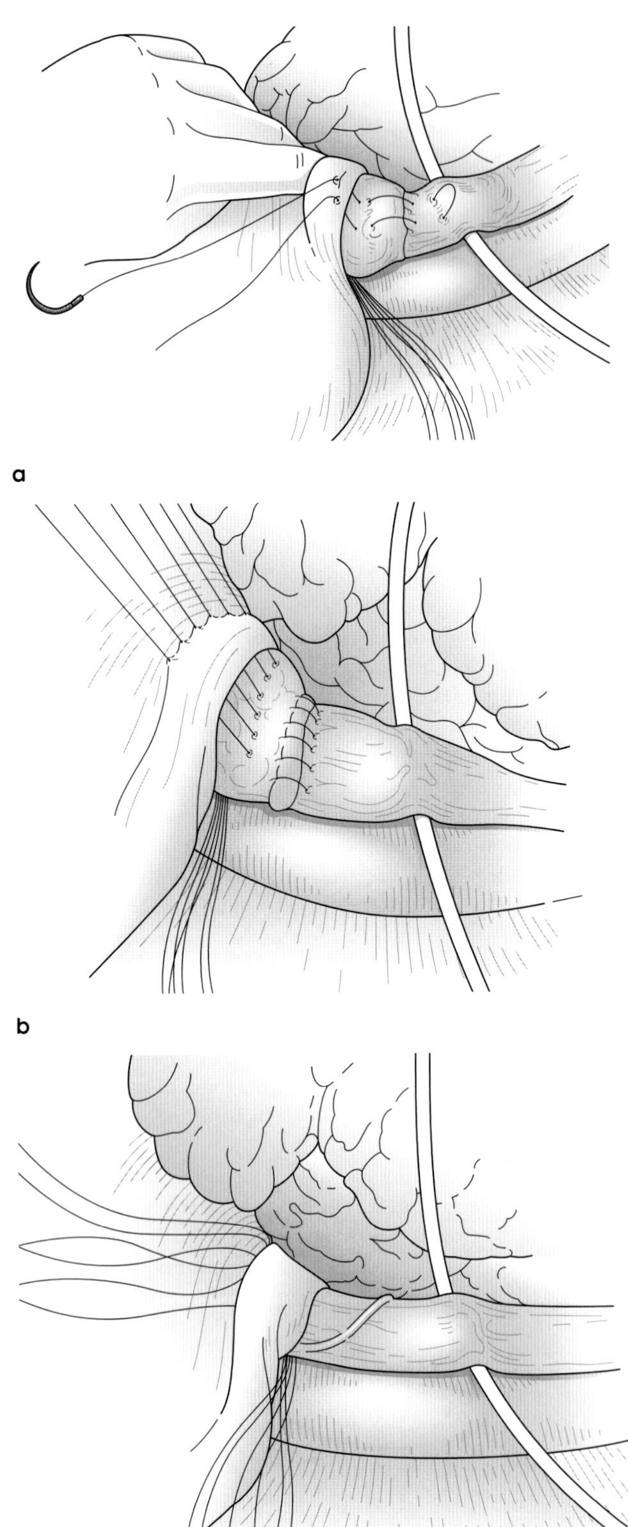

Figure 20.11 Belsey transthoracic antireflux procedure, which involves two layers of invagination sutures to produce a 270° wrap: (**a**) first layer of plication sutures; (**b**) second layer of sutures placed between the diaphragm and the oesophagus; and (**c**) second layer tied.

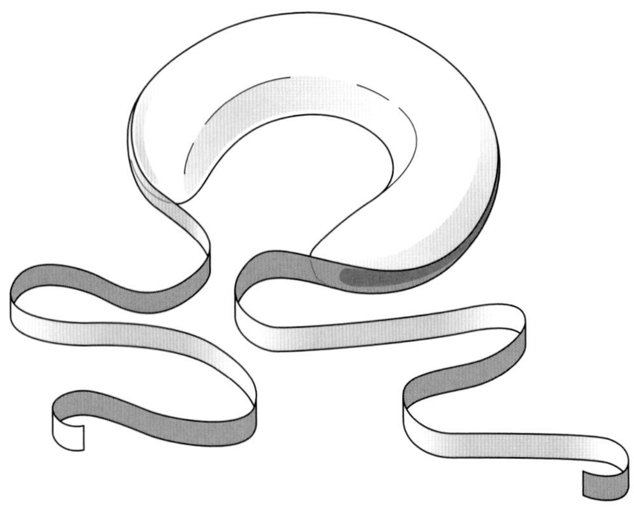

Figure 20.12 Angelchik antireflux prosthesis, which is fixed around the lower oesophagus at the oesophagogastric junction by tying the tapes.

Other antireflux operations

The Belsey mark IV antireflux procedure[73] is carried out through a transthoracic approach, either by formal open thoracotomy or as a minimal access procedure. The repair is sutured to the diaphragm (Fig. 20.11). The main advantage of this approach is in cases of shortening of the oesophagus, where the transthoracic approach allows greater mobilization of the oesophagus with placement of the wrap below the diaphragm. The disadvantages of this approach are the occasional post-thoracotomy neuralgia, which may be troublesome, and a higher rate of postoperative reflux when compared with Nissen fundoplication.

The Hill repair[74] relies on fixation of the partly plicated oesophagogastric junction to the median arcuate ligament, and may be combined with intraoperative manometry to gauge the magnitude of the lower oesophageal sphincter pressure. It has been performed through a laparoscopic approach with good results.[75]

The introduction of the Angelchik prosthesis some years ago offered the prospect of an easier, shorter and more standardized operation. The prosthesis is a silicon 'collar' with two tapes attached (Fig. 20.12). The lower oesophagus is mobilized and any hiatus hernia reduced; the collar is then passed around the lower oesophagus, and the tapes are tied and transfixed to anchor the prosthesis below the diaphragm. The Angelchik was associated with good reflux control and there were many enthusiastic reports on its use. Sporadic reports of migration of the prosthesis into the mediastinum and erosion into the gastrointestinal tract dampened enthusiasm for its use, but the main drawback is the postoperative dysphagia,[76] which occurred in up to 42% of patients and often required removal of the prosthesis. The dysphagia could even persist following removal. For this reason it has been abandoned as an antireflux procedure.

REFERENCES

73. Belsey R. World J Surg 1977; 1: 475–481
74. Hill LD. Ann Surg 1967; 166: 681–692
75. Low DE. Chest Surg Clin North Am 1995; 5: 411–422
76. Maxwell-Armstrong CA, Steele RJ, Amar SS et al. Br J Surg 1997; 84: 862–864

Operations for recurrent gastro-oesophageal reflux

Recurrent reflux occurs because a fundoplication has disrupted or slipped. Revision of a fundoplication for recurrent reflux may be technically demanding, but should have a success rate similar to that of a first-time operation. The operation of partial gastrectomy and Roux-en-Y duodenal diversion (Fig. 20.13) is a reasonable option if there is considerable scarring around the hiatus making oesophageal dissection very difficult. It is well tolerated and has a success rate almost equal to that of fundoplication.[77]

If the previous operation failed because of oesophageal shortening, then a Collis gastroplasty lengthens the oesophagus by constructing a neo-oesophagus from the stomach (Fig. 20.14). Classically, two light vascular clamps are applied to the stomach at the gastro-oesophageal junction with a size 60-FG oesophageal bougie in place. The stomach is incised between the clamps and sutured to form a tube. This allows a tension-free wrap to be carried out below the diaphragm. In this situation a 270° wrap has an unacceptably high failure rate and therefore a 360° Nissen-type wrap is preferred.[78] A Collis gastroplasty can be carried out through an abdominal approach with a stapler, and some surgeons have performed it through a laparoscope.

The efficacy of a totally intrathoracic Nissen has been mentioned in the past, but one report quoted a 33% incidence of gastric ulceration within the intrathoracic wrap;[79] this should mitigate against its use as a routine antireflux procedure. It also shows the importance of carrying out an adequate crural repair to lessen the chances of an abdominal Nissen migrating into the chest.

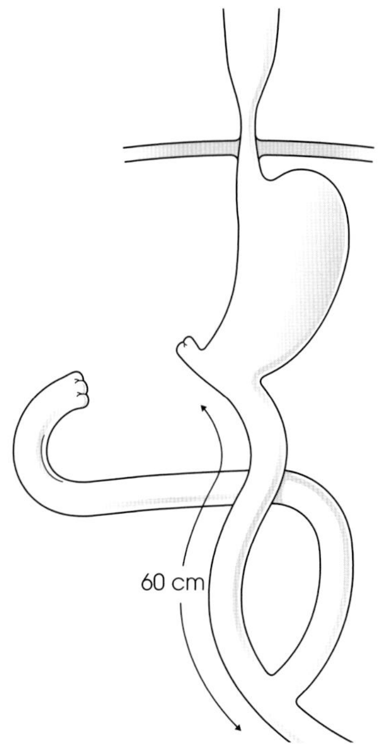

Figure 20.13 Partial gastrectomy and Roux-en-Y duodenal diversion. The vertical loop of jejunum should be at least 60 cm long.

MOTOR DISORDERS OF THE OESOPHAGUS

The passage of a food bolus from the mouth to the stomach is initiated by pharyngeal contraction with simultaneous relaxation of the cricopharyngeus. This allows the bolus to enter the oesophagus. A coordinated peristaltic wave then sweeps the bolus down the body of the oesophagus to reach the lower oesophageal sphincter, which then relaxes to allow the food to enter the stomach. Peristalsis is described as primary when it is initiated by swallowing and therefore follows a pharyngeal contraction, and secondary when it starts in the body of the oesophagus, usually in response to distension of the oesophagus by liquid or a food bolus. Tertiary waves are non-propulsive synchronous contractions of the oesophageal body that are occasionally seen in health, but when they are frequent they signify a motility

REFERENCES

77. Washer GF, Gear MW, Dowling BL et al. Br J Surg 1984; 71: 181–184
78. Orringer MB, Sloan H. Ann Thorac Surg 1978; 25: 16–21
79. Richardson JD, Larson GM, Polk HC Jr. Am J Surg 1982; 143: 29–35

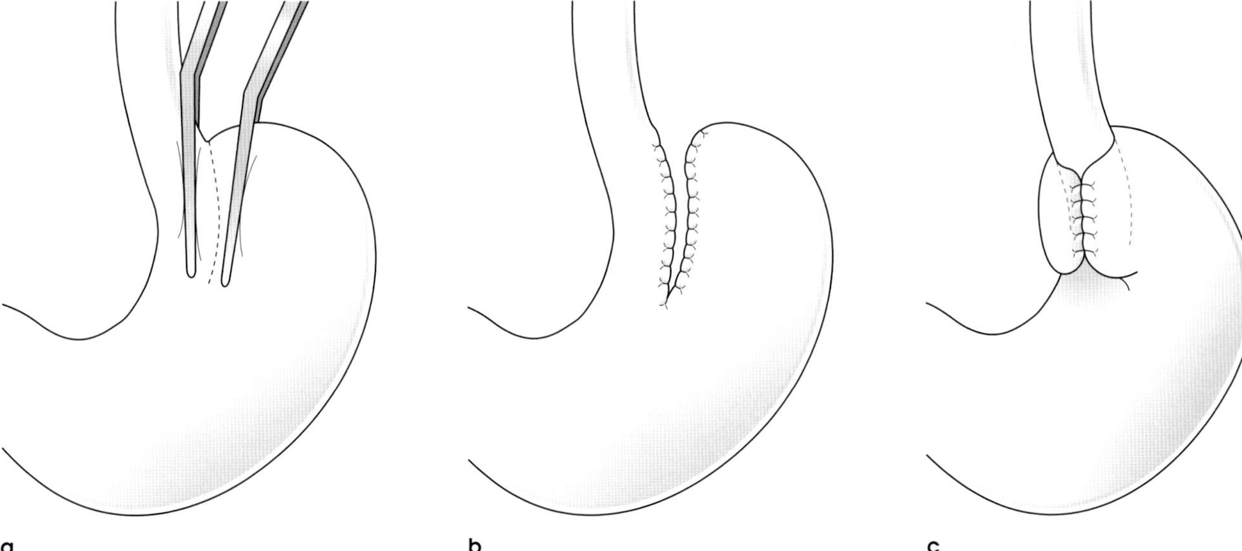

Figure 20.14 Collis Nissen operation. (**a**,**b**) A neo-oesophagus is formed by constructing a gastric tube. (**c**) The fundus is then wrapped around the neo-oesophagus to produce a Nissen wrap below the diaphragm.

disturbance. The term *achalasia* was initially used by Hertz to describe the absence of relaxation of the lower oesophageal sphincter,[80] and this is the commonest primary disorder of motility. Osgood described a condition that he called 'oesophagismus',[81] and which is now known as *diffuse oesophageal spasm*.

OESOPHAGEAL MANOMETRY

Manometry is used to study oesophageal motility and records pressure changes in the upper and lower oesophageal sphincters and in the body of the oesophagus. A manometry catheter is usually passed nasally, with the pressure being measured at multiple points in the oesophagus and also in the upper stomach. Pressure is measured by intraoesophageal minitransducers.

The lower oesophageal sphincter is assessed by gradual withdrawal of the catheter from the stomach into the oesophagus, measuring the rise in pressure in the sphincter zone, from which its length can be estimated. The ability of the sphincter to relax completely in response to a swallow is also noted. The catheter is then withdrawn further into the body of the oesophagus to record the motor activity, which may be peristaltic or non-peristaltic. Finally, the upper oesophageal sphincter is studied, looking for coordinated relaxation of the cricopharyngeus in response to pharyngeal contraction. Oesophageal manometry is a particularly useful investigation in patients with unexplained dysphagia. Achalasia can be recognized by a failure of the lower oesophageal sphincter to relax, combined with absence of peristalsis in the body of the oesophagus. Diffuse oesophageal spasm is identified by the presence of repetitive non-peristaltic multipeaked contractions of the body of the oesophagus. The picture can become blurred by variations in these classical patterns of motility, and very occasionally patients may change from one motility pattern to another over several years. Manometry has also been widely used for the investigation of obscure chest pain, but because it rarely leads to improved management its popularity is on the wane for this purpose.[82]

ACHALASIA

Achalasia affects one per 100 000 of the population and usually presents between the ages of 30 and 60 years. Abnormalities have been found in the dorsal nucleus of the vagus or in the vagal trunks, and there may be either a reduction or total absence of ganglia in Auerbach's plexus.[83] It has been suggested that the condition is caused by a neurotropic virus affecting the vagal nucleus and then travelling down the vagal trunk to the oesophageal ganglia, but this theory remains unproven.[84] In the early phases, before oesophageal dilatation has occurred, the oesophageal body exhibits vigorous non-peristaltic simultaneous contractions (the so-called vigorous achalasia). At this stage, chest pain may be a prominent symptom and may be confused with reflux pain or even anginal pain. Later on, as dilatation of the oesophagus occurs with retention of solids and liquids, dysphagia and regurgitation become prominent symptoms. Regurgitation of food may be delayed for some time after a meal and referred to by the patient as 'vomiting'. This may confuse the clinician into thinking of gastro-oesophageal reflux or even pyloric stenosis. Symptoms may be intermittent and exacerbated by stress, and the swallowing of both liquids and solids often present equal difficulty to the patient.

The classic radiological appearance of achalasia is a dilated oesophagus with a tapering lower oesophageal segment, likened to a bird's beak, which fails to relax (Fig. 20.15). There is no gastric air bubble because the dilated oesophagus never completely empties, and therefore swallowed air cannot pass into the stomach. This classic appearance is now uncommon because achalasia is usually diagnosed before dilatation has occurred. Oesophageal manometry is essential to make the diagnosis. The condition is characterized by the absence of peristaltic waves in the oesophagus, with a high resting intraoesophageal pressure and impaired relaxation of the lower oesophageal sphincter, which may also be hypertensive.

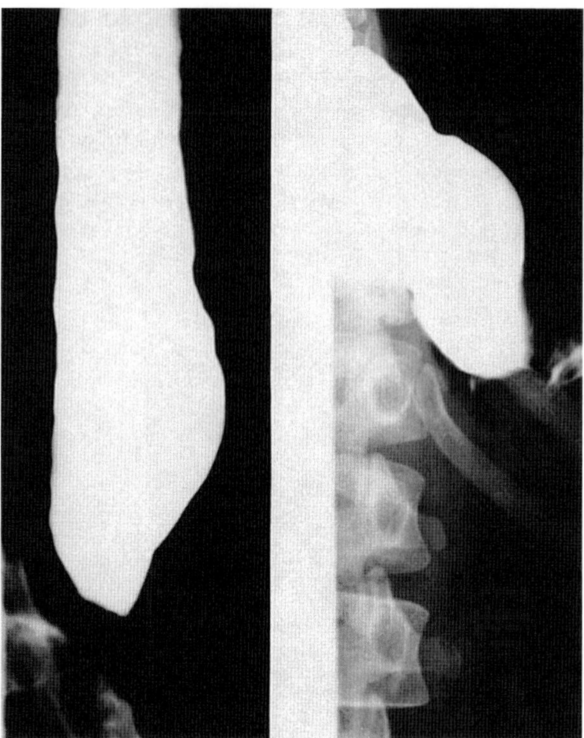

Figure 20.15 Barium swallow in a patient with achalasia, showing a dilated oesophagus with a constriction at the lower oesophageal sphincter.

Pseudoachalasia can cause diagnostic difficulties and occurs typically in patients, over the age of 50 years, with a short history of dysphagia. Cases have all the radiological and manometric features of achalasia. Pseudoachalasia can be caused by a carcinoma of the lower oesophagus, a carcinoma of the cardia, a pancreatic tumour, a lymphoma or a bronchogenic cancer.[85] Oesophagogastric endoscopy may reveal a tumour, but in some cases endoscopy and biopsy may still miss the diagnosis. The endoscope should 'pop' through the lower oesophageal sphincter in true achalasia, and any greater resistance to its passage must put the diagnosis in doubt. A CT scan or endoscopic ultrasonography may be required if doubt remains.

REFERENCES

80. Hertz AF. Q J Med 1915; 8: 300–310
81. Osgood H. Boston Med Surg J 1889; 120: 401–405
82. Storr M, Allescher H-D. Dis Esophagus 1999; 12: 241–257
83. Spiess AE, Kahrilas PJ. JAMA 1998; 280: 638–642
84. Robertson CS, Martin BA, Atkinson M. Gut 1993; 34: 299–302
85. Vantrappen G, Janssens J, Hellemans J et al. Gastroenterology 1979; 76: 450–457

Complications

Overspill from the dilated oesophagus into the bronchial tree may result in nocturnal aspiration, and this may lead to bronchiectasis and lung abscess (see Ch. 21). Carcinoma complicates achalasia in 3% of cases and this is usually a squamous cell carcinoma, developing in midoesophagus as a bulky tumour with a particularly bad prognosis.[86]

Treatment

Treatment is designed to reduce the competence of the lower oesophageal sphincter without producing gastro-oesophageal reflux. Forceful dilatation of the cardia with a balloon was first described by Plummer in 1908.[87] The modern pneumatic oesophageal dilator with an inelastic balloon evolved in the 1980s and is a safe and effective treatment.[88] The dilating balloon is positioned in the lower oesophageal sphincter and inflated to a fixed pressure, usually 20 psi for 1 min. This is successful in relieving dysphagia in about 67% of patients. The success rate increases with the increasing age of the patients.[89] Perforation of the oesophagus should occur in less than 2% of cases. Dilatation therapy is recommended in the first instance, as it is relatively safe and easy. Surgery is reserved for patients who still have symptoms after dilatation, for postdilatation rupture, and for children in whom dilatation seems ineffective. Postdilatation rupture is usually managed conservatively (see p. 433). This is effective provided the oesophagus is empty before the dilatation and the condition is recognized early by means of a contrast examination after the dilatation. When balloon dilatation was compared with myotomy in a specialized centre the results are very similar, except that the myotomized patients had a higher incidence of reflux.[90] It seems sensible, therefore, to recommend balloon dilatation as the primary treatment and to reserve myotomy for those who fail to respond to dilatation. Intrasphincteric injection of botulinum toxin has attracted considerable interest, but suffers from the disadvantage that its effect wears off after a few months.[91]

The standard operation for achalasia is Heller's cardiomyotomy, which was first performed in 1913 as an anterior and posterior myotomy.[92] A single myotomy is now considered to be adequate (Fig. 20.16) and should be about 5 cm in length, extending no more than 1 cm on to the stomach; the oesophagogastric junction is recognized by the presence of small, transverse, extramucosal veins. The operation may be performed through a laparoscope or through a thoracoscopic approach. Controversy exists as to whether an antireflux procedure should be simultaneously performed to avoid postoperative gastro-oesophageal reflux, although if the operation is correctly performed, with only minimal extension of the myotomy on to the stomach and minimal mobilization of the oesophagogastric junction, the incidence of reflux is less than 3%.[93] Vantrappen and Hellemans reviewed a collected series of 1045 cases treated by myotomy and found the incidence of reflux to be 10%.[88] If an antireflux operation is carried out, it is important that any associated fundoplication should be short and loose to avoid postoperative dysphagia in view of the absence of peristalsis in the body of the oesophagus.

CHAGAS' DISEASE

This interesting condition is found in Central and South America and is a manifestation of chronic infection with the parasite *Trypanosoma cruzi*. The disease mainly affects the heart, but gastrointestinal effects are common. It is most prevalent in certain parts of Brazil, where about a quarter of the population show evidence of infection.[94] As in achalasia, the intermuscular ganglion cells are destroyed and motility changes are evident when there is a 50% reduction in the ganglion cell count; dilatation occurs when this figure rises to 90%.[95] The clinical features are identical to achalasia, and the treatment is also by balloon dilatation or cardiomyotomy. Very advanced cases may be complicated by extreme dilatation and tortuosity of the oesophagus, where resection may be necessary. Chagas' disease may also affect other parts of the gastrointestinal tract, producing megacolon (Ch. 28), megaduodenum (Ch. 26) and also possibly megaureter (Ch. 35).[96]

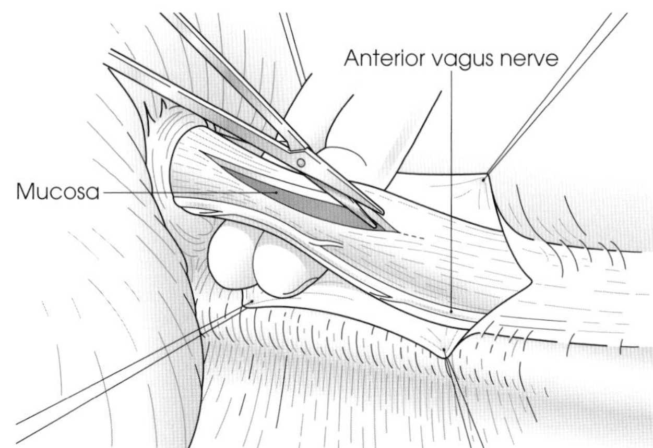

Figure 20.16 Heller's myotomy (transthoracic approach).

DIFFUSE OESOPHAGEAL SPASM AND RELATED DISORDERS

Interest in diffuse oesophageal spasm and related disorders increased following the use of coronary angiography for the investigation of 'presumed' anginal chest pain. In the USA, 30% of these patients were found to have a normal coronary angiogram, and up to half of this group were then found to have an oesophageal abnormality that was considered to be responsible for their symptoms.[97] Management of oesophageal motility disorders in patients with angina-like chest pain, without dysphagia, is disappointing enough to raise doubt about the relevance of the motility disorder.[82] Patients with diffuse

REFERENCES

86. Streitz JM Jr, Ellis FH Jr, Gibb SP et al. Ann Thorac Surg 1995; 59: 1604–1609
87. Plummer HS. JAMA 1908; 51: 549–554
88. Vantrappen G, Hellemans J. Gastroenterology 1980; 79: 144–154
89. Robertson CS, Fellows IW, Mayberry JF et al. Digestion 1988; 40: 244–250
90. Abid S, Champion G, Richter JE et al. Am J Gastroenterol 1994; 87: 979–985
91. Richter JE. Gastrointest Endosc Clin North Am 2001; 11: 359–370
92. Heller E. Med Chir (JENA) 1913; 27: 141–145
93. Ellis FH Jr, Crozier RE, Watkins E Jr. J Cardiovasc Surg 1984; 88: 344–351
94. Earlam RJ. Am Dig Dis 1972; 17: 559–571
95. Koberle F. Adv Parasitol 1968; 6: 63–116
96. de Oliveira RB, Troncon LE, Dantas RO et al. Am J Gastroenterol 1998; 93: 884–889
97. DeMeester TR, O'Sullivan GC, Bermudez G et al. Ann Surg 1982; 196: 488–498

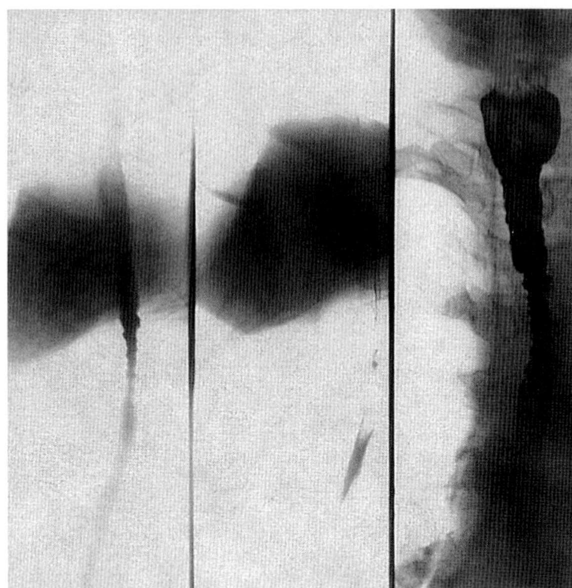

Figure 20.17 Barium swallow in a patient with diffuse oesophageal spasm, showing an area of intense muscle contraction in the midoesophagus.

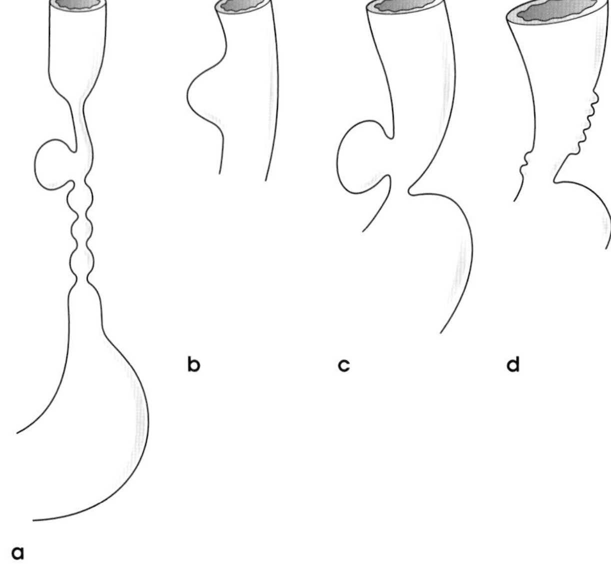

Figure 20.18 Oesophageal diverticula: (**a**) pulsion; (**b**) traction; (**c**) congenital; and (**d**) pseudodiverticula.

oesophageal spasm may certainly have episodic chest pain, but treatment is more effective in relieving dysphagia.

The intermittent nature of diffuse spasm belies the difficulty there may be in making a diagnosis. Barium swallow is abnormal in less than half of the cases (Fig. 20.17),[98] and endoscopy is usually unremarkable. Oesophageal manometry characteristically shows a high proportion of high-amplitude simultaneous contractions of the body of the oesophagus that are of long duration and display multiple peaks. Some peristalsis is maintained, thereby distinguishing it from achalasia.

The 'nutcracker' oesophagus refers to the manometric finding of high-amplitude peristaltic contractions. It has been reported as being associated with chest pain and dysphagia.[99] A number of authorities do not consider this a true pathological condition and question its relevance.

The distinction between abnormalities of oesophageal motility can become blurred with the realization that achalasia may occasionally develop after many years of diffuse spasm. Gastro-oesophageal reflux may be associated with diffuse spasm,[100] but whether there is any causal relationship is debatable. Nevertheless, ambulatory pH monitoring should always be obtained at the same time as manometry to provide a complete diagnostic assessment. Occasionally during manometry a hypertensive lower oesophageal sphincter will be encountered that relaxes normally on swallowing but may nevertheless be associated with dysphagia.

The first line of treatment in a patient with diffuse oesophageal spasm is a thorough explanation of the abnormality that has been found. Calcium channel blockers and nitrates have been used, but rarely help. Balloon dilatation can be helpful if the dysphagia is severe, but it is less effective than in the treatment of achalasia. A long oesophageal myotomy may be useful in an extremely small group of patients with severe dysphagia and gross manometric findings with high contraction amplitudes. Such patients are very rare. Long oesophageal myotomy fell into disrepute when it was widely used in the 1980s as a treatment for non-cardiac chest pain. This period was also characterized by overenthusiastic interpretation of oesophageal manometry. It is important not to forget the lessons learned from this experience.

OTHER NON-NEOPLASTIC DISEASES OF THE OESOPHAGUS

OESOPHAGEAL DIVERTICULA

Oesophageal diverticula have been classified into four types (Fig. 20.18):

1. Pulsion diverticula, which are mucosal and usually caused by high intraluminal pressure, associated with motor disorder of the oesophagus.
2. Traction diverticula, which are less common and historically associated with tuberculous mediastinal glands.
3. Congenital diverticula, which may be a type of oesophageal reduplication.
4. Pseudodiverticula, which usually represent oesophageal ulcers and are therefore devoid of an epithelial lining.

Midoesophageal diverticula are usually of the traction variety, often asymptomatic, and require no treatment. Rarely, they may be complicated by fistula formation into the bronchial tree or into a major vessel. Epiphrenic diverticula are often single and situated just above the diaphragm. They are usually of the pulsion variety and may be associated with achalasia, diffuse spasm, or a hypertensive lower oesophageal sphincter. A large epiphrenic diverticulum may be associated with significant dysphagia, regurgitation, or even nocturnal aspiration into the bronchial

REFERENCES

98. Henderson RD. The Oesophagus Reflux and Primary Motor Disorders. Williams & Wilkins, Baltimore, 1980
99. Benjamin SB, Gerhardt DC, Castell DO. Gastroenterology 1979; 77: 478–483
100. Adler DG, Romero Y. Mayo Clin Proc 2001; 76: 195–200

tree.[101] Bleeding, perforation and malignant change are rare complications.[102] Treatment of the diverticulum is often not required. The symptoms may be relieved by balloon dilatation of the lower oesophagus distal to the diverticulum, as for achalasia. The diverticulum should be excised if this fails and it is large enough to cause a mechanical problem. A myotomy should be performed on the segment of oesophagus distal to the diverticulum.

SCLERODERMA

The oesophagus is involved in approximately 80% of cases of scleroderma, and is typically affected in patients with the calcinosis, Raynaud's, oesophagus, scleroderma and telangiectasis (CREST) syndrome (see Ch. 10). The problems are related to the effects of gastro-oesophageal reflux combined with an adynamic oesophagus, which eventually produce reflux strictures causing dysphagia. Even subtle strictures may cause severe dysphagia in scleroderma, because secondary peristalsis is often completely ineffective. Manometrically, scleroderma is 'diagnosed' by the presence of normal peristalsis in the upper part of the oesophagus and very low-amplitude peristalsis in its lower two-thirds, although these features are not confined to scleroderma. Medical treatment of the associated gastro-oesophageal reflux is usually highly effective. Occasionally a fundoplication may be required for severe regurgitation. Scleroderma has a diffuse effect on the gut, and gastrointestinal symptoms often persist even after a successful fundoplication.

MISCELLANEOUS OESOPHAGEAL CONDITIONS

AIDS and the oesophagus

Dysphagia and odynophagia may be presenting features of AIDS, as the patient is a potential host for *Candida albicans*, herpes simplex virus or cytomegalovirus (see Ch. 4).[103] The same infections can also be seen when patients are immunosuppressed for other reasons, such as after transplantation or during chemotherapy. Barium swallow may show ulceration that can be confirmed by fibre-optic endoscopy, but the routine diagnostic techniques of biopsy and brush cytology may fail to confirm the causative organisms, and in some cases the diagnosis will only be made at post-mortem.

Monilial oesophagitis

Monilial oesophagitis is characteristically seen when an immunocompromised patient complains of painful dysphagia and is found to have oral thrush (see Ch. 13). Oesophagoscopy may reveal white specks of fungus on a friable hyperaemic oesophageal mucosa. The diagnosis may be confirmed by taking biopsies and brushings that should be placed directly into Sabouraud's medium. Oesophageal moniliasis may complicate oesophageal cancer, reflux oesophagitis and achalasia. It can also develop in otherwise normal patients as a side effect of antibiotic therapy or steroid inhalers. Complications include ulceration, fistula and bleeding, and treatment is with an oral antifungal agent. Occasionally fibrous strictures require dilatation.

Other oesophageal infections

Other organisms producing oesophagitis, ulceration or fistulae may occasionally affect the oesophagus. Syphilis is now only of historical importance, but tuberculosis and actinomycosis, diphtheria, lactobacilli, streptococci, histoplasmosis and blastomycosis are rare offenders.

Crohn's disease

Crohn's of the oesophagus is rare, and only a few cases have been described in the literature.[104] The diagnosis should be suspected if a patient with known Crohn's disease at another site (see Ch. 28) develops an oesophageal stricture with ulceration and a 'cobblestone' mucosa. It should also be suspected if a patient has unusually severe 'reflux' oesophagitis that does not respond to a proton pump inhibitor. These appearances must be differentiated from a reflux stricture and from a carcinoma by biopsy. Some of the cases have been operated on in the mistaken belief that they were malignant strictures. There are reports of success with steroid therapy, and one case report describes the use of balloon dilatation of a tight cricopharyngeal stricture in a patient with small-bowel Crohn's disease whose swallowing was restored to normal after two dilatations.[105]

PARAOESOPHAGEAL HIATUS HERNIA

Unlike sliding hiatus hernia, the clinical significance of which is still debated, paraoesophageal (or rolling) hiatus hernia can cause severe mechanical disturbances that may give rise to serious complications. The pure paraoesophageal hernia is a pathological curiosity, confined to museum specimens and personal collections of interesting cases. The vast majority of rolling hernias are mixed hernias in which the cardia is displaced into the chest and a large portion of the stomach rolls up alongside the oesophagus (Fig. 20.19). As the hernia enlarges, the stomach assumes an inverted position and the anatomical distortion of the cardia and the distal stomach is responsible for the symptoms.

The symptom pattern depends on the mechanical effects in the individual case. Distortion of the cardia produces dysphagia. Distortion of the distal stomach as it is drawn through the diaphragm may produce gastric outlet obstruction. Some patients have severe chest pain after eating. They are able to swallow, although with difficulty, but have difficulty belching and have poor gastric emptying. As a result the stomach may become markedly distended. This painful sequence is often eased if attempts to belch are successful. Occasionally the pain is so severe that the patient may be admitted as an emergency with a suspected myocardial infarction. Passage of a large-bore nasogastric tube gives instant relief. Gastric volvulus with strangulation and gangrene is a danger in long-standing cases (see Ch. 26). Respiratory embarrassment may occur, but is uncommon even with very large hernias, unless the patient has concomitant lung disease.

The only effective treatment is operative repair. Unfortunately, many patients are elderly and the risks of operation must then be carefully weighed against the risks of leaving the hernia untreated.

Repair may be performed via the abdominal or thoracic route. Laparoscopy is probably the most common approach, but these

REFERENCES

101. Evander A, Little AG, Ferguson MK et al. World J Surg 1986; 10: 820–829
102. Duranceau AC. In: Jamieson GG (ed). Surgery of the Oesophagus. Churchill Livingstone, Edinburgh, 1988
103. Bonacini M, Laine LA. Gastrointest Endosc Clin North Am 1998; 8: 811–823
104. Geboes K, Janssens J, Rutgeerts P et al. J Clin Gastroenterol 1986; 8: 31–37
105. Cynn WS, Chon H, Gureghian PA et al. Am J Roentgenol Radium Ther Nucl Med 1975; 125: 359–364

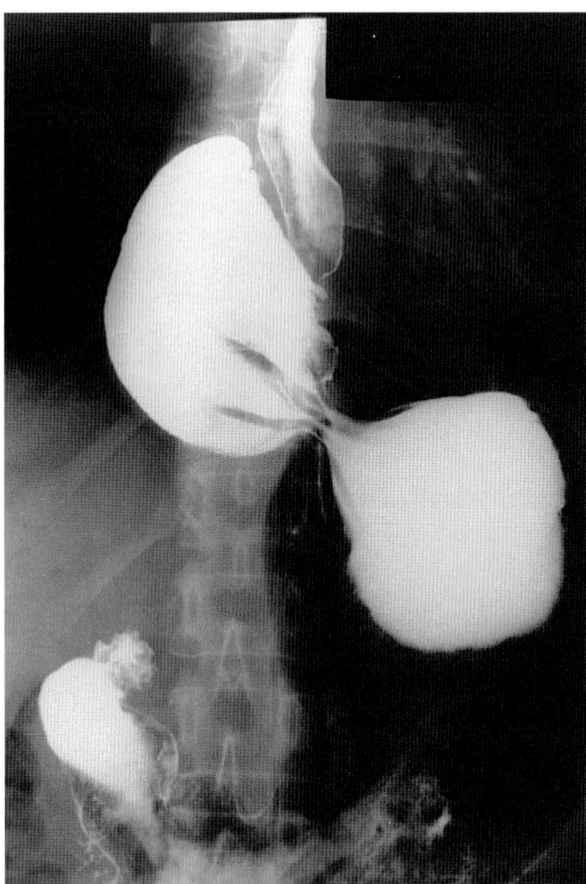

Figure 20.19 Large mixed hiatus hernia.

are often challenging operations.[106] Anatomical reduction is the main priority and may be maintained either by gastropexy, as in the Hill operation, with fixation to the anterior abdominal wall (Boerema gastropexy; see p. 442), or by a formal reflux-preventing operation such as a Nissen fundoplication (see p. 441). Despite opinions to the contrary, reflux symptoms are common,[107] and a formal antireflux procedure is entirely appropriate in many cases. It is possible to do a very simple Boerema type of gastropexy by laparoscopy that may be appropriate for the unfit or elderly.[108]

EXTRINSIC PROBLEMS AT THE CARDIA

After vagotomy

During the vagotomy era, dysphagia was an uncommon but well-recognized complication.[109] It was usually transient and was presumably an effect of denervation and handling the oesophagus. Rarely, considerable fibrosis developed in the tissues around the oesophagus at the hiatus. This produced severe dysphagia. Oesophageal dilatation was often ineffective, and operative release of the oesophagus was required.

After antireflux surgery

Any form of antireflux surgery can produce obstruction of the lower oesophagus. This may be the effect of the operation itself, for example a Nissen wrap that is too tight or too long, or reaction to an Angelchik prosthesis. It can also be caused by overzealous tightening of the diaphragmatic hiatus. Whatever the cause, the obstruction may be difficult to diagnose, because there are other causes of persistent dysphagia following antireflux surgery. It may also be deceptively easy to pass tapered dilators through the obstruction, as it is often elastic. The resistance to passage of a large (at least 50-FG) olive dilator, such as the old-fashioned Eder–Puestow dilator, gives a more accurate appreciation of the problem. As with postvagotomy fibrosis, operative correction is usually required.

TUMOURS OF THE OESOPHAGUS

BENIGN TUMOURS

Benign tumours of the oesophagus are exceedingly rare. Leiomyomas are the most frequent of these unusual lesions.[110] They most often develop in the distal oesophagus and may become quite large before they cause dysphagia. Typically, they can be shelled out of the oesophageal wall at thoracotomy or thoracoscopy[111] without breaching the mucosa.

With the increasing use of endoscopy, small polyps are being found more frequently.[112] They may be squamous papillomas or true adenomas. Fibrovascular polyps have been reported, particularly in the upper oesophagus. They can be large enough to cause symptoms, and in about half of the cases the tumour may be regurgitated into the mouth or even outside the mouth![113] Lipomas,[114] chondromas,[115] granular cell tumours,[116] haemangiomas[117] and lymphangiomas[118] have all been described. Carcinoid tumours may occur, but they usually have malignant potential.[119]

MALIGNANT TUMOURS

Sarcoma

Sarcoma of the oesophagus is excessively rare. Leiomyosarcoma[120] and rhabdomyosarcoma[121] have been reported. Other sarcomas are rarer still, and in most instances are confined to

REFERENCES

106. Freeman RE, Hinder RA. Semin Laparosc Surg 2001; 8: 240–245
107. Walther B, DeMeester TR, Lafontaine E et al. Am J Surg 1984; 147: 111–116
108. Agwunobi AO, Bancewicz J, Attwood SE. Br J Surg 1998; 85: 604–606
109. Spencer JD. Br J Surg 1975; 62: 354
110. Hatch GF III, Wertheimer-Hatch L, Hatch KF et al. World J Surg 2000; 24: 401–411
111. Pross M, Manger T, Wolff S et al. Surg Endosc 2000; 14: 1146–1148
112. Enterline HE, Thompson J. Pathology of the Esophagus. Springer Verlag, Berlin, 1984
113. Jang GC, Clouse ME, Fleischer FG. Radiology 1969; 92: 1196–1200
114. Nora AF. Lipoma of the esophagus. Am J Surg 1964; 108: 353–356
115. Stout AP, Lattes R. In: Atlas of Tumor Pathology, Series 1, Fascicle 20. Armed Forces Institute of Pathology, Washington, 1957
116. Voskuil JH, van Dijk MM, Wagenaar SS et al. Dig Dis Sci 2001; 46: 1610–1614
117. Konstantakos AK, Douglas WI, Abdul-Karim FW et al. Ann Thorac Surg 1995; 60: 1798–1800
118. Armengol-Miro JR, Ramentol F, Salord J et al. Endoscopy 1979; 11: 185–189
119. Rankin R, Nirodi NS, Browne MK. Scott Med J 1980; 25: 245–249
120. Miettinen M, Lasota J. Virchows Arch 2001; 438: 1–12
121. Vartio T, Nickels J, Hockerstedt K et al. Virchows Arch A Pathol Anat Histol 1980; 386: 357–361

single case reports.[122] Neurogenic sarcoma, osteogenic sarcoma and malignant granular cell tumours have all been recorded. The oesophagus may be involved in lymphomas, but this is usually secondary to involvement of adjacent mediastinal lymph nodes. There are few convincing case reports of primary lymphoma of the oesophagus.[123]

A carcinosarcoma with adenomatous elements was described, but is now thought to be a polypoid carcinoma with dominant spindle cell elements.[124] It has a relatively good prognosis.

Carcinoma of the oesophagus

General

Carcinoma of the oesophagus is one and a half to three times commoner in men than in women.[112] Most of the patients are middle-aged or elderly, and the condition is uncommon before the age of 40 years. It is said to be commonest at the points of physiological narrowing of the oesophagus—at its upper limit, at the arch of the aorta, at the level of transit of the left main bronchus, at the diaphragm, and at the cardia—but many tumours are too long to permit precise determination of their site of origin. Multiple cancers are as rare in the oesophagus as in the stomach, although submucosal secondary deposits, usually proximal to the primary tumour, are not uncommon.[125] In parts of the world where squamous cancer is still the dominant cell type, approximately 55% of cases are in the upper and midthoracic oesophagus, 34% in the lower oesophagus, and 8% in the cervical oesophagus. The remainder cannot be classified.[112] In most of the westernized world this traditional distribution has changed markedly in the last 20 years, and oesophageal cancer is now commonest in the lower oesophagus and at the oesophagogastric junction.

Pathology and aetiology

Worldwide, most carcinomas of the oesophagus are squamous cell tumours. Adenocarcinomas account for 0.8–65% of all carcinomas, depending on the local epidemiology, and are now the most common type in westernized countries.[126] Most of these are thought to arise as a result of Barrett's metaplasia.[127] Oat cell carcinoma (small cell undifferentiated carcinoma) is an unusual variant with a very poor prognosis.[128] Other epithelial tumours that have been described include adenoid cystic carcinoma,[129] mucoepidermoid carcinoma,[130] malignant melanoma,[131] and the occasional carcinoid tumour.[112]

The incidence of squamous cell carcinoma of the oesophagus varies widely from one part of the world to another. There is a particularly high incidence in three areas: northern China in the provinces of Henan, Hebei and Shanxi; the regions of Iran and Russia that border on the Caspian Sea; and in the black population of South Africa around Durban and in the Transkei.[112] In these areas the incidence is over 35 per 100 000 people, in contrast to two to eight per 100 000 in most of Europe and the USA. It is thought that diet is very important in the high-incidence areas. Four major factors have been identified: a diet high in nitrosamines; diets that include mouldy foods; foods raised on soils deficient in trace elements, especially molybdenum; and diets deficient in vitamins C and A, riboflavin, protein and caloric content.[112] Cigarette smoking and alcohol consumption are important factors in areas of the world that have a low or moderate risk.

Genetic factors may also play a part. A condition has been described in which oral leukoplakia and tylosis are associated with a high incidence of oesophageal cancer.[132] In most westernized countries the incidence of adenocarcinoma of the oesophagus and cardia has risen sharply in the past 20 years. As a result these are now relatively common lesions. The reason for the change is unknown, but reflux symptoms and obesity appear to be independent risk factors.[133–136]

The poor prognosis of oesophageal cancer is proof of its ability to spread. Spread occurs directly through the wall of the oesophagus to adjacent organs, along the lymphatics in the submucosa or muscularis to form separate nodules, and to regional and distant lymph nodes; the pattern of spread depends on the primary site of the tumour. Blood-borne distant metastases are also common, mainly passing to the liver and lungs, but occasionally also to bone and brain.

Clinical presentation

Dysphagia is the most common presenting symptom. It is relentlessly progressive unless the carcinoma is treated. Unfortunately, this conceals the fact that symptoms may be very subtle at first. There may be minor retrosternal discomfort that the patient dismisses as 'wind' or which is treated as non-specific dyspepsia by a family doctor. Atypical chest pain is another early presentation that may cause difficulty. Pseudoachalasia may occur with intermittent dysphagia and the radiological and manometric appearances of achalasia. The carcinoma in such cases is often a small tumour at the cardia that may be easily missed. Sometimes the initial presentation is with pulmonary symptoms, or frank pneumonia caused by overspill. More advanced cases may develop persistent cough during eating as the result of a tracheo-oesophageal fistula. Extensive cancers of the middle third of the oesophagus may cause a recurrent laryngeal nerve palsy. Anaemia or frank haematemesis is uncommon, but massive haematemesis from an aorto-oesophageal fistula may be a terminal event.

Physical signs are seen only in advanced cases and are those of malnutrition and disseminated cancer. Cervical lymphadenopathy should not be forgotten.

REFERENCES

122. Stein HA, Murray D, Warner HA. Dig Dis Sci 1981; 26: 457–461
123. Golioto M, McGrath K. Am J Med Sci 2001; 321: 203–205
124. Osamura RY, Shimamura K, Hata J et al. Am J Surg Pathol 1978; 2: 201–208
125. Huang GJ, K'ai WY. Carcinoma of the Esophagus and Gastric Cardia. Springer Verlag, Berlin, 1984
126. Allum WH, Griffin SM, Watson A et al. Gut 2002; 50 (Suppl V): 1–23
127. Cameron AJ, Lomboy CT, Pera M et al. Gastroenterology 1995; 109: 1541–1546
128. Briggs JC, Ibrahim HB. Histopathology 1983; 7: 261–277
129. Jacobsohn WZ, Libson Y, Dollberg L. Gastrointest Endosc 1980; 26: 102–104
130. Osamura RY, Sato S, Miwa M et al. Am J Gastroenterol 1978; 69: 467–470
131. Sabanathan S, Eng J, Pradhan GN. Am J Gastroenterol 1989; 84: 1475–1481
132. Howel-Evans W, McConnell RB, Clarke CA et al. Q J Med 1958; 27: 413–429
133. Brown LM, Swanson CA, Gridley G et al. J Natl Cancer Inst 1995; 87: 104–109
134. Lagergren J, Bergstrom R, Lindgren A et al. N Engl J Med 1999; 340: 825–831
135. Lagergren J, Bergstrom R, Nyren O. Ann Intern Med 1999; 130: 883–890
136. Vaughan TL, Davis S, Kristal A et al. Cancer Epidemiol Biomarkers Prev 1995; 4: 85–92

Diagnosis

Endoscopy is the mainstay of diagnosis. It yields material for histology and is a more accurate examination than a barium swallow for small tumours and for those at the cardia. It should, however, be borne in mind that cancers may be missed by both types of investigation. Errors are most likely to occur at the entrance to the oesophagus and at the cardia. Video-endoscopes should be passed under direct vision because they may easily be pushed past a small lesion in the upper oesophagus if this segment is not observed. Sometimes the best views of the upper oesophagus are obtained during withdrawal, and the pharynx and vocal cords should be inspected as the endoscope is removed. The cardia should always be examined with the retroflexed endoscope.

Staging and general assessment

Once the diagnosis has been confirmed, it is essential to assess both the tumour and the patient to determine the best form of treatment.[126] Unfortunately, many patients are only suitable for palliation because of advanced disease, advanced age or their poor general condition.

Locoregional and metastatic disease may be detected by helical CT scanning, endoscopic ultrasonography and laparoscopy, which may be combined with laparoscopic ultrasound. Bronchoscopy may be useful if there is doubt about invasion of the trachea or bronchus. Laparoscopy is particularly useful for assessing adenocarcinomas of the distal oesophagus and cardia to assess transperitoneal spread. Both CT and MRI scanning are relatively inaccurate for assessing nodal spread, and endoscopic ultrasonography provides the most accurate assessment of the local lymph nodes and the depth of invasion of the primary tumour.[137] Oesophageal cancer may metastasize to bone or brain, but these possibilities are usually investigated only in those with suspicious symptoms. Assessment of the cardiovascular and respiratory systems is an essential preliminary to radical treatment.

Preoperative preparation

Preliminary investigation excludes many patients from radical treatment. In general, those with severe malnutrition have incurable disease, and meticulous staging is essential. Patients with adenocarcinoma are usually obese. If some sort of nutritional support seems advisable (see Ch. 2), the simplest method of providing this is to withdraw all solid food and start the patient on a high-protein liquid diet. It is surprising how often severe dysphagia improves once obstructing food material in the oesophagus has been cleared. Fine-bore nasogastric tubes and intravenous feeding have their occasional uses, but neither is a good solution for the severely obstructed oesophagus. Oesophageal dilatation should be avoided because of the risk of perforation. A feeding jejunostomy is probably the best option if a liquid diet cannot be tolerated and a programme of radical treatment is planned.

It is the respiratory system that requires the greatest attention, because postoperative pulmonary problems are common. Most western patients with squamous cell cancers are smokers, and even a short period of abstinence is a help. Good physiotherapy for the lungs and encouragement of exercise free of tubes and other medical encumbrances are beneficial.

TREATMENT OF MALIGNANT TUMOURS

Curative treatment

Surgery

Surgical resection remains the treatment of choice for adenocarcinomas of the oesophagus, which are relatively radioresistant, although the advent of chemoradiotherapy is changing this view. Squamous cell cancers are more sensitive to radiation, and the best form of management is therefore controversial. Unfortunately, no controlled trial has ever been done. The debate was started by Pearson.[138] He compared the results of surgery and radiotherapy in Edinburgh during the period 1948–67. After 5 years, only 11% of those treated surgically were alive, compared with 19% of those treated by radiotherapy. It must be stressed that this was not a controlled trial, but nonetheless the results achieved by radiotherapy were impressive at the time, mainly because the overall mortality was lessened by the absence of a postoperative mortality. Since that time there have been progressive improvements in both radiotherapy and surgery.

While the debate continues, the previously prohibitive operative mortality has been greatly reduced by improved methods of anaesthesia and perioperative care. For more than 20 years, most experienced surgeons have reported mortality rates of 10% or less for oesophageal resection at any level.[139,140] In 1980, Akiyama reported two deaths in 279 resections (0.7%) and. the trend to generally safer surgery continues.[141]

Many techniques have been described for resection of the oesophagus and its subsequent reconstruction. Safe resection usually involves thoracotomy, but some have returned to the older technique of resection of the oesophagus by transhiatal dissection popularized by Orringer.[142] This is appropriate for lesions in the lower oesophagus that can be mobilized by transhiatal dissection. The normal oesophagus above the tumour is then removed by blunt dissection, which is the well-established method of treating postcricoid tumours.[143] Cancers in the midoesophagus may also be extracted by transhiatal dissection, but there are occasional alarming unpublished reports of exsanguination from injury of the azygos vein, which may be infiltrated by tumour.

Tumours at the cardia may be removed via a left thoracotomy or a thoracoabdominal incision made through the sixth interspace. The resection includes the distal oesophagus together with the proximal stomach or the whole stomach. Total gastrectomy is probably preferable because the postoperative function is often better than with proximal gastrectomy, which allows free gastro-oesophageal reflux. Adenocarcinomas at this site are discussed in Chapter 26.

A left thoracotomy gives poor access for adequate clearance and intrathoracic anastomosis if the tumour is above the cardia. In these instances a right thoracotomy through the fourth or fifth interspace is preferable.[126] The aortic arch does not come into play through this approach, and the only structure of note that runs across the oesophagus is the azygos vein, which is easily divided. A midline or oblique laparotomy provides access to the abdomen for mobilization of the stomach, and is usually done as the first stage of the operation. The next step is right thoracotomy, and at least 6 cm of oesophagus should be resected

REFERENCES

137. Botet JF, Lightdale CJ, Zauber AG et al. Radiology 1991; 181: 419–425
138. Pearson JG. Cancer 1977; 39: 882–890
139. Dark JF, Mousalli, Vaughan R. Thorax 1981; 36: 891–895
140. Skinner DB, Dowlatshahi KD, DeMeester TR. Cancer 1982; 50: 2571–2575
141. Akiyama H. Curr Prob Surg 1980; 17: 53–120
142. Orringer MB. Surg Clin North Am 1983; 63: 941–950
143. Ong GB, Lee TC. Br J Surg 1960; 48: 193–200

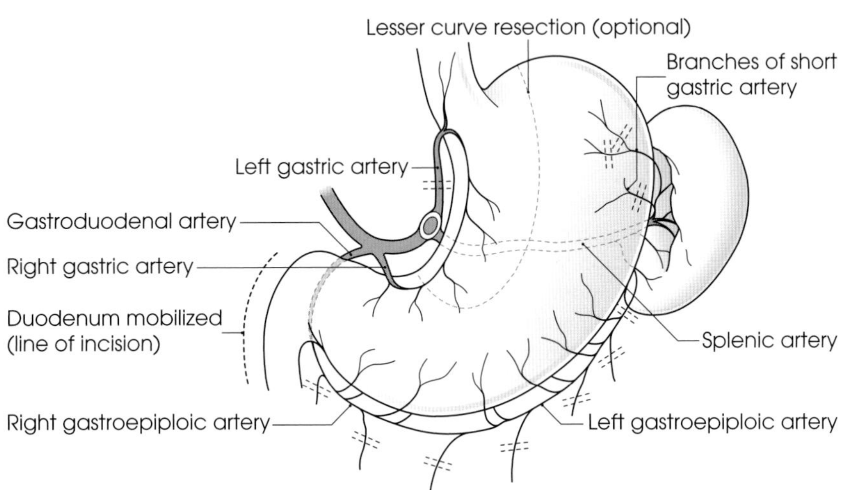

Figure 20.20 Gastric mobilization for oesophageal reconstruction.

proximal to the primary lesion. Because of the potential for submucosal spread, it has been suggested that the entire intrathoracic oesophagus should be removed, in which case a cervical incision may be used to deliver the upper part of oesophagus. This approach also simplifies access for the anastomosis, which need not be done deep in the chest. It is an attractive concept but, even if a cervical incision is used to mobilize the upper oesophagus, a stump is left and the anastomosis eventually lies in the upper thorax.

There is still controversy about the role of extensive lymphadenectomy for oesophageal cancer. Akiyama has reported 5-year survival rates of 55% with three-field dissection in the neck, chest and abdomen[144] compared with 38.3% with conventional two-field dissection. Others feel that there is limited scope for such a major procedure.[145] Nevertheless, systematic two-field lymph node dissection (chest and abdomen) has become much more common. This may improve prognosis, although this is still debated. It does give excellent staging information.

Minimally invasive surgical techniques have been used for oesophageal resection. Completely endoscopic procedures have been performed, but these are still a lengthy tour de force. Thoracoscopic mobilization of the oesophagus is more practical, but has not yet been demonstrated to reduce postoperative mortality.[146] Video-assisted thoracic surgery that allows use of a combination of endoscopic and conventional instruments may be the way ahead (see Ch. 21). An ingenious endoscope for performing transhiatal oesophagectomy under direct vision was developed by Buess,[147] but has not gained popularity.

It is fortunate that lesions of the upper thoracic or lower cervical oesophagus are rare, because adequate removal is usually difficult. A small tumour may be amenable to removal by blunt dissection via a cervical incision, but full exposure is required if the cancer is adherent to the trachea. Injury to the trachea is a formidable complication that should not be risked. Exposure of the thoracic inlet may be through a 'trapdoor' incision with partial division and lateral reflection of the sternum and attached clavicle.

Oesophageal reconstruction

The stomach is the most suitable organ for reconstruction following resection of the oesophagus for cancer. With appropriate mobilization it may be brought up to the neck (Fig. 20.20), unless a partial gastrectomy has been previously carried out. Troublesome postoperative reflux and stricture development are uncommon, but may be a problem after limited resections of the cardia. The anastomosis should therefore be as high in the oesophagus as possible, or a generous gastric resection should be carried out.

More complex reconstructions using colon or jejunum are sometimes indicated, but pose a greater hazard for the debilitated patient.

Radiotherapy

Radiotherapy may be used for the treatment of a small primary squamous carcinoma, as well as for the treatment of cancers that are not amenable to surgical resection. As previously mentioned, the relative indications for surgery and radiotherapy remain controversial, particularly for squamous carcinomas.

There is as yet no evidence that routine pre- or postoperative radiotherapy improves the results of surgical resection. A meta-analysis by the British Medical Research Council of all prospective randomized studies of preoperative radiotherapy has shown identical survival curves in the two groups.[148] Reports of the possible benefit of postoperative adjuvant radiotherapy are mostly anecdotal and uncontrolled. It is still possible that certain relatively favourable subgroups benefit, but further study is required.

Chemotherapy

Cytotoxic chemotherapy is improving steadily and now produces significant clinical benefits. Chemotherapy combined with radiotherapy (chemoradiotherapy) has been shown to improve survival over radiotherapy alone.[149] Preoperative chemotherapy has also been shown to improve survival following surgical resection.[150] A single small trial has shown improved survival

REFERENCES

144. Akiyama H, Tsurumaru M, Udagawa H et al. Ann Surg 1994; 220: 364–372
145. Law SYK, Fok M, Wong J. Br J Surg 1996; 83: 107–111
146. Cuschieri A. Endosc Surg Allied Technol 1994; 2: 21–25
147. Manncke K, Raestrup H, Walter D et al. Endosc Surg Allied Technol 1994; 2: 10–15
148. Arnott SJ, Duncan W, Gignoux M et al. Int J Radiat Oncol Biol Phys 1998; 41: 579–583
149. Herskovic A, Martz K, al-Sarraf M et al. N Engl J Med 1992; 326: 1593–1598
150. Medical Research Council Oesophageal Cancer Working Party. Lancet 2002; 359: 1727–1733

with preoperative chemoradiotherapy, but its use remains controversial.[151]

Palliative treatment

Stenting

Intubation or stenting of malignant strictures has been a simple form of management for those with incurable tumours. Semirigid tubes have largely been replaced by expanding metal stents, of which there are now many designs. These may be inserted at endoscopy or in the radiology department. They are relatively expensive, but provide excellent palliation with a very low complication rate.[152]

Bypass or resection

It is possible to bypass an irresectable lesion, or at least remove part of it. The Kirschner operation has been used for this purpose. In this operation the oesophagus is divided in the neck and the abdomen. The stomach is brought up subcutaneously and anastomosed to the cervical oesophagus. The upper end of the excluded oesophagus is closed, and the distal end is anastomosed to a loop of jejunum. In the years of its popularity the postoperative mortality of this approach was 41.5%, which most would regard as prohibitive.[153]

It is quite true that better palliation of dysphagia may be achieved in those who survive palliative resection or bypass than by intubation. However, the benefit of a major procedure in patients with a limited life expectancy is questionable. Their survival may be so short that it seems inappropriate to spend a large proportion of this time recovering from major surgery, because there are now so many less radical ways that provide effective palliation.

Laser phototherapy

Expanding metal stents have tended to dominate palliative treatment in recent years, but other forms of treatment may still have a place. Laser phototherapy for incurable carcinomas is capable of restoring swallowing to normal. The laser probe is passed down the biopsy channel of a fibre-optic endoscope, and vaporization is carried out under direct vision. A disadvantage of this approach is that it has to be done on several occasions, but eventually fibrosis seems to limit inward growth of the tumour.[154] In general, it works best for lesions that are protuberant, whereas scirrhous lesions are still best treated by intubation. Somewhat similar results to laser phototherapy have been obtained with bipolar diathermy probes[155] or intratumoural injection of alcohol.[156]

Radiotherapy

External beam radiotherapy for palliation is superficially attractive. It is not, however, without morbidity, and the dose may need to be reduced to the tolerance of the patient. This limits its usefulness. Intraluminal radiotherapy, or brachytherapy, is a much more practical approach. A low-penetration radiation source with a suitable delivery system can treat a malignant stricture in 30 min or less. Results are comparable with other methods of intraluminal treatment.[157]

MALIGNANT TRACHEO-OESOPHAGEAL FISTULA

Fistulation of a cancer into the trachea or left main stem bronchus is a very distressing complication. Such cancers are always incurable, and the best form of palliation is to insert an expanding metal stent. If necessary, stents may be placed both in the oesophagus and in the trachea, so-called parallel stenting.[158]

COMPLICATIONS OF RESECTION

Leaks

Leakage from an oesophageal anastomosis is a particularly lethal complication. The best management is not to get a leak in the first place! The low mortality rates following oesophageal resection quoted previously are largely from a reduction of anastomotic leakage by careful surgical technique. Meticulous and generous mobilization of the stomach, with careful preservation of its blood supply, is the best insurance against anastomotic problems. If more complex methods of reconstruction are used, even more care should be taken to ensure that the blood supply of the anastomosis is adequate. Prior angiography, careful inspection of the arterial and venous anatomy, and trial clamping of vessels before division are useful aids when long segments of colon are used.

There is little point in attempting resuture of the anastomosis if leakage does occur; except in the most fortunate circumstances this is doomed to failure. Small leaks may be managed conservatively with antibiotics, but mainly with patience and nutritional support. Leakage of an anastomosis in the superficial part of the neck with a retrosternal reconstruction may produce a local fistula that will heal spontaneously. Intrathoracic leakage is a much more serious problem. Large leaks producing cardiovascular collapse are likely to prove lethal, and if this occurs in a patient with a poor prognosis, radical attempts at salvage may not be worthwhile Exploration of the anastomosis may be worthwhile if the patient is young, or has benign disease or a small cancer. If the leak is relatively small and the tissues are viable, carefully placed drains may control the contamination until healing occurs. Otherwise further resection, with creation of an end cervical oesophagostomy and an appropriate abdominal stoma, is the only effective treatment. Reconstruction is carried out some months later.

Strictures

Anastomotic strictures are the result of either poor technique with the construction of a narrow stoma or postoperative reflux. The latter should be prevented by avoiding known pitfalls in reconstruction, such as a conservative excision of the cardia. Stapled anastomoses may stenose in a rather unpredictable way. Simple dilatation is effective if the stricture is not too fibrous. Mature strictures may require radial division with endoscopic diathermy.

REFERENCES

151. Walsh TN, Noonan N, Hollywood D et al. N Engl J Med 1996; 335: 462–467
152. Laasch H-U, Nicholson DA, Kay CL et al. Clin Radiol 1998; 53: 666–672
153. Wong J, Lam KH, Wei WI et al. World J Surg 1981; 5: 547–552
154. Krasner N, Barr H, Skidmore C et al. Gut 1987; 28: 792–798
155. Jensen DM, Machicado G, Randall G et al. Gastroenterology 1988; 94:1263–1270
156. Nwokolo CU, Payne-James JJ, Silk DB et al. Gut 1994; 35: 299–303
157. Low DE, Pagliero KM. J Thorac Cardiovasc Surg 1992; 104: 173–178
158. van den Bongard HJ, Boot H, Baas P et al. Gastrointest Endosc 2002; 55: 110–115

The chest wall, pleura, lungs, trachea, mediastinum and diaphragm 21

Francis C. Wells, James C. Halstead, Nicholas Screaton

CHEST WALL TUMOURS

Primary chest wall tumours are rare; metastases to the chest wall from a variety of primaries (including breast, thyroid, renal, lung and prostate) are commonplace. Malignant tumours can arise from any of the elements of the chest wall, but most arise from bone or cartilage. Benign disorders occur as often as primary malignant tumours, the commonest being chondroma and fibrous dysplasia.

Tumours of the chest wall usually present with pain and a palpable mass, although some are found incidentally on chest radiography. Most require further imaging with CT and/or MRI.[1] These can be combined with percutaneous biopsy, but often the diagnosis is made only from an open biopsy. For small tumours an excision biopsy can be both diagnostic and curative. Larger tumours may need to have the diagnosis confirmed by an incision biopsy before a radical resection is undertaken. The incision biopsy site should be fully excised at subsequent surgery to avoid the risk of tumour seeding. If the incision biopsy is inconclusive, a radical excision should be performed, because this is the only effective method of treating those tumours that ultimately turn out to be malignant.[2]

BENIGN TUMOURS

Chondromas develop in the ribs and costal cartilages, occasionally becoming huge (giant chondromas).[3] They usually appear as rounded homogenous masses on chest radiographs, although they can contain stippled calcification. All chondromas should be excised, because differentiation from a chondrosarcoma is rarely possible.

Fibrous dysplasia affects the ribs, producing typical radiological appearances of an expanded thin bone cortex with a trabeculated radiolucent core. Excisional biopsy is, however, almost always indicated, because percutaneous needle biopsy is unreliable and resection is usually warranted to alleviate symptoms. Recurrence is extremely rare.

MALIGNANT TUMOURS

Chondrosarcoma is the commonest primary chest wall tumour. Its clinical, radiological and incision biopsy features are often identical to those of benign cartilaginous tumours.[4] The treatment is by surgical resection, because this tumour is not radiosensitive. The prognosis is dependent primarily on the histological grade of the tumour and its completeness of resection.

Fibrosarcomas often produce radiolucent erosions of the ribs. Percutaneous or incisional biopsy is diagnostic when the characteristic features of disorganized collagen formation are present. The prognosis is poor, but reasonable survival can follow wide excision of a low-grade tumour. Postoperative irradiation may be given to try and provide local control of the tumour.

Ewing's sarcoma of the chest wall is rare (see Ch. 42). It is a radiosensitive tumour, and the best management probably combines wide excision and a histologically clear margin[5] with radiotherapy and multiagent chemotherapy.

All malignant tumours should be widely excised (Fig. 21.1), and this will often include the whole of the involved rib(s) and one further rib on either side, because these tumours may extend through the intercostal space. Frozen sections may be sent to confirm tumour-free margins. Sternal tumours should be treated by excision of the whole sternum and its attached costal cartilages. The method of reconstruction depends on the size and site of the defect (Fig. 21.2) and the chest wall vascularity, because this may be affected by previous surgery or radiotherapy. Small defects do not usually need to be reconstructed, especially those that underlie the scapula. Larger defects should be closed to protect the underlying structures and to maintain chest wall mechanics and correct shape. Polypropylene (Marlex) mesh is often used, and this can be constructed in two layers with methyl methacrylate cement between.[6] The bone cement is shaped to the contour of the chest wall and the Marlex mesh is sutured to the surrounding structures. The soft tissue defect can be closed by pectoralis major, latissimus dorsi or rectus abdominis myocutaneous (Fig. 21.3) flaps (see Ch. 9). Pedicled greater omentum or microvascular flaps[7] have also been used for this purpose.

CONGENITAL CHEST WALL LESIONS

PECTUS EXCAVATUM

Pectus excavatum is present when there is posterior depression of the sternum and lower costal cartilages (Fig. 21.4). It is frequently asymmetrical, and while it may appear in infancy it usually presents in adolescence when schoolmates pass comment. There

REFERENCES

1. Knisely BL, Broderick LS, Kuhlman JE. Magn Reson Imaging Clin North Am 2000; 8: 125–141
2. Sabanathan S, Salama FD, Morgan WE et al. Ann Thorac Surg 1985; 39: 4–15
3. Pandey S. J Bone Joint Surg Br 1975; 57: 519–522
4. Somers J, Faber LP. Semin Thorac Cardiovasc Surg 1999; 11: 270–277
5. Incarbone M, Pastorino U. World J Surg 2001; 25: 218–230
6. Lardinois D, Muller M, Furrer M et al. Ann Thorac Surg 2000; 69: 919–923
7. Netscher DT, Valkov PL. Semin Surg Oncol 2000; 19: 255–263

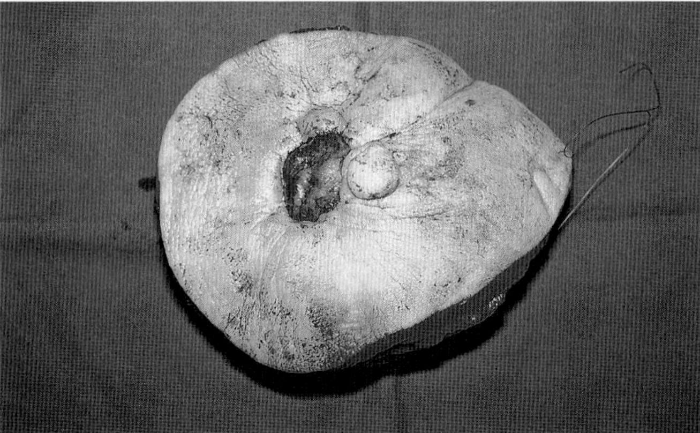

Figure 21.1 Resected ulcerated chest wall sarcoma demonstrating wide macroscopic resection margins.

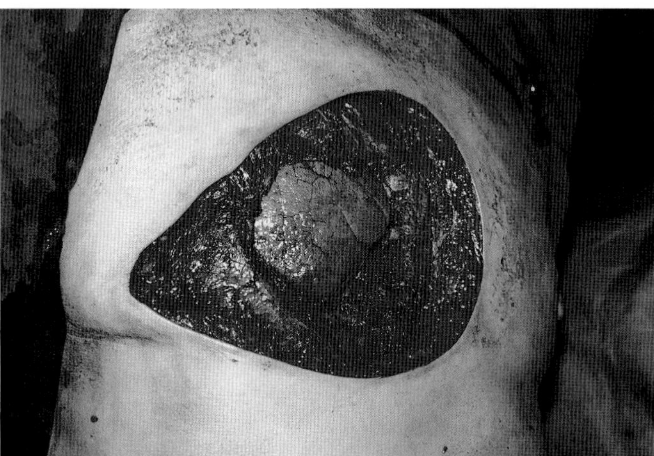

Figure 21.2 The chest wall defect resulting from resection.

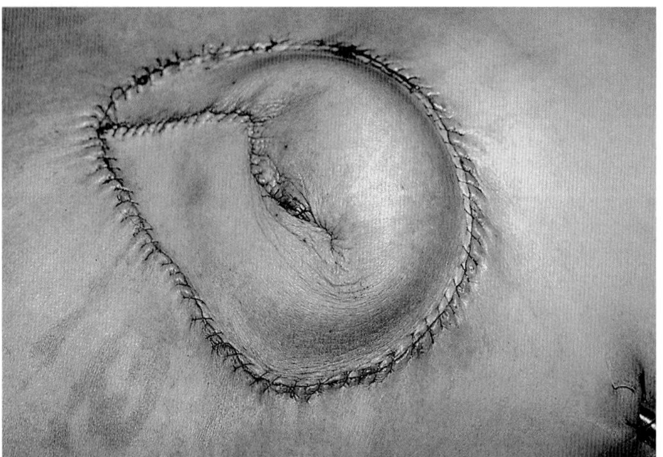

Figure 21.3 Completed reconstruction using a transversus abdominis pedicled flap to cover the defect.

is often a family history of thoracic deformity. Correction is usually undertaken for cosmetic reasons. While overt cardiopulmonary compromise is unusual, many patients have measurable increased exercise tolerance after repair.[8] When associated with congenital heart disease simultaneous repair of defects can be successfully undertaken in infancy.[9]

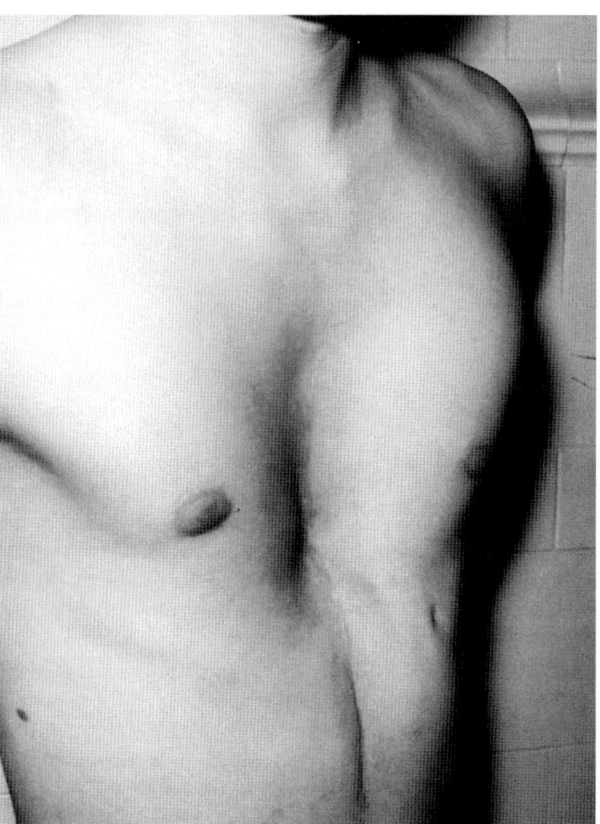

Figure 21.4 Pectus excavatum deformity.

Repair is performed through a vertical or submammary incision (the latter is more cosmetic). The affected costal cartilages are resected with preservation of their perichondrial sheaths, which allows cartilaginous regeneration. The sternum is then lifted forward and fixed in a normal position with an underlying metal (pectus) bar. Occasionally, a transverse osteotomy is needed to achieve this. The metal bar often migrates, necessitating its removal. Up to 10% of those treated surgically develop a recurrence of the deformity. Minimally invasive techniques are being developed[10] in which a curved pectus bar is inserted via a 1–2-cm incision and rotated to push the sternum forwards.[11]

PECTUS CARINATUM

Pectus carinatum is an anterior protrusion of the chest wall, which is less common than pectus excavatum and is usually symmetrical. It is otherwise similar to pectus excavatum and the principles of its repair are identical. An osteotomy is usually needed to return the sternum to a normal position. Mixed defects do exist and often require sternal osteotomies for correction.

REFERENCES

8. Jacobs JP, Quintessenza JA, Morell VO et al. Eur J Cardiothorac Surg 2002; 21: 869–873
9. Hasegawa T, Yamaguchi M, Ohshima Y et al. Eur J Cardiothorac Surg 2002; 22: 874–878
10. Shamberger RC. Chest Surg Clin North Am 2000; 10: 245–252
11. Nuss D, Croitoru DP, Kelly RE Jr et al. Eur J Pediatr Surg 2002; 12: 230–234

OTHER STERNAL DEFECTS

Cleft sternum occurs when a failure of ventral fusion of the developing bars has occurred. It is associated with craniofacial haemangioma and the defect can be closed directly in infancy.[12]

Ectopia cordis describes a sternal defect with the heart lying outside the thorax. Associated cardiac anomalies are common, and surgery to correct the condition is usually unsuccessful.

Poland's syndrome is characterized by hypoplasia or absence of the nipple, hypoplasia of subcutaneous tissue, absence of the costosternal portion of pectoralis major, absence of pectoralis minor, and absence of costal cartilages and/or ribs.[13] Reconstruction should be undertaken in infancy, and can often be achieved by the anterior transaxillary transfer of latissimus dorsi with its attachment to the sternum and clavicle.[14] Breast prostheses can be placed in female patients.

THE PLEURA

The pleural cavity is a potential space occupying each hemithorax and enveloping the lungs. It consists of mesothelial cells on a basement membrane and has two layers: parietal, which is applied to the chest wall; and visceral, which forms the outer layer of the lungs. In health, there is a considerable fluid transport across this space, but because of active reabsorption pleural fluid does not accumulate despite the negative intrapleural pressure.

A variety of pathological processes can lead to the accumulation of air, fluid or solid matter in the pleural space. These abnormal collections produce dyspnoea and can be life-threatening if mediastinal compression develops. The insertion of an intercostal drain will treat most such collections.

PHYSIOLOGY OF THE PLEURAL SPACE AND ITS DERANGEMENTS

Starling's law governs the production and transport of fluid across the pleural space. The hydrostatic pressure of the capillaries, the colloid osmotic pressure gradient, and the pressure generated by the tendency for elastic recoil of the lungs are the major determinants. The hydrostatic pressure of the parietal pleural capillaries is far higher than that of the visceral pleural capillaries, which are part of the pulmonary circulation. The colloid osmotic pressure gradient is uniform for both sets of capillaries and favours the absorption of fluid from the pleural space. The elasticity of the lungs generates a negative intrapleural pressure, which promotes the loss of fluid into the intrapleural space from both pleural surfaces. The summation of these three forces leads to the production of pleural fluid by the parietal pleura and its absorption by the visceral layer. This ensures that only a tiny volume of fluid occupies the space at any one time. There is reserve in the system to guard against the production of excessive pleural fluid, because the absorptive gradient is stronger and the visceral capillary surface area is larger. This mechanism is remarkably efficient given that many litres of fluid cross the space every day. A low colloid osmotic pressure or elevated capillary pressure can lead to the development of a pleural effusion. The presence of a large pleural collection or pneumothorax can lead to the compression of air spaces and the maldistribution of ventilation as the lung becomes less compliant. This produces a venoarterial shunt (perfusion of unventilated lung) with resultant systemic hypoxia. This can be complicated by maldistribution of perfusion, which can aggravate the hypoxia. In most instances these changes are reversible by the insertion of an intercostal drain.

INTERCOSTAL DRAINAGE

An intercostal drain can be used to drain liquid or gaseous collections from the pleural space. An adequately sized conduit that allows one-way drainage of the pleural space must be provided. This is most commonly achieved by a chest drain connected to an underwater seal. This underwater seal serves as a valve, preventing the return of fluid or air to the pleural space providing the hydrostatic pressure gradient is greater than the negative force generated by forceful inspiration. This is achieved by placing the drainage bottle on the floor below the patient's chest. As long as the drain is in the chest and the tube is only just beneath the fluid level in the drainage bottle, fluid and air will escape. A pleural effusion should be fully drained by an apical drain because of the positive pressure generated in expiration. If necessary, two or more drains can be inserted, and this is often routine after thoracic surgical procedures. Suction can be applied to any drains to speed emptying of the pleural space and to overcome the reduced lung compliance following a period of pulmonary collapse.

Insertion of a chest drain should be a relatively painless and straightforward procedure, which begins with an assessment of the patient and the likely diagnosis. Patients are usually stable enough to allow a chest radiograph to be taken. A drain should be placed at the apex when a pneumothorax is suspected. The differential diagnosis of this radiological abnormality, namely bullous emphysema or an intrathoracic viscus, must be considered, because perforation of either of these with a chest drain can be disastrous. A second expiratory film may help when doubt persists. Where a fluid collection is suspected a drain should be placed toward the base of the fluid level. This can be easily performed under ultrasound control, because identification of the diaphragm may be difficult from chest radiographs. A diagnostic needle can often be introduced into the pleural space, and if fluid is easily aspirated a drain can be inserted at the same position.

The safest and most reliable site to insert a chest drain is between the anterior and midaxillary lines above the sixth rib. A posteriorly located drain is uncomfortable, prone to obstruction when the patient lies supine, and difficult to insert through the bulk of latissimus dorsi. Low drains may penetrate the diaphragm and can enter the abdomen, where they can cause damage to other structures. Anterior drains are also uncomfortable and may injure mediastinal structures. A size 28 or 32 French gauge silastic tube drain is appropriate for most conditions. The skin, periosteum and parietal pleura should be infiltrated with local anaesthetic, because these are the most painful layers. A skin incision large enough to admit an index finger is made, and the subcutaneous fat and intercostal muscles are separated with an artery forceps. Blunt dissection through the midpoint of the interspace avoids the intercostal vessels, which bifurcate soon after their origin to give branches that run immediately above and below each rib. Once the pleura is reached this should be

REFERENCES

12. Fokin AA. Chest Surg Clin North Am 2000; 10: 261–276
13. Urschel HC Jr. Chest Surg Clin North Am 2000; 10: 393–403
14. Garcia VF, Seyfer AE, Graeber GM. Surg Clin North Am 1989: 19: 1103–18

carefully breached with the artery forceps. A finger should then be admitted into the pleural space to ensure the underlying lung is not adherent. The drain should then be guided into the pleural space with the trocar partially withdrawn. It is then connected to an underwater seal and secured in place. Prior angulation of the trocar can aid in the correct placement of the drain.

Where a tension pneumothorax (air-filled pleural space under pressure with mediastinal shift) is suspected, there is no time for a chest radiograph and the affected pleura should be immediately decompressed with a cannula inserted through the second intercostal space in the midclavicular line.

Rapid drainage of a large, long-standing pleural effusion may rarely cause re-expansion pulmonary oedema. It is wise to leave the drainage bottle off suction[15] if excessive drainage is encountered, or to clamp the drain and allow 200–300 mL to drain at regular intervals.

Once in situ, chest drains should *never* be clamped. The only exceptions to this are following pneumonectomy or where there is massive exsanguinating haemorrhage down a chest drain following trauma, or where an agent has been instilled into the chest for pleurodesis and there is no air leak. It can also be clamped (as discussed earlier) where intermittent drainage of a chronic, large pleural effusion is being used.

Chest drains are removed when there is no air leak, the drainage is minimal, and the lung is fully expanded. These should be accompanied by a reduction in the size of the swing of the air-fluid level in the tubing. Removal should occur soon after these criteria are fulfilled, because drains act as portals for the entry of bacteria into the chest. Drain removal should be undertaken with the patient performing a sustained Valsalva manoeuvre to prevent the entry of air.

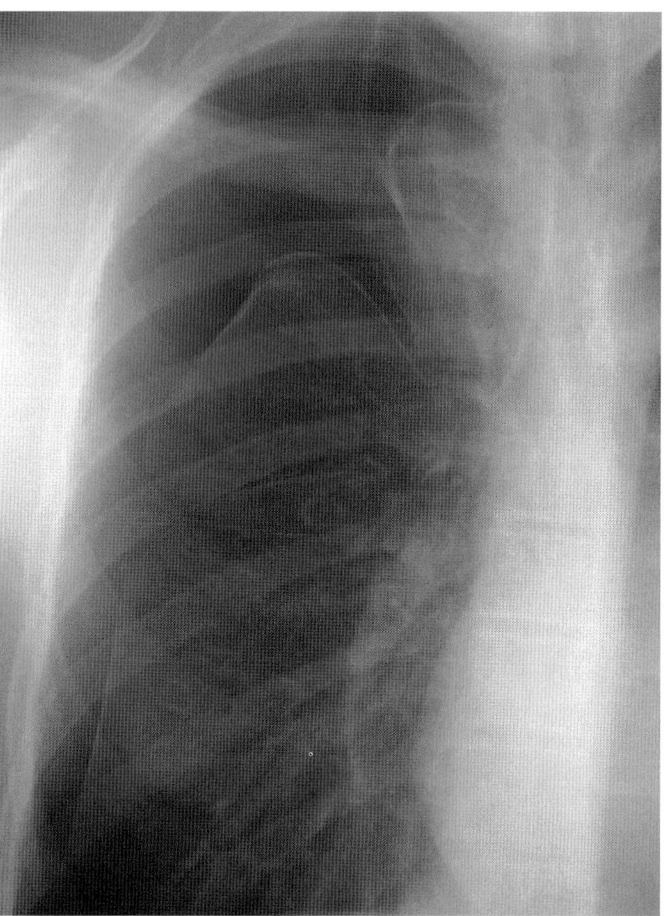

Figure 21.5 Chest radiograph showing absent lung markings peripherally and a pleural edge in a patient with a right pneumothorax and an azygous lobe.

PNEUMOTHORAX

Air can enter the pleural space (Fig. 21.5) through the chest wall or can leak from an intrathoracic structure such as the lungs, tracheobronchial tree or oesophagus. This air leak may occur secondary to injury (blunt or penetrating) or underlying lung disease. Mechanical ventilation with raised pressure can cause barotrauma to the lungs, which may result in a complicated pneumothorax.

Lung diseases associated with pneumothoraces can be classified as either focal or generalized disorders. The commonest focal causes of spontaneous pneumothoraces are small blebs on the visceral pleural surface. These are usually found at the lung apex, but they also occur in the apical segment of the lower lobes or along any of the fissural margins of the lung. Their aetiology is unknown, but they seem to cause pneumothoraces most commonly in tall, thin adolescents. Patients often give a strong family history, and spontaneous pneumothoraces are common in patients with Marfan's syndrome. Connective tissue failure may lead to a pneumothorax following rapid growth in a susceptible individual. Pneumothorax may also complicate emphysema, pulmonary fibrosis, cystic fibrosis, sarcoidosis and asthma. There is a first peak in the incidence of pneumothorax around 20 years of age, associated with the rupture of small apical blebs, and a later peak around 60 years, often the result of chronic obstructive airways disease and associated with cigarette smoking.

Management of a pneumothorax is primarily determined by its size, although the underlying pathology may also influence strategy. Small pneumothoraces, where the lung is less than 2 cm from the chest wall on a chest radiograph (in an adult), can be treated conservatively without drainage. Serial radiographs must, however, be obtained to ensure its resorption. Some advocate repeated aspiration for larger pneumothoraces,[16] but the great majority are treated by the insertion of an intercostal drain. The collapsed lung should expand up to the chest wall, and any air leaks usually seal quite rapidly as the result of adhesions. Occasionally the lung fails to expand and the air leak persists. Surgery may be considered after around 1 week of tube drainage. The aim of the operation is to create a raw surface for the lung to adhere to, thus obliterating the pleural space (a pleurodesis). In addition, pulmonary blebs and bullae should be ligated or stapled. This surgery can be undertaken thoracoscopically or through a limited thoracotomy with similar, excellent results.[17] Recurrent spontaneous pneumothoraces are the usual indication for such surgery, and it is definitely indicated after the third episode (some advocate surgery following the second episode) to prevent further recurrence. Tension pneumothoraces usually occur in injured patients or those receiving intermittent positive-pressure ventilation. They seldom complicate spontaneous pneumothorax.

Catamenial pneumothorax (usually of the right hemithorax) occurs in women around the time of menstruation. It may be

REFERENCES

15. Trapnell DH, Thurston JG. Lancet 1970; 27: 1367–1369
16. Noppen M, Alexander P, Driesen P et al. Am J Respir Crit Care Med 2002; 165: 1240–1244
17. Waller DA, Forty J, Morritt GN. Ann Thorac Surg 1994; 58: 372–376

related to endometriosis and/or pleuroperitoneal connection, or it may be the result of a rupture of an aforementioned apical bleb. As with any pneumothorax, it may be complicated by bleeding that produces a haemopneumothorax, recognized by a horizontal air–blood interface.

An excessive air leak that is incompletely evacuated down an intercostal tube can lead to surgical emphysema, when air accumulates throughout the subcutaneous planes. It can produce gross swelling, which often extends from the eyes down to the perineum, but it is seldom harmful. Very rarely it may cause laryngeal obstruction. The appropriate treatment is to ensure that the pleural space is adequately drained, and occasionally a small skin incision made on the front of the chest allows decompression.

PLEURAL EFFUSION

A pleural effusion is the collection of fluid in the pleural space. They are classified according to their protein content and the underlying aetiology. Transudates have a low protein content (less than 30 g/dL) and are caused by cardiac failure, hypoalbuminaemia and mediastinal fibrosis. Exudates have higher protein content and are caused by infection and inflammation (collagen disorders, arthritides, pancreatitis, pulmonary infarction and malignancy). Pleural effusions cause dyspnoea and can be diagnosed by their dullness to percussion and decreased breath sounds. Bronchial breathing can often be heard at the top of an effusion. Chest radiography shows a homogenous opacity, usually at the lung base, with an upward-curved concave margin. Needle aspiration with biochemical and cytological examination usually provides a diagnosis.

Treatment can be conservative in certain situations (advanced malignancy and small effusions), but large symptomatic effusions require drainage. This is best achieved through an intercostal drain, although the success of this approach is limited when the collection is dense, multiloculated or particulate. In these circumstances, a limited thoracotomy or thoracoscopic procedure usually evacuates the collection and allows the lung to expand.

Malignant effusions associated with primary pleural tumours, invasion from a bronchial primary or metastatic disease, often do poorly with simple drainage. Surgery is often needed to establish the diagnosis when percutaneous needle-based biopsy or cytological analyses have not given an answer. Surgical exploration also enables the effusion to be fully aspirated and the tumour debulked, allowing better lung expansion. This usually leads to pleurodesis and obviates the need for repeated aspiration, which eventually introduces infection.

Parietal pleurectomy can be combined with the instillation of talcum powder, which produces an intense chemical pleuritis and subsequent adhesion formation. Talc slurry can be instilled into the chest through a drain with the same effect. Satisfactory resolution of the effusion by drainage alone is complicated if the lung is trapped by thickened pleura. The use of a pleuroperitoneal shunt can be considered under these circumstances.

CHYLOTHORAX

The presence of chyle in the pleural space is called a chylothorax. The fluid has a milky appearance because of the high concentration of fats, immunoglobulins and lymphocytes. Chylothoraces develop when chyle escapes from the thoracic duct (Fig. 21.6; see Ch. 12). Leaks most commonly occur as a consequence of trauma or iatrogenic injury (e.g. oesophagectomy). Some spontaneous adult chylothoraces may be the result of previous injury.

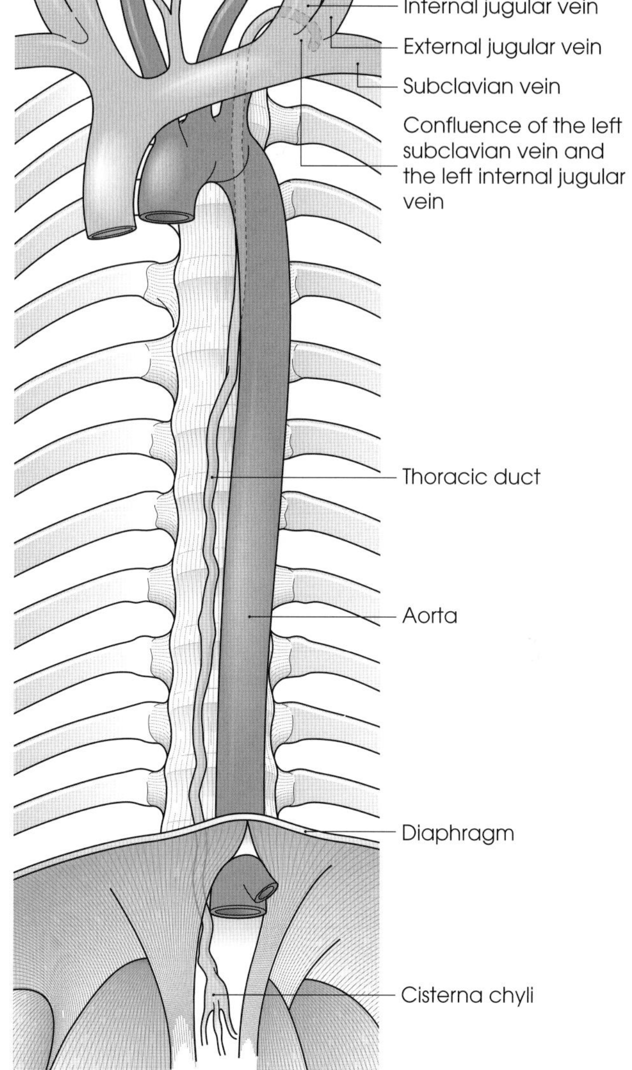

Figure 21.6 Anatomy of the thoracic duct.

Dyspnoea is the usual presenting symptom, although exaggerated tube drainage may occur after recent surgery. The diagnosis is confirmed by biochemical analysis, when chylomicrons and a high triglyceride level are found (of the order of 1 g/L). Chylothoraces can lead to serious nutritional depletion when they are large or persistent.

Conservative treatment includes total parenteral nutrition, drainage of the pleural space with an intercostal drain, and a fat-free diet. Octreotide, the somatostatin analogue, is reported to reduce the drainage of chyle,[18a] but treatment is often protracted and failure is common. At operation the thoracic duct can be litigated just above or below the diaphragm. Early re-exploration is recommended after oesophagectomy, because the opening can be easily visualized and sutured, leading to rapid resolution of the problem. Irradiation may seal the leak[18] if it is the result of malignant infiltration.

REFERENCES

18. Light RW. Curr Opin Pulm Med 2000; 6: 255–258
18a. Rosti L, Bini RM, Chessa M et al. Eur J Pediatr 2002; 161: 149–150.

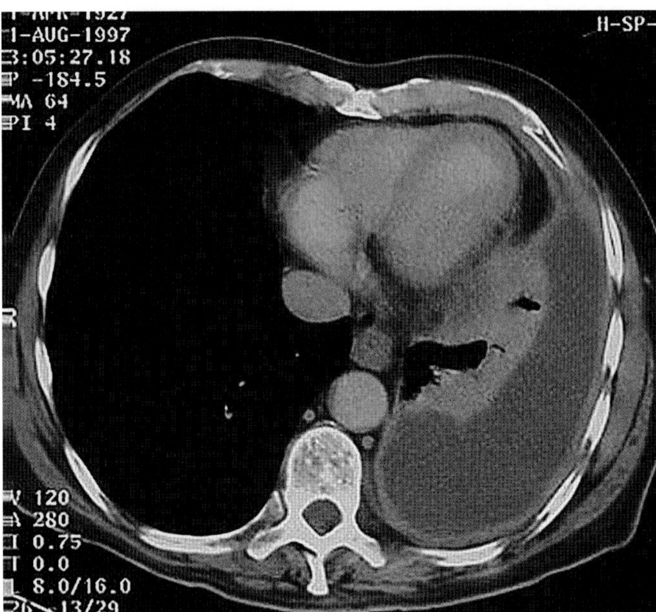

Figure 21.7 Transverse CT image following intravenous contrast medium, demonstrating a large left pleural collection with an enhancing rind of costal pleural thickening and oedema of the extrapleural fat in keeping with an emphysema.

EMPYEMA THORACIS

Empyema thoracis (Fig. 21.7) is a collection of pus in the pleural space and was first described by Hippocrates. It most frequently develops when a pre-existing effusion or haemothorax becomes infected. Such effusions are often parapneumonic in nature, related to bronchial obstruction (foreign body or tumour) or secondary to a subphrenic abscess. Neurological disease, especially if there is bulbar impairment, seems to predispose to empyema development, presumably as a result of aspiration. Haemothoraces often follow chest trauma, which may also cause foreign material to enter the chest. These also predispose to empyemata unless properly drained or evacuated.

A variety of organisms can cause an empyema, with the commonest being lung pathogens such as *Streptococcus pneumoniae*, *Klebsiella* or staphylococcal species. Coliforms may be cultured if there is an oesophageal perforation or subphrenic abscess. Multiple organisms may also be isolated and, if antibiotics have already been administered, cultures may be sterile.

Empyema evolves in stages. Initially, there is contamination of an effusion, with fibrin production and the migration of leucocytes and bacteria into the fluid. Over time the fluid becomes frankly purulent, and the maturation of fibrous tissue leads to the septation of the effusion, with walling off by a thick rind. Empyemata usually lie in a dependent posteroinferior position in the affected hemithorax. The underlying lung is compressed, and the chest wall contracts and becomes increasingly immobile with 'rib crowding'. The septic process of chronic empyema can lead to severe malnutrition.

The treatment depends on the stage of the empyema. Early empyema is usually effectively treated with appropriate antibiotics and drainage of the effusion, either by insertion of a chest drain or thoracoscopically.[19] The use of intrapleural fibrinolytic agents can aid in resolution of early empyemata by breaking down fibrinous loculi, especially in children.[20] When the pus is thick and the loculation mature, such an approach is often unsuccessful. This leaves two choices: thoracotomy with decortication or rib resection and drainage.[21]

A segment of rib (around 5 cm) overlying the empyema is removed, and through this defect the rind is punctured and a large-bore intercostal drain is placed into the cavity. Once the pus has been drained the patient's markers of sepsis improve. The drain does not need to be connected to an underwater seal and can be shortened into a stoma bag. As long as drainage continues, the patient feels better and gains weight. Eventually the cavity starts to close, and the tube is progressively withdrawn. Serial sinograms can demonstrate obliteration of the space.

For fit patients, thoracotomy and decortication should be considered. The lung will only expand if the airway is patent and intact. A bronchoscopy is therefore essential before proceeding to thoracotomy. This is a major procedure, performed through a posterolateral thoracotomy, which removes the visceral and parietal rind together with the enclosed fibrinopurulent material. The aim of surgery is to excise all the infected material and allow the lung to expand. This enables the lung to adhere to the chest wall and prevents recurrence. Success depends on complete removal of the incarcerating visceral rind and normal compliance of the underlying lung. When there is underlying bronchiectasis, lung resection is occasionally necessary. Pulmonary resection should almost never be undertaken if there is an underlying lung abscess.

A tuberculous empyema often has an underlying bronchopleural fistula, and when this is present resection may be necessary. Frequent breakdown of the bronchial stump makes this an unattractive option. All such procedures should be covered with appropriate antibiotics.

Infection of a postpneumonectomy space with bronchopleural fistula is a serious problem and can occur in the early or late postoperative period. The diagnosis is suspected when the fluid level on chest radiograph falls and the patient expectorates brackish watery fluid. The space must be drained.[22] This can be quickly achieved by inserting an intercostal drain before re-exploring the chest to amputate and resuture the bronchial stump, which should then be covered with vascularized tissue. In late cases, drainage can be achieved through a skin-lined tract fashioned after resection of a segment of rib. The space should be regularly irrigated and, once clear fluid is obtained, closed with antibiotic solution instilled in the chest. Alternatively, pedicled muscle flaps can be advanced into the residual space to promote healing. Where a bronchopleural fistula persists, consideration should be given to closure of the bronchial defect. This is best achieved in a long right-sided stump through a trans-sternal transpericardial approach.

PLEURAL TUMOURS

Benign tumours of the pleura are rare. The commonest is a localized (solitary) fibroma, although differentiation from a malignant tumour can be challenging.[23] These tumours are usually pedunculated, arise from the visceral pleura, and can be

REFERENCES

19. Waller DA. Curr Opin Pulm Med 2002; 8: 323–326
20. Thomson AH, Hull J, Kumar MR et al. Thorax 2002; 57: 343–347
21. Forty J, Yeatman M, Wells FC. Respir Med 1990; 84: 147–153
22. Vallieres E. Chest Surg Clin North Am 2002; 12: 571–585
23. Churg A, Colby TV, Cagle P et al. Am J Surg Pathol 2000; 24: 1183–1200

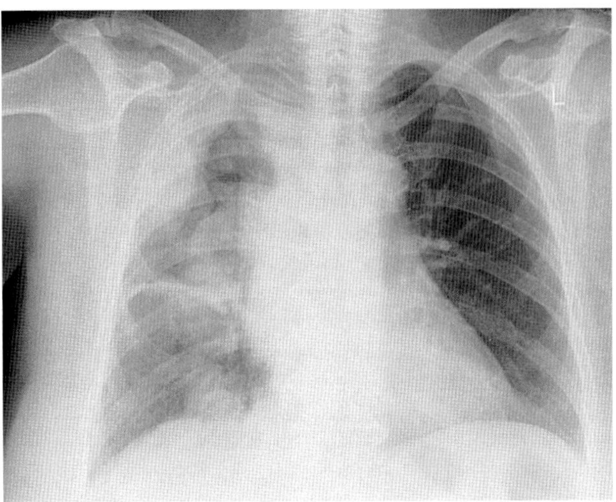

Figure 21.8 Posteroanterior chest radiograph showing volume loss in the right hemithorax, where there is lobulated pleural thickening in the mid- and upper zone involving costal, mediastinal and fissural pleurae.

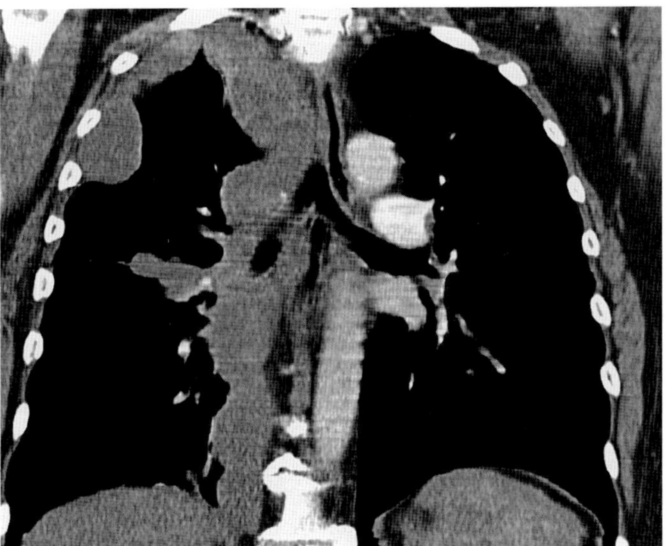

Figure 21.9 Contrast-enhanced CT confirms the extensive nodular pleural thickening, which involves the mediastinal pleural surface and is typical of malignant pleural disease.

associated with hypertrophic pulmonary osteoarthropathy. They are found incidentally on chest radiographs or can present with exertional dyspnoea. Resection is warranted for symptoms and to confirm the diagnosis. This can be safely undertaken thoracoscopically.[24]

A primary malignant tumour of the pleura known as a mesothelioma (Figs 21.8 and 21.9) is an uncommon but rapidly increasing condition. Its incidence is expected to rise over the next 20 years because of the long latent period between asbestos exposure and the development of tumour.[25] Mesothelioma often involves the whole of one hemithorax, with confluent sheets of visceral and parietal pleural tumour. It frequently invades the chest wall, diaphragm and mediastinum, with incarceration of the lung. Because of the insidious nature of its development, patients often present late. They are often dyspnoeic and may have intractable chest wall pain. Metastases occur late. Biopsy is indicated to confirm the diagnosis and to allow compensation claims to go ahead. The best treatment for this condition is not established, because surgical resection and cure is very rare.

Surgical treatment ranges from diagnostic incision biopsies to extensive extrapleural pneumonectomy. The initial reports of radical pneumonectomies showed significant mortality rates with little demonstrable benefit for survivors.[26] More recently, this surgical approach has been combined with high-dose irradiation to produce prolonged survival in early-stage tumours.[27] Unfortunately, the addition of chemotherapy has only benefited a small, low-risk subset.[28] The majority of patients present with advanced disease. Their prognosis is primarily related to cell type (epithelial superior to sarcomatous) and tumour stage. Pleurectomy–decortication procedures have been undertaken through both open and thoracoscopic approaches.[29] They can provide some short-term symptom relief and may prevent recurrent effusion, but as yet no survival benefit has been demonstrated. Compensation is available when previous exposure to asbestos can be demonstrated or presumed. The diagnosis is not absolutely reliant on a histological diagnosis.

Metastatic disease from bronchogenic or breast carcinomas can also produce symptomatic pleural deposits and effusions. These are incurable, but symptoms can be improved by draining the effusion and effecting pleurodesis. Where there is a large bulk of more solid disease, thoracoscopic debulking procedures may improve symptoms.

NEOPLASTIC TUMOURS OF THE LUNG

Carcinoma of the lung increased in incidence exponentially during the first half of the 20th century in relation to an increase in tobacco smoking. Its overall incidence in the UK has now begun to plateau, but it is still the commonest cause of cancer death in men. In women, it is a very close second to breast carcinoma overall, and has overtaken it in certain areas of the country. Although lung cancers form primarily as a result of tobacco smoking, other environmental factors and genetic susceptibility clearly play a role. Many malignant tumours are incurable at presentation because of metastatic spread. For the minority that are localized, the best prospect of cure comes from a complete surgical resection. This is rarely achieved. Resection is curative for all benign tumours. Various screening tests have been targeted to at-risk subgroups, but no clear benefit has yet been demonstrated. Low-dose high-resolution CT scanning shows some promise. Most of the screening regimens have, unfortunately, identified large numbers of indeterminate peripheral lesions, the correct management of which remains a challenge.

REFERENCES

24. Haraguchi S, Koizumi K, Kawamoto M et al. Jpn J Cardiovasc Surg 1998; 46: 664–666
25. Peto J, Hodgson JT, Matthews FE et al. Lancet 1995; 345: 535–539
26. Butchart EG, Ashcroft T, Barnsley WC et al. Thorax 1976; 31: 15–24
27. Rusch VW, Rosenweiz K, Venkatraman E et al. J Thorac Cardiovasc Surg 2001; 122: 788–795
28. Sugarbaker DJ, Flores RM, Jaklitsch MT et al. J Thorac Cardiovasc Surg 1999; 117: 54–63
29. Grossebner MW, Arifi AA, Goddard M et al. Eur J Cardiothorac Surg 1999; 16: 619–623

Primary prevention through antismoking campaigns is the main hope for reducing the mortality from this condition. Unfortunately, many young people continue to smoke.

ENVIRONMENTAL FACTORS AND GENETIC SUSCEPTIBILITY

Some lifelong heavy smokers never develop a bronchial carcinoma, some non-smokers develop lung tumours at a relatively early age and others develop multiple tumours with associated cancer of the mouth and larynx, and so there is clearly an interaction of environmental and genetic effects. In common with many other tumours (e.g. bladder and breast), it is proposed that the exposure to carcinogens leads to changes in the cellular expression of certain genes governing cell growth. This may be either the up-regulation of growth-promoting genes (oncogenes) or inactivation of recessive oncogenes (tumour suppressor genes). Individuals free from environmental exposure who develop tumours do so presumably because of spontaneous genetic mutations.

Tobacco smoking is the commonest environmental factor linked to lung cancer. Other agents include radon, asbestos, uranium, arsenic, nickel and chloromethyl ethers. The evidence for the role of tobacco smoking emerged nearly 50 years ago and has been corroborated many times since.[30] Indeed, passive smoking may also be linked to lung cancer.[31] Radon is an inert gas formed from the radioactive decay of uranium. It diffuses from the soil into buildings and is found in high levels in uranium mines. Cigarette smokers are at higher risk of lung tumours if exposed to radon, as are uranium miners. The other agents listed here are known to cause lung tumours in both smokers and non-smokers.

Relatives of cigarette smokers with lung cancer are at higher risk of the condition than other non-smokers. No single, specific factor accounts for all genetic susceptibility, but various karyotypic abnormalities and changes in gene expression clearly play a role. This is supported by finding chromosome-3 short-arm deletions in small cell tumours and oncogene over-expression (*K-ras* and *Erb-B1*) in non-small cell cancers.

HISTOLOGICAL SUBTYPES OF LUNG TUMOURS

The principal malignant bronchogenic tumours are small cell, squamous, adeno- and large cell carcinomas.

Small cell (oat cell) lung cancer

Small cell (oat cell) lung cancer derives from neuroendocrine cells, which can secrete peptides (e.g. adrenocorticotrophic hormone), causing paraneoplastic syndromes. They are highly malignant, have the poorest prognosis, and—because of extensive extrathoracic disease at presentation—are seldom resected. They grow rapidly and present with cough, chest pain, weight loss and haemoptysis. Small cell cancers usually form a large, central, non-cavitating mass with extensive mediastinal involvement. Local compressive phenomena, such as superior vena caval compression syndrome, are not uncommon (see Ch. 11). The stage of the tumour and the performance status of the patient determines prognosis. Two stages are recognized: disease localized to one hemithorax or more extensive involvement. Even within the earlier stage, most tumours have coexistent pleural effusions or advanced nodal metastases. It is, however, worth pursuing formal staging for oat cell cancers, because the occasional patient with a localized tumour and limited nodal involvement (N1, see later) benefit from resection and postoperative chemotherapy. The majority of patients are treated by chemotherapy, and without this, median survival is 3 months. Where the disease is 'limited' to one hemithorax, survival can extend to 12 or even 18 months with aggressive chemotherapy. The prognosis of more extensive disease is far poorer, even with chemotherapy. Radiotherapy does not prolong survival, either alone or in combination with chemotherapy. It does provide excellent palliation for mediastinal compression syndromes (such as superior vena caval obstruction) and metastases (especially cranial). The benefit of prophylactic cranial irradiation is small. It should be used only where a complete remission has been achieved with chemotherapy. The minority of patients with true stage-1 tumours, suitable for surgical resection and postoperative chemotherapy, may have a 50% 5-year survival. Dispute, however, continues as to whether those in this subgroup actually have atypical carcinoid tumours. Resection of tumours 'down-staged' by chemotherapy is not effective.

Non-small cell lung cancer

Non-small cell lung cancer is a blanket term used to describe the three other main histological subtypes: squamous (epithelioid) carcinoma, adenocarcinoma and undifferentiated large cell carcinoma. This is because, while there are differences in their biological behaviour, the treatment algorithms used to treat these tumours are very similar. Tumours containing mixed histological elements are also common.

Squamous carcinoma is the commonest variant, accounting for 40% of all lung tumours. It has characteristic features of keratinization with pearl formation (concentric swirls of cells) and may be detected while still in-situ. Like small cell tumours, they can also secrete adrenocorticotrophic hormone and parathyroid hormone (see Ch. 18). They usually affect older patients and present as central tumours, which cavitate as the tumour growth outstrips its blood supply. Due to metastases occurring relatively late in comparison with other epithelial tumours, squamous tumours form a high proportion of lung cancers treated by surgical resections. The presenting symptoms are similar to those of small cell tumours. The prognosis depends on the stage and the tumour differentiation, but is better for any given stage than the other histological subtypes. These tumours metastasize to the liver, adrenal glands, bone and brain. Irradiation controls symptomatic metastases; solitary cerebral deposits are occasionally resected. Chemotherapy may be used for incomplete resections, advanced disease, and the adjuvant treatment of borderline-resectable disease. It may also be used in a neoadjuvant manner, which may confer a survival advantage in early-stage disease.

Adenocarcinoma is the second commonest malignant epithelial tumour of the lung. These tumours exhibit glandular features (mucus secretion, acinar architecture) and usually occur in distal airways. A subtype of this variant is bronchoalveolar carcinoma. This demonstrates profuse replication of bland mucus-secreting cells into the air spaces. It grows slowly and can resemble consolidation radiologically. All adenocarcinomas are more common in women, and most are associated with scar tissue, either pre-existing or as a consequence of a desmoplastic response. They can present like small cell tumours, but are more

REFERENCES

30. Doll R, Peto R. Br Med J 1976; 2: 1525–1536
31. Wood AA. Br Med J 1990; 300: 1650

frequently found as solitary non-cavitating nodules on an incidental chest radiograph. Bronchorrhoea can accompany bronchoalveolar cell carcinoma and may be responsible for its intrapulmonary spread. Hypertrophic pulmonary osteoarthropathy (clubbing and periosteal reaction) occurs most often in association with an adenocarcinoma.

Localized tumours should be treated by surgical resection. The prognosis is less favourable than that for squamous tumours, because of the greater proclivity of adenocarcinomas to metastasize (liver, adrenal, bone and brain), and is primarily dependent on stage. Histological differentiation is less important than for squamous tumours. The prognosis for bronchoalveolar tumours is better than that for other adenocarcinomas if localized (because of higher resectability rates), but lower if multifocal and irresectable. Adenomatous deposits in the lungs may be impossible to differentiate from metastatic adenocarcinoma of extrathoracic origin (e.g. colorectal tumours). The presence of scar tissue or mediastinal nodes points to the disease being a lung primary. Most of these tumours are primary lung tumours, even if the patient has had a previous adenocarcinoma elsewhere.

Large cell carcinomas are the least common. Histologically, they are composed entirely of undifferentiated cells, occasionally with giant cell or clear cell features. They usually arise distally in the airways and grow centrally as large tumour masses. They can present on routine chest radiographs, with cough, or with symptoms of distant metastases. Treatment is usually surgical resection, and prognosis is dependent on stage. Survival rates are lower than those for other forms of non-small cell bronchogenic carcinomas and especially poor for the giant cell and clear cell subtypes.

DIAGNOSIS OF LUNG TUMOURS

The presence of a lung cancer can be suspected following the reporting of certain symptoms and focal findings on physical examination and chest radiography. The definitive diagnosis follows histological examination of tumour tissue or cytological examination of the sputum or pleural fluid.

Symptoms arise because of the local effects of the tumour, paraneoplastic phenomena, or the presence of metastases. Local effects include cough, haemoptysis, wheeze and dyspnoea. Pneumonia can result from airway obstruction. Other local effects can follow the involvement of a specific structure by tumour. Examples of this include hoarseness from recurrent laryngeal nerve paralysis (see Ch. 19), chest wall pain, superior vena caval obstruction (see Ch. 11), phrenic nerve paralysis, dysphagia, dysrhythmias, brachial plexus infiltration from an apical tumour (see Ch. 13), and stridor from major airway narrowing (see Ch. 19). Paraneoplastic effects occur outside the lungs but are not caused by metastatic deposits. They are from the secretion of various agents, usually polypeptides, by the primary tumour. Examples include adrenocorticotrophic hormone (Cushing's syndrome; see Ch. 34), antidiuretic hormone, parathyroid hormone (hypercalcaemia; see Ch. 18), thyroid-stimulating hormone (hypermetabolism; see Ch. 17), Eaton–Lambert syndrome (akin to myasthenia gravis), Bowen's disease (dermatosis; see Ch. 3) and hypertrophic pulmonary osteoarthropathy. In addition, cerebral and cerebellar degeneration can occur without intracranial metastases. Most extrathoracic symptoms and signs are a consequence of metastatic disease and include bone pain from osteal deposits, epileptic fits from cerebral secondaries, weight loss and poor appetite.

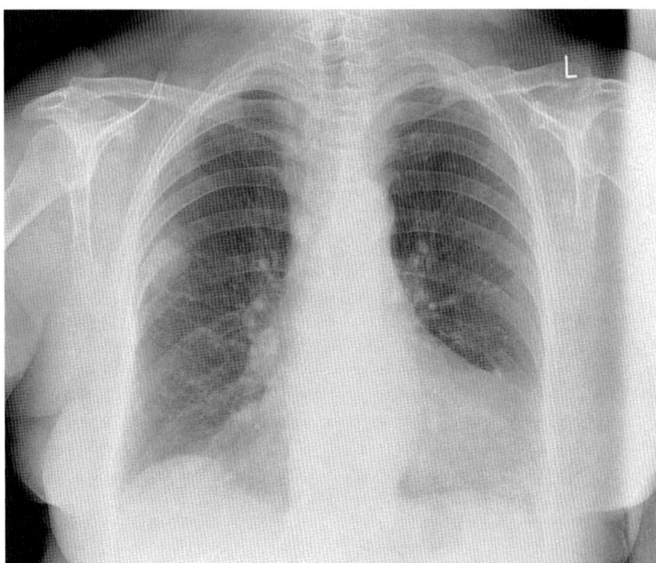

Figure 21.10 Posteroanterior chest radiograph demonstrating a 3-cm mass peripherally in the right midzone.

Chest examination may reveal an area of poor air intake or a monophonic wheeze caused by a tumour. A pleural effusion or supraclavicular nodes may also be detected. Hepatomegaly or focal neurological findings indicate metastatic disease.

Chest radiography is the initial investigation and is inexpensive and sensitive. Any nodule seen should be considered a lung cancer until proven otherwise (Fig. 21.10). The only exception is where a nodule is seen on successive films over several years and is unchanged in size. Many such nodules are also calcified and represent hamartomas or granulomas. Lung cancers can, however, present as calcified nodules. Inflammatory and infectious processes can also give rise to focal lesions. Where there is any doubt, tissue should be obtained for histological analysis.

Computerized tomography scanning is the mainstay in evaluating patients with focal lung lesions. It can visualize nodules (Fig. 21.11), including many too small to be seen on

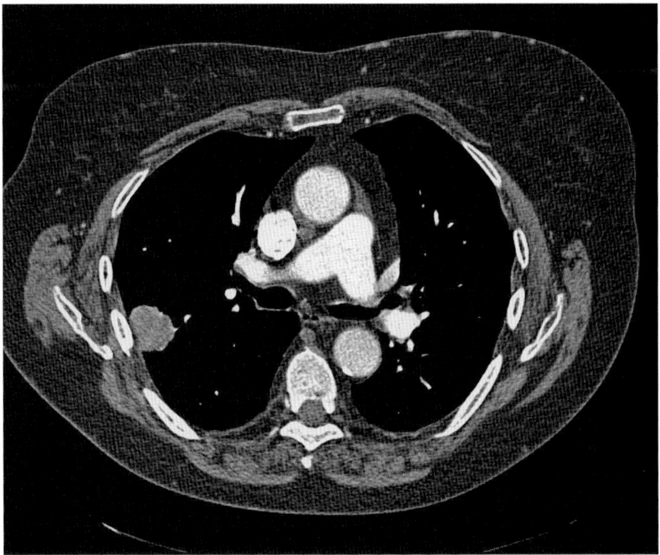

Figure 21.11 Contrast-enhanced CT at the level of the carina, confirming the mass in the posterior segment of the right upper lobe. No associated lymphadenopathy is seen.

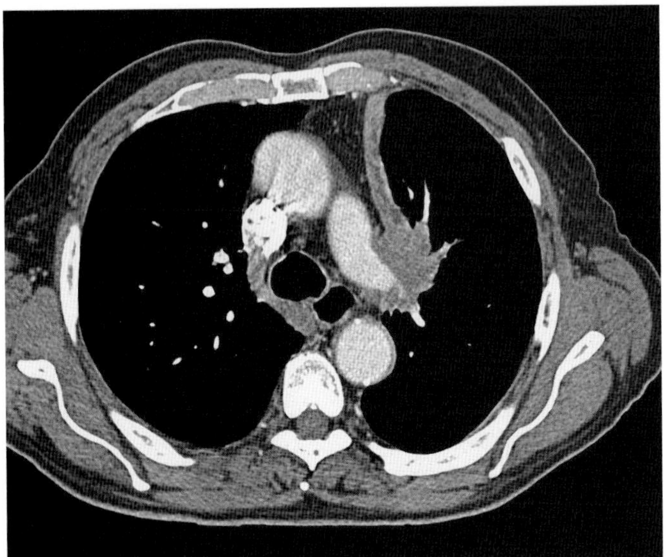

Figure 21.12 Contrast-enhanced transverse CT image demonstrating a 3-cm left hilar mass infiltrating mediastinal fat and abutting the left main pulmonary artery. The left upper lobe bronchus was occluded, with resultant complete left upper lobe collapse.

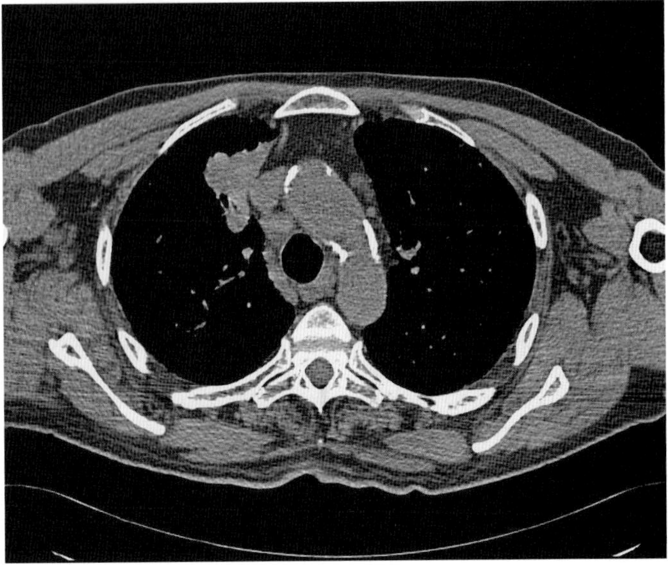

Figure 21.13 Transverse CT image in a patient with a known right upper lobe cancer demonstrates a mass in the right upper lobe and a 1.5-cm right paratracheal node.

a chest radiograph, and characterize them. It is excellent for demonstrating the mediastinal invasion (Fig. 21.12), and associated lymph nodes and their size. Generally, nodes smaller than 1 cm in diameter are considered normal and are not biopsied unless otherwise indicated. The CT scan also shows any liver or adrenal metastases. The commonest cause of adrenal gland enlargement is a benign adenoma (see Ch. 34). Magnetic resonance imaging provides excellent spatial resolution and is used to delineate the involvement of the thoracic inlet in apical tumours and invasion of the thoracic aorta by tumour. Positron emission tomography uses biochemical agents (e.g. 18-fluoro-deoxyglucose), which are differentially taken up by different tissues (Fig. 21.14), to characterize mediastinal nodal enlargement and extrathoracic deposits. Evidence is accruing that it may reduce the rates of unnecessary thoracotomy.[32]

Sputum cytology can confirm a diagnosis of lung cancer in most patients with a productive cough or haemoptysis. It can also provide the cell type in most instances, especially if there is a central tumour. Flexible bronchoscopy can visualize the bronchial tree to around the sixth-order branches. Any abnormalities encountered can be biopsied and washings or brushings can be taken for cytological analysis. Most centrally located lesions can be diagnosed with this technique. Rigid bronchoscopy only visualizes the more central airways but is excellent if a procedural adjunct, such as controlling haemoptysis or debulking a centrally obstructive tumour, is intended. Hypoxia from airway spasm and bleeding are the main complications.

Percutaneous needle biopsy is usually combined with CT or ultrasound guidance for the diagnosis of peripheral lesions. It is a safe and effective technique for abnormalities in the outer two-thirds of the lung parenchyma but is occasionally complicated by the development of a pneumothorax. Occasionally all these techniques fail to yield a diagnosis, and surgery is required to undertake a biopsy for frozen section analysis. If this fails, lobectomy can be undertaken for a suspected lung cancer, but this should never be undertaken where the presumed lung cancer is only resectable by pneumonectomy. Histological confirmation should always be sought before this is undertaken.

PREOPERATIVE EVALUATION OF THE PATIENT

Surgical resection for lung cancer should be considered when the patient is fit enough to tolerate major thoracic surgery with the loss of lung parenchyma, provided the tumour appears resectable on preoperative investigation. Most patients with lung cancer are elderly smokers, and the incidence of associated chronic obstructive airways disease and coronary artery disease is high. Preoperative pulmonary function tests give an idea as to fitness of a patient, but there is no reliable cut-off point of any of these measures. As a general guide, pneumonectomy is feasible if the forced expiratory volume in 1 s (FEV_1) exceeds 1.5 litres. The level of lung function compatible with surgery will, however, depend on both the proposed extent of the resection and the function of the lung tissue to be removed. The removal of an obstructed lobe does not alter the FEV_1 greatly. The finding of hypoxia on arterial blood gas analysis does increase the risk of surgery but does not necessarily preclude it. If a patient can climb a flight of stairs without undue dyspnoea, they will probably tolerate a thoracotomy. A useful general rule is to assign approximately 5% of overall lung function to each segment, and to estimate the percentage of predicted FEV_1 that will remain after the proposed resection. If this is less than 30% postoperative difficulties can be anticipated.

Coronary disease is common in this population, and some will have a history of previous revascularization or myocardial infarction. The ECG may show an old infarct or be normal. Exercise ECG testing should be undertaken in patients with a history of stable angina. Coronary angiography with a view to revascularization before pulmonary resection is indicated in those with unstable angina or an abnormal exercise ECG.

REFERENCES

32. Van Tinteren H, Hoekstra OS, Smit EF et al. Lancet 2002; 359: 1388–1393

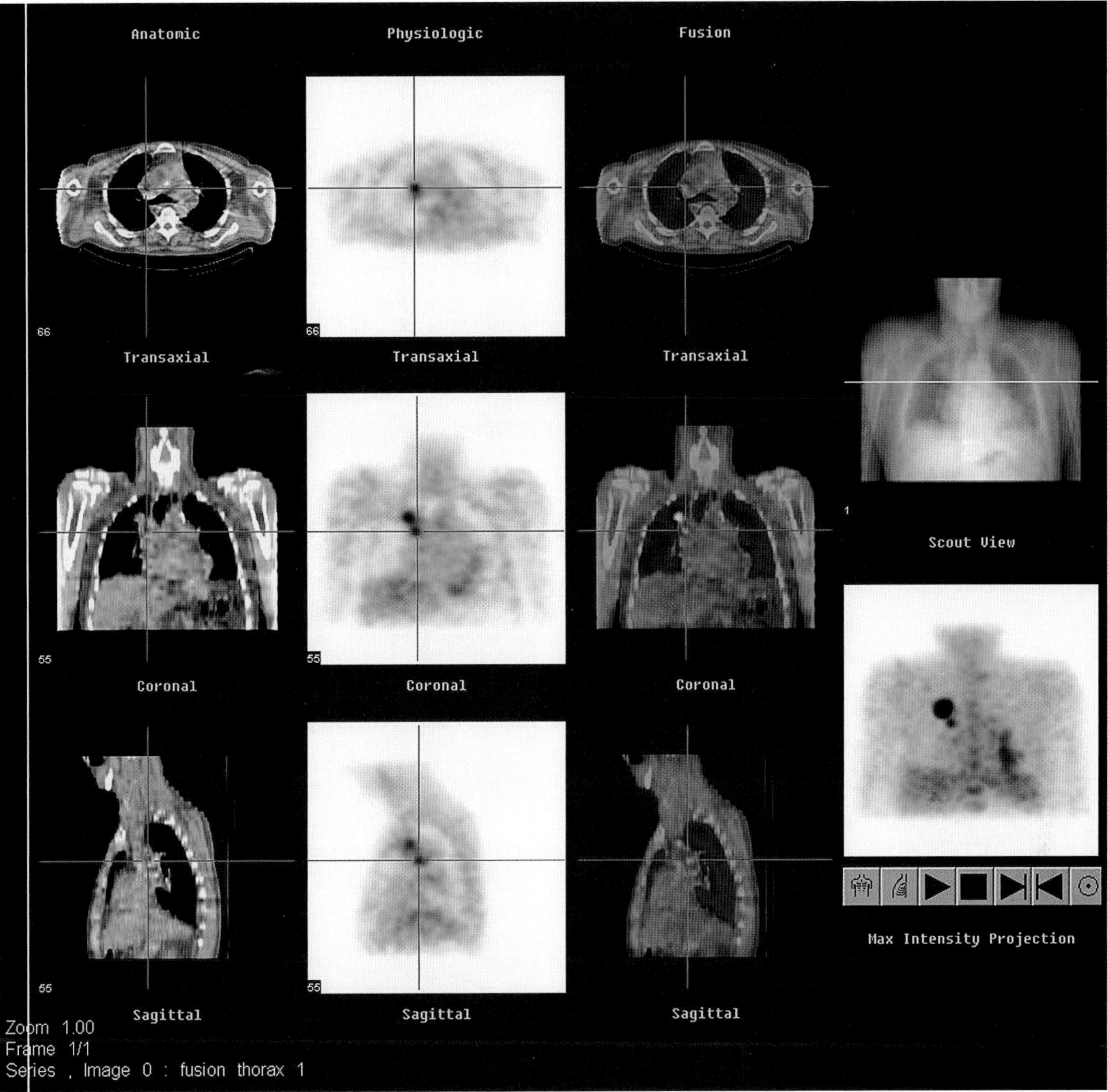

Figure 21.14 Positron emission tomography image and CT–positron emission tomography fusion images showing intense focal uptake of 18-fluorodeoxyglucose in the right paratracheal area consistent with a lymph node metastasis. This was confirmed at mediastinoscopy.

STAGING OF LUNG CANCER

Staging allows selection of the best treatment strategy. It is also an important indicator of prognosis and allows comparison of different hospitals' results and treatment for the purposes of research. A modified tumour node metastasis classification has current acceptance (Table 21.1).[33] The tumour node metastasis subsets are also grouped into stages because of differing prognoses and surgical resectability (Table 21.2). Stage-1 and stage-2 tumours are resectable. Stage 3 is divided according to resectability. Stage 3a should be resectable except for T1-3 N2, which is technically resectable, but this confers no advantage. Where N2 involvement (Table 21.3) is confirmed preoperatively, primary resection is not undertaken, other than for N2 disease from node station 5 or 6 involvement. It may, however, follow if the tumour down-stages with chemotherapy. Stage-3b tumours are generally irresectable, with the exception of localized carinal tumours (T4), where resection and reconstruction confers a 5-year survival of around 25%. Stage-4 tumours have distant metastases and surgery is not indicated. The only exception is the combination of a localized primary tumour with solitary cerebral

REFERENCES

33. Mountain CF. Chest 1997; 111: 1710–1717

Table 21.1 TNM (tumour, node and metastasis) classification

Designation	Definition
T1	Tumour less than 3 cm in greatest dimension, surrounded by the lung or visceral pleura, and located distal to or in a lobar bronchus
T2	Tumour that is > 3 cm, involves a main bronchus more than 2 cm distal to the carina, invades the visceral pleura or causes an obstructive pneumonitis that does not involve the whole lung
T3	Tumour invading chest wall, diaphragm, mediastinal pleura, pericardium, or located in the main bronchus within 2 cm of the carina but not involving the carina or causing obstructive pneumonitis of the entire lung
T4	Tumour invading mediastinum, heart, great vessels, trachea, oesophagus, vertebral body, carina, or malignant pleural or pericardial effusion
N0	No nodal involvement
N1	Ipsilateral peribronchial or hilar nodes
N2	Ipsilateral mediastinal or subcarinal nodes
N3	Involvement of contralateral mediastinal or hilar nodes; supraclavicular or scalene nodes
M0	No distant metastasis
M1	Distant metastasis present

Table 21.2 Lung cancer stage and TNM (tumour, node and metastasis) correlates with 5-year survival

	TNM classification			
Stage	*T*	*N*	*M*	5-Year survival (%)
1	1	0	0	85
1	2	0	0	75
2	1	1	0	55
2	2	1	0	55
3a	3	0–1	0	35–45
3a	1–3	2	0	15–25
3b	4	0–3	0	5*
3b	1–4	3	0	5
4	1–4	0–3	1	< 5†

*Except resectable carinal tumours: 25%.
†Except pulmonary resection and isolated cerebral metastatectomy: 15% at 3 years.

metastasis, where both tumours may be resected with improved survival.[34]

Staging begins with the clinical assessment and non-invasive techniques, such as CT, MRI and bone scans (Figs 21.15 and 21.16). Clinical examination may detect large or abnormal supraclavicular nodes or hepatic deposits, and routine blood tests may show deranged liver function tests. Computerized tomography demonstrates tumour size, mediastinal nodal enlargement, and any deposits in the liver or adrenal glands; CT may not differentiate involvement of the pleurae from deeper chest wall invasion unless bone destruction or obvious muscle invasion is seen. Magnetic resonance imaging may be a useful adjunct for assessing soft tissue involvement and is especially useful for apical tumours. Bone scans and brain CT is undertaken if symptoms or other findings raise the suspicion of metastases. Positron emission tomography scanning is emerging as an effective method for characterizing abnormalities seen on CT[35] and may replace mediastinal nodal biopsy.

Table 21.3 Lymph node stations in lung cancer

Location	Station	Name
Superior mediastinal	1	Highest mediastinal
Superior mediastinal	2	Upper paratracheal
Superior mediastinal	3	Retrotracheal
Superior mediastinal	4	Lower paratracheal
Aortic	5	Subaortic
Aortic	6	Paraaortic
Inferior mediastinal	7	Subcarinal
Inferior mediastinal	8	Paraoesophageal
Inferior mediastinal	9	Pulmonary ligament
N1	10	Hilar
N1	11	Interlobar
N1	12	Lobar
N1	13	Segmental
N1	14	Subsegmental

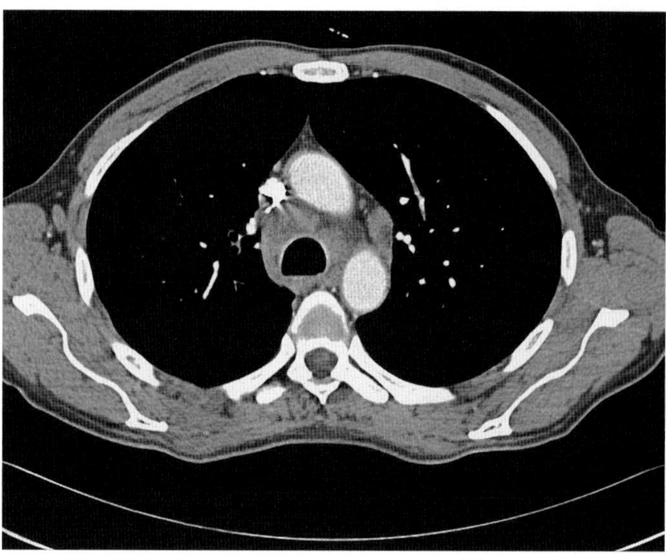

Figure 21.15 Transverse CT image showing extensive mediastinal lymphadenopathy.

REFERENCES

34. Granone P, Margaritora S, D'Andrilli A et al. Eur J Cardiothorac Surg 2001; 20: 361–366

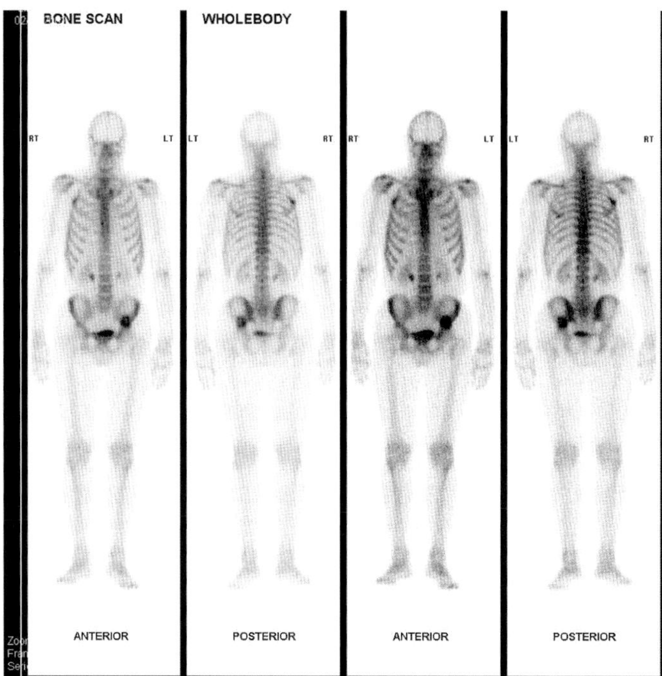

Figure 21.16 Bone scintigram on a patient with non-small cell lung cancer, demonstrating focal uptake in the left acetabulum and the right third anterior rib in keeping with metastatic deposits.

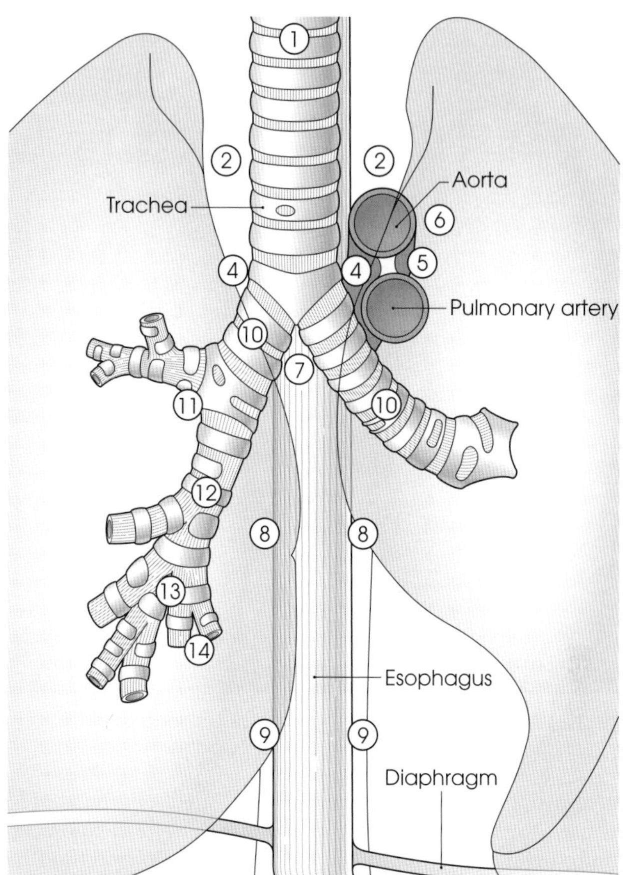

Figure 21.17 Regional lymph node stations.

Invasive staging is undertaken where there is no evidence of extrathoracic disease, to preclude resection, but N2 nodal disease is suspected from the radiological findings. Cervical mediastinoscopy and anterior mediastinotomy are the two principal staging procedures. Cervical mediastinoscopy is performed through a small incision placed in the suprasternal notch. The mediastinoscope is advanced along the anterior wall of the trachea within the pretracheal fascia, and the nodes of the superior and middle mediastinum can be seen and sampled. Most lung tumours metastasize to lymph nodes within the reach of the mediastinoscope (Fig. 21.17). Tumours may, however, spread to other N2 sites. This is especially true of left upper lobe tumours, which spread to the para- and subaortic nodes (stations 5 and 6). However, these sites can be directly assessed and nodes sampled with anterior mediastinotomy, which also allows assessment of mediastinal invasion. This involves a small anterior thoracotomy through the second or third intercostal space just lateral to the sternal edge. Both of these techniques are now routine and provide accurate assessments of the nodal status. They have greatly reduced the incidence of unnecessary thoracotomies. Increasingly, video-assisted thoracoscopic surgery is being used to assess staging. It can provide access to all the areas beyond the reach of the mediastinoscope, but the detection of nodal disease in these sites may not be as potent an indicator of irresectability as superior mediastinal nodal involvement.

THORACOTOMY, ASSESSMENT AND PULMONARY RESECTION

The patient who is fit enough to withstand surgery for a potentially resectable tumour should be offered surgery.[36–38]

Most operations for lung cancer are undertaken through a posterolateral thoracotomy, which provides excellent access to the ipsilateral lung, hilum and mediastinum. The skin is incised from between the medial border of the scapula and the thoracic spine to beyond the anterior axillary fold, usually along the line of the sixth rib. Latissimus dorsi is divided, and the chest is entered through the fifth intercostal space. Other thoracotomy incisions, such as axillary and anterolateral approaches, are muscle sparing but provide poorer access and confer little advantage. Median sternotomy provides excellent access to the trachea but poor access to the lung hilar structures. Video-assisted thoracoscopic surgery allows a minimally invasive approach to lung resection and its role is still being elucidated.[39,40]

Superior sulcus (Pancoast's) lung tumours (Fig. 21.18) often involve structures at the thoracic inlet, such as the first rib, brachial plexus, subclavian vessels, vertebral bodies and sympathetic chain. Ordinarily, such involvement would preclude resection, but because these tumours cause intractable pain that is difficult to palliate they are best treated by surgical resection, often with preoperative radiotherapy. They can be resected via an anterocervical[41] or high posterior approach.

REFERENCES

35. Scott WJ. Surg Clin North Am 2002; 82: 477–495
36. Kohman LJ, Meyer JA, Ikins PM et al. J Thorac Cardiovasc Surg 1986; 91: 551–554
37. Ninan M, Sommers KE, Landreneau RJ et al. Ann Thorac Surg 1997; 64: 328–332
38. Slinger PD, Johnston MR. Anaesthesiol Clin North Am 2001; 19: 411–433
39. Sugi K, Kaneda Y, Esato K. World J Surg 2000; 24: 27–30
40. Kaseda S, Aoki T, Hangai N. Semin Thorac Cardiovasc Surg 1998: 10: 300–304
41. Macchiarini P, Dartevelle PG, Chapelier A et al. Ann Thorac Surg 1993; 55: 611–618

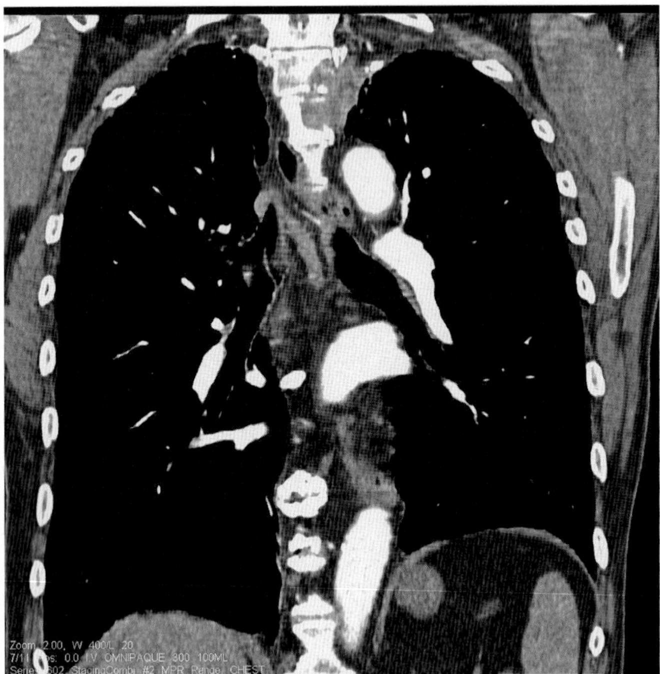

Figure 21.18 Coronally reformed CT image showing a left apical mass that invades two adjacent vertebral bodies.

Once inside the chest, the tumour and mediastinum should be assessed for the local extent of the disease. The relationship of a lung mass to the hilum and fissures of the lung should be determined, and a frozen section can be sent if the diagnosis is not confirmed. The mediastinum should be explored, and any suspicious mediastinal nodes sampled and sent for immediate frozen section analysis. The detection of unsuspected N2 disease at thoracotomy does not usually preclude resection, because the 5-year survival for this group is superior to that of patients with preoperatively identified N2 involvement.[42–44] Resection should proceed if the tumour can be removed and extensive N2 disease is absent. The smallest resection compatible with complete removal of the tumour is undertaken. Lobectomy and pneumonectomy are the main operations for surgical resection of lung cancer. Wedge excision is not anatomical and does not remove the draining lymph node field of the tumour. It should seldom be employed in the treatment of lung cancer.

Lobectomy is the procedure of choice for a lung cancer confined within a lobe.[45] The affected lobe is resected, and the residual space is filled by enlargement of the remaining lobe(s) and contraction of the hemithorax. Bilobectomy is undertaken when a tumour crosses either the transverse or the oblique fissure, or involves the origin of middle and (usually) lower lobe bronchi. The results are better than those of pneumonectomy but not as good as those of lobectomy, probably indicating that more advanced tumours require this approach. Bronchoplastic (sleeve resection) lobectomy is performed for upper lobe tumours extending into the main bronchus, as an alternative to pneumonectomy.[46]

Pneumonectomy removes the entire lung and carries a higher mortality, especially for the right side, because of the larger resected lung volume. They can be undertaken within the pleural space or extended intrapericardially when required.

Segmentectomy is most commonly performed for benign conditions and to prolong survival in metastatic carcinomas of extrathoracic origin, such as osteosarcoma (see Ch. 42) and clear cell renal carcinomas (see Ch. 35). This technique can be used for primary lung tumours if they are localized to one segment and if retention of lung parenchyma is the main priority. In most instances, lobectomy should be the minimum operation for a primary lung tumour, because local recurrence rates are lower.[47]

Mediastinal lymph node excision in preoperatively staged node-negative tumours should be undertaken in all cases. This allows the detection of skip lesions (N2 disease with uninvolved N1 nodes),[48] and provides complete pathological staging. It is not known whether systematic mediastinal lymph node dissection has any impact on survival.[49]

Extensive invasion of the chest wall[50] can be compatible with good 5-year survival rates, and in N0 or N1 disease this may reach 40–55%. N2 disease and mediastinal invasion[51] usually indicates a poor prognosis.

COMPLICATIONS OF SURGICAL TREATMENT

The mortality from lobectomy should be around 2%, and for pneumonectomy approximately 2–4% for left-sided and 8–9% for right-sided procedures.[45,52]

Cardiac complications include dysrhythmia and myocardial infarction. Dysrhythmias are usually supraventricular in nature and can be treated with digoxin, amiodarone[53] or cardioversion as indicated, although amiodarone may precipitate pulmonary fibrosis. Prophylactic digoxin confers no benefit.[54] Because myocardial ischaemia is so common in this population, invasive monitoring and maintenance of haemodynamic stability is important. Despite this, myocardial infarcts do occur and are usually fatal. Selected preoperative revascularization may lower risk.[55]

Respiratory complications are frequent and include atelectasis, pneumonia, and occasionally bronchopleural fistula. Post-pneumonectomy pulmonary oedema is devastating but largely avoidable. It occurs most frequently after right pneumonectomy and may be fatal. It is not cardiogenic and appears to be related to excessive fluid administration. The end result is an adult respiratory distress syndrome-type picture, and there is no

REFERENCES

42. Goldstraw P, Mannam GC, Kaplan DK et al. J Thorac Cardiovasc Surg 1994; 107: 19–27
43. Miller DL, McManus KG, Allen MS et al. Ann Thorac Surg 1994; 57: 1095–1110
44. Pearson FG, DeLarue NC, Ilves R et al. J Thorac Cardiovasc Surg 1982; 83: 1–11
45. Ginsberg RJ. J Thorac Cardiovasc Surg 1978; 94: 673
46. Deslauriers J, Mehran RJ, Guimont C et al. World J Surg 1993; 17: 712–718
47. Ginsberg RJ, Rubinstein LV. Ann Thorac Surg 1995; 60: 615–622
48. Yoshino I, Yokoyama H, Yano T et al. Ann Thorac Surg 1993; 56: 223–236
49. Izbicki JR, Passlick B, Pantel K et al. Ann Surg 1998; 227: 138–144
50. Albertucci M, DeMeester TR, Rothberg M et al. J Thorac Cardiovasc Surg 1992; 103: 8–12
51. Rice TW, Blackstone EH. Surg Clin North Am 2002; 82: 573–587
52. Ginsberg RJ, Hill LD, Eagan RT et al. J Thorac Cardiovasc Surg 1983; 86: 654–658
53. Ciriaco P, Mazzone P, Canneto B et al. Eur J Cardiothorac Surg 2000; 18: 12–16
54. Ritchie AJ, Bowe P, Gibbons JRP. Ann Thorac Surg 1990: 50: 86–88
55. Ciriaco P, Carretta A, Calori G et al. Eur J Cardiothorac Surg 2002; 22: 35–40

specific treatment, although nitric oxide may be of benefit.[56] The best strategy is avoidance through strict fluid management regimen and delaying surgery in patients with recent pneumonia, whose capillary permeability may be altered. Pneumonia is usually bacterial, and its treatment consists of appropriate antibiotics, physiotherapy, and management of airway secretions (including minitracheostomy). Bronchopleural fistulae occur after around 3–5% of pulmonary resections.[57] They are more common after right-sided procedures (usually pneumonectomy), after prolonged mechanical ventilation, an involved resection margin and preoperative radiotherapy.[58] They present early with a productive cough and falling air–fluid level on chest radiograph or later with empyema. If a patient starts to expectorate large volumes of serosanguinous fluid, they should be assumed to have a fistula and laid with their operated side down (to avoid flooding the remaining lung), and the pneumonectomy space should be rapidly drained with an intercostal tube. Early fistulae can be closed directly using local tissue used to cover the bronchus. Bronchopleural fistulae presenting later in association with an empyema may require a trans-sternal approach to reamputate the bronchial stump and insert vascularized tissue into the infected space (e.g. latissimus dorsi flaps). Rib resection and drainage of the space (see *Empyema thoracis* section) can also be used. This may control the infection and ought to relieve any symptoms of chronic productive cough. To reduce the risk of a bronchopleural fistula the blood supply of the carina must be preserved, and the suture line shall be made flush with the remaining airway to avoid a sump, which collects secretions and promotes breakdown.

Other complications include thromboembolus (see Ch. 11),[59] renal failure, stroke and wound infections. Wound infections usually respond to adequate drainage and appropriate antibiotics. An underlying empyema should be suspected if they fail to resolve. Careful barrier nursing of patients infected with methicillin-resistant *Staphylococcus aureus* is essential, because these infections can rapidly spread through the surgical ward.

OTHER LUNG TUMOURS

Carcinoid tumours of the lung have a lower malignant potential than bronchogenic tumours. They arise from the amine precursor uptake and decarboxylase (APUD) cells of the lung (see Ch. 21). Squamous cell tumours also arise from these cells, and overlap occurs with atypical carcinoids. They present with cough, pneumonia or haemoptysis, often over a prolonged time course, and are not related to smoking. Those with typical histological features (90%) are more benign in their behaviour than atypical carcinoids. Neither is as aggressive as squamous cell tumour. Treatment is complete surgical excision, and metastases are rare. A carcinoid syndrome (sweating, bronchospasm and flushing) may result if they occur in the liver. The 15-year survival rate is around 75%.[60]

Hamartomas are the commonest benign tumours affecting the lungs. They are derived from mesenchyme and can contain cartilaginous, fibrous and fatty elements. They usually present as solitary pulmonary nodules, although they can occur endobronchially. Most are symptomless,[61] but excision is recommended to prevent the local effects of their progressive slow growth and to exclude a carcinoma. Where histological examination of a needle biopsy specimen has revealed a clearly benign process, then serial observation may be appropriate. Other primary lung tumours are rare.

SURGICAL MANAGEMENT OF LUNG INFECTION

PULMONARY TUBERCULOSIS

Tuberculosis has declined in developed countries over the second half of the 20th century, but multidrug-resistant tuberculosis associated with HIV infection is now an increasing problem, particularly in Africa. The primary infection causes a localized pneumonitis, which usually settles but can progress to secondary infection through lymph- and blood-borne spread. As a consequence of the sensitivity acquired to the bacillus, reinfection (whether endogenous or exogenous) can lead to the formation of lung abscesses and empyema. The initial treatment is with drugs (isoniazid, rifampicin, pyrazinamide, or ethambutol), but surgery is occasionally required for the treatment of tuberculous lung cavities secondarily colonized with *Aspergillus*. In the past, phrenic nerve crushes, artificial pneumothoraces, plombage and thoracoplasties were used to promote collapse and healing of tuberculous cavities. These are mostly obsolete, although lung resection is still occasionally undertaken to control the disease.[62]

BRONCHIECTASIS

Bronchiectasis is a dilating disorder of the bronchi characterized by excessive pooling of secretions and recurrent sepsis. It is the result of inflammation, usually from infection, but may develop after an inhaled foreign body. The main symptoms are cough and excessive, purulent sputum. Haemoptysis can occur, and if severe may require radiological arterial embolization. The control of this disease has improved with modern antibiotics, and progression to amyloid and brain abscesses are rare. Surgery is required only for intractable symptoms from localized, often unilateral, bronchiectasis or for life-threatening haemoptysis.[63]

LUNG ABSCESS

A lung abscess can develop secondary to pneumonia (especially *Staphylococcus aureus* and *Klebsiella*), but may also develop distal to bronchial obstructions. Abscesses present with cough, swinging pyrexia, and a cavitating lung opacity containing an air–fluid level on chest radiography. Treatment is by intravenous antibiotics and physiotherapy. A percutaneous drain is required if the patient remains septic, and if malignancy is suspected or if infection continues the affected lung should be resected. The rest of the bronchial tree must be protected from the pus during the resection.[64]

REFERENCES

56. Rabkin DG, Sladen RN, DeMango A et al. Ann Thorac Surg 2001; 72: 272–274
57. Sirbu H, Busch T, Aleksic I et al. Ann Thorac Cardiovasc Surg 2001; 7: 330–336
58. Asamura H, Naruke T, Tsuchiya R et al. J Thorac Cardiovasc Surg 1992; 104: 1456–1464
59. Ziomek S, Read RC, Tobler HG et al. Ann Thorac Surg 1993; 56: 223–226
60. Filosso PL, Rena O, Donati G et al. J Thorac Cardiovasc Surg 2002; 123: 303–309
61. Hansen CP, Holtveg H, Francis D et al. J Thorac Cardiovasc Surg 1992; 104: 674–678
62. Souilamas R, Riquet M, Barthes FP et al. Ann Thorac Surg 2001; 71: 443–447
63. Fulimoto T, Hillejan L, Stamatis G. Ann Thorac Surg 2001; 72: 1711–1715
64. Pfitzner J, Peacock MJ, Tsirgiotis E et al. Br J Anaesth 2000; 85: 791–794

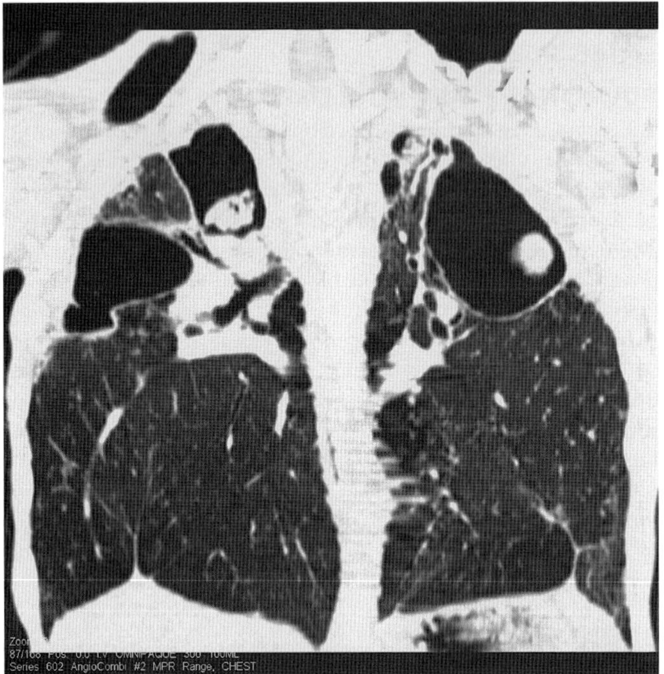

Figure 21.19 Coronally reformatted CT images demonstrating bilateral apical cavities, within which are dependent soft tissue masses with air crescent signs characteristic of aspergillomas. Pleural thickening is also seen at the left lung apex.

ASPERGILLOSIS

Aspergillosis (Fig. 21.19) is the commonest fungal infection of the lung and is caused by *Aspergillus fumigatus*. It has several separate clinical entities: allergic bronchopulmonary aspergillosis, aspergilloma, *Aspergillus* within pulmonary infarcts, and systemic aspergillosis secondary to immunosuppression.

Allergic bronchopulmonary aspergillosis causes an asthma-like syndrome with wheezing and transient pulmonary infiltrates. It resolves with systemic steroids.[65] Aspergilloma is a ball of fungus, which forms in a pre-existing cavity within the lung, usually secondary to tuberculosis or sarcoidosis. Patients present with fever and haemoptysis, which can be massive. The diagnosis is confirmed by the detection of serum precipitins and the definitive treatment is by pulmonary resection.[66] Where this is not possible because of the severity of the associated pulmonary parenchymal disease, antifungal agents and bronchial artery embolization can be effective.[67] Pulmonary infarcts can be secondarily infected with *Aspergillus* if they cavitate.[68] Systemic aspergillosis is often severe and complicates immunosuppression, and this and other fungal infections are a well-recognized cause of anastomotic dehiscence following lung transplantation.

SURGERY FOR EMPHYSEMA

Emphysema is characterized by large distal air spaces, which have formed because of destruction of alveolar wall tissue that has either a panacinar or peribronchial distribution. It produces hyperexpansion of the thorax and dyspnoea. In severe cases it causes right heart failure (cor pulmonale).

In infants, it may occur beyond congenital bronchial abnormalities,[69] and it is often in a lobar distribution. At this age the infant fails to thrive and develops respiratory distress; treatment may include lobectomy.

In adults, emphysema is usually generalized and related to cigarette smoking. Deficiency of α_1-antitrypsin causes severe homogenous emphysema in young adulthood, and is often precipitated by smoking. Patients with emphysema from smoking are often treated expectantly, but severe α_1-antitrypsin deficiency often eventually leads to lung transplantation (usually double lung). Resection of a giant bulla is often associated with considerable symptomatic improvement because of improved ventilation of the remaining, more normal lung. This can now be undertaken thoracoscopically. For patients with widespread emphysema, lung volume reduction surgery can be considered. This is an emerging procedure involving resection of 20% of lung volume (usually from the upper lobes) on both sides of the chest. This can be performed thoracoscopically. The smaller lungs are believed to function better because of less air trapping and reduced splinting of the chest wall and diaphragm. A randomized controlled trial has shown improved objective (FEV_1) and symptoms compared with a control group receiving intensive pulmonary rehabilitation alone.[70] The best candidates appear to be those with heterogenous disease, where the most severely affected segments are peripheral and resectable (Fig. 21.20). This is best evaluated by spiral CT.[71] Patients should not have bullous disease (bullectomy would be preferable here), should have FEV_1 of 20% (or more) of the predicted value, and should be able to cover 500 m (or more) on a shuttle test.

LUNG TRANSPLANTATION

Single-lung, double-lung and heart–lung[72] transplantation have evolved over the past 20 years and are now effective treatments for various forms of end-stage lung disease. Single-lung transplantation is usually selected for fibrotic lung disease and some cases of emphysema where the risk of contamination from the remaining lung is low. In cystic fibrosis or bronchiectasis, where this is not the case, a double-lung transplantation is the usual approach. Where the lung disease has produced irreversible cardiac dysfunction and pulmonary hypertension, then heart–lung transplantation may be required. Heart–lung transplantation is also required when an intracardiac problem has led to increased pulmonary blood flow, the development of pulmonary hypertension, and the eventual reversal of the shunt (Eisenmenger's syndrome; see Ch. 22).[73]

REFERENCES

65. Greenberger PA. J Allergy Clin Immunol 2002; 110: 685–692
66. Regnard JF, Icard P, Nicolosi M et al. Ann Thorac Surg 2000; 69: 898–903
67. Judson MA, Stevens DA. Curr Opin Investig Drugs 2001; 2: 1375–1377
68. Buchanan DR, Lamb D. Thorax 1982; 37: 693–698
69. Warner JO, Rubin S, Heard BE. Br J Dis Chest 1982; 76: 177–184
70. Geddes D, Davies M, Koyama H et al. N Engl J Med 2000; 343: 239–245
71. Cederlund K, Bergstrand L, Hogberg S et al. Eur Radiol 2002; 12: 1045–1051
72. Reichart B, Gulbins H, Meiser BM et al. Transplantation 2003; 75: 127–132
73. Stoica SC, McNeil KD, Perreas K et al. Ann Thorac Surg 2001; 72: 1887–1891

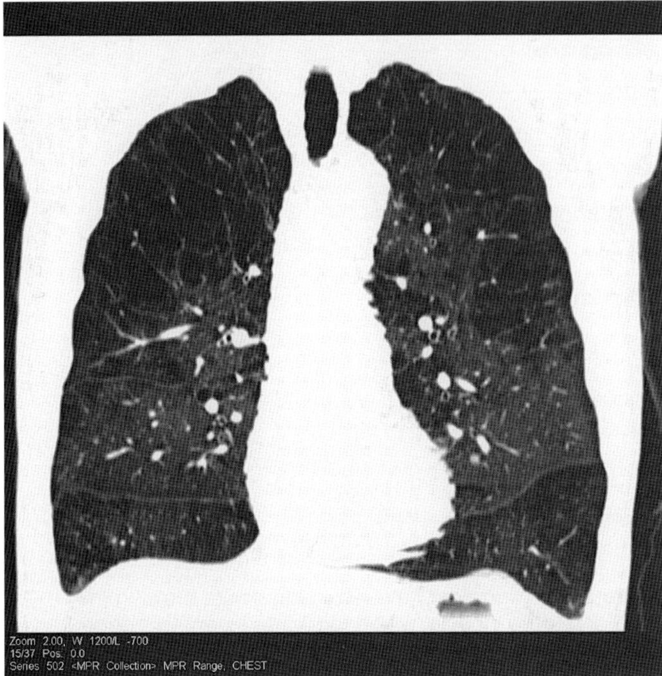

Figure 21.20 Coronally reformatted CT image demonstrating severe emphysema, which predominantly involves the mid- and upper zones with relative sparing of the lung bases. The heterogeneous and upper zone distribution of emphysema makes this a good candidate for lung volume reduction surgery.

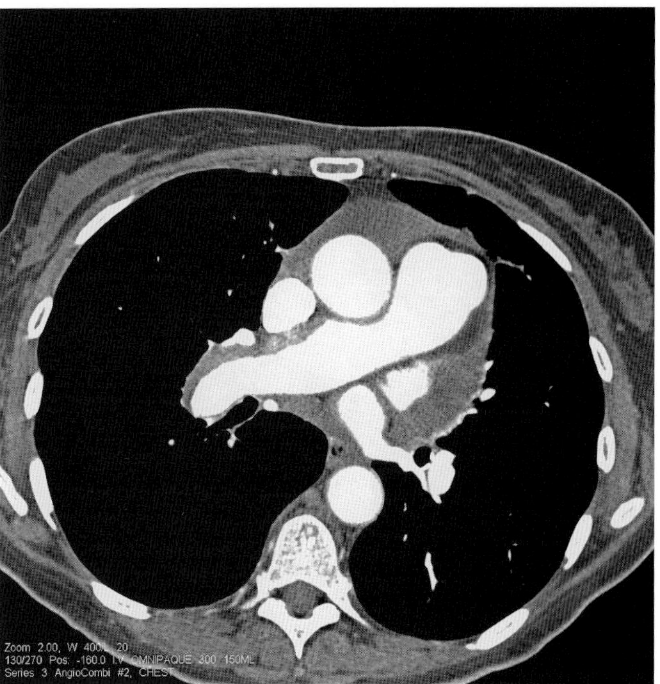

Figure 21.21 Contrast-enhanced CT image demonstrating laminated thrombus in the right main pulmonary artery and a moderate pericardial effusion.

Most organs are procured from cadaveric donors, but experience in living related lobar transplantation is growing.[74] Initial results were poor, but acceptable perioperative mortality rates are now being achieved, and improved immunosuppression is leading to better long-term survival (Table 21.4). The principal limitations of lung transplantation are the limited donor organ supply and the development of obliterative bronchiolitis, which is a form of chronic rejection leading to closure of the airways and death in a high proportion of lung transplant recipients.[75,76]

CHRONIC PULMONARY EMBOLI

Pulmonary emboli can present acutely with chest pain and dyspnoea, but most are symptomless or undiagnosed.[77] Recurrent emboli lead to chronic obstruction of the pulmonary arteries with medial proliferation at truncal, lobar and segmental level. This obstruction produces pulmonary hypertension and right heart failure. The natural history of this condition is extremely poor if left untreated.[78] The presentation of central thromboembolic pulmonary hypertension is with progressive dyspnoea. Affected patients have enlarged central pulmonary arteries, oligaemic lung fields, and right ventricular enlargement. The differentiation of this condition from primary pulmonary hypertension can be made with either a ventilation–perfusion lung scan (primary pulmonary hypertension has a characteristic mottled appearance) or CT pulmonary angiography, which demonstrates the abnormal central arteries (Fig. 21.21). The source of emboli must be dealt with and further emboli prevented. The treatment is by pulmonary thromboendarterectomy, which is performed on cardiopulmonary bypass with deep hypothermic circulatory arrest. The pulmonary arteries are disobliterated of their contained organized thrombus (Fig. 21.22). The operative mortality is less than 10%,[79] and the long-term outlook for these patients is good, especially if their pulmonary artery pressures return to normal following the procedure.[80]

Table 21.4 Survival rates following lung and heart-lung transplantation

Transplant type	1-Year survival (%)	5-Year survival (%)
Single lung	80	65
Double lung	70	45–50
Heart-lung	70	40–50

THE TRACHEA

TRACHEAL TUMOURS

Tumours of the trachea are uncommon. Presentation may frequently be late, because patients are usually symptomless

REFERENCES

74. Barr ML, Schenkel FA, Cohen RG et al. Transplant Proc 1998; 30: 2261–2263
75. Boehler A, Estenne M. Curr Opin Pulm Med 2000; 6: 133–139
76. Heng D, Sharples LD, McNeil K et al. J Heart Lung Transplant 1998; 17: 1255–1263
77. Dalen JE, Alpert JS. Prog Cardiovasc Dis 1975; 17: 259–270
78. Luckraz H, Dunning J. Ann R Coll Surg Engl 2001; 83: 427–430
79. Jamieson SW, Auger WR, Fedullo PF et al. J Thorac Cardiovasc Surg 1993; 106: 116–126
80. Tscholl D, Langer F, Wendler O et al. Eur J Cardiothorac Surg 2001; 19: 771–776

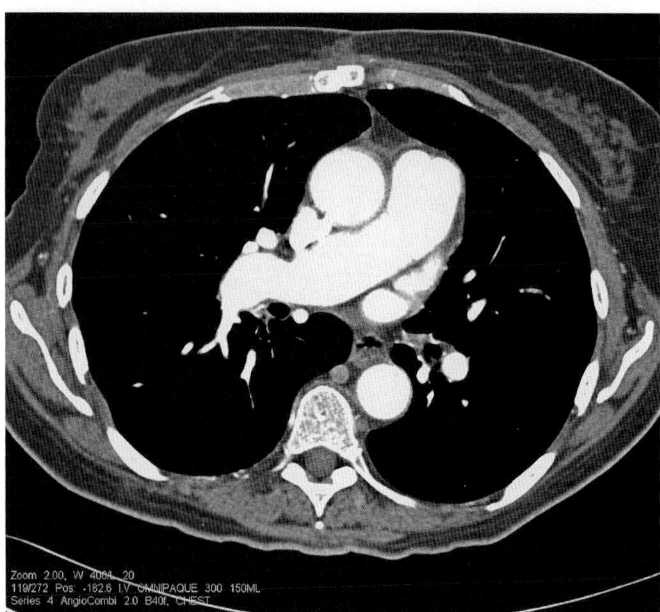

Figure 21.22 Contrast-enhanced CT image showing the successful disobliteration of the pulmonary arteries with reperfusion of the right lower lobar vessels.

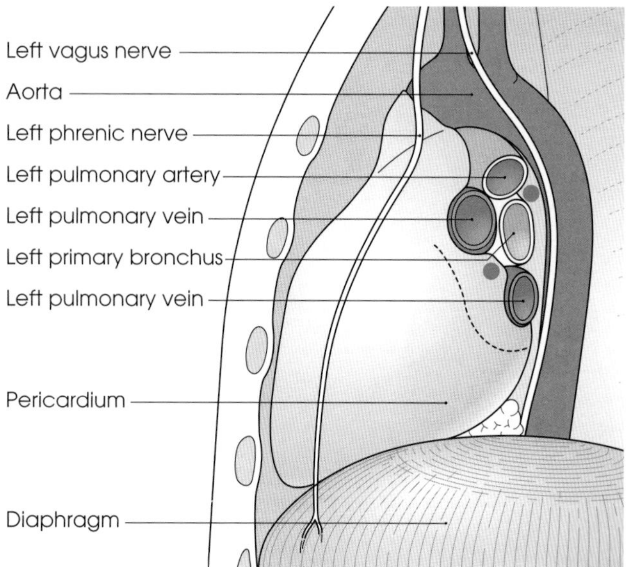

Figure 21.23 Diagram of the left mediastinum showing the perihilar release incision, which facilitates extensive tracheal resection.

until the obstruction is advanced.[81] These tumours can cause dyspnoea, cough, haemoptysis and stridor. The chest radiograph is often normal, and patients are often first diagnosed with asthma. Eventually they develop central airway obstruction and often require emergency intervention.

Primary tracheal tumours are rare. Most are malignant, usually squamous cell or adenoid cystic carcinomas. Benign tumours are usually carcinoid tumours but other growths, such as adenoma, leiomyomas, lipomas and chrondromas, are described. Secondary tumours are far more common and usually arise from direct invasion from lung, oesophageal, laryngeal or thyroid malignancies. Mediastinal nodal deposits from these and other tumours can also invade the central airways.

The principal differential diagnoses are an inhaled foreign body, non-neoplastic tracheal stenosis such as postintubation stricture (rare nowadays), and extrinsic compression from vascular anomalies. The diagnosis is usually made at endoscopy, when biopsies can be taken and, if necessary, the mass can be debulked to remove the threat of impending airway obstruction.[82,83] Proximal and distal mucosal biopsies should be taken to delineate the extent of the tumour in preparation for resection, because squamous tumours may be multiple and adenoid cystic carcinoma has a proclivity for submucosal spread.

Resection is the definitive treatment for a tracheal tumour[82,83] and should be considered when the tumour has not metastasized, is not deeply invasive, and when it occupies a resectable portion of the trachea. Tumours of the upper trachea are best approached through a transverse cervical incision. If necessary this can be extended by division of the upper sternum. The extension of this incision into the fourth interspace can be undertaken if total tracheal exposure is required. A right posterolateral thoracotomy, through the fourth interspace, provides excellent access to the lower trachea. Care should be taken to preserve the lateral segmental blood supply during exposure of the trachea, especially beyond the presumed resection margins. These tumours are unpredictable and are often more extensive than anticipated, but up to one-half of the adult trachea can be resected with a primary reconstruction undertaken. This is facilitated by cervical flexion, suprahyoid release and mobilization of the lower trachea and carina from the great vessels, and division of the perihilar pericardium (Fig. 21.23). Where the involvement is more extensive, a staged approach can be adopted or prosthetic tracheal reconstruction used. Experience with prostheses is limited, and it may be more appropriate to abandon attempts at resection.

Squamous cell carcinoma and adenoid cystic carcinoma of the trachea may be sensitive to external irradiation. This can be used postoperatively for residual disease at the resection margin or where lymph nodes are involved. It can also be used as a primary treatment when the tumour is irresectable. It is seldom curative but can provide good palliation, especially in adenoid cystic carcinoma, and can be delivered as brachytherapy.[84] Laser photoresection can be used to debulk an obstructing lesion but is not curative, because the mural disease often remains.[85] Eventually the bulk of mediastinal disease may lead to collapse of the trachea from extrinsic compression. This advanced disease is best palliated with an airway stent.[86]

TRACHEOSTOMY, TRAUMA AND NON-NEOPLASTIC STRICTURES

Tracheostomy is most frequently undertaken to aid in the weaning of mechanical ventilatory support, because it reduces the dead space (lessens the work of breathing), permits the weaning

REFERENCES

81. Hetzel MR. Clin Oncol (R Coll Radiol) 1993; 5: 272–276
82. Mathisen DJ, Grillo HC. Ann Thorac Surg 1989; 48: 469–473
83. Grillo HC, Mathisen DJ. Ann Thorac Surg 1990; 49: 69–77
84. Spasova I, Petera J. Neoplasma 2001; 48: 234–240
85. Venuta F, Rendina EA, De Giacomo T et al. Ann Thorac Surg 2002; 74: 995–998
86. Vonk-Noordegraaf A, Postmus PE, Sutedja TG. Chest 2001; 120: 1811–1814

of sedation, provides effective tracheal toilet, and enables the patient to communicate.[87] It is also indicated for certain head and neck resections, in maxillofacial trauma, and where transoral intubation has failed (see Ch. 19).

Where possible, it should be performed in an operating theatre with the patient's neck in full extension. A transverse incision is made in the suprasternal notch, a finger's breadth below the cricoid. The incision is carried down, dividing platysma and separating the strap muscles in the midline. Next, the pretracheal fascia is incised and the second and third tracheal rings identified. All vessels encountered should be ligated. A square of the anterior tracheal wall is then removed, with cautery applied to the edges.

Where an endotracheal tube is already present, it should be withdrawn until its tip is just above the opening. The tracheostomy tube is then inserted; its cuff should be inflated to prevent an air leak and it should be firmly secured in place.

Tracheoinnominate artery or tracheo-oesophageal fistulae can complicate tracheostomy. The former is life-threatening and should be treated by immediate direct compression, with oral endotracheal intubation to protect the airway. The neck must then be rapidly explored and the eroded segment of artery excised (neurological sequelae are unusual). It is caused by the tracheal stoma being placed too low and can be prevented by covering any exposed large vessels with neighbouring strap muscles. Tracheo-oesophageal fistulae form as a consequence of pressure necrosis between the tracheostomy cuff and feeding tubes in the oesophagus. The treatment is removal of the nasogastric tube, with insertion of a gastrostomy tube to drain the stomach and a jejunostomy tube to feed the patient. Once the patient is weaned from the ventilator, operative repair can be carried out. This consists of tracheal resection, repair of the oesophageal perforation, and the interposition of healthy muscle. Stenting can be employed for those not fit enough for surgical repair if the defect is low enough in the trachea for the stent to be tolerated.

Percutaneous methods of tracheostomy formation are available, as are minitracheostomies, which provide an effective route for tracheal toilet (see Ch. 19).[88]

Tracheal injury can also occur from blunt and penetrating trauma.[89] Blunt injury to the neck or chest can injure the trachea and is frequently associated with other injuries (cervical spinal, oesophageal, chest wall, lungs, heart and great vessels; see Ch. 7). The commonest cause is a road traffic accident. Penetrating trauma to the airway from gunshot or knife wounds is rare in the UK. The patient may die at the scene from airway obstruction or disruption. Those surviving to hospital present with a spectrum of symptoms from gross respiratory distress through to mild dyspnoea. The diagnosis should always be considered where there has been significant trauma, because an injured but adequate airway may rapidly deteriorate. Surgical emphysema, stridor and hoarseness may be evident on examination, and a chest radiograph may show mediastinal air or pneumothoraces. The most vital step in management is to secure the airway. Usually flexible endoscopy will establish the diagnosis and can aid in intubation. Where this fails a transverse collar incision should be made and a tracheostomy inserted. The distal trachea may have to be located in the mediastinum and intubated directly if the airway is completely disrupted. Primary reconstruction can then proceed if appropriate, but more commonly other concomitant injuries require attention and the definitive airway repair should be delayed.

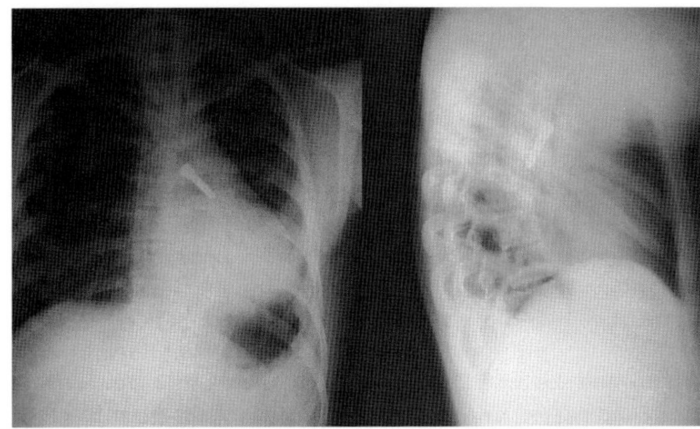

Figure 21.24 A radiopaque foreign body is clearly visible in the left main bronchus on these posteroanterior and lateral chest radiographs.

Burns arise secondary to a thermal or chemical insult (see Ch. 6). Endotracheal intubation is necessary if they acutely compromise the airway. Where this is not possible then a tracheostomy is needed. Once the airway is secure, the inflammation can be left to resolve. Unfortunately, this may lead to scarring, which is often most pronounced in the subglottic larynx and upper trachea. A stent or occasionally surgical resection may be necessary if an adequate airway does not remain.[90]

Foreign bodies can be inhaled into the tracheobronchial tree (Fig. 21.24). This usually occurs in children, but can occur in adults, especially if their conscious level is depressed through alcohol or seizure. The acute presentation is with severe coughing. Chest radiographs demonstrate radiopaque objects, but bronchoscopy is indicated if there is any suspicion of an inhaled non-metallic foreign body.[91] Most objects fall into the right main bronchus, because it is straighter in relation to the distal trachea than the left side. Bronchoscopic removal is almost always possible. Occasionally the acute symptoms subside, leaving the patient unaware of the inhaled foreign body. Distal infection, lung abscess and bronchiectasis can then arise, which may require open surgical treatment.

Postintubation tracheal stenosis can occur at the site of a tracheotomy or lower at the site of an over-inflated cuff (see Ch. 19). They form as a consequence of a fibrotic contracture and may be provoked by infection or excessive mechanical traction. For those fit enough, the best treatment is tracheal resection.[92] Otherwise, they can be managed by dilatation, stenting or the use of a rigid tube in the airway.

REFERENCES

87. Jaeger JM, Littlewood KA, Durbin CG Jr. Respir Care 2002; 47: 469–480
88. Bonde P, Papachristos I, McCraith A et al. Ann Thorac Surg 2002; 74: 196–202
89. Balci AE, Eren N, Eren S et al. Eur J Cardiothorac Surg 2002; 22: 984–989
90. Miller RP, Gray SD, Cotton RT et al. Laryngoscope 1988; 98: 826–829
91. Bodart E, de Bilderling G, Tuerlinckx D et al. Eur J Emerg Med 1999; 6: 21–25
92. Grillo HC, Donahue DM. Semin Thorac Cardiovasc Surg 1996; 8: 370–380

MEDIASTINAL TUMOURS

The mediastinum is located centrally within the thorax between the pleural envelopes. It is bounded inferiorly by the diaphragm, superiorly by the thoracic outlet, and anteroposteriorly by the thoracic cage. It is divided into four compartments. The superior mediastinum lies above a plane transecting the angle of Louis and the fourth thoracic vertebra. The mediastinum beneath this plane is divided into anterior, middle and posterior compartments. The anterior compartment is anterior to the pericardium, the middle compartment contains most of the viscera, and the posterior compartment contains the prevertebral space and paravertebral channels. Understanding the anatomy of these compartments and their relations is important, because the location of a tumour or cyst will give a guide as to its pathology and the surgical access required for its removal.

The common types of mediastinal cysts and primary tumours, together with their usual location, are given in Table 21.5. A posteroanterior chest radiograph, together with a lateral, usually reveals the approximate location of a mass, but its precise location and characterization is best undertaken with contrast CT. Further assessments may be undertaken with MRI, particularly in the case of paravertebral tumours, where accurate delineation of any spinal cord involvement is essential. In addition to these radiological tests, the presence of elevated levels of human chorionic gonadotrophin or alpha-fetoprotein in the blood suggests a tumour of germ cell origin. Biopsy is necessary for the final diagnosis of most tumours and can usually be carried out percutaneously. This avoids formal surgery in a patient whose treatment may be by radiotherapy or chemotherapy. Lymphomas fall into this category, and even where a percutaneous fine-needle aspiration or core biopsy has failed, a mediastinoscopy or mediastinotomy can provide enough tissue for diagnosis. In patients with tumours that appear resectable on CT, surgery should proceed and the mass should be fully excised. For extensive tumours, a percutaneous biopsy may confirm the diagnosis of malignancy, allowing irradiation to proceed in the hope of reducing tumour bulk before resection. Clearly, judgement is vital; the clinical details, the location of the tumour and its features on CT often enable a decision to be taken whether to biopsy or proceed directly to resection.[93]

Table 21.5 Usual location of primary mediastinal tumours and cysts

Location	Tumour
Superior mediastinum	Thyroid goitre, oesophageal masses and cysts, bronchogenic cyst and aneurysm
Anterior mediastinum	Thymic lesions, Morgagni herniae, aberrant thyroid
Middle mediastinum	Aortic aneurysm, cardiomegaly, pleuropericardial cyst, pericardial enlargement
Posterior mediastinum	Neural tumours, oesophageal lesions, Bochdalek herniae, aortic aneurysm
Common to all compartments	Lymphomas, connective tissue tumours

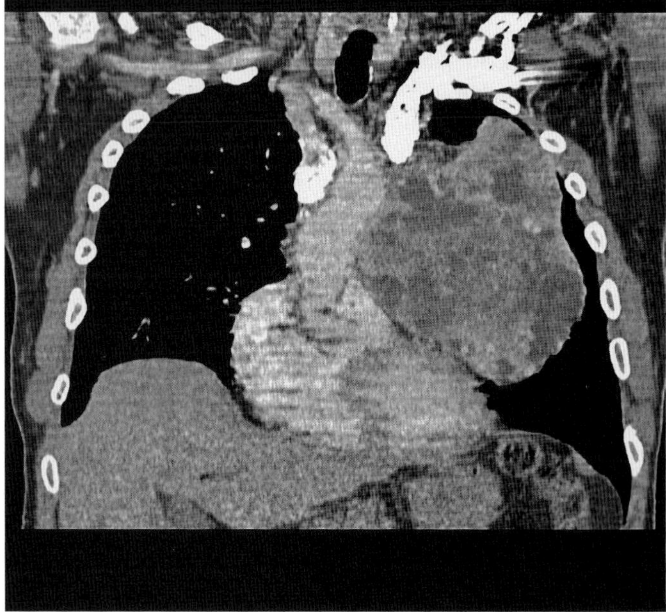

Figure 21.25 Medullary thymoma. Coronal reconstruction from a contrast-enhanced CT, demonstrating a large, heterogeneous, anterior mediastinal mass lying predominantly to the left of midline.

THYMOMA

Tumours of thymic origin account for up to one-half of all masses in the anterior and superior mediastinal compartments (Fig. 21.25). Neoplasia can arise in any of the cell types of the thymus, and so thymoma, thymic carcinoma, and tumours of neuroendocrine origin are all described. Thymomas arise from the epithelial cells of the thymus and are by far the commonest. They can be malignant or benign; the distinction is made by evidence of capsular invasion on microscopic examination of the resected specimen. Malignant thymomas invade locally, but metastases are unusual.

Thymomas have an interesting relationship with the autoimmune disorder myasthenia gravis. This syndrome is caused by antibodies to the acetylcholine receptor at the neuromuscular junction. It leads to excessive fatigability of skeletal muscle, primarily in the ocular and shoulder girdle muscles. A thymoma is present in about 10% of these patients, but thymic hyperplasia is seen in the majority. The thymus, if abnormal on CT, should therefore be resected, because most patients benefit and some may be cured. Myasthenia gravis is present in up to half the patients with a thymoma, and so the two are intricately linked.[94] Resection should be undertaken without biopsy, because this may seed the chest wall with invasive thymoma cells. Plasmapheresis should be used prior to surgery to improve the myasthenic symptoms and avoid problems with respiratory muscle function postoperatively. Surgery should be undertaken through a median sternotomy, and the thymoma should be excised with a wide cuff of normal tissue. This often necessitates the opening of both

REFERENCES

93. Jeung MY, Gasser B, Gangi A et al. Radiographics 2002; 22: S79–S93
94. Persico G, Martignetti A, Imbriani A et al. Ann Med 1999; 31: 70–72

pleurae and excision of the anterior pericardium. Pathological staging based on the extent of macro- and microscopic invasion, and completeness of resection, strongly affect prognosis. Early tumours have a good outlook, with a 5-year survival rate of over 90%. Radiotherapy is indicated for residual tumour and advanced disease, even if it was completely resected.[95]

RETROSTERNAL GOITRE

Thyroid goitres are usually wholly located within the neck (see Ch. 17). They may, however, extend into the superior mediastinum or arise *de novo* in the mediastinum from ectopic thyroid tissue. They can cause symptoms of cough, stridor, dysphagia, or upper body suffusion from local compression. They may also present incidentally on chest radiographs. Continuity with a palpable goitre in the neck indicates the diagnosis, as does evidence of contiguity on CT. The presence of speckled calcification is an additional feature of goitrous thyroid tissue. Uptake of radioactive iodine confirms the diagnosis.

The goitre should be excised in all cases to confirm the diagnosis, exclude malignancy, and to relieve local compressive phenomena. The surgery should be undertaken through a transverse cervical incision. The retrosternal portion of the goitre can be delivered into the wound from the superior mediastinum and excised. All normal thyroid tissue should remain. A proportion of patients may require a partial sternotomy to facilitate resection.[96]

LYMPHOMA

Both Hodgkin's disease and non-Hodgkin's lymphomas can arise in the mediastinum (see Ch. 33). They can occur in lymph nodes in all compartments but are commonest in the superior and anterior mediastinum. Mediastinal lymphoma is usually associated with disease elsewhere, and the diagnosis may be more easily obtained from an excision biopsy of one of these other sites. Where this is not possible, mediastinal nodes can be sampled with mediastinoscopy or anterior mediastinotomy. Percutaneous biopsy should be avoided, because histological examination of an intact node yields far more information. Treatment of these conditions is primarily non-surgical, with radiotherapy and chemotherapy (see Ch. 33). The prognosis is good, even for advanced disease. Surgical resection has been undertaken in selected cases.[97]

GERM CELL TUMOURS

Germ cell tumours usually occur in the gonads but do occur elsewhere on occasion (see Ch. 39). The commonest extragonadal site is the anterior mediastinum. The tumours derive from germ cells and are classified as seminomatous or non-seminomatous, of which the most frequent is teratoma. They usually present with local mass effects and demonstrate characteristic heterogenous density and calcification on CT.[98] Elevated serum tumour markers (alpha-fetoprotein and human chorionic gonadotrophin) are seen in the majority of non-seminomatous tumours. If these are elevated to diagnostic levels then treatment can proceed without biopsy. In other cases, the mass can be biopsied via an anterior mediastinotomy. Seminomas are sensitive to both chemotherapy and irradiation. Benign teratomas are treated by surgical excision, which gives excellent results. Malignant non-seminomatous tumours are treated initially with multiagent chemotherapy. This produces a good response in the majority of patients, and any residual disease should be resected, although this may be technically difficult. Those failing to respond to chemotherapy, as judged by persistently elevated tumour markers, have a poor prognosis.[99]

NEUROGENIC TUMOURS

Neurogenic tumours account for the majority of posterior mediastinal tumours. They particularly arise in children and young adults. Although they may derive from any component of the peripheral nervous system, tumours of the autonomic ganglia and nerve sheath are commonest.

Autonomic ganglion tumours have three variants: ganglioneuroma (benign), ganglioneuroblastoma (malignant) and neuroblastoma (malignant). The latter two occur in childhood and present with cough, chest pain and breathlessness. Ganglioneuromas are usually symptomless and present incidentally in adolescence. The treatment for all these tumours is resection, because the malignant potential cannot be determined on percutaneous biopsy. Irradiation and chemotherapy are considered if resection is incomplete and the lesion is malignant. Occasionally these tumours may extend through the intervertebral foramen as a 'dumb-bell' lesion (see Ch. 48). The patient may even present with or develop paralysis. Resection should be undertaken with thoracic and neurosurgical assistance.

Nerve sheath tumours are usually benign and occur in young adults. Neurilemoma and neurofibroma are the two common types. They usually present incidentally on a routine chest radiograph. Differentiation between the two clinically and even histologically can be difficult. These tumours may also extend into the spinal canal, and neurofibroma may be associated with von Recklinghausen's disease. The presence of symptoms may indicate malignancy. Treatment is by excision of the tumour through an open approach, but thoracoscopic resection for smaller lesions can be considered. Malignant nerve sheath tumours have a very poor prognosis.

BRONCHOGENIC CYSTS

Cysts can arise from the developing foregut and its derivatives. The two commonest sites are the oesophagus (gastroenteric cyst) or tracheobronchial tree (bronchogenic cyst, Fig. 21.26). They can be detected as a mediastinal mass on radiographs or present with compressive syndromes. They can also present with infection or bleeding within the cyst, which may undergo malignant change. Resection is the preferred treatment, because this allows confirmation of the diagnosis and relief of symptoms. This can be undertaken via a thoracotomy or with video-assisted thoracoscopic surgery.[100]

REFERENCES

95. Johnson SB, Eng TY, Giaccone G et al. Oncologist 2001; 6: 239–246
96. Vadasz P, Kotsis L. Eur J Cardiothorac Surg 1998; 14: 393–397
97. Ricci C, Rendina EA, Venuta F et al. J Thorac Cardiovasc Surg 1990; 99: 691–695
98. Wood DE. Semin Thorac Cardiovasc Surg 2000; 12: 278–289
99. Kay PH, Wells FC, Goldstraw P. Ann Thorac Surg 1987; 44: 578–582
100. Lin JC, Hazelrigg SR, Landreneau RJ. Surg Clin North Am 2000; 80: 1511–1533

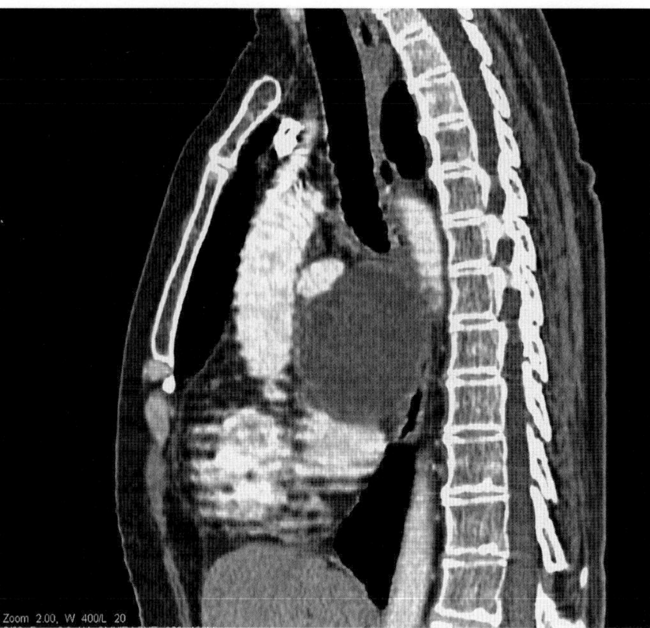

Figure 21.26 Bronchogenic cyst. Sagitally reformatted CT image showing a thin-walled fluid attenuation cyst in the subcarinal region typical of a bronchogenic cyst.

THE DIAPHRAGM

The diaphragm is formed from the fusion of many different elements and is innervated by the phrenic nerves, which have a long intrathoracic course. Thus the commonest diaphragmatic disorders are congenital herniae and paresis. Gastro-oesophageal reflux disease and hiatus hernia will not be dealt with here (see Ch. 20).

CONGENITAL HERNIAE

Congenital herniae arise from a failure of septation of the pleuroperitoneal canal. They are commoner (80%) on the left, because this hemidiaphragm unites later and the developing liver protects the right. The left lung is often hypoplastic, and the condition often presents with neonatal respiratory distress. A right-sided apex beat and abnormal chest radiograph confirm the diagnosis. The child should be resuscitated and then taken to the operating theatre.

The diaphragm is visualized through a subcostal incision, and the edges of the defect mobilized. With the usual posterolateral Bochdalek defect the anterior rim is large, and primary closure can be performed. Occasionally there is insufficient tissue, and a patch has to be inserted. Associated defects, such as malrotation of the gut, can be dealt with if the child is stable (see Ch. 40). The postoperative management can be difficult, especially if there is an associated hypoplastic lung or severe pulmonary hypertension.[101] Extracorporeal membrane oxygenation is occasionally needed.[102] Despite this, the majority of patients survive this condition. Intrauterine surgery is being developed for high-risk cases (severe lung hypoplasia) where there is no associated cardiac anomaly that may preclude survival.[103]

These herniae can present in later life, where the outcome is superior because the defect is not associated with pulmonary hypoplasia. Again, surgical repair is through the abdomen.

Morgagni herniae occur anteriorly through the retrosternal space of Larry. They usually present as an incidental anterior mediastinal mass on chest radiograph. They should be repaired to prevent strangulation, because the defect is often small.

Anterior diaphragmatic defects also occur in the pentalogy of Cantrell. These are more challenging to close and are associated with ectopia cordis, sternal cleft, omphalocoele and congenital heart disease (often Fallot's tetralogy).

DIAPHRAGMATIC PARESIS

The phrenic nerves innervate the muscular component of the diaphragm. Their dysfunction leads to the paresis of the respective hemidiaphragm. It assumes an elevated position within the hemithorax and produces dyspnoea. The causes are myriad, including trauma, neurological diseases (polio, shingles), intrathoracic malignancy, viral infection and surgical division (iatrogenic and therapeutic). Treatment is often conservative, but diaphragmatic pacing or surgical plication may be required.[104]

EVENTRATION

Eventration of the diaphragm is a symptomless laxity of the central tendon. It usually affects the anteromedial aspect of the right hemidiaphragm and may be confused with diaphragmatic rupture, herniae or pleural tumour. Occasionally it causes dyspnoea and can be plicated thoracoscopically.[105]

TRAUMA

Traumatic diaphragmatic disruption (Fig. 21.27) can follow either blunt or penetrating trauma, is often diagnosed late,[106] and usually affects the left side. Symptoms of pain and dyspnoea are common in all thoracic injuries, and a dull, quiet hemithorax usually indicates a haemothorax. Elevation or irregularity of the hemidiaphragm on chest radiography may suggest the diagnosis but are also non-specific. Where there is doubt and the patient is stable, a CT scan with visceral contrast confirms the diagnosis. A bedside ultrasound investigation is less reliable but can be undertaken rapidly in the resuscitation room. The diaphragm can be repaired through a laparotomy or thoracotomy, depending on associated injuries. The former is probably preferable if there are none. Blunt injury usually produces a large stellate tear of the central tendon, while penetrating wounds can affect any area of the diaphragm. In either case, direct suture repair can usually be accomplished once the abdominal organs have been inspected and reduced. Late-presenting traumatic diaphragmatic ruptures require repair via thoracotomy to divide the adhesions between the lung and abdominal viscera.

TUMOURS OF THE DIAPHRAGM

Primary tumours of the diaphragm are rare but may arise from any of its elements. More commonly it is involved by widespread pleural malignancy or secondary disease. Imaging with CT aids

REFERENCES

101. Sokol J, Bohn D, Lacro RV et al. Am J Obstet Gynaecol 2002; 186: 1085–1090
102. Stevens TP, Chess PR, McConnochie KM et al. Paediatrics 2002; 110: 590–596
103. Fowler SF, Sydorak RM, Albanese CT et al. J Paediatr Surg 2002; 37: 1700–1702
104. Higgs SM, Hussain A, Jackson M et al. Eur J Cardiothorac Surg 2002; 21: 294–297
105. Moon SW, Wang YP, Kim YW et al. Ann Thorac Surg 2000; 70: 299–300
106. Iochum S, Ludig T, Walter F et al. Radiographics 2002; 22: S103–S116

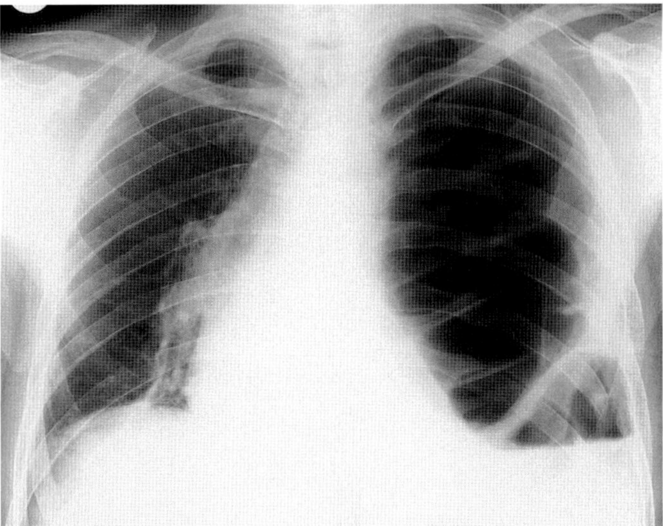

Figure 21.27 Ruptured left hemidiaphragm. Chest radiograph in a patient following a road traffic accident, showing absent lung markings on the left with mediastinal shift to the right. The left hemidiaphragm is not seen. Linear opacities in the left hemithorax are due to haustral folds in the herniated splenic flexure.

the assessment of resectability for primary tumours. Diaphragmatic resection should be undertaken with a wide margin of normal tissue. The resultant defect can be closed with a synthetic patch.

THORACIC TRAUMA

Traumatic injury to the chest can be divided into blunt and penetrating injuries. In the UK, the former is far more common, with the usual cause being road traffic accidents. Overall, thoracic trauma is the commonest cause of death following road traffic accidents (see Ch. 7). Management of these patients begins at the roadside,[107] and thereafter following expeditious transfer to the emergency department. The initial assessment and resuscitation follows the airway, breathing, and circulation (ABC) algorithm of Advanced Trauma Life Support® (see Ch. 7).[108] During the secondary survey the chest should be thoroughly examined. It is important to realize that there can be relatively few external signs of serious intrathoracic injury. Bullets can enter and exit the torso through tiny defects, but injure an essential organ or cause extensive destruction through the effects of cavitation. Following blunt trauma, the elasticity of the chest wall (especially in children) allows a large compressive force to be delivered without necessarily causing rib or sternal fractures.

BLUNT INJURY

Low-velocity injuries, such as those sustained from direct physical violence, frequently cause unilateral fractured ribs and a pulmonary contusion. If the rib punctures the lung there may be a pneumothorax (Fig. 21.28), or if the blow is over the lower thorax then the spleen and liver may be affected. Insertion of a chest drain may be all that is required. The lung will expand, air leaks will usually seal, and any bleeding from intercostal vessels is likely to stop. Anterior injuries that may fracture the sternum are more likely to be associated with a cardiac contusion. Severe low-velocity injuries are sustained from crushing. Here the chest is compressed, usually in the anteroposterior plane. The secondary lateral bulging of the chest can lead to disruption of the carina or main bronchi from stretching.

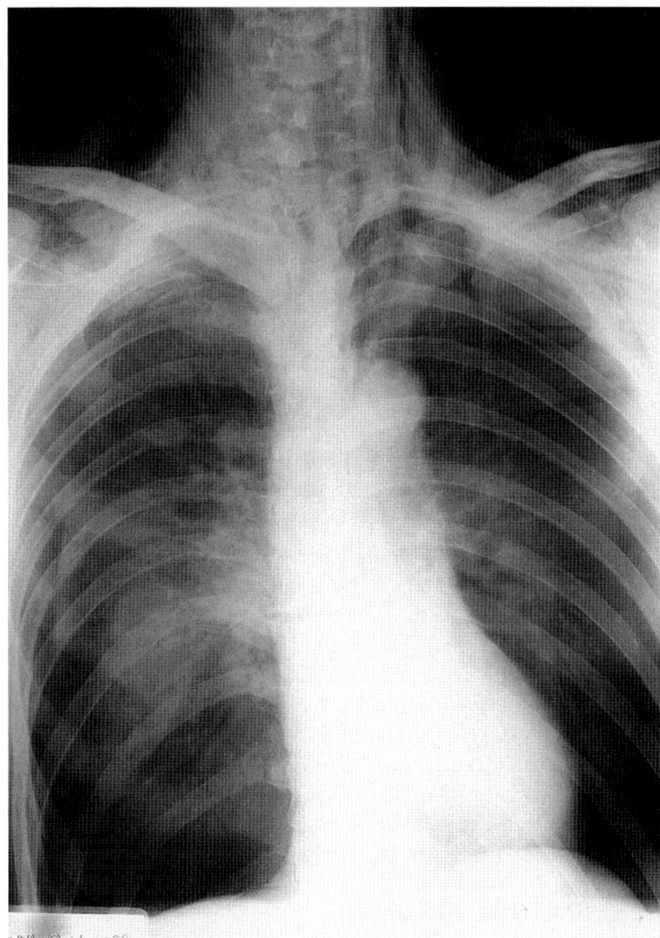

Figure 21.28 Chest radiograph in a patient who ruptured their right main bronchus in a high-speed road traffic accident, showing pneumomediastinum, pneumopericardium, a right pneumothorax and surgical emphysema.

High-velocity injuries, when the chest collides with the steering wheel or dashboard during a road traffic accident, are more serious. The chest wall is often injured at two points, producing ipsilateral double-rib fractures or bilateral rib injuries. Costochondral dislocation can be the second point of injury and will not be seen on a chest radiograph.

Where the force has been sufficient to give rise to these injuries, then underlying trauma can be expected, especially when the upper ribs are fractured. This disruption of the integrity of the chest wall at two levels can give rise to a flail segment, which moves paradoxically during spontaneous ventilation. Intubation and positive-pressure ventilation can usually improve the chest wall mechanics if respiratory distress is present and any haemopneumothoraces are drained. Severe underlying injuries should be sought, such as cardiac, spinal, tracheobronchial and aortic damage. Pericardial tamponade or herniation should be

REFERENCES

107. Pons PT, Honigman B, Moore EE et al. J Trauma 1985; 25: 828–832
108. Vestrup JA, Stormorken A, Wood V. Am J Surg 1988; 155: 704–707

corrected immediately; other cardiac lesions, such as valvar regurgitation[109] or intracardiac communication, need urgent surgical intervention after a period of resuscitation (see Ch. 22). Fluid administration to patients with these injuries should be judicious and accompanied by invasive haemodynamic monitoring to guard against the provocation of further haemorrhage[110] or pulmonary oedema in already contused lungs. Myocardial contusions usually recover spontaneously,[111] but the scar tissue they leave behind can be a focus for ventricular dysrhythmias. Extensive contusion of the anteriorly located and thin-walled right ventricle can lead to fatal right heart failure.

Associated spinal injuries are identified on clinical examination or an abnormal radiograph taken as part of a trauma series; these patients should usually be kept immobilized (see Ch. 7)[112] As a general rule, definitive treatment follows the treatment of life-threatening thoracic, abdominal or intracranial injuries. Tracheobronchial trauma is dealt with in the section on the trachea.

Aortic injury, most commonly transection just beyond the level of the left subclavian artery and ligamentum arteriosum, is usually fatal at the roadside.[113] In some patients the rupture is contained by adventitial tissue and is suspected from the mechanism and the chest radiograph appearance (see Ch. 22).[114] Ideally, it should be confirmed on aortography (Fig. 21.29) or CT[115] before surgery, which is undertaken through a left posterolateral thoracotomy. Control is achieved and the affected aorta is excised; reconstruction is through direct end-to-end repair or the placement of an interposition graft.[116] Endovascular repair is evolving rapidly (see Ch. 10).[117]

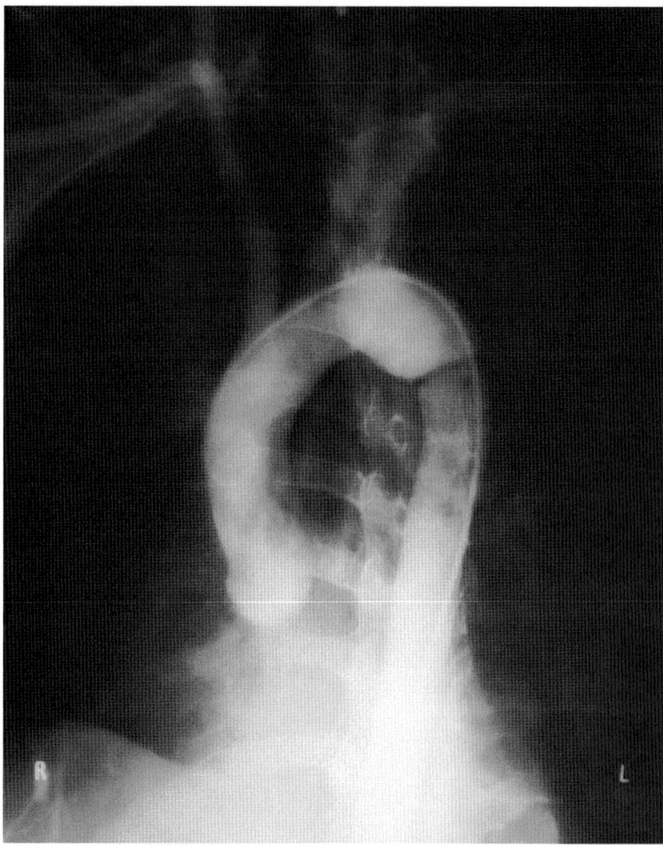

Figure 21.29 Aortogram showing a circumferential aortic transection just distal to the left subclavian artery.

PENETRATING TRAUMA

Penetrating chest injuries usually result from knife and gunshot wounds. Low-velocity injuries, such as knife wounds, cause damage limited to their path. This most frequently results in pneumo- or haemothoraces. Most such cases can be dealt with by the insertion of an intercostal drain. Such injuries are often multiple, and the whole body, including the back, must be examined for entry wounds. If the patient presents in the emergency room with the weapon still embedded then it should not be removed until the patient has been assessed and, if necessary, taken to the operating theatre. Gunshot wounds inflict a wide range of injuries, from those that have similarities to a small knife wound through to extensive destruction secondary to cavitation along the path of the bullet. This latter phenomenon is caused by shock waves from high-velocity bullets.[118]

Thoracotomy is necessary if thoracic bleeding or an air leak cannot be controlled with a chest drain. A median sternotomy provides excellent access if a precordial injury is associated with the suspicion of tamponade or cardiac injury requiring repair. Provided appropriate initial management is given, the results should be excellent.[119] Penetrating wounds of the heart often affect the anteriorly located right ventricle and can usually be repaired with sutures without the need for cardiopulmonary bypass (see Ch. 22).[120]

REFERENCES

109. Halstead J, Hosseinpour AR, Wells FC. Ann Thorac Surg 2000; 69: 766–768
110. Dutton RP, Mackenzie CF, Scalea TM. J Trauma 2002; 52: 1141–1146
111. Lindstaedt M, Germing A, Lawo T et al. J Trauma 2002; 52: 479–485
112. Domeier RM, Swor RA, Evans RW et al. J Trauma 2002; 53: 744–750
113. Avery JE, Hall DP, Adams JE et al. South Med J 1979; 72: 1238–1240
114. Simeone JF, Minagi H, Putman CE. Radiology 1975; 117: 265–268
115. Marotta R, Franchetto AA. Am J Roentgenol 1996; 166: 647–651
116. Sweeney MS, Young DJ, Frazier OH et al. Ann Thorac Surg 1997; 64: 384–387
117. Orford VP, Atkinson NR, Thomson K et al. Ann Thorac Surg 2003; 75: 106–111
118. Fackler ML, Surinchak JS, Malinowski JA. J Trauma 1984; 24: 263–262
119. Biocina B, Sutlic Z, Husedzinovic I et al. Eur J Cardiothorac Surg 1997; 11: 399–405
120. Catarino PA, Halstead JC, Westaby S. Injury 2000; 31: 209–211

Cardiac surgery

22

John Pepper, Tom Treasure, Christopher P. Young

INTRODUCTION

About 38 000 heart operations are performed each year in the UK. The majority are for coronary artery disease and, at a rate of about 400 per million of the population, this represents 65% of all heart surgery.[1] In the context of contemporary surgical methods, the heart is particularly amenable to the mechanistic approach that a surgeon can offer, with restoration of blood supply and correction of mechanical and structural abnormalities.

The increasing complexity of conditions amenable to surgical correction, the extension of surgery into treatment of increasingly severe heart disease, and the steady improvement in results have all depended on refinement of cardiopulmonary bypass techniques. Operations for congenital abnormalities, valve disease and coronary atherosclerosis depend on the skilled application of the basic techniques for supporting the circulation, protecting the brain and preserving myocardial function, and these are therefore outlined first. However, with the development of off-pump techniques, there has been a renewal of interest in operating on the beating heart, so avoiding the necessity to support the circulation with cardiopulmonary bypass and associated potential complications.[2,3]

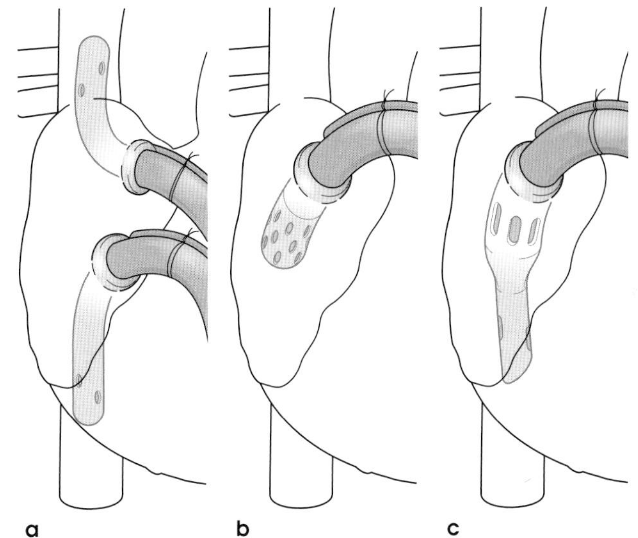

Figure 22.1 (a) The venous return to the heart may be diverted by separate cannulation of the superior and inferior venae cavae, which may be encircled with snares permitting operations to be performed within the right atrium. The coronary sinus venous return must then be collected separately. (b) A Ross basket in the right atrium permits total venous drainage and is the simplest technique for coronary artery surgery when the cardiac chambers are not opened. (c) A refinement with an extension into the inferior vena cava helps ensure that venous drainage is maintained as the heart is displaced to permit surgery to lateral or inferior coronary branches.

CARDIOPULMONARY BYPASS

Credit for the first cardiopulmonary bypass machine used clinically goes to Gibbon in 1953;[4] soon after, Kirklin reported the first series of cases from the Mayo Clinic.[5] Cardiopulmonary bypass is now routine. Blood is drained from the patient by a gravity siphon, either through a single venous cannula in the right atrium or separate cannulation of the superior and inferior venae cavae, depending on how much control of the right heart is required (Fig. 22.1). The blood runs through an oxygenator, in which it is separated from a gas mixture by a system of membranes. The blood is then returned to the patient under pressure through an arterial cannula, which is usually positioned in the ascending aorta (Fig. 22.2). Alternatively, when it is inadvisable (as in aortic dissection), impractical (for example in thoracic aortic surgery), or impossible (in the case of severe adhesions or redo cardiac surgery) to cannulate the aorta, femorofemoral bypass can be employed. Arterial return is via surgical exposure of the femoral artery at the groin. Venous drainage may be from the femoral vein or the right atrium.

The flow during cardiopulmonary bypass is determined by an estimate of the body surface area and is usually set at 2.4 L/m^2. Reduction of the temperature by 5–10°C is common practice, but there are unresolved debates about the ideal pressure limits, the desirability of pulsed perfusion, and the optimum temperature.[6] The surgeon can now isolate the heart from the rest of the circulation with suction pumps to keep the area around the heart clear of blood. A vent suction pump may be used to decompress the heart.

As judged by survival and relief of cardiac disease, results are excellent, but cardiopulmonary bypass is far from perfect.

REFERENCES

1. Society of Cardiothoracic Surgeons of Great Britain and Ireland. National Adult Cardiac Surgical Database Report 1999–2000. Available: http://www.scts.org/file/NACSDreport2000part4.pdf
2. Buffolo E, Andrade JCS, Branco JNR et al. Ann Thorac Surg 1996; 61: 63–66
3. Angelini GD, Taylor FC, Reeves BC et al. Lancet 2002; 359: 1194–1199
4. Gibbon JH. Recent Advances in Cardiovascular Physiology and Surgery. University of Minnesota, Minneapolis, 1953: 107
5. Kirklin JW, DuShane JW et al. Proc Staff Meet Mayo Clin 1955; 30: 201
6. (Various). Perfusion 1989; 4: 83–161

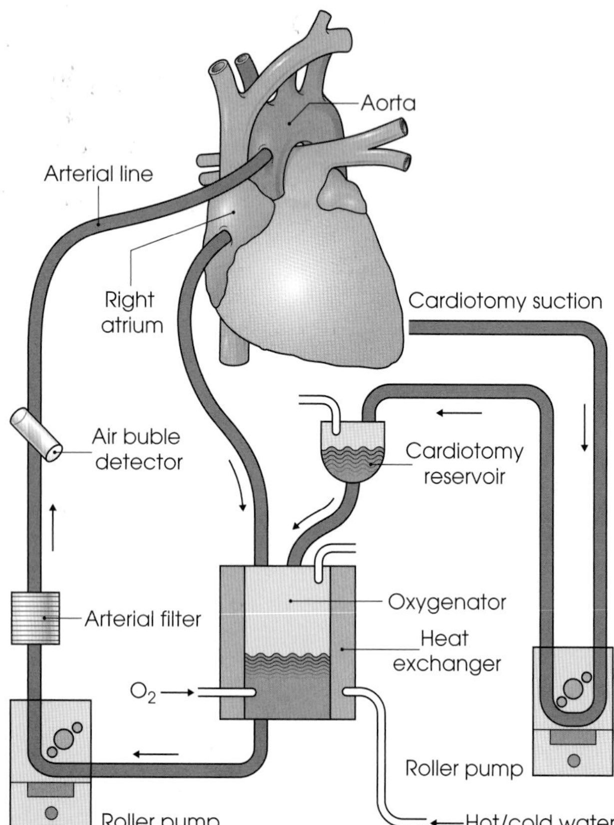

Figure 22.2 Components of a standard cardiopulmonary bypass circuit: the simplest and most commonly used system of venous drainage from the right atrium with arterial return to the ascending aorta, thus bypassing the heart and lungs. The circuit includes a reservoir, an oxygenator, a pump to deliver the blood, and usually a filter of 40-mm pore size to remove gaseous microemboli.

Deleterious effects on end organs including the brain,[7] lungs, kidneys and liver, as well as on the total body inflammatory response, occur with increasing severity with longer bypass time (Box 22.1). There have been many studies showing changes in complement, neutrophil activation, free radical activity and generation of cytokines.[8,9]

MYOCARDIAL PROTECTION

On cardiopulmonary bypass, the myocardium may be perfused normally through the coronary arteries as blood flows from the arterial cannula into the aortic root and the coronary ostia, but for many cardiac operations the perfusion of the heart muscle must be interrupted and a bloodless operative field obtained. The heart must then be protected from the consequences of ischaemia. This may be kept to a minimum by direct cannulation of the coronary ostia during aortic valve surgery, or by intermittently releasing the clamp during mitral valve or coronary surgery.

Myocardial ischaemia seems to be well tolerated for up to about 15 min in a non-working heart, especially with the help of moderate cooling on bypass. More thorough cooling of the heart—especially by intracoronary infusion of solutions containing potassium as the arresting agent (about 20 mmol/L) into the aortic root or directly into the coronary orifices—greatly prolongs the protection and improves working conditions for the surgeon and the subsequent performance of the heart.

Box 22.1 Potential complications of cardiopulmonary bypass

- Neurological dysfunction or stroke
- Renal dysfunction or acute renal failure
- Myocardial depression
- Pulmonary injury or adult respiratory distress syndrome
- Intestinal ischaemia or infarction
- Vascular injury
- Bleeding disorders
- Air embolism
- Microembolization
- Pancreatitis or cholecystitis
- Postcardiotomy syndrome or constrictive pericarditis
- Infection

The use of cardioplegic arrest is widely practised and usually consists of selectively perfusing the heart intermittently with oxygenated blood modified in one of a variety of ways, nearly all of which include raising its potassium content to between 15 and 20 mmol/L to arrest the heart in diastole (St Thomas's solution). Cooling was central to most techniques, but with increasing experience some surgeons have returned to more physiological temperatures.[10] The cardioplegic solution may also be given or supplemented by retrograde perfusion into the coronary sinus. Combined with systemic cooling or induced hypothermia (see *Systematically induced hypothermia*) on cardiopulmonary bypass, a margin of safety is provided, particularly if there are concerns about the degree of myocardial protection. With these techniques, safe cardiac arrest can be sustained for 2 h or more.

A technique called intermittent ischaemic arrest is an alternative method to the use of cardioplegic solutions. With this technique the aorta is cross-clamped, rendering the heart ischaemic, and ventricular fibrillation is induced by a small electrical charge. In ventricular fibrillation the heart becomes relatively still in a non-ejecting state, allowing the construction of a single distal coronary anastomosis. The heart can tolerate short periods (10–20 min) of intermittent ischaemia, providing that it is then reperfused, defibrillated, and allowed to beat while the proximal anastomosis is constructed. The sequence is then repeated for the construction of each graft.

The relative merits of these two techniques—intermittent ischaemic arrest (or cross-clamp fibrillation) and cold cardioplegic arrest—are debated,[11,12] and both techniques have been shown clinically to give excellent results, but the importance of preserving myocardial function cannot be overemphasized.

REFERENCES

7. Smith PLC, Treasure T, Newman SP et al. Lancet 1986; 1: 823–825
8. Treasure T. In: Yacoub MY, Pepper J (eds). Annual of Cardiac Surgery. 7th edn. Current Science, London, 1994: 161–169
9. Kirklin JK, Westaby S, Blackstone EH et al. J Thorac Cardiovasc Surg 1983; 86: 845–857
10. Fremes SE, Tamariz MG, Abramov D et al. Circulation 2000; 102 (Suppl 3): III339–III345
11. Anderson JR, Hossein-Nia M, Kallis P et al. Ann Thoracic Surg 1994; 58: 768–772
12. Sunderdiek U, Feindt P, Gams E. Eur J Cardiothorac Surg 2000; 18: 393–399

SYSTEMICALLY INDUCED HYPOTHERMIA

The protective effect of cooling is largely the result of a reduction in oxygen requirement of the brain. This knowledge was used to permit the earliest successful open-heart operations.

Mild systemic cooling on cardiopulmonary bypass is used routinely, but profound hypothermia with total circulatory arrest can be used when clarity of the operative area is essential, as in surgery of the ascending and arch of the aorta or in some paediatric procedures. It emerged empirically with uncertain time limits; sometimes an hour or more of circulatory arrest was used. More rigorous evaluation of clinical experience and laboratory experiments indicates that the technique allows up to about 40 min if the temperature is below 20°C.[13]

There has been a vogue in recent years to perfuse the brain retrogradely during hypothermic arrest: retrograde cerebral perfusion.[14,15] This is performed by perfusing blood up the superior vena cana cannula, and the return is into the open aortic arch. This has the theoretical advantage of maintaining a 'water jacket' around the brain and scalp; it may provide oxygen to the cerebral tissues and it washes out any debris from the arch vessels. The benefits of retrograde perfusion have been questioned, and there is a move away from the technique.[16] It may, however, still be valuable if the period of circulatory arrest is prolonged (over 30 min).

Antegrade cerebral perfusion is an alternative approach in providing neurological protection during total circulatory arrest during thoracic aortic procedures.[17] The arch vessels are selectively cannulated and perfused. This technique was associated on occasions with embolization of atheromatous debris from the origin of the arch vessels, and air could be entrained around the cannulae and embolize also. These problems have been largely avoided by cannulating the axillary artery directly.[18]

INVESTIGATION OF SURGICAL CARDIAC DISEASE

CLINICAL ASSESSMENT

A clinical history should elicit the presence of symptoms including chest pain, breathlessness, fatigue, swelling, palpitations and syncope. The severity of the symptoms and the extent to which they are interfering with everyday activities are extremely important. Symptoms of breathlessness and angina can be graded according to two universally accepted systems. For dyspnoea the New York Heart Association classification into groups I–IV is used (see Table 22.1), and for angina the Canadian Heart Association classification into groups 0–IV is used (see Table 22.2). In both systems the lowest group is normal and group IV represents symptoms at rest. An assessment of risk factors should also be included. These include advancing age, high cholesterol, diabetes, hypertension, smoking, obesity, and a family history of heart disease. Clinical examination follows and, although often normal, any evidence of myocardial ischaemia or stigmata of associated disease such as diabetes should be noted.

Table 22.1 Classification of heart failure based on the New York Heart Association functional classification of heart failure

Class	Definition
I	No limitation: ordinary physical exercise does not cause undue fatigue, dyspnoea, or palpitations.
II	Slight limitation of physical activity: comfortable at rest but ordinary activity results in fatigue, palpitations or dyspnoea (shortness of breath, particularly after exercise and when lying down).
III	Marked limitation of physical activity: comfortable at rest but less than ordinary activity results in symptoms.
IV	Unable to carry out any physical activity without discomfort: symptoms of heart failure are present even at rest, with increased discomfort with any physical activity.

Table 22.2 Grading of angina using the Canadian Cardiology Society functional grading system

Grade	Definition
0	No angina
I	Ordinary physical activity (e.g. walking or climbing stairs) does not cause angina; angina occurs with strenuous, rapid or prolonged exertion at work or recreation.
II	Slight limitation of ordinary activity, for example angina occurs when walking or stair-climbing after meals, in cold, in wind, under emotional stress, or only during the few hours after awakening, walking more than two blocks on the level, or climbing more than one flight of ordinary stairs at a normal pace and in normal conditions.
III	Marked limitation of ordinary activity, for example angina occurs when walking one or two blocks on the level or climbing one flight of stairs in normal conditions and at a normal pace.
IV	Inability to carry on any physical activity without discomfort: angina syndrome may be present at rest.

ELECTROCARDIOGRAPHY

As a baseline test, a 12-lead resting ECG often provides the first indication of ischaemic cardiac disease and is very helpful in patients admitted as an emergency. Other ECG changes can indicate the presence of left or right ventricular hypertrophy or rhythm disturbances that in association with other clinical and diagnostic tests may suggest underlying valvular heart disease.

EXERCISE TOLERANCE TESTING

The exercise tolerance test is valuable in the preoperative assessment of coronary artery disease and consists of a continuous ECG performed while the patient walks on a moving platform.

REFERENCES

13. Treasure T, Naftel DC, Conger KA et al. J Thorac Cardiovasc Surg 1983; 86: 761–770
14. Usui A, Oohara K, Liu TL et al. Thorac Cardiovasc Surg 1994; 107: 300–308
15. Reich DL, Uysal S, Ergin MA et al. Ann Thorac Surg 2001; 72: 1774–1782
16. Murkin JM. J Thorac Cardiovasc Surg 2003; 126: 631–633
17. Hagl C, Khaladj N, Karck M et al. Eur J Cardiothorac Surg 2003; 24: 371–378
18. Schachner T, Vertacnik K, Laufer G et al. Eur J Cardiothorac Surg 2002; 22: 445–447
19. Bean WB, Nora JJ. Circulation 1976; 54: 522

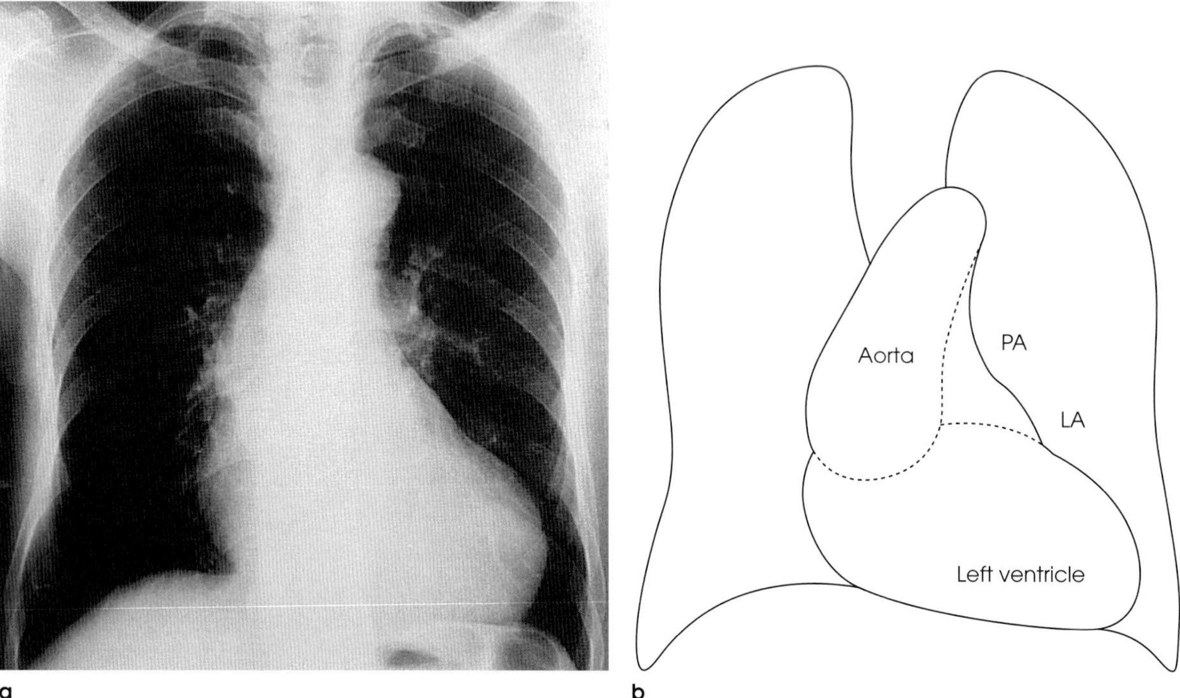

Figure 22.3 Plain posteroanterior chest radiograph of a patient with aortic stenosis. Note that the ascending aorta forms the midportion of the right heart border. The arch of the aorta is prominent on the left, and in this case the concavity of the left border is striking because of the prominent left ventricle but normal-sized pulmonary artery (PA) and left atrium (LA).

This becomes progressively steeper and faster in stages according to a specific protocol (e.g. the Bruce protocol). Symptoms, changes in pulse and blood pressure, and the development of S–T and T wave changes are documented. An abnormal exercise test must, however, be interpreted in the light of the probability of coronary artery disease, and the physiological response to exercise is measured by the percentage of the maximum predicted heart rate achieved. A positive test showing evidence of ischaemia on the ECG (S–T depression of 2 mm) does not always indicate ischaemic heart disease, and a negative test does not always exclude its presence. A positive exercise test in the presence of known coronary artery disease does, however, have significant prognostic value. Although two patients may have the same coronary stenoses, the patient with a positive exercise test is at much greater risk of infarction in the next 12 months and merits earlier treatment. The natural response to exercise is for the blood pressure to rise. Again, in someone with known coronary stenoses, a fall in blood pressure with exercise is associated with a significantly poorer prognosis than if the blood pressure rises.

CHEST RADIOGRAPH

The plain chest radiograph provides a two-dimensional image of the cardiac chambers and great vessels superimposed on each other. It provides information on mediastinal structures as well as the presence of associated heart disease (congestive cardiac failure) or pulmonary pathology (Figs 22.3 and 22.4).

ECHOCARDIOGRAPHY

Transthoracic echocardiography or transoesophageal echocardiography are valuable imaging tools for evaluating ventricular function and regional wall motion abnormalities, as well as valvular lesions. Stress echocardiography can detect regional wall motion abnormalities brought on by exercise or the use of dobutamine. It is a reliable method of identifying viable myocardium. Impaired but recoverable myocardium possesses a functional reserve that allows it to be temporarily recruited into action, whereas scar tissue does not. The resulting improvement can be assessed using stress echocardiography and is therefore a useful diagnostic tool in coronary artery disease. It can also be used to assess prognosis following myocardial infarction.

RADIONUCLIDE INVESTIGATION

In myocardial perfusion scintigraphy (thallium imaging) a gamma camera detects the distribution of intravenously injected thallium-201. This isotope behaves like potassium, entering cells, and its distribution is proportional to blood flow. In the diagnosis of myocardial infarction, technetium pyrophosphate is able to enter infarcted cells and bind to intracellular calcium. For left ventricular studies the technique of ECG gating is employed. The red cells are labelled with technetium-99. At any given moment the scintillation counts over the heart cannot be distinguished from the background. The counts from many cardiac cycles are therefore stored and divided into 16 subdivisions of the R–R interval 'gated' from the ECG. The cumulative counts provide a series of measurements of the volume of the heart in systole and diastole, and from these measurements the ejection fraction can be calculated.

CORONARY ANGIOGRAPHY

Despite the growth of non-invasive methods such as echocardiography, Doppler imaging and nuclear cardiology, coronary angiography remains an important diagnostic technique. Catheters are inserted into the arteries by a Seldinger technique through the groin, wrist or antecubital fossa. All the chambers of the heart and all the significant vessels can be reached.

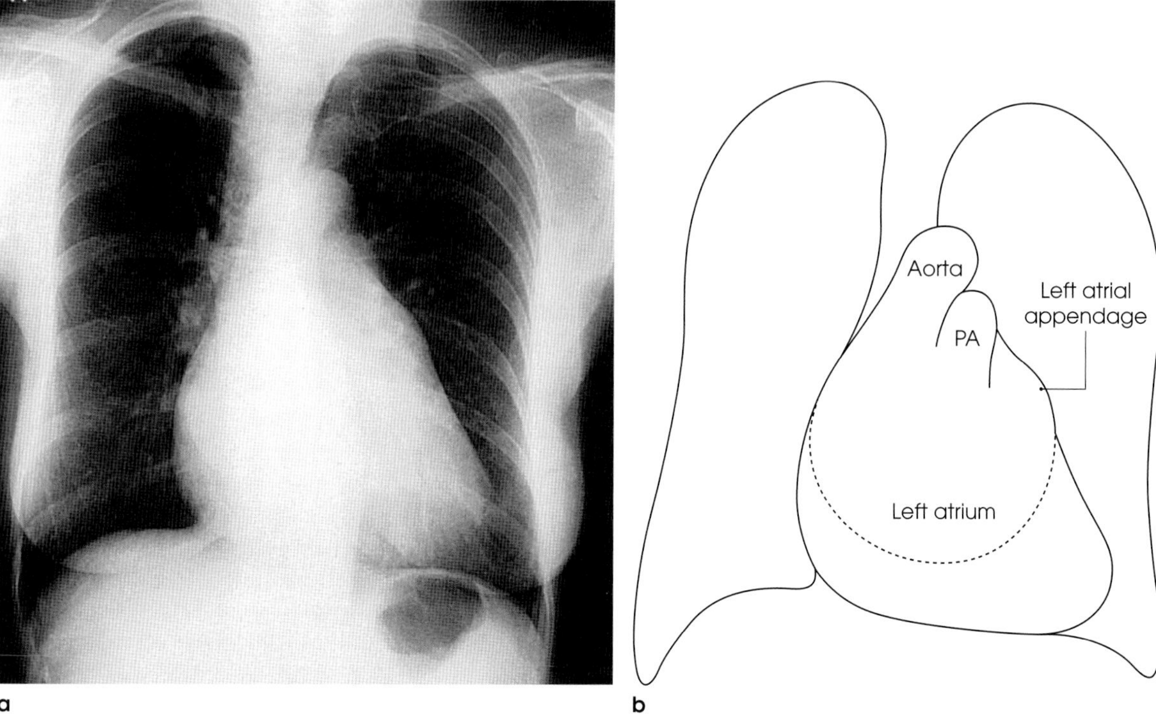

Figure 22.4 Chest radiograph of a patient with mitral stenosis. The left border is filled out by the prominent pulmonary artery (PA) and left atrial appendage. The left atrial enlargement also creates a double shadow on the right.

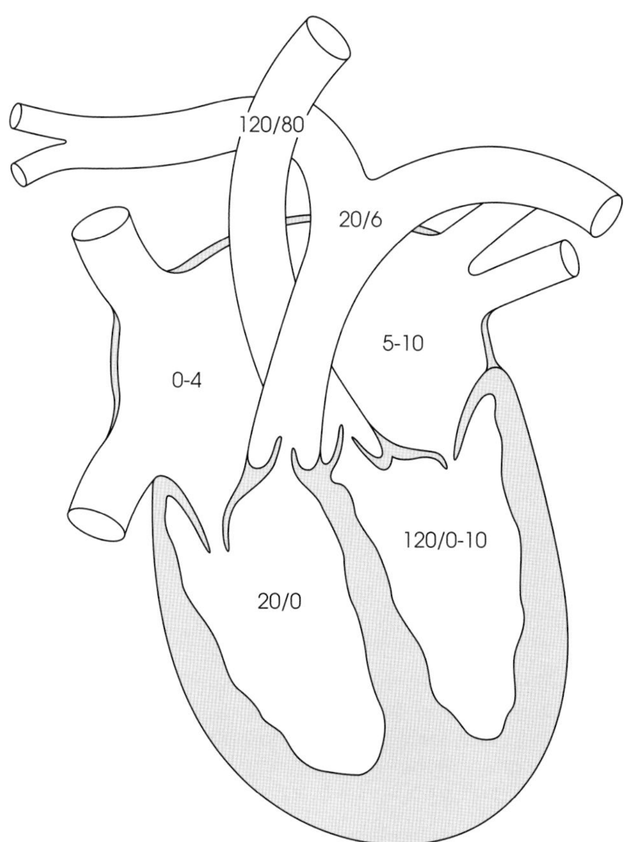

Figure 22.5 Typical normal pressures in mmHg in the cardiac chambers and great vessels.

Pressures are measured, blood is withdrawn for oxygen saturation measurements, and radiopaque contrast media injected and recorded. Complete information can be obtained about stenosed or incompetent valves (Figs 22.5 and 22.6), abnormal shunts between the right and left heart can be demonstrated, and the coronary arteries can be visualized.

CONGENITAL HEART DISEASE

The continuing advance in the surgical correction of many forms of congenital heart disease has realized Souttar's prediction.[20] The surgery is obvious enough in its more simple forms, such as closure of a persistent ductus arteriosus or patching a septal defect. More complex procedures, such as the Senning and Mustard operations (both means of switching the venous inflow in transposition of the great vessels),[21,22] are conceptually brilliant. The surgery requires an appreciation of disordered three-dimensional anatomy and allows little room for error. Congenital heart surgery, apart from simple procedures in older children or adults, is in most countries in the hands of a relatively small number of very expert surgeons working in specialized units.

REFERENCES

20. Souttar HS. Br Med J 1925; 2: 603–606
21. Senning A. Surgery 1959; 45: 966–980
22. Mustard WT. Surgery 1964; 55: 469–472

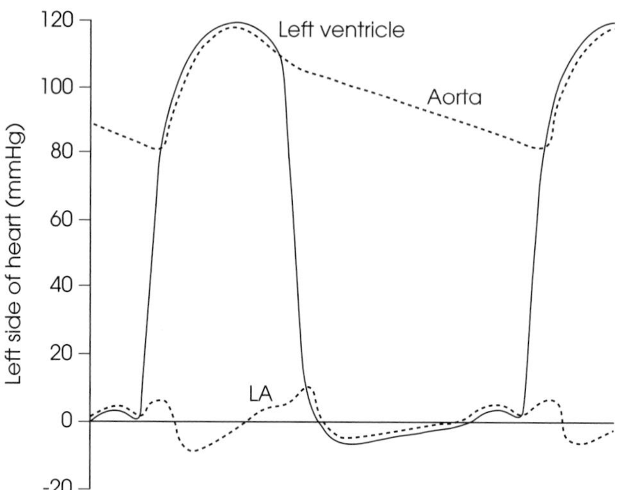

Figure 22.6 The left-sided pressures against a time base marked each 0.1 s. Note that the left ventricular pressure goes from just below left atrial pressure when the mitral valve is open to just above aortic pressure when the aortic valve is opened. As the lines cross, a valve opens or closes. Knowledge of these pressure changes is fundamental to a logical appreciation of valve disease and its symptoms and signs.

PALLIATIVE OPERATIONS FOR CONGENITAL HEART DISEASE

The earliest procedures were palliative. To understand them it must be appreciated that many patients with congenital heart disease fall into two large groups:

- those who are cyanosed either because of inadequate pulmonary blood flow or because of a failure to direct the returning venous blood to the lungs, and
- those in whom pulmonary flow is excessive because of a shunt from the left side of the heart into the more compliant pulmonary circulation.

Palliative procedures are used when the abnormality in the heart is too complex to correct, or if there are reasons to want to improve the situation as a temporizing manoeuvre until the child is bigger.

SYSTEMIC-PULMONARY SHUNT OPERATIONS

(Fig. 22.7)

In cyanotic congenital heart disease, the child's arterial blood may be desaturated because of a reduction in pulmonary blood flow. In Fallot's tetralogy, for example, there is a combination of restricted blood flow into the pulmonary artery (caused by obstruction) and a communication between the ventricles. Desaturated blood flows into the systemic circulation. Because the predominant feature is cyanosis, the label 'blue baby' was almost diagnostic enough for this whole group of conditions before corrective heart surgery was possible. Very effective palliation became possible with the first description of a systemic to pulmonary artery shunt to bypass the obstructive pulmonary lesion and improve pulmonary blood flow. The circulations are still mixed, but the child may derive great benefit from the improvement in systemic oxygenation.

The first technique described was the Blalock–Taussig shunt (Fig. 22.7a).[23] The subclavian artery was mobilized, divided, swung down, and anastomosed to the main right pulmonary artery. Today, a length of vascular graft is often used to make the anastomosis between the two vessels. This has gained popularity as better synthetic material for small-calibre grafts has become available. The size of the anastomosis must be judged so that the patient's condition is improved but flooding of the lungs is avoided.

PULMONARY ARTERY BANDING

If there is a communication between the left and right sides of the heart (e.g. ventricular septal defect), the more compliant pulmonary circulation permits a high left to right shunt and an increased pulmonary blood flow to the detriment of the lungs. The systemic blood flow is maintained and thus the total cardiac output is very much increased. If there is a common ventricle or multiple ventricular septal defects, closure in infancy is often too hazardous and then narrowing (or 'banding') the pulmonary artery to increase the resistance to pulmonary blood flow may provide useful palliation.

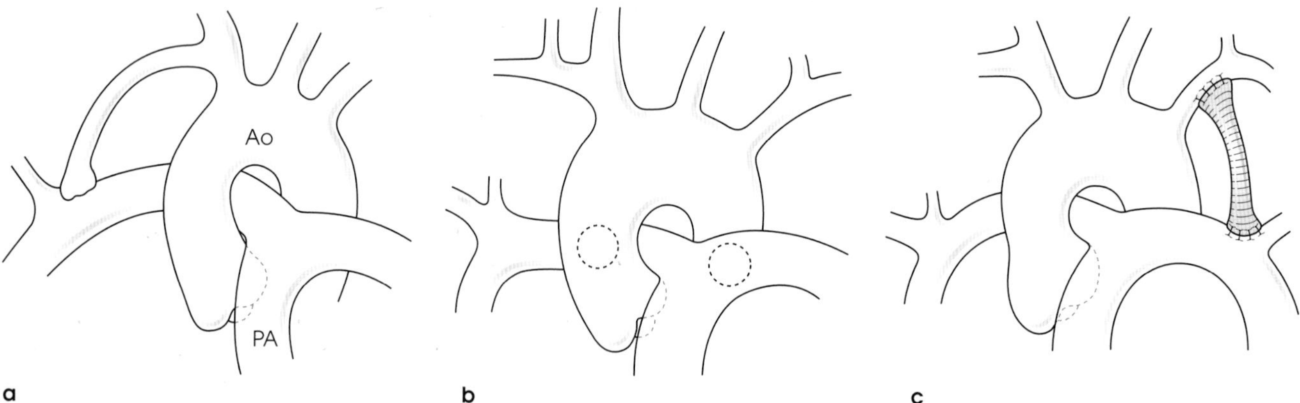

Figure 22.7 Systemic to pulmonary artery shunts for the palliation of cyanotic heart disease. (a) The Blalock–Taussig shunt, in which the subclavian artery is divided just before the vertebral and internal mammary arteries branch off and is anastomosed end to side into the right main pulmonary artery (PA). (b) Direct side to side anastomoses used to be made between the ascending aorta and the right pulmonary artery (Waterston) or the descending aorta and the left pulmonary artery (Potts). Neither is now employed but may be seen in some adults who have had palliation in childhood. (c) Interposition of a tube graft is now used in some cases.

REFERENCE

23. Blalock A, Taussig HB. JAMA 1945, 128: 189–202

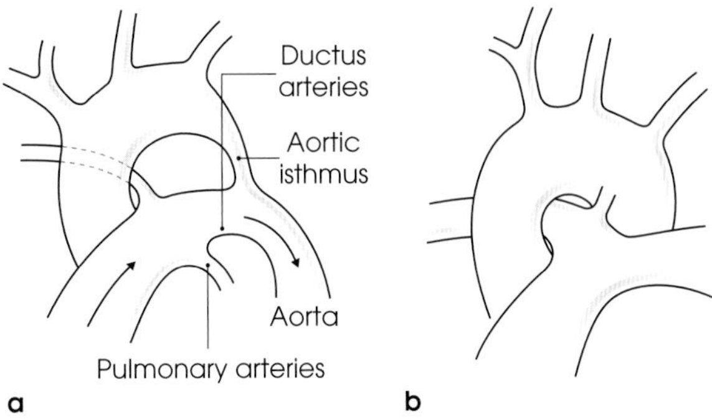

Figure 22.8 (a) In the fetus, the bulk of the desaturated blood passing through the right heart passes in the descending aorta and reaches the placenta via the umbilical artery. Failure of the ductus to close results in the condition of persistent ductus arteriosus. The blood flow reverses, resulting in excessive pulmonary blood flow. (b) The ligamentum arteriosum remains as a fibrous band in the adult; the recurrent laryngeal nerve passes around it.

It has to be noted that paediatric surgeons are increasingly moving towards primary repair of cardiac defects at an earlier stage, and that palliative procedures are becoming less common and reserved for the sickest babies and the most complex defects.

CLOSED CARDIAC OPERATIONS

Operations for patent ductus arteriosus and coarctation were possible before the use of cardiopulmonary bypass and are grouped together to distinguish them from open or intracardiac operations.

Persistent ductus arteriosus

In the fetal circulation, the relatively poorly oxygenated blood from the superior vena cava passes via the right atrium and right ventricle into the pulmonary artery. From the main pulmonary artery the majority of blood bypasses the airless lungs and flows via the ductus arteriosus into the upper end of the descending aorta. These three vessels form a continuous conduit in the fetus (Fig. 22.8).

The ductus contains muscle in its wall and normally closes after birth, largely in response to a rise in oxygen tension as the lungs begin to function. Prostaglandins keep the duct patent and can be used therapeutically for this purpose in cases where, as a consequence of intracardiac abnormalities, the blood flow to the lungs is so poor that survival depends on the presence of the ductal flow. In normal infants the duct closes within about 12 h of birth and is obliterated within a few weeks.

Persistence of the ductus arteriosus is one of the most common forms of congenital heart disease, accounting for approximately 12% of congenital cardiac defects. As the pulmonary vascular resistance falls in the days and weeks after birth, blood flows increasingly from left to right and clinical manifestations depend on how large a shunt results. If the duct is large there is a free flow of blood at arterial pressure into the pulmonary circulation, the pulmonary vasculature is engorged, and the left ventricle runs at high filling pressure and high output. On the other hand, a narrower ductus limits flow and the patient may be symptom-free. The abnormally high blood flow may nevertheless result in pulmonary vascular disease in due course.

The physical signs are a collapsing pulse and a continuous 'machinery murmur'. If the flow is small, resulting in a less than 2:1 pulmonary to systemic flow ratio, the patient may be symptomless throughout life and the only important risk is then of endocarditis.

Gross ligated a ductus arteriosus for the first time in 1938.[24] A simple tie may suffice, or in infants a clip, but these may fail to obliterate the lumen and some advocate division and suturing in all cases. The ductus is fragile and it has a very large vessel at either end! The recurrent laryngeal nerve is very close. The operation is treated with considerable respect by cardiothoracic surgeons because disaster is always close, and yet complete cure of the problem should be possible unless pulmonary vascular disease has supervened. Closure by a balloon, introduced from the femoral artery and passed retrogradely, is now a very successful way of closing the duct.

In the cardiothoracic units of the UK, about 200 operations per year are performed to close a persistent ductus.[1] The mortality is consistently about 1%. Operation for patent ductus arteriosus in the adult has become quite uncommon, but it can be very difficult if there is calcification or aneurysm formation.

Coarctation of the aorta

Almost invariably, the site of coarctation is in the upper aorta opposite the ductus arteriosus. There may be a shelf-like narrowing with a pinhole orifice or a longer, tube-like narrowed segment, or a combination of these two. In severe cases, there is considerable collateral development augmenting blood supply to the lower half of the body.

The problem may present as heart failure in infancy, but in most cases there is then a major associated abnormality. Those patients surviving to childhood are symptom-free, unless they have associated anomalies. The majority are hypertensive. The femoral pulses are delayed and attenuated, and a systolic murmur can be heard over the coarctation. The collateral circulation is between the branches of the subclavian artery, notably the internal mammary arteries and scapular vessels, which arise above the coarctation and feed the intercostal vessels from the third down. These have reversed flow into the descending aorta. They may be felt and heard clinically, and seen as rib-notching on the chest radiograph. Quite a high proportion of patients, at least a quarter, have a congenitally abnormal aortic valve (usually bicuspid), and berry aneurysms in the intracranial vessels are a sometimes fatal association.

Symptoms from left ventricular failure occur in time, but by then the hypertension, which has a renal component, is irreversible (see Ch. 35). For this reason, coarctation should be relieved before symptoms appear. The techniques of repair are end to end anastomosis, patching, and use of the left subclavian artery as a flap (Fig. 22.9). The operation of extended end to end repair is favoured in infants and children. It requires extensive mobilization of the arch and descending aorta, which is relatively straightforward in the young. The anastomosis between the two ends of the aorta is then made obliquely by incising the aorta proximally and distally. This technique reduces the risk of recurrent coarctation (with a simple end to end repair the child may outgrow the anastomosis). The first operation for this condition was performed by Crafoord in 1944.[25] About 250 operations per year are performed in the UK,[1] with a mortality of 1–2%.

REFERENCES

24. Gross RE, Hubbard JP. JAMA 1939; 112: 729–731
25. Crafoord C, Nylin G. J Thorac Surg 1945; 14: 347–361

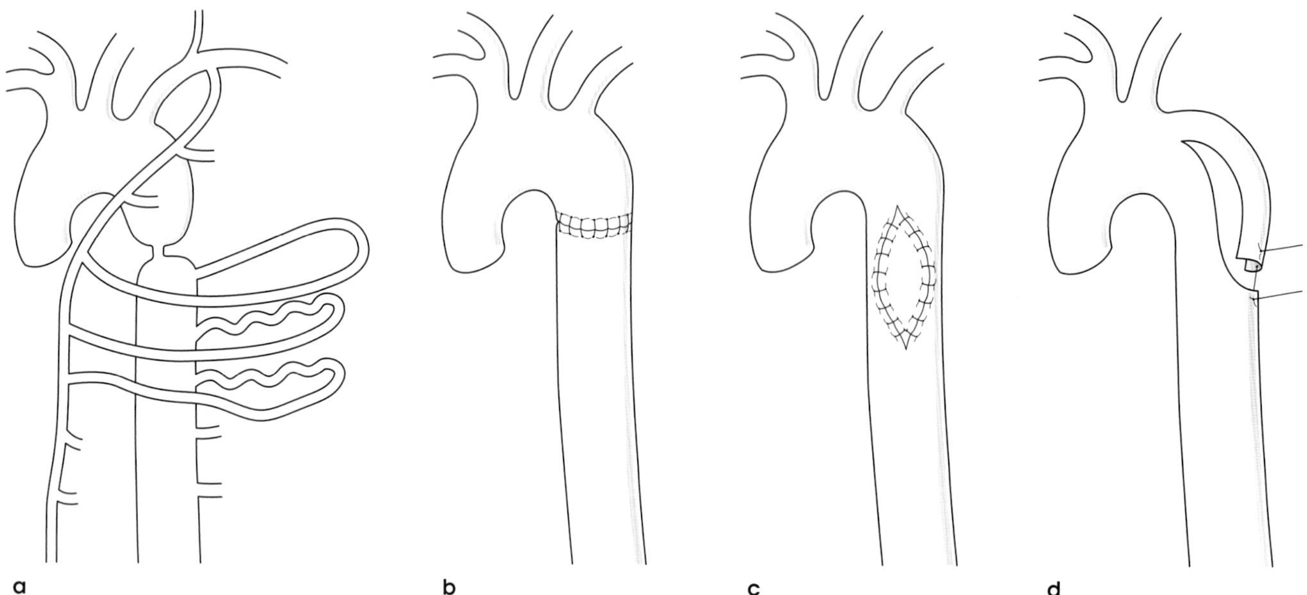

Figure 22.9 (a) Coarctation is a narrowing of the aorta in the area just beyond the left subclavian artery, which probably develops after birth due to abnormal ductus tissue. (b) Excision and end to end repair was the first and probably most common method of surgical management. (c) Widening the area with a gusset is a simpler alternative, particularly if the aorta is immobile or there is need for speed to avoid spinal cord ischaemia. (d) Mobilization of the left subclavian artery permits repair with normal arterial tissue and may allow for natural growth.

OPEN CARDIAC OPERATIONS FOR CONGENITAL DEFECTS

Atrial septal defect

The foramen ovale is a normal communication between the atria up to the time of birth, which remains probe-patent in a proportion of hearts throughout life. It is valve-like and permits a flow of oxygenated blood from the placental vein passing via the hepatic vein to stream through to the left side of the heart. As the lungs expand and the left atrium fills, the valve is held closed and in most cases seals. Blood does not pass through except where there are other abnormalities causing the right atrial pressure to exceed the left, and a patent foramen ovale is rarely a problem, although it can cause problems with right to left shunting in divers.

There are three patterns of atrial septal defect. The most common pattern (about 80%) is defects in the fossa ovalis, also called ostium secundum defects. About 15% are ostium primum defects and are part of the spectrum of atrioventricular septal defects. High defects associated with minor anomalies of pulmonary venous drainage are called sinus venosus defects (Fig. 22.10).

Although the pressures in the atria are low and not very dissimilar, the thin-walled right ventricle is very compliant and permits a large left to right shunt. This is very well tolerated for many years, even when the pulmonary to systemic flow ratio is in excess of 3:1. Heart failure is rare, but a tendency to 'chestiness' in childhood is typical. Gradually the heart size increases, the pulmonary artery pressure may rise, and the heart rhythm may change to atrial fibrillation. On examination, a systolic murmur can be heard as a result of the increased flow through the pulmonary valve. The lung fields are usually plethoric on radiographs. It is usual to advise operation if the pulmonary to systemic flow ratio—as estimated from the measurement of oxygen saturation in the right atrium, pulmonary artery and aorta—is greater than 2:1.

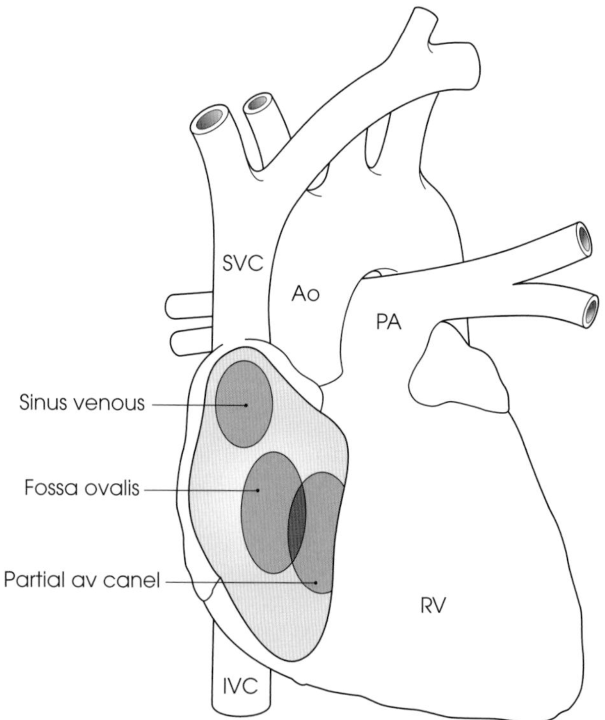

Figure 22.10 Defects in the atrial septum. A defect of the fossa ovalis (also called an ostium secundum defect) is the most common form of atrial septal defect. A *partial atrioventricular canal defect* is also known as an *ostium primum* defect; both terms suggest the supposed embryological abnormality. It is part of a complex of atrioventricular septal defects. A sinus venosus defect may be associated with various anomalies of venous drainage into the atria. SVC, superior vena cava; IVC, inferior vena cava.

There was great enthusiasm for operating on this defect in the early days of cardiac surgery before cardiopulmonary bypass, and some ingenious methods were devised to satisfy Souttar's admonition that we should operate without halting the flow of blood or interfering with the heart beat.[20] These included suturing the free atrial wall on to the defect, placing a purse string externally between the atria, and suturing a well to the atrium and then operating by feel alone. The technique of moderate hypothermia was the most successful, and Holmes Sellors perfected the technique of using surface cooling to about 30°C to permit safe closure of fossa ovalis defects.[26] Cardiopulmonary bypass has replaced all these techniques. In the UK over 500 operations are performed each year, the majority in childhood, with a mortality of under 1%.[1] In fossa ovalis defects (ostium secundum) there is often adequate tissue to permit direct suture. In other, more complex types of atrial septal defect—where suturing would cause distortion of the entry of great veins or interfere with the functioning of the atrioventricular valves—a patch is used to close the defect.

Ventricular septal defect

Defects in the ventricular septum vary widely in site and size. They may coexist with other anomalies—for example with pulmonary stenosis in Fallot's tetralogy or with atrial septal defect in complex atrioventricular defects—when the site is of diagnostic importance. In an isolated ventricular septal defect, the site affects the surgical approach and technical difficulty involved (Fig. 22.11). The size of the defect governs the haemodynamic consequences and therefore symptoms, and is the major determinant of the eventual outcome for the patient.

When a ventricular septal defect is present, there are two routes for blood to exit from the pressure-generating left ventricle; in addition to the normal route through the aortic valve, blood flows through the ventricular septal defect into the right ventricle. The volume of blood passing through the defect depends on both the size of the ventricular septal defect and the pressure generated in the right ventricle during systole, which in turn depends on the vascular resistance in the lungs. If the hole is as large as the aortic orifice, the pressure in the two ventricles equalizes, and flow is governed by the relative resistance of the pulmonary and systemic vasculature. In utero the pulmonary vascular resistance is relatively high in the airless lung, and blood passes preferentially through the ductus arteriosus. This resistance takes some time to fall, and initially there may be little left to right shunt and no murmur. Within a few days the pulmonary vascular resistance falls, and then the ratio of pulmonary to systemic flow may well be over 4:1 in a sick baby. Clinically, the baby is tachypnoeic and fails to thrive. The murmur is pansystolic. If the pulmonary vascular resistance rises again later, the shunt falls and eventually balances or reverses with the development of cyanosis. This is the phenomenon referred to as the Eisenmenger complex, and by this stage the condition is inoperable (except by heart and lung transplantation).

The natural history of ventricular septal defect includes a high incidence of spontaneous closure. A substantial proportion of those detected in infants under 1 month of age eventually close spontaneously. The likelihood of closure diminishes as time passes, and those still open by the time the child is of school age are very unlikely to close. Surgery is therefore indicated in infancy only if heart failure occurs. If the defects are multiple or the infant is very sick, pulmonary artery banding to protect the pulmonary vasculature until the child grows may be a wiser policy, although the combined risks of the palliative operation and its subsequent revision are not inconsiderable. In the UK about 100 babies under 1 year of age are operated on for this condition each year, and nearly twice as many older children, with mortality of under 1%.[1]

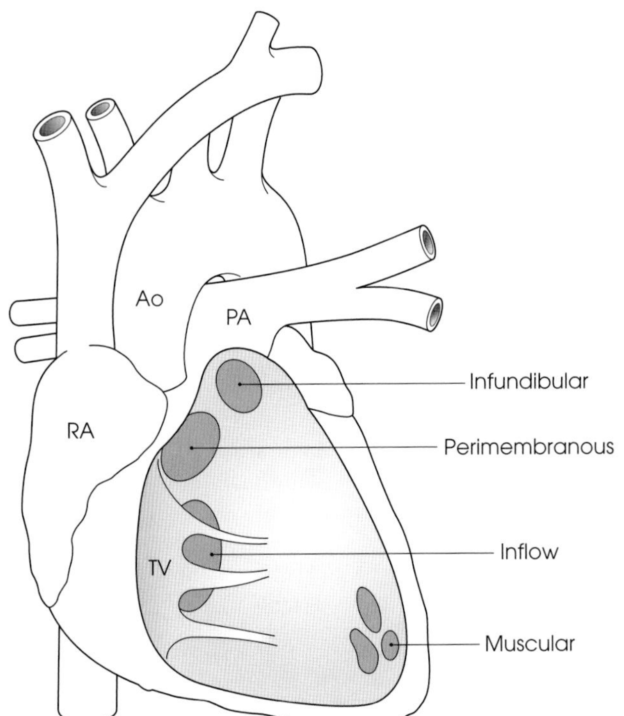

Figure 22.11 Cutaway view of the heart from the right side to show the common sites of ventricular septal defects. TV, tricuspid valve.

Aortic stenosis

Congenital stenosis related to the aortic valve may be valvar, subvalvar or supravalvar. The severe forms, presenting in infancy and childhood, are treated rather unsatisfactorily by an operation designed to open the commissures and relieve obstruction while leaving some competence to the valve. Balloon valve dilatation has replaced surgery as the first treatment for most cases. It is also less than ideal but less invasive.

The mildest form of congenital abnormality is a bicuspid valve where two of the cusps, usually the right and left coronary cusps, have failed to separate. These valves usually function well but tend to calcify and present as aortic stenosis in the seventh decade. They are vulnerable to endocarditis. If this occurs they may present as severe aortic regurgitation at a much younger age. Aortic valve disease is most commonly encountered in adult life, and this is covered later in this chapter.

Complex congenital heart disease

The isolated abnormalities of development already described are relatively easy to understand; the haemodynamic consequences are clear and the mechanics of correction are obvious. In complex lesions, the whole development of the heart is abnormal

• REFERENCE •

26. Bedford DE, Sellors TH, Sommerville W et al. Lancet, 1957; i: 1255

and the description of the morphology itself is contentious. The work of Anderson[27] has done a great deal to clarify this subject, and the system of sequential chamber analysis promulgated in his writing is widely, although not universally, accepted. In essence it recognizes that the terms *right* and *left*, *mitral* and *tricuspid* cease to have clear meanings in the most complex cases, and the system identifies structures by their morphology, irrespective of the actual side of the chest, and by their connections.

The exact mixture of symptoms and signs in an individual case is of limited use in making the final anatomical diagnosis. In most it merely serves to indicate that the heart is the cause of the infant's failure to thrive, and it denotes the relative severity of the physiological abnormality and the urgency with which it must be treated.

Fallot's tetralogy

Fallot's tetralogy is perhaps the best known of the complex congenital heart conditions, largely because of its memorable eponym. Fallot correlated the clinical and anatomical abnormalities. He identified four components:

1. a ventricular septal defect;
2. the aorta overrides it, with the result that it receives desaturated right ventricular blood;
3. obstruction to the right ventricular outflow; and
4. abnormal thickness of the right ventricular wall.

In an extreme form the aorta can arise from the right ventricle: a rare but well-recognized condition called double-outlet right ventricle. Those with a special interest in cardiac morphology describe the anatomy of tetralogy in great detail. The severity and extent of the infundibular, valvar or pulmonary artery obstruction, and the relationship between the ventricular septum and the aorta, must be clearly understood if a surgical correction is to be achieved.

The most severe cases present in infancy, although the condition is associated with a classical clinical presentation at a slightly later age. It is noticed that the normally highly active toddler becomes blue and adopts a characteristic squatting posture after running around in the course of play. The degree of arterial desaturation becomes more severe with exercise, and children learn that squatting will relieve their hypoxia by abruptly raising the resistance to flow in the systemic circulation and thus forcing a little more blood to the lungs. The discovery of the systolic murmur generated by the pulmonary stenosis virtually confirms the diagnosis when this almost pathognomonic history is elicited from the parent or carer.

About 300 operations are performed each year for this and related conditions, and the overall mortality is about 5%.[1] An alternative is to perform palliative surgery; this was the first use of the Blalock anastomosis.[23] The usual approach is to perform total correction when the anatomy is in any way favourable and the child is large enough. Otherwise a carefully planned shunt may be performed to allow the child to grow as the risks then fall. The balance of risks and benefits of one- versus two-stage correction continues to be debated.

Transposition of the great arteries

In transposition the great vessels leaving the heart are reversed in position, with the aorta arising from the right ventricle and the pulmonary artery from the left ventricle. This abnormality occurs once in 2000–3000 live births and accounts for around 5% of congenital heart disease. The pulmonary and systemic circulations are essentially parallel, but if there is enough mixing across the atrial septum through the foramen ovale, and between the great vessels via the ductus arteriosus, the condition is compatible with survival for a time. The condition usually presents at birth with cyanosis, which worsens as the ductus closes. Only 10% of patients survive to 1 year without intervention.

There are usually a number of associated abnormalities, of which pulmonary stenosis and ventricular septal defect are the most common. The presence of a ventricular septal defect permits mixing, and pulmonary stenosis reduces the magnitude of pulmonary blood flow that would otherwise result in heart failure as the pulmonary vascular resistance falls. The diagnosis may be suspected in an infant cyanosed from birth. The diagnosis is confirmed and the anatomy defined by echocardiography. In a particularly interesting form of the condition there is also discordance of the atrioventricular connections, a condition called corrected transposition; in these cases the physiology is essentially normal.

The initial treatment in sick, cyanosed babies is aimed at increasing the amount of mixing of the circulations to permit survival. Rashkind balloon septostomy is a useful palliative measure.[28] A catheter is passed transvenously to the right atrium and then through the foramen ovale into the left atrium. A balloon at its tip is inflated and the catheter sharply jerked back to tear the septum.

The aim of surgery is to correct the anatomical abnormality. The obvious anatomical correction of resiting the great arteries is made difficult by the problem of connecting the child's tiny coronary arteries to the oxygenated systemic outflow. Also, the left ventricle is unprepared to carry the systemic load unless it has remained hypertrophied because of the associated pulmonary stenosis.

Truncus arteriosus

Failure of division of the truncus arteriosus into the aorta and pulmonary artery results in a single great vessel leaving the heart through a common valve before giving rise to systemic and pulmonary branches. This is a rare condition that usually presents with heart failure in infancy.

Atrioventricular septal defects

Abnormalities of development resulting in deficiency of tissue immediately above and below the atrioventricular junction result in a wide spectrum of cardiac abnormalities, which are particularly common in Down's syndrome. At the mildest end of the spectrum, an actual communication is present only between the atria; this is the condition already described under *Atrial septal defect* (p. 484) as an ostium primum atrial septal defect and was also known in the past as partial atrioventricular canal. In the more severe form of atrioventricular defect, commonly known as complete atrioventricular canal, there are deficiencies of atrial and ventricular septation with abnormalities of both atrioventricular valves. These abnormalities are also grouped together as endocardial cushion defects, suggesting at least a nodding acquaintance with the embryological abnormality.

The presentation and clinical course of these cases are similarly diverse. The mild cases are similar in presentation to

REFERENCES

27. Shinebourne EA, Macartney FJ, Anderson RH. Br Heart J 1976; 38: 327–340
28. Rashkind WJ, Miller WW. JAMA 1966; 196: 991–992

atrial septal defect, although the course is less benign and the surgical correction is technically more exacting. Involvement of the ventricular septum results in a natural history more akin to ventricular septal defect, but with a much greater risk of developing severe pulmonary vascular disease. Associated atrioventricular valve regurgitation results in rapidly progressing congestive heart failure. The morphological description and the meticulous techniques involved in reconstructing the heart to create two valves and four chambers from a common atrioventricular canal are very complex.

Total anomalous pulmonary venous connection

In this rare condition, the pulmonary veins carrying oxygenated blood are not connected to the left atrium but instead drain into the right atrium. They most commonly (45%) drain above the heart through a vein reminiscent of a persistent left superior vena cava. In other cases, they drain through the coronary sinus or below the diaphragm into the portal system.

Presentation is with severe cyanosis from birth, without cardiac murmurs. Survival depends on the size of the atrial septal defect, which permits blood to reach the left atrium and thence the systemic circulation. A balloon septostomy therefore helps but early surgery is the treatment of choice. The surgical mortality is around 15%.

Abnormalities of lateralization

The term *dextrocardia* means that the heart points towards or is largely on the right rather than the left. The normal arrangement, with the right atrium inferior vena cava and the liver on the right, is called situs solitus. The reverse is called situs inversus. Situs ambiguus describes states in which there may be right- or left-sided mirror image or isomerism. In right-sided isomerism there is no spleen. Asplenia is known to be associated with bizarre cardiac malformations with mirror image atria, failure of septation, and abnormal connections.

SURGERY OF THE VALVES OF THE HEART

MITRAL VALVE DISEASE

Mitral valve surgery makes up over one-third of all valve surgery performed in the UK, approximately 1400 isolated cases per year.[1] There is increasing emphasis on valve repair as the importance of preserving the mitral valve apparatus has become apparent.[29]

Mitral stenosis

Before cardiopulmonary bypass was available, mitral stenosis was consistently and safely relieved in large numbers of patients in the 1950s by valvotomy performed within the beating heart.[20] Virtually all cases of mitral stenosis, other than a few very rare congenital malformations, are the result of rheumatic fever. Women with the condition outnumber men by about 3:1.

Pathophysiology

Rheumatic fever follows throat infections with β-haemolytic streptococci, the antigens of which cross-react with those of various tissues of the body. The manifestations of acute rheumatic fever include involvement of several of the large joints in sequence—the basal ganglia causing Sydenham's chorea (St Vitus's dance)—and most importantly the heart, including valves, muscle, conducting system and pericardium. It is a disease associated with overcrowding and poor living conditions and has become uncommon in the more affluent nations.[30]

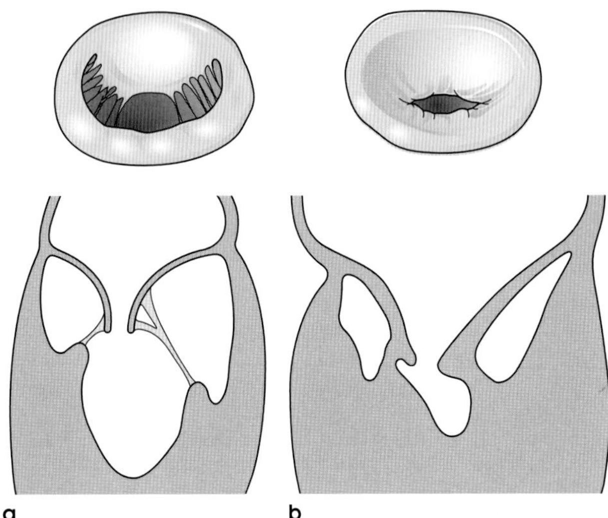

Figure 22.12 (**a**) The normal mitral valve, with a large anterior cusp and a crescent-shaped posterior cusp that can open to the full size of the atrioventricular orifice. (**b**) At its most severe form, the rheumatic valve has fused commissures, thickened immobile cusps, and short matted chordae. Of these, commissural fusion is the only component easily corrected by conservative valve surgery.

After the acute illness there are usually years of freedom from symptoms, during which one or more valves becomes progressively thickened. The mitral valve is most often and most severely affected. The commissures become adherent, the cusps thickened, and the chordae shortened (Fig. 22.12). Left ventricular filling is obstructed and the left atrial pressure rises, producing the symptoms of tiredness, as the result of limited cardiac output, and breathlessness, as the atrial and therefore pulmonary capillary pressures reach the critical point where the drying effect of the intravascular oncotic pressure is exceeded. The alveoli become moist and oxygenation is impaired.

The natural history is of steady deterioration, with 40% of patients dying within 10 years of presentation and only 20% surviving for 20 years, but sometimes deterioration is very slow. In older patients seen now, the history may include a previous conservative mitral valve operation.

Clinical symptoms

The characteristic feature of progressive mitral stenosis is breathlessness that becomes worse on lying flat, because of alterations in the pressure and volume relationships of the pulmonary circulation. Symptoms may progress steadily or appear suddenly with pregnancy or the onset of atrial fibrillation. Patients may also present with symptoms of systemic embolization, most commonly with stroke, but mitral stenosis must always be considered as a source of embolus to the leg or mesenteric arteries.

REFERENCES

29. Carpentier A. J Thorac Cardiovasc Surg 1983; 86: 323–337
30. Hall RJC, Treasure T. In: Julian DG, Camm AJ, Fox KM et al. (eds). Diseases of the Heart. 2nd edn. Saunders, London, 1996

Clinical signs

At some stage atrial fibrillation always develops, but the heart may stay in sinus rhythm for years. The apex beat has a tapping quality because of the abrupt nature of the first sound; on auscultation there is a loud first sound, an opening 'snap', and a rumbling diastolic murmur. The explanation for these sounds and their interpretation is important in making surgical decisions. The diastolic murmur is the result of turbulence as the left ventricle fills through the stenosed valve. Its loudness is related to the severity of stenosis but also to the cardiac output, so it may be very quiet even when the stenosis is severe. The loud first sound and the opening snap are the result of the sudden tensing of the valve to and fro as the ventricular pressure abruptly changes in relationship to the left atrial pressure (Fig. 22.13). The louder the sounds the more mobile is the mitral valve. A mobile valve may be conserved, but if the tissues are rigid from fibrosis or calcification the valve should be replaced.

Investigations

The chest radiograph shows a straight or bulging left border to the cardiac shadow where the enlarged pulmonary artery and left atrial appendage fill out the normal concavity below the aortic knuckle (Fig. 22.5). Other signs of left atrial enlargement are a double atrial shadow and widening of the subcarinal angle to more than 90°. The ECG shows abnormal notched P waves (P mitrale) if atrial fibrillation has not developed. There is evidence of right ventricular hypertrophy and a digitalis effect on S–T segment in advanced disease.

The diagnosis of pure mitral stenosis is made clinically, and investigations are aimed at diagnosing and quantifying other factors such as left ventricular function, pulmonary hypertension, the presence and severity of concomitant aortic valve disease, and the state of the coronary arteries. The usual indication for cardiac catheterization is to establish the state of the coronary arteries, particularly if the patient is male, is above middle age, or has had chest pain. Otherwise echocardiography provides excellent information about the state of the mitral valve leaflets, an estimate of the area of the valve, a calculation of the gradient across the valve, and an estimate of pulmonary artery and right-sided pressures.

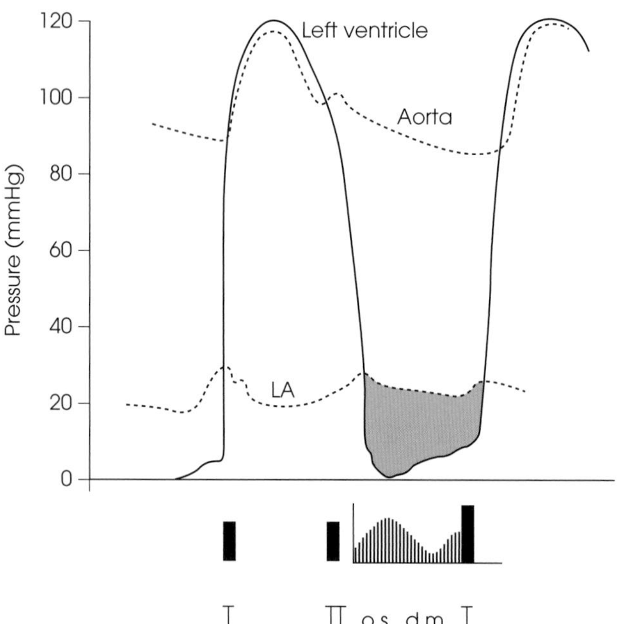

Figure 22.13 The pressure diagram (Fig. 22.6) modified to show the effects of mitral stenosis. There is now a pressure difference between the left atrium and the left ventricle when the valve is opened. This creates a murmur in diastole due to turbulent flow, and the valve opens with a 'snap' as the tension is taken up and closes more noisily, making a loud S1.

Surgical options

Mitral stenosis, unless trivial, should be relieved because of the ever-present risk of arterial embolization and the progressive nature of the condition, with often irreversible changes in pulmonary artery pressure and right heart function. The classical closed operation has lost favour in developed countries—where commissurotomy is most often performed on cardiopulmonary bypass or in the catheter laboratory by balloon mitral valvuloplasty—but closed mitral valvotomy remains an efficient and effective operation for those patients who have pure commissural fusion with a pliable valve, because it spares the patient the deleterious effects of cardiopulmonary bypass.[31]

Increasingly, the surgical option of choice is open mitral valve repair, but when valve repair is not possible—as in patients with severe calcific mitral stenosis who have fused and immobile subvalvular structures, or thickened and inflexible valve leaflets—mitral valve replacement is necessary. This usually involves a median sternotomy and access to the left atrium on cardiopulmonary bypass.

Mitral regurgitation

Rheumatic heart disease may result in acute, severe mitral valve incompetence; but more commonly a mild degree of regurgitation coexists with mitral stenosis. The most common cause of pure mitral regurgitation is now floppy valve disease, where the leaflets become soft and spongy and the chordae elongated because of a biochemical abnormality of the valve collagen.[32] The papillary muscles may infarct as a result of ischaemic heart disease, resulting in varying degrees of regurgitation. When a papillary muscle ruptures after myocardial infarction, this often results in catastrophic regurgitation in an already sick patient. More commonly, mitral regurgitation after infarction is caused by the inability of the inferior wall and inferolateral papillary muscle to shorten. As a result the anterior and posterior leaflets do not coapt in the same plane, causing regurgitation. At operation the valve looks structurally normal. This can make repair difficult because the problem is pathophysiological and functional. Infective endocarditis may involve the mitral valve, causing or exacerbating mitral regurgitation, and this especially occurs in floppy valve disease.

Pathophysiology

In mitral regurgitation the larger proportion of the stroke volume, and therefore the ventricular work, is wasted in blood passing to and fro through the mitral valve. The lungs are subjected to high pressure, although in the early stages this is intermittent and the pressure falls to the ventricular diastolic pressure.

REFERENCES

31. Tutun U, Ulus AT, Aksoyek AI et al. J Heart Valve Dis 2003; 12: 585–591
32. Barlow JB, Pocock WA, Marchand P et al. Am Heart J 1963; 66: 443–452

Clinical symptoms and signs

Symptoms may be mild while the heart compensates by increasing in size. Eventually breathlessness on exertion or attacks of pulmonary oedema occur. On examination the heart is abnormally large and active, and there is a murmur lasting throughout systole, heard all over the chest but not radiating to the neck. The murmur muffles the second heart sound (which distinguishes it from an ejection systolic murmur) as flow into the left atrium continues after the second heart sound (effectively the period of isometric relaxation).

Investigations

The chest radiograph typically shows generalized cardiac enlargement with all four chambers becoming involved, because of the volume load on the left side of the heart and eventually the pressure load on the right side, as the pulmonary artery pressure rises. The left-sided problem is volume-loading of the ventricle. The physiological response to this is ventricular enlargement, initially in diastole but later in systole. Later ventricular hypertrophy occurs (according to the law of Laplace). The ECG therefore may display features of left atrial and left ventricular hypertrophy. Echocardiography usually confirms the diagnosis. Doppler imaging quantifies the severity of regurgitation, and allows the structural abnormalities to be visualized, the ventricular dimensions and function assessed, and pulmonary artery pressures estimated. In addition, any right heart problems (e.g. tricuspid regurgitation) can also be assessed. Cardiac catheterization is needed only to assess any associated coronary artery disease.

Surgical options

The decision to recommend operation may be very difficult. Pulmonary oedema occurs in acute cases with gross regurgitation into a small atrium, and under these circumstances surgery is essential. In chronic cases when mitral regurgitation is relatively mild or has progressed slowly, it is very well tolerated and surgery is hard to justify in a symptom-free patient, especially as the results of mitral valve replacement are far from perfect and the operation includes a risk of thromboembolic problems, which may require the added inconvenience and danger of anticoagulants. Once the heart begins to enlarge on echocardiography, surgery is usually recommended to halt a progressive and eventually irreversible deterioration in the left ventricle. Some increase in the diastolic dimensions of the left ventricle is inevitable, but an increase in the systolic dimensions indicates a heart that is beginning to decompensate; at this stage surgery is usually recommended even if the symptoms are minor.[33]

Mitral valve replacement

The usual approach is through median sternotomy. In revision surgery, however, the valve can be approached through the right chest via an anterolateral thoracotomy. Under these circumstances the right atrium may be very dilated and thin-walled; it may also be in close proximity to the back of the sternum! Cardiopulmonary bypass is established, usually with separate cannulation of the superior and inferior venae cavae (Fig. 22.2). The left atrium is opened from the right side through an incision just behind and parallel to the interatrial septum. Access may be difficult, and attention to details of exposure and operating conditions is important.

The mitral valve is excised, preserving the posterior cusp with its chordae if possible to reduce the risk of posterior ventricular rupture, an uncommon and disastrous complication, and this also preserves left ventricular function. The chords, as well as maintaining mitral valve integrity, also maintain ventricular shape. Occasionally after a mitral valve replacement where the valve and chords are completely resected, the patient's ventricle may balloon a few months later, causing the ventricular function to deteriorate dramatically. A variety of suture techniques can be used: continuous and interrupted, with and without buttresses. A continuous technique has the advantage of speed, but interrupted suturing techniques are easier in that individual stitches are inserted and spaced in the annulus first and then in the sewing ring of the prosthesis. Interrupted sutures are definitely indicated if the valve is infected, when the tissues can be extremely friable. The operative mortality (death within 30 days) is approximately 5–6% for all cases of isolated mitral valve replacement.

Mitral valve repair

There is an increasing trend to return to conservative operations on the mitral valve, reflecting disillusionment with the performance of mitral prostheses. Procedures to refashion the cusp tissue, repair the chordae, and reduce the size of the annulus allow the surgeon to restore the function of the mitral valve.[34] The repair almost always needs to be buttressed by the insertion of an annuloplasty ring. A ring is selected that restores the diameter and shape of the annulus. The approach is the same as for a mitral valve replacement. Valve repair gives better results in patients with mitral regurgitation than in those with mitral stenosis, and repair is more feasible in degenerative mitral lesions than in rheumatic valves or after endocarditis. The risk of operation is 1–3%, with valve repair probably offering better preservation of ventricular function and avoiding prolonged anticoagulation as well as the valve-related complications such as prosthetic valve endocarditis or structural dysfunction.

AORTIC VALVE DISEASE

Despite a reduction in the incidence of rheumatic fever in the western world, aortic valve disease still remains a common indication for referral to a cardiac surgeon, being responsible for nearly two-thirds of all valve surgery performed in the UK.[1]

Aortic stenosis

Aortic stenosis exists when the valve orifice is substantially reduced, producing a pressure gradient across the valve. Aortic stenosis may be congenital, which includes degeneration of a bicuspid valve, and it may also be the result of rheumatic damage and senile degeneration. Congenital bicuspid aortic valves have a variable degree of fusion of the cusps; the right and left coronary sinuses often share a common cusp and as long as this remains flexible there is no significant obstruction to flow. Bicuspid valves tend to stiffen and calcify, and over half of the patients presenting for aortic valve replacement in middle and old age have a congenitally malformed bicuspid valve. Rheumatic heart disease causes progressive commissural fusion and cusp rigidity of the aortic valve. This can occur in isolation or may coexist with mitral valve disease. The third form of aortic stenosis is generalized calcification of an anatomically normal valve, which develops in the elderly (Fig. 22.14).

REFERENCE

33. (Anonymous). J Am Coll Cardiol 1998; 32: 1486–1588

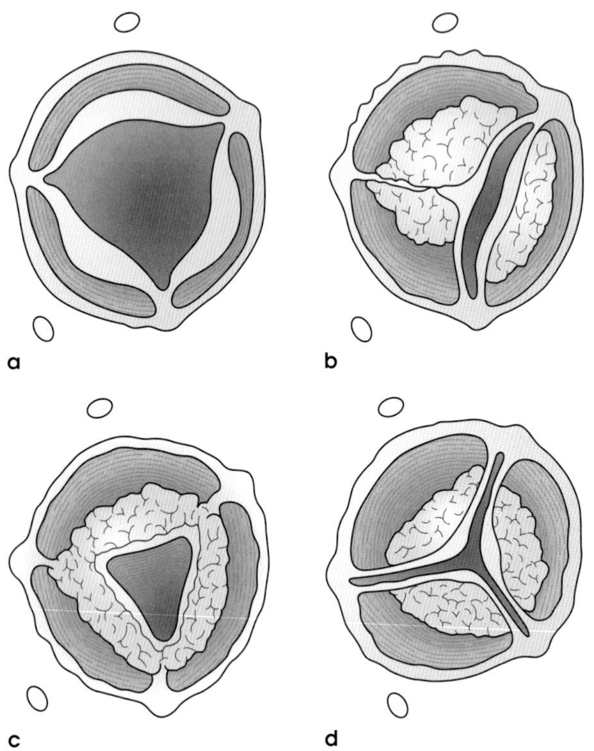

Figure 22.14 Aortic valve. (a) Normal valve, with three cusps opening symmetrically. The right coronary orifice is shown anteriorly and the left coronary posteriorly. (b) A congenitally abnormal valve with failure of development resulting in a bicuspid appearance; it is likely to become calcified and stenotic in later life. (c) Rheumatic fever obliterates the commissures and leads to thickening and later calcification. (d) Some anatomically normal valves become calcified in old age.

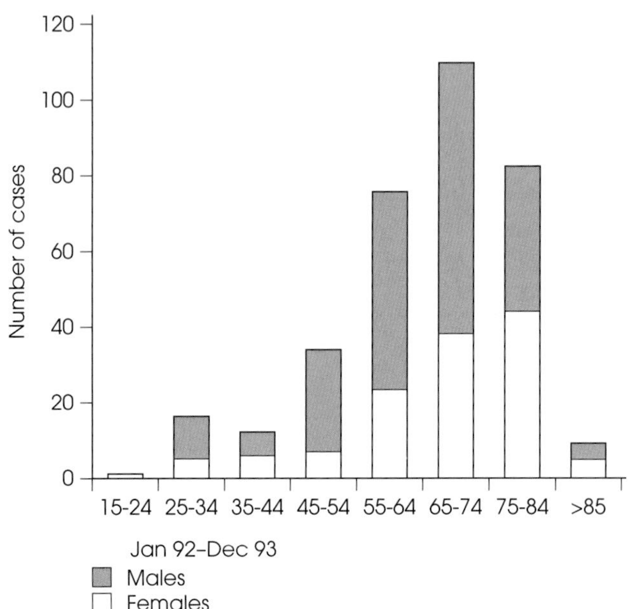

Figure 22.15 Age and gender distribution of a series of our own patients undergoing aortic valve replacement at St George's Hospital, London, UK in 1992 and 1993.

Pathophysiology

The typical orifice area of the adult aortic valve is 2.5–3 cm^2, but once the area is one-quarter of this it causes significant changes in haemodynamics. As a pressure gradient develops between the left ventricle and the aorta, the left ventricle adapts by hypertrophying to overcome the systolic pressure overload. This is a different response to the volume load as in mitral regurgitation, where the initial response is ventricular dilatation. This adaptive process may minimize symptoms for many years, but eventually myocardial function is affected and ventricular contractility becomes impaired.

Clinical symptoms and signs

The characteristic symptoms of aortic stenosis are effort syncope, where the patient suddenly falls to the ground after exertion; angina pectoris, which may occur without any coronary disease; and breathlessness on exertion. Many cases are discovered because a systolic murmur is heard or an abnormality is detected on incidental investigation. Exertional syncope can be the result of an inadequate increase in cardiac output or be a consequence of malignant dysrhythmias. The prognosis is poor following the onset of this symptom.

Investigations

The chest radiograph is often normal, but the heart can have a characteristic shape, with prominence of the aorta and left ventricular apex exaggerating the concavity on the left side. Calcification of the valve may be seen on the lateral chest radiograph. The ECG has the characteristic changes of left ventricular hypertrophy, most easily recognized by increased voltage of the QRS complex in the chest leads (e.g. S in V1 plus R in V5 greater than 35 mm), with flattening and inversion of the lateral chest leads in more advanced cases. The T wave changes represent subendocardial ischaemia. Coronary perfusion occurs from the epicardium down into the myocardium, which makes the subendocardium the most susceptible area to ischaemia as hypertrophy progresses and the wall thickness increases. The ECG combination of hypertrophy and T wave changes is termed *left ventricular strain.* Echocardiography confirms the diagnosis and provides a measure of the left ventricular hypertrophy and function, and the degree of thickening and calcification of the valve. In addition, the severity of the stenosis can be assessed by calculating the gradient across the valve and estimating the effective orifice area. Cardiac catheterization is often performed to assess the coronary anatomy, and also allows direct measurement of the pressure gradient across the valve in certain cases.

Surgical options

Aortic valve replacement is indicated in most cases of aortic stenosis causing symptoms, however well tolerated these are, because of the poor prognosis and the risk of sudden death. The natural history of patients with symptomatic aortic stenosis is very poor, with a 10-year mortality rate of 80–90%. Even in the absence of symptoms, a peak systolic gradient greater than 50 mmHg carries a risk of sudden death and a surgical opinion should be sought. Operation is invariably advised.[33] Surgery improves both the symptoms and the prognosis, and can be performed with a mortality of about 3%.[1] The peak incidence of aortic valve replacement in contemporary practice is around the age of 70 (Fig. 22.15), and more than 25% of patients are over 75. Surgery in patients over 80 years is not uncommon and the results are excellent, with life expectancy often being better than that in the general population of a similar age!

Aortic regurgitation

The causes of incompetence of the aortic valve are classified according to whether the predominant anatomical location of the pathology is in the valve leaflet or the aortic wall. Causes of valve leaflet disease leading to aortic regurgitation include congenital abnormalities, usually a bicuspid valve leading to degenerative changes; infective endocarditis; and rheumatic fever. Pathology of the aortic wall causing aortic regurgitation includes inflammatory and systemic conditions such as syphilis, rheumatoid arthritis, ankylosing spondylitis or Reiter's syndrome; degenerative changes, for example Marfan's syndrome; aortic root dissection; and senile aortopathy causing annular dilatation.

Pathophysiology

Aortic valve incompetence leads to a volume load on the left ventricle because of backflow into the ventricle. Patients can present acutely or insidiously, depending on whether the volume load is acute or chronic. If the progression is insidious (as in senile aortopathy), patients may remain apparently well until the heart is enormously enlarged and the left ventricle is damaged beyond recovery. The natural history is very variable, and some patients with a known regurgitant valve remain well without cardiac enlargement. Because the regurgitation is often well tolerated, these patients may be followed in cardiology clinics for many years before decompensation occurs.

Clinical symptoms and signs

Symptoms include breathlessness, and some patients have a discomfort that is like angina, particularly on lying down. The signs can be very dramatic. The long-standing increased pulse pressure results in a massive arterial pulsation in the neck, and the phenomenon of the collapsing, Corrigan or 'water hammer' pulse is well known to medical students. The heart is abnormally active but the diagnostic high-pitched decrescendo diastolic murmur is easily missed. It should be carefully sought at the left sternal edge, immediately after the second sound. It can be heard more easily by asking the patient to breathe out while sitting forward. The severity of the regurgitation correlates with the length of the murmur as much as with its intensity.

Surgical options

The usually benign but unpredictable course of aortic regurgitation makes timing of surgery difficult. The patient is followed until symptoms justify surgery or there is evidence of left ventricular deterioration, either with increasing ventricular dimensions on echocardiography or cardiac enlargement on the radiograph. Evidence of deterioration of the ECG is another indication that surgery should be considered.[33]

Aortic valve replacement

The operation is performed through a median sternotomy and a single venous cannula is sufficient. Cardioplegic arrest of the heart, which can be achieved or supplemented by direct coronary cannulation, has greatly improved the protection of the hypertrophied and vulnerable left ventricular muscle from ischaemic damage. Again, both interrupted and continuous suture techniques have their proponents. The risk is around 3% for all cases,[1] but it is very low in patients with well-preserved left ventricular function. The addition of coronary artery grafting does not greatly complicate the operation and is safer than leaving unrelieved left ventricular ischaemia.

TRICUSPID VALVE DISEASE

Isolated tricuspid valve disease is rare. The tricuspid valve may be involved with rheumatic fever in association with the mitral valve, or it may become incompetent as a secondary phenomenon consequent on high right-sided pressures as a result of left-sided valve disease (the pulmonary venous circulation possessing no valves). Endocarditis of the tricuspid valve is rarely seen apart from in drug addicts, in whom it is characteristic. Tricuspid incompetence occasionally presents with a large pulsating liver, which is felt as a tender mass in the epigastrium. The characteristic clinical signs are a raised jugular venous pressure with systolic waves and a pulsatile liver. The systolic murmur is not readily distinguishable from mitral regurgitation, with which it may coexist.

The majority (about 85%) of tricuspid valve operations are performed at the same time as mitral valve surgery. These patients have a particularly high operative risk (10–20%), largely because of their preoperative state and the damage done to the pulmonary vasculature and the liver over many years of high pulmonary and systemic venous pressure.

PULMONARY VALVE DISEASE

Pulmonary valve disease is a rare disorder caused by rheumatic fever or carcinoid syndrome. In both conditions other valves are almost always affected. Pulmonary valvotomy may be attempted for pulmonary stenosis; replacement is very rarely performed.

TYPES OF PROSTHETIC HEART VALVE

The indications and techniques for mitral, aortic and tricuspid valve replacement differ considerably, but many aspects of cardiac valve prostheses can be considered in common.

There are two basic types of prosthetic valve: the mechanical valve and the biological valve. These two types of valve can be further divided according to their design, how they are manufactured, and their relationship with the recipient.

Mechanical valves

Ball and cage valve

A spherical occluder is retained within the cage. This valve is one of the first mechanical valve designs used. It has poor haemodynamics because of the centrally placed ball, and has a higher thromboembolic rate than newer valves. The ball and cage valve has certainly stood the test of time and proved durable for over 40 years. It is still available but is now rarely inserted.

Tilting disc valve

The tilting disc valve is a single disc that is restrained by struts. The orifice has a major and a minor orifice with good haemodynamics.

Bileaflet valve

The bileaflet valve is a valve with two semicircular disc occluders. It is now the most commonly used prosthesis. The valve has three orifices when open, including a central orifice between the two leaflets. It has excellent haemodynamic properties and low thromboembolic rates.

Biological valves

Heterograft (or xenograft)

This valve has a basic design of three semilunar leaflets with central flow. These consist of harvested porcine aortic valves or are manufactured from bovine pericardium. In both instances the tissues are tanned using glutaraldehyde. They are now the most commonly used biological valves. Classically, the valves are attached to a flexible sewing ring, but in the past few years stentless aortic bioprostheses (both porcine and bovine pericardial) have been developed and inserted. When compared with the bulkier stented varieties, the stentless models have the theoretical advantage that a larger valve can be inserted into any given orifice. This may be important in patients with a small aortic root. (Note that porcine mitral prostheses are manufactured from larger porcine aortic valves—not porcine mitral valves!)

Homografts (or allografts) aortic valves

These are derived from donor cadavers and are usually cryopreserved; they are limited in their use by availability.

Autografts (for aortic valve replacement)

Autografts are performed using the patient's own valve. The pulmonary valve is harvested and used to replace the diseased aortic valve. The right ventricular outflow tract is then reconstructed with a homograft valve. This operation is called the Ross procedure.[35,36] It is technically demanding but has the advantage that the autograft should be viable. When the operation is performed in a young patient, the valve should continue to grow with the patient.

CHOICE OF PROSTHETIC VALVE

There are advantages and disadvantages to using the two basic types of valve. In essence, mechanical valves have a higher risk of thromboembolic complications, and patients receiving them must be rigorously controlled on anticoagulants for the rest of their lives. The valves, however, should not wear out, but there are sporadic examples of sudden mechanical failure.[37] Warfarin therapy has the extra disadvantage of requiring regular blood testing. Warfarin is interfered with by many factors, including alcohol. Warfarin therapy in the elderly is also associated with an increased risk of serious and sometimes fatal haemorrhages.

The tissue valves are probably safer, needing no long-term anticoagulation, but eventual failure seems inevitable. The median valve life is 12–14 years, leading to reoperation in many patients who live longer than that.[38] One major confounding factor in predicting the likelihood of valve failure in a patient is that bioprosthetic valve durability relates to the patient's age at implantation. Xenograft replacements are not generally recommended in the young, in whom calcification and valve deterioration are accelerated compared with in a patient in their seventies. In a younger patient who wishes to be active, and play sports for example, a homograft valve or a Ross procedure are preferable.

The closing stresses on mitral and aortic valves are very different. The aortic valve closes more gently, even though it is within a higher pressure system. The mitral valve closes with great force as ventricular pressure rapidly rises from end diastolic (*c*.5–10 mmHg) to systemic levels. It is not surprising, therefore, that the durability of bioprosthetic mitral valves is reduced when compared with that of aortic prostheses. Manufacturers are consistently seeking to improve on their valve designs but the haemodynamic characteristics, which include the pressure drop across the valve and the magnitude of any regurgitation, are satisfactory in all the currently available artificial valves. All prosthetic valves share a serious and perpetual risk of endocarditis, although the risk appears to be lowest with homograft and autografts.

COMPLICATIONS OF PROSTHETIC VALVES

Prosthetic valve endocarditis

This occurs in about 2–4% of patients with a prosthetic valve replacement. Like paravalvular leaks, it can occur early and probably arises from contamination at the time of surgery, or late, when it is the result of acquired infection. The condition of any patient with a previous prosthetic valve replacement presenting with a fever and a new murmur must be regarded with great suspicion. The diagnosis is confirmed with echocardiography, and aggressive antibiotic therapy should be commenced. It is very difficult to eradicate the infection with antibiotics alone, and surgery is almost always required. The timing of surgical intervention is important, but the risks in patients with prosthetic valve endocarditis remain high (native valve infective endocarditis is discussed below). Prophylactic antibiotics at the time of certain procedures, such as dental work, should be given to all patients with prosthetic valves.

Paravalvular leak

Paravalvular leaks following prosthetic valve insertion can also occur early or late. Early paravalvular leak is likely to be the result of a technical problem at the time of surgery, whereas leaks occurring late may be related to an episode of endocarditis or leaflet degeneration of a biological valve. Paravalvular leak can lead to haemodynamic problems and require replacement.

Thromboembolism

The risk of thrombus formation on a prosthetic valve with subsequent embolic episodes is about 0.5–3% per patient year with current mechanical valves. Risk is greater for mitral as opposed to aortic valve replacement.

INFECTIVE ENDOCARDITIS

The term *infective endocarditis* includes all infections seated on valvular and congenital abnormalities of the heart and great vessels, and includes the very important group of prosthetic valve endocarditis already discussed. Endocarditis rarely develops on previously normal valves except in drug addicts. The rate of progress varies widely between an acute fulminating course and a slow insidious progression that defies detection for months, making the demarcation into acute and subacute endocarditis unhelpful.

AETIOLOGY

Streptococci remain the most common infecting organism, although many other organisms are also responsible. Microbes are released into the bloodstream in the normal course of life, and in larger numbers during dental treatment. Gram-negative organisms may originate from large bowel disorders. Staphylococci of skin origin, including coagulase-negative staphylococci, are also increasingly important and particularly difficult to treat.

REFERENCES

34. Carpentier A, Chauvaud S, Fabiani JN et al. J Thorac Cardiovasc Surg 1980; 79: 338–348
35. Ross DN. Lancet 1967; 2: 956–958
36. Pillsbury RC, Shumway NE. Surg Forum 1966; 17: 176–177
37. Treasure T. Br Heart J 1991; 66: 333–334
38. Cohn LH, Collins JJ Jr, DiSesa VJ et al. Ann Surg 1989; 210: 435–442

These organisms predominate in prosthetic valve endocarditis occurring within the first year after surgery (when primary infection is suspected). They are also common in drug addicts, when they are related to recurrent dirty injections. Rickettsia or fungi (not just bacteria) may be the infecting agent, therefore making the still familiar term *SBE* (subacute bacterial endocarditis) obsolete.

CLINICAL PRESENTATION

The symptoms are often initially mistaken for influenza, with aching muscles and alternating fever and shivering. The combination of fever with any cardiac lesion on history, clinical examination or suspicion should lead to a working diagnosis of endocarditis. A series of blood cultures should be obtained without delay. The clinical signs include splenomegaly, splinter haemorrhages, and sometimes clubbing in long-standing cases. Anaemia, a high erythrocyte sedimentation rate and leukocytosis are usually present.

MANAGEMENT

Echocardiography confirms the presence of infective endocarditis, and serial examinations indicate the spread of infection into the surrounding myocardial tissues, the development of root abscesses, and the function of the infected valve. Early aggressive intravenous antibiotics are indicated, but this should ideally be started once the complete microbiological work-up has been completed. The condition should be managed in consultation with a cardiologist and a microbiologist. Surgery has a life-saving role in resistant cases, especially in those with prosthetic valve endocarditis, and the surgeon should be involved early.

There are two main indications for surgery. The first is uncontrollable and life-endangering haemodynamic abnormalities that are amenable to surgical correction, for example valve replacement, closure of septal defects, or ligation of a persistent ductus arteriosus. Second, surgery may be required if infection cannot be brought under control by antibiotics, which may be the result of an intracardiac abscess.

PREVENTION

Short or single high-dose prophylactic antibiotics given before predictable episodes of bacteraemia may reduce the incidence of endocarditis in susceptible individuals. All patients with an abnormal heart should take antibiotics before even the most minor dental treatment (including scaling) and probably a number of other events, such as instrumental delivery in childbirth, cystoscopy, and other forms of instrumentation.

CORONARY ARTERY DISEASE

INTRODUCTION

The advances in diagnosis and management of coronary artery disease have been formidable in the last 30 years. When Aird wrote on the subject in 1957, coronary angiography had not been performed and the surgery described, which was aimed at relieving angina, is now of only historical interest. It included creating pericardial adhesions with asbestos, a futile approach because these adhesions are bloodless. Cardio-omentopexy, in which the omentum was brought up through the diaphragm, and Vineberg's operation, where the internal mammary artery was tunnelled into the myocardium,[39] may have had more hope of success but both depended on chance formation of a capillary network without direct access to the coronary system.

Since the late 1960s, bypass grafting for coronary artery disease has become one of the most commonly performed operations. Favaloro described the technique of saphenous vein bypass grafting from the Cleveland Clinic in 1967;[40] in the 1980s, over 10 000 operations per year were performed in the UK and over 200 000 in the USA. Operation rates range from 200 to nearly 1000 per million of the population in developed countries, but after the enormous growth rate in the 1970s there are signs that both the epidemic of coronary artery disease and the numbers of operations performed are now levelling off. Medical management has also improved greatly with the availability of accurate methods of diagnosis and effective drugs. In particular, with the advent of percutaneous methods of treating coronary artery disease, such as coronary angioplasty and stenting, the nature of the patient population undergoing coronary artery bypass grafts has changed.

PATHOLOGY

Deposition of atheroma in the coronary arteries is part of the spectrum of occlusive arterial disease (see Ch. 10). The diet and way of life in developed countries is of clear epidemiological importance, with family history, lipid disorders, smoking, hypertension and diabetes being recognized risk factors.

CLINICAL PRESENTATION

The consequence of occlusive coronary artery disease is myocardial ischaemia; the mode of presentation depends on whether this is reversible, as is the case in patients who suffer recurrent episodes of angina pectoris, or irreversible, resulting in myocardial infarction. Any combination of these clinical states may occur.

ANGINA PECTORIS

Angina pectoris is the key symptom; it may be very characteristic but diagnostic uncertainty is common. Its timescale and its precipitating and relieving factors are of more diagnostic help than the exact site or subjective description of the attack. The sensation is usually described as crushing or choking, but some patients call it sharp or burning, or describe a feeling of breathlessness; pain is often denied. Radiation—which is usually into the left arm, to the elbow or the wrist, or into the jaw—is strongly in favour of the diagnosis, but not essential for it. Onset with exercise, relief by rest, and exacerbation by wind, cold, or a recent large meal should be sought, with specific questioning if necessary.

Unfortunately the history may be inconclusive. There are many patients who are misdiagnosed as suffering from indigestion or from oesophageal or biliary pain; the cardiac condition is overlooked until the patient is admitted with acute infarction. The reverse is also true, and unexpected gallstones have been seen in the corner of a normal coronary angiogram! Clinical examination may not detect any abnormalities, but hypertension and aortic valve disease should be specifically considered and excluded.

The other common and characteristic presentation of myocardial ischaemia is myocardial infarction. The symptoms develop

REFERENCES

39. Vineberg AM, Niloff PH. Surg Gynecol Obstet 1950; 91: 551–561
40. Favaloro RG, Effler DB, Groves LK et al. Ann Thorac Surg 1969; 8: 20–29

over several minutes (not suddenly) and persist for well over an hour with sustained intensity. The sensation may be similar or worse and more persistent than angina attacks that the patient has experienced, or it may be the first-ever experience of cardiac symptoms. It is accompanied by distress, pallor, sweating, nausea and sometimes vomiting. Although the clinical features of myocardial infarction are well known, the differential diagnosis is not always easy, and the various causes of acute chest pain—including aortic dissection, pulmonary embolism, pneumothorax, and oesophageal pain—must be considered in the differential diagnosis. Acute abdominal conditions also have to be considered, especially acute cholecystitis and acute pancreatitis (see Ch. 25). The most valuable diagnostic test is a 12-lead ECG, which usually shows evidence of ischaemia in the presence of evolving myocardial infarction. The immediate management should be active but is rarely surgical.

SURGICAL MANAGEMENT OF ANGINA PECTORIS

Investigations

Clinical examination, chest radiograph and ECG are characteristically normal. The exercise ECG is important for confirming the diagnosis and assessing the severity of the disorder. Nuclear medical techniques can demonstrate perfusion abnormalities and document the state of the left ventricle reasonably well, but coronary angiography is the important investigation that determines management.

Coronary angiography

This technique was developed and pioneered at the Cleveland Clinic, USA. Preformed catheters are passed retrogradely into the aortic root from the femoral, brachial or radial arteries. The ostia of the coronary arteries are selectively cannulated and injected with contrast medium and the angiogram recorded on cine-film or CD-ROM. At least two views, and often more, are taken of each of the coronary arteries to define the exact site and severity of any stenoses or occlusions.

Coronary anatomy

Figure 22.16 illustrates coronary anatomy.

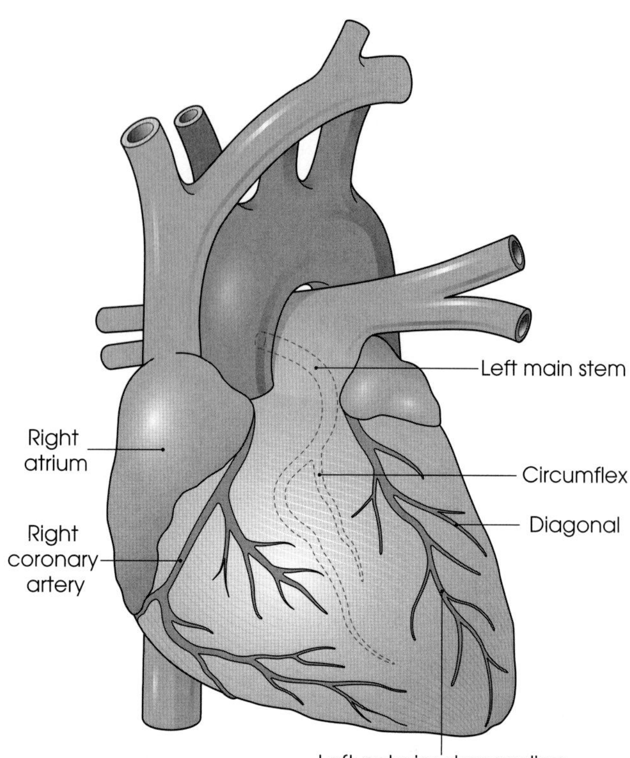

Figure 22.16 In simple terms there are two coronary arteries arising from the aortic sinuses, which, on division of the left coronary artery into its anterior descending (anterior interventricular) and circumflex branches, comprise with the right coronary artery three functional systems supplying the heart approximately in thirds.

Medical management

The initial assessment is clinical. The best care of the patient with angina is holistic and should include removal of known and avoidable risk factors, judicious use of drugs, consideration of relief of obstruction with surgery or angioplasty, and sensible advice about changes in lifestyle. An adverse family history cannot be changed but a smoking habit can. Hypertension, diabetes and hypercholesterolaemia are factors that can be ameliorated to some extent.[41]

Drug treatment of angina is by vasodilator drugs, β-blockers and calcium antagonists. The beneficial effects of vasodilators have been known for many years. The first described was amyl nitrite. Glyceryl trinitrate has been the mainstay for many years; it is used sublingually as tablets and spray, and can also be given percutaneously and intravenously. A wide range of nitrates are now available that can be given orally and in sustained-release preparations. It is likely that the effect on the coronary circulation itself is the least important, and that venous dilatation, reducing the preload or wall stress during diastole, and arteriolar dilatation that reduces after-load (that is, the work done in systole) are more important in relieving angina. Full medical treatment may include all three agents: vasodilators, β-blockers and calcium antagonists.

When the symptoms are readily brought under control with medical treatment and there are no particular features in the history to identify the patient as high risk, no further action may be taken at this stage. Surgery is indicated in symptomless patients only if they have an anatomical pattern of disease known to be an independent hazard (for example left main stem stenosis) that could be neutralized by surgery. Patients whose angina is uncontrolled by medical treatment should be considered for active intervention.

The decision whether to perform surgery or undertake angioplasty (percutaneous transluminal coronary angioplasty, PTCA) with stent insertion is debatable. Certainly there are no trials showing improved survival with PTCA in the same way there are with surgery, except for small specific groups (acute PTCA during infarction). Randomized trials of surgery and PTCA have concluded that survival is similar with both treatment options. Surgery is more invasive but the PTCA cohort had a greater risk of recurrent angina and reintervention.

There are several occasions when PTCA gives suboptimal results, such as in diabetic patients or when the lesion is calcified or eccentric. Certain lesions may be difficult to treat (bifurcation lesions) and left main stem stenoses are not attempted because the risk of complications is high.

REFERENCE

41. ASPIRE Steering Group. Heart 1996; 75: 334–342

Angioplasty techniques have developed remarkably over the past 10 years to allow treatment of difficult lesions and even blocked vessels. Multivessel PTCA is undertaken frequently (usually as a staged procedure), and the advent of drug-eluting stents has reduced the restenosis rates markedly. It is predicted that the number of surgical cases will reduce over the next 5 years as PTCA and stenting are able to achieve more.

Selection of patients for surgery

Surgery produces the most dramatic and rewarding relief of severe disability in a high proportion of patients. The ideal case has tight proximal stenoses and large healthy distal vessels beyond, but surgeons long ago extended surgery to include almost any severity of coronary disease while still gaining symptomatic relief for the great majority. The question of whether surgery can extend life has been the subject of considerable debate. Three large, multicentre, prospective randomized trials have addressed this issue: the Veterans Administration Cooperative Study,[42] the European Coronary Surgery Study Group,[43] and the Coronary Artery Surgery Study.[44] The problem that underlies this debate is that there is little relationship between the symptom (angina) and the fatal consequence of coronary narrowing (myocardial infarction). Some patients live for years with daily angina but have an undamaged left ventricle, while others suffer a massive infarction without warning and without subsequent angina.

Cardiologists and surgeons have used the information from these studies and other published series to formulate rational treatment policies.[45,46] Certain clinical and anatomical descriptors of good and bad prognostic groups have now been defined. Patients with only one or two vessels involved, relatively distal lesions, unimpaired left ventricular function, and stable angina have a very good chance—better than 90% probability—of being alive 5 years later, and this cannot been improved on by operation. The margin of improvement that might be gained by surgery is in any case small because of the age and underlying pathology in these cases. In patients with a good natural history, the decision depends on the severity of symptoms and limitation of the enjoyment of life, after medical measures have been tried. On the other hand, left main stem stenosis, proximal left anterior descending disease, three-vessel involvement, angina coming on at rest (unstable angina), and a left ventricle already damaged by infarction are all predictors of an increased likelihood of death; in these cases an operation significantly improves the probability of survival up to and beyond 5 years. In addition to these specific questions about probability of long-term survival with and without operation, the decision on advisability of revascularization should take into account the various other risks that must be weighed up as the balance of risks and benefits is considered.

Coronary artery surgery

Until recently, the operation was nearly always performed on cardiopulmonary bypass but, because none of the cardiac chambers need be opened, this can be set up in its simplest form (see Fig. 22.2). A single cannula is adequate for venous drainage; an arterial cannula is placed in the ascending aorta and no intracardiac vent is necessary, so the risks of air embolism are minimized. The coronary arteries are about 1.5–2.0 mm in diameter at the sites usually selected for grafting, so a still bloodless heart is ideal. The use of cardioplegia arrest or short periods (5–10 min) of ischaemia and ventricular fibrillation are equally well tolerated. The conduits are sutured to a vertical arteriotomy about 1.2 cm long using 7/0 prolene. With cardioplegic arrest, all distal (cardiac) anastomoses are constructed first. After the aortic cross-clamp is released, proximal anastomoses are constructed with the heart again beating by isolating a portion of the aortic wall with a side-biting clamp. Needless to say, the internal mammary artery grafts do not require a proximal anastomosis unless they are placed as free grafts (for shortage of length etc.). With the cross-clamp–fibrillation technique, a distal anastomosis is constructed during a period of ischaemic arrest; the clamp is then removed and the heart reperfused while the proximal anastomosis is constructed. This pattern is repeated until all grafts have been constructed.

There has been a move to performing these operations without cardiopulmonary bypass. There are few randomized studies, and those reported show little overall benefit from the off-pump technique.[3] Theoretically there may be an advantage in patients who are at higher risk of stroke because the heart beats and ejects throughout. The continuous flow of cardiopulmonary bypass is non-pulsatile and malperfusion can occur. In addition, cannulation of a diseased ascending aorta may embolize atheromatous debris, which is avoided by the off-pump technique. During construction of a distal anastomosis off pump, particularly to inferolateral branches, the cardiac output and blood pressure may fall precipitately, which in itself can cause cerebral hypoperfusion. The off-pump technique reduces the incidence of bleeding postoperatively and reduces the incidence of an acute inflammatory reaction, which is prevalent with conventional bypass.

The use of the left internal mammary artery as the graft of first choice for the left anterior descending coronary artery has become widespread since 10-year follow-up results from the Cleveland Clinic[47] and other centres demonstrated that the long-term results are superior to those for saphenous vein grafts, not only in terms of graft patency but also infarct-free survival. Three or four coronary branches are usually bypassed (Fig. 22.17). Various permutations of conduits are used. These include left and right mammary arteries and other arterial grafts such as the free radial artery (or occasionally the pedicled gastroepiploic artery). Veins still remain the most commonly used conduit, especially long saphenous vein, although short saphenous and cephalic veins can also be used. Endarterectomy is avoided by most surgeons because the risk of perioperative myocardial infarction is increased, but it may be the only means of access in a totally blocked system, most commonly the right coronary artery. The vessel is then grafted at this site, but patency at 1 year is worse than that for grafts anastomosed directly to a more normal segment of the vessel.

REFERENCES

42. Henderson RA, Pocock SJ, Sharp SJ et al. Lancet 1998; 352: 1419–1425
43. Cooperative Study. N Engl J Med 1977; 297: 621–627
44. European Coronary Surgery Study Group. Lancet 1982; 2: 1173–1180
45. Gersh BJ, Kronmal RA, Schaff H et al. N Engl J Med 1985; 313: 217–224
46. Scottish Intercollegiate Guidelines Network. Coronary Revascularisation in the Management of Stable Angina Pectoris: A National Clinical Guideline. SIGN publication no. 32. Available: http://www.sign.ac.uk/pdf/sign32.pdf
47. Eagle KA, Guyton RA, Davidoff R et al. J Am Coll Cardiol 1999; 34: 1262–1347

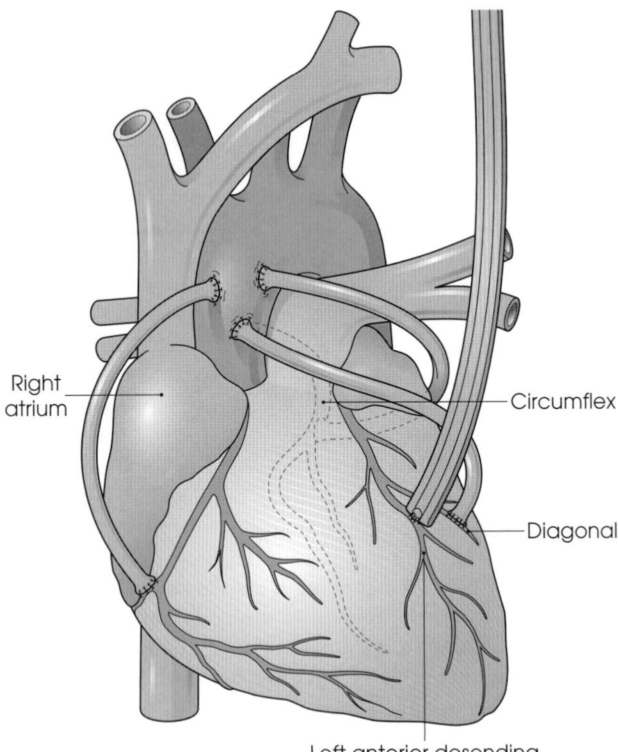

Figure 22.17 A typical coronary operation with a left internal mammary artery anastomosed to the anterior descending coronary artery and aortocoronary vein grafts to three other branches.

The right internal mammary artery has become popular over the past few years as increasing evidence mounts that at 15 years the number of patients with recurrent angina is significantly reduced. The radial artery is also becoming more popular because it has been demonstrated to have better patency than that for saphenous vein. These studies, however, have only medium-term follow-up.[48]

Results of operation

The operative (30-day or in-hospital) mortality rate is 1.5–2.5% for national figures and large multicentre trials. The risk is increased in patients over 70 years of age, in women, in patients with a greater number of grafts (representing more extensive disease), in those with poor left ventricular function, and in individuals with coexistent disease. In men having elective surgery the true risk can be under 1%. The morbidity includes a small risk of major stroke (0.5–1%) and a larger risk of transient focal neurological deficit, probably embolic in origin (2–4%). A considerable proportion of patients undergoing cardiopulmonary bypass have transient neuropsychological impairment, which is usually subclinical but can be detected with sensitive tests.[7] Significant wound infection complicates 2–3% of operations.[46]

The majority of patients have complete relief of angina, but 10–15% have some residual symptoms and a small minority are no better. Failure to relieve angina is associated with failure to bypass all diseased vessels or early graft occlusion. Most patients leave hospital 5–8 days after surgery, but convalescence can take several weeks.

The 1-year patency rate for vein grafts is about 80–90%, with an attrition rate of 3–4% per year thereafter; a similar proportion of patients develop recurrent angina, either from graft occlusion or progression of disease in native vessels. There is evidence that treatment to reduce platelet adherence may improve graft patency. This is usually achieved with low-dose aspirin, although the addition of the newer agent clopidogrel is becoming popular.

Further surgery can be undertaken if symptoms redevelop. Angioplasty (either native vessel or to the bypass conduit) is of great benefit in these circumstances and can often delay the need for further surgical intervention. Although a second sternotomy is associated with a small increase in surgical mortality, often the greater challenge is to dissect and mobilize the heart that has a patent left internal mammary artery graft. Venous grafts are easy to identify, but the pedicled left internal mammary artery is delicate and easily damaged or transected. If trauma occurs early during the procedure, then the heart can become ischaemic, and it may be some time before bypass can be established and the ischaemic area regrafted.

Surgery for the complications of myocardial infarction

By the time a patient presents with an evolving infarction, the area of myocardium beyond the blocked coronary is usually beyond surgical salvage. Immediate thrombolysis (within 3 h) minimizes myocardial damage. Surgery rarely has a useful part to play. Various angioplasty techniques may be applicable in certain cases, although, as with surgery, it is the time to get to this specialized form of treatment that determines how generally applicable it is.

In the days that follow infarction about 3% of patients, often in the group who are doing well, suddenly deteriorate because the infarcted muscle ruptures. The rupture follows one of three characteristic patterns. Rupture of the free wall of the left ventricle results in sudden death with cardiac tamponade. Rupture of the ventricular septum results in a left to right shunt, which if severe (resulting in a pulmonary to systemic flow ratio of over 2:1) is poorly tolerated. The third pattern is the rapid onset of severe mitral regurgitation caused by papillary muscle necrosis. The last two are amenable to surgical correction.

The diagnosis should be suspected in a patient who collapses suddenly with poor cardiac output and develops pulmonary oedema about 3–6 days after a myocardial infarction. Swan–Ganz pulmonary artery catheterization at the bedside is the most valuable approach to the problem, because a step up in saturation will confirm a shunt while the pressure tracing from the pulmonary artery wedge may support the diagnosis of torrential mitral regurgitation. Few patients survive either of these complications without urgent surgery. Echocardiography can delineate the pathology and, if there is a breach in the ventricular septum, estimate pulmonary artery pressures and assess the size of the shunt.

Surgical management of acute myocardial rupture

Investigation and resuscitation must be undertaken urgently and in parallel. At the same time, plans to operate on the patient must be initiated. The information gained from Swan–Ganz catheterization is a valuable first step, but most surgeons prefer to have more information about the number and site of coronary obstructions, the state of the left ventricle, and as much certainty

REFERENCE

48. Loop FD, Lytle BW, Cosgrove DM et al. Cleve Clin J Med 1988; 55: 23–34

as possible about the site and exact nature of the rupture. Modern two-dimensional echo techniques, particularly with the use of intracardiac Doppler flow studies, provide much of the anatomical and haemodynamic information required, but only formal cardiac catheterization provides information about the coronary arteries. A quick, definitive operation may be the only hope of survival, so the surgeon must have as precise a diagnosis and operative plan as possible before embarking on surgery. During cardiac catheterization, it may be useful to place an intra-aortic balloon pump (see Fig. 22.21) to help support the circulation while the patient is being transferred to the operating theatre.

Mitral valve replacement under these circumstances is made a little more difficult by the small, as yet undilated, atrium and the delicate nature of the annulus in an essentially normal valve, but it is otherwise a standard procedure. The operation of repair of ventricular septal rupture is obvious in principle but can be very difficult in practice. The necrotic tissues take sutures extremely badly, and patches must be secured with Teflon® felt buttresses so that they will not tear out, but this must be done without sacrificing functioning myocardium (Fig. 22.19).

Left ventricular aneurysm

In patients who survive a large full-thickness myocardial infarction, the left ventricular scar may begin to stretch and become aneurysmal. This area contributes nothing to ejection, and left ventricular work is wasted in the process. It may therefore be a reversible cause of heart failure. Left ventricular aneurysm may also be a source of embolism and of life-endangering ventricular arrhythmia. Left ventricular aneurysm may present in any of these three ways but the history is often non-specific. Clinical signs are described but are unhelpful. The ECG characteristically has Q waves in the anterior chest leads, absent R waves, and an elevated S–T segment. Echocardiography is a good method of demonstrating left ventricular aneurysms, but angiography is essential to define the coronary anatomy. The ideal case has a large anteroapical aneurysm occurring as a result of proximal left anterior descending coronary artery occlusion, with good functioning muscle elsewhere. Inferior and lateral aneurysms are much less common. Paradoxical filling of the aneurysm during systole can be demonstrated angiographically or by nuclear techniques.

The patients must be carefully selected, because not all will benefit from surgery and the risks are relatively high; a mortality of around 10% is probably still a reasonable figure to quote. Although the ideal case has single-vessel disease, the majority of patients considered for surgery have disease in other vessels. Where these have been grafted at the time of aneurysm resection the mortality is lower in those expected to be at greater risk, which supports this policy.

Operation for resection of left ventricular aneurysm

The aneurysm is resected, leaving a margin of tough scar tissue to take sutures. With careful attention to restoration of the left ventricular architecture this can be a very satisfactory operation, but it requires some judgement (Fig. 22.18). The defect can be closed directly or, if this would reduce ventricular size too much, a Dacron patch closure may be undertaken.

Intra-aortic balloon counterpulsation

The intra-aortic balloon pump is a valuable means of supporting the failing heart. A cylindrical balloon is mounted on the end of

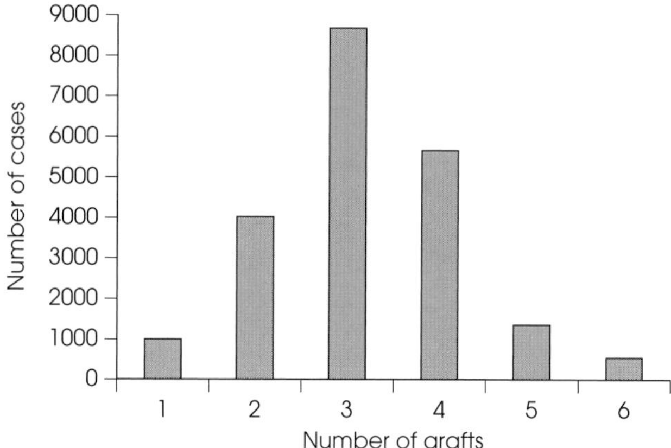

Figure 22.18 (a) Left ventricular aneurysm due to stretching of a full-thickness scar in a survivor of myocardial infarction due to left anterior descending occlusion. (b) Resection and repair of the ventricular aneurysm.

a catheter, through which it can be inflated and deflated abruptly with a low-viscosity gas such as helium. The balloon is inserted via the femoral artery and is located in the descending aorta. The external pump is triggered from the patient's ECG, so that it inflates during diastole and deflates at the onset of systole. It does not generate any cardiac output, but during diastole it displaces its own volume of blood into peripheral vessels and also enhances coronary blood flow (as the myocardium relaxes in diastole and coronary flow is greatest). It also permits the left ventricle to eject against a lowered peripheral vascular resistance because it relaxes abruptly at the onset of systole (it reduces afterload). It should be used only if there is a realistic prospect of the patient's condition improving or of it being improved by surgery. This is the case when septal or papillary muscle rupture occurs after myocardial infarction.

MYXOMA

Primary cardiac tumours are very uncommon, and myxoma is the only one that appears with sufficient frequency to merit discussion in a general clinical textbook. This is a fascinating condition that can manifest itself in a variety of ways and can lead to great diagnostic confusion. Whenever it is considered, echocardiography should be performed and is diagnostic. About 50 cases per annum are operated on in the UK.[1]

PATHOLOGY[49]

In 80% of cases the myxoma is in the left atrium, in 15% it is in the right atrium, and the remainder are ventricular or multiple. Myxomas vary in morphology but usually arise from the atrial septum on a short pedicle. Sometimes they are relatively solid and present late as they begin to obstruct the mitral valve. Others are friable, with a sago pudding appearance, and in this form are particularly likely to present with stroke or other embolic arterial occlusion.

The old debate about whether these are true primary tumours or some form of organizing thrombus can now be

REFERENCE

49. Hasleton PS, Leonard JC. Q J Med 1979; 48: 63–76

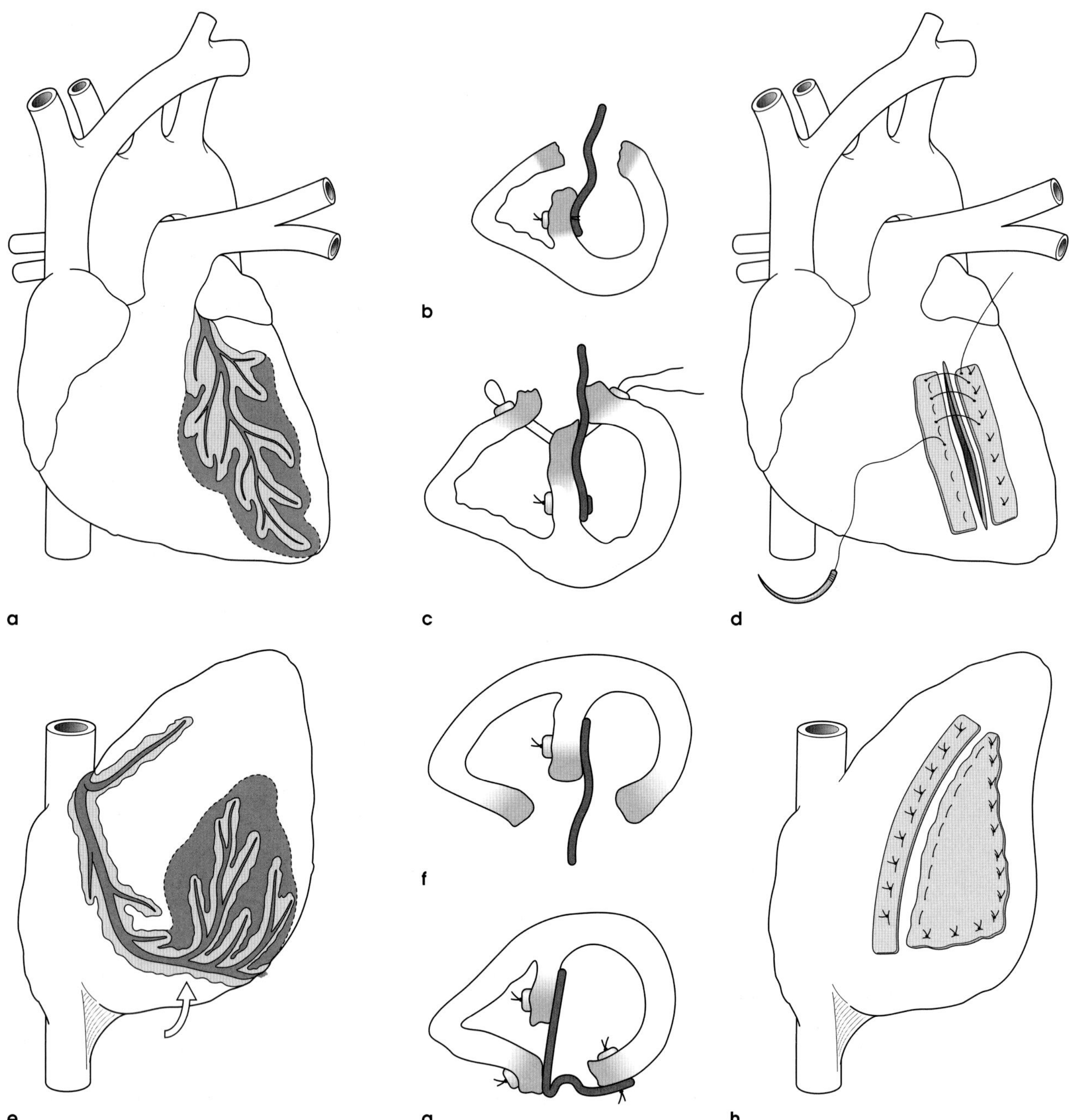

Figure 22.19 Surgical repair of ventricular septal rupture following acute myocardial infarction. Shading shows the affected area. (a) Occlusion of the proximal left anterior descending coronary artery in a patient with little collateral supply results in extensive infarction of the anteroapical portion of the left ventricle and the septum. (b) An incision is made through the area of infarction and a patch sutured to the left side of the septum, with exclusion or excision of infarcted tissue. (c) The patch is brought out through the ventricular incision. (d) The defect is closed with buttressed sutures. (e) Complete occlusion of the right coronary artery results in an inferior infarction. (f,g) Rupture of the posterior part of the septum is much more difficult to close but the principles are similar. (h) Closure of the left ventricle with a patch is required with inferior infarction. Infarction of right ventricle is usually associated and right ventricular function is a determinant of outcome in these cases.

forgotten. Their clinical behaviour and appearance at surgery are sufficiently characteristic for myxomas to be recognized as a discrete pathological entity. Their tendency to recur if incompletely removed and the occurrence of metastasis, albeit extremely rare, confirms that they are a form of tumour.

CLINICAL FEATURES

Myxoma can present in three quite distinct ways. As the tumour enlarges within the atrium it begins to obstruct blood flow and in the most common site, on the left side, mimics mitral stenosis. Breathlessness, orthopnoea, and paroxysmal nocturnal dyspnoea may all occur. On examination the signs tend to support a diagnosis of mitral valve disease, and although characteristic features such as variability of the murmur, postural changes, and a tumour 'plop' are described, it is a very astute clinician who even suspects the diagnosis. Aird's statement, 'Myxoma of the auricle has not been recognized during life', is no longer true but the diagnosis is still clinically elusive.

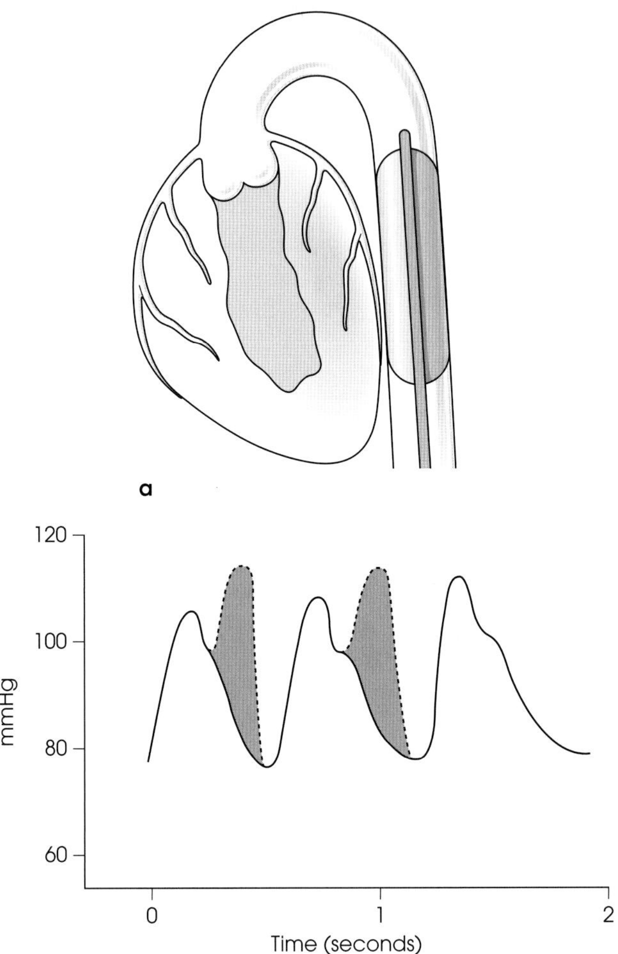

Figure 22.20 (a) The balloon positioned in the descending aorta (see text). (b) The augmentation of the pressure trace (shaded area) due to balloon inflation during diastole, beginning at aortic valve closure.

Embolism should always prompt a search for a cause; if the embolus is removed, histological examination confirms the diagnosis. Stroke is so common that it may not arouse suspicion. Finally, some cases present with rather non-specific systemic effects such as fever, high erythrocyte sedimentation rate, and plasma protein abnormalities, and it may be a long time before the diagnosis is reached. Whichever way the patient presents, if the possibility of a cardiac cause is considered, an echocardiogram makes the diagnosis with ease and certainty (Fig. 22.21).

MANAGEMENT

These tumours are removed as a matter of urgency because there is an ever-present risk of embolism or acute obstruction within the heart. Only about 50 operations per year are recorded for this condition in the UK Cardiac Surgical Register,[1] and although it is a rare condition, it is likely that many more are missed. Operation should include complete excision of the attachment and careful removal of all fragments from the heart.

AORTIC DISSECTION

Dissection is the most common aortic emergency. The patient has little chance of surviving the acute event without surgical repair of the dissection if the ascending aorta is involved in the process. The real incidence of dissection is difficult to ascertain because many cases are diagnosed as myocardial infarction, and the true diagnosis may never be made. Thoracic aortic dissection is two to three times more common than rupture of an abdominal aneurysm, and occurs at a rate of 5–10 per million of the population per year. It presents as an emergency under various guises and may be seen on medical or surgical take.

The condition is rare before the age of 40, and most cases occur between 50 and 70 years of age. Men and women are about equally affected. Hypertension is an important aetiological factor. In Marfan's syndrome there is a propensity for aortic dissection as a consequence of a generalized abnormality in elastic tissue,[50] and it is one of the conditions that produce a histological appearance known rather imprecisely as cystic medial necrosis. Aneurysmal dilatation of the proximal aorta is characteristic and may be seen without the other features. Both pregnancy and a bicuspid aortic valve predispose to aortic dissection, but considering the prevalence of these conditions the association is a weak one.

PATHOLOGY[49,51]

In aortic dissection the intima of the aorta suddenly gives way, producing a transverse tear. Blood then enters the media, tracks longitudinally in the aortic wall, and splits it along a plane of cleavage in the outer part of the media spiralling distally. There is some evidence that an intramural haematoma is the first event and that the tear is secondary.[52] The intimal tear usually extends for half to two-thirds of the aortic circumference. The commonest sites are, in order of frequency:

1. 2–3 cm beyond the aortic valve, the majority, about 65%;
2. the uppermost part of the descending aorta just beyond the origin of the left subclavian—about a quarter occur here; and
3. in the aortic arch itself for the remainder.

The longitudinal component, or dissection, which usually involves half to two-thirds of the aortic circumference, may extend antegradely and retrogradely for a variable distance. Retrograde extension is usually right back to the aortic valve, while antegrade dissection may extend along branches and beyond the aortic bifurcation with or without a re-entry tear. The dissection may obstruct the coronary arteries (particularly the right) or the arch vessels, or it may impair the blood supply to the spinal cord, kidneys or intestine, producing appropriate clinical syndromes.

Aortic dissections are best classified according to their anatomical extent (Fig. 22.22). The diagnostic watershed depends on whether the ascending aorta is involved. If it is, the dissection is of type A irrespective of the site of the tear, which is most commonly in the ascending aorta. If the dissecting process is confined to the descending aorta it is type B. This has largely replaced the time-honoured DeBakey classification (Fig. 22.22). Dissections are further classified as acute or chronic depending on the interval from occurrence to diagnosis, arbitrarily placed at 2 weeks.

REFERENCES

50. Possati G, Gaudino M, Prati F et al. Circulation 2003; 108: 1350–1354
51. Treasure T. Br Heart J 1993; 69: 101–103
52. De Sanctis RW, Doroghazi RM, Austen WG et al. N Engl J Med 1987; 317: 1060–1067

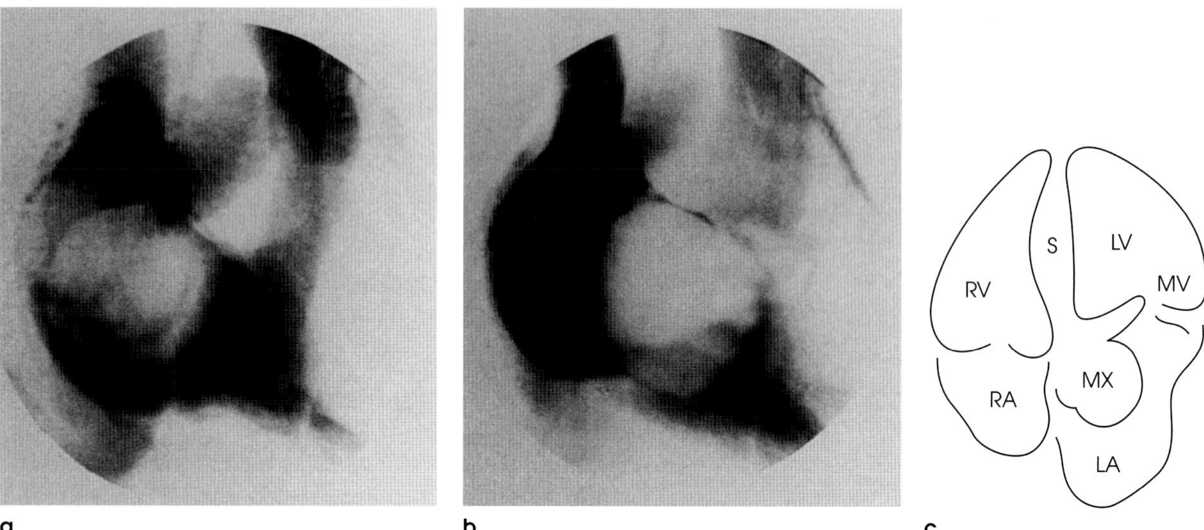

Figure 22.21 Atrial myxoma. Digital subtraction angiogram of a myxoma seen as a white filling defect surrounded by contrast medium (black), which in this uncommon example is in the right atrium (**a**). With atrial systole it prolapses into the ventricle (**b**), seeming to fill the orifice completely. (**c**) Apical four-chamber view of the heart with two-dimensional echocardiography. The four chambers are labelled. RV and LV are the right and left ventricles, respectively, and the septum (S) is easily seen between them. LA and RA are the left and right atria, respectively. The mitral valve (MV) is well seen and the myxoma (MX) is in the most common site, attached to the atrial septum.

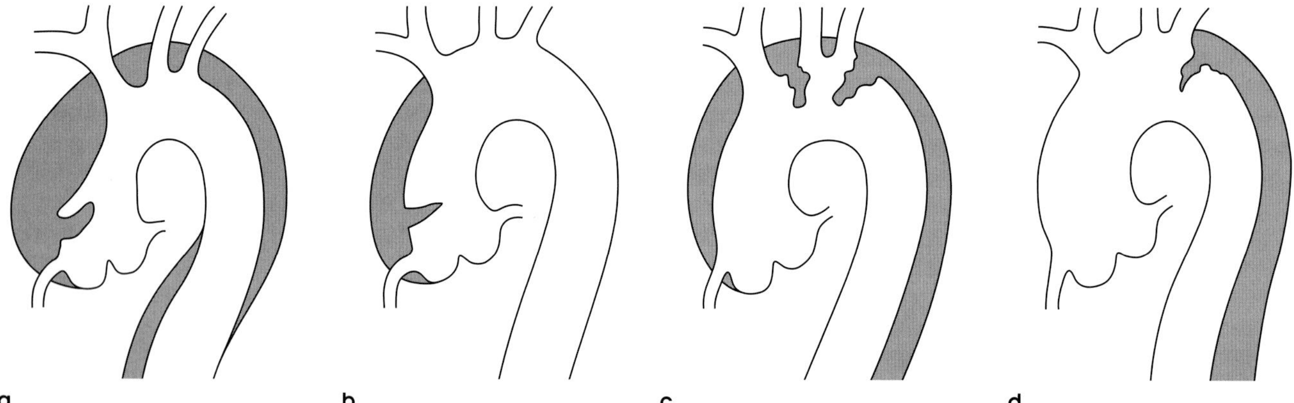

Figure 22.22 (**a**) The commonest pattern of aortic dissection, with a tear in the ascending aorta and dissection extending retrogradely to the aortic valve and antegradely into the descending aorta (type I in DeBakey's classification). (**b**) Sometimes the dissection stops short of the arch (type II in DeBakey's classification). (**c**) Some cases with extensive dissection have a tear in the arch or multiple tears; these do not fall easily into DeBakey's classification. (**d**) The second most common site for the tear is just beyond the left subclavian artery, and then the tear may be confined to the descending aorta (type III DeBakey). In a simpler classification, all cases where the ascending aorta is involved in dissection (irrespective of the site of the tear) are called type A (i.e. a, b and c); these have a very high mortality rate without surgery. Dissection confined to the descending aorta, type B (d), may be managed conservatively in selected cases.

The restraining adventitia may rupture at any time. In the case of type A dissections, rupture occurs within the pericardium and tamponade results. This is the cause of death in most cases. Any of the aortic branches may be occluded as a result of the dissection. In type A the right coronary artery is particularly vulnerable, and the association of a dissection with ECG changes of inferior myocardial infarction may add to the diagnostic difficulty. Stroke may occur if the arch vessels are involved, and paraplegia may result from interference to the arterial supply to the cord via the anterior spinal artery. Less commonly, acute renal failure or intestinal infarction may follow occlusion of visceral arteries (see Ch. 10), and iliac occlusion may produce ischaemia of the lower limbs (see Ch. 10). Retrograde dissection to the aortic root can result in aortic valve regurgitation. This is a very typical and almost diagnostic feature of type A dissection.

The natural history in type A dissection is poor, with 40% of patients dying within 24 h and 90% dead in 2 weeks.

PRESENTATION AND DIAGNOSIS

The usual presentation is with chest pain of very sudden onset, tearing in quality and going through to the back. Collapse is common; the patient may lose consciousness and is often pale, clammy and pulseless. In those who survive to reach hospital, and in whom the diagnosis is suspected, a careful history should be taken of any transient neurological deficit, either cerebral or spinal. Any information about the arterial pressure before the event should be carefully documented.

Examination

Documentation of the pulses is of particular importance because missing and varying pulses lend great weight to the diagnosis of dissection. The blood pressure should be checked in both arms and may well be significantly different. The patients are frequently hypertensive on presentation; the presence of hypotension with aortic dissection is a poor sign. Listen specifically for the soft, early diastolic murmur of aortic regurgitation, which is easily overlooked but may clinch the diagnosis. The findings on neurological examination should be recorded: an evolving stroke is a contraindication to surgery.

INVESTIGATION: RADIOLOGY AND ECHOCARDIOGRAPHY

The majority of patients with an aortic dissection present as emergencies to local general hospitals. The plain chest radiograph shows widening of the mediastinum and relative inward displacement of the crescent-shaped streak of calcification, which marks the atheromatous intima of the aorta in many cases.

The appropriate confirmatory investigations depend to a large extent on where the patient presents. In peripheral hospitals a CT scan with contrast enhancement is often the most effective test. A transverse flap is usually seen lying across the aorta, and there may be different opacification of each lumen. It is often possible to see the flap extending into the origins of the arch branches, and the spiral nature of the tear can be visualized. The tear frequently extends into the abdomen, where each renal artery may arise from a different lumen. It is important to look for contrast enhancement of the kidneys. Because surgical repair requires cannulation of one common femoral artery, the distal extent of the dissection, including whether either or both femoral arteries are involved, should be ascertained. One of the weaknesses of CT scanning is that the patient has to be left unmonitored in the scanner for a significant period of time; the scan time should be kept to a minimum and all patients should be given oxygen therapy. Medical treatment should be instigated before the scan is undertaken if the suspicion of acute dissection is high.

Echocardiography, if available, has much to offer in assessing aortic dissection. Transthoracic echocardiography is non-invasive and gives useful information. Transoesophageal echocardiography provides better images of the ascending and descending aorta. Sedation is required for this investigation, so its value is often intraoperative. Views of the aortic arch are not always clear. Although the dissection flap may not be seen, the presence and degree of aortic regurgitation can be measured. In addition, several other features can be assessed (Box 22.2).[53]

Hypotensive management should be initiated once the diagnosis is suspected. The aim of this therapy is not only to reduce overall blood pressure but also to reduce the shear stresses on the aortic wall. A β-blocker is usually first-line treatment; this reduces both blood pressure and the force of contraction of the ventricle, thus reducing the shear stress. A labetalol infusion (which also has α properties) is usually very effective. If the heart rate drops below 70 beats per minute and the patient remains hypertensive, vasodilating agents can be added. Used in isolation, vasodilators may reduce blood pressure but paradoxically increase shear stress. Sodium nitroprusside should be given by intravenous infusion and titrated against the arterial pressure (ideally this is measured by an intra-arterial cannula).

Steps should be made to transfer the patient for specialist assessment, and although this means transfer to a specialist surgical centre, all patients require intensive medical management initially.

Box 22.2 Features assessed by echocardiography

- Presence of the dissection flap
- Presence of pericardial blood
- Assessment of aortic regurgitation
- Assessment of the degree of left ventricular hypertrophy
- Assessment of regional wall motion (myocardial infarction or RCA involvement)

SURGERY

The demonstration of dissection involving the ascending aorta (type A) is now generally accepted as sufficient indication to operate, because of the otherwise poor outcome if it is left untreated.[54] Operation is contraindicated if there is an established or evolving stroke, or if there is clear evidence of gut infarction (see Ch. 27). Patients should have surgery if they have an initial stroke that has fully resolved by the time that they reach the surgical centre. Relative contraindications to surgery include anuria (because of renal vascular involvement) and paraplegia (from anterior spinal artery involvement), and of course extreme old age and the existence of intercurrent illness are arguments against surgery.

Dissections confined to the descending aorta (type B) are managed conservatively from choice. The exception is a type B dissection with retrograde extension of the process to involve the ascending aorta, by definition converting it to a type A dissection. The medical mortality is significant, but the operative mortality in uncomplicated cases is prohibitively high (*c.*35%). Surgery is reserved for life-endangering progression of the dissection process, as indicated by continued pain, enlargement of the sac, or closure of distal vessels.

Surgical treatment of type A dissections

Bypass is established with a femoral arterial cannula. The patient is cooled on bypass to 15°C. Circulatory arrest is used to avoid clamping a fragile aorta. Distally the layers of the aorta are reconstituted, often with Teflon® felt support. A tube graft is then inserted, the arch deaired and the graft clamped. Every effort is made to conserve the aortic valve, which often requires resuspension of the valve commissures. The valve itself is not damaged by the dissection process but the commissural supports are dissected; their placement back into the original position with a single mattress suture is often enough to restore valve integrity. The tube graft is then inserted into the reconstituted sinotubular junction. When there is dilatation of the aortic root itself, as occurs in Marfan's syndrome, the aortic root and the valve must be replaced and the coronary arteries reimplanted (Fig. 22.23).

Results

The hospital mortality for medically managed type A dissections is over 90%, while the UK Cardiac Surgical Register reports a

REFERENCE

53. Davies MJ, Treasure T, Richardson PD. Heart 1996; 75: 434–435

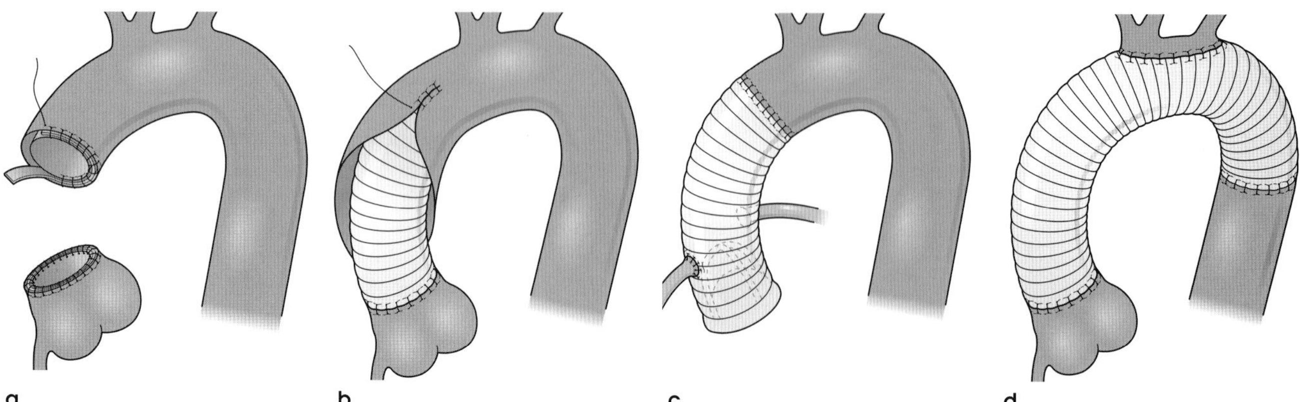

Figure 22.23 Operations for aortic dissection. The operative approach ranges from transection and repair (**a**), through tube graft replacement (**b**) and replacement of aortic root and aortic valve (**c**), to total aortic arch replacement (**d**), depending on the extent of the pathology and the judgement and skill of the surgeon.

mortality of about 25% for operated cases in recent years. There is little doubt that this group of patients stands the best chance of survival if the diagnosis is made promptly and they are referred for urgent surgery.[54]

TRAUMA TO THE HEART AND GREAT VESSELS

The assessment of the multiply injured patient should take into account the pattern of the injury and all the systems that may be involved, whether these are a consequence of the primary injury or as a result of blood loss, hypotension, hypoxia or sepsis. Care of the patient cannot follow a leisurely sequence of assessment, investigation and treatment with each phase completed before the next is embarked on, and the principles of Advanced Trauma Life Support® are widely known and practised. As minutes, then hours and eventually days go by, the team has to reassess priorities, and it is against this background that injury to a particular organ or system should be considered.

BLUNT TRAUMA

In something as apparently random as a motor accident the possible combinations of injuries may seem infinite, and yet there are patterns that occur with sufficient frequency to be recognized. The three cardiothoracic injuries that may confront the trauma team are rupture of the aorta, myocardial contusion, and rupture of cardiac valves.

Rupture of the aorta

In patients who have died after deceleration accidents such as aeroplane crashes or motor vehicle collisions, rupture of the aorta is a common finding.[55] In those who reach hospital alive, the most common site for the tear is in the uppermost part of the descending aorta, just beyond the left subclavian artery, with the aortic adventitia and mediastinal pleura containing the rupture (Fig. 22.24). The likely explanation for the rather constant site of this lesion is that the heart, with the ascending aorta and the arch, swing forwards as the body is brought to an abrupt halt by the impact. The descending aorta, with its pairs of intercostal branches, is a more fixed structure, tethered to the vertebral column, and the tear occurs at the junction of the fixed and mobile portions of the aorta.

The relevant features on examination are absent or weak femoral pulses or unequal blood pressure in the arms. A chest radiograph is usually taken supine under these circumstances, and it is of very little help in making the diagnosis because it always enlarges the mediastinal shadow compared with a postero-anterior view. Fluid in the left chest is also missed or under-estimated. If at all possible, an upright chest radiograph taken under careful supervision greatly helps in diagnosis. Imaging by aortography, digital subtraction angiography or CT confirms the diagnosis in most cases but there may be false negative results, especially with lack of experience in the investigation or its interpretation.

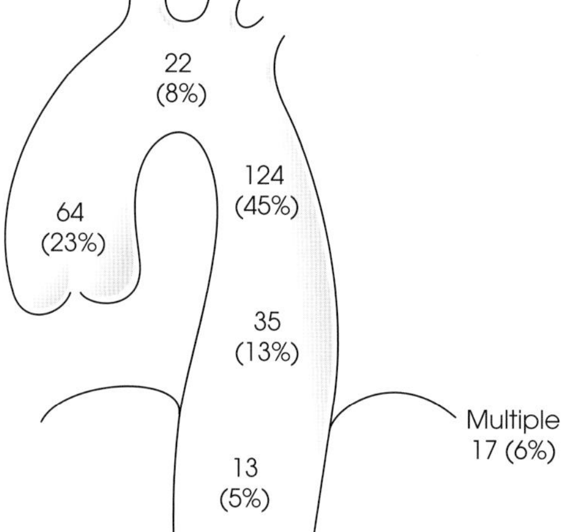

Figure 22.24 The frequency with which various parts of the aorta are involved in traumatic rupture (data from Parmley[56]).

Once the suspicion has been raised, the problem may be an extremely difficult one. The condition is likely to prove fatal and requires emergency surgery, yet the process of investigation and transfer to a cardiothoracic unit has its own hazards. An unnecessary journey for investigation may not be in the best interests of a multiply injured patient, but attempts at local look and see surgery are unlikely to have a good outcome. The best policy is to discuss the case with members of the cardiothoracic unit by telephone so as to plan the logistics of investigation and surgery in the light of the available facilities. The patient who has survived the first few hours has a good chance of surviving long

REFERENCES

54. Treasure T, Raphael MJ. Lancet 1991; 338: 490–495
55. Erbel R, Alfonson F, Boileau O et al. Eur Heart J 2001; 22: 1642–1681
56. Parmley LF. Circulation 1958; 17: 1086

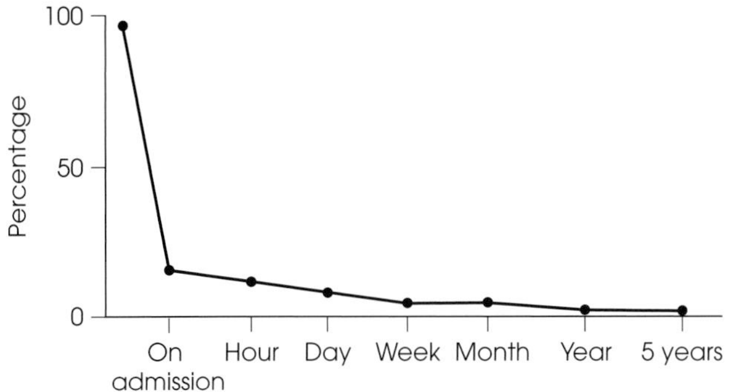

Figure 22.25 Survival after traumatic aortic rupture (see text).

enough to get to expert help, having reached a flatter part of the survival curve (Fig. 22.25). Some patients contain the injury and survive for years, when a calcified false aneurysm is found.

Surgery is performed through a left thoracotomy. The mediastinum is featureless because of a spreading haematoma, and the first manoeuvre is to attempt to cross-clamp the aorta, ideally between the left carotid and the left subclavian artery, without entering the haematoma. This may be very difficult. When the haematoma is large, it may be necessary to open the pericardium and approach the tear by dissecting around the arch. Direct suture may be possible but an interposition graft is placed if this is not possible.

The spinal cord is particularly vulnerable to ischaemic injury. Supportive left heart bypass (perfusing the lower body via the femoral artery with drainage via the left atrial appendage) gives the best chance of avoiding damage, but if the patient has other injuries full heparinization may be contraindicated. Whatever technique is employed, it is important to move the proximal cross-clamp from the native aorta proximal to the left subclavian artery down on to the graft as soon as possible. This improves distal perfusion via subscapular and internal mammary artery collaterals.

Increasingly, intravascular stenting is being used in this setting. The procedure is performed by a surgeon and a radiologist with access via the femoral artery. At present the place of stenting in general is evolving and limited to only a few centres, but its use is becoming increasingly widespread in aneurysms and dissections of the descending aorta.

Blunt cardiac injury

The heart may be compressed between the sternum and the vertebral column. Severe force may rupture the right ventricle, the septum, or the atrioventricular valves. After a complete rupture the patient is likely to die with tamponade before reaching hospital, but there are three patterns that are worth recognizing, as described below.

Myocardial contusion

When the myocardium is contused but remains intact, the consequences are similar to those of myocardial infarction. Changes in ECG are common, with classical Q waves or more usually a generalized S–T segment abnormality. Cardiac enzymes are elevated, but their interpretation is difficult in the presence of other muscle injury. The course is similar to that for myocardial infarction and depends on the area of damage.

When the injury is full thickness it may rupture at some later stage. Direct rupture into the pericardium is likely to be fatal, but if the injury has become contained by pericardial adhesions, or if rupture is delayed, a false aneurysm results that can be assessed and dealt with electively.

Ruptured valves

Rupture of the atrioventricular valves (tricuspid more often than mitral) is likely to occur at the time of the injury. The clinical signs are those of acute valvular regurgitation for any other reason but may well prove difficult to sort out in a multiply injured patient!

SHARP TRAUMA

The management of stab wounds of the heart is a challenge for the emergency surgeon; if the patient arrives alive with a stab wound it should be technically possible to repair the damage.

The history is of interest but is often unavailable or at best incomplete. The site of the wound is important because some thought as to the structures that might have been reached from that entry wound indicates the need for surgery and the site of the incision. Clinical examination and repeated assessment of the state of the patient are vital. If the cardiac output is adequate to maintain consciousness and there is a palpable pulse, an ill-judged exploration may upset a delicate balance. There is nothing to be lost by performing a thoracotomy in the emergency department if the patient is pulseless and apparently dead, but this is very rarely successful.

The two factors that require consideration are as follow.

1. Is the patient at risk from continuing haemorrhage? In this case, in addition to pallor, tachycardia, a weak pulse and arterial hypotension, the veins are empty.
2. Is there cardiac tamponade? In this case the neck veins are engorged and the volume of blood lost may be small.

The clinical distinction between the two is usually dramatic: the aspiration of as little as 50 mL of blood from the pericardium in a case of acute tamponade usually improves cardiac filling and thus cardiac output. The bleeding may be at a low pressure if it is atrial and a temporarily stable equilibrium may be reached. Ventricular bleeding may stop for a while. In the marginal case, where the cardiac output is good and there is debate about the need for emergency surgery, it is wisest to allow a cardiothoracic surgeon to supervise if possible.

SURGICAL MANAGEMENT

The first decision is whether or not to insert a drain. If there is haemopneumothorax an intercostal drain should be inserted, and this may be essential if there is tension. It is best to insert the drain laterally. When there is a major cardiac or vascular injury, the drain will permit copious bleeding, and if the situation was previously balanced because atrial, pulmonary or right ventricular haemorrhage was limited by a rise in intrathoracic pressure, it may quickly spiral out of control and require urgent surgery. Suction should not be used under these circumstances because it may lead to rapid exsanguination, and there may even be circumstances when the drain should be clamped while the chest is rapidly opened to control haemorrhage. This is occasionally justifiable on the grounds that a brief period of tamponade, which is then relieved, may be preferable to exsanguination.

A cardiac surgeon would prefer a median sternotomy for speed and access, but the equipment and expertise to make this incision are not always available. Those who have had even minimal exposure to cardiothoracic surgery will appreciate this incision, which can be made in an emergency using a Gigli saw. The usual emergency incision is a left anterior thoracotomy through which reasonable access can be obtained and that can be made with the patient supine or, more easily, with the chest tilted with sandbags bringing the left side up. The fifth interspace is identified by counting the ribs down from the manubriosternal angle. The skin incision is made in the line of the interspace, usually in the submammary fold, and extending laterally in a gentle curve that passes 2–3 cm below the angle of the scapula. The anterior part of latissimus dorsi should be divided to give the generous access required under emergency conditions. The serratus anterior can be split along the length of its fibres. The periosteum is incised with diathermy along the upper border of the sixth rib, and stripped off with a periosteal elevator as far back as possible. The ribs are spread with some form of geared or ratchet retractor, and the pericardium is incised longitudinally from the apex upwards, 2 cm in front of and parallel to the phrenic nerve.

The left ventricle with its thick walls can be controlled with 3/0 atraumatic sutures. It is important to place the sutures quite deeply into the muscle to avoid picking up only the epicardial fat, which will not control the bleeding. A buttress may be necessary to achieve haemostasis in the thinner-walled right ventricle, but it is wise to avoid foreign material and pledgets constructed from the local pericardium are preferred. The atria can be sutured directly, or controlled with a side-biting clamp to allow more time. Haemorrhage from coronary arteries is a particular problem. Small branches, well away from the interventricular and atrioventricular grooves, can be over-sewn if necessary but it is usually possible to control the haemorrhage by taking delicate bites of epicardium on either side of the vessel with 4/0 sutures, stopping the bleeding without occluding the artery.

When all the bleeding has been controlled, leaving a large hole, the pericardium can be left open, but widely, so that the heart cannot be strangulated if it prolapses. This is most unlikely to occur when the lungs are fully inflated. The pericardium and hemithorax should be drained. If there is any pulmonary injury, which might leak air, drainage should be with underwater seal. The ribs are approximated, and the intercostal muscle and periosteum of the fifth space sutured to the intercostal muscle below the sixth rib. The closure is completed in layers.

CARDIAC TRANSPLANTATION

Heart transplantation has become a standard and accepted surgical technique. Any discussion about indications and patient selection should begin with an awareness that it is strictly limited by an external factor: the availability of donor organs (see Ch. 8).

Donors must have adequate cardiac performance, as judged by adequate arterial pressure at low filling pressure, and good urine flow. This must be without drug support. About 300 such hearts become available for transplantation in the UK each year. The donor heart must be within about 4 hours' retrieval and journey time of the recipient hospital.

Recipients are typically very symptomatic with end-stage left ventricular failure, most commonly from ischaemia or dilated cardiomyopathy. Patients in terminal heart failure, in hospital, on support drugs or technologies, may be saved but are frequently excluded because they are often on the verge of multisystem failure, and the donor heart wastage in these cases is not justified when much better yield can be gained by offering the hearts to a chronically disabled but relatively stable outpatient pool.[57] The latter group of patients has a median survival of about a year without transplantation. Survival rates of over 90% at 1 year in these stable patients are excellent compared with relatively poor rates in patients who require mechanical support to bridge them to transplantation.

THE PERICARDIUM

Pericardial disease is encountered less frequently than it was. The two areas where the surgeon is involved in pericardial problems are cardiac tamponade and constrictive pericarditis.

Cardiac tamponade

Cardiac tamponade occurs when the intrapericardial pressure rises acutely. The usual cause is either postoperative bleeding after open heart surgery when the drains block or bleeding is excessive and trauma (commonly sharp trauma). The rise in intrapericardial pressure causes a rise in venous pressure on both sides of the heart (seen clinically as engorged neck veins). The diastolic pressures within the heart tend to equalize so that atrial pressures, diastolic ventricular pressures, and pulmonary artery diastolic pressure approximate.

In the postoperative setting there has almost always been a significant previous loss of blood, and then the drainage increases. Usually this can be picked up early with signs of hypotension, tachycardia, decreased urine output and rising filling pressures, often with restlessness as a sign of cerebral hypoperfusion.

In the setting of sharp trauma, stab wounds should be sought and urgent surgery undertaken. The incision depends on the location of the stab, but a left anterolateral thoracotomy gives enough access to decompress the pericardium. Only a relatively small amount of blood is enough to obtund the cardiac output, and the removal of 100 mL can be enough to restore the haemodynamics.

If the picture appears to be one of tamponade after a road traffic accident with a blunt injury, then a full assessment of the patient should be made before proceeding to thoracotomy. Clearly, other injuries may play a part and one must be mindful of the possibility of aortic transection. The commonest pathology to mimic tamponade is a major cardiac contusion with ensuing low cardiac output. An echocardiogram and ECG are helpful in distinguishing the two.

Constrictive pericarditis

Constrictive pericarditis is a chronic problem of variable aetiology. The main pathophysiological component of the disease is that left and right ventricular filling pressures increase with time. The problem is that the ventricles are constantly underfilled (reduced preload), despite the fact that the venous pressure may be grossly elevated, and the stroke volume falls due to the reduced ventricular compliance.

The aetiology is frequently unknown. It may have infective origins, but it is rare to see tuberculous pericarditis in the western world today. The diagnosis can be difficult to make. There may be pericardial calcification that can be seen on X-ray, but the usual investigations of echocardiography, CT scanning and MRI

REFERENCE

57. Parmley LF, Manion WC, Mattingly TW. Circulation 1958; 18: 371

imaging will demonstrate the thickened adherent pericardium. Cardiac catheterization is required to confirm that the thickened pericardium is causing constriction. The diastolic pressures in all chambers are elevated and approximate to each other. If there is doubt, then a fluid challenge of 0.5–1.0 L of saline will often confirm the diagnosis.

Surgery is performed via a median sternotomy; only occasionally is cardiopulmonary bypass required. The pericardium is incised with a blade, and the plane between the epicardium and pericardium developed. The dissection is often tedious, and great care must be taken when mobilizing the fragile atria. The pericardium is excised 1–2 cm anterior to both phrenic nerves. The heart is mobilized from the remainder of the pericardium, and often a plane can then be developed to remove most of the thickened pericardium from the pleura and particularly from the diaphragm.

Following surgery the patients are often slow to recover. They usually require high filling pressures in the short term; indeed, because of the chronic venous hypertension the circulation is often converted from having a low preload preoperatively to being overloaded postoperatively.

Breast disease

23

J. Michael Dixon, Helen Sweetland

INTRODUCTION

One in four women at some time in their lives are referred to a breast clinic. Approximately 70% of these women will present with a breast lump or lumpiness, which may be painful (Table 23.1).[1]

ASSESSMENT OF SYMPTOMS

Age is the most important predictor of diagnosis in a woman presenting with a palpable breast lump (Fig. 23.1). In a premenopausal woman benign lumps often vary in relation to the menstrual cycle, whereas patients with cancer rarely report cyclical fluctuation. Although cancer classically presents as a lump or localized nodularity, it can present as nipple discharge, nipple retraction, change in contour and even rarely as breast pain.

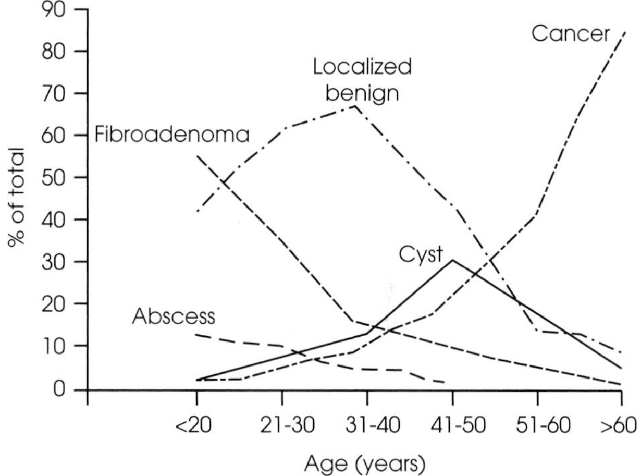

Figure 23.1 Changing frequencies of different discrete breast lumps with age.

INVESTIGATIONS

For clinical examination, the breast should be inspected in a good light with the patient with her arms by her sides, above her head and pressing on her hips. Skin dimpling or change in contour is present in over a quarter of patients with breast cancer. Skin dimpling is also seen following surgery, trauma, infection and a range of benign conditions, or it can occur as part of normal breast involution. The breast is palpated with the patient lying flat. All palpable lesions should be measured with calipers and details, including a diagram, recorded carefully in the medical notes. The regional nodal areas are then checked. Clinical examination of axillary nodes is, however, inaccurate: palpable nodes can be identified in up to 30% of patients with no clinically significant breast disease, and up to 40% of patients with histologically involved nodes have a clinically normal axilla.

Table 23.1 Prevalence of presenting symptoms in patients attending a breast clinic

Symptom	Percentage
Breast lump	56
Painful lump or lumpiness	33
Pain alone	17.5
Nipple discharge	5
Nipple retraction	3
Strong family history of breast cancer	3
Breast distortion	1
Swelling or inflammation	1
Scaling nipple (eczema)	0.5

MAMMOGRAPHY

In patients over the age of 35 presenting with breast symptoms, and in younger women with a strong clinical suspicion of malignancy, mammography is usually performed.[1] Two views are performed: oblique and craniocaudal. Mammography can detect mass lesions, areas of distortion or microcalcification, and is also used to screen for breast cancer in women between the ages of 50 and 69 years.

ULTRASONOGRAPHY

Women under the age of 35 with a lump should have ultrasound as their primary imaging investigation. Older women with a localized mass lesion visible on mammography should also have ultrasound. Cysts show up as transparent objects; benign lesions tend to have well-demarcated edges, whereas cancers usually have indistinct outlines and are hypoechoic (Fig. 23.2). In women of any age with clinically localized nodularity, ultrasound helps in the assessment of whether a localized mass lesion is present. Ultrasound is particularly useful in assessing patients with breast inflammation because it can identify and localize collections of pus. Ultrasound can be used to guide fine-needle aspiration and core biopsy (Fig. 23.3).

REFERENCE

1. Dixon JM, Mansel RE. Br Med J 1994; 309: 722–726

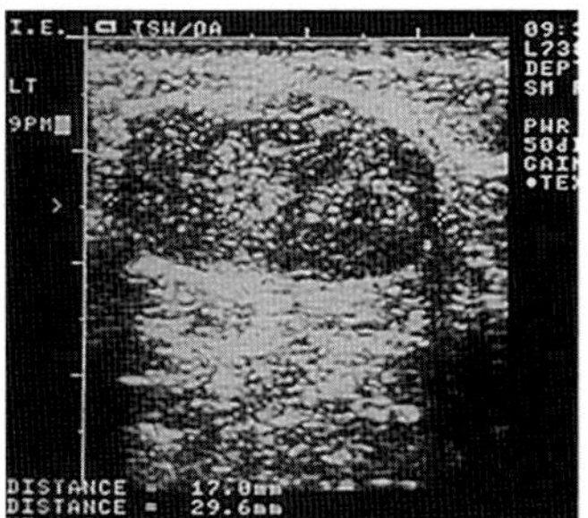

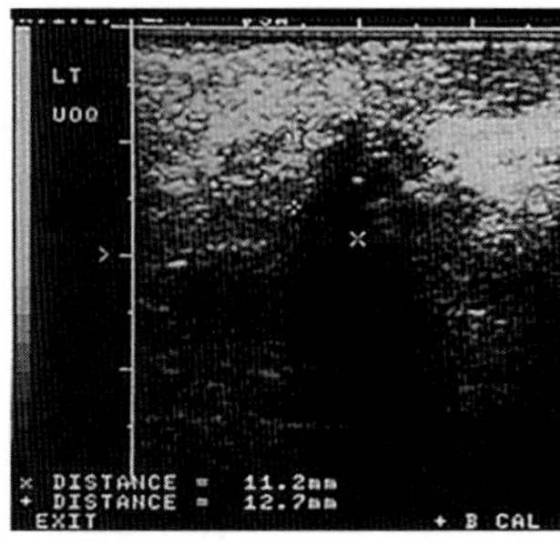

Figure 23.2 Ultrasound scan showing clear edges of fibroadenoma (left) and indistinct outline of carcinoma (right).

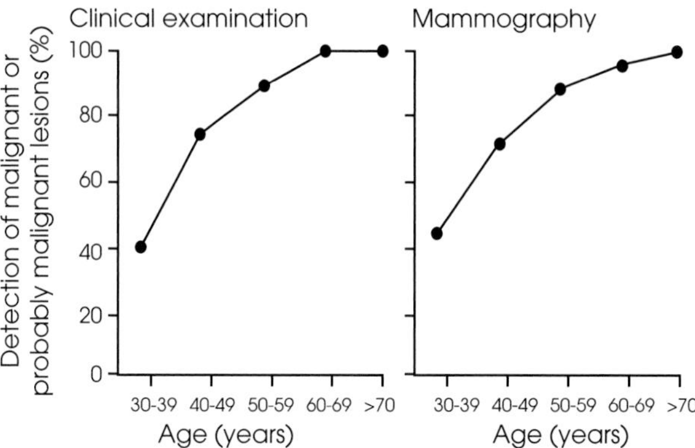

Figure 23.4 Sensitivity of clinical examination and mammography by age in patients presenting with a breast mass. (From Dixon JM, Mansel RE Symptoms, assessment and guidelines for referral. In Dixon JM, ed, ABC of Breast Diseases, 2nd edn, ch. 1, BMJ Books, London. Reprinted with permission of BMJ Books, London.)

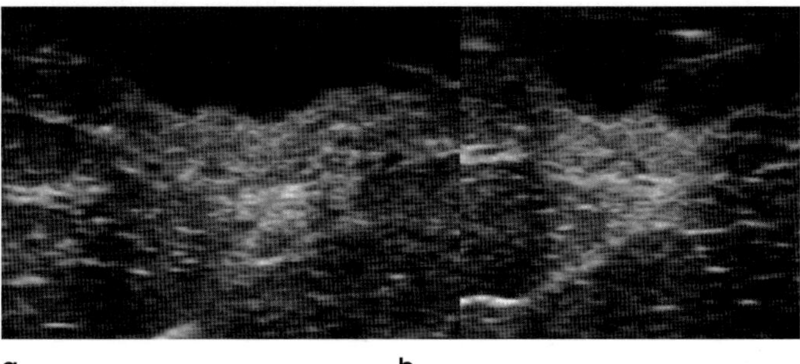

Figure 23.3 Ultrasound of a breast abscess (**a**) and a needle is seen within the abscess prior to aspiration (**b**).

MAGNETIC RESONANCE IMAGING

Magnetic resonance imaging has a high sensitivity for breast cancer. It is of particular value in assessing abnormalities in a previously treated breast, patients with metastatic carcinoma in axillary nodes where no breast primary is visible on conventional imaging, and patients with breast implants; MRI can assess any implant leakage and can assess surrounding breast tissue. It is currently being evaluated as a screening tool for high-risk women between the age of 35 and 50 years.

ASPIRATION CYTOLOGY AND CORE BIOPSY

Fine-needle aspiration cytology can differentiate between solid and cystic lesions. Aspiration of solid lesions can, with a high degree of accuracy, assess whether a lesion is benign or malignant.[2] A 23- or 21-gauge needle is attached to a syringe, the needle is introduced into the lesion and suction applied before making multiple passes through the lesion. The plunger is then released, the needle removed from the breast, and the aspirated material is spread on to microscope slides, which are then viewed by a specialist cytopathologist. In some units a report is available within 30 min.

Core biopsy has now largely replaced fine needle aspiration in the diagnosis of both palpable and impalpable mass lesions and areas of microcalcification visible mammographically. A 14-gauge needle attached to an automated mechanical gun is most commonly used. An alternative option is to remove larger samples using an 11- or 8-gauge needle with vacuum assistance, and this appears more accurate in areas of indeterminate calcification.[3]

FINE-NEEDLE ASPIRATION OR CORE BIOPSY?

These two techniques are complementary. Combining the two increases overall diagnostic accuracy compared with each investigation alone. Fine-needle aspiration cytology can be reported immediately but only core biopsy can differentiate between invasive and in situ disease.

ACCURACY OF INVESTIGATIONS

The sensitivity of clinical examination and mammography varies with age (Fig. 23.4). Only two-thirds of cancers in women aged under 50 are considered suspicious of malignancy or definitely malignant by either clinical examination or mammography.

False positive results occur with all diagnostic techniques. It is acceptable to plan treatment on the basis of a malignant (C5) cytology, providing this is supported by a diagnosis of malignancy on clinical examination and imaging. Nevertheless, if mastectomy is planned it is prudent to confirm this with a histological evidence of malignancy. Patients with cytology reported as highly suspicious of malignancy (C4) require a biopsy before planning definitive surgery. The false positive rate of cytology is approximately two per 1000. The lesions most likely to be misinterpreted are fibroadenomas and areas that have previously been irradiated. Even with core biopsy there are false positives, but these are exceedingly rare.

TRIPLE ASSESSMENT

Triple assessment is a combination of clinical examination, imaging (mammography for women aged 35 or over and ultrasonography for all women), fine-needle aspiration cytology and/or core biopsy. All discrete masses and areas of localized nodularity, even if not discrete masses, should undergo triple assessment.

ONE-STOP CLINICS

Patients attending breast clinics should have all relevant investigations at their initial clinic visit. In some centres, fine-needle aspiration cytology or cytology obtained from rolling a

REFERENCES

2. Dixon JM, Anderson TJ, Lamb J et al. Br J Surg 1984; 71: 593–596
3. Zannis V, Kristina M, Aliano R. Am J Surg 1998; 176: 525–528

core biopsy is reported immediately. One-stop diagnostic clinics reduce patient's short-term anxiety but may increase overall costs,[4] and so may be cost-effective only in centres seeing large volumes of patients.[5]

CONGENITAL ABNORMALITIES

EXTRA NIPPLES AND BREASTS

Between 1 and 5% of women have supernumerary or accessory nipples, or less frequently supernumerary or accessory breasts. The usual site for these is along the milk line, which runs from the axilla to the labia majora. Accessory breasts are most commonly located in the axilla (Fig. 23.5), and accessory nipples are most often seen on the milk line below the breast but above the umbilicus (Fig. 23.6). Accessory breasts have been reported in the groin, the labia majora, the inner side of the thigh and the buttock. Extra breasts and nipples rarely require treatment unless they are unsightly. They are subject to the same diseases as normal breasts and nipples.

ABSENCE OR HYPOPLASIA OF THE BREAST

One breast can be absent or hypoplastic, usually in association with defects in the pectoral muscles.[6] Some degree of breast asymmetry is the norm; the left breast is more commonly larger than the right. Significant breast asymmetry can be treated by augmentation of the smaller breast, reduction or elevation of the larger breast, or a combination of the two procedures.

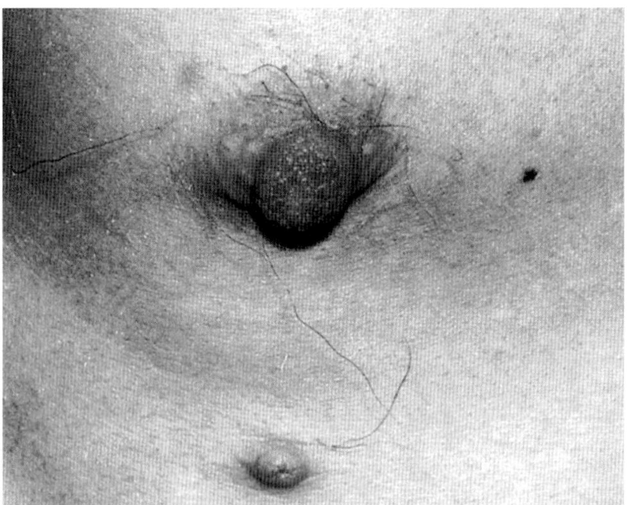

Figure 23.5 Supernumerary or accessory nipple.

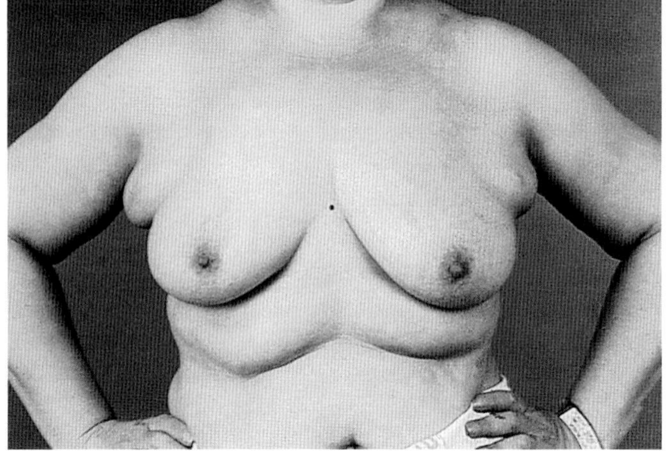

Figure 23.6 Bilateral accessory breasts.

ABSENCE OF A BREAST AND CHEST WALL ABNORMALITIES

Complete absence of a breast is uncommon, and 90% of patients with true unilateral absence of a breast have either absence or hypoplasia of the pectoral muscles,[7] although 90% of patients with pectoral muscle defects have normal breasts.[8] Some patients with abnormalities of the pectoral muscles and absence or hypoplasia of the breast have a characteristic deformity of the upper limb (synbrachydactyly with hypoplasia of the middle phalanges and skin webbing); this cluster of anomalies is known as Poland's syndrome.[9]

BREAST DEVELOPMENT AND INVOLUTION

During the first week or two of life the breast bud enlarges in about 60% of normal newborn babies. Enlargement can be asymmetrical and associated with secretion of a colostrum-like substance known at witches' milk. Enlargement may persist for many months in breastfed babies.

Breast development proceeds identically in boys and girls until puberty. In females, growth of the breast starts at about age 10 and can initially be asymmetrical. A unilateral lump in a 9–10-year-old girl is invariably developing breast tissue, and any surgical interference should be avoided because it can damage the breast bud. The functional unit of the breast is the terminal duct lobular unit or lobule (Fig. 23.7) and this drains via a branching duct network to the nipple. The ductal system is not organized in a linear radial manner and the breast is not separated into well-defined segments. The lobules and branching networks of ducts are supported by fibrous tissue known as stroma. The majority of conditions affecting the breast arise within the terminal duct lobular unit, but some conditions do develop in the ducts or involve the stroma.

Following breast development, regular changes occur in relation to the menstrual cycle. The breast doubles in weight during pregnancy and following cessation of breastfeeding the breast involutes. In nulliparous women, involution starts at a variable age but in some women it is evident by the age of 30. During involution there is a reduction in the number of breast lobules and the breast stroma is replaced by fat; the result is that the breast becomes less radiodense, softer and ptotic (droopy). Other changes occur in the glandular tissue, including development of areas of fibrosis, formation of small cysts (microcysts), and focal increase in glandular elements (adenosis).

The life cycle of the breast involves three main periods: development (and early reproductive life), mature reproductive

REFERENCES

4. Dey P, Bundred NJ, Gibbs A et al. Br Med J 2002; 324: 507–510
5. Dixon JM. Br Med J 2002; 324: 510
6. Dixon JM, Mansel RE. Br Med J 1994; 309: 797–800
7. Trier WC. Plast Reconstr Surg 1965; 36: 430
8. Pers M. Scand J Plast Reconstr Surg 1968; 2: 125
9. Nerakha GJ. In: Gallager HS, Leis HP, Synderman RK et al (eds). The Breast. Mosby, St Louis, 1978: 442–451

Table 23.2 Aberrations of normal breast development and involution

Age (years)	Period	Normal process	Aberration
< 25	Breast development and early reproductive life	Stromal development Lobular development	Juvenile hypertrophy Fibroadenoma
25–40	Mature reproductive life	Cyclical activity	Cyclical mastalgia, cyclical nodularity (diffuse or focal)
35–50	Involution	Lobular involution Stromal involution Ductal involution	Macrocysts Sclerosing lesions Duct ectasia

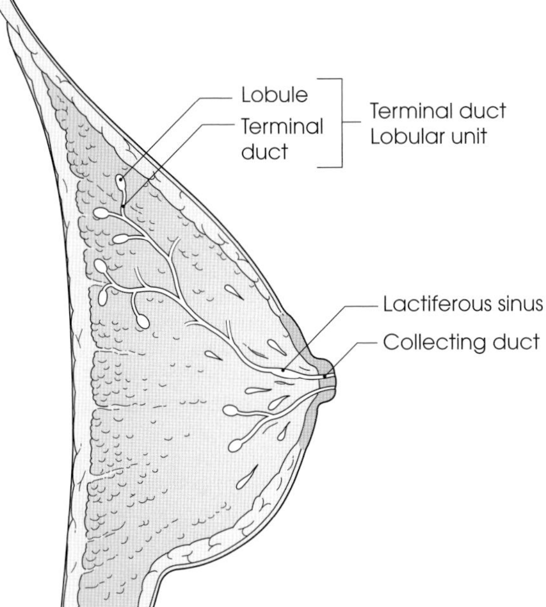

Figure 23.7 Anatomy of breast showing terminal duct lobular units and branching system of ducts.

life and involution. The majority of benign conditions occur during one of these specific periods, and are so common that they are best considered as aberrations of normal breast development and involution rather than diseases (Table 23.2).

ABERRATIONS OF BREAST DEVELOPMENT

Prepubertal breast enlargement in girls is a common occurrence in the absence of other signs of sexual maturation. Only if there are other signs of early and unusual sexual development are hormonal investigations required. Rarely a hormone-secreting ovarian or adrenal tumour is responsible.

Juvenile hypertrophy

Uncontrolled overgrowth of breast tissue is sometimes seen in adolescent girls whose breast development begins normally during puberty but the breasts continue to grow, often quite rapidly. Histologically, overgrowth of periductal connective tissue in association with proliferation and branching of ducts but no lobule formation is seen. These changes are usually bilateral, but can be limited to one breast or even part of one breast. Called virginal or juvenile 'hypertrophy', it is not a true hypertrophy and is not associated with any underlying endocrine abnormality.

Patients present with social embarrassment, pain, discomfort, and an inability to perform regular daily tasks. Reduction mammoplasty—of which there are a variety of techniques, the most common being the inferior dermal pedicle technique—considerably improves their quality of life. Danazol given during rapid breast enlargement has been reported to be of benefit.

Fibroadenoma

Previously considered a benign neoplasm, fibroadenomas are best classified as aberrations of breast development. Each fibroadenoma develops from a single lobule and not a single cell; they are exceedingly common and remain under the same hormonal control as normal breast lobules. They account for 13% of all palpable symptomatic breast lesions and in women aged 20 or younger they account for almost 60% of such masses.[6]

There are three separate types of fibroadenoma: common fibroadenoma, giant fibroadenoma and juvenile fibroadenoma. Because intracanalicular and pericanalicular fibroadenomas behave identically, there is no reason to distinguish between the two. Common fibroadenomas develop most frequently after the period of breast growth, in the 15–25-year age group. The term *giant fibroadenomas* should be reserved for those that measure over 5 cm in diameter.[10] They appear more commonly in certain African countries.[10,11] Juvenile fibroadenomas occur in adolescent girls and can undergo rapid growth; they are often large at diagnosis (Fig. 23.8) and are more cellular than ordinary fibroadenomas. Phyllodes tumours are distinct pathological entities that can be benign or malignant and cannot always be distinguished clinically or on imaging from fibroadenomas.[12]

A definitive diagnosis of a simple or common fibroadenoma can be made by a combination of clinical examination, ultrasonography and fine-needle aspiration cytology, and/or core biopsy. Fibroadenomas have characteristic mammographic features in older women as they tend to calcify. The majority of patients with fibroadenomas have only a single lesion, but a few patients have multiple fibroadenomas. Less than 10% of untreated common fibroadenomas increase in size, and a third get smaller or disappear completely within 2 years while the remainder stay the same size.

Management

Fibroadenomas over 4 cm in size should usually be excised following core biopsy to establish the diagnosis. Large juvenile

REFERENCES

10. Fechner RE. In: Page DL, Anderson TJ (eds). Diagnostic Histopathology of the Breast. Churchill Livingstone, Edinburgh, 1987: 72
11. Azzopardi JG. Problems in Breast Pathology. WB Saunders, London, 1981
12. Hughes LE, Mansel RE, Webster DJT. Benign Disorders and Diseases of the Breast. Baillière Tindal, London, 2001

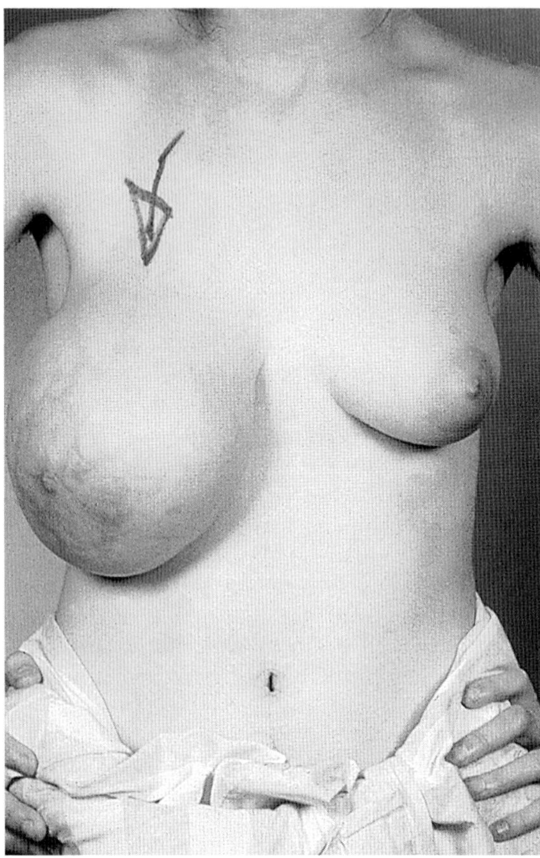

Figure 23.8 Juvenile fibroadenoma of right breast.

fibroadenomas are best removed through an incision in the inframammary crease or inferolaterally. Subsequent revisional surgery may be required if excess skin remains. Common fibroadenomas less than 4 cm need excision only when requested by the patient once a definite diagnosis is established. Excision can be under local or general anaesthesia. Good cosmetic results are obtained by excising fibroadenomas through remote incisions in the circumareolar or axillary region. Mammotome excision of small fibroadenomas is also possible.

Cancer arising in a fibroadenoma is rare; the incidence is approximately one per 1000.[11] It is usually of lobular type and is most commonly non-invasive.[13] The prognosis of invasive cancer limited exclusively or almost exclusively to a fibroadenoma is excellent.[11,13]

Pain and nodularity

Cyclical pain and diffuse or localized painful nodularity is common. Pain that is severe or prolonged is regarded as an aberration.[14] Approximately 10% of all breast cancers, particularly in younger women, present as localized areas of nodularity. Areas of localized nodularity can develop in relation to areas of breast involution. This was previously called fibroadenosis; the preferred pathological term for this condition is *benign breast change.*

Breast pain

Breast pain or mastalgia either alone or in combination with lumpiness is reported in up to half of all women attending breast clinics. Of 8504 patients presenting with pain as their major symptom to the Edinburgh Breast Unit over a 10-year period, 220 (2.7%) were diagnosed as having breast cancer.[14] During this period, 4740 patients were diagnosed with breast cancer, so 4.6%

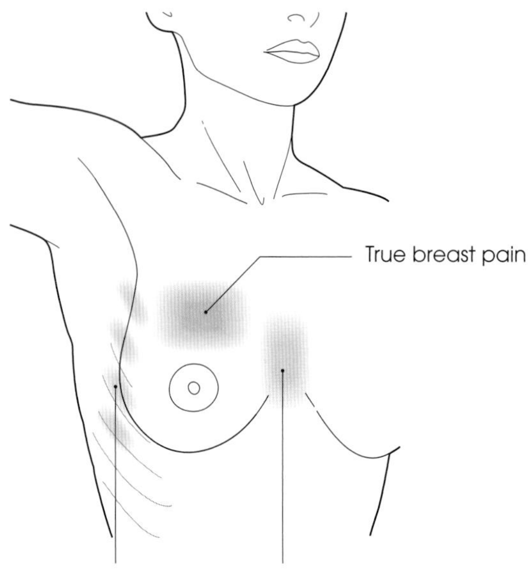

Figure 23.9 Classification of non-cyclical breast pain. Non-cyclical pain can be divided into true breast pain arising from the breast tissue or musculoskeletal pain arising from the ribs or chest wall. Musculoskeletal pain is common medially (costochondritis) or laterally at the edge of the breast. Examining the patient while leaning forward to make the breast fall away from the chest wall allows better differentiation of these subtypes.

of women with cancer had pain as a major presenting symptom. Two-thirds of working women and 77% of women attending for screening reported recent breast pain when directly questioned.[14] Most mastalgia is of minor or moderate degree and is part of the changes that occur in relation to the menstrual cycle. Women with mastalgia are psychologically no different from women attending outpatient clinics for other conditions.

Patients with both cyclical and non-cyclical breast pain should have a careful examination combined with appropriate imaging. Non-cyclical pain is more common than cyclical pain.

Cyclical mastalgia

Cyclical mastalgia affects premenopausal women (average age 34 years) or women on cyclical hormone replacement therapy. Women with cyclical mastalgia of moderate and severe degrees typically report increasing severity of pain from midcycle onwards, with pain improving after menstruation. Classically, the outer half of the breast is affected (Fig. 23.9). This type of breast pain tends to be persistent over many years and is relieved by the menopause. Sometimes pregnancy and starting or changing the type of oral contraceptive can affect breast pain, but these do not have a consistent effect.

Treatment

A low-fat, high-carbohydrate diet may reduce breast pain to a greater degree than general dietary advice, but such diets are difficult to sustain.[15] Evening primrose oil is commonly used to

REFERENCES

13. Oyyello L, Gump FE. Surg Gynecol Obstet 1985; 116: 99–101
14. Mansel RE. Br Med J 1994; 309; 866–868
15. Bundred NJ. In: Clinical Evidence. 7th edn. BMJ Publishing Group, London, 2002: 1631–1638

treat breast pain, but trials to date have been of poor quality and contained small numbers of women.[16,17] One trial did show that pain, tenderness and lumpiness improved in cyclical but not in non-cyclical breast pain with evening primrose oil. Danazol reduces cyclical breast pain but can cause side effects including weight gain, deepening of voice, menorrhagia and muscle cramps.[18] Bromocriptine relieves breast pain but has a high incidence of adverse effects, so it is now rarely used. Tamoxifen is effective in treating breast pain at doses of 10 or 20 mg per day, even when given for only 2 weeks prior to menstruation,[19] but it is not licensed for breast pain. There is no evidence that vitamin B_6, diuretics or antibiotics are effective in treating breast pain.

Non-cyclical mastalgia

Affecting an older age group (mean age 43 years), the most common site of pain is the lateral chest wall (Fig. 23.9), although non-cyclical pain can originate in the breast.[14] It has a random pattern, although it occurs more commonly on exercise and is described as a burning or drawing pain. Chest wall tenderness is assessed by examining the patient on her side and allowing the breast to fall away from the chest wall.

Treatment

Infiltration of local anaesthetic and steroid (40 mg methylprednisolone) produces short-term benefit in most patients with localized chest wall pain and up to 60% get a prolonged effect.

ABERRATIONS OF INVOLUTION

Approximately 7% of women in the western world present with a palpable breast cyst at some time in their life,[20] and these constitute 50% of all discrete masses. Cysts are distended or involuted lobules, and are seen most frequently in perimenopausal women or in older women taking hormone replacement therapy. They present as discrete lumps that can be painful.

Mammographically, cysts have characteristic halos and are easily diagnosed by ultrasound. Women with cysts should have mammography because between 1 and 4% have cancer that is often remote from the cyst (Fig. 23.10). Ultrasound can differentiate between simple cysts and intracystic cancers. Large and painful cysts are treated by needle aspiration, and if the aspirated fluid is not bloodstained it need not be sent for cytology. Asymptomatic cysts require no action. Patients with cysts have a slightly increased risk of developing breast cancer, but the magnitude of this risk is not considered clinically significant.[21] Intracystic cancers are rare but should be suspected if the ultrasound shows a complex, partly cystic or solid lesion, or if the aspirate is bloodstained.

Sclerosis

During stromal involution, areas of fibrosis or sclerosis produce three different groups of lesions: sclerosing adenosis, radial scars and complex sclerosing lesions (previously called sclerosing papillomatosis or duct adenoma and including infiltrating epitheliosis). These lesions cause diagnostic problems during breast screening and on mammography are difficult to differentiate from malignant lesions. Although core biopsy of an area of this type of distortion can indicate the lesion is likely to be benign, excisional biopsy is usually required to exclude malignancy and to make a definitive diagnosis.[22]

Duct ectasia

The subareolar breast ducts dilate and shorten with age and by age 70, 40% of women have a substantial degree of major duct dilatation. Some women have marked dilatation with nipple discharge and/or duct shortening that causes nipple inversion; an aberration of the normal involution process, this is called duct ectasia. The discharge is usually cheesy and the nipple retraction is usually slit-like (Fig. 23.11). Surgery is indicated only if the discharge is troublesome or if the patient wishes the nipple to be everted.[23]

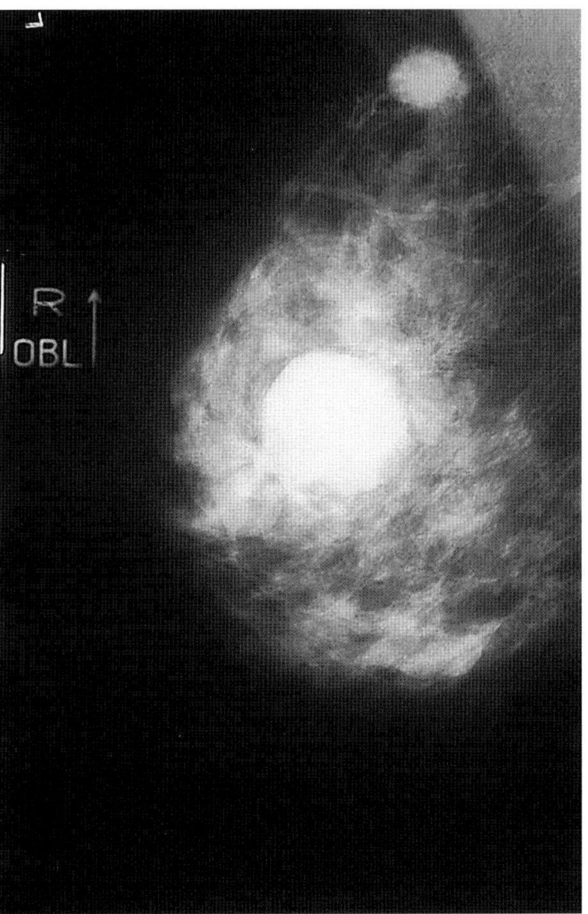

Figure 23.10 Mammogram showing a cyst in the central part of the breast and a carcinoma in the upper part of breast.

Epithelial hyperplasia

An increase in the number of epithelial cells lining the terminal

REFERENCES

16. Pye JK, Mansel RE, Hughes LE. Lancet 1985; 1: 373–377
17. Preece PE, Hanslip JI, Gilbert L et al. In: Horrobin D (ed). Clinical Uses of Essential Fatty Acids. Eden Press, Montreal, 1982: 147–154
18. Kontostolis E, Stefanidis K, Navrozoglou I et al. Gynecol Endocrinol 1997; 11: 393–397
19. Fentiman IS, Caleffi M, Brame K et al. Lancet 1986; 1: 287–288
20. Haagensen CD, Bodian C, Haagensen DE. Breast Carcinoma Risk and Detection. WB Saunders, London, 1981: 55
21. Dixon JM, McDonald C, Elton RA et al. Lancet 1999; 353: 1742–1745
22. Page DL, Anderson TJ. Diagnostic Histopathology of the Breast. Churchill Livingstone, Edinburgh, 1987
23. Dixon JM, Bundred NJ. In: Harris J, Lippman ME, Morrow M (eds). Diseases of the Breast. 2nd edn. Lippincott Williams and Wilkins, Philadelphia, 1999: 47–55

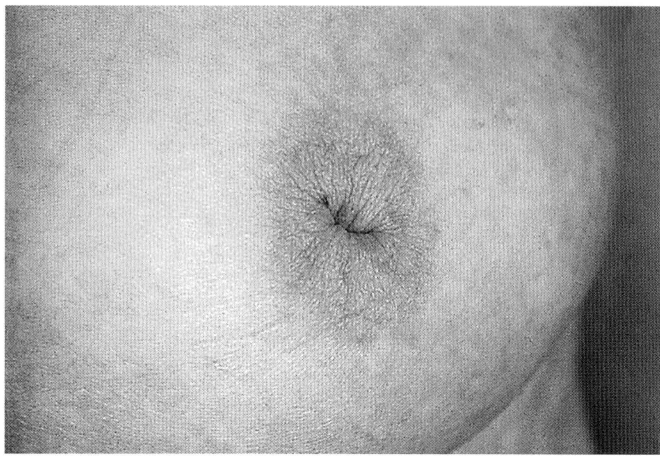

Figure 23.11 Slit-like nipple retraction due to duct ectasia.

duct lobular unit is known as epithelial hyperplasia (previously called epitheliosis or papillomatosis) and is graded as mild, moderate or florid.[24] If the hyperplastic cells also show cellular atypia, the condition is known as atypical hyperplasia. Women with atypical hyperplasia are at significantly increased risk of developing breast cancer (Fig. 23.12); the absolute risk is 8% at 10 years for a woman who does not have a first-degree relative with breast cancer and 20–25% at 15 years for a woman with a first-degree relative with breast cancer.[25] The incidence of subsequent breast cancer can be reduced by the administration of tamoxifen (Fig. 23.13).[26] Yearly mammography up to the age of 50, and yearly or biennial mammography thereafter until 15 years after the original biopsy, is advised for these women.

Nipple discharge

Nipple discharge accounts for 5% of referrals to breast clinics and is a frightening symptom because of the fear of breast cancer. Over 95% of women will have a benign cause for the discharge.[23] Investigation is outlined in Fig. 23.14. Cytology of nipple discharge has a low sensitivity for malignancy, although this may be increased by ductal lavage. Ductoscopy can differentiate between different causes of nipple discharge but is available in only a small number of centres. Treatment depends on whether the discharge is spontaneous and whether it is from a single or from multiple ducts. Single-duct discharge should be tested for haemoglobin. Only moderate or large amounts of blood are significant. Leakage of fluid from the nipple is common, and two-thirds of premenopausal women can be made to produce nipple secretion by cleansing the nipple and applying suction; this discharge varies in colour from white to yellow to green to blue-black.

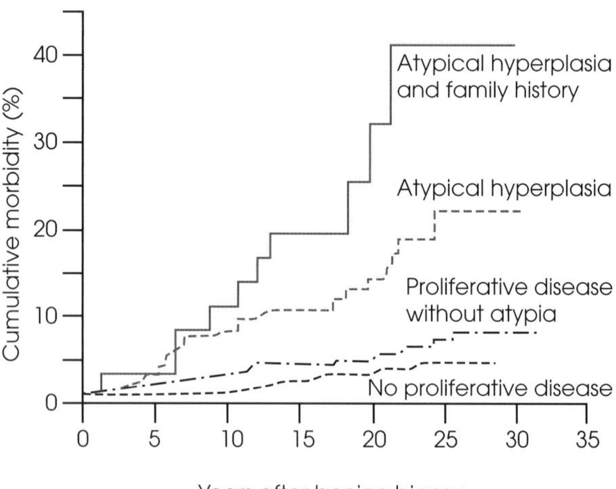

Figure 23.12 Risk of subsequent development of invasive carcinoma in patients with no epithelial proliferation, proliferative disease without atypia (moderate or florid hyperplasia), atypical hyperplasia, or atypical hyperplasia and a family history of cancer. (From Page.[25])

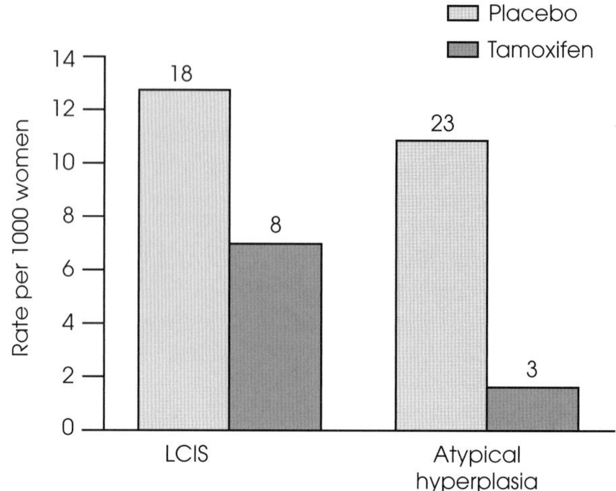

Figure 23.13 Reduction in invasive breast cancer observed in the National Surgical Adjuvant Breast and Bowel Project tamoxifen and breast cancer prevention trial for women with a prior diagnosis of LCIS and atypical hyperplasia. (From Page,[25] with permission of BMJ Books.)

Bloody nipple discharge in pregnancy

Nipple discharge with blood present either visibly or cytologically occurring during pregnancy or lactation is common.[27] This condition is benign and requires no specific investigations or treatment.[28]

Galactorrhoea

Copious bilateral milky discharge not associated with pregnancy or breastfeeding is known as galactorrhoea. Drugs, particularly psychotropic agents, can cause hypoprolactinaemia and galactorrhoea. Blood should be taken to measure prolactin if copious milky discharge is present, and if prolactin levels are elevated greater than 1000 mU/L and there is no obvious drug cause a search for a pituitary tumour should be instituted.[29] Milky discharge from the nipple can persist for many months after stopping breastfeeding, particularly if the nipple is squeezed. It does not require investigation or treatment.

REFERENCES

24. Dupont WD, Page DL. N Engl J Med 1985; 312: 146–151
25. Page DL. Breast 1992; 1: 3–7
26. Fisher B, Costantino JP, Wickerham DL et al. J Natl Cancer Inst 1998; 90: 1371
27. Kline TS, Lash SR. Am J Pathol 1964; 8: 336
28. Lafreniere R. J Surg Oncol 1990; 43: 228
29. Chetty U. In: Smallwood JA, Taylor I (eds). Benign Breast Diseases. Edward Arnold, London, 1990: 85

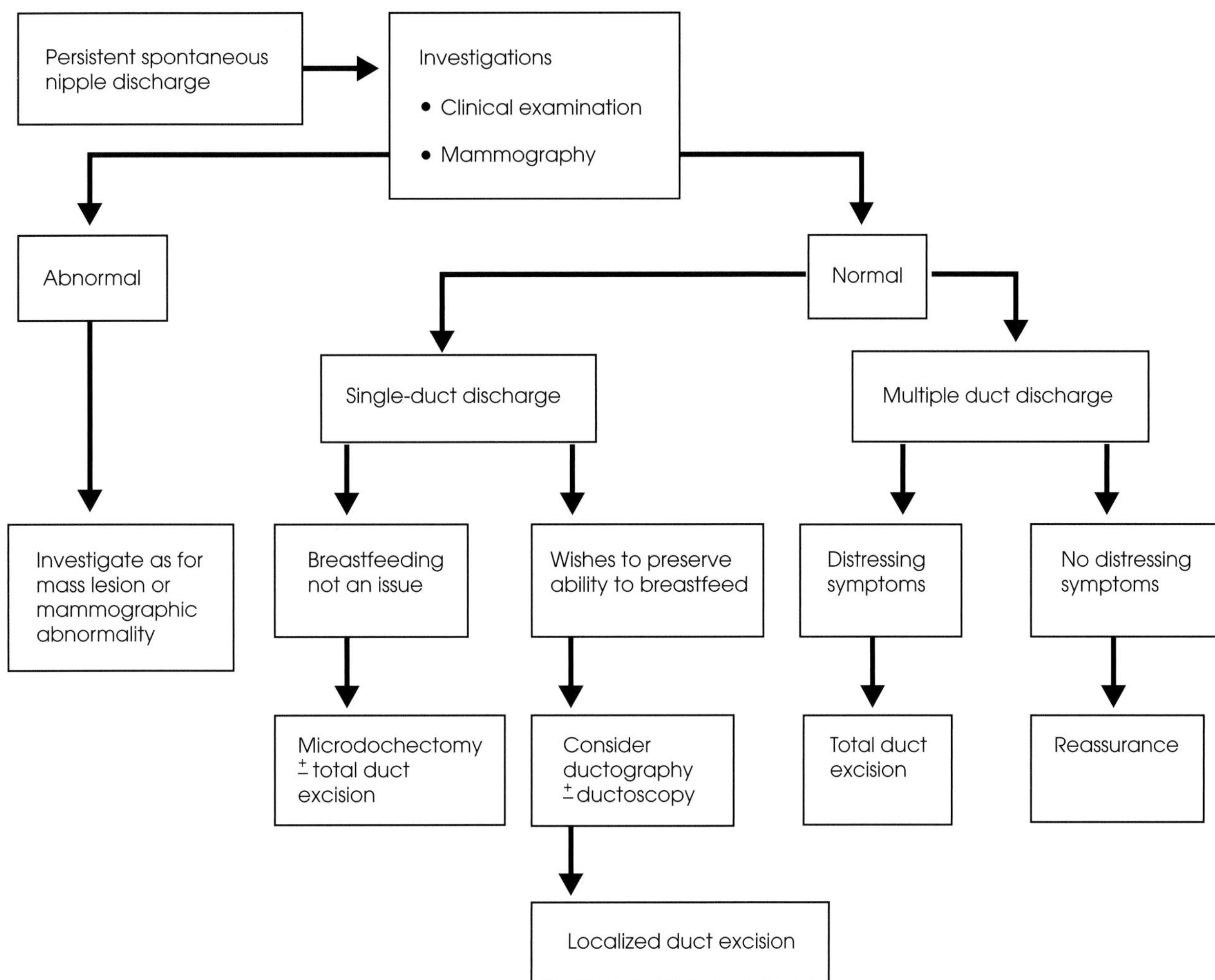

Figure 23.14 Investigation of nipple discharge.

Duct papilloma

Duct papilloma is a common cause of serous or bloodstained nipple discharge; papillomas can be single or multiple, are very common and have minimal malignant potential.

Nipple retraction or inversion

Slit-like retraction of the nipple is characteristic of benign disease, whereas nipple inversion when the whole nipple is pulled in can be congenital or occur in association with breast cancer, inflammatory breast conditions, or as a result of previous surgery. For women with unsightly congenital nipple retraction and those who develop acquired nipple retraction that is unsightly and does not respond to conservative measurements, duct division or total duct excision everts the nipple. An illustration of nipple retraction is shown in Fig. 23.11.

Lipomas

Lipomas are soft, lobulated, radiolucent lesions that are common in the breast. They can be confused with a pseudolipoma, which is a soft mass around a breast cancer caused by in-drawing of the fat surrounding a carcinoma.

Haematoma

Haematoma most frequently follow trauma, such as road traffic accident, fine-needle aspiration, or core biopsy or open biopsy. A haematoma can also develop in an area of the breast affected by malignancy following trauma, so persistent masses after trauma should be fully investigated. Breast haematomas can also follow spontaneous bleeding into a cancer, and they can also occur spontaneously in normal breast tissue in patients on anticoagulant therapy.

Fat necrosis

Often called traumatic fat necrosis, a history of trauma is present only in approximately 40%. Most commonly seen after a road traffic accident as a result of seat belt trauma to the breast (Fig. 23.15), it presents clinically as a firm mass, sometimes with overlying skin dimpling, which is difficult to differentiate from malignancy. A core biopsy usually establishes the diagnosis, but sometimes excision is required.

Spontaneous necrosis of the breast

Spontaneous necrosis of the breast has been reported but is rare and occurs more commonly in women with diabetes.

BREAST INFECTION

Breast infection is now much less common than it used to be. Characteristically seen in women between 18 and 50, it is divided

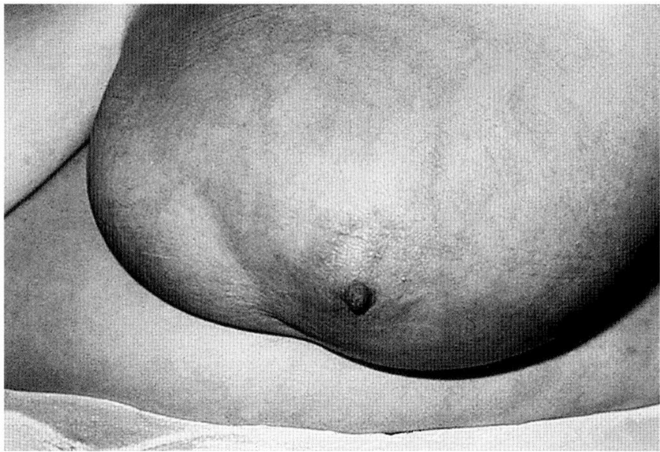

Figure 23.15 Consequence of extensive fat necrosis following a seat-belt injury in a road traffic accident.

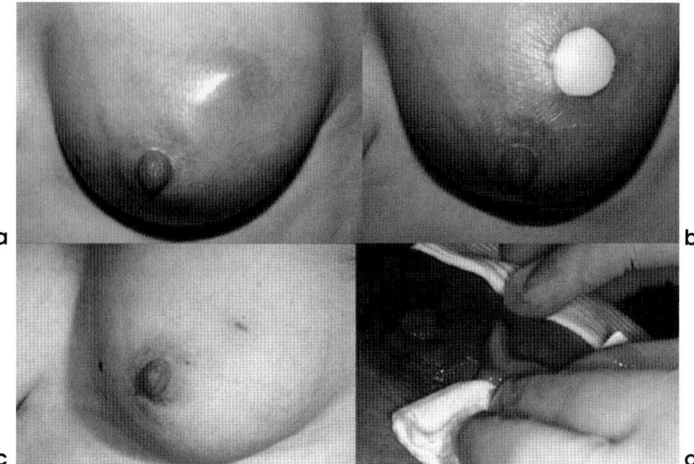

Figure 23.16 A lactating breast abscess in the left breast (**a**), EMLA cream in situ (**b**), postoperative result (**c**), and pus being expressed through a small incision under local anaesthesia (**d**).

Box 23.1 Organisms responsible for breast infection

Neonatal
- *Staphylococcus aureus*
- *Escherichia coli**

Lactating
- *Staphylococcus aureus*
- *Staphylococcus epidermidis**
- Streptococci*

Non-lactating
- *Staphylococcus aureus*
- Enterococci
- Anaerobic streptococci
- *Bacteroides* spp.

Skin-associated
- *Staphylococcus aureus*

*Organisms only occasionally responsible.

into lactational and non-lactational. Infection can affect the skin overlying the breast as a primary event, or it can develop secondary to infection of a sebaceous cyst or underlying skin problem such as hidradenitis suppurativa.

The principles of treating breast infection are as follows.

- Give appropriate antibiotics early to reduce abscess formation (the organisms responsible are shown in Box 23.1).
- If an abscess is suspected, confirm it by ultrasound or aspiration before surgical drainage is performed.
- If an inflammatory lesion does not settle on appropriate treatment, breast cancer should be excluded by cytology or core biopsy.

Almost all breast abscesses can be treated by either repeated aspiration combined with oral antibiotics or by incision and drainage under local anaesthesia (Fig. 23.3). When treating patients by aspiration, this needs to be repeated every 2–3 days until no further pus is aspirated. Ultrasound guidance allows the abscess to be aspirated through normal skin following local anaesthetic infiltration. Pain is further reduced by irrigation of the abscess cavity with local anaesthetic. Very few breast abscesses require drainage under general anaesthesia except those in children; placement of a drain or packing the cavity after incision and drainage are unnecessary (Fig. 23.16).

NEONATAL INFECTION

Neonatal infection occurs in the first few weeks of life when the breast bud is enlarged. If an abscess develops, any incision should be placed peripherally to avoid damaging the breast bud.

LACTATING INFECTION

Improved maternal–infant hygiene has dramatically reduced the frequency of breast infection-associated breastfeeding. Most often seen within the first 6 weeks of breastfeeding, some women do develop it during weaning (Fig. 23.16a). It presents with pain, swelling and tenderness; there is usually a history of a cracked nipple or skin abrasion but this is not the site of entry of organisms. Drainage of milk from the affected segment is often reduced, and resolution of the infection is improved by continuing to breastfeed. Antibiotics given as soon as infection is suspected can stop abscess development. Tetracycline, ciprofloxacin and chloramphenicol should not be used because these drugs enter breast milk and can harm the baby. If infection does not settle after one course of flucloxacillin and no pus or area suspicious of malignancy is present on ultrasound, the patient should be changed to co-amoxyclav to cover other possible pathogens. Lactating breast abscesses can be effectively treated by repeated aspiration unless the overlying skin is thinned or necrotic, when a small incision using a 15 blade (Fig. 23.16d) is made to drain the pus under local anaesthetic. Ultrasound can identify all loculi and allows complete drainage of all pus.

NON-LACTATING INFECTION

Non-lactating infection can be separated into periareolar and peripheral infection.

Periareolar infection

Periareolar infection is seen most commonly in young women (mean age 32); the majority of these patients are smokers. The underlying pathology is periductal mastitis.[30,31] It presents with periareolar inflammation with or without a mass, or as an abscess

REFERENCES

30. Dixon JM. Br Med J 1994; 309: 946–949
31. Dixon JM. Breast 1998; 7: 128–130

or a mammary duct fistula. Nipple retraction is often present, although this may be subtle;[32] nipple discharge, which can be yellow or frankly purulent, can also be present. Treatment of periareolar inflammation is with co-amoxyclav or a combination or erythromycin and metronidazole.[33] Periareolar breast abscesses are treated by recurrent aspiration and oral antibiotics or by incision and drainage under local anaesthesia. Up to half of patients with periareolar infection get recurrence; the only effective long-term treatment for these women is total duct excision performed under peri- and postoperative antibiotic cover; it is usually curative.[34]

A mammary duct fistula is a communication between the skin usually in the periareolar region and a major subareolar breast duct (Fig. 23.17). Treatment is surgical and consists of either opening up the fistula and allowing it to granulate,[35] or excising the fistula and affected duct or ducts (a total duct excision is usually required) and closing the wound primarily under antibiotic cover;[36] the latter is preferred because it produces a more satisfactory cosmetic outcome.[37]

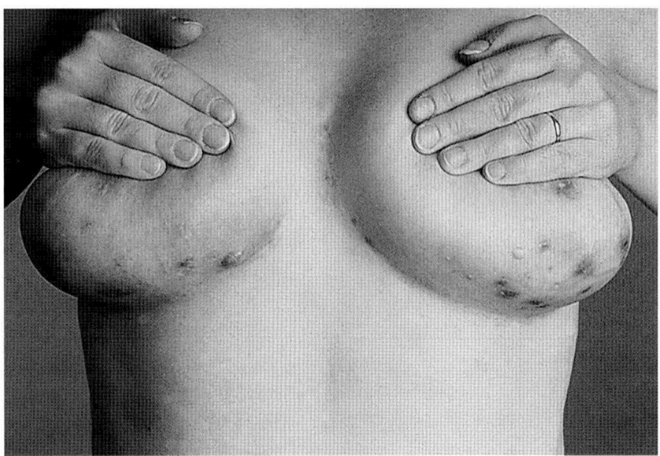

Figure 23.18 Infection of the skin in the lower half of the breasts due to hidradenitis suppurativa.

Peripheral non-lactating breast abscesses

Peripheral non-lactating breast abcesses are much less common than periareolar infection and are sometimes associated with underlying conditions such as diabetes, rheumatoid arthritis, steroid treatment, granulomatous lobular mastitis or trauma. Pilonidal breast abscesses in sheep shearers and hairdressers have been reported. Infection associated with granulomatous lobular mastitis can be a particular problem. This condition, which affects young parous women, may present with large areas of infection or multiple simultaneous peripheral abscesses. There is a tendency for this condition to persist and recur despite surgery. Steroids have been tried but with limited success. It usually settles spontaneously so having established the diagnosis surgery should be avoided. Treatment of a peripheral abscess is by recurrent aspiration or incision and drainage.

Very rarely, subareolar or peripheral non-lactating infection occurs as a consequence of infection of necrotic debris associated with ductal carcinoma in situ (DCIS). For this reason, following resolution of an unexplained abscess in women over the age of 35, mammography should be performed.

SKIN-ASSOCIATED INFECTION

Cellulitis or abscesses developing in the skin of the breast are more common in women who are overweight, have large breasts or have poor personal hygiene; cellulitis also occurs more frequently in patients who have previous surgery or radiotherapy. Treatment of cellulitis is with oral antibiotics, although in irradiated patients i.v. antibiotics may be required. Abscesses should be drained or aspirated. Women with recurrent infections should be advised about weight reduction and keeping the area as clean and dry as possible. Intertrigo in the submammary fold is also common in this same group of patients. If it does not respond to simple hygiene then it is often treated with clotrimazole (Canesten) cream, although the role of fungi and the effectiveness of this treatment in this condition is unclear.

Sebaceous cysts in the skin of the breast can become infected. Recurrent infections in the inframammary fold can occur due to hidradenitis suppurativa (Fig. 23.18), a smoking-related condition. Conservative excision of affected skin is effective in reducing further infective episodes in about half of these patients.

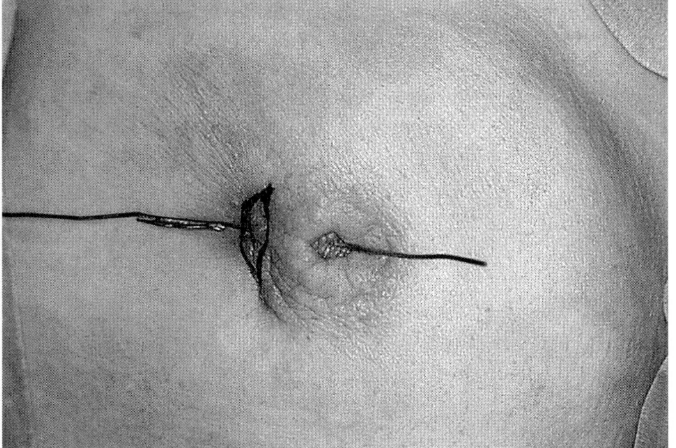

Figure 23.17 Mammary duct fistula.

OTHER INFECTIONS

Tuberculosis, primary actinomycosis, syphilis, and mycotic, helminthic and viral infections occasionally affect the breast but are rare. Herpetic ulceration of the nipple has been reported. Molluscum contagiosum can affect the areola and presents as wart-like lesions.

FACTITIAL DISEASE

Artefactual or factitial disease is created by the patient, often through complex and repetitive actions. This diagnosis should be considered when the clinical situation does not conform to common appearances or pathological processes (Fig. 23.19).

REFERENCES

32. Rees BI, Gravelle IH, Hughes LE. Br J Surg 1977; 64: 577
33. Dixon JM, Lee ECG, Greenall MJ. Br J Clin Pract 1988; 42: 78
34. Dixon JM, Kohlhardt SR, Dillon P. Breast 1998; 7: 216–219
35. Atkins HJB. Br Med J 1955; 2: 1473
36. Dixon JM, Thompson AM. Br J Surg 1991; 78: 1185–1186
37. Schnitt SJ, Connolly JL. In: Harris JR, Lippman N, Morrow M et al (eds). Diseases of the Breast. Lippincott–Raven, Philadelphia, 1996: 39

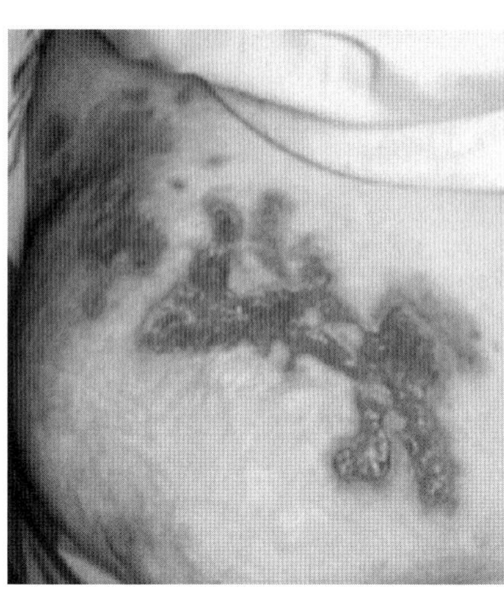

Figure 23.19 A patient with factitial disease.

MISCELLANEOUS LESIONS

FIBROMATOSIS

Fibromatosis is a poorly understood condition and usually presents as a firm mass that is often deep seated, is usually attached to the pectoral fascia, and may distort the breast and cause skin dimpling. It is caused by proliferation of myofibroblasts and it behaves in a similar manner to other extra-abdominal fibromatoses (desmoid tumours). It frequently recurs despite excision. Diagnosis can be established by core biopsy. Treatment is wide excision to clear margins.

NODULAR FASCIITIS

Nodular fasciitis usually develops in the pectoral fascia and presents as a deep-seated breast lump. Like fibromatosis, it is treated by wide excision.

LYMPHOCYTIC LOBULITIS

The pathogenesis of lymphocytic lobulitis is unknown. It can be associated with other autoimmune conditions and presents with a mass that can mimic breast cancer; it is characterized by lymphocytic infiltration around breast lobules with lymphocytic vasculitis and epithelioid fibroblasts in the stroma.[38] Once diagnosed, it requires no specific treatment.

DIABETIC MASTOPATHY

Patients with diabetes can develop dense, keloid-like areas of fibrosis within the breast. The condition is often diagnosed only after open biopsy. The condition is not well understood.[38]

SARCOIDOSIS

Involvement of the breast by sarcoidosis is rare. Patients with sarcoid can present with a single or multiple masses in the breast, which can occur as a first presentation of the disease or in association with sarcoidosis elsewhere. Diagnosis is established by core biopsy or excision.

AMYLOID

Amyloid deposits in the breast, causing a mass, have been reported.[39]

HAMARTOMA

Hamartomas are uncommon breast lesions; they are also known as fibroadenolipomas. Histologically they consist of fibroglandular tissue admixed with fat surrounded by a capsule of connective tissue. The halo of connective tissue can be seen on mammography and helps differentiates these lesions from fibroadenomas.

INTRAMAMMARY LYMPH NODES

Intramammary lymph nodes are common and are often misdiagnosed as fibroadenomas or small carcinomas. Fine-needle aspiration cytology or core biopsy can establish the correct diagnosis. Enlargement of intramammary lymph nodes may be secondary to local pathology, including breast cancer, or may be the result of a systemic or lymphoproliferative disorder.

PARAFFIN AND SILICONE GRANULOMAS

The desire for larger breasts has led women to seek augmentation. Originally accomplished by injecting liquid paraffin or silicone into the submammary space, these substances can migrate into the breast and cause a low-grade inflammatory reaction. The preferred method of augmentation is the placement of silicone gel enclosed in a Silastic envelope in the submammary space. These can rupture and result in a granulomatous reaction within the breast.

BLOCKED MONTGOMERY'S TUBERCLE

Montgomery's tubercles are blind-ending ducts in the areola. Secretions from the lining cells can become inspissated and can cause a periareolar lump that if necessary can be locally excised.

MONDOR'S DISEASE OF THE BREAST

Superficial thrombophlebitis, most commonly of the thoraco-epigastric vein over the breast, is known as Mondor's disease. It is most common after surgery and occurs more frequently in people with an underlying predisposition to thrombosis. It can also occur spontaneously. In the early stages the vein is tender and there is a string-like band that may be associated with skin dimpling. It resolves in a few weeks without specific treatment.

ARTERITIS

Patients with generalized vasculitis can have localized changes in the breast causing a breast lump.

ANEURYSM

Aneuryms or dilatation of vessels within the breast can present as a discrete mass with an audible bruit.

ECZEMA OF THE NIPPLE

Discharge from the surface of the nipple should be differentiated from discharge from the surrounding areola. The common causes are eczema or Paget's disease (Fig. 23.20). Eczema when it affects the breast always affects the areola and only secondarily affects the nipple. This contrasts with Paget's disease, which always involves the nipple first. Removal of the sensitizing agent in patients with eczema can result in rapid resolution. Topical steroids are effective if no sensitizing agent is identified.

REFERENCES

38. Howell JD, Barker F, Gazet J-C. Breast 1994; 3: 119
39. Fernandez BB, Hernandez FJ. Arch Pathol 1973; 95: 102–105

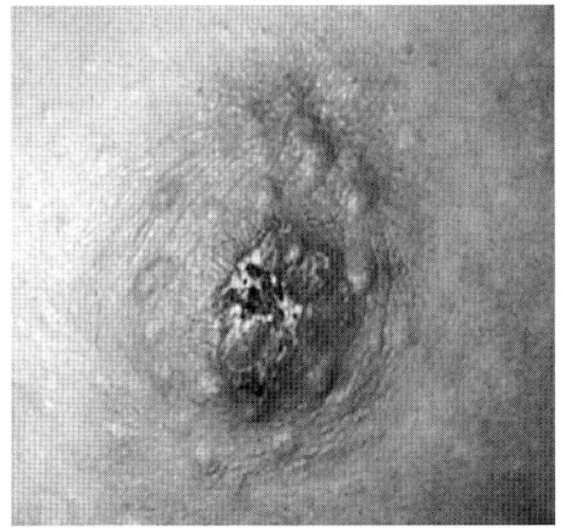
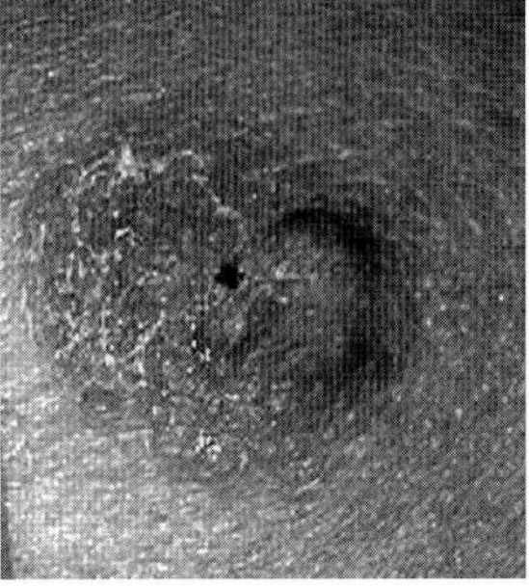

a b

Figure 23.20 Paget's disease of the nipple (a) and eczema (b).

NIPPLE ADENOMA

Nipple adenoma presents as an abnormal ulcerated area on the nipple. Treatment is by wide excision.

NIPPLE TRAUMA

The nipple can be the site of recurrent trauma from friction on an unprotected warm or moist nipple by overlying clothing during jogging or cycling. It is sometimes severe enough to produce bleeding. Tassel dancer's nipple has also been described. Chronic inflammation and chronic infection can also result from cosmetic nipple piercing, particularly in smokers. This does not usually resolve unless the nipple ring is removed, and if there is permanent damage to underlying ducts, total duct excision and rarely removal of the nipple are necessary to cure the infection.

GYNAECOMASTIA

Any enlargement of breast tissue in males at any age is known as gynaecomastia. It is an entirely benign condition and is usually reversible. In extreme cases the breast is similar in size to that seen in the female. In approximately a quarter, it is bilateral. The histological changes are similar to those seen in virginal hypertrophy. Pubertal gynaecomastia affects 30–70% of 10–16-year-old boys and usually requires no treatment because 80% of cases resolve spontaneously within 2 years.

Embarrassment or persistent enlargement are indications for surgical referral. Both tamoxifen and danazol have been reported to produce resolution in approximately half of patients. Surgery is only occasionally required. When performed, a small disc of tissue should be left attached to the undersurface of the nipple and fat should be left on the skin flaps to ensure that the patient is not left with an unsightly depression.

Senescent gynaecomastia affects men between the ages of 50 and 80 years, and in most it is not associated with an underlying endocrine abnormality. It is usually soft or rubbery, involves the whole gland and is often bilateral. A careful history and examination will often reveal the cause. Specific causes include hypogonadism, neoplasm, systemic disease and drugs (Box 23.2). A history of recent progressive breast enlargement without an identifiable cause is an indication for investigation.

Mammography can help differentiate between breast enlargement due to fat or gynaecomastia from malignancy. Fine-needle aspiration cytology and/or core biopsy should be performed where there is suspicion that the breast enlargement could be malignant. Only if no clear cause for the gynaecomastia is apparent should oestradiol, testosterone, luteinizing hormone and follicle-stimulating hormone be measured.

Box 23.2 Drug causes of gynaecomastia

Hormones
- Anabolic steroids (bodybuilders)
- Oestrogenic agonists
- Antiandrogens for treatment of prostate cancer (e.g. cyproterone acetate and goserelin)

Recreational drugs
- Alcohol
- Cannabis
- Heroin

Cardiovascular drugs
- Digoxin
- Spironolactone
- Captopril
- Enalapril
- Amiodarone
- Nifedipine
- Verapamil
- Methyldopa

Antiulcer drugs
- Cimetidine
- Ranitidine
- Omeprazole

Antibiotics
- Ketoconazole
- Metronidazole
- Minocycline

Psychoactive agents
- Tricyclic antidepressants
- Diazepam
- Phenothiazines

Others
- Domperidone
- Metoclopramide
- Penicillamine
- Phenytoin
- Theophylline

Cytotoxic agents

These impair Leydig cell function

- Alkylating agents
- Methotrexate
- Vinca alkyloids
- Combination chemotherapy

MALIGNANT DISEASE

CARCINOMA

Carcinoma of the female breast accounts for 30% of all cases of cancer in women and will affect approximately one in 9 adult women during their lifetime. In 1998, there were almost 35 000 new cases of breast cancer in the UK,[40] and in 2000 a total of 11 340 women died of the disease. The mortality rate from breast

REFERENCES

40. Quinn MJ, Babb P, Brock M et al. Cancer Trends in England and Wales 1950–99. The Stationery Office, London 2001

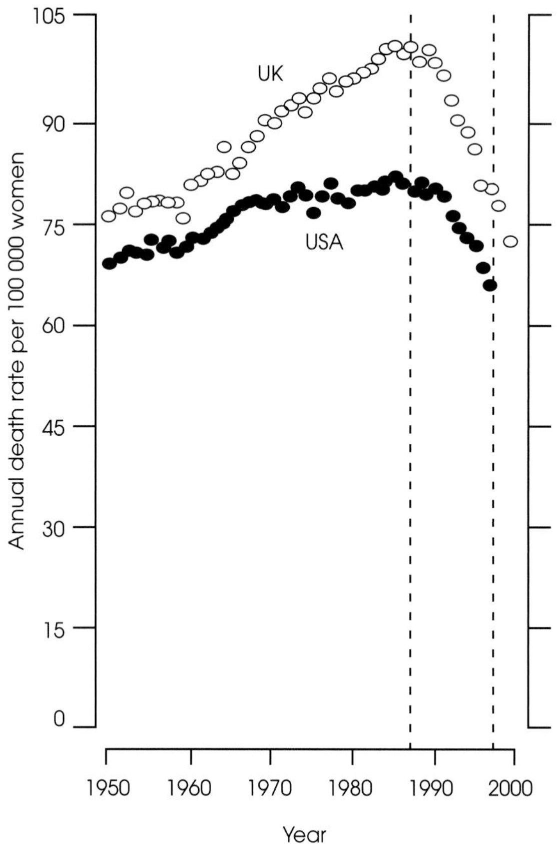

Figure 23.21 The recent decrease in UK and US breast cancer mortality in patients aged 50–69 years. (From Peto 2000,[41] with permission.)

cancer is, however, falling in all age groups, which may be due to earlier diagnosis and improvement in treatment, especially adjuvant treatments (Fig. 23.21).[41]

AETIOLOGY

The aetiology is not known but genetic, endocrine and dietary factors are implicated in its genesis. The development of the disease is probably multifactorial with no predominant cause. The disease is commoner in females who are nulliparous and live in developed countries. Conversely, multiparous women who had their first pregnancy at an early age and who live in underdeveloped countries have a low incidence of the disease. The protective effect of multiparity is almost certainly related to the fact that fecund women tend to have their first child young. The protective effect of breastfeeding is also related to a young age at first birth.

The mechanism by which endocrine events alter the susceptibility of breast tissue to malignant change is unclear, but Korenman has suggested that overexposure to oestrogens unopposed by progesterone—a circumstance that happens in nulliparous women—may be implicated.[42] This oestrogen window hypothesis is consistent with the higher incidence of breast cancer in women who have an early menarche and late menopause. Similarly, an artificial early menopause induced by ovarian irradiation or oophorectomy has been shown to be a protective factor. Hyperoestrogenism has also been thought to explain the observation that obese women have a higher incidence of breast cancer, because it is known that aromatization of androgens to oestrogens occurs in peripheral fat. Nevertheless, direct measurement of oestrogens in the blood has failed to show any differences between women with cancer and control subjects, and no consistent endocrine abnormality has been recorded in women with breast cancer compared with age-matched controls.

Genetic and environmental factors

In the mouse, transmission of breast cancer from one generation to another has been demonstrated but this was found to be caused by transmission of the Bittner virus in the mother's milk. No such mechanism has been shown for human breast cancer. Breast cancer in women is generally a sporadic disease but approximately 5–10% of cases can be considered hereditary,[43] and these are due to germ-line mutations in breast cancer predisposition genes. These mutations are usually associated with a dominant Mendelian pattern of inheritance. A family history of premenopausal breast cancer in a mother or sister certainly carries an increased risk of breast cancer, especially if bilateral. Up to 20% of breast cancer patients have a first-degree relative with breast cancer.

Two major breast cancer genes (*BRCA1* and *BRCA2*) were identified in 1994 and 1995, and these have been shown to be associated with inherited breast cancer in several large affected families.[44,45] *BRCA1* is located on chromosome 11 and is associated with both breast and ovarian cancer development, while *BRCA2* is on chromosome 17 and is mainly associated with breast cancer and less commonly with ovarian cancer. They are large, complex genes and a large number of mutations have been identified. Testing is only relevant to a small number of women with an identified family history of breast and ovarian cancer.

Breast cancer predisposition genes are involved in DNA repair. *BRCA1* and *BRCA2* probably account for up to 85% of all breast or ovarian cancer families and up to 60% of breast only families. In some cases there is incomplete penetrance of the gene, so that an individual with a germ-line mutation may live their entire life without a somatic mutation and so do not develop the disease.[46]

Apart from *BRCA1* and *BRCA2*, there are a number of other syndromes that are associated with an increased breast cancer risk, which include Cowden's, Peutz–Jeghers and Li–Fraumeni syndromes. It is becoming apparent that there are also other genes that have a low penetrance and act together with other susceptibility genes and risk factors, including environmental factors, to increase a woman's risk.[47] These may be responsible for familial clustering of breast cancers without a well-defined pattern of inheritance. These are genes in which subtle sequence variants (polymorphisms) may be associated with a moderate increase in relative risk of breast cancer.[48]

REFERENCES

41. Peto R, Boreham J, Clarke M et al. Lancet 2000; 355: 1823
42. Korenman SG. Lancet 1980; 1: 700–701
43. Easton DF, Petro J. Cancer Surv 1990; 9: 395–416
44. Miki Y, Swenson J, Shattick-Elders D et al. Science 1994; 266: 66–71
45. Wooster R, Bignall J, Swift S et al. Nature 1998; 378: 789–792
46. Ford D, Easton DF, Stratton M et al. Am J Hum Genet 1998; 62: 678–689
47. Antoniou AC, Pharoah PD, McMullan G et al. Genet Epidemiol 2001; 21: 1-18
48. Weber BL, Nathanson KL. Eur J Cancer 2000; 36:1193–1199

It is likely that environmental factors are also influential; this is supported by the observations that it is more common in higher socioeconomic groups and that second-generation Japanese women in Hawaii who eat American-style diets tend to increase their breast cancer incidence.[49] The role of hormones and genes is probably a permissive one in conjunction with an unidentified environmental carcinogen or carcinogens. There is interest in the role of dietary saturated fats and exercise in breast cancer because there is a close correlation of fat intake nationally with breast cancer incidence (Fig. 23.22). Exposure of the breasts to radiation (i.e. after mantle radiotherapy for Hodgkin's disease) also increases the risk of breast cancer.[50]

Previous benign breast disease

Many older reports suggested an increased incidence of breast cancer in women who had been diagnosed as having benign breast disease, but reports by several American pathologists relating the component parts of benign breast histology to future cancer risk have clarified the situation. Dupont and Page have shown that only hyperplasia with atypia is associated with increased risk, especially if a family history of breast cancer is also present.[51] Most of the lesions formerly included in the non-specific umbrella terms of *fibroadenosis* or *fibrocystic disease* have not been shown to have any increased risk of subsequent breast cancer.[52] A consensus conference organized by the American College of Pathologists resulted in a much simpler classification of cancer risk. Only lobular or ductal hyperplasia with atypia are thought to be histological markers of increased cancer risk, but because these histological entities occur in just 4% of breast biopsies they are not useful as population markers; only 15% of women have ever had a breast biopsy.

Exogenous hormones: oral contraceptive

The most important exogenous hormones are the oestrogens and progestogens. The modern oral contraceptive pills are taken by millions of women from their early teens to their fourth decade. The doses of hormones are small and a 1996 overview of all the studies concluded that use of the oral contraceptive is associated with a small increase in the relative risk of breast cancer of about 1.24-fold and that this returns to the normal level of risk 10 years after stopping use.[53] This increased risk is of little significance because it is mainly young women who take the oral contraceptive when they have a low risk of developing cancer. Use of the oral contraceptive is, however, associated with a reduction in benign breast disease.[54]

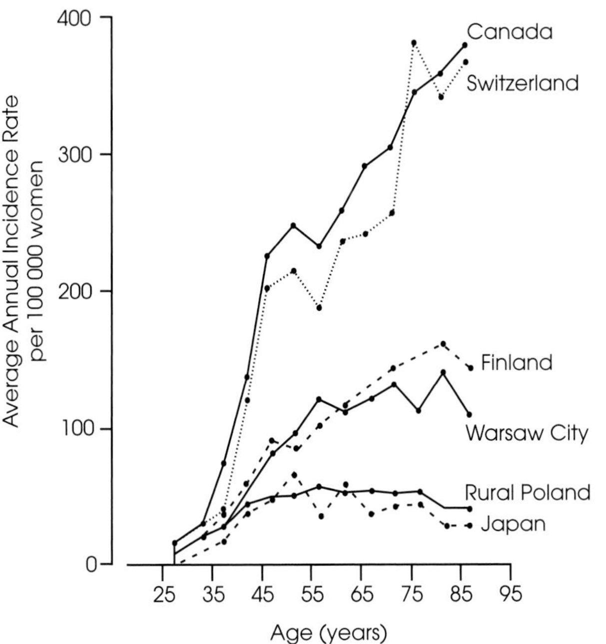

Figure 23.22 The annual incidence of breast cancer by age in different countries. Note the high incidence in Europe and Canada compared with Japan and the continuing rise with age in the high-incidence countries. (After Haagensen et al 1981,[20] with permission.)

Hormone replacement therapy

There has also been much controversy related to the risk of hormone replacement therapy as a cause of breast cancer. One of the problems associated with the use of hormone replacement therapy is the fact that it makes interpretation of mammograms more difficult: the glandular tissue is maintained by the hormone replacement therapy and this decreases the sensitivity of mammograms.[55] In 1997, an overview of all the published studies concluded that there is a small increased risk after 5 or more years of hormone replacement therapy use.[56] Most of the studies were based on women who were taking unopposed oestrogens. A large study conducted in the UK, the Million Women Study, has confirmed that hormone replacement therapy particularly combined therapy is associated with a significant increase in breast cancer incidence (relative risk 1.3 for oestrogen only and 2 for combined preparations).[57] The increased risk starts to occur after 1–2 years use. The risk decreases after hormone replacement therapy has been stopped and returns to the population level after 5 years.

Because of the increased risks of stroke, deep venous thrombosis, pulmonary embolus and in the first few years of their use coronary vascular problems, hormone replacement therapy is advocated for perimenopausal women with significant menopausal symptoms.

BREAST CANCER: CLINICAL FEATURES

Cancer of the breast is seen most commonly in women from their fourth decade of life, but the incidence of the disease continues to increase indefinitely.

Presentation

The commonest presenting feature is a painless dominant breast lump that is usually firm, irregular in outline and may be fixed to adjacent breast tissue, skin or muscle. In early cases there may be no skin changes and the diagnosis rests on the discovery of a

REFERENCES

49. Brinton LA, Hoover R, Fraumeni JF Jr. J Natl Cancer Inst 1982; 69: 817–822
50. Deniz K, O'Mahoney S, Ross G et al. Lancet Oncol 2003; 4: 207–214
51. Dupont WD, Page DL. N Engl J Med 1985; 312: 146–151
52. Page DL, Van der Zwagg R et al. J Natl Cancer Inst 1978; 61: 1055–1063
53. Collaborative Group on Hormonal Factors in Breast Cancer. Lancet 1996; 347: 1713–1727
54. Vessey MP, Baron J et al. Br J Cancer 1983; 47: 455–462
55. Kavanagh AM, Mitchele H, Giles G. Lancet 2000; 355: 270–274
56. Collaborative Group on Hormonal Factors for Breast Cancer. Lancet 1997; 350: 1047–1059
57. Million Women Study Collaborators. Lancet 2003; 362: 419–427

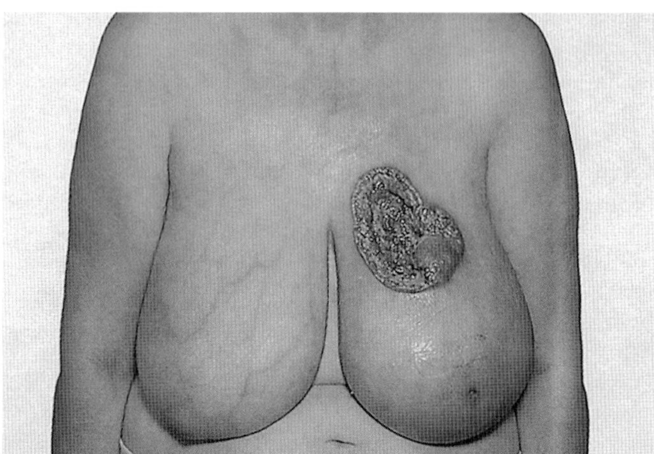

Figure 23.23 Advanced cancer of the left breast, showing ulceration of the skin as well as elevation and retraction of the nipple. The cancer shows the typical rolled edge of a malignant ulcer.

lump. In more advanced cases skin dimpling, nipple inversion, skin ulceration and palpable axillary nodes may be apparent (Fig. 23.23).

Nipple changes such as recent onset of nipple inversion or retraction, irritation and ulceration may also be presenting features of a breast cancer. Nipple retraction of slight degree is best demonstrated by raising the arms and looking for differences in nipple height in the vertical and horizontal planes. More severe degrees of retraction are obvious on simple inspection (Fig. 23.24).

A more subtle change in the nipple caused by the presence of intraepidermal large clear cells, which results in Paget's disease (Fig. 23.20). The early signs can be difficult to perceive because they may be only slight reddening of the skin with mild excoriation, not dissimilar to eczema, but eventually erosion takes place. Ultimately the whole nipple may be destroyed and the process may extend into the areolar skin. Paget's disease is usually associated with in situ or invasive carcinoma, but there may not be a palpable mass or even a radiologically evident cancer in some cases.

Another rare presentation of breast cancer is that of an 'inflammatory' cancer, which is a particularly aggressive form of breast cancer. It presents with signs of inflammation in the breast (i.e. redness, generalized oedema, heaviness and swelling) rather than as a discrete breast lump. There is often palpable axillary lymphadenopathy at presentation despite the short history given by the patient. It is often misdiagnosed as an infection of the breast, and it should be suspected if there is nothing in the history to suggest a cause for any infection, such as postpartum mastitis or periductal mastitis.

Pain in the breast is a fairly uncommon primary presentation of a small breast cancer. Preece and colleagues noted mastalgia as a presenting complaint in about 10% of operable breast cancers.[59] Although it was much less common in a large Edinburgh series (see page 510 of this chapter). Pain may be a more prominent feature in advanced breast cancer.

Occasionally a serosanguinous nipple discharge is produced by underlying ductal carcinoma in situ, but this is more commonly associated with duct ectasia or intraduct papilloma. Both serosanguinous and watery discharges may be seen in association with breast cancer, but in the series of 2437 cancers seen by Leis and coworkers only 3.4% presented with nipple discharge alone.[60]

Locally advanced or a locally recurrent breast cancer developing after initial treatment may give rise to ulceration, signs of oedema or satellite nodules, which can cause extensive infiltration of the skin of the chest, back and neck and is known as cancer en cuirasse. Localized oedema can best be seen in the areolar or dependent skin of the lower half of the breast, and when marked shows the pitted appearance of an orange skin or peau d'orange. Skin oedema is seen on mammograms and can be detected to some degree in a large proportion of cancers. Mammographic skin thickening has been shown to be a prognostic indicator for breast cancer.[61] Very rarely, areas of secondary ulceration may arise from the axillary or supraclavicular nodes.

The final stage of local disease results in destruction of the breast (automastectomy) and ulceration into the pleura with en cuirasse disease over the whole chest, back and neck; fortunately this is not often seen. The tumour may have taken many years to progress to this stage. Patients may be well aware that they have a serious disease but seek medical help only when the offensive smell of their ulcerated cancer attracts attention. Infiltration of the brachial plexus or axillary nerves can make the end stage of the disease very painful.

Breast cancer can present initially as metastatic disease and symptoms such as weight loss, debility, breathlessness, ascites or jaundice with liver secondaries, or central nervous symptoms from cerebral metastases. Rarely, hypercalcaemia as the result of massive osteolysis and leukoerythroblastic anaemia from marrow infiltration are primary presentations. Patients with bony secondaries may present with pathological fractures, especially of long bones and ribs.

An increasingly important presentation of breast cancer is the discovery of an impalpable cancer on routine screening of the breast by mammography. This is seen frequently as a result of the introduction of population screening now available for women aged 50–69 in the UK following the implementation of the Forrest report.[62] Some 20% of the cancers detected by this method are non-invasive. The invasive lesions tend to be smaller, with less node involvement than symptomatic cases, and are presumed to be biologically early lesions.[63] There is good evidence from European and US studies that screening by mammography reduces mortality from breast cancer in women over 50. Long-term follow-up of the Swedish Two Counties Trial of women screened between the ages of 40–74 has shown a 30% reduction in breast cancer mortality.[64]

Diagnosis

Most women will present to diagnostic breast clinics, where they are assessed by taking a history and performing an examination.

REFERENCES

58. MHRA. Curr Probl 2003; 29: 1–3
59. Preece PE, Baum M et al. Br Med J 1982; 284: 1299–1300
60. Leis HP Jr, Greene FL et al. South Med J 1988; 81: 22
61. Shukla HS, Gravelle IJ et al. Br Med J1984; 288: 1338–1341
62. Department of Health and Social Services. Forrest Report: Breast Cancer Screening. HMSO, London, 1986
63. Walls J, Boggis et al. Br J Surg 1993; 80: 436–438
64. Tabar L, Vitak B, Chen H et al. Radiol Clin North Am 2000; 38: 625–651

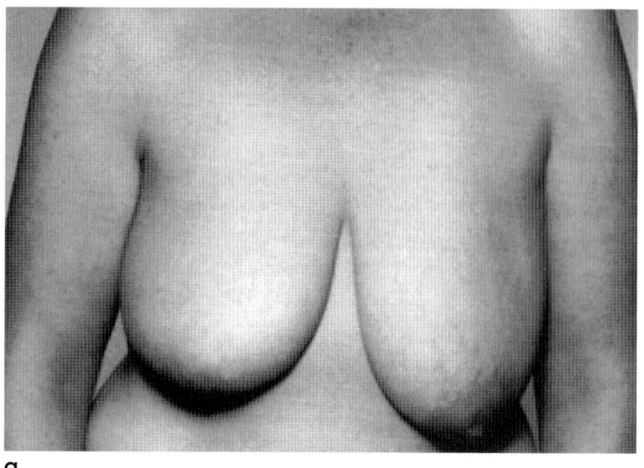

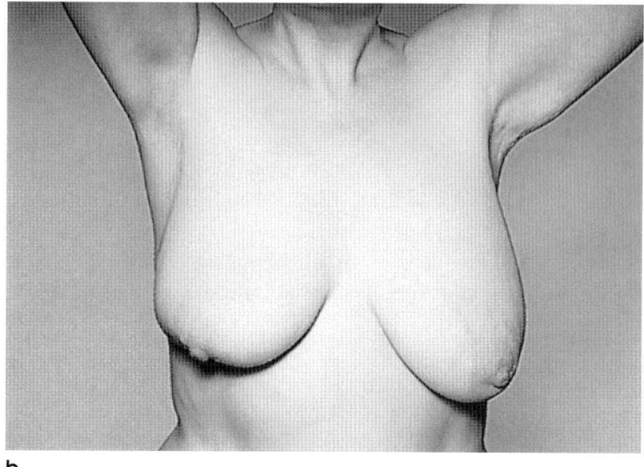

Figure 23.24 Inspection of the breasts with arms by the side (**a**); note the alteration of contour and nipple height in the right breast, which contains the cancer. With arms raised (**b**), the altered contour is exaggerated by elevating the breast.

All breast lumps should undergo triple assessment. In women over 35 years mammography should be performed both as a diagnostic test on the symptomatic breast and as a check on the other breast. It is an accurate diagnostic method in breast cancer, with rates of 80–95% depending on the experience of the radiologist.[65] It is less accurate in younger women with dense glandular breast tissue and in deep-seated or peripherally situated tumours.

The mammographic signs of malignancy are a mass lesion with irregular edges, called spiculation, which may be associated with fine scattered microcalcification. Distortion of the normal parenchymal markings may also be seen, and thickening may be evident in the skin over the quadrant harbouring the cancer. Some cancers may appear as discrete rounded masses with smooth edges and mimic fibroadenomas or cysts. An example of a mammographic cancer is shown in Fig. 23.25, but approximately 10–15% of palpable cancers are invisible on mammography, and this is more common for invasive lobular carcinomas.[66]

Ultrasound examination is also used to define abnormalities and guide biopsies of palpable or impalpable abnormalities. Magnetic resonance imaging is not used routinely for the assessment of breast cancers, but it can be useful to look for impalpable cancers in patients who present with axillary lymphadenopathy or to assess recurrence after previous treatment for breast cancer.[67,68]

Accurate diagnosis requires pathological examination of the tumour, because clinical diagnosis is unreliable even in the presence of signs normally associated with cancer. A preoperative diagnosis of cancer should normally be made before definitive surgery. Diagnosis is usually made by taking a needle core biopsy, which is assessed histologically. If Paget's disease of the nipple is suspected, a punch biopsy of the nipple can be taken under local anaesthetic in the outpatient clinic.

Figure 23.25 Craniocaudal mammographic views of both breasts, showing a mass lesion with irregular margins and spicules in the outer half of the right breast, typical of carcinoma of the breast.

Other investigations

Patients who are diagnosed with early-stage breast cancer do not need any other investigations because detection rates for metastatic disease are extremely low. Patients with locally advanced breast cancers should have a routine chest X-ray and liver function tests performed to exclude pulmonary and hepatic metastases. A bone scan and liver ultrasound scan or CT scan may be helpful if the blood tests for liver and bone profile are abnormal. Focal areas of acute bone pain in the long bones should be radiographed to pick up pathological fractures and lytic or sclerotic deposits. Measurement of serum CA15-3 may be helpful to monitor progress of metastatic disease, but this should not be used as a diagnostic test for breast cancer.

REFERENCES

65. Locker AP, Manhire AR et al. Lancet 1989; i: 887–889
66. Mendelson EB, Harris KM, Doshi N et al. Am J Radiol 1989; 153: 256–271
67. Drew PJ, Turnbull LW, Chatterjee S et al. Ann Surg 1999; 230: 680–685
68. Drew PJ, Chatterjee S, Turnbull L et al. Ann Surg Oncol 1999; 6: 599–603

Special techniques for screen-detected cancers

The small asymptomatic cancers detected on mammography are often impalpable and require localization by ultrasound or stereotactic methods to achieve a biopsy. These cancers show up as small mass lesions, spiculated lesions disturbances of architecture or clustered microcalcifications. Most lesions can be seen by ultrasound and a core biopsy can thus be taken. Microcalcifications are often not associated with a mass lesion and in these circumstances cannot usually be seen by ultrasound, so methods of stereotactic fine-needle aspiration cytology and biopsy may be needed.

If a definitive diagnostic biopsy is required or if a small impalpable cancer requires localization for definitive surgery, the principal method used to guide the surgeon to the impalpable lesion is the hooked wire technique (Figs 23.26 and 23.27). Ultrasound or X-ray with or without stereotactic methods are used to place the needle as close to the abnormality as possible, and a hooked wire is pushed down the needle and engaged in the breast tissue. The wire is left in the breast, mammograms are taken, and the wire acts as a guide to the surgeon as to the location of the radiological abnormality.

The excised tissue is assessed radiographically immediately on removal to confirm that the abnormal area has been excised. Localization biopsies or treatments are always subjected to paraffin histology and not frozen section, because the differentiation between DCIS and hyperplasia is difficult and depends on optimal cytological detail. The margins of the surgical specimen also require careful histological assessment.

Box 23.3 Differential diagnosis of breast cancer

20–30 years
- Fibroadenoma

30–60 years
- Cystic disease
- Aberrations of normal development and involution
- Intraduct papilloma
- Phyllodes tumour

Any age
- Duct ectasia
- Periductal mastitis
- Fat necrosis

Radiological
- Sclerosing adenosis
- Microcystic disease
- Aberrations of normal development and involution
- Radial scars or complex sclerosing lesions
- Fibroadenoma

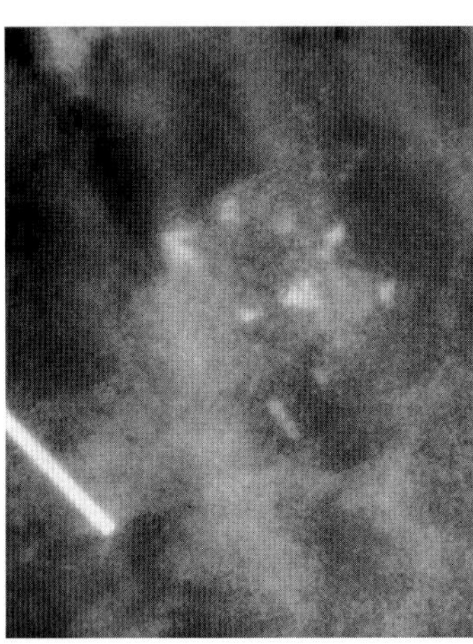

Figure 23.26 Magnification view of a mammogram showing microcalcification caused by DCIS. The wire marker inserted to localize the calcifications is also seen.

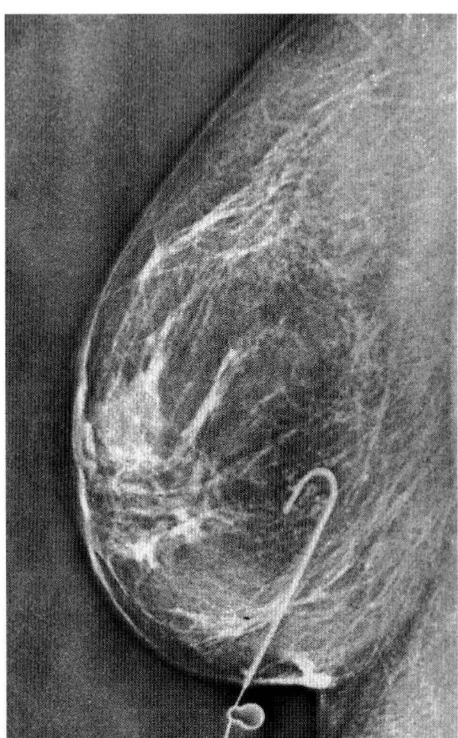

Figure 23.27 Mammogram with a hooked needle in situ before biopsy. The mammographic abnormality is a small cluster of calcifications shown within the head of the hooked wire.

Differential diagnosis

Because breast cancer can occur from the age of 16 years upwards, it may be confused with any of the benign diseases that give rise to a lump or skin changes. The main differential diagnoses are given in Box 23.3, but most confusion occurs in women in the 30–50-year age group, where cysts and breast nodularity can be misdiagnosed clinically as carcinoma. Cysts can be confusing when they are multilocular, with extensive fibrosis, or when they produce skin tethering by distorting the breast architecture. Circumscribed carcinomas in younger women are often mistaken for fibroadenomas. Conversely, well-circumscribed, radiologically benign masses in elderly women may be a mucinous carcinoma. A good mimic of breast cancer is, however, the inflammatory phase of periductal mastitis, which produces induration, redness and nipple retraction and can be indistinguishable clinically from a breast cancer.

Radiologically the most confusing problem is the microcalcification seen in common conditions such as cystic disease or sclerosing adenosis. It can be impossible to differentiate from DCIS—although the number and size of the particles of calcium can be helpful—as numerous small, sharp, irregularly sized and shaped spicules suggest cancer. The stellate appearance of complex sclerosing lesions or radial scars is also difficult to distinguish from small well-differentiated cancers.

Staging

Breast cancer can be staged in a variety of ways, but the two major clinical systems are the Union International Contre le Cancer (UICC) classification, which incorporates TNM (tumour, node and metastasis), and the Manchester classification, which are essentially similar. All the systems describe the clinical staging

Table 23.3 The UICC TNM classification (fifth revision, 1997)[69]

Designation	Definition
Primary tumour	
TX	Not assessable
T0	No primary tumour
TIS	Carcinoma in situ or Paget's
T1	≤ 2 cm
T1a	< 0.5 cm
T1b	0.6–1 cm
T1c	1.1–2 cm
T2	> 2 cm but < 5 cm
T3	> 5 cm
T4	Any size with chest wall or skin extension
T4a	Chest wall
T4b	Oedema, ulceration or nodules
T4c	Both 4a and 4b
T4d	Inflammatory cancer
Nodes	
NX	Not assessable
N0	No node metastasis
N1	Ipsilateral* axillary (mobile) disease
N2	Ipsilateral* axillary (fixed)
N3	Ipsilateral* internal mammary nodes
Distant metastases	
MX	Not assessable
M0	No distant metastases
M1	Distant metastases present

*Any other lymph node metastases are coded M1.
(From the International Union Against Cancer,[69] with permission of Wiley-Liss.)

of the disease by reference to the primary tumour, regional nodal areas and systemic disease, but the more universal and comprehensive UICC system is to be preferred.[69] The UICC system is summarized in Table 23.3 and describes the size of the primary tumour from T0 (subclinical) to T4 (any size with fixity or ulceration).

The approximate equivalent terms of the main staging systems are shown in Table 23.4. The clinical staging systems are accurate for definition of tumour size, but estimation of nodal involvement by palpation is inaccurate because studies show that palpable nodes are frequently not invaded by tumour on microscopic examination and vice versa. In the fifth revision of TNM codes, stages have been added to take account of additional information from sentinel nodes.[69]

Pathology

The classification of breast cancer used to be based on the belief that certain tumours arise from lobules and others arise from ducts, but it has increasingly become clear that it is impossible to say which cells give rise to most tumours. The 1982 revision of the World Health Organization classification simply divides the tumours into those arising from epithelial cells and those arising from connective tissues (Box 23.4).[70] This classification is based on histological appearance alone and thus recognizes the difficulty in determining the cell of origin of each individual tumour. The malignant tumours of epithelial origin are divided into the non-invasive lobular or ductal in situ carcinomas and the invasive tumours have many subgroups. By far the commonest type of all is the invasive ductal carcinoma of no special type,

Table 23.4 Breast cancer staging systems*

TNM	Manchester	Columbia
T0–T1, N0–N1a	Stage I	Stage A
N1b	–	–
T2	Stage II	Stage B
T3–T4	Stage III	Stage C
N2–N3	–	–
M1	Stage IV	Stage D

*These are approximate equivalents because all three sections are different in points of detail.

Box 23.4 The pathology of primary breast cancer: World Health Organization classification

Percentages indicate proportions of all breast carcinomas.

Epithelial tumours

Non-invasive

- Intraductal carcinoma or ductal carcinoma in situ (DCIS)
- Lobular carcinoma in situ (LCIS)

Invasive

- Invasive ductal carcinoma (not otherwise specified) (80–90%)
- Invasive ductal with predominant DCIS component
- Invasive lobular (1–2%)
- Mucinous carcinoma (5%)
- Medullary carcinoma (1–5%)
- Papillary carcinoma (rare)
- Tubular carcinoma (2%)
- Adenoid cystic carcinoma (rare)
- Secretory carcinoma
- Apocrine carcinoma (1%)
- Carcinoma with metaplasia (rare)
- Paget's disease (2%)

Others

- Mixed connective tissue and epithelial
- Miscellaneous (e.g. skin or soft tissue)
- Unclassified tumours

(Based on World Health Organization classification.[70])

which in most symptomatic series forms around 80–90% of all carcinomas of the breast.

The non-invasive tumours are becoming increasingly important as modern screening methods are detecting more of these types. Lobular carcinoma in situ (LCIS) is uncommon, being seen in some 1% of biopsies, and usually occurs as an incidental finding in premenopausal women. It is frequently multifocal and bilateral.[71] The finding of lobular neoplasia (atypical lobular neoplasia, atypical lobular hyperplasia and LCIS) has been shown to be a risk factor for subsequent

REFERENCES

69. International Union Against Cancer. TNM Classification. 5th edn. Wiley-Liss, New York, 1997
70. Azzopardi JG, Chepick OF et al. Am J Clin Pathol 1982; 78: 806–816
71. Lakani SR. Lancet 2003; 361: 96

carcinoma in both breasts. Molecular studies of atypical lobular hyperplasia and LCIS show DNA mutations similar to each other and to those of invasive carcinoma, and they are therefore considered to be premalignant conditions. Long-term follow-up of LCIS treated by simple excision shows that invasive cancer subsequently occurs in up to 40% of women in either breast.[72]

Ductal carcinoma in situ in isolation forms only 3–5% of pathological series of symptomatic breast cancers but is much more common in association with invasive ductal cancers. Series of screen-detected cancers, however, show a much higher incidence of DCIS: up to 30% in some series. This is because it is readily detected as fine microcalcification on mammography. In this condition the cells are packed into the ducts in varying architectural patterns but do not show invasion outside the basement membrane of the duct.

There are several different types of DCIS, such as comedo, cribriform, solid, papillary and clinging, depending on the architectural pattern within the tumour. Mixtures of these subtypes may be seen, but the tumour is classified by the predominant pattern. The comedo type is more likely to be associated with multicentric disease and is thought to have a worse prognosis than the cribriform type. More recent classifications are based on cytonuclear grades, which are described as high, intermediate or low, and the presence or absence of necrosis.[73] These factors are considered in the Van Nuys prognostic index, which has been shown to correlate well with prognosis in locally excised DCIS.[74]

The significance of DCIS is that it is a premalignant condition; some 30% of women who have been followed after incomplete local excision of this entity have gone on to develop ipsilateral invasive carcinoma.[75,76] When DCIS is seen around an invasive cancer the degree of cellular activity of the in situ and invasive cancers are very similar. The risk of metastases in pure DCIS is very low (1%) and is probably due to missed areas of invasion. The rare intracystic carcinoma should also be considered as an in situ cancer.

Invasive ductal cancers form the majority of breast cancers, especially the category of 'not otherwise specified'. This term simply recognizes the fact that most invasive ductal cancers are undifferentiated and cannot be easily classified in terms of morphology. The specified types of invasive ductal cancer are listed in Box 23.4, but invasive lobular, medullary, mucinous and tubular are the commonest variants. These special subtypes form only 10% of all breast cancers. The differentiation between these subtypes is based on microscopy, but the significance of the invasive subtypes is that they tend to be better differentiated and hence have a better prognosis than the 'not otherwise specified' type. Invasive lobular cancer often presents as an ill-defined mass or a thickening that is often diffuse and multifocal. Microscopically, the malignant cells merge with normal tissue and form 'Indian files'.

Paget's disease of the nipple is a special category of DCIS where the nipple skin contains large pale cells and nipple erosion occurs eventually. This condition is usually associated with an underlying invasive cancer or DCIS.

In the mixed connective and epithelial section of the classification, the most common tumour is the phyllodes tumour (formerly known as cystosarcoma phyllodes). This is a circumscribed neoplasm with a leaf-like structure composed of stroma and epithelial elements, which have a spectrum from benign to malignant depending on the varying degrees of cellularity and mitotic rate. Predicting the behaviour of this tumour is difficult, but lesions with a high mitotic rate, cellular atypia and infiltrative margins tend to recur locally after simple excision, and thus should be widely excised.

Pathological prognostic factors

Tumour grade is a good predictor of subsequent prognosis, and is based on cytological and structural patterns in the primary breast cancer. Most systems are based on the Bloom and Richardson classification[77] modified by Ellis and Elston,[78] which allocates three grades from 1 (well differentiated) to 3 (poorly differentiated). This system is based on the amount of tubule formation, pleomorphism and mitotic activity. Low grade breast cancers, such as tubular and lobular carcinomas, have a good long-term prognosis[79] but tend to be uncommon. Some subtypes, such as the medullary tumour, would score grade 3 on the Bloom and Richardson scale but are known to have a good prognosis. Observer variation is a problem in tumour grading. Lymphovascular invasion seen in and around the primary tumour and multicentric tumours within the breast are also pathological markers of poor prognosis.

Cancerous invasion of the regional nodes demonstrated on histology (positive nodes) is an excellent predictor of subsequent prognosis (Fig. 23.28).[80] Fisher and colleagues, in their analyses of 505 patients with known nodal involvement enrolled in the National Surgical Adjuvant Breast and Bowel Project, showed that an increasing number of positive nodes correlated very well with worsening prognosis.[81] Patients with more than five positive nodes had a 5-year survival rate of less than 20%. Histological examination of the regional nodes is the only reliable method of determining lymph node involvement because clinical examination and imaging methods underestimate this.

Modern histological methods can be used to look for micrometastases, which are tumour deposits of less than 2 mm in axillary nodes. Conventional techniques or special techniques, such as immunohistochemistry for cytokeratin-positive cells, can be used. The prognostic significance of these findings is uncertain at the present time.

Several biochemical markers of prognosis have been proposed but few have been demonstrated to be of clinical value. The presence of oestrogen receptor protein in the primary tumour has, however, been found to be useful for predicting response to endocrine therapy and for short term survival.[82,83] Between 50 and 85% of breast cancers express oestrogen receptors. The progesterone receptor, which is itself regulated by the oestrogen

REFERENCES

72. Van Dongen JA, Fentiman IS et al. Lancet 1989; 2: 25–27
73. Shoker BS, Sloane JP. Histopathology 1999; 35: 393–400
74. Silverstein MJ, Lagios MD, Graig PH et al. Cancer 1996; 72: 2267–2274
75. Rosen PP, Brown DW, Kinnie DW. Cancer 1980; 40: 919–925
76. Page DL, Dupont WD et al. Cancer 1982; 49: 751–758
77. Bloom HJG, Richardson WW. Br J Cancer 1957; 11: 359–377
78. Elston CW, Ellis JO. Histopathology 1991; 19: 403–410
79. Dixon JM, Page DL et al. Br J Surg 1985; 72: 445–448
80. Julien JB, Bijker N, Fentiman IS et al. Lancet 2000; 358: 528–533
81. Fisher B, Bauer M et al. Cancer 1983; 52: 1551–1557
82. Clark GM, McGuire WL. Breast Cancer Res Treat 1983; 3 (Suppl): 69
83. Howell A, Barnes DM et al. Lancet 1984; 1: 588–591

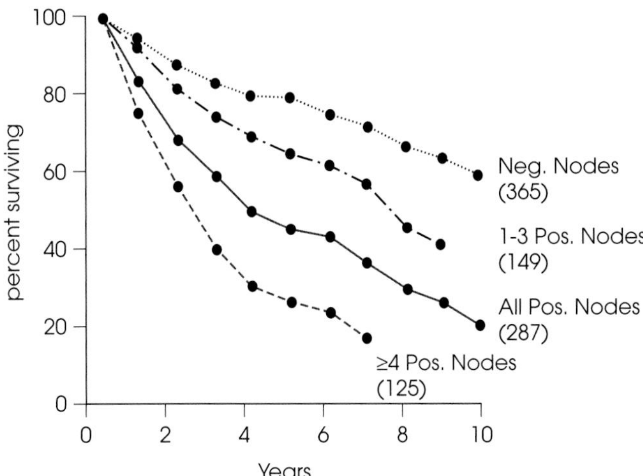

Figure 23.28 Life table survival curve showing the effect of increasing numbers of pathologically involved axillary nodes on survival. Nodal status is the most powerful prognostic factor. Numbers in parentheses indicate patient numbers. Neg, negative; pos, positive.[80]

receptor, was reported to be of even greater prognostic value[84] but there is little evidence that reporting of both adds much more to the prognostic information. Oestrogen receptor status is currently assessed by immunohistochemical techniques and should be assessed routinely on all breast cancer specimens.

Following the identification and production of a humanized monoclonal antibody (trastuzumab) that blocks the HER2 pathway, there has been renewed interest in HER2 or c-erb B-2, which is a member of the epidermal growth factor family. It is over-expressed in about 30% of breast cancers. HER2 amplification is associated with node positivity, oestrogen receptor negativity and a poor clinical outcome. Suitable patients for trastuzumab treatment can be identified using immunohistochemistry showing protein over-expression or by fluorescent in situ hybridization to demonstrate gene amplification.

The different prognostic factors have been incorporated into a single index devised by multifactorial analyses of the individual weighting of each prognostic factor to the whole. The most important prognostic factors are node status, tumour grade and the size of the primary tumour. These three factors are incorporated into the Nottingham prognostic index (NPI).[85] This is calculated using the formula

$$\text{NPI} = 0.2 \times \text{tumour size (cm)} + \text{lymph node stage} + \text{grade (1–3)},$$

where stage is given as 1 for no lymph nodes, 2 for one to three nodes, and 3 for more than three nodes. An NPI of less than 3.4 indicates a good prognosis, 3.4–5.4 a moderate prognosis, and greater than 5.4 a poor prognosis.

TREATMENT OF BREAST CANCER

Treatment depends on the stage of the disease at presentation and has three specific aims:

1. the control of local disease,
2. the control of systemic disease, and
3. the maintenance of cosmesis if possible.

Historical note

The early concept of breast cancer was that it spread from the breast, via lymphatics, to regional nodes and thence systemically. Treatment was directed at removal of the breast, lymphatic pathways and regional nodes in the Halsted mastectomy. The continuing mortality from breast cancer after radical local therapy brought the realization that early spread by the bloodstream was a more common means of dissemination, and that the micrometastases responsible are probably present at the time of diagnosis in most patients with symptomatic breast cancer. The fact that the axillary nodes are involved in some 40–60% of operable breast cancers was realized to be a prognostic marker of systemic metastases rather than a filter mechanism trapping cancer cells escaping from the breast.

Micrometastases may arise from very small invasive cancers, although they are unusual in cancers smaller than 5 mm in diameter. The rate of growth of micrometastases can be quite slow, taking many years to appear as secondary disease. Data from long-term studies suggest that distant disease may appear up to 40 years after removal of the primary tumour by mastectomy,[86] and it could be argued that only some 20% of breast cancer patients are truly cured of their disease.

These considerations and observations have become embodied in the current philosophy that the outlook for most patients with breast cancer is predetermined by the biological fact of early metastatic spread by the bloodstream, that local therapy is therefore likely to affect only the control of the primary disease, and that systemic adjuvant therapy is needed to control micrometastases. Local therapy can be curative when the cancer is truly confined to the breast, but it is not possible to say whether the disease is totally confined (although it is more likely if it is pure DCIS).

Treatment for DCIS

Ductal carcinoma in situ is the preinvasive stage of the disease, so there is potential to treat and cure patients who present at this stage. With the introduction of breast screening the number of cases of DCIS has increased, and most of them are impalpable and asymptomatic. Previously, when symptomatic DCIS was diagnosed it was traditionally treated by mastectomy, but it was thought that mastectomy was over-treatment for localized areas of DCIS when invasive cancers were being treated with breast conservation surgery. Thus a wire-guided wide excision of a mammographic abnormality diagnosed as DCIS can be performed. After breast conservation surgery there is a risk of local recurrence that can be either further DCIS or invasive disease. Several studies have shown that the risk of recurrence is increased if the original lesion is not completely excised with a clear margin, if the lesion is larger than 40 mm, and if it is of high cytological grade with necrosis. These factors have been grouped together by Silverstein to form the Van Nuys prognostic index.[74] Age is another prognostic factor that should be considered because young women have a 25% risk of recurrence, compared with 10% for women older than 50 years.[87]

There have been several trials to assess whether or not radiotherapy can reduce the risk of local recurrence after breast

REFERENCES

84. Clark GM, McGuire WL et al. N Engl J Med 1983; 309: 1343–1347
85. Haybittle JL, Blamey RW, Elston CW et al. Br J Cancer 1982; 45: 361–366
86. Brinkley D, Haybittle JL. Lancet 1984; 1: 1118
87. Szelci-Stevens KA, Kushe RR, Yantsos VA et al. Int J Radiat Oncol Biol Phys 2000; 48: 943–949

Table 23.5 Comparison of DCIS trials[88,89,91]

	B17		EORTC[a] 10853		B-24	
Design	Breast conservation surgery versus breast conservation surgery plus deep X-ray therapy		Breast conservation surgery versus breast conservation surgery plus deep X-ray therapy		Breast conservation surgery plus deep X-ray therapy with or without tamoxifen	
Number enrolled	818		1010		1804	
Number excluded	4		8		6	
Follow-up (years)	8		4		5	
Events	Breast conservation surgery	Plus deep X-ray therapy	Breast conservation surgery	Plus deep X-ray therapy	Placebo	Tamoxifen
Ipsilateral invasive recurrence	53	17[b]	40	24[c]	40	23[c]
Ipsilateral non-invasive	51	30[c]	44	29	47	40
Contralateral invasive cancer	11	11	5	16	23	15
Contralateral DCIS	2	8	3	12	13	3[c]
Regional and distant metastases	5	7	12	12	7	3
Total in group	403	411	506	502	899	899

[a]European Organization for Research and Treatment of Cancer, [b]$P < 0.001$, [c]$P < 0.05$.

conservation surgery. The National Surgical Adjuvant Breast Project (NSABP) 17,[88] European Organization for Research and Treatment of Cancer,[80] and UK DCIS[89] studies have shown a reduction in the number of cases of in situ and invasive recurrences following radiotherapy (Table 23.5). The risk of recurrence is, however, affected by the cytological grade of the DCIS, and therefore areas of low-grade DCIS less than 20 mm may be adequately treated by wide excision alone if they are completely excised. The role of tamoxifen in the management of localized DCIS is less clear, as demonstrated by the results of the UK DCIS study[89] and NSABP 24,[90] which showed a non-significant reduction in risk of invasive recurrence in postmenopausal women but not premenopausal women. Further analysis has shown that this benefit is for oestrogen receptor-positive DCIS.

Mastectomy is, however, still advised for women with multicentric DCIS or an area larger than 40 mm, because even with radiotherapy and tamoxifen there is an unacceptably high rate of recurrence if these patients are treated by breast conservation surgery and larger deep X-ray therapy (XRT) alone.[74]

The management of the axilla in pure DCIS remains controversial. The nodal status should not be assessed where there are localized areas of DCIS treated by breast conservation surgery. If, however, a mastectomy is performed for extensive DCIS many people would advocate sampling the lower nodes in case an invasive focus is subsequently found in the breast specimen.

Women who have been treated for DCIS by breast conservation surgery with or without XRT should be monitored closely in case they develop recurrent disease. A baseline mammogram of the treated side should be performed 6 months after surgery and then bilateral annual mammograms should be taken. If recurrent disease is diagnosed it should be treated by mastectomy. If the recurrence is invasive the nodal status should be assessed and appropriate systemic adjuvant treatment given postoperatively.

The management of DCIS continues to be refined in the light of new evidence, trial results, and the development of new treatment strategies.

Treatment of invasive breast cancer: operable disease

Most women diagnosed with breast cancer bring with them to the consultation many preconceptions—and often misconceptions—about the options for managing the disease. Each patient should be discussed at a multidisciplinary meeting with pathologists, radiologists, surgeons and oncologists. A discussion should then occur between the surgeon and the patient, assisted by a specialist breast care nurse to explain the treatment options that are available. Involvement in the decision-making process is beneficial to the patient's well-being.[91] There is, however, no difference in the psychological outcome between women who have a mastectomy and those who have breast conservation surgery.[92] Women who choose a mastectomy tend to have excessive concern about their illness.[93]

For operable carcinoma—usually defined as T1–3, N0 or N1, and M0 by the UICC staging or stages 1, 2 and some 3 by the Manchester staging—many women can be offered a choice of treatment, i.e. breast conservation surgery, which excises the breast tumour and preserves the breast shape, or mastectomy.

REFERENCES

88. Fisher FR, Dignam J, Tan Chiu et al. Cancer 1999; 86: 429–438
89. UK Coordinating Committee on Cancer Research Ductal Carcinoma in Situ Working Party. Lancet 2003; 362: 95–102
90. Fisher B, Dignam J, Wolmark N et al. Lancet 1999; 353: 1993-2000
91. Deadman JM, Leinster SJ, Owens RG et al. Soc Sci Med 2001; 53: 669–677
92. Fallowfield L, Hall A, Maguire G et al. Br Med J 1990; 301: 575
93. Black W, Pilowsky L, Gill G. Breast 1995; 4: 196–199

Formerly, Halsted radical mastectomy was predominant, especially in the USA, but the modified radical mastectomy (Patey) then became more popular. This in turn was supplanted by simple mastectomy with radiotherapy to the axilla to cover disease in the axillary nodes. A large study carried out by the National Surgical Adjuvant Breast and Bowel Project in the USA compared radical mastectomy with total mastectomy with or without radiation and found no differences in overall survival or local recurrence between the groups at 10 years.[94,95] In this study, 50 Gy were given to the axilla in clinically node-negative patients and a further boost of 10 Gy to the node-positive patients. In general, local recurrence rates of around 8% in node-positive patients and 4% in node-negative patients at 5 years were obtainable by surgical treatment with mastectomy and axillary clearance or by simple mastectomy with adjuvant radiotherapy.[94]

Until the mid 1970s, mastectomy was the standard treatment for women with breast cancer. Mastectomy is still indicated if there is widespread DCIS, if there are multifocal invasive cancers, and if the tumour is larger than 2–3 cm in diameter in a small or moderate-size breast. Central tumours have traditionally been treated by mastectomy, but some small localized tumours can be treated by central excision of the breast, including the nipple–areola complex, with reshaping of the breast.

Breast conservation surgery

Since the 1980s, there has been a move towards breast conservation on the grounds that better cosmesis can be obtained with no difference in survival. Controlled studies were carried out by Veronesi's group in Milan[95] and Fisher's group in the USA.[96] Veronesi and colleagues compared conventional Halsted mastectomy with quadrantectomy, surgical axillary clearance and radiotherapy to the breast (QUART). This trial was run from 1973 to 1980 and involved 701 patients, all with T1 tumours and without palpable axillary nodes. Those who had a quandrantectomy were given a dose of 50 Gy (5000 rad) to the breast, with a local boost using high-energy photons of 10 Gy to the tumour bed. At 8 years, the disease-free survival rate was 77% in the Halsted mastectomy group and 80% in the QUART group, but there was a higher rate of local recurrence within the QUART group, which the researchers attributed to second primary tumours rather than recurrences.

The American trial run by Fisher (NSABP B-06) compared lumpectomy with axillary irradiation against total mastectomy with axillary dissection in 1843 women.[96] In the lumpectomy patients the margins of excision were examined to ensure that they were clear of microscopic tumour. A total mastectomy was carried out if the margins were found to contain tumour, and this occurred in some 10% of the patients. In the lumpectomy and irradiation group, a minimum of 50 Gy was given over 5 weeks, with no boost to the scar. The results of this trial showed that lumpectomy alone did not control local recurrence in the ipsilateral breast because 30% of patients suffered from this problem. When radiation to the breast was added to lumpectomy, the local recurrence rate fell to around 10% at 5 years. No survival differences were, however, shown between the lumpectomy plus radiotherapy and the mastectomy groups.

Several studies have shown no differences in mortality between mastectomy and breast conservation, but local recurrence is slightly higher in the conserved breast. Local recurrence rates after conservation are currently 1% or less per year. Factors that predispose to local recurrence are incomplete excision, poor histological differentiation (grade 3), lymphovascular invasion, and extensive DCIS both within and around the invasive component.[97–100]

The Milan trial and the NSABP B-06 trial showed good results for conservation, but the tumour excision was radical in the conservation arms of both trials because quadrantectomy was performed and clear pathological margins were confirmed in the NSABP B-06 trial; axillary clearance was used in both. These results highlight the need to confirm tumour excision margins pathologically if a policy of breast conservation is adopted. A further Milan trial compared QUART with tumourectomy and radiation, and showed that narrower excision margins resulted in a higher local recurrence (13.3% versus 5.3%), although cosmesis was better and survival was unaffected.[101] The long-term safety and efficacy of breast conservation surgery was confirmed by the publication of the long-term results of these original randomized trials.[102,103]

The guiding principle of all breast conservation surgery should be the complete excision of the invasive tumour and any surrounding DCIS, with confident histological confirmation that the excision margins are free of disease. The tumour should be excised, aiming for a 1 cm margin of macroscopically normal tissue. The specimen should be oriented for the pathologist and the margins should be inked to allow proper histological evaluation. Whether or not a patient is suitable for breast conservation depends on the size of the tumour compared with the rest of the breast, because excision of more than 10% of the breast volume leaves a poorer cosmetic result. This should then be followed by radiotherapy to the rest of the breast (Fig. 23.29).

A further problem is that the anticipated psychological benefits of conservation therapy have not clearly emerged in practice. Some research has shown no differences in psychological debility between mastectomy and conservation patients who were given a choice of therapy. A randomized trial by Schain and coworkers showed that mastectomy patients reported less control over events in their lives, more problems with sexual relations, and more degrees of distress looking at their nude bodies than patients treated by lumpectomy.[104] The expected improvement in psychiatric morbidity in the patients with conserved breasts may be replaced by an increased anxiety regarding recurrence in the conserved breast; the end result appears to be similar short-term morbidity in both conservation and mastectomy groups.[105]

The current trend is towards use of conservation techniques, although careful long-term follow-up of these patients is

REFERENCES

94. Fisher B, Bauer M et al. N Engl J Med 1985; 312: 665–673
95. Veronesi U, Zucali R, Vecchio MD. World J Surg 1985; 9: 676–681
96. Fisher B, Redmond C, Poisson R et al. N Engl J Med 1989; 320: 822–828
97. Locker AP, Elias IO et al. Br J Surg 1989; 76: 890–894
98. Harris JR, Connolly JL et al. Ann Surg 1985; 201: 164–169
99. Bulman A, Lindley RP et al. Ann R Coll Surg Engl 1988; 70: 289–292
100. Veronesi V, Banfi A, Salvador B et al. Eur J Cancer 1990; 26: 668–770
101. Veronesi V, Volterrani F, Luini A et al. Eur J Cancer 1990; 26: 671–673
102. Veronesi U, Cascinelli N et al. N Engl J Med 2002; 347: 1227–1232
103. Fisher B, Anderson S, Bryant J et al. N Engl J Med 2002; 347: 1233–1241
104. Schain WS et al. Cancer 1994; 73: 1221-1228
105. Fallowfield L. Patient Educ Couns 1997; 30: 209–214

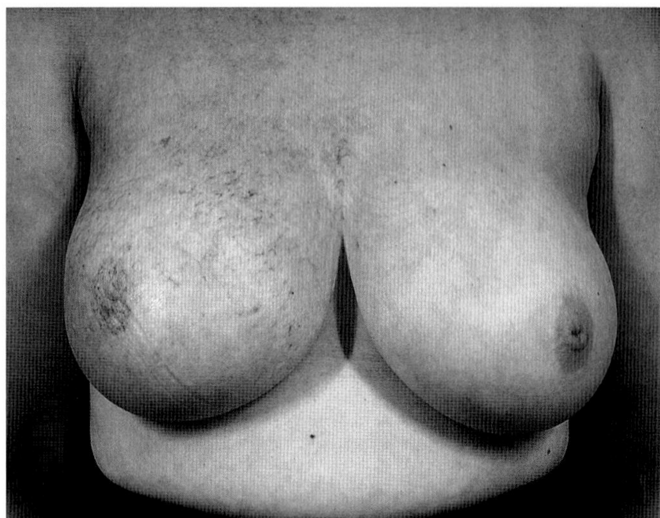

Figure 23.29 Breast conservation surgery, showing preservation of the breast shape.

important because the risk of recurrence can continue for at least 10 years. Risk factors for local recurrence are young age (less than 35 years), high tumour grade, vascular invasion, and presence of extensive intraduct component associated with involved margins.

Detection of a recurrence in an irradiated breast can be difficult because the postradiation fibrosis makes both palpation and mammography difficult to interpret. Magnetic resonance imaging has proved to be useful in detecting recurrence in an irradiated breast.[106] Long-term follow-up also includes surveillance of the contralateral breast by mammography, because there is a risk of developing a second cancer (1% per year).

When local recurrence does occur it is usually treated by mastectomy with or without reconstruction. Salvage mastectomies can be technically difficult and may need a myocutaneous flap to give sound healing in previously irradiated tissues. It is reported that the outlook after salvage mastectomy for local recurrence secondary to conservation is as good as that for the initial conservation group, but so far follow-up is short and series are small. Kurtz and colleagues reported 118 salvage operations for local recurrences in the breast after conservation treatment of stage I and II cancers.[107] They performed mastectomy in 56% and further wide excision in the others. After a median follow-up of 7 years, they reported an actuarial survival of 72% at 5 years and 58% at 10 years. Further local recurrence occurred in 17% of the patients.

Axillary surgery

Management of the axilla is still a controversial area, and options range from axillary clearance, to sampling, to sentinel node biopsy. Complete axillary clearance has been the standard treatment with a radical or modified radical mastectomy. Because this procedure is not without morbidity (lymphoedema, paraesthesia and shoulder stiffness), lesser procedures have been advocated.

Surgical clearance of the axillary nodes has the advantage of accurate staging of lymph node metastases for prognostic purposes, but node sampling or excising the level I and II nodes has been reported to be as accurate.[108] In stage I and II cancers, involved nodes are very common when assessed histologically, even when nodes are not clinically palpable, as shown in the Milan trial.[96] Most series show that if the axilla is cleared and examined pathologically, about 27% will have involved nodes in stage I cases and 40–50% in clinical stage II cases. A large Danish study showed that the extent of the nodal dissection is inversely correlated with the risk of local recurrence.[109]

Nodes can also be obtained by a sampling operation that removes at least four of the lower axillary nodes. A randomized study comparing axillary clearance and sampling with selective use of axillary radiotherapy has shown no difference in time to recurrence or any difference in survival.[110,111] The Danish Breast Cancer Group analysed the number of lymph nodes removed with axillary sampling and the risk of local recurrence.[112] The 5-year probability of axillary recurrence was 19% when no nodes were found, 10% when one or two negative nodes were removed, 5% when three or four negative nodes were removed, and 3% when five nodes were removed. The researchers therefore advise that at least four nodes must be examined to achieve acceptable accuracy for axillary staging. If the nodes are positive then radiotherapy can be given to the axilla, but this should not be done after an axillary clearance because of an unacceptable rate of lymphoedema.

As tumours are detected earlier, the incidence of nodal disease is decreasing, so about 60% of axillas are node-negative. If these patients are all treated by axillary clearance this is overtreatment and exposes them to the risk of complications. A targeted sampling technique using radioisotope and blue dye, known as sentinel node biopsy, has come into practice and is now replacing standard axillary node clearance with clinically uninvolved nodes. A radioisotope is injected around the tumour or into the periareola region a few hours prior to surgery, and then a blue dye is injected around the tumour or the areola at the time of the operation. These travel to the sentinel node or node(s) in the axilla. These node(s) can then be identified by the blue dye or by the presence of radioactivity. If the node is positive for metastatic disease then there may be other positive nodes in the axilla, and either a clearance should be performed or radiotherapy could be given to the axilla. If there is no sign of metastatic disease in the sentinel node or nodes then no further surgery is required. Several large studies in the USA and Europe have been evaluating this new technique for accuracy, complications and recurrence.[113,114] The important figure in these assessments is the false negative rate for such patients who may, in theory, be denied valuable adjuvant therapy if they are considered to be 'node-negative'.

• REFERENCES •

106. Mumtaz H, Davidson T, Hall-Craggs MA et al. Br J Surg 1997; 84: 1147–1151
107. Kurtz JM, Amalrie R et al. Ann Surg 1988; 207: 347–351
108. Steele RJC, Forrest APM et al. Br J Surg 1985; 72: 368–369
109. Graversen HP, Blichert-Joff M et al. Eur J Surg Oncol 1988; 14: 407–412
110. Forrest AP, Everington D, McDonald CC et al. Br J Surg 1995; 82: 1504–1508
111. Chetty U, Jack W, Prescott RS. Br J Surg 2000; 87: 163–169
112. Kjaergaard J, Blitchert-Toft M, Andersen J et al. Br J Surg 1985; 72: 365
113. Veronesi V, Galinberti V, Zurrido S et al. Eur J Cancer 2001; 37: 454–458
114. Giuliano AE, Haigh PI, Brennan MB et al. J Clin Oncol 2000; 18: 2553-2559

Surgical procedures

Excision of tumour

If a diagnostic open biopsy or breast conservation surgery has to be performed, the incisions should be placed in such a way that the scar can be re-excised if a mastectomy is found to be necessary at a later date. Circumferential and skin crease incisions are preferred, but transverse incisions can be used in the medial half of the breast. Radial and vertical incisions should be avoided because these heal poorly, especially in the upper half of the breast. Good haemostasis is essential because haematoma is the major complication of this technique; however, it should occur in less than 5% of cases.

Mastectomy procedures

These operations are performed for tumours that are unsuitable for conservation (such as multicentric tumours and large tumours in a small breast), for widespread DCIS, as a salvage procedure for recurrent or locally advanced cancers, and when the patient prefers this treatment for an operable breast carcinoma after discussion with the clinician and specialist breast care nurse. In the UK, around 30–40% of patients with breast cancer undergo mastectomy,

The terminology can be confusing. Excision of the breast alone should be called *total* rather than *simple* mastectomy; removal of the breast with or without pectoralis minor and the axillary contents is termed a *modified radical* or *Patey* mastectomy; and excision of the breast, with both pectoral muscles and axillary contents termed a *radical* or *Halsted* mastectomy. When only the breast tissue is removed, leaving the nipple and areola, this is called a *subcutaneous* mastectomy, although many variations on this operation are performed. Mastectomy can be combined with a reconstructive procedure, which may be performed immediately or later.

Operative technique Total mastectomy is performed with the patient's arm on a sideboard, but only the chest and axilla are prepared. If an axillary dissection is to be performed it is helpful to be able to move the arm into flexion and abduction, and this is best done by preparing the arm and wrapping it in sterile towels at the start of the operation. Alternatively, an arm board mounted on a universal joint, which allows movement in any plane, can be used.

In all forms of mastectomy, except the subcutaneous, skin flaps are raised and the nipple areola complex is removed with the breast. A transverse elliptical incision is made and the flaps are reflected to the midline, to the clavicle superiorly, to the anterior border of latissimus dorsi posteriorly, and to the rectus sheath inferiorly. The subcutaneous vessels are retained within the flaps to ensure flap survival. The flaps should be thin distally but thicker towards the chest wall. In both total and modified radical operations the breast is removed from the pectoral fascia, and the internal thoracic perforating vessels coming through the second to fourth anterior intercostal space are cauterized.

In a total mastectomy the axillary tail is dissected from the axillary fat and the lower nodes may be taken as a sampling procedure. At this stage, the total mastectomy operation is complete; haemostasis is secured and the flaps are closed with suction drainage. In the total mastectomy no muscles or nerves are sacrificed.

Axillary surgery

In a Patey mastectomy the axilla is dissected free of all nodes; the boundaries of the dissection are the axillary vein superiorly, the latissimus dorsi laterally, the subscapularis muscle posteriorly, and the chest wall medially. The axillary vein is displayed by dissection of the tough anterior layer of the clavipectoral fascia that invests the axillary fat.

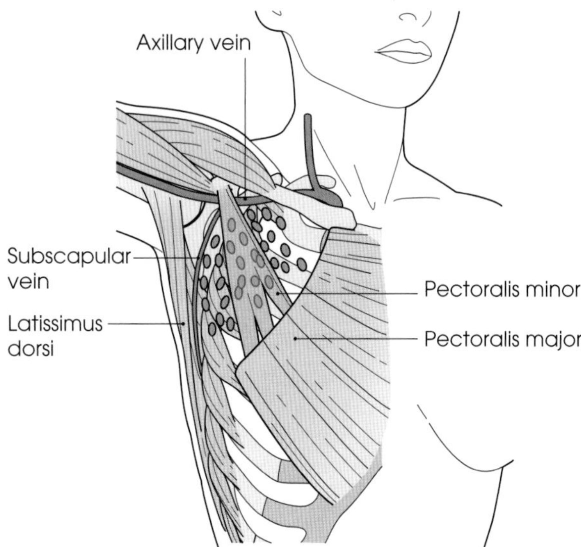

Figure 23.30 Nodal areas in the axilla. Area I lies lateral to the lower border of pectoralis minor muscle, area II lies beneath that muscle, and area III (the apex) lies medial to the upper border of pectoralis minor. In practice, most axillary sampling takes a portion of area I, and full axillary clearance with division of pectoralis minor should clear all three areas and yield upwards of 20 nodes in the specimen.

The nodes are swept downwards from the axillary vein, and the level III or apical nodes (Fig. 23.30) are dissected free from the apex of the axilla. During this phase of the dissection it is important to ligate and divide the branches going to the axillary vein and to avoid damaging the vein. Access to the apex of the axilla is improved by flexing the arm at the shoulder joint to relax the pectoralis major muscle.

The axillary fat and nodal mass are mobilized and then swept downwards. The pectoralis minor can be divided at its origin from the coracoid process and taken with the specimen, but it is usually just retracted because this is only rarely necessary. The medial pectoral nerve running to the pectoralis major muscle is carefully preserved on the underside of the muscle.

During the clearing of the mid axilla, the intercostobrachial nerve may need to be divided as it emerges from the chest wall just posterior to the origin of the pectoralis minor muscle, but most surgeons now try to preserve this nerve.[115] The thoracodorsal pedicle and long thoracic nerves are preserved; very rarely the thoracodorsal pedicle needs to be divided if surrounded by involved nodes. At the end of the procedure the wound is drained by one or two suction drains and the skin flaps are closed.

If an axillary dissection is performed with breast conservation surgery, it can be done simultaneously through the same incision as for upper outer quadrant cancers or via a separate incision in the axilla for tumours located in other parts of the breast. The same principles are followed to remove all the axillary tissue.

References

115. Abdullah JI, Iddein J, Barr L et al. Br J Surg 1998; 85: 1443–1445

The drains are left in for 3–5 days or until the volume of daily drainage falls to less than 50 mL in 24 h. Several studies have shown that patients may be safely sent home with the drain in situ, reducing the hospital stay.[116] Postoperative complications include seromas, which often occur in the axilla and can be treated by simple aspiration, infections and skin necrosis if the flaps are too thin. When the intercostobrachial nerve has been divided the patient should be warned that she may have altered sensation and an anaesthetized patch of skin in the axilla and upper medial part of the arm. Patients should be encouraged to exercise the arm postoperatively to avoid shoulder stiffness.

Subcutaneous mastectomy is performed via a submammary, axillary or circumareolar incision, and is usually indicated for prophylaxis of breast cancer in women at high risk of the disease or those with DCIS. One problem is that it is not possible to guarantee that all the breast tissue has been removed, and instances of late breast cancer have been recorded.[117] After excision of the breast tissue the breast shape can be reformed by using a subpectoral implant or expander, or by using a muscle flap with or without a prosthesis. A variant of subcutaneous mastectomy is known as a skin-sparing mastectomy and may be done with or without preservation of the nipple.[118] All breast tissue removed should be carefully examined for occult carcinoma.

Breast reconstruction

Some 10–20% of women undergoing mastectomy will experience lifelong distress from the damage to the perceived body image that may follow mastectomy. It is not always easy to predict which women will be affected. The option of breast reconstruction should therefore be discussed with most patients. Not all women will wish to undergo reconstruction, particularly if the complications, the need for an implant and the possibility of a second operation are explained. Reconstruction can, however, be performed at the same time as the mastectomy or at a later date. The aim is to produce a mound on the chest wall that resembles the lost breast; the patient should not be given the impression that a normal breast can be reproduced.

The techniques vary from simple placement of an implant or tissue expander under the pectoralis major muscle to the more complicated insertion of a myocutaneous flap into the mastectomy defect. These operations are best performed in consultation with a plastic surgeon or by a breast surgeon with specialist training in reconstruction (i.e. an oncoplastic surgeon).

The techniques employing an implant or expander alone are relatively simple to perform but difficult to achieve symmetry and produce less satisfactory cosmetic results, because a subpectoral implant may lie above the level of the natural inframammary fold, giving a high breast. Enlarging the muscular pocket inferiorly by dissecting underneath the serratus anterior can help to address this problem. If a tissue expander is used, the expander is filled with saline in outpatients over the next 3–6 months until over-expansion of some 100–200 mL over the desired breast size is achieved. Although appearing to be a simple operation, numerous complications have been reported[119,120] and the technique is losing favour. It does, however, offer the patient a reconstruction without an additional donor scar on the back or abdomen.

Myocutaneous flaps, i.e. the latissimus dorsi or transverse rectus abdominis flap, can produce good cosmetic results and are especially useful where skin and muscle are short after an extensive mastectomy or where the skin flaps have been irradiated (Fig. 23.31). These techniques involve longer operating times and greater blood loss. The choice between a latissimus dorsi reconstruction or a rectus flap depends on patient preference and the amount of abdominal fat present. Extensive abdominal scarring precludes the use of a rectus flap because the blood supply to the muscle may have been damaged by the previous surgery. These techniques are also useful for salvage surgery for recurrence after breast conservation surgery or for locally advanced disease (Fig. 23.32).[121,122]

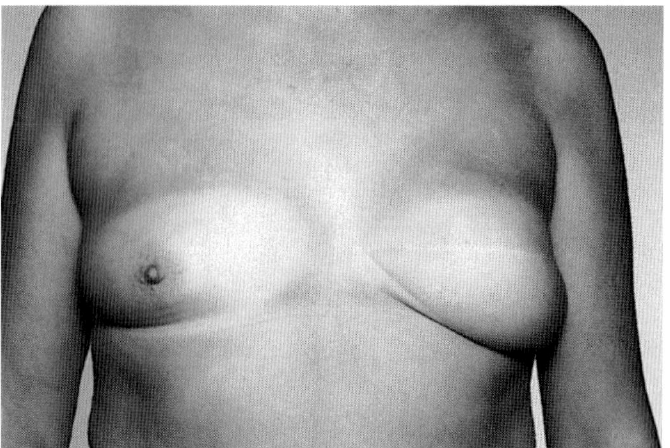

Figure 23.31 Breast reconstruction using a latissimus dorsi myocutaneous flap with a silicone gel implant. This procedure was done as an immediate reconstruction at the same time as the mastectomy.

Further details of these and other reconstructive techniques using free flaps, which are usually performed by plastic surgeons, are included in Ch. 9.

Adjuvant therapy

Postoperative radiotherapy: DXT

All women who have a wide local excision (breast conservation surgery) of an invasive cancer need to have breast radiotherapy to decrease the risk of local recurrence. Dosage regimens vary from one institute to another,[123] and in the UK the results of the Standardization of Breast Radiotherapy (START) trial, which has evaluated different radiotherapy regimens, are awaited. The standard regimen is a total dose of 45–50 Gy given over 3–5 weeks. Long-term follow-up of breast conservation surgery trials has shown that the effects are maintained but that the natural history of local recurrence is protracted, with recurrence rates of 1% or

REFERENCES

116. Holcombe C, West N et al. Eur J Surg Oncol 1995; 21: 604–606
117. Meijers-Heijboer H, Van Geel B, Van Patten WLT. N Engl J Med 2001; 345: 159–164
118. Carlson GW, Bostwick J et al. Ann Surg 1997; 225: 570–578
119. Ringberg A, Tengrup I, Aspergron K et al. Eur J Surg Oncol 1999; 25: 470–476
120. Camilleri IG, Malata CR et al. Br J Plast Surg 1996; 49: 346–351
121. Flook D, Webster DJT et al. Br J Surg 1989; 76: 512–514
122. Sweetland HM, Kartsis P, Rogers K. J R Coll Surg Edinb 1995; 40: 88–92
123. Winfield E, Deighton A, Venables K et al. Clin Oncol 2002; 14: 267–271

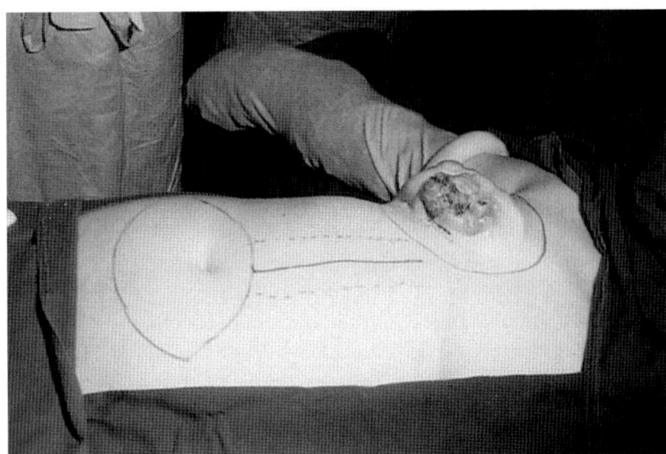

Figure 23.32 Operative photograph of a patient with locally advanced breast cancer about to undergo a radical mastectomy with closure using a rectus abdominis myocutaneous flap. The outlines of the flap and rectus muscle have been drawn on the abdomen at the start of the operation.

less per year over at least 10 years. Most recurrences occur in the index quadrant.[124]

Even after a mastectomy women are at risk of local recurrence, and therefore some women are advised to have chest wall and supraclavicular fossa radiotherapy. Factors that are taken into consideration are tumours larger than 4 cm, grade 3 tumours, four or more positive lymph nodes, lymphovascular invasion, involvement of the pectoral muscle and age less than 35 years. In these high-risk patients, locoregional recurrence occurs in 30–40% and tends to occur within the first 3 years of surgery.

The use of radiotherapy after mastectomy has been shown to decrease locoregional recurrence and increase survival if combined with adjuvant systemic therapy.[125,126] Radiotherapy after mastectomy and reconstruction with implants does, unfortunately, have an adverse effect on the cosmetic result because of fibrosis and capsular contractures.[127]

Radiotherapy is not without complications, as was shown by a review of randomized controlled trials of radiotherapy that were started before 1975. Initial results in 1985 and updated results in 1994 showed that there was an excess mortality rate.[128] If the patients survived 10 years there was a 66% reduction in locoregional recurrence. If patients survived 25 years there was a 42% survival after radiotherapy compared with 51% in the control group, and this difference was due to an increase in cardiac deaths.[128] This was predominantly in patients with left-sided tumours.

A meta-analysis of 40 randomized controlled trials of DXT showed that DXT reduces breast cancer mortality but increases mortality from other causes.[126,129] Overall mortality was influenced favourably when the risk of breast cancer was high in younger patients. In older patients with a lower risk of recurrence, DXT had an unfavourable impact on all-cause mortality.

The methods of giving DXT are now closely calculated and monitored to try to avoid the risk of cardiac damage, and fractionated regimens are used to reduce the risk of late side effects to normal tissues.

Systemic treatments

When it was realized that radical surgery did not cure some women of breast cancer, it became apparent that breast cancer could be a systemic condition from an early stage. The use of adjuvant therapy in operable breast cancer is based on the hypothesis that early treatment by either chemotherapy or hormone therapy destroys the micrometastases that are present but undetectable at the time of surgery on the primary cancer. The results of randomized trials of adjuvant therapy support this concept in part, and this is one area in the therapy of breast cancer that has seen significant advances. The first adjuvant treatments were based on the fact that many breast cancers were thought to be hormone-sensitive, and therefore a surgical oophorectomy or pelvic irradiation, adrenalectomy and hypophysectomy were performed. These were followed by treatments using chemotherapy and drugs causing hormonal change.

The discovery in the 1960s of oestrogen receptors and tamoxifen, an oestrogen receptor blocker, made a significant breakthrough in the management of breast cancer. Initial studies of antioestrogen therapy using tamoxifen for 2 years confirmed an advantage over control patients, especially in postmenopausal patients with positive nodes.[130,131]

The large Nolvadex Adjuvant Trial Organization study of 1285 patients in the UK showed an increased survival in the tamoxifen-treated group, with very low toxicity (Fig. 23.33).[130] This trial treated both pre- and postmenopausal patients with tamoxifen 10 mg twice daily for 2 years, compared against controls who were given no adjuvant treatment. The results suggested that the benefit of tamoxifen was also found in the oestrogen receptor-negative patients, although only about half the patients had their receptors assayed. A trial in Scotland of 1312 patients on tamoxifen 20 mg/day for 5 years showed a highly significant delay in relapse in the treatment group, which was independent of nodal or menopausal status.[131] At this time the beneficial effect was thought to be in all the oestrogen receptor categories, although the greatest benefit was in patients with high oestrogen receptor levels.

An overview in 1996 of ovarian ablation by the Early Breast Cancer Trialists' Collaborative Group (EBCTCG) reported on 2102 premenopausal women and showed an absolute 6% improvement in survival at 15 years for the ovarian ablation group.[132]

The overall 10-year results of adjuvant tamoxifen therapy were summarized by Peto in 1998 in a meta-analysis of 37 000 women in 55 trials. This showed that tamoxifen reduced the annual odds of recurrence by 47% and the annual odds of death by 26%. This gave an absolute improvement of the 10-year survival rate of 10.9% for node-positive and 5.6% for node-negative. There was also a reduction of 47% in contralateral breast cancer after

REFERENCES

124. Fourquet A, Campano F, Zafrani B et al. Int J Radiat Oncol Biol Phys 1989; 17: 719–725
125. Ragaz J, Jackson SM, Le N et al. N Engl J Med 1997; 337: 956–962
126. Overgaard M, Hansen PS, Overgaard J et al. Lancet 1999; 353: 1641–1648
127. Spears T. Plast Reconstr Surg 1995; 96: 116–118
128. Cuzick J, Stewart H, Rutquist L et al. J Clin Oncol 1994; 12: 447–453
129. Early Breast Cancer Trialists' Collaborative Group. Lancet 2000; 355: 1757–1770
130. Nolvadex Adjuvant Trial Organization. Lancet 1985; 1: 836–840
131. Breast Cancer Trials Committee—Scottish Cancer Trials Office. Lancet 1987; ii: 171–175
132. Early Breast Cancer Trialists' Collaborative Group. Lancet 1996; 348: 1189–1196

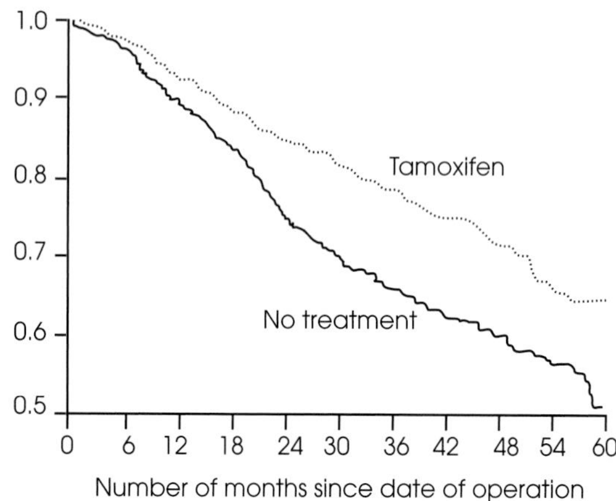

Tamoxifen	562	547	515	489	456	429	354	259	196	106	43
No treatment	567	545	502	470	411	354	288	224	150	81	32

Number of patients at risk

Figure 23.33 Life table of the Nolvadex Adjuvant Trial Organization trial, showing significantly higher event-free levels (events being recurrence or death) in the tamoxifen-treated patients.[130]

5 years of treatment. All these effects were most apparent for women with oestrogen receptor-positive tumours.[133]

Adjuvant chemotherapy

The important studies of chemotherapy were first run in the Milan Cancer Institute by Bonadonna's group[134] and in the USA by Fisher's group,[135] who used the combination of cyclophosphamide, methotrexate and fluorouracil (CMF) in both pre- and postmenopausal patients. The drugs were given for 12 months after surgery in patients with positive axillary nodes. Both trials showed a definite advantage for the treated patients over control patients in both disease-free interval and subsequent mortality. This advantage was greatest in premenopausal patients with one to three metastatic nodes in the axilla. However, the toxicity of the therapy was a problem: some 30% of patients experienced significant side effects.

The EBCTCG overview of 1998 analysed 30 000 women in 69 trials and confirmed that polychemotherapy decreased the odds of recurrence by 35% in patients younger than 50 years and by 20% for those aged over 50 years.[133] The absolute increase in 10-year survival was 7–11% in patients younger than 50 years and 2–3% in those over 50 years. There was evidence that there is no survival advantage for courses of chemotherapy longer than 6 months. There was, however, evidence that in those trials that had included an anthracycline there was an additional benefit so that there was absolute reduction in recurrence of 3.2% and reduction in mortality of 2.7% greater than the effect produced by CMF regimens. Regimens including anthracyclines are now used routinely.

The short-term side effects of all chemotherapy regimens are nausea, vomiting, alopecia, stomatitis, fatigue, bone marrow suppression and decreased quality of life. The long-term side effects are ovarian failure and cardiac toxicities (especially after anthracycline therapy). As more women survive breast cancer the long-term effects of chemotherapy will become more of a problem.

These results suggest that mortality can be reduced modestly by adjuvant chemotherapy in young women and by adjuvant tamoxifen in older women. Patients with negative nodes had been regarded as having such a good prognosis that adjuvant therapy was unnecessary, but a trial of node-negative, oestrogen receptor-positive patients has shown a significant prolongation of disease-free survival in patients treated with tamoxifen 20 mg/day for 5 years; the benefits continue beyond 5 years.[132,136] It is considered that because of the small but real risk of induced uterine malignancy, tamoxifen should not be taken for longer than 5 years; however, this is still being assessed.

Tamoxifen has both oestrogenic and anti-oestrogenic effects because of the presence of alpha and beta receptors in different tissues. The common side effects experienced by patients are hot flushes, vaginal discharge, nausea, and increased thrombotic tendency because of a decrease in plasma concentrations of antithrombin III, protein S and fibrinogen. There is also a risk of endometrial hyperplasia and long-term increased risk of developing uterine cancer, but those that arise are mostly low-grade, stage I tumours. Tamoxifen does help preserve bone density in postmenopausal women[137] and reduces the concentration of total cholesterol and low-density lipoproteins.

New hormonal medications have been developed; these are aromatase inhibitors. Aromatase is the enzyme responsible for the conversion of androgens, such as androstenedione and testosterone, to oestrogens in the ovary of premenopausal women and the extragonadal tissues of postmenopausal women (fat, muscle, skin and breast).

The three new aromatase inhibitors anastrazole, letrozole and exemestane have been evaluated in the adjuvant setting in the Arimidex, Tamoxifen, Alone or in Combination (ATAC) study. This randomized over 9,500 postmenopausal women with early breast cancer to receive tamoxifen, anastrozole, or both. Results have shown a significant improvement in survival with the new drug, with the improvement being seen in oestrogen receptor with positive tumours only. There are less hormonal or gynaecological side effects with anastrazole but there was a small increase in adverse musculoskeletal events.[138] Studies switching patients after 2–3 years of tamoxifen to anastrazole or exemestane have shown improvements in disease free survival for those patients who switched to an aromatase inhibitor. Letrozole given after 5 years of tamoxifen significantly improves chain free and metastatic free survival in all patients and improves overall survival in node positive patients. These new aromatase inhibitors are likely to replace or be resuture combined in sequence with tamoxifen as part of adjuvant, for many postmenopausal women with hormone sensitive breast cancer.

Neoadjuvant chemotherapy

If a breast cancer is operable it is standard practice for surgery to take place first, followed by chemotherapy and then radiotherapy

REFERENCES

133. Early Breast Cancer Trialists' Collaborative Group. Lancet 1998; 351: 1451–1467
134. Bonadonna G, Brussamolino E et al. N Engl J Med 1976; 284: 405–410
135. Fisher B, Carbone P et al. N Engl J Med 1978; 292: 117–122
136. Fisher B, Costantino PH et al. N Engl J Med 1989; 320: 479–484
137. Rowles TJ, Huckish T, Kanis JA et al. J Clin Oncol 1996; 14: 76–84
138. Arimidex, Tamoxifen, Alone or in Combination (ATAC) Trialists' Group. Lancet 2002; 359: 2131

if required. In the 1990s, there were several trials of neoadjuvant chemotherapy (primary chemotherapy before surgery) for women with operable cancers, with the aim of reducing the need for mastectomy and increasing the conservation rate.[139,140] There was a significant downstaging of the tumours and nodes, and a decrease in the mastectomy rate, but long-term follow-up of these patients has shown that there is no difference in local or distant recurrence or overall survival. Neoadjuvant chemotherapy is therefore only recommended routinely for those patients with inflammatory cancers and locally advanced inoperable disease, but it can also be used to downsize tumours and make them suitable for breast conservation surgery. Neoadjuvant endocrine mercq3 with new aromatase inhibitors in selected postmenopausal women is also effective at downstaging and avoiding the need for any in many women.

Indications for adjuvant treatment

Most women who are treated for an invasive breast cancer need some form of systemic adjuvant treatment, unless they have a small, grade 1, node-negative tumour where the risk of systemic recurrence is minimal. Most premenopausal women and many postmenopausal women with grade 2 and 3 tumours that are node-negative or -positive will receive chemotherapy with or without tamoxifen, depending on their oestrogen receptor status. The age for prescribing chemotherapy has gradually increased. Postmenopausal women with oestrogen receptor-negative tumours, especially if they are node-positive, will be advised to have chemotherapy unless there are medical contraindications.

Elderly patients with oestrogen receptor-positive tumours who are unfit for surgery may receive hormonal treatments only. Ovarian ablation or luteinizing hormone-releasing hormone (LHRH) agonists, such as goserelin and tamoxifen, are used in some premenopausal women with oestrogen receptor-positive disease as an additional treatment after chemotherapy or if they develop recurrent disease. There are ongoing trials of the use of LHRH agonists; the advantage is that it is a reversible method of stopping ovarian function.[141]

BREAST CANCER IN THE ELDERLY

In the 1980s, there was a trend to treat elderly patients in a different way to younger patients, in the belief that the disease is less aggressive, that it could all be treated by tamoxifen, and that the overall life expectancy of elderly patients is not so good. Women aged more than 70 years were not offered surgery but just prescribed tamoxifen; however, it controls disease in less than 30% of elderly patients at 5 years.[142] This should not therefore be the treatment of choice today, because life expectancy and general health have improved. All women should be given the same surgical choices and offered appropriate adjuvant treatments unless they have other significant medical problems that put them at high risk from other treatments.

Endocrine treatment with an aromatase inhibitor such as letrozole should be reserved for the elderly and infirm. In these women the disease should still be monitored because progressive disease may require surgical intervention to avoid the sequelae of uncontrolled local progression.

BREAST CANCER IN PREGNANCY

Breast cancer complicates one in 3000 pregnancies.[143] It often presents late because of delay in diagnosis. When deciding on treatment, consideration needs to be given to the oncological aspects and to the pregnancy. The usual treatment is surgery followed by chemotherapy and radiotherapy as needed. Chemotherapy cannot be given during the first trimester and radiotherapy should be avoided throughout pregnancy. This is probably one of the reasons why traditionally women have been advised to have a mastectomy. They may be able to have chemotherapy in the third trimester. The management of breast cancer in pregnancy crucially involves multidisciplinary team working because there needs to be close liaison between the oncologist, surgeon and obstetrician. It may be appropriate to deliver the baby early so that treatment for the breast cancer can begin. Most cancers found during pregnancy are, unfortunately, grade 3, oestrogen receptor-negative, and node-positive, and have evidence of vascular invasion.[144]

INOPERABLE AND ADVANCED DISEASE

Some patients present with locally advanced and inoperable disease as indicated by the presence of skin oedema, peau d'orange, skin ulceration, chest fixation and satellite nodules. Patients who present with inflammatory breast cancer should also not be treated by surgery in the first instance because they are very likely to have metastases at presentation; if surgery is performed, local recurrence occurs very quickly because there are tumour cells within the lymphatics. These patients should be treated initially by neoadjuvant chemotherapy. If there is a clinical response, patients then undergo surgery and usually also need radiotherapy. Unfortunately, many of these women soon develop metastatic disease and have a very poor prognosis.

Patients who present with locally advanced or metastatic disease were previously deemed incurable because local treatment, whether surgical or radiotherapeutic, could not save the patient. When a patient is likely to die within a few months as a result of her breast cancer, then mastectomy should be avoided if possible because this procedure does not help the patient and often increases her distress. Mastectomy may, however, be appropriate to obtain local control of the cancer when used together with radiotherapy or chemotherapy.

When the disease is locally advanced, it is important to ascertain the oestrogen receptor status. If it is oestrogen receptor-negative and the primary tumour is deemed inoperable, or when the patient presents with metastases but is relatively fit, outpatient chemotherapy can be given prior to local treatment in an attempt to reduce the size of the tumour. If there is a good response and there is no metastatic disease, surgery can be performed. If the disease is still inoperable local radiotherapy can be given.

Where the tumour is found to be oestrogen receptor-positive, the history is of a slow-growing tumour, or the patient is unfit, endocrine therapy is often worthwhile as first-line therapy, keeping radiotherapy in reserve for later progression. In

REFERENCES

139. Makris A, Powles TJ, Ashley SE et al. Ann Oncol 1998; 9: 1179–1184
140. Fisher B, Bryant J, Wolmark N et al. J Clin Oncol 1998; 16: 2672–2685
141. Kirkpatrick K, Mokbel K. Endocrine and Biological Therapy of Breast Cancer in the 21st Century. Petroc Press, Newbury, 2001
142. Robertson JFR, Todd JH, Ellis IO et al. Br Med J 1988; 297: 511–514
143. Keurer HM, Cunningham JD, Brower ST et al. Surg Oncol 1997; 6: 93–98
144. Fatherinberry SS. Obstet Gynecol Clin North Am 2002; 29: 225–232

premenopausal women this could be ovarian ablation or LHRH agonists followed by tamoxifen because the combination has produced superior results to single therapy.[145] Endocrine therapy with letrozole 2–5 mg/day should be used in postmenopausal women. There is a potential for an initial complete and partial response rate of 30–40%. This is often the case in elderly patients. Assessment of response is usually defined by shrinkage of measurable disease and the UICC criteria[146] are generally employed. These classify responses as complete, partial, no change or progression; to conform with these definitions response should be maintained for at least 6 months. Even if the primary tumour becomes impalpable, there may still be surviving malignant cells and surgery or radiotherapy may still be required.

METASTATIC DISEASE

Approximately 35% of women with breast cancer will experience recurrence with clinical metastatic disease and 7% will have distant metastases at presentation. When patients have metastatic disease treatment is directed at the relief of symptoms, maintenance of a good quality of life, and stabilization of disease because cure is not possible. This will involve a multidisciplinary team to assess the symptoms, arrange investigations to evaluate the extent of the disease, and then plan the further management of these difficult problems.

The risk of developing metastatic disease relates to the known prognostic factors of the original tumour (size, grade of tumour, nodal status, oestrogen receptor status and presence of HER2). Factors that are associated with a better response to treatment for metastatic disease are a long disease-free interval, oestrogen receptor positivity, and the presence of bone rather than soft tissue disease.

In premenopausal women with oestrogen receptor-positive disease confined to bones and soft tissues, tamoxifen combined with a surgical oophorectomy, ovarian radiation or LHRH agonists to ablate ovarian function should be used. If there is a response with endocrine manipulation, the response tends to be longer lasting than chemotherapy responses.

Combination cytotoxic chemotherapy is usually used as the first-line therapy if the disease is oestrogen receptor-negative, involves viscera, or is likely to be rapidly life-threatening. Combinations of cytotoxic drugs are used; however, many patients may have already received chemotherapy as adjuvant treatment so alternative drugs can be used, such as the taxanes (paclitaxel or docetaxel). These were discovered in the 1990s and are particularly effective for those who have anthracycline-resistant disease, which is described as disease occurring within 6 months of receiving an anthracycline regimen. Treatment with paclitaxel is associated with response rates ranging from 6 to 48%.[147]

In postmenopausal women with oestrogen receptor-positive, metastatic disease, tamoxifen was the standard first-line treatment if it had not been used before, but the newer aromatase inhibitors are more effective and have a very low toxicity.[148–150] On further relapse a second-line hormone therapy such as exemestane or the pure antioestrogen fulvestrant can be used to obtain a further response because a good first endocrine response predicts a better chance of a second response.

New treatments for metastatic disease

Other new treatments are vinorelbine, which is a semisynthetic vinca alkaloid that can give response rates of 20–30% in anthracycline-resistant disease,[147] and capecitabine, which is an oral agent that is converted to 5-fluorouracil after a series of enzymatic reactions. It has low toxicity profile and there have been some promising early results.[151] In general, however, responses to further chemotherapy having relapsed after standard chemotherapy are poor, with objective response rates of 20–30% and a median duration of response ranging from 3–6 months.

Some tumours that are oestrogen receptor-negative overexpress HER2. Those patients whose condition is strongly HER2-positive may respond to newer treatments such as trastuzumab, which is a humanized monoclonal antibody against the HER2 receptor. It has a minimal side effect profile and is well tolerated by patients, but it can be associated with some cardiac dysfunction and this needs to be monitored. A trial of the addition of trastuzumab to chemotherapy showed a longer time to disease progression (7.4 versus 4.6 months), higher objective response, and improved survival (25.1 versus 20.3 months).[152] Trials of monotherapy versus a second- and third-line agent have shown response rates of 10–20%.[153]

BONE METASTASES

Localized painful bony metastases are best treated by a large single fraction of radiotherapy, bisphosphonates and analgesics.[154] The response to DXT of skeletal metastases is 70–90%, but it may take several months to reach the maximal effect. Breast cancer micrometastatic disease causes bone destruction by the stimulation of osteoclasts through the production of substances such as parathyroid-related peptide.[155] As the tumour burden increases and osteolysis increases the bone is weakened, leading to pain and pathological fractures that may need to be surgically stabilized to prevent or treat a fracture.

Bisphosphonates are pyrophosphates, the main mechanism of action of which is to inhibit osteoclastic activity and decrease bone resorption, but they also have a direct action on tumour cells. These drugs can be given intravenously or orally and are effective in treating hypercalcemia and skeletal disease if used with hormonal regimens or chemotherapy. If the patient is symptomatic from bone metastases, 2 years of bisphosphonate treatment is recommended once they are stabilized. Bisphosphonates are well tolerated, although there are some gastrointestinal side effects from oral preparations. Randomised trials have shown a reduction in all skeletal events when bisphosphonates are given with other endocrine or chemotherapy and the effect lasts for at least 2 years.[156]

REFERENCES

145. Klijn JG et al. J Natl Cancer Inst 2000; 92: 903–911
146. Hayward JC, Hewson JC. Cancer 1977; 39: 1289–1294
147. Vermokien JB, Jen Bokkel Huiniet WW. Breast 1996; 5: 304–311
148. Kaufman M et al. J Clin Oncol 2000; 18: 1399–1341
149. Mouridsen H et al. J Clin Oncol 2001; 19: 2596–2606
150. Boneterre J et al. J Clin Oncol 2000; 18: 3748–3757
151. Blum JL, Jones SE, Buzdar AU. J Clin Oncol 1999; 17: 485–493
152. Slamon DJ, Leyland-Jones B, Shak S et al. N Engl J Med 2001; 344: 783–792
153. Vogel CL, Cobleigh MA, Tripathy D. J Clin Oncol 2002; 20: 719–726
154. Breast Specialty Group of British Association of Surgical Oncology. Eur J Surg Oncol 1999: 25: 3–23
155. Guise TA. Cancer 2000; 88: 2892–2898
156. Lepton A, Theriault RL, Hortobagyi GN et al. Cancer 2000; 88: 1082–1090

Cerebral metastases that may produce symptoms such as confusion, headaches, vomiting and fits are treated by fractionated radiotherapy and dexamethasone. Metastatic disease may also produce many other disease states, such as leukoerythroblastic anaemia when the bone marrow is infiltrated, or hypercalcaemia when massive osteolysis occurs. Involvement of the spinal canal may produce cord compression and paresis that will require urgent spinal canal decompression by laminectomy (see Ch. 55). Radiotherapy may also be needed for treatment of locoregional recurrence in the chest wall or for supraclavicular or mediastinal lymphadenopathy.

The place of surgery in advanced disease is limited to salvage mastectomy for local control of residual disease or further localized recurrent disease after radiotherapy or chemotherapy. These salvage operations are often massive, requiring excision of the chest wall as well as the breast and pectoral muscles because the disease has often infiltrated widely. The resulting defect can be filled with a myocutaneous flap or omental graft.[121,122] These large excisions are intended to be palliative and aim to produce local control until the patient dies of distant recurrence. The outlook for most patients with stage IV disease is very poor: only 10% survive 5 years.

When it is clear that the disease is advancing despite treatment, it should be recognized that the doctor's duty is to palliate distressing symptoms. Pain should be managed by adequate and frequent doses of appropriate analgesics (see Ch. 5); locally painful areas can often be usefully palliated by a single dose of radiation. Constipation induced by opiates can be treated by regular laxatives. Pleural effusions can be treated by tube drainage and instillation of bleomycin or talc into the pleural space. Ascites should be tapped, and if chronic can be managed by a peritoneovenous shunt.

When clearly no further active treatment can be given, this should be discussed with the patient and her relatives. The palliative care teams in the community and hospice should be involved in the management of the terminal phase of the disease.

MALE BREAST CANCER

Male breast cancer is 100 times less common than the female variety and represents only 0.7% of all cancers in men.[157] The peak age incidence is 5–10 years older than that in women. The aetiology, like that of female breast cancer, is unknown, but there is an increased incidence in patients with Klinefelter's syndrome and many cases have a family history because there is a relationship with *BRCA2* gene. Gynaecomastia is seen in some 30% of men and is not a risk factor for breast cancer.

The presenting features are identical to those in women; a discoloured and palpable lump, skin or nipple retraction, and occasionally nipple discharge are the main symptoms. The only difference between the sexes is that the male tumour infiltrates skin and nipple at an early stage because of the smaller breast volume and the closer proximity of the chest skin. All the common histological varieties of breast cancer are seen in men, with the exception of lobular carcinoma because no lobular development occurs in the male breast.

The prognosis of male breast cancer is now thought to be identical to that of the female when compared stage for stage but, as noted, men tend to present at a later stage. The preferred treatment in men is mastectomy. Although the hormonal milieu is different in men, breast cancer still appears to respond well to hormonal therapy when it is oestrogen receptor–positive. Men should receive the same adjuvant treatments as women, depending on the pathological results, but consideration should also be given to psychological needs.

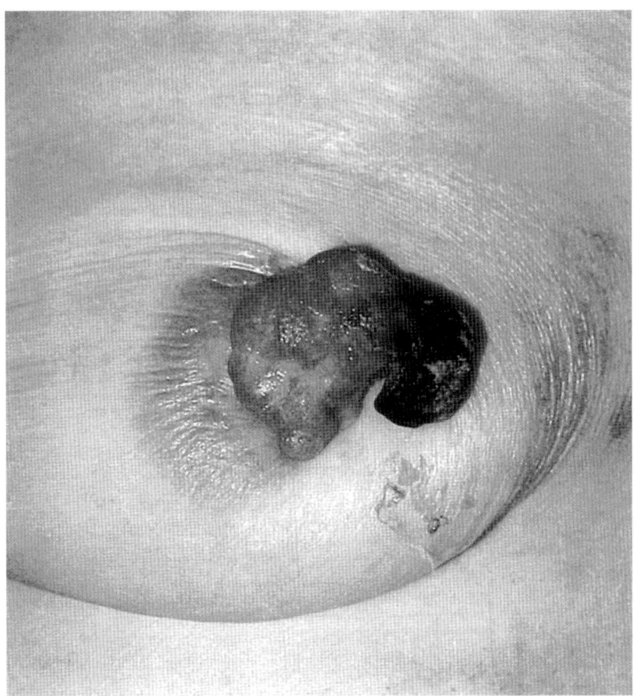

Figure 23.34 Spindle cell sarcoma of the breast presenting as a rapidly growing ulcerating mass destroying the nipple.

NON-EPITHELIAL TUMOURS OF THE BREAST (SARCOMA)

There are several types of non-epithelial tumour, although all are rare in comparison with ductal carcinomas. Sarcomas form the largest group and are divided into fibrosarcomas, leiomyosarcomas, rhabdomyosarcomas and angiosarcomas, depending on the predominant cell type. The angiosarcoma is the commonest subtype, although in 1989 a review of the world literature yielded only 87 cases.[158] The tumour presents as a lump or diffuse infiltration of the skin, and skin discolouration is seen in 30% of cases. There is considerable variation in the size of the primary tumour, with a range from 2 to 11 cm, and macroscopically the tumour may appear spongy with multiple blood-filled spaces. Donnell and coworkers divided the tumour into three groups based on histology, with 12 out of 13 group I patients alive at 5-year follow-up, compared with four out of 18 group III patients.[159] The other sarcomas form less than 1% of malignant tumours and are thus very rare in the breast (Fig. 23.34).

REFERENCES

157. Ravandi-Kashani F, Hayes TG. Eur J Cancer 1998; 34: 1341–1347
158. Chen KTK, Kiregaard DD, Bowan JJ et al. Cancer 1989; 46: 368–371
159. Donnell RR, Rosen PP et al. Am J Surg Pathol 1981; 5: 629–642

Table 23.6 Quality assurance guidelines for the National Health Service Breast Screening Programme

Aspect of screening	Acceptable number
Number of women accepting invitation	> 70%
Number of women recalled for assessment	< 7% at prevalent screen, < 4% at incident screen
Total number of cancers detected	50 out of every 10 000 women screened
Preoperative diagnosis rate	> 70%
Benign malignant biopsies	1:1
Weight of open diagnostic specimens	< 20 g
Availability of nodal status in invasive cancers	> 90%

Fibrosarcoma presents as a poorly defined mass in the breast, and microscopic examination shows the typical spindle cells with multiple mitotic figures. Simple mastectomy is indicated for local control, and node dissection is not indicated because the distant spread is usually via the bloodstream to the liver. The prognosis is poor and chemotherapy is usually ineffective. Nevertheless, one long-term survivor of metachronous bilateral breast tumours has been reported, with disease-free survival up to 13 years after the first tumour.[160]

Occasionally the breast is the site of other primary tumours, with the lymphomas or leukaemia being the most common group. The skin overlying the breast can be affected by any primary skin cancer, and occasionally secondary deposits from adenocarcinomas at other sites are seen in the breast.

BREAST SCREENING

The Health Insurance Plan study, set up in New York as a randomized study of breast screening, was the first to demonstrate a survival advantage for women whose carcinoma was detected by mammography.[161] These findings have been validated in European studies in the Netherlands and Sweden, where screening was performed by mammography alone. The first Dutch study reported 30 000 women over 35 years old screened by a single-view mammogram every 2 years, and demonstrated a halving of the mortality rate from breast cancer in the screened group.[162] Another non-randomized, case–control Dutch study screened 14 000 women by mammography and clinical examination, and showed a significant reduction in mortality.[163] A major randomized study from Sweden studied 134 000 women in a mammographic screening programme and recorded a high attendance rate and a 40% reduction in mortality from breast cancer in women aged 50–74 years screened by a single-view mammogram.[164]

As a result of these and other studies, the British government instituted a population-based screening programme for women aged 50–64 by a single-view mammogram.[62] This programme has been running for 20 years, and all women aged 50–70 years are offered screening every 3 years by two-view mammography.

The latest review of the quality of the national screening programme showed that most targets (Table 23.6) were being met by all the screening clinics.[165] The take-up rate for most units was well above the target of 70% of the population that is needed if the results are to be similar to those achieved by the Swedish Two-Counties Study. This performance is good, but it is difficult to prove that a reduction in breast cancer mortality is due to the screening programme alone and not due to improvement in treatment generally.[166]

FAMILY HISTORY OF BREAST CANCER

With discovery of the *BRCA1* and *BRCA2* genes, there has been considerable interest in family history clinics. These are usually run by geneticists with some surgical input as necessary. Referral guidelines have been developed by the UK Cancer Family History Group to help primary care physicians to make appropriate referrals to specialist clinics (Boxes 23.5 and 23.6).

The indications for screening women with a moderate- or high-risk family history are not proven, but there are many schemes; in most clinics screening by mammography is offered from the age of 40 for women with moderately increased risk, but there is no evidence to say it is of proven value. The role of MRI in high-risk women is being evaluated.

Women who are considered to be at high risk of having a genetic abnormality may be offered genetic testing if there is a living affected relative who agrees to give a blood sample for analysis. This should be done only after extensive genetic counselling because there are implications for those who want to know and to other family members.

Prophylactic mastectomy should be performed only at the request of the patient who is at high risk, preferably after genetic evaluation (although this is not always possible). People who choose surgery tend to have a higher and often inflated perception of their risk of developing breast cancer, and if surgery is advised by a doctor rather than requested by a patient there is a higher level of dissatisfaction.[167] The surgery usually decreases the anxiety levels[168] and significantly decreases the risk of developing

REFERENCES

160. Bundred NJ, O'Reilly K, Smart JG. Eur J Surg Oncol 1989; 15: 263–264
161. Shapiro S, Venet W et al. J Natl Cancer Inst 1982; 69: 349–355
162. Verbeek ACM, Holland R et al. Lancet 1984; I: 1222–1224
163. Colette HJA, Rombach JJ et al. Lancet 1984; 1: 1224–1226
164. Tabar L, Fagerberg G, Gad A. Lancet 1985; 1: 829–832
165. National Health Service Breast Screening Programme Quality Assurance Guidelines. NHSBSP, 1996.
166. Blanks RG, Moss SM, McGahan CE et al. Br Med J 2000; 321: 665–669
167. Borgen P, Hill AD, Tian KN et al. Ann Surg Oncol 1998; 5: 603–606
168. Bebbington Hatcher M, Fallowfield L, A'Kearn R. Br Med J 2001; 322: 1–7

Box 23.5 Family history referral guidelines for a genetic clinic

Breast cancer
- One first-degree relative diagnosed at 40 years or less
- Two first-degree relatives at 60 years or less (on the same side of the family)
- Three first- or second-degree relatives at any age (on the same side of the family)
- One first-degree male breast cancer
- A first-degree relative with bilateral breast cancer

Note: breast cancer can also be inherited through the paternal side of the family.

Breast or ovarian cancer
- Minimum: one of each cancer in first-degree relatives (if only one of each cancer, the breast cancer diagnosed under 50 years)
- A first-degree relative who has *both* breast and ovarian cancer

Box 23.6 Definitions of moderate- and high-risk groups of women

High-risk group
- Breast or ovarian families with four or more relatives on the same side of the family affected, at any age
- Breast cancer (only) families with three affected relatives with an average age at diagnosis of age less than 40 years
- Breast or ovarian families with three affected relatives with an average age at diagnosis of breast cancer and ovarian cancer of 40

Moderate-risk group
- One first-degree relative with breast cancer diagnosed under age 40
- Two first- or second-degree relatives with breast cancer diagnosed under age 60, or ovarian cancer at any age
- Three first- or second-degree relatives with breast or ovarian cancer diagnosed at any age
- A first-degree relative with bilateral cancer under age 60
- A first-degree male relative with breast cancer at any age

The relative risk of breast cancer for women in this group is at least three times that of the general population.

breast cancer,[169] but a surgeon must always state that surgery cannot guarantee removal of all the breast tissue and some risk of malignancy remains.

BREAST CANCER PREVENTION

Another possible approach to decrease the mortality from breast cancer is to try to prevent it by the use of endocrine or other agents. This was based on the fact that tamoxifen decreases the risk of contralateral cancer in women who are receiving tamoxifen as adjuvant treatment. Four studies using tamoxifen have been reported from the USA,[170] Italy,[167] Guy's Hospital in the UK,[168] and the International Breast Cancer Intervention Study (IBIS).[169]

There are differences in the results reported because of differences in the risk levels of the women who were recruited. The US study showed an overall reduction in breast cancer for all ages, but it exceeded 51% for postmenopausal women. There was, however, an increase in the number of cases of endometrial carcinoma and the trial was stopped early because the results were thought to be significant. The Italian trial showed no difference, but the trial had recruited only women who had previously had a hysterectomy, and therefore their risk was different if they had also had an oophorectomy.

The International Breast Cancer Intervention Study studied prevention of breast cancer in women at high risk of breast cancer by randomizing women aged over 40 years to receive tamoxifen or a placebo. Results have shown that there was a 30% reduction in breast cancer cases and a reduced incidence of subsequent cancers in women with atypical ductal hyperplasia and LCIS for those in the tamoxifen group, but there was also an increased incidence of thromboembolic events in those taking tamoxifen.

The case for tamoxifen as a preventative agent is not yet proven. Further studies are being undertaken to assess the role of aromatase inhibitors and raloxifene (a selective oestrogen receptor modulator) in preventing breast cancer in postmenopausal women.

REFERENCES

169. Hartmann L, Schaid DJ, Woods JE et al. N Engl J Med 1999; 340: 77–84
170. Eccles DM, Evans DGR, Mackay J. J Med Genet 2000; 37: 203–209

The abdominal wall and hernias

24

Andrew N. Kingsnorth, Shoo Yee Wong, Paddy J. O'Dwyer

ABDOMINAL INCISIONS

In 1946, Sir Heneage Ogilvie defined a good incision as one that offers access, extensibility and safety to the abdominal structures.[1] Additional features of a good incision include speed of access, ease of closure, security from wound failures (i.e. early dehiscence and incisional hernia), and a good cosmetic appearance.

VERTICAL INCISION

A vertical midline abdominal incision (Fig. 24.1) cuts through the linea alba and is used for most abdominal operations in adults. It provides a relatively bloodless, speedy and extensible access to all four abdominal quadrants. Midline incisions are relatively bloodless and the gastrointestinal tract, which is developed from a midline primitive gut, can be mobilized centrally on its mesentery.

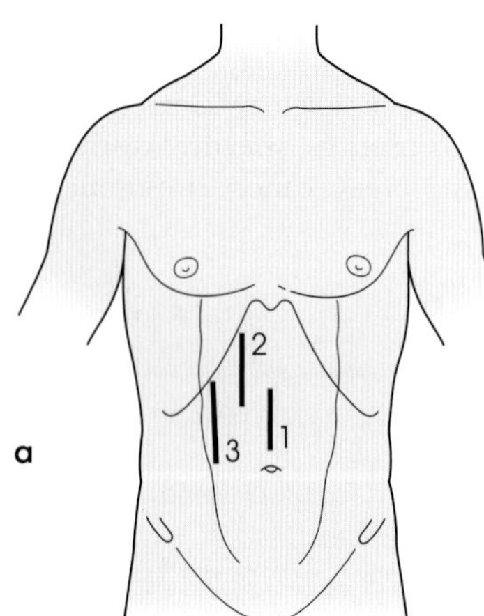

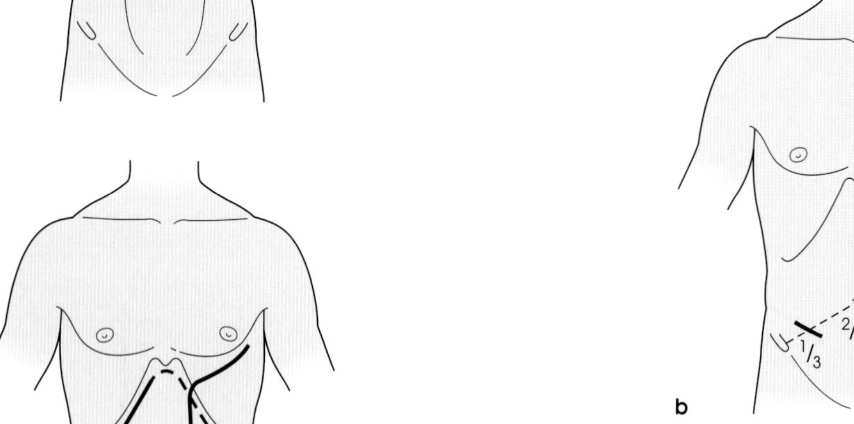

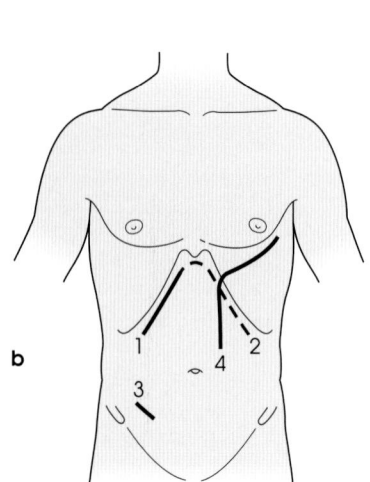

Figure 24.1 (**a**) Vertical incisions: 1, median; 2, paramedian; and 3, lateral paramedian. (**b**) Oblique incisions: 1, Kocher; 1 and 2, Leclerc rooftop; 3, McBurney gridiron; and 4, thoracoabdominal.

Paramedian and lateral median abdominal incisions—1.5 cm and 3.5 cm from the midline, respectively—cut through both anterior and posterior rectus sheaths. They have little advantage over a midline incision, but lateral paramedian incisions develop fewer incisional hernias.[2]

LATERAL AND TRANSVERSE INCISIONS

Lateral and transverse abdominal incisions (Fig. 24.2) are used to gain access to laterally based organs such as the kidneys and liver, and some retroperitoneal organs such as the pancreas. They are reputed to have a low incidence of dehiscence, and reduce post-

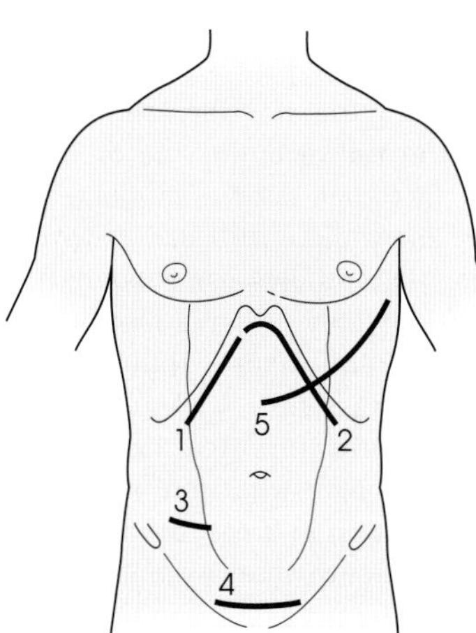

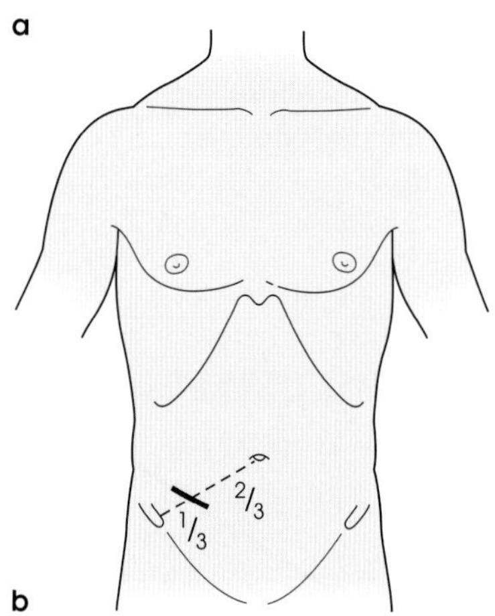

Figure 24.2 Lateral and transverse abdominal incisions (**a**): 1, Kocher subcostal on the right; 2, Leclerc rooftop; 3, Lanz; 4, Pfannenstiel suprapubic; and 5, thoracoabdominal. McBurney gridiron incision (**b**).

REFERENCES

1. Ogilvie H. Proc R Soc Med 1946; 39: 234
2. Guillou PJ, Hall TJ, Donaldson DR et al. Br J Surg 1980; 67: 395–399

operative pain and pulmonary complications. The disadvantages of these incisions are extra blood loss from division of abdominal wall muscles and the potential damage to innervating motor nerves supplying the abdominal wall muscles, causing muscle atrophy and development of an incisional hernia.

A transverse abdominal incision has a cosmetic advantage in neonates and younger children; the wound does not elongate longitudinally as the child grows. At these early ages the sub-diaphragmatic and pelvic recesses do not exist, therefore transverse abdominal incisions give excellent access to the entire abdominal cavity.

The Pfannenstiel suprapubic incision is the most frequently used transverse incision in adults. It allows excellent access to the pelvic organs, including the uterus in caesarean section as well as the ovaries, fallopian tubes, urinary bladder and prostate gland. It is also used in the preperitoneal approach to groin hernia repairs, and for combined repair of infantile hernia and orchidopexy.

The Pfannenstiel suprapubic incision is made on the suprapubic skin crease. The anterior rectus sheath underneath is divided transversely; the exposed rectus muscles are laterally displaced; and the posterior rectus sheath (above the arcuate line of Douglas), transversalis fascia and peritoneum are also divided transversely. The wound is closed in three layers: first, the transversalis fascia and posterior rectus sheath, followed by repositioning of the rectus muscles; second, the anterior rectus sheath; and last, the skin. It is unnecessary to close the peritoneum. The scar is often well hidden by pubic hair.

Other incisions are the Kocher subcostal, Leclerc rooftop, McBurney gridiron, and Rutherford–Morrison lower oblique and thoraco-abdominal oblique incisions. They all have distinct advantages for local access, without the versatility of vertical incisions. Kocher subcostal incisions can be used for cholecystectomy on the right and splenectomy on the left.[3] The incision is placed 2.5 cm below the costal margin and extends obliquely downwards from the midline to the tip of the ninth costal cartilage, sacrificing only the ninth neurovascular bundle. Lateral extension beyond this point divides more neurovascular bundles, which can cause muscle atrophy and incisional hernia. The rooftop or Leclerc incision allows easy access to the liver and spleen. It is also employed for pancreatic and gastric surgery, and bilateral adrenalectomy.

The McBurney gridiron incision was the standard approach to the appendix.[4] It is safe and the scar heals well. The oblique incision lies with its midpoint at the junction of the outer third and medial two-thirds of a line from the anterior superior iliac spine to the umbilicus (Fig. 24.2). The incision can be extended obliquely as a Rutherford–Morrison incision, splitting the external oblique muscle to gain access to the caecum, appendix and right colon.[5] The incision on the left allows access to the left colon but not the rectum.

The Lanz incision is lower, more medial and transverse than the classic McBurney incision, and produces a better cosmetic result. The Lanz incision, however, may damage the iliohypogastric and ilioinguinal herniation.[6]

The thoraco-abdominal incision allows access to the lower thorax and upper abdomen. By dividing the diaphragm from its costal margin, it is relatively simple to expose the aorta in the lower thorax. This incision on the right can be used for liver or complicated biliary surgery and on the left for oesophageal, gastric and aortic surgery.

The small port-site incisions used in laparoscopic surgery for cholecystectomy, antireflux surgery, adrenalectomy and splenectomy greatly reduce incision size and the risk of subsequent herniation.

ABDOMINAL WOUND CLOSURE

APONEUROTIC WOUND HEALING

The process of wound healing is conveniently considered in three stages.[7] The first is the lag or inflammatory phase, during which the blood vessels are plugged, the wound is enmeshed with fibrin, and an inflammatory response occurs. This phase lasts up to 4 days, and in this period the wound draws its strength predominantly from the sutures. The second stage is the proliferative or fibroblastic phase, when macrophages and fibroblasts migrate into the wound and primitive collagen is laid down. This phase continues for 21 days and the wound rapidly gains in strength. The last stage is a long remodelling or maturation phase of collagen realignment. It takes aponeurotic tissue 50 days to regain half its initial strength. Thereafter the process is even slower, and after 1 year the aponeurosis achieves 80% of its initial tensile strength.[8]

The quality and rate of wound healing is adversely affected by infection and comorbidities such as old age, immunosuppression, diabetes, renal and liver failure, malnutrition and vitamin C deficiency.[9] Wound breakdown can be prevented by applying correct surgical technique and using the correct suture.

SUTURE CHOICE

Aponeurotic wounds are slow to heal, and they require the support of the sutures in the first 4 months. Modern sutures cause little in the way of biological response; slowly absorbable polydioxane and non-absorbable polyamides (nylon), polyesters (Mersilene and Ethibond), and polypropylene (Prolene) all fulfil this requirement. Minor complications of non-absorbable sutures include difficulty in applying a secure knot, hence multiple throws are required (which are often bulky and palpable under the scar); persistent infection and suture sinus from infected braided sutures; and sawing through of the tissues and sutures.[10]

CLOSURE TECHNIQUE

Apart from the choice of suture material, the geometry of the suture technique is also important for good wound healing. The normal anatomy must be reconstituted with low tension to allow for better perfusion and better alignment of collagen fibrils which facilitates rapid healing. The peritoneum does not add strength and therefore separate closure is unnecessary.[11] Mass closure, in which all layers of the abdominal wall are taken by each stitch, is recommended for midline incision.[12] Lateral and

REFERENCES

3. Kocher T. Chirurgische Operationslehre. Verlag von Gustav Fischer, Jena, 1907
4. McBurney C. Ann Surg 1894; 20: 38
5. Morrison R. Br Med J 1906; 2: 1005
6. Arnbjornsson E. Am J Surg 1982; 143: 367–369
7. Douglas DM. Br J Surg 1952; 40: 79
8. Van Winkle W. Surg Gynecol Obstet 1969; 129: 819–842
9. Levene CI, Ockleford CD, Barber CL et al. Virchows Arch B 1977; 23: 325–328
10. Krukowski ZH, Matheson NA. Br J Surg 1987; 74: 824–825
11. Ellis H, Heddle R. Br J Surg 1977; 64: 633
12. Pollock AV, Greenall MJ, Evans M. Proc R Soc Med 1979; 72: 889

transverse wounds require layer-by-layer closure of the tendinous, aponeurotic and fascial structures. Continuous sutures are quick and allow tension to distribute evenly along the length of the wound. The ratio of suture to wound length should be at least 4:1, in accordance with the recommendations of Jenkins and Israelsson.[13] This is achieved by taking a bite of the aponeurosis 1 cm from the wound edge and placing stitches at intervals of 1 cm.

ACUTE WOUND DEHISCENCE

Wound dehiscence, an acute wound failure, generally occurs 5–10 days after surgery. It is heralded by a serosanguineous discharge, and the patient may feel 'something is giving way'. The incidence is 2%, and the associated mortality can be as high as 25%. Acute wound failure ranges from superficial skin breakdown to complete failure of the wound, resulting in exposure of the abdominal contents (i.e. burst abdomen).

The wound and exposed abdominal contents may be temporarily covered with clear adhesive sheets to prevent excessive heat and fluid losses. Adequate resuscitation should be carried out before the patient is taken to the operating theatre (see Ch. 2). The wound is resutured using strong non-absorbable monofilament for a mass closure with wide bites (greater than 3 cm) from the wound edges. Deep tension sutures are optional but are rarely necessary. These sutures stay for 3 weeks or more.

The patients may be seriously ill with systemic infection, resulting in multiorgan failure. Sound surgical technique with good haemostasis, minimal tissue destruction, and effective closure of aponeuroses reduces the risk of wound failure.

DISEASES OF THE UMBILICUS

UMBILICAL TUMOURS

A primary umbilical tumour is rare. Irritation from retained sebaceous material and other debris in the umbilicus can cause squamous carcinoma. This should be treated by full-thickness excision of the umbilicus and its surrounding abdominal wall. Metastasis to the inguinal lymph nodes can develop. Primary adenocarcinoma may arise from the urachal remnant at the umbilicus.[14]

Secondary tumours often arise from direct extension of malignant diseases along the ligamentum teres from the liver to the umbilicus (Fig. 24.3).[15] Primary tumours of the breast, stomach, colon, ovary or other intra-abdominal malignancies can spread from the liver into the umbilicus. Endometrioma of the umbilicus resembles a tumour, which enlarges and bleeds at the time of the menstrual bleed.

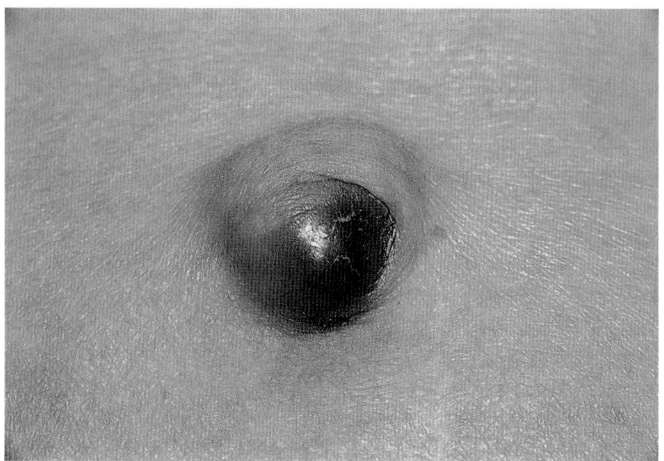

Figure 24.3 Tumour in umbilicus.

UMBILICAL FISTULA

Umbilical fistulas are abnormal communications between the umbilicus and embryonic structures of the urinary or gastrointestinal tracts; they may present as a mass just below the umbilicus. Long-healed urinary fistulas may present again with urine leaking from the umbilicus when patients develop bladder neck outflow obstruction in old age.

UMBILICAL INFECTION IN THE ADULT

Umbilical infection is more common in the obese. It is caused by a local collection of sebum, debris or body hair, and sometimes stenosis of the umbilical orifice. It may spread inwards into the peritoneal cavity. Also, because the umbilicus is the thinnest part of the abdominal wall, any intraperitoneal abscesses may present as umbilical infection. Chronic intrahepatic and subhepatic infection can extend to the umbilicus along the ligamentum teres. Preoperative investigations should exclude developmental abnormalities, abdominal infection and neoplastic diseases. Pilonidal infections are rare. Abscesses should be drained, and occasionally recurrent infections and congenital abnormalities may require the umbilicus to be excised.

UMBILICAL INFECTION IN CHILDREN

Omphalitis in newborn children may give rise to septicaemia or to thrombophlebitis of the portal vein with fatal liver suppuration and jaundice. Tetanus neonatorum can also complicate neonatal omphalitis. Most umbilical infections of the infant heal quickly with adequate hygiene. They are often associated with an umbilical polyp if they persist, which is an overgrowth of granulation tissue that should be destroyed by application of a caustic stick.

Superficial remnants of the omphalomesenteric duct or urachal remnants can lead to local suppuration in children. It is important to screen the intestine and urinary tract for other defects, which frequently coexist if there is an umbilical anomaly. Treatment is by local excision.

DISEASES OF THE ABDOMINAL WALL

TUMOURS OF THE ABDOMINAL WALL

Abdominal wall tumours are rare. They can arise from fibrous septa or muscle.

Desmoid tumours arise in the intermuscular fibrous septa of the rectus, often in women of childbearing age. The tumour is not encapsulated. It can infiltrate the rectus muscle, peritoneum and pubic bones. It presents as an elongated mass within or attached to the lower rectus sheath. Desmoid tumours arise in Gardner's syndrome, which is associated with colonic polyps and multiple osteomata, and familial polyposis coli.[16]

The tumour is treated by a full-thickness wide excision of the abdominal wall, including the skin, muscles and underlying

REFERENCES

13. Jenkins TP. Br J Surg 1976; 63: 873–876
14. Blumenthal NJ. S Afr Med J 1980; 58: 457–458
15. Quenu J, Longuet JP. Rev Chir 1896; 16: 97
16. Parks TG. Ann R Coll Surg Engl 1990; 72: 181–184

peritoneum. The defect is closed by reconstructive techniques (Ch. 9). A CT scan is used to ascertain the size of the tumour prior to surgery. Recurrence is rare following adequate local excision.[17]

Abdominal wall sarcomas are usually large, and the diagnosis is confirmed by core or incision biopsy. Preoperative assessment should include CT or MRI of the abdominal wall and the lungs (to exclude pulmonary metastases). Preoperative radio- and/or chemotherapy may be required to downstage the tumour before surgery. Treatment is by wide excision of the muscle group from their origin to insertion where possible. The abdominal wall is then reconstructed.

HAEMATOMA OF THE RECTUS SHEATH

Haematoma of the rectus sheath is the result of a spontaneous rupture of the inferior epigastric vessels or disinsertion of abdominal wall muscles.[18] Epigastric vessels may bleed following trivial events such as coughing or sneezing, especially in patients with haemophilia or in those on anticoagulation. Seat-belt and sporting injuries are other well-recognized causes of abdominal wall bleeding.

High-velocity injuries causing fractures of the ribs or pelvic fractures can tear the abdominal wall muscles from their insertions. Fractures of the lower ribs can also result in concomitant diaphragmatic injury and diaphragmatic hernia (see Ch. 7).

INJURY AND LOSS OF ABDOMINAL WALL

Abdominal wall injuries are treated by debridement followed by primary or delayed closure. When a defect is too large to be closed directly, a musculo-aponeurotic abdominoplasty can be supplemented by a mesh large enough to overlap the defect margin by 5 cm all round. Direct contact between the mesh and the underlying intestine should be minimized by positioning the omentum between them. The wound may also be closed with myocutaneous sartorius and latissimus dorsi flaps (see Ch. 9).[19]

INGUINAL HERNIA

An inguinal hernia is the protrusion of a peritoneal sac through the deep ring (indirect) or the transversalis fascia of Hasselbach's triangle (direct). It may contain abdominal contents, and indirect hernias may extend into the scrotum.

An indirect hernia is a persistent processus vaginalis that becomes patent, forming the sac of a hernia. The processus vaginalis is a protrusion of peritoneum that accompanies the testis during its descent from the abdomen. An indirect inguinal hernia is caused by a weakening of the transversalis fascia around the internal inguinal ring as a result of degeneration or increased abdominal pressure. The hernial sac follows the path of the inguinal canal through the internal and external inguinal rings before descending into the scrotum or labium majus.

EPIDEMIOLOGY AND AETIOLOGY OF INGUINAL HERNIAS

Indirect inguinal hernias occur in 4% of male infants born in the UK, and more frequently in low birth-weight and premature male infants.[20] Inguinal hernias develop most frequently in the first 3 months of life; thereafter their occurrence falls off with age, and hernias in children after 3 years of age are rare. Infantile hernias represent an intrauterine or periparturition failure of the processus vaginalis to close. At all ages, inguinal hernias are more frequent on the right side than on the left (ratio 5:4); in males this may be because the right testis takes longer to descend, leading to delayed closure of the right processus vaginalis.[21] Inguinal hernias are occasionally associated with other developmental abnormalities, such as an undescended testis.

Indirect inguinal hernias are uncommon in baby girls compared with boys (ratio 1:9), and when they occur conditions such as the testicular feminization syndrome or complete androgen insensitivity should be ruled out by chromosome studies.[22]

In adults, inguinal hernias are 10 times more common in men than in women. Five per cent are direct and 5% are a combination of direct and indirect (saddlebag or pantaloon hernias). Direct inguinal hernias are more common in elderly men as the transversalis fascia progressively weakens, but they are very uncommon in women. Both direct and indirect hernias are more common on the right side in a ratio of 5:4. Recognized predisposing factors include prematurity, twins, low birth weight and race, with Africans having a much higher incidence than Europeans.[23] The African pelvis is more oblique and has a lower arch than the European pelvis. This is associated with a narrower origin of the internal oblique muscle from the lateral inguinal ligament, which therefore fails to protect the deep ring, predisposing to herniation.

Anatomical variation may also predispose to direct inguinal hernia development. The conjoint tendon is the common insertion of the internal oblique and transversus abdominis muscles into the superior medial aspect of the pubic bone. This tendinous insertion normally extends laterally beyond the pubic tubercle for 1–2 cm along the pectineal line, where it is continuous with the iliopectineal ligament of Astley Cooper. When this lateral extension is not present the strength of the posterior wall is reduced, and this predisposes to direct herniation.[24] There is also some association between hernia development, cigarette smoking and aneurysm formation. A collagen defect has been demonstrated in these patients.[25]

Indirect hernias may occasionally develop as a complication of increased intra-abdominal pressure caused by ascites or continuous ambulatory peritoneal dialysis. Presumably, a pre-existing processus vaginalis is opened up by the increased intra-abdominal pressure.

CLINICAL FEATURES

Pain, combined with a variable or constant groin swelling, are the most common presenting symptoms. The pain is usually

REFERENCES

17. Posner MC, Shiu MH, Newsome JL et al. Arch Surg 1989; 124: 191–196
18. Siddiqui MN, Abid Q, Qaseem T et al. J R Soc Med 1992; 85: 420–421
19. Neidhardt JPH et al. In: Chevrel JD (ed). Chirurgie des Parois de l'Abdomen. Springer Verlag, Berlin, 1985
20. Rowe MI, Copelson LW, Clatworthy HW. J Paediatr Surg 1969; 4: 102–107
21. Devlin HB. Management of Abdominal Hernias. Butterworths, London, 1988
22. Berkovitz GD, Brown TR, Migeon CJ. Clin Endocrinol Metab 1983; 12: 155–173
23. Badoe EA. Afr J Med Sci 1973; 4: 51–58
24. Issac RE. Br J Surg 1961; 49: 204
25. Cannon DJ, Read RC. Ann Surg 1981; 194: 270–278

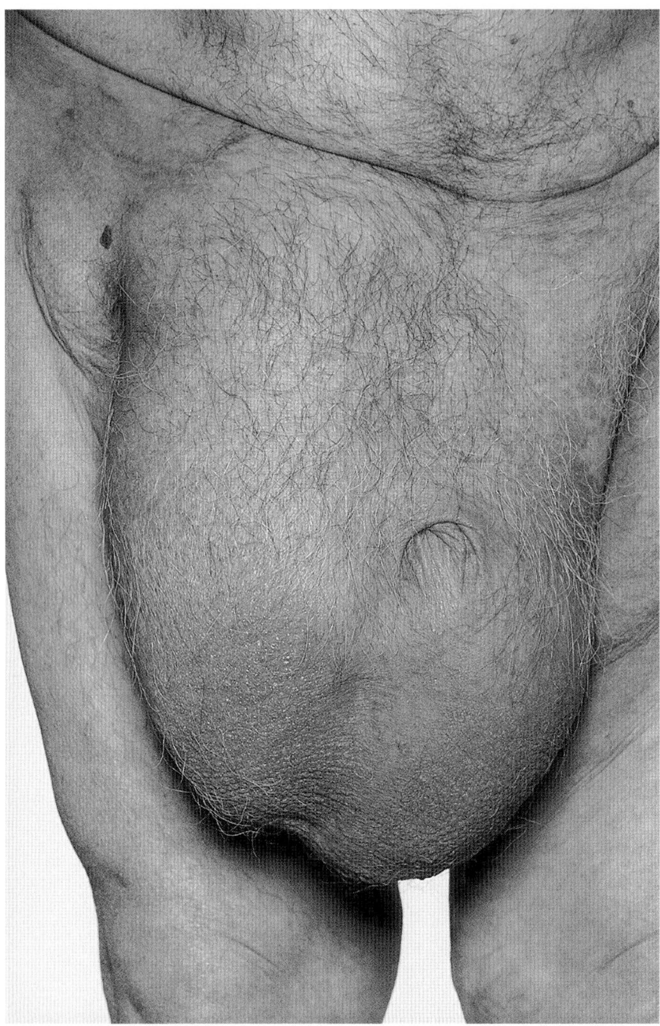

Figure 24.4 Inguinal hernia.

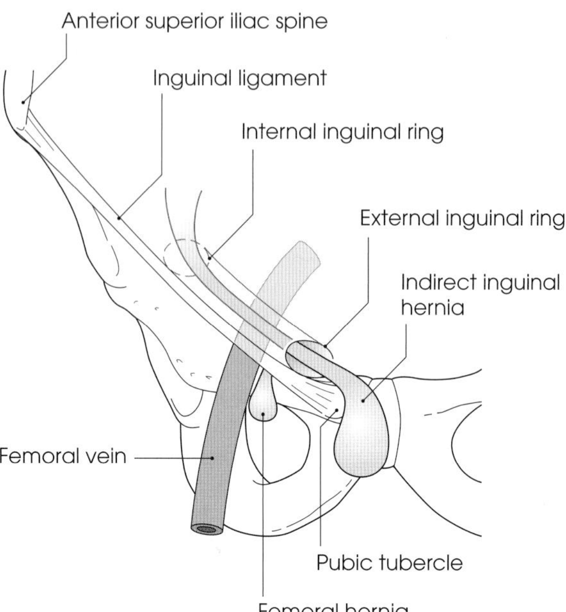

Figure 24.5 The relation of pubic tubercle to inguinal and femoral hernias.

described as a dull, dragging sensation that leads the patient to feel the groin and find the swelling. Severe pain in the groin should suggest the possibility of strangulation. Hernias are initially uncomfortable because the neck of the sac is relatively narrow and, as the neck widens, the pain improves and turns into a vague dragging sensation. The swelling is usually intermittent at first and is most frequently present in the evening or after exertion.

Patients should first be examined while they are relaxed and lying on the couch. Even if an inguinal hernia is not actually present at the time of examination, enlargement of the cord at the superficial inguinal ring may be felt by careful palpation as it emerges from the abdomen. The cord is gripped and its constituents allowed to slip one by one through the examining fingers. Thickening of the cord contents may be detected on the side of the hernia; this is known as the 'rolled skin' sign.

Invagination of the canal with the examining finger thrust up the scrotal wall is uncomfortable and gives useful information only in very large hernias, when the diagnosis is obvious anyway (Fig. 24.4). When the hernia is not obvious, a cough may send the abdominal contents down into the sac and a cough impulse may be felt by a finger placed over the external ring. The groin must be carefully examined to confirm that a hernia is present, to determine reducibility, and to establish its position in relation to the pubic tubercle (Fig. 24.5).

Patients should always be examined while they are standing up. In men, the position and size of the testicles must be checked when they are standing, and in both sexes an inguinal hernia may only be apparent when the patient stands up and coughs. A second hernia, of which the patient is unaware, on the opposite side may be detected only on standing. The abdomen must also be examined to exclude ascites and other coincidental conditions.

The patient's general fitness and any predisposing factors, such as chronic cough, constipation or prostatism, must be assessed. Previous illnesses, drug history, social history and allergies must also be noted.

IMAGING AND THE ABDOMINAL WALL

Groin hernias are usually diagnosed by clinical examination. When there is doubt, especially in obese patients, ultrasound scanning may be helpful.

Herniography is particularly helpful for detecting recurrent hernias that are not demonstrated on clinical examination (Fig. 24.6). It is performed by injecting water-soluble contrast into the peritoneal cavity of the patient in the prone position. The patient is then tilted to allow contrast to fill the hernial sac.[26] This appears as an out-pouching below the line of the peritoneal cavity. Although this investigation is sensitive, a negative investigation does not exclude a small, reducible hernia. Herniography is also useful in the investigation of patients with obscure groin pain.[27]

Computerized tomographic scanning is useful in assessing tumours of the abdominal wall in detail. Its sensitivity is increased by giving oral contrast.

REFERENCES

26. Gullmo A. World J Surg 1989; 13: 560–568
27. Smedberg SGG, Broome AE, Gullmo A et al. Am J Surg 1985; 149: 378–382

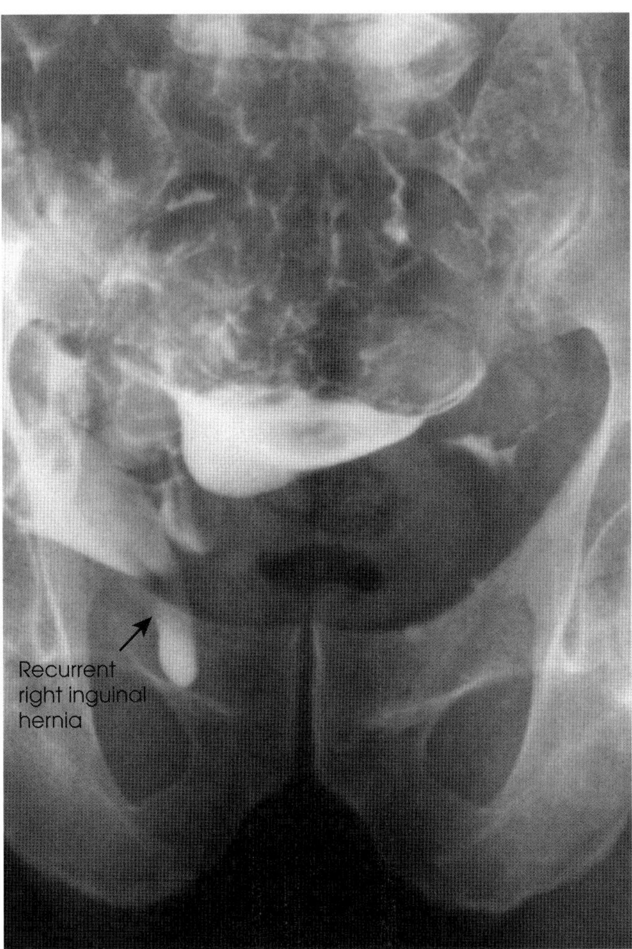

Figure 24.6 Herniography: recurrent right inguinal hernia.

DIFFERENTIAL DIAGNOSIS OF AN INGUINAL HERNIA

A hernia needs to be differentiated from other groin lumps. This depends on demonstrating the clinical features of a hernia, which is a lump of varying size with an expansible cough impulse. Not all hernias are reducible and not all lumps that are reducible are hernias, for example a varicocele.

The anatomy of the hernia should be carefully assessed. While it is usually possible to distinguish inguinal from femoral hernias, there are many inaccuracies in preoperative diagnosis.[28] Some 10% of femoral hernias are misdiagnosed as inguinal.[29] It is not possible to differentiate between direct and indirect herniation.[30] The accuracy of diagnosing a direct hernia is little better than 50%, while an indirect hernia can be correctly diagnosed in 90% of patients.[31]

Other conditions that must be distinguished from hernias in the groin include those listed below.

Hydroceles of the cord or canal of Nuck

Hydroceles of the cord or of the canal of Nuck may appear and disappear. They are usually oval, smooth and transilluminable, and they can be manipulated in the long axis of the cord. When they are pulled the testicle moves too, because it is attached to the cord. The testicle does not move when a hernia is reduced.

Ectopic testicle

An ectopic testicle can easily be mistaken for an inguinal hernia if the patient is inadequately or cursorily examined. The scrotum and its contents must always be examined with the patient lying relaxed on the couch and standing erect. The scrotum is then found to be empty and the lump is irreducible.

Spermatic cord lipoma

A lipoma of the spermatic cord is soft and lobulated, and does not vary with coughing.

Inguinal lymph node swellings

Swellings of inguinal lymph nodes are generally multiple and extend laterally, as well as lying medial to the femoral vessels.

Lipoma of femoral canal fat

A lipoma of the fat in the femoral canal can be differentiated from a femoral hernia only at operation; enlargement of this pad of fat often precedes the development of a femoral hernia and is sometimes said to be responsible for the hernia.

Saphena varix

A saphena varix presents as a smooth, soft swelling that is easily emptied by pressure and disappears when the patient lies down. It usually has a bluish appearance and demonstrable thrill on coughing. A percussion impulse can be felt when dilated veins below the sapheno-femoral junction are percussed. Distal varicose veins are usually present.

Psoas abscess

A psoas abscess may transmit a cough impulse but is usually lateral to the femoral vessels. The patient will have symptoms and signs related to the primary pathology in the spine or retroperitoneum. The abscess is often palpable above and below the inguinal ligament.

Iliofemoral aneurysm

An iliofemoral aneurysm has an expansile pulsation (see Ch. 10) and a false femoral aneurysm has an iatrogenic cause.

Diagnosis

Clinical examination remains the mainstay of diagnosis for inguinal and femoral hernias, but clinical differentiation between these groin lumps is notoriously unreliable. Much greater accuracy can be obtained by ultrasound scanning, and this is recommended whenever there is doubt. Persistent intermittent groin pain in obese women is difficult to diagnose; in these cases ultrasound may demonstrate an impalpable hernia.[32] Other causes of groin pain are shown in Table 24.1.

SURGICAL TREATMENT OF AN INGUINAL HERNIA

Principles of inguinal hernia repair in adults

A careful inspection must be made to rule out a combined hernia and to avoid the possibility of a missed hernia. A small hernial sac,

REFERENCES

28. Hardy JC, Costin JR. J Am Osteopath Assoc 1969; 68: 696–704
29. Glassow F. Ann Surg 1966; 163: 227–332
30. Ralphs DN, Brain AJ, Grundy DJ et al. Br Med J 1980; 1: 1039–1040
31. Cameron AE. Br J Surg 1994; 81: 250
32. Spangen L, Andersson R, Ohlsson L. Am Surg 1988; 54: 574

Table 24.1 Differential diagnosis of groin pain

Painful lymph nodes
- Infective and neoplastic diseases of the pelvic organs, perineal organs (vulva and anus) and lower limbs

Urological conditions
- Stone or neoplastic diseases
- Urinary tract infection

Gynaecological conditions
- Pelvic inflammatory disease

Scrotal conditions
- Epididymo-orchitis
- Torsion of ectopic testis

Hip abnormalities
- Arthritic hip pain
- Septic arthritis
- Slipped femoral epiphysis

Musculoskeletal disorders
- Adductor tendonitis
- Osteitis pubis
- Iliopsoas injury

Enthesopathy
- Inflammation of the insertion (enthesis) of the ligament or tendon

Groin disruption (Gilmore's groin)[33]
- In sportspersons, transversalis fascia

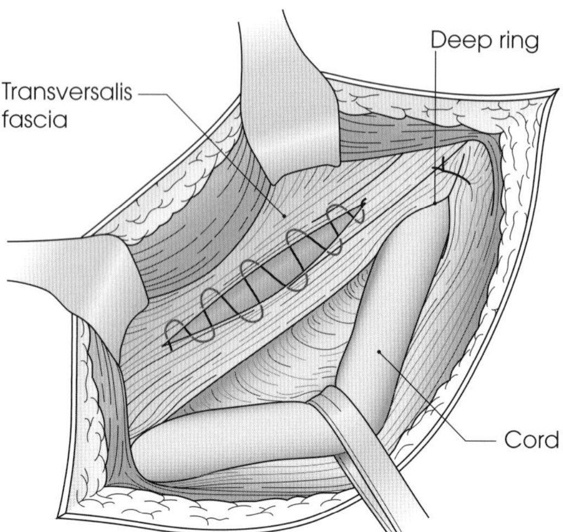

Figure 24.7 A suture is placed laterally to narrow the internal inguinal ring holding back the hernial sac. The transversalis fascia is flattened with a stitch in preparation for the placement of a mesh.

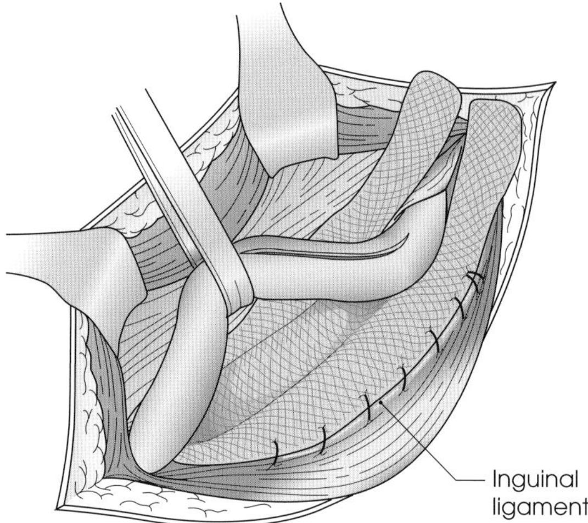

Figure 24.8 A continuous non-absorbable suture to fix the mesh along the inguinal ligament.

especially if it is direct, may be inverted and returned to the peritoneal cavity. A large or inguinoscrotal hernial sac should be opened and the contents returned to the peritoneal cavity. The distal scrotal sac should be left in situ so as not to disrupt the vascular supply to the testis. The repair of the posterior wall of the inguinal canal should be by the Lichtenstein mesh or Shouldice technique once the sac has been excised or inverted. Inguinal hernias are largely the result of a failure in the transversalis fascia of the abdominal wall. The treatment is to repair and reinforce this layer. Non-absorbable sutures and mesh are used because aponeurotic healing is slow. The mesh is sutured only to aponeurotic tissue because red muscle possesses no intrinsic strength. Operations may be carried out under local anaesthetic, regional or general anaesthesia (see Chapter 5). The decision on the type of anaesthetic depends upon the technique of repair being used (e.g. mesh or laparoscopic), the preference of the patient and their fitness for a general anaesthetic.

Lichtenstein mesh repair

Lichtenstein mesh repair may be carried out under local or general anaesthesia. An oblique incision is made 1 cm above and parallel to the medial half of the inguinal ligament, and the external oblique aponeurosis is opened in the line of its fibres into the superficial ring. The spermatic cord is carefully separated from other structures in the inguinal canal by blunt dissection. The cord is then lifted out of the inguinal canal before the sac is carefully dissected free from the cord. When a direct inguinal hernia is present, a search should still be made for an indirect sac by opening the cord coverings. The transversalis fascia over the direct sac is opened before the fascia is closed with a suture to flatten the posterior wall, easing the placement of a mesh (Fig. 24.7).

The mesh is tailored to the patient by trimming it to an appropriate size and cutting a lateral slit to accommodate the cord. The inferior border of the mesh is cut to lie parallel with the inguinal ligament. It should overlap the internal oblique–conjoint tendon by 2–3 cm. A continuous non-absorbable monofilament suture is used to attach the mesh to the inguinal ligament (Fig. 24.8).

The suture begins from medial to the pubic tubercle and is carried laterally beyond the lateral margin of the internal ring. The horizontal slit in its lateral margin is placed around the cord. A suture closes the fishtail around the internal ring securing the lower edge of the upper and lower flap to the inguinal ligament (Fig. 24.9). Interrupted sutures are used to secure the upper edge of the conjoint tendon on to the underlying aponeurosis. The mesh must be tension-free and lie flat on the posterior wall of the inguinal canal. The tails are then trimmed and tucked laterally beneath the external aponeurosis.

REFERENCE

33. Gilmore OJA. In: Kurzer M, Kart AE, Wantz GE (eds). Surgical Management of Abdominal Wall Hernias. Dunitz, London, 1999: 151–157

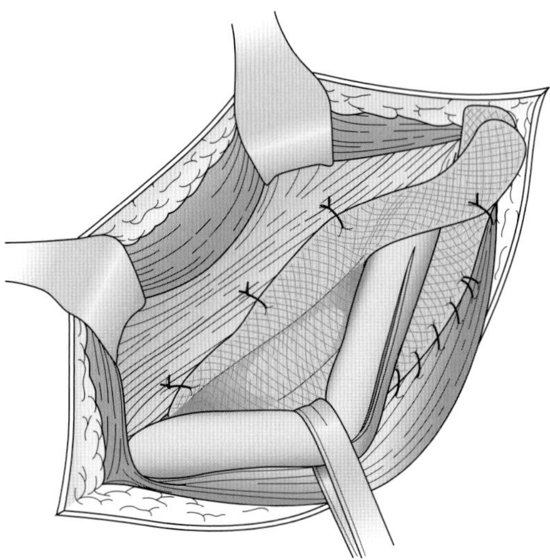

Figure 24.9 The fishtail is closed around the cord. Interrupted sutures are placed to secure the mesh flatly on to the aponeurosis.

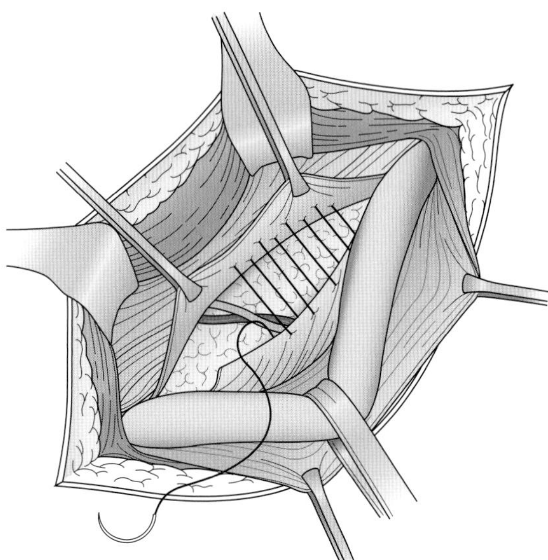

Figure 24.10 The repair is made by suturing the cut margin of the lower lateral flap of transversalis fascia to the undersurface of the upper medial flap along the white line of the conjoint tendon or arch.

Mesh

The mesh should be chemically and biologically inert, and must be incorporated into the tissues without causing a chronic inflammatory reaction, hardening or stiffness. Polypropylene and Mersilene meshes are the most commonly used. Expanded polytetrafluoroethylene mesh has a low incidence of visceral adhesion and is used if the mesh is placed intraperitoneally where contact with the bowel is possible (i.e. incisional hernia and laparoscopic hernia repair). Expanded polytetrafluoroethylene does not become incorporated, and its effectiveness is dependent on the strong non-absorbable sutures used to stitch the mesh to the surrounding tissues. A low weight Vypro mesh, combined polypropylene with absorbable polyglactin 910, does not form a tough scar.

Shouldice operation

A similar oblique incision is made 2 cm above and parallel to the inguinal ligament. The cremaster muscle is removed from the cord to give good access to the internal inguinal ring. The transversalis fascia is opened from the internal ring down to the pubic tubercle. The edges of the divided transversalis fascia are cleared of the preperitoneal fat and repaired in two overlapping layers (Fig. 24.10). This transversalis fascia repair is reinforced with two further lines of suturing between the aponeurotic conjoint tendon and the aponeurosis of the external oblique adjacent to the inguinal ligament (Fig. 24.11).

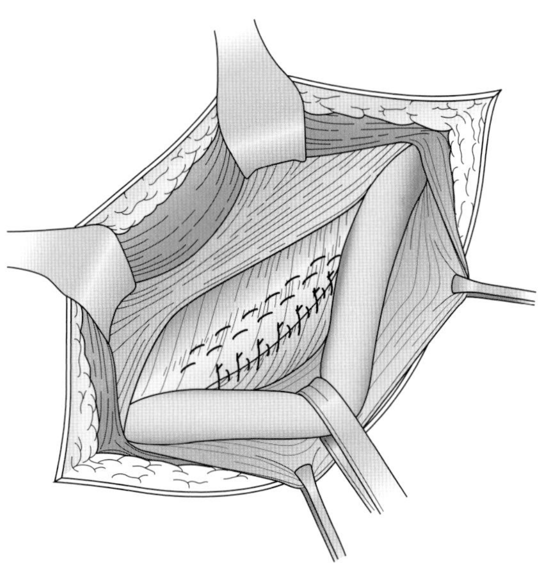

Figure 24.11 The medial repair is reinforced by suturing the cut edge of the upper flap to the lower flap.

The preperitoneal mesh repair

The preperitoneal space, behind the abdominal wall muscles, is approached through a midline or Pfannenstiel incision. The hernial sacs are identified, excised or inverted. The hernia repair and the transversalis fascia are then reinforced with a mesh sutured to Cooper's ligament and the pubis within the preperitoneal space (Fig. 24.12).[34]

Laparoscopic repair of inguinal hernia

Laparoscopic hernia repair requires a general anaesthetic. The National Institute of Clinical Excellence in the UK has recommended that it is only used for recurrent inguinal hernias or bilateral hernias by experienced surgeons. The results of multicentre randomized trials have indicated that laparoscopic repair is associated with less postoperative pain and quicker recovery, with a more rapid return to normal activity. The procedure costs more, however, and has the occasional disastrous complication of visceral injury or bowel perforation.

Laparoscopic repair can be carried out through totally extraperitoneal and transabdominal preperitoneal approaches. The mesh is placed in the preperitoneal space in both approaches (Fig. 24.13). The totally extraperitoneal approach is safer but more difficult to learn. The transabdominal preperitoneal approach is simpler to learn but carries a small risk of visceral and vascular injuries. It has the advantage that both

REFERENCE

34. Stoppa R et al. Chirurgie 1982; 108: 570

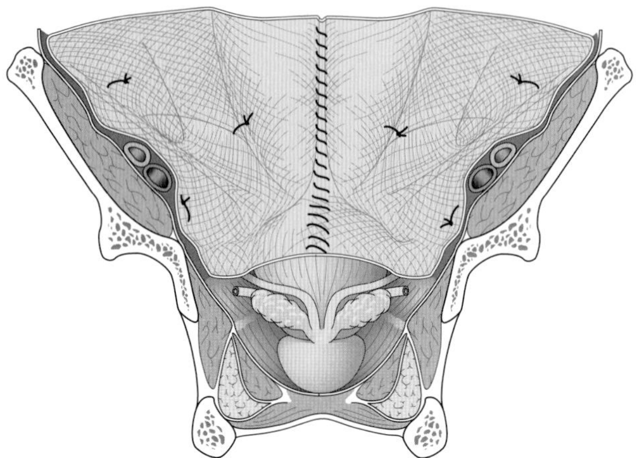

Figure 24.12 The mesh is held in the preperitoneal space by a few sutures and abdominal pressure. All hernia sites are covered.

hernial orifices can be examined if bilateral hernias are suspected.

Many of the early complications of vascular and nerve injury were associated with incorrect placement of staples. Patients are asked to empty their bladder before surgery to avoid injury and to avoid obscuring the operative view.

A totally extraperitoneal approach is performed through an infraumbilical incision of 1–2 cm. The anterior rectus sheath on the side of the hernia is divided and the rectus muscle is retracted laterally. A 10-cm cannula is used to enter the space immediately posterior to the rectus muscle, which is relatively avascular. A combination of gentle blunt dissection with an insufflating pressure of 10–12 mmHg opens the preperitoneal space. Balloon dissection can also be used to open this space. It is important not to injure the inferior epigastric vessels by dissecting close to the rectus muscle. Beneath this space is a thicker posterior layer of the transversalis fascia and the peritoneum.

The hernial sac is dissected from surrounding structures, care being taken not to tear the peritoneum in the process. The potential sites for indirect, direct and femoral hernias are exposed and covered with a 15 × 10-cm open-weave polypropylene mesh, and the transversalis fascia is reinforced. The mesh does not usually need to be fixed, but if this is thought necessary it should be attached only to the pectineal (Cooper's) ligament.

In the transabdominal preperitoneal approach, a pneumoperitoneum is created and the hernial contents are identified and reduced. The preperitoneal space is entered by dividing the peritoneum anterior to the hernia. The space is then enlarged and the vessels and nerves identified. A pocket is dissected in the peritoneal space to enable the mesh to spread out flat. The internal ring may be reinforced with a stitch if an indirect hernia is present, and the transversalis fascia of the direct inguinal hernia may be plicated. The peritoneal opening is then carefully closed to avoid direct contact of the mesh with the bowel, because this may result in erosion with the formation of a fistula. Port sites of more than 1 cm in size must have a fascial closure to prevent the risk of an incisional hernia developing.

Results

The mortality rate for all types of elective hernia repair is close to zero at all ages, and the incidence of recurrence should be under 5%.

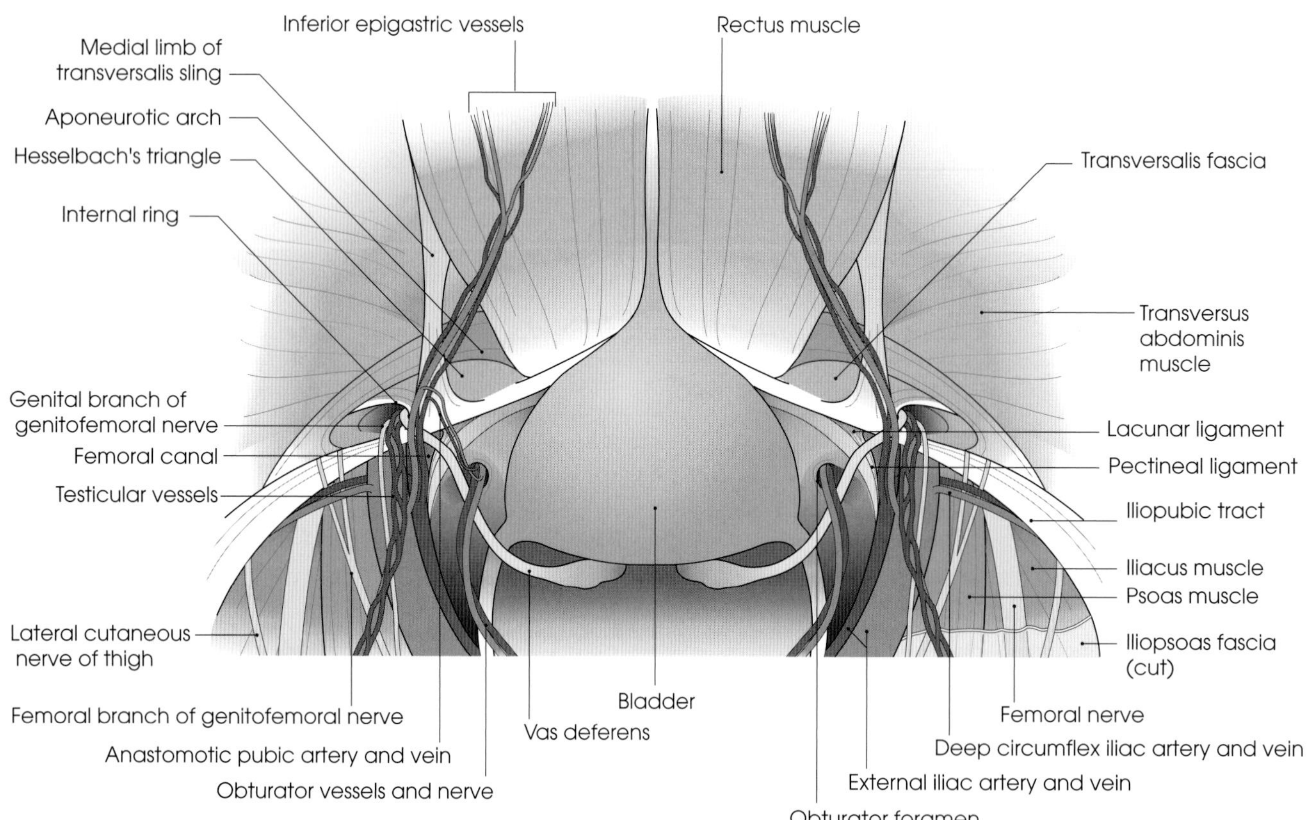

Figure 24.13 Preperitoneal space.

COMPLICATIONS

Recurrent inguinal hernia

The recurrence rate of inguinal hernia has decreased to 1–3% since the development of mesh repair. Recurrence is related to the experience of the surgeon, technical failure and infection. A missed hernia may also present as a recurrent hernia.

Recurrent groin hernias should be repaired by experienced surgeons. A routine Lichtenstein mesh repair is recommended for a first-time recurrence following a sutured repair without complications. The preperitoneal approach is recommended if the primary repair was by the Lichtenstein technique or was complicated by infection, because this obviates the need for extensive dissection and potential damage to the testicular vessels, which may be encased by a thick layer of fibrous tissue.

Any subsequent recurrence should be performed through virgin territory via the peritoneal route, avoiding the fibrosed site. Laparoscopic repair is an attractive option.

Strangulated inguinal hernia

Strangulation occurs when a viscus, normally the small intestine, is trapped within a hernial sac and both the lumen of the bowel and its blood supply are constricted. The constricting agent may be the neck of the peritoneal sac, which is often fibrosed and rigid as it passes through the transversalis surrounding the deep inguinal ring. The external inguinal ring may also be the site of occlusion in many of the large, obstructed inguinoscrotal hernias. Direct inguinal hernias rarely obstruct. The ischaemic obstructed bowel becomes gangrenous if left untreated and patients die from peritonitis and sepsis.

Clinical features

Patients present with a tender irreducible groin lump, and in the early stages there are usually no signs of bowel obstruction, although these often develop over the next few hours if nothing is done (see Ch. 25). Eventually, colicky abdominal pain, distension and vomiting develop, although in a Richter's hernia these symptoms may never arise before the patient develops septicaemic shock.

The differential diagnosis includes other causes of irreducible painful groin lump, such as an infected lymph node, a groin abscess, a femoral false aneurysm, an abdominal abscess pointing to the groin and, of course, a strangulated femoral hernia. Other causes of intestinal obstruction are discussed in Ch. 25. Occasionally a plain abdominal radiograph and groin ultrasound are required, but the diagnosis is usually made from the history and careful examination of the groin. Any irreducible tender swelling in the inguinal region must be considered to be a strangulated hernia unless proved otherwise.

A femoral hernia should be distinguished from an inguinal hernia by the relationship of the neck of the sac to the pubic tubercle, the femoral variety being below and lateral. This distinction, however, is difficult when the neck is overlain by the main body of the hernial sac. A large femoral hernia may extend upwards across the inguinal ligament because the fusion of Scarpa's fascia with the deep fascia of the thigh, prevents extension inferiorly. When this is the case, the neck may be impalpable. By contrast, a small femoral hernia that may be the site of dangerous small bowel obstruction or ischaemia is easily missed unless the groin is meticulously examined.

Management

At an early stage, careful taxis may be attempted to try to reduce the hernia and avoid emergency surgery. This is, however, a risky procedure and should be performed only by an experienced surgeon. Patients who present with painful irreducible hernias require careful assessment and adequate resuscitation before surgery (see Ch. 25).

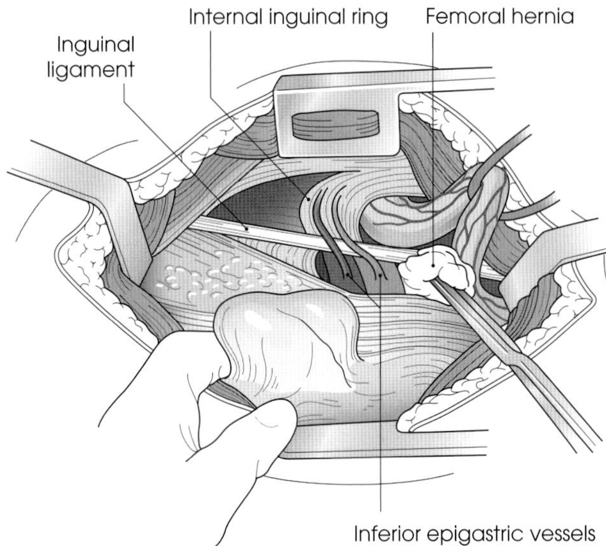

Figure 24.14 A preperitoneal approach to strangulated groin hernias.

There are more than 300 deaths per year from strangulated hernias in England and Wales. Cardiopulmonary comorbidity accounts for most of these. The anaesthetist must be informed of the patient's condition at an early stage and should be encouraged to participate in their resuscitation. The duration of resuscitation depends on the patient's response to treatment, and a failure to respond indicates that the hernia probably contains ischaemic bowel. Emergency surgery must then be carried out to ensure survival.

A full blood count, urea and electrolytes, as well as insertion of a urinary catheter, should assess the fluid requirements that are usually given as normal saline (see Ch. 2). Resuscitation and optimization of any comorbidity is especially important in neonates and the elderly. The mortality of strangulated hernia increases with age: at 60 years it is 3%, at 70 years it is 6%, and at 80 years it is 12%.[35]

A preperitoneal approach is recommended for a strangulated inguinal hernia (Fig. 24.14). A lower midline or unilateral Pfannenstiel incision is used to enter the preperitoneal space behind the rectus muscle. The strangulated hernial sac is identified and its neck opened. The contents are returned to the peritoneal cavity. Warm moist packs are applied to any borderline ischaemic bowel to improve its viability. Infarcted bowel is resected and anastomosed before a mesh is placed in the preperitoneal space, unless there is gross contamination. Laparotomy may be necessary if the strangulated hernia is large. It is not advisable to place a mesh in a grossly contaminated area, when the Shouldice repair should be used.

Incomplete reduction of hernia: reduction en masse

Hernias can be reduced, but this carries risks if they are tender and might be strangulated. Ischaemic bowel can be returned

REFERENCE

35. Ryan EA. Surg Gynecol Obstet 1971; 133: 440–446

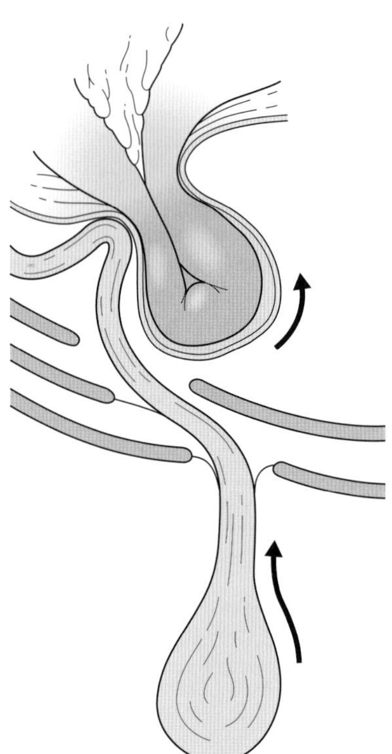

Figure 24.15 Reduction en masse. The hernial content is returned into the peritoneal cavity without relieving the constriction.

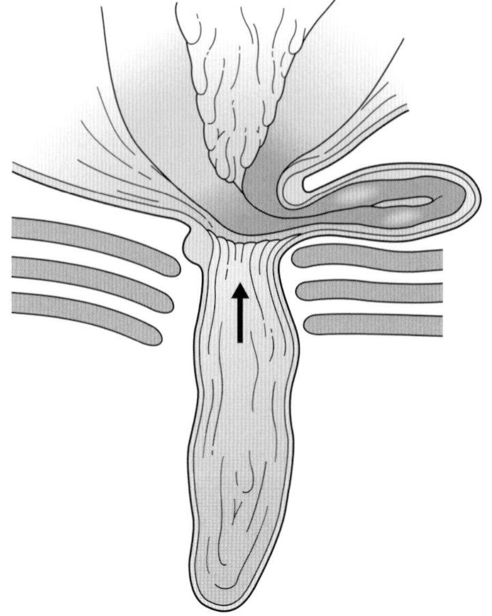

Figure 24.16 Reduction en masse. The hernial content is reduced between the muscle layers of the abdominal wall.

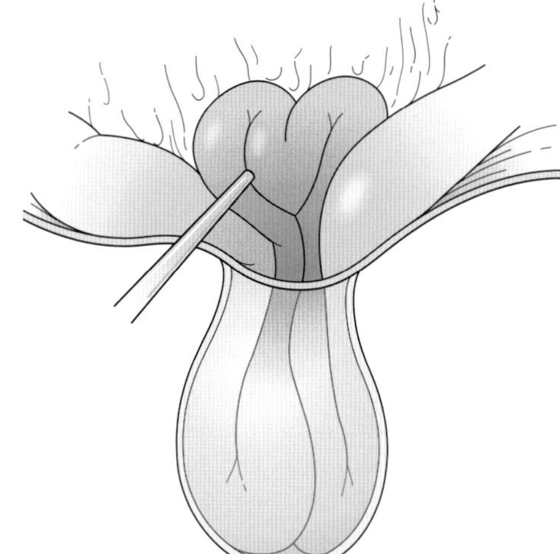

Figure 24.17 Maydl's W-loop hernia strangulation.

to the peritoneum, and the hernial contents may be returned to the abdomen without relieving the constriction (Fig. 24.15) or the contents being reduced between the muscle layers of the abdominal wall (Fig. 24.16). For these reasons, great care must be taken if taxis is attempted.

Maydl's hernia

Maydl's hernia is when a W shape of the small bowel loop lies within the sac and the affected loop is strangulated within the main abdominal cavity by a constriction at the neck of the sac (Fig. 24.17).[36]

Afferent loop strangulation

Afferent loop strangulation occurs when the afferent small bowel entering the hernial sac loops around the afferent and efferent small bowel loops coming into and leaving the sac (Fig. 24.18).[37] This results in strangulation and ischaemia.

Richter's hernia

Richter's hernia occurs when part of the bowel, usually its antimesenteric portion, is strangulated in the sac (Fig. 24.19). Patients may present with symptoms of incomplete bowel obstruction and ischaemia. This complication is more often seen in femoral hernias.

Littré's hernia

Littré's hernia is a rarity.[38] An inflamed Meckel's diverticulum is present within the hernial sac, causing symptoms and signs that cannot be differentiated from strangulation. The pain resolves when local inflammation closes off the diverticulum within the hernial sac.

Sliding hernia

Sliding hernia is a hernia in which part of the sac wall is formed by a viscus, such as the caecum or colon (Fig. 24.20). It occurs when the caecum or sigmoid colon, which are retroperitoneal structures, become detached from the posterior abdominal wall, sliding down the inguinal canal, dragging down their anterior covering of peritoneum. In children the medial wall of the sac may contain the bladder, and an ovary with its fallopian tube may also be present. Large inguinoscrotal hernias in the elderly are likely to be sliding hernias.

At operation, the hernial sac is opened, taking care to avoid opening the bowel by mistake. The hernial contents and the sliding bowel are returned to the abdomen, and the repair carried out in the usual fashion. Redundant sac is excised before the transversalis fascia is reconstituted.

Ischaemic orchitis

A strangulated inguinal hernia can obstruct the testicular vessels at the external inguinal ring. During all hernia surgery, testicular

REFERENCES

36. Bayley AC. Br J Surg 1970; 57: 687–690
37. Philip PJ. Br J Surg 1967; 54; 96–99
38. Treves F. Med-Chir Trans 1887; 52: 149–167

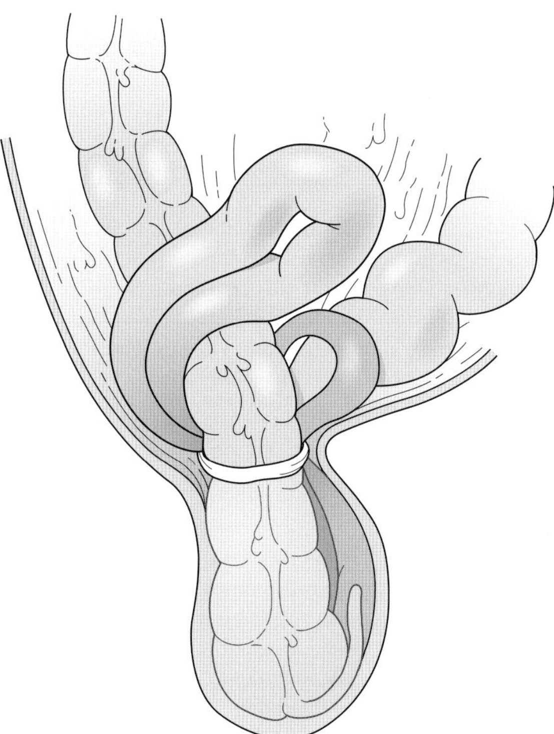

Figure 24.18 Afferent loop strangulation.

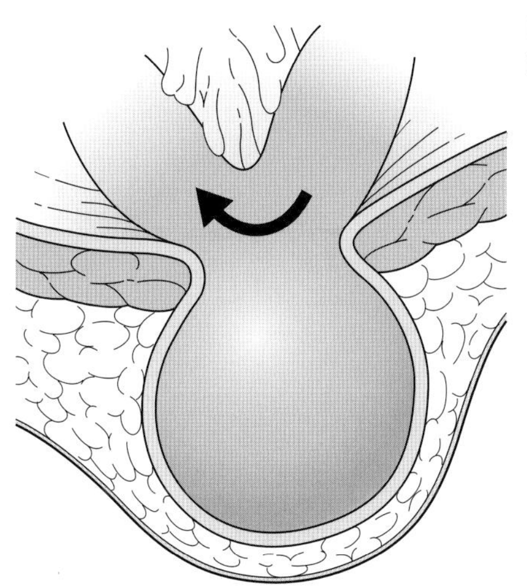

Figure 24.19 Richter's hernia.

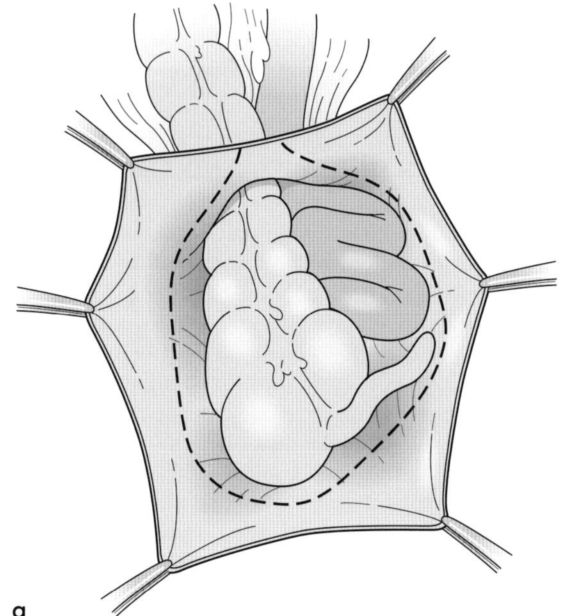

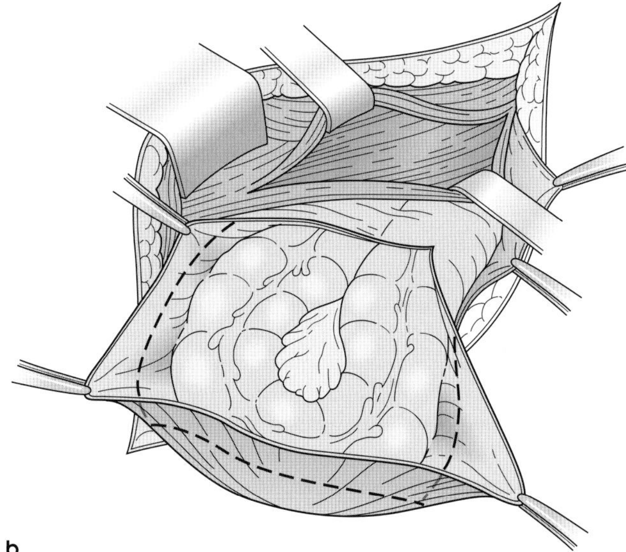

Figure 24.20 A sliding hernia with caecum as part of the hernial sac wall. The caecum is on the right (**a**), the sigmoid colon on the left (**b**).

vessels must be handled with care when the hernial sac is being dissected. The collateral circulation to the testis is preserved if the testes are not displaced from the scrotum.[39] The affected testis may feel hard in the postoperative period, but usually this recovers with adequate endocrine function and cosmetic outcome.

Ischaemic orchitis is slow in onset, causing a painful and swollen testis. A low-grade fever is present and the spermatic cord feels shortened and tender. The symptoms last for 4–5 days and a quarter of affected patients develop testicular atrophy. It is caused by venous infarction following thrombosis or ligation of the pampiniform plexus. Ischaemic orchitis complicates 0.3% of primary inguinal hernia repairs[40] and 2% of recurrent inguinal hernia repairs. Multiple operations increase the risk of developing ischaemic orchitis. The treatment is conservative, with analgesia and scrotal support. Orchidectomy is rarely required but spermatogenesis is usually lost.

Postoperative hydrocele

This is a rare complication of inguinal hernia repair. It is more likely if a large amount of fat is dissected out of the cord and the lymphatics are disrupted. The incidence is less than 0.5% and virtually all resolve spontaneously. Aspiration may help to relieve any discomfort. Operation is rarely required.

Chronic groin pain

Severe, chronic groin pain occurs in about 2% of postoperative patients[41] and is difficult to treat. Nerve injury is usually the cause.

REFERENCES

39. Puri P, Guiney EJ, O'Donnell B. J Paediatr Surg 1984; 19: 44
40. Wantz GE. Surg Clin North Am 1984; 64: 287–298
41. O'Dwyer PJ, Serpell MG. In: Bendavid R et al (eds). Principles and Management in Abdominal Wall Hernia. Springer-Verlag, New York, 2001: 726–730

Patients with pain that persists for 3 or more months after the hernia repair should be referred to a pain clinic. Re-exploration with division of the nerves or removal of the mesh should be considered only as a last resort.

INGUINAL HERNIAS IN BABIES AND CHILDREN

(see Ch. 40)

Ten per cent of children with inguinal hernias present as emergencies with incarceration, which has its highest incidence in the first 3 months of life. Although incarceration is common, strangulation is rare.[42] In infants, prompt elective surgery for inguinal hernia is essential, whatever the age of the child. The probability of incarceration is one in four for all inguinal hernias in boys before the age of 1 year.

Until the inguinal canal develops its obliquity at the age of 11–12 years, simple herniotomy is sufficient to repair the common indirect inguinal hernia. The operation should be carefully performed to avoid testicular vessel damage and to give a good cosmetic scar.[43] A skin-crease incision is made 1 cm cephalad to the external inguinal ring. The cord is defined as it emerges from the inguinal canal, and the fibres of the cremaster are gently opened to display the blue peritoneal sac on the anterosuperior aspect of the cord. The sac is separated from the cord structures, and if the sac is complete, extending into the scrotum and containing the testicle, it is divided across and the distal sac is left in situ without dislocating the testis from the scrotum. The sac is dissected proximally and its neck, with the parietal peritoneum, is identified. Any contents are returned to the peritoneal cavity; this is especially important in females, when the fallopian tube and ovary can be a sliding component of the hernial sac wall. The sac is transfixed and ligated at its junction to the peritoneal cavity, and any redundant sac excised before the wound is closed.

The testicle should not be dislocated from the scrotum during the operation because this causes a higher incidence of testicular ischaemia. The surgeon must check that the testicle is in its proper place in the scrotum at the completion of the operation, to avoid iatrogenic ectopic testicles.

FEMORAL HERNIA

Femoral hernia is two and a half times more common in females than in males in the UK, although in females indirect inguinal hernia is as common as femoral hernia.[44] The incidence of femoral hernias varies around the world; femoral hernias are very rare in native Africans.[45] It is postulated that chronic foot infections lead to repeated inflammation of groin lymph nodes and that the consequent fibrosis of the femoral canal prevents herniation.[46]

The femoral sac is an acquired downwards extension of peritoneum through the femoral canal, which is normally occupied by extraperitoneal fat and Cloquet's lymph node. The sac has inguinal ligament in front, the lacunar ligament medial, the femoral vein lateral, and the pectineal ligament and pectineus muscle behind as it passes through the femoral ring. The anterior layer of the femoral sheath, lying in front of the sac, is a downwards continuation of the transversalis fascia; the posterior wall is a downwards continuation of the fascia iliaca. Thus the femoral sheath is a funnel-shaped extension of the transversalis fascia into the thigh (Fig. 24.21).[47]

The hernial sac is considered to be acquired because a preformed sac has never been found at autopsy on a newborn infant. The hernia commonly arises late in life and it is most frequently seen in multiparous women. Weight loss predisposes to femoral herniation in both sexes. Ten per cent of femoral hernias follow a previous operation for an inguinal hernia, especially in adult men.

Femoral hernia is more common in females than in males because the inguinal ligament makes a wider angle with the pubis in the female, and an increase in the fat of the femoral canal occurs in obese middle-aged women which stretches the femoral sheath. When the obesity disappears in old age, a femoral hernia develops. Pregnancy increases the intra-abdominal pressure and may stretch the transversalis fascia predisposing to femoral herniation.

When a femoral hernia enters the thigh, it lies below the fossa ovalis and enlarges forwards, stretching the cribriform fascia over its fundus. The upper edge of the fossa ovalis has a strong, tight and sharp edge, and the hernia twists over this edge before extending upwards and medially in the superficial fascia, over the inguinal ligament, and into the angle between the superficial external pudendal and superficial epigastric veins. As a femoral hernia enlarges through the cribriform fascia it may obstruct the saphenous vein, which becomes dilated.

A femoral hernia is rarely large, and in an obese patient may be difficult to find. It is not usually reducible, and frequently patients have no cough impulse. It usually contains omentum and rarely contains bowel. Richter's hernia is more common here than at any other site, and more common in the right femoral canal than in the left.

Certain rare varieties of femoral hernia are recognized. They are listed below in order of frequency.

PREVASCULAR HERNIA

A prevascular hernia (Narath's hernia) protrudes as a long narrow sac in front of the femoral artery. It is the prolongation of the transversalis fascia, which constitutes its sheath.[48] Its relation to the inferior epigastric artery is variable. The sac lies lateral to the saphenous opening and shows no tendency to protrude forwards or to ride up over the inguinal ligament. A hernia of this type may complicate congenital dislocation of the hip, or follow surgery on the innominate bones or the external iliac vessels. This type of hernia can complicate any groin wound when the inguinal ligament has been divided.[49]

EXTERNAL FEMORAL HERNIA

An external femoral hernia (Hesselbach[50]) enters the thigh lateral to the deep epigastric vessels and the femoral vessels. It is usually associated with an indirect inguinal hernia.

REFERENCES

42. Nussbaum A. Munch Med Wochenschr 1913; 60: 1434
43. Harvey MH, Johnstone MJ, Fossard DP. Br J Surg 1985; 72: 485–487
44. Glassow F. Ann J Surg 1971; 121: 637–641
45. Cole GJ. Trans R Soc Trop Med Hyg 1964; 58: 441–447
46. Wosornu L. Trop Doct 1974; 4: 59–63
47. McVay CB. Surg Clin North Am 1971; 51: 1251–1261
48. Narath A. Arch Klin Chir 1899; 59: 396
49. Keynes G. Br J Surg 1932; 20: 55
50. Hesselbach FK. Neueste Anatomisch-Pathologische. Baumgartner, Wurzburg, 1814

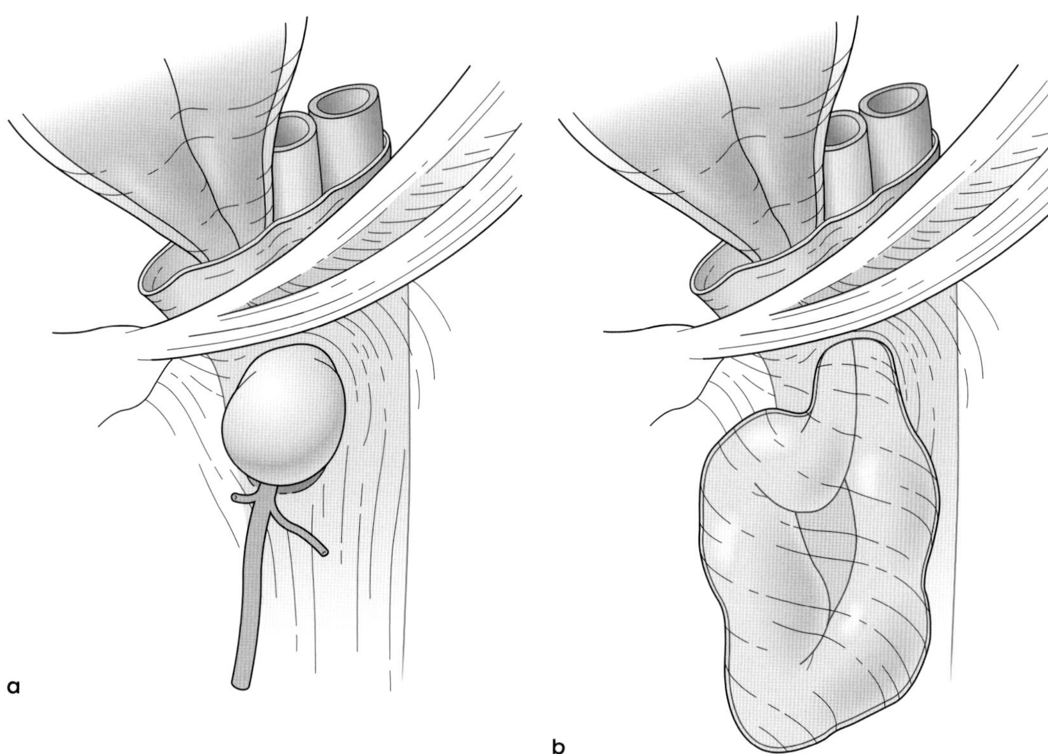

Figure 24.21 Femoral hernia. (a) A femoral hernia exploits the medial femoral sheath to enter the thigh and emerge through the saphenous opening. (b) The sac descends along the femoral sheath to the saphenous opening, where it enters the superficial tissues of the thigh.

TRANSPECTINEAL FEMORAL HERNIA

A transpectineal femoral hernia (Laugier[51]) enters the thigh through a defect in the pectineal part of the inguinal ligament or through the lacunar ligament.

DEEP FEMORAL HERNIA

In a deep femoral hernia (Callisen or Cloquet[52]), the sac descends deep to the femoral vessels and spreads out fanwise under the deep fascia. It cannot protrude through the saphenous opening.

MULTILOCULAR DEEP FEMORAL HERNIA

A multilocular deep femoral hernia enters the thigh deep to the investing deep fascia.[53] Loculi spread out and can be mistaken for an obturator hernia.

VARIANT ASSOCIATED WITH TESTICULAR MALDESCENT

An extremely rare variant of a femoral hernia associated with maldescent of the testicle had been described once in the literature. In this case the testicle descended behind the inguinal ligament, causing a femoral hernia with the testicle as a sliding component of its wall.[54]

DIFFERENTIAL DIAGNOSIS

A femoral hernia must be differentiated from the following.

Inguinal hernia

An inguinal hernia lies above the inguinal ligament. Difficulties may arise when the fundus of a femoral hernia turns upwards and lies in front of the inguinal ligament. The neck of the sac can usually be felt below and lateral to the pubic tubercle.

Saphena varix

A saphena varix, which often has a bluish tinge, is very soft, is associated with a dilated long saphenous vein and disappears on lying down. It frequently has a palpable thrill on coughing and a tap impulse (see Ch. 10).

Enlarged lymph node

An enlarged lymph node may be impossible to diagnose with certainty unless other enlarged nodes are present. Ultrasound or fine-needle aspiration cytology may be useful.

Psoas bursa

A psoas bursa is usually associated with an osteoarthritic hip and disappears on hip flexion. Ultrasound and aspiration confirm the diagnosis.

Psoas abscess

A psoas abscess is normally fluctuant, and there may be cross-fluctuation above the inguinal ligament with an iliac abscess. There are signs in the back, and radiographs of the spine, CT scanning and ultrasound confirm the diagnosis.

Lipoma

A lipoma may be impossible to differentiate from a femoral hernia.

Femoral aneurysm

A femoral aneurysm has an expansile pulsation.

REFERENCES

51. Laugier S. Arch Gen Med Paris 1833; 2: 27
52. Callisen H. Herniaerarioram Hanniae 1777; 2: 321
53. Cooper A. The Anatomy of Hernia. Cox, London, 1804
54. Stirk DI. Br J Surg 1955; 43: 331–332

Sarcoma

A sarcoma usually enlarges rapidly, but slow-growing leiomyosarcomas of the femoral vessels can be difficult to differentiate.

Ectopic testis

An ectopic testis is suspected if the testis is not present in the scrotum. Ultrasound should confirm the diagnosis.

Obturator hernia

An obturator hernia feels deeper and more lateral but can be mistaken for a femoral hernia in a very thin thigh.

TREATMENT OF FEMORAL HERNIA

Operation should always be recommended. Elective operation is advised as soon as possible, because femoral hernias have a considerable risk of strangulation, and elective operations on relatively fit elderly patients have a lower morbidity than emergency operations. An emergency operation for obstruction or strangulation should be preceded by careful resuscitation (see Ch. 2).[55]

A femoral hernia is caused by a defect of the transversalis fascia, which allows a peritoneal protrusion to occur. Repair is by removing the peritoneal sac, repairing the transversalis fascia and reinforcing the aponeurosis. Three approaches to femoral hernia repair are described:

1. the abdominal, suprapubic, retroperitoneal, preperitoneal or extraperitoneal (eponyms Cheatle, Henry, McEvedy);[56]
2. the inguinal or high (eponyms Annandale, Lothiessen or Moschowitz);[57] and
3. the crural or low (eponyms Bassinni or Lockwood).[58]

The extraperitoneal approach utilizes a midline vertical or a Pfannenstiel incision to undertake bilateral repairs. A transverse incision and oblique muscle split can be used for unilateral operations. The extraperitoneal space is opened by blunt dissection; the sac is found and evacuated from the parietes. The peritoneum can be opened to inspect or resect contents.

The inguinal approach opens the inguinal canal and then divides the transversalis fascia forming the posterior wall of the canal to gain access to the femoral canal from above (Fig. 24.22).

The crural approach uses an oblique incision in the groin about 1 cm below and parallel to the medial two-thirds of the inguinal ligament. The femoral sac is found in the subcutaneous tissue; the sac is then cleared, isolated and opened. It is then transfixed or closed, and excised (Fig. 24.23).

The extraperitoneal approach is the most useful approach for a strangulated hernia. The inguinal approach enables inguinal and femoral hernias to be repaired simultaneously, but the posterior wall of the inguinal canal must be repaired to avoid an inguinal hernia developing. The crural operation is easy to do and is best reserved for elective situations. A standard paramedian incision should be made to deal with the devitalized bowel or omentum if it is used on an emergency case.

The parietal repair is achieved by suturing the medial inguinal ligament to the Cooper's pectineal ligament with a non-absorbable monofilament polymer (Fig. 24.23). Care should be taken not to compress or damage the femoral vein, which lies immediately laterally. Iliofemoral vein thrombosis and fatal pulmonary embolism have occurred after femoral hernia repair when the vein has been compressed.[59]

This repair can be reinforced by placing an extraperitoneal mesh or by suturing the lower aponeurotic fibres of the conjoint tendon to the pectineal line. A flap of pectineal fascia can also be turned up and sutured over the defect. Alternatively, the femoral canal can be plugged with a rolled-up mesh secured by sutures placed through its fascial margins.

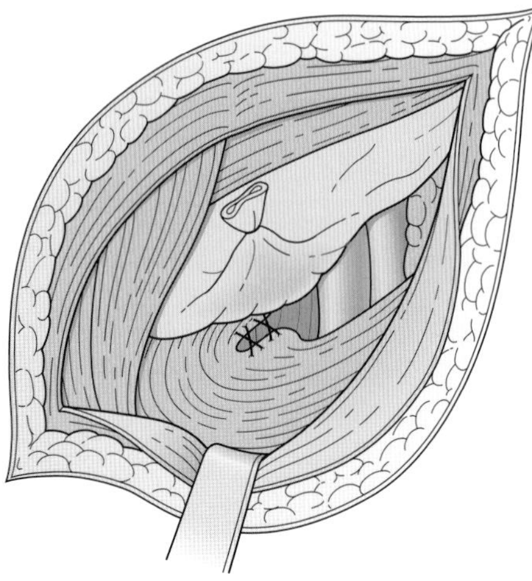

Figure 24.22 The femoral sac has been transferred and the femoral canal closed from above.

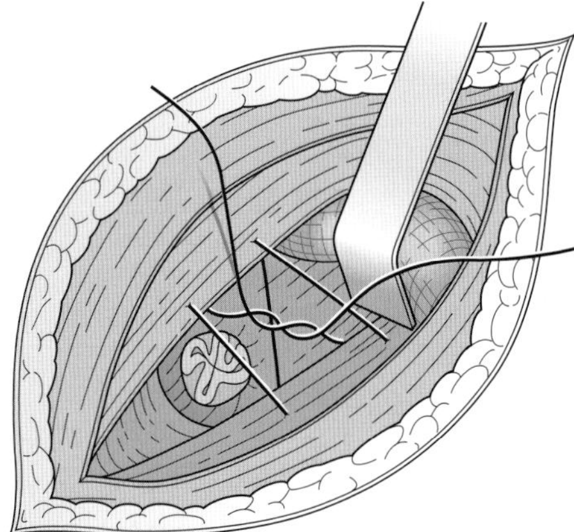

Figure 24.23 The femoral canal is closed by suturing the medial inguinal ligament to the pectineal ligament.

The high extraperitoneal approach is ideal when the hernia is strangulated, and the low crural operation is the simplest for the elective case. The overall recurrence rate for femoral hernia operations by either of these routes is 15%; this doubles to 30% if the inguinal approach is used.[60] When the inguinal approach is used electively and combined with a Shouldice repair of the inguinal canal, an impressively low recurrence rate of under 2% has been recorded.[29,55]

The principles that govern the management of strangulated femoral hernia are the same as those employed in strangulated inguinal hernia. The constricting agent is usually the thickened neck of the sac where it abuts the femoral ring. The neck is then divided, but division of the edge of the lacunar ligament is not required. Rarely, the strangulating agent of a large hernia is the edge of the fossa ovalis. A formal laparotomy should always be carried out if there is any doubt about the viability of the sac contents.

REFERENCES

55. Nicholson S, Keane TE, Devlin HB. Br J Surg 1990; 77: 307–308
56. McEvedy PG. Ann R Coll Surg Engl 1950; 7: 484
57. Moschowitz AV. NY State J Med 1907; 7: 396–400
58. Lockwood CB. Lancet 1893; ii: 1297
59. Brown RE, Kinateder RJ, Rosenberg N. Surgery 1980; 87: 230–232
60. Wheeler MH. Proc R Soc Med 1975; 68: 177–178

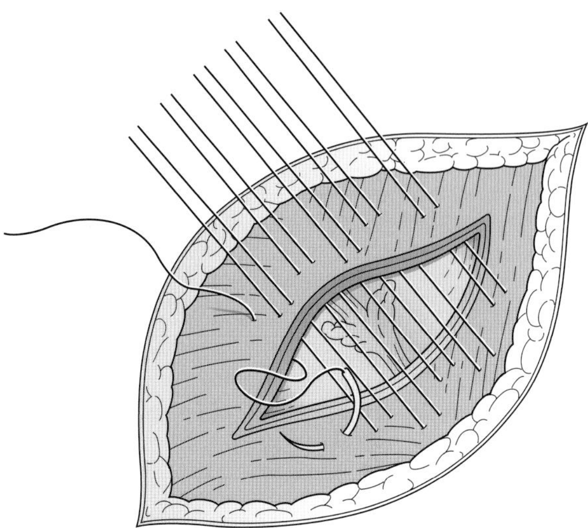

Figure 24.24 Mayo repair.

UMBILICAL HERNIA IN INFANTS AND CHILDREN (see Chapter 40)

Minor degrees of umbilical herniation are present in many neonates, but the majority resolve spontaneously. The number of umbilical hernias that require surgery is about three per 1000 live births in the UK. Risk factors are prematurity, Down's syndrome and a family history.

The hernia is usually noticed when the child cries, and consists of a peritoneal sac protruding through the umbilical cicatrix. Repair can usually be safely delayed until the age of 3 or 4 years. The Mayo operation (Fig. 24.24) is an effective method of repair.

ADULT UMBILICAL HERNIA

Adult umbilical hernias have no gender bias. They can be related to increased intra-abdominal pressure caused by obesity, multiple pregnancies, ascites and continuous ambulatory peritoneal dialysis. The neck of the hernial sac is often surprisingly narrow and fibrous, and the contents often adhere to each other, forming complex multiloculation. The hernial sac may also adhere to the overlying umbilicus and skin, and in some instances it may be difficult to preserve the umbilicus.

Strangulation is common in umbilical hernias. Patients present with abdominal pain and subacute bowel obstruction.

A horizontal incision is made over the hernia and down to the rectus sheath to expose the neck of the sac. The sac is opened near its neck, where adhesions are least likely to be present, and the contents are reduced into the peritoneal cavity. The sac is ligated and excised at the neck. A Mayo repair (Fig. 24.24) is the operation of choice when there is a small fascial defect. The repair is reinforced with mesh if the defect is very large.

EPIGASTRIC HERNIA

Preperitoneal fat protrudes through a small defect in the linea alba and may draw peritoneum after it as a small hernial sac. Preoperative investigations must be carried out if there are symptoms of dyspepsia, reflux or epigastric pain, which are present in a third of patients in some series.[61] The sac should be excised and the linea alba repaired by Mayo's technique (Fig. 24.24).

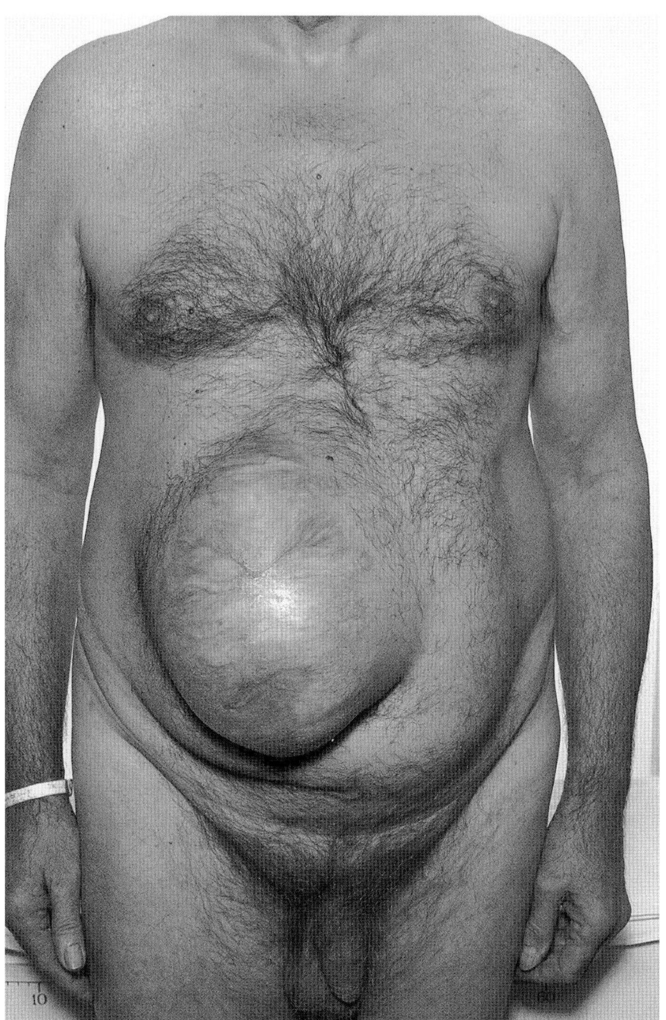

Figure 24.25 Incisional hernia.

INCISIONAL HERNIA (CHRONIC WOUND FAILURE)

Incisional hernia has an incidence of 10–15%. Many do not become apparent until more than 5 years after surgery, and few strangulate. The fascial layer degenerates beneath a healed scar, and the protruding abdominal viscera come to lie in a subcutaneous sac.

The majority of patients (60%) with incisional hernias are symptomless. When symptoms do occur they include disfigurement, discomfort, pain, subacute intestinal obstruction, ischaemic bowel obstruction, skin excoriation, and very occasionally spontaneous rupture of the hernia, exposing its contents.

Patients are examined when they are in the standing position, and once the hernia has been identified, placed in a supine and more relaxed position (Fig. 24.25). Reducibility of the hernia is determined, and the edges of the fascial defect are carefully

REFERENCE

61. Pemberton J de J, Curry FS. Minn Med 1936; 19: 109

Table 24.2 Classification of incisional hernia by Korenkov and colleagues

Location

Vertical
- Midline above or below umbilicus
- Midline including umbilicus
- Paramedian right or left

Transverse
- Above or below umbilicus
- Crossing midline
- Oblique
- Above or below umbilicus

Combination
- Midline, oblique, parastoma, etc.

Size
- Small (< 5 cm)
- Medium (5–10 cm)
- Large (> 10 cm)

Recurrence
- No
- Yes

Reducibility (with or without obstruction)
- Reducible
- Irreducible

Symptoms
- No
- Yes

(From Korenkov et al 2001,[62] with permission of Springer-Verlag.)

palpated. The diagnosis may be difficult in obese patients, when ultrasound examination and CT scan can be helpful. A CT scan also provides useful information on the organs present in massive, complex incisional hernias. The return of the hernial content to the abdominal cavity can result in an increase in the abdominal pressure, with detrimental effects on respiration. Careful preoperative planning is vital to ensure successful outcome. Planning includes considering the use of prosthetic mesh and discussing abdominal wall reconstructive surgery with the plastic surgeons.

CLASSIFICATION

This is shown in Table 24.2 and allows comparisons to be made between different centres.

AETIOLOGY

The causes can be broadly classified into technical or tissue failures. Inadequate surgical technique can cause a broken suture, a slipped knot, wide stitch intervals (greater than 1 cm), excessive tension (resulting in wound edge necrosis), sutures cutting through the fascia, and placement of a drain or stoma through the incision. Patient risk factors (Table 24.3) should be assessed preoperatively and, whenever possible, corrected.

Wound infection is the commonest cause of wound failure and the development of an incisional hernia. The risk of infection is minimized by a late preoperative shave and administration of prophylactic antibiotics perioperatively where there is any risk of contamination.

Postoperative factors such as persistent cough, prolonged ileus, or obstruction and straining at stool increase intra-abdominal pressure.

Table 24.3 Patient-related risk factors for wound failure

- Obesity
- Diabetes
- Pulmonary disease and chronic cough
- Malnutrition
- Liver failure
- Renal failure
- Malignancy
- Emergency operation, faecal peritonitis, drainage of abscess
- Immunosuppression, steroid use

MANAGEMENT OF INCISIONAL HERNIAS

Surgical treatment of an incisional hernia depends on the size of the fascial defect. Primary closure techniques have a recurrence rate of up to 50%. Small hernias can be repaired using the Mayo repair technique, in which the fascial edges are overlapped (Fig. 24.24). Larger fascial defects should be repaired with a prosthetic mesh, which has a recurrence rate of less than 5%. Strangulation and spontaneous rupture are rare complications that require urgent operation.

MESH PLACEMENT IN INCISIONAL HERNIA

Meshes may be placed retromuscularly (**sublay**) covering the posterior rectus fascia; **onlay**, overlying the fascial and muscular structures; and **inlay**, the mesh being sutured to the edges of the fascia within the peritoneum. The best results have been achieved using a sublay or onlay placement.

In the sublay technique for midline incisional hernia, the mesh is placed in the space between the posterior belly of the rectus abdominis and the posterior rectus sheath. Below the arcuate line, the prosthesis is placed in the preperitoneal space. For lateral incisional hernias, the mesh is placed intraperitoneally and sutured to the ribs and cartilages superiorly, and the preperitoneal space inferiorly. In flank incisional hernias mesh should, if possible, be placed in the retroperitoneal space; alternatively, an onlay technique is used. In the onlay technique, the mesh is placed on the anterior rectus sheath after the fascia defect and the rectus sheaths are closed.

OBTURATOR HERNIA

An obturator hernia is six times more common in women than in men, nearly half the patients are over 60 years old, and this hernia is nearly twice as common on the right side as on the left. It particularly affects elderly women who have had recent rapid weight loss.

The hernial sac protrudes through the obturator canal, which is a 3-cm long fibro-osseous canal that contains the obturator nerve. This canal has a rigid margin made up of the lower surface of the pubic ramus and the upper border of the obturator membrane. The hernial sac protrudes forwards into the femoral triangle, where it may be mistaken for a femoral hernia.

The sac usually contains small intestine and less commonly caecum, sigmoid colon, ovary and fallopian tube. A Richter's

REFERENCE

62. Korenkov M, Paul A, Sauerland S et al. Langenbecks Arch Surg 2001; 386: 65–73

hernia is not unusual. A strangulated obturator hernia may cause referred pain in the inner aspect of the knee, by pressing on the geniculate branch of the obturator nerve. Intestinal obstruction with pain and tenderness on the inner side of the groin should raise the suspicion of a strangulated obturator hernia, even when a swelling is not palpable in the thigh. The hernia may be felt as a palpable mass on vaginal examination.

Despite this, the diagnosis is seldom made until laparotomy. At operation the tight obturator foramen must be carefully opened without damaging the obturator vessels and nerve. Once the hernial contents are reduced, the obturator canal can be closed by one or two sutures, or it can be closed by a preperitoneal mesh plug if it is very large.

SPIGELIAN (SEMILUNAR LINE) HERNIA

The aponeurosis of the internal oblique muscle splits at the semilunar line (Fig. 24.13) to contribute to the anterior and posterior rectus sheaths. Herniation can occur through the slits along this line, often aiming below the umbilicus and adjacent to the line of Douglas, where the posterior rectus sheath is at its thinnest. The overlying external oblique muscle may occasionally deflect the hernial sac medially, forcing it between the muscle layers, where the pain and swelling can be confused with ruptured rectus muscle, a caecal tumour or a rectus sheath haematoma.

Spigelian hernias are slightly more common in women than in men, in a ratio of 1.5:1. They are responsible for less than 1% of abdominal wall hernias, and may contain small and large bowel or omentum. The rigid margins of the defect can cause strangulation and tissue pressure necrosis. The diagnosis can be confidently made by ultrasound CT scanning.[61]

The defects are often small and can be easily closed by a Mayo repair using non-absorbable sutures.

LUMBAR HERNIA

These hernias can develop in patients whose muscles have been paralysed by poliomyelitis or spina bifida. They can appear spontaneously through weak points in the lumbar region. The first is the lumbar triangle of Petit, which is bounded by the crest of the ilium, the posterior edge of external oblique muscle and the anterior edge of latissimus dorsi. The neck is nearly always wide and its contents are usually reducible. The second weak point is the superior quadrilateral lumbar space. Its boundaries are the 12th rib, the lower border of the serratus posterior, the anterior border of erector spinae and the internal oblique. A mesh can be used to carry out an extraperitoneal repair. Lumbar hernias may also follow renal surgery and drainage of lumbar abscess.

GLUTEAL AND SCIATIC HERNIA

Gluteal hernias protrude through the greater sciatic notch, and a sciatic hernia passes through the lesser sciatic notch. They are both very rare. A palpable swelling or tenderness in the buttock or pain at the distribution of the sciatic nerve may suggest the diagnosis.

PELVIC HERNIA

A true pelvic hernia of the pouch of Douglas may occur spontaneously in multiparous women or, more commonly, as a result of the trauma of childbirth. The hernia protrudes into the posterior vaginal wall and vulva during intercourse. The patient or her partner may complain of peristalsis or gurgling gas. The swelling has to be differentiated from a rectocele by bimanual vaginal and rectal examination.

A false pelvic hernia is the protrusion of peritoneum with a cystocele, rectocele or prolapse of the rectum. This is a variety of sliding hernia with the viscus forming part of the wall of the sac.

A pelvic hernia can develop after an abdominoperineal resection of the rectum or vaginal hysterectomy. A lateral pelvic hernia is a protrusion of peritoneum and its abdominal contents through a persistent gap between the levator ani and the obturator internus. These hernias, which may appear in the ischiorectal fossa or the labia majora, are therefore called ischiorectal or pudendal hernias.

INTERNAL HERNIAS

Internal hernias can cause recurrent abdominal pain and vomiting secondary to small bowel obstruction. Small bowel contrast enema can help to diagnose an internal hernia, if it is suspected, before surgery (see Ch. 27).

There are numerous potential sites for the formation of internal hernias; a brief description of some known internal hernias is given below.

Hernias into the lesser sac

- Through the epiploic foramen.
- Through a congenital defect in the transverse mesocolon.
- Postoperatively, through the loop of a gastroenterostomy.

Paraduodenal hernias

Paraduodenal hernias are often associated with anomalies of midgut rotation.

- Left paraduodenal hernia: behind the duodenum, extending towards the right of the duodenum.
- Inferior duodenal hernia: behind the duodenum and extending downwards behind the transverse peritoneal fold.
- The mesentericoparietal hernia of Waldeyer,[62] extending behind the mesentery from the left to the right.
- Retroduodenal hernia: behind the ascending fourth part of the duodenum, extending from right to left.

Hernias through mesenteric defects

Defects in the distal ileal mesentery are frequently multiple.

Paracaecal hernias

Paracaecal hernias occur in the various folds around the appendix and caecum.

REFERENCE

63. Waldeyer-Hartz HWG. Hernia Retroperitonealis. Jungfer, Breslau, 1868

Intersigmoid hernias

Intersigmoid hernias occur into the potential space that extends upwards and laterally between its two limbs. They are very rare and may be associated with gut malrotation.

Supravesical hernias

Supravesical hernias are associated with weight loss, which allows the hernial sac to develop anterior to the bladder. It is sometimes associated with symptoms of reduced bladder capacity.

Hernia through the broad ligament

Hernia through the broad ligament is very rare. It usually occurs in elderly women.

THE MANAGEMENT OF INTERNAL HERNIA

At laparotomy for small bowel obstruction the hernia should be identified and its contents reduced. The bowel may have to be decompressed prior to reduction. The defect must be closed to prevent recurrence. Care must be taken when dividing any constrictions because they may contain critical structures, for example the opening for left paraduodenal hernia is bounded by the inferior mesenteric vein, the ascending branch of the left colic artery, and the duodenum.

The acute abdomen and peritoneal cavity

25

Simon Paterson-Brown, Benjamin N. J. Thomson

THE PERITONEUM

STRUCTURE, ANATOMY AND NERVE SUPPLY

Both the visceral and parietal peritoneal membrane lining the intestines and abdominal cavity are formed of a single layer of mesothelial cells, which are flattened and polyhedral in appearance. These cells have microvilli and cilia on their intraperitoneal border, which increase the peritoneal surface area and help to circulate peritoneal fluid towards the diaphragm.[1] The peritoneal surface area is almost 2 m, which is larger than that of all the glomeruli. This allows large fluid and electrolyte movements and provides a semipermeable membrane for dialysis of patients with renal failure. The fluid and particulate matter that enters the vesicles and lacunae of the mesothelial cells passes along the lymphatics towards the diaphragm. This forms an interface with the pleural cavity, which probably accounts for the pleural effusions found in association with some ovarian tumours, a phenomenon described as Meigs syndrome.[2] The peritoneal cells contain many vesicles, which are involved in fluid transport and have lacunae with valves at the entrance of the lymphatics.[3]

The abdomen is bordered by the diaphragm superiorly and pelvis inferiorly. Apart from the openings of the fallopian tubes, the peritoneal cavity is a completely closed sac unless there is a defect in the anterior abdominal wall. The peritoneal cavity is divided into greater and lesser sacs, which communicate through the foramen of Winslow (Fig. 25.1). The peritoneum has a visceral component lining the intra-abdominal organs and a parietal component lining the wall of the abdominal cavity (Fig. 25.2). Both parts of the peritoneum receive visceral innervation, but the parietal peritoneum also has somatic sensation. Thus pain arising from intra-abdominal pathology that involves the parietal peritoneum leads to pain that is experienced in the abdominal wall.[4]

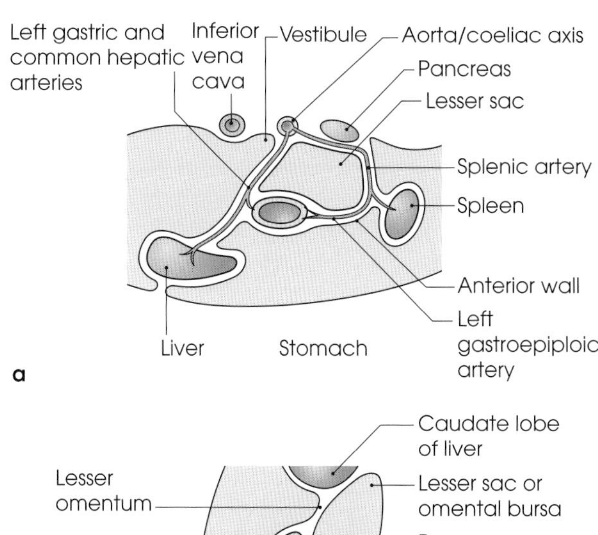

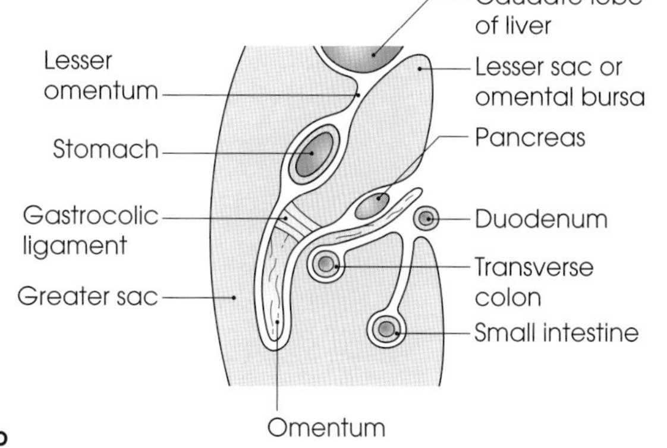

Figure 25.1 Transverse (a) and longitudinal (b) sections through the peritoneal cavity. The greater and lesser sacs are shown.

FUNCTION

The peritoneal membrane provides lubrication for the loops of intestine by secreting a slightly viscous fluid. Under normal conditions the amount of peritoneal fluid that is produced is minimal. The mesothelial cells are also able to secrete lytic enzymes, prostaglandins, interferon and lymphokinase, some of which probably discourage infection.

EMBRYOLOGY

During fetal development the exteriorized intestine elongates and undergoes rotation,[5] before being accommodated within the developing abdominal cavity. Changes also occur in its blood supply, which lead to the formation of a number of common but inconstant peritoneal folds.[6] As the third part of the duodenum becomes fixed to the posterior abdominal wall, the ligament of Treitz is formed.

Occasionally paraduodenal fossae are formed by folds of peritoneum in association with the ligament of Treitz (Fig. 25.3a). A loop of jejunum can herniate into one of these fossae, causing

REFERENCES

1. Andrews PM, Porter KR. Anat Rec 1973; 177: 409–426
2. Meigs JV, Cass JW. Am J Obstet Gynecol 1937; 33: 249
3. Granger HJ, Laine GA et al. In: Stanb NC, Taylor AE (eds). Edema. Raven Press, New York, 1984: 189–228
4. Capps JA, Coleman GH. An Experimental and Clinical Study of Pain in the Pleura, Pericardium and Peritoneum. Macmillan, New York, 1932
5. Haymond HE, Dragstedt LR. Surg Gynecol Obstet 1931; 53: 16
6. Kiewswetter WB, Smith JW. Arch Surg 1958; 77: 483

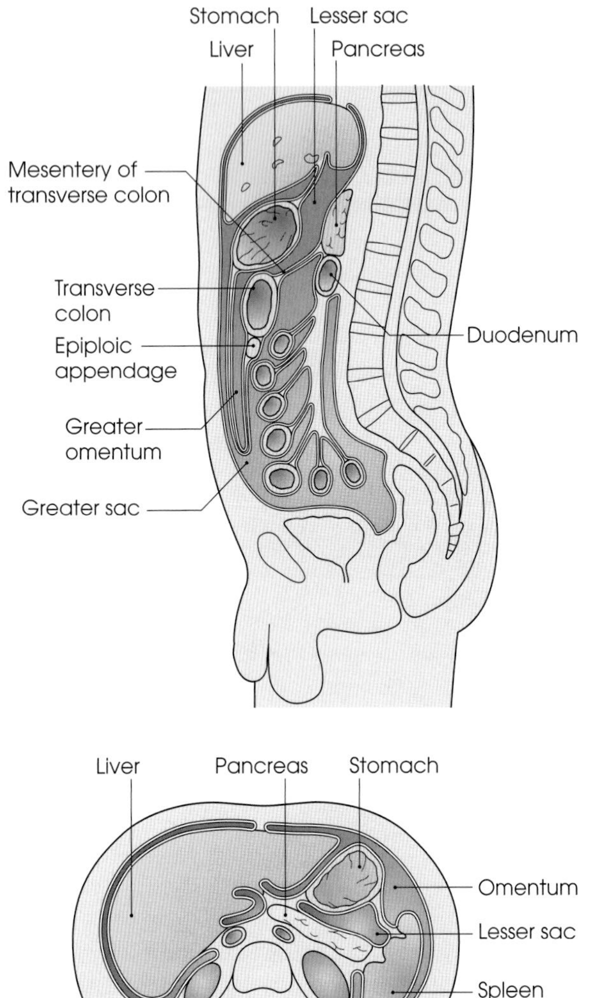

Figure 25.2 (a) Coronal section of the peritoneal cavity, showing peritoneum lining the abdominal cavity (somatic) and surrounding the organs (visceral). (b) Transverse section of the abdominal cavity.

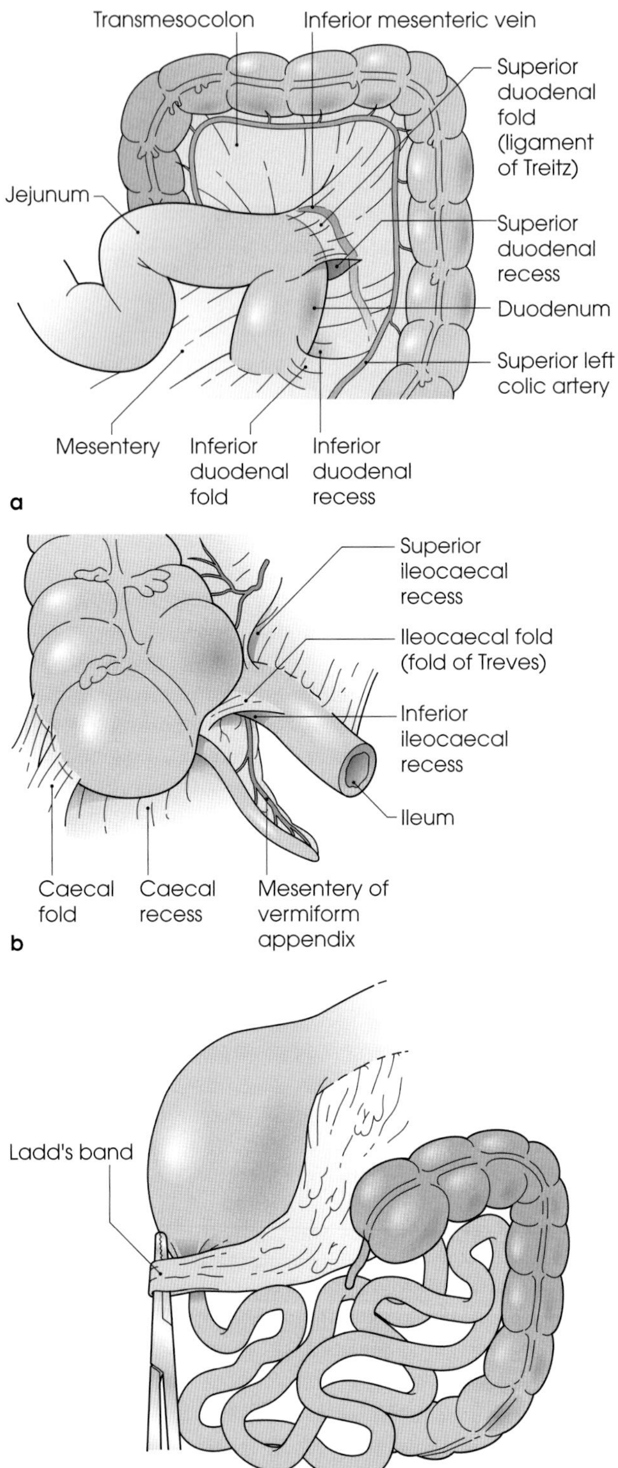

Figure 25.3 (a) The paraduodenal fossae and the ligament of Treitz. (b) The paracaecal fossae and the fold of Treves. (c) Malrotation of the bowel associated with a Ladd's band.

intestinal obstruction.[7] The bloodless fold of Treves[8] develops during fixation of the caecum and may make the appendix difficult to find at operation (Fig. 25.3b). When rotation of the caecum is incomplete, Ladd's band (fold of peritoneum) comes into relationship with the duodenum on the posterior wall of the abdominal cavity (Fig. 25.3c) and can cause small bowel obstruction (see Ch. 27).

PERITONITIS

Although micro-organisms are the commonest cause of peritonitis, bacteria, enzymes and chemicals all cause a similar inflammatory response. Peritonitis may be generalized or localized when anatomical partitions prevent dissemination. The peritoneal cavity is effectively divided into four compartments. The two infracolic compartments situated below the transverse mesocolon and above the pelvic brim are divided into left and right by the longitudinal barrier formed by the lumbar spine, abdominal aorta, inferior vena cava and small bowel mesentery.

REFERENCES

7. Treitz W, Prag FA. Hernia Retroperitonealis. Ein Beitrag zur Geschichle Inner Hernien. Crednar, 1957
8. Treves F. Cassell, London, 1884 (Jacksonian prize essay.)

Table 25.1 Organisms responsible for peritonitis

Organism	Cases (%)
Aerobes	
Escherichia coli	100
Streptococci	33
Proteus	24
Klebsiella	24
Pseudomonas	24
Anaerobes	
Bacteroides fragilis	90
Clostridia	52

The pelvic cavity is situated below the pelvic brim, psoas muscles and iliac vessels. The supracolic compartment is situated below the diaphragm and above the transverse mesocolon.

The greater omentum, which constantly alters its position within the peritoneal cavity, adheres to and surrounds any inflamed viscus with which it comes into contact. Fibrinous peritoneal exudate glues the bowel and omentum to the inflammatory focus, walling it off and preventing a generalized peritonitis. The spread of infection around the peritoneal cavity is further reduced when toxic exudate inhibits intestinal peristalsis.

Infection may reach the peritoneum directly from an abdominal wound, from a suppurative process in one of the intraperitoneal viscera, after an operation on an infected viscus, through the bloodstream, through lymphatic spread from the pleura, or directly via the open ends of the fallopian tubes. Gram-positive organisms, Gram-negative bacilli, mixed synergistic infections and anaerobic organisms can all be pathogenic in the peritoneal cavity. The organisms most commonly isolated in peritonitis are listed in Table 25.1.

The mortality of peritonitis depends on the underlying cause and increases with the bacterial count, the delay in treatment, and the age of the patient. The mortality of peritonitis caused by appendicitis is 10% above the age of 80, but in peritonitis secondary to large bowel perforation the mortality is 20% below the age of 40 and rises to 80% in those over 80 years of age.[9] The overall mortality for perforated peptic ulcer is 26%, but for those over 70 years rises to 34%.[10] When acute suppurative peritonitis is suspected, treatment should be regarded as an emergency before local changes progress to renal failure with secondary cardiovascular collapse and respiratory failure.[11]

VARIETIES OF PERITONITIS

Peritonitis may be classified according to its pathogenesis.

Primary peritonitis

Primary bacterial peritonitis that occurs without any obvious source for the infection being demonstrated is much more common in those with some intercurrent disease, such as children who have undergone a splenectomy or who have a nephrotic syndrome[12] and adults with cirrhosis (see Ch. 29).[13] In true spontaneous peritonitis, only one organism is found in the cultures of the peritoneal fluid. Pneumococci used to be the most commonly isolated organisms, but *Escherichia coli* and *Klebsiella* are now more frequently cultured.[14] In cases where bacteria cannot be identified, raised viral titres are sometimes found. The route of entry of organisms into the peritoneal cavity usually cannot be determined, but transmural spread as well as bloodstream spread have both been postulated. Primary peritonitis is more common in young girls than in young boys, and as a consequence it has been suggested that the female genital tract may be a portal of entry.[15] Aird reported that the pneumococcus could be isolated from the vaginas of many young girls in Edinburgh. Primary pneumococcal peritonitis, however, appears to be declining in incidence, and an intraperitoneal foreign body must always be excluded in cases of primary peritonitis.

Aseptic chemical peritonitis

The most common form of aseptic peritonitis occurs after perforation of a duodenal ulcer, when the gastric contents and bile enter the peritoneal cavity (see p. 593). Secondary overgrowth with intestinal flora occurs if the peritoneal contamination persists for some hours without treatment. Bile escaping from a ruptured gall bladder (see Ch. 30) and pancreatic enzymes collecting in patients with acute pancreatitis can also cause chemical peritonitis (see Ch. 30). Bile peritonitis usually requires drainage. It can also occur when a T tube becomes dislodged or an accessory hepatic duct is inadvertently divided at the time of cholecystectomy. Blunt abdominal trauma can release blood, pancreatic enzymes, bowel contents and urine into the peritoneal cavity following rupture of the relevant organs. Blood within the peritoneal cavity can cause pain and peritonism.

Meconium peritonitis can occur in neonates following intestinal rupture any time after the third month of intrauterine life (see Ch. 40). The term should not be used unless meconium, mucus droplets or lanugo hairs are demonstrated in the peritoneal cavity. The peritonitis is initially sterile but infection may develop later. Usually the bowel perforation causing the condition has closed before birth, but it occasionally persists. In half the cases of meconium ileus, atresia, volvulus or hernia are responsible. In viable infants there are signs of intestinal obstruction, distension and pneumoperitoneum. The meconium may have become calcified and is visible on plain radiographs of the abdomen.

Interventional peritonitis

Following abdominal surgery, bowel and gastric contents, blood and urine may all escape and cause peritonitis. Diagnostic procedures such as percutaneous transhepatic cholangiography or barium enema causing perforation of a diverticulum can give rise to a similar clinical picture. Diagnostic endoscopy may perforate the oesophagogastric junction, the caecum, sigmoid colon and bladder, leading to peritonitis. An increasing number of patients are treated by continuous ambulatory peritoneal dialysis for chronic renal failure, and this is known to predispose to peritonitis despite careful tunnelling and positioning of

REFERENCES

9. Bohnen J, Boulanger M et al. Arch Surg 1983; 118: 285–290
10. Irvin TT. Br J Surg 1989; 76: 215–218
11. Renvall S. Acta Chir Scand 1976; 142: 407–414
12. Rubin HM, Blau EB, Michaels RH. Paediatrics 1975; 56: 598–601
13. Correia JP, Conn HO. Med Clin North Am 1975; 59: 963–981
14. Bartlett JG, Miao PVW, Gorbach SL. J Infect Dis 1977; 135: S80–S85
15. Fraser, McCartney. In: Aird I. Companion in Surgical Studies. Livingstone, Edinburgh, 1958 (Quote.)

the catheters[16] and the use of an aseptic technique when changing bags.

Drugs

A chronic form of plastic peritonitis with the formation of matted loops of bowel and greatly thickened visceral peritoneum (sclerosing peritonitis) resulted from the chronic usage of the β-blocking drug practolol, which has been withdrawn.[17,18]

Foreign bodies

Talc, which is a magnesium silicate powder, and starch may stimulate foreign body granulomata if they are inadvertently introduced into the peritoneal cavity on surgical gloves.[19,20] The associated inflammation encourages adhesion formation. Modern operating gloves are starch- and talc-free, and this condition is now extinct. Starch peritonitis produced abdominal pain, distension and pyrexia. Ascites was present with matted omentum and bowel causing abdominal masses. The diagnosis was confirmed on a wound or peritoneal biopsy, when birefringent granules were seen. Malignant and tuberculous peritonitis have to be considered in the differential diagnosis.

SPECIAL FORMS OF PERITONITIS

The signs of peritonitis may be masked in patients on steroids, in immunosuppressed patients (those with AIDS or on immunosuppressive drugs), in young children, and in the very old and infirm.

COMPLICATIONS

Complications include adhesive obstruction (see *Adhesions*, p. 584) and intraperitoneal abscesses.

INTRAPERITONEAL ABCESSES

An intraperitoneal abscess is formed when peritonitis remains localized or when generalized peritonitis fails to resolve completely. Localization can occur as a result of developmental folds or adhesions between local intestinal loops, or when the omentum prevents the spread of infection. Occasionally a bacteraemia may cause a retroperitoneal infection that leads to a localized peritoneal reaction and abscess formation. Abscesses usually develop close to the original source of infection. Localized abscesses in the peritoneum are most often found in the subphrenic region or in the pelvis. *E. coli* and *Bacteroides* are the commonest organisms to be isolated from these collections of pus (see Ch. 4).

SUBPHRENIC ABSCESSES

There are seven anatomical spaces and potential spaces below the abdominal surface of the diaphragm where pus can collect, three on each side and one placed centrally (Fig. 25.4). In practice, pus is usually bounded by inflammatory adhesions rather than by the ligaments of the liver, but a broad anatomical classification is helpful when considering approaches to drainage.

Right anterior intraperitoneal (right subphrenic) space

This lies in front of the liver and right coronary ligament, below the diaphragm and behind the abdominal wall. Its left boundary is the falciform ligament, and inferiorly it communicates over the liver edge with the general peritoneal cavity. This space is

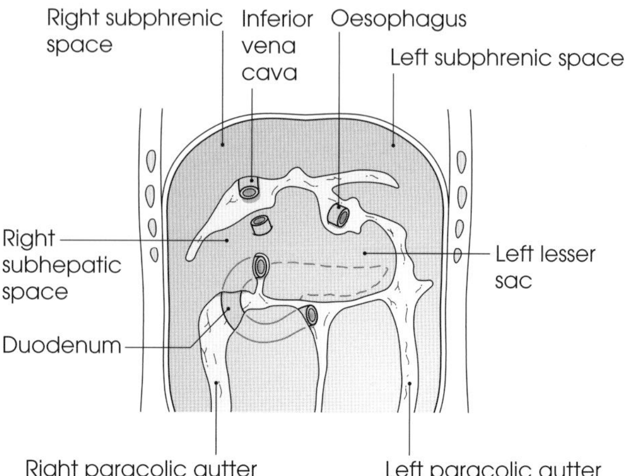

Figure 25.4 The subphrenic spaces beneath the diaphragm.

commonly infected from infection of the gall bladder or from a perforation of the stomach or duodenum. An abscess in this space tends to point towards the right costal margin.

Right posterior intraperitoneal (right subhepatic) space

This is the hepatorenal pouch of Rutherford Morison. It lies behind and below the right lobe of the liver, in front of the peritoneum covering the diaphragm and the kidney. It is bounded above by the posterior leaf of the paracolic gutter. Infection commonly reaches this space from the appendix, the gall bladder, the right colon, the duodenum or the right perinephric tissues. An abscess in this space points towards the loin.

Right extraperitoneal subphrenic space

This is a potential space between the bare area of the liver and the diaphragm. In front and behind are the two layers of the coronary ligament, which fuse in the right corner. On the left, the space is bounded by the inferior vena cava. This space is usually infected by a perinephric abscess arising from the right kidney. Abscesses in this space tend to track forwards in front of the vena cava to a point in the epigastrium between the layers of the falciform ligament. An abscess in this space is unusual.

Left anterior intraperitoneal subphrenic (left subhepatic) space

This is similar to its fellow of the opposite side. Anteriorly is the abdominal wall, superiorly the diaphragm, posteriorly the left triangular ligament, and inferiorly the left lobe of the liver. The falciform ligament lies to the right and the spleen to the left. The space communicates over the liver edge with the anterior peritoneal compartment in front of the omental curtain. This space is infected by an anterior gastric perforation, or from infection associated with the left colon, pancreas or spleen. An abscess in this space points below the left costal margin.

REFERENCES

16. Bengmark S. The Peritoneum and Peritoneal Access. Wright, Bristol, 1987
17. Brown P, Baddeley H et al. Lancet 1974; 11: 1477–1481
18. Eltringham WK, Espiner CWD et al. Br J Surg 1977; 64: 229–235
19. Antapol W. Arch Pathol 1933; 76: 326
20. McAdams GB. Surgery 1956; 39: 329–336

Left posterior intraperitoneal (left subhepatic) space

This is the lesser sac situated between the stomach and lesser omentum anteriorly and the undersurface of the left lobe of the liver superiorly; the peritoneum and the transverse mesocolon and transverse colon lie inferiorly. The lienorenal ligament and the gastrosplenic ligament form the left boundary, and it communicates with the greater sac behind the porta hepatis through the foramen of Winslow on the right. It is usually infected from pancreatitis or following gastric surgery. Abscesses in the lesser sac tend to point anteriorly through the lesser omentum or greater omentum below the greater curvature of the stomach.

Right and left extraperitoneal spaces

These are unimportant, and their names are applied to the areolar tissue around the upper poles of the kidney. An abscess in these spaces is usually classified as a perinephric abscess (see Ch. 35).

MICROBIOLOGY

Subphrenic abscesses are almost always pyogenic, although tuberculous abscesses have been reported complicating tuberculosis of the gall bladder, liver, spleen, kidney and lung.[21]

CLINICAL FEATURES

The clinical picture depends on the site and size of the abscess. The presentation and signs are frequently obscure, when it is described by the surgical aphorism 'pus somewhere, pus nowhere, pus under the diaphragm'. A subphrenic abscess is suspected when a patient develops a swinging pyrexia associated with marked toxaemia after an intra-abdominal infection or operation. A fever and abdominal pain with tenderness that persist and defy diagnosis should suggest the possibility of a subphrenic abscess, especially if there is a raised sedimentation rate and accompanying leukocytosis. Pain may be entirely absent or may be referred to the chest wall, loin, upper abdomen, back or shoulder. Pain may be produced or exacerbated by pressing the rib margins together. Hiccup is common and may be distressing. Tenderness can usually be elicited at one of the points of Vegni:[22]

- the anterior phrenic point at the tip of the 10th rib;
- the posterior phrenic point where the edge of the erector spinae crosses the 11th intercostal space; or
- the superior phrenic point, which is situated over the phrenic nerve between the two heads of sternomastoid.

The liver is usually depressed and its edge is palpable. The signs of a pleural effusion may be present, and occasionally hyper-resonance indicates the presence of gas in the subphrenic space as a result of a perforation or an anaerobic infection. Rarely, a palpable swelling is present in the upper abdomen or lower chest. The extent of the apparent liver dullness is often decreased.

A leukocytosis is invariably present, and a chest radiograph may show a small pleural effusion or even an empyema (Fig. 25.5). Air may be seen in the subphrenic space and occasionally an air–fluid level is seen. Other diagnoses that should be considered include liver abscess, empyema, lung abscess, pelvic abscess, deep vein thrombosis and septic pulmonary embolism, portal pyaemia and pneumonia.

Subphrenic abscesses have in the past been diagnosed by finding reduced movement on screening of the diaphragm, but now most are well demonstrated by ultrasound or CT (Figs 25.6 and 25.7). Radiolabelled leukocytes, using indium, are

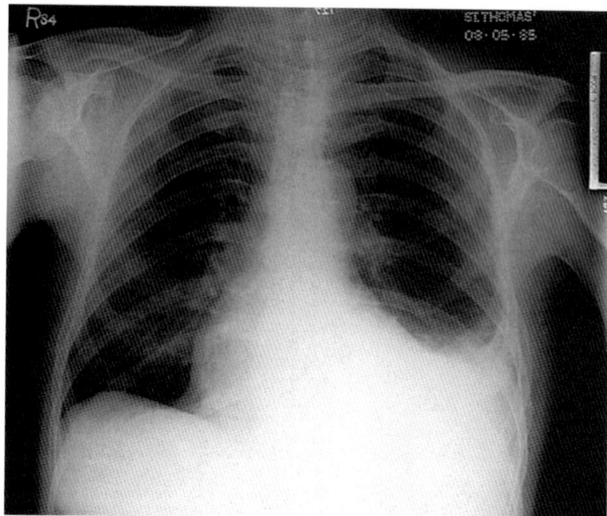

Figure 25.5 Chest X-ray showing a small pleural effusion above a subphrenic abscess.

concentrated in abscess cavities, and this is an alternative means of locating a collection of pus.

TREATMENT

Once a subphrenic abscess has been diagnosed, a decision has to be made between conservative management with antibiotic therapy and drainage. Many abscesses can be treated by ultrasound (Fig. 25.6) or CT-guided placement of a drainage tube inserted under local anesthesia.[23] This drain can be left in place or the pus can be aspirated and antibiotics instilled into the cavity. The aspiration may be repeated on several occasions provided that the clinical picture is improving, but deterioration should indicate the need for open surgical drainage.

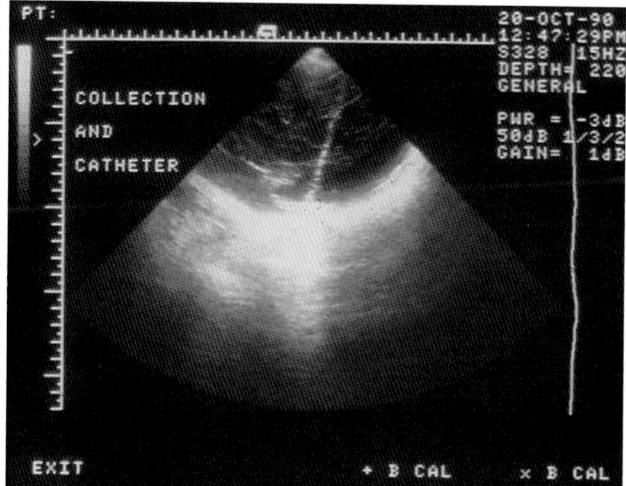

Figure 25.6 An ultrasound scan demonstrating a collection of pus in the subhepatic space (Rutherford Morison's pouch). A catheter can be seen within the abscess for drainage.

REFERENCES

21. Piquand G. Rev Chir 1909; 40: 336
22. Vegni. In: Aird I. Companion in Surgical Studies. Livingstone, Edinburgh, 1958 (Citation.)
23. Russell RCG. J R Soc Med 1987; 80: 471–472

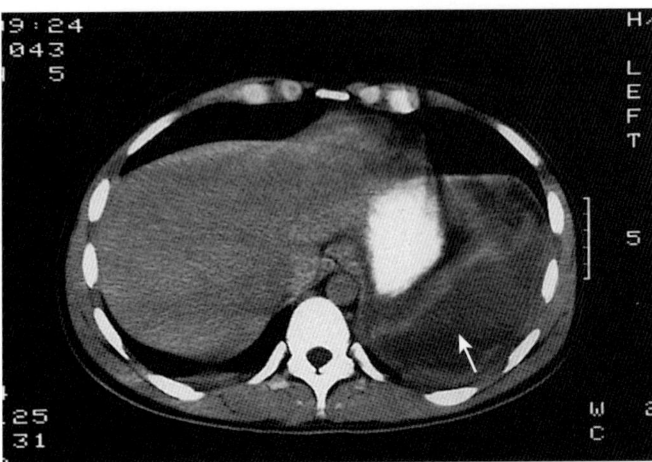

Figure 25.7 A CT scan of a subphrenic abscess.

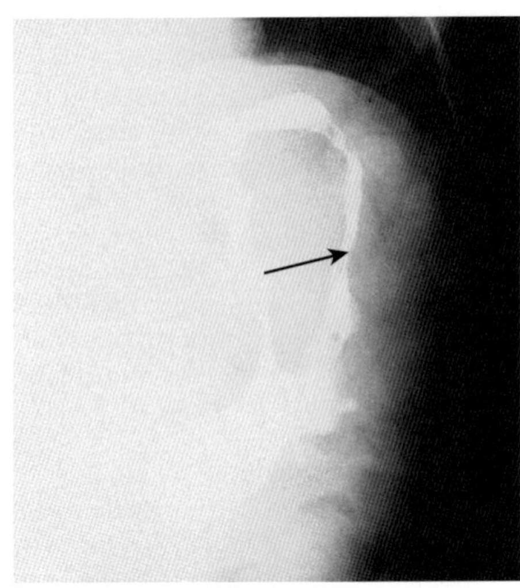

Figure 25.8 Sinogram outlining a subphrenic abscess cavity in the left subphrenic space after a splenectomy.

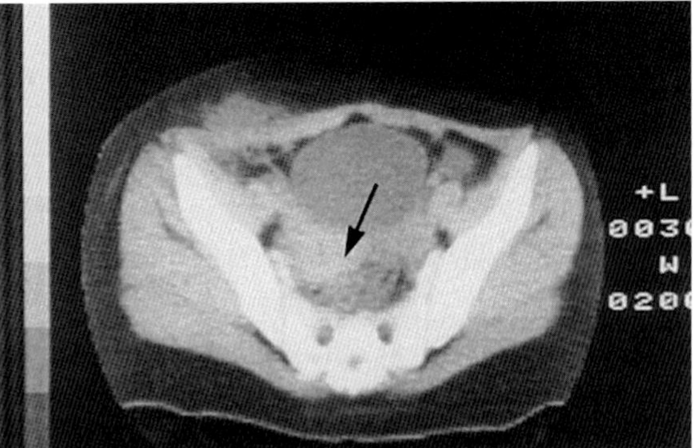

Figure 25.9 A CT scan showing a pelvic abscess developing after acute appendicitis.

Surgical drainage

The presence of a swelling or the position of an abscess on CT scanning or ultrasound may indicate the best approach for drainage. An anterior approach may be used for a right subphrenic abscess; however, both right and left subphrenic abscesses are often best approached from behind through the bed of the 12th rib. Care must be taken to avoid opening the pleura and producing an empyema. The pleura should be pushed gently upwards, and a finger can then be inserted below the diaphragm and above the kidney to explore the subphrenic space. An area of induration may be entered with a resultant satisfying gush of pus. A long wide-bore needle attached to a syringe can be used to explore the subphrenic space if this technique fails to locate the abscess. It is important to stay in the extraserosal plane if possible. Once the abscess cavity is entered it must be widely explored, opened and drained to avoid loculi developing. A large tube drain is left in the cavity. Regular and repeated sinograms down the drainage tube indicate that the cavity is shrinking, and this should be confirmed before the tubes are removed (Fig. 25.8).

PELVIC ABSCESS

Many of the features of a pelvic abscess are similar to those of a subphrenic abscess, from which it must be differentiated. A pelvic abscess is the commonest variety of intraperitoneal abscess. An inflamed appendix, pelvic inflammatory disease, and acute diverticulitis can all cause local pelvic peritonitis and eventually lead to pelvic abscess formation. Pus can also track down into the pelvis from a perforated peptic ulcer.

The condition must be suspected in any patient known to have had one of the predisposing conditions or who has had pelvic surgery and develops a swinging pyrexia some days after the initial event. Pelvic abscesses often cause few symptoms, but a frequent call to stool and the excessive passage of mucus on defecation indicate that the abscess is beginning to point into the rectum. Occasionally urinary frequency occurs. A palpable boggy mass felt on digital examination of the rectum confirms the diagnosis, but this may not be present in the early stages, when rectal examination may only elicit pain. Ultrasound and CT scanning provide a more accurate means of making an early diagnosis (Fig. 25.9). There is usually a marked accompanying leukocytosis.

Many pelvic abscesses drain spontaneously into the rectum, requiring no additional treatment. This can be encouraged by gentle finger pressure at the site of maximal swelling. If spontaneous drainage does not occur, the abscess should be formally drained under general anaesthesia with the patient in the lithotomy position. A proctoscope or operating sigmoidoscope is inserted into the rectum. If the abscess is clearly seen to be pointing, a pair of sinus forceps can be gently pushed into its centre, but if uncertainty exists a large-bore aspirating needle and syringe can be used to locate the pus. Good drainage must be obtained. All loculi should be broken down with a finger. Occasionally, pelvic abscesses can drain through the vagina but rectal drainage is always preferable.

ABDOMINAL TUBERCULOSIS

INTESTINAL TUBERCULOSIS

Intestinal tuberculosis is discussed in Chapter 27.

TUBERCULOUS MESENTERIC ADENITIS

Tuberculous mesenteric adenitis was and still is in some parts of the world a common disease of childhood. It usually follows the entry of bovine bacillus via a Peyer's patch or a solitary lymph follicle. The pathology is similar to tuberculosis of the cervical glands. It is normally discovered incidentally as a calcified symptomless lymph node or on routine abdominal X-ray. Enlarged tuberculous nodes are hardly ever palpable. The bowel occasionally becomes adherent to a tuberculous gland, which can then cause intestinal obstruction. Tuberculous mesenteric glands can caseate and rupture, causing tuberculous peritonitis.

TUBERCULOUS PERITONITIS

Tuberculous peritonitis can develop from miliary tuberculosis, from direct spread from the bowel or the fallopian tubes, or from rupture of a tuberculous mesenteric lymph node. Bloodstream spread to the peritoneum from a focus outside the abdominal cavity—such as the lung, a bone or joint, or the urinary tract—is unusual. Women are affected twice as commonly as men, perhaps because the female genital tract is an important portal of infection. Although the disease has declined in western countries since the early part of the 20th century, it is still common in India and the Far East,[24] and population migration has increased the incidence in many western countries.[25]

Four forms of the disease have been described—ascitic, adhesive, acute and caseous—but these are often not clearly defined and more than one type of response may be present in the same patient.

Ascitic

The ascitic variety is characterized by liberal peritoneal exudate and numerous tubercles. It has an insidious course with vague abdominal symptoms, vomiting, constipation or diarrhoea, weight loss, evening temperature, malaise, night sweats, abdominal distension and congested abdominal veins. Occasionally the ascites fills a hernial sac, causing persistent protrusion. Shifting dullness or a fluid thrill can usually be detected, and a doughy abdominal mass represents the matted greater omentum studded with tubercles. Localized encysted collections can occur and may be mistaken for a mesenteric cyst or an abdominal tumour.

Ascitic tuberculosis has to be distinguished from other types of ascites and if a laparotomy is performed, fat necrosis, starch peritonitis and widespread carcinomatosis are usually considered in the differential diagnosis. A strongly positive Mantoux test supports the diagnosis. Ultrasound and CT scans confirm the presence of ascites and may show irregular soft tissue masses within the peritoneal fluid. A pale yellow fluid is obtained with a high specific gravity if the ascites is tapped for diagnostic purposes. Tubercle bacilli are rarely demonstrated even after centrifugation, but may be confirmed by culture after 6 weeks.

Because of the delay in making a bacteriological diagnosis and starting treatment, laparoscopy and biopsy are usually necessary to establish the diagnosis.[26] Ziehl–Neelsen staining of bacilli in the biopsy specimens and typical histological findings usually confirm the diagnosis. Laparoscopy should be performed with care, preferably using the open Hassan technique (see Ch. 30) because adhesions may make insertion of the Veress needle dangerous, increasing the risk of bowel perforation.

Adhesive

Bowel loops are matted together at first by tubercles and later by fibrous bands. This type usually presents with subacute intestinal obstruction, although acute obstruction can develop. If surgery is required, careful separation of small bowel loops by division of adhesions is preferable, with intestinal resection or bypass being kept in reserve for inoperable disease.

Acute

This form presents as a purulent peritonitis with abdominal pain and distension. It may be suspected if there is a history of tuberculosis or if ascites is detected, although a presumptive diagnosis of carcinomatosis is often made in western countries. At operation the adhesions should be divided and the tubercles biopsied. Carcinomatosis, fat necrosis and starch peritonitis are again the important differential diagnoses.

Caseous

This is a rare variety of abdominal tuberculosis, which presents with large collections of caseous pus within the abdominal cavity. Cold abscesses may develop within the abdomen, and these often point towards the umbilicus or burst into the lumen of the bowel with the development of intestinal fistulae. Previous abscesses may require surgical drainage, and the fistulae require operative closure or bowel resection.

CLINICAL FEATURES

Chronic debility, abdominal pain, fever, night sweats, abdominal distension, weight loss and anorexia are all common complaints, while the presence of ascites, a doughy abdomen and irregular abdominal masses are the most common clinical findings in all forms of abdominal tuberculosis.[27,28]

TREATMENT

Besides the operative measures outlined above, all patients are placed on antituberculous combination chemotherapy for 9–12 months, which usually consists of rifampin (rifampicin), ethambutol and isoniazid (see Ch. 4). This often causes complete relief of the symptoms, although surgery may occasionally be required to divide fibrous adhesions.[25,26]

GRANULOMATOUS PERITONITIS

Yeast, amoebas, fungi and parasites are rare causes of non-specific granulomatous peritonitis.

TUMOURS OF THE PERITONEUM

Solid primary tumours of the peritoneum are rare. The most common tumours are secondary carcinomas, usually derived from transcoelomic dissemination from another abdominal tumour or occasionally by blood or lymphatic spread from an extra-abdominal primary neoplasm. Peritoneal metastases may take the form of discrete nodules, plaque-like masses, diffuse malignant adhesions, flat subperitoneal deposits, cystic masses (usually ovarian), and pedunculated tumours. Bizarre deposits with tufts of hair are associated with secondary teratomas. Ascites is often present.

The differential diagnosis of peritoneal metastases may be extremely difficult. Other conditions that can give similar appearances include tuberculosis, encapsulated foreign bodies, talc granulomata, chronic sepsis, fat necrosis, infestation by parasites (schistosomiasis, cysticercosis or hydatids), polyarteritis

REFERENCES

24. Bhansali SK, Desai AN. Ind J Surg 1968; 30: 218
25. Wells AD, Northover J, Howard ER. J R Soc Med 1986; 79: 149–153
26. Udwadia TE. Ind J Surg 1978; 40: 91
27. Dineeen P, Homan WP, Grafe WR. Ann Surg 1976; 184: 717–722
28. Addison NV. Ann R Coll Surg Engl 1983; 65: 105–111

nodosa, gas cysts, splenosis, actinomycosis, leprosy, and infection with *Pasteurella* and *Brucella*. Carcinomatosis of the peritoneal cavity usually presents with pain, weight loss and abdominal swelling.

The diagnosis is by biopsy, although if ascites is present a cytological diagnosis is possible. The biopsy may be obtained at laparotomy or at laparoscopy (see later text).

Treatment is usually supportive, with measures designed to relieve pain, vomiting, constipation and abdominal distension. Occasionally, intraperitoneal chemotherapy can cause a useful regression.

The best recognized primary tumour of the peritoneum is the mesothelioma or the endothelioma, which occurs in benign and malignant forms and is similar to the well-recognized pleural tumour (see Ch. 21). The malignant variety usually responds to radiotherapy but recurrence is invariable.

PSEUDOMYXOMA PERITONEI

After rupture of a pseudomucinous cystadenoma of the ovary or, more rarely, of a mucocele of the appendix, mucus-secreting cells are liberated into the peritoneal cavity, where they become implanted on the peritoneal surface. The abdominal cavity becomes filled with tumour masses and fluid. Biopsy of the tumours shows a fibrinous network with mucin or pseudomucin in its spaces; the masses may be enclosed by epithelium or may project from the serous surfaces of the viscera into the peritoneal cavity. In places, scattered islands of columnar cells are found.

The symptoms are those of progressive abdominal distension and weight loss. An effort should be made to clear out all the abnormal tissue. If pseudomyxomatosis is found at operation, the causative appendix or ovary should of course be removed. Unfortunately recurrence is common and further laparotomies and peritoneal toilet may be required. It is a condition that is better avoided than treated.

ASCITES

Ascites is the name given to an increased amount of fluid collecting within the peritoneal cavity. Ascites can be the result of either increased production or decreased absorption of peritoneal fluid. It is often a protein-rich exudate resulting from increased capillary and mesothelial permeability following peritonitis or carcinomatous infiltration and irritation, or it may be a transudate in patients with cardiac failure, constrictive pericarditis, tricuspid incompetence (see Ch. 22), or Budd–Chiari syndrome (see Ch. 11). These conditions all cause an increase in the hydrostatic pressure of the local blood vessels and capillary bed. When ascites occurs in cirrhosis of the liver the mechanism is complex, but raised portal venous pressure, hyperaldosteronism, and reduced oncotic pressure from osmotic low albumin levels all play a part. Rupture of hepatic lymphatics may also contribute to fluid formation. Patients with hypoproteinaemia also develop ascites, as do patients with abnormal lymphatic drainage (chylous ascites; see Ch. 12).

CLINICAL FEATURES

Abdominal distension, nausea, constipation and weight loss are the main symptoms. Patients often notice that their clothes no longer fit or that they have to let out their belts. The physical signs are of shifting dullness when the fluid collection is small and a percussion thrill when it is tense. Ascitic fluid must be differentiated from the other five Fs—fetus, faeces, flatus, fat and fibroids—which can also cause abdominal enlargement. A large ovarian cyst is the main differential diagnosis but tuberculous peritonitis must also be considered.

INVESTIGATIONS

The patient must be investigated to confirm the diagnosis and if possible determine the cause. Urea and electrolytes, and liver function tests may confirm the nephrotic syndrome, liver failure or hypoproteinaemia. Plain radiographs of the abdomen usually show a ground-glass appearance with a paucity of gas shadows. Abdominal ultrasound and CT scanning confirm the presence of intraperitoneal fluid. The fluid should be tapped and sent for chemical analysis, microbiological microscopy, and culture and cytology to look for malignant cells. The patient should be re-examined for signs of cardiac disease, hypoproteinaemia, lymphatic disorders, chronic liver disease and tuberculosis. A milky tap suggests chylous ascites and requires lymphography to confirm the presence of megalymphatics and if possible to define the site of leakage (see Ch. 12).

The finding of malignant cells may occasionally encourage the search for the primary tumour, because carcinoma of the ovary has a good long-term prognosis following surgery and chemotherapy.[29] Liver biopsy and laparoscopy may be required to exclude chronic liver disease, tuberculosis and Meigs syndrome (ascites associated with a benign ovarian fibroma).[2] Occasionally, laparotomy functions as the final court of appeal if all other causes have been excluded, but under these circumstances it rarely provides the answer.

TREATMENT

When a cause can be found this should be treated (e.g. heart failure, hypoproteinaemia, tuberculosis and ovarian malignancy). Cirrhotic ascites usually responds to diuretics, and a combination of a thiazide diuretic with an aldosterone antagonist such as spironolactone is usually effective (see Ch. 29). Dietary sodium restriction may also be helpful. Repeated paracentesis became unpopular on the grounds that it induced hypoproteinaemia, although its value has had support.[30] The ascites is tapped through a peritoneal dialysis catheter and great care is taken to avoid introducing infection, which can be rapidly fatal in patients with cirrhosis.

Insertion of a peritoneo-venous shunt between the abdominal cavity and the internal jugular vein has been used to treat patients with a severe refractory ascites. This type of shunting may be unsuccessful in patients with a heavy proteinaceous exudate because the one-way valve mechanism used to prevent venous reflux within the shunt rapidly blocks up, even if the open end of the tubing remains patent. Two types of shunt are commercially available: the Le Veen[31] and the Denver[32] shunts. They are tunnelled subcutaneously from the peritoneal cavity to the internal jugular vein. They are made of Silastic, and contain a non-return valve to prevent blood reflux and allow manual compression in an effort to overcome blockage. Large quantities of ascites must be present and being continuously formed for the

REFERENCES

29. Raju KS, McKinna JA et al. Am J Obstet Gynecol 1982; 144: 650–654
30. (Editorial). Lancet 1988; ii: 475
31. Le Veen HH, Wapnick S et al. Ann Surg 1976; 184: 574
32. Lund RH, NewKirk JB. Contemp Surg 1979; 14: 31

shunt to remain patent. Dangers include fluid overload, cardiac failure, disseminated intravascular coagulation, and bloodstream spread of malignancy.[33]

Chylous ascites may be reduced by ligation of lymphatic fistulae, by resection of abnormal small bowel (leaking lymph from its surface), and by forming a lymphovenous anastomosis to bypass an obstructed thoracic duct (see Ch. 12).[34]

Malignant ascites may improve with intraperitoneal or systemic chemotherapy.

HAEMOPERITONEUM

Blood within the peritoneal cavity may occur from the following causes.

- Traumatic injury to abdominal organs, vessels, omentum or mesentery, or a trivial injury to a diseased organ (e.g. a malarial spleen or a vascular malformation of the liver).
- Ruptured ectopic pregnancy.
- Ruptured ovarian cyst, torted uterine fibroid, torted ovarian cyst or tumour.
- Rupture of splenic or hepatic artery aneurysms.
- Ruptured aortic or iliac aneurysms.
- Rupture of an atherosclerotic mesenteric artery.
- Torted omentum.
- Acute pancreatitis.
- Perforated bleeding peptic ulcer or carcinoma of the stomach.
- Haemorrhage from an intra-abdominal tumour, especially a hepatic adenoma or hepatocellular carcinoma.
- Haemorrhagic disorders such as thrombocytopenia or over-anticoagulation.
- Primary amyloid.

The signs and symptoms of haemoperitoneum depend on the underlying cause but include severe abdominal pain, abdominal distension and hypovolaemic shock. The diagnosis is confirmed by a peritoneal tap, peritoneal lavage or laparotomy. Treatment is that of the underlying condition. Urgent laparotomy after appropriate resuscitation is usually essential, although there is an increasing tendency to manage some cases of traumatic haemoperitoneum conservatively if the patient remains stable (see Ch. 32).

PERITONEAL LOOSE BODIES

Most peritoneal loose bodies arise by torsion and separation of epiploic appendices, but larger ones may originate from tubal abortions. Loose bodies should be distinguished from foreign bodies such as fish or meat bones that have perforated the intestine. All peritoneal loose bodies have a central crystalline core of calcium phosphate with a laminated fibrinoid capsule derived from peritoneal exudate. Loose bodies are usually symptomless.

THE MESENTERY

EMBRYOLOGY

Like the omentum, the mesentery develops from splanchnic mesoderm. The dorsal mesentery of the gastrointestinal tract undergoes a great change during development, as the intestine elongates outside the embryo and subsequently rotates before returning to the peritoneal cavity. In the course of this process, there is an anticlockwise rotation of the small bowel around the superior mesenteric artery. The mesentery fixes the intestines to the posterior wall of the abdominal cavity and allows the vascular and lymphatic vessels access to the bowel. The mesentery also contains lymph nodes, visceral nerve fibres, and fat. The cells covering the mesentery are identical to those that lie in the peritoneal cavity, which have already been described. The mesentery of the small bowel arises from the posterior abdominal wall, passing obliquely from the duodenojejunal flexure to the ileocaecal junction (see Fig. 25.10). Although the root of the mesentery is only about 15 cm in length, it fans out to be attached to the entire length of the small bowel. The ascending colon is usually without a mesentery, but the transverse colon has a long mesocolon fused with the greater omentum (Fig. 25.11). The descending and sigmoid colons also have mesenteries of variable lengths.

PHYSIOLOGY AND ANATOMY

The mesentery acts as another site of absorption from within the peritoneal cavity, having a cell structure and intracellular pore size similar to those of the peritoneum. It also acts as the vascular pedicle for the intestine and allows lymphatic transport to and from the mucosa. The splanchnic bed contained in the bowel and mesentery receives up to 30% of the cardiac output, and large vascular alterations and fluid movements occur during stress and digestion. The superior mesenteric artery passes from behind the neck of the pancreas and in front of the third portion of the duodenum before entering the mesentery (Fig. 25.11). The small bowel is richly supplied with vascular arcades, but the terminal branches of the colonic vessels are less frequent and arise from a marginal artery close to the wall of the colon. The preservation of this marginal artery is therefore of great importance in the blood supply of the colon during resection and anastomosis. The inferior mesenteric artery—which supplies the splenic flexure of the transverse colon, the descending colon, the sigmoid colon, and the proximal part of the rectum—arises from the lower aorta and is not uncommonly compromised by severe atherosclerotic disease. Both the superior and inferior mesenteric veins drain into the portal venous system. The haemorrhoidal veins, which drain into the inferior mesenteric vein, form a communication between the portal and systemic venous systems (Fig. 25.11). The importance of this communication is recognized when abscesses in the perineum and rectum are complicated by development of portal pyaemia.

The lymphatic vessels of the mesentery accompany the arteries and veins. After ingestion of food they are prominently outlined by chylomicrons from fat digestion, and after a fatty meal can be easily observed at operation. They drain lymph to the proximal nodes within the mesentery and thence to the preaortic nodes and cisterna chyli before joining the thoracic duct, which passes to the left subclavian vein in the neck. Mesenteric lymph nodes

REFERENCES

33. Lund RH, Mortz MW. Arch Surg 1982; 117: 924
34. Browse NL, Burnand KG, Moetimist PS. Diseases of the Lymphatics. Arnolds, London, 2003

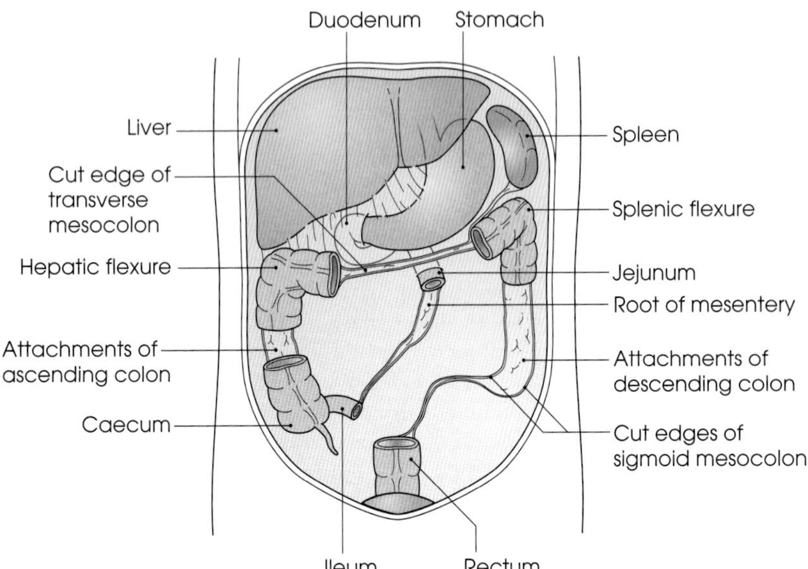

Figure 25.10 The mesenteric attachments to the posterior abdominal wall.

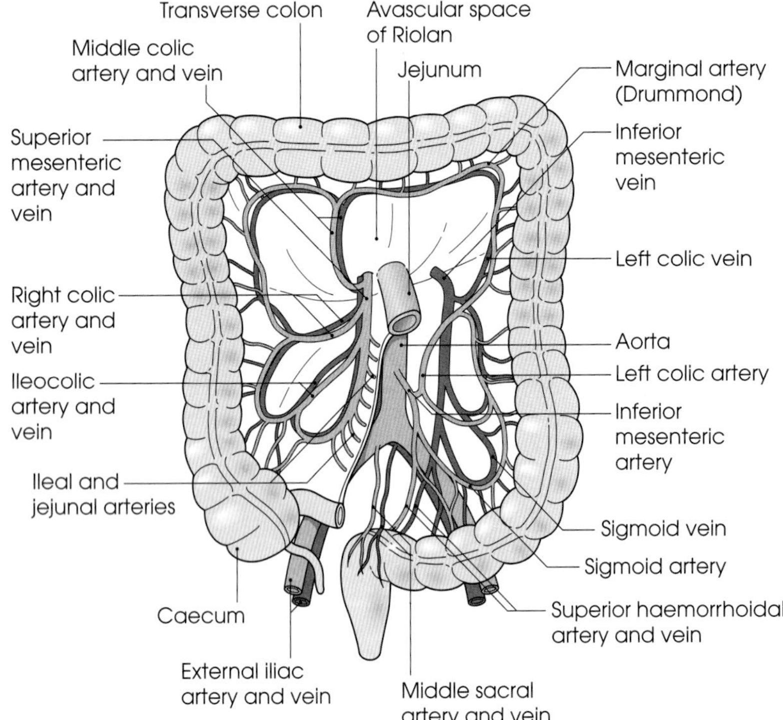

Figure 25.11 The arterial supply and venous drainage of the small and large intestines.

are frequently enlarged and may cause symptoms that have to be differentiated from acute appendicitis, especially in children.[35] Mesenteric adenitis may be the result of both viral and bacterial infection. The mesenteric lymph nodes are a common site for tuberculous infection and are often involved in the secondary spread of malignant disease within the peritoneal cavity.

CONGENITAL ABNORMALITIES

On re-entering the peritoneal cavity, the intestine may fail to rotate and the mesentery may not adhere to the posterior peritoneal wall.[36,37] Abnormal peritoneal folds are common. Intraperitoneal hernias can occur as a result of these anatomical variations. Herniation may take place through congenital defects in the mesentery of both the large and small intestine. Mesenteric defects may also follow injury or surgery. The window through which the bowel herniates may be associated with a vascular pedicle, and care must be taken to avoid damaging blood vessels at the time of surgery to release the herniated bowel. Herniation through the foramen of Winslow has been reported, and bowel may be caught in a congenital fold around the duodenum

REFERENCES

35. Foster AK. Arch Surg 1939; 38: 131
36. Kanagasuntheram R. J Anat 1957; 91: 188
37. Aird I. Br Med J 1945; 2: 680

(paraduodenal herniation) or in a fossa in the sigmoid mesocolon.[38,39] Such patients present with unexplained small bowel obstruction (see *Small bowel obstruction*, pp. 584–588).

VASCULAR DISEASE

Diseases of the mesenteric arteries and veins are described in Chapters 10 and 27. Arteriovenous fistulae are occasionally seen in the mesentery as a result of a penetrating injury or, rarely, following surgery.[40] They are treated by ligation and excision, repair being rarely feasible. Bowel resection may be necessary.

CYSTS

Mesenteric cysts are uncommon in adults and even rarer in children.[41,42] Most are loculated, indicating their origin from several abnormal lymphatic vessels. The walls of the cyst are formed from endothelial cells but may contain fibrous tissue and smooth muscle. The first such cyst was described by Benevieni, the Florentine anatomist, in 1507.[43] Cysts vary in size and may grow to over 20 cm in diameter. They can resemble a reduplication of the bowel, and their contents may be clear or chylous.

Acquired cysts of the mesentery also occur. These may follow trauma and rupture of lymphatic vessels or contain enzyme-rich secretions following rupture of the pancreas. Occasionally, cysts arise from degeneration of a tumour or as a result of certain infections, such as tuberculosis, and infestation, such as hydatid disease (see Ch. 29). Dermoid cysts can also occur in the mesentery.

Many mesenteric cysts are symptomless until the swelling is noticed by the patient. Some cause abdominal pain, which may be colicky in nature, while as many as one-third cause intestinal obstruction or volvulus. Some rupture, some become infected, and some present with anaemia following repeated haemorrhage into the cyst. If the cysts are palpable, the attachment of the mesentery ensures that they are mobile in a transverse direction but restrained from moving vertically. They can be diagnosed with reasonable certainty by ultrasonography or CT, and although needle aspiration under imaging control may be useful for diagnostic purposes, surgical excision is the definitive form of treatment,[44] with or without resection of the adjacent segment of intestine. If the anatomical position of the cyst makes surgical excision hazardous, marsupialization can be performed, leaving the open cyst to drain into the peritoneal cavity.

TUMOURS

Solid primary tumours of the mesentery are rare.[45] They are most commonly sarcomas, desmoid tumours or neurofibromas. The mesentery may also contain deposits of lymphoma and other metastases from intra-abdominal and distant primary carcinomas. Rare benign tumours of the mesentery include lipomas, fibromas and haemangiomas.

THE OMENTUM

The omentum is a fold of visceral peritoneum that is related to the stomach and transverse colon, and is composed of a thin double layer of mesothelium containing a large amount of fat and a rich vascular network. The surface area of the omentum is as much as 1500 cm^2.

The lesser omentum lies between the lesser curve of the stomach and the undersurface of the liver. The greater omentum forms the walls of the lesser sac and becomes fused into an apron of tissue that hangs from the transverse colon. The gastrocolic omentum lies between the greater curvature of the stomach and transverse colon.

ANATOMY

The omentum contains many aggregates of lymphoid tissue in addition to vessels and adipose tissue. The arterial supply of the omentum is from the right and left gastroepiploic arteries, which are derived from the coeliac axis and pass along the greater curvature of the stomach. The gastric branches are more numerous than the epiploic branches. The right gastroepiploic artery is larger and longer than the left. Both arteries diminish in size and usually anastomose about two-thirds of the way along the greater curvature from the duodenum. The venous drainage runs in conjunction with the arterial supply. The right gastroepiploic vein joins the superior mesenteric vein, and the left gastroepiploic vein drains into the splenic vein.

There is an extensive network of lymphatic vessels within the omentum, which drain into the subpyloric, splenic and coeliac nodes. Nerve fibres have been described in connection with the omental vessels, but there is a lack of sensory perception and the nerves probably only subserve vascular reflexes.

PHYSIOLOGY

The omentum adheres to injured and inflamed surfaces.[46] It also provides a large surface area for fluid movement and the absorption of molecular substances from the peritoneal cavity. The overall function of the omentum is encapsulated in the phrase ‘the abdominal policeman’, used originally by Rutherford Morison.[47]

CLINICAL FEATURES OF OMENTAL DISEASE

It is usually difficult, if not impossible, to differentiate between primary omental pathology and omental disease originating from other intra-abdominal organs. Patients who have primary omental pathology present with the signs and symptoms of intra-abdominal inflammation, acute vascular occlusion or space-occupying lesions.

Inflammation of the omentum may develop as the result of any of the acute intra-abdominal infections, such as acute cholecystitis, diverticulitis and appendicitis. Adhesions may then form, which can cause acute or subacute obstruction. Tuberculous peritonitis can cause diffuse omental adhesions. Vascular occlusions can occur in the omentum as a result of torsion, adhesions, trauma, atherosclerosis and embolism. They usually cause non-specific abdominal pain and local tenderness. Primary,

REFERENCES

38. Hansmann GH, Marton SA. Arch Surg 1939; 39: 333
39. Fiddian RV. Br J Surg 1961; 49: 186–188
40. Sumner RG, Kistler PC et al. Circulation 1963; 27: 934
41. Moynihan B. Ann Surg 1897; 26: 1
42. Kurzweg FT, Daron PB et al. Am J Surg 1974; 40: 462
43. Warfield JO. Ann Surg 1932; 96: 329
44. Carpreso P. Arch Surg 1974; 108: 242
45. Weinberger HA, Ahmed MS. Surgery 1977; 82: 754–759
46. Myllainie H. Acta Chir Scand 1967; 377 (Suppl): 1
47. Crofoot DD. Am J Surg 1980; 139: 262–264

solid or cystic lesions in the omentum are rare but may occur at any age. They usually cause abdominal distension and pain. Haemorrhage into a cyst or solid tumour may present as a rapidly increasing abdominal mass.

INVESTIGATION OF OMENTAL DISEASE

Plain abdominal radiographs may show a soft tissue mass or cystic lesion within the abdominal cavity, and if this is seen to be lying anteriorly on the lateral film, an omental lesion should be suspected. Ultrasonography and CT are the main methods of diagnosis. Occasionally, laparoscopy is undertaken to confirm an omental lesion and establish the pathology by biopsy. Laparotomy is required for treatment of omental injuries, inflammatory disease associated with other organs, omental torsion, tumours and cysts.

INJURIES OF THE OMENTUM

Blunt abdominal trauma may lead to omental disruption and haemorrhage. An omental defect may result, through which a loop of bowel may herniate and later obstruct. The omentum may also be injured at operation and by penetrating abdominal injuries such as stab wounds. The defects caused by these injuries are also potential sites for future herniation.

HERNIATION OF OMENTUM

Either small bowel or omentum may herniate into the paraduodenal fossa. Other rare sites of omental herniation include the foramen of Winslow, the transverse mesocolon, the supravesical fossa, and the diaphragm. Omentum may also enter any external hernia, and it is often found within a partial dehiscence of the abdominal wall. A penetrating injury can cause prolapse of the omentum through the abdominal wall, and omentum may herniate through the site of a surgical drain. It is a common finding inside a poorly closed laparoscopy port site. The symptoms depend on the site of the hernia. Treatment is often required to reduce the omentum and repair the defect to prevent future problems.

ADHESIONS

Trauma, ischaemia, inflammation and foreign bodies can cause peritoneal adhesions that often involve the omentum. The symptoms and signs depend on the site and extent of the adhesion formation. Adhesions may be silent or they may cause bowel obstruction (see p. 584).

INFLAMMATION

The inflammation in generalized peritonitis also involves the omentum. Occasionally, the inflammatory process is localized to the omentum and may arise spontaneously in the postoperative period or following injury.[47] Spontaneous inflammation of the omentum usually follows intraperitoneal infection in another viscus. Parasites and tuberculosis can also cause omentitis, and postoperative and post-traumatic omentitis follows the introduction of foreign material.

Laparotomy may be required to exclude another interperitoneal disease if the symptoms and signs are of sufficient severity. Resection of part of the omentum may be necessary if the inflammation is sufficiently severe to produce areas of infarction.

TORSION OF THE OMENTUM

Primary torsion of the omentum is a rare condition that has most often been recorded in men of between 30 and 50 years who are of obese build.[48] Secondary torsion is much more common, accounting for more than half of the reported cases. Adhesions of the omentum to the parietal peritoneum, to any old focus of infection, or to a hernia may lead to torsion.

Clinical features and treatment

Sudden severe abdominal pain, nausea and vomiting are usually present. The twisted omentum may be felt as a mobile mass, or it may be obscured by abdominal rigidity. Sometimes a string of several masses may be felt, which are several twists of omentum. Free fluid is usually present in the peritoneal cavity. Most cases come to operation with a mistaken diagnosis of acute appendicitis. At operation the strangulated omentum should be resected.

TUMOURS

Fibromas, lipomas, haemangiomas and lymphangiomas are benign tumours that have been found to arise in the omentum. Primary malignant tumours account for less than 3% of all malignancy arising in the omentum. Fibrous histiocytoma, malignant haemangiopericytoma, malignant mesothelioma, and a number of sarcomas (including liposarcoma, leiomyosarcoma and rhabdomyosarcoma) have all been described.[49] The majority of malignant tumours of the omentum are secondary deposits. These have been described from almost every site, but deposits from the ovary, stomach and colon are particularly common, and secondaries from malignant melanomas are also well recognized.

Although both primary and secondary tumour deposits in the omentum are often discovered by chance at the time of laparotomy, if sufficiently large or sufficiently numerous, symptoms and signs may arise. These include pain, abdominal distension, intestinal obstruction and ascites. On occasions, large space-occupying tumours cause pressure symptoms on neighbouring organs.

Surgery is often confined to a diagnostic biopsy at the time of laparotomy. Resection of large deposits causing pressure symptoms or obstruction can give symptomatic relief. The omentum is usually excised at the time of radical surgery for gastric and ovarian carcinomata as a debulking manoeuvre, even if it is not involved with tumour. The plane of dissection for omental resection begins at the fusion between the omentum and transverse mesocolon. It should be divided from its attachment to the greater curvature of the stomach in ovarian cancer, and it is removed en bloc with the stomach for gastric cancer (see Ch. 26). The resection of the omentum with deposits of ovarian carcinoma is an important means of reducing tumour bulk before chemotherapy.[50]

RARE TISSUE DEPOSITS

Abnormal fat deposited in the omentum has been described in Christian–Weber disease.[51] Splenic rupture may lead to splenosis (see Ch. 32). Endometriosis of the omentum has also been described.[52] Limited resection of the omentum is undertaken in

REFERENCES

48. Eitel GG. Med Rec NY 1899; 55: 715
49. Braasch JW, Mon AB. Surg Clin North Am 1967; 47: 663–678
50. Berek JS, Hacker NF et al. Obstet Gynecol 1983; 61: 189–193
51. Soergel KH, Hensley GT. Gastroenterology 1966; 51: 529–565
52. Venter PF. S Afr Med J 1980; 57: 895–899

these conditions for diagnosis, but radical omentectomy may be required if symptoms persist.

CYSTS

Lymphatic cysts and lymphangiomas may arise as developmental abnormalities. Diagnostic laparotomy and resection is required if these cysts become large enough to produce symptoms. In addition, rare dermoid and urogenital cysts resulting from tissue displacement have been described.[53,54] Care must always be taken at the time of surgery to remove omental cysts intact, because some may be the result of hydatid disease, which disseminates throughout the peritoneal cavity on rupture (see Ch. 29).

RECONSTRUCTIVE SURGERY

The omentum has increasingly been used for reconstructive surgery. Initially it was used within the peritoneal cavity to repair defects in the intestinal wall at various sites.[55] It can also be used for closing pelvic fistulae, including those of rectum, vagina and bladder.[55] Because of the ability of the omentum to be mobilized on either the left or right gastroepiploic pedicle, it can also be transposed to distant sites outside the peritoneal cavity. It has been used in reconstructive procedures on the chest wall, buttock, groin and leg,[55] and it has also been transposed to the arm for a limited period to revascularize devitalized tissue. Free omental grafts have also been undertaken for head and neck reconstructive surgery using a microvascular anastomosis.

MISCELLANEOUS INTRA-ABDOMINAL USES

Occasionally, the omentum is of value to tamponade hepatic trauma and to obliterate the dead space in the liver after excision of cysts and tumours (see Ch. 29). It may also be used to fill the presacral space after an anterior resection or pelvic exenteration. It is thought to be of value in protecting anastomoses with a poor blood supply and in those threatened by previous or subsequent radiotherapy.[55]

When foreign material such as a vascular prosthesis is inserted within the abdomen, omentum may be used to separate organs from the prosthesis, as for example at the duodenal flexure, where an aortic graft enteric fistula may develop if the prosthesis is allowed to adhere to the duodenal wall (see Ch. 10).

The omentum has also been used in patients with retroperitoneal fibrosis to wrap the ureters after they have been successfully lysed to help prevent further fibrosis from developing (see Ch. 35).

RETROPERITONEAL TUMOURS

Retroperitoneal tumours are listed below.

- Neuroblastomas in the adrenal gland or lumbar sympathetic chain; these are common tumours in children.
- Ganglioneuromas or phaeochromocytomas of the adrenal or lumbar sympathetic chain (see Ch. 34).
- Sarcomas, usually of a small round-celled type, histiocytic, myxomatous or lipomatous (see Ch. 54).
- Lymphoma in the lumbar glands (see Ch. 32).
- Vascular malformations, usually of a cavernous type. These often originate in the pelvis and may cause bleeding from the rectum, bladder or vagina. They may be part of the Klippel–Trenaunay syndrome or consist of congenital arteriovenous fistulae (see Chs 10 and 11).
- Lipoma. This is the commonest retroperitoneal tumour and accounts for as many as 60% of all retroperitoneal masses in some series. Most tumours contain mixed elements of fibrous tissue, myxomatous tissue, and sometimes fibrosarcomatous tissue. The majority start in the perirenal fat; the largest may extend from the diaphragm to the pelvis. Patients often present between 40 and 50 years of age and females out number males.
- Teratoma may occur in the retroperitoneal tissues of both women and men. They may arise from totipotential blastomeric cells misplaced along the cavity of the primitive coelom, or from aberrant germ cells. Like teratomas elsewhere (see Ch. 39), they may develop malignancy in one of their component elements. They usually present as palpable tumours, with pressure effects such as gross oedema of the lower limb. A teratoma is probably responsible for the retroperitoneal chorion epithelioma. Retroperitoneal seminomas or teratomas can develop in undescended testes (see Ch. 39) and may be encountered in hermaphrodites.
- Adrenogenital urinary tumours. These are solid tumours resembling renal or ovarian tissue. Others are neuroblastomas or adrenocortical tumours (see Ch. 34).
- Renal and pancreatic tumours (see Ch. 35 and Ch. 31, respectively) are strictly speaking retroperitoneal but are usually classified individually.

Most retroperitoneal tumours are diagnosed on CT scan and can be confirmed by biopsy. Arteriography may give an indication of resectability.

The surgical approach to retroperitoneal tumours is always difficult. Large retroperitoneal tumours are best approached through a midline abdominal incision or a left-sided thoraco-abdominal incision. The right colon and duodenum are mobilized medially if they lie on the right side, or the left colon, spleen, body and tail of pancreas, and splenic vessels are reflected to the left if the tumour lies on the left side. The prognosis is poor, except in the case of cystic tumours. The only retroperitoneal tumours that can be removed with a confident hope of cure are ganglioneuromas, neurofibromata and lipomas. Unfortunately the lipoma is frequently a liposarcoma, and a teratoma usually contains malignant elements.

Retroperitoneal germ cell tumours can be preoperatively diagnosed if circulating tumour markers are detected (B human chorionic gonadotrophin and alpha-fetoprotein). They are initially treated with aggressive chemotherapy, and if the markers return to normal and the tumour shrinks or disappears on CT scan, surgical resection of residual tissue is attempted to prevent the possibility of recurrence from surviving cell nests in an otherwise dead tumour.

RETROPERITONEAL CYSTS

- Nephrogenic cysts of Wolffian origin, which usually occur in adult women. They are often large, may be unilocular or

REFERENCES

53. Nichols HM. Ann Surg 1947; 126: 340
54. Howarth VS. Br J Surg 1950; 37: 329
55. Liebermann-Meffert D, White H. The Greater Omentum: Anatomy, Physiology, Pathology, with a Historical Survey. Springer Verlag, New York, 1983

multilocular, and are usually situated laterally. The wall is formed of fibrous tissue with a lining of high cylindrical epithelium.
- Epidermoid cysts of Wolffian duct.
- Dermoid cysts.
- Renal cysts (see Ch. 35).
- Pancreatic cysts (see Ch. 31).

TREATMENT

These cysts may be ignored, aspirated or resected.

ACUTE ABDOMINAL PAIN (THE ACUTE ABDOMEN)

The parietal peritoneum is innervated by the somatic nervous system through spinal nerves in the distribution of the overlying dermatomes. The xiphisternum is at the level of T4, the umbilicus at T8, and the inguinal ligament at T12. Pain is sharply localized to the point of inflammation of the parietal peritoneum. For example, acute sigmoid diverticulitis causes irritation of the overlying parietal peritoneum, producing pain in the left iliac fossa.

The viscera and visceral peritoneum are innervated by the autonomic nervous system, with pain travelling in sympathetic fibres and localized to the somatic distribution of the equivalent somatic nerve roots from T1 to L2. The pain is therefore deep, poorly localized, and usually associated with sympathetic symptoms such as sweating and nausea. The gastrointestinal tract is divided embryologically into the foregut, midgut and hindgut, each with its own blood supply and nerve supply. Pain from the foregut is localized to the epigastrium, the midgut to the periumbilical region, and the hindgut to the lower abdomen. As a result, early inflammation of the appendix and small bowel obstruction without parietal inflammation produce periumbilical pain. This is *referred* pain (Fig. 25.12). Another example of referred pain follows irritation of the diaphragm by subphrenic inflammation. Because there is no directly overlying dermatome as there is elsewhere in the abdominal cavity, pain is felt in the dermatome associated with the nerve supply of the diaphragm (C3–5), which is the shoulder tip. Pain from inflammation of the parietal peritoneum, caused by acute cholecystitis, can also *radiate* as it spreads from the right subcostal region around to the back, along the distribution of the overlying spinal somatic nerve.

Inflammation of the retroperitoneum arising from acute pancreatitis, pyelonephritis, or a posterior perforation of a duodenal ulcer causes irritation of the somatic spinal nerves, producing back pain. A retrocaecal appendicitis may inflame the iliopsoas muscle, which can produce pain in the right loin, especially when the psoas muscle is stretched.

Many of the possible causes of the acute abdomen may combine both visceral and parietal pain, and this often produces an evolving picture. Hence the importance of regularly reviewing patients admitted with acute abdominal pain. The pain of acute appendicitis classically starts in the periumbilical region because of irritation of the visceral peritoneum. With further inflammation the parietal peritoneum may become inflamed, and the pain localizes to the right iliac fossa. Pain from a small bowel obstruction might initially be central and colicky, but as the obstructed loop becomes ischaemic and starts to inflame the overlying peritoneum, the pain becomes continuous and more widespread.

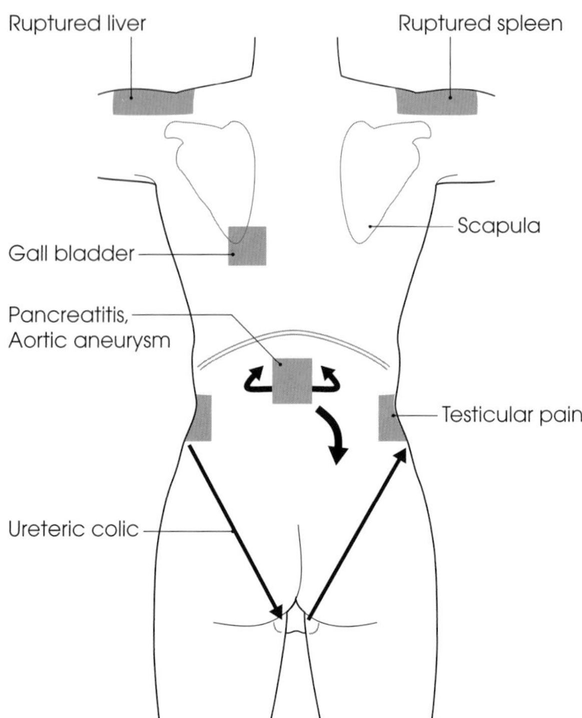

Figure 25.12 Some of the well-recognized sites of referred pain derived from intra-abdominal viscera.

PATHOLOGY

INFLAMMATION AND INFECTION

These conditions are usually characterized by a febrile illness with localized signs of peritonitis. The origin of the inflammation can frequently be determined from the history and onset of the pain, and by the site of maximum tenderness. Common intra-abdominal inflammatory conditions include acute appendicitis, acute cholecystitis, acute diverticulitis, acute pancreatitis, acute salpingitis (pelvic inflammatory disease), and mesenteric adenitis. Other less common inflammatory conditions that can cause abdominal pain are Crohn's disease, Meckel's diverticulitis, pyelonephritis and cystitis. Very occasionally, *Yersinia* infection of the small bowel can also present with an acute abdomen. The pain is often very non-specific to start with, gradually increasing in intensity over a period of several hours or even days (Fig. 25.13).

PERFORATION

Perforation of an abdominal viscus usually results in the sudden onset of severe abdominal pain (Fig. 25.14). Identification of which viscus has perforated may be determined from the history of any preceding abdominal symptoms or illness, such as constipation or peptic ulcer disease. In the early stages, the site of maximum tenderness may also indicate the organ that has perforated. The usual end point of generalized peritonitis is, however, a rigid board-like abdomen where selective tenderness can no longer be elicited. This sign represents widespread involuntary guarding, which will be discussed in more detail. The cause of the perforation must then await the findings at laparotomy. The most common organs that perforate, excluding the appendix, are the stomach and duodenum (from peptic ulcer disease) and the colon (from diverticular disease or severe

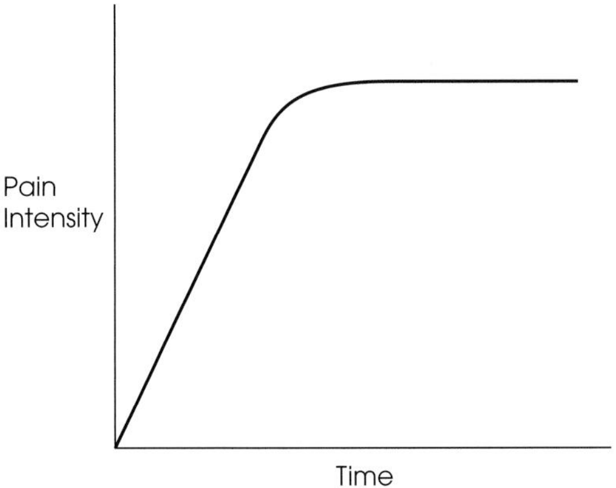

Figure 25.13 Inflammation and pain.

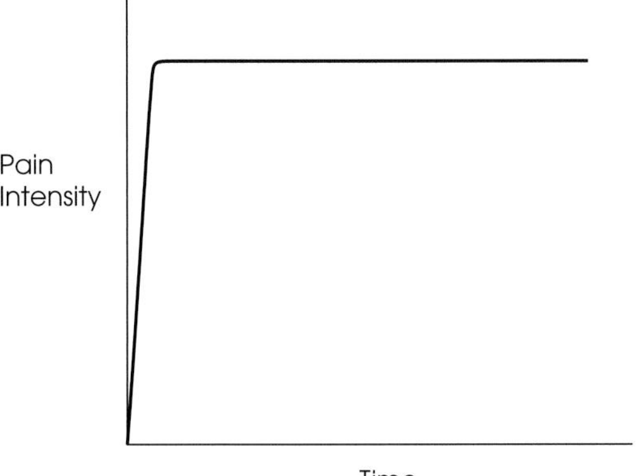

Figure 25.14 Perforation and pain.

constipation). The end point of many of the conditions that produce visceral inflammation is perforation, but generally these patients present with symptoms of the underlying disease first, rather than the short, severe presentation associated with a sudden perforation.

OBSTRUCTION

Obstruction of any hollow viscus within the abdominal cavity usually causes acute abdominal pain. Obstruction of all viscera except the gall bladder tends to produce colicky pain, while obstruction of the gall bladder (inaccurately termed 'biliary colic') usually presents with a more continuous type of pain, often punctuated by acute exacerbations, which is similar to that of inflammation (see Ch. 30). Colicky pain classically resolves between short-lived episodes, and it is only when underlying inflammation or infection set in that a more continuous background element to the pain occurs (Fig. 25.15). This can of course represent the development of a serious complication such as ischaemia of the bowel, and therefore its recognition by the clinician is vital for prompt treatment.

INFARCTION

There are a number of processes that can cause an abdominal viscus to infarct. These include torsion of the viscus, occlusion of its arterial inflow by thrombosis or embolus, venous thrombosis, and haematological disorders that lead to arterial occlusion. The vascular supply of the small bowel may be occluded by an adhesion or a hernial orifice causing a strangulating obstruction

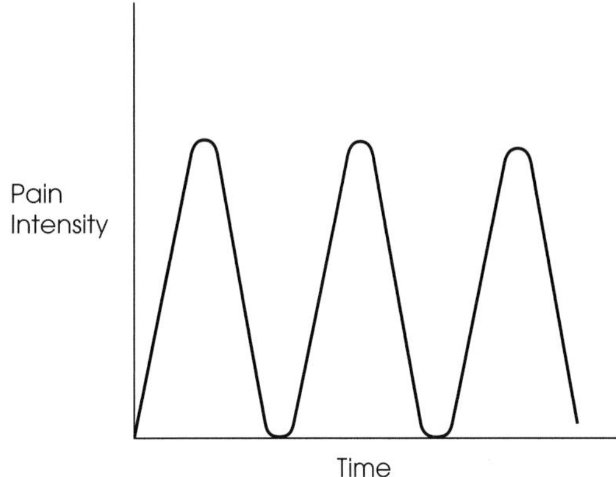

Figure 25.15 Obstruction and pain.

that ultimately leads to infarction and perforation. An acute aortic dissection can occlude the origins of the mesenteric vessels as the false lumen extends (see Ch. 10).

Organs that may undergo infarction include those on mesenteries that can twist, such as the ovaries (usually from torsion of associated cysts), the testes or testicular appendices, and segments of intestine. Others include appendices epiploicae; the omentum; the spleen, usually secondary to haematological disorders such as sickle cell disease but also from processes involving the arterial supply or venous drainage; and the kidney, usually as a result of atherosclerotic disease. Uterine fibroids that twist or outgrow their blood supply may also infarct. In severe cases of acute pancreatitis, infarction and necrosis of the pancreas can occur, as well as infarction of adjacent structures such as the colon and the spleen from involvement of their blood vessels. Pain from infarction has a wide spectrum of presentations, from being poorly localized, relatively non-specific and quite deep-seated to sudden and severe with associated peritonitis.

HAEMORRHAGE

Blood within the peritoneal cavity produces the symptoms and signs of an acute abdomen. This may initially be localized to the site of the bleed but rapidly becomes more generalized. The history and the original site of abdominal pain should again give some indication as to the source of the haemorrhage. In addition to abdominal trauma, conditions causing intraperitoneal bleeding include ruptured abdominal aortic aneurysms, aneurysms of mesenteric vessels (including the splenic, coeliac and hepatic arteries; Fig. 25.16), ruptured ovarian cysts, ruptured ectopic pregnancies, retrograde menstruation, endometriosis, spontaneous rupture of liver tumours, or rupture of a pathologically abnormal spleen.

MEDICAL CAUSES

Medical causes of abdominal pain come from conditions outside the abdomen, from systemic diseases, or from conditions of the abdominal wall and back.

DIAGNOSIS

A thorough history and examination remain the key to an accurate diagnosis of the cause of the abdominal pain. The importance of history-taking combined with a careful

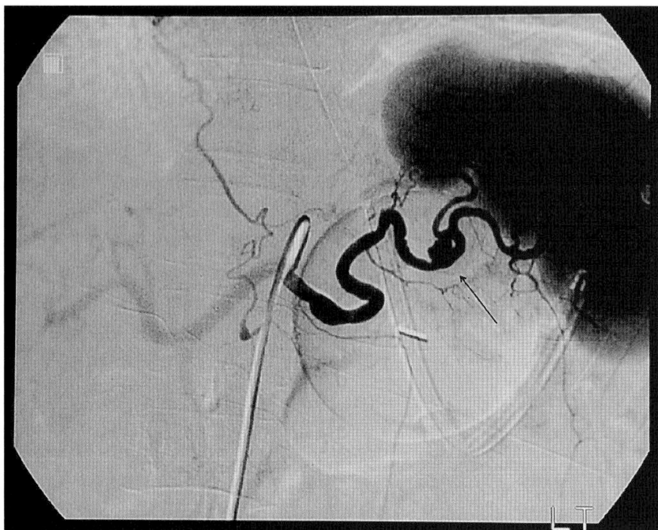

Figure 25.16 Angiogram of a false aneurysm of the splenic artery (arrow) secondary to acute pancreatitis. (Courtesy of Ms Tracey Gillies.)

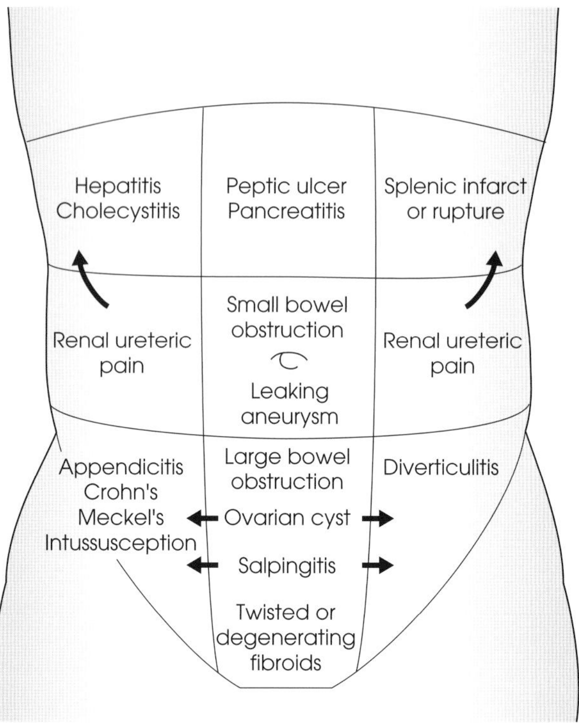

Figure 25.17 The nine regions of the abdomen and some of the commoner conditions responsible for pain in these areas.

examination, emphasized repeatedly by Zachray Cope,[56] was confirmed by the important work carried out by de Dombal[57] and Gunn.[58] Their computer-aided diagnostic systems required a detailed pro forma of the patient's history and examination findings to be completed by the assessing surgeon. These were then entered into a computer and a list of the probable diagnoses was produced. Repeated results throughout the UK demonstrated an improvement in diagnostic accuracy of around 20%.[59] When the influence of computer-aided diagnosis was analysed further, it was shown that much of the improvement was related to using the pro forma or structured data sheets rather than the computer programme.[60]

HISTORY

The site, onset, character and duration of the abdominal pain provide important pointers to the diagnosis. Radiation of the pain, progression or alteration of its site or character, factors that aggravate the pain or relieve it, and any associated symptoms are also helpful in refining the diagnosis. The site of the abdominal pain is usually related to one of nine areas (Fig. 25.17). These regions are demarcated by the midclavicular lines in the vertical axis and by the transpyloric and transtubercular lines in the horizontal axis. Figure 25.17 also indicates some of the common organs and pathological processes that commonly cause pain experienced in these regions.

Obtaining information on aggravating or relieving factors can be particularly helpful to the assessing surgeon. Pain made worse by moving and coughing suggests peritoneal inflammation (peritonism), whereas pain that makes the patient roll around or double up is typical of colic. Factors that aggravate or relieve pain are also important in making a diagnosis, and information on the influence of movement, injury, position, food, antacids, vomiting, bowel action and micturition on the pain must always be sought. A history of previous trauma, however minor, may be important. It is also important to ask about associated symptoms such as vomiting, diarrhoea, dysuria, or a missed period that preceded or followed the onset of the pain because these may again provide important diagnostic clues.

True colic is a gripping pain of sudden onset, which rapidly reaches a crescendo before equally swiftly dying away, usually completely.[61] This description is true of intestinal and renal colic, but biliary colic is a misnomer because patients tend to complain of a continuous pain with exacerbations of severe pain.[62] Strangulation and ischaemia should be suspected when an intestinal colic alters to become a continuous pain.

Common adjectives used by individual patients to describe the character of abdominal pain—including stabbing, wrenching, boring, burning and crushing—rarely help when trying to reach a diagnosis. Specific areas of radiation are characteristic of certain causes of abdominal pain, and some of the classical sites of referral are shown in Fig. 25.12. The history should conclude with details of past illnesses or operations, the family and social history, and details of alcohol intake and any regular medication, in addition to any known allergies. A general systems enquiry should also be made.

It is impossible to list every direct question that could or should be asked to elucidate possible disorders of the gastrointestinal, genitourinary, cardiorespiratory and reproductive systems. Some of these questions will become apparent from

REFERENCES

56. Cope VZ. The Early Diagnosis of the Acute Abdomen. 2nd edn. Oxford University Press, London, 1921
57. de Dombal FT, Leaper DJ, Staniland JR et al. Br Med J 1972; 2: 9–13
58. Gunn AA. J R Coll Surg Edinb 1976; 21: 170–172
59. Adams ID, Chan M, Clifford PC et al. Br Med J 1986; 293: 800–804
60. Paterson-Brown S, Vipond MN, Simms K et al. Br J Surg 1989; 76: 1011–1013
61. Stokes MA, Moriarty KT, Catchpole BN. Lancet 1988; i: 211–215
62. French EB, Robb WAT. Br Med J 1963; ii: 135–141

reading the remainder of this chapter, while others will be learned only by the practical experience of assessing many patients with acute abdominal pain.

EXAMINATION

Anaemia, pallor, cyanosis, jaundice, lymphadenopathy, dehydration, fetor and pyrexia are some of the important physical findings that should be specifically looked for. A rapid pulse and low blood pressure may indicate signs of shock. A rapid or irregular pulse may also be relevant.

The chest should be examined next, looking especially for signs of pulmonary disease, while examination of the cardiovascular system may uncover evidence of cardiac failure, valvular disorders, or peripheral vascular insufficiency.

A careful abdominal examination is obviously essential, and is facilitated by early administration of adequate analgesia.[63] The swellings caused by enlargements of the liver, spleen, kidneys and bladder, or tumours of the bowel or ovary and other intra-abdominal or retroperitoneal structures, may all be visible on careful inspection. The expansile pulsation of an abdominal aneurysm may also be seen. All abdominal scars must be noted and tested for an incisional hernia. Distension (which is usually caused by ascites), intestinal obstruction, or a large intra-abdominal tumour may also be apparent. Skin eruptions caused by herpes zoster, distended veins as a result of portal hypertension or occlusion of the inferior vena cava, hernial swellings and visible peristalsis are other physical signs that may be detected by a careful inspection. The hernial orifices must be specifically examined, as must the male genitalia, looking especially for tenderness and masses within the scrotum.

Palpation should be carried out to establish the site or sites of maximum tenderness, which can be determined by repeated gentle pressure at different points on the anterior abdominal wall. At the same time, the presence of abdominal wall rigidity and involuntary guarding should be assessed. Guarding represents contraction of the abdominal wall muscles over the area of pain. This might occur voluntarily when the patient wishes to avoid the pain from examination, or involuntarily when the muscles go into spasm when the inflamed viscus touches the parietal peritoneum. The presence of rebound tenderness indicates underlying peritoneal inflammation and is best examined by using percussion, although pain on coughing is also indicative of rebound tenderness.[64] Specific pain from abdominal wall tenderness is indicated by an increase in pain at the point of maximal abdominal tenderness, when the abdominal muscles are contracted. This finding is present in nearly a third of patients with non-specific abdominal pain.[65]

Auscultation is used to assess the characteristic bowel sounds produced by an obstructed intestine and the total absence of bowel sounds found in patients with a severe generalized peritonitis or a paralytic ileus. Abdominal bruits may also be detected but are of dubious diagnostic value.

The role of the rectal examination in the assessment of the acute abdomen has changed over the past decade following a large study from Edinburgh, which demonstrated that in patients with right iliac fossa pain no further additional information was obtained if rebound tenderness has already been demonstrated.[66] When a gynaecological diagnosis is suspected or needs to be excluded, a gentle pelvic examination should be carried out.

There are specific signs associated with certain specific diagnoses shown in Table 25.2; these should also be sought where appropriate.

Table 25.2 Named abdominal signs

Sign	Description	Pathology
Cullen	Periumbilical bruising	Haemorrhagic pancreatitis or ectopic pregnancy
Grey–Turner	Bruising of flank	Haemorrhagic pancreatitis
Rovsing	Pain on extension of the hip joint (due to psoas irritation)	Retrocaecal appendicitis
Murphy	Right upper quadrant tenderness without left upper quadrant tenderness	Acute cholecystitis

OBSERVATION AND REVIEW

Following a full clinical assessment, the admitting surgeon must then make one of the three following decisions: an urgent operation is required, an urgent operation is not required, or the need for urgent operation remains uncertain. In the first instance, apart from some basic baseline investigations and adequate resuscitation, nothing else need be done. In the second instance, further investigations and resuscitation can take place at a speed determined by the clinical condition. The third decision is, however, the most difficult and undoubtedly the one in which the majority of errors occur. Further expeditious investigations are obviously essential in this group of patients and are discussed here in some detail. Enough emphasis cannot, however, be placed on the value of continued observation with regular review, which has become an essential part of the early management of patients with acute abdominal pain.[67] The value of this approach was confirmed by a prospective trial of CT in the investigation of abdominal pain. In this study the presumed diagnosis was recorded on admission and after 24 h, with a further review at 6 months. Only half the diagnoses on admission were correct at 6-month follow-up, but 76% of the diagnoses at 24 h were correct. This included patients both in the CT arm and in the standard treatment arm.[68]

DIFFERENTIAL DIAGNOSIS

There are many conditions that can present as an acute abdomen, but there is a much smaller group of conditions that are responsible for around 90% of presentations. These are listed in Table 25.3.[69] On completion of the initial clinical assessment, a working or differential diagnosis should be made. Additional specific investigations may then be ordered to confirm the pre-

REFERENCES

63. Attard AR, Corlett MJ, Kidner NJ et al. Br Med J 1992; 305: 554–556
64. Bennett DH, Tambeur LJ, Campbell WB. Br Med J 1994; 308: 1336
65. Gray DWR, Seabrook G, Dixon JM et al. Ann R Coll Surg Engl 1988; 70: 233–234
66. Dixon JM, Elton RA, Rainey JB et al. Br Med J 1991; 203: 386–388
67. Thompson HJ, Jones PF. Am J Surg 1986; 152: 522–525
68. Chaan SN, Watsin CJE, Palmer CR et al. Br Med J 2002; 325: 1387–1389
69. Irvin TT. Br J Surg 1989; 76: 1121–1125

Table 25.3 Conditions that may present with acute abdominal pain[20]

Condition	Cases (%)
Non-specific abdominal pain	35
Acute appendicitis	17
Intestinal obstruction	15
Urological causes	6
Gallstone disease	5
Colonic diverticular disease	4
Abdominal trauma	3
Abdominal malignancy	3
Perforated peptic ulcer	3
Pancreatitis	2
Exacerbation of peptic ulcer, ruptured abdominal aortic aneurysm, gynaecological causes, inflammatory bowel disease, medical conditions, mesenteric ischaemia, gastroenteritis, and other miscellaneous conditions	≤ 1%

sumptive diagnosis or help to reduce the number of differential diagnoses.

DIAGNOSTIC PROCEDURES

BLOOD TESTS

The presence of anaemia, a leukocytosis, a raised serum amylase level, and abnormal liver and renal function tests are all helpful in reaching a diagnosis but, with the exception of the amylase level, are not diagnostic and must be interpreted in the light of the clinical condition of the patient. An amylase level greater than three times the upper limit of normal is diagnostic of acute pancreatitis (see Ch. 31), but lower levels can be the result of any number of underlying diseases including perforated peptic ulcers, obstruction and mesenteric infarction. In the diagnosis of acute appendicitis, little store should be placed on the initial white cell count, which, like the first temperature reading,[70] is often of little value. Sequential measurements are, however, much more helpful because a trend can be observed.[71] Liver function tests are performed in cases of presumed cholecystitis, not so much for confirmation of the diagnosis but more to identify choledocholithiasis or cholangitis (see Ch. 30).

The desirability of other investigations obviously depends to some extent on the initial working diagnosis or the differential diagnosis reached on completion of the clinical examination. It also depends on the availability of diagnostic equipment and laboratory facilities. Urea and electrolyte measurement is essential if dehydration or renal failure is suspected, and liver function tests are required for all hepatobiliary and pancreatic conditions. Hepatitis A and B antigens may also be tested for, and the Paul–Bunnell test may be obtained if glandular fever is considered. The serum calcium, arterial blood gases, white cell count, blood glucose, lactate dehydrogenase and C-reactive protein may all be helpful in diagnosing and assessing the severity of acute pancreatitis. A sickle test should be obtained if the condition is suspected, and the urinary porphyrins should be measured if acute porphyria is considered.[72] A urinary pregnancy test or serum human chorionic gonadotrophin level should be obtained in any case of lower abdominal pain in a woman of fertile age. Antibody titres may be measured if amoebic or viral disease is suspected.

URINE ANALYSIS

Examination of a urine sample should be performed in *all* patients presenting with abdominal pain, because a urological cause of abdominal pain is responsible for 6% of admissions with an acute abdomen.[69] The finding of urobilinogen in the urine is useful in jaundiced patients and glycosuria in suspected diabetics. Any patient suspected of having urinary tract sepsis or lower abdominal pain should have urine microscopy, culture and sensitivity performed to identify a urinary pathogen and select the appropriate antimicrobial therapy.

PERITONEAL FLUID FOR CYTOLOGY

The aspiration of ascites and its cytological examination in suspected intra-abdominal malignancy is an established technique (see p. 564). Peritoneal cytology has been used over the past few years and provides a relatively simple method of obtaining intraperitoneal information without resorting to laparoscopy. This was first described by Stewart from New Zealand[73] and subsequently verified by other groups.[74–76] A small 14-gauge venous cannula is inserted into the peritoneal cavity halfway between the umbilicus and the symphysis pubis after infiltration with local anaesthesia. An umbilical catheter (size 3.5 Ch) is then passed down the cannula and aspirated. The resultant aspirate is deposited on a glass slide, stained, and the percentage of polymorphonuclear cells in one high-powered field determined by light microscopy. A percentage greater than 50% is indicative of significant inflammation. Although extremely useful in differentiating those patients without an intra-abdominal inflammatory process, peritoneal cytology on its own cannot indicate the need for surgery because some inflammatory conditions—such as pelvic inflammatory disease, which does not require surgery—cannot be differentiated from acute appendicitis.

PLAIN RADIOLOGY

Conflicting evidence exists regarding the role of the plain abdominal radiograph,[77,78] but there is little doubt that the investigation is overused and should be reserved for patients suspected of having intestinal obstruction or renal tract disease, and it is also valuable in those patients who remain a diagnostic dilemma. A supine film (Fig. 25.18) will usually suffice in patients suspected of having bowel obstruction, because the erect abdominal film rarely adds any further information.[79] There are, however, occasions when the erect film can be useful. These

REFERENCES

70. Howie CR, Gunn AA. J R Coll Surg Edinb 1984; 29: 249–251
71. Thompson MM, Underwood MJ et al. Br J Surg 1992; 79: 822–824
72. Stein JA, Tuschudy DP. Medicine 1970; 49: 1–16
73. Stewart RJ, Gupta RK et al. Lancet 1986; ii: 1414–1415
74. Vipond MN, Paterson-Brown S et al. Br J Surg 1990; 77: 86–87
75. Baigrie RJ, Saidan Z et al. Br J Surg 1991; 78: 167–170
76. Caldwell MTP, Watson RGK. Br J Surg 1994; 81: 276–278
77. Lee PWR. Br J Surg 1976; 63: 763–766
78. Stower MJ, Amar S et al. Soc Med 1985; 78: 630–633
79. Field S, Guy PJ et al. Br Med J 1985; 290: 1934–1936

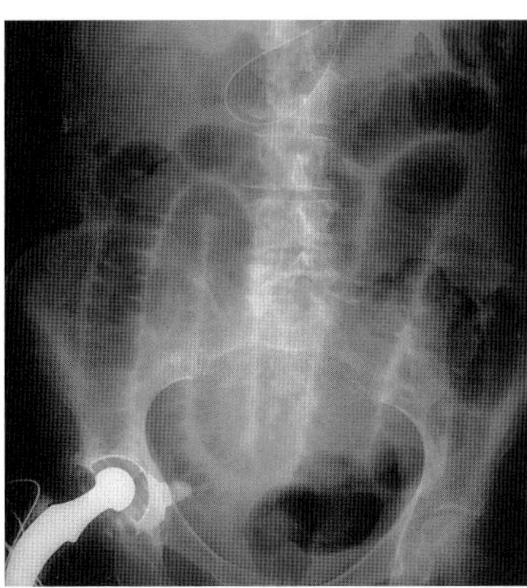

Figure 25.18 Supine abdominal X-ray showing obvious small bowel obstruction.

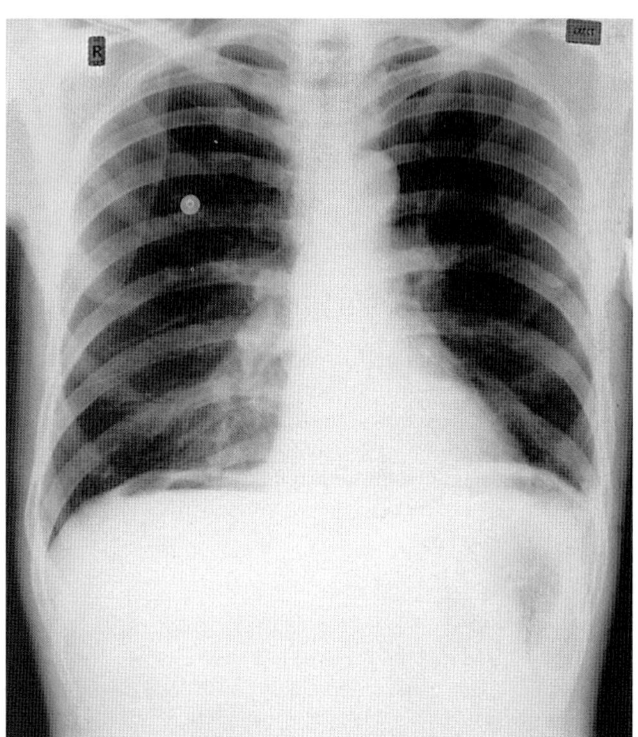

Figure 25.20 An erect chest X-ray showing air under the diaphragm.

include differentiating between a paralytic ileus and mechanical obstruction, particularly in the postoperative period. In the former, the fluid levels within a single loop of bowel on the erect film are at the same level because there is no forward pressure, whereas in the latter the levels are different (Fig. 25.19). Free gas from a perforated intra-abdominal viscus is best seen on the erect chest X-ray[80] or the lateral decubitus abdominal view (Fig. 25.20).[79–81] Gas seen in the biliary tree on the plain abdominal radiograph can clinch the diagnosis of gallstone obstruction of the small bowel.

CONTRAST RADIOLOGY

The use of an intravenous pyelogram in patients with presumed renal colic is well established; however, the role of contrast radiology in the diagnosis of other causes of the acute abdomen is still being refined. There are three pathological processes in which it has a useful role.

Perforated peptic ulcer

Perforated ulcers of the stomach and duodenum can be managed conservatively in patients who have a localized rather than generalized peritonitis.[82] It is, however, important to confirm that the perforation has sealed, and this can be demonstrated only by a contrast meal. In patients in whom the diagnosis is uncertain, a contrast study can confirm that the perforation has not sealed, indicating the need for appropriate surgery. A contrast study is required to confirm the diagnosis if the clinical condition suggests that surgery is indicated because up to half the patients with a perforated peptic ulcer do not have free gas visible on the erect chest X-ray[83] (Fig. 25.21).

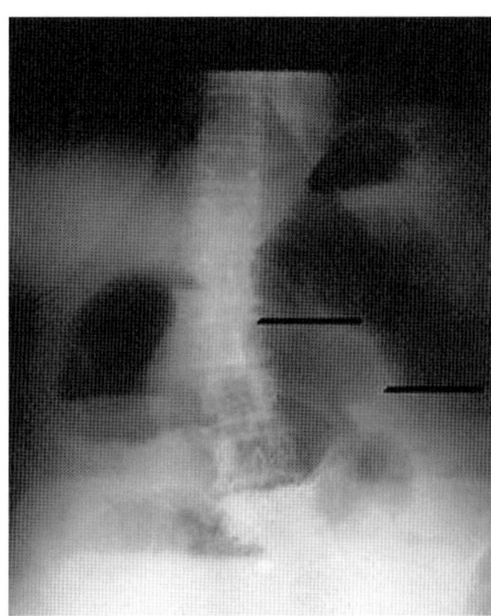

Figure 25.19 Erect abdominal radiograph showing fluid levels (marked with the lines).

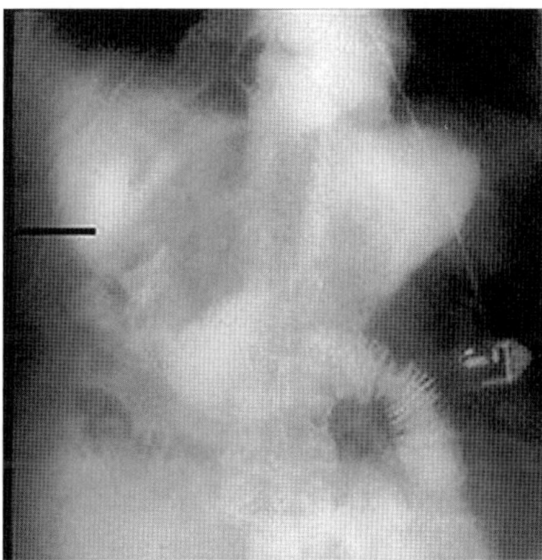

Figure 25.21 Oral contrast demonstrating a large leak (arrow) from the first part of the duodenum.

REFERENCES

80. Miller RE, Nelson SW. Am J Roentgenol 1971; 112: 574–585
81. de Lacey GJ, Wignall BK et al. Clin Radiol 1980; 31: 453–455
82. Crofts TJ, Park KG, Steele RJ et al. N Engl J Med 1989; 320: 970–973
83. Wellwood JM, Wilson AN, Hopkinson BR. Br J Surg 1971; 58: 245–249

Small bowel obstruction

The diagnosis of small bowel obstruction is usually evident from the history and examination, and it is confirmed on a plain abdominal radiograph. The majority of episodes are related to adhesions and settle with conservative management, although those with no previous abdominal surgical procedures may well benefit from earlier intervention. This is discussed in more detail under *Management of small bowel obstruction* (p. 586).

Large bowel obstruction

A contrast enema is indicated for all those patients with symptoms, signs, and an abdominal radiograph demonstrating colonic dilatation to confirm or refute a mechanical obstruction. Colonic pseudo-obstruction cannot be distinguished from a mechanical obstruction on plain abdominal radiographs,[84,85] and because the management of the two conditions is so different, a contrast enema must be performed in all patients with suspected large bowel obstruction.

ULTRASOUND

Ultrasonography has become a vital diagnostic tool in the assessment of the acute abdomen. Its main areas of use are on the diagnosis of hepato-pancreatico-biliary disorders, appendicitis and gynaecological disease. It is also useful in the detection of free intra-abdominal fluid and abscesses (see p. 596).

Ultrasonography is the first radiological investigation for patients with suspected gallstone disease and has a sensitivity of greater than 95% for the detection of acute cholecystitis (see Ch. 3).[86] Because about a quarter of the patients initially thought to have acute cholecystitis following clinical assessment alone are subsequently found to have another non-biliary pathology as the cause of their pain,[87] it is important that any diagnosis of acute cholecystitis is confirmed with an ultrasound examination (Fig. 25.22).

Many gynaecological disorders do not require operations and settle with conservative management. Transvaginal ultrasonography is a good investigation for many gynaecological conditions and is particularly useful for the detection of ovarian cysts and ectopic gestations.

Ultrasound is also useful in the detection of appendicitis and in the detection of free intra-abdominal fluid from trauma, ascites and perforated viscera. It is easily portable, making it particularly useful in the emergency setting.

COMPUTERIZED TOMOGRAPHY

Until recently, CT has not had an important place in the early assessment of patients with acute abdominal pain of non-traumatic origin, with the exception of acute diverticulitis,[88] leaking abdominal aneurysms, and pancreatic necrosis.[89] A 1998 study exploring its role in the diagnosis of acute appendicitis showed it to have a 98% accuracy.[90] Another study on the use of CT in a range of acute abdominal conditions was a prospective randomized trial of CT within 24 h in patients who did not have an indication for immediate laparotomy.[68] When early CT was compared against standard practice, there was a significant reduction in mortality (0 versus 11%, respectively) in the CT group. The improved survival was attributed to the earlier detection by CT of significantly more serious diagnoses (Fig. 25.23).

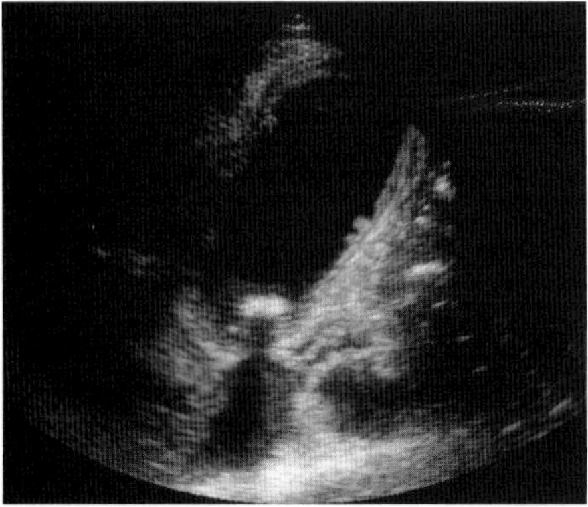

Figure 25.22 Ultrasound scan of gall bladder, showing the thickened gall bladder wall and pericholecystic fluid characteristic of acute cholecystitis along with an obvious gallstone.

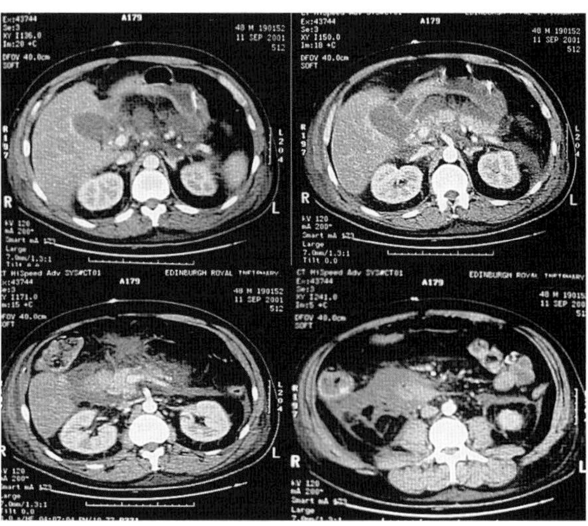

Figure 25.23 A CT scan demonstrating acute pancreatitis with necrosis.

LAPAROSCOPY

Although available and practised by a few enthusiastic surgeons since the turn of the 20th century,[91] laparoscopy remained a gynaecological investigation until the development of video-laparoscopy. The ability to carry out laparoscopic cholecystectomy spread the technique to general surgeons, and this has undoubtedly been the main reason for its acceptance as an important investigation, and now treatment, of other acute abdominal conditions (Fig. 25.24).[92]

When used to assess those patients in whom the decision to operate is uncertain, laparoscopy has been shown to reduce the error rate,[93] particularly when acute appendicitis is suspected in

REFERENCES

84. Stewart J, Finan BJ, Courtney DF et al. Br J Surg 1984; 71: 799–801
85. Koruth NM, Koruth A, Matheson NA. J R Coll Surg Edinb 1985; 30: 258–260
86. Samuels BL, Freitas JE, Bree RL et al. Radiology 1983; 47: 207–210
87. Schofield PF, Hulton NR, Baildam AD. Ann R Coll Surg Engl 1986; 6: 14–16
88. McKee RF, Deignan RW, Krukowski ZH. Br J Surg 1993; 80: 560–565
89. Glazer G, Mann DV on behalf of the Working Party of the British Society of Gastroenterology. Gut 1998; 42 (Suppl 2): S1–S13
90. Rao PM, Rhea JT, Novelline RA et al. N Engl J Med 1998; 338: 141–146
91. Jacobaeus HC. Munch Med Wochenschr 1911; 58: 2017–2019
92. Paterson-Brown S. Br J Surg 1993; 80: 279–283

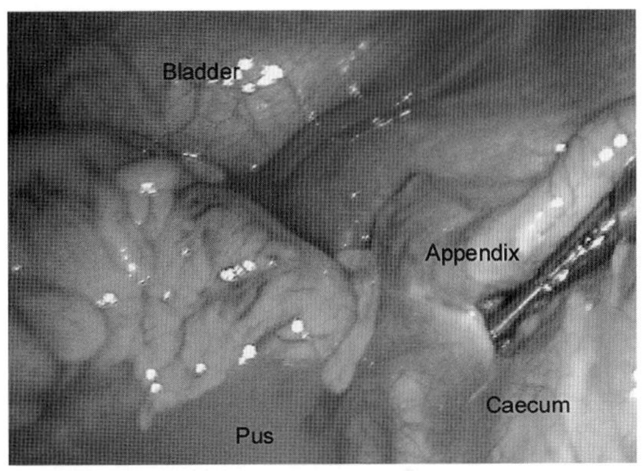

a

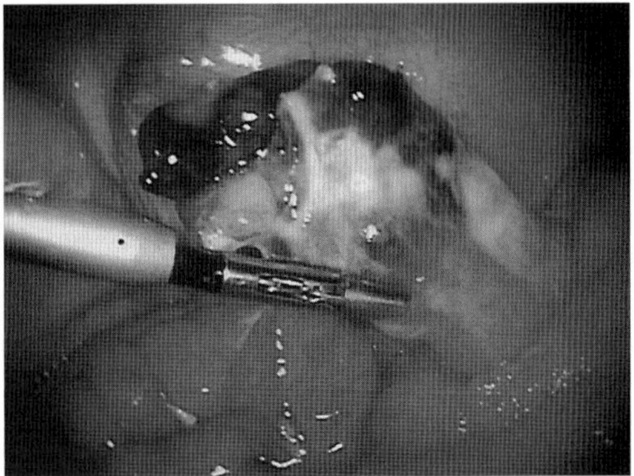

b

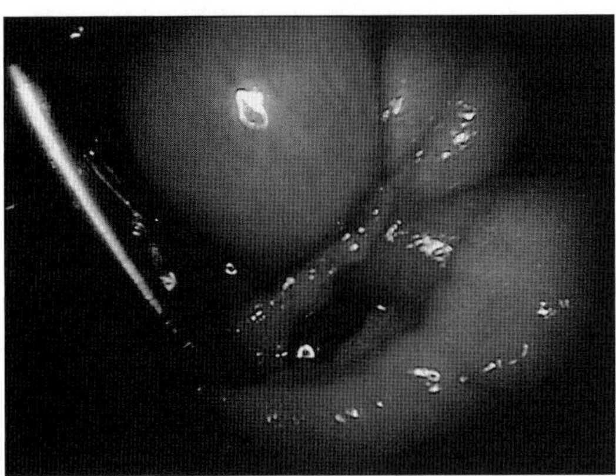

c

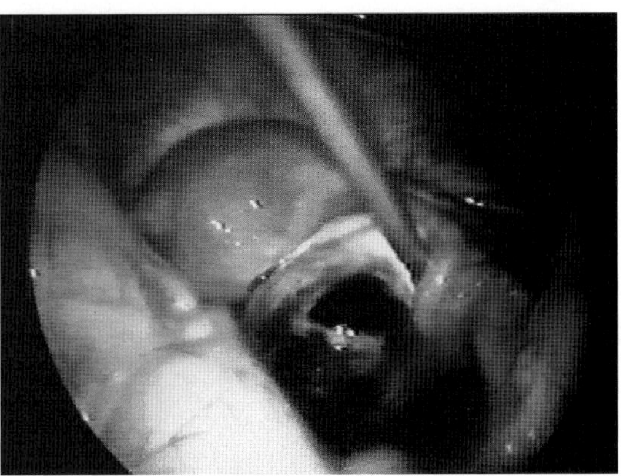

d

Figure 25.24 (a) Laparoscopic appearance of an acute appendicitis, (b) gangrenous appendicitis, (c) band adhesion causing a small bowel obstruction, and (d) haemorrhagic ovarian cyst. (Courtesy of Mr Peter Driscoll (a) and Mr Luigi Sussman (b,c).)

young women.[94] Its obvious advantage over other less invasive investigations is that it can accurately differentiate between acute appendicitis and acute gynaecological conditions, such as pelvic inflammatory disease, which can pose a diagnostic dilemma to the emergency surgeon. Because the conditions of more than 10% of women admitted to a surgical ward with acute abdominal pain have a gynaecological cause,[95] the importance of laparoscopic assessment is clear.

In the acute abdomen, another difficult diagnostic dilemma is differentiating acute appendicitis and other defined pathological conditions from non-specific abdominal pain. In a randomized trial of early laparoscopy versus observation for patients with 'suspected non-specific abdominal pain', laparoscopy had a higher diagnostic accuracy and an improved quality of life 6 weeks after discharge.[96] This study has, however, been criticized because 19% of patients who underwent laparoscopy remained without a surgical diagnosis.[97]

CLINICAL OUTCOMES

Data from a large audit of 1190 patients admitted to hospital with acute abdominal pain reported a 30-day mortality rate of 4%, with a perioperative mortality rate of 8%.[69] The perioperative mortality rate was, not surprisingly, age-related, being 2% for those under the age of 60 years, 12% for those 60–69 years of age, and 20% for those over the age of 80 years. The commonest cause of perioperative mortality was laparotomy for irresectable malignant disease (28%), followed by ruptured abdominal aortic aneurysm (23%), perforated peptic ulcer (16%), and colonic resections (14%).

TREATMENT

GENERAL

The initial treatment of all patients with abdominal pain is similar. The urgency and degree of treatment should be adjusted to the severity of the presentation, and can be initiated at the same time as the history and examination are taking place. Supplemental oxygen may be administered, if indicated, and a review by an intensivist or anaesthetist should be arranged if there is impending respiratory failure. Intravenous access should be obtained with large-gauge cannulae and resuscitation commenced. Regardless of the level of dehydration, many patients benefit from a litre of crystalloid. Further resuscitation should be according to the clinical hydration status of the patient (see Ch. 3). Aggressive resuscitation is avoided in patients with ruptured abdominal aortic aneurysms as hypotension reduces

REFERENCES

93. Paterson-Brown S, Ekersley JR et al. Br J Surg 1986; 73: 1022–1024
94. Paterson-Brown S, Thompson JN, Eckersley JRT et al. Br Med J 1988; 296: 1363–1364
95. Paterson-Brown S, Eckersley JRT, Dudley HAF. J R Coll Surg Edinb 1988; 33: 13–15
96. Decadt B, Sussman L, Lewis MPN et al. Br J Surg 1999; 86: 1383–1386
97. Poulin EC, Schlachta CM, Mamazza J. Lancet 2000; 355: 861–863

Box 25.1 Surgical causes of the acute abdomen

Inflammation and infection
- Acute appendicitis
- Acute cholecystitis
- Acute diverticulitis
- Acute pancreatitis
- Salpingitis
- Septic abortion
- Mesenteric adenitis
- Primary peritonitis
- Crohn's disease
- Meckel's diverticulitis
- Pyelonephritis and cystitis
- *Yersinia* infection

Perforation
- Gastric ulcer
- Duodenal ulcer
- Diverticular disease
- Carcinoma of the colon
- Crohn's disease
- Ulcerative colitis
- Lymphoma
- Foreign body perforation
- Acute cholecystitis with perforation
- Acute appendicitis with perforation
- Perforation of the oesophagus (Boerhaave's syndrome)
- Perforation of a segment of strangulated bowel
- Perforation of the urinary bladder

Obstruction
- Renal colic
- Biliary colic

Small bowel
- Congenital bands or atresia
- Meconium ileus
- Malrotation of the gut
- Adhesions from previous surgery
- Hernia
- Intussusception
- Gallstone
- Tumours
- Crohn's disease

Large bowel
- Tumour
- Volvulus
- Inflammatory stricture

Infarction
- Torsion of a viscus
- Arterial thrombosis or embolus
- Venous thrombosis
- Dissecting aortic aneurysm

Haemorrhage
- Ruptured abdominal aortic aneurysm
- Aneurysms of mesenteric vessels
- Dissecting aneurysm of the aorta
- Ruptured ovarian cyst
- Ruptured ectopic pregnancy
- Ovulatory bleed
- Endometriosis
- Spontaneous rupture of liver tumour
- Rectus sheath haematoma
- Abdominal trauma

further reactive bleeding (see Ch. 11).

The early administration of opiate analgesia does not compromise subsequent surgical assessment and is probably easier in patients who are not in pain.[15] A 2003 review of eight trials of analgesia for undifferentiated abdominal pain concluded that there is 'a common theme suggesting that analgesia is safe'.[98]

Antibiotic treatment is based on the presumed diagnosis. A perioperative dose of antibiotics is appropriate for patients with acute appendicitis and acute cholecystitis. In patients with severe sepsis, broad-spectrum combination antibiotics should be commenced at the earliest opportunity (see Ch. 30).

Resuscitation before surgery is nearly always possible, except in cases of life-threatening blood loss, and there is some evidence that further steps should be taken in some patients to improve their preoperative status. A prospective randomized trial of preoperative 'optimization of oxygen delivery' demonstrated a significant reduction in mortality for the invasively monitored and resuscitated group (3%) compared with the group given routine preoperative care (17%).[99] The mortality in the control group was, however, exceptionally high for the procedures reported.

Prophylaxis against deep venous thrombosis and pulmonary embolus should be considered in all patients (see Ch. 11).

CAUSES OF ABDOMINAL PAIN

Many of the causes of acute abdominal pain are covered in more detail in other chapters. The management of the common causes of acute abdominal pain is now discussed. These are shown in Box 25.1.

NON-SPECIFIC ABDOMINAL PAIN

Many non-surgical disorders result in abdominal pain, creating a diagnostic dilemma. Many patients are eventually categorized as having non-specific abdominal pain, and this diagnosis accounts for as many as one-third of admissions with abdominal pain.[100] The causes are listed in Box 25.2.

CLINICAL FEATURES

The finding of abdominal wall tenderness is an important sign in distinguishing between different causes of non-specific abdominal pain and is present in about a third of patients.[100]

MANAGEMENT

Patients with non-specific abdominal pain should not have signs of peritonitis, and are therefore best treated by a period of observation to allow spontaneous improvement. Although laparoscopy can exclude other surgical conditions,[96] such as acute appendicitis, it should be used sparingly because most patients' symptoms rapidly settle and regular review identifies those with continuing problems.[101] A suggested management algorithm is presented in Fig. 25.25.[102]

REFERENCES

98. Thomas SH, Silen W. Br J Surg 2003; 90: 5–9
99. Wilson J, Woods I, Fawcett J et al. Br Med J 1999; 318: 1099–1103
100. Gray DWR, Collin J. Br J Surg 1987; 74: 239–242
101. Jones PF. Br J Surg 1990; 77: 365–367
102. Gallegos NC, Hobsley M. Br J Surg 1990; 77: 1167–1170

Box 25.2 Causes of non-specific abdominal pain[52]

Viral infections
- Mesenteric adenitis

Bacterial infection
- Acute bacterial gastroenteritis (*Yersinia enterocolitica, Y. pseudotuberculosis*)

Worm infestation
- *Enterobius vermicularis*

Abdominal wall pain
- Abdominal wall haematoma
- Hernia
- Shingles
- Nerve entrapment
- The "rib-tip" syndrome

Irritable bowel syndrome

Gynaecological pain
- Pelvic inflammatory disease
- Mittelschmerz pain
- Ovarian cysts

Psychosomatic pain

Other
- Iatrogenic peripheral nerve injuries
- Myofascial pain syndromes
- Pain of spinal origin
- Lactose intolerance
- Discitis
- Abdominal epilepsy
- Abdominal migraine
- *Clostridium difficile* colitis

ACUTE APPENDICITIS

Acute appendicitis is the commonest cause of the acute abdomen requiring surgery, accounting for 17% of all presentations with abdominal pain.[69] It most commonly develops in children and young adults, with a peak incidence of 30 years of age. Despite this, it should be considered in all age groups because of its frequent occurrence. Its incidence has, however, declined over the past half century.

AETIOLOGY

The underlying cause of this common condition remains uncertain. A number of theories have been proposed, which include abnormalities in the diet, genetic factors, and a variety of infectious agents. The last of these may be related to poor domestic hygiene.

Diet

In the early part of the 20th century, when appendicitis was increasing in incidence, it was suggested that a lack of fibre in the diet might be the cause. The increase in appendicitis occurred during the time that imported flour, which had a low cellulose content, was being used more widely. It was also observed that the upper social classes, who were the major users of white flour, had a higher incidence of acute appendicitis. Acute appendicitis is an uncommon disease in poorer countries where the population consumes a high-fibre diet, but there is an increasing incidence of appendicitis when the diet changes to a low-fibre western-type diet. Burkitt suggested that the high-fibre diet produced bulkier

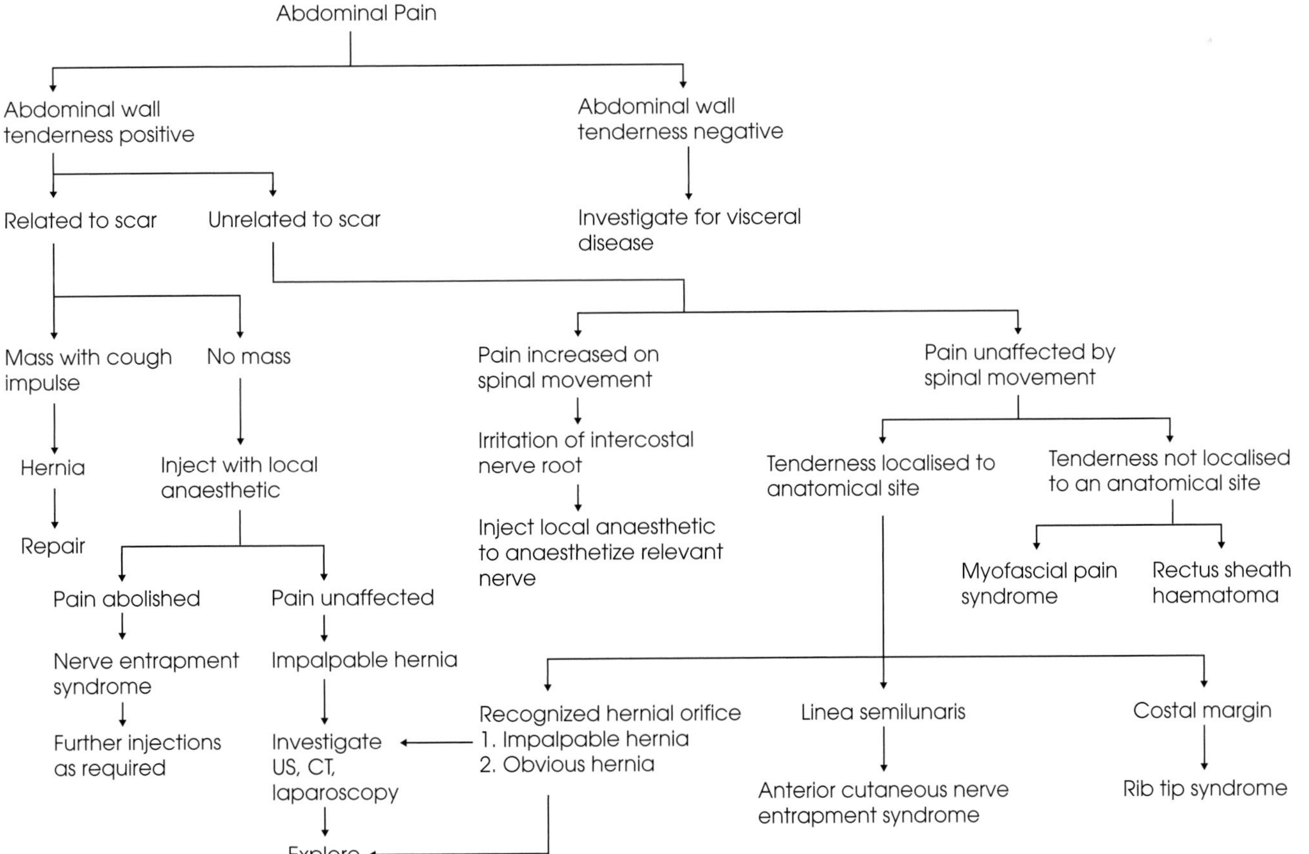

Figure 25.25 Management algorithm for non-specific abdominal pain. (Adapted from Gallegos and Hobsley 1990.[102])

stools, which had a faster transit time through the intestine. It is thought that a slower transit time associated with a low-fibre diet leads to an alteration in the bacterial flora, which may also contribute to a higher incidence of appendicitis.

More recently, the validity of the dietary fibre theory has been challenged. Epidemiological evidence shows that appendicitis in western Europe and the USA has been declining steadily for the past 40 years, although the dietary fibre intake has not altered, and studies performed in South Africa have shown that urban black people continue to have a very low incidence of acute appendicitis despite diets that are lower in fibre than those of the urban white population. A positive correlation has been found between potato consumption and appendicitis, whereas a high intake of fruit and vegetables other than potato is associated with a lower incidence of the condition. The influence of diet in the aetiology of acute appendicitis has not been clarified, and the role of dietary fibre is less convincing than was originally thought.

Genetic factors

A number of authors have demonstrated a familial tendency to develop acute appendicitis. The reason for this is not known, although it has been suggested that shared dietary habits, genetic resistance to bacterial flora, or inheritance of fibrous band anomalies in the appendix may be the cause.

Infection

The relationship between viral infections and acute appendicitis has been based on the findings of raised viral antibody titres, the association between appendicitis and coincidental viral illness, the clustering of appendicitis during particular seasons, and the presence of lymphoid tissue within the mucosa and submucosa of the appendix. Lymphoid hyperplasia is not, however, always present in appendices resected for acute appendicitis, and not all patients have raised viral antibody titres during acute appendicitis.

It has been shown that the incidence of appendicitis closely relates to the percentage of homes without fixed baths and hot water systems, suggesting that the lack of these facilities is associated with domestic overcrowding and a greater risk of respiratory and enteric infection. Continued improvements in hygiene may be responsible for the falling incidence of appendicitis.

PATHOLOGY

For whatever reasons, the wall of the appendix becomes inflamed and oedematous, and pus eventually fills the lumen. This oedema and inflammation cause venous congestion, which may impair the arterial inflow, leading to thrombosis and gangrene. Organisms from the lumen of the appendix then enter the devitalized wall, causing it to liquefy and perforate. If this occurs early, before surrounding adhesions have formed, generalized peritonitis develops, but if the inflammatory process is more gradual, small bowel and omentum adhere to the appendix and localize the sepsis.

It has been thought for many years that occlusion of the appendix is a very significant event in the development of appendicitis. Faecoliths, hyperplasia of the lymphoid tissue, foreign bodies, congenital or inflammatory strictures of the appendix, carcinoid tumours or rare congenital bands may cause obstruction and subsequent appendicitis. The incidence of obstruction by faecoliths and the extent of the lymphoid hyperplasia vary considerably in studies where the cause of appendicular obstruction has been sought.

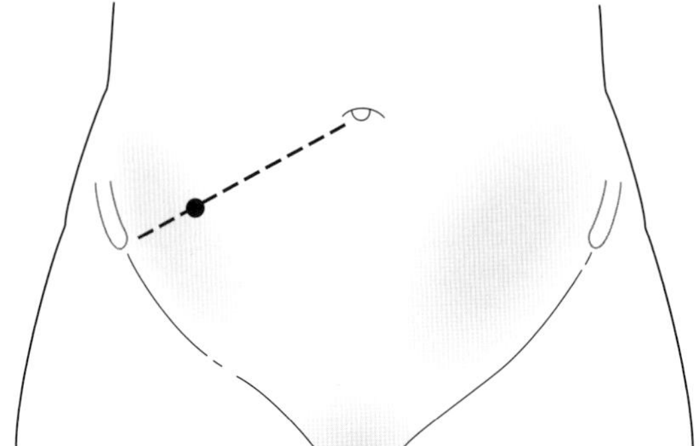

Figure 25.26 McBurney's point.

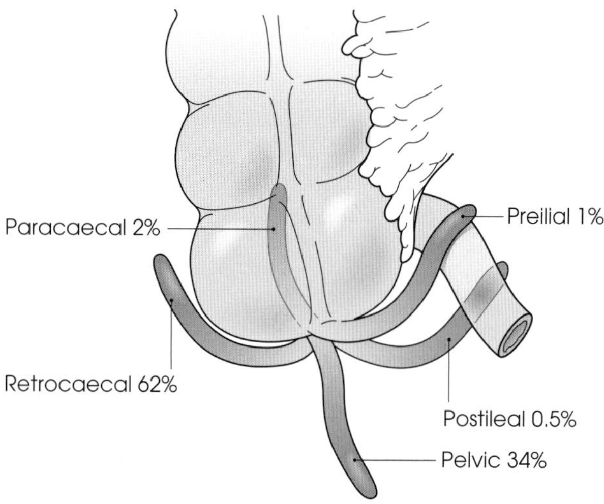

Figure 25.27 The positions where the appendix lies.

CLINICAL FEATURES

Acute appendicitis is one of only a few surgical conditions in which the diagnosis can be made from the history and examination alone. The classical history of acute appendicitis is of 12–24 h of central abdominal pain that moves to the right iliac fossa, with tenderness at McBurney's point (Fig. 25.26). Nausea and vomiting are frequently associated symptoms. Because of the wide variation in the anatomical position of the appendix (Fig. 25.27), a classical history is often absent. A retrocaecal appendix can present with pain in the right loin or right upper quadrant. Because peritoneal irritation does not occur until later, the history may be of a longer duration. A pelvic appendix may present with diarrhoea and increased urinary frequency. Marked tenderness may be elicited on rectal examination. The pre- and postileal positions are less common positions for the appendix. In the preileal or anterior position, the signs of appendicitis may be very obvious because the appendix lies close to the anterior abdominal wall. The retro- or postileal position is possibly the most difficult of all positions for making an accurate diagnosis. The appendix lies behind the ileum and its mesentery, with its tip directed towards the spleen. The symptoms may be very vague, with poorly localized abdominal pain and early vomiting. The abdominal signs may be non-specific, with tenderness located high in the abdomen.

An inflamed appendix can also be situated in the right upper quadrant of the abdomen and may mimic acute cholecystitis or a perforated ulcer. This position is the result of non-descent of caecum, an anomaly of intestinal developmental rotation that leaves the appendix closely related to the liver. With a very long appendix, the inflamed tip can be some distance from McBurney's point and give rise to tenderness in other sites. In very rare instances, transposition of the viscera causes the caecum to lie on the left side and may produce signs in the left iliac fossa. At the extremes of age the diagnosis is often more difficult. The very young cannot give a history and the clinical signs may be difficult to elicit. In the elderly, the differential diagnosis is much larger and the symptoms and signs are often atypical.

DIAGNOSTIC PROCEDURES

The role of ultrasound in the assessment of patients presenting with suspected appendicitis or pelvic pain is changing. Ultrasound has a sensitivity of 81% for appendicitis,[103,104] which is recognized by visualizing a narrow blind-ended lumen of bowel that is not compressible (Fig. 25.28). The sensitivity of detecting a perforated appendix is, however, only 29%. The use of routine abdominal ultrasound in the diagnosis of appendicitis in *all* patients has been shown to be of little benefit,[105,106] and this test should be performed only when the diagnosis is uncertain (this will usually be in women). Computerized tomography has also been advocated as a method for diagnosing appendicitis, with an accuracy of 98%.[90]

Laparoscopy has become an important investigation and therapeutic tool in suspected appendicitis, especially in women of a fertile age and in obese patients.

The Alvarado score is a simple scoring system that is based on eight clinical features shown in Table 25.4.[106] No patients who have a score of less than 6 were found to have a perforated appendicitis.[107] It is always difficult to use scoring systems to decide on individual patient treatment, but it has been suggested that the Alvarado score could be used to select patients for admission with suspected appendicitis.[108]

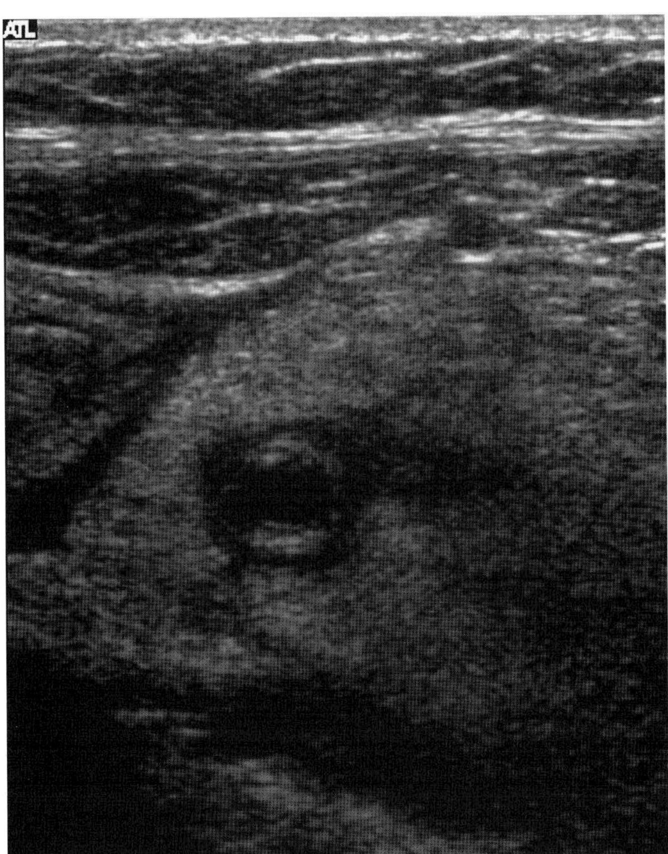

Figure 25.28 Transverse images of a fluid-filled appendix (dark area) with an appendicolith at the end. (Courtesy of Dr Paul Allan.)

Table 25.4 The Alvarado scoring system[58]

Feature	Score
Symptoms	
Migratory right iliac fossa pain	1
Nausea or vomiting	1
Anorexia	1
Signs	
Right iliac fossa tenderness	2
Fever > 37.3°C	1
Rebound pain in right iliac fossa	1
Laboratory tests	
Leukocytosis (> 10 × 10^9 cells/L)	2
Neutrophilic shift to the left > 75%	1
Possible total	10

DIFFERENTIAL DIAGNOSIS OF ACUTE APPENDICITIS

Gastroenteritis/mesenteric adenitis

Vague gastrointestinal upsets are the most common disorders that are confused with appendicitis, and often a specific diagnosis is never established. Occasionally, positive cultures are obtained from the stools. Abdominal tenderness is usually less well localized than in acute appendicitis.

Mesenteric adenitis in children and young adults poses a particular problem, which may be correctly diagnosed if the tenderness is found to shift when the child is placed on his or her side.

Disorders of the female pelvis

An incorrect diagnosis of acute appendicitis is most commonly made in women of childbearing age. The conditions that cause confusion include ruptured ovarian follicle, pelvic inflammatory disease, ruptured ectopic pregnancy, and torsion of an ovarian cyst (see below).

Ruptured ovarian follicle (mittelschmerz)

This diagnosis is suspected if the pain occurs in the middle of the menstrual cycle at the time of ovulation. The pain is initially severe before gradually subsiding over the course of several days. There is usually some tenderness in the right lower quadrant, but there are rarely any gastrointestinal symptoms and the patient does not look unwell.

REFERENCES

103. Puylaert JBCM, Rutgers PH, Lalisang RI et al. N Engl J Med 1987; 317: 666–669
104. Roosevelt GE, Reynolds SL. Acad Emerg Med 1998; 5: 1071–1075
105. Franke C, Bohner H, Yang Q et al. World J Surg 1999; 23: 141–146
106. Alvarado A. Ann Emerg Med 1986; 15: 557–564
107. Owen TD, Williams H, Stiff G et al. J R Soc Med 1992; 85: 87–89
108. Chan MYP, Tan C, Chiu MT et al. Surg J R Coll Surg Edinb Irel 2003; 1: 39–41

Pelvic inflammatory disease (acute salpingitis)

In this condition, the lower abdominal pain is associated with a high fever and tenderness, which is usually most marked in the suprapubic region and in both iliac fossae. A vaginal discharge is often present, although this may be absent in the early stages. On pelvic examination, a discharge may be observed coming from the cervix and bacteria can be cultured from a swab. Cervical manipulation usually exacerbates the pain.

Ruptured ectopic pregnancy

In this condition, there is classically a history of a missed or abnormal period that precedes a sudden pain in the lower abdomen. This pain may be referred to the shoulder tip. On examination, altered blood may be seen coming from the vagina. The patient may be pale and hypotensive, although in the early stages these signs are often not present. Tenderness is present across the lower abdomen, with signs of guarding and rebound tenderness. There may be some periumbilical bruising (Cullen's sign). There is usually pain on movement of the cervix, but vaginal examination should be performed with caution. The diagnosis is supported by a positive pregnancy test and evidence of an abnormality within the fallopian tube on ultrasound or at laparoscopy.

Torsion of an ovarian cyst

Torsion of an ovarian cyst can cause marked pain of sudden onset and a low-grade fever. There are few gastrointestinal symptoms, although the patient will often vomit with the pain. Tenderness is present in the lower abdomen but usually confined to one iliac fossa. A mass may be felt arising from the pelvis if the cyst is large, otherwise there may be no evidence of any mass on palpation. The cyst can sometimes be palpated on pelvic examination, but it can almost always be confirmed by abdominal ultrasound. The torsion involves the ovary, and once the diagnosis has been made surgery is required.

Iliocaecal disorders

There are a number of disorders of the iliocaecal region, which can mimic acute appendicitis.

Meckel's diverticulitis

This diagnosis is rarely made before operation for presumed acute appendicitis. The only differentiating features that occasionally arouse suspicion are a more medial point of maximal tenderness and possibly some evidence of mechanical small bowel obstruction.

Regional ileitis (Crohn's disease)

Acute forms of regional ileitis can be mistaken for acute appendicitis. The presence of a vague, tender mass in the right lower quadrant or symptoms of diarrhoea may suggest Crohn's disease. The appendix should be removed with careful repair of the caecum if Crohn's disease is discovered during an operation for presumed acute appendicitis. Although there is a risk of postoperative fistulation, this is small and the operation removes potential diagnostic uncertainty during subsequent episodes of acute abdominal pain. *Yersinia* infection may cause a condition that appears on microscopic examination to be identical with Crohn's.

Carcinoma of the caecum

Occasionally, carcinoma of the caecum may cause acute appendicitis. It may also present with acute right iliac fossa pain if the caecum ruptures proximal to a carcinoma in the colon or if a local perforation leads to a paracolic abscess (see Ch. 28).

Foreign body perforation

When foreign body perforation occurs in the caecum or distal small bowel, it can mimic acute appendicitis. The diagnosis is not usually made until laparotomy.

GENITOURINARY DISORDERS

Several genitourinary disorders produce symptoms similar to those of acute appendicitis.

Ureteric calculus

Ureteric calculus is usually differentiated from acute appendicitis because the pain of renal colic is quite different to the pain of acute appendicitis (see Ch. 35). It is much more severe, gets worse in waves, and radiates from the loin to the groin. Nausea and vomiting occur with both conditions, and pelvic or retrocaecal appendicitis can be associated with haematuria and white cells in the urine. Haematuria is usually more marked with ureteric colic, and although there may be right iliac fossa tenderness in ureteric colic, this is generally less marked than that found with acute appendicitis and is usually associated with loin tenderness. Plain abdominal X-rays show a radiopacity in the line of the renal pelvis or ureter in 90%, and the presence of obstruction can be determined by an intravenous urogram or CT scan with contrast.

Pyelonephritis

The presentation of this condition is usually with loin pain and urinary frequency associated with a high fever and chills, which are uncommon in acute appendicitis. There is normally some renal tenderness, and sometimes the tenderness is maximal in the right iliac fossa. Under these circumstances the differentiation from retrocaecal or pelvic appendicitis is difficult, especially as white and red cells may be found in the urine of patients with retrocaecal appendicitis. Organisms identified on a Gram stain of the urine will usually help to make the diagnosis, and if a pyonephrosis is present ultrasound will be diagnostic. It is particularly difficult to differentiate between acute pyelonephritis and appendicitis in pregnancy.

Other less common conditions mimicking acute appendicitis

Cholecystitis, perforated ulcer, and a number of medical conditions such as herpes zoster and acute porphyria may be misdiagnosed as appendicitis.

Rupture of the inferior epigastric artery, causing a haematoma in the rectus abdominis muscle, particularly during a fit of coughing or unaccustomed exercise, may occasionally be mistaken for acute appendicitis. Other symptoms of acute appendicitis, such as anorexia and the typical colicky pain moving to the right iliac fossa, are absent.

TREATMENT OF ACUTE APPENDICITIS

In patients without widespread peritonitis, non-operative management is usually successful, but as many as one-third of patients present with recurrent symptoms within 12 months.[109] A

REFERENCE

109. Eriksson S, Granstrom L. Br J Surg 1995; 82: 166–169

policy of observation with antibiotics is therefore perfectly reasonable in borderline cases of appendicitis without obvious peritoneal signs, or when other factors favour a non-operative approach. Appendicectomy should, however, be performed in the majority of patients.

The role of laparoscopic appendicectomy has been examined by two meta-analyses; these studies have confirmed a benefit from the laparoscopic approach, which produces less pain, a faster recovery, and a lower incidence of wound infections. This is at the expense of slightly longer operating times and a trend to a higher incidence of intra-abdominal abscesses.[110,111] Laparoscopic appendicectomy should be carried out by an appropriately experienced surgeon, when laparoscopy has been used to establish the diagnosis and the appendix is mobile and easily visible. Obese patients also appear to benefit from the laparoscopic approach. Care should be taken to remove the inflamed appendix through one of the ports, or within a retrieval bag, to prevent contamination of the wound. It is probably prudent to convert to an open operation if there is gross intra-abdominal soiling or if the appendix is very friable.

The small bowel should be inspected for inflammation or a Meckel's diverticulum if the appendix appears normal (Fig. 25.29). The pelvic organs should also be inspected for evidence of pelvic inflammatory disease and both ovaries inspected for cysts. Laparoscopy provides an excellent view of the pelvic organs. When no other pathology is detected, a decision should be taken as to whether the normal appendix requires removal. Arguments for and against need to be weighed up in each patient before a decision is made.

COMPLICATIONS OF ACUTE APPENDICITIS

The complications of acute appendicitis can be divided into preoperative, and early and late postoperative complications. They include complications that occur after any operative procedure and those that are specific for appendicitis. In a survey of 8651 appendicectomies performed in England and Wales in 1992 the mortality rate was 0.24% and the morbidity 8%.[112,113]

The complications of perforation, generalized peritonitis and appendiceal abscess are considered in detail. Other complications include septicaemia; portal pyaemia; haemorrhage; paracaecal, pelvic and subphrenic abscesses (see *Intraperitoneal abscesses*, p. 560); intestinal obstruction (see *Intestinal obstruction*, p. 584); faecal fistula (Ch. 28); and urinary retention (Chs 36 and 37).

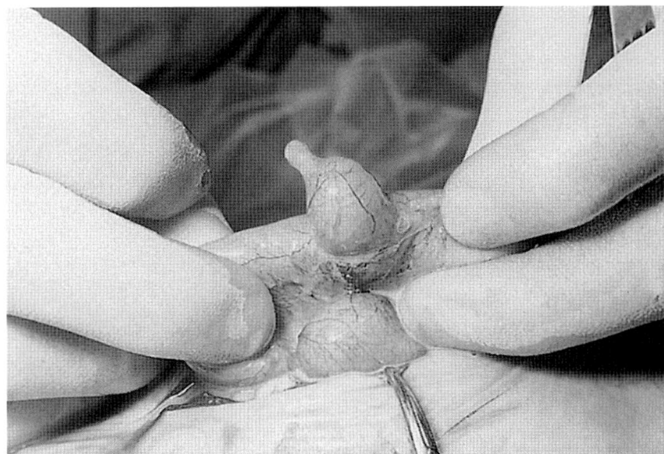

Figure 25.29 A Meckel's diverticulum.

Perforation

Gangrenous appendicitis and perforation usually follow a significantly longer period of pain than experienced by patients with uncomplicated appendicitis. The consequences of perforation are generalized peritonitis and the formation of an intra-abdominal abscess. In young women there may be an increased risk of infertility following perforated appendicitis.

Generalized peritonitis

Perforation of the appendix leads to a generalized peritonitis if the appendix has not been walled off by surrounding omentum and loops of bowel. The abdominal pain becomes more diffuse, with tenderness and guarding over the whole abdomen. The patient has a high fever and appears very unwell, becoming dehydrated and hypotensive. At a later stage, the abdomen becomes distended as a result of a paralytic ileus. Under these circumstances, operation is better performed through a midline or right paramedian incision to enable general peritoneal lavage to be performed and to ensure that there is no other cause of the peritonitis.

Appendiceal abscess

Occasionally, patients may present with an appendiceal abscess with fever and a right iliac fossa mass. The history of pain is often prolonged, and the abdominal signs are localized as the inflammation has been contained by the surrounding structures, especially when the appendix lies in a retrocaecal position. In patients over 50 years of age, a perforated caecal cancer and occasionally a solitary caecal diverticulum or sigmoid diverticulitis can present in a similar fashion (see Ch. 28).

An abscess can be confirmed by ultrasound (Fig. 25.30) or CT (Fig. 25.31) if clinically suspected. As treatment is by drainage and intravenous antibiotics, radiological imaging may proceed to percutaneous drainage. Drainage can also be performed at open surgery; however, the morbidity is significantly lower when abscesses are radiologically drained, with similar early reoperation rates.[114] No attempt should be made to perform an appendicectomy because the surrounding tissues are very friable and easily injured. Gangrenous necrosis can completely destroy the appendix.

Once the abscess has resolved, a colonic malignancy can be excluded by a double-contrast barium enema or colonoscopy. Debate continues about the role of interval appendicectomy because in many patients minimal or no residual appendix is found. A laparoscopic appendicectomy can be carried out if there are recurrent symptoms.

REFERENCES

110. Sauerland S, Lefering R, Holthausen U et al. In: Krahenbuhl L, Frei E, Klaiber CH et al. (eds). Progress in Surgery, Acute Appendicitis: Standard Treatment or Laparoscopic Surgery? Karger, Basel, 1998: 109–114
111. Golub R, Siddiqui F, Pohl D. J Am Coll Surg 1998; 186: 545–553
112. Flum DR, Koepsell T. Arch Surg 2002; 137: 799–804
113. Andersson RE. Br J Surg 2001; 88: 1387–1391
114. Hurme T, Nyalamo E. Ann Chir Gynaecol 1995; 84: 33–36

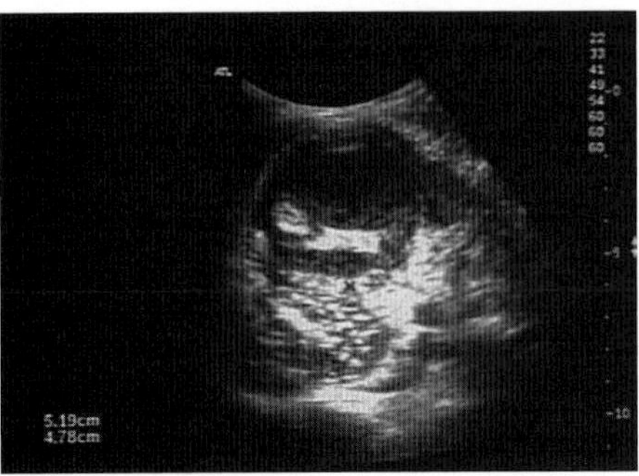

Figure 25.30 Ultrasound scan showing appendix abscess.

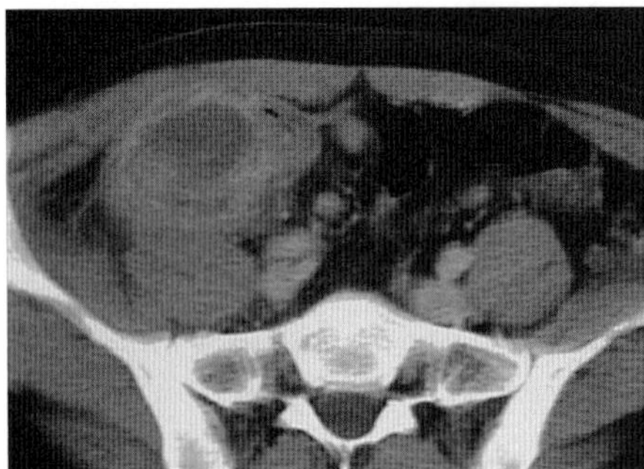

Figure 25.31 A CT scan showing appendix abscess in the same patient as in Fig. 25.30.

MISCELLANEOUS CONDITIONS OF THE APPENDIX

GRUMBLING APPENDIX (CHRONIC APPENDICITIS)

It is doubtful if the condition of chronic appendicitis exists, although appendicectomy is still performed for recurrent attacks of pain located in the right iliac fossa (see Ch. 27). Recurrent attacks of lower abdominal and right iliac fossa pain in childhood and adolescence is a common problem that is sometimes labelled grumbling appendix. Such chronic abdominal pain in childhood rarely has an identifiable cause.

An essential feature of recurrent appendicitis is a clear history that the recurrent abdominal pain followed an attack of acute appendicitis. It is therefore vital to establish the nature of the first attack of pain. Recurrent pains are frequently associated with anorexia, general malaise, and tenderness over the appendix. When this type of story is obtained, the appendix is often found to be inflamed or to show clear evidence of previous inflammation when it is removed.

Some children with chronic recurrent right iliac fossa pain have psychological difficulties, and the over-anxious parent is of real relevance. Others appear to be experiencing genuine attacks of pain that may be related to the irritable bowel syndrome, although this tends to be a problem of later life. Some children are found to have appendices containing *Enterobius vermicularis.* Constipation is the most common cause of abdominal pain in children.

Recurrent right iliac fossa pain in adolescent and adult life can be caused by Crohn's disease, pelvic sepsis, small bowel obstruction by bands or adhesions, irritable bowel syndrome, mittelschmerz (midcycle pain from a ruptured ovarian follicle), constipation, urinary tract infections, and many other conditions that are extremely rare. Sensible investigations after a detailed history and examination will often elucidate a cause, but eventually laparotomy, laparoscopy or appendicectomy may be required. This will occasionally reveal an appendicular carcinoid tumour or clear evidence of prior inflammation.

MECKEL'S DIVERTICULUM

This ilial diverticulum (see Ch. 27) derives its name from Johann Friedrich Meckel the Younger, who described its pathological and embryological features. It is a true diverticulum containing all the layers of the intestinal wall and is the commonest congenital anomaly of the small bowel. It is a remnant of the omphalomesenteric or vitelline duct and is normally found arising from the antimesenteric border of the ileum approximately 50 cm proximal to the ileocaecal valve (although this varies considerably). It may contain ectopic tissue, most frequently gastric or pancreatic mucosa. The incidence in the general population has been variously recorded at 0.6–2.3% in autopsy series, and a figure of 2% is the most widely accepted.

A Meckel's diverticulum may cause abdominal pain in a number of ways. In the adult, the commonest complication is intestinal obstruction. This may result from a volvulus or kinking of loop of small bowel round a congenital band running from the tip of the diverticulum to the umbilicus, the abdominal wall, or the mesentery. Obstruction may also be caused by intussusception, with the diverticulum as the apex of the intussusceptum (see p. 588). The next most common complication is inflammation of the Meckel's diverticulum. This can produce abdominal pain that is clinically indistinguishable from acute appendicitis; the diagnosis is rarely made until operation. The incidence of perforation in the presence of acute inflammation of a Meckel's diverticulum is reported to be as high as 50%. In children the most commonly encountered complications are intestinal obstruction and rectal bleeding.

The diverticulum can usually be treated by simple excision, but in some cases ileal resection is necessary. A broad-based diverticulum may be difficult to excise without narrowing the lumen. Figure 25.32 shows two methods that are commonly used to avoid this problem.

There is no consensus on the correct management of the incidentally discovered Meckel's diverticulum; some surgeons favour surgical excision while others advocate a less aggressive approach. In coming to a decision, it is necessary to weigh up the relative risks of developing a complication compared with the risk of surgical excision. Most complications occur in children and the lifetime risk of a complication from Meckel's diverticulum is thought to be around 4%, although after the age of 16 years the likelihood of developing complications reduces significantly towards zero in old age.

The risk of developing complications from a Meckel's diverticulum is associated with the presence of ectopic mucosa, a length exceeding 4 cm, and a base width less than 2 cm. These factors may be used to select which Meckel's diverticula to resect and which to leave alone.

INTESTINAL OBSTRUCTION

SMALL BOWEL OBSTRUCTION

In developed countries, the majority of small bowel obstructions (see also Ch. 27) are caused by intra-abdominal adhesions (Table 25.5), and around 80% settle with conservative management. Obstruction in a hernia is a less common problem than it was 20 years ago.

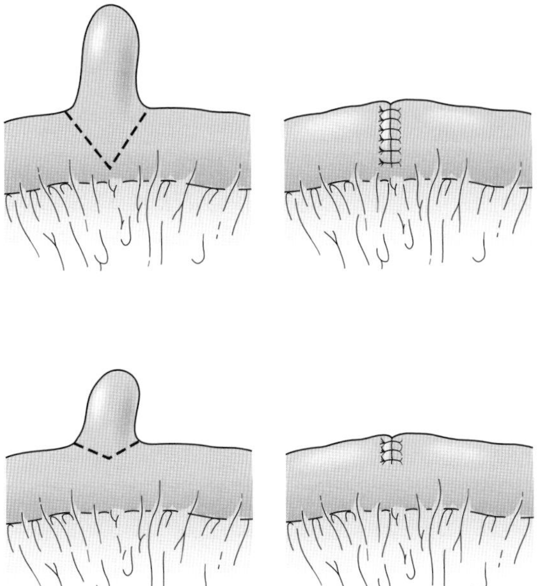

Figure 25.32 Operative techniques for dealing with a Meckel's diverticulum.

Table 25.5 Causes of small bowel obstruction

Cause	Approximate incidence (%)
Adhesion	60–80
Strangulated hernia	10–15
Neoplasm	5–10
Others	< 5

Diagnostic procedures

A plain abdominal radiograph may be diagnostic of a small bowel obstruction (Fig. 25.18); however, the classical picture of dilated small bowel and air–fluid levels may not be present despite clinical suspicion of obstruction. This may be a consequence of fluid filling of the dilated small bowel. Patients with subacute obstruction may not have the same contrast filling, and a contrast small bowel enema or CT may confirm the diagnosis.

Pathophysiology

The small intestine may be considered to have two functional components: a proximal part, which has a predominantly secretory role, and a distal segment for absorption. Table 25.6 shows the average volume of alimentary juice secreted in 24 h by a normal 70-kg man. One-fifth of the total body fluid is secreted and reabsorbed through the intestine each day, and any interference with this process rapidly causes fluid sequestration in the bowel with effective fluid depletion.

SIMPLE OBSTRUCTION

The bowel distal to the point of obstruction is emptied by absorption and evacuation of its fluid and gas content, causing it to shrink as it is no longer kept distended. Peristalsis in this collapsed segment ultimately ceases. This is well illustrated at laparotomy when the bowel distal to an obstruction is found to be empty, collapsed and quiescent. In contrast, the bowel proximal to the obstruction distends with gas and fluid, which is persistently augmented by the continuous secretion of biliary, pancreatic and gastrointestinal juices.

Table 25.6 Approximate amounts of alimentary secretions occurring within 24 h in a 70-kg man

Secretion	Volume (L)
Gastric juice	3
Intestinal secretions	2
Saliva	1
Bile	1
Pancreatic juice	1
Total	8

In the early stages, the major source for the intestinal gas is swallowed air, which is responsible for approximately 70% of the gas in the distended bowel. The major component of atmospheric air is nitrogen, which, unlike oxygen, is poorly absorbed. With time, the amount of oxygen within the bowel steadily falls, and this is associated with a concomitant rise in carbon dioxide. Gas arising from bacterial fermentation becomes increasingly important if the obstruction is not relieved. This process is responsible for the production of other gases such as hydrogen sulphide, ammonia, and a variety of other amines. These gases lower the partial pressure of nitrogen within the bowel lumen, and in so doing establish a gradient for the further diffusion of nitrogen from the congested vessels in the mucosa into the lumen. This provides a third and important source of luminal gas.

Large quantities of isotonic fluid pass into the bowel lumen and, because this fluid is not reabsorbed, it is lost from the extracellular compartment. This loss is augmented by the continual addition of biliary, pancreatic and gastrointestinal juices into the obstructed segment. The colour and nature of the fluid within the lumen of the bowel proximal to the obstruction slowly changes. Although initially the fluid contains recognizable food, this is soon replaced by turbid biliary fluid, and gradually the colour of the intestinal juice darkens. Eventually the intestinal contents become brown or even black as a result of the leakage of blood into the intestine and the continued fermentation and digestion by proliferating micro-organisms. This is responsible for the faeculant odour of obstructed small bowel content.

Under normal circumstances a bidirectional flux of salt and water exists, but this is disrupted in the presence of an obstruction. The movement of salt and water from the blood to the lumen increases, while movement from the lumen to the blood either remains static or decreases. Thus not only is absorption halted but fluid moves in the opposite direction, resulting in further losses of water, sodium and potassium from the extracellular space.

In response to the loss of salt and water, a number of compensatory changes are set in motion. Salt and water excretion in the urine is reduced to maintain plasma volume. This results in oliguria. Fluid moves from the interstitial space into the intravascular space in an endeavour to preserve plasma volume. The blood pressure is maintained for some time by these changes, although the clinical features of dehydration become apparent at a relatively early stage (see Ch. 2).

As well as the loss of sodium ions, potassium loss is usually considerable. This eventually causes a large deficit in the total body potassium, but because of shifts in potassium between the extravascular and intravascular compartments, hypokalaemia develops late. Acid–base control also becomes disrupted as bicarbonate ions are retained to compensate for the loss of chloride ions. Vomiting accentuates fluid and electrolyte deficits and causes further problems with acid–base homeostasis. Profound hypovolaemia is an important cause of death in untreated small bowel obstruction (see Ch. 2). It is essential to understand these fluid and electrolyte changes to achieve optimal resuscitation.

As the bowel becomes progressively more distended with gas and fluid, the intraluminal pressure rises and may reach a peak of 75 cm of water during a peristaltic wave. When the sustained intraluminal pressure reaches 10 cm of water, which is common during an obstructive episode in humans, venous drainage from the bowel wall becomes impaired. This in turn causes congestion and oedema of the mucosa, contributing to further intraluminal fluid losses and additional losses from the serosal surface of the bowel into the peritoneal cavity. Peristalsis becomes more vigorous in an endeavour to overcome the resistance imposed by the obstruction, and audible peristaltic rushes are heard early in the course of an obstruction. Eventually, however, the smooth muscle becomes fatigued, especially when the bowel has become greatly distended, and there is associated hypokalaemia, at which time bowel sounds are no longer heard.

Unobstructed small bowel has low bacterial counts, but micro-organisms proliferate rapidly in the stagnant fluid of an obstructed bowel. Indeed, this overgrowth of anaerobic bacteria is partially responsible for the faeculant nature of the vomitus and nasogastric aspirate. It has never been shown that the absorption of bacterial toxins from the distended loops of bowel is in any way responsible for the disordered physiology of uncomplicated obstruction, although this unquestionably becomes important once strangulation has occurred.

STRANGULATION OBSTRUCTION

Strangulation (Fig. 25.33) occurs when there is an impairment of the blood supply to and from the bowel wall. It is the most feared complication in any mechanical obstruction, but it is

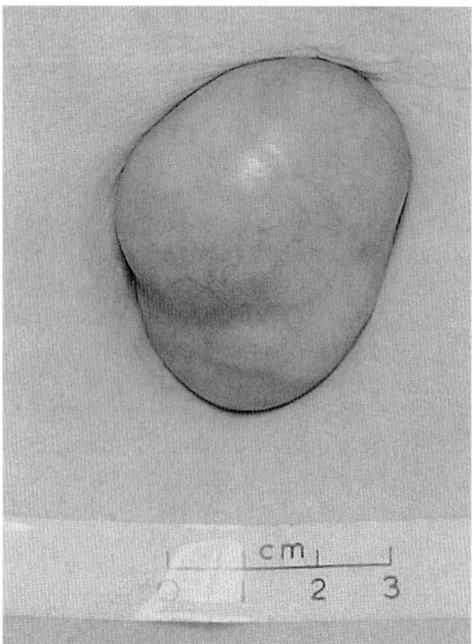

Figure 25.33 A loop of bowel strangulated within a paraumbilical hernia.

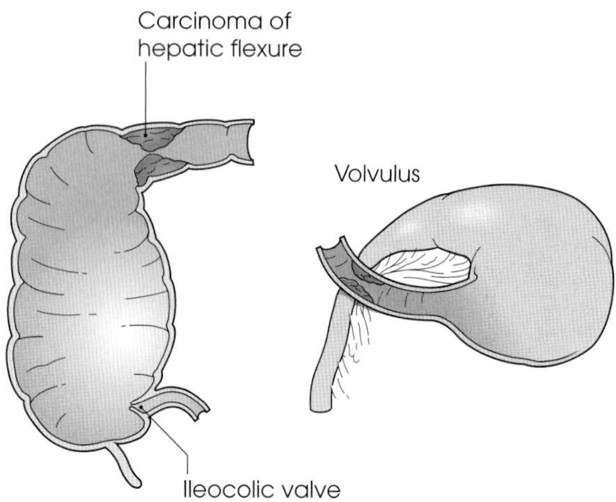

Figure 25.34 Closed-loop obstruction.

especially common in a closed-loop obstruction. The effects of strangulation are rapidly fatal if left untreated. If a segment of bowel becomes caught in a rigid and unyielding space, the venous outflow becomes impaired and causes capillary engorgement. This greatly increases the tension within the bowel wall, which eventually compromises the arterial inflow to the involved segment of bowel, resulting in arterial occlusion. This in turn causes a haemorrhagic infarct of the bowel wall; this is responsible for bleeding into the lumen of the bowel, which can be considerable at times. Bacteria pass through the damaged wall into the peritoneal cavity, causing peritonitis. Eventually frank perforation occurs with signs of generalized toxaemia.

CLOSED-LOOP OBSTRUCTION

A closed-loop obstruction is a form of mechanical obstruction in which a segment of bowel is isolated by closure of both its ends (Fig. 25.34). This may occur as a result of a loop of small bowel becoming trapped in a hernia or twisting about an unyielding band, causing a volvulus. The rapidity of the onset of symptoms and signs depends on the length of the involved segment and the number of organisms present within the lumen. For example, if the intestinal contents are heavily colonized or the length of the affected loop is short, tension rises rapidly before devitalization and rupture swiftly follow.

MANAGEMENT OF SMALL BOWEL OBSTRUCTION

Patients require resuscitation, nasogastric decompression, restriction of their oral intake, and analgesia. A metabolic alkalosis from loss of hydrogen ions can occur if vomiting has been prolonged. Renal compensation leads to an associated hypokalaemia, and both require correction (see Ch. 2).

There are four situations in which surgery is indicated in patients with small bowel obstruction.

1. Any patient in whom intestinal ischaemia is suspected.
2. When the patient has an irreducible abdominal hernia.
3. In patients with no previous history of abdominal surgery, when the obstruction does not resolve promptly.
4. When conservative management fails.

Severe constant pain requiring increasing dosage of opiates, fever, localized or generalized signs of peritonitis, shock, closed-loop obstruction on radiography, or the development of acidosis are all warning signs of impending intestinal strangulation. Patients with these signs or symptoms should proceed

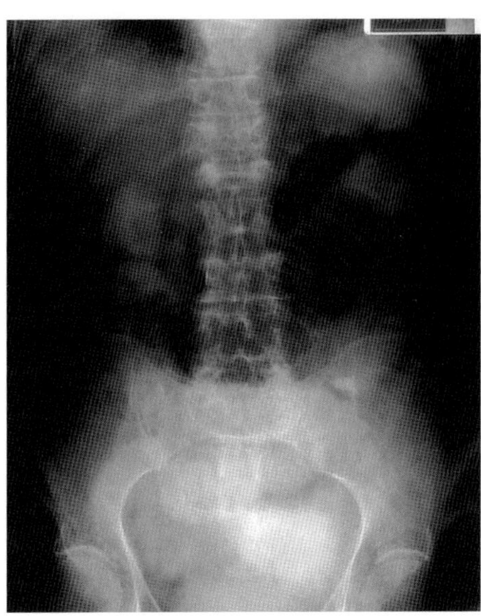

Figure 25.35 Contrast follow-through after 4 h, showing failure of contrast to reach caecum and obviously distended loops of jejunum.

immediately to laparotomy after resuscitation. Surgery is carried out as a scheduled case, usually within 24–48 h if obstruction is unlikely to be caused by adhesions and does not resolve with a trial of conservative therapy.

Surgery is usually delayed for 24–48 h in the majority of patients suspected of having adhesive small bowel obstruction, and patients with known extensive adhesions may benefit from a longer period of conservative treatment. Contrast studies are increasingly being used for both diagnostic and therapeutic reasons if resolution has not occurred by this time. Partial obstruction demonstrated by a contrast study is very likely to resolve, with no patients requiring surgery in two recent studies.[115,116] High-grade or complete obstruction requires surgery. This is thought to be present when the water-soluble contrast material fails to reach the colon by 4 h (Fig. 25.35). Computerized tomography has been demonstrated to be more sensitive (90% versus 50%) than and with a similar specificity (57%) to contrast studies alone;[117] however, its availability may be limited in some hospitals.

Occasionally an adhesional obstruction may be caused by a single band adhesion, especially after an appendicectomy, and if this is suspected laparoscopic treatment may be indicated. This can, however, be very hazardous in the presence of grossly dilated loops of bowel and should be attempted only by experienced laparoscopic surgeons using a direct cut-down approach to the peritoneal cavity.

SPECIAL CAUSES OF SMALL BOWEL OBSTRUCTION

There are several causes of small bowel obstruction where the clinical features and management are so different from the general principles outlined earlier that they warrant separate discussion.

Meconium ileus

Meconium ileus (see Ch. 40), first described by Landsteiner in 1905,[118] is a condition in which the distal small bowel or colon becomes obstructed in the neonatal period as a result of inspissated intestinal contents. This condition occurs in children with the inherited metabolic disorder of cystic fibrosis (mucoviscidosis). Disordered intestinal secretion, including a lack of pancreatic juice, results in the formation of obstructing, firm, putty-like, sticky meconium.

The clinical features and management in childhood are described in Chapter 40. A similar condition, known as meconium ileus equivalent, is now seen in teenagers and young adults who have survived childhood with cystic fibrosis. The lack of digestive enzymes reaching the intestine, combined with reduced mucus secretion, results in indigestible cellulose plugs obstructing the terminal ileum, causing bolus obstruction. These may have to be removed at open operation by milking them on into the large bowel or by extracting them through one or more transverse enterotomies.

Malrotation

Maltrotation of the intestine is an important cause of intestinal obstruction in infancy. Its pathophysiology, clinical features and management are discussed in Chapter 40.

Gallstone ileus

Gallstones are responsible for fewer than 1% of all cases of small bowel obstruction. About 90% of gallstones entering the intestine lodge in the terminal ileum, although impaction at other sites, including the jejunum, duodenum, colon and rectum, has been described. The stone originates in the gall bladder and passes into the intestine through a biliary–enteric fistula, usually between the gall bladder and duodenum (see Chs 27 and 30).

Clinical features

The patients are almost invariably elderly. They may have a history of chronic cholecystitis, but this is often not the case. Patients usually present with symptoms of acute intestinal obstruction, which are sometimes preceded by recurrent attacks of subacute obstruction.

Investigations

The radiological appearances are those of an intestinal obstruction, and in addition a gallstone may be visible in an unusual location. A fistula is usually present if the bile ducts or gall bladder are outlined by gas (Fig. 25.36), and the diagnosis of gallstone ileus can then be made preoperatively. Gas in the biliary tree may also follow a biliary-intestinal bypass or sphincterotomy, and is rarely the result of gas-forming organisms multiplying within the biliary tract.

Treatment

An operation is required to relieve the bowel obstruction. The stone should be milked upwards into the healthy bowel to avoid opening the bowel at the point where the stone has impacted, because this area heals poorly. The cholecystoenteric fistula is always encased in scar tissue and it is best left alone. The risk of further stones impacting is low, and the potential dangers of unpicking the cholecystoenteric fistula and causing peritonitis from a duodenal or binary leak is considerable. Stones that have already passed into the proximal bowel should be sought and removed at the same time. Cholecystectomy is not required.

REFERENCES

115. Chen S, Lin F, Lee P et al. Br J Surg 1998; 85: 1692–1694
116. Choi H, Chu K, Law W. Ann Surg 2001; 236: 1–6
117. Peck JJ, Milleson T, Phelan J. Am J Surg 1999; 177: 375–378
118. Landsteiner KZ. All Pathol Anat 1905; 16: 903

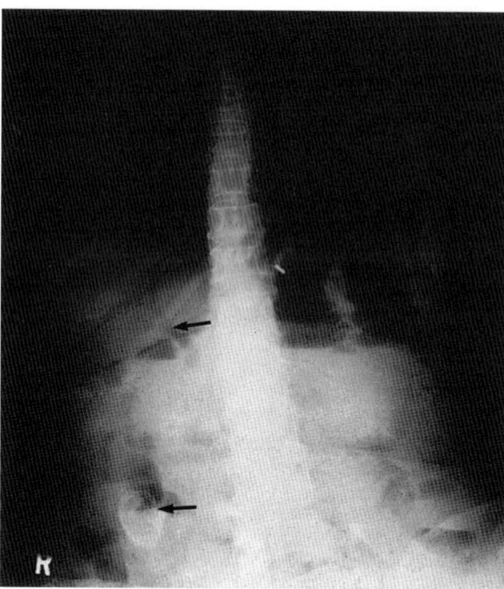

Figure 25.36 Gallstone ileus. Arrows identify gas in biliary tree in right upper quadrant, and the gallstone in the right iliac fossa.

Intussusception

An intussusception occurs when a segment of bowel (the intussusceptum) invaginates into its adjoining lower segment (the intussuscipiens). Intussusception may be caused by the presence of a nidus in the bowel wall, such as a polyp or a Meckel's diverticulum, but often no abnormality is present.

Ileocaecal intussusception

This form of idiopathic intussusception classically occurs in healthy infants aged between 3 months and 2 years (see Ch. 40). It is thought that the development of this type of infantile intussusception may be related either to an exaggerated protrusion of the ileocaecal valve into the caecum or a disproportionate amount of submucous lymphoid tissue in the Peyer's patches of the ileum, which may be grasped and passed on as the apex of an intussusception.

Although intussusception also occurs in children over the age of 2 years, the likelihood of a pathological cause for the intussusception becomes far more likely. The clinical features and management are described in Chapter 40.

Adult volvulus

A volvulus occurs when a segment of bowel twists through 360° (Fig. 25.34). This often compromises the circulation of the affected segment of bowel and always causes a closed-loop obstruction. In 75% of instances it involves the sigmoid, in 22% the caecum, and in 2% the transverse colon.[119]

LARGE BOWEL OBSTRUCTION

There are many possible causes of a large bowel obstruction, but malignant tumours and diverticular disease are the commonest aetiologies (see Ch. 28). The relative incidence is listed in Table 25.7. Colonic cancer presents more frequently with obstruction in the elderly. Sixteen per cent of 4583 patients with a colonic adenocarcinoma presented with obstruction; however, this increased to 25% of those aged over 80 years.[120] Tumours of the splenic flexure are the most likely to obstruct, followed by those in the left colon, right colon and rectosigmoid. Around 10% present with a perforation, which can occur either at the site of the tumour or in the caecum. Caecal perforation is imminent when the caecum measures greater than 12 cm in diameter on plain abdominal radiographs. Tumours that present with obstruction or perforation have a poorer prognosis.[121]

Table 25.7 Causes of colonic obstruction in adults

Cause	Approximate incidence (%)
Carcinoma of the colon	65
Miscellaneous (including pseudo-obstruction)	20
Diverticulitis	10
Volvulus	5

CLINICAL FEATURES

Small and large bowel obstructions are responsible for 15% of admissions with acute abdominal pain.[69] A history of previous colonic surgery or diverticular disease is important. On examination, a mass may be felt, especially in the left iliac fossa, which can be a tumour or a diverticular mass. Severe pain, shock, or signs of peritonitis should raise concerns about colonic infarction or perforation. A tumour may be palpable on rectal examination which often reveals a rectum empty of faeces.

DIAGNOSTIC PROCEDURES

A plain abdominal radiograph is essential and usually demonstrates a dilated colon proximal to the obstruction (Fig. 25.39). There may be partial decompression into the small bowel, with some small bowel dilatation, if the ileocaecal valve is incompetent. The classical appearance of a sigmoid volvulus with an inverted bean shape arising from the left iliac fossa may be seen (Fig. 25.37a,b), and a high-riding caecum containing a fluid level indicates a caecal volvulus (Fig. 25.38). A water-soluble contrast enema is essential in the diagnosis of large bowel obstruction, because it differentiates between pseudo-obstruction (Box 25.3) and a mechanical cause (Figs 25.40 and 25.41).[84,85]

MANAGEMENT OF MALIGNANT LARGE BOWEL OBSTRUCTION

There is nearly always time for adequate resuscitation, which is important because the mortality from emergency surgery for colonic obstruction is at least twice that for elective surgery.[122] The patient is advised about the possibility of a stoma, and patients should preferably be seen by the stoma therapist preoperatively.

The obstruction should be relieved and the tumour resected. Needle decompression of the bowel may be used to make

REFERENCES

119. Phillips RK, Hittinger R, Fry JS et al. Br J Surg 1985; 72: 296–302
120. Griffin MR, Mergstralh EJ, Coffey RJ et al. Cancer 1987; 60: 2318–2324
121. Ashkanani F, Munro A. In: Paterson-Brown S (ed.). Core Topics in General and Emergency Surgery. 2nd edn. WB Saunders, London, 2001: 233–274
122. Gandrup P, Lund L, Baslev I. Eur J Surg 1992; 158: 427–430

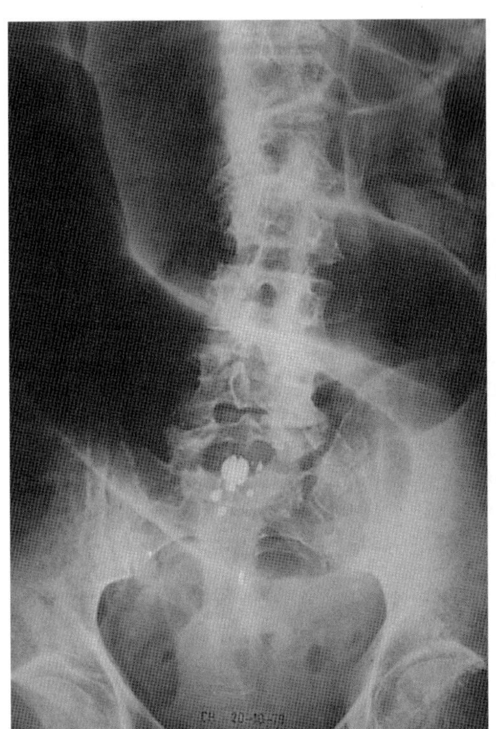

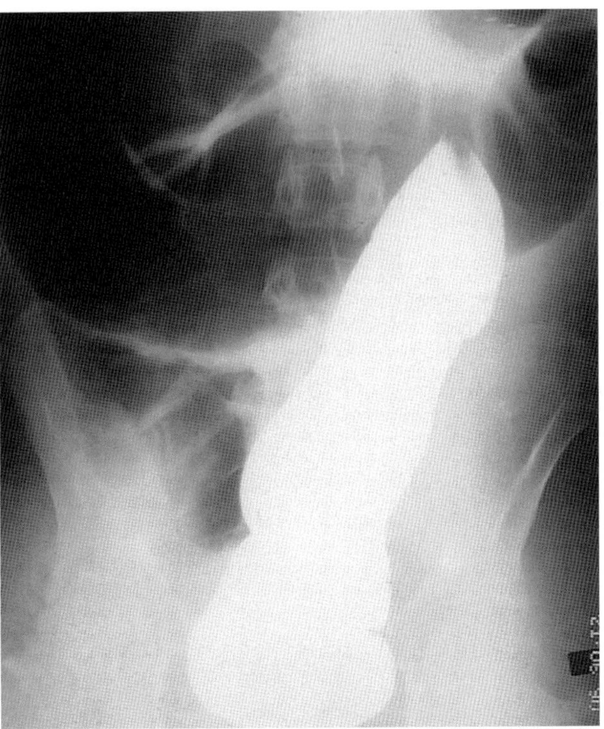

a b

Figure 25.37 (a) Plain X-ray of abdomen and (b) barium enema of a sigmoid volvulus.

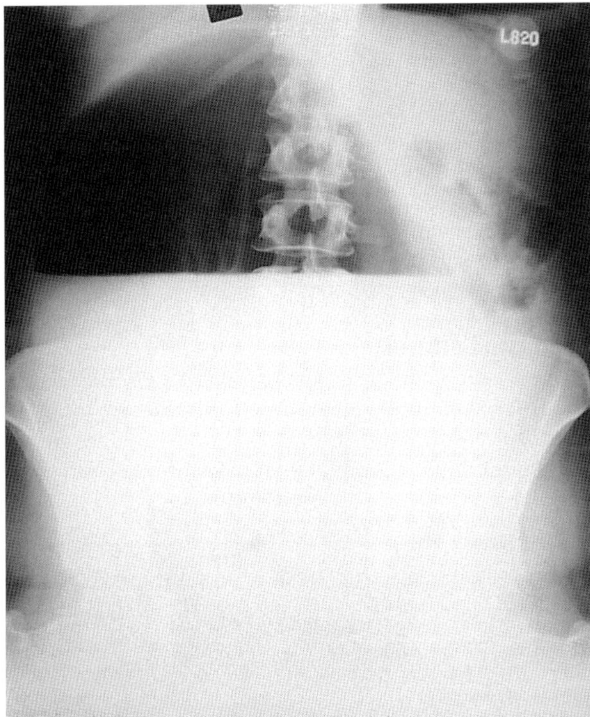

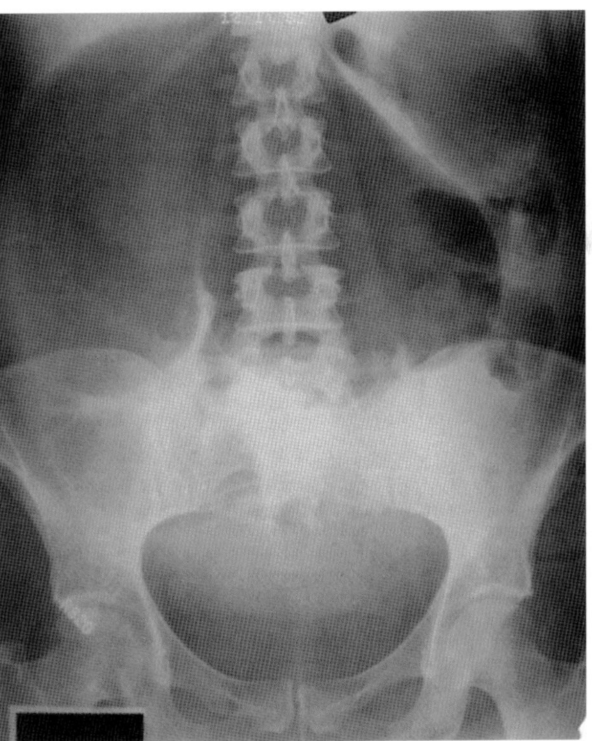

a b

Figure 25.38 Erect (a) and supine (b) films of a caecal volvulus.

handling easier and to reduce the risks of contamination from inadvertent bowel rupture. During laparotomy, the remaining colon should be inspected for a synchronous tumour and the liver palpated for hepatic metastases.

Right-sided or transverse colon obstruction can usually be managed by right hemicolectomy or extended right hemicolectomy (see Chapter 28). An end ileostomy and mucus fistula of the distal colon might be more advisable if there is gross peritoneal contamination from perforation or if the patient is unstable, with reconstruction left for later date.

Left-sided obstruction is more difficult to manage because the proximal bowel is unprepared and usually full of liquid faeces. In the past, treatment was by a three-stage approach: initial defunctioning transverse colostomy followed by resection of the

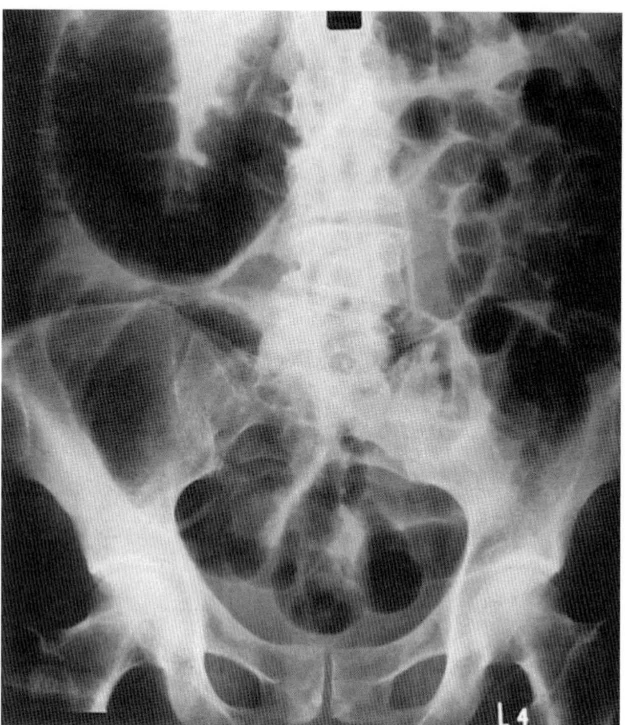

Figure 25.39 Distension of the caecum in a case of large bowel obstruction.

tumour with anastomosis, and finally then reversal of the stoma. This has been replaced by the two-stage and finally the single-stage procedure (see Ch. 28).

Two-stage procedure

The two-stage procedure consists of tumour resection with an end stoma (Hartmann's procedure) and later reversal. This remains very popular among many surgeons and has a mortality rate of around 10%.[123] An anastomosis on unprepared bowel in the presence of sepsis or cardiovascular instability should be avoided, but as many as 40% of patients may never have their stomas reversed.

A two-stage procedure consisting of resection of the tumour with primary anastomosis and defunctioning loop ileostomy, with ileostomy reversal 6 weeks to 3 months later, is now seen as an alternative. A difficult second operation is avoided, and the mortality and morbidity associated with anastomotic leakage is minimized (see Ch. 28).

Single-stage procedure

The single-stage procedure has become increasingly popular, having the twin advantages of a shorter hospital stay and avoidance of a stoma. There are two main techniques employed. The first is resection with on-table lavage[124] and anastomosis, the second is subtotal colectomy with ileo-rectal anastomosis. The operative mortality of both these procedures is similar to that of the two-stage operation.[125] In a subtotal colectomy, the whole dilated colon is resected before the small bowel is anastomosed to the sigmoid colon or upper rectum (see Chapter 28). This is a useful technique if there is perforation or necrosis of the caecum, a synchronous tumour, or a faecally impacted colon but often results in a liquid stool, which can be a major problem, particularly for the elderly. The two techniques have a similar mortality rate (5–9%) and risk of anastomotic leak (4%).[126] In a prospective randomized study of 91 patients who underwent either subtotal colectomy or on-table irrigation and segmental colectomy, there was no difference in the operative mortality, hospital stay, anastomotic leak rate or incidence of wound infection.[127] Diarrhoea and faecal incontinence were more frequent complications of subtotal colectomy. A prospective study of 58 patients with large bowel obstruction managed by simple colonic decompression rather than on-table washout and primary anastomosis resulted in only one leak and one postoperative death.[128]

Endoluminal colonic stents

The successful use of expandable stents for the palliation of malignant oesophageal and biliary strictures encouraged the use of similar techniques to manage large bowel obstruction. Stents can be used as palliative treatment for patients not fit for surgical resection,[129] and they can be used to decompress the obstructed colon before elective resection, when the patient's overall condition has improved.[130] Laser recanalization has also been used to avoid surgery (see Chapter 26).[131]

COLONIC DIVERTICULAR DISEASE

The incidence of diverticular disease increases with age, and by the ninth decade of life is present in half the population.[132] Complicated diverticular disease accounts for 4% of admissions with abdominal pain. Patients may present with diverticulitis, a diverticular abscess, peritonitis, or rarely stricture formation and a large bowel obstruction (see Ch. 28).

Clinical features

Patients usually report increasing left iliac fossa pain, fever, and either constipation or diarrhoea. A previous history of diverticular disease or constipation is common. Occasionally there is a sudden onset of generalized abdominal pain, which is associated with signs of general peritonitis following rupture of a diverticulum or diverticular abscess. These patients are often shocked and require resuscitation.

Diagnostic procedures

An erect chest radiograph may demonstrate free subdiaphragmatic gas from a colonic perforation (Fig. 25.20), and an abdominal ultrasound may show an abscess or free intra-abdominal fluid. Computerized tomography is, however, the best

REFERENCES

123. Dudley HA, Radcliffe AG, McGrechan D. Br J Surg 1980; 67: 80–81
124. Murray JJ, Schoetz DJ, Coller JA et al. Dis Colon Rectum 1991; 34: 527–531
125. Poon RTP, Law WL, Chu KW et al. Br J Surg 1998; 85: 1539–1542
126. The SCOTIA Study Group. Br J Surg 1995; 82: 1622–1627
127. Naraynsingh V, Rampaul R, Maharaj D et al. Br J Surg 1999; 86: 1341–1343
128. Harris GJC, Senagore AJ, Lavery IC et al. Am J Surg 2001; 181: 499–506
129. Mainar A, DeGregorio MA, Tejero R et al. Radiology 1999; 210: 65–69
130. Keifhaber P, Kiefhaber K, Huber F. Endoscopy 1986; 18: 44
131. Parks TG. Clin Gastroenterol 1975; 4: 53–69
132. Gooszen AW, Tollenaar RA, Geelkerken RH et al. Br J Surg 2002; 89: 246–247

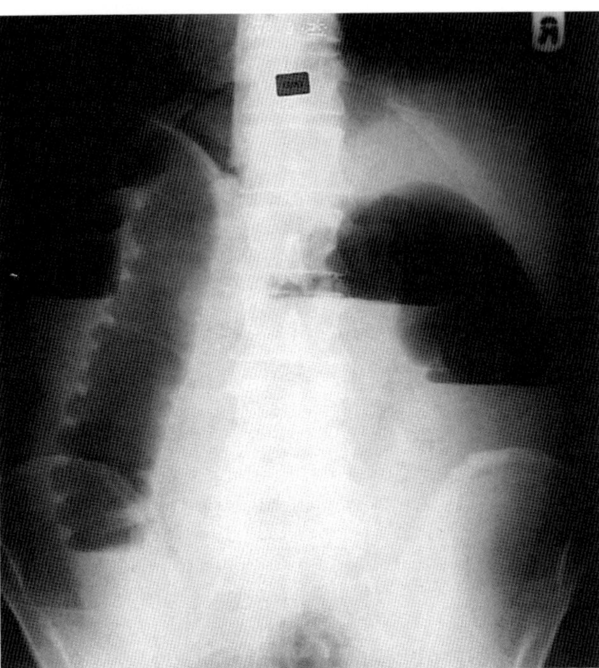

Figure 25.40 Haustral markings in a case of large bowel obstruction.

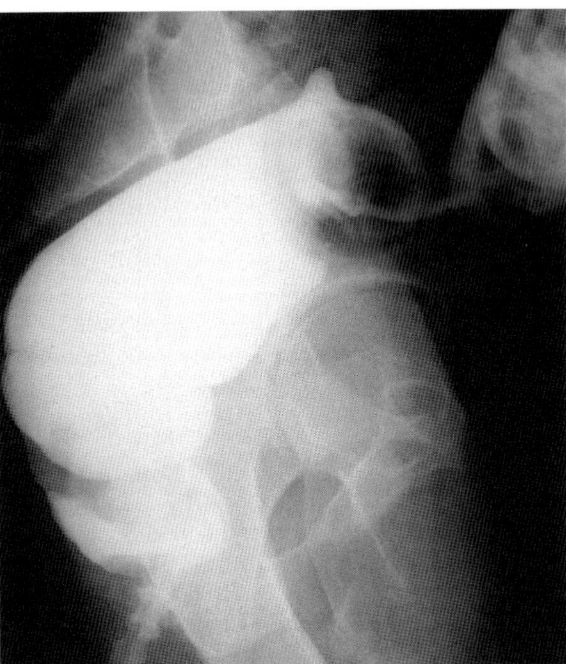

Figure 25.41 Contrast enema of a tumour causing large bowel obstruction.

method of demonstrating an abscess and should be performed early (Fig. 25.29).

Treatment

All patients require resuscitation with intravenous fluids. Analgesia and antibiotics are given to relieve pain and to cover a broad spectrum of colonic flora. A third-generation cephalosporin and metronidazole are a satisfactory combination. These measures with limitation of oral fluid intake can be used to treat most patients with diverticular disease unless there are signs of general peritonitis.

The signs and symptoms will resolve in many patients, and decisions about further definitive management can be made at leisure.

Drainage is required if an abscess is present. Drainage can usually be achieved using ultrasound or CT guidance but some colorectal surgeons prefer to proceed directly to resection and primary anastomosis (see Ch. 28).[133]

When there are signs of peritonitis a laparotomy must be performed after adequate resuscitation. The patient should be advised about the chance of a stoma, and if possible seen by the stoma therapist preoperatively. The aim of surgery is to remove the diseased colon and any associated intra-abdominal sepsis. The commonest procedure performed is a Hartmann's operation, where the sigmoid colon is removed and an end colostomy fashioned (see Ch. 28). The abdominal cavity must be thoroughly washed out, especially the pelvis and subdiaphragmatic spaces, and drains can be placed. Once the patient has recovered, the bowel continuity can be restored after a period of 3–6 months. A resection of the affected segment with primary anastomosis is now often carried out,[134,135] occasionally with an accompanying defunctioning ileostomy.[136] A 1981 study comparing the morbidity and mortality of patients treated by intraoperative colonic lavage followed by resection and primary anastomosis or a Hartmann's procedure demonstrated no statistical difference in outcomes in those with localized or diffuse peritonitis.[137]

SIGMOID VOLVULUS

Volvulus of the sigmoid colon is responsible for approximately 4% of all cases of intestinal obstruction in western Europe and the USA, but it is the major cause of colonic obstruction in parts of eastern Europe, Africa and Asia. The greatest incidence is in the sixth and seventh decades (see Ch. 28).

Predisposing factors

Essential prerequisites are a redundant sigmoid colon and a short mesenteric attachment that serves as the focal point about which the volvulus rotates. Most patients have a long history of disordered bowel habit with chronic constipation and laxative abuse. It commonly develops in psychiatric and senile patients, especially if they eat a diet that contains excessive quantities of fibre. This may explain the high incidence of the condition in Uganda and Russia.

Pathology

The bowel twists in an anti-clockwise direction, and the circulation is not impaired until one and a half twists have occurred. At this point the associated closed-loop obstruction also interferes with the blood supply of the bowel wall, leading to gangrene, perforation, and rapidly fatal peritonitis if left untreated.

REFERENCES

133. Tucci G, Torquati A, Grande M et al. Hepatogastroenterology 1996; 43: 839–845
134. Lee EC, Murray JJ, Coller JA et al. Dis Colon Rectum 1997; 40: 669–674
135. Ferzoco LB, Raptopoulos V, Silen W. N Engl J Med 1998; 338: 1521–1526
136. Biondo S, Jaurrieta E, Martí Ragué et al. Br J Surg 2000; 87: 1580–1584
137. Anderson JR, Lee D. Br J Surg 1981; 68: 117–120

Clinical features

An accurate history may not be forthcoming because patients are frequently senile or psychiatrically disturbed. There is usually a prior history of many years of constipation. The onset of the volvulus is accompanied by abdominal pain, nausea and vomiting. This is followed by absolute constipation, at times with distressing tenesmus if the twist produces traction on the rectum. The abdomen soon becomes very distended and tympanitic as the loop of sigmoid colon fills with gas. A one-way valve seems to exists, which allows faeces and air to continue to enter the volvulus but prevents their onward egress. Tachycardia, toxaemia, and signs of peritonitis are indications of developing gangrene.

Radiological findings

The radiological features of a sigmoid volvulus are often diagnostic. On plain radiographs, a grossly distended loop of large bowel is seen arising from the pelvis and forming an 'omega loop' or 'double cotyledon', with its convexity lying away from the site of obstruction. A 'bird's beak' narrowing of the air-filled colon points towards the site of obstruction. Barium enema is usually not necessary to confirm the diagnosis, but in doubtful cases it may be helpful. Characteristic features indicate narrowing at the site of the torsion, spiral mucosal folds, and the ace-of-spades deformity. This investigation is contraindicated if gangrene is suspected (see Fig. 25.37).

Treatment

Treatment should be prompt to prevent ischaemia of the bowel wall. The initial management of a suspected sigmoid volvulus consists of a rigid sigmoidoscopy at which a twist in the colon may be seen.[138] A soft rectal tube can often be passed though the twist to decompress the volvulus, allowing relief of the obstruction without surgery. The tube should be left in situ for 24–48 h. Flexible sigmoidoscopy is even better because it allows more of the volvulus to be intubated and decompressed. It also allows the wall of the sigmoid colon to be inspected for evidence of necrosis, which indicates the need for surgery.

Surgery is required for any patient in whom colonic perforation or necrosis is suspected. It is also indicated if endoscopic management fails. After preoperative resuscitation and administration of broad-spectrum antibiotics, a laparotomy is performed. The colon should be resected if it is gangrenous. It should be manipulated as little as possible to avoid introduction of toxic metabolites into the portal venous system. The decision on whether to perform a primary anastomosis depends on the colonic viability, the peritoneal soiling, and the patient's condition. Primary resection with anastomosis is the preferred option if all factors are ideal (see Chapter 28). On-table washout can be used to prepare the proximal bowel, which can be decompressed into a bucket before proceeding with anastomosis.

VOLVULUS OF THE CAECUM

This condition is less common than volvulus of the sigmoid colon. It occurs when the caecum and ascending colon have not adhered to the posterior abdominal wall and are freely mobile on a lax mesocolon. It accounts for fewer than 1% of all cases of intestinal obstruction and about 30% of colonic volvuli.

Caecal volvulus presents with the signs and symptoms of a low small bowel obstruction. Patients often describe previous similar minor attacks that resolve spontaneously. The caecum is visible as a distended, palpable and tympanitic swelling, lying centrally and rather to the left of the abdomen, while the right iliac fossa is relatively empty. Plain abdominal radiographs show a grossly distended gas-filled loop of bowel containing a large fluid level in the central abdomen, and an empty left colon (see Fig. 25.38).

The caecum may perforate within a few hours unless it is decompressed. At operation the volvulus is untwisted, and the safest method of preventing recurrent episodes is to perform a right hemicolectomy (see Chapter 28), although this opinion is the subject of controversy. Caecopexy and caecostomy have also been advocated, although recurrence rates of 20% have been reported. Volvulus of the transverse colon can also occur but is incredibly rare.

PSEUDO-OBSTRUCTION

Pseudo-obstruction (see Ch. 28) is a term applied to a condition that presents as colonic obstruction but in which a mechanical cause cannot be found. In 1948, Ogilvie suggested a cause for this functional problem when he described it in two patients with malignant retroperitoneal infiltration of their coeliac plexus.[139] In some parts of the world, it is still just called Ogilvie's syndrome.

Aetiology

A long list of conditions have been reported to be possible causes of pseudo-obstruction, although a substantial number of cases occur spontaneously and are classified as idiopathic. Recognized causes are given in Box 25.3.

Pathophysiology

In the presence of such a diversity of causes, the clinical picture of pseudo-obstruction may often simply be a manifestation of multiple adverse stimuli. The mechanism by which these disorders cause atonia of the large bowel appears to be linked with an imbalance in the parasympathetic and sympathetic innervation, resulting in sympathetic reflex inhibition of colonic motility.

Clinical features

The patient is often elderly and frequently bedridden. The abdomen gradually distends and bowel actions cease, although bowel sounds may still be heard and may even sound obstructive. The abdomen is tympanitic but is not tender, and the clinical picture strongly resembles that of a mechanical colonic obstruction, usually without pain.

Abdominal radiographs do not differentiate the condition from a mechanical obstruction, although they usually show that the colon is distended with gas, with few or no fluid levels. Cut-off points may be noted, and these may be seen to progress distally on serial X-rays. Gas is often present in the rectum. Once it has been considered, the diagnosis can often be made in the context of its clinical setting. There is usually ample time to exclude a mechanical obstruction by a water-soluble enema or by colonoscopy.

Management

The management in most instances is expectant, because pseudo-obstruction is usually a self-limiting condition. Any associated metabolic disorder needs to be corrected once the diagnosis has

REFERENCES

138. Ogilvie WH. Br J Med 1948; 2 :761–763
139. Sontag SJ. Am J Gastroenterol 1997; 92: 1255–1261

Box 25.3 Causes of pseudo-obstruction

Idiopathic

Systemic disease
- Cardiac disease
- Recent cardiac or thoracic surgery
- Renal disease and uraemia
- Hypovolaemia
- Hypoxia
- Liver disease
- Acute stress (e.g. burns)
- Lead poisoning
- Electrolyte abnormalities
- Puerperium
- Myxoedema
- Drugs

Local disease
- Retroperitoneal injuries and tumours
- Pelvic injuries and surgery
- Intra-abdominal sepsis
- Infiltration of intrinsic plexus of bowel wall (e.g. amyloidosis, scleroderma, radiation and strongyloidiasis)

been confirmed. This entails correction of fluid and electrolyte abnormalities, adequate oxygenation and nutritional support. It is not necessary to pass a nasogastric tube, and cautious oral fluid may be continued.

In the early phases, decompression is often successfully accomplished by passage of a sigmoidoscope and flatus tube. Colonoscopic decompression has also been described as a means of not only investigating but also treating this condition. Caecal tenderness should be examined for at regular intervals, because it is still possible for even a functionally obstructed colon to dilate to the point of caecal rupture. A laparotomy may still be required to decompress a grossly distended caecum, especially if there is right iliac fossa tenderness and adequate decompression cannot be achieved by a flatus tube or by colonoscopy. The procedure of choice is caecal exteriorization and decompression, even when the caecum has become gangrenous or a pinhole perforation has occurred. Occasionally resection may be required in advanced cases. Tube caecostomy is dangerous and is not recommended.

PERFORATED PEPTIC ULCER

Peptic ulcer disease (see Ch. 26) is usually associated with *Helicobacter pylori* infection or the use of non-steroidal anti-inflammatory drugs.[140] The need for elective surgery has almost disappeared with the introduction of proton pump inhibitors and *H. pylori* eradication (see Ch. 26). Surprisingly, however, the incidence of perforated peptic ulcer has changed little, and the mortality rate remains around 5–10%.[141] Half the patients have no prior history of ulcer dyspepsia.

CLINICAL FEATURES

Patients complain of sudden onset of severe epigastric pain. Initially there are localized peritoneal signs, but the pain and tenderness usually progress rapidly to produce generalized peritonitis and board-like rigidity on examination. In the immunosuppressed, the elderly, and those with chronic illness the symptoms and signs may, however, be minimal.

DIAGNOSTIC PROCEDURES

An erect chest radiograph should be obtained, although the absence of free subdiaphragmatic air does not exclude a perforation. A water-soluble contrast meal is useful if no air is seen and the diagnosis is still suspected. Laparotomy is performed if a leak is seen. If there is no leak, a non-operative approach can be followed or an alternative diagnosis considered. An ultrasound scan might demonstrate another cause for the pain, such as acute cholecystitis. Computerized tomography is very good at picking up small amounts of intraperitoneal air.

TREATMENT

Patients should be resuscitated with intravenous fluids, antibiotics and analgesia. A non-operative approach is acceptable if the signs are localized, the patient is stable, and a contrast study has excluded a major leak. Under these conditions, a randomized trial of non-operative treatment versus surgery demonstrated a similar mortality but a higher rate of intra-abdominal sepsis in those patients managed non-operatively.[82]

At operation the perforation should be closed by a simple omental patch repair. If the perforation is very large, it can be converted into a pyloroplasty or a Bilroth II distal gastrectomy carried out. Postoperative eradication of *H. pylori* is essential to prevent recurrent ulceration,[142] unless it is obvious that the ulcer is related to non-steroidal inflammatory drugs or steroid therapy. In these patients it is still advisable to perform a breath test and treat *H. pylori* if it is present, even when the ulcer was symptomless prior to perforation. There is no indication for definitive antiacid surgery in the form of vagotomy. A 1996 survey of surgeons working in the UK found that the majority of respondents did not perform vagotomy for perforated peptic ulcer, and more than 80% prescribed postoperative *H. pylori* eradication therapy.[143] Interestingly, fewer than 60% routinely tested the success of *H. pylori* eradication. Laparoscopic closure has the advantages associated with other laparoscopic procedures but does not appear to reduce the postoperative stay, and the morbidity and mortality are similar to those of open repair.[144,145]

BILIARY COLIC AND ACUTE CHOLECYSTITIS

Gallstone disease is responsible for 5% of all admissions with acute abdominal pain (see Ch. 30).[69] Biliary colic is thought to occur when a stone impacts at the gall bladder–cystic duct junction. Acute cholecystitis develops if the stone fails to fall back into the gall bladder, and an acute inflammatory response results. Initially the inflammation is sterile, but bacterial superinfection often occurs. Once this has occurred the condition usually resolves over time, but it may be a prelude to recurrent attacks of chronic cholecystitis or a mucocele formation (see Ch. 30).

REFERENCES

140. Branicki FJ. (Editorial, comment). J Gastroenterol Hepatol 1996; 11: 93–96
141. Chu KM, Kwok KF, Law SY et al. Gastrointest Endosc 1999; 50: 58–62
142. Gilliam AD, Speake WJ, Lobo DN et al. Br J Surg 2003; 90: 88–90
143. Lau WY, Leung KL, Kwong KH et al. Ann Surg 1996; 224:131–138
144. Sui WT, Leong HT, Law BKB et al. Ann Surg 2002; 235: 313–319
145. Cooperberg PL. Radiology 1987; 163: 605–613

It may rarely progress to empyema formation or gangrene and perforation of the gall bladder. Perforation tends to be more common in patients with acalculous cholecystitis.

Clinical features

Biliary or gall bladder colic is a constant pain that starts quite suddenly, is experienced in the right hyperchondrium or epigastrium, and normally radiates around the side to the back. The pain is frequently associated with nausea and occasionally vomiting. Fever, localized right subcostal peritonitis, a palpable mass, and a positive Murphy's sign (pain caused by the examining hand placed on the right upper quadrant, brought on by deep inspiration) all suggest acute cholecystitis (see Ch. 30).

Diagnostic procedures

Ultrasound examination of the biliary tree is the first main investigation for all pancreaticobiliary emergencies and has a sensitivity of greater than 95% for detecting gallstones.[146] The presence of calculi, a thickened gall bladder wall, pericholecystic fluid, free fluid, and a positive radiological Murphy's sign (pain over the gall bladder on pressure from the ultrasound probe)[147] are indicative of acute cholecystitis. Despite a confident clinical diagnosis of acute cholecystitis, confirmation by ultrasonography is essential because up to a quarter of all patients are subsequently shown to have another condition (see Ch. 30).[87]

Treatment

The diagnosis is confirmed following intravenous resuscitation and analgesia. The commonest organisms cultured from the gall bladder are *Klebsiella* and *Escherichia coli* (48%), *Enterococcus* (31%), and anaerobes (15%).[148] A third-generation cephalosporin and metronidazole are therefore a sensible choice to treat acute cholecystitis.

Surgery is indicated if there are signs of generalized peritonitis, because these patients may have a gangrenous cholecystitis and possibly perforation. Most patients should have an early cholecystectomy on the next available operating list. This offers a shorter hospital stay and definitive treatment, which is preferable to non-operative management and interval cholecystectomy 3 months later (see Ch. 30).[149]

A number of randomized controlled trials have assessed early versus delayed laparoscopic cholecystectomy for acute cholecystitis. Early laparoscopic cholecystectomy has been found to be safe, with a significant reduction in overall hospital stay. One study of 99 patients randomized to either early or delayed treatment demonstrated a slightly higher (not significant) conversion rate (23% versus 11%) and higher complication rate (29% versus 13%) in the early laparoscopic group, but a significantly shorter hospital stay (6 days versus 11 days) and a shorter recuperation period (12 days versus 19 days).[150] Another randomized trial demonstrated no difference in conversion rate or morbidity but confirmed a significant reduction in the hospital stay (7.7 days versus 11.6 days).[151] In both studies, however, the operating time was significantly longer in the early group, suggesting that it was a technically more difficult procedure. The optimal timing of the early cholecystectomy remains vague, although most surgeons would consider 7–10 days after the onset of attack probably too late for safety.

Percutaneous cholecystostomy

Consideration should be given to percutaneous cholecystostomy rather than surgery in the critically ill or those with significant comorbidity. This can be successfully performed in 90% of patients, allowing the acute inflammation to settle. It is preferential to pass the drainage tract through the liver parenchyma, because this reduces the risk of bile leakage and allows earlier maturation of the tract.[152] In a prospective randomized trial of cholecystostomy in high-risk patients with acute cholecystitis, 123 patients were randomized to either cholecystostomy (63) or conservative management (60). The cholecystostomy was successfully inserted in 95%. There was no significant difference in the 30-day mortality from sepsis. Surprisingly, half of the cholecystostomy group did not require further surgery.[153]

Coexisting choledocholithiasis

Around 12% of patients presenting with gall bladder stones have coexisting stones within the extrahepatic biliary tree.[154] Abnormal liver function tests or a dilated biliary tree on ultrasound should indicate this possibility. These can be confirmed by an intraoperative cholangiogram at the time of laparoscopic cholecystectomy, or preoperatively by endoscopic ultrasound, endoscopic retrograde cholangiopancreatography (Fig. 25.42), or magnetic resonance cholangiopancreatography. Laparoscopic cholecystectomy combined with a cholangiogram is the most appropriate management if the liver function tests settle rapidly following admission and the ultrasound does not confirm stones in the bile duct. If the liver function tests do not settle, then the preoperative investigations suggested above are appropriate, with endoscopic retrograde cholangiopancreatography used to remove any stones detected. Alternatively, the surgeon can opt for duct stone removal at the time of laparoscopic cholecystectomy following intraoperative cholangiography.[155,156]

ACUTE PANCREATITIS

Acute pancreatitis (see Ch. 31) is responsible for around 2% of all admissions with acute abdominal pain. It has an annual incidence in Scotland of 318 cases per million.[157] The commonest aetiologies are gallstones or alcohol. Rare causes are discussed in Chapter 31. The majority of patients have a mild episode of pancreatitis and settle with conservative management; however,

REFERENCES

146. Laing FC, Federle MP, Jeffrey RB et al. Radiology 1981; 140: 449–455
147. Claesson BEB, Holmund DEW, Martzsch TW. Surg Gynecol Obstet 1986; 162: 531–535
148. Spillers WP, Goldman LI. South Med J 1982; 75: 802–804
149. Lo CM, Liu CL, Fan ST et al. Ann Surg 1998; 227: 461–467
150. Lai PB, Kwong KH, Leung KL et al. Br J Surg 1998; 85: 764–767
151. Hatjidakis AA, Karampekios S, Prassopoulos P et al. Cardiovasc Intervent Radiol 1998; 21: 36–40
152. Hatjidakis AA, Prassopoulos P, Petinarakis I et al. Eur Radiol 2002; 12: 1778–1784
153. Motson RW. In: Motson RW (ed.). Retained Common Duct Stones. Prevention and Treatment. Grune and Stratton, London, 1985: 8–9
154. Cuschieri A, Lezoche E, Morino M et al. Surg Endosc 1999; 13: 952–957
155. Rhodes M, Sussman L, Cohen L et al. Lancet 1998; 351: 159–161
156. McKay CJ, Evans S, Sinclair M et al. Br J Surg 1999; 86: 1302–1306
157. Imrie CW, Carter RC, McKay CJ. In: Hepatobiliary and Pancreatic Surgery. 2nd edn. WB Saunders, London, 2001: 305–347

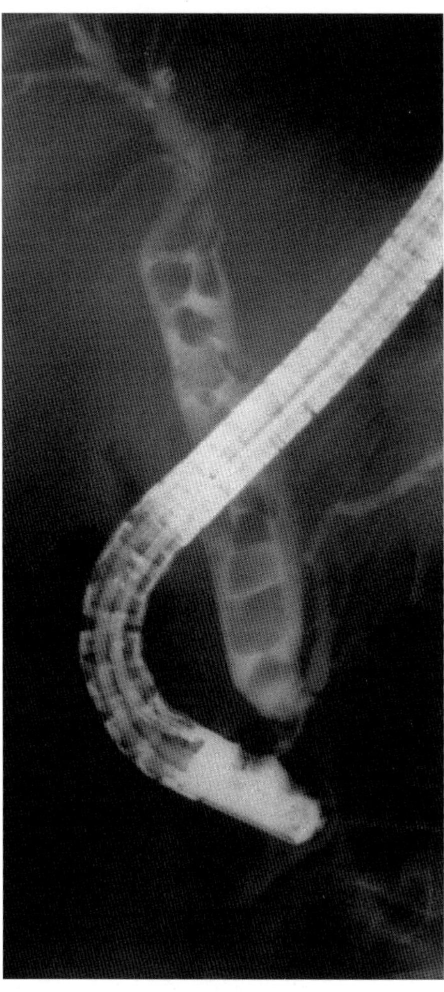

Figure 25.42 Endoscopic retrograde cholangio-pancreatography showing multiple stones in the common bile duct, which were all successfully extracted with a balloon after performing a sphincterotomy.

some present with a severe episode that has a mortality of 50% in those who develop multiorgan failure.[158]

Clinical features

Patients present with severe constant epigastric pain, which often radiates through to the back and is associated with nausea and vomiting. Periumbilical bruising (Cullen's sign) or flank bruising (Grey–Turner's sign) only rarely occur in very severe cases of haemorrhagic pancreatis. The patient may be shocked, with a rapid pulse and low blood pressure, and the condition needs to be differentiated from a perforated peptic ulcer, severe cholecystitis, a mesenteric infarct or a small bowel volvulus.

Diagnostic procedures

An elevated amylase level three times the upper limit of normal confirms the diagnosis. Different assays are available and diagnostic levels vary. After 24 h, the serum amylase level may fall below the diagnostic level, and a serum lipase[159] or a urinary amylase level can then be helpful. A plain abdominal radiograph may demonstrate pancreatic calcification indicative of chronic pancreatitis, or a sentinel loop of bowel. An abdominal ultrasound can confirm the presence of gall bladder stones or a dilated common bile duct that may contain stones. Computerized tomography may help to confirm the diagnosis where doubt persists, or alternatively an upper gastrointestinal contrast study can be used to exclude a perforated duodenal. Computerized tomography is generally used to assess the extent of pancreatic necrosis in cases of severe pancreatitis 3–7 days after the start of the attack (see Ch. 31).

Treatment

The initial management is by resuscitation with intravenous fluids, oxygen, and ranitidine given as prophylaxis against upper gastrointestinal haemorrhage. The severity of an episode of acute pancreatitis is usually assessed to try to identify patients in whom complications are more likely. These patients should be admitted to a high-dependency unit. Severity stratification allows the matching of similar groups when assessing different treatment options. Many scoring systems exist, which include the Glasgow,[160] Ranson,[161] and APACHE II scores,[162] as well as radiological scoring systems[163] and biochemical markers such as C-reactive protein.[164] The modified Glasgow scoring system[165] is straightforward and easy to use (see Ch. 31). Early laparotomy could, if possible, be avoided in patients with severe acute pancreatitis, and is reserved for those patients without a clear diagnosis, in whom other causes of an acute abdomen cannot be excluded. Further management is discussed in Chapter 31.

ABDOMINAL TRAUMA

Abdominal trauma is discussed in detail in Chapter 7 and is not truly part of the acute abdomen unless the injury is so mild that it cannot be recollected by the patient.

CLINICAL FEATURES

Any abdominal tenderness should raise the possibility of an intra-abdominal injury, but conversely the lack of abdominal signs does not reassure the surgeon on the absence of an abdominal injury. A haemoperitoneum may initially produce very few if any abdominal signs, especially in those patients with an associated head injury (see Ch. 7).

The presence of blood on peritoneal lavage does not mandate laparotomy, and an abdominal CT is a better test. High-quality ultrasonography can in experienced hands provide high specificity; however, its low sensitivity usually requires the addition of CT scanning.[166] The problem with both is determining whether the free fluid seen on ultrasound and CT is blood or intestinal contents. There have been some reports advocating laparoscopy in the investigation of abdominal trauma, but with better CT imaging its role is increasingly small.

REFERENCES

158. Dervenis C, Johnson CD, Bassi C et al. Int J Pancreatol 1999; 25: 195–210
159. Osborne DH, Imrie CW, Carter DC. Br J Surg 1981; 68: 758–761
160. Ranson JHC, Rifkind KM, Roses DF et al. Surg Gynecol Obstet 1974; 139: 69–81
161. Knaus WA, Draper EA, Wagner DP et al. Crit Care Med 1985; 13: 818–829
162. Schröder T, Kivisaari L, Somer K et al. Eur J Radiol 1985; 5: 273–275
163. Pezzilli R, Billi P, Miniero R et al. Dig Dis Sci 1995; 40: 2341–2348
164. Blamey SL, Imrie CW, O'Niell J et al. Gut 1984; 25: 1340–1346
165. Stengel D, Bauwens K, Sehouli J et al. Br J Surg 2001; 88: 901–912
166. American College of Surgeons. Advanced Trauma Life Support®. American College of Surgeons, Chicago, 1989: 129

TREATMENT OF BLUNT ABDOMINAL TRAUMA

Immediate laparotomy is indicated for patients with persistent hypotension despite active aggressive resuscitation, and for patients who have signs of peritonitis on examination. The effluent should be analysed if peritoneal lavage is used, and the criteria for laparotomy are a red cell count above 100×10^3 cells/mm^3 or a white cell count above 500 cells/mm^3.[167] The presence of free gas on X-ray or CT also indicates the need for laparotomy. Splenic and liver injuries detected on imaging are increasingly being managed non-operatively in stable patients (see Ch. 7).

ABDOMINAL MALIGNANCY

Abdominal malignancy can present with acute abdominal pain, and in one study 11% of those patients over the age of 55 years who were diagnosed with non-specific abdominal pain were subsequently found to have a cancer, just over half of which were in the colon.[168]

GYNAECOLOGICAL CAUSES OF ACUTE ABDOMINAL PAIN

Gynaecological pathology is a common cause of lower abdominal pain, especially in young women. Pelvic inflammatory disease, ectopic pregnancy, endometriosis and ovarian cysts are common. A full gynaecological history should always be taken, including the dates of the last menstrual cycle, the presence of menorrhagia, vaginal discharge, dysmenorrhoea, and a history of sexually transmitted diseases. The demonstration of cervical irritation on vaginal examination is an important sign of pelvic pathology.

In all patients suspected of a gynaecological condition, a urine or serum chorionic gonadotrophin test to confirm pregnancy and urinalysis are baseline requirements. Often this is supplemented by transvaginal ultrasound or laparoscopy. Occasionally a gynaecological problem is found at laparotomy to be the cause of the acute abdomen. A gynaecologist should then be sought, although a general surgeon still needs to be able to recognize and treat the common gynaecological problems.

PELVIC INFLAMMATORY DISEASE AND TUBO-OVARIAN ABSCESS

Pelvic inflammatory disease is inflammation of the upper genital tract from ascending infection and is frequently poorly treated.[169] After termination of pregnancy 2% of women develop infection, but this increases to 20% in women with sexually transmitted diseases.[170] The commonest organisms include *Neisseria gonorrhoeae, Ureaplasma urealyticum* and *Chlamydia trachomatis.* Broad-spectrum antibiotics that include anaerobic cover will treat the majority of episodes of pelvic inflammatory disease. The combination of cervical excitation and purulent vaginal discharge are diagnostic. Patients are often tender in both iliac fossae, which usually distinguishes the condition from acute appendicitis. It is recognized at operation by the finding of inflamed fallopian tubes draining purulent fluid. The pus should be sampled, the pelvis washed out with saline, and postoperative antibiotics administered.

An unruptured tubo-ovarian abscess should be treated by drainage and antibiotics if recognized at the time of operation. A total abdominal hysterectomy is often recommended for a ruptured tubo-ovarian abscess; however, because it is possible to manage patients with drainage and antibiotics alone, the opinion of an experienced gynaecologist should be sought.

ECTOPIC PREGNANCY

Ectopic pregnancy is an important cause of abdominal pain. Patients are often severely shocked, with marked pallor, tachycardia and hypotension. Ruptured ovarian cyst is the main differential diagnosis. The diagnosis is made by a combination of pelvic ultrasound and measurement of the serum human chorionic gonadotrophin.[171] The traditional treatment of ectopic pregnancy was by unilateral salpingectomy; however, open and laparoscopic tubal sparing techniques now exist, and for this reason a gynaecological surgical opinion should be sought.

ENDOMETRIOSIS

Endometriosis is the presence of functioning endometrial glands and stroma in ectopic locations outside the uterine cavity, and is occasionally found at the time of laparoscopy for the investigation of abdominal pain in women. It may be responsible for pain, formation of adhesions, and infertility. Simple biopsy to confirm the diagnosis is all that is required because resection increases the risk of postoperative adhesions, further symptoms, and impaired fertility.[172] Medical and hormonal therapy alleviate the symptoms in the majority of patients, but there is an eventual recurrence rate of up to 60%.[173]

OVARIAN CYSTS

Ovarian cysts are a common cause of abdominal pain, which often develops when they rupture. The pain is usually of sudden onset and situated in the lower abdomen. Nausea and vomiting are usually absent. There are often signs of lower abdominal peritonism, and these may be accompanied by signs of shock when complicated by severe haemorrhage. The differential diagnosis is from acute appendicitis or a ruptured ectopic. An ultrasound and pregnancy test should be obtained.

When an ovarian cyst is encountered at laparoscopy, it can be aspirated if large. Simple irrigation and aspiration of blood usually relieve pain. In women beyond the fertile age, or if the cyst is greater than 5 cm in diameter, resection is usually indicated because the cyst may be malignant. An experienced gynaecologist's opinion should be sought.

INTESTINAL ISCHAEMIA

Intestinal ischaemia can develop for a number of reasons (Box 25.4). At least half the cases of acute mesenteric ischaemia are related to acute thrombosis of the superior mesenteric artery,

REFERENCES

167. de Dombal FT, Matharu SS, Staniland J et al. Br J Surg 1980; 67: 413–416
168. Pearce JM. Br Med J 1990; 300: 1090–1091
169. Savage W. In: Turnbull AC, Chamberlain GVP (eds). Obstetrics. Churchill Livingstone, Edinburgh, 1989: 430–431
170. Ankum WM. Br Med J 2000; 1235–1236
171. Guzick DS, Rock JA. Fertil Steril 1983; 40: 580–584
172. Shaw RW. In: Shaw RW, Soutter WP, Stanton SL (eds). Gynaecology. 2nd edn. Churchill Livingstone, New York, 1997: 457–474
173. Bradbury AW, Brittenden J, McBride K et al. Br J Surg 1995; 82: 1446–1459

Box 25.4 Aetiology of mesenteric ischaemia

Low-flow states
- Sepsis
- Pancreatitis
- Cardiogenic shock
- Hypovolaemia
- Pharmacological

Arterial
- Thromboembolic
- Atherosclerosis
- Aortic dissection
- Mesenteric arterial thrombosis

Mechanical
- Strangulated hernia
- Adhesions

Venous
- Mesenteric venous thrombosis

while a third are the result of embolic occlusion of the superior mesenteric artery (see Ch. 10). Low-flow states associated with major surgery, myocardial infarction, pancreatitis, renal failure, liver disease or trauma account for the remaining 17%.[174] Patients usually complain of severe constant abdominal pain, but in the early stages there may be no signs of peritoneal irritation, which is often a late sign of mesenteric infarction (see Ch. 27).

Acute mesenteric arterial thrombosis or embolism has at least a 60% mortality rate, and this is 13% for venous infarction.[175] The diagnosis is usually based on a clinical suspicion, because radiological investigations such as 'thumb printing' and intramural gas occur only late in the pathological process. A lactic acidosis is also usually present, but it is also present in other non-surgical conditions such as cardiogenic shock. An angiogram may help to exclude an arterial thrombosis and prevent an unnecessary operation, but because of the diagnostic dilemma most patients undergo an early surgical exploration. Laparoscopy may also prevent unnecessary laparotomy. The decision on whether to operate is particularly difficult in unstable patients in the intensive care unit or following cardiac surgery.

TREATMENT

Initial treatment is by intravenous resuscitation, antibiotics and analgesia. Early diagnosis is critical for successful management because the prognosis is directly related to the degree of infarction.[176] Segmental colonic or small bowel resection can be successful, but widespread irreversible infarction is common. Successful arterial revascularization is ideal (see Ch. 11),[177] but obviously requires early diagnosis and a reasonable length of viable bowel for salvage. Dead bowel should be resected, and an anastomosis carried out between the two remaining ends if their blood supply is good. The safer option if bowel viability is in doubt is to staple off the ends with a planned second-look laparotomy in 24–48 h. At this time, further resection may be required and/or the ends can be joined.

POSTOPERATIVE ACUTE ABDOMEN

It can be difficult to distinguish between postoperative pain and the development of 'new' intra-abdominal pathology. The causes depend on the operation performed, concurrent medical conditions, drugs, and the patient's age. A list of the possible causes is given in Box 25.5. Complications that occur are directly related to the surgery performed or to other factors.

Box 25.5 Causes of postoperative acute abdomen

Complication of surgical procedure
- Anastomotic leak
  Faecal peritonitis
  Biliary peritonitis
  Pancreatic leak
- Intra-abdominal collection
  Haematoma
  Abscess
  Bile
  Pancreatic fluid
  Urine
- Iatrogenic intestinal perforation
- Adhesive small bowel obstruction
- Mesenteric ischaemia
- Burst abdomen

Unrelated to surgical procedure
- Pneumonia
- Urinary tract sepsis
- Pancreatitis
- Perforated peptic ulcer
- Pseudo-obstruction

Bleeding and sepsis can complicate any operation. When a gastrointestinal anastomosis has been fashioned, a postoperative leak must always be suspected if the patient develops any signs of intra-abdominal sepsis. Immediate steps must be taken to confirm or refute this possibility. Intestinal ischaemia and bowel infarction can follow any operation but are obviously more common after aortic surgery, when infarction of the left colon can follow ligation of the inferior mesenteric artery (see Ch. 11). A collection of bile may develop after gall bladder surgery (see Ch. 30), a pancreatic leak can follow injury during splenectomy (see Ch. 32), or faecal peritonitis can occur from an iatrogenic injury during division of adhesions. Pancreatitis is a recognized complication of cardiopulmonary bypass, possibly from the loss of pulsatile flow within the pancreatic end arteries (see Ch. 31). Perforated peptic ulceration occurs after all types of surgery, especially after the chronic use of non-steroidal anti-inflammatory drugs. Pseudo-obstruction is associated with pelvic and spinal surgery (see Ch. 28, Fig. 25.43). Urinary tract sepsis secondary to catheterization may occasionally masquerade as acute abdominal pain. Lastly, pneumonia or a chest infection may present with abdominal pain.

It is important to remember that any patient who develops abdominal pain after laparotomy, even with signs of respiratory tract infection, has an intra-abdominal pathology until proved otherwise. Fever, tachycardia and tachypnoea may be the initial signs of the systemic inflammatory response secondary to an anastomotic leak.

REFERENCES

174. Endean ED, Barned SL, Kwolek CJ et al. Ann Surg 2001; 233: 801–808
175. Haglund U. Gut 1994; 35 (Suppl 1): S73–S76
176. Finan MA, Barton DP, Fiorica JV et al. South Med J 1995; 88: 539–542
177. Rink AD, Goldschmidt D, Dietrich J et al. Eur J Surg 2000; 166: 932–937

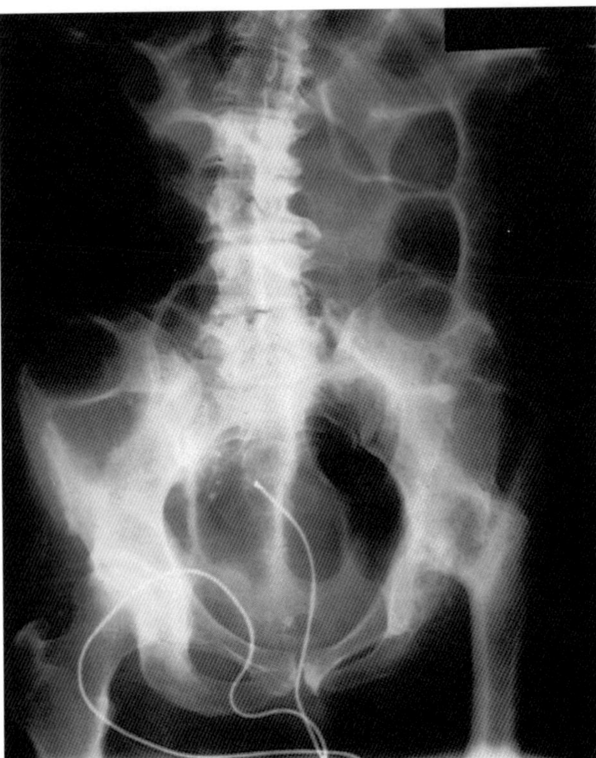

Figure 25.43 A plain X-ray of a patient with pseudo-obstruction. There is generalized dilatation of small and large bowel. A rectal thermometer indicates that the patient is being monitored in the intensive care unit.

CLINICAL FEATURES

The initial assessment is the same as that for a patient presenting 'de novo' with acute abdominal pain, although it must be recognized that the clinical assessment of the postoperative abdomen can be extremely difficult. Tenderness may be from the laparotomy incision or masked by postoperative analgesia, especially if an epidural catheter is being used. At subsequent laparotomy the amount of peritoneal soiling can be extensive, with little in the way of signs. The lack of enteric content, bile, blood or pancreatic fluid coming from an abdominal drain does not provide reassurance that an intra-abdominal problem does not exist. Shoulder tip pain may be an indication of a subdiaphragmatic collection.

DIAGNOSTIC PROCEDURES

Investigation commences with routine biochemistry, liver function tests, and measurement of serum amylase. A haemoglobin estimation may demonstrate blood loss, and an elevated white cell count supports the possibility of intra-abdominal sepsis. Arterial blood gases should be measured in sick patients, and the presence of a lactate acidosis should alert the surgeon to the possibility of intestinal ischaemia. Very high levels of amylase in drain fluid indicate a pancreatic leak or injury.

Because of the difficulties in clinical assessment, a greater reliance is placed on radiological investigations to aid diagnosis. An erect chest radiograph may continue to demonstrate free air for up to 5 days after recent abdominal surgery, although signs of lung consolidation are indicative of atelectasis or pneumonia. An abdominal radiograph may identify an ileus or a small bowel obstruction, and an erect film might differentiate between an ileus and a mechanical obstruction. A water-soluble contrast study can help to differentiate between these condition when doubt remains, although there is no evidence that this will cause earlier resolution of any ileus.[177] In those patients not requiring immediate repeat laparotomy, ultrasonography and CT might reveal an intra-abdominal collection or another cause for the pain, such as acute acalculous cholecystitis. Collections, if present, can be drained using radiological guidance.

TREATMENT

The safest approach may be to re-explore the abdomen if doubt persists and the clinical situation is of concern. Even if little is found, the surgeon is reassured and the associated morbidity is probably very low. A repeat laparoscopy can be performed following laparoscopic operations. Any patient who is 'not right' 2 days after laparoscopic surgery has an intra-abdominal problem unless proved otherwise, and the best course of action is usually to repeat the laparoscopy. In a critically ill patient who requires further surgery for a complication, the key is to drain the sepsis without making any attempt to repair an anastomotic leak or iatrogenic injury. After a colonic anastomosis, proximal diversion or exteriorization achieves this aim. The majority of anastomotic leaks will settle after diversion and drainage, reconstruction being performed at a later date.

RARER (MEDICAL) CAUSES OF ABDOMINAL PAIN

There are many conditions that involve the abdominal, retroperitoneal and intrathoracic organs and mimic the acute abdomen (Box 25.6). The common medical conditions that are mistaken for the acute abdomen but that do not require surgical treatment are discussed below.

ABDOMINAL WALL PAIN

NEUROVASCULAR BUNDLE ENTRAPMENT

Patients with this condition frequently present with recurrent pain in the abdomen, for which no definite cause can be found.[178,179] The features that suggest that the pain is arising from the abdominal wall are the presence of one or two trigger points, which can be accurately localized using one finger.[180] These usually lie just medial to the linea semilunaris of the rectus sheath.[181] Tensing the abdominal wall muscle results in persistence and, on some occasions, accentuation of the abdominal pain, whereas disappearance of the pain during straining is thought to indicate visceral disease.[181] The commonest sites for this pain are in the right iliac fossa and the right hypochondrium. Abdominal scars, felt to be the main source of pain in one series,[182] were thought not to be important in another series, where the site of pain was described as being at least 3 cm from any scar.

REFERENCES

178. Applegate WV. Surgery 1972; 711: 118
179. Gray DWK, Seabrook G et al. Ann R Coll Surg Engl 1988; 70: 233–234
180. Hall PN, Lee ABP. Br J Surg 1988; 75: 917
181. Gallegos NC, Hobsley M. J R Soc Med 1989; 82: 343
182. Tung AS, Tenicela R, Gioranetti J. JAMA 1978; 240: 738

Box 25.6 Medical (non-surgical) causes of the acute abdomen

Intra-abdominal

Disease of the liver
- Liver tumours
- Hepatic abscesses

Primary peritonitis
- Bacterial peritonitis
- Tuberculosis
- *Candida*
- Glove lubricants

Infective conditions
- Acute viral gastroenteritis
- Acute food poisoning
- Typhoid fever
- Mesenteric adenitis
- *Yersinia*
- Fitz-Hugh–Curtis syndrome

Abdominal wall pain
- Rectus sheath haematoma
- Neurovascular enlargement

Retroperitoneal causes
- Pyelonephritis
- Acute hydronephrosis

Intrathoracic causes
- Myocardial infarction
- Pericarditis
- Spontaneous pneumothorax
- Pleurisy
- Coxsackie B virus
- Spontaneous perforation of the oesophagus
- Strangulation of a diaphragmatic hernia
- Dissection of the aorta

Metabolic disorders
- Diabetes
- Addison's disease
- Uraemia
- Porphyria
- Haemochromatosis
- Hypercalcaemia
- Heavy metal poisoning

Neurological causes of the acute abdomen
- Spinal disorders
- Tabes dorsalis

Haematological disorders
- Sickle cell anaemia
- Haemolytic anaemia
- Henoch–Schönlein purpura
- Leukaemia
- Lymphomas
- Polycythaemia
- Anticoagulant therapy

Immunological disorders
- Polyarteritis nodosa
- Systemic lupus erythematosus

Infections
- Infectious mononucleosis
- Herpes zoster

Injection of local anaesthetic is often both diagnostic and curative.[181] The beneficial effect of the local anaesthetic is often considerably longer than its expected duration of action.[182] In some instances a single injection cures the pain, and in others the pain is completely relieved by repeated treatment. Many other methods of treatment have been reported, each with some success. These include injecting a combination of local anaesthetic and steroids,[183] aqueous phenol,[178] the use of radiofrequency sound waves, and surgical decompression of the affected area.

Clearly, in making this diagnosis the clinician needs to be convinced that there is no underlying visceral pathology. The response rates to one injection of local anaesthetic have been reported to be between 55 and 100%.[181,182]

RECTUS SHEATH HAEMATOMA

Rectus sheath haematoma is an uncommon condition that may arise spontaneously, after minor trauma or after bouts of coughing or sneezing.[184–186] The underlying abnormality is thought to be poor elasticity of the arteries, which results in a failure of the vessel to accommodate sudden, marked variations in length as the rectus muscle undergoes contraction and relaxation. When a rectus sheath haematoma occurs spontaneously, it may be associated with an underlying disorder of coagulation, degenerative vascular disease, infectious diseases, or haematological conditions such as leukaemia.

It presents with an acute onset of abdominal pain, and there may be associated symptoms of nausea and vomiting that suggest an intra-abdominal abnormality. Examination frequently reveals exquisite tenderness in the lower abdomen and a sensation of fullness or a mass in the abdominal wall, which can still be felt when the muscles are tensed. The pain is accentuated by tensing the abdominal muscles during palpation. Later bruising and discoloration of the skin over the haematoma may develop. In cases where this is not evident, and a mass is not clearly palpable, a diagnosis of the acute abdomen may mistakenly be made. An ultrasound or a CT scan may confirm the presence of a haematoma if the condition is suspected (Fig. 25.44).

The condition is usually treated conservatively, with the pain settling in 2–3 days, although the mass may take several weeks to resolve. In some patients with severe abdominal pain, evacuation of the haematoma and control of the bleeding point may be considered.

Intra-abdominal causes

Disease of the liver

Any condition that produces stretching of the liver capsule causes acute abdominal pain and signs of tenderness in the right upper hyperchondrium. Acute viral hepatitis often presents in this way, but it is differentiated from acute cholecystitis by finding raised viral antibody titres and altered liver function tests. Congestive cardiac failure causes a similar pain from passive congestion of

REFERENCES

183. Fotergill WE. Br Med J 1926; 1: 941
184. Brodel M. Bull Johns Hopkins Hosp 1937; 61: 295
185. Cullen TS. Bull Johns Hopkins Hosp 1937; 61: 317
186. Crist NR, Bell EJ, Aasaad F. Progress in Medical Virology. Karger, Basel, 1978

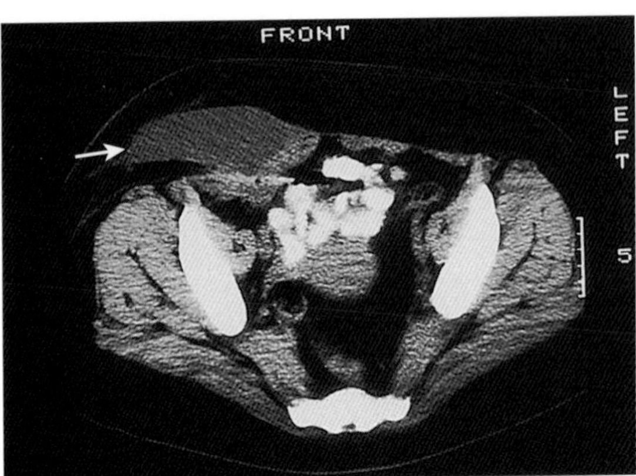

Figure 25.44 A CT scan of a rectus sheath haematoma.

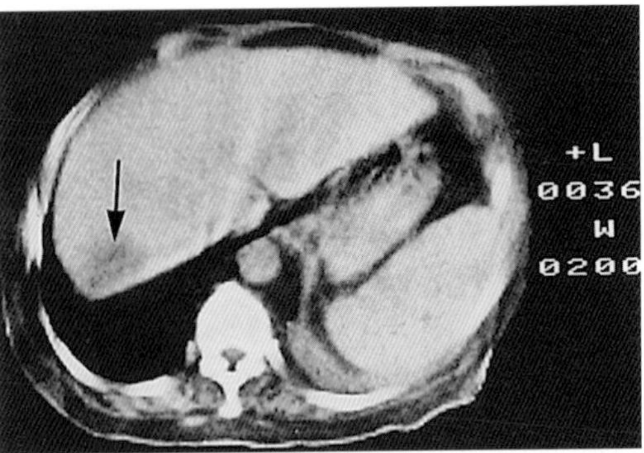

Figure 25.45 A CT scan showing a liver abscess.

the liver, especially if there is tricuspid incompetence, when the liver may be pulsatile. This is suspected when the patient has an elevated jugular venous pressure, peripheral oedema, chest crepitations or gallop cardiac rhythm, and of course a systolic ejection murmur (see Ch. 22).

Primary or metastatic liver tumours may also present with abdominal pain, although these could probably be considered as surgical causes of acute abdominal pain because they occasionally require operations. The pain is caused by sudden enlargement of the liver as a result of rapid tumour growth or by secondary haemorrhage into a necrotic tumour. Free bleeding may also occur into the abdominal cavity. Liver neoplasms can be confirmed by imaging with ultrasound, CT or magnetic resonance (see Ch. 29).

Both pyogenic and amoebic hepatic abscesses (see Ch. 29) may present with abdominal pain, hepatic enlargement and tenderness. The pain is usually in the right upper quadrant but may also be experienced over the right lower chest, where there may be swelling and pitting oedema of the subcutaneous tissues. The pain may be referred to the shoulder if the abscess is in contact with the diaphragm. The upper abdominal signs are generally not as marked as the signs of systemic sepsis. Radiographs reveal an elevated or immobile diaphragm on the right side; the cardiophrenic angle is often obliterated, and if there are gas-producing organisms within the abscess an air–fluid level may be seen within the cavity. Imaging of the liver usually demonstrates the presence of an abscess (Fig. 25.45). An amoebic abscess may be confirmed by a specific complement fixation test or the demonstration of amoebas within stools. The final diagnosis is invariably confirmed by aspiration of 'anchovy' pus from the abscess cavity (see Ch. 29).

Infective conditions

Acute viral gastroenteritis

Acute viral gastroenteritis is a common condition in childhood, when it is self-limiting. The abdominal symptoms are occasionally severe and may mimic the acute abdomen. It is characterized by watery diarrhoea, nausea and vomiting associated with crampy abdominal pain.[187] Tenderness in the abdomen is usually ill-localized.

Acute food poisoning

Acute food poisoning usually produces a similar picture to that of viral gastroenteritis. In some instances the abdominal pain is quite intense and may even be associated with tenderness and rebound. Diarrhoea is common, and the causative organism or its toxin can often be isolated from the stool. Differentiation from other abdominal emergencies may be difficult in some cases. Many patients with viral gastroenteritis or suspected food poisoning are found to have *Campylobacter* in their stools, and giardiasis may also have to be excluded.

Typhoid fever

Typhoid fever may produce symptoms and signs that are similar to those of acute appendicitis (see Ch. 27). The onset is generally less acute, with several days of symptoms. Associated findings include Koplik's spots, a macropapular rash, leukopenia, and at times a marked bradycardia. Patients appear extremely unwell, out of all proportion to their abdominal signs. The diagnosis is confirmed by culture of salmonella from the stools or blood. Perforation of the distal ileum occurs in a small proportion of cases and requires surgical treatment (see Ch. 27).

Mesenteric adenitis

Mesenteric adenitis is an enlargement of the mesenteric lymph nodes caused by an adenoviral infection that particularly affects young children, and can at times be difficult to differentiate from acute appendicitis (see *Acute appendicitis*, p. 579). There is usually a history of an upper respiratory infection, which may either still be present or may have subsided. The upper respiratory tract infection is often associated with fever, pharyngitis and cervical lymphadenitis. The abdominal pain is usually more diffuse than in patients with appendicitis, and tenderness is rarely isolated to the right iliac fossa. The site of maximal tenderness may be altered by re-examining patients on their side. Guarding may be present but rebound tenderness is almost never elicited. A relative lymphocytosis may be present but cannot be relied on to confirm the diagnosis. In most instances, careful observation of the patient and repeated re-examination differentiate mesenteric adenitis from acute appendicitis.

Yersinia

Infection with *Yersinia* has been associated with acute appendicitis, mesenteric adenitis, acute terminal ileitis and non-specific abdominal pain.[188] *Yersinia enterocolitica* has been isolated from patients with gastroenteritis and right iliac fossa pain, while

REFERENCE

187. Attwood SEA, Mealy K et al. Lancet 1987; i: 529–533
188. Weber J, Finlayson NB, Mark JBD. N Engl J Med 1970; 283: 172–174

Y. pseudotuberculosis has been isolated from patients with non-specific abdominal pain. *Yersinia* infection can be confirmed by a rising titre of antibodies to *Y. enterocolitica* and *Y. pseudotuberculosis*. *Yersinia* was found to be present in 31% of a series of patients with acute appendicitis, 12% of cases of non-specific abdominal pain, and two out of six patients with mesenteric adenitis.[189] Despite this study, it is not known how often *Yersinia* causes these conditions. *Yersinia* has also been found in patients with acute terminal ileitis,[190] which may be discovered at the time of appendicectomy and can mimic Crohn's disease of the ileum. This type of ileitis does not go on to produce the recurrent problems associated with Crohn's disease.

Fitz-Hugh–Curtis syndrome[191,192]

Fitz-Hugh–Curtis syndrome was initially thought to be caused by gonococcal salpingitis, but it is now more commonly associated with *Chlamydia trachomatis* infection.[193,194] The pelvic infection tracks up either left or right paracolic gutters to produce perisplenitis or perihepatitis. Patients with this condition may present with both lower and upper abdominal pain, and the epigastric pain often mimics acute biliary disease.[195] The presentation is usually with severe right upper quadrant abdominal pain, which may be associated with anorexia, nausea, and a low-grade fever. The predominant tenderness is in the right upper quadrant. The presence of a pelvic infection must be sought, and high vaginal and cervical swabs sent for culture. The disease is confirmed by the presence of elevated serum levels of specific antibodies. Treatment is by a course of doxycycline. The diagnosis may also be made at laparoscopy or even laparotomy, when adhesions can be demonstrated around the capsule of the liver. The Fitz-Hugh–Curtis syndrome may also occasionally cause diffuse peritonitis and chronic ascites.

Retroperitoneal and renal causes of abdominal pain

Pyelonephritis and other conditions affecting the kidney, such as hydronephrosis and renal colic, can at times present as an acute abdomen.

Renal colic may at times mimic bowel obstruction, especially if there is an associated paralytic ileus. The differentiation between these two conditions relies very much on the history of the pain. Renal colic tends to present with loin pain that radiates to the groin (see Ch. 35). The patient cannot lie still and often rolls around the bed or the floor during the colicky attacks. By contrast, intestinal obstruction produces a central colicky pain, causing the patient to double up, bringing the knees up to their chin. A ruptured abdominal aortic aneurysm causing loin and back pain may also be mistaken for renal colic (see Chapter 11).

Pyelonephritis

Pyelonephritis can also be mistaken for acute appendicitis. Acute pyelonephritis develops fairly rapidly over a few hours and is normally associated with a high fever and rigors. There may also be symptoms of nausea and vomiting. Increased urinary frequency and dysuria usually occur before the onset of the fever, but occasionally they never develop. The pain is experienced in the loin and may radiate to the groin. In some instances the presenting pain appears to be located in the iliac fossa. There is usually marked tenderness in one or both loins, and there is tenderness of varying severity in the iliac fossae. Bacteria and white cells are nearly always present in the urine (Chapter 35).

Acute hydronephrosis

Acute hydronephrosis may present with a pain in the upper abdomen referred from the kidney, and may be difficult to differentiate from other conditions, such as biliary colic. There is usually pain in the loin, and tenderness can generally be demonstrated on bimanual palpation. Ultrasound imaging demonstrates the dilated renal pelvis (Chapter 35).

Intrathoracic causes of abdominal pain

A number of conditions affecting the thoracic organs may cause abdominal pain.

Myocardial infarction

Pain from a myocardial infarction may be localized to the epigastrium and may be associated with nausea and vomiting. This type of cardiac pain is usually of rapid onset, and is a persistent, severe, crushing pain that may radiate to the neck and left arm. Shortness of breath and sweating may also be present. The abdominal muscles may be rigid, but the patient rarely complains of pain during palpation. General examination frequently reveals tachycardia or arrhythmia, sweating and hypotension, with poor peripheral perfusion. Fever and a high white cell count are not normally present in the early stages. The diagnosis is confirmed by characteristic electrocardiographic changes and by finding a subsequent elevation of the cardiac enzymes over the next 48 h. Myocardial infarction must be considered in all patients presenting with severe abdominal pain and shock, and it is one of the differential diagnoses that must be considered in patients suspected of having acute pancreatitis, a perforated peptic ulcer, a ruptured aortic aneurysm, mesenteric infarction, or a small bowel volvulus. Cardiac pain and gall bladder colic may also be confused.

Pericarditis

Pericarditis may also cause abdominal pain, particularly when the inflammation affects the diaphragmatic pericardium (see Ch. 22). This produces severe epigastric pain, which has the peculiar feature of being relieved by sitting and accentuated by taking up other positions. A friction rub is usually present and should be listened for, both over the lung bases and in the precordium. The diagnosis of pericarditis can usually be made on an electrocardiogram, where the widespread elevation of the ST segment differentiates the condition from myocardial infarction. Viral pericarditis, which is the most common form, has no additional symptoms or signs, but other types of pericarditis—associated with uraemia, tuberculosis, rheumatic fever and bacterial infection—may have additional features.

Spontaneous pneumothorax

A spontaneous pneumothorax can occasionally cause abdominal pain as the result of diaphragmatic irritation. Examination of the

REFERENCES

189. Gurry JF. Br Med J 1974; ii: 264–266
190. Curtis H. JAMA 1930; 98: 1221
191. Fitz-Hugh T Jr. JAMA 1934; 102: 2044
192. Muller-Schopp JW, Wang SP et al. Br Med J 1978; 1: 1002
193. Wolner-Hanssen P. Br J Obstet Gynaecol 1986; 93: 619–624
194. Shanahan D, Lord PH, Grogono J et al. Ann R Coll Surg Engl 1988; 70: 44–46
195. Boerhaave H. Lugduni Batavorum Boutesteniana, 1724. Bull Med Lib Assoc 1955; 93: 28

chest and a chest radiograph should confirm the diagnosis. Pain can also be referred to the abdomen from pleurisy, especially when this affects the diaphragmatic pleura (Ch. 21).

Abdominal pain is more frequent when there is an associated pneumonia or pulmonary infarct from a pulmonary embolus. There may be limited chest movement on the affected side, cough and haemoptysis, shortness of breath, signs of consolidation of the lung, a friction rub, and some tightening of the abdominal muscles. Chest radiographs, blood gas and sputum analysis, electrocardiography and lung scanning may be required to confirm the diagnosis (Ch. 11).

Coxsackie B virus

Coxsackie B virus infection (Bornholm disease) or epidemic pleurodynia can present with severe pain in the chest or the abdomen. Other symptoms include shortness of breath, pain on respiration, headache, and a sore throat. The abdominal pain, which is experienced in the upper abdomen and lower thorax, is usually aggravated by movement and respiration. Patients are usually pyrexial, but the white cell count is rarely elevated. The diagnosis is suggested by finding superficial hyperaesthesia over the upper abdomen and by the lack of signs on abdominal examination. An elevation of viral antibodies on repeat testing confirms the diagnosis after several weeks.

Spontaneous perforation of the oesophagus (Boerhaave's syndrome)

Spontaneous perforation of the oesophagus (Boerhaave's syndrome) is a condition in which the oesophagus ruptures and its contents enter the mediastinum and one of the two hemithoraces, usually the left (see Ch. 20).[196] This occurs more commonly in males, and frequently follows an episode of excessive food or alcohol intake associated with violent vomiting or retching. Severe pain rapidly develops in the epigastrium and lower chest, and is aggravated by swallowing and breathing. On examination patients are febrile and tachypnoeic; they may even be cyanotic. Subcutaneous emphysema may be present, and a friction rub may be heard over the left chest. In the early stages the rupture is confined to the mediastinum, which appears widened on a chest radiograph. A pleural effusion may be present in the left chest, and there may also be evidence of mediastinal gas. The diagnosis is confirmed by a water-soluble contrast swallow or by aspirating stomach contents from the pleural cavity; the stomach contents have a low pH or a high amylase content. Oesophageal perforation without associated rupture of the pleura can be managed non-operatively, but when the pleura has been breached the patient needs a thoracotomy, pleural lavage and oesophageal repair, with pleural drainage and antibiotics (see Ch. 20).

Strangulated diaphragmatic hernia

A strangulated diaphragmatic hernia is extremely rare, and other conditions that produce acute mediastinitis can also produce similar symptoms and signs. It requires urgent surgery, especially if it is associated with a gastric volvulus (see Ch. 26).

Aortic dissection

Aortic dissection can also produce chest or abdominal pain, which is similar to that of a myocardial infarction. The original site of the pain is usually in the back between the shoulder blades, but this may spread down into the abdomen even if the blood supply of the intestine is not compromised. The signs of mesenteric ischaemia indicate the need for urgent surgery. The anatomy of the dissection is shown by CT scanning, transoesophageal ultrasound or arteriography (see Ch. 22).

Metabolic disorders

A number of metabolic disorders can produce abdominal pain, which is only occasionally severe enough to be mistaken for a surgical emergency.

Diabetes

Diabetic ketoacidosis can cause severe abdominal pain and tenderness. Nausea and vomiting are frequently associated and the abdomen is diffusely tender on palpation, without evidence of guarding or rebound tenderness. Diabetic ketoacidosis is usually differentiated from other causes of the acute abdomen by the knowledge that the patient has diabetes, although some patients present for the first time with diabetic ketoacidosis.[197] They may, however, give a prior history of polyuria, polydipsia, lassitude, anorexia and weight loss an careful questioning. The general appearance of the patient is characteristic, with laboured breathing from air hunger and a ketoacidotic fetor from acetone on the breath. There is usually evidence of dehydration, with hypotension, a thready pulse and oliguria. The diagnosis is made by testing the urine and the blood for glucose and ketones. It is important to be certain that an acute abdomen is not being overlooked in a patient with diabetic ketoacidosis, and that an acute abdomen has not precipitated the ketoacidotic episode. The abdominal signs of diabetic ketoacidosis resolve once the diabetes is brought under control and fluids have been replaced.

Addison's disease

Chronic deficiency of the adrenal cortex may at times be characterized by gastrointestinal symptoms, which include anorexia, lethargy, weight loss, nausea, vomiting, diarrhoea and ill-defined abdominal pain (see Ch. 34). In an Addisonian crisis, the abdominal symptoms may become intensified. The patient is usually severely dehydrated and hypotensive. A diagnosis of Addison's disease is suggested by the presence of pigmentation, which is a diffuse brown tan or bronze darkening of both exposed and unexposed areas of skin, and severe hypotension, which is out of keeping with the rest of the clinical picture. The diagnosis is confirmed by finding a low plasma cortisol level and the failure of the cortisol to rise in response to stimulation (see Ch. 34).

Uraemia

Patients with chronic renal failure may develop anorexia, nausea, vomiting and bleeding from small ulcers in the gastrointestinal tract. Abdominal pain tends to be associated with severe vomiting and diarrhoea, or with the complications of pericarditis and acute pancreatitis. The pain is not usually severe, but on occasions can be more marked and may be mistaken for an acute abdomen. The clinical picture of a dehydrated patient who is pale, with a yellowish skin and fetor, raises the clinical suspicion of chronic renal failure. The diagnosis is confirmed by finding an elevated blood urea and creatinine level.

REFERENCES

196. Beardwood JT. JAMA 1935; 105: 1168
197. Stein JA, Tuschudy DP. Medicine 1970; 44: 1

Porphyria (acute intermittent porphyria)

Porphyrins are iron-free pigments produced during haemoglobin metabolism.[198] In the porphyrias there is a disorder of pyrrole metabolism, resulting in the formation of large amounts of free porphyrins. Acute intermittent porphyria, which is the most common type, is transmitted as a Mendelian dominant and affects young and middle-aged adults. It is characterized by periodic attacks of intense abdominal pain, which may be associated with nausea and vomiting, constipation, neuromuscular disorders, and abnormal psychological behaviour. Colicky abdominal pain is the presenting complaint in many cases, but fever is rare and the abdominal signs are ill defined. Patients with porphyria may have been erroneously treated in the past for acute appendicitis, cholelithiasis, renal colic or acute pancreatitis. Recurrent abdominal crises can occur for many years before a diagnosis is made. The neurological damage usually causes vague neurotic complaints, but occasionally patients may become comatose, confused or frankly psychotic. They may also develop peripheral neuropathy, neuritic pain in the extremities, paraplegia, quadriplegia and bulbar paralysis.

The diagnosis is confirmed by finding porphobilinogen in the urine. The freshly voided urine is frequently normal in colour, but on standing in sunlight turns to a burgundy or port wine colour (Fig. 25.46). During a remission, the porphobilinogen reaction of heating the urine with the addition of acid is usually positive, but a negative test does not entirely exclude the presence of porphyria.

Haemochromatosis

Haemochromatosis is a disease of iron metabolism, which results in an elevation of the plasma iron and saturation of the iron-binding protein transferrin, leading to iron being deposited in parenchymal cells in the form of ferritin and haemosiderin.[199] Increased amounts of iron are found in almost all body tissues, especially in the liver and pancreas, and to a lesser extent in the heart, kidney, spleen and skin. Symptoms of haemochromatosis are related to skin pigmentation, diabetes, liver impairment and cardiac disease. Abdominal pain occurs in a number of patients with haemodermatosis, and is only rarely severe enough to simulate an acute surgical emergency. The diagnosis is indicated by the presence of high serum iron and iron-binding protein levels, and the definitive diagnosis is made on histological examination of a liver biopsy.

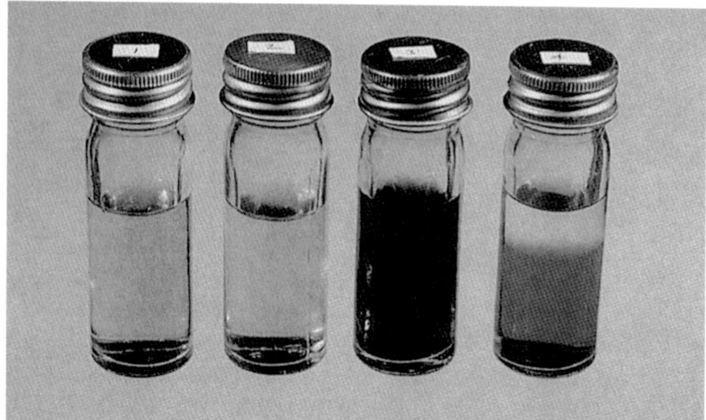

Figure 25.46 Urine from a patient with porphyria. The urine goes dark on standing.

Hypercalcaemia

Hypercalcaemia may be associated with symptoms of muscular weakness, anorexia, nausea, constipation and abdominal pain (Chapter 18). The site of the abdominal pain is variable, and there are very few associated signs. Although it used to be thought that hypercalcaemia could cause acute pancreatitis, it is debatable whether this is true.[200] Hyperparathyroidism may be responsible for the hypercalcaemia, and patients can present with stones (renal colic), bone pain or abdominal pain (Chapter 18).

Heavy metal poisoning

Lead poisoning is the commonest form of heavy metal poisoning to cause abdominal pain.[201] Arsenic and mercury poisoning can cause similar symptoms. Lead is an accumulative poison that is slowly excreted from the body, and acute lead poisoning is virtually non-existent. Lead poisoning is caused by the chronic ingestion of lead-containing materials such as paint and water, or from the inhalation of fumes released by burning lead-containing substances such as solder or batteries. In the early stages the symptoms, which include vague muscular pains, lassitude and weakness, often pass unnoticed. Symptoms usually develop suddenly after chronic exposure. They include generalized abdominal colic, constipation and rigidity of the abdominal wall musculature. The colic is thought to be produced by tonic contractions of the small intestine. The attacks of colic may be exacerbated by intercurrent infections or alcoholic binges, and are often not relieved by narcotic injections. There are usually no signs of infection or inflammation, and abdominal examination is often unremarkable. Other complications include encephalopathy, peripheral neuritis and anaemia. The diagnosis is suspected when a blue line is seen in the gum around the margins of the teeth, and confirmed by finding a raised lead level in the blood.

The pain can be relieved by the intravenous injection of calcium salts. The exposure to lead should be reduced and penicillamine should be administered.[202]

NEUROLOGICAL CAUSES OF THE ACUTE ABDOMEN

Spinal disorders

Any disorder of the spine resulting in compression or irritation of a nerve root can produce abdominal pain (see Ch. 48). Osteoarthritis, osteoporosis, disc degeneration, inflammatory conditions, neoplastic conditions and osteomalacia can all cause root compression. The onset of the pain may be gradual or acute when caused by the prolapse of an intervertebral disc. The pain is usually positional and aggravated by movement or by coughing. It may be eased by adopting specific postures, especially lying down. The pain may be experienced on one or other side and is commonly associated with hyperaesthesia over the relevant dermatome. Abdominal palpation rarely increases the pain and examination of the back usually reveals the source of the pain, which is often associated with a limitation of raising the straight leg. The diagnosis is confirmed by radiographs of the lumbar

REFERENCES

198. Livingstone DJ. Scot Med J 1960; 5: 164
199. Shearer MG, Imrie CW. Br J Surg 1986; 73: 282
200. Dagg JH, Goldberg A et al. Q J Med 1965; 34: 163
201. Catsch A, Harmuth-Hoene AE. Pharmac Ther 1976; Al: 118
202. Harvard CW. Br J Hosp Med 1972; 21: 443

spine, isotopic bone scanning, myelography, radiculography, CT scanning or MRI.

Tabes dorsalis

Approximately 10% of patients with tertiary syphilis develop severe episodes of abdominal pain associated with nausea and vomiting.[203] These episodes, known as gastric crises, can last for several days and lead to dehydration. They usually settle spontaneously, and recur at regular intervals. Other signs of tabes dorsalis, such as ataxia, Charcot's joints, and an alteration in the pupils—Argyll Robertson pupil, meiosis, a poor reaction to light, and a poor response to atropine—may indicate the diagnosis. This is confirmed by serological testing for syphilis, although in the later stages of tabes dorsalis the serology may be negative. This is a rare cause of abdominal pain today.

HAEMATOLOGICAL DISORDERS

Sickle cell anaemia

Sickle cell anaemia is a chronic hereditary haemolytic disease caused by the haemoglobin S gene. Haemolysed red corpuscles become trapped in small vessels, causing deoxygenation and a reduced pH, which in turn favours further sickling and increases blood viscosity. This leads to reduced tissue perfusion, and in the long term may cause infarction and shrinkage of the spleen (see Ch. 32), aseptic necrosis of bone, haematuria, pulmonary infarction, disorders in the central nervous system, chronic leg ulcers, and cholelithiasis. Affected patients often complain of episodic weakness, joint pains and chest pains. Between crises they usually adjust to the chronic haemolytic anaemia and require no specific treatment. Many patients with sickle cell anaemia are poorly developed, often with defective secondary sex characteristics.

During sickle cell crises there are sudden episodes of severe abdominal pain, which are usually experienced in the epigastrium and associated with nausea and vomiting.[204] Patients may have a fever and an elevated white cell count, with signs of tenderness and guarding in the epigastrium. The acute crises are managed by maintaining hydration and electrolyte balance, and by correcting any metabolic acidosis that occurs. The inspired oxygen should be kept at a high level.

Haemolytic anaemia

The onset of any type of haemolytic anaemia can result in an acute illness characterized by severe rigors, fever, malaise, headache, back pain and limb pain. Some patients also develop severe abdominal pain and marked muscular rigidity, simulating an acute abdomen. Severe haemolysis also causes hypotensive shock and anuria. Jaundice tends to develop rapidly, and other symptoms of anaemia may also be present. A haemolytic anaemia is usually normocytic but may be macrocytic during phases of rapid blood regeneration, when many immature cells are present. A raised reticulocyte count is usually present.

Henoch–Schönlein purpura

This form of vascular purpura is characterized by serosanguinous effusions into the subcutaneous, submucous and subserous tissues. These are the result of perivascular inflammation. The pathogenesis of this disorder is obscure, although there is some evidence to suggest that it has an allergic basis.[205] It is more common in children and young adults. The skin haemorrhages vary considerably. They are usually located on the extremities and may be associated with allergic manifestations such as erythema and urticaria. The joint effusions cause swelling and pain. Severe abdominal pain is produced by haemorrhagic effusions developing within the subserosal layer of intestinal wall, and these localized haematomas can lead to intussusception (see Chs 27, 40). Constitutional symptoms such as fever and malaise are present in most cases.

The diagnosis is usually suspected because of the presence of skin haemorrhages. When these are absent, the bouts of abdominal pain—which may be accompanied by fever, leukocytosis and possibly melaena—can be difficult to distinguish from other causes of the acute abdomen. Neutrophilia or eosinophilia may be present but the blood film, differential and coagulation tests are often normal. The diagnosis is made on histological examination of a biopsy taken from a skin lesion, or occasionally by the characteristic appearances at laparotomy.

Leukaemia

Leukaemia can occasionally present with abdominal pain as a result of leukaemic infiltration of the spleen or liver. This can rarely lead to splenic infarction or even rupture. Leukaemic infiltration can also occur in the intestine; in most instances this does not cause abdominal pain, although the involved bowel may very occasionally perforate during vigorous chemotherapy. Leukaemia is usually diagnosed on the peripheral blood film or on bone marrow examination.

Lymphomas

Abdominal pain can similarly be caused by lymphomas as a result of infiltration of the liver and spleen, but more commonly arises from disease in the retroperitoneal lymph nodes or involvement of the gastrointestinal tract (see Ch. 33). There is often evidence of recent weight loss and there may be signs of anaemia. A palpable abdominal mass may be present, and there may be signs of small bowel obstruction. The diagnosis may be surmised if there are other constitutional symptoms or evidence of marked lymphadenopathy elsewhere. Radiological imaging may be required to demonstrate enlargement of the mesenteric or retroperitoneal lymph nodes when the disease is confined to the abdomen. Biopsy is usually required to obtain a histological diagnosis. The association of lymphomas with AIDS has increased the incidence of primary disease of the small bowel, which may perforate or obstruct the affected segment.

Polycythaemia

Polycythaemia can give rise to abdominal pain by causing a thrombosis of the mesenteric vessels. Peptic ulceration is also more common in patients with polycythaemia. The condition is suspected from the patient's dusty red hue, which is most obviously seen in the lips, cheeks and nose. The diagnosis is confirmed by measuring the haemoglobin, haematocrit, red cell count and red cell mass.

Anticoagulant therapy

Poorly controlled anticoagulation can cause retroperitoneal bleeding, which may present with abdominal pain (see Ch. 8).

REFERENCES

203. Tomlinson WJ. Am J Med Sci 1945; 209: 722
204. Silber DL. Pediatr Clin North Am 1972; 19: 1061
205. Carter RI, Penman HG. Infectious Mononucleosis. Blackwell, Oxford, 1969

There is usually some abdominal tenderness on palpation and occasionally a mass may be felt. The diagnosis should be suspected when it is known that the patient is on anticoagulants, especially if the prothrombin ratio is elevated and the haemoglobin has dropped. Computerized tomography scanning confirms the presence of a retroperitoneal blood clot (Fig. 25.47).

The condition should usually be treated conservatively by reversal of the anticoagulation and, if necessary, blood transfusion, while waiting for the haematoma to resolve. Surgical drainage is rarely if ever required and should be avoided.

IMMUNOLOGICAL DISORDERS

Polyarteritis nodosa

Polyarteritis nodosa is a rare condition of uncertain aetiology, in which there is necrotizing inflammation of the blood vessels. The vasculitis can affect arteries, arterioles, and also sometimes adjacent veins in any part of the body. Abdominal symptoms occur in 60–70% of the patients. Ulceration, haemorrhage, perforation and intestinal infarction can develop.[203] Many patients require laparotomy for these complications, but the diagnosis may already be suspected if there are lesions in the skin or evidence of renal or cardiac involvement. Histological examination of the bowel, muscle or kidney usually enables the diagnosis to be made with certainty (see Ch. 11).

Systemic lupus erythematosus

Systemic lupus erythematosus is an immunological disorder of unknown cause that predominantly affects women. Abdominal pain can occur when the vasculitis involves the visceral vessels, and some patients progress to severe mesenteric ischaemia and infarction (see Ch. 11).

INFECTIONS

Infectious mononucleosis

Infectious mononucleosis, or glandular fever, is an acute infection most commonly seen in adolescents and young adults; it is caused by the Epstein–Barr virus.[206] The characteristic clinical picture is one of fever, pharyngitis and lymphadenopathy. Splenomegaly develops in approximately half the patients, and is very occasionally complicated by spontaneous splenic rupture. Patients with hepatomegaly or splenomegaly can also experience abdominal pain, which arises from stretching of the sensitive capsules of these organs. The presence of a tender enlarged spleen or liver is confirmed by abdominal examination, and the diagnosis is made by a Paul–Bunnell test. On occasions this may take some time to become positive, and may therefore have to be repeated.

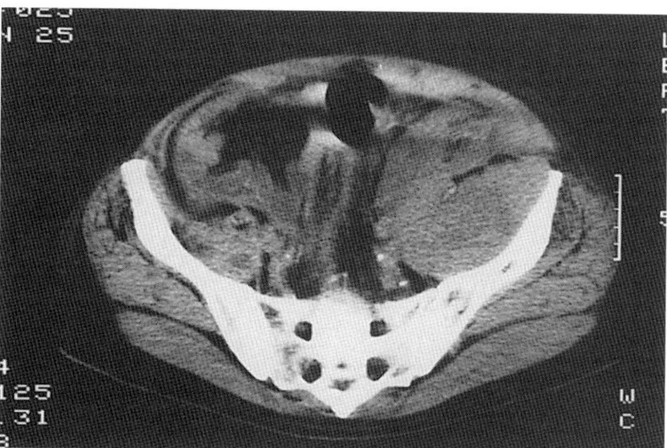

Figure 25.47 A CT scan showing a large retroperitoneal haematoma.

Herpes zoster (shingles)

The virus responsible for this condition primarily affects the nerves of the skin. The thoracic intercostal nerves are involved in approximately half the cases, the cervical nerves in 20%, and lumbar and sacral nerves in 15%. The clinical presentation is usually with fever and pain over the affected dermatomes. A characteristic skin eruption develops over the involved dermatomes, either at the same time as the onset of the pain or up to 4–5 days later. The pain may be very severe, sharp and burning or dull in nature. The skin usually becomes erythematous at first, but then develops red papules that progress to vesicular, pustular and crusting eruptions over the next 2 weeks. The rash usually involves one or two dermatomes on one side of the body. In very rare instances the pain is experienced but the rash never develops. Before the skin eruptions appear, the severe abdominal pain and hyperaesthesia on palpation may be mistaken for an acute abdomen, although careful re-examination rarely demonstrates guarding or rebound tenderness.

Tetanus

The presence of pain, muscular stiffness, and rigidity involving the abdominal musculature may mimic the acute abdomen (see Ch. 3). The clinical manifestations of tetanus follow an injury that occurred from 2 to 56 days before the onset of symptoms, although they usually develop within 14 days of injury. Non-specific symptoms such as restlessness, irritability and headache are the first to occur, and the commonest presenting complaints are stiffness in the jaw, the abdomen and the back, which is accompanied by difficulty in swallowing. There may be a low-grade fever, tachycardia, profuse sweating, brisk tendon reflexes and sustained clonus. Tetanus can usually be differentiated from other causes of intra-abdominal pathology by the presence of symptoms in other muscle groups.

DRUG-INDUCED ABDOMINAL PAIN

Quinine, chlorpromazine and primaquine may produce abdominal pain in the absence of other symptoms, and this may be mistaken for an acute abdomen.[207] Oral contraceptives predispose to mesenteric venous thrombosis, which can also cause abdominal pain (see Ch. 27). Corticosteroids can produce referred pain in the abdomen as a result of osteoporosis and crush fractures of the vertebral bodies.

MÜNCHAUSEN'S SYNDROME

There is a small group of patients with a strange psychological abnormality that leads them to feign symptoms and signs of the acute abdomen to fulfil a desire to expose themselves to surgery.[208–210] Many are itinerant drug abusers who crave attention and delight in baffling their medical attendants. The

REFERENCES

206. Oaton A. Br Med J 1976; 2: 1179
207. Pearson KD, Buchingnal JS et al. Am J Roentgenol 1972; 116: 256
208. Steligmann E, Singer HA. Am J Med Sci 1936; 192: 67
209. Witherbee HR, Oearce ML. Ann Intern Med 1958; 49: 876
210. Loolff L. J Med 1917; 294: 965

condition should be suspected if the level of pain appears out of keeping with the signs, if there are many abdominal scars, or if there is a history of 'failed' operations, unhealed wounds or fistulae, all occurring at another hospital. It is vital to obtain a clear history from the other hospitals visited by Münchausen's patients, because some do the rounds of many institutions before being found out. Psychiatrists appear to be of little help in managing this condition.

The stomach and duodenum

26

Robert C. Mason, John W.L. Fielding

INTRODUCTION

The recognition of the importance of *Helicobacter pylori* and its eradication, together with improved endoscopic techniques, has greatly diminished the role of surgery in the management of peptic ulceration. Recent changes in the distribution of gastric cancer in western countries, with a reduction in antral cancer and an increase in proximal disease, have not reduced the importance of surgery, but have raised questions about the need for adjuvant chemoradiotherapy in their treatment.

CONGENITAL ABNORMALITIES

Congenital abnormalities of the stomach and duodenum, apart from pyloric stenosis, are rare and include duplication, atresia, diverticula, the presence of ectopic mucosa, and megaduodenum or superior mesenteric artery entrapment syndrome.

Diverticula of the duodenum are more common than in the stomach. They develop at the insertion of the ampulla of Vater in 60% of cases, making cannulation of the bile and pancreatic ducts extremely difficult at endoscopic retrograde cholangiopancreatography. They rarely cause symptoms and should be left alone, because surgical excision can be hazardous, especially if the diverticulum lies within the head of the pancreas.[1]

Ectopic pancreatic tissue within the stomach wall rarely produces symptoms, although it can become inflamed and ulcerate. It may be confused with gastric cancer. Ectopic pancreas within the duodenum may encircle the second part of the duodenum as an annular pancreas, and is caused by abnormal rotation of the ventral bud of the pancreas. Patients present with recurrent vomiting, obstruction and, in 20% of cases, peptic ulceration.[2] These symptoms are exacerbated by pancreatitis within the annular tissue. Upper gastrointestinal endoscopy is usually normal, but the diagnosis can be made by a barium meal that demonstrates a smooth, constant constriction of the duodenum. For treatment, see Chapter 31.

Megaduodenum as the result of compression of the third part of the duodenum by the superior mesenteric vessels is another rare cause of a high intestinal obstruction, and the diagnosis is again made by barium meal.[3] Treatment is as for annular pancreas.

The differential diagnosis for both these rare conditions is malignant duodenal obstruction from a primary duodenal carcinoma, pancreatic carcinoma (especially arising in the uncinate process) and renal cell carcinoma.

Rarely, hypertrophic pyloric stenosis can present in adult life with vomiting and the finding of a smooth, narrowed pyloric canal and no ulcer. Malignancy must then be excluded before treatment with balloon dilatation or, if this fails, pyloroplasty.[3]

PEPTIC ULCERATION

The true incidence of gastric and duodenal ulceration is impossible to ascertain, because the majority of acute ulcers never reach medical attention, resolving rapidly or being treated with non-prescription medications. Evidence from autopsies suggests that approximately 20% of men and 10% of women have suffered from peptic ulcers at some time in their life.[4]

Many factors have been associated with the development of peptic ulceration,[5] including socioeconomic class, blood groups, stress, smoking, excess alcohol ingestion, duodenogastric reflux, ingestion of non-steroidal anti-inflammatory agents and steroids, burns (Curling's ulcer and neurotrauma) and Cushing's ulcer, but the most important by far is infection with *H. pylori*. The original observation that 'no acid equals no peptic ulcer' still holds true, and all ulcers originate as the result of an imbalance between the production of luminal acid and pepsin and the ability of the mucosa to resist damage and repair itself.

Before discussing the treatment of peptic ulceration, it is important to understand the basic physiology of the gastric and duodenal mucosa. The factors controlling acid secretion and mucosal defences are summarized in Figs 26.1 and 26.2. Acid secretion is stimulated by the vagus and gastrin by a direct action on the parietal cell or via their joint action on the intermediate enterochromaffin-like cell. Acid secretion is inhibited by the vagus and by the somatostatin cell under the influence of cholecystokinin.[6]

Mucosal defences fall into three categories: extramucosal, mucosal and microvascular. The extramucosal factors include the mucus cap and secreted bicarbonate.[7] It is now thought that the mucus does not form a sheet in normal conditions, but forms ropes that coalesce when the mucosa is damaged to protect the repair processes outlined further in this chapter.[8] Mucosal factors include the increased resistance to acid of the luminal surface of the epithelial cells, mucosal integrity, and the presence of tight junctions between cells.[9] These are influenced by luminal growth factors, which include mucosal integrity peptides (e.g.

REFERENCES

1. Afridi S et al. Am J Gastroenterol 1991; 86: 935
2. Thomford N et al. Ann Surg 1972; 176: 159
3. Hiebert B, Farris A. Am Surg 1966; 32: 712
4. Watkinson G. Gut 1960; 1: 14
5. Langman MJS. In: Misiewicz JJ, Pounder RE, Venables CW (eds). Diseases of the Gut and Pancreas. 2nd edn. Blackwell, London, 1994: 249
6. Hersey SJ, Sachs G. Physiol Rev 1995; 75: 155
7. Rees WDW, Turnberg LA. Clin Sci 1982; 62: 343
8. Morris GP et al. Virchows Arch B Cell Pathol Incl Mol Pathol 1984; 46: 239
9. Sanders MJ et al. Nature 1985; 313: 52

transforming growth factor-α) that maintain epithelial integrity, luminal surveillance peptides (e.g. epidermal growth factor) that act via a receptor on the basal surface of epithelial cells and when damage occurs stimulate proliferation, and rapid response peptides (e.g. the trefoil peptides) that stimulate cell migration.[10] The most important factor governing mucosal resistance is probably the microcirculation.[11] This is responsible for the alkaline tide that neutralizes acid and transports away toxic substances. Prostaglandins, neuropeptides and nitric oxide are important in maintaining this microcirculation, and factors that interfere with them increase ulcer risk.[12]

Damage to the mucosa above the basement membrane repairs by a process of restitution, in which cells migrate from the germinal zone to cover the defect.[13] This process does not require mitosis and can occur in 3–4 h, but is dependent on prostaglandins and an intact microcirculation. Deeper injury, breaching the basement membrane, produces an inflammatory response; healing is then by secondary intention, which involves mitosis in which epidermal growth factor has a role. This produces scar tissue and takes 4–5 days to heal over.[12]

HELICOBACTER PYLORI

The presence of spiral organisms in the gastric mucosa was first recognized over 50 years ago, but the significance of this infection was appreciated only in the early 1980s.[14] *Helicobacter pylori* is an organism that has a worldwide distribution, and its prevalence increases with age, with approximately half of the population over 60 years old showing evidence of infection.[15] It is thought to produce problems as a result of its direct cytotoxic effect on gastric mucosal epithelial cells, which produces an acute inflammatory response. It is also thought to produce hypergastrinaemia and hyperchlorhydria by interference in the somatostatin suppression of gastrin secretion.[16] The association between infection with *H. pylori* and acute gastritis is strong, and antral infection can be demonstrated in over 90% of patients with duodenal ulcers and 66% of patients with gastric ulcers. The means of diagnosis are shown in Table 26.1. Eradication results in substantial ulcer healing and reduces the risk of recurrence. The risk of reinfection in adults is less than 1% per annum.[17] The success for eradication is in excess of 90% and should be confirmed by repeat breath testing.[18]

Debate exists as to whether to eradicate asymptomatic *H. pylori.* To do so would prevent the development of peptic ulceration and possibly reduce the incidence of distal gastric cancer. Eradication does, however, increase the incidence of gastro-oesophageal reflux and thus may well increase the incidence of Barrett's cancer of the gastro-oesophageal junction. Opinion is evenly split.

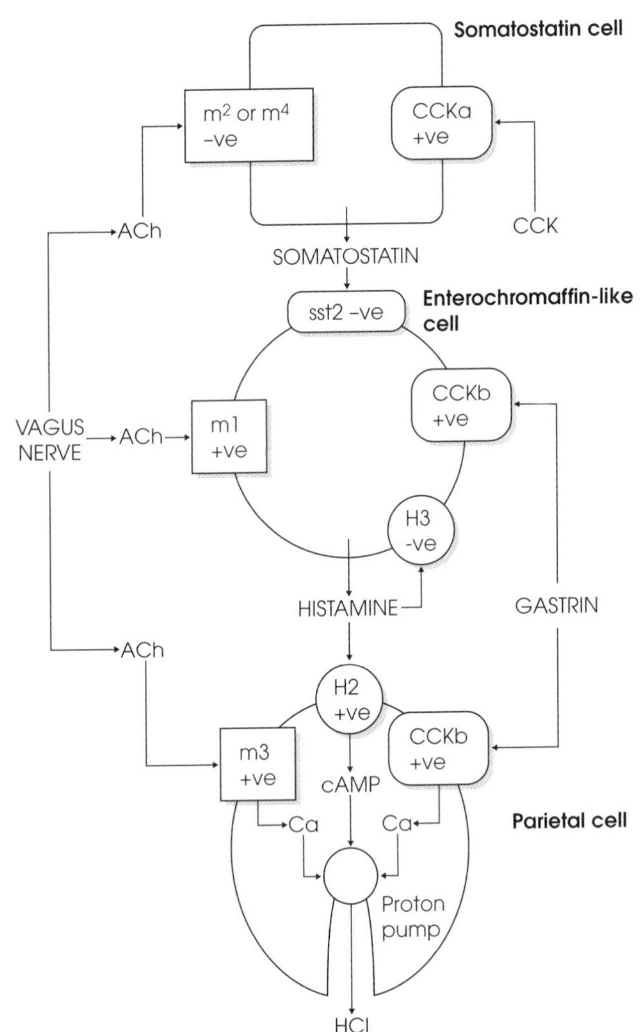

Figure 26.1 Control of acid secretion by the stomach.

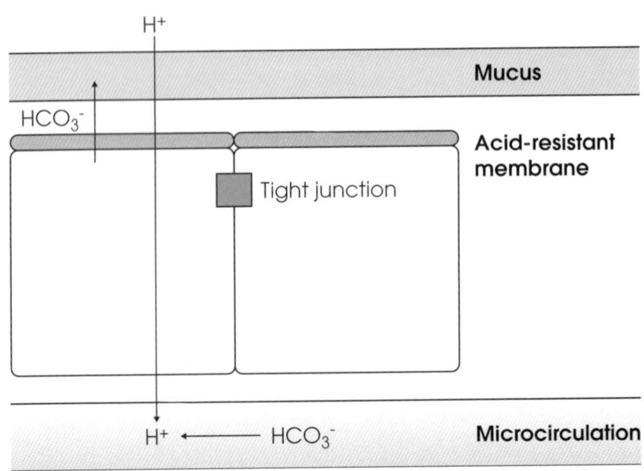

Figure 26.2 Mechanism of the mucosal defence to luminal acid.

DISTRIBUTION

Gastric ulcers classically present at the incisura on the lesser curve at the junction of the body and antral mucosa. They can be divided into:

- type I gastric ulcers, the classical site of which is at the incisura;

REFERENCES

10. Wright NA et al. Nature 1990; 343: 82
11. O'Brien P. In: Splanchnic Ischaemia and Multiple Organ Failure. Edward Arnold, London, 1990: 145
12. Whittle BJR. In: Gustavson S, Kumar D, Graham DY (eds). The Stomach. Churchill Livingstone, Edinburgh, 1992: 81
13. Silen W, Ito S. Ann Rev Physiol 1985; 47: 217
14. Marshall BJ, Warren JR. Lancet 1984; ii: 1311
15. Colin Jones D. In: Misiewicz JJ, Pounder RE, Venables CW (eds). Diseases of the Gut and Pancreas. 2nd edn. Blackwell, London, 1994: 261
16. Moss S, Callum J. Gut 1992; 33: 289
17. Graham DY et al. Ann Intern Med 1992; 116: 705
18. Hosking SW. Lancet 1994; 343: 508

Table 26.1 Tests for *Helicobacter pylori*

	Sensitivity (%)	Specificity (%)
Serology	90	90
^{13}C urea breath test	95	99
Histology	90	95
Urease test	90	99

- type II, which are associated with a duodenal ulcer; and
- type III, which are prepyloric ulcers.

The latter two behave like duodenal ulcers.

Duodenal ulcers normally develop in the duodenal bulb. Ulcers occurring in the second part of the duodenum and beyond should raise the suspicion of Zollinger–Ellison syndrome (see Ch. 31). Peptic ulcers in the distal small bowel result from ectopic mucosa in a Meckel's diverticulum (see Ch. 27).

PRESENTATION AND DIAGNOSIS

Patients with peptic ulcer classically present with dyspepsia. Few patients with gastric ulcer, however, present with the classical picture of pain coming on while eating, which is relieved by vomiting, nor do all patients with duodenal ulcer complain of hunger pain relieved by food, which may wake them in the early hours of the morning. Such dyspeptic symptoms exhibit periodicity and are more common in spring and autumn. Although some patients with peptic ulcer have symptoms that have little association with eating, on close questioning the majority of patients will have some association between their pain and food. When this link is lost and constant background pain and weight loss are present, gastric cancer must be excluded. The fact that early gastric cancer can cause symptoms similar to benign ulceration strengthens the argument for the investigation of all new patients with dyspepsia prior to commencing treatment, especially if they are over 40 years of age.

Other and not infrequent presentations include waterbrash, epigastric tenderness, and the complications of benign peptic ulceration. These complications include haemorrhage, which may be either overt as haematemesis and melaena or occult blood loss presenting with iron-deficiency anaemia. Patients may also present with an acute abdomen as the result of perforation, or gastric outlet obstruction causing vomiting or heartburn. The change of a benign gastric ulcer into a malignant one is now thought to be extremely rare. Such malignant ulcers were probably malignant all along.

DIFFERENTIAL DIAGNOSIS

Almost any condition in the chest and upper abdomen can mimic the symptoms of peptic ulceration, including myocardial infarction, pulmonary embolus and lower lobe pneumonia. Common conditions include gallstones, cholecystitis, acute and chronic pancreatitis, gastric cancer, gastro-oesophageal reflux, non-ulcer or non-gallstone dyspepsia, irritable bowel syndrome and mesenteric ischaemia.

DIAGNOSIS

The clinical diagnosis of peptic ulcer is confirmed by endoscopy (Fig. 26.3). Multiple biopsies must be taken in all cases of gastric ulcer to ensure that a cancer is not missed. This is especially important in cases of gastric ulcer at sites other than the incisura.

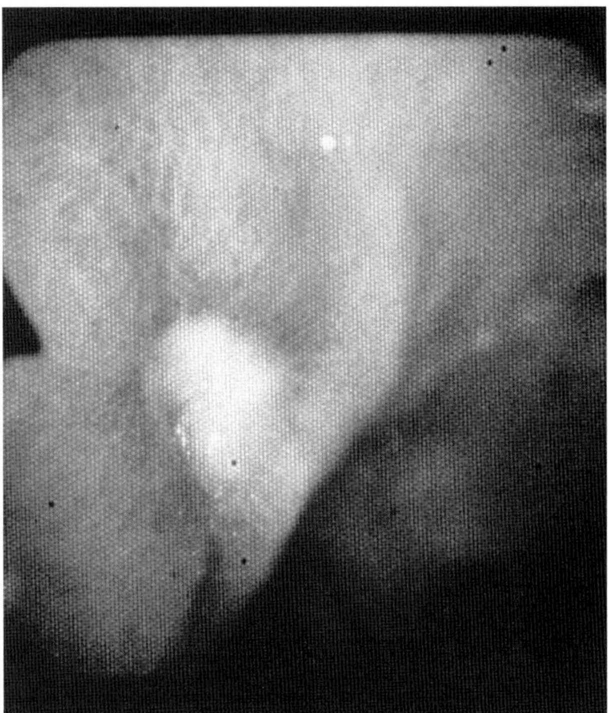

Figure 26.3 A large duodenal ulcer in the first part of the duodenum.

An antral or duodenal biopsy for *H. pylori* should be taken in all cases. The only role for acid secretory studies is in suspected cases of Zollinger–Ellison syndrome (see Ch. 31).

TREATMENT

All peptic ulcers should receive medical treatment with eradication therapy. The current first-line therapy for the eradication of *H. pylori* is 7 days of a proton pump inhibitor (omeprazole or lansoprazole) and any two of amoxicillin, clarithromycin or metronidazole.[19] Other drugs in common use are H_2 receptor antagonists and bismuth, but the success of eradication therapy makes these treatments largely redundant. The main use for H_2 receptor antagonists is to prevent ulceration in patients who have to continue with steroids or non-steroidal anti-inflammatory drugs.

There is no need for surgery in uncomplicated peptic ulcer disease. Patients must be advised to stop smoking and if possible to avoid the use of non-steroidal anti-inflammatory drugs, because failure to do so will increase the incidence of relapse.

SURGERY FOR NON-COMPLICATED PEPTIC ULCER

With the advent of eradication therapy, gastric operations have almost been consigned to history and are used only to treat some of the complications outlined below. The rationale of gastric surgery was to reduce acid secretion by either vagotomy or gastric resection in the case of duodenal ulcer, or to remove susceptible mucosa by gastric resection in the case of gastric ulcer. The operations are shown in Figs 26.4, 26.5 and 26.6.

REFERENCES

19. Malfertheiner P et al. Eur J Gastroenterol Hepatol 1997; 9: 1

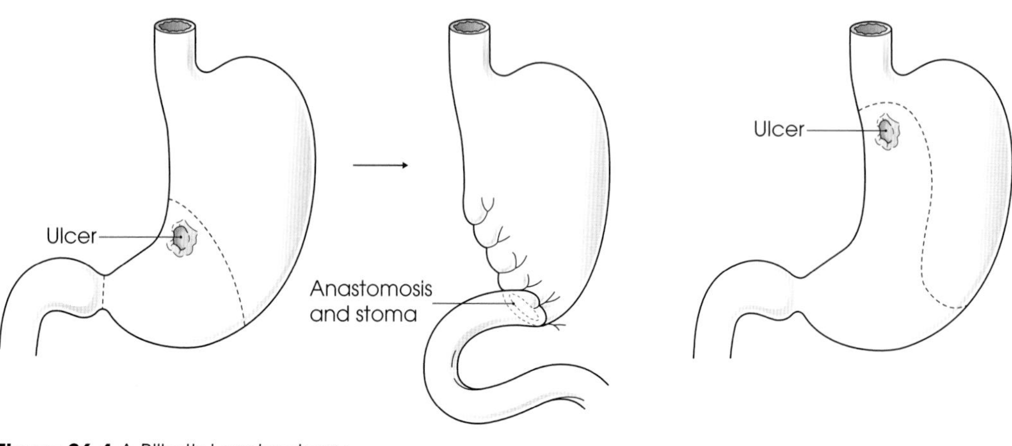

Figure 26.5 Modification of the Billroth I gastrectomy for a high, lesser-curve gastric ulcer.

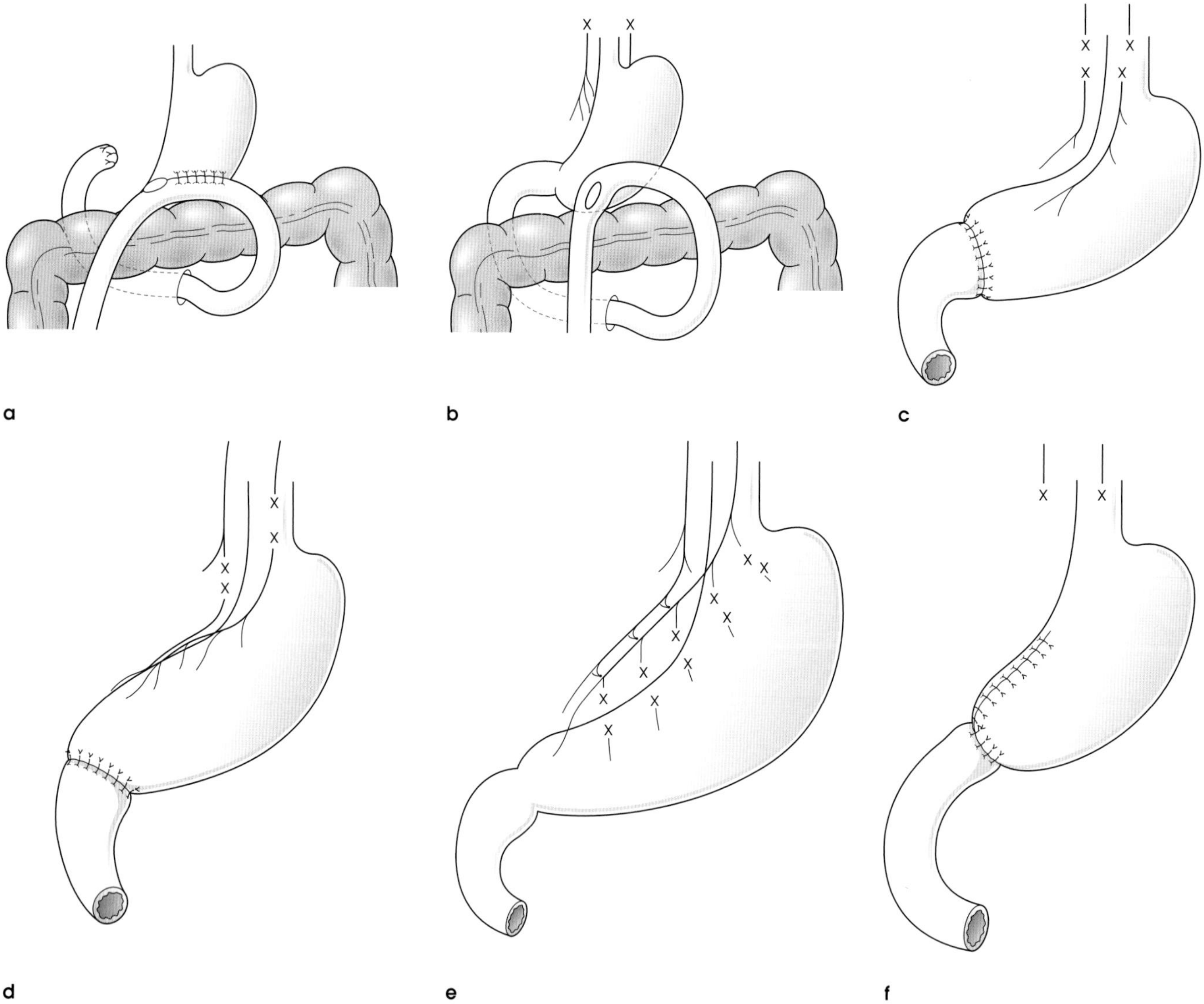

Figure 26.4 A Billroth I gastrectomy.

Figure 26.6 Operations for duodenal ulcer: (**a**) Billroth II gastrectomy; (**b**) truncal vagotomy and gastrojejunostomy; (**c**) truncal vagotomy and pyloroplasty; (**d**) selective vagotomy and pyloroplasty; (**e**) highly selective vagotomy; and (**f**) truncal vagotomy and antrectomy.

COMPLICATIONS OF PEPTIC ULCERATION

Complications of peptic ulcers include ulcer recurrence, haemorrhage, perforation, obstruction, malignant change in a benign ulcer, and fistulation into an adjacent viscus.

RECURRENCE

As mentioned in the earlier section on medical management, it is now possible to heal practically all peptic ulcers with *H. pylori* eradication therapy.[20] It is important to ensure that eradication has been achieved, because this reduces the risk of recurrence to very low levels, especially if causative factors other than *H. pylori* are removed, such as smoking, steroids and non-steroidal anti-inflammatory drugs. In some cases repeat eradication may be required using other combinations of drugs, including bismuth, H_2 receptor antagonists and metronidazole. It is advisable that bacteriological confirmation and sensitivity should be obtained in these cases by sending a fresh biopsy for culture. Recurrence of peptic ulcers after surgery is treated in the same way. When recurrent ulcers do occur after surgery and/or full-dose medical treatment, two possibilities must be considered: the retention of a small area of antrum after gastrectomy (Fig. 26.7) and Zollinger–Ellison syndrome. In the former, this isolated pouch of antrum not exposed to acid will continue to excrete gastrin because of the loss of negative feedback on the G-cells from luminal acid.

ZOLLINGER–ELLISON SYNDROME

Zollinger–Ellison syndrome is characterized by high levels of circulating gastrin and is usually the result of a gastrin-secreting tumour of the islet cells of the pancreas (see Ch. 31). The tumour is rarely in the duodenum or gastric antrum. The condition often presents as intractable duodenal ulceration with a high incidence of bleeding and perforation. Zollinger–Ellison syndrome is associated with multiple endocrine neoplasia type 1, with adenoma of the parathyroids in approximately 25% of cases and hyperplasia of the adrenal and thyroid in 10%. The fasting gastrin level in the blood is in excess of 100 pg/mL. This on its own is not sufficient to make the diagnosis, because any condition producing hypochlorhydria may produce elevated levels of gastrin. The diagnosis is confirmed by acid secretion tests that show high levels of resting acid secretion (greater than 15 mEq/h) that do not increase with administration of pentagastrin. Differentiation between a G-cell tumour and G-cell hyperplasia, in which high gastrin is associated with high acid secretion, can be made by the use of a secretin test, in which a rise in serum gastrin (greater than 200 pg/mL) in response to a bolus of secretin (2 IU/kg body weight) is diagnostic of a gastrinoma.[21]

Gastrinomas can be difficult to localize, because they are frequently invisible on CT scanning of the pancreas. In addition, selective venous sampling has little to offer. The best methods of localization are probably intraoperative or endoluminal ultrasound, or somatostatin receptor scintigraphy.[22]

Treatment is directed towards resection of the pancreatic tumour if it can be localized, because the majority of such tumours are malignant.[23] Blind pancreatectomy is not advised if the tumour cannot be found. Treatment is then directed at the target organ (the stomach) and acid secretion is suppressed by full-dose treatment with proton pump inhibitors. The need for total gastrectomy has largely disappeared.[24]

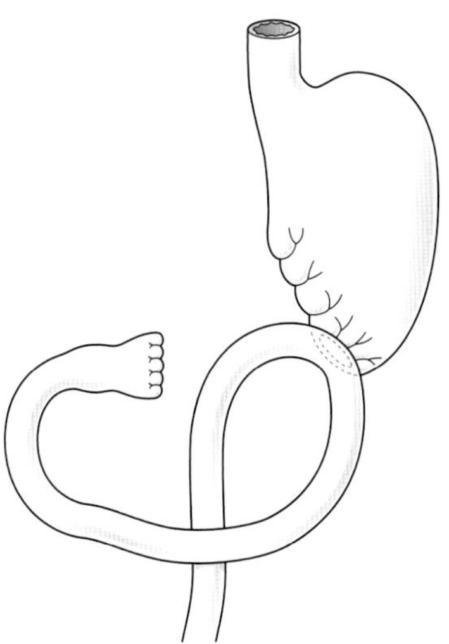

Figure 26.7 Retention of a small antral pouch following Billroth II gastrectomy.

HAEMORRHAGE FROM PEPTIC ULCERS

This complication is now the major cause of death from peptic ulceration.[25] It must be noted that bleeding can be overt (haematemesis and melaena) or occult, presenting with iron-deficient anaemia. It is vital to investigate the large bowel even if a cause for the bleeding is found in the stomach or duodenum, because dual pathology may be present and cancer of the colon is a common finding.[26]

Acute and chronic peptic ulcers and erosions account for over 80% of all cases of upper gastrointestinal haemorrhage (Table 26.2). The other causes include gastric malignancy, angiodysplasia of the stomach, Dieulafoy's syndrome, oesophageal varices, Mallory–Weiss tears, reflux oesophagitis, haemobilia, aortoduodenal fistulae, and medical conditions resulting in thrombocytopenia and coagulopathies. Factors from the history and examination—signs of liver failure (jaundice and ascites); a history of peptic ulceration; ingestion of non-steroidal anti-inflammatory drugs, steroids and anticoagulants; or the presence of blood or melaena on rectal examination—may point to a diagnosis, but it should be remembered that patients with known

Table 26.2 Causes of upper gastrointestinal bleeding

	Cases (%)
Peptic ulcers and erosions	80
Oesophageal varices	8
Oesophagitis	5
Gastro-oesophageal cancer	5
Angiodysplasia	2

REFERENCES

20. Lind T et al. Helicobacter 1996; 1: 138
21. McGuigan JE, Wolfe MM. Gastroenterology 1980; 79: 1324
22. de Kerviler E et al. Eur J Nucl Med 1994; 21: 1191
23. Fraker D et al. Ann Surg 1994; 220: 320
24. Metz DC et al. In: Recent Advances in Research and Management. Karger, Basel, 1995: 240
25. Taylor TV. Br J Surg 1989; 76: 427
26. Cook IJ et al. Br Med J 1986; 292: 1380

cirrhosis and varices are as likely to be bleeding from an ulcer as from varices.[27]

Management of upper gastrointestinal haemorrhage

The immediate management is the same for all patients. The degree of shock should be assessed, and the patient resuscitated. In unstable patients more invasive monitoring is required, and a central venous pressure line and urinary catheter are inserted. A nasogastric tube is passed to empty the stomach and check for evidence of fresh blood.

Investigation

Upper gastrointestinal endoscopy is the most important investigation in these patients. Various stigmata seen on endoscopy can predict for the risk of further haemorrhage. These are the presence of an actively bleeding vessel, a blood clot that is adherent to the ulcer base, and seeing a 'visible vessel'.[28,29]

Debate exists as to when endoscopy should be performed: either immediately or within 24 h.

Endoscopy should be obtained without delay if the patient is actively bleeding, requires continued transfusion of intravenous fluid in excess of 350 mL/h to maintain a satisfactory blood pressure, or has a high likelihood of oesophageal varices. Because of the risk of inhalation of blood and gastric fluids, this should be performed in theatre with adequate suction and resuscitation equipment available, or preferably after a 'crash' general anaesthetic with endotracheal intubation.[30]

In 90% of patients, however, the bleeding stops and the patient responds to simple resuscitation. In this situation it is safe to wait at least 6 h for the stomach to empty before endoscoping the patient under sedation on an elective endoscopy list.

In a small percentage of patients with persistent gastrointestinal haemorrhage, no source of bleeding is found on endoscopy. In this situation, rigid sigmoidoscopy must be performed and, if blood is seen coming from above, the patient is further investigated by radioisotope scanning with chromium-labelled red cells and, if this shows a site of bleeding, with selective mesenteric angiography (Fig. 26.8).[31,32] In young adults, when a Meckel's diverticulum with ectopic gastric mucosa is suspected, a technetium scan is indicated (see Ch. 27).

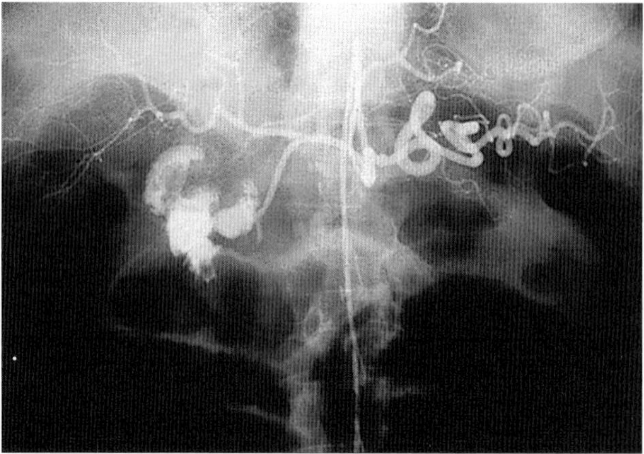

Figure 26.8 Mesenteric angiogram showing bleeding from the gastroduodenal artery.

Treatment of bleeding from peptic ulcers

Medical

The recognition of the importance of eradication therapy dictates that all patients should be treated with these drugs by either the oral or the intravenous route to reduce the incidence of rebleeding by promoting ulcer healing. Non-steroidal drugs should be stopped.

Endoscopic

Endoscopic treatment is the main method of controlling bleeding while ulcer healing is achieved. There are now several techniques by which the endoscopist can arrest haemorrhage from peptic ulcers and prevent rebleeding.[33] These include the use of a heater probe, laser to the ulcer, and injection of sclerosants and adrenaline (epinephrine) to the ulcer base. There are series showing significant improvements in outcome with all these techniques. The simplest technique, and one that should be available in any endoscopy unit, is to inject 1 in 1000 adrenaline (up to 10 mL) in and around the ulcer using a needle used to inject oesophageal varices. This technique is especially useful in treating Dieulafoy's syndrome, which is a localized angiodysplasia where a single vessel projects through apparently normal mucosa.

Radiological

In rare cases where the source of bleeding can be identified only on angiography, selective embolization may be possible, although care must be taken not to produce ischaemic bowel.[34]

Surgery

The decision about on whom to operate and when can be taken only by experienced surgeons. The absolute indication for surgery is persistent uncontrolled haemorrhage. Other indications include rebleeding and the presence of a large chronic ulcer with stigmata, which indicate a high probability of rebleeding, especially if the patient is over 50 years of age. Surgery in this latter group should be undertaken on the first available elective list.

The operation of choice for actively bleeding duodenal ulcers is to open the duodenum and under-run the ulcer with a long-lasting but absorbable suture such as 20-polyglycolate. This must be combined with eradication therapy. Advocates of a Billroth II partial gastrectomy can point to a slight reduction in rebleeding but expose the patient to an increase in mortality.[35]

The operation of choice for bleeding gastric ulcers is a Billroth II partial gastrectomy, but if the patient's condition is too poor, exclusion of the ulcer with large polydioxone sulphate sutures can be life-saving.

PERFORATED PEPTIC ULCERS

The incidence of this complication is approximately 0.5% per year (0.8% in males, 0.3% in females), which compares with 2.8%

REFERENCES

27. Waldram R et al. Br Med J 1974; 4: 94
28. Foster DN et al. Br Med J 1978; 1: 1173
29. Storey DW et al. N Engl J Med 1981; 305: 915
30. Whorewell PJ et al. Digestion 1981; 21: 18
31. Alavi A, Rung EJ. Am J Roentgenol 1981; 137: 741
32. Allison DJ et al. Lancet 1982; ii: 30
33. Steele RJC. Br J Surg 1989; 76: 219
34. Eckstein MR et al. Radiology 1984; 152: 643
35. Schiller KFR. Br Med J 1970; 2: 7

per year for bleeding.[36] The patient usually presents with peritonitis (see Ch. 25), but there are a significant number of silent perforations found on erect chest X-rays, usually in old women taking non-steroidal anti-inflammatory drugs. These should be treated medically. The diagnosis of a perforated peptic ulcer is confirmed by an erect chest X-ray that demonstrates free gas under the diaphragm. At least 10% of patients with a perforated duodenal ulcer do not have any free gas, because only fluid escapes through the perforation. Patients usually also have a small increase in serum amylase (less than 100 units/mL). The differential diagnosis is from acute cholecystitis, acute pancreatitis, perforated appendicitis and acute sigmoid diverticulitis (see Ch. 28).

Treatment

The treatment is surgical, except in cases of silent perforations. The decision to operate is taken on clinical grounds (an acute abdomen), preferably supported by the finding of free gas under the diaphragm. The patient must be fully resuscitated before operation with intravenous fluids, a nasogastric tube, adequate analgesia and intravenous antibiotics. The operation of choice for a perforated duodenal ulcer is patching with greater omentum loosely tied over the hole. This must be associated with full peritoneal lavage and be followed by eradication therapy.[37,38]

The use of the laparoscope to treat perforated duodenal ulcer is now being advocated. It is certainly feasible to close the defect with intracorporeal suturing, but the extent of the lavage remains to be determined.

Perforated gastric ulcers should be treated by Billroth II gastrectomy if the patient's condition permits. The ulcer can be excised if the patient is unfit and the defect closed. The patient is treated with eradication therapy in the postoperative period. In all such cases the ulcer should be biopsied to exclude a cancer.

Complications of perforated peptic ulcer include intra-abdominal abscess formation (especially subphrenic abscess), prolonged ileus and associated haemorrhage.

GASTRIC OUTFLOW OBSTRUCTION (PYLORIC STENOSIS)

Cases of gastric outflow obstruction from peptic ulceration present with weight loss and projectile vomiting. A pyloric stenosis may be caused by a duodenal ulcer adjacent to the pyloric canal or by a prepyloric ulcer of the gastric antrum. Patients with long-standing pyloric stenosis have a hypokalaemic metabolic alkalosis. This must be corrected with intravenous normal saline with added potassium. The metabolic alkalosis corrects itself once the hypokalaemia is corrected. A nasogastric tube is passed to empty the stomach, which may contain over 1 L of gastric contents. The majority of pyloric stenosis resolve by medical treatment and balloon dilatation of the pylorus.[39,40] If this approach fails, the operations of choice are a pyloroplasty or gastrojejunostomy if the stricturing is marked. These are followed by eradication therapy. Prolonged postoperative nasogastric decompression may be needed if the obstruction is of long standing, and peripheral vein intravenous nutrition may also be necessary.

Obstruction of the body of the stomach by large saddle gastric ulcers is a rarity and is treated by gastric resection.

MALIGNANT CHANGE

Duodenal ulcers never turn malignant. Whether gastric ulcers do remains a matter of debate. If they do, the risk is probably less than 1%, although gastric ulcers initially diagnosed as benign may later turn out to be malignant as a result of the initial biopsy being taken from the wrong place.[41]

Table 26.3 Visick grading

Grade	Symptoms
I	No symptoms
II	Mild symptoms relieved by care*
IIIs	Mild symptoms not relieved by care* but satisfactory
IIIu†	Mild symptoms not relieved by care* and unsatisfactory
IV†	Not improved

*'By care' is now meant medical treatment.
†Grade IIIu and IV are considered treatment failures.

Table 26.4 Complications of surgery for peptic ulcer

	Truncal vagotomy and drainage (%)	Billroth II gastrectomy (%)
Diarrhoea	7	16
Dumping	11	14
Bile vomiting	5	10
Anaemia	27	38

FISTULATION

Fistulation is a rare complication of peptic ulcers. Gastric ulcers can fistulate into pancreas and transverse colon and duodenal ulcers into the gall bladder. They should be treated by appropriate surgical resection and anastamosis.

POSTGASTRECTOMY SYNDROMES

Postgastrectomy syndromes include the complications of vagotomy and gastric resection, and those resulting from the excision or bypassing of the pylorus. The presence of these complications, together with the incidence of recurrent ulceration, can be quantified using a Visick grade, which is a subjective scoring system based on the patients' symptoms (Table 26.3).[42] The incidence of these complications is hard to quantify, but they tend to occur more frequently in patients who have undergone gastric resection than in those who have had truncal vagotomy and drainage (Table 26.4). Revisional surgery is a last resort, and the principle that should be applied is to return the anatomy as far as possible to normal.

They fall into the following groups:

- Deficiencies: malnutrition, anaemia (iron and vitamin B_{12}) and calcium deficiency.

REFERENCES

36. Pulvertaft CN. Postgrad Med J 1968; 44: 59
37. Abbasakoor F et al. Irish Med J 1995; 88: 207
38. Ng EKW et al. Ann Surg 2000; 231: 153
39. Griffin SM et al. Br J Surg 1989; 76: 1147
40. Chisholm EM et al. Gastrointest Endosc 1993; 37: 240
41. Mountford RA. Gut 1980; 21: 9
42. Visick AH. Ann R Coll Surg Engl 1948; 3: 266

- Dumping: early and late.
- Diarrhoea.
- Disordered motility: delayed gastric emptying, afferent loop syndrome and increased risk of gallstones.
- Duodenogastric reflux.
- Gastric stump carcinoma.
- Increased incidence of infection.

Deficiencies

Most patients who undergo any type of partial gastrectomy fail to regain their preoperative weight.[43] This is the result of a small stomach and early satiety, together with rapid gastric emptying and rapid intestinal transit. This usually improves with time, and sensible patients alter their eating habit, taking frequent small meals and eating dry food separately from liquids. The need for surgical correction is rare. Any surgery should be delayed for at least a year and only be undertaken after full assessment by barium and gastric-emptying studies. An entero-enterostomy performed below the gastrojejunal anastomosis can help if there is a long afferent loop and failure of the food to mix with the duodenal juices. Patients with a high Billroth II gastrectomy and a tiny gastric remnant preventing any sizeable intake of food may be converted to a total gastrectomy with improvement.[44] Patients with malnutrition following a total gastrectomy combined with a Roux-en-Y reconstruction may be improved by interposing a jejunal pouch between the oesophagus and duodenum (Fig. 26.9).[45,46]

Hypochlorhydria interferes with the absorption of iron and calcium. This can easily be corrected by dietary supplementation. Deficiency of vitamin B_{12} invariably develops after a total gastrectomy but can occur in patients who have undergone partial resection. This is corrected by 3-monthly injections of 1 mg of hydroxocobalamin. This should be started before patients who have had a total gastrectomy are discharged.

Dumping

Dumping is a disabling complication of gastric surgery that affects approximately a fifth of all patients after gastrectomy and a 10th of all patients following a pyloroplasty. There are two main patterns of dumping: early and late.

Early

Early dumping occurs approximately 30 min after eating, and is the result of the rapid gastric emptying of a hyperosmolar meal into the small intestine shortly after or during eating. This results in fluid leaking from the splanchnic circulation into the intestinal lumen, producing third-space losses and hypovolaemia, together with the release of vasoactive peptides. This causes weakness, faintness, dizziness, sweating, palpitations and a sensation of abdominal distension. Late symptoms include cramps and diarrhoea.

This can be confirmed by using a dumping provocation test, which involves serial measurements of the haematocrit in patients given a provocation meal.[47] The complication usually improves with time and is helped by modification of the diet and lying down. There is no role for revisional surgery.[48]

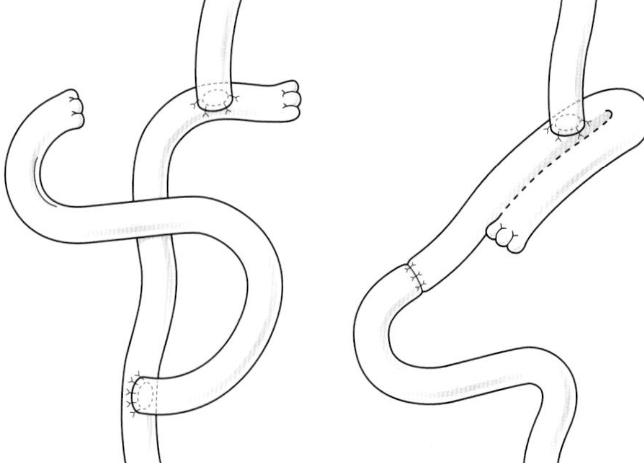

Figure 26.9 Reconstruction following a total gastrectomy and Roux-en-Y by means of a jejunal pouch between the oesophagus and duodenum.

Late

Late dumping results from an inappropriate hyperinsulinaemia after the glucose load has passed, comes on 1–2 h after food, and is the result of hypoglycaemia. This is much less common than early dumping and can be controlled by taking sugar. The symptoms are similar, with weakness, faintness, palpitations and hunger predominating.

Diarrhoea

Mild diarrhoea is a frequent problem after any form of gastric surgery and is usually self-limiting. Severe explosive diarrhoea associated with marked urgency occurs in approximately 20% of patients, and may be the result of early gastric emptying or a small intestine that has lost the controlling influence of the vagus nerve.[43,49] Investigation is by barium meal and follow-through. It may respond to medical management with bulking agents, intestinal sedatives or cholestyramine to bind bile salts. It is worth excluding steatorrhoea, milk allergy and giardiasis. Surgery in the form of reversed loops of jejunum or a reversed ileal patch to slow small bowel transit have been advocated, but the results are disappointing.[50] The risk of developing diarrhoea is substantially increased if a truncal vagotomy is performed in a patient who has previously undergone a cholecystectomy.[51]

Disordered motility

Delayed emptying

Following partial gastrectomy or a vagotomy, many patients experience delayed gastric emptying in the immediate post-operative period.[43] This is a frequent problem following truncal vagotomy, antrectomy and Roux-en-Y anastomosis. The problem is probably related to the loss of the duodenal pacemaker and does not appear to be associated with the size of gastrojejunal anastomosis or, in the case of Billroth II gastrectomy, the type and direction of the gastrojejunal anastomosis. It is also a problem in patients with pre-existing pyloric stenosis who are treated by truncal vagotomy and gastrojejunostomy. Investigation by barium studies can be misleading, because there appears to be a total obstruction at the anastomosis. The investigation of choice is

REFERENCES

43. Tytgat GNJ et al. Hepatogastroenterology 1988; 35: 271
44. Eckhauser FH et al. Ann Surg 1988; 208: 345
45. Cuscheri A. Br J Surg 1982; 69: 386
46. Miholic J et al. Ann Surg 1989; 210: 165
47. Linehan IP et al. Br J Surg 1986; 73: 810
48. Sagar GR et al. Br Med J 1981; 282: 507
49. Condon JR et al. Br J Surg 1975; 62: 309
50. Cuscheri A. Br J Surg 1986; 73: 981
51. Taylor TV et al. Lancet 1978; i: 295

gentle endoscopy at least 1 week after surgery. If there is no physical obstruction encountered at endoscopy, the treatment is to wait and feed the patient parenterally or to insert a long jejunal tube to enable enteral feeding. It can take up to 1 month for the stomach to empty satisfactorily for liquids, and even longer for solids. The temptation to reoperate and refashion the anastomosis should be resisted. Erythromycin, which is a motilium agonist, may be of benefit.

Afferent loop syndrome

Afferent loop syndrome results from kinking or fashioning too long an afferent loop following Polya or Billroth II gastrectomy. The obstruction to the flow of duodenal juices produces sudden epigastric pain, which may be followed by massive bilious vomiting. It should be suspected if a smooth central abdominal mass (the obstructed loop) is felt, and this may be visible on a plain abdominal X-ray. It may be associated with a raised serum amylase. The afferent loop is difficult to enter at endoscopy. Differential diagnoses include acute pancreatitis and high small bowel obstruction.

The condition is corrected by fashioning an entero-enterostomy between the efferent and afferent loops (Fig. 26.10).

Increased incidence of gallstones

This complication appears to result from decreased gall bladder motility following truncal vagotomy. Up to 20% of patients develop this complication 5 years after surgery.[43]

Duodenogastric reflux

Any operation in which the pylorus is bypassed, excised or rendered incompetent can produce duodenogastric reflux. In the majority of cases, this produces no symptoms, but some gastritis is almost always present at the site of reflux.[43] Rarely, this gastritis goes on to produce erosions and bleeds, eventually causing an iron-deficiency anaemia. In a small percentage of cases, reflux of the duodenal contents produces pain in the postprandial period and alkaline gastro-oesophageal reflux. The diagnosis is made by exclusion of other causes of pain, such as recurrent ulcer, and can be confirmed by a provocation test.[52] Revisional surgery should be carried out only if medical treatment with cytoprotective drugs such as sucralfate or cholestyramine, which binds bile salts, have been tried and have failed.

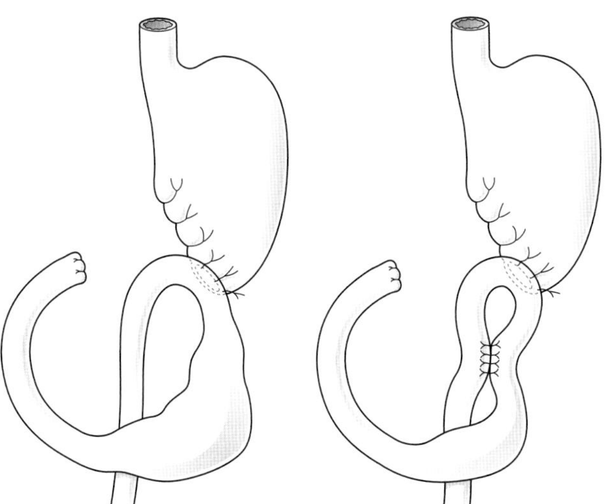

Figure 26.10 Afferent loop syndrome. The afferent and efferent loops are anastomosed side to side below the gastrojejunostomy.

The pyloroplasty can be reversed or a gastrojejunostomy can be taken down in patients who have undergone truncal vagotomy and drainage. This should be carried out only after 1 year has elapsed from the time of surgery, when the stomach will have regained a normal emptying pattern. In patients who have had gastric resection, revisional surgery usually requires conversion to a Roux-en-Y anastomosis with a 50-cm Roux loop to prevent retrograde passage of duodenal contents. This must be combined with a truncal vagotomy or lifetime acid suppression with a proton pump inhibitor to prevent stomal ulceration.

Gastric stump carcinoma

Duodenogastric reflux is associated with an increased incidence of gastric cancer. These cancers occur at the gastrojejunal anastomosis at least 20 years after surgery. The exact cause is unknown but is possibly the result of chronic irritation of the gastric mucosa by duodenal contents.[53] It is also recognized that after a truncal vagotomy there is an increased risk of large bowel cancer, possibly because of excess bile salts reaching the colon.[54]

Increased incidence of infection

There is an association between an increased incidence of pulmonary tuberculosis, gastric mycosis and previous partial gastrectomy. This extremely rare complication is probably the result of a loss of gastric acid, which normally kills the bacterium and fungus.

INFLAMMATION OF THE STOMACH

Acute gastritis can follow any insult to the gastric mucosa by such things as drugs, spicy foods and acute infection with *H. pylori*. This will usually heal when the irritant is removed.

In patients on the intensive care unit, gastrointestinal haemorrhage can occur from acute gastritis, which can progress to widespread superficial gastric erosions. This is the result of mucosal ischaemia failing to sweep away the hydrogen ions that have penetrated the epithelial cells. Prevention of this complication is achieved by maintaining a high intraluminal pH by intravenous proton pump inhibitors, and coating the mucosa with sucralfate or neutralizing the gastric pH with antacids via a nasogastric tube. A total gastrectomy may be required if the bleeding becomes torrential, although the mortality of this is in excess of 80%.[55]

In contrast, chronic gastritis is characterized by a mucosal infiltration with lymphocytes and plasma cells. It is usually persistent and progresses to atrophic gastritis. In most cases this is associated with infection with *H. pylori*. Intestinal metaplasia (type 3) develops in which differentiation is lost; this can be regarded as a form of dysplasia that is associated with an increased risk of gastric cancer.[56,57]

REFERENCES

52. Meshkinpour H et al. Gastroenterology 1980; 79: 1283
53. Clarke CG et al. Br J Surg 1985; 72: 591
54. Mullan FJ et al. Br J Surg 1990; 77: 1085
55. Menguy R et al. Arch Surg 1969; 99: 198
56. Ihamaki T et al. Scand J Gastroenterol 1978; 13: 771
57. Jass JR, Filipe MI. Gastric Carcinoma. Churchill Livingstone, Edinburgh, 1986: 274

The link between the immune system and chronic gastritis has been established in patients with pernicious anaemia in whom anti-intrinsic factor and anti-parietal cell antibodies can be demonstrated. These patients have a fourfold increase in gastric cancer and should have regular surveillance by gastroscopy.[58]

Other forms of gastritis include granulomatous gastritis from Crohn's disease involving the stomach (see Ch. 26) and hyperplastic gastritis of Ménétrier's disease. In Crohn's disease of the stomach there is inflammation and ulceration that may mimic extensive cancer. A biopsy is usually diagnostic if granulomata are seen. Treatment is with high-dose steroids and H_2 receptor antagonists. Ménétrier's disease is characterized by giant enlargement of the gastric rugal folds of the body and fundus of the stomach. The mucosa leaks large volumes of protein; this is associated with reduced levels of acid secretion because of the loss of parietal cells. Patients present with atypical dyspepsia and hypoproteinaemia. They may also, less commonly, develop iron-deficient anaemia as the result of blood loss. There is no increased risk of cancer, and patients are treated symptomatically. Surgery in the form of total gastrectomy is reserved for the few patients with severe hypoproteinaemia.

GASTRIC VOLVULUS

This condition is frequently symptomless and is a chance finding on a barium meal examination. Sudden onset of vomiting and severe epigastric or retrosternal pain are the most common symptoms. Gastric volvulus is invariably associated with a paraoesophageal hiatus hernia, especially if of the organoaxial type (Fig. 26.11). The treatment is surgical and consists of repair of the diaphragmatic defect with fixation of the greater curve of the stomach to the anterior abdominal wall by means of sutures. This can also be achieved by performing a high greater-curve gastrostomy and posterior gastrojejunostomy.[59]

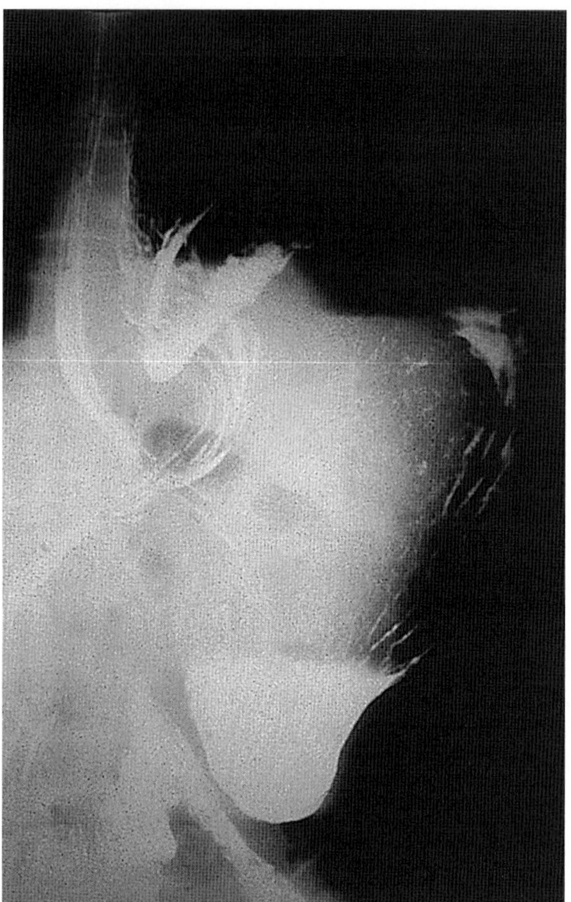

Figure 26.11 Gastric volvulus with associated paraoesophageal hernia.

ACUTE GASTRIC DILATATION

Acute gastric dilatation usually presents as a complication of upper abdominal surgery, especially splenectomy (see Ch. 32). The patient complains of shoulder-tip pain and hiccups. If the condition is not recognized, the patient can rapidly become shocked and may die from massive aspiration of vomit. Treatment is by passage of a wide-bore nasogastric tube. This condition can occur in patients suffering from anorexia nervosa and other psychiatric conditions such as depression, especially when they are prescribed large doses of psychotropic drugs.

TRAUMA TO THE STOMACH AND DUODENUM

These organs are at risk from both sharp and blunt injury (see Ch. 7). In both cases the risk of injury to both stomach and duodenum is increased if the stomach is full at the time of injury. In all cases of gastric and duodenal trauma, care must be taken to exclude injury to other organs.

Sharp injury may be caused by either a stab wound or iatrogenically when a left-sided chest drain is inserted too low. Perforation of the stomach and duodenum by diagnostic and therapeutic endoscopy is virtually never seen, in contrast to oesophageal perforation. Leakage of stomach contents can give rise to local or general peritonitis after a percutaneous endoscopic gastrostomy tube is inserted.

Blunt injury to both the stomach and the duodenum is usually the result of deceleration injuries in road traffic accidents.[60] In the case of gastric trauma, the injury may be full thickness, with a perforation or a contusion presenting with gastric bleeding. This may result in delayed rupture. Repair is dictated by the degree of injury that may require resection.

Duodenal blunt injuries classically involve its third part, which is crushed by the seat belt against the spine. As the escaping contents are contained retroperitoneally, the diagnosis may be delayed. Trauma to the duodenum is invariably associated with injuries to the pancreas (see Ch. 7). If suspected and the patient is stable, contrast-enhanced CT scanning is an important diagnostic tool. If such injury is found it must be repaired surgically, and the stomach drained via a gastrostomy. The patient should receive nutrition via a feeding jejunostomy inserted at operation.

REFERENCES

58. Tytgat GNJ. Misiewicz JJ, Pounder RE, Venables CW (eds). Diseases of the Gut and Pancreas. 2nd edn. Blackwell, London, 1994: 221
59. Otterson MF, Condon RE. In: Wastell C, Nyhus LM, Donahue PE (eds). Surgery of the Esophagus, Stomach and Small Intestine. 5th edn. Little, Brown, New York, 1995: 697
60. Hawkin M, Mullen J. J Trauma 1974; 14: 290

GASTRIC SURGERY FOR MORBID OBESITY

Morbid obesity is defined as a body weight that is 100% greater than the ideal weight. Before contemplating surgery, endocrine disorders and hypothalamic lesions that cause obesity must be excluded. The need to reduce weight is based on the major increase in mortality associated with morbid obesity. There is a 14-fold increase if the patient is 100% above their ideal weight.

The success of diets and psychological modification of eating habits are disappointing in this group. Early surgical procedures to help weight loss are either disappointing (jaw wiring) or have an unacceptable morbidity and mortality (jejunoileal bypass). Current surgical approaches centre on the stomach and are based on suppressing appetite by producing early fullness using a vertical banded gastroplasty or gastric banding. This may be achieved by a combination of reduced gastric capacity with malabsorption produced by a Roux-en-Y gastric bypass or a biliopancreatic bypass.

The importance of full medical and psychological preparation cannot be overstated, and in the postoperative period patients need careful monitoring, because they are at high risk of respiratory and thromboembolic complications. Patients often end up with a degree of malabsorption, and haemoglobin, iron, vitamin B_{12} and calcium should be regularly monitored. All these procedures lead to a loss of excess weight of between 50 and 75% up to 5 years after surgery.[61–63]

NEOPLASMS OF THE STOMACH

Benign and malignant neoplasms originate from any of the elements that make up the stomach or duodenum. The most common neoplasm is adenocarcinoma of the stomach. Because there is a relationship between benign and malignant neoplasms, it is appropriate first to consider adenocarcinoma of the stomach.

ADENOCARCINOMA OF THE STOMACH

Incidence and epidemiology

Unlike other common cancers, the incidence of gastric cancer is falling worldwide. Associated with this fall is a change in distribution, with a reduction in distal antral cancer and a rise in proximal disease. This proximal disease is called Barrett's cancer and has been classified by Siewert into type 1, lower third of the oesophagus; type 2, centred at the oesophagogastric junction; and type 3, proximal gastric.[64] This change affects the intestinal type of cancer, the incidence of diffuse infiltrating disease remaining constant.

These variations in incidence implicate either genetic or environmental factors or both. A study of Japanese migrants to Hawaii demonstrates that the incidence of gastric cancer among first-generation Japanese is similar to that in Japan, but the incidence in second-generation Japanese is significantly lower, although still higher than that seen in North American whites.[65] This alteration may be the result of environmental factors, but because the incidence is not that of the local population it leaves open the question of genetic influences. Insured patients with a family history of gastric cancer have a mortality about a third greater than that of other insured persons, and the risk of stomach cancer is four times greater than among the relatives of non-cancer patients.[66] Gastric cancer is more common in patients with blood group A in the UK, but in Japan is associated with blood group B.[67,68] The existence of a relationship with social class is well established, with the incidence being highest in social classes 3–5.[69]

Aetiology

The role of diet is unclear in the genesis of gastric cancer. In the USA the intake of beef, milk, citrus fruit and green vegetables has increased, while that of potatoes has decreased. In Japan, striking changes in the incidence of gastric cancer have been associated with changes in diet, with a 28-fold increase in the consumption of milk products. There is also a significant inverse relationship between the increase in fatty food and vitamin A and the intake of yellow and green vegetables.[70] There is also a link with the ingestion of nitrate, and a role for nitrate-reducing organisms in the hypochlorhydric stomach is associated with an increased risk of gastric cancer. The Correa hypothesis links the ingestion of nitrate reduced by bacteria to nitrite, which combines with dietary amines to form nitrosamines, which are potent carcinogens. Vitamin C, found in fresh fruit and vegetables, inhibits the bacterial reduction of nitrate as well as being an antioxidant.[71]

There is an association between the incidence of *H. pylori* infection and the incidence of chronic gastritis, intestinal metaplasia, dysplasia and cancer.[72,73] There is no association between *H. pylori* and the proximal gastric or Barrett's cancer, which appears to be associated with gastro-oesophageal reflux and Barrett's metaplasia.[74]

Pathology

Precancerous conditions and lesions

Polyps

Polyps arise in the gastric mucosa and are either hyperplastic or adenomatous. Hyperplastic polyps are covered with well-differentiated glands, and the risk of malignant change is low. In adenomas the epithelium may be dysplastic, and malignant change occurs in 18–75% of these. If the polyp is greater than 2 cm, the incidence of malignant change is increased.[75]

Gastric ulcer

It is now felt that the incidence of malignant change in a benign gastric ulcer is extremely rare (see p. 613) and probably represents an error in diagnosis, with the endoscopic biopsy of the ulcer missing the cancer. In a large Japanese series the incidence of gastric cancer was 7.2% among 1286 patients with gastric ulcer,

REFERENCES

61. Dietel M. World J Surg 1998; 22: 913
62. Scopinaro N et al. Surgery 1996; 119: 261
63. Belachew M. World J Surg 1998; 22: 955
64. Siewert JR et al. Br J Surg 1998; 85: 1457
65. Haenszel W, Karibaru M. J Natl Cancer Inst 1968; 40: 43
66. Lehtola J. Ann Clin Res 1981; 13(3): 144
67. Aird I et al. Br Med J 1953; 1: 799
68. Hirayama T. Early Gastric Cancer. University of Tokyo Press, Tokyo, 1971
69. Stukons M, Doll R. Int J Cancer 1969; 4: 248
70. Hirayama T. In Gastric Cancer. Pergamon, Oxford, 1981, 77–84
71. Correa P et al. Lancet 1975; 2: 58
72. Forman D et al. Br Med J 1991; 302: 1302
73. Farinati F et al. Eur J Cancer Prev 1993; 2: 321
74. Lagergren J et al. N Engl J Med 1999; 340: 825
75. Ming EC. Gastrointest Radiol 1976; 1: 121

with only 2% of 2180 gastric ulcers detected on screening being malignant.[76]

CHRONIC GASTRITIS

Chronic gastritis is frequently found in association with gastric cancer. A total of 94% of superficial cancers are found in areas of gastritis, and carcinomas have been found in 10% of patients with chronic gastritis and intestinal metaplasia.[77] Chronic gastritis can be classified as autoimmune, hypersecretory and environmental, which is associated with infection with *H. pylori*.

Autoimmune gastritis is the gastritis of pernicious anaemia. The inflammatory process involves the body and fundus diffusely, leaving the antrum intact. This type of gastritis increases in prevalence and severity with age and is found more frequently in men than in women. Intestinal metaplasia commonly accompanies autoimmune gastritis and, because it is subject to dysplastic transformation (type 3), there is a high risk of malignancy.[57] Characteristically, when cancers develop they do so in the body of the stomach.

Hypersecretory gastritis is found in association with an ulcer. Histologically, there is distortion of the glandular epithelium, but there is no significant intestinal metaplasia or any association with malignant change.

Environmental chronic gastritis is prevalent in some parts of the world. Its geographical distribution matches areas where there is a high risk of the intestinal type of gastric cancer. For populations with a low incidence of gastric cancer, chronic gastritis is found in less than 20%. This rises to 70% in areas of high incidence. This form of gastritis has a characteristic distribution: it is multifocal, arising in the antrum and body of the stomach. The earliest changes appear on the lesser curve below the incisura. Histologically, the milder areas of inflammation show the characteristic changes of acute gastritis, with a dense inflammatory exudate below the lamina propria. As it progresses, atrophy of the mucosa develops, with a progressive loss of gastric glands. Regeneration produces an intestinal type of mucosa that undergoes dysplasia: intestinal metaplasia type 3.[57] This progresses to an intestinal-type cancer.

The diffuse type of adenocarcinoma is not accompanied by gastritis. Differentiation of gastric carcinoma into intestinal and diffuse types is helpful in relationship to gastritis and geographical variations. The lack of gastritis in the diffuse lesions makes the relationship unclear. It may be that dysplasia is the important feature, because this can occur in foveolar epithelium as well as intestinal metaplasia, and it may be the important premalignant mucosal change.[78]

Microscopic features

Gastric cancer can be classified on the basis of its histological appearance into well, moderately differentiated or poorly differentiated types. The most valuable classification is that described by Lauren, into intestinal and diffuse types.[79] The former are composed of malignant glands and the latter of small groups or single cells. When such cells contain significant intracellular mucus, displacing the nucleus to one side, they are called signet-ring cancers. The prognosis of intestinal-type cancers is better than that of the diffuse type.[80]

THE SPREAD OF CANCER IN THE STOMACH

In 1932, Carnett and Howell described the mechanisms of dissemination of gastric cancer as direct extension into adjacent organs, lymphatic embolization, lymphatic permeation, blood stream embolization and transplantation.[81] Gastric cancer may spread luminally into the duodenum and oesophagus. It is not true that the pylorus is the invariable limit of distal spread. Duodenal involvement occurs in 24–30% of all gastric cancers.[82]

Lymph node metastases are common. The distribution of the nodes is shown in Table 26.5 and Fig. 26.12. They have been simplified into two groups: N1, or within 3 cm of the primary growth, and all others classified as N2. Para-aortic nodes are classified as distant metastases.

Table 26.5 Lymph node groups in gastric cancer

Site of primary lesion	N1 nodes*	N2 nodes*
Upper third	Left cardiac (1) Right cardiac (2) Lesser curve (3) Greater curve (4)	Supra- and infrapyloric (5, 6) Left gastric (7) Common hepatic (8) Splenic artery (9) Splenic hilum (10) Coeliac axis (11)
Middle third	Right gastric (12) Lesser curve (3) Greater curve (4) Supra- and infra pyloric (5, 6)	Splenic artery (9) Splenic hilum (10) Left cardiac (1) Left gastric (7) Common hepatic (8) Coeliac axis (11)
Lower third	Lesser curve (3) Greater curve (4) Supra- and infra pyloric (5, 6)	Right cardiac (2) Left gastric (7) Common hepatic (8) Coeliac axis (11)

*N1 nodes are within 3 cm of the primary; nodes in any of these groups more than 3 cm away become N2 nodes.
Numbers in parentheses represent the node groups shown in Fig. 26.12.

Clinical features

Symptoms

All patients with gastric cancer develop symptoms, yet the diagnosis is often made only when the disease is advanced. The first symptoms are those of dyspepsia, epigastric pain, vomiting, dysphagia and bleeding.[83] These are often impossible to differentiate on clinical grounds from benign peptic ulceration, and the temptation to treat patients medically without confirmation of the diagnosis should be resisted, because these symptoms in early gastric cancer may disappear with acid-reducing treatment. Only later in the disease do the constitutional effects of anorexia, malaise, weight loss and anaemia occur, with the recurrence of epigastric pain, which has lost its association with food.

REFERENCES

76. Yamagatu S, Hisamichi S. World J Surg 1979; 3: 671
77. Freisen G et al. Surgery 1962; 51: 300
78. Morson BC et al. J Clin Pathol 1968; 33: 711
79. Lauren P. Acta Pathol Microbiol Scand 1965; 64: 31
80. Ming SC. Gastric Carcinoma. Churchill Livingstone, Edinburgh, 1986: 197
81. Carnett JB, Howell JC. Surg Clin North Am 1932; 12: 1351
82. Zinniger M, Collin W. Ann Surg 1949; 130: 557
83. Swynnerton BF, Truelove SC. Br Med J 1952; 1: 287

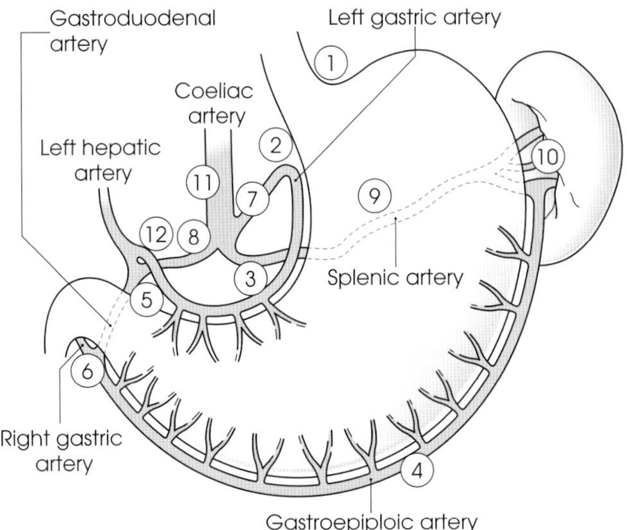

Figure 26.12 N1 and N2 groups of gastric lymph nodes.

Physical signs

The diagnosis should be made before any physical signs are apparent. The presence of a mass indicates spread to the omentum, and a palpable liver, ascites and jaundice imply extensive secondary spread to either the liver or portal nodes. The presence of a Virchow's node, which can be confirmed on fine-needle aspiration cytology, is diagnostic of advanced disease.

Differential diagnosis

Differential diagnosis includes benign conditions, such as peptic ulcer gastritis and Crohn's disease of the stomach, and malignant conditions, such as oesophageal and pancreatic cancer, together with gastric lymphoma and leiomyosarcoma. The generalized presentation of gastric cancer (anorexia, anaemia and aesthenia) can be mimicked by cancer of the bronchus and right colon, together with pernicious anaemia, hypercalcaemia and uraemia.

Diagnosis

The diagnosis is invariably made by endoscopy, with multiple biopsies being taken of all suspicious lesions. Barium meal should be undertaken if endoscopy is apparently normal but the element of suspicion high. It is possible to miss linitis plastica on endoscopy, because the tumour spreads in the submucosa and shallow biopsies may not be diagnostic. An inability to inflate the stomach should arouse suspicions and barium meal is diagnostic, although it cannot differentiate between linitis plastica and lymphoma (Fig. 26.13). The combined accuracy of endoscopy and barium studies is 98%.[84]

Screening

The Japanese have extensive experience of mass screening with indirect radiology followed by endoscopy. This significantly increases the incidence of stage 1 disease, reducing the death rate by a quarter.[85]

Treatment

Ian Aird in the first edition of this book stated that 'the only treatment which offers any prospect of cure is gastrectomy': nothing new has evolved to challenge this approach. Surgery for gastric cancer should accommodate the following factors:

- the stage of disease at time of presentation;

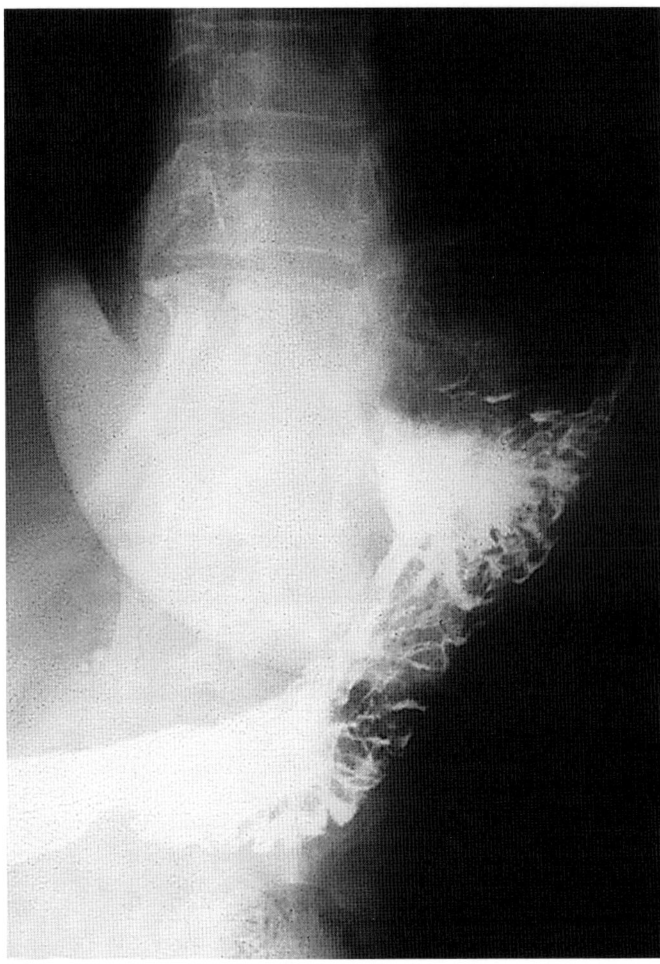

Figure 26.13 A barium meal demonstrating linitis plastica with poor gastric distension.

- the pattern of spread of disease;
- the pattern of failure after resection; and
- the influence of resection on postoperative mortality and long-term survival.

Stage of disease at presentation

Of the current imaging techniques, CT scanning and endoluminal ultrasound offer the best means of staging the disease preoperatively; the two techniques complement each other.[86,87] Computerized tomographic scans can detect liver metastasis, significant thickening of the gastric wall (Fig. 26.14) and lymph nodes over 1 cm in size. The degree of invasion of the gastric wall can best be assessed by endoluminal ultrasound, which will also detect lymph nodes adjacent to the gastric wall, particularly left gastric nodes. Laparoscopy may be of value in detecting small liver metastases and peritoneal deposits.[88] Open and close laparotomy should now be a rare occurrence.

REFERENCES

84. Nagao F, Takahishi MD. World J Surg 1979; 3: 693
85. Hirayama T. In: Bouchier IAD, Allan RN, Hodgson JF, Keighley MB (eds). Textbook of Gastroenterology. Baillière Tindall, London, 1984
86. Mason RC et al. Lancet 1987; 1: 108
87. Rankin S, Mason R. Clin Radiol 1992; 46: 373
88. Shandall A, Johnson C. Br J Surg 1985; 72: 449

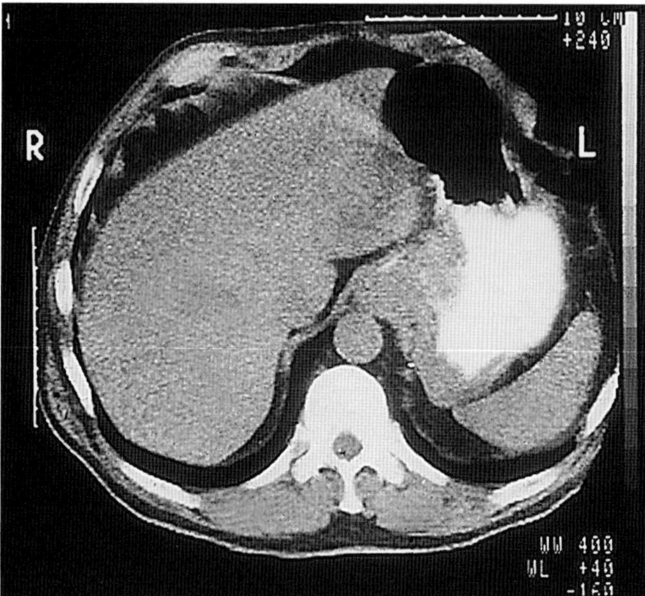

Figure 26.14 A CT scan of the stomach, demonstrating a carcinoma of the lesser curve with significant thickening of the gastric wall.

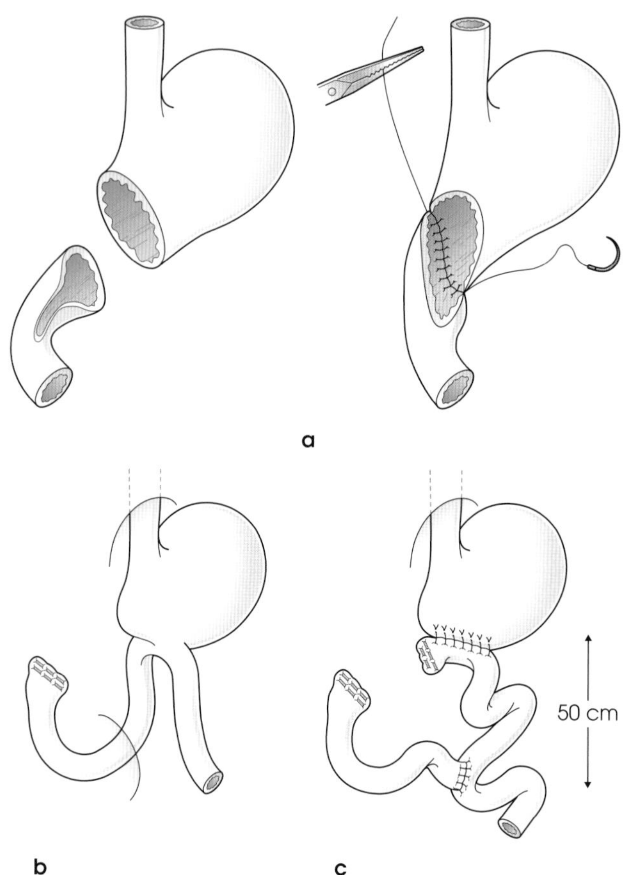

Figure 26.15 Methods of reconstruction after a partial gastrectomy: (**a**) Billroth I; (**b**) Billroth II; and (**c**) Roux-en-Y.

Patterns of spread

Patients who demonstrate features of dissemination or blood stream embolization, such as those with liver or lung secondaries, are suitable only for palliation. Curative resection is only applicable in patients with tumours confined to the stomach and the N1 and N2 nodes.

Patterns of failure after resection

This has important implications for curative surgery. Recurrence occurs in the gastric remnant in 10–50% of cases: an argument for total gastrectomy.[89] The reported 5-year survival rate following a total gastrectomy as a routine operation for gastric cancer is not, however, significantly better than that for subtotal resections. Gundosa and Sosin found that 53% of reoperated cases had recurrent disease either in the gastric remnant or in the gastric bed.[90]

The value of lymphadenectomy is controversial: recent European trials have shown little benefit between D2 resection, which removes all N2 nodes, and D1 resection, in which N1 nodes and some N2 nodes are removed.[91,92] The increased mortality associated with a D2 resection is largely related to the resection of the distal pancreas, which is performed as part of the radical operation and not the splenectomy. Current practice is to undertake resection of N2 nodes preserving the pancreas and, if feasible, the spleen (see Ch. 32). In the Japanese literature a significant survival benefit is demonstrable for D2 over D1 and D0 resection, with an operative mortality as low as 5% for such radical surgery.[93] This has now been replicated in specialist UK centers.[94]

Radical surgery

This operation should remove the part of stomach containing the tumour, with at least 5 cm clearance (excluding the duodenum), and all N1 and N2 nodes. Current practice, however, is to not remove pancreas, but to strip the lymph nodes from the splenic artery and preserve the spleen unless the tumour is in the proximal stomach. The greater omentum is removed in all cases, along with the left gastric, coeliac and common hepatic nodes.[95]

In distal cancers with at least 5 cm (preferably 10 cm) of proximal clearance, the proximal stomach can be preserved. This may be reconstructed as either a Billroth I or II gastrectomy, although in the vast majority of cases the extent of resection necessitates a Billroth II reconstruction. This has the added advantage of removing the stomach and anastomosis from the gastric bed. An alternative is to reconstruct with a Roux-en-Y anastomosis, which prevents bile reflux (Fig. 26.15). This must be combined with truncal vagotomy or lifelong proton pump inhibitors to prevent stomal ulceration.

Following total gastrectomy (performed for body and proximal cancer), the classical method of reconstruction consists of anastomosing a 50-cm Roux-en-Y loop to the oesophagus. Because total gastrectomy is associated with higher morbidity than partial resection, largely as the result of dietary problems, deficiencies and dumping, modifications to the standard Roux

REFERENCES

89. Pichlmayr R, Meyer HJ. In: Gastric Cancer. Pergamon Press, Oxford, 1981: 171–186
90. Gundosa LC, Sosin H. Int J Radiat Oncol Biol Phys 1982; 8: 1
91. Cuschieri A et al. Lancet 1996; 347: 995
92. Sasako M et al. Br J Surg 1997; 84: 1567
93. Kajitani T, Miwa K. WHO-CC Monograph 2. World Health Organization, Tokyo, 1979
94. Sue Ling HM et al. Br Med J 1993; 307: 591.
95. Craven JL. In: Preece PE, Cuschieri A, Wellwood JM (eds). Cancer of the Stomach. Grune & Stratton, New York, 1986: 165

Table 26.6 Staging system for gastric cancer

Stage	Clinical	Pathology
I	Radical resection (T1, N0, M0)	Mucosa +, submucosa +/–, muscularis, propria –, serosa –, node – (T1, N0, M0)
II	Radical resection (T2–4, N0, M0)	Muscularis propria +, serosa +/–, node – (T2–4, N0, M0)
III	Radical resection (TX–4, N1–3, M0)	Muscularis propria +/–, serosa +/–, node + (TX–4, N1–3, M0)
IVA	Palliative resection (TX–4, NX–3, M0 or 1)	Residual disease (TX–4, N0–3, M0 or 1)
IVB	No resection (TX–4, NX–3, M0 or 1)	Positive histology (T4, N0–3, M0 or 1)

loop have been proposed. These are demonstrated in Fig. 26.16. A standard 50-cm Roux loop constructed without kinking and a short proximal jejunal limb offer the best means of reconstruction if the patient takes vitamin and mineral supplements and eats little and often.

Palliative treatment

In the presence of advanced disease, treatment should be directed to the simplest means of alleviating the patient's symptoms, and this should be tailored to the individual. The symptoms most commonly requiring palliation are obstruction, haemorrhage and pain. In distal tumours, resection bypass or stenting can relieve obstruction. In proximal tumours, the results of surgery are poor, and intubation and/or laser ablation offer good palliation with minimum morbidity and mortality.[96,97]

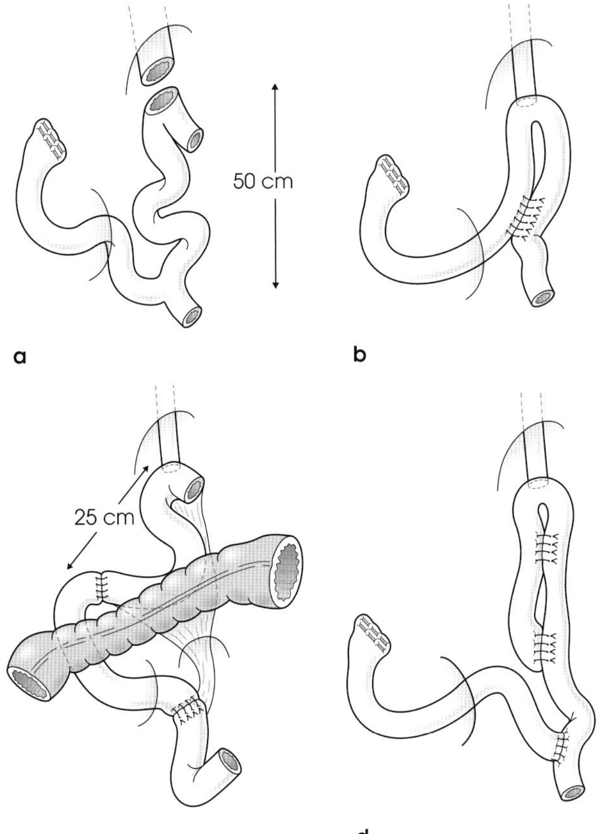

Figure 26.16 Methods of reconstruction after a total gastrectomy: **(a)** Roux-en-Y; **(b)** omega gastrojejunostomy; **(c)** Henley jejunal interposition; and **(d)** Lydidakis modification of Roux-en-Y.

Other therapeutic possibilities

Endoscopic treatment has been advocated for early gastric cancer, either using laser destruction of the tumour or snaring the lesion after elevation of the tumour by injection of saline into the submucosa. This is only applicable to the protruberant or superficial types of early disease, not the ulcerating type, and requires very accurate staging by endoluminal ultrasound.[98]

Until recently, the results of cytotoxic chemotherapy for gastric cancer, both as primary treatment and as adjuvant therapy, have been disappointing.[99,100] The use of regimens based on cisplatin and the continuous infusion of 5-fluorouracil administered via a Hickman catheter and minipump have demonstrated a 60% response rate in advanced disease,[101] and chemoradiotherapy has been shown to prolong survival in the adjuvant setting.[102]

No evidence exists that external beam radiotherapy in gastric cancer is beneficial, but it can be useful in reducing bleeding in patients with advanced disease.

Results of treatment

There are many series demonstrating different survival rates. Series from Europe and North America show curative resection rates of 25–40% with 5-year survival figures of between 10 and 15%.[103,104] This contrasts with Japan, where the curative resection rate is over 50% and 5-year survival figures are between 20 and 30%.[105] The most important determinant of survival is the clinicopathological stage of the disease. The tumour node metastasis staging system (Table 26.6) has been modified to allow identification of the group of patients having palliative resections (stage IVA) as compared with those who have no resection (stage IVB).[106] This system accommodates the important clinicopathological features of gastric cancer:

- resectability;
- depth of penetration of the primary lesion; and
- the presence or absence of lymph node involvement and distant metastases.

REFERENCES

96. Watkinson AF et al. Semin Interv Radiol 1996; 13: 17
97. Mason RC et al. Br J Surg 1991; 78: 1346
98. Hiki Y et al. World J Surg 1995; 19: 517
99. Hockey MSS, Fielding JWL. Gastric Cancer in Randomised Trials in Cancer. Raven Press, New York, 1986: 221
100. Fielding JWL et al. World J Surg 1983; 7: 390
101. Highley MS et al. Br J Surg 1994; 81: 763
102. MacDonald J et al. N Engl J Med 2001; 345: 725.
103. Inberg MV et al. Arch Surg 1975; 110: 703
104. Scott AW et al. Surgery 1985; 97: 55
105. Kajitani T et al. Gann Monogr Cancer Res 1979; 22: 77
106. Fielding JWL et al. Br J Surg 1984; 71: 677

The strength of this system is confirmed in the retrospective study from tumours in the Birmingham Cancer Registry. When international comparisons are made between equivalent-stage disease, similar results are then seen, although the Japanese do report a survival rate for stage 1 disease of 100%. It is likely that the apparent difference in overall results of treatment across the world is related to the variable distribution of stage. In Japan, the incidence of stage 1 disease is as high as 30%.[107]

OTHER EPITHELIAL AND NON-EPITHELIAL TUMOURS

Squamous cell carcinoma and carcinoid tumours of the stomach are exceedingly rare (0.04–0.07% of all gastric cancers) and about four times more common in men than in women. Presentation is similar to adenocarcinoma.[108] Similarly, argentaffinomas are not common, and the diagnosis is frequently established at post-mortem. They occur with equal frequency in both sexes and present in a similar way to adenocarcinoma, although they may have a long preoperative history.

Radiologically, carcinoids appear as polypoid neoplasms. Small tumours with no evidence of metastasis should be locally excised. When the neoplasm is over 2 cm in diameter or where there is evidence of metastasis, operations appropriate to the stage should be performed. The prognosis is good: among the 15 reported cases followed for more than 5 years there were 12 survivors. Among the 90 reported cases, six had malignant carcinoid syndrome, producing high levels of 5-hydroxytryptophan and histamine.[109]

LYMPHOMA

The stomach is the most common extranodal site of non-Hodgkin's lymphoma, but it is still uncommon, accounting for 1.2% of gastric malignancies. The mean age is 60 years, with a male to female ratio of 1.3:1. The presenting symptoms are similar to adenocarcinoma, although a mass is found in 20%. Two-thirds of these lesions are resectable, and the 5-year survival rate is 24%. Significant prognostic factors are tumour node metastasis staging and tumour size. Survival can be doubled by the addition of radiotherapy to resection.[110] The role of chemotherapy regimens used for non-Hodgkin's lymphoma elsewhere remain to be confirmed (see Ch. 33). MALToma is a variant of lymphoma that responds to *H. pylori* eradication therapy.[111]

MESENCHYMAL TUMOURS

Mesenchymal tumours comprise 1–3% of all gastric tumours and were until recently categorized as leiomyoma or leiomyosarcoma. The use of immunocytochemistry has subdivided such tumours into their cells of origin: smooth muscle leiomyoma or sarcoma (positive for desmin and smooth muscle actin), nerve neurofibroma or sarcoma (S100, NSE and PGP9.5), and interstitial cells gastrointestinal stromal tumours (CD37 and CD117, also known as c-KIT positive). Their degree of malignancy is related to the number of mitotic figures per high-powered field. They are most commonly situated on the anterior and posterior gastric walls. Macroscopically they are bulky and vascular, with multiple areas of ulceration. Direct spread is rare, and lymph node metastasis does not occur. The most frequent presenting symptom is bleeding: 75% having either haematemesis or melaena. There may also be epigastric symptoms, and an abdominal mass is found in up to 60% of cases. The diagnosis is established by a combination of endoscopy, CT and positron emission tomography scanning. Surgery consists of wide local excision without lymphadenectomy. The prognosis is quite good, with a 5-year survival rate ranging between 37 and 54%.[112,113] The development of targeted treatment to receptors (imatinib for gastrointestinal stromal tumours) opens the possibility for treatment of metastatic disease.[114]

OTHER RARE TUMOURS OF THE STOMACH

These include Schwannomas, chorionepitheliomas and carcinosarcomas. The diagnosis is usually made only after resection of a gastric mass. They should not be confused with benign hamartomas of the stomach associated with Peutz–Jeghers syndrome.[115]

DUODENAL NEOPLASMS

BENIGN DUODENAL TUMOURS

Benign duodenal tumours are found in 1% of endoscopies. Most are located in the first part of the duodenum, with the risk of malignancy increasing the more distally that they arise. Gastrointestinal haemorrhage is the most frequent presentation. Adenomas are the most common tumours, but villous adenomas do occur. Other rare tumours include Brunner's gland adenomas, leiomyomas, lipomas and carcinoid tumours.[115]

MALIGNANT DUODENAL LESIONS

Duodenal cancers are rare, accounting for only 0.3% of gastrointestinal malignancies. A third of small bowel neoplasms are, however, situated in the duodenum.

Adenocarcinomas are the most frequent tumours, but lymphomas and carcinoids also occur. The presentation depends on the site. In the periampullary region the patient presents with jaundice, whereas elsewhere they present with obstructive symptoms. In a quarter of cases a mass may be felt.[115]

The most effective treatment is pancreaticoduodenectomy. If there is local invasion or distant metastasis, surgical or radiological bypass is indicated. The 5-year survival rate is 25%.

REFERENCES

107. Nishi M. In: Preece PE, Cuschieri A, Wellwood JM (eds). Cancer of the Stomach. Grune & Stratton, New York, 1985: 107
108. Eaton H. Br J Surg 1972; 59: 382
109. Rogers L, Murphy R. Am J Surg Pathol 1979; 3: 195
110. Hockey MS et al. Br J Surg 1987; 74: 43
111. Wotherspoon A et al. Lancet 1993; 342: 578
112. Skandalakis LJ et al. In: Wastell C, Nyhus LM, Donahue PE (eds). Surgery of the Oesophagus, Stomach and Small Intestine. 5th edn. Little, Brown, New York, 1995: 607
113. Levison DA, Shepherd NA. In: Preece PE, Cuschieri A, Wellwood JM (eds). Cancer of the Stomach. Grune & Stratton, New York, 1985: 47
114. Joensuu H et al. N Engl J Med 2001; 344: 1052
115. Otterson MF, Condon RE. In: Wastell C, Nyhus LM, Donahue PE (eds). Surgery of the Oesophagus, Stomach and Small Intestine. 5th edn. Little, Brown, New York, 1995: 691

The small intestine

27

Alastair C. J. Windsor, Alexander G. Heriot

The small bowel extends from the pylorus to the ileocaecal valve and is approximately 300 cm long.[1] The duodenum is C-shaped and lies retroperitoneally. It extends from the pylorus to the duodenojejunal junction where the jejunum begins and develops a mesentery. The jejunum leads into the ileum, which is in turn connected to the colon. The transition from jejunum to ileum is not abrupt, and there is a gradual change from thicker mucosa and larger villi in the jejunum to thinner mucosa and smaller villi in the ileum. The vascular arcades in the jejunum tend to be long and close together, forming high arches, as compared with the ileum, where the arcades tend to be shorter and further apart, although this is often hidden by increasing mesenteric fat.[1]

Although the bowel is sterile at birth, it is rapidly colonized by bacteria. The jejunum is usually sterile, but the ileum has a significant inherent flora including coliforms and bacteroides, which contribute to digestion and absorption of nutrients.

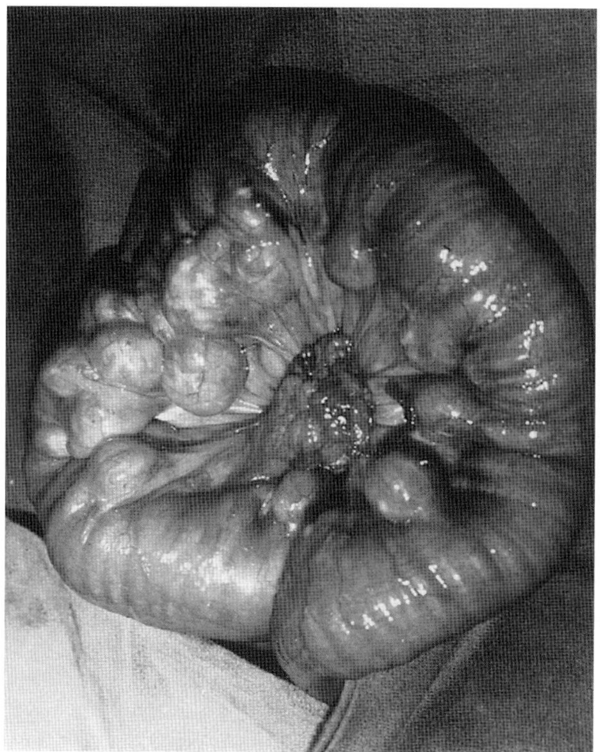

Figure 27.1 Jejunal diverticulosis.

FUNCTIONS

The major function of the small bowel is the digestion and absorption of food. Carbohydrate and protein breakdown occurs in the bowel lumen, catalysed by pancreatic enzymes including amylase, trypsin and chymotrypsin. Enzymes present in the epithelial cells of the small bowel then complete the digestion into monosaccharides and amino acids. These are then absorbed via the villi, which increase the surface area of the bowel substantially. Fats are broken down by pancreatic lipase into glycerol and triglycerides; the latter are converted to chylomicrons and absorbed before passing into the mesenteric lymphatics. Vitamin B_{12} is absorbed in the distal ileum in combination with intrinsic factor. Bile salts are also absorbed in the same region, creating the enterohepatic circulation of bile salts.

EMBRYOLOGY

The small bowel is derived from the midgut, which gives rise to the entire small bowel, and the right colon and proximal third of the transverse colon. This is supplied by the superior mesenteric artery, which is the artery of the midgut. Lymphatic drainage follows the arterial supply, and lymph passes to the mesenteric lymph nodes through the para-aortic nodes and on to the cisterna chyli. In the embryo, the midgut is connected to the yolk sac by the vitellointestinal duct. As the abdominal organs develop, the bowel is extruded from the abdominal cavity. The midgut proximal to the insertion of the vitellointestinal duct, which forms the jejunum and most of the ileum, elongates, and while doing so rotates anticlockwise around the omphalomesenteric or vitelline artery from which the superior mesenteric artery is derived. This rotation places the transverse colon above the jejunum and ileum, anterior to the duodenum. Around the 10th week, the abdominal cavity enlarges and the bowel re-enters the cavity, with the caecum coming to lie in the right iliac fossa. Malrotation can occur. The vitellointestinal duct becomes obliterated and disappears, although a residual portion may be left as a Meckel's diverticulum.

DEVELOPMENTAL ANOMALIES

A number of developmental anomalies may affect the small bowel, including atresia, stenosis, malrotation and duplications. The majority of these will present to paediatric surgeons in infancy (see Ch. 40), but some may not present until adulthood.

REFERENCES

1. McMinn RMH (ed). Last's Anatomy: Regional and Applied. 8th edn. Churchill Livingstone, Edinburgh, 1990

LADD'S BANDS

In 1932, Ladd described duodenal obstruction as a result of the persistence of fibrous bands between the root of the small bowel mesentery and the liver, crossing and obstructing the second part of the duodenum.[2] In the fetus, the bowel rotates 270° anticlockwise around the superior mesenteric artery. Malrotation occurs with a narrow-based mesentery of the midgut, which is prone to volvulus and may also be associated with fibrous bands across the mesentery, named Ladd's bands. These bands can cause compression across the duodenum, resulting in obstruction. This usually presents with bile-stained vomiting during infancy but may present in adulthood.

Treatment is by Ladd's procedure, where the bands are divided and the base of the mesentery widened to prevent further rotation around the mesentery, leaving the small bowel on the right of the abdomen and the colon on the left.[3]

DIVERTICULA OF SMALL INTESTINE

The aetiology is uncertain, but diverticula of small intestine are thought to be acquired rather than congenital. They are often multiple, present on the mesenteric side of the bowel, and confined to the jejunum in 80% of cases (Fig. 27.1). Jejunal diverticulosis is often associated with diverticula elsewhere in the gastrointestinal tract. They may cause diverticulitis, haemorrhage, obstruction or malabsorption, but are usually symptomless.[4] Malabsorption is thought to result from bacterial overgrowth producing a blind loop syndrome.[5] The pathological area of small bowel is resected if it causes symptoms.[6]

MECKEL'S DIVERTICULUM

Meckel's diverticulum is a congenital diverticulum that arises from failure of obliteration of the vitelline duct. This connects the fetal gut to the yolk sac. A Meckel's diverticulum is a true diverticulum containing all layers of the bowel wall. It arises from the antimesenteric side of the distal ileum, around 60 cm from the ileocaecal valve, is present in around 2% of the population, and is on average 5 cm long. Meckel's diverticula may be associated with other anomalies of the vitellointestinal duct. These include persistence of the entire duct, with a fistula from the ileum to the umbilicus; lumen obliteration, resulting in a band from the bowel to the umbilicus; or partial obliteration with a cyst present in a segment of the duct. Ectopic tissue including gastric mucosa may be found within a Meckel's diverticulum.[7]

Meckel's diverticulum is often symptomless, particularly if it has a broad base and no ectopic gastric mucosa, and usually presents only if a complication develops. The commonest presentation is with inflammation, where the symptoms and signs are similar to appendicitis, although the pain may not necessarily be in the right iliac fossa. The diagnosis is rarely suspected prior to surgery until a normal appendix is found. An inflamed Meckel's diverticulum should be excised and the small bowel repaired. Gastrointestinal bleeding may occur in the jejunum adjacent to the Meckel's diverticulum as a result of acid digestion from the ectopic gastric mucosa. This may be suspected following a radioisotope scan (Fig. 27.2). The diverticulum should be resected with a segment of small bowel on either side to remove the source of the bleeding.

Meckel's diverticulum may cause small bowel obstruction, either secondary to a congenital band or from intussusception of the diverticulum.[8] Treatment is again by resection. Excision of a Meckel's diverticulum found incidentally is dependent on the likelihood of it causing problems in the future balanced against the risk of iatrogenic complications resulting from resection. It is reasonable to remove a symptomless diverticulum in patients under 40 years of age or to remove a diverticulum that is either narrow-based or long, because these are more likely to cause future problems.

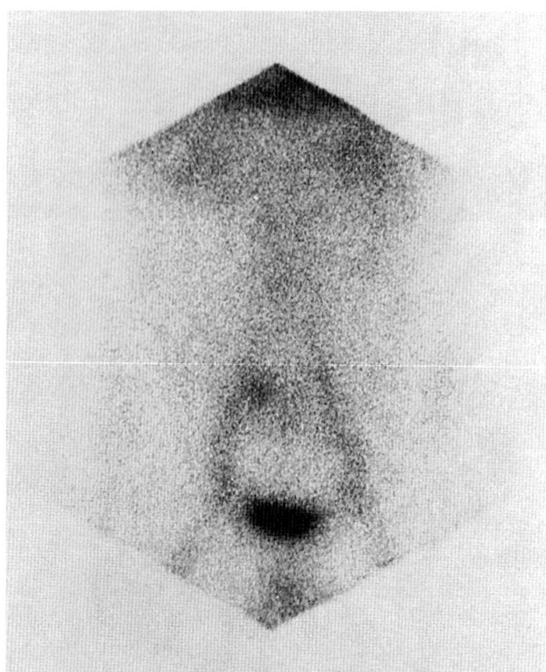

Figure 27.2 Meckel's diverticulum demonstrated by a pertechnetate technetium-99m scan.

Carcinoid tumours are rarely found in Meckel's diverticula and can present with obstruction or haemorrhage.[9]

INFECTIONS AND INFESTATIONS

A large number of organisms can infect the small bowel; many are symptomless but others cause diarrhoea, abdominal pain or malabsorption. A few infections have more serious consequences, causing intestinal obstruction, haemorrhage and perforation.

TYPHOID FEVER

Typhoid fever, or enteric fever, is rare in countries with high standards of hygiene but is endemic in most tropical countries. *Salmonella typhi* produces the most severe symptoms. Typhoid is acquired from contaminated food or water, and organisms that enter the small intestine adhere to epithelial cells and are engulfed. They multiply in these cells before invading the lamina

REFERENCES

2. Ladd WE. N Engl J Med 1932; 206: 277
3. Bill AH, Grauman D. J Paediatr Surg 1966; 1: 127
4. Palder S, Frey CB. Arch Surg 1988; 123; 889–893
5. Donald JW. Ann Surg 1979; 190: 183
6. Wilcox RD, Shatney CH. South Med J 1988; 81: 1386–1391
7. Soltero MJ, Bill AH. Am J Surg 1976; 132: 168
8. Rutherford RB, Akers DR. Surgery 1966; 58: 618–626
9. Weinstein EC et al. Int Abstr Surg 1963; 116: 103–111

propria and submucosa, and are eventually carried by the lymphatics to the mesenteric lymph nodes. This leads to a transient bacteraemia before the organisms are cleared by the macrophages of the reticuloendothelial system. The organisms can then multiply and destroy the macrophages, resulting in a secondary bacteraemia. They may also be carried back in the bile to reinfect the small intestine before becoming localized in the lymphoid tissue of Peyer's patches, where they cause inflammation, necrosis and ulceration, resulting in typhoid ulcers. The patient has severe diarrhoea and systemic illness in the second week of infection. The ulcers usually heal with little fibrosis but may bleed or even perforate,[10] when surgical resection is indicated.[11,12] All patients should receive chloramphenicol to treat the primary infection and to prevent the risk of chronic infection where the patient becomes a carrier of the organism.

TUBERCULOSIS

Abdominal tuberculosis is rare in developed countries but is still comparatively common in India. Intestinal infection produces ulceration of Peyer's patches, with subsequent stricture formation that may result in small bowel obstruction or abscess formation. The most common site of infection is the ileocaecal region, when it must be differentiated from Crohn's disease.

Antituberculous medication may prevent the development of complications. Obstruction or abscess formation requires resection of bowel and drainage of pus.

ACTINOMYCOSES

This chronic inflammatory condition caused by *Actinomyces israelii* is fortunately rare. The condition starts in the cervicofacial area, in 70% of cases usually following dental trauma,[13] but in 20% of cases the organism enters in the ileocaecal region, often following a perforation of the appendix.[14] This causes a chronic inflammatory response with dense fibrosis and multiloculate abscesses, which may eventually discharge through multiple sinuses in the right iliac fossa. The pus characteristically contains the 'sulphur granules', which are dense, matted filaments of organisms surrounded by radially disposed, club-shaped growths. The latter do not appear in artificial culture. From the ileocaecal region the organisms travel in the portal vein to the liver if septicaemia occurs, where multiple abscess formation may result in the characteristic honeycomb appearance. Surgery may be necessary to drain the abscesses, but this may be avoided because the organism is sensitive to a wide variety of antibiotics including penicillin and lincomycin.[15]

OTHER INFESTATIONS

The small bowel may become infested by a number of helminths. *Ascaris lumbricoides* infection results in the presence of multiple worms in the small bowel. This may cause few symptoms other than malabsorption, although in heavy infestations the tangled mass of worms may cause small bowel obstruction.

Hookworm infection is one of the commonest causes of iron-deficiency anaemia worldwide, as a consequence of chronic blood loss from the small bowel after penetration of the bowel wall by the worms.

HUMAN IMMUNODEFICIENCY VIRUS

The appearance of HIV infection and AIDS causes a number of problems in the small bowel. These include opportunistic infections, diarrhoea and malignancies.

Opportunistic infections and diarrhoea

Opportunistic infections most commonly affect the colon, where they cause diarrhoea, but the small bowel may also be involved. *Mycobacterium avium-intracellulare* is an opportunistic infection that usually presents with watery diarrhoea and abdominal pain but may be symptomless. Patients may develop an abdominal mass produced by enlarged mesenteric nodes,[16] associated with small bowel obstruction.[17] This presentation is easily confused with Crohn's disease.[18] Diagnosis is confirmed by finding acid-fast bacilli in a small bowel biopsy. The organisms are often highly resistant to antibiotic treatment, but quinolones or amikacin may be effective.[19]

Cytomegalovirus may infect the small bowel but colonic infection is much more common. Chronic diarrhoea is sometimes associated with chronic HIV infection that causes small bowel enteropathy, and although the precise pathology is uncertain, it may be a consequence of reduced mucosal immune function.[20]

Malignancies

Small bowel malignancies are rare but they are much more common in patients with established AIDS. Kaposi's sarcoma is the commonest malignancy associated with AIDS[21] and predominantly affects the proximal gastrointestinal tract. It may be symptomless, although patients can develop bleeding, obstruction or diarrhoea secondary to a protein-losing enteropathy.[22] The small bowel appearances on barium studies are similar to those of Crohn's disease, with nodules, strictures and skip lesions. Histology provides a definitive diagnosis, although a deep biopsy may be needed to identify the diagnostic spindle-shaped cells and central haemorrhage.[21] Treatment with chemotherapy is disappointing, but malignancy is often a late manifestation of the disease and is rarely the cause of death. Resection of the small bowel is required only if complications develop.

Malignant lymphomas are more common in patients with HIV and these can arise in the small bowel, although the stomach is more commonly affected. Non-Hodgkin's lymphomas[23] are the most common variety. Treatment is by chemotherapy once the diagnosis has been made. Surgical resection may be the only method of making the diagnosis, and small bowel resection may also be required to treat complications.

PNEUMATOSIS CYSTOIDES INTESTINALIS

Pneumatosis cystoides intestinalis is a rare condition that is characterized by the presence of multiple gas-filled cysts in the

REFERENCES

10. Taussig MJ. Processes in Pathology and Microbiology. Blackwell, Oxford, 1984
11. Bitar R, Tarpley J. Rev Infect Dis 1985; 7: 257
12. Butler T et al. Rev Infect Dis 1995; 7: 244
13. Beradi RS. Surg Gynecol Obstet 1979; 149: 257
14. Cope Z. Actinomycosis. Oxford University Press, London, 1938
15. Putnam HC et al. Surgery 1950; 28: 781
16. Waisman J et al. Pathol Res Pract 1987; 182: 729–754
17. Burack JH et al. Arch Surg 1989; 124: 285–286
18. Radin DR. Am J Radiol 1991; 156: 487–491
19. Chiu J et al. Ann Intern Med 1990; 113: 358–361
20. Keating J et al. Gut 1995; 37: 623
21. Rotterdam H, Sommers SC. Pathology 1985; 17: 181–192
22. Macho JR. Gastroenterol Clin North Am 1988; 17: 563–571
23. Joachim HL et al. Cancer 1985; 56: 2831–2842

small bowel wall, but it also occurs in the colon and rectum. The cysts, which may reach a few centimetres in diameter, are often symptomless. They are often identified at laparotomy or by imaging studies, but may cause abdominal pain, intussusception or obstruction. The condition commonly affects men between 30 and 50 years old, and is associated with chronic lung disease.[24] The diagnosis can be made on a barium contrast study that demonstrates radiolucent defects outside the contrast. Symptomless patients do not require treatment. Oxygen therapy has been shown to reduce the size of the cysts that cause symptoms.[25] Surgical resection is required only for complications or very severe symptoms.

CROHN'S DISEASE

In 1932, Crohn and associates published a report describing their findings in 14 young adults with chronic inflammatory bowel disease of the ileum that was not tuberculosis and not neoplastic.[26] Some of these patients developed multiple fistulae, and some developed small bowel obstruction from fibrotic strictures. This condition had almost certainly been described earlier by Dalziel in 1913,[27] and in 1806 a paper (later published in 1813) was delivered at the Royal College of Physicians by Combe and Saunders, entitled 'A singular case of stricture and thickening of the ileum', in which the lower part of the ileum as far as the colon was contracted 'for the space of three feet to the size of a turkey's quill'.[28] In 1907, Moynihan described a possible case of colonic Crohn's disease.[29] The name Crohn's disease has, however, become established in the literature and over the years many thousands of cases have been documented.[30]

Crohn's disease can affect any part of the gastrointestinal tract from the lips to the anus. It is apparently increasing in frequency in western countries but is very uncommon in developing countries. It causes considerable morbidity and some mortality, and its cause remains unknown.

The incidence in the UK is approximately six in 100 000 of the population per year,[31] and the highest prevalence reported is from Scandinavia (75 per 100 000 of population).[32] There is debate over whether the incidence is increasing. In western Europe and North America the incidence is greater in the Jewish population, with a tendency towards a female preponderance.[33] The peak incidence of diagnosis is between 15 and 35 years of age.

AETIOLOGY

Genotype

Although the cause of Crohn's disease remains unknown, there is increasing evidence of a genetic susceptibility. Farmer and colleagues from the Cleveland Clinic reported that 35% of 522 Crohn's patients had an affected family member,[34] but other reports have suggested that the incidence is around 15%. Twin studies also suggest a 35% monozygotic and a 7% dizygotic concordance.[35–37] Family history appears to be the single most important factor in determining an individual's risk of developing the disease. The first Crohn's gene has been found on chromosome 16, the NOD2 or CARD15 gene.[38]

Environment

The phenotype in Crohn's disease is a product of the genotype and the environment, and there is epidemiological evidence that patients with Crohn's disease are more likely to be smokers. There may also be some association with oral contraceptive intake.[39] Attempts to isolate an infective agent in Crohn's disease have so far been inconclusive, although some studies have suggested that a transmissible agent may exist. It has been suggested that *Mycobacterium kansasii* is responsible,[40] but the evidence for this is still weak, as is the evidence that measles infection or paratuberculosis are the cause. The evidence that toothpaste, cornflakes or autoimmunity are important factors is equally improbable.

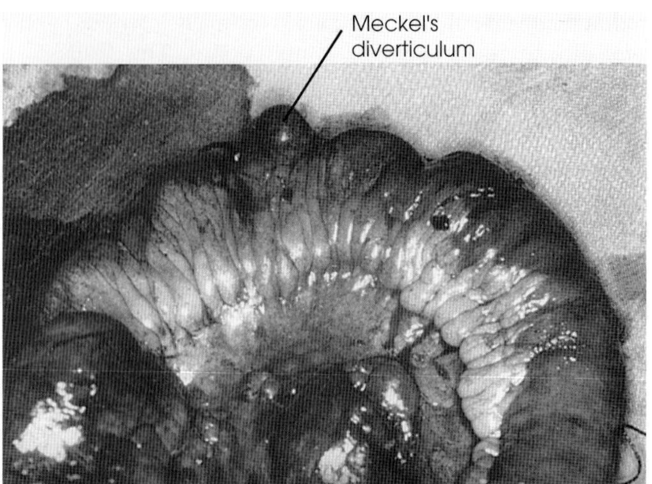

Figure 27.3 Crohn's disease of the ileum, showing the march of fat from the mesentery on to the serosal surface of the bowel. In this case, a Meckel's diverticulum is present and involved in the disease process.

HISTOPATHOLOGY

The primary lesion is a chronic inflammatory reaction in a submucosal lymphoid follicle, leading to overlying ulceration appearing as aphthous-type ulcers. The inflammatory process spreads transmurally, where it can cause deep fissuring ulcers (Fig. 27.3). When these fissures reach the serosal surface the bowel may become stuck to an adjacent organ, often resulting in fistula formation. Thickening of the bowel wall with narrowing of the lumen may eventually cause bowel obstruction. The lymphatic vessels in the bowel wall and mesentery become dilated, and large, fleshy lymph nodes develop. The whole process is often discontinuous, with 'skip' areas of involved bowel separated by normal segments.

REFERENCES

24. Galandiuk S, Fazio VW. Dis Colon Rectum 1986; 29: 358–363
25. Elberg JJ. Acta Chir Scand 1985; 151; 399–400
26. Crohn BB et al. JAMA 1932; 99: 1323
27. Dalziel TK. Br Med J 1913; 2: 1068
28. Combe C, Saunders W. Med Trans Coll Phys 1813; 4: 16
29. Moynihan BGA. Edinburgh Med J 1907; 21: 228
30. Armitage G, Wilson M. Br J Surg 1950–1; 38: 182
31. Hellers GKG. Acta Chir Scand 1979; Suppl: 490
32. Lee FL, Costello FT. Gut 1985; 26: 274
33. Acheson E. Gut 1960; 1: 291
34. Farmer RG et al. Clin Gastroenterol 1980; 9: 271
35. Tysk C et al. Gut 1988; 29: 990
36. Subhome J et al. Gastroenterology 1998; 114: A3113
37. Orholm M. Gut 1996; 59: A187
38. Hugot JP et al. Nature 2001; 411: 599
39. Lesko SM et al. Gastroenterology 1985; 89: 1046
40. Thayer WR et al. Dig Dis Sci 1984; 29: 1080

Non-caseating giant cell granulomas are the diagnostic histological features found in the bowel wall, but they occur only in 60% of the pathological specimens and presumably reflect some aspect of the immunological response to the disease by the patient. These granulomas are often in the subserosal layer, and may be found in rectal biopsies taken from patients with small bowel disease who have no macroscopic evidence of Crohn's disease in the rectum (see Ch. 28). Paneth cell hyperplasia may also develop in response to the chronic inflammatory process. The ileum and ascending colon are affected in two-thirds of patients; the colon alone is involved macroscopically in 20% (see Ch. 28).

CLINICAL PRESENTATION

The onset of the disease may be acute or insidious depending on its site and severity. Abdominal pain is the most common presenting symptom, with diarrhoea, loss of appetite, loss of weight, intermittent fever, nausea, vomiting and lassitude frequently associated. Fistula formation is present in about 15% of patients, and nutritional disturbances causing anaemia (iron, folate or vitamin B_{12} deficiency), hypoalbuminaemia and weight loss are common. These nutritional disturbances may result from anorexia, but are often compounded by the presence of chronic sepsis or malabsorption from involvement of large sections of the small intestine.[41] Anal fissure and fistula formation does occur with ileal Crohn's disease, but isolated anorectal involvement is less common than when the disease is present in the large bowel (see Ch. 28). Chronic blood loss from the ulcerated bowel is common but massive haemorrhage is rare from isolated small bowel disease.

Systemic manifestations of the disease include finger clubbing, large joint arthritis, erythema nodosum, iritis, pyoderma gangrenosum, episcleritis, uveitis and conjunctivitis, sclerosing cholangitis and bile duct carcinoma, although liver problems are much more commonly found in ulcerative colitis. Crohn's disease of the gallbladder has been described, and pathological evidence of Crohn's disease may be found in skin ulcers either directly related to enterocutaneous fistulae or at remote sites such as the scrotum. This may be regarded as metastatic Crohn's disease. Venous thrombosis and arterial occlusion are more common than expected in patients with Crohn's disease, particularly at the time of surgery.[42]

Renal stones have a greater incidence in patients with Crohn's disease than in the general population.[43] Uric acid stones are found particularly in patients who have had an ileostomy, and calcium triple-phosphate stones develop in patients on steroids as the result of calcium mobilization from the bones. Patients with steatorrhoea have an increased colonic oxalate reabsorption, and this may also increase the risk of stone formation.[44] Hydronephrosis can develop in patients with ileocaecal Crohn's disease.

The nutritional consequences of Crohn's disease may be either very severe or very mild, depending on the extent and the severity of the disease. The state of nutrition may also wax and wane with the disease activity, and may act as a useful guide to the extent of the inflammatory process. Anaemia, vitamin deficiencies, electrolyte imbalance, trace element deficiencies and hypoproteinaemia may all occur in association with weight loss.

DIAGNOSIS

The diagnosis is often delayed for some time, because the initial symptoms are often nebulous and non-specific. Confirmation of the diagnosis depends on finding characteristic histological changes in a biopsy taken from an affected area. A small bowel biopsy can be taken at upper gastrointestinal endoscopy using a Crosby capsule, at colonoscopy from the terminal ileum, or at laparotomy following resection. A small bowel enema may demonstrate the characteristic radiological appearances of Crohn's disease, which include areas of luminal narrowing with an irregular thick bowel wall (Fig. 27.4). There may be multiple skip lesions and areas of dilatation associated with obstruction. Deep fissuring ulcers or even fistulae may be demonstrated, and if the terminal ileum is involved the characteristic string sign of Kantor[45] may be present (Fig. 27.5). Between the areas of ulceration the mucosa may be thick and oedematous, giving rise to a cobblestone appearance.

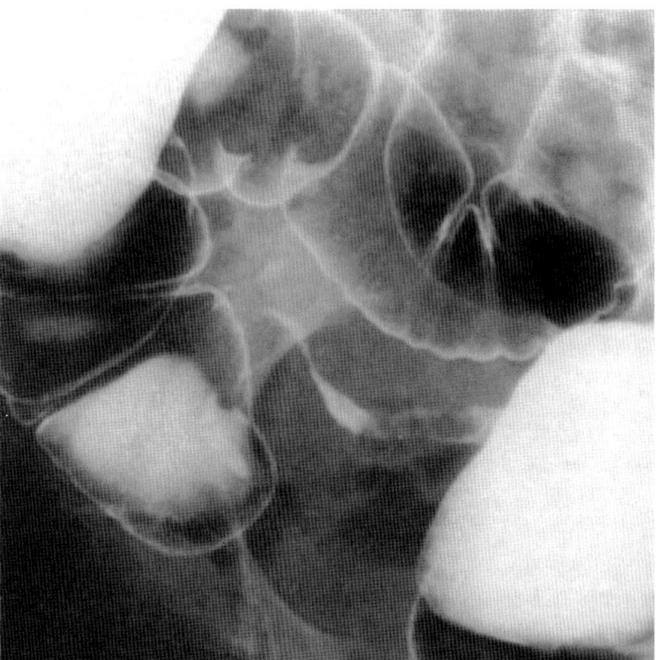

Figure 27.4 Terminal ileal Crohn's disease on barium follow-through examination.

TREATMENT

Because the cause of Crohn's disease is not known, treatment is empirical and aimed specifically at relieving symptoms. A patient with radiological evidence of extensive Crohn's disease but minimal symptoms requires minimal treatment. Medical management is appropriate until specific complications of the disease develop. Many patients, however, experience a long-term remission and better quality of life after early surgical resection (particularly in terminal ileum), rather than struggling on with steroids and immunosuppressive therapy. The best results are obtained when interested physicians and surgeons cooperate in a patient's management.

REFERENCES

41. Dyer NH, Dawson AM. Br J Surg 1973; 60: 134
42. Misiewicz JJ, Pounder RE, Venables CW (eds). Diseases of the Gut and Pancreas. Blackwell Scientific Publications, Oxford, 1987
43. Gelzavd EA et al. Am J Dig Dis 1968; 13: 1927
44. Chadwick VS et al. N Engl J Med 1973; 289: 172
45. Kantor JL. JAMA 1934; 103: 2016

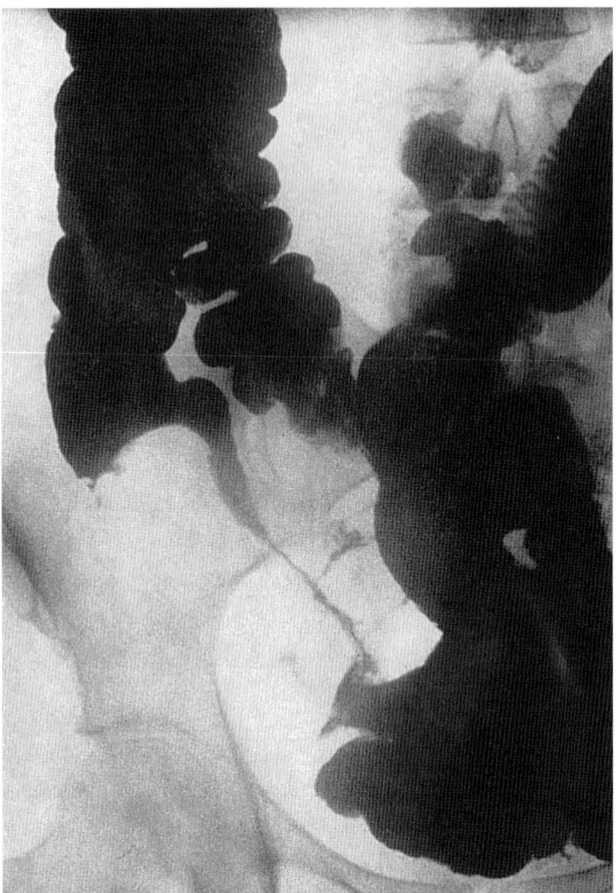

Figure 27.5 Barium follow-through examination (positive print) showing involvement of the terminal ileum with Crohn's disease. The picture shows Kantor's string sign and a deep fissure.

Medical treatment

Most patients with Crohn's disease receive a variable period of medical treatment. This is tailored to the extent and severity of the disease and includes a number of different treatments. These can be subdivided into those compounds that induce remission and others that maintain remission. Unfortunately, because of the complexity and variability of Crohn's disease, many trials have included heterogeneous patient groups and produced inconclusive results. The following is a crude distillate of some of this conflicting evidence.

Compounds that induce remission

Corticosteroids are the most effective and commonly used drugs for moderate to severe Crohn's disease, achieving remission rates of 60–70%. Concern about significant side effects has prompted the development of budesonide, an active steroid with a 90% first-pass metabolism. Clinical trials suggest that it is slightly less effective than conventional steroids but has significantly fewer side effects. Topical steroids are effective for distal colonic or perianal disease (see Ch. 28).

Aminosalicylates can be administered in a number of different ways. Slow-release, bacterial cleavage, pH-responsive delivery systems allow the clinician to target different sites in the gut to provide maximum exposure to the active drug. There is little hard evidence to support the absolute use of different preparations for specific phenotypes of Crohn's disease. Response rates vary greatly between studies, but a remission rate of 40–50% is usual.

Immunosuppression is increasingly used in patients with Crohn's disease. Among the many compounds available perhaps the most robust data are available for the purine metabolites azathioprine and 6-mercaptopurine. Candy and coworkers reported a statistically different remission rate compared with placebo after 15 months of treatment (47% versus 7%), but noted that this effect was not present by 3 months, suggesting a slow onset of action.[46] These drugs therefore tend to be used in combination with other, more rapidly acting compounds.

More selective immunoactive drugs are now available for the management of Crohn's disease. Biological agents such as monoclonal antibodies to tumour necrosis factor-α (infliximab) show great promise. Rapid response rates of up to 80% have been recorded when compared with placebo, following a single infusion.[47] The beneficial effects reported in fistulating Crohn's disease have elevated infliximab to almost magical status, particularly in healing perianal fistulae.[48] Some spectacular early results have sadly disappeared with longer-term follow-up. Combination therapy with infliximab followed by surgery may, however, prove very helpful for longer-term control. Concerns that biological therapy could cause antibodies and lymphoma to appear are as yet unfounded.

Nutritional and dietary alteration are important to address nutritional deficiencies associated with the disease (see Ch. 2), and primary nutritional therapy in difficult Crohn's disease has been shown to be as effective as steroid therapy and without the potential side effects. This is particularly important in children with Crohn's disease. Parenteral therapy provides little or no benefit, and the use of elemental enteral formulae over polymeric formulae does not improve results. Therefore polymeric enteral feeds, which are cheaper and more palatable, are the formulae of choice.

Antibiotics do have a role in Crohn's disease, despite there being little substantial evidence of an infectious cause. They are particularly useful in the management of perianal disease (see Ch. 28). Metronidazole and ciprofloxacin both appear to be effective, and both of these compounds may also have a role in acute disease elsewhere. In addition to its antimicrobial effects, metronidazole appears to have an immunomodulatory effect that may account for some of its efficacy.

Compounds that maintain remission

Unfortunately, many of the compounds that appear to be effective at inducing remission do not seem to maintain this effect. Long-term steroids in particular do not seem to be justified in Crohn's therapy. A meta-analysis has demonstrated that the aminosalicylates do have a moderate effect as maintenance therapy.[49] There is evidence that the purine metabolites can maintain remission, and when these compounds are not tolerated drugs such as methotrexate appear to provide similar clinical benefits. Recurrence following surgical resection may be reduced by maintenance therapy. Metronidazole has been shown to reduce early recurrence after surgery,[50] but was poorly tolerated because of unpleasant side effects. Aminosalicylates appear to

REFERENCES

46. Candy S et al. Gut 1995; 37: 674
47. Targan SR et al. Gastroenterology 1995; 110: A1026
48. Present DH. N Engl J Med 1999; 5: 119
49. Camma et al. Gastroenterology 1997; 113: 1465
50. Rutgeerts P. Gastroenterology 1995; 108: 1817

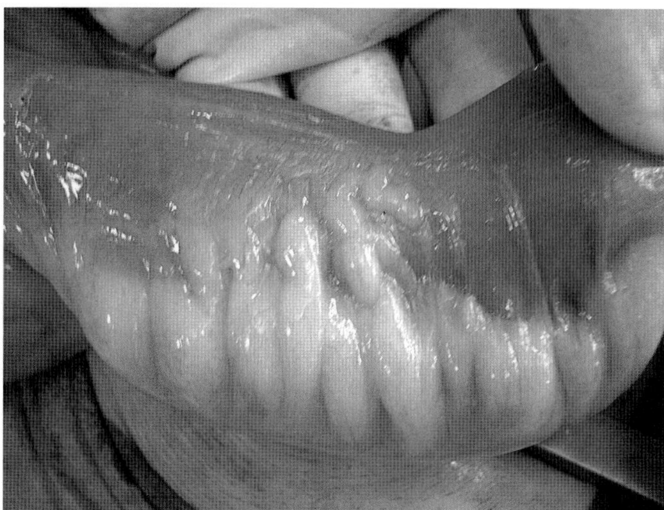

Figure 27.6 Small bowel resection demonstrating classic fat wrapping associated with Crohn's disease.

be effective in preventing recurrence after small bowel resection and azathioprine may also reduce recurrence.

Indications for surgery

Primary disease

Surgery tends to be reserved for patients who have failed medical management or in those who have developed complications of the disease, such as obstruction or fistula (Fig. 27.6). When surgery is delayed until the onset of septic complications such as abscess or fistula, there is a much greater risk that the subsequent operation will result in an extensive resection with the possibility of short bowel syndrome. The complication rate in such patients is significantly higher, and improvements in well-being and quality of life, and a low risk of subsequent recurrence indicate that some patients would clearly benefit from early surgical resection.

Complicated disease

The common indications for surgery are shown in Table 27.1.

Surgery is rarely required as an emergency in Crohn's disease, and there is no doubt that surgical planning and liaison with gastroenterologists improve outcome. Ileocolic Crohn's disease is occasionally noted as an incidental finding at the time of an appendicectomy (see Ch. 28). A lack of informed consent and the expertise of the operating surgeon often determine conservatism. There is, however, evidence to support a favourable outcome if a limited ileocolic resection is performed at the time.

When there is an absolute indication for surgical intervention, the decision to operate is easily made, and the procedure must be tailored to cope with the extent of the disease. In general, the simplest surgical procedure that can solve the problem should be selected. There is now no place for massive resection of the small bowel in an attempt to clear all disease. In a patient with active disease it can be very difficult to determine just how much small bowel is involved. A judicious defunctioning split ileostomy, or appropriate and aggressive preoperative medical or nutrition therapy, may allow inflamed bowel to settle and limit the extent of the subsequent resection.

Acute small bowel perforation or haemorrhage are rare complications occurring in less than 2% of hospital admissions for Crohn's disease, but both must be treated by small bowel resection.[51] The patient with persistent or recurrent pain with or without obstruction who fails to respond to medical treatment is a candidate for excisional surgery if the disease is limited. This is particularly true where ileal disease is causing right ureteric obstruction. Intra-abdominal abscesses should be drained, and in most situations radiologically guided percutaneous drainage of an abscess provides satisfactory resolution, at least in the short term. On many occasions, however, the abscesses are multiloculate and surgical drainage is then more appropriate. Enterocutaneous fistulae and nutritional complications of Crohn's disease are discussed later in this chapter under *Intestinal failure*.

Table 27.1 Indications for surgery for Crohn's disease

- Intestinal obstruction
- Abscess formation
- Fistula formation
- Failure of medical treatment for limited disease
- Nutritional failure
- Small bowel perforation (rare)
- Acute severe haemorrhage (rare)
- Uncertainty of diagnosis

Surgical options

Where surgery is selected, it should be as limited as possible and tailored to meet the particular needs of the patient. It used to be fashionable to examine the margins of bowel resection by frozen section until no evidence of Crohn's inflammatory pathology was found.[52] This has been shown to be unnecessary, and resection only needs to remove macroscopic disease.[53,54]

Surgery should be regarded as 'an incident in a lifetime of disease, rather than an attempt at cure'.[53] At operation, diseased bowel should if at all possible be resected rather than bypassed, because recurrence occurs earlier after bypass surgery.[55] Sometimes a bypass may allow sufficient resolution of the inflamed bowel for resection to be possible 6–12 months later.

The technique of stricturoplasty has been introduced for the management of short chronic strictures of the small bowel. The stricture is divided longitudinally before being sutured horizontally.[56] Balloon dilatation of multiple strictures may also be undertaken at operation.[57]

It is difficult to distinguish operative mortality from the mortality of the disease itself. The operative mortality is probably about 3%,[58] and there is a twofold increase in the overall mortality compared with the general population at all ages.[59] Following any first or subsequent resection for small bowel Crohn's disease, recurrence requiring further surgery occurs

REFERENCES

51. Greenstein AJ et al. Am J Gastroenterol 1985; 80: 682
52. Kyle J. Br J Surg 1972; 59: 821
53. Lee ECG. Gut 1984; 25: 219
54. Cooper JC, Williams NS. Ann R Coll Surg Engl 1986; 68: 23
55. Homan WP, Dineen P. Ann Surg 1978; 187: 530
56. Alexander Williams J. Int J Colorectal Dis 1986; 1: 54
57. Alexander Williams J et al. Ann R Coll Surg Engl 1986; 68: 95
58. Brooke BN et al. Crohn's Disease. Macmillan, London, 1977
59. Higgens CS, Allan RN. Gut 1980; 21: 933

in 40% at 10 years and in 50% at 15 years, figures that are considerably higher than those for Crohn's colitis (see Ch. 30).[60]

CARCINOMA IN CROHN'S DISEASE

Adenocarcinomas may develop in a small intestine that has been affected by chronic long-standing Crohn's disease. In two-thirds of cases the ileum is the site of the tumour, although it is still very rare.[61] The prognosis is poor, with over 70% of patients dying within 8 months of the diagnosis, despite surgery. The reason for this probably relates to a delay in diagnosis, because the symptoms may initially be ascribed to 'recurrent' Crohn's disease. These tumours do, however, tend to be diffuse and infiltrating, arising in areas of epithelial dysplasia. There is no evidence that there is an increase or a decrease in non-intestinal malignant tumours in patients with Crohn's disease.

OTHER INFLAMMATORY CONDITIONS

BACKWASH ILEITIS

In patients with severe ulcerative colitis with total involvement of colon, the terminal ileum may occasionally be affected by an acute or a chronic non-specific inflammatory change (see Ch. 28). It is important to recognize this possibility when surgery is undertaken for ulcerative colitis, and not to confuse the condition with Crohn's disease. The ileum can be preserved, and the inflammation will resolve once the diseased colon has been resected.

SARCOIDOSIS

Involvement of the small intestine by sarcoid is very rare, but if the lymph nodes of the mesentery are involved a protein-losing enteropathy can result.[62]

HENOCH–SCHÖNLEIN PURPURA

Henoch–Schönlein purpura occasionally affects the small intestine, usually in children. It usually presents as an 'acute abdomen' with the signs of peritonitis or with obstruction associated with an intussusception at the site of a haemorrhage in the wall of the intestine (see Ch. 25). It is important to recognize the condition at laparotomy, because reduction or resection of an intussusception may be necessary.

SYSTEMIC SCLEROSIS

Any of the connective tissue disorders may affect the small intestine, but the best recognized is scleroderma, producing systemic sclerosis. If the gastrointestinal tract is affected, about half of cases involve the duodenum, where the smooth muscle is replaced by fibrous tissue.[63] Involvement of the small intestine results in bacterial overgrowth, malabsorption, malnutrition, abdominal pain, bloating and eventually functional obstruction, often erroneously referred to as 'pseudo-obstruction'. It may be difficult to distinguish mechanical obstruction from this form of functional obstruction, and occasionally the diagnosis is found only at laparotomy.

INTESTINAL FAILURE

Intestinal failure is defined as the reduction in functional gut capacity below a level that enables adequate digestion and absorption of nutrients.[64] The pathophysiology was experimentally described by Senn in 1888,[65] and clinically by Flint in 1912 and Hammond in 1935.[66,67] The vast majority of cases of intestinal failure are temporary, straightforward, and can be managed without difficulty in district general hospitals. There are, however, a small number of difficult cases that tax even the most experienced and specialized teams.

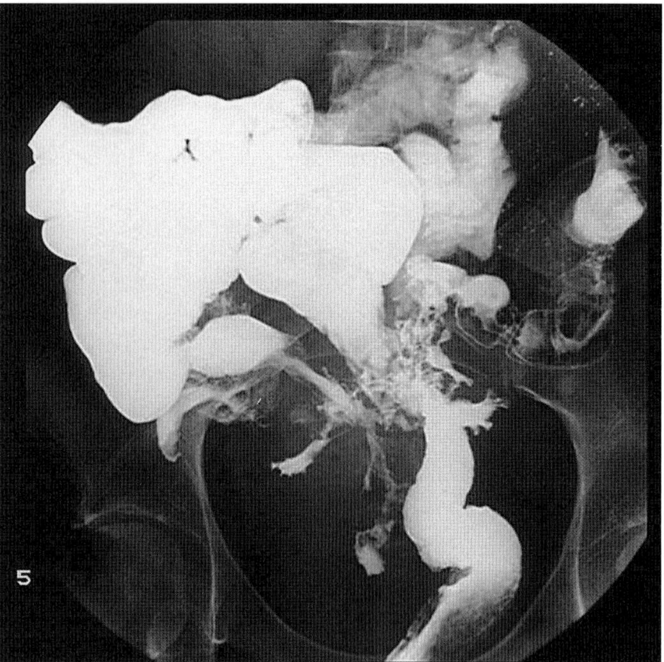

Figure 27.7 Enterocolocutaneous fistula demonstrated on barium follow-through.

The underlying cause of the intestinal failure may be divided into four classes:

1. Short bowel syndrome, defined as a malabsorptive state that follows massive resection of small intestine.
2. Fistulous disease resulting in bypass of functional small intestine by an enterocutaneous fistula, occasionally by an enterocolic tract (Fig. 27.7).
3. Inflammatory conditions of the small bowel that result in non-functioning enterocytes, such as sprue, coeliac disease or radiation enteritis.
4. Dysmotility conditions that occur acutely in postoperative ileus and chronically in pseudo-obstruction and visceral neuropathies.

The detailed management of these classes is complex, and only the principles of management and nutritional support are described.

EPIDEMIOLOGY

There are few studies on the prevalence of short bowel syndrome. Pilot studies suggest that two patients per million require long-

REFERENCES

60. deDomball FJ et al. Gut 1971; 12: 519
61. Hawker PC et al. Gut 1982; 23: 188
62. Popovic OS et al. Gastroenterology 1980; 78: 119
63. Bluestone R et al. Gut 1969; 10: 185
64. Ladefoged K et al. Gut 1989; 30: 943–949
65. Senn N. Ann Surg 1888; 7: 99–115
66. Flint JM. Bull Johns Hopkins Hosp 1912, 127–144
67. Hammond HE. Surg Gynecol Obstet 1935; 61: 693–705

term parenteral nutrition. Half of these may be suitable for small bowel transplantation.

AETIOLOGY OF SHORT BOWEL SYNDROME

The underlying causes of chronic intestinal failure differ between adults and children.

AETIOLOGY OF FISTULOUS DISEASE

The majority of fistulae occur in postoperative patients,[68,69] and are most commonly associated with anastomotic dehiscence. The risk factors for this include the age of the patient, the state of the bowel undergoing anastomosis, the preoperative nutritional status of the patient, and the site of the anastomosis. When associated with malignancy the extent of tumour fixity, the presence of obstruction, previous radiotherapy, an associated abscess and surgical technique all determine the risk. The other common causes of fistulae are Crohn's disease, colorectal cancer and diverticular disease.[70] Rarer conditions include congenital fistulae, such as a patent vitellointestinal tract, traumatic wounding, and inadvertent unrecognized iatrogenic damage occurring during surgery. Tuberculosis may fistulate, and actinomycosis is an alternative possibility. Radiation damage may cause complex and entero-enteric fistulae, which have a high mortality.

CLINICAL PRESENTATION

The syndrome is characterized by diarrhoea from a stoma or fistula, fluid and electrolyte abnormalities, malabsorption and weight loss.[71] Typically there are three stages of intestinal failure.

First, there is a period of diarrhoea or high output from a fistula or stoma. This results in fluid and electrolyte loss, and lasts up to 2 weeks. In this phase, fluid and electrolyte balance are the most immediate concerns. Food is usually restricted, because it contributes to gastric hypersecretion and raised ileal effluent.

Second, there is a period of adaptation lasting up to a year. During this phase, the intestine adapts by dilatation of the bowel, lengthening of the villi and deepening crypts, thus increasing surface area for absorption. Enteral or luminal nutrition, essential for adaptation, is slowly reintroduced and parenteral supplementation is weaned as far as possible.

Finally, the third phase of maximum adaptation is reached. A steady state is achieved, ideally without total parenteral nutrition or enteral feeding.

ENTEROCUTANEOUS FISTULAE

Enterocutaneous fistulae often arise from surgical complications, especially in patients with Crohn's disease. Early reoperation, in an attempt to fix the problem, often results in more fistulae and a worse outcome. The keys to successful management are described below.

Sepsis

Untreated sepsis is the commonest cause of death in patients with enterocutaneous fistulae. Identification and treatment of intra-abdominal and other sources of infection with antibiotics and adequate surgical or radiological drainage is essential (Fig. 27.8).

Nutrition

Replacement of fluid and electrolytes to counter the fistula losses, and parenteral or enteral nutritional support to maintain an adequate nutrition are equally important (see Ch. 2).

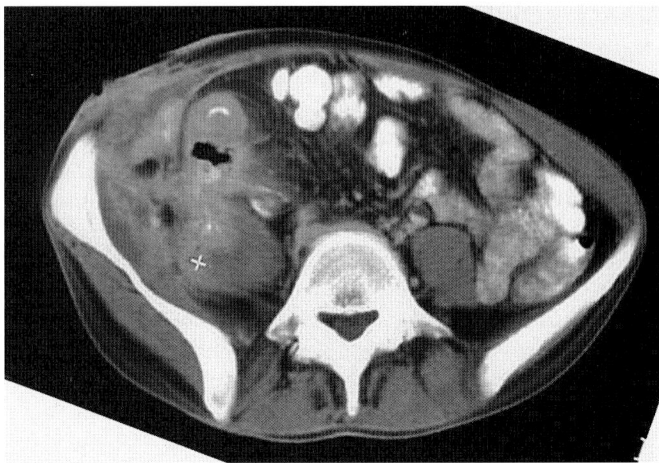

Figure 27.8 Psoas abscess with lateral enterocutaneous fistula on CT scan.

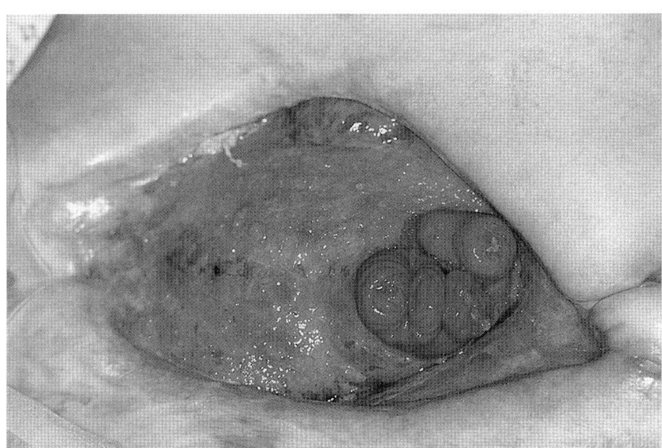

Figure 27.9 Multiple enterocutaneous fistulae.

Protection of the skin

The enzyme content of the fistula fluid may produce severe excoriation of the surrounding skin, which requires skill and ingenuity to treat. Stomahesive, corya paste, and aluminium paste and suction may all be helpful in providing protection.

Planned surgery

Once the patient is stable, the skin protected, and the fluid balance and nutrition returned to normal, the anatomy of the fistula can be determined by appropriate radiology. Under most circumstances, small bowel fistulae heal spontaneously without requiring further surgery. When there is complete intestinal disruption, loss of mucocutaneous continuity, active disease at the fistula site or distal intestinal obstruction, further surgery is going to be required to close the fistula (Fig. 27.9). Definitive surgery should be delayed for approximately 6 months from the onset of the fistula to allow time for the adhesions to settle and for a neoperitoneum to form.

REFERENCES

68. Reber H et al. Ann Surg 1978; 188: 460–467
69. McIntyre PB et al. Br J Surg 1984; 71: 293–296
70. Irvin TT, Goligher JC. Br J Surg 1973; 60: 461–464
71. McIntyre PB. Br J Surg 1985; 72 (Suppl): S92–S93

SMALL BOWEL TRANSPLANTATION

Home parenteral nutrition is essential for patients with significant chronic intestinal failure. In some patients, this becomes impossible because of inadequate vascular access or because hepatic failure develops as a complication of parenteral feeding. These patients require intestinal transplantation if they are to survive. The long-term outlook for small bowel transplant is poor (see Ch. 8). Small bowel is very susceptible to rejection and has the potential to induce graft-versus-host disease. The powerful immunosuppressive regimens required to prevent rejection increase the risk of sepsis and subsequent lymphoproliferative disorders, with sepsis and lymphoma accounting for some 70% of deaths in these patients.

TRAUMA

OPEN WOUNDS

Wounds of the abdomen that are presumed to be penetrating were always thought to require exploration, because the consequences of adopting a policy of careful observation were known to occasionally be fatal. This view has been challenged by reports suggesting that careful observation of the patient, combined with intravenous fluids and antibiotics, might result in a better selection of patients requiring laparotomy (see Ch. 7).[72] These reports have come from hospitals dealing with so many cases of abdominal injury that the workload overwhelms the capacity to provide care; in hospitals where fewer abdominal injuries are seen, a policy of laparotomy for all patients with likely penetrating wounds of the abdomen is probably still more appropriate. The rising incidence of stab injuries in many parts of the UK[73] may result in a change in policy in the future.

When the small intestine is examined during an operation for a penetrating wound of the abdomen, it may be found to be contused, perforated or transected. The mesentery may be damaged with the bowel, or it may be damaged alone. The viability of the bowel depends on the extent to which the mesenteric vessels, and particularly the vessels of the peripheral arcade, have been divided or thrombosed.[74]

Small perforations may be closed with one or two layers of absorbable sutures inserted so that the line of closure is transverse. Large perforations and multiple perforations placed close together usually require resection, with reconstitution by end-to-end anastomosis.

Occasionally the intestine is perforated from within (Fig. 27.10), and the patient presents with a peritonitis (see Ch. 25). Toothpicks, bristles, fishbones, meat bones, nails, wood splinters and other sharp objects have all been described as perforating agents.

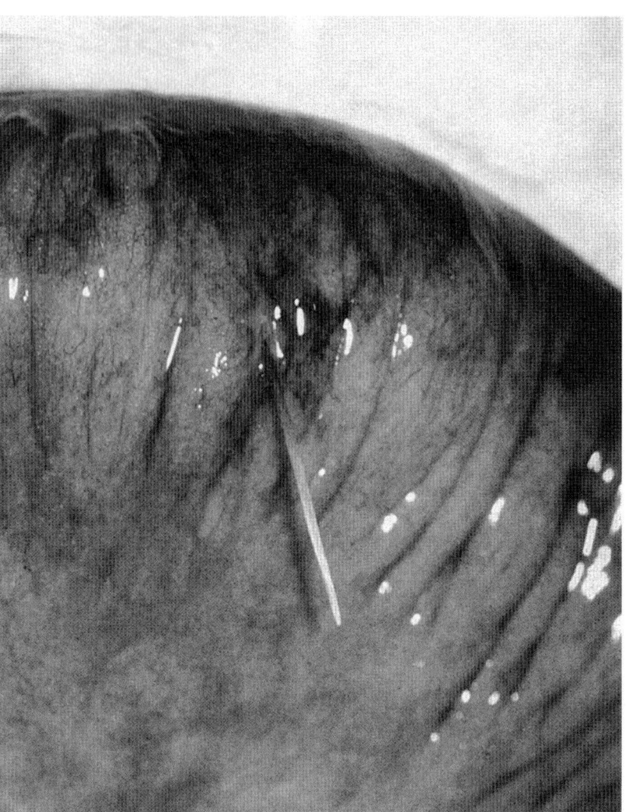

Figure 27.10 A fishbone penetrating the small bowel and presenting in a patient as peritonitis.

BLUNT TRAUMA

The small intestine may be contused or divided by abdominal trauma, without penetration (see Ch. 7). Small intestine partially fixed by adhesions is particularly prone to this type of injury. The normal, non-adherent bowel is injured only by sudden trauma to the abdominal wall, which catches the patient unprepared and with the abdominal muscles uncontracted, allowing the bowel to be squeezed between the traumatizing agent and the vertebral column.

The upper jejunum and lower ileum are most commonly injured, because these are the segments that are prevented from escaping by their relatively fixed attachments to duodenum and caecum. Injury to the duodenum is potentially the most serious, because it is often associated with pancreatic injury (see Ch. 26). This may not be immediately obvious, and serious retroperitoneal sepsis may develop before the diagnosis is made. Blunt trauma was responsible in 14 out of 131 patients with duodenal injury in one large series.[75] The liver was coincidentally damaged in 38% of cases, the pancreas in 28% and the inferior vena cava in 17%.

The diagnosis of duodenal injury is often difficult at laparotomy, although bile staining of the retroperitoneal tissues may provide a clue. The duodenum should be mobilized by a Kocher manoeuvre, and the ligament of Treitz should be divided if there is doubt about a duodenal injury. The presence of a large retroperitoneal haematoma may be caused by an injury of the vena cava, and mobilization of the duodenum may release tamponade and result in torrential venous haemorrhage. A catheter may be introduced into the duodenum through a gastrotomy and water-soluble radiopaque medium introduced. On-table radiographs are then taken to determine if there is a duodenal perforation. When the duodenum appears to be intact and the retroperitoneal haematoma is not expanding, it is probably wiser not to mobilize the duodenum and simply to institute gastric aspiration. When the duodenum is shown to be ruptured, mobilization is necessary and preparations must be made for dealing with a potential injury to the inferior vena cava (see Ch. 11).

REFERENCES

72. Oreskovich MR, Caricco CJ. Ann Surg 1983; 198: 411
73. Mariadson JG et al. Ann Surg 1988; 207: 335
74. Murless BC. Br J Surg 1942–3; 30
75. Morton JR, Jordan GL. J Trauma 1968; 8: 127

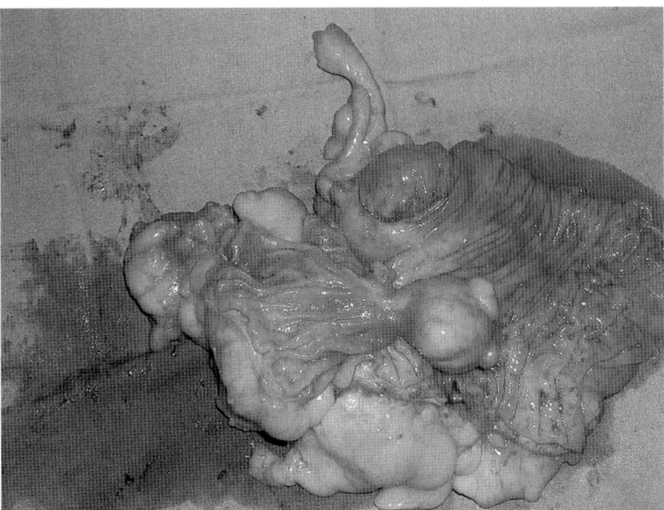

Figure 27.11 Resection specimen demonstrating a terminal ileal polyp that was identified on colonoscopy as it prolapsed through the ileocaecal valve.

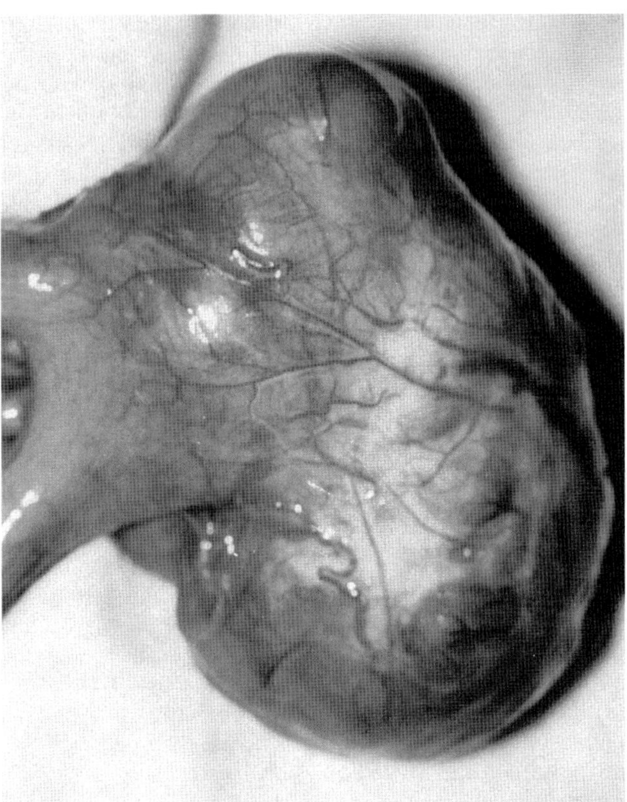

Figure 27.12 An exenteric leiomyoma of the terminal ileum.

TUMOURS

The small bowel accounts for approximately 75% of the length of the gastrointestinal tract and 80–90% of its surface area, but only 1.5–6% of gastrointestinal neoplasms are found in the small intestine, with a quarter of these arising in the short duodenal segment.[76] Small bowel tumours are therefore rare but may demonstrate a variety of pathologies, ranging from benign, through intermediate lesions with strong malignant potential, to frankly malignant lesions (Figs 27.11 and 27.12, Table 27.2).[77]

Table 27.2 Classification of small bowel tumours

Benign tumours

Epithelial
- Tubular adenoma
- Villous adenoma
- Polyposis syndromes (adenomas)
- Brunner's gland adenoma

Stromal
- Adipose tissue: lipoma
- Connective tissue: leiomyomas, neurogenic or fibroma

Endothelial
- Vascular
- Lymphatic

Hamartomas
- Peutz–Jeghers syndrome

Intermediate tumours
- APUD tumours: carcinoid or gastrinomas

Malignant tumours
All the benign and intermediate tumours may develop malignant potential.

Primary
- Adenocarcinoma
- Sarcoma: leiomyosarcoma, fibrosarcoma, liposarcoma or angiosarcoma
- Lymphoma

Secondaries

CLASSIFICATION OF SMALL BOWEL TUMOURS

Presentation

Small bowel tumours are frequently symptomless, only being detected as incidental findings at laparotomy or autopsy. For example, half the patients who died from metastatic malignant melanoma were found to have small bowel secondaries at post-mortem.[79] Small bowel tumours can cause non-specific symptoms that include nausea, bloating and abdominal pain; they may also cause anaemia, haemorrhage and obstruction. The last of these is the presenting feature in over half of the cases and may be partial or complete, be acute or chronic, and result from intussusception, volvulus or stenosis. Haemorrhage, which may be acute or more commonly chronic, is the presenting feature in up to a half of the cases.[79] In gastrinomas or carcinoid tumours, the presenting symptoms can be with persisting treatment-resistant peptic ulceration in the case of gastrinomas (see Ch. 26), or carcinoid syndrome.

Investigation and management

Imaging of the small bowel beyond the third part of the duodenum, or proximal to the terminal ileum, is difficult. Upper

REFERENCES

76. Williamson RCN et al. Ann Surg 1983; 197: 172
77. Dial P, Cohn I Jr. In: Scott HW Jr, Sawyers JL (eds). Surgery of the Stomach, Duodenum and Small Intestine. Blackwell Scientific Publications, Boston, 1987: 937–951
78. Das Gupta TK, Brasfield RD. Arch Surg 1964; 88: 969
79. Ashley SW, Wells SA Jr. Semin Oncol 1988; 15: 116–128

gastrointestinal endoscopy and colonoscopy allow inspection of the proximal and distal small bowel but does not assess the majority of the jejunum or ileum. Radiographic imaging performed and interpreted by an experienced radiologist, by either small bowel follow-through or small bowel enema with contrast installed directly and rapidly into the duodenum via a nasoduodenal tube, is still the best method for assessing this part of the bowel. Direct endoscopic inspection of the bowel is possible via small bowel enteroscopy. A 5-mm scope can be passed into the duodenum and moved through the small bowel, although intubation times can take up to 6 h and its availability is limited to specialized centres.[80] A novel technique that consists of swallowing a capsule containing a small camera provides intermittent images as peristalsis passes it through the small bowel. The images can then be analysed.[81]

Laparotomy may often be required to diagnose and treat small bowel tumours. They may be obvious on external inspection but it may be necessary to inspect the lumen of the bowel.

Isolated tumours may be removed by a limited small bowel resection. Multiple polyps that occur in Peutz–Jeghers syndrome may be removed by endoscopic snare resection.[82]

Carcinoid tumours and other neuroendocrine tumours

Carcinoid tumours are derived from neural crest cells and are part of the amine precursor uptake and decarboxylation (APUD) group of cells, which includes gastrinomas (Fig. 27.13). The term *carcinoid* was introduced by Obendorfer in 1907 to describe a tumour of the small intestine with a capacity to metastasize but which was slow-growing and had a good prognosis.[83] Seventy-five per cent of primary carcinoid tumours occur in the gastro-intestinal tract, with the majority occurring in the small intestine or in the appendix, where it accounts for 85% of appendicular neoplasms.[84] Midgut carcinoids can be identified by their capacity for staining with ammoniacal silver nitrate (argentaffin). They usually secrete high levels of serotonin, and may also secrete a variety of other peptides including gastrin, glucagon and somato-statin. Carcinoids can be considered to have an intermediate malignant potential and with a spectrum ranging from benign to frankly malignant.

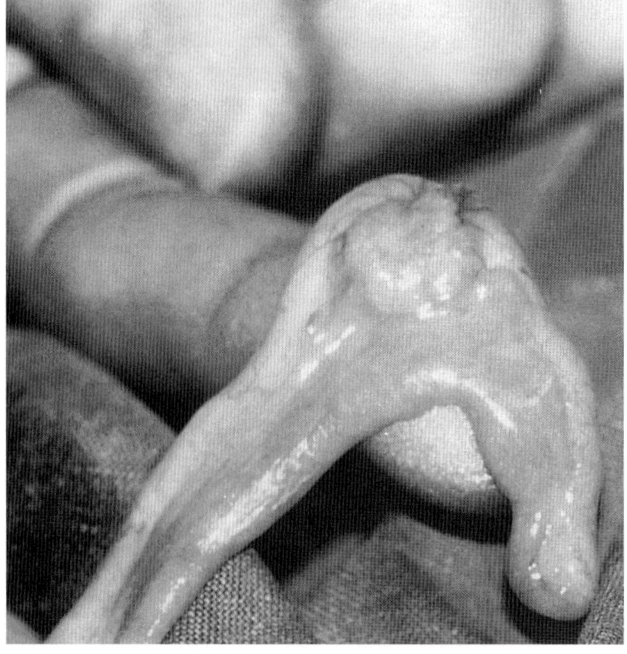

Figure 27.13 A carcinoid tumour of the appendix.

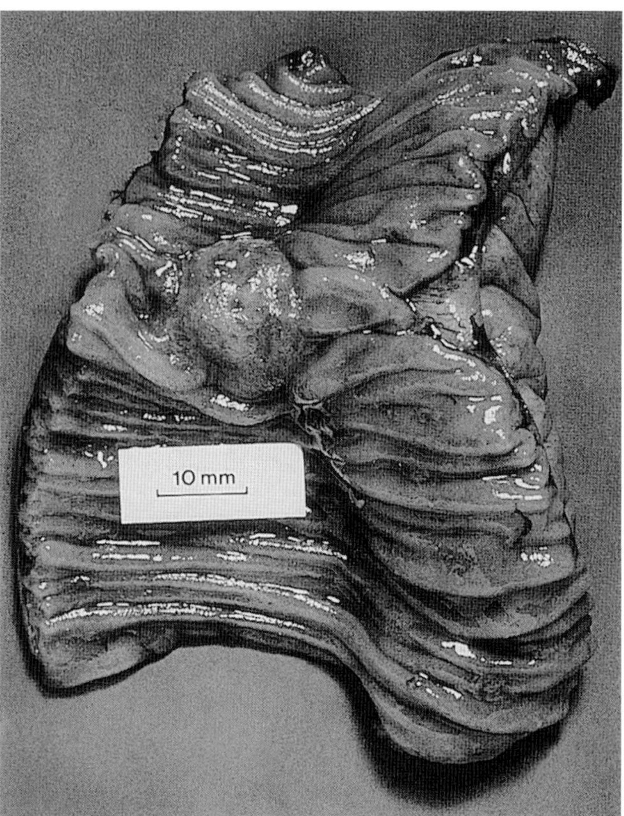

Figure 27.14 A resected specimen of ileum opened to show a carcinoid tumour.

Small bowel carcinoids are usually symptomless or present with non-specific abdominal pain (Fig. 27.14). Differential diagnoses include irritable bowel syndrome, peptic ulcer disease, gastritis or Crohn's disease, because symptoms are often present for 4–5 years prior to diagnosis.[85] The tumours can be recognized by the intense cicatrization that they produce, and when the bowel is opened they appear as raised, yellow submucosal tumours, sometimes with a central area of mucosal ulceration.

Four per cent of patients with small bowel carcinoid tumours develop the carcinoid syndrome from systemic dissemination of vasoactive secretions. This is not a manifestation of non-metastastic carcinoid because serotonin is metabolized in the liver, and it is only when the tumour has metastasized to the liver that serotonin is secreted into the systemic circulation. Symptoms include flushing, diarrhoea and bronchospasm. Identification of 5-hydroxyindoleacetic acid (a breakdown product of serotonin) in the urine is a marker of the syndrome. OctreoScan®, a radioscintigraphic technique using indium-111-labelled octreo-

REFERENCES

80. Cotton PB, Williams CB. Practical Gastrointestinal Endoscopy. 4th edn. Blackwell Scientific Publications, Oxford, 1996
81. Swain P. Gut 2003; 52: 48–50
82. Ishida H, Murata N, Tada M et al. Surg Today 1999; 29: 581–583
83. Obendorfer S. Frankf Z Pathol 1907; 1: 426
84. Modlin IM, Sandor A. Cancer 1997; 79: 813–834
85. Bax NDS et al. World J Surg 1996; 20: 142–146

tide, has demonstrated good accuracy in identifying the location of suspected carcinoid tumours.[86]

Carcinoid tumours should be widely excised with their draining mesenteric lymph nodes. Once the primary tumour exceeds 2 cm in diameter, there is an 80% chance of metastases developing. Appendicular carcinoids may be found incidentally at appendicectomy, but a formal right hemicolectomy is indicated if they exceed 2 cm in diameter.[87] In 40% of cases metastases are found at laparotomy. Cure can be achieved only if all the tumour can be resected, and in some cases this may necessitate hepatic resection. Surgery must inevitably be palliative if complete resection cannot be attained, and the aim of treatment is to relieve the local and distant effects caused by the tumour and its secretions. After surgical debulking the administration of octreotide often abolishes the effects of the carcinoid syndrome, and administration of radiolabelled octreotide and chemotherapy may provide good palliation.[88] The prognosis is dependent on the tumour characteristics, and patients may survive for an extended period of time with metastatic carcinoid tumour.

Gastrinomas and other APUD tumours may be found in the duodenum and the rest of the small bowel but are much more commonly found in the pancreas (see Ch. 31). They may be very small and localization can be difficult. Presentation depends on the active product secreted, but very small tumours can produce full syndromes such as recurrent ulceration (Zollinger–Ellison syndrome secondary to gastrin; see Ch. 26).[89] One half of tumours are malignant, and 50–80% are found to have metastatic lymph nodes at operation.

Surgery is indicated only if a complete resection is thought possible, which may not be apparent until surgery. Otherwise tumours may be palliated by proton pump inhibitors in Zollinger–Ellison syndrome (see Ch. 26).[90]

Lymphoma

Primary lymphomas of the small bowel are rare and may occur at any age or at any site in the small bowel. Patients with coeliac disease are at increased risk, and deteriorating symptoms in a coeliac patient should raise concern. Lymphomas complicating coeliac disease are usually T-cell lymphomas as compared with the usual B-cell lymphoma. Other groups at increased risk include patients with AIDS and those who have undergone small bowel transplantation.

The presentation tends to be non-specific, as with other small bowel tumours, although obstruction is the commonest symptom and some patients present with an abdominal mass. Abdominal CT may identify a mass but the diagnosis is usually made only at laparotomy. Treatment is by small bowel resection, although in some cases only bypass is possible. Patients may receive chemotherapy but the prognosis remains poor, with a 5-year survival rate of less than 20%.[91]

A diffuse lymphoma (Mediterranean type) may develop and result in profound malabsorption. The diagnosis is made by small bowel biopsy combined with demonstration of free alpha chains in the serum, saliva or urine.[92]

Peutz-Jeghers syndrome

Peutz–Jeghers syndrome is an inherited autosomal dominant condition. Multiple hamartomatous polyps develop throughout the stomach, the small bowel and the large bowel, and patients usually have speckled pigmentation around the oral and buccal mucosa (Fig. 27.15).[93,94] The polyps eventually develop symptoms such as obstruction or anaemia secondary to chronic bleeding. Malignant change may occur in the polyps.[95] Identification of the syndrome is important, and genetic markers may contribute to this.

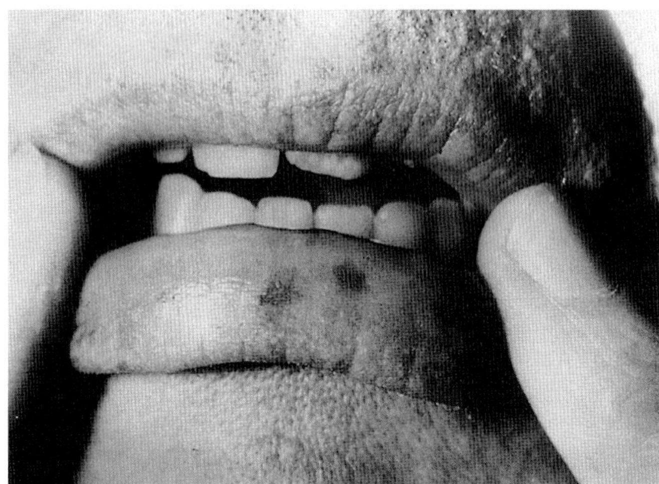

Figure 27.15 Circumoral pigmentation of the Peutz–Jeghers syndrome.

Surgery for small bowel polyps is indicated if the patient becomes symptomatic or if the polyps exceed 1.5 cm in diameter. On-table enteroscopy with endoscopic snare resection is the intervention of choice for small bowel polyps (Fig. 27.16).[96]

Duodenal tumours

Duodenal neoplasms are rare and are most common in the first part of the duodenum. The risk of malignancy increases as they become more distal. The presentation is usually with gastrointestinal haemorrhage, and adenomas are the most common tumours. Malignant lesions are rare and account for only 0.3% of gastrointestinal neoplasms, with adenocarcinoma the most common pathology. Presentation may be with obstructive symptoms or an abdominal mass, although if the lesion is periampullary the patient may present with jaundice (see Ch. 30). If the lesion is resectable, pancreaticoduodenectomy is the procedure of choice. More commonly, however, radical resection is contraindicated because of local invasion or metastatic disease. Biliary stenting or surgical bypass if there is biliary obstruction, or a surgical gastrojejunostomy for duodenal obstruction provide useful palliation.

REFERENCES

86. Krenning EP et al. Eur J Nucl Med 1993; 20: 716–731
87. Memon MA, Nelson H. Dis Colon Rectum 1997; 40: 1101–1118
88. Otte A et al. Lancet 1998; 351: 417–418
89. Zollinger RM, Ellison EH. Ann Surg 1955; 142: 709
90. Lamers C et al. N Engl J Med 1984; 310: 758
91. Awrich AE et al. Surg Obstet Gynecol 1980; 151: 9
92. Al Saleem TI. Lancet 1978; ii: 709.
93. Peutz JLA. Ned Maandschr Geneesk 1921; 10: 134
94. Jeghers H. N Engl J Med 1944; 231: 88
95. Cochet B et al. Gut 1979; 20: 169
96. Spigelman AD et al. Br J Surg 1995; 82: 1311–1314

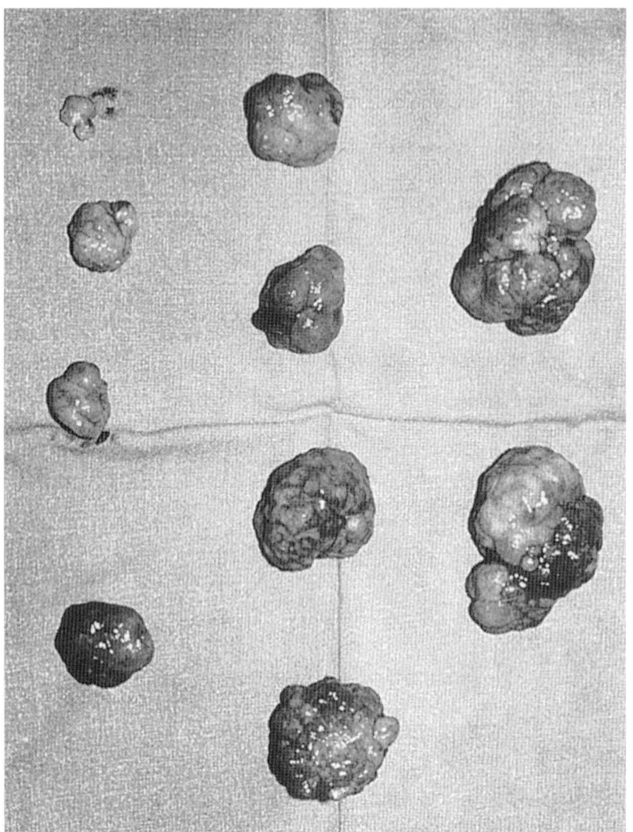

Figure 27.16 Multiple hamartomas removed endoscopically from the small intestine through a single enterostomy made at the time of laparotomy.

Duodenal disease in familial adenomatous polyposis

Familial adenomatous polyposis was previously known as familial polyposis coli, the change in name reflecting the recognition of extracolonic polyps and cancers (see Ch. 28).

Table 27.3 Aetiology of small bowel ischaemia

Arterial thrombosis
- Atherosclerosis
- Thrombotic conditions

Arterial embolism
- Atrial fibrillation
- Mural thrombus
- Vegetations
- Atherosclerotic plaque

Venous thrombosis
Predisposed by
- Hypercoagulable states
- Malignancy
- Inflammation (e.g. pancreatitis or inflammatory bowel disease)
- Mechanical venous occlusion (e.g. volvulus or intussusception)

Rare causes
- Aortic dissection
- Cardiac bypass
- Low-flow states (e.g. cardiogenic shock or septicaemia)
- Interventional radiology

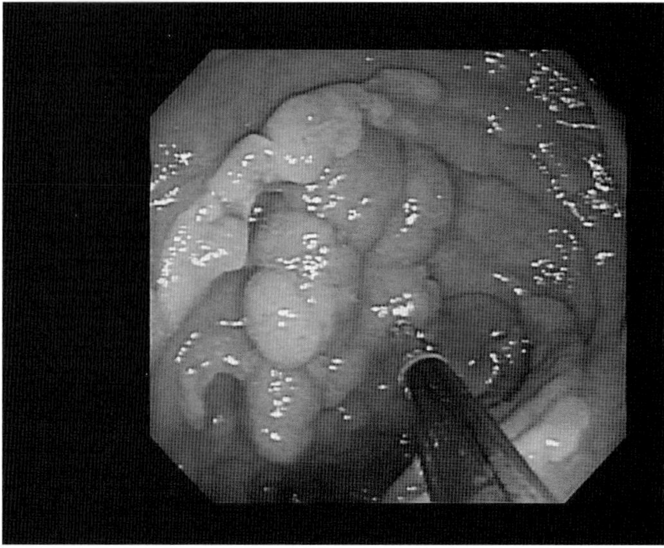

Figure 27.17 Duodenal carcinoma demonstrated on endoscopy.

Epidemiology and natural history

Adenomas tend to be noted in the duodenum approximately 15 years after colonic polyps occur,[97] but this may simply reflect the time when they are sought.

Adenomas are distributed throughout the duodenum and small bowel, the majority being found in clusters around and distal to the ampulla of Vater.[98] Very few are found proximal to the ampulla compared with the number found in the second part of the duodenum. This distribution of polyps closely mirrors the pattern of mucosal exposure to bile.

Duodenal cancer is rare, with an incidence of 0.01–0.04% in the general population (Fig. 27.17).[99] Men are more often affected, usually in the sixth decade. Polyposis is associated with a high frequency of duodenal or periampullary cancer, with estimates of between 1 and 12%,[100] and men and women are equally affected.

Treatment

The aim is to control duodenal polyposis and thereby prevent the development of malignancy. The outcome after surgery for already established duodenal, periampullary or pancreatic malignancy is relatively poor.

ISCHAEMIA OR INFARCTION

Small intestinal ischaemia or infarction occurs from a variety of causes, all resulting from an impairment of the arterial supply (Table 27.3). The speed of development and the degree of arterial impairment determine the clinical presentation, whether acute or chronic.

REFERENCES

97. Sarre RG et al. Gut 1987; 28: 306–314
98. Debinski HS et al. Eur J Cancer 1995; 31A: 1149–1153
99. Lillemoe K et al. Surg Gynecol Obstet 1980; 150: 822–826
100. Jones TR, Nance FC. Ann Surg 1977; 185: 565–573

AETIOLOGY OF SMALL BOWEL ISCHAEMIA

Acute ischaemia

Aetiology

Acute ischaemia is most common in the elderly and is caused by the pathologies shown in Box 27.3. Mesenteric embolism accounts for 25–30% of patients with acute intestinal ischaemia.[101] The most common site of origin is the heart, often from atrial thrombus secondary to atrial fibrillation, but valvular pathology and mural thrombus secondary to myocardial infarction may also embolize (see Ch. 22). The amount of infarcted small bowel depends on the site of impaction of the embolus in the mesenteric arterial tree. Although coeliac embolism may occur, the superior mesenteric artery is the most common site of impaction. The collateral circulation of the bowel is adequate to maintain arterial perfusion if the embolus passes some distance down the superior mesenteric artery, although the collateral circulation is likely to be reduced in elderly patients with atherosclerotic disease. Emboli often impact just beyond the middle colic branch of the superior mesenteric artery, hence sparing the upper jejunum and transverse colon (Fig. 27.18).

Thrombosis of the superior mesenteric artery superimposed on atherosclerosis accounts for 10–15% of cases of acute intestinal ischaemia. The thrombosis usually occurs at the origin of the superior mesenteric artery, and as a consequence the infarction is usually extensive from just beyond the ligament of Treitz to the splenic flexure. Any low-flow situation can result in mesenteric ischaemia, with infarction more likely if there is an underlying arterial stenosis of the splanchnic vessels. Arteriovenous bypass during cardiac surgery is a recognized cause of 'low flow'.

Venous thrombosis is responsible for around 10% of cases of ischaemia and may have no identifiable cause. It may, however, result from any factor or combination of factors producing increased coagulability. This includes inherited thrombophilias such as protein C or S deficiency or neoplastic disease and may be induced by dehydration or sepsis.

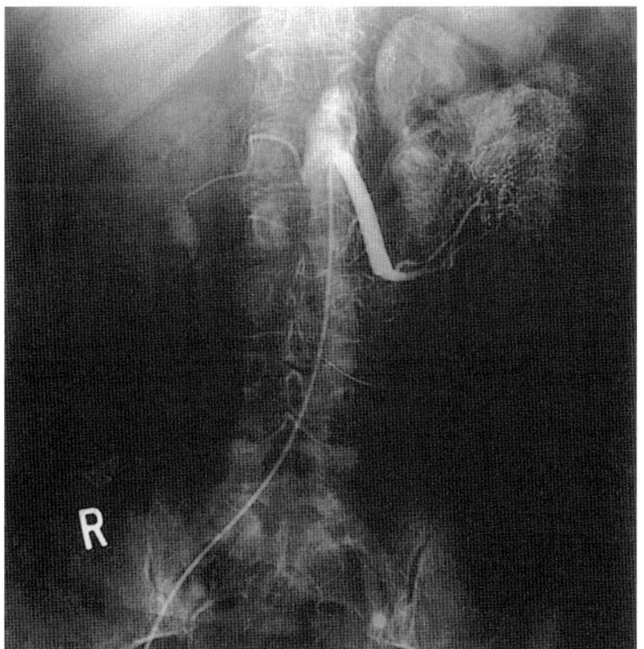

Figure 27.18 Selective superior mesenteric arteriogram showing an embolus lodged just beyond the first jejunal branch of the artery. This 74-year-old woman was suffering from atrial fibrillation.

Diagnosis

The symptoms of small bowel ischaemia or infarction tend to outweigh the signs. Patients complain of severe abdominal pain. The acuteness of onset depends on the aetiology, ranging from minutes in the case of arterial embolus to hours in the case of venous thrombosis. Copious vomiting and diarrhoea usually follow. Signs tend to be limited early in the condition to abdominal distension and minimal tenderness. 'Peritonism' develops only once full-thickness bowel infarction has occurred. Patients may have tachycardia or atrial fibrillation, which should raise suspicion, and they often develop cardiovascular instability, shock and systemic collapse as infarction develops.

A leukocytosis may be present, and arterial blood gas analysis often shows acidosis, a raised base excess and raised lipase, although these are all non-specific. The serum amylase is raised in half the patients, and a plain abdominal radiograph may demonstrate non-specific small bowel gaseous dilatation. The diagnosis may be confirmed by mesenteric arteriography, but suspicion in a patient with signs of peritonism indicates early laparotomy. In patients with minimal abdominal signs mesenteric arteriography may be diagnostic. The entire superior mesenteric artery may be missing if there is a thrombus arising at its ostium, whereas the proximal artery may be clearly visualized in the case of arterial embolism (Fig. 27.18).

Management

The patient is resuscitated, given intravenous antibiotics, and heparin is started. Radiological intervention with angioplasty or arterial thrombolysis is possible if the condition is picked up early, but laparotomy is usually indicated because the possibility of infarcted bowel remains. At laparotomy the whole bowel is inspected for viability, assessing bowel colour, peristalsis, arcade pulsation and bleeding when cut. Ischaemic bowel is grey and does not peristalse, and infarcted bowel is black and friable. Assessment may, however, be difficult and decisions over viability and the amount of bowel that needs to be resected are crucial to the long-term outcome. Often the ischaemia is so extensive that bowel resection is not attempted. Obviously, dead bowel is resected before revascularization is attempted. When sufficient potentially viable bowel is present, it should be revascularized through superior mesenteric artery embolectomy, or reconstruction by reimplanting the superior mesenteric artery into the aorta or by bypass grafting to it from the aorta.

Proximal superior mesenteric artery pulsation suggests embolism rather than thrombosis. The bowel is then reassessed for viability and dead bowel is resected. Short bowel syndrome is often inevitable, and marginally viable bowel should be left and reassessed at a second- (and third- if required) look laparotomy at 24–48 h.[102] Patients are likely to require intensive care support and often require parenteral nutrition for short or long periods.

The procedure is similar for venous thrombosis, but venous thrombectomy tends to be of little value and long-term anticoagulation is vital because the risk of recurrence is high.

REFERENCES

101. Marston A (ed). Vascular Disease of the Gut. Arnold, London, 1986
102. Davis M, Dawson K, Hamilton G. In: Beard JD, Gaines PA (ed). Vascular and Endovascular Surgery. WB Saunders, London, 2001

Low-flow states should be managed by resecting dead bowel and optimizing cardiac output, but mortality remains high at between 70 and 80%.[103]

Chronic ischaemia

Chronic intestinal ischaemia is rare despite the prevalence of visceral atherosclerotic disease, which is the predominant aetiology. Patients complain of severe upper or midabdominal pain around half an hour after eating, which is called 'mesenteric angina'. Patients develop profound weight loss as a result of avoiding food, vomiting and eating smaller meals. They are often female, heavy smokers, with evidence of extensive arterial disease. Mesenteric arteriography may demonstrate osteal stenoses or occlusions of the coeliac, superior or inferior mesenteric arteries, but it may still be difficult to prove that mesenteric ischaemia is the cause of the patient's symptoms.[104]

Revascularization is possible in selected patients if the patient is sufficiently symptomatic, although this is not without risk because patients tend to be chronically malnourished. Balloon dilatation is possible, and although objective data are limited, a long-term success rate of 76% with a mortality of 2% has been achieved.[105] Surgical revascularization is the alternative, either by bypass grafting, usually involving multiple rather than single vessels, or by endarterectomy of the visceral vessels (see Ch. 10). Adequacy of flow must be confirmed following the procedure once the bowel is returned to the abdominal cavity, and the patient should be nursed on intensive care.[106]

SMALL INTESTINAL RESECTION AND ILEOSTOMY

TECHNIQUE

The wide variation of techniques available for small bowel resection are described elsewhere,[107] but the general principles are accepted. The segment of small bowel to be removed is resected with a wedge of mesentery. The vessels in the mesentery should be individually ligated to leave the best possible blood supply to the ends of the bowel requiring anastomosis. The bowel ends should be seen to bleed after removal of any clamps, and if there is any doubt about the blood supply, for example in radiation-damaged small intestine, it is better to avoid applying clamps. When the viability of the bowel is in doubt, it is wiser to bring the two ends of the small intestine out on to the abdominal wall rather than anastomosing them. There are a variety of techniques for anastomosis, including single-layer extramucosal, two-layer or stapled; the general principles of a good blood supply, no tension, and minimal discrepancy in luminal size are important. Size discrepancy may be overcome by taking bites of varying thickness, by creating a Cheatle slit, or by creating an end-to-side or side-to-side anastomosis with a linear stapler having closed off both bowel ends.

ILEOSTOMY

There are a variety of indications for forming an ileostomy, which include diversion of the faecal stream from a more distal anastomosis; avoidance of an anastomosis in conditions of ischaemia, infection or poor nutrition; and as a definite stoma following excision of all the bowel distal to the small bowel in cases where formation of an ileoanal pouch is contraindicated (see Ch. 28). The technical aspects of ileostomies were developed by Brian Brooke.

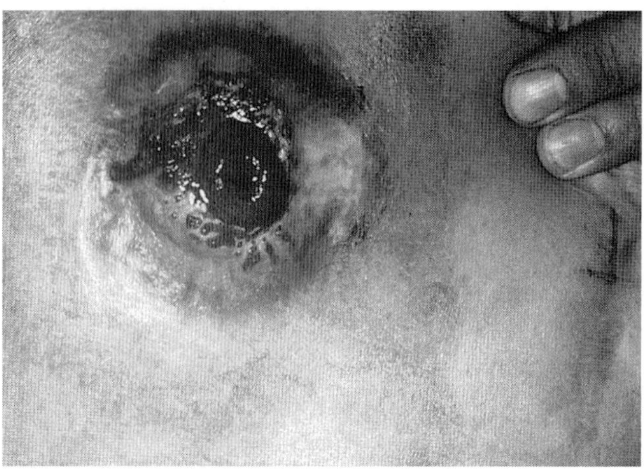

Figure 27.19 Varices developing around an ileostomy in a 50-year-old man who developed portal cirrhosis and portal hypertension 15 years after panproctocolectomy for ulcerative colitis.

Ileostomies may be either a 'loop' or an 'end'. A loop ileostomy is usually formed in the terminal ileum and used to divert the faecal stream from a downstream anastomosis that is considered to have a significant risk of leaking, for example a low anterior resection. A loop ileostomy allows almost complete diversion of the faecal stream and closure can usually be performed without the need for a laparotomy.

An end stoma is constructed when a permanent ileostomy is planned following a proctocolectomy for Crohn's disease or when anastomosis is contraindicated.

The stoma site should be marked on the abdominal wall preoperatively by an experienced stoma nurse to ensure correct positioning; the abdominal opening should be similar to the size of the bowel being delivered; the blood supply to the bowel should be good (the bowel should not be under tension); and in the case of ileostomies, whether loop or end, the stoma should be spouted. The spouted erected bowel avoids the skin unless as the effluent is diverted directly into the ileostomy bag; it also prevents stenosis of the mucocutaneous junction from developing.

Complications

Ileostomy output is significantly greater than that from colostomies, and water and electrolyte depletion can occur. Antidiarrhoeal medication such as loperamide may reduce the output, which should ideally be less than 1000 mL each day. Skin irritation may occur, although this should be avoided by a well-constructed stoma. Ischaemia of the stoma is rare because the blood supply is good. Patients may develop intestinal obstruction as either an early or a late complication from torsion of the bowel or adhesions. The latter can often be managed conservatively.

REFERENCES

103. Rhee RY et al. J Vasc Surg 1994; 20: 688–697
104. Croft RJ et al. Br J Surg 1981; 68: 316–318
105. Matsumoto AH et al. J Vasc Interv Radiol 1995; 6: 165–174
106. Taylor LM, Porter JM. In: Rutherford RD (ed). Vascular Surgery. 4th edn. WB Saunders, Philadelphia, 1995: 1301–1311
107. Keighley MRB, Pemberton JH, Fazio VW et al. Atlas of Colorectal Surgery. Churchill Livingstone, Edinburgh, 1996

Retraction or stenosis of an ileostomy may occur, causing severe skin irritation. Closure or revision is then required. The stoma may prolapse, which is more common in a loop than in an end stoma. This may be treated conservatively by reduction or by stoma closure, or by the formation of an end stoma. A parastomal hernia may also develop, and if the stoma cannot be closed it must be revised. Acute symptoms of ischaemia require correction, and stomas should be closed if possible, or they may be repaired or resited.

Rarely patients develop fistulae associated with the stoma or ulceration of the surrounding tissues. The latter may be the result of pyoderma gangrenosum in association with inflammatory bowel disease. Parastomal varices may occur in patients with portal hypertension (Fig. 27.19). These may bleed heavily and require oversewing or stoma relocation.[108] The portal hypertension should be relieved (see Ch. 29).

BLEEDING

The majority of patients with either acute or chronic blood loss into the gastrointestinal tract are either bleeding from the upper gastrointestinal tract or from the colorectum. A source of bleeding within the small bowel must be sought if no other source of the blood loss is found.

Lower gastrointestinal haemorrhage refers to bleeding distal to the ligament of Treitz. It is classified as massive (profuse bleeding resulting in acute hospital admission), minimal (minor bleeding resulting in outpatient presentation), or occult (no identifiable bleeding but a persistent anaemia considered to be secondary to chronic gastrointestinal loss despite a normal upper gastrointestinal endoscopy and colonoscopy). In half the cases the bleeding is defined as obscure when no preoperative diagnosis is made.

ACUTE HAEMORRHAGE

Aetiology

Patients with acute small bowel haemorrhage may present with melaena (black stools) or fresh bleeding per rectum. Small bowel haemorrhage cannot be distinguished clinically from acute bleeding from an upper gastrointestinal source or from the colon or rectum. All patients with acute gastrointestinal haemorrhage must therefore be actively resuscitated and investigated to identify and treat the source of bleeding.

Table 27.4 Causes of small bowel haemorrhage

- Meckel's diverticulum
- Jejunal diverticula
- Intussusception
- Angiodysplasia
- Peutz–Jeghers syndrome
- Leiomyoma or leiomyosarcoma
- Lymphoma
- Non-specific ulceration (cytomegalovirus or fungus)
- Haemangiomata (Rendu–Osler–Weber syndrome)
- Aortoenteric fistula

Patients require prompt assessment and resuscitation (see Chs 26 and 30). Two main patterns of bleeding are seen: the haemorrhage may stop after an initial significant bleed, or there may be continued bleeding or multiple repeat episodes. The investigations are determined to a degree by the type of presentation (Fig. 27.20).

Acute bleeding from the small bowel is rare in comparison with colonic bleeding, usually from diverticula or angiodysplasia, or from upper gastrointestinal causes. Possible causes are listed in Table 27.4.

Investigation and management

Acute oesophagogastroduodenoscopy is important to exclude a source of upper gastrointestinal bleeding. Colonoscopy is indicated if this is negative. This is often difficult because of the presence of stool and clot, although blood may act as a cathartic. In the presence of active haemorrhage, colonoscopy has been shown to be diagnostic in up to 76% of cases.[109] If nothing is found on either of these tests, further investigation depends on the condition of the patient. Radioisotope scintigraphy is indicated if the patient is continuing to bleed but is stable. Mesenteric angiography is indicated if the patient continues to bleed torrentially, although if it is impossible to stabilize the patient it is better to proceed directly to laparotomy.

Technetium-99m-labelled sulphur colloid is given intravenously before the abdomen is scanned (Fig. 27.21). Following

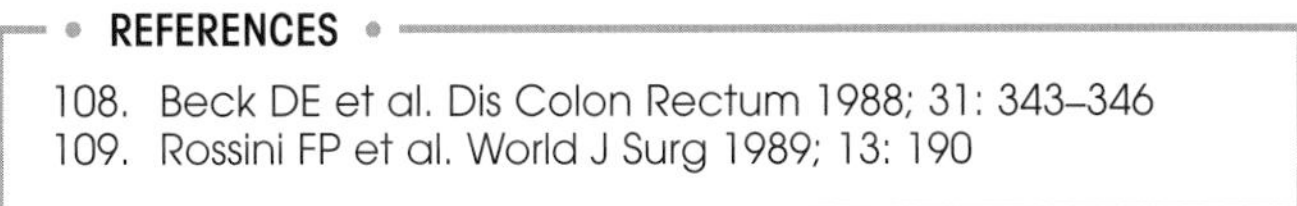
REFERENCES
108. Beck DE et al. Dis Colon Rectum 1988; 31: 343–346
109. Rossini FP et al. World J Surg 1989; 13: 190

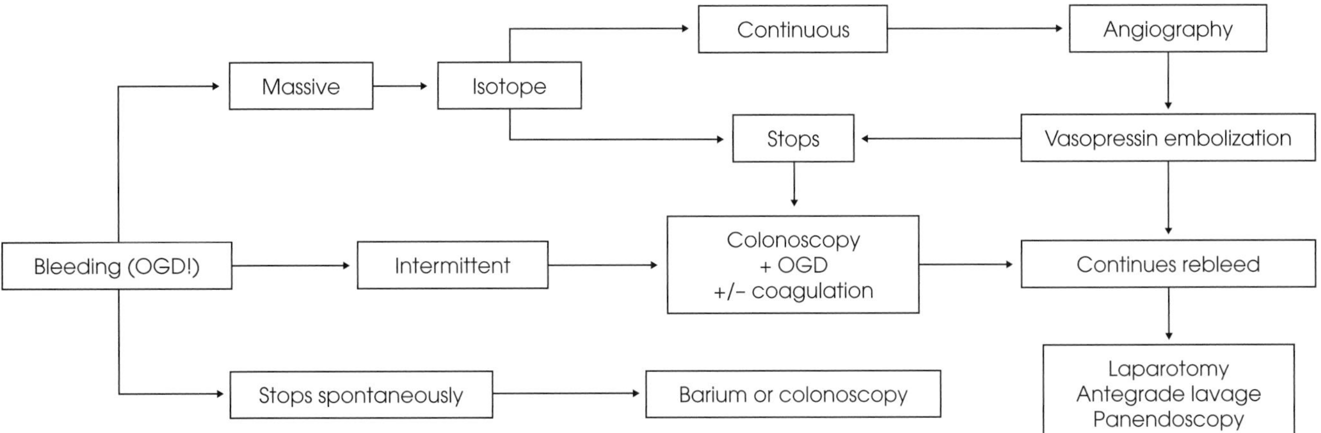

Figure 27.20 Algorithm for lower gastrointestinal haemorrhage.

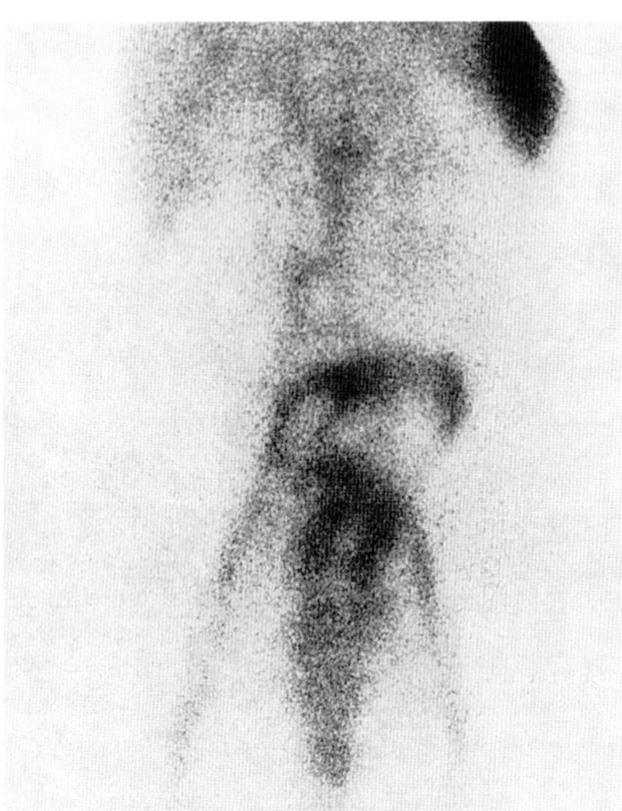

Figure 27.21 A technetium-99m pertechnate red cell scan showing extravasation into the bowel, which subsequently proved to be the terminal ileum. This was the result of non-specific ulceration in a patient with chronic renal failure on dialysis.

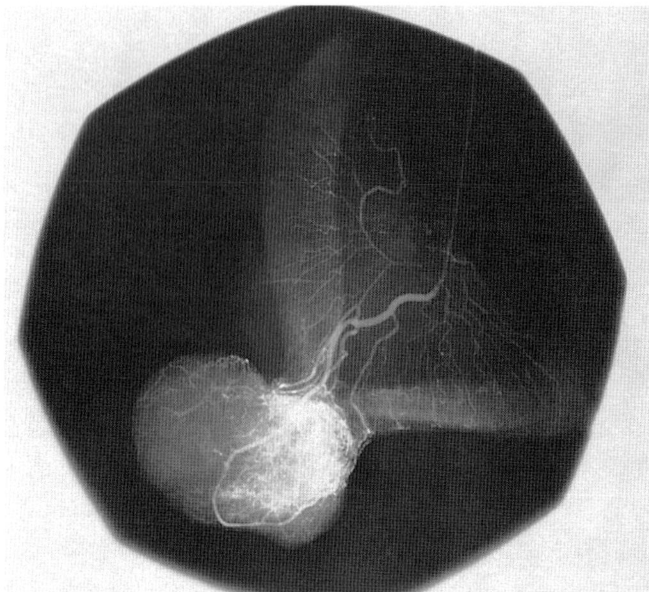

Figure 27.22 Arteriogram performed on a resected portion of terminal ileum containing a leiomyoma.

rapid clearance from the blood by the liver, the technetium-99m marker accumulates at any site of active bleeding into the bowel lumen, and this point can be identified on the scan. The patient must be actively bleeding at the time of the scan for this test to be diagnostic, because the clearance is so rapid. It will, however, demonstrate active bleeding as low as 0.1 mL/min. Technetium-99m-labelled red blood cells may also be used and may indicate the site of bleeding on repeat scanning over the next 48 h. Unfortunately its accuracy is less than 50%.

Mesenteric angiography requires selective cannulation of the coeliac, superior mesenteric and inferior mesenteric arteries (Figs 27.22 and 27.23), and the patient must be actively bleeding 1–1.5 mL/min if it is to be diagnostic. The site of bleeding is most commonly within the distribution of the superior mesenteric artery. The site of bleeding is identified in 58–86% of cases,[110] although supraselective angiography may be required. Therapeutic embolization of the bleeding vessel is possible, and if this is unsuccessful the catheter may be left in situ to aid the identification of the bleeding point by the surgeon.

Laparotomy is indicated if the patient continues to bleed. When the site has been identified by preoperative imaging, the appropriate segment of bowel can be opened or resected. If the diagnosis is uncertain, the patient can undergo repeat colonoscopy on the table, in combination with on-table lavage. If this fails to determine a source, the small bowel may be examined over an endoscope passed through the mouth or anus. An enterotomy can be made to pass the endoscope through the small bowel. Dilated vessels and angiodysplasia can be identified by

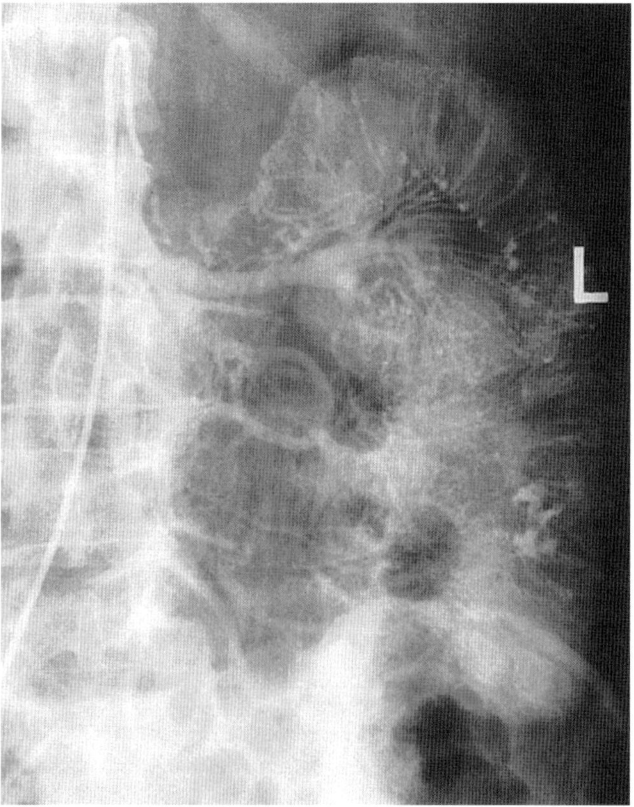

Figure 27.23 Selective superior mesenteric arteriogram showing leakage of contrast into the upper jejunum. This proved to be the site of an area of ulceration associated with angiodysplasia.

REFERENCES

110. Browder W et al. Ann Surg 1986; 204: 530–536

transillumination of the bowel wall. Any bleeding lesion should be resected. The commonest cause of small bowel bleeding is a Meckel's diverticulum.

Aortoenteric fistula

Aortoenteric fistula is a rare but potentially catastrophic cause of small bowel haemorrhage (see Ch. 10).

The possibility of an aortoenteric fistula must always be considered in a patient with gastrointestinal haemorrhage who has had an aortic graft. The diagnosis and management of this condition is described in Ch. 10.

CHRONIC BLEEDING

Chronic bleeding from the small bowel usually presents with iron-deficiency anaemia. Possible pathologies include any of the causes of acute bleeding plus small bowel neoplasms, connective tissue disorders such as Ehlers–Danlos syndrome, vascular malformations such as cavernous haemangioma, and Crohn's disease. The bleeding is usually occult, with a normal upper and lower gastrointestinal endoscopy but positive faecal occult blood testing. Investigation of the small bowel for a source of bleeding is difficult and usually requires a number of investigations. Angiography may be useful but will identify only active bleeding occurring at the time of the investigation. Radioimmunoscintigaphy such as technetium-labelled red blood cell scanning is useful, and a technetium pertechnate scan can identify a Meckel's diverticulum. A small bowel follow-through may identify space-occupying lesions within the bowel, as can abdominal CT scanning. Direct imaging of the small bowel lumen is possible with enteroscopy, although this is limited to the proximal half of the small bowel. The 'pill cam' or video capsule endoscopy described earlier provides direct images of the small bowel lumen.

Often no diagnosis is made and the decision whether to proceed to laparotomy must be taken. At operation an external inspection of the small bowel is followed by an inspection of its lumen through an endoscope as described earlier.

NEUROMUSCULAR DISORDERS

The term pseudo-obstruction is a bad one but has gained acceptance by common usage. It implies a failure of forward propulsion of intestinal contents in the absence of a mechanical cause. The obstruction that this produces is, however, very real. Acute colonic pseudo-obstruction is common (see Ch. 28), occurring in elderly patients with chronic obstructive airway disease, cardiac disease or pneumonia, but involvement of the small bowel is less commonly seen.

Acute postoperative paralytic ileus much less frequently occurs in surgical wards today. The attention to fluid and electrolyte – and particularly potassium – balance (see Ch. 2),[111] and the enormous improvements in anaesthesia appear to have reduced the incidence of this complication, which is believed to be caused by an overactivity of the sympathetic nervous system. The combination of a ganglion-blocking agent, guanethidine, with a parasympatheticomimetic drug, bethanechol[112] was used to stimulate peristalsis in patients with a paralytic ileus, but has now been discontinued because of unpleasant side effects. Following operation, the small intestine usually regains normal motility within 24 h,[113] while the stomach and colon may take several days to recover.[114]

RADIATION ENTERITIS

The purpose of therapeutic radiation is to destroy malignant cells while leaving normal cells unaffected. Normal tissues are relatively resistant to radiotherapy and have a greater capacity for recovery than malignant cells. Radiotherapy is usually fractionated to allow normal tissues time to recover, but it may result in both acute and chronic damage to normal tissues, including the small bowel.

The pelvis is the most common site to be irradiated as this therapy is used to treat solid organ malignancies of the bladder, prostate, cervix and anus. It may be used radically as primary treatment, or as adjuvant therapy. There has been increasing use of radiotherapy as adjuvant therapy for rectal cancer (see Ch. 28).

PATHOLOGICAL CHANGES AND PRESENTATION

The effects of radiotherapy can be considered as early, late and remote. Early effects include inflammatory changes and a temporary loss of cells with a high turnover, such as small bowel mucosa. This may result in colic and diarrhoea, and can rarely cause perforation.

Late effects are from vascular insufficiency, with endarteritis obliterans occurring in medium-sized vessels in the bowel wall.[115] This may cause thickening of the small bowel wall and mucosal ulceration, but is more commonly found in the rectum.

Remote changes occur years after radiotherapy and include fibrous strictures, which may result in obstruction (Fig. 27.24). The obstructive episodes are often recurrent and become progressively more severe. Metabolic problems secondary to ileal disease may cause vitamin B_{12} deficiency, bacterial overgrowth or bile salt-induced diarrhoea.[116]

MANAGEMENT

Treatment depends on the severity of the injury, and a grading system has been devised by Pilepich.[117] A small bowel contrast study is the investigation of choice but often underestimates the extent of disease. The patient should if possible be optimized prior to intervention, and feeding may be very helpful (see Ch. 2). Adhesions should be divided and abnormal bowel excised or bypassed. It is rare for a small bowel resection to be less than 40 cm.[118] Anastomotic breakdown remains a risk.

CHRONIC CONDITIONS AFFECTING THE APPENDIX

The most common appendiceal pathology is acute appendicitis, which is discussed in Chapter 25 along with its sequelae. Other pathologies affecting the appendix are rare.

REFERENCES

111. Ebrill D, Naftalin L. Lancet 1953; ii: 411
112. Neely J, Catchpole B. Br J Surg 1971; 58: 21
113. Ross B et al. Gut 1963; 4: 77
114. Wilson JP. Gut 1975; 16: 689
115. Carr ND et al. Histopathology 1985; 9: 517–534
116. Schofield PF. In: Nicholls RJ, Dozois RR (eds). Surgery of the Colon and Rectum. Churchill Livingstone, Edinburgh, 1997
117. Pilepich MV et al. Am J Clin Oncol 1983; 6: 485–491
118. Carr ND et al. Gut 1984; 25: 1448–1454

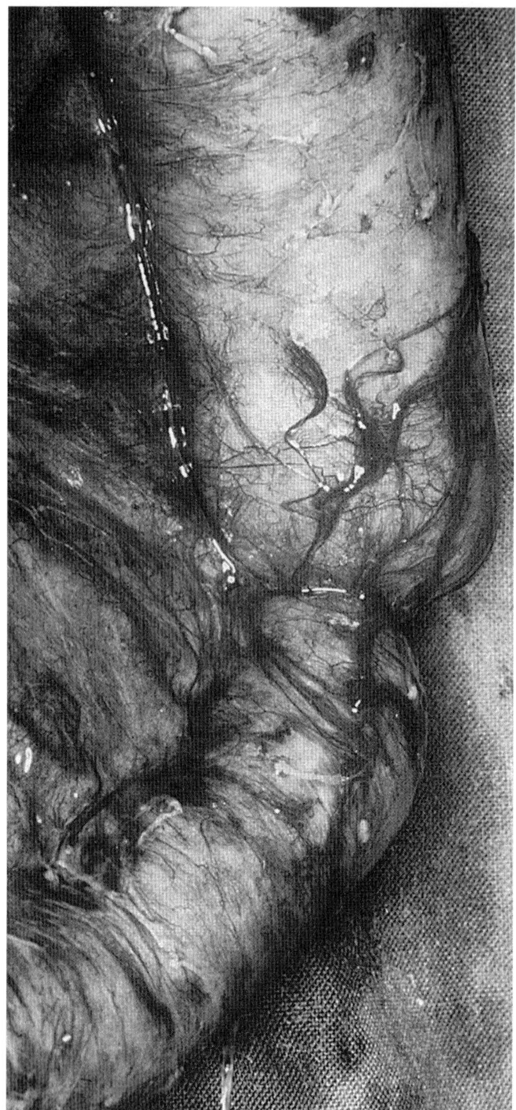

Figure 27.24 A radiation stricture of the ileum.

CONGENITAL ANOMALIES OF THE APPENDIX

Congenital absence of the appendix has been reported.[119] This is permissible if the taeniae coli are followed to a point of junction in the caecum where not even a tiny vestige of an appendix exists, providing of course that the patient has not been subjected to a previous abdominal operation. A double appendix has been recorded.[120]

Congenital diverticula of the appendix differ from the acquired variety in that they are intramuscular, having a lining of smooth muscle in their walls.

Intussusception and torsion of the appendix have also both been recorded.

CHRONIC APPENDICITIS

Some patients complain of recurrent right iliac fossa pain that resolves when the appendix is removed. The macroscopic appearance of the appendix is often abnormal, and this can be identified on laparoscopy prior to removal of the appendix.[121] Many patients presenting with chronic right iliac fossa pain, however, continue to complain after appendicectomy, and this is usually the result of irritable bowel syndrome.

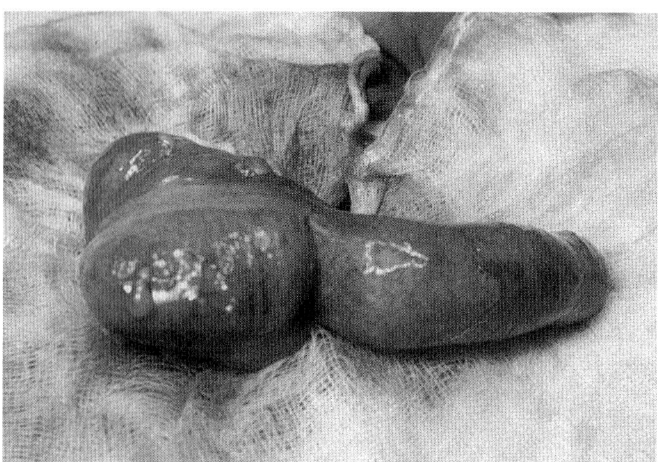

Figure 27.25 Mucocele of the appendix.

MUCOCELE OF THE APPENDIX (Fig. 27.25)

Sometimes obstruction occurs at the mouth of the appendix without producing acute appendicitis. Mucus may accumulate in the appendiceal lumen, and the slow distension results in a thickening of the wall of the appendix.[122] A mucocele of the appendix needs to be distinguished from the rare papilliferous cystadenoma or cystadenocarcinoma that can arise from the appendix, producing a mucoid tumour that, if it ruptures, may result in pseudomyxoma peritonei. Calcification and even heterotopic bone have rarely been described in appendix mucoceles,[123] and intussusception into the caecum has also been recorded.[124]

Chronic inflammation of the appendix without obstruction, followed by subsequent fibrosis, seems to occur, and this is often seen incidentally during laparotomy for some other problem. The appendix may also become blocked by foreign bodies such as lead pellets (Fig. 27.26), fruit seeds, pins and *Ascaris* worms. The patient illustrated in Fig. 27.26 had a history of recurrent colicky lower abdominal pains, and appendicectomy was associated with relief of symptoms: a true example of appendicular colic?

TUMOURS OF THE APPENDIX

CARCINOID TUMOUR

The first tumour of the appendix was described by Von Pommer Esche,[125] and the first undoubted primary adenocarcinoma by Beger.[126] The peculiarities of the carcinoid tumours were not

REFERENCES

119. Robinson JO. Br J Surg 1952; 39: 344
120. Cave I. J Anat 1936; 70: 283
121. Barber MD et al. Br J Surg 1997; 84; 110–112
122. Wilson RR. Br J Surg 1950; 38: 65
123. Juvara U, Borcesou O. Br Med J Surg 1948; I: 931
124. Ward McQuaid JN. Br J Surg 1949; 37: 109
125. Von Pommer Esche W. Med Zeid 1837; 6: 133
126. Beger A. Berlin Klin Wochenschr 1882; 19: 616

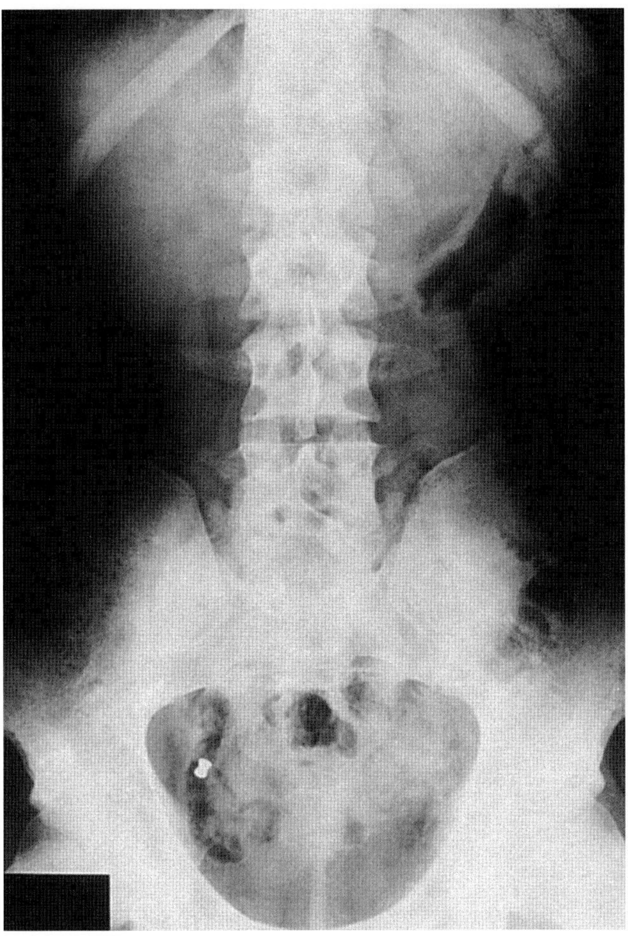

Figure 27.26 Plain abdominal radiograph in a young man with intermittent colicky abdominal pain. The airgun pellet is seen to be in the appendix. Appendicectomy relieved his symptoms. A case of true appendicular colic?

appreciated until the work of Obendorfer,[83] who introduced the term carcinoid. The incidence of carcinoid tumour of the appendix is about 0.5%.

Carcinoid tumours of the appendix are most frequently found in the third decade, and appear to be commoner in women than in men. In 70% of cases the tumour lies near the tip of the appendix,[128] and in only 2% of cases is there any evidence of metastasis to regional lymph nodes. Usually these tumours are discovered incidentally at laparotomy, and there is always some difficulty in deciding the best course of action. On those rare occasions where obvious metastases have occurred, right hemicolectomy is indicated. The general opinion for the remaining cases is that tumours less than 1 cm in diameter should be removed by appendicectomy, but that the larger tumours require a limited right hemicolectomy to remove the draining lymph nodes.

ADENOCARCINOMA

Adenocarcinoma is the second most common tumour of the appendix, and 10% of patients have widespread dissemination by the time of operation. Following right hemicolectomy the 4-year survival rate is 60%.

Lymphoma may affect the appendix, and the regional lymph nodes are usually involved.[128] Benign tumours such as fibroma, myxoma, angioma, adenomatous polyp, myoma, myofibroma and neurofibroma have also been recorded. Endometriosis may also involve the appendix.

REFERENCES

127. McCartey A, McGrath C. Ann Surg 1914; 59: 675
128. Gallaway S, Owens B. Br Med J 1949; ii: 1387

The colon, rectum and anus

28

Neil J. Mortensen, Matthew G. Tytherleigh

INTRODUCTION

The colon is no longer regarded as pathologically distinct from the rectum as a result of new developments in the understanding of the pathophysiology, diagnosis, medical and surgical treatments of colorectal disease. Colonoscopy, introduced in the late 1960s, has enabled precise diagnosis and surveillance of the large bowel and, together with snare polypectomy, has greatly diminished the need for surgical operations for polyps. Radiological imaging of the bowel has progressed rapidly. The double-contrast barium enema continues to be an important investigation, but less invasive imaging, such as CT and MRI, is used routinely. New methods of imaging, such as positron emission tomography and virtual colonography, will in the future play a greater role in the diagnosis of colorectal diseases.

Genetic and epidemiological data for colorectal cancer are accumulating rapidly, and for population screening may eventually reduce the mortality of this condition. The strategy for screening depends on an appreciation of the adenoma–carcinoma sequence, and a greater understanding of risk factors and the natural history of colorectal cancer. The treatment of colorectal cancer by sphincter-preserving operations, avoiding the need for a colostomy, is another major advance. New anastomotic techniques have been established and properly assessed by prospective studies. Adjuvant treatments, including radiotherapy and chemotherapy, are an important new field of clinical research.

Crohn's colitis has been defined as an entity, and the existence of anal disease in this condition established. The natural history, liability to recurrence and indications for surgery are now more fully appreciated. Bypass procedures have been replaced by stricturoplasty, and resections have become increasingly more limited. Clinical trials have rationalized the medical management of colitis, and operations to treat ulcerative colitis can now avoid ileostomy in most cases with the use of an ileal pouch anal anastomosis. The indications for surgery and the choice of operation in both emergency and elective cases have been defined.

Important developments in the treatment of diseases of the anus, including haemorrhoids, fissure, carcinoma and sexually transmitted diseases, have taken place. The management of anorectal sepsis has been simplified by the employment of an effective classification. Increased knowledge of disordered function of the pelvic floor through physiological, radiological and pathological investigation has led to improvements in treatment of constipation and prolapse, and anal ultrasound has transformed the investigation of incontinence and obstetric injuries. An improved understanding of the pharmacology of the anorectum has and will lead to new medical therapies for common anal conditions.

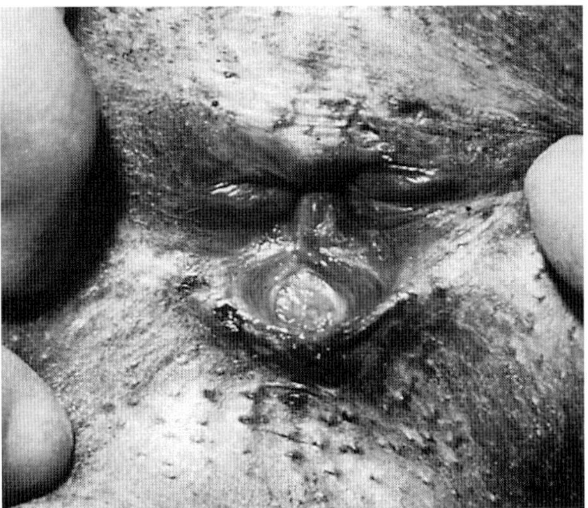

Figure 28.1 Chronic anal fissure seen on displaying distal anal canal. The fissure has a thickened margin and granulating base.

FISSURE IN ANO

Fissure in ano is a common condition and accounts for about 15% of referrals to a rectal clinic. A fissure is a longitudinal tear in the anoderm of the lower third of the anal canal, extending from the dentate line to the anal margin. It is usually situated in the midline. In males about 90% are posterior, while in females anterior fissures are more common, comprising 20% of cases. In approximately 5% of cases, an anterior and a posterior fissure coexist. The condition is most common in young adults, when the sex ratio is approximately equal. Fissures occasionally occur in infants and children but are rare in the elderly.[1]

The aetiology is unknown. Only 20% of patients give a history of constipation, which may in fact have been the result of the fissure rather than the cause. Indeed, sometimes a fissure occurs after a bout of diarrhoea. Fissure is the most common anal abnormality in Crohn's disease and ulcerative colitis.[2] It often occurs in pregnancy, and there is an association with chronic intersphincteric abscess in about 5% of cases.[3] This suggests that the fissure may be the result of anal crypt infection, especially given the midline distribution of both the fissure and the internal

REFERENCES

1. Bennett RC, Goligher JC. Br Med J 1962; 2: 1500
2. Lockhart Mummery HE. Br J Surg 1985; 72 (Suppl): 595–596
3. Parks AG, Thomson JPS. Br Med J 1983; ii: 537

openings of anal fistulae. A further suggestion is that a fissure arises from ischaemia as a result of impaired mucosal blood flow.

The fissure probably starts as a simple linear ulcer. Chronic inflammation then leads to undermining of the edges, and the base deepens to expose the fibres of the internal sphincter.[4] A papilla may form at its upper limit, level with the dentate line, and a skin tag or *sentinel pile* develops at its distal end. The sphincter becomes hypertonic, probably in response to the pain produced by the fissure.

CLINICAL FEATURES

Pain on defecation occurs in 90% of patients and lasts for 1–2 h. The fear of defecation may lead to constipation. Bleeding frequently occurs and is usually seen on the toilet paper on wiping. Other symptoms include pruritus (50%), a watery discharge (20%) and constipation (20%).[5]

The diagnosis is made on inspection by gently parting the anal margin (Fig. 28.1). In 20% of cases a simple split is seen. Chronicity is seen in 80% and is recognized by the presence of any of the following: skin tag or papilla, undermining of the edges of the fissure, or visible sphincter fibres in its base. Digital examination is contraindicated at this stage, because it is very painful and unhelpful.

DIFFERENTIAL DIAGNOSIS

Other causes of severe anal pain include a thrombosed perianal varix, an anorectal abscess, an anal carcinoma, leukaemic ulceration and sexually transmitted diseases such as warts, herpes simplex and a syphilitic chancre.

TREATMENT

Over half of the simple acute fissures heal spontaneously.[5] A 2–3-week trial of conservative treatment should, therefore, be considered when pain is not severe. Most fissures in pregnancy and childhood can be managed in this way. A laxative and a local anaesthetic ointment are prescribed. If this fails, topical glyceryl trinitrate ointment 0.2% used three times daily for 6 weeks heals half the anal fissures and controls anal pain.[6] Calcium channel antagonists such as diltiazem ointment may also be used.[7] Botulinum toxin has recently been introduced as a first-line treatment for anal fissures.[8] It is injected into the anal sphincter and produces sphincter relaxation. Surgery is reserved for fissures that have failed to heal following medical treatment. Surgery does carry a small risk of incontinence, and for this reason a careful history of obstetric sphincter injury should be sought. Anal dilatation under anaesthesia produces healing in 80–90% of cases. The incidence of incontinence, however, has been reported in up to a third of cases, and hence the anal stretch has fallen from favour.[9] Lateral sphincterotomy consists of division of the distal internal sphincter, and 95% of cases heal in 2–3 weeks.[10] There is a small risk of incontinence. Anal fissure in Crohn's disease should be treated conservatively, because the majority (70%) heal spontaneously. Sphincterotomy risks sepsis and should be avoided.[11,12]

ANORECTAL SEPSIS AND ANAL FISTULAE

Infection in the anorectal region can lead to abscess or fistula formation. Acute anorectal abscess is one of the most common surgical emergencies. Drainage or spontaneous rupture results in resolution of the acute inflammation. Recurrence is common, and about 80% of recurrences are associated with the formation of a fistula in ano.[13]

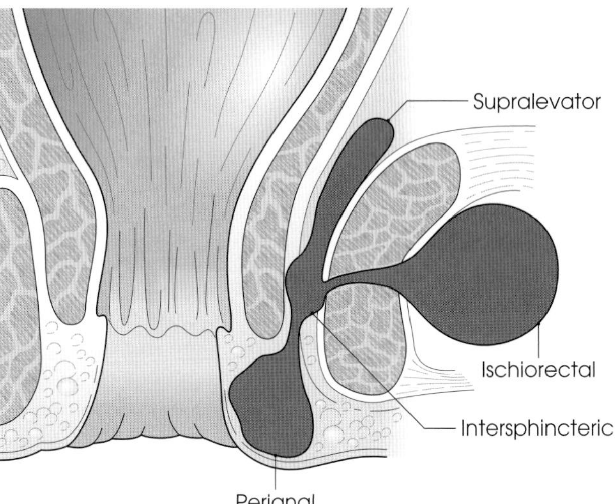

Figure 28.2 Pathogenesis of anorectal abscesses. Pus may track to various sites after initial formation of an intersphincteric abscess.

AETIOLOGY

Anorectal sepsis originates from infection of an anal crypt gland[14] and is associated with other diseases including Crohn's disease, ulcerative colitis and hidradenitis suppurativa. Up to 70% of patients with rectal Crohn's disease have an anal fistula.[15] In some cases, a perianal abscess is caused by a simple furuncle arising from perianal skin. Microbiological culture of the pus distinguishes between enteric and skin flora.

PATHOGENESIS

The 10–12 anal glands are simple glands with a duct draining into the crypts of Morgagni. Anorectal sepsis starts with infection of a gland body lying within the intersphincteric space, causing an intersphincteric abscess. It is already in anatomical communication with the crypt via the gland duct. As the abscess expands, pus may track longitudinally in various directions to present as a perianal, an ischiorectal or a supralevator abscess, as shown in Fig. 28.2. Tracking can also occur circumferentially, leading to a 'horseshoe' extension, which can spread into the ischiorectal

REFERENCES

4. Eisenhammer S. S Afr Med J 1953; 27: 266
5. Lock MR, Thomson JPS. Br J Surg 1977; 64: 355–358
6. Lund JN, Scholefield JH. Dis Colon Rectum 1997; 40: 468–470
7. Carapeti EA, Kamm MA et al. Gut 1999; 45: 719–722
8. Maria G, Cassetta E et al. N Engl J Med 1998; 338: 217–220
9. Watts JM, Bennett RC, Goligher JC. Br Med J 1984; 11: 342–343
10. Hoffman DC, Goligher JC. Br Med J 1970; 111: 673–675
11. Buchmann P, Keighley MRB et al. Am J Surg 1980; 14: 642
12. Sweeney JL, Ritchie JK, Nicholls RJ. Br J Surg 1988; 75: 56–57
13. Chabrot CM, Prasad ML, Abcarian H. Dis Colon Rectum 1983; 26: 105
14. Gordon-Watson C, Dodd H. Br J Surg 1935; 22: 303
15. Lockhart Mummery HE. Br J Surg 1985; 72 (Suppl 595)

fossa (most commonly), the intersphincteric space or the supralevator space.

A fistula in ano usually has a single internal opening connected by the primary track to an external opening, which may be multiple. Upward extensions of pus within the intersphincteric space to the supralevator space or within the ischiorectal fossa are referred to as secondary tracks.

CLASSIFICATION

Anorectal abscesses or fistulae can be classified according to the relationship of the primary track to the external sphincter and puborectalis muscle.[16] About 60% of cases are intersphincteric in type. Here the pus tracks within the intersphincteric space to appear at the anal verge as a perianal abscess, and drainage results in an intersphincteric fistula. Occasionally an intersphincteric abscess becomes walled off by fibrosis and forms a chronic intersphincteric abscess, which may cause intermittent pain.[17]

In about 35% of cases, pus from the focal intersphincteric abscess penetrates the external sphincter to enter the ischiorectal fossa,[18] forming an ischiorectal abscess. After drainage this results in a trans-sphincteric fistula. Rarely (in 5% of cases or less) the pus from the intersphincteric focus extends upwards to the supralevator space and then enters the ischiorectal fossa by penetrating the levator ani muscle. Drainage of this type of ischiorectal abscess results in a suprasphincteric fistula.[16] The rare extrasphincteric fistula occurs when there is a direct communication between the rectum and the perineum lateral to the puborectalis.

CLINICAL FEATURES

Anorectal abscess

Pain occurs in the anal region and is often very severe, being aggravated by defecation. The patient may have a fever and inguinal lymphadenopathy. Swelling and erythema of the perianal skin with tenderness are usual. When an abscess is suspected, digital examination of the rectum should not be performed until a general anaesthetic is given, when a full assessment can be made and appropriate drainage carried out.

Chronic intersphincteric abscess

This condition causes episodic attacks of anal pain without evident discharge, usually resolving spontaneously after a few days. There is an absence of perianal swelling and redness, and the diagnosis is made on digital examination of the rectum. About two-thirds of chronic intersphincteric abscesses lie in the midline posteriorly. The abscess is identified on bidigital palpation and usually measures about 1 cm in diameter. It is usually tender, and an internal opening into the crypt may be found.[17]

Fistula in ano

Fistula in ano is characterized by a discharge of pus from the external opening. This may be intermittent and associated with exacerbations of acute abscess formation, causing pain that resolves when pus discharges from the external opening. Finding the internal opening identifies the primary track. This is usually felt as an area of induration at the level of the anal crypts. In two-thirds of patients the internal opening lies in the midline posteriorly. In the remainder the internal opening lies in the anterior quadrant. Lateral openings are very rare in fistulae not associated with Crohn's disease. Goodsall's rule generally applies

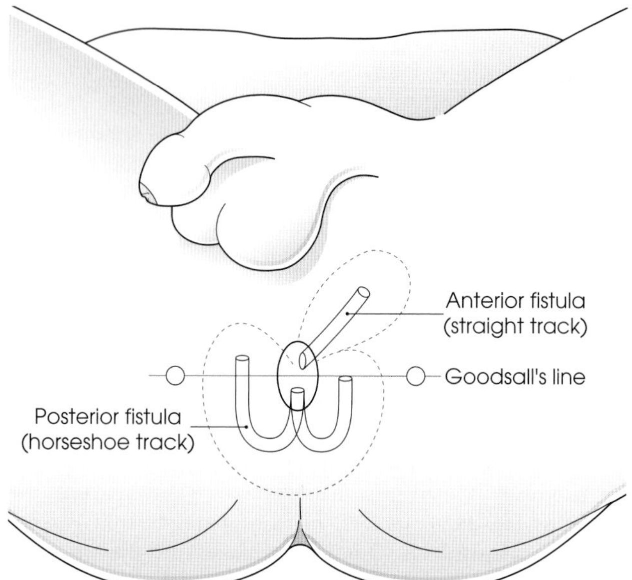

Figure 28.3 Goodsall's rule.

(Fig. 28.3).[19] This states that if the external opening of a fistula lies behind a line drawn transversely across the anus, the track should curve in a horseshoe-like manner towards the internal opening in the midline posteriorly. The track tends to pass radially in a straight line towards the internal opening if the external opening is in front of the transverse anal line.

TREATMENT

Abscess

An anorectal abscess should be drained under general anaesthesia. It is also essential to sigmoidoscope the patient to exclude proctitis, which is suggestive of Crohn's disease. During anorectal examination, pus can sometimes be seen coming from an internal opening, but no attempt should be made to find the internal opening. The abscess is drained by an incision over the point of maximal fluctuation, which is usually in the perineum. A finger is gently inserted into the cavity, and loculi broken down to release pus, which is sent for culture. A small disc of skin should be removed at the point of incision to prevent early closure of the wound. The cavity is then kept open by a short corrugated drain, which may be removed after 24 h. Antibiotics should be given only to patients who are at high risk of infection.

It is inadvisable to lay open an apparent fistula at this stage, because the anatomy of the anal sphincter may not be easily identified. A routine examination under anaesthetic has been advocated to look for an associated fistula when the pus culture has shown the presence of an enteric organism.[20]

REFERENCES

16. Parks AG, Gordon PH, Hardcastle JD. Br J Surg 1976; 63: 1–12
17. Parks AG, Thompson JPS. Br Med J 1983; ii: 537
18. Marks CG, Ritchie JK. Br J Surg 1977; 64: 84–91
19. Goodsall DH. In: Goodsall DH, Miles WE (eds). Diseases of the Anus and Rectum. Longmans, London, 1900
20. Grace RH, Harper IA, Thompson RG. Br J Surg 1982; 69:401–403

Chronic intersphincteric abscess

In cases where an internal opening is evident, it is possible to pass a probe into the abscess, which can then be laid open. Alternatively, the intersphincteric plane can be explored, starting at the inferior border of the sphincter, and the abscess dissected out.

Anal fistula

The principle is to lay open the primary track and to drain any secondary tracks. It is essential to assess patients preoperatively, when they can voluntarily contract their sphincters. This allows the surgeon to determine the level of the internal opening. Faecal continence is maintained provided the puborectalis muscle and the majority of the external sphincter are preserved. Most anal fistulae are either intersphincteric or trans-sphincteric in type, where the primary track enters at the level of the anal crypts, well below the main part of the sphincter, allowing the track to be safely laid open.[18]

The primary track is gently and carefully probed with Lockhart–Mummery's specially designed probes, which are inserted from either the external or the internal opening, and the tissue between the probe and the perineal skin is divided. Any abscess cavity associated with the track is curetted. The probes are then passed into secondary tracks, which are curetted and widened. Curettings from the track are sent for histological examination to exclude Crohn's disease. The wound is trimmed to encourage healing from its base. The dressings are changed after about 24 h, and the wound is then dressed twice daily after baths until healing occurs.

High trans-sphincteric and suprasphincteric fistulae should not be laid open immediately. Instead, a length of suture material, a seton (Latin: seta = bristle), is passed through the fistula track from the external to the internal opening. The seton can either be tied tightly with the aim of producing a slow ischaemic division of the muscle over a period of weeks,[21] or alternatively it can be left loose to act as a drain while any secondary tracks heal. After several weeks or months, the primary track may heal on removal of the seton, although this occurs only in about 40% of cases.[22] The primary track can be laid open with the expectation that the surrounding fibrosis will prevent retraction of the anal sphincter if healing does not occur. An alternative method of managing high fistulae is to drain the primary track externally while repairing the internal opening using an anorectal advancement flap.[23] Early results from the use of fibrin tissue glue inserted into the track are promising.

PRURITUS ANI

Irritation is very common in the lower anal canal and the perianal region, and can be extremely difficult to treat. Pruritus ani is a symptom, not a disease, and there are many causes.

AETIOLOGY

The causes of pruritus ani are listed in Table 28.1. The most common single cause is anal moisture and faecal soiling. Faecal bacteria produce highly irritant metabolites (e.g. neuramidases) and this, combined with moisture through sweat or mucus, leads to maceration and excoriation of the skin. The resulting irritation leads to scratching, causing further damage to the skin and initiating a vicious circle. Any condition that causes an anal discharge can therefore cause pruritus.

Table 28.1 Causes of pruritus ani

Primary

Generalized dermatoses
- Eczema
- Psoriasis
- Lichen planus
- Allergic eruptions

Perianal disease
- Local lesion: fissure, carcinoma, Crohn's disease
- Infection: fungal, yeast, worms, sexually transmitted diseases (condylomata acuminata, chancre, herpes)
- Contact dermatitis: local anaesthetics, antibiotic ointment

Secondary

Skin damage due to moisture and irritants
- Sweat: poor anal hygiene
- Mucus: prolapse (rectal, haemorrhoids), mucus overproduction (adenoma, carcinoma, solitary ulcer)
- Pus: fistula in ano
- Faeces: diarrhoea, incontinence, poor anal hygiene

General medical diseases
- Diabetes mellitus
- Myeloproliferative disorders
- Obstructive jaundice
- Lymphoma

Idiopathic

Eyers and Thomson identified a group of patients in whom an abnormality of the internal sphincter seems to be present.[24] In these patients, internal sphincter relaxation occurs at a lower threshold of rectal distension and remains more profound than in normal subjects. This ready sphincter relaxation may result in subclinical leakage of irritant faecal material. More often, however, poor anal hygiene is the result of inadequate cleaning after defecation. This may be difficult in hairy people or where there are skin tags or prolapsing haemorrhoids. Patients with diarrhoea often have anal soreness, presumably caused by frequent exposure of the perianal skin to liquid faeces. Infestation with threadworm is a common cause of pruritus, especially in children.

DIAGNOSIS

The history should aim to determine the existence of any allergy, the use of allergenic cream or ointment, anogenital contact and symptoms suggesting any of the conditions listed in Table 28.1. The general examination with appropriate investigations aims to exclude dermatoses and general medical diseases. On anorectal examination any moisture and soiling of the perianal region, maceration or excoriation of the skin, or the presence of perianal lesions and prolapse should be noted. Full rectal examination should identify an anal fistula, haemorrhoids, mucus-producing rectal lesions, and sphincter incompetence. An anal skin scraping should be sent for a microbiological

REFERENCES

21. Parnaud E. Int J Colorectal Dis 1987; 2: 56
22. Thompson JPS, Ross AH. Int J Colorectal Dis 1989; 4: 247
23. Aguilhar PS, Plaseucia G et al Dis Colon Rectum 1985; 28:496–498
24. Eyers AA, Thomson JPS. Br Med J 1979; 11: 1549–1551

examination to exclude fungal infection. Worm infestation can be diagnosed by examination of the stool or of a swab from the perianal skin for ova. Often no underlying explanation for pruritus is found.[25]

MANAGEMENT

Management involves general measures and specific treatment of any underlying cause. General measures include advice to avoid scratching or rough wiping after defecation. The anal region should be kept clean and dry, and preparations such as zinc starch dusting powder can be helpful. Local anaesthetic preparations and soap should be avoided. The anus should be carefully washed after defecation and gently dried. Most cases will respond to this approach. Operations on the perianal skin or local injections have not been found to be effective.

PILONIDAL SINUS

The term *pilonidal sinus* may be applied to any subcutaneous sinus that contains hair. There is usually associated chronic inflammation with acute episodes of abscess formation. It is most commonly found in the natal cleft, but other sites have been described. These include the webs of barbers' fingers, the umbilicus, the axilla, the scar in the perineal wound after rectal excision, and within pits in the anal canal. The condition is common and affects young adults, with males predominating in a ratio of about 4:1.[26] It is rare in children, adolescents and in patients over the age of 40 years.[27]

A pilonidal sinus developing between the buttocks consists of one or more primary openings, which communicate via the primary track with a subcutaneous cavity (Fig. 28.4). The primary track lies in the natal cleft and at its origin is lined by cutaneous epithelium. This soon peters out, and the cavity itself is lined by chronic inflammatory granulation tissue, often containing foreign body giant cells. The cavity may ramify in various directions to open on to the surface via one or more secondary tracks. Secondary openings are usually found on either side of the midline. Hairs are almost always found in the primary track. Some are detached and lying loose, but others may still be rooted in hair follicles in the surrounding skin. There are no hair follicles in the primary track itself.

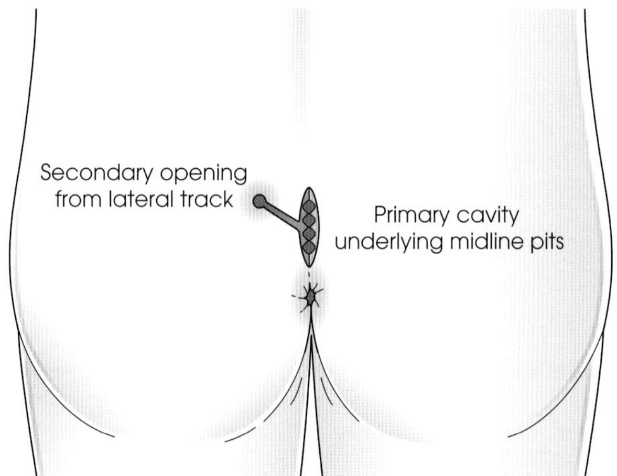

Figure 28.4 Pilonidal sinus: primary openings and secondary tract.

PATHOGENESIS

Pilonidal sinuses were originally thought to be congenital in origin. Patey produced evidence, however, to support an acquired cause.[28] He suggested that the sinus starts by penetration of the skin by hairs. Most patients are hirsute, with considerable hair growth in the natal cleft region. Penetration may occur by the point of a hair still rooted in the surrounding skin, which is propelled inwards by movement of the buttocks[29] and its own growth.[30] Hairs found in the sinus are usually detached and are lying with their tips projecting from the opening. Some are too long to have originated from the buttock area and may well be detached capital hairs. Subsequent infection leads to abscess formation within the subcutaneous tissue. This may drain via the primary point of entry of the hairs or more often it may track laterally.

CLINICAL PRESENTATION

Pilonidal sinus usually presents as an acute abscess or as a chronic discharging sinus. It occasionally presents with discomfort, and the sinus opening may be found by the patient or an observant doctor. A pilonidal abscess produces pain and swelling in the natal cleft region. Occasionally it settles spontaneously but more often bursts to form a chronic sinus. A chronic pilonidal sinus is characterized by relapsing and remitting pain and discharge. The diagnosis is clinched by finding one or more pits within the natal cleft, usually accompanied by an area of induration, where the chronic granulation tissue forms around the hairs. The differential diagnosis includes anal fistula, hidradenitis suppurativa, a simple furuncle or an infected sebaceous cyst.

TREATMENT

An acute abscess should be drained through a laterally placed incision. Occasionally complete healing occurs, but much more often the residual pilonidal sinus requires treatment. Treatment of the sinus depends on the severity of symptoms. A chronic pilonidal sinus giving no trouble should probably be managed conservatively by keeping the area clean, dry, and free of hairs by shaving or using depilatory cream. In many cases, however, an operation is necessary. Many operations have been employed, and none are satisfactory. Wide local excision of the diseased natal cleft with primary closure frequently results in wound breakdown and a prolonged period of healing by secondary intention. Bascom's operation uses lateral incisions and curettage of abscess cavities. Midline pits are excised with a minimal amount of surrounding tissue.[31] Karydakis has described asymmetrical excision and closure of the natal cleft wound with low recurrence rates.[32] Major surgery to obliterate the natal cleft, such as skin flaps and Z plasty, have been employed, but lesser surgery is generally equally efficacious.

REFERENCES

25. Friend WG. Dis Colon Rectum 1977; 20: 40–42
26. Buie LA, Curtiss RK. Surg Clin North Am 1952; 9: 44
27. Allen Mersh TG. Br J Surg 1990; 77: 123
28. Patey DH. Br J Surg 1969; 56: 463
29. Brearley R. Br J Surg 1955; 42: 62
30. Millar DM. Proc R Soc Med 1970; 63: 19
31. Bascom J. Surgery 1980; 87: 567–572
32. Karydakis GE. Lancet 1973; 2: 1414–1415

HAEMORRHOIDS

Haemorrhoids (Greek: haima = blood, rhoos = flowing), or piles (Latin: pila = a ball), are an extremely common condition in all western countries. It is highly likely that aspects of western culture, particularly the refined diet, low in fibre, play a part in their aetiology. The Valsalva effect resulting from excessive straining at stool engorges the anal cushions, and the shearing force of hard stools disrupts these cushions to cause piles. There may be a congenital deficiency of the supporting tissues in some patients, and the progestogenic effect on smooth muscle and the stretching of parturition explain the presence of haemorrhoids in women. Traditionally piles have been classified into first degree, never prolapsing—bleeding only; second degree, spontaneously reducing after defecation; third degree, needing manual replacement; and fourth degree, permanently prolapsed.

PATHOLOGICAL ANATOMY

The normal anal canal contains three cushions of vascular tissue underlying the mucosa of its upper third.[33] When internal piles develop, this tissue hypertrophies and tends to be extruded downwards as the attachments to the underlying internal sphincter weaken over time, ultimately resulting in prolapse through the anus.[34] As these internal piles enlarge, their base extends below the dentate line, producing interoexternal piles.

CLINICAL FEATURES

The most common symptom is bleeding. This is usually painless, fresh, and confined to a smear on the toilet paper on wiping, although it is sometimes more spectacular and may rarely cause anaemia. A tendency to mucous discharge may be noticed, perhaps leading to the complaint of pruritus. Prolapse may occur on defecation or occasionally just with exercise and may require digital replacement. Persistent prolapse can cause interference with venous drainage, which can lead to strangulation and acute thrombosis. This presents with marked pain and swelling, and may occasionally progress to gangrene. This condition must be differentiated from thrombosed perianal varices (perianal haematoma).

It should be noted that there is a considerable symptom overlap between piles and other more serious anorectal conditions, in particular neoplastic diseases. Thorough physical examination of the anorectum is therefore necessary.

When the anus is inspected it may look normal, although there are often skin tags around its margin. Piles may be seen to be prolapsed at rest or on the command to strain; when prolapsed, they usually conform to the triple pattern (three, seven and 11 o'clock) and include tissue from above and below the dentate line becoming continuous with the external haemorrhoidal plexus. Prolapsed piles are usually dark red or purple and, if subject to frequent prolapse and trauma, may be covered by variable pale areas of squamous metaplasia.

Proctoscopy in a patient with non-prolapsing piles demonstrates enlarged submucosal vascular swellings in the three, seven and 11 o'clock positions as the instrument is drawn down into the upper anal canal. These often enlarge on straining.

TREATMENT

There is a tendency to over-treat piles. Until the last half century, surgery formed the mainstay of treatment in the UK. The results of all forms of treatment for haemorrhoids can be seen in Table 28.2. Symptomless piles do not require treatment. Piles that cause occasional spotting of blood can be managed with bulking agents. Non-reducing piles with a large skin component do usually require a formal haemorrhoidectomy. All other piles can be treated by injection of sclerosant or banding.

Bulking agents

Many patients with minor piles respond to this simple measure.[44] Failure to maintain treatment usually leads to relapse.

Injection sclerotherapy

The sclerosant (usually 3 mL of 5% phenol in arachis or almond oil) is injected via a proctoscope, just above each pile at the three, seven and 11 o'clock positions. The needle is inserted firmly into the submucosal layer; if the tip is correctly placed a bleb appears, covered in semitransparent mucosa containing visible blood vessels. The patient should be seen again 6 weeks later to check the result. Further injection is required only if symptoms persist. The most serious potential complication is injection of sclerosant into the prostate or seminal vesicles, which can lead to urinary symptoms and abscess formation.

Rubber band ligation

This procedure was described by Barron[45] and probably produces a longer-lasting effect than sclerotherapy.[46] The proctoscope should be positioned so that the dentate line can just be seen. The pile to be banded is grasped with forceps inserted through the circular metal ring of the bander, which is slid over the pile. The rubber band is then released by pushing down on the handle (Fig. 28.5). It is important to place the band above the dentate line to avoid severe pain. All three piles can be treated in turn. Suction banders have simplified the procedure. The patient should be reviewed 6 weeks later to assess the result. Rarely secondary haemorrhage may occur, and a few cases of fatal portal pyaemia have been reported.

Surgery

Only around 5% of piles need to be treated by operation. Of the many methods available, the one most widely applied in the UK is the open, or Milligan–Morgan, haemorrhoidectomy (Fig. 28.6).[47] This method involves the dissection, transfixion and

REFERENCES

33. Thompson WHF. Br J Surg 1975; 62: 542–552
34. Haas PA, Fox TA, Hass GP. Dis Colon Rectum 1984; 27: 442–450
35. Keighley MRB, Williams JA et al. Br Med J 1979; ii: 967
36. Cheng FCY, Shum DWP, Ong GB. Aust NZ J Surg 1981; 51: 458
37. Greca F, Hares MM et al. Br J Surg 1981; 68: 250
38. Murie JA, Sim AJW, Mackenzie I. Br J Surg 1982; 69: 536
39. O'Callaghan JD, Matheson TS, Hall R. Br J Surg 1982; 69: 157
40. Hancock B. Ann R Coll Surg Engl 1982; 64: 397
41. Leicester RJ, Nicholls RJ, Mann CV. Dis Colon Rectum 1981; 24: 602
42. Templeton JL, Spence RAJ et al. Br Med J 1983; i: 1387
43. Ambrose NS, Hares MM et al. Br Med J 1983; i: 1389
44. Senapati A, Nicholls RJ. Int J Colorect Dis 1988; 3: 124–126
45. Barron J. Am J Surg 1963; 105: 563–570
46. McRae M, McLeod RS. Dis Colon Rectum 1995; 38: 687–694
47. Milligan ETC, Naunton Morgan C et al. Lancet 1937; ii: 1119–1124

Table 28.2 Haemorrhoids: results of clinical trials

Reference	Follow-up (months)	Symptom	No. of symptomless patients/no. of patients followed						
			Injection	RBL	MDA	IR	C	LS	H
Keighley et al (1979)[35]	12	Not specified	–	16/35	11/37	–	4/36	6/34	–
Cheng et al (1981)[36]	12	Bleeding	14/21	15/20	19/22	–	–	–	18/19
		Prolapse	4/9	10/10	5/8	–	–	–	11/11
Greca et al (1981)[37]	12	Not specified	13/33	15/28	–	–	–	–	–
Murie et al (1982)[38]	42	Bleeding	–	27/38	–	–	–	–	32/38
		Prolapse	–	17/25	–	–	–	–	27/29
O'Callaghan et al (1982)[39]	48	Not specified	–	–	–	–	65/89	–	64/88
Hancock (1982)[40]*	60	1st, 2nd degree	–	–	19/22	–	–	–	–
		3rd degree	–	–	12/26	–	–	–	–
Leicester et al (1981)[41]	12	Bleeding	17/35	–	–	20/38	–	–	–
		Prolapse	–	12/34	–	17/43	–	–	–
Templeton et al (1983)[42]	3–12	Not specified	–	33/62	–	34/60	–	–	–
Ambrose et al (1983)[43]	12	1st degree	–	6/17	–	8/22	–	–	–
		2nd degree	–	20/62	–	26/68	–	–	–

RBL, rubber band ligation; MDA, maximal dilatation of the anus; IR, infrared coagulation; C, cryotherapy; LS, lateral sphincterotomy; H, haemorrhoidectomy.
*Non-controlled trial.

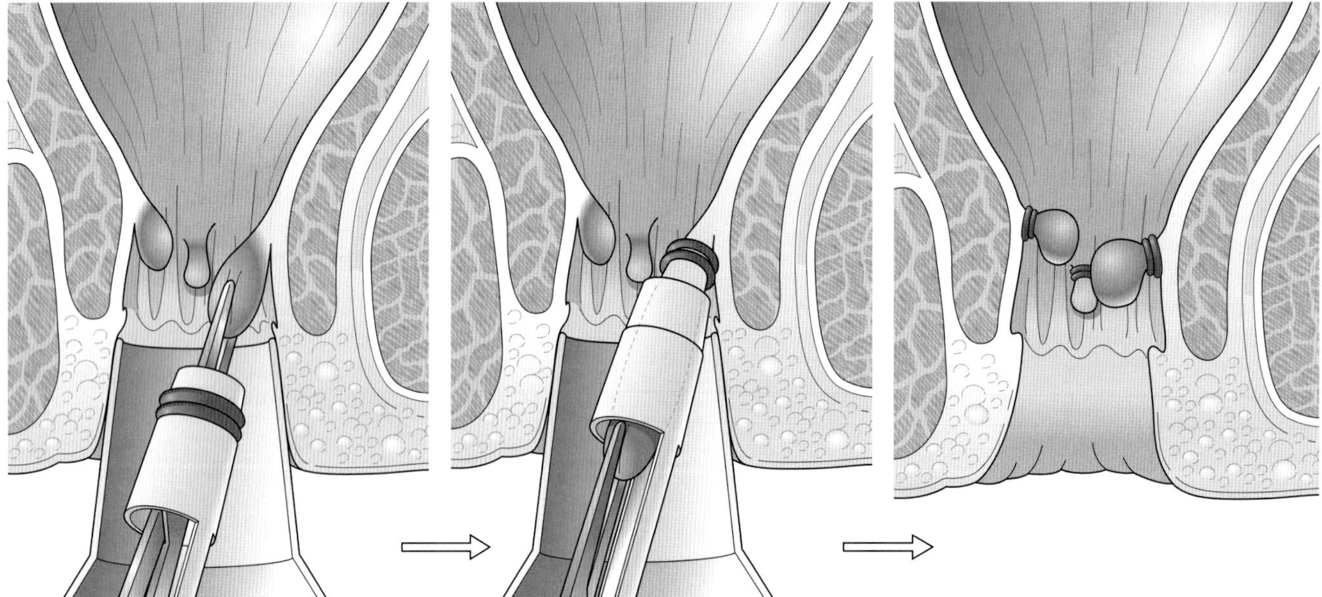

Figure 28.5 Rubber band ligation. Care must be taken to avoid including sensitive skin (below the dentate line) in a band.

excision of the three main piles, preserving the intervening skin and leaving the wounds open. Closed haemorrhoidectomy involves closure of the defects in the lining of the canal after pile excision. This procedure is widely practised in the USA.[48]

A new technique of stapled haemorrhoidectomy has been developed. A circumferential 'doughnut' of rectal mucosa and submucosa is excised from above the dentate line and then closed with a circular staple gun.[49] This procedure causes less pain, and an earlier return to work is possible than after the Milligan–Morgan haemorrhoidectomy. Long-term results are not yet available. Haemorrhoidal surgery is painful, and adequate analgesia needs to be given. A 7-day course of metronidazole, in combination with standard analgesics, has been shown to provide good pain relief.[50]

REFERENCES

48. Ferguson JA, Heaton JR. Dis Colon Rectum 1959; 2: 176–179
49. Mehigan BJ, Monson JR et al. Lancet 2000; 355: 782–785
50. Carapeti EA, Kamm MA et al. Lancet 1998; 351: 169–172

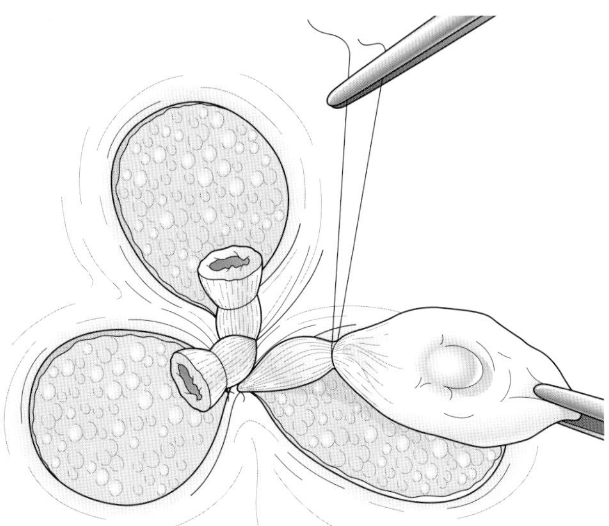

Figure 28.6 Open (Milligan–Morgan) haemorrhoidectomy.

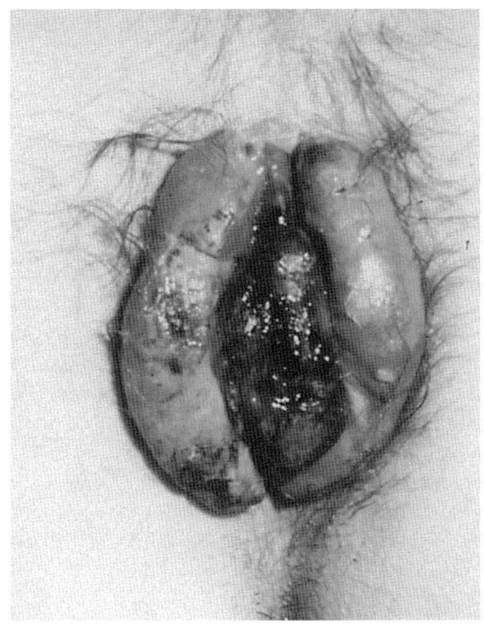

Figure 28.7 Prolapsed strangulated piles.

TREATMENT OF STRANGULATED HAEMORRHOIDS

This condition (Fig. 28.7) can be treated conservatively or by immediate haemorrhoidectomy. The latter has the advantage of rapid symptomatic relief and also ensures that the piles are permanently excised. Conservative management is by bed rest, analgesia, and local application of ice and local anaesthetic cream.

THROMBOSED PERIANAL VARIX (PERIANAL HAEMATOMA)

This condition is caused by a thrombosis in a subanodermal venous saccule and probably occurs as a result of sudden tearing of the anal margins by diarrhoea or constipation.[51]

It presents acutely with severe anal pain, difficulty with defecation, and a perianal lump. It develops over 24–48 h, and the pain gradually subsides over the subsequent 3–5 days. On examination there is a blue, smooth, firm, tender lump at the anal margin. The lump settles over a period of 1–3 weeks, often leaving a small nodule. It is usually around 1 cm in diameter and occupies one lateral half of the anal circumference (Fig. 28.8).

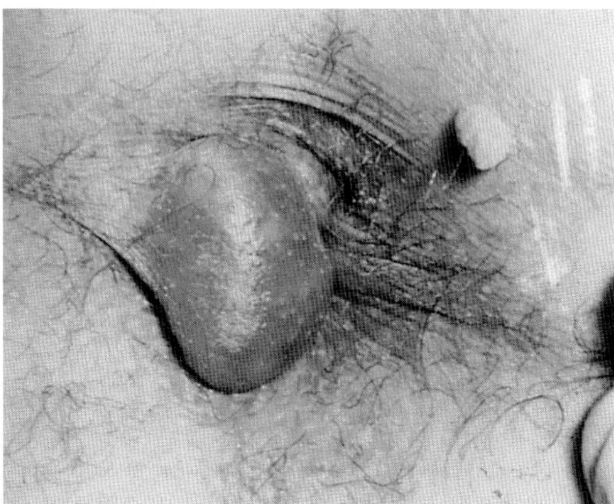

Figure 28.8 Thrombosed perianal varix.

The condition is self-limiting. If it has been present for several days, and the pain seems to be improving, it is best treated conservatively with bed rest, cold compresses or topical local anaesthesia. If it is acutely painful, then surgery should be performed under either local or general anaesthesia. The affected area is incised and the haematoma expressed, thus avoiding the formation of a skin tag when the haematoma resolves.

SEXUALLY TRANSMITTED DISEASES

Although sexually transmitted diseases involving the anorectum affect both sexes, they are most prevalent among homosexual men. Promiscuity and anal sexual practices have led to an increasing incidence, and many affected individuals carry multiple infections.

ANORECTAL GONORRHOEA

This infection may be symptomless and is very common among homosexual men.[52] The symptoms are usually mild, but include constipation, tenesmus and a mucopurulent discharge. Sigmoidoscopy reveals mildly erythematous areas, perhaps with small ulcers and mucopus. Diagnosis is made by Gram stain of a rectal swab. Treatment is by single doses of intramuscular procaine penicillin and oral probenecid.[53]

ANORECTAL HERPES SIMPLEX

Anorectal herpes simplex is another common condition of the male homosexual population. It presents with pain, constipation, discharge and perianal ulceration. Clusters of vesicles or ulcers are seen perianally and in the rectum. The diagnosis can be confirmed by identifying the virus on electron microscopy. Oral

REFERENCES

51. Thompson WHF. Lancet 1982; ii: 467
52. Quinn TC. Med Clin North Am 1986; 70: 611–633
53. Centers for Disease Control. Sexually transmitted diseases: treatment guidelines. MMWR Morb Mortal Wkly Rep 1982; 31: 355

or topical aciclovir (acyclovir) shortens the clinical course of what is a naturally remitting infection.[54]

CHLAMYDIA TRACHOMATIS PROCTITIS

Patients may present with one of two forms of this infection: those with positive lymphogranuloma venereum serology and those who are serum-negative.[55] This condition produces anorectal pain, tenesmus and discharge. Examination of the rectum reveals a friable rectal mucosa with discrete ulcers. In severe cases, fistulae and rectal strictures can mimic cancer or Crohn's disease.[56] Diagnosis is by culture and lymphogranuloma venereum serology. Tetracycline remains the treatment of choice.

ANORECTAL SYPHILIS

Anorectal syphilis presents with a painless anal ulcer, the primary chancre, which can be mistaken for a fissure or a traumatic injury. Untreated, the chancre disappears to be replaced by a condyloma latum, proctitis or mucosal polyps. Serology is the most dependable method for confirming the diagnosis. Penicillin remains the best treatment.

ANAL WARTS (CONDYLOMATA ACUMINATA)

Human papilloma virus types 6 and 11 causes anal warts.[57] Around 70% of those affected report anal sexual practices. The typical warty lesions may be confined to the perianal skin but may also involve the anal canal (Fig. 28.9). Numbers vary from one or two to hundreds of separate warts, giving the appearance of a continuous carpet of wart tissue. Small numbers of discrete perianal warts can be treated with topical podophyllin. More widespread warts are best treated by scissor excision following subcutaneous infiltration with local anaesthetic containing dilute adrenaline (epinephrine; 1:300 000).[58] It is important not to miss malignant change in extensive perianal warts.

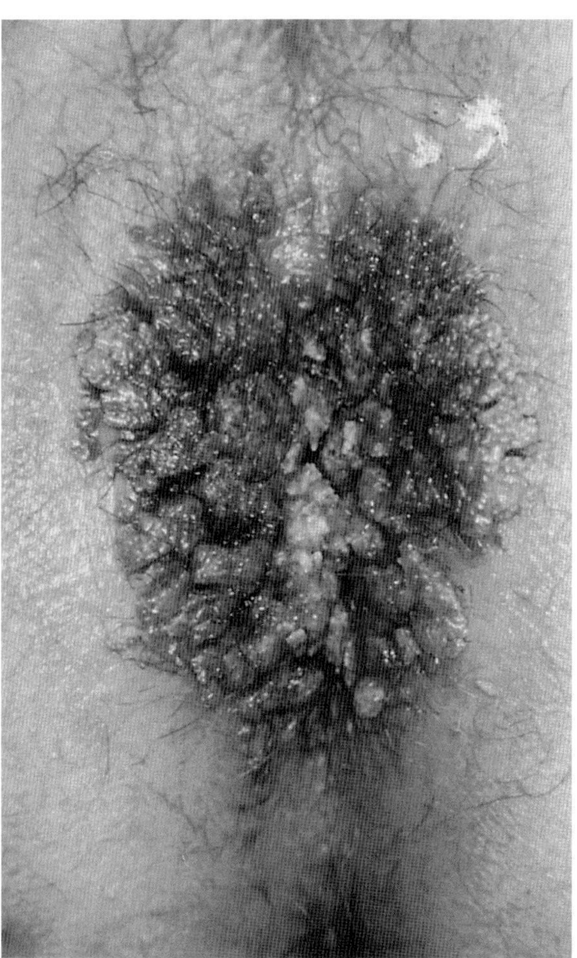

Figure 28.9 Condylomata acuminata.

ACQUIRED IMMUNE DEFICIENCY SYNDROME

This condition has several anorectal manifestations. The patient may have a fissure or perianal sepsis indistinguishable from the standard conditions. Alternatively, more florid lesions such as severe ulceration, rectal lymphoma[59] or Kaposi's sarcoma[60,61] can occur.

CONGENITAL DISEASES

HIRSCHSPRUNG'S DISEASE

First described by Hirschsprung in 1888,[62] this disorder is caused by an absence of ganglia in Auerbach's plexus and an increase in unmedullated innervation of the bowel wall muscle.[63,64] Although there is usually a well-demarcated abnormal segment in the rectum, very occasionally the affected segment is ultrashort and confined to the anal canal. In some cases the affected segment is much longer, extending proximally into the colon.[65] The aganglionic segment creates a functional obstruction.

Although the condition usually presents at birth, the diagnosis may not become apparent until the child is older. Rarely, the patient does not present until adulthood.[66] The incidence is one in 5000 births, and males are affected about four times more often than females.[67] The condition is suspected when a neonate fails to pass meconium in the first 24 h. Abdominal distension, feeding difficulties and vomiting may develop. Rectal examination may reveal a mucous plug, dislodgement of which leads to a dramatic decompression. The older child fails to thrive and has a chronically distended abdomen with refractory constipation.[68] Unlike other forms of chronic constipation, however, faecal soiling does not occur (see Ch. 45).

Barium studies show a megacolon above a narrow, aganglionic segment. Manometry demonstrates the absence of the rectosphincteric inhibition reflex on rectal distension,[69] while biopsy,

REFERENCES

54. Rompalo AM, Mertz GJ et al. Clin Res 1985; 33: 58A
55. Quinn TC, Goodell SE et al. N Engl J Med 1981; 305: 195–200
56. Levine JS, Smith PD, Brugge WE. Gastroenterology 1980; 79: 563
57. Krzyzek RA, Watts SC et al. J Virol 1980; 36: 236
58. Thomson JPS, Grace RJ. Proc R Soc Med 1978; 71: 180–185
59. Burkes RL, Meyer PR et al. Arch Intern Med 1986; 146: 913–915
60. Kaposi M. Arch Dermatol Syphilol 1872; 4: 265
61. Stern JO, Deiterich D et al. Gastroenterology 1982; 82: 1189
62. Hirschsprung H. Jahresbericht Kinderheilk 1888; 27: 1
63. Dalla Valle A. Pediatria Napoli 1924; 32: 569
64. Bodian M, Stephens FD, Ward BLH. Lancet 1949; i: 6
65. Nixon HH. In: Goligher J (ed). Surgery of the Anus, Rectum and Colon. 5th edn. Baillière Tindall, London, 1984: 305
66. Todd IP. Br J Surg 1977; 64: 311
67. Kleinhaus S, Boley SJ et al. J Pediatr Surg 1979; 14: 588
68. Wyllie GG. Lancet 1957; i: 847–850
69. Lawson JON, Nixon HH. J Pediatr Surg 1964; 2: 544

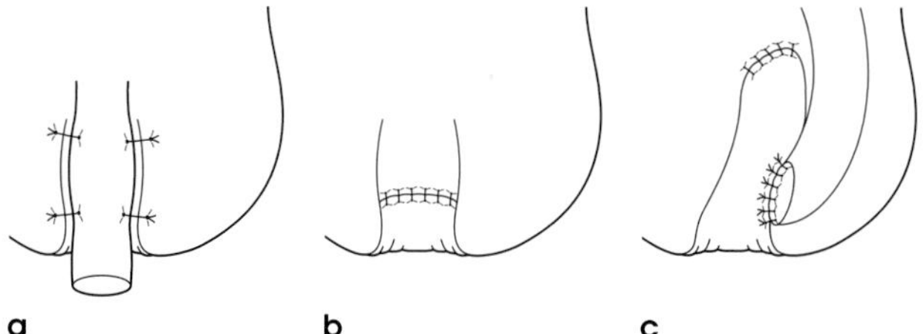

Figure 28.10 Principal operations in Hirschsprung's disease: (**a**) Soave, (**b**) Swenson and (**c**) Duhamel.

preferably by the simple suction method, confirms the absence of submucosal ganglia with proliferation of cholinergic nerve fibres.[70]

In the neonate, meconium ileus associated with cystic fibrosis and infective gastroenteritis can produce similar features to Hirschsprung's disease. In the older child chronic constipation without aganglionosis is the most important differential diagnosis.

Three main curative procedures are available: Swenson's,[71] Duhamel's,[72] and Soave's[73] operations (Fig. 28.10; see Ch. 45). Their aim is to resect the aganglionic segment and to construct an anastomosis between the normal proximal bowel and the anal canal. A preparatory colostomy allows the child to be made fit and ensures that the dilated colon returns to normal calibre, making anastomosis easier.

CONGENITAL ANAL ANOMALIES

Anal anomalies occur in around one in 5000 births. They can be divided into two broad categories—low (e.g. ectopic anus) and high (e.g. anorectal agenesis)—depending on whether the abnormality extends below the pelvic floor.[74] In girls, most anomalies are of the low variety, while in boys there are more high anomalies (see Ch. 45).[75]

INJURIES OF THE COLON, RECTUM AND ANUS

COLONIC INJURIES

Road traffic accidents are the most common cause of blunt bowel injuries from abdominal trauma,[76] but a fall or blow on the abdomen at work or during sport is also a well-recognized cause. The colon is usually torn near a point of fixation, crushed against the vertebral column, or burst by a rise in the intra-abdominal pressure. Damage to its blood supply may cause serious haemorrhage or ischaemic necrosis of the colonic wall. Seat belt injuries, which usually damage the caecum and splenic flexure, can cause discrete perforations of the antimesenteric border or a complete transection of the colon (see Ch. 7).[77] Iatrogenic injury from colonoscopic and radiological examinations can also occur.

The outcome and severity of a penetrating wound usually depends on the nature of the injury. While stab and gunshot wounds are the most common causes of colonic or rectal damage, bomb blast injuries may not only result in blunt trauma but may also drive fragments of shrapnel, clothing and masonry into the abdominal cavity. High-velocity bullets entering through a small wound can cause massive cavitating injuries of the colon and surrounding tissues before passing out through a larger exit wound. Low-velocity bullets, shotgun pellets and shrapnel may by contrast lodge in the abdomen.

Management

After initial resuscitation, a rapid overall assessment must be made. Physical signs usually determine the management of a patient with blunt large bowel trauma, and repeated reassessment is essential. Peritoneal lavage is less useful in diagnosing peritonitis than haemorrhage and may be misleading where there is retroperitoneal injury.[78] It may, however, be valuable in an unconscious patient. An urgent CT scan is now the investigation of choice for most patients with abdominal trauma (see Ch. 7).

Although selected cases of abdominal stab injury can be managed conservatively,[79] gunshot wounds should always be explored. At laparotomy, the full extent of any bowel injury must be carefully assessed through a long midline incision. It may be necessary to mobilize the colonic flexures to exclude retroperitoneal injury. Every injury is different, and it is difficult to propose didactic and specific surgical treatment. There are a range of surgical options depending on the state of the patient and the expertise of the surgeon.

In general, right-sided colonic injuries can be managed more safely by primary suture, or resection and immediate anastomosis, than those on the left side. Primary colonic closure is reasonable if there is a discrete injury of less than 4-h duration, with minimal peritoneal soiling, no major blood loss, and few associated injuries. It is absolutely contraindicated when there is frank peritonitis, extensive contamination, blunt trauma, a high-velocity bullet wound, shattering of multiple bowel loops from an explosion or shotgun injury, severe mesenteric injury or associated damage of multiple organs, especially the pancreas and duodenum. Under these circumstances, exteriorization or resection is preferable.[80,81]

Wounds of the transverse colon are best treated by exteriorization, converting the perforated area into a defunctioning colostomy. Injuries of the descending colon that are treated by primary suture or resection should be protected by a proximal stoma. An anastomosis is best deferred if there has been extensive bowel damage, and the proximal bowel end should be brought out as a colostomy, with closure of the distal stump or formation of a mucous fistula. The sigmoid colon is often mobile enough to be managed by exteriorization when the injury is at the apex of the loop, but wounds near the peritoneal reflection require resection.

The mortality and morbidity from colonic injuries are generally high, especially when there is associated haemorrhagic shock, gross peritoneal contamination, multiple visceral injuries, or delay in diagnosis.

REFERENCES

70. Noblett HR. J Pediatr Surg 1969; 4: 406–409
71. Swenson O. Ann Surg 1964; 160: 540–550
72. Duhamel B. Presse Med 1956; 64: 2249
73. Soave F. Arch Dis Child 1964; 39: 116–124
74. Stephens FD, Smith ED. Anorectal Malformations in Children. Year Book Medical Publishers, Chicago, 1971: 133
75. Nixon HH. In: Goligher J (ed). Surgery of the Anus, Rectum and Colon. 5th edn. Baillière Tindall, London, 1984: 285
76. Towne JB, Coe JD. Am J Surg 1971; 122: 693
77. Falcone RE, Carey LC. Surg Clin North Am 1988; 68: 1307
78. Soderstrom CA, DuPriest RW, Cowley RA. Surg Gynecol Obstet 1980; 151: 513–518
79. Feliciano D. Trauma. Appleton & Lange, Norwalk
80. Parks TG. Br J Surg 1981; 68: 725
81. Kirkpatrick JR, Rajpal SG. Am J Surg 1975; 129: 187

INJURIES OF THE RECTUM AND ANAL CANAL

The rectum and anal canal can be injured in a variety of ways. These include swallowed foreign bodies and objects inserted per anum. Surgical and obstetric procedures may injure the rectum and anal canal, as can the trauma associated with pelvic fractures.

Pneumatic injuries are rare but highly dangerous. They usually result from practical joking in which compressed air is passed up the victim's anus. The sudden increase in pressure results in rupture of the intraperitoneal rectum.

Clinical features

The site of injury is more accessible than in the colon, and a careful examination of the pelvis, perineum and anal margin is important. In gunshot wounds rectal injury should be suspected if the path of the projectile is anywhere near the rectum. It should also be suspected if there is blood in the lumen of the bowel, or if there is an associated sacral fracture. It is important to exclude damage to adjacent organs, especially the bladder and urethra.

Impalement injuries are usually more serious than they at first appear, and when a patient presents with a stake or other foreign body in situ it should be removed only in the operating theatre under a general anaesthetic with the abdomen open.[77] On removal of the transfixing object, there may be brisk haemorrhage, and the direction of the track is seen more easily through a laparotomy incision.

Management

A proximal colostomy is advisable if the injury is above the peritoneal reflection. For wounds below the peritoneal reflection, debridement and repair are still best achieved from the abdomen. When the anal sphincters are damaged, as much sphincter as possible should be preserved, and a primary or delayed primary repair carried out. Unless the injury is minor, a colostomy is necessary, and the rectum must be washed out thoroughly.[82]

FOREIGN BODIES IN THE RECTUM

Most foreign bodies have been inserted through the anus and can be difficult to remove. Extraction is best achieved under general anaesthetic, and the use of obstetric forceps, retractors and snares may be necessary. A catheter passed alongside larger objects high in the rectum allows enough air to be insufflated into the proximal bowel to facilitate removal.[83] Occasionally the foreign body has to be pushed upwards and removed through a colotomy.

VASCULAR MALFORMATIONS

Vascular malformations are a rare cause of colonic bleeding and are often very difficult to identify by conventional investigations. Aneurysms and malformations of the major colonic blood vessels are extremely rare.

ANGIODYSPLASIA

Angiodysplasia has been increasingly identified since the introduction of colonoscopy. It is a condition of unknown aetiology but is occasionally associated with aortic valve stenosis (see Ch. 22) or the vascular malformations of hereditary telangiectasia (Osler–Weber–Rendu disease; see Ch. 10).

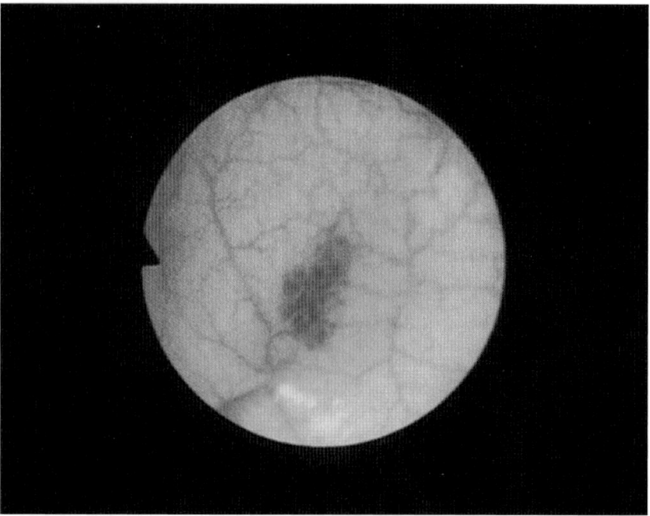

Figure 28.11 Angiodysplasia. A group of abnormal small vessels in the colonic mucosa is clearly seen via a colonoscope.

Histologically there is debate as to whether angiodysplasia is a degenerative, hamartomatous or neoplastic condition.[84]

Clinical features

Rectal bleeding is the most common presenting symptom. On occasions, this is torrential but is more often a series of repeated small bleeds or persistent occult bleeding resulting in anaemia. Angiodysplasia can occur anywhere in the colon but is most common in the right colon of elderly patients.[85]

At colonoscopy, the angiomatous lesions can usually be seen as multiple mucosal abnormalities up to 1 cm in diameter, resembling spider naevi (Fig. 28.11). When there is a major haemorrhage, colonoscopy may be impractical, but selective mesenteric arteriography often demonstrates the characteristic blush of a malformation (Fig. 28.12).[86] Radiolabelled scintigraphy (red cell scan) may also be useful in localizing the site of bleeding, but only if the bleeding rate is greater than 0.5 mL/min.

Management

Small numbers of angiodysplastic malformations can be treated through the colonoscope by coagulation with hot biopsy forceps.[87] Extensive areas of angiodysplasia often require resection. Intraoperative colonoscopy with transillumination of the colonic wall can be helpful in determining the extent of resection.[88] Torrential haemorrhage may require a total colectomy and ileorectal anastomosis if the bleeding site cannot be clearly identified preoperatively.

REFERENCES

82. Haas PA, Fox TA. Dis Colon Rectum 1979; 22: 17
83. Eftaiha M, Hambrick E, Abcarian H. Dis Col Rectum 1977; 112: 691
84. Price AB. Int J Colorect Dis 1986; 1: 121
85. Boley SJ, Di Biase A et al. Am J Surg 1979; 137: 57
86. Sheedy PF, Fulton RE, Atwell DT. Am J Roentgenol 1975; 123: 338
87. Danesh BJZ, Spiliadis C et al. Int J Colorectal Dis 1987; 2: 218
88. Campbell WB, Rhodes M, Kettlewell MG. Ann R Coll Surg 1985; 67: 290

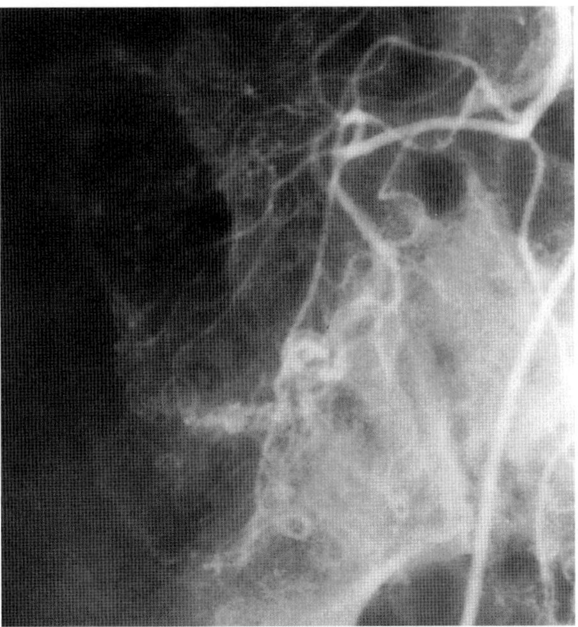

Figure 28.12 Angiodysplasia. A group of abnormal small vessels in the blush seen in the abnormal vessels in the caecum.

OTHER VASCULAR MALFORMATIONS

These are usually cavernous or giant haemangiomata. The most common site is the rectum, but they may extend proximally to involve the colon. The angioma can usually be seen on endoscopy as a prominent red area or as a collection of dilated tortuous submucosal vessels with a bluish tinge (see Ch. 11).

Smaller lesions may be managed by electrocoagulation. Injection sclerotherapy with phenol may give temporary control. A large rectal cavernous haemangioma that is diffuse and symptomatic can be successfully treated surgically. Patients with Klippel–Trenaunay syndrome may also develop pelvic venous abnormalities, which can cause troublesome bleeding (see Ch. 11).

ISCHAEMIC DISEASE OF THE LARGE BOWEL

Ischaemic bowel disease has become more prevalent as the elderly population increases. Two distinct clinical syndromes can be recognized in the colon: colonic gangrene and ischaemic colitis (see Ch. 10 and Ch. 27).[89,90]

AETIOLOGY

Arterial thrombus or embolus

The inferior mesenteric artery may be occluded by a thrombus, an embolism arising from the heart or an aortic dissection (see Ch. 22). The outcome is dependent on the collateral supply and can vary from ischaemic colitis to colonic gangrene. Ligation of the inferior mesenteric artery at its origin during aneurysm repair or colonic surgery occasionally results in left colonic ischaemia.

Small vessel disease

Vasculitides such as polyarteritis, Buerger's disease and systemic lupus erythematosus, together with microemboli from atheromatous disease, can give rise to colonic ischaemia (see Ch. 10).

Low flow states

In patients with severe heart failure or those with septic or hypovolaemic shock the colonic blood supply may fail, allowing metabolically active bacteria, especially pathogenic strains of *Clostridia*, to invade the colonic wall and induce necrosis, toxaemia and shock.[90]

Intestinal obstruction

Blood flow in the colonic wall is not only influenced by its blood supply, but also by intraluminal pressure and the radial tension and diameter of the colon. Sometimes ischaemic changes are seen proximal to an obstructing carcinoma of the colon.

Venous occlusion

The inferior mesenteric vein may be ligated without any obvious effect, but extensive venous thrombosis causes haemorrhagic infarction closely resembling an arterial injury.

Idiopathic infarction

Bowel infarction can occur without any obvious precipitating cause.

PATHOLOGY

Colonic ischaemia follows a characteristic evolution, whatever the cause. There is progressive destruction of the bowel wall ending in full-thickness necrosis, sloughing and perforation after severe prolonged ischaemia. In contrast, a transient episode causes a limited degree of congestion and inflammation, which usually resolves completely. An intermediate degree of ischaemia does not usually threaten the integrity of the bowel wall but does cause ischaemia of the mucosa and muscle. The inflammatory response is followed by mucosal ulceration, haemorrhage and fibrosis extending into the muscle coat. The end result may be a stricture, which can be confused with an annular carcinoma or a segment of Crohn's disease (Fig. 28.13).

COLONIC GANGRENE

Clinical features

A middle-aged or elderly patient, often with a history of cardiovascular disease, presents with symptoms of sudden, severe, generalized abdominal pain that is at first colicky and later becomes constant with associated vomiting and sometimes diarrhoea (see Ch. 25). Rectal bleeding is unusual. The patient's condition rapidly deteriorates, with abdominal distension and shock.

On examination the patient is pale, sweaty and dyspnoeic with a tachycardia and hypotension, and appears gravely ill. There are signs of generalized peritonitis, and on rectal examination dark blood may be present on the glove. This picture may be indistinguishable from small bowel infarction, severe pancreatitis, ruptured abdominal aneurysm, perforation or strangulation obstruction, and the diagnosis is only made with certainty at laparotomy (see Ch. 25). The plain radiograph may be normal at first, but later shows progressive colonic dilatation resembling a volvulus or toxic megacolon. There is often an early and often marked leukocytosis and a metabolic acidosis. Serum enzymes, including the amylase and transaminases, may be elevated.

REFERENCES

89. Abel ME, Russell TR. Dis Colon Rectum 1983; 26: 113
90. Marston A. Intestinal Ischaemia. Edward Arnold, London, 1977

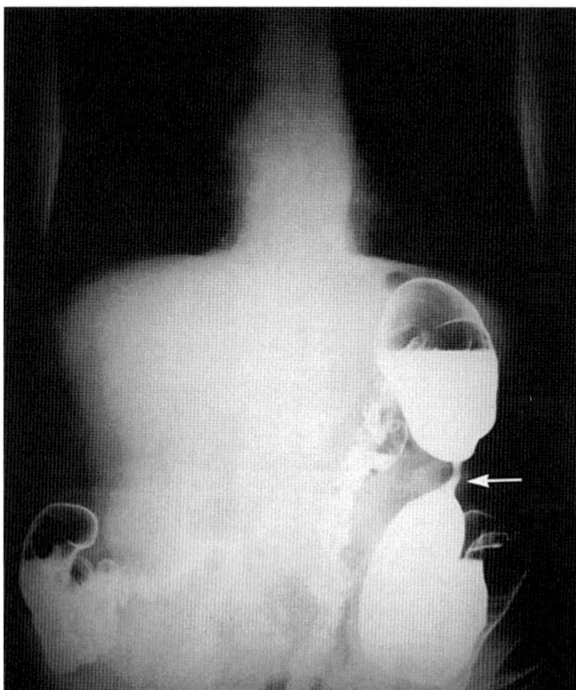

Figure 28.13 Ischaemic stricture. This barium enema shows the smooth stricture, typically situated near the splenic flexure.

Management

The first step is resuscitation while the patient is prepared for an emergency exploration of the abdomen. On opening the abdomen, the presence of a length of necrotic colon and occasionally, small bowel (see Ch. 22) is immediately apparent. The affected colon may have a deep red, purple, black or green blotchy appearance extending for a variable distance between sigmoid and caecum. The rectum is usually spared. A characteristic odour pervades the operating room. The colon is resected widely, ensuring that the cut ends are viable. The proximal bowel is brought out as a colostomy, and the distal colon brought out as a mucous fistula or closed off as a Hartmann's operation if viable bowel cannot reach the abdominal wall. There is absolutely no place for a primary anastomosis in the management of this condition.[90] Colonic gangrene is an abdominal catastrophe with a high mortality in excess of 80%.

ISCHAEMIC COLITIS

Clinical features

The typical patient is middle-aged or elderly with a history of cardiovascular disease but no previous intestinal symptoms. There is usually an acute onset of pain in the left iliac fossa, spreading across the abdomen up to the epigastrium. Diarrhoea often develops, and the stool is characteristically dark, containing blood clots.

On examination there is tenderness in the left iliac fossa and dark blood on rectal examination but often little in the way of systemic disturbance. The differential diagnosis includes complicated diverticular disease, carcinoma of the large bowel, sigmoid perforation, acute inflammatory bowel disease, left-sided renal colic, leaking abdominal aneurysm, and acute infective gastroenteritis.

Colonoscopy can be used to take biopsies for histology in mild cases. The colon has a heaped-up, oedematous, bluish purple mucosa, sometimes with ulceration and contact bleeding. The white cell count is usually raised. A plain abdominal radiograph may reveal 'thumbprinting' (oedematous mucosa) or signs of small bowel obstruction. Arteriography may occasionally be helpful, but the most useful investigation is a barium enema.

Management

Once the diagnosis is established, the management is conservative, with careful monitoring by repeated examination and the administration of intravenous fluids and antibiotics. The condition usually resolves, although it may progress to gangrene or to a late stricture. Surgery is rarely required.

IRRADIATION BOWEL DISEASE

Irradiation for uterine or bladder cancer can result in proctitis, ulceration and stricture formation in the rectum. It can also cause fistulation into the vagina or bladder. The diagnosis should be considered in all patients presenting with rectal bleeding and a change in bowel habit who have previously been treated by radiotherapy. The differential diagnosis includes ischaemic and inflammatory bowel disease and carcinoma of the colon. The full effects of irradation may take years to develop.[91] Radiation proctitis can cause severe bloody diarrhoea, and a diverting colostomy may be necessary. Provided the sphincter has not been damaged, and a recurrent tumour has been excluded, rectal resection with coloanal anastomosis bringing down non-irradiated left colon may be successful. A defunctioning colostomy is advisable, because the healing of irradiated tissues is notoriously poor. Where there is local destruction of the sphincter, an abdominoperineal excision is required.[92]

INFLAMMATORY BOWEL DISEASE

When a patient presents with diarrhoea, two broad groups of diseases must be considered. These include infective and non-infective inflammatory bowel disease. It is important to bear the infective causes in mind when considering the management of patients with severe diarrhoea so that inappropriate surgery can be avoided. Although altered bowel function with blood in the stool following foreign travel is likely to be caused by bacillary or amoebic dysentery, or schistosomiasis, other diseases such as ulcerative colitis, Crohn's colitis and a colonic carcinoma must be considered.

AMOEBIC DYSENTERY

The disease is caused by the protozoan *Entamoeba histolytica*, which when ingested as a cyst causes colonic ulceration with bloody diarrhoea, and occasionally brisk bleeding. Without treatment, it may progress to chronic dysentery, amoebic appendicitis or an amoeboma. Fresh stool specimens must be rapidly examined for protozoa. Treatment with metronidazole is highly effective but must be supplemented with a contact amoebicide such as diloxanide furoate.

REFERENCES

91. Allen-Mersh TG, Wilson EJ, Hopestone HF et al. Surg Gynecol Obstet 1987; 164: 521–524
92. Cooke SAR, Wellsted MD. World J Surg 1986; 10: 220

BACILLARY DYSENTERY (SHIGELLOSIS)

This is often an epidemic disease, and a contact history can usually be obtained. The *Shigella* organisms rapidly multiply in the colon. In severe cases, endotoxins can cause a coagulopathy or haemolytic anaemia.[93] Inflammation of the colon leads to necrosis of epithelium and desquamation with formation of a membrane and discrete ulcers. The diagnosis is usually made by stool culture. Most cases will settle with supportive measures, and treatment with the antibiotics ampicillin or tetracycline is usually reserved for resistant cases.

SCHISTOSOMIASIS

The infective agent is a trematode worm. Repeated stool specimens have to be examined for parasites. Sigmoidoscopy may demonstrate ulceration, and a rectal biopsy is often diagnostic. Barium enema shows an immobile irregular colon. Treatment of schistosomiasis has been simplified with the introduction of a very effective drug, praziquantel.[94]

PSEUDOMEMBRANOUS COLITIS

Pseudomembranous colitis[95] is a severe form of antibiotic-induced diarrhoea caused by *Clostridium difficile*, the toxin of which can be measured in stool. It may occur up to 2 months after any course of broad-spectrum antibiotics.[96] The clinical picture varies from simple diarrhoea to a severe colitis with epithelial necrosis characterized by a white membrane, which can be seen on sigmoidoscopy. Rectal biopsy shows the characteristic histology of a pseudomembrane (Fig. 28.14). Treatment is with oral metronidazole (preferred) or vancomycin, but occasionally colectomy is required for severe necrotizing disease.[97]

OTHER SPECIFIC COLONIC INFECTIONS

Campylobacter and *Yersinia enterocolitica* infections predominantly involve the small intestine (see Ch. 27) but may occasionally cause colitis with a characteristically infective clinical picture.[94]

ULCERATIVE COLITIS

Ulcerative colitis usually develops between the ages of 15 and 40 years. Its prevalence of 40 per 100 000 is static.[98] Genetic factors, immune mechanisms, and environmental and dietary causes have all been considered, but the aetiology remains obscure.[99] About 15% of patients with an onset before 21 years of age have immediate family members with the disease, but careful studies have failed to confirm anything other than polygenic inheritance.[100] Although HLA B27 is associated with ankylosing spondylitis, no blood group antigens have been linked to inflammatory bowel disease. Ankylosing spondylitis is probably an associated disorder, although some consider it to be a complication of the colonic disease.[101] Its incidence in ulcerative colitis is much higher than in the general population. A causative organism has not been identified, but immune responses or an autoimmune aetiology in response to bacteria have been suggested. Dietary antigens, especially milk products, have been implicated, but no direct causal relationship has been established.[102]

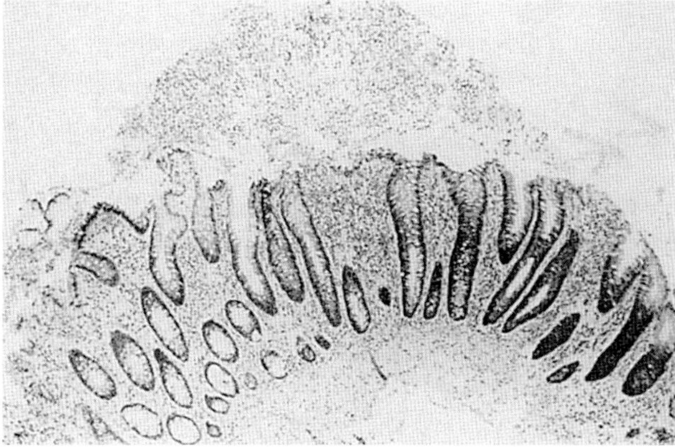

Figure 28.14 Pseudomembranous colitis. Histological section to show epithelial necrosis and pseudomembrane.

PATHOLOGY

Ulcerative colitis is a mucosal disorder, which almost invariably involves the rectum and then spreads more proximally. It may relapse and remit, during which time its distribution can become extensive and then decrease with successful treatment. Inflammation is confined to the mucosa except in patients with acute and severe colitis, where fissures and transmural changes can make the distinction between severe ulcerative colitis and Crohn's colitis very difficult. The disease is confined to the rectum and distal sigmoid in 60% of cases, extension to the splenic flexure is seen in a further 25%, and in the remaining 15% inflammation extends beyond the splenic flexure. This last group is said to have total or near total colitis and is at greater risk of developing severe acute colitis, possibly with toxic dilatation.[103] The cancer risk is also much greater in patients where it is not possible to differentiate ulcerative colitis from Crohn's disease by histology.[104] These are designated as *indeterminate colitis*.[105] It appears that indeterminate colitis behaves more like ulcerative colitis than Crohn's disease.[106]

In colons with ulcerative colitis, there is a diffuse infiltration of acute and chronic inflammatory cells, which are limited to the mucosa. Numerous crypt abscesses are present with distortion of the glandular pattern and goblet cell depletion. In long-standing colitis epithelial dysplasia may develop and, when severe, carcinoma is frequently found at other sites in the colon.[107] A proctocolectomy should be considered if severe dysplasia is found on rectal or colonic biopsies.

REFERENCES

93. Keasch G. J Clin Gastroenterol 1979; 8: 645
94. Jewkes J, Larson HE et al. Gut 1981; 22: 388
95. (Anonymous). Br Med J 1979; 2: 349
96. Klingler PJ, Metzger PP et al. Dig Dis 2000; 18: 147–160
97. Keighley MRB, Burdon DW et al. Br Med J 1978; 2: 1667
98. Langman MJS, Burnham WR. In: Allan RN, Keighley MRB et al (eds). Inflammatory Bowel Diseases. Churchill Livingstone, Edinburgh, 1983
99. Kirsner JB, Shorter RG. N Engl J Med 1982; 306: 775–837
100. Farmer RG, Michener WH, Mortimer EA. Clin Gastroenterol 1980; 9: 271
101. Macrae I, Wright V. Ann Rheum Dis 1973; 32: 16
102. Wright R, Truelove SC. Br Med J 1965; 2: 142
103. Edwards FC, Truelove SC. Gut 1963; 4: 299
104. de Dombal F, Watts J et al. Br Med J 1966; i: 1442
105. Price AB. J Clin Pathol 1978; 31: 567
106. Wells A, McMillan I et al. Br J Surg 1991; 78: 179–181
107. Morson BC, Dawson IMP et al. Gastrointestinal Pathology. 3rd edn. Blackwell Scientific Publications, Oxford, 1990

Table 28.3 Extraintestinal manifestations of inflammatory bowel disease

	Manifestation
Related to disease activity	
Skin	Pyoderma gangrenosum, erythema nodosum
Mucous membranes	Aphthous ulcers of mouth and vagina
Eyes	Iritis
Joints	Activity-related arthritis of large joints
Unrelated to disease activity	
Joints	Sacroiliitis, ankylosing spondylitis
Liver	Chronic active hepatitis, cirrhosis
Biliary tree	Sclerosing cholangitis, bile duct carcinoma
Renal	Amyloidosis in Crohn's disease
Integument	Fingernail clubbing

CLINICAL FEATURES

The most common presentation is bloody diarrhoea in an otherwise fit patient. Patients with a limited proctitis may be constipated, but they still complain of the passage of blood and mucus. In severe cases there may be almost constant diarrhoea with cramping abdominal pain, and urgency to defecate may be accompanied by episodes of incontinence. In severe disease, systemic symptoms include anorexia and weight loss, together with anaemia, and water and electrolyte loss. The recognized extraintestinal associations are listed in Table 28.3.

Rectal examination usually reveals blood and mucus on the glove, and the mucosa may feel velvety. Sigmoidoscopy shows a diffuse proctitis with contact bleeding, ulceration and granularity. It is important to recognize patients with severe acute colitis. Local symptoms are severe, with bowel frequency often exceeding more than ten stools in 24 h, blood and mucus with each stool, and an urgent desire to defecate. Systemic symptoms, such as wasting, pallor, tachycardia and pyrexia, are usually present. Abdominal signs of tenderness or distension are present only in patients with severe disease, and patients with severe colitis may progress to acute toxic dilatation of the colon, ultimately leading to perforation.

The differential diagnosis includes Crohn's colitis, ischaemic colitis, diverticular disease, carcinoma, irritable bowel syndrome, pseudomembranous colitis, *Shigella* and amoebic colitis.

INVESTIGATION

Investigation aims first to make the diagnosis and second to assess the severity of the disease. Sigmoidoscopy enables a biopsy to be taken, but it also permits an assessment of the proximal extent of the disease in cases with inflammation limited to the rectum. Even in mild chronic cases there may be difficulty in differentiating ulcerative colitis from Crohn's disease. The anatomical extent is related to the severity of the disease. A double-contrast barium enema demonstrates the extent of macroscopic disease (Fig. 28.15). Colonoscopy can be helpful as a primary investigation and is also invaluable for assessing strictures and doubtful radiology. It also enables biopsies to be taken from multiple sites throughout the colon. Neither investigation should be employed in patients with severe acute colitis, because there is an increased risk of bowel perforation. Blood samples are taken for haemoglobin and markers of inflammation such as the erythrocyte sedimentation rate, C-reactive protein and the serum albumin.

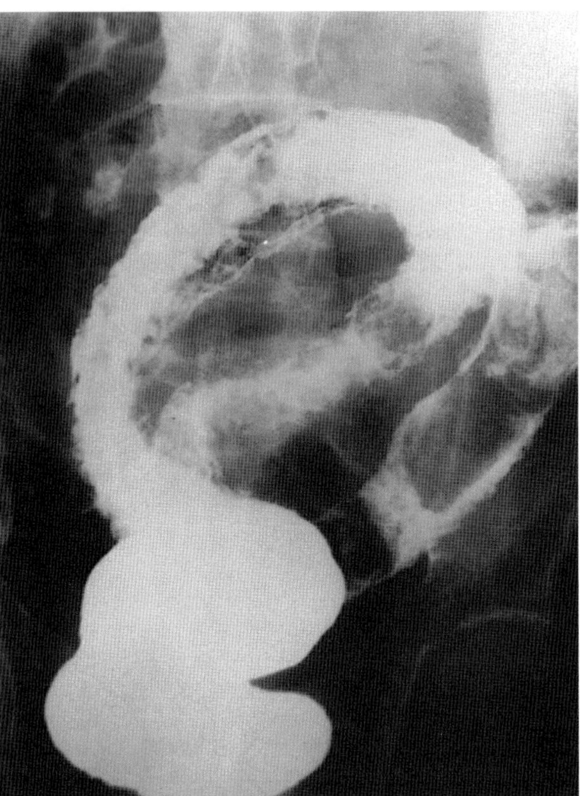

Figure 28.15 Barium enema appearance in severe ulcerative colitis. Undermining of mucosa by ulceration produces epithelial pseudopolyps.

MEDICAL MANAGEMENT

Medical management has several aims, which include reducing inflammation, controlling symptoms, correcting any water and electrolyte imbalances, and nutritional replacement (see Ch. 2).

Anti-inflammatory drugs

Sulfasalazine (sulphasalazine) is a combination of sulphapyridine and 5-aminosalicylic acid. It was one of the first treatments for ulcerative colitis but had a number of side effects. The active moiety has been shown to be 5-aminosalicylate, and new oral aminosalicylate drugs (such as mesalamine and balsalazide) have become first-line treatment for mild or moderate ulcerative colitis.[108] A major advance was the introduction of topical formulations of these drugs. Rectal administration, via suppositories, foams and liquid enemas, is the preferred treatment for mild or moderate distal ulcerative colitis.

The new glucocorticosteroid, budesonide, may be used for distal colitis. It is rapidly absorbed by the colonic mucosa when given as a rectal preparation but, because it is removed by extensive first-pass hepatic metabolism, it does not have the systemic side effects associated with other steroids.

In severe acute ulcerative colitis intravenous hydrocortisone is used, and three-quarters of the patients respond and avoid surgery.[109] In less severe cases, prednisolone is given by mouth. Ciclosporin (cyclosporin) may also be used in severe acute colitis,

REFERENCES

108. Campieri M. Gut 2002; 50 (Suppl 3): III 43–46
109. Truelove SC, Willerby CP et al. Lancet 1978; ii: 1086

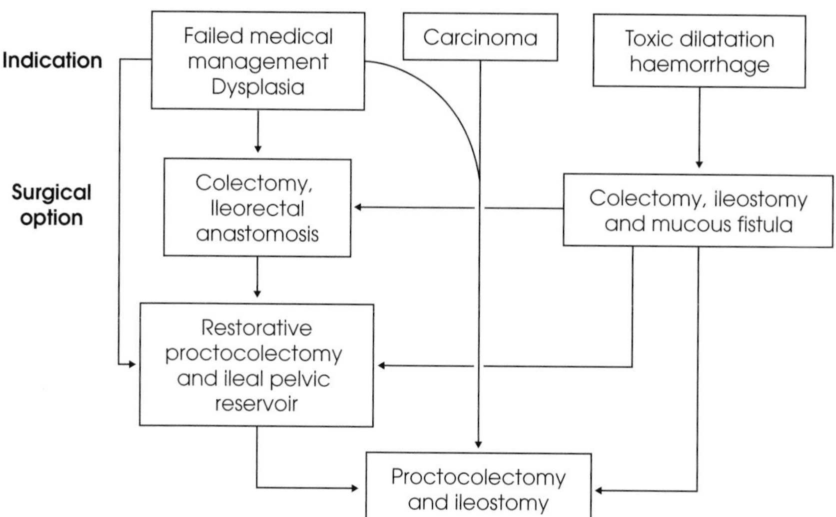

Figure 28.16 Algorithm for surgical management of ulcerative colitis. (From Pounder R (ed). Recent Advances in Gastroenterology 6. Churchill Livingstone, Edinburgh: 1986, with permission.[113])

with 60–80% of patients avoiding an operation.[110] Remission is then maintained using azathioprine, which can also be given to patients who are steroid-intolerant.

Other new therapies include probiotics (a mixture of live commensal organisms given orally), which have been used to treat both ulcerative colitis and 'pouchitis'.[111] Anti-tumour necrosis factor antibody therapies (infliximab) are also being used in trials to treat acute colitis and show early promise.[112]

Symptomatic control

Antidiarrhoeal agents, including codeine phosphate and loperamide, can be used to reduce the number of bowel actions. They are relatively bland and can be given in maximal dosage.

Nutrition

Patients who are acutely ill with associated malnutrition require nutritional supplements (see Ch. 2). Whether the enteral or parenteral route is chosen depends on the severity of disease.

SURGICAL MANAGEMENT

The indications for surgery are rarely absolute, the ideal solution being joint management between an aggressive physician and a conservative surgeon (Fig. 28.16).[113,114] Surgery is essential if the patient develops perforation, severe haemorrhage or toxic dilatation. When a severe attack fails to respond to medical therapy, surgery should be considered, particularly if the patient has: more than eight bloody stools per day, a tachycardia of more than 100 beats/min, a fever above 38.5°C, dilatation of the transverse colon greater than 5 cm, and a falling serum albumin.[109]

Chronic disability or ill health can be an indication for surgery, as can growth retardation in children.[115] There is a definite risk of cancer developing in patients who have long-standing total colitis. The degree of risk is controversial,[116] but it appears to be negligible up to 10 years from diagnosis. Thereafter there is a cumulative incidence of about 1% per annum, so that about 10% of a cohort of patients diagnosed 20 years previously will have developed cancer.[117] The risk is thought to be greater when the whole bowel is affected.

Proctocolectomy with ileostomy

A proctocolectomy is performed, mobilizing the rectum either in the perimuscular 'close rectal' plane or in the mesorectal plane. The anal canal is removed from below in the intersphincteric plane, and the pelvis and perineum closed. A Brooke spouted ileostomy[118] is brought out at the stoma site.

Kock continent ileostomy

There are fewer indications now for this procedure[119] than 10–20 years ago, because of the development of restorative proctocolectomy. It still has a place for patients who have had a proctocolectomy with excision of the anal canal and who are keen to improve their quality of life. It is especially suitable for patients with an unsatisfactory Brooke ileostomy who are having difficulty in keeping an appliance in place. The distal ileum is invaginated into an ileal reservoir to create a nipple valve, which the patient can evacuate by self-catheterization (Fig. 28.17).

Colectomy and ileorectal anastomosis

This avoids the need for an ileostomy but has become less popular since the advent of restorative proctocolectomy.[120] A successful result depends on there being only mild disease in the rectum. It is particularly good for younger patients, allowing them to mature through adolescence without a stoma. Persisting disease in the rectum is responsible for a high relapse rate, with failure, defined by conversion to a permanent ileostomy, being reported in 10–70% of cases.[121–123] Malignant change in

REFERENCES

110. Cohen RD, Stein R et al. Am J Gastroenterol 1999; 94: 1587–1592
111. Farrell RJ, Peppercorn MA. Lancet 2002; 359: 331–340
112. Sands BE, Tremaine WJ et al. Inflamm Bowel Dis 2001; 7: 83–88
113. Pounder R (ed.). Recent Advances in Gastroenterology, Vol 6. Churchill Livingstone, Edinburgh, 1986
114. Jewell DP. Int J Colorect Dis 1988; 3: 186
115. Berger M, Gribetz D, Korelitz B. Paediatrics 1975; 55: 459
116. Dickinson RJ, Dickson MC, Axon ATR. Lancet 1980; i: 620
117. Lennard Jones JE, Morson B et al. Gastroenterology 1977; 73: 1280
118. Brooke BN. Lancet 1952; ii: 102
119. Kock NG. Ann Surg 1971; 173: 545
120. Dozois RR et al. Int J Colorectal Dis 1986; 1: 2–19
121. Jones PF, Munroe A, Ewen SWB. Br J Surg 1977; 64: 615
122. Aylett SO. Br Med J 1966; i: 1001
123. Hawley PR. Br J Surg 1985; 72 (Suppl): S75

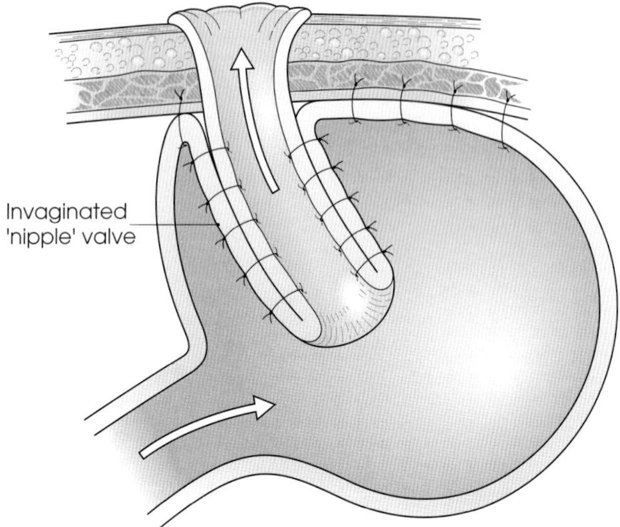

Figure 28.17 The Kock continent ileostomy.

the retained rectum occurs in 5–15%, although this risk may have been overemphasized.[100,121,124] Long-term follow-up by sigmoidoscopy and biopsy at 6-monthly intervals should be undertaken.

Restorative proctocolectomy

The patient avoids a permanent stoma in this procedure, but all the diseased tissue is removed. It is rapidly becoming the procedure of choice in the surgical treatment of ulcerative colitis.[120] Well-motivated patients under the age of 60 years who do not have Crohn's disease and are aware of the possible complications and problems are suitable candidates.[125] The procedure consists of a colectomy combined with a rectal excision, either by close dissection along its wall or within the mesorectal plane, preserving the pelvic nerves. Some advocate anal mucosectomy from the level of the dentate line upwards, while others preserve the whole anal canal.

Various designs of reservoir have been described (Fig. 28.18).[126–128] A two-loop construction, or J pouch, can be easily performed using a 90-mm linear stapling instrument. An ileal pouch to anal anastomosis is performed, with either an endoanal hand-sewn technique or a stapled anastomosis. A loop ileostomy is raised as near to the pouch as possible and placed in the right iliac fossa. This can be closed after 8–10 weeks provided the ileoanal anastomosis and pouch have healed uneventfully. The final result is shown in Fig. 28.19.

The most common complication is pelvic sepsis, usually the result of dehiscence of the ileoanal anastomosis. It is reported to occur in 8–25% of published cases. It does not always drain freely, and the resulting fibrosis and scarring may affect the eventual clinical result. A stricture develops in 10% of patients but usually responds to simple dilatation. Adhesive obstruction is the other major problem and can usually be managed conservatively. Three-quarters of patients do not have any complications from pouch formation.[125]

Following ileostomy closure, patients have a normal desire to evacuate faeces, and in three-quarters this can be deferred without urgency. While there is a range of frequency of defecation after the operation, a mean of three to six actions per 24 h can be expected. Frank incontinence is unusual, but around 10% have minor leakage of mucus, especially at night. Outright failure occurs in around 5% of patients, because of pelvic sepsis, undiagnosed Crohn's disease or unacceptable stool frequency.[125]

No serious nutritional problems have emerged, but the long-term consequences of the pouch are not known. A syndrome of acute pouch inflammation (pouchitis) develops in approximately 10% of patients and is characterized by excessive stool frequency.[129] This complication usually responds to treatment with metronidazole, ciprofloxacin, steroids or pouch drainage.

REFERENCES

124. Baker WNW, Glass RE et al. Br J Surg 1978; 65: 862
125. Mortensen NJ. Gut 1988; 29: 561
126. Parks AG, Nicholls RJ. Br Med J 1978; ii: 85
127. Utsunomiya J, Iwama T et al. Dis Colon Rectum 1980; 23: 459
128. Fonkalsrud EW. Surg Gynecol Obstet 1980; 150: 1
129. Handelsman JC, Fishbein RH et al. Surgery 1983; 93: 247

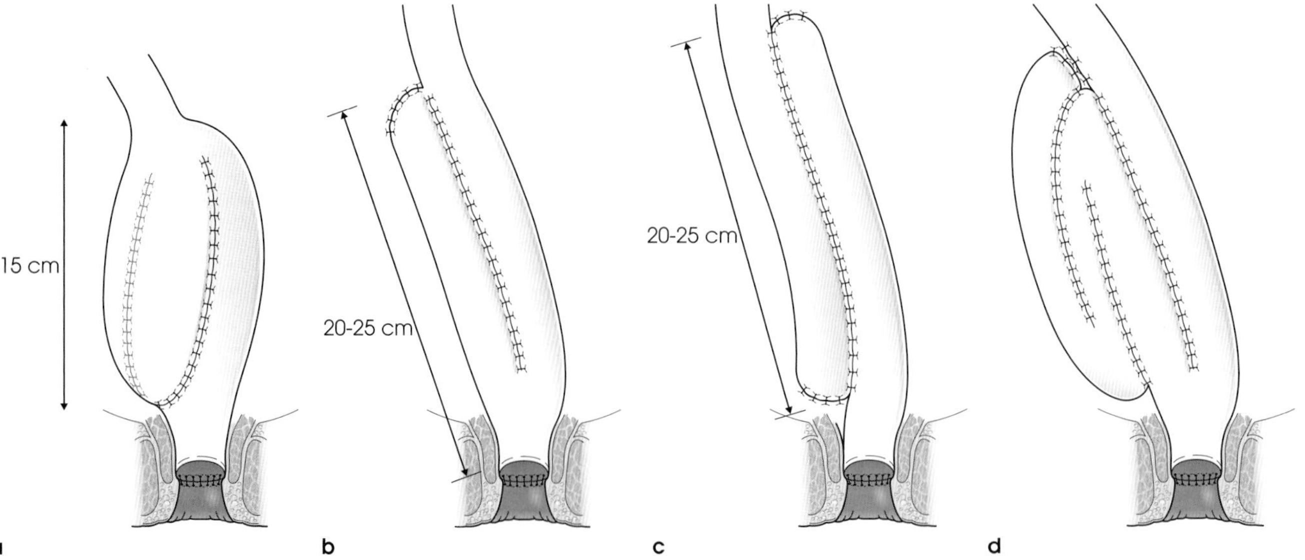

Figure 28.18 Various designs for ileal reservoir in restorative proctocolectomy: (**a**) S pouch, (**b**) J pouch, (**c**) H pouch and (**d**) W pouch.

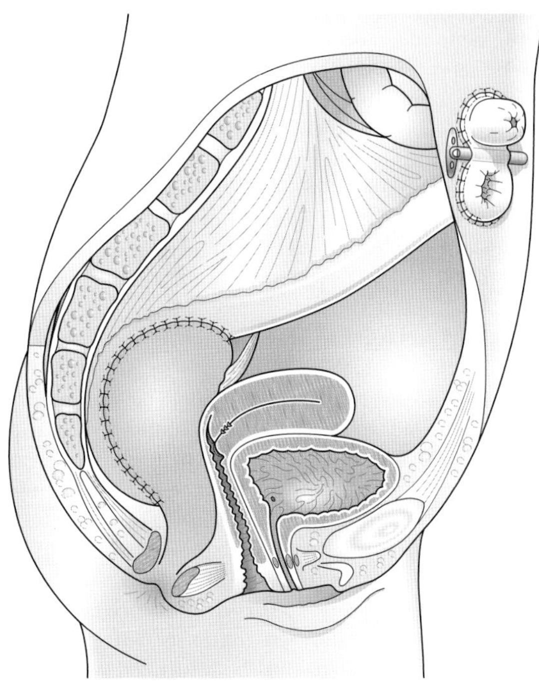

Figure 28.19 Ileal reservoir in situ in the pelvis. The loop ileostomy is closed at about 8 weeks after the pouch operation. (From Pounder R (ed). Recent Advances in Gastroenterology 6. Churchill Livingstone, Edinburgh: 1986, with permission.[113])

Probiotics are also producing promising results in the treatment of pouchitis.[130]

ACUTE SEVERE COLITIS AND TOXIC MEGACOLON

Patients with fulminating colitis should be jointly managed by a physician and surgeon, and reviewed on a daily basis. A sigmoidoscopy, biopsy and stool cultures are essential, but colonoscopy and barium enema examination are contraindicated. Daily plain abdominal films are taken to assess the degree of colonic dilatation, with any increase in diameter greater than 5 cm indicating the development of toxic megacolon.

When surgery is necessary, a subtotal colectomy with an ileostomy and mucous fistula is the preferred option. The rectum and anal sphincter are left undisturbed, hence future restorative surgery is possible. The surgical specimen may allow the histopathologist to make a firm diagnosis, but in severely diseased bowel the distinction between ulcerative colitis and Crohn's disease may be difficult. In about 10% of cases the pathologist will report that the colitis is indeterminate in type.[105]

CROHN'S DISEASE

Crohn's disease can involve any part of the gastrointestinal tract from mouth to anus and cannot be cured. The most frequent site of involvement is the terminal ileum (see Ch. 27). Over 60% of patients have both small and large bowel disease, and 20% only have large bowel disease.[131]

AETIOLOGY

The presence of granulomata suggests a mycobacterial infection, but attempts to prove that *Mycobacterium paratuberculosis* is the causative organism have not been successful. Many other infectious agents (viruses and cell wall-deficient pseudomonads) have been proposed. A popular theory that Crohn's is a measles virus-induced vasculitis is not supported by any convincing evidence. Intriguingly, smoking appears to accelerate recurrence after resection, and in small bowel Crohn's recurrences invariably involve the ileal side of an ileocolic anastomosis.[107] Whatever the initiating factor, immunological mechanisms play a part in the eventual pathogenesis of the disease. The familial incidence of Crohn's disease is around 10–15%.

HISTOPATHOLOGY

The disease is a chronic discontinuous granulomatous condition with transmural aggregates of inflammatory cells, and deep penetrating fissures and ulceration. In the colon it differs from ulcerative colitis, which is confined to the mucosa except in very severe cases.[132] In Crohn's disease, the bowel wall is thickened and featureless, with strictures and fistulae into adjacent small bowel, colon or other organs such as the bladder. There are large fleshy lymph nodes in the mesentery, and the mucosa is oedematous with linear ulceration, giving a cobblestone appearance (Fig. 28.20). Areas of normal mucosa separate involved segments ('skip lesions'), but diffuse disease does occur in the colon. In less severely affected areas, aphthous ulcers are the earliest sign, beginning as ulcerating lymphoid follicles.

CLINICAL FEATURES

Small bowel disease is discussed in detail in Chapter 27. Colorectal Crohn's disease presents with diarrhoea, bleeding, obstruction or perianal disease. In the large bowel both stricture formation and fistulation can also occur. The disease often causes extensive mucosal inflammation, which presents as a colitis. This can have a very similar presentation to ulcerative colitis, but the clinical and endoscopic differences shown in Table 28.4 allow a distinction to be made between the two diseases in the majority of cases. The most useful distinguishing clinical features of Crohn's disease are the segmental involvement the presence of anal disease and rectal sparing. Anal disease is common in cases with large bowel involvement. An anal lesion is present in 50–70% of patients with large bowel Crohn's disease,[133] the most common being an anal fissure and anorectal sepsis.[134,135] Ulceration, oedematous skin tags, stenosis (usually at the anorectal junction) and rectovaginal fistulae can also occur. Patients with large bowel Crohn's disease may present with acute colitis, which can occasionally progress to a toxic dilatation.[136] As with ulcerative colitis, patients with chronic Crohn's disease may develop extra-alimentary manifestations, which are listed in Table 28.3.

INVESTIGATION

A barium enema examination may demonstrate skip lesions and

REFERENCES

130. Gionchetti P, Rizzello F et al. Gastroenterology 2000; 119: 305–309
131. Allan RN. In: Bouchier IAD, Allan RN et al (eds). Textbook of Gastroenterology. Baillière Tindall, London, 1983: 941
132. Lockhart-Mummery HE, Morson BC. Gut 1960; 1: 87
133. Hellers G, Bergstrand O et al. Gut 1980; 21: 525–556
134. Lockhart Mummery HE. Br J Surg 1985; 72 (Suppl): S95
135. Buchanan P, Keighley MRB, Allan RN. Am J Surg 1980; 140: 642
136. Buzzard AJ, Baker WNW et al. Gut 1974; 15: 416

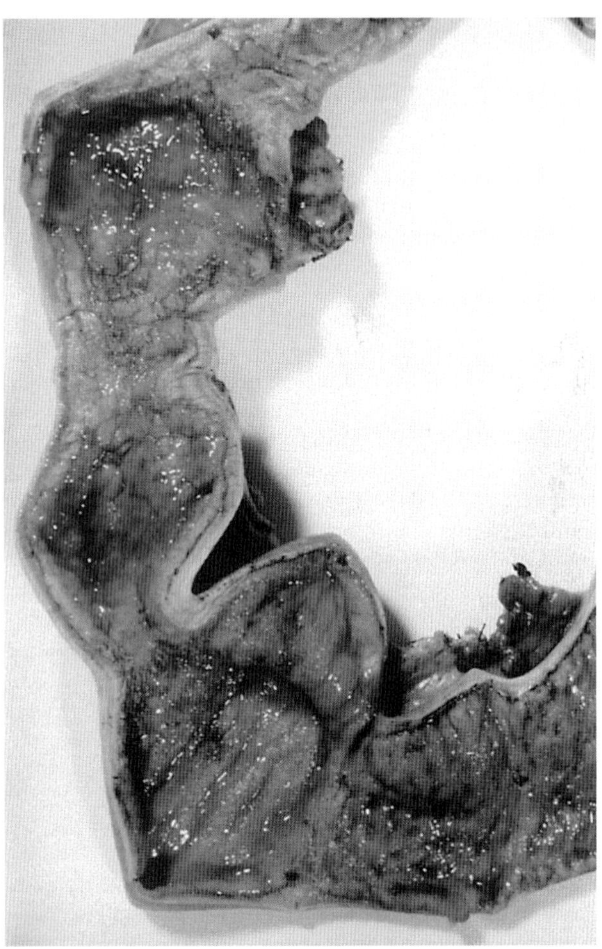

Figure 28.20 Crohn's disease. 'Skip lesions' are separated by normal segments. Diseased areas are characterized by cobblestoning and linear ulcers.

stricture formation. Mucosal changes indicating aphthous ulceration, deep ulceration with fissure formation, and fistulation may also be seen (Fig. 28.21). Colonoscopy provides a view of the mucosa and may confirm terminal ileal disease if the ileocaecal valve can be passed. It also enables multiple biopsies to be taken. Blood tests, including the erythrocyte sedimentation rate and C-reactive protein, give an indication of disease activity. In cases with poor nutrition, the serum albumin level is low. The presence of small bowel Crohn's disease should be confirmed or excluded by a small bowel enema or follow-through study (see Ch. 27).

MEDICAL MANAGEMENT

A flare-up of disease activity giving rise to mucosal ulceration and oedema is likely to respond to medical treatment, which must include steroids and occasionally azathioprine. In patients with strictures causing obstruction, or in those with fistulae or abscesses, medical treatment is unlikely to give long-lasting relief and surgery is invariably necessary. There is no evidence that long-term treatment with steroids or sulfasalazine (sulphasalazine) reduces the likelihood of surgery.[137] The new anti-tumour necrosis factor drug infliximab has been used to induce remission in patients with unresponsive Crohn's, particularly when this is associated with fistulating complications.[138]

Patients with extensive intestinal involvement or sepsis may be severely nutritionally depleted. The serum albumin and the amount of weight loss are a rough guide to the degree of nutritional failure. Intravenous nutrition or, in some suitable cases, enteric feeding may be necessary.

REFERENCES

137. Summers RW, Switz DM et al. Gastroenterology 1978; 77: 847
138. Bell S, Kamm MA. Lancet 2000; 355: 858–860

Table 28.4 Clinical differences between Crohn's disease and ulcerative colitis

	Crohn's disease	Ulcerative colitis
Symptoms		
Bleeding	Sometimes	Very common
Abdominal pain	Common	Sometimes
Urgent defecation	Sometimes	Very common
Abdomen		
Abdominal mass	Sometimes	Rare
Spontaneous fistulae	Sometimes	Never
Anal region		
Fissure	Common	Occurs
Ulceration	Common	Rare
Infection	Common and often complicated	Occurs
Lesions preceding bowel symptoms	Sometimes	Never
Endoscopy		
Rectal involvement	50%	> 95%
Appearance	Oedema, ulcers, granular, friable	Uniform, continuous, normal patches
Prognosis		
Medicine	Inadequate in 80%	80% successful
Surgery	Often recurrence	'Cure' possible
Cancer risk	Slight	Definite

SURGICAL MANAGEMENT

Surgery is indicated for the complications of Crohn's disease, including intestinal obstruction, fistula, bleeding, abscess and intractable diarrhoea. Because the disease cannot be cured, minimal surgery aims to restore bowel function and excise the active inflammation without removing any more bowel than is necessary.

TERMINAL ILEAL AND ILEOCOLIC DISEASE

This is the most common form of Crohn's disease and presents with either obstructive symptoms or abscess. A right hemicolectomy, preserving as much right colon as possible, is usually necessary.[139] Recurrence requiring further resection is unfortunately common, being necessary in 40–60% of cases over a 5–10-year period.[140–142] The risk of recurrence may be reduced when the ileocolic anastomosis is stapled, producing a wide join.[143] Strictureplasty (Fig. 28.22) offers relief of obstruction without the need for resection in patients with multiple strictures in whom resection might lead to the possibility of short bowel syndrome. In this procedure the affected segments are left in situ, and the stricture opened along the long axis of the bowel and sewn transversely to widen the lumen. There is as yet no effective adjuvant drug treatment, which reduces the long-term recurrence rate.[137]

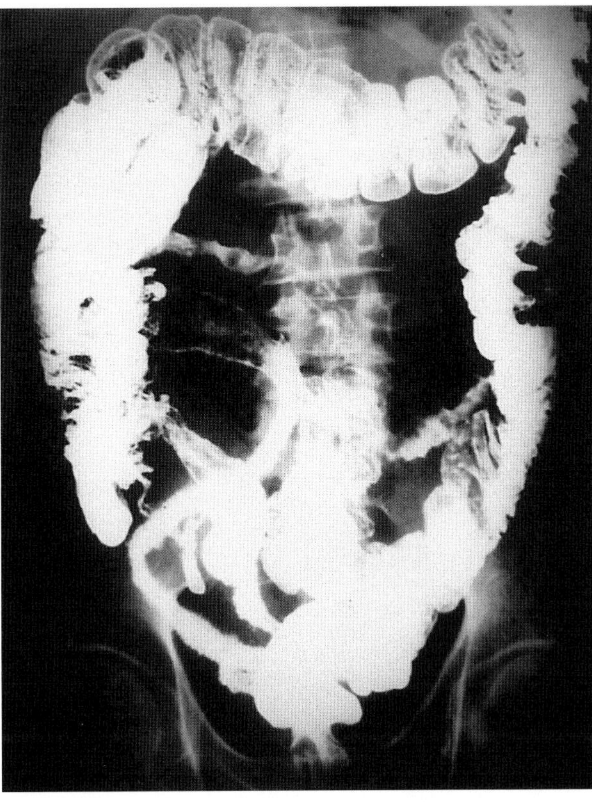

Figure 28.21 Crohn's disease. Barium enema with reflux into small bowel, showing extensive narrowing of the distal ileum, with deep ulceration, wall thickening and cobblestoning.

COLONIC DISEASE

The medical management of colonic Crohn's disease is similar to that for ulcerative colitis. Surgical treatment is different, however, in a number of respects. In patients with diffuse or multifocal colonic disease, a defunctioning ileostomy may allow the disease to resolve, and about one-quarter can subsequently have their gut continuity restored.[144] There is evidence, however, that after this procedure long-term recurrence rates are high and any improvement is short-lived. Segmental resection in patients with localized strictures or discrete areas of involvement may be successful.[145]

Where there is rectal sparing and a normal anus, an ileorectal anastomosis saves the patient an ileostomy, but there is a recurrence rate at 5–10 years of 30%, and more than half require further resection or conversion to a proctocolectomy.[146–148] In patients with widespread colonic disease a proctocolectomy and ileostomy may be indicated, and the surgical technique is similar to that for ulcerative colitis.[149]

REFERENCES

139. Lee ECG. Gut 1984; 25: 217
140. Hellers G. Acta Chir Scand 1979; 490 (Suppl): 1
141. Lock RM, Farmer RG et al. N Engl J Med 1981; 304: 13
142. Higgens CS, Allan RN. Gut 1980; 21: 933
143. Munoz-Juarez M, Yamamoto T et al. Dis Colon Rectum 2001; 44: 20–25
144. Harper PH, Truelove SC et al. Gut 1983; 24: 106
145. Allan A, Andrews H et al. World J Surg 1989; 13: 611–614
146. Flint G, Strauss R et al. Gut 1977; 18: 23
147. Goligher JC. Surg Gynecol Obstet 1979; 148: 1
148. Allan RN, Steinberg DM et al. Gastroenterology 1977; 73: 72
149. Scammell BE, Andrews H et al. Br J Surg 1987; 74: 671

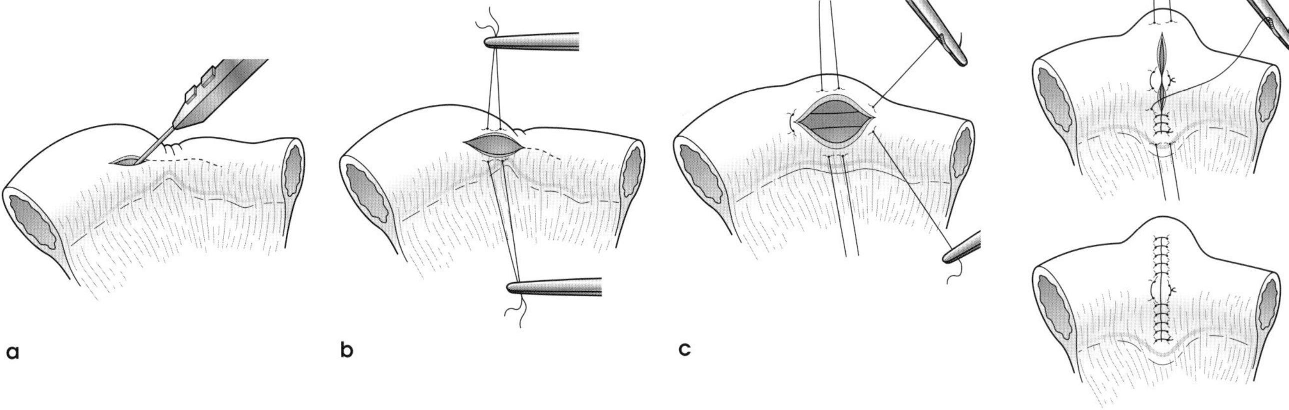

Figure 28.22 Stages in ileal strictureplasty for Crohn's disease.

ANORECTAL DISEASE

Over half the patients with large bowel Crohn's disease have an anal lesion, the most common being anal fissure. Fissures may heal with medical management or become chronic, when they can become the site of fistula formation.[150,151] Sometimes the pain is so severe that faecal diversion is necessary. Haemorrhoidectomy should be avoided, because it may lead to anorectal sepsis, sometimes requiring rectal excision.[152] Many patients' symptoms settle spontaneously or with local steroid applications.

A fistula in ano may develop either directly as a result of Crohn's disease or secondary to its effects on the anal gland anatomy. Conservative surgery with drainage of abscess cavities and insertion of a long-term seton is appropriate. Sometimes treatment with metronidazole will control recurrent episodes of sepsis in otherwise symptomless fistulae. Incontinence as a consequence of a rectovaginal fistula is often severe, and the condition is difficult to manage. Patients without symptoms need no treatment, although a low fistula can be laid open.[153]

DIVERTICULAR DISEASE

In its mildest form, diverticular disease is one of the most common afflictions of western people. It has been estimated that around a third of all British adults over the age of 60 years are affected.[154] There have been great efforts over the past few decades to confirm the link between a low-fibre intake and diverticular disease.[155] It has not been possible to produce an animal model of the condition, nor to perform long-term prospective dietary manipulation trials in human volunteers. There seems little doubt, however, that the causal connection is valid.

PATHOPHYSIOLOGY

Diverticula, or 'wayside inns of ill repute', develop as mucosal extrusions at weak points in the bowel wall, presumably as a result of raised intraluminal pressure produced by the uncoordinated action of hypertrophied circular muscle (Fig. 28.23).[156,157] Most diverticula develop where blood vessels penetrate the colonic muscle at the edges of the antimesenteric taeniae (Fig. 28.24).[158] By far the most common site for diverticula is the sigmoid colon, although any part of the colon can be involved. The rectum never develops diverticula.

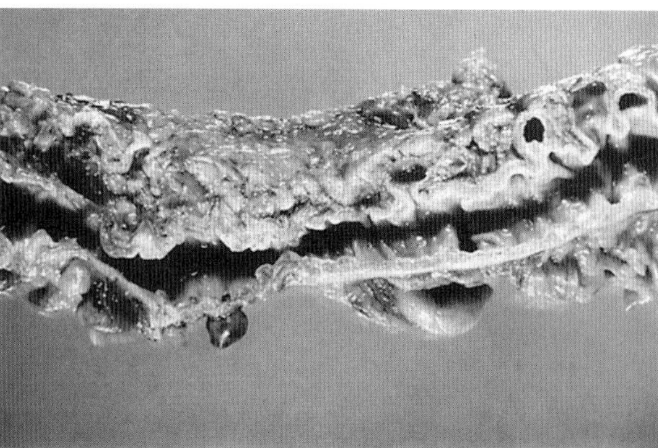

Figure 28.23 Diverticular disease. Marked thickening of the muscle layer and resultant diverticula formation.

When diverticula are present but not inflamed (so-called diverticulosis), the individual is usually unaware of the condition. At most there may be episodic lower abdominal pain.[156] Diverticula are narrow-necked mucosal pouches and likely to collect inspissated faeces within them. This may cause ulceration within the diverticula, leading to pericolic inflammation, perforation or bleeding from the associated penetrating artery. The inflammatory changes can produce a chronic painful condition, an acute exacerbation of disease (acute diverticulitis), or a pericolic abscess, which may rupture into the general peritoneal cavity or into a neighbouring viscus to produce a fistula.

CLINICAL PRESENTATION

Elective presentations

Painful diverticular disease

Painful diverticular disease is the most common and least serious clinical presentation, and some even doubt its existence.[159] The patient usually complains of episodic lower abdominal pain, which may be associated with a change of bowel habit and a feeling of abdominal bloating. The symptoms are akin to those of the irritable bowel syndrome. Physical examination is usually unremarkable, but barium enema reveals the presence of diverticula and the concentric indentations of muscle hypertrophy (Fig. 28.25). Treatment consists of a high-fibre diet and a trial of mebeverine or liquorice extract.[160]

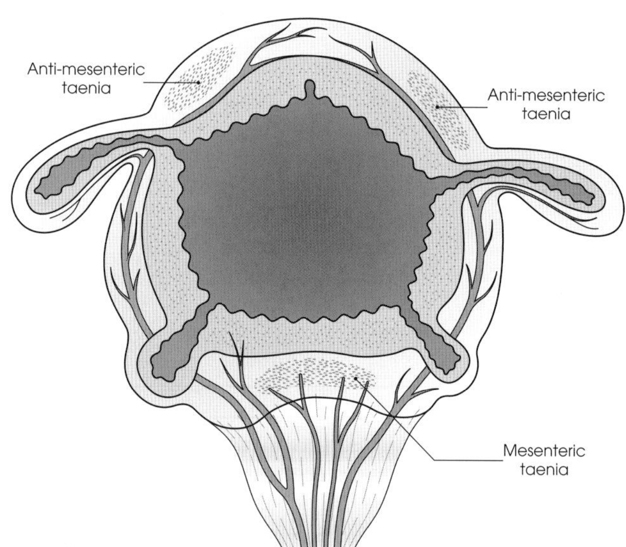

Figure 28.24 Diverticular disease. Transverse section of sigmoid colon showing sites of predilection for diverticula formation.

REFERENCES

150. Buchmann P, Allan RN et al. Am J Surg 1980; 140: 462
151. Sweeney JL, Ritchie JK, Nicholls RJ. Br J Surg 1988; 75: 56–57
152. Jeffrey PJ, Ritchie JK, Parks AG. Lancet 1977; i: 1084
153. Francois Y, Descos L, Vignal J. Int J Colorectal Dis 1990; 5: 12
154. Parks TG. Proc R Soc Med 1968; 61: 932
155. Painter NS, Burkitt DP. Br Med J 1971; 2: 450–454
156. Arfwiddson S. Acta Chir Scand (Suppl) 1964; 342
157. Painter NS. Ann R Coll Surg Engl 1964; 34: 98–114
158. Slack WW. Br J Surg 1962; 50: 185–190
159. Thompson WG. Am J Gastroenterol 1986; 81: 613–614
160. Brodribb AJM. Lancet 1977; i: 664

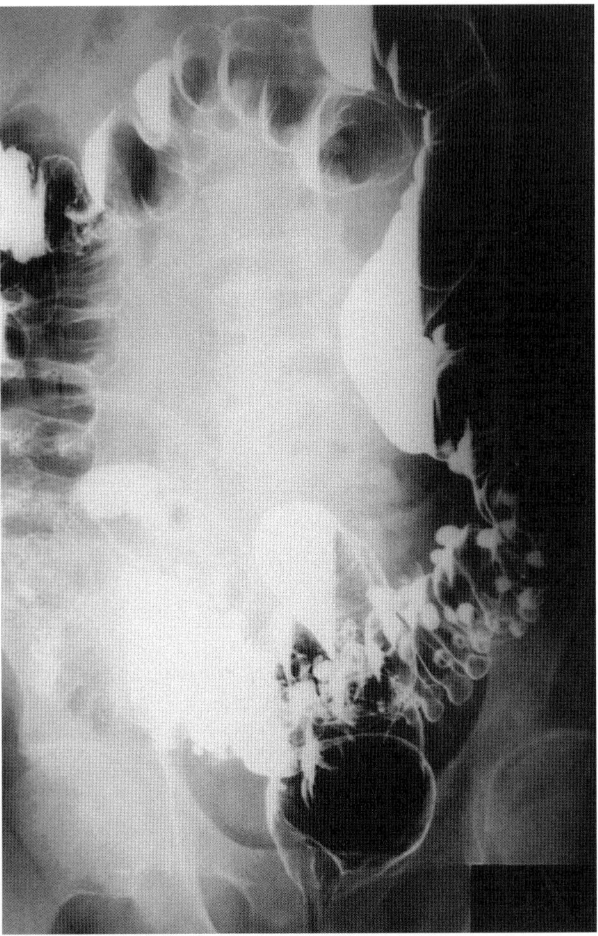

Figure 28.25 Diverticular disease. Barium enema showing concentric muscle hypertrophy and diverticula formation.

Fistulae

Colovesical fistula is the most common type and affects males more than females, presumably because the uterus intervenes between the two organs and has a protective effect. The patient usually complains of recurrent cystitis, pneumaturia, or the presence of solid (i.e. faecal) matter in the urine. Rarely the patient may pass urine per rectum. A lower abdominal inflammatory mass may be palpable. The differential diagnosis includes Crohn's disease; carcinoma of the colon, bladder or uterus; radiation damage; tuberculosis; actinomycosis and trauma. Contrast radiological investigations may not demonstrate the communication, although contrast or plain radiographs may show gas in the bladder or the upper urinary tract. Fibre-optic endoscopy of the bladder and rectum with biopsy is worthwhile before a laparotomy is carried out.

Sigmoid colectomy with a primary bowel anastomosis and repair of the bladder is the procedure of choice when the bowel has been adequately prepared.[161] A defunctioning stoma may be indicated if there is severe local sepsis. A urinary catheter should be left in situ for at least 10 days postoperatively.

Colovaginal and colocutaneous fistulae from diverticular disease present with faecal discharge from the vagina or skin of the lower abdomen, respectively.[162] Coloileal fistulae present with frequent loose excoriating stools, because small bowel contents pass directly into the rectum. Primary colonic resection and anastomosis with closure of the fistula remains the best treatment.

Emergency presentations

Acute diverticulitis

The patient complains of severe lower abdominal pain, which is often accompanied by the frequent passage of loose stools. There are usually associated constitutional symptoms, which may include sweating, nausea and vomiting. The temperature and pulse are invariably raised, and there is marked tenderness and guarding in the left lower quadrant, where a mass may be palpable.

Treatment should be conservative in the absence of signs of generalized peritoneal irritation. Oral intake should be withheld and fluids given intravenously. Broad-spectrum antibiotics (metronidazole and a cephalosporin) and analgesia are administered. Only if the patient's condition deteriorates, particularly if signs of spreading peritonitis develop, is surgical intervention indicated. Failure to improve suggests the development of a pericolic abscess, which may be further suspected if there is a persistent leukocytosis and swinging pyrexia. Ultrasound or CT should demonstrate the pericolic fluid collection.

Pericolic abscess

Drainage is required if this complication develops. Percutaneous catheter drainage, guided by CT or ultrasound, should be used as the first-line treatment.[163] Usually the acute episode resolves satisfactorily, but elective resection to prevent recurrent complications is a sensible precaution if the patient is sufficiently fit.

Generalized peritonitis

Generalized peritonitis (see Ch. 25) may be caused by rupture of a pericolic abscess or by direct perforation of a diverticulum. The patient often presents in septicaemic shock. After initial resuscitation, the patient is taken to theatre and the affected segment of bowel is resected. It is usually prudent to avoid primary anastomosis in the presence of gross contamination with faeces or pus. Bringing out a mucous fistula or over-sewing of the rectal stump with a left iliac fossa colostomy (Hartmann's operation) is recommended.[164] Reanastomosis can then be performed when the patient has made a satisfactory recovery. A primary anastomosis may be performed if there is minimal contamination. When the proximal bowel is loaded with faeces it should be cleared by on-table lavage, and the anastomosis may be defunctioned by a proximal ileostomy.

Intestinal obstruction

Intestinal obstruction can develop as a result of steadily advancing chronic diverticulitis with the development of pericolic fibrosis, but it may also be caused by the adhesion of a loop of small bowel to an acutely inflamed diverticular segment. It is treated by resection and either Hartmann's procedure or a protected primary anastomosis. Obstruction is not common in diverticular disease, and its presence should make the clinician suspect a hidden carcinoma (see Ch. 25).[165]

REFERENCES

161. Rao PN, Knox R et al. Br J Surg 1987; 74: 362–363
162. Fazio VW, Church JM et al. Dis Colon Rectum 1987; 30: 89–94
163. Neff CC, van Sonnenberg E et al. Radiology 1987; 163: 15–18
164. Krukowski ZH, Koruth NM, Matheson NA. Br J Surg 1985; 72: 684–686
165. Hughes LE. Clin Gastroenterol 1975; 4: 147

Haemorrhage

For many years it was felt that diverticular disease was a relatively common cause of fresh rectal haemorrhage. More recently, investigation during such episodes has suggested that vascular malformations (angiodysplasia) are a more common cause.[166] Acute bleeding episodes are usually self-limiting and best treated conservatively. When bleeding does not stop and surgery is required, a total colectomy with ileostomy and preservation of the rectal stump is the procedure of choice if the source cannot be identified by angiography or on-table colonoscopy.

BENIGN TUMOURS OF THE COLON AND RECTUM

POLYPS

A polyp is an abnormal elevation from an epithelial surface and may be pedunculated (on a stalk) or sessile (flat). A sessile polyp may be flat or villous. Polyps may be acquired or inherited, symptomatic or symptomless; they may be single, occur in clusters, or occupy virtually all of the large bowel mucosa. When the latter occurs, the term *polyposis syndrome* is applied. There are numerous histological types of polyp, which are best divided into neoplastic and non-neoplastic.

NEOPLASTIC POLYPS

Adenoma

Adenoma is a benign neoplasm of the large bowel glandular epithelium and is the most common neoplastic polyp. Adenomas are believed to be the precursor of colorectal cancer. Histologically, adenomas are split into three categories: tubular, villous or tubulovillous.

Pathology

A tubular adenoma is generally less than 2 cm in diameter. It may be pedunculated or sessile and is usually darker in colour than the surrounding mucosa owing to its vascularity. Microscopically, it consists of closely packed epithelial tubules, separated by normal lamina propria, which grow and branch horizontally to the muscularis mucosae. The tubules may branch in a regular or an irregular pattern. In a pedunculated adenoma, the pedicle consists of normal mucosa and submucosa.

A villous adenoma is often large and sessile with a shaggy surface made up of numerous fronds. It may be flat or protrude into the bowel lumen and may extend over a considerable area of the bowel wall, hence the term *carpet-like.* Microscopically, it consists of a core of connective tissue bearing numerous delicate frond-like branches or villi. Between the villi, the mucosa rests directly on the muscularis mucosae with no intervening connective tissue.

The tubulovillous adenoma is an intermediate form containing features of both morphological types.

Dysplasia and malignant transformation

The epithelial cells may show an increase in mitotic figures; they may form several layers and their nuclei may become pleomorphic, with loss of polarity. The term *dysplasia* is applied to these changes. Any invasion of these abnormal epithelial cells through the muscularis mucosae to enter the submucosa constitutes malignant transformation. Dysplasia may be classified as mild, moderate or severe.[167–169]

Approximately 60% of adenomas show mild dysplasia, about 30% exhibit moderate dysplasia, and the remaining 10% contain areas of severe dysplasia. It is generally believed that there is a gradual transformation through the various grades of dysplasia to frank malignancy: the so-called 'adenoma–carcinoma sequence'.[170]

Incidence and anatomical distribution

A prospective autopsy study in a population with a high incidence of colorectal cancer showed prevalence rates of adenomas of around 35% in men and about 30% in women.[171] Colonoscopic and autopsy studies demonstrated that approximately two-thirds of all colorectal adenomas occur distal to the splenic flexure.[172,173] Villous adenomas are more common in the rectum.

Age and sex incidence

Adenomas may occur at any age, but they increase in frequency with advancing age. Males seem to be more commonly affected than females. The average age at presentation is 55–60 years.[171,173,174]

Adenoma–carcinoma sequence

The evidence that there is a link between adenoma and colorectal cancer is most persuasive, yet it is still circumstantial. Virtually all pathologists believe that adenomas can develop into carcinomas, but whether all carcinomas start life as an adenoma remains debatable. Adenomas and carcinomas have a similar topographical distribution.[175–177] Three-quarters of the patients presenting with two synchronous carcinomas had associated adenomas.[178] Similarly, patients with polyps associated with a carcinoma of the colon are twice as likely to develop a subsequent carcinoma after operation, compared with patients who had no polyps at the time of surgery.[179]

Epidemiological data also support the adenoma–carcinoma sequence, in that both conditions are more prevalent in a westernized society in which a low-fibre, high-meat diet predominates. Experimental carcinogens, such as azoxymethane, which are capable of producing colorectal cancers also induce adenoma formation. Careful histological studies of carcinomas frequently show elements of benign adenomas within the tumour. Similarly, there is an incidence of 3–4% of carcinomas in

REFERENCES

166. Goligher J. Surgery of the Anus, Rectum and Colon. 5th edn. Baillière Tindall, London, 1984
167. Potet F, Soullard J. Gut 1971; 12: 468
168. Ekelund G, Lindstrom C. Gut 1974; 15: 654
169. Kozuka S. Dis Colon Rectum 1975; 18: 483
170. Morson BC. The Pathogenesis of Colorectal Cancer. WB Saunders, Philadelphia, 1978: 33–42
171. Williams AR, Balasoorya BAW, Day DW. Gut 1982; 23: 835–842
172. Shinya H, Wolff WI. Ann Surg 1979; 190: 679–683
173. Gillespie PE, Chambers TJ et al. Gut 1979; 20: 240–245
174. Minopoulos GL, McIntyre RLE et al. Br J Surg 1983; 70: 51–53
175. Ekelund G. Acta Pathol Microbiol Scand 1963; 59: 165–170
176. Helwig EB. Dis Colon Rectum 1959; 2: 5–17
177. Berge T, Ekelund G et al. Acta Chir Scand 1973; 4 (Suppl): 38
178. Heald RJ, Bussey HJR. Dis Colon Rectum 1975; 18: 6–10
179. Bussey HJR, Wallace MH, Morson BC. Proc R Soc Med 1967; 60: 208

apparently benign adenomas.[180] Finally, there is the condition of familial adenomatous polyposis, in which all patients eventually develop carcinomatous change within their polyps if left untreated.

The circumstantial evidence for the adenoma–carcinoma sequence is convincing, but there is no definite proof that all carcinomas develop from adenomas. Routine colonoscopic removal of adenomas should reduce the incidence of carcinoma within a population if the theory is correct. Gilbertsen and colleagues followed 18 000 subjects over a 25-year period who underwent regular sigmoidoscopic surveillance.[181] All detected polyps were removed. This population was predicted to develop 75–80 rectal carcinomas during the period of follow-up. In fact, only 11 carcinomas developed, and each of these was an early growth. This lends further support to the idea that many carcinomas develop from adenomas.

The malignant adenoma

Malignant change within an adenoma is diagnosed when there is invasion by malignant cells deep to the muscularis mucosae. The incidence in colonoscopically removed polyps is about 5%, and this incidence increases with increasing polyp size. Villous adenomas are far more likely to develop malignant change. Approximately 10% of malignant polyps that can be colonoscopically removed have lymph node metastases. Certain pathological characteristics (e.g. a sessile polyp, villous architecture, poor differentiation, and lymphatic invasion) help to identify those polyps that have nodal spread.

Clinical features

Adenomatous polyps are often symptomless and may be detected on routine screening after a positive occult blood test. Rectal bleeding may occur, and its hue will depend on the distance of the polyp from the anus. The larger rectal polyps may cause a change in bowel habit, with diarrhoea and the passage of mucus being prominent. Occasionally a rectal polyp may prolapse through the anus on straining. Rarely, abdominal colic may be the result of a colocolic intussusception of a polyp.

Large villous adenomas of the rectum frequently present with tenesmus or the passage of copious mucus, often tinged pink by blood. Incontinence is not infrequent. The fluid and electrolyte loss may be so great that the patient may develop severe metabolic disturbance.

Diagnosis

Villous tumours of the rectum may be palpated on digital rectal examination, but can be difficult to feel because of their soft consistency. Occasionally a pedunculated adenomatous polyp may be palpable. Digital examination may detect areas of hardness within the polyp, suggesting the possibility of focal malignant invasion. Sigmoidoscopy should be performed; polyp detection is three times as great with the flexible instrument.[182] Carcinoma of the colon is the main differential diagnosis and can commonly coexist.

After a polyp has been detected, the rest of the bowel should be examined. Colonoscopy, rather than barium enema, is the better method of investigation, because it is more sensitive and it allows the polyp to be removed at the same time.[183]

Management

Once a polyp has been detected, it should be removed so that its histological type can be determined. Clearly, however, common sense should prevail; it would be wrong to pursue the removal of a 2-mm colonic polyp in a frail, elderly patient. Most adenomas can be removed via the flexible sigmoidoscope or colonoscope using a diathermy snare. Every attempt must then be made to retrieve the whole polyp in order that an adequate histological examination can be made. Large whole sessile polyps can rarely be removed satisfactorily and are done so usually by piecemeal resection. Even if this technique is necessary, it is still important to retrieve as much of the polyp as possible. For very small polyps that look entirely innocent, the 'hot biopsy' technique may be used. In this, an electric current is applied to the biopsy forceps, which coagulates the base of the polyp, while that part of the polyp grasped by the jaws of the forceps is preserved for histological examination.

Surgical excision should generally not be undertaken without first attempting colonoscopic polypectomy, because some polyps that look sessile or malignant on barium enema prove to have small stalks on endoscopy. If it proves impossible to remove a polyp through the colonoscope, many now prefer the technique of operative colonoscopic removal in preference to resection. In this procedure, the colonoscope is passed at laparotomy, and with the help of the surgeon the polyp is removed. This manoeuvre allows polypectomy to be performed without opening the bowel.

Larger sessile, usually villous, rectal adenomas are best removed surgically via the transanal route. The submucosal plane beneath and around the tumour is infiltrated with 1:300 000 adrenaline (epinephrine) solution. By a combination of sharp dissection and diathermy, the whole of the tumour can be excised from the underlying rectal muscle.

Transanal endoscopic microsurgery is a new intraluminal technique for the full-thickness excision of villous lesions in the mid and upper rectum. A 40-mm diameter rectoscope is placed in the anal canal, the rectum insufflated with carbon dioxide and, through gas-sealed ports, long-handled instruments are manipulated to carry out the procedure and repair the defect. For more extensive adenomas, anterior resection may be necessary.

An alternative to surgical excision of a villous adenoma of the rectum is diathermy fulguration. This technique should, however, be regarded only as a second-line treatment, because it is unlikely that the whole tumour can be destroyed and adequate histopathological assessment cannot be made. Nevertheless, the technique can be used as a palliative procedure in a patient who is unfit for a major procedure. The recurrence rate after transanal excision or diathermy has been reported to vary between 7 and 27%.[184–186]

REFERENCES

180. Nivatvongs S, Goldberg SM. Dis Colon Rectum 1978; 21: 8–11
181. Gilbertsen V. Cancer 1974; 34: 931–939
182. McCallum RW, Meyer CT et al. Am J Gastroenterol 1984; 79: 433–437
183. Durdey P, Weston P, Williams NJ. Lancet 1987; ii: 549
184. Jahadi MR, Baldwin A. Am J Surg 1975; 130: 729–732
185. Thomson JPS. Dis Colon Rectum 1977; 20: 467–472
186. Adair H, Everett W. J R Coll Surg Edinb 1983; 28: 318–323
187. Williams CB. Endoscopy 1973; 5: 215

Complications of polypectomy

The incidence of haemorrhage requiring transfusion after colonoscopy is approximately 2%.[188–190] Perforation occurs in 0.2–0.7% of polypectomies.[191,192] The overall mortality rate from perforation and haemorrhage following polypectomy is about 0.05%.

Follow-up after polypectomy

There are no firm data on which to base a follow-up policy. Colonoscopy may be carried out every 3–5 years if the patient remains symptom-free. Exceptions are patients who have had several adenomas removed, or whose adenoma, although benign, was greater than 2 cm in diameter. Those who have had a malignant adenoma removed should also be included in a different category. All these patients should undergo endoscopy annually.

Management of a malignant adenoma removed via the colonoscope

Management of malignant adenomas is controversial but should probably be based on histological criteria. Pedunculated adenomas containing cancer limited to the head of the polyp may be treated by polypectomy alone. An adenoma with a poorly differentiated carcinoma, lymphatic invasion or carcinoma at the resection margin requires surgical resection, as do sessile malignant adenomas.[193]

Table 28.5 Classification of polyposis syndromes

Neoplastic
- Familial adenomatous polyposis
- Turcot's syndrome
- Lymphosarcomatous (lymphomatous) polyposis
- Leukaemic polyposis

Inflammatory
- Ulcerative colitis
- Crohn's disease
- Other inflammatory polyposis: amoebiasis, schistosomiasis, eosinophilic, granulomatous polyposis, diffuse histoplasmosis

Hamartomatous
- Juvenile polyposis
- Peutz–Jeghers syndrome
- Neurofibromatous polyposis
- Lipomatous polyposis
- Cronkhite–Canada syndrome
- Cowden's disease

Unclassified
- Metaplastic polyps
- Pneumatosis cystoides intestinalis

After Morson BC. Some peculiarities in the histology of intestinal polyps. Dis Colon Rectum 1962; 5: 337–344. © 1962 Springer-Verlag.

Other benign neoplastic polyps

These are rare and include benign lymphoma, lipoma, leiomyoma, fibroma and haemangioma.

Benign lymphoma

Benign lymphoma is the most common non-epithelial benign tumour. It occurs in the large intestine and is usually seen in the rectum as a single, reddish purple or grey, rounded polyp varying in diameter from several millimetres to 3–4 cm. The differentiation between benign and malignant is difficult, but if the pathologist is sure of the diagnosis, the benign lesion can be treated by local excision.

Lipoma

A lipoma is the second most common non-epithelial benign tumour, with an incidence of 0.2–0.3% in autopsy studies.[194] It is more commonly present in the caecum and right colon.[195] Most lipomas are situated in the submucosal layer, but some lie subserosally. They vary in size from a few millimetres to 6 cm or more. They usually present with symptoms that are indistinguishable from an adenocarcinoma. A barium enema shows a narrow line of barium surrounding a smooth lobulated filling defect, and colonoscopy shows a pedunculated, lobulated, spherical tumour projecting into the lumen. Ulceration of the mucosa normally takes place, and the lipoma then looks like a carcinoma. A diathermy snare can sometimes remove a polypoid lipoma, but surgery is required for larger lipomas.

NON-NEOPLASTIC POLYPS

Metaplastic or hyperplastic polyps

These are the most common type of polyp found in the rectum, but they occur throughout the large bowel. They are usually small in size, being around 2–5 mm in diameter, plaque-like and the same colour as normal mucous membrane. They are often seen at sigmoidoscopy in the elderly, but can occur at all ages. These polyps are usually symptomless, being discovered only on routine sigmoidoscopy. There is no evidence to suggest that they may develop dysplastic or neoplastic change.[196]

Hamartomatous polyps

The juvenile polyp occurs in infants and children, although occasionally adults are affected. It has characteristic appearances, being 1–2 cm in diameter, with a smooth surface. It has a slender stalk covered with normal colonic epithelium that, as it extends over the head of the polyp, becomes granulation tissue. These polyps are usually found in the rectum and may sometimes present by prolapsing through the anus. Torsion or intussusception may also occur. Such polyps should be treated by either transanal excision or colonoscopic polypectomy. The rest of the colon must be checked by colonoscopy, because a third of patients have multiple polyps.[197] Peutz–Jeghers polyps are considered later in this chapter and in Ch. 27.

POLYPOSIS SYNDROMES

There are several forms of polyposis syndrome: all are rare. They are best classified according to their histological types (Table 28.5).

REFERENCES

188. Berci G, Panick JF et al. Gastroenterology 1974; 67: 584–585
189. Frumorgen P, Demling L. Endoscopy 1979; 11: 146–150
190. Williams CB, Tan G. Gut 1979; 20: A903
191. Roseman DM. Gastrointest Endosc 1973; 20: 36
192. Rogers BHG, Silvis E et al. Gastrointest Endosc 1975; 23: 73–75
193. Cooper H. Am J Surg Pathol 1983; 7: 613–623
194. Haller D, Roberts TW. Surgery 1964; 55: 773–781
195. Pemberton J, McCormack CJ. Am J Surg 1937; 37: 205–218
196. Grand Quist S, Gabriellson B, Sundelin P. Endoscopy 1979; 11: 36–42
197. Mazier P, Mackeigan JM et al. Surg Gynecol Obstet 1982; 154: 829–832

Familial adenomatous polyposis

Familial adenomatous polyposis is a dominantly inherited condition, the gene for which has been shown to be located on the short arm of chromosome 5.[198] Characterized by myriad colorectal adenomas, together with widespread extracolonic stigmata, it affects around one in 10 000 live-born and is responsible for the development of approximately 1% of all colorectal cancers.

Pathology

The key feature is the development, usually during the teenage years, of hundreds or thousands of adenomas on the mucosa of the colon and rectum. Left untreated, progression to malignancy is inevitable within about 20 years. Hamartomatous polyps in the stomach, adenomas in the duodenum (see Ch. 26), mandibular osteomas, dental cysts (see Ch. 13), epidermoid cysts, retinal pigmentation and desmoid tumours are other features of this condition. Duodenal adenomas may progress to malignancy. Desmoid tumours may develop after any type of abdominal trauma, for example bowel surgery or pregnancy. Desmoid tumours may cause no symptoms, or they may expand or invade locally, causing intestinal or ureteric obstruction, ulceration through the abdominal wall, bleeding from the bowel or severe abdominal pain. The term *Gardner's syndrome* has been assigned to patients with polyposis coli harbouring extracolonic lesions, but it has become apparent that most, if not all, individuals affected by familial adenomatous polyposis exhibit some of these features, so the eponym has been dropped.

Clinical features

This condition is increasingly diagnosed before symptoms develop by screening the children of affected individuals. When it is not identified in this manner, symptoms are likely to occur in the late teens or twenties. The passage of loose stools and blood or mucus per rectum is usually the presenting complaint.

Diagnosis

Gene markers are being used increasingly at a prephenotypic stage, even before birth. In the children of known patients, it is usual to examine the rectum by rigid sigmoidoscopy in the mid teens. Annual repeat examination is necessary until middle age (rarely the adenomas do not appear until later in life) or until genotyping excludes the condition. New mutations are responsible for cases with no family history. Conventionally, familial adenomatous polyposis is assumed in the presence of a hundred or more adenomas. The finding of other stigmata, including skin cysts and jaw abnormalities, adds strength to the diagnosis.

Management

Prophylactic surgery involves a colectomy with ileorectal anastomosis or proctocolectomy and ileal pouch anal anastomosis. This restorative proctocolectomy is favoured on the grounds of cancer prevention when the rectum is badly affected, or if regular follow-up is for any reason likely to be difficult to implement. The duodenum should also be examined on a regular basis to try to identify and remove large or severely dysplastic adenomas.[199,200]

MALIGNANT TUMOURS OF THE COLON AND RECTUM

Colorectal cancer is the second most common malignancy in Western societies and the second leading cause of death related to cancer. There are approximately 35 000 new cases of colorectal cancer and 19 000 deaths per year in the UK.[201]

Ninety-eight per cent of malignant tumours of the colon and rectum are adenocarcinomas. Carcinoids and squamous cell carcinomas are rare tumours of colonic epithelial origin. Tumours of mesenchymal origin, sarcomas and malignant melanoma are relatively rare.

Table 28.4 Incidence of colorectal cancer in different countries*

Area	Colonic	Rectal	Colorectal
Nigeria	1.3	1.2	2.5
India	4.6	4.4	9.0
Osaka, Japan	6.3	6.9	13.2
East Germany	13.6	12.0	25.6
Vas, Hungary	9.1	11.0	20.1
Connecticut, USA	30.1	18.2	48.3
Detroit, USA			
White	26.2	16.0	42.2
Black	24.5	13.8	38.3
Birmingham, UK	16.5	16.1	32.6
Oxford, UK	15.7	15.4	31.1
Ayrshire, UK	16.6	14.0	30.0
Denmark	16.2	16.7	32.9
Finland	7.9	7.7	15.6
New Zealand			
Maori	7.4	4.6	12.0
Non-Maori	23.0	15.4	38.4
Hawaii			
Japanese	22.4	16.3	38.7
Caucasian	23.9	13.5	37.4
Hawaiian	14.1	9.4	23.5

*Per 100 000, age-adjusted to world population.
Adapted from Waterhouse JAH, Muir CS et al (eds). Cancer Incidence in 5 Continents, Vol III. International Agency for Research in Cancer, Lyons, 1976, with permission.[202]

GEOGRAPHICAL DISTRIBUTION

The highest incidence of colorectal cancer is seen in Western Europe and North America, whereas intermediate rates prevail in Eastern Europe (Table 28.6).[202] The lowest rates are seen in Asia, Africa and South America. The incidence of rectal cancer varies less in different parts of the world than that of colonic

REFERENCES

198. Bodmer WF, Bailey CJ, Bussey HSR. Nature 1987; 328: 614–616
199. Jones JR, Nance FC. Am Surg 1977; 185: 565
200. Jagelman DG, De Cosse JJ, Bussey HJR. Lancet 1988; i: 1149–1150
201. Boyle P, Langman JS. BMJ 2000; 321: 805–808
202. Waterhouse JAH, Muir CS et al (eds). Cancer Incidence in 5 Continents, Vol III. International Agency for Research in Cancer, Lyons, 1976

cancer. The disease is more common in urban areas than in rural areas.[203]

AETIOLOGY

The precise causes of colorectal carcinoma are unknown, but both genetic and environmental factors seem to be involved. It is believed that the latter are more important. Support for this thesis comes from the fact that migrants who move from an area of low incidence to one of high incidence become just as prone to develop cancer of the colon as the indigenous population of the high-risk area.[203]

ENVIRONMENTAL FACTORS

Dietary and digestive factors

Lack of fibre

From epidemiological studies, it appears that populations that consume a high-fibre diet are protected from cancer of the large intestine. Burkitt believed that this is because the high-fibre intake speeds transit and reduces the exposure of the gut mucosa to potential carcinogens.[204]

Increased fat

There is some evidence suggesting that a western diet, rich in animal fat, is an important risk factor. The concept is that fat favours the development of a bacterial flora containing organisms that are capable of degrading bile salts to carcinogens.

Bile acids

Evidence suggests bile acids have a direct toxic effect on colonic mucosa, which is capable of promoting the neoplastic process. Human epidemiological studies have found higher concentrations of bile acids in the faeces of high-risk populations.[205,206]

Previous cholecystectomy

A previous cholecystectomy (see Ch. 30) may increase the risk of colorectal cancer, particularly carcinomas of the right colon.[207–209] Although such studies are of considerable interest, the case as yet remains unproven. Cholecystectomy does increase the production and turnover of degraded bile salts.

Inflammatory bowel disease

The risk of colorectal cancer developing in patients with long-standing ulcerative colitis is well appreciated and has already been discussed. The relationship between cancer and Crohn's colitis, however, is far more tenuous. Although diverticular disease and carcinoma frequently coexist, there is no evidence to link the two disorders.[210] Evidence from China suggests that there may be a link between schistosomiasis and colorectal cancer.[211,212]

Ureterosigmoidostomy

Although this technique is rarely performed for urinary diversion, patients who have undergone the procedure seem to be at considerable risk of developing a carcinoma of the sigmoid.[213,214] Presumably, certain constituents of the urine are carcinogenic to colonic mucosa (see Chs 35 and 36).

Irradiation

Patients who have received pelvic irradiation appear to be at higher risk of developing rectosigmoid carcinoma compared with the normal population.[215]

GENETIC FACTORS

Although environmental factors seem to be the most significant in colorectal carcinogenesis, there is evidence to suggest that genetic factors are more important than was previously realized. The most obvious genetic link is with familial adenomatous polyposis, although it accounts for less than 0.5% of all colorectal cancers. Hereditary non-polyposis colorectal cancer is an autosomal dominant cancer predisposition syndrome caused by germ-line mutations in DNA mismatch repair genes, and this accounts for 5–10% of all colorectal cancers. The clinical syndrome may be defined by the Amsterdam criteria, which require the presence of colorectal cancer in at least three family members, one of whom is a first-degree relative of the other two, spanning two generations, with one or more cases diagnosed before the age of 50 years.[216] Patients with hereditary non-polyposis colorectal cancer (Lynch type I) are susceptible to colorectal cancer, but not cancer of other organs. Lynch type II also has an increased incidence of other gastrointestinal, urinary tract, breast and gynaecological malignancies.

PATHOLOGY

Approximately half of all large bowel tumours are situated in the rectum. Of those developing in the colon, approximately half occur in the sigmoid and a quarter occur in the caecum and ascending colon. The remaining quarter is distributed in order of frequency as follows: transverse colon, splenic flexure, descending colon and hepatic flexure. The number of neoplasms arising in the right colon is steadily increasing.[217]

Synchronous tumours are those that are present at the time of presentation in addition to the primary carcinoma. Approximately 3% of patients have synchronous carcinomas. Metachronous carcinomas are those cancers that develop subsequently to the primary carcinoma; they occur in roughly 10% of patients.

Macroscopic appearances

Bowel cancers may be polypoid or ulcerating, and may spread around the circumference of the colon as a scirrhous, an obstructing or an annular type of tumour.

Microscopic features and histological grading

Both Dukes[218] and Grinnell[219] introduced grading systems in

REFERENCES

203. Blot WJ, Fraumeni JF et al. J Natl Cancer Inst 1976; 57: 1225
204. Burkitt D. Cancer 1971; 28: 3–13
205. Crowther JS, Drasar BJ et al. Br J Cancer 1976; 34: 191–196
206. Hill MJ. Gut 1983; 24: 871–875
207. Linos DA, O'Fallon WM et al. Lancet 1981; ii: 379–381
208. Turunen MJ, Kivilaakso EO. Ann Surg 1981; 194: 639–641
209. Vernick LJ, Kuller LH. Am J Epidemiol 1982; 116: 86–101
210. Stewart M. Lancet 1931; ii: 669–674
211. Cheng M, Chuang C et al. Cancer 1980; 46: 1661
212. Cheng M, Chuang C et al. Lancet 1981; ii: 971–973
213. Thompson P, Hill J et al. Br J Surg 1979; 66: 65
214. Harford F, Fazio V et al. Dis Colon Rectum 1984; 27: 321–324
215. Sandler R, Sandier D. Gastroenterology 1983; 84: 51–57
216. Vasen HF, Mecklin JP. Dis Colon Rectum 1991; 34: 424–425
217. Welch CE, Hedberg SE. In: Dunphy JE, Ebert PA (eds). Polypoid Lesions of the Gastrointestinal Tract. 2nd edn. WB Saunders, Philadelphia, 1979
218. Dukes CE. Proc R Soc Med 1937; 30: 371–376
219. Grinnell RS. Ann Surg 1939; 109: 500

which tumours were graded I–IV according to the degree of dedifferentiation of the cells, grade I being well differentiated and grade IV anaplastic. Grade IV also includes all colloid tumours. Ten per cent of tumours are colloid, producing excessive mucus within the tumour. Approximately 60% of tumours are moderately differentiated (average grade), and the remaining 40% are divided up equally between well differentiated (low grade) and poorly differentiated (high grade or anaplastic).

SPREAD

DIRECT SPREAD

Direct lateral spread is far more common than spread in the longitudinal axis. The circumferential resection or mesorectal margin has gained importance as a predictor of local recurrence and survival.[220] Distal intramural spread is particularly pertinent to rectal cancer, when the length of the resection may determine whether the patient retains or loses the anal sphincter. Most studies suggest that distal intramural microscopic spread is rare, but when it is present it usually extends for less than 1 cm.[221] In those cases where it exceeds this distance, the tumour is advanced, and the patient is highly likely to die from widespread metastases without developing local recurrence.[221–223] As a result of these findings, the traditional 5-cm margin of clearance distal to a rectal cancer can be reduced to 1–2 cm if necessary, thus enabling more sphincter-saving operations to be accomplished.

LYMPHATIC SPREAD

Lymphatic spread of rectal cancer is usually proximal, with distal spread occurring rarely. Lateral lymphatic spread is unusual in tumours of the intraperitoneal rectum, being more common in extraperitoneal growths.

BLOOD-BORNE SPREAD

Liver metastases were considered to develop late in patients with colorectal cancer, but more recent data have shown that up to 30% of patients have occult liver metastases at the time of presentation.[224] Pulmonary metastases occur in about 5% of cases,[225] and the adrenal glands, kidneys and bones are involved in about 10% of cases. Neoplastic cells have been found in the circulation at the time of surgery, but their viability is uncertain.

TRANSPERITONEAL SPREAD

Spread by this route occurs in approximately one in 10 patients after resection. Spread to the ovaries may also occur by this route, resulting in Krukenberg tumours.

SPREAD BY IMPLANTATION

Several reports have suggested that this method of spread is possible, although uncommon. Thus implantation metastases have been described in anal fistulae, haemorrhoidectomy wounds, abdominal incisions and around colostomies. Suture line recurrences may also be explained on the basis of implantation. There is considerable debate about the viability of cells released into the lumen of the bowel during surgery.[226] They may be an important mechanism of spread in patients having laparoscopic colonic resections, where port site recurrence is now well recognized and may limit the feasibility of this type of surgery in cancers of the colon and rectum.[227]

STAGING

PATHOLOGICAL STAGE

The standard method of staging patients with colorectal cancers is based on the pathological characteristics of the resected specimen, and this is achieved using Dukes' system,[228,229] originally described for rectal tumours only, and the TNM (tumour, node and metastasis) classification.[230]

Dukes' staging system

Stages of Dukes' system are:

- Stage A: the tumour is confined to the bowel wall with no involvement of lymph nodes.
- Stage B: the tumour extends through the wall of the bowel without spread to lymph nodes.
- Stage C: lymph node metastases. When the apical lymph node is involved, the tumour is a Dukes' stage C2; otherwise, the tumour is said to be a Dukes' stage C1.

Since Dukes originally described his system, it has been customary also to include stage D for those patients with distant metastases.

TNM classification

For primary tumours:

- TX: primary tumour cannot be assessed.
- T0: no evidence of primary tumour.
- Tis: carcinoma in situ; intraepithelial or invasion of lamina propria.
- T1: tumour invades submucosa.
- T2: tumour invades muscularis propria.
- T3: tumour invades through muscularis propria into subserosa, or into non-peritonealized pericolic or perirectal tissue.
- T4: tumour directly invades other organs or structures and/or perforates visceral peritoneum.

For regional lymph nodes:

- NX: regional lymph nodes cannot be assessed.
- N0: no regional lymph nodes.
- N1: metastasis in one to three regional lymph nodes.
- N2: metastasis in four or more regional lymph nodes.

Distant:

- MX: distant metastasis cannot be assessed.
- M0: no distant metastasis.
- M1: distant metastasis.

CLINICAL STAGE

Patients can be classified into three broad prognostic groups following surgery. Patients may have had a curative operation

REFERENCES

220. Wibe A, Rendedal PR. Br J Surg 2002; 89: 327–334
221. Quer EA, Dahlin DC, Mayo CW. Surg Gynecol Obstet 1953; 96: 24–30
222. Black WA, Waugh JM. Surg Gynecol Obstet 1948; 87: 457–464
223. Grinnell RS. Surg Gynecol Obstet 1954; 99: 421–430
224. Finlay IG, Meek DR et al. Br Med J 1982; 284: 803–805
225. Cole WH, Packard D, Southwick HW. JAMA 1954; 155: 1549–1554
226. Umpleby HC et al. Dis Colon Rectum 1984; 27: 803–809
227. Berends FJ, Kazemier G et al. Lancet 1994; 344: 58
228. Dukes CE. Br J Surg 1930; 17: 643–648
229. Dukes CE. J Pathol Bacteriol 1940; 50: 527
230. Sobin LH, Wittekind C. TNM Classification of Malignant Tumours. 6th edn. Wiley-Liss, New York, 2002

where all demonstrable tumour has been removed. They may be incurable because of the presence of distant metastases, or incurable because of the presence of residual local disease.

CLINICAL FEATURES

Patients usually present in the sixth to eighth decade, although the disease may occur at any age. Approximately 250 patients below 35 years of age present each year with a colorectal cancer in the UK, and a small proportion are children. Colon cancer occurs with equal frequency in men and women, but rectal cancer is more prevalent in men.[231] In its early stages an uncomplicated carcinoma of the colon is usually symptomless. Symptoms include a change in bowel habit, bleeding per anum (which is often dark in colour), the passage of mucus, and abdominal discomfort or distension. Anorexia and weight loss are rarely early features but may occur if the tumour becomes disseminated.

The site of the carcinoma often dictates the symptoms. Carcinoma of the right colon is soft and friable, and bleeds easily. Thus the patient may present with symptoms of anaemia from occult bleeding, which is mixed within the stool and invisible by the time it reaches the rectum. Sometimes the patient complains of abdominal pain if the tumour obstructs or infiltrates, and a mass may be palpable in the right iliac fossa.

Tumours in the left colon are more likely to constrict and cause obstruction, particularly so because the intraluminal contents are more solid on the left. Constipation, therefore, is a frequent initial symptom and is often accompanied by abdominal colic. Overt bleeding and the passage of mucus per anum are more common with tumours on the left side.

Carcinoma of the rectum often produces a classic symptom complex. Bleeding is common and resembles that coming from haemorrhoids in being bright red, although often it is darker. A change in the bowel habit is frequent, with patients often suffering from explosive episodes of diarrhoea punctuated by periods of relative constipation. Tenesmus, the painful and repeated call to stool, is usually a late feature and indicates an advanced tumour. These symptoms are often present in the morning and improve as the day wears on. The patient may also present with symptoms referable to the organ or organs invaded, if local spread has occurred. Posterior invasion into the sacral plexus may cause back pain and sciatica, and extension downwards into the anal canal may produce anal pain reminiscent of a fissure in ano. Invasion of the ureters, bladder or prostate may produce urinary tract symptoms, and extension of a rectal tumour into the vagina may cause a rectovaginal fistula.

DIFFERENTIAL DIAGNOSIS

The differential diagnosis includes diverticular disease, irritable bowel syndrome, Crohn's disease, ulcerative colitis, ischaemia, solitary rectal ulcer, radiation enteritis and other tumours, including polyps, lymphoma and melanoma.

DIAGNOSIS

A combination of history, clinical examination, sigmoidoscopy, and either barium enema or colonoscopy, or both, will invariably determine the diagnosis. Seventy per cent of rectal tumours are situated within 12 cm of the anal verge, as measured on sigmoidoscopy, and are palpable on digital examination. There is some debate as to whether a colonoscopy or a barium enema should be the initial investigation if rectal examination and sigmoidoscopy are normal. Colonoscopy is more accurate in detecting neoplasms and more comfortable for the patient,[232] and as a consequence many feel that this procedure should be the first investigation. A satisfactory compromise is to combine flexible sigmoidoscopy with a double-contrast barium enema. Once a tumour has been identified, it should be biopsied to confirm the diagnosis.

SCREENING

The earlier detection of colorectal carcinoma by screening populations might be expected to improve the long-term survival of patients with colorectal cancer. Screening can be divided into selective screening of high-risk groups and general screening of individuals of average risk. The high-risk group includes patients with a long history of ulcerative colitis, a past history of an adenoma or a colon cancer, female genital cancer, and those with a strong family history.[233–237] This group should have a regular barium enema and/or colonoscopy every 1–5 years.

It is not yet known whether the cost of screening the general population justifies the benefit for the few positive cases identified. Using faecal occult blood testing, a carcinoma is detected in about one or two cases per 1000 screened, with a false-positive rate of approximately 2%. Several studies have shown that carcinomas can be detected at an earlier pathological stage by this method of screening.[238–241] The National Polyp Study Workgroup has published evidence that confirms that colonic screening, combined with polypectomy, reduces the incidence of colorectal cancer, and that the disease-specific mortality is reduced by about 15%.[242] The Italian Multicentre Study Group has replicated these results.[243] The UK trial of once-only flexible sigmoidoscopy has published their early results and shown that it is a safe, acceptable screening tool. Distal neoplasia (adenomas or cancers) was detected in 12% of the 40 674 people screened.[244] The evidence continues to mount for a national colorectal screening policy.

REFERENCES

231. Offices of Population Censuses and Surveys. Cancer Statistics: Registration 1976. HMSO, London, 1981
232. Durdey P, Weston P, Williams NJ. Lancet 1987; ii: 549
233. Anderson DE, Ramsdahl MM. In: Mulvihill JJ, Miller RW, Fraumeni JF Jr (eds). Progress in Cancer Research and Therapy: Genetics of Human Cancer, Vol 3. Raven Press, New York, 1977
234. Devroede G. In: Winawer SJ, Sherlock P, Shottenfeld D (eds). Colorectal Cancer: Epidemiology and Screening. Progress in Cancer Research 1980. Raven Press, New York, 1980
235. Kushin SZ, Lipkin M, Winawer SJ. Am J Gastroenterol 1979; 72: 448–453
236. Lynch HT, Lynch J, Lynch P. In: Mulvihill JJ, Miller RM, Fraumeni JF Jr (eds). Progress in Cancer Research and Therapy: Genetics of Human Cancer, Vol 3. Raven Press, New York, 1977: 235
237. Winawer SJ, Sherlock P et al. Gastroenterology 1976; 70: 783–788
238. Winawer SJ. In: de Cosse JJ (ed). Large Bowel Cancer. Churchill Livingstone, Edinburgh, 1981
239. Hardcastle JD, Farrands PA et al. Lancet 1983; ii: 1–4
240. Siba S. Hepatogastroenterology 1983; 30: 27–29
241. Gilbertsen VA, Church TR, Grewe FJ. J Chron Dis 1980; 33: 107–114
242. Winawer SJ, Zauber AG. N Engl J Med 1993; 329: 1977–1981
243. Citarda F, Tomaselli G et al. Gut 2001; 48: 812–815
244. UK Flexible Sigmoidoscopy Screening Trial Investigators. Lancet 2002; 359: 1291–1300

COMPLICATIONS

OBSTRUCTION

Carcinomas of the left colon are more likely to cause obstruction than those of the right, because they are often of the constricting variety and the faecal matter is more solid (see Ch. 25). A carcinoma may cause obstruction from a colocolic intussusception. Half of all such intussusceptions in adults are caused by a carcinoma.[245]

PERFORATION

Perforation may occur either through the carcinoma itself or, more commonly, at a site proximal to it. The latter occurs late, and the most common area to perforate is the caecum, as a result of a closed loop obstruction. Despite improvements in resuscitation and antibiotic therapy, the mortality from faecal peritonitis is still high. A perforated carcinoma is unlikely to be curable.

FISTULA FORMATION

A colorectal carcinoma may adhere to and eventually penetrate any abdominal or pelvic viscus, although it is a rare occurrence. The organ most commonly involved is the bladder, and the carcinoma usually develops in the sigmoid colon. The resulting vesicocolic fistula may produce pneumaturia, faecuria and frequent urinary tract infections. The diagnosis is often difficult, and the differentiation from diverticular disease as a cause of the fistula may be impossible until the pathologist has examined the excised specimen.

Rectal cancer may invade the vagina and produce a rectovaginal fistula. A fistula may also develop between a tumour in the transverse colon and the stomach or duodenum, when the patient may present with faecal vomiting. Rarely, an external spontaneous fistula may develop, but this is more commonly associated with Crohn's disease.

RARE COMPLICATIONS

Although a tumour frequently causes minor bleeding, massive haemorrhage can occur. Occasionally a large caecal carcinoma obstructs the base of the appendix and causes acute appendicitis (see Ch. 25).

TREATMENT

GENERAL PRINCIPLES

Surgical resection is the standard treatment for colorectal cancer, although further improvements in survival rates are likely to come from adjuvant therapy. The aim of a curative excision is to eradicate the disease and also to remove the regional lymphovascular drainage. Excision of the tumour should be attempted whenever possible, even if it is considered that an operation is only palliative, because it may prevent intestinal obstruction developing and avoid distressing symptoms.

Laparoscopic techniques for colorectal surgery have been developed. Initial reports suggested an increase in complications, but in expert hands the operative morbidity is similar to that of the open operation. There does remain a question of trocar site tumour recurrence, which seems greater than would have been expected. The majority of laparoscopic colorectal resections are performed as laparoscopic assisted procedures where the colon or rectum is mobilized laparoscopically and an extracorporeal anastomosis is undertaken through a small transverse incision. Prospective, randomized, multicentre trials of laparoscopic versus open colorectal resections are underway in the UK and USA.

PREOPERATIVE PREPARATION

Patients must be carefully assessed before operation to determine their fitness for surgery and the extent of the spread of their disease. Preoperative staging is important, because it may change the patient's management; an elderly patient with liver metastases and a relatively small rectal tumour may best be served by a local procedure rather than a major resection. Similarly, a large rectal tumour with extensive local invasion should best be managed by a course of preoperative radiotherapy, which will help to reduce the bulk of the tumour and often convert an inoperable growth to an operable lesion, although it may not necessarily improve the chances of survival.[246] Local spread of a rectal cancer should be investigated with a CT or an MRI scan together with transrectal ultrasound. Spread of colorectal cancer to the liver is best shown by CT portography. Intraoperative liver ultrasound may also be used.

BOWEL PREPARATION

The chief source of sepsis is the endogenous bacteria within the bowel lumen. Mechanical clearance for left sided colonic and rectal resections is desirable, because it reduces the possibility of contamination at operation. Bowel prepartion for right sided colonic resections is unnecessary.[247] Two sachets of sodium picosulfate are taken in the 24 h before operation, together with clear liquids only. In patients who have obstructive symptoms, on-table bowel irrigation is safer and more effective, because a purgative may cause massive bowel dilatation above the tumour, increasing the risk of caecal rupture.[248]

The other main advance has been the use of prophylactic antibiotics to reduce septic complications. Systemic antibiotic cover has dramatically reduced the incidence of postoperative wound infection. A combination of metronidazole and a cephalosporin is now most popular. The administration of either one dose on induction of anaesthesia or three doses perioperatively reduces the risks of drug resistance and side effects, while providing satisfactory prophylaxis (see Ch. 4).[249]

COUNSELLING

It is important to inform the patient and relatives of the intended procedure, particularly if a stoma is a possibility. A stoma therapist or experienced senior nurse must be available to indicate the ideal site for the stoma, explain precisely how it will function, and provide advice and reassurance.

SURGICAL TECHNIQUES FOR ELECTIVE CASES

The type of operation depends on the site of the tumour. Because the lymphatic drainage accompanies the main blood vessels, the length of bowel resected depends on the extent of the lymphatic clearance that is required. A large bowel anastomosis can be made in one or two layers with interrupted sutures using a non-

REFERENCES

245. Sanders GB, Hazen WH, Kinnaird PW. Ann Surg 1958; 147: 796–801
246. Gerard A, Berrod J et al. Rec Res Cancer Res 1985; 110: 130–133
247. Guenaga KF, Matos D et al. Cochrane Database Syst Rev 2003; 2: CD001544
248. Dudley H, Phillips R. In: Fielding LP, Welch J (eds). Intestinal Obstruction. Churchill Livingstone, London, 1984
249. Herter FP. Surg Clin North Am 1972; 52: 859–870

absorbable material (e.g. silk or nylon) or long-lasting absorbable material (e.g. polyglycolic acid, polyglactin, polydioxanone sulphate or Maxon). Staple guns are commonly used to form anastomoses in the pelvis.

The colon

Right hemicolectomy

Right hemicolectomy is used for growths of the caecum, the ascending colon, the hepatic flexure, and the right half of the transverse colon (Fig. 28.26). Intestinal continuity is restored by an ileocolic anastomosis. An extended right hemicolectomy can be used for the resection of a distal transverse colon or splenic flexure carcinoma, with the terminal ileum being anastomosed end-to-end to the mobilized splenic flexure or descending colon. Transverse colonic lesions are usually managed by an extended right hemicolectomy.

Transverse colectomy

A tumour situated in the middle of the transverse colon may be removed by transverse colectomy. The anastomosis is made between the ascending colon and the descending colon.

Left hemicolectomy

This operation is used to treat cancers of the splenic flexure, and descending and sigmoid colon (Fig. 28.27). Segmental resection of the sigmoid colon is also possible (Fig. 28.28). A colocolic or colorectal anastomosis is constructed.

The rectum

Historically, rectal cancers required an abdominoperineal excision. It is now known that a safe distal clearance of 1 cm is possible, and continence can be achieved even if the whole rectum is excised. Together with new techniques to allow safe anastomoses deep in the pelvis, excision of the rectum is possible, with continuity being restored by a colorectal or coloanal anastomosis.[250]

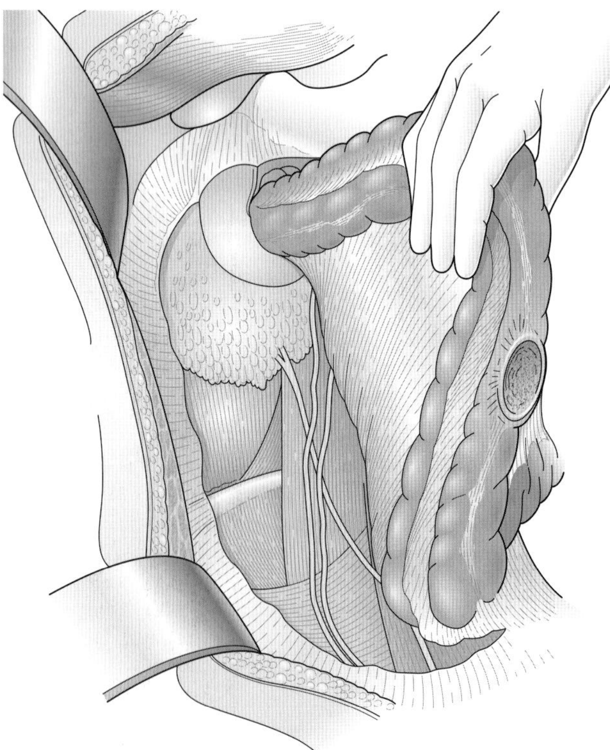

Figure 28.26 Right hemicolectomy. Mobilization reveals the duodenum, right ureter and gonadal vessels.

Anterior resection

Excision of the lower two-thirds of the rectum should be undertaken with a total mesorectal excision to produce low local recurrence rates.[251] A stapled anastomosis is usually performed, using a transverse stapler to close the distal bowel and a circular stapling gun to form the anastomosis (Fig. 28.29). The formation of a defunctioning loop ileostomy or colostomy is recommended if the anastomosis is low in the pelvis or if there have been technical difficulties. When the tumour lies at the anorectal junction or even extends into the anal canal, it is possible to continue the pelvic dissection, either via the abdomen or transanally. A stapled ultralow colorectal or hand-sewn transanal coloanal anastomosis is then performed (Fig. 28.30).

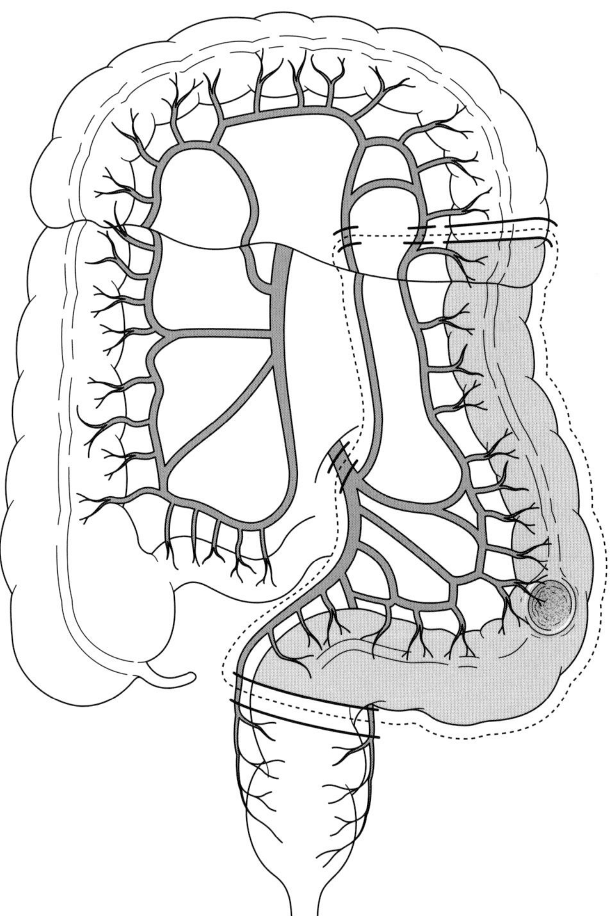

Figure 28.27 Standard left hemicolectomy. An extended left hemicolectomy would involve extension of the resection proximal to the splenic flexure.

REFERENCES

250. Tytherleigh MG, Mortensen NJ. Br J Surg 2003; 90: 922–923
251. Heald RJ, Husband EM, Ryall RDH. Br J Surg 1982; 69: 613

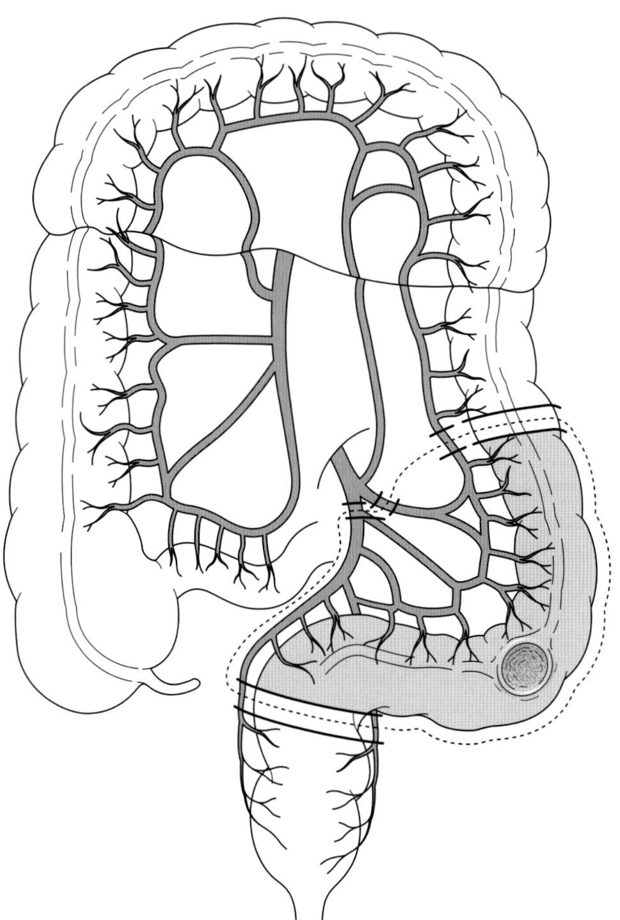

Figure 28.28 Sigmoid colectomy.

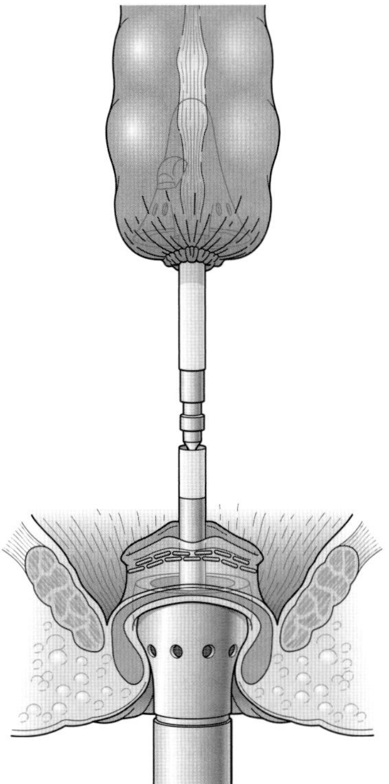

Figure 28.29 Low anterior resection using a Premium CEEA stapling gun.

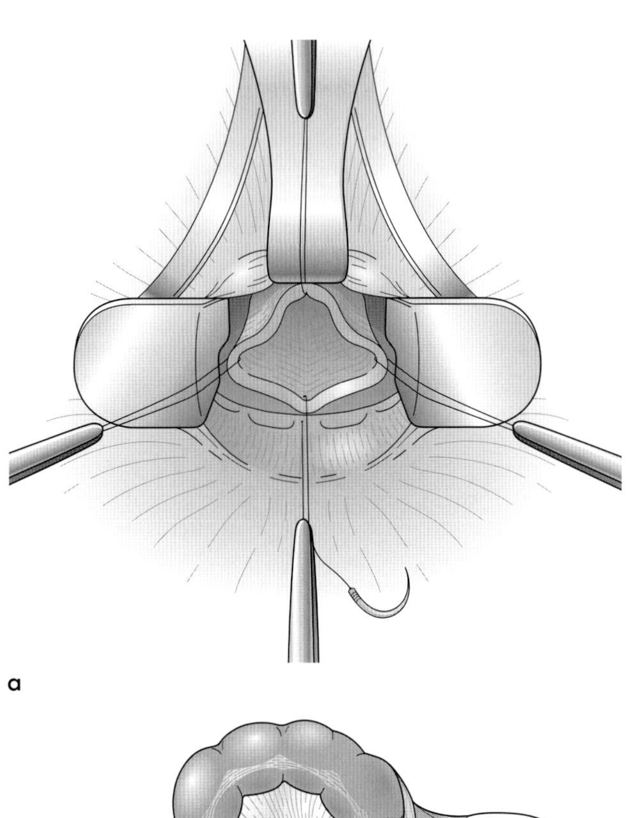

a

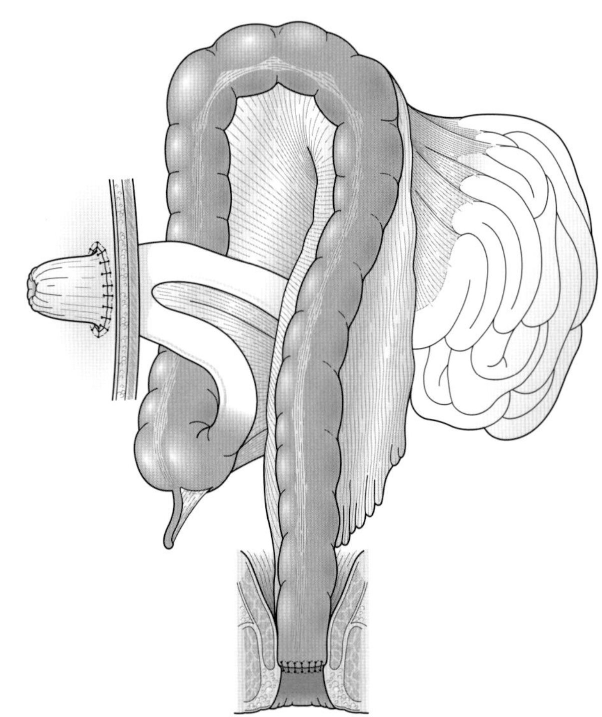

b

Figure 28.30 Abdominotransanal coloanal anastomosis. (**a**) The rectum has been excised, and the mucosa of the upper part of the anal canal has been removed. The colon is brought down through the denuded anal canal and is anastomosed transanally to the dentate line. (**b**) On completion of the procedure a covering ileostomy is fashioned to protect the healing anastomosis.

Abdominoperineal excision

This operation is necessary if the cancer is invading the anal sphincter or if the formation of an anastomosis is technically impossible, usually because of a narrow pelvis in an obese man (Fig. 28.31). Both abdominal and perineal dissections may be performed simultaneously. The perineal wound is closed, and an end sigmoid colostomy is brought out in the left iliac fossa.

POSTOPERATIVE CARE AFTER COLORECTAL RESECTION

Intravenous fluids maintain hydration until a normal oral intake has been re-established. Two further doses of prophylactic antibiotics are given, usually 6 and 12 h after operation. The patient should receive adequate systemic analgesia, which may be administered as epidural opiates (see Ch. 5). The urethral catheter is kept in situ for several days until the patient is relatively mobile. Normal micturition is often delayed after rectal excision. The patient must be encouraged at the earliest stage to take an interest in their stoma, if one has been formed, and be taught under supervision how to change the appliance.

COMPLICATIONS

Anastomotic dehiscence

Anastomotic dehiscence is the most dangerous complication and may present in a number of ways. Generalized peritonitis develops if there is a perforation into the peritoneal cavity, while a pelvic abscess develops if the leak remains localized. The abscess may subsequently perforate into the peritoneal cavity, and once again peritonitis will result. Alternatively, the abscess may drain spontaneously through the defect in the anastomosis back into the intestinal lumen, resulting in the passage of pus per anum. The abscess may also track to the skin and discharge through either the main wound or the drain track. The discharge of pus is then almost always followed by a discharge of faeces, indicating an established fistula. Most fistulae close spontaneously provided there is no distal obstruction.

Anastomotic dehiscence is related to two main factors: the level of the anastomosis and the surgeon. After high anterior resection the leak rate is around 5%. This rises significantly where the anastomosis is constructed below the peritoneal reflection. After low anterior resection, anastomotic leakage has been reported to range from 5% to more than 25% of cases.[252–254] These rates refer to a clinical dehiscence; radiological examination of the anastomosis using a water-soluble contrast medium demonstrates some degree of leakage in a much higher proportion.[255]

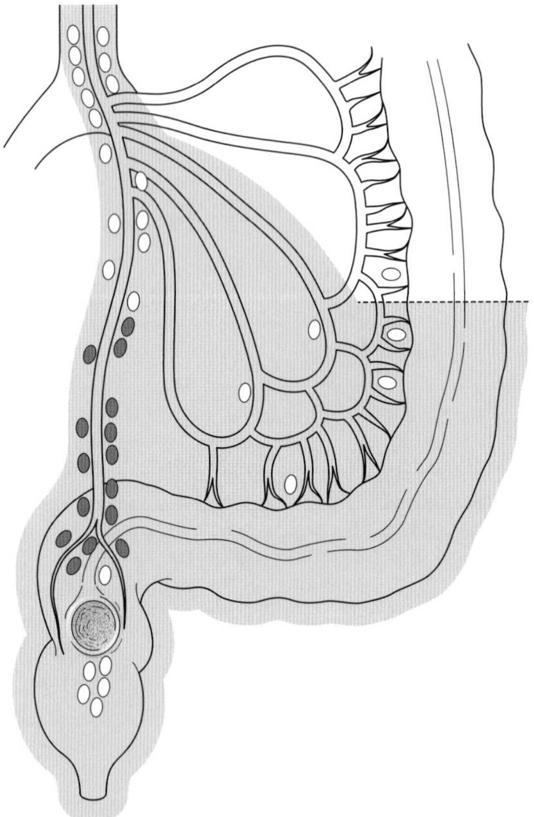

Figure 28.31 Abdominoperineal excision of the rectum: extent of excision.

Intestinal obstruction

Small bowel obstruction may occur from herniation of small intestine lateral to the colostomy loop or through the pelvic peritoneal wound closure. Small intestine may also become adherent to the pelvic peritoneal closure. After sphincter-saving resections, a small dehiscence in the anastomosis may become plugged by a loop of small bowel, which may then become obstructed. The large bowel may become temporarily obstructed, either as the result of oedema of the colostomy or from a bolus of faeces. The former settles in time, the latter may need suppositories or a gentle enema. It is unwise to treat this problem until at least 7 days have elapsed.

Urinary complications

Acute retention may be the result of denervation of the bladder or prostatic obstruction (see Ch. 37 and Ch. 38). Direct injury to the ureters may lead to hydronephrosis, pyonephrosis or urinary fistula. The bladder may be opened during the anterior dissection, and the urethra may be injured in the perineal phase of abdominoperineal excision, leading to fistula or stricture at a later date.

Sexual dysfunction

Damage to pelvic nerves may also result in impotence or failure of ejaculation. The former is caused by injury to the nervi erigentes, the latter by damage to the presacral nerves. Impotence is more common after abdominoperineal excision (around 50%) than after anterior resection (20–50%).[256] In females, fibrosis around the vagina may result in dyspareunia.

Perineal wound

Primary, reactionary or secondary haemorrhage may occur. Infection is probably the most frequent complication: if drainage is not satisfactory, an abscess may form in the deep recesses of the cavity. Pressure necrosis of the wound edges may develop if the patient is not turned frequently. A perineal sinus may form if the wound fails to heal completely, and at a later date a perineal hernia may develop.

REFERENCES

252. Beart RW, Kelly KA. Am J Surg 1981; 141: 143–147
253. Weakley FL. Dis Colon Rectum 1981; 24: 231–246
254. Blamey SL, Lee PWR. Br J Surg 1982; 69: 19–22
255. Goligher JC, Simpkins KC, Lintott DJ. Br J Surg 1977; 64: 609
256. Williams N, Johnston D. Br J Surg 1983; 70: 460–462

Phantom rectum

Phantom rectum is a condition akin to phantom limb (see Ch. 10), which may develop after amputation. About half of the patients feel that the rectum is still present, and this can produce a distressing sensation.[257]

Colostomy complications

The stoma may bleed, prolapse, retract or stenose if it has not been correctly made. The skin around the colostomy may become excoriated, or a fistula may develop between the stoma and the skin. A paracolostomy hernia may also develop, although this complication was more frequent when the colostomy was brought out lateral to the rectus sheath, with an incidence of around 25% at 5 years.

Bowel frequency

Increased bowel frequency and incontinence are more likely the lower the colorectal anastomosis. After coloanal anastomosis, the mean bowel frequency is around three or four times per 24 h, but some patients go considerably more often. Continence is normal in around 70%, with some soiling (usually minor) in the remainder.[258] Function tends to improve with time up to almost 1 year from operation. The addition of a colonic pouch to coloanal reconstruction appears to improve bowel function significantly.[259,260] The coloplasty reservoir is functionally similar to the J pouch but is technically easier to construct. A longitudinal incision is performed in the distal colon, which is then closed transversely.[261,262]

RESULTS OF SURGERY FOR COLORECTAL CANCER

The results for carcinoma of the colon and rectum are similar. Survival rates are linked to the Dukes' stage (see Table 28.7).

Local recurrence

The local recurrence rate is a good indicator of the completeness of surgical excision. Local recurrence rates approaching 40% occur after abdominoperineal excision. Total mesorectal excision performed during an anterior resection has brought local recurrence rates down to about 5%. Approximately 80% of all local recurrences develop within the first 2 years after surgery.[263] Patients may develop an increase in serum carcinoembryonic antigen concentration before they develop clinical recurrence, although the measuring of carcinoembryonic antigen postoperatively is controversial.[264] Imaging of local recurrence has improved with positron emission tomography.[265,266] The Swedish radiotherapy trial has unequivocally shown that a short course of neoadjuvant radiotherapy reduces rates of local recurrence and improves survival among patients with rectal cancer.[267]

Table 28.7 Corrected 5-year survival for rectal cancer according to modified Dukes' classification

Dukes' stage	Corrected 5-year survival (%)
A	91.9
B	71.3
C1	40.0
C2	26.5
D	16.4

Patients with local recurrence often complain of persistent pelvic pain, which may radiate down the legs if the sacral nerve roots are involved. Urinary symptoms develop if the bladder or urethra is invaded. A swelling or some induration may be visible or palpable in the perineum if there is a local recurrence after an abdominoperineal resection. Alternatively, an abscess or a discharging sinus may develop. Bilateral leg oedema may arise from invasion and obstruction of the lymphatics and veins.

Local recurrence after anterior resection may also cause a change in bowel habit or the passage of blood per rectum. The best method of treating recurrence is by further surgical excision, but this is often not possible because of the advanced stage of the tumour. Radiotherapy and chemotherapy are merely palliative.

LOCAL TECHNIQUES FOR RECTAL CANCER

Patients who are unfit for major surgery may receive useful palliation by electrocoagulation,[268] contact irradiation,[269] local excision, and Nd YAG laser therapy. These techniques can also be used as the primary treatment for low-grade carcinomas that are confined to the bowel wall. These tumours account for only around 5% of all rectal cancers and can be identified and assessed by a combination of digital examination, biopsy and rectal endoluminal ultrasound.[270,271] Five-year survival rates of over 90% have been reported in these low-grade tumours. Histopathological examination must confirm that the tumour is confined to the rectal wall. A curative resection should be undertaken if there is evidence of local spread beyond the bowel wall.

Self-expanding metal stents are being used for the palliation of primary tumours and recurrences.[272] They are also used to relieve malignant obstruction so that bowel preparation can be achieved before elective surgery. They are placed during colonoscopy under radiological screening.

ADJUVANT THERAPY

Much attention has been focused on radiotherapy and chemotherapy, because there has been no significant improvement in survival rates after surgery alone in the past 30 years. The Swedish Rectal Cancer Trial showed that preoperative radiotherapy does confer a survival benefit and reduces the risk of local

REFERENCES

257. Druss RG, O'Connor JF, Stern L. Q Arch Gen Psychiatry 1969; 20: 419–426
258. Parks A, Percy J. Br J Surg 1982; 69: 301–304
259. Lazorthes F, Faget P et al. Br J Surg 1986; 73: 136–138
260. Parc R, Tiret E et al. Br J Surg 1986; 73: 139–141
261. Z'Graggen K, Maurer CA et al. Dig Surg 1999; 16: 363–366
262. Mantyh CR, Hull TL. Dis Colon Rectum 2001; 44: 37–42
263. Morson BC, Vaughan EG, Bussey HJR. Br Med J 1963; 2: 13
264. Macdonald JS. Semin Oncol 1999; 26: 556–560
265. Bomanji JB, Costa DC et al. Lancet Oncol 2001; 2: 157–164
266. Arulampalam TH, Costa DC et al. Br J Surg 2001; 88: 176–189
267. Swedish Rectal Cancer Trial. N Engl J Med 1997; 336: 980–987
268. Strauss A, Strauss S et al. JAMA 1935; 104: 1480
269. Papillon J. Proc R Soc Med 1973; 66: 1179
270. Nicholls RJ, York Mason A et al. Br J Surg 1982; 69: 404–409
271. Hildebrandt U, Feifel G. Dis Colon Rectum 1985; 28: 42–46
272. Rey JF, Romanczyk T et al. Endoscopy 1995; 27: 501–504

recurrence.[267] Unfortunately, radiotherapy cannot be used for colonic cancer because of the unwanted effects of radiotherapy on the small bowel. Preoperative radiotherapy may also convert a growth deemed inoperable on clinical examination into an operable one.[273]

Postoperative chemotherapy is now standard therapy for patients with node-positive colorectal cancer. A combination of 5-fluorouracil and leucovorin given as intravenous boluses over 6 months has been shown to reduce cancer mortality by a third in these node-positive patients.[274] New chemotherapeutic agents, such as irinotecan, capecitabine and the monoclonal antibodies Edrecolomab, Letuximab and Bevacizumab, are undergoing evaluation.

SURGICAL TREATMENT FOR METASTATIC COLORECTAL CANCER

In appropriately selected patients, single or even multiple hepatic metastases may be resected. Survival rates of 30% at 5 years are possible.[275] Pulmonary metastases may also be resected. The possibility of ovarian metastases has encouraged some surgeons to perform an oophorectomy at the time of the original surgery.

RARE MALIGNANT TUMOURS

CARCINOID

Carcinoid is a rare tumour of the large bowel derived from the Kulchitsky cells of the crypts of Lieberkühn. Large bowel carcinoid tumours do not secrete serotonin (5-hydroxytryptamine), even when spread to the liver has occurred.[276,277]

The tumour usually arises as a polyp of yellowish hue, which often becomes ulcerated. The clinical presentation and treatment are the same as for adenocarcinoma, but the prognosis is usually better.[278] Somatostatin analogues can successfully treat diarrhoea caused by metastatic carcinoid.

PRIMARY MALIGNANT LYMPHOMA

This tumour is also rare, accounting for only 0.1% of all malignant tumours of the large bowel. Malignant lymphomas occur more commonly in the caecum than in the left colon or rectum. The tumour may develop in patients with long-standing ulcerative colitis.

The degree of malignancy depends on the cell type and extent of spread at the time of diagnosis. Both Hodgkin's and non-Hodgkin's lymphomas can occur (see Ch. 34). Their clinical presentation is similar to that for adenocarcinomas. Radiotherapy and chemotherapy play an important adjuvant role to surgical excision, particularly when there is lymph node involvement.

LEIOMYOSARCOMA

These neoplasms, which originate from the muscularis propria, project either into the bowel lumen or on to its external surface. They are usually large, rubbery, lobulated tumours and ulcerate through the overlying mucosa. Microscopically, they are often difficult to differentiate from their benign counterparts. The symptoms are similar to those of other tumours, but massive rectal haemorrhage is characteristic. Treatment is by surgical resection. Postoperative radiotherapy may prevent recurrence.

OTHER MALIGNANT TUMOURS

Fibrosarcoma, haemangiopericytoma, plasmacytoma, endothelioma and malignant lymphomatous polyposis are very rare tumours of the large bowel.[278–283] Very occasionally a malignant melanoma or squamous cell carcinoma may arise in the colorectum, but these are much more common in the anal canal.

ANAL TUMOURS

Anal tumours are rare. The incidence of epidermoid squamous cancers, the most common type, is only 300 new cases per annum in the UK.[284]

BENIGN ANAL TUMOURS

Leiomyomas, lipomas and other mesodermal tumours can arise in the anal region.[285] The diagnosis should be confirmed by biopsy, and treatment is by local excision.

MALIGNANT ANAL TUMOURS

SQUAMOUS CELL TUMOURS

The term *squamous cell tumours* refers to tumours variously known as epidermoid, basaloid and cloacogenic. Neoplasms at the anal verge are more common in men, while tumours in the anal canal more frequently affect women. Evidence suggests that anal tumours occur more frequently in homosexual men and are related to anal sexual practices.[286] Human papilloma virus has been shown to be associated with anal cancer in the majority of cases.

These tumours present with bleeding, anal pain and discharge; sometimes the patient may notice a lump. The tumour may look like a typical skin cancer, appearing as a raised ulcer or as an irregular plaque. It may have invaded the anal sphincters or have spread upwards to involve the rectum. The inguinal nodes should be palpated for evidence of spread, although distant metastases are uncommon.

Combined chemoradiotherapy treatment has become first-line treatment; it has an approximately 60% 5-year survival rate and avoids a colostomy in most patients. Abdominoperineal excision is reserved for failed primary treatment and recurrence.[287] Local excision may have a role in treating small anal margin lesions.

REFERENCES

273. Gerard A, Berrod JL et al. Cancer 1985; 55: 2373–2379
274. Dube S, Heyen F. Dis Colon Rectum 1997; 40: 35–41
275. Fong Y, Salo J. Semin Oncol 1999; 26: 514–523
276. Goligher JC. Surgery of the Anus, Rectum and Colon. 4th edn. Baillière Tindall, London, 1984
277. Peskin GW, Orloff MJ. Surg Gynecol Obstet 1959; 109: 673–678
278. Orloff MJ. Cancer 1971; 28: 175–180
279. Stout AP. In: Turell R (ed). Diseases of the Colon and Anorectum, Vol 1. WB Saunders, Philadelphia, 1959
280. Morgan CN. Proc R Soc Med 1932; 25: 1020–1025
281. Norbury LEC. Proc R Soc Med 1952; 25: 1021–1026
282. Orda R, Bawbik JB et al. Dis Colon Rectum 1976; 19: 626–631
283. Pack GT, Miller TR, Trinidad SS. Dis Colon Rectum 1963; 6: 1–6
284. Offices of Population Censuses and Surveys. Registration 1976. HMSO, London, 1983
285. Morson BC, Dawson IMP. Gastrointestinal Pathology. Blackwell, Oxford, 1990: 754
286. Daling JR, Weiss NS et al. N Engl J Med 1987; 317: 973–977
287. Ryan DP, Compton CC et al. N Engl J Med 2000; 342: 792–800

LEUKOPLAKIA

Leukoplakia is a premalignant condition of the anorectum, which is similar to the oral disorder (see Ch. 13). The firm white plaques may be circumscribed or confluent around the anus. Local excision often fails to prevent further disease, and careful surveillance is required to detect invasive malignancy.

MALIGNANT MELANOMA

This anal tumour is extremely rare. It presents as a pigmented lump, with bleeding and fluid discharge. The results of surgery are often so poor that many feel a palliative local excision is preferable to radical excision.

LYMPHOMA

Lymphoma can arise in the anal region, usually as part of a generalized disease. More recently, it has been described as a complication of AIDS.[288]

KAPOSI'S SARCOMA

Kaposi's sarcoma is now recognized as another complication of AIDS[289] and can cause rectal bleeding. Kaposi's sarcoma appears dark red and slightly raised. Histology shows the typical haemangiomatous changes.

FUNCTIONAL DISORDERS OF THE LARGE BOWEL AND PELVIC FLOOR

There are a number of conditions in which symptoms arise from failure of rectal function. These include certain forms of constipation and diarrhoea. Abnormalities in intestinal transit or rectal capacitance are demonstrable in these patients. Abnormalities of the pelvic floor can cause incontinence, difficulty in evacuation, perineal discomfort and pain. Conditions encompassed by the term *functional disorders* are common, and the physiological mechanisms that are responsible are largely unknown.

TECHNIQUES OF INVESTIGATION

COLORECTUM

Intestinal transit time can be estimated by following the passage of a known number of ingested radiopaque markers by plain radiographs. Delay is diagnosed when more than 80% of the markers are still present in the bowel after 5 days.[290] Dynamic evacuating proctography is used to video the rectum during defecation after instillation of barium paste. The rate of emptying, the presence of internal prolapse, pelvic floor descent and spasm, and the size of the anorectal angle can be estimated by this method (Fig. 28.32).

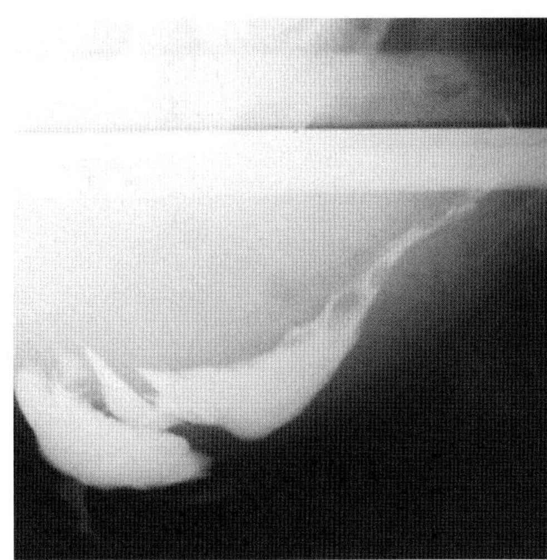

Figure 28.32 Defecating proctogram, lateral view. The coccyx can be seen to the right, highlighting the gross perineal descent during straining.

PELVIC FLOOR

The levator muscles support the abdominal contents while the puborectalis is responsible for maintaining the anorectal angle at about 90°. The external sphincter contributes to anal canal closure. Branches of the sacral plexus from segments S2 to S4 supply levator ani, the puborectalis and the external anal sphincter. The internal sphincter, which is the splanchnic component, lies concentrically within the external sphincter and is continuous above with the circular smooth muscle of the rectum. The somatic component is in a constant state of tonic contraction maintained by muscle sphincter reflex activity.[291] The anal tone can be increased by voluntary contraction and sudden rises in intra-abdominal pressure, and is inhibited during defecation.[292,293] The internal sphincter is in a state of maximal contraction at rest and relaxes during defecation. Rectal distension produces a reflex relaxation of the internal sphincter, known as the rectosphincteric reflex.[294]

MANOMETRY

A balloon probe, an open-tip tube, or a pressure transducer connected to a suitable recording device can measure anal canal pressure.[295] Normal resting pressure is 50–100 cm of water, 80% of which is derived from internal sphincter activity.[296] On voluntary contraction, the anal pressure increases by 60–120 cm of water, as the result of external sphincter activity. A low resting anal pressure suggests internal sphincter weakness. A low voluntary contraction pressure indicates a weak external sphincter.

CHRONIC CONSTIPATION

Constipation is a symptom that is often treated with levity, yet undoubtedly there are patients with severe intractable constipation who warrant surgical attention. Some are subsequently found to be suffering from Hirschsprung's disease, while others have a megacolon demonstrated on radiological investigation. The remaining patients, with normal investigations, are the group most likely to be labelled as having a psychosomatic disorder, yet this is a group in which surgery may occasionally have a role. The label *idiopathic slow-transit constipation* has been used if all defined causes of constipation have been excluded and the symptoms continue despite an adequate high-fibre diet.[297]

REFERENCES

288. Burkes RL, Meyer PR et al. Arch Intern Med 1986; 146: 913
289. Stern JO, Deilerich D et al. Gastroenterology 1982; 82: 118
290. Hinton JM, Lennard-Jones JE, Young AC. Gut 1969; 10: 842–847
291. Floyd WF, Walls EW. J Physiol Lond 1953; 122: 599–609
292. Parks AG, Porter NH, Melzack J. Dis Colon Rectum 1962; 5: 407–414
293. Porter NH. Ann R Coll Surg Engl 1962; 31: 379–404
294. Gowers WR. Proc R Soc (Lond) 1877; 26: 77–84
295. Miller R, Bartolo DCC et al. Br J Surg 1988; 75: 40–43
296. Bennett RC, Duthie HL. Br J Surg 1964; 51: 335–357
297. Hinton JM, Lennard-Jones JE, Young AC. Gut 1969; 10: 842–847

Typically the patient is a young adult woman. Some can trace their symptoms back to childhood, while others remember that symptoms started at puberty or following a hysterectomy. Bowel evacuation without strong laxatives is often very infrequent, perhaps once every several weeks. In addition, the patient may complain of abdominal discomfort and bloating.

Initially, treatment should consist of the regular use of osmotic laxatives such as magnesium sulphate. Patients whose quality of life remains significantly affected by their symptoms should be offered a total colectomy and ileorectal anastomosis. This results in a marked improvement of constipation in 60–70%, but in the remainder diarrhoea may occur and the abdominal pain and bloating are not relieved.[298]

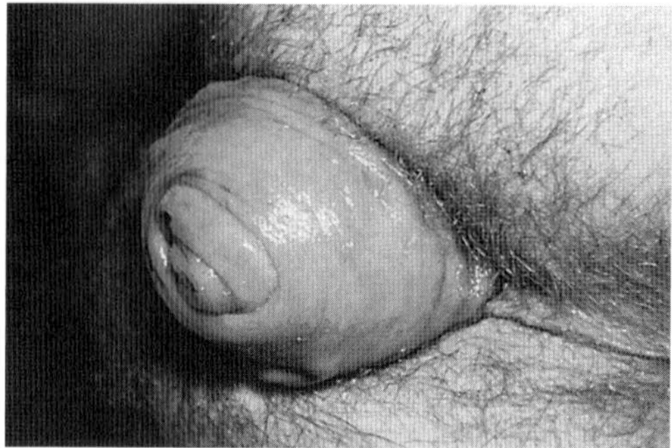

Figure 28.33 Full-thickness rectal prolapse.

RECTAL PROLAPSE

COMPLETE RECTAL PROLAPSE

There is an increased incidence of prolapse in infancy and in those over the age of 75 years. In old age, women are affected 20 times more often than men.[299] Predisposing factors include increased rectal and colonic mobility, and weakness of the pelvic floor musculature. Progressive neuropathic pelvic floor weakness is a normal process occurring after the age of 65 years but may also result from obstetric injury and possibly from chronic straining.[300]

Often patients with prolapse give a history of long-standing chronic constipation. Some, particularly in the younger age group, have learning difficulties or personality disorders[301] and are prone to episodes of faecal impaction. There is an association between rectal prolapse and the solitary ulcer syndrome, in which difficulty in defecation and straining are major aetiological factors.[302] The apex of the prolapse may become ulcerated, and mucus production from the irritated mucosa is increased. Usually the prolapse reduces spontaneously, but it can occasionally become incarcerated, when strangulation and gangrene may develop.

Clinical features

In infants, the prolapse is usually noticed by the parent and may be accompanied by the passage of blood and mucus. Prolapse in infants can be distinguished on digital examination from intussusception, in which the finger enters the rectum lateral to the intussuscipiens. Adults complain of the presence of the prolapsing mass itself, the passage of blood and mucus, and faecal incontinence (Fig. 28.33). The prolapse may descend only during defecation and reduce spontaneously afterwards, but in more severe cases it occurs on standing or walking, and sometimes it is permanently present. About half the patients have some degree of faecal incontinence; this is more common in the older patient.[303–305] Often it is necessary to ask the patient to strain down to demonstrate the prolapse.

Treatment

Correct bowel training can almost always treat infants successfully. The parent should pot the child regularly for short periods, and a mild laxative may be prescribed to avoid straining. The prolapse should be digitally replaced when it occurs. In a few children where this management fails, submucous injection of a sclerosant such as phenol in arachis oil may be effective.

In adults rectal prolapse should be treated surgically. Operations for rectal prolapse include simple excision of the protruding bowel, improvement of the anal sphincter mechanism, or fixation of the rectum. Rectosigmoidectomy is the best example of the first.[306] The prolapse is delivered and excised via a perineal approach. The bowel is anastomosed outside the anus before being reduced. Delorme's procedure is similar, but only the mucosa of the prolapse is resected. The operation is well tolerated even by the frailest patient. Recurrence may occur but the operation can be repeated. Combined rectosigmoidectomy with pelvic floor repair has a low recurrence rate.[301,307] Abdominal rectopexy involves mobilization of the rectum followed by fixation. Many methods of fixation have been described, and it is increasingly performed laparoscopically. Some use an implant of foreign material, for example polyvinyl alcohol (Ivalon sponge), polypropylene (Marlex) or polyfluorine (Teflon®) to provoke fibrosis around the rectum (Fig. 28.34). Infection of the implant is rare (less than 5%), but it is a serious complication and antibiotic cover is obligatory. Recurrence rates of around 5% have been reported.

PARTIAL (MUCOSAL) PROLAPSE

Mucosal prolapse of the lower rectum may be overt, when it emerges from the anus, or it may be occult, when it is only detectable by proctoscopy. As a result, the condition is often associated with prolapsing haemorrhoids and also with abnormal perineal descent and uterine prolapse in women.

Clinical features

The symptoms include bleeding, a protruding swelling, pruritus ani, anal discomfort and mucus leakage. The discomfort is often described as heaviness in the perineum, similar to a feeling of incomplete evacuation. Some patients admit to straining at stool,

REFERENCES

298. Kamm MA. Int J Colorectal Dis 1987; 4: 229
299. Kupfer CA, Goligher JC. Br J Surg 1970; 57: 34
300. Snooks SJ, Swash M et al. Lancet 1984; ii: 546–555
301. Altemeier WA, Cuthbertson WR et al. Ann Surg 1971; 173: 993–1006
302. Kennedy DK, Hughes ESR, Masterton JP. Surg Gynecol Obstet 1977; 144: 718–720
303. Morgan CN, Porter NH, Klugman DJ. Br J Surg 1972; 59: 841
304. Holmstrom B, Ahlberg J et al. Acta Chir Scand 1978; 482 (Suppl): 51
305. Keighley MRB, Fielding JWL, Alexander-Williams J. Br J Surg 1983; 70: 229–232
306. Gabriel WB. The Principles and Practice of Rectal Surgery. 4th edn. HK Lewis, London, 1948
307. Watts JD, Rothenberger DA et al. Dis Colon Rectum 1985; 28: 96–102

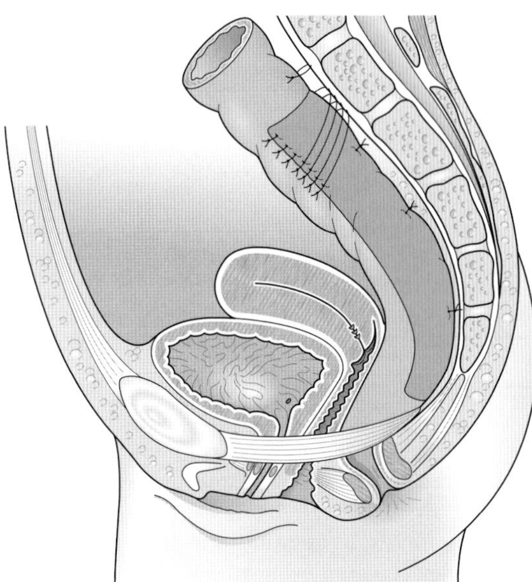

Figure 28.34 Wells' operation or Ivalon rectopexy.

and there may be an evacuation disorder in these cases. The prolapse may be seen on direct inspection of the perineum but is more likely to be evident on proctoscopy. The prolapsing mucosa may be reddened and is occasionally ulcerated. Anal sphincter weakness and perineal descent are present in many cases, as are haemorrhoids.

Treatment

The treatment involves correction of associated constipation by laxatives or suppositories. The nature of the condition should be explained to the patient, who should be advised against straining. Injection or rubber band ligation of the prolapse may improve the symptoms of bleeding and mucus discharge.

SOLITARY ULCER SYNDROME

This rare condition most commonly affects young adults, although the age range extends from childhood to old age. The peak incidence occurs in the third to fourth decades of life. There is clinical, radiological and histological evidence to link the solitary ulcer syndrome with rectal prolapse. Both complete and mucosal rectal prolapse have been reported to occur in 16–60% of patients with a solitary ulcer.[308–310] Proctographic studies have demonstrated a rectal intussusception to be a common finding (between 70% and 58%) in patients with a solitary ulcer syndrome.[311,312] The aetiology of the condition remains unknown. There is undoubtedly a disorder of defecation that leads to a vicious cycle of straining, producing internal prolapse and further difficulty in defecation, leading on to further straining.

Almost all patients complain of bleeding (more than 90%) and the passage of mucus (70–90%). Some also have pain (20%), and many report episodes of incontinence (57%). One of the most notable symptoms, however, is that of difficulty with evacuation, which on detailed questioning may have preceded the other symptoms.

The term *solitary ulcer* is inaccurate, because the pathological abnormalities may be multiple[308,309] and ulceration is not always present. Redness and oedema of the mucosa, varying in length from a few millimetres to several centimetres, are present in all cases and may be the only physical sign in about 20%. In over half, however, frank ulceration occurs, and in a further 20% the mucosa is elevated to give a polypoid appearance, which is easily mistaken for a carcinoma. The majority (more than 60%) of ulcers lie anteriorly at 7–10 cm from the anal verge, often on the fold of a valve of Houston.

Conservative treatment includes the prescription of laxatives and advice to avoid straining. Biofeedback defecation retraining can lead to symptomatic relief. Abdominal rectopexy may be necessary when conservative measures have failed, and are associated with long-term improvement in approximately half of patients affected.[313]

FAECAL INCONTINENCE

Anal incontinence is defined as the involuntary loss of control of flatus or faeces. It can be subdivided into three orders of severity: incontinence to flatus only, to fluid faeces, and to solid faeces. Continence depends on the competence of the anal sphincter mechanism. This serves two main functions: first, the maintenance of the anorectal angle at rest by the forward pull of the puborectalis; and second, closure of the anal canal by the combined action of the internal and external anal sphincters. There may be a sensory component dependent on sensory receptors in the upper anal canal mucosa, which influence external sphincter activity when stimulated by contact with faeces in the rectum.[314]

Defecation involves propulsive activity of the left colon. Incontinence can occur when propulsive activity is excessive, when rectal capacitance is reduced (e.g. by inflammation),[315] or when rectal sensation is diminished.[316]

AETIOLOGY

The causes of incontinence are listed in Box 28.3. Diarrhoea associated with urgency is common and may cause incontinence even in the presence of a normal pelvic floor. The anal sphincter mechanism may be weak as the result of neurological diseases such as multiple sclerosis, cauda equina lesions, and denervation of the somatic pelvic floor, which occurs with ageing.[317] Physiological changes indicative of transient denervation have been demonstrated in the immediate postpartum period after vaginal delivery.[318] Studies using anal ultrasound have shown an alarming incidence of occult and more obvious injuries to both the external and internal anal sphincters as a result of obstetric

REFERENCES

308. Madigan MR, Morson BC. Gut 1969; 10: 871–881
309. Martin CJ, Parks TG, Biggart JD. Br J Surg 1981; 68: 744–757
310. Schweiger M, Alexander-Williams J. Lancet 1977; i: 70–71
311. Mahieu PHG. Int J Colorectal Dis 1986; 1: 85–90
312. Kuijpers HC, Schreve RH, Hoedemakers H. Dis Colon Rectum 1986; 29: 126–129
313. Vaizey CJ, van den Bogaerde JB et al. Br J Surg 1998; 85: 1617–1623
314. Miller R, Bartolo DCC et al. Br J Surg 1988; 75: 44–47
315. Varma JS, Smith AN, Bussutil A. Br J Surg 1985; 72: 875–878
316. Goligher JC, Hughes ESR. Lancet 1951; i: 543–548
317. Neill ME, Parks AG, Swash M. Br J Surg 1981; 68: 531–536
318. Snooks SJ, Swash M et al. Lancet 1984; ii: 546–550

Box 28.3 Causes of incontinence

Diarrhoea
- Inflammatory bowel disease
- Functional bowel disease

Neurological
- General neurological diseases (e.g. multiple sclerosis)
- Dementia
- Age
- Spinal trauma (cauda equina lesion)
- Pudendal nerve neuropathy
- Faecal impaction

Mechanical
- Sphincter ring disruption
- Trauma
- Congenital
- Fistula
- Extrarectal
- Rectovaginal

trauma, and many third-degree tears are probably inadequately repaired.[319]

A similar weakness of the sphincter occurs in patients with rectal prolapse,[317] which may itself be responsible for stretching of the sphincter.[320] The sphincter may be damaged by direct trauma, most commonly after surgery for anal fistula. In cases of faecal impaction, rectal distension produces reflex relaxation of the internal sphincter, leading to faecal leakage. Incontinence may also be associated with dementia.

CLINICAL FEATURES

The severity and frequency of incontinence, including the amount lost on each occasion, must be determined from the history. It is also important to ascertain whether the stool is liquid, semiformed or solid. Any previous anal operations, radiotherapy, and spinal or perineal trauma must be documented, and a full obstetric history taken, including details of the duration of labour, forceps delivery and tears.

Inspection and palpation of the anal canal can determine an obvious reduction in the resting anal tone or an inability to sustain a voluntary contraction, and this may also determine whether the weakness is diffuse or whether it is localized to a specific point in the sphincter ring, indicating trauma. Anorectal functional tests, including manometry and electromyography, give an objective assessment of anal canal pressure and the presence and severity of any neuropathic changes. Anal ultrasound is a good technique for demonstrating structural abnormalities in the sphincters.

TREATMENT

The cause of any diarrhoea should be treated. The patient should start a low-fibre diet and, if necessary, add in constipating agents such as loperamide. Suppositories or enemas may be helpful. Conservative treatment often improves the patient's symptoms and surgery is not required. Conditions resulting in persistent debilitating symptoms that do not resolve with conservative measures should be treated surgically. Localized trauma to the sphincter ring can be treated by identification of the divided ends of the muscle, and then repaired using an overlapping technique (Fig. 28.35). Seventy-five per cent of a series of 97 patients were rendered continent by this procedure.[321]

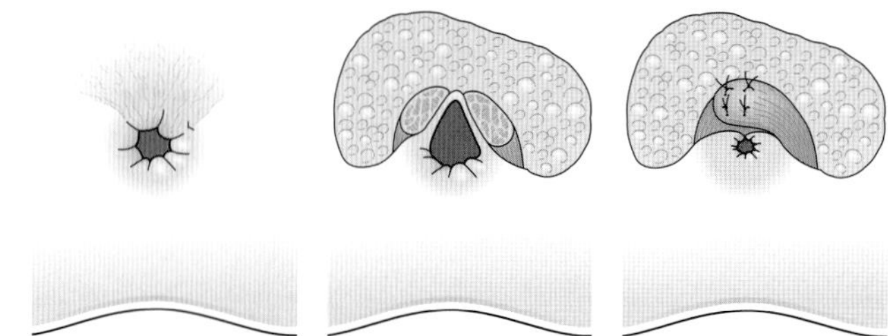

Figure 28.35 Anal sphincter repair.

Treatment of patients with pudendal neuropathy depends on the severity of the incontinence. Mild incontinence often associated with a loose stool is treated conservatively. Biofeedback techniques have been reported to improve up to 90% of patients treated by this method.[322] More severely affected patients require surgery. Postanal repair attempts to re-establish the anorectal angle and lengthens the anal canal,[323] but is now infrequently performed. Other operations for incontinence include the gracilis sling procedure,[324] in which the gracilis muscle tendon is placed around the anal canal and sutured to the contralateral ischial tuberosity.[325] The muscle tone of the gracilis may be maintained postoperatively by long-term electrical stimulation of the muscle by an implanted electrode and power unit.[326] The artificial bowel sphincter employs a plastic balloon device that encircles the anal canal and, when inflated, closes the anus.[327] In cases where surgical repair fails, a colostomy may be the final resort.

REFERENCES

319. Sultan AH, Kamm M et al. Br J Surg 1994; 81: 463–465
320. Broden G, Dolk A, Holmstrom B. Int J Colorectal Dis 1988; 3: 23–28
321. Browning GGP, Motson RW. Br Med J 1983; 28: 1873–1875
322. Cerulli MA, Nikoomanesh P, Schuster MM. Gastroenterology 1979; 76: 742–746
323. Parks AG. Proc R Soc Med 1975; 68: 681–690
324. Pickrell LE. Ann Surg 1952; 135: 853–859
325. Corman ML. Dis Colon Rectum 1980; 23: 552–555
326. Williams NS, Hallan RI et al. Br J Surg 1989; 76: 1191
327. Vaizey CJ, Kamm MA. Lancet 1998; 352: 105–109

The liver and portal circulation

29

Jake E. J. Krige, Stephen J. Beningfield, Philippus C. Bornman

ANATOMY

Surgery of the liver and portal circulation is based on a clear understanding of the detailed anatomy of the liver, and its arterial and portal blood supply, as well as the biliary and venous drainage. Overlap with details of biliary anatomy covered in Chapter 30 is inevitable.

The obvious surface markings of the liver that divide it into the anatomical right and left lobes conceal a functional system of liver segments divided vertically by the scissurae demarcated by the planes of the right, middle and left hepatic veins. Within each of the resulting four liver sectors there is a segmental arrangement defined by the portal and arterial blood supply. This system of eight structurally and functionally independent liver segments has now been universally accepted (Fig. 29.1). Segment I (caudate lobe) lies posteriorly, between the fissure for ligamentum venosum and the inferior vena cava. Segments II and III lie to the left of the left-most vertical hepatic scissura and are separated by the horizontal scissura, with segment II lying superiorly and segment III inferiorly. Segment IV (quadrate lobe) lies between the left and middle hepatic scissurae, and is subdivided into segments IVa (superior) and IVb (inferior) by the horizontal scissura. Segments V and VIII lie between the middle and right hepatic scissura, with segments VI and VII lateral to the right vertical hepatic scissura. Segments VII and VIII lie superiorly, separated from segments V and VI by the horizontal scissura.

Major resections of the liver are possible provided that whole segments are left intact with their associated blood supply, biliary apparatus and venous drainage. Identification of segmental anatomy is essential in patients with focal lesions being considered for surgery, because this aids planning of liver resections. Accurate localization of individual lesions by preoperative imaging and intraoperative ultrasound may allow segmental anatomical resections that reduce blood loss and loss of hepatic functional reserve. Although the size of the liver segments is variable, there is little variation in their arrangement.[2] This is not true of the biliary tree, particularly around the region of the confluence of the main segmental hepatic ducts, and knowledge of these variations is important during major liver and biliary surgery.[3]

The venous drainage of the liver comprises three main hepatic veins that drain into the suprahepatic inferior vena cava, and smaller accessory hepatic veins that drain into the retrohepatic vena cava. The right hepatic vein is single in 90% of cases.[4] The middle hepatic vein runs in the principal portal fissure and forms a common trunk with the left hepatic vein in 85% of cases. The left hepatic vein arises from the confluence of a transverse vein that drains segment II, and a sagittal vein that drains segment III and has contributions from segment IV.[5]

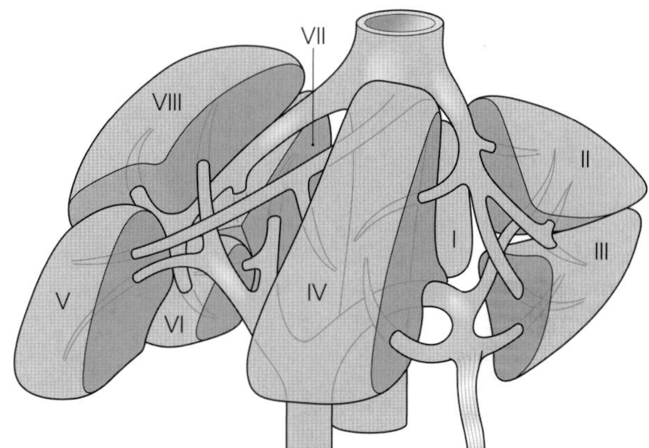

a

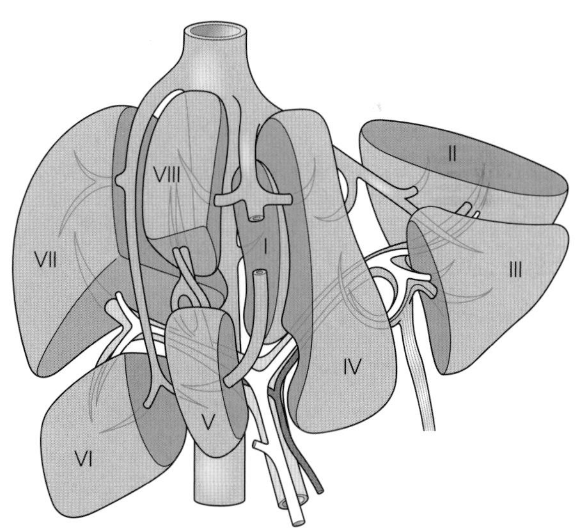

b

Figure 29.1 Functional division of the liver and liver segments according to Couinaud's nomenclature: **(a)** as seen in the patient, **(b)** in the ex vivo position. (From Blumgart and Fong 2000,[1] with permission.)

REFERENCES

1. Blumgart LH, Fong Y (eds). Surgery of the Liver and Biliary Tract. 3rd edn. WB Saunders, Baltimore, 2000
2. Bismuth H, Houssain D, Castaing D. World J Surg 1982; 6: 10–24
3. Deshpande RR, Heaton ND, Rela M. Br J Surg 2002; 89: 1078–1088
4. Nakamura S, Tsuzuki T. Surg Gynecol Obstet 1981; 152: 43–50
5. Delattre JF, Avisse C, Flament JB. Surg Clin North Am 2000; 80: 345–362

Important variations in hepatic venous drainage can affect liver resection. Short accessory right hepatic veins from segments VI and VII drain directly into the retrohepatic vena cava. A prominent inferior right hepatic vein that drains directly into the vena cava via a very short trunk from the posterior aspect of segment VI may be present. In some patients it may be possible to isolate a sufficient length of right hepatic vein between the liver and vena cava to allow separate control of this vessel during resection of the right lobe of the liver. More frequently, the entire length of the hepatic vein is within the liver, which may preclude early, safe hepatic venous isolation during hepatic resection. The hepatic veins have fragile, thin walls, and inadvertent injury may result in major bleeding and considerable difficulty in isolating and controlling the injury. The junction between the left and middle hepatic veins and the inferior vena cava is not constant and must be carefully defined during left lobe resections. The caudate lobe (segment I) drains directly into the vena cava through a variable number of short veins.

The portal vein divides at the hepatic hilum into right and left pedicles on which the right and left lobes of the liver are based. A theoretical plane through the main portal fissure separates the two lobes.[5] The right portal vein, the shorter of the two, lies anterior to the caudate process and enters the liver through the hilar plate to divide into anterior and posterior branches. The anterior branch divides into segments VIII and V. The posterior branch supplies segments VII and VI. The left portal vein is longer than the right, and runs transversely in the hilum and then superiorly in the base of the umbilical fissure to supply segments II, III and IV, and the caudate lobe.[6] The anatomy of the left portal venous system is remarkably constant.

The common hepatic artery, usually a branch of the coeliac trunk but occasionally arising from the superior mesenteric artery, supplies the liver with arterial blood through its right and left hepatic branches. Accessory hepatic arteries arising from the left gastric artery are frequently present.[7] The common hepatic artery may divide into its terminal branches anywhere between its origin and the hilum of the liver, but usually arises to the left of the hilum. The right hepatic artery passes behind the common bile duct and right hepatic duct to enter the liver parenchyma. The left hepatic artery runs along the inferior margin of the quadrate lobe with the left hepatic duct and left portal vein, before entering the left lobe in the umbilical fissure.

LIVER PHYSIOLOGY

The liver has a key role in the metabolism of carbohydrates, lipids, proteins and vitamins. It produces bile, has an important role in the detoxification of both exogenous and endogenous blood-borne substances, and has an important immune function through the reticuloendothelial system of Kupffer cells. There is no single comprehensive test of liver function and the term *liver function tests* covers a wide variety of investigations used for different purposes. The most commonly performed blood tests include the serum bilirubin, a measure of conjugation and excretion of bile pigment; alkaline phosphatase, an enzyme associated with cholestasis; and the transaminases, alanine aminotransferase (ALT) and aspartate aminotransferase (AST), which are elevated by liver cell injury. Gamma-glutamyl transpeptidase (or gamma-glutamyl transferase, GGT) provides a sensitive measure of enzyme induction, including that associated with alcohol abuse. Albumin concentration is a measure of hepatocellular protein synthesis, as is the prothrombin time. These tests give a broad assessment of underlying liver pathology, and are also used in gallbladder disorders (see Ch. 30).

Jaundice becomes clinically apparent when plasma bilirubin exceeds 50 μmol/L, which is three times the upper limit of normal. Routine bilirubin levels reflect total bilirubin, but in some circumstances it is useful to measure conjugated and unconjugated bilirubin separately.[5] Unconjugated hyperbilirubinaemia is caused by an overproduction of bilirubin, usually as a result of haemolytic diseases such as congenital spherocytosis. It may also be caused by decreased hepatocyte uptake in sepsis or decreased conjugation caused by drug reactions, jaundice of prematurity, cirrhosis, hepatitis or Gilbert's syndrome. An increase in conjugated bilirubin may be the result of decreased biliary secretion caused by drug reactions, cirrhosis, hepatitis, cholestasis of pregnancy or Dubin–Johnson syndrome, but more often is the result of biliary obstruction. Excess conjugated bilirubin in the urine, resulting from extra- or intrahepatic biliary obstruction, produces the dark urine and pale stool of obstructive jaundice. In contrast, excessive urobilinogen in the urine implies an increased load or failure of extraction.

An increase in the serum alkaline phosphatase in hepatobiliary disease is a sensitive marker of biliary obstruction and is also elevated in patients with space-occupying lesions in the liver. Activity of GGT is induced by a variety of drugs, including ethanol, and may be markedly elevated even after a single episode of excessive alcohol intake. In combination with raised transaminase levels and increased mean corpuscular volume, it is a sensitive although non-specific indicator of chronic alcohol abuse. Less commonly used is 5′-nucleotidase, which is more specific than alkaline phosphatase in detecting liver disease.

Some elevation of the liver enzymes is found in almost all forms of liver disease. Both AST and ALT are significantly elevated in the presence of hepatocyte necrosis, although there is no direct relationship with the degree of functional liver impairment. High values of AST and ALT are found in acute hepatitis, but high levels without a raised alkaline phosphatase suggest a hepatocellular rather than an obstructive cause for jaundice.

Albumin is one of the most important plasma proteins produced by the liver. Patients with cirrhosis and ascites frequently have low plasma albumin levels. Albumin levels are affected not only by liver disease but also by nutrition, osmotic pressure, acute-phase reaction stimuli and alcohol. Thus the serum albumin concentration per se is not an accurate prognostic indicator in liver disease, although it is a useful component of the Child–Pugh scoring system.

The liver is the major synthetic site for all coagulation proteins except von Willebrand factor. The synthesis of factors II, VII, VIII and X is dependent on normal liver function and on adequate vitamin K levels. Because vitamin K is fat-soluble, deficiency develops in the presence of biliary obstruction with fat malabsorption. The prothrombin time must always be checked before invasive procedures are undertaken in patients with suspected liver disease. Parenteral administration of vitamin K usually corrects deficiencies caused by biliary obstruction but is not effective in patients with prolonged or severe hepatocellular

REFERENCES

6. Ger R. Surg Clin North Am 1989; 69: 179–192
7. Michels NA. Am J Surg 1966; 112: 337–347

disease, in whom fresh frozen plasma or cryoprecipitate should be given.

The tests described above are static indicators of individual components of liver function. More sensitive information may be obtained by quantitative or semiquantitative dynamic tests, including antipyrine, aminopyrine, lidocaine (lignocaine) and galactose clearance tests. Arterial ammonia levels are sometimes measured in patients with suspected liver failure and portal systemic encephalopathy. The indocyanine green dye clearance test is used in some specialist units to predict complications after hepatic resection and rejection after liver transplantation.

Specific tests for liver disease include screening for hepatitis A, B and C. Antimitochondrial, smooth muscle and antinuclear antibodies are used to investigate suspected primary biliary cirrhosis and autoimmune chronic active hepatitis. Iron, iron-binding capacity and serum ferritin are used in the diagnosis of haemochromatosis. Caeruloplasmin and urinary copper levels are used to diagnose Wilson's disease. The enzyme α_1-antitrypsin is measured when a deficiency is suspected. Specific markers for neoplasms include alpha-fetoprotein and carcinoembryonic antigen levels. Infectious serological markers include cytomegalovirus and Epstein–Barr virus antibodies, leptospiral agglutination tests, and amoebic and hydatid complement fixation tests.

SCORING SYSTEMS IN LIVER DISEASE

Scoring systems have been used to monitor the progression of conditions such as primary biliary cirrhosis and sclerosing cholangitis, and to predict the need for and timing of transplantation. The most commonly used is the Child grading system, modified by Pugh (Table 29.1)[8] Originally designed to predict mortality and encephalopathy following portal–systemic shunting, it has been extended to grade liver function and to assess risk in patients with liver disease.

DIAGNOSIS OF LIVER DISEASE

The clinical history, physical examination, urine investigation, and stool and haematology tests are important, and combined with the liver biochemical tests and radiographic imaging allow an initial differential diagnosis as well as triage and supplementary investigations.

Details of any anorexia, nausea, jaundice, pruritus, fever and pain, as well as previous operations, drug use (especially alcohol), toxins and exposure to infection should be sought. Fever and pain are common in alcoholic hepatitis; rigors and sudden severe pain suggest cholangitis. Relentless progression of jaundice with weight loss, pruritus and pale stools points to malignant extrahepatic obstruction. Prior biliary surgery directs attention to the bile duct (see Ch. 30). Transfusion, injections, polypharmacy, promiscuity, contact with dialysis patients or jaundiced persons, intravenous drug use and tattooing raise the possibility of hepatitis.

Stigmata of chronic liver disease, including palmar erythema, spider naevi, finger clubbing, white nails, gynaecomastia, muscle wasting, spontaneous bruising and scratch marks from pruritus, should be specifically sought. Skin bruising may be present, reflecting the clotting defects characteristic of vitamin K deficiency in severe liver disease. Testicular atrophy, gynaecomastia, parotid enlargement and Dupuytren's contracture suggest an alcoholic aetiology. Intellectual deterioration, flapping tremor and foetor hepaticus indicate marked liver decompensation. Liver size, consistency and tenderness should be noted. Greater enlargement tends to occur with extrahepatic biliary obstruction. Jaundice and a palpable gallbladder suggest periampullary cancer (Courvoisier's law). A cirrhotic liver may be large, medium-sized or small, with blunt, lobulated and firm edges. A liver with hepatocellular cancer is often large, hard and nodular. A systolic bruit over the liver may indicate hepatocellular cancer or alcoholic hepatitis. Dilated abdominal wall veins draining away from the umbilicus signify portal hypertension. Splenomegaly and ascites are other indicators of portal hypertension.

Table 29.1 Child–Pugh grading system for liver disease

Variable	Number of points 1	2	3
Bilirubin (μmol/L)	< 34	34–51	> 51
Albumin (g/L)	> 35	28–35	< 28
Prothrombin time	< 3	3–10	> 10
Ascites	None	Mild	Moderate to severe
Encephalopathy	None	Mild	Moderate to severe

Grade A, 5 or 6 points; grade B, 7–9 points; and grade C, 10–15 points.

IMAGING

X-rays

Liver size may be indicated by bowel displacement. Calcification in gallstones (10–15%) and chronic pancreatitis or mass effects of tumours, or hydatid cysts can sometimes be seen. Gas in intrahepatic bile ducts or abscess cavities (Fig. 29.2) can aid in diagnosis.

Ultrasound

Ultrasound is the first-line radiological test used for hepatobiliary disease, especially jaundice. It is quick, cheap and patient-friendly, and can be used to guide invasive procedures such as drainage of fluid collections and biopsies. Intrahepatic duct dilatation is usually indicative of biliary obstruction; ultrasound establishes the presence and level of biliary obstruction in over 90% of cases, and is less expensive than CT. Parenchymal liver disease or sclerosing cholangitis may prevent biliary dilatation, and obesity and bowel gas can limit visibility. Use in the intensive care unit and in theatre extends its role. Duplex Doppler combines greyscale ultrasound images with Doppler to evaluate blood flow in vessels, tumours and shunts.

Computerized tomography scanning

Computerized tomography scanning is extremely helpful in evaluating liver disease and masses, often complementing ultrasound (Fig. 29.3). Spiral CT allows the rapid acquisition of high-quality images during various intravenous contrast

REFERENCES

8. Pugh RNH, Murray-Lyon IM, Dawson JL et al. Br J Surg 1973; 60: 646–649

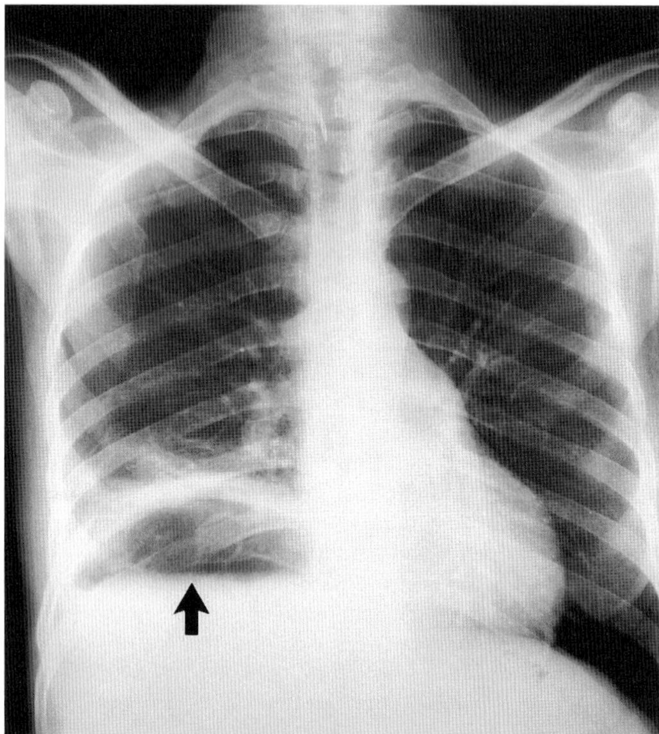

Figure 29.2 Chest radiograph showing a large air–fluid level (arrow) in a right lobe liver abscess.

phases. Lipiodol™, an iodized oil suspension, has some value in detecting small primary hepatocellular carcinomas.

Magnetic resonance imaging

The MRI technique images hydrogen nuclei in water using magnetic fields and radiowaves. Different sequences may provide valuable information for evaluating the nature of liver tumours.

Biliary imaging

Endoscopic retrograde cholangiopancreatography and percutaneous transhepatic cholangiography can both be used to depict biliary strictures, tumours or calculi (see Ch. 30).

Hepatic angiography

Hepatic angiography is particularly useful before liver resection. Arterial portography with digital subtraction angiography can be used in patients with portal hypertension.

Arterial embolization

Selective transcatheter arterial embolic occlusion with a variety of materials including metal coils and gelfoam sponge can used to treat arterial injuries. Shrinkage of tumours by occlusion or chemo-embolisation of the arterial blood supply is also used in selected cases. Transhepatic portal venous embolization is used to produce atrophy of a liver lobe and allow hypertrophy of the remaining liver before resection.

Isotope scanning

Nuclear medicine studies may be of value in diagnosing certain liver masses and the causes of postoperative jaundice, and in evaluating the success of biliary drainage procedures. Positron emission tomography is a new investigation that may enable better detection of hepatic primary and secondary tumours, by means of the increased glucose metabolism in neoplasms.

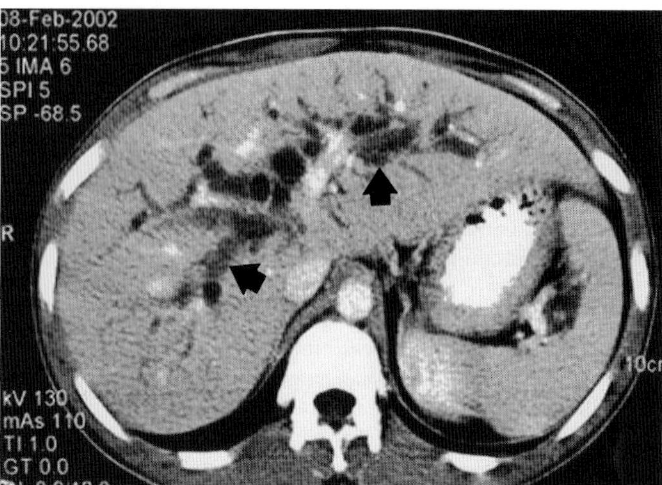

Figure 29.3 A CT scan showing dilated intrahepatic ducts (arrows) due to extrahepatic biliary obstruction.

ASSESSMENT OF A LIVER MASS

This common problem merits separate consideration. The objectives in assessing a liver mass are:

- to establish a likely diagnosis;
- to determine whether surgery or alternative treatment are indicated; and
- to judge whether resection is possible (i.e. the extent of the lesion and its relation to vascular and biliary structures).

The importance of a careful history and examination has already been emphasized. Particular attention is given to details of previous surgery, malignancy or liver disease. The clinical features of the mass should be assessed. Large right adrenal, kidney or pancreatic tumours may mimic liver tumours. Liver function tests and serum tumour markers (alpha-fetoprotein, carcinoembryonic antigen and CA 19-9) should be obtained if a liver mass is suspected. Gastrointestinal hormones and urinary 5-hydroxyindoleacetic acid for carcinoid tumours are measured when appropriate. Patients with primary fibrolamellar liver tumours often do not express alpha-fetoprotein, but the presence of neurotensin and an elevated vitamin B_{12}-binding capacity in the serum are relatively specific for this type of tumour. Rapid recourse to percutaneous biopsy of a liver mass without careful diagnostic evaluation and planning of possible treatment is often inappropriate, may be dangerous, and is often not necessary.

IMAGING

Radiological imaging is the main method of diagnosing focal liver lesions (Table 29.2). Various algorithmic approaches have been described, all starting with an ultrasound scan (Fig. 29.4). The initial questions to determine are whether lesions are single or multiple, solid or cystic. Cystic lesions of the liver are considered later in this chapter.

The solitary or potentially resectable liver 'tumour' is best evaluated by CT and, when appropriate, MRI scanning. Each of the benign and malignant tumour types has typical but seldom diagnostic appearances. The CT evaluation of the tumour appearance and behaviour during the various phases of contrast injection may be helpful. It should be possible to distinguish most cavernous haemangiomas from other tumours by this means, although some vascular tumours may create difficulty. It is important to remember that chest radiographs, and possibly CT

Table 29.2 Imaging methods for liver lesions

Lesion	Abdominal X-ray*	Ultrasound and duplex Doppler	CT†	MRI‡	Other§
Cysts					
Simple	Mass effect	Anechoic, rounded, well-defined	Low density, rounded, well defined	T1 dark, T2 bright (fluid signal)	Aspiration will not cure cysts
Hydatid	Mass effect, calcification	Membranes, daughter cysts, hydatid 'sand', calcification, multiple	Membranes, daughter cysts, hydatid 'sand', calcification , multiple loci, debris, complications	Fluid, membranes, daughter cysts	Can be treated percutaneously
Abscesses					
Amoebic	Mass effect, chest inflammatory changes	May be echogenic, mass-like, halo possible, slow resolution	Mixed or low density, adjacent inflammatory changes	Fluid, debris	Aspiration or drainage if indicated
Pyogenic	Gas may be present	Hypoechoic, gas bubbles, echogenic fluid	Fluid density, debris, gas	Rounded, fluid, debris, gas	Aspiration, drainage
Fungal	None	Small target lesions, splenic	Small target lesions, splenic	Rounded, fluid	Diagnostic aspiration
Tumours					
Cavernous haemangioma	Mass effect	Echogenic if small, mixed/not homogenous if large with thrombosis or fibrosis	Well-defined, rounded, low-density, possible central thrombosed or fibrosed portions, peripheral nodular enhancement with isodense fill-in after i.v. contrast	Bright T2 'light bulb', contrast behaviour as for CT	Red cell scan photopoenic area that fills in later, biopsy limited role
Focal nodal hyperplasia	None, unless large	Difficult to see because similar to liver, possible scar	Isodense, transient, arterial-phase enhancement, possible enhancing scar	Similar to liver, T2 bright scar	Sulphur colloid, biopsy limited role
Hepatic adenoma	None, unless large	May be echogenic, mixed if haemorrage	Isodense or echogenic, mixed high density with haemorrhage	Usually similar to liver	May take up sulphur colloid, avoid biopsy because of bleeding risk
Malignant					
Hepatocellular carcinoma	Mass effect, calcification	Usually hypoechoic, may be mixed or poorly seen, portal vein invasion	Hypodense or mixed density, transiently enhancing, multiple nodules in or around lesion, portal vein invasion, Lipiodol™ CT may be helpful in Asian or western variations.	T2 bright, portal vein invasion, occasionally T1 bright due to fat	Biopsy only if irresectable; percutaneous treatment options
Fibrolamellar hepatocellular carcinoma	Mass effect	Central scar	Mild enhancement, calcification, nodes, non-enhancing scar	Scar T2 dark, non-enhancing	Serum markers (see text)
Cholangiocellular carcinoma	Mass effect if nodular type	Usually hypo- or isoechoic	May exhibit mild delayed enhancement	Mild enhancement	Biopsy limited role
Secondary (e.g. colorectal)	Mass effect	Usually hypoechoic	Usually hypodense, best seen during portal enhancement, occasionally cystic or fine calcification, some others hypervascular	T2 slightly bright, T1 slightly dark, usually poor enhancement	Biopsy limited role

*Chest X-ray, especially if inflammatory or malignant. †Use of i.v. contrast in different phases is important. ‡Most pathology T1 dark, T2 bright, reflecting water content. §Including nuclear medicine, lesions all photopoenic unless otherwise stated.

scans of the lungs, may avoid unnecessary investigations by demonstrating that the patient has metastatic disease, rendering further investigation and surgery futile.

Solid lesions that are multiple and bilobar are unlikely to be treated by liver resection and may reasonably be biopsied under ultrasound guidance, provided there are no other contraindications. Biopsy of a liver mass may be performed percutaneously with or without CT or ultrasound guidance, laparoscopically, or at laparotomy. The biopsy may be for cytology only (fine-needle aspiration) or for histology (larger-bore core biopsy).

Early biopsy of a solitary lesion, or of lesions likely to be resected, is not advised. Not only is there a risk of bleeding from vascular tumours, but tumour dissemination into the peritoneal cavity and along the needle track following percutaneous needle biopsy may occur.[9] Sampling and interpretational errors, and

REFERENCES

9. Quaghebeur G, Thompson JN, Blumgart LH et al. J R Coll Surg Edinb 1991; 36: 127

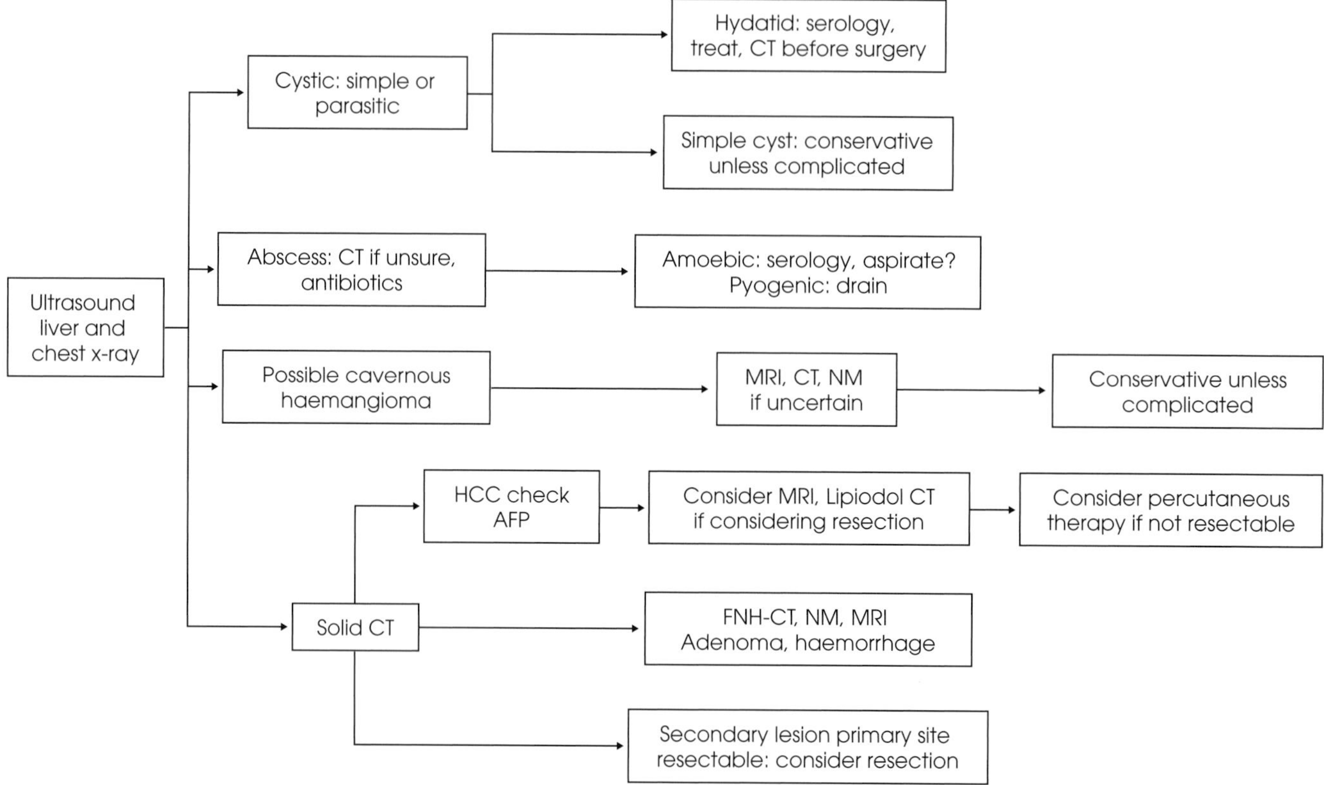

Figure 29.4 Algorithm for imaging a liver mass. NM, nuclear medicine; HCC, hepatocellular carcinoma; AFP, alpha fetoprotein; FNH, focal nodular hyperplasia.

infection, can also occur. Fine-needle aspiration cytology is safer, but is more difficult to interpret and has a higher false negative rate for diagnosing tumours.[10] Hypervascular masses, coagulopathy and ascites are contraindications to percutaneous core biopsy. Fine-needle aspiration biopsy is generally safe under these circumstances.

In the evaluation of any liver mass, percutaneous biopsy should be performed only if it can reasonably be expected to obviate the need for exploratory laparotomy. Most patients with symptomatic masses would be considered for laparotomy, making preoperative histology superfluous. However, biopsy of an irresectable primary or metastatic malignancy can spare the patient an unnecessary laparotomy. Laparoscopic biopsy can also be used to evaluate liver masses and to avoid laparotomy.

LIVER INJURIES

A third of patients undergoing laparotomy for abdominal trauma have liver injuries (see Ch. 7); road traffic accidents dominate as a cause in the UK and in Europe, while in the USA gunshot and stab wounds are more common.[11] The injuries range from inconsequential lacerations to lethal crush injuries and lacerations of the vena cava or hepatic veins.[12] Blunt trauma causes lacerations from shearing stresses; high-velocity and crush injuries cause marked liver fragmentation, lacerated vessels and massive intraperitoneal haemorrhage. Blunt injuries generally produce more severe damage with a higher mortality. Low-velocity injuries and stab wounds may cause bleeding without major devitalization.

CLASSIFICATION

The American Association for the Surgery of Trauma classification is the most widely used (Table 29.3). Classifying he differing degrees of haematoma or laceration are important. Mortality rates depend on the extent of the liver injury, the number of segments involved, and especially any associated vena caval or major hepatic vein injury.

DIAGNOSIS AND ASSESSMENT

The general principles of management are discussed in Chapter 7 and follow standard Advanced Trauma Life Support® (ATLS®) principles. A liver injury should be suspected in patients with evidence of blunt trauma or with knife or gunshot wounds in the right upper quadrant or epigastrium. Physical signs may be minimal. Gunshot entry and exit wounds can appear to be deceptively distant from the liver.

Major liver injury manifests with hypotension, tachycardia, decreased urine output, a low central venous pressure, and abdominal distension with guarding and tenderness. Altered

REFERENCES

10. Ferrucci JT, Wittenberg J, Mueller PR et al. Am J Roentgenol 1980; 134: 323–330
11. Terblanche J, Krige JEJ. In: Williamson RCN, Cooper MJ (eds). Emergency Abdominal Surgery. Clinical Surgery International, Vol 17. Churchill Livingstone, London, 1990: 21–35
12. Terblanche J, Krige JEJ. In: Bircher J, Benhamou J-P, McIntyre N et al (eds). Oxford Textbook of Clinical Hepatology. Oxford Medical Publications, Oxford, 1998: 2029–2038

Table 29.3 American Association for the Surgery of Trauma liver surgery scale

Grade	Injury	Description
I	Haematoma	Subcapsular, non-expanding, < 10% of surface area
	Laceration	Capsular tear, non-bleeding with < 1-cm deep parenchymal disruption
II	Haematoma	Subcapsular, non-expanding, 10–50%; intraparenchymal, non-expanding, diameter < 10 cm
	Laceration	Parenchymal depth < 3 cm, length < 10 cm
III	Haematoma	Subcapsular, > 50% of surface area or expanding; ruptured subcapsular haematoma with active bleeding; intraparenchymal haematoma > 10 cm
	Laceration	Parenchymal depth > 3 cm
IV	Haematoma	Ruptured central haematoma
	Laceration	Parenchymal destruction 25–75% of hepatic lobe
V	Laceration	Parenchymal destruction involving > 75% of hepatic lobe
	Vascular	Juxtahepatic venous injuries (retrohepatic cava or major hepatic veins)
VI	Vascular	Hepatic avulsion

sensorium, and head or spinal cord injuries may interfere with clinical assessment, and the insidious onset of shock can easily be missed. Intra-abdominal haemorrhage and liver damage may be detected by diagnostic peritoneal lavage, abdominal ultrasound or CT scanning. Ultrasound readily identifies free fluid (blood) in the peritoneal cavity and may show major hepatic or other visceral lacerations; CT scans are more accurate but are restricted to stable patients. Peritoneal lavage is used in the unconscious, inebriated or multiply injured patient. Laparoscopy offers little advantage over diagnostic peritoneal lavage.

TREATMENT

The most important decision after initial resuscitation is whether or not urgent surgery is needed (see Ch. 7). Patients who respond to resuscitation and who remain stable without clinical evidence of associated hollow viscus injury should be closely observed, investigated and re-evaluated regularly. Persisting shock despite 3 L of intravenous fluid usually indicates continued bleeding and requires urgent laparotomy.

STABLE PATIENTS

Large intrahepatic haematomas with an intact liver capsule can often be treated by careful observation and regular re-examination with imaging over several days. The same approach can be used for limited capsular tears with small amounts of intraperitoneal blood (Table 29.4). Larger capsular tears with continued intraperitoneal bleeding require surgery. Computerized tomography can contribute by showing the extent of lacerations, the size of liver haematomas, and the amount of intraperitoneal blood; however, the extent of injury on CT alone is not an indication for surgery. When a non-operative policy is used, the intensive care unit and operating theatres must be readily available should the patient become unstable.

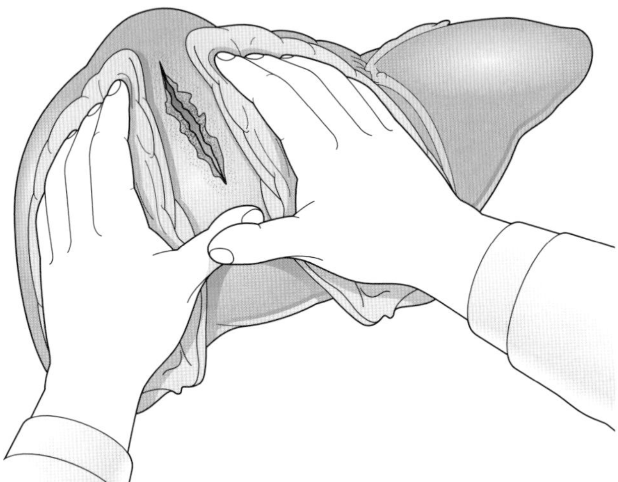

Figure 29.5 Liver injury compressed manually with packs to control bleeding.

Table 29.4 Criteria for non-operative management of liver injuries

- Haemodynamically stable after resuscitation.
- No persistent or increasing abdominal pain or tenderness.
- No other peritoneal injuries that require laparotomy.
- Less than 4 units of blood transfusion required.
- Haemoperitoneum less than 500 mL on CT scan.
- Simple hepatic parenchymal laceration or intrahepatic haematoma on CT scan.

SURGICAL PRINCIPLES

The priorities are to control bleeding, remove dead or devitalized tissue, and to oversew or repair damaged blood vessels and bile ducts. Most liver injuries are simple and can be treated without difficulty. Complex injuries need to be identified early and may require specialist surgical treatment.[13] The patient is routinely prepared from the sternal notch to the pubis, permitting a median sternotomy if more proximal vena caval or aortic control is required. A midline incision is used, and intraperitoneal blood and clot rapidly removed.

The next priority is to identify the source of active bleeding. Bleeding from liver lacerations is controlled by packing. Time should then be taken to complete resuscitation. A thorough exploratory laparotomy is performed to exclude other injuries, and any other sources of major haemorrhage are controlled (see Ch. 7).

Most liver injuries will have stopped bleeding at operation. These wounds should not be sutured and merely require drainage to prevent collections. Liver bleeding can usually be stopped by compressing the laceration with abdominal packs while summoning experienced surgical and anaesthetic help (Fig. 29.5). When bleeding continues after release of pressure, vessels in the laceration must be carefully sought and sutured, aided by temporary occlusion of the hepatic artery and portal vein with a vascular clamp (Pringle manoeuvre) for up to 20 min. Repacking may be required if bleeding continues.

REFERENCES

13. Krige JEJ. Br J Surg 2000; 87: 1615–1616

The management of all grades of liver injury has been revolutionized by perihepatic packing between the liver and diaphragm, as well as placing packs under the liver.[14] The packs should not be inserted into the liver injury (Fig. 29.6) because this often causes further bleeding when the packs are removed (Box 29.1). Bleeding must be controlled before the abdomen is closed. The packs should be removed after 48–72 h, although this may be carried out after the patient has been transferred to a specialist centre. When bleeding continues, hepatic angiography can be used to determine the potential value of therapeutic embolization, which can then be used to prevent further bleeding.

Serious injuries to the inferior vena cava and hepatic veins require vascular isolation with caval clamping below the liver, combined with a Pringle manoeuvre, and suprahepatic caval clamping (Box 29.2). Suturing of the lacerated hepatic veins or the inferior vena cava can then be performed. Rarely, a formal hepatic lobectomy is required for severe crush injury.[15] Packing has dramatically altered the management of major liver injuries,[13] and it has reduced the need for emergency liver resection.

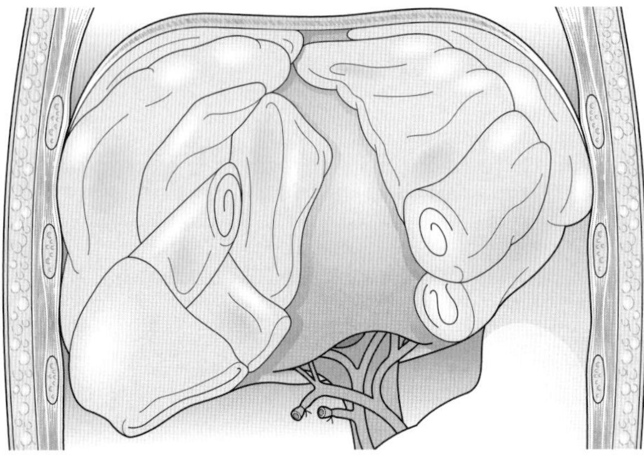

Figure 29.6 Packs placed to compress liver injury and stop bleeding.

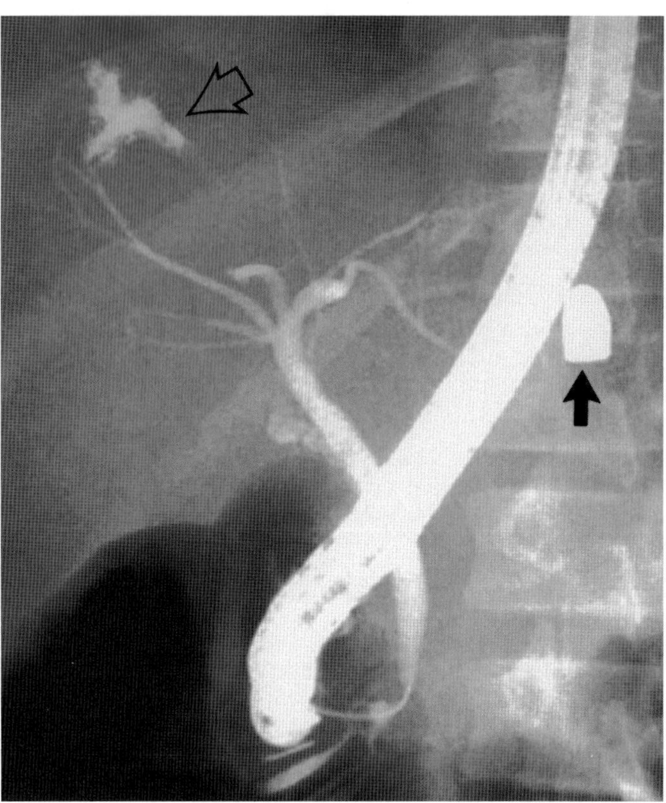

Figure 29.7 Endoscopic retrograde cholangiopancreatography showing peripheral bile leak (open arrow) caused by a bullet (arrow).

Box 29.1 Liver packing technique: the 'Ten Commandments'

1. Use dry-gauze packs.
2. Pack above and below the liver.
3. Avoid packing into the laceration.
4. Use sufficient packs ('six-pack').
5. Restore liver contour to normal by reapproximating the edges of the defect.
6. Avoid excessive packs, which may cause increased intra-abdominal pressure, caval compression or acute renal failure.
7. Ventilate patient until packs are removed.
8. Anticipate sepsis, especially if there is bile leakage or bowel contamination.
9. Give i.v. antibiotics.
10. Remove packs in the operating theatre within 48–72 h once coagulation abnormalities are corrected.

Box 29.2 Advanced operative techniques for control of bleeding from liver parenchyma and vessels

- Hepatorrhaphy with absorbable sutures for compression
- Hepatotomy with selective vascular suture
- Resectional debridement
- Segmentectomy
- Lobectomy
- Perihepatic packing
- Absorbable mesh wrap
- Total hepatic isolation

POSTOPERATIVE COMPLICATIONS

Rebleeding, bile leaks, segmental liver ischaemia and infected fluid collections are the main complications. Coagulation should be corrected before laparotomy if possible. Angiography with selective embolization is useful to treat recurrent arterial bleeding or haemobilia.[16] Computerized tomography scanning is used to define intra-abdominal collections that are best drained by ultrasound-guided needle aspiration or percutaneous catheter drainage. Perihepatic sepsis complicates about 10% of major injuries and is usually related to bile leaks, ischaemic tissue, undrained collections or bowel injury.[17] Endoscopic retrograde cholangiopancreatography can localize bile leaks, which can then be treated by endoscopic sphincterotomy and stenting (Fig. 29.7).

REFERENCES

14. Krige JEJ, Bornman PC, Terblanche J. Br J Surg 1992; 79: 43–46
15. Strong RW, Lynch SV, Wall DR et al. Surgery 1998; 123: 251–257
16. Corr P, Beningfield SJ, Krige JEJ. Injury 1992; 23: 347–349
17. Marr JDF, Krige JEJ, Terblanche J. Br J Surg 2000; 87: 1030–1034

PROGNOSIS

The overall mortality after liver injury ranges from 10 to 15%, and depends largely on the type of injury and the extent of any associated injuries to other organs.[17] Only 1% of penetrating civilian wounds are lethal, while 20% of blunt injuries are. The mortality is 10% if only the liver is injured, whereas if three major organs are damaged the mortality approaches 70%.

PYOGENIC LIVER ABSCESS

Liver abscesses are caused by bacterial, parasitic or fungal infections. Pyogenic abscesses account for three-quarters of hepatic abscesses in developed countries. Elsewhere, amoebic abscesses are more frequent and worldwide are the commonest cause of liver abscesses.

AETIOLOGY

Most pyogenic liver abscesses are secondary to infection originating elsewhere in the abdomen. Cholangitis associated with biliary stones or strictures is the commonest cause, followed by abdominal infection from diverticulitis or appendicitis (Box 29.3). In 15% of cases, no cause can be found (cryptogenic abscesses) but host defences may be compromised.

BACTERIOLOGY

Most pyogenic liver abscesses are polymicrobial, with Gram-negative aerobic and anaerobic organisms predominating.[18] Enterogenous *Escherichia coli*, *Klebsiella pneumoniae*, *Bacteroides*, enterococci, anaerobic streptococci and microaerophilic streptococci are the most common pathogens. Staphylococci, haemolytic streptococci, and *Streptococcus milleri* usually arise from bacterial endocarditis or dental sepsis. Immunosuppression from AIDS, from intensive chemotherapy, or after transplantation has increased the incidence of abscesses caused by fungal and opportunistic organisms.[19]

CLINICAL FEATURES

Upper abdominal pain, swinging fever and nocturnal sweating are common, and are often associated with vomiting, anorexia, malaise and weight loss. The onset of symptoms may be insidious or occult in the elderly. Single abscesses, which are often cryptogenic, tend to have a more gradual onset; multiple abscesses tend to be associated with acute systemic features and a cause that is more often identified. Clinically the liver is enlarged and tender; jaundice occurs only at a late stage, unless there is suppurative cholangitis. Some patients present with a fever of unknown origin.

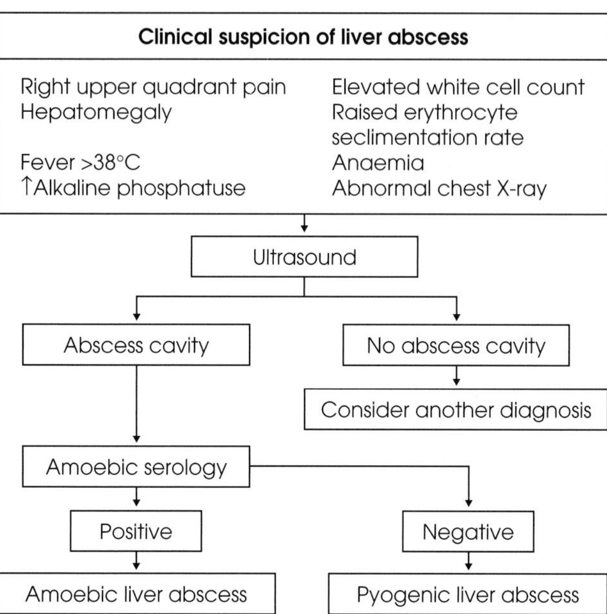

Figure 29.8 Diagnostic scheme for suspected liver abscess.

INVESTIGATIONS

Two-thirds of patients have leukocytosis, raised sedimentation rate and an anaemia of chronic infection. Alkaline phosphatase levels are usually raised, hypoalbuminaemia is present, and serum aminotransferase activity may be marginally elevated. Plain abdominal radiographs may show hepatomegaly with gas in the abscess cavity (Fig. 29.2). The right diaphragm is often raised with a pleural reaction and basal lung consolidation. Ultrasound is an excellent initial investigation and can be used to guide diagnostic aspiration (Fig. 29.8). A CT scan is used to assess complicated cases (Fig. 29.9). Endoscopic retrograde cholangiopancreatography can be used to define the site and cause of any biliary obstruction, which can be treated by biliary stenting and drainage.

TREATMENT

Liver abscesses should be treated by intravenous antibiotics, and any large abscess should be drained by ultrasound-guided percutaneous aspiration, percutaneous catheter drainage or formal surgical drainage.[20] Broad-spectrum combined parenteral antibiotics such as penicillin, aminoglycosides and metronidazole are adequate for *E. coli*, *K. pneumoniae*, *Bacteroides*, enterococcus and anaerobic streptococci. In the elderly and those with renal failure, a third-generation cephalosporin should be used instead

Box 29.3 Origin and causes of pyogenic liver abscesses

Biliary tract
- Stones
- Strictures
- Stent occlusion
- Sclerosing cholangitis
- Cholangiocarcinoma

Portal vein
- Appendicitis
- Diverticulitis
- Crohn's disease
- Pelvic sepsis

Hepatic artery
- Dental infection
- Bacterial endocarditis
- Intravenous drug abuse

Direct extension
- Gallbladder empyema
- Perforated peptic ulcer
- Subphrenic abscess
- Perinephric abscess

Trauma
- Penetrating injuries
- Blunt liver trauma

Iatrogenic
- Liver biopsy
- Postembolization

Cryptogenic

Secondary infection
- Liver cyst
- Amoebic abscess
- Hydatid cyst

REFERENCES

18. Krige JEJ, Beckingham IJ. Br Med J 2001; 322: 537–540
19. Huang CJ, Pitt HA, Lipsett PA et al. Ann Surg 1996; 223: 600–609
20. Krige JEJ, Bornman PC, Terblanche J. Curr Surg 1995; 52: 395–400

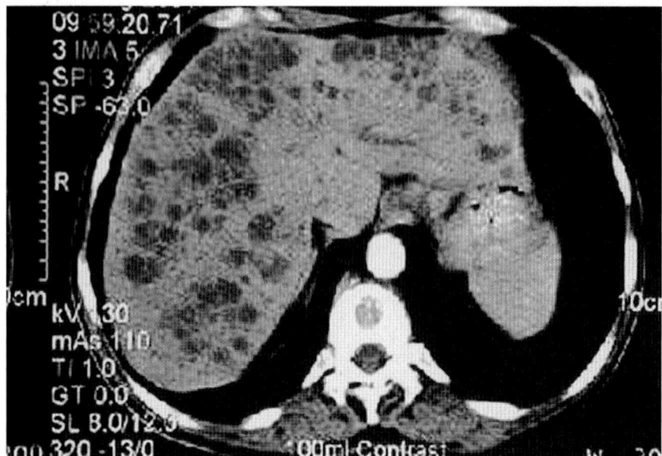

Figure 29.9 A CT scan showing multiple cholangitic liver abscesses.

of an aminoglycoside. Metronidazole is effective against both anaerobes and amoebiasis. Penicillin is the drug of choice for *S. milleri* infections, which are usually resistant to metronidazole. In patients allergic to penicillin, the combination of vancomycin, an aminoglycoside and metronidazole is effective. Ampicillin should be added if *S. faecalis* is cultured.

Plasma levels of aminoglycosides and renal function, especially in septic and jaundiced patients, should be monitored. Prolonged antibiotic administration may occasionally cure multiple small cholangitic abscesses where focal drainage is not possible, providing there is effective biliary drainage. The duration of antibiotic therapy is based on the number of abscesses, the clinical response and any potential toxicity. Patients with multiple biliary abscesses should receive 4 weeks of antibiotic therapy. Shorter courses may suffice for small, solitary abscesses that have been adequately drained. Oral agents may be started after 2 weeks of systemic therapy.

Most pyogenic liver abscesses require ultrasound- or CT-guided percutaneous aspiration (Fig. 29.10) or catheter drainage.[21] The percutaneous route avoids general anaesthesia, reduces the time spent in hospital, and is preferred by patients. Open surgical drainage is reserved for failed percutaneous aspiration or catheter drainage. It may also be selected for very large, multiloculated abscesses, or if there is associated intra-abdominal sepsis requiring surgery. An underlying cause should always be sought and treated. Acute biliary obstruction with cholangitis must be relieved urgently, and this can usually be achieved by an endoscopic papillotomy and placement of a temporary biliary stent.

A transabdominal approach is preferable if surgical drainage becomes necessary. The site of the abscess in the liver is identified using intraoperative ultrasound if necessary, and the liver is isolated with abdominal swabs to avoid contamination of the abdomen. The abscess is approached at its most superficial point, and the contents are aspirated through a wide-bore trocar and cannula. A large irrigating sump drain is inserted into the cavity and retained until drainage ceases. Regular ultrasound or sinograms are used to determine the progress of resolution of the cavity before any drains are removed.

The mortality has been substantially reduced by early diagnosis, treatment with appropriate antibiotics, and selective drainage. Adverse prognostic factors include shock, adult respiratory distress syndrome, disseminated intravascular coagulation, immunodeficiency states, severe hypoalbuminaemia, diabetes, ineffective surgical drainage and associated malignancy.[20]

AMOEBIC LIVER ABSCESS

Approximately 10% of the world's population is chronically infected with *Entamoeba histolytica*, which is the third commonest parasitic cause of death, surpassed only by malaria and schistosomiasis. The prevalence varies widely, and amoebiasis occurs most commonly in tropical and subtropical climates, where overcrowding and poor sanitation are the main predisposing factors.

REFERENCES

21. Krige JEJ. In: Kirsch R, Robson S, Trey C (eds). Diagnosis and Management of Liver Disease. Chapman and Hall Medical, London, 1995: 196–202

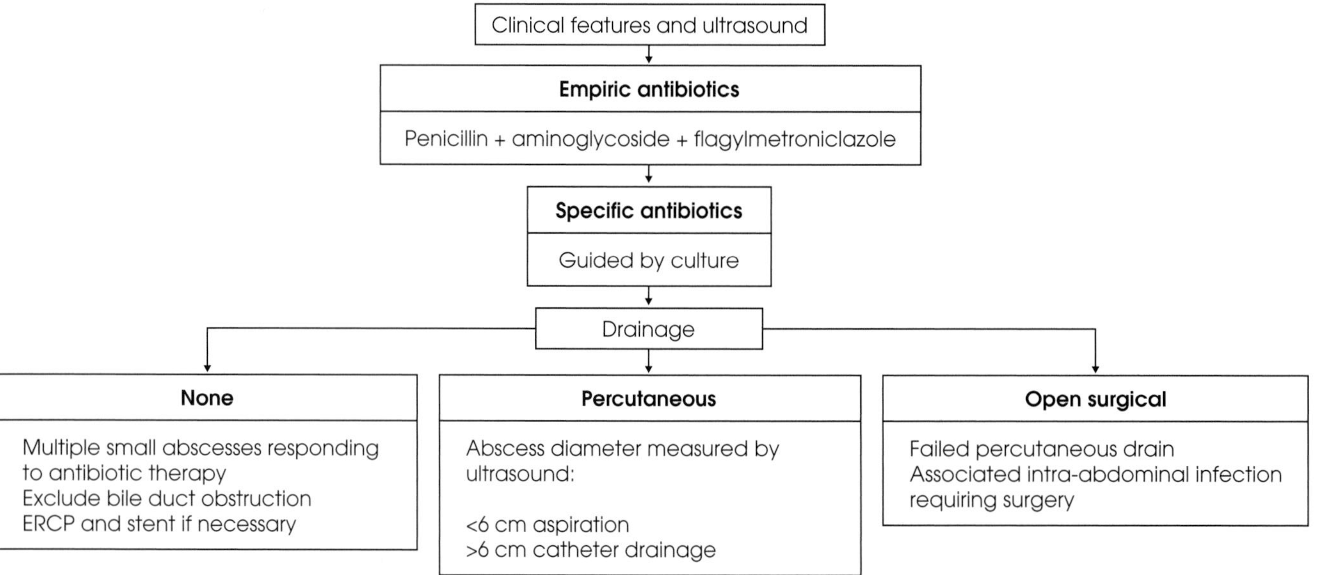

Figure 29.10 Treatment scheme for pyogenic liver abscesses.

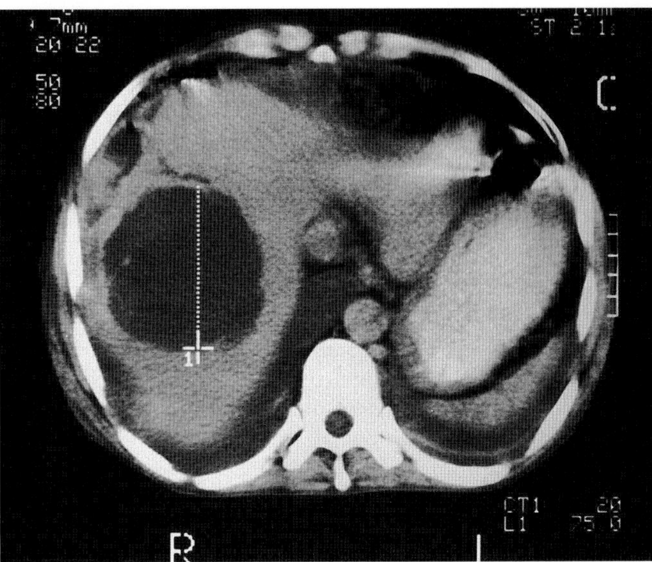

Figure 29.11 A CT scan showing a large, single, right lobe, amoebic liver abscess.

PATHOGENESIS

The parasite is transmitted via the faecal–oral route with the ingestion of viable protozoal cysts, the walls of which disintegrate in the small intestine, releasing motile trophozoites. These migrate to the large bowel, where pathogenic strains may cause mucosal invasion into the portal venous system. The typical amoebic liver abscess is solitary, affecting the right lobe in 80% of cases (Fig. 29.11). The abscess contains sterile pus and reddish brown, liquefied, necrotic liver tissue ('anchovy paste').

CLINICAL PRESENTATION

Symptom duration varies from a few days to several weeks. The patient appears in pain and is toxic, febrile and chronically ill. The diagnosis is based on the clinical features combined with serological and radiological tests. The patient is usually resident in or has visited an endemic area recently, although there is often no history of diarrhoea. Leukocytosis with 70–80% polymorphs (eosinophilia is not a feature), a raised sedimentation rate and moderate anaemia are common. In patients with severe disease and multiple abscesses, alkaline phosphatase activity and bilirubin concentrations are raised. Stools may contain cysts or, in the case of dysentery, haematophagous trophozoites. Chest radiographs may show a raised right diaphragm with atelectasis or a pleural effusion. Ultrasonography shows the size and position of the abscess and is useful when aspiration is necessary. It also allows the response to treatment to be monitored.[22]

Serological tests provide a rapid means of confirming the diagnosis, but the results may be misleading in endemic areas because of a previous infection. Indirect haemagglutination titres for *Entamoeba* are raised in over 90% of infected patients. In areas where amoebiasis is uncommon, a failure to consider the infection may delay diagnosis. Serious complications occur as either a result of secondary infection or rupture into adjacent structures such as pleural, pericardial or peritoneal spaces. Two-thirds of ruptures occur intraperitoneally and one-third intrathoracically.

TREATMENT

Adequate nutrition and pain relief are important. Metronidazole 800 mg three times a day for 5 days is effective treatment, curing 95% of patients. Clinical symptoms usually dramatically improve within 24 h. Lower doses of metronidazole are often effective in invasive disease but may not eliminate intraluminal infection, and clinical relapses can occur. Diloxanide furoate 500 mg 8 hourly for 7 days is used to eliminate intestinal amoebae.

Ultrasound-guided needle aspiration is performed if the serology is negative, or if the abscess is large (greater than 10 cm) or has bacterial superinfection. It is also used if there is no satisfactory response to treatment, or there is impending peritoneal, pleural or pericardial rupture. Surgical drainage is required only if the abscess has ruptured and caused amoebic peritonitis, or if there is no response to medical treatment despite needle aspiration or catheter drainage. It is also used if the abscess is not accessible to percutaneous drainage. Although most abscesses respond to medical treatment and resolve by 6 months, 10% of cavities may persist for up to 1 year. It is therefore important to recognize that radiographic evidence of a cavity does not indicate a need for drainage.[22]

Box 29.4 Classification of liver cysts

Congenital cysts
- Simple cysts
- Polycystic liver disease

Traumatic cysts

Parasitic cysts
- Hydatid

Biliary cysts
- Choledochal cysts (type IVa)
- Caroli's disease

Neoplastic cysts
- Biliary cystadenoma
- Biliary cystadenocarcinoma

CYSTIC LIVER LESIONS

Liver cysts are commonly seen on ultrasound, although most are symptomless and discovered by chance. The classification of liver cysts is shown in Box 29.4.

Congenital simple cysts are intrahepatic cysts lined by cuboidal epithelium derived from the biliary system, without a biliary communication. These are the most common liver cysts and range in size from a few millimetres in diameter to more than 20 cm (Fig. 29.12). Symptoms are uncommon but include dull right upper quadrant pain. Spontaneous rupture and haemorrhage are exceptional, but bleeding following trauma may cause a sudden increase in the cyst size, producing pain.

Polycystic liver disease is a genetic disorder. The majority of those affected also have autosomal dominant polycystic kidney disease (see Ch. 35).[23] Most patients present in early to mid adult life with gradual onset of progressive abdominal distension. Liver function is usually well preserved. Computerized tomography scans give the best anatomical information, and there is a wide

REFERENCES

22. Krige JEJ, Adams S, Simjee A. In: Kirsch R, Robson S, Trey C (eds). Diagnosis and Management of Liver Disease. Chapman and Hall Medical, London, 1995: 186–195
23. Chen MF. J Gastroenterol Hepatol 2000; 15: 1239–1242

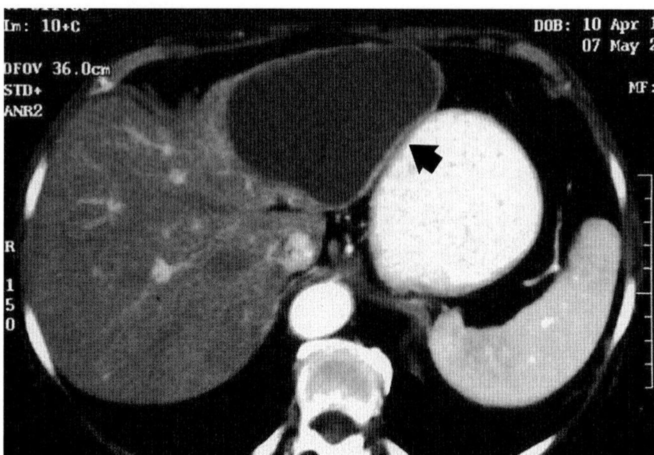

Figure 29.12 A CT scan of a large, simple, left lobe liver cyst (arrow).

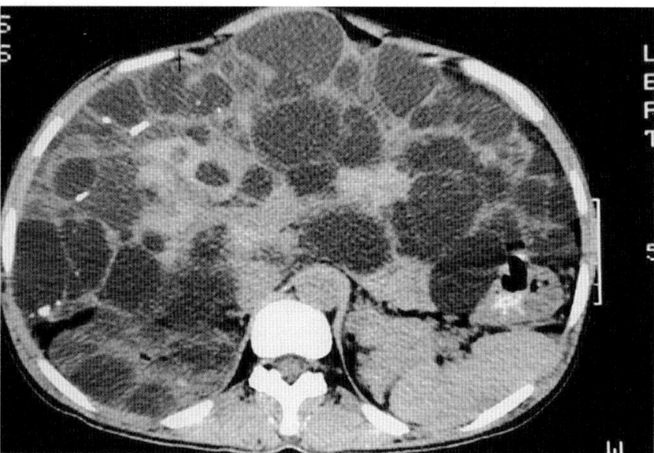

Figure 29.13 A CT scan showing polycystic disease of the liver.

variation in the distribution, size and number of the cysts (Fig. 29.13). The prognosis is usually determined by progression of the renal disease to end-stage renal failure rather than by the polycystic liver.

Traumatic cysts develop following intrahepatic or subcapsular haematomas. Most resolve spontaneously but some may persist and require drainage. An assessment must be made of any biliary communication.

Neoplastic cysts, although uncommon, are important because they must be distinguished from simple cysts. Cystadenoma and cystadenocarcinomas are multiloculated cysts lined with cuboidal or columnar mucus-producing epithelium. The malignant elements often have a papillary appearance in cystadenocarcinoma, and careful histological examination is therefore important after excision.

MANAGEMENT

Symptomless cysts should be left alone. Percutaneous aspiration is invariably followed by refilling. Percutaneous aspiration followed by instillation of sclerosing agents is also frequently followed by recurrence if the cysts are large. Surgical deroofing or fenestration is effective for large cysts in which a large section of the superficial surface is removed. Deroofing can be performed laparoscopically in selected cases.[24] This treatment is most successful for medium-sized or large cysts. Diffuse, symptomatic polycystic disease requires a combination of partial liver resection and fenestration.[25] Reoperation may be difficult because of adhesions if multiple fenestrations have been performed. Orthotopic liver transplantation is reserved for severe adult polycystic liver disease.[23,25]

HYDATID DISEASE

Hydatid disease is common in Mediterranean countries, the Middle and Far East, Africa, Australia and South America. It is endemic in many sheep-raising countries. Increasing migration and world travel have made hydatidosis a global problem. *Echinococcus* is the smallest of all adult tapeworms, measuring 6 mm in length. Four closely related species of *Taenia echinococcus* have the potential to cause hydatid disease in humans: *E. granulosus* is cosmopolitan and *E. multilocularis* is limited to the northern hemisphere, while *E. vogeli* and *E. oligarthrus* are indigenous to Central and South America.

BIOLOGY OF THE PARASITE

Echinococcus granulosus, the commonest species, infects dogs but also wolves and foxes as definitive hosts. The definitive host harbours the adult worm, and an intermediate host carries the larval stage. The mature parasite lives in the definitive host's small bowel, attached to mucosa, and sheds its eggs in the intestine. Humans are unwitting, accidental intermediate hosts when ova are swallowed after contact with infected dog faeces. Sheep, the intermediate host, ingest the ova through pasture. The eggs develop into embryos, which are called *oncospheres*. The oncospheres are released in the human duodenum and pass through the portal vein to the liver, the lung and other tissues, where they lodge and develop into their larval form, the hydatid cyst.

Hydatid cysts can develop anywhere in the body, but two-thirds occur in the liver and one-quarter involve the lungs (see Ch. 21). The brain, kidneys, spleen and bones are infrequently involved. The mature cyst has three layers: an inner germinal lining (endocyst), a middle acellular laminated layer (ectocyst), and an outer fibrous host pericyst layer. In older cysts the laminated and pericyst layers may become calcified. The germinal layer produces daughter cysts and brood capsules containing scolices capable of spreading the disease.[26]

CLINICAL FEATURES

Hydatid cysts may remain latent and symptomless for years. A liver hydatid may present either with liver enlargement and right upper quadrant pain from cyst pressure, or acutely with a complication. These include cyst rupture into the peritoneal cavity and may result in urticaria, anaphylactic shock, eosinophilia and implantation into omentum and other viscera. Cysts may compress or erode into a bile duct, causing pain, jaundice

REFERENCES

24. Martin IJ, McKinley AJ, Currie EJ et al. Ann Surg 1998; 228: 167–172
25. Ammori BJ, Jenkins BL, Lim PC et al. World J Surg 2002; 26: 462–469
26. Milicevic M. In: Blumgart LH (ed). Surgery of the Liver and Biliary Tract, Vol 79. Churchill Livingstone, Edinburgh, 1994

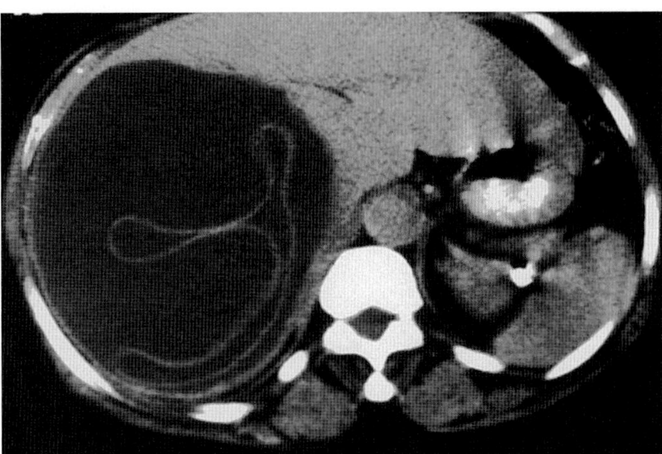

Figure 29.14 A CT scan showing a delaminated membrane in a hydatid cyst of the liver.

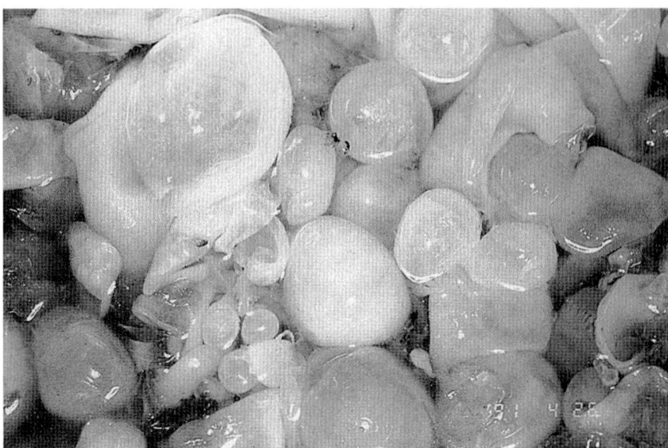

Figure 29.15 Operative photograph of multiple hydatid daughter cysts.

and cholangitis, or the cyst may become infected secondary to a bile leak. Perforation through the diaphragm and communication with the lung and bronchus is uncommon, leading to the patient coughing up 'grape skins'.

DIAGNOSIS

The diagnosis may be confirmed by haemagglutination and complement fixation tests.[27] Plain abdominal radiographs may show elevation of the right hemidiaphragm or calcification of the cyst wall. In 10% of patients, the chest radiograph also shows lung hydatids. Ultrasonography may detect a variety of appearances, including a well-defined cyst lined by a laminated membrane, daughter cysts and echogenic content. Computerized tomography scanning is a good means of imaging hydatid cysts and can clearly demonstrate daughter cysts and intraperitoneal spread (Fig. 29.14); CT also provides clear anatomical information on the relations of the cyst, facilitating subsequent operative planning. Endoscopic retrograde cholangiopancreatography may be of value in patients who have intrabiliary rupture.

TREATMENT

Surgery

Small, densely calcified cysts with a 'golf ball' appearance signify the death of the parasite and require no further treatment. Surgical treatment should be withheld if there is a single, small (less than 4 cm), symptomless cyst that is deeply situated in the liver. Cysts of this size rarely cause symptoms or complications and require extensive surgery to remove them because of their location. If left to grow under regular observation, they almost always extend to the periphery of the liver capsule, making the eventual surgical approach easier. All symptomatic cysts require surgery to prevent complications.

A subcostal incision is used. The operative field is carefully isolated with abdominal swabs soaked in scolicidal fluid to prevent spillage and implantation of hydatid contents. Because the wall may be fragile, care must be taken to avoid rupturing the cyst. The cyst fluid is initially aspirated and replaced by a scolicidal agent such as 0.5% sodium hypochlorite or 0.5% silver nitrate solution. Scolicidal solutions are not injected if there is a bile leak (suggested by yellow staining), because of the risk of chemical injury to the biliary epithelium. The use of a large-bore gynaecological curettage apparatus facilitates aspiration of membranes and daughter cysts, and reduces the risk of spillage. After aspiration, deroofing of the cyst permits removal of residual cyst content (Fig. 29.15). The cyst is shelled out by peeling the endocyst off the ectocyst layer along its cleavage plane. The fibrous wall of the residual cavity is examined for bile leaks, and if present these are sealed with sutures.

Management of the residual cavity depends on its size, depth and position. Superficial cysts are treated by resection of the visible pericyst wall, leaving a shallow remnant of pericyst exposed to the peritoneal cavity. Deep cavities are filled with omentum and a suction drain is inserted. Conservative surgery is effective in most cysts; formal liver resection is seldom necessary. Regular postoperative ultrasound scanning is useful for follow-up to detect recurrent disease.[28]

Medical treatment

Medical treatment alone cannot control hydatid disease, and it should be used only in elderly, high-risk patients; in those with small cysts; or as adjuvant therapy in disseminated disease.[29] Albendazole, flubendazole and praziquantel are given for 2 weeks postoperatively to prevent or limit recurrence after surgical excision. Drug therapy is also used in patients who are unfit for surgery; in those with disseminated, recurrent or inoperable disease; and as an adjuvant to complex surgery. These drugs must be used cautiously, because side effects include bone marrow depression, and hepatic and renal toxicity.[29]

LIVER TUMOURS

Liver tumours are benign or malignant, which may be either primary or secondary, the latter arising from a variety of malignant sources. Primary liver tumours are classified as shown in Box 29.5.

REFERENCES

27. Biava MF, Dao A, Fortier B. World J Surg 2001; 25: 10–14
28. Sielaff TD, Taylor B, Langer B. World J Surg 2001; 25: 83–86
29. Morris DL. Gut 1994; 35: 1517–1518

Box 29.5 Classification of primary liver tumours

Benign
- Hepatic adenoma
- Focal nodular hyperplasia
- Cystadenoma
- Mesenchymal hamartoma
- Haemangioma
- Haemangioendothelioma

Other rarities
- Fibroma
- Lipoma
- Leiomyoma
- Teratoma

Malignant
- Hepatocellular carcinoma
- Hepatoblastoma
- Cholangiocarcinoma
- Angiosarcoma

Rare primary tumours
- Malignant lymphoma
- Malignant teratoma
- Carcinoid and other endocrine tumours
- Fibrosarcoma
- Leiomyosarcoma
- Adenomatous hyperplasia
- Partial nodular transformation
- Inflammatory pseudotumour

Rare regenerative or inflammatory mass lesions

Figure 29.16 Dynamic T_1-weighted MRI scan through a haemangioma of the liver after intravenous gadolinium contrast injection, showing peripheral nodular filling (arrows).

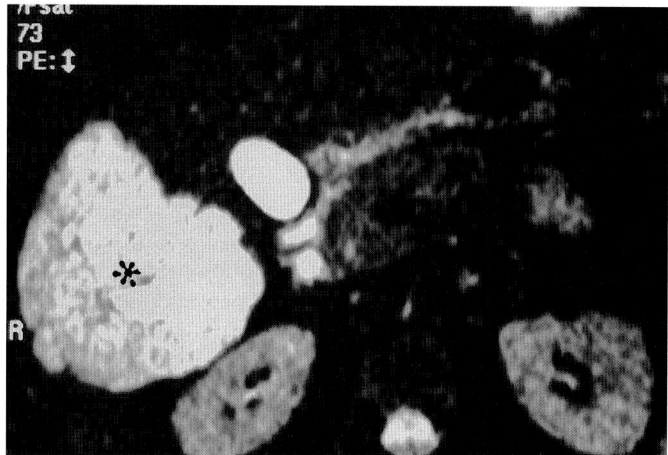

Figure 29.17 A T_2-weighted MRI scan showing the characteristic bright white 'light bulb' sign (*) in the same patient seen in Fig. 29.16.

BENIGN LIVER MASSES

Benign liver masses occur in 9% of the population. Incidental liver 'tumours' are found on imaging performed for other reasons. An understanding of their natural history allows rational management and limits unnecessary investigations, including biopsies and inappropriate resections.[30] The differential diagnosis includes cavernous haemangioma, focal nodular hyperplasia and hepatic adenoma. Most symptomless, solid, benign liver masses can be managed conservatively, the exception being hepatic adenomas because of their risk of rupture and bleeding.

BENIGN TUMOURS

Cavernous haemangioma

Cavernous haemangioma is the most common benign mesenchymal liver tumour, occurring in 4% of normal adults. Most are detected incidentally on ultrasonography and are small, single and symptomless. Haemangiomas are congenital hamartomas with a soft, spongy consistency, and consist of large, well-defined vascular channels separated by fibrous septa and lined by flattened endothelium. Areas of organized thrombus and sometimes dystrophic calcification may be present. Haemangiomas range in size from 1 cm to more than 20 cm in diameter. Giant haemangiomas are those greater than 10 cm in size. Platelet trapping in giant haemangiomas can result in thrombocytopenia in children.

The characteristic hyperechoic appearance of small haemangiomas on ultrasound is suggestive but not diagnostic. Computerized tomography and MRI after intravenous contrast scans often show characteristic peripheral nodular enhancement, progressing slowly to almost complete isodense filling of the tumour (Fig. 29.16). Technetium-99m-labelled red blood cell scans or T2-weighted MRI showing the classic 'light bulb' sign improve diagnostic confidence (Fig. 29.17). Haemangiomas are not premalignant but have a tendency to grow. Spontaneous rupture is rare, but thrombosis or growth producing stretching of the liver capsule may cause symptoms. Large haemangiomas should be resected if treatment is required, but enucleation is often feasible in smaller lesions.

Focal nodular hyperplasia

Focal nodular hyperplasia is a well-circumscribed abnormality of uncertain origin. It is usually found in women of reproductive age and is the second commonest benign liver lesion. An apparent increase in its incidence over the past two decades probably reflects improved ultrasound and CT imaging. The condition is a regenerative hyperplastic response to a localized hepatic vascular malformation. The hyperplastic liver parenchyma containing hepatocytes, bile ducts and Kupffer cells is arranged around a central stellate scar sometimes visible on CT scanning. A large artery branches into radiating smaller vessels, producing a 'spoke wheel' appearance. The condition is rarely symptomatic and bleeding seldom occurs. The majority of cases are discovered incidentally during radiological studies or at laparotomy. It has no malignant potential and the treatment depends on the certainty of diagnosis. No further investigation or treatment is required other than follow-up if the imaging appearances are typical. Resection is reserved for lesions that enlarge or become symptomatic.

REFERENCES

30. Little JM. In: Terblanche J (ed). Hepatobiliary Malignancy. Edward Arnold, London, 1994

Hepatic adenoma

Hepatic adenoma is a benign neoplasm of hepatocytes, occurring predominantly in women aged 20–40 years. Oral contraceptive usage has increased its incidence. This tumour also occurs 10 times less commonly in males. The adenoma usually consists of solitary nodules that are very vascular. The portal tracts, hepatic veins and bile ducts are absent internally. Approximately 10% of patients with adenoma have multiple lesions. Hepatic adenomatosis is a distinct entity with an equal gender incidence. A hepatic adenoma may be discerned as an incidental finding at laparotomy or found in patients undergoing imaging for other reasons. Localized upper abdominal pain may be a consequence of bleeding into a tumour. On imaging, adenomas may appear as well-demarcated and hyperechoic masses because of their high lipid content. Colour Doppler ultrasound may show large intratumoral veins without a central arterial signal, which helps to differentiate them from focal nodular hyperplasia. Biopsy is dangerous because bleeding may occur.

The malignant potential of these 'benign' tumours is controversial. Small adenomas less than 3 cm in size can generally be observed with 6-monthly ultrasounds. Some adenomas regress on withdrawal of oral contraceptive agents. Larger, enlarging, symptomatic or doubtful adenomas should be resected with a margin of clearance.[31] Patients presenting with rupture or bleeding require resection of the tumour. Hepatic arterial embolization can be a useful but temporary life-saving intervention if bleeding is severe.

Rare benign tumours

Rare benign tumours include nodular regenerative hyperplasia, adenomatous hyperplasia, and various fatty tumours (including myelolipoma and angiomyolipoma), as well as inflammatory pseudotumours, which can be confused with malignant tumours. Mesenchymal hamartomas present during the first 2 years of life and may cause considerable diagnostic difficulty because of rapid enlargement. They are therefore often resected. Partial nodular transformation, a localized form of adenomatous hepatocyte hyperplasia, produces large and small nodules containing sheets of regenerating hepatocytes and fibrous bands. In the porta hepatis it may cause portal venous obstruction and extrahepatic portal hypertension.

MALIGNANT TUMOURS

Hepatocellular carcinoma

This common cancer accounts for 90% of all primary hepatic malignancies. It tends to occur in older patients with long-standing alcoholic cirrhosis in low-incidence geographical areas. In many high-incidence parts of Africa and Asia, tumours occur in younger patients with chronic hepatitis B or C virus infection and macronodular cirrhosis.[32] Alcohol and haemochromatosis also increase the risk of hepatocellular carcinoma, as do crop contamination by aflatoxin and *Aspergillus flavus* mould, which acts synergistically with the hepatitis virus by inducing mutation of the tumour suppressor gene p53.[33]

Three morphological types of this tumour are described: solitary, a single large mass with or without small satellite nodules; multifocal, in which multiple discrete nodules are present; and diffuse, where multiple, minute, indistinct nodules occur throughout the liver. Hepatocellular carcinoma spreads by centrifugal growth, parasinusoidal extension into the surrounding parenchyma, invasion into the portal and hepatic veins, and distant lymphatic and vascular spread. It can also invade the biliary tract, causing obstructive jaundice.

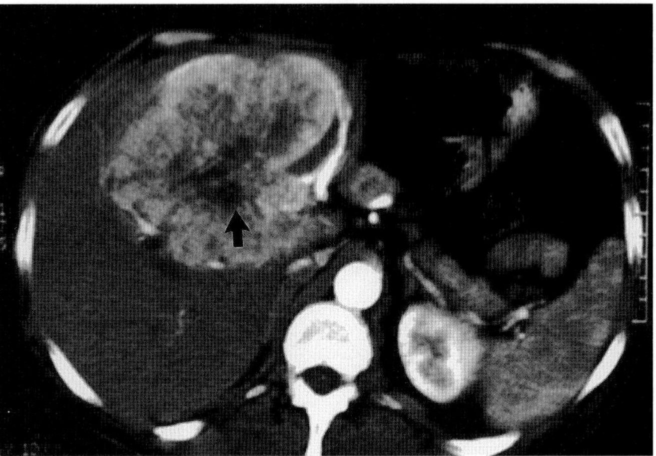

Figure 29.18 A CT scan of a large vascular hepatocellular carcinoma with a prominent central scar (arrow).

Fibrolamellar hepatoma is a distinct histological type with large eosinophilic cells and a fibrous stroma, which usually occurs as a solitary tumour in younger patients without any underlying liver disease or other known risk factors. The mean age at presentation is younger, and there is no male preponderance.

Most hepatocellular carcinomas are diagnosed late, and the average survival in the West is less than 1 year from diagnosis. Dull, persistent upper abdominal discomfort or pain, and weakness associated with weight loss and low-grade fever are common presenting features. Hepatomegaly, splenomegaly, ascites and jaundice may be present. Sudden onset of pain and shock is indicative of intraperitoneal haemorrhage following tumour rupture. Manifestations of portal hypertension, such as bleeding varices, are infrequent but ominous symptoms. Rapid deterioration in patients with cirrhosis or haemachromatosis suggests the development of a hepatocellular carcinoma. Since the advent of liver transplantation (see Ch. 8), many small hepatocellular carcinomas are found incidentally after removal of cirrhotic livers.

The diagnosis of hepatocellular carcinoma depends on tumour markers and imaging. Eighty per cent of patients with hepatocellular carcinoma produce plasma alpha-fetoprotein. Fibrolamellar hepatomas seldom express alpha-fetoprotein, but an elevated level of plasma neurotensin may be present.[34] Vitamin B_{12}-binding capacity may also be increased in fibrolamellar tumours. Biopsy can cause tumour implantation and should be avoided if curative resection is being considered. Ultrasound can be used as a screening tool in high-risk patients, and Doppler can aid in characterization. Computerized tomography (Fig. 29.18) and MRI allow more exact demonstration of tumour and complications, and angiography can demonstrate small hypervascular tumours, which can be embolized (Fig. 29.19).

REFERENCES

31. Leese T, Farges O, Bismuth H. Ann Surg 1988; 208: 558–564
32. Schafer DF, Sorrell MF. Lancet 1999; 353: 1253–1257
33. Hsu IC, Metcalf RA, Sun T et al. Nature 1991; 350: 427–428
34. Collier NA, Weinbren K, Bloom SR et al. Lancet 1984; i: 538–540

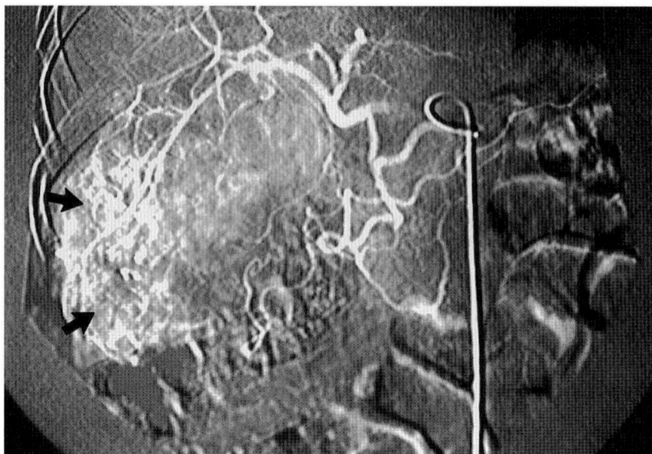

Figure 29.19 Selective hepatic angiogram showing neovascularity (arrows) in a hepatocellular carcinoma.

Late presentation and coexistent cirrhosis limit management options. The only curative treatment for hepatocellular carcinoma is by surgical excision,[35] which in most instances is a limited resection. Major resections are often impossible, because the associated cirrhosis prevents adequate regeneration. Intra-operative ultrasound has aided limited resections, particularly in cirrhotic patients. Resection of solitary tumours in non-cirrhotic patients produces 5-year survival rates between 20 and 40%, which rises to 50% for the fibrolamellar variant.[36] Transplantation may be the best choice for lesions smaller than 5 cm in cirrhotic livers, particularly in the presence of progressive liver disease.[37] Percutaneous ultrasound-guided injection of ethanol, chemo-embolization using Lipiodol™ bound to a chemotherapeutic agent such as epirubicin, radiofrequency ablation or cryotherapy are newer alternatives to surgery.[38] Systemic chemotherapy is of little value.

Liver metastases

Metastases are the most common malignant tumours of the liver, and half the patients dying of gastrointestinal cancer have hepatic metastases. Metastatic tumours reach the liver by four possible routes: they may enter the portal venous circulation, the lymphatic system, or the hepatic arterial system, or they can directly invade the liver.

Metastases appear in the liver at varying times after detection of the primary tumour. Precocious metastases, however, are present before the primary tumour has been detected, for example a carcinoid tumour of the ileum. Synchronous metastases are detected at the same time as the primary tumour, and metachronous metastases appear after the primary tumour has been removed. Liver metastases from the lung, breast, stomach or pancreas are usually widespread and have a poor prognosis. Surgery is beneficial in selected patients with colorectal, neuroendocrine and carcinoid tumours.

Colorectal liver metastases are important because of their frequency. About half of the 30 000 new cases of colorectal cancer annually in the UK have liver metastases, and most are present at the time of diagnosis of the primary tumour (see Ch. 28).[39] Long-term survival beyond 5 years is rare without surgery, whereas 5-year survival rates of 35% are reported after liver resection. Although isolated colorectal liver metastases occur more frequently than other tumours, less than 10% of all patients with colorectal metastases benefit from liver resection. Resection is considered only if the primary tumour has been controlled and there are no systemic or intra-abdominal metastases. The patient must be able to tolerate a major operation, and complete resection of the metastases must be feasible. The most important determinants of survival after resection are adequate tumour clearance and no residual extrahepatic disease. Dukes' stage, degree of differentiation and number of tumour deposits, particularly if greater than four, also influence survival. Metastatic size may have an effect on morbidity but has surprisingly little impact on survival.

There is now good evidence that combination chemotherapy produces a useful but still limited survival benefit in both resectable and unresectable tumours.[40] Other treatments have been introduced for irresectable lesions. The tumour may be ablated either by heat, e.g. radiofrequency ablation, or by cryotherapy using a liquid nitrogen-cooled probe at −80°C during operation. Despite clear evidence of major necrosis, no survival benefit has yet been shown. Some of these techniques may extend the role of liver resection by dealing with otherwise untreatable and residual tumours.

Neuroendocrine metastases are also worth resection, because they are usually slowly growing tumours that exert their effects through associated endocrine syndromes such as the carcinoid syndrome (see Ch. 27). Unlike colorectal metastases, multiple metastasectomies performed by 'shelling out' tumours from the liver may relieve symptoms and prolong survival.[41] Liver transplantation is also an option in these patients (see Ch. 8).

Locoregional chemotherapy

Dissatisfaction with the results of systemic chemotherapy, and in particular with high rates of systemic toxicity, led to the use of intra-arterial infusion for liver metastases.[42] Various techniques have been used for this, but the most common method is to introduce a catheter through the gastroduodenal artery at laparotomy to allow direct infusion of cytotoxic agents into the hepatic circulation. This procedure may be limited by the existence of multiple hepatic arterial vessels, such as the anomalous right hepatic artery arising from the superior mesenteric artery. The catheters can be led to a subcutaneous port into which intermittent infusions can be given, or attached to a permanent pump for long-term constant-rate infusion.

Liver resection

The major advances in liver resection have followed improvements in metabolic, haemodynamic and respiratory support, although there have also been advances in technology and surgical technique. A detailed knowledge of the liver anatomy is

REFERENCES

35. Lau WY. J R Coll Surg Edinb 2002; 47: 389–399
36. Rosen CB, Nagorney DM. In: Terblanche J (ed). Hepatobiliary Malignancy. Edward Arnold, London, 1994
37. Wong LL. Am J Surg 2002; 183: 309–316
38. Dick EA, Taylor-Robinson SD, Thomas HC et al. Gut 2002; 50: 733–739
39. McArdle CS, Hole D, Hansell D et al. Br J Surg 1990; 77: 280–282
40. Kemeny N, Huang Y, Cohen AM et al. N Engl J Med 1999; 341: 2039–2048
41. Benjamin IS. In: Terblanche J (ed). Hepatobiliary Malignancy. Edward Arnold, London, 1994
42. Clavien PA, Selzner N, Morse M et al. Surgery 2002; 131: 433–442

essential. The use of vascular control to reduce intraoperative blood loss, intraoperative ultrasound, ultrasonic dissection, argon beam coagulation and fibrin glue have reduced the postoperative morbidity and mortality.

Anatomical liver resection follows the segmental anatomy of Couinaud. The common resections are right hepatectomy (removing segments V–VIII), left lateral segmentectomy (segments II and III), left hepatectomy (segments II–IV, with or without segment I), and extended right hepatectomy (segments IV–VIII, with or without segment I). The overriding principle is to stay within the anatomical plane while obtaining optimal tumour clearance, and to preserve inflow and outflow structures to the residual segments. Improvements in operative technique allow the removal of multiple segments from different parts of the liver, and resections such as central hepatectomy and extended left hepatectomy.[43] These technically challenging procedures should, however, be restricted to specialist centres.

The liver is mobilized by dividing the ligamentum teres, and the falciform, triangular and coronary ligaments, and the inflow vessels are controlled, either outside or within the liver substance. Dissection of the porta hepatis identifies the branches of the hepatic artery, portal vein and biliary system supplying the segment(s) or lobe(s) to be removed. These are individually temporarily occluded depending on the type of resection. By rotating the liver, the hepatic veins may be isolated and controlled at their junction with the inferior vena cava. Some surgeons routinely ligate the relevant hepatic veins outside the liver, while others approach them from within the liver substance.

Glisson's capsule is incised along the resection line and the hepatic parenchyma is divided to expose the larger ducts and vessels, which are individually ligated and divided. Parenchymal division is performed either with a crushing clamp or using a Cavitron ultrasonic surgical aspirator. The parenchymal transection is continued posteriorly until the major hepatic veins are identified, sutured and divided. Intraoperative ultrasound is very useful for locating the intraparenchymal major vessels. Blood flow to and from the remaining segments is carefully preserved. Oozing from the resection margin is controlled with diathermy or fine monofilament sutures, and the cut parenchymal surface is sealed using an argon beam and the application of a fibrin tissue sealant (Tisseel).

The sequence described does not need to be used for every liver resection, and the steps may need to be modified depending on the size, position and number of tumours, and their proximity to the hepatic vasculature. Blood flow into the liver can be reduced by cross-clamping the hepatoduodenal ligament intermittently for periods up to 60 min using a vascular clamp. It may be possible to avoid occluding the vascular inflow to the liver remnant for long periods because this results in less postoperative liver dysfunction. Many surgeons routinely perform major liver resection without blood transfusion using these modern techniques. The mortality of elective liver resections should now be less than 3%, although the long-term survival ultimately depends on the underlying pathology.

Particular care is taken in the postoperative period to avoid hypoglycaemia, coagulopathy and hypoalbuminaemia. The larger the hepatic resection, the greater the probability of postoperative complications. The most frequent major complications are blood or bile collections after partial hepatectomy and intra-abdominal sepsis. Percutaneous drainage of perihepatic collections and endoscopic stenting of biliary leaks can avoid the need for reoperation.

REGENERATION OF THE LIVER

The liver has a unique capacity to recover its normal mass and function through DNA synthesis and mitosis after partial resection or injury.[44] The residual tissue regenerates until the original mass has been restored. The process is highly efficient after resection of normal liver, and the timescale is more rapid than was previously thought. The human liver begins to regenerate within 3 days and reaches its original size by 3 months. In most cases, liver function is restored to almost normal levels within 2–3 weeks.

The mechanisms that control regeneration are complex and subtle. Loss of functional liver mass stimulates the release of cytokines, including tumour necrosis factor and interleukins 1 and 6, which initiate DNA synthesis. Once the cell has been primed, progression is dependent on continued stimulation by mitogens such as epidermal growth factor, transforming growth factor-α, and insulin and glucagons, as well as growth factor.[44] The physical direction of liver growth is determined by the anatomy of the resection and the position of the liver remnant in relation to the surrounding structures. Interruption of the portal blood supply to segments of the liver, segmental biliary obstruction, or combinations of both cause atrophy and fibrosis in affected segments and regenerative hyperplasia in the remaining liver. This may lead to gross distortion of the liver anatomy, and in the case of right-sided atrophy and left-sided hyperplasia the liver may rotate around its axis, producing distortion of the bile ducts and portal vein in the porta hepatis, and causing a potential hazard during operations in this area.

Patients with cirrhosis may have insufficient hepatocyte function to meet the increased metabolic demands after major resection and have significantly reduced levels of hepatic regeneration after liver resection, making them extremely vulnerable to posthepatectomy liver failure. Hyperbilirubinaemia tends to be prolonged, with extreme rises in serum bilirubin in patients who ultimately do not survive resection. Cirrhotic patients also become severely protein-deficient after operation, a feature that is not usually seen in patients with normal liver function.

PORTAL HYPERTENSION

An increase in the portal venous pressure over 10 mmHg (normal range 5–10 mmHg) causes portal hypertension with compensatory portosystemic collaterals, increased splanchnic flow, and a disturbance of the intrahepatic circulation. These factors cause the important complications of chronic liver disease, which consist of variceal bleeding, hepatic encephalopathy, ascites, hepatorenal syndrome, recurrent infection and coagulopathy. The coronary and short gastric veins draining towards the azygos system produce oesophagogastric varices. These varices are the major source of gastrointestinal haemorrhage and mortality, but bleeding from congestive gastropathy and anorectal varices also occurs. The epigastric and abdominal wall vessels may enlarge through recanalization of the umbilical vein, and multiple retro-

REFERENCES

43. Scheele J, Stangl R. In: Blumgart LH (ed). Surgery of the Liver and Biliary Tract, Vol 2. 2nd edn. Churchill Livingstone, Edinburgh, 1994
44. Court FG, Wemyss-Holden SA, Dennison AR et al. Br J Surg 2002; 89:1089–1095

Box 29.6 Causes of portal hypertension

Presinusoidal

Extrahepatic

- Increased splenic blood flow
- Arterial–portal venous fistula
- Portal vein thrombosis
- Splenic vein thrombosis

Intrahepatic

- Schistosomiasis
- Sarcoidosis

Sinusoidal

- Cirrhosis
- Other (Wilson's disease or haemochromatosis)
- Congenital hepatic fibrosis

Postsinusoidal

- Budd–Chiari syndrome
- Congestive heart failure
- Veno-occlusive disease

peritoneal collaterals may develop, complicating any surgical intervention. Splenomegaly and hypersplenism result from impeded splenic vein outflow.

AETIOLOGY

Increased portal resistance and increased portal blood flow lead to portal hypertension. Increased resistance to flow is classified as presinusoidal, sinusoidal or postsinusoidal (Box 29.6). Increased flow is caused by either arteriovenous fistulae or increased splenic arterial flow. Portal hypertension has a wide variety of causes and geographical prevalences: while cirrhosis dominates in the Western world, schistosomiasis is a more common cause worldwide.

NATURAL HISTORY

Management of portal hypertension depends on understanding the risks of bleeding and rebleeding, and the response to therapy. One-third of compensated cirrhotic patients have varices at the time of diagnosis. The bleeding risk can be predicted by the presence of varices, a portal pressure over 12 mmHg and advanced liver disease. Thirty per cent of patients with varices will bleed, and of these, one-third die. There is a 70% chance of rebleeding, which carries a similar mortality. Variceal location, hepatic function, systemic disease, continuing drug or alcohol abuse, and splanchnic vein patency determine therapy. In addition, many patients with acute variceal bleeding develop liver decompensation with encephalopathy, ascites, coagulopathy, bacteraemia and malnutrition.

Assessment of the hepatic functional reserve is necessary before selecting the appropriate treatment. Dynamic tests of hepatocellular function – which include the aminopyrine breath test, the galactose elimination capacity and the hepatic amino acid clearance – have been used, but the Child–Pugh classification is the most useful and practical predictor of survival (Table 29.1). The operative mortality for Child's A patients is less than 5%, while for Child's class C it is over 25%.

ACUTE OESOPHAGEAL VARICEAL BLEEDING

Variceal bleeding is the most lethal complication of portal hypertension, causing one-third of deaths in cirrhotic patients. In Western countries, variceal bleeding accounts for 7% of all cases of upper gastrointestinal bleeding, although this varies geographically (11% in the USA, 5% in the UK) depending on the prevalence of alcoholic liver disease.

Box 29.7 Management of acute variceal bleeding

Treatment options

Pharmacological agents

- Somatostatin
- Octreotide
- Glypressin®
- Vasopressin plus nitroglycerin

Endoscopic therapy

- Band ligation
- Injection sclerotherapy: sclerosants, cyanoacrylate ('superglue') or thrombin

Balloon tamponade

Transjugular intrahepatic portosystemic shunt

Surgery

- Oesophageal transection
- Shunt procedures

Management

Many techniques have been used to control acute variceal bleeding and these include medication, balloon tamponade, endoscopic therapy, transjugular intrahepatic portosystemic shunts (TIPS) and emergency surgery (Box 29.7). All patients suspected of having acute variceal bleeding require admission to intensive care or high-dependency units. Emergency treatment includes haemodynamic stabilization with blood volume replacement to prevent hypovolaemic shock and liver failure. Although bleeding stops spontaneously in two-thirds of patients, it is not possible to predict which patients will continue to bleed and require further measures. Patients should be transferred to a centre with appropriate facilities as soon as they have been stabilized (Fig. 29.20).

Initial measures

The severity of the bleeding determines the urgency and extent of the therapy. Stable patients with intermittent bleeding benefit from endoscopic measures, while exsanguinating bleeding may require balloon tamponade before endoscopy. Securing the airway and prompt restoration of blood volume is vital, superceding any diagnostic studies. Crystalloid solution, followed by blood when available, is rapidly infused until the blood pressure and urine output are adequate (see Ch. 3). Saline infusions may aggravate ascites and should be avoided. Overzealous volume expansion can precipitate further bleeding and a central venous pressure line should be placed. The central venous pressure should be maintained at 2–5 cm H_2O. Unstable patients with associated cardiac or pulmonary disease may require insertion of a pulmonary artery wedge catheter, because excessive crystalloids and vasoactive drugs can cause oedema, ascites and hyponatraemia. Fresh frozen plasma, vitamin K and occasionally platelet transfusions may be necessary to correct clotting (see Ch. 3). Sedatives should be avoided, other than haloperidol for alcohol-withdrawal symptoms.

Emergency endoscopy

Several drugs can be used to try to control acute bleeding before proceeding to emergency endoscopy. Somatostatin (250 μg/h) or

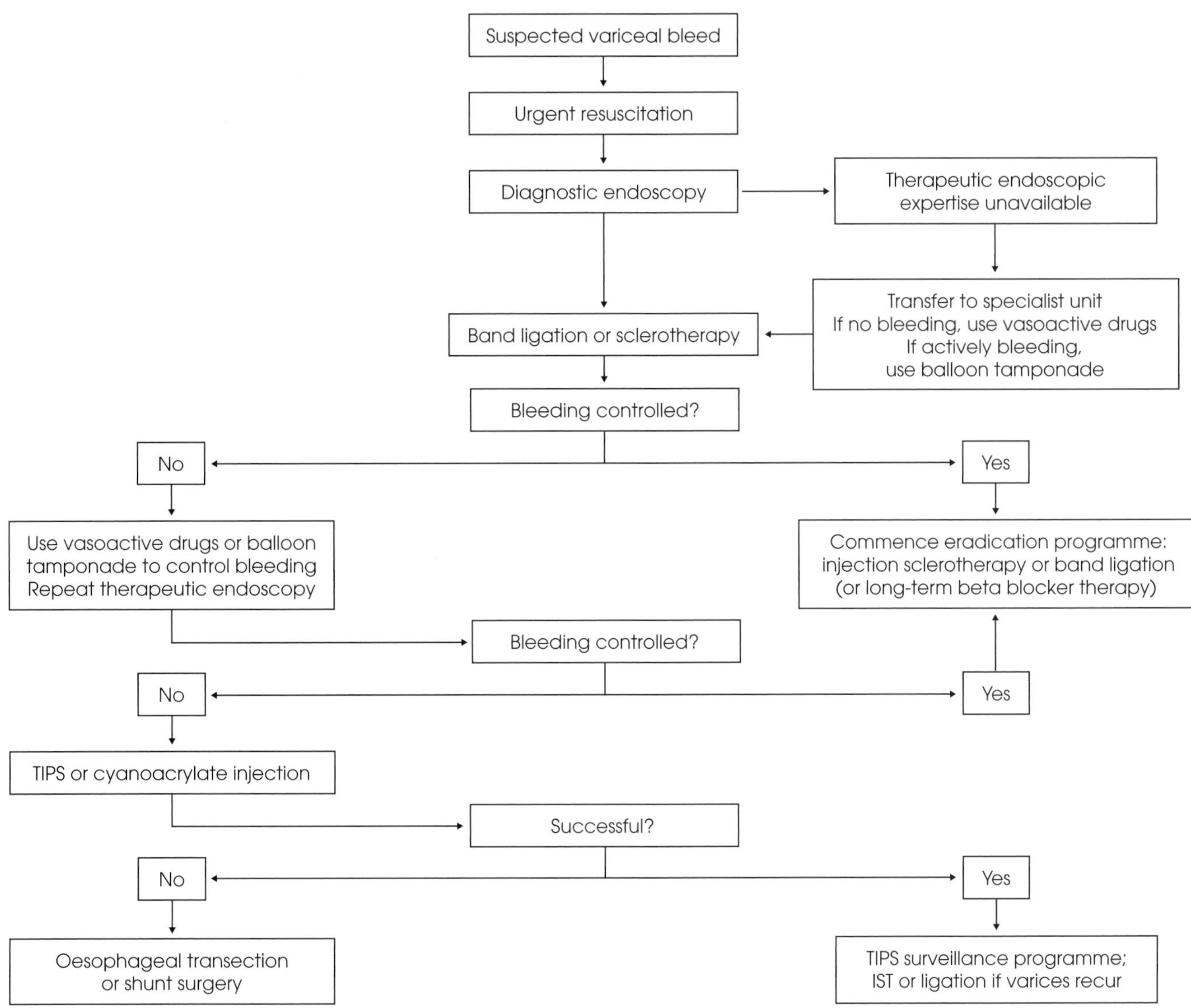

Figure 29.20 Algorithm for the management of acute variceal bleeding. IST, injection sclerotherapy.

octreotide (50 μg/h) given intravenously are safe and effective, and have superseded vasopressin. Emergency endoscopy is essential to confirm that oesophageal varices are the source of bleeding.[45] Most varices will have stopped bleeding before endoscopy, with or without treatment. Endotracheal intubation may be required in actively bleeding, encephalopathic or unstable patients. Intravenous analgesia and sedation should be administered in the smallest effective doses. Ninety per cent of varices bleed from the lower 5 cm of the oesophagus. Gastric varices on either the lesser curve or the fundus, and occasionally portal hypertensive gastropathy, account for the rest. Actively bleeding oesophageal varices are either injected with sclerosant or have elastic bands applied to them.

Sclerotherapy

Emergency sclerotherapy effectively controls acute variceal bleeding but requires an experienced endoscopist. A 23-gauge needle on a long catheter is passed through the endoscopic channel, and sclerosant solution (ethanolamine oleate or sodium tetradecyl sulphate) is injected into the bleeding varix (intravariceal injection) to cause thrombosis, or into the overlying and adjacent submucosa (paravariceal injection) to produce sclerosis. A combination of both techniques can also be used (Fig. 29.21). Control is achieved in 80% of patients, and if bleeding recurs injections are repeated. Four or five injection sessions may be required to eradicate the varices.[46] Minor complications related to the sclerosant include transient fever, dysphagia, chest pain and oesophageal ulceration at the injection site. Oesophageal strictures are uncommon and perforations are rare. Bleeding gastric varices are more difficult to inject and 'superglue' or thrombin is often used.

Band ligation

Endoscopic placement of a rubber band around the base of an ensnared oesophageal varix, as for internal haemorrhoids, is

REFERENCES

45. Krige JEJ, Terblanche J. In: Carter D, Russell RCG, Pitt H et al (eds). Rob and Smith's Operative Surgery: Surgery of the Liver, Pancreas and Bile Ducts. 5th edn. Chapman and Hall Medical, London, 1996: 163–172
46. Terblanche J, Stiegmann GV, Krige JEJ et al. World J Surg 1994; 18: 185–192

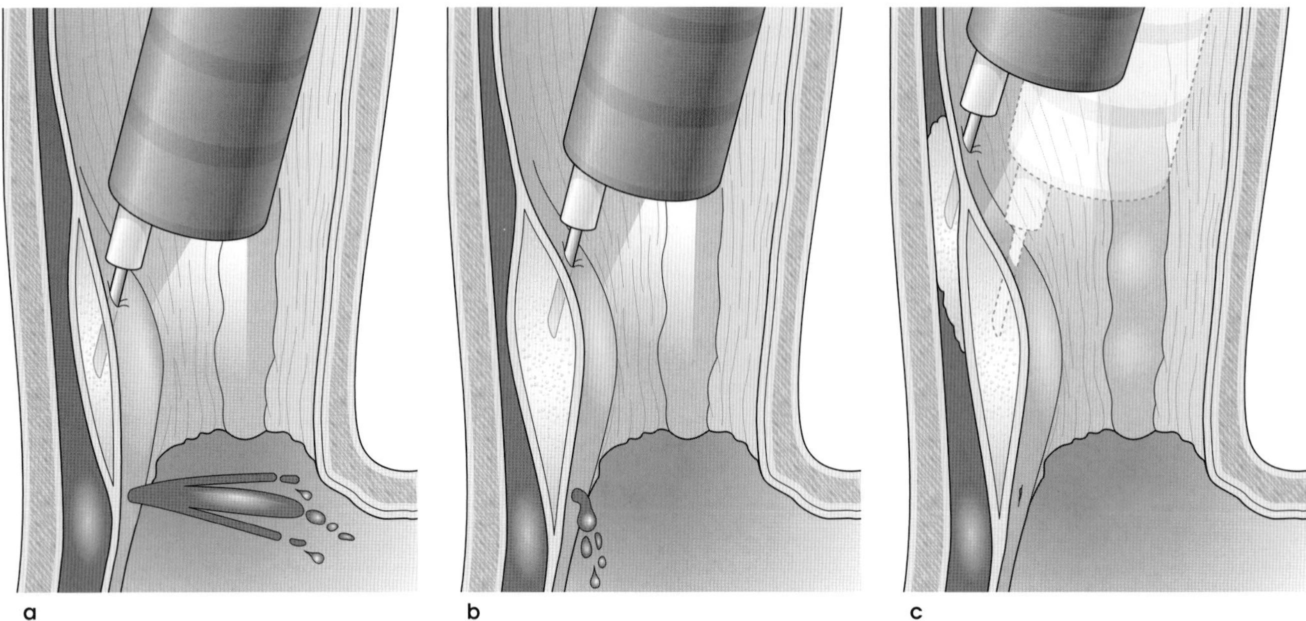

Figure 29.21 The combined paravariceal and intravariceal injection technique used during emergency sclerotherapy: (**a**) initial paravariceal injection proximal to the bleeding point; (**b**) bleeding controlled by the paravariceal injection; and (**c**) an intravariceal injection completes the procedure.

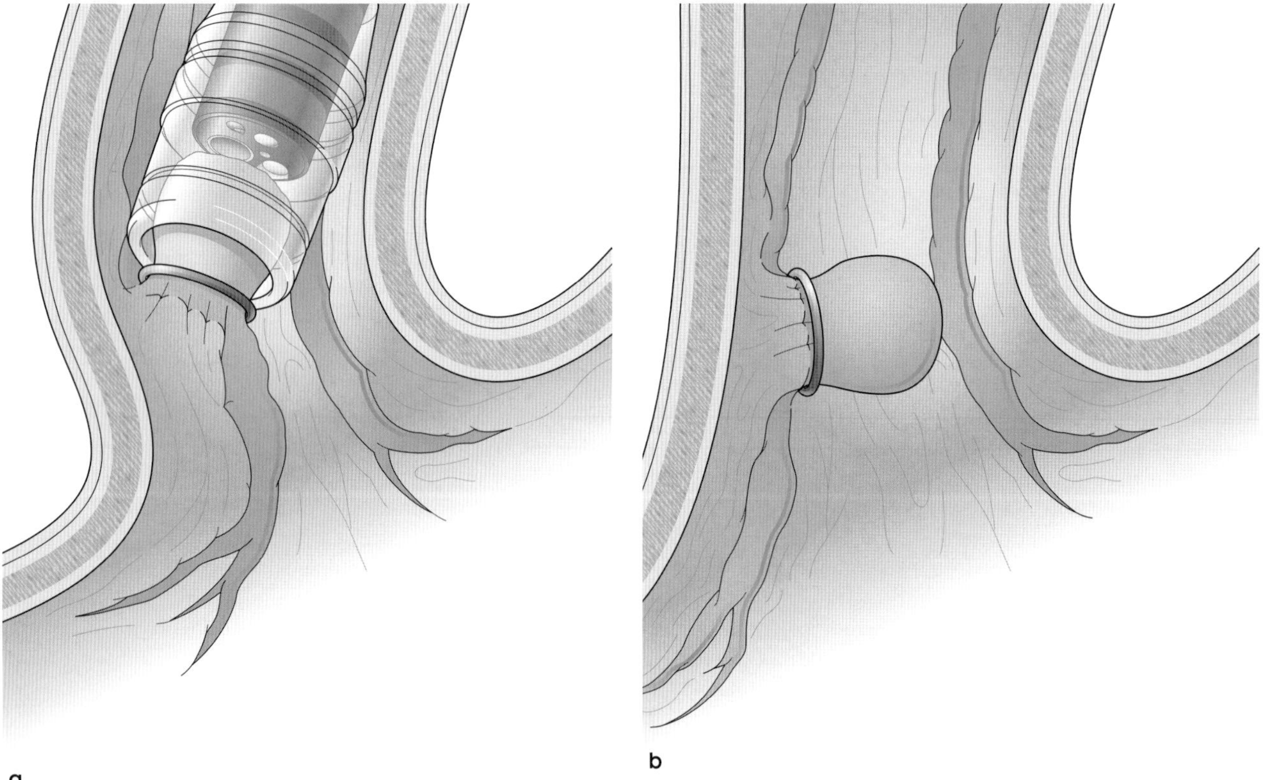

Figure 29.22 Endoscopic ligation of oesophageal varices: (**a**) the endoscopist aspirates the varix into the ligating device mounted on the end of the scope and the trip wire is pulled, displacing the elastic band to encircle the base of the varix; and (**b**) the elastic band causes thrombosis of the ligated varix.

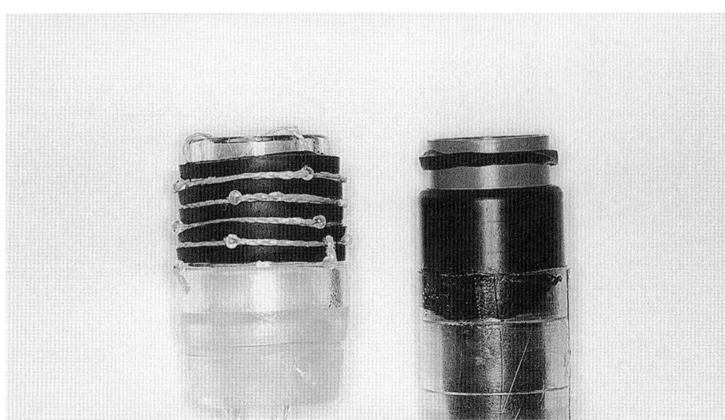

Figure 29.23 Multiple (left) and single (right) endoscopic banding devices.

a newer alternative.[47] The banding device, attached to the endoscope tip, allows the varix to be sucked into the banding chamber (Fig. 29.22). A tripwire dislodges a rubber band, ligating the entrapped varix. One to three bands are applied to each variceal column. The banded varix thromboses and sloughs after a week, leaving a shallow mucosal ulcer that heals with scar tissue. The band ligation procedure is repeated until all the varices are obliterated. Band ligation eradicates oesophageal varices with fewer sessions and less complications than sclerotherapy. Two different types of ligating devices are used: the original Stiegmann single-band device, which requires the use of a cumbersome over-tube, has been replaced by newer multi-banding devices that require no over-tube and allow delivery of 6, 8 or 10 bands (Fig. 29.23). The cost of these disposable units ($200 each) may, however, limit their widespread use.

Failure to control bleeding after two emergency endoscopic sclerotherapy or banding treatments during a single admission for acute bleeding indicates that balloon tamponade or a TIPS procedure is probably required.

Balloon tube tamponade

Balloon tube tamponade is used if emergency sclerotherapy or banding fails, or if active bleeding fails to stop. An endotracheal tube should be inserted before the oesophageal balloon tube is passed. Both the modified Sengstaken–Blakemore tube and the newer Minnesota balloon tube have four lumens: one for gastric aspiration, one each to inflate the gastric and oesophageal balloons, and one secretion–aspiration channel above the oesophageal balloon to prevent aspiration.[48] Only new tubes should be used, and all the balloons should be tested by inflation under water before insertion.

The tube is passed through the patient's mouth and its position in the stomach is confirmed by abdominal X-ray. The gastric balloon is inflated with 200 mL of air in 50-mL increments, and resistance to this or pain on insufflation points to incorrect tube placement. The fully inflated gastric balloon is pulled up snugly against the oesophagogastric junction, compressing the submucosal varices. Tension is maintained by strapping a split tennis ball to the tube outside the patient's mouth, and a bite guard prevents pressure necrosis of the lip (Fig. 29.24). The main complications of balloon tamponade are oesophageal perforation, gastric and oesophageal ulceration, and aspiration pneumonia. The tube is removed to allow repeat endoscopy within 12 h to avoid these complications. Continued bleeding after inflation indicates an incorrectly positioned tube or bleeding from another source.

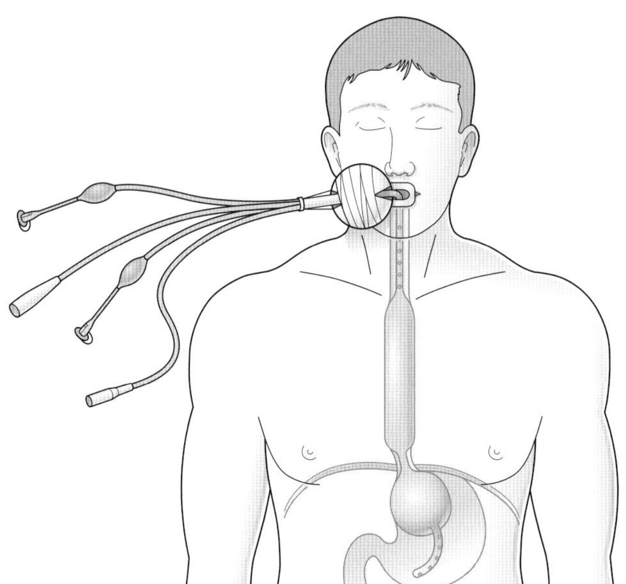

Figure 29.24 Four-lumen balloon tube. The gastric balloon filled with air is held firmly against the oesophagogastric junction by fixing a split tennis ball to the tube at the patient's mouth.

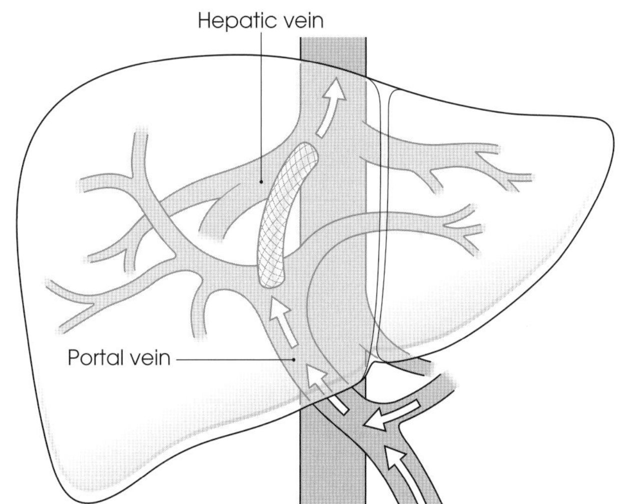

Figure 29.25 Transjugular intrahepatic portosystemic shunt.

Alternative management

Transjugular intrahepatic portosystemic shunt

The TIPS procedure is now the salvage procedure of choice for bleeding that cannot be controlled by endoscopy.[48] A fluoroscopically placed intrahepatic shunt has advantages over surgical shunts. Usually TIPS is performed through the right internal jugular vein, under local anaesthesia and neuroleptic analgesia. The right or middle hepatic vein is cannulated, and a tract is created with a needle through the liver parenchyma between the hepatic and portal veins (Fig. 29.25). An expandable metal stent

REFERENCES

47. Tait IS, Krige JEJ, Terblanche J. Br J Surg 1999; 86: 812–817
48. Krige JEJ, Terblanche J. In: Blumgart L, Fong Y (eds). Surgery of the Liver and Bile Ducts. 3rd edn. WB Saunders, Baltimore, 2000: 1885–1906

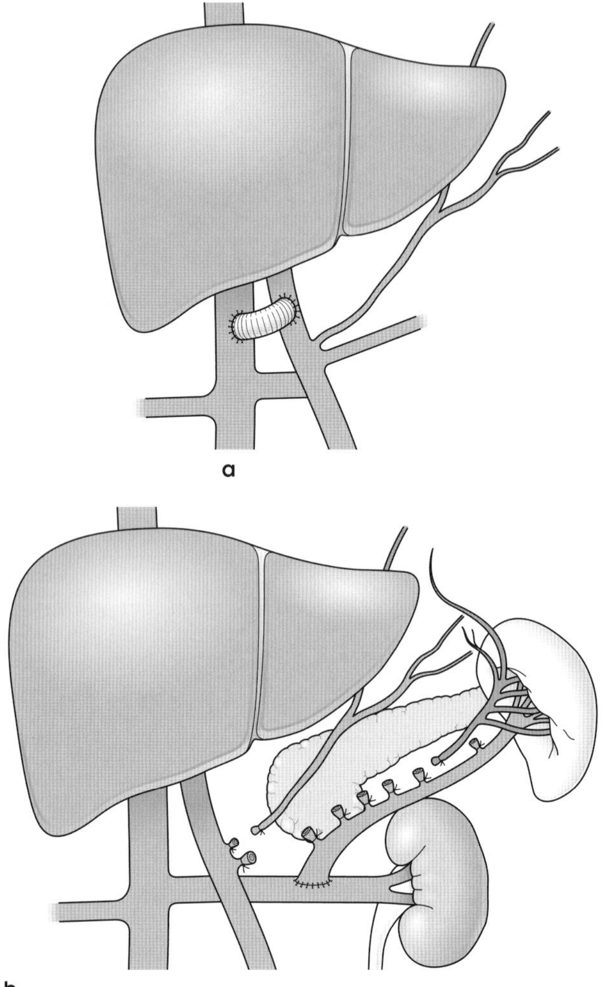

Figure 29.26 (**a**) Side-to-side portocaval shunt and (**b**) distal splenorenal shunt (Warren shunt).

creates an intrahepatic portosystemic shunt, with good short-term success rates and equivalent haemodynamic effects to surgical shunts but with a lower morbidity and mortality. In patients who have failed medical and endoscopic therapy, TIPS stops acute bleeding from oesophageal and gastric varices, and congestive gastropathy. Encephalopathy unfortunately still develops in nearly a quarter of the patients, and half the shunts occlude by 1 year. The primary role of the procedure is to rescue patients who have failed endoscopic therapy and to act as a bridge to subsequent liver transplantation.[49]

Operative shunts

The standard 8-mm side-to-side portocaval H-graft shunt is the preferred emergency shunt (Fig. 29.26a). This halts acute variceal bleeding and prevents recurrent bleeding. The operative mortality of this procedure in poor-risk patients is high. Progressive liver decompensation and unpredictable postoperative encephalopathy develop, and emergency operative shunts are now seldom used because of better endoscopic therapy and the availability of TIPS.

Oesophageal transection

Anastomotic staple gun oesophageal transection is the simplest emergency operation for failed endoscopic therapy when TIPS or operative shunts are not suitable (Fig. 29.27a).

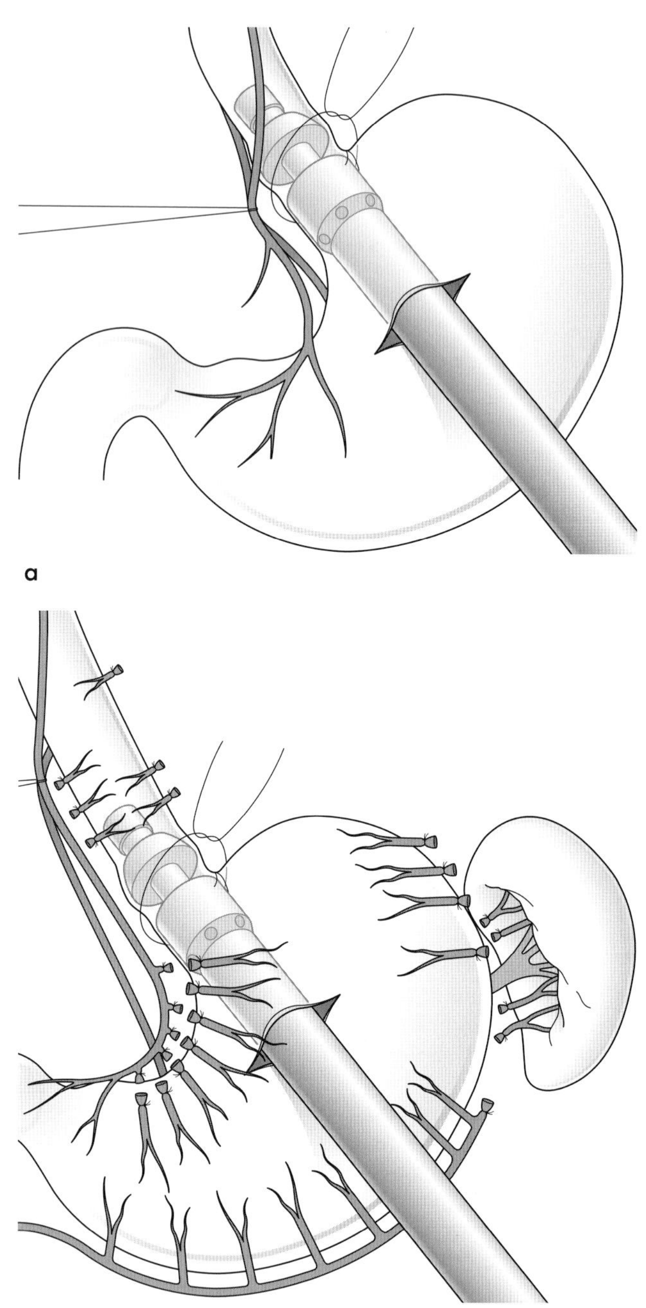

Figure 29.27 (**a**) Oesophageal transection and (**b**) oesophagogastric devascularization and transection (modified Sugiura procedure).

Long-term management after variceal bleeding

There is a 70% risk of rebleeding following successful control of the initial haemorrhage. The cause of the portal hypertension and the severity of the liver disease should be determined in the interim because this will dictate the choice of subsequent treatment (Box 29.8).

REFERENCE

49. Rössle M, Siegerstetter V, Huber M et al. Liver 1998; 18: 73–89

Box 29.8 Long-term prevention of variceal rebleeding: treatment options

Endoscopic therapy
- Injection sclerotherapy
- Variceal band ligation

Pharmacotherapy
- Beta blockers
- Isosorbide mononitrate

Surgery
- Shunt: distal splenorenal or portocaval
- Non-shunt: oesophageal transection and oesophagogastric devascularization or splenectomy for gastric varices due to splenic vein thrombosis

Transjugular intrahepatic portosystemic shunt

Liver transplantation

Repeated endoscopic therapy

This low-risk technique is effective and durable, and does not damage liver function or increase the risk of encephalopathy. Regular surveillance endoscopy is required after the varices have been eradicated. Recurrent varices usually appear as single channels and are easily treated.[50]

Pharmacological therapy

Several meta-analyses show that long-term beta blockers, principally propanolol, reduce recurrent bleeding and increase survival. Beta blockade dose is titrated to lower portal pressure below 12 mmHg or to achieve a reduction of 20% below baseline. Because invasive monitoring is not feasible in every patient, a reduction in heart rate of 20% or to less than 60 beats/min is used as a surrogate marker of adequate beta blockade.

Contraindications to beta blockade include asthma, chronic obstructive airways disease, peripheral vascular disease, congestive cardiac failure and unstable insulin-dependent diabetes mellitus. The most common side effects are tiredness, dyspnoea, depression, cold extremities, impotence and headaches. These side effects, however, rarely require discontinuation of treatment. Unfortunately, an appreciable number of patients may not be suitable for treatment with beta blockers or stop taking the drug as a result of side effects. In addition, approximately a third of patients treated with standard doses of beta blockers do not achieve a significant reduction in portal venous pressures.

While long-term propanolol therapy remains an alternative option to endoscopic management of varices, it should be restricted to compliant patients. Recurrent bleeding despite beta blockade requires alternative treatment, which is usually endoscopic therapy.

Surgical shunts

The only indication to use these as first-time treatment is in patients with good liver function who fail endoscopic management. They may also be indicated where endoscopic treatment is unavailable and in those who are unsuitable for beta blockade.

Surgical shunts are classified as total or partial, and selective or non-selective. Total shunts have diameters greater than 10 mm and divert all the portal flow into the systemic circulation, usually into the inferior vena cava. Liver function deteriorates rapidly and encephalopathy occurs faster because of the major diversion of blood away from the hepatocytes. Partial portosystemic shunts use 8-mm interposition grafts placed in mesocaval or portocaval positions. These lower portal pressure while maintaining portal blood flow to the liver, thus preserving liver function. A successful portosystemic shunt effectively prevents recurrent variceal bleeding, but it is a major operation with a substantial morbidity and mortality in poor-risk patients.

Selective shunts decompress oesophageal varices rather than the entire portal system while preserving portal flow and liver perfusion, thus preventing liver atrophy and encephalopathy. The distal splenorenal shunt is the preferred selective shunt, but this is a technically demanding operation (Fig. 29.26b) and is now done less frequently because other effective, non-operative alternatives are available. Good results are reported in non-alcoholic cirrhosis, but results in alcoholic cirrhosis are equivalent to standard portocaval shunts. Venous patency, individual experience and urgency dictate the technique used to make the shunt.

Devascularization procedures

Portal and splenic vein thrombosis causing repeated gastric and oesophageal variceal bleeding despite endoscopic and pharmacological therapy can be treated by the Sugiura procedure, which consists of splenectomy, proximal gastric and oesophageal devascularization, selective vagotomy, pyloroplasty and oesophageal transection. Devascularization reduces inflow to oesophageal varices, eliminating bleeding while maintaining portal flow and minimizing encephalopathy. Modifications without splenectomy, pyloroplasty or vagotomy, or using an automatic circular stapling gun appear equally effective (Fig. 29.27b).

Liver transplantation

Liver transplantation (see Ch. 8) is the only treatment that cures the underlying liver disease and eradicates the portal hypertension. All patients presenting with variceal bleeding and liver decompensation should be considered for transplantation. Organs are a scarce resource, and ultimately only a small proportion of patients will have a liver transplantation. If endoscopic therapy fails to control acute variceal bleeding, an emergency TIPS procedure should be considered as a bridge to transplantation.

Prevention of initial bleeding

Attempts to identify patients at high risk for variceal haemorrhage by measuring the size or appearance of varices at endoscopy have been largely unsuccessful. Most patients with portal hypertension never bleed, and it is difficult to predict those who will. The best indicators are chronic decompensated liver disease, the presence of 'cherry red spots', red and white streaks, and the size of the varices on endoscopy. Varices rarely bleed at pressures below 11 mmHg, but above this level pressure is a poor predictor of the likelihood of a bleed. Sclerotherapy is not used for primary prophylaxis because of the substantial incidence of complications, but beta blockers are used in selected cases.[51]

REFERENCES

50. Lebrec D. J Hepatol 1998; 28: 896–907
51. Shahi HM, Sarin SK. Am J Gastroenterol 1998; 93: 2348–2358

Gastric varices and portal hypertensive gastropathy

Gastric varices are the source of bleeding in 5–10% of patients with variceal haemorrhage. Higher rates are reported in patients with left-sided portal hypertension from splenic vein thrombosis. Endoscopic treatment of gastric varices is difficult unless these are located on the proximal lesser curve in continuity with oesophageal varices. Endoscopic application of cyanoacrylate monomer (superglue) can be used to treat gastric varices.

Portal hypertensive gastropathy accounts for 2–3% of bleeding episodes in cirrhotic patients. Although major bleeding is uncommon, its diffuse nature precludes endoscopic therapy. Treatment by beta blockers, TIPS or surgery is dictated by the severity of bleeding and liver impairment.

Portal and splenic vein obstruction

Portal vein thrombosis is the commonest cause of portal hypertension in children. Tumours, chronic pancreatitis, abdominal sepsis and hypercoagulable states cause thrombosis of this vein in adults. In children, omphalitis, umbilical vein catheterization or neonatal septicaemia may be responsible, but it usually remains unnoticed until variceal bleeding or splenomegaly and pancytopenia occur. Liver function tests are normal and the diagnosis is made by duplex Doppler. Treatment is initially by endoscopic therapy.

Splenic vein thrombosis is rare and is also caused by chronic pancreatitis, pseudocysts, trauma or pancreatic tumours. Splenic blood flow is diverted through the short gastric veins and produces sinistral (or left-sided) portal hypertension, although only fundal gastric varices may be present. Splenectomy is curative.

Budd–Chiari syndrome

This uncommon syndrome is caused by obstruction to hepatic venous outflow, leading to increased sinusoidal pressure, hepatocyte necrosis and progressive liver damage. Myeloproliferative disorders, hypercoagulable states, tumours of the liver, kidney and adrenal gland; caval or hepatic vein webs; and intrahepatic veno-occlusive disease may cause thrombosis of hepatic veins. Acute, subacute or chronic forms occur depending on the pathophysiology.

The clinical presentations depend on the rapidity of the hepatic vein occlusion. Ultrasound, duplex Doppler, CT, hepatic venography and liver biopsy are used to make the diagnosis and plan treatment. Hepatic decompression with a TIPS, or side-to-side portocaval or mesocaval shunt treats the obstruction if it only involves the hepatic veins. A mesoatrial shunt using a prosthetic graft may be necessary if the inferior vena cava is obstructed by caudate lobe hypertrophy. Liver transplantation provides excellent results in patients with liver decompensation (see Ch. 8).

ASCITES

The formation of ascites in cirrhosis arises from a combination of increased sinusoidal pressure and hepatic insufficiency. The pathophysiology is complex. Elevated hepatic sinusoidal pressure leads to a transudate of high-protein fluid from the liver into the peritoneal cavity. Ascites accumulation causes decreased intravascular volume, increased aldosterone secretion, redistribution of renal blood flow, and salt retention. Rapid onset of ascites in patients with cirrhosis may be caused by infection, portal venous thrombosis, or the development of hepatocellular carcinoma. Ascites can also develop during a period of heavy alcohol misuse or excessive sodium intake in food or medication.

Box 29.9 Analysis of ascitic fluid

- Evaluate macroscopic appearance (straw-coloured, turbid, bloody or chylous)
- Cell count and differential
- Chemistry profile (protein, albumin and amylase)
- Cytology
- Gram stain and bacterial culture

Tests to consider ordering

- Adenosine deaminase (if tuberculosis is suspected)
- pH, lactate, lactate dehydrogenase (if bacterial peritonitis suspected)

Ultrasonography is used to confirm the presence of minimal ascites and to guide diagnostic paracentesis. Paracentesis with ascitic fluid analysis is the most rapid and cost-effective method of diagnosis, especially in patients with recent-onset ascites, cirrhotic patients with ascites admitted to hospital, or those with clinical deterioration. The ascitic fluid is submitted for quantitative cell counts, fluid culture, and calculation of the serum:ascites albumin gradient, which reflects differences in oncotic pressures and correlates with portal venous pressure (Box 29.9). It is important to exclude malignant ascites and chylous ascites.

The principal aim of treatment of symptomatic ascites in cirrhotic patients is to improve their general comfort and quality of life. Treatment includes restriction of sodium and water intake, the promotion of sodium and water excretion by diuretics, and the correction (where possible) of precipitating factors. It is important to convince patients with alcoholic cirrhosis to abstain from alcohol, because – in a period of months – abstinence can result in a substantial improvement in the reversible component of alcoholic liver disease.

A low-sodium diet of 1–1.5 g of salt (40–60 mmol/day) usually produces a net sodium loss, which may be sufficient to treat mild ascites. Fluid restriction is not essential; however, marked hyponatraemia (serum sodium less than 120 mmol/L) does warrant fluid restriction. Most patients need diuretics as well as dietary restrictions. A single morning dose of oral spironolactone (an aldosterone antagonist) and furosemide (frusemide; a loop diuretic), beginning with 100 mg of spironolactone and 40 mg of furosemide, is prescribed initially. Both oral diuretics can be increased simultaneously, maintaining the 100 mg:40 mg ratio, if weight loss and natriuresis are inadequate on the lower doses. Maximum doses are 400 mg/day of spironolactone and 160 mg/day of furosemide. Dietary sodium restriction and dual diuretic therapy is effective in 90% of patients.

The patient's weight, electrolytes and renal function should be carefully monitored. Ascites that is refractory to diuretics can be managed by repeated paracentesis; however, this suggests that decompensation and liver transplantation should be considered. In the past, peritoneojugular Denver or Le Veen shunts were inserted for the management of refractory ascites but are now seldom used. Recently, TIPS has been used to treat refractory ascites with some success.

HEPATIC ENCEPHALOPATHY

Hepatic encephalopathy is a metabolic neuropathy that occurs in patients with liver disease or portal systemic shunts. It presents

Box 29.10 Events precipitating hepatic encephalopathy in cirrhosis

Electrolyte imbalance
- Diuretics
- Vomiting
- Diarrhoea

Gastrointestinal bleeding
- Oesophageal and gastric varices
- Gastroduodenal erosions

Drugs
- Alcohol withdrawal
- Benzodiazepines

Infection
- Spontaneous bacterial peritonitis
- Urinary
- Chest

Constipation
- Dietary protein overload

as a reversible state of impaired cognitive function or altered consciousness ranging from minor mental changes to lethargy and coma. The typical features include monotonous speech, a flat affect, tremor, muscular incoordination and impaired handwriting. On examination foetor hepaticus, up-going plantar responses, hypo- or hyperactive reflexes, and decerebrate posturing may be elicited. Hepatic coma, especially in alcoholic patients, should be diagnosed only after other causes of unconsciousness have been excluded.

Hepatocellular insufficiency and portosystemic shunting may act separately or in combination to cause encephalopathy. Almost all cases of clinically apparent encephalopathy occur in patients with cirrhosis. While less than 5% of non-cirrhotic portal hypertensive patients develop encephalopathy, it develops in a disproportionately large proportion of patients with surgical shunts or TIPS (Box 29.10). Drugs and gastrointestinal tract haemorrhage may precipitate encephalopathy, and a small proportion of cases are precipitated by excess dietary protein, hypokalaemic alkalosis, constipation, and deterioration of liver function secondary to drugs, toxins, viruses or hepatocellular carcinoma.

The treatment of hepatic encephalopathy is empirical and relies largely on establishing the correct diagnosis; identifying and treating precipitating factors; emptying the bowels of blood, protein and stool; attending to electrolyte and acid–base imbalance; and the selective use of benzodiazepine antagonists. Non-absorbable disaccharides such as lactulose are used to empty the bowels. Antibiotics and protein restriction (40 g/day) can be used if there is no response to this treatment, and in intractable cases closure of surgical shunts or TIPS or liver transplantation should be considered.

THE HEPATORENAL SYNDROME

The hepatorenal syndrome is characterized by acute oliguric renal failure due to intense renal vasoconstriction in otherwise normal kidneys in patients with liver disease.[52] A clinical cause is often not found, treatment is often ineffective, and the prognosis is poor. The syndrome is prevented by avoiding excessive diuresis and by early recognition of electrolyte imbalance, bleeding or infection. Potentially nephrotoxic drugs such as aminoglycosides should be avoided.

Patients who develop hepatorenal syndrome should have blood cultures taken and bacteraemia treated. The diagnosis is one of exclusion and should not be made until all potentially reversible causes of renal failure have been excluded.[53] Most patients with liver disease who develop renal failure have prerenal failure or acute tubular necrosis. The more common potentially reversible causes are sepsis, excessive diuresis or paracentesis, and nephrotoxic drugs. All patients suspected of having hepatorenal syndrome should be given an intravenous colloid infusion to exclude intravascular hypovolaemia as a cause of prerenal failure. Liver transplantation, if feasible, is ultimately the only consistently effective treatment.

SPONTANEOUS BACTERIAL PERITONITIS

Spontaneous bacterial peritonitis is usually a consequence of bacteraemia caused by defects in the hepatic reticuloendothelial system and defective peripheral destruction of bacteria by neutrophils. This allows secondary seeding of bacteria into the ascitic fluid, which is deficient in antibacterial activity.

Clinical signs may be minimal, although other causes of peritonitis may need to be excluded (see Ch. 25). Diagnostic paracentesis should be performed in any cirrhotic patient with ascites who rapidly deteriorates or presents with fever or abdominal pain. A white cell count greater than 500 cells/mm^3 is indicative of peritonitis. Treatment with intravenous broad-spectrum antibiotics should be started while awaiting the ascitic fluid culture results. Although the mortality of the condition decreases with early treatment, it remains high (over 50%) and is usually related to the severity of the underlying liver disease.

REFERENCES

52. Dagher L, Moore K. Gut 2001; 49: 729–737
53. Moreau R. J Gastroenterol Hepatol 2002; 17: 739–747

The gall bladder and bile ducts

30

Ian J. Beckingham

ANATOMY AND PHYSIOLOGY

NORMAL ANATOMY

Gall bladder

The gall bladder is a pear-shaped organ that lies on the visceral inferior surface of the liver between segments IV and V of the liver. The first and second parts of the duodenum lie behind it and the transverse colon lies below. It is covered with peritoneum except where it is adherent to a depression in the liver surface known as the gall bladder fossa. The expanded lower end of the gall bladder, or fundus, may or may not project beyond the inferior border of the liver in the region of the right ninth costal cartilage, and the body of the organ narrows to form the neck, which terminates in the cystic duct. The dilated area proximal to the junction of the neck and cystic duct is known as Hartmann's pouch.

The cystic duct arises from the neck of the gall bladder and joins the common hepatic duct. It is typically 1–3 mm in diameter, although may be much wider in some individuals. The mucosa is arranged in spiral folds known as the valve of Heister. It most frequently is 3–4 cm in length and joins the common hepatic duct at a slight angle.

The main blood supply to the gall bladder is provided by the cystic artery, which commonly arises from the right branch of the hepatic artery posterior to the common hepatic duct (Fig. 30.1). The cystic artery runs above and behind the cystic duct to reach the neck of the gall bladder, where it divides into an anterior and a posterior branch. The gall bladder also receives a variable blood supply from the liver through its bed. A major portion of the venous drainage passes directly to the liver through the gall bladder fossa, but veins may be seen around the cystic artery and these drain directly into the portal vein.

The cystic lymph node lies adjacent to the cystic artery where it meets the gall bladder wall, and is therefore a useful landmark during cholecystectomy. Lymph from the gall bladder and bile ducts passes through the cystic node and into other intrahepatic nodes in the edge of the lesser omentum.

Bile ducts

The right and left hepatic bile ducts fuse at a variable distance below the liver to form the common hepatic duct. The area between the common hepatic duct, which lies within the edge of the lesser omentum, the liver and the cystic duct, is called Calot's triangle. Its contents are the cystic artery and lymph node, and its accurate identification and dissection are crucial to the safe performance of cholecystectomy. (Note: Calot actually described the triangle lying between the cystic artery, cystic duct and hepatic duct, but the above description is the one usually referred to and of more practical relevance.[1])

The hepatic artery lies on the left of the common hepatic duct, and the portal vein lies posteriorly. The cystic duct joins the common hepatic duct to form the common bile duct approximately 2 cm above the duodenum. As it passes behind the first part of the duodenum and the head of the pancreas, the bile duct loses its peritoneal covering, and it enters the duodenum through the posteromedial wall to join the main pancreatic duct within the ampulla of Vater, which then opens into the duodenum via a papilla in the second part of the duodenum approximately 10 cm beyond the pylorus. Circular muscle fibres are present around the terminal portion of the bile and pancreatic ducts and their confluence at the ampulla. The combination of all these sphincteric mechanisms is known as the sphincter of Oddi.[2]

The blood supply to the bile ducts is complex, and branches are received from the gastroduodenal, hepatic and cystic arteries as well as the coeliac and superior mesenteric vessels.[3] Two vessels run along the lateral borders of the supraduodenal segment and 60% of their blood supply is provided from arteries below, mainly from the retroduodenal and retroportal vessels. The right hepatic artery provides most of the blood supply of the main bile duct from above, and only 2% of the blood is derived from the common hepatic artery. This arrangement of the blood supply suggests that bile duct damage during surgery can be minimized by restricting dissection at the lateral margins of the common bile duct so as to avoid damaging the axial vessels. Flush ligation of the cystic duct on the common bile duct is also best avoided for the same reason. Anastomotic complications after transplant surgery may also be related to arterial damage.[3]

The nerves to the extrahepatic bile ducts are derived from segments 7–9 of the thoracic sympathetic chain and from the parasympathetic vagi. Afferent nerves, which include pain fibres from the biliary tract, run in sympathetic nerves and pass through the coeliac plexus and the greater splanchnic nerves to reach the thoracic spinal cord via the white rami communicantes and dorsal ganglia. The preganglionic efferent nerves from the spinal cord relay with cell bodies in the coeliac plexus, and the postganglionic fibres run with the hepatic artery to supply the biliary tract. A small contribution of pain afferents may travel within the right phrenic nerve and peritoneum below the right diaphragm.[4] These fibres may account for the radiation of gall bladder pain to the right shoulder tip during attacks of biliary colic. Vagal fibres supply the hilum of the liver and the bile ducts. Although vagal stimulation results in gall bladder contraction and relaxation of

REFERENCES

1. Wood D. Am J Surg 1979; 138: 746
2. Hand BH. Clin Gastroenterol 1973; 2: 3
3. Northover JMA, Terblanche J. Br J Surg 1979; 66: 379
4. Burnett W, Cairns FW, Bacsich P. Ann Surg 1964; 123: 8

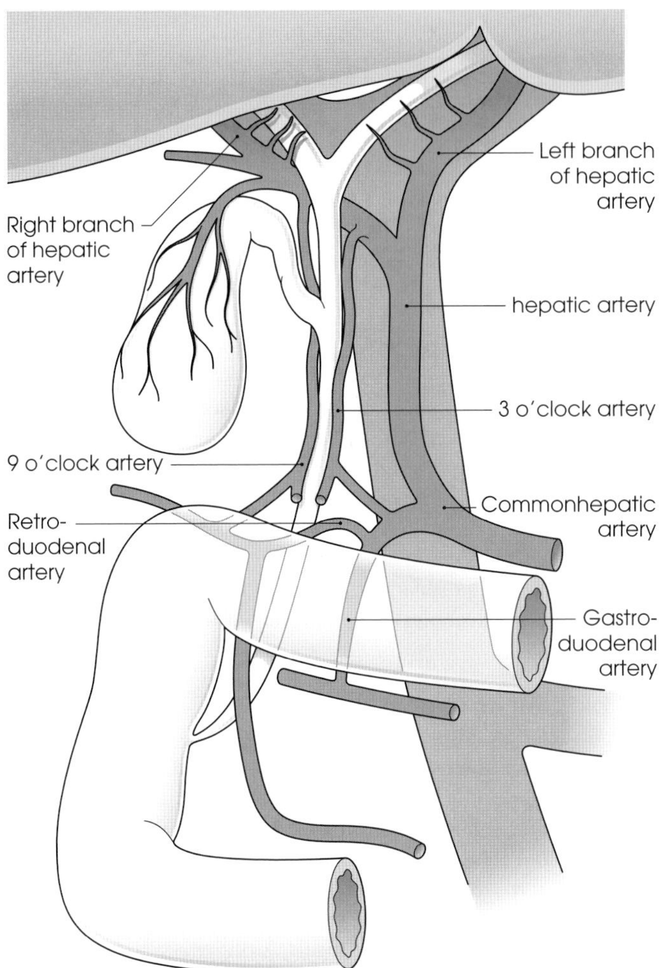

Figure 30.1 The blood supply of the gall bladder and bile ducts.

the sphincter of Oddi, the effects are overshadowed by the action of gastrointestinal hormones such as cholecystokinin.

VARIATIONS AND ANOMALIES OF ANATOMY

Gall bladder

The gall bladder is rarely absent or rudimentary,[5] but when this occurs it may be associated with other congenital anomalies such as tracheo-oesophageal fistula or imperforate anus. Left-sided or intrahepatic gall bladders, and double and triple gall bladders have also been reported. Discovery of duplications at operation, usually by operative cholangiography, should be followed by removal of both gall bladders. A second operation may be necessary later if only one organ is removed.[6]

The gall bladder may be abnormal in structure, for example the body may be divided completely or partially by a septum. Complete division may result in two separate cavities fused at their necks to form a single cystic duct, or they may drain by two separate ducts. Partial separation of the fundus from the body seen at surgery or during preoperative imaging is known as a Phrygian cap,[7] and is caused by a localized thickening of the gall bladder wall. It is of little significance and gall bladder function is usually normal.

Complete investment of the gall bladder with peritoneum can predispose to torsion around its associated mesentery,[8] particularly when this is restricted to the neck of the organ so that the body and fundus remain free.

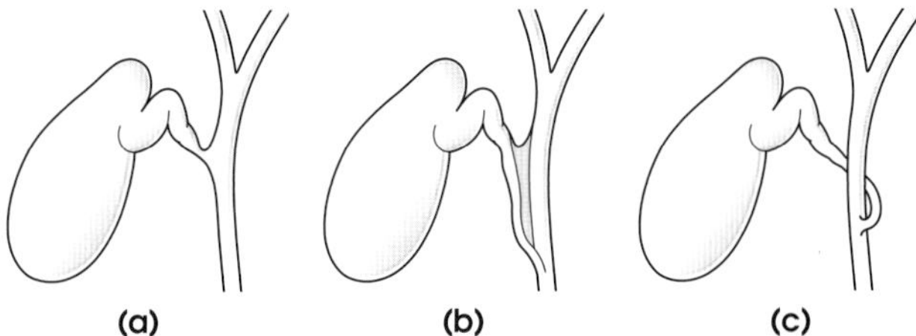

Figure 30.2 The normal variations of the cystic duct junction: (a) direct joining from the right side (75%), (b) running parallel before entering from the right side (20%), and (c) spiralling behind the hepatic duct and joining from the left side (5%).

Bile ducts

Major variations in bile duct anatomy are common,[9] and their frequency has been analysed in a large series of operative cholangiograms.[10] The most important anatomical variations from an operative viewpoint are those pertaining to the cystic duct (Fig. 30.2). The most important, and potentially dangerous, variations involve different types of right subsegmental ducts and their drainage into the biliary tract via or close to the cystic duct (Fig. 30.3). A few examples of the commoner variations include the following:

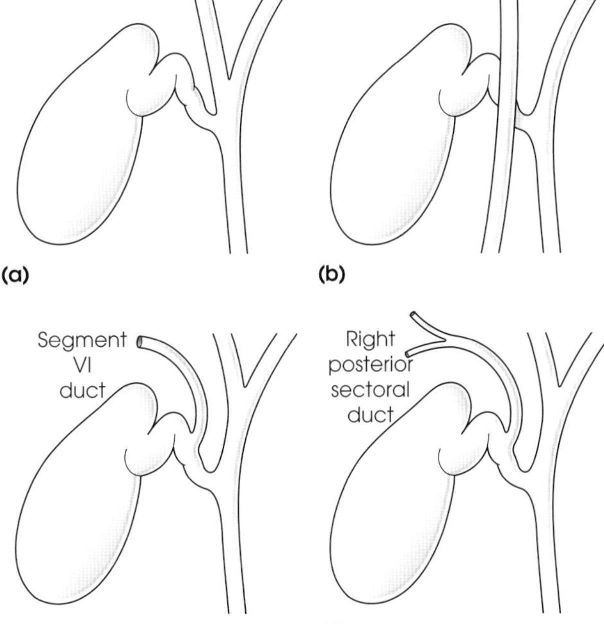

Figure 30.3 Main variations in ectopic drainage of intrahepatic ducts into the cystic duct: (a) drainage of the cystic duct into the biliary confluence, (b) drainage of the cystic duct into the left hepatic duct associated with no biliary confluence, (c) drainage of the segment VI duct into the cystic duct, and (d) drainage of the right posterior sectoral duct into the cystic duct.

REFERENCES

5. Ferris DO, Glazer IM. Arch Surg 1965; 91: 359
6. Harlaftis N, Gray SW, Skandalakis JE. Surg Gynecol Obstet 1977; 145: 928
7. Joseph AEA, Grundy A. In: Wilkins RA, Nunnerley HB (eds). Imaging of the Liver, Spleen and Pancreas. Blackwell Scientific Publications, Oxford, 1990: 309
8. Ashby BS. Br J Surg 1965; 52: 182
9. Benson EA, Page RE. Br J Surg 1976; 63: 853
10. Kullman E, Borch E et al. Br J Surg 1996; 83: 171

- A high insertion of the cystic duct into the region of the common bile duct bifurcation (3.1%).
- An accessory hepatic duct, defined as a separate channel draining a segment of the right lobe of the liver into the common hepatic duct, cystic duct or gall bladder. The incidence is between 1 and 4%,[11] and it may be the only drainage from the relevant segment. An injury can easily occur to these ducts during cholecystectomy and may result in partial or total occlusion of a portion of the biliary tract, because there is a lack of interductal communications within the liver.
- The cystic duct entering the right hepatic duct. This is an uncommon variation (0.2%), but it increases the risk of transection or ligation of the right duct during surgery.
- The right and left hepatic ducts may join the common hepatic duct in a variable manner, and occasionally this junction may be truly intrahepatic. The right duct occasionally fuses with the cystic duct.
- Duplication of the cystic ducts has been described.

Intraoperative cholangiography is used for the recognition of the above anomalies. Accessory ducts may be tied off if small, but larger ducts should be preserved and implanted into a Roux loop if necessary. Bile peritonitis or fistula may be a consequence of the unrecognized division of such a duct. Anomalies of the common bile duct itself are very rare, but ectopic drainage of accessory ducts into the stomach has been described on five occasions,[12] including an original report by Vesalius in 1543. The anomaly has been associated with symptomatic biliary gastritis.

Hepatic and cystic arteries

Major anomalies of vessel origin are particularly important during hepatectomy and pancreatectomy (see Ch. 29 and Ch. 31). The left hepatic artery arises from the left gastric, splenic or superior mesenteric in 3–6% of the population and may be especially at risk during gastrectomy (see Ch. 26). The right hepatic artery arises from the superior mesenteric artery in 10–20%, and an accessory right hepatic artery arising from the superior mesenteric is found in 5% of patients.

The right hepatic artery is particularly at risk during cholecystectomy if it takes a tortuous course close to the cystic duct and neck of the gall bladder, because the cystic artery may be very short in this variation. Anatomical variations of the cystic artery itself are common, and it may arise from the left, common or accessory hepatic arteries and pass anterior or posterior to the main bile duct. More than one cystic artery is present in some patients. The cystic artery not uncommonly runs in front of the common bile duct, increasing the risk of damage to the bile duct during cystic artery dissection and ligation.

PHYSIOLOGY OF THE BILIARY TRACT

Composition and functions of bile

Bile is made up of bile salts (0.7%), bile pigments (0.2%), cholesterol (0.1%) and lecithin (0.1%) dissolved in an alkaline electrolyte solution (97% water). About 500 mL are excreted into the gastrointestinal tract per day. Bile pigment is conjugated bilirubin derived from effete red blood cells. Bile salts are sodium and potassium salts of bile acids conjugated to taurine and glycine. Bile salts aid lipid absorption in the gastrointestinal tract by activating lipases, and by combining directly with lipids to form water-soluble micelles. Bile salts are 95% reabsorbed in the terminal ileum entering the portal vein and excreted in the bile, constituting the enterohepatic circulation. When bile is excluded from the intestine, a quarter of the ingested fat appears in the stool.

Bile is transported from the liver to the duodenum through the biliary tract. Some 50–60% of bile enters the gall bladder in the fasting state,[13] where it is concentrated and modified in composition. Normal bile secretion pressures range from 12 to 15 cm of water. The papillary sphincter provides a resistance to bile flow between meals, although the flow never ceases completely. Bile secretion is inhibited when the bile duct pressure reaches 20 cm of water.[14]

Gall bladder resorption

The gall bladder capacity is approximately 40 mL, and its function includes the active absorption of sodium, chloride and bicarbonate ions, which is followed by the passive absorption of water.[15] Lipid-soluble substances pass across the epithelium easily, and there is slow absorption of conjugated bile salts. The absorption of unconjugated bile salts appears to be speeded up by mucosal damage, and therefore deconjugation by bacterial activity within the gall bladder may result in a significant loss of bile salts, reduced cholesterol solubility, and possibly gallstone formation.

Gall bladder contractility

Both gall bladder contraction and relaxation of the sphincter of Oddi are under hormonal control. Cholecystokinin is released during absorption of fat and essential amino acids from the duodenum and small bowel mucosa,[16] and it causes contraction of the gall bladder and relaxation of the sphincter of Oddi. It has a direct action on the gall bladder muscle and is the major stimulus for contraction.[17] Secretin decreases contractility and motilin alters motility between meals. Motility is also affected by gastrin and prostaglandins. Hormone production from the gastrointestinal tract is inhibited by bile salts, and this mechanism may allow the gall bladder to fill between meals.

In contrast to the hormonal effects on the biliary tract, neurological control is more difficult to measure. Reciprocal reflex activity between the gall bladder and the duodenum has been demonstrated in dogs during vagal stimulation, but vagal effects are complicated by gastrointestinal secretion and hormone release. No direct vagal influence has been found on either the sphincter of Oddi[18] or on gall bladder contractility.[19] Vagotomy does not appear to affect gall bladder emptying in response to either cholecystokinin or a fatty meal.

Bile is stored and concentrated in the gall bladder but passes through the common bile duct in a passive manner. Common

REFERENCES

11. Knight M, Smith R, Sherlock S (eds). Surgery of the Gall Bladder and Bile Ducts. Butterworth, London, 1981
12. Sieber WK, Wiener ES, Chang J. J Pediatr Surg 1980; 15: 817
13. Watts M, Dunphy JE. Surg Gynecol Obstet 1966; 122: 1207
14. Strasberg SM, Dorne BC et al. Gastroenterology 1971; 61: 357
15. Diamond IM, Tormey IM. Nature 1966; 210: 817
16. Bouchier IAD. In: Smith R, Sherlock S (eds). Surgery of the Gall Bladder and Bile Ducts. Butterworths, London, 1981: 67
17. Vagne M, Grossman MI. Am J Physiol 1968; 215: 881
18. Pitt HA, Doty JE et al. J Surg Res 1982; 32: 598
19. Sandblom P, Poegtlin WL, Ivy AC. Am J Physiol 1935; 113: 175

bile duct emptying is controlled by gall bladder activity and contractions in the sphincter of Oddi. Substantial common bile duct dilatation does not occur after cholecystectomy unless there is either mechanical or functional obstruction in the distal duct.

RADIOLOGICAL INVESTIGATION OF THE GALL BLADDER AND BILE DUCTS

X-RAY INVESTIGATIONS

Approximately 10% of gallstones are radiopaque (Fig. 30.4), and very occasionally the gall bladder itself is calcified (porcelain gall bladder). Enlargement of the gall bladder may be recognized as a soft tissue mass above the hepatic flexure of the colon. Air within the bile ducts may be associated with a spontaneous biliary–intestinal fistula or gas-forming organisms, particularly in severe cholangitis. Previous endoscopic or surgical procedures (e.g. sphincterotomy or choledochojejunostomy) will also allow the free passage of air into the bile ducts.

Oral cholecystography was used to diagnose gall bladder stones and to assess gall bladder contractility and function. Both these roles have now been replaced by ultrasonography. Intravenous cholangiography was also used extensively in the past to investigate the common bile duct, but high false negative rates of stone detection in the common bile duct[20] and the risks of anaphylactic shock have led to its replacement.

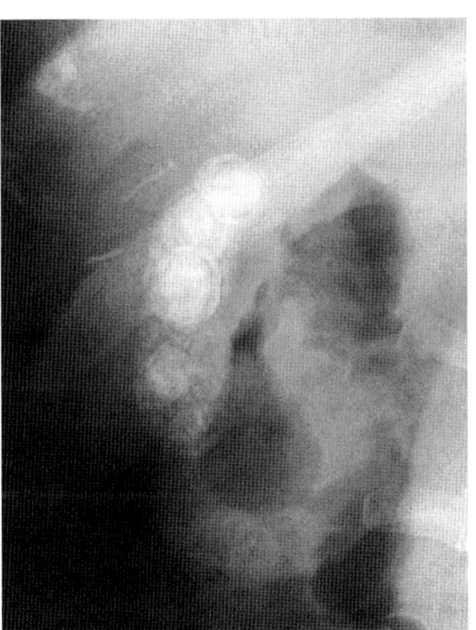

Figure 30.4 Gallstones are visible on plain X-ray in 10% of cases.

ULTRASONOGRAPHY

Ultrasound is the simplest and least invasive means of assessing the biliary system. It is an extremely sensitive test for demonstrating gall bladder stones and detecting bile duct dilatation. It is very specific for stones down to a few millimetres in diameter.[21] The examination is performed with the patient fasting, so that the biliary tract is distended with bile and the stomach and duodenum empty of gas. Stones are visualized as echogenic foci with acoustic shadowing; movement of the patient changes their position. Stones in the cystic duct are poorly visualized because of reflections from the spiral valve,[22] and stones can be confused for small polyps, particularly when the polyps are calcified. A small shrunken gall bladder with stones but little fluid within it may be missed on ultrasound, and stones may be misinterpreted for bowel gas or vice versa.

The technique is often poor for visualizing the lower common bile duct, because gaseous distention of the duodenum or transverse colon obscures the head of the pancreas. This explains its low sensitivity for demonstrating common bile duct stones (56% sensitivity and 65% specificity[22]). The presence of gall bladder wall thickening, distension, and the presence of stones together with a sonographic Murphy's sign are suspicious of acute cholecystitis.[23] Gall bladder polyps and tumours are well visualized and liver tumours may be demonstrated.

Biliary obstruction with dilated bile ducts is readily identifiable with ultrasound, and the level and cause of obstruction can be determined in 70–90% of cases, again limited in the lower bile duct by the frequent presence of overlying bowel gas. Duplex ultrasound is highly accurate at predicting vascular involvement and resectability in hilar cholangiocarcinoma, particularly in assessing invasion of the portal vein.[24]

COMPUTERIZED TOMOGRAPHY

Computerized tomography (CT) imaging can be used to assess biliary duct dilatation and intrabiliary calcification, but both of these are better seen with ultrasound scan, which is less expensive and avoids the radiation exposure. The place of CT is in visualizing the extrahepatic bile duct and its relationship to adjacent viscera, and in imaging the liver and pancreas for causes of obstruction and tumour staging. Scans need to be with oral and intravenous contrast and of thin collimation (3–5 mm). Computerized tomography is less good than ultrasound at visualizing gall bladder stones but better than ultrasound in visualizing common bile duct stones (75–88% sensitivity and 97% specificity for CT[25,26]) because of its ability to consistently image the lower common bile duct. Newer multislice scanners with faster acquisition times and higher attenuation are likely to improve CT images. Reconstruction of CT images can give cholangiogram-like pictures, but these are no better than magnetic resonance cholangiopancreatography (MRCP).

MAGNETIC RESONANCE IMAGING AND MAGNETIC RESONANCE CHOLANGIOPANCREATOGRAPHY

Magnetic resonance imaging is non-invasive and has no radiation hazard. It is contraindicated in patients with cardiac pacemakers and ferrous metal intracranial aneurysm clips, but appears to be safe in pregnancy. A small proportion of patients (around 5%) are unable to tolerate the procedure because of claustrophobia.

Magnetic resonance cholangiopancreatography (MRCP) is an imaging technique used to evaluate the biliary system. Heavily T2-weighted images show stationary fluid (including bile and

REFERENCES

20. Goodman MW. Gastroenterology 1980; 79: 642
21. De Graaff CS, Dembner AG, Taylor KJW. Arch Surg 1978; 113: 877
22. Tobin MV, Mendelson RM, Lamb GH et al. Br Med J Clin Res 1986; 293: 16–17
23. Rails PW, Colletti PM et al. Radiology 1985; 155: 767
24. Hann LE, Greatrex KV, Bach AM et al. Am J Roentgenol 1997; 168: 985–989
25. Barakos JA, Ralls PW, Lapin SA et al. Radiology 1987; 162: 415–418
26. Neitlich JD, Topazian M, Smith RC et al. Radiology 1997; 203: 753–757

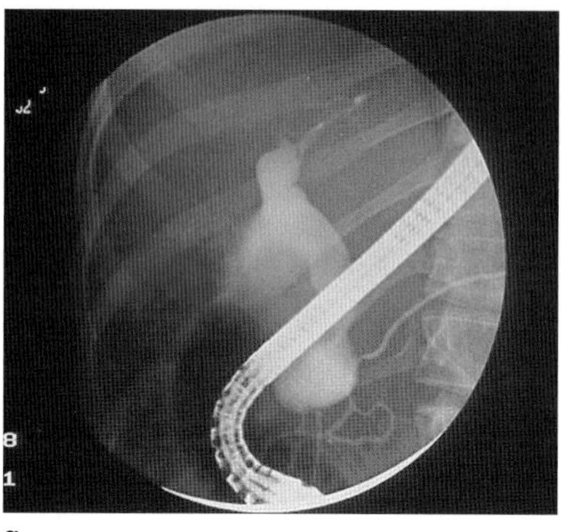

a

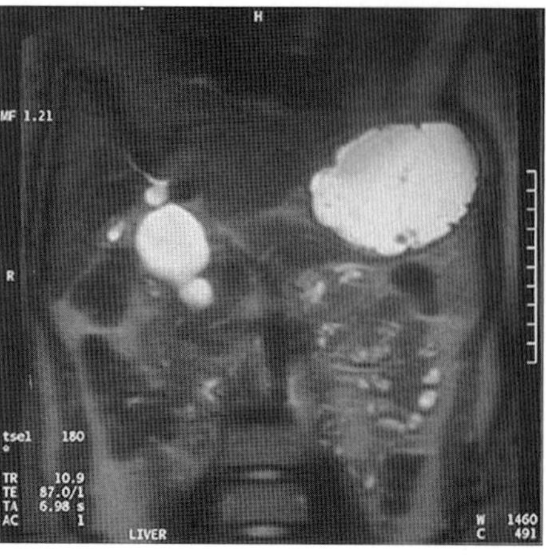

b

Figure 30.5 Choledochal cyst: (a) endoscopic retrograde cholangiopancreatography and (b) magnetic resonance cholangiopancreatography.

pancreatic fluid) as high signal intensity compared with surrounding tissues. The technique has a 95% sensitivity for the detection of obstruction,[27] and has been shown to be of equal accuracy to endoscopic retrograde cholangiopancreatography (ERCP) in the determination of the level and cause of the obstruction.[28,29] Standard magnetic resonance images with intravenous gadolinium can be used to assess the vascular system in biliary tumours and also to look for liver metastases, allowing an all-in-one staging assessment. In choledocholithiasis, MRCP has a sensitivity of 91–98%.[30–32]

ENDOSCOPIC ULTRASOUND

An endoscope with an ultrasound head can be passed via the mouth into the duodenum under conscious sedation. Imaging of the porta hepatis and extrahepatic biliary tract is possible because of their close proximity to the gastric antrum and duodenum, eliminating the disadvantages of transabdominal ultrasound (i.e. bowel gas and obesity). Two types of echoendoscopes are available: mechanically rotating transducers, which obtain 360° images perpendicular to the end of the instrument, and electronic convex linear array probes producing an ultrasound beam parallel to the endoscope working channel. The circumferential view enables easier anatomical and pathological orientation, whereas the radial view permits targeted biopsying. Intrabiliary probes 1.4–3.2 mm in diameter are also available and can be inserted through the duodenal papilla for assessment of cholangiocarcinomas.

Endoscopic ultrasound is of similar sensitivity and specificity to ERCP in the detection of common bile duct stones[33] but may well be more accurate. In patients with idiopathic pancreatitis, endoscopic ultrasound detected small quantities of biliary sludge in 60%.[34,35] The technique is highly sensitive in detecting abnormalities of the bile duct, although it is unable to distinguish between benign and malignant thickening in early lesions.[36,37] It is as sensitive as ERCP in detecting small bile duct tumours and superior to ultrasound, CT and angiography.[38,39] The staging of extrahepatic cholangiocarcinomas is 72–81% accurate compared with resected specimens, but nodal assessment only 61% reliable.[40,41] Nodal assessment with all imaging techniques relies on equating size, internal structural patterns and border profiles with malignancy, for which imaging appearances are unreliable. The addition of fine needle aspiration using the curvilinear array echoendoscope improves the accuracy of nodal assessment to 91%.[42]

ENDOSCOPIC RETROGRADE CHOLANGIOPANCREATOGRAPHY

Used extensively to investigate the bile ducts by retrograde injection through the duodenal papilla, the diagnostic role of ERCP is being largely replaced by MRCP (Fig. 30.5) but it remains a valuable method of treating biliary pathology. Patients should have preprocedure coagulation studies before being sedated and placed semiprone. A side-viewing duodenoscope is inserted orally and passed into the second part of the duodenum to locate the papilla. A cannula is then passed into the papilla, and water-soluble contrast is injected to demonstrate the bile ducts and/or pancreatic duct. Failure to cannulate the papilla occurs in 5–10% of procedures. The presence of periampullary diverticula or a previous Polya gastrectomy increases the failure rate up to 50%.

REFERENCES

27. Guibaud L, Bret PM, Reinhold C et al. Radiology 1995; 197: 109–115
28. Lee MG, Lee HJ, Kim MH et al. Radiology 1997; 202: 663–669
29. Soto JA, Barish MA, Ferrucci JT. Semin Roentgenol 1997; 32: 188–201
30. Becker CD, Grossholz M, Becker M et al. Radiology 1997; 205: 523–530
31. Chan YL, Chan AC, Lam WW et al. Radiology 1996; 200: 85–89
32. Reinhold C, Taourel P, Bret PM et al. Radiology 1998; 209: 435–442
33. Prat F, Amouyal G, Amouyal P et al. Lancet 1996; 347: 75–79
34. Ros E, Navarro S, Bru C et al. Gastroenterology 1991; 101: 1701–1709
35. Lee SP, Nicholls JF, Park HZ. N Engl J Med 1992; 326: 589–593
36. Tamada K, Tomiyama T, Ichiyama M et al. Gastrointest Endosc 1998; 47: 28–32
37. Gress F, Chen YK, Sherman S et al. Endoscopy 1995; 27: 178–184
38. Yasuda K, Nakajima M, Kawai K. In: Kawai K (ed). Endoscopic Ultrasonography in Gastroenterology. 1st edn. Igaku-Shoin, Tokyo, 1988: 96–105
39. Sugiyama M, Hagi H, Atomi Y et al. Abdom Imaging 1997; 22: 434–438
40. Mukai H, Nakajima M, Yasuda K et al. Gastrointest Endosc 1992; 38: 767–683
41. Qilian Z, Weidong N, Lando Z et al. Chinese Med J 1996; 109: 622–625
42. Hoffman BJ, Hawes RH. Gastrointest Endosc Clin North Am 1995; 5: 587–594

The main complication is acute pancreatitis, which occurs in 5% of patients and is severe in 10–20% of these, occasionally resulting in the patient's death (procedural mortality rate about one in 1000). Bleeding and perforation occur in around 1 in 100 and are usually associated with therapeutic sphincterotomy (division of the sphincter of Oddi with diathermy to allow stone removal).

Endoscopic retrograde cholangiopancreatography allows visualization of stones and strictures within the main bile ducts and intrahepatic ducts, and it allows removal of stones with baskets or balloons, or the insertion of plastic or metal wall stents. It also allows cytological and histological specimens to be obtained from pathology within the bile ducts, pancreas or duodenum.

PERCUTANEOUS TRANSHEPATIC CHOLANGIOGRAPHY

The procedure consists of insertion of a thin needle into the liver substance through the seventh or eighth intercostal space under local anaesthesia. Water-soluble contrast is injected into the liver as the needle is slowly withdrawn until a bile duct is entered. Contrast often outlines the hepatic or portal veins and lymphatics but quickly clears. Contrast within bile ducts persists for a longer period. Access can be achieved in 95% of dilated ducts, and even 80% of non-dilated bile ducts can be entered.[43] Bacteraemia and occasionally septic shock are rare complications of the technique and are most common in patients with strictures or stones. Peritoneal bile leaks and bleeding are now rare since the use of ultrathin needles. Antibiotic prophylaxis and preprocedure coagulation studies are essential.

Percutaneous transhepatic cholangiography, like ERCP, has become almost entirely a therapeutic procedure as a result of the development of MRCP. Once access to the bile ducts has been established, the needle is exchanged for a guide wire over which the tract can be dilated to admit an external drain, internal–external drain, internal plastic pigtail stent, or expanding metal wall stent. Some centres still use percutaneous transhepatic cholangiography to assess hilar cholangiocarcinomas preoperatively.[44]

RADIONUCLIDE (HIDA) SCANS

Technetium-99-labelled derivatives of 2,6-dimethyl phenylcarbamoylmethyl-iminodiacetic acid (HIDA) administered intravenously enter the biliary tract within 15 min, where it can be imaged using a gamma camera. The technique is useful for the diagnosis of acute cholecystitis and bile duct anomalies in childhood (discussed later in this chapter). The passage of radionuclide into the bowel is also useful in diagnosing bile leaks and iatrogentic biliary obstruction after biliary–enteric anastomosis (Fig. 30.6).[45]

Acute cholecystitis is diagnosed when there is a failure of uptake of HIDA into the gall bladder because the cystic duct is obstructed. This is diagnostic in 97% of patients with pathological signs of gall bladder inflammation,[46] and hepatobiliary scintigraphy is the best test if there is diagnostic uncertainty.[47]

JAUNDICE

Jaundice is the yellow discoloration of the skin, sclera and other tissues caused by excess deposition of bilirubin. It is normally visible only when the serum bilirubin rises above 35–40 μmol/L (2 g/dL).

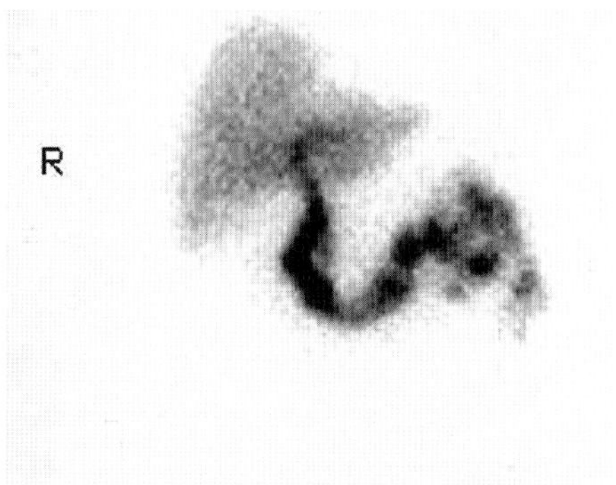

Figure 30.6 A normal HIDA scan following successful biliary reconstruction with hepaticojejunostomy, showing radionuclide passing from liver into roux loop.

THE BILIRUBIN PATHWAY

Bilirubin is formed from the breakdown of senescent red blood cells (80%), myoglobins, and hepatic haemoproteins such as cytochrome P450. In its unconjugated state, it is highly insoluble and is transported to the liver bound to albumin (Fig. 30.7). Within the hepatocytes it is conjugated by ursodeoxycholic acid–glucuronyl transferase to bilirubin glucuronides, which are subsequently excreted into the canalicular lumen. A small amount refluxes back into the circulation. Virtually all the bilirubin in normal individuals is unconjugated, with less than 5% being in the conjugated form. Bilirubin is degraded to stercobilinogen within the bowel, a small proportion of which is reabsorbed and subsequently excreted in the urine as urobilinogen.

CLASSIFICATION AND CAUSES OF JAUNDICE

Jaundice can be classified into three groups: prehepatic (caused by increased haemolysis), hepatic (from defective hepatic metabolism of bilirubin), and posthepatic (from obstruction of the bile ducts).

Prehepatic jaundice

In the prehepatic group of disorders the liver is presented with an excessive load of unconjugated bilirubin, which being insoluble is therefore absent from the urine. Increased haemolysis from spherocytosis, thalassaemia and sickle cell disease is the commonest cause. A normal liver can handle up to six times the normal daily load of bilirubin before jaundice develops. Patients may exceed this threshold and develop an unconjugated hyperbilirubinaemia after major trauma associated with large haematoma formation. In children the Crigler–Najjar syndrome, a rare conjugation defect inherited as an autosomal recessive (type I) or dominant (type II) disorder,[48] interferes with conjugation of bilirubin.

Gilbert's syndrome is a common disorder in which there is a deficiency of glucuronyl transferase, resulting in a poor uptake of bilirubin into hepatocytes.[49] When stressed patients develop an

REFERENCES

43. Jaques PF, Mauro MA, Scatliff JH. Radiology 1980; 134: 33–35
44. Nimura Y. Endoscopy 1993; 25: 76–80
45. Reichelt HG. Chirurgica 1978; 49: 167–171
46. Suarez CA, Block F et al. Ann Surg 1980; 191: 391
47. Shea JA, Berlin JA, Escarce JJ et al. Arch Intern Med 1994; 154: 2573–2581
48. Crigler JF, Najjar VA. Pediatrics 1952; 10: 169
49. Foulk WT, Butt HR et al. Medicine 1959; 38: 25

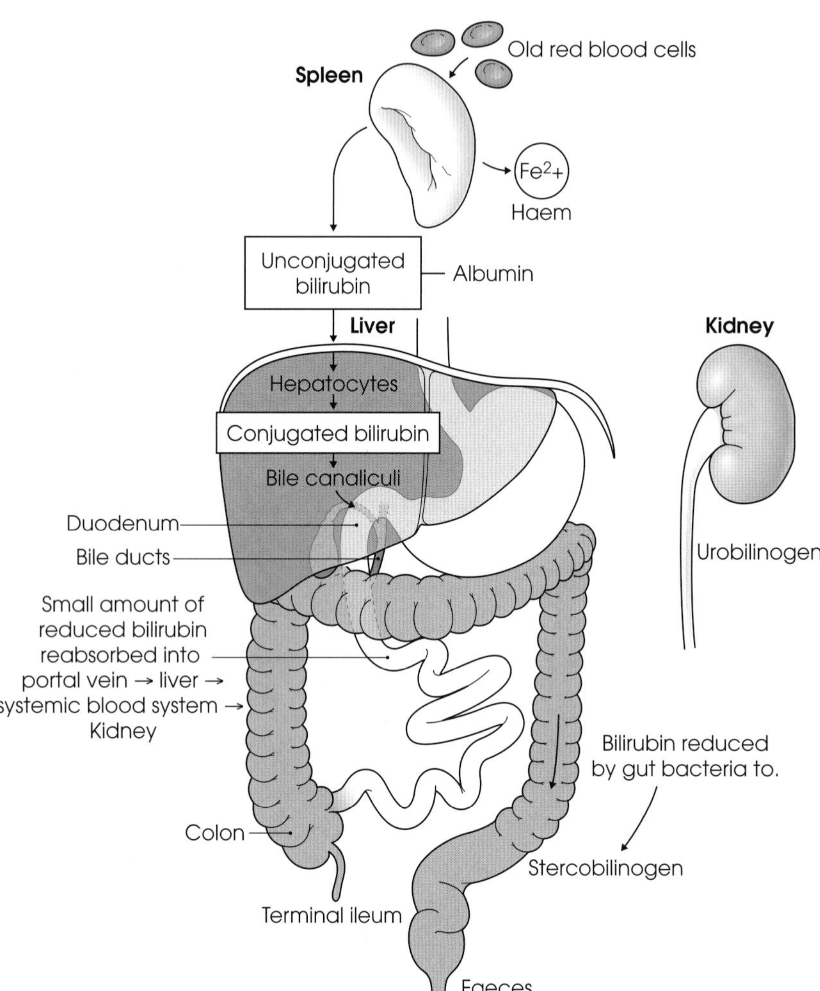

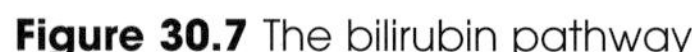
Figure 30.7 The bilirubin pathway.

isolated hyperbilirubinaemia with otherwise normal liver function tests. This occurs after surgery or viral illness. It is a benign condition and patients have a normal life expectancy.

Hepatic jaundice

Hepatocytes may be damaged by a wide variety of causes including viral infection and ingested toxins such as alcohol and drugs. Inherited metabolic disorders and autoimmune disorders can also cause hepatic damage (Table 30.1). Patients can present with acute liver failure or chronically with cirrhosis and the associated features of chronic liver disease. The serum bilirubin may be unconjugated because the damaged hepatocytes are unable to process bilirubin, or it may be conjugated because of a failure to excrete bilirubin into the cannaliculi. Often there is a mixture of both, depending on the cause of liver damage. Conjugated bilirubin is water-soluble and therefore excreted in the urine. Surgery plays no role in the management of prehepatic and hepatic jaundice except to transplant the failing liver (see Ch 29).

Table 30.1 Common Hepatic (Parenchymal) causes of Jaundice
Viral Hepatitis (Hepatitis A–E, CMV, FBV, Infectious Mononucleosis
Alcoholic hepatitis
Drug induced (eg Paracetamol overdose, idiosyncratic drug reactions)
Metabolic (eg Haemochromatosis, Wilsons Disease)
Autoimmune (eg Primary Biliary Cirrhosis, Primary Sclerosing Cholangitis, Autoimmune hepatitis)

Posthepatic jaundice

Bile duct obstruction causes a conjugated hyperbilirubinaemia with bilirubin in the urine and pale stools. With complete obstruction of the biliary tract there is an absence of urobilinogen in the urine. The commonest causes are bile duct calculi and malignancies of pancreatic, bile duct and ampullary origin. Less frequent causes include sclerosing cholangitis, chronic pancreatitis, choledochal cysts and metastatic portal lymphadenopathy. In developing countries, parasitic infestations with *Ascaris lumbricoides* or *Clonorchis sinensis* may cause obstructive jaundice.

INVESTIGATION OF THE JAUNDICED PATIENT

History and examination

The diagnosis and treatment of the jaundiced patient begins with the clinical history and examination. Recent travel (which may indicate hepatitis, malaria, alcohol consumption and drug usage), recent blood transfusion, family history (Gilbert's syndrome, Wilson's disease, autoimmune conditions and inherited haemoglobinopathies) should be enquired about. Infective hepatitis is more common in intravenous drug abusers. An intermittent or fluctuating history of jaundice suggests the possibility of common bile duct stones, sclerosing cholangitis, autoimmune hepatitis, or Gilbert's syndrome.

Obstructive jaundice typically presents with dark urine, pale stools and pruritis. Accompanying pain and rigors, experienced as alternating hot sweats and chills, suggest the presence of stones in the common bile duct. Constant back pain and weight loss are suggestive of pancreatic cancer. Intermittent severe pains radiating to the tip of the right scapula and lasting several hours are suggestive of gallstone disease.

Pruritis is an important feature of both hepatic and posthepatic cholestasis. It is related to bile salt deposition within the skin and is experienced most severely on the extremities, being worse in warm weather. Severe bruising is the result of hypoprothrombinaemia from either hepatocellular damage or malabsorption of vitamin K.

General examination should detect the stigmata of chronic liver disease if present, such as spider naevi, palmar erythema, finger clubbing, leukonychia, gynaecomastia and ascites. The presence of splenomegaly and prominent veins of the abdominal wall suggest portal hypertension and cirrhosis. Features of specific types of liver disease include xanthomata in biliary cirrhosis and Kayser–Fleischer rings in Wilson's disease.[50]

Enlargement of the liver is recognized by palpation of its lower margin below the rib cage and percussing over the right lower ribs to assess its upper limit, which is normally in the fifth intercostal space. The character of the liver edge and surface may be diagnostic; for example the irregular hard edge of malignant disease.

When jaundice is caused by a stone in the common bile duct, dilatation of the gall bladder is rare because the gall bladder is thickened, fibrotic and less able to distend in the presence of stones. Conversely, when the duct is obstructed by a carcinoma of the pancreas, non-tender dilatation of the gall bladder is common (Courvoisier's sign).[51] The obstruction must be below the confluence of the cystic and common hepatic ducts. Gall bladder distention together with signs of sepsis and tenderness suggests acute cholecystitis or empyema of the gall bladder.

Blood and urine tests

The initial investigation of jaundice is by urinary, biochemical and serological tests. When taken with the history and examination, these allow classification of the jaundiced patient into the three categories outlined above in around 70% of cases.

Patients with prehepatic causes of jaundice usually have a low haemoglobin level, and examination of the blood film identifies reticulocytosis and abnormal erythrocytes.

Alkaline phosphatase is expressed mainly in liver and bone, with smaller amounts derived from the kidney and intestine. It is produced by the cholangioles in the brush border of the canna-liculi, and synthesis is increased with obstruction of the bile ducts.

Gamma glutamyltranspeptidase is present in many organs besides the liver but not in bone. It is elevated in bile duct obstruction but also increased by many drugs, including alcohol. It is useful in differentiating the source of an elevated alkaline phosphatase as being of liver origin rather than bone.

Transaminases are useful indicators of hepatocellular damage. The two most commonly used in clinical practice are alanine aminotransferase, which is localized mainly in the liver, and aspartate aminotransferase, found in liver, heart, kidney and muscle. The alanine aminotransferase can reach very high levels in viral hepatitis but is less marked in alcoholic hepatitis. An aspartate aminotransferase:alanine aminotransferase ratio greater than 2 is highly suggestive of alcohol as the aetiology of parenchymal liver disease.[52,53] Transaminase levels are not specific, however, and can be elevated in congestive heart failure and in biliary obstruction with or without cholangitis.

The liver is the major site where blood-clotting factors are produced. Factors II, VII, IX and X are produced in the liver and are dependent on absorption of the fat-soluble vitamin K. Impaired synthetic capacity or failure of absorption because of bile obstruction can cause a coagulopathy.

Albumin is produced solely in the liver. It has a relatively long half-life of 20 days and is therefore not a very sensitive indicator of synthetic function. Hypoalbuminaemia is seen in patients with chronic liver disease and hepatic malignancy, and like the clotting time is useful in prognostic scoring systems for chronic liver disease.

Normal urine contains small amounts of urobilinogen but no bile pigments. The presence of bilirubin occurs with elevated levels of conjugated bilirubin within the blood in patients with obstructive jaundice, hepatitis and cirrhosis. Urobilinogen is absent in the urine of patients with complete biliary obstruction, and is elevated in patients with non-obstructive jaundice. Urine analysis is cheap and provides a quick answer but unfortunately has a high proportion of false negative results.

Sequence of investigations in obstructive jaundice

When the biochemical, serological and urinary tests suggest that the patient has a cholestatic jaundice, an ultrasound scan should be obtained to demonstrate any ductal dilatation, gallstones or intrahepatic lesions. Ultrasound can determine the level of biliary obstruction in 92% of cases and the cause in 71%.[54] Its main failing is in the lower common bile duct, which is often obscured by the presence of overlying bowel gas from the duodenum or colon. Computerized tomography will determine the cause and level with 95% accuracy.[55]

Further management depends on the level of obstruction and its cause, the degree of jaundice, and locally available resources and expertise. Further non-invasive definition of the biliary tract can be obtained by MRCP, which has the ability to visualize the biliary tract both above and below a complete obstruction, without risk to the patient and without contamination of the obstructed system. In patients with a high serum bilirubin (greater than 150 mmol/L), it is reasonable to proceed directly to ERCP because stone removal or stent placement is likely.[56] Hilar obstruction is generally better assessed and easier drained with percutaneous transhepatic cholangiography than with ERCP. Ideally, all staging investigations should precede intervention to allow a single interventional treatment: surgical, endoscopic or percutaneous transhepatic cholangiography drainage. Patients with biliary sepsis or very high levels of jaundice (greater than 300 mmol/L) require endoscopic or percutaneous drainage to achieve biliary decompression prior to definitive staging.

A liver biopsy to identify the cause should be considered in patients with liver function tests indicative of cholestasis in the

REFERENCES

50. Nazer H, Ede RJ et al. Gut 1986; 27: 1377
51. Taylor I, Wright R. In: Blumgart LH (ed). Surgery of the Liver and Biliary Tract. 2nd edn. Churchill Livingstone, Edinburgh, 1994: 184
52. Cohen JA, Kaplan MM. Dig Dis Sci 1979; 24: 835–838
53. Williams AL, Hoofnagle JH. Gastroenterology 1998; 95: 734–739
54. Laing FC, Jeffrey RBJ, Wing VW et al. Radiology 1986; 160: 39–42
55. Pedrosa CS, Casonova R, Lezana AH et al. Radiology 1981; 139: 635–645
56. Brown JJ, Naylor MJ, Yagan N. Radiology 1997; 202: 1–16

absence of biliary tract dilatation. This may be obtained percutaneously or, if coagulopathy is present, via the transhepatic route.

GALLSTONE DISEASE

CLASSIFICATION OF GALLSTONE TYPE, COMPOSITION AND DEVELOPMENT

Gallstones are classified as black pigment stones, brown pigment stones or cholesterol stones.

Black pigment stones

Black pigment stones occur commonly in patients with haemolysis (from any cause) or in patients with cirrhosis. Unconjugated bilirubin is absent from the bile of normal individuals;[57] in patients with black pigment stones, a small amount of the excess bile escapes conjugation and 'spills' into the bile. It becomes polymerized and coprecipitates with free ionized calcium to form sludge, and then coalesces to form stones.[58] Up to half the individuals who are homozygous for sickle cell disease have sludge in their gall bladders by the age of 10 years.[59]

Brown pigment stones

Brown pigment stones are found more often in the bile ducts than in the gall bladder and are rare in the western hemisphere, accounting for less than 5% of stones. They are most common in the Far East, along with small areas of high incidence in Kashmir and various parts of South America and southern Africa.[60,61] Their formation is not fully understood, but they are associated with the high prevalence of *Ascaris lumbricoides* in all these areas and *Clonorchis sinensis* (found only in the Far East). Bacterial infection is also thought to be part of the complex development of these soft, friable stones, and it may be that fragments of the parasites act as a nidus for subsequent stone formation with bacterial glucuronidase, which breaks down conjugated bilirubin to its insoluble unconjugated form.

Cholesterol stones

Cholesterol-rich stones are the commonest gallstones in western society, accounting for over 80% of stones. Their appearance varies from pure white crystalline solitaires to multifaceted grey-green mixed stones. They consist of 70–90% cholesterol. Cholesterol is a normal constituent of bile, and the formation of cholesterol stones is dependent on the relative presence of three components: supersaturation of bile with cholesterol; the nucleation defect, i.e. an imbalance of promoters (such as mucin and ionized calcium) and inhibitors (such as phospholipids and apolipoproteins) of microcrystal precipitation; and gall bladder stasis. The precipitation of cholesterol stones almost always occurs in the gall bladder.

Epidemiological studies have demonstrated a familial tendency in patients with cholesterol gallstones, with 37% of patients having a first-degree relative with stones.[62] Cholesterol lithogenic genes have been identified in Hispanics and Amerindians with a high incidence of stones.[63] Obesity is a major risk factor for gallstones because of increased total body cholesterol synthesis,[64] as well as increased biliary cholesterol excretion.[65] Gall bladder motility is also decreased in obese individuals.[66] Cholesterol-lowering agents such as fibrates can cause gallstone formation by increasing the bile cholesterol levels.[67] Crohn's disease and ileal resection may result in bile salt malabsorption and a reduction in bile acids, and they are associated with an increased rate of cholelithiasis.[68]

Many of the risk factors associated with development of gallstones—such as pregnancy, total parenteral nutrition, octreotide, rapid weight loss and high spinal injury—cause gall bladder stasis, which has been clearly shown to occur in both animals[69] and humans[70] before the formation of stones.

THE NATURAL HISTORY OF GALLSTONES AND ASYMPTOMATIC GALLSTONES

It is estimated that 10–15% of the adult population has gallstones in the USA,[71] with similar figures of 12% of men and 24% of women reported from post-mortem studies in the UK.[72] This equates to around 7.5 million Britons and 20 million Americans with gallstones.

In a population study of 30 000 Italians, the incidence of gallstones was 10% in men and 19% in women, with a linear incidence by age group of 10 per 1000 individuals per year.[73] Less than 15% of patients had experienced symptoms attributable to gallstones. The incidence of developing biliary symptoms in patients with symptomless gallstones has been estimated as 1–4% per annum, or about a third of patients over 20 years.[74] Patients with symptomless gallstones rarely develop complications of gallstone disease.[75] On the basis of these and other studies, it is recommended that patients with symptomless gallstones should not undergo cholecystectomy. Exceptions to this are in populations with a genetically determined early development of gallstones and gall bladder cancer (e.g. Pima Indians of USA[76]

REFERENCES

57. Goresky CA, Gordon ER, Hinchey EJ et al. Hepatology 1995; 21: 373–382
58. Werlin SI, Scott JP. J Pediatr 1996; 129: 321–322
59. Webb DHK, Darby JS, Dunn DT et al. Arch Dis Child 1989; 64: 693–696
60. Beckingham IJ, Cullis SNR, Krige JEJ et al. Br J Surg 1998; 85: 907–910
61. Beckingham IJ, Krige JEJ, Bornman PC. Br J Surg 1998; 85:1360–1363
62. Sarin SK, Negi VS, Dewan R et al. Hepatology 1995; 22: 138–141
63. Miquel JF, Covarrubias C, Vallaroel L et al. Gastroenterology 1998; 115: 937–946
64. Nestel PJ, Schreibman PH, Ahrens EH Jr. J Clin Invest 1973; 52: 2389–2397
65. Reuben A, Maton PN, Murphy GM et al. Clin Sci 1985; 69: 71–79
66. Hendel HW, Hojgaard L, Andersen T et al. Int J Obes Relat Metab Disord 1998; 22: 294–302
67. Read AE. In: Millward-Sadler GH, Wright R, Arthur MJP (eds). Wright's Liver and Biliary Disease. 3rd edn. WB Saunders, London, 1992: 1252
68. Heaton KW, Read AE. Br Med J 1969; 3: 494
69. Pauletzki JG, Xu Q-W, Shaffer EA. Hepatology 1995; 22: 325–331
70. Van der Linden. Tijdschr Gastro 1974; 17: 121–128
71. (Anonymous). NIH Consensus Statement 10, No. 3. Gallstones and Laparoscopic Cholecystectomy. National Institutes of Health, 1992; 10: 1–28
72. Godfrey PJ, Bates T, Harrison M et al. Gut 1984; 25: 1029–1033
73. Attili AF, Carulli N, Roda E et al. Am J Epidemiol 1995; 141: 158–165
74. Friedman GD. Am J Surg 1993; 165: 388–404
75. Gracie WA, Ransohoff DF. N Engl J Med 1982; 307: 798–800
76. Lowenfels AB, Walker AM, Althaus DP et al. Int J Epidemiol 1989; 18: 50–54

and Mapuche Indians of Chile[63]), and young symptomless patients with gallstones associated with haemoglobinopathies such as homozygous sickle cell disease, where the majority will become symptomatic.[77] Patients with diabetes have not been shown to have a higher incidence of gallstones, and again there is no clear benefit of cholecystectomy in symptomless patients in this group.[78]

PRESENTATIONS OF GALLSTONE DISEASE

Biliary colic

The commonest way that gallstone disease presents is with biliary colic that starts suddenly in the epigastrium or right upper quadrant and may radiate round to the back to the tip of the right scapula. Contrary to its name, the pain often does not fluctuate but persists from 15 min up to 24 h, subsiding spontaneously or with opiate analgesia. Nausea or vomiting often accompanies the pain, which is visceral in origin and occurs as a result of gall bladder distension consequent on obstruction or the passage of a stone through the cystic duct. Examination may demonstrate some tenderness in the right upper quadrant. Blood tests are normal, and abdominal radiographs may show gallstones in around 10% of patients. The differential diagnosis of severe biliary colic includes peptic ulcer disease, oesophageal spasm, acute pancreatitis, myocardial infarction and right lower-lobe pneumonia. Management is with appropriate analgesia and antiemetics. There is no evidence that smooth muscle relaxants such as scopolamine butylbromide (Buscopan) have any effect. Recurrent attacks may be prevented by avoiding dietary fat, which provokes gall bladder contraction, but this is helpful in only 30–50% of patients. Definitive treatment is by cholecystectomy.

Gall bladder (flatulent) dyspepsia

Many vague abdominal symptoms have been attributed to gallstones. These include poorly localized upper abdominal pain, early satiety, fat intolerance, nausea and bowel symptoms. These symptoms have been shown to occur with similar frequency in patients with and without gallstones,[79] and they respond poorly to inappropriate cholecystectomy.[80,81] In many of these patients the symptoms are from another cause, such as peptic ulcer or irritable bowel syndrome.

Acute cholecystitis

Right upper quadrant or epigastric pain lasting longer than 24 h or accompanied by fever suggests acute cholecystitis. There may be a history of previous attacks of biliary pain. Acute cholecystitis is more common in diabetic individuals (20% of all cases), occurring predominantly in men. Movement exacerbates the pain, and examination reveals tenderness in the right upper quadrant and cessation of breathing on deep inspiration (Murphy's sign).

Symptoms are from impaction of a stone within the cystic duct. Secretion of mucus causes distension of the gall bladder and pain. Release of prostaglandins causes an acute inflammatory response that results in fever, toxicity, and a rise in neutrophils. Ultrasound typically shows gallstones within a tender, thick-walled, oedematous gall bladder with adjacent inflammatory fluid, or a distended obstructed gall bladder. A mild derangement of liver enzymes is often present in patients with acute cholecystitis. Secondary bacterial infection occurs in up to 20% of patients. Occasionally there is secondary infection with a gas-forming organism (e.g. *Clostridium perfringens* and anaerobic streptococci), and gas may be identified within the gall bladder wall as emphysematous cholecystitis on a plain radiograph.

The diagnosis is straightforward in many cases but may be confused with perforated peptic ulcer, acute pancreatitis, pleurisy, cardiac pain, Curtis–Fitz-Hugh syndrome, and occasionally with the pain caused by liver secondaries. A HIDA scan gives the most accurate confirmation of the diagnosis but is rarely necessary in practice.

Patients generally require admission for analgesia and intravenous fluid rehydration. Non-steroidal anti-inflammatory agents such as diclofenac or indomethacin have been shown to reduce inflammation and speed recovery.[82] Broad-spectrum antibiotics such as a second-generation cephalosporin are given to prevent secondary bacterial infection.

Around 20% of patients require emergency surgery because of generalized peritonitis, which can be caused by gangrenous cholecystitis or perforation, or because of deterioration despite medical therapy. The timing of surgery in the other 80% has been the subject of much debate throughout the open as well as the laparoscopic era.[83] It has been traditional to delay surgery where possible for a period of 6–12 weeks to allow inflammation to settle and facilitate subsequent cholecystectomy.[84] It is now clear from several randomized studies that early surgery within the first 3–4 days of onset of symptoms avoids the complications associated with failed conservative management, reduces the time spent in hospital, and has a lower rate of complication and conversion to open surgery when compared with patients in whom surgery is deferred for the traditional 6 weeks.[85–87] There remains a significant conversion to open procedure (10–30%), and surgeons operating on this group of patients must have the full repertoire of techniques and equipment (e.g. cholangiography and choledochoscopy), and be prepared to perform a subtotal cholecystectomy or cholecystostomy.

The optimal treatment for acute cholecystitis should be adequate resuscitation and initiation of parenteral antibiotics, followed by laparoscopic cholecystectomy on the next available list.

Empyema of the gall bladder

Infection of gall bladder contents after stone impaction can result in a pus-filled gall bladder and symptoms of persisting inflammation. The patient appears toxic, with a high swinging temperature and a high white cell count. Omental adherence, thickening and inflammation of the gall bladder often result in a

REFERENCES

77. Serafini AN, Spoliansky G, Sfakianakis GN et al. Arch Intern Med 1987; 147: 1061–1062
78. Aucott JN, Cooper GS, Bloom AD et al. Arch Intern Med 1993; 153: 1053–1058
79. Price WH. Br Med J 1963; ii: 138–141
80. Black NA, Thompson E, Sanderson CF. Gut 1994; 35: 1301–1305
81. Fenster LF, Lonborg R, Thirlby RC et al. Am J Surg 1995; 169: 533–538
82. Akriviadis EA, Hatzigavriel M, Kapnias D et al. Gastroenterology 1997; 113: 225–231
83. Indar AA, Beckingham IJ. Br Med J 2002; 325: 639–643
84. Du Plessis DJ, Jersky J. Surg Clin North Am 1973; 53: 1071–1077
85. Lai PB, Kwong KH, Leung KL et al. Br J Surg 1998; 85: 764–767
86. Lo CM, Liu CL, Fan ST et al. Ann Surg 1998; 227: 461–467
87. Elder S, Eitan A, Bickel A et al. Am J Surg 1999; 178: 303–307

palpable large tender mass. Broad-spectrum antibiotics and percutaneous ultrasound-guided drainage of the gall bladder allow control of sepsis prior to definitive surgery in most patients.

Ischaemia and infection can lead to patchy gangrene that may be walled off by the omentum, duodenum and small bowel, or this may progress to a pericholecystic abscess. Occasionally, especially in elderly patients, the gall bladder perforates. This usually presents as generalized peritonitis of unknown cause. Mortality rates as high as 50% have been reported.[88]

Mucocele of the gall bladder

An attack of biliary colic or acute cholecystitis may be followed by persistent discomfort or pain in the right hypochondrium, indicating the development of a mucocele. Examination reveals a large, tense gall bladder caused by the impaction of a stone in the neck, without infection. Bile pigment is absorbed but mucus secretion continues. The gall bladder may become very large, thick-walled and tortuous.

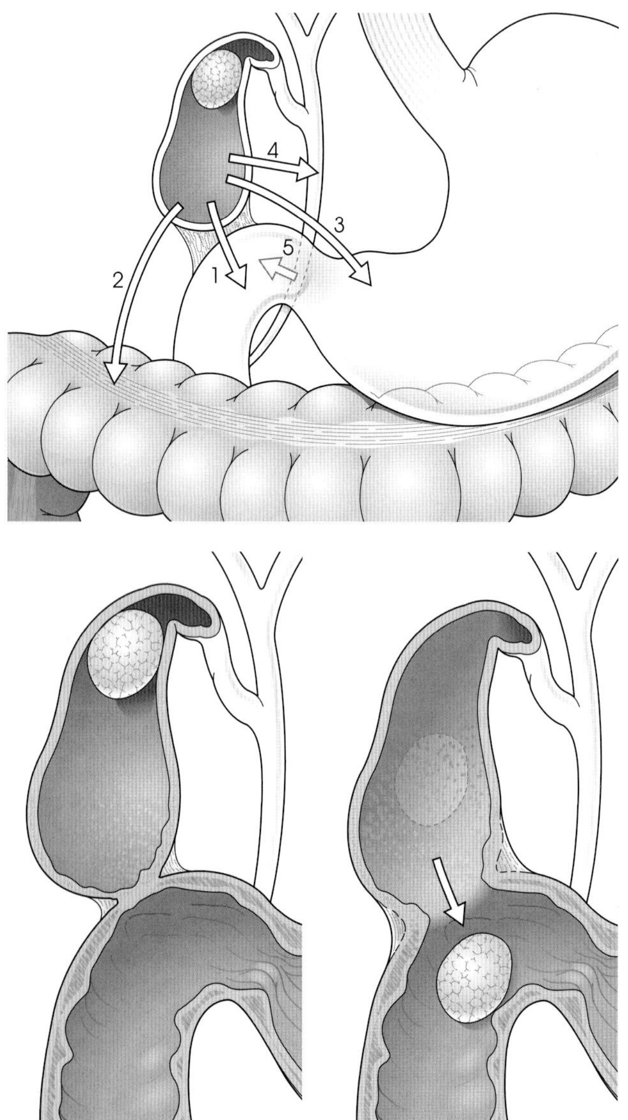

Figure 30.8 (a) Cholecystenteric fistulae can arise in the stomach, duodenum or colon. Stages in the development of a choleduodenal fistula: (b) the gall bladder inflamed, distended, and adhering to the duodenum, and (c) the fistula formed (the stone has passed into the duodenum).

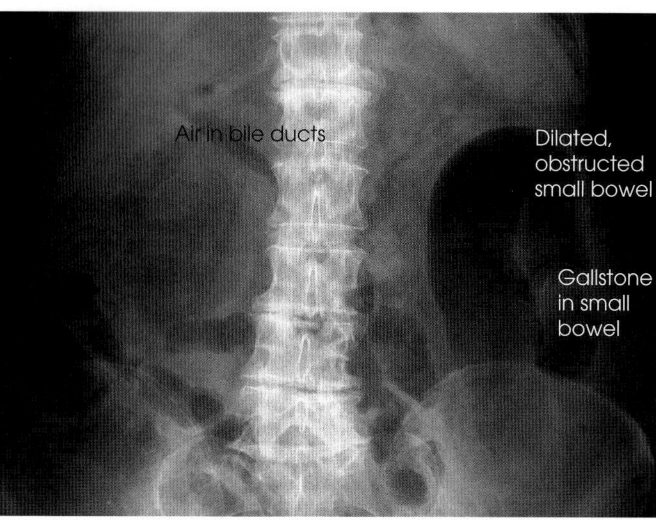

Figure 30.9 Gallstone ileus with air visible within the bile ducts (pneumobilia) and a large gallstone seen in the left iliac fossa, with bowel dilatation proximal to it.

Cholecystenteric fistula and gallstone ileus

A cholecystenteric fistula follows adherence of an acutely inflamed gall bladder to the stomach, duodenum or colon, with the development of pressure necrosis (Fig. 30.8). There may be a history of acute cholecystitis but this is surprisingly uncommon. The presentation depends on the size of the stone. Many are small and do not obstruct the bowel, when the fistula is found only as an unpleasant surprise at cholecystectomy. Larger stones may block the small bowel, causing small bowel obstruction, most commonly at the ileocaecal valve or occasionally within the duodenum, resulting in gastroduodenal obstruction (Bouveret's syndrome).

Elderly women over 70 years of age are most commonly affected. Gallstone ileus accounts for 20% of older patients with small bowel obstruction who do not have a history of a hernia or previous abdominal surgery (see Ch. 27)[89] Plain radiographs may show the triad of small bowel obstruction, a gallstone in the bowel, and gas in the biliary tract (Fig. 30.9). Often the diagnosis is made only at laparotomy for small bowel obstruction.

Choledocholithiasis and jaundice

Gallstones can migrate from the gall bladder into the bile duct, especially if the cystic duct is short and wide. The prevalence of bile duct stones in European patients is around 12%;[90] it is more common in the elderly. Many are symptomless and some pass spontaneously.[91–93] Impaction of the stone within the lower common bile duct or ampulla may lead to the development of obstructive jaundice. The diagnosis is made on the basis of liver

REFERENCES

88. Cuschieri A. In: Blumgart L (ed). Surgery of the Liver and Biliary Tract. Churchill Livingstone, Edinburgh, 1988: 535
89. Clavien PA, Richon J et al. Br J Surg 1990; 77: 737
90. Motson RW. In: Motson RW (ed.) Retained Common Duct Stones. Prevention and Treatment. Grune and Stratton, London, 1985: 8–9
91. Way LW, Admirand WH, Dunphy JG. Ann Surg 1972; 176: 347
92. Stubbs RS, McCloy RF, Blumgart LH. Clin Gastroenterol 1983; 1: 179
93. Perisat J, Huibregtse K et al. Br J Surg 1994; 81: 799

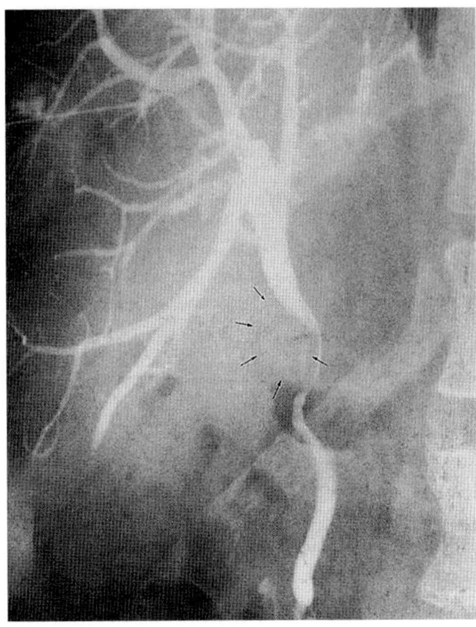

a

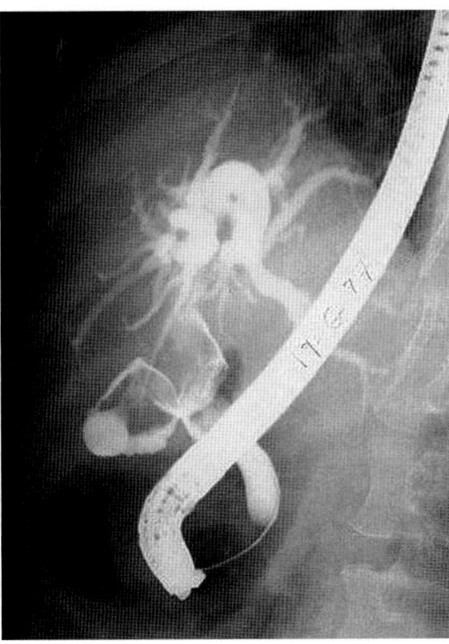

b

Figure 30.10 Endoscopic retrograde cholangiopancreatography films showing (a) type I Mirrizi's syndrome (without connection to bile ducts), and (b) type II Mirrizi's syndrome with two large stones seen within the gall bladder eroding into the common bile duct and contrast seen within the gall bladder via the cholecyst-choledochal fistula.

function tests confirming an obstructive or mixed picture that is not clearly obstructive or hepatic in origin, together with finding dilated bile ducts on ultrasound. Common bile duct stones are visible with transabdominal ultrasound in only 30–50% of patients. Magnetic resonance cholangiopancreatography, endoscopic ultrasound or ERCP can be used to confirm the diagnosis.[94]

Acute cholangitis

Normal bile is sterile, but bacteria are frequently found when stones are present within the biliary tract. In the presence of partial or complete biliary obstruction, bacterial infection leads to acute cholangitis, the most frequent cause of this being bile duct stones. The commonest bacteria are enteric in origin and include *Escherichia coli*, *Klebsiella* spp. and enteroccocci (see Ch. 4).[95]

Acute cholangitis commonly presents as a combination of right upper quadrant pain, rigors (which consist of swinging fevers associated with rigors and chills), and jaundice. This combination is called Charcot's triad, although the full triad may not be present. It is caused by complete or partial biliary obstruction and ascending infection of the biliary tree. It in turn may lead to septicaemia and multiple hepatic abscesses. Treatment is with broad-spectrum antibiotics such as a second-generation cephalosporin or ciprofloxacin. The diagnosis should be confirmed and an early ERCP performed to decompress the bile ducts. A plastic biliary stent should be inserted if pus is present, reserving definitive clearance of the bile duct until the patient's condition has improved.

Acute pancreatitis

Gallstones are responsible for 60% of all episodes of acute pancreatitis (see Ch. 31),[96] although in some individual published series, most notably from inner city areas, alcohol may predominate. The most popular theory of pathogenesis asserts that partial or complete impaction of a small gallstone within the common channel of the duodenal ampulla, or spasm of the sphincter of Oddi following extrusion of the stone through the papilla, allows reflux of duodenal and/or biliary fluid into the pancreatic duct, which activates pancreatic enzymes, initiating pancreatitis.[96,97]

The diagnosis is based on the presence of severe central or epigastric abdominal pain, which often radiates through to the back. A significantly raised serum amylase or lipase is confirmatory. Ultrasound demonstration of gall bladder stones and the absence of alcohol ingestion or other causes of pancreatitis confirm the aetiology. An increasing proportion of up to 60% of the so-called 'idiopathic' group of acute pancreatitis patients have small stones within the bile ducts on endoscopic ultrasound.[34,35] The further management and treatment of gallstone pancreatitis is dealt with in Chapter 31.

Mirrizi's syndrome

Mirrizi's syndrome occurs when there is partial obstruction of the common hepatic duct from impaction of a large gallstone within Hartmann's pouch. The stone induces chronic fibrosis and this, together with the obstruction by the stone itself, causes obliteration of the cystic duct. The inflammatory process fuses the gall bladder to the common hepatic duct, and obstruction of the main bile duct ensues over time. The most useful classification recognizes two types of Mirrizi's syndrome: type I, where there is no communication between the gall bladder and the bile duct, and type II, where the gallstone has eroded into the bile duct, resulting in a cholecyst–choledochal fistula (Fig. 30.10).[98] The condition may be difficult to differentiate from gall bladder cancer or cholangiocarcinoma, and CT and ERCP are the

REFERENCES

94. Beckingham IJ. Eur J Hepatol 2003; 15(7): 809–13
95. Keighley MRB. In: Blumgart LH (ed.). The Biliary Tract. Churchill Livingstone, Edinburgh, 1982
96. Mayer AD, McMahon MJ, Benson EA et al. Ann R Coll Surg Engl 1984; 66: 179–183
97. Neoptolemos JP, Hall AW, Finlay DF et al. Br J Surg 1984; 71: 230–233
98. McSherry CK, Fertenberg H, Virshup M. Surg Gastroenterol 1982; 1: 219–225

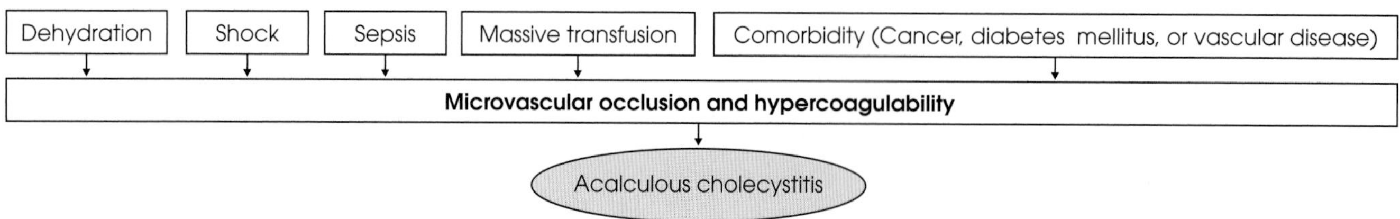

Figure 30.11 Pathogenesis and risk factors for acute acalculous cholecystitis.

most useful investigations when the diagnosis is suspected preoperatively.

Other diseases of the gall bladder

Acalculous cholecystitis

Acute acalculous cholecystitis is a life-threatening condition that occurs in critically ill patients. It accounts for 5–14% of all cases of cholecystitis. The diagnosis is often elusive and is associated with considerable mortality (up to 50%). It tends to occur in patients admitted with multiple trauma or other severe acute non-biliary illness. Risk factors include severe trauma or burns, major surgery (such as cardiopulmonary bypass), long-term fasting, total parenteral nutrition, sepsis, diabetes mellitus, atherosclerotic disease, systemic vasculitis, acute renal failure and AIDS (Fig. 30.11). The condition is thought to be caused by microvascular occlusion of end arteries within the gall bladder wall, resulting in ischaemia and (in up to 60% of cases) gangrene.[99] Over 70% of patients have atherosclerotic disease, which might explain the higher prevalence of the condition in elderly men.[100]

The diagnosis of acute acalculous cholecystitis is often hindered by obtundation of the patient and the presence of pre-existing diseases or recent abdominal surgery, and it requires a high index of suspicion. Ultrasound confirms the diagnosis within the intensive care unit and also allows immediate percutaneous cholecystostomy, which has become the preferred alternative to cholecystectomy in the treatment of the condition in severely ill patients.[101] Early cholecystectomy may be appropriate depending on the patient's clinical condition, because gangrene can develop within the gall bladder and perforation may occur.

Primary infections of the gall bladder

Primary infective cholecystitis is rare and is more commonly seen in immunocompromised patients. Typical causative organisms include *Salmonella typhi*, *Campylobacter jejuni*[102] and *Vibrio cholera*.[103] The presentation is similar to that in patients with acute acalculous cholecystitis, but there is often an antecedent history of a gastroenteritis-like illness.

Patients with AIDS are susceptible to opportunistic gastrointestinal infections including acute cholecystitis and cholangitis, especially when the CD4 count falls below 200 mm^3. In half the cases, there are no associated gallstones within the biliary tract. The most common infecting agents are cytomegalovirus and *Cryptosporidium*, and less commonly *Candida*, fungi and *Mycobacterium tuberculosis*. The 30-day mortality in AIDS patients with acute cholecystitis is 20%.

Treatment is by appropriate intravenous antibiotics followed by laparoscopic cholecystectomy.

MANAGEMENT OF GALLSTONE DISEASE

Medical treatment of gallstones

An alternative treatment to cholecystectomy for gallstone disease has long been sought. Treatments are centred on agents that dissolve cholesterol back into the bile. These are either directly injected into the gall bladder (such as methyl-tert-butyl ether) or given by oral administration, in which case the agent (such as ursodeoxycholic acid) is subsequently excreted into the bile and concentrated in the gall bladder. These agents are capable only of dissolving cholesterol stones and are of no use in treating calcified or pigment stones. Extracorporeal lithotripsy has been used to shatter cholesterol stones and increase the surface area for dissolution, but this can be used only when there are less than four stones that are greater than 10 mm in diameter. Reliable identification of cholesterol stones is difficult and depends on cholecystography, while CT remains the most reliable way of identifying calcification within stones. Patients must also have a functioning gall bladder and patent cystic duct to clear the debris. Only around 10–20% of patients with gallstones fit the criteria for dissolution therapy.

Controlled trials of patients with few stones (of less than 20 mm in diameter) and functioning gall bladders, receiving doses of ursodeoxycholic acid of 8–10 mg/kg for 6–24 months, have achieved dissolution rates of around 40%.[104] Recurrent stones occur in 50–100% of patients when treatment is stopped. Ursodeoxycholic acid is expensive, and a significant proportion of patients suffer with diarrhoea. Direct instillation of methyl-tert-butyl ether in appropriately selected patients achieves dissolution in 80–90%,[105,106] but with recurrent stone formation in 40–70% over 5-year follow-up.[107] Complications include nausea, vomiting, bradycardia and hypotension, leakage and peritonitis, gall bladder injury, duodenal erosions and ulceration.

The development of laparoscopic cholecystectomy has led to abandonment of these procedures in all but the most surgery phobic patients.

Cholecystectomy

Karl Langenbuch first described cholecystectomy in 1882. One hundred years later, the procedure was revolutionized by the

REFERENCES

99. Kalliafas S, Ziegler DW, Flancbaum L et al. Am Surg 1998; 64: 471–475
100. Savoca PE, Longo WE, Pasternak B et al. J Clin Gastroenterol 1990; 12: 33–36
101. Indar AA, Beckingham IJ. Br Med J 2002; 325: 639–43
102. Landau Z, Agmon NL, Argas D et al. Isr Med Sci 1995; 31: 696–697
103. Gomez NA, Leon CJ, Gutierrez J. Surg Endosc 1995; 9: 730–732
104. Roda E, Bazzloi F, Morselli J et al. Hepatology 1982; 2: 804–810
105. Van Sonnenberg E, Casola G, Zakko SF et al. Radiology 1988; 169: 505–509
106. Thistle JU, May GR, Bender CE et al. N Engl J Med 1989; 320: 633–639
107. Hellstern A, Leuschner U, Benjaminov A et al. Dig Dis Sci 1998; 43: 911

development of the laparoscopic approach. By 1992, over 80% of the 600 000 cholecystectomies performed in the USA were carried out laparoscopically.[71] In the UK, some 50 000 cholecystectomies are performed per annum. There has been a rise in the incidence of cholecystectomy since the introduction of the laparoscopic technique, although it is not clear whether this is from a lowering of the threshold for offering surgery or because patients are more willing to undergo the minimally invasive approach.

The indications for cholecystectomy remain unchanged: documented cholelithiasis with symptoms attributable to the presence of gallstones or a diseased gall bladder. Symptomless gallstones should not be removed unless there are established indications (see earlier text).

Laparoscopic cholecystectomy

The first laparoscopic-assisted cholecystectomy was performed by Muhe in Boblinghen, Germany, in 1985. Following the development of the solid-state image sensor in 1985, it was possible for the first time to transmit the pictures from the laparoscope to a television monitor to enable assistants to hold the camera and participate in the operation. The first early laparoscopic cholecystectomy as we would recognize it today was performed by Phillip Mouret in Lyons in 1987, and shortly after in 1988 by McKernan and Saye in Georgia, and Reddick and Olsen in Nashville. The technique was introduced into the UK the following year.

Contraindications

The number of absolute and relative contraindications have diminished over the past 10 years as equipment and skills have improved. Absolute contraindications are an inability to tolerate general anaesthesia, refractory coagulopathy, and suspicion of gall bladder cancer. Laparoscopy in patients with gall bladder cancers is associated with a 20% incidence of port-site metastases. Relative contraindications are dictated primarily by the surgeon's philosophy and experience, and include previous upper abdominal surgery with extensive adhesions, portal hypertension, and third trimester of pregnancy.[108] Severe cardiopulmonary disease and morbid obesity, initially deemed to be contraindications, have been demonstrated to be associated with a lower morbidity when surgery is performed laparoscopically.

Advantages and disadvantages

The advantages of the laparoscopic over the traditional open technique are now well established and include earlier return of bowel function, less postoperative pain, a lower incidence of incisional hernias and adhesions, improved cosmesis, a shorter hospital stay, an earlier return to full activity, and a decrease in the overall cost.[109–115] The procedure is now routinely carried out as a day-case procedure in many centres.

The major disadvantage is cited as a higher risk of bile duct injury. The true incidence of major bile duct injury (defined as injury affecting over 25% of the circumference of the common bile duct) in the open cholecystectomy era was poorly documented, but it was in the order of 0.1–0.5%.[116–118] Initial results from small series of laparoscopic cholecystectomies demonstrated an increase in these rates,[119,120] but subsequent large multicentre and single-centre prospective studies show that bile duct injury rates are similar to those in the open era: 0.2% of 1200 patients,[108] less than 0.01% of 1236 patients,[121] and 0.3% of 6865 patients.[122] A number of studies have shown that the incidence of bile duct injuries is proportional to the surgeon's experience with the technique.[123] When bile duct injuries do occur, however, it appears that they are more proximal and more extensive (i.e. complete transection or excision of the bile duct).

Operative technique

Preparation

Patients fast for 4 h prior to surgery. Antiembolic prophylaxis is used: full-length compression stockings, prophylactic-dose low-molecular-weight heparin, and calf compression boots (see Ch. 11). A general anaesthetic is administered, with full muscle relaxation. A nasogastric tube is not routinely required. Routine antibiotic prophylaxis has been shown to be unnecessary, but it should be used in patients with biliary tract infection or when there is intraoperative bile spillage.

Set-up and port placement

A pneumoperitoneum is established. The author's preferred technique is an open longitudinal cut down below the umbilicus, permitting insertion of a blunt 10-mm trocar. A Veress needle can be used, but there is increasing evidence to suggest that the incidence of bowel (0.083 versus 0.048%) and vascular (0.075% versus 0) injuries is higher with the Veress needle,[124] and furthermore, there are no apparent disadvantages of the open technique. A 10-mm laparoscope is inserted through the umbilical port. Two 5-mm ports are then inserted under direct vision below the costal margin, at the levels of the anterior axillary line and the midclavicular line. A second 10-mm port is inserted in the midline, approximately 5 cm away from the xiphisternum. The aim is to be able to work comfortably on both sides of the gall bladder. Reverse Trendelenburg position and lateral tilt are not routinely required but may be helpful in obese patients.

REFERENCES

108. Underwood RA, Soper NJ. In: Bumgart LH, Fong Y (eds). Surgery of the Liver and Biliary Tract. WB Saunders, London, 2000
109. Bass EB, Pitt HA, Lillemoe KD. Am J Surg 1993; 165: 466–471
110. McMahon A, Russell I, Baxter J et al. Lancet 1994; 343: 135–138
111. McMahon A, Russell I, Baxter J et al. Surgery 1994; 115: 533–539
112. Soper N. Curr Probl Surg 1991; 28: 585–655
113. Soper NJ, Stockmann PT, Dunnegan DL et al. Arch Surg 1992; 127S: 917–921
114. Soper N, Barteau J, Clayman R et al. Surg Gynecol Obstet 1992; 174: 114–118
115. Soper N, Hunter J, Petrie R. Surg Endosc 1992; 6: 115–117
116. Blumgart LH, Kelley CJ, Benjamin IS. Br J Surg 1984; 71: 836–843
117. Andren-Sandberg A, Alinder A, Bengmark S. Ann Surg 1985; 201: 328–333
118. Banting S, Carter DC. In: Paterson-Brown S, Garden J (eds). Principles and Practice of Surgical Laparoscopy. WB Saunders, London, 1994: 53–66
119. Steele RJ, Marshall K, Lang M et al. Br J Surg 1995; 82: 968–971
120. Dunn D, Fowler S, Nair R et al. Ann R Coll Surg Engl 1994; 76: 269–275
121. Cuschieri A, Bobois F, Mouiel J et al. Am J Surg 1991; 161: 383–388
122. Croce E, Azzola M, Golia M et al. Surg Endosc 1994; 8: 1088–1089
123. Moore M, Bennett C. Am J Surg 1995; 170: 55–59
124. Bonjer HJ, Hazebroek EJ, Kazemier G et al. Br J Surg 1997; 84: 599–602

Dissection of Calot's triangle

The gall bladder fundus is grasped with an atraumatic grasper through the most lateral port and pushed cephalad. The assistant holds this instrument and the camera. The surgeon stands on the patient's left side with the monitor on the patient's right side. The surgeon grasps the lower part of Hartmann's pouch and applies lateral and caudal traction to open out Calot's triangle (Fig. 30.12). The peritoneum investing Calot's triangle is opened, staying close to the gall bladder at all times. This can be done with a combination of blunt dissection and short accurate bursts of the diathermy hook. Blunt dissection alone can result in oozing and bleeding from small vessels; overzealous use of the diathermy may result in damage to the bile duct. The gall bladder is flipped medially, and the process repeated on the lateral aspect of the gall bladder. In this way exposure of the cystic duct and artery is achieved with the development of a 'window' posterior to the cystic artery.

Intraoperative cholangiography

Intraoperative cholangiography may be performed routinely or on an occasional basis when a bile duct stone is suspected or when there is uncertainty over the biliary anatomy. All surgeons performing laparoscopic cholecystectomy should be capable of performing the procedure, and patients should be routinely set up on a radiolucent table with facilities available to perform the procedure in the event of a problematic dissection.

The cystic duct is opened with scissors, and any small stones within the duct 'milked' back and removed. A 14-Fr Abbocath

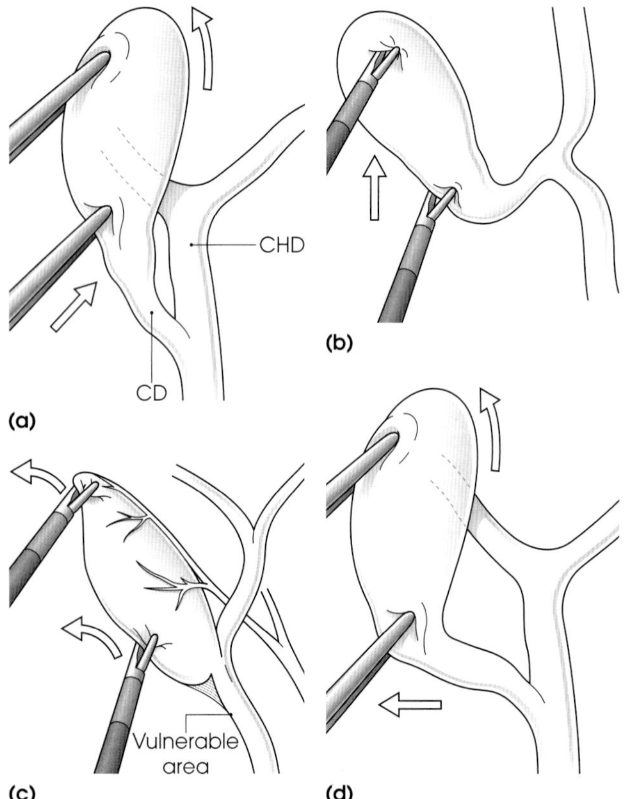

Figure 30.12 Causes of bile duct injury at cholecystectomy. Incorrect traction of Calot's triangle with excessive caudal elevation can cause tenting of the common bile duct (**a**), especially when the cystic duct is short (**b**). Adhesions within Calot's triangle can hide the cystic duct (**c**). Correct inferolateral traction of Hartmann's pouch (**d**) allows Calot's triangle to be opened up and reduces the risk of bile duct injury.

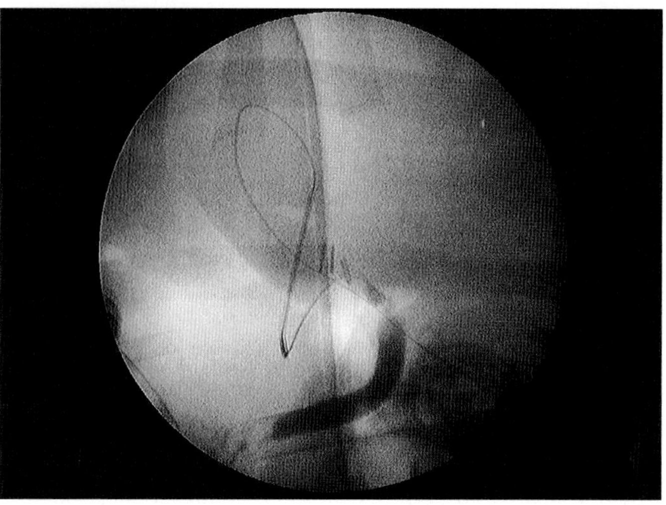

Figure 30.13 Intraoperative cholangiogram showing failure to visualize common hepatic duct due to occlusion by proximal clip. Conversion to open procedure and correct identification of anatomy avoided major biliary injury.

cannula is inserted into the abdomen under the costal margin in the midclavicular area, and a 4-Fr umbilical feeding tube (flushed with saline to remove bubbles) inserted through this and into the cystic duct. A metal clip is used to hold it in place. An image intensifier is used to obtain contrast images using dilute non-ionic contrast media, with care to ensure that no bubbles are within the lumen of the catheter. Use of the image intensifier avoids the problems of misplacement of the machine or X-ray plate, saves time, uses less radiation exposure, and enables real-time imaging, giving much more information than plain film imaging. Four points should be established.

- The entry point of the cholangiogram catheter (marked by the metal clip) should be through the cystic duct and not the common hepatic duct.
- These must be cephalad and caudal flow along the main bile duct, with opacification of right (anterior and posterior branches) and left ducts (Fig. 30.13).
- No stones must be present in the bile duct.
- Contrast should flow into the duodenum.

The debate over whether all patients should have intraoperative cholangiogram has continued through the open and laparoscopic eras, based largely around whether routine cholangiography prevents bile duct injury. There is conflicting evidence to support both arguments. Most surgeons adopt a middle ground, accepting a low threshold for performing cholangiography in patients with an intermediate or a high risk of having common bile duct stones, or when there is any uncertainty in the biliary anatomy. A routine cholangiogram itself does not prevent all bile duct injuries, but performing one should allow early recognition of injury and prevent conversion of an inadvertent choledochotomy into a more major excision of the bile duct.

Evaluation of the common bile duct by laparoscopic ultrasound in experienced hands is more sensitive than cholangiography for detecting bile duct stones and can be performed more rapidly.[125] It is, however, less good at defining ductal anomalies,

REFERENCES

125. Steigmann G, Soper N, Filipi C et al. Surg Endos 1995; 9: 1269–1273

and the two methods of duct imaging are likely to develop differing roles as its use becomes more widespread.[126]

Removal of the gall bladder

Two or three clips are applied to the cystic duct and artery, well away from the portal structures. The vessels are then divided (not diathermied, which may cause necrosis and allow clip slippage). The gall bladder is then removed using the diathermy hook or scissors, staying close to the gall bladder itself. Care should be taken to neither enter the liver, with resultant bleeding, nor the gall bladder, with bile spillage and possible stone leakage into the abdomen. With the gall bladder remaining attached by a small portion near the fundus, a check is made (with gentle suction and irrigation if necessary) to ensure that the clips are still intact and that no bleeding points or bile leaks are present. Finally, the final few attachments of the gall bladder are divided. The camera is moved to the upper port, and a large grasper passed through the umbilical port and applied across the neck of the gall bladder. A tissue-spreading device is slid around the grasper to stretch the umbilical port as the gall bladder is withdrawn through the abdominal wall. The linea alba is closed with absorbable sutures and the skin incisions closed with glue, Steristrips or sutures.

As with all operations, there are many variations on the exact technique, but the one described is safe and reliable.

DEALING WITH OPERATIVE DIFFICULTIES

Obesity

There is good evidence that obese patients have better results with laparoscopic than with open cholecystectomy, both in terms of ease of access within the abdomen and reduced postoperative respiratory problems. Extra-long ports are only rarely needed but ports may need to be inserted more cephalad, particularly the camera port, which is best sited above the umbilicus in morbidly obese patients. A 30° laparoscope improves views in Calot's triangle. Insertion of a fifth port in the left upper quadrant, and use of an atraumatic retractor to push down the omentum and duodenum, improves views in Calot's triangle.

Bleeding

Bleeding from the cystic artery should be controlled with the grasper in the left hand, allowing suction with the right hand and subsequent identification of the bleeding point prior to careful application of a clip. Grasping or pressure together with diathermy, without identification of the bleeding point vessel, is dangerous and runs the risk of damage to the bile duct or its blood supply, causing a delayed bile leak or stricture. Blind firing of multifeed clip appliers should also be avoided. A small swab inserted through the 10-mm port can be used to control bleeding, while the sucker is used to identify the artery before it is grasped with atraumatic forceps. Failure to achieve rapid control of bleeding necessitates immediate conversion to open procedure, with insertion of a pack and direct pressure until adequate wound retraction can be achieved to safely locate the bleeding point.

Gallstone spillage

Inadvertent opening of the gall bladder should be controlled by moving the assistant's grasper to close the defect where possible. Clips are rarely successful in containing the leak. If stones cannot be contained, a bag should be inserted and the gall bladder emptied to prevent further stone spillage and loss. Most retained stones will cause no harm,[127] but efforts should be made to retrieve dropped stones where possible because a small proportion may cause intra-abdominal abscesses.

Difficulty grasping the gall bladder

A mucocele or empyema can be decompressed by inserting a Veress needle or cannula connected to the suction tubing, followed by grasping the drainage point with the assistant's grasper to prevent intra-abdominal leakage. Very thick-walled gall bladders or others packed with stones may necessitate replacing the lateral port with a 10-mm port to insert an endo-Babcock or similar wide-jawed instrument.

Difficult dissection: acute cholecystitis

The dissection should always be started on the gall bladder wall. Use of a harmonic scalpel allows safe dissection of dense adhesions by reducing oozing and allowing division of vessels without the risk of inadvertently knocking off clips. If no progress can be made in Calot's triangle, a retrograde dissection must be considered or subtotal cholecystectomy performed by opening the gall bladder, removing the stones in a preplaced bag, and closing Hartmann's pouch with an endoloop or purse-string suture. Conversion to open cholecystectomy is the safest option in inexperienced hands.

Wide or thick-walled cystic duct

The duct must be confirmed to be the cystic duct by cholangiogram before it is divided. Endoloops should be used to close the duct rather than clips, which are likely to come off as the inflammation resolves.

Difficulty extracting the gall bladder

The gall bladder should be opened and bile aspirated. Desjardins stone forceps are used to carefully remove any stones without perforating gall bladder. Large stones may be crushed with Kocher forceps within the gall bladder, then extracted. Otherwise the wound can be extended by inserting an artery clip between the gall bladder and linea alba to allow a reversed knife blade to extend the midline incision. When multiple stones are present, it is wise to put the gall bladder into a bag to prevent spillage during extraction.

Operative technique of open cholecystectomy

A transverse incision is made over the gall bladder at the site of the intersection of the rectus semilunaris with the costal margin. The use of a small 5–7-cm transverse incision is known as a minicholecystectomy, and in this technique the exact position of the gall bladder should be identified preoperatively by ultrasound.[128] The muscle layers are divided with diathermy and the peritoneum opened. A self-retaining retractor is inserted, and dissection proceeds by grasping Hartmann's pouch and using blunt dissection to dissect out the cystic artery and duct, staying close to the gall bladder wall. The cystic duct and artery can be clipped or tied with ligatures.

REFERENCES

126. Wu J, Dunnegan D, Soper N. J Gastrointest Surg 1998; 2: 50–59
127. Memon MA, Deeik RK, Maffi TR et al. Surg Endosc 1999; 13: 848–857
128. Downs SH, Black NA et al. Ann R Coll Surg (Engl) 1996; 78 (Part 2): 241

Although the minicholecystectomy has the advantage of allowing familiarity, tactile feedback and standard open instrumentation, the views of Calot's triangle are inferior to those obtained laparoscopically, particularly in obese patients or when inflammation is present. It is also very difficult for assistants to get any view inside the abdomen, making training in the technique difficult. It appears to offer no advantages over the laparoscopic technique and has not been widely performed despite two randomized trials demonstrating similar outcomes to those of laparoscopic cholecystectomy.[129] The wound is closed with absorbable sutures in two layers.

Cholecystostomy

Cholecystostomy is a useful method of treating severe acute gall bladder disease in the gravely ill and may be carried out percutaneously using ultrasound guidance. At operation it may be useful when the anatomy is obscured by severe inflammatory disease, particularly when less experienced surgeons are called on to operate in an emergency.

The gall bladder is usually under tension and should be aspirated before an incision is made in the fundus. Infected bile and stones are removed, but stones impacted in the cystic duct may be impossible to dislodge at this stage. The gall bladder is closed around a large Foley catheter, which is brought out through a separate skin incision and allows the drainage of bile and pus. The Foley catheter should be left in situ for 4–6 weeks to ensure adherence to the abdominal wall prior to its removal.

In the long term, there is a 75% incidence of recurrent stone formation following cholecystostomy,[130] and patients should undergo definitive cholecystectomy once their overall condition has improved.

MANAGEMENT OF CHOLEDOCHOLITHIASIS

The management of common bile duct stones has become increasingly complex with the increase in diagnostic and therapeutic measures now available. Few randomized trials are available, and the solution for many patients is largely dictated by the available equipment and expertise in any particular unit.

Techniques for common bile duct stone removal

Endoscopic stone management

Endoscopic retrograde cholangiopancreatography allows access to the bile duct without requiring a general anaesthesia. Access to the papilla can be achieved in 95% of patients but may be impossible with large periampullary diverticula or after Polya gastrectomy. Following the demonstration of stones within the bile ducts, the cannula is exchanged over a guide wire for a sphincterotome. A sphincterotomy is performed using diathermy to allow extraction of stones less than 3 mm in diameter. Stones can then be extracted using a Dormia basket or balloon catheter. Larger stones can be broken with a mechanical lithotripter. In the presence of suppurative cholangitis, or occasionally when multiple or large stones are present, a plastic stent is inserted to prevent stone impaction and allow drainage of bile or pus. Various techniques are available for dealing with the occasional large stone that is too big for mechanical lithotripsy, including contact electrohydraulic lithotripsy[131] and extracorporeal shockwave lithotripsy.[132] This allows removal of 98% of stones without surgery.[133]

There are a number of situations in which ERCP remains the best option for removal of common bile duct stones. These include acute cholangitis, acute gallstone pancreatitis in the presence of biliary obstruction, stones causing obstructive jaundice, postcholecystectomy common bile duct stones, and bile duct stones in elderly patients considered unfit for cholecystectomy.

Open choledocholithotomy and choledochoscopy

The standard approach to the common bile duct is from the supraduodenal route. Intraoperative cholangiography is obtained via the cystic duct, noting the number and site of stones, diameter of the main bile duct, position of entry of the cystic duct, and ease of flow of contrast into the duodenum. The gall bladder is removed and the duodenum mobilized medially (Kocher's manoeuvre) to allow palpation of the lower common bile duct and facilitate choledochoscopy. The choledochotomy should be performed in the lowest part of the bile duct to preserve as much duct as possible should a further procedure be necessary. The duct is opened vertically between fine stay sutures.[134] The cystic duct may overlay the bile duct and be opened in error.

Exploration of the duct should be as atraumatic as possible. Palpation of the lower duct between the fingers of the left hand can often milk stones back into the choledochotomy. A flexible choledochoscope and Dormia baskets or Fogarty balloon catheters allow removal of stones under direct vision with minimal trauma. Avoiding passage of the choledochoscope or instruments into the duodenum reduces the risk of postoperative pancreatitis. The scope should then be passed up into the intrahepatic ducts to look for further stones. Continuous irrigation through the scope flushes small stones out through the choledochotomy.

The duct can be primarily closed with fine absorbable sutures if there has been minimal trauma, few stones were present, all stones identified on the cholangiogram have been removed, and there is no evidence of cholangitis. In the presence of multiple stones, cholangitis or a large duct, a T tube should be placed through the choledochotomy site. The limbs of the tube should be cut short to prevent passage into the duodenum, because this avoids duodenal reflux into the bile or pancreatic ducts and segmental obstruction of the smaller intrahepatic ducts. Fine interrupted absorbable sutures are used to close the choledochotomy to achieve a watertight seal on testing. A drain should always be left following a choledochotomy for a period of 24–48 h and can be removed if no bile is present.

Stones can be removed blindly with palpation, Desjardin forceps and a Fogarty balloon catheter if no choledochoscope is available, but care should be taken to avoid damaging the bile duct wall, creating a late stricture or creating false passages. A T tube should be inserted and a completion cholangiogram taken to confirm removal of all stones and good flow of contrast into the duodenum. It can be very difficult to remove all the air from

REFERENCES

129. Squirrell DM, Majeed AW, Troy G et al. Surgery 1998; 123: 485–495
130. Norby S, Schonebeck J. Acta Chir Scand 1970; 136: 711
131. Hixson LJ, Fennerty MD, Jaffee PE et al. Am J Gastroenterol 1992; 87: 296–299
132. Ponchon T, Martin X, Barkun A et al. Gastroenterology 1990; 98: 726–732
133. Schumacher B, Frieling T, Haussinger D et al. Hepatogastroenterology 1998; 45: 672–676
134. Dudley HAF (ed.). Alimentary Tract and Abdominal Wall, Vol 11. 4th edn. Butterworths, London, 1983

the biliary system, and differentiation between air bubbles and stones is often difficult.

Laparoscopic common bile duct stone removal

Stones identified on the intraoperative cholangiogram at laparoscopy can be removed either via the cystic duct or through a choledochotomy. The transcystic route can be used only for removal of stones of similar diameter to that of the cystic duct itself. These may be removed by fluoroscopic Dormia basket extraction or more commonly by introduction of an ultrathin choledochoscope (3.0–3.5 mm in diameter) with Dormia basket extraction. It is not usually possible to pass the choledochoscope proximal to the entry point of the cystic duct because of its angled entry into the common hepatic duct. Occlusion of the common bile duct with a balloon and flushing after an intravenous injection of glucagons or Buscopan to open the sphincter of Oddi can sometimes be successful in flushing small stones through the duodenal papilla. The main advantage is relative simplicity without the need to open the bile duct. It is, however, limited to a small group of patients and excludes those with small cystic ducts, tortuous spiral valves within the cystic duct, multiple or large stones, and stones in the proximal ducts.

In patients not suitable for transcystic stone removal, a choledochotomy is made in the distal bile duct of a size just bigger than the largest stone. A flexible choledochoscope is introduced through the midaxillary or epigastric port into the bile duct, and the stones are removed with a Dormia basket or balloon catheter. When multiple stones are present, it is useful to place a bag beneath the porta hepatis to ensure stones are not lost. From an ergonomic viewpoint, the procedure is easier to perform with the surgeon standing between the patient's legs, the so called 'French' position for laparoscopic cholecystectomy. Insertion of a fifth port in the middle of the left upper quadrant also improves the position for suturing. As in open surgery, the choledochotomy may be closed primarily or over a T tube and a drain left for 24–48 h. Stone extraction rates of 70–95% are achievable using the laparoscopic approach.[135–137] Failure is usually because of impaction of the stone in the lower common bile duct, necessitating conversion to an open procedure.

Management of T tubes

T tubes should be left on free drainage, avoiding kinking in the postoperative period, and great care should be taken to avoid inadvertent removal, which necessitates replacement surgery.[138] Patients should have a T-tube cholangiogram performed before discharge from hospital. This should be performed under antibiotic cover, by a single dose of intravenous cephalosporin given 30 min before the procedure, to prevent bacteraemic episodes associated with flushing the T-tube under pressure back into the bile ducts. If there are no stones present, no leaks, and good passage of contrast into the duodenum, the T-tube can be spigotted and strapped to the abdominal wall, preventing unnecessary bile loss and reducing the risk of contamination or infection and accidental removal. The patient can then come back on the ward 14 days postoperatively for T-tube removal with gentle traction. If the tube will not dislodge, it is left for a further 2–4 weeks before attempting its removal again.

If stones are found at T-tube cholangiography, they may be removed by either radiological percutaneous techniques or endoscopy. The T-tube is left in situ on free drainage for 6 weeks to allow a sinus tract to develop. It is then removed under fluoroscopy and a steerable catheter and Dormia basket inserted along its tract to capture the stone. Stones larger than 6–8 mm will not pass through a 14-Fr tract but can be either crushed or pushed into the duodenum. Stone clearance rates of 88–97% can be achieved.[139,140] Alternatively, ERCP can be performed at the same time, which has the advantage of avoiding several weeks with an open T-tube.

Choledochoduodenostomy

Anastomosis of the common bile duct to the first part of the duodenum may be performed when stones are impacted at the papilla, or when the duct is large and contains multiple stones, making it uncertain that all the stones have been removed.[141,142] With the advent of ERCP and the laparoscopic approach to cholecystectomy and choledocholithiasis, the procedure is less frequently performed nowadays.

A side-to-side anastomosis between a longitudinal choledochotomy in the bile duct and the adjacent portion of the duodenum is performed using absorbable sutures. To reduce the risk of stenosis of the opening, the duodenum is fully mobilized and an anastamosis greater than 2 cm in diameter is made. The main use of the procedure is in the elderly patient with a large bile duct and when there has been difficulty in establishing complete clearance of calculi from the bile ducts (Fig. 30.14). There is a high stenosis rate when the procedure is performed on younger patients and patients with strictures in the lower common bile duct and is rarely performed these days. These patients should undergo formal Roux-en-Y choledochojejunostomy.

Management of Mirrizi's syndrome

Mirrizi's syndrome is usually associated with the presence of dense fibrosis in Calot's triangle. Opening the gall bladder at the fundus with removal of stones allows identification of absence of a connection with the bile duct. Type I Mirrizi's syndrome is managed by a subtotal cholecystectomy avoiding dissection of the bile duct. A drain should always be left in case a subsequent bile leak occurs. Type II Mirrizi's syndrome, which is associated with the presence of a cholecyst–choledochal fistula, is best managed by a choledochojejunostomy. Primary closure of the clinically inflamed bile duct or closure over a T-tube should be avoided because this inevitably results in bile leaks or later stenosis.[143]

Management of gallstone ileus or cholecystoenteric fistula

At laparotomy, palpation of the bowel reveals the large gallstone at the site of obstruction, most commonly the ileocaecal valve. It may be possible to crush or milk the stone into the colon, obviating the need for enterotomy. Usually an enterotomy is required, which should be closed transversely to reduce stricturing. The cholecystoenteric fistula may be managed by

REFERENCES

135. Rhodes M, Sussman L, Cohen L et al. Lancet 1998; 351: 159–161
136. Cuschieri A, Croce E, Faggioni A et al. Surg Endosc 1996; 10: 1130–1135
137. Petelin JB. Am J Surg 1993; 165: 487–491
138. Lygidakis NJ. Surg Gynecol Obstet 1986; 163: 153
139. Burhenne HJ. Am J Roentgenol 1980; 134: 88–898
140. Geisinger M, Owens DB, Meaney JF. Am J Surg 1989; 158: 222–227
141. Lygidakis NJ. Surg Gynecol Obstet 1982; 155: 679
142. Parilla P, Ramirez P et al. Br J Surg 1991; 78: 470
143. Baer HU, Matthews JB, Schweizer WP et al. Br J Surg 1990; 77: 743–745

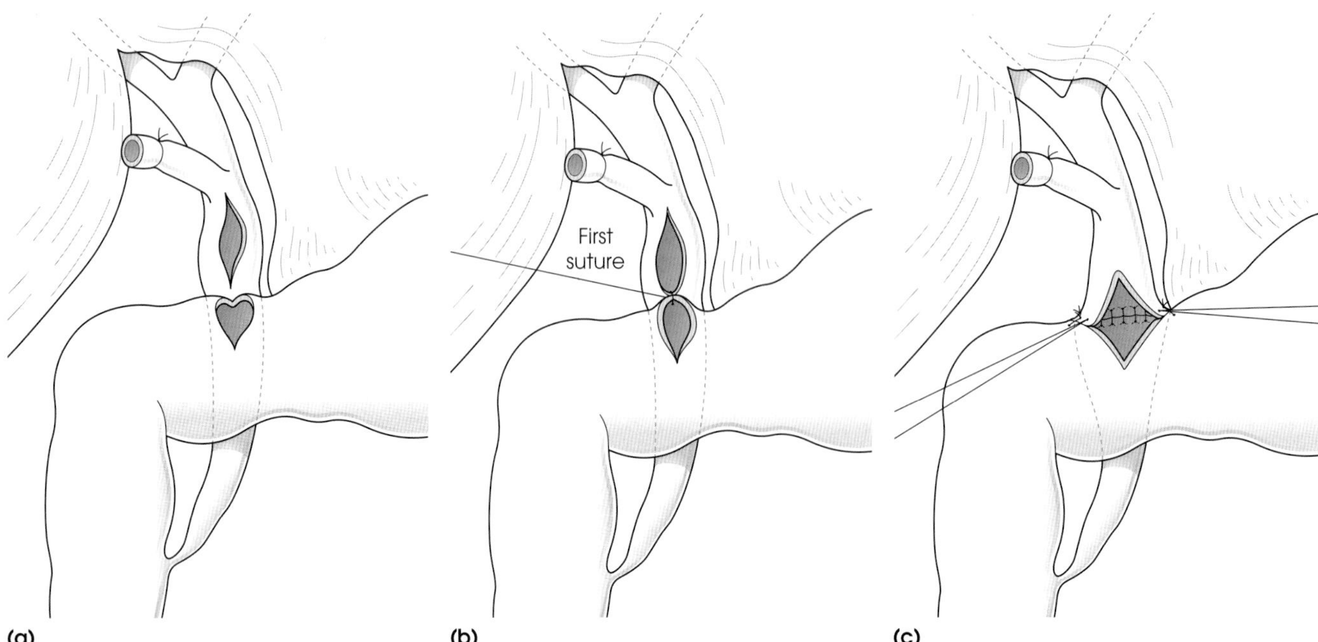

Figure 30.14 External choledochoduodenostomy. (a) The creation of a stoma in the duodenum and a stoma in the supraduodenal part of the common bile duct. (b) The first suture in position tied on the mucosal side. (c) The posterior layer of sutures in situ and the start of the insertion of the anterior layer sutures. (From Dudley HAF (ed). Alimentary Tract and Abdominal Wall, 4th ed, vol 11. Reproduced with permission from Elsevier.[134])

stapling or suturing across the gall bladder fistula tract, avoiding narrowing of the bowel lumen, with removal of the gall bladder. In the presence of severe inflammation and adhesions, particularly in an obstructed elderly patient, it is sensible to simply relieve the bowel obstruction by removal of the stone and leave the gall bladder and fistula alone.

Decision making for patients with possible common bile duct stones

There are several different preoperative diagnostic techniques and intraoperative techniques for imaging and treating common bile duct stones. There are few data to support one or other approach, and it is therefore important to develop a strategy for the preoperative and operative treatment of patients with gallstones dependent on the local availability of techniques and skills.

Most clinicians attempt to stratify their patients in some way, according to the probability of bile duct stones being present. Patients with normal liver function tests, non-dilated bile ducts on ultrasound, and no history of jaundice will have a less than 1.5% chance of having a retained bile duct stone.[144] This group can undergo laparoscopic cholecystectomy without the need for further preoperative imaging or intraoperative cholangiography.

Patients at high risk of bile duct stones can be identified preoperatively. If the presence of one of the criteria is used—presentation with jaundice, bilirubin level greater than 20 mmol (2 g/dL), common bile duct greater than 10 mm and/or common bile duct stone seen on ultrasound, alkaline phosphatase level of 150 mmol/L—the presence of ductal stones is 56%.[144] These criteria may be used to identify patients for preoperative ERCP or for referral to a surgeon performing laparoscopic bile duct exploration. Two randomized trials have shown similar duct clearance rates with either strategy but with shorter hospital stay in the single-stage surgery arm.[135,136]

Patients in the intermediate group with a mild derangement of liver function test, or a history of acute pancreatitis in which 90% will have passed their stones, present more of a dilemma. The incidence of stones in this group is around 5%. Preoperative ERCP is no longer justified in this group without prior demonstration of stones, because the risk of complications is likely to exceed the rate of demonstration of bile duct stones. Preoperative imaging with MRCP or endoscopic ultrasound will demonstrate most stones,[145] but at a high financial cost because 95% of the procedures will be negative. A more pragmatic approach is to perform intraoperative cholangiography or laparoscopic ultrasound on this group to demonstrate stones at the time of surgery. Stones can then be removed laparoscopically or by open bile duct exploration. A third alternative, particularly when the bile duct is small (and therefore at risk of stricturing following choledochotomy), is to tie the cystic duct with an endoloop, complete the cholecystectomy, and arrange a postoperative ERCP. This strategy relies heavily on ERCP expertise, because failed ERCP requires referral on to a more experienced endoscopist or a second operative procedure. Intraoperative ERCP at the time of discovery of bile duct stones has also been performed by a few groups, but this is cumbersome and time-consuming. The choice between the various strategies in this intermediate group of patients depends largely on the quality of the surgical and endoscopic therapy available.

BILE DUCT INJURY

CLASSIFICATION OF BILE DUCT INJURIES

The most widely used and comprehensive classification is Strasberg's modification of the Bismuth classification

REFERENCES

144. Somnay K, Carr-Locke DL. In: Blumgart LH, Fong Y (eds). Surgery of the Liver and Biliary Tract. WB Saunders, London, 2000
145. Griffin N, Wastie ML, Dunn WK et al. Eur J Gastroenterol Hepatol 2003; 15: 809–813

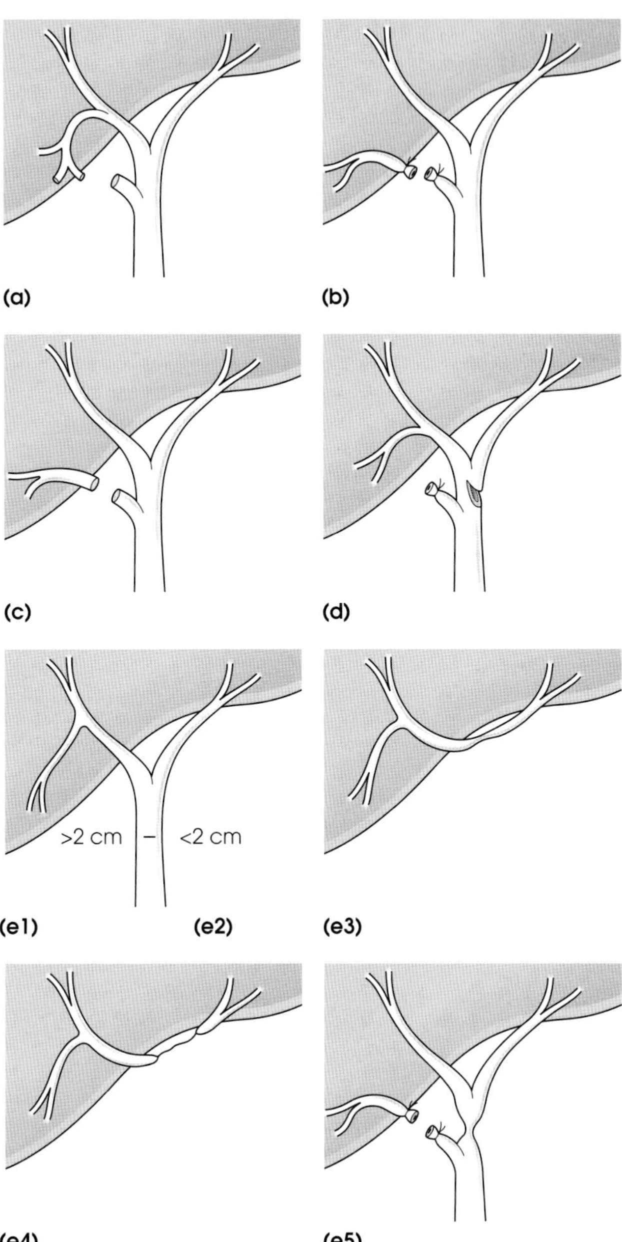

Figure 30.15 Strasberg's classification of bile duct injuries stratified from A–E, with type E injuries further subdivided into E1–E5 (based on Bismuth's classification of hilar strictures).

(Fig. 30.15).[146] Type A injuries occur following cystic duct clip slippage or division of an accessory subvesical duct of Luschka (Fig. 30.16). Type B and C injuries involve damage to an aberrant right sectoral duct with division and occlusion of biliary drainage (type B) or division and leakage (type C). Type D injuries are partial division of the main bile duct. Type E injuries involve the main bile duct (E1 and E2), or the common hepatic duct with maintenance of the biliary confluence (E3) or with loss of the confluence (E4). E5 lesions are complex injuries involving the right sectoral duct and common hepatic duct. These injuries may be transections, excisions or strictures.

Mechanisms of injury and prevention

Risk factors have been identified and include inexperience on the part of the laparoscopic surgeon, inadequate training, a difficult dissection in Calot's triangle, failure to recognize the correct anatomy, and operations performed on patients who have had recent acute cholecystitis.[147–151] The classical injury occurs where the operator mistakes the common bile duct for the cystic duct, with the result that the bile duct is clipped in two places and to achieve removal of the gall bladder a segment of the duct is resected as well (Fig. 30.17).[152] When the upper clip is correctly placed on the cystic duct, the proximal bile duct will not be obstructed and a bile leak will be present (variant classical injury, Fig. 30.18). These injuries and many of the partial transections with clips applied to the common bile duct occur as a result of excessive traction on Hartmann's pouch or the gall bladder fundus. This allows tenting up of the common bile duct and misidentification. It is notable that young slim women with small common bile ducts feature heavily in the injured bile duct group.

Safe surgery requires clear visualization of the anatomy, which itself demands proper exposure. Avoiding these injuries requires use of caudal and lateral traction on Hartmann's pouch and always dissecting as close to the gall bladder wall as possible. No structure should be clipped or divided unless its identity is certain, and an intraoperative cholangiogram should be performed if any uncertainty exists. Conversion to open surgery should not be seen as a failure and should be performed if doubts persist.

A second group of injuries occur as a consequence of abnormal anatomy where a low-entry right sectoral hepatic duct is mistaken for the cystic duct and is clipped or divided (Fig. 30.15-e5). Segmental ducts (ducts of Luschka) can be damaged by dissection drifting away from the gall bladder wall during dissection of Calot's triangle or by inadvertent dissection into the liver parenchyma during removal of the gall bladder (Fig. 30.16).

Ischaemic injury to the main bile ducts or clip placement across a main bile duct usually occur with haemorrhage in Calot's triangle.[153,154] Over-dissection of the bile duct and damage to the coaxial vessels may be other factors in ischaemic injuries. At laparoscopy even a small amount of blood obscures the field and hinders dissection. Precise control of haemorrhage is required and injudicious application of diathermy and clips avoided. Early conversion to open surgery should be considered in the presence of bleeding around the porta hepatis.

Presentation and management of bile duct injuries

A proportion of injuries are recognized at surgery. Advice should be obtained from an experienced hepatobiliary surgeon, and major biliary reconstruction in this charged setting should not be undertaken by surgeons unfamiliar with high biliary anastamosis. Large-bore drainage tubes placed in the right upper quadrant and transfer to a tertiary referral unit for definitive surgery may

REFERENCES

146. Strasberg SM, Hertl M, Soper NJ. J Am Coll Surg 1995; 180: 101–125
147. Fullarton GM, Bell G. Gut 1994; 35: 1121
148. Metzler P, Camal EM. Int Surg 1995; 80: 328
149. MacMahon AJ, Fullarton G et al. Br J Surg 1995; 82: 307
150. Windsor JA, Vaux DE. Br J Surg 1994; 81: 1208
151. Scholl FPG, Go PMN, Gouma DJ. Br J Surg 1994; 81: 1786
152. Richardson MC, Bell G, Fullarton GM. Br J Surg 1996; 83: 1356–1360
153. Davidoff AM, Pappas TN, Murray EA et al. Ann Surg 1992; 215: 196–208
154. Rossi RL, Schirmer WJ, Braasch JW et al. Arch Surg 1992; 127: 596–602

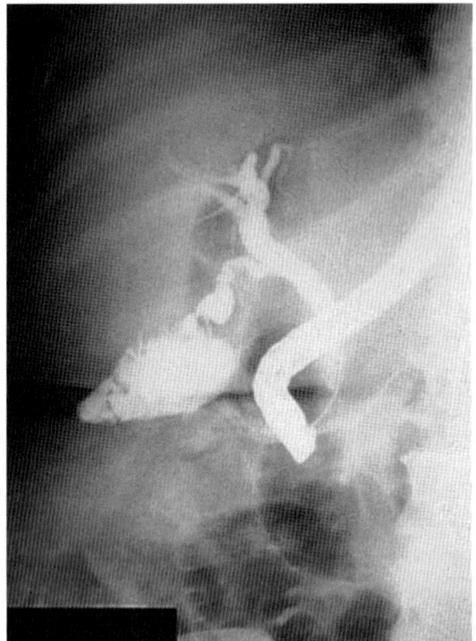

a

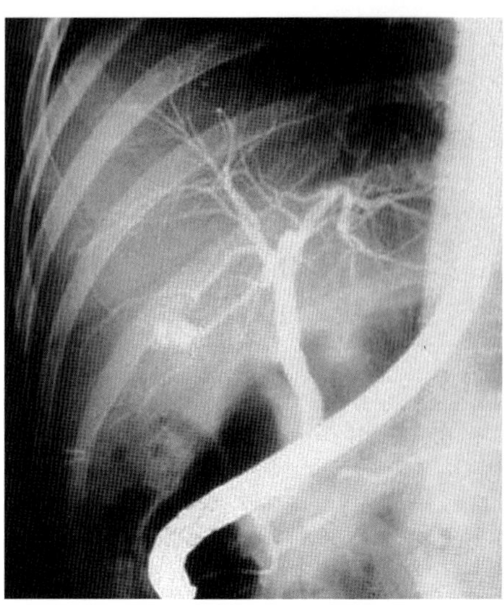

b

Figure 30.16 Strasberg type A injuries, which occur in around 1% of cholecystectomies: (**a**) cystic duct clip slippage and (**b**) duct of Luschka injury.

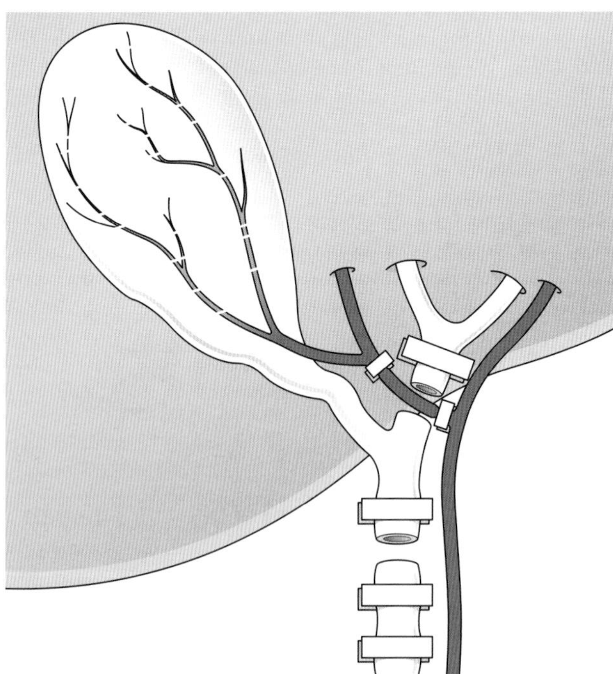

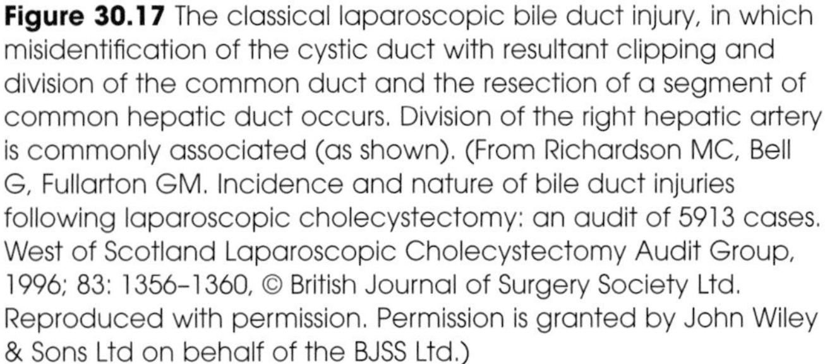

Figure 30.17 The classical laparoscopic bile duct injury, in which misidentification of the cystic duct with resultant clipping and division of the common duct and the resection of a segment of common hepatic duct occurs. Division of the right hepatic artery is commonly associated (as shown). (From Richardson MC, Bell G, Fullarton GM. Incidence and nature of bile duct injuries following laparoscopic cholecystectomy: an audit of 5913 cases. West of Scotland Laparoscopic Cholecystectomy Audit Group, 1996; 83: 1356–1360, © British Journal of Surgery Society Ltd. Reproduced with permission. Permission is granted by John Wiley & Sons Ltd on behalf of the BJSS Ltd.)

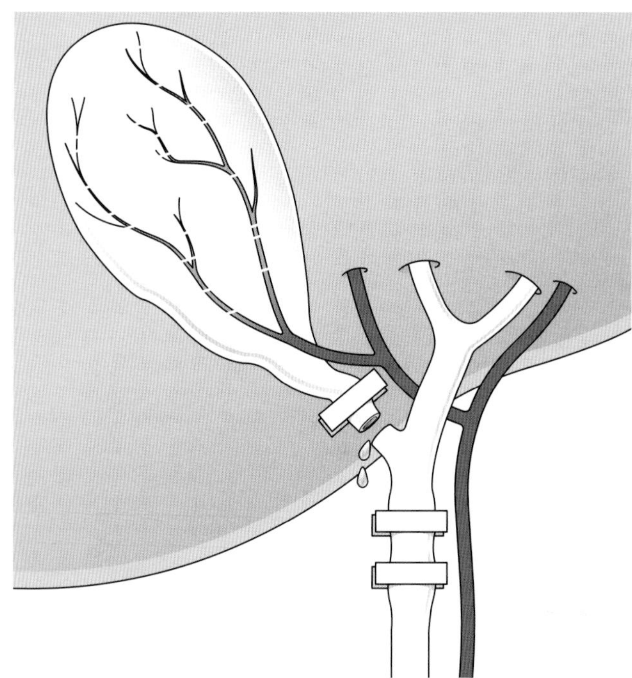

Figure 30.18 Variant classical bile duct injury, with misidentification of the common bile duct for the proximal cystic duct but correct identification of the upper cystic duct, resulting in a bile leak. (From Richardson MC, Bell G, Fullarton GM. Incidence and nature of bile duct injuries following laparoscopic cholecystectomy: an audit of 5913 cases. West of Scotland Laparoscopic Cholecystectomy Audit Group, 1996; 83: 1356–1360, © British Journal of Surgery Society Ltd. Reproduced with permission. Permission is granted by John Wiley & Sons Ltd on behalf of the BJSS Ltd.)

be more appropriate. The importance of repairing the injury at the first attempt cannot be overemphasized. Around two-thirds of patients have undergone a failed repair by the original surgeon before referral for definitive surgery.[155,156] Each failed repair is inevitably accompanied by a further loss of bile duct length, requiring a higher anastamosis. In skilled hands, immediate reconstruction has good results. End-to-end anastamosis and choledochoduodenostomy have a high stricture rate and are not appropriate repairs in this setting.[157] Partial division of the bile duct (type D injury) may be closed primarily if the bile duct is sufficiently large and there is minimal diathermy injury. This is rare, and usually there is more extensive injury requiring insertion of a T-tube. Subsequent stricturing may occur but this often causes ductal dilatation, making reconstruction easier. Injuries affecting more than half the circumference of the bile duct require hepaticojejunostomy.

The majority of patients present within the first 2 weeks of surgery with a combination of pain, sepsis and jaundice, and a failure to progress in their recovery. Blood investigations show abnormalities in the liver function tests, most notably a rise in bilirubin and an elevated white cell count in the presence of sepsis. An ultrasound scan or CT scan shows a fluid collection with non-dilated ducts if a bile leak is present, or may show dilated ducts with a complete bile duct obstruction. Fluid collections should have a percutaneous drain inserted to confirm bile leakage and establish drainage. Further management depends on the presence or absence of sepsis and the level and extent of injury. In a septic patient, drainage of intra-abdominal collections and establishment of adequate biliary drainage is the first priority.

In the absence of sepsis, further investigation of the extent of the bile duct injury should be obtained. Magnetic resonance cholangiopancreatography has the advantage of being able to visualize above and below any obstructing lesion. Endoscopic retrograde cholangiopancreatography will delineate the lower level of an obstructive lesion (Fig. 30.19), diagnose and sometimes treat type B and C injuries, and is the standard treatment for type A and D injuries. Some of the type D injuries may require later surgery if stricturing develops.

Type E injuries are more difficult to manage. Establishment of the level of injury may be facilitated by MRCP, radionuclide scanning or percutaneous transhepatic cholangiography. The last of these can be used to establish external drainage of an obstructed system. At surgery, diathermy damage to the duct may indicate that the injury is more extensive than identified preoperatively. Division of the right hepatic artery is found in around 20% of patients. Surgical repair of the bile duct is by proximal hepaticojejunostomy on to healthy ductal tissue. Successful outcome, defined as requiring no further intervention following specialist repair, in units reporting more than 40 cases ranges from 76 to 95% with follow-up of 6–9 years.[155,158,159]

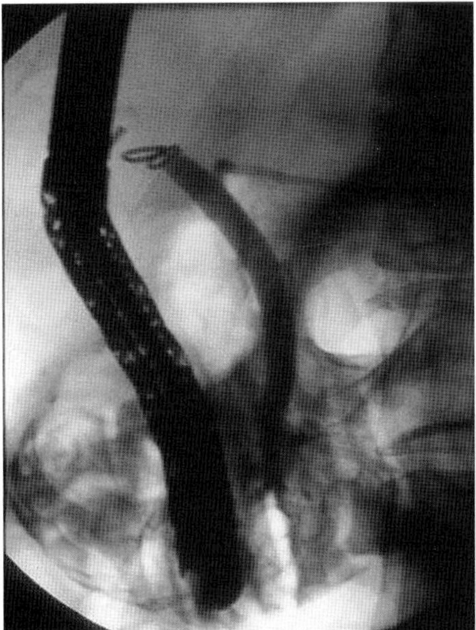

Figure 30.19 Endoscopic retrograde cholangiopancreatography of a Strasberg type E injury with complete transection of the common bile duct and occlusion by clips.

NON-SURGICAL TRAUMA

Blunt injury to the biliary tract from road traffic accidents is rarely an isolated injury and frequently involves other intra-abdominal viscera, particularly the liver, pancreas and duodenum (see Ch. 7). It is often associated with head and thoracic injuries. The prognosis is usually determined by the extent and severity of the associated injury. Injury to the portal vein and hepatic artery is infrequent.[148,154] The presence of retroperitoneal bile, or the infiltration of periportal structures with blood and bile, strongly suggests injury to the duodenum or bile duct. Delayed diagnosis is quite common, and abdominal tap and lavage may be helpful. HIDA scans may be extremely useful in demonstrating bile accumulation.

Penetrating injuries by gunshots or stab wounds may occasionally directly involve the bile ducts. Most patients require immediate laparotomy, but in a few (5%) laceration of the bile ducts leads to slow bile leakage that may give rise to difficulty in diagnosis and to delayed surgery. Blunt or penetrating injury to the liver parenchyma may result in transection of intrahepatic bile ducts and presents as a bile leak.

Transected peripheral bile ducts can be ligated or, if not directly visible, will usually settle following insertion of a drain. Injuries in the hilum to the main ducts require Roux-en-Y hepaticojejunostomy, usually as a delayed secondary procedure after the patient's condition has been stabilized.

POSTCHOLECYSTECTOMY PAIN

Cholecystectomy results in improvement or cure of pain in over 90% of patients, and the incidence of postcholecystectomy pain, excluding wound pain, following laparoscopic cholecystectomy appears to be similar to that following open cholecystectomy.[160–162] The term *postcholecystectomy syndrome* was widely used in the 1970s but should be avoided because the implication is that the removal of the gall bladder itself is the cause of symptoms, which is not the case.

REFERENCES

155. Chapman WC, Halevy A, Blumgart LH et al. Arch Surg 1995; 130: 597–604
156. Stewart L, Way LW. Arch Surg 1995; 130: 1123–1129
157. Rossi R, Tsao J. Surg Clin North Am 1994; 74: 825–841
158. McDonald ML, Farnell MB, Nagorney DM et al. Surgery 1995; 118: 582–591
159. Tocchi A, Costa G, Lepre L et al. Ann Surg 1996; 224: 162–167
160. Wilson RG, Macintyre IM. Br J Surg 1993; 80: 439–441
161. McMahon AJ, Ross S, Baxster RN et al. Br J Surg 1995; 82: 1378–1382
162. Vander-Velpen GC, Shimi SM, Cuschieri A. Gut 1993; 34: 1448–1451

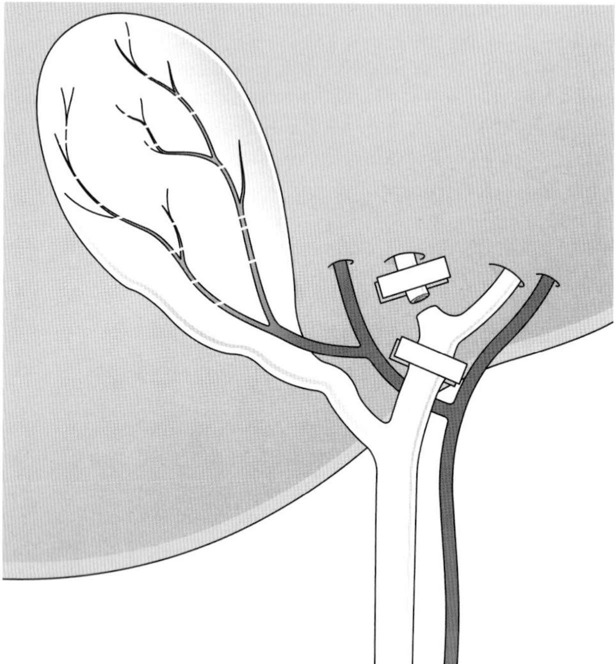

Figure 30.20 Misidentification of the right hepatic duct for the cystic duct. Clipping and division around the confluence result in a high, severe injury. (From Richardson MC, Bell G, Fullarton GM. Incidence and nature of bile duct injuries following laparoscopic cholecystectomy: an audit of 5913 cases. West of Scotland Laparoscopic Cholecystectomy Audit Group, 1996; 83: 1356–1360, © British Journal of Surgery Society Ltd. Reproduced with permission. Permission is granted by John Wiley & Sons Ltd on behalf of the BJSS Ltd.)

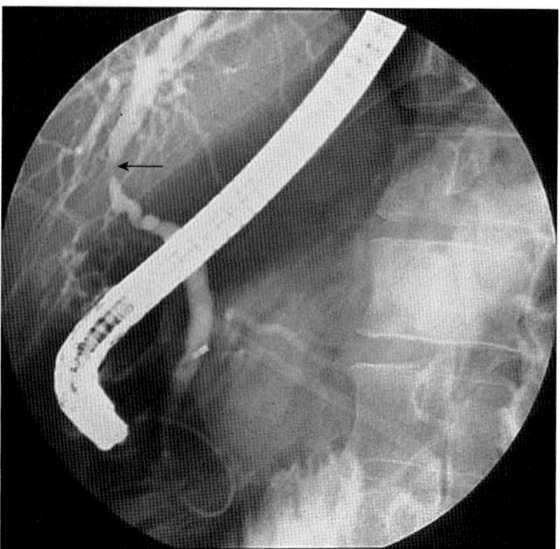

Figure 30.21 High common hepatic duct stricture following laparoscopic cholecystectomy (type E2).

Because 90% of people with gallstones are symptomless, it is perhaps to be expected that some symptoms attributed to the gallstones do not resolve following cholecystectomy and were in fact from concomitant pathology. An accurate preoperative history is important to identify an alternative diagnosis, and all patients must give fully informed consent.

Investigation of postcholecystectomy pain requires exclusion of operative complications (bile collections or leaks and biliary strictures), other biliary pathology (missed or retained common bile duct stones), and non-biliary-related conditions (gastroduodenal disease and chronic pancreatitis) and functional bowel disorders (irritable bowel syndrome and non-ulcer dyspepsia). Depending on the degree of disability and the index of suspicion, liver function tests, ultrasound scanning, gastroscopy and MRCP will allow non-invasive identification of the majority of patients with organic pathology. A small group of patients may require investigation for sphincter of Oddi syndrome.

SPHINCTER OF ODDI DYSFUNCTION

Sphincter of Oddi dysfunction remains a diagnostic and therapeutic challenge. The syndrome is poorly defined, incompletely understood, and difficult to diagnose. A number of terms have been used to describe the same entity (e.g. *papillary stenosis, sclerosing papillitis, biliary spasms, biliary dyskinesia* and *postcholecystectomy syndrome*). Pathologically distinct entities exist. Papillary stenosis with chronic inflammation and fibrosis is usually associated with gallstone migration through the sphincter or previous surgical or endoscopic intervention. Papillary dyskinesia is caused by an intermittent functional blockage. The distinction is useful because it correlates well with outcome.

The diagnosis of sphincter of Oddi dysfunction is suspected in patients with pain of a biliary or pancreatic nature in the absence of a demonstrable gallstone cause (i.e. after cholecystectomy or in patients without gall bladder stones). Patients may have a dilated bile duct or abnormal liver function tests, and these patients respond better to treatment compared with those patients with normal liver function tests and normal bile duct diameter. Investigations include the morphine–neostigmine provocation test (Nardi test),[163] dynamic biliary scintigraphy, and sphincter of Oddi manometry.[164]

Treatment is by endoscopic sphincterotomy or surgical division of the sphincter (transduodenal sphincteroplasty and transampullary septectomy.[165] Endoscopic sphincterotomy has the advantage of minimal access, and 43–57% of patients become pain-free following treatment.[166,167] Surgery has the advantage of a more complete division of the sphincter complex, allowing resection of the transampullary septum and drainage of the pancreatic duct, and allows accurate apposition of the duodenal mucosa and duct lining, reducing restenosis,[168] with 55–68% reported as pain-free.[169,170]

BENIGN STRICTURES OF THE BILE DUCTS

The causes of strictures that may be encountered in the bile duct are summarized in Table 30.2.

REFERENCES

163. Nardi GL, Acosta JM. Ann Surg 1966; 164: 611–621
164. Toouli J. Gut 1989; 30: 353
165. Moody FG, Becker JM, Potts JR. Ann Surg 1983; 197: 627–636
166. Geenen JE, Hogan WJ, Dodds WJ et al. N Engl J Med 1989; 320: 82–87
167. Bozkurt T, Orth KH, Butsch B et al. Eur J Gastroenterol Hepatol 1996; 8: 245–249
168. Beckingham IJ, Rowlands BJ. In: Blumgart LH, Fong Y (eds). Surgery of the Liver and Biliary Tract. WB Saunders, London, 2000; 799–814
169. Kelly SB, Rowlands BJ. HPB Surg 1996; 9: 199–207
170. Stephens RV, Burdrick GE. Am J Surg 1986; 152: 621–627

Table 30.2

a) Post-Traumatic
   - Damage at time of cholecystectomy
   - Following CBD store renal or t-tube insertion
   - Abdominal injury
   - Suture of duodenal ulcer

b) Post-Inflammatory
   - Minizzo Sundrome
   - Parasitic infestations
   - Chronic pancreatitis
   - Sclerosing cholangitis
   - Pseudotumours

PRIMARY SCLEROSING CHOLANGITIS

Primary sclerosing cholangitis is a chronic fibrosing inflammatory condition of the biliary tree, which affects both the intrahepatic and extrahepatic ducts and may involve the gall bladder and pancreas. It is of unknown origin,[171,172] but there is increasing evidence that it has an autoimmune aetiology.[173] It is associated with inflammatory bowel disease, usually ulcerative colitis, in 50–70% of cases.[171,172]

The patient, who is commonly between 20 and 50 years of age, presents with a progressive cholestatic disorder with right upper quadrant discomfort, jaundice, pruritus and fever. Investigation reveals an elevation of the alkaline phosphatase level, which often predates development of symptoms. An ERCP is the most sensitive diagnostic test and shows an irregular beaded appearance of the bile ducts, focal dilatation, and in more advanced cases multifocal stricturing of the intra- and extrahepatic ducts (Fig. 30.22). Immunological studies may show elevated levels of IgM (50%), perinuclear antineutrophil cytoplasmic antibody (75%) and anti-smooth muscle antibodies (10%), but no rise in the antimitochondrial antibodies, which differentiates the condition from primary biliary cirrhosis. In 80% of patients both the intra- and extrahepatic ducts are involved, but in 20% only extrahepatic involvement is present. Liver biopsy may show typical features of periductal and portal fibrosis: bile ductular proliferation, with a reduction in the number of normal bile ducts, piecemeal necrosis and copper accumulation.[172]

Treatment aims to relieve episodes of cholangitis, pruritis, jaundice and discomfort. Antibiotics, vitamin K, cholestyramine, steroids and azathioprine do not usually help. Proctocolectomy does not alter the prognosis.[172] Ursodeoxycholic acid (7 mg/kg) improves liver function tests, but randomized studies have not shown a difference in time to treatment failure.[174] Disease progress is highly variable, and treatment is generally supportive until there is a need for endoscopic or surgical intervention.

There is a strong association between sclerosing cholangitis and cholangiocarcinoma, and the radiological features are usually indistinguishable. The cumulative risk for biliary malignancy is 11%,[175] with 75% occurring in the extrahepatic biliary tract. Two-thirds of patients have metastatic disease at the time of diagnosis of their cholangiocarcinoma, reflecting the insidious nature of the tumour and the difficulty in diagnosis.[176] Endoscopic retrograde cholangiopancreatography is used for diagnosis and to obtain cytology in suspicious strictures, but its sensitivity is only 50%. Elevations of tumour markers Ca19-9 and CEA lack sensitivity and specificity in early diagnosis. Positron emission tomography scanning has been shown to identify small tumours accurately and may become a useful diagnostic tool.[177]

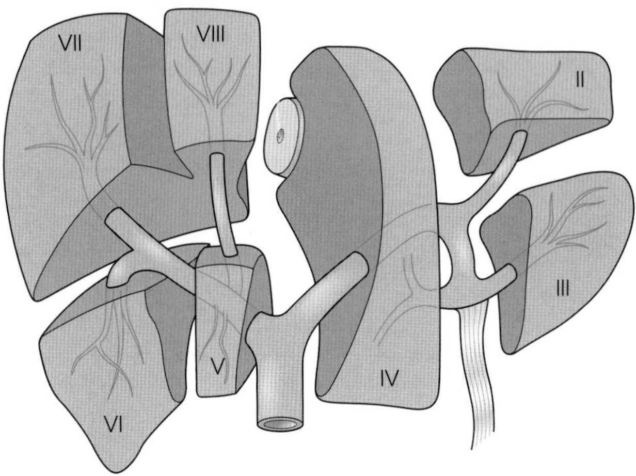

Figure 30.22 Segmental structure of the liver, demonstrating that the left portal triad is always extrahepatic beneath the quadrate lobe. (From Hepaticojejunostomy in benign and malignant high bile duct stricture: approaches to the left hepatic ducts. Blumgart LH, Kelley CJ. Br J Surg. 1984 Apr; 71(4): 257–261, © British Journal of Surgery Society Ltd. Reproduced with permission. Permission is granted by John Wiley & Sons Ltd on behalf of the BJSS Ltd.)

Occasionally a dominant extrahepatic biliary stricture can be dilated with an endoscopic balloon or managed surgically with a hepaticojejunostomy with or without an access loop. Before the availability of liver transplantation, the median survival from diagnosis was 12 years, with death usually from deteriorating liver function. Liver transplantation for end-stage sclerosing cholangitis is promising, with survival rates at 1 and 5 years of 92% and 86%, respectively, reported from the Mayo Clinic for this subgroup.[178]

POSTINFLAMMATORY STRICTURE

Narrowing of the distal common bile duct may be transient during acute pancreatitis, and is the result of compression by oedema of the head of the pancreas. Bile duct stricture is a well-recognized feature of chronic pancreatitis and may lead to progressive derangement of liver function.[179] A long tapering stricture (rat's tail stricture) seen on MRCP or ERCP is typical. Endoscopic retrograde cholangiopancreatography stenting may be used as a temporizing procedure in patients with obstructive jaundice, but definitive treatment with choledochojejunostomy is inevitably required. Patients often have very tight, symptomless strictures with minimal derangement of liver function, and therapy should not be instituted until they are symptomatic,

REFERENCES

171. Lefkowitch JH. Arch Intern Med 1982; 142: 1157
172. Chapman RWG, Arborgh BAM et al. Gut 1980; 21: 870
173. Chapman RW, Kelly PM, Heryet A et al. Gut 1988; 29: 422–427
174. Lindor KD. N Engl J Med 1997; 336: 691–695
175. Kornfield D, Ekbom A, Ihre T. Scand J Gastroenterol 1997; 32: 1042–1045
176. Rosen CB, Nagorney DM. Semin Liver Dis 1991; 11: 26–30
177. Keiding S, Hansen SB, Rasmussen HH et al. Hepatology 1998; 28: 700–706
178. Prall RT, Wiesner RH, LaRusso NF. In: Blumgart LH, Fong Y (eds). Surgery of the Liver and Biliary Tract. WB Saunders, London, 2000: 877–894
179. Smits ME, Rauws AS et al. Br J Surg 1996; 83: 764

jaundiced, or have a persistently elevated alanine aminotransferase level of three times normal.

Inflammatory non-neoplastic lesions of the bile ducts, called pseudotumours, may develop throughout the bile duct and present with jaundice or cholangitis. They are most common in the hilum, where they are often indistinguishable from cholangiocarcinomas. They are usually only identified histologically, following resection for a presumed cholangiocarcinoma, and most large series of hilar resections for presumed cholangiocarcinoma record the presence of benign pathology in 10–15% of resected lesions.[180,181,182] The operative and histological findings in these series have reported a mixture of pathologies including benign pseudotumour, benign granulomas, idiopathic benign focal stenosis, inflammation secondary to gallstones (including Mirrizi's syndrome), sclerosing cholangitis and tuberculosis. Brush cytology and endoscopic biopsy and staging cannot reliably exclude these patients preoperatively. A positive cytology diagnosis of malignancy is helpful, but a negative report cannot be regarded as proof that malignancy is not present. All these patients require surgical management of their hilar strictures, although hepatectomy for what is ultimately shown to be benign disease remains unfortunate. Radical resection is the only way to avoid the tragedy of not resecting a potentially curable lesion, and every surgeon should be prepared to accept the occasional benign pathology report.

POST-TRAUMATIC STRICTURE

The majority of bile duct injuries present intraoperatively or in the early postoperative period when the patient presents with bile leakage and peritonitis or progressive jaundice (see *Presentation and management of bile duct injuries*, p. 727). A small proportion of patients present with jaundice secondary to a bile duct stricture some months or years after cholecystectomy, probably as a result of a thermal injury or ischaemia to the bile duct during the original procedure (Fig. 30.21). Some patients with sectoral duct ischaemic or clip damage may present some time after cholecystectomy with atrophied segments or abscess formation. Choledochotomy and biliary drainage procedures including choledochoduodenectomy and choledochojejunostomy may all present with biliary stricturing. Presentation in all cases is typically with recurring episodes of abdominal pain, jaundice and cholangitis.

Untreated, strictures lead over a period of several years to the development of liver fibrosis, secondary biliary cirrhosis, and portal hypertension. A proportion of these patients may also have had portal venous damage at surgery or underlying parenchymal liver disease and should undergo transjugular liver biopsy as part of their assessment. Patients with biliary strictures and portal hypertension have a poor outcome following surgical intervention.[116,155]

Investigation of patients following initial liver function tests and ultrasound is with MRCP to delineate the upper and lower extent of the stricture. When biliary sepsis is present, ERCP and stenting or percutaneous transhepatic cholangiography and external biliary drainage are required. Classification of the injury depends on the length of undamaged hepatic duct that remains and the extent of the involvement of the biliary confluence (see Fig. 30.15, e1–4).

SURGICAL TREATMENT OF BENIGN BILIARY STRICTURES

For benign strictures the initial operation offers the best chance of cure. Routine preoperative percutaneous transhepatic catheter drainage has not been shown to reduce mortality and morbidity because the high incidence of infective complications following the procedure (10%) outweighs any possible benefits.[183–186] It also causes an electrolyte disturbance that can be serious and difficult to manage (see Ch. 2).

For a successful outcome, an accurate mucosa-to-mucosa anastomosis must be achieved, with a good blood supply and without tension. This rules out end-to-end repair in the majority of cases.[185] Long-term results of end-to-end repair are disappointing, with a high incidence of recurrent stricture,[185,187–189] and this approach should not be used. For the low stricture, a hepaticojejunostomy Roux-en-Y procedure may be fashioned without undue difficulty. For the higher strictures the left hepatic duct approach, originally described by Hepp and Couinaud in 1956,[187] allows a safe and satisfactory biliary enteric anastomosis. The left hepatic duct is really an extrahepatic structure (Fig. 30.22) that can be lowered from the inferior surface of the liver by dissection within the hilar plate, which is a condensation of Glisson's capsule.

THE TECHNIQUE OF HEPATICOJEJUNOSTOMY

A bilateral subcostal incision and a table-mounted retractor, such as a Grays liver retractor or an Omni-Tract, give good access to the hilum of the liver. The ligamentum teres is divided, tied, and pushed cephalad to elevate the hilum. The base of segment IV is now identified as well as the plane between Glisson's capsule and the peritoneal reflection encasing the portal triad (the portal plate) (Fig. 30.23, see Ch. 29). The dissection is deepened, and the structures of the left portal triad are lowered from the inferior surface of segment IV. The dilated left duct is then opened between stay sutures and the incision extended proximally to the stricture. The stricture is excised and the distal end of the bile duct closed with absorbable sutures. The standard technique as described by Voyles and Blumgart aims to achieve mucosal apposition.[190] Fine interrupted absorbable sutures (4/0 Vicryl or PDS) are preplaced along the upper margin of the bile duct, allowing elevation and improved exposure of the lower border of the duct. A Roux-en-Y loop is fashioned and an incision made along the antimesenteric border, slightly shorter than the opening in the bile duct to permit a side-to side anastamosis. A row of interrupted sutures is placed between the lower borders of the duct and the Roux loop and tied (Fig. 30.24). Finally, the upper border sutures are placed in the Roux loop and tied. Stents are not routinely used, but a drain is left adjacent to the

REFERENCES

180. Gehards MF, Vos P, Van Gulik TM et al. Br J Surg 2001; 88: 48–51
181. Hadjis NS, Collier NA, Blumgart LH. Br J Surg 1985; 72: 659–661
182. Wetter LA, Ring EJ, Pellegrini CA et al. Am J Surg 1991; 161: 57–62 (discussion 62–63)
183. Lai ECS. Br J Surg 1990; 77: 604
184. Dawson JL, Heaton ND. Surgery 1992; 64: 84
185. Blumgart LH, Kelley CJ. Br J Surg 1984; 71: 257
186. Pogany AG, Kerlan RK, Ring E. J Clin Gastroenterol 1985; 14: 387
187. Bismuth H. In: Blumgart LHB (ed). The Biliary Tract. Churchill Livingstone, Edinburgh, 1982
188. Dooley JSJ. Hepatology 1985; 1: 681
189. Pellegrini CA, Thomas MJ, Way LW. Am J Surg 1984; 147: 175
190. Voyles CR, Blumgart LH. Surg Gynecol Obstet 1983; 154: 885–887

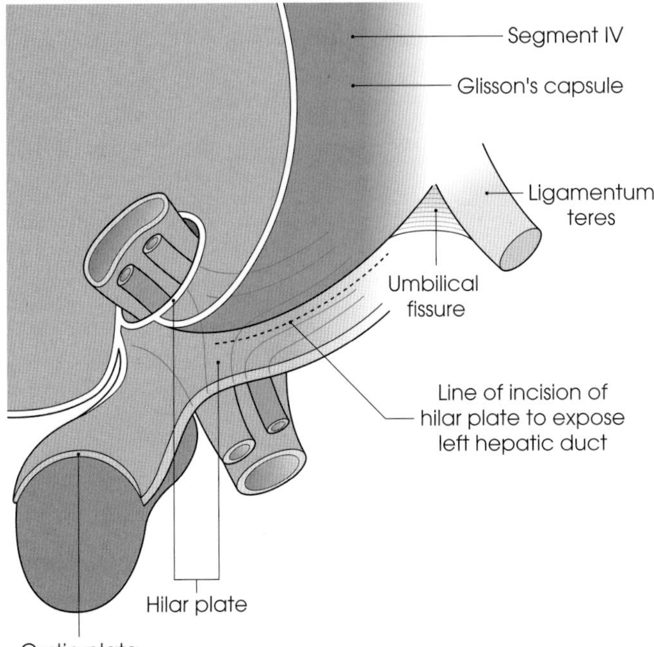

Figure 30.23 The peritoneum overlying the portal structures (the portal plate) merges with Glisson's capsule. Division of the portal plate is necessary to adequately expose the biliary confluence.

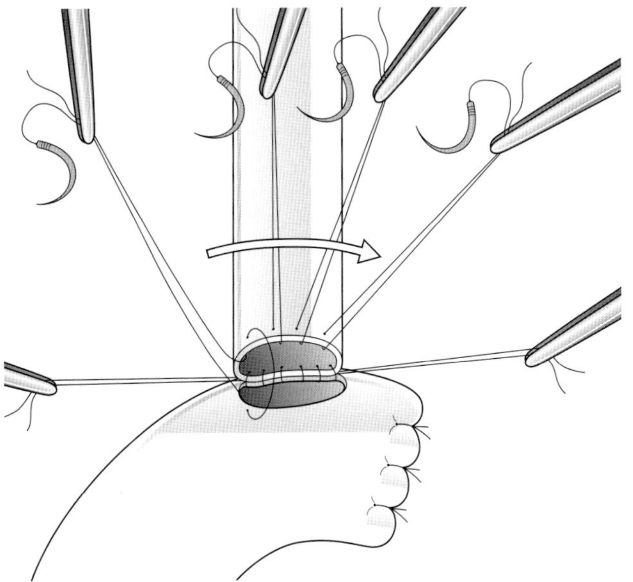

Figure 30.24 The technique of hepaticojejunostomy.

anastamosis. The continuity of the bowel is restored by entero–entero anastamosis 70 cm from the biliary anastamosis.

Results of surgery for benign strictures using the Hepp–Couinaud approach have been reported to have a good outcome in 93% at 10 years, but 2% developed restenosis and 5% died from secondary biliary cirrhosis.[187] Recurrent episodes of cholangitis after biliary surgery may be the result of stenosis of the hepaticojejunostomy with or without the presence of intrahepatic stones. Episodes of cholangitis may also occur after biliary reconstruction in the absence of stenosis.[191] Hepaticojejunostomy patency may be assessed by the presence of air within the intrahepatic ducts, by finding a stenosis on MRCP or a HIDA scan, and by a delay in emptying on a HIDA scan.

PARASITIC INFESTATION AND INVOLVEMENT OF THE BILE DUCTS

INTRAHEPATIC STONE DISEASE (RECURRENT PYOGENIC CHOLANGITIS)

Recurrent pyogenic cholangitis is a condition characterized by repeated attacks of bacterial infection of the biliary tract as a result of stones and strictures in the bile ducts, especially the intrahepatic segments. It has many synonyms in different countries, including hepatolithiasis, oriental cholangiohepatitis and intrahepatic stone disease. It is most prevalent in South-East Asia,[192] but is also seen in areas of deprivation in southern Africa, Kashmir, and Central and South America. It has been linked to the Chinese liver fluke *Clonorchis sinensis* and to the roundworm *Ascaris lumbricoides*. However, *Clonorchis*, obtained by ingesting contaminated raw fish, does not occur outside South-East Asia, and in countries such as Japan, where *Clonorchis* is endemic, recurrent pyogenic cholangitis is on the decline. Furthermore, stool isolated from patients contained *Clonorchis* in 25% and *Ascaris* in 5%,[193] and it may simply be that the diseases coexist in areas of poor sanitation.

Acute episodes present with the typical features of cholangitis—right upper quadrant pain, high swinging fevers, and jaundice progressing to septic shock and confusion—with 100% mortality if left untreated. Emergency decompression has now replaced surgery as the treatment of choice. Disimpaction of the stone and drainage of the bile duct is accompanied by drainage of pus.[194] Insertion of a plastic stent maintains drainage, allowing later sphincterotomy and stone retrieval or elective surgical drainage.

Subsequent definitive surgical management aims to clear the biliary tract of stones, provide adequate biliary drainage, and where necessary provide adequate access to the biliary duct. When there are extrahepatic duct or hilar duct strictures a hepaticojejunostomy is performed, leaving the afferent loop long and fixing it to the abdominal wall as an access loop that permits subsequent percutaneous or endoscopic management of recurrent stones and strictures.[61,195] A proportion of patients require resection of an atrophied portion of the liver containing multiple stones. The disease more frequently affects the left lobe than the right. Patients with intrahepatic stone disease have a 10% risk of developing a cholangiocarcinoma.[196]

ASCARIS LUMBRICOIDES

The roundworm *Ascaris lumbricoides* is endemic in large parts of Africa, Asia and Central America, and in parts of the world where poor socio-economic conditions and bad sanitation exist. It is estimated that over 600 million people are infested with the worm. Adult worms live in the human intestine and may enter the papilla into the pancreatic duct, causing acute pancreatitis, or into the bile ducts, causing biliary pain, partial obstruction, and

REFERENCES

191. Goldman LD, Steer ML, Silen W. Am J Surg 1983; 145: 450
192. Wong J, Choi TK. Prog Clin Biol Res 1984; 152: 175–192
193. Ong GB. Arch Surg 1962; 84: 199–225
194. Ikeda S, Tanaka M et al. World J Surg 1981; 5: 587
195. Fan ST, Mok FPT, Zhang SS et al. Am J Surg 1993; 165: 332–335
196. Chu KM, Lo CM, Liu CL et al. Hepato-Gastroenterology 1997; 44: 352–357

cholangitis with complications such as liver abscesses, perforation and stricture of the bile duct.[197]

Children are most frequently affected. The diagnosis is based on the identification of worms in the biliary tree on ultrasound, on intravenous cholangiography, or at ERCP. Treatment is with antibiotics, parenteral fluids, and antispasmodics to relax the sphincter of Oddi and allow egress of the live worms from the biliary tree. Anthelminthics such as mebendazole are given orally to kill the worms, but reinfestation occurs in a third of patients. Persistent intraductal worms or dead worms and ova can be removed endoscopically.[60] Surgery may also be required for persistent worms in the gall bladder (Fig. 30.25) and for stones or worms trapped behind an inflammatory biliary stricture.[197] Liver abscesses can be drained percutaneously under ultrasound guidance. The association between ascariasis and intrahepatic stone disease is unclear, but fragments of dead worms or their ova probably act as initiators of stone formation in some cases.

HYDATID DISEASE

The biliary tree may be involved when a hydatid cyst either compresses or ruptures into a biliary radical, causing severe cholangitis (see above). Compression by a hydatid cyst usually requires surgical drainage of the cyst. Care must be taken to avoid spillage of the cyst contents and to oversew any open bile duct radicals. When rupture into the biliary tree has occurred, hydatid debris may be removed by endoscopic sphincterotomy and either extraction with a Dormia basket or flushing through a cannula.[198] The scolicidal agents formalin and hypertonic saline used during surgical procedures can cause strictures if they enter the biliary tract.[198]

HAEMOBILIA

Haemobilia occurs when there is an abnormal communication between blood vessels and the bile ducts. Minor degrees of haemobilia may pass unnoticed because clots are normally lysed by the fibrinolytic action of free-flowing bile, but major bleeding leading to clot formation may cause biliary obstruction. Major haemobilia presents with the classical triad of gastrointestinal bleeding (melaena in 90%, haematemesis in 60%, biliary colic in 70%, and jaundice in 60%).[199] Investigation should begin with an upper gastrointestinal endoscopy to exclude alternative bleeding, with direct visualization of the papilla, where blood clot or fresh blood may be seen.[200] It may be combined with ERCP, which may show clots within the bile duct or identify causative intraductal pathology. Ultrasound, endoscopic ultrasound, CT or MRI may visualize pathology and blood within the biliary tract. Selective hepatic angiography reveals the source of bleeding in most cases by indicating a tumour blush or filling an aneurysm sac.

The causes of major haemobilia in order of frequency are iatrogenic trauma from liver biopsy, cholecystectomy or endoscopic sphincterotomy; penetrating and blunt accidental trauma; bile duct infestation from *Ascaris* and *Clonorchis*; and hepatic artery aneurysms. Gallstones, liver and biliary tumours, and coagulopathies rarely cause major bleeds.

Treatment of major bleeding is by selective embolization of involved hepatic artery branches with Gel-foam or coils.[201] Significant liver necrosis occurs in less than 5% of cases.[202]

Bleeding from the papilla may also arise from the pancreatic duct, where it is termed *haemosuccus pancreaticus*;[203] this is usually seen in patients with chronic pancreatitis and an associated pseudocyst and pseudoaneurysm.

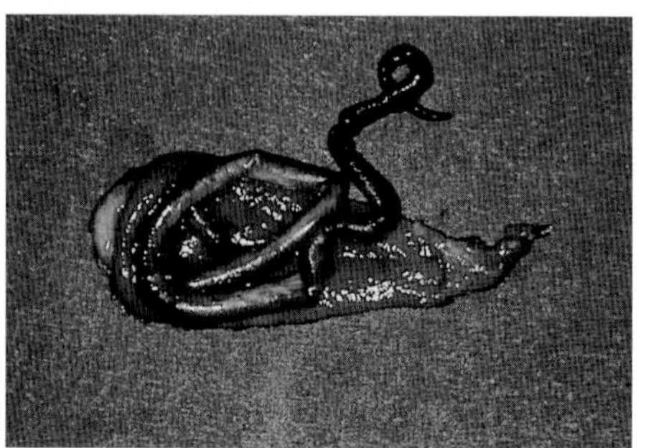

Figure 30.25 *Ascaris lumbricoides* infestation of gall bladder treated by laparoscopic cholecystectomy.

DISORDERS OF THE BILIARY TRACT IN CHILDHOOD

Conjugated hyperbilirubinaemia in infancy may be caused by structural changes within the biliary tract associated with extrahepatic biliary atresia or choledochal cysts. The presentation and biochemical abnormalities of these conditions may be difficult to distinguish from infective and metabolic causes of jaundice in infancy. Rarer surgical conditions of the bile ducts in children include inspissated bile syndrome, spontaneous perforation of the bile ducts, gallstones and tumours.

EXTRAHEPATIC BILIARY ATRESIA

Extrahepatic biliary atresia is the commonest cause of childhood biliary tract obstruction. The incidence is approximately one per 14 000 live births, and the sexes are equally affected.[204] The extrahepatic bile ducts are progressively destroyed by an inflammatory process, which starts around the time of birth. Intrahepatic changes also occur and eventually result in biliary cirrhosis and portal hypertension. The untreated child dies before 3 years of age of liver failure or haemorrhage.

The aetiology is unknown, although a viral infection has been proposed[176] and studies of the pancreaticobiliary junction in eight infants with atresia revealed a long common channel at the ampulla in all cases.[176] Associated anomalies are present in approximately 20% of cases and include cardiac lesions, polysplenia, situs inversus, absent vena cava and preduodenal portal vein.[204] The condition is classified into three main types (Fig. 30.26).[206]

REFERENCES

197. Lloyd DA, White JAM. In: Blumgart LH (ed). The Biliary Tract. Churchill Livingstone, Edinburgh, 1982
198. Khodadadi DJ, Kurgan A, Schmidt B. Int Surg 1981; 66: 361
199. Sandblom P, Saegesser F, Mirkovitch V. World J Surg 1984; 8: 41
200. Carr-Locke DL, Westwood CA. Am J Gastroenterol 1980; 73: 162
201. Horak D, Guseinov E, Amanyan A et al. J Biomed Mater Res 1996; 33: 193
202. Wagner W, Lundell C, Donovan A. Arch Surg 1985; 120: 1241
203. Sandblom P. Ann Surg 1970; 171: 61–66
204. Howard ER. In: Howard ER (ed). Surgery of Liver Disease in Children. Butterworth-Heinemann, London, 1991: 39
205. Morecki R, Glasser JH, Horwitz MS. In: Daum F (ed). Extrahepatic Biliary Atresia. Marcel Dekker, New York, 1983
206. Hays DM, Kimura K. Curr Probl Surg 1981; 18: 546

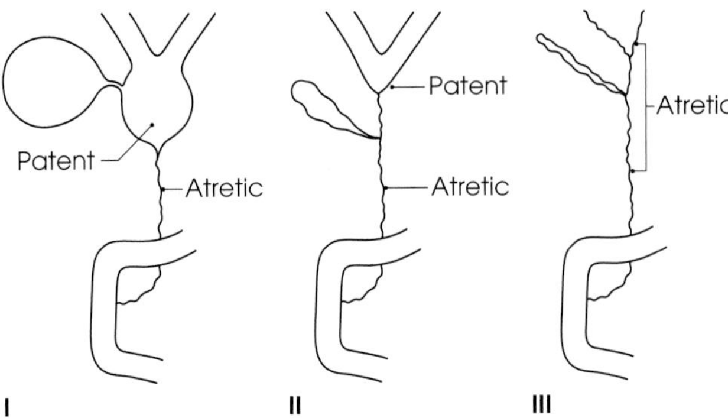

Figure 30.26 Classification of biliary atresia: type I, patent common hepatic duct; type II, patent hepatic ducts; and type III, atresia of all extrahepatic ducts.

1. Type I: atresia restricted to the common bile duct.
2. Type II: atresia of the common hepatic duct.
3. Type III: atresia of right and left hepatic ducts.

Histology of the obliterated atretic bile ducts shows fibrosis and variable numbers of inflammatory cells. Small segments of partially obliterated hepatic ducts can sometimes be identified but are usually replaced by ductules lined by either cuboidal or columnar epithelium. Intrahepatic changes include portal fibrosis, bile duct proliferation, and giant cell change in the hepatocytes. Hepatic fibrosis increases with age.[205]

Investigations include screening tests for infective and metabolic causes of jaundice. The stools are white as a consequence of the absence of bile pigment. Liver biopsy and radionuclide excretion scans are essential, and some centres aspirate duodenal juice for bile analysis.

Patent segments of proximal bile ducts are found in less than 10% of cases (type I lesions). A conventional biliary–enteric anastomosis may be possible in this group, and an analysis of 64 such cases showed satisfactory postoperative bile flow in 75%.[207] Progressive liver disease, however, results in a more disappointing long-term survival rate, which varies between 25 and 50% at 5 years.

Type II and type III lesions—in which the atretic process affects more proximal portions of the extrahepatic bile ducts—are not amenable to conventional surgery. The affected tissue at the porta hepatis, however, frequently contains ductular structures that can communicate with intrahepatic bile ducts. These communications were first demonstrated by Kasai,[208] and the operation of portoenterostomy was developed from his observations. Portoenterostomy consists of a radical excision of all bile duct tissue up to the liver capsule. A Roux-en-Y loop of jejunum is anastomosed to the exposed area of liver capsule above the bifurcation of the portal vein (Fig. 30.27). The chances of achieving effective bile drainage after portoenterostomy are maximal when the operation is performed on infants before the age of 8 weeks, and approximately 90% of the children whose bilirubin falls to within the normal range can be expected to survive for 10 years or more.[209] Early referral to specialist paediatric units for surgery is therefore critical.[210] There are now an increasing number of adolescents and adults with successfully treated biliary atresia, and Laurent and colleagues reported 40 patients who had survived for more than 10 years.[211]

Postoperative complications of portoenterostomy include bacterial cholangitis, which complicates the postoperative course in approximately 40% of cases.[204] Repeated attacks of infection cause increasing hepatic fibrosis. Portal hypertension also affects approximately half the long-term survivors, with variceal bleeding occurring in 20–30%.[212] Reduced bile flow may be associated with poor growth and deficiency of fat-soluble vitamins such as vitamin D.

Liver transplantation (see Ch. 8) may be considered when portoenterostomy fails to relieve jaundice,[213] and most transplants are required within the first 2 years of life when it becomes clear that bile drainage has not been achieved. Transplantation may be indicated in older patients with atresia for progressive liver failure or severe portal hypertension and secondary biliary cirrhosis.

Liver transplantation is not regarded as the primary treatment for biliary atresia in the UK but is considered to be complementary to the portoenterostomy operation.

CHOLEDOCHAL CYSTS

Benign bile duct cysts (choledochal cysts) are a rare condition, with 80% of cases presenting in infants or children. The classical triad of jaundice, pain, and a mass in the right hypochondrium is present in around only 40% of cases.[214] A third have the clinical features of pancreatitis, with a raised amylase at diagnosis.[215] When diagnosed in adults, 15% are found to have overt evidence of cirrhosis or hepatic fibrosis. More than 80% of cysts occur in females, and the condition is more common in Japan.

The aetiology can be explained by a congenital weakness of the bile ducts associated with a functional obstruction at the lower end. Anomalous junctions of the biliary–pancreatic junction are frequently observed, and long common channels result in high levels of biliary amylase in 70–80% of cases. Common pancreaticobiliary channels may be associated with repeated attacks of pancreatitis (Fig. 30.28).

Cysts are classified by their site within the biliary tract (Fig. 30.29). A survey of 1433 patients showed that 51% of cases were type I cystic, 11% were type I fusiform, and 28% were type IV.[216] Type II and III cysts and isolated intrahepatic cysts (Caroli's disease) were rare collectively, constituting less than 10% of the total. The diagnosis can usually be made with ultrasound and MRCP in most cases, with ERCP and radionuclide scans reserved for indeterminate cases. Complications of the cysts include pancreatitis, spontaneous rupture, liver abscess, cirrhosis and portal hypertension. Carcinoma of the biliary tract is a well-recognized complication[217] and carries a poor prognosis, probably because of the difficulty of early diagnosis. The

REFERENCES

207. Ohi R. In: Ohi R (ed.). Biliary Atresia. Professional Postgraduate Services, Tokyo, 1987: 125
208. Kasai M. (Citation). In: Howard ER. Br J Surg 1983; 70: 193
209. Ohi R, Hanamatsu M et al. World J Surg 1985; 9: 285
210. Mieli-Vergani G, Howard ER et al. Lancet 1989; 1: 421
211. Laurent J, Gauthier F et al. Gastroenterology 1990; 99: 1793
212. Stringer M, Howard ER, Mowat AP. J Pediatr Surg 1989; 24: 438
213. Beath S, Pearmain G et al. J Pediatr Surg 1993; 28: 1044
214. Flanigan DP. Ann Surg 1975; 182: 635
215. Nagorney DM, McIlrath DC, Adson MA. Surgery 1984; 96: 656–663
216. Yamaguchi M. Am J Surg 1980; 140: 653
217. Kagawa Y, Kashihara S, Kuramoto S. Gastroenterology 1978; 74: 1286

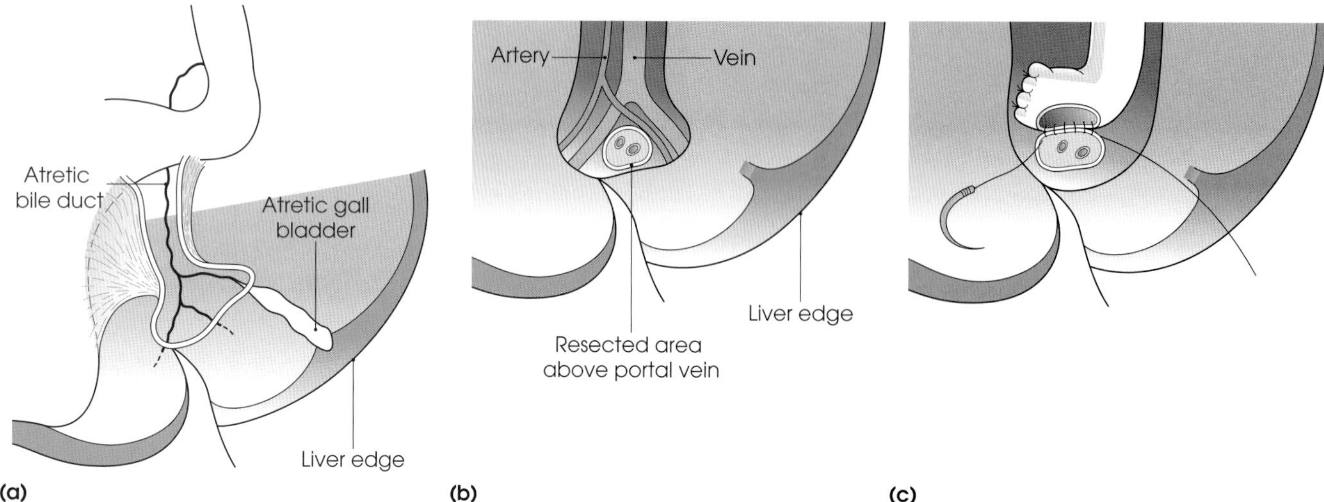

Figure 30.27 Kasai portoenterostomy: **(a)** atretic ducts exposed by dissection, **(b)** residual ductal tissue completely excised to above the level of the portal vein bifurcation, and **(c)** anastamosis of Roux-en-Y loop of jejunum to edges of excised tissue.

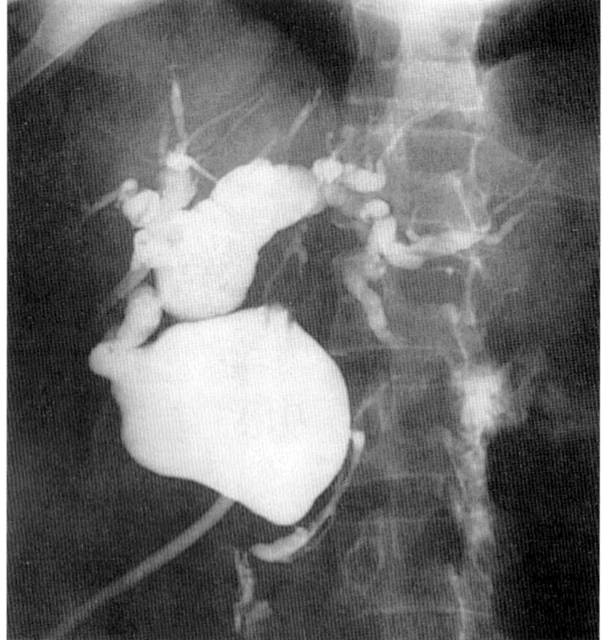

Figure 30.28 Operative cholangiogram of cystic dilatation of the extrahepatic bile ducts in an adult woman. The terminal portion of the narrow pancreatic duct forms a common channel with the bile duct.

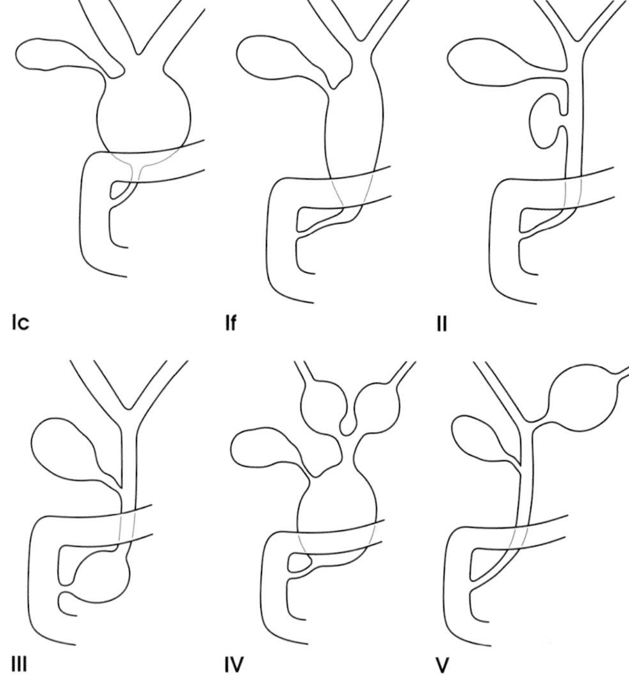

Figure 30.29 Classification of choledochal cysts: Ic, extrahepatic cystic dilatation; If, fusiform dilatation; II, diverticulum; III, choledochocele; IV, intrahepatic and extrahepatic dilatation; and V, intrahepatic dilatation (Caroli's disease).

incidence of cholangiocarcinoma rises with age, from less than 1% in the first decade to more than 14% after 20 years of age.[218] The mean age of presentation of cholangiocarcinoma is 32 years.[219] It is, however, a very rare complication in children who have undergone complete surgical excision.

Internal drainage, once advocated for biliary cysts, is complicated by recurrent cholangitis and anastomotic stenosis in approximately 40% of cases, and patients remain at risk of malignant change.[220] Treatment is by radical excision of the

REFERENCES

218. Voyles CR, Smadja C, Shands C et al. Arch Surg 1983; 118: 986–988
219. Ono J, Sakoda K, Akita H. Ann Surg 1982; 195: 203–208
220. Trout HH, Longmire WP. Am J Surg 1981; 121: 68

extrahepatic biliary tract from the biliary confluence down to the junction with the pancreatic duct. Care is taken to avoid narrowing the main pancreatic duct. Reconstruction is with a standard Roux-en-Y hepaticojejunostomy.

Management of Caroli's disease is difficult and determined by the presence of congenital hepatic fibrosis or secondary biliary cirrhosis. Disease confined to one lobe can be managed with hepatic resection with or with extrahepatic biliary resection, and hepaticojejunostomy if the main bile ducts are involved.[221,222] Diffuse disease is treated with long-term antibiotics, analgesics and litholytic agents, which may improve symptoms but rarely eliminates them completely. The natural history of Caroli's disease is progression to secondary biliary cirrhosis, portal hypertension and liver failure. Liver transplantation offers the best management (see Ch. 8), and interventional procedures prior to this should be avoided.[223]

INSPISSATED BILE SYNDROME

Obstructive jaundice in early infancy is occasionally associated with inspissated bile within the common bile duct. It is sometimes secondary to haemolysis caused by blood group incompatibility. Dilatation of the proximal bile ducts and gall bladder is observed at laparotomy. The inspissated material is removed through a choledochotomy, but occasionally an additional sphincterotomy is necessary.[217]

SPONTANEOUS PERFORATION OF THE COMMON BILE DUCT

This rare condition should be suspected when an infant of a few weeks of age develops fluctuating jaundice, pale stools and dark urine. Less specific signs include weight loss, irritability and occasional vomiting. Examination shows biliary ascites, which may cause a dark staining of the umbilicus or scrotum. More than 50 cases have been reported.[224,225] Investigations show raised serum bilirubin levels of between 100 and 120 mmol/L and normal liver enzymes. Radionuclide scans demonstrate the intraperitoneal bile and provide images of the peritoneal cavity, confirming the diagnosis.

The perforation occurs at the junction of the cystic and common bile ducts. The cause is unknown, but the condition may be associated with inspissated bile at the lower end of the common bile duct.[225] The diagnosis is usually made at laparotomy, and operative cholangiography via the cystic duct confirms the site of perforation, which is drained by insertion of a T-tube. The addition of a cholecystenterostomy has been suggested, but in most cases the perforation heals satisfactorily with drainage alone.[225]

GALL BLADDER DISEASE IN CHILDHOOD

Acute gall bladder distension known as hydrops of the gall bladder, which is unrelated to gallstones or inflammation, occurs in early childhood with a mean age at presentation of 5 years.[226] The condition often follows respiratory tract infection and may be related to cystic node enlargement. Abdominal pain, vomiting, and tenderness and a mass in the right hypochondrium are typical signs. Ultrasonography confirms the diagnosis. Tube cholecystostomy is the treatment of choice and the postoperative recovery is usually uncomplicated.

Acalculous cholecystitis in children may follow burns and trauma, and it may also be seen as a postoperative complication of abdominal surgery. It occurs at any age from 1 month to 15 years[227] and is frequently misdiagnosed as appendicitis. Cholecystostomy is the treatment of choice in these children.

Haemolytic anaemias and congenital anomalies may predispose to gallstone formation in children. Cholesterol stones also occur occasionally, with presenting symptoms, complications, and management with laparoscopic cholecystectomy similar to that of adults.[228] Common bile duct stones are the commonest surgical cause of jaundice in children.

TUMOURS OF THE BILE DUCT

SOLITARY BENIGN TUMOURS

Solitary benign tumours are very rare, representing less than 0.1% of all biliary tract operations and only 6% of all biliary tumours.[229] They present with obstructive jaundice, and when diagnosed preoperatively can be managed by local resection. Histologically, papilloma and adenoma are the commonest tumours, but granular cell myoblastoma, neural tumours and leiomyoma have all been reported.

BILIARY PAPILLOMATOSIS

This rare condition is characterized by the presence of multiple soft, fragile, papillary, mucus-secreting tumours of the biliary epithelium, distinguishing them from a solitary polyp or a papillary adenocarcinoma that does not secrete mucus.[221] They are more common in elderly women. The presentation simulates calculus disease with intermittent biliary obstruction and biliary pain. The diagnosis is made on preoperative or intraoperative cholangiography; this demonstrates a scalloped edge to the bile duct, which may be associated with filling defects.[221] The finding of copious mucus on opening the bile duct is strongly suggestive of papillomatosis, and choledochoscopy with biopsy is confirmatory.[221] Occasionally the diagnosis is made preoperatively by the presence of mucus seen extruding from the duodenal papilla on ERCP.

A number of treatments have been tried but all are unsatisfactory, including curettage, internal bilioenteric anastomosis, and external U-tube drainage. When there is sparing of part of the biliary tract, radical resection of the involved liver and bile ducts with hepaticojejunostomy to the remaining healthy liver may achieve control.[221] Although the condition is non-malignant, its often extensive involvement of the biliary tract results in recurrent biliary obstruction and sepsis, with a mean survival of 3 years.[230] Liver transplantation may be the best treatment.

REFERENCES

221. Mercadier M, Bodard M et al. World J Surg 1984; 8: 30
222. Mercadier M, Chigot JP, Clot JP et al. World J Surg 1984; 8: 22–29
223. Scharschmidt BF. Hepatology 1984; 4: 95S–101S
224. Howard ER, Johnston DI, Mowat AP. Arch Dis Child 1976; 51: 883
225. Davenport M, Howard ER. In: Howard ER (ed). Surgery of Liver Disease in Children. Butterworth-Heinemann, London, 1991: 91
226. Chamberlain JW, Hight DW. Surgery 1970; 68: 899
227. Ternberg JL, Keating JP. Arch Surg 1975; 110: 543
228. Kirtley JA, Holcomb GW. Am J Surg 1966; 111: 39
229. Burhans R, Myers RT. Am Surg 1971; 37: 161–166
230. Hubens G, Delvaux G, Willems G et al. Hepato-gastroenterology 1991; 38: 413–418

BILIARY CYSTADENOMA AND CYSTADENOCARCINOMA

A cystadenoma of the biliary tract is a rare tumour. Most are single large mucinous tumours arising from the intrahepatic (85%) or extrahepatic bile ducts or from the gall bladder (15%). Although usually benign they tend to recur with incomplete resection, and there may be progression to cystadenocarcinoma. They are most commonly seen in women over the age of 40 years and present with abdominal pain, a palpable abdominal mass, nausea and vomiting. The diagnosis is based on ultrasound and CT findings of fluid-filled masses with internal echoes from multiple septa, mucinous fluid contents, and papillary projections. Differentiation from malignant cystadenocarcinoma is not usually possible, although calcification is more common in the latter. Biliary obstruction can occur by compression of neighbouring bile ducts. The differential diagnosis includes simple cysts, hydatid disease, and polycystic liver disease.

Drainage and biopsy should be avoided to prevent risk of infection, haemorrhage and tumour dissemination. Treatment of all cases should be by complete excision, because malignancy cannot be confidently excluded preoperatively and benign cystadenomas can become malignant. Five-year survival following resection of cystadenocarcinoma is around 55%.[231]

CHOLANGIOCARCINOMA (CARCINOMA OF THE BILE DUCT)

Cholangiocarcinoma can occur anywhere within the biliary tract, but around 50% occur at the biliary confluence, where they are called hilar cholangiocarcinoma or Klatskin tumour (Fig. 30.30).

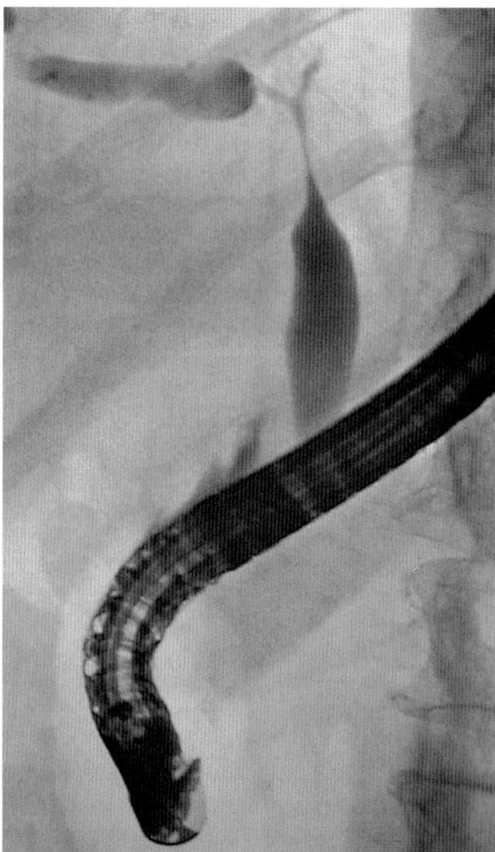

Figure 30.30 Hilar cholangiocarcinoma involving confluence and extending into left and right hepatic ducts (Bismuth type IV).

Around 10% occur within the intrahepatic biliary tract, presenting as an intrahepatic mass. Less than 10% present with multifocal or diffuse involvement of the biliary tract. Direct invasion of liver or perihepatic structures is common. Neural and perineural spread is common, as is lymphatic spread, with a third having nodal metastases at presentation. Haematogenous spread is uncommon.

Cholangiocarcinoma is uncommon in Europe and the USA, with an incidence of one or two in 100 000,[232] or around 500 new cases per annum in the UK. The disease is more common in South-East Asia, with rates of 90 per 100 000 in some parts of Thailand.[233] Most patients are over 65, with a 2:1 male preponderance. Untreated, most patients die within 6 months. Patients with sclerosing cholangitis, choledochal cysts, Caroli's disease and intrahepatic stone disease each have around a 10% risk of developing cholangiocarcinoma.

Three distinct macroscopic subtypes occur: sclerosing, nodular and papillary. Sclerosing tumours account for the majority of cases and are more common in the hilum. They are firm annular thickenings of the bile duct, often with diffuse infiltration and periductal fibrosis. Nodular tumours are characterized by an irregular nodule projecting into the lumen of the duct. Features of both subtypes are seen together, leading to the term *nodular–sclerosing*. The papillary variant accounts for only 10% of tumours and is most commonly seen in the distal bile duct. They are soft and friable and often arise from a stalk. They have little transmural invasion and may grow quite large before causing problems. They tend to cause expansion of the duct rather than narrowing, and are thus more likely to be resectable and have a better prognosis. Longitudinal spread along the duct wall and periductal tissues is common, and submucosal extension may reach 2 cm proximal to the main lesion.[234] Although most cholangiocarcinomas are adenocarcinomas, a few may arise from other malignant cell types, such as carcinoid tumours.

Early symptoms are non-specific, with abdominal pain and discomfort, anorexia and weight loss, and pruritis. The usual presentation is with progressive jaundice. Segmental obstruction may present without jaundice in patients with non-specific illness investigated for abnormal liver function tests. Cholangitis is uncommon in these patients.

Staging and assessment for resection

Surgery remains the only curative option for cholangiocarcinoma. Patients must be fit for major surgery, which usually includes partial hepatectomy. Major comorbidity, chronic liver disease, and portal hypertension preclude resection. There are four critical determinants to resectability: the extent of tumour within the biliary tract, vascular invasion, liver atrophy and metastatic disease.[235] Lobar atrophy is associated with biliary or portal vein involvement, and its presence often precludes treatment. The radiological criteria preventing resection are shown in Table 30.3.

REFERENCES

231. Barthet M, Garcia T, Payan MJ et al. Dig Surg 1992; 9: 285–287
232. Carriaga MT, Henson DE. Cancer 1995; 75: 171–190
233. Watanapa P. Br J Surg 1996; 83: 1062–1064
234. Shimada H, Niimoto S, Matsuba A et al. Int Surg 1988; 73: 87–90
235. Burke EC. Ann Surg 1998; 228: 385–394

Table 30.3 Radiological criteria defining irresectability of cholangiocarcinoma

- Hepatic duct involvement up to secondary biliary radicles bilaterally
- Encasement or occlusion of main portal vein proximal to its bifurcation
- Atrophy of one hepatic lobe with encasement of contralateral portal vein branch
- Atrophy of one hepatic lobe with contralateral involvement of secondary biliary radicles
- Distant metastases (peritoneum, lung, liver)

Cholangiography has been the mainstay of investigation, with percutaneous transhepatic cholangiography preferred to ERCP because the proximal extent of the lesion usually defines resectability.[236,237] Many centres now, however, perform preoperative staging with non-invasive MRCP and duplex ultrasound. In patients operated on without previous intervention, bacterial contamination of the bile duct occurs in less than 30% compared with 100% in patients who have had ERCP or percutaneous transhepatic cholangiography.[238] Patients who have cholangitis, which usually follows biliary intervention, should wait until the sepsis has resolved before undergoing resection. Duplex ultrasound has been shown to be as accurate as angiography and CT portography in predicting vascular invasion.[24] Both MRCP and MRI scanning can provide information on patency of hilar vessels, presence of nodal or distant metastases, and lobar atrophy.

Surgical management of hilar cholangiocarcinoma

The surgical management of cholangiocarcinoma depends on its location. Tumours within the intrapancreatic segment of bile duct require a pancreatoduodenectomy. They present like pancreatic head neoplasms and are discussed in Chapter 31.

Tumours involving the supraduodenal segment of common bile duct require complete excision of the extrahepatic biliary tract above the duodenum with en bloc resection of the tissues within the hilum, followed by Roux-en-Y reconstruction.

Hilar cholangiocarcinoma usually requires additional resection of the ipsilateral liver and the caudate lobe to achieve a complete resection margin. Resectability rates, negative resection margins, and long-term survival rates are all higher in series where liver resection has been incorporated.[235,239,240] Biliary reconstruction without hepatectomy should be considered only when there is no liver atrophy and no involvement of the second-order ducts or portal vein on either side.

Technique for resection of hilar cholangiocarcinoma

The initial assessment of the liver surface and peritoneum is undertaken to exclude peritoneal disease. This may be performed laparoscopically. The lower part of the bile duct is divided and the bile duct, tumour, and all lymphatic and neural tissue dissected from the portal vein and hepatic artery towards the hilum. A portion of the distal duct is sent for frozen section. Careful assessment can now be made of the tumour in relation to the portal vein and artery. If resection is not possible at this stage, a palliative hepaticojejunostomy to the segment III duct is performed. Relief of jaundice will be achieved if at least a third of the functioning liver parenchyma is drained.[241] Once it has been established that resection is feasible and will leave behind a tumour-free liver remnant with an intact blood supply and biliary drainage, the inflow to the lobe that is to be removed is controlled and divided. The contralateral hepatic duct above the tumour should be divided extrahepatically, and the cut edge sent for frozen section. The hepatic vein draining the portion of liver to be excised is divided. Parenchymal transection is commenced and usually requires a trisectionectomy and excision of the caudate lobe. Tumour invasion was found in 44 of 46 caudate lobes in resection specimens in one series.[240] Once resection is complete, a Roux-en-Y hepaticojejunostomy is fashioned to the remaining bile duct (Fig. 30.31).

Results depend on obtaining clear resection margins. In the high-volume centres, a mortality rate of 6%, median survival of 40 months, and 5-year survival rates of 40–56% have been reported.[235,240]

PALLIATIVE CARE

The majority of patients with hilar cholangiocarcinoma are not suitable for resection. Chemotherapy, internal and external radiotherapy, and photodynamic therapy have all been tried but none have shown any clear benefit as yet. Liver transplantation is associated with early disseminated tumour recurrence and should no longer be performed (see Ch. 8). Those that do best have very early lesions that would anyway be suitable for resection in most cases.

The majority of patients with cholangiocarcinoma require biliary decompression to relieve pruritis, and this is usually best achieved by insertion of a metal wall stent either by percutaneous transhepatic cholangiography for hilar lesions or by ERCP. Jaundice may be caused not only by bile duct obstruction but also by portal vein occlusion with hepatic dysfunction, which will not improve with biliary drainage. Drainage of atrophic liver segments incurs no benefit and should be avoided. Elderly patients with significant comorbidity and without significant pruritis may be best treated with supportive care alone.

CARCINOMA OF THE GALL BLADDER

Gall bladder cancer is the most common biliary tract malignancy and the fifth most common gastrointestinal malignancy, with an incidence of 1.2 cases per 100 000 of population. It has a wide geographical variation, with higher incidences in Chile, Japan, and north-eastern Europe. It is also common in American Indians. It is two to six times more common in women. It is invariably associated with gallstone disease (75–95% of cases, Fig. 30.32), although it is uncertain whether this is cause or effect or the result of common risk factors.[242] The risk of developing gall

REFERENCES

236. Pitt HA, Dooley WC, Yeo CJ et al. Curr Probl Surg 1995; 32: 1–90
237. Pitt HA, Nakeeb A, Abrams RA et al. Ann Surg 1995; 221: 788–798
238. Hochwald SN, Burke EC, Jarnagin WR et al. Arch Surg 1999; 134: 261–266
239. Klempnauer J, Ridder GJ, von Wassiuelewski R et al. J Clin Oncol 1997; 15: 947–954
240. Nimura Y, Kayakawa N, Kamiya J et al. World J Surg 1990; 14: 535–544
241. Baer HU, Rhyner M, Stain SC et al. Hepato-Biliary Surg 1994; 8: 27–31
242. Zatonski WA, Lowenfels AB, Boyle P et al. J Natl Cancer Inst 1997; 89: 1132–1138

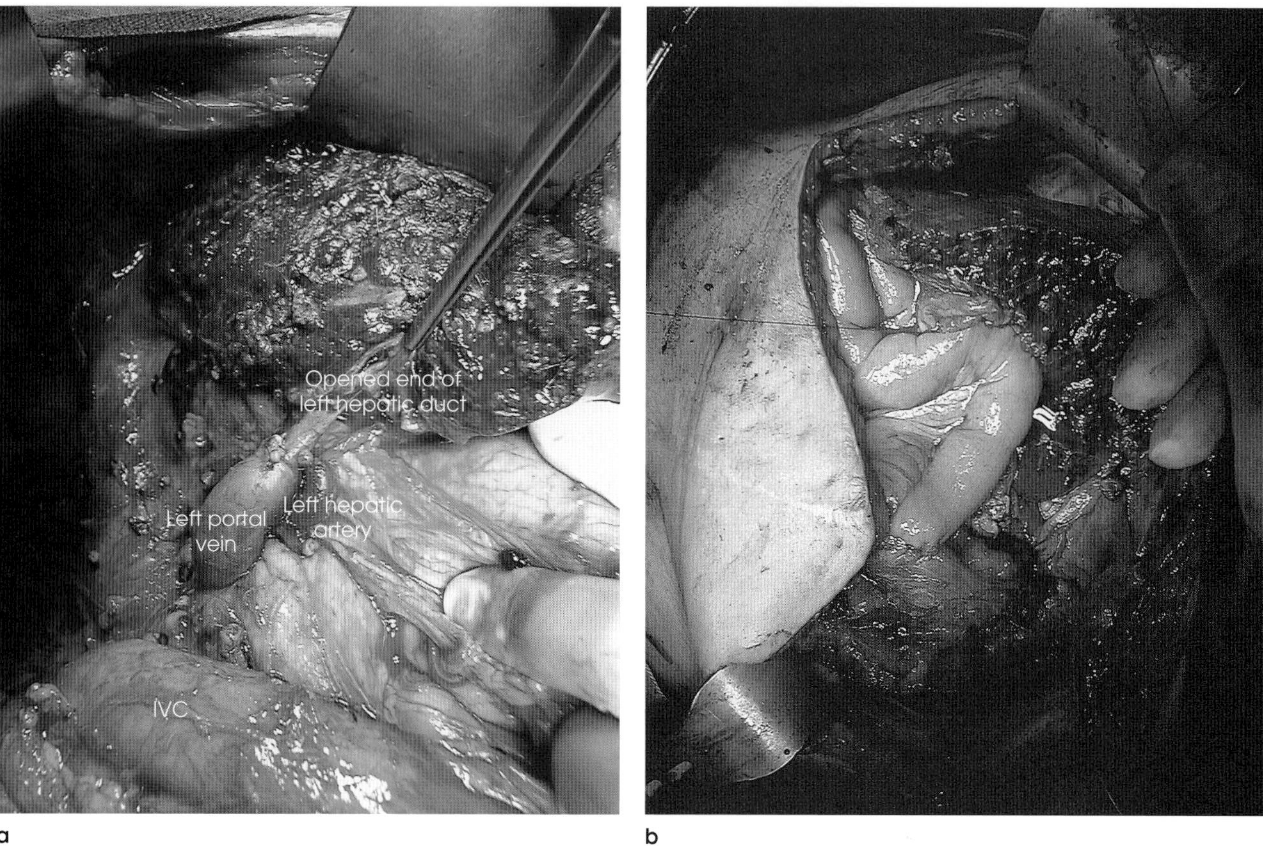

Figure 30.31 (a) Extended right hepatectomy for hilar cholangiocarcinoma. (b) The same patient following hepaticojejunostomy to left heptic duct.

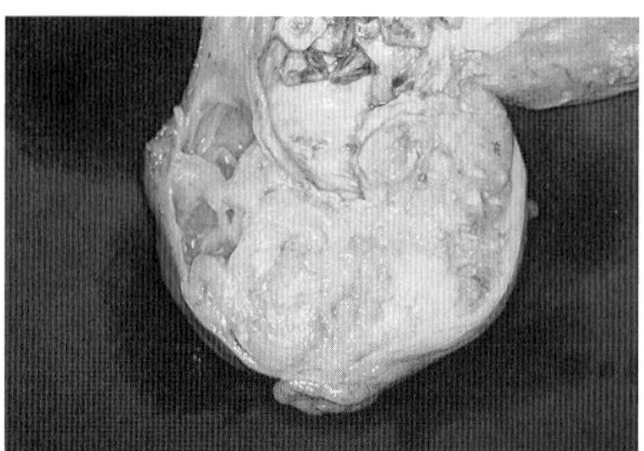

Figure 30.32 Gall bladder cancer in the presence of multiple gallstones.

bladder cancer in patients with gallstone disease is low, estimated as 0.5–1%,[243–245] and prophylactic cholecystectomy is not therefore justifiable in symptomless patients with gallstones. Calcification of the gall bladder (a porcelain gall bladder) is, however, associated with a high incidence of gall bladder cancer, present in up to 25% of cases.[246] These patients should therefore have a prophylactic cholecystectomy. There is a fivefold increased risk of cancer of the gall bladder in smokers, probably as a result of excretion of carcinogens in bile.[247,248]

Histologically, 97% of tumours are adenocarcinomas or undifferentiated, 2% squamous, and 1% sarcoma or metastatic in origin. There is good evidence to support the hypothesis that it changes from dysplasia through carcinoma in situ to invasive carcinoma. The role of adenomatous polyps in the development of gall bladder cancer is less clear, but the presence of carcinoma in polyps greater than 1 cm in diameter in several series suggests recommending cholecystectomy for patients with polyps of this size.[249] Incidental carcinoma of the gall bladder is found in up to 1–2% of cholecystectomy specimens.[250,251] Spread of gall bladder cancer is by direct invasion into the liver (segments IVb and V; 60%), early lymphatic spread (94%), and haematogenous venous spread (65%).[250] Liver metastases are common (35%), and peritoneal metastases are seen in 60% of patients in post-mortem studies. Only 10% of patients have disease confined to the gall bladder wall.[252]

REFERENCES

243. Brossart PA, Patterson AH, Zintel HA. Am J Surg 1962; 103: 366
244. Maram ES, Ludwig J, Kurland LT et al. Am J Epidemiol 1979; 109: 152–157
245. Comfort MW, Gray HK, Wilson JM. Am Surg 1948; 128: 931–936
246. Berk RN, Armbuster TG, Saltzstein SL. Radiology 1973; 106: 29–31
247. Bevan DR, Sadler VM. Carcinogenesis 1992; 13(3): 405–407
248. Scott TE, Carroll M, Cogliano FD et al. Dig Dis Sci 1999; 44: 1619–1625
249. Aldridge MC, Bismuth H. Br J Surg 1990; 77: 363–364
250. Kimura W, Nagai H, Juroda A et al. Cancer 1989; 64: 98–103
251. Silk YN, Douglas JHO, Nava HR et al. Ann Surg 1989; 210: 751–757
252. Boerma EJ. Eur J Surg Oncol 1994; 20: 537–544

Table 30.4

Stage	Pathological Findings	Management
I	Mucosal or muscular invasion.	Simple cholecystetomy (usually incidental finding).
IIA	Transmural invasion	Radical Choleystectomy with resection of extrahepatic bile ducts and segment IVb and V liver resection
IIB	Liver invasion < 2 cm	
III	Liver invasion 72 cm; NI disease	Extended light hepatectomy and excision of extrahepatic bile ducts and lymphadenectomy
IV	Distant metastases	Palliative care

The presentation is similar to that of gallstone disease. The upper abdominal pain may be more constant and associated with weight loss. Patients with gall bladder cancer present on average 10 years later than those with gallstones. Presentation with jaundice is invariably associated with advanced inoperable tumours. Ca19-9 and CEA tumour markers are frequently elevated. Ultrasound scan evidence of a mass in the gall bladder or extending from the gall bladder wall into the liver is highly suggestive of carcinoma. Contrast-enhanced CT provides good staging information, although its sensitivity for lymph node metastases is low.[253] There are a number of staging systems used, with the most useful in terms of management protocols and survival being the Sloan-Kettering modification of the tumour, node, metastasis (TNM) system.[254] Patients with early gall bladder cancer are invariably diagnosed following histological examination of cholecystectomy specimen for calculus disease.

Management of gall bladder cancer

Patients with early gall bladder cancer (stage Ia and Ib) who have had a cholecystectomy have no evidence to suggest that further, more radical surgery is of any benefit so long as resection margins are clear (Table 30.4).[254,255] Stage II tumours (with invasion into the liver) require partial hepatectomy in addition to cholecystectomy. This should ideally be carried out as a single procedure, but in some patients the diagnosis will only have been made by histological examination of a cholecystectomy specimen. Further surgery is advocated in this group because an improvement in survival has been demonstrated.[256] Surgery should involve en bloc resection of the gall bladder and segments IVb and V, with frozen section of the cystic duct stump to ensure a clear resection margin. Resection of the bile duct and Roux-en-Y anastamosis should be performed if the margin is involved.

The majority of patients present with stage III or IV disease, and treatment of this group of patients remains controversial, with most large series reporting 5-year survival rates of 0–8% regardless of the extent of resection, the use of intraoperative radiotherapy, and chemotherapy.[257–259] The overall outcome for this group has been dismal, although a few centres have reported long-term survivors after aggressive radical surgical management involving extended right hepatectomy, bile duct excision and lymphadenectomy, and achieved 5-year survival rates of 67% (stage IIIb) and 37% (stage IV),[254] and 45% in patients with N1 positive nodes,[260,261] albeit with very small numbers of patients. Complication rates for these major surgical procedures are high, with a morbidity rate of 26–54% (bile leaks, liver failure, intra-abdominal abscesses and respiratory failure) and mortality rate of 0–18%,[254,257] with patients undergoing hepatic lobotomy or bile duct reconstruction most at risk.

The situation is further complicated in patients who have undergone laparoscopic cholecystectomy prior to the diagnosis of gall bladder cancer, because of the well-documented high incidence of wound metastases in these patients of around 17%.[262] In many of these patients, the metastases developed in wounds other than those used for the gall bladder extraction, and in some patients the gall bladder had been extracted within a bag. It is recommended therefore that patients in whom there is any suggestion of a gall bladder carcinoma should undergo an open procedure, with an immediate potentially curative procedure if confirmed. Patients who undergo secondary resection after laparoscopic cholecystectomy may benefit from excision of the previous laparoscopic port sites.[263]

Palliative treatment

The median survival of patients presenting with carcinoma of the gall bladder is 3 months, with a 1-year survival of less than 5%.[264,265] The goals of palliation should be the relief of pain, jaundice and bowel obstruction, and the prolongation of life. Jaundice is usually best treated via percutaneous transhepatic

REFERENCES

253. Ohtani T, Shirai Y, Tsukada K et al. Abdom Imaging 1996; 21: 195–201
254. Bartlett DL, Fong Y, Fortner JG et al. Ann Surg 1996; 224: 639–646
255. Shirai Y, Yoshida K, Tsukada K et al. Ann Surg 1992; 216(5): 565–568
256. De Aretxabala X, Roa OIS, Burgos LA et al. Eur J Surg 1997; 163: 419–426
257. Ogura Y, Mizumoto R, Isaji S et al. World J Surg 1991 15: 337–343
258. Matsumoto Y, Jujii H, Aoyama H et al. Am J Surg 1992; 63: 239–245
259. Todoroki T, Iwasaki Y, Orii K et al. World J Surg 1991; 15: 357–366
260. Shirai Y, Yoshida K, Tsukada K et al. Ann Surg 1992; 216: 565–568
261. Shirai Y, Yoshida K, Tsukada K et al. Br J Surg 1992; 79: 659–662
262. Paolucci V, Schaeff B, Schneider M et al. World J Surg 1999; 23: 989–997
263. Fong Y, Brennan MF, Tuyrnball A et al. Arch Surg 1993; 128: 1054–1056
264. Oertli D, Herzog U, Tondelli P. Eur J Surg 1993; 159: 415–420
265. Wanebo HJ, Castle WN, Fechner RE. Ann Surg 1982; 196: 624-631

cholangiography with metal wall stent insertion or, if not possible, by surgical segment III bypass.[266] In jaundiced patients with advanced disease and without itching, it may be best to avoid any intervention. Chemotherapy has been used but has poor response rates and no proved benefit on survival. Radiotherapy may improve symptoms and may have some improvement in survival in selected patients.[267]

REFERENCES

266. Bismuth H, Corlett MB. Surg Gynecol Obstet 1975; 140: 170–176
267. Houry S, Schlienger M, Huguier M et al. Br J Surg 1989; 76: 448–450

The pancreas

31

Richard M. Charnley, Paul V. Gallagher

INTRODUCTION

The pancreas is a relatively inaccessible retroperitoneal organ with intimate relations to surrounding structures. It has an exocrine function in the form of secretion of digestive enzymes and endocrine functions including glucose homeostasis. Management of pancreatic disease has been assisted in recent years by improved techniques of imaging and the development of new laboratory tests.

EMBRYOLOGY

The morphology of the pancreas is largely established by the eighth week of gestation.[1] In the fourth week of gestation, endodermal buds develop on the ventral and dorsal aspects of the foregut. The ventral bud becomes the liver, biliary tree, gallbladder and ventral pancreas, which consists of the future uncinate process and caudal part of the head of the pancreas. The dorsal bud becomes the dorsal pancreas, which makes up the future cranial part of the head of the pancreas, and the body and tail. In the sixth week, the duodenum rotates to the right. The bile duct and ventral pancreas then rotate behind the foregut tube and superior mesenteric vessels to come to lie posterior to the dorsal pancreas (Fig. 31.1). The duct of the ventral pancreas, the duct of Wirsung, drains into the future ampulla of Vater with the bile duct. The duct of the dorsal pancreas forms the accessory duct of Santorini and drains into the duodenum via the minor papilla. In the adult, the main pancreatic duct is formed by all the ventral system and the distal part of the dorsal system. The accessory duct usually becomes obliterated, but in 10% of individuals this does not occur and a double duct system persists. The islets of Langerhans develop from the pancreatic parenchyma and begin to produce insulin in the fifth month of intrauterine life.

CONGENITAL ANOMALIES

Several congenital abnormalities of the pancreas can occur. These may present with specific symptoms, they can cause pancreatitis, or they may be found incidentally during the course of investigations. Complete agenesis is fatal, while hypoplasia may produce a short pancreas. Accessory ectopic pancreatic tissue may develop at any site in the gastrointestinal tract but most commonly in the stomach, in the duodenum, or in a Meckel's diverticulum (see Ch. 27). It rarely causes symptoms but can cause nodules in the bile or pancreatic ducts. Congenital pancreatic cysts have also been described. Pancreas divisum and annular pancreas are the two most important congenital anomalies.

PANCREAS DIVISUM

In the normal pancreas, the ventral and dorsal duct systems fuse and the main pancreatic duct empties into the duodenum at the major papilla (Fig. 31.2). Pancreas divisum occurs in approximately 5% of people and is caused by failure of the dorsal

REFERENCE

1. Androulakis J, Colborn GL et al. Surg Clin North Am 2000; 80: 171–199

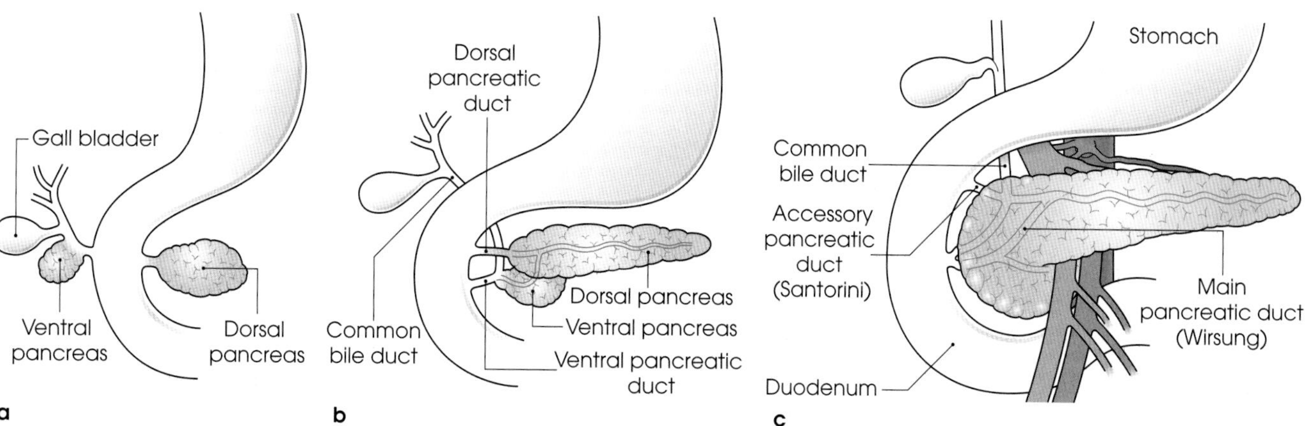

Figure 31.1 The development of the pancreas. (**a**) Endodermal buds from the dorsal and ventral border of the foregut form during the fourth week. (**b**) The ventral bud rotates behind the foregut to lie posterior to the dorsal pancreas. (**c**) The duct systems fuse during the sixth week.

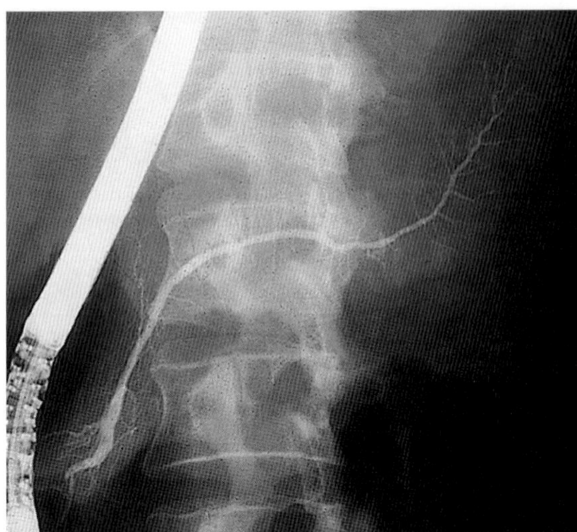

Figure 31.2 ERCP: a normal pancreatogram.

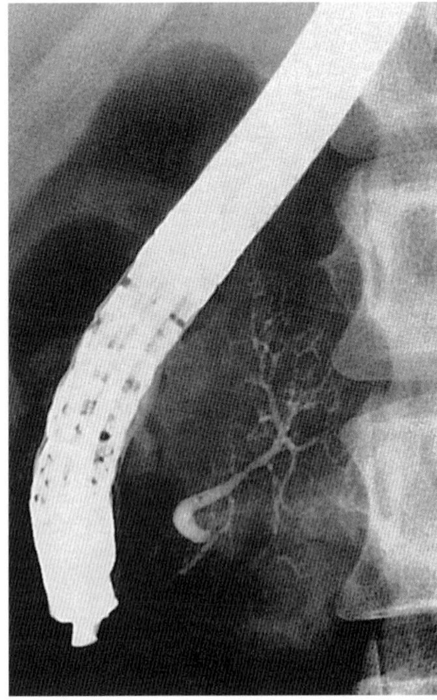

Figure 31.3 Pancreas divisum.

and ventral buds to fuse. Ductal imaging by magnetic resonance cholangiopancreatography or endoscopic retrograde cholangiopancreatography (ERCP) demonstrates a small ventral remnant draining with the common bile duct at the major papilla, while the main duct system (the dorsal duct) drains more proximally via the smaller accessory papilla (Fig. 31.3).

The vast majority of individuals with pancreas divisum are symptomless. Other patients with pancreas divisum have a clear relationship between pain, which is usually caused by recurrent acute pancreatitis, and obstruction of the minor papilla. This is probably related to the small size of the pancreatic orifice draining the main pancreatic duct. In this group of patients, treatment by accessory duct sphincterotomy (surgical or endoscopic) gives good results, particularly in those with recurrent acute pancreatitis. Unfortunately there is also an intermediate group of patients with pancreas divisum who have symptoms of chronic abdominal pain but no evidence of obstruction of the minor papilla on imaging. These patients are difficult to treat because it is difficult to prove that the pain is caused by the pancreas divisum. Surgery or endoscopic treatment is less successful.[2]

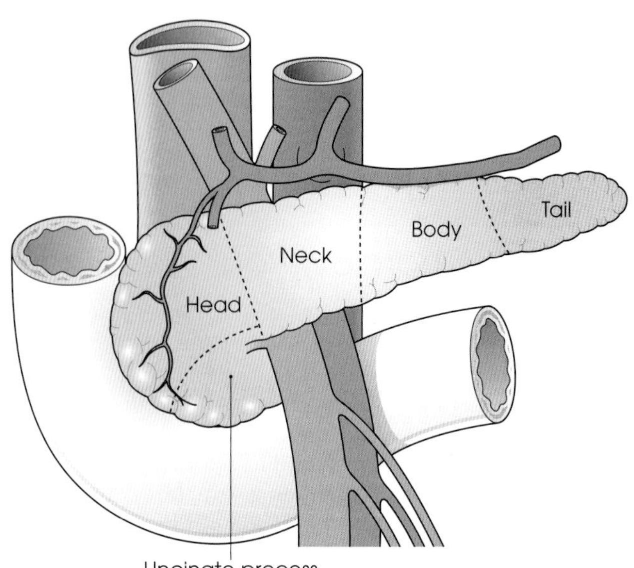

Figure 31.4 Gross anatomy of the pancreas.

ANNULAR PANCREAS

Annular pancreas occurs when the duodenum is completely encircled by pancreatic tissue. It is the result of abnormal rotation of the ventral pancreatic bud as the duodenum rotates, and may be associated with congenital abnormalities of other organs. The neonate may present with vomiting if duodenal obstruction is significant (see Ch. 40). Plain X-rays show the characteristic double-bubble sign. In adults, annular pancreas may be associated with peptic ulceration and chronic pancreatitis, although it is often symptomless. Treatment is by duodenoduodenostomy or duodenojejunostomy to bypass the obstruction.

SURGICAL ANATOMY

The pancreas has a head bound by the curve of the duodenum, a neck, a body and a tail extending to the splenic hilum. The head and neck are intimately related to the superior mesenteric vessels that pass behind the neck of the pancreas, but anterior to the pancreatic uncinate process and third part of the duodenum (Fig. 31.4).

The arterial supply of the pancreas is shown in Fig. 31.5. The splenic artery runs along the superior border of the pancreas, while the splenic vein lies behind the pancreas. The splenic vein and superior mesenteric vein unite behind the neck of the pancreas to form the portal vein. The right hepatic artery arises from the superior mesenteric artery rather than the coeliac axis in 10% of individuals, and when this occurs it usually then runs close to the posterior aspect of the head of the pancreas.

Peripancreatic lymph vessels drain to the coeliac and superior mesenteric nodes. The tail of the pancreas drains, into nodes

REFERENCE

2. Pathak R, Cooperman AM. Surg Clin North Am 2001; 81: 479–482, xiii

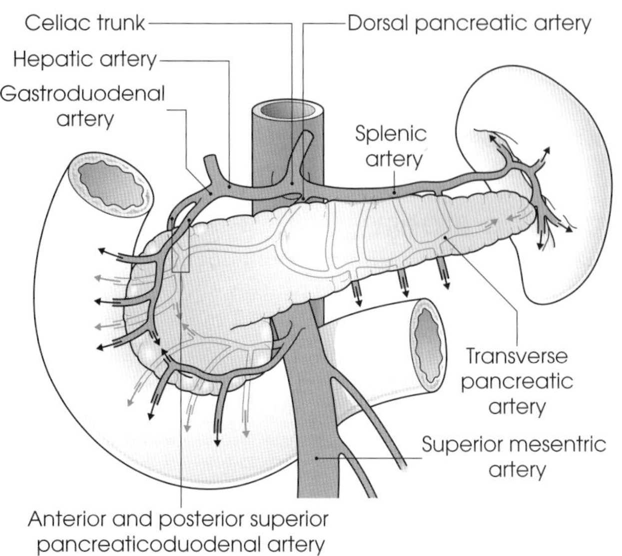

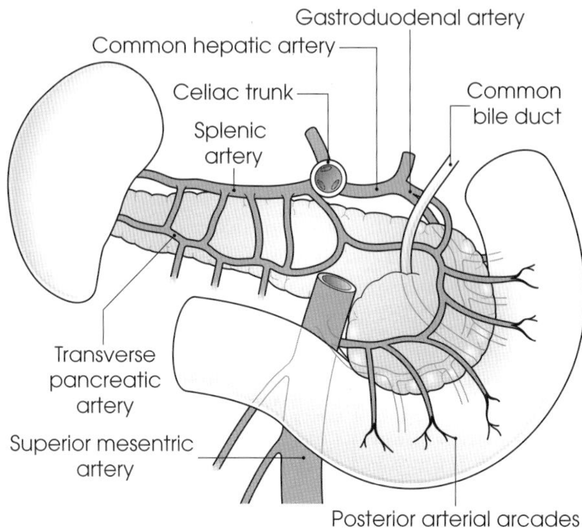

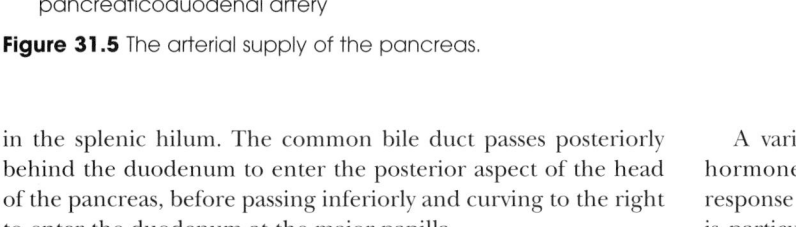

Figure 31.5 The arterial supply of the pancreas.

in the splenic hilum. The common bile duct passes posteriorly behind the duodenum to enter the posterior aspect of the head of the pancreas, before passing inferiorly and curving to the right to enter the duodenum at the major papilla.

The pancreas is innervated from the sympathetic and parasympathetic nervous systems through the coeliac plexus. Sympathetic nerves travel via the greater and lesser splanchnic nerves arising from the sympathetic chain in the thorax. Parasympathetic innervation is through the vagus nerve.

The functional unit of the exocrine pancreas is the acinus. Each acinus surrounds the terminal portion of a pancreatic duct. The acinar cells are arranged so that the zymogen granules containing enzymes empty into the lumen. The endocrine pancreas is closely related to blood vessels and consists of islets of Langerhans, which are nests of cells that synthesize insulin, glucagon and other hormones.

PHYSIOLOGY

Pancreatic acinar cells produce a variety of substances that are important for the digestion and absorption of nutrients. The acinar cells secrete into lobular ductules, which eventually drain via the main pancreatic duct into the duodenum. Approximately 1–1.5 L of exocrine secretions are produced each day. The ionic composition and pH varies with the flow rate.

Proenzymes are produced for protein digestion (trypsinogen, chymotrypsinogen, proelastase and procollagenase), fat digestion (prolipase and prophospholipase) and carbohydrate digestion (alpha-amylase). When these proenzymes reach the lumen of the duodenum, they are activated by enterokinase produced by the enterocytes of the small intestine to produce active enzymes. Proteins are broken down into polypeptides and amino acids, lipids into free fatty acids, and complex carbohydrates into oligosaccharides and monosaccharides. These end-products are then absorbed by the small bowel mucosa.

Pancreatic secretion is rich in bicarbonate, which is secreted by the epithelial cells of the pancreatic ducts. Bicarbonate neutralizes gastric acid and is important for the absorption of iron, calcium and phosphate ions in the upper small bowel.

A variety of mechanisms control pancreatic secretion. The hormones cholecystokinin and secretin are released in response to food and acidity in the duodenum. Cholecystokinin is particularly important in stimulating proenzyme release, and secretin stimulates bicarbonate production. Gastrin is secreted by the stomach in response to distension and as well as causing gastric acid secretion it also stimulates the pancreatic acinar cells to produce enzymes. Pancreatic enzymes are released by direct stimulation of duodenal stretch reflexes by the duodenal contents and this is facilitated by vagal tone.

The endocrine pancreas produces a variety of hormones, which are involved in glucose homeostasis and control of the digestive system, from the islet cells, the density of which is higher in the body and tail of the pancreas. Islet cells are divided into glucagon-producing alpha cells, insulin-producing beta cells, and somatostatin-producing delta cells. Pancreatic polypeptide and other substances are also produced.

Pancreatic insufficiency, from either disease or surgery, causes a number of problems. Lack of proteolytic proenzymes impairs protein digestion and results in protein malnutrition and weight loss. Impaired lipid digestion worsens calorie malnutrition and weight loss, impairs fat-soluble vitamin absorption, and causes steatorrhoea. Colonic bacterial overgrowth increases, causing excessive flatus. Iron deficiency and osteoporosis result from inadequate iron absorption. Glucose intolerance or diabetes may develop, and total pancreatectomy results in a very brittle form of diabetes, as the counter-regulatory effects of glucagon are also lost.

INVESTIGATION OF PANCREATIC DISEASE

INVESTIGATIONS OF PANCREATIC FUNCTION

Faecal elastase, a pancreatic enzyme that passes through the intestine unaltered, is a useful test of exocrine function and can be detected by ELISA.[3] It gives an accurate assessment of exocrine

REFERENCE

3. Löser C, Möllgaard A et al. Gut 1996; 39: 580–586

function in patients with severe and moderate dysfunction, but is less useful in identifying patients with slight derangement of exocrine function. The ELISA detects only human elastase and is therefore not confounded by porcine enzymes present in pancreatic enzyme supplements. It is a useful test in patients with pancreatic insufficiency, who can remain on enzyme supplements during collection of the faecal samples.

There are a number of duodenal intubation tests, which are invasive but provide a good discrimination between normal and abnormal exocrine pancreatic function in the early stages of chronic pancreatitis. The output of pancreatic enzymes and bicarbonate is measured in duodenal aspirate after placement of a nasoduodenal tube following pancreatic stimulation by intravenous injection of secretin and cholecystokinin. Duodenal intubation tests are, however, rarely used outside specialist pancreatic centres. Other tests of exocrine function are less accurate than the faecal elastase assay and are now rarely used.[4]

Pancreatic endocrine function tests aim to identify patients with abnormal glucose tolerance, and all patients with pancreatic disease should have estimation of their fasting blood sugar and glycosylated haemoglobin. An oral glucose tolerance test may be obtained in those patients with borderline diabetes.

IMAGING INVESTIGATIONS OF THE PANCREAS

Transabdominal ultrasound

Transabdominal ultrasound is usually the first imaging investigation to be carried out in a patient with symptoms suggestive of pancreatic disease. The presence of overlying fat and bowel gas usually obscures some of the pancreas unless the patient is very thin.

Computerized tomography

Computerized tomography of the pancreas gives the best images if a helical or multislice scanner is used with 3-mm slice reconstruction. Intravenous and oral contrast should be given, and this usually provides good views of the whole pancreas. The information obtained should assist in the diagnosis and staging of suspected pancreatic tumours, and in identifying the severity of acute pancreatitis and the complications of chronic pancreatitis.

Magnetic resonance imaging

Magnetic resonance imaging is of most value in imaging the bile duct and pancreatic duct (see Ch. 30). This technique outlines the duct systems without injection of contrast medium, and is used for determining the cause of obstructive jaundice and for identifying strictures and stones within the main pancreatic duct. Intravenous injection of secretin accentuates any abnormality during this test, and this is useful in evaluating patients with chronic pancreatitis.

Endoscopic ultrasound

Endoscopic ultrasound improves the resolution of pancreatic ultrasound (see Ch. 30). A high-frequency transducer is used and this gives better images. Endoscopic ultrasound provides good images of the gallbladder, bile duct and pancreas. It is useful for identifying pancreatic tumours and chronic pancreatitis. It is safer than ERCP, with a reduced incidence of postprocedure pancreatitis.

Endoscopic retrograde cholangiopancreatography

Experience and familiarity with this technique, and improvements in instrumentation have led to reduced complication rates of this procedure. The use of ERCP for diagnostic purposes can, however, be reduced by investigating patients with endoscopic ultrasound or magnetic resonance cholangiopancreatography, and reserving ERCP for those patients who are likely to require a therapeutic procedure such as endoscopic sphincterotomy or insertion of a biliary or pancreatic stent (see Ch. 30).

PANCREATIC BIOPSY

An image-guided biopsy using either ultrasound or CT scanning enables tissue to be obtained from patients with a suspicious mass in the pancreas. A biopsy is not required if surgical exploration is indicated, and many surgeons will operate on a distal bile duct stricture because a negative biopsy does not rule out malignancy (see Ch. 30). Endoscopic ultrasound-guided biopsy is more accurate, and is useful in those patients in whom the diagnosis is uncertain and surgery can be avoided.

ACUTE PANCREATITIS

INTRODUCTION

Acute pancreatitis is a commonly encountered surgical emergency, the annual incidence in the UK ranging in various studies from 21 to 283 per million. Gallstones and alcohol are the major causes of acute pancreatitis in the western world. Seventy-five per cent of patients have a mild case, but in 20% the condition is severe, the overall mortality being 10%. A mild attack of pancreatitis has a limited inflammatory response, which usually resolves spontaneously. With a more profound response, necrosis of all or part of the gland occurs, and this causes severe pancreatitis. Severe pancreatitis is associated with greatly increased mortality and morbidity. Treatment is largely supportive, with operative management generally reserved for patients with complications.

PATHOPHYSIOLOGY

Acute pancreatitis represents a spectrum of diseases (Table 31.1). Definitions used in acute pancreatitis conform to an internationally agreed terminology.[5] Mild acute pancreatitis is a self-limiting inflammatory condition. The severe form usually results from necrosis of pancreatic parenchyma and causes a systemic inflammatory response syndrome. The condition may further deteriorate and cause organ failure known as multiple organ dysfunction syndrome. Organ failure is more likely to occur if the sterile necrosis becomes infected, in which case mortality is quadrupled.

Many factors have been reported to cause acute pancreatitis, but gallstones and alcohol are responsible for over 70% (Box 31.1). It was originally thought that gallstone pancreatitis was caused by bile reflux into the pancreatic duct by obstruction of the ampulla of Vater. This theory has been superseded following studies in animal models, where reflux of bile was not found to be a prerequisite for the development of pancreatitis.[6] Gallstone pancreatitis is associated with small gallstones, a wide cystic duct, and a common channel formed by fusion of the pancreatic duct

REFERENCES

4. Glasbrenner B, Kahl S et al. Eur J Gastroenterol Hepatol 2002; 14: 935–941
5. Bradley EL III. Arch Surg 1993; 128: 586–590
6. Runzi M, Saluja A et al. Gastroenterology 1993; 105: 157–164

Table 31.1 Terms used in acute pancreatitis

Term	Definition
Mild acute pancreatitis	Acute inflammation of the pancreas, characterized by interstitial oedema; recovery is uneventful
Severe acute pancreatitis	Pancreatitis associated with distant organ dysfunction or local complications: necrosis, pseudocyst or abscess
Acute fluid collection	Fluid collections that appear within or adjacent to the pancreas in the early course of the disease: they lack a wall compared with pseudocysts
Pancreatic necrosis	Non-viable areas of pancreatic parenchyma, which may be focal or diffuse
Infected pancreatic necrosis	Necrosis associated with isolation of organisms from necrotic tissue or blood cultures, or implied by free gas in pancreas on imaging
Acute pseudocyst	A fluid collection of pancreatic juice, surrounded by a wall of granulation or fibrous tissue that takes at least 4 weeks to develop
Pancreatic abscess	A collection of pus with little or no necrosis as a result of pancreatitis

Box 31.1 Main causes of acute pancreatitis

- Gallstones and microlithiasis
- Alcohol
- Trauma: accidental and iatrogenic (e.g. ERCP and surgery)
- Metabolic: hyperlipidaemia and hypercalcaemia
- Hereditary pancreatitis
- Anatomical abnormalities: pancreas divisum
- Infection: viral (coxsackievirus B or mumps) or parasitic (*Clonorchis sinensis* or *Ascaris lumbricoides*)
- Medications: azathioprine, steroids, thiazides, (frusemide) (furosemide) or sodium valproate
- Obstructive pancreatitis: ampullary tumours and cancer of the head of the pancreas

and bile duct.[7] Pancreatic duct obstruction by a small stone is likely to be the initiating cause that results in activation of proenzymes within pancreatic duct acinar cells. A cascade of mediators then results in inflammation and predisposes towards necrosis.[8] Elevated intracellular calcium levels may also play an important role. Alcohol-induced pancreatitis is thought to be caused by direct damage of the acinar cells, allowing escape of enzymes into surrounding tissues and also into the systemic circulation. The reason why necrosis should develop in some patients and not others remains unclear.

CLINICAL FEATURES

History

Pain is the cardinal symptom in an attack of acute pancreatitis, and is usually severe and of relatively sudden onset. It is felt in the epigastrium or left hypochondrium and often radiates into the back. The pain is constant but may be eased by sitting upright. It can often become generalized to the whole abdomen. Vomiting will usually be present but is rarely profuse.

A history of precipitating factors should be sought. Rarer causes should be considered, especially when gallstones and alcohol have been excluded. Attacks of biliary colic may precede the attack of pancreatitis. Associated jaundice usually indicates the presence of a common bile duct gallstone, although recurrent exacerbations of alcohol-induced chronic pancreatitis may also cause biliary obstruction from an inflammatory mass or fibrosis in the head of the pancreas. Important comorbid factors should also be sought, such as ischaemic heart disease, and pulmonary and renal disease, because these are likely to influence the outcome of the acute attack.

Patients can present atypically, and the condition can mimic many other causes of abdominal pain (see Ch. 25). The serum markers of pancreatitis should always be checked in all patients with an acute abdomen, although they cannot always be relied on. Pancreatitis may also mimic extra-abdominal emergencies such as myocardial infarction. Confusion, general deterioration or renal failure are less obvious presentations. An attack of acute pancreatitis should always be considered in a sedated patient on the intensive care unit who develops abdominal signs.

Examination

The patient is usually distressed and in obvious pain. Tachycardia, tachypnoea and cold sweaty peripheries indicate the presence of shock, and after a few hours hypotension may develop. Mild pyrexia may be present but a reduced temperature can occur in shocked patients, especially if they are elderly. Upper abdominal tenderness with accompanying guarding and rebound tenderness is usually present, and the signs may be generalized. Bruising in the flank (Grey Turner's sign) or in the periumbilical region (Cullen's sign) is uncommon but indicates severe pancreatitis with retroperitoneal tracking of haemorrhagic exudate. A mass or ascites may be present, as may a reactive pleural effusion.

Repeated clinical assessment

Repeated assessment is essential in gauging the course of the disease and in detecting the first signs of complications, particularly infection. This is the best method of deciding the necessity and timing of investigations and interventions.

DIAGNOSIS AND ASSESSMENT OF AETIOLOGY

The diagnosis of acute pancreatitis is usually made from the clinical history and signs, and confirmed by the detection of an elevated serum amylase or lipase. Serum lipase is slightly more accurate in the detection of pancreatitis,[9] but amylase estimation is in more widespread use. The serum amylase, however, often may not reach the diagnostic level of four times the upper limit of normal, especially in patients with alcoholic pancreatitis. Urinary amylase levels are valuable and remain elevated for longer than serum levels.

A perforated viscus, such as a peptic ulcer, ischaemic bowel or ruptured aortic aneurysm, may mimic acute pancreatitis. These conditions may also cause an elevation of the serum amylase, but usually not to the level of that seen with acute pancreatitis. Myocardial infarction and pneumonia should also be considered in the differential diagnosis (see Chs 21 and 22). A salivary gland tumour, which should be palpable, may cause an elevated amylase without abdominal pain. A chest X-ray should be performed

REFERENCES

7. Armstrong C, Taylor T et al. Br J Surg 1985; 72: 551–555
8. Karne S, Gorelick FS. Surg Clin North Am 1999; 79: 699–710
9. Keim V, Teich N et al. Pancreas 1998; 16: 45–49

to rule out the possibility of a perforation and to assess for pulmonary complications such as pleural effusions.

Occasionally the diagnosis of acute pancreatitis cannot be made until an exploratory laparotomy has been performed. Features of acute pancreatitis at laparotomy include the presence of ascites, fat necrosis and inflammation of the pancreas.

A careful history of alcohol and drug use is essential to try to identify the cause. An ultrasound examination should be done as soon as possible to demonstrate the presence of gallstones and biliary dilatation. Elevated liver function tests also suggest a biliary aetiology. Other conditions must be considered if there is no definite history of gallstones or alcohol before presuming that a patient has idiopathic pancreatitis (see *Recurrent acute pancreatitis*, p. 751).

Severity stratification

Once the diagnosis has been made, the disease should be stratified into mild (uncomplicated) or severe (complicated), so that the patient's condition may be managed appropriately. Clinical assessment[10] and the levels of amylase or lipase,[9] although important for diagnosis, are not useful prognostic indicators. A pleural effusion detected on chest X-ray is associated with severe necrosis. Several multifactorial scoring systems have been devised, which indicate physiological derangement and attack severity. These are based on the results of a number of blood tests. If three or more factors in the modified Glasgow criteria (Table 31.2)[11] are present within 48 h of admission, severe pancreatitis is predicted. Unfortunately it may take 48 h for the genuine score to become apparent, and it has a low sensitivity (50–70%).

The acute physiology, age and chronic health evaluation (APACHE) II score, which is another scoring system that takes chronic illness as well as acute physiological changes into account, can be used at the time of admission, although its accuracy improves over 48 h. The APACHE II score has the advantage of being easy to perform. Patients over 65 years old tend to be over-scored by APACHE II.[12]

The C-reactive protein level can be used as a single factor and is a useful predictor of severe pancreatitis, with a cut-off level of 150 mg/L at 48 h indicating that severe pancreatitis is likely. Combining the C-reactive protein with other scoring systems may also be useful.[11] Determination of the APACHE II score and C-reactive protein level can be repeated over time to monitor disease progression. The ideal test would predict the severity of the pancreatitis at the time of presentation. No such test is available at present, but estimation of levels of inflammatory mediators (such as interleukin-6) or peptides (such as trypsinogen activation peptide) may provide a genuinely predictive test in the future.[13]

Table 31.2 Modified Glasgow criteria

Variable	Value
P_AO_2	< 60 mmHg (8kPa)
Albumin	< 32 g/L
Calcium	< 2.0 mmol/L
White cell count	> 15 × 10^9 cells/L
Aspartate transaminase	> 100 units/L
Lactate dehydrogenase	> 600 units/L
Glucose	> 10 mmol/L*
Urea	> 16 mmol/L

*In non-diabetic patients

On admission, patients with acute pancreatitis should be scored by the modified Glasgow system, by APACHE II, or by levels of C-reactive protein. A dynamic contrast-enhanced CT scan should be performed between 3 and 10 days after the onset of pain, if the patient is classified as having severe pancreatitis, to detect the presence of necrosis. This allows sufficient time to elapse from admission for the necrosis to develop. The CT scan often needs to be repeated depending on the initial findings and the clinical course; Fig. 31.6a shows a contrast-enhanced CT scan at 3 days, and Fig. 31.6b a scan at 18 days showing more pronounced difference between enhancing pancreatic tissue and necrosis. The proportion of necrosis in relation to viable pancreas can be used to predict mortality and morbidity.[14]

The most difficult decision is to determine whether the necrosis seen on CT is infected, because this largely dictates the need for operative necrosectomy. Gas in the peripancreatic tissues on CT is usually produced by gas-forming organisms (Fig. 31.7), although occasionally a fistula into the stomach or colon can produce a similar picture. Infection may also be diagnosed on blood cultures and suggested by pyrexia and a high white cell count. A fine-needle aspiration of the pancreas under CT guidance should be carried out if the presence of infected necrosis is suspected.[15] This procedure should be done with great care under sterile conditions, because it risks introducing infection into sterile necrosis.

TREATMENT

Mild pancreatitis

Almost all mild cases of acute pancreatitis have an uncomplicated course. Intravenous fluids are administered until oral intake can be resumed, and nasogastric aspiration may be required to prevent vomiting. Antithromboembolic prophylaxis should be given. Careful clinical observation is essential, and the blood glucose concentration should be measured repeatedly. Some patients predicted as having mild pancreatitis may cross over into the severe group. It is essential that the cause of the acute pancreatitis is identified to prevent further and perhaps more serious attacks. When the patients have recovered, a cholecystectomy should be performed for gallstones or microlithiasis before they are discharged from hospital (see Ch. 30). Abstinence from alcohol is essential, although this may be difficult to achieve even with appropriate support and counselling.

Severe pancreatitis

Patients stratified as having severe pancreatitis should be monitored in high-dependency or intensive care units. Because of large fluid shifts, invasive monitoring is valuable. Fluid balance

REFERENCES

10. Corfield AP, Cooper MJ et al. Lancet 1985; 2: 403–407
11. Imrie CW. In: Buchler MW, Uhl W, Friess H et al (eds). Acute Pancreatitis: Novel Concepts in Biology and Therapy. Blackwell Science, Oxford, 1999: 199–208
12. Wilson C, Heath DI et al. Br J Surg 1990; 77: 1260–1264
13. Neoptolemos JP, Kemppainen EA et al. Lancet 2000; 355: 1955–1960
14. Balthazar EJ, Robinson DL et al. Radiology 1990; 174: 331–336
15. Buchler MW, Gloor B et al. Ann Surg 2000; 232: 619–626

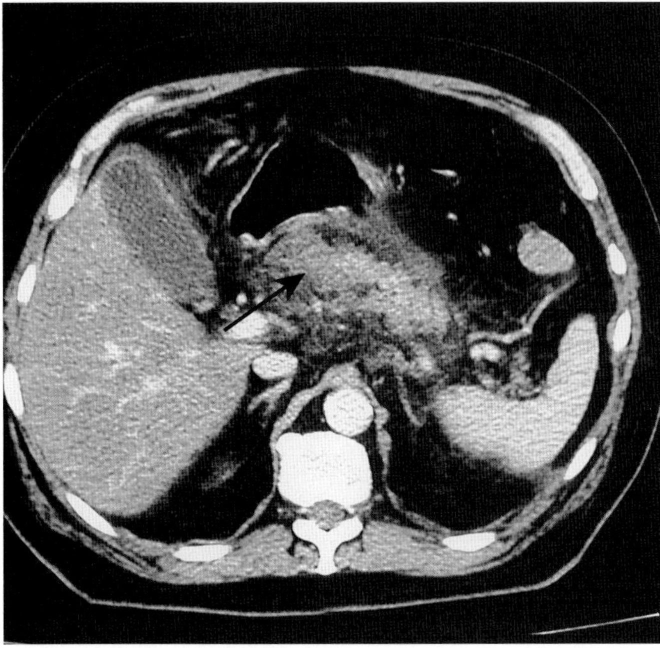

a

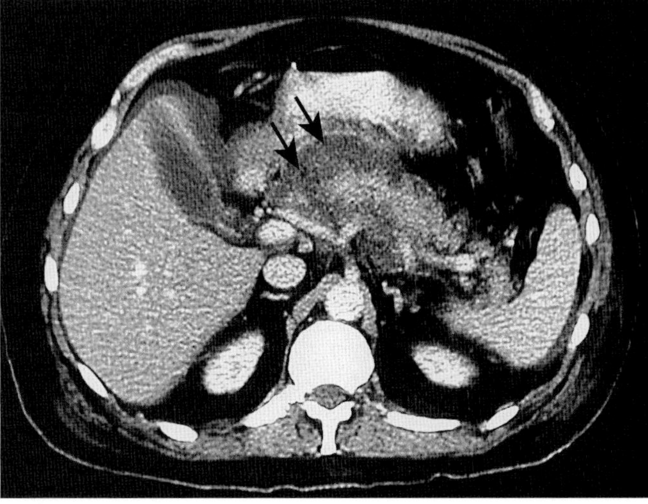

b

Figure 31.6 (**a**) A CT scan at 3 days in a patient with severe acute pancreatitis, showing acute inflammation and oedema of pancreas (arrowed). (**b**) A CT scan at 18 days in the same patient, showing demarcation between necrotic (arrowed) and viable pancreas.

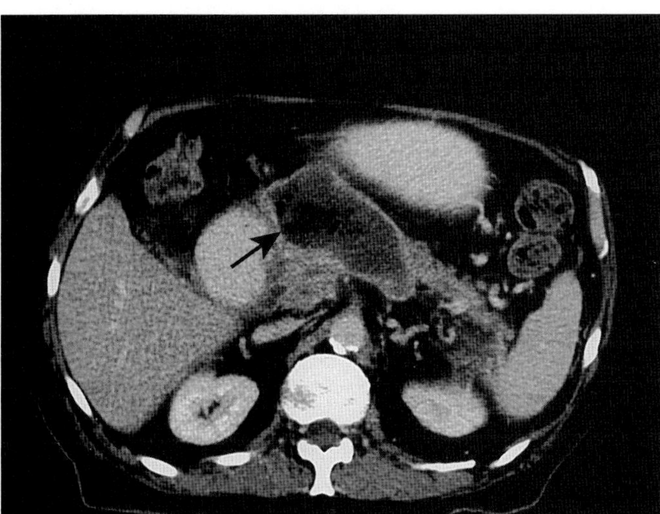

Figure 31.7 A CT scan showing infected pancreatic necrosis (arrowed).

and oxygen delivery should be optimized in an attempt to prevent the development of multiple organ failure; ventilation, inotropes and dialysis may be required. The reduction of pancreatic secretion, inhibition of pancreatic enzymes, and down-regulation of systemic inflammatory response syndrome[16] have all proved ineffective as a means of overcoming deterioration in severe pancreatitis.

The mortality quadruples if pancreatic necrosis becomes infected. Attempts to prevent infection have proved difficult. The use of prophylactic antibiotics remains contentious because they cause an increased incidence of fungal infections.[17,18] A 7-day course of a broad-spectrum antibiotic such as imipenem or ciprofloxacin is, however, widely used for subjects with severe pancreatitis.[19,20] At the end of that period, antibiotics should be given only in response to positive bacteriological cultures or as prophylaxis at the time of surgery or other procedures. The use of antifungal treatment may become necessary. Oral gut decontamination has no clear benefit.[21] Enteral feeding should theoretically reduce bacterial gut translocation, but this has not been proven. Enteral feeding can, however, be introduced early in severe pancreatitis and should certainly be used in preference to parenteral nutrition (see Ch. 2).[22]

Endoscopic retrograde cholangiopancreatography and sphincterotomy should be performed if there is evidence of cholangitis. Early ERCP has also been investigated in patients with severe acute biliary pancreatitis in several studies. These demonstrated that ERCP and sphincterotomy, carried out within 48 h, improves the outcome of a significant proportion of patients with severe gallstone pancreatitis.[23]

Acute serous fluid collections in acute pancreatitis (Fig. 31.8) do not usually require specific treatment unless they are large enough to compromise respiration. Pseudocysts are walled-off collections and become spherical as they mature. Small pseudocysts less than 6 cm in diameter are unlikely to require treatment, but if they enlarge they may compress the stomach and cause vomiting. Drainage can be performed percutaneously – although this may result in recurrence once the drain is removed – or endoscopically using the transgastric route. Occasionally a

REFERENCES

16. Johnson CD, Kingsnorth AN et al. Gut 2001; 48: 62–69
17. Grewe M, Tsiotos GG et al. J Am Coll Surg 1999; 188: 408–414
18. Gloor B, Muller CA et al. Arch Surg 2001; 136: 592–596
19. Pederzoli P, Bassi C et al. Surg Gynecol Obstet 1993; 176: 480–483
20. Nordback I, Sand J et al. J Gastrointest Surg 2001; 5: 113–118, discussion 118–120
21. Luiten EJT, Bruining HA. In: Buchler MW, Uhl W, Friess H et al. Acute Pancreatitis: Novel Concepts in Biology and Therapy. Blackwell Science, Oxford, 1999: 411–421
22. Windsor AC, Kanwar S et al. Gut 1998; 42: 431–435
23. Neoptolemos JP, Carr-Locke DL et al. Lancet 1988; 2: 979–983

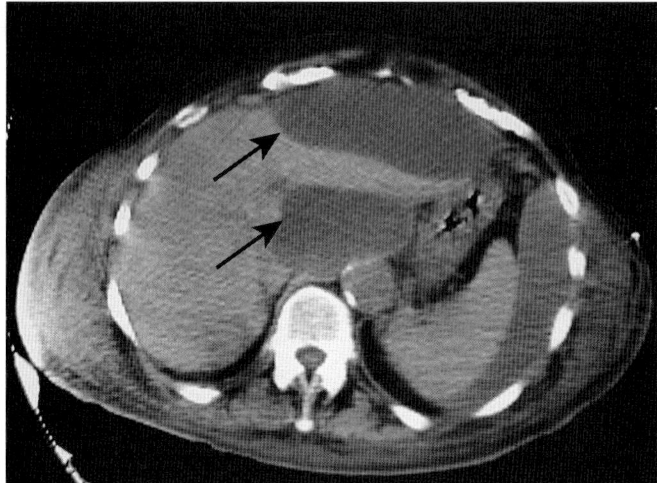

Figure 31.8 A CT scan of acute fluid collections in acute pancreatitis (arrowed).

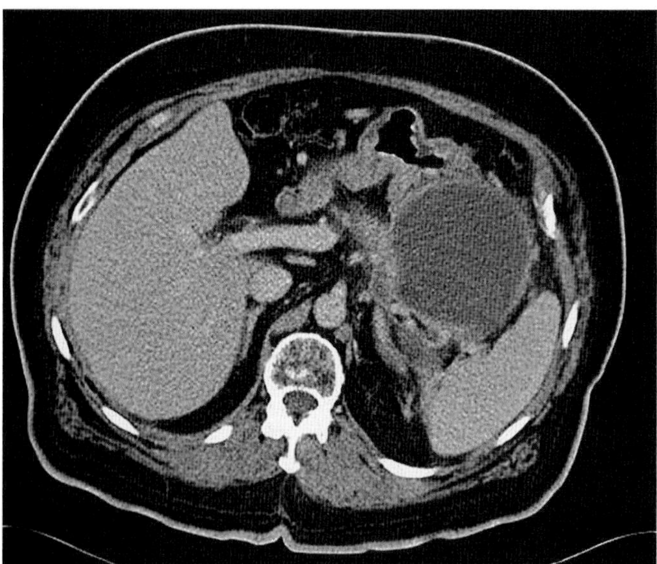

Figure 31.9 A CT scan of pseudocyst following acute pancreatitis.

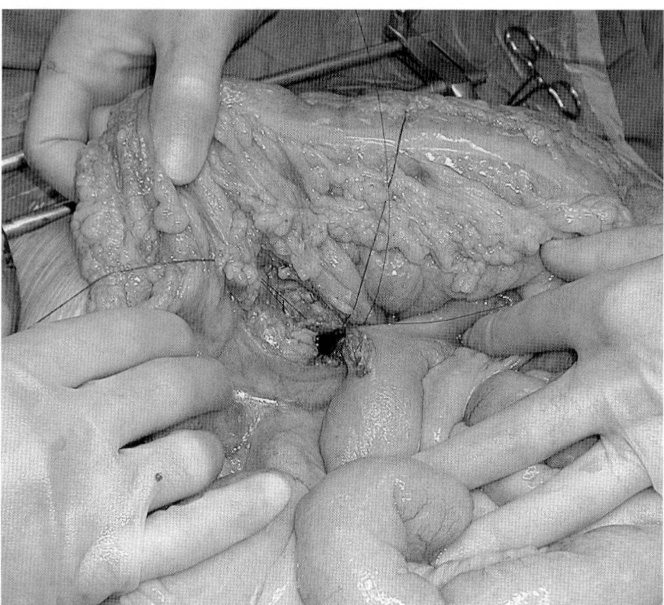

Figure 31.10 Pancreatic cyst-jejunostomy. A pseudocyst of the pancreatic head has been opened inferiorly through the transverse mesocolon and is being anastomosed to a Roux loop of jejunum.

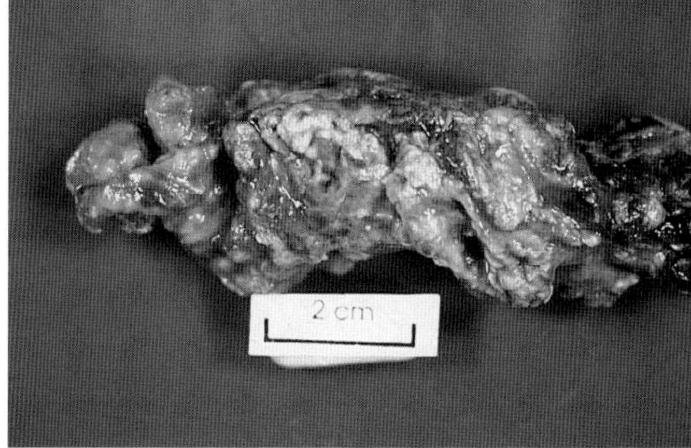

Figure 31.11 Specimen of necrotic pancreas removed at open operation.

larger cyst (Fig. 31.9) may need to be surgically drained by cyst-gastrostomy or cyst-jejunostomy (Fig. 31.10). A laparoscopic approach may be used.

Surgery for necrotizing pancreatitis is associated with a high mortality and morbidity because of the underlying sepsis and ongoing necrosis. Surgery should probably be reserved for infected necrosis, because non-operative treatment has a better outcome in sterile necrosis.[15] It may, however, be difficult to definitely isolate an organism, and the patient's condition may dictate surgery. Necrosectomy involves the blunt debridement of necrosis. Attempts to perform formal pancreatic resections result in haemorrhage and a poorer outcome. The necrotic cavity can usually be entered through the thickened gastrocolic omentum. All non-viable tissue is then gently removed and fluid collections are evacuated. All the necrotic tissue must be removed, and this may entail extensive debridement of the retroperitoneum including the muscles of the posterior abdominal wall, which are involved in some patients (Fig. 31.11). A thorough lavage is performed. The abdomen is then closed, with continuous irrigation to the pancreatic cavity through drains placed at the time of surgery.[24] Repeat laparotomy is quite often necessary to allow further sequential debridements, and sometimes the abdominal wound may be better left open as a laparostomy.[25]

A transperitoneal laparoscopic approach can be used to remove pancreatic necrosis. Alternatively, a procedure akin to percutaneous nephrolithotomy may be performed. This allows evacuation of the necrosis through a nephroscope via a retroperitoneal approach.[26] This method is particularly useful in patients unlikely to survive major abdominal surgery, but may

REFERENCES

24. Beger HG, Isenmann R. Surg Clin North Am 1999; 79: 783–800, ix
25. Bradley EL III. Surg Gynecol Obstet 1993; 177: 215–222
26. Carter CR, McKay CJ et al. Ann Surg 2000; 232: 175–180

Table 31.3 Investigations in patients with idiopathic pancreatitis

Tests	Causes under investigation
Phase 1 tests	
Detailed alcohol, drug and family history	Alcohol, drugs and hereditary pancreatitis
Fasting serum lipids and serum calcium	Hyperlipidaemia and hypercalcaemia
Phase 2 tests	
Endoscopic ultrasound (with duodenoscopy)	Biliary microlithiasis or ampullary tumour
Magnetic resonance cholangiopancreatography	Pancreas divisum
Phase 3 tests	
ERCP	Minimal change chronic pancreatitis
Sphincter of Oddi manometry	Sphincter of Oddi dysfunction

need to be repeated on several occasions until all the necrotic material is removed. Radiologically guided drainage has been used for acute fluid collections and sterile necrosis.[27] Retroperitoneal haemorrhage is often a fatal complication, and is usually the result of a ruptured false aneurysm of the splenic vessels. Surgery or embolization of the splenic artery may be life-saving.

CLINICAL OUTCOMES IN ACUTE PANCREATITIS

The overall mortality of acute pancreatitis should be less than 10%, and less than 30% with severe necrosis.[28] All patients should be diagnosed and stratified within 48 h, and a definite aetiology established wherever possible. Urgent therapeutic ERCP should be performed in patients proven to have severe acute biliary pancreatitis. All patients with biliary pancreatitis should undergo definitive management of gallstones during the same hospital admission.

RECURRENT ACUTE PANCREATITIS

The cause of a single attack of acute pancreatitis remains unknown in 15–20% of cases. In these patients a repeat abdominal ultrasound should be carried out. If this fails to show anything, further investigation is required (Table 31.3). After the first attack patients require only phase 1 tests. After a second attack, however, the aetiology should be keenly sought. Biliary microlithiasis is the most common cause of recurrent acute pancreatitis (Fig. 31.12).

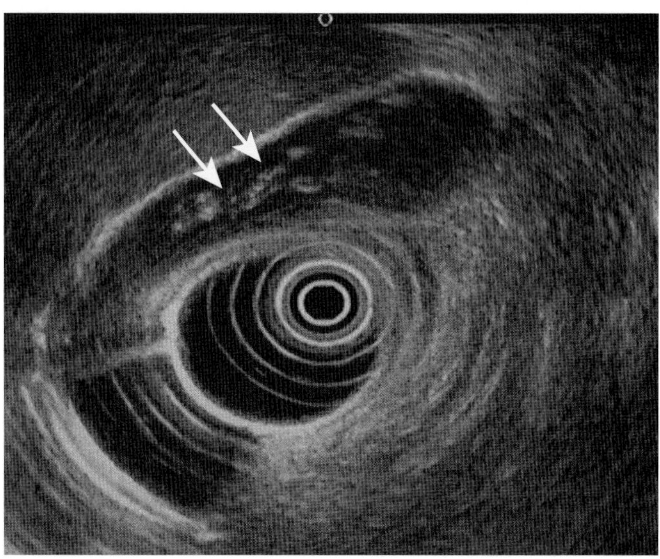

Figure 31.12 Endoscopic ultrasound scan of gallbladder, showing biliary microlithiasis (arrowed) not identified by external ultrasound.

CHRONIC PANCREATITIS

INTRODUCTION

Chronic pancreatitis is a continuing inflammatory disorder of the pancreas, characterized by irreversible changes of inflammation and fibrosis. It usually presents with abdominal pain but may occasionally be painless. Exocrine and endocrine pancreatic insufficiency often coexist.

INCIDENCE AND AETIOLOGY

The yearly incidence of chronic pancreatitis is approximately five new cases per 100 000 of the population in Western Europe. The average age of onset is between 36 and 55 years, and the male to female ratio approximately seven to one.

Box 31.2 Causes of chronic pancreatitis

Main causes
- Alcohol
- Idiopathic

Less common causes
- Tropical
- Hypercalcaemia
- Hyperlipidaemia
- Hereditary pancreatitis
- Gallstones
- Pancreatic tumours
- Pancreas divisum

Alcohol is an important factor in approximately 70% of patients in developed countries. There is, however, no definitive threshold for the toxic effects of alcohol on the pancreas, so patients who give a history of regular alcohol consumption probably have alcohol-induced disease. In the UK the next most common aetiology is idiopathic, accounting for 20–30% of cases. These patients quite understandably resent a label of 'alcoholism', which is often unfortunately applied.

Fewer than 10% of patients with chronic pancreatitis have one of the less common causes (Box 31.2). Hereditary pancreatitis, an autosomal dominant disorder, is increasingly recognized and must be suspected in patients who have a family history of pancreatitis or diabetes.[29] Gallstone disease is only rarely implicated, when chronic obstructive pancreatitis results from pancreatic duct stenosis after an attack of acute gallstone pancreatitis. Tropical chronic pancreatitis is a juvenile form of

REFERENCES

27. Ashley SW, Perez A et al. Ann Surg 2001; 234: 572–579, discussion 579–580
28. Glazer G, Mann DE. Gut 1998; 42 (Suppl 2): S1–S13
29. Charnley RM. World J Gastroenterol 2003; 9: 1–4

Table 31.4 Complications of chronic pancreatitis

Complication	Comment	Treatment
Pancreatic insufficiency	Exocrine and endocrine	Pancreatic enzyme supplements and diabetic therapy
Biliary obstruction	May produce cholangitis or exceptionally secondary biliary stenosis	Stent as temporary solution then consider isolated biliary bypass (choledochojejunostomy) or resection
Duodenal stenosis or colonic stricture	Intestinal obstruction	If does not resolve, surgical resection required
Pseudocyst	Usually mature and connected to ductal system, so resolution is unlikely	Endoscopic or surgical drainage
Inflammatory mass in head of pancreas	May cause recurrent attacks of pain	Consider surgical resection (Frey or Beger procedure)
Portal hypertension	Splenic vein thrombosis, although high alcohol intake may cause hepatic cirrhosis	Supportive
Haemorrhage	Splenic artery erosion causing pseudoaneurysm or variceal bleeding	Surgical or endoscopic control; angiography or embolization may be useful for postprocedural bleeding
Pancreatic ascites	From ductal disruption or ruptured pseudocyst	Optimize nutrition, consider octreotide and percutaneous drainage; surgery required if persistent
Pancreatic cancer	Risk of pancreatic cancer is increased in chronic pancreatitis	Consider suitability for resection

chronic pancreatitis that occurs in certain parts of the tropics, most notably in southern India.[30] Pancreas divisum and pancreatic tumours cause chronic pancreatitis by obstruction of the main pancreatic duct. Drug-induced chronic pancreatitis is extremely rare.

Different theories have been proposed to explain the pathogenesis of chronic pancreatitis. A direct toxic effect of alcohol in combination with abnormal nutrition is postulated in many cases. This results in an increase in protein secretion with production of insoluble abnormal forms of protein, combined with an increase in ductal permeability to calcium, resulting in protein plug formation and intraduct calcium deposition. Repeated acute attacks cause irreversible fibrosis and distortion of interlobular ducts, with a loss of pancreatic parenchyma and fibrosis of the gland, which may be either focal or diffuse. During acute exacerbations the pancreas is inflamed and oedematous, and pseudocysts may form within the pancreas or in its proximity. Pseudocysts in chronic pancreatitis are usually connected to the ductal system, unlike those of acute pancreatitis, and are therefore less likely to resolve spontaneously. An inflammatory mass in the head of the pancreas may be a direct cause of pain and can cause duodenal or biliary obstruction.

The pathogenesis of the severe pain that is a major feature of the condition is not fully understood, although oedema causing a compartment syndrome, tissue hypoxia and acidosis may all be factors. Pancreatic insufficiency because of the parenchymal loss may exacerbate malnutrition, and diabetes may also develop. Splenic vein thrombosis may occur and result in left-sided portal hypertension (see Ch. 29).

CLINICAL FEATURES

History

Pain is the principal presentation of chronic pancreatitis, although patients can present with pancreatic insufficiency without pain. Patients have often had chronic abdominal pain for months or years prior to seeing a specialist. Characteristically the pain is in the epigastrium and radiates through to the back. It is eased by sitting upright or by drawing the knees up into the jackknife position. Abstinence from alcohol initially improves the episodic attacks of pain, but as the pain becomes more chronic, the beneficial effects of abstinence are reduced. Pain may decrease in some patients after several years as the disease burns out, but this is not predictable. It is often difficult to assess the pain in alcoholic patients because of their manipulative personalities and dependency. Loss of sleep, interference with work or family responsibilities, and hospital admissions may be useful indicators of the severity of pain.

Pancreatic insufficiency tends to develop 10–15 years after the onset of pancreatitis. Endocrine deficiency results in diabetes, which is ultimately insulin-dependent. Nephropathy and retinopathy are less likely to develop than in other diabetic patients because of the shorter life expectancy associated with chronic pancreatitis. Exocrine deficiency results in steatorrhoea and poor nutrition.

The patient with established chronic pancreatitis may present with a variety of complications (Table 31.4). Jaundice and duodenal obstruction can be caused by an inflammatory mass. Haemorrhage may present as a gastrointestinal bleed or with shock and an acute abdomen (see Chs 25 and 26).

Examination

Examination may not reveal any specific features. Weight loss and malnutrition may be apparent and can be monitored from serial measurements. Erythema ab igne on the epigastrium or back is indicative of attempts to relieve pain by the application of topical heat. Anaemia, jaundice, ascites and splenomegaly may be detected. Signs of liver stigmata and failure should be looked for in alcoholic patients (see Ch. 29).

The principal differential diagnosis is with pancreatic cancer, which is discussed later in this chapter. Chronic pancreatitis should be considered in all patients with malnutrition and diarrhoea. A careful history and appropriate tests of exocrine function should reveal the underlying diagnosis.

REFERENCE

30. Petersen JM. J Clin Gastroenterol 2002; 35: 61–66

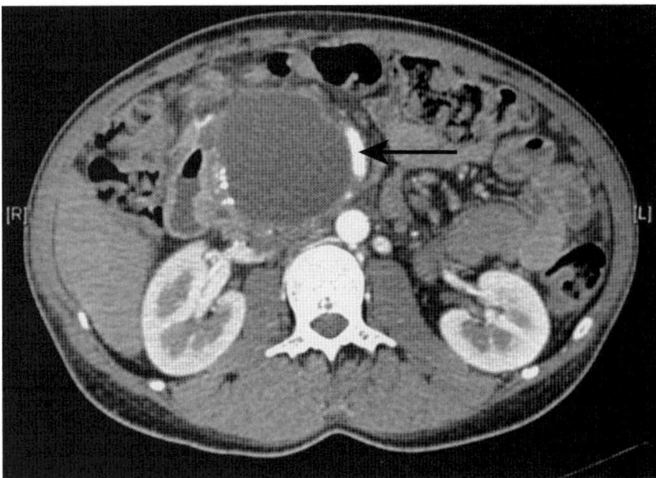

Figure 31.13 Pancreatic cyst with calcification in the wall abutting the superior mesenteric artery (arrowed), typical of chronic pancreatitis.

DIAGNOSIS

Diagnosis of the early stages of chronic pancreatitis may be difficult, whereas at an advanced stage it is more obvious. Blood tests are unhelpful, with the serum amylase usually being normal even during an acute exacerbation. Liver function tests may indicate biliary obstruction, while thrombocytopenia may suggest a splenic vein thrombosis. The urine should be tested for glucose, and the glycosylated haemoglobin should be measured. Tests of pancreatic exocrine function do not differentiate chronic pancreatitis from pancreatic cancer. All chronic pancreatitis patients should, however, have pancreatic function tests (see earlier in this chapter) to determine what replacement therapy is necessary.[4]

The diagnosis is almost always made on imaging studies. Calcification may be seen on a plain X-ray, while enlargement of the pancreas, duct dilatation and pseudocysts may be seen with ultrasound. Computerized tomography is more accurate in defining ductal morphology and the presence of pseudocysts (Figs 31.13 and 31.14). Traditionally ERCP has been used to define the degree of ductal abnormality. This role has diminished with the advent of improved spiral CT scanning and magnetic resonance cholangiopancreatography.[31] Cytological analysis of brushings taken by ERCP cannot make a positive diagnosis of chronic pancreatitis. Endoscopic ultrasound is also developing an increasing role because it is extremely sensitive in detecting the subtle early pathological changes of chronic pancreatitis.[32,33] When chronic pancreatitis is strongly suspected but unproven, endoscopic ultrasound is the investigation of choice and ERCP should rarely be necessary. Endoscopic ultrasound-guided biopsy is now known to be very valuable in definitively diagnosing the condition,[34] although it may be difficult to obtain a good sample from an indurated gland.

TREATMENT

Cases without complications can be managed expectantly. Abstinence from alcohol must be emphasized, and psychiatric and psychological support may be required. Pain relief is the major problem for most patients, and analgesics are required during acute exacerbations and continuously in a minority of patients. The introduction of regular opiate analgesia treads a difficult path between pain relief and addiction. Pancreatic

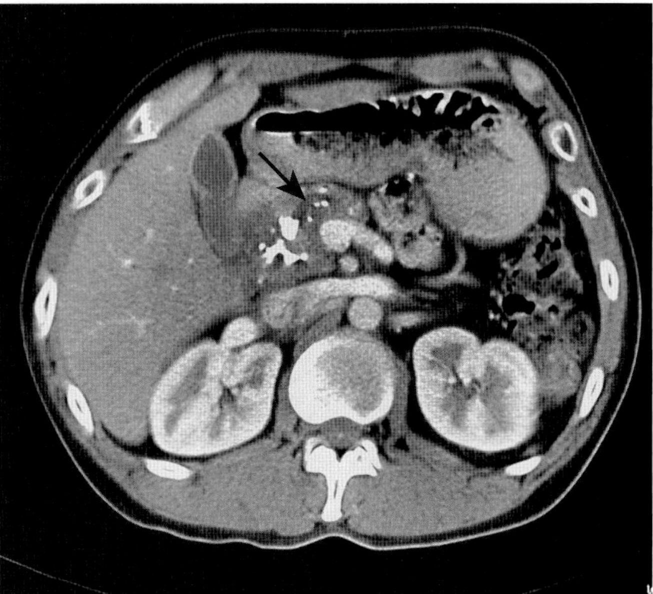

Figure 31.14 A CT scan showing calcification within the head of the pancreas and a dilated pancreatic duct (arrowed).

enzyme supplements, particularly in large doses, can produce a reduction in the pain of some patients with chronic pancreatitis.[35] Octreotide therapy is beneficial only in a minority, and trials have given conflicting results. The long-term results of neurolytic treatments such as coeliac plexus block or thoracoscopic splanchnicectomy have also proved disappointing.[36] Acute exacerbations requiring hospital admission should be treated by resting the intestine, with supplemental nutrition. The decision to perform surgery for intractable pain is difficult, and the advice of a pain specialist and clinical psychologist is essential.

Exocrine failure can be improved by pancreatic enzyme replacements, and a variety of preparations exist that are extracts of porcine pancreas. The enzymes are inactivated by gastric acidity, so patients should be counselled to take them with food. Proton pump inhibitors may also be taken to aid digestion, although newer enzyme preparations come in the form of enteric-coated microspheres, which allow delivery of enzymes to the duodenum. Dosage is dictated by the stool size and frequency, and varies widely between patients, from 30 000 to 200 000 units of lipase per adult per day. The starting dose is usually 20 000 or 25 000 units with each meal and 10 000 units with a snack. Steatorrhoea can also be helped by controlling the daily fat intake. Reasons for an apparent failure of treatment include poor compliance, an inadequate prescription, excessive heating of the supplements if mixed in with food, or an incorrect diagnosis. Endocrine failure tends to be progressive and requires insulin.

REFERENCES

31. Varghese J, Masterson A et al. Clin Radiol 2002; 57: 393–401
32. Wiersema M, Wiersema LE. Gastrointest Endosc Clin North Am 1995; 5: 487–496
33. Kahl S, Glasbrenner B et al. Gastrointest Endosc 2002; 55: 507–511
34. Hollerbach S, Klamann A et al. Endoscopy 2001; 33: 824–831
35. Ramo O, Puolakkainen P et al. Scand J Gastroenterol 1989; 24: 688–692
36. Buscher H, Jansen J et al. Br J Surg 2002; 89: 158–162

Compared with patients with idiopathic diabetes, hypoglycaemia occurs more easily because there is a lack of endogenous glucagon. This is worse in alcoholic patients with a poor calorific intake, and higher blood glucose levels should be allowed to avoid hypoglycaemia.

Interventional non-surgical treatment can be used to treat pseudocysts and dilate duct strictures and stones in the main pancreatic duct. Pseudocysts only need treatment if they cause symptoms. Percutaneous pseudocyst aspiration or drainage risks an external pancreatic fistula or infection, and internal drainage is preferable. Assessment by CT or endoscopic ultrasound is important and if the cyst is applied to the stomach, endoscopic cyst-gastrostomy can usually be carried out using ERCP-type stents. This is ideally performed under endoscopic ultrasound guidance to avoid hitting vessels within the cyst wall. Alternatively a laparoscopic approach can be used. Open drainage may be necessary if the cyst is not in contact with the stomach or duodenum, either by cyst-gastrostomy or cyst-jejunostomy using the most dependent part of the cyst. If a successful communication is established, resolution of the cyst should be successful in 80–90%.[37] Endoscopic retrograde cholangiopancreatography can relieve jaundice in patients with chronic pancreatitis by biliary stenting, but most patients eventually require surgery in the form of a choledochoduodenostomy or choledochojejunostomy. The benefits of treating ductal hypertension by stenting dominant strictures in the pancreatic duct and removing ductal calculi are well recognized, but pancreatic endotherapy can be demanding for the endoscopist,[38] and it is possible to eradicate long-term symptoms in only a few patients.

Surgical management for chronic pancreatitis is reserved for patients with complications (Table 31.4). The role of surgery to treat intractable pain or to preserve pancreatic function depends on the calibre of the main duct and the distribution of disease in the pancreas. A variety of drainage procedures have been described in the case of a dilated pancreatic duct, which should be about 7 mm in diameter. These procedures work either by reducing ductal pressures or by a fasciotomy effect.

Lateral pancreaticojejunostomy (a modified Puestow or Partington–Rochelle procedure) involves exposure of the gland, opening of the length of the pancreatic duct to the ampulla, and anastomosis of the duct to a Roux loop of jejunum. The disadvantage of this operation is that the inflammatory tissue of the head of the pancreas is left in situ and the disease can progress in the head, giving rise to further complications such as biliary obstruction or portal vein thrombosis. If the head of the gland is partially excised in addition to a lateral pancreaticojejunostomy (Fig. 31.15), as described by Frey,[39] a better result can be obtained. Alternatively a duodenum-preserving resection of the head of the pancreas, as described by Beger, may be performed. This is similar but with a more extensive resection of the head of the pancreas, with duodenal preservation,[40] and gives similar results to the Frey procedure in terms of relief of pain. These duodenum-preserving resectional procedures provide good relief from recurrent attacks of pain[41] and are superior to pancreaticoduodenectomy,[42] which is only rarely required for chronic pancreatitis.

The main indication for pancreaticoduodenectomy is suspicion of a tumour in the head of the pancreas. Focal chronic pancreatitis in the tail of the pancreas is best managed by a distal pancreatectomy. Total pancreatectomy is rarely indicated in patients with chronic pancreatitis. Because autonomic nerve pathways are damaged, it abolishes pain in only half the patients.

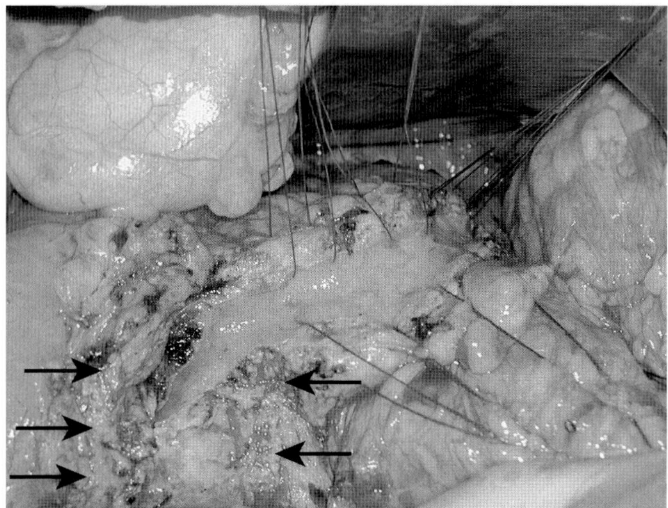

Figure 31.15 Surgery for chronic pancreatitis: partial duodenum-preserving resection of head of pancreas and lateral pancreaticojejunostomy (Frey's procedure). The mass in the head of the pancreas has been resected, and the pancreatic duct has been laid open from the tail to the ampulla and is seen held open by stay sutures. Arrows indicate the edges of the head of the pancreas, to which a Roux-en-Y loop of jejunum will be anastomosed.

The main complication is instability of diabetic control, which results in unpredictable hypoglycaemia.[43]

COMPLICATIONS AND CLINICAL OUTCOMES

Patients with chronic pancreatitis do not have a normal life expectancy, and complications of the disease account for some deaths. Many alcoholic patients have a significant tobacco intake, and smoking-related deaths are more common than in the general population. Surgery should be undertaken in carefully selected individuals. Resectional procedures have a perioperative mortality rate of up to 5%, although this is less for those procedures that are combined with drainage.

TUMOURS OF THE PANCREAS

Pancreatic ductal adenocarcinoma is the most common and the most lethal primary tumour of the pancreas. There are, however, many other types of pancreatic tumour, which have a variety of modes of presentation and have much better prognosis. These include periampullary tumours, benign and malignant cystic pancreatic tumours, intraductal papillary mucinous tumours, and neuroendocrine tumours of the pancreas (which include insulinomas, gastrinomas and non-functioning islet cell tumours).

REFERENCES

37. Binmoeller K, Seifert H et al. Gastrointest Endosc 1995; 42: 219–224
38. Kasmin FE, Siegel JH. Surg Clin North Am 2001; 81: 421–430
39. Frey C, Amikura K. Am Surg 1994; 220: 492–507
40. Beger H, Krautzberger W et al. Surgery 1985; 98: 467–472
41. Bloechle C, Izbicki J et al. Pancreas 1995; 11: 77–85
42. Izbicki J, Bloechle C et al. Ann Surg 1998; 228: 771–779
43. Flemming W, Williamson R. Br J Surg 1995; 82: 1409–1412

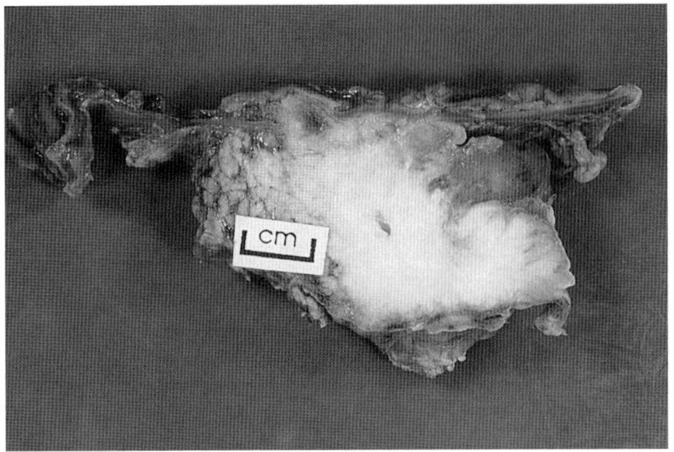

a

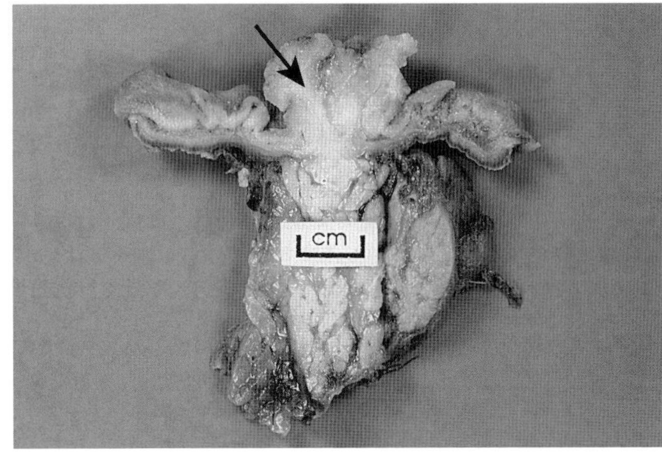

b

Figure 31.16 Surgical specimens of (**a**) carcinoma of the head of the pancreas, showing tumour as a white mass and impression of portal vein on inferior aspect, and (**b**) periampullary carcinoma (arrowed).

Secondary tumours of the pancreas are unusual but occasionally arise from carcinoma of the breast, kidney or melanoma by haematogenous spread. Direct extension of adjacent tumours, such as the stomach into the pancreas, may also occur (see Ch. 26). Although a proportion of cystic tumours are benign (discussed further in this chapter), solid tumours of the pancreas, unless neuroendocrine tumours (see further), are almost universally malignant. Rare benign tumours such as haemangioma, fibroma or neurilemmoma can also occur.

MALIGNANT PANCREATIC EXOCRINE TUMOURS

Pancreatic exocrine cancers are classified by where in the gland they arise. Tumours of the head, including the uncinate process, are the commonest, with 90% being ductal adenocarcinomas (Fig. 31.16a). Other histological types of malignant exocrine pancreatic cancers also exist, including mucinous non-cystic carcinoma (mucinous adenocarcinoma), adenosquamous carcinoma, anaplastic carcinoma, acinar cell carcinoma and clear cell carcinoma. Lymphoma and stromal cell tumours may also arise from the pancreas.

Tumours arising from the ampulla of Vater or nearby structures are known as periampullary tumours (Fig. 31.16b) and are a special subset of cancers. They have a different pathological distribution (ductal adenocarcinoma 80%, ampullary cancer 5%, distal bile duct cancer 5%, duodenum 5%, and rarer tumours or unclassified 5%), but their surgical management is similar to head of pancreas cancers. Duodenal and bile duct cancers are discussed elsewhere in this book (see Ch. 30).

Pancreatic adenocarcinoma

Pancreatic cancer is more common in developed countries. There is evidence of an increasing incidence in recent years in North America. Racial factors appear to be important, although migrant studies indicate that environmental factors also have an important part to play. A list of factors associated with an increased risk of developing pancreatic cancer is shown in Box 31.3. Smoking is the most important.

The majority (80%) of pancreatic cancers arise within the head of the pancreas. Tumours of the neck, body and tail of the pancreas are less common and tend to present at an advanced stage, causing symptoms only when they invade a structure outside the pancreas, such as the coeliac plexus. Many different histological types of pancreatic cancer have been described, but the recognition of rarer forms is not easy and requires specialist histopathological expertise. Certain types, such as cystic tumours, generally have a better prognosis.[44] Spread of the tumour may occur via the lymphatic, transcoelemic or haematogenous routes, or by direct extension to other organs such as the duodenum, stomach, colon or liver.

Box 31.3 Aetiological factors in the development of pancreatic cancer

Lifestyle and dietary
- Smoking
- High fat consumption

Occupational exposure
- Napthylamine
- Ethylene dichloride

Hereditary
Mostly sporadic but increased risk in families with familial pancreatic cancer and hereditary pancreatitis.

Others
- Diabetes: possible effect rather than cause
- Chronic pancreatitis
- Gastrectomy

Clinical features

History

Obstructive jaundice is the commonest presentation of tumours of the head of the pancreas. The jaundice progressively deepens from yellow to orange to an almost brown colour over the course of a few weeks as bile duct compression worsens. Fluctuant jaundice suggests incomplete obstruction by gallstones or an inflammatory process, although ampullary tumours may occasionally undergo partial necrosis, producing a temporary improvement. Bile duct obstruction may also occur from cholangiocarcinoma or from metastatic lymph nodes in the

REFERENCE

44. Warshaw A, Compton C et al. Ann Surg 1990; 212: 432–445

hepatoduodenal ligament (see Ch. 29). Patients will notice the passage of dark urine and pale stools, and steatorrhoea may be present if there is pancreatic insufficiency. Newly diagnosed adult-onset diabetes is a well-recognized presentation, and in older patients an unexplained episode of acute pancreatitis may be secondary to a pancreatic or periampullary tumour.

Epigastric pain is a common feature of pancreatic malignancy. It is usually aching in nature, is progressive in its severity, and may be aggravated by eating. As the tumour enlarges, invasion posteriorly often produces severe aching back pain, which is an ominous symptom suggesting that the tumour is irresectable. Tumours in the uncinate process are situated posteriorly and may therefore present with back pain before jaundice develops. Weight loss has occurred in most patients by the time of diagnosis. Anorexia and malabsorption are common. Relief of jaundice improves nutrition and weight gain can occur. Gastric outlet obstruction from duodenal invasion causes anorexia and vomiting, and exacerbates malnutrition.

Examination

Signs of weight loss may be apparent. Jaundice is common, while pallor may be the result of an ulcerated bleeding ampullary tumour. The paraneoplastic syndrome thrombophlebitis migrans may occasionally be present (see Ch. 11). Abdominal examination may demonstrate a palpable primary tumour or para-aortic lymphadenopathy in a thin patient. Courvoisier's law states that in the presence of obstructive jaundice a palpable gallbladder is unlikely to be the result of gallstones (see Ch. 30). A tumour of the head of the pancreas initially causes a painless obstructive jaundice with an enlarged gallbladder. Common bile duct gallstones are usually associated with a shrunken, fibrotic gallbladder from previous episodes of inflammation. Exceptions to the rule, however, occasionally occur. Metastatic deposits in the greater omentum may be felt as an omental cake, and ascites may be detectable. Gastric outlet obstruction is indicated by epigastric fullness and a succussion splash. The presence of cervical lymphadenopathy should always be sought.

Investigations

Liver function tests may show an obstructive picture, with a progressively rising serum bilirubin and alkaline phosphatase. Serum amylase levels are usually normal. Anaemia may be present, especially if the tumour is invading the duodenum. The tumour antigen CA 19-9 is the most specific marker for pancreatic cancer, but it is also elevated in obstructive jaundice and pancreatitis. In non-jaundiced patients, if an upper limit for normal of 120 U/mL is used this test has a positive predictive value of 85% and negative predictive value of 100%.[45]

Patients presenting with upper abdominal pain or jaundice should have an ultrasound scan. Occasionally a pancreatic mass may be found as an incidental finding on imaging. In obstructive jaundice the ultrasound findings give an indication of the underlying cause (see Ch. 30). The presence of extrahepatic bile duct dilatation and the absence of gallstones suggest a tumour causing distal biliary obstruction.

If the patient is a surgical candidate, staging of the suspected tumour is best carried out before a biliary stent is inserted to relieve the jaundice. Features that suggest that the tumour is going to be irresectable include peritoneal or liver metastases, involved lymph nodes other than peripancreatic nodes, and vascular invasion into the superior mesenteric vein or artery, portal vein or hepatic artery.

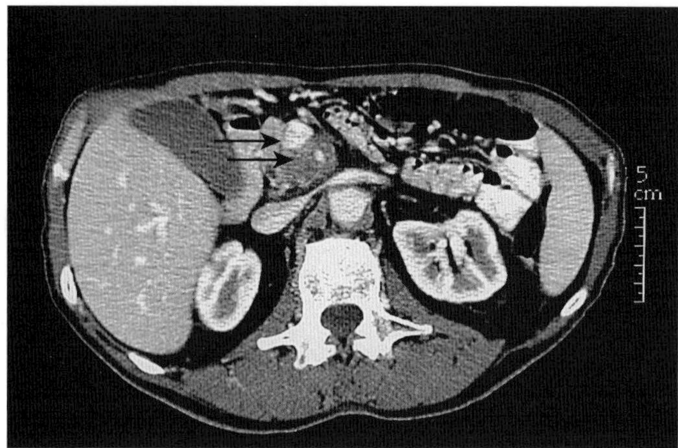

Figure 31.17 A CT scan showing the relationship of a pancreatic carcinoma to the superior mesenteric vein (upper arrow) with encasement of the superior mesenteric artery (lower arrow).

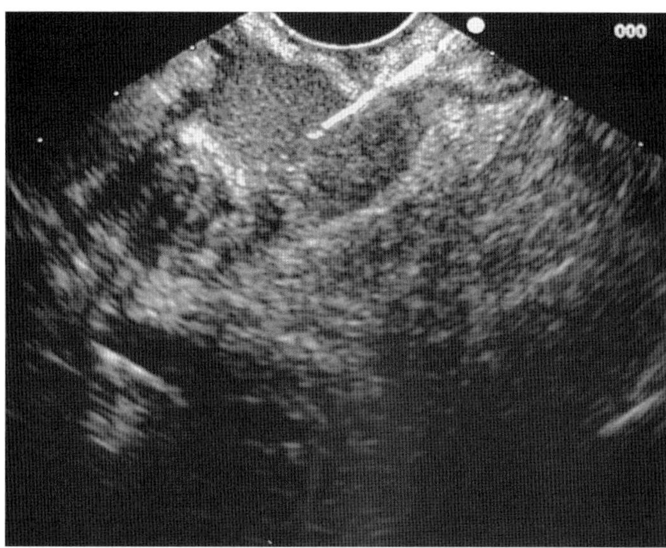

Figure 31.18 Endoscopic ultrasound–guided biopsy (fine-needle aspirate for cytology) of a pancreatic cancer, showing the needle entering the tumour mass.

Triple-phase CT with intravenous and oral contrast enhancement is the means of staging the tumour. This will demonstrate the tumour, its relationship to surrounding structures (including the major vessels; Fig. 31.17), and the presence of nodal and liver metastases.[46] The CT scan should include the lungs to exclude pulmonary metastases.

Endoscopic ultrasound is used to assess small tumours and provides excellent images. It may be combined with ultrasound-guided biopsy (Fig. 31.18). Laparoscopic assessment is useful for excluding peritoneal involvement and small liver metastases in patients with larger tumours, but in less than 15% of people does this prevent an unnecessary laparotomy from being done.[47]

REFERENCES

45. Malesci A, Montorsi M et al. Pancreas 1992; 7: 497–502
46. Midwinter M, Beveridge C et al. Br J Surg 1999; 86: 189–193
47. Hennig R, Tempia-Caliera A et al. Dig Surg 2002; 19: 484–488

Laparoscopic ultrasound and MRI do not add sufficient additional information to CT to be worthwhile in every patient.

Endoscopic retrograde cholangiopancreatography can demonstrate a distal ductal stricture, and has the advantage that a biliary stent can be inserted at the time of investigation. Brushings from the stricture can be analysed cytologically and this has an accuracy of 70%. A patient with a distal bile duct stricture who has no previous history to suggest a benign process (e.g. previous cholecystectomy or sclerosing cholangitis) has a 95% chance of having a malignant stricture (see Ch. 30). Efforts to prove that it is benign or malignant are likely to result in a delay in carrying out a surgical resection. Such patients should be counselled accordingly and advised to undergo resection in the absence of histological evidence.

Other causes of obstructive jaundice are usually clarified by investigation. Patients without jaundice may occasionally have had abdominal pain investigated for some time before a pancreatic tumour is visualized. The most difficult differential diagnosis is between pancreatic cancer and chronic pancreatitis, especially in the head of the pancreas. Both may present with pain, jaundice or a mass visible on imaging. Features suggesting chronic pancreatitis are a younger patient with a longer history, which consists of exacerbations and remissions. Gross elevation of tumour markers makes cancer likely, although intermediate levels may be caused by benign biliary obstruction. Pancreatic calcification suggests chronic pancreatitis, although tumours may arise within chronic pancreatitis.

Generalized oedema of the head of the pancreas may be visible on CT without a discrete mass being present. A small tumour may be visible only on endoscopic ultrasound. Previously, patients who survived for long periods with a supposed diagnosis of advanced pancreatic cancer but without confirmatory histology were almost always suffering from chronic pancreatitis. This is less likely with modern imaging techniques. Differentiation between a pseudocyst and a cystic tumour may be difficult, but a clear history of an attack of severe pain strongly suggests a pseudocyst secondary to previous acute pancreatitis, whereas no history of pain and the presence of septation within a cyst should suggest a tumour. Sometimes the diagnosis is not resolved until the lesion has been resected.

Patients with pancreatic cancer tend to be of an older age group and are likely to have coexistent cardiorespiratory disease that may preclude major surgery. A full preoperative assessment with an evaluation of cardiac function, including an exercise ECG, an echocardiogram and pulmonary function tests, may be required if pancreatic resection is planned.

Treatment

Surgery offers the only hope of cure for pancreatic adenocarcinoma. Although 50–60% of periampullary tumours and over 75% of pancreatic cystic tumours are resectable, only 15–20% of ductal adenocarcinomas can be resected. The majority of these patients therefore require some form of palliative treatment. The mortality following major upper abdominal surgery has been shown to be lower in those hospitals treating larger numbers of patients.[48]

Curative pancreatic resection

Curative resection should be considered when preoperative investigations suggest a localized primary pancreatic tumour. Resection should include the primary tumour and draining lymph nodes. For resectable tumours in the body and tail (which rarely occur), resection is by distal pancreatectomy with splenectomy. This is, however, rarely feasible. For tumours in the head of the pancreas the operation of choice is pancreaticoduodenectomy. The first successful pancreaticoduodenectomy was performed by Kausch in 1912, but it is Whipple who was given the credit for describing it in 1935. The operation involves excision of the pancreatic head, distal stomach and duodenum, upper jejunum, omentum, common bile duct and gallbladder.[49] This operation has been modified to preserve the distal stomach and pylorus; this is known as a pylorus-preserving pancreaticoduoenectomy and gives better functional results. Concerns have been raised that this results in a lesser degree of cancer clearance, but this does not appear to have any importance in terms of survival.[50]

There is debate over operating on patients who are jaundiced or performing biliary drainage preoperatively.[51,52] Balanced against the deleterious consequences of jaundice are the risks of biliary stent insertion, causing infected bile at the time of resection. Operating on a patient with a bilirubin level of less than 300 μmol/L and serum albumin within the normal range is unlikely to increase the risk of complications.

The operation of pancreaticoduodenectomy is preferably performed through a bilateral subcostal incision, although a long midline incision is an alternative. A careful laparotomy is conducted to evaluate the presence of metastases and coincidental disease. Intraoperative ultrasound can be used to examine the liver (see Ch. 30), but is unlikely to yield any further information than modern cross-sectional imaging. A decision must then be made on whether the cancer is resectable. This follows a trial dissection, with the decision usually resting on whether the superior mesenteric or portal veins are invaded by tumour or whether tumour extends posteriorly into the dorsal pancreatic space.

The operation of pylorus-preserving pancreaticoduodenectomy proceeds as follows.

The hepatic flexure of the colon and duodenum is mobilized by an extended Kocher's manoeuvre. The gastrocolic omentum is divided outside the gastroepiploic arcade to expose the body and tail of the pancreas. The superior mesenteric vein is identified as it passes from the small bowel mesentery up to the neck of the pancreas. The gallbladder is mobilized and the common hepatic duct is divided. A palliative bypass can be performed to the transected common hepatic duct if the cancer is subsequently found to be irresectable. The hepatic arteries and portal vein must be identified, and any invasion of these structures and aberrant arterial anatomy must be clarified. Connective tissue and lymph nodes must be dissected off these vessels while the right gastric artery is preserved. The right gastroepiploic vessels are divided, and the duodenum is transected 2 cm distal to the pylorus. The gastroduodenal artery is also ligated and divided. The first loop of jejunum and its mesentery are transected, which allows the third and fourth parts of the duodenum to be passed posteriorly behind the small bowel mesentery. The neck of the

REFERENCES

48. Ho V, Heslin M. Ann Surg 2003; 237: 509–514
49. Tait IS. J R Coll Surg Edinb 2002; 47: 528–540
50. Seiler CA, Wagner M et al. J Gastrointest Surg 2000; 4: 443–452
51. Pisters P, Hudec W et al. Ann Surg 2001; 234: 47–55
52. Povoski S, Karpeh MJ et al. J Gastrointest Surg 1999; 3: 496–505

pancreas is divided, taking care to avoid damaging the portal vein or its tributaries. The uncinate process and pancreatic head are then dissected from the portal vein, superior mesenteric vein and superior mesenteric artery, and the specimen is removed. The pancreatic stump is gently mobilized off the posterior structures, particularly the splenic vein, for a distance of 2 cm to facilitate the pancreatic anastomosis.

Reconstruction begins by anastomosing the pancreas to the jejunum. This is the most critical anastomosis because leakage accounts for most of the operation-specific complications. The following principles reduce complications: careful mobilization of 2 cm of pancreatic stump off the splenic vein, with ligation of small vessels; preparation of the proximal jejunum for an end (pancreas) to side (jejunum) anastomosis; an inner layer of fine interrupted absorbable monofilament sutures between the pancreatic duct and parenchyma and the full thickness of the jejunum; and an outer layer of stronger interrupted absorbable monofilament sutures between capsule, with parenchyma of pancreas and serosubmucosa of jejunum placed posteriorly and anteriorly (Fig. 31.19). A free-lying pancreatic soft plastic stent with side holes is used in a patient with a narrow pancreatic duct.

A hepaticojejunostomy should then be performed as an end-to-side anastomosis using fine absorbable monofilament interrupted sutures. A duodenojejunostomy is then performed by making an end-to-side anastomosis with absorbable monofilament continuous sutures. This anastomosis is performed 30 cm distal to the biliary anastomosis. A feeding jejunostomy is inserted for nutritional support and two silastic drains are left near the pancreatic anastomosis.

The order of the dissection may vary depending on the morphology of the tumour and the surgeon's preference. When there is invasion of the portal vein some surgeons favour resection followed by reconstruction. This may be by excision of a cuff of vein or as a circumferential resection. This does not appear to increase the operative morbidity or mortality.[53] Survival is unaffected in patients who have an isolated portal vein resection to achieve tumour clearance.[54]

Radical lymphadenectomy with skeletonization of the coeliac and superior mesenteric vessels has resulted in higher mortality and morbidity. This may cause diarrhoea because of resection of autonomic nerves and has not been shown to confer any additional survival benefit.[55] Total pancreatectomy may occasionally be considered if the tumour is close to the neck of the pancreas or if the remaining pancreas is unsuitable for anastomosis.

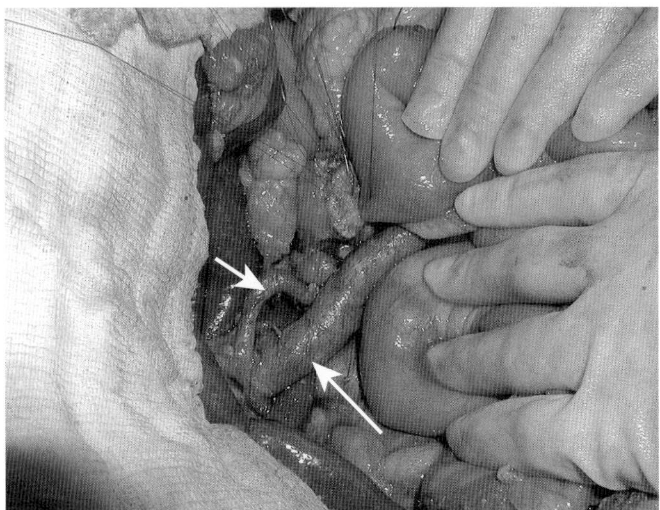

Figure 31.19 Anastomosis of the neck of the pancreas to the jejunum in two layers: hepatic artery (short arrow) and portal vein (long arrow).

The mortality rate of pancreaticoduodenectomy has reduced over the last 20 years to 3–6%, but the complication rate remains high at 20–30%. Management of the complications has improved, the most important being leakage from the pancreatic anastomosis. A clinically significant leak carries a mortality rate of about 25% and is more likely to occur in patients with a soft pancreas without pancreatic duct obstruction.[56] Perioperative octreotide may reduce the leak rate.[57]

A leak should be suspected if there is anything other than a normal recovery from surgery. Daily estimates of drain amylase are routinely performed and may indicate a biochemical leak. If there is no systemic upset, a CT scan can be used to confirm the diagnosis and allow percutaneous drainage of any collections. A patient with a suspected leak should be starved, placed on total parenteral nutrition, and treated with a high-dose octreotide infusion for a minimum of 10 days. An early laparotomy is indicated if there is any sign of clinical deterioration. At laparotomy a completion pancreatectomy is usually necessary,[58] although a localized leak into a well-defined cavity can be treated by surgical drainage and postoperative irrigation of the cavity. Anastomotic leak from the biliary or gastric anastomoses is uncommon but usually requires an operative repair rather than conservative treatment.

Distal pancreatectomy is the operation of choice for patients with resectable tumours of the body and tail of the pancreas. After distant spread has been excluded, the lesser peritoneal sac is opened so that the pancreas can be examined from the hilum of the spleen to the duodenum. The spleen and tail of the pancreas are mobilized forward by entering the plane between the pancreas and the posterior abdominal wall. The omentum is taken off the splenic flexure of the colon, and the left gastroepiploic artery and short gastric vessels are divided and ligated. The splenic artery is divided close to the coeliac axis, and the splenic vein is divided flush with the inferior mesenteric vein and oversewn. The neck of the pancreas is then divided on the anterior surface of the portal vein. This can be done using a linear stapler, or alternatively the duct and pancreatic stump can be oversewn.

Although removal of the whole pancreas is a more radical cancer operation and avoids a pancreatic anastomosis, the mortality rate is higher[59] and the long-term morbidity of diabetes is 15%.

Adjuvant therapy following resection

Surgical resection alone has a 5-year survival rate of 10–20% for ductal adenocarcinoma of the pancreas. Several studies have been carried out to determine whether adjuvant radiotherapy or chemotherapy might improve the survival rate. The European

REFERENCES

53. Leach S, Lee J et al. Br J Surg 1998; 85: 611–617
54. Sasson A, Hoffman J et al. J Gastrointest Surg 2002; 6: 147–158
55. Pedrazzoli S, Di Carlo V et al. Ann Surg 1998; 228: 508–517
56. Sakorafas G, Friess H et al. Dig Surg 2001; 18: 363–369
57. Li-Ling J, Irving M. Br J Surg 2001; 88: 190–199
58. van Berge Henegouwen M, De Wit L et al. J Am Coll Surg 1997; 185: 18–24
59. van Heerden J, McIlrath D et al. World J Surg 1988; 12: 658–660

Study Group for Pancreatic Cancer – Trial 1 randomized patients to adjuvant chemoradiotherapy with or without maintenance chemotherapy (5-fluorouracil and folinic acid) against resection alone.[60] The most recent analysis of this study has shown no benefit for chemoradiotherapy but a definite advantage for adjuvant 5-fluorouracil chemotherapy, with an improvement of the median survival from 15 to 21 months. Further trials evaluating the role of other chemotherapeutic agents, including gemcitabine, are under way.

Palliation

The majority of patients (between 80 and 85%) will not be able to undergo curative resection. Pancreatic supplements may be helpful in reducing steatorrhoea, and relief of obstructive jaundice also provides good palliation. Relief of duodenal obstruction prevents vomiting. It is still contentious whether obstructive jaundice should be relieved by endoscopic biliary stenting or by surgery. Biliary stenting by ERCP is probably all that is required for patients with advanced disease and a predicted survival of less than 6 months. Metal stents take longer to occlude and give better palliation but are more expensive.

A palliative biliary and duodenal bypass should be performed at the time of exploratory surgery if a tumour is found to be unresectable and there is no evidence of hepatic or peritoneal metastases. The duodenal bypass can be performed laparoscopically and the obstructive jaundice relieved by biliary stenting. An operative bypass gives good palliation if the patient is relatively fit. A Roux loop of jejunum anastomosed to the common bile duct gives better results than an anastomosis to the gallbladder.[61] A prophylactic gastroenterostomy should be performed at the same time to reduce the potential risk of duodenal obstruction.[62] A coeliac plexus block performed at the time of bypass surgery reduces pain from nerve invasion.

Patients with unresectable and recurrent pancreatic cancer are treated by chemotherapy, but before this is started the diagnosis should be confirmed histologically or cytologically, because chronic pancreatitis may be misdiagnosed as pancreatic cancer. The diagnosis may be confirmed by biliary brushings, endoscopic ultrasound-guided biopsy, percutaneous biopsy of pancreas or liver, or laparoscopic biopsy. Gemcitabine, which is given as an intravenous bolus, is the agent of choice and has been shown to be superior to bolus 5-fluorouracil.[63] Gemcitabine is well tolerated and has been shown to improve patients' quality of life, providing good pain control and weight gain. Palliative radiotherapy is occasionally indicated, and novel treatments such as gene therapy are currently being evaluated.[64]

Pancreatic enzyme supplements should always be given to patients with advanced pancreatic cancer because they help to maintain weight and lead to an improved quality of life.[65] Pain may be difficult to control as the tumour infiltrates the retroperitoneal nerve plexuses. Although escalating doses of opiates are given to many patients, both coeliac plexus block[66] and thoracoscopic splanchnicectomy[67] have been shown to reduce pain from pancreatic cancer. Other symptoms, including vomiting, ascites, diarrhoea and constipation, must be treated appropriately with the aid of the palliative care team.

PANCREATIC ENDOCRINE TUMOURS

Introduction

Pancreatic endocrine tumours are usually characterized by the hormones they produce and are rare in comparison with pancreatic cancer (Table 31.5). The commonest of the tumours are insulinomas, glucagonomas, gastrinomas and somatostatinomas. Rarer varieties, including secreting vasoactive intestinal peptide, parathyroid hormone, growth hormone releasing hormone and adrenocorticotrophic hormone, may occasionally occur. Carcinoid tumours may also occur, particularly in the ampulla.

Table 31.5 Pancreatic endocrine tumours

Tumour	Hormone produced	Manifestation
Insulinoma	Insulin	Hypoglycaemia
Glucagonoma	Glucagon	Diabetes mellitus
Gastrinoma	Gastrin	Zollinger–Ellison syndrome
Somatostatinoma	Somatostatin	Diabetes mellitus and diarrhoea
PPoma	Pancreatic polypeptide	Non-functioning

Pancreatic endocrine tumours arise from neuroendocrine cells known as amine precursor uptake and decarboxylation (APUD) cells. Neuroendocrine tumours must be correctly diagnosed, localized and then surgically excised if possible. Localization can be difficult because the tumours may be only a few millimetres in diameter. Most pancreatic endocrine tumours are malignant, except for insulinomas. Non-functioning islet cell tumours are quite frequent and usually present as a mass in the pancreas that may reach a large size before metastases develop (Fig. 31.20). Although non-functioning islet cell tumours do not secrete hormones, they are similar to functioning endocrine tumours, being generally slow-growing. Occasionally aggressive tumours are encountered.

Multiple endocrine neoplasia syndrome type 1

Multiple endocrine neoplasia syndromes are inherited conditions with a propensity to produce endocrine tumours. Multiple endocrine neoplasia type 1 is characterized by parathyroid hyperplasia, different pancreatic islet cell tumours, pituitary and adrenal tumours, and lipomas,[68] while multiple endocrine neoplasia type 2A rarely and type 2B never involve the pancreas. Patients may provide a family history and endocrine tumours elsewhere must be excluded.

Insulinoma

Insulinomas arise from beta cells in the pancreatic islets. They have an incidence of one per million of the population and nearly always arise in the pancreas, with approximately 10% being

REFERENCES

60. Neoptolemos JP, Dunn JA et al. Lancet 2001; 358: 1576–1585
61. Watanapa P, Williamson R. Br J Surg 1992; 79: 8–20
62. Lillemoe KD, Cameron JL et al. Ann Surg 1999; 230: 322–328
63. Burris HR, Moore M et al. J Clin Oncol 1997; 15: 2403–2413
64. Gilliam AD, Watson SA et al. In: Johnson C, Taylor I (eds). Recent Advances in Surgery, Vol 25. Royal Society of Medicine Press, London, 2002: 87–98
65. Bruno MJ, Haverkort E et al. Gut 1998; 42: 92–96
66. Rykowski J, Hilgier M. Anesthesiology 2000; 92: 347–354
67. Ihse I, Zoucas E et al. Ann Surg 1999; 230: 785–790
68. Mignon M, Ruszniewski P et al. World J Surg 1993; 17: 489–497

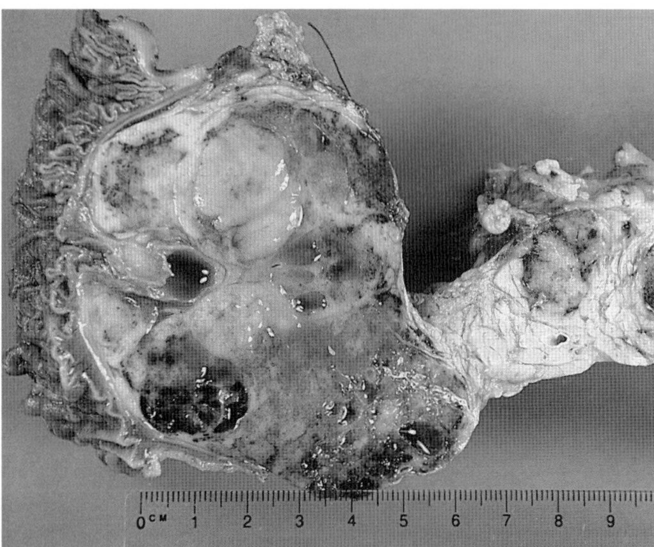

Figure 31.20 Non-functioning islet cell tumour of the head of the pancreas, which reached 7 cm in diameter.

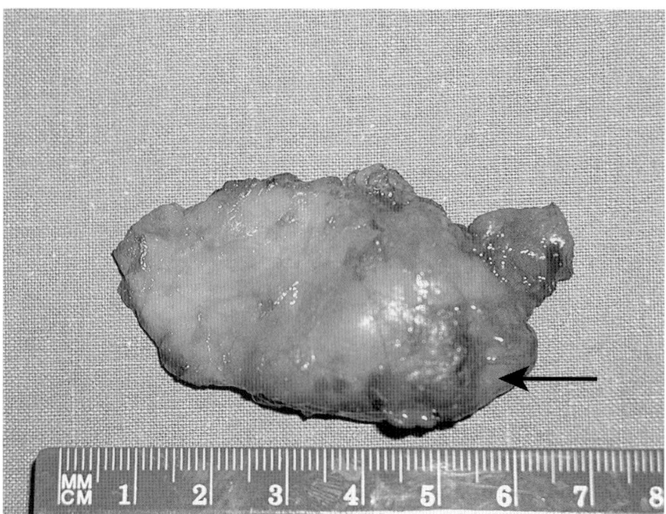

Figure 31.21 Insulinoma 1.5 cm in diameter (arrowed) resected as a limited spleen-preserving distal pancreatectomy.

multiple and 5–10% having metastases at the time of diagnosis. Ten per cent of patients with multiple endocrine neoplasia type 1 may develop an insulinoma.

Clinical features

Patients may present with a variety of neurological or psychiatric symptoms caused by hypoglycaemia, such as anxiety, confusion, convulsions and coma. These symptoms usually occur in the morning, when glucose stores are low after overnight fasting, or after exercise. Many patients are initially thought to have neurological or psychiatric conditions. Some patients may present with hunger, abdominal pain and diarrhoea. Patients often feel well between attacks and weight gain is common.

Diagnosis

Patients present with clinical features which occur in association with fasting hypoglycaemia and are relieved by glucose. A supervised in-patient fasting test confirms the diagnosis.[69] Serum levels of glucose, insulin and C-peptide are measured for up to 72 h while the patient is given only non-calorific fluids. The diagnosis is confirmed by finding high serum insulin in the presence of hypoglycaemia. Sulphonylureas are known to increase the secretion of endogenous insulin and C-peptide, and therefore a sulphonylurea screen should be conducted at the time of a hypoglycaemic episode in all patients with suspected insulinoma.

The location of the tumour within the pancreas must be identified once the diagnosis has been proven. This may be difficult prior to surgery. Computerized tomography is better than transcutaneous ultrasound but may detect only larger tumours. Somatostatin receptor scintigraphy is not helpful. Endoscopic ultrasound has good sensitivity for detecting these tumours and is the preoperative investigation of choice.[70] Selective hepatic venous sampling in combination with selective arterial injection of calcium can be used to localize the tumour more precisely. A catheter is placed in the hepatic vein and blood insulin concentrations are measured as different areas are stimulated. This technique has a high success rate but should probably be reserved for patients whose insulinoma has not been identified at the first operation.[71]

Treatment

Surgical excision is the best treatment because symptoms are poorly controlled by medical means. Hypoglycaemia can be avoided in the preoperative period by eating frequent meals, especially at night-time. Diazoxide inhibits insulin secretion in some patients and may be a useful means of preventing hypoglycaemia. It can, however, cause oedema, and a concomitant diuretic, such as bendrofluazide, should be given. Treatment with a synthetic somatostatin analogue may also be beneficial.

At operation the site of the tumour must be confirmed. The pancreas must be fully mobilized and assessed by bimanual palpation and intraoperative ultrasound. Ideally the tumour is enucleated with a small rim of normal pancreas, but if the tumour invades other structures, especially the pancreatic duct, formal pancreatic resection is required (Fig. 31.21). Lymph node and liver metastases should also be excised if possible, to improve symptom control. Patients with multiple endocrine neoplasia type 1 syndrome invariably have multiple insulinomas, one of which often predominates. Distal pancreatectomy should be performed if the tumour is in the tail of the pancreas because of the likelihood of multiple tumours.

The tail of the pancreas should be resected and subjected to immediate frozen section histological analysis to exclude islet cell hyperplasia if the tumour is not found at operation despite the use of careful palpation and operative ultrasound. The serum glucose should be measured during surgery, and levels should rise immediately the tumour is resected.

Even if patients have liver metastases, the primary and as many metastases as possible should be resected. Radiofrequency tumour ablation may also be tried (see Ch. 29). Chemotherapy and the medical treatments described earlier can be tried when surgical excision is not possible.

REFERENCES

69. Pasieka J, McLoed M et al. Arch Surg 1992; 127: 442–447
70. Glover J, Shorvon P et al. Gut 1992; 33: 1721–1722
71. Doppman J, Miller D et al. Radiology 1991; 178: 237–241

Complications

Care must be taken to ensure that simple enucleation will not damage the pancreatic duct, and if this occurs resection is indicated.

Clinical outcomes

The long-term survival of patients with sporadic benign insulinomas is normal. Patients with multiple endocrine neoplasia type 1-associated insulinomas also usually remain symptomless, but missed insulinomas or metastases may occasionally cause further problems.

Gastrinoma

Basic science summary

Gastrinomas secrete excessive amounts of gastrin, which stimulates the chief cells in the stomach to increase acid production, resulting in multiple duodenal and jejunal ulceration. These tumours also cause increased gastrointestinal motility. Approximately two-thirds of gastrinomas are found in the pancreas and a third in the duodenum. At least two-thirds are malignant, but the tumours tend to be slow-growing. Twenty per cent of gastrinomas arise as part of the multiple endocrine neoplasia type 1 syndrome, while 80% are sporadic.

Clinical features

Gastrinomas produce the Zollinger–Ellison syndrome as a consequence of excessive gastric acid secretion. Oesophagitis, epigastric pain or watery diarrhoea may be presenting symptoms, but the diagnosis should always be considered in patients with peptic ulcer disease (see Ch. 26). Any pattern of ulcer disease may be present, but severe ulcer disease, ulcers in unusual positions, and recurrence after ulcer surgery or *Helicobacter pylori* eradication should raise the possibility of Zollinger–Ellison syndrome. Twenty per cent of patients do not have peptic ulceration at the time of presentation, the majority of these presenting with diarrhoea.

Diagnosis

The diagnosis is dependent on demonstrating hypergastrinaemia and increased gastric acid output. Fasting gastrin levels less than 100 pg/mL make the diagnosis unlikely. Less than 1% of those with the syndrome have a normal fasting serum gastrin. The most useful measure of gastric acid secretion is finding that the basal acid output is greater than 15 mEq/h in patients without previous gastric surgery or 5 mEq/h in patients who have had previous gastric operations.[72] The secretin provocation test is reliable and has a sensitivity of 85% for diagnosing Zollinger–Ellison syndrome. The fasting serum gastrin is measured before and at 2, 5, 10, 15 and 20 min after a bolus of (2 U/kg) intravenous secretin. The condition is diagnosed if the serum gastrin increases by greater than 200 pg/mL.[73]

The differential diagnosis includes achlorhydria associated with pernicious anaemia or atrophic gastritis. These conditions are associated with hypergastrinaemia but basal acid output is decreased.[74] Gastric outlet obstruction and massive gastric distension may also mimic Zollinger–Ellison syndrome, but although they can cause hypergastrinaemia and hyperchlorhydria, the secretin provocation test does not cause any rise in fasting gastrin levels.

Localization studies are essential because 25% of patients have metastases at the time of diagnosis. Imaging of the liver as well as the pancreas and duodenum is important. Despite the wide availability of different imaging techniques, 50% of gastrinomas are not identified preoperatively.[75] Endoscopic ultrasound is the most accurate method for detecting gastrinomas.[76] Hepatic venous gastrin concentrations can be measured at rest and at 20, 40, 60, 90 and 120 s after a bolus injection of 2–3 U/kg of secretin is given into the gastroduodenal artery, superior mesenteric artery or splenic artery. This is the selective arterial secretin injection test, and if the serum gastrin concentrations increase by more than 80 pg/mL within 40 s to at least 120% of the basal level, it is considered that the artery concerned must be feeding a gastrinoma.[77]

Computerized tomography and MRI are the first 'localizing' investigations to be used, followed by endoscopic ultrasound. The selective arterial secretin injection is used only if the tumour is still not found. The majority of gastrinomas express somatostatin receptors, and somatostatin receptor scintigraphy is now frequently used to detect both the primary tumour and the metastases.[78]

Treatment

Proton pump inhibitors control symptoms and heal ulcers in almost all patients (see Ch. 26). Prior to the development of these drugs, total gastrectomy was often used to heal ulcers; however, curative resection of the primary tumour should be attempted to avoid the risk of hepatic metastases. Resection of limited hepatic metastases should also be considered (see Ch. 29).

The primary tumour in the pancreas or duodenum may be small and difficult to detect. At operation gastrinomas are usually found within a triangle bounded by the neck and body of the pancreas, the junction of the cystic duct with the common bile duct, and the second and third portions of the duodenum. This is called the gastrinoma triangle. The pancreas should be fully mobilized if the tumour is not present within this region. Intraoperative ultrasound of the pancreas can be used in addition to palpation. The most sensitive technique for identifying duodenal gastrinomas is duodenal transillumination using an endoscope passed orally into the duodenum during surgery, and this detected 75% of gastrinomas less than 10 mm in diameter.[79] A duodenotomy should be carried out to expose gastrinomas of the medial wall of the duodenum. The primary tumour must be enucleated when found, and a formal resection is sometimes required. All involved lymph nodes should be removed. Hepatic metastases should also be enucleated or ablated if these are present.

The 5-year survival for a sporadic gastrinoma is 60–75%. The extent of tumour at the time of diagnosis is an important prognostic factor, and 5-year survival in patients with unresectable metastatic disease is only 28%.[80]

REFERENCES

72. Deveney C, Deveney K et al. Ann Surg 1978; 188: 384–393
73. Frucht H, Howard J et al. Ann Intern Med 1989; 111: 713–722
74. Wolfe M, Jensen R. N Engl J Med 1987; 317: 1200–1209
75. Zeiger M, Shawker T et al. World J Surg 1993; 17: 448–454
76. Zimmer T, Scherubl H et al. Digestion 2000; 62 (Suppl 1): 45–50
77. Imamura M, Takahashi K. World J Surg 1993; 17: 433–438
78. Jensen R, Gibril F. Ital J Gastroenterol Hepatol 1999; 31: S179–S185
79. Frucht H, Norton J et al. Gastroenterology 1990; 99: 1622–1627
80. Carty S, Jensen R et al. Surgery 1992; 112: 1024–1032

CYSTIC TUMOURS OF THE PANCREAS

Most cysts of the pancreas are pseudocysts that have developed as a result of acute or chronic pancreatitis (see earlier). There is, however, a small but very important group of neoplastic cysts. These are important to identify because they are usually resectable and carry a better prognosis than solid tumours of the pancreas.

Cystic tumours have been classified into two distinct entities. One is the microcystic adenoma, also known as serous cystadenoma, which is almost universally benign.[81] The other is the mucinous cystic tumour, which can be benign, premalignant or an invasive carcinoma.[82] Both types cause a cystic pancreatic mass. A new entity of 'cystic' tumour, the intraductal papillary mucinous tumour, has been recognized in the past 10 years (see under *Intraductal papillary mucinous tumour*.[83] Other rarer lesions have also been identified, including the uncommon papillary cystic neoplasm.

Cystic tumours of the pancreas are more common in women, with a ratio of 4:1. The mean age at diagnosis of mucinous cystic tumours is 60 years, whereas serous cystadenomas tend to occur in older patients at a mean age of 65 years.[44,84] The mean age of females with cystic tumours is about 20 years younger than that for males. Most patients with cystic tumours present with abdominal pain or discomfort, weight loss or a palpable mass; vomiting may occasionally be present. A third of cystic tumours are symptomless and are discovered incidentally, usually as the result of a radiological investigation for another symptom.

Although mucinous cystadenocarcinomas tend to be less aggressive than ductal adenocarcinomas, they do occasionally present with metastases and rapidly progressive disease. Serous cystadenomas may cause symptoms from pressure on other organs. Serous cystadenomas occur in patients with von Hippel–Lindau syndrome, an autosomal dominant condition that manifests itself by the development of retinal angiomas, cerebellar haemangioblastomas, renal cell carcinoma, phaeochromocytoma and multiple pancreatic cysts. Twenty per cent of patients have pancreatic pathology, which occasionally progresses to adenocarcinoma.

Diagnosis of cystic tumours

The most important point to determine from the history is whether the patient has had a genuine previous attack of acute pancreatitis. When this is not present the diagnosis is likely to be a cystic tumour.[85] Patients with cystic tumours rarely have a history of an acute illness but are more likely to complain of dull pain. Cystic tumours should be suspected on imaging, when septa and loculations are seen on CT and ultrasound.[86] Calcification is seen in about a third of cystic tumours but is not present in the wall of a pseudocyst. It is, however, very common within the duct and parenchyma in patients with chronic pancreatitis (see earlier).

Serous cystadenomas usually appear as a sponge-like mass on CT (Fig. 31.22). Occasionally a central area of 'sunburst' calcification can be seen. Mucinous cysts tends to have thick walls with septa, but any solid components should raise the suspicion of malignancy. Serous cystadenomas are not found to communicate with the pancreatic duct on ERCP, but mucinous tumours may have duct communication or duct obstruction.[87] Unfortunately up to a third of tumours are misclassified as pseudocysts before they are correctly diagnosed.

Endoscopic ultrasound and ultrasound-guided aspiration have improved the diagnosis of cystic tumours. The amylase of the cyst fluid is usually elevated in pseudocysts but is low in cystic tumours. Tumour markers, particularly carcinoembryonic antigen and CA 19-9, are usually raised in mucinous tumours but are normal in serous cystadenomas and pseudocysts.[88] Cytology of cyst fluid is less helpful as a diagnostic tool.

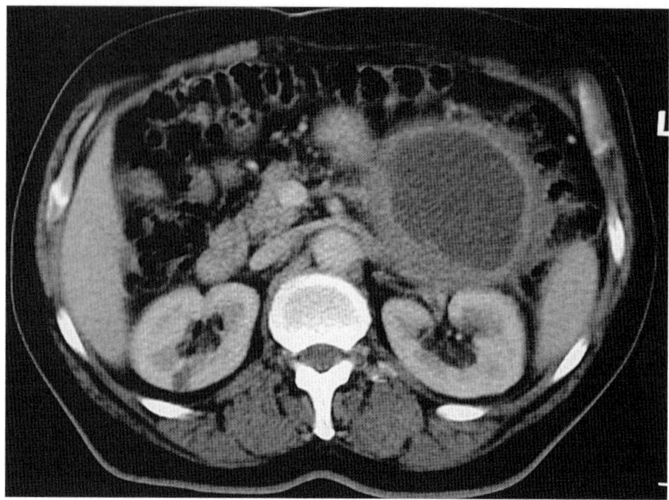

Figure 31.22 A CT scan of a serous cystadenoma of the tail of the pancreas.

Surgical resection should be performed for symptomatic cystic tumours. For left-sided tumours a distal pancreatectomy is appropriate, while for tumours of the head of the pancreas a pancreaticoduodenectomy is the operation of choice. When the diagnosis is known from a previous biopsy or from an endoscopic ultrasound-guided biopsy it is reasonable to avoid surgery in symptomless serous cystadenomas, particularly in the elderly. All tumours suspected of being mucinous cystic neoplasms should be considered malignant and resected if possible. Even if metastases are present they should also be resected if possible, because long-term cures have been reported. Mucinous cystic neoplasms considered to be benign should have 5-year survival rates of over 95%. For resected cystadenocarcinomas the long-term survival rate is between 50 and 75%. There are few data available on the use of chemotherapy on these tumours.

Intraductal papillary mucinous tumour

Intraductal papillary mucinous tumour is a type of pancreatic tumour previously known as mucin-producing tumour of pancreas or mucinous ductal ectasia. It is characterized by dilatation and filling of the main pancreatic duct or its side branches with thick mucus. The hyperplastic epithelium of the duct, which is responsible for the overproduction of mucus,

REFERENCES

81. Compagno J, Oertel J. Am J Clin Pathol 1978; 69: 289–298
82. Compagno J, Oertel J. Am J Clin Pathol 1978; 69: 573–580
83. Yamada M, Kozuka S et al. Cancer 1991; 68: 159–168
84. Albores-Saavedra J, Gould EW et al. Pathol Ann 1990; 25: 19–50
85. Martin I, Hammond P et al. Br J Surg 1998; 85: 1484–1486
86. Johnson C, Stephens D et al. Am J Roentgenol 1988; 151: 1133–1138
87. Yamaguchi K, Hirakata R et al. Acta Chir Scand 1990; 156: 553–564
88. Bounds B, Brugge W. Int J Gastrointest Cancer 2001; 30: 27–31

forms papillary projections into the duct lumen.[83] The epithelium may be normal, dysplastic or contain infiltrating carcinoma. The tumour grows along the duct before invading the parenchyma of the pancreas, and patients present with a long history of recurrent acute pancreatitis or symptoms of chronic pancreatitis including exocrine and endocrine insufficiency.

Duodenoscopy usually demonstrates mucus exuding from the papilla and the pancreatic duct system, which is dilated and filled with mucus plugs. The head of the pancreas is frequently affected, causing dilatation of the duct system in the body and tail of the pancreas. The process may be benign or malignant, but benign lesions may take many years to progress to frank malignancy. Endoscopic ultrasound is of value only in diagnosing these lesions, and endoscopic ultrasound-guided fine-needle aspiration and cytology provide useful information.[89]

The condition should be treated by pancreatic resection, which relieves symptoms and removes a malignant or potentially malignant tumour. Most tumours are situated in the head of the pancreas, and therefore pancreaticoduodenectomy is the treatment of choice. The pancreatic duct resection margins should be examined by frozen section. Total pancreatectomy is required if the resection margin is involved.

PANCREATIC TRAUMA

INTRODUCTION

Iatrogenic pancreatic trauma can occur at the time of ERCP or at open or laparoscopic surgery. A severe attack of acute pancreatitis may follow ERCP, and although good technique can reduce its incidence mortality does occasionally occur; ERCP is therefore justified only if therapy is planned. An alternative, less invasive procedure, such as endoscopic ultrasound or magnetic resonance cholangiopancreatography, should therefore be used for diagnosis if possible. The management is the same as for any patient with acute pancreatitis (see p. 749).

The tail of the pancreas is liable to injury during splenectomy, gastrectomy or any other surgery where the pancreas is mobilized. Management should follow the principles outlined in the section on the postoperative complications of pancreatic surgery (see p. 758).

The pancreas is usually injured by a blow to the midabdomen (see Ch. 7). Isolated pancreatic injury is uncommon because the pancreas is surrounded by other organs, which are often also injured. Duodenal and bile duct injury are often associated with injuries to the head of the pancreas. Although pancreatic trauma is discussed here in isolation, other injuries should also be managed in an appropriate order (see Ch. 7). Retroperitoneal injuries often have poor outcomes because of delay in diagnosis.

CLINICAL FEATURES

Penetrating injuries can produce any pattern of injury depending on their magnitude. Stab injuries rarely damage the duct. Two particular mechanisms of blunt injury are associated with transection of the pancreas, which is caused by the pancreas being crushed against the vertebral column. These occur in children falling from bicycles and landing on handlebars, and follow a steering wheel injury to the epigastrium. There are few signs initially. Children who are often well compensated initially should be actively observed for some time. Patients who present with multiple organ injuries can have a simultaneous pancreatic injury that is missed. Pancreatic injury should be considered in any patient with a major thoracic or abdominal injury. A midthoracic vertebral injury is an especially useful pointer to the likelihood of a pancreatic injury.

DIAGNOSIS

After abdominal trauma, a high index of suspicion must be maintained to allow a prompt diagnosis of pancreaticoduodenal injuries. The signs may be subtle, and the diagnosis should be reconsidered if there is any deterioration in a patient who has sustained trauma to the chest or abdomen. Laparotomy may be necessary for injuries to other organs. The presence of fat necrosis, bile staining, air bubbles or haematoma in the retroperitoneum at laparotomy indicates the possibility of a pancreatic injury. The serum amylase and lipase should not be relied on to make a diagnosis, although later estimations can be useful.[90]

Ultrasound is a poor method of imaging the retroperitoneum. Contrast-enhanced CT scan (Fig. 31.23) is valuable, but the patient's overall condition must be carefully taken into account when interpreting the images. The presence of pancreatic or duodenal haematomas indicates the need for active observation, repeat scanning or operative exploration. Pancreatic disruption or retroperitoneal gas indicate the need for a laparotomy, but CT is poor in diagnosing duct disruption.[91] A non-ionic contrast swallow may show duodenal leakage and enhances the diagnostic ability of CT. Pseudocysts or pancreatic abscesses can develop in patients with a delayed presentation. Amylase levels are usually high, and cross-sectional and pancreatic ductal imaging usually defines the anatomy of the injury.

Stratification

It is important to determine if the main pancreatic duct has been transected. In the stable patient, this may be assessed by ERCP, although magnetic resonance cholangiopancreatography may also be effective. These investigations are likely to be unsatisfactory in the emergency situation.

Different classifications have been used to stratify pancreatic trauma. One such classification has been proposed by the American Association for the Surgery of Trauma.[92] A simpler classification divides the degree of injury into three groups:[93]

- Minor: minimal parenchymal disruption without duct disruption.
- Intermediate: significant injury to the body or tail, such as laceration, perforation or transection.
- Major: injury involving the head such as crush or transection, or combined pancreaticoduodenal injury.

TREATMENT

Control of bleeding and prevention of contamination are the initial goals in trauma laparotomy (see Ch. 7). It may be necessary to perform damage control surgery and a second look laparotomy when the patient is in a more stable condition.[94] The

REFERENCES

89. Aithal G, Chen R et al. Gastrointest Endosc 2002; 56: 701–707
90. Takishima T, Sugimoto K et al. Ann Surg 1997; 226: 70–76
91. Bradley EL III, Young PR Jr et al. Ann Surg 1998; 227: 861–869
92. Moore EE, Cogbill TH et al. J Trauma 1990; 30: 1427–1429
93. Lucas CE. Surg Clin North Am 1977; 57: 49–65
94. Botha A. In: Brooks A, Loosemore T (eds). Definitive Surgical Trauma Skills. Royal College of Surgeons of England, London, 2002: 60–81

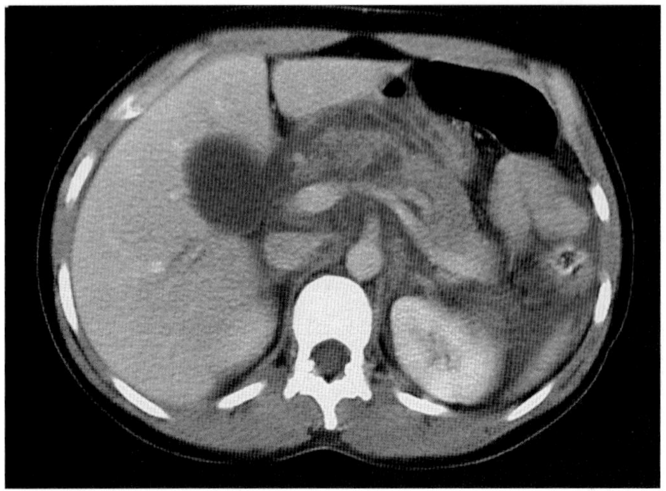

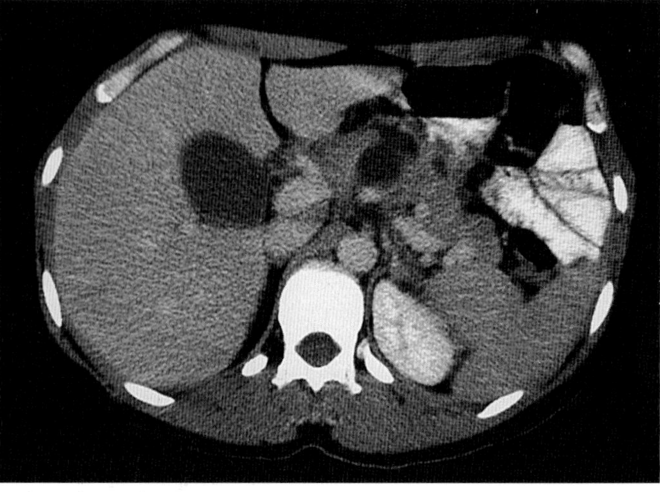

a b

Figure 31.23 (a) A CT scan following blunt pancreatic trauma, showing oedema around the head of the pancreas and a laceration of the neck of the pancreas. (**b**) Three weeks later, a localized collection has formed at the site of the laceration. The patient recovered without surgery.

duodenum must be kocherized to allow inspection of the head. The body and tail can be inspected through the lesser sac, and this can be aided by splenic mobilization.

The presence of an injury to the pancreatic duct determines the operative strategy.[95] Injuries of the body and tail without pancreatic duct disruption can be managed by placing large drains to the injured area. The body and tail should be resected if the duct is injured. When the spleen is clearly not involved in the injury it can usually be preserved. Injuries to the head are more difficult to manage because of associated vascular and duodenal injuries. Minor and intermediate injuries may be treated by drainage and haemostasis. A Whipple procedure for major injuries of the head is associated with a very high mortality (see Ch. 7). A Roux loop of jejunum may be sutured over the area of injury as an alternative. Depending on the experience of the surgeon, simple drainage or stapling across the pylorus to exclude gastric contents may be more appropriate than resection. A Whipple resection with or without delayed anastomosis is beset by problems, not least of which is performing a pancreatico-jejunostomy anastomosis to a normal soft pancreas.[96]

COMPLICATIONS

Patients with multiple organ injuries often have a protracted course. Pancreatic fistula or duodenal leakage, pancreatic necrosis, sepsis and haemorrhage can all follow pancreatic injury. Some complications may be managed conservatively with minimally invasive means, but further laparotomy is often necessary. When injuries are missed or their severity is not appreciated, they can present at a much later stage, often with a pseudocyst.

CLINICAL OUTCOMES

The mortality is often related to associated injuries rather than pancreatic injury. The outcome should be good as long as an isolated pancreatic injury is treated appropriately. Pancreatic fistula is the chief cause of morbidity.[95]

REFERENCES

95. Farrell RJ, Krige JE et al. Br J Surg 1996; 83: 934–937
96. Koniaris LG, Mandal AK et al. J Gastrointest Surg 2000; 4: 366–369

The spleen

32

Thomas W.J. Lennard, Anne L. Lennard

INTRODUCTION

The importance of the spleen and its recognition as part of a large integrated system of immunologically functional organs within the body have only recently been recognized. In the past, it was considered as an isolated organ of little significance, disposable and of no major consequence. Now it is recognized as part of the reticuloendothelial system, and it plays a crucial role in response to infection and overall management of the haematopoietic system. This role has led to a greater reluctance to consider the spleen as dispensable and an increasing desire to conserve it wherever possible. This applies not only after trauma, but also in procedures such as spleen-preserving distal pancreatectomy. The routine removal of the spleen as part of staging for various lymphoproliferative disorders has long since been abandoned and superseded by imaging. Specific indications for splenectomy do remain, however, and splenectomy remains a technically challenging operation, particularly when the spleen is diseased or badly traumatized. The short- and long-term consequences of removing the spleen need to be understood, and preventative measures taken to minimize long-term, dangerous sequelae.

BASIC SCIENCE SUMMARY

In adults the spleen normally lies in the left hypochondrial region between the fundus of the stomach and the diaphragm, although ectopic locations are described. It weighs approximately 150 g. It receives its blood supply via the splenic artery that arises from the coeliac axis and characteristically follows a tortuous course along the superior border of the pancreas.[1] Near the hilum of the spleen, the splenic artery divides into two (or rarely three) branches: the superior and inferior splenic arteries. Subsequent subdivisions give rise to segmental arteries supplying individual splenic segments and its upper and lower poles. The venous drainage of the spleen follows a parallel course to the arterial supply, with segmental veins uniting to form the splenic vein. Ultimately this joins with the superior mesenteric vein to form the portal vein. Efferent lymphatics from the spleen follow the same route.[2] Considerable anatomical variation in the arterial supply and venous drainage of the spleen can occur, and this may have important surgical consequences.

The capsule of the spleen has two layers: an outer serous peritoneal layer and an inner layer of more fibrous material that gives rise to trabeculae extending into the organ towards the hilum. The trabeculae provide support for branches of the splenic artery and vein passing to and from the hilum. The parenchymal tissue of the spleen is organized into red and white pulp within the structural framework provided by the trabeculae and the arteriovenous bundles.

WHITE PULP

Blood entering the spleen from the splenic artery travels along segmental arteries to trabecular arteries, and from there outwards into the parenchyma of the spleen via pencillar arteries and arterioles. These small vessels are sheathed by lymphoid tissue: periarterial lymphoid sheaths.[3] The periarterial lymphoid sheaths contain T lymphocytes and are clearly demarcated from the surrounding red pulp. At intervals along the periarterial lymphoid sheaths, there are expansions of lymphoid tissue forming lymphoid follicles with the same histological characteristics as nodal lymphoid follicles (i.e. germinal centres, mantle zones and marginal zones). The branching arrangement of the pencillar arteries causes some separation of blood components to occur during transit through the spleen. Plasma containing the majority of the white cells is skimmed off laterally into the perpendicular arterioles and is directed towards the marginal zones, where some arteriolar branches terminate. Others containing the red cells that have been propelled forwards discharge into the sinusoids of the red pulp.

RED PULP

The red pulp consists of sinuses and sinusoids lined by endothelial cells. Cellular cords (cords of Billroth) containing resident macrophages separate the sinusoids from each other.[3] Lymphocytes, plasma cells, neutrophils, monocytes and red blood cells circulate through the cords. Blood entering the sinusoids can either return directly to efferent capillaries, and thence leave the spleen quickly (the rapid transit pathway), or first percolate through the cords, resulting in prolonged exposure to phagocytic cells. Cells taking this pathway must also negotiate the basement membrane and endothelial lining of the efferent sinuses if they are to rejoin the general circulation. Red blood cells that do not have the necessary deformability to complete this obstacle course can be detained and destroyed. It appears to be a matter of chance whether abnormal red cells move straight through the spleen in the rapid transit pathway or are directed to the slower route. The spleen has no known way of selecting abnormal cells

REFERENCES

1. Michels NA. Blood Supply and Anatomy of the Upper Abdominal Organs. JB Lippincott, Philadelphia, 1955: 208–210
2. Redmond HP, Redmond JM, Rooney BP et al. Br J Surg 1989; 76: 198–201
3. Wilkins BS, Wright DH. Illustrated Pathology of the Spleen. Cambridge University Press, Cambridge, 2000: 13–17

to percolate through the cords and thus enhance their chances of destruction.

NORMAL SPLENIC FUNCTIONS

Normal splenic functions have been described as follows.[4]

The major function of the spleen is to clear from the blood senescent or defective red cells, micro-organisms and other foreign particles using simple filtration and/or phagocytosis as described earlier.

Red cells that contain inclusion bodies, for example nuclear remnants (Howell–Jolly bodies), denatured haemoglobin (Heinz bodies), siderotic granules or malarial parasites, are not as deformable as normal red cells. Portions of the red cell containing the inclusion bodies can be pinched off as the red cell tries to pass between the endothelial cells to enter the venous sinuses. This process is known as pitting. The red cell membrane rejoins and the cell is returned to the circulation while the inclusion body is phagocytosed.

The spleen also plays a part in immunoregulation and contains the largest collection of lymphoid cells in the body. Immune functions include production of antibody, removal of antigens from the blood, and proliferation of lymphocytes.

In normal human subjects the spleen has a minor role in the storage of red blood cells, storing some 20–30 mL, but this capacity can be increased in certain pathological conditions. The human spleen, unlike that of some animals, does not have the capacity to 'transfuse' the circulation when haemorrhage occurs.

The spleen normally contains a considerable proportion of the body's total platelet mass (around 30%). In conditions causing splenomegaly the proportion of the body's platelet cell mass stored in the spleen can increase to as much as 95%, and this may be associated with peripheral thrombocytopenia.

In comparison with the liver, the spleen plays only a minor role in haematopoiesis in the human fetus. Under normal circumstances there is no haematopoietic function in the adult, but in certain pathological conditions, most notably the myeloproliferative disorders, the spleen is a favoured site for extramedullary haematopoiesis.

Regarding iron reutilization, phagocytic cells remove iron from the haemoglobin of ingested red cells and normally return it to circulating plasma transferrin, the iron transport protein.

ABNORMAL SPLENIC FUNCTION

HYPERSPENISM

Hypersplenism is a term used to describe anaemia, thrombocytopenia or neutropenia in the presence of normal or increased blood cell production by the bone marrow and an enlarged spleen.[5] Almost any cause of splenomegaly may give rise to hypersplenism. The mechanism is multifactorial, and the following factors may all play a role: increased filtration and/or phagocytic activity, increased pooling of cellular blood components, or reduced blood cell lifespan.

HYPOSPLENISM

Hyposplenism is a term that encompasses all causes of reduced splenic function. Clearly patients who have congenital asplenia or those who have had a splenectomy will have hyposplenism. However, there are many other disease states that can lead to reduced splenic function, sometimes in the presence of a normal-sized spleen, for example sickle cell anaemia, various autoimmune conditions, and gastrointestinal disorders such as coeliac disease. The diagnosis may be suggested by examination of a blood film that shows increased numbers of deformed red cells, red cell inclusion bodies and target cells.[6] Patients with functional hyposplenism (that is, those whose spleen is not absent) are at the same increased risk of overwhelming sepsis as those whose spleen is congenitally absent or has been surgically removed.[7]

TRAUMA AND INJURY

Tearing of the spleen most commonly occurs after a closed and blunt abdominal injury, often in association with significant trauma to the chest. The spleen can also be damaged following apparently trivial injury, and spontaneous rupture of the spleen has been described. Damage to the spleen must be carefully considered in any patient who has undergone significant polytrauma, for example following a road traffic accident. Associated injuries in this setting can divert the attention of the attending clinician, and bleeding from a ruptured spleen must always be thought about and excluded. The spleen may rupture spontaneously or after minimal trauma as a result of disease within it, such as vascular malformation, splenic enlargement from malaria and infectious mononucleosis, splenic abscess, and necrosis of treated lymphoma within the spleen.

The spleen is also at risk in surgical operations where the operation field is in close proximity, particularly gastric and pancreatic surgery and occasionally adrenal surgery.

In children and adolescents trauma remains the leading cause of death, accounting for up to 40% of all deaths in those aged 1–15 years in the UK.[8] The recognition that in children splenic trauma can be treated conservatively is gaining support, and there are guidelines designed to identify those individuals who need a laparotomy and those whose condition can be safely managed by observation.[9] Non-operative treatment of children with blunt liver and/or splenic injuries can be recommended provided that haemodynamic stability can be achieved after no more than 40 mL/kg of intravenous fluid replacement.

In children, therefore, a policy of meticulous observation and fluid replacement should be instituted, and laparotomy reserved for those who show evidence of continued bleeding or failure to respond to conservative management. As in the adult, in the stable child with suspected splenic injury, a CT scan will be helpful in identifying those with splenic trauma (Fig. 32.1). Diagnostic peritoneal lavage is insensitive for the exclusive diagnosis of a ruptured spleen (see *Diagnosis and diagnostic procedures* section, p. 768).

REFERENCES

4. Pippard MJ. In: Cuschieri A, Forbes CD (eds). Disorders of the Spleen. Blackwell Science, Oxford, 1994: 30–40
5. Bowdler AJ. Clin Haematol 1983; 12: 467–488
6. Hoffbrand AV, Lewis SM. Postgraduate Haematology. 3rd edn. Blackwell Scientific Publications, Oxford, 1989: 20
7. Working Party of the British Committee for Standards in Haematology – Clinical Haematology Task Force. Br Med J 1996; 312: 430–434
8. Advanced Life Support Group. Advanced Paediatric Life Support. The Practical Approach. 3rd edn. BMJ Publishing, London, 2000
9. Godbole P, Stringer MD. Ann R Coll Surg Engl 2002, 84: 106–108

a
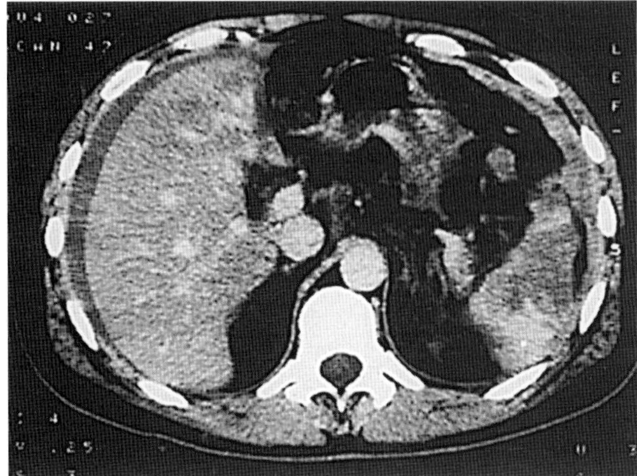

b
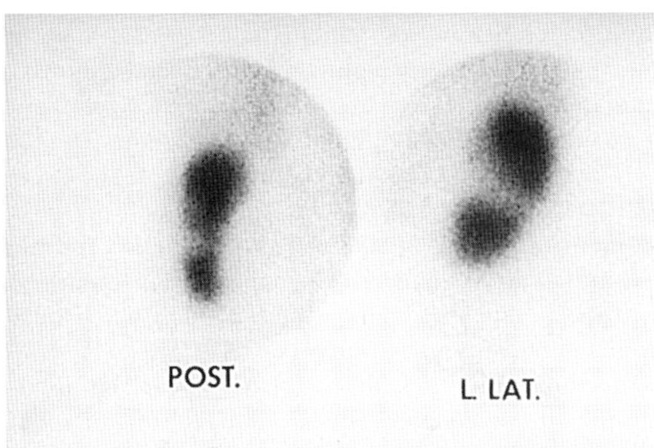

c
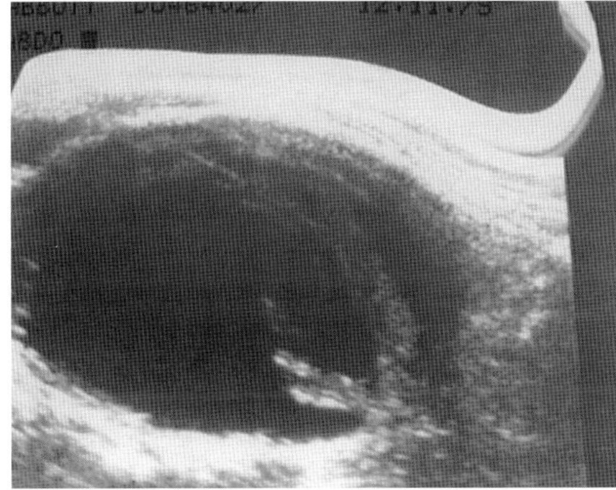

Figure 32.1 Ruptured spleen: (**a**) CT scan; (**b**) isotope scan; and (**c**) ultrasound scan.

CONSERVATIVE MANAGEMENT OF THE RUPTURED SPLEEN IN ADULTS

Patients who are clinically stable following trauma may be suitable for observation and a conservative approach, as favoured in children. Such patients will, by nature of their clinical stability, have been candidates for imaging on suspicion of splenic injury. A CT scan and/or abdominal ultrasound examination are helpful, the former especially so to evaluate other potential damage in the abdomen. Subcapsular haematoma, minimal disruption of the spleen, intrasplenic haematoma and polar tears may all lend themselves to a conservative approach if the patient is clinically stable and other organ damage does not dictate the need for laparotomy. Major disruption of the spleen, evidence of extensive free fluid in the abdomen suggesting significant blood loss despite clinical stability, or other organ damage will tend to mitigate against a conservative approach.

If operation is not immediately required then regular observations of pulse and blood pressure, clinical assessment, and scanning to look for evidence of continued bleeding are mandatory.

Clinical symptoms and signs such as increasing abdominal pain, distension or flank dullness are signs to be wary of. The development of shock, falling blood pressure and urine output, or tachycardia are all warning signs of continued bleeding and should lead to early operative intervention. The decision to abandon a watch policy and move to an operation should be based mainly on clinical grounds, and while repeat scans and blood tests have a role to play they can be unreliable on their own in either confirming or refuting continued bleeding.

Observation should continue for 7 days to exclude delayed bleeding; in practice, patients who have had significant trauma to damage the spleen are commonly going to be observed carefully for such a time in any event. There are no data to inform an evidence base for the decision on when to discharge patients after conservatively managed splenic trauma, but 7–10 days would be in keeping with observations after splenic repair, and the incidence of delayed complications after this time interval is very small.

CLINICAL FEATURES

Disorders of the spleen producing symptoms and signs can present as emergencies (almost exclusively trauma) or in the more common elective setting. Enlargement of the spleen is not always symptomatic, and the old surgical adage that palpable spleens are not always abnormal and abnormal spleens are not always palpable is worth remembering. Where the spleen is enlarged, the patient will often complain of a sense of abdominal fullness. The spleen itself may be a source of pain, and it may press on other organs, inducing early satiety if the stomach is compressed, or significant constipation or change in bowel habit if the colon is compromised. The occasional patient will discover an abdominal mass on self-examination.

Enlarged spleens have an increased risk of infarction. Patients present with acute left hypochondrial pain that may be pleuritic in character and/or associated with fever and referred diaphragmatic shoulder pain. Auscultation may reveal a friction rub. Infarction of the spleen will commonly lead to quite dense adhesions between the spleen and the diaphragm and peritoneum, making operative mobilization difficult. Large infarcts may go on to produce sterile or contaminated abscesses, and spleens enlarged by tumour, which have been treated with chemotherapy, may also develop abscesses as the tumour liquifies in response to treatment.

The large blood flow through a diseased spleen may significantly increase cardiac work and even precipitate cardiac failure.

In addition to symptoms specifically arising from the diseased spleen, patients may have systemic symptoms as a result of the disease process that has caused the splenomegaly. In lymphoma patients additional symptoms may include nocturnal sweating, weight loss, anorexia and itch. If the patient has hypersplenism there may be abnormal bruising and increasing transfusion requirements. Patients suffering from idiopathic thrombocytopenic purpura, HIV infection, haemolytic anaemia, thalassaemia and the leukaemias may all exhibit symptoms related to their underlying primary medical condition.

After trauma to the spleen the physical signs and symptoms can be misleading. Patients with marked abdominal pain and discomfort in the left upper quadrant may have nothing more than chest wall bruising with or without rib fractures, and patients with minimal physical signs and symptoms may have complete disruption of the spleen. In the setting of suspected ruptured spleen the first priority is maintenance of the airway, breathing and circulation; a careful history as to the mechanism of the injury that has taken place; and a thorough clinical examination. In the stable patient immediate transfer for CT scanning of the abdomen, with or without contrast, is the optimal way of making the diagnosis. In the unstable patient a laparotomy, following initial resuscitation, may be both the investigation of choice and the gateway to the ultimate treatment, namely splenic repair or splenic removal. In patients who have multiple injuries, careful consultation with multidisciplinary teams will be necessary to prioritize and coordinate management of the patient.

The patient with splenic trauma and rupture will commonly have signs compatible with shock, namely a low blood pressure and a rapid pulse, and if there is free blood in the peritoneal cavity there will be evidence of marked peritoneal irritation. Unless the spleen is otherwise diseased, it will be unlikely to be palpable in the trauma setting, but the patient will be tender in the left upper quadrant, and significant clot there may also produce dullness, displacement of other organs, and a pseudo-mass effect.

Clinical features of the enlarged, non-ruptured spleen include the presence of a mass arising from beneath the left costal margin, with a palpable notch sometimes felt on its medial border. The mass may extend down towards or even beyond the umbilicus to the right iliac fossa. There will be dullness over the upper abdomen, particularly in the left upper quadrant, and the mass will feel firm and comparatively non-mobile. It can normally be distinguished from a renal mass because it descends on inspiration.

DIAGNOSIS AND DIAGNOSTIC PROCEDURES

The process of diagnosing any condition affecting the spleen begins with a detailed history and a careful physical examination (as described in the previous section). Additional radiological or nuclear medicine investigations may be necessary to reach a definitive diagnosis.

Radiology

Plain abdominal radiographs are of limited value in assessing splenic size, although larger spleens may alter the colonic or gastric gas shadows, or even displace the left kidney inferiorly. Calcification within the spleen can also be noted, but no specific diagnosis can be reached.[10]

Ultrasound (Fig. 32.1c)

Abdominal ultrasound is the test most frequently employed to assess splenic size. Alterations in the echo pattern from the organ may be diagnostic of cysts or tumour deposits.[11] In good ultrasound subjects it may be possible to identify any associated intra-abdominal lymphadenopathy. Doppler studies can give useful information about blood flow in the splenic and portal veins, and after trauma can help in diagnosing rupture of the spleen and free intraperitoneal blood.

Computerized tomography scanning (Fig. 32.1a)

Computerized tomography scanning can readily assess splenic size and volume. Cystic lesions and tumour deposits are readily distinguishable, although a definitive diagnosis of underlying pathology is rarely possible.[11] Computerized tomography scanning is part of the routine staging investigations of many intra-abdominal tumours, in particular lymphomas, and is valuable in diagnosing trauma or disruption of the spleen.

Magnetic resonance imaging

Magnetic resonance imaging is becoming more widely available. However, access to scanners is still limited in some areas. In several studies, MRI has shown promise in assessing splenic (and marrow) involvement by Hodgkin's disease.[12] Prospective studies comparing MRI with CT for diagnosis of other splenic disorders are needed.

Positron emission tomography scanning

Positron emission tomography with 2-fluorine-18-fluoro-2-deoxy-D-glucose is not yet widely available and is therefore not a part of the routine evaluation of patients with splenic disorders. 2-Fluorine-18-fluoro-2-deoxy-D-glucose has been shown to concentrate in both nodal and extranodal lymphoma sites and is useful as a tool in lymphoma staging[13] and restaging.

Radioisotope studies (Fig. 32.1b)

The assessment of splenic uptake of isotope-labelled red blood cells is no longer part of the routine preoperative investigation of a patient with haemolytic anaemia, because it is not a reliable predictor of a good response to surgery.

Presplenectomy, indium-labelled platelets can be used to determine the site of platelet sequestration. Results of splenectomy are better in those patients in whom the spleen is shown to be the major site of consumption, but the investigation is not available in many centres.[14]

Technetium-99-labelled red cells are occasionally employed in the postsplenectomy evaluation of patients with relapsed idiopathic thrombocytopenic purpura to identify accessory splenic tissue that may be amenable to further surgery (Fig. 32.2).

DIFFERENTIAL DIAGNOSIS

Generally speaking, a diseased spleen is always enlarged, although not always palpable. In contrast, a palpable spleen is a relatively common clinical finding that need not necessarily indicate a pathological process. Studies have shown that 3% of normal students and 2% of all adults have palpable spleens.[15] Nevertheless, in the great majority of cases a palpable spleen indicates an underlying pathological process.

There are numerous causes of splenomegaly. A classification is suggested in Box 32.1. In most of the diseases listed the spleen is only modestly enlarged, and in some splenomegaly is only an

REFERENCES

10. Chapman S, Nakielny R. Aids to Radiological Differential Diagnoses. Ballière Tindall, London, 1984: 192
11. Costello P, Kane RA, Oster J et al. J Can Assoc Radiology 1985; 36: 22–28
12. Bangerter M, Griesshammer M, Binder T et al. Ann Oncol 1996; 7 (Suppl 4): 55–59
13. Partridge S, Timothy A, O'Doherty MJ et al. Clin Positron Imaging 1999; 2(6): 323
14. Najean Y, Rain JD, Billotey C. Br J Haematol 1997; 97: 547–550
15. McIntyre OR, Ebaugh FG Jr. Ann Intern Med 1967; 66: 301–306

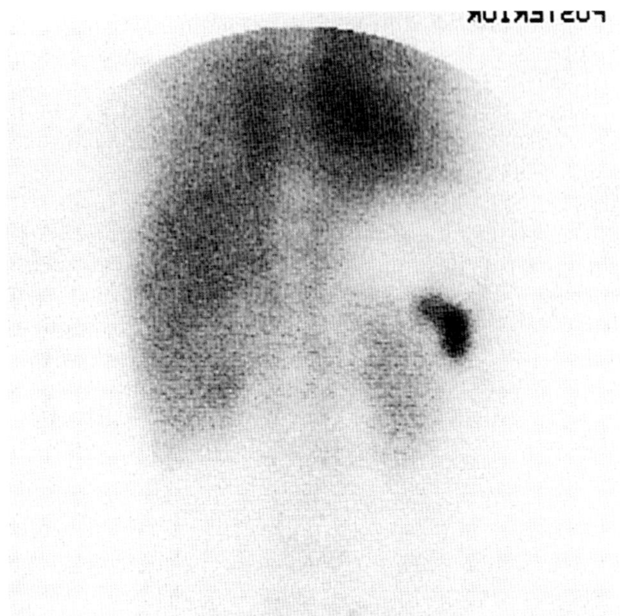

Figure 32.2 Isotope scan showing regrowth of splenic tissue after splenectomy for trauma. Such tissue may derive from implanted cells shed from the ruptured spleen or from hypertrophy of a small accessory spleen.

occasional finding. An asterisk indicates those disorders that are associated with massive splenomegaly, defined as an enlarged spleen extending into one or both lower quadrants.

A detailed description of all disorders listed in Table 32.1 is beyond the scope of this chapter. Only those conditions where splenectomy is indicated for either diagnostic or therapeutic purposes will be described in more detail.

Table 32.1 Disorders of the spleen

Infections
- Acute: infectious mononucleosis, subacute bacterial endocarditis, septicaemia, splenic abscess.
- Chronic: tuberculosis, *malaria, brucellosis, *leishmaniasis (kala-azar), schistosomiasis and hydatid disease

Systemic diseases
- Amyloidosis
- Sarcoidosis
- Collagen vascular disorders, rheumatoid arthritis (Felty syndrome), systemic lupus erythematosis

Storage diseases
- *Gaucher's disease
- Neimann–Pick disease
- Other inborn errors of metabolism disorders

Congestion
- Cirrhosis of the liver
- Budd–Chiari syndrome
- Portal vein thrombosis
- Congestive heart failure

Haematological
- Myeloproliferative disorders: *chronic myeloid leukaemia, *idiopathic myelofibrosis, polycythaemia rubra vera
- Lymphoproliferative disorders: *chronic lymphocytic leukaemia, *prolymphocytic leukaemia, *hairy cell leukaemia, *splenic lymphoma with villous lymphocytes, other malignant lymphomas
- Acute leukaemias
- Haemolytic anaemias: hereditary spherocytosis, hereditary elliptocytosis, pyruvate kinase deficiency, acquired autoimmune haemolytic anaemia
- Idiopathic thrombocytopenic purpura
- *Thalassaemia major
- Sickle cell anaemia (in infants)

Other
- Secondary tumours
- Cysts

*Denotes conditions associated with massive splenomegaly.

Chronic myeloid leukaemia

Chronic myeloid leukaemia is a myeloproliferative disorder affecting predominately patients over the age of 50 years; it is characterized by hepatosplenomegaly, a high peripheral blood white cell count, and a bi- or triphasic course terminating in acute transformation.[16] Median survival is around 5–7 years. The diagnosis is suggested by examination of a peripheral blood film, which will reveal large numbers of mature neutrophils, increased numbers of basophils and some immature white cell precursors.

Cytogenetic examination of peripheral blood or bone marrow for the Philadelphia chromosome will confirm the diagnosis.

Splenectomy is only rarely indicated for relief of pain from repeated splenic infarcts or discomfort related to splenic size in patients with accelerated-phase disease. Splenectomy has no role in the routine management of patients with chronic myeloid leukaemia.[17]

Myelofibrosis (agnogenic myeloid metaplasia)

Myelofibrosis may be a primary myeloproliferative disorder or can arise secondary to polycythaemia rubra vera, essential thrombocythaemia, or chronic myeloid leukaemia. Primary myelofibrosis is a disease of elderly patients, with a median survival of 3–5 years. It presents usually with abdominal discomfort related to massive splenomegaly, early satiety and/or symptoms of anaemia. The majority of patients have associated thrombocytopenia. A peripheral blood film will show aniso-poikilocytosis (variation in the size and shape of the red blood cells), and the presence of immature white cells (myelocytes) and nucleated red blood cells: a leukoerythroblastic picture. Bone marrow aspiration may be impossible, but trephine biopsy will show gross distortion of architecture and deposition of reticulin fibres. The spleen and liver are enlarged by extramedullary haemopoiesis.[18]

Splenectomy will not influence the course of the disease but may be indicated in a minority of patients with debilitating symptoms, for example unacceptable transfusion requirements, splenic pain or high-output cardiac failure.

Chronic lymphocytic leukaemia

Chronic lymphocytic leukaemia is the most common adult leukaemia in western societies. It is a disease of the elderly, 90% of patients being over the age of 50 years at diagnosis.[19] Between 20 and 25% of patients present incidentally during investigation

REFERENCES

16. Kantarjian HM, Deisseroth A, Kurzrock R et al. Blood 1993; 82: 691–703
17. The Italian Cooperative Study Group on Chronic Myeloid Leukemia. Cancer 1984; 54: 333
18. Messinezy M, Pearson TC. Br Med J 1997; 314: 587–590
19. Litz CE, Brunning RD. Baillières Clin Haematol 1993; 6: 767–783

of another problem or after routine blood count at well person screening clinics. Such patients may have few if any abnormal clinical findings, and the only abnormalities on investigation are peripheral blood lymphocytosis and lymphocytic infiltration of the bone marrow.

More advanced cases present with lymph node enlargement, fatigue, weight loss or symptomatic anaemia that is autoimmune in 8% of patients. Easy bruising due to thrombocytopenia may also occur. The thrombocytopenia is secondary to extreme marrow infiltration by leukaemic cells or may be autoimmune in origin. Abdominal examination may reveal mild to moderate splenomegaly.

The clinical course is variable, and treatment is not curative. Therapeutic options include chemotherapy, steroids and occasionally radiotherapy. Splenectomy is indicated only rarely for symptoms associated with splenic size. It can, however, be extremely helpful in controlling the secondary autoimmune complications of haemolytic anaemia or thrombocytopenic purpura.

Pro-lymphocytic leukaemia

Pro-lymphocytic leukaemia is a variant of chronic lymphocytic leukaemia, with distinct clinicopathological features.[19] The typical patient is a middle-aged or elderly man who presents with constitutional symptoms of weight loss and fatigue. There is little or no lymph node enlargement except in those patients with the T-cell variant, but abdominal examination reveals massive splenomegaly. Full blood count shows lymphocytosis, with counts often in the hundreds of thousands. In 75% of cases the cells mark as B cells, and in 25% as T cells.

Response to chemotherapy is disappointing. Splenectomy is often indicated for relief of pain and discomfort related to splenic size. Median survival is 3 years in B-cell disease and 6–9 months in the T-cell subtype.

Hairy cell leukaemia

Hairy cell leukaemia is an uncommon low-grade B-cell lymphoproliferative disorder, accounting for 2% of all adult leukaemias.[20] It occurs in middle-aged patients, and the male:female ratio is 4:1. Presenting symptoms include weight loss, fatigue, abdominal discomfort, early satiety or infection, which may be of an atypical nature. In 25% of cases the diagnosis is made incidentally after routine blood count. Lymph node enlargement is rarely present, but 70–80% of patients have splenomegaly at diagnosis, which may be moderate or massive.

Full blood count shows pancytopenia with absolute neutropenia and monocytopenia. Examination of a blood film may show the typical lymphoid cells with hairy cytoplasmic projections that give the disease its name. The diagnosis is confirmed by demonstrating typical histological appearances on the bone marrow trephine and immunophenotyping the abnormal cells.

Most patients with hairy cell leukaemia used to be treated by splenectomy, but this is no longer the case. The nucleoside analogues pentostatin and cladribine both induce high rates of complete response that may be prolonged, and they have become the treatments of choice. Interferon alpha may be used on a short-term basis in patients with severe pancytopenia to improve the blood count prior to treatment with purine analogues. Splenectomy may still be indicated for a small minority of patients with large spleens and little bone marrow infiltration, or for those with symptomatic splenomegaly who do not respond to primary therapy.

Splenic lymphoma with villous lymphocytes

This syndrome is a disease of the spleen and bone marrow, which has numerous features in common with hairy cell leukaemia. Its incidence and its age and sex distribution are similar to those of hairy cell leukaemia, and patients present with non-specific symptoms and significant, sometimes massive, splenomegaly. However, although there may be features of hypersplenism in the peripheral blood count, there is no significant neutropenia or monocytopenia. Peripheral blood white cell count is typically in the range of $10–30 \times 10^9$ cells/L. A blood film may show the characteristic lymphoid cells with villous projections at one or both poles. The diagnosis is usually confirmed by immunophenotypic studies on the peripheral blood and by histological examination of a bone marrow trephine biopsy.[21] In some cases with little marrow infiltration the diagnosis is made only after splenectomy.

The disease follows an indolent course, and patients are often followed without treatment for extended periods of time. When indicated by progressive symptomatology, splenectomy is the treatment of choice.

Hereditary haemolytic anaemias

Hereditary spherocytosis is the commonest inherited red cell membrane defect. It is usually transmitted as an autosomal dominant. Clinical presentation is very variable, and the condition may be diagnosed at any age.[22] Many cases present in the neonatal period with mild anaemia, jaundice and splenomegaly. The diagnosis is suggested by spherocytes on a peripheral blood film, increased osmotic fragility of the red cells, and a positive family history. The spherocytic red cells are less deformable than normal red blood cells. They become trapped in the splenic cords and are removed by phagocytosis. Pigment gallstones may develop at any age, and aplastic crises can be a feature, particularly with parvovirus B19 infection.

Mild cases require supportive treatment only, for example folic acid supplementation to support the increased red cell turnover. Aplastic crises or severe haemolytic episodes require transfusion support.

Splenectomy should be performed in patients with symptomatic anaemia, but the operation is usually delayed until after the age of 7 years to minimize the risks of postsplenectomy sepsis. Splenectomy improves red cell survival and reduces anaemia but will not cure the underlying red cell defect.

Hereditary elliptocytosis is a heterogeneous group of conditions with variable red cell morphology. Most patients are asymptomatic and compensate their chronic haemolysis well. Severe cases will benefit from splenectomy.

Pyruvate kinase deficiency is an autosomal recessive condition. There is deficiency of the enzyme pyruvate kinase, resulting in a congenital non-spherocytic haemolytic anaemia.[23] The abnormal red cells are culled prematurely by the spleen, leading to chronic

REFERENCES

20. British Committee for Standards in Haematology. Guidelines on Diagnosis and Therapy of Hairy-Cell Leukaemia. BCSH, Darwin folders, 2000
21. Catovsky D, Matutes E. Semin Haematol 1999; 36: 148–154
22. Bolton-Maggs PH. Baillières Best Pract Clin Haematol 2000; 13: 327–342
23. Zanella A, Bianchi P. Baillières Best Pract Clin Haematol 2000; 13: 57–81

haemolysis. The anaemia may be improved by splenectomy, and a family history of response to splenectomy can prove helpful.

Glucose-6-phosphate dehydrogenase deficiency is inherited in an X-linked fashion. The resultant enzyme deficiency leads to acute haemolytic episodes after exposure to certain drugs, infections or after ingestion of fava beans.[24] Although splenomegaly is not a usual clinical finding, splenectomy may occasionally be indicated in cases where haemolytic episodes are frequent and severe.

Autoimmune haemolytic anaemia

This type of anaemia occurs when the body produces antibodies (most frequently those of the IgG subtype) against its own red cells. Red cells coated with antibody are taken up by macrophages of the reticuloendothelial system, particularly in the spleen, and are removed from the circulation. In the laboratory, IgG on the red cells can be detected using an anti-IgG antibody, which causes the coated cells to agglutinate. This is the principle of the diagnostic test for autoimmune haemolytic anaemia: Coombs' test. This type of autoimmune haemolytic anaemia is also called warm antibody autoimmune haemolytic anaemia, because the antibody reacts best with cells at 37°C. Autoimmune haemolytic anaemia may have an associated underlying cause, such as chronic lymphocytic leukaemia, lymphoma, a coexisting autoimmune condition, or ingestion of certain drugs,[25] or it may be idiopathic.

Presentation is highly variable. Patients may be asymptomatic, or severely anaemic and jaundiced. Modest splenomegaly is common. Assuming any underlying cause has been removed (e.g. fludarabine), treatment usually includes steroids and/or intravenous immunoglobulin. Splenectomy is considered for those patients who fail to maintain satisfactory haemoglobin levels with conventional treatments or whose disease relapses frequently.

In cold antibody haemolytic anaemia splenectomy is not indicated.

Immune thrombocytopenic purpura

This condition may be diagnosed in children and adults with a low platelet count and normal bone marrow appearances. Autoantibodies against platelet antigens cause accelerated platelet destruction by phagocytic cells in the liver and spleen. Associated causes, such as coexisting autoimmune conditions, drug ingestion (heparin, quinine and gold), recent transfusion, and HIV infection, should be excluded, particularly in adults. In most cases no underlying cause is identified, and idiopathic thrombocytopenic purpura is diagnosed.

Immune thrombocytopenic purpura presents with easy bruising, mucous membrane bleeding or a purpuric rash. In children there may be a history of a recent viral illness.[26] In the absence of purpura, physical examination is usually normal.

A full blood count will confirm a low platelet count. Platelets may be morphologically normal or increased in size.

In children the disease is frequently self-limiting, and no treatment may be indicated if the platelet count is above 20×10^9cells/L and there are no haemorrhagic manifestations. Between 70 and 80% of children eventually recover spontaneously, but those in whom the disease becomes chronic are treated along the same lines as adults.[27] In adults spontaneous resolution is rare, and in many patients the disease follows a relapsing and remitting course.

For those patients requiring treatment, steroids are the first-line therapy of choice. The majority of patients respond, but only in 15% of adults will it be complete and persisting. Patients failing steroid treatment may go on to receive intravenous gamma globulin, immunosuppression with azathioprine, cyclophosphamide, vincristine, or anti-CD20 monoclonal antibodies.

Splenectomy is reserved for patients remaining symptomatic after failure of other treatments and is only rarely indicated in children. The timing of splenectomy is important; the platelet count should be optimized, vaccination completed, and repeated courses of unsuccessful treatment (e.g. steroids), which may compromise the patient's operative course, should be avoided.

Thalassaemia

The thalassaemias arise as a result of inherited mutations or deletions in the genes coding for the globin chains. The net result is a disturbance in the normal balance of chain production, leading to precipitation of excess chains within the red blood cells. The affected cells either die within the bone marrow or are prematurely removed from the circulation by the spleen. These disorders are common in Mediterranean countries, the Middle East, South-East Asia, India and parts of Africa.

The clinical presentation is determined by the globin chain affected and the number of genes involved.[28]

Production of the α-globin chain is controlled by four genes. Patients may have deletion of one, two, three or all four genes. Deletion of one or two genes leads to a largely asymptomatic carrier state, while deletion of all four genes is a common cause of stillbirth in areas of the world with a high incidence of alpha-thalassaemia. Deletion of three α-genes gives rise to the clinical syndrome of haemoglobin H disease, and such patients occasionally require splenectomy for control of hypersplenism.

Production of the β-globin chain is controlled by two genes. Abnormality in one β-globin gene leads to a carrier state that requires no treatment, whereas abnormality in both genes leads to a severe illness characterized by presentation in early childhood with anaemia and failure to thrive.

The only curative treatment is bone marrow transplantation, but for patients without a suitable donor, regular transfusions to suppress ineffective erythropoiesis should be undertaken. Such a programme allows normal growth and development to occur. Iron overload begins to cause serious problems in the second decade if a rigorous chelation schedule is not instituted. Splenectomy may be indicated for massive splenomegaly or for increasing transfusion requirements.

SPLENIC TUMOURS

A primary tumour presenting in the spleen is an uncommon finding, but occasionally lymphomas of various histological subtypes may present in this fashion. Involvement may be diffuse or as a solid tumour mass. In splenic lymphoma with villous lymphocytes, splenomegaly may be the only clinical finding.

Other tumours that may involve the spleen include malignant haemangiosarcomas, Kaposi's sarcoma and metastases. The

REFERENCES

24. Mehta A, Mason PJ, Vulliamy TJ. Baillières Best Pract Clin Haematol 2000; 13: 21–38
25. Petz LD, Garratty G. Clin Haematol 1975; 4: 181–197
26. Bolton-Maggs PH. Arch Dis Child 2000; 83: 220–222
27. Reid MM. Arch Dis Child 1995; 72: 125–128
28. Weatherall DJ, Provan AB. Lancet. 2000; 335: 1169–1175

incidence of metastatic carcinoma in the spleen is of the order of 4%.[29] The most frequent primary tumours are breast, lung and malignant melanoma.

SPLENIC CYSTS

Splenic cysts are classified as primary (cysts with a proper cyst wall or lining) or secondary (cysts without a proper cyst wall or lining).[30] Primary cysts may be congenital, neoplastic or parasitic.

Congenital cysts can be single or multiple, and are often discovered incidentally during investigation of unrelated symptoms. Other intra-abdominal organs may be similarly affected. The commonest parasitic cause is hydatid disease: *Echinococcus*. Such parasitic cysts may be very slow-growing and largely symptomless. Occasionally they become large enough to cause detectable splenomegaly and abdominal discomfort, or they may rupture into the abdominal cavity. The treatment of choice is splenectomy.

Secondary cysts most commonly arise as a result of trauma or inflammation.[30] They can be of any size, and although usually symptomless can become infected or rupture spontaneously. Some cysts are amenable to resection without the need for total splenectomy.[31]

SPLENIC ABSCESS

In western societies splenic abscesses are rare. They can occur as a result of haematogenous spread from an infection elsewhere in the body, for example bacterial endocarditis or lung abscess. These are classified as secondary splenic abscesses. Alternatively, they may arise primarily in the spleen if a subcapsular haematoma or necrotic tumour becomes infected. Aerobic organisms such as *Streptococcus* and *Staphylococcus* are the most frequently identified pathogens, although in the immunocompromised host more unusual bacteria, yeasts or fungi may be implicated.

The patient presents with fever. Pain in the left hypochondrium or vague abdominal discomfort is present in 40–60% of cases. Splenomegaly is present in around half the patients. Diagnosis is by blood culture and appropriate imaging. Splenectomy has been the treatment of choice, but advances in imaging have made percutaneous drainage a viable alternative, particularly in the patient deemed too elderly or frail for surgery, or in the immunocompromised.[32]

SPLENECTOMY

Splenectomy is normally undertaken as an open operation, but in selected cases in experienced centres may be performed laparoscopically.

It is a truth to say that there is no such thing as an easy splenectomy. In the injured patient with a ruptured spleen there are commonly other injuries, the patient's condition by definition will be unstable, the anatomy is displaced, and anatomical planes are disrupted. The diagnosis and procedure will often be carried out with a degree of haste.

The incision and approach to the injured spleen will depend on the suspicion or knowledge of other intra-abdominal injuries that may need to be dealt with at the same time. A long midline incision is a good starting point, but the operating surgeon should have no hesitation in extending the incision to get good access to the spleen if required. The priority will be to control haemorrhage early in the operation. Adequate suction and lighting are essential, as is adequate assistance. With good exposure, good lighting and suction, a rapid assessment of damage to the spleen can be undertaken, and a decision made as to whether the spleen is repairable or whether it will have to be removed.

Conservation of the spleen should be performed if at all possible. Conserving the spleen may be possible by packing with either absorbable materials, which will remain within the patient, or external packing, which can be removed at a second laparotomy 24 h later. Reported conservation techniques include suture repair of the spleen, partial splenectomy, and wrapping the damaged organ in absorbable mesh (Fig. 32.3).

Success in preserving the spleen will depend largely on the extent of the injury to it and the skill and experience of the operating surgeon. If it is decided that splenectomy is the best course of action, then the spleen may need to be mobilized, although often this has already been achieved as a result of the trauma. Dividing the peritoneum laterally (the lienorenal ligament) allows the spleen to be lifted forwards. Care must be taken in the trauma setting to ensure that no damage occurs to the pancreatic tail or to the stomach wall when the short gastric vessels are secured. Both of these manoeuvres can be difficult if there is a lot of blood clot, retroperitoneal blood or free blood in the peritoneal cavity. A plane of dissection close to the hilum of the spleen should minimize the risk of damaging the pancreas, and gentle and careful dissection under vision should also make damage to other retroperitoneal organs, such as the adrenal gland or the kidney, unlikely (Fig. 32.4).

If the spleen does have to be removed autotransplantation of splenic fragments has been described, but the success of this in producing functioning splenic tissue of future value to the patient is not guaranteed.

At the end of the procedure a closed suction drainage system should be passed down to the splenic bed, and the abdomen should be lavaged and all clot removed.

In elective splenectomy the organ may be enlarged or of normal size. In the former category, a careful history will indicate whether or not the spleen is likely to be adherent through adhesions to the underside of the diaphragm. A history suggestive of splenic infarction should alert the surgeon to the possibility of adhesions between the diaphragm and the surface of the spleen. The incision for splenectomy will depend somewhat on the general habitus of the patient and the position of the enlarged spleen. On occasions a midline incision will be the most appropriate, on others a left subcostal incision may afford the best exposure.

If the spleen is moderately enlarged and not adherent to the diaphragm, then it may be mobilized by dividing its peritoneal attachments posteriorly, thus allowing it to be lifted upwards and the vessels ligated under direct vision. These will include the splenic artery and vein, which may be in several branches, and the short gastric vessels. Dissection for these vessels should remain close to the hilum of the spleen, and care should be taken to

REFERENCES

29. Marymount JH. Am J Clin Pathol 1963; 40: 58–66
30. Dawes LG, Malangoni MA. Am J Surg 1986; 52: 333–336
31. Tagaya M, Oda M, Furihata M et al. Surg Laparosc Endosc Percutan Tech 2002; 12: 279–282
32. Green BT. Am Surg 2001; 67: 1014–1015

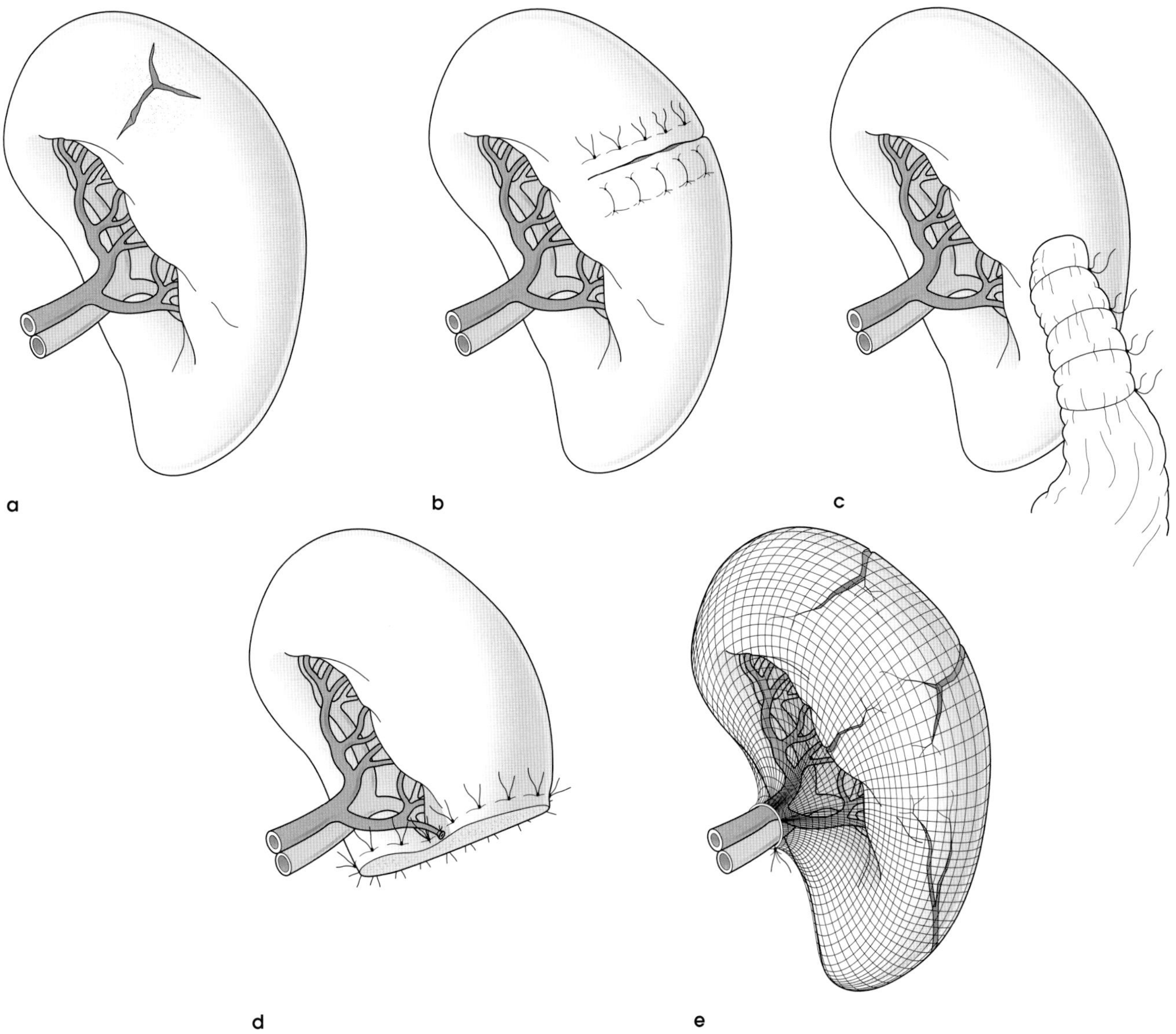

Figure 32.3 Techniques of splenic conservation: (**a**) capsular tear treated with thrombogenic agent; (**b**) rent in spleen closed with deep mattress sutures, buttressed if necessary; (**c**) ragged tear packed with omentum; (**d**) traumatized pole amputated; and (**e**) fragmented spleen packed together in an absorbable mesh bag.

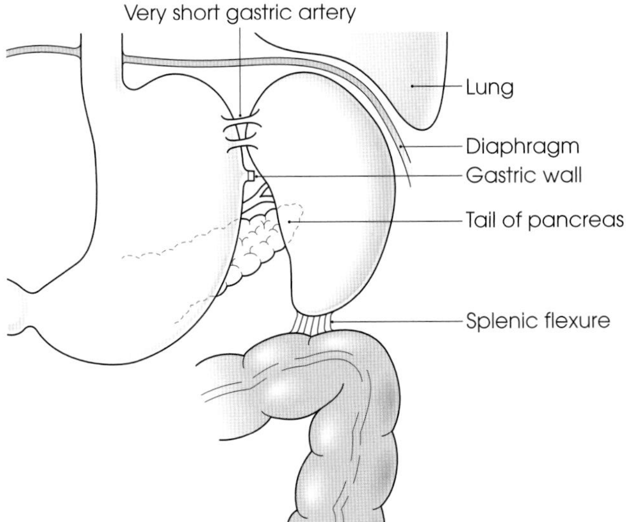

Figure 32.4 Points of danger during excision of a large spleen.

identify the pancreas. This can often be difficult, because of the size and fragility of the vessels in the hilum and also because of occasional coexistent lymphadenopathy around these vessels. The spleen enlargement may be such that it envelops the tail of the pancreas. Meticulous attention to haemostasis, coupled with gentle handling of the tissues, should ensure that the pancreas is clearly seen and protected. Once the vessels of supply have been doubly secured with absorbable ties, preferably in continuity, the spleen can be removed. A closed suction drainage system down to the splenic bed is placed before the wound is closed.

The grossly enlarged spleen or one adherent to the diaphragm may present a major surgical challenge. The optimal approach for such spleens is often first to divide the short gastric vessels so as to obtain access to the lesser sac. The highest short gastric is frequently the largest, shortest and most inaccessible.

Once the lesser sac is entered, the splenic artery may be ligated in continuity and in situ on the upper border of the pancreas. Subsequent manoeuvres to mobilize the spleen are now much less likely to cause dangerous haemorrhage.

In the non-enlarged spleen the patient may well be undergoing the operation because of a clotting or haematological disorder, which can further add to the demands of the operation. Correction of clotting factors, transfusion of platelets and availability of blood should be ensured, as in all cases of splenectomy, and the spleen mobilized by dividing the peritoneal attachments laterally and posteriorly and lifting it forwards. Careful display of the hilar vessels with ligation in continuity is advised to minimize the risk to the pancreas, and securing the short gastric vessels, ensuring that the stomach wall is well clear of the ligatures, is also essential.

When splenectomy is performed for haematological diseases, a search should be made for accessory spleens in the gastrocolic omentum and along the line of the splenic vein. Points of danger during excision of a large spleen are shown in Fig. 32.4.

LAPAROSCOPIC SPLENECTOMY

First reported in 1991, laparoscopic splenectomy is now firmly established in the repertoire of operations on the spleen. The development of technology and instrumentation to achieve this has been a major part in the success story of laparoscopic splenectomy, and for the patient the advantages are less pain, reduced hospital stay, and possibly reduced risk of adhesions in later life.[33] Typical operating times are around 120 min, length of stay postoperatively 2 days, and conversion to open operation occurs in less than 5% of cases in experienced hands.[34] Laparoscopic splenectomy has been shown in several series to be equal in efficacy to the open operation, and complication rates are equivalent between the two procedures, 5% of cases developing minor complications that resolve spontaneously and 5% potentially life-threatening complications that require intervention (iatrogenic injuries and bleeding).[33]

Most of the indications for splenectomy are suitable for laparoscopic splenectomy,[35] although most authors advise caution in the massive spleens and the shocked patient with trauma. Early ligation of the splenic artery and hand-assisted techniques may facilitate laparoscopic splenectomy in the very large spleen.

Use of an endoscopic stapling device with a vascular cartridge (e.g. the Endo GIA 30-2.5 mm, US Surgical Corporation, or the Endopath 35-2.5 mm, Ethicon Endosurgery) is advised for the vessels in the splenic hilum. The principles of laparoscopic splenectomy are otherwise similar to those of the open operation, namely division of splenocolic and lienorenal ligaments, the lienogastric ligaments, the short gastric vessels and the main vascular pedicle. A careful search for accessory spleens should be undertaken. Use of the harmonic ultrasonic scalpel (LCS, Ethicon Endosurgery) allows careful haemostasis and dissection to proceed synchronously. For laparoscopic splenectomy the patient will usually be best positioned in the right lateral decubitus position, and the 12-mm ports placed close to the umbilicus for the camera and either side of this for the main operating instruments, but close to the costal margin to permit access to the dome of the diaphragm. At the end of the procedure the spleen can be fragmented in a bag to facilitate removal, or if histology is vital then an incision made to remove it.

COMPLICATIONS

Complications of splenectomy can be classified as immediate or delayed.

Immediate complications

In the short term haemorrhage and haematoma are significant risks. This is particularly so if the patient has a coexisting haematological abnormality. Bleeding postoperatively may lead to a collection in the subphrenic space and subsequent development of a subphrenic abscess.

Damage to organs anatomically close to the position of the spleen can occur. Part of the stomach wall may be incorporated in the ties securing the short gastric vessels, and damage to the pancreas can occur as a result of its close proximity to the hilum of the spleen. Splenic vein and ultimately portal vein thrombosis can occur through propagated clot along the splenic vein. The area of dissection in the region of the left hemidiaphragm can reduce movement of the diaphragm, particularly if there have been adhesions there, and thus increase the risk of atelectasis of the basal part of the left lung, with subsequent chest infection. Postoperative pancreatitis can occur due to mobilization of the pancreas, even if the integrity of that gland is intact. Gastric stasis can occur as a result of handling of the stomach and ligation of the short gastric vessels, and it is good practice, therefore, to have a nasogastric tube inserted for the first 24 h postoperatively.

The inevitable rise in platelet count following splenectomy, for whatever reason, leads to an increased thromboembolic risk of deep venous thrombosis and pulmonary embolism, especially in elderly or immobile patients. A careful check should be made of the platelet count in the postoperative period, but intervention is rarely necessary because the count usually corrects itself given time. The leukocyte count may also rise dramatically, and care must be taken not to misinterpret this as sepsis.

Wound infection and breakdown should be uncommon following splenectomy but, as with any operation, can occur. Prolonged ileus and adhesion formation are uncommon, given the position of the organ in relation to the other abdominal contents.

In the long term the most serious risk of splenectomy remains overwhelming postsplenectomy sepsis. The syndrome probably occurs at the rate of 1–2% in children splenectomized for trauma and 0.5% or less for adults.[7]

A seemingly innocuous illness can develop very rapidly into a fulminating and rapidly fatal illness complicated by disseminated intravascular coagulation. The risk is highest in small children, and hence the need to delay therapeutic splenectomy in some inherited disorders until the risk lessens with age.

Infections caused by capsulated organisms, namely the meningococci, *Haemophilus* species and the pneumococci, are the most dangerous and life-threatening, but all febrile infections should be treated seriously and antibiotics started promptly. The British Committee for Standards in Haematology guideline recommends preoperative vaccination against *Pneumococcus*, *Haemophilus influenzae* B and *Meningococcus* C in the elective setting and as soon as possible postoperatively in the emergency setting. Patients should also be advised to remain on prophylactic lifelong penicillin at a dose of 250 mg twice daily to minimize the risk, and dental work should be covered with additional antibiotics. Erythromycin can be used in patients who are penicillin-sensitive. The patient's name should be added to the splenectomy register, and an alert card issued that should be

REFERENCES

33. Rescoria EJ. Semin Paediatr Surg 2002; 11; 226–232
34. Park AE, Birgisson G, Mastrangelo MJ et al. Surgery 2000; 126: 660–667
35. Rosen M, Brody RM, Walsh M et al. Surg Endosc 2002; 16: 272–279

carried at all times. Patients are advised to have an influenza vaccination every year.

CLINICAL OUTCOMES

When a patient with an enlarged spleen has symptoms and splenectomy is performed, the desired clinical outcome could include abolition of constitutional or systemic symptoms, pain relief, and improvement in appetite and performance score. Reduction in transfusion requirements in the hypersplenic patient can significantly improve quality of life, because the patient is no longer tied to such a rigorous programme of hospital attendances. In such instances the primary intention of surgery is not to extend life, but to make it more tolerable by relief of symptoms.

In other circumstances splenectomy is performed for diagnostic purposes, and here the main positive outcome is an accurate diagnosis for the patient and thence appropriate treatment.

In conditions such as splenic lymphoma with villous lymphocytes, hairy cell leukaemia or prolymphocytic leukaemia, splenectomy is a valuable debulking exercise that can increase survival and abrogate the need, albeit temporarily, for other therapeutic strategies.

In patients with autoimmune haemolytic anaemia who fail steroids, splenectomy should be seriously considered. Splenectomy removes the principal site of red cell destruction, and although antibody still coats the red cells, fewer of them are destroyed, and transfusion requirements are reduced or abolished as the haemoglobin rises. Approximately two-thirds of patients have a complete or partial response to splenectomy.

In idiopathic thrombocytopenic purpura, response rates to splenectomy vary from 50 to 92% in reported series.[36] It remains controversial whether preoperative prediction of splenic sequestration of platelets has a role in patient management. Around 10% of patients relapse after an initially successful splenectomy, usually within the first year. However, long-term outlook may still remain good, with a substantial proportion of patients eventually recovering a clinically useful platelet count.

Surgery for splenic tumours, cysts and abscesses is curative if the lesions are confined to the spleen. Careful preoperative evaluation should establish which patients will benefit from splenectomy, and a multidisciplinary approach including surgeons, haematologists, anaesthetists, pathologists and radiologists should ensure correct case selection and good clinical outcomes.

REFERENCES

36. Karpatkin S. Lancet 1997; 349: 1531–1536

Lymphoma

33

Adrian R. Timothy, Paul A. Fields

INTRODUCTION

The lymphomas are relatively uncommon and account for less than 5% of all new malignancies diagnosed annually in the UK. However, they hold a far greater importance than their incidence suggests due to recent advances made in classification, biology and treatment. Over the past 10 years the classification has been refined and facilitated by advances in diagnostic techniques, and treatment options are increasing with the advent of immunotherapies.

There are two principal forms of lymphoma, namely Hodgkin's disease and the non-Hodgkin's lymphomas. Each group has different histological appearances and clinical manifestations, demanding different approaches to their management. They are therefore discussed separately in this chapter. Additionally, site-specific lymphomas are discussed as the final part of this review.

HODGKIN'S DISEASE

In western countries, Hodgkin's disease accounts for approximately 1% (annual incidence approximately two in 100 000) of newly diagnosed cancers. Over the past two decades there has been a slight increase in incidence, but this has been accompanied by a clear reduction in mortality, reflecting the increasing success of treatment. The disease demonstrates a classic bimodal age incidence (Fig. 33.1).[1] Although uncommon in children, the incidence reaches a peak in the late teens and mid twenties, and falls during the middle years but increases again with advancing age, particularly in the male population. The disease is more common in men and in higher social classes.

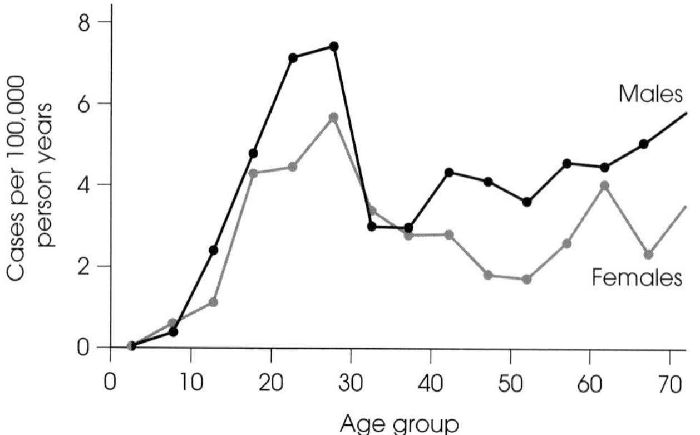

Figure 33.1 Age-specific incidence rates for Hodgkin's disease.

Epidemiological work suggests that Hodgkin's disease may occur as an unusual effect of infection with a common virus. In young people the increased risk is associated with factors that increase susceptibility to common childhood infections, such as higher social class, smoking in families and later birth position.[2] This is not the case for older patients with the disease. Despite reports of clustering of cases, there is no evidence at the present time that Hodgkin's disease is contagious.

PATHOLOGY

The aetiology of Hodgkin's disease has been debated for many years since the original description of the disease by Thomas Hodgkin in 1832.[3] There is an ongoing debate about whether Hodgkin's disease is a true malignancy or whether it represents an atypical response to infection. The debate centres around the possible association of Hodgkin's disease with Epstein–Barr infection, which can be detected in up to 40% of cases. Additionally, the cell origin of the Reed–Sternberg cell (Fig. 33.2) has proved a source of debate, although clonality studies suggest that the cell is derived from the B-cell lineage.[4]

Interestingly, in many cases of Hodgkin's disease malignant cells form only a small proportion of the tumour, the rest being made up of lymphocytes, granulocytes, macrophages, eosinophils and fibrous tissue. This is due in part to the wide variety of cytokines secreted, which act as stimulants and growth factors that attract these cells. These cytokines also mediate many of the systemic features observed in this disease.

The characteristic malignant cells are the mononuclear Hodgkin's cells, which by themselves are insufficient to establish the diagnosis, and the definitive binucleate or multinucleate Reed–Sternberg cells. Reed–Sternberg cells are not pathognomonic of Hodgkin's disease, however, and have been identified in certain virus infections, for example infectious mononucleosis and postvaccinial lymphadenopathy, and in drug reactions, especially to phenylhydantoins.[5] Nevertheless it is essential to identify Reed–Sternberg cells to establish a diagnosis of Hodgkin's disease. At the Ann Arbor Symposium in 1971, it was agreed that where there is a firm diagnosis of Hodgkin's disease, the presence of Reed–Sternberg cells is not essential to the diagnosis if there are mononuclear Hodgkin's cells in an appropriate cellular

REFERENCES

1. Gutersohn N, Cole P. N Engl J Med 1981; 304: 136
2. Mueller NE. In: Selby P, McElwain TJ (eds). Hodgkin's Disease. Blackwell Scientific Publications, Oxford, 1987: 68–93
3. Hodgkin T. Med Chir Trans 1832; 17: 68–114
4. Kuppers R, Rajewsky K et al. Proc Natl Acad Sci USA 1994; 91: 10962–10966
5. Sloane JP. Baillières Clin Haematol 1987; 1: 1–44

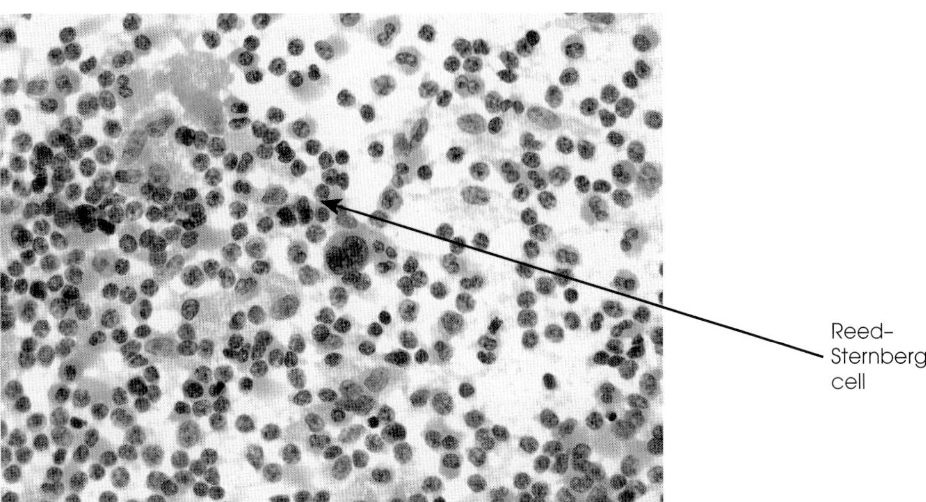

Figure 33.2 Reed–Sternberg cell.

environment.[6] In the absence of either mononuclear cells or Reed–Sternberg cells the disease should not be diagnosed.

CLASSIFICATION

The most recent clinicopathological literature is dominated by the Rye classification system published in 1966.[7] This system is a modification of the preceding Lukes–Butler classification, which was based on the idea of varying host responses to the malignant Reed–Sternberg cells as judged by the number of lymphocytes and other reactive cells. The advent of immunophenotyping has facilitated a stricter diagnosis of Hodgkin's disease, and as a result has led to a decrease in the number of erroneous diagnoses. A major change has been the recognition of the importance of the distinction between lymphocyte-predominant Hodgkin's disease and the other types (classical Hodgkin's disease). Therefore five histopathological entities are now described, lymphocyte-predominant disease differing in histological characteristics, the immunophenotype of the malignant cells, and clinical behaviour:

- Lymphocyte-predominant Hodgkin's disease
- Classical Hodgkin's disease: nodular sclerosing, mixed cellularity, lymphocyte-rich or lymphocyte-depleted

Lymphocyte-predominant Hodgkin's disease

Lymphocyte-predominant Hodgkin's disease is an unusual type of Hodgkin's disease and accounts for 3–5% of all cases. This form differs in its histological characteristics, the immunophenotype of the malignant cells, and its clinical behaviour. Classic Reed–Sternberg cells are usually absent or exceedingly rare. The neoplastic cells are called L and H (or popcorn) cells. They have a lobulated contour that looks like popcorn, dispersed chromatin and vague or inconspicuous nucleoli.

Classical Hodgkin's disease

The universally accepted pathological classification of Hodgkin's disease is based on the Rye system published in 1966.[7] The Rye classification describes four histological subtypes:

- Nodular sclerosing (65–70% of all Hodgkin's lymphoma). This type is characterized by thickening of the lymph node capsule together with interconnecting bands of collagenous connective tissue. Lacunar cells (variants of Reed–Sternberg cells) are found in nearly all cases of nodular sclerosing Hodgkin's disease but are not exclusive to the nodular sclerosing subtype.
- Mixed cellularity (20% of all Hodgkin's lymphoma). Here the appearances are variable. This subgroup includes those cases that lack sclerosis but have too many Reed–Sternberg cells to be classified as lymphocyte-predominant.
- Lymphocyte-rich (5% of all Hodgkin's lymphoma). This is relatively uncommon. Reed–Sternberg cells are rare and the predominant cells in the lymph node are lymphocytes or histiocytes, or a mixture of the two.
- Lymphocyte-depleted (1–2% of all Hodgkin's lymphoma). There are two variants of lymphocyte-depleted Hodgkin's disease – diffuse fibrosis and reticular – which tend to show general cellular depletion, although with the presence of numerous Reed–Sternberg cells. Both types may be present in the same section.

The features of classical-type Hodgkin's disease are as follow.

- Morphology: classical- or lacunar-type Reed–Sternberg cells in a background of T and B lymphocytes, macrophages and eosinophils. Nodular formation and fibrosis characterize the nodular scelerosing types.
- Immunophenotype: $CD30^+$, $CD15^+$, $CD45^-$, $CD3^-$ and $BLA36^+$. Rosettes of adherent T cells are often present.
- Cytogenetic: no specific abnormality
- Pattern of disease: contiguous nodal spread beginning in the neck or mediastinum.

The distinct histopathological differences between lymphocyte-predominant and classical Hodgkin's disease are described in Table 33.1.

CLINICAL FEATURES

Lymphocyte-predominant Hodgkin's disease

Most cases present with cervical lymphadenopathy, which may be localized and of large size. Few patients show disease progression beyond stage II. If there is evidence of infiltration of the spleen or marrow, the diagnosis should be carefully reviewed, with T cell-rich B-cell lymphoma being the main differential diagnosis.

REFERENCES

6. Carbone PP, Kaplan HP et al. Cancer Res 1971; 31: 1860–1861
7. Lukes RJ, Craver LF et al. Cancer Res 1966; 26: 1311

Table 33.1 Comparison of phenotypes of classical and lymphocyte-predominant Hodgkin's lymphoma

Phenotypes	Classical Hodgkin's lymphoma Reed–Sternberg cells	Lymphocyte-predominant Hodgkin's lymphoma atypical lymphocytic and histiocytic cells
CD20	Rarely positive	Usually positive
Other B-cell antigens	Usually negative	Usually positive
CD30	Positive	Negative
CD15	Usually positive	Negative
Immunoglobulin expression	Absent	Present

Lymphocyte-predominant Hodgkin's disease may occur at any age, although the median age of onset is in the fourth decade, with a small number of cases described in young children.

Classical Hodgkin's disease

The usual presenting feature is painless enlargement of lymph nodes with single sites usually located in the cervical and supraclavicular area. About two-thirds of patients have a mediastinal mass at presentation, with the most common association being the nodular sclerosing phenotype. In some patients the diagnosis is made following the discovery of a symptomless mediastinal mass on routine chest radiograph (Fig. 33.3). The disease spreads contiguously to adjacent nodes, with late involvement of bone marrow and extranodal sites.

In making the diagnosis, the pattern of disease at presentation should be considered together with the biopsy features. Approximately one-third of patients present with systemic B symptoms, which include weight loss, fever and drenching night sweats. Generalized pruritus, and occasionally pain in involved sites following alcohol ingestion, is also reported: this occurs as a consequence of eosinophilic degranulation by alcohol. The fever may be intermittent, with a prolonged afebrile period separating febrile episodes. However, the classic manifestation of Hodgkin's disease, so-called Pel–Ebstein fever, is rare. Other rarer presentations include pericardial tamponade from pericardial effusion, bone pain from bony involvement, superior venal caval obstruction, and flank or back pain from retroperitoneal adenopathy. Paraneoplastic syndromes may also be seen, including hypercalcaemia, dermatological lesions (erythema nodosum and dermatomyositis), and neurological syndromes (Guilllain–Barré).

Noted laboratory abnormalities include thrombocytosis, granulocytosis, eosinophilia, raised erythrocyte sedimentation rate and anaemia. When there are atypical features the clinical course and response to treatment may be unpredictable. Additionally, the diagnosis should be reconsidered if the patient has early-stage nodal disease but evidence of bone marrow, splenic or hepatic infiltration. Experienced histological review is required to differentiate between Hodgkin's disease, anaplastic lymphoma or T-cell–rich B-cell lymphoma. Infradiaphragmatic presentations are uncommon and account for approximately 10% of patients with clinically localized disease. Extranodal presentation is rare, occurring in less than 5% of all cases. The diagnosis is confirmed in the majority of cases by lymph node biopsy. Where there is no evidence of lymph node enlargement, great care must be taken in establishing a diagnosis of classical Hodgkin's disease based on tissue obtained from other sources. All new cases should be reviewed at a multidisciplinary team meeting.

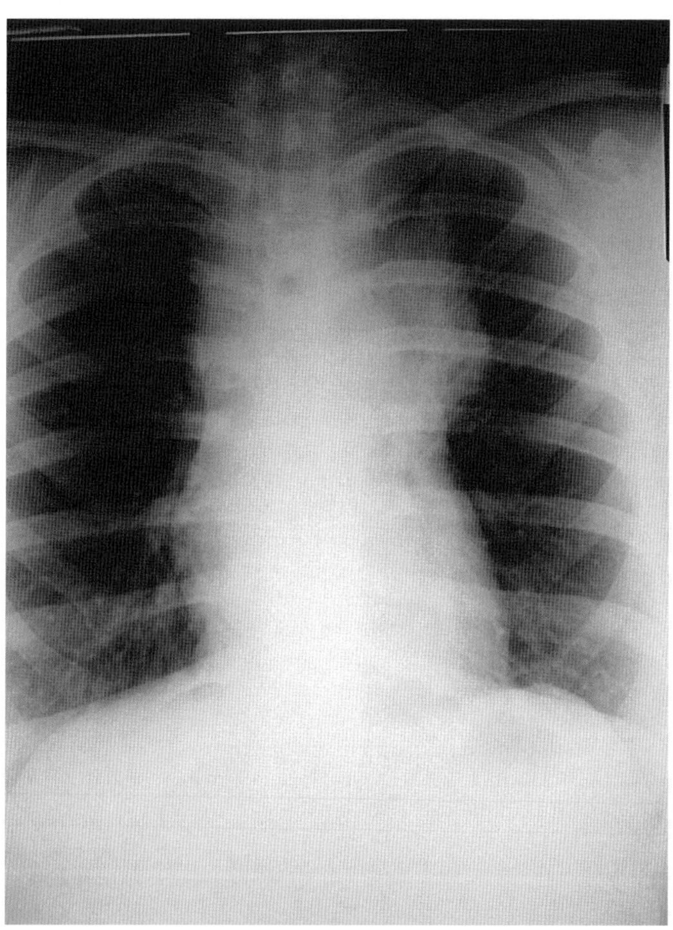

Figure 33.3 Chest X-ray of a patient with Hodgkin's disease, demonstrating extensive mediastinal lymphadenopathy.

AETIOLOGY

No consistent genetic abnormalities have been found in Hodgkin's disease, which underscores the model of genetic instability as one pathogenic factor in Hodgkin's disease.

PATHOGENESIS

The ability to isolate individual Hodgkin Reed–Sternberg cells from frozen lymph node sections has facilitated molecular studies and genetic analysis on these cells. This has confirmed the monoclonal B-cell origin of Reed–Sternberg cells; however, the mechanism of transforming events is unclear. Cytogenetic abnormalities can be demonstrated, and although these are not consistent they may represent a pathogenetic factor in this disorder.

Patients who have had infectious mononucleosis have a two- or threefold increased risk of developing Hodgkin's disease. Elevated IgG and IgA titres against viral capsid antigen have been shown to be correlated with an increased risk for Hodgkin's disease. Weiss and colleagues were the first to demonstrate Epstein–Barr virus DNA in lymph nodes affected with Hodgkin's disease using southern blotting.[8] Epstein–Barr virus infection can be demonstrated in about 50% of the population in industrialized countries and 95% in developing countries.

The pattern of expression of viral proteins and its relationship to the cellular fractions present in the lymph nodes is interesting. Epstein–Barr virus-positive Reed–Sternberg cells express the viral latent membrane protein (LMP) with transforming as well as T-cell immunogenic functions. Activated T lymphocytes (helper cells) represent the majority of lymphocytes surrounding the Hodgkin Reed–Sternberg cells. The Hodgkin Reed–Sternberg cells themselves all express the necessary accessory molecules needed for T-cell recruitment. In the initial stages of the disease, a pronounced but inefficient T-cell reaction against a target antigen (LMP in Epstein–Barr virus-positive cases) expressed on Hodgkin Reed–Sternberg cells seems to take place.

Characterization of the Reed–Sternberg cell

The mononuclear cells and their polymorphonuclear counterparts, the Reed–Sternberg cells, are considered to represent the malignant cell of classical Hodgkin's disease, which incorporates the NS subtype, the MC subtype and the lymphocyte-depleted subtype. Hodgkin Reed–Sternberg cells represent only 0.10–1.0% of the entire cell population in classical Hodgkin's disease and express the activation markers Ki-1 (CD30), the Leu-M1 antigen (CD15), the interleukin receptor (CD25), the transferrin receptor (CD71) and HLA class II molecules, but not surface antigens, which might otherwise help to determine the cell of origin.

STAGING

The Ann Arbor classification (Table 33.2), which defines four principal stages of spread of Hodgkin's disease, has provided a useful basis for management and enabled comparisons to be made between treatment schedules from different centres and individuals. It is apparent, however, that within individual stages defined by the Ann Arbor system, prognosis is influenced by a variety of clinical factors. For example, the extent of mediastinal involvement in patients with stage II disease is crucial in determining whether or not such patients may be cured by radiotherapy; where the mass exceeds one-third of the thoracic diameter, high relapse rates occur with radiotherapy alone. Similarly, the number of lymph node sites involved, the presence or absence of systemic symptoms, and the extent of abdominal disease may all have an adverse influence on prognosis within a given stage. Any definition of stage must therefore take into account not only the anatomical distribution of disease but also these other clinical features. The management is determined on the basis of the 'complete' clinical picture.

Over the past few years the staging approach to Hodgkin's disease has become simplified as most treatment protocols involve patients receiving systemic chemotherapy at the outset. This, coupled to the development of more sophisticated and sensitive imaging techniques such as CT gallium and positron emission tomography scanning, has removed the requirement for intensive pathological staging procedures such as surgical laporotomy, and in particular has rendered splenectomy obsolete in the staging process.

Table 33.2 The Ann Arbor staging system and later amendments

Term	Definition
Stage I	Disease in one lymph node area only
Stage II	Disease in one or more lymph node areas on the same side of the diaphragm
Stage III	Disease in lymph node areas on both sides of the diaphragm (the spleen is considered to be nodal)
Stage III_1	Involvement of splenic, coeliac or portal nodes*
Stage III_2	Involvement of para-aortic, iliac or mesenteric nodes*
Stage IV	Extensive disease in liver, bone marrow or other extranodal sites
Substage E	Localized extranodal disease
Symptom status A	Absence of fevers, sweats or weight loss
Symptom status B	Unexplained fevers (> 38°C), drenching night sweats, weight loss > 10% in preceding 6 months
Bulk	Mediastinal mass greater than one-third of the maximum diameter of the chest*, nodal mass > 10 cm

*Cotswold classification.

INVESTIGATIONS

History and physical examination

The introduction of increasingly sophisticated imaging techniques has tended to overshadow the fundamental value of a detailed history and thorough physical examination in patients with Hodgkin's disease. For example, the presence of significant symptoms, including weight loss of more than 10% over the preceding 6 months, unexplained fever of greater than 38°C and drenching night sweats, invariably relegates an individual to the B category of the Ann Arbor classification, implying a poorer prognosis and thereby allocation to more intensive first-line therapy. Similarly, careful documentation of all clinical sites of involvement (including Waldeyer's ring) not only provides a measure of predicted response to treatment but more importantly may allow, by a simple biopsy procedure, confirmation of more extensive spread of disease. Such information may determine a change in management from localized to systemic therapy, thereby avoiding further unnecessary (and often unpleasant) staging investigations.

Clinical assessment of the spleen is unreliable. An enlarged spleen may not be involved, while approximately 30% of clinically or radiologically normal spleens are found to be infiltrated when examined after splenectomy.

Laboratory investigation

In the majority of untreated cases the blood count is normal. Anaemia is uncommon at presentation; when present it suggests bone marrow involvement and the need for a bone marrow trephine examination. A proportion of patients will have a

REFERENCES

8. Weiss LM, Movahed LA. N Engl J Med 1989; 320: 502

neutrophil leukocytosis, which appears to have no prognostic significance; however, lymphopenia may be associated with a poor prognosis. Eosinophilia is occasionally seen but is of no prognostic significance. The erythrocyte sedimentation rate is elevated in 30–50% of cases, often in association with B symptoms, and can provide a useful marker for assessing remission and relapse.

Abnormalities of liver function tests, particularly elevation of alkaline phosphatase levels, may be found at the time of presentation of Hodgkin's disease without liver involvement. Experience has demonstrated the poor correlation of parenchymal liver involvement with liver size or tests of liver function, and every effort should therefore be made to obtain tissue for histological confirmation before therapy when involvement is suspected.[9] The serum lactate dehydrogenase is a useful marker, which when elevated indicates the degree of tumour bulk. Impairment of renal function, either by direct infiltration or secondary to obstructive nephropathy or nephrotic syndrome, is extremely uncommon at presentation, as is hypercalcaemia.

Bone marrow examination

Bone marrow involvement occurs in between 5 and 15% of previously untreated cases of Hodgkin's disease and automatically indicates stage IV disease. Marrow involvement is closely associated with the presence of systemic (B) symptoms, anaemia and a raised alkaline phosphatase level. The focal nature of bone marrow infiltration and the high incidence of associated fibrosis require a bone marrow trephine biopsy to be performed, because marrow aspiration alone is of very limited value. Bilateral biopsies or the use of wide-bore biopsy needles significantly increase the likelihood of a positive yield.

Chest radiograph

Hodgkin's disease frequently affects the mediastinum, although this is often in association with cervical or supraclavicular lymph-

REFERENCES

9. Filly RA, Marglin S, Castellino RA. Cancer 1976; 38: 2143–2148

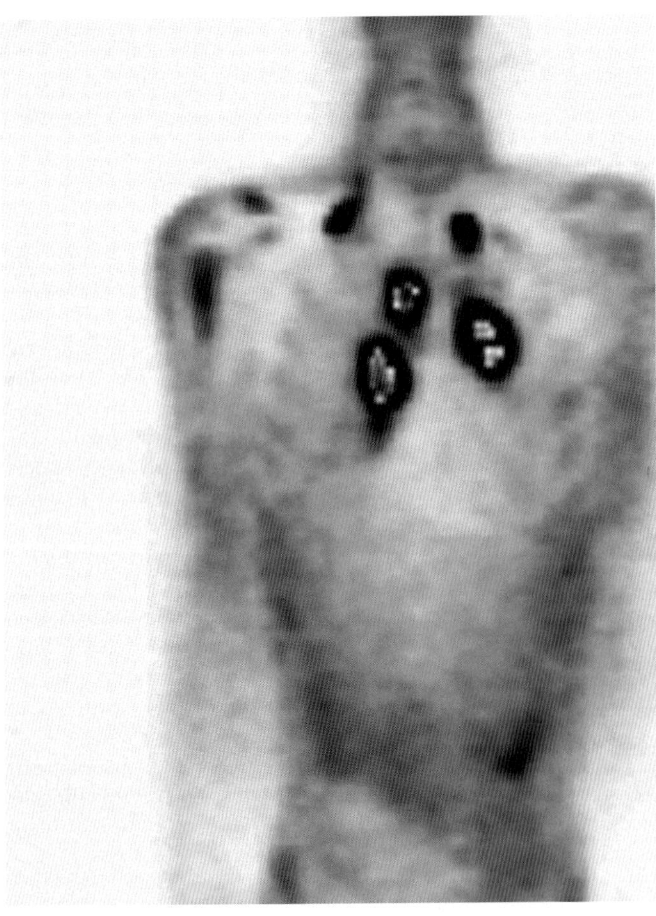

a

Figure 33.4 (a) Mediastinal uptake in Hodgkin's disease. This investigation is especially useful when trying to detect whether masses post treatment are active. A patient with stage II Hodgkin's disease (**b(i)**) pretreatment. *Continued*

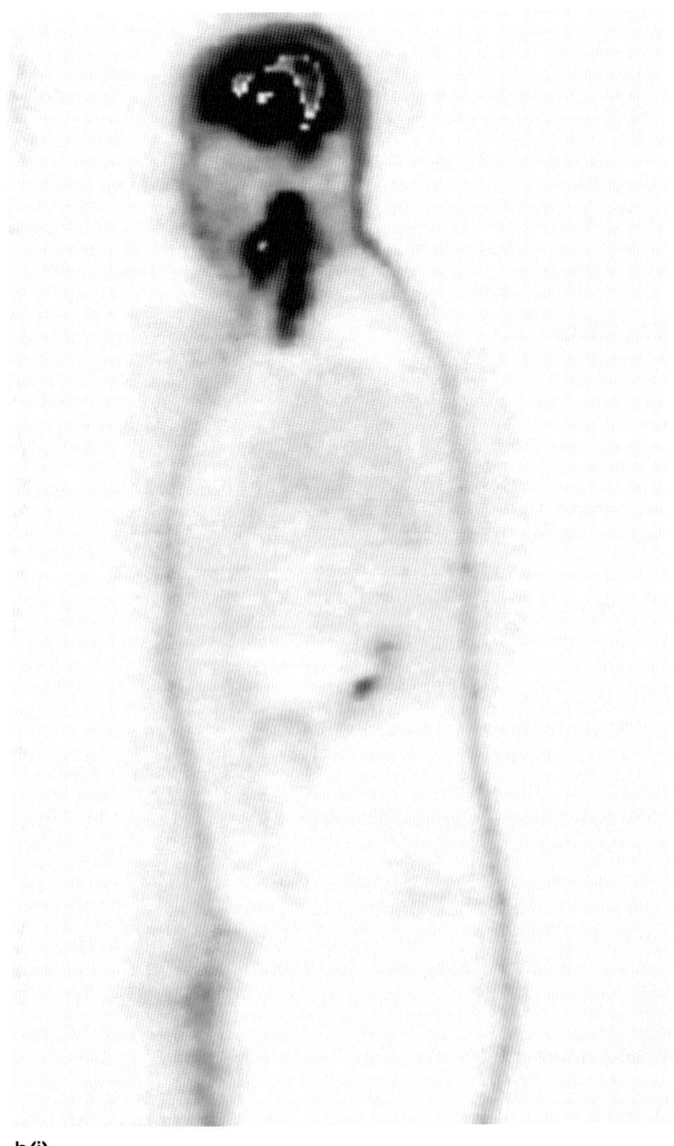

b(i)

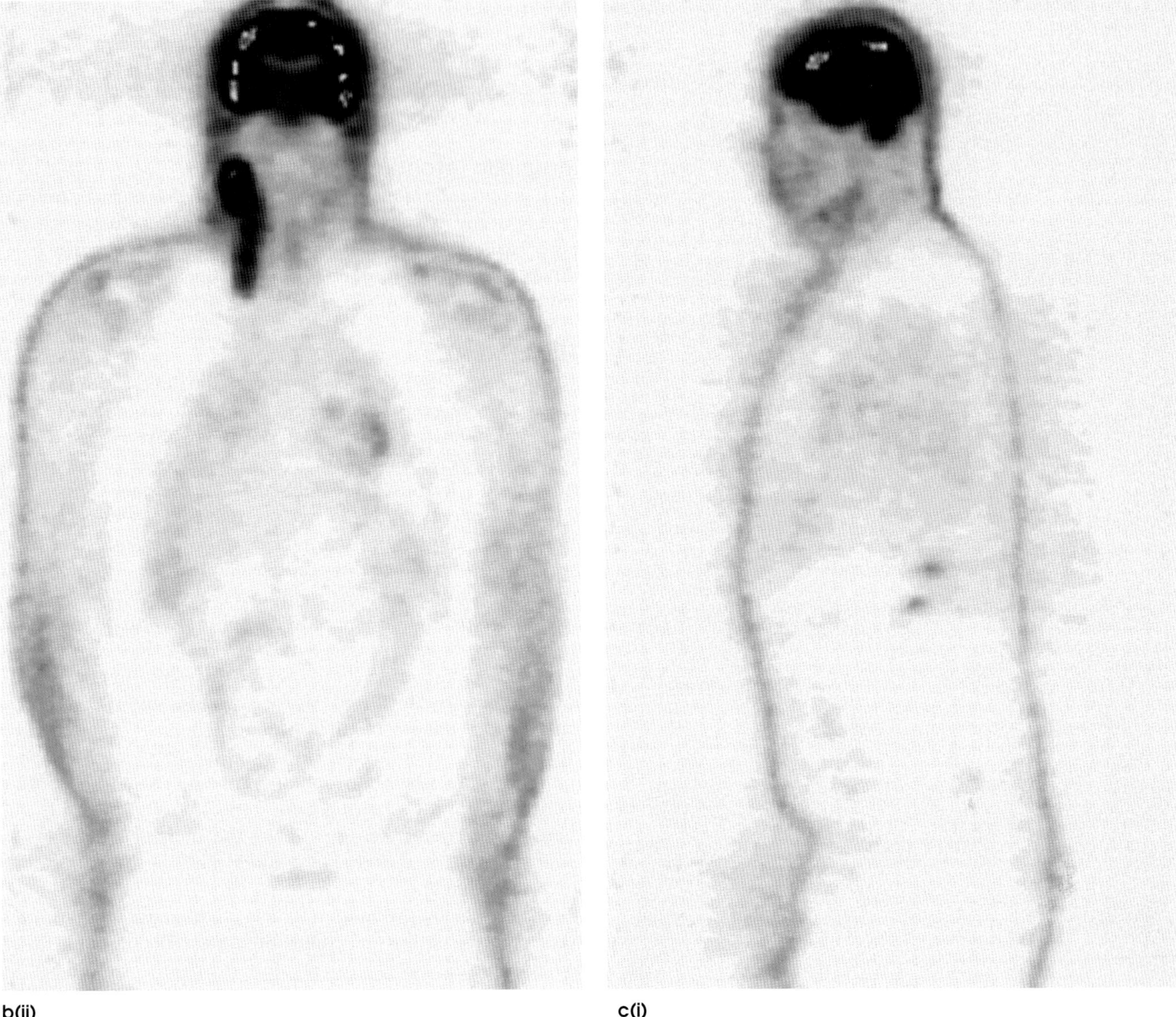

Figure 33.4, *cont'd* (b(ii)) pretreatment and (**c**) post-treatment, sagittal and coronal sections. The echodense areas in the brain reflect the normal high physiological activity. Courtesy of the Clinical Positron Emission Tomography Centre, Guy's and St Thomas's Hospital, London, UK.

adenopathy. Changes on routine chest radiograph range from minimal superior mediastinal distortion to massive enlargement of mediastinal and hilar nodes with adjacent parenchymal infiltration (Fig. 33.4). Computerized tomography is of value in assessing hilar node involvement, particularly in the presence of extensive mediastinal disease.

Computerized tomography scanning

At presentation all patients should have a CT scan performed of the neck, thorax, abdomen and inguinal areas. Although providing confirmation of lymph node enlargement (greater than 1 cm), unfortunately CT scanning cannot demonstrate involvement of normal-sized nodes or microscopic infiltration of the parenchyma of the liver or spleen with any degree of accuracy.

Radiographic skeletal survey

Bone involvement occurs in 5% of patients, usually those with advanced disease, and involvement may be sclerotic, lytic or mixed in appearance. The differentiation between bone involvement and aseptic necrosis occurring after treatment is often resolved only by surgical biopsy.

Ultrasound scanning

Diagnostic ultrasound is a quick and efficient method of assessing lymphomatous involvement in the abdomen, pelvis and retroperitoneal area. Its greatest potential is in the demonstration of enlarged nodes in the porta hepatis, in the splenic hilum or around the pancreas; however, the technique is limited by the inability to detect involved nodes less than 1.5 cm in diameter or to differentiate reactive hyperplasia from malignant infiltration. Splenic enlargement is readily detected by ultrasound scan even when not apparent clinically, but although large discrete filling defects may be demonstrated, routine scanning is not able to separate diffuse involvement by lymphoma from enlargement from other causes. Similar problems arise when scanning the liver. In the kidney, mass lesions, diffuse enlargement from infiltration, or hydronephrosis secondary to lymph node compression may all be identified by routine ultrasound examination.

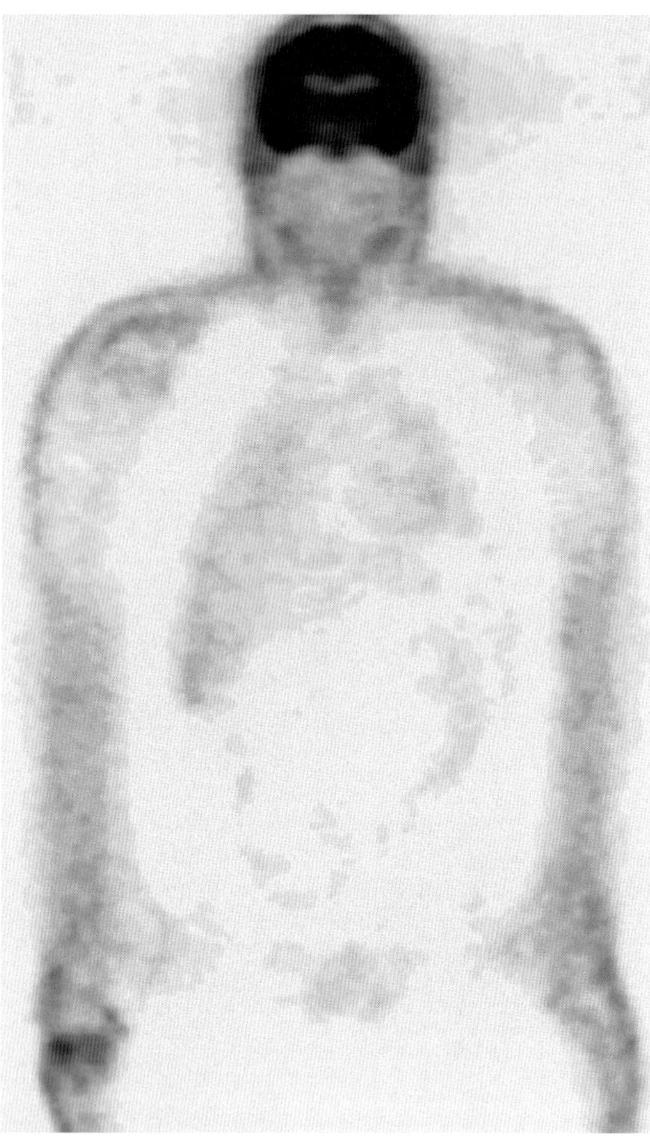

c(ii)

Figure 33.4, *cont'd.*

Radioisotope scanning

Radioisotope scanning has an increasing role in the investigation of patients with Hodgkin's disease. Technetium bone scans are sensitive but they do not differentiate from other pathological processes. Isotopic liver and spleen scans occasionally show a clear filling defect but diffuse involvement is usually missed.

The discovery that gallium-67 localizes well within tissues involved by Hodgkin's disease prompted great interest in its possible role in staging. Gallium-67 has proved a useful isotope in high doses in assessing involvement of the mediastinum, but interpretation of abdominal gallium-67 scans is compromised by interference from uptake of the isotope in the liver, colon and marrow.[10] Whole-body positron emission tomography using 2-deoxy-2-[^{18}F]fluoro-D-glucose (FDG) has shown encouraging results in pretreatment staging and remission assessment in both Hodgkin's disease and non-Hodgkin's lymphoma. The FDG concentrates preferentially in metabolically active tissue including lymphoma, and initial studies show a high degree of sensitivity and specificity for this technique. Prospective studies to assess the role of FDG positron emission tomography scanning in the management of lymphoma are in progress.[11] The potential advantages of positron emission tomography scanning are in pretreatment staging, the ability to determine response to chemotherapy at an early stage, and the evaluation of residual masses post treatment.

Magnetic resonance imaging

The expectation that MRI scanning would replace surgical staging in the detection of abdominal Hodgkin's disease has not been realized. Magnetic resonance imaging has not yet been shown to be useful in the detection of splenic disease and is of only marginal value in the examination of the liver.[12]

TREATMENT

The goal in Hodgkin's disease is to cure the disease with minimal short- and long-term morbidity, taking into account the side effects of each treatment modality. The last three decades have witnessed a steady improvement in the prognosis of patients at all stages of Hodgkin's disease. Several factors have contributed to this change, including better pretreatment staging, improvements in radiotherapy equipment and technique, and the introduction of effective systemic chemotherapy. The euphoria associated with these dramatic advances must be tempered, however, by the realization that only 70% of those with disseminated disease may expect a cure. Similarly, despite intensive staging investigations and optimal radiotherapy, a proportion of patients with apparently localized disease relapse after treatment. Patients who relapse require systemic high-dose chemotherapy and possible consolidation with peripheral blood stem cell transplantation. Combining radiotherapy and chemotherapy may reduce relapse rates but does not improve overall survival, and there is continuing concern about the increased risk of late complications, in particular second malignancy, with more intensive treatment.

The growing appreciation of the late iatrogenic complications has led to use of less toxic chemotherapy schedules and lesser radiation fields and doses. This underscores the importance in any treatment policy for Hodgkin's disease of employing the minimum amount of initial therapy compatible with the highest probability of cure. It has now been possible to stratify treatment according to prognostic group and the number of risk factors for each patient. The intensity of treatment increasingly uses prognostic indices, for example the Hasenclever Index,[13] which is based on stage of disease, the performance status, and indices based on blood tests (lymphocyte count and haemoglobin).

Given the inherited limitations of CT scanning in differing sites of active disease, there is increasing enthusiasm to measure response to treatment more effectively by positron emission tomography scanning before and after two cycles of chemotherapy.[14] If the position emission tomography scan after the second cycle of chemotherapy shows complete remission,

REFERENCES

10. Anderson KC, Leonard RCG, Canellos GP. Am J Med 1988; 75: 321–327
11. Timothy AR, Ahern V et al. Ann Oncol 1996; 7 (Suppl 3): 3
12. Reznek RH, Richards MA. Clin Haematol 1987; 1: 77–108
13. Hasenclever D, Dielhl V et al. N Engl J Med 1998; 339: 1506–1514
14. Mikhaeel NG, Timothy AR et al. Ann Oncol 2000; 11 (Suppl 1): S147–S150

position emission tomography is not repeated after completion of treatment but CT scan is. It is recommended that post-treatment CT and positron emission tomography scans should be done 6 weeks after the last chemotherapy and 12 weeks after the last radiotherapy treatment. Clinical follow-up should be every 3 months for the first year, every 4 months for the second year, every 6 months for up to 5 years, every 12 months in years 6–10 and alternate years thereafter.

PROGNOSTIC GROUPS IN HODGKIN'S DISEASE

For early-stage disease, prognostication is based on stage and the presence or absence of risk factors. The division of these prognostic groups may be into nodular lymphocyte-predominant Hodgkin's disease, and for classical disease, early favourable, early unfavourable and advanced disease. The risk factors are as follow and constitute four factors:

A. large mediastinal mass (greater than one-third transverse chest diameter) at T5–6 level on chest radiograph or bulky disease (any single tumour mass at least 7 cm in greatest dimension);
B. extranodal disease;
C. Erythrocyte sedimentation rate 50+ (30+ with B symptoms); and
D. Three or more sites.

The prognostic groups are:

- nodular lymphocyte-predominant disease stage I or II with no risk factors;
- early favourable (stage I or IIA with no risk factors);
- early unfavourable (stage I or IIA with risk factors and stage IIB with C or D risk factors); and
- advanced (stage IIB with A or B risk factors)

Early favourable disease

Because of the risk of long-term complications that may arise as a result of mantle-field radiotherapy (i.e. the increased incidence of breast carcinoma and cardiac disease) – with the exception of patients with stage IA high neck disease – with favorable histology, radiotherapy is now commonly given in combination with chemotherapy (combined modality treatment) using smaller radiation fields and doses. Wide-field irradiation to include all lymph node areas above or below the diaphragm has generally been superseded by a combination of three or four cycles of chemotherapy (ABVD: doxorubicin, bleomycin, vinblastine and dacarbazine) and involved-field (smaller volume and lower dose) radiotherapy.

Early unfavourable disease

Stage I and II disease with poor prognostic factors is classified as early unfavourable disease.

Patients with apparently localized disease but adverse prognostic factors – large mediastinal mass, multiple sites of disease, high erythrocyte sedimentation rate or B symptoms – have high relapse rates with radiotherapy alone and are therefore best treated with combined modality therapy, typically ABVD × 4 plus involved-field radiotherapy.

Advanced disease

Advanced disease is stage IIIA with risk factors C or D, stage IIB with risk factors A or B, stage IIIB or stage IV.

These patients should be treated with chemotherapy from the outset because this produces excellent results (Fig. 33.5) with

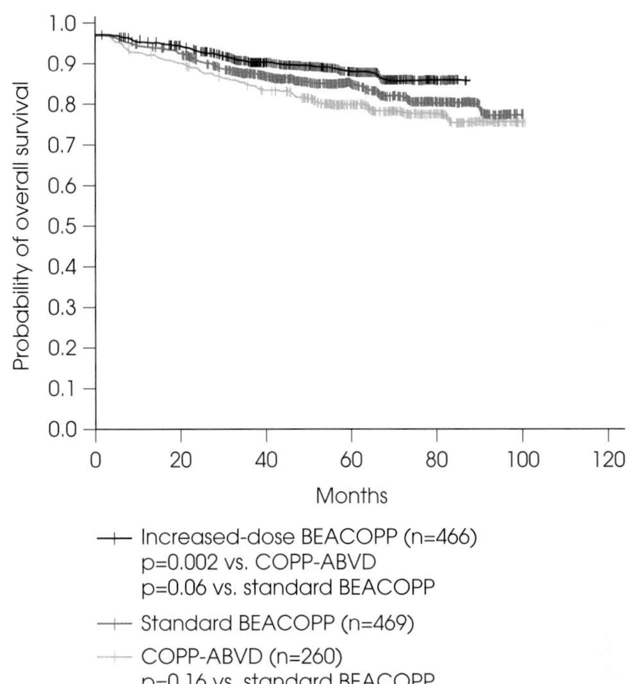

Figure 33.5 Overall survival for advanced Hodgkin's disease.

minimal long-term morbidity. In patients with residual bulk disease, at the end of the chemotherapy course consolidation-involved field therapy may be considered; however, although this may improve disease-free survival it has little effect on overall survival rates. Positron emission tomography scanning may be useful here to differentiate between active and inactive disease.

The treatment schedules typically use ABVD in the chemotherapy regimens of choice, because this type of chemotherapy has been shown to be associated with a reduced risk of sterility and late malignancy when compared with other regimens that include alkylating agents, such as MOPP (mechlorethamine, vincristine, procarbazine and prednisone). Although ABVD remains the gold standard, German studies are yielding results that may be superior in poor-risk patients using dose intensification regimens such as escalated BEACOPP (bleomycin, etoposide, doxorubicin, cyclophosphamide, vincristine, procarbazine and prednisone).[15]

Relapsed or refractory disease

For patients with primary refractory disease or those who fail to attain a complete remission, the prognosis is very poor (8-year survival 0–8%).[16] Patients less than 65 years old should be considered for high-dose chemotherapy and consolidation autologous stem cell transplantation.[17] For patients who relapse after attaining remission the prognosis depends on the duration of remission and the extent of relapse. The recommended treatment in these cases is to administer initial salvage chemotherapy

REFERENCES

15. Diehl V, Franklin J et al. N Engl J Med 2003; 348: 2386–2395
16. Longo DL, Duffey PL et al. J Clin Oncol 1992; 10: 210–218
17. Sweetenham JW, Taaphipour G, Milligan D et al. Bone Marrow Transplant 1997; 20(9): 745–752

to assess disease sensitivity, and to proceed to a consolidation autologous stem cell transplant. If appropriate, in certain young patients who fail these measures newer experimental treatments, such as the use of low-intensity and full allograft transplants, may be an option providing that a compatible donor is found.

TREATMENT MODALITIES AND SIDE EFFECTS

Radiotherapy

With the introduction of high-energy cobalt units and linear accelerators during the 1950s and 1960s, the delivery of wide-field irradiation to major lymph node areas above and below the diaphragm, without significant morbidity, became a practical proposition. Experience with this type of radiotherapy established that the optimal tumoricidal dose for Hodgkin's disease lay in the range 30–40 Gy (3000–4000 rad), given in 20 daily fractions, treating 5 days a week with appropriate shielding of the lungs and spinal cord. There is no evidence that significantly increasing the dose of radiation above these levels does anything other than increase the risk of late morbidity, and studies suggest that doses of 20–30 Gy are sufficient, particularly when used in combination with chemotherapy. The question remains whether it may be possible to omit radiation entirely in many patients with Hodgkin's disease.

Acute side effects of radiotherapy

The acute effects of radiotherapy are those occurring up to 12 weeks after completion of treatment. The occurrence and intensity of these reactions are unpredictable in the individual patient, although debilitating side effects are rare. Fatigue, particularly towards the end of treatment, is common but usually improves within a few weeks of completing irradiation. Occasionally patients may suffer persistent lassitude for several months.

Anorexia is common and may be accompanied by nausea (rarely vomiting), although this can usually be controlled with simple antiemetic medication. Nausea and vomiting are more commonly a problem with infradiaphragmatic rather than supradiaphragmatic irradiation. Patients should be advised that they may lose weight during a routine course of radiotherapy, and attention should be paid to adequate nutritional intake. Radiotherapy fields in Hodgkin's disease do not routinely include the oral cavity but may encompass the sublingual, the submaxillary and a large proportion of the parotid glands. This inevitably results in reduced saliva production, and the saliva becomes more viscous, producing a dry mouth with altered taste sensation. Taste perception usually returns within 3 months but dryness of the mouth may persist.

Modern megavoltage radiotherapy equipment, with its skin-sparing properties, has reduced the incidence of skin reactions to a minimum. However, erythema within the radiation fields does occur on occasions, and moist desquamation may rarely be seen in skin folds. Thoracic irradiation may be accompanied by mucositis in the pharynx and occasionally dysphagia starting from the second or third week of treatment. These reactions are self-limiting, and patients should be reassured that they are a normal part of the treatment.

Temporary alopecia overlying the occiput is invariable with mantle radiation, together with a similar loss of beard hair (Fig. 33.6). Hair regrowth usually commences within 3 months of stopping treatment and should be complete, although the texture and the color of the hair may change within the irradiated area.

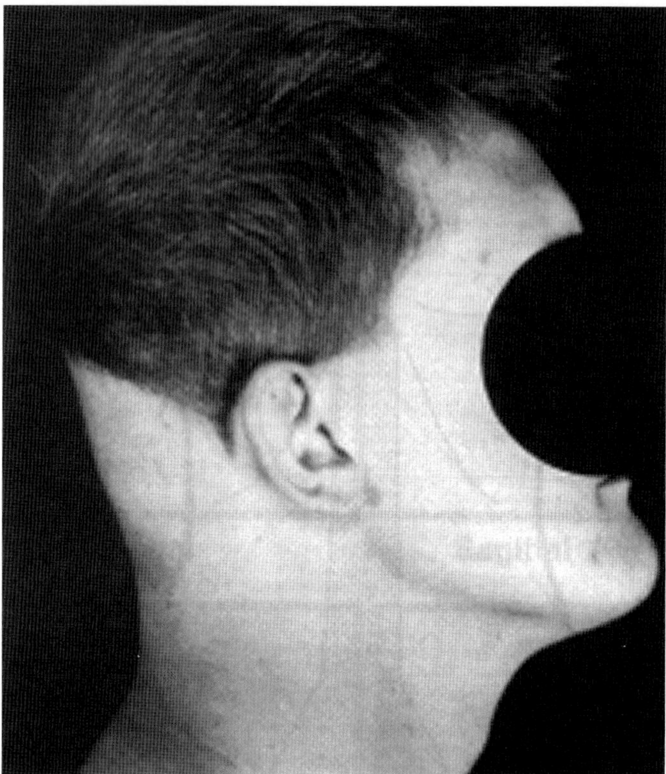

Figure 33.6 Temporary alopecia associated with mantle radiation.

Wide-field irradiation rarely causes significant haematological depression but regular monitoring of blood counts is important. The risk of haematological toxicity is increased when patients have received chemotherapy prior to radiation, and extra care must be exercised. With infradiaphragmatic irradiation gastrointestinal side effects such as cramps, flatulence and occasionally diarrhoea may occur but can usually be adequately controlled with appropriate medication. Patients are advised to avoid milk products, spiced foods or raw vegetables during abdominal treatment because these may accentuate any side effects.

Late side effects of radiotherapy

The late effects of radiotherapy reflect normal tissue damage, which may occur months or even years after treatment and is usually permanent. Irradiation to the thorax given to excessive volumes or with very high doses may produce transient pneumonitis, which in rare cases may progress to permanent respiratory disability. The risk of pulmonary damage is increased with prior or concomitant chemotherapy with drugs such as bleomycin or doxorubicin, and great care must be taken in planning thoracic radiotherapy.

Late cardiac problems following radiotherapy are a continuing concern, especially in younger patients, and every effort must be made to keep to a minimum the volume and dose of radiation applied.

Lhermitte's syndrome, the onset of numbness, paraesthesia or electric shock sensations in the lumbar region, or upper or lower limbs 2–4 months after completion of mantle radiotherapy is well documented. The symptoms may last up to 6 months but settle without intervention. The syndrome is thought to be due to transient demyelinization and does not presage permanent neurological damage. Transverse myelitis is, however, a risk when separate thoracic (mantle) and abdominal (inverted Y) and radiation fields are matched incorrectly and overdose occurs on the spinal cord. Exceptional care must be exercised when matching radiation fields.

Extending abdominal irradiation to include the spleen and upper part of the left kidney has not been associated with any long-term sequelae on prolonged follow-up.[18] Care must be taken, however, to exclude an adequate volume of renal tissue from the radiation field to avoid chronic renal damage.

The potential for radiation to damage the gonads is of obvious importance in a disease that predominantly affects the young, a large percentage of whom will have a normal life expectancy. Fractionated radiotherapy to the testis above the level of 200 cGy will produce prolonged and often permanent azoospermia. With appropriate testicular shielding, radiation doses to the testis may be reduced by 95%, to levels at which a reasonable probability of germinal epithelial recovery might be expected. It should be noted that a significant proportion of males will be azoospermic before therapy as a consequence of their disease. Semen analysis and storage should be undertaken prior to any treatments as appropriate.

For the ovary, doses above 800 cGy are associated with a high risk of permanent amenorrhoea. The associated hormonal dysfunction in female patients leads to menopausal symptoms, and in a young patient severe social and psychological sequelae may result unless appropriate hormone replacement therapy is instituted.

For both men and women receiving radiation to the abdomen and pelvis for Hodgkin's disease, full discussions must take place with patients and their partners, and the possibility of sterility and hormonal side effects must be fully explained before treatment is begun.

Chemotherapy

Studies of cytotoxic chemotherapy in the late 1940s demonstrated that Hodgkin's disease showed a peculiar sensitivity to these drugs, and a small proportion of patients obtained worthwhile remission of their disease. Among the most active drugs were the alkylating agents, particularly nitrogen mustard and the vinca alkaloids.[19] By giving several of these agents together at one time the response rates increased significantly, and the MOPP combination developed at the National Cancer Institute in the USA produced complete remissions and 'cures' in some 50% of patients, including those with advanced disease.[20] Several modifications of the MOPP schedule have subsequently been reported, many introduced in an attempt to reduce the potential for acute and long-term toxicity now recognized to be associated with alkylating agents.

Doxorubicin-based schedules, particularly ABVD (Table 33.3), show not only similar response and relapse-free survival rates to MOPP but, more importantly, reduced risks of late toxicity, particularly with regard to infertility and the induction of second malignancies.[21] The majority of patients who relapse will do so within 36 months of treatment; late relapses after more than 5 years are uncommon.[22]

Combining radiotherapy and chemotherapy may increase complete remission rates but the potential advantages must be balanced against the risk of increased acute and late toxicity.

Acute side effects of chemotherapy

Chemotherapy may cause nausea and vomiting and, less commonly, diarrhoea occurring within a few hours of administration but rarely lasting more than 24 h after treatment. Premedication with domperidone or prochlorperazine continued for a short period after chemotherapy is usually sufficient to control nausea and vomiting. In severe cases the newer 5-HT_3 antagonists such as ondansetron or granisetron may be required. Anticipatory vomiting as a prelude to chemotherapy can be a problem and may prove more difficult to overcome; however, these side effects are rarely severe enough to cause patients to reject treatment.

Table 33.3 ABVD schedule

Drug	Dose
Doxorubicin	25 mg/m^2
Bleomycin	10 units/m^2
Vinblastine	6 mg/m^2
Dacarbazine	375 mg/m^2

Each drug administered on days 1 and 15.

The effect of suppression of normal bone marrow function is a major factor influencing the dosage and schedule of cytotoxic chemotherapy. With the standard combinations (e.g. ABVD) the white cell and platelet counts characteristically fall to a nadir 10–12 days after the start of treatment. In the absence of complicating factors, the blood count will usually return to normal within 14 days and allow further chemotherapy to be given, although treatment may need to be delayed in the face of persistent neutropenia or thrombocytopenia. In severe cases the use of granulocyte stimulating factor is necessary to allow successful delivery of chemotherapy.

Cytotoxic drugs are immunosuppressive, especially in patients with lymphoma who are already compromised by their disease. The risk of severe and occasionally life-threatening infections must be anticipated and warned against, particularly in splenectomized subjects, for whom long-term precautions must be taken. Any patient on chemotherapy who presents with signs of infection should have an immediate blood count, and if shown to be severely neutropenic should be started on broad-spectrum intravenous antibiotic therapy while blood cultures are awaited. Likewise, patients developing signs and symptoms of herpes zoster infection should be treated promptly with antiviral agents. Patients on chemotherapy should also be warned to report any untoward fevers or evidence of bruising or bleeding so that platelet blood counts can be checked and appropriate action taken.

One major cause for concern among patients due to receive chemotherapy is the prospect of alopecia. The incidence of hair loss varies depending on the cytotoxic agents used and to some

REFERENCES

18. Le Bourgeois JP, Meignan M et al. Br J Radiol 1979; 52: 56–60
19. Goodman LS, Wintrobe MM, Dameshek W. JAMA 1946; 132: 126–132
20. De Vita VT Jr, Serpick AA, Carbone PP. Ann Intern Med 1970; 73: 881–895
21. Selby P, McElwain TJ, Canellos G. In: Selby P, McElwain TJ (eds). Hodgkin's Disease. Blackwell Scientific Publications, Oxford, 1987: 269–300
22. De Vita VT, Simon RM, Hubbard SM. Intern Med 1980; 92: 587–595

extent on the individual. Scalp cooling may be useful to prevent hair loss.

Late side effects of chemotherapy

The increasingly successful outcome for patients treated with chemotherapy has revealed the potential risk of long-term side effects, prompting the investigation of less toxic drug combinations.

Schedules such as MOPP, which include alkylating agents, render the majority of men azoospermic; this is usually permanent when six or more cycles of treatment are given. Similar treatment in women produces ovarian ablation in approximately 50%, but this effect appears to be age-related. Patients over the age of 30 have a 20% chance or less of remaining fertile. Recent experience has shown that non-alkylating drug combinations such as ABVD have a significantly reduced incidence of azoospermia immediately after treatment, with complete recovery in the majority of cases. As with radiotherapy, patients undergoing chemotherapy should be counselled fully and the need for appropriate contraceptive precautions should be emphasized to avoid the misfortune of an untimely pregnancy during treatment and the psychological trauma associated with subsequent termination.

An issue of major concern in patients surviving successful treatment for Hodgkin's disease has been the development of second malignancies. Radiation and cytotoxic agents are potentially mutagenic and carcinogenic in experimental systems. The alkylating agents, particularly procarbazine, appear to be particularly implicated. In one series of over 1500 patients treated for Hodgkin's disease at Stanford University, California, there was a significant increase in second 'cancers', including leukaemia, non-Hodgkin's lymphoma, lung and stomach cancers, melanoma and connective tissue malignancy.[23] At 15-year follow-up the overall risk for a second cancer was 17.6% compared with 2.6% in the general population.

The risk of developing leukaemia appears to reach a plateau 10 years after treatment. Although there appears to be a small risk of secondary leukaemia in patients treated by radiotherapy alone, the major risk comes from the alkylating agent-based chemotherapy regimens such as MOPP. There does not as yet appear to be a similar risk with the ABVD schedules.

The risk of solid cancers continues to increase with time, even after 10 years, and is related to the intensity of treatment, being highest in those who have received both alkylating chemotherapy and radiation. Every effort should be made to minimize the amount of treatment given to patients with Hodgkin's disease, but the risk of second malignancies should not be a justification for avoiding intensive therapy. Patients should be fully informed about the potential risks of therapy and kept under close surveillance. Any untoward feature must not be automatically regarded as recurrent lymphoma: every effort should be made to obtain a histological diagnosis to exclude other forms of malignancy.

NON-HODGKIN'S LYMPHOMA

INTRODUCTION

The non-Hodgkin's lymphomas comprise a complex group of diseases with a wide heterogeneous clinical presentation and patterns of behavior, which reflect complex varying histological subtypes. Non-Hodgkin's lymphoma represents about 2.4% of all cancers registered in England and Wales, and accounts for approximately 3% of deaths from malignant disease in western countries. Non-Hodgkin's lymphoma is a tumour with an increasing incidence in the western world and currently stands in the UK at 11 in 100 000, a figure that has risen dramatically since the 1970s and is in part accounted for by HIV-related lymphomas. In contrast to Hodgkin's disease, the non-Hodgkin's lymphomas have a peak incidence in the fifth and sixth decades, are less commonly localized at presentation, and more frequently involve extranodal sites.

The members of the non-Hodgkin's group of lymphomas are distinctive clonal neoplasms, which represent malignant perturbations of the cellular components of normal lymph nodes, primarily of lymph node follicles. Hence non-Hodgkin's lymphomas are mainly B-cell tumours (80%), with 15% being of the T-cell lineage and the remainder being made up from natural killer cells and macrophages. The two most common B-cell types are follicular cell lymphoma and diffuse large B-cell lymphoma (Fig. 33.7).

These disorders encompass a heterogeneous group of diseases that is based on a multiplicity of histological subtypes, clinical presentations (nodal or extranodal), tumour behaviour (localized versus disseminated), and the presence or absence of concomitant disease that impacts on treatment options. As with Hodgkin's disease, experience over the past three decades following the introduction of intensive cytotoxic chemotherapy has clearly shown that with appropriate management many patients with non-Hodgkin's lymphoma now have a real prospect for cure. Treatment, however, must be carefully tailored to the patient's individual circumstances and depends on the extent and histological subtype of the lymphoma concerned.

DIAGNOSIS: THE MULTIDISCIPLINARY TEAM MEETING

The incidence of the tumour is increasing and the tumour may present many challenges for the histopathologist and the clinician managing patients with this disease. The reasons for this are in part due to the varying complexity of the disease subtypes – there are over 30 subtypes as defined in the Revised European–American Lymphoma classification[24] – and the demands this brings to make a watertight diagnosis with the subsequent correct management. For this reason, before deciding on treatment and with the advent of best possible practice guidelines, it is strongly recommended that all lymphomas should be managed under the auspices of a multidisciplinary team. The multidisciplinary team should consist of a haemato-oncologist, a clinical oncologist, a histopathologist, a radiologist, nurses qualified in haemato-oncology and designated pharmacists.

Adequate sampling and biopsy preparation

The management of de novo non-Hodgkin's lymphoma starts with obtaining an adequate biopsy specimen, which ideally should be taken by a designated surgeon. In the case of head and neck disease, an ear, nose and throat surgeon should obtain the material, while for other biopsy sites a general surgeon is used. The actual material should be sent to the histopathology

REFERENCES

23. Tucker MA, Coleman CN et al. N Engl J Med 1988; 318: 76–81
24. Harris NL, Jaffe, Stein H et al. Blood 1994; 84: 1361–1392

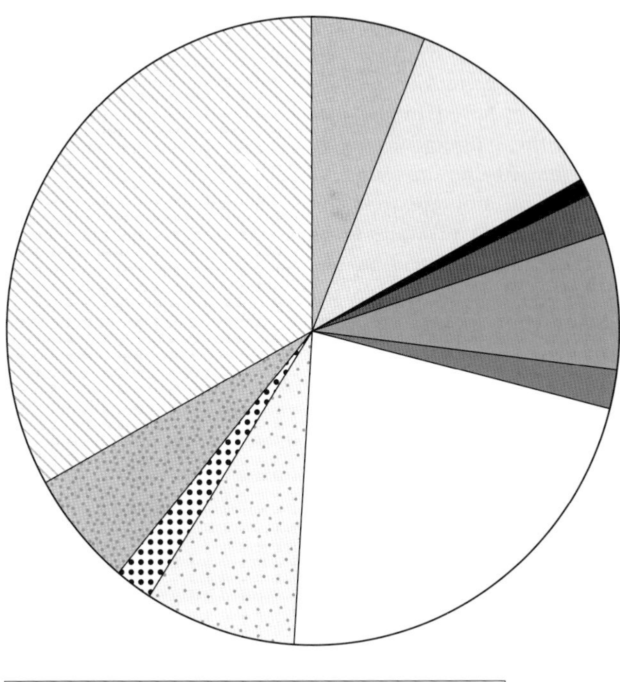

Figure 33.7 Non-Hodgkin's lymphoma incidence (Revised European–American Lymphoma classification): non-Hodgkin's lymphoma classification project.

laboratory unfixed as soon as possible after surgery. A consistent fixation time of approximately 24 h will aid reproducibility in immunostaining. Consideration should also be given to taking fresh tissue for microbiology and cytogenetics, and to storage of samples for future molecular analysis.

PATHOLOGY AND CLASSIFICATION

For many years the most widely adopted classification for the non-Hodgkin's lymphomas has been that of Rappaport (Box 33.1).[25] This classification divided lymphomas based on the pattern of cell growth and the size and shape of the tumour cells. Although useful clinically, the lack of detail and imprecise terminology led to the classification becoming outdated when it became apparent that all non-Hodgkin's lymphomas are tumours of lymphocytes and that lymphocytes could be divided into those of T-cell origin and those of B-cell origin.

Other classifications have been proposed to overcome the deficiencies of the Rappaport system: the Revised Working Formulation, the Kiel classification,[26] and more recently the Revised European–American Lymphoma classification.[24]

Box 33.1 Rappaport classification of non-Hodgkin's lymphoma

Nodular
- Lymphocytic and well differentiated
- Lymphocytic and poorly differentiated
- Mixed lymphocytic and histiocytic
- Histiocytic

Diffuse
- Lymphocytic and well differentiated
- Lymphocytic and poorly differentiated
- Mixed lymphocytic and histiocytic
- Histiocytic

The majority of malignant lymphomas are derived from B lymphocytes, although there are now varieties of distinctive T-cell lymphomas, such as peripheral T-cell lymphomas and adult T-cell lymphoma or leukaemia, which do not fit well into most classifications. From the clinician's point of view, the value of any classification is the division of the lymphomas into low-, intermediate- and high-grade, which will form the basis of a rational treatment policy. This marked variation in behaviour and prognosis between the different subgroups of non-Hodgkin's lymphoma demands that a comprehensive and easily comprehensible histological classification should be available to provide the clinician with an insight into the expected behaviour of a given patient's disease and also serve as a guide to treatment.

Over the past 30 years there have been repeated attempts to reclassify the non-Hodgkin's lymphomas based on morphological and, more recently, on immunological criteria. The difficulties of experienced specialist histopathologists in producing a uniform classification have only served to compound the problems for clinicians dealing with these diseases, and led to increasing frustration and the temptation to provide frivolous alternative classifications (Box 33.2).[27] Since Rappaport's 1966 classification, many classifications have been proposed but only two, the Kiel classification and the 1982 Working Formulation for Clinical Usage (Table 33.4), have been in use for many years in Europe and the USA. These classifications were based on cell morphology and its prognostic implications (small cell lymphoma was indicative of a good prognosis and large cell lymphoma a poor prognosis).

In 1994, the International Lymphoma Study Group proposed a classification based on morphology, immunology, genetics and clinical presentation of the various disease entities.[24] This Revised European–American Lymphoma classification was modified to become the World Health Organization classification (Table 33.5).[28]

STAGING AND INVESTIGATION

The Ann Arbor staging system (Table 33.2) has traditionally been used for the non-Hodgkin's lymphomas but, as with Hodgkin's disease, it is clear that factors other than just clinical (or pathological) stage, such as tumour bulk, histology, age and serum lactate dehydrogenase values, are of major importance in

REFERENCES

25. Rappaport H. Atlas of Tumour Pathology. Armed Forces Institute of Pathology, Washington, 1966
26. Rosenberg SA et al. Cancer 1982; 49: 2112–2351
27. Higby D. N Engl J Med 1979; 300: 1283
28. Jaffe ES, Harris NL. Ann Oncol 1998; 9 (Suppl 5): 525–530

defining therapy and predicting prognosis. New staging systems that take account of these other important characteristics will be required.

Despite the introduction of more sophisticated imaging, a careful history and clinical examination still provide important information in patients with non-Hodgkin's lymphomas. The presence of systemic symptoms and the duration of lymph node enlargement may influence the decision whether or not any treatment is required in the low-grade lymphomas. Symptoms such as deafness, diplopia, bone pain or altered bowel habit may indicate that further investigation is required to exclude sites of involvement not apparent on initial clinical examination. Careful inspection of Waldeyer's ring and examination of the epitrochlear and popliteal lymph nodes may also yield valuable information on the extent of spread. It is also important to remember the established associations of specific sites, for example disease in the postnasal space is associated with enlarged upper cervical lymph nodes; intestinal lymphoma may be associated with certain head and neck presentations; and central nervous system disease is associated with lymphomatous involvement of the paranasal and nasal sinuses.

Box 33.2 The Higby classification of lymphomas

Good ones
Includes non-convoluted diffuse centrilobulated histioblastoma, immune binucleolar hyperbolic folliculated macrolymphosarcoma, T_2-terminal transferase-negative bimodal prolymphoblastic, leukosarcoma, Jergen–Kreuzart–Munier–Abdullah syndrome and reticulated histioblastic pseudo-Sezary IgM-secreting folliculoma.

Characteristics
Small tumour that does not recur after treatment.

Not so good ones
Formerly 'hairy cell' pseudoincestuoblastoma, quasiconvoluted binucleate germinoma, sarcoblastiocytoma, Syrian variant of heavy-chain disease and German grossobeseioma.

Characteristics
Such tumours disappear on treatment but return and cause appreciable mortality.

Really bad ones
Includes farsical mononuclear diffuse convoluted pseudoquasihistiolymphosarcomyeloblastoma, immunoglobulin variant of fragmented plasmatic gammopathy, triconvoluted ipsilateral rhomboid fever, Armour's hyperthermic carcinoma and Hohner's harmonica.

Characteristics
Regardless of treatment such tumours keep growing.

Laboratory investigations

Haematological

Approximately 40% of patients with non-Hodgkin's lymphoma have bone marrow involvement at presentation, with 80% of patients with 'low-grade' small cell lymphomas having evidence of marrow infiltration compared with less than 15% of those with more aggressive, high-grade malignancies. Examination by bone marrow aspiration alone is inadequate and a bone marrow trephine is required. Peripheral blood involvement occurs in the presence of marrow infiltration and is found most commonly in patients with small cell lymphomas, although up to 80% of patients with highly malignant lymphoblastic lymphomas have tumour cells in the peripheral blood at some time during their illness. Half of the patients with abnormal blood counts will have a normal bone marrow examination.

Table 33.4 Comparison of Working Formulation for Clinical Usage and Kiel classification of non-Hodgkin's lymphoma

Working Formulation for Clinical Usage	Kiel equivalent
Low grade	
Malignant lymphoma, small lymphocytic consistent with chronic lymphocytic leukaemia plasmacytoid	Malignant lymphoma, lymphocytic; malignant lymphoma, lymphoplasmacytic, lymphoplasmacytoid
Malignant lymphoma, follicular predominantly small cleaved and large cell, diffuse, sclerosis	Malignant lymphoma, centroblastic, centrocytic (small) follicular +/– diffuse
Malignant lymphoma, follicular, mixed, small cleaved and large cell, diffuse areas, sclerosis	–
Intermediate grade	
Malignant lymphoma, follicular predominantly large cell, diffuse, sclerosis	Malignant lymphoma, centroblastic or centrocytic (large), follicular or diffuse
Malignant lymphoma, follicular predominantly small cleaved, sclerosis	Malignant lymphoma, centrocytic
Malignant lymphoma, follicular predominantly mixed small and large cell, epithelioid cell	Malignant lymphoma, centroblastic or centrocytic (small), diffuse; malignant lymphoma, lymphoplasmacytic or -cytoid, polymorphic
Malignant lymphoma, diffuse, large cell, cleaved cell, non-cleaved cell, sclerosis	Malignant lymphoma, centroblastic or centrocytic (large), diffuse; malignant lymphoma, centrocytic (large); malignant lymphoma, centroblastic
High grade	
Malignant lymphoma, large cell, immunoblastic, plasmacytoid, clear cell, polymorphous, epithelioid cell component	Malignant lymphoma, immunoblastic; T-zone lymphoma; lymphoepithelioid cell lymphoma
Malignant lymphoma, lymphoblastic, convoluted cell, non-convoluted cell	Malignant lymphoma, lymphoblastic, convoluted cell type; malignant lymphoma, lymphoblastic, unclassified
Malignant lymphoma, small non-cleaved, Burkitt's follicular areas	Malignant lymphoma, Burkitt type and other B lymphoblastic

Table 33.5 World Health Organization classification of lymphoma

Type	Precursor: B lymphoblastic	Precursor: T lymphoblastic
Lymphoma or leukaemia	Leukaemia or lymphoma Chronic lymphocytic leukaemia Small lymphocytic lymphoma • +/– monoclonal component • +/– plasmacytoid differentiation B prolymphocytic leukaemia Lymphoplasmacytic lymphoma Lymphoplasmacytic lymphoma or immunocytoma	Lymphoma or leukaemia Prolymphocytic leukaemia Large granular lymphocyte leukaemia • T-cell type • Natural killer cell type Natural killer cell leukaemia Mycosis fungoides or Sezary syndrome (cutaneous T cell lymphoma) Variants Pagetoid reticulosis Follicular mucinosis Granulomatous chalazodermia
Indolent nodal or extranodal lymphomas	Marginal zone B-cell lymphoma • MALT-type lymphoma • Splenic marginal zone +/– villous lymphocytes Nodal lymphomas Follicular lymphomas • Grade 1 (< 15% centroblasts) • Grade 2 (15–50% centroblasts) • Grade 3 (> 50% centroblasts) Cutaneous Gastrointestinal Mantle cell lymphoma Classic variant with round cells Blast variant with large cells	T-cell, natural killer cell or gamma delta T Subtypes: nasal Nasal type Subcutaneous panniculitis Intestinal Gamma or delta T-cell hepatosplenic • Peripheral T cell Lymphoepithelioid T-zone lymphoma Angioimmunoblastic • Anaplastic large cell Lymphohistiocytic Small cell • CD30+ T-cell cutaneous lymphoproliferative • Human T lymphotropic virus-1-associated
Aggressive nodal or extranodal lymphomas	Diffuse large B-cell lymphoma Variants • Centroblastic • Immunoblastic • B-cell lymphoma rich in T cells • B-cell rich in histiocytes • Anaplastic large B cell • Burkitt-like • Lymphomatoid granulomatosis • Pyothorax-associated lymphoma Subtypes • Mediastinal • Intravascular • Serous lymphoma Burkitt's lymphoma or leukaemia Variant • Plasma cell type	–

Thrombocytopenia may be a reflection of associated hypersplenism, but thrombocytopenia coupled with anaemia is strongly suggestive of marrow disease. In 70% of patients with lymphoma cells in the bone marrow, the spleen and liver will be involved at laparotomy. There is a high correlation between bone marrow infiltration and central nervous system involvement in patients with high-grade lymphomas, especially those of the Burkitt type.

Biochemical

Routine biochemical analysis is essential to exclude major organ dysfunction prior to treatment, although such abnormalities by themselves are not reliable indicators of direct infiltration. Raised immunoglobulin levels may be found in lymphoplasmacytoid lymphomas and hyperviscosity may occur as a result. Measurement of plasma viscosity in these patients may demonstrate the need for urgent corrective therapy to prevent additional complications. Serum lactate dehydrogenase should be performed in new cases because raised levels correlate with tumour bulk. The serum lactate dehydrogenase now forms one of the prognostic factors in the International Prognostic Index (discussed later). Rapid tumour lysis of highly chemosensitive tumours following therapy can produce severe metabolic disturbance, including electrolyte imbalance, uric acid nephropathy and renal failure. Preventive measures, including regular allopurinol, high fluid intake and alkalinization of the urine, are necessary before starting chemotherapy. Close monitoring of urea and electrolytes should be carried out to detect this complication.

Microbiological investigations

A full search should be made for infectious aetiological factors, including Epstein–Barr virus, cytomegalovirus and toxoplasmosis serology. In suspected cases HIV serology should be screened for because the incidence of HIV-related lymphoma has risen dramatically since the 1970s.

Radiology

Plain X-rays

Even in the advanced stages of non-Hodgkin's lymphoma, intrathoracic disease is less common than in Hodgkin's disease. However, approximately 25% of patients with non-Hodgkin's lymphoma will show some abnormality on routine chest radiograph. Hilar or mediastinal adenopathy is the most common finding, followed by pleural effusion and parenchymal involvement. Parenchymal disease may show up as ill-defined miliary mottling or discrete nodules with or without central cavitation. A malignant pleural effusion may be present in the absence of other intrathoracic disease.[29]

Computerized tomography scanning

Computerized tomography scanning has become the optimal staging method on non-Hodgkin's lymphoma, and has largely replaced more cumbersome invasive methods such as lymphangiography and surgical laporotomy. In the abdomen and pelvis, lymph nodes up to 1 cm are usually considered normal; in non-Hodgkin's lymphoma involved nodes tend to be significantly enlarged, with mesenteric node involvement in more than 50% of cases. Computerized tomography scanning of the chest may provide additional information when the chest radiograph is equivocal, but adds little when the plain chest radiograph shows no obvious mediastinal or lung involvement. Computerized tomography scanning has become routine in the assessment of response to treatment.

Intravenous urogram

Renal involvement may be found at post-mortem in up to 30% of patients with disseminated lymphoma but it is rarely diagnosed clinically. Renal involvement or obstructive uropathy may be shown on routine intravenous urogram, and displacement of the ureters may raise the suspicion of enlarged para-aortic lymph nodes; however, the intravenous urogram has been generally replaced by CT scanning, which is a more accurate method of demonstrating renal involvement in non-Hodgkin's lymphoma.

Radioisotope scanning

Technetium liver and spleen scanning is an unreliable indicator of organ involvement by lymphoma. The discovery that gallium-67 localizes well within lymphoma tissue (particularly in high-grade lymphoma) has prompted considerable interest in the role of this isotope in scanning for occult sites of involvement. Uptake by gallium is not restricted to areas of lymphoma but also occurs in inflammatory tissue and in normal organs.[30] Detection rates have been increased by using high doses of gallium (7–10 mCi) and more sensitive imaging equipment. Scanning may be highly specific in the chest, particularly in differentiating fibrosis following treatment from active lymphoma, but within the abdomen the rate of detection is poor, with an accuracy of less than 50% for both liver and spleen. Scanning by FDG positron emission tomography has been shown to be very useful in the prediction of response to chemotherapy, and has become incorporated where this resource exists into assessment of disease response.[14]

Magnetic resonance imaging

Magnetic resonance scanning offers a further method for staging of patients with non-Hodgkin's lymphoma, with the advantage that no contrast medium is required and no ionizing radiation is involved. Richards and coworkers reported that low field strength MRI is a very sensitive method of detecting liver disease, although not specific for lymphoma.[31] Preliminary data suggested that MRI scanning at low strength may also be useful to detect bone marrow infiltration, but at the present time this investigation offers no advantage in detecting splenic involvement.

Staging laparotomy

Staging laparotomy and splenectomy have no place in the routine management of non-Hodgkin's lymphoma patients, who are in general an older and less fit population. Because truly localized non-Hodgkin's lymphoma is rare, local radiotherapy alone is appropriate treatment for very few patients; the majority require some form of systemic therapy from the outset, thereby rendering laparotomy unnecessary.

ASSIGNATION OF PROGNOSIS

The increasing importance of an accurate diagnosis reveals that the disease in itself is very heterogeneous, and that different subgroups of the disease do not respond equally to therapy. New ways have been developed to predict treatment outcome. Given the multiplicity of prognostic parameters in multivariate studies, major centres have developed indices incorporating the most important among them, essentially comprising tumour volume and stage of disease at diagnosis. In 1990, it was decided to put forward an international index for aggressive lymphomas.[32] The resulting International Prognostic Index incorporates five factors; the adverse prognosis for each of these is as follows:

1. Age: older than 60 years
2. Ann Arbor stage: III or IV
3. Serum lactate dehydrogenase: above normal
4. Number of extranodal sites: more than two
5. Performance status: over Eastern Cooperative Oncology Group 2 or equivalent

In young patients a simplified index, the age-adjusted index, is based on performance status, stage and lactate dehydrogenase level. The two indices are used to identify four prognostic groups: low risk, low intermediate risk, high intermediate risk and high risk. In both models, the increased risk of death is due to both a lower complete remission rate and higher relapse rate.

The International Prognostic Index has also been applied to the low-grade group of non-Hodgkin's lymphoma, with equal success. The International Prognostic Index and age-adjusted International Prognostic Index are more accurate than the Ann Arbor staging in predicting long-term survival (Fig. 33.8). Patients are assigned one point for each adverse prognostic factor, and it is important for the managing clinician to take these into account when deciding on treatment options. Once the diagnosis is confirmed and the disease staged with all prognostic factors taken into account, a decision has to be made as to what is the optimal treatment.

TREATMENT OF NON-HODGKIN'S LYMPHOMAS

Once the diagnosis has been made and the disease staged, the treatment given depends on the subtype of non-Hodgkin's

REFERENCES

29. Filly RA, Marglin S, Castellino RA. Cancer 1976; 38: 2143–2148
30. Anderson KC, Leonard RCG, Canellos GP. Am J Med 1988; 75: 321–327
31. Richards MA, Webb JAN et al. Br Med J 1986; 293: 1126–1128
32. International Non-Hodgkin Lymphoma Prognostic Factors Project. N Engl J Med 1993; 329: 987–994

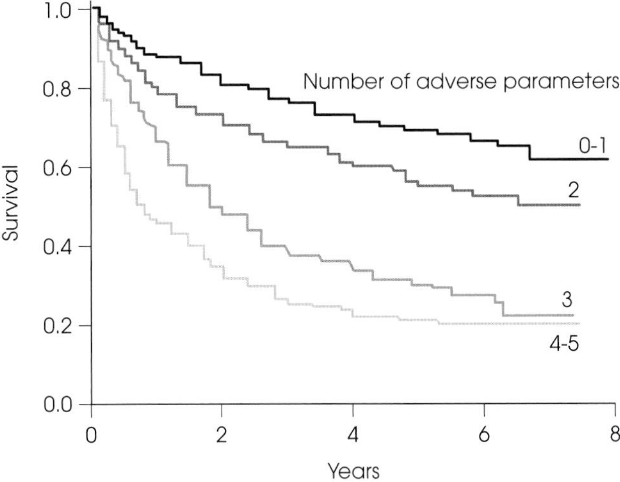

Figure 33.8 Correlation of overall survival and International Prognostic Index factors.

Table 33.6 Treatment modalities in non-Hodgkin's lymphoma

Treatment	Comment
Chemotherapy	Mainstay of most protocols
Radiotherapy	May be curative alone in early-stage non-Hodgkin's lymphoma
Stem cell transplantation: autograft or allograft transplant	Usually reserved for relapsed non-Hodgkin's lymphoma as a consolidation treatment after salvage chemotherapy; allograft transplants with low-intensity conditioning regimens are being increasingly used
Immunotherapy	Anti-CD20 is licensed in relapsed follicular cell lymphoma and aggressive high-grade lymphoma

lymphoma, and the age and performance status of the patient. Because of heterogeneity in the disease, some subtypes carry a worse prognosis than others and may require more aggressive treatment regimens. The mainstay of most treatment protocols includes the use of chemotherapy, but other modalities may also be used in combination with chemotherapy, as shown in Table 33.6.

General treatment principles

Low-grade lymphomas

The non-Hodgkin's lymphomas may be divided histologically into a low-grade subgroup (erroneously classified as 'good prognosis'); here the disease tends to run an indolent course characterized by frequent periods of relapse. Although these low-grade lymphomas have a median survival of between 5 and 10 years, the majority of patients ultimately die of their lymphoma or associated complications. In patients with such low-grade lymphomas aggressive treatment has not been rewarded by improvements in cure rates. In fact, the converse is often true: many patients die early of treatment-related complications. Despite the low cure rates, patients with low-grade non-Hodgkin's lymphoma may maintain an excellent quality of life over several years without active treatment or with the use of minimal intervention with radiation or chemotherapy.

Follicular cell lymphoma is the most common subtype of low-grade lymphoma, and treatment issues relating to this disease centre around the age at diagnosis and the risk factors associated with the International Prognostic Index. The distinguishing features of indolent lymphoma are the high sensitivity to initial therapy, inevitable relapse, and a gradual reduction in sensitivity to chemotherapy after successive courses.[33]

For this disease it should be borne in mind that the disease is frequently incurable and the median survival for patients is 6–8 years. Therefore clinical-based decisions should consider these endpoints because treatment may not always need to be started early and be aggressive. The clinical course typically follows a pattern of multiple remissions and relapse, with responses becoming less durable with successive courses of chemotherapy. Cumulative toxicity becomes rate-limiting with successive treatment courses, and therefore fine judgement is required when to intervene while trying to maintain maximal longevity. Treatment of early-stage disease may simply require local radiotherapy, while more advanced disease is usually treated by intermittent therapies administered over many years. Treatment may not even be required at all at diagnosis, and a watch and wait policy pursued in those patients who have no symptoms and a favourable prognosis.[34,35] It is possible for patients to delay treatment for up to 3 years, and treatment only needs to begin after disease progression, development of systemic symptoms, bone marrow decompensation or critical organ involvement.

Treatment of relapse

The initial response to chemotherapy is the most important factor in subsequent treatment strategy. A short-lived response to treatment is an ominous sign, and generally subjects the patient to increasingly toxic regimens with no guarantee of success. The choice of second-line treatments for this disease may use anthracycline therapy or incorporate the use of purine analogues, either as single agents or in combination regimens such as FMD (fludarabine, mitoxantrone and dexamethasone), which has been reported to induce an over 90% response rate and over 47% complete responses in patients with recurrent lymphoma.[36,37] For patients with further relapsed and refractory disease the use of rituximab has been shown to be effective in this setting and has been approved by the National Institute for Clinical Excellence for use in this group of patients.[38]

High-grade lymphomas

At the other end of the disease spectrum, the high-grade, biologically aggressive lymphomas tend to pursue a rapid and relentless course when untreated, with median survival times of

REFERENCES

33. Non-Hodgkin's Lymphoma Classification Project. Blood 1997; 89: 3903–3918
34. Young RC, Longo DL, Glatstein E et al. Semin Haematol 1988; 25: 11–16
35. Horning SJ, Rosenburg SA. N Engl J Med 1984; 311: 1471–1475
36. Keating NJ, McLaughin P, Cabinillas F et al. J Cancer Care 1997; 6 (Suppl 4): 21–26
37. Mclaughin P, Hagemeister FB et al. J Clin Oncol 1996; 14: 1262–1268
38. National Institute for Clinical Excellence. Technology Appraisal Guidance 65. NICE, London, 2003

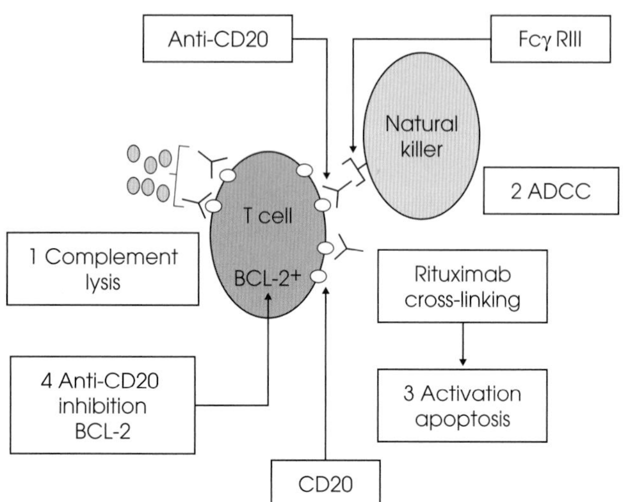

Figure 33.9 Mechanisms of anti-CD20 (rituximab). ADCC, antibody dependent cellular cytotoxicity.

12–24 months. This group of lymphomas, previously referred to as 'poor prognosis', have witnessed a treatment revolution in the past 5 years with the advent of immunotherapies. This has been facilitated by the characterization of suitable cells, such as the CD20 antigen, which is specifically expressed on the surfaces of normal and malignant pre-B and B lymphocytes but not on pluripotent stem cells. The monoclonal antibody rituximab (anti-CD20) is a chimeric antibody consisting of the constant region from human IgG and the variable region derived from mouse immunoglobulin. The mechanism of action of anti-CD20 antibody is multiple (Fig. 33.9) and includes the following:[39]

- induction of antibody cell-mediated cytotoxicity;
- induction of complement-mediated lysis;
- induction of apoptosis (programmed cell death); and
- sensitization of resistant human lymphoma cells to certain cytotoxic agents.

The most common type of high-grade non-Hodgkin's lymphoma is diffuse large B-cell lymphoma. Treatment decisions in this disease are more straightforward than in follicular cell lymphoma, and the results of large randomized trials have established standard therapies for these patients based on stage and the International Prognostic Index.

Patients with stage I and II non-bulky disease (less than 10 cm) should receive combined modality therapy with CHOP (cyclophosphamide, doxorubicin, vincristine and prednisone) plus involved-field radiotherapy. Long-term progression-free survival of 60–70% and overall survival of 80% have been achieved with this approach.[40] All other patients should be treated according to the International Prognostic Index group. Low- and intermediate-risk patients should receive six to eight courses of CHOP chemotherapy, and consideration should be given for entry into clinical trials where the use of new agents is being investigated.

Clinical results with rituximab have shown that the addition of rituximab to standard CHOP chemotherapy (R-CHOP) in aggressive non-Hodgkin's lymphoma diffuse large B-cell lymphoma obtains higher response rates (76% with R-CHOP compared with 63% with CHOP alone).[41] R-CHOP also demonstrated significant superiority in event-free survival and overall survival at 36-month follow-up compared with CHOP alone. The improved survival figures represent the most significant advance in the management of high-grade lymphoma for over 20 years.

For patients with relapsed and refractory disease, autologous stem cell transplantation is standard for those patients who respond to second-line, non-cross-resistant chemotherapy, i.e. IVE (ifosfamide, vincristine and etoposide) or ESHAP (etoposide, methylprednisolone, cytarabine and cisplatin).[42]

Mantle cell lymphoma

Mantle cell lymphoma accounts for approximately 5–8% of all lymphomas. This type of lymphoma is most frequent in males, especially those aged over 50 years. Most patients present with stage IV disease. Proliferation is generally widespread at diagnosis, with extensive hypertrophy of lymph nodes and spleen, infiltration of the marrow and blood, and extranodal and nodal sites of involvement, particularly the gastrointestinal tract, with presentation sometimes as lymphomatoid polypomatosis.

Historically, although classed as an indolent or intermediate-grade tumour, the prognosis is poor, with a 25–30% 5-year survival rate. Because of this, newer intensive chemotherapy strategies have been sought, with combinations of fludarabine and cyclophosphamide with or without rituximab yielding encouraging results in ongoing European studies.

Burkitt's lymphoma

Burkitt's lymphoma consists of medium-sized monomorphic cells with a round nucleus, multiple nucleoli and relatively abundant cytoplasm. The tumour shows multiple mitoses and the presence of many effete dead cells on histological analysis, giving rise to the characteristic starry sky appearance.

The cells are positive for surface immunoglobulin (IgM^+), express B-cell antigens, and are $CD5^+$ and $CD10^+$. Most cases show translocation of the c-myc gene on chromosome 8 to the immunoglobulin heavy chain region on chromosome 14, t(8;14), or to the light chain region on chromosome 2, t(2;8), or chromosome 22, t(8;22).

Burkitt's lymphoma is more common in children but accounts for 55% of cases in adults. Most patients present with an abdominal tumour involving the caecum and mesentery, but some cases develop in an ovary, breast, testis or peripheral lymph node. Bone marrow or meningeal involvement carries a very poor prognosis. Interestingly, the treatment of this form of lymphoma has been revolutionized by the use of high-intensity chemotherapy regimens such as CODOX-M IVAC (cyclophosphamide, vincristine, doxorubicin, methotrexate, ifosfamide, etoposide and cytarabine), which has significantly improved survival rates.

SPECIAL SITE LYMPHOMAS

TESTICULAR LYMPHOMA

Testicular lymphoma has a predilection to spread to unusual extranodal sites and to relapse after achieving remission, and shows an overall poor prognosis. The tumour itself is uncommon,

REFERENCES

39. Male et al. Advanced Immunol 1996; 1: 1
40. Miller TP, Dahlberg S, Cassady R et al. N Engl J Med 1998; 339: 21–26
41. Coiffier B, Lepage E, Briere J et al. N Engl J Med 2002; 346: 235–242
42. Philip T, Guglielmi C et al. N Engl J Med 1995; 333: 1540–1545

accounting for only 1–9% of all testicular neoplasms and 1% of all non-Hodgkin's lymphoma. It is prevalent in the elderly population and is the most common testicular tumour after the age of 60.

As with other extranodal lymphomas, malignant lymphoma of the testis is prone to occur in the setting of immunosuppression. Data suggest that 25% of patients with testicular non-Hodgkin's lymphoma are HIV-positive. In this specific subgroup the lymphoma tends to occur at an earlier age and to behave aggressively. In contrast to primary testicular non-Hodgkin's lymphoma, secondary involvement of the testis during the clinical presentation of systemic lymphoma is more common and has the highest prevalence in patients with high-grade lymphomas, especially Burkitt's lymphoma.

The most common clinical presentation is with a unilateral, painless scrotal swelling. On physical examination there is usually a non-tender, firm mass inseparable from the testis. The testis varies from normal size too, as large as 16 cm. The epididymis, when involved, is enlarged, firm and nodular. In a significant number of patients, testicular lymphoma is associated with hydrocele (43%), which may mask the underlying testicular parenchymal lesion. Involvement of both testes occurs in up to a fifth of cases, and a careful examination must be made of the contralateral side. The tumour itself has a propensity to metastasize to a variety of unusual extranodal sites involving the central nervous system, Waldeyer's ring, skin and lung. Central nervous system involvement may manifest as symptoms of headache, cranial nerve palsy, focal motor weakness, sensory deficits and gait abnormalities.

For any clinical abnormality of the testis, ultrasound is the initial investigation of choice. For pathological diagnosis, a high inguinal orchidectomy is the optimal method of obtaining tissue. Following a histological diagnosis a thorough evaluation to determine the extent of lymphomatous involvement of nodal and extranodal sites is indicated.

Because of histological similarity between malignant lymphoma and some germ cell tumours, cases of lymphoma have been misdiagnosed as seminoma and less often as embryonal cell carcinoma. Careful histological examination is required as defined by the criteria of Gowing.[43] Other diseases that may lead to diagnostic confusion include granulomatous orchitis, pseudolymphoma, plasmacytoma and rhabdomyosarcoma. Immunohistochemistry should resolve these issues.

Treatment has not been formally standardized, but there is universal agreement that orchidectomy is the initial treatment of choice, particularly for stage IE and IIE disease. Although long-term survival has been achieved in stage IE disease with orchidectomy alone, the majority have relapsed in the first 2 years at various nodal and gonadal sites. After intensive staging the majority of patients have at least stage II disease, and chemotherapy offers the only hope for cure for high-grade tumours.

LYMPHOMAS OF THE BREAST

Lymphomas of the breast are uncommon, and a broad variety of histological subtypes have been described. They may arise as a primary or in the setting of systemic lymphoma. Clinically and pathologically they must be distinguished from benign lymphoid infiltrates and non-lymphoid neoplasms of the breast. The breast normally contains some lymphoid tissue and functions during lactation as part of the mucosal immune defence, and lymphomas in the breast may be related to lymphomas of the mucosa-associated lymphoid tissue (MALT).

Primary and secondary lymphomas of the breast are defined according to the criteria of other extranodal lymphomas. Primary lymphomas of the breast can be diagnosed when:

- clinically the breast is the site of first or major manifestation of the lymphoma; and
- there is no documentation of lymphoma elsewhere, excluding the presence of ipsilateral axillary node involvement.

Regional node involvement is accepted, provided that both mammary and lymph nodal lesions developed simultaneously. The incidence of primary breast lymphomas ranges from 0.5 to 1.0% of malignant breast neoplasms in most series.

There appears to be geographical variation, with a higher incidence seen in western countries compared with Asian countries.[44] Several clinicopathological presentations are seen; the most frequent scenario is that of a unilateral breast mass in a middle-aged woman (median age 55–60 years) or as massive bilateral breast enlargement occurring in young women of childbearing age during or immediately after pregnancy. Histology of the latter often reveals a Burkitt's or Burkitt-like lymphoma.

This particular disease carries a grave prognosis because dissemination is rapid, with prominent ovarian and central nervous system involvement.[45] The diagnosis of breast lymphomas is made in most cases by core or excision biopsy. Most primary breast lymphomas are of B-cell type.[45] There is no uniform approach to the treatment of primary breast lymphoma. In many of the cases, treatment is according to that given for systemic lymphomas; that is, usually based on histological grade. Mastectomy has no place in management, and wide local excision is usually unnecessary because the tumours are sensitive to both chemotherapy and radiotherapy.

The 5-year overall survival for all cases of breast lymphoma is 40%. For patients with stage I disease, the 5-year freedom from progression and overall survival is 50 and 60%, respectively, whereas for stage II disease the figures are 26 and 27%, respectively.[46,47]

HEAD AND NECK LYMPHOMA

Approximately 10% of patients with non-Hodgkin's lymphoma present with extranodal disease in the head and neck region. The distinct sites within this area included Waldeyer's ring, the salivary glands, nasal cavity, paranasal sinuses, thyroid gland and orbit.[48] Although they are in close proximity, lymphomas arising from these particular areas each have distinct clinical characteristics. The average age of presentation is between 50 and 60 years, with a slight male predominance (1.6:1). More than half of these tumours occur in Waldeyer's ring, which comprises lymphoid tissue located in the nasopharynx, tonsil and base of the tongue.

Presenting symptoms are similar to those of squamous cancers: for the tonsils, tonsillar swelling or throat pain; for the naso-

REFERENCES

43. Gowing NFC. Malignant Lymphoma of the Testis: Pathology of the Testis. Blackwell Scientific Publications, London, 1976: 334–355
44. Aozoa K, Ohsawa M et al. Am J Clin Pathol 1992; 97: 699–704
45. Arber DA, Simpson JF et al. Am J Surg Pathol 1994; 18: 288–295
46. Cohen PL, Brooks JJ. Cancer 1991; 67: 1359–1369
47. Giardini R, Piccolo C et al. Cancer 1992; 69: 725–735
48. Jacobs C, Hoppe RT. Int J Radiat Oncol Biol Phys 1985; 11: 357–364

pharynx, cervical mass, nasal obstruction or decreased hearing; and for the base of the tongue, sensation of a foreign body or sore throat. About one-third of head and neck lymphomas occur in extralymphatic sites, including the paranasal sinuses, nasal cavity, salivary gland, oral cavity, larynx and orbit. Sinus lymphomas usually present with symptoms of sinusitis, with diplopia and with exophthalmos. The distribution of subtypes correlates with the site, with paranasal and nasal cavity lymphomas almost always intermediate- or high-grade lymphomas, whereas half of the patients with salivary gland lymphomas have a low-grade histology. Staging should include whole-body CT scan and bone marrow biopsy.[49] A lumbar puncture should be performed because these patients have a high propensity for central nervous system involvement.

For stage IE disease staged by lymphogram and bone marrow, 5-year survivals exceed 75% with radiotherapy alone, compared with less than 40% for stage IIE patients. Radiotherapy fields should encompass the primary disease and uninvolved cervical nodes. With the rare exception of those patients with low-grade histology who achieve long-term disease-free survival with radiotherapy alone, all other patients with stage IIE head and neck lymphoma should receive chemotherapy as primary treatment.

Lymphomas arising in the nasal area must be differentiated from other midline or midfacial destructive lesions such as Wegener's granulomatosis, infections, sarcoidosis and idiopathic midline destructive disease (Table 33.7).[50,51]

Primary lymphoma of the central nervous system (reticulum cell sarcoma, microgliomatosis and malignant reticuloendotheliosis) predominantly involves the brain and only rarely the spinal cord. The incidence of primary central nervous system lymphoma has increased in recent years, particularly in patients with chronic immunosuppression in association with either AIDS or following organ transplantation.[52]

Presenting symptoms are similar to those of other intracranial tumours and include headache, nausea and vomiting, seizures and localized weakness. The origin and histological classification of primary central nervous system lymphomas has caused considerable controversy, but it appears that they are largely of B-cell origin and of the high-grade type. Involvement of the brain is usually multifocal and the disease infiltrates widely. Whole-brain irradiation may produce good palliation, but survival to 5 years is exceptional even with high-dose radiotherapy and with combination chemotherapy. Given the appalling prognosis of this disease, alternative treatment strategies need to be explored.

SECONDARY CENTRAL NERVOUS SYSTEM INVOLVEMENT

Central nervous system involvement occurs in up to 30% of patients with disseminated non-Hodgkin's lymphoma, the incidence being highest in those with high-grade disease and bone marrow or liver infiltration. The disease primarily affects the meninges, and less commonly the spinal cord and brain parenchyma. Patients with high-grade lymphoma achieving complete remission after chemotherapy show central nervous system relapse rates of between 5 and 8%, but this is rarely the only site of recurrent disease.

THYROID

Lymphomas of the thyroid gland constitute 2.5–3.0% of all non-Hodgkin's lymphomas and 5% of all thyroid malignancies. Women are affected more commonly than men, and the mean age at presentation is over 60 years.

The presentation is usually characterized by a rapidly enlarging neck mass causing local obstructive and infiltrative symptomatology, but patients may also present with symptoms of dysphagia, hoarseness, choking or a cold thyroid nodule. Primary thyroid carcinomas are frequently associated with Hashimoto's thyroiditis, and thyroid lymphoma should be suspected in such patients who show signs of rapid thyroid enlargement.

The most common histological subtype is diffuse large B-cell non-Hodgkin's lymphoma. The management of this type of tumour is combined modality therapy with radiotherapy and CHOP. Overall, survival rates at 5 years range from 40 to 75%, with relapse-free survival rates of 38–64%. Radiotherapy alone may still be considered appropriate therapy for patients with limited small bulk disease confined to the thyroid gland.

PRIMARY GASTROINTESTINAL LYMPHOMAS

The gastrointestinal tract is the most frequently involved extranodal localization in non-Hodgkin's lymphoma. Gastrointestinal non-Hodgkin's lymphoma accounts for 4–20% of all non-Hodgkin's lymphoma, and it is the most common of all the extranodal lymphomas (30–40%).[53] In the western world the most common locations are the stomach (50–60%) and the small intestine (30%). It is the most common stomach malignancy after adenocarcinoma, and accounts for approximately 25% of all small intestinal tumours but less than 0.5% of colorectal neoplasms.

A number of risk factors have been associated with gastrointestinal non-Hodgkin's lymphoma, such as infection with *Helicobacter pylori* and HIV, immunosuppression after solid organ transplantation, coeliac disease and inflammatory bowel disease. Prognostic factors that have been associated with a poor outcome include advanced stage, involvement of para-aortic lymph nodes, tumour size, serosal penetration, and an intestinal as opposed to a gastric presentation.[54]

Gastrointestinal lymphomas include a number of discrete clinicopathological entities that have undergone many revised classifications. Those seen frequently or exclusively in the

Table 33.7 Summary of treatment options for head and neck lymphoma

Histology	Stage	Treatment options
Low grade	I or II	IFRT
Intermediate grade	I or II	CHOP × 3 plus IFRT
	III or IV	CHOP or other combination chemotherapy
High grade	I–IV	Combination chemotherapy

REFERENCES

49. Aisenberg AC. J Clin Oncol 1995; 13: 2656–2675
50. Weiss LM, Arber DA, Strickler JG. Ann Oncol 1994; 5: 39–42
51. Li YX, Coucke PA, Li JY et al. Cancer 1998; 83: 449–456
52. Penn I. In: Toledo-Pereyra LH (ed). Complications of Organ Transplantation. Marcel Dekker, New York, 1987: 237–251
53. d'Amore F, Christensen BE, Brincker H et al. Eur J Cancer 1991; 27: 1201–1208
54. Radaszkiewicz T, Dragosics B, Bauer P. Gastroenterology 1992; 102: 1628–1638

Table 33.8 Clinical features of primary gastrointestinal non-Hodgkin's lymphoma

Feature	Stomach	Small intestine	Colon or rectum
Symptoms	Pain, nausea, vomiting, weight loss, bleeding	Pain, obstruction, weight loss, malabsorption	Pain, bleeding, diarrhoea
Proportion of gastrointestinal non-Hodgkin's lymphoma (%)	55–65	25–35	10–15
Predominant histology	MALT, diffuse large B cell	Diffuse large B cell, T cell, Burkitt's or lymphoblastic	Diffuse large B cell, MALT
Stage at presentation			
I (%)	50	25	30
$II_{1,2}$ (%)	20	30	20
IV	30	45	50
5-year survival			
Stage I (%)	70–85	40–60	30–40
Stage II (%)	35–60	20	–

gastrointestinal tract include mantle cell lymphoma, intestinal T-cell lymphoma and MALT type of extranodal marginal zone lymphoma. The symptoms and signs depend on the anatomical location of the presenting tumour, as summarized in Table 33.8.

Patients with localized gastrointestinal non-Hodgkin's lymphoma should undergo examination to exclude Waldeyer's ring involvement, bone marrow aspiration, and biopsy for immunophenotyping and histology (Table 33.9). Patients who have not had a surgical exploration should have barium studies performed to exclude multifocal disease (10–25% of cases). Associated disease of HIV, inflammatory bowel disease and coeliac disease should be excluded.

The most appropriate management for these patients needs to be decided on a case-by-case basis. Where possible all diseased bowel should be resected at laporotomy to allow adequate histological assessment and to minimize the risk of haemorrhage and perforation during subsequent treatment. Because the majority of these patients have high-grade malignancy they will require intensive combination chemotherapy after surgery.[55]

Table 33.9 Staging of gastrointestinal non-Hodgkin's lymphoma

Stage	Description
I	Tumour confined to the gastrointestinal tract; single primary site or multiple non-contiguous lesions
II	Tumour extending in abdomen from primary gastrointestinal site; nodal involvement; II_1 local (paragastric or paraintestinal), II_2 distant (mesenteric, para-aortic, paracaval, pelvic or inguinal)
IIE	Penetration of serosa to involve adjacent organs or tissues
IV	Disseminated extranodal involvement or gastrointestinal tract lesion with supradiaphragmatic nodal involvement

GASTRIC MALT LYMPHOMA

Between 20 and 30% of gastric lymphomas are of low grade and arise specifically within organized extranodal lymphoid tissue. Gastric MALT and its association with *H. pylori* is well established: several lines of evidence suggest that chronic gastritis caused by *H. pylori* provides the immunological stimulus for T-cell-dependent B-cell proliferation. Both low- and high-grade MALT lesions are seen, the latter usually arising as a consequence of overexpression of BCL6 or p53, or deletion of the p16 tumour suppressor gene. Regression of primary low-grade gastric MALT lymphoma following treatment with antibiotics raises the possibility that eradication of *H. pylori* may be sufficient therapy for selected patients with early MALT lymphoma. The recommended anti-*Helicobacter* therapy is amoxicillin 1 g twice daily, clarithromycin 250 mg twice daily and omeprazole 20 mg twice daily for 7 days. The expected rate of eradication is over 90%, and although eradication may occur within a month of the completion of drug therapy, disappearance of lymphoma usually takes several months, and delays of up to 18 months are documented.

All patients with low-grade gastric MALT treated only with antibiotics to eradicate *H. pylori* should be followed up with careful endoscopic examination. Those cases that are refractory to antibiotic therapy may be treated with radiotherapy alone. An alternative approach is to use chlorambucil alone or in combined modality therapy.

PRIMARY INTESTINAL T-CELL LYMPHOMA

Between 10 and 25% of primary intestinal lymphomas have a T-cell phenotype. The presenting symptoms are weight loss, abdominal pain, diarrhoea and bowel obstruction. Patients with coeliac disease have a 200-fold increase in the risk of developing small bowel lymphoma. Epstein–Barr virus has also been implicated, although the exact pathogenesis is not known. The management of these patients is difficult and should follow protocols designed for aggressive lymphoma.

PRIMARY BONE LYMPHOMA

Primary non-Hodgkin's lymphoma of bone accounts for approximately 5% of all extranodal non-Hodgkin's lymphomas and 7% of primary bone tumours. The peak incidence is in the fifth decade, with a slight male preponderance. The presenting symptoms usually consist of localized bone pain (most commonly in a long bone) and occasionally a palpable mass. The vast

REFERENCES

55. Timothy AR, Sloane J, Selby P et al. In: Sikora K, Halnan HE. Treatment of Cancer. 2nd edn. Chapman &Hall, London, 1990: 695–736

majority of patients present with localized disease and without systemic symptoms. The differential diagnosis includes other round cell tumours including metastatic carcinoma, Ewing's sarcoma and eosinophilic granuloma.

To establish a histological diagnosis of primary non-Hodgkin's lymphoma of bone, tissue from the bony lesion or, if present, the associated tissue mass is usually obtained by fine-needle aspiration or by open surgical biopsy. However, fine-needle aspiration is often unsuccessful because of crush artefact. By the criteria of the Revised European–American Lymphoma classification the majority of tumours are of the diffuse large B-cell type. Staging is based on the Ann Arbor classification and should include plain X-rays and MRI scanning.

The mainstay of treatment of primary non-Hodgkin's lymphoma of bone is radiation therapy and chemotherapy. The role of surgery in primary non-Hodgkin's lymphoma of bone is limited to the diagnostic biopsy and to the repair of fractures that either present at initial diagnosis or arise during treatment. For the treatment of localized non-Hodgkin's lymphoma it appears from several studies that induction chemotherapy followed by consolidation radiotherapy achieves better results in terms of progression-free and overall survival. Combined radiation and chemotherapy is currently the preferred option, with 5-year survival rates in the order of 50%.[56]

REFERENCES

56. Barr J, Burke R. Cancer 1994; 73: 1194

The adrenal glands

34

Gregory P. Sadler, Kumar Ravi

INTRODUCTION

The adrenal glands were first described by the Roman anatomist Bartholomaeus Eustachius in the sixteenth century.[1] In 1856, following Addison's clinical observations, Charles Brown-Sequard demonstrated that the glands were essential for life.[2] Adrenaline (epinephrine) was first identified in 1897 as a medullary extract causing vasoconstriction, and in the early 19th century a cortical extract (cortin) was successfully used to treat Addison's disease.[3,4] Since these early discoveries, the nature of the adrenal hormones and their complex role in both normal body function and the pathogenesis of disease have been fully elucidated.

ANATOMY

The adrenals are retroperitoneal structures situated either side of the vertebral column, enclosed by Gerota's fascia. Inferiorly they are intimately related to the superior poles of the kidneys, and posteriorly to the crura of the diaphragm. The pyramidally shaped right adrenal is also related to the bare area of the liver and the inferior vena cava. The left adrenal is a semilunar shape and related to the stomach, the spleen and the pancreas.

The aorta, and the renal and inferior phrenic arteries provide the arterial blood supply to each gland. The right adrenal drains through a small short vein directly into the inferior vena cava. The left adrenal vein drains into the left renal vein. Additional small veins drain into the inferior vena cava, and hepatic and phrenic veins.

The coeliac plexus supplies the sympathetic innervation to the gland. However, the preganglionic splanchnic nerves also supply the adrenal medulla.

Macroscopically the glands are golden yellow in colour. On cut section each gland has an outer cortex (85%), which is yellowish and mesodermal in origin, and an inner medulla, which is reddish brown and arises from the neuroectoderm. Histologically there are three distinct cortical layers: an outer zona glomerulosa, a middle zona fasciculata, and an inner zona reticularis.

PHYSIOLOGY

Cholesterol is the principal substance utilized in the synthesis of adrenocortical hormones. A series of specific enzymatic reactions results in the conversion of cholesterol, via intermediates such as pregnenolone and progesterones, to the different adrenocortical hormones (Fig. 34.1).

The mineralocorticoid aldosterone, produced by the zona glomerulosa, is primarily responsible for maintaining the plasma volume by promoting reabsorption of sodium ions in the renal tubules in exchange for potassium and hydrogen ions. The rate of exchange of these ions depends directly on the concentration of sodium in the tubules. Thus plasma concentration of sodium and potassium, together with angiotensin, regulates the synthesis and secretion of aldosterone. A fall in plasma volume stimulates the juxtaglomerular apparatus in the afferent renal tubules, triggering the release of renin. Renin splits angiotensinogen to angiotensin I, which is then converted to angiotensin II by angiotensin-converting enzyme.

The zona fasciculata mainly produces cortisol and small amounts of corticosterone. Secretion is regulated by adrenocorticotrophic hormone (ACTH) produced by the anterior pituitary, which is in turn controlled by corticotrophin-releasing hormone produced by the hypothalamus. A negative-feedback mechanism exists by which the corticosteroids suppress the secretion of both ACTH and corticotrophin-releasing hormone. Steroid synthesis demonstrates significant diurnal variation. The highest levels are demonstrated in the early morning, and the lowest levels at night.[5] The corticosteroids exert metabolic, vascular, immune and permissive functions essential for life.

Androgens produced by the zona reticularis are also under the control of ACTH and have a role in growth and sexual differentiation.

ADRENAL INSUFFICIENCY

Thomas Addison first described primary adrenal insufficiency in 1855.[2] The term *Addison's disease*, however, was coined the following year by Armand Trousseau, a French physiologist. The incidence of this rare condition has risen in recent years, due to the re-emergence of tuberculosis and AIDS.

AETIOLOGY

More than 60% of patients with adrenal insufficiency have an autoimmune cause, with autoimmune thyroiditis, pernicious

REFERENCES

1. Rolleston HD. The Endocrine Organs in Health and Disease. Oxford University Press, Oxford, 1936
2. Addison T. On the Constitutional and Local Effects of Disease of the Supra Renal Capsules. Samuel Highley, London, 1855
3. Oliver G, Sharpey-Shafer EA. J Physiol (Lond) 1895; 18: 230
4. Welbourn RB (ed). The History of Endocrine Surgery. Praeger Publishers, New York, 1990
5. Veldhuis JD, Iranmanesh A, Lizarralde G et al. Am J Physiol 1989; 257: E6–E14

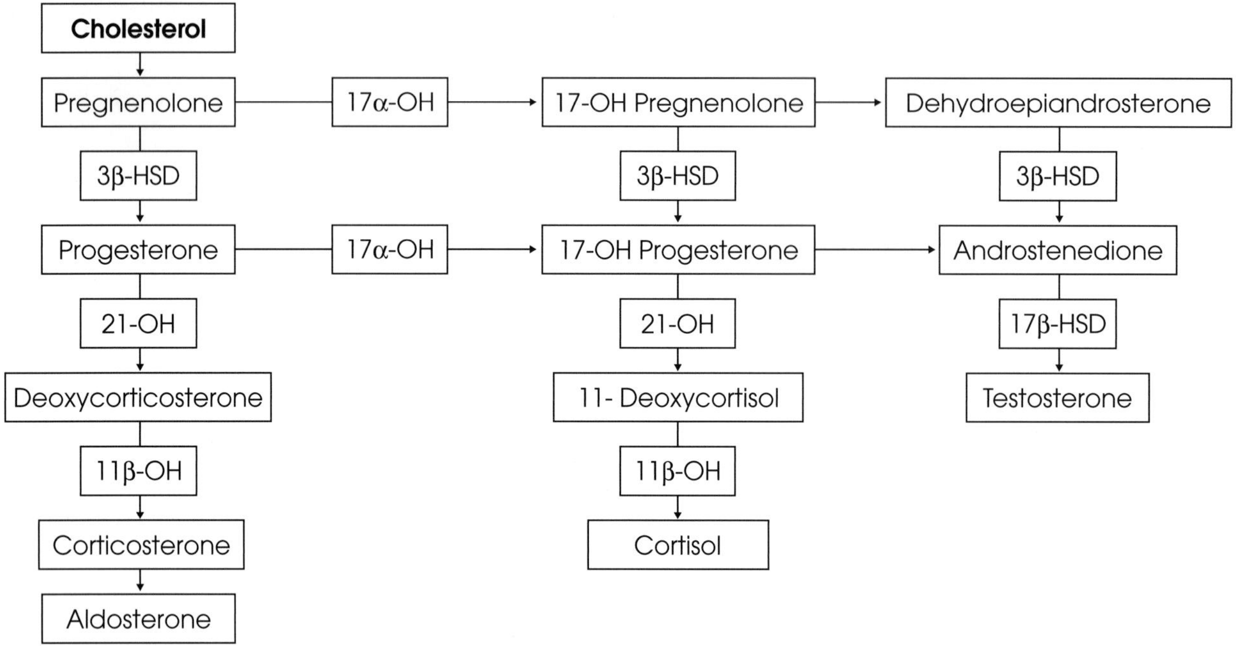

Figure 34.1 Mechanism of steroid synthesis.

anaemia and insulin-dependent diabetes being commonly associated conditions. Tuberculosis, sarcoidosis, amyloidosis, metastatic carcinoma, sarcoma, lymphoma, histoplasmosis, haemochromatosis, AIDS, drugs (antivirals, antifungals, rifampicin and phenytoin), abrupt corticosteroid withdrawal, and bilateral adrenalectomy are among the other causes of adrenal insufficiency.[6] Bilateral adrenal haemorrhages may occur in a neonate due to prolonged labour (adrenal apoplexy of the newborn), and in meningococcal septicaemia (Waterhouse–Friderichsen syndrome), postoperative states and anticoagulated patients, and lead to hypoadrenalism.

CLINICAL PRESENTATION

Addison's disease has an equal sex distribution, predominantly affecting patients in the third and fourth decades. Symptoms include lethargy, muscle weakness, anorexia and amenorrhoea coupled with signs of hypotension, pigmentation of buccal mucosa (particularly in the pressure areas), vitiligo and loss of body hair. In the acute presentation patients may present with drowsiness, confusion and eventually coma. Death may follow if patients are not treated promptly. Adrenal insufficiency associated with sepsis may present with cutaneous petechial haemorrhages, hyperpyrexia, rigors and cardiovascular collapse. A history of long-term steroid use and the scars of surgical adrenalectomy should be sought if this condition is suspected clinically. Patients may also present with features of pituitary and hypothalamic disease.

DIAGNOSIS

Lack of plasma cortisol elevation at 30 and 60 min following an injection of 250 μg of tetracosactide (tetracosactrin), the short synacthen test, will confirm the diagnosis.[6] Primary adrenal disease may be differentiated from adrenal disease secondary to pituitary causes by a depot test (the long synacthen test).

Determination of the exact aetiology requires other investigations, such as chest and abdominal radiographs and autoantibody screening.

TREATMENT

Acutely ill patients need rapid resuscitation with normal saline and 100 mg of hydrocortisone immediately; 100 mg of hydrocortisone should then be administered every 6 h until the patient is stable. Oral steroids such as dexamethasone or hydrocortisone may be started when the patient can tolerate oral medications. Intravenous antibiotics and other constitutional treatments may also be necessary, depending on the exact cause for the adrenal insufficiency.

Maintenance therapy for chronic adrenal insufficiency is usually 10 mg of hydrocortisone in the morning, 5 mg in the afternoon, and 5 mg in the evening. Additional fludrocortisone 0.05–0.1 mg may be required, particularly in patients unable to retain salt.[7]

Suggested steroid replacement therapy

The following are guidelines to steroid replacement therapy in differing surgical situations.[8] An outline of equivalent dosage regimens is detailed in Table 34.1.

Hypoadrenal states

Hypoadrenal states result from previous bilateral adrenalectomy and adrenal suppression due to long-term steroids.

For *major surgery*, hydrocortisone sodium succinate 100 mg IM or IV with premedication, followed by further 100 mg IV perioperatively. Thereafter, 100 mg every 6 h IV until oral intake of replacement dose is reinstituted. If oral intake is delayed for a long time, intravenous steroids may have to be weaned off gradually before starting the oral replacement therapy.

REFERENCES

6. Neumann PJ. In: Clark OH, Duh QY (eds). Textbook of Endocrine Surgery. WB Saunders, Philadelphia, 1997
7. Werbel SS, Ober KP. Endocrinol Metab Clin North Am 1993; 22: 303–328
8. Plumpton FS, Baser GM, Cole PV. Anaesthesia 1969; 24: 12–18

Table 34.1 Potency of steroids in relation to cortisol

Compound	Equivalent dose (mg)
Hydrocortisone (cortisol)	20
Cortisone	25
Prednisone	5
Prednisolone	5
Methylprednisolone	4
Dexamethasone	0.75
Betamethasone	0.6

For *minor surgery*, intramuscular steroids for 24 h in the perioperative period or a single preoperative dose of 100 mg of hydrocortisone for minimal procedures.

Patients undergoing bilateral adrenalectomy

Hydrocortisone sodium succinate 100 mg IM or IV given with premedication, followed by a further 100 mg during gland removal. This is continued postoperatively every 6 h for 48–72 h. Thereafter, the dose is reduced to 50 mg every 6 h, simultaneously introducing 20 mg of hydrocortisone orally in the morning and 10 mg at night, reducing the IV dose until oral replacement has been established. Oral fludrocortisone acetate 0.05–0.1 mg may be required after stopping parenteral steroids.

Patients undergoing unilateral adrenalectomy

Patients with Cushing's syndrome due to an adrenal adenoma may have their normal adrenal suppressed. Steroid therapy in these patients follows the same protocol as for bilateral adrenalectomy. However, oral replacement is gradually weaned off over a period of months, by which time the suppressed adrenal should have fully recovered.

HYPERCORTISOLISM

CUSHING'S SYNDROME

In 1932, American neurosurgeon Harvey Cushing described the features of this syndrome in patients who were found to have basophil adenomas of the pituitary gland.[9] The syndrome results from abnormally high levels of circulating glucocorticoids. Cushing's syndrome may be ACTH-dependent or non-ACTH-dependent. Strictly, the pituitary ACTH-dependent is described as Cushing's disease.

Adrenocorticotrophic hormone-dependent Cushing's syndrome

Cushing's disease

The majority (70%) of patients with Cushing's syndrome have an ACTH-producing pituitary tumour (Cushing's disease). Tumours are either adenomas or microadenomas (usually smaller than 1 cm); malignant tumours are rare. The primary defect may be excessive production of corticotrophin-releasing hormone by the hypothalamus. The negative-feedback mechanism is set to a higher level than normal, with the persistently high levels of ACTH leading to bilateral hyperplasia of the adrenal cortex. Over-production of corticosteroids by the adrenals results in the clinical features of Cushing's syndrome.[10] The disease is more prominent in the third and fourth decades, with women affected four times more commonly than men.

Ectopic adrenocorticotrophic hormone syndrome

Liddle coined the term *ectopic ACTH syndrome* in 1962.[11] Approximately 10% of patients with Cushing's syndrome have an ectopic source of ACTH production. Tumours implicated in this syndrome include neuroendocrine tumours, small cell carcinoma of the bronchus, medullary thyroid cancer, phaeochromocytoma, thymoma, pancreatic endocrine tumours and bronchial carcinoid. Gastric and ovarian cancer, and pancreatic carcinoid are also rare causes.[12] The peak incidence is also in the third and fourth decades. In contrast to Cushing's disease, men are affected twice as commonly as women.

Non-adrenocorticotrophic hormone-dependent Cushing's syndrome

There are a number of causes of non-ACTH-dependent Cushing's:

- Iatrogenic: administration of corticosteroids (such as prednisolone) is undoubtedly the most common cause of Cushing's syndrome.
- Adrenal tumours: 20% of patients with Cushing's syndrome have either a benign adrenal adenoma or a carcinoma. Adenoma is more common in adults and carcinoma in children.
- Macronodular adrenocortical hyperplasia: an uncommon condition of unknown aetiology leading to excessive cortisol production, independent of ACTH.
- Primary pigmented nodular adrenocortical disease (Carney's syndrome): cardiac, breast, cutaneous myxoma and peripheral nerve tumours may be associated with autonomous hypersecreting nodular adrenals secondary to primary pigmented nodular adrenocortical disease.[13] Neuroendocrine tumours and pituitary adenomas may also be associated. Nodules in this rare condition are usually small and may be difficult to localize.

CLINICAL FEATURES OF CUSHING'S SYNDROME

The clinical features and their causative factors are outlined in Table 34.2 and illustrated in Fig. 34.2. The differential diagnosis in Cushing's syndrome includes diabetes, polycystic ovarian disease, alcoholism and hirsuitism.

Diagnosis of Cushing's syndrome involves establishing biochemical hypercortisolism, identifying the cause of the disease, and localizing the source of the excess hormone production.

CONFIRMATION OF HYPERSECRETION OF CORTISOL

Plasma cortisol levels

In normal individuals, plasma cortisol exhibits a diurnal variation; highest levels are recorded at 9.00 a.m. (140–180 nmol/L) and

REFERENCES

9. Cushing H. Johns Hopkins Hosp Bull 1932; 50: 137–195
10. Edwards CR, Besser GM. Clin Endocrinol Metab 1974; 3: 475–505
11. Liddle GW, Island D, Meador CK. Recent Prog Hormone Res 1962; 15: 125–166
12. Azzopardi JG, Williams ED. Cancer 1968; 22: 274–286
13. Grant CS, Carney JA, Carpenter PC et al. Surgery 1986; 100: 1178–1184

Table 34.2 Clinical features of Cushing's syndrome[14-16]

Symptoms and signs	Cause	Comment
Obesity	Cortisol stimulation of appetite and gluconeogenesis; glucose is liberated for fat synthesis	Truncal fat distribution. Limbs wasted, in contrast to generalized distribution of simple obesity.
Striae and thin skin	Reduction in skin collagen	Purple-coloured striae on abdomen, breasts and flanks. Plethoric moon face.
Excessive bruising and haematomas	Vessel wall collagen depletion	Clotting is normal.
Hypertension and oedema (seen in 30% of cases)	Salt and water retention due to cortisol excess	Significant cause of mortality.
Muscle weakness	Toxic effect of cortisol on muscles	Primarily affects proximal muscle groups.
Back pain	Osteoporosis	Collapse of vertebral bodies and pathological fractures of ribs and long bones may occur.
Skin pigmentation	Concomitant hypersecretion of ACTH and melanocyte stimulating hormone	Common in ectopic ACTH syndrome due to malignancy, when rapid weight loss and generalized muscle wasting may dominate. Also a feature of pituitary tumour with high ACTH levels (Nelson's syndrome).
Psychiatric illness		Wide range of symptoms from depression to psychosis.
Glucose intolerance	Action of cortisol on carbohydrate metabolism	Diabetes mellitus may result.
Hirsutism, virilism	Adrenal androgen secretion	Adrenal carcinoma should be suspected if virilism is pronounced. Acne on face and trunk.
Growth retardation	Reduced release and action of growth hormone	Important feature of Cushing's syndrome in children.
Poor wound healing	Cortisol effect on collagen synthesis; increased protein catabolism	Important surgical consideration, particularly when anterior approach is used
Menstrual and sexual dysfunction	Increased testosterone in females and decreased in males	Amenorrhoea or irregular menstruation. Impotence and loss of libido in men.

lowest at midnight (less than 190 nmol/L).[6] In Cushing's syndrome both these levels are raised, and the diurnal variation is lost.

Urinary free cortisol

The 24-h secretion of cortisol in urine is raised in patients with Cushing's syndrome (less than 360 nmol/day for men and less than 280 nmol/day for women).[17]

Dexamethasone suppression tests

Exogenous administration of a steroid (such as dexamethasone) will suppress ACTH and thereby cortisol in normal individuals. This effect is much less marked in Cushing's syndrome.[18] This test can be performed either as an *overnight test* (2 mg of dexamethasone given orally at midnight and cortisol levels measured at 9.00 a.m.) or as a *low-dose suppression test* (measurement of plasma and urinary free cortisol before and after administration of 0.5 mg of dexamethasone every 6 h for 2 days). Plasma cortisol is rarely suppressed in Cushing's syndrome.[18]

Insulin-induced hypoglycaemia

This test is helpful in differentiating patients with depression, who have elevated cortisol levels, from those with Cushing's syndrome, where insulin fails to cause a rise in cortisol levels.

IDENTIFICATION OF THE CAUSE OF HYPERCORTISOLISM

This test helps differentiate between ACTH-dependent and non-ACTH-dependent disease.

Plasma adrenocorticotrophic hormone

Plasma ACTH can be measured by radioimmunoassay. Patients with adrenal lesions demonstrate low or undetectable ACTH levels (less than 10 pg/mL); in contrast, patients with pituitary lesions will have normal or raised ACTH levels. Patients with ectopic ACTH syndrome are found to have extremely high levels (greater than 200 pg/mL).[19]

High-dose dexamethasone suppression test

Two milligrams of dexamethasone is administered every 6 h for 2 days, and cortisol levels are measured before and after suppression. Pituitary disease (ACTH-dependent) will result in suppression of cortisol levels, whereas adrenal lesions and ectopic ACTH sources (non-ACTH-dependent) will show little or no suppression.[20] Adrenal nodular hyperplasia and ectopic ACTH syndrome may give false positive results.

REFERENCES

14. Cutroneo KR, Rokowski R, Counts DF. Collagen Relat Res 1981; 1: 557–568
15. Nelson DH, Meakin JW, Thorn GW. Ann Intern Med 1960; 52: 560
16. Favio G, Lumachi FN. In: Clark OH, Duh QY. Textbook of Endocrine Surgery. WB Saunders, Philadelphia, 1997
17. Crapo L. Metab Clin Exp 1979; 28: 955–977
18. Liddle GW. J Clin Endocrinol Metab 1960; 20: 1539
19. Thompson NW, Cheung PS. Surg Clin North Am 1987; 67: 423–436
20. Young AE, Smellie WJB. In: Farndon JR (ed). A Companion to Specialist Surgical Practice: Endocrine Surgery. 2nd edn. WB Saunders, London, 2001

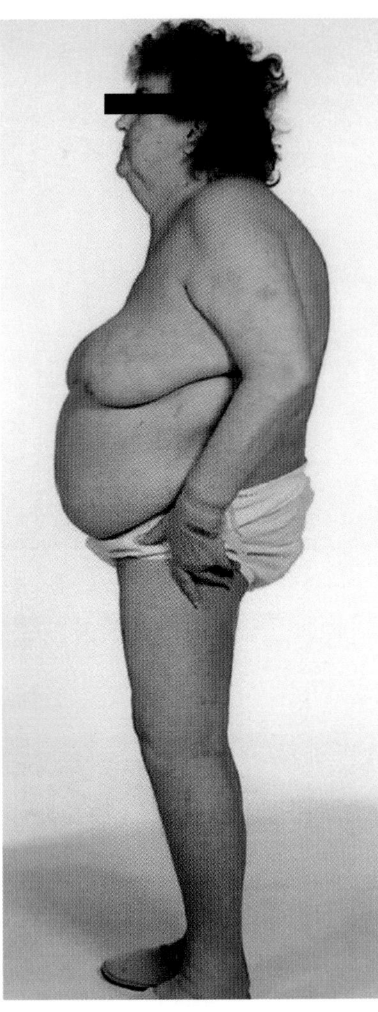

Figure 34.2 Clinical features of Cushing's syndrome demonstrated in a patient with adrenocortical carcinoma.

Metyrapone test

The metyrapone test is performed only rarely, in case of diagnostic difficulty. It also helps differentiate ACTH-dependent diseases from non-ACTH-dependent ones.

LOCALIZING INVESTIGATIONS

Pituitary disease (Cushing's disease)

Plain X-rays of the skull are not helpful. A CT scan will identify only 50% of tumours and has been replaced by MRI, which may localize up to 85% of the tumours.[21] Microadenomas (5–10 mm in size) may be missed on MRI. When suspected, these tumours are best detected by selective petrosal venous sampling for ACTH following corticotrophin-releasing hormone stimulation.[22]

Adrenal disease

A CT scan is the investigation of choice for localizing adrenal lesions. Tumours as small as 1 cm can be detected. Magnetic resonance imaging does not have any added advantage but may be useful for very small or large tumours with suspicion of malignancy.[20] Selenium cholesterol scintiscan is now avoided due to the persistence of the isotope and thus unacceptable doses of radiation.

Ectopic adrenocorticotrophic hormone

These tumours are often small and may be difficult to locate. A chest radiograph may demonstrate bronchial and pulmonary lesions, although CT and MRI may be more sensitive investigations. Thymic and pancreatic lesions may also be seen on CT scan. Bilateral adrenal enlargement is seen with all ectopic ACTH lesions.

TREATMENT OF CUSHING'S SYNDROME

Medical therapy

Metyrapone inhibits the synthesis of cortisol from 11-deoxycortisol. It is used to treat patients in whom surgery is contraindicated, and also in preparation of patients prior to surgery for Cushing's syndrome.[23] Ketoconazole, aminoglutethimide, bromocriptine and mitotane have also been used in the management of this condition.

PITUITARY DISEASE

The treatment of choice for pituitary adenomas is selective excision by trans-sphenoidal microsurgery. Partial or total hypophysectomy may be necessary for larger tumours. Cure rates up to 90% have been achieved following excision of microadenomas.[24] Pituitary replacement therapy tends to be necessary only following total excision, which is associated with lower cure rates.

Pituitary irradiation using an external beam, linear accelerator, or interstitial gold-198 or yttrium-90 may also be used. Pituitary insufficiency in children is seen less commonly than in adults with this form of treatment.[25] Resolution of symptoms may take over a year.

Improved techniques in pituitary surgery mean that bilateral adrenalectomy is now performed less commonly. It is reserved for:

- failed pituitary surgery or when surgery is not an option;
- palliation of ectopic ACTH syndrome;
- primary adrenal hyperplasia; and
- rapid progressive or severe hypercortisolism.

Bilateral adrenalectomy for ACTH-dependent Cushing's syndrome results in remission in 65% of patients at 5–15 years, and 50% of patients are alive at 20 years.[26] These patients need steroid cover during the operation and replacement on a long-term basis.

NELSON'S SYNDROME

Nelson and his colleagues described this condition in 1960.[15] It is characterized by the effects of continued growth of the ACTH-producing pituitary tumour following bilateral adrenalectomy. Features include skin hyperpigmentation, headache, visual field defects and hypopituitarism. Prophylactic pituitary irradiation may reduce the incidence of this condition.[27] The established syndrome requires surgery or irradiation.

REFERENCES

21. Dwyer AJ, Frank JA, Doppman JL et al. Radiology 1987; 163: 421
22. Oldfield EH, Chrousos GP, Schulte HM et al. New Engl J Med 1985; 312: 100–103
23. Jeffcoate WJ, Rees LH, Tomlin S et al. Br Med J 1977; 2: 215–217
24. Burke CW, Adams CB, Esiri MM et al. Clin Endocrinol 1990; 33: 525–537
25. Welbourn RB, Manolas KJ. Endocrine Surgery. Butterworth, London, 1983
26. Montgomery DAD, Welbourn RB. Br J Surg 1978; 65: 210–220
27. Rovit RL, Duane TD. Am J Med 1969; 46: 416–427

ECTOPIC ADRENOCORTICOTROPHIC HORMONE SYNDROME

Tumours (benign or malignant) identified as the source of ectopic ACTH should be excised, because this offers the only hope of symptom resolution. Radiotherapy and/or chemotherapy can also be considered for malignant tumours. Most tumours have a poor prognosis. For unresectable malignant tumours and non-localized tumours, bilateral adrenalectomy may help control symptoms. Metyrapone and mitotane may be used as palliative treatment.

ADRENAL TUMOURS

When facilities permit, unilateral adrenalectomy via a laparoscopic approach is the current favoured treatment of choice for adrenal adenomas. However, tumours greater than 7 cm should be removed via an open approach, because of the increased incidence of malignancy.

Excellent cure rates and long-term survival can be achieved.[26] Steroid replacement is necessary perioperatively, and for up to a year or more subsequently, to allow the contralateral suppressed adrenal to recover.

MACRONODULAR ADRENOCORTICAL HYPERPLASIA AND PRIMARY PIGMENTED NODULAR ADRENOCORTICAL DISEASE

The treatment for these rare conditions is bilateral adrenalectomy.

ADRENOCORTICAL CARCINOMA

Carcinoma of the adrenal glands is rare. It accounts for 10% of all patients with Cushing's syndrome. The peak incidence is between the fourth and fifth decades. These aggressive cancers may be functioning (60%) or non-functioning (40%). Functioning tumours are more common in the younger patients (under 40 years), with a 4:1 female preponderance. Non-functioning tumours occur in the older patients (over 40 years), and males are more commonly affected (2:1).

Pathology

Tumours can grow to a large size, and non-functioning tumours are frequently over 5 cm at the time of diagnosis. Macroscopically they are greyish pink and appear lobulated. Areas of haemorrhage and necrosis may be seen. Microscopically, it may be difficult to establish their malignant nature unless there is clear evidence of vascular or capsular invasion. Spread is by direct invasion of pancreas, kidney, diaphragm, liver and bowel, or metastasis through veins and lymphatics to liver, lungs, bones and skin.

Clinical features

Functioning tumours usually present with syndromes specific to the hormone produced.

- Glucocorticoid-producing: Cushing's syndrome. Development of this syndrome in a child is usually due to a carcinoma rather than a benign lesion.
- Androgen-producing: virilization, hirsutism and amenorrhoea in females and precocious puberty in males.
- Oestrogen-producing: gynaecomastia and testicular atrophy in males, precocious puberty and menstrual irregularities in females; this is a rare condition.
- Aldosterone-producing: Conn's syndrome. Most aldosterone-producing adrenal tumours are benign. Malignancy should be suspected only when a patient with Conn's syndrome presents with a tumour greater than 3–5 cm in diameter.

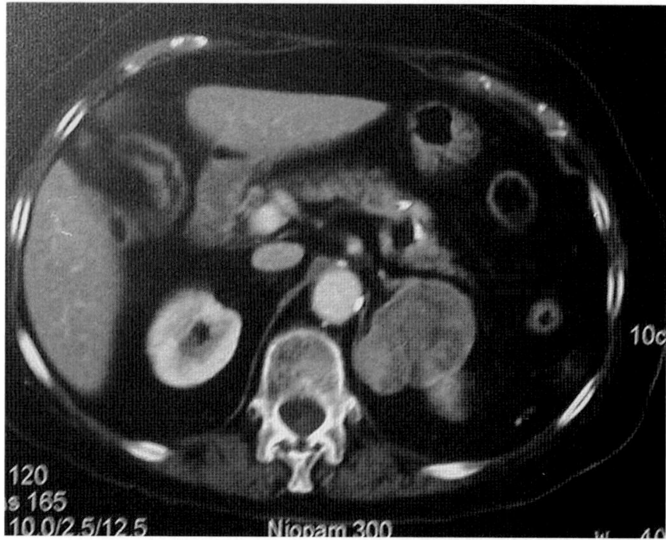

a

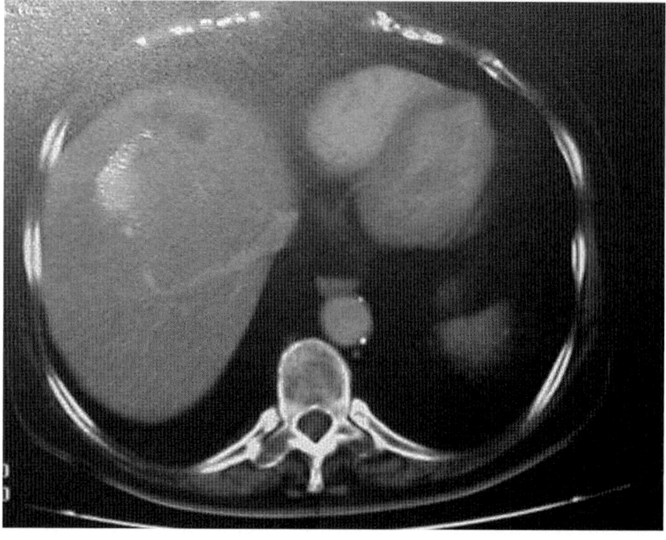

b

Figure 34.3 Computerized tomography scans revealing a left-sided adrenocortical carcinoma and liver metastases.

Non-functioning tumours usually present with weight loss, weakness, malaise, unexplained fever and an abdominal mass. Haemorrhage may present with acute pain and collapse.

Investigations

Urinary 17-ketosteroids and 17-hydroxysteroids are raised in functioning tumours. Dehydroepiandrosterone measurements may be diagnostic in non-functioning malignant adrenal tumours.[27] Computerized tomography and/or MRI localize tumours and provide valuable information regarding direct invasion and resectability (Fig. 34.3). Selenocholesterol scintigraphy may show poor or absent bilateral uptake.

Treatment and prognosis

Surgical resection is the mainstay of treatment. Surgical debulking may be performed in advanced tumours, and resection of adjacent organs such as spleen, kidneys, liver and pancreas is justified (Fig. 34.4). Repeated resection for recurrence also helps prolong survival. A thoracoabdominal approach may be necessary for large tumours (Fig. 34.5).

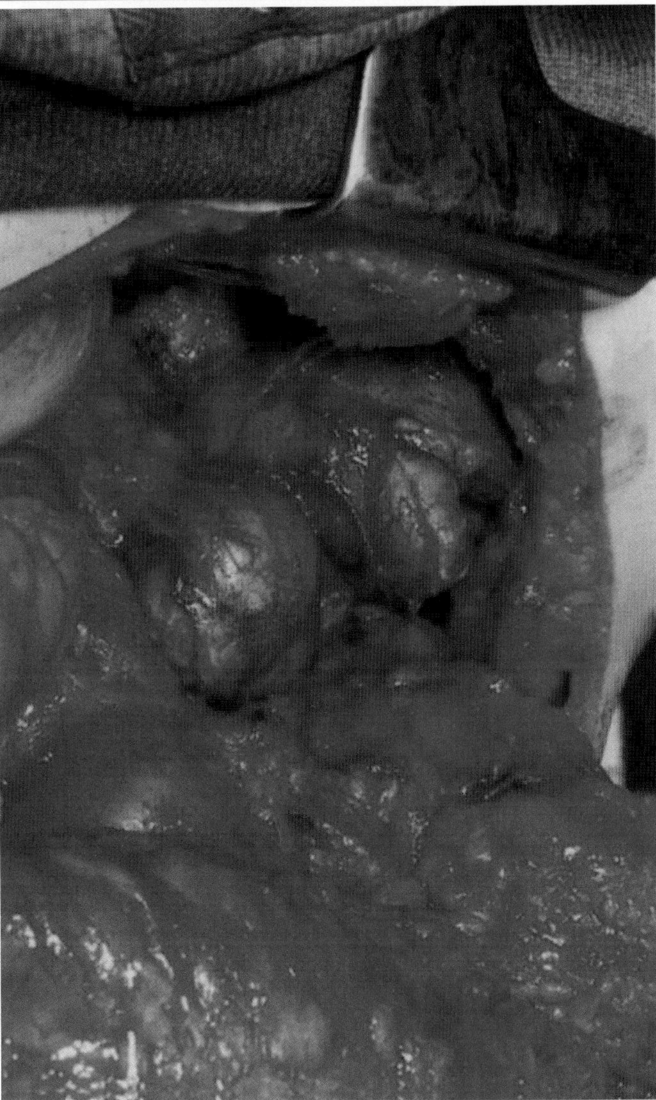

a

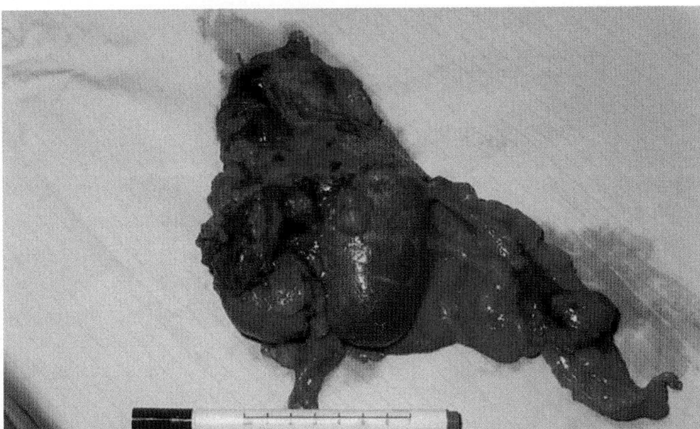

b

Figure 34.4 Extensive local recurrence of adrenal carcinoma, with deposits in the adrenal bed, tail of pancreas and splenic flexure, and local invasion into the left kidney. No distant disease was demonstrated. The tumour was excised en bloc with the left kidney, spleen and adjacent lymph nodes. Three years on, the patient was maintained on mitotane and remained well and disease-free.

Box 34.1 Causes of primary and secondary hyperaldosteronism

Causes of primary hyperaldosteronism
- Aldosterone-producing adenoma (Conn's tumour): this is the most common cause of hyperaldosteronism (85%)
- Bilateral adrenocortical hyperplasia (idiopathic hyperaldosteronism)
- Aldosterone-producing carcinoma (very rare)
- Glucocorticoid-suppressible: familial type 1 (autosomal dominant)
- Non-glucocorticoid-suppressible: familial type 2 (inheritance not yet defined)
- Aldosterone-producing ovarian carcinoma.

Causes of secondary hyperaldosteronism
- Cirrhosis
- Nephrotic syndrome
- Cardiac failure
- Diuretic therapy
- Renal artery stenosis and renin secreting renal tumours

Radiotherapy has not been shown to be useful in treating these tumours and has only a palliative role. Mitotane has been used as an adjuvant treatment, and has a limited role in recurrent disease and in patients who have early-stage disease with no metastases.[28,29] Mitotane, however, also destroys the contralateral adrenal cortex. Steroid replacement is essential with this treatment. Overall prognosis in patients with adrenal cancer is poor. Five-year survival rates are as low as 16%. Early-stage disease, tumours with no local invasion or metastases, have better prognosis (50% 5-year survival).[29]

HYPERALDOSTERONISM

Primary aldosteronism is due to excessive secretion of aldosterone by the zona glomerulosa. This leads to salt and water retention and a fall in renin secretion, with consequent loss of potassium and hydrogen ions in urine. The syndrome was first described by Jerome Conn in 1955.[30]

Secondary aldosteronism follows diminished plasma volume, resulting in angiotensin-mediated stimulation of the cortex and raised plasma renin activity. The causes of primary and secondary hyperaldosteronism are listed in Box 34.1.

CONN'S TUMOUR OR ALDOSTERONE-PRODUCING ADENOMA

Conn's tumours are usually discrete, less than 2 cm in size, unilateral, project from the surface of the gland, and are bright yellow (Fig. 34.6). They are more commonly located on the left side.[31] Approximately 10% of tumours are bilateral.[32] Between 40 and 50% of patients may have associated macroscopic or microscopic nodular hyperplasia.[31,33]

REFERENCES

28. Schteingart DE, Motazedi A, Noonan RA et al. Arch Surg 1982; 117: 1142–1146
29. Pommier RF, Brennan MF. Surgery 1992; 112: 963–970, discussion 970–971
30. Conn JW. Lab Clin Med 1955; 45: 3
31. Young WFJ Jr, Klee G. Endocrinol Metab Clin North Am 1988; 17: 367–395
32. Granberg PO, Adamson U, Cohn KH et al. World J Surg 1982; 6: 757–764
33. Hunt TK, Schambelan M, Biglieri EG. Ann Surg 1975; 182: 353–361

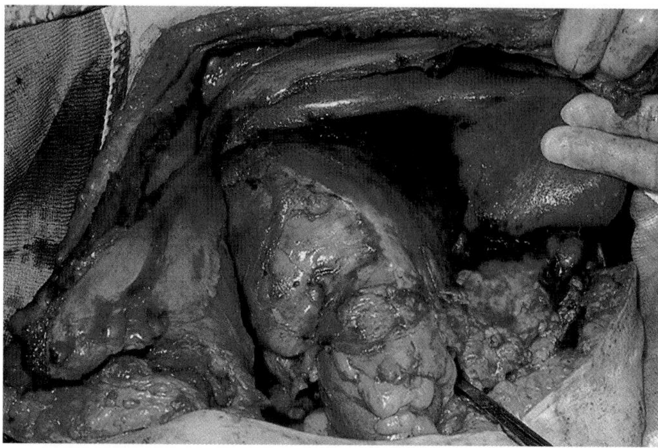

a

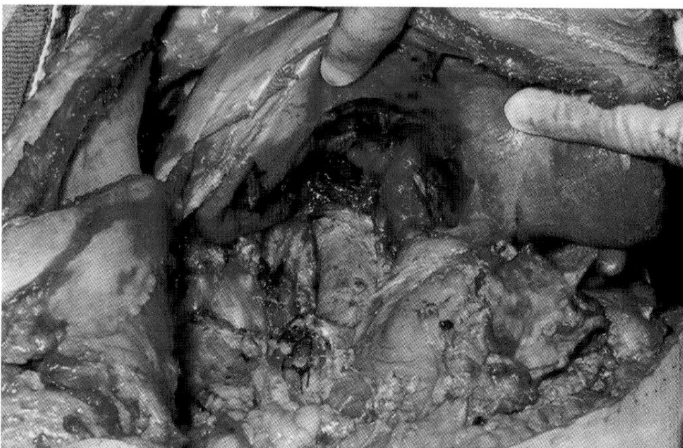

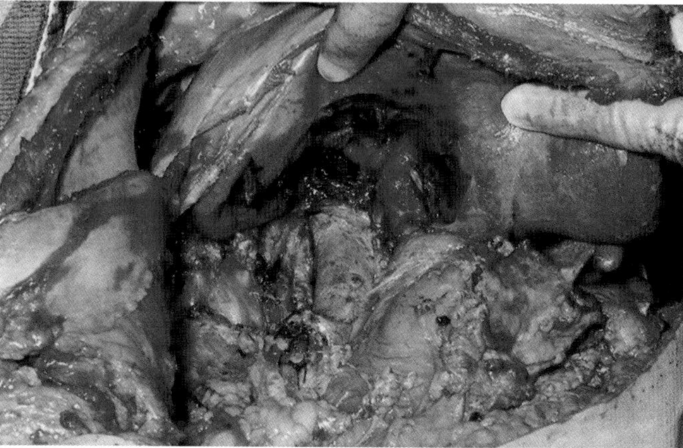

c

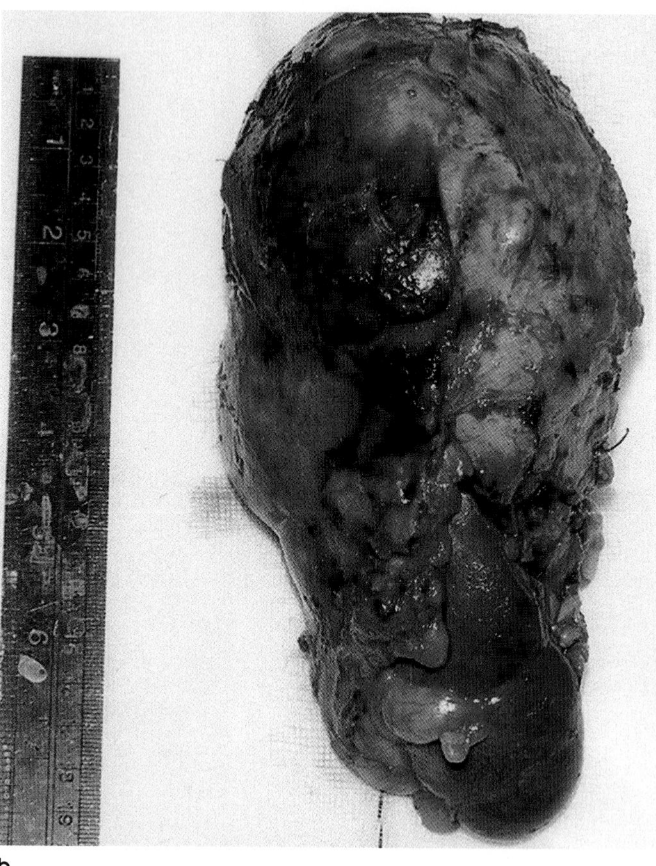

b

Figure 34.5 A right thoracoabdominal approach for a large, locally recurrent, adrenal carcinoma. The tumour had invaded locally into the liver, and was adherent but not invading the inferior vena cava.

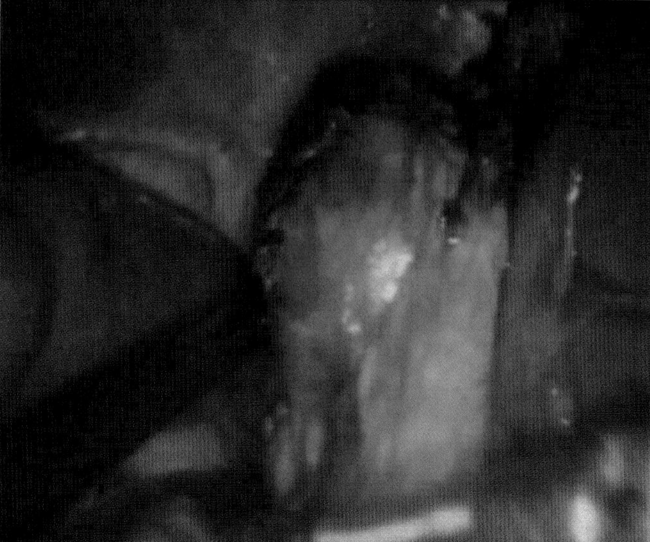

Figure 34.6 Laparoscopic view of a Conn's tumour in a mobilized adrenal gland. The tumour was removed by performing a subtotal adrenal resection.

Idiopathic hyperaldosteronism is identified in 10–15% of patients with hyperaldosteronism. It is characterized by both focal and diffuse areas of hyperplasia of the zona glomerulosa, leading to the formation of nodules.

Clinical features

The peak incidence for this condition is between the third and fifth decades. Conn's tumours are more common in women (2:1). Idiopathic hyperaldosteronism is equally distributed between the sexes and tends to occur at a later age.

Persistent hypertension that is usually resistant to antihypertensive therapy characterizes this syndrome. The duration of symptoms prior to diagnosis is often around 7 years. Hypokalaemia causing muscle weakness, cramps, and in severe cases flaccid paralysis and tetany may be seen. Hypokalaemia may be unmasked by the administration of diuretics for the treatment of the hypertension. Polyuria, polydipsia and nocturia may also be associated. Occasionally patients are asymptomatic and diagnosis is only established on biochemical tests.

Investigations

Serum and urinary potassium levels

Primary aldosteronism should be suspected if serum potassium is less than 3 mmol/L and urinary potassium excretion is greater than 40 mmol/L per day.[34] Any potassium deficit should be corrected and spironolactone, angiotensin-converting enzyme inhibitors and diuretics should be discontinued 4–6 weeks before testing.

REFERENCES

34. Young WF Jr. Endocrinol Metab Clin North Am 1997; 26: 801–827

Plasma aldosterone concentration and plasma renin activity

Aldosterone is elevated in all cases (normal level 2.2–15 ng/dL), but in primary hyperaldosteronism the plasma renin activity (normally 0.2–0.5 ng/dL) is suppressed. In contrast, the plasma renin activity is raised in secondary hyperaldosteronism. A plasma aldosterone concentration:plasma renin activity ratio of greater than 50 is diagnostic for primary hyperaldosteronism.

Aldosterone suppression test

Failure to suppress urinary aldosterone secretion following a sodium load confirms primary aldosteronism. Oral sodium (9 g/day for 3 days) and 0.5 mg of fludrocortisone are administered, and a 24-h urine sample is obtained for analysis. Sodium values in excess of 200 mEq (indicating adequate sodium load) with aldosterone levels over 12 μg are diagnostic.[31] Normokalaemia should be ensured prior to testing, because the test may precipitate hypokalaemia.

Differentiation between aldosterone-producing adenoma and idiopathic hyperaldosteronism

Patients with aldosterone-producing adenoma will benefit from surgery, patients with idiopathic hyperaldosteronism will not. Differentiating between aldosterone-producing adenoma and idiopathic hyperaldosteronism is therefore important.[31,34] Plasma aldosterone concentration changes with posture. This is used as a reliable test, because aldosterone-producing adenomas are sensitive to ACTH. Plasma aldosterone concentration is measured at 8.00 a.m. following overnight recumbency and 4 h later following mobilization. Plasma aldosterone concentration falls in patients with aldosterone-producing adenoma but rises in patients with idiopathic hyperaldosteronism. Accuracy of 86% has been reported for this test.[13]

Localization

Adenomas greater than 1 cm can be readily localized in 90% of patients with a CT scan. Smaller lesions may occasionally be localized with MRI.[35,36] Iodocholesterol scintigraphy may occasionally be useful in difficult cases and in differentiating aldosterone-producing adenoma from idiopathic hyperaldosteronism. However, the test requires suppression with steroids prior to scanning and administers a large dose of radiation; it is not widely favoured.

Selective venous sampling

This technique is highly accurate but invasive and potentially dangerous, because it can precipitate adrenal haemorrhage and necrosis.[37] It may be useful for tumours not localized by other modalities. Both aldosterone and cortisol levels are measured.

Treatment and prognosis

Treatment of choice for adrenal adenomas is unilateral adrenalectomy by experienced endocrine surgeons, with a laparoscopic approach. When technically possible a subtotal adrenalectomy may be performed, removing only the tumour. Spironolactone is used to correct hypokalaemia and hypertension prior to surgery. The average cure rate for these patients is 70% at 1 year.[38] Younger patients tend to fare better. Women also have a better long-term prognosis, probably because of the protective effect of female hormones. The longer the period of hypertension prior to surgery, the less successful is the surgery.

Surgery is not appropriate for idiopathic hyperplasia, and these patients are therefore treated with long-term spironolactone or amiloride. Patients who are unfit for surgery, or those who have recurrent hypertension following removal of an adenoma, should also be treated with medication. Glucocorticoid-suppressible aldosteronism can be treated with dexamethasone or spironolactone.

CONGENITAL ADRENAL HYPERPLASIA (ADRENOGENITAL SYNDROME)

Deficiency in the enzymes responsible for the synthesis of corticosteroids results in excessive production of androgenic steroids. Lack of the corticosteroid negative-feedback mechanism results in high levels of ACTH and bilateral adrenal hyperplasia. The most common deficiency (90% of cases) is lack of 21-hydroxylase, inherited as an autosomal recessive disorder.[39] Various other deficiencies of both hydroxylases and dehydrogenase have also been reported.

Clinical presentation

Congenital adrenal hyperplasia is rare. The reported incidence is between 1:5000 and 1:15 000.[40] Aldosterone deficiency results in salt wasting and presents in the newborn with vomiting, failure to thrive and poor feeding. Excessive androgen production in females leads to virilization, ambiguous external genitalia, enlargement of clitoris and pseudohermaphroditism. In males, androgen excess is not usually obvious, but precocious puberty and penile enlargement may ensue. Patients may have a short stature due to early epiphyseal closure (infant Hercules).

Diagnosis

The diagnosis is reliably confirmed by radioimmunoassay of plasma levels of 17-OH progesterone.[41]

Treatment

The primary aim of treatment is to correct the lack of corticosteroids and thus suppress ACTH drive. Administration of 5 mg of hydrocortisone daily in divided doses is usually successful. Plasma and urine levels of 17-OH progesterone are closely monitored, and the dose of hydrocortisone adjusted as necessary.[42]

In the newborn with salt wasting, early recognition and prompt treatment with intravenous saline and mineralocorticoids is vital in preventing the sequelae of this syndrome.[40] Genital manifestations may require corrective surgery.

PHAEOCHROMOCYTOMA

INTRODUCTION

The term *phaeochromocytoma* was first used by Pick in 1912. The term stems from the Greek for dusky (*phaeo*) and colour (*chromo*).

REFERENCES

35. Cirillo RL Jr, Bennett WF, Vitellas KM et al. Am J Roentgenol 1998; 170: 429–435
36. Herrera MF, Grant CS, van Heerden JA et al. Surgery 1991; 110: 1014–1021
37. Grant CS, Carpenter P, van Heerden JA et al. Arch Surg 1984; 119: 585–590
38. Ferriss JB, Brown JJ, Fraser R et al. Br Med J 1975; 1: 135–138
39. Finkelstein M, Shaefer JM. Physiol Rev 1979; 59: 353–406
40. Edis AJ, Grant CS, Egdahal RH (eds). Manual of Endocrine Surgery. 2nd edn. Springer-Verlag, New York, 1984
41. Savage MO. Clin Endocrinol Metab 1985; 14: 893–909
42. Hughes IA, Winter JS. J Clin Endocrinol Metab 1978; 46: 98–104

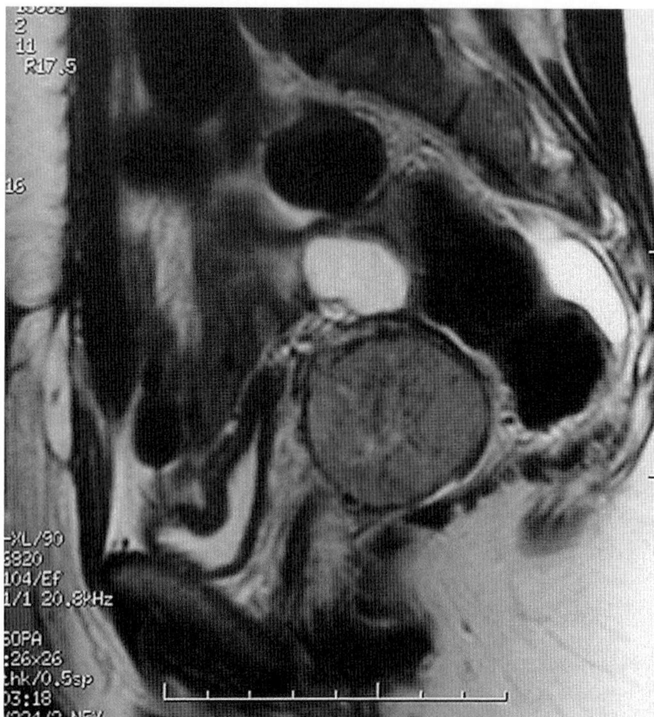

Figure 34.7 An MRI scan of pelvis, demonstrating a rare example of a malignant phaeochromocytoma adjacent to the rectum.

It is a functioning tumour of the chromaffin cells of the medulla, and is characterized by excess secretion of catecholamines.[43] Roux in Lausanne, Switzerland (1926) and Mayo in the USA (1927) are credited with the first successful surgical excisions of this tumour.[44,45]

Phaeochromocytoma was found in 0.3% of post-mortems at the Mayo Clinic.[46] The tumour accounts for 800 deaths annually in the USA, but remains undiagnosed in 35% of patients during their lifetime.[46] A raised index of suspicion, improved preoperative imaging, and judicious perioperative medical management have resulted in significantly improved outcomes.

PATHOLOGY

Tumours arise predominantly from the neuroectodermal chromaffin cells of the adrenal medulla (80–90%). Extra-adrenal tumours are normally close to the adrenals. They arise in the paraganglionic system along the course of the organ of Zuckerkandl, which extends from the pelvis to the base of the skull in the retroperitoneal and retropleural spaces. Rare sites include the pelvis (Fig. 34.7), kidneys, bladder, scrotum, neck and thorax (Fig. 34.8).

Phaeochromocytoma has been called the '10% tumour', because 10% of lesions are bilateral, 10% extra-adrenal, 10% multiple, 10% malignant, and 10% associated with familial syndromes such as multiple endocrine neoplasia types 2A and 2B, von Recklinghausen's syndrome and von Hippel–Lindau syndrome.[47]

Children are more often affected by multiple and extra-adrenal tumours, and are therefore more likely to have malignant tumours (40% of paraganglionomas are malignant). Multiple tumours are more frequent in familial disease (50–70%).

Tumours vary in size from 1 to 15 cm, and can weigh between 50 and 200 g. Macroscopically they are thinly encapsulated and show a pinkish grey surface. They are very vascular and may contain areas of haemorrhage and necrosis, and thus are often very soft.

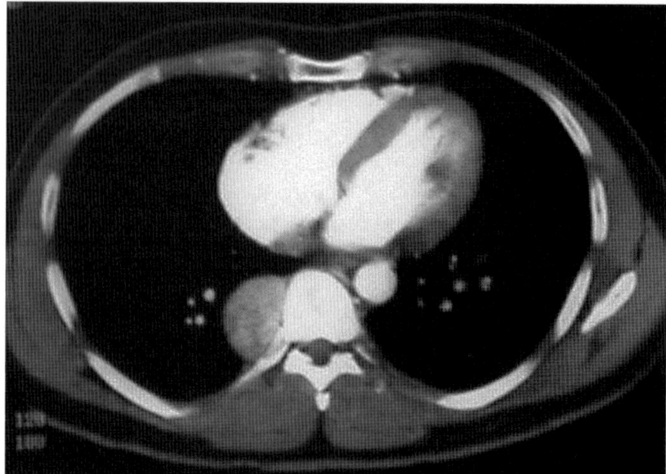

a

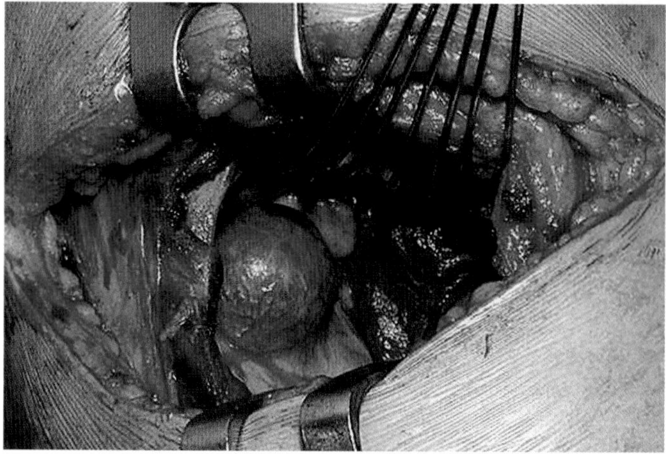

b

Figure 34.8 (**a**) A CT scan of the thorax, detailing a phaeochromocytoma in the right chest. (**b**) Operative picture of the tumour.

Histological confirmation of malignancy can be difficult, because benign tumours frequently demonstrate capsular and vascular invasion. Malignancy is usually confirmed if there is direct local invasion or signs of metastatic disease.

CLINICAL PRESENTATION

Hypertension in association with palpitation, sweating and headache is central to the diagnosis of phaeochromocytoma.[47] Hypertension may be persistent (50% of patients) or paroxysmal and associated with tachycardia, angina, arrhythmias and myocardial infarction. The incidence of hypertensive encephalopathy, cerebrovascular accidents and cardiomyopathy is also

REFERENCES

43. Manger WM, Gifford RW Jr. Pheochromocytoma. Springer-Verlag, New York, 1977
44. Roux. Thesis Lausanne. Cited by Barbeau A, Marc-Aurele J, Brouillet J et al. J Union Med Can 1958; 87: 165–172
45. Mayo CH. JAMA 1927; 89: 1047
46. St John Sutton MG, Sheps SG, Lei JT. Mayo Clin Proc 1981; 56: 354–360
47. Daly PA, Landsberg L. Baillières Clin Endocrinol Metab 1992; 6: 143–166

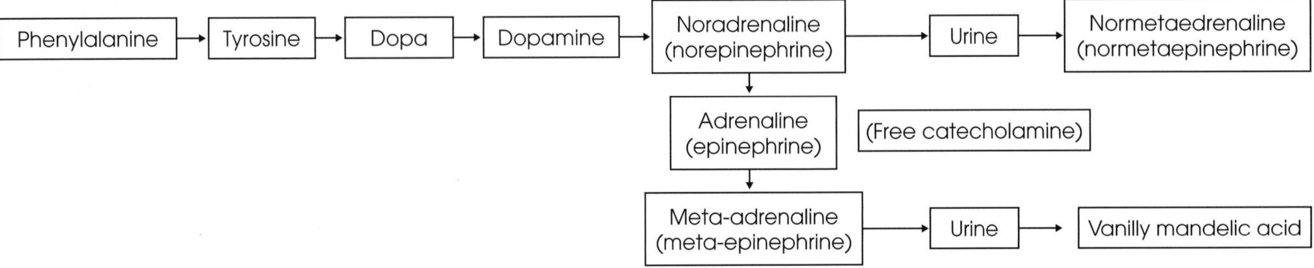

Figure 34.9 Biosynthesis and metabolism of catecholamines.

increased in patients with phaeochromocytoma. On occasion patients may present with malignant hypertension and need emergency treatment; if untreated, coma and death may ensue. Many of these symptoms are secondary to catecholamine release, although dopamine-secreting tumours may not be associated with hypertension.

Activities that raise intra-abdominal pressure – palpation, defecation, exercise, micturition, labour, invasive procedures (angiography and surgery), and sexual activity – may precipitate an attack. Other factors, such as drugs (tricyclic antidepressants), alcohol, and foods containing tyramine, may also provoke symptoms.

Other described manifestations include flushing, pallor, pupillary dilatation, Raynaud's phenomenon, fever, tremors, nausea, vertigo, weakness and a feeling of impending doom. Gastrointestinal symptoms including abdominal pain, pseudo-obstruction, ileus, ischaemic colitis, and megacolon have also been reported. Malignant tumours may cause severe hyperglycaemia. Rupture of a phaeochromocytoma may mimic a leaking aortic aneurysm, presenting acutely with abdominal pain and shock.

Examination may reveal a pale, thin and anxious patient. Severe hypertension with a postural drop is characteristic. A small number of patients have a palpable abdominal mass. The characteristic features associated with the various syndromes detailed above may also be seen.

DIFFERENTIAL DIAGNOSIS

Phaeochromocytoma may present with a wide range of symptoms, rendering differential diagnosis difficult. This includes essential hypertension, anxiety neurosis, diabetes mellitus, hyperthyroidism, functional bowel disorders, carcinoid syndrome and the menopause.

INVESTIGATIONS

The synthesis of catecholamines from phenylalanine (as described by Armstrong) is outlined in Fig. 34.9 and forms the basis for biochemical testing.[48] Hypersecretion of catecholamines provides the biochemical diagnosis of phaeochromocytoma, but further localization studies are needed prior to surgical resection.

Urinary metanephrines, catecholamines and vanillylmandelic acid

Two separate 24-h urine collections should be made. The 24-h urinary levels of metanephrines (0–6.5 μmol/24 h) have a 95% sensitivity compared with 60% sensitivity for vanillylmandelic acid levels (0–35 μmol/24 h) and 90% sensitivity for free catecholamine levels (adrenaline [epinephrine] less than 35 μg/L and noradrenaline [norepinephrine] less than 170 μg/L). Foods containing tyrosine, monoamine oxidase inhibitors, stress, haemorrhagic shock, sepsis and severe illness may result in false positive results.

Plasma free catecholamine levels

Plasma free catecholamine levels may be markedly elevated after acute hypertensive episodes but are not generally reliable as a diagnostic test.

Fasting plasma catecholamine levels

Plasma catecholamine levels may be assayed by high-pressure liquid chromatography with a sensitivity of over 90%. Drugs and severe illnesses may affect levels.

LOCALIZATION

Magnetic resonance imaging is the investigation of choice in localizing phaeochromocytoma.[35] Tumours display with low signal intensity on T1-weighted images and as hyperintense signals on T2-weighted images (Fig. 34.10). Magnetic resonance imaging helps differentiate lesions from non-functioning adrenal adenomas, which have the same MRI characteristics as normal adrenals. Also, MRI is of particular help in localizing extra-adrenal paraganglionomas. Computerized tomography scanning has an accuracy of over 90% but has the potential disadvantage of precipitating a contrast-induced hypertensive crisis. Ultrasound scans are useful as a preliminary investigative test where suspicion is raised, but are poor in defining smaller tumours (less than 3 cm). Metaiodobenzylguanidine or indium-111 pentetreotide scans may be helpful in identifying lesions or metastatic disease in difficult cases (Fig. 34.11).[35] Scans have been reported to have a specificity of 100% if several scans are done over 72 h after administration of the isotope, but they have a false negative rate of 5–10%.[49,50] Angiography and selective venous sampling are no longer used, because they may precipitate a hypertensive crisis.

TREATMENT

Surgery is the mainstay of treatment, providing a cure of hypertension in the majority of patients. Exceptions are patients who are unfit for surgery or who have metastatic disease from a malignant lesion. Prior to surgical resection, preoperative stabilization of blood pressure is critical, because both anaesthesia and tumour manipulation may result in hypertensive crises. These patients have a constricted circulation, and blockade allows the blood volume to rise preoperatively.

REFERENCES

48. Armstrong MD, McMillan A, Shaw KNF. Biochem Biophys Acta 1957; 25: 422–428
49. Troncone L, Rufini V, Montemaggi P et al. Eur J Nucl Med 1990; 16: 325–335
50. Peplinski GR, Norton JA. Surgery 1994; 116: 1101–1110

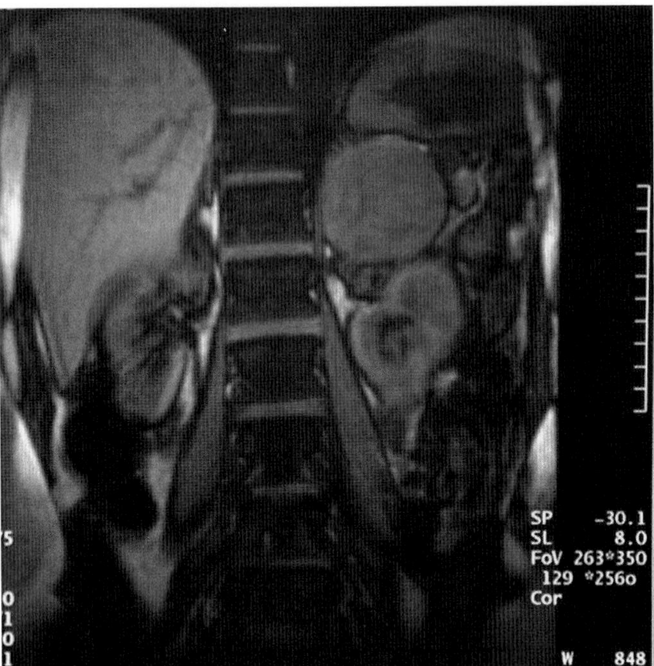

Figure 34.10 An MRI scan of a large left-sided phaeochromocytoma. The lesion was successfully removed laparoscopically.

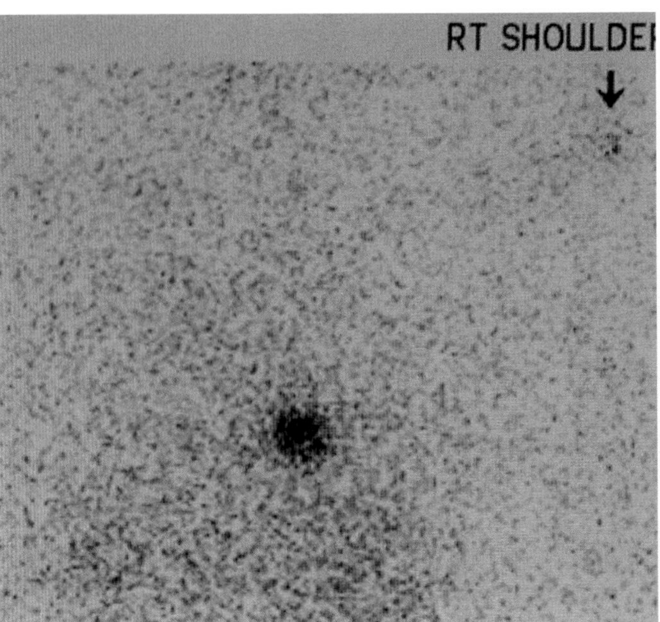

Figure 34.11 Metaiodobenzylguanidine scan demonstrating a right intrathoracic phaeochromocytoma.

PREOPERATIVE CONTROL OF HYPERTENSION

Preoperative control of hypertension should be commenced soon after the diagnosis is established and prior to localization studies. Treatment should precede surgery by at least 10–14 days. The α-adrenergic blocker phenoxybenzamine is the agent of choice. The initial dose is 10 mg b.d., increasing up to a maximum of 160 mg/day until hypertension is well controlled. Side effects of phenoxybenzamine include weakness, lassitude, nasal congestion, nausea, sedation and orthostatic hypotension. Additional beta blockade with propanolol (40–60 mg/day) may also be necessary in patients with pure adrenaline (epinephrine)-secreting tumours and tachyarrhythmia. Asthma, cardiac failure, and incomplete or lack of alpha blockade are contraindications to beta blockers; unopposed vasoconstriction can cause severe hypertension. Selective α_1-receptor blockers, such as prazosin, terazosin and doxazosin, may help control hypertension without reflex tachycardia.[51] Other drugs, including labetalol (alpha and beta blocker), nifedipine (calcium channel blocker), and α-methyl-*p*-tyrosine (which inhibits catecholamine synthesis), have a limited role only.

ANAESTHESIA FOR PHAEOCHROMOCYTOMA

A coordinated experienced team approach is essential. This should include an endocrinologist, a surgeon and an anaesthetist to ensure optimal preparation of the patient prior to surgery, a smooth surgical course and a safe outcome. Patients usually need central venous monitoring along with invasive arterial pressure monitoring. Swan–Ganz catheters may be required in patients with cardiac compromise. Isoflurane rather than halothane is used in maintaining anaesthesia to minimize cardiac arrhythmia. Phentolamine, sodium nitroprusside, lidocaine (lignocaine), propranolol, dopamine and noradrenaline (norepinephrine) must be available to control blood pressure and treat arrhythmia. Facilities for cardioversion should also be available. In cases of bilateral adrenalectomy, steroid cover and replacement will also be required. Because alpha blockade renders the vascular bed refractory to vasopressors, careful expansion of plasma volume with fluids is necessary perioperatively.

SURGERY FOR PHAEOCHROMOCYTOMA

Laparoscopic adrenalectomy is the favoured surgical approach for phaeochromocytoma in suitably sized tumours.[52,53] For larger tumours, a transabdominal approach via a subcostal or midline incision may be employed. When tumours are bilateral, a 'rooftop' incision may be employed. During the surgical procedure, special consideration should be given for minimal handling of tumour and good haemostasis. Extra-adrenal tumours are managed by a variety of surgical approaches depending on the location of the tumour.

POSTOPERATIVE MANAGEMENT

Careful monitoring of central venous pressure, blood pressure and urine output is essential. Loss of vasoconstrictor drive following surgical removal of the tumour (secondary to a fall in catecholamine levels) usually requires large amounts of fluid in the postoperative period. However, persistent hypotension should be suspected as possible haemorrhage rather than refractory vasodilatation. Blood glucose levels must also be carefully monitored, because dangerous hypoglycaemia can occur. Persistent hypertension may be due to residual or metastatic tumour, or chronic hypertensive renal vascular damage.

Following surgery, urinary catecholamine and vanillylmandelic acid levels should be monitored on a long-term basis, because malignancy may become apparent only many years later. With

REFERENCES

51. Bravo EL. Endocrine Rev 1994; 15: 356–368
52. Dudley NE, Harrison BJ. Br J Surg 1999; 86: 656–660
53. Smith CD, Weber CJ, Amerson JR. World J Surg 1999; 23: 389–396

good preoperative preparation and careful surgery, excellent cure rates can be achieved, with low morbidity and mortality.[54]

PHAEOCHROMOCYTOMA IN SPECIAL CIRCUMSTANCES

Unsuspected phaeochromocytoma encountered during surgery

This rare scenario presents both surgeon and anaesthetist with a difficult and potentially life-threatening challenge. Unexplained tachycardia, arrhythmia or hypertension during induction of anaesthesia or during surgery for an unrelated condition should be met with a high degree of suspicion. Untreated, pulmonary oedema and cardiac arrest may follow. Alpha blockade should be instigated immediately, and surgery terminated as quickly as is feasible to allow proper diagnosis, localization and preoperative preparation.

Phaeochromocytoma in pregnancy

Maternal mortality of 40% and fetal mortality of 40–56% have been reported with phaeochromocytoma.[55] Pregnant woman with hypertension (particularly in early pregnancy) and a positive family history should be investigated for possible phaeochromocytoma. Labour and anaesthesia precipitates the symptoms. Early diagnosis helps reduce mortality.[55] During early pregnancy, MRI is the localization procedure of choice. In the first and second trimesters, surgical excision should be performed after the usual preoperative preparation. In the third trimester, Caesarian section followed by excision of tumour under the same anaesthetic is appropriate.[56] Vaginal delivery is associated with significant mortality and is thus contraindicated.

Phaeochromocytoma in children

Twenty per cent of all phaeochromocytomas are found in children. Bilateral, extra-adrenal and multiple tumours are more common because of familial multiple endocrine neoplasia type 2 syndromes, and other members of the family should be screened. Adrenal tumours are less likely to be malignant, and surgery gives excellent results.

Phaeochromocytoma and inherited syndromes

Multiple endocrine neoplasia type 2 syndromes are inherited in an autosomal dominant manner.[57] They result from germ-line mutations in the *RET* proto-oncogene located on chromosome 10. The syndrome is characterized by medullary thyroid carcinoma, seen in all patients, and phaeochromocytoma, seen in some. In the type 2A variant, primary hyperparathyroidism is also associated, and in type 2B characteristic facies, marfanoid habitus, mucocutaneous ganglioneuromas and skeletal abnormalities may be seen.

Other inherited disorders giving rise to phaeochromocytoma include von Hippel–Lindau syndrome and familial neurofibromatosis (von Recklinghausen's disease).

MALIGNANT PHAEOCHROMOCYTOMA

Ten per cent of adrenal phaeochromocytomas are malignant. The incidence of malignancy rises to 40% if the lesion is extra-adrenal.[47] Histological diagnosis of malignancy may be difficult. Complete surgical excision after accurate localization offers the best chance of a cure. Recurrent disease should be resected or debulked, or occasionally even ablated. Metaiodobenzylguanidine may have a therapeutic role. Chemotherapy is ineffective. Radiotherapy may provide useful palliation. In selected patients, α-methyl-*p*-tyrosine may help alleviate symptoms of catecholamine excess. Prognosis is generally poor, but 5-year survival rates of 40% have been reported; the prognosis for extra-adrenal lesions is much worse.[58]

OTHER ADRENAL TUMOURS

Incidentaloma

Advances in imaging and the increasing use of radiology have resulted in a large number of incidental lesions of the adrenal glands being identified. Incidental lesions are now diagnosed in 0.5–4.5% of patients undergoing imaging for reasons other than adrenal disease. 'Incidentaloma' is identified in 1.5–5.7% of post-mortem examinations.[59] These lesions pose a diagnostic problem.

Having excluded the possibility of the lesion simply being a metastasis from a known primary malignancy, the next step in management is to determine its functional status. Serum electrolytes, 24-h urinary catecholamine and metanephrine levels, 9.00 a.m. and midnight serum cortisol and aldosterone levels should be checked.

Approximately 35–95% of lesions are benign, non-functioning adenomas. Magnetic resonance imaging may help distinguish lesions from cysts or secondary malignant deposits. Selenocholesterol scanning may aid in diagnosis of functioning adenomas (5%) and malignancy, but to protect the patient from examination, radiation should not normally be used. Fine-needle aspiration is only of limited value.

The incidence of malignancy in these lesions increases with size. Previously, surgical resection was recommended for all lesions greater than 4 cm in patients under the age of 50 years; however, with the introduction of laparoscopic adrenalectomy, this has fallen to 3 or 3.5 cm in many centres. In older patients the risk of malignancy is less (Fig. 34.12).[36]

Suspicious radiological features may render the size criteria irrelevant in all age groups. Smaller lesions should be regularly monitored, and excised if they increase in size.

SECONDARY ADRENAL METASTASES

Breast, bronchial and melanoma malignancies are the most common cause for secondary deposits in the adrenal glands. They can destroy the adrenal tissue and may precipitate an Addisonian crisis.

OTHER ADRENAL MEDULLARY AND EXTRA-ADRENAL TUMOURS

These are classified, according to the international World Health Organization classification, as follows:

Neuroendocrine lesions

- Phaeochromocytoma.
- Sympathetic paraganglionoma: tumours arise from non-chromaffin tissue and are rarely functional.

REFERENCES

54. Van Heerden JA, Sheps SG, Hamberger B et al. Surgery 1982; 91: 367–373
55. Schenker JG, Granat M. Austral NZ J Obstet Gynaecol 1982; 22: 1–116
56. Fudge TL, McKinnon WM, Geary WL. Arch Surg 1980; 115: 1224–1225
57. Mulligan LM, Kwok JB, Healey CS et al. Nature 1993; 363: 458–460
58. Javadpour N, Woltering EA, Brennan MF. Curr Prob Surg 1980; 17: 1–52
59. Peppercorn PD, Grossman AB, Reznek RH. Clin Endocrinol 1998; 48: 379–388

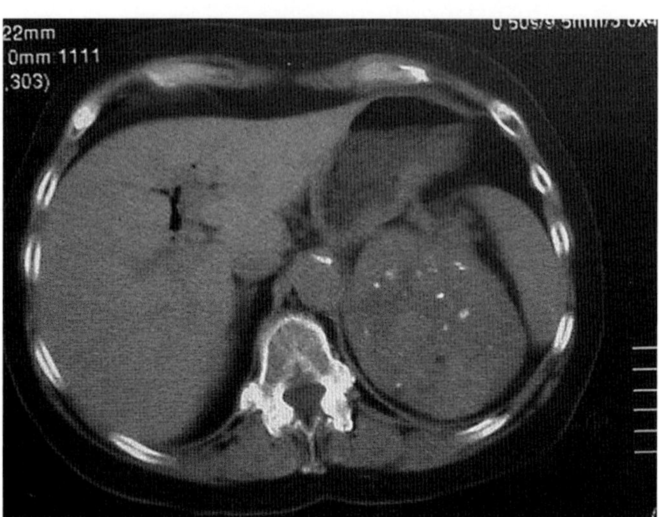

Figure 34.12 A CT scan of a patient presenting with upper abdominal pain and a palpable mass. The lesion was thought to be a large adrenal carcinoma and removed via an open approach. In fact, the lesion was an adrenal haemangioma (extremely rare).

- Parasympathetic paraganglionoma: usually found in carotid or aortic bodies (chemodectoma) and glomus jugulare.

Neural lesions

- Neurofibroma and ganglioneuromas.
- Ganglioneuroblastoma: malignant lesion of neuroblasts and ganglion cells.
- Neuroblastoma.

NEUROBLASTOMA

Neuroblastoma is a malignant tumour of neuroblasts, affecting mainly the adrenal medulla. It may also affect the adjacent retroperitoneal tissue and sympathetic ganglia. It is the commonest extracranial malignant tumour of childhood, with over 60% of lesions presenting within the first year of life.[58]

Clinical presentation

Boys are affected slightly more than girls. Approximately 75% of cases present with an abdominal mass, the remainder occurring in thorax (20%) and neck (5%). Associated features may include anorexia, nausea, vomiting, diarrhoea (due to vasoactive intestinal peptide) and flushing. Hypertension may also be present. Dumb-bell-shaped tumours extending into the spinal cord may present with neurological symptoms. They are aggressive malignancies and are spread by direct invasion, the lymphatic system and the bloodstream. Metastases are frequently present at the time of diagnosis. Two distinct types of metastatic disease patterns are seen:

- Pepper's type: tumour on the right side, with metastatic spread to liver.
- Hutchinson's type: left-sided tumour producing metastases to orbit, skull and long bones.

Nephroblastoma (Wilms' tumour) needs to be differentiated from these lesions.

Investigations and staging

Chest X-ray, intravenous urograms, and CT, MRI and metaiodobenzylguanidine scans are used to diagnose and stage lesions. Lesions are classified from stages 1 to 4, depending on whether the tumour is confined to the adrenal gland or is extra-adrenal, whether it extends across the midline, and the extent of lymph node involvement.

Treatment

For stages 1 and 2 – lesions confined to the adrenal gland or extra-adrenal lesions not extending across the midline – surgery is the treatment of choice. For stages 3 and 4, surgery may still be used to debulk the tumour prior to radiotherapy and/or combination chemotherapy with vincristine, cyclophosphamide and dacarbazine. Radiotherapy is helpful in palliation of bony metastases.

Prognosis

Prognosis is dependent on the patient's age and tumour stage. The 2-year survival rate for stages 1 and 2 is 86%, with an overall 2-year survival rate of 32%. Children below the age of 2 years have a better 2-year survival rate (77%) compared with older children (38%).

SURGICAL APPROACHES TO THE ADRENAL GLANDS

The adrenal glands can be approached either by an open technique or by a minimally invasive, endoscopic technique. Each method has its own advantages, and the choice of the approach depends on a number of factors, including the patient's physique; a history of previous surgery; tumour size, type and location; and the expertise of the surgeon. The introduction of laparoscopic techniques has undoubtedly resulted in an increasing number of referrals, especially of incidentaloma, but the indications for surgery have not changed.[60]

OPEN ANTERIOR APPROACH

Separate bilateral subcostal incisions, transverse upper abdominal incision (rooftop), or an upper midline incision may be employed. This approach is useful for large tumours (which are potentially malignant), phaeochromocytomas, and lesions with equivocal localization. It provides excellent exposure of both adrenals and enables the surgeon to search for extra-adrenal lesions. It also provides an opportunity to examine the intra-abdominal and pelvic organs. This approach, however, carries an increase in morbidity and mortality, with high incidence of wound-related complications.

OPEN POSTERIOR OR POSTEROLATERAL APPROACH

A unilateral or bilateral oblique incision is used, and the 11th or 12th ribs are removed extrapleurally. This technique is suitable for small Conn's adenomas, bilateral adrenal hyperplasia of Cushing's syndrome, and well-localized small phaeochromocytomas or adrenal adenomas. It is associated with a low morbidity and mortality.[61]

THORACOABDOMINAL APPROACH

An oblique thoracoabdominal incision is used across the costal margin in the ninth intercostal space to provide exposure for very

REFERENCES

60. Micolli P, Rafaelli M et al. Br J Surg 2002; 89: 779–782
61. Proye CA, Huart JY, Cuvillier XD et al. Surgery 1993; 114: 1126–1131

large malignant tumours. Although it provides an excellent access, the procedure is associated with increased risk of complications.

LAPAROSCOPIC ANTERIOR APPROACH

The laparoscopic anterior approach is becoming more popular.[62–64] Recent reports suggest that this should be the gold-standard technique. The most common approach is a four-port lateral flank technique. It is an ideal approach for Conn's tumours, bilateral hyperplasia of Cushing's, and small phaeochromocytomas (less than 8 cm). It has major advantages in that the postoperative recovery is quick, in-patient stay is short, and it dramatically reduces the wound-related complications. It is contraindicated for large adrenal masses and malignant lesions.

POSTERIOR ENDOSCOPIC APPROACH

The posterior endoscopic approach is a modification of the open posterior approach. The retroperitoneal space is developed by a minimally invasive technique, using a balloon to allow insertion of ports and visualization of the gland.[65] It may be useful where the anterior laparoscopic approach is not possible due to extensive abdominal surgery. The approach has not proved popular because of the limited access and the technical difficulty of the procedure.

REFERENCES

62. Horgan S, Sinanan M, Helton WS et al. Am J Surg 1997; 173: 371–374
63. Duh QY, Siperstein AE, Clark OH et al. Arch Surg 1996; 131: 870–875, discussion 875–876
64. Thompson GB, Grant CS, van Heerden JA et al. Surgery 1997; 122: 1136
65. Walz MK, Peitgen K, Hoermann R et al. World J Surg 1996; 20: 769–774

The kidneys and ureters

35

Vivek Kumar, Christopher R. Chapple

GROSS ANATOMY

The adult kidney measures 10–12 cm in length, 5–7 cm in breadth and 3 cm in thickness, and it weighs 135–150 g. The kidneys are covered with a tough fibroelastic capsule. At birth, the kidneys are irregular in contour due to fetal lobulations (Fig. 35.1) that usually disappear in the early years of life. On the medial surface of either kidney is the renal hilum that opens into the renal sinus. The urinary collecting system and vessels occupy the renal sinus.

The renal parenchyma is divided into a cortex and a medulla (Fig. 35.2). The medulla consists of multiple distinct conical segments called pyramids. The apex of each pyramid is the renal papilla, which is cupped by an individual minor calyx of the collecting system. The intrapyramidal extension of cortex is called the column of Bertin. The minor calyces (8–12 in number) unite to form two or three major calyces, which in turn join to form the renal pelvis. The renal pelvis, which may be intrarenal or extrarenal, tapers to form the ureter. The adult ureter is about 30 cm long, following a smooth S curve as it descends down into the pelvis to join the bladder.

Radiologically, the ureter may be divided into three parts:

1. Upper one-third: portion lying above the sacroiliac joint.
2. Middle one-third: portion lying over the sacroiliac joint.
3. Lower one-third: portion lying below the sacroiliac joint.

A normal ureter has three areas of narrowing:

1. at the pelviureteric junction;
2. at the point where the iliac vessels cross the ureter; and
3. where it courses through the bladder wall.

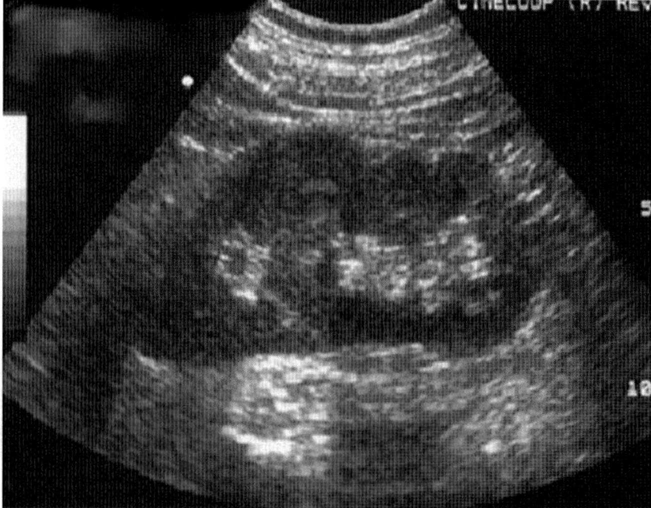

Figure 35.1 Fetal lobulation on ultrasound.

The kidneys and adrenals are surrounded by perinephric fat, and these together are enclosed by Gerota's fascia, which remains open inferiorly and contains the ureter and gonadal vessels. Fat surrounding the Gerota's fascia is called the pararenal fat. Gerota's fascia forms an important barrier around the kidneys, limiting spread of renal malignancy as well as benign perinephric collections in the form of urinoma, abscess or blood.

HISTOLOGY

A nephron is the functioning unit of the kidney, and is composed of a tubule that has both secretory and excretory functions (Fig. 35.3). The secretory portion is contained largely within the renal cortex, and consists of a renal corpuscle and the secretory part of the renal tubule. The excretory portion lies in the medulla. The renal corpuscle is composed of a vascular glomerulus, which projects into Bowman's capsule. Bowman's capsule is continuous with the proximal convoluted tubule that, along with the loop of Henle and the distal convoluted loop, forms the secretory portion of the renal tubule. The distal convoluted tubule drains into the collecting tubule, which forms the excretory portion of the nephron.

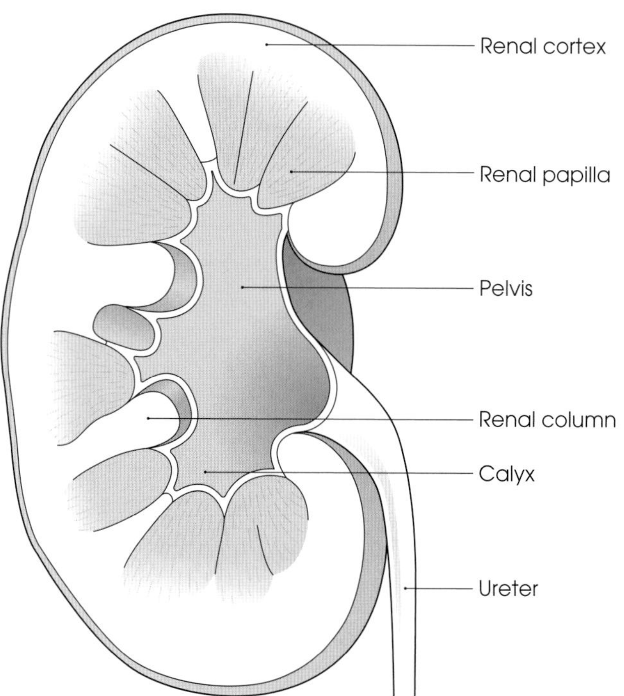

Figure 35.2 Renal anatomy.

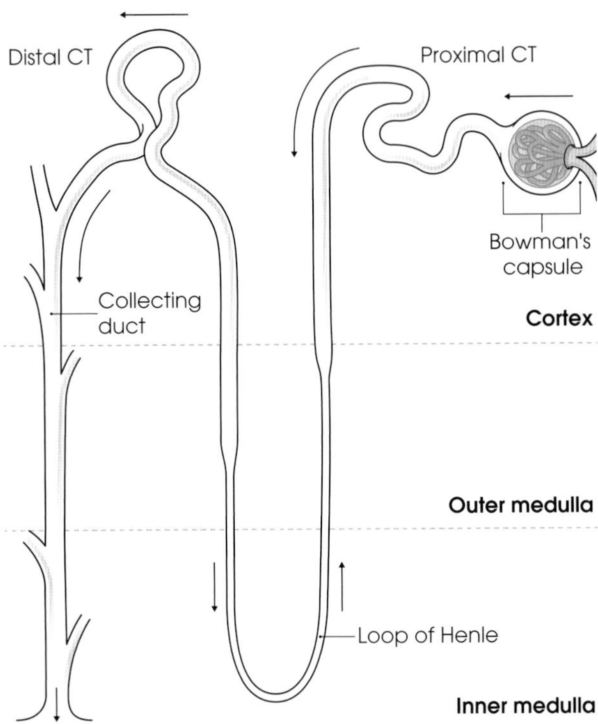

Figure 35.3 Nephron. CT, convoluted tubule.

The calyces, pelvis and ureters are lined by transitional cell epithelium overlying lamina propria. External to these are a mixture of helical and longitudinal smooth muscles.

RELATIONS

Posteriorly the diaphragm covers roughly the upper third of both kidneys. The pleural reflection follows the diaphragm very closely, and therefore there is always a risk of this being injured with any surgical approach to the kidneys. The 12th rib on either side crosses the kidney at the lower extent of the diaphragm. The lower two-thirds of either kidney is related to psoas, quadratus lumborum and the aponeurosis of transversus abdominis, in this sequence, when we move laterally from the hilum.

Anterior, the right kidney is related to liver very closely, separated by a fold of peritoneum, leaving only a small bare area where it lies in direct contact with liver. The medial aspect, along with the hilum and the hilar vessels, is related to the third part of duodenum. The hepatic flexure of the colon crosses the lower pole of the right kidney. The adrenal glands cover the supero-medial aspect of the upper pole of both the kidneys. The upper two-thirds of the anterior surface of left kidney is closely related to spleen and pancreatic tail. Above the pancreatic tail lies the posterior wall of the stomach, and below the tail lies a loop of jejunum. The lower pole is crossed by the splenic flexure of the colon. The spleen and left kidney are separated by a peritoneal reflection, forming an avascular lienorenal ligament. During any surgical procedure involving the left kidney, undue tension on this ligament may result in a splenic tear, necessitating a splenectomy.

The renal pelvis lies on the lateral border of the psoas muscle and on the quadratus lumborum muscle. In the hilum, the pelvis lies posteriorly, with the renal artery and vein lying in front, in this order. The ureters lie on the psoas muscle, passing medially to the sacroiliac joint, swinging laterally near ischial spine before passing medially to penetrate the base of the bladder. In females, the uterine arteries are closely related to the juxtavesical portion of the ureter.

EMBRYOLOGY

The urinary system develops progressively as three distinct entities.

The *pronephros* is the earliest nephric stage, and consists of tubules that extend caudally, reach and open into the cloaca that eventually disappears completely by the fourth week of embryonic life.

The *mesonephros* is the principal excretory organ during early embryonic life (4–8 weeks). Most of the mesonephros disappears; however, the mesonephric tubules form the glomerular complex.

The ureter and rest of the collecting system arise from the *metanephros* as a ureteric bud, which in turn arises from the mesonephric duct.

PHYSIOLOGY

FLUID AND ELECTROLYTE BALANCE

The main physiological function of the urinary tract is the maintenance of fluid, acid–base and electrolyte balance, and the excretion of waste products. A subsidiary but extremely important role is that of the production of certain hormones.

Approximately one-fifth of the cardiac output passes through the kidneys each minute, resulting in a renal blood flow of up to 400 mL per 100 g of kidney per min (650 mL/min per kidney). The renal blood pressure remains extremely constant, despite profound changes in systemic blood pressure, and the survival advantage of this mechanism is apparent on reflection.

A total of 170–180 L of plasma is filtered through the glomeruli, at an approximate rate of 125 mL/min. The glomerular membrane acts as a main filtration mechanism and is impermeable to molecules larger than 4 nm in diameter. The ultrafiltrate of plasma then passes down to the tubules.

The proximal tubule

The proximal tubule decreases the volume of glomerular filtrate by 75–80%, with active resorption of glucose, phosphate, bicarbonate, potassium and chloride. It is important to realize that glucose is reabsorbed entirely from the proximal tubule, unless the glucose load exceeds the capacity for absorption. The majority of filtered sodium and bicarbonate is reabsorbed from the proximal tubules, and sodium is actually pumped via hydrogen- or potassium-linked pump mechanisms. The proximal tubular filtrate is iso-osmotic as a consequence of passive absorption of both water and urea. Sulphates, amino acids and low-molecular-weight proteins are reabsorbed, as is potassium.

Loop of Henle

Sodium chloride and water are reabsorbed passively. The water is reabsorbed from the more proximal part (descending limb) in combination with sodium, while the distal part (ascending limb) is impermeable to water, with active sodium resorption. This produces a concentration gradient in the renal medulla, which is important in maintaining water balance. Loop diuretics, for example furosemide (frusemide), inhibit chloride and sodium resorption from the ascending loop.

Distal tubule and collecting duct

The filtrate is hypotonic when it leaves the loop of Henle, entering the distal tubules, where water resorption is under the control of antidiuretic hormone. Sodium is actively pumped out of the distal tubules, and resorption is modified by aldosterone secretion. The collecting tubules pass through the renal medulla, and the water resorption is independent of sodium resorption and is regulated by antidiuretic hormone secretion. Sodium is actively pumped out of the collecting tubules against a concentration gradient to maintain the hypertonicity of the renal medulla, with associated passive resorption to a small degree. Large amounts of urea also are reabsorbed passively from the collecting tubules. A number of substances are secreted in the distal tubule, including potassium, hydrogen and drugs. Seventy-five per cent of the potassium content of urine results at this level, due to tubular secretion. Potassium secretion is linked with sodium and hydrogen concentrations, and is modified by aldosterone secretion. Hydrogen secretion occurs in the distal tubules against a concentration gradient.

MAINTENANCE OF WATER BALANCE

The osmolality of urine varies between 50 and 1200 mOsm/L and depends on the amount of water in the collecting tubule, which also is related to an appropriate corticomedullary osmotic gradient and the permeability of the collecting ducts under the control of antidiuretic hormone. Sodium and chloride are transported out of the ascending limb of the loop of Henle, and the sodium concentration falls progressively as the distal tubule is reached. The remainder of the loop of Henle is in osmotic equilibrium with the substance of the kidney. As the iso-osmolar filtrate reaches the bottom of the loop of Henle, the contents of the descending limb become more concentrated as a result of being pushed towards the ascending limb. Further concentration occurs due to active sodium resorption in the ascending limb, resulting in an osmolar gradient in the renal medulla.

Any increase in medullary blood flow results in dissipation of medullary osmolality, decreased water resorption, and the production of large quantities of dilute urine. Dehydration results in release of antidiuretic hormone, increasing permeability in the distal nephron, and results in increased water resorption. Antidiuretic hormone is released from the posterior lobe of pituitary gland. The endogenous control of antidiuretic hormone release is under the regulation of osmoreceptors adjacent to the supraoptic nucleus, which is under the influence of sodium and chloride concentration in the plasma. There are also volume receptors in the atria and great veins, which are under the control of the vagus nerve.

MAINTENANCE OF ACID–BASE BALANCE

The kidneys cannot excrete urine of pH less than 4.5. Maintenance of acid–base relies on a complex series of buffer mechanisms. In the proximal tubules the predominant buffer system is dependent on bicarbonate (HCO_3^-, H_2CO_3), while in the distal tubules the predominant buffer is phosphate (HPO_4^{2-}, $H_2PO_4^-$) and the weakest is the NH_4^+ system. The phosphate buffer system is the most important during normal renal function, but the NH_4^+ system has a particular advantage in that it allows excretion of acid without loss of metallic cations such as sodium ions.

HORMONE PRODUCTION BY THE KIDNEY

A number of important hormones are produced within the kidney. The renin–angiotensin system is important, with renin being released from juxtaglomerular cells in response to sympathetic nerve stimulation, via a decrease in afferent arteriolar pressure and hyponatraemia. Renin acts on circulating angiotensinogen to produce angiotensin I, which is converted by a circulating enzyme to angiotensin II. Angiotensin II stimulates the zona glomerulosa of the adrenal gland to produce aldosterone, which increases the sodium resorption by the kidneys and also produces vasoconstriction. These effects feed back in a negative fashion and switch off renin secretion, and therefore maintain homeostasis. This mechanism is essential to maintain a smooth blood pressure, and to compensate for changes in extracellular fluid volume and sodium excretion.

Kallikrein, produced in the distal nephron, is an important vasodilator; kallikrein is shown to have a motor effect within the lower urinary tract and may be involved in sensorimotor mechanisms within the bladder.

The kidney is also involved in calcium metabolism and produces 1-α-hydroxylase in response to low circulating levels of calcium, which acts to convert 25-hydroxycholecalciferol into the active metabolite 1,25-dihydroxycholecalciferol, which then promotes calcium reabsorption and decreases urine excretion to maintain homeostasis.

Erythropoietin is produced by the kidney in response to hypoxia (either due to anaemia or respiratory causes), high circulating levels of the products of red cell destruction, and vasoconstriction. It is produced in smaller amounts by the liver and spleen. Erythropoietin stimulates an increase in the number of nucleated red cells in the haemopoietic tissue, thereby raising red cell and reticulocyte counts in the peripheral blood.

The renal cortex and medulla synthesize a number of prostaglandins, the exact function of which remains obscure.

SIGNS AND SYMPTOMS OF KIDNEY DISEASE

PAIN

Pain of renal origin is usually located in the ipsilateral costovertebral angle, just lateral to the sacrospinalis muscle and beneath the 12th rib. Pain is usually caused by acute distension of the renal capsule that may result from inflammation or obstruction. This pain may radiate across the flank anteriorly and towards the upper abdomen, umbilicus and testis. There may be associated gastrointestinal symptoms caused by reflex stimulation of the coeliac ganglion and the proximity of the visceral organs.

Ureteric pain is usually acute and secondary to obstruction, often by a stone or a clot. While pain caused by an upper ureteric obstruction resembles that of renal origin, pain originating from the midureter is referred to the ipsilateral iliac fossa, simulating appendicitis or diverticulitis. This pain may also be referred to the scrotum in males and the labia in females. Lower ureteric obstruction frequently produces symptoms of vesical irritability, causing frequency, urgency and suprapubic pain radiating to the tip of the penis. These features may help in predicting the site of obstruction. Slow onset obstruction is often symptomless.

Loin pain associated with fever or rigors is suggestive of infection or inflammation, and patients with this history may develop septicaemia from an acutely obstructed infected kidney.

HAEMATURIA

Haematuria (blood in the urine) may be macroscopic or microscopic. Haematuria of any degree should never be ignored, and in adults it should be regarded as a symptom of urological malignancy until proven otherwise. The character of haematuria may indicate the site of origin. Bleeding from urinary bladder or the upper urinary tract usually results in haematuria throughout the stream. In terminal haematuria, bleeding usually arises from the bladder neck or prostate. Initial haematuria is a result of a urethral bleed, although the history may not be as clear as this. The presence of proteinuria and casts in urine in association with microscopic haematuria strongly suggests a nephrological cause for the haematuria.

CHYLURIA

Chyluria is passage of milky white urine containing lymphatic fluid or chyle. This results from fistulous connections between the lymphatics of kidneys, ureters or bladder and the urinary tract, which in turn results from lymphatic obstruction or megalymphatics. Filariasis, trauma, tuberculosis and malignancies of the retroperitoneum may result in chyluria (see Ch. 12).

LOIN MASS

Normal kidneys are protected by the costal margin and are seldom palpable. In thin individuals, however, the lower pole of the right kidney may be palpated during deep inspiration. A bimanually palpable mass in the loin, which is ballottable and descends with inspiration, is likely to be a renal mass, which may be the result of cysts, tumour or obstruction.

INVESTIGATION OF URINARY TRACT DISEASE

MIDSTREAM SPECIMEN OF URINE

The specimen should be obtained prior to genital or rectal examination to avoid contamination. Urine obtained from a collecting device, such as a sheath, chronic catheter or conduit drainage bag, is *not* a proper specimen for analysis. In uncircumcised men the foreskin must be retracted and the glans cleaned prior to providing the specimen. The first 50 mL should be discarded. In women a clean catch specimen is obtained. Sample collection can be difficult in children, and often a sterile pad is placed in the nappy to get a specimen. Ideally the sample should be obtained from suprapubic puncture or through a catheter. If there is likely to be delay in transport of the sample it should be collected in a container with boric acid (1.7–2%) or should be refrigerated (not frozen). This type of sample can provide useful data up to 24–36 h.

Colour

Red urine does not always suggest haematuria. Methyldopa, L-dopa and metronidazole may turn the urine reddish brown. Whereas nitrofurantoin turns it brown, rifampicin and pyridium will make it orange. Beetroot ingestion and myoglobinuria following muscle trauma may produce red urine.

Specific gravity

The normal specific gravity of urine is 1.003–1.030. It may be low if there is an inappropriate secretion of antidiuretic hormone, in diabetes insipidus or in renal failure. It may be falsely raised by the presence of glucose, proteins, plasma expanders, and intravenous contrast agents.

pH

Patients with uric acid stones rarely have a urinary pH of over 6.5, and those with calcium stones, nephrocalcinosis or both may have renal tubular acidosis and are unable to acidify the urine below pH 6.0.

Protein

Normally, 80–150 mg of protein is excreted per day. A maximum excretion of 300 mg/day can occur transiently following severe exercise. Protein excretion that exceeds 300 mg/day is significant proteinuria and indicates the presence of renal disease. Dip-strips containing bromphenol measure albumin but does not detect the present of Bence–Jones proteins. Large numbers of leukocytes, vaginal contamination and concentrated urine may give false positive results. Persistently raised protein levels usually indicate glomerular damage.

Glucose

The glucose oxidase–peroxidase in a dip-strip is specific for urinary glucose. False positive results have been seen when large amounts of ascorbic acid, aspirin and cephalosporins have been ingested.

Haemoglobin

The dip-strip test for haemoglobin is not specific for erythrocytes and should be used only once, to screen for haematuria.

Bacteria and leukocytes

Dip-strips are used to determine the number of bacteria (nitrite) or leukocytes (leukocyte esterase) in urine specimens. A positive nitrite test suggests the presence of greater than 100 000 organisms/mL. The presence of more than 10^5 organisms/mL indicates a bacteriological urinary infection. Leukocyte esterase can detect 10–12 leukocytes per high-power field. These tests, used in combination, maximize the chances of predicting urinary tract infection. More than five leukocytes per high-power field are considered abnormal. A routine bacterial culture is advisable in all suspected cases of urinary tract infection. Persistent sterile pyuria may indicate underlying urinary tuberculosis, a stone or a tumour.

Cellular casts

The presence of cellular casts implies the presence of renal disease; granular and red cell casts are seen in proliferative glomerulonephritis, and white cell casts are associated with active pyelonephritis. The use of phase-contrast microscopy distinguishes glomerular red cells from lower urinary tract red cells (dysmorphic and isomorphic red cells) and can help differentiate urological from nephrological haematuria.

Crystals

Crystals of urate, oxalate and phosphate may be seen on microscopy in normal urine, but the presence of the hexagonal benzene ring-like crystals of cystine is diagnostic of cystinuria.

OTHER URINE TESTS

Urinary cytology is useful in cases of high-grade transitional cell carcinomas and carcinoma in situ. Other tests that can be used for an early detection of urothelial malignancy include the bladder tumour antigen test, nuclear matrix protein 22, Aura-Tek FDP and the Quanticyt system (these are currently being investigated and are not recommended in routine clinical practice).

RENAL FUNCTION TESTS

Serum creatinine

Creatinine, which is the end product of metabolism of creatine in skeletal muscle, is mainly excreted by the kidneys. The normal level of serum creatinine is 60–120 mmol/L. The creatinine level remains within this range until approximately half of the kidney function is lost.

Blood urea

Urea is the primary metabolite of protein catabolism and is excreted entirely by the kidneys. In contrast to creatinine, blood urea is influenced by dietary protein intake and hydration, and is therefore a remarkably insensitive indicator of renal function. Approximately two-thirds of renal function must be lost before there is a significant rise in the blood urea.

Creatinine clearance

The fact that daily creatinine production is remarkably constant, and that it is filtered through the glomerulus, makes the creatinine clearance approximately equal to the glomerular filtration rate. Therefore the creatinine clearance test is an accurate and reliable measure of renal function. It can be calculated by using the equation

$$\text{Creatinine clearance} = (U \times V)/P$$

where U is urinary creatinine level; P, plasma creatinine level; and V, the urinary volume in 24 h.

The creatinine clearance is a highly reliable estimate of renal function; however, the values may be falsely low, and the most common cause of this is an incomplete urine collection.

A rough estimation of creatinine clearance can be made using the formula

$$\text{Creatinine clearance} = \frac{(140 - \text{age in years}) \times \text{body weight (kg)}}{72 \times \text{serum creatinine (mg/mL)}}$$

For females the creatinine clearance will be 15% less than the calculated one.[1]

RADIOLOGICAL ASSESSMENT OF THE URINARY TRACT

Plain film of the abdomen

Frequently referred to as the 'KUB' (kidney, ureter, and bladder), the plain X-ray of the abdomen is the simplest uroradiological investigation. It is generally a part of a more extended radiological examination (e.g. an intravenous urogram or angiogram). Clinically relevant findings on a plain film include:

- Bony abnormalities, such as deformity of the spine and lytic or sclerotic patches suggestive of secondary deposits from a urological malignancy.
- Soft tissue shadows of the kidneys and psoas muscles.
- Calcification in the renal parenchyma, lymph nodes, or the wall of an aortic aneurysm (see Ch. 10).
- Radiopaque shadow suggestive of a urinary tract calculus.
- Pelvic phleboliths, often mistaken for lower ureteric calculi. Features such as round shape, central lucency and peripheral location of such calcification are all suggestive of a phlebolith.

Intravenous urography

Ionic contrast media have largely been replaced by non-ionic media, which produce better images and have a lower incidence of allergic reactions.[2] This iodine-containing contrast medium is given as an intravenous injection, and films are taken at timed intervals. An immediate film shows a nephrogram when the contrast is present in the renal tubules. The sequence of filming should demonstrate a nephrogram, the collecting system, the

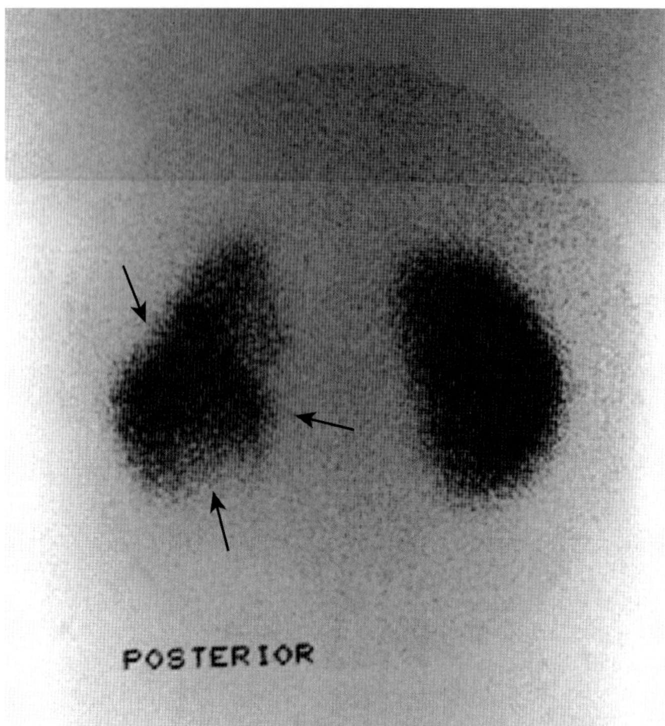

Figure 35.4 Renal scarring.

ureters and the bladder by tailoring the examination according to the clinical history and findings in the early images.

A high serum creatinine indicates that excretion of contrast may not be sufficient to delineate the urinary system, and this examination is of little value. There is a small risk of a hypersensitive reaction with contrast media, which can have a nephrotoxic effect, especially if there is pre-existing renal damage. Transient renal failure, characterized by a rise in serum creatinine, may occur in about 10% of the high-risk cases.[3] Patients on metformin with a raised creatinine have a high risk of developing renal failure. Tomography significantly increases the recognition of renal masses, renal calcification and paranephric structures, but it may not be of much help in patients less than 40 years of age.

Retrograde ureteropyelogram

Retrograde urography is a moderately invasive procedure that requires cystoscopy and placing catheters in the ureteric orifices. Bubble-free contrast medium is then injected, while the whole of the ureter and collecting system is screened by fluoroscopy. This examination may be helpful if the intravenous urogram has failed to demonstrate the urinary tract clearly.

Renal angiography

The indications for renal angiography are limited to:

- Diagnosis of renovascular hypertension, when it can be combined with simultaneous balloon angioplasty.

REFERENCES

1. Cockcroft DW, Gault MH. Nephron 1976; 16: 31–41
2. Morcos SK, Thomsen HS, Webb JA. Eur Radiol 2001; 11: 1720–1728
3. Golman K, Almen T. In: Sovak M (ed). Radiocontrast Agents. Springer-Verlag, New York, 1985: 153–156

- Embolization of a bleeding vessel, for example in trauma cases prior to surgery, especially where renal parenchymal preservation is being attempted.
- Mapping the renal vessels before nephron-sparing surgery is attempted in a patient with renal mass.

Isotope renography

This very useful investigation depends on the ability of the kidney to filter and secrete radiopharmaceuticals. A computerized traced plot of isotope activity in an area of interest can then be made. The commonly used isotopes are:

- technetium-99m dimercaptosuccinic acid (DMSA);
- technetium-99m diethylenetriaminepenta-acetic acid (DTPA); and
- mercaptoacetyltriglycine (MAG3)

Each of these is handled differently by the kidney, and therefore gives different information. The isotope DMSA is secreted by the tubules and is the most commonly used agent for renal cortical imaging. This is particularly useful when segmental renal abnormalities, such as renal scarring (Fig. 35.4), tumours or evidence of trauma, are being assessed. It also provides useful information on the function of each kidney relative to the other, commonly referred to as the 'split renal function'. This is especially important if a nephrectomy is contemplated in a patient with pre-existing renal failure. In addition, DMSA scanning gives an indication of the potential of renal function to recover following a procedure to relieve an obstructed kidney. It is often used to determine whether there is sufficient function in a diseased kidney to merit its conservation.

On the other hand, DTPA and MAG3 are the agents most commonly used for excretory imaging, because they are rapidly excreted in the urine. Their main value lies in identifying an obstructed kidney. A diuretic is administered 15 min before performing the test, stressing the affected kidney to the maximum. Failure of excretion of the isotope from the kidney demonstrates increased activity above the site of obstruction, and a rising curve is seen on the renogram.

The agent MAG3 is also secreted by the kidney and is one of the most commonly used isotopes in radionuclear departments, when the overall renal function is poor.

Isotope renography is a good method of imaging the genitourinary tract, because the radiation dose is much less from isotopes than conventional radiographs. It is also used to diagnose and monitor the progress of renal damage associated with vesicoureteric reflux.

Ultrasonography

Ultrasonography is the most commonly performed investigation of the urinary tract. In cases of renal failure it is used to diagnose an obstructive renal failure. It is an excellent investigation for diagnosing hydronephrosis and assessing the nature of mass lesions in the kidney, whether cystic, solid or infective (abscess). The technique is operator-dependent but is non-invasive and inexpensive. It does not carry any risk of irradiation. Its diagnostic and therapeutic uses include the following.

Renal failure

Ultrasonography helps in distinguishing an obstructed kidney. The presence of a dilated urinary tract on ultrasound is not, however, diagnostic of obstruction; conversely, acute obstruction may not give rise to a hydronephrotic system.

Trauma

Perirenal haematomas and renal parenchymal damage can be assessed and renal blood flow visualized with Doppler ultrasound. Urinomas can be visualized and drained percutaneously.

Infections

The presence of pyonephrosis or a perirenal abscess can be easily identified.

Calculus disease

Ultrasound not only detects radiolucent stones in the kidney but is also used to provide real-time imaging during lithotripsy.

Renal tumours

Ultrasound can be used for both diagnosing and staging of patients with renal tumour. Needle biopsy of renal masses, and aspiration of cysts from the kidney for cytological and histological assessment, can safely be performed under ultrasound guidance.

Renal transplants

Ultrasound can provide evidence of acute rejection in the form of bright echoes in transplanted kidneys (see Ch. 8). It also detects invasive obstruction or the presence of urinomas. The transplant can be biopsied under ultrasound guidance or percutaneously drained if obstructed.

Computerized tomography

Computerized tomography provides excellent anatomy of the upper urinary tract and surrounding structures. The CT attenuation values for different soft tissues in the body provide better resolution in imaging, and therefore clearer identification of structures such as fat, kidney, liver, spleen and vessels. Renal masses can be identified and characterized, and renal tumours can be staged. Angiomyolipoma, a benign tumour of the kidney, can be diagnosed and followed up by CT imaging. It is extremely useful in assessing the extent of renal parenchymal damage, and ureteric integrity and function in patients with renal injuries. It is also useful in the diagnosis of retroperitoneal fibrosis. In many centres, a non-contrast spiral CT scan has replaced an intravenous urogram as a first-line investigation in suspected stone disease.

The renal vasculature can be visualized using newer spiral CT scans with three-dimensional reconstruction. These advances in CT imaging allow for digital subtraction and reconstruction to give unsurpassed pictures of the renal and ureteric anatomy; this is useful in cases where a partial nephrectomy is planned.

Magnetic resonance imaging

Magnetic resonance imaging remains a research tool in urology; it has, however, been shown to have a role when renal cell carcinoma is suspected and CT is unhelpful, or when the patient is sensitive to contrast. It can demonstrate the local spread of stage IV renal cell carcinoma better than CT, and can also show the extent of tumour thrombus in the renal vein and inferior vena cava more clearly than a CT scan.[4] It is better than CT in determining the haemorrhagic component of a cystic mass, and is currently being evaluated in renal vascular hypertension, where

REFERENCE

4. Kabala JE. Br J Radiol 1991; 64: 683

it has been found to be 100% sensitive, and will pick up 76% of significant renal artery stenoses, in the proximal 3 cm of the renal artery.

CONGENITAL ANOMALIES OF THE KIDNEY AND URETER

AGENESIS

Bilateral renal agenesis is extremely rare and incompatible with life. Prenatal suspicion of the existence of the anomaly is raised by oligohydramnios. It is associated with pulmonary hypoplasia and a characteristic 'Potter' facies. Abdominal ultrasound usually establishes the diagnosis.

Unilateral agenesis is seen in one in 1100 births.[5] The fault most probably lies with the ureteric bud: either a complete absence of the ureteric bud is present or it fails to reach the metanephros. Half of those with unilateral renal agenesis will have an absent ipsilateral ureter, while the other half would have a blind-ending ureter. Associated anomalies include the absence of the vas deferens on the same side in men. An abnormality of the internal genitalia is seen in a third of the women with unilateral renal agenesis.[6] Unilateral renal agenesis is symptomless, but there may be other associated anomalies of the heart, vertebral column and anal canal.

SUPERNUMERARY KIDNEY

Supernumerary kidney is again an extremely rare anomaly. Approximately 75 cases have been reported in the literature to date.[7] The supernumerary kidney has its own separate capsule and blood supply. Approximately half of all supernumerary kidneys have their own completely independent ureter. They are located caudal to the dominant kidney and are usually smaller than the main ipsilateral organ. In a quarter of cases the condition remains completely symptomless.[8]

RENAL HYPOPLASIA

Renal hypoplasia is a term that should be strictly restricted to small kidneys that have less than the normal number of calyces and nephrons, but are neither dysplastic nor have embryonic remnants within them. They have a uniformly narrow renal artery. When the hypoplasia is bilateral, failure to thrive, renal insufficiency or associated respiratory problems can occur, with the urine being of low specific gravity.

ANOMALIES OF ASCENT

The kidney may be arrested either in the pelvis, in the iliac fossa (Fig. 35.5), or in the abdominal cavity. Occasionally it may be ectopic, as in a thoracic kidney.[9] This must be differentiated from renal ptosis, where the kidney is initially located in the renal fossa but is excessively mobile. An ectopic kidney has an ectopic blood supply. There is a slight risk of developing hydronephrosis and calculi in a pelvic or a malrotated kidney. Thoracic kidneys have completed their rotation and have no predilection for specific renal diseases attributable to their position.

Crossed renal ectopias are present when the kidney is located on the opposite side to the side where the ureter enters the bladder. The possibilities are a bilaterally crossed renal ectopia or a simple crossed ectopia with or without fusion to the ipsilateral kidney. Fusion is present in 90% of crossed ectopic kidneys. The diagnosis is usually incidental and the prognosis is good, with normal longevity.

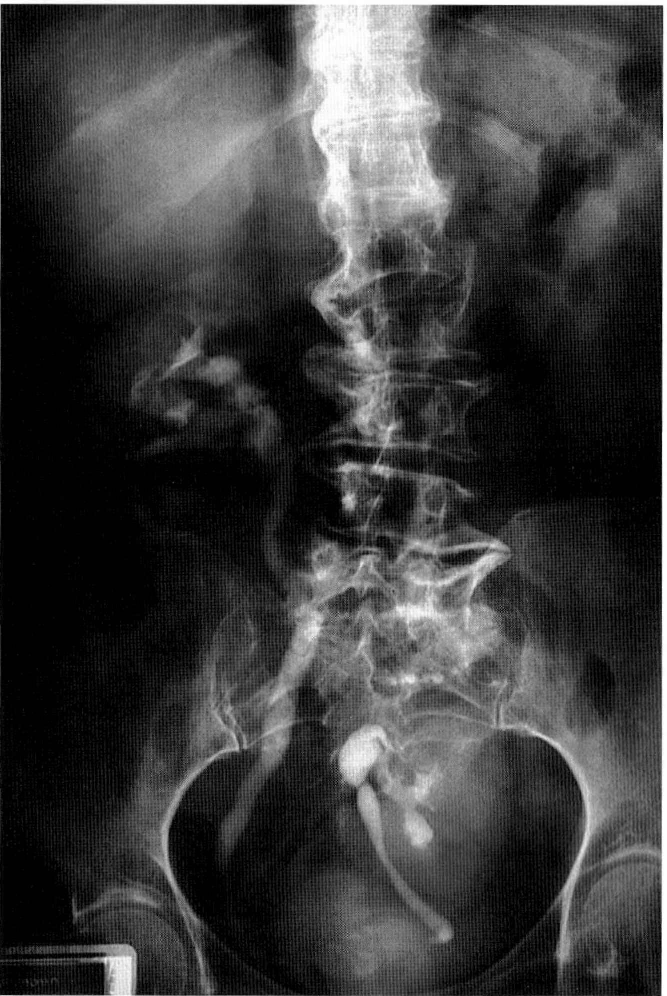

Figure 35.5 Pelvic kidney.

HORSESHOE KIDNEY

Horseshoe kidney is the most common of all renal fusion anomalies and occurs in one in 400 of the population,[10] occurring twice as commonly in men. The metanephric masses lie closely together, and a development disturbance leads to their fusion. The inferior mesenteric artery prevents its full ascent, causing low-lying kidneys. Fusion occurs between the lower poles in 95% of cases. The connecting isthmus usually consists of parenchymal tissue with an independent blood supply.[11] Occasionally, it may be a bridge of fibrous tissue at the level of the third and fifth lumbar vertebrae. The calyces are normal in number but abnormal in orientation, because the kidneys fail to rotate. The ureter enters the bladder normally. The isthmus may receive its blood supply from the main renal arteries, but not

REFERENCES

5. Doroshow LW, Abeshouse BS. Urol Surv 1961; 11: 219
6. Thompson DP, Lynn HB. Mayo Clin Proc 1966; 41: 538
7. McPherson RI. Can Assoc Radiol J 1987; 38: 116
8. Hoffman RL, McMillan TE. Trans South Central Sec Am Urol Assoc 1948; 40: 82
9. Kirshenbaum KS, Puri HC, Rao BR. J Urol 1981; 125: 412–413
10. Dees J. J Urol 1941; 46: 659
11. Glenn JF. N Engl J Med 1959; 261: 684

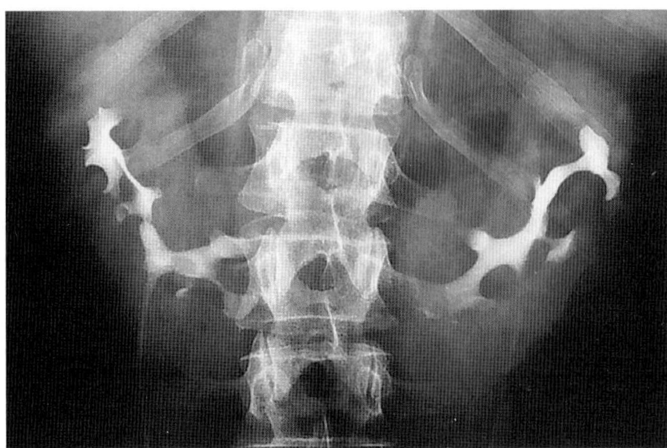

Figure 35.6 Horseshoe kidney.

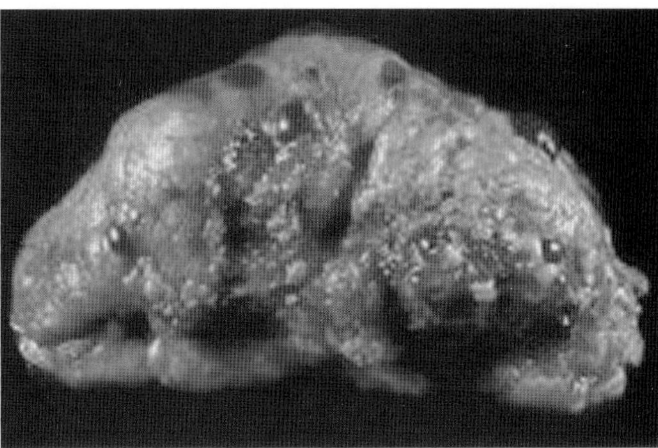

Figure 35.7 Polycystic kidney.

infrequently also receives a blood supply from the inferior mesenteric, common external iliac or sacral arteries.[12]

One-third of patients remain symptomless.[11] Symptoms are usually caused by a hydronephrosis, infection or stone formation. About 5–10% of horseshoe kidneys are palpable.

A plain radiograph may show a soft tissue mass connecting the two kidneys, and an intravenous urogram usually shows an abnormal but characteristic orientation of the collecting system, giving rise to a flower vase appearance (Fig. 35.6). A CT scan may be necessary for confirmation of the diagnosis.

Ureteric obstruction with hydronephrosis, recurrent infections and recurrent stone formation are indications for surgical correction. This can be achieved by performing an isthmusectomy.

CYSTIC DISEASES OF THE KIDNEY

The kidney is one of the most common sites of cysts. The cysts may or may not communicate with the collecting system. They were classified by the American Academy of Pediatrics Section of Urology in 1987.

POLYCYSTIC RENAL DISEASE

Infantile polycystic kidney

Infantile polycystic kidney is caused by an autosomal recessive gene; cystic changes occur in both the kidneys and liver.[13] It is associated with periportal fibrosis, leading to portal hypertension and subsequent development of oesophageal varices. The onset of renal failure is rapid and, although attempts may be made to improve renal function, the development of progressive liver disease is usually fatal. There is no cure for this condition; however, treating the associated cardiac, hepatic and renal failure can prolong survival.

Adult polycystic kidney

Adult polycystic kidney (Figs 35.7 and 35.8) is an autosomal dominant hereditary condition affecting both the kidneys in 95% of cases, and is much more common. It is the third most common cause of end-stage renal failure. It may be associated with cysts of the liver, pancreas and spleen. The cysts enlarge and compress the surrounding parenchyma, causing its ischaemic necrosis and resulting in progressive renal functional impairment. The condition generally presents in the third or fourth decade of life.

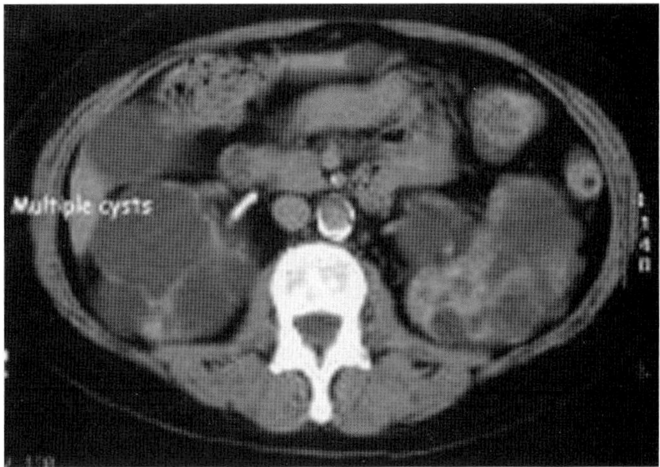

Figure 35.8 A CT scan of polycystic kidney.

Patients present with pain over one or both the kidneys as a result of the weight of the heavy kidneys, infection, obstruction or haemorrhage. Hypertension is present in 60–70% of cases, and renal failure eventually develops. Recurrent urinary tract infections occur in 20% of cases, and some patients have gross haematuria that may give rise to clot colic. Occasionally a palpable renal mass is picked up on routine examination.

Investigations

A plain radiograph may demonstrate enlarged renal shadows. An intravenous urogram shows the renal calyces stretched out by the cysts, giving rise to a 'spider' deformity. Ultrasound confirms large bilateral multicystic kidneys with a normal renal pelvis. Computerized tomography scanning has an accuracy of around 95% in detecting cysts. Amniocentesis can be used to diagnose intrauterine disease, and counselling for termination can be offered.

REFERENCES

12. Boatman DL, Cornell SH, Kolln CP. Am J Roentgenol 1971; 113: 447
13. Kissane JM, Smith MG. Pathology of Infancy and Childhood. 2nd edn. CV Mosby, St Louis, 1975: 587

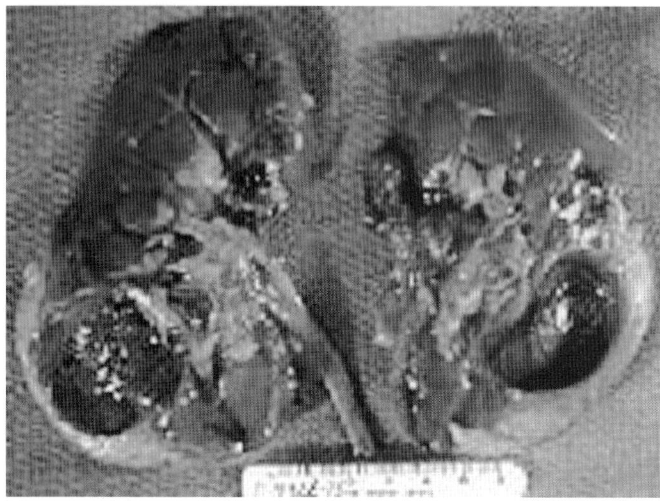

Figure 35.9 Simple cyst.

Management

Cases are increasingly diagnosed early, either by sonography or by genetic testing. Treatment is mainly conservative and aimed at controlling hypertension, treating infections and monitoring for renal failure. It is considered that the chance of developing renal failure is lower than was formerly thought, and half the affected patients have developed renal failure at the age of 73 years.[14] Surgery to the cysts is seldom indicated unless there is troublesome bleeding or loin pain. There is no evidence to suggest that Rovsing's operation, which consists of deroofing the cysts, improves renal function. Patients with renal failure may require dialysis and eventually renal transplantation (see Ch. 8). This may be combined with bilateral nephrectomy if the renal masses are causing symptoms.

SIMPLE CYSTS

Despite being a common entity and 20–30% of the population having simple renal cysts (Fig. 35.9), their origin remains obscure. Simple cysts are mostly detected incidentally on sonography, CT or intravenous urogram, and are usually asymptomatic. However, they can give rise to pain due to haemorrhage or urinary tract obstruction, and hypertension due to segmental ischaemia. Large renal cysts may be palpable on abdominal examination.

Ultrasonography is the baseline investigation for a renal cyst, and the features of a classical benign cyst would be:

- spherical shape with sharply defined, smooth and distinct margin;
- absence of internal echoes; and
- good transmission of sound waves through the cyst, with consequent acoustic enhancement behind the cyst.

A CT scan is better in defining the individual cysts; however, in case of doubt, a further needle aspiration or MRI is indicated. Bosniak divided cysts into four categories, as shown in Table 35.1.[15]

A benign cyst does not require any surgical intervention unless complications ensue. An infected cyst will require percutaneous drainage. Pain may be relieved by aspiration; however, for cysts causing obstruction, surgical excision is the definite solution.

MEDULLARY SPONGE KIDNEY

This condition results from cystic dilatation of the terminal collecting ducts as they cross the medulla. In 75% of the patients

Table 35.1 Bosniak's classification of renal cysts

Class	Description
I	Simple benign cysts. These lesions are round or oval in shape, are unilocular with the uniform density of water, have no perceptible wall, and exhibit no enhancement on radiographs taken after the administration of contrast medium.
II	Probable benign simple cystic lesions that are minimally complicated. These lesions include septated cysts, minimally calcified cysts, infected cysts and high-density cysts.
III	More complicated cystic lesions. These lesions exhibit some findings seen in malignancy, such as thick, irregular calcifications, irregular borders, multilocular form, thickened or enhancing septa, uniform wall thickening or small non-enhancing nodules.
IV	Clearly malignant cystic masses. The appearance of these lesions results from necrosis and liquefaction of a solid tumour or a tumour growing in the wall. These lesions are heterogeneous, with a shaggy appearance, thickened walls or enhancing nodules.

the disease is bilateral.[16] A characteristic pattern is seen on intravenous urography: the dilated ducts are invariably filled with small calculi, which are secondary to stasis and sepsis in the ducts. There is also a persistent medullary opacification. The patient may present with pain, infection or haematuria; however, most cases are asymptomatic. Treatment is aimed at specific complications such as infection and stones.

CALYCEAL CYSTS

These are small cystic spaces adjoining the calyces or renal pelvis. They may be found on routine urography. Intervention is required only if secondary stone formation occurs.

HYDATID CYSTS

This is parasitic infection with *Echinococcus*, an intestinal tapeworm of dogs, wolves and foxes. The liver is much more commonly affected, and less than 2% of patients with hydatid disease develop a renal cyst.

The intravenous urogram may show a space-occupying mass, which can be confirmed on ultrasound. Serological testing is generally diagnostic. Medical treatment of hydatid disease is unsatisfactory, although α-mebendazole may provide some benefit. Surgical removal of the cyst by partial nephrectomy is the best treatment. Spillage of infected particles can produce severe anaphylactoid reactions. Patients are often given a prolonged course of α-mebendazole postoperatively to prevent recurrence.

CONGENITAL ANOMALIES OF THE URETER

URETERAL ATRESIA OR AGENESIS

Bilateral ureteral agenesis is incompatible with life. A true unilateral agenesis is associated with an absent kidney on that side

REFERENCES

14. Churchill DN, Bear JC, Morgan J et al. Kidney Int 1984; 26: 190
15. Bosniak MA. Radiology 1986; 158: 1
16. Kuiper JJ. Perspect Nephrol Hypertens 1976; 4: 151

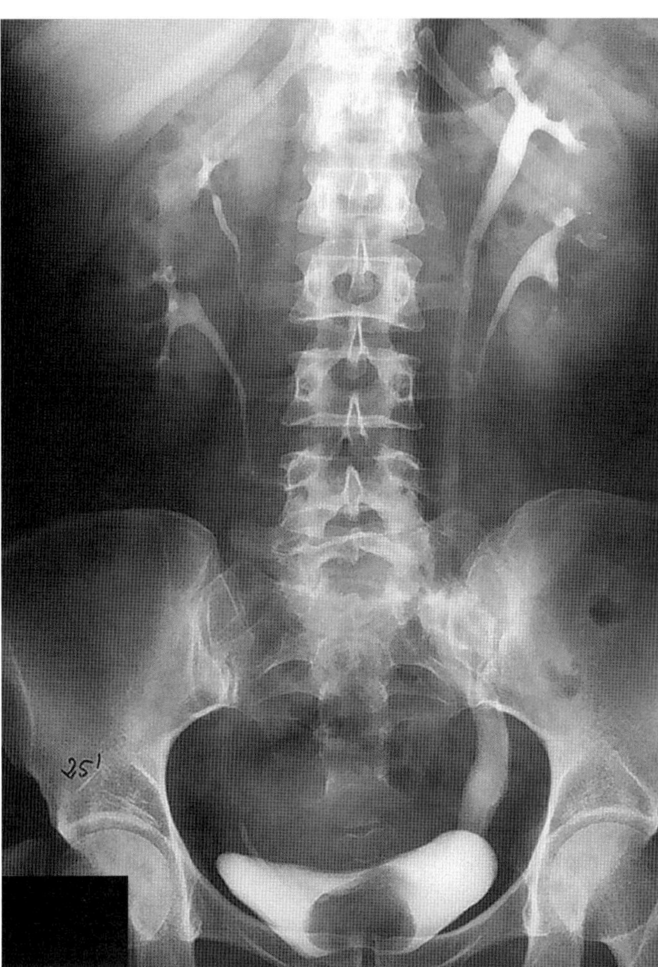

Figure 35.10 Bilateral ureteral duplication with ureterocele.

because of a failure of induction of the ipsilateral metanephros. Most clinicians feel observation is the best management.

URETERIC DUPLICATION

Complete or incomplete duplication of ureter is one of the most common congenital malformations of the urinary tract. The overall incidence of complete duplication is less than 1%.[17] A duplicated ureter usually drains a duplex kidney (Fig. 35.10). Many forms of ureteric duplication exist. The most common is an incomplete ureteric duplication with a Y junction in the ureter, which may result in 'yo-yo' reflux between the two moieties of a duplex kidney, causing stasis, ureteric dilatation and infection.

Complete ureteric duplication is invariably associated with vesicoureteric reflux, and it is usually the lower pole ureter that refluxes. The upper pole ureter drains distally and medially, and this feature is so consistent that it has been termed the *Weigert–Meyer law*.[18,19] Because the lower pole drains laterally and cranially, it has a shorter intravesical length, thereby causing reflux. Occasionally, the insertion of the upper pole ureter into the bladder is situated at the bladder neck or urethra. In females this may cause urinary incontinence if the ectopic opening is beyond the sphincter or in the vagina.[20]

The condition results from duplication of the ureteric bud.

Clinical features

Most patients are diagnosed in childhood when they present with recurrent urinary infections. Intravenous urography shows

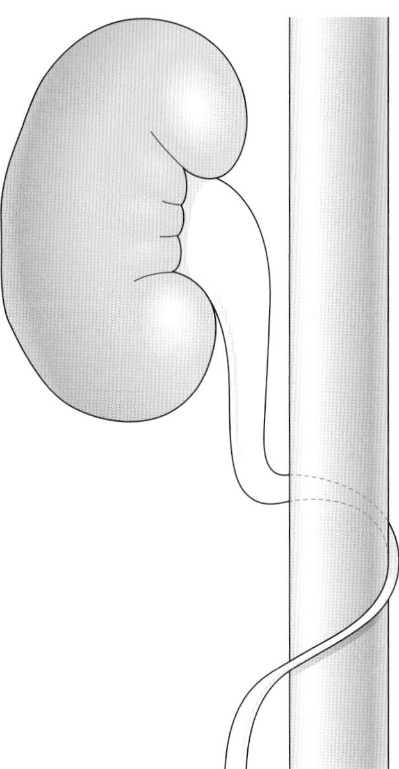

Figure 35.11 Retrocaval ureter.

duplication of the collecting system, and a micturating cystourethrogram confirms the presence of reflux.

Management

The management of refluxing duplex ureters is usually conservative. However, for major reflux, recurrent infections and upper pole obstruction, surgery is indicated. It may vary from ureteric reimplantation to uretero-ureterostomy or to partial nephrectomy.

URETERIC DIVERTICULUM

Ureteric diverticulum is an extremely rare cause of urinary infection or pain; local excision or uretero-ureterostomy is the treatment of choice.

RETROCAVAL URETER AND RETROILIAC URETER

The inferior vena cava is formed from the supracardinal vein while the subcardinal vein atrophies. If subcardinal vein persists, the ureter is trapped dorsal to it (Fig. 35.11). The finding of a retrocaval ureter is often incidental, but occasionally it causes loin pain and tenderness due to obstruction. Intravenous urography usually shows fullness of the upper ureter and fails to demonstrate the retrocaval part of the ureter. This can be visualized well on a retrograde pyelogram. A CT scan is required for a definitive diagnosis. Symptomatic cases may need surgical intervention in the form of repositioning of the ureter by ureteric division.

REFERENCES

17. Nation EF. J Urol 1944; 51: 456
18. Meyer R. Anat Rec 1946; 96: 355
19. Weigert C. Virchows Arch (Pathol Anat) 1877; 70: 490
20. Ellerker AG. Br J Surg 1958; 45: 344

ECTOPIC URETER

Ectopic ureter is a ureter that does not open at its normal location on the trigone. It may be a part of a duplex system, in which case it is associated with the upper pole moiety. The orifice may be found at any number of possible sites. The condition is 10 times more common in females, and 20% of ectopic ureters are bilateral.[20] It is commonly associated with hypoplasia or dysplasia of renal tissue.

If the opening of the ectopic ureter is below the distal sphincter mechanism of the urethra, there is a complete urinary incontinence. In the male it is invariably suprasphincteric. When the opening is intrasphincteric, the ectopia is associated with upper tract obstruction, and reflux may also occur. One-third of ectopic ureters in the female open into the vagina.

In the male, an ectopic ureter may drain into the epididymis, seminal vesicles, vas deferens or posterior urethra. Epididymitis may occur; this anomaly accounts for virtually all cases of prepubertal epididymitis.[21] The diagnosis is extremely difficult, requiring a combination of intravenous urography, ultrasound and cystoscopy.

The type of surgical correction depends on the amount of renal function remaining in the affected kidney. Upper pole partial nephroureterectomy is frequently required, although a ureteropyelostomy or a uretero-ureterostomy may be performed if the function of the upper pole is good.

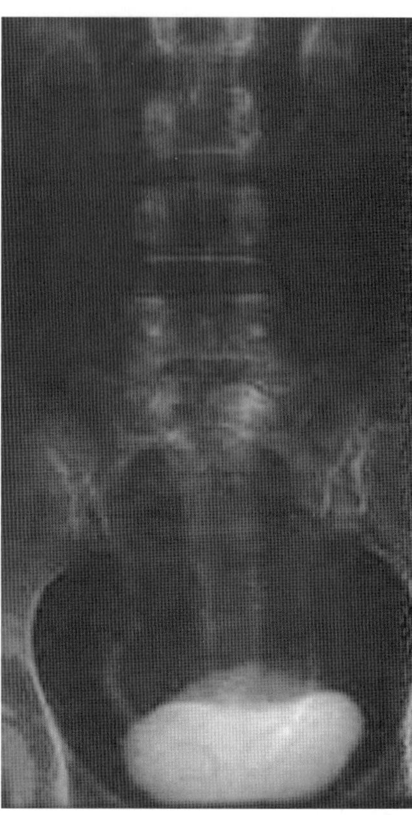

Figure 35.12 Bilateral ureterocele.

URETEROCELE

A ureterocele is a sacculation of the terminal portion of the ureter. It may be either intravesical or ectopic, the latter being the more common form. It is commonly seen in the ureter draining an upper pole moiety in patients with complete ureteric duplication. The wall of the ureterocele generally contains patchy muscle and collagen. Ureteroceles are more common in women, and are bilateral in 10% of cases (Fig. 35.12).[22] Many ureteroceles in adults are incidental findings and, provided they are symptomless, do not require treatment.

The management of ureteroceles in children is highly complex, depending on the presence of symptoms, associated infection, the anatomy and other urinary tract anomalies, and the amount of functioning renal tissue. If the ureterocele is small and well supported, an endoscopic incision in the lower lip of the ureteric meatus may relieve obstruction, while leaving a flap of mucosa that may prevent reflux. This procedure may, however, cause reflux, which then requires correction by ureteric reimplantation.

RENAL FAILURE

ACUTE RENAL FAILURE

Acute renal failure is an abrupt decline in renal function, with a loss of normal activity. A daily urine output of less than 500 mL is termed *oliguria*; the absence of urine formation is *anuria*. The underlying cause of acute renal failure is usually a persistent fall in renal blood flow to levels 30–40% of normal, with a consequent reduction in glomerular filtration to less than 5 mL/min. The causes of acute renal failure can be divided broadly into prerenal, renal and postrenal. Prerenal acute renal failure usually results from dehydration or circulatory collapse, producing hypovolaemia associated with conditions such as blood loss, septicaemia or trauma. Renal causes can be broadly considered to be interstitial (drugs or infection), glomerular (autoimmune conditions or diabetes), tubular damage (antibiotics, drugs or toxic chemicals), or renal (vasculitis or thrombosis).

The routine biochemical investigations that are useful in diagnosis of acute renal failure are summarized in Table 35.2.

An ultrasound along with a plain abdominal X-ray is useful in excluding an obstructive cause. The main aim of the treatment of patients with acute renal failure is to identify a cause and to institute appropriate treatment. Fluid intake is restricted to 500 mL/day (equivalent to insensible loss). Sodium intake is restricted to 20–30 mmol/day, and careful monitoring of metabolic and nutritional status is important. H_2-receptor antagonists and antacids are often used, because of the associated incidence of upper gastrointestinal haemorrhage. Dialysis is indicated if conservative measures fail to control the situation, and usually in the acute situation it is instituted via haemodialysis. Indications of haemodialysis include hyperkalaemia, metabolic acidosis and fluid overload.

The clinical course of acute renal failure is highly variable, depending on the aetiology, and can be considered to comprise of oliguric, diuretic and postdiuretic phases. The oliguric phase is seen early in acute renal failure. A diuresis can occur at any time and is often a sign of recovery. It is important to maintain vigilance, particularly during this time, because of the potential for loss of fluid and electrolytes. Acute renal failure is a condition with a high mortality, the worst prognostic features being haemorrhage, trauma, peritonitis, advanced age and infection.

REFERENCES

21. Schnitzer B. J Urol 1965; 93: 576
22. Mandell J, Colodny AH, Lebowitz R et al. J Urol 1980; 123: 921

Table 35.2 Biochemical recognition of established acute renal failure

	Physiological oliguria	Established acute renal failure
Urine volume	Low (?high)	Low
Urine specific gravity	> 1020	1010
Urinary osmolality (mOsm/kg H_2O)	> 500	250–300
Urinary sodium (mmol/L)	< 15	> 60
Urinary urea (mmol/L)	> 250	< 160
Urine/plasma osmolality	> 1.3	≤ 1.1
Urine/plasma urea	> 10	< 10
Response to fluid load	Always	Occasional

(From Bullock N, Sibley G, Whittaker R (eds). Essential Urology. Edinburgh: Churchill Livingstone: 1989, with permission.[23])

CHRONIC RENAL FAILURE

Chronic renal failure is an end-stage renal failure resulting most commonly from chronic glomerulitis and pyelonephritis. Polycystic renal disease accounts for approximately 5% of cases and hypertension approximately 10%.

Patients with chronic renal failure usually have polyuria with loss of normal concentrating ability. Nocturia is often said to be an early sign, and the urine contains protein with granular casts and white blood cells. Sodium is gradually retained in chronic renal failure, although the serum sodium level is a poor reflection of this. In end-stage chronic renal failure potassium levels may rise, and acidosis is inevitable due to decreased ammonium ion excretion and decreased excretion of buffer phosphate, the urine pH usually being less than 5. Because calcium levels may fall secondary parathyroidism is not uncommon, and osteomalacia may occur, which is sometimes vitamin D-resistant. Magnesium levels may rise because of the inability to excrete a magnesium load. Characteristically the urea, uric acid and creatinine levels rise. Anaemia is normochromic and normocytic, and is likely to be due to marrow suppression with reduced red cell survival.

Appropriate investigation of patients with chronic renal failure in addition to biochemical investigations includes ultrasound scan of the upper tract and a check on postvoiding residual urine. Up to a third of patients with chronic retention of urine present with chronic renal failure.

The aim of conservative treatment is to delay the progressive deterioration of renal function and its consequences. Fluid intake should be controlled to produce a urine output of approximately 1 L/24 h, blood pressure is controlled by use of antihypertensive drugs, and cardiac failure is treated using standard measures. The anaemia of chronic renal failure may be treated successfully by exogenous erythropoietin or transfusion. In some patients the protein intake is restricted to 40 g/24 h to reduce the production of nitrogenous waste products.

When conservative measures fail dialysis is instituted, and this is usually in patients in whom the serum creatinine has risen above 1000 mmol/L or if the creatinine clearance is less than 1 mL/min. The options for dialysis lie between haemodialysis and peritoneal dialysis. Peritoneal dialysis is particularly useful in the home situation and is cheaper than haemodialysis. However, it is less efficient and associated with a higher incidence of infection.

RENAL AND URETERIC TRAUMA

Renal injuries may be classified as penetrating or blunt. All penetrating injuries should be carefully evaluated. Blunt trauma accounts for more than 80–85% of all renal injuries, and kidneys with existing pathological conditions such as hydronephrosis or tumour are more susceptible.

Renal injuries may be graded as suggested by Moore and colleagues into five grades.[24] Grades I and II are considered minor and the rest are regarded as major:

- Grade I: renal contusion or contained subcapsular haematoma with no parenchymal laceration.
- Grade II: non-expanding, confined perirenal haematoma or cortical laceration less than 1 cm deep with no urinary extravasation.
- Grade III: parenchymal laceration extending more than 1 cm without urinary extravasation.
- Grade IV: parenchymal laceration extending to the collecting system, leading to an extravasation.
- Grade V: thrombosis of the main renal artery, multiple lacerations resulting in a shattered kidney or a pedicle avulsion.

CLINICAL FINDINGS

Pain may be localized to the affected flank, or it may be generalized. Retroperitoneal bleeding may cause abdominal distension and ileus, with associated nausea and vomiting.

Haematuria may be gross or microscopic; however, the degree of renal injury does not correspond to the degree of haematuria.

Bruising in the flank may be associated with fracture of lower ribs.

An abdominal swelling may be occasionally palpable if the trauma is associated with a large perirenal haematoma.

Profound hypotension with tachycardia is usually associated with major renal trauma.

REFERENCES

23. Bullock N, Sibley G, Whittaker R (eds). Essential Urology. Churchill Livingstone, Edinburgh, 1989
24. Moore EE et al. J Trauma 1989; 29: 1664

INVESTIGATIONS

Diagnosis and assessment of the extent of injury can be made successfully by imaging the kidneys. However, not all cases would require imaging. As per the recommendations made by Miller and McAninch,[25] patients who require radiographic assessment are those with:

- gross haematuria;
- microscopic haematuria with shock (systolic blood pressure less than 90 mmHg);
- suspicion of renal injury following a physical examination; and
- children with gross or microscopic haematuria.

A preliminary plain abdominal X-ray may suggest a significant renal injury in the presence of the following signs:

- obliteration of the psoas shadow;
- an enlarged renal outline;
- fractured lower ribs;
- fractured transverse processes of first, second and third lumbar vertebrae; and
- scoliosis to the injured side.

The nephrotoxic effect of contrast in shocked patients and the inevitable delay in obtaining a renal angiogram, which exceeds the viability time of an ischaemic kidney following a pedicle injury, limits the use of arteriography in cases where a major renal injury is suspected.

A normal intravenous urogram requires no further radiological studies. The findings on an intravenous urogram that suggest a renal trauma are:

- extravasation of contrast (Fig. 35.13), and
- non-visualization of the affected kidney.

A CT scan is the preferred investigation modality, because it better defines the renal and associated visceral injuries. Both small amounts of extravasation and infarction can be picked up, and it provides a precise idea of blood flow to the renal parenchyma.

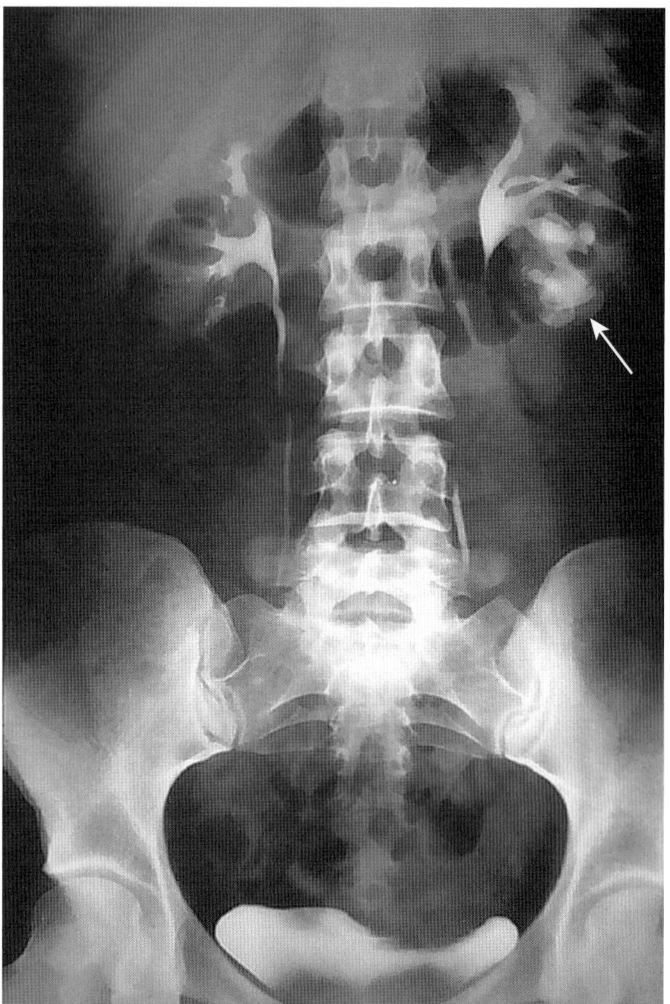

Figure 35.13 Extravasation on the left.

COMPLICATIONS

Early complications

Haemorrhage with heavy retroperitoneal bleed may result in shock. Bleeding ceases spontaneously in over 80% of cases; however, careful monitoring of blood pressure and haematocrit is essential.

Extravasation of urine may lead to formation of a urinoma in the retroperitoneum. This may expand, get infected and form an abscess. Such a perinephric abscess causes flank tenderness and a spiking temperature, and requires formal drainage.

Late complications

The important late complications following renal trauma include hypertension, hydronephrosis, arteriovenous fistula, calculus formation and recurrent kidney infections. Blood pressure should be monitored carefully every few months. A follow-up CT scan or an intravenous urogram should be performed at 3–6 months to assess the degree of renal scarring, any resulting hydronephrosis or vascular compromise. Renal atrophy may result from ischaemia.

MANAGEMENT

Following renal trauma caused by a blunt injury, approximately 80% of the patients will require no surgical exploration. A further 5–10% will require surgical exploration and reconstruction, while in the remaining 5% the kidney will be non-salvageable.[26] Minor injuries (grades I and II) are best managed conservatively with bed rest until the gross haematuria settles. Routine use of prophylactic antibiotics is not necessary, and they should be prescribed only in the event of a high fever and raised white cell count, or in cases of perirenal extravasation. Percutaneous drainage of a urinoma may be required. In patients with a minor or moderate degree of renal injury and perirenal haematomata, serial ultrasound scans help to determine whether or not the haematoma is expanding.

An exploration is carried out in cases of the patient being haemodynamically unstable due to a persistent retroperitoneal bleed, urinary extravasation, evidence of non-viable renal parenchyma, or an avulsion injury to the hilum. An exploration may have to be carried out in cases of penetrating injuries to rule out injury to other organs. The kidney is explored via the transabdominal route if open exploration is necessary. A careful search must be made for any associated injuries. In the presence of a large retroperitoneal haematoma, the renal pedicle should be controlled first, followed by examination of the kidney and repair. Nephrectomy is frequently necessary in the case of high-velocity missile wounds, but it is often possible to conserve part of

REFERENCES

25. Miller KS, McAninch JW. J Urol 1995; 154: 352–355
26. Carlton CE Jr. In: Harrison JH, Gittes RF, Perlmutter AD et al (eds). Campbell's Urology. 4th edn. WB Saunders, Philadelphia, 1978

the kidney after stab injuries. If the renal pedicle is damaged nephrectomy is usually required, although there are reports of successful conservative operations for renal injury.

TREATMENT OF COMPLICATIONS

Urinomas and abscesses can be drained via a percutaneous route. Hypertension caused by ischaemia, renal artery stenosis, or perirenal constriction from capsular fibrosis is the most serious late sequel. Surgery is seldom indicated because this hypertension is transient in most patients. Perirenal fibrosis may also cause pelviureteric junction obstruction, which may require surgical correction.

URETERIC INJURIES

Injuries to the ureter are uncommon and are usually iatrogenic, occurring during the course of ureterorenoscopy, or intra-abdominal, pelvic, or laparoscopic surgery. They are mostly associated with surgery that is particularly difficult, such as hysterectomy for severe pelvic inflammatory disease or endometriosis, a large bulky fibroid uterus or an ovarian tumour, when the ureter may be cut or ligated. Interference with the ureteric blood supply during a Wertheim hysterectomy or during pelvic surgery following previous pelvic irradiation may result in an ischaemic and subsequently necrotic ureter. A large pelvic mass may displace the ureter, and malignant or inflammatory mass may involve it, making recognition of the ureter extremely difficult during the surgical procedure. Occasionally, ureteric injuries may result from gunshot or stab wounds. In thin children, ureteropelvic junction disruption may occur following an acute hyperextension of the spine and blunt trauma.

Clinical features

A ligated ureter would present as pain in the flank with associated nausea and vomiting in the postoperative period. An ultrasound

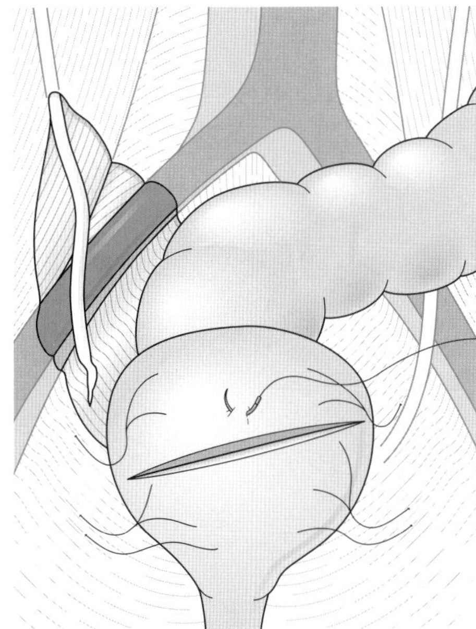

a

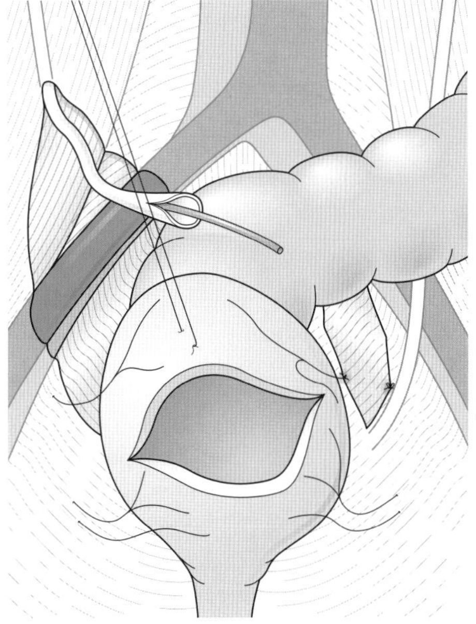

b

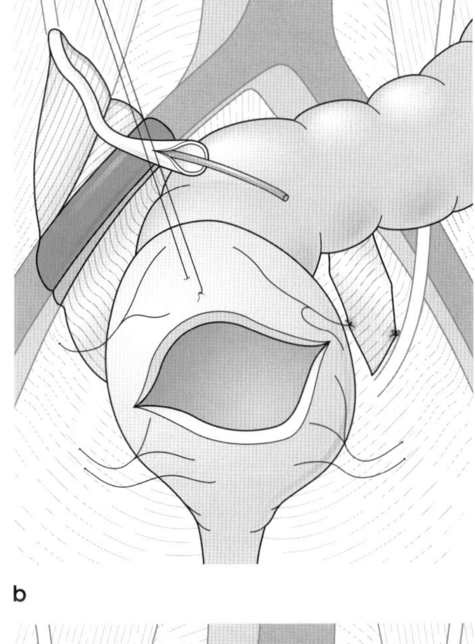

c

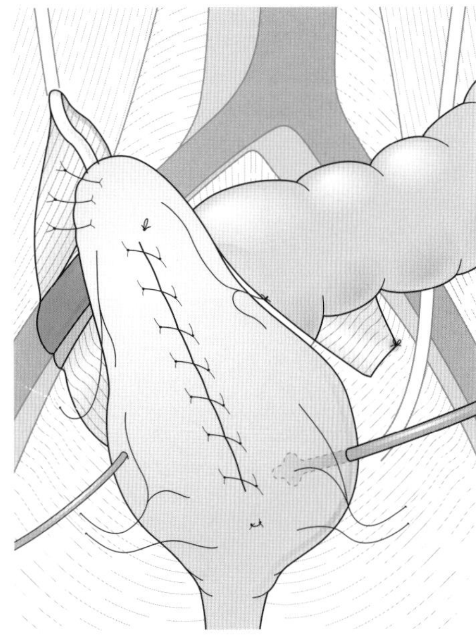

d

Figure 35.14 'Psoas hitch'.

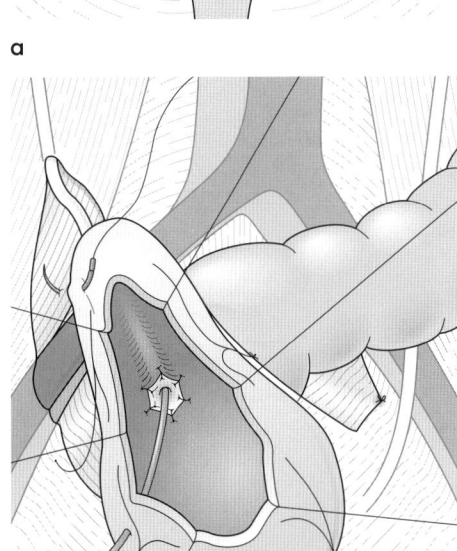

will confirm a hydronephrosis on the affected side. If both the ureters are ligated, anuria will result. In contrast, the cut ureter will lead to an extravasation of urine, forming a urinoma that may present as a swelling in the flank. A high-grade temperature indicates an infection of the urinoma. Occasionally, a watery discharge from the wound may be the only indicator of a ureteric injury. A high creatinine level in the discharge fluid will confirm the diagnosis. An intravenous injection of 10 mL of indigo carmine will turn the fluid blue if it is urine.

Investigations

An intravenous urogram will show extravasation of contrast from the injured segment. It may show a dense nephrographic phase and later a dilated pelvicalyceal system, where the ureter has been ligated. Retrograde ureteropyelogram will show the exact site of obstruction or extravasation.

Treatment

Best results following ureteric repair are seen if the injury is recognized during the operation and repaired immediately. If the injury is recognized late, proximal urinary drainage by percutaneous nephrostomy or formal nephrostomy should be considered. Proximal drainage is also a safer option if, for some reason, immediate repair is not possible. The treatment is also dictated by the location of the injury and the length of the devitalized segment of the ureter.

INJURIES OF LOWER URETER

The procedure of choice in cases of injuries to the lower third of the ureter is reimplantation of the proximal segment into the bladder, which is elongated by closing vertically a transverse incision on the dome of the bladder. The anastomosis is non-refluxing and is usually combined with 'psoas hitch' to minimize the tension at the anastomotic site (Fig. 35.14). If it is not possible to perform a ureteric implantation because of infection and inflammation, a transuretero-ureteric anastomosis may be performed.

INJURIES OF MIDURETER

Injuries of midureter usually occur following an external injury rather than being iatrogenic. These are best repaired by a primary uretero-ureteric anastomosis in a spatulated fashion (Fig. 35.15). The anastomosis is performed over a double-J stent, which can be removed in 4–6 weeks' time. If the defect is large and a primary uretero-ureterostomy is not possible, a segment from small bowel or the appendix can be interposed between the two ends. In some cases it may be possible to perform a transuretero-ureteric anastomosis (Fig. 35.16).

INJURIES TO UPPER URETER AND THE PELVIURETERIC JUNCTION

Upper ureteric injuries are best managed by a primary uretero-ureteric anastomosis. If the defect is large, bowel segment can be interposed to provide continuity. Autotransplant of the kidney is another option.

LATE RECOGNITION

Some ureteric injuries may not be recognized at the time of surgery. If they are recognized within 24 h of surgery they should be explored and repaired using a suitable reconstructive

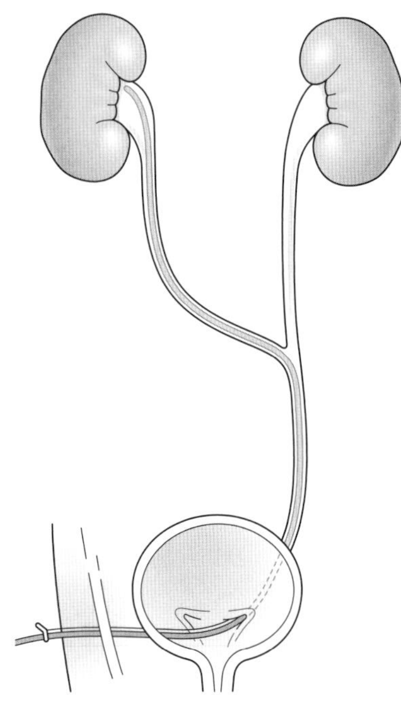

Figure 35.16 Transuretero-ureteric anastomosis.

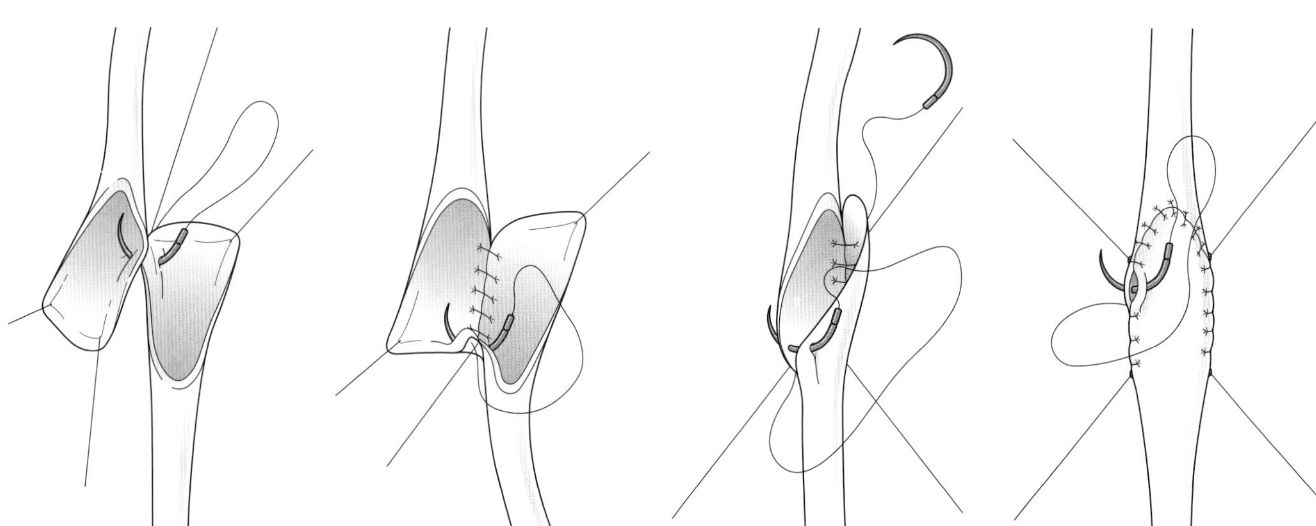

Figure 35.15 Uretero-ureteric anastomosis.

procedure (as mentioned earlier), provided that the patient's condition permits this. It is impossible to generalize about the correct timing of repair of ureteric injuries, because this depends on the underlying condition and the skill of the surgeon. If the injury is recognized late, or if the patient's condition is not stable enough for a re-exploration, a proximal urinary drainage in the form of a nephrostomy should be considered (Fig. 35.17). This is particularly true in the case of patients with a ligated ureter, where a delay can result in considerable loss of renal function. Patients in whom a fistula or urinary leak develops should have an intravenous urogram followed by a cystoscopy and ascending ureterogram to delineate the exact site of the injury. In such cases it may be possible to place a double-J stent across the injured segment. Occasionally, the fistula may heal, but generally it requires a formal reanastomosis. Ureteric strictures from ischaemia following ureteroscopic surgery may be treated by endoscopic incision or by balloon dilatation. Occasionally, when a fistula develops after pelvic radiotherapy in a patient who is unfit for surgery, symptomatic relief may be obtained by percutaneous transcatheter embolization of the affected kidney: 'radiologist's nephrectomy'. Rarely, ileal conduit urinary diversion may be the only available option in a case of massive postirradiation injury.

The prognosis for ureteric injury is excellent if the diagnosis is made early and an early exploration with suitable repair is undertaken. There are higher incidences of complications such as infection, hydronephrosis and renal damage following delay in diagnosis.

INFECTIONS OF KIDNEY AND URETERS

Infection of the renal pelvis, calyces and parenchyma due to bacteria may affect the kidney diffusely or in a patchy fashion. Extensive bacterial infection may result in renal cortical abscesses or 'carbuncles'. If the outflow of the kidney is obstructed, a pyonephrosis will develop, and if left untreated may discharge into the surrounding perirenal tissues, producing a perinephric abscess.

ACUTE PYELONEPHRITIS

Acute pyelonephritis is a bacterial infection, which in over 80% of cases is caused by *Escherichia coli.* Other organisms responsible for similar infections include *Klebsiella, Proteus, Pseudomonas,* and *Serratia.* Occasionally it may be caused by *Enterococcus* and *Staphylococcus aureus.*

Acute pyelonephritis is usually an ascending infection from the lower urinary tract.[27] The presence of vesicoureteric reflux helps in the spread of infection from the bladder to the upper tract, giving rise to pyelonephritis. Less frequently, acute pyelonephritis may occur as a result of haematogenous spread and is often associated with staphylococcal bacteraemia.

Clinical features

Patients are systemically ill, with the abrupt onset of high-grade fever and unilateral or bilateral loin pain. Lower urinary tract symptoms suggesting a urinary infection, such as dysuria, frequency and urgency, may be present. Nausea and vomiting are frequently associated. There is tachycardia and loin tenderness on examination. Occasionally there are signs of bacteraemic shock.

Investigations

Polymorphonuclear leukocytosis is usual, but renal function is rarely compromised. The urine analysis will typically show numerous leukocytes, as well as accompanying bacteria, proteins and red cells. Urine cultures are usually positive and guides the antimicrobial therapy. Blood cultures should always be taken prior to the start of antibiotic therapy, because there is a coexisting bacteraemia in up to one-third of patients.[28]

Previously, intravenous urogram used to be the standard investigation for such cases. The positive findings may include a general or focal renal enlargement due to interstitial oedema, cortical striations in the nephrogram, delay in excretion of contrast due to local vasoconstriction, and non-obstructive dilatation of the collecting system.[29] An ultrasound scan is a simple radiological tool that can help rule out an obstruction, and therefore an obstructed infected system, which is sometimes difficult to distinguish from pyelonephritis on a clinical basis. However, it is poor at demonstrating inflammation,[30] and 70% of patients with acute pyelonephritis will have normal kidneys on sonography. A CT scan and radioisotope scan have yet to prove their usefulness in such cases.

Management

On the basis of the presenting clinical picture, patients should be started on antibiotics. If there is an associated bacteraemia, intravenous antibodies (e.g. cephalosporins or aminoglycosides) are recommended for 72 h and then followed with appropriate oral antibiotics for 2 weeks. Approximately 10–30% of patients will have a relapse, and occasionally patients with recurrent episodes may require a 6-week course of a suitable antibiotic. If the pyelonephritis is secondary to a stone, the stone should be extracted once the acute inflammation has resolved. The infection may result in a renal abscess, which may require percutaneous drainage under ultrasound guidance.[31]

CHRONIC PYELONEPHRITIS

Chronic pyelonephritis refers to a small, contracted, shrunken kidney or to the coarsely scarred kidney that has been produced by bacterial infection, whether recent or remote. In contrast to acute pyelonephritis, the chronic pyelonephritis is usually diagnosed by radiological or pathological investigations.

In many patients the condition is asymptomatic and discovered incidentally. In others, it may present as a urinary tract infection or as a complication of chronic pyelonephritis, such as hypertension or renal failure.

The urinary sediments may show leukocytes, proteinuria, and rarely leukocyte casts. The characteristic feature on an intravenous urogram is a small, atrophic kidney with focal renal scarring and clubbing of the underlying calyces. The renal cortex in the affected area is especially thin. These findings may be unilateral or bilateral. A voiding cystourethrogram is useful, particularly in children, to show vesicoureteral reflux, which may be associated with focal renal scarring when it is referred to as reflux nephropathy.

REFERENCES

27. Mitsumori K et al. J Urol 1997; 158: 2329
28. Behr MA et al. Am J Med 1996; 101: 277
29. Teplick JG et al. Clin Radiol 1978; 30: 59
30. Talner LB, Davidson AJ, Lebowitz RL. Radiology 1994; 192: 297
31. Fernandez JA, Miles BJ, Buck AS. Urology 1985; 25: 142

The renal damage incurred by chronic pyelonephritis is, unfortunately, irreversible. However, identifying and correcting the structural abnormalities that are responsible for the recurrent infections can limit the damage. The infection can be checked by using suitable antibiotics or, in some cases, low-dose antibiotics on a long-term basis. Rarely, a partial polar nephrectomy may be required. In patients with unilateral renal atrophy and renin-mediated hypertension, nephrectomy is an option.

PERINEPHRIC ABSCESS

An abscess in the perinephric region is usually contained within the Gerota's fascia, and can result from an extension of a renal abscess or from a distant source via the haematogenous route. It presents with high-grade fever, flank pain and lower urinary tract symptoms. The patient may experience a pleuritic type of chest pain, with irritation of the diaphragm. A flank mass and an associated skin erythema may be present in about half of the patients.[32] There may be an associated reactive pleural effusion.

Blood tests would show raised inflammatory markers. Urinalysis is normal in up to 25% of cases. Urine culture is positive in only one-third of patients, and blood culture in about 40%. A CT scan is the most helpful imaging tool; however, percutaneous aspiration of the pus under CT or ultrasound guidance provides the definitive diagnosis.

Antibiotic therapy along with percutaneous drainage of the abscess is the treatment of choice.

PYONEPHROSIS

Pyonephrosis results from an infection in an obstructed and hydronephrotic kidney. There is a rapid destruction of renal parenchyma and loss of renal function. The resulting sepsis may be life-threatening.

The patient is usually very ill, with high-grade fever, chills, flank pain and tenderness. A previous history of urinary stones, infections or surgery is common. However, a non-specific picture of loss of weight and few clinical signs can be seen, and here the diagnosis of pyonephrosis can be delayed unless considered at an early stage.

Urinalysis is normal in cases of complete obstruction. Ultrasound is the most useful procedure to diagnose pyonephrosis.

Rapid treatment of pyonephrosis is essential and includes early drainage combined with appropriate antibiotics (Fig. 35.17).

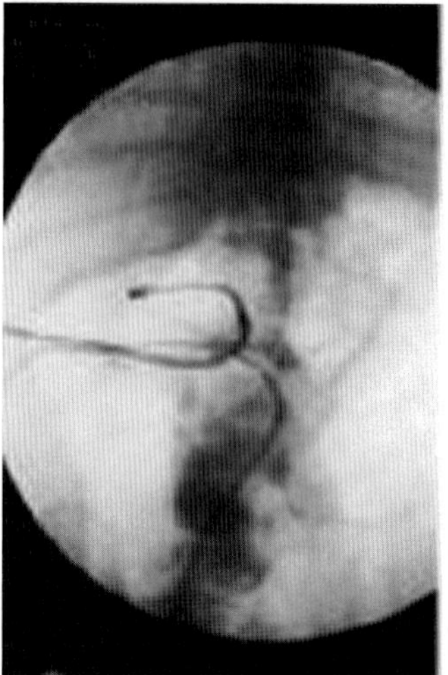
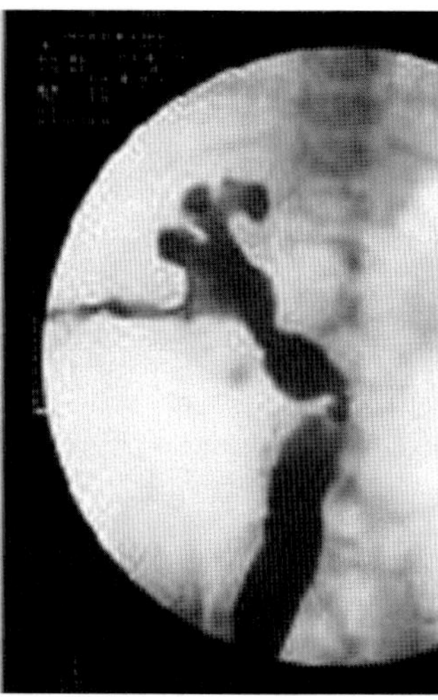

Figure 35.17 Percutaneous nephrostomy.

XANTHOGRANULOMATOUS PYELONEPHRITIS

Xanthogranulomatous pyelonephritis is an extremely rare condition, which is usually associated with stone disease.[33] Its importance lies in differentiating the mass it forms from a renal tumour.

It is usually seen in association with a *Proteus* urinary infection in the presence of renal stones. The renal stone causes urinary obstruction and infection, resulting in accumulation of macrophages called *xanthoma cells*, which eventually obliterate the renal parenchyma. The xanthoma cells may be confused with those seen in the renal clear cell carcinoma. The inflammatory process can spread beyond the kidney. It may present as flank pain, fever and a palpable renal mass.

The intravenous urogram shows a non-functioning kidney and the presence of stones. On ultrasound or CT examination it may be very difficult to differentiate this condition from a renal tumour.

Nephrectomy is usually required; however, it may be difficult because of the extent of the inflammatory process and associated fibrosis.

TUBERCULOSIS

Genitourinary tuberculosis occurs via the haematogenous route, the primary site usually remaining unrecognized and asymptomatic. The incidence of genitourinary tuberculosis has shown a notable decline in the past two decades. However, the condition remains a serious problem in developing countries and in immigrants to the UK from these countries, and in recent years strains resistant to standard treatment have emerged, along with a significant incidence of tuberculosis in immunosuppressed patients.

Management

Most patients can be treated as outpatients. Short-course chemotherapy lasting 4–6 months is particularly applicable in the management of genitourinary tuberculosis, because high concentrations of antituberculous drugs are excreted in the urine. The main aim of treatment is to preserve renal parenchyma and function, as well as to render the patient non-infectious. Standard treatment is rifampicin, isoniazid, pyrazinamide plus ethambutol for 2 months, then rifampicin plus isoniazid for another 4 months, unless resistance to rifampicin or isoniazid exists. Follow-up involves culture and sensitivity reports, and the regimen is changed if necessary. In HIV-positive patients treatment should be continued for a total of 9 months. Severe bladder symptoms and involvement of the pelvicalyceal system, resulting in stricture formation, are indications for prescribing steroids. High-dose prednisone for 4–6 weeks is recommended, because rifampicin reduces the effectiveness and bioavailability of prednisone by 66%.

Although chemotherapy is the mainstay of treatment, surgical intervention, either ablation or reconstruction, is often required. As a general rule, if immediate surgery is not necessary at least 4–6 weeks of prior chemotherapy with appropriate agents is instituted. Renal function may be preserved in the presence of upper tract obstruction by the insertion of a double-J silicone

REFERENCES

32. Saiki J, Vazira ND, Barton C. West J Med 1982; 136: 95
33. Parsons MA et al. Diagn Histopathol 1983; 6: 203

stent, although frequently this is poorly tolerated because of the associated bladder symptoms. Surgery often consists of nephrectomy for the non-functioning kidney. For extensive disease involving the whole of the kidney and ureter, nephroureterectomy is advisable. Reconstructive surgery, including ureteric replacement, urinary diversion or bladder augmentation, may be required.

OTHER INFECTIONS

Schistosomiasis or bilharzial infection primarily affects the bladder and ureter, causing strictures of the ureter and a small contracted bladder. Effective treatment to control the disease and prevent its complications is by using praziquantel, metrifonate or oxamniquine. The ureteric scarring may produce obstruction and reflux, and reimplantation of the ureter may be required. In cases of severely contracted bladders, a bladder augmentation may be carried out. Treatment of squamous cell carcinoma resulting from schistosomiasis is discussed elsewhere.

Filariasis caused by *Wuchereria bancrofti* affects the lymphatics, resulting in inflammation, which obstructs the lymphatics. There is generally a history of a systemic illness, malaise, fever, rigors and pain, especially in the groin. On examination, there is tenderness and swelling of the affected lymph nodes. It may be associated with giant hydroceles. Diethylcarbamazine is the drug of choice. The lymphatic obstruction may result in a fistulous connection between the pelvicalyceal system and the lymphatics. This results in chyluria. Intravenous urography is performed to define the anatomy. A retrograde ureteropyelogram or a lymphangiogram may identify the renolymphatic connections. Approximately 50% of cases with chyluria require no treatment and there is spontaneous remission. The fistulous channels may be sealed off by using 2% silver nitrate. In persistent cases, renal decapsulation and resection of renal lymphatics may be required.

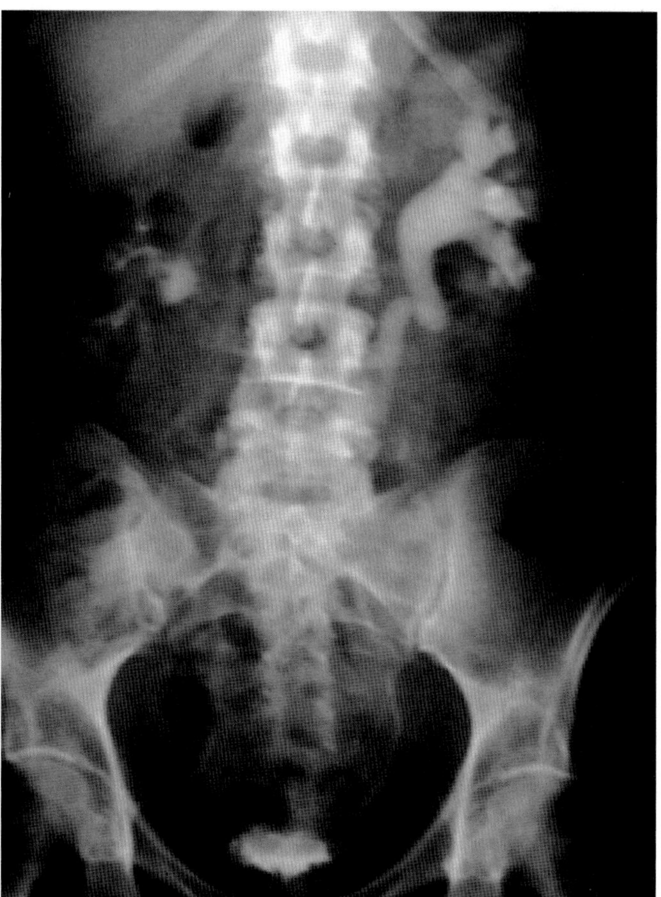

Figure 35.18 Left hydronephrosis.

UPPER URINARY TRACT OBSTRUCTION

Upper urinary tract obstruction may result from obstruction to the ureter, which may arise from lesions outside the ureter, for example tumours (cervical carcinoma); problems arising within the ureteric wall, such as strictures and pelviureteric junction obstruction; or within the ureteric lumen, for example back-pressure from the bladder in chronic retention or severe detrusor overactivity associated with neurogenic disease, and the presence of ureteric stones. The obstruction may be complete or incomplete. It results in dilatation of the pelvicalyceal system. Untreated upper urinary tract obstruction, whether complete or incomplete, will eventually destroy renal function. The resulting hydronephrosis (Fig. 35.18) is graded as follows:

- Grade 0: normal kidney with no hydronephrosis.
- Grade 1: slightly dilated renal pelvis without caliectasis.
- Grade 2: moderately dilated pelvis with mild caliectasis.
- Grade 3: large renal pelvis, dilated calyces, and normal renal parenchyma.
- Grade 4: very large renal pelvis, large dilated calyces, with thinning of the renal parenchyma.

PATHOPHYSIOLOGY

Secondary to back-pressure resulting from reflux or from obstruction, the ureteral musculature thickens in its attempt to push the urine down; this is commonly referred to as the stage of compensation. There is increased peristaltic activity accompanied by elongation and some tortuosity of the ureter. With continuing obstruction, periureteral fibrous bands develop, which result in further angulation of ureter, causing secondary ureteral obstruction. In such cases, relieving the obstruction from below may not prevent progressive damage to the kidney due to the presence of secondary obstruction. This is followed by the stage of decompensation, when the ureteric muscle loses contractile power.

The pressure within the renal pelvis is normally close to zero. As a result of obstruction this pressure rises and results in dilatation of renal pelvis and calyces. Proximal obstruction and presence of an intrarenal pelvis favour the early development of hydronephrosis. The renal pelvic muscle undergoes changes similar to those in ureter, showing stages of compensation and decompensation. The changes in the calyces mark the initiation of hydronephrosis. A normal calyx is sharp and concave, due to projection of renal papilla into it. The calyces become blunt and later on 'clubbed' with raised intrapelvic pressure. Persistently high intrapelvic pressure results in ischaemic atrophy of renal parenchyma. Unlike other organs of the body, kidneys continue to form urine despite complete obstruction. The secreted fluid exits the renal pelvis by:

- pyelolymphatic back-flow with low pressures;
- pyelovenous back-flow with higher pressures; and
- pyelointerstitial back-flow resulting from extravasation into the perirenal spaces.

Recovery of renal function may occur after up to 4 weeks of complete obstruction, as shown by experimental studies. It is difficult to determine the extent of recovery following incomplete obstruction. Percutaneous drainage via a nephrostomy tube, followed by a DMSA scan, provides the best form of assessment of renal function.

PELVIURETERIC JUNCTION OBSTRUCTION

Pelviureteric junction obstruction can be congenital or acquired. It is probably the most common congenital abnormality of the ureter. Congenital pelviureteric junction is more common in boys than in girls, with a ratio of 5:1. In 10–15% of cases the obstruction is bilateral.

Congenital pelviureteric junction obstruction is mostly the result of an intrinsic disorder. Frequently, there is a segment of aperistaltic ureter at the junction that results in failure of the normal peristaltic waves to progress from renal pelvis to the ureter.[34] This segment, despite being of normal calibre, causes a functional obstruction. Less commonly, there is a true stricture at the site, which results from an excessive collagen deposition.

The most important extrinsic cause resulting in a pelviureteric junction obstruction is an aberrant renal artery. As the pelvis fills, the upper part of the ureter becomes kinked and obstructed by the aberrant vessels, while the renal pelvis balloons up in its anterior wall. Besides this, a high insertion of the ureter into the renal pelvis may cause kinking of the ureter just below the pelviureteric junction, resulting in dilatation of the renal pelvis. The persistence of fetal ureteric folds is a rare cause of obstruction.

Pelviureteric junction obstruction may be secondary to a peripelvic cyst or a retroperitoneal tumour. Other causes include trauma, surgery and infection, such as tuberculosis.

Clinical features

Fetal hydronephrosis is the most commonly diagnosed antenatal abnormality on ultrasound. In children, pelviureteric junction obstruction may be a cause of failure to thrive, especially if associated with recurrent urinary infections. It may present as an abdominal mass, with or without pain. The pain may develop or worsen after consumption of alcohol (Dietl's crisis). A bilateral obstruction may result in renal failure. Patients may also present with infection or septicaemia due to the development of a pyonephrosis. However, many cases are discovered incidentally during the development of an investigation of other symptoms.

Investigations

Ultrasound may be used to differentiate a hydronephrotic kidney from a Wilms' tumour or neuroblastoma in children. In adults the diagnosis is often obvious on the intravenous urogram. However, confirmation must be sought with the help of radioisotope studies, e.g. an F-15 MAG3 renogram (this involves the administration of furesemide 15 min prior to the renogram). Rarely, Whitaker's test[35] involving a pressure flow study is necessary to establish the diagnosis beyond all doubt.

The intravenous urogram often shows characteristic appearances:

- delayed excretion of contrast, resulting in a dense nephrogram (Fig. 35.19);
- hydronephrosis of the affected side (Fig. 35.20); and
- ureter either not visualized or of normal calibre.

In some patients the symptoms can be intermittent, and an intravenous urogram performed in between the painful episodes may not show any abnormality. In such patients, provocation of the obstruction by intravenous administration of 40 mg of furosemide (frusemide) may produce the characteristic radiological findings.[36]

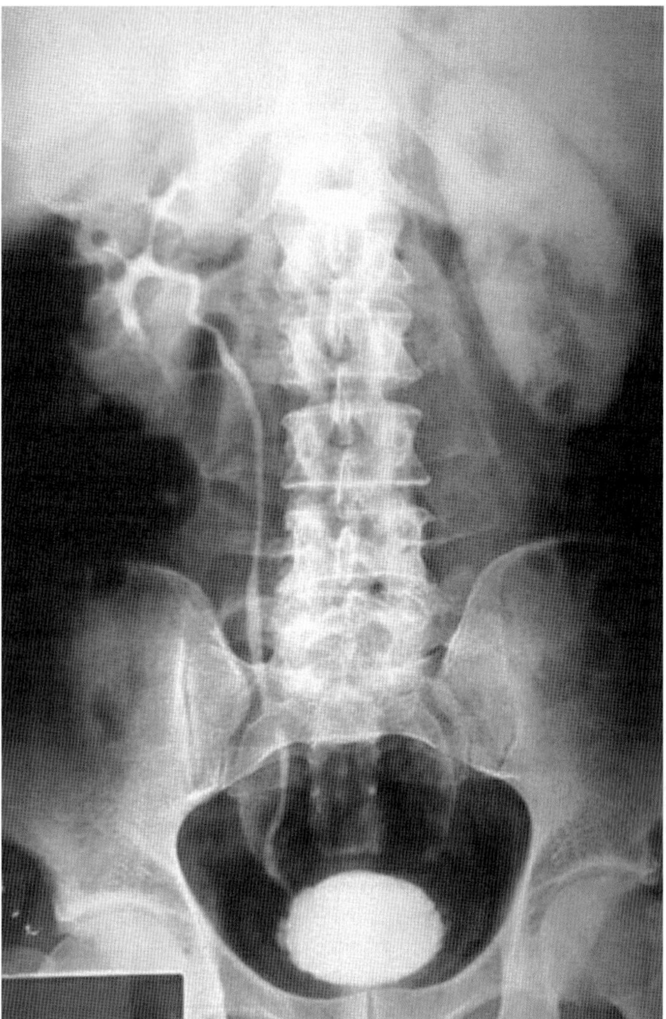

Figure 35.19 Dense nephrogram on the left side.

Radioisotope studies should be used to confirm pelviureteric junction obstruction and to assess the differential renal function (Figs 35.21 and 35.22). A retrograde ureterogram may be required to define the ureteric anatomy (Fig. 35.23), especially if a reconstruction is planned, and should always be performed in the older patients, newly diagnosed, to distinguish other pathology in the ureter that is mimicking pelviureteric junction obstruction.

Indications of intervention include:

- presence of symptoms;
- impairment of renal function; and
- development of complications, such as stones or infection.

If the contribution to overall renal function is 15% or more, corrective surgery is indicated, whereas below these levels nephrectomy may be the most appropriate option. Asymptomatic cases with preserved renal functions can be followed up with periodic DMSA scans. About 25% of such patients will eventually require intervention in due course.

REFERENCES

34. Hanna MK et al. J Urol 1976; 116: 718–725
35. Whitaker RH. Br J Urol 1973; 45: 15
36. Malek RS. J Urol 1983; 130: 863

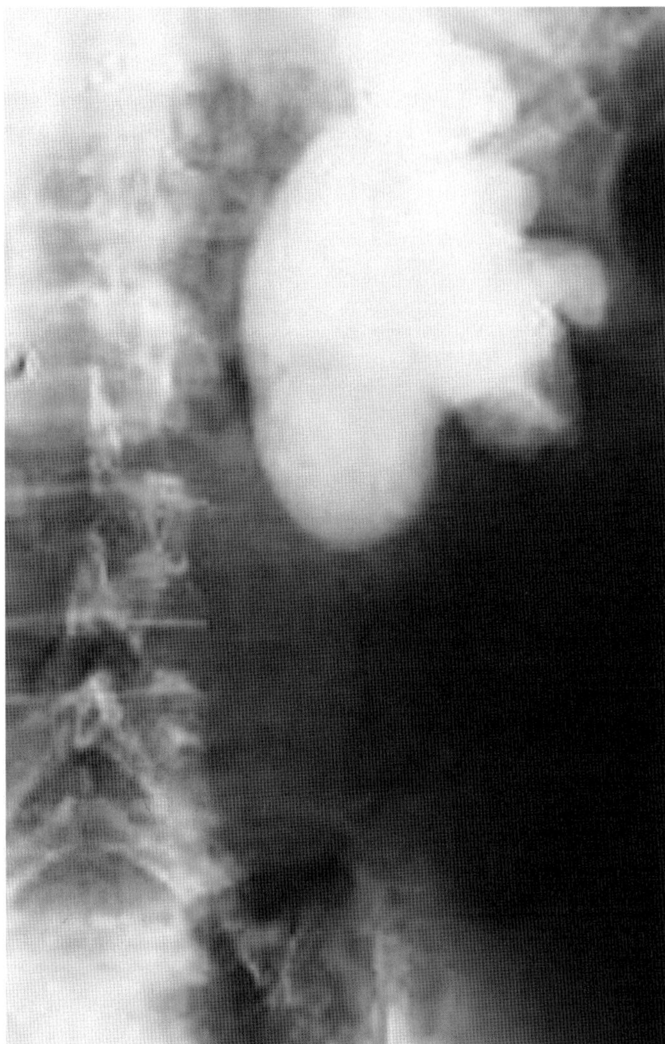

Figure 35.20 Hydronephrosis.

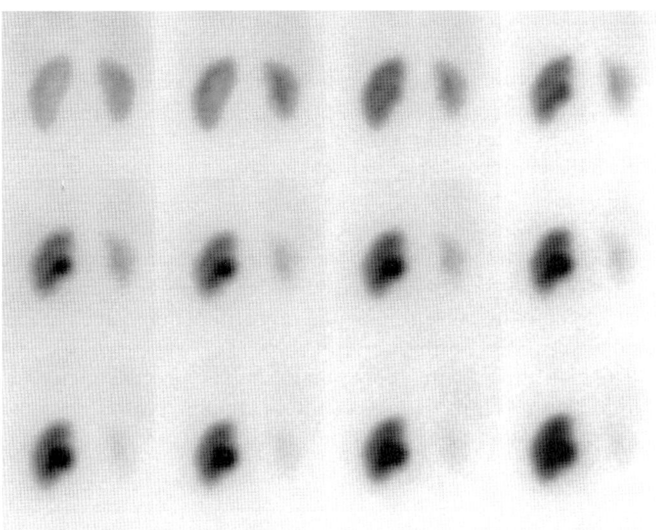

Figure 35.21 Renogram showing obstruction on the right side.

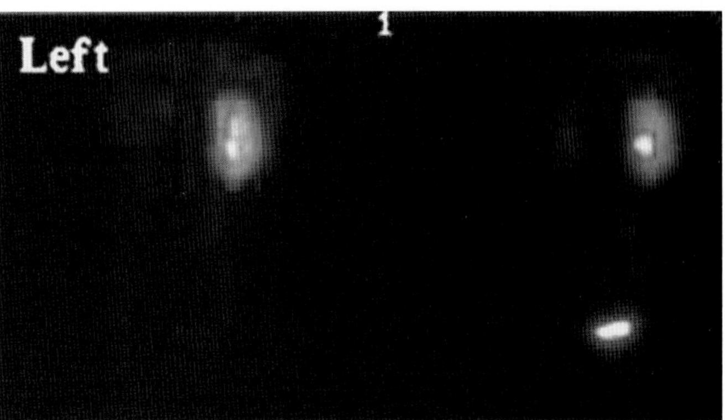

Figure 35.22 Right pelviureteric junction obstruction.

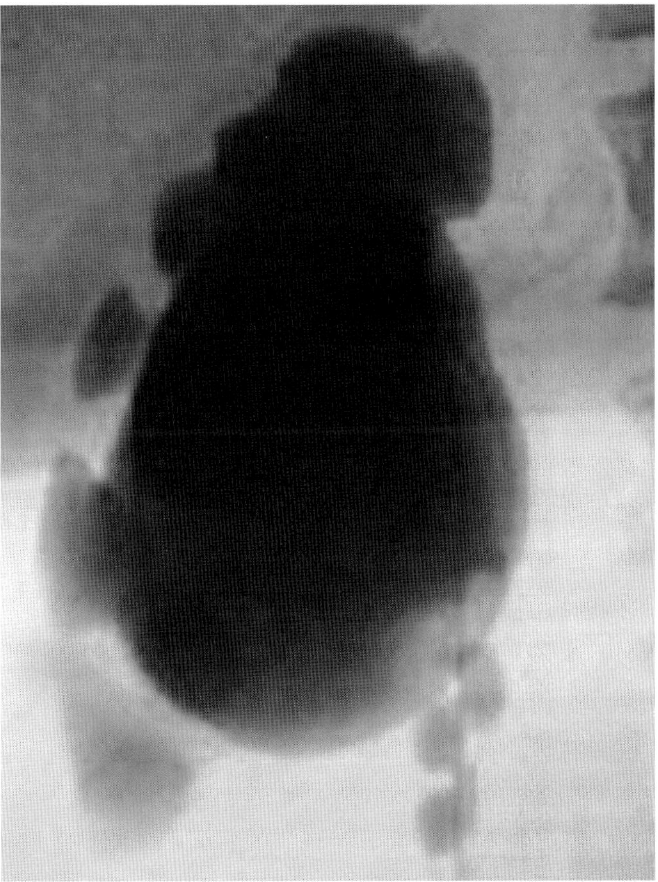

Figure 35.23 Retrograde ureteropyelogram.

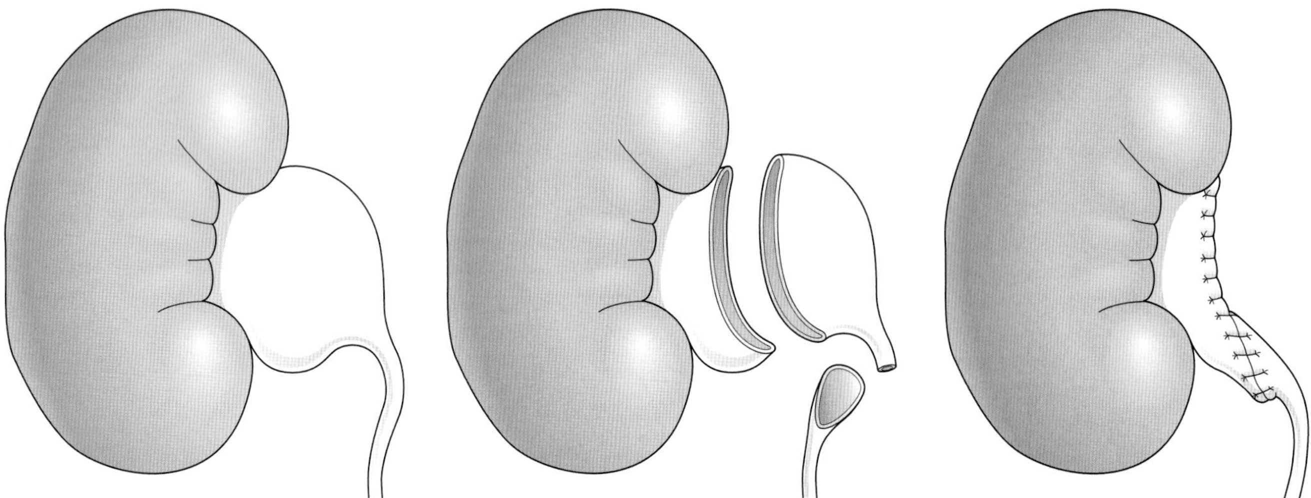

Figure 35.24 Dismembered pyeloplasty.

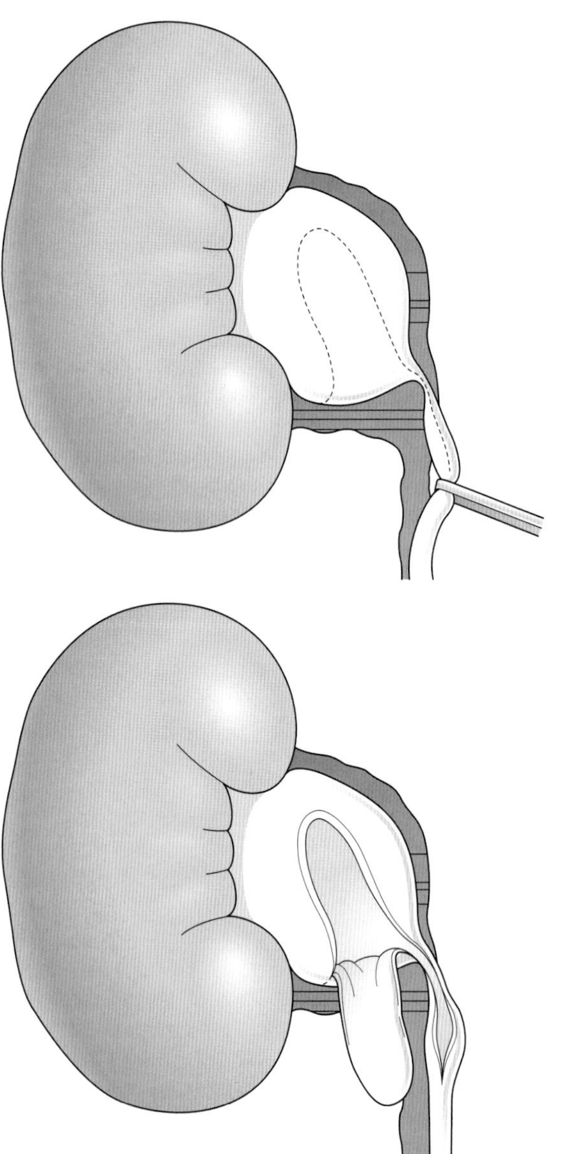

Figure 35.25 Culp–DeWeerd flap pyeloplasty.

Treatment

The overall aim of treatment is to relieve the symptoms and preserve renal function. In neonates, infants and children an early repair is desirable. The procedure of choice is traditionally an open repair, referred to as a pyeloplasty. Open pyeloplasty can be classified as dismembered and non-dismembered. The dismembered pyeloplasty[37] can be employed regardless of the anatomy of the pelviureteric junction (Fig. 35.24). The aims of dismembered pyeloplasty are:

- Removal of the dyskinetic segment.
- Reduction of redundant pelvis.
- Straightening of a lengthy and tortuous proximal ureter.
- Making the pelviureteric junction dependent.
- Proper repositioning of the pelviureteric junction; this can be carried out in the presence of an aberrant renal artery that may be contributing to the obstruction.

To carry out a dismembered pyeloplasty, the pelviureteric junction is exposed properly and the abnormal segment is excised. The proximal ureter is spatulated laterally, and this spatulated ureter is anastomosed to the pelvis over a stent, using non-absorbable sutures. The stent can be removed in 4–6 weeks' time. If the pelvis is large and redundant, a reduction pyeloplasty can be performed. In cases where there is an aberrant renal vessel contributing to the obstruction, the anastomosis can be repositioned to minimize this.

Non-dismembered pyeloplasty implies that the abnormal segment stays and the pelviureteric junction is made wider. A vertical (Scardino–Prince)[38] or a spiral flap (Culp–DeWeerd; Fig. 35.25)[39] can be taken from the pelvis and rotated down on to the pelviureteric junction to make it wider. This may be an option in cases where the pelviureteric junction is dependent and/or the vascular supply is compromised.

The pelviureteric junction repair can be carried out endoscopically using either a percutaneous technique or ureteroscopy. An endopyelotomy can be performed endoscopically. Alterna-

REFERENCES

37. Anderson JC. Hydronephrosis. Heinemann, Oxford, 1963
38. Scardino PL, Prince CL. South Med J 1953; 46: 325
39. Culp OS, DeWeerd JH. Mayo Clin Proc 1951; 26: 483

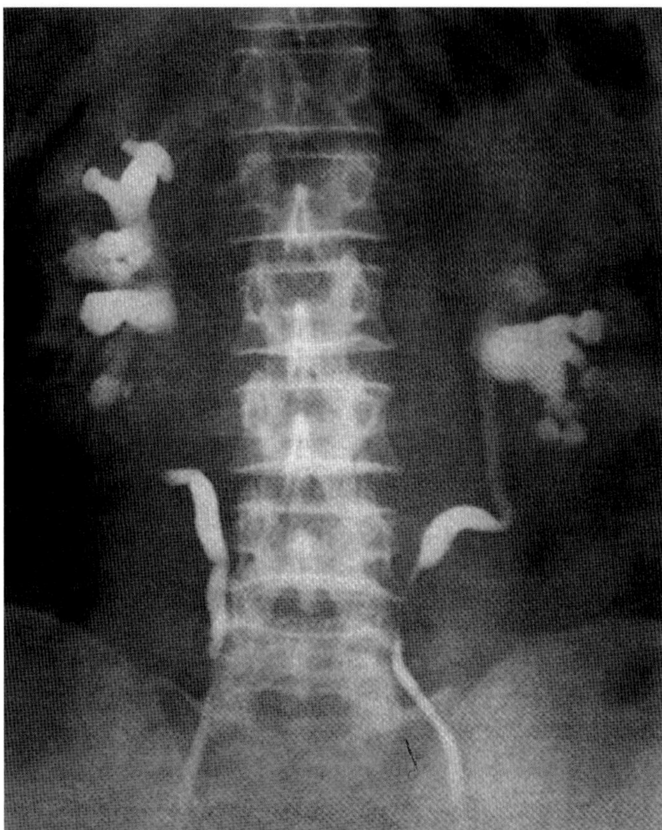

Figure 35.26 Retroperitoneal fibrosis. The ureters are drawn together by the fibrosis and there is obstruction of the upper ureter and pelvis on each side.

tively a balloon dilatation can be carried out under fluoroscopic control. Endopyelotomy dilatation has a success rate of around 80%[40] as compared with 98% with open pyeloplasty.[41] Laparoscopic pyeloplasty is a recent and promising development.

Nephrectomy is sometimes required if the kidney has no function or if there is an extensive stone disease with significant loss of function. Asymptomatic patients with a non-functioning, hydronephrotic kidney should be offered a nephrectomy, because there is a risk of pyonephrosis.

RETROPERITONEAL FIBROSIS

The ureters may be obstructed by a chronic inflammatory process affecting the retroperitoneum, usually in the region of the lower lumbar vertebrae (Fig. 35.26). It may result from malignancy (primary or secondary) affecting lymph nodes or lymphatics, an aortic aneurysm[42] or inflammatory bowel disease,[43] or it may be associated with drug therapy, classically methysergide.

Many patients have no symptoms, and the condition is diagnosed incidentally. Some patients present with non-specific symptoms of malaise, fever, weight loss, anorexia and nausea, and many complain of poorly localized backache. Occasionally patients may present with renal failure.

A raised erythrocyte sedimentation rate is invariable, and anaemia is frequently noted. Medial deviation of one or both ureters with proximal dilatation is characteristic on an intravenous urogram. A retrograde pyelogram may be required to better define the anatomy if the intravenous urogram fails to show the typical features. The diagnosis can be confirmed by CT or MRI scan, which may show related pathology as well.[44]

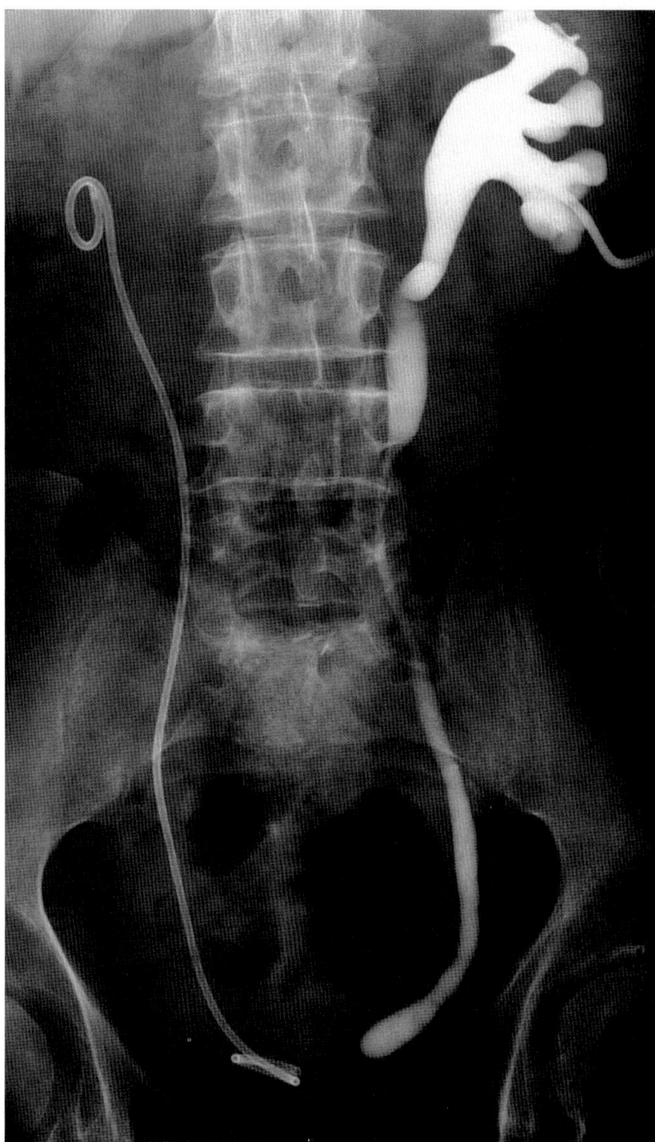

Figure 35.27 Double-J stenting of an obstructed system on the right, note the nephrostomy tube on the left, with a nephrostogram showing obstruction of the ureter at the vesico-ureteric junction.

Management

The best way of managing the renal failure is by draining the kidneys by either double-J stenting (Fig. 35.27) or a percutaneous nephrostomy. Once the renal function has stabilized, formal treatment can be planned, provided the kidney is salvageable. In most cases steroids should be tried as the initial therapy.[45] Failing a response to this, some will require formal surgical dissection of the fibrous plaque with an omental wrap.[46]

REFERENCES

40. Aslan P, Preminger GM. Urol Clin North Am 1998; 25: 295
41. Bogaert GA et al. J Urol 1996; 156: 734
42. Brock J, Soloway MS. Urology 1980; 15: 14
43. Siminovitch JM, Fazio VW. Am J Surg 1980; 139: 95
44. Hricak H, Higgins CB, Williams RD. Am J Roentgenol 1983; 141: 35
45. Moody TE, Vaughan ED. J Urol 1979; 121: 109
46. Lepor H, Walsh PC. J Urol 1979; 122: 1

RETROCAVAL URETER

Persistence of the posterior cardinal vein, to form the inferior vena cava below the level of the renal vein, results in the ureter passing behind the vena cava before running distally. The finding of a retrocaval ureter is often incidental, but occasionally it causes loin pain and tenderness. The reverse J pattern on intravenous urography is characteristic. In the majority of patients no treatment is necessary, but in those who develop pain a reanastomosis of the ureter in front of the vena cava may be required.

VESICOURETERIC REFLUX IN ADULTS

The condition occurs as a result of malfunction of the physiological valve at the vesicoureteric junction, and it may be primary (i.e. congenital) or secondary. Secondary vesicoureteric reflux occurs in the presence of obstruction to the bladder neck, prostate or urethra, but may also occur after certain surgical operations, such as transurethral resection of the prostate or bladder tumour, or ureteric meatotomy for stone or ureterocele. It may also occur after radiotherapy and other conditions causing an inflammatory reaction in the bladder, such as urinary infection, tuberculosis, bilharzia, interstitial cystitis and stones. It is also a complication of the neuropathic bladder.

Clinical features

The condition most commonly presents with recurrent urinary infections or loin pain. There may also be a history of infection in childhood. Hypertension, renal failure or incidental proteinuria are less common presentations.

Investigations

The midstream urine specimen may show evidence of infection. Intravenous urography demonstrates a variety of changes from normal (in approximately one-third of patients) to a non-functioning kidney. There may be features of chronic pyelonephritis with blunting of the calyces, cortical scarring or atrophy. A micturating cystourethrogram is diagnostic, showing contrast refluxing up into one or both kidneys (Fig. 35.28). At cystoscopy the ureteric orifice may be laterally placed and widely open. Assessment of renal function by urea and creatinine estimation, and a renal isotope scan to determine the differential renal function and the presence of scarring, are also usually necessary.

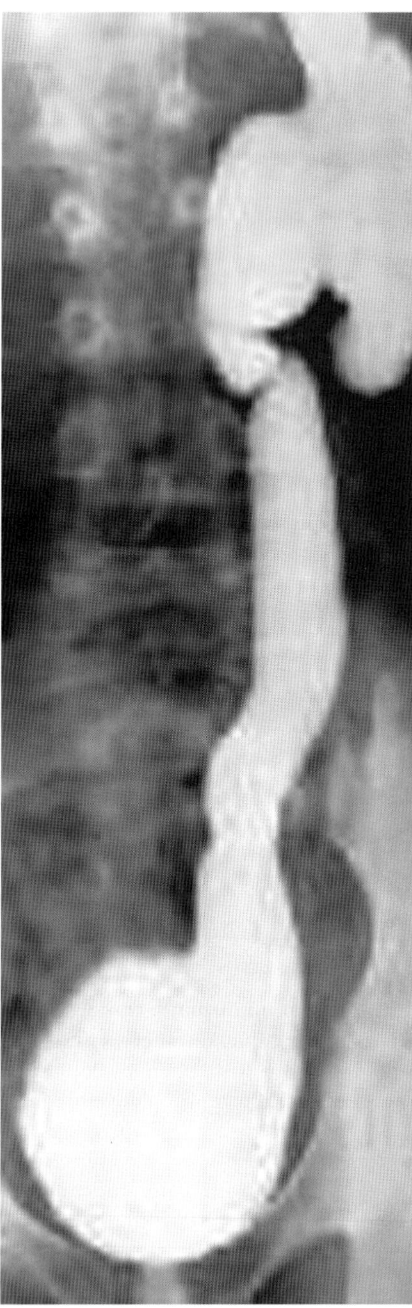

Figure 35.28 Marked left vesicoureteric reflux.

Management

The long-term effects of primary vesicoureteric reflux in adults are unknown. This is in contrast to vesicoureteric reflux in children, where the condition is self-correcting before puberty in 80% of patients. Low-dose prophylactic antibiotics are advised in patients with primary reflux and recurrent urinary infections in whom there is no evidence of renal damage. Ureteric reimplantation should be reserved until there is objective evidence of deterioration of the upper tract.

In most cases where recurrent urinary infections occur, antibiotic prophylaxis is sufficient and it is rarely necessary to carry out ureteric reimplantation. An endoscopic submucosal injection of a bulking agent may prevent reflux in children, with good medium-term results at 4–10 years.

STONE DISEASE

Urinary calculi are one of the common urinary tract afflictions, second only to infection and pathology related to the prostate. They are four times more common in men than in women. In children, however, this ratio is more or less in unity. Stone recurrence rates can be as high as 50% within 5 years. Despite being a common problem, the aetiology of urinary stones remains largely speculative in the majority of cases.

AETIOLOGY AND PATHOGENESIS OF STONES

Urinary stone formation is a multifactorial process, which is affected by genetic factors, environment, hydration status, diet and metabolic variations. The hypothesis behind formation of stone suggests that it occurs in three steps:

1. Crystal formation.
2. Growth of the crystal.
3. Aggregation of similar crystals to form the stone.

The pathogenesis of uric acid, cystine and magnesium ammonium phosphate (struvite) can be explained, to some extent, on the basis of supersaturation and crystallization. If predominantly acidic urine becomes oversaturated with either cystine or uric acid, these substances will precipitate and form stones. Similarly, in urinary infections with organisms having the urea-splitting enzyme (e.g. *Proteus* and *Klebsiella*), urea is split into ammonia in an alkaline pH, and when the product of concentration of ammonium, magnesium and calcium phosphate exceeds the saturation product, struvite stones are formed. Xanthine calculi are the result of hereditary xanthinuria and are extremely rare.

However, supersaturation alone is not sufficient to explain stone formation, because it may result in crystal formation but not necessarily in crystal growth, which is believed to be linked to a deficiency of crystal-inhibiting factors. These inhibitors can be organic (peptide inhibitor[47] and nephrocalcin[48]) or inorganic (urinary citrate[49]). Matrix is the non-crystalline protein part of the urinary stone, which is thought to be a beneficial inhibitor of stone formation. However, on undergoing a qualitative change, it may *promote* stone formation.

Crystals and foreign bodies present in the urine may act as a nidus for crystal formation, as suggested by the 'nucleation theory'.

Normal urine is not a static solution. While nucleation and aggregation occur rapidly, crystal growth takes longer. Stagnant urine predisposes to infection and precipitation of triple phosphate crystals. When the drainage of the kidney is impaired by congenital abnormalities such as horseshoe kidney, medullary sponge kidney, pelviureteric junction obstruction or megaureter, then the resultant sluggish or stagnant urine facilitates crystal formation. Once formed, the crystal can then grow, adding layers of crystals that are not necessarily of the same type to form a calculus. The varieties of urinary stones are listed here.

Calcium oxalate

Calcium is a major cation present in urinary crystals. Many patients with calcium oxalate stones show no abnormality of calcium metabolism. In those patients in whom an abnormality is present, this is usually hypercalciuria, which may be dietary, absorptive, resorptive or tubular in origin. The absorption of calcium is increased by high dietary phosphorus, sugars and animal protein intake, and is reduced by phytate and high dietary fibre. Reduction in dietary calcium alone, however, offers no benefit in reducing the risk of recurrent stone formation. Normally 98–99% of filtered calcium is reabsorbed in the renal tubules. Resorptive hypercalciuria occurs when the renal tubules fail to reabsorb the filtered calcium. Resorptive hypercalciuria may also occur in patients who are immobilized for a long time, when there is an increased mobilization of calcium resulting in a higher calcium load on the tubules. A higher load may also occur in conditions such as osteoporosis, hyperparathyroidism, bony metastasis and multiple myeloma, where there is a higher bone turnover. There is a high fasting urinary calcium:creatinine ratio, urinary hydroxyproline excretion is elevated, and the serum calcium is raised.

Urinary oxalate is now considered to be at least 10 times more important in calcium lithiasis than either calcium or phosphate. Hyperoxaluria is seen in 20–30% of patients with stone disease. An increase in the dietary oxalates is the main culprit in hyperoxaluria and calcium lithiasis, and diet regulation is the key to reducing the risk of recurrent stone formation. Primary hyperoxaluria occurs as an autosomal recessive genetic disorder in which glyoxalase or hydroxypyruvate fails to metabolize oxalates. Renal failure develops early in the disease and is associated with a poor prognosis. More commonly, however, hyperoxaluria is the result of extensive small bowel resection or malabsorption syndromes and is the reason for the association of urinary calculi with Crohn's disease.

An increased uric acid excretion is important, because this inhibits the production of acid mucopolysaccharides and thus increases the overall tendency to crystal formation. Additionally, it may form a nidus for calcium oxalate stones.

Hyperparathyroidism is present in 2–3% of calcium stone formers. The increased production of parathyroid hormone results in an increased intestinal calcium absorption. This may lead to an increased secondary hyperoxaluria. With hyperparathyroidism, there is an increased excretion of bicarbonate by the kidney, and therefore the urinary pH is high.

Renal tubular acidosis results in an inability to excrete acid urine. It is the type I (distal) disorder that is associated more commonly with stone disease. The failure to secrete hydrogen ions by the distal tubule is compensated by an increased secretion of potassium, sodium and calcium. The body conserves sodium via the aldosterone mechanism, resulting in hypercalciuria. This results in the formation of calcium phosphate stones. These patients fail to produce a urinary pH lower than 5.3 in response to an acid load.

Triple phosphate stones

Urinary infection with a urea-splitting organism (usually *Proteus*) produces an alkaline urine that increases the precipitation of calcium phosphate and magnesium ammonium phosphate. Precipitation is further increased by the high ammonium concentration in the urine. The concentration of citrate and pyrophosphate, which is a potent inhibitor of calcium phosphate crystallization, is low.

Uric acid stones

The incidence of uric acid stones is increasing. The majority are idiopathic and occur in patients who do not have elevated plasma uric acids, although they do have a persistently acidic urine. A quarter of all patients with gout develop urate stones, as do 40% of patients with myeloproliferative disorders. The urinary excretion of uric acid is high, and there is an associated low urinary pH and acid mucopolysaccharide concentration.

Cystine stones

Cystine stones occur as a result of an autosomal recessive disorder in which there is a defect in the tubular reabsorption of cystine, lysine, arginine and ornithine. The solubility of cystine is doubled at a pH of 7.8.

CLINICAL FEATURES

Stone disease may be symptomless, the presence of stone being an incidental finding during the investigation of some other symptom; alternatively, it may present as an emergency with acute ureteric colic. Between these two extremes there may be varying degrees of pain, haematuria, urinary infection and renal failure.

REFERENCES

47. Howard JE, Thomas WC, Barker LM et al. Johns Hopkins Med J 1967; 120: 119
48. Nakagawa Y, Ahmed MA, Hall SL. J Clin Invest 1987; 79: 1782
49. Thomas WC. Md Med. J 1988; 37: 861

The severity and amount of pain associated with stones depend on their size, position and mobility. Thus, paradoxically, a small mobile stone may produce more symptoms than a large immobile staghorn calculus. Other features that influence symptoms are urinary tract obstruction and urinary infection. There may be a history of previous stone disease, urinary infection, or a family history of stones. The patient's dietary habits should be elucidated, especially with regard to intake of animal protein and calcium-containing foods such as milk and alkalis. There may also be a history of other illnesses, such as osteoporosis or a recent prolonged period of recumbency.

If a stone gets impacted at the neck of a calyx, at the pelviureteric junction or in the ureter, it may produce a hydrocalycosis, hydronephrosis or hydroureter, which may get infected, resulting in pyonephrosis. Xanthogranulomatous pyelonephritis is an important sequela of renal stones, which can present as a loin mass and may be mistaken for carcinoma.

Rarely, a patient with bilateral ureteric obstruction may present with renal failure

EXAMINATION

In acute ureteric colic, the patient is often unable to lie still and may be vomiting. Tenderness in the renal angle may be elicited. Fever, hypotension and cutaneous vasodilatation may be apparent in cases of urosepsis. Such cases need immediate attention, with resuscitation and decompression of the obstructed system. The urine should always be tested to determine the presence of blood, leukocytes and nitrites where possible.

DIFFERENTIAL DIAGNOSIS

Stone disease must be distinguished from other urinary tract pathologies such as idiopathic hydronephrosis, pyelonephritis or perinephric abscess. The presence of a fever, pus cells in the urine, and a raised white cell count may be suggestive of infection, but in all patients presenting with renal pain further investigation is necessary to establish the diagnosis. Ureteric colic must also be distinguished from biliary colic, appendicitis, small or large bowel obstruction, and a leaking abdominal aortic aneurysm. In these conditions additional features in the history, together with additional physical signs such as the presence of abdominal tenderness, distension or peritonism, are often useful indicators of the cause of the pain. Differentiation from muscular pains related to spinal disorders is also important, and a full examination of the spine, reflexes and straight leg raising is helpful.

INVESTIGATIONS

Investigations are necessary to confirm the primary diagnosis and to establish the aetiology and risk of recurrent stone formation. Intravenous urography is the ideal primary investigation. A plain abdominal radiograph may suggest a radiopaque shadow in the line of ureter. However, uric acid stones are radiolucent and not seen on plain X-ray. An intravenous urogram may suggest the presence of a radiolucent stone (Fig. 35.29), which may be confirmed on a CT scan.

In patients with suspected ureteric colic, urgent intravenous urography will confirm the presence of urinary tract stones. If the urogram is delayed until the pain has settled, the radiographic appearances may well have returned to normal, and the opportunity to make the diagnosis with certainty is lost.

A non-contrast spiral CT scan is emerging as the investigation of choice in cases of an acute ureteric colic. It can be performed easily, without any risk of contrast allergies, and it is less expensive than an intravenous urogram. It can give information on the other visceral organs when the diagnosis is not definitive and will diagnose other pathology that may be present. It is equally useful for radiolucent stones.

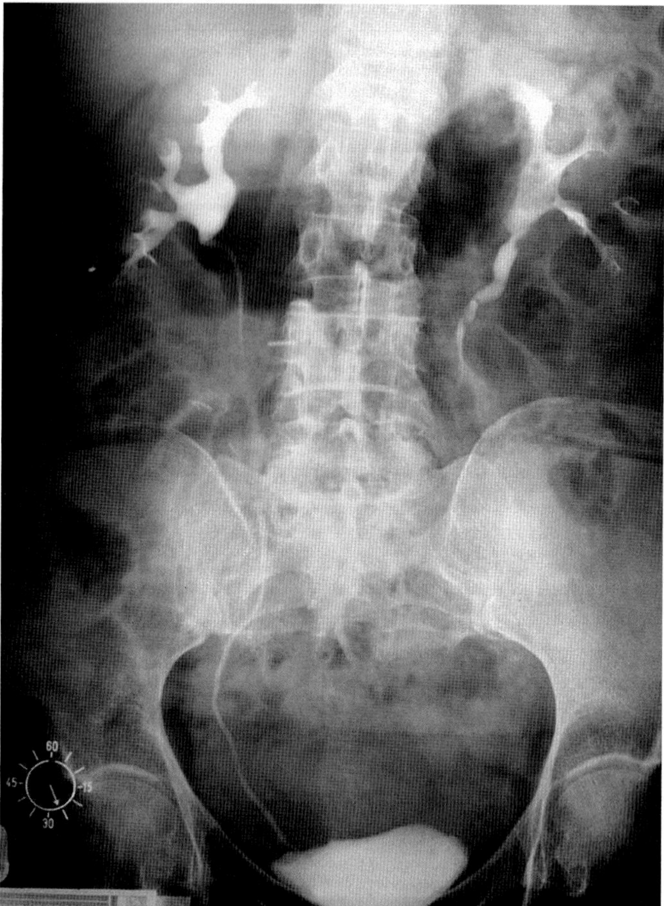

Figure 35.29 Radiolucent stone.

A retrograde ureteropyelogram may be required to better define the anatomy when no stone has been identified on the radiological investigations in a patient where there is a high clinical suspicion of ureteric colic.

A radioisotope scan may be used to assess the degree of function and degree of obstruction in patients in whom these appear to be impaired on the intravenous urogram. However, it does not delineate the upper tract anatomy well.

The renal function is assessed by estimation of the urea, electrolytes, creatinine and creatinine clearance where appropriate. Serum calcium, phosphate and uric acid levels are obtained to try to find a cause for the stone formation. A midstream specimen of urine is sent for culture to determine the presence of infection. A 24-h urine collection for assessing the levels of urates, calcium, phosphates and oxalates should be made to determine whether or not there are any underlying biochemical abnormalities and to determine the risk of further stone formation.

TREATMENT

The management of patients with renal stones is aimed at the specific treatment of the stone and the correction of anatomical or metabolic abnormalities that may predispose to recurrent stone formation. It is important to identify the underlying abnormality, because up to 50% of patients may have recurrence of stones within 5 years.

Conservative management

Most small (less than 5 mm in diameter), symptomless renal stones in an unobstructed non-infected kidney do not require removal. Patients should be followed by annual plain radiographs of the urinary tract to monitor the size and position of the stones. Exceptions are professional pilots or divers, who will require removal of even symptomless stones to continue their occupation. An increase in the size of the stone or the development of symptoms may alter the decision to treat it expectantly.

There are no rules governing whether a ureteric calculus will pass spontaneously. Half the patients with symptomatic ureteric stones pass their stones within 48 h of the onset of symptoms, and most have passed within 7 days. In general terms, 90% of stones that are less than 4 mm in diameter pass spontaneously,[50] two-thirds of those between 4 and 6 mm pass spontaneously, and over three-quarters of stones greater than this size fail to pass. The lower the position of stone in the ureter, the higher are the chances of it being passed spontaneously. There should, therefore, be a trial of expectant therapy in all patients with ureteric stones less than 6 mm in diameter, providing the ureter is unobstructed. Analgesics and antiemetics are usually required. There is no evidence that a forced diuresis increases the likelihood of the spontaneous passage of the stone, because the contralateral normal kidney excretes the bulk of the fluid load. In the absence of significant obstruction or increasing symptoms, such expectant therapy may be continued indefinitely.

It is permissible to carry out a trial of expectant therapy in patients with small stones in the presence of obstruction, but the period for which it should be continued is ill defined. The degree of obstruction may be monitored by radioisotope renography. Although complete functional recovery may occur even after complete obstruction has been present for 10 days, it is more prudent to recommend early removal of ureteric stones in the presence of even mild degrees of obstruction (Fig. 35.30), especially in view of the newer and less invasive methods of stone removal. Intervention is necessary in cases of significant obstruction resulting in progressive renal deterioration, refractory pyelonephritis or unremitting pain; paradoxically, in cases of upper tract obstruction where nephrostomy drainage is necessary, a stone may subsequently pass following insertion of the nephrostomy tube.

Medical management of stone disease

For all patients, and especially those in whom no underlying metabolic disorder is found, an increased fluid intake is the single most important factor in minimizing recurrent stone disease. The recurrence rate is of course higher if the patient is not initially stone-free.

Idiopathic hypercalciuria may be controlled by the use of a thiazide diuretic: bendroflumethiazide (bendrofluazide) 5 mg/day. Thiazide diuretics act on the renal tubules by impairing calcium excretion. Sodium cellulose phosphate combines with calcium in the intestine, preventing absorption of dietary calcium and so reducing urinary calcium. To be effective this treatment must be taken approximately 30 min before a meal and is associated with the development of diarrhoea in a quarter of patients. When the urinary or plasma urate levels are elevated in association with hypercalciuria, a small dose of allopurinol may lower the stone recurrence rate. Potassium citrate may also be effective. Hypercalcaemia is often caused by primary hyperparathyroidism, which will need treating to reduce stone recurrence. Patients with recurrent urinary infection and stones should be treated for the infection, which is often by a Gram-negative coliform organism. Predisposing factors should be sought and corrected.

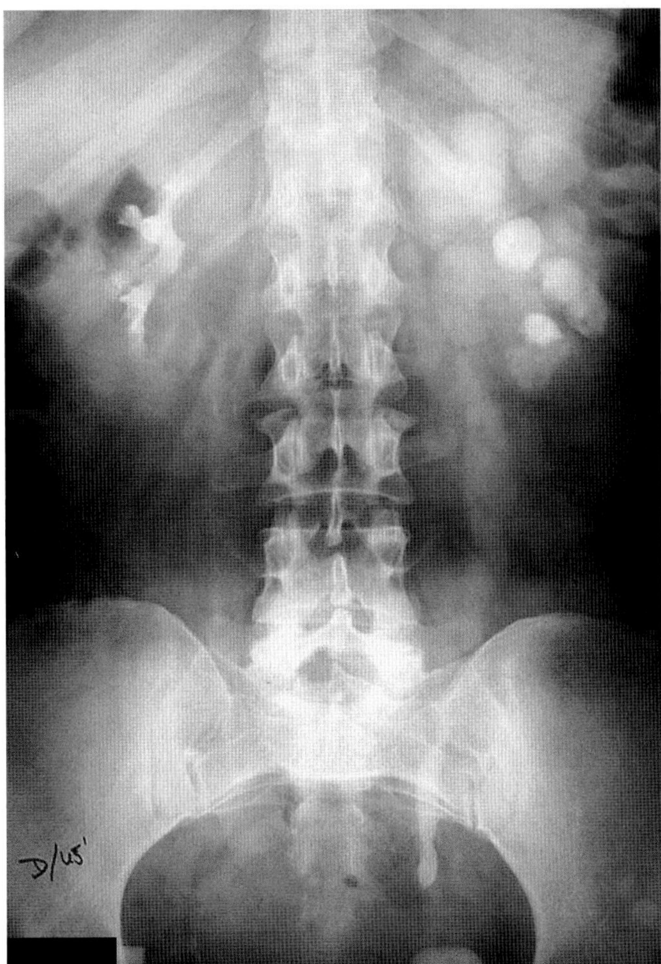

Figure 35.30 Lower left ureteric stone with obstruction.

Uric acid stones are uncommon in the UK, accounting for approximately 8% of all stones. It is usually possible to prevent further uric acid stone formation and also to dissolve existing stones by increasing the fluid intake, restricting purine-rich foods, and alkalinizing the urine with sodium bicarbonate 3–6 g daily. Allopurinol at a dose of 200–400 mg/day reduces both the plasma and the urinary urate, and can be prescribed. An intrarenal alkalinization may be achieved by irrigation with bicarbonate solution via a nephrostomy tube.

Cystine stones may be dissolved in situ by increasing the patient's fluid intake, by alkalinizing the urine, and by the administration of penicillamine or α-mercaptopropionylglycine, which has fewer side effects. This is the one type of stone for which medical treatment is unequivocally effective. Struvite stones may be dissolved by making the urine acidic. Stone

REFERENCE

50. Drach DW. Urol Clin North Am 1983; 10: 709

dissolution is a slow process, with approximately 1 cm of stone dissolving per month with active treatment. Careful assessment of the metabolic aspects of renal stone disease, together with an integrated surgical approach, should result in high stone-free rates with a reduced risk of stone recurrence.

Interventional management

In the past 10 years the active approach to the management of urinary stone disease has undergone a dramatic change. This applies equally to the management of renal and ureteric stones.

The options available are listed here.

Extracorporeal shock-wave lithotripsy

Renal calculi less than 2 cm are best treated by extracorporeal shock-wave lithotripsy. Patients undergoing extracorporeal shock-wave lithotripsy need to be followed up regularly. Stone-free rates vary, but approximately 85% of patients can be expected to be stone-free at 3 months. Stones between 2 and 3 cm in diameter may be treated by extracorporeal shock-wave lithotripsy or percutaneous nephrolithotomy. However, the best results for stones larger than 3 cm in diameter are obtained by primary percutaneous nephrolithotomy, reserving extracorporeal shock-wave lithotripsy to treat residual fragments. Stones in the upper or middle third of the ureter may be treated with lithotripsy in situ as first choice, employing ureteroscopy and intracorporeal lithotripsy or the push-bang technique (pushing the stone back into the kidney and then fragmenting it with extracorporeal shock-wave lithotripsy) if this fails. However, poorly visualized stones overlying the sacroiliac joint may not be amenable to this treatment method. In cases of obstruction, a double-J stent may be required to ensure kidney drainage.

There may be transient haematuria, flank pain, ecchymosis at the skin site, intrarenal haematomata, or oedema of the treated kidney. These settle in 3–7 days, and the incidence of these complications is dependent on the total number of shock waves delivered. The glomerular filtration rate drops immediately after lithotripsy but returns to baseline after 3 weeks. In the long term, the initial fear of producing a higher risk of hypertension has not been proven. Lithotripsy is contraindicated in pregnancy. Patients with pacemakers can be treated with lithotripsy, but adequate precautions must be taken. Patients on anticoagulant or aspirin therapy should stop it prior to lithotripsy to allow platelet and coagulation function to return to normal. A quarter of the patients develop ureteric colic from stone fragments, and transient haematuria is inevitable. Occasionally, stone fragments obstruct the ureter (steinstrasse) and require endoscopic removal. The risk of this complication can be minimized by the insertion of a self-retaining ureteric stent before commencing treatment of stones greater than 2 cm in size.

Percutaneous nephrolithotomy

This technique permits the removal of stones from the kidney and ureter by the creation of a track between the skin surface and the collecting system of the kidney. The track is dilated to allow the introduction of a rigid nephroscope into the kidney, and the stone is then removed intact with forceps or reduced in size by the use of direct application of intracorporeal ultrasound or electrohydraulic lithotripsy. Renal stones over 3 cm in size (Fig. 35.31) are best treated with percutaneous nephrolithotomy. Complications of percutaneous nephrolithotomy relate mainly to bleeding during the procedure and perforation of the renal pelvis.

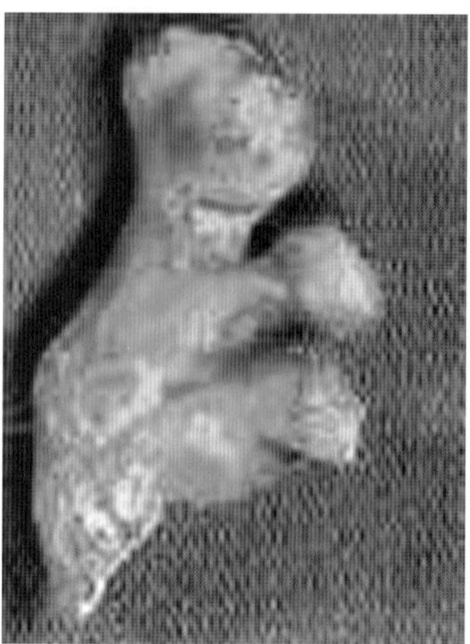

Figure 35.31 Staghorn calculus.

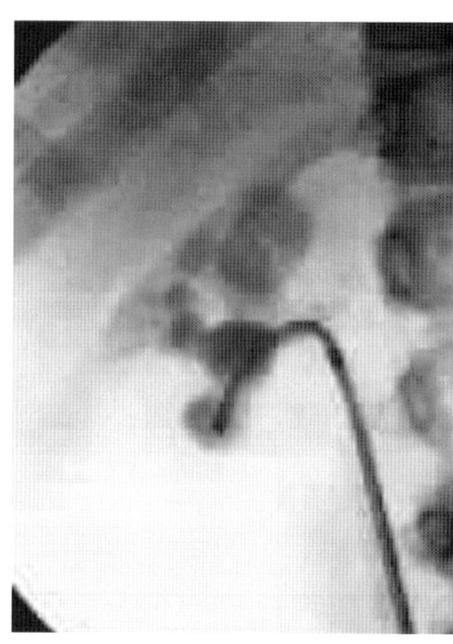

Figure 35.32 Flexible ureteroscopy.

Ureterorenoscopy

The development of the rigid ureteroscope has allowed the removal of many ureteric calculi from the lower third of the ureter under vision. If the stone is too large to be removed in this way, then it may be disintegrated with intracorporeal laser, ultrasound or electrohydraulic lithotripsy. The fragments may be allowed to pass or are extracted under vision using a stone basket or graspers. Newer fibre-optic flexible ureteroscopes (Fig. 35.32) are now available that permit the removal of stones in the upper and middle third of the ureter. For lower-third ureteric calculi both lithotripsy and ureteroscopy are reasonable options, although higher stone-free rates are obtained with primary ureteroscopy. The most significant complication following ureteroscopy is the development of a ureteric stricture, which is generally the result of a traumatic introduction of the ureteroscope. Perforation of the ureter, if it occurs, should be managed by ureteric stenting and generally does not cause long-term problems.

Stone baskets

The technique of 'blind basketing' of ureteric stones has a number of disadvantages. The success rate using this technique is considerably lower than that using ureteroscopy, and there is a much greater risk of perforating the ureter, causing mucosal stripping or even avulsion. It is possible to push the stone back into the kidney with fluoroscopic control under anaesthesia if it proves impossible to remove a ureteric stone by the methods outlined in this chapter. The stone can then be removed by percutaneous nephrolithotomy or disintegrated with extracorporeal shock-wave lithotripsy (the push-bang technique).

Laparoscopic surgery

More complex renal and ureteric stones that are not suitable for an endoscopic extraction are more commonly treated with a laparoscopic approach. A laparoscopic pyelolithotomy or ureterolithotomy can be carried out safely and with much less morbidity compared with the classical open methods.

Open surgery

Open surgery includes an open pyelolithotomy, an anatropic nephrolithotomy, or an occasional nephrectomy for a non-functioning kidney. Open surgery is reserved for complex stones (Fig. 35.33) for which other treatment options either do not exist or have been tried without success. An anatropic nephrolithotomy implies a near bisecting of the kidney along the least vascular plane, as represented by the Brodel's line.

An open ureterolithotomy may be required in cases of large and impacted ureteric calculi where other options have failed. When a stone is impacted in the upper third of the ureter, it is best exposed through a loin incision; for stones in the mid third the approach should be similar. The lower third is the most difficult portion of the ureter to reach and is best approached extraperitoneally through a paramedian, Pfannenstiel or oblique muscle-cutting incision. The stone is removed through a longitudinal incision in the ureter.

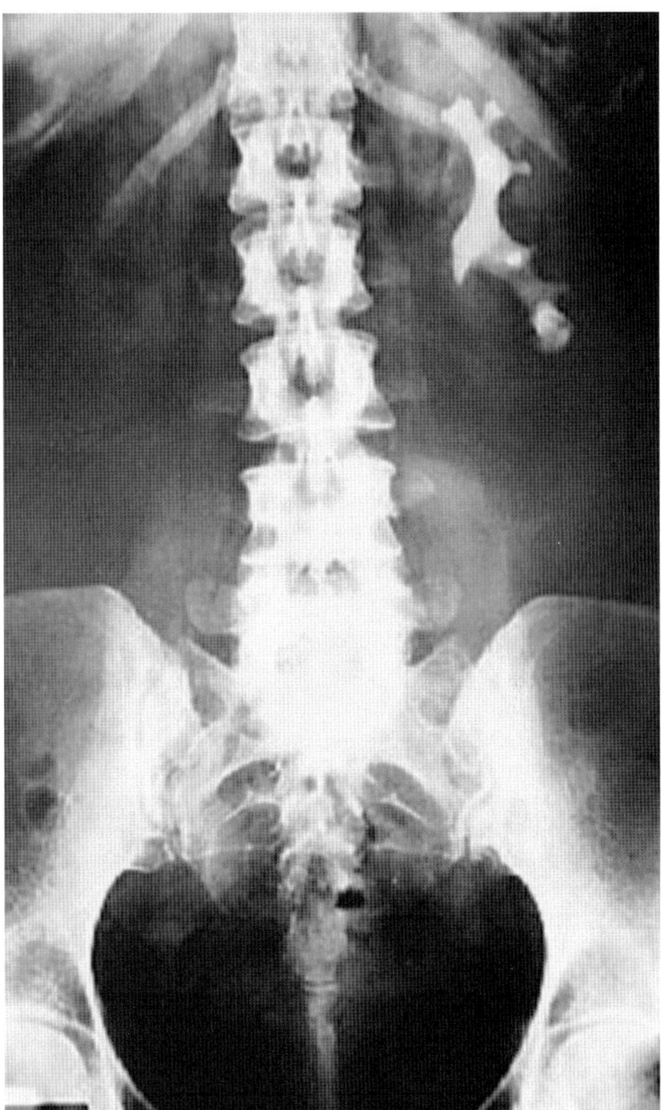

Figure 35.33 Staghorn calculus.

RENAL TUMOURS

Renal tumours may be classified according to the aggressiveness of the tumour. Most renal tumours should be regarded as malignant; there are very few benign kidney tumours. This section initially concentrates on the two most common renal tumours: Wilms' tumour and renal cell carcinoma. A brief description of the rarer types of renal tumour is then given.

NEPHROBLASTOMA (WILMS' TUMOUR)

Incidence

Wilms' tumour is the most common tumour of the urinary system in childhood, accounting for roughly 5% of childhood cancers. The peak incidence is between 3 and 4 years of age, and in 5 and 10% of the cases the tumour is bilateral. There is no sex predilection.

Aetiology

Nephroblastoma may occur in familial and non-familial forms, the familial form accounting for only 1% of cases. There is an abnormal proliferation of the metanephric blastema which fails to differentiate into tubules and glomeruli. In the hereditary group, the tumour is thought to result from a loss of maternal chromosome 11 alleles and a loss of function of a recessive tumour suppressor gene in the 11p13 region. Approximately 10% of cases are associated with congenital malformations such as hypospadias, non-familial aniridia, hemihypertrophy of the body, and Beckwith–Wiedemann syndrome (macroglossia, omphalocele, mental retardation and organomegaly).

Pathology

Gross features

The tumour is large and is frequently separated from the remainder of the kidney by a fibrous pseudocapsule. In aggressive tumours the capsule is breached, so that the tumour invades the kidney and adjacent structures. The tumour is often lobulated, with areas of necrosis and haemorrhage.

Microscopic appearances

There is considerable variation in tumour composition, but nephrogenic (tubuloglomerular pattern) and stromagenic cells are seen. A typical nephroblastoma consists of blastemal, epithelial and stromal components in varying proportions. The rhabdoid type, the clear cell sarcoma type and the anaplastic type are the three histological subtypes that are associated with a poor

Table 35.3 Staging of Wilms' tumour

Stage	Description
1	Tumour limited to kidney and completely excised with no tumour rupture.
2	Tumour extending outside the kidney but completely excised.
3	Tumour incompletely excised at operation with positive lymph nodes.
4	Distant metastases.
5	Bilateral renal tumour.

prognosis.[51] Although they constitute only 10% of all Wilms' tumours, they account for 60% of deaths. The rhabdoid type is now being increasingly identified as a separate and different type of tumour, distinct from Wilms' tumours. Nephroblastoma has been staged by the National Wilms' Tumour Study Group (Table 35.3).[52]

Clinical features

The tumour commonly presents as an abdominal swelling. Haematuria and pyrexia may occur, with pain from the local spread of the disease. On examination the child often appears well, with a firm non-tender mass that does not cross the midline. This tumour must be differentiated from a neuroblastoma, where the child looks ill and the mass is more nodular and irregular, and usually crosses the midline.

Investigations

The plain X-ray of the abdomen may show an eggshell calcification from old haemorrhage; stippled calcification suggests a neuroblastoma. Intravenous urography, once the first-line investigation for the diagnosis of a Wilms' tumour, has been replaced by CT scan and MRI. On an intravenous urogram, distortion of calyces as the result of an intrarenal mass is characteristic. The contralateral kidney is assessed for function and the possibility of a bilateral Wilms' tumour. The solid nature of the tumour can be confirmed by ultrasound scanning, and the vena cava and renal veins assessed for tumour thrombus. A CT scan is used for staging the disease. A neuroblastoma can be excluded by assessing urinary catecholamine levels and examining a bone marrow aspirate for neuroblastoma cells.

Treatment

An improved understanding of the disease and a multidisciplinary approach to the management of Wilms' tumours has resulted in a progressive increase in the survival rate of children with this tumour. The best results are obtained if children are treated in specialist centres.

Patients less than 2 years of age and with favourable histology are treated with radical nephrectomy. Patients with stage I who are over 2 years of age and those with stage II tumours (early-stage tumours) are treated by radical nephrectomy followed by chemotherapy but no radiotherapy. Children with stages III and IV (late-stage) tumours or those with unfavourable histology also have a radical nephrectomy, receive radiotherapy to the bed of the renal tumour, and are given more aggressive chemotherapy than those with early-stage tumours. Survival rates for children with favourable histology and stage I–IV tumours are 97% and 83%, respectively; for those with unfavourable histology and stage I–III tumours the rate is 68%. Of patients with unfavourable histology and stage IV disease, 55% will be alive 4 years after nephrectomy. Many chemotherapeutic regimens have been used: vincristine, actinomycin D, doxorubicin and cyclophosphamide have all been shown to be effective.

RENAL CELL CARCINOMA

Renal cell carcinoma accounts for 3% of all adult cancers and 85% of all primary malignancies of the kidney. In the UK about 2300 patients die of renal cell carcinoma each year. It is more common in the fifth and sixth decades of life, with a male to female ratio of 2:1.

Aetiology

Cigarette smokers and coffee drinkers appear to be at increased risk of developing renal cell carcinomas; the presence of dimethylnitrosamine in tobacco smoke has been shown to induce renal parenchymal tumours in rats. Occupational contact with cadmium and tanning products have also been blamed.

Renal cell carcinoma can occur in familial or sporadic forms. There is increasing interest in chromosomal abnormalities found in association with renal cell carcinoma, with a fairly constant finding of deletions or translocations in the short arm of chromosome 3 (3p) in the familial type. In the sporadic type of renal cell carcinoma, a particular allele in the 3p locus has been found to be consistently deleted in most tumour tissue, suggesting that there is a suppressor cancer gene at that locus. There is an increased risk of developing renal tumours in patients with von Hippel–Lindau syndrome.

Pathology

Renal cell carcinoma arises from the cells of the proximal convoluted tubule,[53] and is an adenocarcinoma in a mixed form containing clear cells, granular cells, and occasionally sarcomatoid cells. Grossly, the tumour is characteristically orange to yellow because of lipid content. These tumours have a pseudocapsule of compressed renal tissue surrounding them.

Spread of the tumour occurs into the veins, and it may extend into the renal vein and inferior vena cava. Occasional retrograde spread into the spermatic or ovarian vein may produce secondary deposits in the testis or ovary. Direct spread occurs into the perinephric fat and overlying muscle. Metastases occur in bones, brain and lungs, where they are often solitary and large (cannonball). There is debate about the relative degree of malignancy of smaller renal tumours, which have often been described as benign adenomas when they are less than 3 cm in diameter. It is now recognized that some carcinomas start as small adenomas and, while metastases from such tumours are rare, the distinction between benign and malignant tumours on the grounds of size alone is somewhat artificial. The tumour staging is as shown in Table 35.4.

Clinical features

The most common presenting features of renal cell carcinoma include haematuria, loin pain or a palpable mass, or a combination of all three. The systemic immunological response to malignant disease produces a number of features. Many of these

REFERENCES

51. Beckwith JB, Palmer NF. Cancer 1978; 41: 1937
52. D'Angio GJ et al. Cancer 1989; 64: 349–360

Table 35.4 Tumour staging for renal cell carcinoma

Stage	Description
Primary tumour (T)	
Tx	Primary tumour cannot be assessed.
T0	No evidence of primary tumour.
T1	Tumour 7 cm or smaller in greatest dimension, limited to the kidney.
T2	Tumour larger than 7 cm in greatest dimension, limited to the kidney.
T3	Tumour extends into major veins or invades adrenal gland or perinephric tissues but not beyond the Gerota fascia.
T3a	Tumour invades adrenal gland or perinephric tissues but not beyond the Gerota fascia.
T3b	Tumour grossly extends into the renal vein(s) or vena cava below the diaphragm.
T3c	Tumour grossly extends into the renal vein(s) or vena cava above the diaphragm.
T4	Tumour invading beyond the Gerota fascia.
Regional lymph nodes (N)*	
Nx	Regional lymph nodes cannot be assessed.
N0	No regional lymph node metastasis.
N1	Metastasis in a single regional lymph node.
N2	Metastasis in more than one regional lymph node.
Distant metastasis (M)	
Mx	Distant metastasis cannot be assessed.
M0	No distant metastasis.
M1	Distant metastasis.

*Laterality does not affect the N classification.

effects are non-specific and are produced by the body's response to the tumour. These include fever (15%), anaemia (30%), raised erythrocyte sedimentation rate (50%), and abnormal liver function (30%). Myopathy and amyloid deposition may also occur. With the exception of amyloid, these features are potentially reversible on removal of the tumour. Some renal cell carcinomas are associated with a variety of paraneoplastic syndromes that result from hormone secretion by the tumour. Hypertension may occur in a quarter of these patients, but it is uncertain whether this is caused by renin excretion or ischaemia. Erythropoietin secretion produces polycythaemia, and occasionally parathormone is excreted by renal tumours, producing hypercalcaemia. Patients may also present with bone pain from metastases or from the secondary effects of obstruction of the vena cava or renal vein. An acutely developing left-sided varicocele is a mode of rare presentation.

Diagnosis

Urine

The majority of patients with renal tumours have evidence of haematuria on microscopy or on chemical testing. Patients with urothelial tumours may have tumour cells seen on urine cytology.

Radiological investigations

The mainstay of investigation used to be the intravenous urogram. The characteristic feature on the intravenous urogram is distortion of the calyces, with a space-occupying lesion expanding the cortex. This abnormality is more clearly seen on nephrotomography after a large dose of contrast medium. The differential diagnosis in such cases lies between a renal tumour or cyst, and further investigations are utilized to establish this.

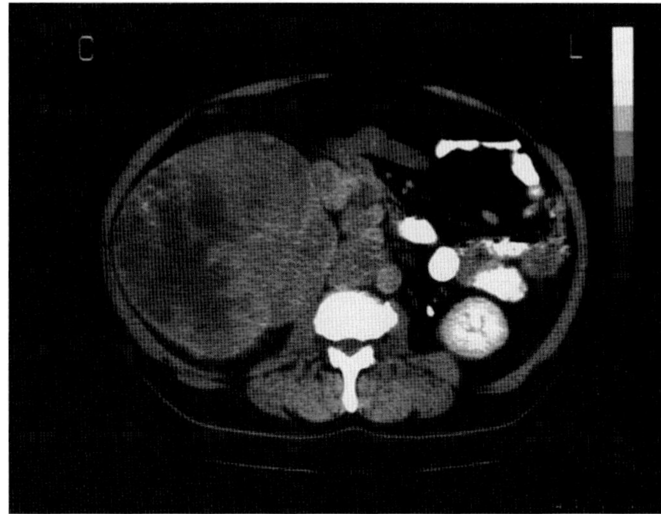

Figure 35.34 Renal cell carcinoma.

Urothelial tumours are seen as distortions of the calyces or a luminal filling defect in the renal pelvis on the urogram.

Ultrasound examination differentiates between solid and cystic space-occupying lesions with an accuracy approaching 98%. An ultrasound scan is sufficient to make a diagnosis in the majority of patients in whom a space-occupying lesion is an incidental finding during intravenous urography.

Computerized tomography scanning of abdomen (Fig. 35.34) and chest is considered to be a standard investigation for both diagnosis and staging of the disease. It also helps in assessment of the lymph nodes. Magnetic resonance imaging is more or less equally informative as the CT scan; however, it is superior to CT for assessment of vascular extension of the tumour thrombus.

Treatment

Radical nephrectomy is the classical treatment for localized renal cell carcinoma. Classically, this involves removal of kidney along with removal of the perinephric fat, Gerota's fascia, ipsilateral adrenal, proximal half of the ureter, and lymph nodes around the renal pedicle[53] to increase the chance of cure. This concept has altered recently with the more routine use of partial nephrectomy, where only the affected pole or segment is removed to preserve renal function. The adrenal may be left intact in lower pole tumours. The role of lymphadenectomy also remains controversial. There are different approaches to kidney for performing an open radical nephrectomy:

- an abdominal transperitoneal approach through a transverse incision;
- an anterior thoracoabdominal approach; or
- a posterior approach.

More recently, with the introduction of advanced laparoscopic techniques there has been an increased interest in a minimally invasive surgical approach to the tumour.

Partial nephrectomy

Nephron-sparing surgery in the form of partial nephrectomy may be considered for small (less than 4 cm) tumours in the upper or lower pole of the solitary kidney especially in patients with impaired renal function prior to surgery.

REFERENCE

53. Robson CJ. J Urol 1963; 89: 37

Radical nephrectomy in patients with metastatic disease

The 1-year survival rate for metastatic renal cell carcinoma is 7–35%. There is little evidence to support the role of nephrectomy in inducing spontaneous regression of metastases, with one series reporting a 0.8% incidence of disease regression following nephrectomy.[54] Patients with a solitary metastasis that is amenable to surgical removal may be offered a combined nephrectomy and removal of the metastasis (metastatectomy). This has produced long-term disease-free survival, but some of the beneficial response claimed for treatment may relate more to tumour biology than to the surgical procedure.

Nephrectomy as a palliative procedure can be helpful in managing patients with severe haemorrhage and unremitting pain, and also in those with paraneoplastic syndromes. Renal embolization prior to surgery may be attempted in such cases.

Control of primary symptoms may also be achieved by embolization of the renal artery supplying the tumour.

Radiation therapy

Radiotherapy remains an important tool for palliation in patients with metastatic renal cell carcinoma. Effective palliation may be achieved in up to two-thirds of the patients with metastasis to brain, bone and lungs.[55] Tumours may be reduced in size by preoperative radiotherapy.

Other options

Renal tumours should be regarded as chemoresistant, with up to only 6% response rate. Regression has, however, been seen following immunotherapy with interferon, which may have a role in the management of metastatic disease. A response rate of up to 30% has been demonstrated.[56] Because of the severe side effects, it is reserved for young patients with metastatic disease. Hormone therapy with medroxyprogesterone acetate has shown a response rate of around 1–2%, which is partial and of brief duration.

Prognosis

Renal cell carcinoma is slow-growing, and occasionally patients present with metastatic disease up to 20 years after nephrectomy for the primary tumour. When the tumour is confined to kidney, the prognosis following radical nephrectomy is excellent, with up to 93% of patients surviving 5 years. However, survival figures from reported series vary; in patients with locally invasive tumour and involved lymph nodes a more realistic expectation is that 30% will survive 5 years.

TRANSITIONAL CELL CARCINOMA OF THE RENAL PELVIS AND URETER

Carcinoma of renal pelvis and ureter are rare, accounting for only 4% of all urothelial cancers. In these cases there is thought to be a widespread abnormality of the urothelium. Patients with single, upper tract urothelial cancer have a 30–50% chance of developing a bladder cancer, and a 2–4% risk of developing a contralateral transitional cell carcinoma.

The risk factors for development of a transitional cell carcinoma of the kidney and ureter are the same as those responsible for a bladder cancer: smoking, exposure to industrial dyes and solvents, and analgesic abuse.

Gross haematuria is noticed in about 90% of cases. There may be an associated flank pain resulting from the ureteric obstruction. Irritative voiding symptoms may be present in approximately 5–10% of cases. A flank mass resulting from the tumour itself or due to an associated hydronephrosis may be present.

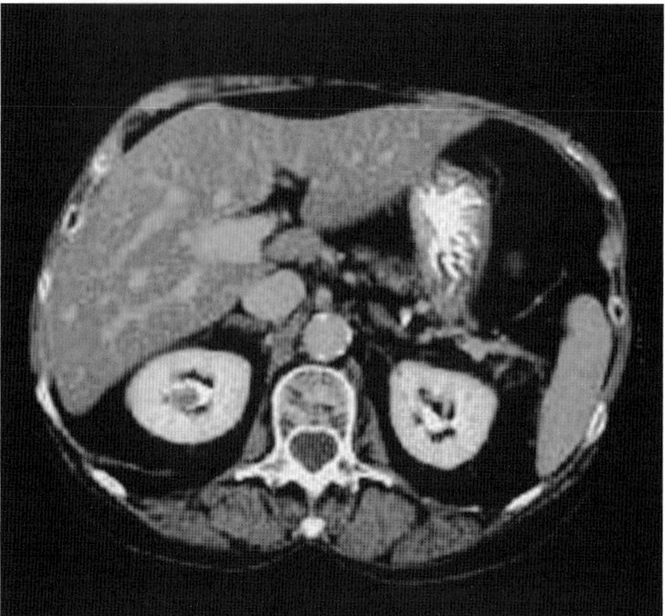

Figure 35.35 Transitional cell carcinoma of the left renal pelvis on a CT scan.

An intravenous urogram shows a filling defect in the renal pelvis or the ureter, often with some degree of obstruction. A CT scan gives a clear anatomical picture (Fig. 35.35).

The standard treatment of both ureteric and renal pelvic transitional cell carcinomas is a nephroureterectomy. This includes removing the whole length of the ureter, along with a cuff of the bladder wall. These patients should be carefully followed up, because they are at significant risk of developing a bladder cancer.

The role of chemotherapy and radiotherapy is very limited.

BENIGN TUMOURS

Renal oncocytoma

Renal oncocytoma is a well-differentiated, eosinophilic granular cell renal tumour associated with a good prognosis. Oncocytomas arise from the proximal convoluted tubules. They are large and impossible to differentiate from renal cell carcinomas preoperatively. Treatment usually consists of nephrectomy.

Angiomyolipoma

Angiomyolipoma is a benign lesion consisting of smooth muscle, blood vessels and fat. Very occasionally this tumour is malignant and involves local lymph nodes. It is found in association with tuberous sclerosis in half of the cases. In such patients the lesions are generally bilateral and multiple. Lesions less than 4 cm and not producing symptoms may be followed up yearly with an ultrasound scan. Lesions larger than 4 cm and producing only mild symptoms may be followed up at 6-monthly intervals. Symptomatic patients with lesions over 4 cm may be offered a nephrectomy.

REFERENCES

54. Montie JE et al. J Urol 1977; 117: 272
55. Aulitzky W et al. J Clin Oncol 1989; 7: 1875
56. Kjaer M. Cancer Treat Rev 1988; 15: 195

Other benign renal tumours

Other rare benign tumours of the kidney are leiomyoma, lipoma, fibroma, mesoblastic nephroma, adenoma and haemangiopericytoma.

METASTASES

Primary tumours metastasizing to the kidney include those of lung, breast and uterus and are commonly bilateral. Treatment depends on the nature of the primary tumour.

The bladder

36

Christopher Blake, Paul Abrams

STRUCTURE AND FUNCTION

The bladder is a hollow muscular organ lined by a mucous membrane, surrounded by smooth muscle (the detrusor muscle), and covered on its outer aspect partly by peritoneal serosa and partly by fascia. The functions of the bladder are the storage and controlled elimination of urine. These are under the control of the autonomic nervous system. Sympathetic supply is from the lower two thoracic and upper two lumbar segments of the spinal cord, via the hypogastric plexus. Parasympathetic fibres arise from the second to fourth sacral segments and are carried in the pelvic nerves.

The epithelial lining of the bladder (the urothelium) is urine-proof and can accommodate large changes in surface area without losing its integrity. The urothelium has three to seven layers of cells; the most superficial is adapted to be urine-proof, with a characteristic asymmetrical unit membrane on the luminal surface covered with a glycosaminoglycan layer. The urothelium has a slow turnover but is also capable of a rapid proliferation in response to injury. It lies on a basement membrane and is separated from the detrusor muscle by the lamina propria.

The normal detrusor muscle accommodates an increase in volume during filling of the bladder with no increase in tone and therefore without a concomitant rise in intravesical pressure. It only contracts to provide the expulsive force for voiding. The detrusor is richly supplied with cholinergic receptors, except in the trigone, and has β-adrenergic receptors situated predominantly in the dome and α-adrenergic receptors in the bladder neck region.[1]

CONGENITAL ANOMALIES

AGENESIS OF THE BLADDER

Complete agenesis of the bladder is one of the most rare anomalies of the urinary tract. It is more likely to occur in a non-viable fetus and is usually associated with multiple other congenital anomalies. In those rare patients who survive urinary diversion is required.

BLADDER EXSTROPHY (ECTOPIA VESICAE)

This defect of the bladder and lower abdominal wall occurs in approximately three per 100 000 live births and is more common in males.[2] Exstrophy occurs as part of a spectrum of anomalies ranging from cloacal exstrophy at its most severe to pseudo-exstrophy at its mildest. Exstrophy of the bladder is the most common abnormality, comprising an open bladder with a defect in the abdominal wall, separation of the pubic bones anteriorly, and epispadias of the penis or bifid clitoris. The upper tracts are usually normal at birth but are at risk of deterioration as a result of ureteric reflux, obstruction or infection consequent on efforts to close the bladder or divert the urine.

Exstrophy is rarely diagnosed prenatally,[3] but the deformity is usually easily recognized at birth: the dark-red bladder mucosa bulges from the lower abdomen. The upper part is rugose and the lower part, representing the trigone, is smooth. From the apex to the lower part a gutter runs down the dorsum of the penis as an epispadic urethra, the testes are commonly undescended, and the scrotum may be poorly developed. In girls the clitoris is bifid. The mucosa of the bladder rapidly becomes oedematous, making it hard to judge the size of the bladder before an attempt at primary closure, and glandular metaplasia develops. When the bladder cannot be closed there is a risk of adenocarcinoma developing, and patients treated by urinary diversion should have the bladder remnant removed.

Surgical reconstruction of the bladder is the treatment of choice and is possible in almost all cases. This comprises closure of the pelvic ring, often necessitating iliac osteotomies, closure of the bladder, reconstruction of the bladder neck, and reconstruction of the epispadic penis. On becoming adult, 18% of patients with closed bladders have been reported to be continent. A quarter had renal damage but social and sexual functions were good. Late failure of both the detrusor and the urethra in adult life is significant and requires prolonged follow-up.[1]

THE URACHUS

The urachus is an embryological structure that arises from the dome of the anterior wall of the bladder and extends to the umbilicus. It closes by involution, and arrest of this normal process results in the disorders that occur (Fig. 36.1):

- patent urachus;
- urachal sinus;
- urachal cyst; and
- urachal diverticulum.

A patent urachus results in a communication between the bladder and umbilicus, and presents at birth with a wet umbilicus associated with granulation tissue. The diagnosis can be confirmed by demonstrating that the fluid is urine or by demonstrating a patent sinus on a cystogram. Complete excision of the tract is required. Urachal sinus may present in childhood

REFERENCES

1. Wallace DMA. In: Burnand KG, Young AE (eds). The New Aird's Companion in Surgical Studies. 2nd edn. Churchill Livingstone, Edinburgh, 1998: 1069–1087
2. Lancaster PAL. Teratology 1987; 36: 221–227
3. Mirk P, Calisti A, Fileni A. J Ultrasound Med 1986; 5: 291–293

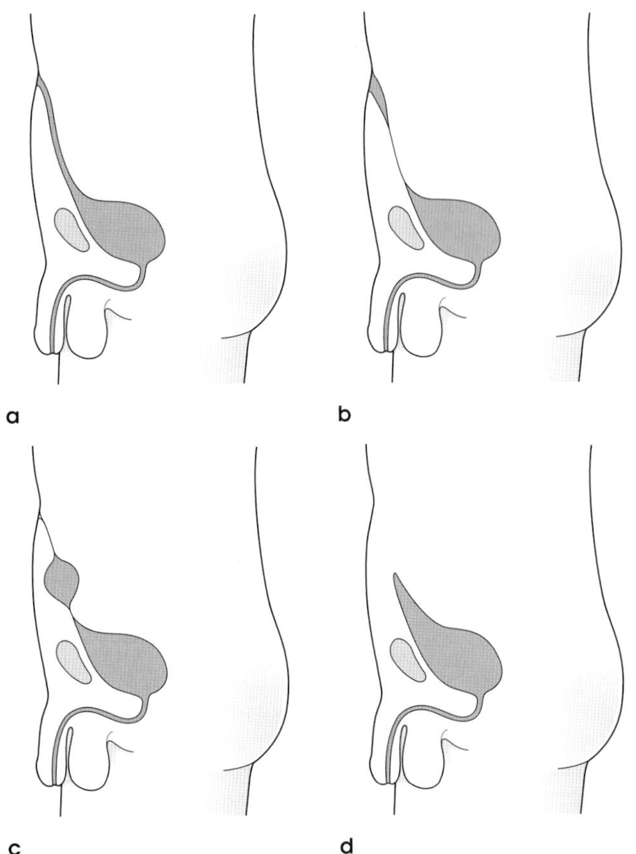

Figure 36.1 Urachal anomalies: (**a**) patent urachus; (**b**) urachal sinus; (**c**) urachal cyst; and (**d**) urachal diverticulum.

or adult life with a discharge from the umbilicus and may become chronically infected. A sinogram should be performed to demonstrate the whole tract before surgical excision. Urachal cysts may present at any age with a mass and signs of infection. They tend to develop in the lower third of the urachus. Urachal diverticula are usually an incidental finding and do not require treatment unless they interfere with voiding of urine. With all urachal abnormalities a patent omphalomesenteric duct must be considered in the differential diagnosis. Rarely, urachal remnants are associated with the development of adenocarcinomas in adults.[1,4]

DISORDERS OF BLADDER FUNCTION

PATIENT ASSESSMENT

Lower urinary tract symptoms may be divided into *storage* symptoms, such as daytime frequency, urgency and nocturia, and *voiding* symptoms, such as hesitancy, slow stream and terminal dribbling.[5] It is important to ascertain any neurological symptoms and details of any previous surgery. Physical examination should determine the presence of a palpable bladder, or abdominal or pelvic masses. Neurological signs in the lower limbs must be assessed, including the loss of perianal sensation or anal tone (supplied by S2–4, the nerve roots carrying parasympathetic innervation to the bladder and urethra). In men, the presence of a meatal stenosis or epididymitis should be excluded, and prostatic size and consistency should be assessed. In women, a pelvic examination should be carried out to assess evidence of prolapse.

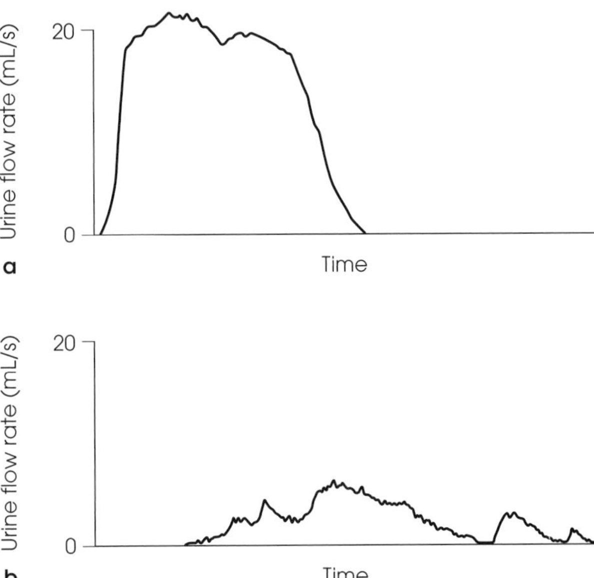

Figure 36.2 Urine flow rate. (**a**) Normal flow with a peak flow of over 20 mL/s and a normal voiding pattern. (**b**) An obstructed voiding pattern, with a low peak flow, hesitancy, interrupted stream and a prolonged voiding time.

Other baseline investigations include a midstream urine specimen to exclude infection, urine cytology, assessment of renal function, and imaging of the upper tracts.

Urodynamic studies

Urodynamics are the investigations carried out to evaluate patients with lower urinary tract symptoms. The simplest of these techniques is uroflowmetry. This non-invasive test gives information on flow rate and pattern but cannot supply information on detrusor function (Fig. 36.2). Flow rates should be performed with a full bladder.

Conventional cystometry requires insertion of filling- and pressure- (p_{ves}) recording catheters into the bladder. Abdominal pressure (p_{abd}) is also recorded using a rectal catheter. True detrusor pressure (p_{det}) is derived by the subtraction of abdominal pressure from bladder pressure ($p_{det} = p_{ves} - p_{abd}$) (Fig. 36.3). Filling cystometry is used to look for evidence of detrusor overactivity, which may lead to urge incontinence, and evidence of urodynamic stress incontinence, which may be provoked by coughing and movement. Voiding cystometry assesses detrusor function and outlet obstruction.

Videourodynamics combines cystometry with videocystography and allows the definition of bladder anatomy as well as detrusor/outlet coordination and the presence of ureteric reflux.

Ambulatory urodynamic studies are more physiological and utilize natural filling of the bladder. All these urodynamic techniques can be carried out using either urethral or suprapubic catheters to measure intravesical pressure.

Electromyography is used in some patients to study pelvic floor and sphincter function, particularly in neurogenic disorders.

REFERENCES

4. Caldamone A. In: Fitzpatrick J, Krane R (eds). The Bladder. Churchill Livingstone, Edinburgh, 1995: 493–500
5. Abrams P, Cardozo L, Fall M et al. Neurourol Urodynamics 2002; 21: 170–181

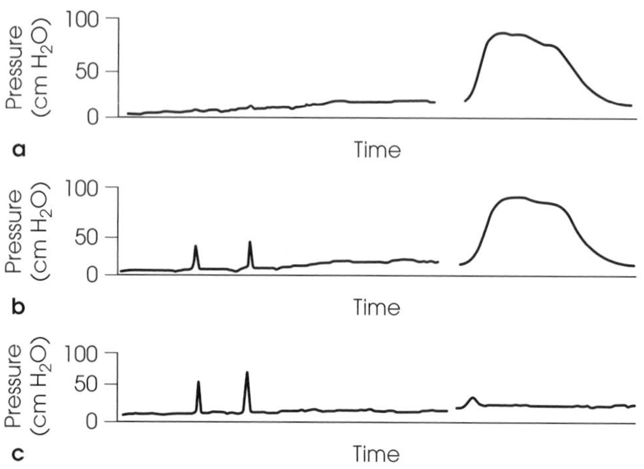

Figure 36.3 A normal cystometrogram. **Left side:** during filling; **right side:** during voiding. **Lower trace:** rectal pressure; **middle trace:** intravesical pressure; **upper trace:** detrusor pressure, produced by subtracting the rectal pressure from the intravesical pressure. The peaks produced by coughing are subtracted out of the detrusor pressure. The detrusor pressure does not rise above 15 cm of water during filling.

CLASSIFICATION OF DISORDERS OF BLADDER FUNCTION

Following urodynamic investigation it should be possible to classify patients into categories of storage or voiding dysfunction.

Vesicourethral storage function

Disorders of bladder sensation during filling

Sensation may be absent, reduced, normal or increased.

Disorders of detrusor function during filling

Detrusor overactivity (previously called detrusor instability) is the urodynamic observation of involuntary detrusor contraction during the filling phase, which may be spontaneous or provoked. This may be neurogenic, in the presence of neurological disorders, or idiopathic. Such involuntary contractions may lead to *detrusor overactivity incontinence*. Bladder compliance describes the relationship between change in bladder volume and change in detrusor pressure; the normal bladder has high compliance, i.e. a large change in volume during filling with minimal change in pressure.

Disorders of urethral function during filling

The urethral closure mechanism during storage may be competent or incompetent. If incompetent it will allow leakage of urine in the absence of a detrusor contraction. *Urodynamic stress incontinence* (previously genuine stress incontinence) is a urodynamic diagnosis where there is involuntary leakage of urine during increased abdominal pressure, in the absence of a detrusor contraction.

Vesicourethral voiding dysfunction

Abnormal detrusor activity

The detrusor muscle may be underactive or non-contractile, leading to a prolonged void or failure to achieve complete bladder emptying.

Abnormal urethral function

Abnormal urethral function may be either caused by obstruction, which may occur at any point between bladder neck and external urethral meatus (such as an enlarged prostate or urethral stricture), or by urethral overactivity. *Bladder outlet obstruction* is the generic term for obstruction during voiding and is characterized by increased detrusor pressure and reduced urine flow rate demonstrated by urodynamic pressure or flow studies. *Dysfunctional voiding* is an intermittent or fluctuating flow rate caused by involuntary contractions of the periurethral striated muscles in neurologically normal individuals. *Detrusor sphincter dyssynergia* is where a detrusor contraction occurs concurrently with an involuntary contraction of the urethral or periurethral striated muscles; this typically occurs in patients with suprasacral lesions of the spinal cord and is uncommon in lesions of the lower cord. *Non-relaxing urethral sphincter obstruction* usually occurs in patients with sacral or infrasacral lesions of the cord and is characterized by a non-relaxing, obstructing urethra, resulting in reduced urine flow.[5]

THE NEUROGENIC BLADDER AND SPINAL CORD INJURY

Neurological conditions can affect the innervation of both the bladder and the urethra, and can therefore affect both storage and voiding functions. A variety of conditions can cause such problems, for example strokes, Parkinson's disease, multiple sclerosis, spinal cord injury and spina bifida. In spinal cord injury, lower urinary tract dysfunction is a major cause of late morbidity and mortality.[6] Bladder function may also be affected by major pelvic surgery, and may take weeks or months to recover. Management of these patients must take into account their locomotor disability to find the best solutions for their problems.

In the acute phase after spinal cord injury, there is a period of spinal shock lasting several weeks, where there is no reflex activity and the bladder is unable to contract. Bladder drainage by intermittent catheterization is preferred, although suprapubic or indwelling urethral catheters may be used.[7] Reflex contractions return after 6–12 weeks.

AIMS OF TREATMENT

In many neurological conditions the low-pressure storage function of the bladder is lost, leading to high intravesical pressures and reflux into the upper tracts. If the bladder fails to empty completely or if an indwelling catheter is present, there will be an increased risk of stone formation. All these factors predispose to urinary infection. Recurrent reflux and infection can result in renal damage. Urinary incontinence may also be a problem as a result of overflow incontinence or neurogenic detrusor overactivity. It is therefore important to assess both the bladder and sphincter function using videourodynamics.[8]

The main aims of treatment are:

- protection of the upper tracts and renal function; and
- to achieve social continence.

REFERENCES

6. Wyndaele JJ. Paraplegia 1995; 33: 305–307
7. Wyndaele JJ, Madersbacher H, Kovindha A. Spinal Cord 2001; 39: 294–300
8. Shenot P, Rivas D, Watanabe T et al. Neurourol Urodynamics 1998; 17: 25–29

TREATMENT OPTIONS FOR THE NEUROGENIC BLADDER

Conservative measures

Drug treatment

Neurogenic detrusor overactivity is one of the commonest problems. This may be improved by the use of oral anti-cholinergic agents combined with bladder emptying by clean intermittent self-catheterization.[9] The goal is to inhibit detrusor muscular overactivity. The first anticholinergic used was oxybutynin, which is effective but compliance is often poor because of the high incidence of side effects. Newer agents, such as tolterodine, trospium and a long-acting oxybutynin preparation, have similar efficacy with reduced side effects.[10] Intravesical oxybutynin and capsaicin have also been used to treat neurogenic overactivity, with some success.[9]

Clean intermittent self-catheterization

Clean intermittent self-catheterization is indicated in cases with detrusor underactivity or ineffective bladder emptying because of detrusor sphincter dyssynergia. Self-catheterization should achieve complete bladder emptying and should be carried out at regular intervals. This reduces the risks and consequences of infection, and an aseptic technique is not necessary. The patient must be sufficiently mobile and have the manual dexterity to be able to perform the procedure.[1]

Indwelling catheter

This has advantages for some patients and their carers, but eventually there may be many problems with infection, catheter blockage and catheter expulsion. Bladder stones and squamous cancers may develop later.[11] In men and women urethral erosion can occur, and in women this can lead to dilatation of the urethra with catheter expulsion and profound incontinence. Inserting a larger catheter merely exacerbates this problem. If an indwelling catheter is essential then a suprapubic catheter is preferable. Drinking two glasses of cranberry juice a day appears to reduce catheter complications.

Condom catheters

Condom catheters can be useful in male patients troubled with incontinence. They collect urine into an external device, which can give better hygienic control as well as a better quality of life. They are not suitable in all patients, particularly those with small or retractile penises, and they can lead to problems with skin damage and latex allergy.[7]

Surgical treatments

Despite conservative measures, for some patients results remain poor. They may continue to suffer incontinence or retention, and rising bladder pressures may threaten the upper tracts. In these patients operations may be considered.

Bladder surgery

In the presence of detrusor overactivity or decreased bladder compliance, the aims are to increase bladder capacity or lower the intravesical pressure. In enterocystoplasty a segment of detubularized bowel[12] on its pedicle is used to either augment the bladder (such as the 'clam' procedure; Fig. 36.4) or, if this is impossible, to replace it with a 'neobladder' such as the Studer pouch (Fig. 36.5).[13] Following enterocystoplasty, bladder emptying may be ineffective and intermittent catheterization may be necessary. Other complications include excessive mucus

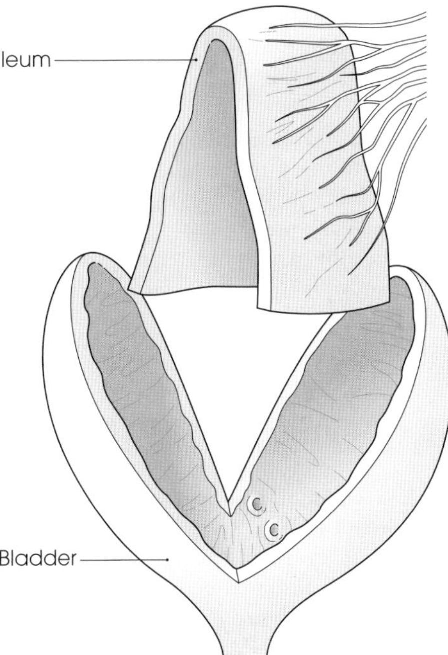

Figure 36.4 The 'clam' augmentation cystoplasty. The bladder must be almost completely bivalved and the correct length of opened-out ileum used. It is wise to protect the ureters with catheters while suturing the lower part of the bladder.

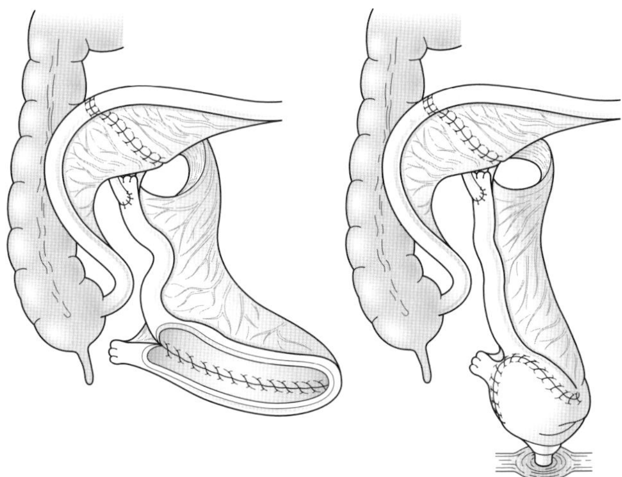

Figure 36.5 A segment of the ileum approximately 60 cm long is isolated and formed into a pouch using the method described by Studer.

production, stone formation, and a metabolic acidosis from reabsorption of urine. In young patients there is impairment of bone formation and mineralization. Late development of malignant tumours has been described, and this risk appears

REFERENCES

9. Madersbacher H. Curr Opin Urol 1999; 9: 303–309
10. Dmochowski RR, Appoll RA. Advancements in pharmacologic management of the overactive bladder. Urology 2000; 56(6 Suppl 1): 41–49
11. Kohler-Ockmore J, Feneley RC. Br J Urol 1996; 77: 347–351
12. Greenwell TJ, Venn SN, Mundy AR. BJU Int 2001; 88: 511–525
13. Studer U. In: Fitzpatrick J, Krane R (eds). The Bladder. Churchill Livingstone, Edinburgh, 1995: 461–474

greater if colon is used instead of ileum.[14,15] Yearly flexible cystoscopy after 10 years is therefore advised.

Outlet surgery

Incision of the external sphincter or bladder neck can be used when bladder outlet obstruction is a problem. This renders the patient incontinent, but in some patients this option combined with condom drainage may still be preferable.

Implantation of an artificial urinary sphincter (Fig. 36.6) may be used if urethral pressure is very low and severe stress incontinence is a problem. The main complications are erosion into the urethra, infection and mechanical failure.

INCONTINENCE OF URINE

Urinary incontinence is a common and distressing problem. It is defined as an involuntary leakage of urine. Stress urinary incontinence occurs on effort, exertion, sneezing or coughing. Urge urinary incontinence is accompanied or immediately preceded by a sudden, compelling desire to pass urine, which is difficult to defer.[5]

INCONTINENCE IN CHILDREN

Few children are investigated for incontinence before the age of 5 years. Recurrent urinary infections and persistent bedwetting (nocturnal enuresis), with or without daytime symptoms suggestive of detrusor overactivity, are the main reasons for referral. Behavioural modification, including star charts and enuresis alarms, together with pharmacotherapy, including analogues of antidiuretic hormone and antimuscarinic drugs, are the mainstays of conservative treatment.[16]

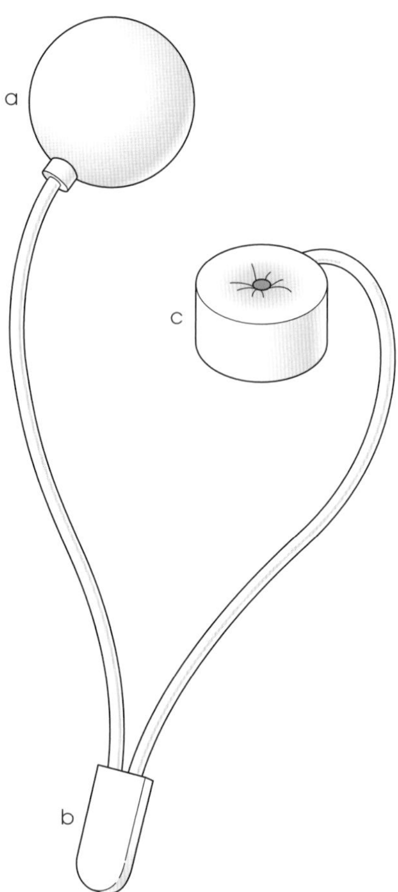

Figure 36.6 The AMS artificial urinary sphincter. This has three main components; the reservoir (**a**) contains the fluid at a set pressure. The control valve and pump (**b**) is squeezed to empty the cuff (**c**), which is usually placed around the bladder neck but can be placed around the bulbar urethra.

INCONTINENCE IN MEN

Incontinence is largely a condition of elderly men and commonly occurs as urge incontinence or postmicturition dribble. A small proportion of men undergoing prostatectomy have postoperative incontinence, which may be stress incontinence secondary to sphincter damage, urge incontinence associated with detrusor overactivity, or 'overflow' incontinence associated with chronic retention. Postmicturition dribble can be treated by pelvic floor exercises and manual compression of the bulbar urethra behind the scrotum. Urge incontinence associated with detrusor overactivity can often be improved or alleviated by bladder training, pelvic floor exercises, reduction in caffeine intake, and anticholinergic drugs.[16] Stress incontinence associated with sphincter weakness may improve with pelvic floor exercises over a period of months but may require the placement of an artificial urinary sphincter. Incontinence associated with chronic retention may be treated with clean intermittent self-catheterization or an indwelling catheter.

INCONTINENCE IN WOMEN

The causes of incontinence in women differ markedly between developed and less developed countries. In less well off countries such as those in sub-Saharan Africa, incontinence is commonly the result of parturition injury leading to urinary fistulae. In more developed countries many women complain of stress and urge incontinence. History taking and physical examination should classify women as having stress, urge or mixed incontinence. The patient's oestrogen status should be assessed by examination of the perineum and introitus, and any deficiency corrected with topical oestrogen preparations. Urinary infection should be treated.

Conservative management includes the suggestion to lose weight, cease smoking, and regulate fluid and food intake. Pelvic floor exercises are recommended for stress incontinence. For urge incontinence pelvic floor exercises, bladder training, reduction in caffeine intake, and antimuscarinic drugs are tried.[17]

Surgery may be considered for women with stress incontinence in whom conservative treatment has failed. The aims of continence surgery in women are to stabilize the bladder neck, support the midurethra or increase urethral resistance. This can be done using a variety of procedures, such as injection of urethral bulking agents, open colposuspension, sling operations, and the insertion of an artificial urinary sphincter. New techniques such as laparoscopic colposuspension and tension-free vaginal tape are being evaluated in randomized controlled trials. Urethral bulking agents are suitable for those with mild stress incontinence and those unfit for surgery. Laparoscopic

REFERENCES

14. Hohenfellner M, Dahms S, Pfitzenmaier J et al. Curr Opin Urol 1999; 9: 309–314
15. Mast P, Hoebeke P, Wyndaele JJ et al. Paraplegia 1995; 33: 560–564
16. Abrams P, Lowry S, Wein A et al. Lancet 2000; 355: 2153–2158
17. Burton G. Neurourol Urodynamics 1999; 18: 295–296

colposuspension is less invasive compared with an open procedure; however, it has been shown to be about 20% less successful.[17,18] The less invasive needle suspension procedure also appears less effective, in the long term, than open operations but offers the advantages of a reduced morbidity and recovery time.

In detrusor overactivity with associated incontinence, clam enterocystoplasty is highly effective at abolishing contractions and may be considered if conservative treatments have failed. The risks of major abdominal surgery and long-term complications – such as infection, mucus production and need for self catheterization – need, however, to be balanced against the benefits of curing urgency and urge incontinence. Failure rates of bladder augmentation are higher in idiopathic detrusor overactivity than in neurogenic patients.[12] Detrusor myomectomy (autoaugmentation) consists of incising and removing the bladder muscle to allow the bladder mucosa to form a pseudo-diverticulum. This procedure also appears to be more successful in neurogenic patients. Sacral nerve neuromodulation may also be used in patients with detrusor overactivity that has failed to respond to pharmacotherapy. This may be applied and tested by a variety of non-invasive techniques before invasive sacral nerve stimulation of S3 is considered.[19]

INJURY TO THE BLADDER

Bladder injury may be traumatic, blunt, penetrating or iatrogenic. Traumatic injury to the bladder is uncommon but is usually associated with significant morbidity and mortality related to concurrent severe injuries, such as abdominal injuries or pelvic fracture.

Bladder rupture may be classified as intraperitoneal or extraperitoneal. Extraperitoneal rupture, associated with pelvic fracture, usually occurs at the anterolateral aspect of the bladder in the region of the bladder neck. Intraperitoneal ruptures classically consist of a tear in the dome of the bladder.[20] Bladder rupture should be suspected in patients with suprapubic tenderness, an inability to urinate, or macroscopic (rarely microscopic) haematuria. If a bladder rupture is suspected, the entire urinary tract should be assessed with an intravenous urogram, and the bladder itself should be assessed by ascending cystourethrogram.

Intraperitoneal bladder perforations resulting from external trauma should be managed by open exploration and repair.[20] Some extraperitoneal ruptures may be treated conservatively with catheter drainage and broad-spectrum antibiotics; however, patients with severe haematuria or those undergoing laparotomy for concurrent injury should undergo surgical closure.[21]

A more common form of bladder perforation is following transurethral resection of bladder tumours. These are usually extraperitoneal and can be treated conservatively with antibiotics and catheter drainage. Intraperitoneal perforations usually require surgical exploration and closure.

VESICAL FISTULAE

Fistulae of the bladder involve the genital or gastrointestinal tracts. The commonest examples of these are vesicovaginal and colovesical fistulae.

Vesicovaginal fistulae occur as the result of surgical or obstetric trauma or from pelvic irradiation for malignant disease. Continuous urinary incontinence is the usual presenting symptom. The diagnosis may be made on physical examination, intravenous urography, cystogram, and cystoscopy and retrograde pyelography. Fistulae resulting from obstetric or surgical trauma may be primarily repaired with omental interposition, either by a vaginal or an abdominal route. Urinary diversion should be considered when fistulae are associated with pelvic irradiation; primary healing may not be possible.

Vesicouterine fistulae are an uncommon complication of caesarean section.[22] Patients present with urinary incontinence with or without 'menouria' (Youssef's syndrome).[23]

Colovesical fistulae are usually related to pathology arising in the large bowel, such as diverticular disease, colonic carcinoma and Crohn's disease. Patients usually present with recurrent urinary tract infections and may complain of pneumaturia. Investigation is by endoscopy and contrast radiology of both the urinary tract and the colon. Treatment is by surgical exploration and repair, with resection of the diseased bowel, closure of the bladder defect, and omental interposition.

BLADDER CALCULI

Bladder stones are now rare in the UK. They occur in three main groups of patients: children in developing countries, patients with bladder outlet obstruction, and those who have undergone bladder reconstruction or augmentation.

CHILDREN IN DEVELOPING COUNTRIES

The incidence in this group is thought to be related to malnutrition. The stones seen in this group tend to be of ammonium acid urate or calcium oxalate.

BLADDER OUTLET OBSTRUCTION

Obstruction may be caused by prostatic enlargement, urethral stricture or neurogenic problems. Stones develop because of urinary stasis in association with a high urinary salt concentration. Stasis may also lead to chronic infection with urease-producing organisms and the development of 'infection stones'.

POST BLADDER RECONSTRUCTION OR AUGMENTATION

Where bowel segments are used mucus production continues, and this may form a nidus for stone formation. These also tend to be infection stones.[24]

Any stone passed from the upper tracts may form a nidus for bladder stone formation. Equally, any foreign body introduced by the patient or iatrogenically (suture material or the eggshell calculus formed around the balloon of an indwelling catheter) may present a nidus for further stone formation.

REFERENCES

18. Su T, Wang K, Hsu C et al. Acta Obstet Gynaecol Scand 1997; 76: 576–582
19. Abrams P, Cardozo L, Khoury S et al (eds). Incontinence: 2nd International Consultation on Incontinence. 2nd edn. Health Publications, London, 2002
20. Bodner DR, Selzman AA, Spirnak JP. Semin Urol 1995; 13: 62–65
21. Kotkin L, Koch MO. J Trauma 1995; 38: 895–898
22. Tancer M. Obstet Gynaecol Surg 1986; 41: 73
23. Youssef A. Am J Obstet Gynaecol 1957; 73: 759
24. Westenberg A, Harper M, Zafirakis H et al. Hosp Med 2002; 63: 34–41

Bladder calculi usually present with frequency and urgency, with or without frank haematuria. There may also be suprapubic pain or penile tip pain from a stone sitting against the trigone. Stones impacting in the bladder neck may cause interruption of urine flow or retention of urine. Stones in the bladder are often symptomless.

The diagnosis of a bladder stone may be made on ultrasound, plain abdominal radiograph, an intravenous urogram or cystoscopy. Further investigation should be directed towards the underlying cause, such as obstruction, and urine should be sent for culture.[25]

Treatment of the bladder calculus depends on its size. Small stones may be removed endoscopically via the urethra. Larger stones may be fragmented using either a stone punch or a mechanical, ultrasonic or laser lithotripter. Huge stones are not amenable to endoscopic removal and may have to be removed by open cystotomy. Treatment of any underlying cause should also be addressed.

BLADDER DIVERTICULA

Bladder diverticula may be either congenital or acquired. True congenital diverticula are rare, often situated close to a ureteric orifice, and are not associated with trabeculation. They are usually symptomless but if large can result in stasis, infection, hydronephrosis or reflux, and are treated by diverticulectomy, often combined with ureteric reimplantation.[25]

Acquired diverticula occur as a result of increased intravesical pressure, most commonly associated with bladder outlet obstruction[26] or detrusor overactivity against a closed sphincter.[27] These diverticula may be single or multiple, of variable size, and are composed of bladder mucosa with no overlying muscle layer. Large diverticula may cause incomplete bladder emptying, frequency and infection. They should be excised if they are causing symptoms, and the underlying cause also needs to be treated.

Approximately 4% of bladder diverticula undergo malignant change,[28] and the management of these tumours may be complicated. Transurethral resection may result in bladder perforation because of the absence of a muscle layer in the wall of the diverticulum. Solitary tumours in large diverticula may be excised as part of a partial cystectomy, but the risk of recurrence is high, particularly in invasive, poorly differentiated tumours.

URINARY INFECTION AND INFECTIVE CYSTITIS

Bladder infection may result from colonic bacteria, mycobacteria, viruses, fungi and parasites. Symptoms of urinary infection include dysuria, frequency, urgency, nocturia, incontinence, suprapubic or pelvic pain, and occasionally macroscopic haematuria. Infection may not be associated with any symptoms. Urinalysis usually shows the presence of pyuria and often haematuria. The diagnosis is usually confirmed by urine microscopy and culture. In the majority of cases the responsible organism is *Escherichia coli*, a member of the Enterobactericeae, *Staphylococcus saprophyticus* or an enterococcus (see Ch. 4 for treatment).[29]

URINARY INFECTION IN CHILDHOOD

Urinary infection may present in neonates and young children, with fever, vomiting and feeding problems. Up to 3 months it is more common in male infants. Above 1 year it is nine times more common in girls.[30] At least 8% of girls develop an overt infection in childhood compared with only 1–2% of boys.[31] Clean catch urine specimens may be difficult to obtain in children and are often contaminated; suprapubic aspiration or catheterization may be needed. Children presenting with a proven urinary tract infection for the first time should be investigated for any underlying pathology or upper tract anatomical abnormality. Approximately half will have no significant abnormality.[32] Vesicoureteric reflux is diagnosed in 25–50% of children with infection and is more frequent in those under the age of 1 year.[30] Other abnormalities include ureteroceles and stones. Ultrasound is the imaging method of choice,[33] and in children with reflux a voiding cystourethrogram enables grading of the reflux and definition of the anatomy.[34] Recurrent infections, particularly in young children, may lead to renal scarring, usually as a result of reflux.

Vesicoureteric reflux

Vesicoureteric reflux is the retrograde flow of urine from the bladder into the ureter and usually the pelvicalyceal system. It provides a pathway for the ascent of bacteria from the bladder to the kidney, and results in an aliquot of stagnant urine remaining in the urinary tract after voiding.[35] Reflux occurs in 1–2% of apparently healthy children. In those with infection approximately 30% have radiological evidence of renal scarring, which is secondary to congenital dysplasia, postinfection damage, or both. This ‘reflux nephropathy’ is a major cause of hypertension in children and young adults, and can lead to chronic renal failure.[36] Acquired reflux is the result of bladder outlet obstruction or a neuropathic bladder.

Reflux may be graded according to its severity. Grading systems use the degree of dilatation of the ureter, the pelvicalyceal system and the calyceal fornices (Fig. 36.7).[37] Investigation is with a voiding cystourethrogram.

Reflux has a tendency to resolve with time, although the rate of resolution is dependent on its grade. Low-grade reflux has a resolution rate of 85%, but for severe reflux the figure may be less than half this. The grade also tends to improve with time.

The main aim of treatment is to prevent secondary pyelonephritis. This may be achieved either with long-term prescription of antibiotics or with surgical reimplantation of the ureters. Studies have shown little difference in outcome between these treatment options.

REFERENCES

25. Pengelly A. In: Fitzpatrick J, Krane R (eds). The Bladder. Churchill Livingstone, Edinburgh, 1995: 183–187
26. Fox M, Power R, Bruce A. Br J Urol 1962; 34: 286–298
27. Gillon G, Nissenkorn I, Servadio C. Eur Urol 1988; 14: 34–36
28. Peterson L, Paulson D, Glenn J. J Urol 1973; 110: 62–68
29. Ronald AR. Med Clin North Am 1984; 68: 334
30. Shapiro E, Elder J. Urol Clin North Am 1998; 4: 725–734
31. Larcombe J. Br Med J 1999; 319: 1173–1175
32. Smellie JM, Normand IC, Katz G. Kidney Int 1981; 20: 717–722
33. Kangarloo H, Gold R, Fine R et al. Radiology 1985; 154: 367
34. Riccabona M. Curr Opin Urol 2000; 10: 25–28
35. Lebowitz R. J Urol 1992; 148: 1640–1642
36. Smellie JM, Barratt TM, Chantler C et al. Lancet 2001; 357: 1329–1333
37. Lebowitz R, Olbing H, Parkkulainen K et al. Paediatr Radiol 1985; 15: 105

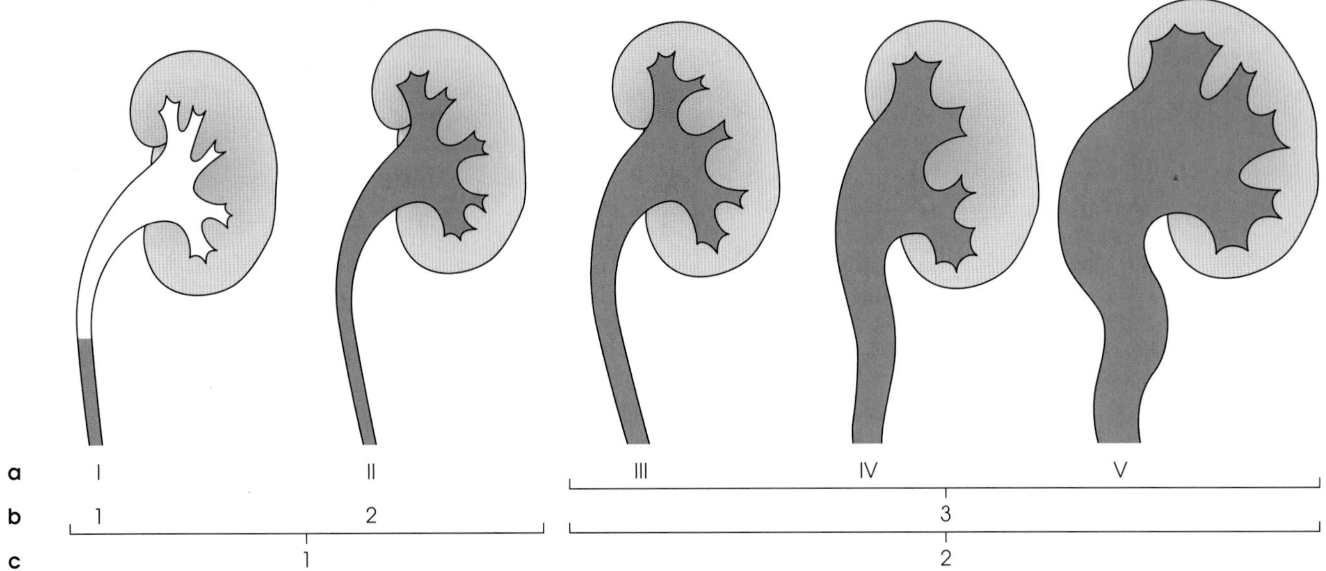

Figure 36.7 The grading of vesicoureteric reflux. **(a)** The five grades of the International Reflux Study Committee. **(b)** The three grades of the Medical Research Council Bacteriuria Committee. **(c)** The two grades according to calibre of the ureters (normal and dilated). The black area shows the distance to which urine refluxes.

URINARY INFECTION IN ADULTS

Bacterial infection is more common in women and affects a fifth of women during their lifetime.[38] In women urinary infection is less likely to be secondary to a functional or anatomical abnormality. It rarely causes severe upper tract complications, and only recurrent infections need be investigated. In men, however, all urinary tract infections should be investigated to exclude an underlying cause. Common causes are bladder outlet obstruction, instrumentation, congenital abnormalities, tumours, stones and foreign bodies. Investigation should include urinary tract ultrasound, which can provide information on the whole urinary tract. Measurement of the flow rate should be made in all. Cystoscopy is indicated if there is suspicion of a tumour, and urodynamics if obstruction or bladder neuropathy is suspected.

Nosocomial infection

The urinary tract is responsible for approximately 40% of nosocomial infections,[39] and is the most common source of infection acquired in both hospitals and nursing homes; it is usually associated with catheterization.[40] The duration of catheterization is the most important risk factor for the development of catheter-associated bacteriuria.[41]

Organisms may enter the urinary tract either at the time of catheterization or by ascending into the bladder via the lumen of the drainage system. Bacteria may also enter between the external catheter surface and the urethral mucosa. Organisms survive in the catheterized urinary tract because a biofilm develops over the catheter surface or when a long-term catheter becomes encrusted even in the presence of antibiotics.[42]

To prevent bacteriuria, the catheter drainage system should remain closed and urine should be drained via the bag outlet. All catheters should be removed as soon as possible.[40]

TUBERCULOUS CYSTITIS

The worldwide prevalence of tuberculosis has remained almost unchanged in the past century. Despite a decrease in industrialized countries there has been an increase in the developing world. There is also an increased prevalence associated with HIV infection. Genitourinary tuberculosis is the commonest extrapulmonary manifestation of the disease.[43]

Tuberculous cystitis presents with the usual features of cystitis (frequency and dysuria) and storage symptoms, or prostatitis or epididymitis in men.[44] There may also be systemic symptoms, such as fever, weight loss and sweats, or a previous history of tuberculous infection. Tuberculous cystitis always results from downward spread of renal mycobacteria.

A midstream urine specimen often shows a sterile pyuria, and at least three complete early morning samples should be sent for culture. Cystoscopy may aid diagnosis. The typical appearance is of a contracted erythematous bladder, with an oedematous and ulcerated wall with bullous granulations. Tubercles may be seen as yellow elevated spots. These changes are usually most marked around the ureteric orifices.

Management of genitourinary tuberculosis is by an appropriate multiple drug regimen of antibiotics given for 6–9 months. The end result of tuberculous cystitis may be a severely contracted bladder requiring an augmentation cystoplasty or a urinary diversion.

REFERENCES

38. Johnson J, Stamm W. Ann Intern Med 1989; 111: 906
39. Paradisi F, Corti G, Mangani V. Crit Care Clin 1998; 14: 165–180
40. Warren JW. Int J Antimicrob Agents 2001; 17: 299–303
41. Platt R, Polk B, Murdock B et al. Am J Epidemiol 1986; 124: 977–985
42. Liedl B. Curr Opin Urol 2001; 11: 75–79
43. Lenk S, Schroeder J. Curr Opin Urol 2001; 11: 93–96
44. Wechsler H, Westfall M, Latimer J. J Urol 1960; 83: 801

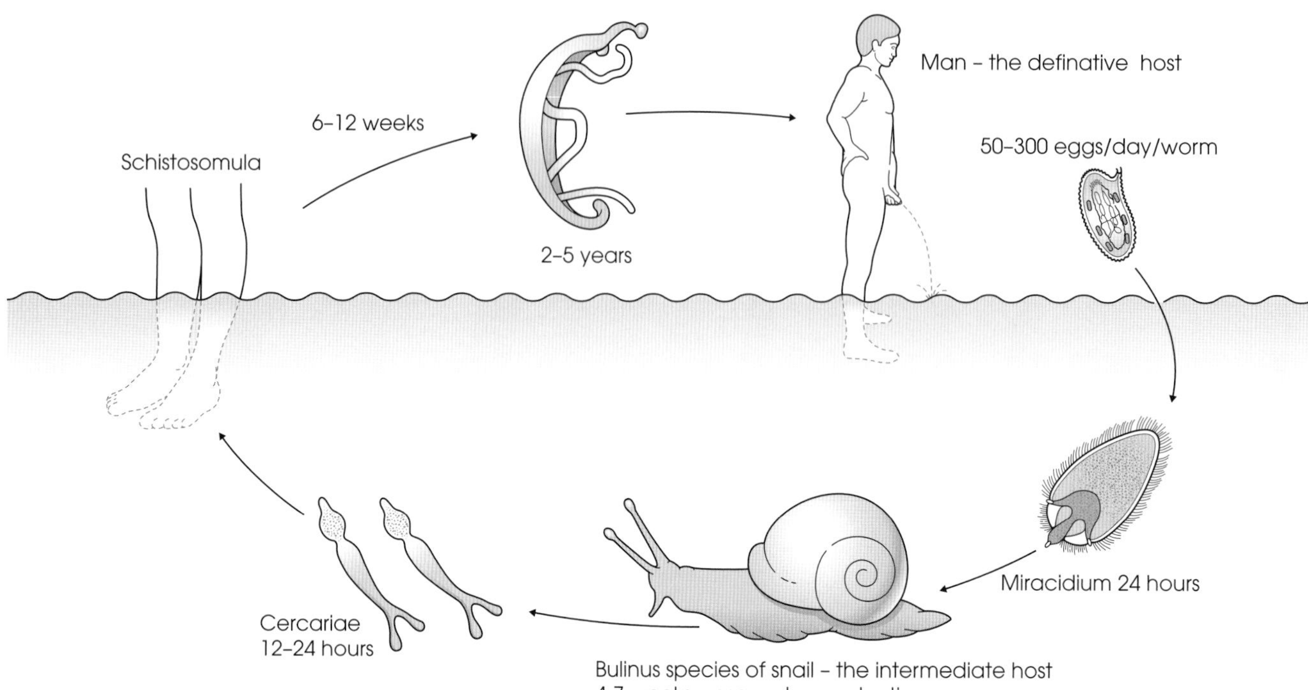

Figure 36.8 The life cycle of *Schistosoma haematobium.*

BILHARZIA OF THE BLADDER

EPIDEMIOLOGY

After malaria, schistosomiasis is the second most prevalent human parasitic disease. It affects an estimated 200 million people worldwide, with the main endemic areas being in Africa and the Middle East.[45,46] It is caused by infestation with digenetic parasitic trematodes (flatworms and flukes). Five species infect humans, the most important being *Schistosoma japonicum*, *S. mansoni* and *S. haematobium*. *Schistosoma haematobium* is almost entirely responsible for urinary bilharzia.

LIFE CYCLE

The *S. haematobium* worms live in the perivesical venous plexus in humans, where they undergo sexual reproduction. The female lays 200–500 eggs a day for 3–6 years in the vesical and pelvic venules.[47] The eggs then migrate into the lumen of the bladder and are excreted in the urine. When the eggs enter fresh water they hatch into miracidia. The miracidia are short-lived and must enter the intermediate host, the *Bulinus* species of freshwater snail. The miracidia undergo asexual reproduction via successive sporocyst stages to become cerceriae. The cerceriae are shed by the snail and penetrate the unbroken skin of the definitive human host. When they fail to do this within a few hours the cerceriae exhaust their energy supplies and die. At penetration the cerceriae become schistosomula and migrate through the portal vein to end up as mature worms in the pelvic veins after 5–6 weeks (Fig. 36.8).

PATHOLOGY

The bladder pathology represents a reaction of the host against deposition of schistosomal eggs. These elicit a granulomatous inflammatory reaction in the bladder wall. Atrophic changes lead to ulceration of the urothelium, and hyperplasia results in polypoid cystitis. Squamous metaplasia commonly occurs, and leukoplakia, dysplasia, carcinoma in situ and invasive cancer may develop as a result of chronic irritation. Eggs that die before they are shed calcify and become covered with epithelium. This results in sandy patches, which are visible cystoscopically. The associated calcification may be seen on plain X-ray. A late complication of the chronic inflammation is fibrosis, which leads to a contracted, non-compliant bladder and strictures of the ureters and urethra. Secondary bacterial infection is almost invariable, and this contributes greatly to the morbidity of the condition, with ascending infection of the upper tracts leading to deterioration in renal function.

Urinary bilharzia is associated with a raised incidence of bladder cancer, particularly squamous cell carcinomas. Carcinogenesis is a multistep process; tumours originate in the areas of highest egg burden within the bladder, metaplastic change alters the histological differentiation into squamous cell tumours, and secondary bacterial infection produces carcinogenic nitrosamines from nitrates and nitrites in urine.[47]

CLINICAL FEATURES

Urinary schistosomiasis may progress through five clinical stages: swimmer's itch, followed by acute, active, chronic active and finally chronic inactive schistosomiasis.

REFERENCES

45. Bichler KH, Feil G, Zumbragel A et al. Curr Opin Urol 2001; 11: 97–101
46. Dunne DW, Hagan P, Abath FG. Lancet 1995; 345: 1488–1491
47. Hazen Smith J, von Lichtenberg F. In: Walsh P et al (eds). Campbell's Urology. WB Saunders, Philadelphia, 1998: 733–778

Swimmer's itch

Swimmer's itch is a result of cercarial penetration from infested fresh water into the human host.

Acute schistosomiasis

Also known as Katayama fever, acute schistosomiasis is less commonly found in endemic populations. It causes fever, lymphadenopathy, splenomegaly, eosinophilia and urticaria. Katayama fever corresponds with egg laying and occurs at about 3–9 weeks, although this may be delayed. It is the result of a profound antibody response generated by the host.

Active schistosomiasis

This stage occurs as the eggs are shed into the bladder and the urine, and gives rise to the classic features of active bilharziasis, namely urinary frequency, dysuria and terminal haematuria.

Chronic active schistosomiasis

After several years of active infection a more quiescent phase may be reached. Although the clinical disease is not apparent, silent fibrotic change may occur, leading to irreversible damage to bladder and ureters with associated upper tract obstruction.

Chronic inactive schistosomiasis

Viable eggs are no longer detected in the urine, and most of the features of this stage are those of the long-term sequelae of the infection, such as obstructive uropathy with or without superadded infection and urothelial cancer.

DIAGNOSIS

The presence of schistosomal eggs in the urine is diagnostic of infection. In the presence of a low infective load, however, no abnormalities may be present in the urine, and infection may be diagnosed only on bladder biopsy. In chronic infection, where egg excretion is reduced or absent, immunological, radiographic and cystoscopic diagnosis may be more accurate.

Radiographic investigation should include a plain abdominal radiograph, which may reveal calcification within the urinary tract, and intravenous urography to look for the presence of ureteric obstruction. Cystoscopic findings vary but include the presence of tubercles, polyps, sandy patches, ulcers, cystitis cystica, leukoplakia and carcinoma in situ.

TREATMENT

Medical treatment

The two main antimicrobials used in the treatment of schistosomiasis are metrifonate and praziquantel. They are cheap, well tolerated and effective. They are given in short or single-dose courses. Metrifonate is effective against *S. haematobium* but not against *S. mansoni* or *S. japonicum*. Praziquantel, however, is effective against all three species and is the drug of choice.

Surgical treatment

A large number of surgical procedures are used to treat the various complications of urinary schistosomiasis. Functional bladder outlet obstruction may be treated by urethral dilatation or transurethral resection of prostate; bladder contractions by ileocystoplasty or urinary diversion; ureteric stricture by dilatation, reimplantation or urinary diversion; and bladder carcinoma by radical cystectomy with or without orthotopic bladder substitution.

NON-INFECTIVE CYSTITIS

INTERSTITIAL CYSTITIS

Interstitial cystitis is a chronic and debilitating inflammatory condition of the bladder leading to storage urinary symptoms associated with pelvic and perineal pain.[48] Its reported prevalence varies between four and 70 per 100 000 female patients. It is between six and nine times more common in women, and there is an increasing prevalence with age. Some chronic pelvic pain syndromes in women and chronic prostatitis and prostadynia in men may be part of the same disease process.[49]

The pathogenesis of the condition is not known and may well be multifactorial. Alteration in bacterial flora, mast cell activation, increased permeability in bladder epithelial cells, and an abnormal inflammatory response have all been suggested as possible aetiological factors.[50]

The diagnosis is made by excluding other diseases and may be aided by cystoscopy. Typical cystoscopic findings include bladder inflammation, glomerulations, submucosal haemorrhages and stellate ulcers (Hunner's ulcers). There is a reduced bladder capacity and distension, even under light anaesthesia, is painful, even though it may be helpful therapeutically. The bladder histology may show an inflammatory infiltrate, increased fibrosis, and an increase in mast cell numbers. The potassium sensitivity test is a minimally invasive outpatient diagnostic test advocated by some, and urodynamic testing may be useful to exclude detrusor overactivity.[51]

A large number of conservative treatments have been described, with variable success. Simple hydrodistension of the bladder at the time of cystoscopy may help to relieve symptoms in the short term. Oral amitriptyline and sodium pentosan polysulfate have both been used with some success, as has intravesical instillation of dimethyl sulfoxide (DMSO), lidocaine (lignocaine) with dexamethasone and bacillus Calmette–Guérin (BCG).[50] Discrete areas of disease may be treated by transurethral resection or fulguration. In less than 10% of patients, cystectomy with urinary diversion or orthotopic bladder substitution is required for intractable symptoms or failed medical treatment.[50]

EOSINOPHILIC CYSTITIS

Eosinophilic cystitis is rare, being roughly as common in women as in men.[52] It is of uncertain aetiology, although infection, parasitic infestation, and reaction to food and drug allergens have all been implicated. The clinical presentation varies between mild bladder involvement with associated storage symptoms, haematuria and suprapubic pain with erythematous bladder lesions, to serious, painful, haemorrhagic masses and associated upper tract obstruction.[53] Biopsy shows a heavy eosinophilic infiltration of the bladder wall. The mainstays of treatment are oral antihistamines, non-steroidal anti-inflammatory drugs and steroids. Antibiotics should be used if secondary infection is present. In the majority of cases the course of the disease is benign, but it can occasionally

REFERENCES

48. Wesselmann U. Interstitial cystitis: a chronic visceral pain syndrome. Urology 2001; 57(6 Suppl 2): 32–39
49. Kusek JW, Nyberg LM. Urology 2001; 57 (Suppl 1): 95–99
50. Sant GR, Theoharides TC. Curr Opin Urol 1999; 9: 297–302
51. Sant GR, Hanno P. Urology 2001; 57 (Suppl 6A): 82–88
52. van den Ouden D. Eur Urol 2000; 37: 386–394
53. Itano NM, Malek RS. J Urol 2001; 165: 805–807

lead to serious progressive bladder disease with upper tract deterioration.[53]

RADIATION CYSTITIS

Radiation cystitis may result if the bladder is included in a field of radiation, most often given for treatment of prostate or cervical cancer. Complications may be early or late, and range from an acute cystitis with associated storage symptoms, dysuria and sometimes haematuria, to fibrosis of the bladder and fistula formation. Haematuria may be microscopic or severe. Cystoscopic findings include fibrotic change, haemorrhagic cystitis and telangiectasia. Persistent bleeding may be treated with transurethral diathermy but may require instillation of intravesical alum or silver nitrate. Occasionally salvage cystectomy is required for severe bleeding. Salvage cystectomy or urinary diversion may also be required in cases of a severely fibrotic and contracted bladder.

CYCLOPHOSPHAMIDE CYSTITIS

This condition is caused by a metabolite of cyclophosphamide, acrolein, which is an aldehyde that is toxic to the bladder urothelium. Severe haemorrhagic cystitis may result, as can fibrosis of the bladder, causing storage symptoms. Oral cyclophosphamide treatment is less likely to cause severe cystitis than the intravenous drug. Use of mesna (2-mercaptoethane sulfonate) is also protective. Secondary bladder cancer may occur many years after cessation of treatment.[54]

RESPONSES OF THE BLADDER TO INJURY AND INFLAMMATION

Cystitis cystica and *cystitis glandularis* result from recurrent and chronic bladder infection. Subepithelial islands of transitional cells degenerate and invaginate to form cysts, which may be visible on cystoscopy. Proliferation in the walls of these cysts gives a more glandular appearance called cystitis glandularis. These conditions are benign and no treatment is required.

Non-keratinizing squamous metaplasia, also called pseudomembranous trigonitis, is a common and normal finding in women, and is entirely benign. Cystoscopically it is visible as raised patches over the trigone. *Keratinized squamous metaplasia* appears as white patches and is premalignant.

Malakoplakia is a granulomatous process usually associated with chronic infection with *E. coli*. There may be associated storage symptoms; endoscopic changes vary from small brown patches to a large granulomatous mass. Treatment is with a long course of intracellular antibiotics, such as trimethoprim (see Ch. 4).

Nephrogenic adenoma is a metaplastic change giving rise to red patches in the bladder. These may have a papillary appearance and can be mistaken for cancer. They usually occur after trauma. Rarely, they may undergo malignant change.

Chronic granulomas usually contain a foreign body, and again may be mistaken for cancers. Some are amenable to endoscopic resection, but others require complete excision.[1,54]

CARCINOMA OF THE BLADDER

INCIDENCE

Bladder cancer is the commonest tumour of the urinary tract. It is the fifth most common malignancy in Europe and the fourth commonest in the USA.[55] It accounts for 6–8% of all malignancies in males and 2–3% of those in females. It has a peak incidence during the sixth and seventh decades of life, although it is becoming increasingly prevalent in younger patients.[56] It is approximately twice as common in the white population as in the black population, although black people are more likely to present with advanced disease.[57]

AETIOLOGY

Bladder cancer is strongly linked to occupational and environmental exposure to chemicals. The development of the disease is associated with the excretion of carcinogenic metabolites in the urine.[55] Aromatic amines and nitrosamine compounds are potent urothelial carcinogens in humans. There may be a long latent period of up to 30 years between exposure to a carcinogen and subsequent tumour occurrence.

Smoking

Cigarette smoke contains numerous aromatic amines and nitrosamines, and is the most significant environmental carcinogen today. Smokers have a fourfold increase in risk for developing bladder cancer. This is a dose–response relationship, with ex-smokers having a reduced risk compared with current smokers. It has been estimated that one-third of bladder cancers are related to cigarette smoking.[55,57]

Occupational bladder cancer

An increased prevalence of bladder cancer in aniline dye workers was first noted at the end of the 19th century. Subsequently, β-naphthylamine, benzidine and 4-aminodiphenyl were all shown to be associated with an increased risk of bladder cancer. The main occupational exposure to these chemicals has been in the chemical-, dye- and rubber-manufacturing industries, the plastic industry and in some laboratories.

Infections

Cystitis and chronic urinary tract infection predispose to bladder cancer. In areas where schistosomiasis is endemic there is a high incidence of epithelial tumours, mostly of squamous cell type.[56]

Drugs

Cyclophosphamide has been associated with a ninefold increase in prevalence of bladder cancer over the general population.[58] Long-term use of the analgesic phenacetin has also been implicated in the development of the disease.[59]

Genetic linkage

A number of genetic alterations have been observed in the different types of carcinoma. Abnormalities in chromosome 9 have been associated with the development of superficial lesions confined to the mucosa.[60] Defects in the *p53* gene on chromo-

REFERENCES

54. Quinlan D. In: Fitzpatrick J, Krane R (eds). The Bladder. Churchill Livingstone, Edinburgh, 1995: 161–174
55. van der Meijden AP. Br Med J 1998; 317: 1366–1369
56. Macvicar AD. Bladder cancer staging. BJU 2000; 86(Suppl 1): 111–122
57. Hassen W, Droller MJ. Curr Opin Urol 2000; 10: 291–299
58. Stillwell T, Benson RJ. Cancer 1988; 61: 451
59. Bengtsson U, Angervall L, Ekman H et al. Scand J Urol Nephrol 1968; 2: 145
60. Hopman A, Moesker O, Smeets A. Cancer Res 1991; 51: 646–651

some 17 and the retinoblastoma gene (*RB*) on chromosome 13 have been found in more invasive tumours.[61]

PATHOLOGY

Transitional cell carcinoma accounts for 90% of all cases of bladder cancer. These tumours range from small, solitary, non-invasive tumours through to invasive and metastasizing disease. Approximately 70% of newly diagnosed tumours are superficial and limited to the lamina propria and mucosa. Twenty-five per cent are invading the detrusor muscle at presentation, and about 5% are in situ changes.[62] Superficial tumours confined to the mucosa, which have not penetrated the lamina propria, have a high recurrence rate (50–70%) but few progress (2–4%).[63] Those that invade the lamina propria appear to have a different malignant potential, and 30–50% will progress, particularly if poorly differentiated. Superficial tumours are generally papillary in appearance, whereas muscle-invasive tumours tend to be solid and ulcerating. These transitional cell carcinomas are histologically graded G1–3: G1 tumours are well differentiated, G2 moderately differentiated, and G3 poorly differentiated or anaplastic carcinoma. The grade correlates well with disease progression and prognosis.[64]

Two theories have been proposed to explain the multifocal and recurrent nature of bladder cancer: the 'field change' and 'clonality' theories. The field change theory suggests that exposure of the entire urothelium to carcinogens, through various exogenous and endogenous routes, leads to multiple areas of transformed cells that may progress at varying times to develop clinical cancer. The clonal theory suggests that mutations in urothelial stem cells, caused by environmental carcinogens or by genetic instability, lead to DNA damage and the development of progenitor cells that have undergone malignant transformation. Implantation of such tumour cells during resection or spontaneous intravesical dissemination may account for multiple recurrences of tumours sharing identical chromosomal changes.[57]

CLINICAL FEATURES AND DIAGNOSIS

The most common presenting feature of bladder cancer is haematuria. This may be macroscopic or microscopic and is generally painless, although some patients may have associated bladder pain or dysuria. There is no correlation between the amount of haematuria and the extent of the cancer.[57] Between 16 and 22% of adults presenting with macroscopic haematuria are found to have malignant disease of the urinary tract. Over 90% of these have bladder tumours.[1] Between 9 and 18% of normal patients have microscopic haematuria;[57] however, 5–10% of patients over 50 years old with microscopic haematuria will have bladder cancer.[62] It is therefore important to follow up all cases of adult haematuria.

The patient must be assessed by a history and an examination. Urine samples should be sent for culture to exclude infection, and for cytology to look for the presence of malignant cells. Cytology is relatively insensitive for low-grade carcinoma, and a negative result does not exclude the presence of disease. For high-grade disease and carcinoma in situ, it is both sensitive and specific.[57,65] A number of tumour markers found in the urine have been suggested and studied to try and improve diagnostic accuracy; however, at present no chemically useful marker has been identified.[65,66]

Examination of the urinary tract should be undertaken with intravenous urography or ultrasound to exclude upper tract tumours. Ultrasonography is simple, safe and quick to perform, and is superior to intravenous urography in detecting renal parenchymal carcinoma; however, it will miss small renal pelvis and ureteric tumours. Intravenous urography detects most but not all upper tract urothelial tumours; however, it also exposes the patient to a small dose of ionizing radiation. Renal failure and anaphylactic reactions to contrast media have been reported. Each imaging technique therefore has its limitations.[67]

Table 36.1 The Jewett-Strong-Marshall classification for bladder tumours

Class	Characteristic
0	Preinvasive
A	Submucosal invasion
B1	Superficial muscle
B2	Deep muscle
C	Extravesical spread
D1	Fixed to or invading prostate, uterus, vagina or pelvic lymph nodes
D2	Spread to extrapelvic lymph nodes or distant metastases

Cystoscopy is the best investigation for diagnosing bladder cancer. Flexible cystoscopy under local urethral anaesthesia allows direct visualization of the entire urethra and bladder mucosa. It allows the tumours to be characterized as papillary or solid. It also allows identification of areas of carcinoma in situ and an estimation of the stage of disease to be made.[57] Once a tumour has been identified, further cystoscopy under general anaesthetic is undertaken. Tumours should be completely resected endoscopically, ensuring detrusor muscle is included in the biopsy specimen. This allows accurate staging by the pathologist, who should be able to provide information on the depth of invasion of the tumour. Bimanual examination should be performed following resection of the tumour to assess for a residual mass or induration. The presence of these findings may indicate the presence of residual invasive disease.

One-stop haematuria clinics, providing rapid consultation, ultrasonography and flexible cystoscopy on the same day, have been shown to speed diagnosis and definitive treatment.[68]

CLASSIFICATION AND STAGING

Two main classifications are used for evaluating bladder cancer: the Jewett–Strong–Marshall system (Table 36.1)[69,70] in the USA

REFERENCES

61. Grossman H, Liebert M, Antelo M et al. Clin Cancer Res 1998.; 4: 829–834
62. Leung HY, Griffiths TR, Neal DE. Postgrad Med J 1996; 72: 719–724
63. Lutzeyer W, Rubben H, Dahm H. J Urol 1982; 127: 252–256
64. Griffiths D. In: McGee J, Isaacson P, Wright N (eds). Oxford Textbook of Pathology. Oxford University Press, Oxford, 1992: 1524–1531
65. Kausch I, Bohle A. Eur Urol 2001; 39: 498–506
66. van der Poel H, Debruyne F. Curr Opin Urol 2001; 11: 503–509
67. Britton JP. Br J Urol 1993; 71: 247–252
68. McFarlane JP, Ellis BW, Harland SJ. Br J Urol 1996; 78: 372–378
69. Jewett H, Strong G. J Urol 1946; 55: 366–372
70. Marshall V. J Urol 1952; 68: 723

Table 36.2 The TNM (tumour, node and metastasis) classification for bladder cancer

Stage	Characteristic
Ta	Non-invasive papillary carcinoma
Tis	Carcinoma in situ: 'flat tumour'
T1	Tumour invades subepithelial connective tissue (lamina propria)
T2	Tumour invades detrusor muscle (muscularis propria)
T2a	Tumour invades superficial muscle (inner half)
T2b	Tumour invades deep muscle (outer half)
T3	Tumour invades perivesical tissue:
T3a	microscopically
T3b	macroscopically
T4	Tumour invades any of the following: prostate, uterus, vagina, pelvic wall, abdominal wall
T4a	Tumour invades prostate or uterus or vagina
T4b	Tumour invades pelvic or abdominal wall
N0	No regional lymph node metastases
N1	Metastasis in a single lymph node < 2 cm in greatest dimension
N2	Metastasis in a single lymph node > 2 cm but < 5 cm in greatest dimension, or multiple lymph nodes none > 5 cm in greatest dimension
N3	Metastasis in a lymph node > 5 cm greatest dimension
M0	No distant metastases
M1	Distant metastases

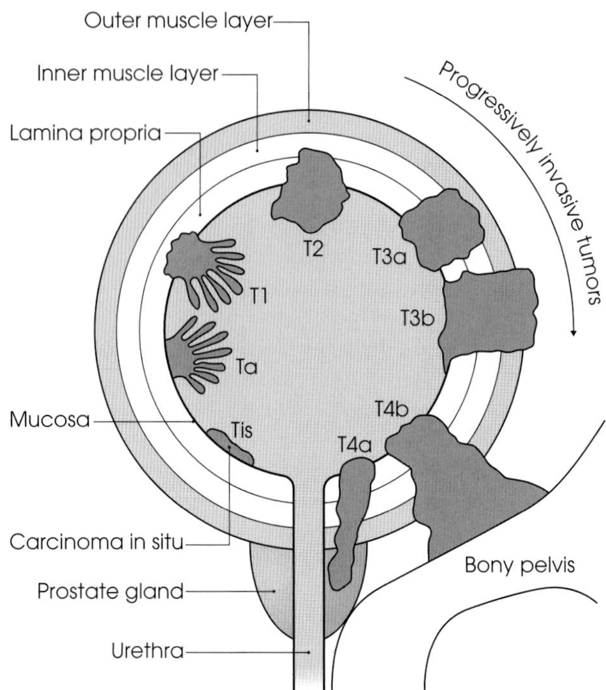

Figure 36.9 Tumour staging in bladder cancer according to the 1997 TNM system. (From van der Meijden AP. Bladder cancer. Br Med J 1998; 14: 1366–1369, by permission of BMJ Publishing Group.[55])

and the International Union Against Cancer (UICC) TNM (tumour, node and metastasis) system (Table 36.2; Fig. 36.9), which is accepted and used elsewhere.[56]

Patients with bladder cancer should be staged at presentation. The identification of those with muscle-invasive disease is one of the most important factors, because these patients, for the most part, are not suitable for endoscopic follow-up. Those with invasive disease may benefit from radical treatment. Clinical staging with cystoscopy, histological examination of biopsy specimens, and bimanual examination has been shown to be inaccurate, with errors of 25–50%.[69,71]

At the time of presentation approximately 30% of patients have multifocal disease. Carcinoma in situ is associated with an increased risk of recurrence and an increased likelihood of developing invasive disease. A third of patients have lymph node deposits when the deep muscle is involved, and approximately two-thirds will have lymph node metastases if extravesical invasion is present. The presence of lymph node metastasis has prognostic significance; patients with invasive tumours and no nodal involvement have a 5-year survival of 28%, those with nodal involvement have a 5-year survival of 11%. Distant metastatic spread occurs late in the clinical course of the disease.[56]

When the histological findings demonstrate muscle-invasive disease or if the patient is considered high risk for the development of such disease, then staging of local disease spread and lymph node involvement should be undertaken using CT or MRI, although both these techniques have a limited success in distinguishing between superficial and muscle-invasive disease.[72]

SUPERFICIAL TUMOURS AND CARCINOMA IN SITU

Between 50 and 70% of superficial tumours recur following initial treatment. Risk factors for recurrence or progression of superficial tumours include:

- large tumours,
- bladder neck tumours,
- carcinoma in situ,
- multifocality,
- poor differentiation, and
- T1 disease.

Initially all bladder tumours should be completely excised by transurethral resection. This allows the tumour to be staged accurately and a decision to be taken on the need for further therapy. Patients with solitary low-grade Ta tumours are followed by regular cystoscopy. High-risk patients with multiple primary tumours, frequent recurrences, or G3, T1 or Tis tumours should have regular intravesical instillation of either a chemotherapeutic agent, such as mitomycin, epirubicin or doxorubicin, or an immunotherapeutic agent, such as BCG. These agents have been shown to reduce recurrence rate, although there is no convincing evidence that they affect tumour progression.[73] Chemotherapeutic agents appear to be of most benefit in low-grade disease.

REFERENCES

71. Whitmore WJ, Batata M, Ghonein M et al. J Urol 1977; 118: 184–187
72. Gschwend JE, Fair WR, Vieweg J. Eur Urol 2000; 38: 121–130
73. Oosterlink W. Recent clinical trials in superficial bladder cancer. Curr Opin Urol 2001; 11(5): 511–515

Compared with chemotherapy, BCG has more local side effects,[57] including severe cystitis and systemic toxicity. Cystoscopic surveillance is essential to assess the effectiveness of treatment.

Small localized areas of carcinoma in situ may be successfully resected. Diffuse carcinoma in situ, especially if there is severe dysplasia in normal-looking urothelium, should be treated with intravesical BCG, which appears to reduce the risk of disease progression. Intravesical treatment can give an 80% remission after one or two 6-week courses.[74]

More aggressive surgical intervention, such as radical cystectomy, should be considered in patients with T1 disease or carcinoma in situ that is refractory to intravesical therapy.[57]

MUSCLE-INVASIVE TUMOURS

Invasive bladder cancer can be treated by radical cystectomy with pelvic lymph node dissection, followed by ileal conduit diversion or orthotopic bladder reconstruction; or alternatively by radical radiotherapy, with salvage cystectomy in patients whose tumours fail to respond.[62] Neither of these approaches is suitable for those patients with locally advanced or metastatic disease, who only require palliative treatment. Various techniques are available for bladder preservation, which use a combination of transurethral resection, radiotherapy and chemotherapy. The combinations have been shown to produce similar results to radical cystectomy. This approach involves a complex treatment schedule and is associated with significant morbidity and mortality. It is only possible in hospitals in which radiotherapy and oncological facilities are available, and at present radical surgery remains the standard care for invasive bladder cancer.[75]

Radical cystectomy

Radical cystectomy is the definitive curative option for carcinomas that have not spread outside the bladder.[76] The 5-year survival is dependent on the stage of the tumour at presentation. The reported survival rate at 5 years varies from 63 to 83% for T2 tumours, between 53 and 71% for T3a tumours, and from zero to 28% for T4b tumours. Lymph node resection may improve outcome, particularly in patients with tumours confined to the bladder; however, involved lymph nodes at the time of pelvic lymph node resection predict a poor prognosis.[72] Improved surgical technique has led to a fall in the incidence of perioperative complications and local recurrence rates. The presence of micrometastases at the time of surgery still presages a poor outcome.

Radical cystectomy consists of an anterior pelvic exenteration with inclusion of the perivesical and pelvic lymph nodes. The ureters are anastamosed to an ileal conduit or to a reservoir constructed from bowel (which may be connected to the urethra, as an orthotopic neobladder, or to the abdominal wall, as a continent diversion).[62] In men the prostate is excised, and in women the ovaries, fallopian tubes and the uterus are often removed. Nerve-sparing cystectomy in men and sparing of the internal genitalia in women have been considered, but no long-term data on survival are available.[77]

Urethral recurrence may occur in up to 18% of patients after cystectomy, often when there is prostatic invasion. Tumour present on frozen section of the urethral resection margin or proven transitional cell carcinoma of the anterior urethra is a contraindication to orthotopic urinary diversion or preservation of the urethra.[72] Urethrectomy may be performed synchronously with cystectomy or as a secondary procedure.

Radiotherapy

Radical radiotherapy aims to give a total dose of 60–65 Gy to the bladder tumour over a period of 4–6 weeks. Reported 5-year survival rates are 35–71% in patients with T1 tumours, 27–59% with T2 tumours, 10–38% with T3 tumours, and 0–16% with T4 tumours.[78] A review of the results of both forms of treatment showed no statistical difference in survival for patients treated by radiotherapy and by cystectomy; however, pretreatment staging inaccuracies, principally with radiotherapy, makes comparison difficult.[79] Approximately a third of invasive tumours can be cured by radiotherapy alone,[62] but up to half of the patients treated in this way will require a salvage cystectomy.[57]

The aim of radiotherapy is to treat the tumour while avoiding damage to the surrounding tissues. Complications of radiotherapy include haematuria and bladder contracture, which may require palliative cystectomy. Damage to the rectum and small bowel is also well recognized (see Ch. 28 and Ch. 27, respectively).

Chemotherapy

Chemotherapy for invasive cancer may be used as sole treatment, as an adjuvant to conservative surgery, as an adjuvant to radical cystectomy or radiotherapy, or for treatment of metastatic disease.[62] Combination therapy, especially with methotrexate, vinblastine, doxorubicin and cisplatin (MVAC), has been widely used and has been shown to have proven efficacy, with a response rate of up to 65%.[80] Two trials looking at 5-fluorouracil and cisplatin in combination with radiotherapy and bladder preservation have shown response rates of 50–67%.[81,82] Metastatic bladder cancer is generally regarded as incurable, although some response rates to MVAC have been encouraging, with a number of series reporting a complete response rate of 10–15%.[62] These regimens are toxic but should be offered because they may prolong survival and relieve symptoms.

SQUAMOUS CARCINOMA OF THE BLADDER

Squamous carcinoma of the bladder constitutes approximately 5% of urothelial malignancies, except in areas that have a high prevalence of bilharzia, where this proportion rises to 50%. These tumours are related to chronic bladder irritation secondary to persistent urinary tract infection, stones or urinary stasis in diverticula. Tumours are usually infiltrating by the time of presentation.[64] Radical cystectomy is the treatment of choice when the tumour is operable. Squamous cell carcinomas are not sensitive to cisplatin or methotrexate, but hexamethylamine and

REFERENCES

74. Hall RR. Br Med J 1994; 308: 910–913
75. Kim HL, Steinberg GD. J Urol 2000; 164: 627–632
76. Bassi P. Curr Opin Urol 2000; 10: 459–463
77. Bassi P. Outcomes of radical cystectomy for invasive bladder cancer. Curr Opin Urol 2000; 19(5): 459–463
78. Sengelov L, der-Maase H. Radiother Oncol 1999; 52: 1–14
79. Shelley MD, Barber J, Mason MD. Cochrane Database Syst Rev 2001; 3: CD002079
80. Akaza H. Curr Opin Urol 2000; 10: 453–457
81. Kaufman D, Winter K, Shipley W et al. Oncologist 2000; 5: 471–476
82. Hussain M, Glass T, Forman J et al. J Urol 2001; 165: 56–61

4-epi-doxorubicin have been shown to produce some remission.[83] Squamous carcinomas are not as radiosensitive as transitional cell carcinomas.

ADENOCARCINOMA OF THE BLADDER

The majority of bladder adenocarcinomas are found around the dome of the bladder and are probably of urachal origin. Secondary tumours may arise from prostatic, colonic or ovarian origin. Primary tumours tend to be infiltrating and prognosis is poor. Surgery is considered the treatment of choice, because these tumours are relatively insensitive to radiotherapy.[84]

SARCOMAS OF THE BLADDER

The most common sarcoma of the bladder is the leiomyosarcoma, which constitutes 0.5% of all bladder tumours. Survival depends on the degree of differentiation and the stage of the disease. Rhabdomyosarcoma occurs almost exclusively in children under 6 years of age. They tend to grow rapidly and are locally aggressive. Advances in combination therapy have improved the outlook for children with these tumours.[64] Sarcomas of the bladder, however, usually have a poor prognosis.

REFERENCES

83. Newling D, Denis L, Gerard J et al. In: Peckham M, Pinedo H, Veronesi U (eds). Oxford Textbook of Oncology. Oxford University Press, Oxford, 1995: 1459–1479
84. Gill H, Dhillon H, Woodhouse C. Br J Urol 1989; 64: 138–14

The prostate

37

David P. Shipstone, John B. Anderson

INTRODUCTION

The prostate is a fibromuscular accessory sex gland located just below the bladder, and is transversed by the posterior urethra and distal ejaculatory ducts. It has a role in seminal emission and ensuring antegrade ejaculation, and its secretions form part of the ejaculate. Both prostate cancer, which is the second most common malignancy in western men, and benign prostatic enlargement are among the most common disorders that affect the ageing male, while prostatitis may affect men of all ages.

BASIC SCIENCE

ANATOMY

The adult prostate is composed of epithelium, smooth muscle and collagen. On average it is 3 cm long, 4 cm wide and 2 cm in depth, and it grows by 1.6% per year from middle age.[1] It is an ovoid pyramid in shape, with anterior, posterior and lateral surfaces narrowing to a distal apex.

Denonvilliers' fascia lies immediately posterior to the prostate, separating it from the rectum and acting as a natural barrier to the direct extension of disease from either aspect. Laterally, the prostate lies on the pubococcygeal part of levator ani, with the endopelvic fascia intervening. At the apex of the gland, the fascia thickens to form the paired puboprostatic ligaments binding the prostate (and membranous urethra) to the posterior aspect of the pubis. The dorsal vein runs between these ligaments while lying directly anterior to the urethra just beyond the prostatic apex. The prostatic urethra is 3–4 cm long, and its internal posterior midline is raised to form the urethral crest with a sulcus on each side, which receives all glandular secretions.[2] The verumontanum is an expanded portion of the urethral crest on which lies a 5-mm slit called the prostatic utricle, a remnant of the Müllerian system. The prostatic urethra is lined by transitional epithelium and surrounded by two muscular components: an inner longitudinal and an outer circular layer that is thickened to form the internal urethral sphincter. The common ejaculatory ducts open on each side of the verumontanum.

The prostate is divided into transitional, central and peripheral zones that make up 5–10%, 25% and 70% of the glandular tissue, respectively (Fig. 37.1). Benign prostatic enlargement occurs exclusively in the transitional zone and the periurethral area near the bladder neck. Seventy per cent of prostate cancers arise in the peripheral zone, 20% in the transitional zone, and 5% in the central zone.

The prostatic artery leaves the inferior vesical artery at the bladder neck and divides into urethral and capsular branches. Its urethral branches perforate the vesicoprostatic junction posterolaterally and then travel inwards, perpendicular to the urethra, towards the bladder neck. They then turn caudally to supply the urethra, periurethral glands and transitional zone. The vessels are largest posterolaterally, and during transurethral resection of the prostate are mainly encountered at the four and eight o'clock positions as viewed through the endoscope.

PHYSIOLOGY

The prostate plays an important physiological role during the reproductive years, contributing around 0.5 mL (20%) of the seminal ejaculate. Its secretions contain a number of substances thought to be necessary for maintaining sperm viability and motility. Prostate-specific antigen (PSA), a glycoprotein protease, is responsible for the liquefaction of semen after ejaculation, while zinc, spermine and immunoglobulins have an antimicrobial action.

Seminal emission and ejaculation are controlled by the sympathetic and somatic nervous systems. Emission of seminal fluid into the prostatic urethra is achieved by consecutive contraction of the epididymides, vasa, seminal vesicles and prostate in response to appropriate stimuli. This is under sympathetic control via adrenergic fibres terminating on α_{1a} receptors of smooth muscle. Subsequent contraction of bladder neck smooth muscle and the internal urethral sphincter close the retrograde route into the bladder, thereby allowing antegrade ejaculation, which is achieved by rhythmic contractions of the bulbospongiosus muscle under somatic (pudendal nerve) control.

ENDOCRINOLOGY AND GROWTH FACTORS

The hypothalamus releases gonadotrophin-releasing hormone (in pulses), which stimulates the release of luteinizing hormone from the anterior pituitary gland. This in turn acts on the Leydig cells of the testes, which then release testosterone. Testosterone forms a negative-feedback loop inhibiting further release of luteinizing hormone. Once released by the Leydig cells, serum testosterone is transported in the serum bound to sex steroid–binding globulin and albumin, with only 2% of the hormone remaining unbound.

Prostate stromal and epithelial cells possess both 5α-reductase and androgen receptors, and both cell types produce growth factors. Although prostatic growth factors can behave in both an autocrine and a paracrine fashion, in general they tend to act as paracrine agents, being produced by stromal cells and acting on epithelial cells.

REFERENCES

1. Rhodes T, Girman CJ, Jacobsen SJ et al. J Urol 1999; 161: 1174–1179
2. McNeal JE. Prostate 1981; 2: 35–49

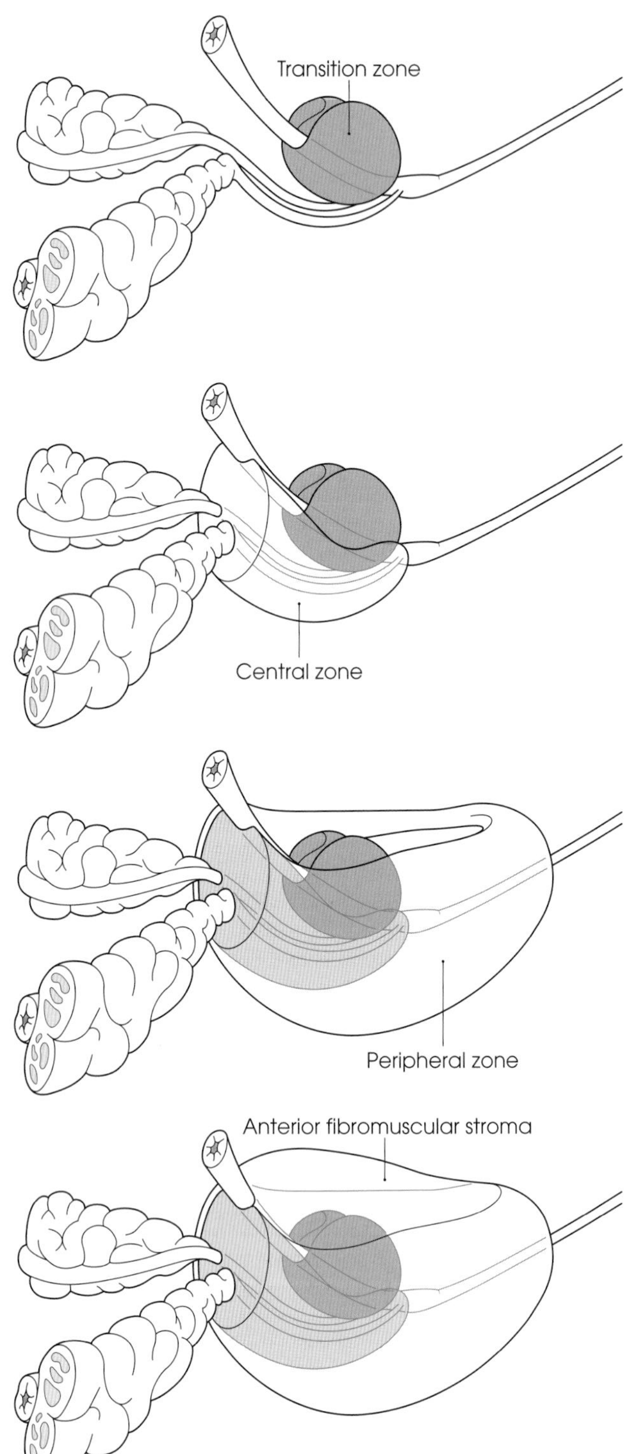

Figure 37.1 The anatomical zones of the prostate.

In prostate cancer the selective response of the epithelial cells to paracrine stromal transforming growth factor is less marked, and autocrine epithelial growth factor becomes up-regulated, which enhances metastasis and invasion. Fibroblast growth factor is up-regulated, enhancing metastasis by several mechanisms including altering extracellular matrix production, an immunosuppressive effect on lymphocytes, and increasing angiogenesis. Other growth factors are also up-regulated with less specifically known effects.[3]

TRAUMA AND INJURY

Trauma in the region of the prostate is usually associated with pelvic fracture, and is discussed together with urethral trauma in Chapter 36.

BENIGN PROSTATIC ENLARGEMENT

Lower urinary tract symptoms is the preferred term for the symptom complex commonly referred to as 'prostatism', because it is well recognized that these symptoms may occur in both women and men with increasing age,[4] and in men with no evidence of bladder outflow obstruction. At any given time the bladder is either filling or emptying, and these symptoms can therefore be divided into filling or storage symptoms and voiding symptoms. The terms *irritative symptoms* and *obstructive symptoms* are often used, suggesting that a specific pathophysiological process is responsible for each, but this is an artificial distinction. As history alone is an unreliable guide to the final clinical diagnosis, it is reasonable to describe filling and voiding symptoms because no diagnosis is implied by these terms.[5] Filling symptoms are frequency, nocturia (night-time frequency), urgency and urge incontinence. Voiding symptoms are hesitancy, urinary retention, a slow urinary stream, intermittency (a stop–start flow), postmicturition dribble, and a sensation of incomplete bladder emptying.

Benign prostatic enlargement refers to the finding of an enlarged prostate with no malignant features on digital examination or imaging studies, whereas *benign prostatic hyperplasia* is a histological diagnosis characterized by glandular and stromal hyperplasia. Benign prostatic hypertrophy is an unusual histological finding in patients with benign prostatic enlargement.

Bladder outflow obstruction is a urodynamic diagnosis indicating an increased resistance to voiding, defined by the measurement of flow rate and detrusor pressure, although a poor flow rate alone may be used to infer bladder outflow obstruction. When benign prostatic enlargement results in outflow obstruction the term *benign prostatic obstruction* is preferred.

The functional bladder capacity is the volume of urine present in the bladder when an intense urge to void occurs.

CLINICAL FEATURES OF BENIGN PROSTATIC ENLARGEMENT

Epidemiology

Benign prostatic enlargement and its associated symptoms may be common clinical problems, but their actual prevalence depends on the definitions used in different epidemiological studies. The presence of lower urinary tract symptoms, prostate size, reduced urinary flow rate, urodynamically proven bladder outflow obstruction, and histological evidence of benign prostate hypertrophy have all been reported in this context. Individual studies may employ one or more of these criteria in defining the prevalence of benign prostatic enlargement. In addition, increased awareness of prostate disease may heighten the perception of symptoms in a given community.

REFERENCES

3. Hellawell GO, Brewster SF. BJU Int 2002; 89: 230–240
4. Lepor H, Machi G. Urology 1993; 42: 36–40
5. Abrams P. Br Med J 1994; 308: 929–930

Autopsy studies on prostates from men not dying of prostate disease reveal an almost linear age-stratified relationship, independent of ethnic and geographical origin, with the prevalence of benign prostatic hyperplasia ranging from nil in men younger than 30 years to over 50% in the 51–60 years age group, and over 85% in men in their eighties.[6] The mean prostatic volume increases with age, from around 25 mL for men in their thirties to 45 mL in men in their seventies.[6] The prevalence of benign prostatic enlargement is therefore absolutely dependent on whichever arbitrary criterion is used to define the clinical problem.

The international prostate symptom score allows men with lower urinary tract symptoms to be categorized into mild, moderate and severe symptom groups. Using a definition of a total prostatic volume greater than 20 mL and a flow rate of less than 15 mL/s in the presence of any lower tract symptoms gave an incidence of 25% in a 40–79-year-old Scottish cohort, rising from 14% in those aged 40–49 years to 43% in the 60–69 years age group. In the USA, an international prostatic symptom score of 8 or more and a prostatic volume of over 30 mL yielded a prevalence of 19% in a 55–74-year-old cohort.[7]

Aetiology

Functioning testes and ageing are prerequisites for the development of benign prostatic hypertrophy.[8] There is strong evidence for a genetic component in its aetiology. This is evidenced by familial benign prostatic hypertrophy, which is a relatively rare syndrome where prostate size is on average 67% greater and treatment is required at an earlier age.[9] A higher concordance rate has been found for benign prostatic hyperplasia in monozygotic compared with dizygotic twins.[10] The aetiology for prostate enlargement remains unknown. It has been suggested that androgen–oestrogen imbalance causes activation of cells in the embryonic state,[11] and a recent review suggested that some of the transitional zone tissue has an origin from the Müllerian duct, and is therefore more sensitive to a relative increase in oestrogen activity with ageing.[12] Modest associations have been found between prostatic hyperplasia and intakes of protein and specific long-chain polyunsaturated fatty acids.[13] Lipids in the form of butter and margarine may increase the risk of hyperplasia, while an increased fruit intake may reduce this risk.[14]

Clinical findings

Men with benign prostatic enlargement may experience lower urinary tract symptoms that usually progress with time,[15,16] but commonly wax and wane in severity.[17] These symptoms can be assessed objectively by the international prostate symptom score, although this is of no diagnostic value.[4] This instrument may be self-administered but does not obviate the need for a direct clinical consultation with the patient about his symptoms. The history should confirm and clarify a number of further facts.

Benign prostatic enlargement may cause haematuria, and further investigation is then essential to exclude urinary tract cancer. Patients should be questioned about dysuria, incontinence, abdominal pain and weight loss. A history of urinary tract infections and previous urological or pelvic surgery is also important. Patients should be asked to complete a voiding diary for up to 1 week prior to the consultation, detailing fluid intake and the frequency and volume of voiding.

Other comorbid conditions should be assessed. Cardiac, endocrine and neurological symptoms should be ascertained. Symptoms of frequency and nocturia[18] may occur when the functional bladder volume is normal but the patient has polyuria as a consequence of diabetes mellitus, polydipsia or diabetes insipidus. When polyuria occurs exclusively at night, the patient is likely to experience nocturia but not daytime frequency. This can occur when third-space fluid loss is returned to the intravascular compartment during recumbency. This may be an early sign of cardiac failure and can be alleviated by rest and diuretics taken during the afternoon.

The blood pressure must be measured and a digital rectal examination performed. The purpose of the rectal examination is to exclude overt prostate and lower rectal cancer, and to elicit the sacral cord reflexes. The assessment of prostate size has little diagnostic value but may sometimes influence therapy. A focused neurological examination and examination of the abdomen and external genitalia should also be performed.

Investigations include urine dipstick analysis for blood, protein, glucose, leukocyte esterase and nitrite. Urine culture and sensitivities should be performed if an abnormality is detected by microscopy. The maximal urinary flow rate is recorded and the postvoid bladder volume estimated by an ultrasound scan. The serum PSA may also be measured. The National Screening Committee in the UK recommends that the test should be available to all men on request but that full counselling should first be undertaken. This is discussed further in the section on prostate cancer. Ideally two or three urinary flow rates should be recorded.[19] In men with lower urinary tract symptoms performing a single flow test, a maximum flow rate of less than 10 mL/s has a positive predictive value of 70% and sensitivity of 47% for urodynamically proven outflow obstruction.[20] The combination of clinical assessment and uroflowmetry has a positive predictive value of 80–95% in the context of selection for transurethral prostatectomy.[21] The measurement of postvoid residual bladder volume is of limited value, because it has been found to have poor reproducibility and is neither diagnostic nor

REFERENCES

6. Berry SJ, Coffey DS, Walsh PC et al. J Urol 1984; 132: 474–479
7. Bosch JL, Hop WC, Kirkels WJ et al. Urology 1995; 46 (Suppl A): 34–40
8. Glynn RJ, Campion EW, Bouchard GR et al. Am J Epidemiol 1985; 121: 78–90
9. Sanda MG, Doehring CB, Binkowitz B et al. J Urol 1997; 157: 876–879
10. Partin AW, Page WF, Lee BR et al. Urology 1994; 44: 646–650
11. Bierhoff E, Vogel J, Benz M et al. Eur Urol 1996; 29: 345–354
12. Cai Y. BJU Int 2001; 87: 177–182
13. Suzuki S, Platz EA, Kawachi I et al. Am J Clin Nutr 2002; 75: 689–697
14. Lagiou P, Wuu J, Trichopoulou A et al. Urology 1999; 54: 284–290
15. Jacobsen SJ, Girman CJ, Guess HA et al. J Urol 1996; 155: 595–600
16. Logie JW, Clifford GM, Farmer RD et al. Eur Urol 2001; 39 (Suppl 3): 42–47
17. Barry MJ. Urol Clin North Am 1990; 17: 495–507
18. Donovan JL. BJU Int 1999; 84 (Suppl 1): 21–25
19. Reynard JM, Peters TJ, Lim C et al. Br J Urol 1996; 77: 813–818
20. Reynard JM, Yang Q, Donovan JL et al. Br J Urol 1998; 82: 619–623
21. McLoughlin J, Gill KP, Abel PD et al. Br J Urol 1990; 66: 303–305

predictive of the natural history or treatment outcome.[22,23] Whenever there is doubt about the diagnosis, urodynamic pressure flow studies are valuable.

The serum creatinine should be measured, because renal insufficiency is detected in 14% of men with lower urinary tract symptoms.[24] Imaging of the upper tracts by either an intravenous urogram or ultrasound is unnecessary[25,26] unless dictated by a specific symptom, sign or investigation such as biochemical renal impairment.[27] Cystourethroscopy should always be performed when there is a history or finding of haematuria and usually obtained if there has been previous bladder, prostate or urethral surgery.

The symptom severity often correlates poorly with urinary flow rates,[20,28,29] urodynamically assessed outflow tract obstruction,[20,28] prostate volume,[29] and postvoid residual bladder volume.[29] When individual symptoms are considered in isolation, only urgency and urge incontinence have any relationship to urodynamically proven bladder outflow obstruction.[28,29]

PATHOPHYSIOLOGY OF BENIGN PROSTATIC HYPERPLASIA

The classic progression described by Hunter, of prostatic enlargement leading to obstructive uropathy, renal failure and death, is rare. The majority of patients with benign prostatic hyperplasia do not develop renal failure, and most do not develop retention.[30] It is debatable whether patients with either low- or high-pressure chronic retention are actually at the end stage of this pathway or should be considered as a separate subgroup of patients when prostatic hyperplasia and bladder pathology coexist.

Benign prostatic hyperplasia is initially demonstrable only by the microscopic examination, and consists of a proliferation of fibroblast-like stromal cells in the periurethral region of the prostate. These form micronodules near the bladder neck. In the transitional zone, epithelium buds off existing ducts to form new glands taking on a nodular form. There is little stromal proliferation in this region, and any that does occur clearly has smooth muscle morphology. The micronodules coalesce and macroscopic changes may be apparent on endoscopy. The most common appearance is of enlargement of both lateral lobes, which often 'kiss' in the midline. An enlarged median lobe at the six o'clock position often protrudes into the bladder, causing a 'ball valve' type of obstruction. The lateral lobes are due to transitional zone enlargement, while the median lobe is a consequence of periurethral stromal proliferation.

Benign prostatic hyperplasia consists of 50% connective tissue, 25% smooth muscle and 25% epithelium.[31] It is not fully understood how prostatic enlargement causes bladder outflow obstruction, because there is usually little difficulty passing a urethral catheter. It has been suggested that prostatic enlargement may alter the urethral alignment, leading to 'kinking' during micturition.[32]

Increased outflow resistance initially gives rise to the symptoms of hesitancy, reduced flow and an intermittent urinary stream. The detrusor muscle is required to generate more power and responds by undergoing hypertrophy,[33] giving rise to characteristic appearances on cystoscopy. The hypertrophied and fibrosed muscle fibres appear as trabeculations and sacculations. Weakness between the muscle bundles results in mucosal outpouchings or diverticula. The combination of detrusor muscle hypertrophy and raised bladder pressure may cause detrusor ischaemia. Initially the detrusor compensates to the increased resistance provided by the prostate. The contractile apparatus is altered to produce more efficient tension generation. Hypertrophied detrusor muscle has been found to exhibit an increase in anaerobic oxidation, indicated by an increased concentration of lactic acid and lactate dehydrogenase. The contractile responses of hypertrophied bladder have also been shown to be more resistant than those of the normal bladder to the effects of hypoxia.[34] These compensatory changes may lead to detrusor overactivity and the irritative or filling symptoms of frequency, nocturia and urgency.

This situation may remain unchanged for a variable period of time before the detrusor enters the next phase of decompensation. There has been considerable debate as to whether decompensation is a part of the natural history of benign prostatic hypertrophy or an independent ageing process. Experimental models of bladder outflow obstruction produce high-pressure overactive bladders, not chronic retention.[35] The relief of obstruction improves both the symptoms and the morphology of detrusor hypertrophy,[36] but it rarely reverses poor detrusor contractility. By contrast, detrusor decompensation is known to be associated with the release of free radicals stimulated by long-term ischaemia. Free radicals attack the membranes of nerves, sarcoplasmic reticulum and mitochondria.[37] As more muscle is damaged, the detrusor fails and incomplete emptying ensues. Chronic urinary retention is usually associated with a high end-void bladder pressure that interferes with ureteric drainage, leading to renal dysfunction.[38]

COMPLICATIONS OF BENIGN PROSTATIC ENLARGEMENT

Men with prostatic enlargement may go on to develop urinary tract infections, bladder stones, urinary retention and renal

REFERENCES

22. Dunsmuir WD, Feneley M, Corry DA et al. Br J Urol 1996; 77: 192–193
23. Roehrborn CG. Urol Clin North Am 1995; 22: 445–453
24. McConnell JD, Barry MJ, Bruskewitz RC. Clin Pract Guidel Quick Ref Guide Clin 1994; 8: 1–17
25. Koyanagi T, Artibani W, Correa R et al. Initial Diagnostic Evaluation of Men with Lower Urinary Tract Symptoms. Fourth International Consultation on Benign Prostatic Hypertrophy, 1997
26. Wilkinson AG, Wild SR. Br J Urol 1992; 70: 53–57
27. Koch WF, Ezz el Din K, de Wildt MJ et al. J Urol 1996; 155: 186–189
28. de la Rosette JJ, Witjes WP, Schafer W et al. Neurourol Urodynamics 1998; 17: 99–108
29. Barry MJ, Cockett AT, Holtgrewe HL et al. J Urol 1993; 150: 351–358
30. McConnell JD, Bruskewitz R, Walsh P et al. N Engl J Med 1998; 338: 557–563
31. Shapiro E, Hartanto V, Lepor H. Prostate 1992; 20: 259–267
32. Mundy AR, Fitzpatrick JM, Neal DE et al. The Scientific Basis of Urology. Isis Medical Media, Oxford, 1999
33. Buttyan R, Chen MW, Levin RM. Eur Urol 1997; 32 (Suppl 1): 32–39
34. Levin RM, English M, Barretto M et al. Neurourol Urodynamics 2000; 19: 701–712
35. Dixon JS, Gilpin CJ, Gilpin SA et al. Br J Urol 1989; 64: 385–390
36. Malkowicz SB, Wein AJ, Elbadawi A et al. J Urol 1986; 136: 1324–1329
37. Levin RM, Levin SS, Zhao Y et al. Eur Urol 1997; 32 (Suppl 1): 15–21
38. George NJ, O'Reilly PH, Barnard RJ et al. Br Med J Clin Res Ed 1983; 286: 1780–1783

impairment. The prevalence of bladder stones at autopsy was 3.4% in men with histological evidence of prostatic enlargement, compared with 0.4% in controls.[39] However, only one man out of 276 developed a bladder stone over a 3-year follow-up period in the observation arm of a randomized study of men suitable for prostatectomy.[40] Urinary tract infections are more common in men with prostatic enlargement and a significant postvoid bladder volume.

Retention of urine

Retention of urine is defined as the inability to pass urine and may be classified into five distinct categories, as described below.

Acute painful retention

Acute painful retention of urine occurs when the patient is unable to pass urine and has suprapubic pain with a tender palpable bladder. The residual urine volume on catheterization is usually less than 1 L. A 60-year-old man has a 23% chance of developing acute retention if he lives to the age of 80, and men with symptoms have a 1–2% risk per year.[30,41] The risk of developing painful retention increases with age, the severity of pre-existing lower tract symptoms, a family history of prostatic hyperplasia, a clinically enlarged prostate,[41] an elevated PSA,[42] and a previous history of urinary retention.[43] Urinary retention may be precipitated by excessive consumption of fluid, forcible delayed micturition, and anticholinergic medication. The underlying cause is prostatic hyperplasia in about half the cases with urethral stricture and prostate cancer, accounting for 7.5% and 7%, respectively.[44] There is often a history of lower urinary tract symptoms.

Only a quarter of men void following initial removal of the catheter, although those with a urinary tract infection, those with no previous symptoms, and those with gross constipation have a better chance following correction of the precipitating cause.[43] The majority of recurrent retention episodes occur within 1 week of the initial trial without catheter.[45] On this basis, those men with pre-existing lower tract symptoms should ideally be offered surgery to correct their bladder outflow obstruction, while those with little or no prior symptoms and a reversible precipitating cause should be offered a trial without catheter followed by surgery if this is unsuccessful. There is some evidence to support the use of α_1-adrenergic antagonists before a trial without catheter in these patients.[46]

Acute painless retention

Acute painless retention is rare and usually the result of an acute neurological event, such as a central disc prolapse or spinal metastatic disease causing cord compression. Urgent evaluation, including MRI of the spinal cord (see Ch. 48), and appropriate intervention are required.

Postoperative urinary retention

Postoperative urinary retention is usually caused by a combination of factors, and bladder outflow obstruction by an enlarged prostate is rarely the main cause.[47] Outflow tract surgery should not be offered in the first instance. Intermittent self-catheterization is the optimal therapy or, if this is not feasible, an indwelling catheter may be inserted. Normal voiding usually returns within days unless the surgery caused iatrogenic neurological damage to the pelvic autonomic nerves. When patients fail to recover a normal pattern of voiding, pressure flow studies identify those with bladder outflow obstruction who are likely to benefit from surgery.

Low-pressure chronic retention

Low-pressure chronic retention is typically painless and characterized by a large residual urine volume, often in excess of 1 L. It occurs as a consequence of detrusor failure, and may be caused by long-standing bladder outflow obstruction from benign prostatic enlargement or an atonic bladder secondary to neurological causes. Intermittent self-catheterization is the optimal treatment, although a long-term indwelling catheter is appropriate for patients who are unable to catheterize. Transurethral resection of the prostate may allow normal voiding in some patients. Pressure flow studies can be used after a period of catheter drainage to identify recovery of detrusor function and to identify patients who are most likely to benefit from outflow tract surgery.

High-pressure chronic retention

In high-pressure chronic retention the resting pressure of the bladder remains high after micturition,[38] resulting in impaired drainage of the pelvicalyceal systems, hydronephrosis and obstructive uropathy. The condition is painless, and patients may present with dribbling overflow incontinence, especially at night. Patients may have an easily palpable bladder or symptoms of renal failure. At presentation, 20% of patients have evidence of fluid overload and half are hypertensive.[48] Catheter drainage of the bladder usually results in a marked postobstructive diuresis until the renal tubules are able to concentrate urine again. Significant intravenous fluid replacement may be required until the diuresis has settled. Urine output in excess of 200 mL/h for the first 12 h usually indicates patients at risk. Renal function should be monitored regularly, and once the serum creatinine and electrolytes have returned to normal, transurethral resection of the prostate should be carried out. It is unsafe for the patient to undergo a trial without catheter with this type of presentation. Transurethral resection of the prostate produces spontaneous voiding in most cases.[38,49] When surgery is not possible because of significant comorbidity, a long-term indwelling catheter or intermittent self-catheterization is a safe alternative, but strict compliance must be ensured.

The differential diagnosis of urinary retention

Although the distinction between retention of urine and anuria is usually clear, the presentation of acute abdominal pain together with a palpable pelvic mass and oliguria may be confused with acute urinary retention. An abdominal ultrasound

REFERENCES

39. Grosse H. Z Urol Nephrol 1990; 83: 469–474
40. Wasson JH, Reda DJ, Bruskewitz RC et al. N Engl J Med 1995; 332: 75–79
41. Jacobsen SJ, Jacobson DJ, Girman CJ et al. J Urol 1997; 158: 481–487
42. Lieber MM, Jacobsen SJ, Roberts RO et al. Prostate 2001; 49: 208–212
43. Hastie KJ, Dickinson AJ, Ahmad R et al. J R Coll Surg Edinb 1990; 35: 225–227
44. Choong S, Emberton M. BJU Int 2000; 85: 186–201
45. Klarskov P, Andersen JT, Asmussen CF et al. Scand J Urol Nephrol 1987; 21: 23–28
46. McNeill SA, Daruwala PD, Mitchell ID et al. BJU Int 1999; 84: 622–627
47. Anderson JB, Grant JB. Br Med J 1991; 302: 894–896
48. Jones DA, George NJ. Br J Urol 1992; 69: 337–345
49. George NJ, Feneley RC, Roberts JB. Br J Urol 1986; 58: 290–295

or catheterization usually confirms the diagnosis, and ultrasound has the added advantage of providing an assessment of any upper tract obstruction in cases of anuria. All patients presenting with acute retention should be reassessed once the bladder has drained. Persisting abdominal pain should raise the concern of an alternative or additional diagnosis.

TREATMENT OF BENIGN PROSTATIC OBSTRUCTION

The treatment of benign prostatic obstruction depends not only on the severity of symptoms and the presence of complications, but also on the patient's concern over their symptoms. Treatment ranges from simple reassurance and observation, through medical management with alpha blockers and 5α-reductase inhibitors, to minimal surgical intervention utilizing different techniques to produce tissue necrosis or major operations to remove the prostate through a transurethral or open surgical approach. In general, treatments that remove prostatic tissue by surgery (open prostatectomy, transurethral resection of the prostate, and laser resection) are more effective at relieving obstruction than those that rely on tissue necrosis and sloughing over time (contact laser ablation, transrectal microwave therapy and transurethral needle ablation), and these in turn are more effective than alpha blockade or 5α-reductase inhibitors. The morbidity associated with each treatment tends to correlate with its efficacy.[50,51]

Observation

While lower urinary tract symptoms tend to progress with time,[15,16] there is good evidence to suggest that patients managed by observation alone do not develop serious complications. An early and important retrospective study of 107 patients with symptoms of benign prostatic obstruction, many confirmed by urodynamics, found that only 1.9% developed urinary retention and 10% required surgery within 5 years.[52] More recent prospective studies comparing treatment with placebo and treatment with observation have demonstrated that observation usually provides a sustained improvement in symptom scores and a reduced risk of urinary retention. Patients in the observation or placebo arms of these trials very rarely developed dangerous complications such as renal failure.[30,40,53]

Medical therapy

Urinary outflow tract resistance caused by benign prostatic enlargement consists of a static component related to the physical increase in the bulk of the prostate, and a dynamic component related to variations in smooth muscle tone within the gland. The α_1-adrenergic antagonists reduce muscle tone by an antagonistic action on α_{1a} receptors, but may also modify symptoms by their effect on the α_{1d} receptors of the spinal intermediary neurons. The α_{1b} receptors are generally found on blood vessels throughout the body, and the antagonism of these receptors is responsible for the hypotensive episodes that are a recognized side effect of these drugs.

Alfuzosin, doxazosin and terazosin are non-selective α_1-adrenergic antagonists, while tamsulosin is considered to be selective for α_{1a} receptors. A meta-analysis of placebo-controlled studies involving 6840 men demonstrates that all these drugs produce similar improvements in lower tract symptoms and urinary flow rate. The mean symptom score is improved by 2.6–9.6 points (30–40%) and maximum urinary flow by 1.4–4 mL/s (16–25%).[54,55] Their side effects include postural hypotension (2%), dizziness (7%), asthenia (2%) and abnormal ejaculation (0.8–4.5%). Alfuzosin (especially the sustained-release formulation) and tamsulosin (the modified-release formulation 0.4 mg) are better tolerated than terazosin and doxazosin. Tamsulosin has less effect on blood pressure than alfuzosin, especially in elderly patients, and causes less symptomatic orthostatic hypotension during stress testing than terazosin. Four to ten per cent of patients on alfuzosin and tamsulosin 0.4 mg do not tolerate treatment, whereas 8–20% cannot tolerate terazosin or doxazosin.[55,56]

In comparison with the α_1 antagonists, 5α-reductase inhibitors such as finasteride reduce prostatic mass, but several months of treatment may be required for this to occur.[57] Although finasteride therapy has been shown to reduce symptom scores marginally (by 2 points), the effect on symptoms[58] and pressure flow studies[59] is more marked in a subgroup of men with larger prostates. The side effects include decreased libido (6%), impotence (8%) and diminished ejaculation (4%), although at 1 year the rates are equivalent to placebo.[30]

Studies have shown that finasteride has another role in reducing bleeding during prostate surgery.[60,61]

Minimally invasive therapy

Laser energy can be used to induce coagulative necrosis or to resect prostatic tissue. Coagulative ablation using a neodymium: YAG side-firing technique has less impact on improving symptom scores, flow rate and the quantity of residual urine than holmium laser resection, where the results are equivalent to transurethral resection at 2 years. Longer-term follow-up is awaited.[62,63] Microwave treatment may be delivered by a transrectal or transurethral route. Recently, equipment has been available to deliver transurethral microwave therapy at higher intensities, and while the effects on symptom scores compare favourably to transurethral resection in the short term, the effect on the urinary flow rates is less marked.[64–67]

REFERENCES

50. Madersbacher S, Marberger M. BJU Int 1999; 83: 227–237
51. Schatzl G, Madersbacher S, Djavan B et al. Eur Urol 2000; 37: 695–701
52. Ball AJ, Feneley RC, Abrams PH. Br J Urol 1981; 53: 613–616
53. Flanigan RC, Reda DJ, Wasson JH et al. J Urol 1998; 160: 12–16
54. Chapple CR. Eur Urol 1996; 29: 129–144
55. Djavan B, Marberger M. Eur Urol 1999; 36: 1–13
56. Hofner K, Claes H, De Reijke TM et al. Eur Urol 1999; 36: 335–341
57. Marks LS, Partin AW, Gormley GJ et al. J Urol 1997; 157: 2171–2178
58. Roehrborn CG, Boyle P, Bergner D et al. Urology 1999; 54: 662–669
59. Abrams P, Schafer W, Tammela TL et al. J Urol 1999; 161: 1513–1517
60. Sandfeldt L, Bailey DM, Hahn RG. Urology 2001; 58: 972–976
61. Hagerty JA, Ginsberg PC, Harmon JD et al. Urology 2000; 55: 684–689
62. Donovan JL, Peters TJ, Neal DE et al. J Urol 2000; 164: 65–70
63. Gilling PJ, Kennett KM, Fraundorfer MR. J Endourol 2000; 14: 757–760
64. Bosch JL. J Urol 1997; 158: 2034–2044
65. Djavan B, Roehrborn CG, Shariat S et al. J Urol 1999; 161: 139–143
66. Roehrborn CG, Preminger G, Newhall P et al. Urology 1998; 51: 19–28
67. Ahmed M, Bell T, Lawrence WT et al. Br J Urol 1997; 79: 181–185

Transurethral needle ablation delivers low-level radio frequency to the prostate gland and is less efficacious than transurethral resection.[68] High-intensity focused ultrasound is delivered by a transrectal probe, and although the initial improvement in symptom scores and flow rates is impressive the effect is short lived.[69]

Surgical resection of the prostate

Transurethral resection of the prostate is performed using a diathermy wire loop under direct vision. The enlarged adenomatous tissue of the transitional zone of the prostate is removed in a systematic fashion, guided by the anatomical landmarks of the bladder neck proximally, the verumontanum distally, and the capsule and bladder neck muscle deeply. Prostatectomy dramatically reduces the mean symptom score from 20.1 to 7.4, with 63.5% of men improving by more than 9 points and 23% by 3–9 points; 10% show no change and 4% are worse.[70] Failure to produce a symptomatic improvement is usually because of persistent storage symptoms causing the bladder to remain overactive. When a transurethral resection is carried out to treat acute urinary retention, 90% of men will void after their catheter is removed and 99% will achieve spontaneous voiding in the longer term.[71]

The complications include a mortality of 0–0.5%, septicaemia in 1.5%, blood loss requiring transfusion in 0.4–6.4%, erectile dysfunction in 0–10%, retrograde ejaculation in 70% and incontinence in 1%. Bladder neck stenosis develops in 2.1%, urethral stricture in 1%, and 1–2% of patients per year require reoperation.[53,72–74] Intravascular absorption of irrigating fluid can result in cardiovascular and neurological symptoms in 0.5–2% of patients having a transurethral resection, and this risk is increased in patients having prolonged resections. Hypertension from fluid overload is the first sign. The intravascular irrigating fluid causes an osmotic diuresis leading to sodium and water excretion, but it also diffuses into cells where it is metabolized, attracting water molecules by osmosis. This causes intracellular oedema, and extracellular sodium and water depletion. Diuretic therapy may not always help and can lead to further circulatory collapse. Hypertonic saline should be administered to correct the profound hyponatraemia and intracellular oedema, but this must be carefully monitored in an intensive care unit. The use and complications of irrigating fluids have been comprehensively reviewed by Hahn.[75]

The risks associated with prolonged transurethral resection of very large prostatic enlargement may justify an open surgical enucleation of the adenomatous tissue. The patient usually recovers rapidly following an extraperitoneal open approach, and the long-term complications are similar to those of transurethral surgery, including a mortality of less than 1%. The risks of septicaemia, blood loss requiring transfusion, erectile dysfunction, retrograde ejaculation, incontinence and bladder neck stenosis are also very similar to those of transurethral resection.

Long-term catheterization

Elderly, infirm patients who present with severe symptoms or urinary retention may be unfit for any form of surgery, and a long-term silastic catheter placed via the urethral or suprapubic route may be a safer option. A long-term suprapubic catheter is easier to change and is less likely to inhibit sexual activity, but has a greater risk of complications. Patients with long-term catheters should have their catheters changed every 3 months. Half of these patients develop catheter blockage, and this risk is increased by bladder stone formation, a high urinary pH, and the presence of *Proteus* in the urine.[76] Frequent catheter changes, intermittent bladder irrigation, and the use of silicon catheters may reduce the frequency of blockages. The skin and catheter at the urethral meatus should be cleansed with water every day to prevent encrustation by dried urethral secretions, and care should be taken to avoid undue traction on the catheter, which can cause a traumatic hypospadias. Symptomless bacteriuria is usual and does not require treatment, although clinical infections should be treated by antibiotics. Bladder spasms occur in 37% of all patients on long-term catheterization, and these may cause urinary incontinence around the catheter. This usually responds to anticholinergic therapy.

PROSTATE CANCER

EPIDEMIOLOGY, AETIOLOGY AND RISK FACTORS

The incidence of prostate cancer in the UK in 1999 was 74.3 per 100 000, with 21 400 new registrations and a mortality rate of 32.5 per 100 000.[77] The incidence increases with age, and in the UK in 1998 there were 150.1, 448.4 and 802.2 new registrations per 100 000 in the 60–64, 70–74 and 80–84-year-old age groups, respectively. There are also significant ethnic and racial differences, with the highest incidence and mortality rates in African Americans and the lowest in Asian men.[78]

Little is known about the aetiology of prostate cancer, but both environmental and genetic factors are known to be contributory. Immigrants to the USA from Japan, where the disease is rare, develop incidence rates that are intermediate between their country of origin and their adopted country. These rates reach that of the host country with successive generations, suggesting that there is an environmental cause.[79] Diet appears to be the most likely explanation for this difference, but it is not clear whether a high-fat, low-fibre, western diet promotes prostate cancer or a low-fat, high-fibre, eastern diet is protective. It has been suggested that the high content of plant oestrogens in a typical eastern diet may modify the carcinogenic process.[80]

Individual genetics also appear to have an important bearing on the aetiology of prostate cancer. In 5–10% of cases there is a dominantly inherited susceptibility to prostate cancer, but to date

REFERENCES

68. Roehrborn CG, Burkhard FC, Bruskewitz RC et al. J Urol 1999; 162: 92–97
69. Mulligan ED, Lynch TH, Mulvin D et al. Br J Urol 1997; 79: 177–180
70. Emberton M, Neal DE, Black N et al. Br J Urol 1996; 77: 233–247
71. Pickard R, Emberton M, Neal DE. Br J Urol 1998; 81: 712–720
72. Mebust WK, Holtgrewe HL, Cockett AT et al. J Urol 1989; 141: 243–247
73. Neal DE. Br J Urol 1997; 79 (Suppl 2): 69–75
74. Borboroglu PG, Kane CJ, Ward JF et al. J Urol 1999; 162: 1307–1310
75. Hahn RG. Br J Urol 1997; 79: 669–680
76. Kohler-Ockmore J, Feneley RC. Br J Urol 1996; 77: 347–351
77. Office for National Statistics. Cancer Trends in England and Wales 1950–1999. Online. Available: http://www.statistics.gov.uk/statbase
78. Farkas A, Marcella S, Rhoads GG. Ethn Dis 2000; 10: 69–75
79. Shimizu H, Ross RK, Bernstein L et al. Br J Cancer 1991; 63: 963–966
80. Meyer JP, Gillatt DA. BJU Int 2002; 89: 250–254

the gene has not been identified. Epidemiological studies confirm that a family history of prostate cancer is a definite risk factor. A first-degree relative with prostate cancer doubles the risk for any given individual, and if diagnosed under the age of 60 years this risk trebles. The risk is quadrupled if a brother and father are affected, and there is a fivefold increase in men from families with hereditary prostate cancer.[81]

Many other possible aetiological agents have been investigated, including vasectomy, smoking, and the role of heavy metals such as cadmium. While a few studies have suggested a link between prostate cancer and vasectomy,[82] most do not support this association. One study suggested that vasectomized men are more likely to present with earlier-stage and lower-grade tumours.[83,84] Population studies have failed to demonstrate a causative link with cigarette smoking. Epidemiological and animal studies have demonstrated a carcinogenic effect of cadmium on the prostate,[85] and work is continuing to identify the underlying mechanisms.[86]

DIAGNOSIS

Since the introduction of serum PSA estimation in the late 1980s, the early diagnosis of symptomless prostate cancer has become standard practice. Prior to this, patients often presented with symptoms from locally advanced or metastatic disease when potentially curative treatment was not possible.

Prostate-specific antigen

Prostate-specific antigen is a protease consisting of a 34-kDa glycoprotein. It is synthesized by prostatic glandular acini and drains into the prostatic urethra at the time of ejaculation. It acts by lysing a protein called seminogelin, resulting in dissolution of the seminal coagulum, thereby aiding sperm migration through the female genital tract.

The prostate concentration of the antigen is between a thousand and a million times greater than that found in serum. Anything that affects the prostate can cause the serum PSA to be elevated. Transient increases are caused by ejaculation, prostatic massage and cycling! Urethral instrumentation and catheterization, transrectal ultrasound and prostatic biopsy also cause an elevation in serum levels.[87] Serum PSA is also raised by prostate cancer, prostatic hyperplasia, prostate trauma, prostatitis, urinary tract infection or retention, and the presence of pelvic inflammation and sepsis. Therefore an elevated reading must be carefully interpreted, and this is important in selecting those patients who will benefit from further investigation to exclude prostate cancer.

Population studies have provided important information on the probability of having prostate cancer for a given PSA level. The normal serum PSA is related to the age of the patient and the size of the prostate. Depending on the cut-off level for the upper limit of the normal range, further investigation yields a diagnosis of cancer in varying proportions. A serum PSA level of 4–10 nmol/mL indicates a 22% risk of prostate cancer and above 10 nmol/mL a 63% risk.[88] The PSA density (which is the PSA level divided by the prostate volume), age-related reference ranges, doubling time and PSA velocity (the rate of PSA change over time), and the ratio of free to bound PSA all improve specificity.[89–91] Because PSA-detected prostate cancer has a mean survival of 10 years, it is crucial to test only those men in whom further evaluation and radical treatment is appropriate. The National Screening Committee has stressed the importance of counselling symptomless men who request the investigation.

Digital rectal examination

Digital rectal examination remains an important part of any clinical examination. Prior to the measurement of PSA, it was the standard means of detecting and staging prostate cancer, although it has major limitations. Although rectal examination has only a 7–9% specificity for diagnosing cancer and a 52–56% predictive value for staging organ-confined disease, it has an 81–93% predictive value for widespread disease. It is therefore a poor diagnostic test for early prostate cancer, but it is highly likely to be abnormal in patients with advanced disease.[92]

Transrectal ultrasound scan

Transrectal ultrasound scanning of the prostate using a 7- or 8-mHz multiplanar probe to allow targeted prostate biopsies is now the best method of diagnosing prostate cancer. The transrectal ultrasound is used to guide the biopsy, but more sensitive scanning equipment, including MRI, now allows accurate staging of the disease.[93] Six, eight, ten or more biopsies are performed, mainly in the peripheral zone of the gland.[94–96] The sensitivity of ultrasound-guided biopsies in detecting prostate cancer is 77%.[97] Between 24 and 60% of patients develop immediate complications of mild haematuria, although this is severe only in under 1%. Mild rectal bleeding and vasovagal fainting can also occur in a few patients. Delayed morbidity comprises fever in 3%, haemospermia in 10%, recurrent mild haematuria in 16% and persistent dysuria in 7.2%, with a urinary tract infection developing in 10%. Major complications are rare and include urosepsis and rectal bleeding.[98]

CLINICAL FEATURES

Routine opportunistic measurement of the PSA in men with lower tract symptoms is often responsible for the detection of

REFERENCES

81. Bratt O. BJU Int 2000; 85: 588–598
82. Emard JF, Drouin G, Thouez JP et al. Health Place 2001; 7: 131–139
83. Stanford JL, Wicklund KG, McKnight B et al. Cancer Epidem Biomarkers Prev 1999; 8: 881–886
84. Bernal-Delgado E, Latour-Perez J, Pradas-Arnal F et al. Fertil Steril 1998; 70: 191–200
85. Ye J, Wang S, Barger M et al. J Environ Pathol Toxicol Oncol 2000; 19: 275–280
86. Martin MB, Voeller HJ, Gelmann EP et al. Endocrinology 2002; 143: 263–275
87. Tchetgen MB, Oesterling JE. Urol Clin North Am 1997; 24: 283–291
88. Catalona WJ, Richie JP, Ahmann FR et al. J Urol 1994; 151: 1283–1290
89. Potter SR, Horniger W, Tinzl M et al. Urology 2001; 57: 1100–1104
90. Catalona WJ, Southwick PC, Slawin KM et al. Urology 2000; 56: 255–260
91. Djavan B, Zlotta AR, Remzi M et al. Urology 1999; 54: 846–852
92. O'Dowd GJ, Veltri RW, Orozco R et al. J Urol 1997; 158: 687–698
93. Wilkinson BA, Hamdy FC. BJU Int 2001; 87: 423–430
94. Borboroglu PG, Comer SW, Riffenburgh RH et al. J Urol 2000; 163: 158–162
95. Babaian RJ, Toi A, Kamoi K et al. J Urol 2000; 163: 152–157
96. Ravery V, Billebaud T, Toublanc M et al. Eur Urol 1999; 35: 298–303
97. Rabbani F, Stroumbakis N, Kava BR et al. J Urol 1998; 159: 1247–1250
98. Djavan B, Waldert M, Zlotta A et al. J Urol 2001; 166: 856–860

early, 'symptomless' prostate cancer. When symptoms are present they can be either local or related to distant metastases. Local urinary symptoms from prostate cancer usually indicate more advanced disease. They include those of bladder outflow obstruction and bladder overactivity, which can be secondary to outflow tract obstruction from the direct effects of the expanding cancer on the bladder base. There is, however, no evidence that men with lower tract symptoms are at increased risk from prostate cancer.[99] Other local effects may include tenesmus and very rarely bowel obstruction or rectal bleeding, as Denonvilliers' fascia usually functions as an efficient natural mechanical barrier to the spread of the tumour. Upper urinary tract obstruction may occur from bladder outflow tract obstruction or from direct invasion and compression of the ureters.

More distant symptoms may occur from bony metastases, when pain, pathological fracture and spinal cord compression may result. Spinal cord compression may be from bony or soft tissue (dural) metastases. Marrow failure gives rise to the symptoms of anaemia and thrombocytopenia, and pelvic lymph node metastases can cause lower limb oedema and lower abdominal pain.

PATHOLOGY

Adenocarcinoma of the prostate is usually heterogeneous. Pathological grading of the tumour is based on the Gleason system, which depends on both the cytological features and the degree of glandular organization. Grades range from 1, which is a well-differentiated tumour, to 5, which is anaplastic. The most common tumour pattern is given a grade, and this is then combined with the next most common pattern to produce a Gleason sum score ranging from 2 to 10.[100]

Tumour staging is based on the 1997 version of the TNM (tumour, node and metastasis) system for urological tumours (Table 37.1).

Table 37.1 The 1997 TNM (tumour, node and metastasis) staging system for prostate cancer

Stage	Description
Tx	Primary tumour cannot be assessed
T0	No evidence of primary tumour
T1	Non-palpable and/or not detectable on imaging
T1a	Incidentally detected at transurethral resection of the prostate and present in less than 5% of the specimen
T1b	Incidentally detected at transurethral resection of the prostate and present in more than 5% of the chippings
T1c	Biopsy detected
T2	Palpable and/or detectable on imaging but not invading the capsule
T2a	One lobe involved
T2b	Both lobes involved
T3	Extracapsular
T3a	Extracapsular extension but not invading the seminal vesicles
T3b	Invasion of the seminal vesicles
T4	Fixed or invading adjacent structures
N0	No lymph node involvement
N1	Regional lymph nodes
Mo	No metastatic spread
M1a	Non-regional lymph nodes involved
M1b	Bone metastases
M1c	Metastases at additional or other sites

INVESTIGATIONS

Full blood count analysis and the estimation of serum urea, electrolytes, liver enzymes and alkaline phosphatase are helpful baseline investigations once prostate cancer has been diagnosed. A technetium-99 radionuclide bone scan is the most sensitive method of detecting bony metastases and should be obtained in all men with prostate cancer and skeletal pain, or a serum PSA of greater than 20 ng/mL. Omitting the bone scan in symptomless men with a PSA of less than 20 ng/mL will miss 1% of patients with bony metastastatic disease.[93]

Radioimmunoscintigraphy and positron emission tomography are other imaging techniques under investigation for the detection of lymph node metastases.[93]

Tables combining PSA, stage and grade are available that indicate the probability and 95% confidence limits of finding organ-confined prostate cancer, capsular penetration by the tumour, seminal vesicle involvement and lymph node spread. These are commonly used as an adjunct for therapeutic planning.[101]

TREATMENT AND CLINICAL OUTCOMES

The treatment of prostate cancer is best considered by categorizing patients into three broad groups consisting of early, locally advanced and metastatic prostate cancer.

Early disease is where the cancer is confined to the prostate gland and there is no evidence of metastatic spread (T1N0M0 to T2bN0M0). The serum PSA is usually less than 20 nmol/mL. Because prostate cancer is a relatively slow-growing tumour and it may be many years before it becomes symptomatic, radical potentially curative therapy with either surgery or radiotherapy is indicated only in patients with a life expectancy of 10 years or more. Simple observation or hormone manipulation is indicated for patients unsuitable for or not wishing radical treatment.[102]

Locally advanced disease implies tumour extension beyond the prostatic capsule, with possible regional lymph node involvement (T3 or 4, N0 or 1, M0). Few surgeons suggest radical surgery under these circumstances but radical radiotherapy, with or without adjuvant hormone manipulation, or hormone manipulation alone as palliation may be considered.

In *late disease*, once there is evidence of distant metastatic spread the tumour is considered to be incurable; hormone manipulation with supportive palliative care is the only possible treatment.

REFERENCES

99. Young JM, Muscatello DJ, Ward JE. BJU Int 2000; 85: 1037–1048
100. Algaba F, Epstein JI, Aldape HC et al. Cancer 1996; 78: 376–381
101. Partin AW, Kattan MW, Subong EN et al. JAMA 1997; 277: 1445–1451
102. Steineck G, Helgesen F, Adolfsson J et al. N Engl J Med 2002; 347: 790–796

Comparative studies of the different treatments are very limited. The results from a tumour registry suggest that the 10-year prostate cancer-specific survival rate for low-grade disease that has not metastasized is 94% after radical prostatectomy, 90% after external beam radiotherapy and 93% with conservative management. The corresponding survival rates in patients with moderate-grade tumours are 87%, 76% and 77%, and for those with high-grade cancer are 67%, 53% and 45%.[103] These figures are derived from over 60 000 men in the North American cancer registry, and because these groups are not randomized, comparisons must be interpreted with caution.[104] The only comparative trial has shown that radical prostatectomy can reduce the cancer-specific mortality rate compared with simple observation, but the overall survival rates for patients remain unchanged.[105]

Seventy per cent of men with palpable, clinically localized, moderately differentiated prostate cancer do not develop symptomatic disease progression by 5 years, and 40% are still symptom-free at 10 years.[106] The risks of disease progression are, however, significantly greater for men with poorly differentiated disease.[107]

Radical prostatectomy

Radical removal of the prostate, with full assessment of lymph node status, through a suprapubic approach has been developed and popularized by Walsh.[108] A similar resurgence of interest in radical prostatectomy via the perineal approach came about because of the current drive to reduce medical costs and because of the increased detection of localized prostate cancer. The selected use of lymphadenectomy and the development of laparascopic techniques to perform node sampling have also encouraged enthusiasm for surgical resection.[109] Although the perineal technique provides a cost-effective, low-morbidity, and efficacious means of resecting localized prostate cancer, the risk of rectal injury is increased and the neurovascular bundles are less easily identified. The majority of surgeons continue to use the abdominal approach. Laparoscopic radical prostatectomy has now started to gain popularity.[110] The learning curve for this procedure is steep, and advantages in terms of outcomes and efficacy have yet to be demonstrated.

A retropubic radical prostatectomy is performed via a retropubic, extraperitoneal, lower midline abdominal incision. Pelvic lymphadenectomy and frozen section is advisable when the PSA is above 10 ng/mL, when high-grade cancer is present in the biopsy (Gleason score 8 or above), or when enlarged or suspicious lymph nodes are palpable.[111] Some favour performing a laparascopic node dissection before definitive surgery so that the results can be discussed with the patient. The whole prostate is resected and the bladder neck is anastomosed to the urethral stump. The neurovascular bundle containing the cavernosal nerves responsible for erectile function should, if possible, be preserved. Early complications include mortality of around 0.1% and a small risk of pulmonary embolus, myocardial infarction, and bleeding requiring surgical re-exploration.[112] The late complications are specific to the operation and include early incontinence in up to a third of patients and erectile dysfunction in at least half.[113,114] Significant stress incontinence occurs in less than 5% of men by 12 months and can be effectively treated by inserting an artificial urinary sphincter,[115] while erectile dysfunction often responds to treatment with sildenafil (see Ch. 38).[116]

Neoadjuvant hormone manipulation prior to surgery may result in pathological down-staging of more extensive tumours and better local cancer control, but has not been shown to confer any advantage in survival.[117,118] When a PSA rise occurs after radical prostatectomy, the median time to metastases is 5 years and the median time to death is 13 years.[119]

Radical external beam radiotherapy

Traditionally up to 6000 cGy have been used to treat prostate cancer, but studies have shown that increased doses up to 7800 cGy administered daily over a 5-week period are more effective at achieving disease control.[120] The PSA is an important predictor of outcome, and cure has been defined as maintenance of PSA below 0.5 ng/mL.[121]

Early side effects are experienced by most patients and include urinary frequency, dysuria, proctitis and fatigue. Late complications include persisting radiation cystitis and proctitis,[122] incontinence,[123] and erectile dysfunction developing in roughly a third of those treated.[116] Efficacy is improved and side effects, particularly proctitis, reduced by the use of conformal radiotherapy.[122,124]

Although neoadjuvant hormone therapy does not delay PSA progression or the development of distant metastases, continuing adjuvant hormone treatment certainly delays progression and may prolong survival when combined with external beam radiotherapy.[117,118,125]

REFERENCES

103. Lu-Yao GL, Yao SL. Lancet 1997; 349: 906–910
104. Barry MJ, Albertsen PC, Bagshaw MA et al. Cancer 2001; 91: 2302–2314
105. Holmberg L et al. N Engl J Med 2002; 347: 781–789
106. Adolfsson J, Steineck G, Hedlund PO. Urology 1997; 50: 722–726
107. Johansson JE, Holmberg L, Johansson S et al. JAMA 1997; 277: 467–471
108. Walsh PC. J Urol 1998; 160: 2418–2424
109. Scolieri MJ, Resnick MI. Urol Clin North Am 2001; 28: 521–533
110. Guillonneau B, Cathelineau X, Doublet JD et al. J Endourol 2001; 15: 441–445
111. Fergany A, Kupelian PA, Levin HS et al. Urology 2000; 56: 92–95
112. Lepor H, Nieder AM, Ferrandino MN. J Urol 2001; 166: 1729–1733
113. Catalona WJ, Carvalhal GF, Mager DE et al. J Urol 1999; 162: 433–438
114. Fowler FJ Jr, Barry MJ, Lu-Yao G et al. Urology 1993; 42: 622–629
115. Klijn AJ, Hop WC, Mickisch G et al. Br J Urol 1998; 82: 530–533
116. Vale J. Radiother Oncol 2000; 57: 301–305
117. Lawton CA, Winter K, Murray K et al. Int J Radiat Oncol Biol Phys 2001; 49: 937–946
118. Bolla M, Gonzalez D, Warde P et al. N Engl J Med 1997; 337: 295–300
119. Pound CR, Partin AW, Eisenberger MA et al. JAMA 1999; 281: 1591–1597
120. Pollack A, Zagars GK. Urology 1998; 51: 258–264
121. Critz FA, Levinson K, Williams WH et al. Urology 1997; 49: 668–672
122. Dearnaley DP, Khoo VS, Norman AR et al. Lancet 1999; 353: 267–272
123. Nguyen LN, Pollack A, Zagars GK. Urology 1998; 51: 991–997
124. Zelefsky MJ, Fuks Z, Hunt M et al. J Urol 2001; 166: 876–881
125. Pilepich MV, Winter K, John MJ et al. Int J Radiat Oncol Biol Phys 2001; 50: 1243–1252

Brachytherapy

Brachytherapy, or interstitial radiotherapy, consists of the insertion of multiple radioactive pellets (seeds) into the prostate. A perineal approach is used, and the seeds are placed in a pattern previously determined by transrectal ultrasound. This therapy cannot be used to treat high-grade cancers, large prostates, patients with a PSA above 10 mmol/L, and patients who either have undergone a previous transurethral resection or have significant bladder outflow obstruction. Morbidity from the procedure is not insignificant, and complications include urinary retention in 6–8% and incontinence in 13–18%. Cystitis or urethritis, and proctitis affect about 10% of those treated and erectile dysfunction occurs in up to a half.[126,127]

Hormone manipulation

In over 80% of cases prostate cancer depends on testosterone for its growth.[128] Any treatment that lowers or blocks testosterone therefore arrests the growth of the cancer and provides effective palliative treatment for the disease, often for several years.

Hormone manipulation is the standard treatment for early or locally advanced prostate cancer and has always been used to treat metastatic disease. There is good evidence that initiation of hormone manipulation at the time of diagnosis, rather than waiting for the patient to become symptomatic, prolongs survival in men with advanced prostate cancer.[118,129] To defer hormone manipulation until the patient becomes symptomatic doubles the patient's risk of presenting with a pathological fracture, spinal cord compression, ureteric obstruction or extraskeletal metastases.[129] Hormone therapy is being used to treat early prostate cancer and is also commonly used as an adjunct to radiotherapy for locally advanced disease. It has been shown to confer a survival advantage when it is used to treat men with metastatic lymph nodes following radical prostatectomy.[130]

Hormone therapy given in early prostate cancer has been prompted by the use of tamoxifen in the analogous situation of hormone-dependent breast cancer. Early adjuvant treatment with bicalutamide has been shown to have similar benefits in treating early prostate cancer. Bicalutamide has been shown to delay the progression of the disease, as judged by bone scan and PSA progression, when used in combination with all other forms of treatment for early prostate cancer.[131]

Hormone manipulation by bilateral orchidectomy is cost-effective but is less popular with patients than a chemical castration. Testosterone levels fall to castrate levels within hours, making this form of treatment ideal when a rapid response is required, such as in a patient with impending spinal cord compression.

Luteinizing hormone-releasing hormone (LHRH) analogues (goserelin and leuprorelin) are the main alternative to surgical castration and act by providing a continuous serum level of synthetic gonadotrophin. The pituitary gland normally requires a pulsed stimulation by LHRH to produce luteinizing hormone, which in turn stimulates testosterone production by the Leydig cells in the testis. The LHRH analogues produce castrate levels of testosterone within 2 weeks.

Lowering testosterone inevitably results in a loss of libido with erectile dysfunction, and may cause other less specific side effects including energy loss, weight gain, osteoporosis and impaired cognitive function.

Antiandrogens provide effective control of prostate cancer by competing with endogenous testosterone at the androgen receptors and thereby blocking its activity. There are two main classes of antiandrogens: steroidal and non-steroidal. Cyproterone acetate is a steroidal drug that acts both centrally, as a progestogen inhibiting luteinizing hormone release, and peripherally, blocking the effect of testosterone at the androgen receptor. Following several cases of severe hepatotoxicity, cyproterone acetate is no longer recommended as first-line hormone treatment for the long-term control of prostate cancer, and should certainly be used with caution in patients with liver disorders or in those with a history of thromboembolic disease. It still has a useful role in preventing the testosterone-mediated tumour flare that occurs when LHRH analogues are initially commenced, and these drugs are also useful at lower doses to treat hot sweats associated with orchidectomy or LHRH analogue therapy.

Bicalutamide, flutamide and nilutamide are non-steroidal antiandrogens that act exclusively on the androgen receptor as competitive antagonists. They do not lower serum testosterone levels and hence have fewer side effects. Sexual function and libido are maintained in up to 80% of patients,[132] but gynaecomastia can be a significant problem caused by these drugs. Bicalutamide can be used as monotherapy in the treatment of locally advanced prostate cancer and has equivalent efficacy to castration.[133] Non-steroidal antiandrogens can also be used to prevent tumour flare.

Antiandrogens have been used extensively in combination with orchidectomy or gonadotrophin-releasing hormone analogues to provide a total androgen blockade. The concept of a total androgen blockade is to achieve castrate testosterone levels and also to block the effects of adrenal androgen that are not under the control of the pituitary gland. The evidence for additional benefit is conflicting, and extensive meta-analysis suggests that at best it confers a 5% survival advantage.[134,135]

Chemotherapy

There is no established role for chemotherapy in the treatment of prostate cancer, but a number of cytotoxics are the subject of continuing clinical trials.

COMPLICATIONS OF PROSTATE CANCER

Complications from prostate cancer are commonly seen once the tumour escapes from hormone control but may be encountered at initial presentation or in men under surveillance. Androgen deprivation is the first-line therapy for men not previously treated, but in those presenting with spinal cord compression or ureteric obstruction additional intervention may be required.

REFERENCES

126. D'Amico AV, Whittington R, Malkowicz SB et al. JAMA 1998; 280: 969–974
127. Henderson A, Cahill D, Laing RW et al. BJU Int 2002; 90: 567–572
128. Huggins C, Hodges CV. Cancer Res 1941; 1: 293
129. Medical Research Council Prostate Cancer Working Party Investigators Group. Br J Urol 1997; 79: 235–246
130. Messing EM, Manola J, Sarosdy M et al. N Engl J Med 1999; 341: 1781–1788
131. See WA, Wirth MP, McLeod DG et al. J Urol 2002; 168: 429–435
132. Iversen P, Melezinek I, Schmidt A. BJU Int 2001; 87: 47–56
133. Iversen P, Tyrrell CJ, Kaisary AV et al. J Urol 2000; 164: 1579–1582
134. Prostate Cancer Trialists' Collaborative Group. Lancet 2000; 355: 1491–1498
135. Prostate Cancer Trialists' Collaborative Group. Lancet 1995; 346: 265–269

Pain from bony metastases

Radiotherapy can be given to individual sites, and hemibody treatment can be used for more extensive disease. It can be given systemically as intravenous strontium-89 or samarium-153. External beam radiotherapy provides pain relief in 70% of men.[136] Hemibody and local radiotherapy provide equivalent symptom control when compared with strontium, but fewer patients report new pain sites after strontium treatment.[137]

Systemic mitoxantrone has been shown to provide useful palliation,[138] but biphosphonate therapy has a more limited benefit.[139]

Ureteric obstruction

Ureteric obstruction may cause loin pain, renal failure and ultimately death. Patients who have not undergone previous hormone manipulation should be actively treated by nephrostomy, urinary diversion and androgen deprivation. A trial of nephrostomy clamping may be considered after a period of weeks. An initial short course of systemic corticosteroids may avoid the need for nephrostomy diversion in some patients.[140] Careful consideration must be given before active treatment is selected for men whose cancer has escaped hormone control, because their prognosis is poor.[141]

Spinal cord compression

Symptoms of spinal cord compression from spinal metastases may be acute or progressive, and consist of sensory and motor deficits, radicular pain and bladder dysfunction. The spinal pathology is best delineated by MRI when the diagnosis is suspected.[142] Immediate treatment with systemic steroids and androgen deprivation by orchidectomy are indicated. Urgent radiotherapy, surgical decompression, or both should follow. Surgery and radiotherapy are equally effective in relieving symptoms,[143] but radiotherapy is the standard initial approach.[144] Sixty per cent of paralysed men walk again, with a mean survival of 115 days; a quarter survive 2 years.[142]

PROSTATITIS

INTRODUCTION

Acute bacterial prostatitis is caused by an acute infection of the lower urinary tract and usually has no long-term sequelae. Chronic prostatitis and the chronic prostatitis syndromes, on the other hand, are usually idiopathic and are associated with long-term morbidity and a reduced quality of life.[145]

EPIDEMIOLOGY

It has been estimated that 8% of all genitourinary consultations in the USA are for complaints of prostatitis, making it the most common urological diagnosis in men under 50 years of age and the third most common condition in those over 50 years.[146] The prevalence of moderate to severe symptoms of prostatitis in men aged 20–74 years is 6.6%, with no apparent relationship to age,[147] although others have suggested that men under 66 years old are twice as susceptible as those over this age. A previous diagnosis of prostatitis is a significant risk factor.[148]

DIAGNOSTIC PROCEDURES

Lower urinary tract localization studies

Culture of aliquots of urine collected at different times during voiding and after prostatic massage can be used to confirm the presence and the location of infection. The Meares–Stamey four-glass test localization technique is still used. The four aliquots are the first 10 mL voided (from the urethra), a late midstream sample (from the bladder), urethral secretions following prostatic massage, and the first 10 mL voided following prostatic massage. They are labelled VB1, VB2, EPS (expressed prostatic secretions) and VB3, respectively. In bacterial prostatitis the colony counts from EPS and VB3 are at least 10-fold greater than from VB1. A higher colony count from VB1 compared with VB2 suggests urethritis.[149]

A simpler procedure is to collect urine specimens just before and after a prostate massage.[150] The presence of bacteria and leukocytes in the postmassage specimen that are not present in the premassage specimen indicates chronic bacterial prostatitis (type IIa), whereas leukocytes alone indicate inflammatory prostatitis (type IIIa) and neither bacteria nor leukocytes suggest a diagnosis of prostadynia (type IIIb).

Classification of prostatitis

The traditional classification[151] has now been replaced by the National Institutes of Health classification.[152] The latter system recognizes the fact that prostadynia may not arise from the prostate and has introduced the term *chronic pelvic pain syndrome.* A comparison of these classifications and the relative frequency of each type of prostatitis are shown in Table 37.2.

AETIOLOGY

Bacterial prostatitis

Enterobacteriaceae are responsible for the majority of infections, with *Escherichia coli* accounting for 65–80% and *Pseudomonas aeruginosa*, *Serratia* species, *Klebsiella* species and *Enterobacter aerogenes* a further 10–15%. The Gram-positive enterococci account for 5–10% of infections. Risk factors that allow bacterial colonization of the prostate include intraprostatic ductal reflux, phimosis, unprotected anal intercourse, urinary tract

REFERENCES

136. McQuay HJ, Carroll D, Moore RA. Clin Oncol (R Coll Radiol) 1997; 9: 150–154
137. Quilty PM, Kirk D, Bolger JJ et al. Radiother Oncol 1994; 31: 33–40
138. Tannock IF, Osoba D, Stockler MR et al. J Clin Oncol 1996; 14: 1756–1764
139. Bloomfield DJ. J Clin Oncol 1998; 16: 1218–1225
140. Hamdy FC, Williams JL. Br J Urol 1995; 75: 782–785
141. Paul AB, Love C, Chisholm GD. Br J Urol 1994; 74: 642–645
142. Huddart RA, Rajan B, Law M et al. Radiother Oncol 1997; 44: 229–236
143. Constans JP, Divitiis E, Donzelli R et al. J Neurosurg 1983; 59: 111–118
144. Osborn JL, Getzenberg RH, Trump DL. J Neurooncol 1995; 23: 135–147
145. Wenninger K, Heiman JR, Rothman I et al. J Urol 1996; 155: 965–968
146. Collins MM, Stafford RS, O'Leary MP et al. J Urol 1998; 159: 1224–1228
147. Nickel JC, Downey J, Hunter D et al. J Urol 2001; 165: 842–845
148. Roberts RO, Lieber MM, Rhodes T et al. Urology 1998; 51: 578–584
149. Meares EM, Stamey TA. Invest Urol 1968; 5: 492–518
150. Nickel JC. Tech Urol 1997; 3: 38–43
151. Drach GW, Fair WR, Meares EM et al. J Urol 1978; 120: 266
152. Krieger JN, Nyberg L Jr, Nickel JC. JAMA 1999; 282: 236–237

Table 37.2 Comparison of the classifications of prostatitis, its features and their relative frequency

Traditional classification	US National Institutes of Health classification	Features	Frequency
Acute bacterial prostatitis	Category I	Acute infection of the prostate gland	Rare
Chronic bacterial prostatitis	Category II	Recurrent urinary tract infection or chronic infection of the prostate	5–15%
Not applicable	Category III or chronic pelvic pain syndrome	Discomfort or pain in the pelvic region, variable voiding and sexual symptoms, and no demonstrable infection	–
Non-bacterial prostatitis	Category IIIa or inflammatory chronic pelvic pain syndrome	Significant number of white cells in semen/EPS/VB3	50%
Prostadynia	Category IIIb or non-inflammatory chronic pelvic pain syndrome	Insignificant number of white cells in semen/EPS/VB3	40%
Not applicable	Category IV or asymptomatic inflammatory prostatitis	No symptoms but evidence of inflammation and/or infection in prostate biopsy/semen/EPS/VB3	–

EPS, expressed prostatic secretions; VB3, the aliquot of urine following prostatic massage (see text).

infection, epididymitis, indwelling catheters, condom urinary drainage and urethral instrumentation. Acute bacterial prostatitis is caused by an acute infection of the lower urinary tract. While proven infection accounts for only around 14% of all diagnosed cases of chronic prostatitis,[153] there are several other aetiological theories.

Non-bacterial prostatitis or chronic pelvic pain syndrome

The role of non-pathogenic micro-organisms and those not detectable by standard microbiological techniques in the aetiology of chronic prostatitis has been fully investigated. *Chlamydia trachomatis* has received most attention but the evidence is conflicting. Other organisms investigated include *Staphylococcus saprophyticus*, *S. aureus*, haemolytic streptococci, anaerobes, *Ureaplasma urealyticum* and *Trichomonas*. The role of fastidious non-culturable organisms also remains unclear.[154]

Some investigators have suggested that dysfunctional voiding leads to chronic pelvic pain syndrome. Anatomical abnormalities of the bladder neck, urethra and prostate may predispose some to prostatitis,[155] and many patients with prostadynia have obstructed urodynamics[156] or vesicourethral dyssynergia.[157,158] Dyssynergic voiding may lead to chronic pain and intraprostatic duct reflux. Reflux mainly affects the peripheral zone of the prostate[155] and allows urate, urea, creatinine and micro-organisms to enter the prostate. The resulting inflammation may be infective, chemical[159] or immunological. Bacterial prostatitis produces a transient prostatic immune response,[160] which might be prolonged, or an autoimmune phenomenon.[161]

CLINICAL FEATURES

Acute prostatitis

Acute prostatitis is a rare but well-recognized condition. The patient presents with lower abdominal, pelvic, and perineal pain and dysuria associated with voiding difficulty or acute urinary retention. Systemic symptoms include fever, nausea and vomiting, and there are sometimes signs of septicaemia. On examination the prostate is swollen, 'boggy' and exquisitely tender. The urine and blood should be sent for culture, and bacteria are almost always isolated. The development of a prostatic abscess is indicated by a failure to respond to antibiotics.

Chronic bacterial prostatitis

The symptoms of chronic prostatitis are usually long-standing but are often intermittent and variable. Both filling and voiding lower urinary tract symptoms may be present. The pain is typically perineal and deep in the pelvis, but pain may also be experienced in the penis, testicles, inguinal area, suprapubic area and back. The pain is often exacerbated by ejaculation, and sexual dysfunction is common. There are usually no abnormalities to be found on physical examination other than variable prostatic tenderness. Some patients experience anal sphincter spasm, which leads to an uncomfortable digital rectal examination and should not be confused with prostatic tenderness. Urine is taken for microscopy and culture, and localization studies may be performed. It can be difficult to distinguish chronic bacterial prostatitis from chronic pelvic pain syndrome, but a history of urinary tract infections is indicative of a bacterial aetiology. The National Institutes of Health Chronic Prostatitis Symptom Index has been developed. Nine questions address symptom severity: pain, lower urinary tract symptoms and quality of life.[162]

TREATMENT

Bacterial prostatitis

Broad-spectrum intravenous antibiotics (e.g. a cephalosporin and gentamicin) are given for acute prostatitis, and the fever and

REFERENCES

153. Nickel JC, Downey J, Johnston B et al. J Urol 2001; 165: 1539–1544
154. Walsh PC, Retik AB, Darracott Vaughan E Jr et al (eds). Campbell's Urology, Vol 1. 8th edn. WB Saunders, Philadelphia, 2002
155. Blacklock NJ. Infection 1991; 19 (Suppl 3): S111–S114
156. Barbalias GA, Meares EM Jr, Sant GR. J Urol 1983; 130: 514–517
157. Kaplan SA, Santarosa RP, D'Alisera PM et al. J Urol 1997; 157: 2234–2237
158. Kaplan SA, Te AE, Jacobs BZ. J Urol 1994; 152: 2063–2065
159. Persson BE, Ronquist G. J Urol 1996; 155: 958–960
160. Kumon H. Infection 1992; 20 (Suppl 3): S236–S238
161. Alexander RB, Brady F, Ponniah S. Urology 1997; 50: 893–899
162. Litwin MS, McNaughton-Collins M, Fowler FJ Jr et al. J Urol 1999; 162: 369–375

acute symptoms usually settle within 2 or 3 days. A prostatic abscess is suspected when the signs and symptoms do not settle and prostatic fluctuance can be felt on digital rectal examination. The abscess may be confirmed by transrectal ultrasound scan but this may not be tolerated by the patient. Antibiotics against anaerobic bacteria should be added, and the abscess drained endoscopically following urethroscopy under anaesthetic. A suprapubic catheter is placed if the patient has urinary retention.

Chronic bacterial prostatitis is treated by a quinolone for 4 weeks, which appears superior to trimethoprim for 3 months.[154]

Chronic pelvic pain syndrome

The vast array of treatment options for this condition is a reflection of the lack of understanding of its aetiology and pathogenesis, and the high failure rate of its treatments. Some prefer to categorize patients using localization studies and adopt a different treatment plan for each group. Others take a more pragmatic approach on the basis that the same therapeutic path will be followed for most patients irrespective of their diagnostic category. Evidence supports the pragmatic approach,[155] and 80% of urologists rarely or never utilize localization tests.[163]

A number of different forms of treatment are in routine use.

Antimicrobial agents

Prospective placebo-controlled randomized trials are yet to report,[164] but observational data show that 40% of men have some symptomatic relief.[165,166]

Alpha blockers

Reducing outflow resistance in theory relieves some of the symptoms if prostatitis is secondary to dysfunctional voiding, with or without intraprostatic duct reflux. Small randomized placebo-controlled studies and a larger, non-randomized study with phenoxybenzamine, alfuzosin, tamsulosin and terazosin lend support to this approach to treatment.[167–169] Some advocate the simultaneous use of muscle relaxants such as diazepam and baclofen.[170]

Anti-inflammatory drugs

Non-steroidal anti-inflammatory drugs and the cyclo-oxygenase 2 inhibitors may provide symptom relief but never achieve complete resolution. It has been suggested that some cases of prostatitis may be part of the spectrum of interstitial cystitis (see Ch. 36). One prospective study has demonstrated the efficacy of pentosan polysulfate in some patients with chronic prostatitis,[171] and a randomized placebo-controlled trial of this agent is underway.[154]

Phytotherapy

Some plant extracts have 5α-reductase activity and anti-inflammatory effects, and marginally improve voiding parameters. Cernilton, a bee pollen extract, and quercetin, a natural bioflavonoid, show some promise.[172,173]

5α-Reductase inhibition

In a small, poorly conducted randomized trial, finasteride reduced benign prostatic hyperplasia and prostatitis symptoms but not pain scores.[174] A larger trial has begun.[154]

Allopurinol

Intraprostatic reflux of uric acid may contribute to prostatitis, and one randomized study showed a beneficial effect of allopurinol versus placebo, although the results were not substantiated in a later analysis.[175–177]

Microwave hyperthermia

Between 50 and 70% of men experience an improvement in symptoms in small, sham-controlled randomized trials.[178,179]

Surgery

Surgery plays only a minor role in the treatment of prostatitis. Although radical transurethral prostatic resection and radical prostatectomy have been tried, there is only limited anecdotal evidence to support their use and they cannot be recommended.

Biofeedback

Biofeedback has been shown to be helpful in ameliorating symptoms.[180]

A practical treatment plan for chronic pelvic pain

An initial empirical course of a quinolone antibiotic is commenced, and the patient reviewed after 8 weeks. When this produces symptomatic improvement, the antibiotic should be continued for a further 6 weeks. When there is no improvement, second-line treatment consists of alpha blockade and non-steroidal anti-inflammatory drugs. If these fail, third-line therapy such as finasteride, pollen extract and pentosan polysulfate may be tried. Biofeedback may provide useful support; although time-consuming it benefits many patients.

REFERENCES

163. McNaughton Collins M, Fowler FJ Jr, Elliott DB et al. Urology 2000; 55: 403–407
164. Shoskes DA. Can J Urol 2001; 8 (Suppl 1): 24–28
165. Naber KG, Busch W, Focht J. Int J Antimicrob Agents 2000; 14: 143–149
166. Weidner W, Ludwig M, Brahler E et al. Drugs 1999; 58 (Suppl 2): 103–106
167. Lacquaniti S, Destito A, Servello C et al. Arch Ital Urol Androl 1999; 71: 283–285
168. de la Rosette JJ, Karthaus HF, van Kerrebroeck PE et al. Eur Urol 1992; 22: 222–227
169. Barbalias GA, Nikiforidis G, Liatsikos EN. J Urol 1998; 159: 883–887
170. Zermann DH, Ishigooka M, Doggweiler-Wiygul R et al. World J Urol 2001; 19: 173–179
171. Nickel JC, Johnston B, Downey J et al. Urology 2000; 56: 413–417
172. Rugendorff EW, Weidner W, Ebeling L et al. Br J Urol 1993; 71: 433–438
173. Shoskes DA, Zeitlin SI, Shahed A et al. Urology 1999; 54: 960–963
174. Leskinen M, Lukkarinen O, Marttila T. Urology 1999; 53: 502–505
175. Persson BE, Ronquist G. Eur Urol 1996; 29: 111–114
176. Nickel JC, Siemens DR, Lundie MJ. Lancet 1996; 347: 1711–1712
177. Persson BE, Ronquist G, Ekblom M. J Urol 1996; 155: 961–964
178. Liatsikos EN, Dinlenc CZ, Kapoor R et al. J Endourol 2000; 14: 689–692
179. Nickel JC, Sorensen R. J Urol 1996; 155: 1950–1954
180. Clemens JQ, Nadler RB, Schaeffer AJ et al. Urology 2000; 56: 951–955

The urethra and penis 38

Kay Thomas, Nicholas A. Watkin

THE URETHRA

ANATOMY AND APPLIED PHYSIOLOGY

THE MALE URETHRA

The male urethra extends from the bladder neck to the external meatus at the tip of the glans penis (Fig. 38.1). It may be divided into four parts: prostatic, membranous, bulbar, and penile. The former two parts are posterior, the latter two parts anterior.

The veru montanum is an important landmark within the prostatic urethra (Fig. 38.2). It is a crest of tissue arising from the posterior aspect of the prostatic urethra on the surface of which the ejaculatory ducts open. The membranous urethra is very short and is that part of the urethra that traverses the perineal membrane. It is encircled by the distal or external sphincter mechanism. The bulbar urethra is that portion of urethra covered by the bulbospongiosus muscle. The penile (pendulous) urethra is about 15 cm long and is contained within the corpus spongiosum. It terminates at the external meatus, and just before it opens there is a slight dilatation, the navicular fossa.

Continence in the male is maintained by two mechanisms: the external urethral sphincter and the bladder neck (internal urethral sphincter). The external sphincter surrounds the membranous urethra and is composed of circular smooth and striated muscle fibres. These are slow-twitch fibres, which can therefore remain contracted for prolonged periods without fatigue. The pudendal nerve innervates both the external sphincter and levator ani muscles. The external sphincter also has an autonomic nerve supply via the pelvic plexus. The internal sphincter or bladder neck is composed of smooth muscle fibres that actively contract with the bladder neck during ejaculation to prevent retrograde emission of semen. Adrenergic receptors in the bladder neck control muscle tone. These receptors can be blocked by α-blocker drugs, which cause relaxation of the internal sphincter mechanism and relieve lower urinary tract symptoms in men with bladder outflow obstruction.

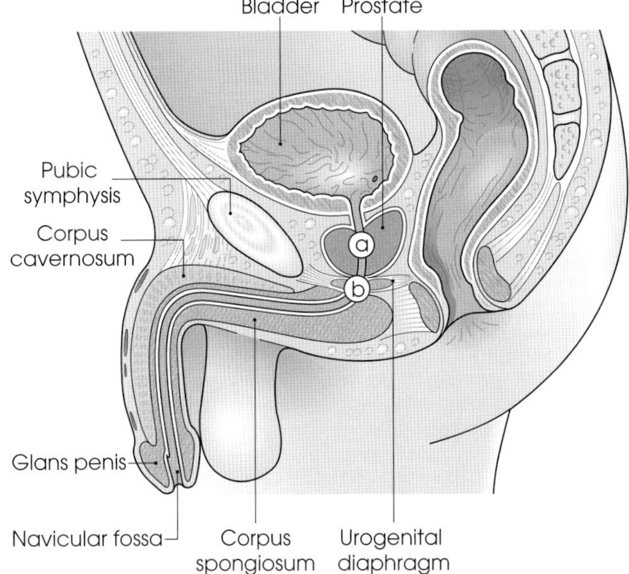

Figure 38.1 Anatomy of the male urethra.

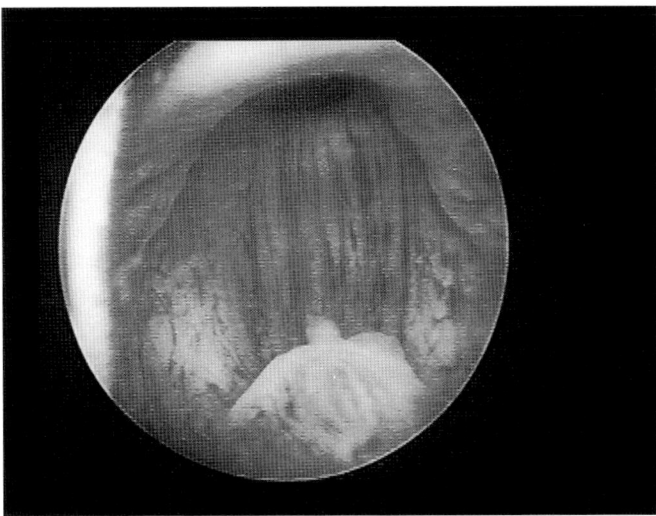

Figure 38.2 Endoscopic view of the veru montanum.

The proximal internal sphincter is usually disrupted during a transurethral resection of the prostate. Continence is then dependent on the distal sphincter mechanism, hence the importance of the veru montanum because this is used to define the boundary of the sphincter during prostatic resection.[1–4]

THE FEMALE URETHRA

The urethra is much shorter in the female (4 cm) compared with the male (20 cm). It is surrounded along its length by a circular layer of striated and smooth muscle, which is thickest in the

REFERENCES

1. Tanagho EA, McAnninch JW (eds). Smith's General Urology. 14th edn. Appleton and Lange, Connecticut, 1995
2. Walsh PC, Retik AB, Stamey TA et al (eds). In: Campbell's Urology. 6th edn. Saunders, Philadelphia, 1994
3. Mundy AR, Fitzpatrick JM, Neal DE et al (eds). The Scientific Basis of Urology. ISIS Medical Media, Oxford, 1999
4. Blandy JP. Lecture Notes on Urology. 5th edn. Blackwell Science, Oxford, 1998

middle third. In combination with the pelvic floor, this diffuse layer of muscle is responsible for maintaining urinary continence.

THE MALE URETHRA

CONGENITAL CONDITIONS

Posterior urethral valves

Posterior urethral valves are abnormal congenital folds of mucosa in the prostatic urethra, which cause outflow obstruction in male children. They occur in between one in 5000 and one in 8000 male births. Three types of these valves were originally described; however, it is now recognized that only two of these varieties (types I and III) are clinically important.[5] Type I are the most common (95%) and are thought to arise because of the anterior insertion of the mesonephric ducts into the cloaca. During separation of the cloaca these ducts are thought to fuse. Type III valves are formed because of incomplete dissolution of the urogenital membrane.

Because of the increasing use of antenatal ultrasound, posterior urethral valves may be diagnosed in utero as a cause of bilateral hydronephrosis and a distended bladder.[6] In the newborn they may present with a palpable bladder, renal mass, ascites, or respiratory distress secondary to pulmonary hypoplasia. In older boys they can cause febrile urinary tract infections or daytime incontinence. The diagnosis is usually made by obtaining a micturating cystogram (Fig. 38.3). Initial treatment should ensure adequate drainage of the bladder via a urethral catheter or vesicostomy, correction of renal impairment, and treatment of sepsis. Endoscopic ablation or hook resection can then be used to treat the valves. Although this treatment is relatively simple, irreversible renal damage secondary to the obstruction may already have occurred if a child presents late.[7–9]

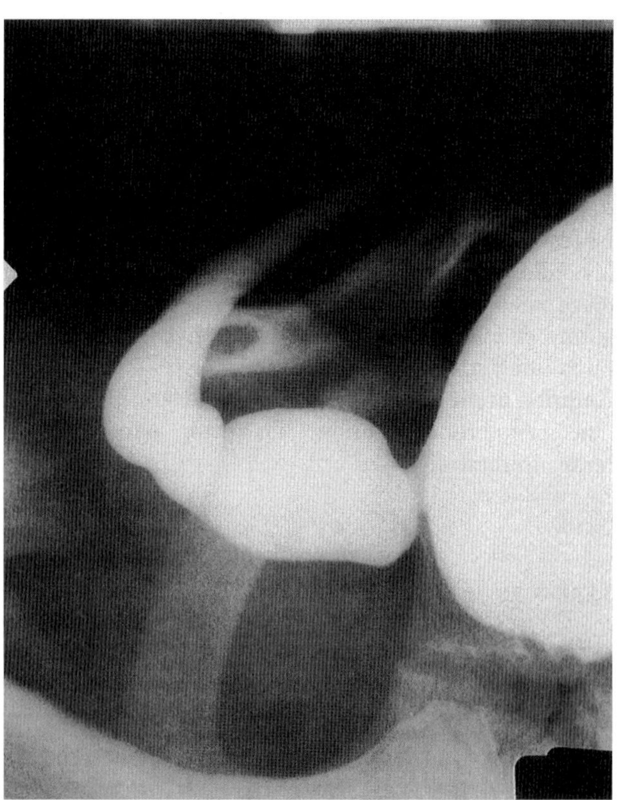

Figure 38.3 Micturating cystogram of posterior urethral valves.

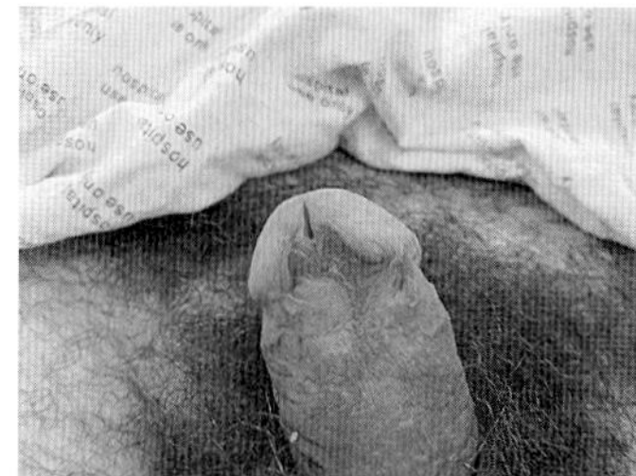

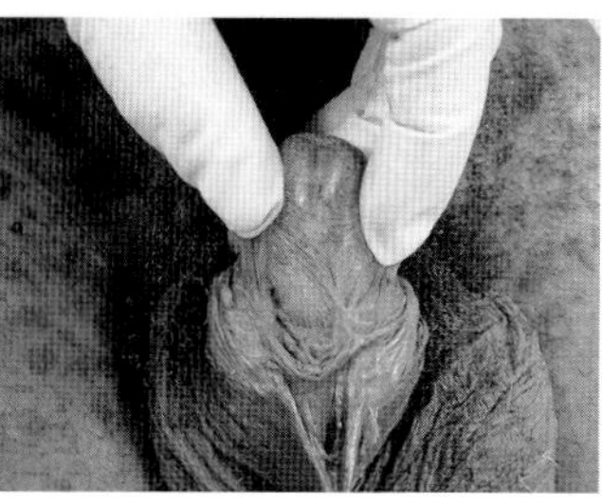

a b

Figure 38.4 (a) Coronal hypospadias and (b) penoscrotal hypospadias.

Hypospadias

Hypospadias describes a condition where the meatus or opening of the urethra occurs on the underside (ventral) aspect of the penis rather than at its tip. It is associated with chordee of the penis and a hooded foreskin (Fig. 38.4). A genetic component may influence the development of hypospadias because children who have an affected parent or sibling are more likely to have the condition. The incidence of hypospadias is one in 200, but this appears to be increasing, possibly secondary to environmental factors such as dietary oestrogens. The apparent increase may, however, simply be a reflection of enhanced awareness of the condition among physicians and parents.[10–12] Hypospadias can be classified according to the site of the meatus (Fig. 38.5, Table 38.1).

Hypospadias can be associated with other congenital abnormalities, such as testicular maldescent, persistence of female structures (e.g. the utricle), and sexual ambiguity (e.g. testicular feminization). Treatment is usually surgical and has two aims: cosmesis and restoration or preservation of normal function (i.e. voiding and straightness of erection). The surgical procedure performed depends on the site of the hypospadias (Table 38.2). Over the years many operations have been described, each called by a surgeon's name.[13–15] The number of procedures and modifications reflects the suboptimal results often obtained. The most durable procedures currently used are listed in Table 38.2.

Circumcision should be avoided in a child with hypospadias, because the foreskin may subsequently be required as a skin flap for repair. Complications of hypospadias surgery are urethra–cutaneous fistula, stricture, meatal stenosis, urethral diverticulum, chordee, and breakdown of repair.[16] These

REFERENCES

5. Young HH, Frontz WA, Baldwin JC. J Urol 1919; 3: 289
6. Mergurian PA, McLorie GA, Churchill BM et al. J Urol 1992; 148: 1499–1503
7. Parkhouse HF, Barratt TM, Dillon MJ et al. Br J Urol 1988; 62: 59–62
8. Warshaw BL, Hymes LC, Trulock TS et al. J Urol 1985; 133: 240–243
9. Tejani A, Butt K, Glassberg K et al. J Urol 1986; 136: 857–860
10. Gatti JM, Kirsch AJ, Troyer WA et al. BJU Int 2001; 87: 548–550
11. Silver RI. Del Med J 2000; 72: 343–347
12. Toppari J, Kaleva M, Virtanen HE. Hum Reprod Update 2001; 7: 282–286
13. Snodgrass W. J Urol 1994; 151: 464–465
14. Humby GA. Br J Surg 1941; 29: 84–92
15. Metro MJ, Wu HY, Snyder HM III et al. J Urol 2001; 166: 1459–1461
16. Hensle TW, Tennerbaum SY, Reiley EA et al. J Urol 2001; 165: 77–79

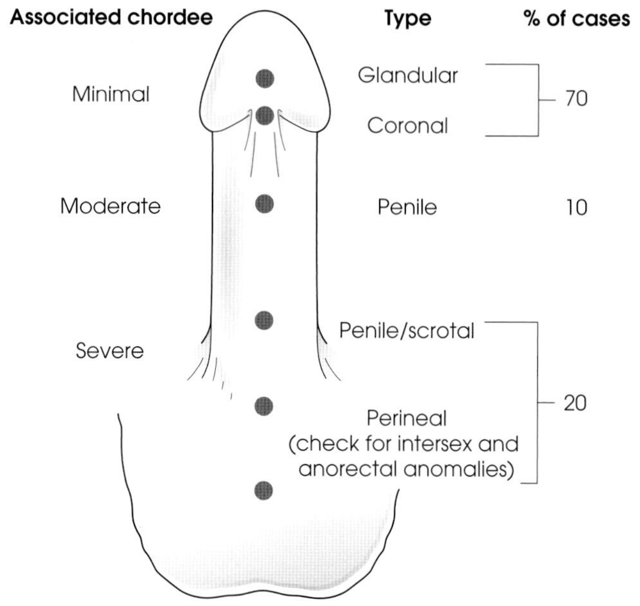

Figure 38.5 Types of hypospadias.

Table 38.1 Classification of hypospadiac deformities

Traditional	Duckett	Koyanagi	Cases (%)
Glandular	Anterior	–	70
Coronal			
Anterior penile			
Middle penile	Middle	Distal	10
Posterior penile	Posterior	Proximal	20
Penoscrotal			
Scrotal			
Perineal			

Table 38.2 Types of hypospadias repair

Site of hypospadias	Repair
Distal	Tubularization of urethral plate Meatal advancement or glanduloplasty incorporated Meatal advancement flap
Middle or proximal	Island skin flap Onlay tubularized skin flap Free graft (buccal mucosa or postauricular Woolfe graft)

complications are best avoided by using well-vascularized tissues. The tissues should be handled as little as possible and always with the utmost care during the procedure. Redo surgery has a higher complication rate because the tissues are often unhealthy. Mobilization must be adequate to allow tension-free anastomosis but not so extensive as to impair the vascular supply. Meticulous haemostasis should be achieved, and where possible the suture lines should not overlap. Ideally, associated chordee should be corrected at the time of the hypospadias repair.

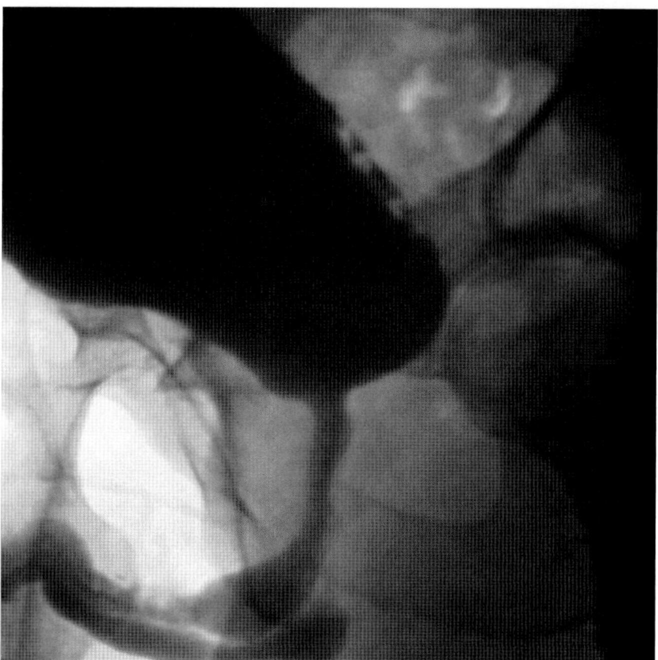

Figure 38.6 Urethral false passage secondary to traumatic catheterization.

ACQUIRED DISORDERS

Urethral injury

Iatrogenic

In the UK this is one of the most common causes of urethral injury. Unskilled instrumentation of the urethra with either a catheter or an endoscope can result in a false passage with the potential for stricture formation in the future (Fig. 38.6).[17,18] The treatment and management of this is described in the section on urethral strictures (see *Urethral strictures*, p. 877).

Traumatic

About 10% of pelvic fractures have an associated urethral injury, usually of the membranous portion (Fig. 38.7). The most common cause of this is a road traffic accident. After resuscitating and stabilizing the patient, any life-threatening injuries should be treated. Once the patient's condition is stable the urethral injury can be considered. Broad-spectrum antibiotics should be administered, and a gentle attempt made by a suitably trained person at passing a urethral catheter. A suprapubic catheter should be inserted if this fails. When a urethral catheter cannot be inserted, the site of injury inevitably strictures or completely obliterates. Treatment of the stricture should be delayed for 6 months after the initial injury to allow the scar tissue to stabilize.[19–22]

REFERENCES

17. Hammarsten J, Lindqvist K, Sunzel H. Br J Urol 1989; 63: 397–400
18. Balbay MD, Ergen A, Sahin A et al. Int Urol Nephrol 1992; 24: 49–53
19. McAninch JW. J Trauma 1981; 21: 291–297
20. Colapinto V, McCallum RW. J Urol 1977; 118: 575–580
21. Webster GD. Urol Clin North Am 1989; 16: 303–312
22. Webster GD, Mathes GC, Selli C. J Urol 1983; 130: 898–902

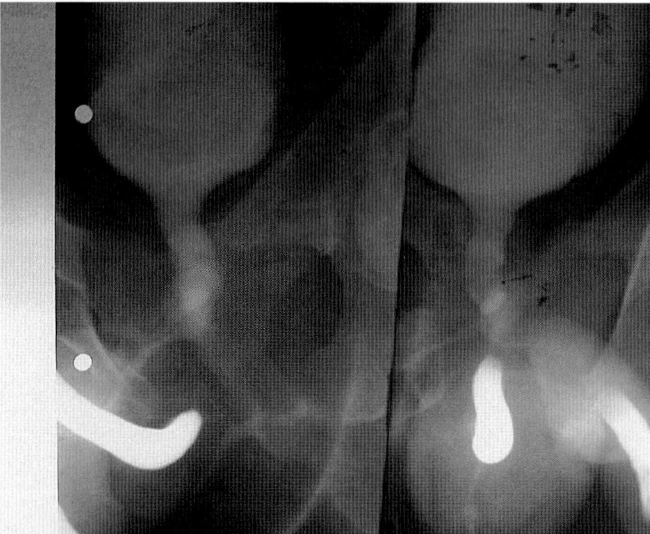

Figure 38.7 Pelvic fracture with urethral disruption. A 2-cm gap is present between the blind-ending bulbar and the prostatomembranous urethra.

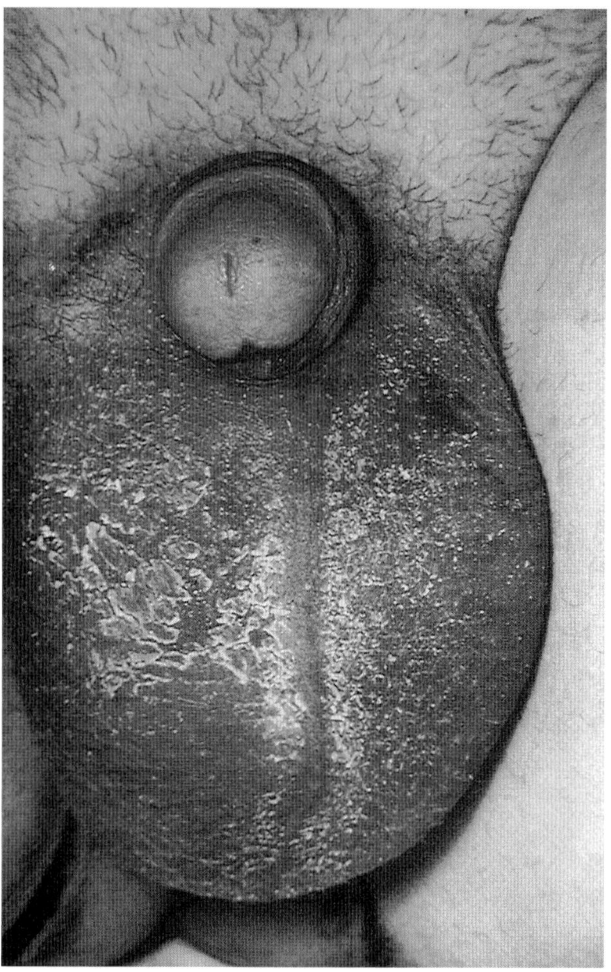

Figure 38.8 Scrotal bruising from a ruptured urethra.

Injury of the urethra can be partial or complete, regardless of the site. Clinical signs are the development of haematoma in the perineum and scrotum, and the presence of frank blood at the external urinary meatus. A high-riding prostate may be detected on rectal examination when there is an associated pelvic fracture. The patient may still be able to void urine or they may develop urinary retention. Extravasation of urine and a swollen scrotum may occur if they are still voiding (Fig. 38.8). Because of the fascial attachments, urine can spread backwards towards the perineal body and superiorly up the anterior abdominal wall but not down the thighs (Fig. 38.9).

The bulbar urethra is injured when it is crushed against the pubic arch. This can occur in a fall astride for example a bicycle crossbar or tree branch, especially in young boys. The bulbar urethra is also commonly injured by a kick in the crotch in young men (Fig. 38.10). Traumatic injuries of the penile urethra are uncommon and nearly always occur as the result of violence to the erect penis, when the penoscrotal angle is the usual site of injury.

Insertion of suprapubic catheters

The two main methods of inserting a suprapubic catheter are percutaneously under local anaesthetic (Banano or Add-a Cath catheter) or at open cystotomy.

The contraindications to placing a suprapubic catheter include a known transitional cell cancer of the bladder (where

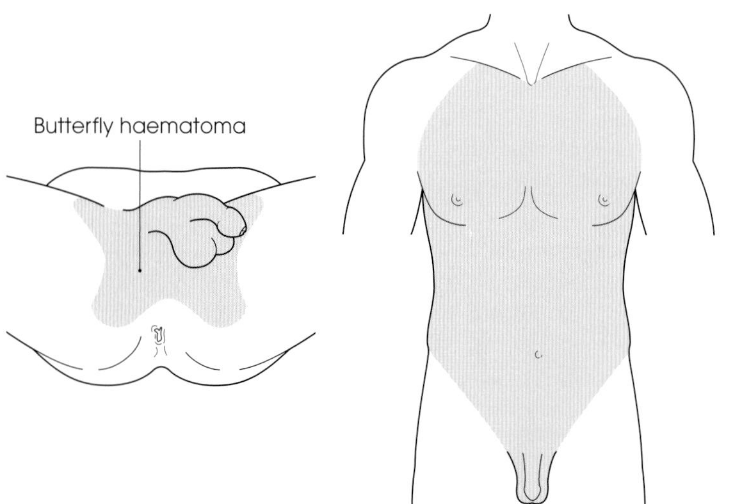

Figure 38.9 Potential areas of extravasation following attachments of Colles' fascia.

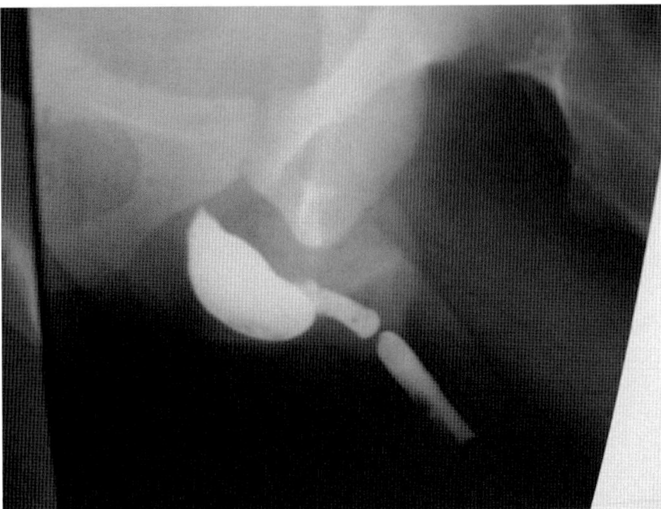

Figure 38.10 Stricture secondary to fall astride injury, a very tight stricture that requires urethroplasty because of dense scar tissue surrounding the site of the stricture.

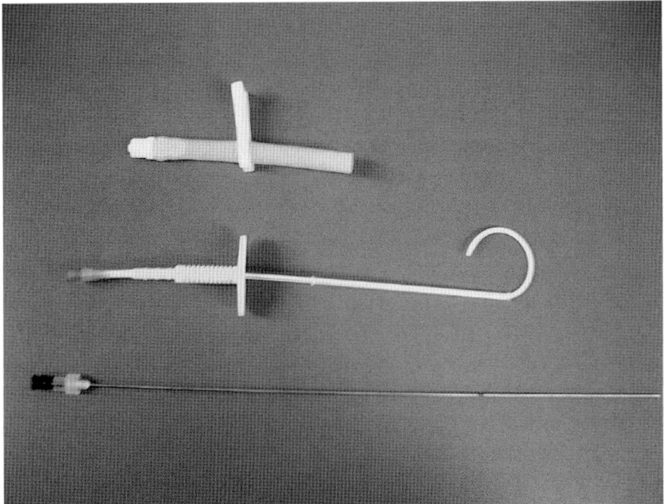

Figure 38.11 The Banano suprapubic catheter.

there is a risk of seeding tumour), and this includes patients with haematuria of unknown cause. There is also the risk of injuring a femoro-femoral crossover bypass graft (see Ch. 10).

Caution should be used when patients are on warfarin or have a known coagulopathy (see Ch. 3). Other relative contraindications include patients with augmented bladders and those with lower midline scars from previous bowel surgery, when there is an increased risk of injuring or perforating the bowel.

Percutaneous insertion under local anaesthetic

Banano catheters are useful as a temporary measure. The device consists of a 22-gauge needle covered by a plastic sheath (Fig. 38.11). The sheath has plastic wings attached to it at its midpoint and a pigtail distal end to retain it in the bladder. The wings have to be sutured to the skin to hold the catheter in place. The Add-a Cath catheter merely consists of an introducer and a sheath with a conventional urinary catheter (Fig. 38.12).

Both catheters are inserted using the same basic principles. The patient is laid as flat as possible. The skin is prepped with antiseptic from the umbilicus to the groins. Local anaesthetic,

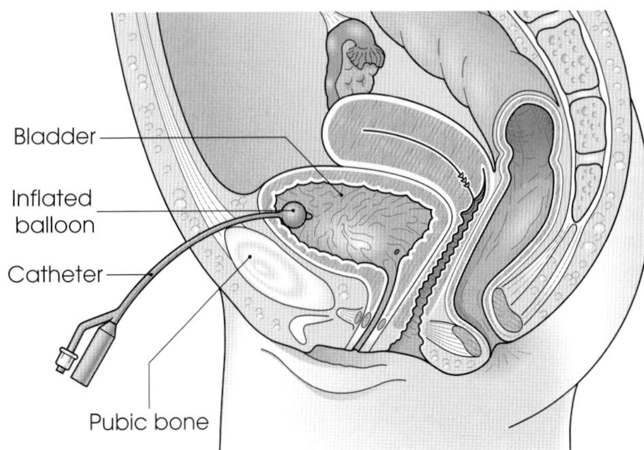

Figure 38.12 The Add-a-Cath suprapubic catheter: side view of suprapubic catheterization in a female patient.

with or without adrenaline (epinephrine), is infiltrated into the skin two fingers' breadth above the symphysis pubis. The underlying tissue is then infiltrated, advancing towards the bladder. Once urine is aspirated infiltration ceases. NO attempt to place a suprapubic catheter should be made unless urine can be aspirated first.

When a Banano catheter is used, it is important to remember the angle used to aspirate urine before pushing the sheath into the bladder using the introducer. Once the sheath is well inside the bladder the introducer is removed, allowing the pigtail to curl, preventing displacement. The sheath is held in place by suturing the wings to the skin.

For the Add-a-Cath catheter, the sheath is again pushed into the bladder using the introducer in the direction of the aspirating needle. The introducer is removed once the sheath is well into the bladder, and the catheter is then advanced down the sheath. The balloon is inflated and a strip is peeled off the sheath, allowing it to be removed over the catheter. The catheter is connected to a urine bag and the output measured.[23–25]

Insertion at open cystotomy

Suprapubic catheter insertion under cystoscopic guidance or placement via open cystotomy may be required if there are scars from previous abdominal surgery where adhesions are suspected. This technique should also be used if there is a small-capacity bladder that cannot be filled, or if the patient cannot hold a full bladder because they are incontinent.

Urethral strictures

A narrowing of the urethra secondary to scar tissue from a variety of causes (see Box 38.1) is called a stricture.[26] Patients present with poor urinary flow, double micturition, recurrent infections caused by residual urine, incontinence secondary to overflow, epididymitis, and occasionally renal failure or impairment. A history of an underlying cause should be sought, remembering that the original insult may have occurred many years previously. Examination should be directed towards establishing the

REFERENCES

23. Horgan AF, Prasad B, Waldron DJ et al. Br J Urol 1992; 70: 149–151
24. Ischan J, Hunt DR. Aust N Z Surg 1987; 57: 33–36
25. Abrahams PH et al. J R Soc Med 1980; 73: 845–848
26. Singh M, Blandy JP. J Urol 1976; 115: 673–676

Box 38.1 Causes of urethral strictures

Trauma
- External: pelvic injury, fall astride
- Internal: foreign body

Iatrogenic
- Instrumentation: urethral catheter, endourology (e.g. transurethral resection of the prostate)
- Postoperative: hypospadias repair, penectomy (partial or total)

Neoplastic
- Primary: urethral carcinoma

Inflammatory
- Gonorrhea, non-specific urethritis, balanitis, xerotica obliterans

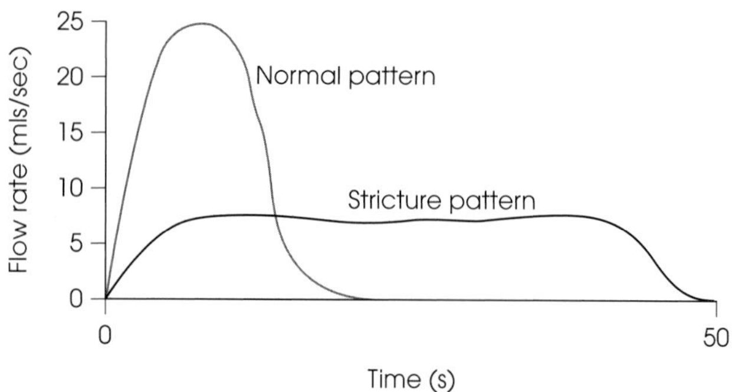

Figure 38.13 Typical flow rate for a stricture.

presence of chronic retention (an enlarged bladder) and any abnormality of the genitalia or prostatic size. Appropriate investigations are obviously influenced by the clinical history, and examination should include a midstream urine taken for culture and sensitivities, and measurement of the urea and electrolytes, the flow rate, and the volume of the postvoid residual (Fig. 38.13).

Treatment is dependent on the age, comorbidity and previous history of the patient. In patients over 60 years old, treatment is primarily endoscopic with either urethral dilatation or incision by optical urethrotomy.[27] These procedures can be repeated as often as necessary to control the stricture. Patients who form recurrent strictures should be kept on regular follow-up; some surgeons encourage their patients to regularly self-dilate their urethra to reduce the frequency of stricture formation, although others feel that this promotes rescarring and stricture recurrence.[28]

Younger patients should have one attempt at endoscopic management because they have a 50% chance of success. If this fails, however, they should be offered a urethroplasty.[29,30] The exact type of procedure chosen will depend on the site and extent of the stricture and on any previous surgery. Prior to planning surgery, an ascending and descending urethrogram should be obtained to clearly define the stricture (Fig. 38.14). Short (less than 2 cm) bulbar or membranous strictures are best managed by excising the stricture and joining the ends by an anastomotic urethroplasty (Fig. 38.15).[31] A graft or flap may be required if the stricture is in a different site or is more extensive. The penile or preputial skin can be used as a flap. Grafts are usually taken from behind the ear (postauricular Woolfe) as a full-thickness skin graft or from inside the mouth (buccal mucosa). The procedure may have to be done in two stages separated by 6 months, with the patient voiding through a temporary urethrostomy if a large area is grafted.[32–38]

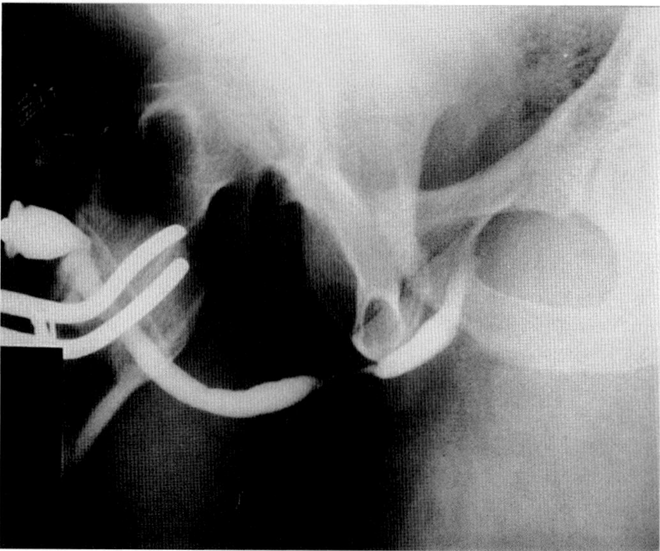

Figure 38.14 An ascending urethrogram.

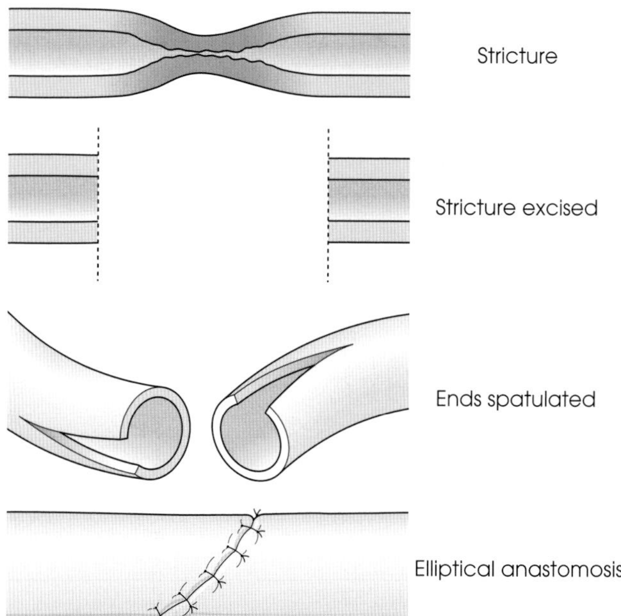

Figure 38.15 Anastomotic urethroplasty.

REFERENCES

27. Pansadoro V, Emilozzi P. J Urol 1996; 156: 73–75
28. Lapides J, Diokno AC, Silber SJ et al. J Urol 1972; 107: 458–461
29. Barbagli G, Palmminteri E, Lazzeri M et al. J Urol 2001; 165: 1918–1919
30. Johanson B. Acta Chir Scand 1953; 176: 1–103
31. Orandi A. J Urol 1972; 107: 977–989
32. Pansadoro V, Emilozzi P. Curr Opin Urol 2002; 12: 223–227
33. Webster G, Ramon J. J Urol 1991; 145: 744–748
34. Rogers HS, McNicholas TA, Blandy JP. Br J Urol 1992; 69: 621–628
35. Burger RA, Muller SC et al. J Urol 1992; 147: 662–664
36. Bbarbagli G, Selli di Cello V et al. Br J Urol 1996; 78: 929–932
37. Andrich D, Mundy AR. J Urol 2001; 165: 1131–1134
38. Duckett JW, Coplen D, Ewalt D et al. J Urol 1995; 153: 1660–1663

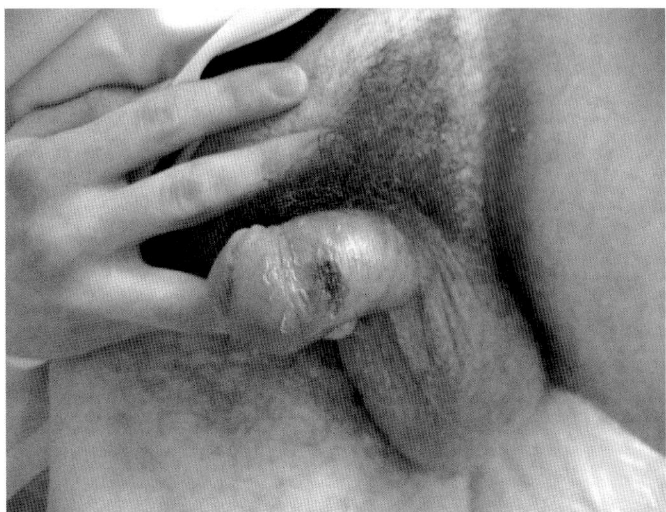

Figure 38.16 Urethral fistula secondary to stricture repair.

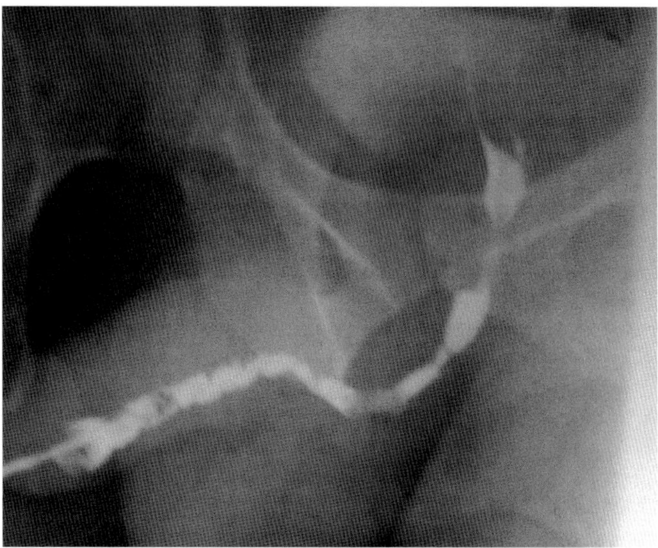

Figure 38.17 An advanced postinfectious panurethral stricture.

Table 38.3 Causes of urethritis

Pathogen	Antibiotic therapy
Sexually transmitted pathogens	
Gonorrhoea	Penicillin
Trichomonas	Metronidazole
Chlamydia (non-specific urethritis)	Tetracycline or doxycycline
Urinary tract pathogens	
Escherichia coli, Proteus	Trimethoprim, cephalosporin, nitrofurantoin, penicillin

The main potential complications of urethroplasty are failure of the graft or flap restricturing, fistula formation, or the development of a diverticulum (Fig. 38.16). Anastomotic repairs have better long-term success when compared with those using flaps or grafts.

Urethritis

Urethritis is an inflammatory condition of the urethra and may be secondary to infection from either a sexually transmitted or urinary tract pathogen (Table 38.3).

Urethritis secondary to urinary tract pathogens needs investigation with a midstream urine test, urinary tract radiography and ultrasound, flexible cystoscopy, and appropriate antibiotic treatment (Table 38.3).[39] Sexually transmitted infections are divided into gonococcal and non-gonococcal. These can often be distinguished by the amount of urethral discharge, because gonorrhoea typically produces a profuse urethral discharge. Patients are usually referred to a special clinic, where investigations include a urine culture and a urethral swab. Treatment is with antibiotics appropriate to the organism (Table 38.3). Contact tracing is important, and all contacts should be treated. To ensure that this is done adequately, patients should be referred to a genitourinary medicine physician. Patients may present with a urethral stricture many years after the original infection (Fig. 38.17).[40–42]

URETHRAL TUMOURS

Benign tumours

Urethral warts (or condylomata acuminata) are benign tumours of the urethra, usually of viral origin (human papilloma virus types 6, 11, 16, 18, 31, 33 and 35), which are sexually transmitted. They occur in the urethra or on the surface of the penis (Fig. 38.18). Treatment is initially by topical applications of podophyllin or imiquimod cream. Urethral warts are, however,

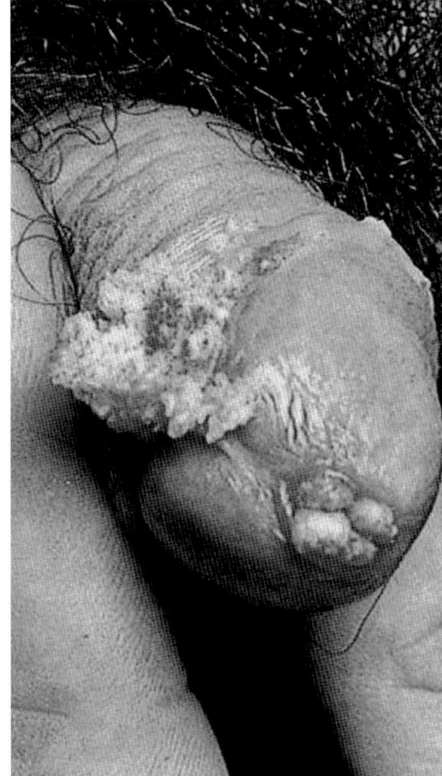

Figure 38.18 A proliferation of viral warts extending from the coronal sulcus on to the glans and urethral meatus.

REFERENCES

39. Trulus E, Bjerklund J. Curr Opin Urol 2002; 12: 39–43
40. Joly-Guillou ML, Lasry S. Drugs 1999; 57: 743–750
41. Bowie WR. Drugs 1992; 44: 207–215
42. Mogabgab WJ. Am J Med 1991; 30: 140–144

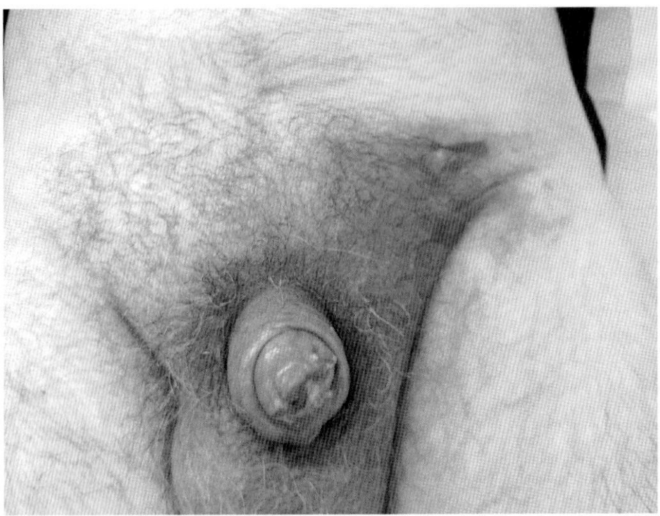

Figure 38.19 Squamous carcinoma of the penis, involving the left inguinal nodes (there is also evidence of superadded infection).

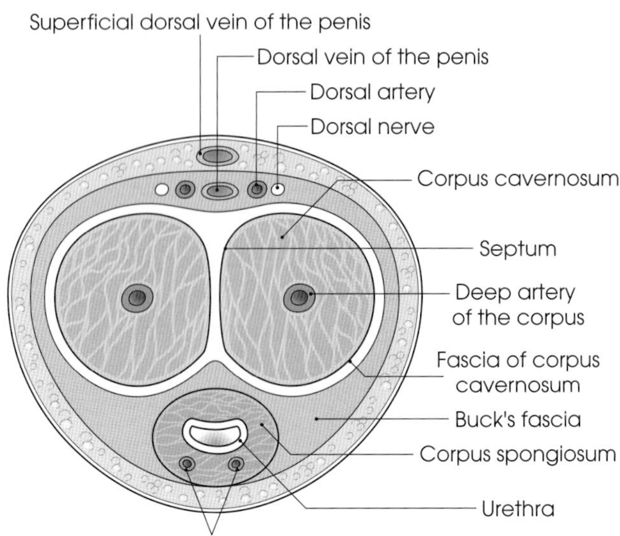

Figure 38.20 Transverse section of the penis.

often resistant and commonly recur. Treatment is then by excision, laser ablation or 5-fluorouracil cream.[43–46]

Malignant tumours

Primary tumours of the urethra are rare. They are either squamous cell carcinomas of the penis invading the external meatus and distal urethra, or transitional cell carcinomas of the more proximal urethra. They present with haematuria, haematospermia, a fistula, priapism, dysuria or urethral discharge.

The management depends on the histological type of the tumour. A urethrectomy is required for a transitional carcinoma, combined with a cystectomy if indicated. Squamous cell carcinomas should be managed as a penile tumour, with local excision, partial or total penectomy, and lymphadenectomy as required (Fig. 38.19).

THE FEMALE URETHRA

URETHRAL CARUNCLE

The urethral mucosa may prolapse, particularly if a submucosal haematoma is present. This produces a urethral caruncle. The patient may present with haematuria, pain, dysuria or dyspareunia. Treatment is by surgical excision of the redundant mucosa.

DIVERTICULUM

A diverticulum is an out-pouching of the urethral mucosa inferiorly. Infection or birth trauma causes most diverticula. Patients present with symptoms of dysuria, dribbling, and occasionally dyspareunia. On examination, pus may appear at the meatus when pressing on the urethra. The diagnosis is made by obtaining a micturating cystogram and an MRI scan. It is a cause of urinary tract infection that can be cured by surgical excision of the diverticulum.

HYPOSPADIAS

Hypospadias is a much rarer condition in female compared with male patients. The urethra opens on the anterior vaginal wall, which leads to recurrent urinary tract infections because of its shorter length. Treatment is by surgical lengthening of the urethra using a tube of vaginal mucosa. Any resultant urethral stenosis can be treated by urethral dilatation.

TRAUMA

The female urethra is much less prone to injury than in the male because of its shorter length. A fall astride, however, may crush the urethra against the pubic arch and require a vaginal mucosal tube for reconstruction.

THE PENIS

ANATOMY AND APPLIED PHYSIOLOGY

The penis is composed of three blood-filled spaces. The paired corpora cavernosa on the dorsal surface communicate and are surrounded by tough fibrous tissue. Ventrally the corpus spongiosum surrounds the urethra, distally forming the glans penis (Fig. 38.20). It does not communicate with the corpora cavernosa. The outer layer of the corpora cavernosa is called the tunica albuginea and is tough, fibrous and relatively indistensible.

The corpora are supplied by the penile arteries, which are branches of the pudendal arteries arising from the internal iliac arteries. The penile artery divides into two: the dorsal and deep penile artery. The deep penile artery gives branches that open directly into the cavernous spaces (helicine arteries), which form shunt arteries and end as capillaries within the corpus cavernosa. The dorsal artery of the penis pierces the perineal membrane and passes along the dorsum of the penis to supply the prepuce and the glans.

REFERENCES

43. Schneede P. Curr Opin Urol 2002; 12: 57–61
44. Wikstrom A, Popescu C, Forslund O. Int J AIDS 2000; 11: 80–84
45. Fife KH, Ferenczy A, Douglas JM et al. Sex Transm Dis 2001; 28: 226–231
46. Von Krogh G, Lacey CJN, Gross G. Sex Transm Infect 2000; 76: 162–168

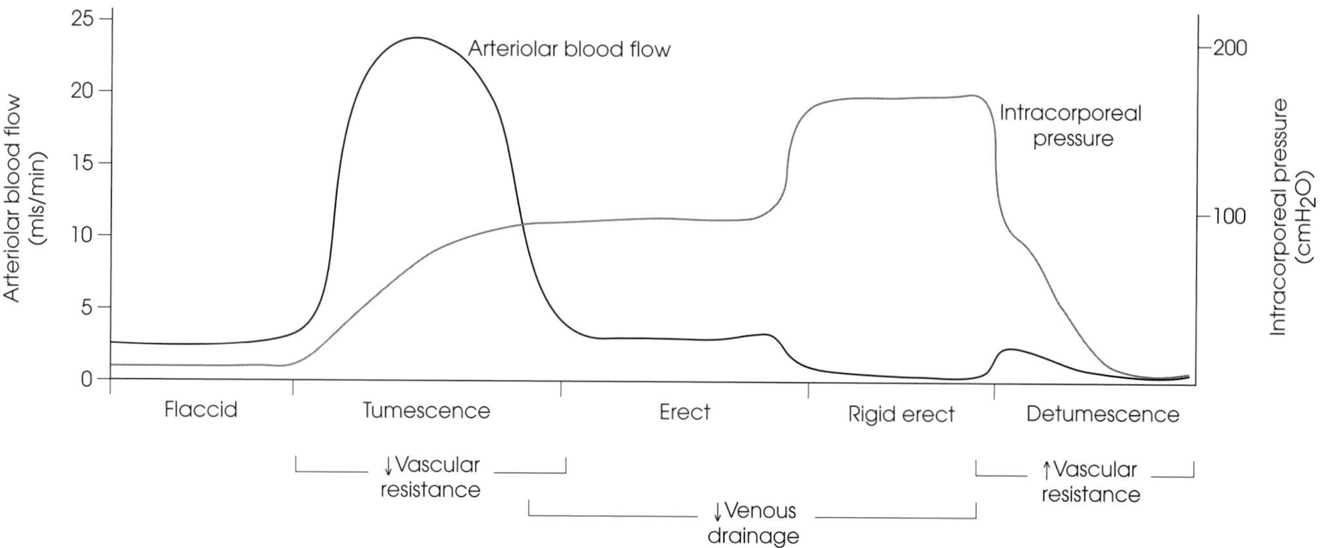

Figure 38.21 Physiology of erection: changes in arteriolar blood flow and intracorporeal pressure of the penis, are demonstrated during erection and detumescence.

The nerve supply is from the second, third and fourth sacral nerve roots; the parasympathetic controls erection and the perineal nerve sensation. The lymphatic drainage of the penis is from the prepuce and penile skin to the superficial inguinal nodes, which then drain to the deep inguinal nodes.

The mechanism of erection is secondary to increased arterial inflow and decreased venous outflow. It is dependent on decreased vascular resistance within the arterioles, which then cause blood to pool in the penis and make it erect (Fig. 38.21). As the corpora fill, the draining veins are compressed, maintaining the erection.

PARAPHIMOSIS

Paraphimosis is a relatively common problem. The foreskin is normally a little tight, but after intercourse or an intervention such as catheterization or cystoscopy, it may remain retracted behind the glans. This forms a tight band around the coronal sulcus, causing the glans to become engorged and preventing the patient from replacing the foreskin to its normal position.[47–49]

A number of steps can be taken to relieve the situation. The initial treatment is to attempt digital reduction. The fingers of both hands should be placed along the length of the shaft and thumbs gently but firmly should press on the glans. The oedema is gradually squeezed out, enabling the foreskin to be reduced. If this fails, the foreskin may be split along its dorsal surface under local anaesthetic. Some patients may wait many hours or days, usually because of embarrassment, before seeking help. Digital reduction is too painful and is not tolerated. A penile block with 10 mL of 1% plain lidocaine (lignocaine), with no adrenaline (epinephrine), can be infiltrated circumferentially around the base of the penis, as for a ring block. Digital reduction can be attempted again, and if it is still not possible a dorsal slit performed. This is done by cutting the tight band around the coronal sulcus. This method may fail if the band is incompletely divided, which is not uncommon because most of these patients will have very oedematous tissues.

It may be necessary in some patients, especially children, to perform either of the above procedures under general anaesthetic. Patience is required for digital reduction because it may take up to 15 min to squeeze all of the oedema out of the glans. A circumcision may be performed, but the cosmetic result is often suboptimal because of the swollen, oedematous tissues. The technique is described on p. 882.

PHIMOSIS

A phimosis occurs when the foreskin is too narrow to retract. The foreskin may then tear, especially during intercourse, and each time this happens further scarring worsens the condition. The foreskin may narrow to a pinhole, which in children causes ballooning of the foreskin during micturition. Balanoposthitis, which is infection of the glans and prepuce, can sometimes be the initial presentation of diabetes.

Phimosis may be caused by balanitis xerotica obliterans (see *Balanitis xerotica obliterans*, p. 882), and if long-standing is associated with cancer of the penis (Fig. 38.22). Treatment is by formal circumcision unless the patient is too infirm, when a dorsal slit under local anaesthetic may be used.

CIRCUMCISION

Circumcision is usually performed for medical indications in the UK, although occasionally it may be undertaken for religious reasons. It may be performed under local anaesthetic using a penile block as described earlier but using 10 mL of 1% plain lidocaine (lignocaine) and 10 mL of 0.05% Marcain with or without intravenous sedation (depending on the patient's age, weight and build). Some patients prefer local anaesthetic, but it is usually best reserved for the older age group.

Regardless of the anaesthetic, the operative technique remains the same. The sleeve technique is described here but there are

REFERENCES

47. Waters TC, Sripathi V. Br J Urol 1990; 66: 666
48. Saxena A. Br J Urol 1992; 69: 220
49. King PA. BJU Int 2001; 88: 305

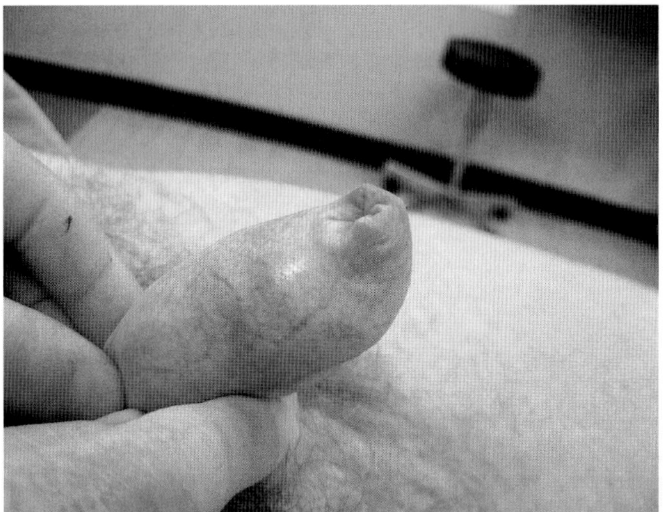

Figure 38.22 Balanitis xerotica obliterans phimosis.

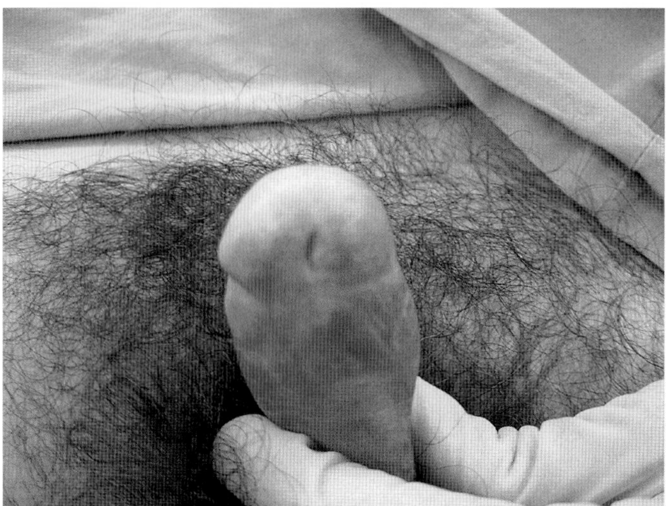

Figure 38.24 Balanitis xerotica obliterans meatal stenosis.

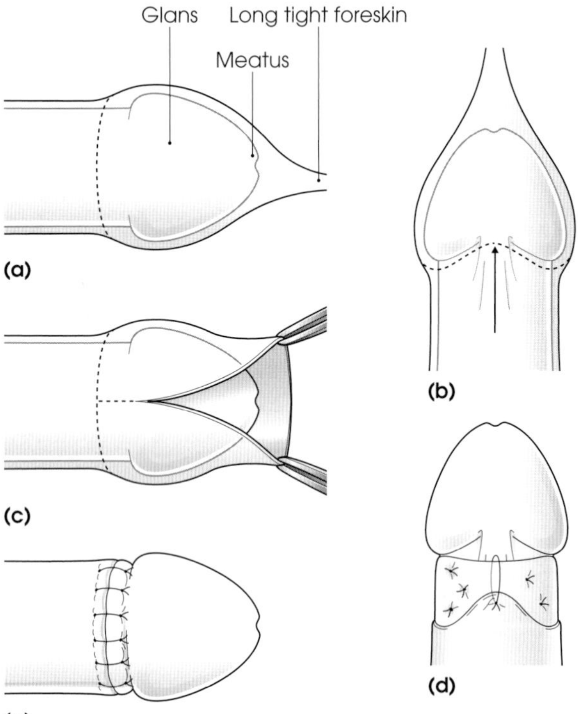

Figure 38.23 Circumcision: (a) line of incision, (b) small ventral extension by the frenulum, (c) dorsal slit, (d) bleeding points are ligated with absorbable sutures, and (e) skin–mucosal apposition with interrupted absorbable sutures.

many variations of this. The line of the skin incision is marked around the coronal sulcus with the skin under no tension (Fig. 38.23). The skin is incised and the foreskin retracted. A dorsal slit may be performed initially if this is not possible. The mucosal surface is incised 5 mm from the coronal sulcus, and the foreskin is then excised. If there is any pathology suspected the foreskin should be sent for histological diagnosis, and some surgeons do this routinely.[50] Haemostasis is secured using bipolar diathermy or by artery forceps and absorbable sutures before the skin edges are apposed with 4–5.0 absorbable sutures. Haemorrhage, usually from the frenular artery, is the main immediate complication and may necessitate a return to theatre. Late complications are loss or altered sensation of the glans.[51–53] Penile damage from poor surgical technique remains a major cause of litigation.

BALANITIS XEROTICA OBLITERANS

Balanitis xerotica obliterans is a disease of unknown aetiology and is histologically identical to lichen sclerosis. It is a dyskeratotic lesion caused by inflammatory changes, which in turn lead to fibrosis and atrophy. It can result in phimosis and scarring, which may require a circumcision (Fig. 38.24). The disease process can involve the foreskin, glans and urethra (causing urethral stricturing). Regardless of its site, treatment is by excision, but the condition often recurs.[54,55]

PRIAPISM

Priapism is a rare but important condition. It is the maintenance of an erection despite the absence of sexual stimulation. The glans and corpus spongiosum are not involved and remain flaccid. Predisposing conditions include sickle cell disease, leukaemia, extensive pelvic malignancy, and haemodialysis. It can also follow iatrogenic intracavernosal injection of vasoactive drugs for erectile dysfunction.[56]

REFERENCES

50. Pearce I, Payne SR. Ann R Coll Surg Engl 2002; 84: 325–327
51. Fink KS, Carson CC, DeVillis RF. J Urol 2002; 167: 2113–2116
52. Tucker SC, Cerqueiro J, Sterne GD et al. Ann R Coll Surg 2001; 83: 121–125
53. Holman JR, Stuessi KA. Am Fam Physician 1999; 59: 1514–1518
54. Das S, Tunuguntla HS. World J Urol 2000; 18: 382–387
55. Deppasquale I, Park AJ, Bracka A. BJU Int 2000; 86: 459–465
56. Keoghane SR, Sullivan ME, Miller MA. BJU Int 2002; 90: 149–154

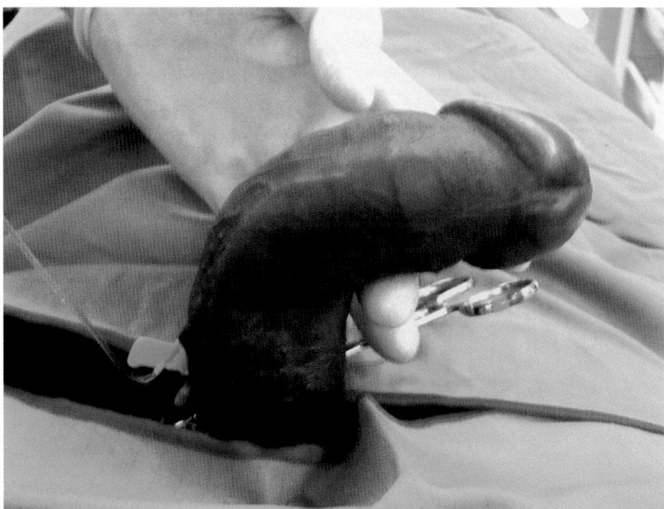

Figure 38.25 Congenital penile curvature demonstrated by an artificial saline erection.

When the erection has been present for more than 6 hours, permanent erectile failure may result. Patients should be warned of this prior to commencing treatment, otherwise they may blame the treatment used. If caused by a sickle cell crisis, patients should also undergo an exchange transfusion.[57] The following treatments can be used in sequence for low-flow priapism.

The corpora can be aspirated using a 21-G butterfly or cannula, and the old blood washed using normal saline. Vasoconstrictive agents can be infused into the corpora to aid detumescence, with care being taken to monitor for hypertension and arrhythmias. A caverno-spongiosal shunt can be performed by passing an 18-G TruCut needle through the glans and into the corpora. Subsequent failure of erections can be managed by placement of a penile prosthesis.[58] Surgical shunts anastomosing long saphenous vein to the corpora are rarely performed now.

PEYRONIE'S DISEASE

Peyronie's disease is of unknown aetiology, characterized by plaques of fibrosis in the tunica albuginea or within the corpora, which cause pain and deformity during an erection (Fig. 38.25).[59–61] The penis usually has a dorsal curvature and the disease is self-limiting. The curvature may be so severe that it renders intercourse impossible or very painful.

Treatment is initially by reassurance if the curvature is mild and intercourse is acceptable. The plaque must be allowed to stabilize before considering any intervention, and patients are usually monitored for a year. Vitamin E, steroid injection, tamoxifen, lithotripsy and radiotherapy have all been tried but with limited success, and the best option remains surgical.[62–64] There are several operations that have been described, but before they are performed it is important to assess the extent of the disease by producing an artificial erection by injecting normal saline into the corpora with a tourniquet around the penis.[65,66] Following this assessment, the plaques can be excised or the tunica albuginea plicated to straighten the shaft (Nesbitt's procedure) (Fig. 38.26). Patients should be counselled that the procedure may not be effective, that penile sensation may be altered, and that the penis will be shorter (however, because it is straight this is rarely noticed).

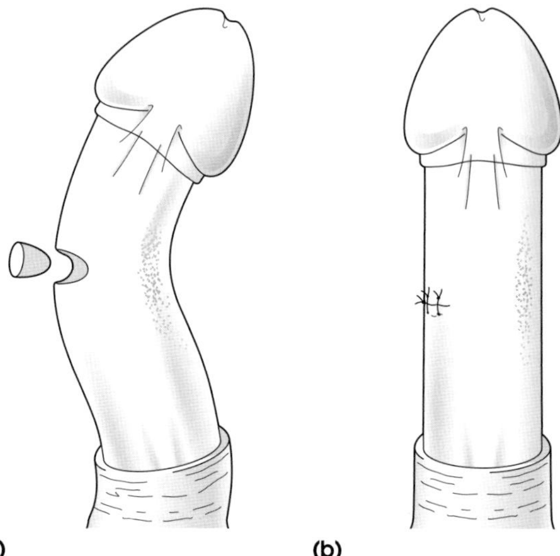

Figure 38.26 Nesbitt's procedure to correct penile curvature in Peyronie's disease: **(a)** an ellipse of tunica albuginea of corpus (about 1 cm) is excised, and **(b)** haemostatic closure of the corporeal defect is performed.

CARCINOMA OF THE PENIS

Carcinoma of the penis is an uncommon tumour that usually arises in an uncircumcised male and is associated with phimosis.[67] It can present as a warty growth or ulcer on the glans penis or prepuce, which may be hidden under the foreskin (Fig. 38.27). Patients may sometimes present with a red patch on the penis, when it can be hard to differentiate between benign pathology and carcinoma in situ of the penis (Figs 38.28 and 38.29).[68] A biopsy may then be required to establish the diagnosis. Some patients present at a late stage, when the tumour extends into the penile shaft and enlarged inguinal nodes are palpable (see Fig. 38.19).

Biopsy and/or circumcision may be required to confirm the diagnosis. Treatment is then by radiotherapy (which may be by brachytherapy or external beam) or surgery. Surgery may be local excision, or partial or total penectomy. Enlarged lymph nodes may be irradiated or removed by surgical block dissection to the

REFERENCES

57. Adeyoju AB, Olujohungbe AB, Morris J et al. BJU Int 2002; 90: 898–902
58. Rees RW, Kalsi J, Minhas S et al. BJU Int 2002; 90: 893–897
59. La Peyronie FG. Mem Acad R Chir 1743; 1: 337–342
60. Pryor JP, Ralph DJ. Int J Impot Res 2002; 14: 414–417
61. Sommer F, Schwarzer U, Wassmer G et al. Int J Impot Res 2002; 14: 379–383
62. Scardino PL, Scott WW. Ann NY Acad Sci 1949; 52: 390–393
63. Ralph DJ, Brooks MD, Bottazzo GF et al. Br J Urol 1992; 70: 648–651
64. Manikandan R, Islam W, Srinivasan V et al. Urology 2002; 60: 795–799
65. Ralph DJ, Al-Akraa M, Pryor JP. J Urol 1995; 154: 1362–1363
66. Seftel A. J Urol 2002; 168: 2324
67. Dillner J, von Krogh G, Horenblas S et al. Scand J Urol Nephrol 2000; 205: 189–193
68. Buechner SA. BJU Int 2002; 90: 498–506

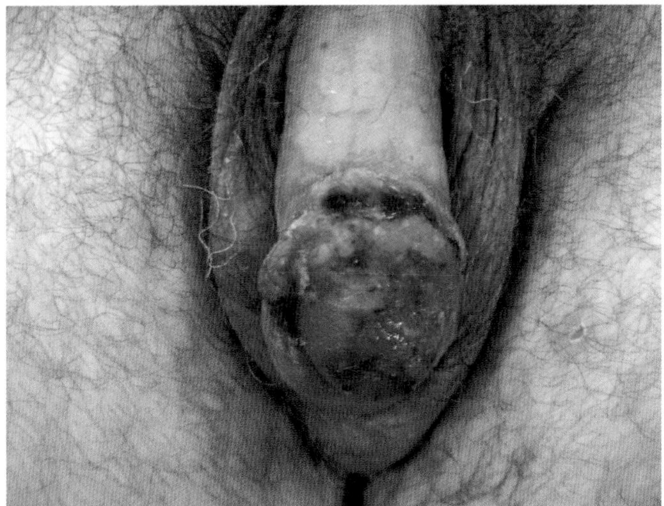

Figure 38.27 Penile carcinoma: a large fungating penile squamous carcinoma.

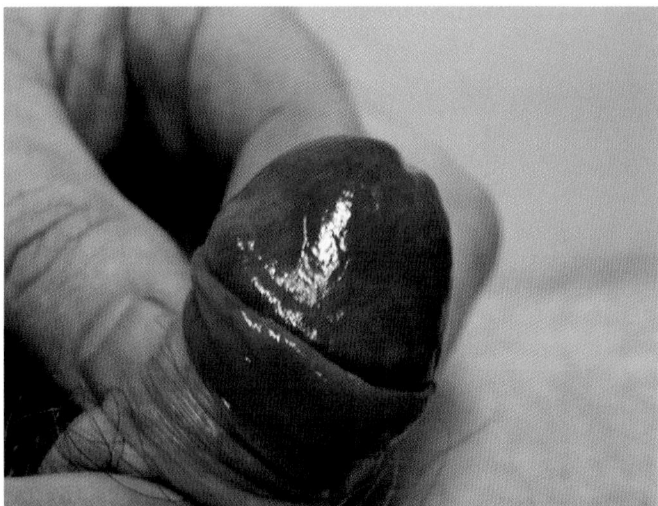

Figure 38.28 Zoon's balanitis: florid erythematous glans with features that were suspicious of malignancy, but biopsy confirmed benign histology.

primary lesion and any lymph nodes.[69,70] The choice of treatment depends on the stage and extent of the primary lesion. Advanced disease can be treated with chemotherapy, but by then the patient has a poor prognosis.

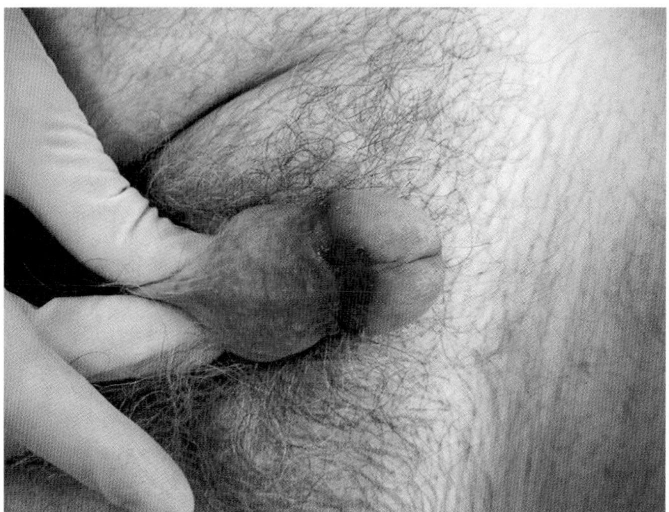

Figure 38.29 Carcinoma in situ of the penis: red patch at coronal sulcus confirmed as in situ carcinoma (erythroplasia of Queryat).

Box 38.2 Drugs that can cause erectile dysfunction

Antihypertensives
- Thiazide diuretics
- Beta blockers
- Angiotensin-converting enzyme inhibitors
- Calcium channel blockers

Antidepressants
- Tricyclic antidepressants
- Monoamine oxidase inhibitors

Major tranquillizers
- Phenothiazines
- Haloperidol

Antiandrogens
- Cyproterone acetate
- Luteinizing hormone–releasing hormone analogues

Anxiolytics
- Benzodiazepines

Miscellaneous
- Cimetidine
- Digoxin
- Metoclopramide

ERECTILE DYSFUNCTION

The causes of erectile dysfunction can be divided into organic or psychological, although it is now recognized that elements of both coexist in most patients. There are specific illnesses, and also certain drugs, known to be associated with erectile dysfunction (Box 38.2).

Investigation of erectile dysfunction begins with a thorough sexual history. Spontaneous nocturnal or early morning erections and masturbation suggest a psychological cause, especially when the problem started suddenly on a background of relationship difficulties and recent stresses. Symptoms more suggestive of an organic origin are a gradual onset with loss of early morning erections and a normal libido. Risk factors should be sought; these include drugs, chronic disease, previous surgery (especially aortic aneurysm repair, and pelvic or prostatic surgery), tobacco use and alcohol consumption.

The blood pressure should be taken, the abdomen examined for scars and masses, the penis for plaques, and the testicles for size and consistency. The peripheral pulses should be palpated, a rectal examination performed, and the anal sphincter tone noted.

REFERENCES

69. Horenblas S, van Tinteren H, Delemarre JF et al. J Urol 1992; 147: 1533–1538
70. Horernblas S, van Tinteren H, Delemarre JF et al. J Urol 1993; 149: 492–497

The urine should be tested for sugar to exclude undiagnosed diabetes. Blood tests should include the serum testosterone, sex hormone-binding globulin, and prolactin. Special investigations consist of Doppler ultrasound of the cavernosal arteries to assess arterial inflow, and the more invasive cavernosography to look at the venous outflow. These tests are usually reserved for younger patients without obvious risk factors whose condition has failed to respond to conventional therapy.

There are an increasing number of treatments for erectile dysfunction. Psychological advice and support may be all that is required for some patients. Patients with complex problems may need a structured programme of relearning sexual behaviour under the guidance of a counsellor, who may be a psychotherapist or specially trained GP. This may be the only treatment required or it can be given in tandem with a physical treatment.

The serum testosterone level is known to decrease with age, although the relevance of this is unclear because the level often remains within the normal range. Patients can be treated with testosterone if the testosterone level is low. This is available in various preparations, although these are not without risk and patients must be counselled over the potential increased risk of prostate cancer. Its benefit is most pronounced in men with a low libido.

ORAL THERAPY

Sildenafil is the most successful oral therapy and acts by inhibiting phosphodiesterase-5, which is an isoenzyme specific to the penis. This prevents the breakdown of cyclic GMP, a mediator of cavernosal smooth muscle relaxation that acts via nitric oxide.[71–74] Sildenafil is contraindicated in patients with serious cardiac conditions or those taking nitrates. Flushing, headache, indigestion and myalgia are some of the side effects. There are several new phosphodiesterase-5 inhibitors undergoing final trials, which have similar side effects and will be available soon.

Apomorphine hydrochloride acts centrally to enhance the nervous control of erection.[75] It is taken sublingually 20 min before intercourse is anticipated. The most common side effects are nausea, headache and dizziness.

INTRACAVERNOSAL INJECTIONS

Alprostadil is a prostaglandin E_1 injected by the patient into the corpora cavernosa, and acts by relaxing the cavernosa smooth muscle and adrenergic tone in the penis; it has an 80% response rate.[76,77] Alprostadil has replaced papaverine, which was the original agent injected intracorporeally, because it is safer to use. The risk of priapism with papaverine was 8% and is 1% with alprostadil.

The main disadvantage is the technical difficulty some patients (e.g. those with failing sight or Parkinson's disease) may have in administering the drug. Injections are not recommended for patients with sickle cell disease, leukaemia or hepatitis, nor those who are anticoagulated. Lessons in administration and titration of the dose are often performed in a specialist clinic. The main complication from administration is priapism, and patients should be warned of this complication. After administration of the drug, the patient must be given both written and verbal advice to go to a casualty department immediately if an erection lasts over 4 h. They then require aspiration of blood to achieve detumescence and avoid permanent ischaemic damage.

A new and promising treatment, still undergoing trials, is the combination of vasoactive intestinal peptide (a neurotransmitter) with phentolamine mesylate, which has been found to produce erections in patients resistant to other forms of intracavernosal therapy.

Prostaglandin E_1 is also available as a pellet, for administration into the urethra.[78,79] This is a more acceptable form of treatment for some patients who are unable to cope with injections, although it has only a 40% response rate. The low incidence of side effects, including priapism, make it a simple and effective treatment.

MECHANICAL DEVICES

The application of a vacuum to the penis creates an erection, which is then maintained by placing a constricting ring around the base of the penis. This device is successful, with a response rate of 70% and few side effects, but unfortunately many patients find it unacceptable. The device costs more than £100 and is not available on the National Health Service.

There is a diminishing role for the use of a penile prosthesis. Suitable patients should have an organic cause for their erectile dysfunction, which is resistant to all other treatments. The two main types of prosthesis are the inflatable or semirigid rods. The implants are placed in the corpora cavernosa through an incision in the tunica albuginea. The main problems with prostheses are the risk of infection and erosion. There is also a risk of technical failure when an inflatable prosthesis is inserted.

REFERENCES

71. Goldstein I, Lue TF, Padma-Nathan H et al. N Engl J Med 1998; 338: 1397–1404
72. Rendell MS, Raifer J, Wilson P et al. JAMA 1999; 281: 421–426
73. Jarow JP, Burnett AL, Geringer AM. J Urol 1999; 152: 722–725
74. Kloner RA, Zusman RM. Am J Cardiol 1999; 84: 11–17
75. Dula E, Keating W, Isami PF et al. Urology 2000; 56: 130–135
76. Virag R. Lancet 1982; 23: 938
77. Shabsigh R, Padma-Nathan H, Gittleman M et al. Urology 2000; 55: 477–480
78. Padma-Nathan H, Hellstrom WJ, Kaiser FE et al. N Engl J Med 1997; 336: 1–7
79. Williams G, Abbou CC, Amar ET et al. Br J Urol 1998; 81: 889–894

The testis, epididymis and scrotum

39

Prokar Dasgupta, Richard C. Tiptaft

THE TESTIS

INTRODUCTION

The word *testis* is derived from Latin, meaning *witness*; perhaps it is a witness to the creation of life.[1] The two main functions of the testis are to generate and maintain masculinity through testosterone production and to produce sperm, so ensuring fertility.

EMBRYOLOGY

The testis is first recognizable as the genital ridge in about the fifth week of fetal life, when the embryo is only 4–5 mm in length. This lies in the coelomic epithelium adjacent and medial to the mesonephros; hence the observed association between congenital testicular and renal anomalies. The descent of the testis within the coelomic cavity relies on growth of its feeding vessels and the gubernaculum, which is attached to the inferior pole. As it descends towards the scrotum it carries with it a fold of peritoneum. The peritoneum passes through the developing anterior abdominal wall via the undeveloped inguinal canal and forms the tunica vaginalis. Normally this 'diverticulum' of the peritoneum becomes obliterated. If it fails to obliterate, it becomes known as a patent processus vaginalis. The testis would normally arrive in the scrotum at about the eighth month of development. Three groups of factors are thought to influence development and descent of the testis.

Hormonal factors

Anencephaly or pituitary aplasia causes a total lack of hormones, and testicular development does not occur. The gubernaculum and the testis are thought to act and migrate under hormonal influence.

Genetic factors

Bilateral cryptorchidism is always a feature of the prune belly syndrome. Cryptorchidism is also more common in boys with spina bifida, imperforate anus and cloacal abnormalities. There is an association with urinary tract abnormalities and also splenogonadal fusion.[2]

Mechanical factors

Descent is dependent on the growth of the gonadal vessels and lengthening of the processus vaginalis, which may become fibrosed.[3] Failure of the correct attachment of the testis to the gubernaculum has been postulated as a cause of maldescent.[4]

CONGENITAL ABNORMALITIES OF THE TESTIS

Agenesis

Bilateral anorchia is very uncommon in an otherwise normal male infant; unilateral agenesis is, however, more common. Absent testicles may have infarcted or even torted *in utero*. The vas deferens may be absent even when the testis is present.

The investigation of an impalpable testis is considered later, but the testis is hypertrophied in children with only one testis. A wide inguinal surgical exploration has been recommended to search for an impalpable testis, and often only a streak gonad is found. Children with anorchia should have hormone replacement to stimulate puberty and maintain their secondary sexual characteristics.

Dysgenesis

Dysgenesis is characterized by a tiny nodule of testicular tissue that contains abnormal seminiferous tubules and some undifferentiated cells. These rudimentary testes are best removed, because they may theoretically undergo malignant change.

Polyorchism

This very rare anomaly has been described in 30 patients.[5] It occurs as a result of splitting of the genital ridge in the embryo and is more common on the left side. The abnormality is found at surgical exploration of an undescended testis or as an incidental finding when exploring a hernia. The accessory testes may exhibit spermatogenesis but sometimes have no ductal drainage. They are best removed.

Synorchism

This extremely rare anomaly is characterized by fusion of the testicles, which normally have their own vas deferens. The condition may be associated with renal fusion.

Inversions

Occasionally the epididymis lies anterior to the testis, which is called retroversion of the testis. Other anomalies affecting the lie of the epididymis are rare.

Ductal abnormalities

The vas deferens takes its origins from the mesonephric duct, so absence of the vas deferens and epididymis may be associated with ureteric and renal anomalies or even agenesis of the kidney.

REFERENCES

1. Anderson WR, Hicks JA, Holmes SA. BJU Int 2002; 89: 910–911
2. Cortes D, Thorup JM, Visfeldt J. Br J Urol 1996; 77: 285–290
3. Backhouse KM. Ann R Coll Surg Eng 1964; 35: 15
4. Scorer CG. Br J Surg 1962; 49: 357
5. Westcott JW, Dykhuizen RF. J Urol 1967; 98: 479

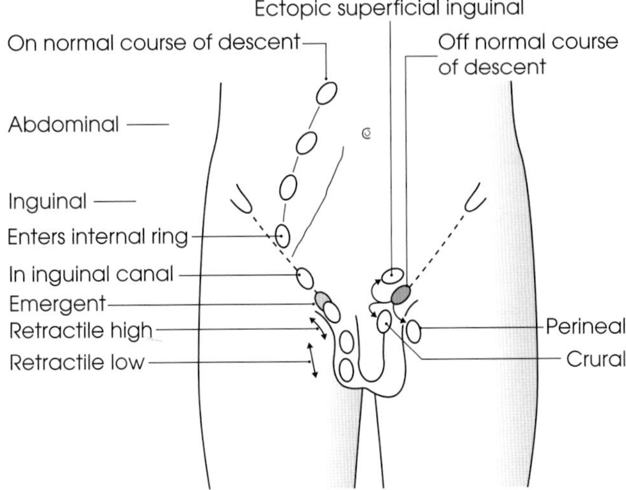

Figure 39.1 The ectopic positions possible for an incompletely descended or maldescended testicle.

Malposition of the testis

The most common congenital abnormality affecting the testis is related to its descent. It may become arrested along its normal route to the scrotum, when it is a truly undescended testis, or it may go off course, when it is a maldescended testis (Fig. 39.1).

The undescended testis

Having started life as an intra-abdominal organ, the testis normally passes down the retroperitoneum through the inguinal canal and into the scrotum, where it normally remains. The testis has been observed to lie in the scrotum at birth and then subsequently has ascended.[6] This may follow inguinal surgery, usually for hernia or hydrocele repair.

The main anatomical sites of arrested descent are described as:

- intra-abdominal;
- inguinal;
- intracanalicular;
- emergent; and
- high scrotal.

The testis is impalpable when it is within the abdomen or inside the inguinal canal. Once through the canal the testis should be palpable, although if it is maldescended it is usually smaller than its normal counterpart.

Incidence

The true incidence of undescended testis in a normal full-term child at birth is between 1.8%[6] and 2.7%.[7]

The overall incidence at 1 year is, however, about 0.8%.[6–8] There seems to be good evidence that an undescended testis at birth can still descend into the scrotum, and this usually occurs within the first few weeks of life. Descent after 1 year is rare. The incidence of unilateral or bilateral undescended testis in premature infants is much higher, between 17.2[6] and 21%,[7] but the majority descend within the first few months of life. Campbell found an incidence of 0.55% undescended testes in a huge number of American military recruits.[9]

Ectopic testis

Once the testis leaves its normal course it is regarded as being ectopic. The anatomical abnormality responsible for this derangement is not a patent processus vaginalis nor is the testis found to be lying within a hernial sac. Backhouse suggested the testis might follow the aberrant tails (Lockwood) of the gubernaculum, causing it to lie in one of four recognized sites (Fig. 39.1):[3]

1. the superficial inguinal pouch;
2. the base of the penis;
3. the perineum; or
4. the femoral region.

The superficial inguinal pouch is by far the most common site for the testis to be found, and it usually lies just lateral and above the superficial inguinal ring under Scarpa's fascia. It cannot be drawn into the scrotum preoperatively.

Spermatogenesis

The main function to be affected is spermatogenesis. The development of a normal testis seems to depend on its being maintained in an environment cooler than the core body temperature. Histology of biopsies taken from undescended testicles have shown varying degrees of hypoplasia, and these changes are established by the age of 2 years.[10] The risk of infertility in unilateral cryptorchidism is 15–30%, which increases to 50% or more for bilateral cryptorchids.[11]

Clinical features

All newborn children are examined shortly after birth. The possibility of a chromosomal or endocrine abnormality should be considered if neither testis is palpable, and other congenital anomalies might be present. This examination is important because if an absent testis is not discovered, and later missed by the parents, the child may not be examined again until the age of 4 or 5 years when he starts school.

The scrotum on the side in question is not developed and remains empty. When the testis lies outside the inguinal canal and is reasonably well formed, it may be observed as a tiny nodule in a slim child. Careful palpation in quiet conditions determines if the testis is palpable. The hand should be warm and be gently passed from just above the inguinal region down towards the scrotum; the other hand is placed on the inguinoscrotal region to see if it can palpate the testis. The child may register slight discomfort as the testis is trapped or pushed by the examiner. A retractile testis can be correctly diagnosed and differentiated from a maldescended or ectopic testis by careful examination. The scrotum is developed and full and, as the observer approaches to palpate the area, the testicles shoot up under influence of the overactive cremaster. It sometimes takes more than one examination to be confident of making this diagnosis, but it is important because no specific treatment is required other than the reassurance of the parents.

REFERENCES

6. Villumsen AL, Zachau-Christiansen B. Arch Dis Child 1966; 41: 198
7. Scorer CG. Arch Dis Child 1964; 39: 605
8. Cour-Palais IJ. Lancet 1966; i: 403
9. Campbell HE. J Urol 1959; 81: 663
10. Scorer G, Farrington GH. Congenital Deformities of the Testis and Epididymis. Appleton-Century Crofts, New York, 1971
11. Gough MH. Br J Surg 1989; 76: 109–112

INVESTIGATION OF THE IMPALPABLE TESTIS

The testicle is impalpable in 20% of children with an undescended testis.[12] Neither testis is palpable in a much smaller proportion.

Human chorionic gonadotrophin stimulation test

In an otherwise normal child with bilateral absence of a palpable testis, the testicles may be within the abdomen or inguinal canal, they may have undergone infarction, or they may simply be hypoplastic. The administration of human chorionic gonadotrophin causes a rise in the serum testosterone if functioning testicular tissue is present. This test is, however, thought not to be wholly reliable,[13] and so some form of imaging is probably indicated even when the result is negative.

Radiological investigation

Ultrasound may be better able to detect an intracanalicular testis or one just inside the inguinal canal; however, it has been claimed that ultrasound is no better than a careful examination by an experienced surgeon.[14] For the impalpable testis MRI and laparoscopy are the next steps.[15]

Laparoscopy

This examination is safe and may be therapeutic. It was first described by Cortesi and colleagues as a means of localizing the undescended testis.[16] Cores described three variations identified by laparoscopy:[17]

1. An absent testis with a blind-ending vas and spermatic vessels above the inguinal ring.
2. An intra-abdominal testis.
3. Normal or atretic spermatic structures entering the inguinal ring.

The inguinal region was surgically explored in the third group, and this accounted for 21% of their overall series.

TREATMENT OF UNDESCENDED TESTIS

The use of hormone treatment to promote descent of the testis in a normal child is not acceptable, because it may result in premature puberty, premature epiphyseal fusion, and degeneration of the other testis. The aim of treatment is to anchor the testis in the scrotum in the hope of preventing progressive hypoplasia. This must be done safely, and the decision on the age that the child should be operated on depends very much on the experience of the surgeon, the anaesthetist, and the whole team involved with the child's care.

Orchidopexy is normally carried out through an inguinal skin crease incision, through which the testis and its associated peritoneal coverings are identified. The cremaster is then opened, and the testicular vessels and vas deferens are dissected free from the peritoneum. When the suspensory ligament of Browne[18] is divided, considerable lengthening of the cord is obtained. The small associated hernial sac is closed once the mobilization is sufficient to bring the testis into the scrotum without tension. A pouch is then fashioned between the skin and the dartos muscle, and the testicle is pulled through a small blunt puncture to lie within this artificially created cavity. If this is done correctly the dartos itself anchors the testis and there is no need for holding sutures.[19] The skin of the dartos is then closed over the testicle.

A success rate of over 95% should be achieved for straightforward cases. Undue tension on the delicate vessels must be avoided. When the testis cannot be brought down into the scrotum easily and it is of reasonable size, there is a place for anchoring the organ as low as possible and re-exploring 6 months later. This is called a staged orchidopexy.

The Fowler–Stephens manoeuvre of ligating the testicular vessels[20] may be appropriate when the testis lies higher, for instance inside the inguinal ring, and the vessels are too short to permit mobilization. The testis then relies on the blood supply of the vasal artery. This manoeuvre can be done laparoscopically.[21,22]

Orchidectomy should be performed when a streak testis is found or if there is difficulty in mobilizing a poorly developed organ, and the other testis is normally placed in the scrotum.

In older children (over 15 years) or the young adult, the testis should also be removed. Spermatogenesis is most unlikely at this age and the risk of developing a tumour is increased, although this risk is quoted at less than 10%.[23]

The Keatley–Tourek procedure of fixing the testis beneath the fascia lata of the thigh, and Ombredannes' procedure of fixation by passing the testis through the scrotal septum, are now only of historical interest.[24]

TORSION OF THE TESTIS

This condition was first described by Delasiauve in 1840. Although it can occur at any age from the neonatal period to late middle age, the peak incidence is between 14 and 20 years. A congenital abnormality of the investing tunica, which lies higher than normal, is usually present. This allows excessive mobility of the testis, predisposing to torsion. In neonates torsion often occurs extravaginally, but in later years it is usually intravaginal, when it is invariably associated with a horizontally lying testis. Although excessive movement and perhaps mild trauma may be additional factors, many torsions occur while the patient is asleep, and there is often a history of one or two short prodromal episodes of pain, when the testis almost certainly twisted but managed spontaneously to untwist itself. Rarely the testis alone may rotate, when the epididymis and testis are joined only at the upper pole of the testis. This accounts for less than 5% of all cases of torsion.[25]

Clinical features

Patients present with sudden severe pain in the scrotum, which is often accompanied by nausea and vomiting. Despite the severity of the pain, most delays in diagnosis are the result of failure by

REFERENCES

12. Jones PG. Aust Paediatr J 1966; 2: 36–38
13. Boddy SAM, Gordon AC, Thomas DFM et al. J Urol 1991; 68: 199–202
14. Weise RM, Seashore JH. J Urol 1987; 138: 382–384
15. Siemer S, Humke U, Ucler M et al. Eur J Pediatr Surg 2000; 10: 114–118
16. Cortesi N, Ferrari P, Zambarda E et al. Endoscopy 1976; 8: 33–34
17. Cores D, Thorup JM, Kenz BL et al. Br J Urol 1995; 75: 281–287
18. Browne D. Proc R Soc Med 1949; 42: 643
19. Frank JD, O'Brien M. BJU Int 2002; 89: 331–333
20. Fowler R, Stephens FD. Aust N Z J Surg 1959; 29: 92
21. Gheiler E, Spencer Barthold J, Gonzalez R. J Urol 1997; 148: 1498–1551
22. Esposito C, Cariponi V. J Urol 1997; 148: 1951–1955
23. Jones PF. Br J Urol 1995; 75: 693–696
24. Tiptaft RC. In: Rains AJ, Mann CV (eds). Short Practice of Surgery. 20th edn. Chapman & Hall, London, 1988
25. Johnston JH. In: Williams DI, Johnston JH (eds). Paediatric Urology. 2nd edn. Butterworth, London, 1982

the patient to seek advice, although occasionally doctors fail to consider the diagnosis.[26] Rarely pain may be experienced only in the abdomen, usually in the loin of the affected side. The twisted testis lies at a higher level in the scrotum than a normal testis and is acutely tender when palpated. Doppler ultrasound has been used to check blood flow in the testicular artery.[27] False positives and negatives can occur with this technique, and it can be used only as an adjunct to clinical diagnosis. The skin may have a bluish tinge over a gangrenous testis, and examination of the other testis usually reveals a horizontal lie (a bell-clapper testis).

Differential diagnosis

A number of other conditions can cause testicular pain. Torsion of the hydatid of Morgagni, or of the other appendages of the testis or epididymis, is more common in boys under 11 years of age than torsion of the testis. Idiopathic scrotal oedema occurs in boys under the age of 5 years. An inflammatory testicular tumour is important to rule out because of its lethal potential. Ultrasound and isotope scanning may be helpful if this diagnosis is suspected, provided treatment is not delayed while they are being obtained. An inguinal approach must be used to explore the testis if this diagnosis is entertained. Acute epididymo-orchitis may provide diagnostic difficulties in the older age group, but there is often a history of dysuria or urethral discharge and pus cells can usually be seen in the urine.

Treatment

Early operation remains the only means of salvaging a viable testis. After 7 h the seminiferous tubules are permanently damaged, although the Leydig cells, which produce androgens, appear to be relatively spared.[28] It is always worth trying to untwist the testis at once; the patient will quickly inform you if you are exacerbating rather than alleviating the symptoms! This is occasionally possible in the robust individual but not normally possible in a casualty department.

The scrotum should be explored without delay. The tunica vaginalis is opened and blood-stained fluid is often released. The testis usually looks dusky blue and the cord is seen to be twisted. The torsion is then released and the viability of the testis assessed during the next 5–10 min (Fig. 39.2).

There is still considerable controversy over whether an apparently non-viable testis should be removed. Animal studies have shown that autoantibodies are released from an infarcted

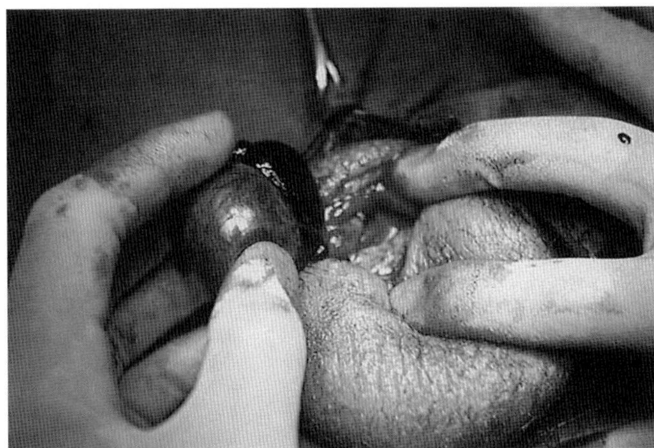

Figure 39.2 A gangrenous twisted testis.

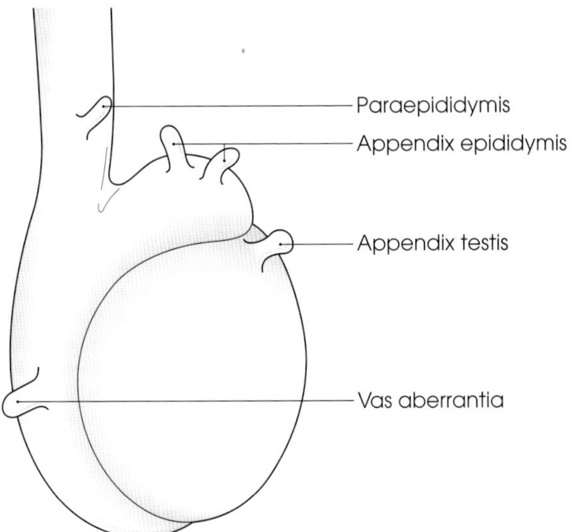

Figure 39.3 The appendages of the testis.

testis, and these may react with the contralateral testis, inhibiting spermatogenesis;[29] however, this has not been confirmed by human studies.[28] An infarcted testis may slough or form an abscess if it is left in situ. This is a rare occurrence, and most testes simply atrophy over the course of the next few weeks. A testis that has been ischaemic for longer than 12 h should normally be excised because it is unlikely that it will continue to function, but if the history appears to be less than 12 h the testis should be retained unless it is frankly gangrenous.[25]

It is important to fix the contralateral testis at the same time to prevent future torsion. This is easily performed by invaginating the tunica vaginalis and fixing the testis to the dartos with a couple of sutures. Most advocate the use of absorbable sutures for fixation, but recurrent torsion has been reported when absorbable sutures have been used. This is, however, a rare problem and non-absorbable sutures can give rise to problems by forming a permanent sinus.

TORSION OF THE APPENDAGES OF THE TESTIS

The appendages of the testis are four in number (Fig. 39.3).

Although it is actually pedunculated, the *appendix testis* (the sessile hydatid of Morgagni) is a vestige of the Müllerian duct and is morphologically analogous to the fimbriated end of the fallopian tube. It is normally a reddish lobule, 2–15 mm long, attached to the front of the upper pole of the testis or situated in the groove between the testis and epididymis. It consists of capillaries fed by a large artery and vein clothed in the tall epithelium and indented in gland-like ciliated epithelium.

The *paradidymis* (organ of Giraldès) is a remnant of the Wolffian body, analogous to the parovarium, and is a collection of tubules lying in front of the spermatic cord above the globus major of the epididymis.

The *vasa aberrantia* are also Wolffian tubules lying within the epididymotesticular groove.

REFERENCES

26. Parker RM, Robinson JM. J Urol 1971; 106: 243
27. Wang Y, Mack L, Kreiger J. J Urol 1990; 143: 197A
28. Bartsch G, Frank S, Narberger H et al. J Urol 1980; 124: 375–378
29. Krarup T. Br J Urol 1978; 50: 43

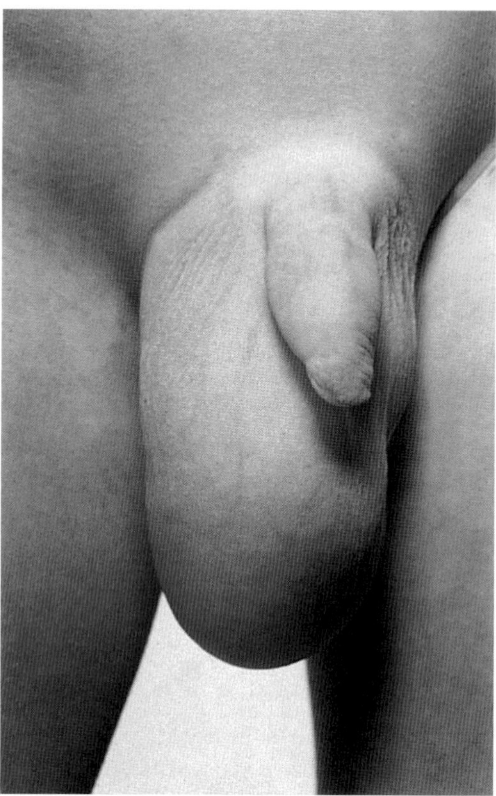

Figure 39.4 A right-sided hydrocele in a child. The testis cannot be separated from the swelling.

The *appendix epididymis* (pedunculated hydatid) lies in front of the globus major and is a collection of blind fragmentary canals lined by columnar epithelium and surrounded by vascular connective tissue.

The appendix testis is the appendage that undergoes torsion in 90% of cases. There is usually sudden pain in the scrotum, with oedema and congestion of the cord, testis and epididymis. Sometimes a 'blue dot sign' may be visible. The treatment is by operative removal of the appendix, which is always followed by complete relief of symptoms. Eversion of the tunica vaginalis prevents a postoperative hydrocele from developing. Occasionally, if symptoms are not too severe and of several days duration, the condition may be treated conservatively, provided there is confidence in the diagnosis.

HYDROCELE

A hydrocele is produced when an excessive amount of fluid accumulates in some portion of the processus vaginalis (Fig. 39.4). Hydrocele fluid is straw-coloured and serous in character. It contains water, electrolytes, plasma proteins such as albumin and fibrinogen, and cholesterol.

The most common form is the vaginal hydrocele, when the fluid collects in the tunica vaginalis that surrounds the testis but does not extend up into the cord (Fig. 39.5). Rarely fluid may collect in a more proximal portion of the processus, producing a hydrocele that does not envelop the testis. Such a hydrocele of the cord may be mistaken for an irreducible inguinal hernia (Fig. 39.6).

Congenital hydrocele

The sac communicates with the peritoneal cavity because the proximal part of the processus vaginalis fails to obliterate. It distends with the peritoneal fluid and may appear to be intermittent if there is a narrow neck.

Infantile hydrocele

Infantile hydrocele occurs when the processus vaginalis is obliterated only at or near the deep inguinal ring, but remains patent in the cord and scrotum.

Complications

Hydroceles may rupture, usually after trauma, and haemorrhage may occur into them either spontaneously following trauma or iatrogenically following aspiration. Rarely they may become infected and require drainage, and mesotheliomata can arise within them. Calcification of the sac and herniation of the dartos muscle have also been reported.

Treatment

Aspiration is the simplest and easiest method of treatment and, although the hydrocele fluid inevitably re-accumulates, it allows the testis to be palpated. Injections of sclerosing agents (sodium tetradecyl sulphate) at the time of aspiration have been used to prevent recurrence,[30] but this can cause severe pain and has not gained general acceptance.

REFERENCES

30. Maloney GE. Br Med J 1973; 3: 170

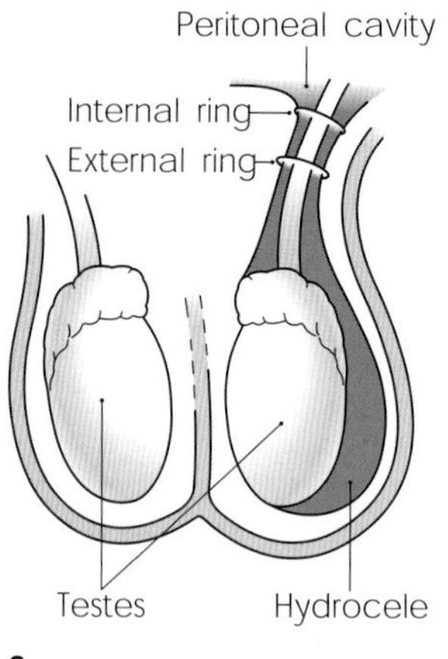

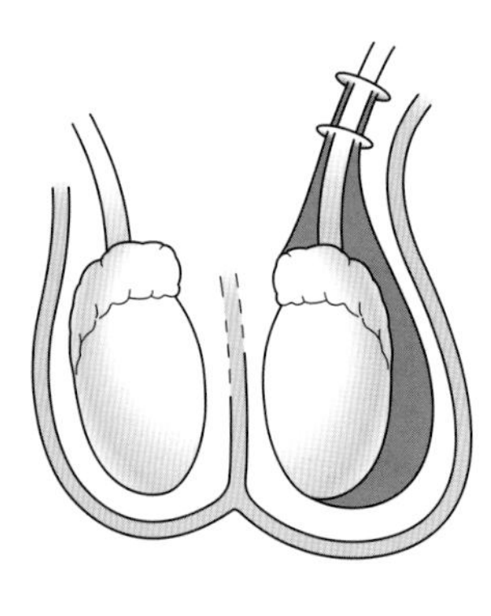

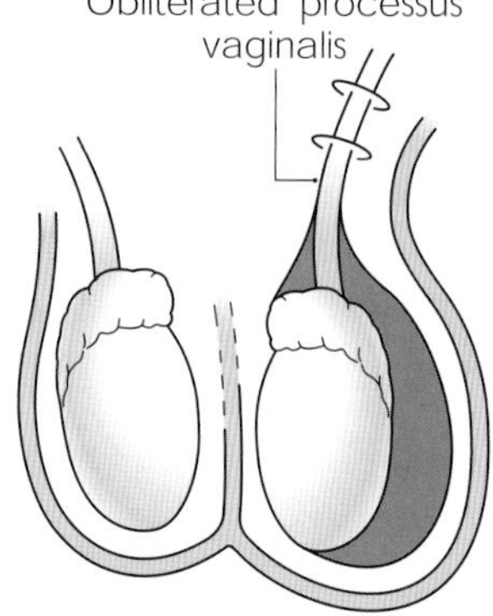

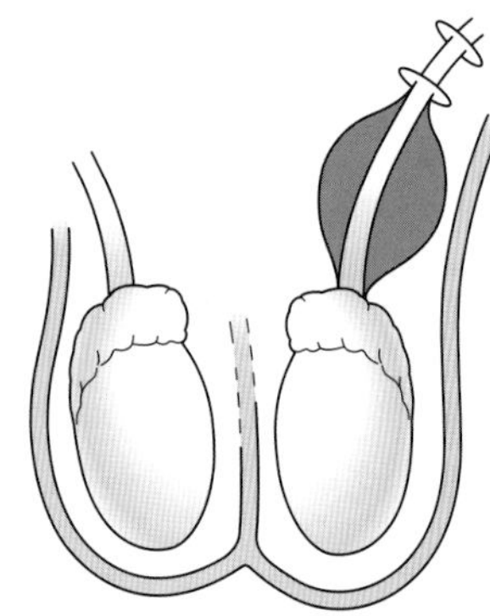

Figure 39.5 Hydrocele: (a) congenital hydrocele; (b) infantile hydrocele; (c) vaginal hydrocele; and (d) hydrocele of the cord.

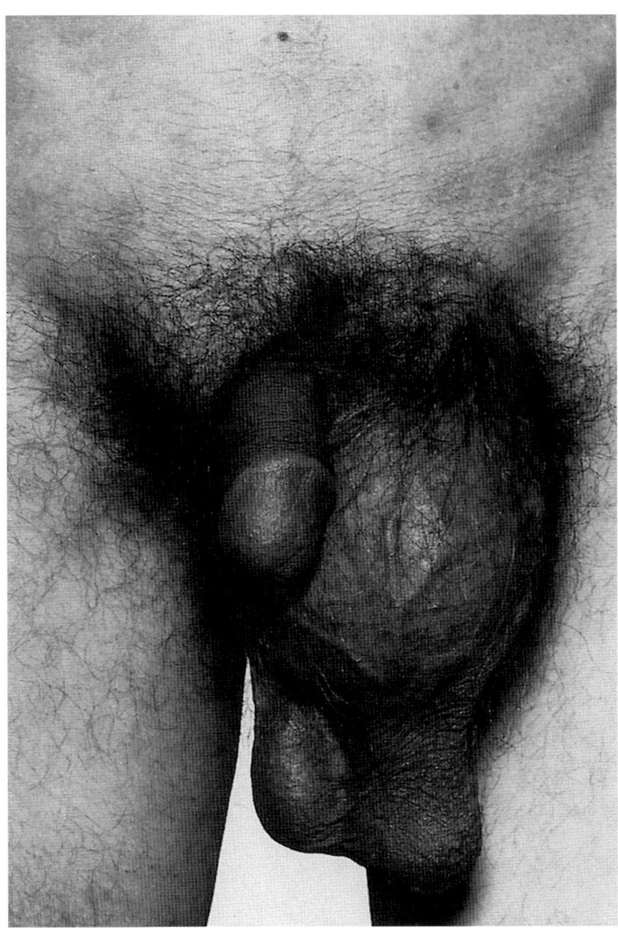

Figure 39.6 Hydrocele of the cord. The testis is seen to be separate from the swelling.

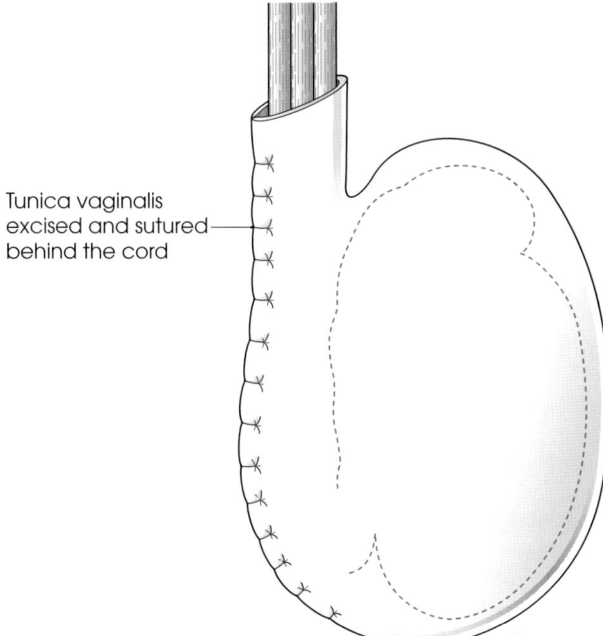

Figure 39.7 Jaboulay's procedure for repair of a hydrocele.

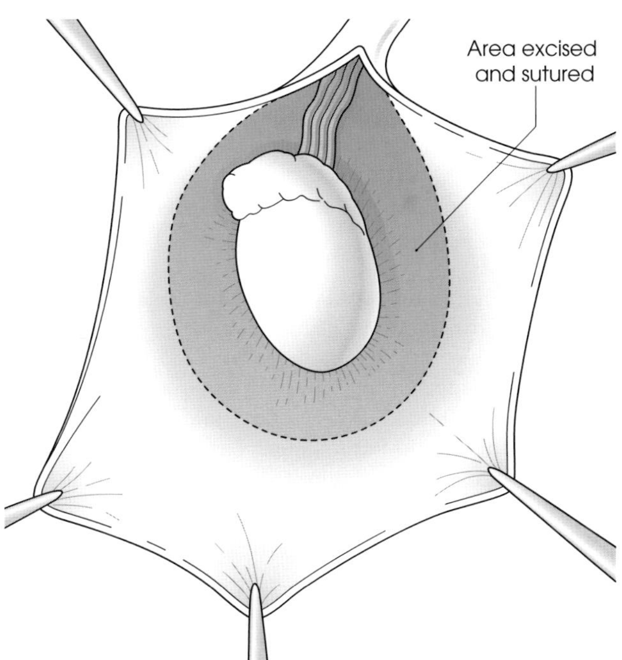

Figure 39.8 Excision of a redundant hydrocele sac.

In a young man it is prudent to organize an ultrasound of the scrotal contents in case there is an underlying tumour. In such cases aspiration is contraindicated.

Surgical excision should lead to a permanent cure. This may be carried out by Jaboulay's operation (Fig. 39.7),[31] in which the sac is incised longitudinally and everted. A variable proportion is then excised and the remaining sac is reapproximated behind the cord. Alternatively, after the tunica has been delivered, the sac can simply be excised from around the testis with the free margin oversewn to achieve haemostasis (Fig. 39.8).

Lord's operation involves a small incision through the scrotum and tunica, allowing the testis to be lifted from the sac and scrotum.[32] The sac is then plicated to the junction of the testis and epididymis. This procedure involves less dissection (Fig. 39.9).

Recurrences may occur after any of these operations, although they are uncommon. The Jaboulay procedure, because of the dissection required to expose and deliver the hydrocele, has a greater risk of haematoma formation than Lord's procedure; Lord's procedure is really only suitable for small- or medium-sized hydroceles and leaves a palpable mass adjacent to the testis. Postoperatively, haematomata are common but their incidence can be reduced by careful haemostasis and effective support bandaging. Some people advocate drains; these certainly cause no harm, and if left in for 24 h do appear to be helpful on occasions.

CYSTS OF THE EPIDIDYMIS

Cysts of the epididymis are variable in size and position, but usually arise from the head of the epididymis. They are probably simple retention cysts of one of the tubules of the epididymis, and may contain either clear fluid or a varying number of spermatozoa, when they appear opalescent and are called

REFERENCES

31. Howards SS. In: Walsh PC et al (eds). Campbell's Urology. 5th edn. WB Saunders, Philadelphia, 1986
32. Lord PH. Br J Surg 1964; 51: 914

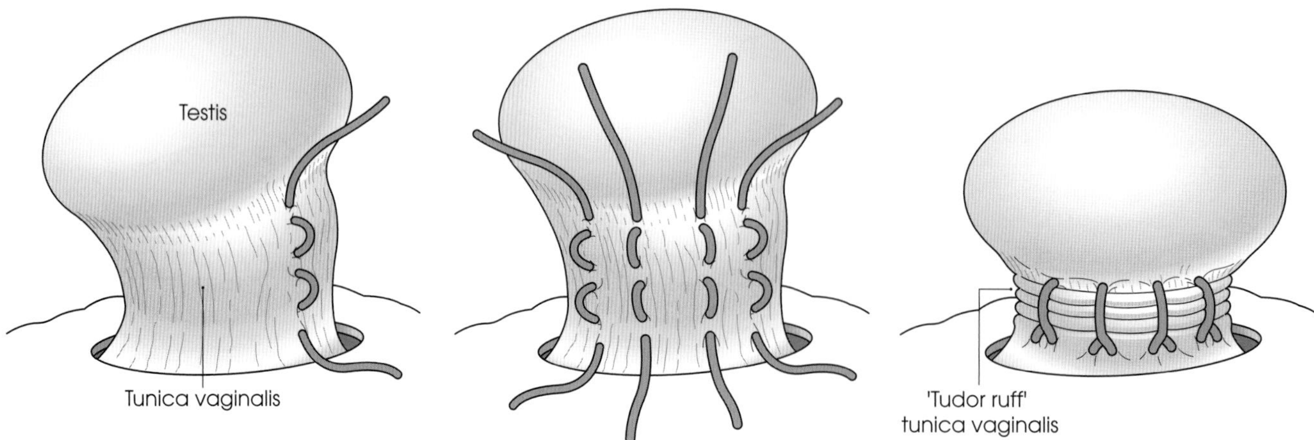

Figure 39.9 Lord's procedure for repair of a hydrocele.

spermatoceles. They cause smooth and often loculated swellings that are situated above and behind the testis. On occasions they can be extremely large, making a differential diagnosis from hydrocele difficult. They are often bilateral and occur disynchronously. They are brilliantly transilluminable unless they contain spermatozoa.

Treatment

Treatment is conservative unless the cyst becomes large or causes symptoms of pain or discomfort, when it may be enucleated. Cyst enucleation should be avoided in young men before they have fathered children, because epididymal function and sperm transfer may be impaired by postoperative fibrosis. New cyst formation can occur, and occasionally epididymectomy is necessary to avoid operating on frequent recurrences.

VARICOCELE

Varicocele is a collection of dilated and tortuous veins in the pampiniform plexus and is usually found in young adults (Fig. 39.10). The aetiology is often obscure; 98% of varicoceles occur on the left side, although this condition may be bilateral. The reasons for a left-sided preference are said to be:

- The left spermatic vein forms a more vertical angle with the left renal vein than the right does when it enters the vena cava.
- The left renal vein is crossed and may be compressed by the pelvic colon.
- The left testicular vein is longer than the right.
- The terminal venous valve is frequently absent on the left side.

A varicocele is a rare clinical finding under the age of 10 years,[33] and it seems the venous dilatation appears after puberty. At least 10% of the male population have a varicocele, and these are almost exclusively left-sided. When a varicocele is present on the right side, venous occlusion must be suspected higher up from a renal carcinoma or another invasive retroperitoneal process.

Varicoceles are associated with infertility as a consequence of poor sperm count, poor-quality sperm and poor motility. There has been no clear answer as to why this should occur. Increased intrascrotal temperature,[34] relative hypoxia as the result of retrograde flow of venous blood, and toxic metabolites have all been suggested as causes.

The sudden appearance of a varicocele in a middle-aged man should always raise the suspicion of retroperitoneal disease. A

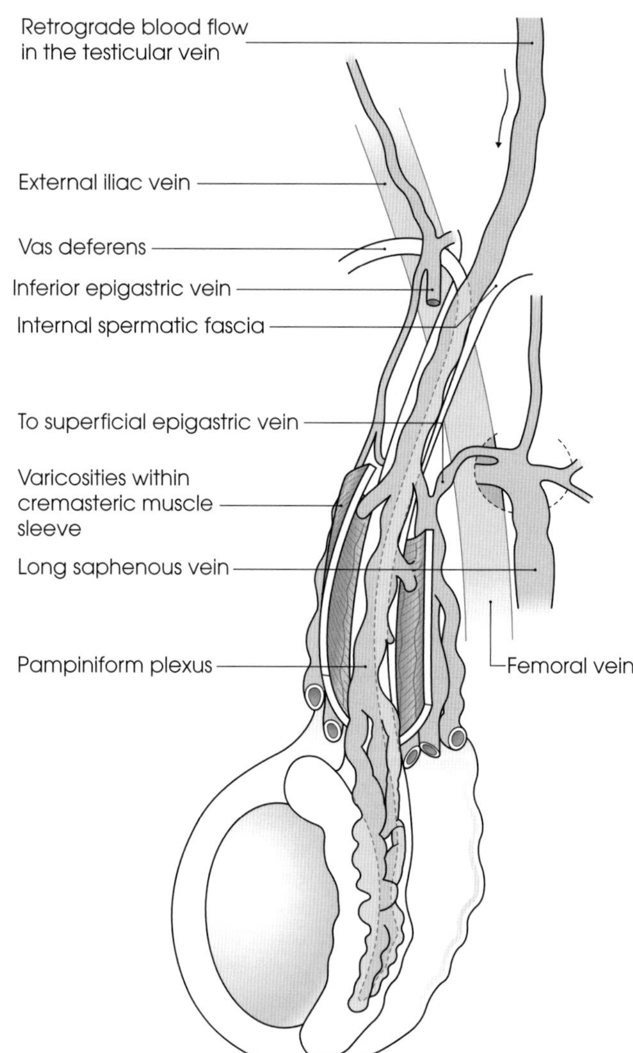

Figure 39.10 The venous drainage of the testis.

REFERENCES

33. Oster J. Scand J Urol Nephrol 1971; 5: 27
34. Davidson HA. Br Med J 1954; 2: 12

Table 39.1 Principles related to acute epididymitis

	Child	Young man	Older man
Aetiology	Bacterial	Venereal	Bacterial
Organism	Gram-negative bacillus	*Chlamydia trichomatis* (70%)	Gram-negative bacillus
Urinary tract abnormality	Possible	Unlikely	Bladder outflow obstruction
Investigation	Ultrasound urinary tract	Partner: urethral swab	Ultrasound urinary tract, urinary flow rate
Treatment	Broad-spectrum antibiotic	Tetracycline, broad-spectrum antibiotic	Relief of outflow obstruction

renal carcinoma extending into the left renal vein, causing an obstruction to the testicular vein, is a rare cause of varicocele but must be excluded if the varicocele remains tense with the patient lying supine. Most varicoceles occur in young men around puberty and are rarely noticed by the patient.

Clinical features

In many patients varicoceles are symptomless. The collection of varicosities feels like a bag of worms within the scrotum. The diagnosis can be confirmed by examining the patient standing, when the varicosities will become more prominent, and lying him down, when the mass disappears or decreases in size. The venous return is occluded when the patient bends forwards. The varicocele may become palpably softer as the obstruction is relieved.

Patients occasionally present because they notice a lump in the scrotum or because of an aching pain. The scrotum on the side of the varicocele may be seen to hang lower than on the normal side, and a cough impulse may be present.

Management

The treatment of a young man presenting with a varicocele is controversial. Not all will prove to be infertile; however, if, a decade later, they are still having difficulty initiating a pregnancy, the medicolegal implications are clear-cut. A World Health Organization varicocele trial confirms that men presenting with a varicocele and poor sperm quality have achieved a higher pregnancy rate after immediate varicocele ligation than when the operation was delayed for a year.[35] Varicocele ligation should probably be advised if there is any sign that the left testis is smaller than the right.

A varicocele may be removed or ligated by the inguinal, retroperitoneal or microvascular approaches. The last of these requires the use of an operating microscope.

When the high retroperitoneal approach is used, an incision is made just above the anterior superior iliac spine, which allows the testicular artery and its accompanying one or two veins to be clearly seen. Segments are excised from the veins, which are then ligated.

The identification of the artery is probably more difficult through the inguinal approach, but the dissection is simpler than the retroperitoneal dissection. Once again the dilated veins should be ligated and divided. Recurrence is usually the result of development of obturator collaterals.

It is important to warn the patient that after ligation the varicocele will initially become more prominent and feel harder until the thrombosis organizes. Varicocele ligations can also cause hydrocele formation, and the patient should be warned that this might occur, although it is uncommon.[36]

It is possible to embolize the filling veins via the transfemoral route under local anaesthetic. This was done initially with sclerosants[37] and more recently with spring coils. The main hazard is migration of the coil and potential embolic problems with the coils ending up in the lower limb veins.

ACUTE EPIDIDYMITIS

The aetiology of this condition varies with the age of the patient. The infection may be bacterial, viral or secondary to *Chlamydia trachomatis* (Table 39.1). In childhood it is usually a bacterial infection and may be associated with an underlying anatomical abnormality. The infection should be treated with antibiotics and an ultrasound obtained of the urinary tract. A cystogram and radionucleotide imaging may be indicated if an abnormality is demonstrated by ultrasound. Very occasionally chickenpox can cause an epididymal swelling and pain.

In young men epididymitis is most commonly venereal in origin, and in 70% it is the result of chlamydia. It is often difficult to make the diagnosis.[38] Chlamydia can be identified by cell culture or by an ELISA method of antigen detection. Ligase chain reaction and PCR are now the best methods of detecting chlamydia,[39] and these techniques can be used for examining either a urethral swab or the first voided urine sample, collecting the first 20 mL.

Acute gonorrhoea has been increasing in frequency, and a small proportion of affected men develop a secondary epididymitis. About 26% of the young men have a positive urine culture, so this investigation must not be omitted.

In men older than 60 years presenting with acute epididymitis, lower urinary tract obstruction due to benign prostatic hypertrophy, prostate cancer or a urethral stricture is identified in about 56%.[39]

Acute epididymitis can follow any instrumentation of the urinary tract by catheter, urethral sound or cystoscope. Retrograde spread of organisms appears to occur down the vas deferens, and it is postulated that this is the result of abdominal straining. Prophylactic vasectomy used to be advocated at the time of open prostatectomy, although this is not routinely practised today.

REFERENCES

35. Hargreave TB. Br Assoc Urol Surg Meeting, Edinburgh, 1996
36. Leny M, Kersting-Sommerhoff B, Bary W. Radiology 1996; 19B: 425–431
37. Porst H, Bahren W, Lenz M et al. Br Med J 1984; 56: 73
38. Robinson AJ, Grant JBF, Spencer RC et al. Br J Urol 1990; 66: 642–645
39. Luzzi GA, O'Brien TS. BJU Int 2001; 87: 747–755

Any type of epididymitis may lead on to a secondary prostatitis and seminal vesiculitis.

Clinical features

Adults complain of pain and swelling in the scrotal region, which usually develops over a period of several hours or even a day or two. The slow onset helps to differentiate the condition from testicular torsion, where the pain develops much more rapidly.

The pain is usually constant and throbbing in nature, and is made worse by moving about. There may be associated urinary symptoms of burning, frequency and difficulty passing urine, which can even lead on to retention. An associated urethral discharge may be present if the infection is sexually transmitted. Quite often these patients are unwell, with a high fever, rigors and lethargy.

A tender swollen epididymis may be palpable and, as the process becomes more advanced, the epididymis enlarges and erythema may be present in the scrotal skin, which becomes tense. The testis and epididymis often become fused together in an inflammatory mass. The spermatic cord may also become tender and swollen, and the patient is pyrexial and systemically unwell.

It is important to establish the correct diagnosis and exclude testicular torsion. This can usually be achieved by taking a careful history, performing a proper physical examination, and looking for pyuria and bacteriuria. A Doppler ultrasound can be helpful in excluding testicular torsion but should not be allowed to outweigh the clinical features. Occasionally scrotal exploration is necessary to exclude torsion of the testis.

Complications

An abscess may develop in the scrotum or the testis. This is suggested by a high swinging pyrexia and the presence of a scrotal mass that fails to settle with antibiotics. It is not always possible to detect fluctuation because the tissues are so tense and painful to touch. Testicular ultrasound confirms the diagnosis. The pus must be released by formal surgical drainage under general anaesthesia.

There may be a secondary prostatitis or seminal vesiculitis, and the inflammation may later lead to blockage of the epididymal tubular network, which usually occurs towards the head of the epididymis.

Treatment

A urine culture and urethral swab should be obtained. Bed rest, scrotal elevation and support, and non-steroidal anti-inflammatory drugs may be helpful.[39] For children and older men a broad-spectrum antibiotic is indicated (e.g. amoxicillin and clavulanate potassium or ciprofloxacin). Doxycycline 100 mg twice daily is prescribed for 10–14 days in men younger than 35 years with probable chlamydial infection. The patient should be reviewed with their culture results and sensitivities. The bladder should be drained if there is associated urinary retention.

CHRONIC EPIDIDYMITIS

The commonest cause of true chronic epididymitis is tuberculosis, but it may occasionally be a result of an incompletely resolved acute infection. Sarcoidosis and coccidioidomycosis are rare causes of chronic inflammation.

Clinical features

Tuberculous epididymo-orchitis often arises in the tail of the epididymis, and less frequently involves the head. It begins as a painless nodule that persists before eventually the whole epididymis becomes hard and enlarged. When the tuberculosis caseates, the inflammatory mass surrounds and buries the testis, and often an associated hydrocele further obscures the nature of the swelling. Fluctuation is then usually detectable before the skin of the scrotum reddens and breaks down, often with fistula formation. The general health of the patient is not usually affected, but if the condition remains untreated there may be additional symptoms of tuberculous cystitis before there is widespread genitourinary tuberculosis. The ductus deferens is hard and nodular in the cord, and on rectal examination the prostate is enlarged and firm. Tuberculosis of the lung is present in three-quarters of the patients, and organisms can be cultured from the urine of about half the patients with epididymitis.[40] A chest radiograph may demonstrate evidence of apical lung disease. Polymerase chain reaction is the most accurate method of establishing the diagnosis.[41]

Treatment

In some patients this condition resolves with antituberculous chemotherapy, but bilateral epididymectomy is often required.

Epididymectomy

Epididymectomy is performed through a transverse incision. The tunica vaginalis is opened and the vas is isolated and followed to the inferior pole of the epididymis. As the upper pole of the epididymis is reached, it is necessary to identify the main branch of the testicular artery and its bifurcation, where the branch to the epididymis is found and separately ligated. The upper pole of the epididymis can then be excised.

ORCHITIS

Orchitis is usually the result of an extension of an epididymitis, but can occur as a separate entity from viral infections such as mumps, Coxsackie virus or adenovirus. All these viral conditions can cause patchy infarction of the seminiferous tubules and render the patient sterile.

In the tertiary stage of syphilis, diffuse orchitis or a circumscribed testicular gumma may occur, but these are now rarely seen in western countries. The affected testis feels wooden, hard and painless. On palpation the testis is swollen, while the epididymis feels entirely normal. Positive serological tests differentiate the condition from a tumour. Treatment with penicillin produces resolution of the inflammatory mass but function rarely returns.[42]

Actinomycosis, filariasis and sarcoidosis have all been described as rare causes of testicular inflammation. Malacoplakia (von Hanseman's disease) is another rare inflammatory condition of the testis of unknown aetiology. It is difficult to differentiate from a tumour and is usually treated by orchidectomy.[43]

REFERENCES

40. Medlar EM, Spain DD, Holiday RW. J Urol 1949; 61: 1078–1088
41. Hemal AK, Gupta NP, Rajeev TP et al. Urology 2000; 56: 570–574
42. Whitaker RH. In: Blandy JP (ed). Urology. Blackwell, Oxford, 1976
43. Dasgupta P, Womack C, Turner AG et al. BJU Int 1999; 84: 464–469

Granulomatous orchitis is occasionally the end result of a recurring *Escherichia coli* infection.[44] The testis turns into a tender mass that then becomes hard. Such a testis often has to be removed to exclude a tumour and relieve the chronic pain.

TESTICULAR PAIN

Testicular pain may be caused by disease in the testis or adjacent organs, and is experienced either within the scrotum or referred up to the abdomen, loin or back. The pain may also be produced elsewhere and referred to the scrotum.

The pain produced and felt within the scrotum is a result of epididymitis, orchitis, torsion of the testis or its appendages, and occasionally discomfort from a varicocele. Patients with prostatitis frequently experience pain within the epididymis, which may be referred pain or may be caused by true inflammation of the epididymis. Ureteric colic may be referred to the scrotum, with pain passing down the genital branch of the genitofemoral nerve, producing pain on one or both sides of the scrotum. Small hernias protruding through the deep inguinal ring may also cause a testicular ache. The pain of epididymitis is often felt within the inguinal canal or occasionally within the perineum. Cremaster spasm can cause non-specific testicular pain, and occasionally division of the cremaster muscle brings relief to patients in whom no other cause can be found. It is helpful to perform either a nerve or spermatic cord block to confirm that the pain can be abolished before any operation is undertaken.[45]

Scrotal pain can occur after a vasectomy. Sperm granulomata develop between 2 and 4 months after this procedure, and they may be felt as tender, painful nodules that can be excised.[46] Immediately after vasectomy it is often difficult to disentangle the discomfort caused by operative bruising from the pain produced by distension of the epididymis. Most early pain responds to simple analgesics, but persistent pain and discomfort within the epididymis may eventually require epididymectomy to provide relief. It is worthwhile, however, giving an extended course of non-steroidal anti-inflammatory agents before resorting to operation.

There is a small but distinct group of patients who have an ache in the testis and inguinal area as their only symptom. They may be found to have a definitive and sometimes quite large fibrocystic nodule in the gluteal fascia, situated lateral to the posterior superior iliac spine. Pressure on this point reproduces the discomfort in the scrotum, and infiltration with local anaesthetic provides temporary relief. Excision of this nodule provides a lasting cure.

In young men, testicular pain may be caused by distension of the epididymis following sexual activity that stops short of ejaculation, but in many cases no cause can be found.

Surgery for testicular pain is fraught with hazards and should be undertaken only for removal of definitive pathology in which pain can be abolished by local anaesthetic infiltration. Even then, relief cannot be guaranteed, and pain may often progress to the other testis, to other sites, and sometimes to other organs.[47]

TESTICULAR INJURY

Blunt trauma of the testis is a common occurrence. Direct injury leads to small linear tears in the tunica albuginea with haematocele formation. More extensive testicular damage is caused by the testis being driven hard against the pubic arch or the thigh. This can result in gross equatorial disruption of the testis, leading to extrusion and necrosis of testicular tissue, often eventually causing loss of viability.

Clinical features

There is almost always a clear history of injury. Significant scrotal bruising may be present, and a firm, slightly tender mass that does not transilluminate can usually be palpated within the scrotum. It is important to remember that testicular tumours may present with a history of injury, and whenever there is any doubt an ultrasound of the testis should be obtained. Biopsy may also be needed in cases where the swelling does not resolve.

Treatment

All severe cases of testicular injury should be explored. Any haematocele that is found is evacuated, and small linear tears in the tunica should be sutured. Orchidectomy is preferred where there has been gross equatorial disruption and it is unlikely that the testis is viable. Occasionally severe trauma may lead to dislocation of the testis into the superficial fascia or even into the inguinal canal. The testis then needs to be relocated within the scrotum.

TESTICULAR TUMOURS

Testicular tumours are relatively rare, accounting for about 1% of all cancers in males.[48] The incidence in England and Wales is rising, and about one in 500 men can expect to develop this type of tumour by the age of 50 years.[49] The majority of testicular neoplasms are malignant and 90% originate in germ cells.

Approximately 10% of tumours occur in maldescended testes, and of those with bilateral maldescent who develop a tumour in one testis, 25% develop a contralateral tumour. The age when orchidopexy was performed does not appear to have an effect on the risk of cancer,[50] although fixation of the testis in a subdartos pouch makes subsequent detection of cancer much easier. A number of other factors, such as torsion, trauma, herniotomy, prenatal exposure to exogenous hormones and radiation, have been considered. Using microarrays, growth factor receptor-bound protein 7 and junction plakoglobin on chromosome 17 have been shown to be the most highly expressed genes in testicular germ cell tumours.[51]

Testicular cancer is more common in males of the upper social classes and lowest among manual workers. It is very common in Denmark and much less so in men of African descent.[52] Teratomas tend to occur in a younger age group (20–30 years) compared with seminomas (30–40 years).

The incidence of tumours in contralateral testis is 2.5–5%.[53] A prospective study from Denmark suggests that carcinoma in situ can be found in the contralateral testis in 5% of men with a testis

REFERENCES

44. Morgan AD. Br J Urol 1964; 36 (Suppl): 95
45. Smith DR. J Urol 1941; 46: 74–76
46. Sternberg J, Straus R. J Urol 1947; 57: 498–503
47. Padmore DE, Norman RW, Millard GH. J Urol 1996; 155: 95–96
48. Clemmensen AJ. Acta Pathol Microbiol Scand A 1974; (Suppl 247): 1
49. Hendry WH, Horwich A. In: Whitfield HN et al (eds). Textbook of Genitourinary Surgery. Blackwell Science, Oxford, 1998
50. Pike MC, Chilvers C, Pekham MJ. Lancet 1986; 1: 1246–1248
51. Skotheim RI, Monni O, Mousses S et al. Cancer Res 2002; 62: 2359–2364
52. Blandy JP. In: Blandy JP (ed). Urology. Blackwell, Oxford, 1976
53. Collins DH, Pugh RCB. Br J Urol 1964; 36 (Suppl): 1–11

tumour.[54] Because at least half of these men go on to develop testis tumours,[55] it is prudent to biopsy the opposite testis in patients aged less than 30 years with a history of maldescent or testis size less than 12 cc.[56]

Pathological classification

Testicular tumours can be broadly divided into germ cell and non-germ cell tumours (which are discussed later in this chapter). The former are further classified into seminomatous and non-seminomatous germ cell tumours. For the germ cell tumours, a modification of the histological classification described by the British Testicular Tumour Panel[57] (with corresponding American terminology in parentheses) is described here:

Seminoma (39.5%)
  Classic seminoma
  Spermatocytic seminoma
  Anaplastic seminoma
Teratoma (31.7%)
  TD: teratoma differentiated (teratoma)
  MTI: malignant teratoma intermediate (teratocarcinoma)
  MTU: malignant teratoma undifferentiated (embryonal carcinoma)
  MTT: malignant teratoma trophoblastic (choriocarcinoma)
Combined tumour (13.5%)
Yolk sac tumour

Tumour markers

The contribution of tumour markers to the diagnosis of patients with testicular tumours is now established. A central assay laboratory should be used so that the correlation, clinical course and usefulness of markers can be established. Alpha-fetoprotein, β-human chorionic gonadotrophin, lactate dehydrogenase and placental alkaline phosphatase can all be measured in peripheral blood (Table 39.2). The two most widely applied are alpha-fetoprotein and β-human chorionic gonadotrophin, and one or the other is elevated in most non-seminomatous germ cell tumours.[58] Alpha-fetoprotein is a major protein in the human fetus and is elevated in hepatocellular carcinoma and testicular teratomas. Syncytiotrophoblastic cells of the normal placenta produce human chorionic gonadotrophin, and its α subunit is very similar to luteinizing hormone. Placental alkaline phosphatase is raised in the majority of active seminomas but gives false positive results in about a third of patients in remission, which is probably attributable to concomitant smoking.

Clinical presentation

The longest delay in the management of patients with testicular tumours is from the time the patient observes an abnormality within the testis until he seeks medical advice.[59] Testicular self-examination among young men should be encouraged. In a Medical Research Council study the 3-year survival for those with a history of less than 3 months was 81%, compared with 69% in those with a history more than 3 months.[60]

Most men present with a painless testicular swelling and a sensation of heaviness in the testis or groin. A history of trauma may be recorded in about 20% of cases, coinciding with the discovery of the lump. Some 10% present with an acutely painful testis, which may be the result of a small bleed into the tumour. The commonest error is to mistake a tumour for epididymitis. Abnormal firmness in the body of the testis is the most reliable finding, and testicular sensation is lost at a relatively early stage. A small hydrocele may be present and should not be tapped. Some patients present with low back pain due to enlargement of the para-aortic lymph nodes. Other patients develop gynaecomastia or chest symptoms from pulmonary metastases. A palpable abdominal swelling may sometimes be detected. Some tumours spread rapidly and are classified as 'hurricane' type, while others, the encapsulated type, grow slowly.

Table 39.2 Testicular tumour markers

Tumour marker	Alpha-fetoprotein	β-Human chorionic gonadotrophin
Seminoma	0%	7%
Non-seminomatous germ cell tumours	55%	60%
Half life	4–6 days	1–2 days

Investigations and initial management

An urgent testicular ultrasound[61] usually confirms the diagnosis (Figs 39.11 and 39.12). Blood samples for tumour markers (Table 39.2) must be obtained before and after surgery, and a preoperative chest radiograph should also be obtained (Fig. 39.13, Table 39.3).[62] The patient should be informed of the possible diagnosis and consent obtained for radical inguinal orchidectomy. Sperm banking is recommended for future use in young men who may wish to have a family.

Orchidectomy should be through an inguinal incision with soft clamping of the cord at an early stage. The testis is delivered and inspected; if doubt remains about the diagnosis the testis may be bivalved through a vertical incision (Chevassu's manoeuvre).[63] A biopsy may subsequently be sent for frozen section to confirm the diagnosis. In bilateral tumours and those in a solitary testis, the German Testicular Tumour Group has reported successful outcomes with testis-sparing surgery. This involves early clamping of the cord, testicular cooling with ice, tumour excision, and biopsies for frozen section from the tumour edges and a normal testis. The procedure is successful in tumours less than 20 mm, and normal serum testosterone can be maintained in 85% of men after surgery. About 82% need adjuvant radiotherapy to the residual testis for carcinoma in situ.[64]

REFERENCES

54. Berthelsen JG, Skakkebaek NE, Nogensen P et al. Br Med J 1979; 2: 363
55. Giwercman A, von der Masse H, Skakkebaek NE. Eur Urol 1993; 23: 104–114
56. Harland SJ, Cook PA, Fossa SD et al. J Urol 1998; 160: 1353–1357
57. Pugh RCB, Cameron K. In: Pugh RCB (eds). Pathology of the Testis. Blackwell Scientific Publications, Oxford, 1976
58. Scardino PT, Cox HD, Waldmann TA et al. J Urol 1977; 118: 994–999
59. Jones WG, Appleyard I. Br Med J 1985; 290: 1550–1551
60. MRC Working Party on Testicular Tumours. Lancet 1985; 1: 8–11
61. Tiptaft RC, Nicholls BM, Hatley W et al. Br J Urol 1982; 54: 759–764
62. Klein EA. Urol Clin North Am 1993; 20: 67–73
63. Chevassu P. Tumeurs Testicule. These de Paris. No. 193. G Steinheil, Paris, 1904
64. Heidenreich A et al for the German Testicular Cancer Study Group. J Urol 2001; 166: 2161–2165

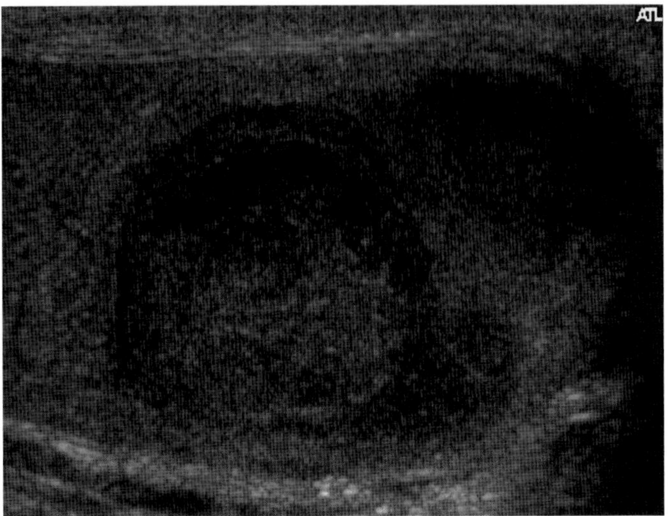

Figure 39.11 Ultrasound showing testicular tumour treated by radical orchidectomy.

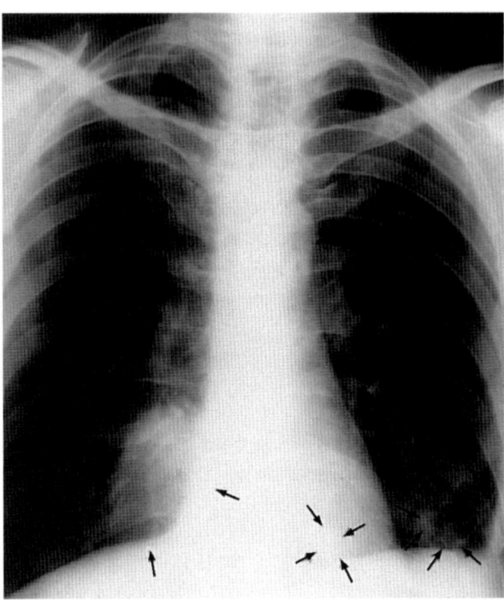

Figure 39.13 Chest radiograph showing metastatic testicular teratoma.

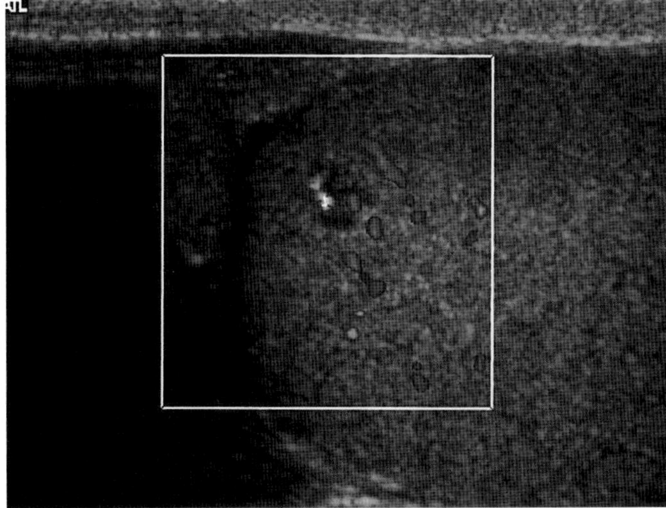

Figure 39.12 Ultrasound showing testicular tumour treated with testis-sparing surgery.

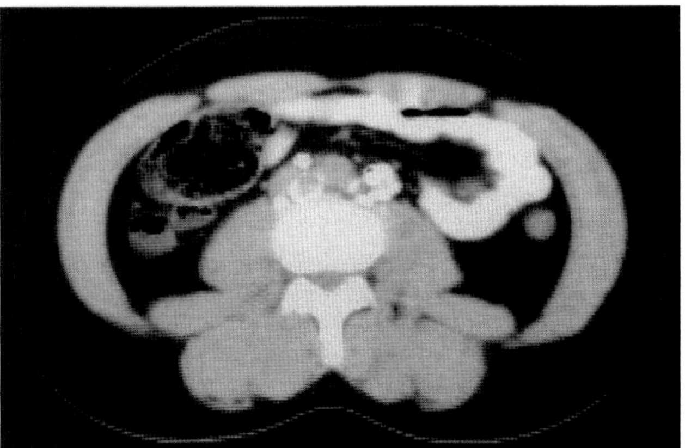

Figure 39.14 A CT scan of the upper abdomen showing a small pulmonary metastasis from a testicular teratoma.

After orchidectomy, the staging process is then completed by arranging tumour markers and CT scans (Fig. 39.14). In some instances delayed orchidectomy following chemotherapy has been advocated in advanced testis cancer, with no adverse impact on survival. Like all cancers, the management of testicular cancers should be discussed at multidisciplinary team meetings. There is evidence to suggest that the risk of dying is more than doubled if the patient is not managed in a specialist tumour unit.[65]

Staging of testicular cancer

The Royal Marsden Hospital staging described by Peckham in 1979 has helped plan logical therapy:[66]

- Stage I: tumour confined to the testis.
- Stage IM: rising serum markers with no other evidence of metastases.
- Stage II: abdominal lymph nodes.
- Stage IIA: less than 2 cm.
- Stage IIB: 2–5 cm.
- Stage IIC: greater than 5 cm.
- Stage III: supra- and infradiaphragmatic lymph nodes.
- Stage IV: extralymphatic metastases.

Treatment of seminomas

Seminomas are exquisitely radiosensitive, and those with stage I and IIA,B disease are treated with 30 Gy radiotherapy to the para-aortic lymph nodes. More than 95% of these men are alive at 5 years.[67] There is considerable interest in the use of a single dose of cisplatin or carboplatinum.[68]

For more advanced disease (stage IIC and above), combination chemotherapy with BEP (bleomycin, etoposide and cisplatin) or carboplatin as a single agent can achieve a rate of

REFERENCES

65. Harding MJ, Paul J, Gillis CR et al. Lancet 1993; 341: 999–1002
66. Peckham MJ, Barre H et al. Lancet 1979; ii: 267–270
67. Walther PJ, Paulson DF. World J Urol 1984; 2: 68–72
68. Oliver RTD, Ong J, Blandy JP et al Br J Urol 1996; 78: 119–124

Table 39.3 Testicular tumour investigations

Preoperative	Postoperative
Ultrasound of testis[61]	CT abdomen, pelvis, chest[62]
Alpha-fetoprotein, β-human chorionic gonadotrophin, lactate dehydrogenase	Alpha-fetoprotein, β-human chorionic gonadotrophin, lactate dehydrogenase
Chest X-ray Haemoglobin, creatinine, LFTs	Creatinine clearance, lung function tests
	Intravenous urogram, ?positron emission tomography scan

91% disease-free at 3 years.[69] Postchemotherapy residual masses are densely fibrotic and attempted surgical excision is fraught with difficulty.

Treatment of non-seminomatous germ cell tumours

Studies coordinated by the Medical Research Council have confirmed that surveillance alone allows two-thirds of patients with stage I teratoma to escape further treatment after orchidectomy. In this group of patients four key factors—invasion of testicular lymphatics, vascular invasion, presence of undifferentiated cells and absence of yolk sac elements—are associated with a 50% risk of recurrence.[70] Two cycles of BEP chemotherapy prevents relapse in the vast majority of these high-risk patients.[71] A trial between Nijmegen and Amsterdam showed no difference in survival between surveillance and retroperitoneal lymph node dissection in patients with stage I teratoma.[72]

The excellent response of disseminated testicular cancer to bleomycin, vinblastine and cis-platinum reported by Einhorn and Donohue in 1977 is the best for any metastatic cancer.[73] Vinblastine has been replaced by the less toxic etoposide, and BEP chemotherapy is the treatment of choice for those with stage IIC, III and IV disease, with an 80% survival rate at 3 years.[74] There is some controversy regarding the management of patients with stage IIA,B disease, in that they are managed with initial retroperitoneal lymph node dissection in the USA[75] and BEP chemotherapy followed by retroperitoneal lymph node dissection for residual masses in the UK.[49] In the latter approach, residual masses are excised 4–6 weeks after completion of four cycles of chemotherapy, provided that serum tumour markers have returned to normal. Histology of excised tissue reveals TD in half the specimens, fibrosis or necrosis in a quarter, and active disease in the remainder.[76] The last of these groups of patients has a poor prognosis, as do those with incomplete excision of residual masses. Sparing of the sympathetic nerves passing over the great vessels has led to significant reduction in ejaculatory dysfunction after retroperitoneal lymph node dissection. This operation has been performed laparoscopically.[77]

OTHER TUMOURS OF THE TESTIS AND ADNEXA

Leydig cell tumours

Leydig cell tumours account for 3% of the remaining testicular tumours. Young boys develop virilism and precocious puberty, becoming infant Hercules. Approximately 10% of these tumours are malignant. Smaller Leydig cell tumours can be managed with testis-sparing surgery. The finding of Reinke crystals is pathognomonic.

Sertoli cell tumours

Sertoli cell tumours produce gynaecomastia in adult men and may histologically be mistaken for seminoma on some occasions.[78] Bilateral Sertoli cell tumours, myxoma, spotty pigmentation and endocrine overactivity may be part of the Carney's complex.[79] They are best managed by excision.

Lymphomas

Lymphomas usually occur in older patients and are often bilateral. The prognosis relates to the stage of the disease but is usually poor.

Secondary tumours

The most frequent primary sites are bronchus, prostate, kidney and colon.

Adnexal tumours

Adenomatoid tumours may arise from the epididymis, tunica vaginalis, and rarely the spermatic cord itself. They are usually less than 5 cm, benign, and thought to be of mesonephric origin.

Papillary cystadenoma

Mostofi and Price feel that this is often a form of generalized von Hippel–Lindau syndrome[80] and may occur in the epididymis.

Nodular fibrous periorchitis

Nodular fibrous periorchitis is a hyalinized, fibrous condensation located on the tunica, which may be mistaken for a testicular tumour.

Rhabdomyosarcoma

Rhabdomyosarcoma develops in the spermatic cord of children, although there is a secondary peak incidence around the age of 19 years. Treatment is by excision, radiotherapy and chemotherapy. Leiomyomas, leiomyosarcomas and liposarcomas of the cord are extremely rare.

CONTRACEPTION AND INFERTILITY

In the latter part of the 19th century, vasectomy was performed for urinary outflow obstruction and obviously achieved some success, perhaps by inadvertently performing orchidectomy by

REFERENCES

69. Peckham MJ, Barrett A, Husband JE et al. Lancet 1982; ii: 678–680
70. Freedman LS, Jones WG, Peckham MJ et al. Lancet 1987; ii: 294–298
71. Cullen MJ, Cook J, Woodroffe C et al. Br J Cancer 1994; 69: 14
72. Spermon JR, Roeleveld TA, van der Poel HG et al. Urology 2002; 59: 923–929
73. Einhorn LH, Donohue JP. Ann Intern Med 1977; 87: 293–298
74. Ravi R, Oliver RTD, Ong J et al. Br J Urol 1997; 80: 647–652
75. Donohue JP, Einhorn L, Williams S. J Urol 1980: 123: 876–880
76. Cels ME, Nijboer AP, Hoekstra HJ et al. Br J Urol 1997; 79: 263–268
77. Janetschek G. Urol Clin North Am 2001; 28: 107–114
78. Henley JD, Young RH, Ulbright TM. Am J Surg Pathol 2002; 26: 541–550
79. Washecka R, Dresner MI, Honda SA. J Urol 2002; 167: 1299–1302
80. Mostofi FK, Price EB. Atlas of Tumour Pathology. Series 2. Armed Forces Institute of Pathology, Washington, 1973

including the testicular artery in its excision.[81] Vasectomy is now the preferred permanent method of contraception.

Vasectomy

In this operation (Fig. 39.15), the thumb and index finger of the non-dominant hand are used to isolate the cord. The vas is located within the cord as the only solid structure. It is possible to fix the vas over the middle finger, between the index finger and the thumb. Local anaesthetic is infiltrated directly into the skin around the vas. An incision is made directly over the vas, and the covering fascia is divided before the vas is pulled free. The artery to the vas may be ligated and divided, or it may be pushed away with the adventitia before the vas is isolated and divided. It is debatable whether the preservation of the artery to the vas enables a more successful vasovasostomy if this becomes necessary at a future date. Spontaneous reanastomosis of the vas is uncommon, but the chance of this occurring is reduced if a portion of the vas is removed and one end buried beneath the adventitia.

In the great majority of patients, bruising and discomfort are minimal and they can return to normal activities within 48 h. Haematoma formation is the only important immediate complication and on occasion this may be gross, extending up as far as the axilla. Evacuation of the haematoma is usually ineffective unless performed early, and rest is the only remedy. A haematoma, however, may become secondarily infected and occasionally abscesses need to be drained.

Sperm granulomata may develop after 2 or 3 months. They are caused by a reaction between sperm that have escaped from the proximal end of the vas and the surrounding tissue. This usually settles with anti-inflammatory drugs, but occasionally excision of the nodule is necessary. Vasectomy has a significant morbidity. Some patients have pain and discomfort for several weeks and bruising may occur; occasionally this may require admission to hospital. Fit young patients may lose time from work. These risks need to be explained to the patient before the procedure is carried out.

Before contraceptive precautions are abandoned, it is essential that the patient provides two seminal samples in which no spermatozoa are seen. This must also be clearly explained prior to operation. It is customary to ask them to provide specimens at 10 and 12 weeks, because most patients will be sterile at about this time. The continuing presence of spermatozoa indicates a failed operation, and re-exploration should be offered.

Vasovasostomy

Vasovasostomy is being performed with increasing frequency, although patients are counselled that a vasectomy is an irreversible procedure with little or no chance of a successful reanastomosis or subsequent pregnancy. Technically the procedure is not difficult, and many methods of reanastomosing the vas have been described (Fig. 39.16).

These include end-to-end, side-to-side (with or without splints), using the operating microscope, using multilayer anastomosis, or just a naked-eye single-layer anastomosis. Some 70–80% of patients obtain sperm in their ejaculate using any of the above techniques, although successful pregnancy is achieved in a significantly smaller percentage. It is believed that many of the failures are the result of ischaemia of the vas caused by fibrosis, and occlusion because of possible damage to the artery to the vas at the time of the vasectomy. Anti-sperm antibodies may also be an important cause of sterility when they are present. A successful operation can produce spermatozoa within a couple of weeks, but if a further seminal analysis is repeated the spermatozoa have often disappeared. It is sound policy only to ask for samples 2 months after the operation. Royle and Hendry recommend a second procedure after a failed first operation,[82] and there is some evidence that this carries an equal chance of success. It does not, however, appear that multiple reoperations

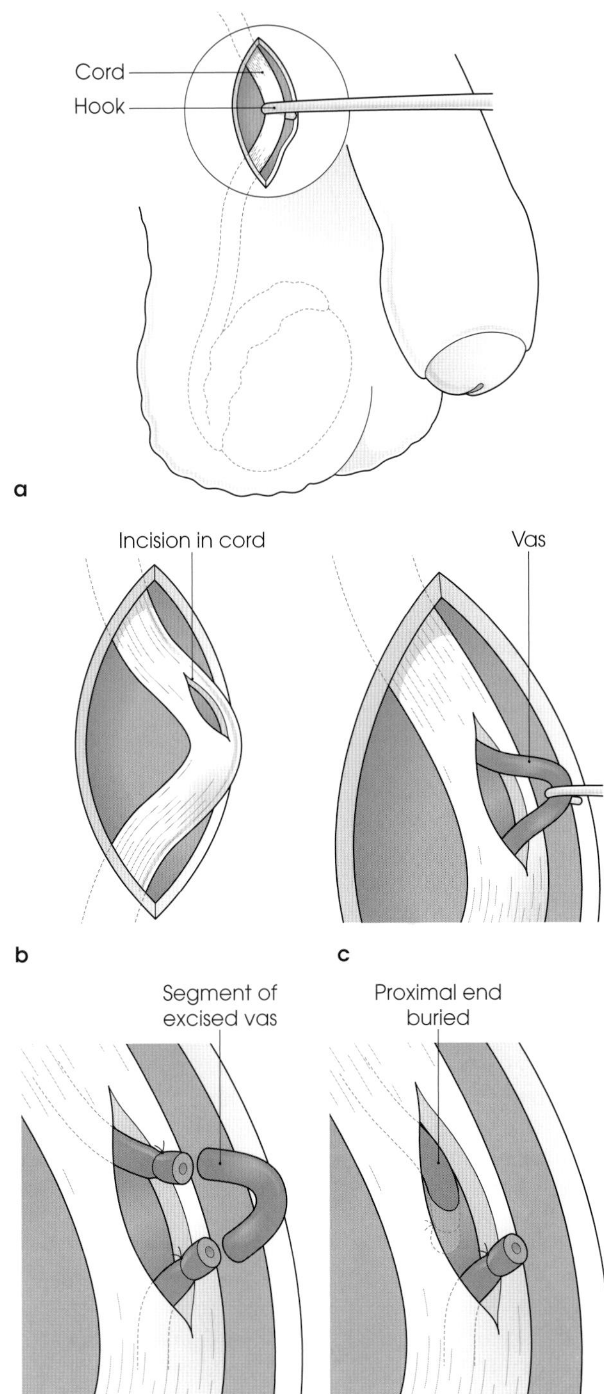

Figure 39.15 The operation of vasectomy shown in five stages (**a**–**e**).

REFERENCES

81. Clark PB. Br J Urol 1987; 60: 549–559
82. Royle MG, Hendry WF. Br J Urol 1980; 57: 780

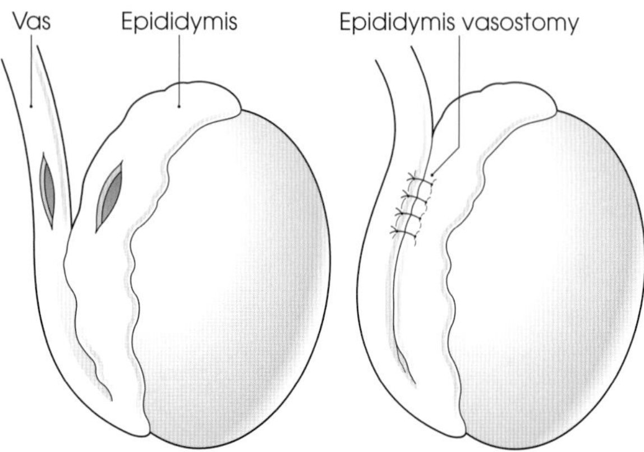

Figure 39.16 The vas is anastomosed side-to-side to the epididymis in epididymovasostomy.

increase the chances of success, and it would seem sensible to limit the patients to two procedures at most.

Infertility

Infertility, defined as failure of conception after at least 1 year of unprotected intercourse, affects approximately 15% of couples and is the result of male factors in about half. Infertile men may be divided into those who are oligospermic and those with azoospermia.

The infertile couple should ideally be seen together. History should include age, occupation, medical conditions, family history, infections, cryptorchidism, previous groin surgery and the use of tobacco, alcohol or drugs. Secondary sexual characteristics, voice and genitals (particularly testicular size and the presence or absence of vasa) should be examined, followed by two semen analyses and a hormonal screen (testosterone, luteinizing hormone, follicle-stimulating hormone and prolactin). Other tests, such as karyotype, transrectal ultrasound of the prostate and seminal vesicles, scrotal thermography, MAR/TAT test for antisperm antibodies, postcoital test, testicular biopsy and vasography may be necessary. Biopsies should be performed in the presence of an embryologist in centres equipped to store sperms.[83]

Genetic disorders

Genetic factors occur in up to 17% of men with azoospermia[84] or severe oligozoospermia. The commonest are Klinefelter's syndrome and cystic fibrosis, in which there may be congenital bilateral absence of vas deferens. A PCR-based analysis can detect abnormalities of the deleted azoospermia gene, which has been completely sequenced as a result of the Human Genome Project.[85] Although intracystoplasmic sperm injection[86] has given new hope, the risk of transmitting genetic defects is a real concern and needs to be discussed with these couples. Preimplantation diagnosis may allay such anxiety.

Primary spermatogenic failure

These men present with non-obstructive azoospermia and elevated follicle-stimulating hormone levels. Spermatozoa are found in testicular biopsies in about 60% and should be stored for assisted reproduction.[87]

Obstructive azoospermia

Epididymal obstruction is the commonest cause (40%), although ejaculatory duct obstruction is seen in 1–3%. The diagnosis can be established by clinical examination, semen analysis, transrectal ultrasound and vasography. End-to-end or end-to-side microsurgical epididymovasostomy should be performed in acquired epididymal obstruction. Some spermatozoa should be aspirated and stored.[87] Likewise vasovasostomy may be performed for more distal obstruction. There is no difference in the results between one- or two-layer microsurgical anastomoses.[88]

Idiopathic oligoasthenoteratozoospermia

Although a number of empiric drug therapies have been suggested, there is consensus that only randomized controlled trials with the outcome of pregnancy can be accepted for efficacy analysis.[87] Antioxidants and mast cell blockers may be worth further evaluation. The use of high-dose steroids against antisperm antibodies is controversial, and a meta-analysis showed no influence on pregnancy rates.[89]

Varicocele

Varicoceles (see *Varicocele* section, p. 892) are present in about 15% of adult men and 40% of infertile males. While a World Health Organization trial indicated a benefit in pregnancy rates, meta-analysis of randomized trials showed no benefit after varicocele ligation in adults, although restoration of spermatogenesis has been reported.[90] This controversial issue should be fully discussed with the patient prior to treatment.[87] Treatment is recommended for adolescents with progressive failure of testicular development and ipsilateral testicular atrophy. Retrograde embolization and open operation (inguinal or microsurgical) are equally effective, and the type of intervention depends on the available expertise. Patients should be informed of the risks of testicular atrophy and hydrocele formation.

THE SCROTUM

The scrotum is a cutaneous and fibromuscular sac containing the testes and the lower part of the spermatic cords. It lies dependently below the pubis, in front of the upper parts of the thighs. Very rarely a prepenile scrotum is seen, when the scrotum is suspended from the mons pubis anterior to the penis. The scrotal skin is red-brown and is normally thrown into folds or rugae. It contains numerous sebaceous glands, as well as sweat glands and pigment cells. Beneath the subcutaneous adipose tissue is a thin layer of dartos muscle fibres.

TRAUMA

An avulsion injury may be caused by road traffic accidents, industrial accidents, or occasionally a blast injury. Significant skin may be lost from the scrotum, and half or more may be lost and still be satisfactorily reconstituted. Most scrotal injuries are 'dirty', and the primary treatment consists of wide excision and delayed

REFERENCES

83. Bates C. EUUS 1997; 6: 91–96
84. Rucker GB, Mielnik A, King P et al. J Urol 1998; 160: 2068–2071
85. Dasgupta P, Corr J. Urol News 2001; 5: 6–10
86. Van Steirteghem A, Nagy P, Joris H et al. Hum Rep 1996; 11 (Suppl 1): 59–72
87. EAU Guidelines on Infertility 2001: 1–57
88. Belker AM, Thomas AJ Jr, Fuchs EF et al. J Urol 1991; 145: 505–511
89. Kamischke A, Nieschlag E. Hum Reprod 1999; 14: 1–23
90. Evers JL. In: Templeton A, Cooke ID (eds). 35th RCOG Study Group. RCOG Press, London, 1998

primary suture. This procedure should be covered by a broad-spectrum antibiotic.

Pinch grafts may be used to cover large defects, but when the whole of the scrotum has been degloved and the testes hang free, pedicle skin grafts may be raised from either the thigh or the lower abdomen to provide complete skin cover.

ACUTE INFECTIONS (FOURNIER'S GANGRENE)

Acute cellulitis of the scrotal skin, following either surgical incision or trauma, usually responds rapidly to broad-spectrum antibiotics. A rare but more sinister problem is that of necrotizing subcutaneous infection of the scrotum, originally reported by Fournier in 1883.[91] In this paper, five patients were described in whom there appeared to be three common characteristics:

1. An acute onset in a young healthy male.
2. Rapid progression to gangrene.
3. Absence of a discernible cause.

Clinical features

A painful, tense, glossy oedema develops suddenly in the scrotum. This may spread to the base of the penis. Crepitation may develop in the subcutaneous tissue, and may spread rapidly before subcutaneous gangrene develops between 12 h and 3 days later. The gangrene follows the same path as extravasation of urine, spreading out along the inguinal areas and up over the lower abdominal wall (Fig. 39.17). A line of demarcation forms around the eschar that, if left untreated, separates to leave the testes hanging naked, healthy, painless and unaffected.

Jones and coworkers reviewed all the cases of Fournier's gangrene reported before 1979.[92] They found that Fournier's description remained true before the antibiotic era, but patients described since 1945 were older (usually in their fifties), and frequently there were local contributing factors such as perineal surgery and urinary tract, perianal or retroperitoneal infections. Many were diabetic.

The condition appears to arise from the bacterial synergism between relatively non-pathogenic organisms—usually a streptococcus and *Clostridium perfringens* (*welchii*)—derived from faecal flora, which initially induces vascular thrombosis, then subcutaneous tissue necrosis, and eventually dermal gangrene.

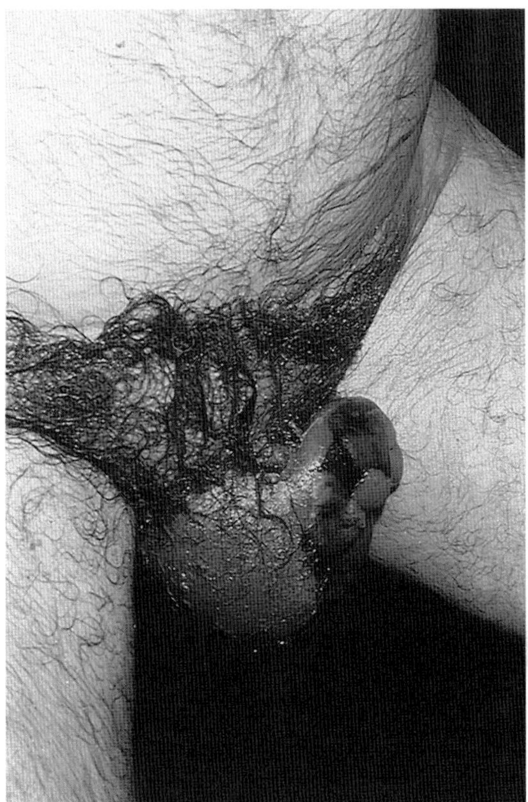

Figure 39.17 Fournier's gangrene.

Treatment

Broad-spectrum antibiotics, such as amoxicillin and clavulanate potassium, gentamicin and metronidazole, which are active against both anaerobic Gram-negative bacilli and facultative bacilli are started immediately. Early, wide surgical excision is also essential. Excision may have to be repeated, as further areas of gangrenous skin become evident. Once the gangrenous area has become well demarcated and has been fully excised, the underlying tissue remains healthy and free from infection. Delayed primary suture, split-skin grafting, or the use of pedicle skin flaps raised from the thigh or lower abdomen can again be used to provide skin cover (Fig. 39.18).

Unless they are obvious, sources of infection must be carefully pursued and patients should have an intravenous pyelogram, a barium enema, sigmoidoscopy and cystoscopy as part of this quest. The mortality rate in 267 patients treated before the antibiotic era was 22%, while in the 119 cases reported since antibiotics were developed the mortality remains about 30%.[93]

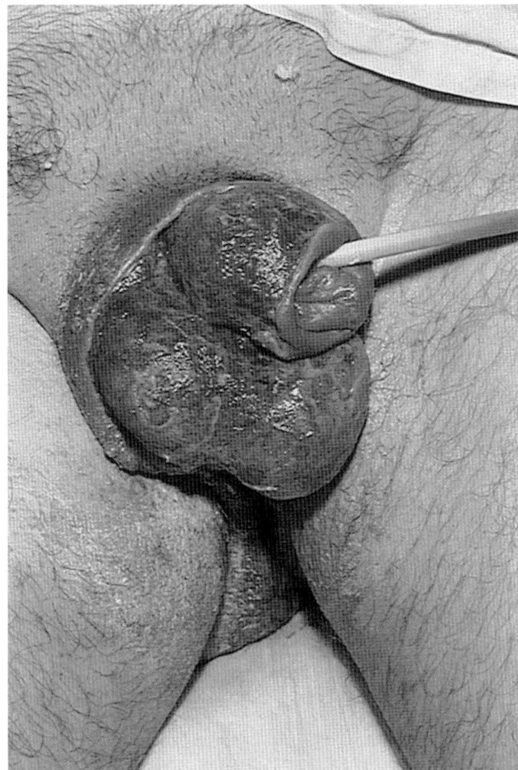

Figure 39.18 Fournier's gangrene. The same patient as in Fig. 39.17 after excision of affected tissues.

CHRONIC INFECTIONS

The commonest chronic infection of the scrotum worldwide is filariasis. This is caused by *Wuchereria bancrofti*, which lives part of

REFERENCES

91. Fournier AJ. Semain Med 1883; 3: 345
92. Jones RB, Hirshman JV, Browning S et al. J Urol 1979; 122: 279–282
93. Tan R. J Urol 1964; 92: 508–510

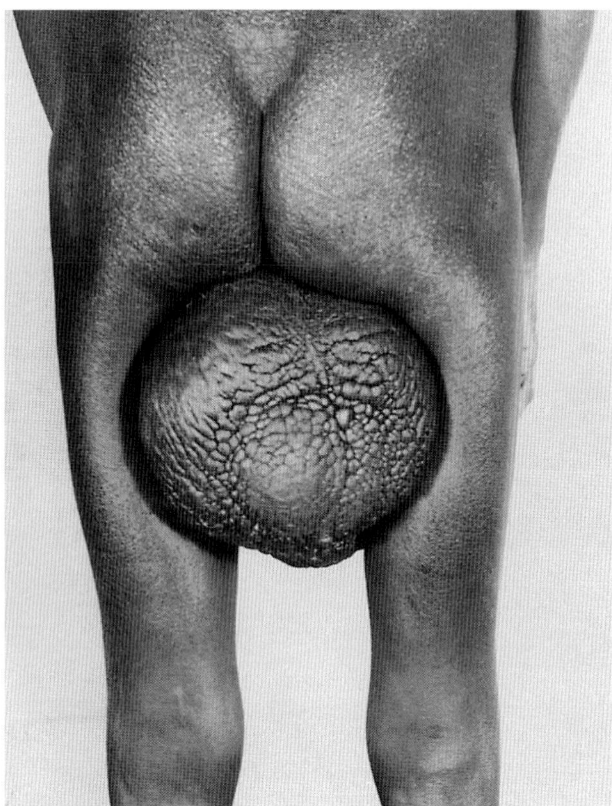

Figure 39.19 Elephantiasis of the scrotum.

its life cycle in the lymphatic system of humans and the other half in the *Culex* mosquito. There is an acute inflammatory stage, which takes the form of scrotal lymphangitis, and this can lead to gangrene of the scrotal skin that is indistinguishable from Fournier's gangrene. The filaria may also cause a retroperitoneal lymphangitis, which is often the start of a reactive process that obliterates the lymphatics and eventually causes lymphoedema and elephantiasis of the scrotum and penis (see Ch. 38; Fig. 39.19). Hydroceles of the testis and lymphoceles of the cord may develop later. Ultrasonography has emerged as the primary diagnostic test, because living adult worms may be identified by their movements within the lymphatics; this is known as the 'filarial dancing sign'.[94]

The World Health Organization has set up a Global Alliance to eliminate lymphatic filariasis.[94] Drug therapy consists of diethylcarbamazine or ivermectin, either alone or in combination with albendazole.[94] Radical excision of the oedematous fibrofatty tissue (scrotal reduction) is the only practical way to deal with the problem (see Ch. 12).

ACUTE IDIOPATHIC LYMPHOEDEMA (IDIOPATHIC SCROTAL OEDEMA)

This is a rare disease of children and must be differentiated from torsion of the testis, epididymitis, and torsion of a testicular appendage. It presents with reddening and oedema of the whole scrotum, and although antibiotics are sometimes given it appears to resolve spontaneously. The diagnostic feature is that the testes may be palpated through the oedematous scrotum and are relatively painless.

LIPOCALCIFICATION OF THE SCROTUM

This results from extravasation of urine into the tissues of the scrotum. Carlson documented a typical case history of an elderly horseman who had sustained repeated injuries while breaking in young horses.[95]

WATERING CAN PERINEUM

This condition arises as the result of a urethral stricture. There is usually a history of acute gonorrhoea some 10–20 years earlier. The patient presents with a thickening fibrosed scrotum with a number of fistulous tracts extending on to the scrotum. This often causes chronic retention. In the acute phase, there may be a grossly swollen scrotum that contains a mixture of extravasated urine and pus, and patients are often extremely toxic.

The treatment is to insert a suprapubic cystostomy, which must be left in situ for some weeks and sometimes even months. Once the inflammatory process has resolved, a urethroplasty is normally performed to treat the stricture.

SEBACEOUS CYSTS OF THE SCROTUM

These are quite common and may be worrying to the adolescent. Dozens of cysts may occur on the scrotal skin and are usually small. Although there is no absolute indication to remove these surgically unless they become infected, many request treatment on aesthetic grounds. The cysts may be individually enucleated or the central area of skin containing the cysts may be excised.

SCROTAL TUMOURS

Squamous carcinoma of the scrotal skin has been known to be associated with exposure to tar products since its first description in chimney sweeps by Percival Pott in 1775.[96] The disease has been linked with mineral oil products, associated especially with those used in the metal and cotton industries (mule-spinners). In the Haute-Savoie region of France, metal workers have a very high incidence of squamous cell carcinoma, and in this part of France scrotal cancer was among the three most common cancers to occur in males.[97]

The growth usually starts as an ulcer, but it may appear as a plaque or papilloma. The spread is to the inguinal nodes, which become palpably enlarged. The primary treatment is wide surgical excision of the scrotal ulcer or plaque, and in addition some recommend prophylactic lymphadenectomy on the side of the tumour.[98]

Patients with advanced disease may benefit from a combination of radiotherapy and bleomycin, and this can occasionally be followed by delayed lymphadenectomy if there has been a good response. Survival appears to be related to the stage of the disease at presentation. One study reported a 70% survival rate at 5 years.[98]

Other tumours that may arise in the scrotum include basal cell carcinoma, malignant melanomas and sweat gland tumours. These tumours are all treated by wide local excision in the first instance.

REFERENCES

94. DeVries CR. BJU Int 2002; 89 (Suppl 1): 37–43
95. Carlson HE. J Urol 1964; 100: 656
96. Pott P. Chirosurgical observations relative to the cataract, polyps of the nose, the cancer of the scrotum, the different kinds of receptors. Hames, Clark & Collins 1775. Roy Coll Surg Library
97. Lafontaine M. Huiles Minerales et Cancer Catane. Instituto National de Recitercite et de Securite, Paris, 1978
98. Ray B, Whitmore WF. J Urol 1977; 117: 741

Paediatric surgery

40

David Lloyd, Simon E. Kenny

PAEDIATRIC SURGERY

The speciality of paediatric surgery is defined by the age of the patient and is not confined to a specific organ system or disease. It covers a broad range of disorders, some apparent at birth while others manifest later. Demographically, the child is defined as aged 16 years or less.

THE NEWBORN INFANT

The traditional definition of a newborn infant as an infant of 4 weeks of age or less does not take into account the gestational age of the infant at birth. A newborn infant is now defined as an infant whose postconceptional age (the sum of the gestational age plus the post-natal age) is equal to or less than 44 weeks. The fetus changes anatomically and physiologically as it develops. These differences are apparent in newborn infants of different gestational ages and weights, and have an important influence on their management and outcomes. Premature infants are defined as those less than 37 weeks' gestational age; subgroups are low birth weight (less than 2500 g) and very low birth weight (less than 1500 g).

Premature infants lack the nutritional reserves of full-term infants, notably in respect of energy stores.[1] Their organs are not fully mature and are vulnerable to the demands of the extra-uterine environment and supportive treatment. For example, lung function is compromised by surfactant deficiency and the pressure effects of mechanical ventilation.[2] The immature gut is vulnerable to the osmotic effects of enteral feeding and fluctuations in mesenteric blood flow; these may compromise the mucosal barrier, predisposing to bacterial translocation.[3] These patients therefore must be cared for in specialist units by appropriately trained staff who understand their special needs.

An infant is not just a small adult, and it behoves the surgeon to understand the principles of care of the surgical neonatal infant. Key factors are temperature control, respiration, fluid balance and nutrition. Incubators provide a controlled thermo-neutral environment, but infants are susceptible to hypothermia when exposed for procedures. In the radiology department, measures for avoiding heat loss include a warm ambient temperature and overhead heating, and in the operating theatre use of forced-air warming together with covering the infant's head and limbs with impermeable drapes will minimize water and heat loss. Risk factors for inadequate postoperative respiration are prematurity, young postconceptional age, anaemia and prior apnoeas.[4] Abdominal distension may restrict ventilation by impairing diaphragmatic movement.

Table 40.1 Guidelines for maintenance fluid requirements for neonates (ml/kg/h)

Age	Term infant	Premature*
Day 1	2–3	3–4
Day 2	3–4	4–5
Day 3	3–4	4–5
Then	4–5	5–6

*Requirements are often higher for low birth weight infants

The normal neonate contains an excess of water, and thus fluid requirements are limited in the first 3 days of life (Table 40.1). Standard maintenance fluid is provided as 0.18% saline with 20 mmol/L potassium and 10% dextrose. Accurate monitoring is essential because the ability of the neonatal kidney to excrete excess fluid or sodium is restricted. This is further discussed later in this chapter. The circulatory volume approximates to 80 mL/kg.

Enteral feeding is often inappropriate after operation, and intravenous nutrition has an important role in preventing under-nutrition.[5] The hyperosmolar solutions must be delivered into a central vein via a percutaneous peripheral 'long-line', or a Hickman–Broviac catheter inserted directly into a major vein percutaneously or by open operation.

RECOGNIZING CONGENITAL ANOMALIES

Prenatal ultrasound scanning will identify many anomalies, including abdominal wall defects; gastric or small bowel distension suggestive of intestinal obstruction; bladder distension due to outlet obstruction; lung abnormalities; and congenital diaphragmatic hernia. Polyhydramnios raises the possibility of oesophageal atresia and upper gastrointestinal obstruction. Oligohydramnios may indicate a renal disorder. Elevated maternal serum alpha-fetoprotein levels should prompt investigation for a neural tube defect or teratoma. Karyotyping of the

REFERENCES

1. Chwals W. In: O'Neill J, Rowe MI, Grosfeld JL et al (eds). Pediatric Surgery. 5th edn. Mosby, St Louis, 1998: 57–66
2. Bjorklund LJ, Ingimarsson J, Curstedt T et al. Pediatr Res 1997; 42: 348–355
3. Dai D, Walker WA. Adv Pediatr 1999; 46: 353–382
4. Cote CJ, Zaslavsky A, Downes JJ et al. Anesthesiology 1995; 82: 809–822
5. Pierro A, Jones MO, Donnell SC. Biochem Soc Trans 1998; 26: 131–136

fetus may be considered in abnormalities with a high risk of chromosomal disorders, such as exomphalos.

Some conditions are apparent at birth, including abdominal wall defects and spina bifida, while others (such as intestinal obstruction) may not be suspected until symptoms develop. Preoperative assessment includes a family history and a full examination of the infant. More than one congenital abnormality may coexist, sometimes as well-defined associations such as the vertebral, anorectal, cardiac, tracheo-oesophageal, renal and limb (VACTERL) anomalies sequence discussed later in this chapter.[6]

TRANSPORTING THE SURGICAL NEWBORN INFANT

Ideally, infants known from prenatal screening to have a major surgical anomaly should be delivered in a specialist centre. Postnatal transfer is nevertheless safe provided that attention is paid to the key points in Table 40.2.[7]

SURGICAL CAUSES OF RESPIRATORY DISTRESS IN THE NEWBORN INFANT

Surgical causes of respiratory distress in the newborn (Table 40.3) are relatively uncommon in comparison with medical causes. Respiratory distress is characterized by tachypnoea (respiratory rate greater than 60 breaths/min), expiratory grunting, chest wall retraction or recession, nasal flaring and central cyanosis. After initial resuscitation and clinical examination, a chest X-ray is obtained and, if indicated, echocardiography and blood cultures.

Table 40.2 Key points for neonatal transfer

- Trained nursing and, if necessary, medical staff must accompany the patient.
- Temperature control using a transport incubator to prevent hypothermia.
- Intubation and ventilation must be established before transfer of infants with respiratory distress.
- Nasogastric drainage is essential for abdominal disorders, with the tube on open drainage and regular aspiration during transport.
- Intravenous fluids appropriate for the needs of the infant.

Send with patient:

- Maternal blood sample for cross-matching.
- Documentation of medications given, notably vitamin K and antibiotics.
- Results of investigations and copies of radiographs.
- Written consent by the mother for operation where appropriate.

Table 40.3 Surgical causes of respiratory distress

Upper airway causes

- Choanal atresia
- Pierre Robin syndrome
- Subglottic stenosis
- Laryngeal web or atresia
- Laryngomalacia or tracheomalacia
- Laryngeal and laryngotracheal cleft
- Vascular compression anomalies

Lower airway causes

- Oesophageal atresia and tracheo-oesophageal fistula
- Congenital diaphragmatic hernia
- Congenital cystic adenomatoid malformation
- Congenital lobar emphysema

Upper airway causes

Choanal atresia

Choanal atresia occurs in one in 8000 newborns and results from failure of the choanal plate to perforate. The atresia is usually bony and unilateral but may be bilateral or membranous. Because neonates are obligate nasal breathers they may present as a neonatal emergency.[8] Keeping the mouth open with an oropharyngeal airway will allow the infant to breathe; definitive treatment involves operative perforation of the choanal plate and stenting.

Pierre Robin syndrome

Pierre Robin syndrome is characterized by micrognathia and relative glossoptosis with or without cleft palate. This condition is self-correcting by the age of 3 months, but acute airway obstruction can occur when infants are placed in the supine position, because the tongue occludes the airway. Feeding is also difficult, and specialized nursing care is required during the early months.[9]

Lower airway causes

Oesophageal atresia

The incidence of oesophageal atresia is approximately one in 4000 births. The aetiology remains uncertain, due in part to incomplete knowledge of the mechanisms of early oesophageal development.[10] Separation of the foregut and lung is a relatively early phenomenon, and associated anomalies are common; 30–40% of children have an associated cardiac or gastrointestinal malformation, often as part of the VACTERL association of anomalies.[6]

Affected neonates present with choking episodes due to accumulation of saliva in the pharynx, relieved by suction. Up to 50% of infants have an antenatal history of polyhydramnios, and on ultrasound scan the stomach bubble may be absent.[11] Inability to pass an orogastric tube and obtain acid gastric aspirates points to the diagnosis, which is confirmed by a chest radiograph showing the gastric tube held up in the upper oesophageal pouch (Fig. 40.1). Delayed diagnosis, especially if feeding is attempted, increases the risk of aspiration pneumonia and compromises the outcome.[12] Oesophageal atresia can occur with or without tracheo-oesophageal fistula (Fig. 40.2). In 85% of patients the upper oesophagus ends blindly and the distal oesophagus communicates with the trachea (tracheo-oesophageal fistula). Absence of gastro-intestinal air on the X-ray is indicative of pure atresia without a fistula, which occurs in 5% of infants. Rare anomalies include H-type tracheo-oesophageal fistula without atresia.

Immediate management includes nursing the infant in a prone position to minimize the risk of aspiration. A large-bore nasogastric catheter or double-lumen Replogle tube is passed

REFERENCES

6. Khoury MJ, Cordero JF, Greenberg F et al. Pediatrics 1983; 71: 815–820
7. Lloyd DA. Semin Neonatol 1996; 1: 241–248
8. Friedman NR, Mitchell RB, Bailey CM et al. Int J Pediatr Otorhinolaryngol 2000; 52: 45–51
9. Wagener S, Rayatt SS, Tatman AJ et al. Cleft Palate Craniofac J 2003; 40: 180–185
10. Kluth D, Fiegel H. Semin Pediatr Surg 2003; 12: 3–9
11. Sparey C, Jawaheer G, Barrett AM et al. Am J Obstet Gynecol 2000; 182: 427–431
12. Sharma AK, Shekhawat NS, Agrawal LD et al. Pediatr Surg Int 2000; 16: 478–482

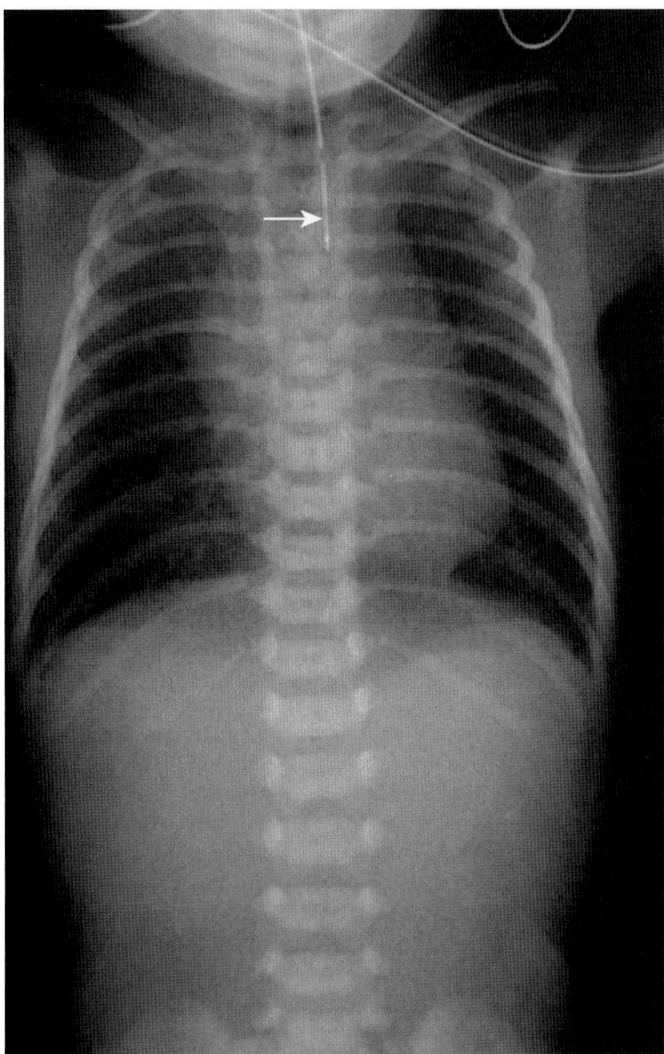

Figure 40.1 Oesophageal atresia showing nasogastric tube in the upper pouch. Absence of air below the diaphragm indicates the absence of a tracheo-oesophageal fistula.

for continuous suctioning. Assessment for associated malformations should include echocardiography and renal ultrasound. The operative principles include disconnecting the tracheo-oesophageal fistula and either primary or delayed oesophageal anastomosis depending on the gap between proximal and distal oesophageal pouches.[13] Rarely, oesophageal substitution is necessary using colon[14] or stomach.[15] Overall survival is 80–90%; associated cardiac malformations and low birth weight are the leading causes of death.[16]

Congenital diaphragmatic hernia

The diaphragm develops between the 8th and 10th weeks of gestation by fusion of the dorsal pleuroperitoneal membrane with the ventral septum transversum, thus separating the pleural and peritoneal cavities. Congenital diaphragmatic hernia through a posterolateral (Bochdalek) defect results from failure of this process. The cause is unknown. The high mortality is due to the associated lung hypoplasia and pulmonary hypertension.[17] Major associated anomalies such as cardiac defects occur in 25% of patients.[18] Congenital diaphragmatic hernia remains one of the challenges in paediatric surgery, with a mortality of 30–50% despite therapeutic advances.[17] The incidence is one in 2500

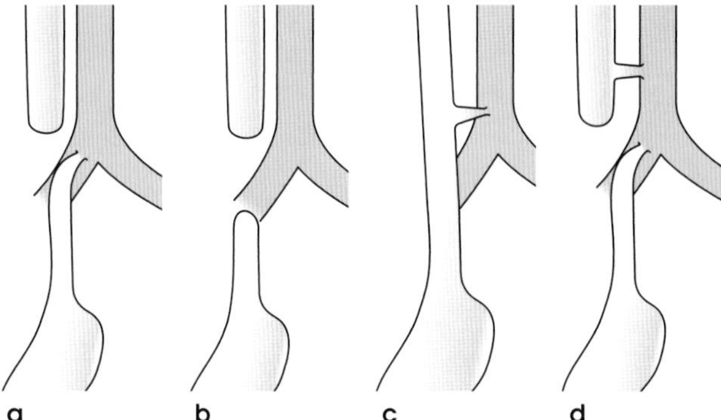

Figure 40.2 (**a**) Oesophageal atresia with distal tracheo-oesophageal fistula (87% incidence); (**b**) isolated oesophageal atresia (8%); (**c**) isolated H-type fistula (4%); and (**d**) oesophageal atresia with proximal and distal fistulae (1%).

births, and diagnosis is often made on antenatal ultrasound. Affected infants present with respiratory distress, cyanosis, tracheal deviation and diminished breath sounds on the side of the hernia. A chest X-ray will show abdominal viscera in the chest cavity (Fig. 40.3).

Initial management centres on optimizing gas exchange. Early endotracheal intubation and ventilation avoiding high ventilatory pressures, followed by transfer to a specialist neonatal intensive care facility are essential.[19] Opinion favours preoperative stabilization of the infant prior to operative reduction of the hernia, through a subcostal incision, and repair of the diaphragmatic defect.[20] For a large defect a synthetic patch is used. High-frequency ventilation, inhaled nitric oxide, extracorporeal membrane oxygenation and partial liquid ventilation have been used to ameliorate the pulmonary hypertension and to minimize iatrogenic pulmonary barotraumas, but no consistent benefit has been demonstrated.

ABDOMINAL WALL DEFECTS

Exomphalos and gastroschisis

Exomphalos is a midline developmental defect of the anterior abdominal wall (Fig. 40.4). As a result, some of the abdominal organs, notably the intestine, stomach, liver and spleen, lie outside the abdominal cavity within a membranous sac derived from the amniotic membrane. Up to 75% of infants have associated congenital cardiac defects and chromosomal anomalies, notably trisomy 13, 18 or 21, which may determine the outcome. In the Beckwith–Wiedemann syndrome of exomphalos, macro-

REFERENCES

13. Beasley S. In: Stringer MO, Mouriquand PDE, Howard ER (eds). Pediatric Surgery and Urology: Long-term Outcomes. WB Saunders, London, 1998: 166–180
14. Ure BM, Slany E, Eypasch EP et al. Eur J Pediatr Surg 1995; 5: 206–210
15. Ludman L, Spitz L. J Pediatr Surg 2003; 38: 53–57
16. Driver CP, Shankar KR, Jones MO et al. J Pediatr Surg 2001; 36: 1419–1421
17. Smith NP, Jesudason EC, Losty PD. Paediatr Respir Rev 2002; 3: 339–348
18. Witters I, Legius E, Moerman P et al. Am J Med Genet 2001; 103: 278–282
19. Sakurai Y, Azarow K, Cutz E et al. J Pediatr Surg 1999; 34: 1813–1817
20. Nio M, Haase G, Kennaugh J et al. J Pediatr Surg 1994; 29: 618–621

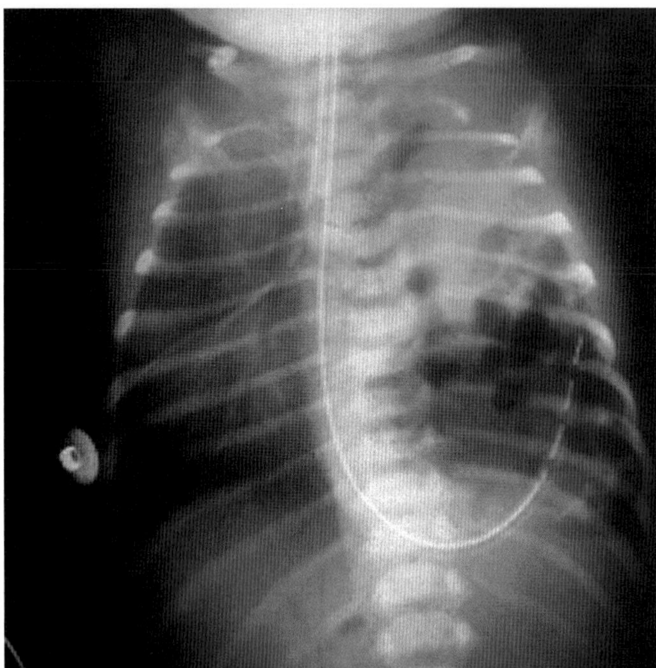

Figure 40.3 Congenital diaphragmatic hernia: note the bowel and nasogastric tube in the left thoracic cavity.

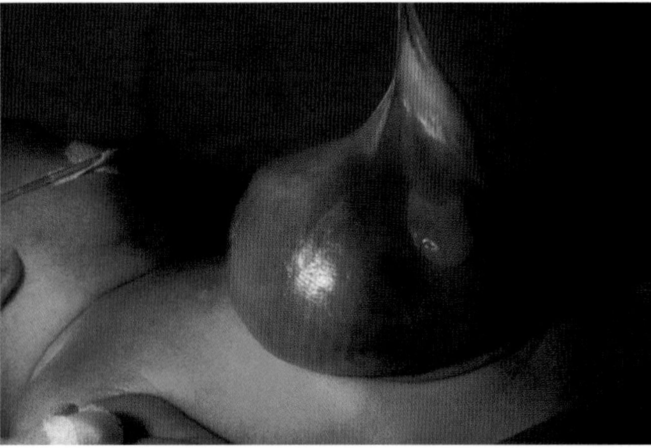

Figure 40.4 Exomphalos. (Reproduced with permission from Lloyd DA, Kenny SE. Congenital Anomalies. In: Walker WA et al (eds) Pediatric Gastrointestinal Disease. BC Decker Inc. 2004; 561–572.)

glossia and hypoglycaemia, early recognition is essential to prevent complications from hypoglycaemia.[21]

With gastroschisis, the stomach and intestine are eviscerated through a defect to the right of the base of the umbilical cord (Fig. 40.5). There is no enveloping sac and evisceration of other organs is rare. A possible mechanism, supported by evidence from serial ultrasound scans, is prenatal rupture of a small hernia at the base of the umbilical cord. Abnormalities of the intestine, notably atresia, occur in about 10% of infants but chromosomal and extra-abdominal anomalies are rare.[22]

Accurate diagnosis is possible with antenatal sonography.[23] Amniocentesis and karyotyping may be appropriate for exomphalos.[23] Delivery should take place in a specialist unit. Stable infants with a gastroschisis or a small exomphalos may be delivered safely per vaginam. Eviscerated bowel is wrapped in 'cling' film to prevent water and heat loss, particularly if the

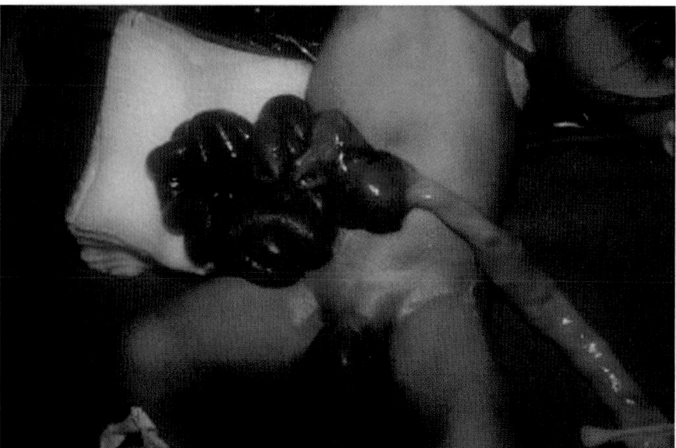

Figure 40.5 Gastroschisis. (Reproduced with permission from Lloyd DA, Kenny SE. Congenital Anomalies. In: Walker WA et al (eds) Pediatric Gastrointestinal Disease. BC Decker Inc. 2004; 561–572.)

infant is to be transferred. Pre-operative correction of hypovolaemia is essential and boluses of normal saline 20 ml/kg or albumin 10 ml/kg may be required.

Primary closure of the defect may be possible depending on the volume of the herniated viscera; postoperative ventilation is usually required because the increased intra-abdominal pressure restricts diaphragmatic movement. Alternatively, the eviscerated organs are placed in an artificial bag (silo) attached to the abdominal wall.[22] This is progressively reduced in size each day, allowing secondary closure of the abdomen by 7–10 days. Infection is a major cause of morbidity, and antiseptic care and prophylactic antibiotics are important. Intravenous feeding is required via a central venous catheter. With a large intact exomphalos there is no urgency for repair provided infection is not a concern.

Overall survival for gastroschisis is greater than 90%; postoperative problems include adhesive obstruction and short gut syndrome. For exomphalos the outcome depends on the associated abnormalities; in the absence of these, most infants survive to lead a normal life.[24]

Umbilical abnormalities

Umbilical granuloma

Umbilical granuloma is a mass of pink granulation tissue at the umbilicus caused by low-grade infection of the umbilical cord stump. It must be distinguished from an omphalomesenteric duct remnant. Topical treatment suffices, with local cleansing and applications of either steroids or silver nitrate. The latter carries a risk of damage to the adjacent skin, which must be protected.

Omphalomesenteric duct remnants

The omphalomesenteric duct (vitellointestinal duct) normally regresses between the fifth and seventh weeks of gestation.[25]

REFERENCES

21. Elliott M, Maher ER. J Med Genet 1994; 31: 560–564
22. Driver CP, Bruce J, Bianchi A et al. J Pediatr Surg 2000; 35: 1719–1723
23. Langer JC. World J Surg 2003; 27: 117–124
24. Langer JC. Semin Pediatr Surg 1996; 5: 124–128
25. Vermeij-Keers C, Hartwig NG, van der Werff JF. Semin Pediatr Surg 1996; 5: 82–89

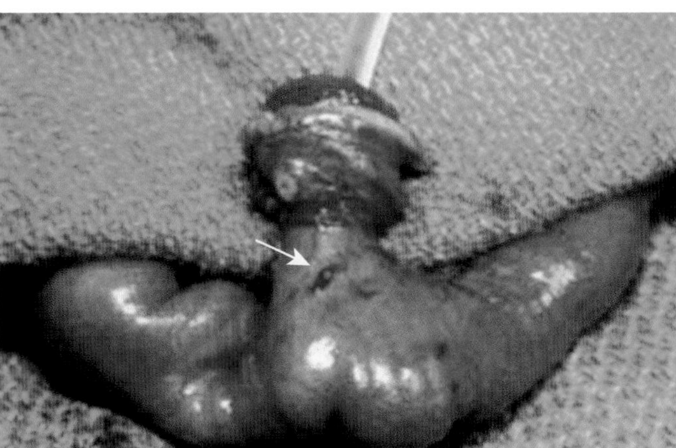

Figure 40.6 Patent omphalomesenteric duct with tube inserted. Note the ectopic mucosa at the umbilicus and the Meckel's diverticulum (arrow).

Failure of this process results in a fistula that presents with a persistent umbilical discharge, often with ectopic intestinal mucosa at the umbilicus (Fig. 40.6). The diagnosis is confirmed by passing a nasogastric tube through the fistula and aspirating small bowel content or injecting radiopaque contrast. The entire fistula is resected through a subumbilical incision. The obliterated omphalomesenteric duct may persist as a solid band.

Remnants of the omphalomesenteric duct may persist, of which the most common is the Meckel's diverticulum.[26] Meckel's diverticulitis is indistinguishable from acute appendicitis and is diagnosed at operation. Acid secretion from ectopic gastric mucosa within the diverticulum may lead to mucosal ulceration, bleeding or perforation. Ectopic gastric tissue may be identified by technetium-99m scanning, which has 85% sensitivity and 95% specificity.[26] Intestinal obstruction may result from intussusception of the diverticulum or from volvulus around a connecting band to the umbilicus. In all situations the diverticulum is resected with the adjacent segment of ileum. There is no sound evidence to support routine resection of an asymptomatic diverticulum encountered incidentally at operation.

An isolated mucosal remnant at the umbilicus must be distinguished from an umbilical granuloma, and is suspected when the 'granuloma' fails to respond to topical treatment. Treatment is excision of the ectopic mucosa; a limited exploration beneath the umbilicus is advisable to exclude an omphalomesenteric band.

Patent urachus

Persistence of the embryonic communication between the bladder and the allantois presents as a watery discharge at the umbilicus or as an infected cyst. Excision of the fistulous remnant through a subumbilical incision is curative.

GASTROINTESTINAL OBSTRUCTION IN THE NEWBORN INFANT (Table 40.4)

Clinical features

Vomiting

Bilious (green) vomiting is characteristic of intestinal obstruction distal to the ampulla of Vater. Non-bilious vomiting may be due to obstruction at the pylorus or in the proximal duodenum, and must be distinguished from gastro-oesophageal reflux.

Table 40.4 Causes of gastrointestinal obstruction

Vomiting in the newborn infant
- Duodenal atresia
- Malrotation
- Jejunoileal atresia
- Meconium ileus
- Duplication cyst
- Incarcerated inguinal hernia

Failure to pass stool
- Anorectal malformation
- Hirschsprung's disease
- Meconium plug syndrome
- Colonic atresia

Abdominal distension

Abdominal distension will depend on the level of obstruction, and is most marked in the case of distal large bowel obstruction.

Failure to pass stools

The normal infant should pass meconium within 36 h of birth. Failure to pass stool in association with abdominal distension suggests colonic, rectal or anal obstruction.

General principles of management

Gastric drainage

An 8–10 French nasogastric tube is inserted to prevent vomiting and aspiration, and to reduce abdominal distension, which in the newborn infant may restrict diaphragmatic movement and compromise ventilation. The tube must be left open for continuous gravity drainage, and regularly flushed with air or water and aspirated to confirm that it is patent.

Intravenous fluids

With intestinal obstruction, fluid losses into the stomach and intestine are not adequately compensated for by standard maintenance solutions. In anticipation of these additional requirements we use 0.45% sodium chloride (half normal) with 20 mmol/L potassium chloride. A 10% dextrose solution reduces the risk of hypoglycaemia, but regular monitoring of the blood sugar level is important. Fluid volume is increased for the same reason, starting from day 1 at 4–5 mL/kg per hour for full-term infants and 5–6 mL/kg per hour for premature infants, depending on the level of obstruction and the degree of dehydration. For severe hypovolaemia, boluses of saline 20 ml/kg or albumin 10 ml/kg may be required. Measured gastric aspirates are replaced with 0.9% sodium chloride (normal saline).

Hydration is monitored by clinical assessment of the peripheral circulation, skin turgor and anterior fontanelle tension, and by accurately monitoring the urine volume (normal for a neonate is 2 mL/kg per hour) and concentration (normal specific gravity is 1008–1012). Based on these findings the volume of intravenous fluid is increased or decreased every 4–8 h, the frequency of assessment depending on the individual clinical situation.

• REFERENCE •

26. Moore TC. Semin Pediatr Surg 1996; 5: 116–123

Laparotomy

The neonatal abdomen is square rather than rectangular, and the umbilical to pubic symphysis length is relatively short. A transverse supraumbilical incision provides excellent access for most situations and vertical incisions should be avoided.

Vomiting in the newborn infant (Box 40.4)

Non-obstructive causes of vomiting must be excluded, including feeding difficulties (under- or over-feeding), food allergy, systemic infection, urinary tract infection, raised intracranial pressure, and adrenogenital syndrome. Non-bilious vomiting may be due to pyloric stenosis and gastro-oesophageal reflux (see further in this chapter).

Duodenal atresia

The site of obstruction typically is at the level of the ampulla of Vater, and may take the form of complete obstruction due to an atresia or an intact membrane, or partial obstruction due to stenosis or a fenestrated membrane. The common bile duct usually opens on to the membrane and is vulnerable if an attempt is made to excise the membrane. The pancreas may encircle the atretic site (annular pancreas). Distal to the level of the atresia there is a marked decrease in the calibre of the duodenum, unless an intact membrane bulges distally, forming the 'windsock' anomaly.

The incidence of duodenal atresia ranges from one in 6000 to one in 10 000 live births. Prematurity is common, and associated anomalies include trisomy 21 (Down's syndrome), congenital cardiac disease, oesophageal atresia, anorectal abnormalities and malrotation. The cause of the anomaly is not understood; its occurrence at the complex site of development of the duodenum, pancreas, and biliary and pancreatic ducts, and the association with trisomy 21, suggest a genetic origin.[27]

The prenatal ultrasound scan shows hydramnios and a distended stomach; this may prompt fetal karyotyping to exclude trisomy 21 if termination of pregnancy is a consideration.[28] Following birth, the typical presentation is with bilious vomiting and epigastric distension. A plain abdominal X-ray showing the characteristic 'double bubble' representing the distended stomach and proximal duodenum is diagnostic (Fig. 40.7). When gas is present distal to the dilated proximal duodenum, malrotation must be distinguished from duodenal stenosis by ultrasound scan or contrast study. Partial duodenal obstruction may not be recognized for months or years until persistent postprandial vomiting prompts investigation.

Preoperative management includes gastric decompression and correction of fluid and electrolyte abnormalities. Because of the risk of injury to the ampulla of Vater, the preferred operative procedure is a duodeno-duodenostomy to bypass the obstruction.[29] For a fenestrated diaphragm a longitudinal incision is extended across the diaphragm, taking care to avoid the ampulla of Vater by placing the incision anterolaterally. Postoperative ileus may be prolonged and intravenous feeding is often needed. If this is not available, a transanastomotic nasoduodenal feeding tube is passed at operation under direct vision to enable early postoperative enteral feeding. Survival rates are over 95%, and depend largely on the associated anomalies.[30]

Midgut malrotation

Malrotation describes a situation where the intestine does not lie in a normal position. The common form is midgut malrotation, in which there are two components: the third part of the duodenum lies to the right of the vertebral column instead of crossing to the left, and the caecum lies in the upper abdomen, adjacent to the duodenum (Fig. 40.8). As a result, the mesentery of the midgut (small intestine and right half of the colon) is not attached in the usual manner across the posterior abdominal wall but is freely suspended from the base of the superior mesenteric artery. It is liable to twist around this narrow pedicle at any time. A volvulus of more than 270° may lead to irreversible midgut ischaemia (Fig. 40.9). Traditionally, malrotation is attributed to failure of the intestine to 'rotate' to its normal position when it returns to the peritoneal cavity from the normal umbilical cord hernia during the first month of gestation. This is probably an over-simplification, and the true mechanism is not understood.[31]

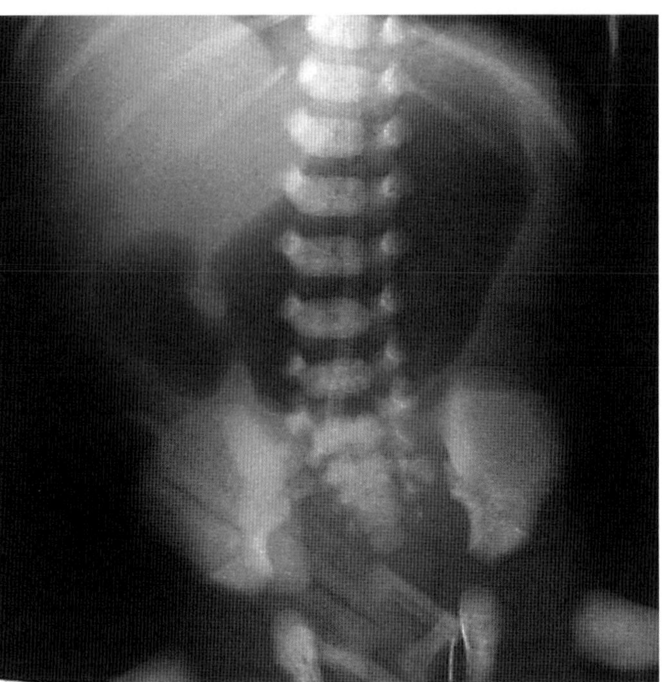

Figure 40.7 Abdominal X-ray showing the 'double bubble' sign (stomach and duodenum) characteristic of duodenal atresia.

The risk of acute volvulus is highest during the neonatal period, but malrotation may remain asymptomatic throughout life. Recurrent volvulus may present at any age and must be suspected when there is a history of chronic intermittent abdominal pain with or without vomiting. A contrast X-ray will show the characteristic features of malrotation, but may appear to be normal if the patient is asymptomatic at the time the X-ray is done and should be repeated if symptoms persist.

In the infant, acute midgut volvulus presents with bilious vomiting, abdominal distension and tenderness, and altered

REFERENCES

27. Torfs CP, Christianson RE. Am J Med Genet 1998; 77: 431–438
28. Lawrence MJ, Ford WD, Furness ME et al. Pediatr Surg Int 2000; 16: 342–345
29. Kimura K, Mukohara N, Nishijima E et al. J Pediatr Surg 1990; 25: 977–979
30. Murshed R, Nicholls G, Spitz L. Br J Obstet Gynaecol 1999; 106: 1197–1199
31. Kluth D, Kaestner M, Tibboel D et al. J Pediatr Surg 1995; 30: 448–453

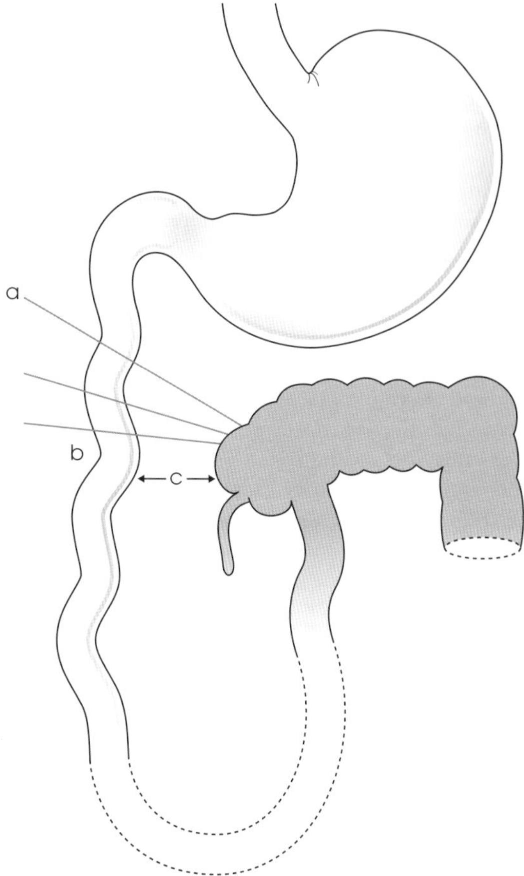

Figure 40.8 Malrotation with (**a**) Ladd's bands and (**b**) the duodenum to the right of the midline. (**c**) The narrow base of the mesentery predisposes to volvulus.

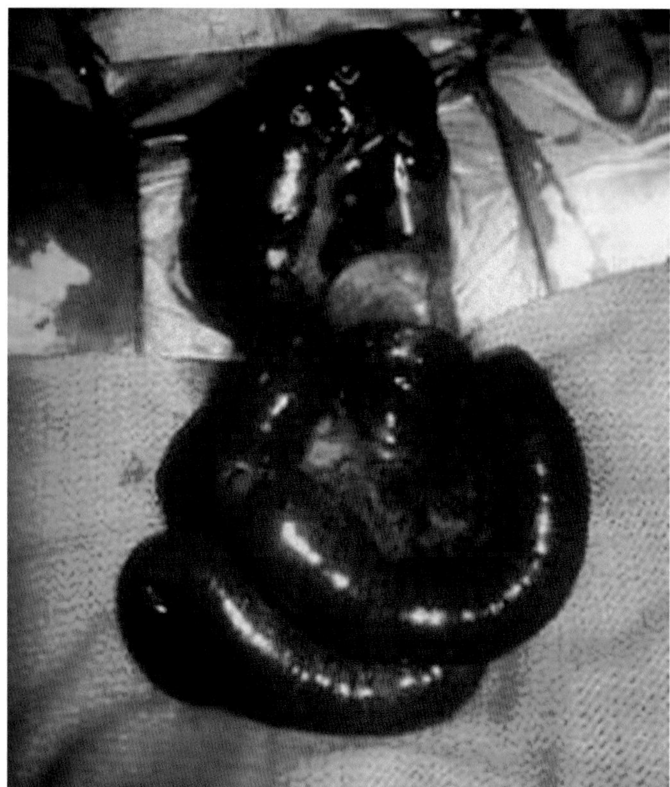

Figure 40.9 Midgut malrotation with irreversible ischaemia.

blood in the stools. With progressive midgut ischaemia the infant rapidly deteriorates, with increasing abdominal distension, hypovolaemia and metabolic acidosis. A plain abdominal X-ray shows features of duodenal obstruction; beyond this the bowel may contain more fluid than air, with resultant opacification of the abdominal cavity.

Urgent laparotomy is required after rapid correction of fluid and electrolyte abnormalities, and nasogastric drainage. A generous supraumbilical transverse incision is important to enable easy delivery and inspection of the whole of the small and large bowel. The volvulus is derotated, usually in an anticlockwise direction, to allow restoration of the mesenteric circulation and to reveal the caecum lying adjacent to the duodenum. The peritoneal folds extending from the caecum across the duodenum (Ladd's bands, Fig. 40.8) are divided and the caecum is mobilized towards the left, thus widening the base of the mesenteric. The small intestine is displaced to the right. The appendix may be removed to avoid future diagnostic confusion. When the viability of the bowel is uncertain, only the obvious non-viable bowel is resected and stomas are made; the bowel is re-examined at a second laparotomy after an interval of 24–36 h. If the entire volvulus clearly is not viable, resection inevitably will result in severe short gut syndrome with significant morbidity and mortality.[32]

Jejunoileal atresia

Congenital obstruction of the jejunum or ileum due to atresia or stenosis develops as a result of sterile ischaemic infarction of a segment of fetal intestine. This was first demonstrated experimentally in a fetal dog model in 1955 by Louw and Barnard.[33] Presentation is with bilious vomiting and abdominal distension. Meconium stool may be passed. The diagnosis is confirmed by plain abdominal X-ray showing multiple dilated loops of intestine with air fluid levels. A contrast enema may be required to distinguish distal ileal atresia from meconium ileus, long segment Hirschsprung's disease or colonic atresia.

At operation, the site of obstruction is easily identified by the abrupt change in calibre from the dilated proximal intestine to the narrow empty distal small bowel. The dilated proximal bowel is resected and continuity is restored by end-to-end or end-to-back anastomosis. Postoperative recovery may be prolonged and parenteral nutrition may be required. Survival rates over the past two decades have ranged from 78 to 100%.[34]

Meconium ileus

As a result of pancreatic enzyme deficiency, the ileum is obstructed by viscid pigmented meconium with a high albumin content. With rare exceptions this is associated with cystic fibrosis. Up to 20% of newborn infants with cystic fibrosis present with meconium ileus. The diagnosis is confirmed by chromosomal analysis, which in 85% of patients will demonstrate the ΔF508 mutation, a three base pair deletion from chromosome 7.[35]

REFERENCES

32. Hwang ST, Shulman RJ. Clin Perinatol 2002; 29: 181–194, vii
33. Louw JH, Barnard CN. Lancet 1955; 2: 1065–1067
34. Grosfeld J. In: O'Neill JA, Grosfeld JL, Fonkalsrud EW et al (eds). Pediatric Surgery. 5 edn. Mosby, St Louis, 1998: 1145–1158
35. Kerem B, Buchanan J, Markiewicz D et al. Am J Hum Genet 1989; 44: 827–834

Mutations result in defective chloride transport in the apical membrane of epithelial cells and an abnormally high excretion of chloride from the skin.[36] This can be measured by iontophoresis (the sweat test), an alternative diagnostic test in mature infants.

The characteristic abnormality is a narrow terminal ileum containing multiple pellets of meconium, with an abrupt transition proximally to dilated ileum containing meconium that is abnormally tenacious and adherent to the intestinal mucosa. The colon is empty and contracted (microcolon). Presentation is with distal ileal obstruction, which must be distinguished from ileal atresia and long segment Hirschsprung's disease. Abdominal X-rays show air fluid levels in the proximal small bowel, while in the right iliac fossa the dilated meconium-filled ileum contains multiple translucencies due to fat globules, the 'soap bubble' appearance.

Following nasogastric decompression and correction of fluid and electrolyte imbalances, the diagnosis is confirmed by water-soluble contrast enema, which will show the microcolon, the meconium pellets in the distal ileum, and the dilated proximal dilated ileum (Fig. 40.10). By changing the contrast to gastrograffin it is possible to clear the obstructing meconium in over 50% of patients.[37] Gastrograffin has an osmolality of approximately 1700 mOsm/L, and great care must be taken to anticipate and replace fluid losses into the intestine.

At operation for uncomplicated meconium ileus the proximal dilated ileum is opened and the meconium removed using saline irrigation. Simple enterostomy or resection of the dilated intestine with primary anastomosis is safe when bowel wall is healthy and the obstruction can be cleared distally with certainty. Alternatively, proximal and distal stomas should be created. Pancreatic enzyme replacement is essential once feeding commences.

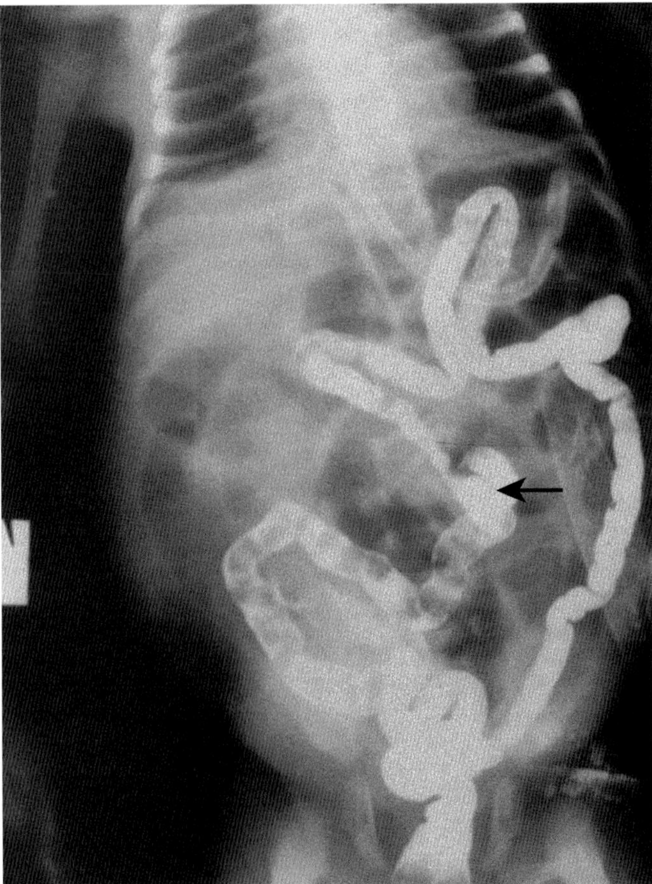

Figure 40.10 Meconium ileus: contrast enema showing a microcolon, displaced caecum (arrow) and filling defects in the terminal ileum. (Reproduced with permission from Lloyd DA, Kenny SE. Congenital Anomalies. In: Walker WA et al (eds) Pediatric Gastrointestinal Disease. BC Decker Inc. 2004; 561–572.)

The survival rate for meconium ileus has improved from 30% in the 1960s to over 90%. This is attributed to the overall improvement in perioperative respiratory care, increasingly successful non-operative management, and avoidance of stomas.[37] In older children, episodic obstruction due to inspissated meconium may occur (meconium ileus equivalent or distal intestinal obstruction syndrome), possibly associated with under-hydration and altered enzyme replacement needs. Presentation is with colicky pain and tenderness, and typically a mass in the right iliac fossa, which must be distinguished from appendix mass, ovarian tumour and inflammatory bowel disease. In most children oral gastrograffin will relieve the obstruction.[38]

Duplication cysts

Duplication cysts are congenital tubular or spherical cysts attached to the alimentary canal anywhere between the mouth and the anus, most commonly in the ileocaecal region. The cysts have a muscle layer and an epithelial lining resembling the adjacent gastrointestinal tract, with which the blood supply is shared. Thoracic duplications may communicate through the diaphragm with the intra-abdominal gastrointestinal-tract, from where the blood supply is derived (a potential pitfall for the unwary surgeon). Abdominal duplications lie on the mesenteric side of the small intestine and on the antimesenteric side of the large bowel. Tubular duplications, in which islands of ectopic gastric mucosa may be present, may communicate with the intestinal lumen.[39]

The diagnosis may be suspected on prenatal ultrasound scan. Postnatal presentation is with an abdominal mass or obstruction of the adjacent intestinal lumen. In a tubular cyst, peptic ulceration secondary to acid secretion from ectopic gastric mucosa may lead to rectal bleeding or perforation. Ultrasound and technetium-99m scanning may be diagnostic. Computerized tomography or MRI scanning may help to distinguish the duplication from ovarian or other cystic lesions. Complete excision is the treatment of choice. Where this is not possible, partial excision with removal of the mucosa from the remaining cyst wall or resection of the duplication and adjacent intestine are options.

Omphalomesenteric duct remnants

Intestinal volvulus may occur around a vestigial omphalomesenteric band between a Meckel's diverticulum and the umbilicus (see p. 907).

Failure to pass stool in the newborn infant (Table 40.5)

Anorectal anomalies

Anorectal anomalies (imperforate anus) occur in approximately one in 5000 live births. The development of the hindgut remains

REFERENCES

36. Schwiebert E, Egan M, Hwang T et al. Cell 1995; 81: 1063–1073
37. Kao S, Franken E. Pediatr Radiol 1995; 25: 97
38. O'Halloran SM, Gilbert J, McKendrick OM et al. Arch Dis Child 1986; 61: 1128–1130
39. Wardell S, Vidican DE. J Clin Gastroenterol 1990; 12: 681–684

Table 40.5 Classification of anorectal anomalies

Males defects
- Low defects: cutaneous fistula, anal stenosis, anal membrane, 'bucket handle' malformation
- Recto-urethral bulbar fistula
- Recto-urethral prostatic fistula
- Rectovesical (bladder neck) fistula
- Imperforate anus without fistula
- Rectal atresia and stenosis

Females defects
- Cutaneous (perineal) fistula
- Vestibular fistula
- Imperforate anus without fistula
- Rectal atresia or stenosis
- Persistent cloaca

poorly understood. The cloaca forms at approximately 21 days gestation and is a cavity into which hindgut, allantois and mesonephric ducts open. By 6 weeks, a combination of programmed cell death and differential growth results in the formation of an anterior urogenital cavity and a posterior anorectal cavity. When this process is disrupted, an anorectal malformation may result. The cause of anorectal anomalies is unknown. Although prenatal dosing of rats with the antimitotic agent doxorubicin can cause anorectal malformations,[40] there is little evidence that environmental factors play a major causative role in humans.

The anatomical findings in children with anorectal malformations vary considerably, from simple anterior malposition of the anus to complex anal agenesis, in which the anus is absent or represented by a shallow pit, the buttocks are flattened, and the sacrum and anorectal innervation are deficient. The simplified classification of Pena (Box 40.5) summarizes the most commonly encountered variants.[41]

Anorectal anomalies are most often detected during routine postnatal examination, although with some the perineum may appear relatively normal to casual inspection. When the rectum terminates as a fistulous communication to the genitourinary tract, meconium may be discharged from the vagina or urethra. Up to 60% of infants will have malformations affecting other organ systems, most commonly cardiac, gastrointestinal, genitourinary or vertebral in origin. These may coexist as the VACTERL sequence. Assessment must include echocardiography, renal tract and spinal ultrasound scanning, plain spinal radiography and karyotyping.

The principles underlying the initial management of infants with imperforate anus are relief of the distal bowel obstruction, protection of the anal sphincter mechanism, and assessment of associated anomalies. Surgical options are to form a colostomy or to perform definitive reconstruction. Only 'low' (perineal) lesions, such as cutaneous fistula, where the anomaly is distal to the anal sphincter, are amenable to perineal reconstructive procedures without diverting colostomy. The cutaneous fistula discharges meconium and can occur anywhere in the midline from the presumptive site of the anus to the scrotum and penis (Fig. 40.11). Because of the risk of damaging the anal sphincter, for all other anomalies or in case of doubt it is advisable to perform a temporary diverting colostomy followed by staged reconstruction. A sigmoid colostomy is suitable for most cases of imperforate anus, but for a cloacal anomaly a transverse colostomy is recommended.

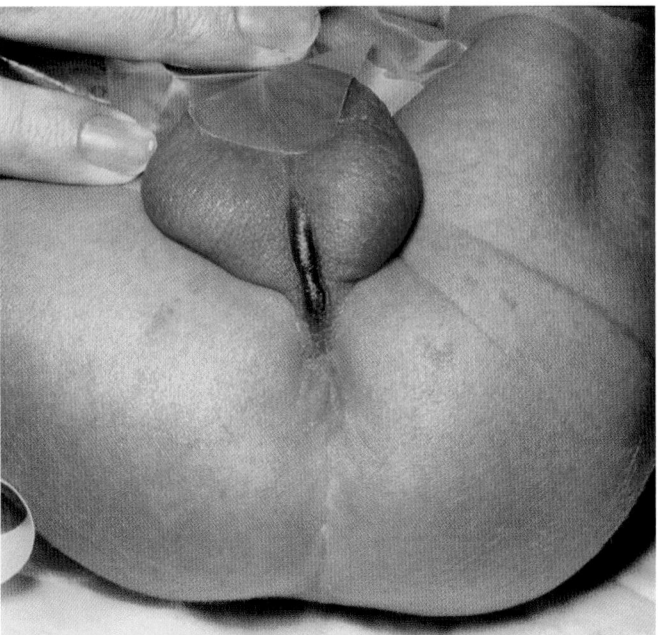

Figure 40.11 Anorectal malformation: cutaneous fistula. The anus is absent and meconium is tracking along the fistula anteriorly in the midline on to the scrotum. (Reproduced with permission from Lloyd DA, Kenny SE. Congenital Anomalies. In: Walker WA et al (eds) Pediatric Gastrointestinal Disease. BC Decker Inc. 2004; 561–572.)

The two main steps in definitive reconstruction are mobilization and ligation of the fistula followed by creation of the neoanus; with a cloacal anomaly, genitourinary reconstruction is also required. The posterior sagittal approach (Pena) has been adopted by most surgeons, and more recently, laparoscopic anorectal reconstruction has been advocated with high anomalies.[42] Following reconstruction the parents are taught to dilate the anus to avoid stenosis of the neoanus.

The long-term outcome of children with anorectal malformations is variable and to a large extent depends on the initial anatomical anomaly and clinical management. Children with 'high' malformations tend to have a poorer outcome with higher rates of faecal incontinence.[41] Troublesome constipation can also occur in children with 'low' lesions. Careful follow-up and parental support are necessary to ensure that constipation is effectively managed and development of a dilated megarectum is avoided. The psychological effects of incontinence and constipation on the child and the family are considerable.[43] The antegrade continence enema procedure, developed over the past decade,[44] has proved to be valuable for achieving independent continence. Adolescent girls will need specialist obstetric assessment and advice regarding pregnancy and the most appropriate form of delivery. In some, vaginal reconstruction may be necessary.

REFERENCES

40. Merei JM. Pediatr Surg Int 2002; 18: 36–39
41. Pena A, Hong A. Am J Surg 2000; 180: 370–376
42. Georgeson KE, Inge TH, Albanese CT. J Pediatr Surg 2000; 35: 927–930
43. Ludman L, Spitz L. J Pediatr Surg 1995; 30: 495–499
44. Malone PS, Curry JI, Osborne A. World J Urol 1998; 16: 274–278

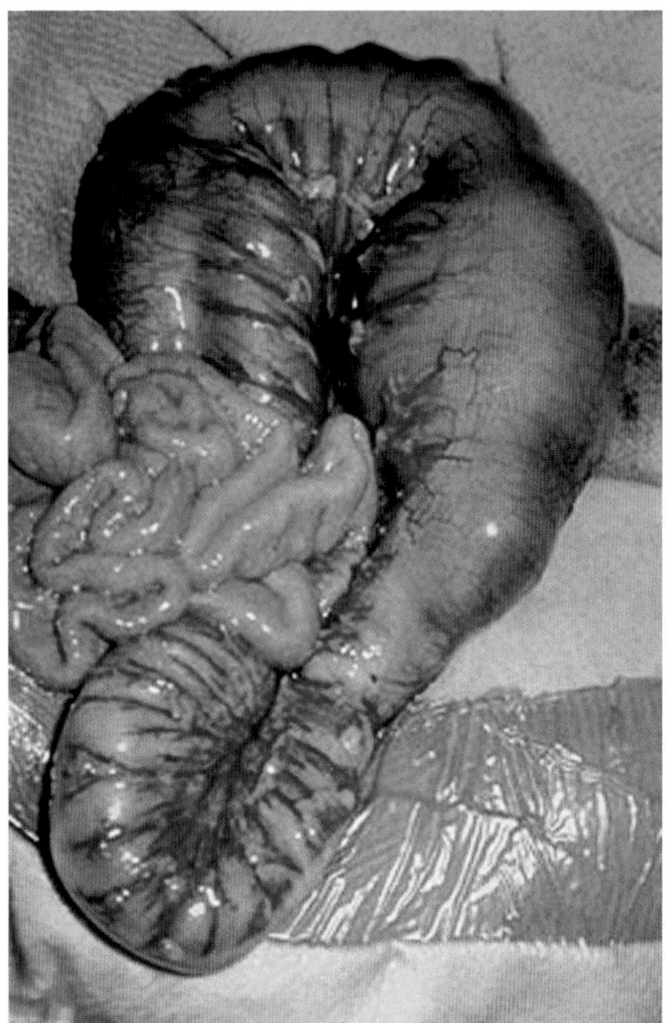

Figure 40.12 Hirschsprung's disease: macroscopic appearance of the transitional zone with dilated proximal ganglionic colon and contracted distal aganglionic colon.

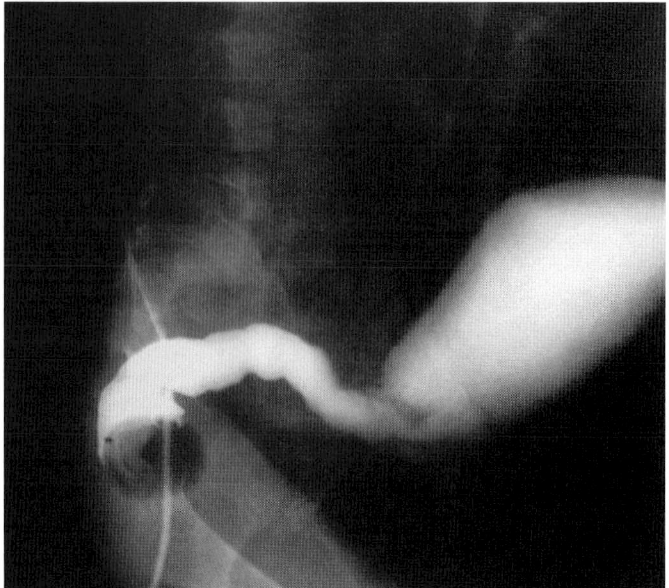

Figure 40.13 Hirschsprung's disease: contrast enema showing the transitional zone.

Hirschsprung's disease and related disorders

Hirschsprung's disease affects one in 5000 newborn infants and is defined as absence of ganglion cells (aganglionosis) in a variable length of distal bowel. In 70% of infants the aganglionosis is confined to the rectum and sigmoid, including the internal sphincter (short segment disease), but may extend to involve the entire colon (total colonic disease) and rarely the entire intestine. The affected gut looks macroscopically normal but is unable to relax, causing a functional bowel obstruction with dilatation of the proximal ganglionic intestine (megacolon) and an intervening transitional zone (Fig. 40.12).

Ganglion cells of the enteric nervous system are derived from the vagal neural crest, and during the first trimester migrate from the vagal neural crest into the oesophagus and then distally to colonize the developing gut in a craniocaudal direction. Aganglionosis results from a failure of migration, differentiation or survival of these cells and is associated with mutations in several genes, most commonly the receptor tyrosine kinase gene *RET*. Mutations in *RET* occur in multiple endocrine neoplasia syndrome types 2A and 2B, and familial medullary thyroid carcinoma; a family history must therefore be taken and genetic counselling offered to affected families.[45] There is also an increased risk of Hirschsprung's disease in children with trisomy 21 (Down's syndrome).

Hirschsprung's disease should be suspected in all infants who have not passed meconium within 48 h of birth and infants presenting with signs of distal bowel obstruction, notably constipation and abdominal distension. Children may also present acutely with vomiting, loose stools and cardiovascular collapse due to Hirschsprung's enterocolitis. A minority of children will present later in life with chronic constipation. Plain abdominal X-rays will show distended loops of bowel, although in neonates it is often impossible to distinguish large from small bowel obstruction.

In neonates, the diagnosis is confirmed by suction rectal biopsy of the submucosal plexus on the ward, using custom-made biopsy forceps. Histopathological examination will reveal absence of ganglion cells, thickened nerve trunks extending into the lamina propria, and increased acetylcholinesterase staining. In the older child a full-thickness biopsy that includes the myenteric plexus is obtained under general anaesthetic. A contrast enema is useful for determining the extent of aganglionosis if the transitional zone is seen (Fig. 40.13); however, false positives can occur and a contrast enema alone is not diagnostic. Anorectal manometry can be diagnostic in older children on the basis of an absent rectoanal inhibitory reflex, but this cannot be performed reliably in neonates.

Initial management includes intravenous fluids and nasogastric drainage. When the abdomen is very distended, gentle anal dilatation and rectal washouts with 0.9% saline solution often result in dramatic decompression and improvement in the physical condition of the infant. The principles of definitive surgical reconstruction are excision of the aganglionic colon and 'pull through' of ganglionic colon with a coloanal anastomosis. Traditionally, a colostomy is made at the distal limit of ganglionic

REFERENCES

45. Decker RA, Peacock ML. J Pediatr Surg 1998; 33: 207–214

bowel followed by the definitive pull-through procedure at 3–9 months of age. Frozen section biopsies are used to confirm the presence of ganglion cells at the level of resection. Increasingly, infants are being managed by rectal washouts alone until the definitive procedure within the first few weeks of life. Initial data suggest little difference in outcome from either approach.[46] Advances have been laparoscopic assisted or a purely transanal approach.[47]

Earlier outcome studies of surgery for Hirschsprung's disease reported excellent continence. However, subsequent more objective studies have not confirmed this. Impaired continence has been reported in up to 75% of children compared with age-matched peers; 10% required a permanent colostomy and a further 10% were severely incontinent.[48,49] The reasons for these poor results are multifactorial; incomplete excision of the aganglionic segment, internal sphincter dysfunction, external sphincter damage, and dysmotility of the apparently normal ganglionic bowel may all play a role and children need careful follow-up into adulthood.

Hirschsprung's enterocolitis, characterized by malaise, pyrexia, abdominal distension, constipation or severe diarrhoea, is a potentially life-threatening complication that can occur before or following surgery. The pathological basis of Hirschsprung's enterocolitis is poorly understood, but causal factors include relative gut stasis, alterations of bacterial flora, and impaired mucosal or neuronal immunity. Treatment is empirical, consisting of rectal washouts, systemic antibiotics (vancomycin and metronidazole), probiotics and sodium cromoglycate. Urgent colostomy may be necessary. Chemical (botulinum toxin) or surgical internal sphincterotomy may be of benefit.

Meconium plug syndrome

Occasionally when a rectal examination or contrast enema is performed in neonates with symptoms suggestive of Hirschsprung's disease, a grey 'plug' of epithelial cells is passed, followed by meconium and flatus, with relief of symptoms. This is the meconium plug syndrome and is common in premature infants, possibly due to relative immaturity of their ganglion cell development. Cystic fibrosis and Hirschsprung's disease must be positively excluded in children with meconium plug syndrome.

RECTAL BLEEDING IN THE NEWBORN INFANT

In the neonate, coffee ground vomitus may result from maternal blood swallowed during delivery. Ingested red dyes or pigments in food, drink or food (e.g. beetroot) may give the appearance of blood in the stool.

Fissure in ano

Fissure in ano is a common cause of rectal bleeding in the newborn infant, usually following the passage of a large, but not necessarily hard, stool. The fissure is seen on gently everting the anus. In most infants no treatment is required (see p. 917).

Necrotizing enterocolitis

Necrotizing enterocolitis almost exclusively affects premature infants. Typically there is patchy progressive ischaemic necrosis of the intestine. Predisposing factors include low birth weight, congenital heart disease, sepsis and umbilical vein catheterization. Necrotizing enterocolitis presents with the passage of blood per rectum and refusal to feed. As the disease progresses, bilious vomiting, abdominal distension and signs of generalized sepsis develop. Pneumatosis intestinalis (Fig. 40.14) and portal venous gas are diagnostic radiological features. Pneumoperitoneum indicates advanced disease with intestinal perforation.

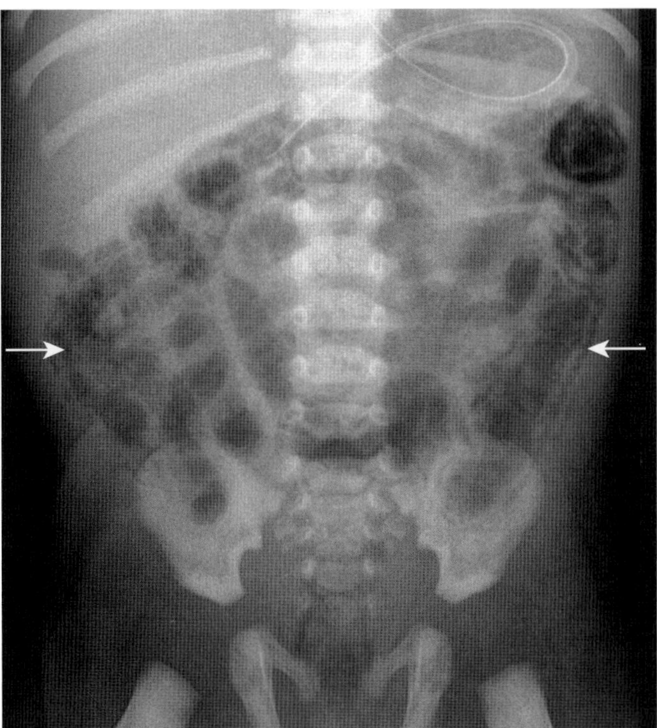

Figure 40.14 Necrotizing enterocolitis: there is intramural gas in the colon (arrows).

In the early phase of the disease, most infants will respond to withholding feeds, parenteral nutrition and broad-spectrum intravenous antibiotics. Operation is indicated for complications, notably perforation and gangrene. Percutaneous peritoneal drainage is a useful adjunct to resuscitating the low birth weight infant with perforation;[50] subsequent surgical options include resection of non-viable bowel with stoma formation or primary anastomosis. The indications for operation and the choice of intervention remain controversial.

INGUINOSCROTAL AND GENITAL CONDITIONS IN THE NEWBORN INFANT

Congenital hernia and hydrocele

Congenital inguinal hernia and hydrocele are common abnormalities of childhood, with a peak incidence in the neonatal period. They result from persistent patency of the processus vaginalis, an extension of the peritoneal cavity that passes through the inguinal canal within the spermatic cord in boys and along the round ligament in girls. Normally the processus vaginalis begins to obliterate once testicular descent is complete;

REFERENCES

46. Teitelbaum DH, Cilley RE, Sherman NJ et al. Ann Surg 2000; 232: 372–380
47. Georgeson KE, Cohen RD, Hebra A et al. Ann Surg 1999; 229: 678–682
48. Ludman L, Spitz L, Tsuji H et al. Arch Dis Child 2002; 86: 348–351
49. Baillie C, Kenny S, Williams J et al. J Pediatr Surg 1999; 34: 325–330
50. Demestre X, Ginovart G, Figueras-Aloy J et al. J Pediatr Surg 2002; 37: 1534–1539

it follows that obliteration does not occur when the testis is undescended. It is essential to distinguish between a congenital hernia and hydrocele because the natural history and management of each is radically different in the newborn period.

Congenital inguinal hernia

Congenital inguinal hernia is the presence of an abdominal viscus in the processus vaginalis (hernia sac), usually small intestine but occasionally an ovary, which presents as a firm mobile inguinal mass often confused with a lymph node. Spontaneous resolution does not occur, and because of the high risk of incarceration (10–28%) during the first 3 months of life,[51] and hence strangulation, prompt operation is advised, if possible within a week of diagnosis, provided that the infant is well enough for general anaesthesia. The infant with an incarcerated hernia is admitted to hospital and sedated; if the hernia can be gently reduced, it is repaired after an interval of 2 days to allow the tissue oedema to resolve. If easy reduction is not possible, immediate operation is required through an inguinal or preperitoneal approach.[52] When strangulation has occurred, the infant is ill and shows features of intestinal obstruction. Urgent resuscitation is followed by emergency repair of the hernia, potentially an extremely difficult operation. Compression of the spermatic cord by a strangulated hernia may result in testicular ischaemia and atrophy.

Congenital hydrocele

Congenital hydrocele is associated with a narrow processus vaginalis that becomes distended distally by accumulation of peritoneal fluid. Most hydroceles will spontaneously resolve in the first 6 months of life, and because there is no risk of incarceration, treatment is expectant. After 2 years of age a hydrocele is not likely to close spontaneously and operative closure of the processus vaginalis is advised.

Testicular torsion

Torsion of the testis in the newborn infant occurs pre- or postnatally and presents with a firm, purple, indurated and often tender swelling in the scrotum or groin. It is commonly extravaginal but may be intravaginal. The diagnosis is clinical. In the groin, torsion must be distinguished from a strangulated inguinal hernia, which will be associated with evidence of intestinal obstruction. Although salvage of the testis is rare in the neonate, operation is recommended to remove the infarcted testis to avoid the risk of infection, and for fixation of the contralateral testis.

INFANTS AND CHILDREN

VOMITING IN INFANCY

Hypertrophic pyloric stenosis

Hypertrophic pyloric stenosis is the commonest condition requiring operation in the first 2 months of life. The incidence is approximately three per 100 000 births and is four times higher in boys than in girls.

The underlying mechanism for hypertrophic pyloric stenosis is spasm of the pyloric muscle, which progresses to hypertrophy and evolution of the obstructive pyloric mass. Relaxation of the pyloric muscle appears to be dependent on inhibitory innervation through the non-adrenergic, non-cholinergic neural system, mediators of which have been shown to be reduced or absent, notably certain neuropeptides and nitric oxide.[53] Other neural components have also been shown to be abnormal, including the interstitial cells of Cajal,[54] neurotrophins, synapse formation and neural supporting cells. An increase in extracellular matrix proteins associated with increased collagen deposition in the intermuscular septum has also been demonstrated, but whether these are cause or effect is not clear.[55] None of these findings explain the transient nature of hypertrophic pyloric stenosis.

The aetiology of pyloric stenosis is not known, but a higher incidence in infants with a family history of hypertrophic pyloric stenosis and a lower incidence among Asian ethnic groups point to a genetic predisposition. Hypertrophic pyloric stenosis is characterized by elongation and narrowing of the pyloric lumen; secondary gastritis and mucosal oedema result in virtually complete obstruction.

Typically, infants are well for the first 2–3 weeks of life. Non-bilious vomiting begins intermittently after feeds, progressively increasing in frequency and volume, often projectile, leading to dehydration, weight loss and constipation. The vomitus may contain altered blood from secondary oesophagitis or gastritis. On examination, peristaltic waves may be seen traversing the epigastrium from left to right. Palpation of the pyloric tumour is diagnostic. Examination must be done with the stomach empty and the infant relaxed. This is achieved by aspirating the stomach through a nasogastric tube; the hungry infant is relaxed by allowing it to drink an electrolyte solution while the abdomen is palpated above and to the right of the umbilicus, the fingers probing under the liver. If the clinical findings are inconclusive, the diagnosis may be confirmed by ultrasonography (Fig. 40.15) or contrast meal.

Preoperative correction of fluid, electrolyte and acid–base abnormalities, typically hypochloraemic alkalosis, is essential. A nasogastric tube is passed to empty the stomach and for saline irrigations to alleviate the gastritis by removing residual feeds. Intravenous fluids are given as 0.45% saline with 10% dextrose and potassium chloride 20 mmol/L. Nasogastric aspirates are replaced with equal volumes of normal saline. Because of the risks of postoperative apnoea and cardiac arrhythmia, operation should not be undertaken until the serum electrolyte and blood gas levels have returned to normal.

Ramstedt's pyloromyotomy, introduced in 1912, remains the treatment of choice. The pylorus is approached through a transverse right upper quadrant or a periumbilical incision.[56] An incision across the pyloric tumour is deepened by blunt dissection to expose the mucosa. The incision must be extended proximally on to the gastric antrum and distally to a point just proximal to the pyloric vein. Accidental perforation of the duodenal mucosa must be excluded by inspecting the incision for air bubbles while the anaesthetist distends the stomach with air. If present, simple transverse closure of the perforation with interrupted absorbable

REFERENCES

51. Rescorla FJ, Grosfeld JL. J Pediatr Surg 1984; 19: 832–837
52. Turnock RR, Jones MO, Lloyd DA. Br J Surg 1994; 81: 251
53. Kusafuka T, Puri P. Pediatr Surg Int 1997; 12: 576–579
54. Vanderwinden JM, Liu H, De Laet MH et al. Gastroenterology 1996; 111: 279–288
55. Ohshiro K, Puri P. Pediatr Surg Int 1998; 13: 243–252
56. Tan KC, Bianchi A. Br J Surg 1986; 73: 399

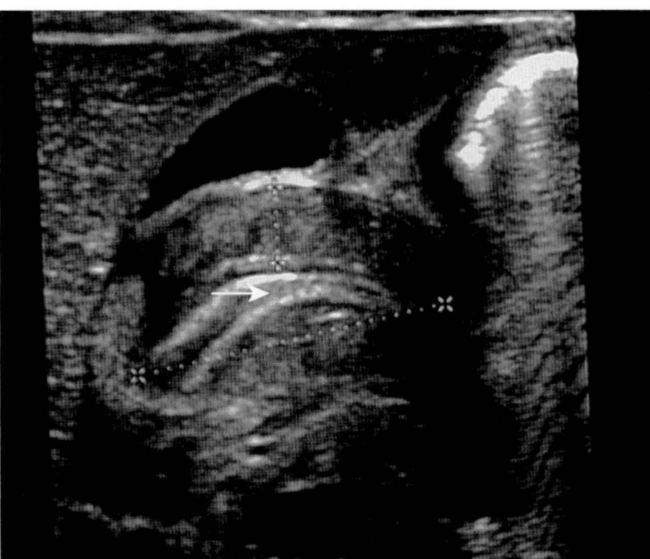

Figure 40.15 Pyloric stenosis: the ultrasound scan shows the elongated thickened pyloric muscle and narrow lumen (arrow). (Reproduced with permission from Lloyd DA, Kenny SE. The Surgical Abdomen. In: Walker WA et al (eds) Pediatric Gastrointestinal Disease. BC Decker Inc. 2004; 742.)

sutures and an omental patch will suffice. Laparoscopic pyloromyotomy is an established option.[57]

Postoperatively, oral feeds are given on demand, beginning with a small volume, and increased progressively as tolerated. Most infants can be discharged 24–48 h after operation. Postoperative complications include wound infection and dehiscence. Persistent vomiting after operation is usually due to persistent gastritis and rarely to unrecognized duodenal perforation or inadequate pyloromyotomy.

Gastro-oesophageal reflux

Most newborn infants have gastro-oesphageal reflux to a lesser or greater degree, and in most this will resolve spontaneously within weeks or months. In a few infants the frequency and volume of reflux episodes becomes clinically significant. Such infants typically present with non-bilious vomiting after feeds, which may at times be projectile. Infants may present with complications of gastroesophageal reflux, notably failure to thrive, recurrent aspiration pneumonitis, apnoeic episodes and near-miss sudden infant death syndrome. Stridor due to reflex laryngobronchospasm, and dysphagia or haematemesis are associated with reflux oesophagitis. Infants with central neurological impairment or who have had repair of oesophageal atresia are particularly susceptible to gastroesophageal reflux.

Investigations include an upper gastrointestinal contrast study to exclude gastroduodenal obstruction. The diagnosis is confirmed and quantified by oesophagogastroscopy and oesophageal pH monitoring. The condition of most infants is successfully managed medically, paying attention to posture (currently a supine position is recommended, with the head elevated unless there is a risk of sudden infant death syndrome) and feeding (small, frequent, thickened feeds) supported by antacids and prokinetic agents, depending on the severity of reflux. Fundoplication is indicated for intractable reflux not responsive to medical therapy.

Table 40.6 Causes of abdominal pain in childhood

Common Causes:
- Gastroenteritis
- Appendicitis
- Urinary Tract Infection
- Constipation
- Mesenteric adenitis
- Ovulatory/perimenstrual pain
- Non-specific abdominal pain (NSAP)

Serious causes:
- Intussusception
- Malrotation
- Bacterial enterocolitis
- Ovarian/testicular torsion
- Pancreatitis
- Intestinal obstruction (adhesion/volvulus/strangulated hernia)

THE CHILD WITH ABDOMINAL PAIN

Successful evaluation of the child with abdominal pain requires good interaction between the surgeon, child and parents. Patience is needed to gain the confidence of the child. No diagnostic information can be gleaned from abdominal examination of a crying child who is not relaxed. Common and serious causes of abdominal pain in children are listed in Table 40.6. The clinical skills required to differentiate between them should not be underestimated.

Appendicitis

Appendicitis can be difficult to diagnose in the very young and the neurologically impaired. Presentation is invariably late, and in most children under the age of 5 years perforation has occurred by the time of presentation and they may be very ill.[58] Abdominal signs may be subtle and true peritonism may be absent; abdominal distension is a common finding. Ultrasound and/or CT may provide useful diagnostic information in equivocal cases and save unnecessary operation. Management includes intravenous fluid resuscitation, adequate intravenous opiate analgesia, and intravenous antibiotics when necessary. The choice between open or laparoscopic appendicectomy in children usually depends on the training and experience of the surgeon. A recent systematic review concluded that laparoscopic appendicectomy was ‘likely to be beneficial’ when performed by an experienced laparoscopist.[59]

Urinary tract infection

Urinary tract infections are common in children, affecting 4% of boys and 12% of girls by the age of 16. Of children presenting with a first urinary tract infection, 4.5% have been shown to have renal scarring, regardless of age, sex or symptoms.[60] Ongoing reflux nephropathy can lead to hypertension or end-stage renal failure, and all children presenting with a urinary tract infection should be screened with renal tract ultrasound and technetium-

REFERENCES

57. Downey EC Jr. Semin Pediatr Surg 1998; 7: 220–224
58. Nance ML, Adamson WT, Hedrick HL. Pediatr Emerg Care 2000; 16: 160–162
59. Simpson J, Speake W. Clin Evid 2002; 7: 386–391
60. Coulthard MG, Lambert HJ, Keir MJ. Br Med J 1997; 315: 918–919

99m dimercaptosuccinic acid scans, regardless of age. The risk of renal scarring is greatest in the first 4 years of life.

Predisposing factors to renal scarring are infection in the presence of vesicoureteric reflux and intrarenal reflux within compound papillae.[61] The diagnosis of urinary tract infection is based on demonstration of bacteria on microscopy of a fresh urine specimen or pure culture of more than 10^7 bacteria per mL; the urine white cell count alone is not reliable. The gold standard test for determining the presence or absence of vesicoureteric reflux is a micturating cystourethrogram, but this requires catheterization. The optimal treatment of vesicoureteric reflux remains controversial; options include long-term antibiotic prophylaxis, endoscopic injection of a bulking agent at the ureterovesical junction (the subureteric Teflon® injection or STING procedure), or ureteric reimplantation. A randomized trial of medical versus reimplantation surgery failed to show a difference in the progression of renal scarring.[62] The role of the STING procedure, a minimally invasive procedure with a 70% success rate in abolishing vesicoureteric reflux, remains unclear.[63]

Intussusception

With intussusception, a segment of bowel telescopes into distal bowel, causing obstruction and compromising blood flow to the intussuscepted bowel segment. The peak incidence of intussusception is between 4 and 14 months, when most cases are idiopathic. Enlarged gut-associated lymphoid tissue (Peyer's patches) secondary to increased exposure to novel antigens ingested during weaning may play a role as a lead point. In older children, a pathological lead-point such as Meckel's diverticulum or small bowel lymphoma may be found.

Typically infants will experience colicky abdominal pain and bilious vomiting with bloody mucoid stools. Most morbidity and mortality from intussusception arise from delays in diagnosis, and a high index of suspicion should be maintained.[64] Between bouts of colic, infants are quiet but irritable, with evidence of hypovolaemia. A mobile sausage-shaped abdominal mass may be palpated. Some children present atypically with lethargy but no colic; mild abdominal tenderness and mucoid rectal blood may be the clue to the cause. The diagnosis can be confirmed by ultrasound scanning (Fig. 40.16). Vigorous fluid resuscitation with supplemental oxygen is often required. Treatment is by either pneumostatic or hydrostatic reduction through a rectal Foley catheter under controlled pressure conditions by an experienced radiologist, with ultrasound or X-ray screening. During the procedure children must be adequately resuscitated and monitored by staff trained in paediatric life support. Complications include intestinal perforation and tension pneumoperitoneum. In a minority of patients reduction is unsuccessful and open surgical reduction is then required. Enema reduction is contraindicated in children who are hypovolaemic or have signs of peritonitis. In advanced cases the necrotic intussusception will need to be resected.

Constipation

Childhood constipation, defined as the infrequent painful passage of stools, is extremely common in the West as a consequence of both diet and parental or societal attitudes to toileting. It can be difficult to determine the pathological basis of constipation in an infant or child, and good history taking is important. Although most cases are idiopathic, constipation may be a presenting feature of a range of disorders.

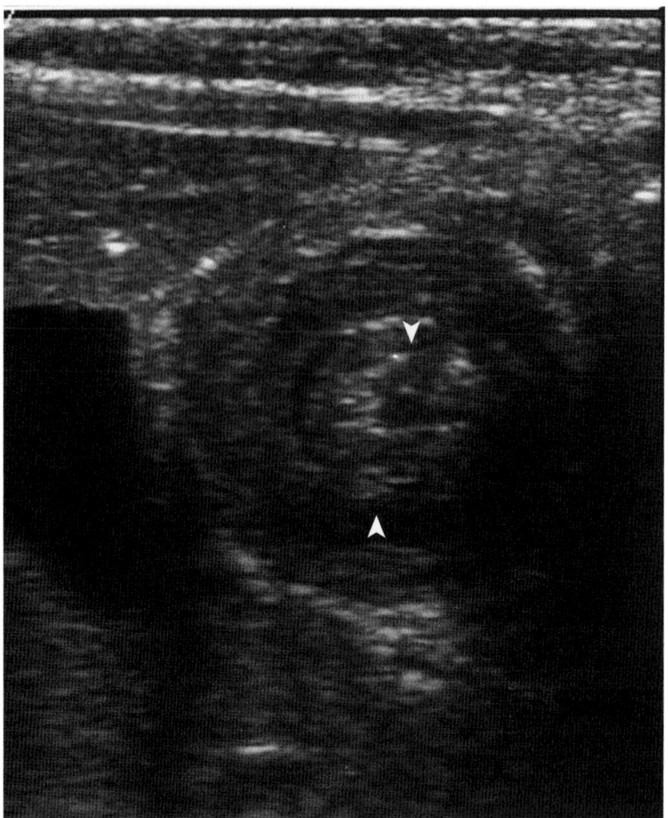

Figure 40.16 Intussusception: this ultrasound scan shows the intussuscepted bowel 'doughnut' sign (arrowheads). (Reproduced with permission from Lloyd DA, Kenny SE. The Surgical Abdomen. In: Walker WA et al (eds) Pediatric Gastrointestinal Disease. BC Decker Inc. 2004; 742.)

Examination should include evaluation for a pelvic mass, anorectal pathology and neurological deficit, including examination of the lumbar sacral spine. When constipation first develops after the first few months of life, the likelihood of Hirschsprung's disease and related congenital disorders is very low. Childhood constipation is characterized by avoidance of stooling and retention of faeces, which become increasingly firm and bulky, making defecation painful and provoking further retentive behaviour. Faecal soiling due to paradoxical overflow incontinence is common. Therapy should be centred on a clear explanation to the family of the nature of the problem and its management. Initial clearance of faecal loading, which may require enemas or manual evacuation, is followed by maintenance treatment including diet, toileting, and stimulant and osmotic laxatives. Cognitive psychotherapeutic approaches may provide short-term benefits.[65] The key to successful treatment of childhood constipation is a good relationship and clear communication between the clinician, child and the parents.

REFERENCES

61. Ransley PG, Risdon RA. Contrib Nephrol 1979; 16: 90–97
62. Smellie JM, Barratt TM, Chantler C et al. Lancet 2001; 357: 1329–1333
63. Chertin B, De Caluwe D, Puri P. J Urol 2003; 169: 1847–1849
64. Stringer MD, Pledger G, Drake DP. Br Med J 1992; 304: 737–739
65. Sunic-Omejc M, Mihanovic M, Bilic A et al. Coll Antropol 2002; 26 (Suppl): 93–101

GASTROINTESTINAL BLEEDING

Gastrointestinal bleeding is uncommon in childhood and emergency surgery is only occasionally indicated. It is essential to remember that children have a considerable physiological reserve in response to hypovolaemia. Increasing heart rate, prolonged capillary return, and widening core–periphery temperature differences are early signs of significant blood loss, and changes in blood pressure and conscious state are late indicators of hypovolaemic shock. Vascular access can be difficult in the child in hypovolaemic shock, and an intraosseous needle may be invaluable.

A good history will usually provide valuable clues as to the source of the bleeding, which may present as haematemesis, melaena, fresh rectal bleeding or anaemia. As in the neonate, confirmation of blood in the vomitus or stool is advisable using the Hemoccult® test or equivalent. A family history of clotting disorders or history of previous bleeding may raise suspicions of a congenital clotting disorder. Milk allergy may present with significant fresh rectal bleeding.[66] Physical examination may provide clues, such as stigmata of liver disease, the perioral pigmentation of Peutz–Jeghers disease, or generalized lymphadenopathy from lymphoma.

Haematemesis

The principal causes of haematemesis in children are listed in Table 40.7. Following appropriate resuscitation and haematological investigations, diagnostic upper gastrointestinal endoscopy should be performed by an experienced paediatric endoscopist.

Rectal bleeding

The appearance of the rectal blood will often suggest the origin of bleeding in proximal or distal bowel. Bloody mucus is characteristic of intussusception. The diverse causes of rectal bleeding are listed in Table 40.8. Investigations will depend on the likely pathology, and may include colonoscopy for suspected chronic inflammatory bowel disease or juvenile polyp, ultrasound scanning for suspected intussusception or intra-abdominal cyst, and isotopic scanning for Meckel's diverticulum.

Table 40.7 Causes of haematemesis

- Reflux peptic oesophagitis
- Oesophageal varices
- Acute gastric 'stress' ulcer
- Peptic ulcer
- Trauma
- Swallowed blood (e.g. following epistaxis)
- Gastritis

Table 40.8 Causes of rectal bleeding

- Infective gastroenteritis or colitis
- Anal fissure
- Intussusception
- Polyp
- Meckel's diverticulum
- Duplication cyst
- Inflammatory bowel disease
- Volvulus
- Milk allergy
- Vascular malformations

Fissure in ano

Fissure in ano is the commonest cause of rectal bleeding in childhood. A history of painful defecation associated with bright red rectal bleeding not mixed in with stool is highly suggestive. The fissure or a 'sentinel' skin tag can often be seen on gentle eversion of the anus. The goal of treatment is the painless passage of a soft stool. In most patients this can be achieved by attention to the diet, in particular the fibre content, and a combination of osmotic and stimulant laxatives. In practice, children often need to remain on such treatment for several months until they have 'unlearnt' the avoidance behaviour that leads to accumulation of bulky hard stools.

Meckel's diverticulum

A Meckel's diverticulum is an uncommon source of rectal bleeding, particularly during the first 2 years of life (see earlier).

HEPATOBILIARY DISORDERS

Biliary atresia

Transient physiological jaundice is common in newborn infants, in particular premature infants and infants small for their gestational age. The hyperbilirubinaemia peaks at 3–4 days and resolves in 7 days. Hyperbilirubinaemia persisting beyond the neonatal period may be due to hepatic disorders, including infections (notably the TORCH group: toxoplasmosis, rubella, cytomegalic virus and herpes); α_1-antitrypsin deficiency; or biliary obstruction due to extrahepatic biliary atresia. Diagnostic studies for biliary atresia include ultrasound and radionuclear scanning and liver biopsy. If biliary atresia is suspected, intraoperative cholangiography is followed by Roux-en-Y portoenterostomy (Kasai operation). Diagnosis is urgent because the best results are obtained when biliary drainage is established within 90 days of age, after which the inevitable cholestatic liver disease is so advanced that liver transplantation may be a better option.[67]

ABDOMINAL MASSES IN INFANCY AND CHILDHOOD

A faecal bolus is the most commonly palpated mass; typically the mass can be indented and there is a history of constipation. For other masses, ultrasound scanning will distinguish cystic from solid lesions and may identify the organ of origin. Subsequent investigations will depend on these findings. Important solid tumours are nephroblastoma, neuroblastoma and hepatoblastoma, while cystic masses include hydronephrosis and cysts arising in the ovary, kidney and liver. It is important that a solid tumour is assessed by a paediatric surgeon or oncologist before any operation is performed, including biopsy.

GENITAL CONDITIONS IN CHILDHOOD

Undescended testis

The testis migrates from the abdominal cavity during the third trimester, so it is not surprising that 30% of premature infants have undescended testes in comparison with 3% of full-term infants. Spontaneous descent of the testis may occur during the

REFERENCES

66. Willetts IE, Dalzell M, Puntis JW et al. J Pediatr Surg 1999; 34: 1486–1488
67. McKiernan PJ, Baker AJ, Kelly DA. Lancet 2000; 355: 25–29

first year of life, but more than 2% of boys have undescended testes after 1 year.

Careful history taking and examination allows discrimination between retractile testes, undescended testes and ectopic testes. Retractile testes are a normal variant and often there is a history of the testis having been felt in the scrotum. A brisk cremasteric reflex is common in young boys, so that local stimulation or stress may result in the testes being retracted into the groin. A quiet, warm environment and calm manner are necessary to demonstrate retractile testes. Examination requires the use of both hands; one hand palpates the testis and manipulates it from the inguinal region into the lower scrotum, where it is received into the other hand. The testis should remain in this location without traction. No treatment is required and in most cases the testes will have descended permanently by puberty.

In contrast, the testis that cannot be manipulated into the scrotum is classed as undescended, either ectopic if the testis is palpable outside the line of normal descent (e.g. lateral to the external ring or in the perineum, thigh or femoral region), or incompletely descended if in the normal line of descent. In 20% of patients the testis is impalpable due to an intracanalicular or abdominal location, or because it is atrophic or absent. Orchidopexy is advised for undescended testes during the second year of life to prevent deterioration of the spermatogenetic capacity of the testis.[68] In addition, orchidopexy reduces the risk of trauma and torsion, and allows surveillance for testicular tumour. The testicular malignancy rate of males following orchidopexy for intra-abdominal testes may be up to five times greater than the background male population.[69] A testicular germ cell tumour susceptibility gene that also predisposes to undescended testis has been located on chromosome Xq27.[70] The inguinal approach is favoured for palpable undescended testes, and a laparoscopic or open two-staged approach is generally advocated for boys with impalpable testes.

Circumcision

A common parental concern is that their son's foreskin is non-retractile; this is due to misconceptions as to the natural history of the foreskin. Although the foreskin is developed by 16 weeks' gestation, there is no plane of separation between foreskin and glans until late gestation. Separation of foreskin and glans is a slow and variable process, and only 30% of 5-year-old boys have a fully retractile foreskin.[71]

The only indication for circumcision is phimosis. High-dose topical steroid cream may be used to promote separation of foreskin and glans in cases of 'physiological' phimosis, and preputioplasty and division of the frenulum are useful options. Pathological causes of phimosis, notably balanitis xerotica obliterans and recurrent balanoposthitis, are rare under the age of 5 years and thus the medical indications for circumcision of boys under the age of 5 are rare. Potentially serious complications of circumcision include bleeding, infection and injury to the glans or urethra. There are ethical issues surrounding a procedure of dubious medical efficacy where the child is often unable to give his assent.

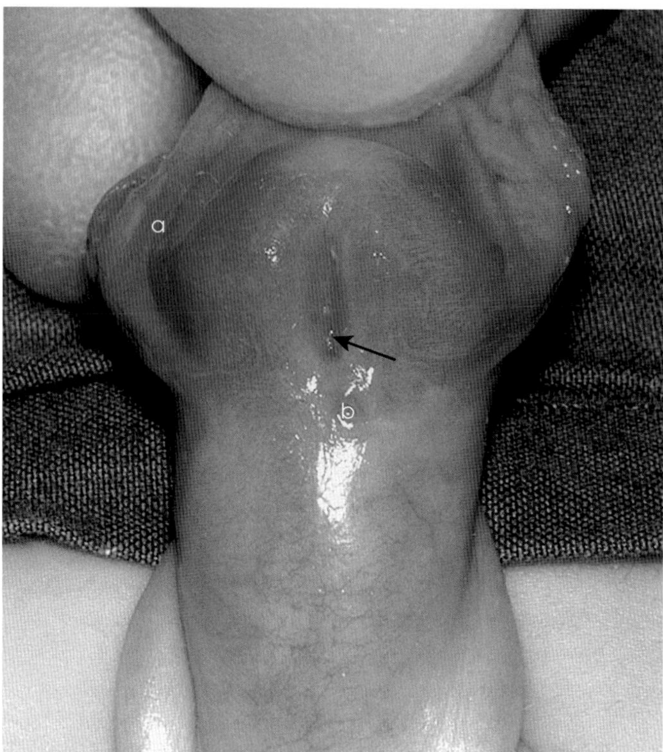

Figure 40.17 Hypospadias: **(a)** the arrow indicates the urethral opening on the penile shaft; **(b)** ventral deficiency of the foreskin gives a 'hooded' appearance to the foreskin.

Hypospadias

The commonest congenital penile disorder, affecting one in 300 male infants, is hypospadias, an abnormally sited urethral meatus on the ventral surface of the penile shaft. The anomalies range from mild glandular hypospadias to perineal hypospadias (Fig. 40.17). Associated anomalies include a hooded foreskin and ventral curvature of the penis (chordee). In the newborn infant with severe forms of hypospadias, careful assessment is required before gender assignment because such appearances can occur in virilized females in association with congenital adrenal hyperplasia. In addition to the cosmetic appearance, functional problems may occur, with downward misdirection of the urinary stream and with penetrative sexual intercourse. Operation to correct all these abnormalities is usually performed before the boy is out of nappies, and may be a one- or two-stage procedure depending on the nature of the hypospadias.

REFERENCES

68. Leissner J, Filipas D, Wolf HK et al. BJU Int 1999; 83: 885–891
69. Stang A, Ahrens W, Bromen K et al. Int J Epidemiol 2001; 30: 1050–1056
70. Rapley EA, Crockford GP, Teare D et al. Nat Genet 2000; 24: 197–200
71. Gairdner D. Br Med J 1949; 2: 1433–1437

Orthopaedic pathology

41

Ann Sandison

INTRODUCTION

This chapter describes non-neoplastic disorders of bones and joints commonly encountered in orthopaedic practice and includes the histological features.

The pathology of the musculoskeletal system comprises diseases of bone and joints, including associated soft tissues such as tendon ligament, nerve and skeletal muscle.

Bones are not inert: they are dynamic structures. Like other organs they can respond to systemic changes, they can become infected, and they will die if deprived of their blood supply. They atrophy with disuse and they can repair themselves. Diseases of bone may be categorized into one of seven major categories common to all diseases: congenital, metabolic, traumatic, circulatory, neoplastic, infectious and change due to systemic disease. Congenital disorders, neoplasms and trauma are dealt with elsewhere in this book.

Disease of the joints or 'arthritis' may be generally divided into two main categories: degenerative (or non-inflammatory) and inflammatory. In degenerative or non-inflammatory disease, the pathological changes begin at the articular surface. In inflammatory disease the pathological changes begin in the synovial membrane. The articular or hyaline cartilage is relatively avascular, and degenerative changes in this tissue are thought to be brought about by mechanical pressures, wear and tear, rather than being mediated by inflammation. Changes in the synovium in degenerative joint disease are secondary and represent a non-specific inflammatory response to the articular changes. In contrast, in inflammatory arthropathy the highly vascular synovium responds to damage by becoming intensely inflamed; the articular changes are directly related to the inflammation and are not, therefore, essentially degenerative.

JOINTS

ARTHRITIDES

NON-INFLAMMATORY JOINT DISEASE

Osteoarthritis (synonyms include degenerative joint disease and, less commonly, hypertrophic arthritis and osteoarthrosis) is characterized by focal degeneration of articular cartilage and secondary changes in the subchondral bone. The bone changes include cyst formation, and new bone formation with sclerosis of subchondral bone and the development of osteophytes at the joint margins. Multiple joints may be affected, the main sites being vertebrae, hips and knees. Pain and joint stiffness are the principle symptoms, and the radiological findings may not correlate with the severity of the symptoms. The disease may be primary, usually associated with elderly patients, or secondary, occurring at any age and related to a previously damaged or congenitally abnormal joint.

Primary osteoarthritis

Primary disease (Figs 41.1–41.3) may be subdivided into:

- localized osteoarthritis, i.e. Heberden's nodes, marginal bony exostoses on the dorsal aspect at the base of the terminal phalanges, with no other joint involvement;
- generalized osteoarthritis, with three or more joints or joint groups involved; and
- erosive osteoarthritis, sometimes called inflammatory osteoarthritis, which may represent end-stage disease and may overlap with rheumatoid arthritis.[1]

Incidence

Osteoarthritis is the most common joint disease and affects elderly people of all racial and ethnic groups. It is rare in people younger than 40 years and common over the age of 60 years. Overall, women are affected more often than men, but between the ages of 40–55 years and in osteoarthritis of the hip, the sex incidence appears to be equal. In women, particularly postmenopausal women, many if not all of the terminal interphalangeal joints may be affected. Heberden's nodes are 10 times more common in women than in men.

Pathogenesis

The forces exerted on a joint during motion or weight bearing are dispersed between cartilage, subchondral bone, and surrounding joint capsule and muscle. Hyaline articular cartilage has the unique properties of compressibility and elasticity. It is composed of a three-dimensional network of cross-linked type II collagen fibres with aggregates of proteoglycan molecules attached as side chains. The proteoglycan molecules can bind a large amount of water, which is lost when the cartilage is compressed and recaptured when the pressure is released. This gives cartilage the ability to undergo reversible deformations.

The joint constituents of bone, cartilage and synovium are variably affected in primary osteoarthritis. The aetiology is uncertain and likely to be multifactorial. Two main theories about the mechanism of the disease process exist. The first is that a defect in cartilage matrix leads to premature failure. The other theory is that the primary defect is in the subchondral bone and the cartilage failure is secondary. It is postulated that changes in the shape or hardness of subchondral bone may subject the

REFERENCE

1. Pincus T. Curr Rheumatol Rep 2001; 3: 524–534

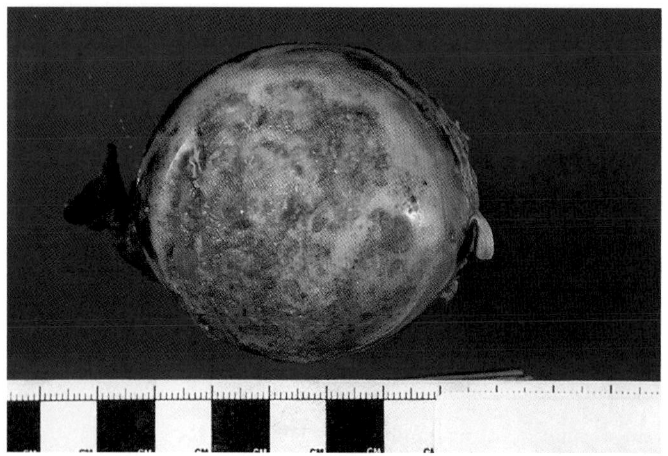

Figure 41.1 Macroscopic picture of a femoral head with erosion of surface cartilage exposing underlying subchondral bone.

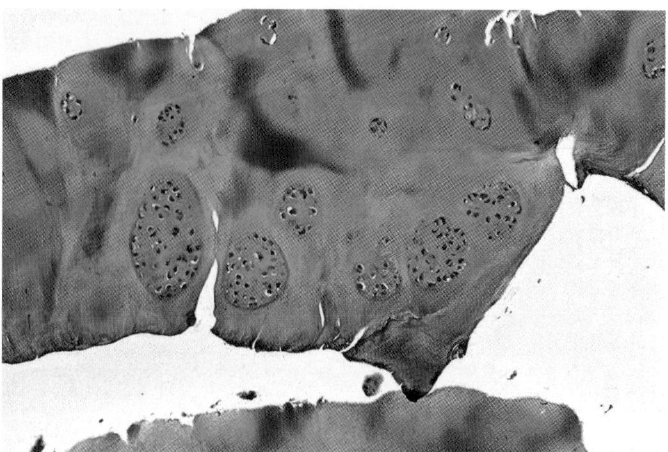

Figure 41.3 Low-power view of saffronin-stained cartilage, showing fissuring of the surface and regenerating chondrocytes growing in small clones.

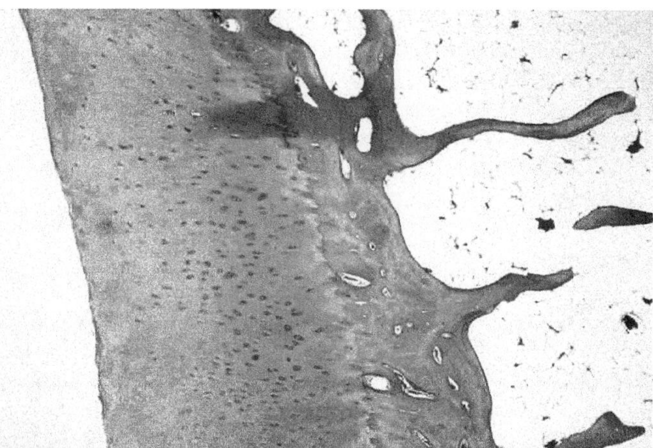

Figure 41.2 Low-power haematoxylin and eosin–stained section, showing normal articular cartilage overlying subchondral bone and fatty marrow.

articular cartilage to abnormal biomechanical stresses and trauma, resulting in failure even with normal use. The following factors have been thought to play a role.

Ageing

There is a strong association of osteoarthritis with ageing, but senescent changes alone are not now believed to be causal. Many elderly people show radiological changes of joint space reduction and osteophyte formation but do not have clinical symptoms. Also, the ankle, a weight-bearing joint, is rarely involved, even in old age. The ability of cartilage to withstand fatigue testing diminishes with age in human cartilage, but the number of chondrocytes and their normal metabolism appear to be preserved. The ends of the bones change shape with ageing, partly due to constant remodelling, which may be non-uniform and result in subtle changes in the joint contour. Ageing bones contain less water and become harder and less compliant, which may contribute to trauma to the overlying articular cartilage.

Mechanical factors (overuse or wear and tear)

Occupational osteoarthritis, such as that seen in the metacarpophalangeal and shoulder joints of boxers and in the spines of miners, may result from accumulated episodes of microtrauma, which alter the quality of the subchondral bone and reduce the ability of the joint to withstand impulse loading. However, excessive use of the joints does not inevitably lead to osteoarthritis. Athletes and dancers for example, although they may develop traction spurs and soft tissue symptoms related to overuse, do not develop premature osteoarthritis. Soft tissue injuries in ligaments or tendons, such as occur commonly in athletes, are thought to alter the joint biomechanics and result in secondary osteoarthritis.

Genetic factors

Family studies have shown that hereditary factors are important in the development of Heberden's nodes. Collagen content of cartilage and the ability to synthesize prostaglandins has been shown to be genetically determined. A type II collagen gene mutation, substituting an arginine for a cysteine in type II procollagen chains, has been demonstrated in families with premature osteoarthritis. Similar body habitus and gait patterns are seen within multiple generations of families.[2] This may reflect the inheritance of a particular joint shape, which results in abnormal stresses on articular cartilage and the subsequent development of osteoarthritis in these families.

Biochemical factors

Early in the disease the cartilage shows reduced proteoglycans, which result in decreased elasticity and stiffness. Later the collagen breaks down and is lost due to increased matrix metalloproteinase activity.

Secondary osteoarthritis

In secondary osteoarthritis, cartilage damage may occur due to abnormal loading of cartilage, instability of joints, or direct chemical damage of the cartilage. Abnormal loading of the articular cartilage may occur, for instance, as a consequence of malunited fractures leading to distortion of the normal joint anatomy, leading to point loading. Instability of a joint leading to

REFERENCE

2. McCarthy EF, Frassica FJ (eds). Pathology of Bone and Joint Disorders with Clinical and Radiographic Correlation. WB Saunders, 1998

progressive disorganization of the joint and articular damage, and the development of a Charcot joint, may occur as a consequence of tubes dorsalis or syringomyelin. Direct chemical damage of articular cartilage occurs in alkaptonuria and crystal deposition disease.

Histology

The histopathological changes in degenerative joint disease include surface fibrillation and fissuring of articular cartilage, with subsequent erosion and loss of articular cartilage. Clones of regenerating chondrocytes appear adjacent to cracks in the cartilage matrix. The subchondral bone may crack or show reactive thickening or sclerosis due to deposition of new bone on subchondral trabeculae. In areas where the cartilage is completely eroded, the subchondral bone may appear polished due to contact with the opposing denuded joint surface. This process is known as eburnation, and the friction between two eburnated bones is painful. The marrow spaces between bony trabeculae contain reparative granulation tissue. Foci of myxomatous change in this granulation tissue coalesce to form subchondral cysts. Adjacent bone and cartilage may fragment and collapse into the cysts, and nests and islands of cartilage and fibrous tissue may be seen extending into the subchondral bone. Osteophytes form at the margins of the joint by enchondral ossification within the articular cartilage or by cartilage metaplasia in areas near capsule or ligament insertions. This is reflected in the radiographic changes that are seen with loss of joint space due to the loss of the articular catilage, subchondral cysts, sclerosis and osteophyte formation (Fig. 41.4).

NEUROPATHIC ARTHROPATHY

Neuropathic arthropathy is a chronic progressive degenerative disorder that develops as the result of a disturbance in the normal sensory (pain or proprioceptive) innervation of joints. Movement that is uninhibited by pain results in traumatic damage to the bones and joints, as well as other soft tissues. Diabetes mellitus, syphilis (tabes dorsalis) and syringomyelia are the most commonly associated clinical entities. Approximately 5–10% of patients with tabes dorsalis will develop neuroarthropathy or neuropathic fracture. The lower limbs are more often affected (75%), with the knee being involved in 50% of cases. The hip, shoulder, ankle and elbow comprise 35% of cases, and the vertebral column and foot account for most of the remainder. Commonly, one joint is affected and multiple joint involvement is often bilateral. Patients with syringomyelia show neuroarthropathy in 25–35% of cases.

Typical findings on imaging include joint destruction, disorganization and effusion with osseous debris. Other findings include resorption of the ends of tubular bones and neuropathic fracture. Clinically, the progression of destruction may appear more rapid in comparison with advanced osteoarthritis.

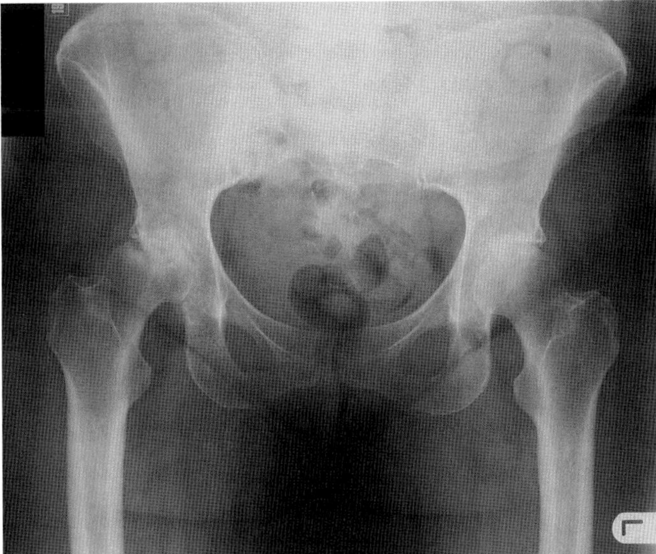

Figure 41.4 Anteroposterior X-ray of the pelvis, showing severe osteoarthritis of both hips with complete loss of joint space, subchondral cysts, sclerosis and osteophyte formation. (Sclerosis is derived from the Greek *sklerosis*, meaning 'harden'.)

ACUTE RHEUMATIC FEVER

Acute rheumatic fever follows a pharyngeal infection with group A streptococcal organisms. It is a systemic inflammatory disease characterized by an acute painful polyarthritis of large joints, and the heart, blood vessels, serous membranes and nervous system may be affected.

Pathogenesis

Tissue damage results from an abnormal, exaggerated, host immune response to the infecting organism because of cross-reactivity between streptococcal antigens and antibodies in host tissue. For example, antigens to the hyaluronic capsule of the streptococcus and streptococcal M proteins cross-react with cardiac tropomyosin and myosin. A genetic predisposition for the disease appears to exist, and family studies suggest the mode of transmission is autosomal recessive or autosomal dominant with incomplete penetrance. Some association with major histocompatibility alleles (HLA-DR4 and HLA-DR2) has been reported but this is controversial. In all the patients with rheumatic fever tested, B-lymphocytes have been shown to express a monoclonal immunohistochemical marker called D8/17.

The disease is rare in developed countries, but in poor socioeconomic areas may be as high as 60 in 100 000 children aged 5–14 years. The streptococcal throat infection usually precedes the onset of symptoms by 2–3 weeks. There may be fever that resolves quickly with non-steroidal anti-inflammatory drugs. Arthritis with fever occurs in 50–70% of patients presenting with acute rheumatic fever. Any joint may be affected, but usually the knees and the ankles. The arthritis occurs within 5 weeks of the throat infection, when antistreptococcal titres are high, and settles spontaneously, rarely causing joint deformity. Carditis occurs less frequently in cases with severe arthritis.

Arthralgia in the absence of clinical evidence of joint inflammation may precede synovitis, and migratory arthralgia may be an important clinical sign.

Histology

The histological finding associated with rheumatic fever is the Aschoff body, which is a specific type of granuloma formed in response to deposition of fibrinoid deposits of immunoglobulin in connective tissue. The granulomas are composed of fibroblasts, macrophages and multinucleate giant cells. The fibrinoid deposits in joint disease are found in collagen deep in the fibrous capsule.

The macroscopic and microscopic findings in the joints of patients with rheumatic fever are unimpressive. There is congestion and oedema of the synovium, with no abnormality of surface articular cartilage. There may be a mild effusion, which does not usually appear turbid but if analysed will show 7000–10 000 cells/mL. The cells are usually degenerate polymorphs and synoviocytes.

OCHRONOSIS

Ochronotic arthropathy is the musculoskeletal manifestation of alkaptonuria. This is an uncommon, inherited metabolic disorder associated with various clinical and radiological abnormalities resulting from the deposition of homogentisic acid pigment in connective tissues.[3] Homogentisic acid forms in the metabolism of phenylalanine and tyrosine, and accumulates in the absence of homogentisic acid oxidase. So-called alkapton bodies are deposited, particularly in the matrix of hyaline and fibrocartilage, and sometimes in other poorly vascularized connective tissue. Oxidation of the homogentisic acid results in the discolouration of the tissues, which may appear yellow, brown or black. The intervertebral discs may appear calcified on radiographs and the urine becomes dark with oxidation.

Histology

The cartilage surface is eroded, and black pigment is seen in chondrocytes and the intracellular matrix. Degenerate fragments of pigmented cartilage may be seen in association with granulation tissue and macrophages. The bone changes are less severe. Pigment is seen in the calcified matrix and in a few osteocytes. There may be degenerative changes in the osteocytes. Pigment is also seen in osteoclasts but not in osteoblasts. Black specks of ochronotic cartilage may be seen in synovial fluid, and cells containing pigment may be present. There may be calcium pyrophosphate crystal deposition in the synovial membrane.

INFLAMMATORY ARTHROPATHY

Rheumatoid arthritis

Rheumatoid arthritis (Figs 41.5–41.7) is a severe chronic relapsing synovitis, which follows an unpredictable course. There is a variable degree of extra-articular involvement. The disease causes joint damage within the first 2 years, with a significant loss of function by 5 years, and an estimated reduction in life expectancy of 5–7 years.

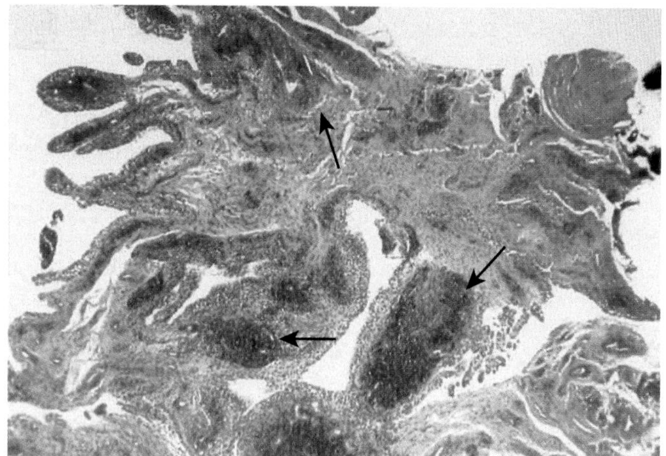

Figure 41.5 Synovium from a joint affected by rheumatoid arthritis. There is villous hyperplasia with a prominent lymphoid infiltrate.

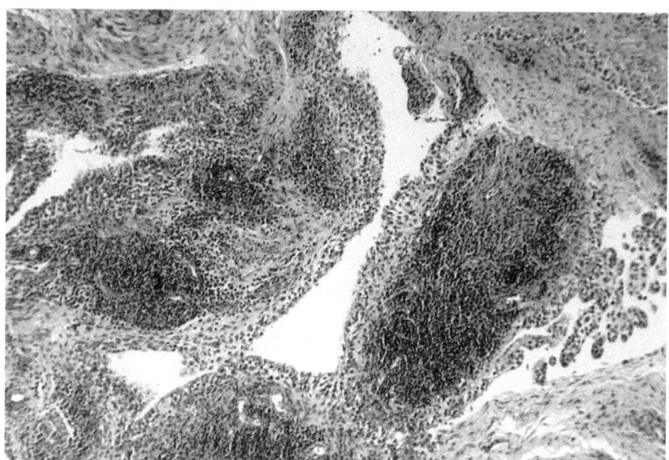

Figure 41.6 High-power view of synovium from a rheumatoid joint, showing lymphoid follicle formation in subsurface tissue.

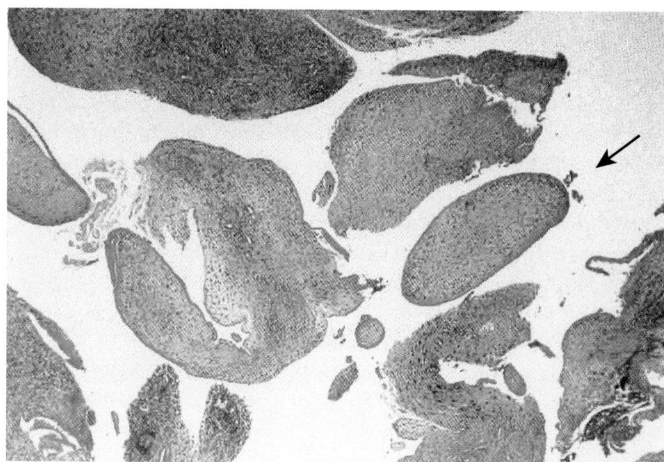

Figure 41.7 Low-power view of rheumatoid synovium, showing fibrinoid 'rice body' formation on the surface.

Incidence

Rheumatoid arthritis is the most common inflammatory arthropathy, affecting about 1% of the population of the world. Females are more commonly affected (ratio 3:1), and the age of onset is commonly between 40 and 60 years. However, about one-third of patients may present after the age of 60 years and the sex incidence approaches equal in the older age group. The disease is often symmetrical and affects small joints in the hands and feet, sparing distal interphalangeal joints. It may affect the larger joints: wrists, elbows, ankles and knees.

There appears to be a genetic predisposition for this disease. Family studies have shown an increased incidence among first-degree relatives, and a degree of concordance of 12% in monozygotic twins and 4% in dizygotic twins. The major histocompatibility complex (MHC) is a group of genes on the short arm of chromosome 6, which produce proteins that provide a system of demonstrating antigenic peptides to T lymphocytes. These proteins are called human lymphocyte antigen (HLA)

REFERENCE

3. Borman P, Bodur H, Ciliz D. Rheumatol Int 2002; 21: 205–209

class I and class II, and there are several subtypes. Rheumatoid arthritis has been associated with haplotypes HLA-DR4 and HLA-DR1. These MHC genes are associated with not only the initiation of the disease but also the course and severity. Patients without the HLA-DR4 gene are more likely to have a milder form of the disease.

Aetiology

No clear aetiology for this disease has been established. It is most likely autoimmune, and 80% of patients are serum rheumatoid factor-positive. Immune responses initially generated against an immunogen (e.g. an infectious agent) could be sustained by cross-reactivity in the host synovium and joint tissues. This would eventually result in a chronic destructive autoimmunity. Destruction of cartilage tissue results from the action of proteases produced in rheumatoid arthritis synovium, chondrocytes and pannus. Cytokines released by these tissues are thought to induce osteoclast resorption of bone.

Several infectious agents have been implicated and include parvoviruses B19 and Epstein–Barr virus, mycoplasma and bacteria, including streptococci. It has been postulated that antibodies could cross-react with type II collagen, proteoglycan, chondrocytes, heat shock proteins and immunoglobulins. The rheumatoid factor is mostly IgM and is an autoantibody against the Fc portion of an IgG molecule. Rheumatoid factor may form immunocomplexes with IgG. These circulating immune complexes may underlie associated extra-articular disease.[4–6]

Clinical presentation

Over half of patients present with a chronic symmetrical polyarthropathy, and 10–25% will report an acute onset. The disease may be monoarticular and episodic. Extra-articular manifestations such as subcutaneous nodules may be the presenting complaint. Four of seven disease criteria used by the American College of Rheumatology for the classification of rheumatoid arthritis (Box 41.1) should have been present for at least 6 weeks before a patient is diagnosed as having rheumatoid arthritis.

Constitutional symptoms, such as fatigue and general malaise, may be the first manifestation of the disease and the extra-articular symptoms, including sclerosis, serositis and vasculitis, may be prominent or even life-threatening. Rheumatoid nodules are seen in 20–30% of seropositive patients and occur over pressure points such as fingers and elbows. They can occur in Achilles tendon or scalp, usually associated with more severe disease. Pulmonary disease is common and effects include pleurisy, pleural effusion, parenchymal nodules, interstitial alveolitis, fibrosis, bronchiolitis obliterans and organizing pneumonia. Cardiac manifestations include inflammation of pericardium, myocardium and valves; nodule formation with arrhythmia; amyloidosis; and vasculitis. Other extra-articular manifestations include ocular keratoconjunctivitis sicca and peripheral neuropathy secondary to nerve entrapment or vasculitis. Sjögren's syndrome and Felty's syndrome (granulocytopenia, splenomegaly and rheumatoid arthritis) may occur in association with rheumatoid arthritis, often in patients with severe active disease.

Characteristic joint deformities include radial deviation of wrist, ulnar deviation of the metacarpophalangeal joints, 'swan neck' and boutonnière deformities of the fingers. Flexor tenosynovitis can result in carpal tunnel syndrome, 'triggering' of the fingers and eventually tendon rupture, usually of the extensor tendons.

Box 41.1 American College of Rheumatology clinical criteria for the classification of rheumatoid arthritis

- Morning stiffness or stiffness after rest lasting more than 1 h.
- Polyarthritis affecting at least three joints in 14 areas including right and left proximal interphalangeal joints, metacarpophalangeal joints, wrists, elbow, knees, ankles and metatarsophalangeal joints.
- Arthritis of hands, wrists, metacarpophalangeal or proximal interphalangeal joints, or symmetric arthritis.
- Simultaneous arthritis in both sides of the body.
- Subcutaneous rheumatoid nodules.
- RF positive (rheumatoid factor).
- Radiographic changes typical of rheumatoid arthritis in the hand, including bone erosions or periarticular osteoporosis.

Histology

Synovial biopsy will show a proliferative synovitis with thickening of synovial membrane. There is hyperplasia of surface synoviocytes, possibly with syncytia formation. An intense inflammatory cell infiltrate of plasma cells and lymphocytes with or without lymphoid follicles is characteristically present in the subsurface layer. There may be fibrin deposition and necrosis. These features are not specific to rheumatoid arthritis and may be seen in association with other types of inflammatory arthropathy, such as psoriatic arthropathy or Reiter's syndrome. Pannus, which is a mass of exuberant inflamed synovium covering the articular surface and eroding joint tissues, is characteristic of rheumatoid arthritis.

Juvenile rheumatoid arthritis

Juvenile rheumatoid arthritis, also known as juvenile chronic arthritis, comprises three main disease groups differentiated according to the onset of the illness, pattern of symptoms and disease progression. These are systemic (20%), polyarticular (50%), and pauciarticular or oligoarticular (30%). The diagnostic criteria for the classification of juvenile rheumatoid arthritis according to the American College of Rheumatology guidelines are given in Box 41.2.

Incidence

The exact frequency of the disease is difficult to determine because the pauciarticular disease may be unrecognized or undiagnosed. There is no geographic or racial predilection. About six in 10 000 children per year are thought to be affected in the UK. Unlike adult rheumatoid arthritis, juvenile rheumatoid arthritis is characterized by involvement of the large joints, particularly those of the lower extremities. Amyloidosis may complicate the disease in 4–6% of patients, mainly those with systemic disease, and this is a relatively frequent cause of death. The overall mortality rate is 10%.

REFERENCES

4. Firestein GS. Nature 2003; 423: 356–361
5. Yamanishi Y, Firestein GS. Rheum Dis Clin North Am 2001; 27: 355–371
6. Golding SR. J Rheumatol Suppl 2002; 65: 44–48

Box 41.2 American College of Rheumatology criteria for the classification of juvenile rheumatoid arthritis (revised in 1989)

- Age of onset less than 16 years.
- Arthritis in one or more joints (defined as swelling or effusion, or a combination of two or more of the following: pain on movement of the joint, limitation of movement or increased heat in the joint).
- Disease duration greater than 6 weeks.
- Pattern of disease in the first 6 months: systemic (arthritis with intermittent fever), polyarticular (five or more joints involved), or pauciarticular (four or less joints involved).
- Exclusion of other forms of juvenile arthritis.

Clinical features

Systemic juvenile rheumatoid arthritis affects 20% of patients and starts in early childhood. It is characterized by fever, exanthema, hepatosplenomegaly, polyserositis and leukocytosis. Joint involvement is said to be 60% polyarticular, associated with more severe joint destruction, and 40% oligoarticular. Large and small joints may be affected symmetrically.

Patients with polyarticular juvenile rheumatoid arthritis may be seropositive (10% of all patients) or seronegative (25% all patients). Girls are predominantly affected. There may be mild generalized symptoms. The joints affected are similar to those seen in adult-onset rheumatoid arthritis and include large joints of the upper and lower extremities. The distal interphalangeal joints seem to be spared in seropositive disease but may be involved in seronegative disease. Rheumatoid factor can be demonstrated in the serum of all seropositive patients, and there is an association with HLA-DR4. Disease progression and joint destruction is more severe in seropositive patients.

The oligoarticular type of juvenile rheumatoid arthritis is rarely associated with generalized symptoms, but 50% of patients may develop iridocyclitis and there is a risk of defective healing and blindness. Two subtypes in this disease category have been described: type I, associated with HLA-DR5 and HLA-DR8 and affecting predominantly girls, and type II, associated with HLA-B27 and affecting mainly boys. In type I disease, joint involvement is asymmetric and usually limited to one large joint, commonly the knee. Type II disease affects both large and small joints asymmetrically, and progressive involvement of both sacroiliac joints over time is pathognomic. The clinical picture may develop into that of alkylosing spondylitis.

Pathology

The appearance of the synovium in adult rheumatoid arthritis and juvenile rheumatoid arthritis is similar. However, the hyperplasia is less in juvenile rheumatoid arthritis and the surface proliferation of synoviocytes is usually seen only in seropositive polyarticular disease. Rheumatoid nodules in skin occur commonly in children with seropositive disease, in 20% of patients with seronegative systemic disease, and in 10% of other patients with seronegative disease. These are histologically indistinguishable from those seen in adult-onset disease.

Relapsing polychondritis

Relapsing polychondritis is a rare autoimmune disease characterized by recurrent inflammation of cartilage, predominantly elastic cartilage of ear, nose and larynx but hyaline cartilage of joints may also be involved. There may be ocular manifestations. The most common presentation is with inflammation of the cartilaginous portion of the ears with sparing of the ear lobes.

Incidence

The disease is most commonly seen in middle-aged adults and affects both sexes equally. There is an association with HLA-DR4, and up to one-third of patients suffer from other autoimmune disorders. There is an overlap with Behçet's disease in patients with mouth and genital ulcers with inflamed cartilage (MAGIC) syndrome.

Clinical presentation

Three of the following symptoms are required for the diagnosis of relapsing polychondritis: bilateral auricular chondritis, non-erosive seronegative polyarthritis, nasal chondritis, audio-vestibular damage and ocular inflammation.

The disease affects only one ear in any given episode. Destruction of auricular cartilage can occur with repeated episodes and result in fibrosis and 'cauliflower ear'. If the inner ear is affected nausea, tinnitus and sensorineural deafness may occur. Nasal cartilage involvement results in rhinitis with inflammatory crusting and bleeding. The saddle nose deformity may occur in long-standing disease. Inflammation of tracheo-bronchial cartilage may cause hoarseness, coughing and dyspnoea. Laryngeal or bronchial cartilage collapse may require insertion of a stent or positive-pressure respiratory support. Examination of the eyes may show conjunctivitis, keratitis, episcleritis or iritis. Migratory arthritis affecting one or more large or small joints is often present. There may be skin lesions associated with leukocytoclastic vasculitis, and aortic aneurysm can occur. Medications include colchicine, indomethacin and dapsone. Systemic glucocorticoids may be indicated in severe cases, and cyclosporine and methotrexate may be used as steroid-sparing agents. The disease follows a chronic relapsing course with a variable outcome. Symptoms may resolve in a few weeks but typically recur after a few weeks or months. There is a 30% mortality rate, and death is usually due to respiratory collapse or cardiovascular involvement.

Aetiology

In 50% of patients, IgG antibodies to type II collagen can be detected either in serum or bound to cartilage. The titres correspond to disease activity. The antibodies may cross the placenta, resulting in neonatal chondritis.

SYSTEMIC LUPUS ERYTHEMATOSIS

Systemic lupus erythematosis is a broad-spectrum systemic disease with variable manifestation and a course characterized by exacerbations and remissions. Multiple autoantibodies, which may participate in tissue injury, may be detected in the serum of patients. Commonly anti-nuclear antibodies, especially those to native DNA, are found.

Incidence

The disease can present at any age but usually begins in the second to fourth decade. There is a strong female predominance (ratio 9:1). The disease is more common in persons of Afro-Caribbean and Hispanic ethnicity than in Caucasians is more common in the USA than in the UK, and the prevalence in Afro-Caribbean women is as high as 1 in 2500. The disease appears to be more severe in Afro-Caribbean and Hispanic patients. There appears to be a genetic predisposition, with increased incidence of the disease in first-degree relatives and up to 50% concordance in monozygotic twins. Systemic lupus erythematosis is associated with the MHC class II alloantigens HLA-DR2 and HLA-DR3, and mutations in MHC class III genes for complement components have been identified in lupus and lupus-like diseases. Variations in other non-major histocompatibility genes, including those coding for various cytokines, have also been reported in association with systemic lupus erythematosis.

Clinical presentation

The nature of the disease means that there is a very wide spectrum of disease manifestation and severity. A whole constellation of clinical and laboratory findings are required to confirm the diagnosis. The presence of a 'butterfly' rash in a malar distribution and serum antibodies to double-stranded DNA are characteristic. A list of criteria have been established by the American College of Rheumatology, of which four are required to establish the diagnosis of systemic lupus erythematosis. The four symptoms need not occur simultaneously. These symptoms are a combination of skin rash, oral or nasal ulceration, non-erosive arthritis, renal disease, pleuritis or pericarditis, psychosis, convulsions, and haematological or immunological disorders.

Fever and skin rashes are common at presentation, with facial erythema being more usual than the characteristic butterfly rash. Arthritis is common and may affect large and small joints in a symmetrical distribution. The spine is not involved. There is usually no bone erosion, even with long-standing disease. Joint deformity and tendon rupture may occur. Osteonecrosis or infection may cause symptoms asymmetrically in large weight-bearing joints. Systemic lupus erythematosis is associated with inflammatory myositis in 10–20% of patients. Pericarditis is the most common cardiovascular problem in systemic lupus erythematosis, but the greatest morbidity is from accelerated atherosclerosis and ischaemic heart disease.

Aetiology

The causes of systemic lupus erythematosis are unknown. In susceptible individuals, it is thought that the disease may be initiated or exacerbated by exposure to sunlight, emotional stress and viral infection.

Histology

No histological feature is diagnostic of systemic lupus erythematosis but several features are very suggestive, including fibrinoid necrosis of blood vessels and connective tissue, haematoxylin bodies present in the so-called lupus erythematosis cells, concentric ('onion skin') thickening of arterioles in the spleen, and Libman–Sacks verrucous endocarditis. Synovial biopsy may show villous hypertrophy and chronic inflammation. In contrast with rheumatoid arthritis, pannus formation and bone and cartilage erosion are usually not seen.

SPONDYLOARTHROPATHIES

The family of seronegative spondyloarthropathies includes ankylosing spondylitis, psoriatic arthritis and reactive arthritis. They are linked by the fact that nearly all patients are positive for HLA-B27, an antigen that is normally present in only 8% of the population. There is thought to be a common pathogenesis. It has been suggested that infection by *Salmonella, Klebsiella* or *Yersinia* organisms may play a role because these organisms are known to cause a reactive arthritis, and antibodies produced against these organisms may cross-react with the HLA-B27 molecule.[7]

Ankylosing spondylitis

Ankylosing spondylitis is an inflammatory arthritis syndrome that primarily affects the spine, although the hips, knees and shoulder joints may be affected in 30% of patients. The skeletal abnormalities are largely explained by changes that occur at sites of tendon insertion. The pathological process, which is known as enthesopathy, results in ossification and bony fusion at these sites. Enthesopathy in the spine results in vertebral body fusion, which is characteristic of the disease.

Incidence

The disease is thought to affect at least one in 1000 people, and predominantly affects boys and young men in the second to fourth decades (average age 26 years). Onset after 40 years is rare. There is a male:female ratio of 3:1. Ninety per cent of patients are HLA-B27-positive, and the disease is less common in populations that are negative for this antigen (e.g. Africans and Japanese). There is a spectrum of severity of disease ranging from mild or asymptomatic sacroiliitis to the rare but characteristic immobilizing fusion of the entire spine, the so-called 'bamboo' spine.

Clinical features

The most common scenario at presentation is a male patient aged between 15 and 40 years old who complains of gradual onset of intermittent low back pain and stiffness. There are bony erosions on both sides of the sacroiliac joint, best seen on CT scan, and serum analysis shows a raised erythrocyte sedimentation rate. Later, the joint fuses. During the course of the disease, 50% will experience peripheral arthritis, usually in the hip and shoulder joints. There may be extraskeletal manifestations such as anterior uveitis (25–30%), and rarely aortic valve regurgitation (3–5%) secondary to inflammation of the wall of the aortic root. Restriction of the thoracic cage may result in reduced lung function, and thoracic pain may mimic angina pectoris.

In most cases the disease is mild and self-limiting. In those severe cases where the disease progresses up the spine the patients are stooped forward, a posture brought about by curvature of the spine and flexion deformities of the hip. Treatment is usually conservative, with non-steroidal anti-inflammatory drugs and physiotherapy. The aim is to control the pain and preserve function. Long-term corticosteroid therapy is not considered appropriate because of the side effects and its failure to modify the disease process.

Pathology

There is an erosive inflammatory response centred on fibrocartilage at the site of ligament insertions. An overgrowth of new bone then fills in the defect in the eroded bone and the eroded end of the ligament becomes ossified. A new insertion site develops, overlying the original cortical bone. Eventually an irregular bony prominence forms and there is reactive sclerosis of underlying cancellous bone. In the spine, fusion of adjacent vertebral bony prominences results in an osseous bridge that is level with the vertebral body. In peripheral joints there is a histological picture similar to that seen in rheumatoid disease. There is severe synovitis and destructive pannus formation may be present. There may be an acute chondrolysis secondary to

REFERENCE

7. Wollheim FA. Curr Opin Rheumatol. 2001; 13: 305–309

inflammation of subchondral bone, with erosion of the articular cartilage from below.

Reactive arthritis and Reiter's syndrome

Reactive arthritis is a seronegative, asymmetric, non-purulent inflammatory arthritis that occurs in association with an infection anywhere in the body. Patients may have extra-articular symptoms of conjunctivitis, skin lesions of erythema nodosum and painful tendon insertions (enthesopathy). The disease usually follows a gastrointestinal or urogenital infection. The triad of conjunctivitis, urethritis and arthritis is known as Reiter's syndrome.

Incidence

The disease is usually seen in young adults and there is a male predominance. There is a strong association with HLA-B27. The clinical course is similar, irrespective of affected site and infecting organism. The initial infection resolves and is followed a few weeks later by an asymmetric oligoarthritis. In 5–20% of patients only one joint is affected. The weight-bearing joints of the lower limb are mainly involved, which become swollen, stiff and painful. There is pain at tendon insertion sites, with Achilles tendon and plantar fascia being most commonly affected. Initially the arthritis resolves but may recur in up to 50% of patients. The disease becomes chronic in 5–30% of cases.

Pathology

The pathogenesis of reactive arthritis is not clearly understood. It is likely that migration, deposition and persistence of microbial antigens in synovium cause the joint inflammation. Possible mechanisms include an exaggerated autoimmune response due to cross-reactivity between host and microbial antigens; an altered cellular immune response to the organism, mediated by HLA alleles; or an altered microbial–host cell interaction by which certain HLA alleles affect the host response to 'arthritogenic' pathogens. The pathogens implicated are *Yersinia*, *Salmonella*, *Shigella*, *Campylobacter* and *Chlamydia*. Despite the association with HLA-B27, a positive family history is unusual. The histological picture is indistinguishable from other inflammatory joint diseases.

Psoriatic arthropathy

Psoriasis is a skin disorder, affecting 1–2% of the population, which usually appears in the second or third decade of life. Psoriatic arthropathy is a rheumatoid factor-negative inflammatory arthropathy affecting 5–7% of patients with psoriasis. It affects both sexes equally. The arthropathy usually develops slowly, but it can be acute and may precede the skin symptoms by months or years.

Clinical features

Several patterns of disease are recognized. Most patients (70%) present with oligoarticular disease, which is usually asymmetric, affecting the knee and one or more interphalangeal or metacarpophalangeal joints. There may be associated diffuse swelling of the affected hands and feet, the so-called 'sausage digit'. The next most common pattern is the symmetric polyarthritis (15%), which resembles rheumatoid disease and is associated with morning stiffness and fatigue. The classic symptoms of asymmetric involvement of distal interphalangeal joints affect only 10% of patients. The affected fingers and toes may show the pitted nails characteristic of psoriasis. Patients with this form of the disease may develop the oligoarticular pattern. Up to 5% of patients have a severe disabling erosive arthropathy of the fingers and toes known as arthritis mutilans, which results in osteolysis and severe joint deformity. Finally, up to 5% of patients suffer from psoriatic spondyloarthritis, which is a sacroiliitis radiologically indistinguishable from idiopathic sacroiliitis or ankylosing spondylitis. There is an association with HLA-B27 in 40% of patients with psoriatic spondyloarthritis. The temperomandibular joint is commonly affected in psoriatic arthropathy.

Extra-articular symptoms are unusual, although up to 30% of patients may have inflammatory eye disease.

Pathology

The pathogenesis of the disease is unknown. There is a 70% concordance in monozygotic twins and family studies show a high risk in first-degree relatives, suggesting that there may be a genetic component. Because psoriatic skin lesions are associated with a high incidence of bacterial infection, it has been suggested that altered T-cell immunity and antigen cross-reactivity may also play a role.

The histological changes are similar to those seen in other inflammatory arthropathies.

Enteropathic arthropathy

Enteropathic arthritis occurs in association with inflammatory bowel disease such as ulcerative colitis or Crohn's disease. Approximately 50–100 people in 100 000 suffer from inflammatory bowel disease. Between 10 and 25% of these patients may develop a migratory arthritis, usually peripheral but which can affect the axial skeleton.

Clinical features

The peak age of onset is in the third and fourth decades. There is an equal sex incidence and the arthritis is more common in association with Crohn's disease. There is no association with HLA-B27 in patients with peripheral arthropathy but up to 50% of patients with spinal involvement are HLA-B27-positive.[8]

Pathology

There are no specific histological changes to distinguish enteropathic arthritis from other inflammatory arthritides. However, granulomas may be seen in synovium of patients with Crohn's disease.

CRYSTAL DEPOSITION ARTHROPATHIES

The crystal-induced arthropathies are a group of metabolic diseases that result in the deposition of crystals in and around joints. Three main types of crystals are deposited: monosodium urate associated with gout, and calcium pyrophosphate and calcium hydroxyapatite in pseudogout.

Gout

Gout occurs as a result of prolonged hyperuricaemia due to abnormal purine metabolism or impaired excretion of uric acid. High blood uric acid level is defined as a serum urate level more than two standard deviations above the mean, or 0.42 mmol/L (7 mg/100 mL) for adult men and 0.36 mmol/L (6 mg/100 mL) for adult women. Uric acid is an end product of purine metabolism. The vast majority of cases (90%) are primary, and

REFERENCE

8. Zachariae H. Am J Clin Dermatol 2003; 4: 441–447

Box 41.3 Conditions associated with hyperuricaemia and gout

Overproduction of urate
- Myeloproliferative disorders
- Lymphoma
- Haemoglobinopathies
- Haemolytic anaemia
- Psoriasis
- Chemotherapy for cancer

Under-excretion of urate
- Chronic renal failure
- Lead nephropathy
- Drugs (e.g. diuretics and cyclosporine)
- Lactic acidosis (alcohol and pre-eclampsia)
- Ketosis (diabetes and starvation)
- Hyperparathroidism
- Hypertension

Unknown mechanism
- Sarcoidosis
- Obesity
- Hypoparathyroidism
- Paget's disease
- Down's syndrome

10% are secondary associated with a variety of diseases that cause hyperuricaemia or impaired excretion of uric acid (see Box 41.3).

Most of the cases of primary gout are idiopathic, but in about 1% of patients a specific enzyme defect has been identified. The best characterized of these defects are decreased hypoxanthine-guanine phosphoribosyltransferase activity and increased phosphoribosylpyrophosphate synthase activity.

Clinical features

The majority of patients are men, with a peak age of onset in the fifth decade. It is rare in women before the menopause. The American College of Rheumatology have 13 criteria, and the presence of six or more of these suggests the diagnosis of gout (see Box 41.4). The disease is characterized by an intensely painful acute arthritis, usually in one joint (70%) but multiple joints may be affected. Repeated attacks may result in chronic tophaceous arthritis and crystalline deposits or tophi in soft tissue (Fig. 41.8). Any joint may be affected but the great toe is involved in 90% of cases. The disease is usually limited to the lower extremities, the dorsum of the foot, the ankle and the knee being commonly affected. There is a precipitate of needle-shaped crystals into the joint. Predisposing factors include recent surgery, rapid weight loss, chronic renal disease, alcohol abuse, infection, and drugs including diuretics, cyclosporine and cancer chemotherapy agents. Heberden's and Bouchard's nodes may be involved in elderly women on diuretics. The tophus is the pathognomonic lesion, and the lesions usually appear after at least 10 years of repeated attacks. The tophi are usually situated in the olecranon bursa, finger joints and helix of the ear.

Pathology

The disorder is diagnosed by the demonstration of needle-shaped urate crystals in synovial fluid or synovium. The crystals are 5–25 μm long and can be seen in smear preparations made from synovial fluid samples in 85% of cases. The smears are viewed under polarized light and the crystals show a strong negative birefringence. Uric acid dissolves in aqueous solutions, therefore

Box 41.4 American College of Rheumatology criteria for gout

- More than one attack of acute arthritis.
- Maximum inflammation developed within 1 day.
- Monoarthritis attack.
- Redness observed over joints.
- First metatarsophalangeal joint painful or swollen.
- Unilateral first metatarsophalangeal joint attack.
- Unilateral tarsal joint attack.
- Tophus (proven or suspected).
- Hyperuricemia.
- Asymmetric swelling within a joint on X-ray.*
- Subcortical cysts without erosions on X-ray.
- Monosodium urate monohydrate microcrystals in joint fluid during attack.
- Joint fluid culture negative for organisms during attack.

*This criterion could logically be found on examination as well as on X-ray. However, the protocol did not request this information in regard to examination. (After Wallace et al 1977,[9].)

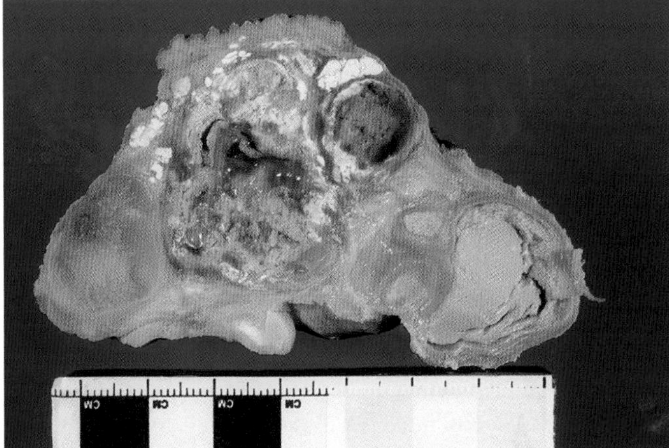

Figure 41.8 Macroscopic picture of gouty tophus from olecranon.

ordinary formalin fixation is contraindicated for synovial biopsies where gout is suspected. The specimens are best fixed in absolute alcohol or transported to the histopathology laboratory fresh and in a dry pot with the suspected diagnosis clearly indicated on the request form.

Crystals are thought to be deposited in joints because the synovial fluid is a poorer solvent than plasma, and because the lower peripheral temperature (e.g. in the feet) favours crystallization. Chemotactic factors induced by the crystals themselves via complement, and by incoming inflammatory cells such as neutrophils and macrophages, intensify the inflammatory response.

The synovial biopsy may show variable features depending on the stage of disease. There may be an acute inflammatory infiltrate of polymorph neutrophils associated with lymphocytes and macrophages in the early stages. Crystals may be difficult to identify, but with appropriate fixation they may be demonstrated in the cytoplasm of the inflammatory cells. In chronic disease there may be joint erosion and tophi may develop in soft tissue.

REFERENCE

9. Wallace SL, Robinson H, Masi AT et al. Arthritis Rheum 1977; 20: 895–900

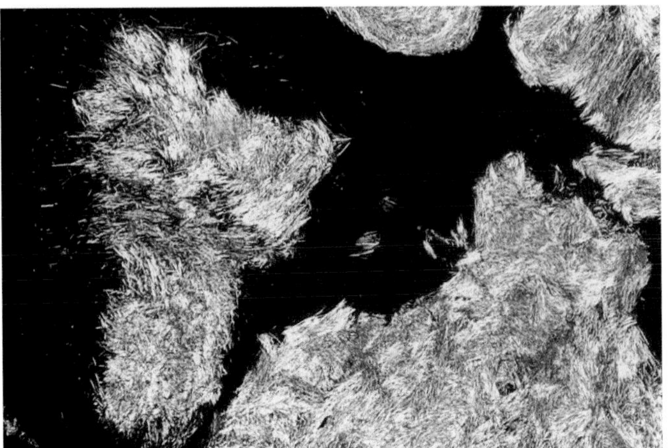

Figure 41.9 Needle-shaped sodium urate crystals seen at high power under polarized light.

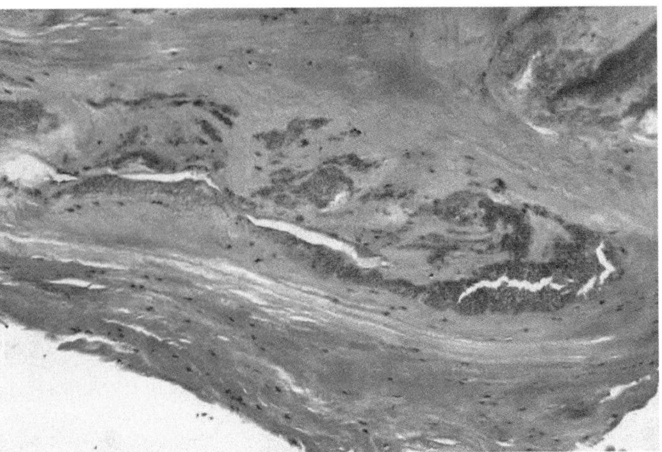

Figure 41.10 Low-power haematoxylin and eosin stain of tissue from a joint affected by pseudogout. There are irregular deposits of amorphous grey material.

The tophi are masses of monosodium urate surrounded by fibrous tissue and inflammatory cells including foreign body-type giant cells. Early lesions are microscopic, but large white chalky masses several centimetres in diameter can develop (Fig. 41.9).

Treatment

In the acute phase the aim is to reduce pain and inflammation, mainly using non-steroidal anti-inflammatory drugs. Oral colchicine is used but there can be severe side effects, with gastrointestinal disturbances. Long-term strategies include lifestyle and dietary changes as well as drugs to reduce blood urate levels.

Calcium crystal deposition disease (pseudogout or chondrocalcinosis)

Calcium crystal deposition disease is an inflammatory arthropathy that may be acute or chronic and is caused by the deposition of calcium pyrophosphate dihydrate crystals in synovium. Patients can be classified into groups with two overlapping syndromes. The first syndrome is pseudogout, an acute synovitis caused by a release of a shower of crystals from the hyaline cartilage (Fig. 41.10). It is most common in the elderly and affects one or more joints, usually the knee. The second syndrome, called chronic pyrophosphate arthropathy (Fig. 41.11), mimics primary osteoarthritis. Less commonly the disease may mimic rheumatoid arthritis. Rarely there may be tumoural deposits of calcium pyrophosphate in soft tissue, and this is known as tophaceous pseudogout.

Chondrocalcinosis is a common cause of joint pain and arthritis, which is found in the majority of patients with pseudogout and is caused by the deposition of calcium-containing crystals in articular cartilage. Calcified cartilage is seen on radiographs. Punctate or linear intra-articular calcification is present in menisci, intervertebral discs, and articular cartilage or tendon insertions. The knee is commonly affected but the changes may also be seen in hip, symphysis pubis, spine and wrist. The prevalence of this disease is unknown, but 8% of people over 60 years have evidence of chondrocalcinosis; this increases to 28% of the population in the ninth decade.

Pathology

The underlying problem is thought to be an inherited metabolic defect that results in the inability of hyaline cartilage to maintain the extracellular matrix. This results in the deposition of calcium pyrophosphate dihydrate crystals in synovium, cartilage and juxta-articular tissue.

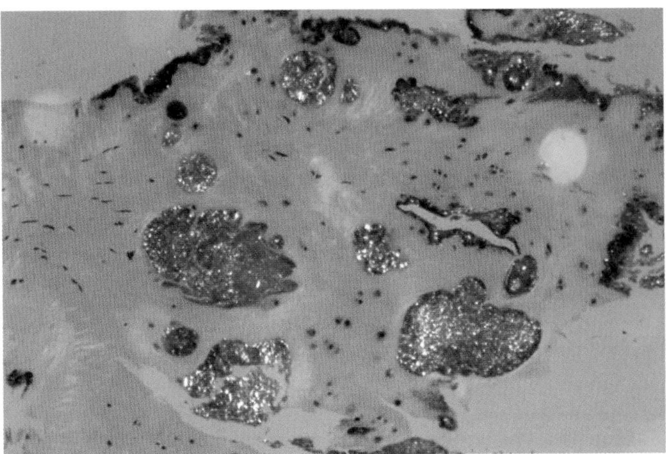

Figure 41.11 Low-power view of tissue from a joint affected by pseudogout viewed under polarized light. Polygonal crystals of calcium pyrophosphate are seen within deposits.

Calcium crystal deposition disease can be seen in several settings. Most cases are sporadic, but rare familial forms have been identified that have been linked to gene mutations on chromosome 8 (*CCAL1*) or the short arm of chromosome 5 (*CCAL2*).[9] Among the loci on the short arm of chromosome 5 is the *ANKH* gene, which is the human homologue of a gene that causes progressive ankylosis in the mouse. The *ANKH* gene codes for a transmembrane protein that appears to regulate the transport of inorganic phosphate. Abnormalities in this gene have been associated with familial calcium crystal deposition disease. The mode of inheritance is unclear, but an autosomal dominant pattern has been described in some populations in which the disease may begin in childhood, be polyarticular and progress rapidly.[10]

REFERENCE

10. Pendleton A, Johnson MD, Hughes A et al. Am J Hum Genet 2002; 71: 933–940

Calcium crystal deposition disease may follow joint trauma or surgery such as meniscectomy or major illness such as stroke. Other metabolic or endocrine diseases—such as hyperparathroidism, haemochromatosis, hypophosphatasia, gout and neuropathic arthropathy—have all been associated with calcium crystal deposition disease. These conditions are thought to enhance deposition of calcium pyrophosphate dihydrate crystals in synovium. Most commonly, calcium crystal deposition disease is associated with increasing age.

The crystals shed into the joint undergo phagocytosis by leukocytes and induce an acute inflammatory response. If the inflammation persists there may be a lymphocytic infiltrate and fibrosis. Calcium pyrophosphate crystals may be seen histologically in samples of intervertebral discs or joint arthroplasty specimens removed for degenerative disease. They may also be seen in biopsies taken at arthroscopy. The crystals appear as well-defined clusters of deeply basophilic material. In synovium there may be an associated inflammatory response that is absent in tendon or cartilage. Under polarized light the crystals are polygonal, are 1–5 μm long, and show a weakly positive birefringence.

Treatment is symptomatic. Non-steroidal anti-inflammatory drugs help to reduce the symptoms but crystal deposition cannot be prevented.

INFECTIOUS ARTHRITIS

Rarely, a blood-borne pathogen will infect the synovium and joint space without bony involvement. The joint may also become infected from an intracapsular focus of osteomyelitis or from trauma by puncture wound or surgery. The resulting acute septic arthritis is a medical emergency because the condition progresses rapidly and may cause extensive destruction of articular cartilage and permanent joint damage.

Clinical features

Infectious arthritis is most commonly caused by *Staphylococcus aureus* organisms. In infants and young children, *Haemophilus influenzae* and *Streptococcus* organisms are also important pathogens. *Salmonella* is a well-recognized causative organism in patients with sickle cell disease. In young adults (younger than 30 years) *Neisseria gonorrhoeae* is the most common cause of septic arthritis. An estimated one in 200 patients with gonorrhoea develops a septic arthritis, usually involving wrist, knee or ankle.

Acute septic arthritis is primarily a disease of children. There is a swollen painful joint, usually the knee, associated with fever and leukocytosis. The hip is the most common site of pyogenic arthritis in infants and the pain may not localize there. The symptoms and signs are often non-specific, and the only clue may be that the child does not move the affected limb.

The most commonly affected sites are the knee in adults and hip, but in intravenous drug abusers the sternoclavicular, sacroiliac or shoulder joints may be affected. Bacterial pathogens usually affect one joint but polyarticular symptoms are present in 10% of patients, which may reflect associated bacteraemia. Systemic sepsis and septic shock can occur with virulent pathogens in vulnerable patients. Extra-articular infection, underlying inflammatory or degenerative arthropathy, chronic illness (e.g. diabetes mellitus) and immunosuppression are all predisposing factors.

Pathogenesis

The causative organisms seed the synovial membrane and cause an acute purulent synovitis. The pus tacks into the joint space and distends the joint capsule (pyarthrosis). Bacterial and inflammatory cell enzymes degrade the articular cartilage. The speed of progression of the disease is determined by the nature of the pathogen, the inflammatory response and the host vulnerability. Cytokines from polymorph neutrophils play an essential role in tissue destruction.

Joint aspiration is virtually mandatory, and fluid should be sent for culture and sensitivity, microscopy with Gram stain, cell count and differential, and glucose level analysis. Synovial biopsy is often non-specific and will show acute inflammation. Occasionally, causative organisms can be demonstrated with special stains.

Tuberculous arthritis

Mycobacterium tuberculosis is a rare cause of arthritis. An estimated 5% of patients with tuberculosis have bone or joint involvement. The most common presentation is with involvement of the spine (tuberculous spondylitis in more than 50% of cases). Other presenting complaints include a chronic monoarthritis, usually of hip or knee, or tenosynovitis of hands or feet. Skeletal disease is usually mixed osteomyelitis and arthritis. Haematogenous spread of the organism from the primary site can cause the joint disease, but in the spine the organisms are thought to spread directly from the lungs via lymphatics. Tuberculous spondylitis commonly results in vertebral collapse with associated infection of disc and soft tissue, and development of paravertebral abscesses. About 60% of patients with vertebral collapse develop kyphosis, which can be severe and become associated with paraplegia—a syndrome known as Pott's disease.

There is often no sign of systemic disease and chest X-ray is clear in 50% of patients. The tuberculin test on skin is usually positive. Synovial fluid analysis shows an elevated white blood cell count with neutrophil predominance. The Zeil–Neelson stain for acid-fast bacteria is positive in only 27% of fluid samples, and although culture is positive in over 80% of cases, the results take 4–6 weeks. Therefore synovial biopsy is the investigation of choice. Granulomas have been shown to be present in 95% of cases, with associated caseation necrosis in 55%, and demonstration of the organism with special stains in 10%.

Fungal arthritis

Fungal organisms can cause bone and joint infection, mostly in immunocompromised patients or those on long-term steroid therapy. The spine is most commonly affected. Fungal arthritis usually presents as a chronic monoarticular infection, but acute polyarticular disease can occur with and without the skin lesions of erythema nodosum. Diagnosis is made by synovial biopsy sent for microbiological and histopathological investigation. *Blastomyces* organisms spread from the lungs to skin and bone. The knee, ankle and elbow joints are the usual sites. Synovial fluid culture is positive in 90% of cases. *Candida* species cause septic arthritis by haematogenous dissemination in immunosuppressed individuals. Two-thirds of patients present acutely, 40% have polyarticular disease and 65% also have osteomyelitis. *Coccidioides* and *Histoplasma capsulatum* species may cause septic arthritis in people with normal immunity.

Lyme disease

Lyme disease is an inflammatory arthropathy that resembles juvenile arthritis clinically, but that is part of a complex multisystem illness resulting from a tick bite and subsequent infection by the spirochaete *Borrelia burgdorferi.* The first epidemiological study of the disease described an epidemic form of arthritis in young people in a group of rural communities in Connecticut, USA (Lyme, Old Lyme and Haddam), with an onset between May and November. The organism is named after the microbiologist Burgdorfer, who first isolated the organism from the tick species *Ixodes dammini* in 1982. The tick bite had been previously associated with a skin rash called erythema chronicum migrans, also known as erythema migrans, and the organisms were seen in samples of the skin lesions. A neurological manifestation of the disease, meningopolyneuritis, was also recognized. Soon after the organism was discovered, it was linked serologically to patients suffering from Lyme disease.

Lyme disease affects both sexes equally, and although people of any age may be affected there appears to be a peak incidence in children of 5–9 years and in adults over 30 years old.

Clinical features

The disease may be roughly divided into three stages that may merge into each other or be divided by symptom-free intervals.

Stage 1 (early, localized) disease begins after the tick bite and injection of the spirochaete. The characteristic skin rash develops in 90% of patients between 3 and 32 days (typically 7–10 days) after the bite. This begins as a red macule or papule at the site, which expands over days and weeks to between 1 and 50 cm in diameter. The site may be anywhere but is frequently thigh, groin and axilla, with ear lobe being a common site in children. There may be associated lymphadenopathy and mild general malaise.

Stage 2 (early, disseminated) disease starts within days or weeks and marks the spread of the spirochaete in blood or lymphatics. Many organs may be affected, in particular the musculoskeletal system, nervous system and heart. There may be associated severe headaches and neck stiffness, as well as secondary erythema chronicum migrans in skin, in which the lesions are smaller and migrate less. The neurological complications include Bell's palsy, peripheral neuropathy and aseptic meningitis. The cardiac manifestations include heart block and arrhythmia. The joint involvement is usually considered to be a late-stage complication, but acute attacks may develop early in the disease. There is usually an asymmetric involvement of four or fewer joints. Usually larger joints are affected, commonly the knee. The infective organism may be isolated from synovial fluid or tissue biopsy.

Stage 3 (late, persistent) infection is dominated by arthritis. There may be prolonged attacks of acute arthritis, and development of chronic arthritis (episodes lasting more than 1 year) occurs in less than 10% of patients. It has been suggested that HLA-DR4 serology and a poor response to antibiotic treatment may be predisposing factors for the development of chronic disease. The skin may show localized scleroderma-like lesions, and there may be chronic neurological complications of chronic radiculopathy and encephalopathy.

Treatment

Treatment is based on prevention, with protection against the organism. Vaccines are available. Antibiotic therapy is used for proven disease where possible. Prophylactic treatment is thought to be ineffective.

Pathology

The diagnosis of Lyme disease is a clinical one. The histological features in biopsy of synovium are not specific. The organisms can rarely be demonstrated, and positive immunohistochemistry or PCR analysis for organism antigens are not diagnostic of the acute disease because they will remain positive once the infection is eradicated. Culture of the organism is virtually 100% specific. It is difficult to classify Lyme arthritis because it appears to be a mixture of infectious and reactive arthritis. The organism can be demonstrated in joint tissues, consistent with an infectious arthritis, but the pattern of joint involvement most resembles the seronegative spondylarthropathies. However, there is no association with HLA-B27 and no involvement of the sacroiliac joint as is usually seen in this group.

ARTHROPATHY RELATED TO HAEMATOLOGICAL DISORDERS

Haemophilia

Haemophilia is an inherited, recessive, sex-linked disorder of blood coagulation. Females are asymptomatic carriers of the mutated gene on the X chromosome. There are several subtypes of the disease. Broadly, haemophilia A is caused by a deficiency of factor VIII (Von Willebrand factor) and haemophilia B (Christmas disease) is associated with deficiency of factor IX. There may be recurrent haemorrhage into joints, with associated synovial proliferation and inflammation, which are thought to be responsible for the arthropathy associated with this disease.

Pathology

The pathogenesis of haemophilia-associated arthropathy is not clearly understood. There is deposition of iron pigment (or haemosiderin) in synovium, which is thought to elicit an inflammatory response with subsequent pannus formation and degenerative changes. These features of haemosiderotic synovitis may also be seen in biopsies from patients with a traumatic haemarthrosis or those on anticoagulant therapy.

Clinical features

Three stages of the disease are recognized. The initial phase is that of acute haemarthrosis, and the frequency and severity of attacks reflect the severity of the coagulation disorder. Repeated acute attacks result in the development of subacute haemophilic arthropathy manifested by persistent synovitis and joint effusion, synovial proliferation and variable pain. Last, chronic haemophilic arthropathy results in severe degenerative changes with joint deformity, fibrous ankylosis and osteophyte formation. There may be associated intramuscular haemorrhage or cysts, and formation of osseous pseudotumours. Treatment involves a multidisciplinary team approach with fast appropriate replacement of coagulation factors and symptomatic relief (Fig. 41.12).

Sickle cell disease and β-thalassaemia

Arthritis associated with haemoglobinopathy usually occurs as a result of ischaemia or infarction of synovium or periarticular bone. In sickle cell crises there may be a painful arthritis of the large joints with associated non-inflammatory effusion. Venous occlusion due to sickling of the erythrocytes may cause local bone necrosis, and this involves the femoral head in up to 33% of sickle cell patients. Dactylitis secondary to bone ischaemia in the hands and feet of affected children may be the first sign of sickle cell disease. Treatment is aimed at relieving symptoms and includes rehydration, analgesia and folate supplementation. Sickle cell disease is associated with infectious arthritis and osteomyelitis due to *Salmonella*.

β-Thalassaemia minor is associated with recurrent asymmetric arthritis. β-Thalassaemia major is associated with osteoporosis, pathological fracture and epiphyseal deformities largely due to expansion of the marrow space.

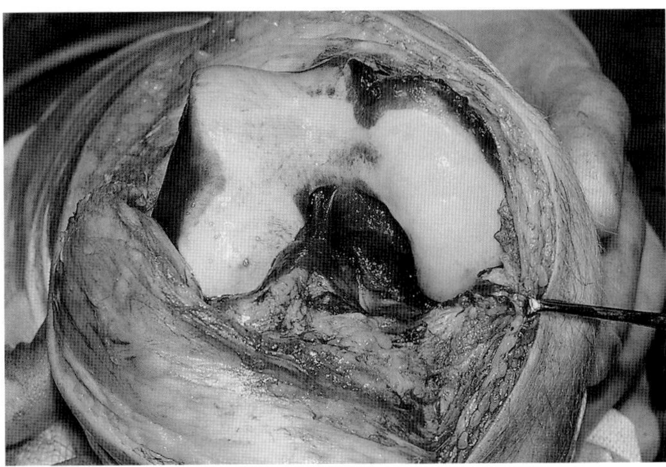

Figure 41.12 Haemophilic arthropathy of the knee, with peripheral erosions produced by pannus.

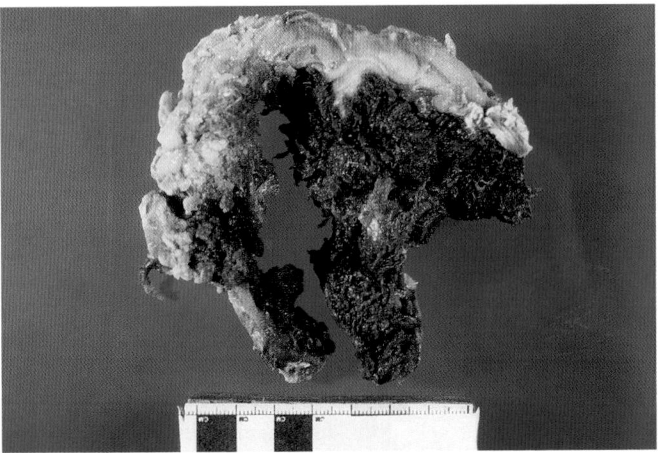

Figure 41.13 Macroscopic view of hyperplastic pigmented synovium from an affected knee joint.

Pigmented villonodular synovitis

Pigmented villonodular synovitis (synonyms include giant cell tumour of tendon sheath and nodular tenosynovitis) is a benign disease of synovium that may be locally aggressive. The synovium is thickened and hyperplastic. It may appear nodular or villous and shows brown discolouration. The synovium involved may be intra-articular or extra-articular involving bursae or tendon sheaths. The disease usually affects only one joint, most commonly the knee (Fig. 41.13). Polyarticular cases have been described but these are usually young patients with a positive family history.

Clinical features

The disease usually affects adults in the third or fourth decade. The disease is rarely seen in children. There appear to be three distinct clinical forms. The first is a nodular localized form occurring as a painless swelling in the hands. This is more common in women. The second is a diffuse intra-articular form that presents as a chronic monoarticular arthropathy affecting young adults and usually involving the knee. The hand, shoulder, wrist or vertebra may also be affected. This is usually slowly progressive and the symptoms may mimic rheumatoid arthritis. The third clinical presentation is with locking of the knee, secondary to a localized pedunculated swelling usually involving the knee and confined to the medial or lateral compartment.

Treatment is by surgical excision, which is of variable success. Recurrences may be multiple and treatment with radiotherapy has been advocated.

Pathology

Synovial biopsies characteristically show a proliferation of mononuclear cells in the subsurface tissue together with a variable number of multinucleate giant cells, foamy histiocytes and haemosiderophages (Fig. 41.14). Numerous mitotic figures may be present. The localized nodular form of the disease tends to show marked hyalinization of the stroma. The mononuclear cells stain positively with immunohistochemical markers for histiocytic cell lineage. The aetiology of the disease is uncertain. Cytogenetic analysis has demonstrated trisomy 7 and aneuploidy in the mononuclear cells, which suggests they may be neoplastic.

Diagnostic difficulty may arise in distinguishing between pigmented villonodular synovitis and haemosiderotic synovitis, or pigmented villonodular synovitis and giant cell tumour of bone.

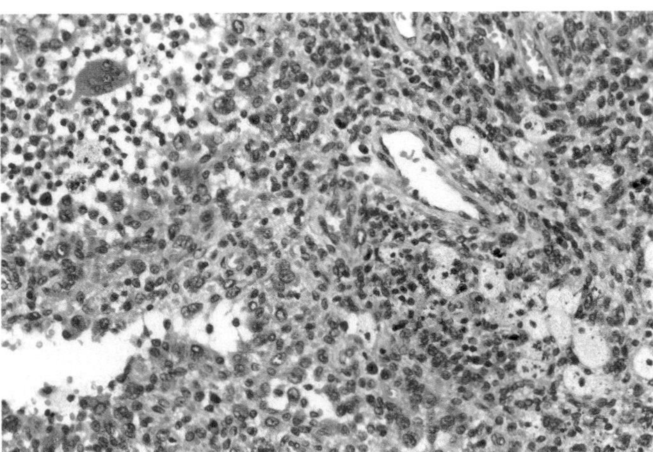

Figure 41.14 Medium-power view of haematoxylin and eosin-stained section of synovium with features of pigmented villonodular synovitis. There are scattered multinucleate giant cells associated with a proliferation of bland spindle to polygonal cells and pigment deposition in the stroma.

The mononuclear proliferation and the giant cells are usually not a feature of haemosiderotic synovitis, which is most often seen in association with haemophilia or anticoagulation therapy, or following trauma. Bone erosions on both sides of the joint are a feature of pigmented villonodular synovitis but not giant cell tumour of bone, and the heavy haemosiderin deposition characteristically seen in pigmented villonodular synovitis is not a feature of giant cell tumour of bone.

BONE

GENERAL CONSIDERATIONS

The structure of bone reflects its function. Bone needs to be strong for protection and to support soft tissues, and light for mobility. It is the main storage site for calcium and the chief site for haemopoiesis. Dense compact or cortical bone functions mainly as mechanical support and for protection. Compact bone is very dense, with few spaces, and comprises 70% of the bone in the body. Cancellous (spongy or trabecular) bone (e.g. in vertebra) has a large surface area and has a main function in calcium metabolism. Lamellar bone is characteristic of adult bone, compact and cancellous. It is so-called 'mature' bone, while woven bone is immature and usually pathological. Periosteum histology covers cortical surface and delivers the blood supply.

Microscopically, bone consists of cells and an abundant extracellular matrix of collagen impregnated with calcium hydroxyapatite. The collagen matrix resists tension forces and the crystals withstand compression; a similar arrangement is seen in reinforced concrete.

There are three types of bone cell: osteoblasts, osteoclasts and osteocytes (Fig. 41.15).

Osteoblasts

Osteoblasts are bone-forming cells that line endosteal surfaces. They are cuboidal cells with an eccentrically placed nucleus. They deposit osteoid at a rate of about 1 μm a day. They possess receptors for 1,25-$(OH)_2$ vitamin D and parathyroid hormone. Osteoblasts also produce alkaline phosphatase, and this enzyme can be demonstrated histochemically. Increased serum alkaline phosphatase is associated with excess osteoblastic activity seen in association with diseases such as Paget's disease and bone-forming neoplasms.

Osteoclasts

Osteoclasts are multinucleate cells, part of the macrophage family, involved in bone resorption. They are 20–100 μm in diameter and are found on the bone surface in resorption craters known as Howship's lacunae. Their ability to resorb bone is reflected in their structure. They have a ruffled border seen ultrastructurally, which vastly increases the surface area. They possess lysosomes containing proteases and osteoclast-specific, tartrate-resistant acid phosphatase that can be detected histochemically.

Resorption takes place in stages, and the osteoclast must be in direct contact with the mineralized bone. Therefore the surface-lining cells must contract and the surface layer of osteoid must be resorbed. This may occur as a result of parathyroid hormone stimulation or under the influence of local factors. The osteoclasts then secrete protons to acidify the local environment and digest the matrix mineral, and proteases to digest matrix proteins. Finally, osteoclasts undergo fission into mononuclear cells to complete the resorption process.

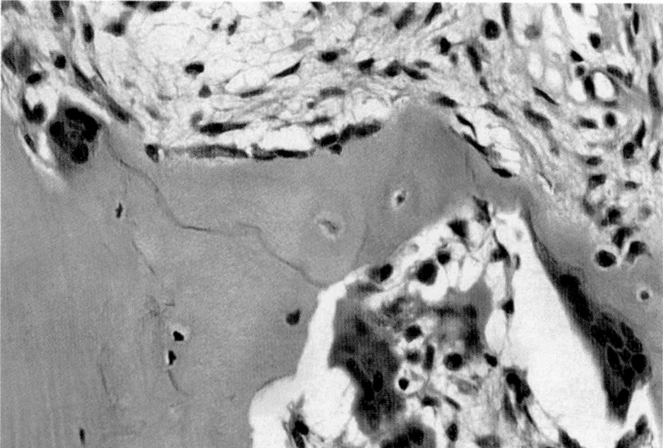

Figure 41.15 High-power view of haematoxylin and eosin-stained section of lamellar bone with multinucleate osteoclasts and mononuclear osteoblasts on the surface. Osteocytes are present in lacunae within the bone.

Osteoclasts do not possess parathyroid hormone receptor, and bone resorption is mediated by osteoblasts. Interleukins, prostaglandins and vitamin D induce osteoclast proliferation and bone resorption, and this is also most likely mediated by osteoblasts. Osteoclasts do have receptors for calcitonin, which inhibits bone resorption by causing retraction of the osteoclasts from the bone surface. Persistent exposure to calcitonin results in the osteoclast becoming resistant due to down-regulation of the surface receptors.

Osteocytes

Osteocytes are osteoblasts that have become trapped in the bone matrix. They are in contact with other bone cells and the bone surface. Cytoplasmic processes extending between osteocytes and cells lining the bone surface form the osteocytic membrane system. This has two functions. First, in response to parathyroid hormone, osteocytes release calcium from the matrix into the extracellular tissue; this process, known as osteocytic osteolysis, raises blood calcium levels almost immediately, even before osteoclasts can be recruited to digest bone. Second, the osteocytic membrane system transmits electronic signals in response to bone deformation, which ensures even distribution of forces and active bone remodelling in areas under most stress.

BONE BIOPSY

Indications for bone biopsy include:

- suspected tumour or infection,
- suspected metabolic bone disease (e.g. osteomalacia or Paget's disease),
- diagnostic classification of renal osteodystrophy,
- evaluation of therapy, and
- research.

The multidisciplinary team approach is essential to the practice of orthopaedic pathology. The biopsy should be planned to obtain representative tissue from the most appropriate site and to ensure that any appropriate special stains are carried out. The options include closed-needle biopsy with or without image guidance and open biopsy.

Closed-needle biopsies are preferable wherever possible, because general anaesthesia is usually not required and the complications are few and rare. High diagnostic accuracy rates have been reported in biopsy series taken under CT guidance by radiologists in specialist centres. The drawback is that the small amount of tissue obtained may preclude ancillary studies, including cytogenetic and molecular analysis. The small-needle core biopsies obtained are easily crushed and distorted. To achieve diagnostic accuracy with such small tissue samples, full and accurate clinical information is essential to the pathologist, as are specialist laboratory techniques.

Open biopsies are necessary for densely calcified lesions and lesions in particularly inaccessible sites. Frozen section analysis is rarely used for diagnostic purposes in specialist centres in the UK. It is not possible to cut frozen sections of undecalcified bone, and the technique is usually reserved for cases where the diagnosis is almost certain or to confirm recurrence or metastasis.

INFECTIONS

Bone infection (or osteomyelitis) may be primary, resulting from haematogenous spread of micro-organisms, or secondary, as a result of trauma, surgery (introduced osteomyelitis) or direct spread from adjacent soft tissue. It has been classified also as acute, subacute or chronic, which may be useful for therapeutic purposes. Bacteria usually cause osteomyelitis but any type of organism may be implicated. The main clinical considerations are that infection causes bone destruction, which predisposes to deformity and pathological fracture, and that the organisms encased in bone are difficult to eradicate.

Primary osteomyelitis (haematogenous bacterial osteomyelitis)

The causative organism is usually *S. aureus*, and patients are usually children less than 15 years old. However, the site of bone involvement and the infective organism is age-dependent. The long bones (tibia, femur and humerus) are preferential sites from birth to puberty. There is a rich blood supply to these bones during development. Other causative organisms include *H. influenzae*, especially in children under 3 years, and group B streptococci and coliforms in neonates. In sickle cell anaemia the disease process may affect multiple sites and may be caused by *Salmonella* species.

Infection may be difficult to distinguish from bone infarction. In adults, the lumbosacral and thoracic spine are more commonly affected and there is relatively more blood flow to these sites, with maturation. Organisms reach the vertebral bodies via arterial blood or via backflow from the perivertebral venous plexus of Batson. The process affects the more vascular anterior end plates, and commonly involves adjacent vertebrae and the intervertebral disc.

The causative organism reflects the micro-organism causing the bacteraemia, and streptococci, Gram-negative bacteria, mycobacteria, anaerobes and fungi can cause osteomyelitis in a variety of clinical situations. For example, Gram-negative bacteria or streptococci may be associated with urinary tract infection or instrumentation, and *M. tuberculosis* with an underlying respiratory infection.

Patients with AIDS may develop bacillary angiomatosis of bone, which is related to infection with the cat scratch bacillus and which can mimic an aggressive neoplasm radiologically. Chronic haemodialysis patients may develop osteomyelitis presumed secondary to infected catheter sites. The ribs and thoracic spine are commonly affected. The symptoms in these patients may be mistaken for renal osteodystrophy, a common complication of end-stage renal disease.

Pathology

Bacteraemia results in seeding of the bone, usually in the metaphysis adjacent to the physis. The bacteria pass from the blood via fenestrated capillaries and adhere to the bone using receptors to surface sialoproteins and collagen. The organisms then secrete a thick coat of mucopolysaccharide (the glycocalyx), which assists adhesion and protects against antibiotics and host immunity. A purulent acute inflammatory reaction results, which seeps through trabecular bone into cortical bone, where a subperiosteal abscess may form. The epiphysis usually acts as a barrier to infection, but infants have a transphyseal blood supply and the epiphysis may not be spared. As the disease progresses there is bone destruction by osteoclasts, which are activated by cytokines such as tumour necrosis factor, interleukin-1 and prostaglandin E_2. There is some evidence that the inflammatory cells themselves may be able to resorb bone.

Extension of the subperiosteal abscess may lift the periosteum, thus disrupting the blood supply to the cortical bone and producing segments of necrosis (sequestra). Reactive new bone (involucrum) is produced by the viable periosteum.

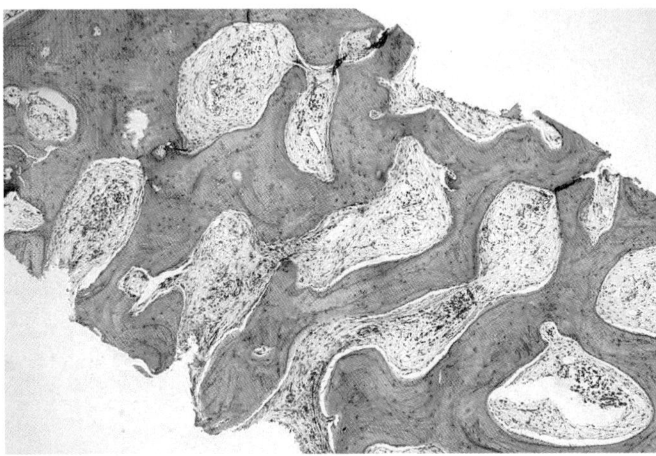

Figure 41.16 Lower-power view of haematoxylin and eosin-stained section of core biopsy of bone with features of osteomyelitis. The marrow is fibrotic and contains a mixed inflammatory cell infiltrate.

Histology

Osteomyelitis is characterized by bone destruction, inflammatory cells in marrow, and reparative new bone formation (Fig. 41.16). Acute, subacute and chronic osteomyelitis cannot be distinguished histologically. The features are not specific and clinicopathological correlation is essential.

Radiology

The most sensitive modality is the bone scan, which is positive within 48–72 h after the onset of symptom; however, the findings are not specific. The plain radiograph is more specific but signs may not develop until 10–14 days after the onset of symptoms.

Subacute osteomyelitis

Sometimes the initial infection in bone may be contained by the body's defences but not eradicated. Mild systemic symptoms with vague pain and fever may be present for months. Plain radiographs may show a well-defined lytic area in the metaphysis with a rim of reactive bone (Fig. 41.17). The syndrome is known as subacute osteomyelitis or Brodie's abscess. The tibia is the most common site but femur and tarsal bones may be involved.

Secondary osteomyelitis

Direct inoculation of micro-organisms into bone causes secondary osteomyelitis. This may result from infection of adjacent soft tissue, contaminated open fracture or puncture wound. Patients are at risk of introduced osteomyelitis whenever trauma or surgery breaches the skin or soft tissues overlying bone. Adequate debridement and prophylactic antibiotics keep infection rates down between 2 and 9%.

Any bone may be affected, and symptoms may be vague and non-specific. Osteomyelitis secondary to diabetes-related chronic foot ulcers might develop in 33–66% of patients.

Chronic osteomyelitis

Failure to eradicate primary or secondary osteomyelitis results in chronic symptomatic infection. Most cases result from compound fracture, and an estimated 5% of open fractures are complicated

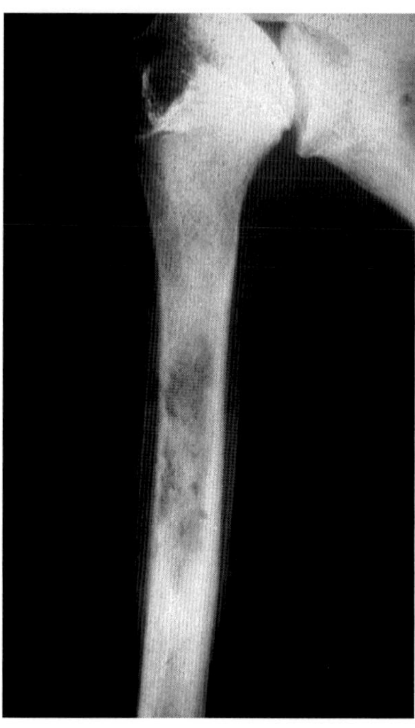

Figure 41.17 Plain radiograph of a humerus, showing lytic lesion in the diaphysis with perioneal reactions and causing osteomyelitis.

Box 41.5 Hormones that influence calcium metabolism

- 1,25-dihydroxy vitamin D increases intestinal absorption of vitamin D and augments the parathyroid hormone recruitment of osteoclasts, which then resorb bone.
- Parathyroid hormone responds to low ionic calcium levels by stimulating calcium retention (and phosphate excretion) by the kidneys, and indirectly promotes intestinal absorption of calcium and bone resorption.
- Calcitonin decreases both the number and activity of osteoclasts, primarily decreasing bone resorption (and increasing bone formation transiently).
- Oestrogen and progesterone influence bone mass; oestrogen appears to inhibit bone resorption and oestrogen receptors are present in osteoblast-like cells.
- Glucocorticoids impair osteoblast activity and decrease bone formation; calcium excretion is increased and gut absorption decreased, leading to hypocalcaemia (which induces secondary hyperparathyroidism).
- Thyroid hormone induces a net loss of bone, which may be partially reversed by oestrogen.

by chronic osteomyelitis. The characteristic feature is the persistence of micro-organisms, harboured and protected by necrotic bone. Patients have intermittent episodes of pain and systemic symptoms that may be separated by months or years. Recurrent infection may result in spread through overlying soft tissue and production of a sinus tract from bone to skin. Sequestra and pus may drain through these sinus tracts during bouts of active inflammation. Rare complications of chronic osteomyelitis include the development of squamous cell carcinoma in sinus tracts and amyloidosis.

METABOLIC BONE DISEASE

Metabolic bone diseases result from disordered bone turnover under the influence of chemical imbalances in the body. The chemicals include hormones, vitamins, minerals and other factors that alter the bone constituents of calcium and inorganic matrix. Metabolic bone disease almost always results in reduced bone mass (osteopenia) and a tendency to fracture spontaneously or with minimal trauma. Therefore although treatment for the underlying disease is in the realm of the endocrinologist, the patient may present first to the orthopaedic surgeon (Box 41.5).

There are three main categories of disease: those related to endocrine abnormalities, particularly those involved in calcium homeostasis (parathyroid hormone and vitamin D; Fig. 41.18); those unrelated to endocrine abnormalities, such as age-related osteoporosis; and osteopenia related to disuse.

The usual biopsy for the investigation of metabolic bone disease is a needle biopsy taken from the anterior iliac crest.

To investigate metabolic bone disease, a patient is given two doses of demeclocycline 10–14 days apart before bone biopsy, because mineralization lags behind osteoid formation by about 10 days (Fig. 41.19). The specimen must not be decalcified and needs to be embedded in resin to cut sections. Special stains are then used to demonstrate osteoid or uncalcified bone matrix (Fig. 41.20). Histomorphometry is the quantitative analysis of undecalcified bone.

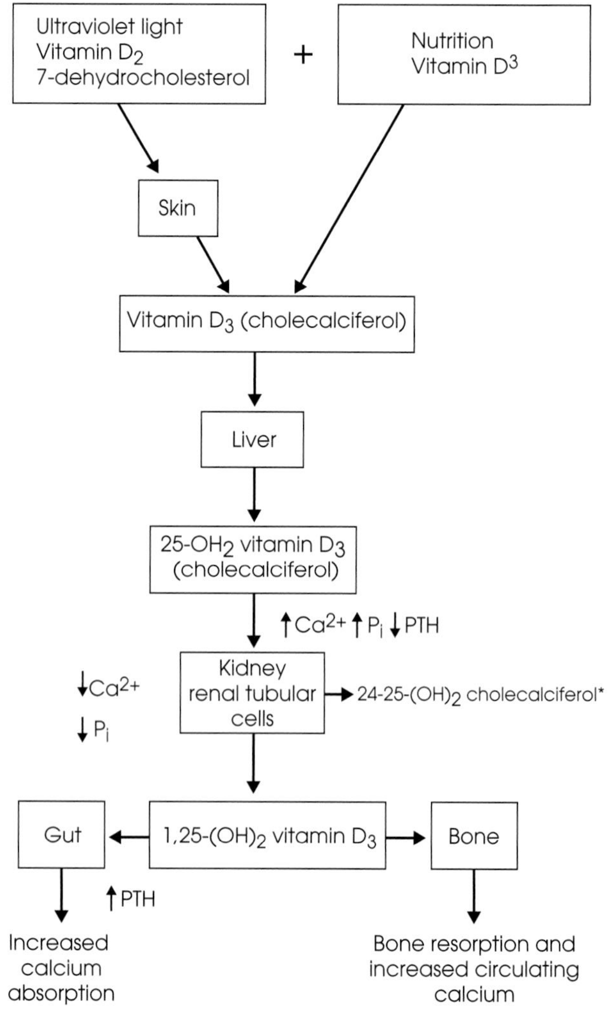

Figure 41.18 The metabolic pathway of vitamin D. P_i, inorganic phosphate; PTH, parathyroid hormone. 24–25-$(OH)_2$ cholecalciferol is the inactive form of vitamin D.

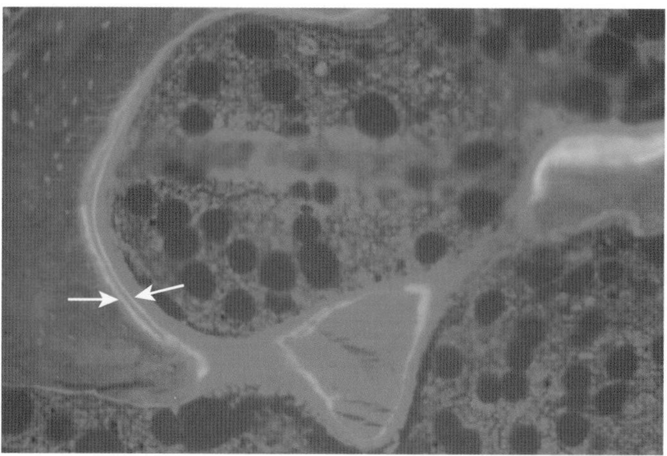

Figure 41.19 Section of normal bone after tetracycline labelling viewed at high power under fluorescent light showing double 'tramlines' indicating newly formed bone on the surface.

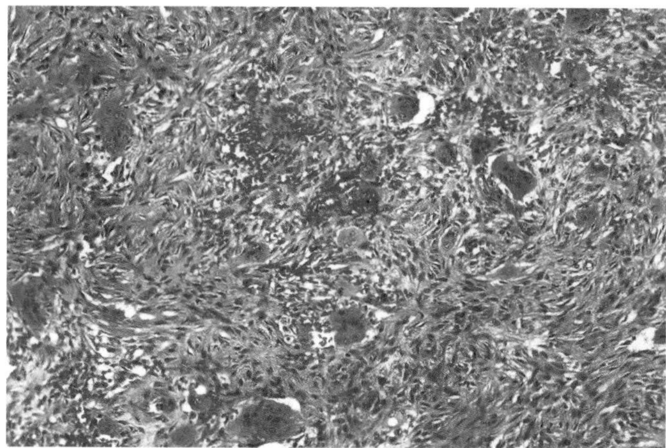

Figure 41.21 Medium-power haematoxylin and eosin-stained section of a brown tumour, showing numerous giant cells on a background of spindle cells in a richly vascular stroma.

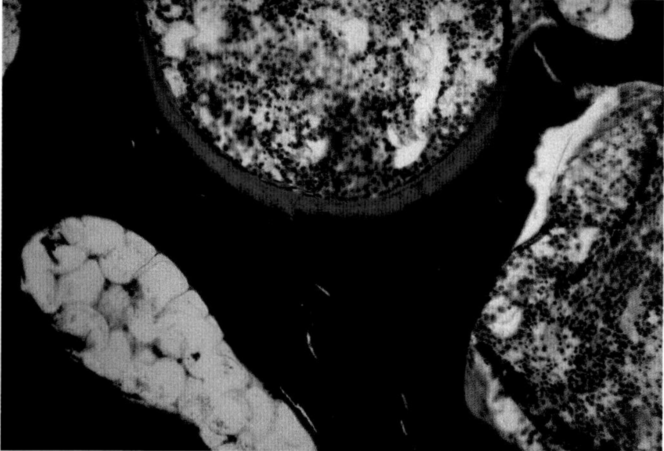

Figure 41.20 Medium-power view of normal undecalcified bone, stained green with Goldner's method, showing a thin rim of osteoid (orange) on the surface.

Hyper- and hypoparathyroidism

Hyperparathyroidism is caused by excess secretion of parathyroid hormone by the parathyroid glands, and the overall effects on bone, kidney and intestine result in hypercalcaemia. There is associated hypophosphataemia and increased excretion of calcium and phosphorus in urine. The detection of the disorder increased in the 1970s with the advent in clinical chemistry laboratories of the autoanalyser, which automatically screened serum calcium levels. Historically, hyperparathyroidism was a rare disease associated with florid skeletal complications of massive bone decalcification and fibrosis (osteitis fibrosa cystica). The incidence today is as many as one in 500 persons, and skeletal manifestations are seen in less than 5%. Many patients may have gone undiagnosed in their lifetime.

Hyperparathyroidism may be primary or secondary. The majority of cases of primary hyperparathyroidism (85–90%) result from a benign tumour or adenoma of one of the four parathyroid glands. It may occur at any age but is most common in the sixth decade. There is a female predominance (ratio 3:1), so the majority of patients are postmenopausal women. Most patients are asymptomatic but there may be vague symptoms of fatigue and muscle weakness. When the disease is more advanced there are symptoms related to the target organ, most commonly nephrolithiasis (20%) and more rarely nephrocalcinosis, and in the gastrointestinal tract peptic ulcer disease and pancreatitis. There may also be psychological disturbances.

The most characteristic skeletal changes associated with hyperparathroidism are seen in plain radiographs of the hand. There is subperiosteal bone erosion seen in the tufts of the distal phalanges or along the ulnar border of the proximal phalanges. These changes are detectable in about 17% of patients. The skull may show granular mottling. Localized lytic lesions, known as brown tumours, caused by intense bone resorption are rarely seen in primary hyperparathyroidism and are more often associated with severe secondary disease (Fig. 41.21). Bone densitometry studies are more sensitive and detect demineralization of predominantly cortical bone in up to 50% of patients.

Aetiology

Most cases of primary hyperparathyroidism (85–90%) are associated with a benign parathyroid adenoma in one of the parathyroid glands. The next most common cause is chief cell hyperplasia, which affects all four parathyroid glands and may be asymmetrical. The hypercalcaemia is less marked in cases of chief cell hyperplasia.

Secondary hyperparathyroidism

Chronic renal insufficiency, vitamin D deficiency and malabsorption may increase parathyroid hormone secretion sufficiently to produce marked skeletal changes. The renal insufficiency causes reduced urinary phosphate excretion, elevation of serum phosphate, and depression of serum calcium levels. In turn, there is hyperplasia of parathyroid glands and excess parathyroid hormone secretion. Under the influence of parathyroid hormone there is increased osteoclast activation, increased resorption of calcium by the renal tubule, increased synthesis of dihydroxycholecalciferol (1,25-$(OH)_2$ vitamin D) by kidney, and increased resorption of calcium from gut.

Histology

The biopsies are best evaluated with histomorphometric techniques. The hallmark of the disease is increased osteoclast activity and bone resorption, the so-called 'high turnover state', eventually resulting in progressive bone demineralization and fibrosis. Histomorphometry demonstrates increased bone resorption surfaces and osteoid surfaces. In hyperparathyroidism, bone resorption equals bone formation and there is preservation of trabecular bone architecture, but most patients show loss of cortical bone with reduced thickness and increased porosity seen with histomorphometric techniques. The more advanced cases may show features of tunnelling resorption, where the centre of the bony trabecula is being eroded because the osteoclast cannot digest the thick layer of osteoid on the surface. There may also be paratrabecular fibrosis and increased woven bone formation. Focal haemorrhage and aggregates of osteoclast giant cells constitute the brown tumour of hyperparathyroidism. Haemorrhage and necrosis may result in cyst formation.

Renal osteodystrophy, progressive bone disease associated with chronic renal failure, was rare prior to the use of dialysis. The principal cause is hyperphosphataemia that causes decreased serum calcium. The pathological effects are mainly secondary to hyperparathyroidism, although a marked increase in unmineralized matrix also presents; this is probably because hyperphosphataemia indirectly reduces synthesis of 1,25-$(OH)_2$ vitamin D, which in turns reduces calcium absorption from the gut. Fifty-four per cent show features of hyperparathyroidism alone, while 34% show features of both hyperparathyroidism and osteomalacia.

Osteoporosis

Osteoporosis (Fig. 41.22) is a general term for a symptomatic decrease in bone mass. Bone is normal in quality but reduced in quantity (density). The condition results when increased osteoclastic activity exceeds osteoblastic activity.

Three categories of the disease are recognized: primary, secondary and idiopathic. Primary osteoporosis is a generalized reduction in bone mass associated with increasing age. It is associated with bone loss that begins in middle age and continues until death. Maximum bone density is in the third decade, and the rate of loss averages 0.7% per year. A subset of patients in this category are postmenopausal women in whom dramatic bone loss associated with decreased oestrogen is superimposed on the effects of ageing. The decreased oestrogen associated with the menopause is thought to result in increased levels of interleukin-1, which subsequently causes increased interleukin-6 release by osteoblasts; this activates osteoclasts.

Osteoporosis can be secondary to drugs or systemic disease, for example corticosteroid therapy, Cushing's disease, hyperparathyroidism or primary amenorrhoea. It may be localized, for example following immobilization post fracture, or adjacent to a rheumatoid joint.

Rarely, young adults or even children may become osteoporotic, and if this occurs in the absence of endocrine abnormality or predisposing factors the disorder is called idiopathic. The greatest loss is in the spine and femoral neck.

OSTEOMALACIA

Mineralization of bone and cartilage requires sufficient serum calcium and serum phosphorus; a deficiency in either results in defective bone mineralization. The resulting diseases are known as rickets and osteomalacia (or 'soft bones'; Fig. 41.23). Rickets is a disease of children, results from defective mineralization of the growth plate, and is associated with growth retardation and deformity. Osteomalacia can affect adults or children and is characterized by weak bones caused by the lack of mineralization of surface osteoid.

These conditions are classified into two types depending on the abnormality: first, deficiency of vitamin D, and second, deficiency of phosphate (PO_4^-). Deficiency may result from a myriad of causes, including congenital defects affecting synthesis of vitamin D itself or synthesis of receptors for vitamin D, inadequate diet, malabsorption, lack of exposure to sunlight, chronic liver disease, chronic renal disease and anticonvulsant therapy. The sequelae is of bone pain, fracture, proximal weakness and bone deformity. Childhood rickets is now rare in developed countries; however, adult osteomalacia is not uncommon. The reason is related to increased longevity, with associated problems in old age of decreased exposure to sunlight, impaired synthesis of vitamin D, and inadequate diet. Gastrointestinal surgery and subsequent malabsorption is common in developed countries and some drugs cause osteomalacia.

As well as affecting the elderly, osteomalacia is associated with certain ethnic and dietary customs. Women who follow the custom of purdah and cover the entire body, preventing exposure to sunlight, may develop osteomalacia. Consumption of large quantities of chapatti flour in India and Pakistan is associated with osteomalacia because the flour contains chemicals that bind calcium and inhibit absorption of calcium.

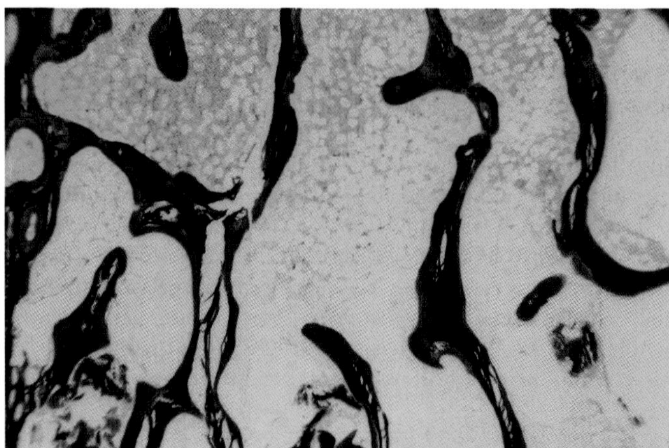

Figure 41.22 Low-power view of undecalcified osteoporotic bone and marrow stained using Goldner's method. The trabeculae are thin and show normal mineralization (green) and a thin layer of osteoid (orange) on the surface.

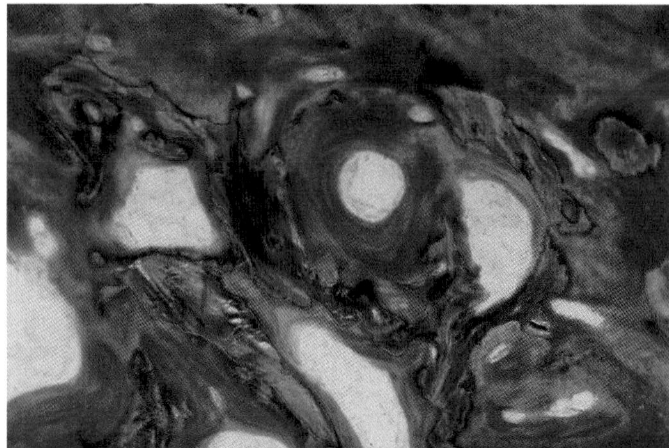

Figure 41.23 Medium-power view of undecalcified bone, stained using Goldner's method, from a patient with osteomalacia. The normally mineralized bone is scanty (green) and there is abundant osteoid (orange) bone.

Clinical features

Osteomalacia may be asymptomatic but most patients complain of vague muscular aches and pains and/or bone pain or tenderness. The serum biochemical profile is characteristic. Calcium level is normal or low, there is elevated parathyroid hormone, raised alkaline phosphatase and low vitamin D. The low serum calcium distinguishes the disorder from hyperparathyroidism. However, not all patients show the characteristic blood profile. Radiographic studies characteristically show reduced bone density, and there may be symmetrical, linear, horizontal stress fractures known as Looser's zones (Fig. 41.24). These Looser's zones may be seen in only 18% of patients with osteomalacia (Fig. 41.25). Diagnosis is made via the histomorphometric analysis of an undecalcified bone biopsy. The positive biopsy will show increased total osteoid thickness and broad, ill-defined tetracycline label, which is narrow and crisp on normal bone. There is demonstrable low mineralization and low bone formation rate. The disease is usually treated with vitamin D therapy with or without calcium supplements.

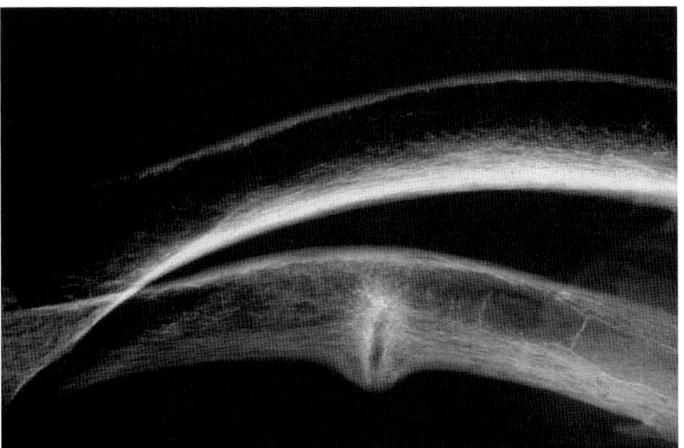

Figure 41.24 Plain radiograph of forearm bones, showing bowing and a horizontal linear lucency or Looser's zone.

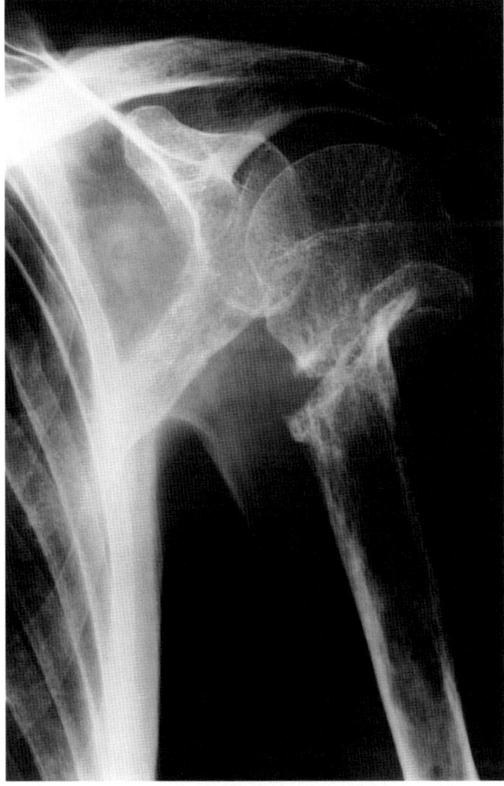

Figure 41.25 Osteomalacia fracture of the proximal humerus.

Oncogenic osteomalacia

Certain soft tissue and bone tumours are associated with osteomalacia. These lesions are thought to secrete phosphatonin, which reduces phosphate resorption and inhibits vitamin D synthesis by the kidneys. Polyostotic fibrous dysplasia, neurofibromatosis and metastatic prostate carcinoma may also cause osteomalacia. Stress fractures are common in these patients. Blood analysis shows normal serum parathyroid hormone, low 1,25-$(OH)_2$ vitamin D and normal 25-(OH) vitamin D. The symptoms resolve after complete removal of the lesion.

PAGET'S DISEASE

Paget's disease of bone is a focal disorder of bone turnover, structure and architecture that is common in middle-aged and elderly persons. It is the second most common metabolic bone disease in the UK after osteoporosis. It is only rarely diagnosed before the age of 40 years but the incidence increases rapidly with age. The estimated prevalence is estimated at 5% of those aged 55 years and over to 10% in patients aged 95 years. There appears to be a slight male predominance. There has been an apparent decrease in the incidence and severity of Paget's disease over the past two decades. The reason for the decline is uncertain, but it suggests there may be an environmental factor causing the disease.

Pathology

Paget's disease results in focal increased bone resorption by osteoclasts, associated with a marked osteoblast response resulting in abundant new bone formation and increased vascularity. The new bone may be of the woven or lamellar type but with abnormal spatial orientation and structural organization. This renders the new bone weaker and less resistant to deformation. The affected bone becomes enlarged, which suggests that there is abnormal bone remodelling. The effect of biomechanical forces on the abnormal bone accounts for the clinical symptoms and complications associated with Paget's disease.

The exact aetiology remains uncertain. Paramyxoviral-like inclusions have been found in osteoclasts from pagetic bone, and infection by the measles or canine distemper virus has been implicated. The virus is thought to increase osteoclast activity and bone resorption by inducing interleukin-6. However, no viral material has yet been isolated and this theory remains unproved.

Thirty to forty per cent of patients with Paget's disease have an affected first-degree relative. Several studies have shown an autosomal dominant pattern of inheritance. Possible gene loci on chromosomes 2, 5, 6, 9, 10 and 18 have been identified by linkage analysis. The receptor activator of nuclear factor-κB gene (*RANK*) and its ligand (*RANKL*) are members of the tumour necrosis superfamily and have been shown to be essential for osteoclast formation. The *RANK* gene has been mapped to chromosome 18, and mutations within this gene have been shown to segregate with Paget's disease in one family. Genetic screening of sporadic cases of Paget's disease has not, however, demonstrated *RANK* mutations, and Paget's disease has not been associated with polymorphisms at this gene locus.[11]

The histological appearance of Paget's disease is variable and depends on disease activity. It is effectively divided into three stages: osteolytic, osteolytic–osteosclerotic, and quiescent osteosclerotic. Macroscopically, the affected bone is thickened and coarsened. In places the bone may be compacted, with a pumice-like architecture, and there may be obliteration of the corticomedullary junction.

In active disease the microscopic features are difficult to distinguish from hyperparathyroidism. There is marked osteoclast resorption and increased osteoblastic activity, evidenced by the deposition of new bone. The marrow is fibrotic and there is chronic inflammation (Fig. 41.26). In the more quiescent stages there is less osteoclastic activity and fibrosis. Osseous tissue is more prominent, which shows a characteristic mosaic pattern with prominent irregular cement lines.

Clinical features

There is a wide spectrum of disease from asymptomatic to life-threatening. The majority of cases are asymptomatic, and are diagnosed as a result of high serum alkaline phosphatase with normal calcium and phosphate levels or when imaging demonstrates characteristic bone changes. The severity of the symptoms is dependent on disease activity and the site affected. Any bone may be affected but the most common sites are pelvis, femur, lumbar spine, skull and tibia. The disease is mostly polyostotic but a single bone is affected in 15% of patients.

Complications are numerous and arise as a result of local and systemic effects. Local effects include bone pain, enlargement and deformity; secondary osteoarthritis; and sometimes dental abnormalities. Deafness, hydrocephalus, and nerve root or spinal cord compression may occur. There may be pathological fracture, and 1% of patients develop a primary bone sarcoma in an affected site. Systemic manifestations of the disease include high-output cardiac failure secondary to increased vascularity, hypercalcaemia and/or hypercalciuria associated with immobility, secondary hyperparathyroidism and increased risk of vertebral fracture.

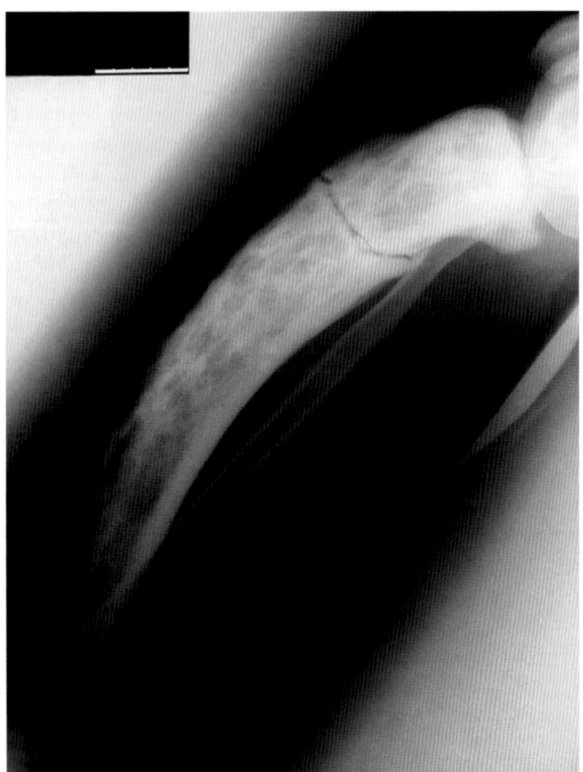

Figure 41.26 Paget's disease of tibia showing bowing of the bone and proximal fracture.

Most patients present with pain thought to be due to bone enlargement and stretching of the periosteum and increased vascularity. Fracture usually occurs with minimal trauma and in sites under high mechanical stress. The majority occur in the subtrochanteric region or shaft of femur, and the proximal tibia (upper third) is less commonly involved (Fig. 41.26). Immobilization causes increased bone loss and should be avoided. Sudden onset of pain in pagetic bone may be indicative of malignancy. Other signs of malignancy are rapid swelling and a rise in serum alkaline phosphatase. Sarcomas associated with Paget's disease are difficult to treat and have a poor prognosis.

Treatment is aimed at relieving symptoms, suppression of abnormal osteoclast activity, and control of bone turnover. Drug therapy includes the use of calcitonin and bisphosphonates. Surgery may be necessary for patients with severe complications and most commonly involves joint arthroplasty. All patients with Paget's disease are best treated at specialist centres.[12]

OSTEOPETROSIS

Osteopetrosis is a genetic disorder that is mentioned here because it results in decreased osteoclast activity and radiodense bones. The control of osteoclast differentiation and activity is multifactorial. It depends on the competence of haematopoietic stem cells as well as cell–cell and cell–matrix signals. The disease varies in severity depending on the cause of the reduced osteoclast function. In some cases numerous osteoclasts may develop, but their function is impaired and they are unable to resorb bone. In other cases they are markedly reduced in number.

There are at least nine forms of the disease, ranging from a mild autosomal dominant form of the disease to a severe autosomal recessive form. The latter is associated with severe pancytopenia, hepatosplenomegaly, blindness, deafness and hydrocephaly. The genetics of osteopetrosis are poorly understood in all but one of the phenotypes. Mutations in multiple genes including c-*src* and c-*fos* have been implicated. In some phenotypes there is a defect in osteoblasts that are unable to synthesize the cytokine macrophage colony factor, which is important in the stimulation of osteoclast differentiation.

The presence of the viral protein reverse transcriptase in some patients is suggestive that viral infection may play a role. There is a form of the disease that is associated with renal tubular acidosis. Affected persons carry a mutation that results in very low levels of carbonic anhydrase II, which is necessary for bone resorption. These patients have cerebral calcification that may result in mental retardation.

Clinical presentation

Symptoms relate to the lack of bone resorption and resulting disorder of bone architecture. The bones are very dense but

REFERENCES

11. Williams CJ. Curr Opin Rheumatol 2003; 15: 326–331
12. Keen RW. Hosp Med 2003; 64: 230–232

fragile, and fractures are common. Obliteration of the marrow causes anaemia, and narrowing of the foramina in the skull causes cranial nerve compression and palsies. Osteopetrosis patients are prone to infection, and the underlying immunological disorder may be related to the defect that causes impaired osteoclast function. There may be growth retardation, and radiologically the bones show diffuse symmetrical sclerosis. Transverse metaphyseal sclerotic bands may be seen in the long bones. In severe forms there may be widening of the bones in the diametaphyseal regions, giving the appearance of an Erlenmeyer flask.

Pathology

The most marked histological changes are seen in the vicinity of the metaphysis. The metaphysis and the diaphysis are filled with broad streams of cartilage encased by bone. The bone is usually woven type, and in severe cases the marrow cavity is obliterated by unresorbed bone. Where osteoclasts are present, they are not sitting in Howship's lacunae and ultrastructural analysis shows an absent ruffled border.

Treatment

Bone marrow transplant has been used to treat severe forms of the disease but matched donors may be found for only 40% of patients. Up to 45% of patients survive this treatment, and of these only 50% may be cured. Some patients (up to 25%) may respond to high doses of calcitriol, and interferon-alpha may be useful in some patients because it stimulates osteoclast superoxide.

BONE NECROSIS

Impairment of blood supply to bone, resulting in bone death, may be due to a number of mechanisms. These include infection, neoplasms, trauma and primary vascular occlusion. Infiltrative processes such as infection and neoplasms destroy or compress vessels, and so interrupt the vascular supply to isolated portions of cortical or medullary bone. Peculiarities of blood supply render several bones susceptible to infarction following trauma. For example, necrosis of the femoral head may complicate fracture of the neck of the femur in up to 75% of cases. The talus and carpal navicular bones are also prone to focal infarction following fracture. Severe trauma to a joint may result in portions of cartilage and bone being sheared off, a condition known as osteochondritis dissecans.

Primary vascular occlusion also results in segmental bone death known as osteonecrosis or bone infarction. Segmental infarction also occurs in other organs, such as the heart or brain, and the underlying pathology is usually vascular occlusion secondary to atherosclerosis. In contrast, bone infarction results from intravascular coagulation in small arterioles or venules.

Pathogenesis

Osteonecrosis may affect any bone at any site. The subchondral areas are sites of predilection because there is little or no collateral circulation. The femoral head is most commonly affected but the proximal humerus, scaphoid, distal femur and talus are also often affected.

Patients usually have an underlying systemic disease that may result in focal intravascular coagulation blocking terminal arterioles or postsinusoidal venules. The predisposing factors include vascular stasis, fat embolism or blood hypercoagulability. Conditions associated with bone infarction and necrosis include steroid therapy, alcohol abuse, sickle cell disease, decompression sickness and Gaucher's disease. Hyperlipidaemia and bone necrosis are also associated with pancreatitis and pregnancy. Smoking is a risk factor, with smokers having a four- to fivefold increased risk of osteonecrosis.

Histology

Bone necrosis is recognized histologically by empty osteocyte lacunae and fat necrosis of adjacent marrow. The features take some time to manifest themselves. Marrow takes about 5 days to show necrosis, and osteocyte drop-out may take between 2 days and 4 weeks to become apparent. The histological interpretation is further compromised by the fact that the bone and marrow cells show different sensitivity to anoxia. Haemopoietic cells are most sensitive and will undergo irreversible damage after only 6 h, bone cells may survive between 6 h and 2 days, and marrow survives from 2 to 5 days.

A reparative reaction may be seen after a few weeks. The necrotic marrow is replaced by granulation tissue and collagenized fibrous tissue. New bone is deposited on the surface of pre-existing necrotic bone and viable new bone is formed in resorption cavities within the necrotic bone, a process called creeping substitution. The necrotic subchondral bone may fracture and collapse, causing the articular cartilage to separate from the bone. This corresponds to the crescent sign seen radiologically.

Clinical features

Symptoms depend on the site of infarction and the resulting alteration of the affected bone structure. Medullary infarcts occur frequently in association with sickle cell disease and steroid therapy, and are usually asymptomatic. Occasionally patients present with pain, and radiological signs may be misdiagnosed as infection or neoplasia. Treatment depends on the aetiology, extent and stage of the lesion. Avoidance of predisposing factors such as alcohol, steroid therapy and trauma is recommended.

OSTEONECROSIS OF THE FEMORAL HEAD

Osteonecrosis of the femoral head deserves special mention because it is a common condition occurring most frequently in

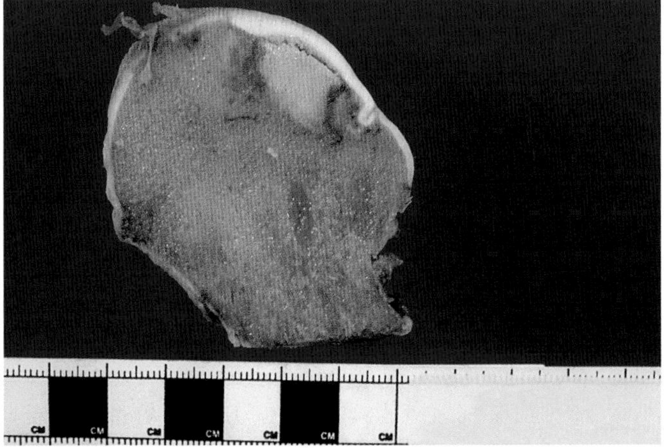

Figure 41.27 Macroscopic picture of a bisected femoral head with features of avascular necrosis. The cartilage is lifting from subchondral bone, and there is a well-delineated pale zone of infarction.

relatively young patients (20–40 years) and causes significant disability. Treatment usually requires total hip arthroplasty. Surgery may not be successful because the prosthesis tends to fail earlier and may not last the patient's lifetime.

The disorder is classified into five stages (0–IV) by Ficat according to pain symptomatology and radiological appearances on plain films and MRI. Most patients do not present until stage III. Surgery is delayed until later stages, when there is evidence of structural failure of the femoral head. Because 50% of patients with osteonecrosis of the femoral head will develop bilateral disease there should be close follow-up with examination of the contralateral hip (Fig. 41.27).

Sarcomas of bone and soft tissue

42

Justin Cobb

INTRODUCTION

This chapter aims to give the essentials of sarcoma management. The pathological processes behind the different tumours are described, followed by the diagnostic algorithms necessary for safe early management. The differential diagnoses are discussed before brief sections on the methods of diagnosis, treatment, complications and outcomes. Where references are given, they are usually to a single paper of an author whose other publications will guide the interested student. In this field as in many others, the questions raised in recent research far outstrip the answers, so many of the classifications and names given to tumours today will be supplanted by more informed and intelligent diagnoses tomorrow. For this reason above all, the doctor caring for a patient with a sarcoma must be sure that the clinical picture fits with the diagnosis, and not embark on treatment of any kind without establishing the confidence with which the diagnosis is made.

BASIC SCIENCE SUMMARY

Sarcomas are malignant tumours arising in connective tissue. They may develop anywhere, but there is a bimodal distribution with primary bone tumours occurring mainly in childhood, adolescence and young adulthood, while soft tissue tumours are commoner in older people (Table 42.1).

For most doctors, the lesion that they encounter should simply be ascribed a tissue type and a clinical grade. The fine print of the diagnosis will be negotiated with the pathologist, but informed by the clinician's knowledge of the history and findings on examination.

DIAGNOSIS

There are three different presentations that need to be discussed:

- a swelling,
- pain, and
- a chance finding on radiograph.

A SWELLING

A patient presenting with a swelling may have a sarcoma. The clinical criteria on which they may be assessed for probability of malignancy are five, as discussed below.

Length of history

A long history suggests a benign process, while a short one implies that there may be a neoplastic process present. Other pathologies are not excluded in this circumstance of course.

Pain

Any lesion that has given rise to pain or even discomfort should be considered potentially malignant until proved otherwise.

Depth

A superficial lesion in the subcutaneous tissues may be well examined clinically, and confidently assessed for size and mobility. In lesions deep to the deep fascia, these factors are much less easily assessable clinically so caution should be used.

Size

Lesions that are small are less likely to be malignant. In the London Bone and Soft Tissue Service we use the cut-off point of 5 cm. Lesions less than this size are considered to be 'small'. The factor of course is a continuous variable, however, and judgement must be used in the interpretation.

Mobility

If a lesion is in one compartment and not fixed to others, it is considered more likely to be benign. If a lesion is in the soft tissue of the thigh, but cannot be moved on the femur, then clinically it involves two compartments. The same applies if the lesion is now fixed to the subcutaneous tissues. An osteochondroma pushing into the muscles of the calf will not cause any loss of function in that muscle group, so cannot be considered to be within it. An osteosarcoma may well invade a muscle and cause significant weakness or restriction of excursion of that muscle, causing stiffness without joint involvement.

Use of these factors

If these five factors are borne in mind when assessing any mass that presents to clinic, the following strategy is suggested.

If all factors are benign, this implies that the lesion has been there for a long time, is painless, superficial, small and mobile. The lesion is clinically benign. It may be managed by excision biopsy, usually under local anaesthesia, or by review. If it has grown on review after 3 months, then it should be excised while it is still easy to do so. If not, the patient may be left to perform their own surveillance if they do not wish it to be removed, on the understanding that they should return if it enlarges.

Should any of the five factors not be benign, then more information is required before a safe management strategy can be implemented. This will first involve two steps:

1. Imaging: a plain radiograph may suffice in bony lesions but is rarely sufficient in soft tissue lesions, and axial imaging with ultrasound, CT or MRI will be needed in most cases to confirm the site and dimensions, and relation to other structures, MRI being the imaging investigation of choice.

Table 42.1 Tumours of four principle grades

Grade	Bone	Cartilage	Connective tissue	Fat	Muscle
Very low	Osteoid osteoma	Osteochondroma	–	Lipoma	–
Low	Osteoclastoma	Grade 0.5 chondrosarcoma	–	Intramuscular lipoma	–
Intermediate	Parosteal osteosarcoma, adamantinoma	Well-differentiated chondrosarcoma	Musculoaponeurotic fibromatosis	Myxoid liposarcoma	–
High	Osteosarcoma, Ewing's sarcoma, malignant fibrous histiocytoma, bone lymphoma	Dedifferentiated chondrosarcoma	Synovial sarcoma	Dedifferentiated liposarcoma	Embryonal or alveolar rhabdomyosarcoma

2. Biopsy: an image-guided biopsy will enable the pathologist to provide a good estimate of the grade of the lesion 95% of the time.[1] This in turn will enable the surgeon to advise the patient on the right strategy in relation to the lesion.

PAIN

From this discussion it will be appreciated that benign tumours should not cause pain, while malignant tumours may hurt because they are growing, even if only slowly. This is not a rule, but many patients with a sarcoma will have attended several doctors or other allied professionals complaining of pain before diagnosis.[2] The pattern of pain in many people is indistinct, and sarcomas are rare, but it is the duty of attending doctors to provide a safe surveillance to exclude a sarcoma when a patient presents with musculoskeletal pain. Safe practice will always exclude an occult sarcoma if the following algorithm is followed:

- History: if the pain has any features that are worrying, specifically night pain or pain that is unrelieved by rest, then a sarcoma cannot be excluded.
- Examination: if there is any tenderness, swelling or wasting then a sarcoma cannot be excluded.
- Investigation: an erythrocyte sedimentation rate and bony chemistry will help exclude occult metastatic disease and multiple myeloma.

An ultrasound of the suspicious area if a mass is not easily discernible in soft tissue, or an X-ray if it is bony, will document the presence and size of a lesion. Ultrasound is preferable to MRI or CT if the diagnosis of a soft tissue mass is unclear, because it is interactive. The patient is able to guide the ultrasonographer and help demonstrate the site of the tenderness or swelling. If nothing is found, an isotope bone scan provides a good screening test for occult lesions elsewhere in the skeleton. Should there be nothing to find on examination, screening bloods and X-ray, or ultrasound, the chances of missing an occult sarcoma are extremely low. The average delay of 4 months in patients reaching an appropriate treatment centre would be obliterated if this algorithm had been followed.

A CHANCE FINDING ON A RADIOGRAPH

As many as 5% of referrals to sarcoma units come as the result of chance findings on radiographs of a lesion in a bone adjacent to the area of interest. If they are asymptomatic – and this is sometimes difficult to establish in the presence of local joint pain – then they are extremely unlikely to be anything more than a very low-grade lesion indeed. A repeat X-ray taken 3–6 months later may be a satisfactory way to manage the problem if there are no radiographic features of concern.

Imaging

Each potential sarcoma will have an optimal imaging strategy. The images will be used for several purposes:

- diagnosis;
- staging;
- baseline for response to treatment;
- planning of resection; and
- planning of reconstruction.

At the entry point into the healthcare system, a minimum of time and effort should be spent on imaging. This will prevent needless waste of time and resources.[3] The precise images needed for these several purposes will be determined best by the treating doctors. The doctor at point of diagnosis should perform only those images needed to confirm the clinical suspicion. Often a plain radiograph or ultrasound will suffice. But axial imaging with a CT or MRI scan will help in the confidence with which a patient is referred. The imaging for the other purposes, on which important decisions will rest, are best organized by the doctors who will be responsible for carrying out the treatment on which those decisions are based.

Plain radiography

These films will provide most of the information needed to classify bony lesions. The features that the doctor requesting a plain film should consider are discussed below.

Site of the lesion within the bone

Some lesions occur only at certain sites. A lytic lesion in the epiphysis of an adolescent will probably be a chondroblastoma, for instance. Osteosarcoma will usually develop in the metaphysis, while Ewing's sarcoma more commonly develops in the axial or paraxial skeleton or diaphysis of long bones. A destructive lesion that extends right beneath the joint surface may be a giant cell tumour or osteoclastoma (Fig. 42.1).

Effect of the lesion on the bone

The extent of replacement of the inside of a bone should be documented, and most importantly whether it has crossed from inside the bone to outside, or vice versa.

REFERENCES

1. Dupuy DE et al. Am J Roentgenol 1998; 171: 759–762
2. Wurtz LD, Peabody TD, Simon MA. J Bone Joint Surg Am 1999; 81: 317–325
3. Ashwood N et al. Ann R Coll Surg Engl 2003; 85: 272–276

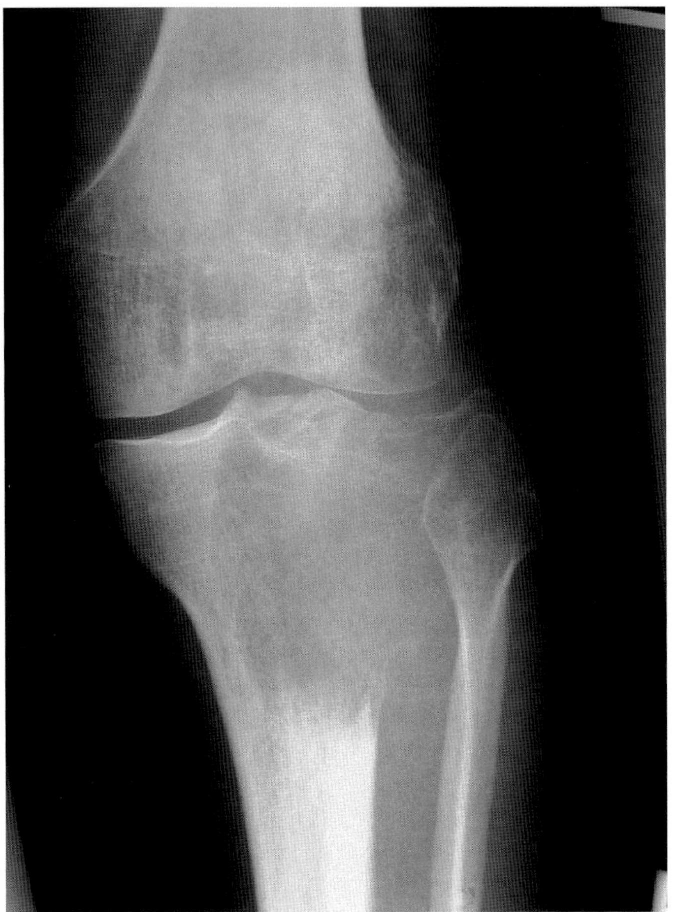

Figure 42.1 Giant cell tumour of the proximal tibia in a 30-year-old man.

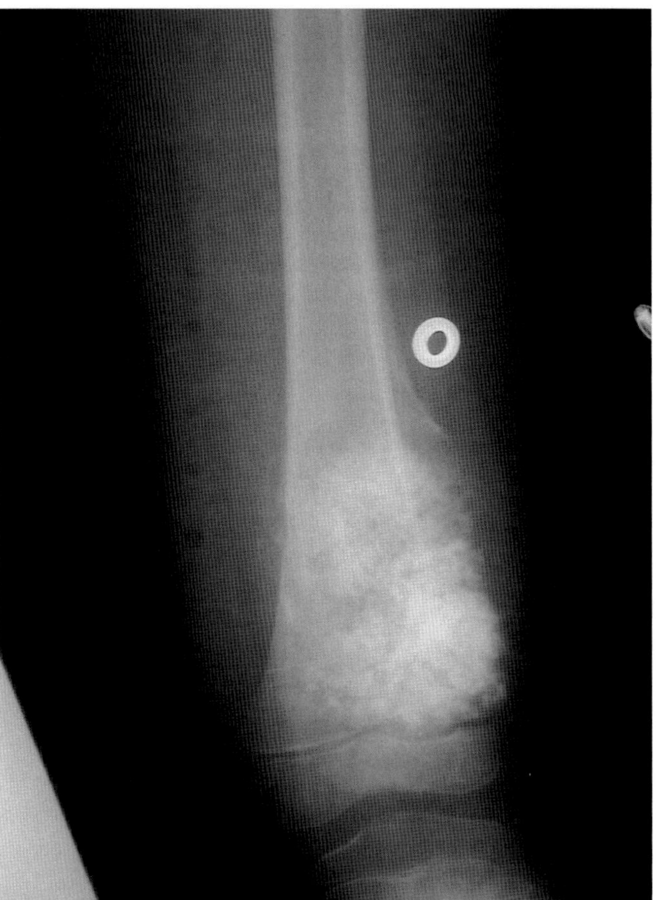

Figure 42.2 Osteosarcoma of the distal femur with Codman's triangle above it.

REACTION BY THE BONE TO THE LESION

Bone responds to changes in strain and stress according to Wolf's Law. When a lesion is of very low grade, the surrounding bone will retain the normal strength of the bone by surrounding the lesion with a rim of normal bone. On the other hand, a rapidly growing lesion will not permit any surrounding reaction of bone to the lesion, and the boundary between lesion and bone is less well defined. Radiologists refer to this boundary as the zone of transition. A well-defined sclerotic line, as typified in a Brodie's abscess, suggests an entirely benign process, while a wide zone of transition, in which it is difficult to be sure where the lesion begins and ends, suggests a malignant tumour. Outside the bone, the maximum extent of the tumour will be demonstrated by the surrounding cortex and periosteum. A high-grade bone tumour breaking out of the bone will lift the periosteum, and layers of bone will be laid down, forming a Codman's triangle of normal reactive bone indicating the boundary of normal bone at that time (Fig. 42.2).

In a low-grade lesion such as an osteochondroma, there may be a wide stalk of entirely normal reactive bone. It is not lesional, and only needs to be considered insofar as it may contribute to the abnormal shape of the bone after removal of the lesion. This same phenomenon may occur in high-grade lesions, causing the 'onion skinning' around a Ewing's sarcoma, as shown in Fig. 42.3.

ANY CHARACTERISTICS OF THE LESION

On plain radiograph some lesions have characteristic appearances. An osteochondroma will show the calcified head, an osteosarcoma may show malignant bone formation, and a chondrosarcoma may have popcorn-like calcification within it and be best assessed using plain films over MRI (Fig. 42.4).[4]

CT and MRI scanning

All lesions in which malignancy is suspected should have axial imaging performed. Depending on access, both MRI and CT may be used because they provide different information to the surgeon. Both these imaging modalities have the huge drawback of having edges: the radiographer will limit the extent of the investigation depending on the request of the doctor. Usually the treating centre will have to repeat these tests, so no time should be wasted waiting for them at the referring hospital.

Magnetic resonance imaging is the imaging modality of choice for the sarcoma surgeon when trying to determine the extent of the tumour in soft tissue, and in particular the intra-medullary extent.[5] It is not particularly sensitive when dealing with the relationship between an expanding tumour and the neurovascular bundles close to it, and even experienced radiologists will be unable to detect the mobile and uninvolved layers of adventitia between a tumour and vessels that may appear next to or even invaginated into it.

REFERENCES

4. De Beuckeleer LH et al. Eur J Radiol 1995; 21: 34–40
5. Redmond OM et al. Radiology 1989; 172: 811–815

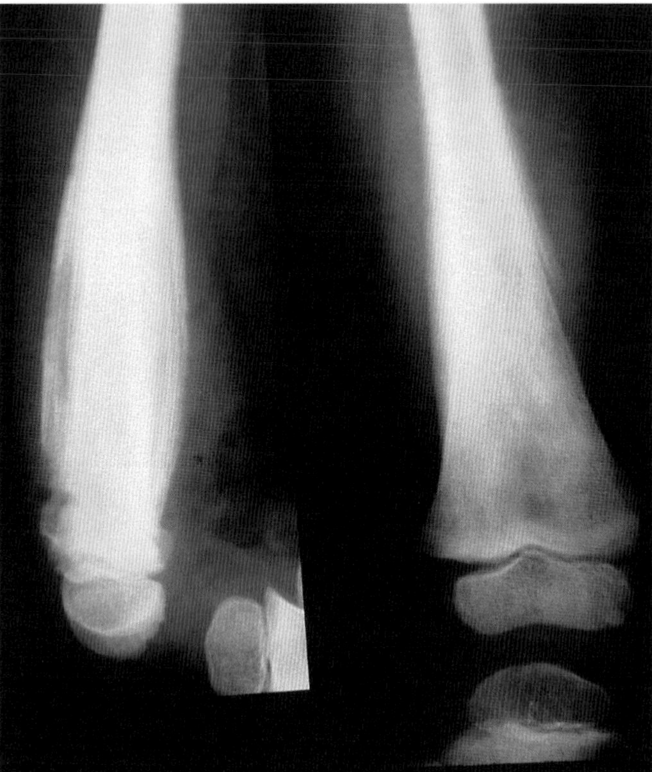

Figure 42.3 Ewing's sarcoma in the distal femur of a 6-year-old. The periosteal reaction is obvious.

CT scanning

This is needed to determine the presence or absence of pulmonary metastases. It is also of great help in the planning of complex resection and reconstruction using three-dimensional modelling for sarcomas of the pelvis.

Nuclear Medicine

Bony metastases, whether local ones (described as skip lesions) or distant ones in sites remote from the primary, occur in 10% of patients,[6,7] sometimes in the absence of pulmonary disease. Technetium scanning of the entire body is therefore mandatory in the work-up of bone tumours. Soft tissue tumours are much less likely to metastasize to bone and may not be shown up on bone scan, so the yield of bone scans in their staging is much lower. In the London Bone and Soft Tissue Sarcoma Service, the policy is to perform bone scans on all high-grade soft tissue sarcomas, because it does act as a baseline. Some sarcomas, notably myxoid liposarcomas, do metastasize to bone in a substantial number of cases, making this policy defendable.

Positron emission tomography scanning now exists as a service rather than a research tool. It is not yet of proven benefit in sarcoma management because the sensitivity and specificity are still far from established.

Biopsy

The biopsy of lesions in the musculoskeletal system should be a straightforward matter, and is only of concern for the surgeon who will manage the patient going forward. Surgeons who will refer the patient on if the pathology confirms malignancy should seriously consider referral prebiopsy. There are four approaches to obtaining biopsy material, as discussed below.

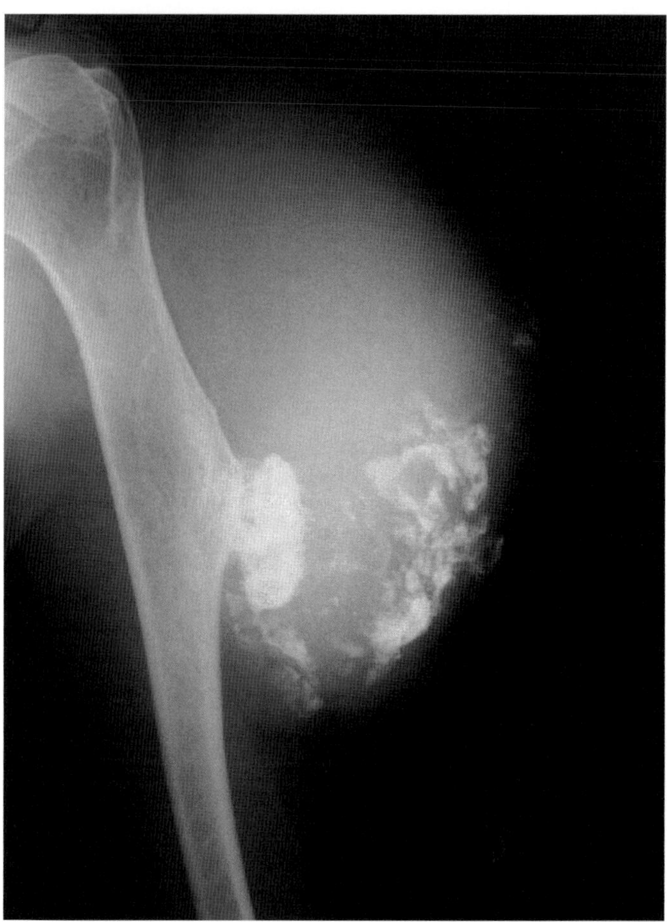

Figure 42.4 Chondrosarcoma arising from an osteochondroma of the proximal humerus.

Excision biopsy

Excision biopsy should be reserved for lesions that are entirely benign in nature.

Incision biopsy

While still favoured by some centres around the world, this is not the first line for the majority of sarcoma specialists. There is no place for incision biopsy or exploration of a suspicious lesion by anyone other than a surgeon who is actively managing malignancy.[8] The impact of ill-placed scars on patients' outcome has been repeatedly stated, and yet amputations continue to be necessary simply to gain clearance of tissue contaminated by a surgeon exploring a tumour through an ill-considered incision (Fig. 42.5).[9]

REFERENCES

6. Wuisman P, Enneking WF. J Bone Joint Surg Am 1990; 72: 60–68
7. Enneking WF, Kagan A. Clin Orthop 1975; 111: 33–41
8. Mankin HJ, Lange TA, Spanier SS. J Bone Joint Surg Am 1982; 64: 1121–1127
9. Mankin HJ, Mankin CJ, Simon MA. J Bone Joint Surg Am 1996; 78: 656–663

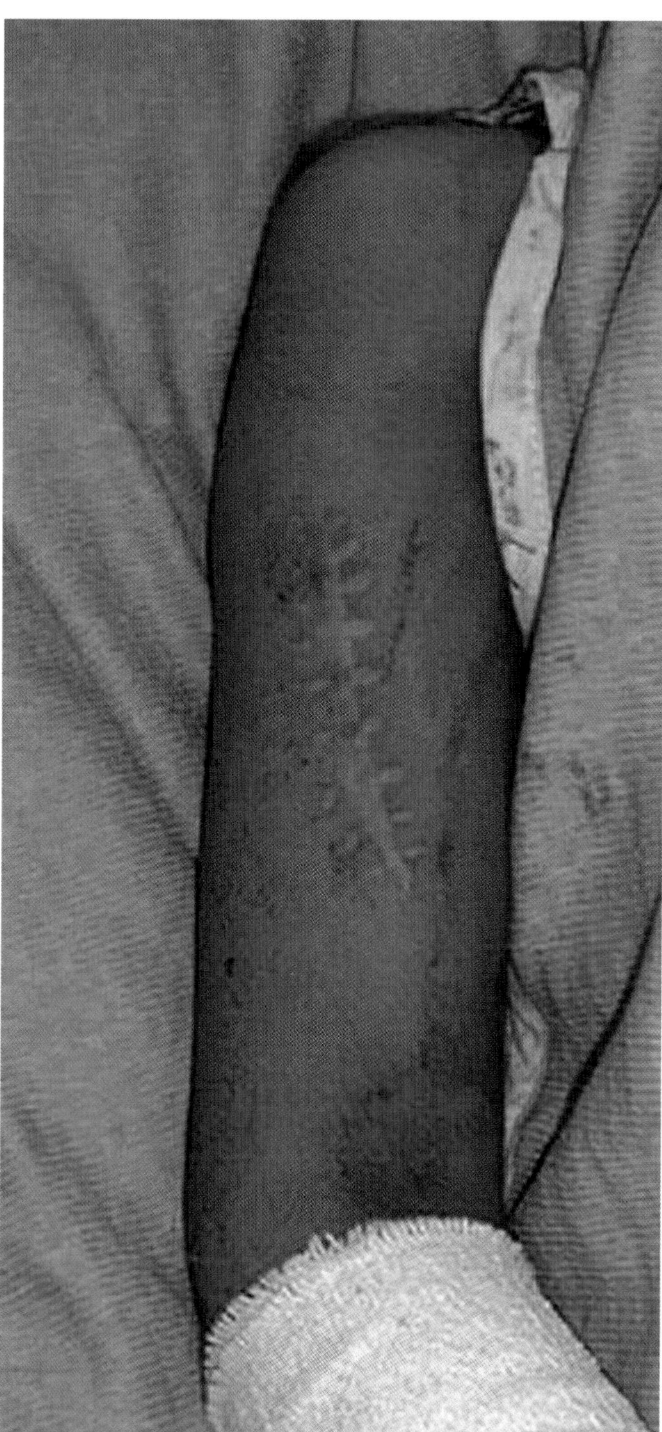

Figure 42.5 An open biopsy scar that will need damaging re-excision.

Image-guided needle biopsy

Needle biopsy, whether by 'tru-cut' of a soft tissue lesion or core biopsy of a bony lesion, is now the biopsy method of choice.[10] It is best performed with image guidance. This may be simply using ultrasound for soft tissue lesions or fluoroscopy for lesions in the limbs. Computerized tomography or MRI guidance will be used for choice in deeper-situated lesions. It need hardly be said that the reason for using guidance is to maximize the hit rate of the procedure.[11] Using these techniques, sensitivity and specificity of over 95% is realistic.[12]

Fine-needle aspiration cytology

Fine-needle aspiration cytology has attraction in a large sarcoma unit with a pathologist in clinic who will perform the cytology on the spot.[13] This is less accurate than core biopsy.[14]

Pathology

Our understanding of the pathological processes involved in malignant transformation remains incomplete in sarcoma, as in other areas of oncology. In chondrosarcoma, within a single lesion there may be several stages of dedifferentiation present, with varying degrees of cellular atypia and polyploidy suggesting a stepwise increase in malignancy. The molecular biology of some sarcomas has become better established: synovial sarcoma is now defined by mutation of a gene involved in apoptosis. There are two common mutations: SSX1, with a 5-year survival rate of 50%, and SSX2, with a 5-year survival rate of 75%.[15,16] Ewing's sarcoma has also been characterized: a translocation between the p arm of chromosomes 11 and 22 causes the tumour. This gene has a fusion transcript, EWS–FLY1, which can be identified in the tumour.[17] It can also be looked for in peripheral blood or bone marrow. Other tumours, such as osteosarcoma, are not characterized by a single mutation.[18]

Staging

Before concluding the assessment of a tumour, its extent should be defined by staging. This will include both the extent to which local structures are involved, and the number and site of any distant metastases (Table 42.2).

The local extent of a tumour

The local extent of a tumour is defined by its size within its host compartment and the number of other anatomical structures it has involved. Initially the local stage was described as bounded by the cortex.[20] The periosteum can now be imaged, and may be considered a more substantial boundary to a compartment.[21] An osteosarcoma of 80 mm in diameter arising in the proximal tibia may have pushed the periosteum away from the bone, but still remains essentially within the bony compartment. A similar-sized tumour developing within the fibula will have surrounded nerves and vessels, and infiltrated several muscles. Its local stage is therefore considerably more advanced and more damaging, and the life expectancy is substantially worsened (Fig. 42.6).[21]

REFERENCES

10. Stoker DJ, Cobb JP, Pringle JA. J Bone Joint Surg Br 1991; 73: 498–500
11. Heare TC, Enneking WF, Heare MM. Orthop Clin North Am 1989; 20: 273–285
12. Anderson MW et al. Am J Roentgenol 1999; 173: 1663–1671
13. Kilpatrick SE et al. Am J Clin Pathol 2001; 115: 59–68
14. Heslin MJ et al. Ann Surg Oncol 1997; 4: 425–431
15. Ladanyi M et al. Cancer Res 2002; 62: 135–140
16. Skytting B. Acta Orthop Scand Suppl 2000; 291: 1–28
17. Papadopoulos N et al. In Vivo 2001; 15: 359–364
18. Ragland BD et al. Lab Invest 2002; 82: 365–373
19. Enneking WF, Spanier SS, Goodman MA. J Bone Joint Surg Am 1980; 62: 1027–1030
20. Enneking WF, Spanier SS, Goodman MA. Clin Orthop 1980; 153: 106–120
21. Spanier SS, Shuster JJ, Vander Griend RA. J Bone Joint Surg Am 1990; 72: 643–653

Table 42.2 Tumour staging

Stage	Extent	Histology	Example
1a	Within a compartment	Low grade	Endochondroma
1b	Within a compartment	High grade	Intraosseous osteosarcoma
2a	Involving two compartments	Low grade	Parosteal osteosarcoma invading muscle
2b	Involving two compartments	High grade	Conventional osteosarcoma invading muscle, tendon or ligament
3	With metastases	–	–

(After Enneking 1980,[19] with permission)

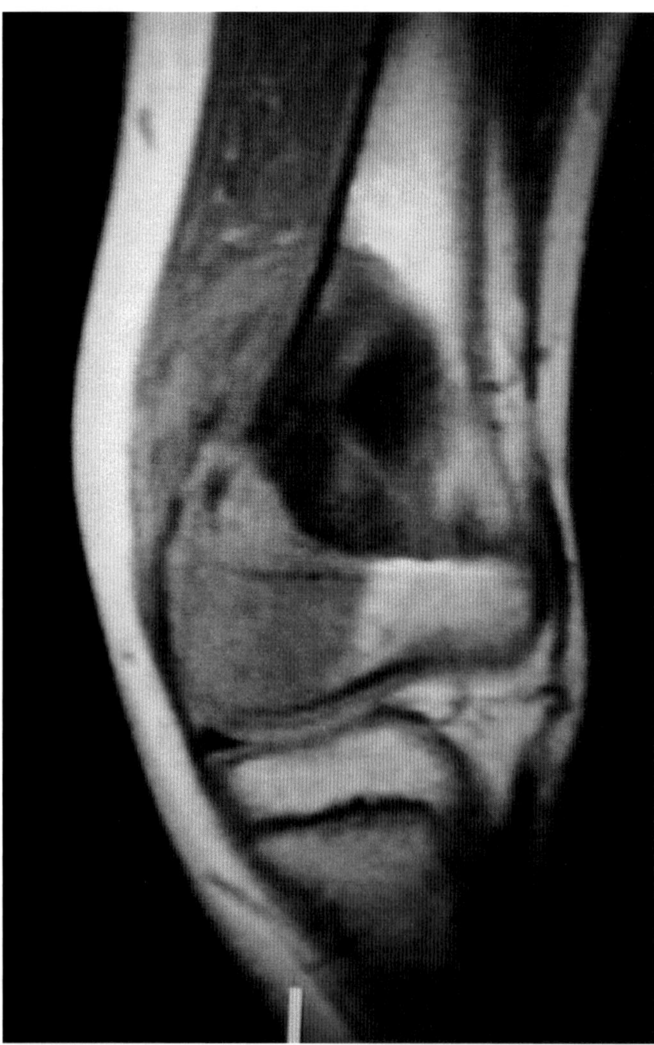

Figure 42.6 An osteosarcoma crossing the distal femoral growth plate and invading the muscle of a 14-year-old.

Distant spread

Distant spread will be documented by a CT scan of the chest and an isotope bone scan, although metastases in the skeleton and soft tissues are not always picked up by these investigations.[22] Positron emission tomography is more sensitive in some tumours,[23] but its place is not yet established in routine use.

Table 42.3 Tumours of four principle grades

Stage	Soft tissue	Bone
1a	Observe or shell out	Observe or ablate intralesionally
1b	Excise	Curette and phenolize or excise
2a	Excise with margin of normal tissue	Excise with margin of normal tissue
2b	Excise with wide margin and consider adjuvant radiotherapy	Excise with wide margin after neoadjuvant chemotherapy

Treatment

Surgical excision is the mainstay of sarcoma management. Small, lower-grade lesions may be treated by intralesional ablation using radiofrequency or laser ablation.[24,25] Giant cell tumours and low-grade intraosseous chondrosarcomas may be treated by curettage alone,[26] but more effectively if an adjuvant such as phenol is used. If the lesion is malignant, then a complete margin of normal tissue surrounding it should be removed with the specimen.[27] The operation should be planned to allow the surgeon to gain sufficient access to permit this excision. Lower-grade lesions may be shelled out or treated intralesionally.[26]

When a lesion is known to be malignant, the aim of the surgeon should be to excise the tumour complete with a cuff of normal tissue. If this result is obtained there should be a negligible chance of local relapse.[28] A contaminated field, even if re-excised, is less satisfactory.[29] There is abundant evidence that an inadequate margin predisposes to a higher local recurrence rate,[30] and many authors also feel that local relapse actually reduces survival,[31] while hard evidence for this remains elusive (Table 42.3).[32]

REFERENCES

22. Khurana JS et al. Clin Orthop 1989; 243: 204–207
23. Franzius C et al. Eur J Nucl Med 2000; 27: 1305–1311
24. Witt JD et al. J Bone Joint Surg Br 2000; 82: 1125–1128
25. Dewar JA, Duncan W. Clin Radiol 1985; 36: 629–632
26. Bauer HC et al. Acta Orthop Scand 1995; 66: 283–288
27. Bergh P et al. Cancer 2001; 91: 1201–1212
28. Campanacci M et al. J Bone Joint Surg Br 1984; 66: 313–321
29. Virkus WW et al. Clin Orthop 2002; 397: 89–94
30. Sheth DS et al. Cancer 1996; 78: 745–750
31. Lindner NJ et al. Clin Orthop 1999; 358: 83–89
32. Bacci G et al. Acta Orthop Scand 1998; 69: 230–236

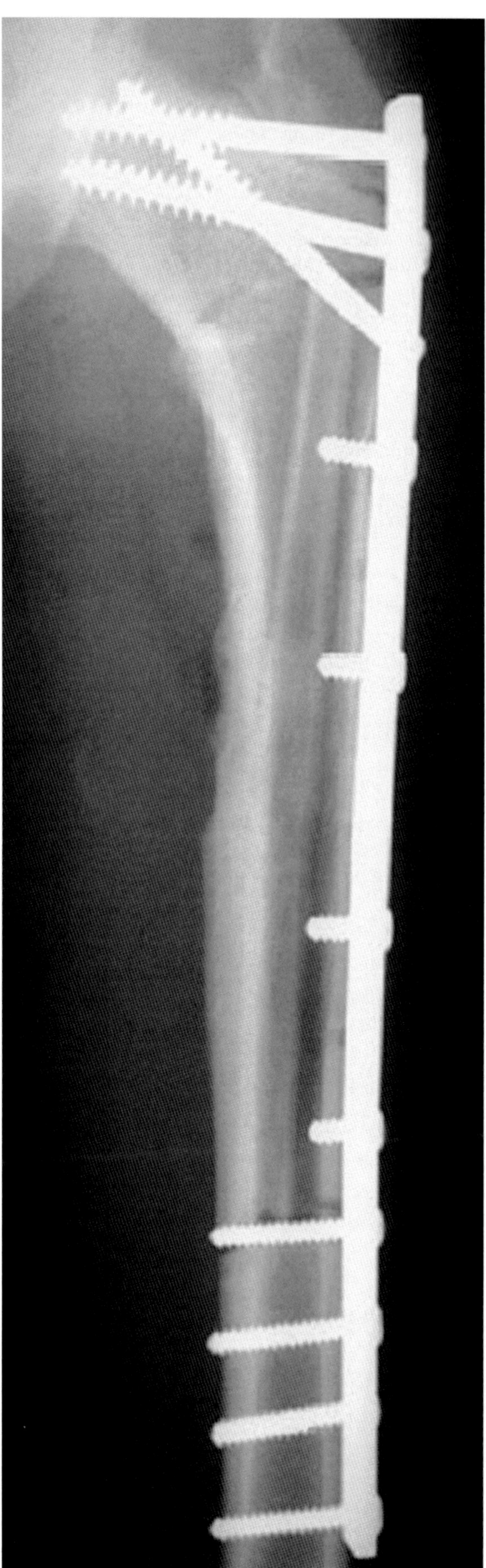

Figure 42.7 Vascularized fibula and irradiated autograft reconstruction for Ewing's sarcoma in a 12-year-old boy.

Chemotherapy

High-grade sarcomas of bone are responsive to chemotherapy, and so patients are routinely offered preoperative combination chemotherapy. A good response, in addition to improving outcome, will make the surgery significantly easier by reducing the tumour bulk.[32] This will be demonstrated by the post-chemotherapy, preoperative MRI scan, when the final decisions regarding surgical margins are made.[33] Soft tissue sarcomas are not so responsive, and so chemotherapy is not offered to all patients with high-grade lesions

Radiotherapy

Soft tissue sarcomas are less responsive to chemotherapy, and so patients will more often be offered adjuvant radiotherapy to improve local disease control.[25,34] Radiotherapy is also helpful if the surgical margins have been compromised, reducing local recurrence rates from 40 to 20%.[35]

Reconstruction

Soft tissue sarcomas

Following resection of a soft tissue tumour, the muscle defect is usually left alone but tendon transfers may be effected. Occasionally an arthrodesis is necessary, but only for secondary instability.

Bone tumours

The segmental defect left following the resection of a bone tumour may be filled in a variety of ways. Biological reconstructions offer the theoretical advantage of leaving the patient with a living segment after healing of the graft. Several centres have popularized the use of vascularized fibulas inserted into an allograft or irradiated autograft (Fig. 42.7).[36]

Increasingly in the developed world the use of massive replacement, even in the young, is accepted as having lower complication rates.[37] It has the attraction of also permitting expansion of the prosthesis to compensate for growth of the other limb in children and adolescents.[38] If the tumour has spared the last 25 mm or so of bone, joint-sparing massive replacement is now the treatment of choice (Fig. 42.8).

Other options, such as resection arthrodesis,[39] remain an option but reoperation rates for complications such as graft failure are as high as 50% in most series.[40,41] Rotationplasty is still recommended by some surgeons for young males.[42–44] It has the

REFERENCES

33. Hogeboom WR et al. Eur J Surg Oncol 1989; 15: 424–430
34. Le Pechoux C et al. Int J Radiat Oncol Biol Phys 1999; 44: 879–886
35. Zlotecki RA et al. Int J Radiat Oncol Biol Phys 2002; 54: 177–181
36. Manfrini M et al. Clin Orthop 1999; 358: 111–119
37. Unwin PS, Cobb JP, Walker PS. J Arthroplasty 1993; 8: 259–268
38. Grimer RJ et al. J Bone Joint Surg Br 1999; 81: 488–494
39. Wada T et al. J Bone Joint Surg Br 2000; 82: 489–493
40. Enneking WF, Shirley PD. J Bone Joint Surg Am 1977; 59: 223–236
41. Gottsauner-Wolf F et al. J Bone Joint Surg Am 1991; 73: 1365–1375
42. Winkelmann WW. J Bone Joint Surg Am 2000; 82: 814–828
43. Winkelmann WW. J Bone Joint Surg Am 1986; 68: 362–369
44. Winkelmann WW. J Bone Joint Surg Br 1991; 73: 697

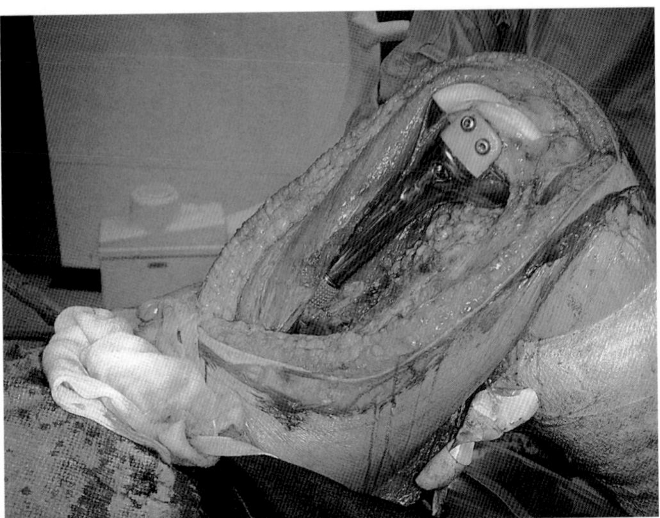

Figure 42.8 Expandable distal femoral joint-sparing prosthesis for osteosarcoma in a 13-year-old boy.

advantage of converting an above-knee amputation into a below-knee one, at no detectable extra cost to the body image.[45] Most surgeons worldwide do not offer this operation because of the psychological morbidity in the early stages, but those who do are increasingly reserving it for revision of failed massive replacement in survivors of sarcoma.[46]

Complications

The complications of surgery for sarcoma are of three main types:

1. oncological,
2. biological, and
3. mechanical.

Oncological

Local relapse is a bad prognostic sign but is usually caused by skip metastases rather than poor surgery. Following limb salvage for a high-grade tumour, the local recurrence rate should be under 10% in the limbs but over 20% in the pelvis.[47]

Biological

Infection of prosthetic devices is a major issue following reconstruction, with 2% of distal femoral replacements becoming infected and requiring massive revision.[37] In the proximal tibia, where wound healing is a problem, this figure rises to over 10%.[38] After radiotherapy, early wound breakdown is an issue in up to 15%, and late fractures of long bones in the radiation field occur in 10% by 5 years.[48] For allograft reconstructions, bony remodelling continues for many years.[49] Non-union rates are high, at 30% or more.[50]

Mechanical

Massive implants fail, like ordinary hips and knee replacements. If patients avoid the early problems of infection and local recurrence, a massive replacement may last for a long time, with a 50% chance of avoiding revision within 20 years,[37] with smaller resections faring better.[51]

Clinical outcome

The relapse rates for sarcomas depend principally on the tumour itself. High-grade tumours, such as osteosarcoma and Ewing's sarcoma, have a 5-year survival rate of about 65% with multiagent chemotherapy in combination with surgery to remove the primary lesion.[31,52,53] The surgical strategy may affect local recurrence rate but is rarely an independent factor determining outcome, because 95% of patients who do relapse locally will also have systemic relapse.[54] The quality of life after limb salvage surgery depends principally on the extent of the resection. The method of reconstruction is a matter of choice dictated not only by the prevailing economic and technical environment but also on social pressures, which for instance may reject or embrace the functionality of a rotationplasty.[45]

REFERENCES

45. Rodl RW et al. Acta Orthop Scand 2002; 73: 85–88
46. Hillmann A et al. Arch Orthop Trauma Surg 2000; 120: 555–558
47. Evans R et al. Int J Radiat Oncol Biol Phys 1985; 11: 129–136
48. Brant TA et al. Int J Radiat Oncol Biol Phys 1990; 19: 899–906
49. Enneking WF, Campanacci DA. J Bone Joint Surg Am 2001; 83A: 971–986
50. Hazan EJ et al. Clin Orthop 2001; 385: 176–181
51. Unwin PS et al. J Bone Joint Surg Br 1996; 78: 5–13
52. Carrie C et al. Med Pediatr Oncol 1999; 33: 444–449
53. Hoffmann C et al. Cancer 1999; 85: 869–877
54. Bacci G et al. Oncol Rep 2000; 7: 1129–1133

The peripheral nerves

43

David T. Gault, Paul J. Smith

INTRODUCTION

Peripheral nerves are subject to a variety of insults. Leprosy is the commonest cause of loss of sensation worldwide;[1] in the UK, troublesome neuropathy is more likely to result from diabetes and peripheral vascular disease.[2] Progressive loss of function with pain as a complication of radiotherapy for malignant disease is greatly underestimated, probably because the onset of symptoms may be delayed for several years.

More acute damage to peripheral nerves usually results from direct mechanical injury; that caused by sharp objects is the most common. Other types of open injury include crush and gunshot wounds, and compound fractures. Displaced fractures of the long bones or dislocation of the joints also cause closed injuries. Ruptures of the brachial and lumbosacral plexuses or their branches occur when traction forces are applied to the limbs in high-velocity road traffic accidents. The radial nerve may be crushed against the humerus by a badly fitted crutch or by the back of a chair over which the arm is draped during a profound, usually intoxicated sleep.[3] A poorly applied splint may contuse the common peroneal nerve against the neck of the fibula, and pressure on an ulnar nerve unprotected during surgery can result in a painful neuritis, or even a nerve palsy.[4]

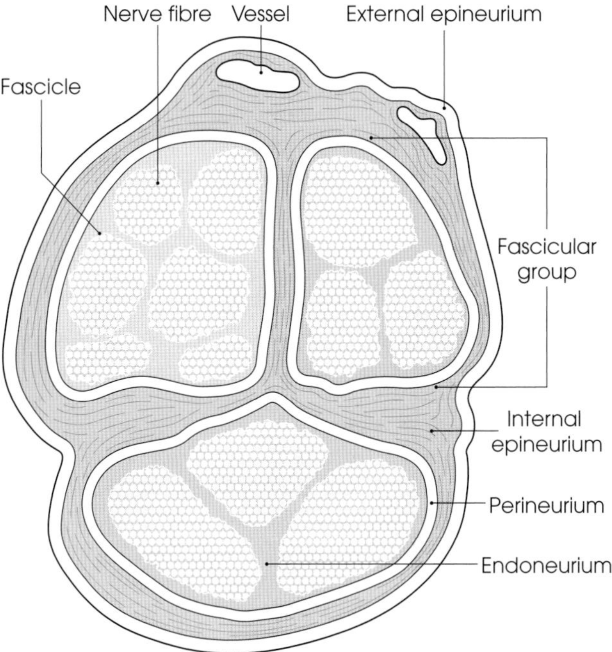

Figure 43.2 Cross-section of a peripheral nerve.

ANATOMY

A sound knowledge of internal topography of peripheral nerves is vital for their successful repair, release and grafting. They emerge from plexuses around the limb roots on which converge nerve roots from several contiguous segments of the spinal cord. As they leave the spinal cord, motor, sensory and sympathetic fibres intermingle and within the peripheral nerves become grouped into bundles or fascicles. Each fascicle may contain motor, sensory or sympathetic elements. There are a variable number of fascicles within a nerve, and their arrangement varies along its course (Fig. 43.1).

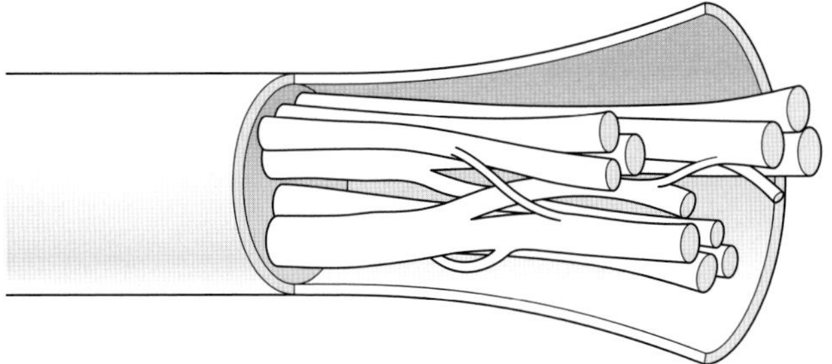

Figure 43.1 The arrangement of the fascicles varies along the course of the nerve within the epineurium.

Packed between the individual nerve fibres within a fascicle is connective tissue called endoneurium (Fig. 43.2). It forms a series of tubes, each occupied by an axon, its Schwann cell sheath and myelin. The endoneurium resists elongation and protects the delicate nerve fibres within it. In a nerve graft, it provides hollow channels down which sprouting axons can grow.

A tough sheath of perineurium surrounds each fascicle. It protects the contents of the endoneural space, acting as a mechanical barrier against trauma, and maintains the intrafascicular pressure so important in promoting proximal-to-distal flow of axoplasm within nerve fibres. The perineurium also acts as a diffusion barrier, protecting the fascicle from a dangerous influx of ions, proteins and other hazardous agents; peripheral nerves can even traverse pyogenic foci without their function being in any way influenced.[5] When the perineural sheath is

REFERENCES

1. Antia NH, Dastur DK (eds). Symposium on Leprosy. Bombay University Press, Bombay, 1967
2. Dyke PJ, Thomas PK, Lambert EH. Peripheral Neuropathy. WB Saunders, Philadelphia, 1983
3. Seddon HJ. Surgical Disorders of the Peripheral Nerves. Churchill Livingstone, Edinburgh, 1975
4. Bonney GJ. Bone Joint Surg 1986; 68B: 9–13
5. Lundborg G. Nerve Injury and Repair. Churchill Livingstone, Edinburgh, 1988

disrupted, however, the conduction properties of the contained nerve fibres are impaired, a point to remember when releasing a nerve trapped in scar tissue.

The outermost layer of connective tissue is the epineurium; it can account for between 25 and 75% of the cross-sectional area of a peripheral nerve and is often more abundant around joints. The epineurium binds the fascicles loosely together and is condensed at the surface of the nerve to form a distinct investing sheath.

Surrounding it is a layer of loose areolar tissue that allows the nerve to glide within its bed. In addition, the fascicles can slide within the deeper layers of the epineurium. The greatest excursion of peripheral nerves during motion occurs at the wrist, where the median and ulnar nerves travel up to 15 mm during a full range of flexion and extension.[6] If a nerve divided at the wrist is repaired under tension with the wrist flexed, there is little chance that gliding during normal movement will be preserved.

CLASSIFICATION OF NERVE LESIONS

An injured nerve may be completely divided or may simply suffer temporary loss of conduction. The types of nerve injury have been categorized by Seddon,[7] but it is important to appreciate that the demarcation between different types is often not clear-cut, and that many lesions represent intermediate grades of injury.

NEURAPRAXIA

Neurapraxia describes a local conduction block at a discrete site along the course of a nerve, the continuity of which is not disrupted. To the naked eye, the nerve appears normal. There is no degeneration of axoplasm, and if there is any anatomical damage, it is restricted to segmental areas of demyelination.

The impairment of nerve function is often partial. The predominant effect depends on the proportions of motor and sensory fibres in the affected nerve. For example, in radial nerve damage motor impairment predominates, whereas in early carpal tunnel syndrome sensory impairment predominates.

Recovery is eventually full, but its completion may vary from minutes or days to several weeks. Examples of this type of injury are tourniquet palsy and the radial nerve paralysis caused when the arm is draped over the back of a chair during a profound sleep. Pressure on the nerve may lead to ischaemia, with damage of its myelin sheath and local oedema. This usually causes a neurapraxia and recovers within days or weeks. If the pressure is prolonged, it may eventually lead to axonotmesis.

A full recovery still occurs but at a slower rate. In very early nerve entrapment syndromes, the injury is neurapraxia. The diagnosis is made with certainty only when the length of the recovery period is known. The recovery rate and long-term effect are proportional to the duration and severity of the compression force.

Neurapraxia comprises a range of pathological events. Early neurapraxia follows intermittent ischaemic episodes, for example the nocturnal symptoms in carpal tunnel syndrome, which respond to attempts to improve the circulation such as elevation and shaking the hand. More severe compression may lead to swelling of the myelin sheath and intussusception of one sheath within another, producing more severe symptoms such as the permanent numbness seen in severe carpal tunnel syndrome. Prolonged compression may lead to intraneural fibrosis with more severe symptoms such as motor wasting, as seen in the thenar eminence in long-standing cases of carpal tunnel syndrome.

AXONOTMESIS

In axonotmesis the continuity of the axons is disrupted, although the endoneural tubes are still intact. Axonotmesis may result from, for example, a closed stretch injury. The injured nerve recovers once the cause is removed, because its architecture has not been destroyed, and the regenerating neurons are able to traverse an intact scaffold to reach their peripheral connection. The axoplasm and myelin sheath degenerate distal to the level of the lesion; recovery occurs at the classic rate of nerve regeneration (1–1.5 mm/day).[8,9] Tinel's sign develops at the level of injury and advances distally with time. Until recovery in axonotmesis begins, it is clinically and physiologically indistinguishable from neurotmesis.

NEUROTMESIS

In neurotmesis, the nerve is severed or so seriously disorganized that spontaneous regeneration is impossible. If not repaired, it is often complicated by the development of a neuroma at the site of injury.

THE PATHOLOGY OF NERVE DIVISION

Within 4–20 days of acute transection of a peripheral nerve, the central nerve cell body enlarges as a result of increased metabolism.[10] Proteins are manufactured and migrate along the axon to the site of injury, where they are used in repair. The enlargement persists for as long as there is active regeneration of the damaged axon. When conduction is re-established, the cell body slowly returns to a normal size. Within the proximal nerve stump, marked oedema, both intracellular and extracellular, develops within 1 h of nerve division; the cross-sectional area of the nerve increases as much as threefold. The oedema persists for a week or more after the injury and then slowly subsides.

Several days after nerve transection, the axons start to sprout. After clean cuts, this begins a few millimetres proximal to the last intact node of Ranvier, but after blast injuries, the axonal sprout may develop 2–3 cm proximal to the severed end. The budding of the axons occurs concomitantly with the anabolic phase of the cell body in the spinal cord or dorsal ganglion. The axon sprouts attempt to locate and grow down an empty endoneural tube in the distal segment of the injured nerve. When the axon sprouts (filopodia) reach out into an empty space and make no contact, they then withdraw to advance again, seeking an appropriate substrate. By contrast, if they contact the basal lamina of a Schwann cell they attach to this structure and draw the growth cone of the nerve distally.[11]

Separated from their cell body, the neuronal elements in the distal nerve die, Wallerian degeneration. Small segments of axon may survive intact for up to 2 weeks, but the majority are broken down within 1 week by the digestive enzymes they contain. The surrounding myelin fragments are digested by Schwann cells. By

REFERENCES

6. Wilgis EFS, Murphy R. Hand Clin 1987; 2: 761–766
7. Seddon HJ. Brain 1943; 66: 237
8. Seddon HJ, Medawar PB, Smiths H. J Physiol (Lond) 1943; 102: 191–201
9. Sunderland S. Arch Neurol Psychiatry 1947; 58: 1–14, 251–256
10. Lehman RA, Hayer GJ. Brain 1967; 90: 285
11. Letourneau PC. Dev Biol 1983; 95: 212

6 weeks, this natural debridement is complete. The fascicular anatomy persists for a while, but in time the endoneural sheaths shrink and this then minimizes the chances of regeneration.

Timely nerve repair is important if the axons are to reach a muscle in good condition. When muscle cells no longer receive repeated stimuli, they shrink: the endomysium and perimysium thicken, the muscle spindles atrophy, and fibrous tissue forms around the motor endplates. The sooner a nerve re-establishes connection with the muscle cells, the more likely it is that normal function will return. If reinnervation is delayed for 1 year, function will at best be poor. A delay for 2 years allows irreversible changes to take place in the muscle cells, and any hope of return of motor function is then unlikely.[12]

In contrast, the sensory end organs survive without nerve connections, although protective sensibility is the best result that can be achieved after a long delay. The quality of sensation is greatly dependent on the ability of the brain to decode messages from the sensory end organs. These messages are usually altered after nerve repair, and whereas young people can accomplish some natural central reorganization, older people need sensory retraining.[13]

MANIFESTATIONS OF NERVE INJURY

An accurate history and careful clinical examination are very important in the diagnosis of peripheral nerve lesions. The site and extent of a wound hint at the possibility of nerve damage. It is important to remember that after glass injuries, extensive internal damage may have occurred despite a small skin puncture wound. Bleeding from major vessels such as the axillary, brachial or ulnar arteries suggests division of the adjacent nerves.

Nerve injury may produce disturbances of motor, sensory and sudomotor function. When a nerve is completely divided, the muscles no longer contract voluntarily. They become flaccid and wasted, and reflexes disappear. The power of both the prime movers and the synergists must be carefully tested. Examination of muscle power may be difficult because of pain or associated injuries to the skeleton, and the examiner may be fooled by the patient's use of subsidiary muscles and trick movements. Examples of such trick movements are the abduction of the fingers by the extensor muscles in an ulnar nerve palsy, flexion of the knee by gracilis in a sciatic nerve palsy, and extension of the interphalangeal joints by the interossei in a radial nerve palsy.

Certain key muscles should be examined. The power of wrist extension reflects radial nerve function, and crossing of the fingers requires an intact ulnar nerve. The median nerve consistently supplies the abductor pollicis brevis, which can be seen and palpated when the position of the abducted thumb is maintained against resistance.

In nerve compression, the muscles supplied may still function, but weakness is apparent. As axons degenerate, the number of nerve fibres supplying a muscle is reduced and wasting occurs. Weakness can be quantitatively measured, and the degree of wasting should be noted.[14]

A divided nerve may also present with loss of light touch, vibration and pinprick sensation. Some patients with divided nerves can still perceive sensation on pinprick testing: the explanation is controversial. It was thought that when the ends of a divided nerve remained in contact, then for several hours impulses can jump across the gap.[15] This has recently been called into question. Any distortion of sensation rather than complete anaesthesia is the key to diagnosis in the first 24 h. In such circumstances the nerve should be explored and, if it is found to be divided, should be repaired.[15]

It is usual that, after nerve division, complete sensory loss occurs in that nerve's exclusive territory. Surrounding this zone is an intermediate area in which sensation is altered. This zone of hypoaesthesia cannot be demonstrated by routine clinical testing with a needle (which gives only maximal stimulation), but it does show a limited response to light touch.[16] Thus the area where light touch is lost is usually greater than the area where pinprick is diminished, which is in turn less than the area where deep pressure is disturbed.

Disturbance of sympathetic function is an important early feature of nerve damage. Transection of a digital nerve interrupts the nerve fibres to the sweat glands of the fingertips, where the combination of sweat and dermal ridges (fingerprints) is important for grip. When sweating is eliminated, grip is lost, and the plastic casing of a ballpoint pen drawn across the affected digit will slide and slip in comparison with an adjacent normal finger where sweating is preserved. This loss of tactile adherence is a useful sign of nerve transection because it can be elicited in a child or an uncooperative adult.[17] As pinprick testing is both uncomfortable and unreliable, it is best avoided.

As well as sudomotor paralysis, pilomotor paralysis occurs. An absence of tone in the muscles surrounding hair follicles leaves the skin abnormally smooth, and the hairs lack uniform orientation.

Vasomotor disturbance is often apparent. A denervated limb may become blue, cold and oedematous after nerve division. It must, however, be remembered that disuse alone, as seen in hemiplegia, leads to coldness, cyanosis and oedema. Denervated skin does not demonstrate a normal inflammatory response. Both the impairment of the neurogenic inflammatory response to injury and the loss of protective pain sensation may contribute to the development of the slow-healing trophic ulcers often seen after nerve injury.[18]

Nerve compression causes changes in the sensory threshold. A very early lesion may cause a hypersensitive response (hyperpathia); later in the course of nerve compression, the threshold rises and a greater stimulus intensity is required.[19,20] With further compression, nerve fibres are actually damaged. Loss of two-point discrimination is then a sign of decreased innervation density.

As the damaged fibres attempt to regenerate, so Tinel's sign may be detected (a tingle on tapping over the advancing fibres).[21]

REFERENCES

12. Bowden REM, Gutman E. Brain 1944; 67: 273
13. Dellon AL, Curtis RM, Edgerton MT. Plast Reconstr Surg 1974; 53: 297–305
14. MRC Memorandum No. 45: Aids to the Examination of the Peripheral Nervous System. HMSO, London, 1980
15. McAllister RMR, Calder JS. Br J Plast Surg 1995; 48: 384–395
16. Trotter W, Davies HM. J Physiol 1909; 38: 134
17. Harrison SH. Hand 1974; 6: 148–149
18. Parkhouse N, LeQuesne PM. N Engl J Med 1988; 318: 1306–1309
19. Dellon AL. Plast Reconstr Surg 1980; 65: 466–476
20. Dellon AL, Schnieder R, Burke R. Plast Reconstr Surg 1983; 72: 208–216
21. Tinel J. Presse Med 1915; 23: 388

ELECTRICAL ASSESSMENT OF MUSCLE DENERVATION (ELECTROMYOGRAPHY)

Electrical tests are used to detect peripheral nerve damage and to determine the level of the lesion. Information can be obtained by direct nerve stimulation, by detection of the potentials that occur when a nerve and muscle are active, or by measuring nerve conduction velocity. Electrical tests are used to confirm a diagnosis, and they also indicate the rate and completeness of recovery after a nerve injury. They are no substitute for clinical examination but do have the outstanding advantage of being objective, and they do not require the close attention or cooperation of the patient. Conversely, they are time-consuming and sometimes unpleasant for the patient. Another drawback is that many of the changes characteristic of muscle denervation are not present immediately after an injury but take some days to develop.

STIMULATION

For a rapid assessment of a patient with suspected nerve involvement, the simplest form of electrodiagnosis is stimulation of the nerve above and below the site of the suspected lesion. Using bipolar surface electrodes, short pulses (0.1 ms) of current of increasing intensity are applied over the nerve until visible or palpable contractions are elicited in the muscles supplied. The threshold and the nature of the peripheral response are noted and are compared with the normal side.

Stimulation of the nerve above the lesion indicates whether conduction is normal or interrupted. A nerve undergoing Wallerian degeneration becomes unresponsive to stimulation below the lesion after 4 days.[22] In compression syndromes, proximal stimulation may cause the patient to feel discomfort at the site of the nerve compression. Stimulation proximal to the compression may fail to evoke distal motor function, while distal stimulation will normally produce function, hence localizing the problem area.

DETECTION

Normal muscle function is dependent on normal innervation, and thus activity in the motor unit reflects the condition of the motor nerve.[23] A close contact between the recording electrode and the muscle under study is essential to detect contraction in normal muscles or fibrillation potentials in denervated muscles.

Two types of electrodes are available: surface electrodes in the form of a metal cup placed on the skin can record information from superficial muscles, while needle electrodes establish the closest possible contact with muscle fibres and provide more detailed information.

A muscle that is denervated cannot be activated voluntarily. For several days after denervation stimulation of the distal nerve causes contraction, until fragmentation of the axons occurs, losing continuity with the muscle.

From 3 weeks after a nerve injury, there is no response to electrical stimulation of the nerve. Both axons and motor nerve terminals disintegrate, and the muscle fibres themselves are left as the sole excitable element. No longer under the control of the motor nerve, nor synchronized with their neighbours, they become hyperexcitable and begin to fibrillate. This is seen as regular action potentials of low amplitude (20–300 μV) and short duration (0.5–2 ms), with a frequency of 2–20 per second.[22] Thus resting muscle that is normally silent becomes the site of spontaneous activity.[24] Fibrillation persists for many months and shows that the muscle fibres are still alive and in principle capable of being reinnervated. Eventually, however, the fibrillatory activity dies down and the muscle atrophies. Fibrillation is not found after neurapraxia, and if a muscle is partially denervated there is reduced electrical activity on voluntary contraction.

VELOCITY

The time interval between stimulation of the nerve and the detection of a muscle action potential at a distant site can be accurately measured in milliseconds. This total conduction time includes the time taken for the stimulus to evoke the nerve action potential, the propagation time, and the terminal delay for the impulse to cross the motor endplate and excite muscle fibres. By stimulating the nerve at two sites a known distance apart, it is possible to calculate the true nerve conduction velocity. Such studies are of particular value in chronic nerve lesions such as compression. Stimulating the nerve above a compression reveals a prolonged conduction time and reduced muscle action potential amplitude. Stimulating the nerve below the lesion gives a normal response in terms of conduction velocity and muscle action potential. Reverse conduction velocity may be measured by applying a stimulus to a finger and recording the sensory action potentials over the proximal nerve.

Whether or not the conduction is slowed is determined by comparison with standard data. The data relate to the largest calibre and most rapidly conducting α motor nerve fibres. Nerve conduction velocity is influenced by many factors, including the age and temperature of the patient. The mean rate of conduction is of the order of 57 m/s in the median nerve, and this is reduced to 49 m/s in cases of carpal tunnel syndrome.[25] Electromyography is not, however, a cut and dried test, and one report has stressed that patients with normal electrodiagnostic studies but an abnormal clinical evaluation do well after surgical decompression.[26]

TREATMENT OF NERVE INJURIES

To maximize the chances of motor and sensory recovery, the repair of divided nerves and the release of compressed nerves should be performed without delay. Wounds in which an associated nerve injury is suspected should be explored, both to confirm the diagnosis, where this is uncertain, and to repair the nerve. The type of injury gives a clue to the likely amount of recovery that can be expected, and this is important to the surgeon who may need to plan palliative tendon transfers. Skin loss, vascular insufficiency and fractures must be dealt with prior to nerve repair. Such serious injuries do not augur well for the limb as a whole, and the scarred tissues that develop after a compound fracture, missile injury or sepsis interfere with nerve regeneration.

Ideally, the neurorrhaphy should be enveloped in a well-vascularized bed of healthy muscle and fat. Adherence of the repaired nerve to moving tendons or to a cutaneous scar interferes with axonal regrowth and stimulates collagen deposition at

REFERENCES

22. Sunderland S. Nerves and Nerve Injuries. Churchill Livingstone, Edinburgh, 1978
23. Bralliar F. Orthop Clin North Am 1981; 12: 229
24. Raimbault J. Clin Plast Surg 1984; 11: 53–58
25. Thomas P K Neurology 1960; 10: 1045
26. Louis DS, Hawkin FM Orthopedics 1987; 10: 434–436

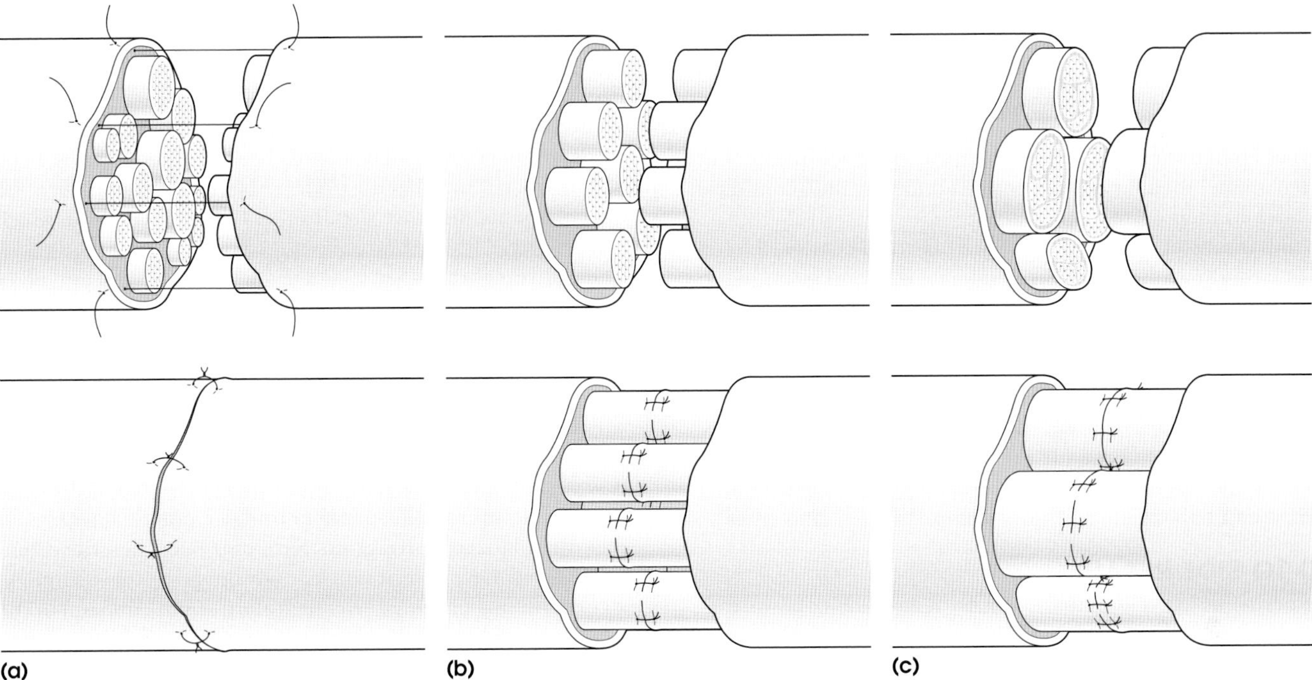

Figure 43.3 (a) Epineural repair; (b) fascicular repair; and (c) grouped fascicular repair.

the site of the repair. Soft tissue defects should be repaired with muscle flaps or local fasciocutaneous flaps. As an alternative, the nerve can be transposed to a different location to avoid such problems.

Primary repair or grafting of a divided nerve appears to give better results than delayed repair.[27] It should be emphasized, however, that this is the experience of those expert in this field, and for the surgeon relatively unversed in handling nerves it may be better to ensure a meticulous debridement of the wound, proper treatment of associated injuries, and sound primary healing, thus ensuring that the ground is prepared for delayed repair in the best possible circumstances. Where delayed exploration is anticipated, it is helpful to mark the nerve ends with fine non-absorbable sutures. Careful coaptation of the severed ends with 6/0 nylon, so as to orient the nerve stumps accurately, is especially useful because the shape of the nerve and the passage of the longitudinal vessels within the epineurium are better defined at this stage rather than later, when the anatomy is distorted by scar tissue. This manoeuvre also prevents retraction of the nerve ends.[28]

Primary repair is the treatment of choice in the ideal circumstances of a cleanly cut nerve in an uncontaminated wound treated by an experienced surgeon. There are four techniques for coapting nerve ends (Fig. 43.3): epineural, fascicular, grouped fascicular or mixed repair, involving several of these techniques.[28] A sound knowledge of the tissue planes in the limbs is essential, particularly in proximal lesions, where a tourniquet cannot be used to help find the nerve ends. Bipolar coagulation should be used to minimize damage to the nerves when securing haemostasis, and a nerve stimulator is also helpful.

The ideal nerve repair should be performed as a primary procedure between viable nerve ends, with no tension and perfect alignment of the fascicles. There should be no foreign bodies in the vicinity, no infection, and the nerve should glide freely in the surrounding tissues. To avoid the foreign body reaction associated with suture material, coaptation with fibrin glue has been used.[29,30] Laser 'spot welding' to bond nerve ends has also been practised experimentally. Practically speaking, nerve repair varies only in suture placement, and each attempts to align the fascicles accurately.

EPINEURAL REPAIR

This is the traditional method.[31] The use of either magnifying loupes or the operating microscope improves suture placement.[32] The nerve ends are trimmed to leave fascicles mushrooming from the end with the epineurium slightly retracted (Fig. 44.3a). The goal of an epineural repair is to restore continuity in the proper rotational alignment without tension. Longitudinal blood vessels in the epineurium and the arrangement of the fascicles may assist in orienting the nerve ends. The neurorrhaphy is carried out using fine non-absorbable sutures.

FASCICULAR REPAIR

When a nerve has very few fascicles, it may be possible to align the individual fascicles with fine sutures. The cut ends are freshened to reveal undamaged tissue. The cross-sectional anatomy is then inspected and the fascicles are apposed with interrupted 10/0 nylon sutures using the operating microscope.[28] (Fig. 44.3b). Individual dissection of the fascicles tends to confuse the situation and is not recommended.

REFERENCES

27. Grabb WC. J Bone Joint Surg 1968; 50A: 964–972
28. Wilgis EFS. In: Green DP (ed). Operative Hand Surgery. Churchill Livingstone, Edinburgh, 1988
29. Bonnard C, Narakas A. Presented to the Third Annual Meeting of the American Society for Reconstructive Microsurgery, San Antonio, Texas, September 1987
30. Seddon HJ, Medawar PB. Lancet 1942; ii: 87
31. Orgel M G Clin Plast Surg 1984; 11: 101–104

GROUPED FASCICULAR REPAIR

Within a large nerve, a number of fascicles are often grouped together.[33] These fascicular groups have different sizes and shapes and they can be separated and the internal epineurium sutured (Fig. 44.3c). It is helpful to suture together a posterior flap of external epineurium first to take the tension off the repair.[34] In this technique, the margin of error is reduced as the axons tend to remain in their correct groupings.[28]

Comparisons of epineural and fascicular repairs of peripheral nerves have shown no conclusive evidence that one technique is better than another.[31,32,35] The potential benefits of fascicular alignment are probably not realized because of the increased surgical manipulation required in order to execute the repair, and the potential to mismatch fascicles is still present. Although the epineural repair is not as precise, it may allow for neurotrophic effects to influence the direction of nerve fibre growth.[32] This is the preference of a motor axon to grow towards a distal motor stump rather than a sensory stump.[36]

END TO SIDE REPAIR

In experiments on laboratory animals, it has been shown that when a nerve is joined end-to-side to a donor nerve without disruption of the axons of the donor nerve but rather after simply making a window in the epineurium, axonal growth can follow. There is also some clinical evidence that this can be effective in restoring muscle power.[37] In other cases, however, the results were less impressive.

It can also be useful to join proximal nerve stump end-to-side to an adjacent nerve after resection of a neuroma, thus providing potentially wayward axons with an appropriate path.

NERVE GRAFTING

In secondary repair, the scar surrounding the area of nerve injury has to be resected to reveal healthy tissue with axons pouting out of the proximal end. A gap in the nerve is inevitable. The true nerve gap is measured with scar tissue removed and with joints extended. If it is possible to perform a comfortable repair with minimal mobilization, and without extensive joint flexion or tension on the nerve, then direct suture can be considered. When the gap cannot be closed without tension, a nerve graft is required. In a digit, defects of only a few millimetres should be grafted. In the forearm, a gap of several centimetres may close directly. Even a minimum of tension on the nerve repair will jeopardize the ultimate functional result.[38,39] The effect of tension on the intraneural blood supply is easily demonstrated by observing the circulation to a peripheral nerve under the operating microscope. Very little tension is required to blanch the nerve.

It is essential that the florid overgrowth of epineurium and adventitial tissue is resected from the nerve ends before grafting is undertaken.

Several nerves can be used to provide nerve graft material. The sural nerve provides a 30–40-cm length of nerve graft.[32] This leaves the patient with an area of numbness on the lateral aspect of the foot, which diminishes with time. The medial and lateral cutaneous nerves of the forearm can also be used as nerve grafts. Prior to the surgery, the patient should be warned of the likely need for a graft, of the additional scar, and of the sensory loss that will occur. The grafts are cut to bridge the nerve gap without tension, and they should be routed through as healthy a bed as possible. For a major nerve, strands of graft are sewn in loosely, using magnification to bridge the gap between groups of fascicles. For gaps in smaller nerves, a single strand of nerve graft may suffice.

To avoid sacrifice of a cutaneous nerve, segments of muscle have been successfully interposed between nerve ends. The muscle is frozen and thawed prior to insertion to denature the cellular elements and leave a scaffold of hollow tubes down which axons can grow.[40,41]

Alternative conduits, such as Dexon tubes or a segment of vein, have been used instead of a nerve graft. This technique is best applied to short gaps only. For gaps in excess of 2 cm, nerve grafting remains the method of choice.

Elongation of a peripheral nerve using slow tissue expansion techniques (cf. stretching of fascicles by a slow-growing schwannoma) has also been used to bridge the nerve gap.[42]

It is possible experimentally to preserve nerve blood flow and function while stretching a nerve to bridge a potential gap.[43]

Free vascularized nerve grafts have also been described, but some surgeons have shown no clear advantage to this technique over conventional grafting.[44] Nerve grafts from the dorsum of the foot, vascularized by the dorsalis pedis artery, have been used to restore sensibility in anaesthetic scarred digits.[45] This technique is most applicable when the bed is unacceptable for conventional grafting.

Preliminary surgery to improve the quality of the bed in which the grafts will lie is sometimes required. Free flaps of muscle or skin provide a bed of well-vascularized tissue. To avoid the repaired nerve becoming enmeshed in scar tissue, a free fascial flap taken from the temporalis area or over the serratus anterior surface can be wrapped around a nerve graft that would otherwise lie in a scarred bed.[46,47] This surrounds the repaired nerve with well-vascularized loose areolar tissue and allows it to glide when the limb is moved. When a normally functioning nerve becomes slowly enmeshed in scar tissue after trauma, good results can be achieved by removing the scar tissue alone (neurolysis) without resort to excision of the damaged segment and nerve grafting or primary repair. When the scarred

REFERENCES

32. Mackinnon S E, Dellon A L Surgery of the Peripheral Nerves. Thieme Medical Publishers, New York 1988
33. Sunderland S Nerves and Nerve Injuries. Williams & Wilkins, Baltimore 1968
34. Jabaley M E J Hand Surg 1984; 9B: 14
35. Lilla J A, Phelps D B, Boswick J A Ann Plast Surg 1979; 2: 24–31
36. Brushert T M, Seiler W A Exp Neurol 1987; 97: 289–300
37. FreyM, Giovani P. Eur J Plast Surg 2003; 26: 89–94
38. Terzis JK, Faibisoff BA, Williams B. Plast Reconstr Surg 1975; 56: 106
39. Millesi H. Hand Clin 1986; 2: 651
40. Glasby MA, Gilmour JA et al. Br J Plast 1990; 43: 169–178
41. Norris RW, Glasby MA et al. J Bone Joint Surg 1988; 70: 530
42. Manders EK, Saggers GC et al. Clin Plast Surg 1987; 14: 551
43. Van der Wey LP, Polder TW et al. Plast Reconstr Surg 1996; 97: 568–576
44. Gilbert A. Clin Plast Surg 1974; 2: 73–77
45. Rose EH, Kowalski TA, Norris MS. Plast Reconstr Surg 1989; 83: 593–604
46. Wintsch K, Helaly P. J Reconst Microsurg 1986; 2: 143–150
47. Millesi H, Zoch G, Rath T. Ann Hand Upper Limb Surg 1990; 9: 87–97

epineurium is removed, the presence of intact fascicles needs to be confirmed. Once neurolysed, the nerve must be placed into a bed of well-vascularized tissue if further scarring is to be prevented. The pronator quadratus muscle has been mobilized at the level of the wrist to wrap around median or ulnar nerves.[48]

Once grafts are in place, the extremity is splinted in a comfortable position for 10–14 days. The patient can be discharged from hospital within 1 or 2 days of the operation. Once the splint is removed, exercises are commenced, avoiding hyperextension for several weeks. A more prolonged period of splintage is not necessary when the nerve repair is not under tension.

Large nerve grafts from cadavers have been used successfully in combination with immunosuppression techniques. The chances of rejection are reduced when nerves are kept in cold storage for a few weeks prior to transplantation.

THE DELAYED NERVE INJURY

Patients presenting at a late stage are difficult to manage. The restoration of lost function is not easy. All too often, treatment is directed towards overcoming fixed deformity that should never have occurred, or at healing the trophic sores that follow neglect of insensate skin. Pain may be difficult to treat in these circumstances. If the delay is considerable – over 6 months in the case of a radial or common peroneal nerve injury – or if the original injury caused extensive nerve damage, as is likely in missile wounds, then an appropriate muscle transfer may be a more satisfactory way of improving the patient's prospects.[49] The treatment plan is determined by the extent of scarring in the limb and the extent of ischaemic fibrosis in the paralysed muscles.

A precise assessment of the patient's functional disability provides the key to the most satisfactory treatment plan. Repair of the nerve itself may form only one step in such a plan.

PATTERNS OF RECOVERY

ADVANCING TINEL'S SIGN

A valuable sign of nerve regeneration is that of Tinel.[21] As the course of a nerve trunk is percussed from distal to proximal, the patient may complain of pins and needles over the area of nerve regeneration. This is caused by the irritability of fine regenerating nerve fibres, which are not fully myelinated. There is a delay of several days before regenerating axons sprout from the cut end of a divided nerve, and Tinel's sign is often difficult to detect until 2 months after an injury. The level of the Tinel should be measured from a fixed bony point to minimize observer error. Tinel's sign first occurs at the site of injury, and then advances at a rate of 2.5 cm/month or 1 mm/day.[9] The rate is faster in more proximal injuries. Without a satisfactory nerve repair, the Tinel's sign will not advance: a Tinel's sign that has progressed beyond the level of the injury is an important indicator of success, and one that does not advance suggests failure of repair. Cohorts of axons advance at differing rates, and it is possible to have a Tinel's sign at two or three positions in the same nerve.

DISAPPEARANCE OF THE TINEL'S SIGN

Shortly after the advancing Tinel reaches a neuromuscular junction or sensory end organ, it disappears. At this stage, gentle stroking of the skin may elicit tingling. In assessing the progress of nerve recovery, it is important to relate the advancing Tinel to the original site of injury. A strong advancing Tinel associated with a diminishing static Tinel indicates a good prognosis. A weak advancing Tinel in the presence of a persistently strong, static Tinel is an indication of a poor prognosis.

Table 43.1 Highet's scheme[50]

Stage	Description
S0	No sensibility in the autonomous zone of the nerve
S1	Recovery of deep cutaneous pain in the autonomous zone of the nerve
S2	Recovery of superficial pain and some touch
S2+	Over-response to painful stimuli and touch
S3	Return of superficial pain and touch throughout the autonomous zone of the nerve
S3+	Some return of two-point discrimination
S4	Complete recovery

Table 43.2 The 0–5 scale for recording muscle power

Stage	Description
M0	No contraction
M1	Flicker or trace of contraction
M2	Active movement with gravity eliminated
M3	Active movement against gravity
M4	Active movement against gravity and resistance
M5	Normal power

ESTABLISHMENT OF SENSATION

Protective sensation then develops, and the patient can withdraw from painful stimuli. More discriminatory sensation often follows. Measurement of the quality of sensory recovery is difficult. A useful test is that of two-point discrimination. The smallest gap between two blunt wires at which the patient perceives the two endings as separate is noted in millimetres. Functional recovery is graded according to Highet's scheme, shown in Table 43.1.[50]

The recognition of early signs of recovery is important. Electromyography may detect early reinnervation of paralysed muscles, and could tip the scales against exploring a motor nerve. Accurate charting of muscle power is also important to assess motor nerve recovery (Table 43.2).[50]

SENSORY RE-EDUCATION

Sensory re-education is a method or combination of techniques that help the patient with sensory impairment to learn to reinterpret the altered profile of neural impulses reaching a

REFERENCES

48. Dellon AL, Mackinnon SE. Plast Reconstr Surg 1986; 77: 427
49. Zachary RB. In: Seddon H (ed). Peripheral Nerve Injuries. HMSO, London, 1954
50. Highest WB, Holmes W. Br J Surg 1943; 30:212

conscious level when the injured hand is stimulated. At a cortical level, sensory information is associated with previous experiences to allow a recognition pattern to develop.[32] After nerve division, the neural impulses from a given stimulus find no match in the associated cortex. The sensation is therefore new and may even pass unnoticed. When sensation reaches the fingertips after nerve repair, the training is begun. The patient repeatedly feels a variety of objects and textures, each session lasting 10–15 min. A rubber (eraser), keys, coins, buttons, rice and other items are used with the eyes closed and open until a reliable recognition pattern develops. Such a programme of retraining has been shown to improve two-point discrimination markedly in adults following sensory nerve repair.[13,51]

PROGNOSIS

Two factors remain within the control of the surgeon. The first is the timing of the nerve repair. There is a decline in the quality of results with progressive delay, so much so that repair of a high ulnar nerve lesion after 6–9 months is barely worthwhile.[49–52] The second is the skill with which the repair is carried out, not only of the nerve but also of the associated injuries. Ulnar nerve repair at the wrist or distal forearm yields better results if the adjacent ulnar artery is repaired at the same time.[53,54] The meticulous repair of tendons and tendon sheaths reduces adhesions between the nerve and nearby tendons. It is preferable for the neurorrhaphy to be surrounded by the minimum of scar tissue, because adherence of a repaired nerve to moving tendons or to a cutaneous scar may interfere with axonal regrowth and encourage the development of a painful neuroma. Nerve and bone injuries are often associated, particularly in gunshot wounds. The presence of an un-united fracture may involve the nerve in callus or cause friction neuritis if the nerve crosses a roughened surface. Successful fixation of fractures allows early gentle movement of joints and reduces stiffness.

The age of the patient also influences prognosis. A good primary repair of the median nerve in a 7-year-old child should be followed by a truly excellent result; such a result is extremely rare in even a young adult. In 1962, Onne evaluated the results of primary nerve repair 5 years after surgery, and found that the degree of static two-point discrimination recovered in millimetres was proportional to the patient's age in years.[55] The more proximal injuries, being further from motor endplates and sensory receptors, are less likely to achieve good functional recovery, especially in the motor system, where successful reinnervation of the muscle fibres is time-dependent.[32]

The level of the lesion is also significant: return of good-quality sensation is rare after repair of a median nerve injured in the axilla, and return of function in the intrinsic muscles of the hand cannot be hoped for after repair of an ulnar nerve injured at the same level.[56] The outlook for repair of a major mixed motor and sensory nerve, such as the ulnar, is worse than for repair of a nerve that contains chiefly motor fibres, such as the axillary or musculocutaneous nerve. This is due to mismatching, with regeneration of nerve fibres to inappropriate distal connections. If a proximal injury occurs in an extremity where motor and sensory nerves are adjacent to each other in the same fascicle, abnormal sensory and motor recovery is likely. More distally, the fascicles may be entirely motor or sensory, with little admixing. At this level, appropriate alignment of the nerve is likely to result in a better recovery.[22]

TENDON TRANSFER

In motor paralysis, there is a temptation to prolong observation in the hope that recovery may occur. Muscle reinnervation is most likely when the injury is close to the muscle group. Where one muscle group is paralysed because of failed nerve recovery, tendon transfers should be considered. In some circumstances, tendon transfers should be undertaken at an early stage if it is clear that the likelihood of recovery is remote, for example a severe injury to the nerve over a wide area in an older patient. It should, however, be remembered that if an early tendon transfer is undertaken and the nerve subsequently recovers, very abnormal movements may develop that may necessitate taking down the transfers. An assessment of how nerve recovery is proceeding can be made by examining the first muscle distal to the injury and assessing when it recovers. If its recovery has not occurred by 6 months in excess of its expected recovery time – assessed by judging the distance between the site of injury and the first muscle to be reinnervated, and assessing the time of axonal growth at a maximum of 1 mm/day – nerve exploration or tendon transfers should be undertaken.

Tendon transfer is a redistribution of the remaining functional parts.[57] Certain basic principles must be adhered to for a successful outcome:

- The tendon to be transferred must be of adequate strength. In practice, this means normal muscle power.
- The direction of transfer must be as close to the original direction of pull as possible.
- The excursion of the tendon chosen must be as close as possible to that of the original muscle it is replacing.
- The route through which the transfer passes must be a well-vascularized bed capable of allowing a tendon to slide. In practice, this means healthy subcutaneous tissue without overlying scars or skin grafts.
- The limb to be operated on must be soft and supple, with a full passive range of motion and no joint contractures.
- The tension of the transfer must be perfect. In practice, this means that the transfer must be tight enough to produce the desired function yet still allow complete reversal of the functional position during passive movement.
- Only one tendon should be used to produce one function (tendons used to produce two functions always fail in one of them).
- If possible, the tendon chosen should be synergistic with the one it is replacing.

In assessing which transfers are to be undertaken, it is useful to draw up a list of the functions that are missing, then a list of the tendons that are available to replace them, and a list of those that can afford to be used. Appropriate choices can then be made. Even for experienced surgeons, this rather basic approach will

REFERENCES

51. Wynn Parry CB, Salter M. Hand 1976; 8: 250–257
52. Woodall B, Beebe GW. Peripheral Nerve Regeneration (American) Veterans Administration Monograph. US Government Printing Office, Washington, 1956
53. Leclercq DC, Caliert AJ et al. J Hand Surg 1985; 10A (Suppl): 997–999
54. Merle M, Amend P et al. Periph Nerve 1986; 2: 17–26
55. Onne L. Acta Chir Scand 1962; 300 (Suppl): 1–70
56. Gaul JS. J Hand Surg 1982; 7: 502
57. Beasley RW. Orthop Clin 1970; 1: 433

guarantee consistently good choices. There are, however, certain examples where tendon transfers work well.

RADIAL NERVE PALSY

Under normal circumstances, tendon transfers for patients with radial nerve palsy work well, for example for wrist extension, the pronator teres can be transferred to extensor carpi radialis brevis. Finger extension can be achieved by transferring flexor carpi ulnaris to the extensor digitorum, and thumb extension by transferring palmaris longus to extensor pollicis longus.

MEDIAN NERVE PALSY

An opponensplasty may be indicated; examples are extensor indicis proprius or the sublimis to the ring finger.

ULNAR NERVE PALSY

In a low ulnar nerve palsy, a loss of thumb adduction can be overcome by using the sublimis from the ring finger. Abduction of the index finger may be achieved by inserting extensor indicis into the interosseous insertion. Clawing, which rarely requires correction following a simple low ulnar nerve division with good repair, may in exceptional circumstances be corrected by either advancing the volar plate or by using the sublimis tendon and forming a loop or lasso around the A2 pulley. Both of these procedures are designed to prevent hyperextension of the metacarpophalangeal joint, which is responsible for the clawing.

COMPLICATIONS OF A NERVE INJURY

A nerve injury may be complicated by loss of sensation, paralysis, loss of sympathetic function, and pain. The most important consequence of loss of sensation is a trophic ulcer from inadvertent injury.[22] The ulcer may become infected. Patients must be warned of the hazards to insensitive skin and advised about proper clothing and footwear. A lack of attention for even a short period can cause many months of disability. In severe cases of ulceration of the foot, amputation may be the only treatment option, especially when osteomyelitis of the underlying bones develops.

Loss of sweating and turgor of the finger pulps increase the vulnerability of the skin of the hand to thermal damage. What is tolerated by the normal hand will not necessarily be tolerated by the insensitive hand.

Paralysis of some muscles, and the unopposed action of others, may lead to a fixed deformity. Common examples include the fixed internal rotation of the shoulder from a brachial plexus lesion, fixed extension of the metacarpophalangeal joint from ulnar nerve injuries, and the equinus deformity of the foot from a severed sciatic nerve.[22] It is essential to prevent fixed deformity after a peripheral nerve injury by splintage and manipulation. Such deformities represent a failure of adequate care.

When the sprouting axons from a divided or partially divided nerve do not make appropriate distal connections, then a swelling of the nerve or neuroma can develop. If injury to the Schwann cells no longer confines the axons to their endoneural tubes, regenerating axons escape into the surrounding tissue in a disorganized fashion, where they mix with fibroblasts, Schwann cells and blood vessels. Partial nerve division usually results in a lateral neuroma or neuroma in continuity. A terminal neuroma usually results from a complete nerve division.

Not all neuromas are painful, and it is not known why one neuroma should be clinically symptomatic and another not so. One of the first goals in preventing neuromas is to use meticulous microsurgical technique to direct appropriate functional axonal regeneration.[32]

PAIN

The pain complicating a nerve injury may be of several different types. *Neuromatous pain* is a discrete area of tenderness at the site of a previous nerve injury; percussion of the neuroma produces paraesthesia in the distribution of the injured nerve.

The wide variety of techniques described to treat peripheral neuromas underlines the fact that this condition is difficult to cure. Where the nerve end is trapped in scar tissue, cutting back the nerve to a more proximal level is useful. Implantation of the transected nerve into a muscle has also proved helpful.[48,58,59] The underlying principle is to move the neuroma to a well-padded area where repeated stimulation is unlikely. In some cases, where both proximal and distal nerve ends can be found, direct repair or nerve grafting to restore nerve continuity is effective.[60] If a neuroma is not trapped in scar tissue, then non-surgical techniques may be helpful. Regular tapping of the point to desensitize the nerve is helpful. Transcutaneous nerve stimulators or local anaesthetic blocks may also help to break the pain cycle.

Causalgia is the burning pain and hyperalgesia in the distribution of an injured peripheral nerve.[61] Even a light touch on the skin produces exquisite pain, which may be exacerbated by a gust of air, loud noises and even emotional output. The lesion responsible is usually a partial injury to a major mixed nerve in the proximal part of a limb. There is a high incidence after injuries to the brachial plexus and sciatic nerves.

Reflex sympathetic dystrophy or regional pain syndrome is characterized by diffuse pain, joint stiffness, swelling and discoloration. The pain may occur after a variety of injuries and is not unique to nerve division or nerve entrapment. Affected limbs may at various times be blue or pink. The skin is often tight and glossy, and there may be excessive sweating, osteoporosis and atrophy of the fat pads of the fingertips. These changes are thought to be due to sympathetic overactivity.

The shoulder–hand syndrome is a form of reflex sympathetic dystrophy caused by proximal limb trauma or a visceral lesion such as a heart attack, stomach ulcer or Pancoast tumour. The pain and swelling in the upper limb are associated with limited shoulder movement.

Reflex sympathetic dystrophy, including causalgia and the shoulder–hand syndrome, is best treated as early as possible. Interruption of the sympathetic reflex can be achieved with repeated stellate ganglion blockade using local anaesthetic. This procedure warms up the limb and causes a temporary Horner's syndrome. Because peripheral nerves carry sympathetic efferent fibres, brachial plexus blockade also interrupts the sympathetic reflex. Continuous slow infusion of local anaesthetic to a trigger point, should there be one, can also quell the pain reflex.[62]

REFERENCES

58. Moskowicz LP. Zentralbl Chir 1918; 45: 547
59. Teneff S. J Int Coll Surg 1949; 12: 16
60. Van Beek AL. In: McCarthy J (ed). Plastic Surgery. WB Saunders, Philadelphia, 1990
61. Mitchell SW, Morehouse GR, Keen WW. Gunshot Wounds and Other Injuries of Nerves. JB Lippincott, Philadelphia, 1864
62. Omer GE, Thomas S. Tex Med 1971; 67: 93–96

The use of intravenous regional sympathetic blockade using guanethidine is another standard treatment.[63] Guanethidine displaces the sympathetic neurotransmitter noradrenaline (norepinephrine) from its storage and receptor sites in sympathetic nerve endings to give a prolonged sympathetic blockade. Surgical sympathectomy is of some value in patients with causalgia[64] but, surprisingly, is often not helpful in other forms of sympathetic dystrophy.[65]

Cold intolerance is a common feature of nerve injuries, even if repaired successfully. There is always a permanent degree of cold intolerance following a crush injury, but it does also temporarily develop after other nerve injuries. Cold intolerance is usually at its worst for 18 months after a simple nerve transection, after which it gradually settles. Regeneration of both somatic and autonomic function occurs after repair, but poor thermoregulation may explain the feeling of numbness and discomfort in cold weather.

IATROGENIC NERVE INJURY

Inadvertent damage to nerves is not uncommon (Fig. 43.4).[4] Irritant drugs may be injected into the sciatic or axillary nerves when the intramuscular route is used.[66,67] Ill-fitting crutches or splints can cause foot or wrist drop.[22] The brachial plexus may be damaged when local anaesthetic is injected to effect a brachial block. The greatest damage is, however, caused during minor surgical procedures. Restricted anatomical knowledge combined with poor technique will place a peripheral nerve at risk. The median nerve has been mistaken for palmaris longus when a tendon graft is required,[68] the accessory nerve is at risk when a neck lump is excised, and branches of the sciatic nerve have been damaged during varicose vein surgery.

When faced with a significant neural deficit after a wound has been made over the course of a nerve, the proper course of action is to assume that the nerve has been divided. If sensation, motor power and sympathetic function are absent, then the wound should be re-explored urgently. It is unnecessary to prevaricate by passing the burden of diagnosis on to a neurologist; neurophysiological signs of nerve injury will not be evident for several weeks after injury.

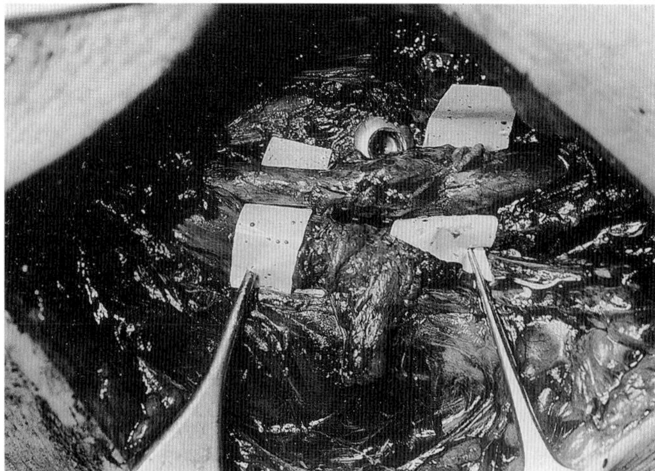

Figure 43.4 Iatrogenic nerve damage: a screw used to secure a humeral fracture fixation plate has eroded through the radial nerve to cause a complete palsy.

BRACHIAL PLEXUS INJURIES

The brachial plexus arises from the lowest four cervical and highest thoracic spinal nerve roots: C5, 6, 7, 8 and T1. The roots unite to form three trunks (Fig. 43.5): the upper contains fibres of spinal elements C5 and 6, the middle C7, and the lower C8 and T1. The trunks lie in the supraclavicular fossa just distal to the scalene muscles. The upper trunk gives origin to the suprascapular nerve. The trunks then divide into anterior and posterior divisions to carry fibres to the dorsal and ventral aspects of the limb (Fig. 43.5).

Patients with severe and multiple injuries from road traffic accidents have an increased chance of survival as a result of the use of helmets by motorcyclists, rapid transport to hospitals from the roadside, and recent advances in medical care. This may explain the marked increase in the number of patients with traction lesions of the brachial plexus being referred to specialist units.[70] The treatment of head, chest and abdominal injuries takes precedence over the management of a peripheral nerve injury. It is, however, important to remember the possibility of a brachial plexus injury in an unconscious patient, especially when there are fractures of the shoulder girdle, the proximal humerus or the first rib.

The prognosis relates to the level of the lesion. There are three main types of injury:

1. In root avulsion, the nerve roots are avulsed from the spinal cord within the vertebral column. Spontaneous improvement is unlikely, and the injury is not amenable to surgical repair.
2. Rupture of the brachial plexus outside the vertebral column. Spontaneous improvement is unlikely, but the injury may benefit from surgical repair.
3. Nerve damage without rupture. A neurapraxia or axonotmesis with preservation of the nerve sheaths is likely to improve spontaneously. In road traffic accidents, low-velocity injuries tend to be associated with neurapraxia and axonotmesis, while a high-velocity impact is more likely to produce a complete disruption of the plexus.

A preganglionic injury where the spinal nerves have been torn directly from the spinal cord presents with deep bruising in the posterior triangle of the neck, loss of sensation above the clavicle, pain in an insensitive hand, and a Horner's syndrome (miosis, enophthalmos, anhidrosis and ptosis). The loss of function of muscles innervated by branches coming directly from the roots of the brachial plexus is highly suggestive of proximal root avulsion. Winging of the scapula and paralysis of the ipsilateral hemidiaphragm on chest X-ray are bad prognostic signs. Lower limb hyper-reflexia may also occur when a root avulsion occurs at cord level.

With a preganglionic lesion, the motor fibres have been separated from their cell bodies in the anterior horn cells, but

REFERENCES

63. Hannington-Kiff JG. Lancet 1974; i: 1019–1020
64. Jebara VA, Saade BJ. Trauma 1987; 27: 519
65. Evans J. Ann Intern Med 1947; 26: 417
66. Gentili F, Hudson AR et al. Neurosurgery 1979; 4: 244
67. Gentili F, Hudson AR, Hunter D. Can J Neurol 1980; 7: 143
68. Vastamaki M. J Hand Surg 1987; 12B: 187–188
69. Walton J. Brain's Diseases of the Nervous System. 9th edn. Oxford University Press, Oxford, 1985
70. Narakas AO. In: McCarthy JG (ed). Plastic Surgery. WB Saunders, Philadelphia, 1990

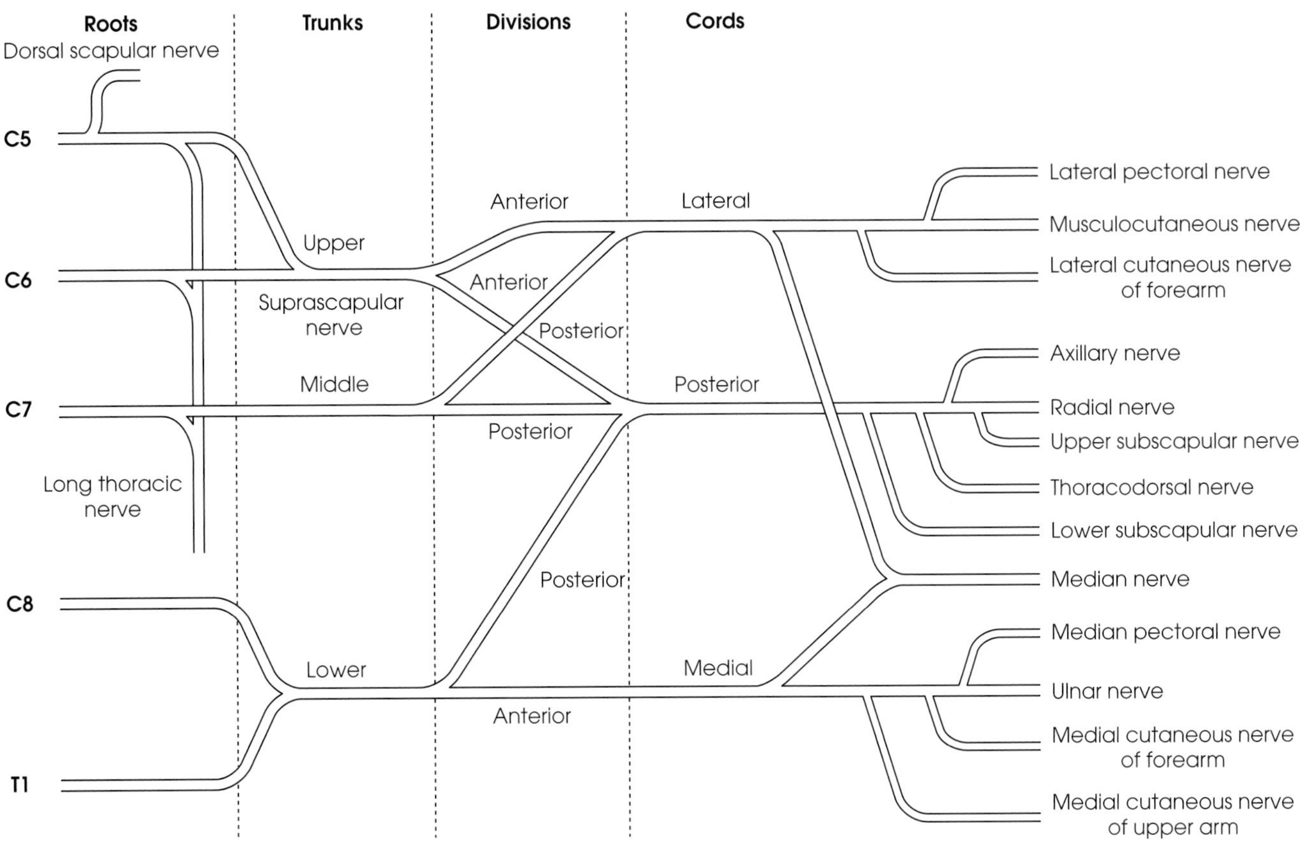

Figure 43.5 The brachial plexus. (Reproduced with permission from HMSO (London).)

the sensory fibres are still connected to their cell bodies in the dorsal root ganglion. Thus, although the patient will not be able to appreciate sensation, there will be no Wallerian degeneration in the sensory fibres, and sensory nerve conduction studies will be normal when tested 4 weeks after injury.[71] The axon flare reflex of Lewis in response to histamine also remains intact. Myelograms are useful to confirm the diagnosis, although deformity of the root sleeve is not an acid test for root avulsion.[72] When the roots have been avulsed directly from the spinal cord, there is no proximal peripheral nerve tissue and surgical repair is not possible.

By contrast, in postganglionic injuries there are normal nerve fibres proximal to the lesion. Should spontaneous recovery of a traction injury not occur, then surgical repair is possible.

Open wounds of the brachial plexus and those associated with damaged vessels merit urgent exploration, both to restore the circulation to the limb and to determine the extent of nerve damage. Clean sharp lacerations of the brachial plexus should be treated by primary epineural repair. The quality of results diminishes markedly if nerve repair or grafting is delayed more than 2 months.[70]

Closed traction injuries account for the majority of brachial plexus injuries seen. An advancing Tinel's sign and electromyographic evidence of reinnervation are favourable signs. Even in axonotmesis, physiotherapy is important to maintain a passive range of movement in involved joints. Should arm function show no signs of spontaneous recovery, then the brachial plexus is explored and divided nerves are repaired. Because of the nature of traction injuries, neurolysis is often required. Although direct nerve suture may on occasion be possible, autogenous nerve grafting of the damaged segments is more often required.

The outcome of an extensive repair of a supraclavicular rupture of the brachial plexus is not good. An improvement in shoulder function and restoration of elbow flexion may be achieved, but recovery of sensation and power in the forearm and hand is unlikely.[73] While striving to restore sensation and movement to the upper limb, it must be remembered that pain is a very important feature of brachial plexus injuries. Patients with root avulsions are especially prone to severe pain, and up to 80% of them suffer with paroxysms of sharp burning pain of several seconds duration.[74] There may be a background of dull pain that the patients are able to endure, while they are defenceless against the severe attacks. Transcutaneous nerve stimulation and thalamic stimulation are often helpful. For those who continue to suffer despite such treatment, coagulation of the dorsal root entry zone has proved helpful.[75] Irritative painful nerve lesions in the absence of root avulsion are also common, but they respond well to nerve repair.[70]

Where spontaneous recovery is not anticipated, close supervision is necessary to prevent contractures, to relieve pain, and to fit functional braces. Arthrodesis of the glenohumeral joint can improve shoulder function when the glenohumeral muscles are paralysed, yet the scapulothoracic group is function-

REFERENCES

71. Bonney G. Brain 1954; 77: 588–609
72. Jelasic F, Peipgras U. Eur Neurol 1974; 11: 158
73. Birch R. Curr Orthop 1987; 1: 316–323
74. Eversmann WW Jr. In: Green DP (ed). Operative Hand Surgery, vol 2. 2nd edn. Churchill Livingstone, New York, 1988
75. Nashold BS, Ostdahl RH. J Neurosurg 1979; 51: 59

ing. Several tendon transfers can be used to restore elbow flexion. In one, the sternocostal portion of pectoralis major is mobilized, preserving its neurovascular supply. When the muscle is swung into the upper arm and joined to the biceps tendon, it acts on the elbow effectively.[76] The shoulder should be of normal power or stabilized by an arthrodesis. In an upper root lesion, where the forearm muscles are functioning, the common flexor origin can be shifted to a more proximal point on the humerus so that the movement of elbow flexion is increased.[77] The presence of a flail anaesthetic upper limb may require the patient to retrain in a new occupation.[78] In some patients the limb becomes the site of chronic infection and multiple fractures, with little hope of functional recovery. The final solution – amputation of the limb – is still a potential means of rehabilitation in some patients.

If the plexus is disrupted at cord level, the spinatus muscles, the serratus anterior, the pectoral muscles and the cervical sympathetic chain are usually spared. Sensation in the forearm and hand is lost after a complete disruption of the plexus, and reflexes cannot be elicited at any point in the upper limb. Complete plexus lesions can be caused by traumatic damage of the cervical spine, by neoplasms involving cervical nerve roots, by prolapsed intervertebral discs, by cervical spondylosis, and by tuberculosis of the spine. In the neck, gunshot wounds, stabbings, fractures of the clavicle, dislocations of the humerus, and motorcycle accidents in which the shoulder and neck are forcibly pulled apart cause disruption of the plexus. The lower plexus can be compressed in patients with the thoracic outlet syndrome, usually by a cervical rib; it may be invaded by a Pancoast tumour or by malignant lymph nodes in the neck. Most commonly, part rather than the whole of the brachial plexus is involved. This invariably involves either the upper or the lower nerve roots.

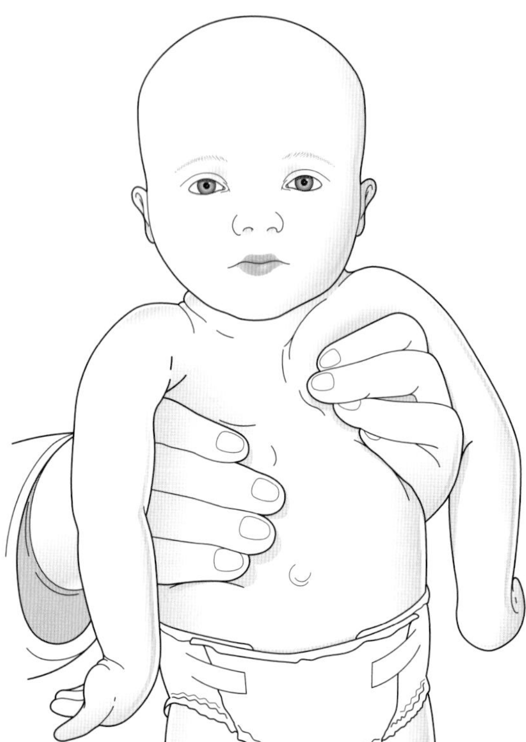

Figure 43.6 Erb's palsy: tip position.

UPPER BRACHIAL PLEXUS INJURY (ERB–DUCHENNE TYPE C5 AND 6)

The upper part of the plexus is most commonly torn as a result of forcible separation of the head and shoulder. This was originally common at parturition when excessive traction was applied to the head to deliver the shoulder. This is now extremely rare. It is most commonly seen in adults following a fall on the shoulder forcing the head to one side. This is particularly common in motorcycle accidents. The muscles supplied by C5 include the biceps, deltoid, brachialis, brachioradialis, supra- and infraspinatus, and rhomboids. The sixth cervical segment supplies serratus anterior, latissimus dorsi, triceps, pectoralis major and extensor carpi radialis. As a result of paralysis of these muscles, the limb hangs at the side, internally rotated at the shoulder due to the unopposed action of subscapularis, with the forearm pronated in the so-called 'tip' position (Fig. 43.6). Patients are unable to abduct the shoulder as a result of paralysis of the deltoid. They cannot flex the elbow because biceps, brachialis and brachioradialis do not function, and external rotation of the shoulder is impossible because the spinati are also denervated. Biceps and supinator reflexes cannot be elicited. There is minor sensory loss over the insertion of the deltoid on the outer part of the arm (see Fig. 43.13).

LOWER PLEXUS INJURY (DEJERINE–KLUMPKE T1 AND C8)

This is produced by traction on an already abducted arm, and often follows an attempt to prevent falling by clutching hold of a strap above the head with a raised outstretched hand. This type of injury occurs to standing passengers on buses and underground trains during sudden stops and starts. It results in paralysis of all the small muscles of the hand, producing a claw hand from the unopposed action of the long flexors and extensors of the fingers. There is sensory loss in the C8 and T1 dermatomes on the ulnar side of the arm, forearm, wrist and fingers (see Fig. 43.13). The cervical sympathetic ganglion chain is also often damaged, resulting in a Horner's syndrome.

CORD INJURIES

The lateral, posterior and medial cords may also be damaged by various fractures and dislocations around the shoulder joint. Injury of the lateral cord usually results in paralysis of the biceps and coracobrachialis muscles, together with all the muscles supplied by the median nerve, except those of the thenar eminence. Posterior cord damage results in axillary and radial nerve damage, while division of the medial cord results in paralysis of the muscles supplied by the ulnar nerve and the intrinsic muscles of the hand, which are supplied by the median nerve.

COMPRESSION SYNDROMES

When nerves pass over a bony prominence or through a narrow osseofascial tunnel, they run the risk of being compressed. A variety of structures including osteophytes, soft tissue swellings, or congenital anomalies such as a cervical rib may contribute to a compression syndrome. As a general rule, unless an entrapment

REFERENCES

76. Clark JMP. Br J Surg 1946; 34: 180
77. Steindler A. NY State Med J 1918; 108: 117–119
78. Yeoman PM, Seddon HJ. J Bone Joint Surg 1961; 43B: 493

neuropathy is severe or long-standing, release of the compression effects a good recovery.

According to many authors, the primary lesion is a vascular compromise.[79–81] When a nerve is subject to pressure, there is obstruction to the flow of blood in the fine plexus of vessels within the nerve. The slowing of the circulation causes venous congestion in the involved segment, which in turn results in anoxia and dilatation of the small vessels. The endoneurium may become oedematous, and this then compounds the circulatory obstruction. If the situation persists, fibroblasts proliferate within the nerve, causing internal scarring that further inhibits the exchange of nutrients between the bloodstream and nerve fibres. The ischaemic nerve fibres are less able to produce high-energy phosphates, so restricting the efficiency of the sodium pump and cell transport systems. This eventually impairs nerve conduction and causes the patient discomfort. The rapid recovery and restitution of a normal conduction velocity after carpal tunnel release favour this vascular theory of nerve damage.[79]

The many compression syndromes have a number of features in common. Pain, usually in the territory of the affected nerve, is by far the most usual complaint. Nerve conduction studies are used to confirm the diagnosis.

THE MEDIAN NERVE

The median nerve is most commonly compressed at the wrist, where it passes through the carpal tunnel.[74] The carpal tunnel syndrome is seen most frequently in women between 40 and 60 years of age. Although often there is no obvious predisposing cause, a multitude of conditions have been associated with this syndrome. They include rheumatoid arthritis, myxoedema, nephrotic syndrome, acromegaly, multiple myeloma, amyloidosis, diabetes mellitus, alcoholism, haemophilia, pregnancy, gout, lipomas, ganglia, anomalous musculature, wrist fractures and the menopause.

The symptoms vary from mild paraesthesia in the distribution of the median nerve to constant sensory impairment, pain and atrophy of the thenar muscles, which causes a pronounced hollow in the thenar eminence (Fig. 43.7). The hand is often weak or clumsy, and numbness of the fingers and pain in the wrist or distal forearm may awaken the patient from sleep. Shoulder and upper arm pain are also common features. Although pain and paraesthesia should be experienced in the thumb, the index finger, the middle finger and the radial side of the ring fingers, this is often not the case. The thumb and index finger are often spared. Relief is obtained by elevating or shaking the limb.

Exaggerated flexion of the wrist[82] (Phalen's test) or percussion of the median nerve at the wrist (a Tinel's sign) usually reproduces the symptoms, and delayed nerve conduction confirms the diagnosis.[83] Application of a forearm tourniquet inflated above arterial pressure may also reproduce the symptoms.[84] Nerve conduction studies may help differentiate the carpal tunnel syndrome from the thoracic outlet syndrome and compression of the cervical nerves in spondylitis.[85]

Splinting the wrist in a neutral position or slight extension will often afford relief,[68] but where this is unhelpful surgery should be advised. The injection of steroid into the carpal tunnel can help, but once again relief is often temporary.[86]

The surgical treatment consists of division of the transverse carpal ligament (flexor retinaculum) under tourniquet control. Particular care must be taken to avoid damage to the palmar cutaneous nerve, which lies superficial to the ligament, and the motor branch to the thenar muscles, which may pass through it. The precise course of these nerves often varies,[87] and it is prudent to place the incision on the ulnar side of the palmar crease, where even the rare variations can be protected. The full extent of the ligament is divided, but care is required because the median nerve may be adherent to the undersurface. It is advisable to secure haemostasis before skin closure. Postoperatively, the wrist is splinted for 10 days in slight extension to prevent the median nerve from adhering to the undersurface of the skin wound. Pain relief is usually immediate, and sensation to the fingers returns quickly.

The median nerve can also be trapped as it courses between the ulnar and humeral heads of pronator teres. This produces an aching pain, which is often elicited by repetitive rotatory movements of the arm.[88]

The nerve may also be kinked against the edge of flexor digitorum superficialis[89] or displaced by the ligament of Struthers.[90] This is a fibrous band arising from the supratrochlear region of the humerus, which passes upwards and medially to attach to the bone at a higher level.

THE ULNAR NERVE

The ulnar nerve may be compressed as it runs in the cubital tunnel behind the elbow joint and between the two heads of flexor carpi ulnaris.[91] Compression generally presents with pain

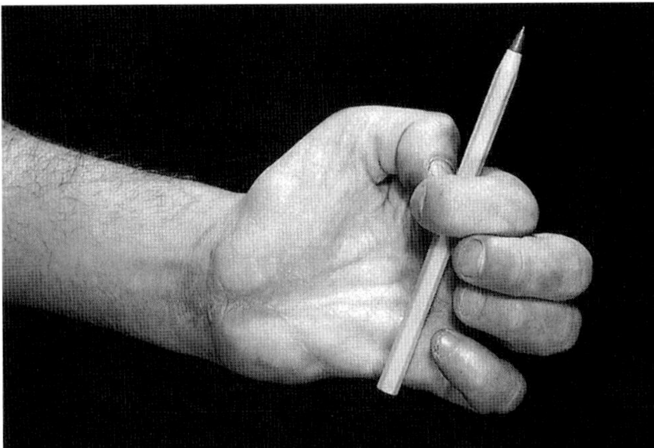

Figure 43.7 Wasting of the thenar and hypothenar eminence due to division of the ulnar and median nerves at the wrist.

REFERENCES

79. Eversman WW, Ritsick JA. J Hand Surg 1978; 3: 77–81
80. Lundborg G. Scand J Plast Reconstr Surg 1970; 6 (Suppl): 1–113
81. Lundborg G, Gelbermann RH et al. J Hand Surg 1982; 7: 252–259
82. Phalen GS. J Bone Joint Surg 1966; 48A: 211–228
83. Simpson JA. J Neurol Neurosurg Psychiatry 1956; 19: 275
84. Gilliatt RW, Wilson TG. Lancet 1953; ii: 595
85. Melvin JL, Schuckmann JA, Lanese RR. Arch Phys Med Rehab 1973; 54: 69
86. Foster JB. Lancet 1960; i: 454–456
87. Lanz V. J Hand Surg 1977; 2: 44–53
88. Kopell HP, Thompson WAL. N Engl J Med 1958; 259: 713–715
89. Kopell HP, Thompson WAL. Peripheral Entrapment Neuropathies. Williams & Wilkins, Baltimore, 1963
90. Nankano KK. Muscle Nerve 1978; 1: 264
91. James GGH. J Bone Joint Surg 1956; 38B: 589

and tingling on the medial side of the forearm and hand. There may also be evidence of weakness in the intrinsic muscles of the hand. A positive percussion test over the ulnar nerve at the elbow, or increased numbness when the elbow is fully flexed, supports the diagnosis. There is weakness of the flexor digitorum profundus to the little finger, and confirmation of delayed nerve conduction is once again helpful in confirming the diagnosis.[92]

The condition may be associated with cubitus valgus, supracondylar fractures of the humerus, osteophytes around the elbow joint, and inadvertent compression of the nerve during anaesthesia.[93] Chronic nerve irritation may cause oedema and restricted gliding as the elbow moves. Elbow splintage in a slightly flexed position may help to reduce this inflammatory reaction and provides relief.[94] Simple surgical decompression is achieved by splitting the cubital tunnel, the arcade of the flexor carpi ulnaris, and the medial intermuscular septum above the elbow.

Transposition of the ulnar nerve is reported by some to be more effective than simple release.[95] The nerve is widely and carefully mobilized so that it can be transposed in front of the medial epicondyle. Care must be taken to preserve motor branches. If the patient has an abundance of subcutaneous fat, the nerve may be left in the subcutaneous plane. In most patients, however, it is necessary to locate it deep to the flexor–pronator muscles by mobilizing then repositioning the common flexor origin.[96]

Occasionally the ulnar nerve is compressed at the wrist as it passes through Guyon's canal.[97] Symptoms include pain and paraesthesia in the little finger and weakness in those intrinsic hand muscles innervated by the ulnar nerve. The condition can be caused by chronic repetitive trauma, and may be seen in mechanics, pipe-cutters, metal polishers and cyclists.[98–100] Lipomas, ganglia, cysts, ulnar artery thrombosis and anomalous muscles may compress the nerve.[101–103] If the hand is rested, most cases recover; open decompression is sometimes required.

THORACIC OUTLET SYNDROME

The mechanism of symptom production is complex, and not simply the result of compression by the scalene muscles (scalene syndrome) or by the rib and clavicle.[104] It is usually caused by a cervical rib that may be rudimentary or complete. It may also result from an abnormal first rib or an enlarged C8 transverse process with a fascial band extending to join the first rib. All these anatomical abnormalities cause the T1 nerve root to be hooked up, compressed and irritated by the anatomical anomaly during movement of the upper limb. Compression of the T1 root is commonly associated with compression of the subclavian artery and vein. It tends to be more common in women than in men, and is maximal between the third and fifth decades. Drooping of the shoulder due to the constant carrying of heavy weights (shopping bags) may be a factor. It is interesting to note that cervical ribs only cause symptoms in between 5 and 10% of all those affected by this anomaly.

Symptoms may be sensory, motor or vascular. Patients normally present with pain along the ulnar border of the hand and distal forearm, often associated with paraesthesiae that can be relieved by raising the hand above the head. Occasionally patients present with pain in the neck, situated over the rib, and at a late stage they may present with weakness and wasting of the muscles in the hand. On examination, there is normally hyperalgesia or analgesia over the C8 and T1 dermatomes. There is weakness of the small muscles of the hand, and a coincidental Horner's syndrome may be present. In some patients there is a palpable rib with a bruit. Other patients experience symptoms in response to local pressure over the origin of the rib.

Thoracic inlet X-rays may show the cervical rib, and nerve conduction studies may show impairment in nerve conduction along the T1 root. It is important to consider the possibility of motor neuron disease in the differential diagnosis, but this is not usually accompanied by pain and there is no sensory loss. Syringomyelia is usually associated with some long tract signs. A Pancoast's tumour must be excluded by appropriate chest radiographs or CT scans. Lesions of the ulnar and median nerve usually have a different distribution of sensory loss.[105] The treatment is by resection of the cervical rib or band.

NERVE TUMOURS

Nerve tumours are uncommon and are often mistaken for other benign soft tissue swellings.[106] Significant peripheral nerve damage may occur if they are removed by inexperienced surgeons. These tumours comprise fewer than 5% of tumours of the hand and upper extremity.[107,108] The tumours most commonly arise from the nerve sheath, but tumours of nerve cell origin also occur (Box 43.1).

BENIGN INTRANEURAL SWELLINGS

Traumatic neuroma

The traumatic neuroma is the most common tumour-like lesion of a peripheral nerve. They develop in approximately 4% of digital amputations. Traumatic neuromata form after nerve injury when regenerating axons grow in an uncontrolled fashion into neighbouring tissue rather than down appropriate distal endoneural tubules. Pain is caused by compression and tethering of nerve twigs by fibrous tissue.

Treatment by resection is helpful, but sometimes the relief of pain is only short-lived. It is thought that earlier treatment is more successful. Resection should be carried out to allow the freshly cut proximal end to retract into an uninjured bed. Alternatively, after resection the nerve can be split longitudinally and the distal ends of each joined to the other end to end (Fig. 43.8).

REFERENCES

92. Payan J. J Neurol Neurosurg Psychiatry 1970; 33: 157–163
93. Ekerot L. Scand J Plast Reconstr Surg 1977; 11: 225–229
94. Diamond ML, Lister G. J Hand Surg 1985; 10A: 430
95. MacNicol MF. J Bone Joint Surg 1979; 61B: 159–164
96. Learmonth JR. Surg Gynecol Obst 1942; 75: 792
97. Dupont C, Cloutier GE et al. J Bone Joint Surg 1965; 47A:757–761
98. Hayes JR, Mullholland RC, O'Connor BT. J Bone Joint Surg 1969; 51B: 469–472
99. Eckman PB, Perstlein G, Altocchi PH. Arch Neurol 1975; 32: 130–131
100. Dawson DM, Hallett B, Millender LH. Entrapment Neuropathies. Little, Brown, Boston, 1983
101. Dell PC. J Hand Surg 1979; 4: 468–473
102. Turner MS, Caird DM. Hand 1977; 9: 140–141
103. Lister G. The Hand: Diagnosis and Indications. 2nd edn. Churchill Livingstone, Edinburgh, 1984: 192
104. Lascelles RG, Mohr PD et al. Brain 1977; 100: 601
105. Gilliatt RW. Peripheral Nerve Compression and Entrapment. Pitman, London, 1975
106. Brooks D. Peripheral Neuropathy 1984; 2: 2236–2253
107. Stack HG. Br Med J 1960; 1: 919–922
108. Harkin JC, Reed RJ. Tumours of the Peripheral Nervous System. Armed Forces Institute of Pathology, Washingston, 1968

Box 43.1 Classification of peripheral nerve tumours

Benign intraneural swellings
- Traumatic neuroma
- Morton's neuroma (compressive neuroma)
- Lipofibromatous hamartoma
- Intraneural ganglion

Benign nerve sheath tumours
- Schwannoma
- Neurofibroma

Malignant nerve sheath tumours
- Malignant schwannoma
- Nerve sheath fibrosarcoma

Tumours of nerve cell origin
- Neuroblastoma
- Ganglioneuroma
- Phaeochromocytoma

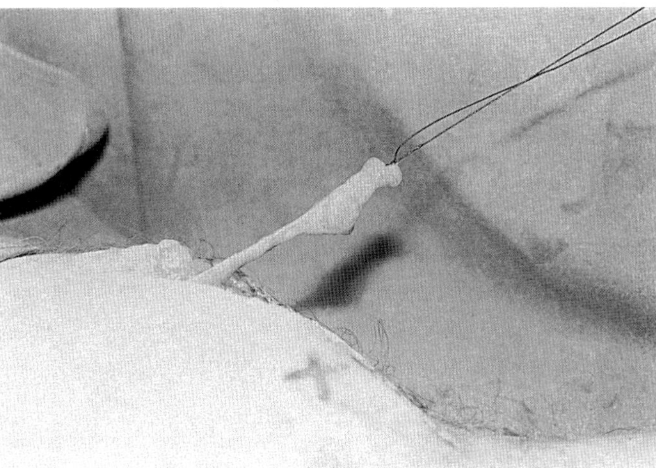

Figure 43.8 A traumatic neuroma: this swelling on a cut nerve was the source of severe pain.

Morton's neuroma (compressive neuroma)

This is not a true neuroma. Histological examination shows that it comprises a number of small fascicles surrounded by dense intraneural fibrosis. Wallerian degeneration is found within the fascicles. Typically between the third and fourth toes, the lesion presents with pain. Resection of the swelling is usually curative.

Lipofibromatous hamartoma

This swelling is also sometimes called intraneural lipoma or fibrofatty infiltration. It commonly involves the median nerve and is often associated with macrodactyly. The tumour usually presents as a soft mass in the palm of children and young adults. Carpal tunnel compression may occur secondary to the tumour mass. Pain, sensory disturbance and motor weakness can occur. If surgery is required, the fibrofatty mass is resected under magnification while preserving strands of nerve tissue.

Intraneural ganglion

It is a rare event for a ganglion cyst to form in a nerve sheath. It is thought that such cysts form when there is degeneration within connective tissue secondary to chronic mechanical irritation. These lesions usually arise in the common peroneal nerve and may present as a mass or with a spontaneous foot drop. The cysts may be several centimetres in diameter. It is usual to excise the ganglion while preserving the nerve, but when the lesion is multiloculated, incision and drainage of the cyst may be thought safer. Recurrence is possible.

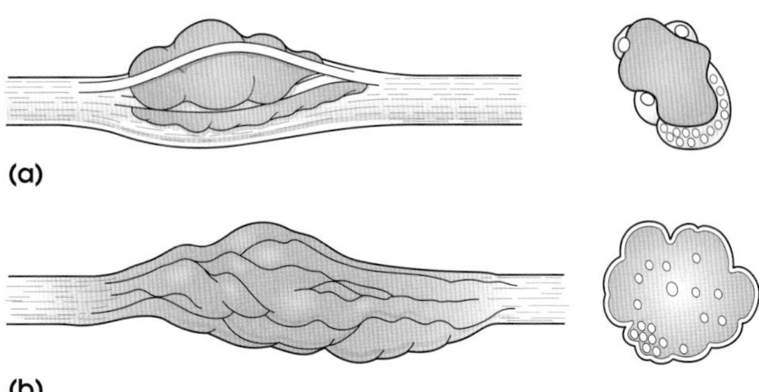

Figure 43.9 (**a**) Schwannoma (intraneural tumour separate from the nerve tissue); and (**b**) neurofibroma (nerve fibres are found within the neurofibroma).

BENIGN NERVE SHEATH TUMOURS

Schwannoma

The most common tumour is the benign schwannoma (neurilemmoma). The median, ulnar and radial nerves are most often affected. The patient presents with a lump but usually has no loss of sensation or power. The lump itself is usually mobile from side to side, but is relatively fixed in the longitudinal axis of the limb. A particularly reliable sign is that percussion induces painful paraesthesia in the territory of the nerve. The tumour usually lies eccentrically within the nerve trunk, displacing fascicles to one side (Fig. 43.9a). Most of these tumours can be enucleated with careful dissection to preserve the conducting elements (Fig. 43.10). Excision of the nerve to remove the tumour is not acceptable treatment. Solitary schwannomas that are enucleated rarely recur, and malignant change in a solitary schwannoma is very rare.[109,110]

Schwannomas arising within the brachial plexus are, however, frequently more infiltrative in nature and their removal may be difficult. In such cases magnification is essential. When this tumour affects the eighth cranial nerve, it is known as an acoustic neuroma. Because access to such tumours is restricted by the surrounding bone, it is occasionally impossible to excise the tumour without damaging part of the nerve. On gross examination the tumour is encapsulated and on cut section may be either solid or cystic.

Neurofibroma

Neurofibroma may occur as a solitary nerve tumour or in association with neurofibromatosis. It may present as a solitary mass in the subcutaneous tissue or along the course of a major peripheral nerve. Like the schwannoma, the neurofibroma arises from the nerve sheath, but unlike the schwannoma, it is intimately associated with the nerve and has nerve fibres running through the tumour (Fig. 43.9b). There is usually little nerve dysfunction and, because excision runs the risk of nerve damage,

REFERENCES

109. Ghosh BC, Ghosh L et al. Cancer 1973; 31: 184–190
110. Dodge HW, Craig WM. Minn Med 1957; 40: 294

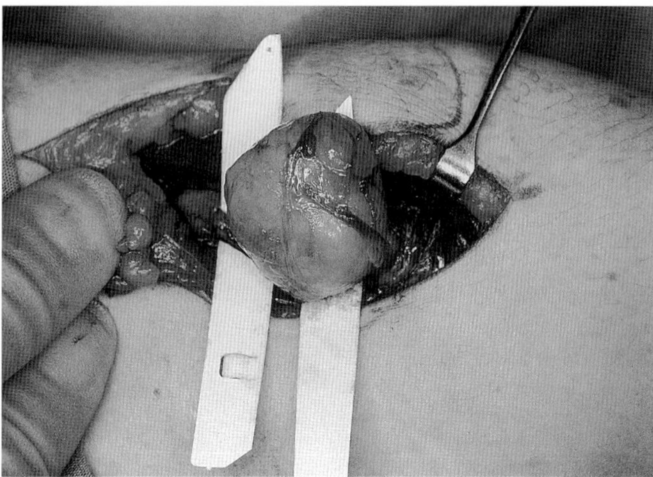

a

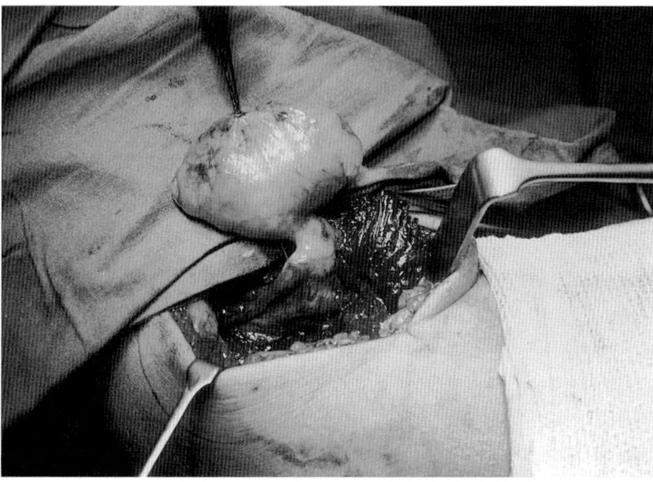

b

Figure 43.10 This schwannoma was resected to leave the main body of the nerve intact.

surgical treatment is usually limited to a biopsy to establish the tissue diagnosis.[32] A neurofibroma in the skin may be completely excised without risk of nerve damage.

Neurofibromatosis

Neurofibromatosis type I is an autosomal dominant genetic disorder with variable gene expression and a quote incidence of one in 3000 live births.[111] The disorder was first reported by von Recklinghausen in 1882[112] and is associated with his name. The clinical diagnosis is made on the presence of two out of seven criteria shown in Box 43.2. The neurofibromas may be widespread cutaneous tumours (Fig. 43.11) or plexiform neurofibromas (Fig. 43.12). Malignant degeneration can occur in lesions of neurofibromatosis with an incidence of 3–10%, but rarely, if ever, in cutaneous neurofibromas.[111]

Neurofibromatosis type II is characterized with bilateral 8th nerve schwannomas, although it may affect other cranial nerves. It is also associated with the development of meningiomas.

MALIGNANT NERVE SHEATH TUMOURS

Malignant nerve sheath tumours are rare and are most often associated with neurofibromatosis.[113] Although there are two types, the malignant schwannoma and the nerve sheath fibrosarcoma, it is difficult to distinguish between them. It is estimated that between 3 and 5% of patients with neurofibromatosis will develop a malignant nerve sheath tumour. The lesions are often central. The peak decade for presentation is 20–30 years. Malignant peripheral nerve sheath tumours also develop in sites that have been previously irradiated.

These malignant peripheral nerve sheath tumours may have a false capsule or be diffusely infiltrative. Central necrosis and numerous mitoses are seen. The tumours typically present with pain and loss of both sensation and power. Palpation of the lump usually causes more pain than is the case when the tumour is benign. If the lump is fixed to adjacent structures, CT and MRI may demonstrate tumour extension into surrounding tissues (e.g. bone or muscle). The regional lymph nodes are rarely affected, but pulmonary metastasis is frequent. These are very aggressive tumours with a tendency to local recurrence and metastasis. Wide excision of these radioresistant tumours is essential. Treatment at specialist centres is recommended.

Box 43.2 Neurofibromatosis type I: clinical diagnosis

Two of the following criteria define the diagnosis:

- Six or more café au lait spots
- Two or more cutaneous neurofibromas or one plexiform neurofibroma
- Lisch nodules, two or more iris lesions on slit-lamp examination
- Axillary or inguinal freckling
- Optic glioma
- Osseous lesion, splenoid dysplasia of bone
- Family history of neurofibromatosis

TUMOURS OF NERVE CELL ORIGIN

Neuroblastoma is a tumour of the sympathetic chain and adrenal medulla that usually presents in childhood. This bulky, soft, cellular tumour tends to destroy the adrenal and spread to the upper abdominal lymph nodes.

Ganglioneuroma is a rare tumour found arising from the sympathetic chain in the abdomen, thorax and cervical region. It is usually a benign encapsulated mass.

Phaeochromocytoma is a tumour of the chromaffin cells in the adrenal medulla. The tumour is usually benign but the cells secrete noradrenaline and adrenaline. The tumour may present with paroxysmal hypertension.

INDIVIDUAL PERIPHERAL NERVE LESIONS

Nerves are commonly damaged by injury or entrapment. They may also be damaged by ischaemia, inflammation (mononeuritis multiplex) and infiltration, or occasionally compressed by benign or malignant tumours. Peripheral nerve lesions must be differentiated from root lesions and upper motor neuron lesions. The cutaneous areas of distribution are shown in Fig. 43.13.

REFERENCES

111. Hope DG, Mulvihill JJ. Adv Neurol 1981; 29: 33–54
112. von Recklinghausen FD. Ueber die multiplen Fibrome der haut und ihre Beziehung zu den multiplen Neuromen. Verlag v. A. Hirschwald, Berlin, 1882
113. Ducatman BS, Scheithauer BW et al. Cancer 1986; 57: 2006–2021

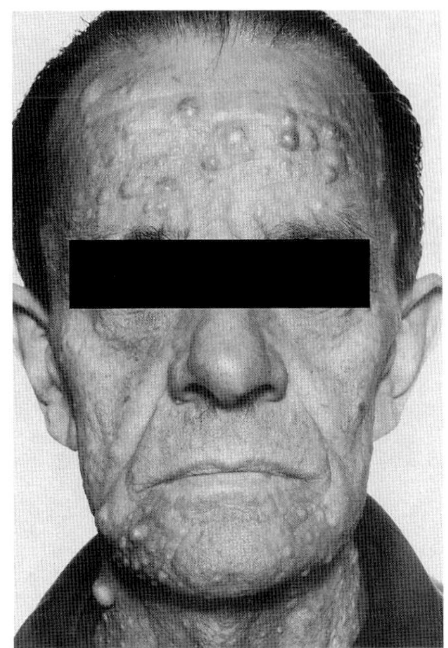
a

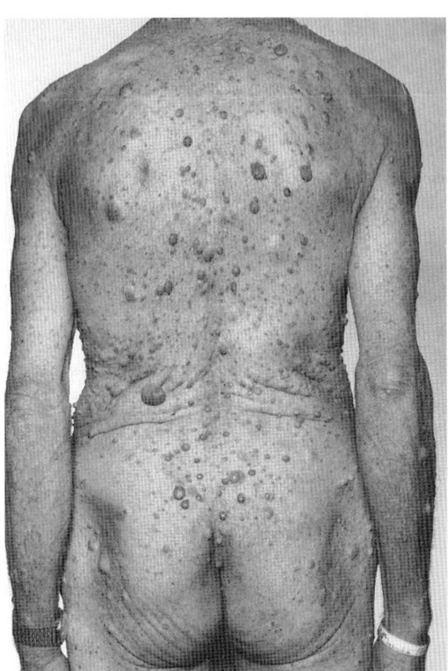
b

Figure 43.11 Neurofibromatosis (von Recklinghausen's disease).

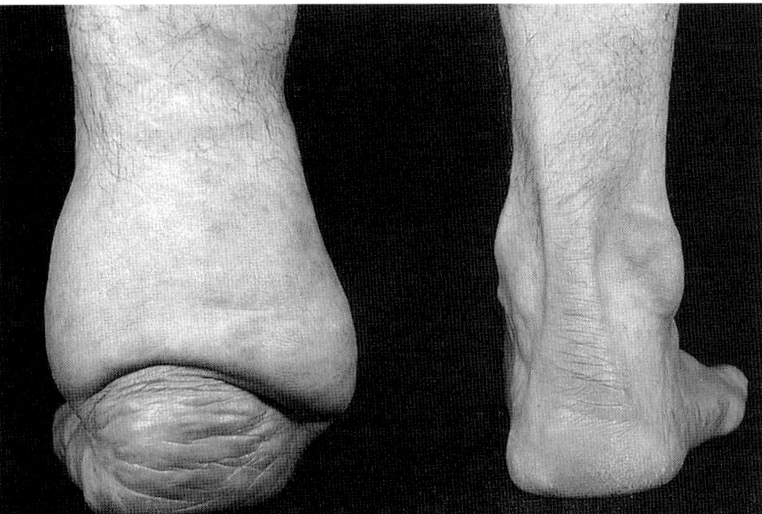
a

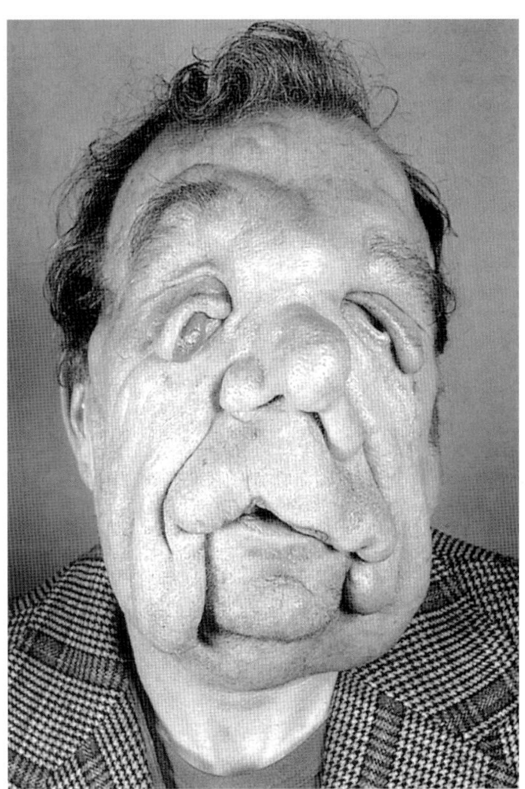
b

Figure 43.12 Plexiform neurofibromatosis of (**a**) the foot and (**b**) the face.

PHRENIC NERVE (C3, 4 AND 5)

The phrenic nerve provides the motor supply of the diaphragm, which becomes paralysed if the nerve is damaged or divided. Irritation of the phrenic nerve causes hiccups or a dry unproductive cough. Diaphragmatic palsy may present with exertional dyspnoea and can be complicated by the development of basal pneumonia. The phrenic nerve may be affected by poliomyelitis and is at risk of injury during operations on the root of the neck, especially cervical sympathectomy, cervical rib resection, block dissection, and surgery on the subclavian artery. It may also be damaged during thoracic surgery and may be infiltrated by carcinoma of the bronchus.

If it is known to be divided at the time of surgery, it can be carefully resutured, but on most occasions diaphragmatic palsy is untreatable and causes few problems unless the patient has severe chronic bronchitis and emphysema.

LONG THORACIC NERVE (C5, 6 AND 7)

The long thoracic nerve supplies the serratus anterior. Although it is reported to have been injured by blows or by the carrying of

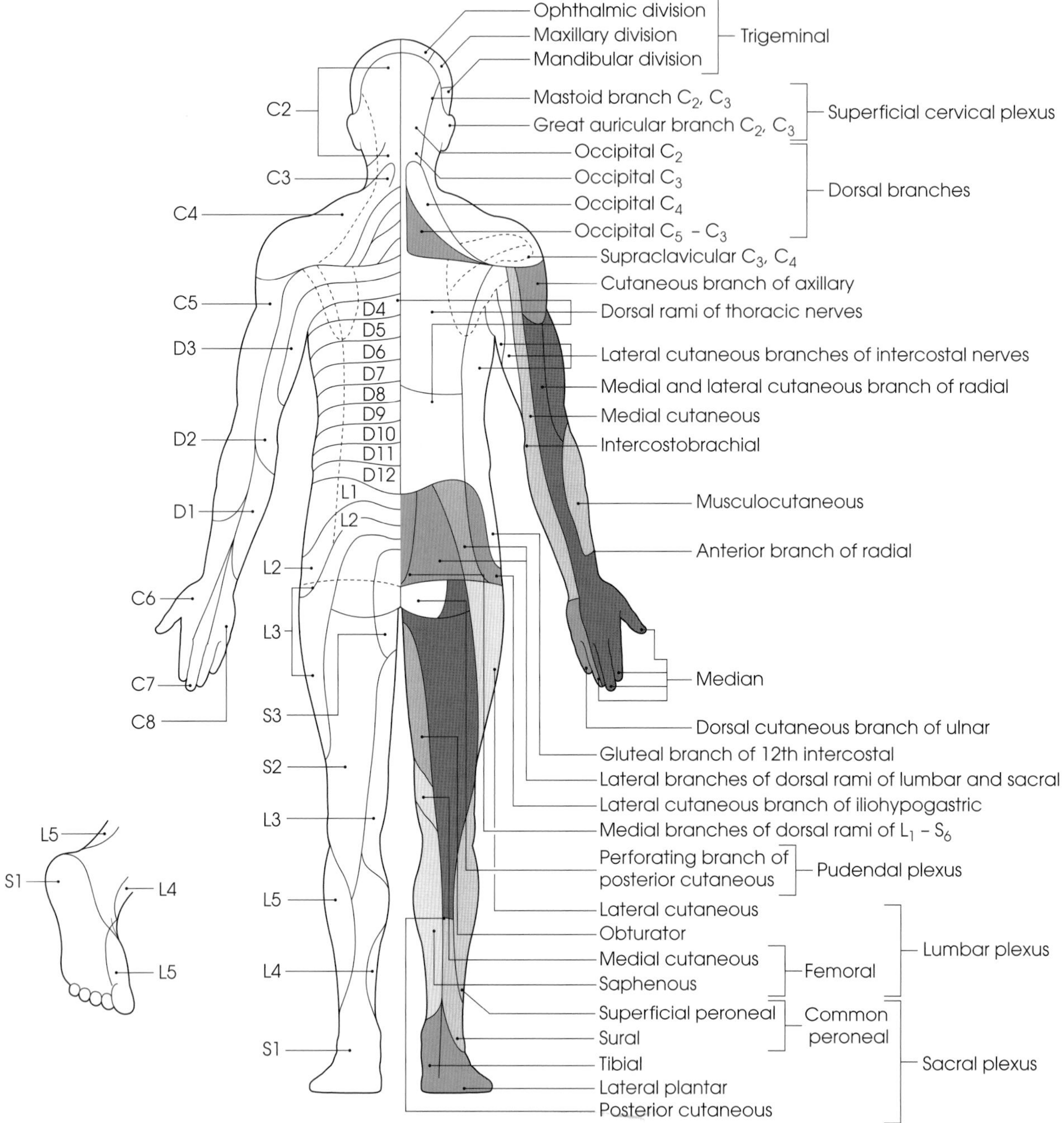

Figure 43.13 Cutaneous areas of distribution of spinal segments and of sensory fibres of the peripheral nerves: (**a**) anterior aspect and (**b**) posterior aspect.

weights, it is most often damaged during axillary operations (either block dissection or mastectomy) combined with axillary clearance. Serratus anterior fixes the scapula to the chest wall, and when forward pressure is exerted on the upper limb, the scapula appears to come away from the thoracic wall ('winging' of the scapula); this is demonstrated by asking the patient to lean forward with outstretched hands against a wall. In addition, patients are often unable to raise the limb in front of the body to 180°. There is usually poor recovery of nerve function, although the nerve should be directly sutured if division is recognized at the time of surgery.

SUPRASCAPULAR NERVE (C5)

The suprascapular nerve supplies the supraspinatus and infraspinatus muscles, which anchor the head of the humerus during abduction of the shoulder. It is rarely damaged, although nerve injury has been reported after scapular fractures.[3] The suprascapular nerve may become entrapped,[89] and this may be responsible for the considerable shoulder pain experienced after certain injuries of this region.[114]

AXILLARY (CIRCUMFLEX) NERVE (C5 AND 6)

The axillary nerve (Fig. 43.14) passes backwards through the quadrilateral space before winding around the humerus beneath the deltoid muscle. Wasting and weakness of the deltoid result

REFERENCES

114. Nankano KK, Lundergau C, Okhiro MM. Acta Neurol (Chicago) 1977; 34: 477

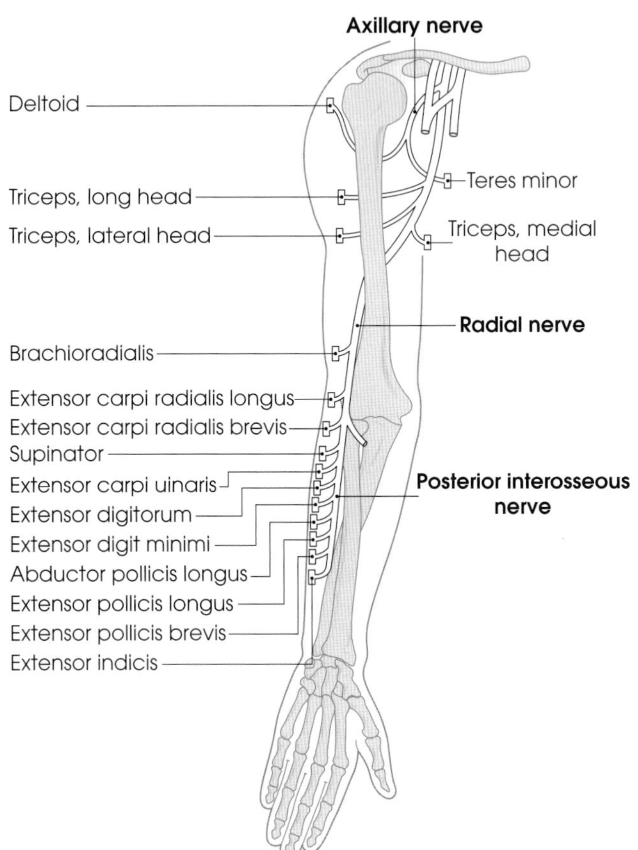

Figure 43.14 Muscles supplied by the radial and axillary nerves. (From the MRC 1980.[14])

in a loss of shoulder abduction together with a small area of cutaneous sensory loss over the insertion of the deltoid (Fig. 43.13), the 'shoulder badge' area. This nerve is most commonly injured in anterior dislocation of the shoulder.

RADIAL NERVE (C5, 6, 7, 8 AND T1)

The radial nerve is the motor nerve to triceps, anconeus, brachioradialis, extensor carpi radialis longus and, through its posterior interosseous branch, to extensor carpi radialis brevis, supinator, extensor digitorum longus, extensor digiti minimi, extensor carpi ulnaris, and extensor pollicis longus and brevis (Fig. 43.14). It supplies sensation to the lower half of the radial aspect of the arm and the middle of the posterior forearm. In addition, it supplies sensation to the back of the hand and the posterior aspect of the three radial fingers (Fig. 43.13). This nerve may be damaged at any point along its course.

Crutch palsy was an important cause of high radial nerve lesions in the axilla in the past. With damage at this level all the muscles supplied by the nerve become paralysed. Patients are unable to extend the elbow because of triceps denervation; they cannot flex the semiprone elbow because the action of brachioradialis is lost. Supination is weak, although still present because the biceps still acts. There is wrist and finger drop as the extensors of the wrist and fingers are all paralysed and the thumb will not extend (Fig. 43.15). The fingers are able to be extended in a supported hand because the small muscles of the hand function normally. These contract synergistically and cause flexion of the metacarpophalangeal and extension of the interphalangeal joints. The radial nerve may also be damaged at the axillary level when an anaesthetized patient is allowed to hang the arm over the edge of an operating table. This type of injury can also occur in a 'Saturday night paralysis', when the patient falls asleep with the arm hanging over the edge of a chair or bed after a surfeit of alcohol. Conduction studies confirm the level of the lesion.[115]

If the radial nerve is injured further down the arm, the triceps escapes, as may the brachioradialis and extensor carpi radialis longus. With this picture, the patient has the signs of an isolated posterior interosseous nerve lesion. The posterior interosseous nerve is damaged directly on occasions by an isolated fracture dislocation of the upper radius, but radial nerve injury in the arm is usually associated with a fracture of the shaft of the humerus. The radial nerve may also be damaged by intramuscular injections, or by the prolonged application of a tourniquet. The posterior interosseous nerve may be compressed by the fibrous edge of extensor carpi radialis brevis[89] or where it passes between the two layers of the supinator. When the posterior interosseous nerve alone is damaged, it has the appearances of a distal radial nerve without any accompanying sensory loss.[116]

The radial nerve usually recovers well after suturing. If an electromyograph confirms interosseous nerve compression, surgical exploration and decompression are indicated. A patient with an irreparable radial nerve palsy needs wrist extension, finger extension (of the metacarpophalangeal joints), and a combination of thumb extension and abduction to open up the hand. Some of the extrinsic muscles innervated by the median and ulnar nerves can be transferred to effect this. It is important to maintain a full passive range of motion in all joints to prevent contractures; dynamic splints with outriggers are often helpful.

The flexor carpi ulnaris can be transferred to power the finger extensors,[117] while palmaris longus is rerouted to effect thumb extension and the pronator teres is used to extend the wrist.[118]

MUSCULOCUTANEOUS NERVE (C5 AND 6)

The musculocutaneous nerve is the motor nerve to biceps and also innervates part of the brachialis. Both these muscles are elbow flexors, and the biceps is the principle supinator of the forearm. It also supplies sensation to a small area on the radial border of the forearm, extending down to the carpometacarpal joint of the thumb (Fig. 43.17). Weakness results in a loss of elbow flexion, which may be partly compensated by the fact that the median nerve supplies part of brachialis.

MEDIAN NERVE (C5, 6, 7, 8 AND T1)

The median nerve is formed from two heads – one from the lateral cord and the other from the medial cord of the brachial plexus (see Fig. 43.9). It is the motor nerve of the anterior compartment of the forearm supplying pronator teres, flexor carpi radialis, palmaris longus, flexor digitorum superficialis, flexor pollicis longus, flexor digitorum profundus and flexor carpi radialis, and in the hand it supplies the two radial lumbricals, opponens pollicis and abductor pollicis brevis. It also supplies the radial half of flexor pollicis brevis and may supply the

REFERENCES

115. Critchlow JF, Seybold ME, Jablecki CJ. J Neurol Neurosurg Psychiatry 1980; 43: 929
116. Spinner M. Injuries to the Major Branches of Peripheral Nerves of the Forearm. WB Saunders, Philadelphia, 1972
117. Jones R. Am J Surg 1921; 35: 333–335
118. Scuderi C. Surg Gynecol Obstet 1949; 88: 643–651

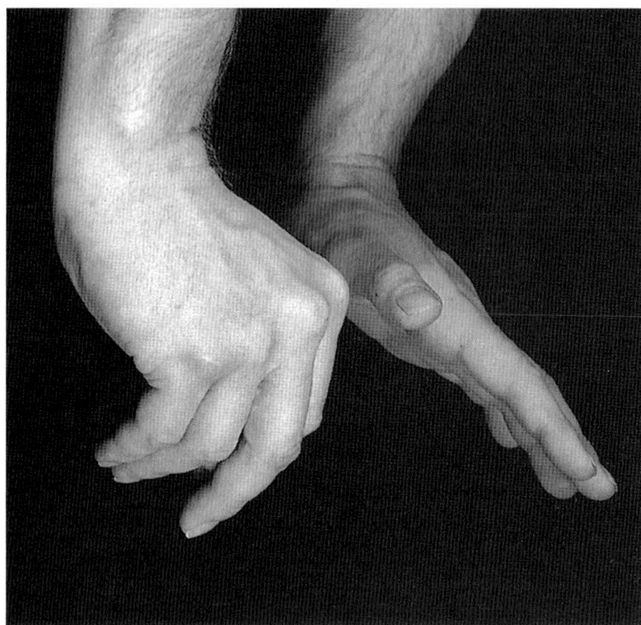

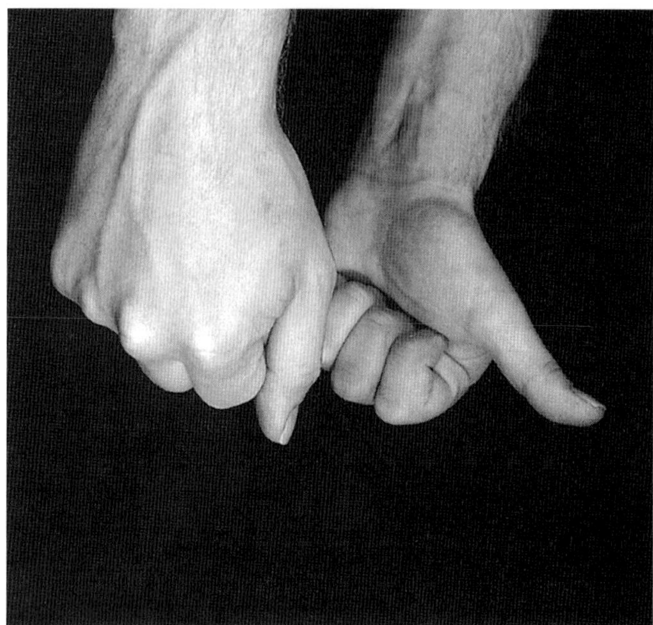

Figure 43.15 The effect of posterior interosseous nerve palsy, showing loss of extension of (**a**) fingers and (**b**) thumb.

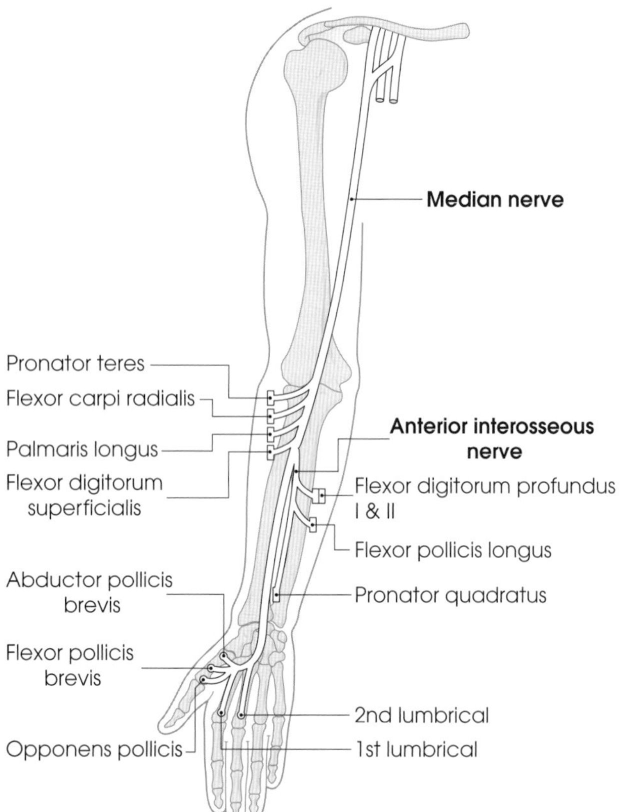

Figure 43.16 The muscles supplied by the median nerve. (From the MRC 1980.[14])

first dorsal interosseous (Fig. 43.16). It provides sensation to the radial three-and-a-half digits, the radial half of the palm, and the dorsal tips of the same three-and-a-half digits (Fig. 43.13).

High median nerve division

High median nerve division results in an inability to pronate the forearm and flex the wrist, thumb or index finger (Fig. 43.17).

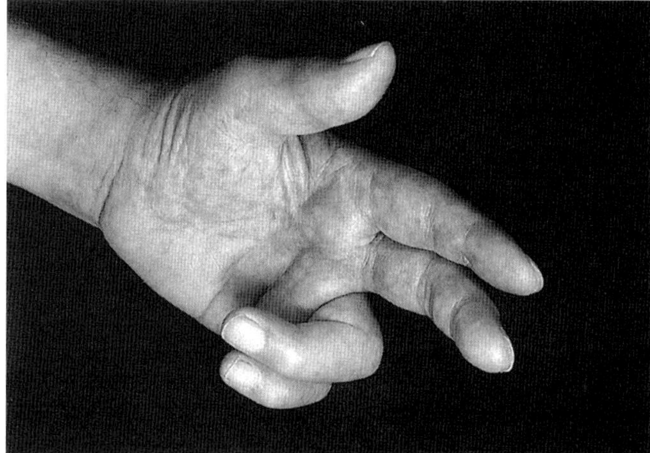

Figure 43.17 High median nerve lesion showing loss of flexion of the index finger (past pointing).

The median nerve is damaged by fracture dislocations, overzealous application of tourniquets, or malplaced injections. It may be damaged during operations on the brachial artery, and it may obviously be lacerated or damaged by knife or gunshot wounds.

When the median nerve is damaged in the upper arm, the hand goes into ulnar deviation when flexed against a resistance, because the radial flexor is paralysed while the ulnar flexor is normally unaffected. Patients with a median nerve injury are unable to flex the terminal phalanx of their thumb or any of the phalanges of their index finger. Flexion of the phalanges of the remaining fingers, especially the middle one, is weak. The other fingers can be flexed because flexor digitorum profundus receives a dual nerve supply. Flexion at the metacarpophalangeal joints is not affected because the interossei and lumbricals function normally. The thenar muscles become wasted, and there is a weakness of thumb abduction that should be tested by asking the patient to elevate the thumb at right angles to the palm.

There is also a weakness of opposition. As a result of the wasting of the thenar eminence, the first metacarpal becomes more prominent.

Low median nerve division

The nerve is more often damaged at the wrist, where glass lacerations and attempts at suicide are common modes of injury. It may also be damaged by venepuncture.[119] With a complete median nerve laceration at the wrist, there will be no function in abductor pollicis brevis or the opponens muscle. Opposition can, however, be simulated by a combined contraction of adductor pollicis and flexor pollicis longus, but the thumb stays flat and does not swing over the palm. Sensation to the thumb, index and middle fingers will also be lost, with a lack of sweating and loss of tactile adherence.

ULNAR NERVE (C8 AND T1)

The ulnar nerve does not give branches above the elbow, at which point it lies subcutaneously, as it passes behind the medial epicondyle of the humerus. In the forearm, it supplies motor fibres to flexor carpi ulnaris and half of flexor digitorum profundus. In the hand, it supplies palmaris brevis, the hypothenar muscles, the two medial lumbricals, all the interossei, adductor pollicis and part of flexor pollicis brevis (Fig. 43.18).

Ulnar nerve lesion at the elbow or above

Lesions above the elbow are rare and occur from the usual causes of local trauma and fracture dislocations. At the elbow, the nerve is also often damaged as a result of fracture dislocations. It may be damaged at a much later stage if cubitus valgus complicates the fracture (the so-called Tardy palsy[105]). Osteophytes, Charcot's joints, and compression beneath flexor carpi ulnaris can also cause nerve damage.[88,116] The nerve may also be injured by constant leaning on the elbow (student's elbow), and repetitive trauma may result in a thickened nerve, which must of course be differentiated from leprosy. Benign tumours may also compress the nerve.

If the wrist is flexed against resistance, radial deviation results from the unopposed action of the radial flexor. The small muscles of the hand are paralysed, resulting in a claw deformity due to loss of flexion of the metacarpophalangeal joint, while the long flexors are still active. The claw hand has a hyperextended metacarpophalangeal joint with flexion of the proximal and distal interphalangeal joints, particularly in the little and ring fingers.

Loss of abduction and adduction of the fingers is the result of paralysis of the interossei and lumbricals. This should be tested with the hand on a flat surface as the long extensors and flexors can achieve some abduction and adduction as a synergistic movement. There is a loss of thumb adduction, shown by the fact that the thumb cannot be squeezed hard against the index finger. The hand is obviously wasted as a result of the loss of small muscle bulk. Froment's sign is present.[120] This is seen when the patient squeezes a piece of paper between the thumb and the side of the index finger. The terminal phalanx of the affected thumb is seen to flex, because weakness of the adductor pollicis results in overaction of flexor pollicis longus (Fig. 43.19). Pinprick sensation is reduced over the little finger, the ulnar border of the palm, and the ulnar side of the ring finger on both its dorsal and palmar aspects (Fig. 43.13).

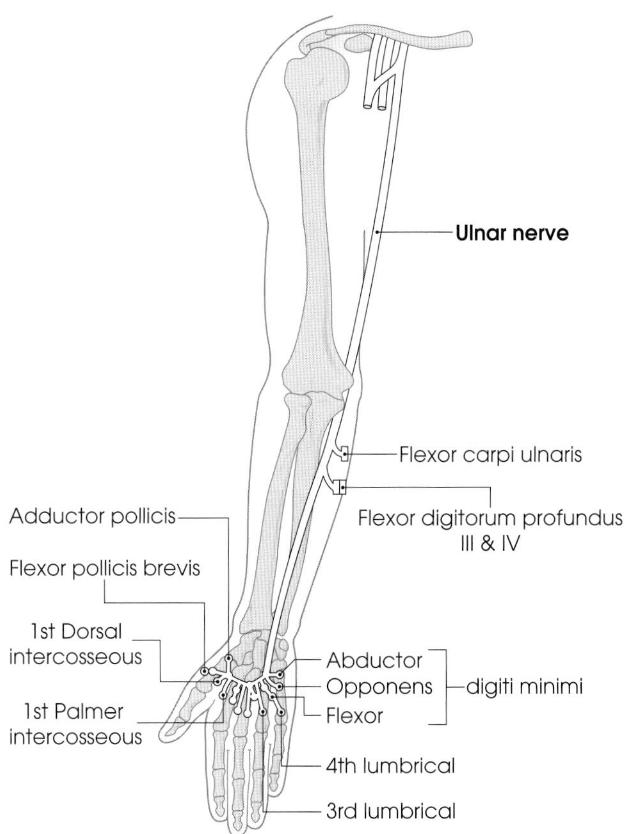

Figure 43.18 The muscles supplied by the ulnar nerve. (From the MRC 1980.[14])

Ulnar nerve lesions at the wrist

The flexor carpi ulnaris and flexor digitorum profundus escape damage with injuries at this level. Sensory loss is mild, but the small muscles of the hand are obviously affected. A lack of adduction of the fingers is easily tested by placing a piece of paper between two fingers and showing that the paper can be easily extracted by gentle pressure, despite the patient's best efforts to prevent this from happening.

Clawing can be prevented by a 'knuckleduster' splint. This maintains flexion at the metacarpophalangeal joint and extension of the interphalangeal joint.[121] Should the nerve require suture, a return of sensation is likely but the small muscles of the hand do not always recover.

Differential diagnosis of median and ulnar nerve lesions

A number of conditions have to be considered in a patient presenting with paralysis and sensory loss in the hand, particularly if the small muscles are wasted. These conditions include acute poliomyelitis, Guillain–Barré syndrome, spinal cord injury or thrombosis of a spinal artery, motor neuron disease and spinal muscular atrophy. Syringomyelia, cervical disc prolapse and spondylosis may also be responsible. A cervical rib may produce sensory and motor abnormalities.

REFERENCE

119. Berry PR, Wallis WE. Lancet 1977; i: 1236
120. Rouillet J. In: Michon J, Moberg E (eds). Traumatic Nerve Lesions of the Upper Limb. Churchill Livingstone, Edinburgh, 1975
121. Highet WB. Lancet 1942; i: 555

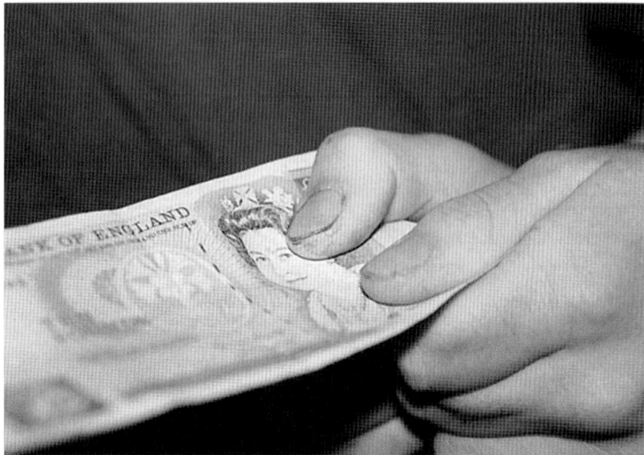

Figure 43.19 Froment's sign for right ulnar paresis.

LOWER LIMB

The lumbosacral plexus is derived from T12, L1, 2, 3 and 4 (lumbar plexus) and L4, 5, S1, 2 and 3 (sacral plexus). The lumbar plexus gives rise to the femoral and obturator nerves, and the sacral plexus to the sciatic and gluteal nerves. The plexuses themselves may be involved in the metastatic spread of pelvic malignancy, compressed at their roots by a disc prolapse, damaged by the fetal head or by the application of forceps,[122] and by pelvic operations including rectal resections, bladder surgery and vascular bypasses.

LATERAL CUTANEOUS NERVE OF THE THIGH (L2 AND 3)

This nerve arises from the lumbar plexus and enters the thigh beneath the lateral part of the inguinal ligament (Fig. 43.13). It pierces the fascia lata 10 cm down the thigh, supplying sensation to the anterolateral thigh. This nerve occasionally becomes entrapped in middle-aged women and is responsible for numbness and hyperalgesia (meralgia paraesthetica). Operative decompression should be considered.[123]

OBTURATOR NERVE (L2, 3 AND 4)

The obturator nerve arises from the lumbar plexus and passes into the thigh through the obturator canal. It supplies motor fibres to pectineus, gracilis, the adductor longus, magnus and brevis, and the obturator externus. It provides sensation to the hip and knee, and to the skin of the medial thigh (Fig. 43.13). It is occasionally injured during hip dislocations, hip replacements, and during a difficult labour. It may also be compressed by an obturator hernia.[83]

GENITOFEMORAL NERVE (L1 AND 2)

The femoral compartment of the nerve (L1) supplies the skin over the femoral triangle. The genital component (L2) enters the spermatic cord to supply the cremaster muscle and sensation to the tunica vaginalis and the spermatic fascia. Injuries to this nerve may be responsible for pain after hernia operations. If the nerve is trapped by a suture, then local anaesthetic infiltration will relieve the discomfort. Neurolysis or nerve section is then indicated.

SAPHENOUS NERVE

This is the sensory part of the femoral nerve running down to the medial malleolus alongside the saphenous vein. It is commonly damaged at the time of varicose vein surgery or femoropopliteal

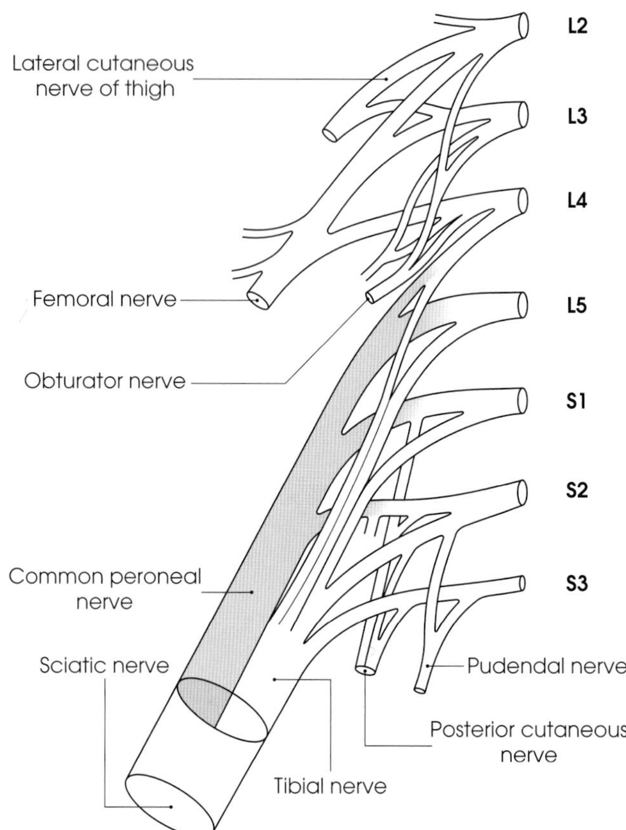

Figure 43.20 The lumbosacral plexus.

bypass surgery. It results in an annoying patch of anaesthesia on the medial calf (Fig. 43.17). This can be avoided if the long saphenous vein is not stripped below the knee.

FEMORAL NERVE (L2, 3 AND 4)

The femoral nerve also arises from the lumbar plexus and passes into the thigh beneath the inguinal ligament lateral to the femoral artery. It supplies motor fibres to iliacus in the abdomen, and in the thigh supplies the quadriceps femoris muscles and sartorius. It carries some sensory fibres from the hip and knee joints and supplies sensory branches to the anteromedial thigh and the medial side of the lower leg.

Damage to the femoral nerve by a psoas abscess, fractured pelvis, hip dislocation or local trauma is quite common because of its relatively exposed position. The nerve is also commonly affected by diabetes and lumbar spondylosis.

Nerve damage results in weak hip flexion because of the weak iliacus muscle and reduced knee extension from the quadriceps denervation. The patient finds that the knee gives way on walking and finds climbing up stairs difficult. Nerve suture or nerve grafting may be helpful.

SCIATIC NERVE (L4, 5, S1, 2 AND 3)

The sciatic nerve (Fig. 43.20) is composed of the tibial (or medial popliteal) nerve and the common peroneal (or lateral popliteal)

REFERENCES

122. Donaldson J. The Neurology of Pregnancy. WB Saunders, Philadelphia, 1977
123. Stevens H. Arch Neurol Psychiatry Chicago 1957; 77: 557

nerve. These nerves can be separated all the way up the main sciatic trunk. The sciatic nerve leaves the pelvis through the greater sciatic notch, and passes straight down the back of the thigh to end in the popliteal fossa by dividing into its two main branches. It provides the motor supply to the hamstrings, to part of adductor magnus, and to all the muscles below the knee.

The common peroneal nerve supplies the muscles of the peroneal compartment through its superficial branch and those of the anterior compartment through its deep branch.

The tibial nerve supplies the gastrocnemius, soleus, the long flexors of the toes, tibialis posterior, and the small muscles of the foot via the medial and lateral plantar nerves.

A lesion of the main sciatic nerve causes loss of the knee flexion, a foot drop, and inability to walk. Patients with sciatic nerve lesions drag their feet behind them and are often unable to stand for long periods. This is accompanied by wasting of the lower leg muscles. Sensation is lost from the knee downwards, except for a strip on the medial side of the leg, which is supplied by the saphenous nerve (a branch of the femoral nerve). A normal knee jerk can be elicited, but the ankle jerk is missing. Trophic ulcers and vasomotor disturbances are common.

The sciatic nerve is injured in association with fractures of the pelvis and femur, and may also be damaged by a misplaced injection. Nurses inject in the safe upper outer quadrant of the buttock to avoid the nerve. Its relatively superficial course also makes it liable to damage by gunshot wounds and other forms of direct trauma. It may occasionally be compressed by the pyriformis muscle or by a large Baker's cyst.[90]

If the nerve is inadvertently divided, it is always worth suturing it. Nerve recovery is, however, slow and usually incomplete.[124]

COMMON PERONEAL NERVE (L4, 5, S1 AND 2)

The common peroneal nerve is damaged nine times more often than the tibial nerve. The peroneal and anterior tibial muscles are usually paralysed, giving a loss of dorsiflexion and a foot drop. Sensation is lost over the dorsum of the foot and lateral part of the lower limb. This nerve is usually damaged as it winds round the neck of the fibula. It is very superficial at this point and wounds, plasters, splints and fractures of the fibula are common sources of nerve injury. In addition, the nerve may be inadvertently damaged during varicose vein surgery or reduction operations for lymphoedema. It may also be compressed occasionally in the anterior tarsal tunnel, causing a foot drop.

TIBIAL NERVE (L4, 5, S1, 2 AND 3)

The tibial nerve supplies the flexor muscles of the calf. Injury results in talipes calcaneovarus. After nerve division, the plantar and ankle jerks cannot be elicited. The sole of the foot is anaesthetic, and trophic ulcers are common. The nerve may be divided or damaged during popliteal dissections to ligate the short saphenous vein at its termination or during operations on the popliteal artery. It may also be damaged by posterior dislocations of the knee and posteriorly displaced fractures of the tibia. The posterior tibial nerve can occasionally be compressed behind the medial malleolus by the posterior tarsal tunnel.

SURAL NERVE (L5, S1 AND 2)

The sural nerve can be damaged at the time of short saphenous surgery. Its division is of little significance but causes an annoying patch of anaesthesia on the outer border of the foot. Because of the minor nature of symptoms following sural nerve resection, it is commonly used as a source of nerve grafts.

AREAS OF POTENTIAL PROGRESS

Diagnosis

The quality of ultrasound imaging has improved. It is now possible to diagnose carpal tunnel syndrome ultrasonically, for example, on finding a significant increase in the cross-sectional area of the median nerve. This, the opposite of what might be expected, is possibly due to venous compression which causes swelling of the distal nerve. In posterior interosseous nerve compression, ultrasound may detect ganglia within the supinator muscle.

Therapy

Neurotrophic factors have been shown to be useful in research situations and have potential. In limb lengthening procedures, expansion of nerves at a rate of about 1mm per day has been shown to be possible. Expansion of individual nerves may allow nerve gaps to be bridged without traditional grafting. The use of botulinum toxin to suppress excess muscle activity in children with cerebral palsy has proved to be highly effective.

REFERENCES

124. Seddon HJ. Surgical Disorders of the Peripheral Nerves. Williams & Wilkins, Baltimore, 1972

Muscles, ligaments and tendons 44

James Bliss

MUSCLES

Skeletal striated muscle generates the force required for all locomotor movement. In addition to striated skeletal muscle, there are broadly two additional forms of muscle found in the body: involuntary smooth muscle and cardiac striated muscle fibres. Striated cardiac muscle contraction generates arterial pressure providing circulatory flow. Smooth muscle contraction provides tone and subsequent movement of contents within the gastrointestinal and urogenital tracts. Smooth muscle is identified within all organ systems, including the skin, and is seen in vessel walls throughout the vascular tree where it provides vascular tone and controls vessel diameter. Striated muscle will be considered in this chapter only.

BIOLOGY OF STRIATED SKELETAL MUSCLE

Muscle acts to generate force, which is transferred through the end tendon and across the joint to produce movement. The muscle itself is surrounded by a thick, loose connective tissue layer, the epimysium. Muscle tissue is made up of muscle fibres, or myofibres, which are themselves aggregates of contractile elements, or myofibrils. Individual myofibrils are bundled together to form a fasciculus, which is encased in a connective layer, the perimysium. Each muscle cell, or myofibre, is surrounded by a complex cell membrane, the sarcolemma, and contains multiple peripheral nuclei. The cell membrane (sarcolemma) is highly specialized and incorporates a system of membrane-bound sacs, which are involved in calcium storage, and hence in the initiation of muscular contraction, on calcium release (Fig. 44.1).

Myofibres have a distinct appearance of alternating light and dark bands when viewed on light microscopy, hence are referred to as striated muscle. The muscle cell contains the contractile proteins actin (thin filament) and myosin (thick filament). It is the interaction between the contractile proteins of actin and myosin, through troponin–tropomyosin binding under the influence of calcium, which generates muscle tension and subsequent muscular contraction (Fig. 44.2).

Muscle fibre types may be subdivided according to physiological properties. Type I fibres are slow-twitch fibres, which have a high myoglobin content and a high fatigue resistance. Type II fibres are fast-twitch fibres, with type IIA fibres having a fast contraction time with a moderate fatigue resistance and type IIB fibres having the fastest contraction time, the largest fibre diameter and the lowest fatigue resistance. Depending on the physiological requirements of the muscle group, differing percentages of each fibre type are seen depending on the fatigue requirements of the muscle and the rapidity of contraction needed. In addition, differing individuals have varying percentages of fibre types, with athletes excelling at sports requiring fast, explosive muscle activity (such as sprinters) having a higher percentage of type II fibres in muscle groups compared with endurance athletes, who have more type I fibres.

ANATOMY OF SKELETAL MUSCLES

Skeletal muscles can be classified according to muscle fibre orientation. Fusiform (or unipennate) muscles have parallel fibres with a tendon or origin at one end and an insertion at the other. Bipennate muscles, such as the biceps brachii, have a split muscle belly with two heads of origin. Multipennate muscles (e.g. the deltoid muscle) have a complex origin, with convergent fibres from the broad origin to the tendon of insertion.

The macroscopic orientation of muscle fibres has an influence on the mechanical properties, with fusiform muscles having the potential for the greatest tendon excursion and multipennate muscles producing the least tendon excursion. However, the orientation of multipennate fibres allows a greater number of contractile elements to act on the tendon of insertion, thus exerting the maximal possible force of contraction. Therefore multipennate muscles are found in locations where great force generation is required, such as from the gluteus maximus, pectoralis major and deltoid muscles.

NEURONAL CONTROL OF MUSCULAR CONTRACTION

Striated skeletal muscle is under voluntary control and contraction, initiated by neuronal activity, under primary control of the α-motor neuron. The α-motor neuron passes out from the ventral root of the spinal cord, through the peripheral nerve, to arrive at its target organ, the skeletal muscle, where it forms a specialized synapse with the muscle tissue, the motor end plate. On arrival at the neuromuscular junction, the action potential releases acetylcholine into the synaptic cleft, which releases stored calcium from the specialized vesicles of the sarcolemma (or cell membrane). Calcium release into the myofibre cytoplasm results in muscular contraction (Fig. 44.3).

In addition to the primary α-motor neuron initiating muscular contraction, skeletal muscle is subject to feedback control through receptor organelles in the muscle itself and the attached tendon, and also through neuronal pathways within the spinal cord.

FORCE GENERATION

The force generated by skeletal muscle is influenced by the orientation of the muscle fibres, fibre preload, muscle geometry and muscle training.

The maximal contractile force generated by any given muscle is governed by the cross-sectional area. For a fusiform muscle, doubling the cross-sectional area has the capability of generating twice the contractile force. Due to the differing directions of pull

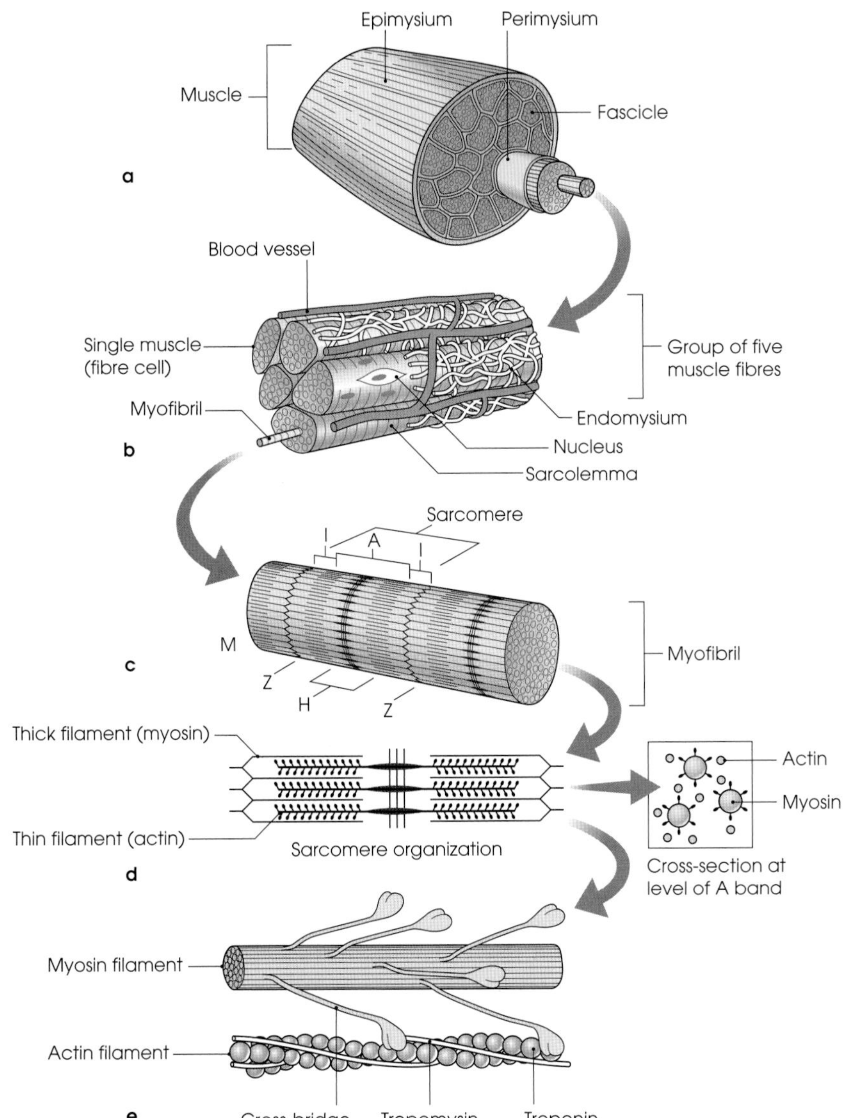

Figure 44.1 The structural organization of muscle. (a) A fibrous connective tissue fascia (the epimysium) surrounds the muscle, which is composed of many bundles (or fascicles). The fascicles are encased in a connective tissue sheath, the perimysium. (b) The fascicles consist of muscle fibres, which are long, cylindrical, multinucleated cells. Between the individual muscle fibres are capillary blood vessels. Each muscle fibre is surrounded by a loose connective tissue called the endomysium. Just beneath the endomysium lies the sarcolemma, a thin elastic sheath with infoldings that invaginate the fibre interior. Each muscle fibre comprises numerous delicate strands (myofibrils), the contractile elements of muscle. (c) Myofibrils consist of smaller filaments that form a repeating banding pattern along the length of the myofibril. One unit of this serially repeating pattern is called a sarcomere. The sarcomere is the functional unit of the contractile system of muscle. (d) The banding pattern of the sarcomere is formed by the organization of thick and thin filaments composed of the proteins myosin and actin, respectively. The actin filaments are attached at one end but are free along their length to interdigitate with the myosin filaments. The thick filaments are arranged in a hexagonal fashion. A cross-section through the area of overlap shows the thick filaments surrounded by six equally spaced thin filaments. (e) The lollipop-shaped molecules of each myosin filament are arranged so that the long tails form a sheaf with the heads, or cross-bridges, projecting from it. The cross-bridges point in one direction along half of the filament and in the other direction along the other half. Only a portion of one half of a filament is shown here. The cross-bridges are an essential element in the mechanism of muscle contraction, extending outward to interdigitate with receptor sites on the actin filaments. Each actin filament is a double helix, appearing as two strands of beads spiralling around each other. Two additional proteins, tropomysin and troponin, are associated with the actin helix and play an important role in regulating the interdigitation of the actin and myosin filaments. Tropomysin is a long polypeptide chain that lies in the grooves between the helices of actin. Troponin is a globular molecule attached at regular intervals to the tropomysin. (After Williams and Warwick 1980.[1])

created within the muscle by the differing orientations of the multipennate muscle fibres, there is not such a direct relationship between cross-sectional area and force of contraction.

Muscles may act as agonists or antagonists. For any given movement agonist muscle groups are the prime movers, for example the quadriceps muscle group acting to generate knee extension, with the antagonist group (hamstrings) undergoing eccentric stretching with an increase in tone but allowing muscle elongation. In this manner, the action of the quadriceps is balanced to produce coordinated and controlled knee extension. The interplay between agonist and antagonist groups may be influenced by proprioceptive feedback during athletic training.

Muscle activity may be described as concentric, when contraction produces a shortening of the muscle, or eccentric, with increased tone but an elongation of the muscle (as in antagonist activity). Isometric contraction refers to a muscle undergoing contraction but with no change in muscle length (Fig. 44.4).

The prestimulation length, or stretch, of a muscle dictates isometric contractile force generated. Preload serves to enhance the cross-bridging between the actin and myosin contractile proteins within the myofibre. However, overstretching of the muscle reduces the contractile force produced, due to slight

REFERENCE

1. Williams PL, Warwick R (eds). Gray's Anatomy. 36th edn. Churchill Livingstone. 1980

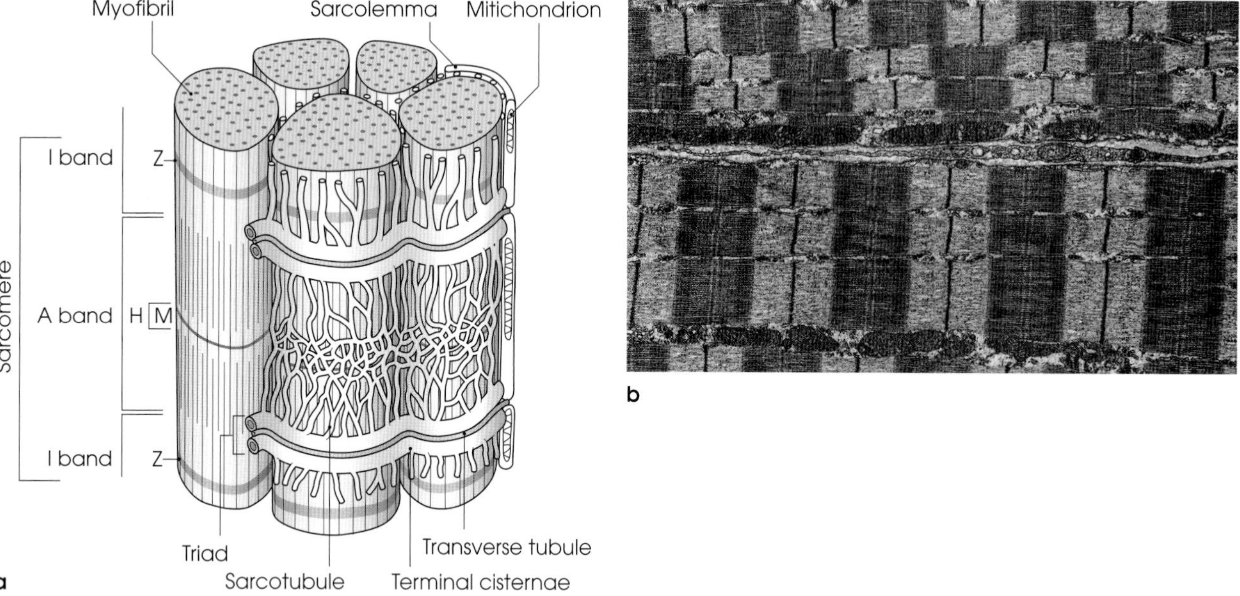

Figure 44.2 (a) A portion of skeletal muscle fibre illustrating the sarcoplasmic reticulum that surrounds each myofibril. The various regions of the sarcomere are indicated on the left myofibril to show the correlation of these regions with the sarcoplasmic reticulum, shown surrounding the middle and right myofibrils. The transverse tubules represent an infolding of the sarcolemma, the plasma membrane that encompasses the entire muscle fibre. Two transverse tubules supply each sarcomere at the level of the junctions of the A band and I bands. Terminal cisternae are located on each side of the transverse tubule, and together these structures constitute a triad. The terminal cisternae connect with a longitudinal network of sarcotubules spanning the region of the A band. (b) Low-power electron micrograph of skeletal muscle in longitudinal section, showing myofibrils. (After Ham and Cormack 1979,[2] (b); the micrograph was taken by Brenda Russell, University of Illinois at Chicago, USA.)

actin–myosin dissociation. Therefore the force of contraction of a given muscle is optimized for its physiological working length.

THE EFFECT OF TRAINING ON SKELETAL MUSCLE

Skeletal muscle may be significantly influenced by athletic training, depending on the form that the training takes. Differing training patterns produce different responses within skeletal muscle.

Endurance training, with an emphasis on long periods of repetitive, low-intensity exercise, produces an increase in mitochondrial activity in all myofibre types, thereby improving the oxidative capacity of the muscle tissue. Prolonged endurance training improves the muscle's capacity to utilize fatty acids through aerobic metabolism, thereby sparing muscle glycogen stores at the expense of fat utilization.

High-resistance, short-duration exercise of high intensity serves to initially increase the contractile protein levels within muscle; therefore initially there is a response to produce increased strength. With protracted high-resistance, high-intensity training, fibre hypertrophy occurs with further contractile protein synthesis, which generates increased force of contraction. In addition, increased contractile velocity is seen, thereby allowing an increased force to also be applied more rapidly.

The individual's response to exercise regimens is highly variable, with some persons demonstrating a more rapid and sustained response to high-intensity, high-resistance programmes, with subsequent muscle hypertrophy.

The influence of anabolic steroid ingestion on skeletal muscle response to exercise is not clear-cut. Irrespective of the central nervous system, cardiovascular and hepatic effects of anabolic steroid usage, the musculoskeletal effects may show an improved recovery time following heavy resistance activity. This allows a more intense regimen to be followed, which in turn sees an increase in contractile protein synthesis and muscle hypertrophy. Collagen synthesis, particularly of tendons, lags behind the response to the contractile elements and therefore tendon ruptures are seen, particularly of the biceps, pectoralis and quadriceps mechanisms. Bilateral patellar tendon and quadriceps tendon ruptures, in the absence of inflammatory joint disease, are usually indicative of anabolic steroid use.[6]

MUSCLE INJURY

Muscle may be overloaded either acutely or as part of a spectrum of chronic microtrauma, which usually presents as an end-organ failure of tendinosis. As a response to an episode of unusual muscular activity, muscular pain is noted between 1 and 34 days after the increased activity, with discomfort predominantly at the muscle–tendon interface. This reversible injury resolves after a couple of days; however, the maximal contractile force that the muscle can generate is reduced during the recovery period. If following muscle recovery activity is repeated, then as a result of adaptation a greater intensity will be possible before muscle soreness recurs.

REFERENCES

2. Ham AW, Cormack DW (eds). Histology. 8th edn. Lippincott. 1979
3. Williams PL, Warwick R (eds). Gray's Anatomy. 36th edn. Churchill Livingstone. 1980
4. Prichard R. Am J Pathol 1979
5. Brobeck JR (ed). Best and Taylor's Physiological Basis of Medical Practice. 10th edn. Williams and Wilkins. 1979
6. Karpakka JA, Pesola MK, Takala TE. Am J Sports Med 1992; 20: 262–266

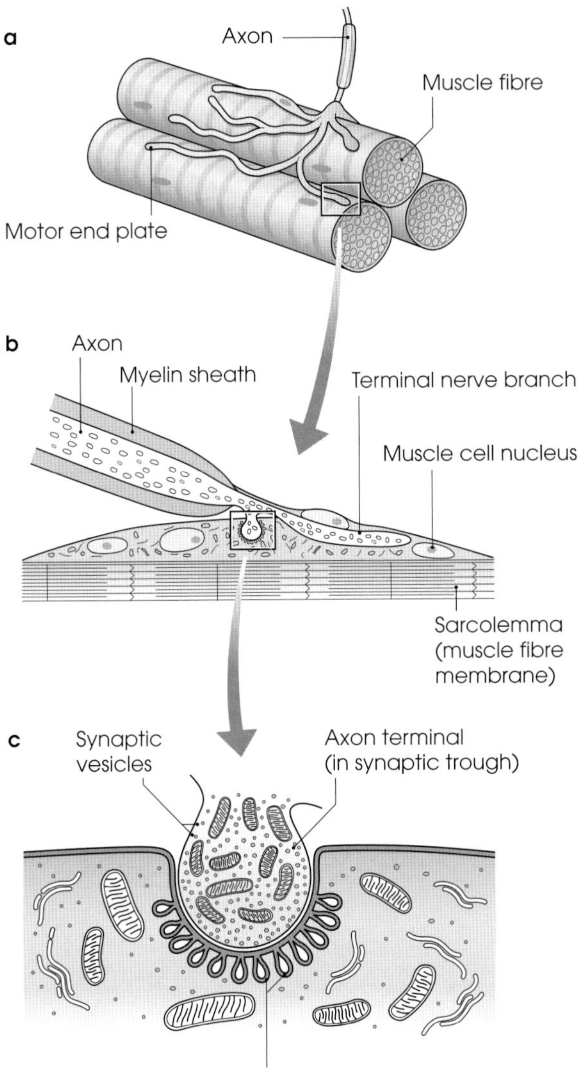

Figure 44.3 The innervation of muscle fibres. (a) An axon of a motor neuron (originating from the cell body in the anterior horn of the spinal cord) branches near its end to innervate several skeletal muscle fibres, forming a neuromuscular junction with each fibre. The region of the muscle membrane (sarcolemma) lying directly under the terminal branches of the axon has special properties and is known as the motor end plate (or motor end-plate membrane). (b) The rectangular area shown in detail; the fine terminal branches of the nerve (axon terminals), devoid of myelin sheaths, lie in grooves on the sarcolemma. The rectangular area in this section is shown in detail in (c): ultrastructure of the junction of an axon terminal and the sarcolemma. The invagination of the sarcolemma forms the synaptic trough into which the axon terminal protrudes. The invaginated sarcolemma has many folds, or subneural clefts, which greatly increase its surface area. Acetylcholine is stored in synaptic vesicles in the axon terminal. (After Prichard 1979,[4] (a) and Brobeck 1979,[5] (b and c).)

Muscle strain consists of a mild degree of fibre disruption, usually as a result of muscle overload, during eccentric activity. The degree of muscle strain is variable, comprising complete muscle disruption at the extreme. Mild muscle strains are managed with initial rest and analgesia, followed by a progressive return to the preinjury level. Modification in exercise programmes may be included in the rehabilitation protocol, to limit the possibility of repeated occurrence.

Muscle tears may be intrasubstance, or more commonly may occur at the muscle–tendon interface. Complete disruption of the muscle–tendon interface requires anatomical repair to allow effective restitution of muscle function. Partial disruption of the muscle–tendon interface may be non-operatively managed but may require imaging to confirm the continuity of the interface.

Complete tears through the muscle belly are classically managed with ice, rest, analgesia, and a progressive return to normal activity levels. Following significant disruption of muscle fibres, muscle strength is reduced, with up to 50% of muscle contractile force being lost following complete sectioning of a fusiform muscle belly. For complete midsubstance disruption the distal portion of the muscle is denervated and is isolated, due to fibrous scar tissue interposition, from the main motor trunk proximally. However, surgical intervention with suturing of the epimysium of disrupted biceps brachii muscles in paratroopers has shown improved functional and cosmetic outcome when compared with non-operative management.[7]

Direct muscle injury due to non-penetrating trauma generates muscle contusion, with a variable degree of fibre disruption depending on the severity of impact. As a result of fibre disruption, haemorrhage occurs at the site of contusion, which generates swelling and bruising. In rare instances swelling may be so great as to produce a localized acute compartment syndrome, which requires decompression, particularly in persons predisposed to bleeding, those on antithrombotic therapy, or those taking non-steroidal anti-inflammatory medication.

Haemorrhage within contused muscle tissue predisposes to myositis ossificans, which produces prolonged pain, swelling and incapacity; this may be long term if the site of myositis affects tendon or ligament excursion or interferes with joint movement. Suspicion of myositic changes prevents early mobilization, and instead the injured region should be rested, with a more prolonged immobilization period.

LIGAMENTS

Ligaments are formed from condensations of fibrous tissue. They provide mechanical support, acting as a physical constraint to tensile loads. In the broadest sense they include peritoneal and pericardial condensations, which provide structural restraint for internal organs within the thorax, abdomen and pelvis, anchoring organs to their surrounding structures. However, within the musculoskeletal system ligaments are composed of condensations of fascial tissue attached at either end to bone. They provide a proprioceptive role, providing joint position sense, in addition to providing mechanical constraint. Therefore ligaments can be thought of as both passive and active devices to provide joint stability.

BIOLOGY OF LIGAMENTS

Ligaments are composite tissues containing cells, a fibrillar component, extracellular matrix and tissue fluid. It is the differing components that provide ligaments with their specific biological and mechanical properties.

Between 60 and 80% of the wet weight of ligaments consists of water. The fibrillar component of the extracellular matrix

REFERENCES

7. Kragh JF, Basamania CJ. J Bone Joint Surg Am 2002; 84-A: 992–998

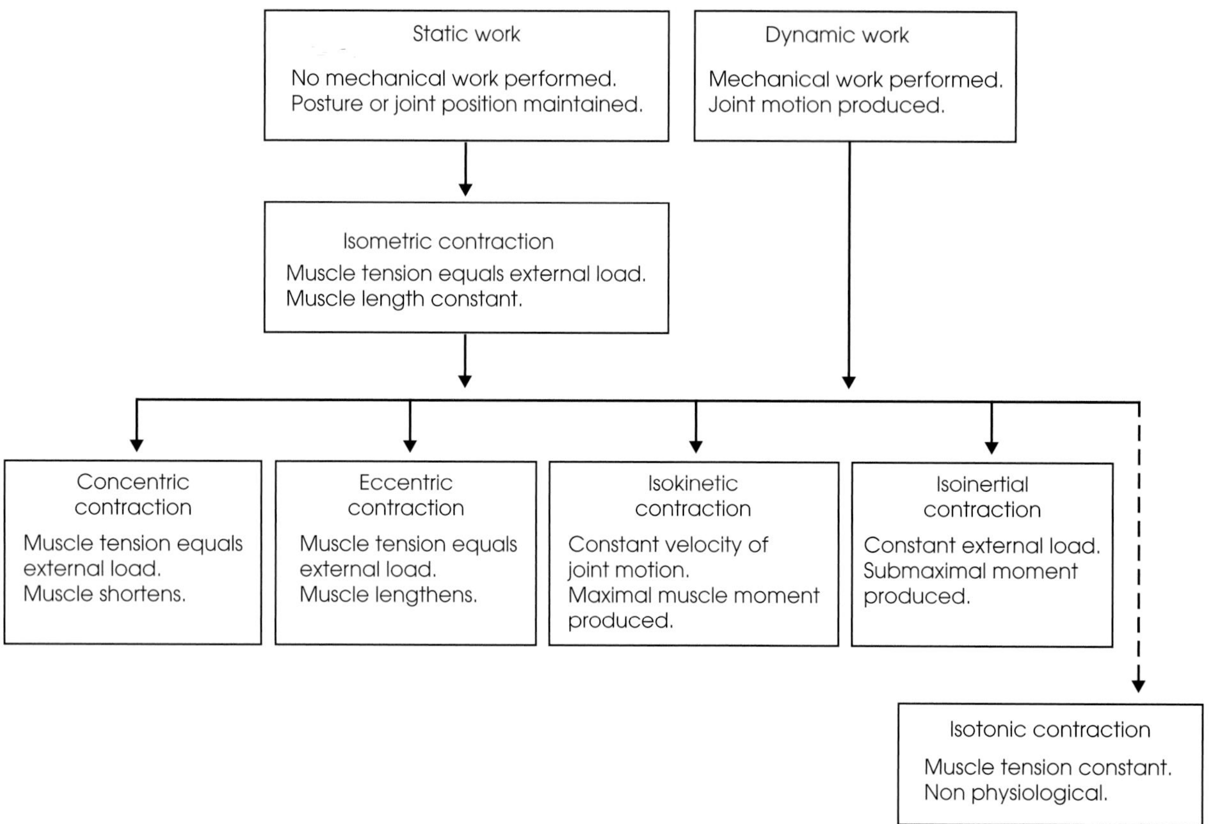

Figure 44.4 Types of muscle work and contraction.

comprises collagen in the main, with up to 70% of the dry weight composed of collagen (of which 90% is type I). In addition to type I collagen, type III is also seen (less than 10%), with type VI in smaller amounts. In addition to collagen, approximately 1% of the fibrillar component consists of elastin, with higher amounts being seen in the spinous ligaments. The fibrillar component is organized into fibrils, which in turn are organized into fibres that coalesce to form bundles oriented along the direction of the tensile load. Ligaments are relatively acellular structures, with the predominant cell type being the fibroblast, which is responsible for the synthesis of the extracellular matrix. The fibroblasts are organized between the rows of collagen fibres. In addition to synthesizing the fibrillar component of the extracellular matrix, fibroblasts also produce the proteoglycan component, which is responsible for retaining water and which influences the viscoelastic properties of the ligament (Fig. 44.5).

Ligaments are relatively avascular tissues, with vessels penetrating the surface and passing longitudinally between the collagen fibrils. The vast majority of ligaments receive penetrating vessels along their length, supplied by the soft tissues around the ligament substance. However, some (such as the anterior cruciate ligament) receive relatively little vessel penetration into their midportions, and instead receive vascular inflow from either end, with a more organized series of small anastomoses along their length, as a result of their intra-articular position.

As a consequence of their role as proprioceptive organs, ligaments contain sensory nerve fibres, which include mechanoreceptors. The proprioceptive mechanoreceptor nerve endings are involved in the ligamentomuscular reflex loop, and they may be damaged should injury occur to the ligament itself.

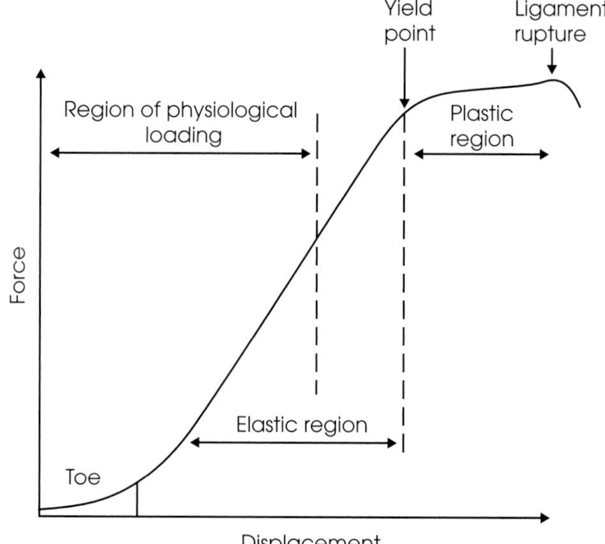

Figure 44.5 Collagen fibrils, fibres and bundles in tendons and collagenous ligaments. Collagen molecules, triple helices of coiled polypeptide chains, are synthesized and secreted by the fibroblasts. These molecules (depicted with heads and tails to represent positive and negative polar changes) aggregate in the extracellular matrix in a parallel arrangement to form microfibrils and then fibrils. The staggered array of the molecules, in which each overlaps the other, gives a banded appearance to the collagen fibrils under the electron microscope. The fibrils aggregate further into fibres that come together into densely packed bundles.

Ligaments are attached to bone by either direct or indirect insertions. In direct insertions, which are the more common of the two forms, the deep collagen fibres attach to the underlying bone at right angles through four distinct zones, which have a combined depth of approximately 1 mm. Zone 1 contains extracellular matrix with collagen and fibroblasts. Both zone 2 and zone 3 contain fibrocartilage, with the mineralization tidemark distinguishing the two zones and zone 3 being mineralized. Zone 4 consists of a rapid change to bone. In indirect insertions, the deep layer of collagen within the ligament anchors through collagen fibres that run directly into the bone (Sharpey's fibres), whereas the superficial layer blends with the periosteal covering of the bone. The medial collateral ligament of the knee demonstrates both forms of insertion, attaching in a direct form at its femoral side and in an indirect form at its tibial side.[8]

MECHANICAL PROPERTIES OF LIGAMENTS

Ligaments are viscoelastic structures, and their physical properties are therefore influenced by the rapidity of load application. In addition to the collagen fibres, they contain further fibrillar components, the predominant substance being elastin. The amount of elastin present is usually around 1%. However, in some of the interspinous and supraspinous ligaments this figure may be significantly higher.

When unloaded, the collagen bundles line up with a slight wave or crimp. This is partly as a result of the elastin content exerting a contractile force within the ligament. As a tensile load is applied, the elastin component is stretched out and the ligament is elongated until such time as the collagen bundles are parallel and straight such that the crimp is removed. At this point, the mechanical property changes and the stiffness of the ligament significantly alter as the collagen fibres are loaded. This change in physical property—as the collagen fibres are suddenly straightened out and then loaded—accounts for the toe in a graphical representation of a stress–strain curve of a ligament as it moves from a low-stiffness to a high-stiffness value. As the ligament is progressively loaded, it undergoes elastic deformation until such time as the applied load exceeds the yield point, after which it undergoes plastic (or non-recoverable) deformity, which will be accompanied by some failure of collagen fibrils. If the applied load is further increased, the load will exceed the ultimate tensile strength of the ligament and rupture occurs (Fig. 44.6).

EFFECT OF TRAINING ON LIGAMENTS

In contrast to that on skeletal muscle and tendons, the effect of athletic training on ligaments is less profound and less well documented. Training has an important effect of protecting ligaments by improving muscle function and subsequent proprioceptive feedback, so reducing ligament overload. However, a direct effect on the ligamentous tissue itself is less clearly defined. In contrast, immobilization has a rapid and profound effect, with a reduction of up to 66% ultimate load to failure in the rabbit medial collateral ligament following immobilization.[9]

The effects of ageing are more clearly established, with a reduction in ligament stiffness with increasing age. In addition, the ultimate strength reduces, with a reduction from 2160 ± 157 N to 658 ± 129 N on comparing young skeletally mature with elderly persons' anterior cruciate ligaments in a cadaveric human study. In the skeletally immature, the ligament tissue matures at more rapid rate than its bony attachment, such that in the skeletally immature, bony avulsion injuries are more common than intra-substance ligament failures.[10]

LIGAMENT INJURY

When ligaments are loaded within their physiological range, they undergo initial elastic deformation as their elastin element is loaded and the collagen fibres are progressively aligned. The collagen fibres are not uniformly aligned within ligaments, as a result of differing regions of the ligament being loaded in differing joint positions. Accordingly, different regions of the ligament are aligned in slightly different directions to best resist the specific direction of tensile load applied when that region is loaded at a given joint position. If the applied load is increased and it exceeds the elastic limit then plastic deformation occurs, with progressive fibre disruption, until ultimately complete failure occurs, with ligament rupture. This is clinically graded as shown in Table 44.1.

REFERENCES

8. Hildebrand KA, Frank CB. In: Dee R, Hurst LC, Gruber MA et al (eds). Ligaments: Structure, Function and Response to Injury and Repair. 2nd edn. McGraw Hill, 1997: 109–117
9. Woo SL, Gomez MA, Sites TJ et al. J Bone Joint Surg Am 1987; 69: 1200–1211
10. Amiel D, Kuiper SD, Wallace CD et al. J Gerontol 1991; 46: B159–B165

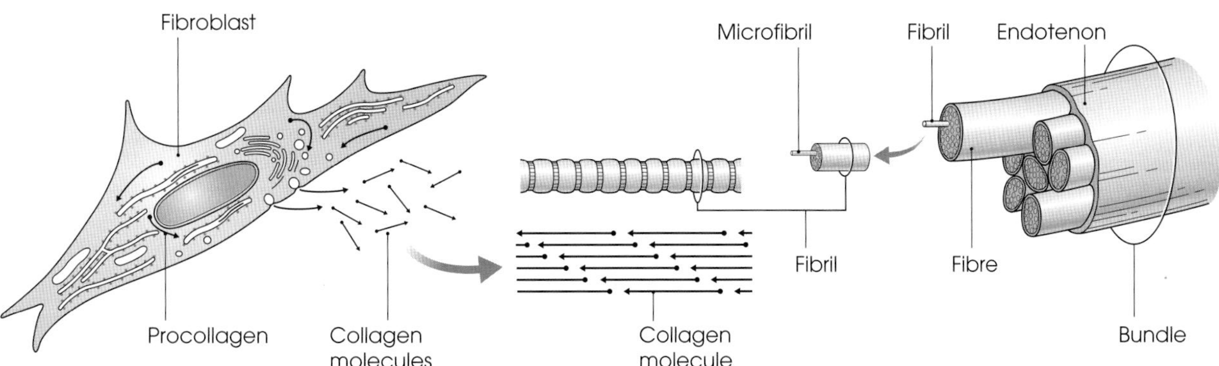

Figure 44.6 Graph of ligament displacement against force.

Table 44.1 Clinical grading of ligament rupture

Grade of injury	Physical findings
1	Tenderness and bruising; no loss of constraint
2	Tenderness and bruising; increased laxity, but with an end point
3	Complete disruption with no resistance on stressing

The healing response of ligaments requires the production of collagen by fibroblasts to restore the mechanical function of the ligament and its ability to resist tensile loads. As in all musculoskeletal tissues, immediately following injury there is initial haematoma formation, followed by organization of the haematoma under the influences of platelets and the acute inflammatory cells recruited to the site of injury. Under the influence of cytokines, the acute inflammation cell population is displaced by angiogenic tissues, and granulation tissue is formed. Collagen is produced at the site of scar formation; the collagen is initially type III. The proportion of type I collagen formation increases in the early stages of scar formation, and there is an increased production of type I collagen in the ligament region surrounding the site of injury.

Maturation and remodelling of the injured region occurs, with a reduction in the cellularity of the scar region and a return to the preinjury proportion of type I to type III collagens. As the cellularity reduces, the collagen density of the site slowly increases, and further maturation of the ligament tissue occurs accompanied by cross-linking of the collagen fibres.

The healing potential of ligaments is site-specific to a certain degree, and thought to be due to both the vascular supply and the presence of synovial fluid. Synovial fluid acts to first physically wash away any formed haematoma from the site of ligament injury and also to inhibit the action of procoagulant molecules, limiting the aggregation of platelets. The anterior cruciate ligament, which is an intra-articular structure, is covered by a thin layer of synovium at most and is bathed in synovial fluid. At the time of anterior cruciate ligament overload and subsequent rupture, the haematoma produced is washed away by the synovial fluid surround and is prevented from undergoing organization. Accordingly, as haematoma organization is inhibited, the healing potential of the anterior cruciate ligament is somewhat limited, and complete fibre disruption is highly unlikely to be followed by effective healing with reconstitution of effective anterior cruciate ligament function.

In contrast, the healing potential of the medial collateral ligament of the knee is significantly better than that of the anterior cruciate ligament, in part due to its extra-articular site and also as a result of its broad, band-like orientation, which presents a significant surface area for new collagen formation to allow effective healing and reconstitution of function.

For the ligament to act effectively it should heal without significant laxity, which may be minimized by avoiding significantly loading the ligament during the healing process until it has sufficient mechanical strength to resist applied load without undergoing additional plastic deformation. A ligament that has undergone a grade 2 or grade 3 injury may approach the mechanical strength of the preinjury ligament but will always show a slight deficit. However, this may not have any functional significance.

For both mechanical constraint and proprioceptive functions to be fully restored, rehabilitation should incorporate proprioceptive feedback and re-education exercises. By undergoing proprioceptive reinforcement, muscle control is optimized to restore joint function and also to reduce the likelihood of further repeated injury to the joint. To give an example, injuries to the lateral ligament complex of the ankle and subtalar joint should be rested until the early swelling resolves. Depending on pain levels, and the extent and severity of the injury to the lateral ligament complex, either early mobilization (for grade 1 injuries) or else initial splintage followed by progressive mobilization (for grade 2 and 3 injuries) should be instituted. As swelling settles and healing occurs, with restoration of ligament constraint, then proprioceptive feedback rehabilitation should be instituted. To assist the restoration of muscular control across the ankle and subtalar region, the patient is encouraged to stand and balance on a wobble board (a foot plate mounted on a hemisphere, producing an intrinsically unstable surface) to restore coordinated muscle activity, particularly of the peroneus longus and peroneus brevis muscles, so reducing the likelihood of further inversion injuries and episodes of ankle and subtalar instability.

THE GENERAL MANAGEMENT OF LIGAMENT INJURIES

Management of ligament injuries depends on the site of the ligament and the degree or grade of injury. Grade 1 injuries are managed using temporary reduction in activity levels, analgesia, application of ice and elevation to limit swelling. As the acute episode settles, then a return to normal activity levels is permitted.

Grade 2 injuries require a more prolonged reduction in activity levels. They may require external support in the form of splintage to limit further damage until healing has occurred.

The management of grade 3 injuries is dependent on the specific ligament involved, such that complete injuries to the lateral collateral ligament of the knee require early operative intervention and repair, often in association with augmentation. In contrast, isolated grade 3 medial collateral ligament injuries of the knee may be effectively managed with bracing and early mobilization in the majority of cases.[11]

Ligaments may rupture in the midsubstance of the tissue at the region adjacent to the bony attachment or else at the insertion site itself. The site of rupture has an influence on the likelihood of surgical intervention being required and the form of repair that may be necessary. Therefore a midsubstance tear requires direct repair of the two ends, usually using sutures, to restore ligament continuity. This direct repair may require augmentation from local tissues or using more distant autograft tissue. An injury towards the insertion of the ligament may be surgically addressed by reattaching the avulsed ligament end to the underlying bone, using bone anchors, staples or screws. In direct ligament insertions, the ligament avulsion may be associated with an avulsed segment of cortical bone. Such bony avulsions may be secured using conventional interfragmentary screws with washers.

Of the three types of ligament failure, the intrasubstance failure is most usually accompanied by a degree of ligament laxity

REFERENCE

11. Gomez MA, Woo SL, Inoue M et al. J Appl Physiol 1989; 66: 245–252

following repair and healing; this is due to a degree of plastic deformation occurring within the body of the ligament tissue prior to complete failure. Ligament failure accompanied by a significant bony avulsion has the least likelihood of laxity following secure anatomical fixation.

By way of example, the lateral collateral ligament of the knee may undergo intrasubstance rupture requiring early operative intervention to correct varus stress instability. Intrasubstance ruptures may be corrected by direct repair augmented by local tissue such as the biceps femoris tendon. In this application, the anterior half of the biceps femoris tendon is left attached to the fibula head, with the tendon being split along its length to the musculotendinous junction. The anterior half is then turned forwards, and the proximal end of the divided anterior portion is secured to the lateral femoral epicondyle as a reinforcing tissue strip to augment the direct repair of the lateral collateral ligament. Alternatively, the distal semitendinosus tendon, harvested from its anteromedial insertion on the proximal tibia, may be used as a free autogenous tendon graft, being passed through a bone tunnel in the fibula head and secured proximally to the lateral femoral epicondyle to augment the direct repair.

The lateral collateral ligament may alternatively fail by avulsing the bony attachment to the fibula head, which can be recognized on plain radiographs. Failure in this manner may be surgically corrected by reattaching the bony avulsion using interfragmentary screws, tension band wiring or any similar construction.

In addition to the use of biological augmentation of ligament repairs (be they autograft, allograft or xenogaft), non-biological augmentation devices have also been utilized in an attempt to provide a scaffold for new collagen production while avoiding the problems of donor site morbidity with autografts and possible viral cross-infection with allografts. Among the many materials and devices assessed have been filamentous carbon, Gore-Tex (polytetrafluoroethylene), Dacron mesh (polyethylene terephthalate) and braided polypropylene yarn (as the Kennedy ligamentation augmentation device). To date, all materials that have undergone trials at intra-articular sites, such as in anterior cruciate ligament reconstruction, have shown a failure to provide any improvement in outcome, while possessing disadvantages including chronic effusions, bone cyst formation, wear debris production and premature failure. The results for extra-articular applications are more favourable, but production of bone cysts and poor orientation of ingrown collagen has been observed.

The theoretical ideal of a biological off-the-shelf ligament graft is yet to be realized. However, the use of commercial type I collagen tissue implants, as a biologically compatible material, shows potential as an implantable that could be used to circumvent the problems seen with autografts and non-biological implants. The future of such tissue-engineered collagen devices is subject to evaluation, but the advantages of implanting a ready-made graft of the desired size and shape to optimize its mechanical function are numerous.

TENDONS

TENDON STRUCTURE

Tendons provide the mechanical link between muscle contraction and subsequent joint movement. To fulfil this role they are flexible but essentially inextensible structures, so enabling muscle forces to pass across joints, often in an indirect line. Tendons, like ligaments, are composite tissues, being made up of a cellular component, fibrillar material, extracellular matrix and water.

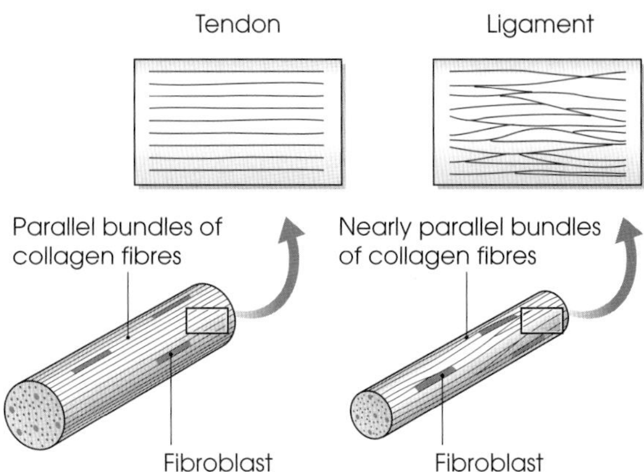

Figure 44.7 The structural orientation of the fibres of tendon and ligament; insets show longitudinal sections. In both structures the fibroblasts are elongated along an axis in the direction of function. (After Snell 1984.[12])

BIOLOGY OF TENDONS

Tendons are relatively acellular, with a fibroblast population existing around the collagen fibrils. The collagen is mainly of type I (86%), with type III also being present at around 5% of the dry weight. The collagen is organized into fibrils, which themselves are surrounded by small amounts of proteoglycan matrix; this is hydrophilic in nature and is responsible for water retention within the tissue and the subsequent viscoelastic properties of the tendon. In contrast to ligaments, which have collagen bundles in slightly differing alignments, within the tissue the collagen fibres in tendons are parallel with the axis of load. In addition to the collagen fibres being parallel, there is very little crimp (or wave) within the collagen, in contrast to the collagen configuration in ligaments (Fig. 44.7).

Tendons are of two broad types. The first type pulls in virtually a direct line and is surrounded by a loose connective tissue, the paratenon. The tendo Achilles is of this type; it receives a blood supply from the paratenon, which sends vessels into the periphery of the tendon and which are themselves linked by a system of longitudinal capillaries.

The second type of tendon is that which is required to bend around bony prominences, or pulleys, such as the long flexors of the fingers and thumb. These tendons are surrounded by a tendon sheath, which guides the tendon motion and is thickened at points to form encircling pulleys. The tendons are surrounded by synovial fluid, which is produced by the synovial membrane lining the tendon sheath, the epitenon. These tendons receive their blood supply from the periosteal insertion at one end and from the perimysium at the muscle belly end. The intervening portion of tendon receives a blood supply through the short and long vinculae, which comprise bridging extensions from the tendon surround to the tendon tissue itself.

MECHANICAL PROPERTIES OF TENDONS

On initial axial loading, tendons deform less than ligaments, thus providing a more effective mechanical link between the

REFERENCE

12. Snell K. Adv Enzyme Regul 1984; 22: 325–400

contractile fibres of the muscle belly and the bony insertion. Tendons possess a toe region to their stress–strain characteristics, but it is shorter than that of ligaments, therefore minimizing energy loss during muscle contraction, which would be wasted on tendon elongation. This shorter toe region is partly as a result of the collagen bundles being straight and parallel in tendons, with an absence of the crimp appearance seen in ligaments. This difference between the stiffness values of tendons and ligaments has implications when tendon grafts are utilized for ligament reconstruction, as is the case using the medial hamstring tendons as a free autograft for anterior cruciate ligament reconstruction. After the initial short toe region, the load–elongation curve for tendons has a similar appearance to that of ligaments.

EFFECT OF TRAINING ON TENDONS

Exercise has an effect on the mechanical properties of tendons, serving to increase the stiffness and the ultimate load to failure through the effects of both increased collagen production and collagen cross-linking, thus producing larger, stiffer tendons.

The effect of immobilization is to have the opposite effect, with a loss of tensile strength and stiffness, these changes occurring within 1–2 weeks of a reduction in normal tendon loading. On recommencing the normal loading pattern of previously immobilized tendons, over time the biological and mechanical properties return to their normal values. However, the time course for recovery is much longer than that of deterioration. Accordingly, as with most aspects of the musculoskeletal system, tendon immobilization should be reduced in both magnitude and duration wherever possible.

The effects of both training and immobilization are dependent on the site of the tendon in question, with the flexor tendons on the carpus and digits being more susceptible than those of the extensor compartment.

TENDON FAILURE AND HEALING

Tendon failure occurs through three broad mechanisms. The first is a direct injury to a normal tendon, such as occurs with a laceration or penetrating injury. The second mechanism is an overload failure of an otherwise normal tendon, which may fail within the tendon substance or else at the bony attachment. The third is an overload injury of a pathological tendon. The three different mechanisms may have differing management, healing mechanisms and outcomes, with failure of a pathological tendon more likely to occur bilaterally (although not necessarily simultaneously) and recurrently.

For a lacerated tendon, the healing mechanism varies slightly depending on whether the tendon is surrounded by a tendon sheath and synovial fluid, such as a long flexor tendon in the hand, or whether it is surrounded by a paratendon, such as the patellar tendon. In tendons surrounded by a paratenon, the tendon gap is filled with haematoma and inflammatory cells, which results in the release of chemoattractants. Capillaries sprout from the enclosing paratenon, and the gap between the tendon ends becomes filled with capillaries surrounded by fibroblasts, which produce collagen (predominantly type I). Within 1–2 weeks the tendon gap is filled by a tissue mass, with collagen fibres connecting the two tendon ends. Over the next 4–6 weeks the collagen mass becomes more organized and gentle loading accelerates this process of realignment. The healing mass continues to mature over months and the tissue bridge further consolidates, with gradual collagen cross-linking occurring to restore tendon strength.

In synovial sheath-enclosed tendons, the healing process involves the synovial lining cells of the sheath, the epitenon. The healing process in synovial tendons is markedly affected by postoperative management of the repaired tendon, with controlled movement promoting intrinsic healing of the tendon through the epitenon, accompanied by collagen formation and subsequent reorganization and remodelling. However, if the tendon is immobilized, then granulation tissue is formed and the endotenon undergoes cellular proliferation, thus increasing the likelihood of adhesions being formed between the tendon and the surrounding tendon sheath. Accordingly, most rehabilitation regimens governing flexor tendon repair promote the ideal of controlled early passive mobilization to reduce the possibility of adhesion formation and subsequent reduction in tendon excursion, while not allowing overloading of the tendon repair and subsequent gap formation while healing occurs.

In overload injuries, failure may occur within the tendon substance or at the bony attachment. In paratenon tendons, overload failure most commonly occurs within the tendon substance itself, such as is seen in the patellar tendon or the Achilles tendon. Midsubstance rupture is often accompanied by microangiopathic histological changes seen at the site of rupture. Accordingly, midsubstance rupture usually occurs in pathological tendons, although the presence of pathology may not be clinically apparent until rupture. Midsubstance rupture of paratenon tendons may be promoted by anabolic steroid usage, where bilateral tendon rupture is often seen (classically of patellar tendon, pectoralis major or triceps), systemic corticosteroid therapy, local corticosteroid injection and fluoroquinolone ingestion. Avulsion of the bony attachments of these tendons is also seen but is less common.

In synovial tendons, avulsion of the bony attachment is relatively more common, particularly of the profundus flexor tendon of the digits. In avulsion injuries in this setting, depending on the size of the bone avulsion the bone fragment may be fixed, as with any form of fracture. For smaller avulsed bony insertions, the small bone fragments may be excised and the tendon secured to the underlying bone surface to restore the tendon–bone interface

To promote tendon healing, various biological manipulations and influences have been assessed. These manipulations have applications in both the repair of tendons themselves and also in promoting healing of the tendon–bone interface in rotator cuff repair surgery, zone 1 tendon injuries in the hand, anterior cruciate ligament reconstruction and posterior cruciate ligament reconstruction. Among the manipulations that have shown promise are platelet-derived growth factors, insulin-like growth factor-1, bone morphogenetic proteins and low-intensity, long-wave ultrasound.[13]

TENDON PATHOLOGY

Intrinsic tendon pathology results from repetitive microtrauma that initially induces an acute inflammatory response, which may settle with no significant long-standing adverse histological changes. However, if the microtrauma continues then chronic changes are produced within the tendon; these changes consist of fibroblastic proliferation and capillary invasion, producing

REFERENCE

13. Bliss J, Svehla M, Bruce W et al. J Orthop Surg (Hong Kong) 2001; 5: S65

tendinosis. Chronic inflammatory changes within the tendon result in the degradation of collagen and matrix components of the tissue, with subsequent microtears. As the pathology progresses, the surviving tissue is progressively overloaded as the microtears occupy an increasing proportion of the tendon. Consequently, the tendon may suddenly undergo an acute or chronic failure with complete rupture. The usual sites for chronic tendinosis are the rotator cuff region, the quadriceps tendon, the origin of the extensor carpi radialis longus and the lateral epicondyle, the patellar tendon and the Achilles tendon.

Management of tendinopathy is problematic and consists initially of reducing activity levels to break the chronic repetitive microtrauma cycle. Non-steroidal anti-inflammatory analgesics may be taken for both their analgesic and anti-inflammatory properties. In established chronic cases, a localized corticosteroid injection may be utilized to control the process of microvascular invasion into the tenopathic region. However, in addition to the effect of subtending the microangiopathic element of the process, corticosteroid also alters the production of polypeptide chains, including collagen and extracellular matrix. In this manner, the use of corticosteroid injection may precipitate catastrophic tendon failure, and due warning must be given to reduce activity levels for 2–4 weeks following injection to reduce the possibility of rupture. Physical therapy, including local ultrasound, has been advocated. However, the most effective physical therapy intervention is the institution of eccentric stretches to reduce the chronic inflammation while not exacerbating the level of microtrauma as the bone–tendon-muscle unit is rehabilitated.

STENOSING TENOSYNOVITIS

The tenosynovium, or epitenon, lubricates the tendon to optimize tendon gliding. If the lining becomes persistently inflamed as a result of subclinical repetitive microtrauma or acute trauma, or as a response to a collagen disease, then a constriction may occur at a point where the synovial sheath thickens slightly to form a fibrous pulley. Therefore, as the constriction occurs in the region of a fibrous pulley, stenosing tenosynovitis occurs at a point where a tendon changes direction, classically the extensor compartment of the wrist, or as the long flexor tendons pass through the A1 pulley on the palmar surface of the metacarpal heads, such as in a snapping or triggering finger. Trigger finger, or triggering thumb, comprises a nodule on the digital long flexor, just proximal to the distal palmar crease, which catches on the first annular pulley, bound to the proximal aspect of the metacarpal, as the tendon moves during flexion and extension.

The stenosing tenosynovitis may respond to a corticosteroid injection into the tendon sheath to address the accompanying synovitis and to allow the nodule to pass without catching. If injection fails, then a release of the A1 pulley may be advocated to allow free passage of the tendon.

When the stenosing tenosynovitis affects the first dorsal compartment of the wrist, containing the extensor policis brevis and abductor policis longus tendons, the presentation is given the eponym De Quervain's disease. This is characterized by pain and tenderness in the radial border and radial styloid of the wrist, which may be accompanied by palpable crepitus in this region. Pain in this region may be exacerbated by passive flexion of the thumb with the wrist held in ulnar deviation: Finkelstein's test. As with all presentations of tendinosis, initial management involves rest with activity modification and the use of a wrist splint, accompanied by anti-inflammatory medication. Failure to respond to activity modification may be addressed by the injection of corticosteroid injection into the tendon sheath, which is successful in up to 80% of cases. The conditions of patients unresponsive to local steroid injection may be managed with surgical release of the first dorsal compartment.

Paediatric orthopaedics

45

Jonathan D Lucas

INTRODUCTION

The term *orthopaedic*—from the Greek *orthos*, meaning straight, and *paedion*, meaning child—was developed in 1741 by Nicholas Andre, professor of medicine at the University of Paris, to describe the speciality of treating crippled children, literally to straighten the deformities of children.[1] The term was subsequently adopted for the speciality of surgery for diseases of the musculoskeletal system, because this is principally what orthopaedic surgeons do, which is to correct bony deformities to relieve pain and restore function. The aims of this chapter are to outline the normal variations, especially of gait, that occur in the normal growing child to be able to differentiate these from abnormal growth patterns that will develop into significant deformities, as well as to outline the common orthopaedic conditions of children.

NORMAL VARIANTS OF GROWTH: INTOEING, BOW LEGS AND KNOCK KNEES, AND FLAT FEET

Many children present to orthopaedic clinics with concerns for their gait or perceived lower limb deformity. The majority of these children are normal, and the lower limb deformity is a normal development as the child grows and matures.

INTOEING

Intoeing is one of the commonest presentations of children to paediatric orthopaedic clinics by concerned parents. Parents or carers complain that the child is clumsy and falls over a lot, although on watching the child in the clinic, the child moves about the clinic without any apparent concerns. There are three main causes of intoeing at different levels of the lower limb, the foot, the tibia and the femur, which appear at different ages.

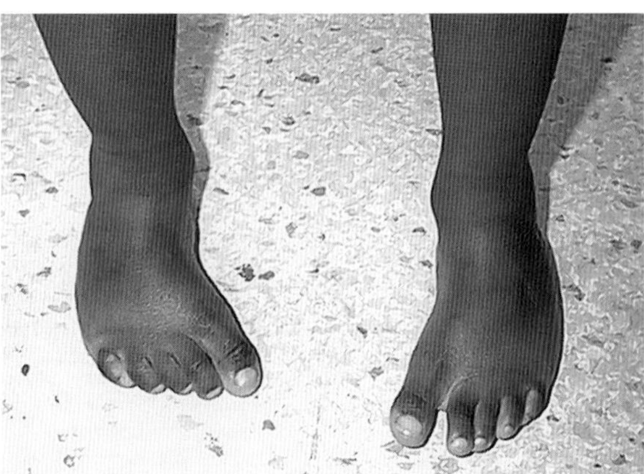

Figure 45.1 Metatarsus adductus: the forefoot is adducted and the heel is normal, which differentiates it from congenital talipes equinovarus.

Metatarsus adductus or varus

This is apparent in the first 3 months of life. The forefoot, especially the hallux, is adducted; the deformity is mobile and usually bilateral but asymmetrical with a normal heel, which differentiates it from congenital talipes equinovarus (Fig. 45.1). The aetiology is of an interuterine packaging defect and is continued by the child sleeping prone. There is an association of metatarsus adductus with developmental dysplasia of the hip, and therefore careful examination of the hip is mandatory.

The condition is self-resolving in approximately 85% of cases by the age of 3–4 years.[2] In those that are slow to resolve, serial splinting may be required; rarely is any form of surgery necessary.

Internal tibial torsion

Internal tibial torsion is common in children between the ages of 1 and 3 years. It may be confused with genu varum but is self-resolving and requires no treatment.

Internal femoral torsion or anteverted femoral necks

This is seen in children between the ages of 3 and 10 years and is bilateral. It is characterized by marked internal rotation of the hip (up to 80°) with marked loss of external rotation (less than 10°), and hence children being comfortable sitting in the W position (Fig. 45.2).

The majority resolve spontaneously with growth; those with less than 10° of external rotation have a poorer prognosis and require surgical intervention, but this should not be performed at a young age (i.e. less than 8–10 years) because the deformity may spontaneously resolve or even recur following surgery. In some children, the femoral neck anteversion is compensated by the development of external tibial torsion, which gives rise to the unsightly inward-looking or squinting patellae. Surgery for this deformity is rarely indicated (Fig. 45.3).

GENU VARUM AND GENU VALGUM

Mild genu varum (bowed legs) is normal to the age of 2–3 (Fig. 45.4), when the knees become progressively valgus to produce genu valgum or knocked knees, up to the age of approximately 6–8 years, when the knees straighten to the normal

REFERENCES

1. Andre N. Orthopedie ou l'Art de Preventir et de Corriger dans les Enfants. Paris, 1741
2. Rushforth GF. J Bone Joint Surg 1978; 60-B: 530–532

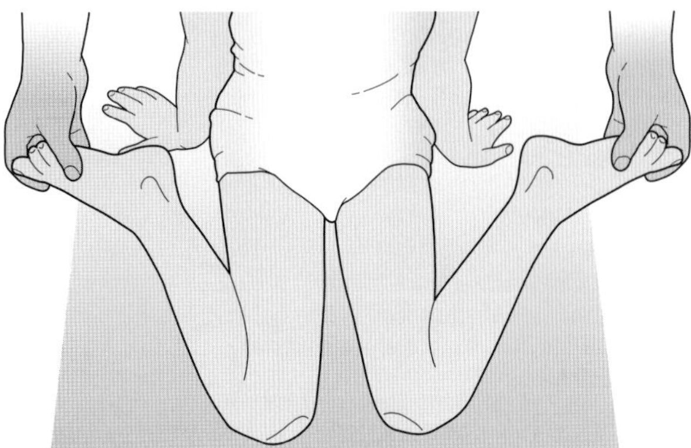

Figure 45.2 A child sitting in the W position.

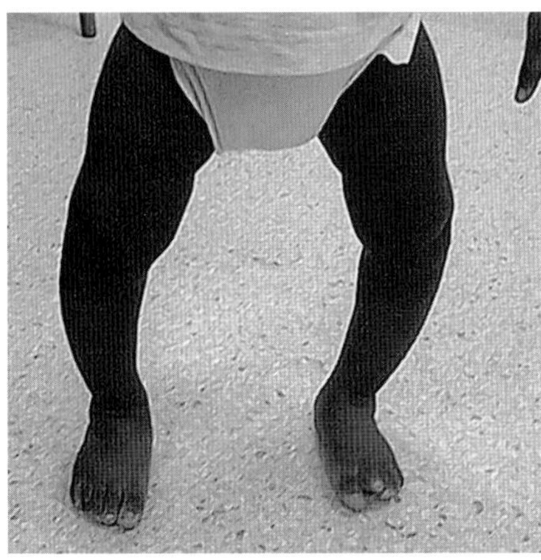

Figure 45.4 Physiological genu varum or bowing of the lower limbs in a 2½-year-old child.

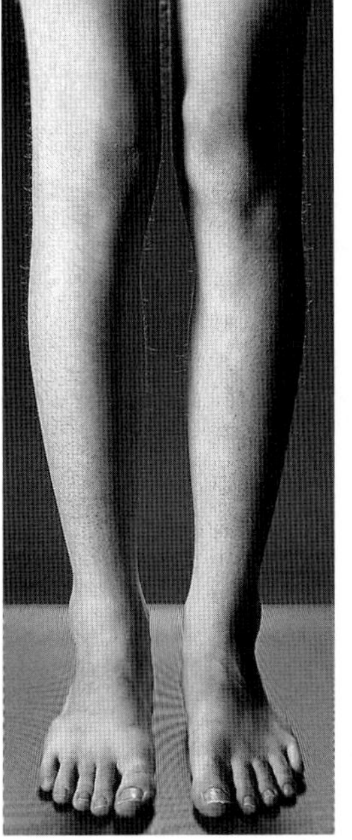

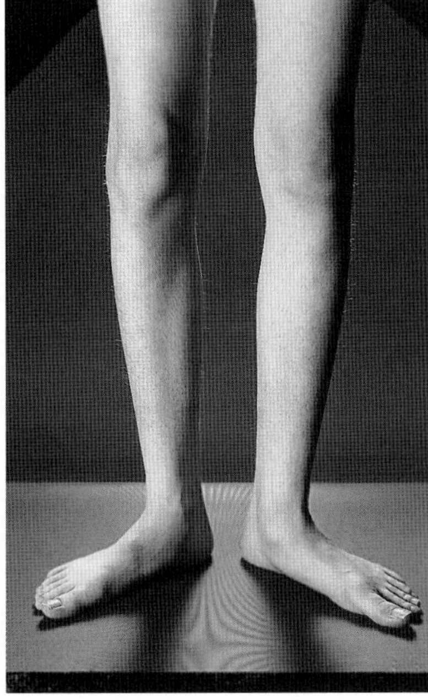

a b

Figure 45.3 Persistent femoral anteversion causing the knees to squint inwards (**a**); external tibial torsion (**b**) develops as a compensation.

degree of valgus seen in the adult. Pathological genu varum is characterized by being either asymmetrical, severe, progressive or failing to resolve, or associated with a child of short stature, and it may be caused by Blount's disease, rickets, trauma and/or skeletal dysplasia, respectively. Pathological genu valgum is also characterized by being asymmetrical, severe and progressive, and causes include trauma, rickets, skeletal dysplasia and congenital limb deficiencies.

PES PLANUS OR FLAT FEET

Flat feet are common and are usually normal. Initially, all infants have the appearance of flat feet due to a fat pad obliterating the medial longitudinal arch. A recognizable medial arch develops by the age of 6 years. In the older child with a flexible flat foot, the medial longitudinal arch is demonstrated by asking the child to stand on tiptoe or by passively dorsiflexing the great toe (the toe-raising test of Jack). Very rarely is any treatment required, and no form of orthotic has been shown to change the natural history of the condition.[3]

Box 45.1 Causes of flat feet

Congenital
- Congenital talipes calcaneovalgus
- Congenital vertical talus

Painless
- Flat foot associated with ligamentous laxity
- Flat foot associated with tight tendo Achilles
- Paralytic flat foot (cerebral palsy or spina bifida)

Painful
- Tarsal coalition → peroneal spastic flat foot
- Subtalar pathology e.g. sepsis, tumour, inflammatory arthritis (e.g. juvenile chronic arthritis)

Pathological causes of a flat foot are shown in Box 45.1. Flat feet associated with hyperlaxity syndromes such as Marfan's syndrome may usually be managed conservatively with appropriate foot orthoses. Surgery may be required for severe deformities that become painful, and a subtalar fusion may be performed. Pes planus is also associated with a tight tendo Achilles; this is generally managed conservatively with stretching and orthoses, but occasionally a tendo Achilles-lengthening procedure is required. A paralytic flat foot is managed on its merits, depending on its severity, pain and the disability.

Peroneal spastic flat foot is due to tarsal coalition. Subtalar movement is restricted and painful, which causes the peronei to go into spasm (hence the name). The commonest bridge is of a calcaneonavicular coalition (Box 45.2). The clinical features are of a child aged between 9 and 13 years who complains of pain on exercise, with a possible history of minor trauma initiating the pain. The child has an antalgic gait with a stiff flat foot and peroneal spasm. Plain X-rays of the foot, especially a 45° oblique view of the foot (Fig. 45.5), usually confirm the clinical diagnosis, and a CT scan is the investigation of choice to define the exact anatomy of the coalition. Treatment is determined by severity of the pain, with no intervention required or else orthoses, a period in plaster, surgical excision of the coalition to an arthrodesis being performed, all being treatment options.

REFERENCE

3. Wenger D, Maudlin D, Speck G et al. J Bone Joint Surg 1989; 71A: 800–810

Box 45.2 Tarsal coalition

- Calcaneonavicular (60%)
- Talocalcaneum (30%)
- Calcaneocuboid
- Cuboid navicular

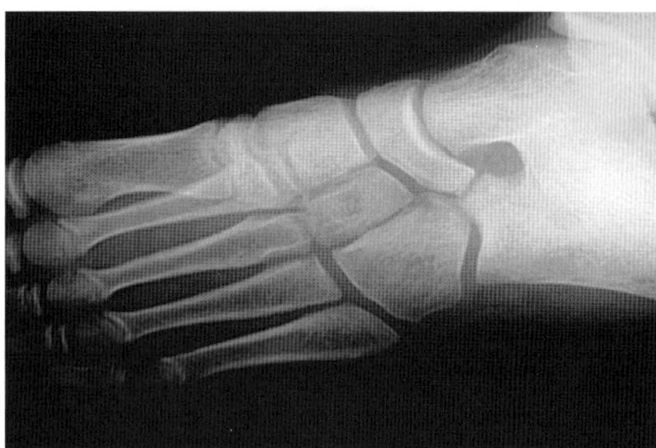

a

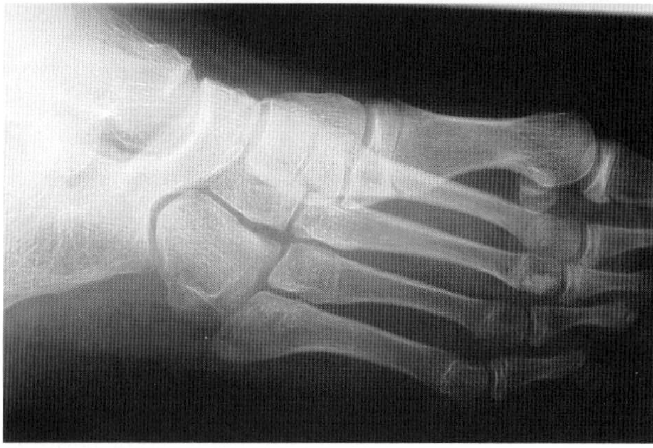

b

Figure 45.5 Oblique X-ray of the foot showing (a) calcaneonavicular and (b) talocalcaneum condition.

CONDITIONS OF THE HIP

DEVELOPMENTAL DYSPLASIA OF THE HIP

Developmental dysplasia of the hip was formerly known as congenital dislocation of the hip, but the name was changed to reflect the spectrum of the disease; not all cases presenting with dislocated hips at birth. The spectrum being the hip: dislocated and irreducible, dislocated and reducible, located but able to be reduced, or located and unable to be reduced but have a developmental abnormality of the acetabulum.

The incidence of unstable hips at birth, i.e. hips that are located but may be reduced, is approximately 5–20 per 1000 live births; the majority of these resolve, become stable by 6 weeks and require no intervention. This leaves an incidence of two per 1000 to one in 400 with significant hip dysplasia.[4] The risk factors are being a first-born girl, breech presentation and/or delivery by Caesarean section, oligohydramnios and a positive family history (Box 45.3).

Developmental dysplasia of the hip is unilateral in 80% of cases (affecting the left hip more than the right) and bilateral in 20% of cases. The extreme form of the condition, in which there is complete dislocation of the hip at birth (which is irreducible), is known as teratogenic; it may not be managed non-operatively and is usually associated with an underlying syndrome.

The aetiology of the condition is unclear, but ligament laxity and a neuromuscular imbalance are thought to be major components contributing to the condition; once the hip is dislocated and there is failure to relocate the femoral head, there is progressive deformity of the hip joint as it fails to develop normally due to abnormal forces through the deformed hip.[5]

Box 45.3 Developmental dysplasia of the hip: risk factors and associations

- Female:male ratio 3–7:1
- Breech presentation, especially extended breech
- First-born
- Positive family history
- Oligohydramnios
- Delivery by Caesarean section
- Northern Italian or North American Indian ethnicity
- Congenital deformities, torticollis, plagiocephaly
- Metatarsus adductus
- Calcaneovalgus

Box 45.4 Neonatal hip assessment for developmental dysplasia of the hip

Inspection/look
- Asymmetrical skin folds
- Leg length discrepancy

Feel/move
- Assess range of motion, especially abduction, which is limited in the dislocated hip.

Barlow's test[6]

The hip is located but unstable
- The pelvis is stabilized, and the hip and knee are flexed to 90°. Longitudinal pressure is exerted, and the hip is subluxed posteriorly and reduced by abducting the hip.

Ortolani's test[7]

The hip is dislocated
- Both hips and knees are flexed to 90° and abducted while lifting the greater trochanter forwards. As the hip is abducted, it relocates (usually with a 'clunk').

Initial assessment of the newborn

In the UK, all children's hips are assessed for stability in the neonatal period (Box 45.4). Those with significant risk factors have an ultrasound of both hips to assess the location of the femoral head and the shape of the acetabulum. Certain ultrasound measures have been determined that are able to assist in predicting prognosis and so are useful in determining definitive management. Plain X-rays of the hip become useful only in children aged between 3 and 6 months once the ossific nucleus of the head of the femur has appeared. The ossific nucleus should lie within Perkin's line and below Hilgenreiner's line, with Shenton's line in continuity (Fig. 45.6). If the head is

REFERENCES

4. Macnicol MF. J Bone Joint Surg 1990; 72-B; 1057–1060
5. Benson

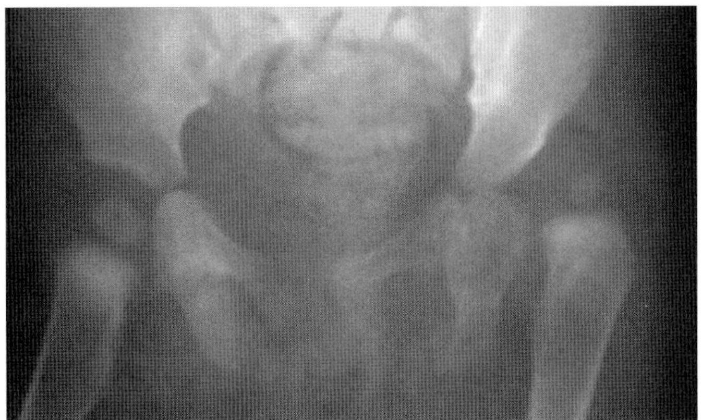

a

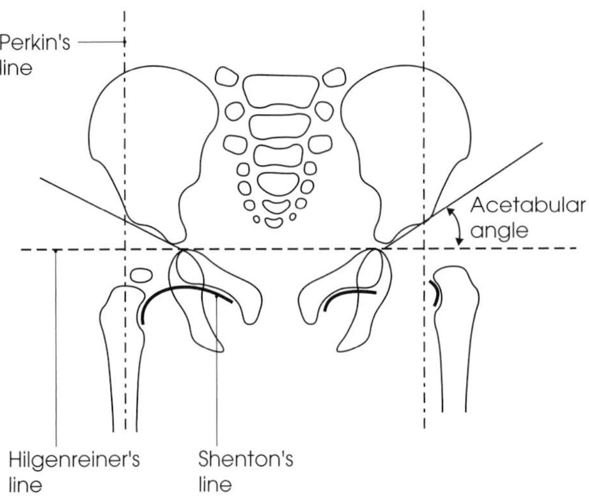

b

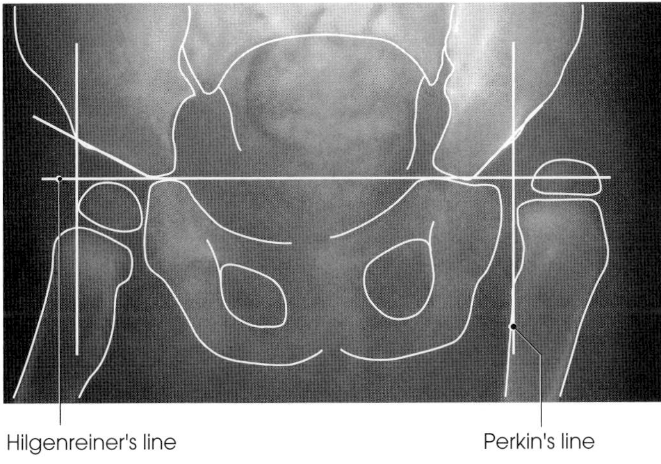

c

Figure 45.6 Developmental dysplasia of the hip. The left hip is dislocated and illustrates the delayed development of the ossific nucleus (which lies lateral to the Perkins line and above Hilgenreiners line), the increased acetabular angle (normally less than 25°), and the break in the Shenton's line.

dislocated there is delay in development of the ossific nucleus and so appearance in the X-ray is also delayed, and when it is apparent it is smaller and less rounded than the normal side (Fig. 45.7).

Management from 0 to 6 months

All neonates are examined within the first 48 h of delivery. Those with unstable hips require no initial treatment because the majority will stabilize by 10–14 days, but each child needs to be reviewed at this time to ensure that the hips have stabilized. Some physicians advocate the use of double nappies but there is very little evidence for this. Those with high risk factors require an ultrasound of the hips, because this will define the level of hip instability and guide further treatment.

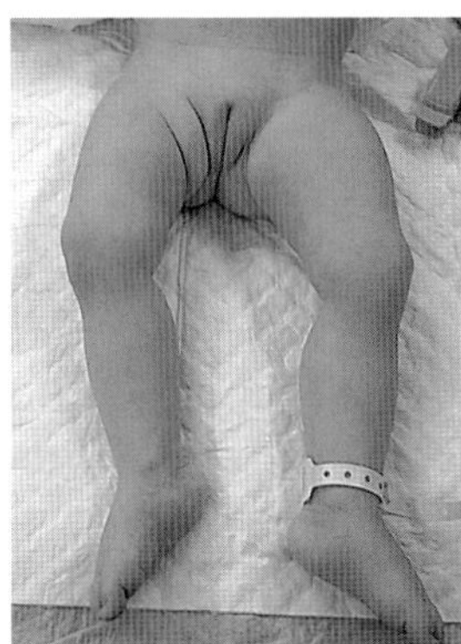

Figure 45.7 A child with a dislocated right hip at 6 months, with right leg shortening and increased groin skin creases.

In those patients with persistent instability of the hip an abduction brace is applied; the commonest type is the Pavlik harness. The child needs to be assessed regularly in the harness to ensure that the hip is located; this is usually done with ultrasound. If the hip is satisfactorily located, the harness is required to be worn for between 3 and 4 months until the hip is stabilized and satisfactory development of the hip joint is occurring. If the hip is not located in the harness there is the risk of the head developing avascular necrosis. If the head is not able to be satisfactorily reduced into the acetabulum, then an examination under anaesthetic is performed, with image-intensifier guidance, and an arthrogram carried out to assess if a satisfactory concentric reduction is able to be achieved. If this is the case then a hip plaster of Paris spica is applied for approximately 3 months. If satisfactory reduction is not able to be achieved, then surgical open reduction is required.

Management from 6 to 12 months

Between 6 and 12 months is the characteristic age for children to present with developmental dysplasia of the hip that has not been identified in the neonatal period or that has developed subsequently. An examination under anaesthetic and a hip arthrogram are performed; if the hip is able to be concentrically reduced, a hip spica is applied for 6–12 weeks. Postoperative X-rays are performed to check that the reduction is satisfactory. Once the hip spica has been removed, an abduction brace is applied to ensure that the hip remains located and that the acetabulum develops normally. If the hip is not able to be reduced, then an open reduction and stabilization procedure is required.

Management from 1 to 3 years

Open reduction is usually required at this stage, and this may or may not have to be combined with some form of acetabular or femoral osteotomy, such as the Salter osteotomy for the acetabulum or a femoral derotation varus osteotomy, or both. Some centres advocated the use of lower limb traction prior to surgical reduction because it is believed that it makes the ease

REFERENCES

6. Barlow TDJ. J Bone Joint Surg 1962; 44: 242
7. Ortolani M. Clin Orthop 1976; 119: 6–10

of reduction simpler, but this is not proved and carries the risk of avascular necrosis of the head if too much abduction is used.

Management after 3 years

This requires surgical management and almost invariably requires some form of acetabular and/or femoral osteotomy to increase the cover of the femoral head. Up to the age of 4 years the acetabulum, if loaded satisfactorily, still has significant remodelling potential, and therefore better results may be achieved once maximum possible cover of the femoral head is achieved before the age of 4 years.

In conclusion, the best outcome of treatment is determined by early detection of the unstable or dislocated hip and by undertaking prompt action to ensure that the head is reduced within the acetabulum to promote normal development of the hip. If this is achieved the outcome is generally satisfactory, with minimal pain and disability requiring further intervention in latter life.[8]

TRANSIENT SYNOVITIS OF THE HIP (IRRITABLE HIP SYNDROME)

Transient synovitis is the commonest cause for a limp in a child aged between 2 and 8 years and affects up to 3% of children in this age group. Boys are affected more commonly than girls and it is rarely, if ever, bilateral. The condition is poorly understood; it consists of a non-specific inflammation of the hip joint synovium accompanied by an effusion. It is of limited duration (a number of days) and appears to have no long-term sequelae, although 5–10% may have a second episode. There is a high association with either recent or concurrent viral illness, such as an upper respiratory tract infection or minor trauma; however, in approximately a third of children there are no associated factors.

Clinically, the child presents with pain in the groin and a limp, and is generally unwell with a mild fever, although this does not usually exceed 38°C. Examination of the hip reveals an irritable hip held in slight flexion, abduction and external rotation, with all movements being painful. There are no other associated signs. Plain X-rays are usually not helpful except to exclude more serious pathology; ultrasound will reveal a joint effusion that on aspiration, the synovial fluid is clear with few if any polymorphs and no organisms.

Management consists of symptomatic relief with appropriate analgesias, including non-steroidal anti-inflammatory drugs and bed rest. The most important part of the management is to exclude other serious causes of the hip pain, principally septic arthritis; differential diagnoses are shown in Box 45.5. The differentiation between an irritable hip and a septic arthritis can be difficult, and various algorithms have been devised to take into account clinical signs, ability to bear weight, raised temperature (above 38°C), raised white cell count, raised erythrocyte sedimentation rate and C-reactive protein.[9,10] If the child is unwell, with a high temperature and raised white cell count, erythrocyte sedimentation rate and C-reactive protein, an ultrasound-guided aspirate of the hip is required to allow examination of the synovial fluid; if organisms are present, an urgent wash out of the joint is required as well as (usually) drilling of the proximal femoral metaphysis, because there is usually an associated osteomyelitis.

Box 45.5 Differential diagnoses of transient synovitis of the hip

- Septic arthritis or proximal femoral osteomyelitis
- Perthes' disease
- Slipped upper femoral epiphysis
- Benign tumours (e.g. osteoid osteoma)
- Occult trauma

LEGG–CALVÉ–PERTHES DISEASE

The initial description of this condition was made in approximately 1910 by Legg in Boston, Calvé in France and Perthes in Germany, but it is usually known under the single eponym of Perthes' disease. The condition is considered one of the osteochondritis juvenilis in which there are avascular changes within bone.

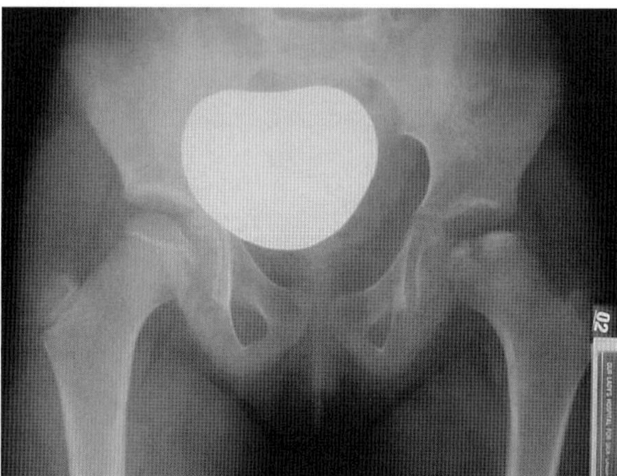

Figure 45.8 Perthes' disease: an anteroposterior X-ray of the pelvis, demonstrating Perthes' disease of the left hip with flattening and fragmentation of the femoral epiphysis.

Perthes' disease is characterized by regions of avascular necrosis of the femoral head, with areas of bone fracturing, head collapse, revascularization, creeping substitution and remodelling. This leads to flattening of the head and subsequent loss of the normal range of movement of the hip joint, with the subsequent development of secondary degenerative change within the hip as it fails to develop normally. The incidence is one in 9000 children, with a sex ratio of four boys to one girl (one in 8000 for boys and one in 30 000 for girls); 80% of cases occur between 4 and 9 (or 10) years of age. Between 12 and 15% are bilateral. Those children with a low birth weight, delayed bone age, short disproportionate stature with disproportionately short distal limb segments, a positive family history and of lower socioeconomic groups are more commonly affected.

The clinical presentation is of a child with limp (which may be relatively painless) with loss of abduction. Approximately 60% of cases resolve and do not require any form of intervention. Poor prognostic features are age over 8 years (girls more so than boys) and development of the head-at-risk signs described by Catterall (Fig. 45.8, Box 45.6),[11] and it is this group of children that requires treatment.

REFERENCES

8. Malvitz TA, Weinstein SL. J Bone J Surg 1994; 76-A: 1777–1792
9. Kocher MS, Zurakowski D, Kasser JR. J Bone Joint Surg 1999; 81-A: 1662–1670
10. Jung ST, Rowe SM, Moon ES et al. J Pediatr Orthop 2003; 23: 368–372
11. Catterall A. J Bone Joint Surg 1971; 53-B: 37–53

Box 45.6 Perthes' disease: the head-at-risk signs

Clinical
- Progressive loss of abduction
- Adduction contracture
- Flexion with abduction
- The overweight child

Radiological
- Gage's sign, a lytic area in the lateral part of the epiphysis and adjacent metaphysic
- Calcification lateral to epiphysis
- A diffuse metaphyseal reaction
- Lateral subluxation
- Horizontal growth plate

Box 45.7 Differential diagnoses of Perthes' disease

Unilateral
- Sequelae of a septic arthritis
- Growth disturbance following treatment of developmental dysplasia of the hip
- Sickle cell disease
- Lymphoma
- Gaucher's disease

Bilateral
- Hypothyroidism
- Multiple epiphyseal dysplasia
- Spondyloepiphyseal dysplasia

The aim of treatment is to restore normal, pain-free hip movements, which require a reduced head within the acetabulum. It is essential that the diagnosis is confirmed; the differential diagnoses are listed in Box 45.7. A bone scan and/or an MRI scan of the hip may be helpful. Treatment consists of either abduction bracing or surgery—in the form of either femoral or pelvic osteotomies, or both—to achieve satisfactory covering or containment of the head in the acetabulum to allow both to develop as normally as possible. This treatment could be considered as salvage treatment because the deformity will never be able to be fully corrected. The aim is to restore the hip biomechanics to as near normal as possible to allow a maximum range of pain-free movement and to delay as long as possible the development of significant secondary degenerate changes in the hip that require treatment in the fourth to sixth decades. Over 80% of patients will develop osteoarthritis by the age of 65, and a significant number will require hip replacements.[12,13]

SLIPPED UPPER FEMORAL EPIPHYSIS

Slipped upper femoral epiphysis occurs as a result of shearing through the hypertrophic zone of the physis, with progressive posterior and inferior displacement of the femoral head relative to the neck of the femur. The condition affects three in 100 000 children, with boys being affected more commonly than girls (ratio 4:1). It occurs at between 12 and 14 years of age in boys and between 11 and 13 years of age in girls. The left hip is more commonly affected but 30% of cases are bilateral, although not necessarily at the same time; up to 60–70% will show some changes in the contralateral hip. The child is typically skeletally immature and overweight. Other aetiological factors are shown in Box 45.8.[14] The classification of slipped upper femoral epiphysis is shown in Tables 45.1 and 45.2. The majority of children (80%) present with mild to moderate chronic or acute on chronic slips.

Box 45.8 Aetiology of slipped upper femoral epiphysis

- Endocrine disorders
  Hypothyroidism
  Hypopituitarism
  Hypogonadism
  Growth hormone therapy
  Adipogenital syndrome
- Head injuries
- Craniopharyngioma
- Renal osteodystrophy
- Marfan's syndrome
- Down's syndrome
- Chemotherapy
- Radiotherapy

Table 45.1 Classification of slipped upper femoral epiphysis-degree of slip

Extent of slip classification	Angle	Degree of slip
Mild	< 30°	Less than one-third
Moderate	30–50°	One-third to one-half
Severe	> 50°	Greater than one-half

Table 45.2 Classification of slipped upper femoral epiphysis - chronological

Category	Definition
Acute	Symptoms for < 3 weeks
Acute on chronic	An acute exacerbation of pre-existing symptoms
Chronic	Symptoms lasting > 3 weeks

The primary symptom is an insidious onset of pain located in the groin or the knee. Any child complaining of knee pain must have careful examination of the spine, hips and feet. The gait may be antalgic, and on lying the hip is held in external rotation and in severe case may be adducted. There is loss of flexion and most particularly internal rotation of hip, which also precipitates pain. Radiological examination of the hip is mandatory, with an anterior–posterior view of the pelvis and either a true lateral of the hips or a frog lateral (Fig. 45.9).

The aims of treatment are to prevent further displacement before physeal closure and to cause no further complications as a result of treatment. The child is admitted to hospital immediately and put on strict bed rest. Children with mild to moderate acute, acute on chronic, or chronic slips are treated with in situ pinning, and this is usually with a single cannulated 6.5–7.5-mm partially threaded cancellous screw.

REFERENCES

12. McAndrew MP, Weinstein SL. J Bone Joint Surg 1984; 66: 860–869
13. Thompson GH, Price CT, Roy D et al. Instr Course Lect 2002; 51: 367–387
14. Weiner D. J Pediatr Orthop B, 1996; 5: 67–73

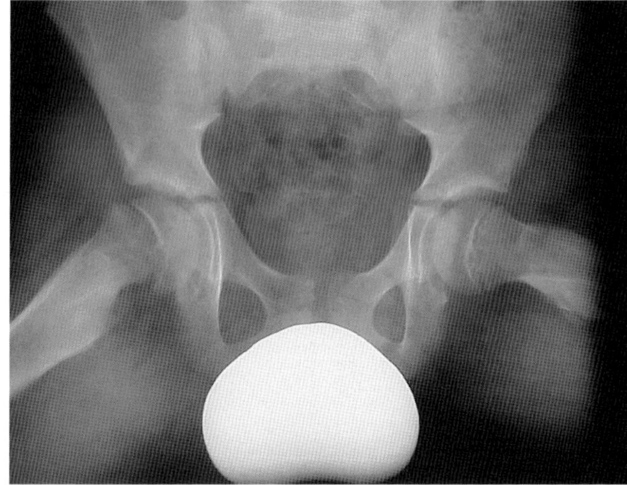

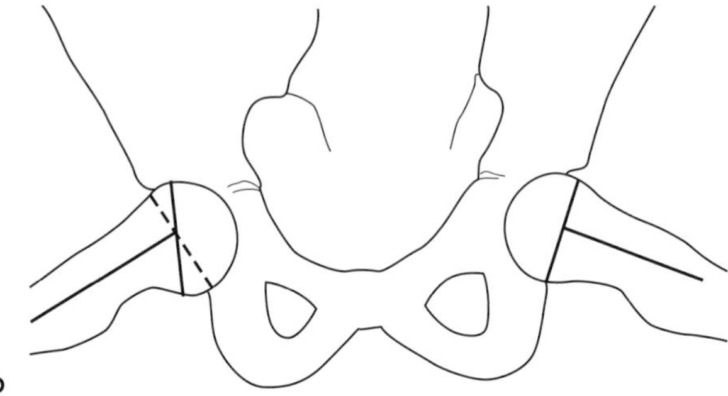

Figure 45.9 Froglateral of both hips demonstrating the moderate slipped upper femoral epiphysis on the right.

There is some controversy as to the best management of the severe chronic slipped upper femoral epiphysis: either reduction of the epiphysis or realignment of the upper femoral anatomy by an osteotomy. Reduction of the epiphysis in moderate slipped upper femoral epiphysis has been abandoned due to the high incidence of avascular necrosis. In acute severe slips there may be a role for slow reduction with traction, but this is also controversial because of the risk of avascular necrosis to the head. The other specific complication of the treatment of slipped upper femoral epiphysis is the development of chondrolysis, in which global loss of the head articular cartilage has been reported in 15–20% of cases. It occurs predominately in cases that have been manipulated or in which either guide wire or the screw or pin has perforated the articular cartilage into the joint during the operation to pin the epiphysis.

Treatment of the chondrolysis is of non-weight bearing, maintenance of range of movement of the hip with physiotherapy, and appropriate analagesia. Approximately 50% of patients will recover; the other half may go on to develop early degenerative changes.[15] Fixation of the contralateral side is indicated in children who have an underlying abnormality that has contributed to the cause of the slipped upper femoral epiphysis (this is usually endocrine); in children who are particularly unreliable at reporting symptoms in the other hip, which may indicate a contralateral slipped upper femoral epiphysis; or in children who are part of a family that would not act appropriately to seek medical advice on such symptoms occurring.[16] Removal of the screws should be performed once the physis has fused.

THE KNEE

CONGENITAL ANOMALIES OF THE KNEE

Congenital dislocation of the knee

At birth the knee is hyperextended, with the tibia displaced anteriorly and laterally on the femur, and is associated with absent cruciate ligaments. The quadriceps and capsule are tight. Congenital dislocation of the knee is rare, with an incidence of two per 100 000 live births. Girls are affected more than boys (ratio 2:1) and 35% of cases are bilateral. The condition is associated with developmental dysplasia of the hip, Larsen's syndrome, arthrogryposis and Down's syndrome.

Treatment is difficult; the knee is usually not able to be reduced closed and requires open reduction at 3–6 months with capsular release, quadriceps lengthening and postoperative splintage. Long-term outcome is unpredictable, with some degree of instability of the knee in adult life.[17]

Congenital recurvatum of the knee

The knee is held in extension at birth but some flexion is possible. Flexion is achieved with serial splintage in progressive degrees of flexion followed by use of a Pavlik harness. The prognosis is good.

PATELLAR DISLOCATIONS

Congenital dislocation of the patella is rare and presents with fixed flexion deformity of the knee with external rotation of the tibia. It is associated with arthrogryposis, Down's syndrome and other syndromes. Plain X-rays are initially unrewarding till the age of 3 years, when the patellar ossific nucleus appears; ultrasound is the initial investigation of choice to confirm the diagnosis.

Treatment is of soft tissue releases and reefing procedures. Outcome is never entirely satisfactory due to the flat shape of the patella and the hypoplastic femoral trochlear.

Acute and recurrent patellar dislocation

Patellar dislocation occurs as a result of a twisting, weight-bearing injury of the knee. The patient is in significant pain, unable to bear weight with a fixed flexion of the knee and the patella is palpable laterally. All traumatic dislocations are lateral, occur more commonly in girls (ratio 2:1), are recurrent in 50% of cases, are often bilateral, and with a familial tendency. Patellar dislocation is associated with hyperlaxity syndromes, patella alta, hypoplastic lateral femoral condyle, poor vastus lateralis function and a Q angle greater than 20° (Fig. 45.10).

Treatment in the acute setting is expeditious reduction of the patella, which is achieved relatively easily under appropriate sedation and analgesia. Postreduction X-rays are performed to exclude an intra-articular loose body or fracture, which may require further treatment. The knee is splinted in extension and rehabilitation is commenced when symptoms allow, principally to strengthen and improve the function of vastus medialis. Surgical

REFERENCES

15. Loder RT, Aronsson DD, Dobbs MB et al. Instr Course Lect 2001; 50: 571–575
16. Castro FP Jr, Bennett JT, Doulens K. J Pediatr Orthop B 1999; 8: 216–222
17. Broughton NS (ed). A Textbook of Paediatric Orthopaedics. WB Saunders, London, 1997

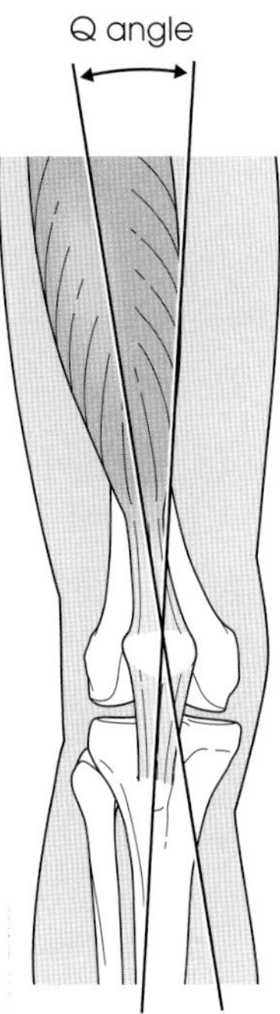

Figure 45.10 The Q angle, the angle of bisection, the line of quadriceps and the patellar tendon at the centre of the patella; this angle should be less than 20°.

realignment procedures are reserved for patients with recurrent dislocation of the patella.

IDIOPATHIC ANTERIOR KNEE PAIN

Anterior knee pain is a descriptive term for pain at the front of the child's knee for which no obvious cause may be found and is usually attributed to the patellar femoral joint. Chondromalacia patellae, softening of the patellar articular cartilage, is often put forward as being the diagnosis giving rise to the pain, but arthroscopic findings on many occasions show no abnormalities of the cartilage at all. A contributing factor may be increased pressure on the lateral facet of the patella, causing microscopic cartilage damage that gives rise to the pain. Twenty per cent of all adolescents report some anterior knee pain, girls more commonly than boys. The pain is often exercise-related and is rarely present at night.

Other causes of anterior knee pain need to be excluded, principally patellar malalignment, traction apophysitis (such as Osgood–Schlatter disease or Larsen–Johannson disease), meniscal tears, and in very rare cases tumours. The majority of symptoms resolve as the child reaches skeletal maturity; on occasion, arthroscopic examination of the knee is indicated and occasionally realignment procedures are required.[18]

DISCOID LATERAL MENISCUS

The lateral meniscus is D-shaped rather than C-shaped and is thought to be caused by the meniscus being hypermobile due to absence or attenuation of the normal meniscal ligaments. It affects one or two per 100 and presents with clicking and pain on the lateral side of the knee. Treatment should be delayed under the child is skeletally mature, and the treatment of choice is arthroscopic debridement of the meniscus to leave a stable rim.[19,20]

OSTEOCHONDRITIS DISSECANS OF THE KNEE

This is a region of avascular necrosis that is normally located on the lateral aspect of the medial femoral condyle and is best seen on a tunnel-view X-ray of the knee. The aetiology is poorly understood; repeated microtrauma, a single traumatic event, abnormalities of ossification, or mild forms of a coagulopathy have all been submitted as theories for the cause. The incidence is between one and four per 1000. The condition is more common in males than in females and presents between the ages of 10 and 20. The presentation is pain within the knee, with features of a loose body, of swelling, giving way, and either intermittent locking or a locked knee.

Treatment is arthroscopic, with the aim of removal of the bony fragment if it has become detached from the medial femoral condyle, and includes manoeuvres to stimulate cartilage healing or reattachment of the fractured fragment.[21]

BLOUNT'S DISEASE AND TIBIA VARA

Blount's disease is a disorder of growth of the posteromedial proximal tibia, leading to tibia vara.[22] The condition is commonest in West Indian and African people and in overweight children. There are two main types: infantile, affecting children up to the age of 8 years and tending to be bilateral, and adolescent, which occurs in children over the age of 8 and is generally unilateral. The cause is unknown.

Surgery is indicated for those with a progressive deformity and is a corrective osteotomy. If the condition is unilateral and requires surgery, contralateral epiphysiodesis may be considered with the aim of minimizing the leg length discrepancy.

TIBIAL BOWING

POSTEROMEDIAL TIBIAL BOWING

Posteromedial tibial bowing is usually physiological and due to a packaging problem. It occurs in the middle third of the tibia and is associated with calcaneovalgus feet. Spontaneous correction usually occurs, but children should be monitored for the development of a leg length discrepancy, which may occur with this condition.

ANTEROMEDIAL TIBIAL BOWING

Anteromedial tibial bowing is typically caused by fibular hemimelia, which is an absence or partial absence of the fibula, the commonest longitudinal congenital anomaly of the lower limb. It is associated with shortening of the femur, ankle instability, missing rays and tarsal coalition.

ANTEROLATERAL TIBIAL BOWING

Congenital pseudarthrosis of tibia is the commonest cause of anterolateral tibial bowing (Fig. 45.11). The commonest cause is neurofibromatosis type; however, it must be noted that less than 10% of children with neurofibromatosis have tibial pseudarthrosis.

Treatment is aimed at avoiding fractures and achieving union of the pseudarthrosis. This requires resection of the soft tissue, and bone grafting and stabilization either by means of external

REFERENCES

18. Jackson AM. J Bone Joint Surg 2001; 83-B; 937–948
19. Kelly BT, Green DW. Curr Opin Pediatr 2002; 14: 54–61
20. Ahn JH, Shim JS, Hwang CH et al. J Pediatr Orthop 2001; 21: 812–816
21. Schenck RC Jr, Goodnight JM. J Bone Joint Surg 1996; 78-A; 439–456
22. Blount WP. J Bone Joint Surg 1937; 19: 1–29

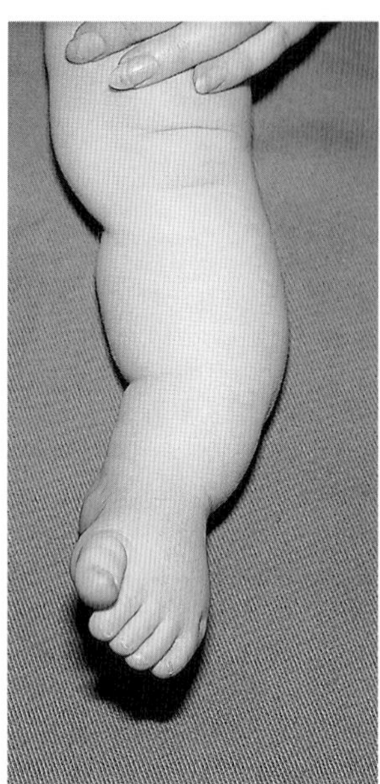

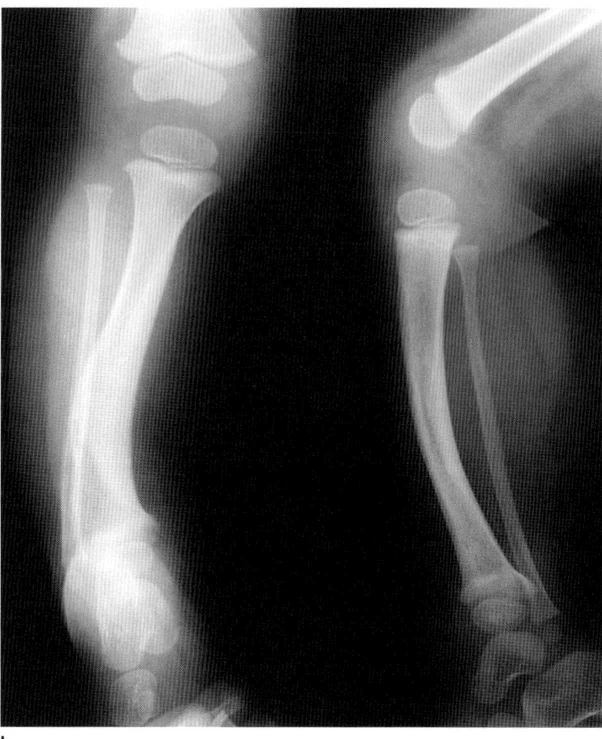

a b

Figure 45.11 Anterolateral tibial angulation (a); radiographic appearance (b).

frames (such as Ilizarov frames) or intramedullary devices.[23] Sometimes amputation is required.

THE FOOT

CONGENITAL TALIPES CALCANEOVALGUS

At birth, the foot is hyperdorsiflexed with the heel in valgus. In severe cases the dorsum of the foot lies against the lateral aspect of the tibia. The condition is an interuterine packaging problem associated with oligohydramnios and developmental dysplasia of the hip in 5% of cases. It is benign and resolves by 3–6 months with gentle physiotherapy stretching. Failure to resolve by approximately 3 months should prompt a very careful re-examination of the child to exclude a neuromuscular abnormality or generalized condition.

CONGENITAL TALIPES EQUINOVARUS (CLUB FOOT)

Congenital talipes equinovarus is characterized by forefoot and midfoot adduction, hind foot equinus and varus. The incidence is one to three per 1000 live births. Fifty per cent of cases are bilateral, and the male to female ratio is 2.5:1. There is a strong familial tendency, suggesting a polygenic inheritance.

The aetiology is not fully understood but is thought to be a combination of the effects of interuterine moulding, a neurological imbalance and delayed development. The talus is laterally oriented in the ankle mortice with an equinus and medially angulated neck. The calcaneum is in varus under the talus and displaced medially. The navicular is angled and displaced medially. The cuboid is also displaced medially, and it is this that leads to adducted, supinated forefoot. There are associated capsule, ligamentous and tendon contractures (Fig. 45.12).

Congenital talipes equinovarus is associated with hand anomalies (Streeter's dysplasia), spina bifida, arthrogryposis and diastrophic dwarfism.

Assessment is by means of careful clinical examination, to measure the flexibility of the foot and assess the degree of passive correction achievable, and radiological examination with plain X-rays (detailed description of the plain X-rays is beyond the scope of this chapter). Management is dependent on the flexibility of the deformity and comprises strapping, serial casting, splinting or surgery. Surgery may consist of soft tissue release and bony procedures depending on the degree and stiffness of the deformity. It must be remembered that even following successful treatment with satisfactory restoration of the foot architecture the deformity can recur, therefore careful follow-up is required.[24]

CONGENITAL VERTICAL TALUS (ROCKER BOTTOM FOOT)

This is a rare condition associated with arthrogryposis, spina bifida, Down's syndrome and developmental dysplasia of the hip. The talus is in a vertical position, with lateral displacement of the calcaneum. The talonavicular joint is dislocated, with the navicular lying dorsally on the neck of the talus. The calcaneum is in equinus. The forefoot is adducted and there are capsule, ligament and tendon contractures giving rise to the deformity being fixed. As the deformity is fixed serial splintage or casting are of little value, and surgery is usually required and undertaken at about 3 months of age.

PES CAVUS AND CAVOVARUS FOOT

Pes cavus is a high medial longitudinal arch with the hind foot in normal alignment. The condition is usually idiopathic, with a positive family history. A cavovarus foot has a high arch with a varus hind foot and is usually caused by a neuromuscular abnormality. The terms are sometimes used interchangeably,

REFERENCES

23. Baker JK, Cain TE, Tullos HS. J Bone Joint Surg 1992; 74-A: 169–78
24. Macnicol MF. J Bone Joint Surg 2003; 85-B: 167–170

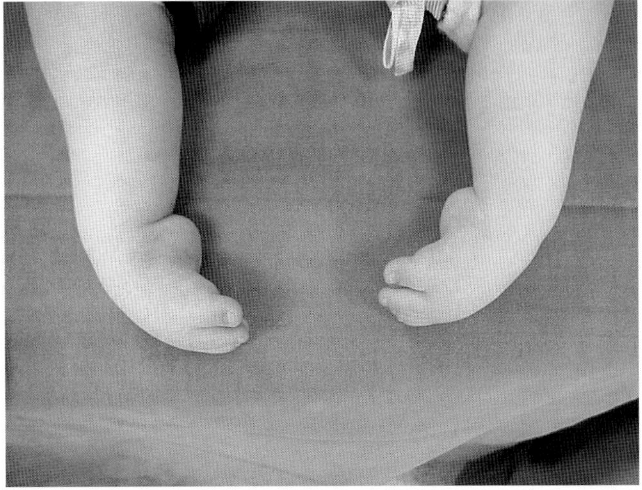
a

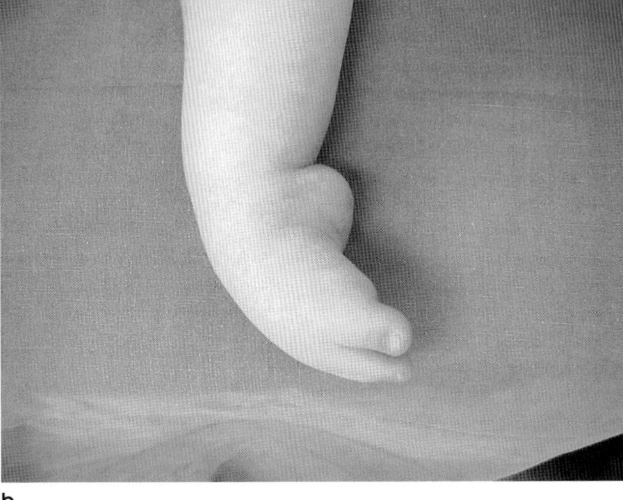
b

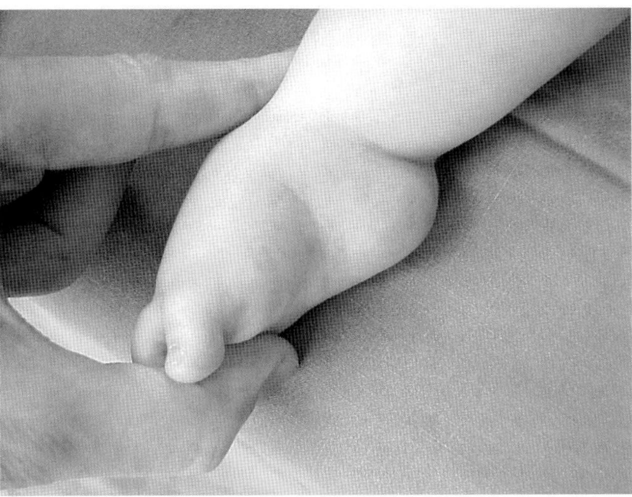
c

Figure 45.12 Congenital talipes equinovarus. This demonstrates the foot equinovarus of the hindfoot with an adducted toefoot (**a** and **b**). The deformity is fixed (**c**).

Box 45.9 Examples of causes of pes cavus or cavovarus foot

Idiopathic (25%)

Muscular

- Duchenne's muscular dystrophy
- Post compartment syndrome: Volkmann's contracture

Neurological

Lower motor neuron

- Peroneal muscular dystrophy or Charcot–Marie–Tooth syndrome
- Spinal muscular atrophy
- Polio

Upper motor neuron

- Cord level: spinal dysraphism
- Central: cerebral palsy
- Friedreich's ataxia

with *pes cavus* being used as a blanket term for all high arched feet regardless of the position of the hind foot.

A classification for pes cavus is shown in Box 45.9. The clinical features are of hind foot in varus, a cavus midfoot, a pronated adducted forefoot, and clawing of the toes. Crucial to the examination is a full and careful neurological examination including an examination of the spine. The assistance of a paediatric neurologist may be required.

The management depends on the accurate diagnosis of the underlying condition. Surgery is rarely indicated for the idiopathic form because this can be managed with footwear inserts and adjustments. If the deformity is severe with significant disability then surgical correction is indicated.

CONDITIONS OF THE TOES

HALLUX VALGUS

Hallux valgus is relatively rare and has a strong familial association, which is probably a much more important factor in the aetiology than inappropriate footwear. There is usually significant metatarsus primus varus, with great toe lateral deviation and a bunionette. Surgery should be avoided until skeletal maturity has been reached, and a scarf osteotomy is probably the operation of choice.

CURLY TOES

Children are born with significantly flexed toes that straighten out as the child starts walking. Residual curly toes are very common, affecting the third, fourth and fifth toes; they run in families and are often bilateral (Fig. 45.13). Treatment is confined to those toes that are symptomatic, significantly deformed and under-riding the medial toe, causing it to be displaced dorsally. Strapping has been demonstrated not to work and is difficult to do. Surgery is of division of the flexor tendons and generally gives very satisfactory results.

SKELETAL DYSPLASIAS

ABNORMALITIES OF STATURE

Skeletal dysplasias may display themselves as abnormally short or tall stature.

Short stature (dwarfism)

Short stature may be proportionate or characterized by short limbs or a short trunk. The causes of proportionate dwarfism

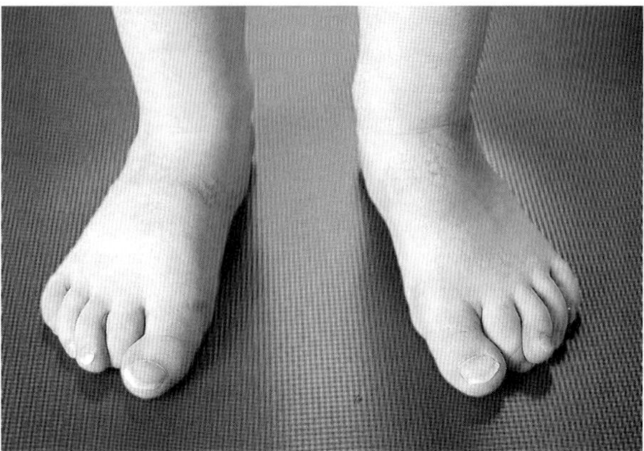

Figure 45.13 Curly second toes.

include the mucopolysaccharidoses, such as Hurler's and Morquio's syndrome; osteopetrosis; metabolic rickets from renal, alimentary, hepatic and pancreatic disorders; and pyknodysostosis,[25] which may have affected Toulouse-Lautrec.[26] This dwarfism is associated with frontal bossing, blue sclerae, and an increased risk of pathological fracture.

The short-limb forms of dwarfism include achondroplasia and hypochondroplasia, osteogenesis imperfecta, metatrophic and diastrophic dwarfism, and lethal forms of short-limb dwarfism.[27] Short-trunk dwarfism occurs in spondyloepiphyseal dysplasia.

Abnormally tall stature

Abnormally tall stature occurs in Marfan's syndrome[28] and acromegaly. The former is an autosomal dominant condition that causes disproportionately long limbs, arachnodactyly, and generalized joint laxity with flat feet and herniae. Scoliosis develops in half of those affected, and spondylolisthesis can also occur. A high arched palate and poor muscular development are also common. Eye problems include lens dislocation, myopia, retinal detachment and squint. Aortic dilatation, dissection and aneurysm are all important life-threatening complications (see Ch. 10).

When considering these skeletal dysplasias it is simplest to consider the portion of the skeleton involved (see Box 45.10).

Box 45.10 Classification of skeletal dysplasias

Epiphyseal
- Multiple epiphyseal dysplasia
- Dysplasia epiphysealis hemimelica
- Chondrodysplasia punctata
- Hereditary arthro-ophthalmopathy
- Cretinism

Metaphyseal
- Classical achondroplasia
- Hypochondroplasia
- Metaphyseal chondroplasia
- Chondroectodermal dysplasia

Diaphyseal
- Progressive diaphyseal dysplasia
- Spondyloepiphyseal dysplasia
- Pseudoachondroplasia

Altered bone density

Reduced
- Osteogenesis imperfecta
- Idiopathic juvenile osteoporosis
- The osteolyses

Increased
- Osteopetrosis
- Paget's disease
- Pyknodysostosis
- Scleronterosis
- Hypophosphatasia
- Pachydermoperiostitis

Anarchic skeletal development
- Diaphyseal aclasis
- Dyschondroplasia
- Ollier's disease or Maffucci's syndrome
- Polyostotic fibrous dysplasia
- Melorheostosis
- Osteopoikilosis
- Osteopathia striata

Epiphyseal dysplasias

The most common abnormality is multiple epiphyseal dysplasia, which is usually an autosomal dominant condition. It develops after childhood. There is mild stunting of growth, and the joints are enlarged and become painful and stiff. Flexion contractures may develop and osteoarthritis is almost inevitable. The child's intelligence is normal. The radiographic features include late-appearing, mottled epiphyses, shortened rays in the hands and feet, and a relatively normal spine.

The epiphysis is also abnormal in dysplasia epiphysealis hemimelica, where there is swelling of one part of an epiphysis in one limb and chondrodysplasia punctata. Hereditary arthro-ophthalmopathy and cretinism can also cause epiphyseal abnormalities, but these are rare conditions that cause facial and vertebral abnormalities.

METAPHYSEAL DYSPLASIAS

Classical achondroplasia, which may be either an autosomal dominant or a sporadic genetic condition, is characterized by widened metaphyses with normal epiphyses; squaring of the iliac wings (elephant ears); widening of the interpedicular distance in the lumbar spine; and flattening of the anteroposterior diameter of the thorax, vertebral canal and pelvis. Achondroplasia is the most common form of dwarfism, affecting three per 100 000 of the population.[29] The clinical features include short limbs, a bulging forehead, lumbar lordosis, stubby and splayed fingers, trident hands and normal intelligence.

Other forms of metaphyseal dysplasia include hypochondroplasia, where the skeletal changes are less severe than in achondroplasia, and metaphyseal chondrodysplasia.

DIAPHYSEAL DYSPLASIAS

Diaphyseal changes occur primarily in progressive diaphyseal dysplasia, which is a sex-linked recessive condition affecting only males and appearing in late childhood with dwarfism, backache

REFERENCES

25. Elmore SM. J Bone Joint Surg 1967; 49A: 153
26. Maroteaux P, Lamy M. JAMA 1965; 191: 715–717
27. Wynne-Davies RW, Hall CM, Apley AG (eds). Fairbank's Atlas of Skeletal Dysplasia. Churchill Livingstone, Edinburgh, 1985
28. McKusick VA. The Marfan Syndrome in Heritable Disorders of Connective Tissue. 4th edn. Mosby, St Louis, 1972
29. Wynne-Davies RW, Walsh WK, Gormley J. J Bone Joint Surg 1981; 63B: 508–515

and a prominent sternum. The radiographic features include platyspondyly, a small pelvis, and mildly abnormal large joints that become osteoarthritic.

Vertebral, epiphyseal and metaphyseal involvement characterize spondyloepiphyseal dysplasia congenita; pseudoachondroplasia, where the skull is normal and dwarfism is more pronounced than in achondroplasia; and metatrophic and diastrophic dwarfism.

ALTERED BONE DENSITY

Decreased bone density

Decreased bone density is a feature of osteogenesis imperfecta, idiopathic juvenile osteoporosis and the osteolyses.

Osteogenesis imperfecta

Sillence and colleagues classified osteogenesis imperfecta into:[30]

- type I, an autosomal dominant with blue sclerae and normal teeth;
- type II, an autosomal dominant that is lethal, with multiple fractures present at birth and associated major malformation of the skeleton;
- type III, an autosomal recessive causing progressive deformity, with fractures at birth and normal sclerae but with dentinogenesis imperfecta; and
- type IV, an autosomal dominant with white sclerae and either normal or abnormal teeth.

The bones are fragile in all types and readily fracture. They are usually slender with a wide medullary cavity and a thin cortex. Occasionally cysts are present.

Increased bone density

Increased bone density is seen in osteopetrosis, an autosomal recessive condition affecting both sexes equally. It is also seen in Paget's disease, pyknodysostosis, melorheostosis, osteopoikilosis and osteopathia striata (candle bones, spotted bones and striped bones), sclerosteosis, hyperphosphatasia and pachydermoperiostitis.

Paget's disease (osteitis deformans)

The bones are thickened, coarsened and enlarged in Paget's disease (Fig. 45.14). It is probably an acquired condition, although there is a possibility that it has an autosomal dominant inheritance. It affects the sexes equally and is rare before middle age. The disorder is common in Europe, Australasia and the USA but rare in Africa and Asia. The finding of inclusion bodies in osteoclasts suggests that a virus may be responsible.[31] The bone architecture is abnormal, and the bones are very brittle and liable to fracture. The process starts at the ends of one or more long bones—the pelvis and tibia are the most commonly affected bones, followed by the femur, skull and spine—and spreads along their shafts. It may remain localized to one bone for many years.

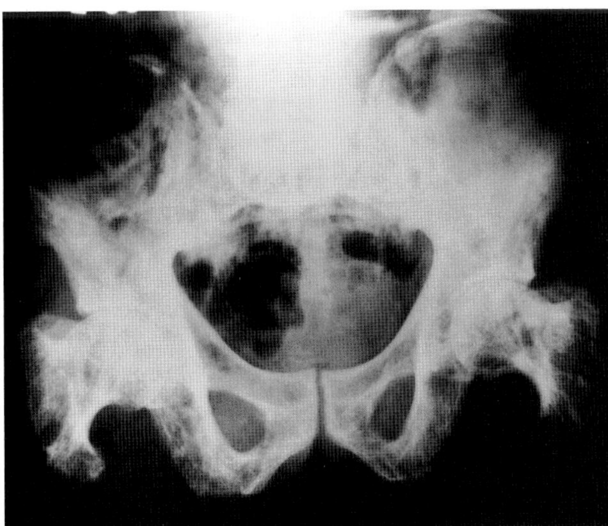

Figure 45.14 Paget's disease of the pelvis.

There is an increase in both osteoblastic and osteoclastic activity with zones of osteolysis, filled with vascular fibrous tissue, adjacent to zones of osteogenesis, where osteoblasts rapidly form new woven and lamellar bone. This is, in turn, digested and reformed on both the periosteal and endosteal surfaces of the bone, increasing its thickness. The newly formed bone is, however, weaker than the normal bone and liable to bend and fracture. Eventually osteoclastic activity ceases and new lamellar bone is deposited in an irregular fashion. The irregular pattern that this produces gives a mosaic appearance with increasingly sclerotic bone, which also makes it more liable to fracture.

Many patients have no symptoms and the disorder is diagnosed by chance on a radiograph. The most common symptoms are pain associated with bony enlargement, and deformity. Patients may also present when complications develop. The pain is a dull constant ache that is worse at night. Severe pain usually indicates the development of a fissure fracture. Deformities are most commonly seen in the lower limb bones; tibial thickening with anterior bowing is characteristic of the disease. The skull also enlarges, and although hats are not commonly worn these days they may no longer fit! Spinal disease causes a short neck, which is often associated with kyphosis. As the bones enlarge, nerve compression may occur. This is particularly true in the skull, where most of the cranial nerves can be damaged or compressed, especially the eighth nerve, causing deafness. At a late stage, patients may develop high-output cardiac failure from shunting through highly vascular bones.

Bone sarcomas develop in 1% of patients and should be suspected if pain increases or if a lump appears. The prognosis for these tumours is very poor. Hypercalcaemia may cause thirst, dehydration and confusion, and pathological fractures need to be appropriately managed. The serum alkaline phosphatase is markedly elevated, and hydroxyproline excretion in the urine is increased. Radiographs show coarse trabeculae in the bones, with an irregular cortical layer. Zones of osteolysis appear as 'bone cysts', and fissured fractures are often seen as a series of fine cracks on the convex surface of bone, unlike in osteomalacia. The skull is thickened and mottled, and the bones are widened and deformed.

Very few patients require treatment; non-steroidal anti-inflammatory agents control most pain satisfactorily. Calcitonin and diphosphonates reduce pain, cardiac failure and hypercalcaemia by reducing osteoclastic activity. This can be monitored by a fall in the serum alkaline phosphatase and urine hydroxyproline levels. Pathological fractures usually require internal

REFERENCES

30. Sillence DO, Senn A, Danks DM. J Med Genet 1979; 16: 101–116
31. Rebel A, Malkani K et al. Rev Rhum 1974; 41: 767

fixation and nerves may have to be decompressed. Osteosarcomas should be resected if possible.

Anarchic development of the skeleton

Anarchic development of the skeleton occurs in diaphyseal aclasis (multiple hereditary osteochondromata), Ollier's disease (multiple enchondromata) and polyostotic fibrous dysplasia.

Diaphyseal aclasis

Diaphyseal aclasis is an autosomal dominant condition with equal sex distribution, causing the symmetrical production of exostoses (osteochondroses), typically at the knees, ankles, elbows, wrists and shoulder girdles. The ribs and pelvis may be involved, and the child is usually slightly short but has reasonably satisfactory limb function. There is a minor risk of a later chondrosarcomatous change in the osteochondromata, particularly if they are subjected to trauma. They can be removed if they cause pressure symptoms or look unsightly.

Dyschondroplasia or Ollier's disease

This is a sporadic disorder that affects the sexes equally. The multiple enchondromata cause swelling in the long bones and fingers, where the deformity may be quite pronounced. Pathological fractures and growth arrest may occur, and the radiographs show irregular lucencies in the metaphyses, with gradual enlargement of these cartilaginous masses and mottling of the epiphyses.

Maffucci's syndrome

Marfucci's syndrome is the rare combination of enchondromatosis and haemangiomata.

Polyostotic fibrous dysplasia

Polyostotic fibrous dysplasia was described by Albright in girls but affects both sexes sporadically. The fibrous dysplasia causes oval areas of 'ground glass' rarefaction in the long bones and there is also skin pigmentation and sexual precocity. Pathological fractures can occur, and patients with this condition may develop coxa vara. Polyostotic fibrous dysplasia may also be associated with diabetes mellitus, acromegaly, hyperthyroidism and Cushing's syndrome.

MISCELLANEOUS CONDITIONS

There are a number of other conditions that can affect the skeleton, including neurofibromatosis, the nail patella syndrome, cleidocranial dysplasia and myositis ossificans progressiva. Hypermobility of the joints and ligaments is a feature of Marfan's syndrome, Down's syndrome, osteogenesis imperfecta, Ehlers–Danlos syndrome and Larsen's syndrome. There are a number of localized skeletal abnormalities that are not genetically transmitted. Vertebral abnormalities are common and consist of agenesis, hemivertebrae, fusions and dysraphism, which is commonly associated with spina bifida or meningomyelocele. Other localized abnormalities include the Klippel–Feil syndrome, where vertebral abnormalities are associated with a short neck and an elevated scapula, and Sprengel's syndrome, where only the scapula is elevated.[32]

Various storage diseases also affect the skeleton. These include the mucopolysaccharidoses, the mucolipidoses and histiocytosis X. This last condition includes eosinophilic granuloma of bone, in which there are tumours of the pelvis, skull or vertebrae with pathological fractures or vertebral flattening. Other rare storage diseases that affect the skeleton include Hand–Schüller–Christian disease—which consists of hepatosplenomegaly and lymphadenopathy, with growth retardation, multiple lytic bone lesions, and the rare triad of exophthalmos, diabetes insipidus and skull defects—and Letterer–Siwe disease, which is characterized by a severe and generalized infiltration during infancy, including pulmonary, visceral and skeletal involvement.

REFERENCE

32. Sprengel O. Langenbecks Arch Klin Chir 1891; 42: 545

The shoulder and elbow

46

Roger J. H. Emery

SHOULDER GIRDLE

A prerequisite for efficient upper limb function is a stable yet dynamic fulcrum with the axial skeleton. This is achieved by the scapular suspension mechanism that, with the stabilizing muscles, allows rotation combined with retraction and protraction. In the erect position, the trapezius and levator scapulae support the entire weight of the upper extremity (Fig. 46.1). On raising the arm, the upper fibres of trapezius and levator scapulae pull in a cephalad direction, while at the same time the lower fibres of trapezius acting with the rhomboids and latissimus dorsi pull the arm backwards, allowing the upper fibres of trapezius to rotate the scapula.

Functional impairment of the upper limb is seen when there is disruption of the bony or ligamentous structures, weakness of an isolated muscle, or global loss of function of the scapular stabilizing muscles.

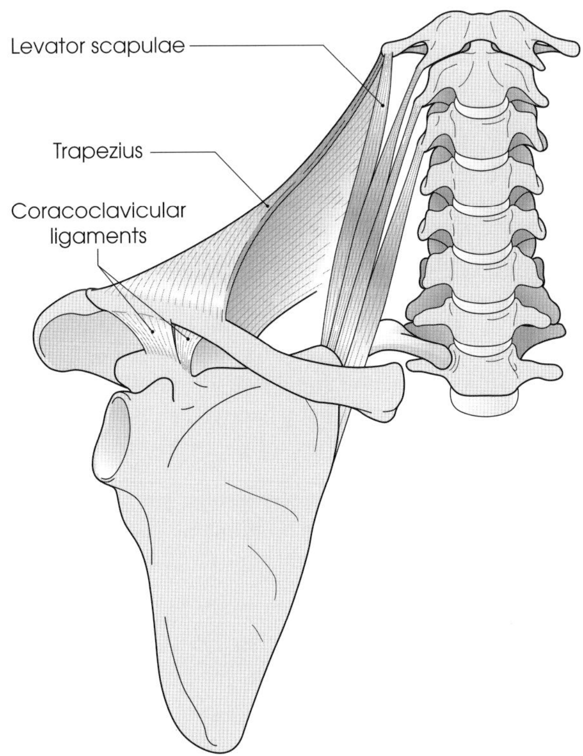

Figure 46.1 The suspensory mechanism of the shoulder.

WINGING OF THE SCAPULA

Trapezius palsy

The major cause of trapezius palsy is injury to the spinal accessory nerve resulting in 'winging' of the scapula. Although the dangers of an iatrogenic nerve injury cannot be over-stressed, it is important to appreciate that this palsy is commonly seen when the nerve is sacrificed intentionally during radical neck dissection for malignant disease. The ensuing disability can be so great that preservation of the nerve should be encouraged if at all possible.

The spinal accessory nerve is the major nerve supply to trapezius. It leaves the base of the skull through the jugular foramen, and passes obliquely through the sternocleidomastoid muscle in its upper third before crossing the posterior triangle of the neck to enter trapezius. It is vulnerable to injury, because it lies very superficially and is at risk with even the simplest surgical operation in the neck region (see Ch. 16). The injury is usually not recognized at the time of surgery, and the diagnosis is often delayed until the patient finds that it is impossible to abduct the arm without pain. Electromyographic examination may be of help to identify the few palsies caused by a neurapraxia that recover spontaneously, but if there is no recovery by 10 weeks the nerve should be explored. If the nerve is found in continuity lying in scar tissue, neurolysis may be successful, but if there is obvious discontinuity, suture or grafting is necessary (see Ch. 43). Should the nerve repair be unsuccessful or not possible, surgical reconstruction with muscle transfer should be considered.

Muscle transfer is the only therapeutic option if the accessory nerve has been excised during a radical neck resection. The degree of disability in these patients is extremely variable; this may be partly because of trapezius's dual innervation from C2 and C3 (occasionally C3 and C4). The indications for surgery must also reflect the activity level, age and life expectancy of the patient.

In every case of shoulder girdle dysfunction, it is important to consider the secondary effect on the soft tissues and the nerves around the shoulder. A trapezius palsy may be associated with pain from neurological denervation, and an adhesive capsulitis of the shoulder joint may also develop. Ptosis of the scapula may cause discomfort as the result of traction radiculitis of the brachial plexus. More commonly the pain appears to be from fatigue and functional impingement or even attrition of the supraspinatus tendon within the subacromial space because of its failure to rotate and retract the scapula. Conservative treatment is invariably unsuccessful, apart from improving any concomitant adhesive capsulitis. Surgical reconstructions must correct not only the winging of the scapula but also the ptosis caused by the loss of the scapular suspension mechanism. The intention is to improve the deformity, which may be severe. The Eden–Lange tendon transfer of levator scapulae and the rhomboids

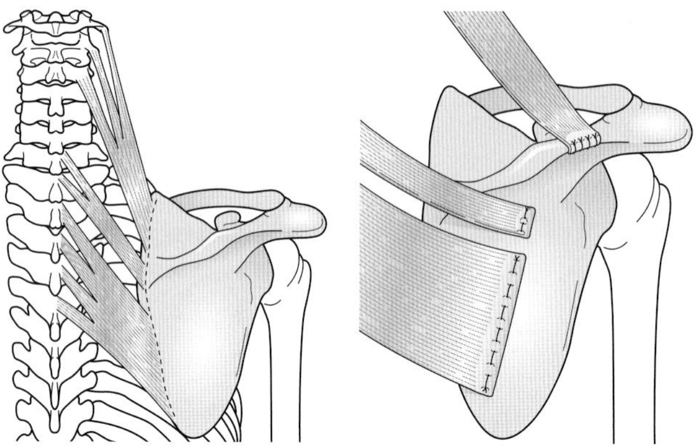

Figure 46.2 The muscle transfers used in the Eden–Lange procedure.

(Fig. 46.2) is probably the best method of achieving near normal function.[1–3] These three muscles are used to replace the upper, middle and lower parts of trapezius, respectively.

Alternative procedures, such as fascial slings passed from the vertebral border of the scapula to the spinous processes of the second and third thoracic vertebrae, in place of the middle and lower parts of trapezius, have significant disadvantages as they stretch with time. If soft tissue reconstruction fails, the only alternative option is scapulothoracic fusion. The lateral transfer of the levator scapulae muscles improves cosmesis, and head and neck surgeons must be cautioned against transposing this important suspensory muscle to cover the carotid artery after radical neck dissection.

Loss of serratus anterior function

The serratus anterior assists the upper fibres of trapezius in upward and forward rotation of the scapula, and also keeps the vertebral border of the scapula in firm apposition with the chest wall in all positions. Loss of this muscle may limit active shoulder elevation, but more frequently presents as deformity with fatigue pain on elevation of the arm. The glenohumeral joint has been aptly described as a 'golf ball on a tee' (the glenoid is the tee); the scapula must be positioned so that the glenoid centre line and the axis of the humeral head are closely aligned. This is particularly important during vigorous shoulder activities, for example a boxer's punch, bench press, throwing action or tennis shot. Power is lost and fatigue occurs if the glenoid centre line and humerus are not aligned.

A long thoracic nerve palsy is the major cause of serratus anterior weakness, because rupture of serratus anterior is extremely rare. The long thoracic nerve is formed from the roots of C5, 6 and 7 immediately after leaving their intervertebral foramina (see Ch. 43). It runs beside the main brachial plexus and is often spared in traction lesions. The cause of an isolated serratus anterior palsy is often difficult to explain but may follow viral illness, carrying objects on the shoulder, recumbency for a prolonged period of time, immunization, open iatrogenic injury in the axilla, and lying on the operating table for long periods. Iatrogenic causes are seen following first rib resection, mastectomies with axillary clearance, scalenotomies, surgical procedures for spontaneous pneumothorax, and infraclavicular plexus anaesthetic blocks. These cases only rarely recover spontaneously; by contrast, palsies occurring after closed trauma are usually traction lesions and recovery can be anticipated. Recovery is usually seen by 1 year, and if palsy persists beyond this time the prognosis is poor, although some patients may still recover after 2 or 3 years.

The major problem is pain associated with difficulty lifting the arm, particularly with weights. Additionally, there may be discomfort from the winging when sitting against a chair back. The shoulder may also be painful at rest from an associated subacromial bursitis, usually as a consequence of functional impingement within the subacromial space. There is little useful treatment; jackets and braces to prevent winging are uncomfortable and rarely tolerated. Many patients learn to live with the disability, and thus few come to surgery. There is no place for nerve repair: the only option is tendon transfer. Pectoralis major transfer with a fascia lata graft through the axilla to the lower pole of the scapula can give satisfactory results.[4]

Global weakness of the scapular stabilizers

Generalized weakness of the scapular stabilizing muscles is commonly associated with many injuries and conditions affecting the shoulder joint. Careful examination often demonstrates minor winging of the scapula even in the absence of stiffness of the glenohumeral joint. However, if the weakness is severe, the relative strength of the deltoid muscle is much greater, and on elevation of the arm this imbalance allows the deltoid to pull up the scapula, causing it to wing.

Muscle dystrophies should be considered in all cases of unexplained weakness and atrophy of these shoulder stabilizers occurring in the first and second decades. The commonest type is facioscapulohumeral dystrophy. The condition is autosomal recessive and a family history may be elicited. This is a bilateral condition, but it is usually unilateral on presentation. The other side may not be affected until months or even years later. Involvement of the facial muscles may be detected early, with the child's inability to whistle or blow out candles on a birthday cake. This condition has variable muscle involvement and prognosis: there is usually slow deterioration and a good life expectancy. The deltoid is spared but loses its stable origin and tilts the scapula rather than raising the humerus. There is a characteristic deformity caused by the selective muscle loss.

Muscular dystrophies involve a number of muscles, and muscle transfer is therefore not applicable. A scapulothoracic fusion should be considered if the disability increases with preservation of the deltoid muscle function. This operation recreates a stable origin by anchoring the scapula to the fourth, fifth and sixth ribs. The procedure has been well described by Copeland and Howard.[5] There are many technical variations but the principles remain the same. The shoulder should be immobilized in a spica for 3 months in 50° of abduction and 30° of forward flexion, with sufficient internal rotation to allow the hand to be placed in front of the mouth.

Other causes of winging

Obligatory winging is seen after glenohumeral fusion. This is rarely of significance except after arthrodesis for brachial plexus

REFERENCES

1. Lange M. Langenbecks Arch Klin Hir 1951; 270: 437–439
2. Langenskiold A, Ryoppy S. Acta Orthop Scand 1973; 44: 383–388
3. Bigliani LU, Compito CA, Duralde XA et al. J Bone Joint Surg 1996; 78A: 1534–1540
4. Marmor L, Bechtol CO. J Bone Joint Surg 1942; 24: 699
5. Copeland SA, Howard RC. J Bone Joint Surg 1978; 60B: 547

injury and should be assessed prior to surgery. The upper part of serratus anterior may be denervated in some cases of C5 and C6 root avulsion. Injuries to the upper roots of the brachial plexus during birth may also cause winging of the scapula. Anterior contracture and capsular tightness develop with posterior subluxation of the humeral head. The glenohumeral joint becomes fixed in abduction so that, when the shoulder is forced into adduction, superior winging occurs: this is known as the scapular sign of Putti.

An abduction contracture of the deltoid may cause secondary winging. This is quite common in developing countries, where it is often bilateral and usually affects the anterior part of deltoid. Two types occur: congenital and secondary to multiple intramuscular injections. The treatment is release of fibrous bands and manipulation. A defect in the deltoid may result, requiring closure by anterior transfer of posterior deltoid. Large subscapular osteochondromata can cause displacement of the scapula, producing pseudowinging.

THE STERNOCLAVICULAR JOINT

The suspensory mechanism requires a stable sternoclavicular joint and an intact clavicle, acromioclavicular joint and coracoclavicular ligaments. These important static suspensory structures not only prevent the scapula from dropping but also prevent posterior displacement of the clavicle and protraction of scapula. The sternoclavicular joint is remarkable for its lack of bony congruity and its dependence on the surrounding ligaments for stability. This saddle type of diarthrodial joint contains the curious intra-articular disc ligament (Fig. 46.3). It is covered by the sternoclavicular ligaments lying within the capsule, but the major structural support is derived from the costoclavicular (rhomboid) and interclavicular ligaments.

Disruption of these ligaments results in instability of the medial end of the clavicle. The disruption is usually from an indirect force in which either the torso is compressed and rolled backwards causing an ipsilateral anterior dislocation, or compressed and rolled forwards causing posterior dislocation. The vast majority of these injuries occur in road traffic accidents or sporting injuries.

Other conditions affecting this joint present as pain or swelling. These conditions unrelated to trauma may be classified into the following categories:

- Spontaneous subluxation or dislocation.
- Congenital or developmental subluxation or dislocation.

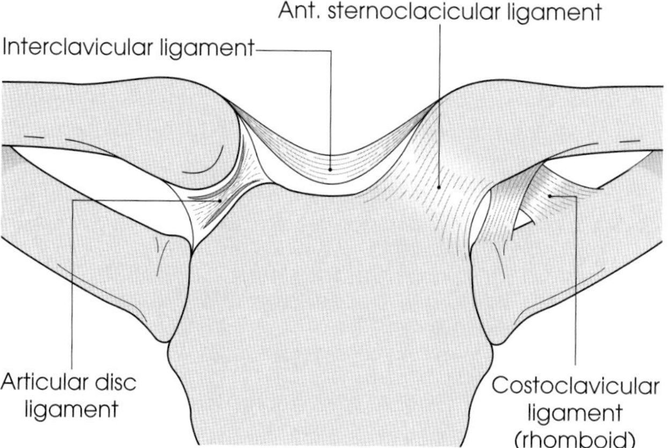

Figure 46.3 The anatomy of the sternoclavicular joint.

- Arthritis:
  osteoarthritis;
  arthropathies;
  condensing osteitis of the medial clavicle;
  sternocostoclavicular hyperostosis; or
  postmenopausal arthritis.
- Infection.
- Tumours.

Evaluation of these conditions may be significantly hindered by the difficulties of imaging the joint. The history and clinical findings may be diagnostic, but imaging is often required. For example, not all cases demonstrate the typical appearances of anterior or posterior dislocation, and even assessment of the direction of displacement may be difficult. Plain radiology may be of limited value, even with special views including the 40° cephalad tilt or 'serendipidity' view advocated by Rockwood.[6] If any doubt persists, tomograms or a CT scan are required. Ultrasound scanning is usually a simpler and quicker method of observing displacement. Magnetic resonance scans show the intra-articular disc ligament very well, and isotope studies are particularly helpful in identifying infection, inflammation and rare tumours.

Spontaneous subluxation or dislocation is usually a self-limiting condition and almost never requires surgery.[6] Arthritis of the sternoclavicular joint may also become symptomless with time and conservative management should be tried, including a limited number of intra-articular steroid injections. If surgery is required, excision arthroplasty alone is recommended; resection of 2 cm of medial clavicle does not compromise its stability because the costoclavicular ligaments are left intact. Particular care must be taken when dividing the clavicle; a blunt retractor should be placed behind the clavicle before making a series of drill holes. The osteotomy is completed with an osteotome. The clavicular head of sternocleidomastoid is released and sutured into the space created by the resected clavicle. Despite the rarity of these injuries and conditions, the complications associated with surgery to this joint are important. Surgery to the sternoclavicular joint is potentially dangerous because of its immediate posterior relations, which include the arch of the aorta, the superior vena cava, the innominate vein and the subclavian vessels. The use of any type of pin is dangerous and unwarranted. Its insertion risks injuring these structures, and migration of pins is well documented. Their persistent use still generates even more bizarre case reports of pins found as far away as the liver and spinal cord, and in some incidences the pinning caused death.

Condensing osteitis of the medial clavicle, sternocostoclavicular hyperostosis and postmenopausal arthritis are poorly defined conditions with many similar features. There is little guidance on management from the small numbers of cases reported. Infections are occasionally encountered, and culture will reveal a wide range of organisms. Although needle biopsy may help with the diagnosis, anterior arthrotomy is usually required for treatment.

THE ACROMIOCLAVICULAR JOINT

The articulation at the lateral end of the clavicle allows as much as 20° of angulation and 40–50° of rotation. This diarthrodial

REFERENCE

6. Rockwood CA Jr, Odor JM. J Bone Joint Surg 1989; 71A: 1280–1288

joint has a fibrocartilaginous disc that may be complete or meniscoid. The stability of the acromioclavicular joint is maintained by the acromioclavicular and coracoclavicular ligaments. Rockwood demonstrated from cadaver studies that horizontal stability was controlled by the acromioclavicular ligaments, whereas vertical stability was dependent on the coracoclavicular ligaments.[7] The superior acromioclavicular ligaments are relatively weak and blend with the fascia of deltoid and trapezius. It is the conoid and trapezoid parts of the coracoclavicular ligament that function as suspensory ligaments of the scapula and the primary supports of the acromioclavicular joint.

Symptomless degenerative arthritis of the acromioclavicular joint is extremely common, and narrowing of the disc space can be considered a normal ageing process after the age of 40 years. Symptomatic cases can be treated by excision of the distal end of the clavicle together with the adjacent osteophytes.[8] This procedure can be effectively performed arthroscopically, and it is also indicated in type I and type II injuries with persistent pain or secondary post-traumatic arthritis (Fig. 53.2). At least 1½ cm of bone should be removed, and clearance should be assessed on the operating table. Particular care should be taken not to remove too much clavicle or destabilize the coracoclavicular ligaments, and the operation should be completed by a strong repair of the overlying fascia.

A common cause of acromioclavicular arthrosis is a previous injury to the joint followed by attempted reduction of the dislocation. There is in fact a higher incidence of post-traumatic arthritis following surgery than there is after conservative treatment, particularly in patients treated by transarticular wires.

Late reconstructions for vertical instability of the distal clavicle are difficult. A Bosworth screw from the clavicle to the coracoid process alone is inadequate, and most of these cases require a coracoacromial ligament transfer.[9] Ligament transfer was originally proposed by Cadenet in 1917,[10] and it has continued to provide good results.[11] The technique is often modified, but the principle is to transfer the coracoacromial ligament from the acromion to the excised end of the clavicle. Probably the most important aspect of the reconstruction is a firm repair of the trapezius fascia. Postoperatively, a broad arm sling is worn for 4 weeks, allowing gentle circumduction exercises. This procedure is equally effective in early and late cases.[12]

Occasionally the coracoacromial ligament is not substantial enough to act as a stabilizer, and alternative techniques are required. The coracoclavicular ligaments cannot be reliably repaired but should be opposed to achieve some reconstitution by fibrous scarring. Coracoclavicular banding with either polydioxanone sulphide cord or tape is preferable to the use of non-absorbable materials such as Dacron or wire, which may cause erosion and subsequent fracture of the bone.

Transfer of the coracoid process to the clavicle provides dynamic stabilization should these procedures fail. In horizontal instability, the important superior acromioclavicular ligament is deficient and may require reconstruction by transfer of the coracoacromial ligament to the upper surface of the clavicle.[13]

The acromioclavicular joint is often affected by rheumatoid arthritis, and a trial of local anaesthetic injections can identify the joint as a major source of pain even in patients with severe glenohumeral or rotator cuff disease. In these patients the acromioclavicular joint may be the only restraint against upward migration, and a dome-type arthroplasty may be preferable to conventional excision.

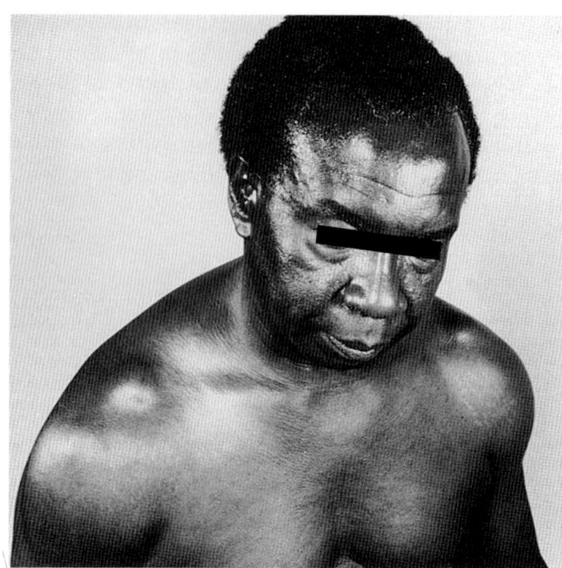

Figure 46.4 Patient with typical acromioclavicular joint cysts due to degenerative change in the underlying joint.

Acromioclavicular joint cysts are associated with degenerative changes in the joint and underlying rotator cuff tears (Fig. 46.4). Simple excision is unpredictable, and resection of the outer end of the clavicle is preferable. Another uncommon condition is osteolysis of the distal clavicle. This is usually seen in men, particularly in weightlifters. It is commonly unilateral and usually resolves with rest and local injections. Curiously, the clavicle may even reconstitute itself. The acromioclavicular joint is also a rare site for septic arthritis, with many case reports describing infection with a variety of organisms.

Plain radiographs are the essential investigation for this joint. It is important to request anteroposterior and axillary views of the acromioclavicular joint and *not* the glenohumeral joint to avoid over-penetration. Stress views may be of value in distinguishing a type II from a type III acromioclavicular dislocation. This is potentially useful because the distinction changes the management of the injury. The stress views compare the coracoclavicular space of the affected joint with that of the normal contralateral joint. The widening of the interspace can be demonstrated by applying weights suspended by loops from the wrists. It is thought that as little as 40% displacement probably reflects some disruption of the coracoclavicular ligaments.

SUBACROMIAL SPACE AND ROTATOR CUFF

IMPINGEMENT SYNDROME

The acromioclavicular joint and adjacent lateral acromion form the roof of the subacromial bursa. This bursa forms an

REFERENCES

7. Rockwood CA Jr. In: Fractures in Adults, Vol 1. 2nd edn. Lippincott, Philadelphia, 1984: 860–910
8. Mumford EB. J Bone Joint Surg 1941; 23: 799–802
9. Bosworth BM. Surg Gynecol Obstet 1941; 73: 866–871
10. Cadenet FM. Internat Clin 1917; 1: 145–169
11. Weaver JK, Dunn HK. J Bone Joint Surg 1972; 54A: 1187–1194
12. Warren-Smith CD, Ward MW. J Bone Joint Surg 1987; 69B: 715–718
13. Neviaser JS. Clin Orthop 1968; 58: 57–68

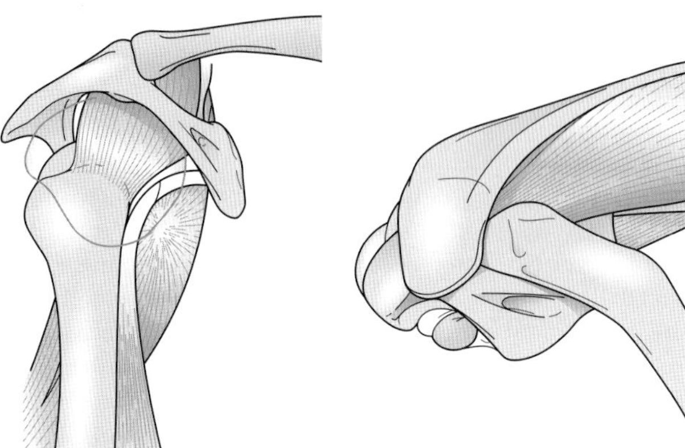

Figure 46.5 The supraspinatus outlet and subacromial bursa.

'articulation' and is the most common site of pathology within the shoulder, largely from conditions affecting the rotator cuff forming its floor. Subacromial bursitis has been recognized since the mid 19th century, but its association with subacromial impingement has been increasingly recognized over the past 60 years. The impingement occurs between the upper surface of the biceps and the rotator cuff with the anterior edge of acromion, coracoacromial ligament, or undersurface of acromioclavicular joint (Fig. 46.5). Symptoms may occur in a normal shoulder following a period of overuse, particularly with repetitive loaded activities in the overhead position. This early stage usually resolves spontaneously.

Supraspinatus involvement was described by Codman in 1927. The prevailing concept is that these tendons are too thick, or more commonly that the supraspinatus outlet is too small. The outlet stenosis is usually caused by an acromial spur developing at the origin of the coracoacromial ligament, or by encroachment of a degenerate acromioclavicular joint. The term 'impingement syndrome' was coined,[14] and Neer also described 'a characteristic ridge of proliferative spurs and excrescences on the undersurface of the anterior process of the acromion, apparently caused by repeated impingement of the rotator cuff and the humeral head, with traction of the coracoacromial ligament... Without exception it was the anterior lip and undersurface of the anterior third that was involved'. Prior to this important description emphasizing the site of impingement, the surgical treatment had been acromionectomy, a mutilating operation with poor results because of loss of the deltoid origin. Current practice is to increase the size of the outlet by resection of the coracoacromial ligament and removal of the spur by undercutting the acromion. This procedure, termed *acromioplasty*, provides good results.

The hallmarks of this condition are the pathological changes in the coracoacromial ligament, with 'crab meat fraying' at the anterior margin as the result of mechanical impingement and injection within its coverings. In addition, alteration of the acromial morphology from spur formation at the enthesis of the coracoacromial ligament can be easily observed. These changes have been described by Bigliani and colleagues[15] and classified into flat (type I), curved (type II) and hooked (type III). The significance of these findings in relation to the development of rotator cuff tears is disputed, because many of the earliest pathological changes are found in the tendons of the rotator cuff. These partial thickness articular side tears suggest that the acromial changes may be a secondary phenomenon.

In practice the presentations of these cases give the clinical impression of a far more imprecise group of conditions; it is now

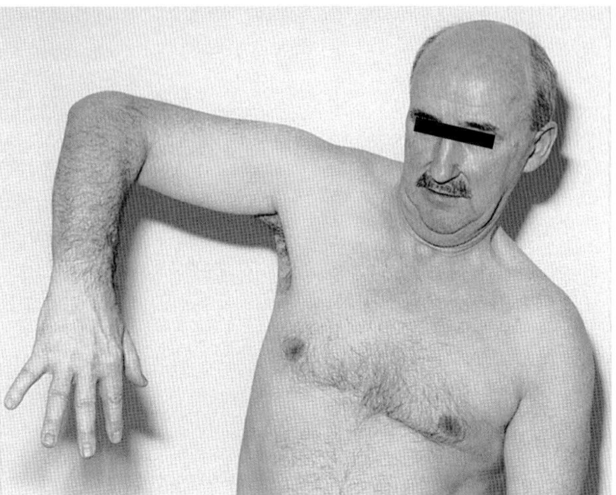

Figure 46.6 Demonstration of a positive impingement sign.

recognized that the causes are diverse and include structural abnormalities of the acromion and acromioclavicular joint, inflammation of the bursa, congenital abnormalities or fracture malunions of the humerus producing prominence of the greater tuberosity, and even functional factors. For example, it has already been discussed how winging of the scapula can cause impingement of the supraspinatus. In addition, alterations in glenohumeral movement caused by changes in the capsule may cause a functional impingement. For example, in the stiff shoulder, the tightness of the posterior shoulder capsule forces the humeral head to ride up against the acromion during flexion. Conversely, capsular laxity can cause impingement from excessive upward translation of the humeral head during sporting activities. This accounts for many of the disappointing and unpredictable results of anterior acromioplasty in athletes and young patients.

The clinical presentation of impingement syndrome is characteristic; there is a history of pain, usually in the periacromial or epaulette area, with additional pain experienced in the lateral aspect of the arm, the anterior aspect of humerus biceps, and the muscle belly of supraspinatus itself. The onset may be associated with overuse in the overhead position or with athletic activity. The pain is usually reproduced on activities requiring forward flexion and internal rotation. Night pain is characteristic and distressing. The physical signs include muscle atrophy of supraspinatus and infraspinatus, slight tenderness over the rotator cuff, and crepitus and clicking as the supraspinatus tendon is passed under the coracoacromial arch. This last effect is also the cause of the characteristic midrange painful arc on abduction and forward flexion. This is made worse by internal rotation and forms the basis of the impingement sign and test (Fig. 46.6). Diminished strength of abduction and external rotation can usually be demonstrated. Relief of pain with subacromial local anaesthetic injection, called the impingement test, is a simple and effective diagnostic manoeuvre.

Plain radiographs may identify bony causes of the outlet stenosis and signs of the rotator cuff disease, such as calcification

REFERENCES

14. Neer CS. J Bone Joint Surg 1972; 54A: 715–718
15. Bigliani LU, Morrison D, April AW. Orthop Trans 1986; 10: 228

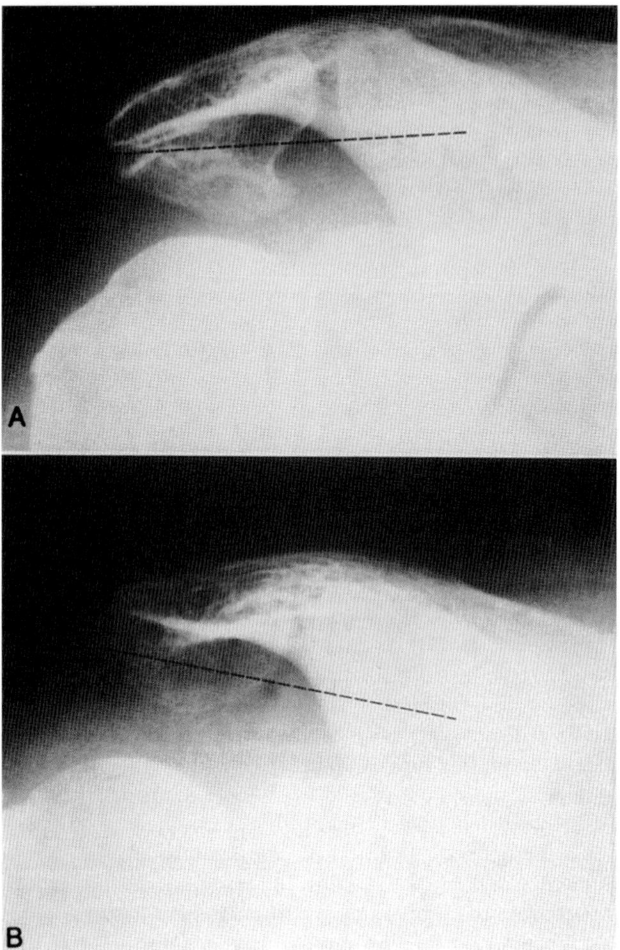

Figure 46.7 A 30° caudal tilt anteroposterior radiograph showing a subacromial spur.

or erosions at the tendon insertion. The axial view shows the degree of degenerative change within the acromioclavicular joint and the presence of an os acromiale. The outlet view is useful but requires skilful and careful radiography. An alternative is the 30° caudal tilt anteroposterior view devised by Rockwood, which allows the spurs to be classified into type I and type II (Fig. 46.7).

Further investigations seek to define whether the rotator cuff is torn. Double-contrast arthrography is invasive but identifies full thickness tears with a high degree of accuracy. Ultrasound and MRI scanning are non-invasive and have replaced arthrography in many centres. With skilled interpretation, these investigations have a greater than 90% sensitivity and specificity. Caution must be exercised, however, because many abnormalities are seen in symptomless individuals, particularly with advancing age. These tests must be used to answer specific questions and are helpful in confirming the diagnosis after careful clinical evaluation.

The majority of impingement syndromes respond to time and rest. Modifications to daily and sporting activities together with exercises to re-educate and strengthen the shoulder muscles are helpful. There is no evidence of benefit from heat, cold, massage, electrotherapy or acupuncture. Non-steroidal anti-inflammatory drugs and the judicious use of subacromial hydrocortisone injection can decrease inflammation and relieve pain.

The indications for surgical decompression by acromioplasty are symptoms of impingement with disability for more than 1 year in patients aged more than 40 years. Stiffness is a contraindication to surgery. The impingement test should be positive, and a full thickness rotator cuff tear must be excluded. Certain patients less than 40 years old can be considered, but extreme caution should be made when confirming the diagnosis.

The principles of the Neer acromioplasty are preservation of the acromial origin of deltoid with secure reattachment after the open procedure, because dehiscence not only compromises function but is also extremely difficult to correct surgically. The use of either No. 1 non-absorbable or polydioxanone suture through drill holes is recommended. Acromionectomy or excessive removal of anterior acromion must also be avoided because this also presents major difficulties for reconstruction. Smooth resection of the undersurface of the anteroinferior acromion and insertion of the coracoacromial ligament is performed.[14] Coracoid impingement is a rarer but well-recognized condition with specific symptoms and signs of impingement.

Careful inspection for other sources of impingement, such as acromioclavicular joint arthritis, is important. This may be primarily degenerative but is also seen after a recent or remote injury.[16,17] It is important to remember that arthritis with osteophytes on the undersurface of the joint, even with encroachment on to the supraspinatus, is common; more than a third of symptomless shoulders in patients over 40 demonstrate these features on MRI scanning. Undercutting of the joint is recommended, or it should be excised if it is symptomatic and irritable on examination.

The importance of awareness of the presence of an os acromiale and of the risks of destabilizing the fragment during acromioplasty cannot be overstated. A similar situation can arise if the acromion is fractured by excessive resection of bone. This needs to be fixed to allow mobilization, in order to reduce bursal scarring without causing malunion or non-union of fragments. Fixation can be performed either with K wires and a tension band or lag screws.

Careful rehabilitation after acromioplasty is imperative. The aim is to regain the movement of the glenohumeral joint and subsequently strengthen the rotator cuff muscles. Early mobilization prevents bursal adhesions and stiffness, but premature strenuous activity can result in increased pain. It is important also to include a strengthening programme of the scapular muscles. A common error is to judge the result too early; one should wait at least 6 months before considering the procedure to have failed.

The same operation can be done arthroscopically, and this makes rehabilitation easier.[18] The results of open or arthroscopic subacromial decompression are good, with total resolution of symptoms in approximately 70% and no improvement in 10%.

Many causes of failure have been proposed after both open and closed procedures. Often an incorrect diagnosis rather than a failure to relieve impingement is responsible. The most common cause of failure to relieve subacromial compression is incomplete division of the coracoacromial ligament. Fibres may be left attached, particularly to the anterior capsule of the acromioclavicular joint. Inadequate resection of bone, usually at the anterior margin and lateral acromion, may also explain continuing impingement.

REFERENCES

16. Kessel L, Watson M. J Bone Joint Surg 1977; 59B: 166–172
17. Petersson CJ, Gentz CF. In: Surgery of the Shoulder. BC Decker, Burlington, 1984: 129–133
18. Ellman H, Kay SP. J Bone Joint Surg 1991; 73B: 395–398

Disappointing results of acromioplasty may also be obtained when there is untreated bicipital tendinitis or rotator cuff tears. Calcification within the tendon may not only cause distortion of the tendon but may also cause pain from local inflammation. Irritability from the acromioclavicular joint, which is distinct from the compressive effect, may also cause persistent symptoms.

Probably the most common cause of pseudoimpingement is instability. This is seen in athletes in whom overuse leads to microtrauma, causing instability, subluxation, impingement and possibly even a rotator cuff tear. This is often compounded by constitutional hyperelasticity. These patients can be made worse by an arthroscopic subacromial decompression and should have their joint instability treated. Pseudoimpingement may also occur with other types of internal derangement within the glenohumeral joint, such as synovitis, and from irritability caused by labral tears.

The most common source of referred pain in the shoulder is the cervical spine in, for example, an intervertebral disc prolapse, but occasionally pain may be referred from the pleura (Pancoast's syndrome), thoracic outlet syndrome, and rarer abdominal causes mediated through the phrenic nerve.

ROTATOR CUFF TEARS

Many of the patients presenting with impingement have either partial or full thickness rotator cuff tears. This condition embraces a progression of changes from bursitis to tearing by persistent attrition. In 1927, Codman noted thin strips of supraspinatus separated from the tendon and suggested that they 'seemed to be worn as if from friction'.[19]

The bursal side partial thickness injury can be easily explained, but many of the changes involve intrinsic rotator cuff damage, and rotator cuff tension failure without evidence of impingement. It is generally believed that partial thickness tears can progress to full thickness damage by further attrition, tendon injury and failure. Once the tendon is detached, retraction and atrophy of the muscle develops. The vast majority of tears are confined to the supraspinatus, but may also involve the neighbouring biceps, subscapularis, infraspinatus, and occasionally even the teres minor tendons. It is important to appreciate that there is a small but significant incidence of both partial and full thickness tears in the symptomless population above the age of 60 years.

The tear can be classified according to its location, according to its depth for partial thickness tears, and according to the size of the defect for full thickness tears. These classifications are of value because they determine treatment as well as the anticipated results from attempts at repair.

The clinical presentation reflects the loss of tendon function, with weakness, a drop arm sign, and even inability to lift the arm. As with impingement, there is often relentless night pain. Many patients respond to the non-operative treatment described for impingement. Partial thickness tears can be treated by decompression and debridement alone. The results of this approach are unpredictable, and many deep partial thickness and full thickness tears require formal repair. This is achieved by mobilization of the retracted tendon to its insertion, division of capsular contractures, and direct repair. This is difficult and painstaking surgery, and large tears may require the tendon insertion to be moved medially by creating a trough into the articular cartilage of the superolateral humeral head. Local and even distant muscle transfers such as latissimus dorsi can be deployed. Tendon reattachment is complicated by disuse osteoporosis, which makes the greater tuberosity a weak point of fixation for transosseous suture techniques. Very few tears are small enough to be amenable to arthroscopic repair.

The results of repair worsen with the size of the tear, and in the very large tears repair may not be possible. Secure fixation without a gap must be achieved if rehabilitation is to be successful. In these cases decompression alone may help to reduce the pain. In these large defects the humeral head migrates superiorly and forms a pseudoarticulation with the acromion, which leads to loss of concentricity and eventual arthropathy of the glenohumeral joint.

GLENOHUMERAL JOINT

ARTHRITIS

The major causes of degenerative changes affecting the glenohumeral joint are similar to those affecting other major joints and include primary osteoarthritis, rheumatoid arthritis, post-traumatic arthritis and avascular necrosis. The non-operative treatment is also similar, with many patients tolerating more severe joint destruction than would be tolerable in the hip. The surgical treatment is joint replacement, because arthroscopic lavage has yet to be evaluated in advanced joint destruction.

The shoulder was the first joint to be replaced with a metallic prosthesis. The operation took place in March 1892 at the Hôpital St Louis in Paris by Dr Jules Péan on a young man with a massive tuberculous abscess of the humerus. The prosthesis was made of a platinum tube and a rubber ball hardened by boiling in paraffin. The muscles were reattached to holes in the tube by horse hair. The prosthesis is reported to have functioned well for 2 years but was finally removed because of a persistent draining sinus.[20]

Modern shoulder replacement has its origins in the 1950s as treatment for fractures of the neck of the humerus with dislocation of the head fragment, an injury normally treated by simple excision at that time. Charles S. Neer from New York and surgeons from France developed prosthetic hemiarthroplasties based on the favourable results obtained by replacement arthroplasty in cases of subcapital fracture of the femur. Twenty years elapsed before a series of 48 replacement arthroplasties for glenohumeral arthritis was reported in 1974.[21] This publication and the subsequent work by Dr Neer created the foundations of our current knowledge of the indications, surgical technique, rehabilitation and results of shoulder replacement.

The articular surfaces are replaced with a stemmed humeral component and high-density polyethylene glenoid (Fig. 46.8). The implants are designed to mimic the complex anatomy of the proximal humerus, in which the correct placement of the centre of rotation and tensioning of the rotator cuff muscles is crucial. This can be achieved with a modular component. Variations in the head size and the angle of inclination between the head and shaft, as the head lies eccentrically in relation to the humeral shaft with a variable degree of posterior offset, must be accommodated. At operation the shoulder is approached through the deltopectoral groove with division and reflection of the subscapu-

REFERENCES

19. Codman EA. Boston Med J 1927; 196: 381
20. Bankes M, Emery RJH. J Shoulder Elbow Surg 1995; 4: 259–262
21. Neer CS. J Bone Joint Surg 1974; 56A: 1–13

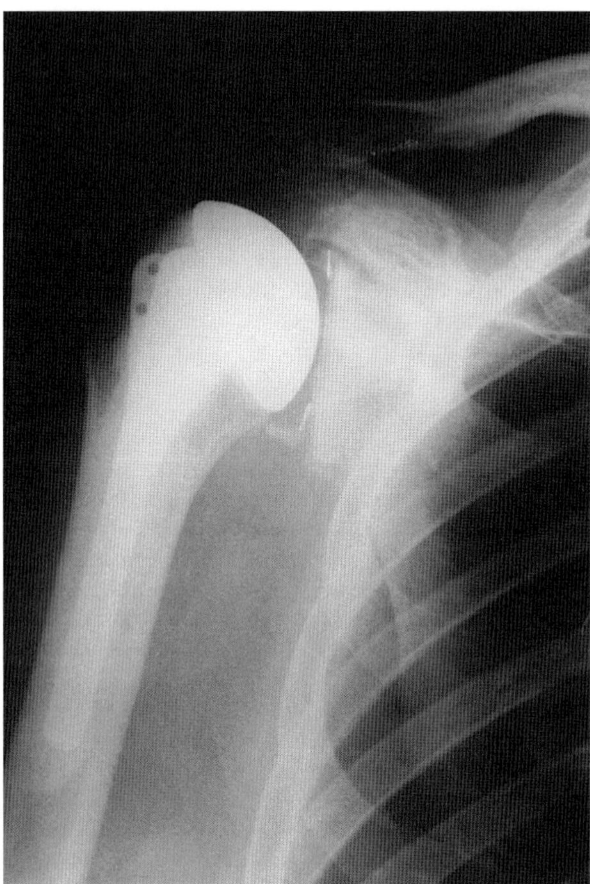

Figure 46.8 Radiograph showing a total shoulder arthroplasty.

laris tendon. The humeral component is usually implanted with cement to prevent loosening and subsidence, particularly in rheumatoid patients. The implantation of the glenoid component is technically difficult, with a significant peri- and postoperative complication rate. The long-term revision rate for loosening can be as high as 5%. The addition of a glenoid component corrects the posterior wear seen in many patterns of arthritis and may be more successful in the relief of pain than a hemiarthroplasty.

The current challenge concerns the design and fixation of the glenoid component. The shoulder is often incorrectly described as a non-weight-bearing joint, but loads of more than body weight are transmitted through the glenoid on lifting the arm. These extreme forces are usually centred on the face of the glenoid but, in the absence of a functional rotator cuff, shear forces in a superior direction can cause progressive glenoid loosening. This potential biomechanical problem is compounded by the small amount of cancellous bone available for fixation. In rheumatoid arthritis, large synovial cysts and medial erosion may result in a glenoid neck less than 1 cm in length. In Larsen stage IV and V rheumatoid arthritis, subchondral plate erosion, low-density trabecular bone, and destroyed internal architecture are encountered. In these cases glenoid replacement may not be possible, but a hemiarthroplasty can provide good results.

Patients can now expect reliable and good relief of pain with restoration of function by either hemiarthroplasty or total shoulder replacement. The modern prostheses are durable and can be offered with confidence, so they should not just be considered for end-stage destructive disease. Earlier referral when there is preservation of bone stock and rotator cuff function makes normal shoulder function a realistic goal rather than a rare achievement.

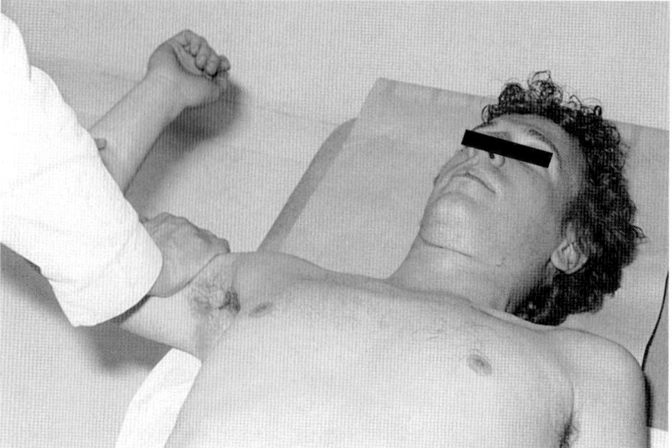

Figure 46.9 Apprehension test for anterior instability. Relocation by applying pressure posteriorly reduces discomfort (Jobe's relocation test).

INSTABILITY

The small surface area of the glenoid, and the incongruency between the radii of curvature of the glenoid and of the humeral head give minimal constraint or intrinsic stability. In the normal joint, glenohumeral movement – which is a combination of rotation, translation and rolling – is accompanied by precise alignment of the humeral head on the face of the glenoid. This is achieved by the parascapular muscles and the compressive action of the rotator cuff; any failure of this mechanism may result in shoulder instability. The majority of dislocations or subluxations are, however, traumatic and occur in an anteroinferior direction. In these circumstances the labrum becomes detached at the insertion of the inferior glenohumeral ligament. This is known as a Bankart lesion, after a surgeon from the Middlesex Hospital. Prior to failure, the inferior glenohumeral ligament stretches, leading to the attenuation and capsular redundancy found at surgery. The other pathological hallmark of shoulder instability is an impression fracture on the posterosuperior aspect of the humeral head, known as a Hill–Sachs defect. These findings are reversed in the rarer posterior subluxations and dislocations.

The diagnosis of shoulder instability is made from the history, supported by physical signs and plain radiology. The physical signs are predominantly the demonstration of apprehension in potentially unstable positions (Fig. 46.9). An appreciation of the degree of generalized joint laxity, and of signs of translation in both the affected and the symptomless shoulder, is important in understanding the underlying pathology and in assessing the need for surgical treatment. Occasionally more complex cases are encountered, in which there may be doubt about the direction of the instability or its cause. In these patients, more sophisticated methods of imaging or diagnostic arthroscopy may be required. Computerized tomography arthrography can identify labral tears and Bankart lesions with 10% error. The disadvantages are that this technique is invasive and attenuation of the inferior glenohumeral ligament cannot be evaluated. Magnetic resonance scanning is a controversial technique for assessing shoulder instability. There are many anatomical variants of the labrum, and changes are frequently found in symptomless volunteers. A number of studies have suggested that MRI alone is insensitive and non-specific, with substantial intra- and interobserver errors. The addition of contrast or gadolinium enhancement has, however, significantly increased its accuracy.

Arthroscopy allows direct visualization of the stabilizing structures of the glenohumeral joint at rest and in motion. Labral lesions and discrete chondral defects can be assessed, and even a subjective quantification of the inferior glenohumeral ligament tension can be made. Arthroscopy is, however, an invasive and expensive procedure with limited indications, which include complex and suspected subtle instability. Arthroscopy is also indicated in shoulder pain in a competitive athlete, particularly when there is an atypical history and examination with inconclusive imaging studies. Evidence of a subtle shoulder instability is often demonstrated.

Arthroscopy has identified many different types of labral tear. The majority are anteroinferior associated with instability; however, a few may be superior with damage to the biceps insertion (superior labral anterior posterior or SLAP lesions). These tears may cause symptoms even in a stable shoulder, and are probably traction injuries that are the result of large forces generated during the deceleration phase of throwing. They have been categorized by Synder and Karzel.[22] These tears are rarely diagnosed preoperatively with conventional imaging. Current treatment is repair or excision of the tear depending on its degree of severity, and the results of surgery are variable.

Symptomatic patients with anteroinferior labral tears or Bankart lesions require surgery if they fail to respond to a programme of shoulder muscle-strengthening exercises. Many surgical procedures have been devised and rely for their success on a variety of mechanisms. Reattachment of labrum with or without inferior glenohumeral ligament insertion (the Bankart operation) and with shortening of the capsule is widely practised, with good results.[23] This procedure is performed through the standard anterior deltopectoral approach. Postoperatively, it is followed by a period of immobilization for at least 4 weeks and careful rehabilitation. Contact sport should be avoided for at least 6 months.

The same Bankart procedure can be performed arthroscopically. Original procedures used metallic devices such as screws or staples, but at present suture techniques and biodegradable devices are widely used. The results are difficult to interpret, because most studies report small series with short follow-up and with very different pathologies. Studies show that failure is undoubtedly more common with arthroscopic repair than with conventional open surgery. A number of contraindications have been identified, and it is clear that not all patients are suitable. The techniques do allow satisfactory reattachment of the labrum, but there is concern about their ability to treat attenuation of the inferior glenohumeral ligament and capsular redundancy.

The arthroscope will undoubtedly play a major role in future shoulder surgery. At present, it is the technique of choice for synovial biopsy, removal of loose bodies, irrigation for septic arthritis, release of acute calcific deposits, and synovectomy. In skilled hands it has been used for posterior capsulorrhaphy, treatment of multidirectional instability, and even arthrodesis.

THE ELBOW

The elbow allows positioning of the hand close to the body, as well as extending the reach of the hand. This flexibility is frequently lost following fractures and dislocations, and with other disorders involving the elbow. Before conditions affecting the elbow joint are discussed, there are some important and relatively common conditions that affect the forearm muscles and the olecranon bursa.

EXTRA-ARTICULAR CONDITIONS

Tennis elbow or lateral epicondylitis involves the origins of the extensor carpi radialis brevis, the anterior edges of the extensor communis, the extensor carpi longus and the extensor carpi ulnaris in descending frequency. Medial epicondylitis, often inappropriately termed ‘golfer’s elbow’, involves the flexor pronator origin. Although frequently associated with racket sports, it also occurs in other sports and occupational activities in which the forearm muscles are overused. The majority of patients are between 35 and 50 years of age, with an equal sex ratio in the sports-related cases. Many cases are associated with or confused with ulnar nerve neurapraxia, carpal tunnel syndrome, radial nerve entrapment or proximal nerve root entrapment.

The pathology of epicondylitis is poorly understood, but characteristic features are usually present. Angiofibroblastic hyperplasia with an absence of inflammatory cells has been described in the affected tendons.[24] Non-operative treatment encompasses rest, modification of activity, pain relief, high-voltage electrical stimulation, and a limited number of steroid injections. The surgical treatment is controversial, with many different procedures of varying magnitude having been described. The majority involve creating an additional injury to the extensor carpi radialis brevis origin, as in simple lateral release, and waiting for healing to occur. The results are good; misdiagnosis accounts for many of the failures.

There are a number of bursae located around the elbow that, with the exception of the olecranon bursa, rarely cause disability. The olecranon bursa may become inflamed or even infected. This is usually as a result of trauma and overuse but may be a complication of inflammatory arthritis. Excision of the bursa is rarely required.

INTRA-ARTICULAR CONDITIONS

Minor repetitive injuries or overuse, particularly in patients with above-average generalized joint laxity, may result in instability of the posterolateral type. This is rare and is normally only encountered in high-grade throwing athletes. Stiffness is more common because of the development of soft tissue contractures. These may be post-traumatic or accompany arthritis, particularly of the rheumatoid type. Prevention is far easier than treatment, with physiotherapy, manipulation and splintage giving limited benefits. Surgical release with removal of osteophytes and heterotopic bone can be achieved by various approaches. The application of a hinged external fixator allows radical release, not only of the capsule but also of the shortened collateral ligaments, without creating joint instability. These devices allow distraction of the joint surfaces in cases where the articular cartilage is damaged.

Degenerative arthritis of the elbow is relatively rare and is usually seen following injury, although it can affect heavy manual labourers, such as steel workers and miners. Erosive arthritis

REFERENCES

22. Synder S, Karzel RO. Arthroscopy 1990; 14: 274–279
23. Bankart ASB. Br J Surg 1938; 26: 23–29
24. Nirschi RP, Pettrone F. J Bone Joint Surg 1979; 61A: 832

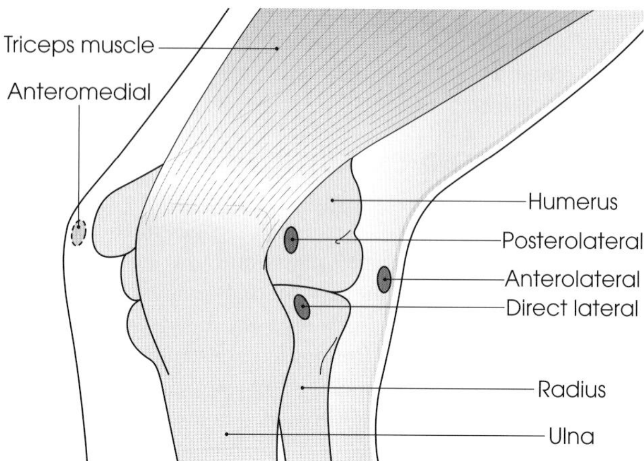

Figure 46.10 Portals for elbow arthroscopy.

is characteristic of rheumatoid arthritis but is also found in seronegative polyarthropathy. The loss of joint movement is accompanied by pain and sometimes instability in advanced cases of rheumatoid arthritis. The diagnosis is made from plain radiographs and the changes can be visualized at arthroscopy.

Elbow arthroscopy permits removal of loose bodies, synovial biopsy, and assessment and treatment of osteochondritis dissecans and of synovial chondromatosis. Debridement of the osteoarthritic elbow and arthroscopic synovectomy in rheumatoid arthritis are technically demanding new techniques. The latter may have significant advantages in the rheumatoid patient, because many areas of synovium are inaccessible at open surgery. Contraindications to arthroscopy include bony or fibrous ankylosis, severe elbow stiffness, mobile subluxation, or previous anterior transposition of the ulnar nerve.

The procedure is usually performed under general anaesthesia in the lateral position, with the arm exsanguinated and a tourniquet inflated to 250 mmHg. The placement of ports requires a clear understanding of the neurovascular anatomy, because the most frequent complication is damage to the surrounding nerves. The direct lateral, posterolateral, anterolateral and anteromedial ports should be marked (Fig. 46.10) and the joint distended before introducing the arthroscope. Other complications include persistent synovial leakage, iatrogenic damage to the articular surfaces, instrument breakage and infection. Neurovascular observations should be continued for 24 h postoperatively, during which time the arm is elevated. The dressings are then reduced and movement allowed as tolerated.

Two other surgical procedures are of value in moderately diseased joints. In the rheumatoid patient, the symptoms may arise from disease in the radiohumeral joint and be efficiently alleviated by excision of the radial head. In osteoarthritis, an adequate debridement of the posterior compartment can be made through a small arthrotomy in the triceps. By making a window in the olecranon fossa, access to the anterior part of the joint is possible. This useful technique is termed the Outerbridge–Kashiwagi procedure.[25]

For severely destroyed joints there is little alternative to elbow replacement. Modern designs have proved successful, with good restoration of movement and low revision rates for rheumatoid patients. The original hinge joints have been superseded by unlinked, non-constrained, resurfacing prostheses or linked sloppy hinges; both types incorporate flanges on the humeral condyles to distribute the torsional loads (Fig. 46.11). The results in cases of osteoarthritis or post-traumatic arthritis are less favourable, with a higher complication and revision rate for aseptic loosening.

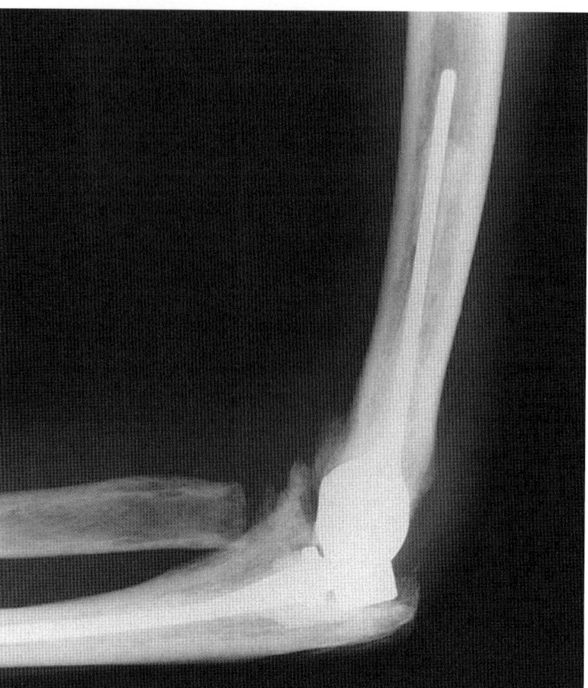

Figure 46.11 A GSB III elbow replacement.

STIFFNESS OF THE UPPER LIMB

The rate of recovery and final functional result after injuries and operations of the upper limb are often adversely affected by the development of stiffness. Reflex sympathetic dystrophy, Sudek's algodystrophy, and adhesive capsulitis of the shoulder are poorly defined conditions with many similar features. Loss of the range of movement with reduced passive range of movement on examination is characteristic. It is often associated with pain at extremes of the range from soft tissue stretching.

Stiffness may be the result of reversible self-limiting conditions such as adhesive capsulitis, with the potential for total functional and structural recovery. The stiffness may improve to expose significant anatomical and pathological abnormalities. Examples include rotator cuff tears and fractures involving the tuberosities or articular surfaces. Occasionally the stiffness is irreversible because of capsular (including coracohumeral ligament) contracture or postsurgical shortening of the rotator cuff muscle tendon units.

Investigation aims to identify any underlying pathology. Primary adhesive capsulitis may be associated with diabetes, and routine urine analysis is a rewarding technique for identifying new cases. Treatment of adhesive capsulitis starts by controlling pain mediated by the associated synovitis of the capsule or bursal layer covering the rotator cuff. Rest, analgesia, anti-inflammatory agents, local physiotherapy techniques, transcutaneous nerve

REFERENCES

25. Kashiwagi D. In: Kashiwagi D (ed). Elbow Joint. Elsevier, Amsterdam, 1985: 177–188

stimulation, and a course of biweekly suprascapular nerve blocks are helpful. Once the pain has been controlled, physiotherapy and a home exercise programme can be employed to increase the range of movement by the application of stretching and mobilization techniques. Manipulation under anaesthesia may be performed but requires careful timing; manipulation attempted before the synovitis has settled is likely to be unsuccessful and may even exacerbate the condition. The value of arthroscopy and hydrostatic distension is uncertain. Occasionally capsular restriction may be so severe and refractory as to merit surgery, with release of the coracohumeral ligament and rotator interval. All cases treated by surgery require early restoration of movement, initially under an interscalene block and subsequently aided by a physiotherapist.

TUMOURS AND INFECTION

Fortunately, both tumour and infection of the shoulder and arm are rarely encountered. Soft tissue and bone tumours require investigation and treatment in specialized centres. Injudicious biopsy may significantly limit the chances of preventing recurrence and eradicating the disease (see Ch. 42). The treatment of infection follows the general principles, but both diagnosis and treatment can be aided by arthroscopy in cases of infection of the subacromial space, and the glenohumeral and elbow joints. Repeated copious irrigation through the arthroscope is effective at treating joint infection and limiting damage to the articular cartilage.

The wrist and hand

47

Frank D. Burke, L. Christopher Bainbridge

THE PRINCIPLES OF THE MANAGEMENT OF HAND INJURIES

The sophisticated mechanisms in the hand are easily disturbed by injury or disease. Frequently, a return to total normality cannot be achieved, but adherence to certain principles of management can ensure a return to optimal function.

Specialized tissues require specialist management at the earliest stages after injury or at the onset of disease. Aird noted in the first edition of this book that the hand was of sufficient complexity to justify specialist centres for the management of hand conditions. Skilled immediate treatment can dramatically affect both short-term and ultimate disability.[1] The principal challenge here is organizational, but it also places a requirement on generalists or surgeons in training to refer cases of concern to specialists immediately. This is particularly important in cases of major hand injury, flexor tendon laceration, or in situations where skin has been lost. When there is late referral, local stiffness, oedema, infection and scarring may have lost ground that cannot be regained.

Even the simpler hand surgery procedures should be performed in operating theatres with satisfactory assistance and lighting, and suitably delicate instruments. Delayed primary or secondary reconstructive surgery should not be compromised by inexpert extension of the original injury.

THE TIMING OF SURGERY

There are three stages during collagen maturation when surgical intervention is appropriate:

1. *At the time of injury*, when most structures can be repaired. Massive injury or gross contamination contraindicates primary repair of all structures, but satisfactory skin cover is essential within a few days.
2. *Delayed primary repair* is particularly valuable in situations where specialist skills are not immediately available and there are injuries to tendons or nerves. At the time of injury the laceration is cleaned and explored, and damaged structures are identified. The skin is carefully sutured, and the hand splinted and elevated to minimize oedema and stiffness. The patient is then referred for specialist treatment, which is performed as an elective procedure within 2–3 weeks of injury. The immediate surgery must be meticulous, for even a superficial wound infection will compromise the success of delayed primary repair.
3. *Reconstructive surgery*. The opportunity for early intervention may have been missed because of either late diagnosis or late referral; alternatively, damage or contamination may have been so severe that late reconstruction is preferred. If delayed reconstruction is necessary, the swollen hand is splinted in a position of optimal function (see below), and then mobilized by active and passive movements in association with static and dynamic splintage. When collagen maturation is complete and the hand is again soft and supple, attention may be turned to reconstructive surgery.

THE POSITION OF OPTIMAL FUNCTION

Experience has shown that the hand posture most favourable to the avoidance of finger stiffness is metacarpophalangeal joint flexion and interphalangeal joint extension (Fig. 47.1); the thumb is held in extension abduction to avoid a first web contracture. The mechanism by which joint mobility is lost in a swollen hand is a complex process that is not fully understood. At the metacarpophalangeal joints the collateral ligaments are taut in flexion and lax in extension (Fig. 47.2). The painful swollen hand will tend to take up a position of metacarpophalangeal extension and proximal interphalangeal joint flexion. Oedema fluid around the lax metacarpophalangeal joint collateral ligaments will lay down fibrin. The foreshortened ligaments will produce a joint held in extension with flexion obstructed. Fibrin laid down around the flexed proximal interphalangeal joint

REFERENCES

1. Smith P. In: Smith P (ed). Lister's The Hand: Diagnosis and Indications. Churchill Livingstone, Edinburgh, 2002: 1

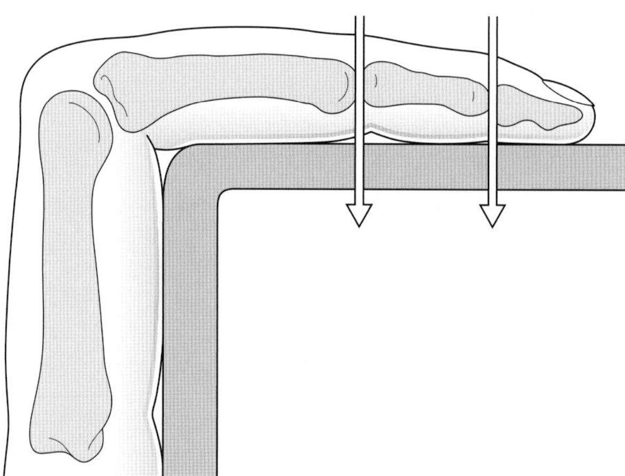

Figure 47.1 The position of function.

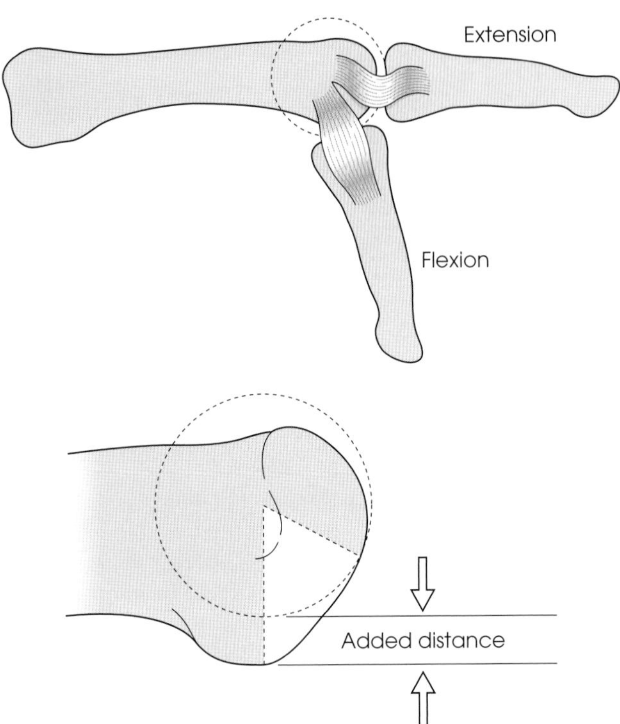

Figure 47.2 The collateral ligaments of the metacarpophalangeal joint.

causes adhesions around the proximal portion of the volar plate, which normally concertinas during joint flexion.

The most satisfactory way to hold the swollen hand in metacarpophalangeal joint flexion and interphalangeal joint extension is with the use of a volar slab.[2] The plaster is ridged as it sets, holding metacarpophalangeal joints flexed and interphalangeal joints and wrist extended. When the plaster is firm, the joint position is maintained using an elasticated bandage (Fig. 47.3). The dressings tend to loosen, with loss of position, and should be checked once a week.

A crushed hand presenting as an emergency without fracture or injury to skin may at first sight appear not to be a significant problem. The patient has, however, a potentially catastrophic condition that if poorly treated may progress to permanent stiffness with a reduced grip. Such patients urgently require splintage in the position of optimal function with elevation of the upper limb. Immediate or early intensive physiotherapy will be required to regain motion.

SKIN LOSS AND FINGERTIP INJURIES

Fingertip injuries are common and are usually a combination of crush, avulsion and amputation. The complications seen include prolonged wound healing, poor cushioning of the bone distally, painful neuromas and insensate fingertips.

Superficial pulp loss without bone exposure should be allowed to granulate and heal by secondary intention. This has the advantage that the final scar will often lie under the nail, and quality pulp skin will be drawn up to cover the fingertip. Children are a special case: the amputated part should either be replaced (within 3–4 h) as a free graft or the wound should simply be dressed with a non-adherent dressing.

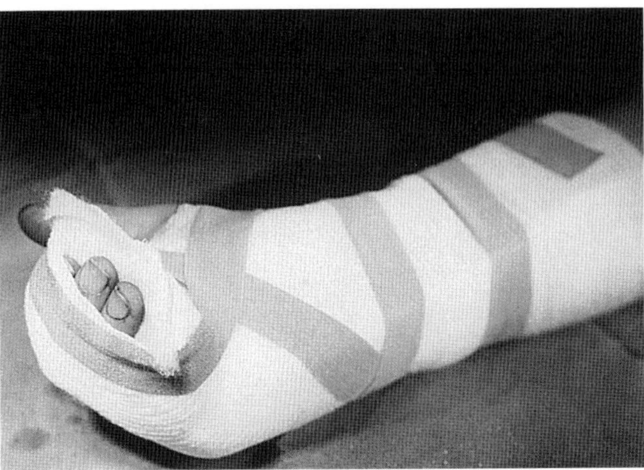

Figure 47.3 The volar slab.

Optimal management is conservative for those cases without exposed bone, or aggressive with flaps for those patients with substantial tissue loss or loss of nail, bone and pulp. Flaps can be taken from either the same finger more proximally (homodigital flaps), another finger (cross-finger) or the toes (toe pulp transfer).

DORSAL OBLIQUE LOSS

Dorsal oblique loss is the most favourable variety of tissue loss. The important volar tissues are intact but there is damage to the nail bed. Trimming of the distal phalanx permits primary closure. If the residual nail is less than half the normal length, nail bed ablation may be preferred.

TRANSVERSE LOSS

Equal amounts of dorsal and volar tissue are lost. Closure is best achieved with a flap, probably with the homodigital flap[3] or one of the variants (for example the Atasoy flap). These flaps seem simple but require a detailed understanding of the anatomy of the finger to make them safe and reliable, and should be undertaken by experienced surgeons in properly equipped theatres.

VOLAR OBLIQUE LOSS

The nail bed is intact but there is extensive loss of the pulp, with exposed distal phalanx and possibly exposed tendon and even joint. A cross-finger flap from an adjacent finger is a safe choice for these injuries, possibly with coaptation of the digital nerve to a dorsal branch supplying the flap. The flap is divided, under anaesthetic, 10–14 days later.

PROXIMAL INJURIES

More proximal injuries can usually be covered quite simply, depending on the tissue lost. On the dorsum, most wounds can be covered with split skin grafts so long as the epitenon is intact. If the tendon is exposed or missing then a flap will be required. Similarly, on the volar aspect the majority of wounds will need a full thickness graft, but if the tendon sheath is breached then a flap will be required.

REFERENCES

2. Varian JPW. Hand 1975; 7: 78
3. Foucher G et al. J Hand Surg (Br) 1989; 14: 204–208

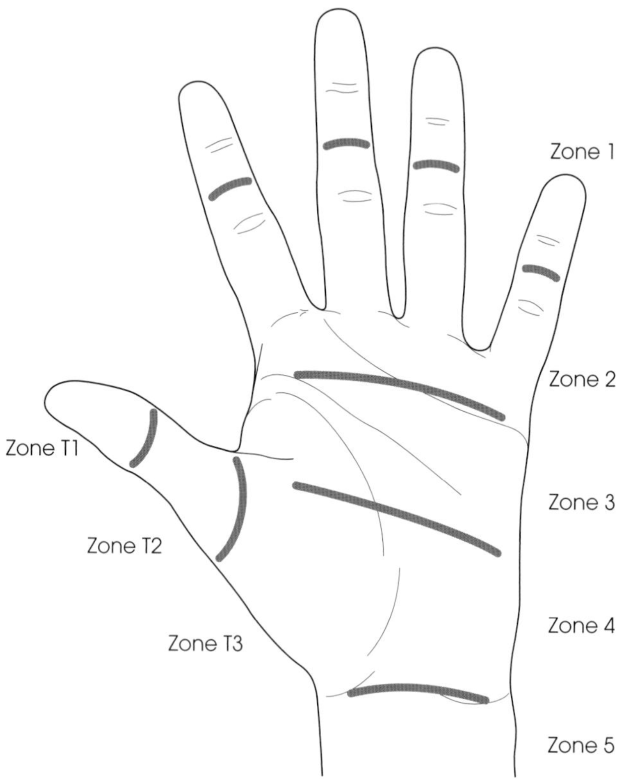

Figure 47.4 Flexor tendon zones.

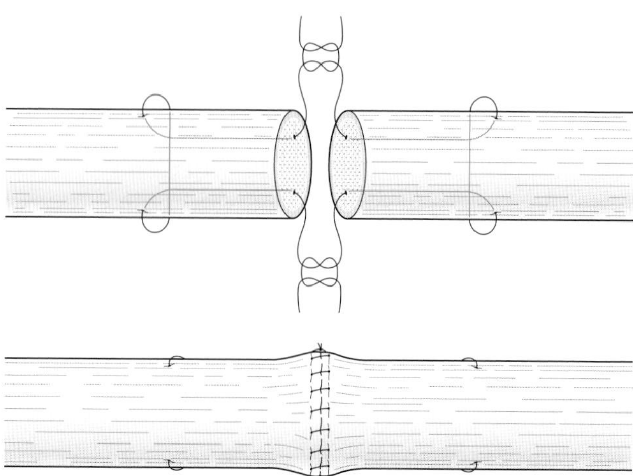

Figure 47.5 The modified Kessler suture.

FLEXOR TENDON INJURIES

Flexor tendon division is usually revealed by an alteration in the normal cascade posture of the fingers, with increasing flexion towards the ulnar border of the hand as it lies in a relaxed posture. The involved finger will be unduly extended. Profundus tendon function can be confirmed by active flexion of the distal interphalangeal joints. The superficialis tendons have individual muscles, unlike the profundus, which has a composite muscle to middle, ring and little finger. The profundus tendon to each of these digits can be immobilized if the other two rays are held in full extension. If the patient can flex the proximal interphalangeal joint of the ring finger with middle and little fingers held fully extended, then a competent superficialis tendon is present. Each finger is tested in this way, seeking proximal interphalangeal joint flexion of one finger with the remainder held in full extension.

The challenge to flexor tendon surgery lies in the digital flexor sheath (zones 1 and 2, Fig. 47.4), where the tendon ends must be opposed but not bunched, and satisfactory healing obtained without significant adhesions to the surrounding sheath or adjacent tendon. The results of repair in zone 2 are at best moderate.

SURGICAL TECHNIQUE

A modified Kessler technique (Fig. 47.5) using a 4/0 nonabsorbable suture grasps the tendon adequately with minimal impairment of its vascularity. The repair is further strengthened with a continuous 6/0 nylon suture, which adds both strength and smoothness to the repair. Where possible, repair of the sheath is advocated. Subsequent management can then follow three broad paths:

1. *Controlled active motion.* This technique[4] relies on controlled active motion of the repair to allow movement without rupture. This technique requires a motivated patient and highly skilled physiotherapists. However, the results with this technique can be superb and reward the amount of work involved.
2. *Early passive mobilization* using the Kleinert regimen. This technique[5] relies on reflex relaxation of the long flexors when the finger is actively extended against elastic band traction. The extensors are then relaxed and the finger passively flexes. This permits some excursion of the repaired tendon but applies minimal load to the repair. However, there is a significant risk of permanent proximal interphalangeal joint contracture.
3. *Immobilization of the wrist and hand.* The wrist and metacarpophalangeal joints are held in some flexion to take load off the repair for 4 weeks. Physiotherapy is then started to break down the adhesions without disrupting the repair. This is mainly used for children or those who are unable to cooperate with the other techniques.

EXTENSOR TENDON INJURIES

The results of extensor tendon repairs in the forearm are generally satisfactory. If division occurs under the extensor retinaculum, the repair should be coupled with a release of the sheath. Repairs to the dorsum of the hand and fingers are also usually satisfactory, but two areas require special mention: the proximal interphalangeal and the distal interphalangeal joint.

The level of the proximal interphalangeal joint

Lacerations in this area may divide the central slip and damage the delicate lateral fibres that maintain the lateral bands on the dorsal aspect of the joint. At the initial assessment, the patient will be able actively to extend the proximal interphalangeal joint, but the lateral bands will migrate in a volar direction over the next 2–3 weeks until they are beyond the centre of rotation of the

REFERENCES

4. Duran RJ, Houser RG. In: AAOS Symposium on Tendon Surgery in the Hand. CV Mosby, St Louis, 1975
5. Kleinert HE, Scheppel D, Gill A. Surg Clin North Am 1981; 61: 267

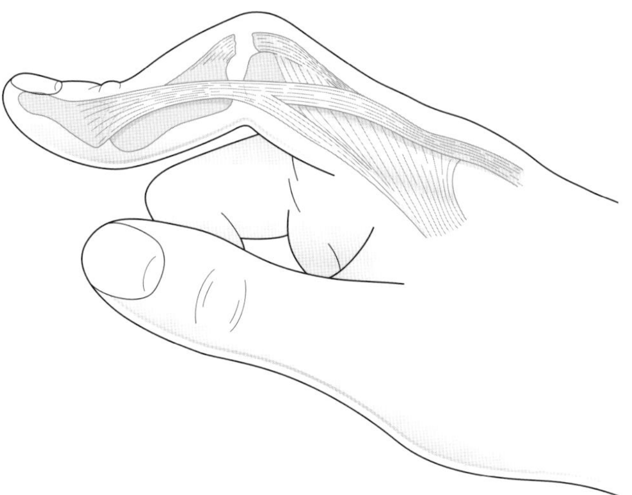

Figure 47.6 The boutonnière deformity: proximal interphalangeal joint flexion with distal interphalangeal joint hyperextension.

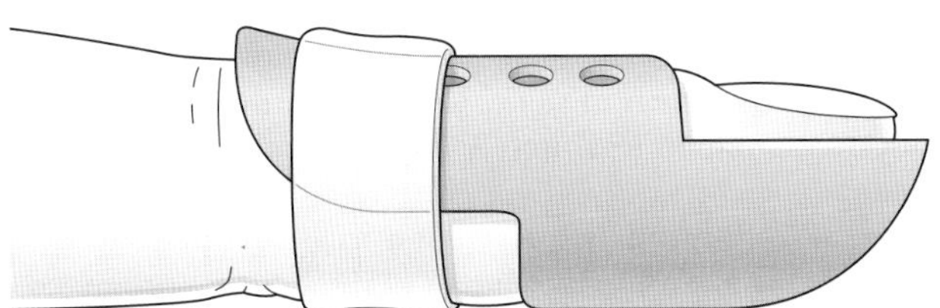

Figure 47.7 The Stack splint.

joint, thus producing the characteristic boutonnière deformity of proximal interphalangeal joint flexion and distal interphalangeal joint hyperextension (Fig. 47.6). Once established, the deformity is difficult to rectify. Because of the difficulty in confirming a central slip injury by clinical examination alone, a full exploration of a wound should be carried out if central slip damage is considered possible.

The level of the distal interphalangeal joint: mallet finger

Injury to the extensor tendon at its insertion produces an extensor lag (a mallet finger deformity). A Stack-type splint (Fig. 47.7) applied and maintained for 6 weeks will usually produce a satisfactory result, although there may be a mild residual extensor lag. Frequently, a fragment of the bone remains attached to the tendon. If it is very large and joint subluxation is present, open reduction and internal fixation of the fragment may be appropriate. Conservative management with a Stack splint remains, however, the preferred treatment in most cases.

NERVE INJURY

Recovery of sensory and motor function after nerve division and repair (see Ch. 43) is inevitably incomplete. The patient should be advised that recovery to total normality should not be anticipated. Even at best, the nerve distal to the repair has a reduced number of axons, which remain less well myelinated and have a prolonged conduction time. The single most important factor affecting the quality of the result, beyond the accuracy of the approximation of the nerve ends, is the patient's age. Under the age of 12 years, adequate results are usually obtained

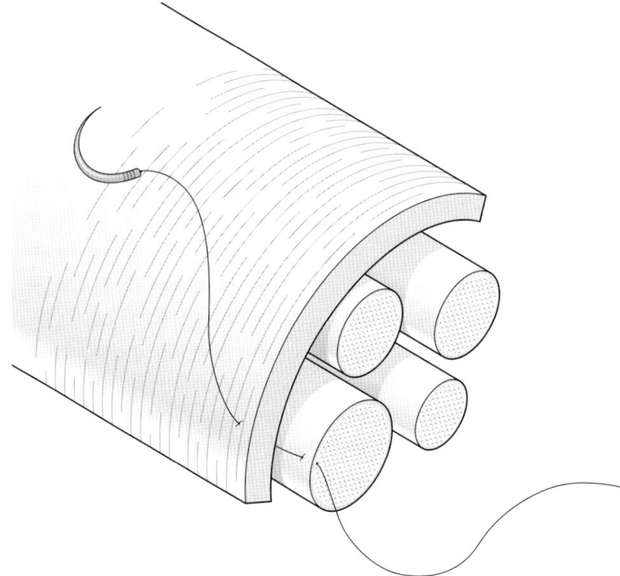

Figure 47.8 The epiperineurial suture.

if careful nerve repair is performed soon after injury.[6] However, as age increases nerve recovery diminishes and perhaps central adaptations are also less readily made.

DIAGNOSIS

Nerve injury is frequently overlooked in accident and emergency departments. Ask the patient to compare the sensations produced when the affected part and the contralateral digit are gently stroked. Sweating in the territory of the nerve is lost immediately. This affects the dermal adherence, which can be demonstrated by the plastic pen test. Reduced adherence of the skin to the pen when it is drawn across the digit is an early reliable indication of nerve division. There is also loss of or impaired two-point discrimination as compared with the normal side.

MANAGEMENT

Primary repair is the treatment of choice[7] unless there are inadequate facilities, or there has been major tissue loss or gross contamination. Delayed repair frequently requires a nerve graft to bridge the gap. Magnification is beneficial during repair, and sutures should be of nylon and not of a thicker gauge than 8/0. Epiperineurial sutures (Fig. 47.8) probably offer the best compromise in that they are easy to perform yet accurate in alignment of fascicles.[8] The repair is rested with adjacent joints held in a position that minimizes tension for 4 weeks. The limb may then be mobilized. Progress is assessed by the Tinel's sign (distal to proximal percussion over the course of the nerve until tingling is experienced by the patient in the line of the nerve). Nerve regeneration proceeds at a speed of approximately 1 mm/day.

REFERENCES

6. Breidenbach WC, Gill RS. In: Gupta A, Kay SPJ, Scheker LR (eds). Peripheral Nerve Injuries in Children in the Growing Hand. Mosby, St Louis, 2000: 643
7. Merle M, Foucher G et al. Bull Hosp Joint Dis Orthop Inst 1984; 44: 338
8. Williams HB, Jabalay ME. Hand Clin 1986; 2: 689

FRACTURES

In many parts of the body, non-union of a fracture is the most feared complication. This is rarely a difficulty in the hand, where the greatest risk is stiffness arising from joint contracture or tendon adhesions. Rotational deformity is an uncommon but significant complication causing increasing malalignment of a finger as it flexes. Rotational deformity is best assessed by comparison of the alignment of the fingernails when viewed end on.

Most hand fractures are managed by immobilization in the optimal position for function on a volar slab for 3–4 weeks until the fracture is stable. The hand is then mobilized to overcome residual stiffness. Some fractures (distal tuft or those that are judged to be stable) may be mobilized from the time of injury. Assessment of a stable fracture is not always easy; they are usually associated with a crack in the bone without displacement. If a programme of immediate mobilization is followed, it is prudent to have a check X-ray after a week to confirm that the position is maintained.

A minority of fractures require internal fixation. Such fractures are either intra-articular with joint incongruity or subluxation, or shaft fractures that cannot be maintained in a satisfactory position on a volar slab. The decision to fix a fracture internally should never be taken lightly; it turns a closed fracture to an open one, and the necessary dissection inevitably further devascularizes the fragments. These disadvantages are acceptable only if, following fixation, the fracture is satisfactorily reduced and sufficiently stable to permit early mobilization. The most rigid form of fixation is by the use of mini fragment screws or plates.[9] Interosseous wiring is used for transverse phalangeal fractures. Kirschner wires alone may be used for internal fixation of fractures, but it should be appreciated that the bone interface is not as well stabilized, nor is there intrafragmentary compression.

REPLANTATION AND REVASCULARIZATION

Replantation problems arise abruptly and demand contingency planning and an understanding of the indications for replantation, because swift referral improves the chances of success. The local replantation centre should be contacted immediately, because they will need time to marshal staff and open a theatre. The amputated part should be wrapped in a damp saline-soaked swab and placed in a clean, dry plastic bag. This bag should be sealed and placed in a container with ice and water.

WHAT ARE THE INDICATIONS FOR REPLANTATION?[10]

Upper arm

There is only one bone, the humerus, to stabilize and it tolerates shortening well. Vessel diameter is large and there are few muscles to repair. The ischaemic time is of critical importance, because there is a risk of Volkmann's ischaemic contracture or gas gangrene in distal musculature. Reinnervation, except in the very young, is often disappointing but body image is preserved. All distal muscle groups should have a formal fasciotomy performed.

Forearm

Amputations distal to the motor endplates of the forearm muscles greatly increase the potential for a good result. The more distal the repair in the forearm, the easier tendon repair becomes. At wrist level mobility may be impaired, but the area remains favourable for replantation.

The metacarpal area

The thumb plays such a key role in hand function that amputation of it at any level should give rise to thoughts of replantation. The same is also true if a composite of all the fingers is amputated, particularly if the thumb remains intact. This region is one of the most gratifying areas for replantation. While amputation of the tip of the thumb is not catastrophic, replantation should provide improved function and cosmesis. More proximal thumb amputations should always be replanted, because the loss of a thumb is important functionally. When replantation is not possible, then alternative methods have to be considered for reconstruction of the thumb.

The digits

Indications for finger replantation depend on the level of injury and the number of fingers injured. If a single digit is involved, then the decision must be made in conjunction with the patient. Many will opt for completion of the amputation at a cosmetic level and an early return to work. The average time to return to work after replantation is around 9–12 months after injury. Distal replantation is technically difficult, often requiring 11/0 sutures and high magnification. However, if successful they are very rewarding, especially if the movement of the finger is preserved.

HAND INFECTIONS

The incidence and severity of hand infections have dropped in developed countries over the past three decades. Nevertheless, inadequate treatment will either extend short-term malfunction or, on occasion, cause permanent disability. The possibility of secondary contributing factors should always be considered. A reduced host response from treatment with steroids or immunosuppressive drugs, malignancy or immune infection (HIV) may be responsible. Any condition that impairs peripheral circulation (e.g. vasculitis associated with rheumatoid arthritis or scleroderma) will reduce the host's ability to overcome infection. The most frequent contributing disease is, however, diabetes mellitus. Infections arising in diabetics are common, often involve Gram-negative organisms, and are slow to resolve. Debilitation, poverty and poor personal hygiene are all contributing factors, and the possibility of drug addiction should also be considered.

Although a course of antibiotics may be of benefit, their effect in most properly treated cases is almost incidental to the resolution of infection. Antibiotic therapy should never be used as an alternative to correct surgical management.

Pulp space infections usually arise from minor penetrating injuries. Pressure in the infected compartment rapidly rises, causing increasing pain. Early incision and drainage is required, for extensive sloughing of pulp tissue will permanently reduce the cushioning of the distal phalanx.

REFERENCES

9. Heim U, Pfeifer KM. Internal Fixation of Small Fractures. 3rd edn. Springer Verlag, Berlin, 1986
10. Tamai S. J Hand Surg 1982; 7: 549

A *paronychia* is an infection of the nail fold, which may extend proximally to involve the eponychium. The condition settles well if treated with a course of antibiotics associated with nail avulsion. A normal nail grows out in the weeks that follow, and there is no scarring to the nail fold.

Infection of the flexor tendon sheath is fortunately uncommon, because even prompt and appropriate treatment may leave the finger with residual stiffness. The cruciate portions of the flexor tendon sheaths lie close to the skin at the proximal and distal interphalangeal joints. Superficial laceration in this area may breach the sheath and introduce infection. There is slowly increasing discomfort in the finger, often several days after a trivial laceration. The finger is held in a semiflexed position, and there is tenderness over the flexor sheath. Attempted movement is extremely painful, especially passive extension of the interphalangeal joints.

The sheath is drained and irrigated with a saline solution, and the hand is rested on a splint in the position of function with intravenous antibiotics. As soon as it is apparent that the infection is controlled, physiotherapy is begun to overcome finger stiffness.

Paronychia, pulp and sheath infections are usually caused by *Staphylococcus aureus*. Infected material should be cultured and treatment started with an appropriate antibiotic, usually flucloxacillin. Treatment can subsequently be altered to a more suitable antibiotic if tests reveal a different organism or sensitivity.

Streptococcal cellulitis does not require incision and drainage because infection is not localized and there is no collection of pus. There is diffuse swelling and erythema of the skin and subcutaneous tissue, usually associated with ascending lymphangitis. Treatment consists of in-patient admission, elevation, intravenous penicillin in large doses, and rest on a volar slab. Signs of resolution are usually apparent within 24 h, and physiotherapy can usually be started after 3–4 days to overcome local stiffness.

Human bites are usually caused by a blow to an opponent's mouth in a brawl. The clenched knuckle strikes a tooth, which penetrates skin, extensor tendon and capsule. The cause of injury is rarely admitted to the casualty officer, and presentation is often delayed. The hand is usually examined in extension, and the extent of the injury may not be appreciated. A high index of suspicion is required in all cases presenting with penetrating injuries over the dorsum of the metacarpophalangeal joints. A polymicrobial inoculation usually occurs at the time of injury; this requires early joint lavage, splintage, and combination antibiotic therapy covering Gram-negative as well as Gram-positive organisms.

High-pressure injection injuries have become increasingly common in recent years as the pressures in industrial sprays and hydraulic systems have risen.[11] Oils, solvents and paints may be driven through the intact skin to disperse within the soft tissues. Management requires immediate transfer to a specialist surgeon, because early exploration may reduce ultimate inflammation and stiffness. Amputation may commonly be required even when early management has been satisfactory; delayed diagnosis or referral only increases this risk.

DUPUYTREN'S DISEASE

Dupuytren's disease remains an ill-understood condition. The tendency to contracture is probably inherited, with the majority of patients having a positive family history. Associations with epilepsy (or anticonvulsant therapy) and diabetes seem certain. Fibromatosis of the plantar fascia in the foot and Peyronie's disease (penile involvement) are, on occasion, seen in those with a strong diathesis. Such patients are likely to develop the condition in their thirties and forties, with relentless progression and recurrence after surgery. Presentation in the sixties and seventies is more common, with more gradual progression and a smaller likelihood of recurrence. The patient should be aware that recurrence rates after surgery lie between 40 and 60% (depending on age and disease activity).[12]

Thickening is usually first seen in the palmar fascia; nodules and bands develop with progressive contracture to metacarpophalangeal or proximal interphalangeal joints. The ring and little fingers are involved most frequently, but any digit may be affected.

MANAGEMENT

Resection of the band (partial fasciectomy) with Z-plasty of the overlying skin is required if the patient is unable to lay the involved hand flat on a table. Night splintage for several months postoperatively to maintain the extensor gain is probably beneficial during the phase of collagen maturation.

A prominent band in the palm may simply be divided (fasciotomy) rather than resorting to band excision. This is particularly valuable in the elderly patient whose contracture is principally at the metacarpophalangeal joint.

Skin excision may be necessary if the tissues are extensively scarred by previous surgery. A full thickness graft is required to cover the defect. Dermofasciectomy is the most extensive surgical option but has the lowest risk of recurrence.

Late presentation or repeated recurrence may require arthrodesis of the proximal interphalangeal joint in a semi-extended position, or even amputation of the ray if finger function cannot be salvaged by reconstructive surgery.

TUMOURS RELEVANT TO THE HAND

Lumps on the hand are commonly site-specific, making diagnosis straightforward in the majority of cases (Fig. 47.9). The word *tumour* in this context refers to local swellings rather than neoplasms, which are an uncommon cause of hand lumps.[13]

GANGLION

Ganglia arise most commonly on the dorsum of the hand over the scapholunate ligament. They are most evident when the wrist is held in a flexed position. The swelling transilluminates. Half of ganglia presenting for an opinion will disappear spontaneously over 6 years, and a quarter to a third will recur if excised (sometimes with tender scars or residual wrist stiffness). Aspiration of the ganglion will resolve a minority and is useful for those concerned about possible malignancy. Excision is restricted to

REFERENCES

11. Neal NC, Burke FD. Injury 1991; 22: 467
12. McGrouther DA. In: Macfarlane RM, McGrouther DA, Flint MH (eds). Recurrence and Extension in Dupuytrens Disease. Churchill Livingstone, Edinburgh, 1990: 383
13. Fleegler E. In: Bogumill GP, Fleegler E (eds). Tumours of the Hand and Upper Limb. Churchill Livingstone, Edinburgh, 1993: 64

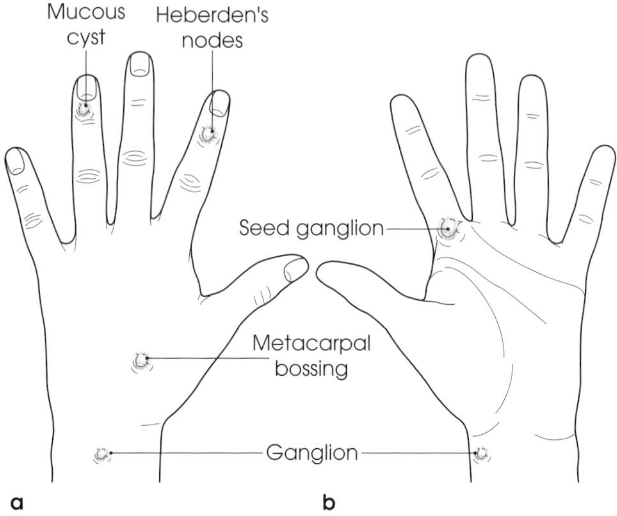

Figure 47.9 Site-specific tumours of the hand.

large or symptomatic ganglia, or where there is a persistent fear of malignancy. The ganglion sac is dissected through the dorsal capsule of the wrist, leaving a small window into the joint.

Volar ganglia also usually arise from the scapholunate ligament or from the scaphotrapezial joint. The radial artery commonly lies closely attached to the ganglion wall. Great care must always be taken during dissection to preserve the radial artery and the palmar cutaneous nerve. A pneumatic tourniquet is essential. The indications for surgery are limited (as described previously), with most patients offered reassurance.[14]

METACARPAL BOSSING

An exostosis develops at the second or third carpometacarpal joint. It lies under the extensor carpi radialis longus or brevis tendons close to their insertion, and may be associated with a small ganglion. Most patients with the condition require reassurance rather than surgery.

MUCOUS CYST

Mucous cysts usually arise from the distal interphalangeal joints (occasionally the more proximal row). The cyst is often a blow-out of an osteoarthritic joint. The cyst may indent the germinal nail matrix, producing distal nail deformity. The cyst will usually settle after excision, but a local skin flap may need to be raised to cover the defect.

SEED GANGLION OF THE FLEXOR TENDON SHEATH

These commonly arise over the A1 pulley and are usually slightly eccentrically placed. The cyst feels like a firm pea, which does not move on digital flexion. The lump is uncomfortable when hard objects are grasped. The ganglion and a segment of the pulley are excised en bloc, leaving a small window in the sheath. Recurrence is exceptional.

ENCHONDROMA

There is a slowly growing mass within a phalanx, which may present acutely with a fracture through the weakened cortex. Diagnosis is made on the characteristic appearance of the radiograph. The cavity is clear with stippled calcification. The interface between cartilage and bone is distinct, indicating its benign nature (malignant neoplasms infiltrate normal bone with a sinister diffuse interface). Curettage followed by cancellous bone graft is the best form of treatment, particularly if cortical thinning has weakened the bone.

INCLUSION DERMOID

Inclusion dermoids are most commonly seen on the volar surface of the fingers and palm. A penetrating injury drives a fragment of dermis into the deeper layers, where it continues to grow. The lump is firm and smooth, and is attached or lies close to the skin, which may be scarred. The mass is not multilobulated and expansion is slow. The entire wall must be excised if recurrence is to be avoided.

RHEUMATOID SYNOVITIS

Rheumatoid synovitis is usually obvious in an established case with other stigmata of the disease. Synovitis under the extensor retinaculum may, however, be a presenting feature and can be mistaken for a wrist ganglion. The opportunity for histological confirmation of an early rheumatoid process should not be missed.

HEBERDEN'S NODES

Heberden's nodes are nodular deformities at the distal interphalangeal joints, and are commonly seen in the index and middle fingers of elderly patients. The deformity is due to bony osteophytes and synovial thickening at the margin of an osteoarthritic joint. Satisfactory function is usually preserved, although the patients do experience some local discomfort and stiffness.

DEQUERVAIN'S SYNDROME

DeQuervain's syndrome may present with pain and thickening to the extensor retinaculum over the wrist. There is myxomatous degeneration to the walls of the first extensor compartment surrounding extensor pollicis brevis and abductor pollicis longus tendons. Abductor pollicis brevis often travels through an additional anomalous tunnel. The condition should be considered a separate entity from tenosynovitis. Symptoms may occur spontaneously or possibly follow unaccustomed use. Non-steroidal anti-inflammatory medications and wrist splintage may relieve the condition. Local steroid injections will resolve some of the more resistant cases, but the remainder may require surgical decompression of the compartment.

TRIGGERING OF FINGERS AND THUMB

Triggering of fingers and thumb may be caused by a nodule on the flexor tendon at the mouth of the A1 pulley. The nodule may be palpated in the palm and noted to excurse proximodistally in flexion and extension. A steroid infiltration to the area will usually relieve mild cases, but surgical release of the proximal portion of the A1 pulley may be required.

ARM PAIN AND THE WORKPLACE

In recent years considerable interest has arisen over the relationship of work to the development of upper limb complaints.

REFERENCES

14. Dias J, Buch K. Palmar Wrist Ganglions. J Hand Surg 2003; 28B: 172

There is no doubt that forceful, awkward activities at work can cause some upper limb complaints, for example tennis elbow. Prolonged static loading of joints or very repetitive activities without adequate rest intervals may also cause difficulties. Tool and workstation design should maintain upper limb joints in midrange during most activities. Poor ergonomics at the workplace may encourage unsatisfactory posture leading to neck discomfort, perhaps with referred pain to the upper limb.

Tenosynovitis is a much abused diagnosis in this context. The diagnosis is frequently loosely applied to arm pain in the absence of physical signs. It is inappropriate to apply the term *tenosynovitis* in the absence of confirmatory physical signs (local heat, swelling and crepitus).

The offer of an ill-informed opinion as to the causation of the patient's complaints is also unwise. Informed opinion concerning causation commonly requires detailed knowledge of the ergonomics of the workplace. It is very unhelpful to the patient to be encouraged into misplaced expectations as to the causation of symptoms and possible compensation. At any given time, 10% of the population are experiencing arm pain.[15] Most complaints are unrelated to work. Great care is always required in this area of practice. The situation requires detailed examination, adequate documentation and careful opinion.

REFERENCES

15. Hadler NM. J Hand Surg 1985; 10A: 451

The spine and spinal cord

48

Brian J. C. Freeman

CLINICAL ANATOMY

THE SPINE

The normal thoracic kyphosis is between 20 and 50° (mean 35°) and increases with age. The normal lumbar lordosis is between 40 and 80° (mean 60°). Most lumbar lordosis occurs between L4 and S1, and it decreases with age. In standing, the normal sagittal vertical axis (sagittal plumb-line) falls from the odontoid process through the C7–T1 disc space, and crosses the spinal column at the T12–L1 disc space before reaching the posterior superior corner of the S1 vertebral body. The relationship of the sagittal plumb-line to the spine is brought about by the normal cervical lordosis, thoracic kyphosis and lumbar lordosis.

The blood supply of the spinal cord is derived from the vertebral, deep cervical, intercostal and lumbar arteries. The arteries of the spinal cord include the anterior spinal artery and the two posterior spinal arteries. In the cervical spine, the anterior spinal artery arises from the vertebral artery. The vertebral artery enters the transverse foramen of C7 and travels cephalad to pass through the foramen magnum. Radicular arteries enter the vertebral canal through the intervertebral foramen and divide into anterior and posterior radicular arteries, which in turn supply the anterior and posterior spinal arteries. The most significant radicular artery to the cervical cord arises from the deep cervical artery and travels with the left C6 spinal nerve. The radicular artery of Adamkiewicz makes a major contribution to the anterior spinal artery supplying the lower spinal cord. It originates on the left in 80% of people, usually accompanying the ventral root of T9, 10 or 11, but can originate anywhere from T5 to L5. Ligation of segmental vessels over the midpoint of the vertebral body will minimize the risk of injury to this important artery.

The spinal nerve roots include eight cervical, twelve thoracic, five lumbar, five sacral and one coccygeal. Dorsal and ventral roots join to form the spinal nerve. The ventral root and the dorsal root ganglion lie within the intervertebral foramen. The neural foramen is bounded superiorly and inferiorly by pedicles, anteriorly by the disc, and posteriorly by the facet joint. Degenerative changes of these structures may lead to neural compromise. Disruption of the medial or inferior pedicle cortex with pedicle instrumentation should be avoided to minimize the risk of injury to nerve root or dura. It is useful to divide each lumbar vertebra into axial and parasagittal subdivisions to assist in the localization of spinal pathology. The first storey is at the level of the disc, the second is the infrapedicular level, and the third is the pedicular level.[1] Further parasagittal subdivision into central, lateral recess, foraminal and extraforaminal zones is also helpful when correlating radiological findings with operative findings. Laminar overlap within the lumbar spine decreases from L1 to S1. So an L5–S1 discectomy requires less bone removal than a more cephalad discectomy.

ILIAC GEST

The superior gluteal artery enters the sciatic notch above piriformis and penetrates the gluteus maximus. Injury to the superior gluteal artery and cluneal nerves can occur during bone graft harvest from the posterior iliac crest. The incision therefore should stay within 70 mm of the posterior iliac crest. An incision made parallel to the cluneal nerves and perpendicular to the posterior iliac crest decreases the morbidity. The lateral femoral cutaneous nerve may be injured when harvesting bone from the anterior iliac crest. By operating at least 2 cm posterior to the anterior superior iliac crest and harvesting from the outer cortex of the ilium the risk is reduced.

HISTORY AND PHYSICAL EXAMINATION

The history and physical examination are never more important than in the management of conditions of the spine. This is especially true in the era of MRI when this is, on occasions, used as a substitute for good clinical skills. The specific site of pain should be enquired about. If the pain is deep, unrelieved by rest and present at night the clinician must consider tumour or infection in the differential diagnosis. Visceral disease, such as pancreatitis and abdominal aortic aneurysm, may produce low back pain. Profound morning stiffness implies an inflammatory arthropathy. It is helpful to grade the pain intensity on a visual analogue scale between 1 and 10. If leg pain is present, is it truly radicular or is it referred? What is the ratio of back to leg pain? Pain aggravated by sitting is more likely to be discogenic. Back pain caused by hyperextension may be related to facet joint arthropathy or due to a defect in the pars interarticularis. Leg pain in extension is usually the result of spinal stenosis. Psychosocial factors, such as ongoing litigation and poor job satisfaction, should be considered. Spinal deformity may present with asymmetry in shoulder heights, leg length discrepancy, rib on pelvic impingement or a noticeable rib hump. Rarely patients may report truncal imbalance or, in the case of kyphosis, loss of forward gaze.

Symptoms in the arms or legs suggestive of radiculopathy should be characterized precisely. In particular, enquiry should be made regarding pain, hyperaesthesia, numbness, tingling or burning, and weakness. Claudication is quantified by walking

REFERENCES

1. McCulloch JA, Young PA. In: McCulloch JA, Young PA (eds). Essentials of Spinal Microsurgery. Lippincott-Raven, Philadelphia, 1998: 250

distance and may be either neurogenic or vascular. Patients with spinal stenosis often stoop or sit to relieve symptoms. Patients may describe numbness, tingling, or heaviness in their legs on walking. They may have no difficulty pedalling a bicycle or walking uphill, because the spine is flexed during these activities thereby increasing the anteroposterior space available for the neural structures. Radicular pain reproduced by coughing, sneezing or straining at stool suggests a lesion in the spinal canal, because these actions increase the intrathecal pressure. Patients with cervical cord pathology may complain of sudden electric shocks down the arm and legs, with flexion of the neck (L'hermitte's sign). Numbness in the radial three and half digits, particularly at night, may indicate carpal tunnel syndrome. Loss of bowel continence, urinary retention with overflow, and saddle anaesthesia suggest cauda equina syndrome. Use of a self-reported questionnaire such as the Oswestry Disability Index can be invaluable in assessing disability.[2] The history should generate a differential diagnosis to be challenged in the physical examination.

The examination should include 'red flag' tests for common important spinal disorders, and should exclude pathology of the hips, knees, sacroiliac joints and vascular system. The normal range of motion in the cervical spine is 45° flexion, 55° extension, 70° rotation and 40° lateral bend. Spurling's test for radiculopathy is the reproduction of arm pain by hyperextension and lateral rotation towards the symptomatic side. This manoeuvre decreases the size of the intervertebral foramen. The tone, power, coordination, reflexes and sensation should be checked (Table 48.1). Tinel's and Phalen's signs should be assessed to rule out compressive syndromes of the median or ulnar nerves in the carpal or cubital tunnel. Myelopathy or upper motor neuron (UMN) lesion is suggested by hyper-reflexia, a positive Hoffman's sign (if the middle finger is flicked into extension the thumb and other fingers flex briskly), up-going plantar responses and, in the case of a high cervical myelopathy, a positive scapulohumeral reflex (tapping on the spine of the scapula or tip of the acromion in the caudal direction will lead to elevation of the scapula or abduction of the humerus). Other manifestations of hyper-reflexia include ankle and patellar clonus. Typical signs of radiculopathy—lower motor neuron (LMN) lesion—include flaccid paralysis, muscle atrophy, loss of reflexes and muscle fasciculation.

Lumbar movement should be assessed. Schober's test determines the degree of actual excursion in flexion and extension and is decreased in ankylosing spondylitis. Functional testing by observation of heel walking (ankle dorsiflexion L4), toe walking (ankle plantar flexion S1), and deep knee bend (quadriceps L3 and 4) can give a quick assessment of lower limb power; however, formal testing of all five myotomes should be performed (Table 48.2). The knee, ankle and Babinski reflex should be assessed. A positive passive straight leg raise test produces radicular pain distal to the knee at less than 70° of elevation. If the contralateral straight leg raise is positive for radicular pain in the symptomatic leg, this is strongly suggestive of nerve root compression. Lasegue's sign denotes straight leg raise radiculopathy aggravated by ankle dorsiflexion, while the bowstring sign denotes straight leg raise radiculopathy aggravated by applying pressure over the popliteal fossa. The femoral stretch test is less specific than the sciatic straight leg raise. When positive it produces anterior thigh symptoms and indicates L3 or L4 nerve root pathology. The patient is examined in the prone position with the knee flexed; the hip is then passively hyperextended. The hips should be examined to assess the range of movement. The sacroiliac joints can be assessed by applying manual compression across the iliac wings and by performing the FABER (flexion, abduction, external rotation) figure-of-four test of the hip to rule out sacroiliac instability and pain.

Examination for thoracolumbar deformity involves inspection of the patient standing and in forward flexion (Adams test) to assess rib prominence. Relative shoulder heights and waist asymmetry should be noted. The skin should be examined for cutaneous neurofibromata, café au lait patches or axillary freckles commonly present in neurofibromatosis. A complete neurological assessment including abdominal reflexes should be performed. Leg lengths should be measured. In the case of kyphosis, the sagittal alignment and forward gaze should be assessed.

Table 48.1 Neurological evaluation of the upper limb

Neurological level	Motor	Sensation	Reflex
C5	Deltoid	Lateral arm	Biceps
C6	Wrist extensor Extensor carpi radialis longus	Lateral forearm	Brachioradialis
C7	Triceps	Middle finger	Triceps
C8	Long finger flexors	Medial forearm	No reflex
T1	Interossei muscles	Medial arm	No reflex

REFERENCES

2. Fairbank JCT, Pynsent PB. Spine 2000; 25: 2940–2953

Table 48.2 Neurological evaluation of the lower limb

Neurological level	Motor	Sensation	Reflex
L2	Hip flexion	Anterior thigh, groin	No reflex
L3	Knee extension	Anterior and lateral thigh	Patellar (L3, 4)
L4	Ankle dorsiflexion	Medial leg and foot	Patellar (L3, 4)
L5	Extensor hallucis longus	Lateral leg and foot	No reflex
S1	Ankle plantar flexion	Lateral foot, little toe	Achilles (S1, 2)

A psychosocial assessment is valuable when patients complain of low back pain. Waddell developed and validated a series of signs and tests that have proven helpful in identifying individuals who are magnifying or exaggerating symptoms.[3] The signs include three observations of pain behavior (pain in a non-anatomical distribution, pain out of proportion to the stimulus, and exaggerated pain behavior such as grimacing) and four tests (skin roll produces radicular symptoms, pain on simulated spinal rotation, back pain on axial compression of the head, and variable straight leg raise in supine and sitting position). Waddell's signs of incongruency do not explain why a patient is exaggerating. A patient may be seeking some secondary gain. Patients with three or more of these signs typically respond poorly to either surgery or physiotherapy unless the underlying cause of the abnormal pain behavior is corrected.

CONGENITAL DISORDERS

Congenital disorders of the spine and cord can be divided into primary neurological disorders (e.g. spina bifida, Arnold–Chiari malformation, and spinal dysraphism) and primary bony disorders (e.g. congenital scoliosis and kyphosis). Primary bony disorders are discussed in the spinal deformity section.

SPINA BIFIDA

Spina bifida is caused by a failure of fusion of the vertebral arches and possibly the underlying neural tube. Two subdivisions exist:

1. Spina bifida occulta: the vertebral anomaly exists in isolation and usually causes no specific problem.
2. Spina bifida manifesta (cystica): the incidence of one in 300 live births is now decreasing as a consequence of folic acid supplementation, antenatal ultrasound, and the measurement of alpha-fetoprotein levels. There are two types:
   a. Meningocele: the meninges herniate through the bony defect and are covered by skin.
   b. Myelomeningocele: the roof of the defect is formed by exposed neural tissue; 75% of cases develop hydrocephalus.

Spina bifida cystica is obvious at birth. A neurological examination of the structures below the defect should be carefully performed. The head should be examined for evidence of hydrocephalus, such as a bulging fontanelle or excessive head circumference.

A meningocele with good-quality skin over the defect may be treated conservatively. A meningocele with a more prominent sac can be excised at 3–6 months. The management of myelomeningocele is more controversial. The enthusiasm for closing all defects has been replaced by a more selective approach with the recognition that it was inappropriate to operate on children with severe hydrocephalus, a large open defect, and no distal neurological function. The majority of these children die in their first year from hydrocephalus or an infection if closure is not attempted. With antibiotics, early surgical closure, and shunts to prevent hydrocephalus, half the children who survive the first 24 h will reach school age. The aims of surgery are to return the nervous tissue to the spinal canal, to preserve the cerebrospinal fluid absorption capacity, and to cover the defect with fascia and skin. After operation, regular examinations are required to detect hydrocephalus. Long-term problems include skin, bone and joint deformity, and the complication of a neuropathic bladder.

ARNOLD–CHIARI MALFORMATION

Arnold–Chiari malformation occurs when the medulla and cerebellar tonsils extend through the foramen magnum into the cervical spinal canal, causing pressure on the lower medulla. Hydrocephalus and impaired neurological function are common, and there is a strong association with spina bifida and syringomyelia.

The presentation is variable because of its complex aetiology. Hydrocephalus and cerebellar ataxia are common. Neck stiffness can occur when the tonsils impact in the foramen magnum. Plain radiographs show a small posterior fossa, but the condition is best demonstrated by MRI or CT myelography. Management consists of decompressing the foramen magnum and usually the posterior arch of the atlas to restore normal cerebrospinal fluid flow (Fig. 48.1).

SPINAL DYSRAPHISM OR CORD TETHERING

This is a group of disorders arising from abnormal embryological formation of tissues; all are associated with a progressive neurological deficit as the result of cord tethering and traction or cord compression. There is a strong association with spina bifida.

Diastematomyelia

In this condition there is an abnormal bony or cartilaginous spur projecting across the middle of the vertebral canal, dividing the dural tube and the spinal cord into two. Between 50 and 70% of patients may have a skin naevus, dimple or hairy patch. Diastematomyelia is more common in females and most commonly occurs in the thoracolumbar region. It often presents during the growth spurt with lower limb weakness, abnormal gait, urinary incontinence or spinal deformity.

SYRINGOMYELIA

PATHOLOGY

In 1824, Olivier d'Angers described a spinal cord cavity in continuity with the fourth ventricle, which he called syringomyelia. Initially, spinal cord lesions were classified into syringomyelia and hydromyelia. Syringomyelia was believed to result from a traumatic cystic dilatation of the spinal cord following trauma. Hydromyelia describes obstruction of the central canal by a tumour, inflammation or mechanical process that causes hydrocephalus. Patients may present with sensory disturbance, weakness of the hands, loss of pain and temperature sensation, or progressive kyphoscoliosis. Hindbrain herniation can lead to headache, neck ache, ataxia, spasticity and lower cranial nerve palsies.

TREATMENT

If outflow obstruction is implicated, then posterior cranial fossa decompression (Fig. 48.1) is indicated to restore cerebrospinal fluid flow through the foramen of Magendie. If the cause is an intramedullary spinal cord, excision of the tumour should restore cerebrospinal fluid communication with the central canal. If the origin of the syrinx is post-traumatic, the obstruction should be relieved by decompression. Fluid diversion should not be the primary or only treatment of syringomyelia. Notwithstanding

REFERENCES

3. Waddell G, McCulloch JA, Kummell E et al. Spine 1980; 5: 117–125

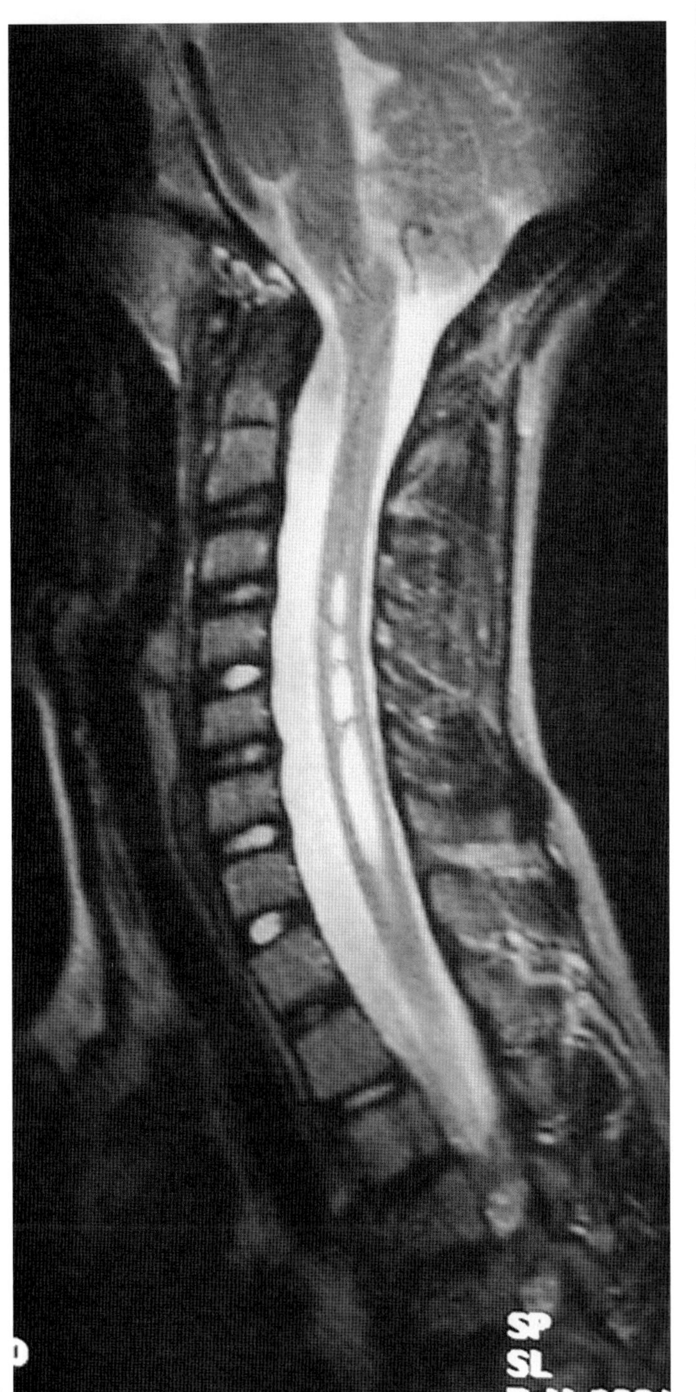

a

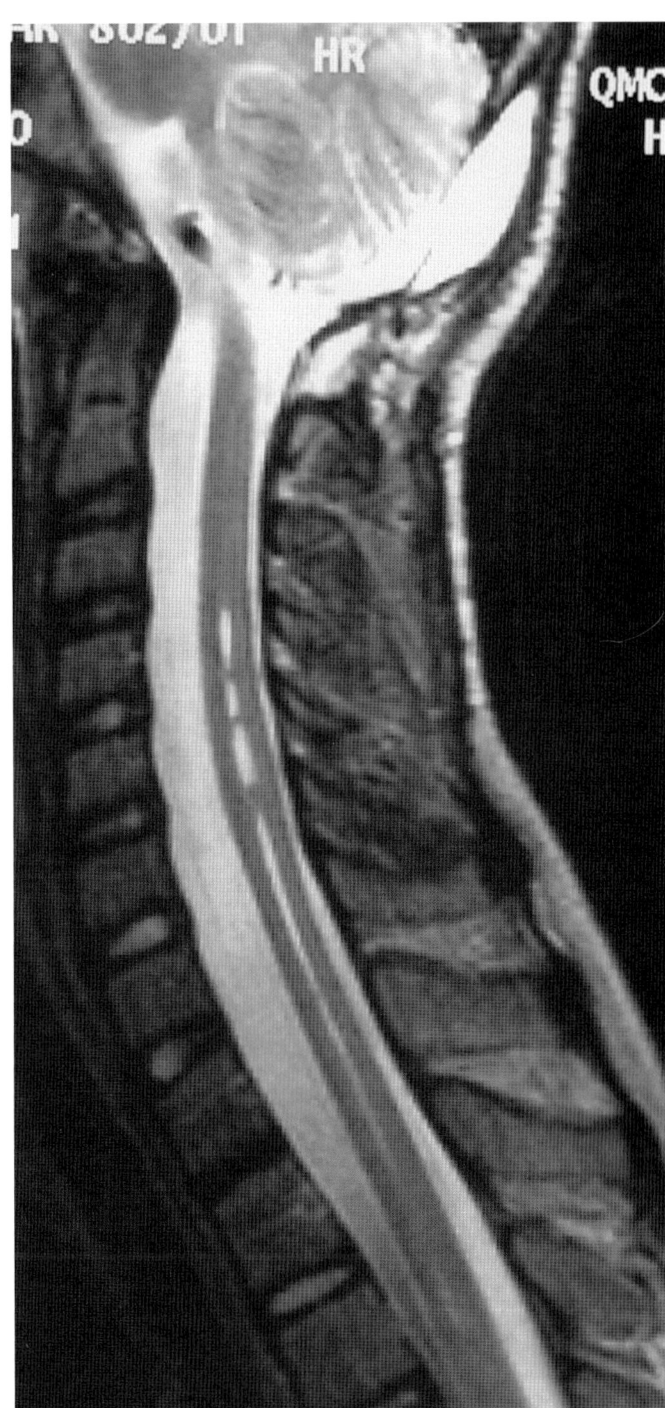

b

Figure 48.1 Arnold–Chiari malformation. (**a**) T2-weighted sagittal MRI scan of the cervical spine; note the cerebellar tonsillar herniation and associated syrinx. (**b**) The same patient following posterior cranial fossa decompression; note regression of syrinx.

this, diversion to the peritoneum (syringoperitoneal) or pleural spaces (syringopleural) has been used with moderate success.

SPINAL TUMOURS

EXTRADURAL TUMOURS

The majority of extradural tumours are metastatic from breast, lung, prostate, kidney or haemopoietic primary malignancies. Non-mechanical pain, weight loss and symptoms of cord compression are the usual presenting features. A histological diagnosis is obviously important if the primary is unknown. Plain radiographs are often normal, but occasionally bony erosion, especially of the pedicles, or vertebral collapse may be present. An isotope bone scan usually shows the tumour before it is visible on plain radiographs. An MRI scan of the whole spine will show the site and nature of the tumour and the presence of any further spinal metastases.

Osteoid osteomas are benign tumours less than 2 cm in diameter. The typical patient is a man in his second or third

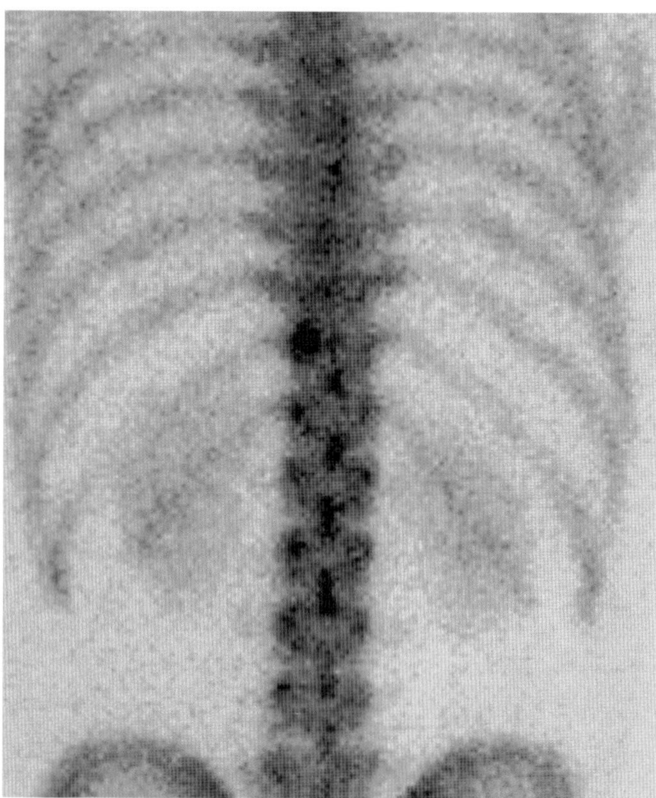

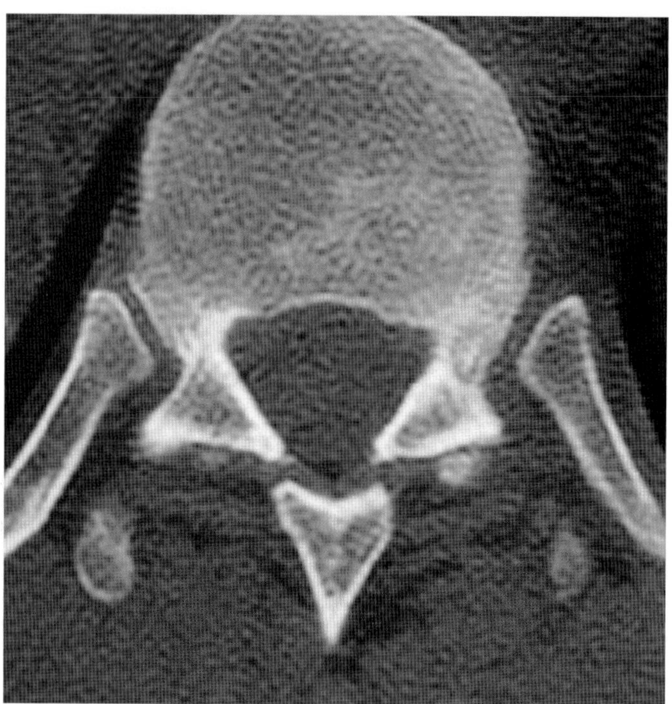

Figure 48.2 Osteoid osteoma. (**a**) Isotope bone scan demonstrating increased uptake in the left T11 pedicle in a 30-year-old man. (**b**) Axial CT scan showing nidus within the left T11 pedicle.

decade presenting with a painful scoliosis. Often there is a delay in diagnosis. Up to one-third of patients report pain relief with salicylates. Radionuclide bone scan and CT scan are helpful in the diagnosis and localization (Fig. 48.2). Treatment consists of complete excision of the nidus. Preoperative injection of isotope with use of a mobile gamma counter assists with intraoperative localization.

Treatment

Metastatic spinal disease without neurological compression, and minor axial pain can be managed with radiotherapy, chemotherapy or hormone manipulation. A scoring system to assess prognosis may assist in choosing excisional or palliative methods.[4] Isolated spinal metastasis with a good life expectancy may be treated by anterior and posterior excision with spinal stabilization. Patients with a poor prognosis (e.g. those with carcinoma of the lung) may be treated by posterior decompression and stabilization only. Patients with a complete spinal cord lesion for more than 24 h or those with widespread disease are unlikely to benefit from surgery.

INTRADURAL TUMOURS

Intradural tumours are rare. They may be intramedullary (within the substance of the cord) or extramedullary (outside the cord). Most are extramedullary and benign, the commonest being meningiomas or neurofibromas. Intramedullary tumours include ependymomas and astrocytomas. Intradural tumours can be multiple, occurring as part of a systemic syndrome, for example von Recklinghausen's syndrome (neurofibromas type I) and von Hippel–Lindau syndrome (multiple haemangioblastomas). Any malignant tumour can metastasize via the normal cerebrospinal fluid pathways. Patients usually show progressive neurological deficits with little pain.

Plain radiographs may reveal scalloping of the vertebral body and pedicles, or an enlarged intervertebral foramen. Myelography can discriminate between intramedullary and extramedullary tumours; however, MRI is the investigation of choice. Occasionally it is impossible to distinguish between syringomyelia and multiple sclerosis on MRI scan: cerebrospinal fluid protein immunoelectrophoresis and visual-evoked responses may help in this situation.

Treatment

Ependymomas are treated by surgical resection, with radiotherapy reserved for malignant or incompletely resected lesions. Astrocytomas are often infiltrative, with variable histology. They may be treated surgically using the carbon dioxide laser or ultrasonic aspirator to assist in their resection, while others believe radiation therapy to be important and the treatment of choice.

DEGENERATIVE CONDITIONS OF THE SPINAL COLUMN

CERVICAL DISC HERNIATION

Cervical disc herniation commonly presents with neck and arm pain (brachalgia), paraesthesia and motor weakness in the distribution of the compromised nerve root (radiculopathy). Rarely the patient may present with a cervical myelopathy in the case of a large disc prolapse. For radiculopathy, surgery is rarely

REFERENCES

4. Tokuhashi Y, Matsuzaki H, Toriyama S et al. Spine 1990; 15: 1110–1113

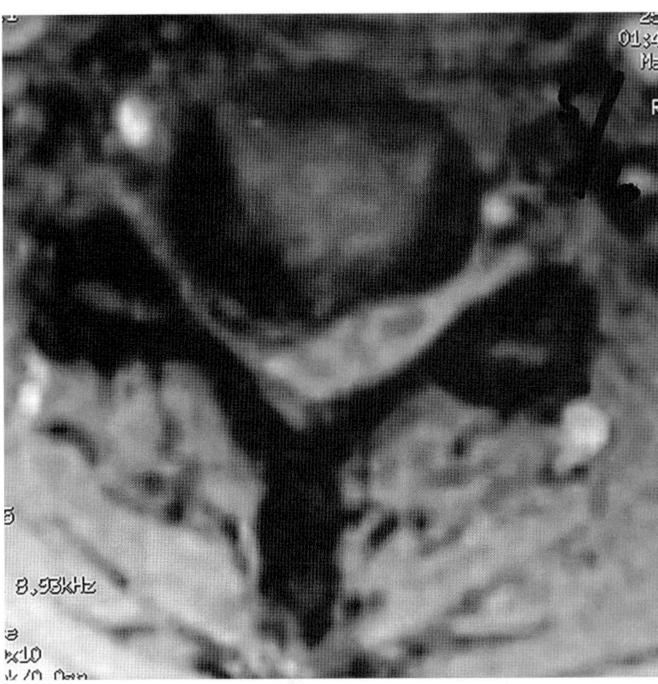

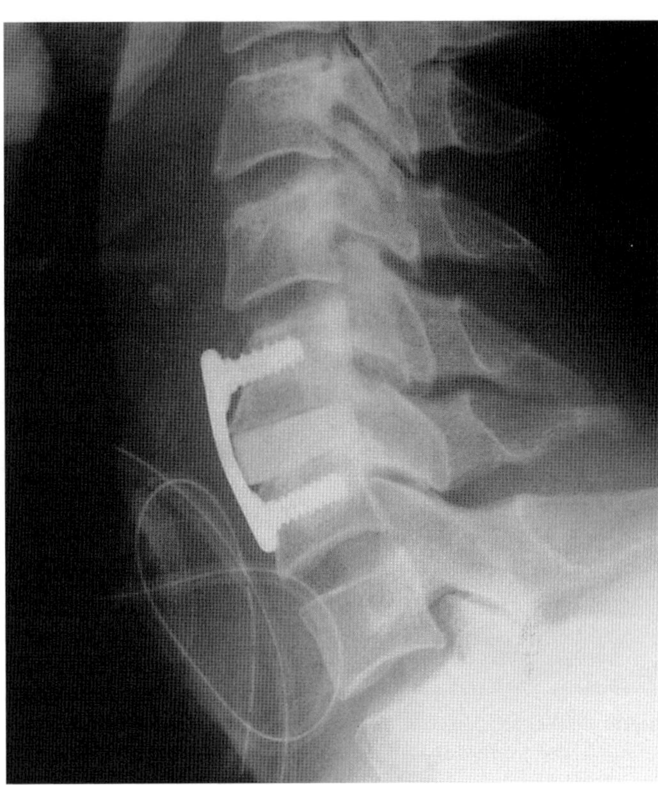

Figure 48.3 Cervical disc prolapse. (**a**) Axial T2-weighted MRI scan showing right C5–6 disc prolapse. (**b**) Post-C5–6 discectomy: interbody fusion with tricortical graft and cervical plate.

indicated in the first 12 weeks, because 90% of patients settle within this time. Intractable pain or functional neurological deficit is an indication for surgical intervention. The natural history of myelopathy is less favourable, and if the degree of spinal cord dysfunction (unsteady gait, hand dysfunction, or neurogenic bladder or bowel disturbance) impairs daily activities then surgical intervention is appropriate. Surgery for pure axial neck pain is controversial, with variable outcomes.

Currently the most prevalent operation is anterior cervical discectomy and fusion for cervical disc herniation (Fig. 48.3). There is no strong evidence that a left- or right-sided approach reduces the risk of injury to the recurrent laryngeal nerve. Bone graft is harvested from the anterior iliac crest, and a cervical spine locking plate applied to immobilize the segment and achieve fusion. Posterior laminoforaminotomy is practised by some to decompress the nerve root for a soft disc herniation in a relatively lateral position, but its use remains limited.

CERVICAL SPINAL STENOSIS

Cervical spinal stenosis may present with radiculopathy, myelopathy, or a combination of both. Careful history and physical examination supplemented by plain radiographs, nerve conduction studies and MRI examination are often required to reach an accurate diagnosis. For isolated radiculopathy, a fluoroscopically guided corticosteroid nerve root block injection may provide significant relief.[5] The method of surgical decompression depends on where the pathology is located. For multilevel disease, a cervical laminectomy from C3 to 6 is commonly performed. If the cervical spine is kyphotic, additional instrumentation (lateral mass screws and posterior rods) is added to restore cervical lordosis and achieve a fusion. An alternative to laminectomy is a canal expansive laminoplasty. This procedure gained popularity in Japan, where the incidence of ossification of the posterior longitudinal ligament remains high. Anterior surgical options include anterior corpectomy and strut grafting.

THORACIC DISC HERNIATION

Thoracic disc herniations are relatively rare, accounting for less than 2% of all discectomy procedures. Disc protrusions predominantly occur in the distal thoracic segments from T8 to 12. Herniations may be soft or calcified. Typically they present with axial pain, radiculopathy or myelopathy. Magnetic resonance scanning is invariably required to demonstrate protrusions and the degree of neural compromise. Thoracic disc protrusions identified on MRI may be asymptomatic.

Non-surgical treatment should be considered if there is no evidence of spinal cord compression. Non-steroidal anti-inflammatory drugs, physiotherapy and general fitness are important. Discectomy and interbody fusion is an appropriate surgical treatment for progressive spinal cord compression. The procedure may also be used to treat selected patients with radicular or axial pain. Surgery may be performed via a thoracotomy or, for a soft disc prolapse, via a thoracoscopic approach.

LUMBAR DISC HERNIATION

A symptomatic lumbar disc herniation occurs during the lifetime of approximately 2% of the population. Risk factors include male gender, age (30–50 years), heavy lifting or twisting, stressful occupation, lower income and cigarette smoking.

Herniations may be described as a protrusion (contained by the annular fibrosis), an extrusion (disc material migrating

REFERENCES

5. Vallee JN, Feydy A, Carlier RY et al. Radiology 2001; 218: 886–892

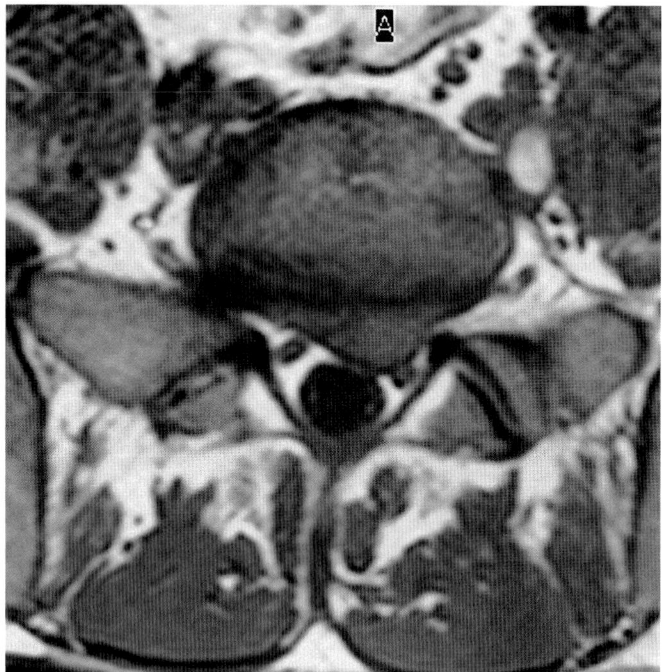

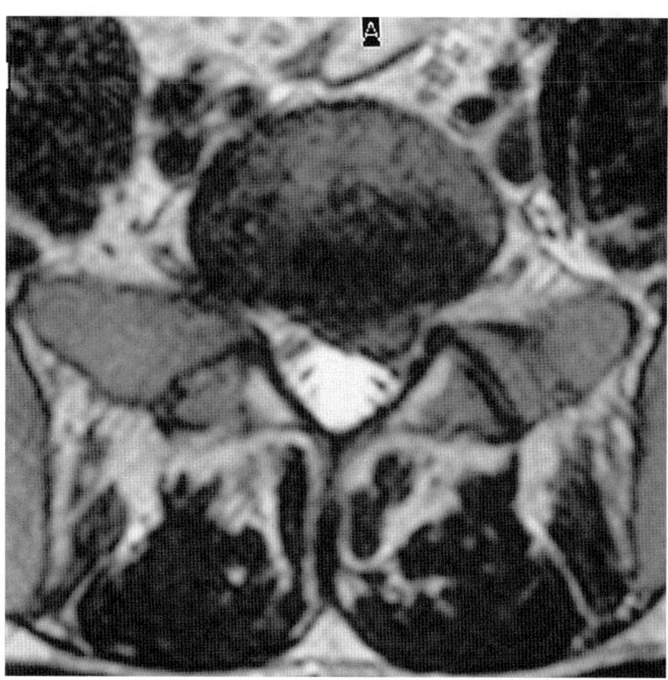

Figure 48.4 Lumbar disc prolapse. (**a**) T1-weighted axial MRI showing L5–S1 disc prolapse leading to compromise of the left S1 nerve root. (**b**) T2-weighted axial MRI scan showing the same.

through the annulus fibrosis but contained by the posterior longitudinal ligament) or sequestered (disc material free in the spinal canal). Disc material may be central, posterolateral, foraminal or extraforaminal. The two commonest levels of disc herniation are L4–5 and L5–S1. A posterolateral disc protrusion will affect the traversing root (e.g. L5–S1 disc protrusion affects the S1 nerve root; Fig. 48.4). A far lateral disc protrusion (extra-foraminal) will affect the exiting nerve root (e.g. a far lateral L4–5 disc protrusion affects the L4 nerve root). Symptoms typically commence with a period of back pain followed by sciatica. There may be paraesthesia, motor weakness, loss of reflexes, and reduction in straight leg raise. A large midline hernia may compress the cauda equina, leading to a syndrome defined by bowel and bladder difficulties, saddle anaesthesia, and lower limb sensory and motor deficits (Fig. 48.5). Surgery for cauda equina syndrome should be performed within 24 h of onset of symptoms to allow the best recovery of neural elements.

For simple sciatica, a period of 6–12 weeks of conservative treatment is advised, with the majority of patients settling spontaneously. Epidural steroid injections may be helpful. Prolonged bed rest is not recommended. Open microdiscectomy is the standard surgical intervention for those in whom conservative treatment has failed. Surgical excision removes both the source of pressure and the initiator of the inflammatory response.

SPINAL STENOSIS

Spinal stenosis is characterized by back, buttock or leg pain. Symptoms are often provoked by exercise. The symptoms of spinal stenosis can be distinguished from vascular claudication because they are frequently associated with neurological symptoms, are often worse in extension and pedal pulses are present on examination. Physical examination may often be normal, with unlimited straight leg raise tests. Plain radiographs may show degenerative changes with or without degenerative

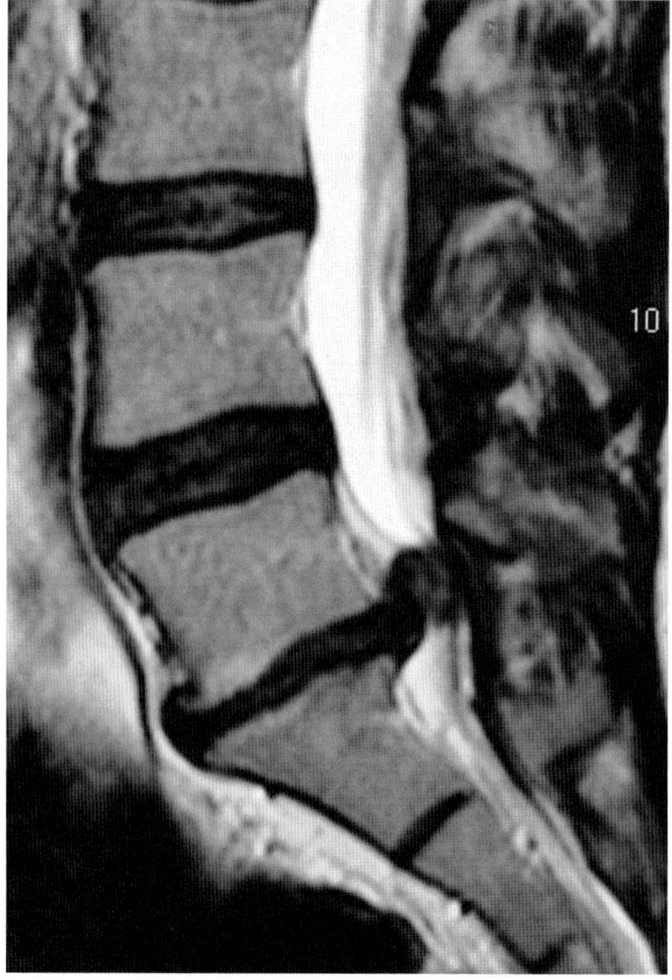

Figure 48.5 Cauda equina syndrome. T2-weighted sagittal MRI scan showing large disc prolapse at L5–S1 leading to a cauda equina syndrome.

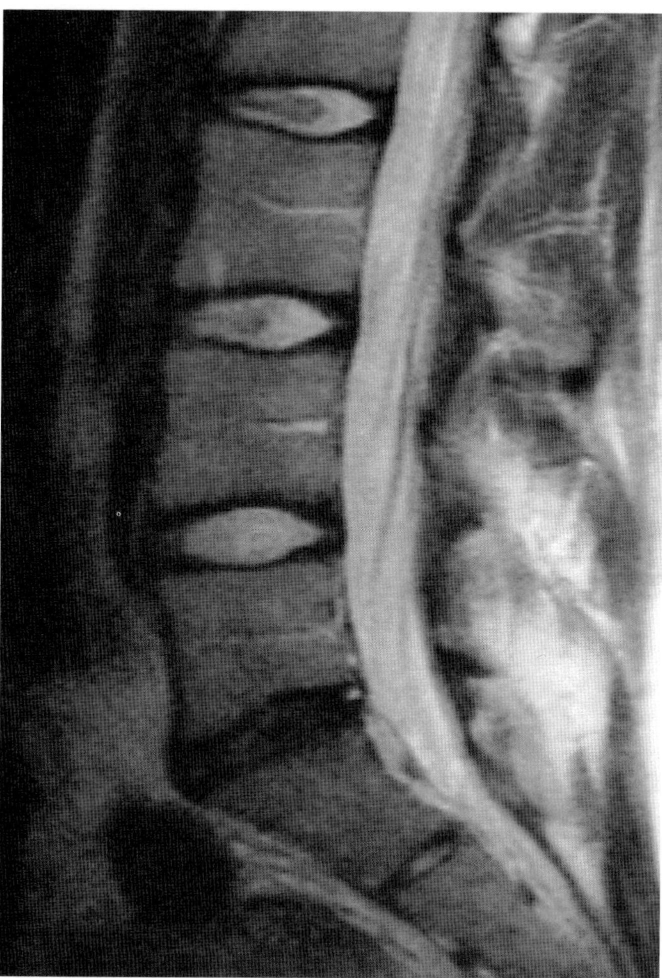

Figure 48.6 Disc degeneration. T2-weighted sagittal MRI scan showing a degenerate L5–S1 disc. A high-intensity zone is visible posteriorly.

spondylolisthesis, and MRI scanning will reveal neural compromise. Stenosis is usually caused by a combination of facet joint hypertrophy, disc bulge and ligamentum flavum thickening.

Review of existing literature suggests that symptoms progress in approximately 20% of patients who receive no treatment. The condition can be successfully treated by surgical spinal decompression. Laminectomy with preservation of the facet joints is a reasonable option, particularly when normal lumbar lordosis is preserved. Others prefer multilevel laminotomies with undercutting of the facet joints, trimming of the ligamentum flavum, and removal of disc bulges. Such a segmental procedure is considered less destabilizing than laminectomy. For patients with associated degenerative spondylolisthesis, concomitant fusion with instrumentation is generally recommended.

CHRONIC DISCOGENIC LOW BACK PAIN

Approximately 10% of patients with acute low back pain become chronic pain sufferers. In a recent study, 40% of patients with chronic low back pain were found to have internal disc disruption. Magnetic resonance imaging may show decreased or absent T2-weighted signal from the disc. An increased signal intensity (high-intensity zone) may be seen within the posterior annulus, suggestive of an annular tear (Fig. 48.6). Type II modic changes may be evident in the adjacent endplates. In one study, over 30% of normal asymptomatic subjects under 40 years of age

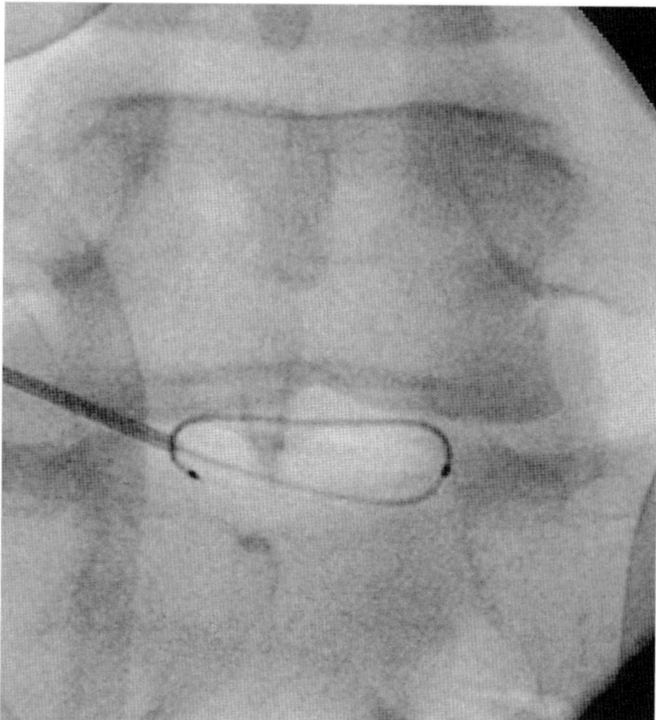

Figure 48.7 Intradiscal electrothermal therapy: anteroposterior radiograph showing IDET catheter deployed in the L5–S1 disc.

had abnormal MRI scans.

A small but significant number of patients fail to improve with conservative measures such as activity modification, non-steroidal anti-inflammatory medication, and physiotherapy (trunk stabilization). These patients should be investigated further with lumbar discography. This provides additional information on the pattern of annular disruption[6] and pain concordance during injection of contrast. Discography, particularly when a negative control is identified, helps decide which patients will benefit from surgical intervention.

Intradiscal electrothermal therapy (IDET) is a new technique developed for the treatment of this condition. Intradiscal electrothermal therapy is a minimally invasive procedure where a catheter is introduced percutaneously into the disc to produce controlled coagulation of collagen and possibly disruption of nociceptors in the posterior annulus (Fig. 48.7). Attempts to evaluate its efficacy remain premature. Another option is total disc replacement; preliminary results for degenerative disc disease remain encouraging, although it is still early on in the advent of such technology (Fig. 48.8). The long-term results of such replacements remain obscure.

Lumbar spinal fusion remains the treatment of choice for patients who have not responded to conservative therapy of at least 6 months. In one randomized study, lumbar fusion diminished pain and decreased disability more efficiently than commonly used non-surgical treatment.[7] Many techniques, including non-instrumented fusion, instrumented posterolateral

REFERENCES

6. Agorastides ID, Lam KS, Freeman BJ et al. Eur Spine J 2002; 11: 76–79
7. Fritzell P, Hagg O, Wessberg P et al. Spine 2001; 26: 2521–2534

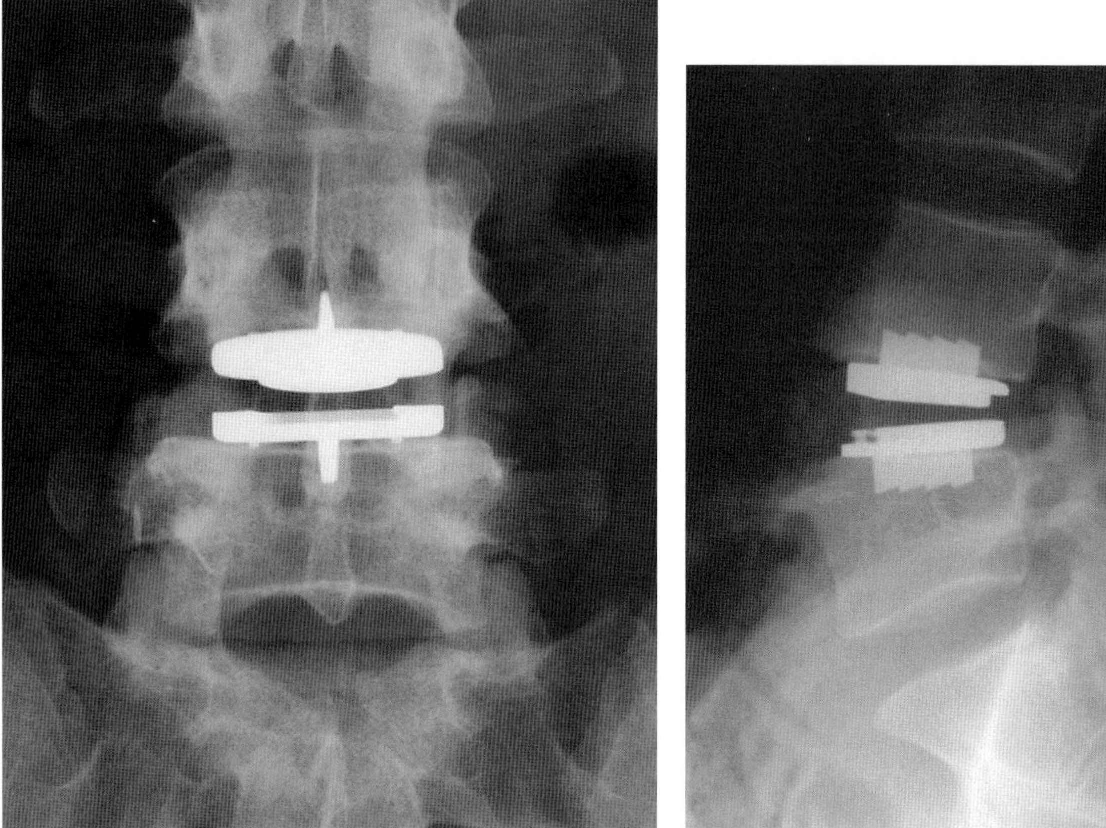

Figure 48.8 Total disc replacement: (**a**) anteroposterior radiograph and (**b**) lateral radiograph showing total disc replacement at L4–5.

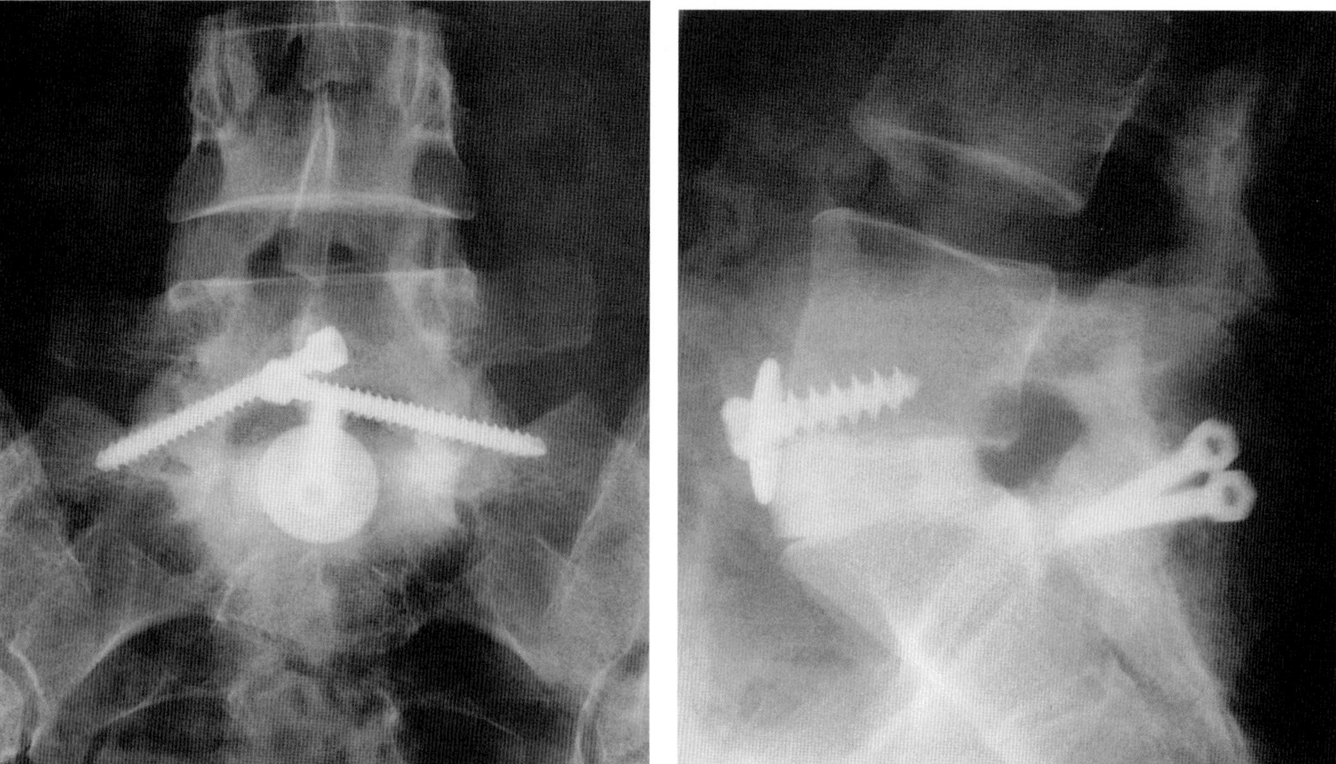

Figure 48.9 Lumbar fusion. (**a**) Anteroposterior radiograph showing circumferential fusion of L5–S1. (**b**) Lateral radiograph of circumferential fusion (femoral ring anteriorly and translaminar screws posteriorly).

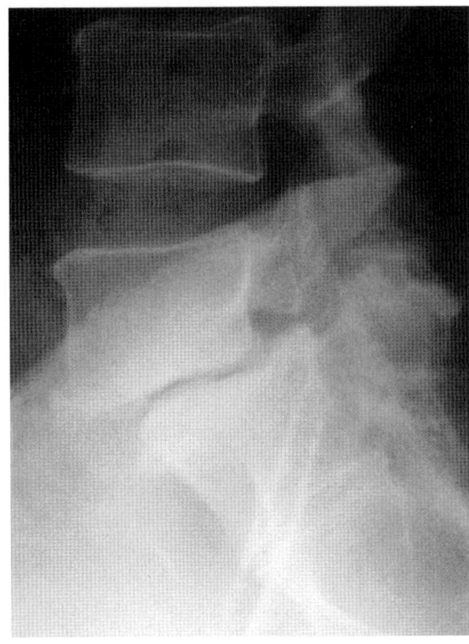
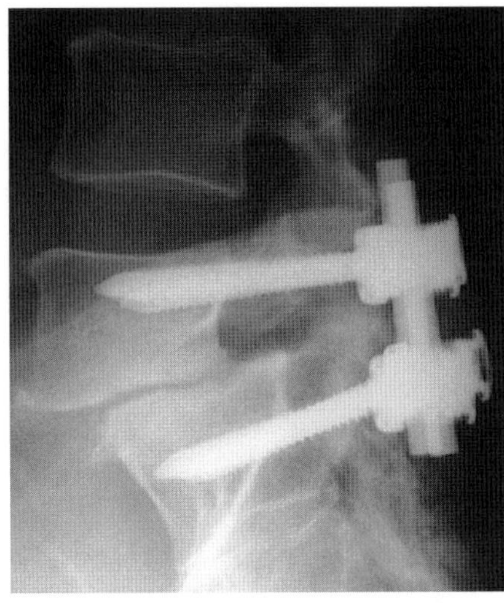
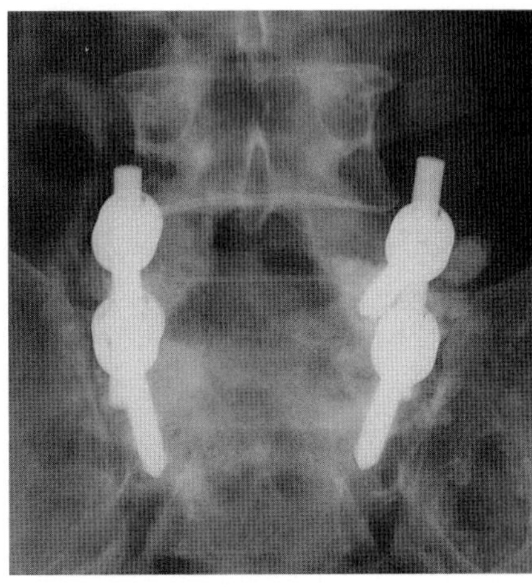

a b c

Figure 48.10 Spondylolisthesis (**a**) Lateral radiograph showing a Meyerding grade II spondylolisthesis at L5–S1. (**b**) Lateral radiograph of instrumented fusion in situ. (**c**) Anteroposterior radiograph; note decompression of both L5 nerve roots.

fusion, posterior lumbar interbody fusion, and combined anterior and posterior (circumferential) fusion (Fig. 48.9), have been used. The literature remains confusing on the best method for lumbar fusion; however, it seems apparent that lumbar interbody fusion, by either anterior or posterior technique, provides a higher success rate when compared with posterolateral fusion.

SPONDYLOLYSIS AND SPONDYLOLISTHESIS

SPONDYLOLYSIS

The pars interarticularis of the posterior lumbar vertebral arch is a narrow bridge of cortical bone joining the lamina and inferior articular facet to the pedicle and superior facet. Repeated stress injury of the pars may lead to fatigue failure producing a fracture. Persistent motion through the fracture may result in a pseudarthrosis. The incidence of symptomatic defects varies between 15 and 47% in the young athletic population and is 6% in the general population.

The diagnosis is usually made with a reverse gantry CT scan and a SPECT scan. Oblique radiographs are no longer acceptable because of the high radiation dose. Treatment depends on the age of the patient, the severity of symptoms, and level of sporting involvement. Avoidance of sporting activity and bracing should be considered before surgery. Provided there is no associated disc degeneration, attempts may be made to repair the defect. Commonly used methods include the direct repair described by Buck, the Morscher hook screw, and Scott's wiring technique. Reports of clinical outcome and return to sport in athletes following Buck's fusion have been very encouraging.[8] If disc degeneration is established then an instrumented spinal fusion is advised.

SPONDYLOLISTHESIS

Spondylolisthesis is a forward slippage of the vertebral body engendered by a break in the continuity or an elongation of the pars interarticularis. The Meyerding classification grades the slip progressively from 1 to 4. One vertebra may sublux completely on the underlying vertebra, a condition called spondyloptosis. Spondylolisthesis has been classified by Marchetti and Bartolozzi into developmental and acquired types. The acquired types include traumatic, postsurgical, pathological and degenerative.

Patients may present with back pain, an associated L5 nerve root pain and/or hamstring spasm. For patients past the third decade of life, it is unusual for spondylolisthesis to produce pain, and more commonly the pain results from secondary degenerative changes in the discs and facet joints. An MRI scan is essential in any patient with neurological symptoms.

A lumbosacral spinal fusion may be indicated for spondylolisthesis that has not settled with conservative treatment (Fig. 48.10). If there is evidence of neural compression this may be combined with a spinal decompression. There is controversy regarding the management of high-grade spondylolisthesis and spondyloptosis. Although some surgeons still perform reduction before spinal fusion, the risks of this procedure are generally considered high and the benefits of reduction before fusion remain unproven. Neurological complications may be avoided by slow reduction with an external fixator followed by definitive fusion.

SPINAL INFECTION

PYOGENIC VERTEBRAL OSTEOMYELITIS

Pyogenic vertebral osteomyelitis is primarily a lesion of the disc and its osseous margins. Infection begins at the vertebral endplates, with deposition of septic emboli and bacterial seeding leading on to subsequent disc penetration. Risk factors include advancing age, obesity, smoking, malignancy, irradiation, malnutrition, diabetes, immunodeficiency, recent infections and trauma. *Staphylococcus aureus* accounts for 30–55% of infections; however, the incidence of Gram-negatives has increased recently. *Pseudomonas* is commonly the causative agent in intravenous drug

REFERENCES

8. Debnath UK, Freeman BJC, Gregory P et al. J Bone Joint Surg 2003; 85B: 244–249

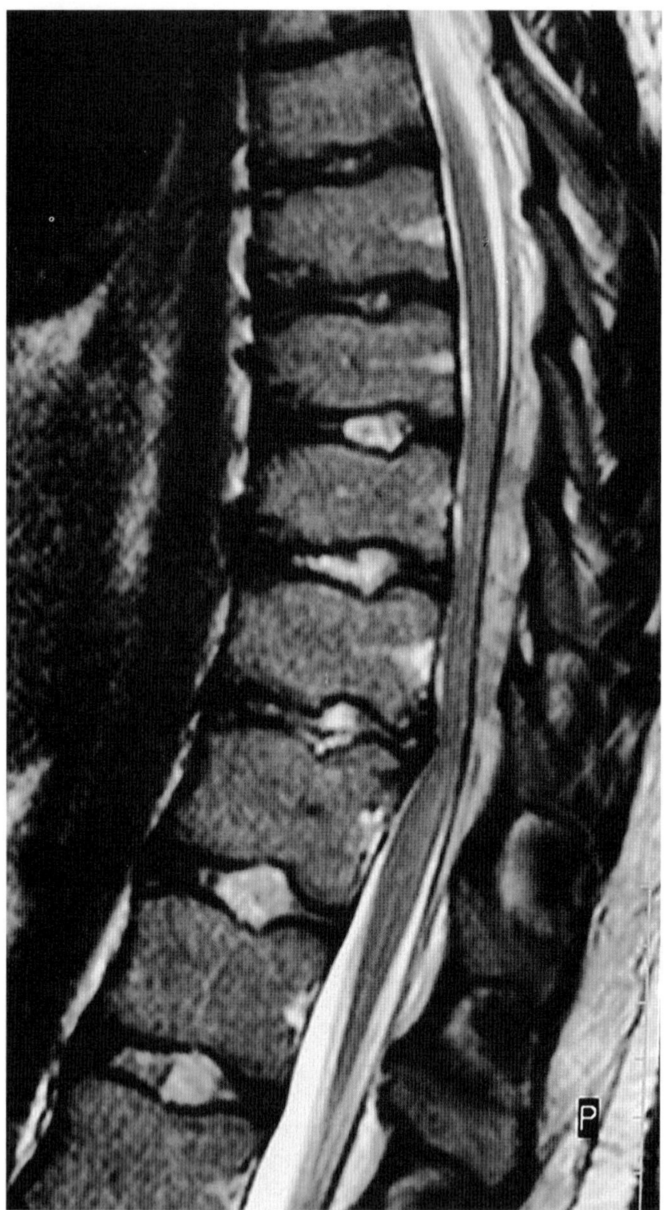

a

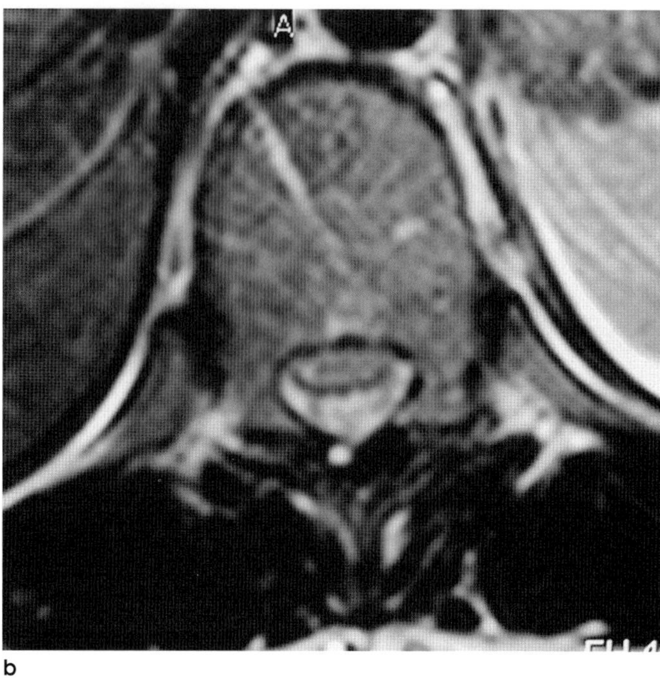

b

Figure 48.11 Epidural abscess. (**a**) T2-weighted sagittal MRI showing posterior collection. (**b**) Axial MRI. The abscess is displacing the cord anteriorly.

abusers. The source of infection is usually the respiratory tract, genitourinary tract or soft tissue infections.

Clinical presentation

Presenting symptoms include pain, sensory disturbance, motor weakness, gait disturbance, fever and sphincter disturbance.[9] Extension of vertebral body osteomyelitis may produce an epidural abscess with possible neurological sequelae. Epidural abcesses are usually found anteriorly in the cervical spine and posteriorly in the thoracic (Fig. 48.11) and lumbar spine.

Diagnosis

Obtaining tissue for culture is the ideal. A full blood count may show a raised white cell count. The erythrocyte sedimentation rate is normally elevated (mean 50–55 mm/h). The C-reactive protein is slightly more sensitive and specific, and may be elevated sooner than the erythrocyte sedimentation rate. Blood cultures may identify an organism, obviating the need for a tissue biopsy. Plain radiographs will be negative for at least 2–4 weeks, following which disc space narrowing will be evident. Radionuclide studies allow survey of the entire skeleton and therefore can detect multifocal involvement (present in 3–5% of cases). An MRI will reveal the presence of a coexisting epidural abscess. Magnetic resonance imaging usually allows the distinction between malignancy and infection, because tumour rarely involves the disc space. Definitive diagnosis is best achieved by CT-guided or percutaneous biopsy. Tissue from the biopsy should be sent for Gram stain, cultures (including aerobes, anaerobes and mycobacteria) and histology to rule out malignancy.

TUBERCULOSIS

The incidence of tuberculosis is higher in the immunocompromised host and in those from underdeveloped countries. Most active cases are a reactivation of quiescent lesions produced and disseminated during an earlier infection. Spinal lesions are

REFERENCES

9. Rezai AR, Woo HH, Errico TJ et al. Neurosurgery 1999: 44: 1018–1026

typically seen following haematogenous spread from a pulmonary source, although direct extension has been reported. The disc spaces are more resistant to invasion by granulomatous infection than they are in pyogenic disease. Therefore disc involvement, if seen, appears much later. The thoracic spine is the most common location, closely followed by the lumbar spine. Multifocal disease ranges from 1 to 24% of patients and is closely related to nutritional status and immune competence. Large paraspinal abscesses are more common when compared with pyogenic infections.

Clinical presentation

The onset of symptoms is typically insidious, with patients complaining of back pain, fever with night sweats, weight loss, malaise, neurological involvement and spinal deformity.

Diagnosis

Typically the erythrocyte sedimentation rate is elevated; often the white cell count is not. Sputum and urine culture may be diagnostic of mycobacterium but take 8–10 weeks. A definitive diagnosis is often achieved by CT-guided or percutaneous biopsy. Polymerase chain reaction is the single best diagnostic modality.

TREATMENT OF VERTEBRAL INFECTION

Initial treatment is medical, with appropriate intravenous antibiotics for a minimum of 4 weeks. C-reactive protein and erythrocyte sedimentation rate are used to monitor the response to treatment. Immobilization with bed rest followed by orthosis for 3 months to assist with pain control and prevention of deformity are the standard of care. Spontaneous fusion of adjacent vertebrae is common. Tuberculosis infections are treated with rifampicin, isoniazid and pyrazinamide for 12 months.

Surgery may be indicated for:

- obtaining tissue biopsy;
- correction of deformity;
- progressive neurological deficit; or
- failure of medical management.

A complete and thorough anterior debridement is the cornerstone of treatment. Reconstruction of the anterior column with tricortical iliac crest bone graft is possible. For larger defects, autologous rib[10] or fibular graft may be used. Use of instrumentation raises concerns because pathogens capable of producing glycocalyx or biofilm may adhere to metallic implants. The anterior column should be supported with extrafocal posterior instrumentation to allow early mobilization.

INFLAMMATORY SPONDYLOARTHROPATHY ANKYLOSING SPONDYLITIS

Ankylosing spondylitis is an inflammatory spondyloarthropathy that primarily affects the axial skeleton, beginning with sacroiliitis. It is associated with formation of syndesmophytes and eventual ankylosis with kyphosis of the spine. It presents with chronic low back pain and stiffness in early adulthood. It is more common in males, and there is an association with the HLA-B27 antigen. Non-spinal manifestations include arthritis of peripheral joints, acute anterior uveitis, renal amyloidosis, cardiac valve and cardiac conduction disturbances. Hip contractures can also result in significant sagittal imbalance and should be corrected prior to spinal osteotomy. Should a patient with ankylosing spondylitis present following trauma, a high index of suspicion for occult fractures must be present. It is not uncommon for patients to develop epidural haematomas with subtle neurological deficit.

Patients with a significant fixed flexion deformity at the cervicothoracic junction limiting forward gaze, eating and swallowing may be treated with an extension osteotomy of the cervical spine. Surgery is performed under general anaesthesia after an awake fibre-optic intubation. The spinal cord is monitored with somatosensory- and motor-evoked potentials. A halo is applied and the osteotomy carried out at the C7–T1 level. The osteotomy is closed under precise control and stabilized with instrumentation and a posterior fusion.[11]

Primary thoracic kyphosis can be corrected by multiple thoracic osteotomies, or the overall spinal deformity can be corrected by a compensatory osteotomy in the lumbar spine. Lumbar osteotomy is best performed by a transpedicular closing wedge osteotomy at the second or third lumbar vertebra, i.e. below the conus and held in place by rigid posterior instrumentation and fusion.

RHEUMATOID ARTHRITIS

Rheumatoid arthritis is a chronic progressive systemic inflammatory disease primarily affecting synovial joints. The most common sites for involvement are hands, feet and the cervical spine. Resultant cervical instability and pannus formation can lead to spinal cord compromise and neurological deficit. Involvement of the cervical spine can lead to subaxial subluxation, basilar invagination, damage to the transverse ligaments, alar and apical ligaments, and capsule of the C1–2 joints leading to atlantoaxial subluxation. Cranial migration of the dens is described when the tip of the dens is above the transverse diameter of the foramen magnum (McRae's line). Subaxial subluxation occurs from erosion of the facet joints, laxity of the interspinous ligaments, and disc degeneration. Neurological symptoms may occur as a result of direct compression by bone or soft tissue, or from neural ischaemia.

Table 48.3 Ranawat classification of neurological deficit

Class	Description
I	No neurological deficit
II	Subjective weakness, dysaesthesia, hyper-reflexia
III	Objective weakness with long tract signs
IIIa	Ambulatory
IIIb	Non-ambulatory

The Ranawat classification of neurological deficit is useful for categorizing patients with rheumatoid arthritis and myelopathy (Table 48.3). Recommendations for surgery include:

- Atlantoaxial subluxation with a posterior atlantodental interval (PADI) of 14 mm or less.
- Atlantoaxial subluxation with at least 5 mm of basilar invagination.

REFERENCES

10. Kamat AS, Freeman BJ, Cain CMJ et al. Eur Spine J 2001; 11: 465–466
11. Mehdian SMH, Freeman BJC, Licina P. Eur Spine J 1999; 8: 505–509

- Subaxial subluxation with a sagittal canal diameter of 14 mm or less.

Rheumatoid patients who develop myelopathy often have a poor prognosis. In one series, 100% became bedridden within 3 years of onset of myelopathy and one-third died suddenly. Early surgical stabilization for those patients with rheumatoid arthritis and cervical myelopathy is therefore recommended. The morbidity is very high, with only 25% of patients (Ranawat IIIb) who underwent surgical decompression having a favourable outcome.[12] Patients with severe rheumatoid arthritis often have very poor bone quality. Techniques of occipitocervical fixation now employ bicortical screw fixation to the occiput, transarticular fixation across the C1–2 joint, and lateral mass screws in the subaxial cervical spine. Bone graft is traditionally harvested from the iliac crest, although good results have been achieved with occipital calvarial bone graft.[13]

SPINAL DEFORMITY

Spinal deformity is categorized into coronal plane deformity (scoliosis) and sagittal plane deformity (kyphosis). Further classification on the basis of aetiology can be made into congenital, neuromuscular, syndrome-related and idiopathic. The appropriate radiograph for scoliosis is a standing posteroanterior projection of the whole spine. When surgery is contemplated, lateral bending radiographs are performed to assess flexibility of the curve. Curve magnitude is assessed using the Cobb method, where the superior endplate of the most cranial vertebra pointing in towards the concavity is chosen, and the inferior endplate of the most caudal endplate pointing in towards the concavity is chosen. The angle between the two is then measured.

Skeletal maturity should be assessed radiographically using the Risser sign, which assesses the degree of ossification of the iliac apophysis. The status of the triradiate cartilage of the acetabulum may also be useful to assess growth potential. The triradiate cartilage closes before the iliac apophysis appears (Risser 0) at about the time of peak growth velocity. Patients with abnormal neurological examination (e.g. asymmetric abdominal reflexes) or patients for whom surgical correction is planned should have an MRI examination of the whole spine to look for intraspinal pathology (e.g. syringomyelia, low-lying conus, diastematomyelia or a tethered cord). These findings may well change the operative strategy.

IDIOPATHIC SCOLIOSIS

The prevalence of curves with a Cobb angle greater then 10° is between 0.5 and 3%. The prevalence for curves greater than 30° is between 1.5 and three per 1000. Idiopathic scoliosis can be divided into early onset (before 7 years of age) and late onset (typical adolescent scoliosis). Severe curves in the early-onset group have a higher chance of respiratory compromise. Risk factors for progression include female gender, remaining skeletal growth, curve location and curve magnitude. Not all curves stabilize when skeletal maturity is reached. In long-term studies, 68% experienced curve progression. The most marked progression of 1° per year was observed in thoracic curves between 50° and 75°.[14]

Treatment

Idiopathic curves of less than 25° are monitored with clinical and radiographic examination. In growing children a brace may be indicated when a curve progresses to 25–30°. Bracing will not reverse a curve, rather it will maintain it at the degree of severity when bracing commenced. Curves beyond 45° are not amenable to brace treatment. In one prospective study, brace treatment was successful in 74%.[15] Surgery in the form of corrective instrumentation and spinal fusion is indicated for curve progression beyond 40°, truncal imbalance and unacceptable cosmesis (Fig. 48.12). During surgery, continuous electrical spinal cord monitoring is used in the form of somatosensory evoked potentials and more recently motor-evoked potentials. The risk of permanent neurological injury for such patients is 0.02% (one in 5000); the risk for incomplete neurological injury is 0.4% (one in 250).

CONGENITAL SCOLIOSIS

Congenital scoliosis is the result of abnormally formed vertebral elements leading to deviation in spinal alignment. These deficiencies occur in the first 6 weeks of intrauterine development and may be associated with cardiac and renal anomalies. Hemivertebrae can readily be detected on antenatal ultrasound at 20 weeks.[16]

Congenital spinal anomalies can be classified into failures in formation, failures of segmentation or both. Radiographs may show asymmetry in the number of pedicles, absent ribs or rib fusions. An unsegmented bar is suggested when the corresponding ribs and/or pedicles are conjoined. Block or wedge vertebrae have a low chance of progression. Hemivertebrae, however, increase between 1° and 2.5° per year. Unilateral unsegmented bars progress at the rate of up to 6–9° per year, and unilateral unsegmented bar with contralateral hemivertebrae are at the greatest risk of progression, at times exceeding 10° per year.

Treatment

Close monitoring of spinal growth is required until skeletal maturity is reached. Brace treatment is ineffective for the primary structural curve, which is often short and rigid, but may have a role in the control of compensatory curves. Investigations should include renal ultrasound, cardiac echo, and MRI of the whole spine (intraspinal pathology is present in up to 25%). Surgical options include posterior fusion in situ, combined anterior and posterior fusion, convex hemiepiphysiodesis, and hemivertebrae excision with correction (Fig. 48.13). The risk of spinal cord injury due to vascular insufficiency seems greatest in congenital scoliosis surgery compared with surgery on other curve types.

NEUROMUSCULAR SCOLIOSIS

Neuromuscular disorders are either neuropathic or myopathic. A progressive spinal deformity producing disturbance in quality of life, or threatening compromise of cardiorespiratory function, can be treated by correction and fusion via a posterior approach.

REFERENCES

12. Casey AT, Crockard HA, Bland JM et al. J Neurosurg 1996; 85: 574–581
13. Robertson SC, Menezes AH. Spine 1998; 23: 249–255
14. Weinstein SL, Ponseti IV. J Bone Joint Surg 1983; 65A: 447–455
15. Nachemson AL, Peterson LE. J Bone Joint Surg 1995; 77A: 815–822
16. Freeman BJ, Ouellet JA, Twining P et al. Eur Spine J 2001; 10 (Suppl 1): S12

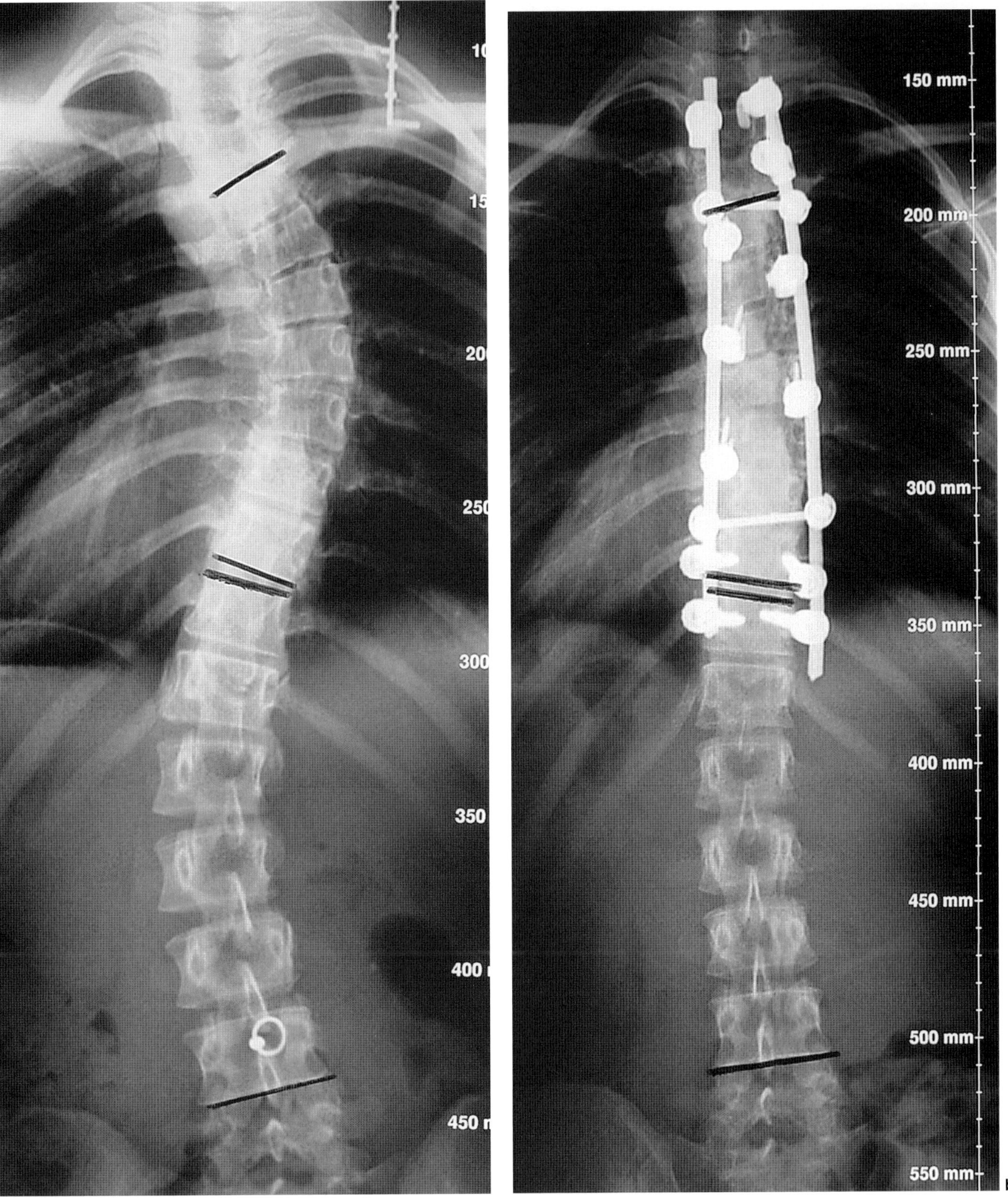

Figure 48.12 Idiopathic scoliosis. (**a**) Anteroposterior radiograph showing right thoracic curve Cobb angle 54°, left lumbar curve 30°. (**b**) Postoperative radiograph: right thoracic curve corrected to 20°; the compensatory curve has corrected spontaneously.

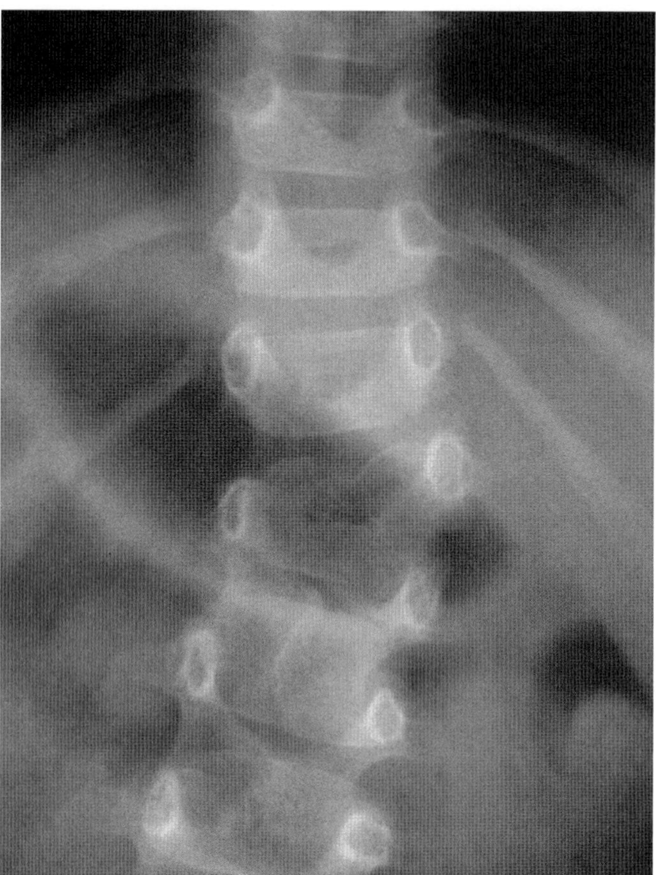
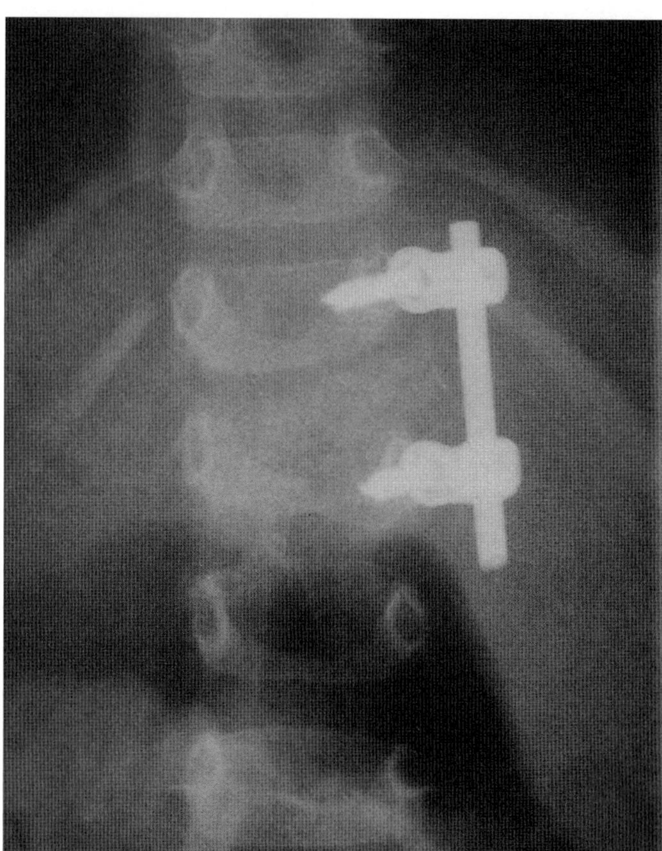

Figure 48.13 Congenital scoliosis. (**a**) Anteroposterior radiograph showing partially segmented hemivertebra at T12–L1. (**b**) Postoperative radiograph following excision and correction with instrumentation.

There is good evidence that stabilization of the spine in children with Duchenne's muscular dystrophy who are unable to walk, before the respiratory compromise is too severe to allow a general anaesthetic, may increase their lifespan by several years.[17] Other common neuromuscular conditions requiring spinal stabilization include cerebral palsy, myelomeningocele, and the sequelae of poliomyelitis.

SCHEUERMANN'S DISEASE-THORACIC KYPHOSIS

Scheuermann's disease was initially described as a rigid kyphosis associated with wedged vertebral bodies occurring in late childhood. At least three adjacent vertebrae must be wedged by at least 5° each. Typically a thoracic kyphosis of 50–90° may exist. The incidence has been estimated at 1–8% of the population. The condition is more common in males.

Physiotherapy directed at postural improvement and hamstring release may be useful. Bracing for skeletally immature patients with kyphosis up to 65° may be effective in arresting progression. Indications for surgery include pain, progressive deformity greater than 70°, unacceptable cosmesis, and neurological and cardiopulmonary compromise. Neurological deficits have been reported relating to thoracic disc herniation, epidural cysts or hyperkyphosis.

If surgery is contemplated, a hyperextension lateral radiograph (over a bolster) is required. If the kyphosis fails to correct to less than 50°, an anterior release and disc excision is required. This may be carried out via a thoracotomy or an endoscopic approach,[18] to be followed by a posterior correction and fusion, typically from T2 to L2 (Fig. 48.14). Care should be taken, however, if the curve has a low apex (e.g. T10–11), when consideration should be given to extend the fusion to the first lordotic disc.

REFERENCES

17. Galasko CSB, Delaney C, Morris PJ. J Bone Joint Surg 1992; 74B: 210–214
18. Neimeyer T, Freeman BJC, Grevitt MP et al. Eur Spine J 2000; 9: 499–504

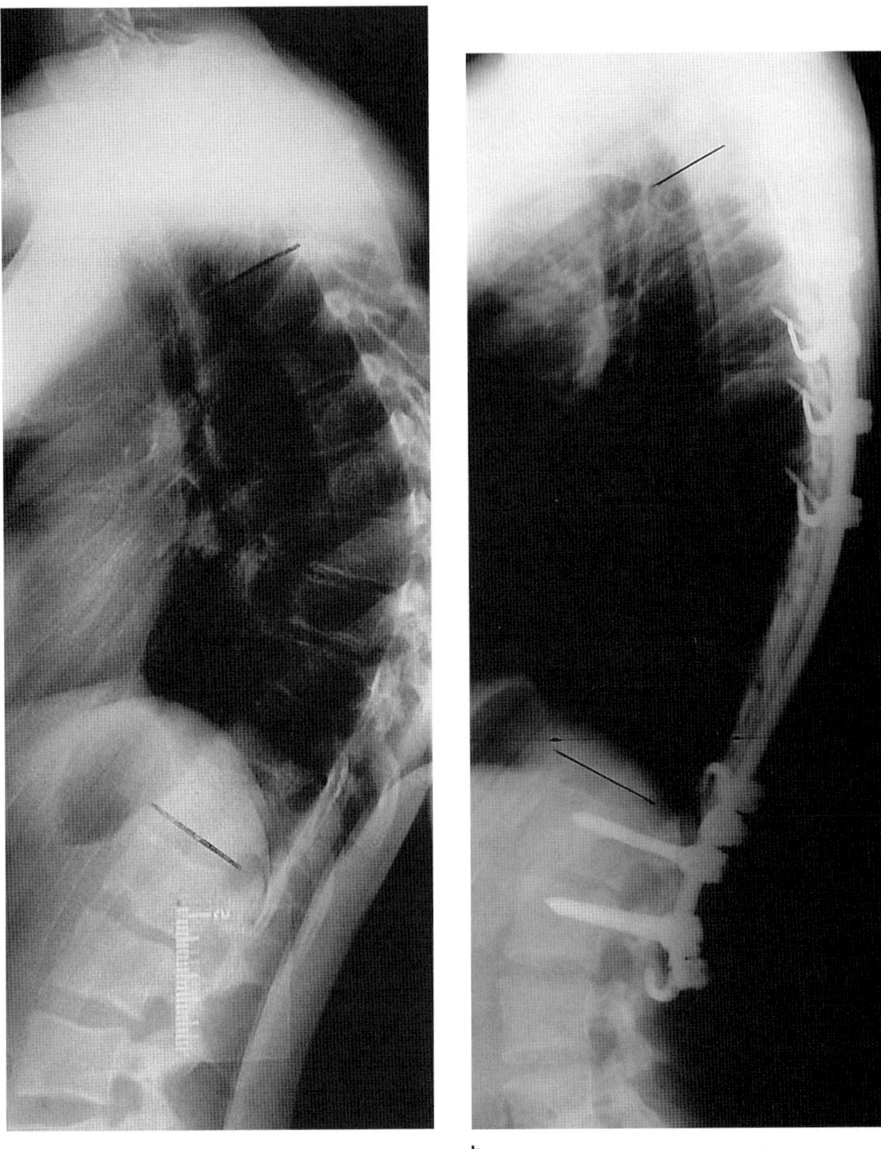

a b

Figure 48.14 Scheuermann's kyphosis. (**a**) Lateral radiograph showing 70° kyphosis between T4 and T12. (**b**) Postoperative radiograph correction to 55°.

The hip and pelvis

49

Marcus Bankes

HISTORY

History taking should concentrate not only on symptoms but also their effect on the patient's lifestyle and activities of daily living; the sole carer of a disabled relative may not endure symptoms that are tolerated by a patient with a sedentary lifestyle and plenty of social support.

Pain from the hip joint may be felt in the groin, buttock and upper lateral thigh, radiating down the front of the thigh to the knee and ankle. Determining the origin of buttock pain may be difficult because it may originate from the lumbar spine, a common coexisting site of osteoarthritis. Severity of pain may be quantified by the frequency of night pain, the range and quantity of analgesics consumed, and whether the patient feels their symptoms warrant surgery. Enquiries should be made about walking distance, stair-climbing ability, limping and effects on leisure activities. Stiffness is indicated by difficulties with putting on socks, tying shoelaces, pedicure and using a bath. Early degenerative symptoms may be episodic, with periods of almost normal hip function between exacerbations. Progressive shortening of the leg may indicate bony destruction of the hip joint, fixed adduction, or gross loosening of a prosthesis. Multiple joint involvement, early morning stiffness and systemic symptoms may indicate inflammatory arthritis.

A history of previous hip problems in childhood or in the family, or past injury or surgery to the hip should be sought. It is also essential to assess general health, especially in elderly patients, who often have concurrent cardiovascular and respiratory ailments. Surgery in these individuals can be a major undertaking, and the benefits must be carefully weighed against the risks. Risk factors for thromboembolic disease should also be identified.

CLINICAL EXAMINATION OF THE HIP

Much information can be gained as the patient walks in, by observing the presence of a limp, use of walking aids, shoe modifications, the ability to carry bags, difficulty getting in and out of a chair, and the amount of assistance needed with shoes and socks. Patients should be suitably undressed to allow adequate inspection and palpation of bony landmarks. In addition, note is taken of the patient's general appearance, their size, and whether there are signs of systemic arthritis or generalized ligamentous laxity.

GAIT

Movements of the lower limb during normal walking can be divided into a swing phase (38%) and a stance phase (62%). An *antalgic* gait results from the patient spending as little time as possible on a painful lower limb, with shortening of the stance phase (i.e. limping). During the swing phase of normal gait, the pelvis and the other leg support the rest of the body. To maintain balance and give the swinging leg ground clearance, the pelvis must tilt towards the stance side leg. This is achieved by the abductor muscles pulling on the pelvic brim from the greater trochanter. This abductor mechanism may be impaired by pain, or muscular weakness or deficiency (i.e. following transgluteal approaches to the hip or polio), or be due to loss of the fulcrum action of the hip joint (i.e. hip dislocation or absent femoral head). Patients compensate for this by either using a walking stick in the opposite hand or swinging the upper body over the weight-bearing foot, producing the lurching *Trendelenburg* gait. A *short leg* gait is characterized by a drop in the shoulder during stance phase and can easily be demonstrated on normal subjects by walking with one shoe. A *stiff hip* gait describes reduction in hip flexion and extension during the swing phase of gait. These gait patterns may exist alone or in combination. Neurological gaits (e.g. drop foot or spastic) may also be associated with hip disease.

INSPECTION OF PATIENT STANDING

Note scars from previous surgery, including old anterior approaches, sinuses from infection or tuberculosis, and swellings. Viewing the patient from in front, pelvic obliquity, knee deformity, wasting of the quadriceps, the flexed knee of a long leg, or the equinus ankle of a short leg may be seen. From the side, the prominent buttock and lumbar lordosis of a hip with fixed flexion should be noted, and from behind, buttock and hamstring wasting, spinal deformity and spinal stiffness should be sought. The Trendelenburg test is then performed by holding the pelvic brim from behind and asking the patient to stand sequentially on the good leg and then on the bad leg by flexing the knee but without flexing the hip. A positive test is indicated by the pelvis dropping towards the normal side from a deficient abductor mechanism on the affected side ('the sound side sags'; Fig. 49.1).

EXAMINATION ON THE COUCH

First observe any difficulty the patient has getting on to the couch, and then look for signs of peripheral vascular disease (ulcers contraindicate implant surgery) or venous hypertension (increased risk of thromboembolic disease). A painful hip lies in flexion, adduction and external rotation, because this is the position when the hip joint has the largest volume. Flexion of the knee may in fact be a consequence of fixed flexion of the hip.

Leg length inequality

Leg length discrepancy is an important indicator of disease severity due to bone loss or fixed adduction, and its presence

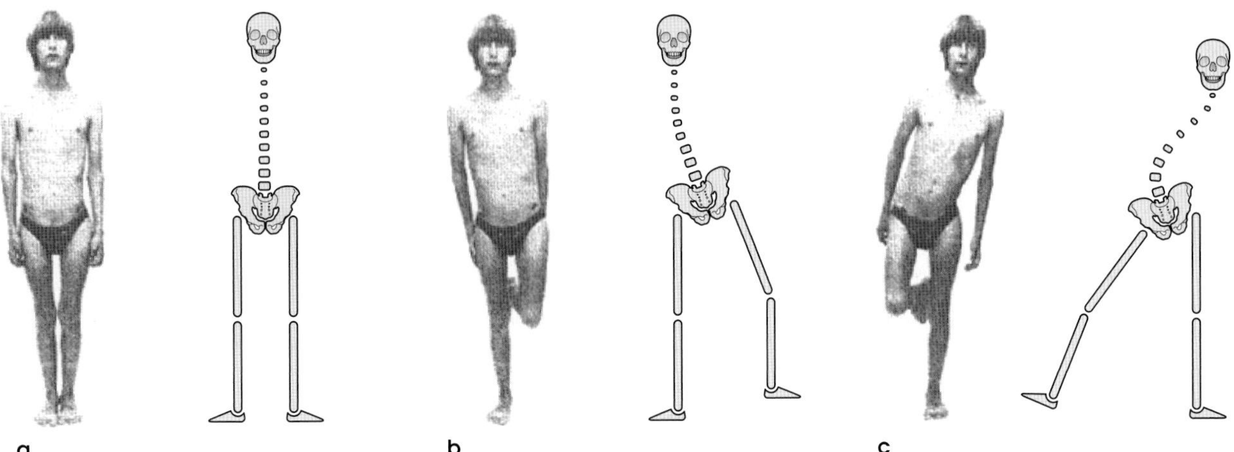

Figure 49.1 Trendelenburg's sign. (**a**) Standing normally on both legs. (**b**) Standing on the right leg; the abductor muscles of the normal hip transfer the weight correctly. (**c**) Standing on the left leg; the hip is faulty and cannot achieve abduction, so the pelvis drops on the unsupported side and the shoulder swings over to the left.

must be determined accurately. The presence or absence of a discrepancy is diagnosed by inspection and palpation.

Real shortening is caused by changes in the bones, apparent shortening results from movements in joints. The length of the femur, tibia, and height of the acetabulum in the pelvis determine real leg length. Normal individuals can appear to make one leg shorter than the other by tilting the pelvis, adducting the hip, or flexing the hip or knee, even though there is no change in the real length. Each of these manoeuvres, alone or in combination, is responsible for *apparent* shortening of the lower limb when the heels are compared when the patient lies 'uncorrected' on the couch.

Squaring the pelvis usually ensures both hips are in the neutral position and corrects discrepancies purely due to adduction and abduction of either hip. In the presence of fixed adduction, it may not be possible to level the pelvis, although an estimate of the position of the limbs relative to the pelvis can still be made. If one lower limb has a 20° fixed adduction deformity at the hip and a 40° fixed flexion deformity at the knee, then the other limb must be put in the same position to exclude the apparent shortening effect of joint position. It can be seen that differences in the real lengths can be assessed only when both limbs lie in the same position (Fig. 49.2). If the painful hip is on the side of the longer leg, consider fixed abduction or shortening of the other leg. If there is a true leg length inequality, the knees should then be flexed to 90° and the heels placed together.

The levels of the knees are then inspected: when observed from the short side, if one knee is lower than the other, then the shortening is in the femur; when observed from the feet, the lower knee indicates shortening in the tibia (Galeazzi's test). If the shortening is in the femur, palpation of the greater trochanters relative to the anterior superior iliac spine will indicate whether the shortening is above or below the trochanter. The trochanter may almost be at the level of the iliac crest in cases of old tuberculosis of the hip and congenital dislocation. In cases of severe shortening, telescoping should be sought.

Only if a leg length discrepancy is demonstrated is measurement required; even then it may be difficult to accurately measure discrepancies of less than 2 cm, particularly in overweight patients. Real length is measured between the anterior superior iliac spine and the medial malleolus. Alternatively, the

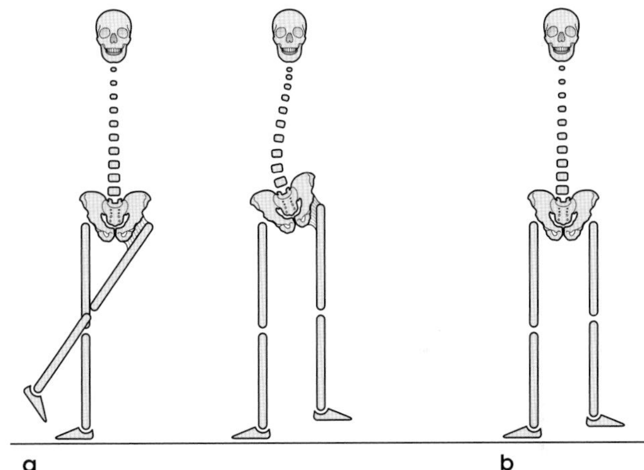

Figure 49.2 (**a**) With adduction of the left hip, the patient must hitch up the pelvis to uncross the legs; the leg then *appears* short. (**b**) Without hip deformity, it is possible to stand or lie with the legs at right angles to the pelvis; the leg *is* short.

patient may be asked to stand with the short leg on blocks or books of known thickness until a level pelvis is obtained.

Fixed deformities and passive movements

Movements of the pelvis and lumbar spine can counteract the effect of lost hip movements. Forward tilting of the pelvis at the lumbosacral junction compensates for loss of hip extension, and this produces a lumbar lordosis.

Thomas's test reveals fixed flexion by obliterating the lumbar lordosis. The left hand is placed under the lumbar spine, and both hips are flexed up maximally until the spine is flat on the hand. While holding the 'good' hip in the maximally flexed position, the affected hip is allowed to extend. The angle between the thigh and the couch is the angle of fixed flexion. If the affected hip is then maximally flexed again (making certain the lordosis remains obliterated) and the good hip allowed to extend, it can be seen that the range of flexion of both hips has been measured (normal range 0–130°). Hip flexion accompanied by abduction and external rotation is seen in osteoarthritis, Perthes' disease, and slipped upper femoral epiphysis.

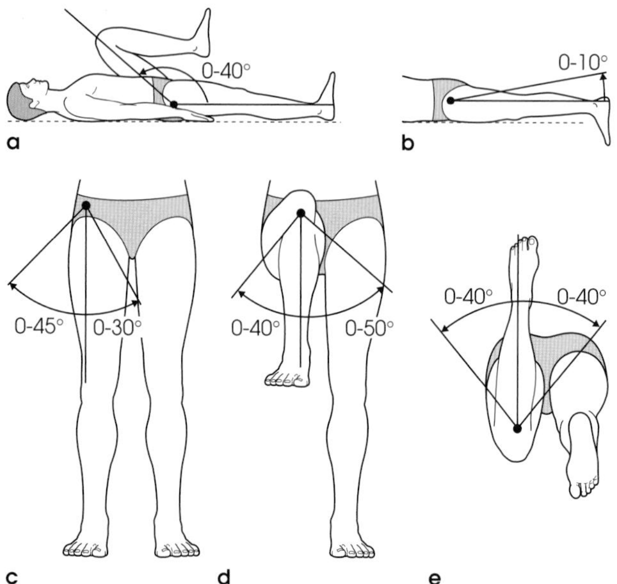

Figure 49.3 The normal range of movements. (**a**) Hip flexion and (**b**) extension. (**c**) Abduction is greater than adduction. Relative internal and external rotation depend on whether the hip is (**d**) flexed or (**e**) extended.

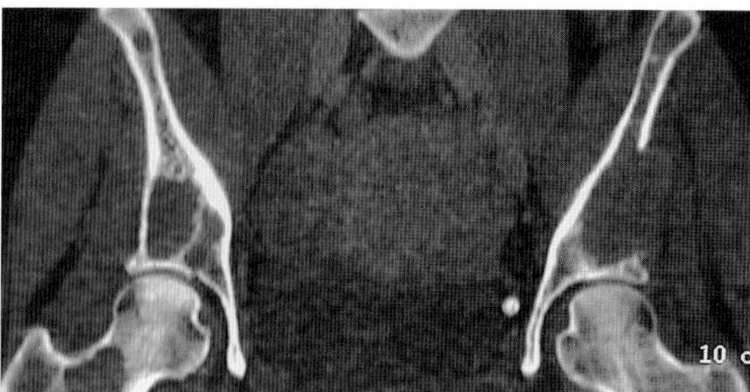

Figure 49.4 CT scan showing metastatic breast carcinoma in the roof of both acetabula.

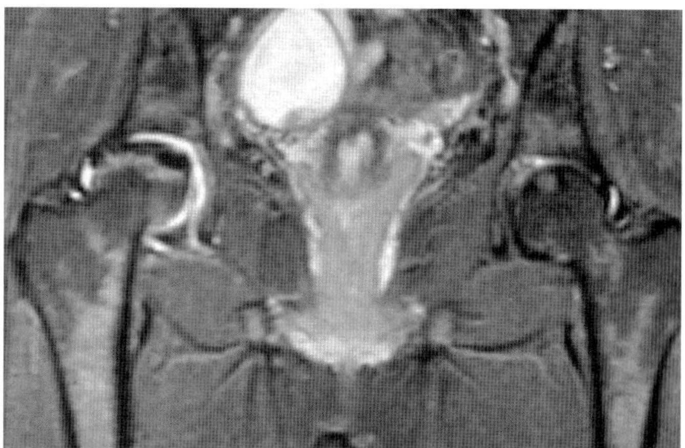

Figure 49.5 MRI scan showing avascular necrosis of the right hip.

Extension of the hips is rarely estimated but can be done so easily with the patient prone (normal range 0–30°). Movements in the coronal plane can be determined by moving the leg first into abduction (0–40°), then adduction (0–25°), while steadying the pelvis with the left hand on the opposite anterior superior iliac spine. The presence of fixed deformities in the coronal plane would have been identified while determining leg lengths. Rotation is measured by cupping both heels from the end of the couch and asking the patient to turn their feet in and out, while watching the patellae. Normal range of internal rotation is 35° and external rotation 45° (Fig. 49.3).

IMAGING

The standard radiographic views provide sufficient information in the majority of patients. These consist of an anteroposterior view of the pelvis and a lateral view of the affected hip. A single anteroposterior view of the affected hip is *not* adequate, because it provides no information on leg length, fixed deformities, the lower lumbar spine, the sacrum and sacroiliac joints, or the presence of disease in the other hip. A 'shoot-through' lateral radiograph is taken with the patient supine, by flexing the other hip out of the beam and firing a horizontal beam through the groin to a vertical plate on the outer aspect of the hip. This view is vital to identify medial osteoarthritis and anterior femoral osteophytes, and to ensure adequate canal dimensions if arthroplasty is considered. The less satisfactory but quicker 'frog leg' lateral view is taken using a vertical beam, and the patient's hip flexed and externally rotated. Special acetabular views (Judet views) are vital to determine the configuration of an acetabular fracture, and are also helpful in estimating bone loss prior to acetabular revision surgery. For accurate assessment of pelvic ring displacement, pelvic inlet and outlet views should be obtained. The inlet view is taken by directing the beam 60° from the head to midpelvis, and demonstrates displacement of the hemipelvis.

Computerized tomography is complementary to and does not replace plain radiography in the management of pelvic and acetabular trauma and deformity. A CT scan can demonstrate loose bodies, tumours and sacroiliac joint problems as well as being useful for planning complex hip reconstructions and osteotomies (Fig. 49.4).

Magnetic resonance imaging can demonstrate avascular necrosis of the hip before changes on the plain films (Fig. 49.5) and, when combined with intra-articular gadolinium injection, shows tears of acetabular labrum. Bone scans using technetium-99m methylene diphosphonate are useful in the diagnosis of tumours, metabolic bone disease and infection but lack specificity when used to distinguish between septic and aseptic loosening in joint replacements.

SURGICAL APPROACHES TO THE HIP (Fig. 49.6)

Early approaches to the hip utilized planes between muscles: the anterior approach (Smith–Petersen) separates the interval between sartorius and tensor fascia lata; the anterolateral (Watson–Jones) that between the gluteus medius and tensor fascia lata; and the intermuscular intervals either side of adductor longus in the medial approaches (Ludloff). With the advent of arthroplasty, strategies were developed to overcome muscular obstructions to enable better visualization of the acetabulum. Some or all of the gluteus medius and minimus are detached in lateral approaches (Hardinge, transgluteal and modified Watson–Jones), and the gluteus maximus is split and short external rotators divided in posterior approaches (Southern and Kocher–Langenbeck). The uses, advantages and disadvantages of the various approaches to the hip are shown in Table 49.1.

Table 49.1 Surgical approaches to the hip

Approach	Indication	Advantages	Disadvantages
Lateral	Total hip replacement, hip hemiarthroplasty	Quick and easy, low incidence of dislocation	Greater blood loss, abductor dehiscence, prolonged limp
Posterior	Total hip replacement, posterior wall and column acetabular fractures	Abductors unmolested, extensile	Meticulous repair of capsule and external rotators required to prevent dislocations
Anterolateral	Open reduction displaced intracapsular hip fractures	Muscle separating approach	Not extensile
Anterior	Open reduction of developmental dysplasia of the hip, innominate osteotomy	Low rates of avascular necrosis	Abductor dehiscence, blood loss
Ilioinguinal	Anterior and both column acetabular fractures, periacetabular osteotomy	Excellent view of the inner side of pelvis	Femoral vessels at risk
Medial	Open reduction of developmental dysplasia of the hip	Allows bilateral surgery	Higher rates of avascular necrosis

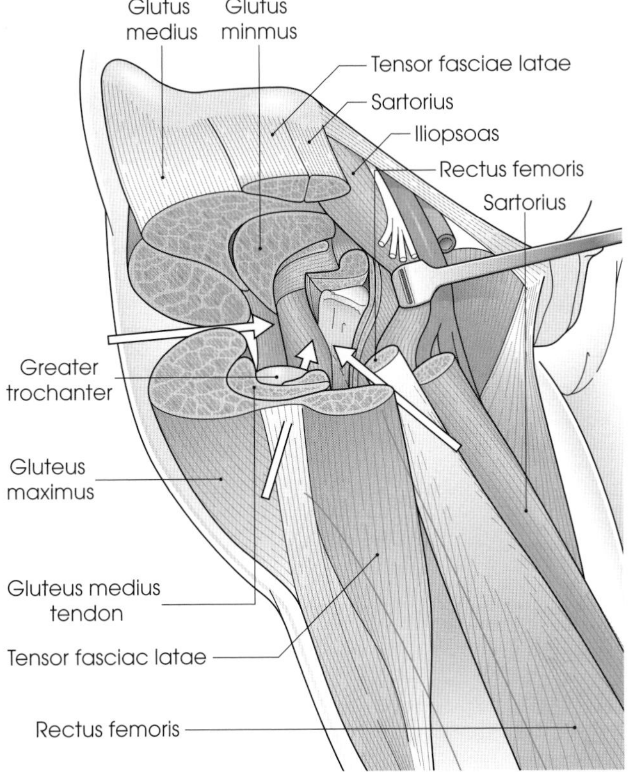

Figure 49.6 The intermuscular intervals used in the anterior, lateral and posterior approaches to the hip.

OSTEOARTHRITIS OF THE HIP

Osteoarthritis is the most common cause of pain and disability affecting the hip. The prevalence increases steadily with age, with radiographic changes present in 5% of subjects over 65. Osteoarthritis is a disease of articular cartilage (type II collagen), which undergoes progressive fibrillation and fragmentation with loss of chondrocytes until subchondral bone is exposed. Microfractures lead to formation of subchondral cysts. Synovitis and capsular thickening result from intra-articular debris. Attempts at healing with proliferation of fibroblasts and formation of fibrocartilage (type I collagen) may occur in the early stages. The degenerating cartilage has reduced strength and is therefore less able to withstand the loads placed on it during normal daily activities. Osteophytes form to protect the diseased cartilage by increasing the surface area available for load transfer. The cartilage changes in osteoarthritis are different from those of normal ageing.

Box 49.1 Causes of secondary osteoarthritis of the hip

Congenital
- Developmental dysplasia of the hip

Acquired
- Avascular necrosis (primary or secondary)
- Trauma (acetabular or femoral head fracture)
- Slipped upper femoral epiphysis
- Perthes' disease
- Paget's disease

Primary osteoarthritis describes the generalized predisposition to cartilage degeneration in previously normal joints, with age, and positive family history being risk factors. Primary hypertrophic osteoarthritis is a particular familial form, characterized by marked osteophyte formation in the lumbar spine, the thumb carpometacarpal joints, the hips, the first metatarsophalangeal joints and the distal interphalangeal joints of the hands. In contrast to osteoarthritis of the knee, obesity is not a risk factor. Secondary osteoarthritis occurs when normal cartilage degenerates in response to abnormal loading due to loss of the spherical congruency between ball and socket (Box 49.1). Careful examination of radiographs may show a cause for osteoarthritis in up to 40% of cases.[1] End-stage inflammatory, metabolic, haemorrhagic or infective arthritis will also produce very similar changes to osteoarthritis due to the destruction of the articular cartilage (Fig. 49.7).

TREATMENT OF HIP OSTEOARTHRITIS

Many patients, particularly in a primary care setting, are content with a clear diagnosis and education about the progression of the disease. Patients should be advised to keep as active as possible and reassured that this does not hasten the 'wear and tear' in the

REFERENCES

1. Harris WH. Clin Orthopaedics Relat Res 1986; 213: 20–33

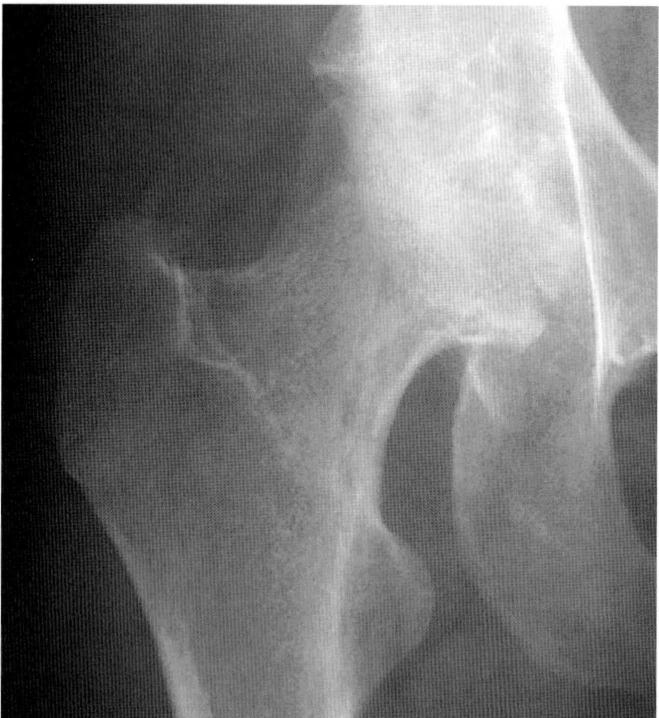

Figure 49.7 Cystic change in both femoral head and acetabulum and loss of joint space from pigmented villonodular synovitis (PVNS).

Table 49.2 Indications for total hip replacement

Indication	Details
Non-inflammatory arthritis	Primary osteoarthritis, secondary osteoarthritis, avascular necrosis
Inflammatory arthritis	Rheumatoid arthritis, juvenile chronic arthritis, systemic lupus erythematosus, spondyloarthropathy, crystal arthropathy
Infection	Old tuberculosis or septic arthritis
Haemorrhagic	Haemophilia, sickle cell disease, pigmented villo-nodular synovitis
Failed reconstruction	Fracture fixation, Girdlestone, hemiarthroplasty, osteotomy, arthrodesis
Tumour	–

joint. Weight loss and use of a walking stick in the contralateral hand reduce joint reaction force and relieve pain. Physiotherapy and hydrotherapy may also be useful. Analgesics form the mainstay of conservative treatment, although prolonged and excessive use of non-inflammatory anti-inflammatory drugs may increase the rate of collapse of the femoral head.

Total hip replacement surgery should be offered when conservative measures have failed and symptoms become severe enough to warrant major surgery, with its attendant small but significant risks. Unremitting pain, especially at night, and loss of mobility are the usual indications, although potential loss of livelihood or difficulty looking after young children may be indications in younger adults. Pain relief is the main indication for total hip replacement (Table 49.2) and, while it can be extremely effective at improving range of movement and correcting leg lengths and fixed deformities, these should not be the primary goals of surgery (Fig. 49.8). When osteoarthritis coexists in the hip and knee, surgical treatment of the hip takes priority.

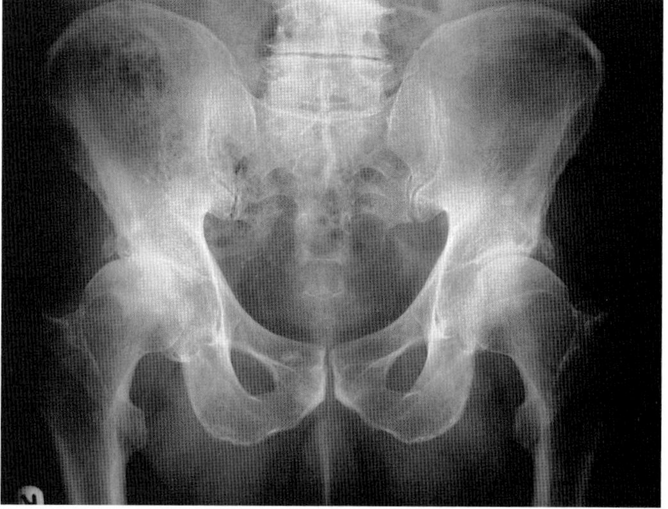

a

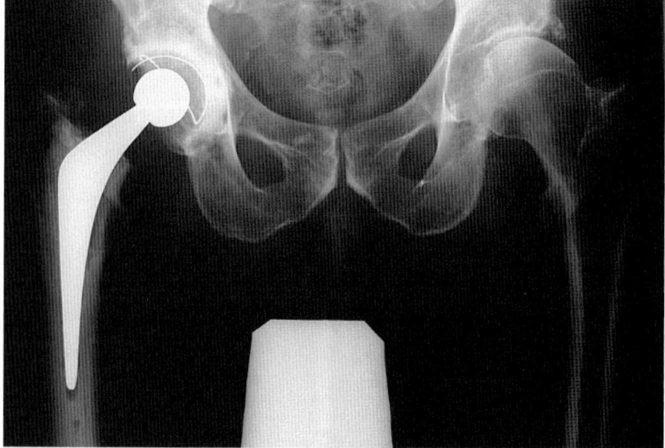

b

Figure 49.8 Primary osteoarthritis of the right hip. (a) Note loss of joint space, osteophytes and sclerosis. Cysts are not a big feature in this case. There is also degenerative change in the lumbar spine. (b) Treatment with a cemented total hip replacement.

TOTAL HIP REPLACEMENT

There were many unsuccessful attempts to invent a successful hip replacement before the advent of Sir John Charnley's low friction arthroplasty in 1962. This consisted of a socket of high-molecular-weight polyethylene articulating with a stainless steel head of 7/8" diameter. Acrylic bone cement was used to secure the implants to the host skeleton, and surgery was performed with meticulous aseptic technique in a clean-air enclosure. By these means he introduced one of the most consistently successful operations in any branch of surgery.

Such is the success of Charnley's implant that it still remains popular over 40 years later, with only minimal design modifications. Pain relief is predictable because the arthritic joint is removed, and careful positioning of implants can restore leg length. Enormous healthcare resources are required for the estimated 50 000 hip replacements performed in the UK annually. There are large numbers of designs of total hip replacement, but in general terms any joint replacement consists of a bearing surface, which allows the new joint to move, and some means of fixing the bearing surface to the host skeleton.[2]

THE BEARING SURFACE

Wear debris, primarily from the bearing surface, is responsible for aseptic loosening of hip replacements. Wear particles are constantly being produced in enormous numbers from prosthetic bearings, with approximately 38 000 submicron particles of ultra-high molecular weight polyethylene (UHMWPE) released per step. These particles exert their biological activity by being phagocytosed by macrophages, stimulating the release of soluble proinflammatory mediators, including cytokines and prostaglandins.[3] Mediators released near to bone cause osteolysis, which may lead to aseptic loosening and ultimate failure of the prosthesis by stimulating osteoclastic bone resorption and eroding bony support for the implant. Other sources of wear debris include abraded cement, metallic and host bone fragments.

The relationship between acetabular wear and aseptic loosening has been demonstrated in observational studies.[4,5] Higher rates of wear and loosening are found with large head diameters (32 mm or more), scratched femoral heads (particularly titanium), thin UHMWPE (8 mm or less),[6] and in younger patients. Excessive wear can easily be identified on radiographs and may lead to catastrophic failure if undiagnosed or neglected.

Despite problems with wear, metal-on-polyethylene still remains the gold standard bearing combination because of its track record and cost-effectiveness. Recognizing its limitations, Charnley limited his new operation to patients of retirement age who were not likely to outlive their implant. However, expanding indications for total hip replacement, particularly in younger, more active patients, have led to the search for alternative bearing surfaces. Ceramics are harder and smoother than metal, but are expensive, difficult to manufacture, and prone to fracture. Ceramic heads demonstrate lower wear rates when used with polyethylene[7] but still produce UHMWPE wear debris, albeit in smaller quantities. Ceramic-on-ceramic bearings wear very slowly, and what little wear debris that is produced is much less biologically active. Early problems with implant manufacture and fixation have been largely overcome and long-term results are awaited.

Wear-resistant UHMWPE has also been developed,[8] although previous efforts to improve this material have proved disastrous.[9] Improvement in manufacturing processes and materials have also led to a resurgence in metal-on-metal bearings, either with conventional head sizes or as part of hip resurfacing. Wear rates are very low, the particles do not stimulate macrophages, and the implants are self-polishing, although concern remains about the potential harmful effects of released metal particles.[10]

FIXATION OF THE BEARING SURFACES TO BONE

Cement

Polymethylmethacrylate (PMMA) bone cement achieves rapid and durable implant fixation. The doughy cement is created by mixing the liquid monomer with the powdered polymer, producing an exothermic reaction. Cement takes 5–15 min to harden, depending on manufacturer and ambient temperature. Optimal fixation is achieved by microinterlock of the cement into the trabecular bone. Contemporary cementing and technique therefore includes hypotensive anaesthesia, pulsed lavage, and adrenaline- (epinephrine-) or peroxide-soaked swabs to exclude blood and debris from the interface. Cement pressurization is achieved on the femoral side using a cement restrictor and cement gun, and on the acetabular side using a pressurizing device and flanged cup. An even cement mantle of at least 2 mm around both components is required to provide adequate strength and protect the bone around the implant from wear debris migrating from the bearing surface.

Biological (uncemented)

The impetus for cementless fixation of implants came predominantly from the USA due to delay in US Food and Drug Administration approval of bone cement, dissatisfaction with obtaining reproducible cement technique, and the once popular but erroneous belief that cement was the main cause of osteolysis.

Three criteria must be satisfied for successful bony incorporation of an implant. First there must be no movement between the bone and implant. On the acetabular side, this is achieved by reaming the acetabulum 1 or 2 mm less than the outer diameter of the shell to 'press-fit' the component. This relies on the elastic properties of bone for initial fixation. On the femoral side, stability is achieved with a combination of precise canal preparation and design features, such as a collar. Second, the host bone must be in intimate contact with the implant. Finally, the component must have some kind of bioactive surface that encourages host bone on-growth. The simplest of these is roughened, usually grit-blasted, titanium, although porous coatings of fine beads or mesh allow bone to actually grow into the surface of the implant. Coatings of hydroxyapatite, the mineral content of bone, speed up bony incorporation and allow on-growth to occur with slightly greater stem movement and gaps between the stem and host bone.

COMPLICATIONS OF TOTAL HIP REPLACEMENT

Hip replacement is performed to improve a patient's quality of life, and many patients look forward to their surgery, often having seen the effect of it on their friends and relatives. In the context of such high patient expectations, any major complication is a disaster.

REFERENCES

2. Learmonth ID (ed). Interfaces in Total Hip Arthroplasty. Springer-Verlag, Heidelberg, 1999
3. Archibeck MJ, Jacobs JJ, Roebuck KA et al. J Bone Joint Surg (Am) 2000; 82-A: 1478–1489
4. Dowd JE, Sychterz CJ, Young AM et al. J Bone Joint Surg (Am) 2000; 82-A: 1102–1107
5. Wroblewski BM, Siney PD. Clin Orthopedics Relat Res 1993; 292: 191–201
6. Morrey BF, Ilstrup D. J Bone Joint Surg (Am) 1989; 71-A: 50–55
7. Wroblewski BM, Siney PD, Dowson D et al. J Bone Joint Surg (Br) 1996; 78-B: 280–285
8. Muratoglu O, Bragdon C, O'Connor D et al. J Arthroplasty 2001; 16 (Suppl): 24–30
9. Livingston BJ, Chmell MJ, Poss R. J Bone Joint Surg (Am) 1997; 79-A: 1529–1538
10. Sieber HP, Rieker CB, Kottig P. J Bone Joint Surg (Br) 1999; 81-B: 46–50

Intraoperative complications

Blood loss

With modern techniques, average blood loss during a standard total hip replacement should be less than 500 mL, having previously been 900–1800 mL. Hypotension, usually provided by epidural or spinal anaesthesia, provides a clear operative field and allows efficient surgery. Allogeneic blood transfusion is expensive and not without its risks,[11] and often oral iron therapy, which allows the haemoglobin to rise 2 g/dL every 3 weeks, is all that is required. Blood loss is increased with the longer operating times encountered in obese patients, and complex primary and revision surgery. Preoperative blood donation and salvage of the patient's own blood with cell savers and reinfusion drains can dramatically reduce transfusion requirements in this group. The role of human recombinant erythropoietin therapy has yet to be defined.[12]

Component malposition

The optimum implant positions are 45° of abduction and 10–25° of anteversion for the cup, and 10–20° anteversion for the stem. Deviations from this lead to instability, because the neck of the femoral component is more likely to impinge on the edge of the cup during normal activities, levering the head out. It is vital that the patient is set up on the operating table with the pelvis held firmly and adequate surgical exposure obtained to avoid malposition. Leg length is determined by the depth of insertion of the stem and length of the neck of the modular head. Too short and there may be inadequate tension in the muscles to prevent dislocation, whereas lengthening produces great dissatisfaction, particularly in women.

Periprosthetic fracture

With the use of cemented stems, the incidence of intraoperative fracture in primary arthroplasty has been reported to be less than 1%. With cementless implants, intraoperative fracture has been reported to occur in 3–20%. Regardless of whether the implant is cemented or cementless, there is a markedly increased incidence of fracture in revision arthroplasty, with rates as high as 6.3% in cemented revisions and 17.6% with cementless implants.[13]

Neurovascular injury

The incidence of nerve palsy after primary total hip replacement ranges from 0 to 3%, and from 3 to 8% after revision surgery. The sciatic nerve is the most vulnerable, but the femoral, superior gluteal and obturator nerves are also at risk. Nerve injuries are usually in continuity and result from excessive lengthening (greater than 4 cm), injudicious use of retractors, compression by wound haematoma, or rarely thermal injury from cement.

Cement complications

Hypotension induced by pressurization of cement in the femur and insertion of the stem is not uncommon during total hip replacement. While the cement monomer was initially implicated, embolization of marrow contents into the pulmonary capillaries is now known to be the cause. The anaesthetist must therefore always be warned whenever cement is inserted. Cement hardening in the femur before the stem has been inserted far enough is a disaster. It is more likely with inexperienced staff, an unfamiliar brand of cement, and warm operating theatres. Because the cement has usually obtained an excellent bond with the bone, on-table revision is challenging. For those without adequate expertise or implants available, it is safer to remove the stem and return to the problem another day.

Anaesthetic complications

Anaesthetic complications are covered in Chapter 5.

Early complications

Wound problems

Wound haematomas are more common in obese patients and those on anticoagulants. They should be evacuated promptly to reduce the risks of superadded infection. Suction drains seem to make little difference to the incidence of wound complications.[14] While serious infections superficial to the fascia lata can occur, this diagnosis should be made only after exploration of the hip. If an early deep infection is encountered it should be treated with radical debridement, exchange of modular bearing surfaces, and intravenous antibiotics for 4–6 weeks. This technique gives success rates of 50–70% provided it is performed within 4 weeks of the original total hip replacement.[15]

Thromboembolic disease

Thromboembolic disease is the commonest reason for emergency readmission to hospital after total hip replacement,[16] with pulmonary embolism responsible for 68% of deaths in patients with total joint replacements.[17,18] Despite these alarming statistics, the role of thromboprophylaxis in lower limb joint replacement is a controversial area in orthopaedic surgery.[19] This is because the majority of cases of deep vein thrombosis are asymptomatic, and fatal pulmonary embolism after lower limb arthroplasty is rare. Without prophylaxis the approximate incidence of radiological deep vein thrombosis is 20–40%, clinical deep vein thrombosis 1–3%, symptomatic pulmonary embolism 1%, and fatal pulmonary embolism 0.3%.[19]

With the current evidence, a reasonable approach would be to stop use of oral contraceptives or hormone replacement therapy at least 6 weeks before surgery. Physical methods reduce risk without bleeding complications, and so patients should be mobilized early and encouraged to exercise in bed. Knee-length elastic stockings should be worn for at least 6 weeks after surgery, and use made in hospital of additional intermittent mechanical compression devices if available. The most effective chemical agents are the low-molecular-weight heparins and adjusted-dose warfarin, which reduce the incidence of deep vein thrombosis by 40–60%. Once-daily low-molecular-weight heparin is given while

REFERENCES

11. Mortimer P. Br Med J 2002; 325: 400–401
12. Mears DC, Durbhakula SM, Miller B. Orthopedics 1999; 22 (Suppl): S151–S154
13. Garbuz DS, Masri BA, Duncan CP. Instructional Course Lectures 1998; 47: 237–242
14. Ritter MA, Keating EM, Faris PM. J Bone Joint Surg (Am) 1994; 76-A: 35–38
15. Tsukayama DT, Estrada R, Gustilo RB. J Bone Joint Surg (Am) 1996; 78-A: 512–523
16. Seagroatt V, Tan HS, Goldacre M et al. Br Med J 1991; 303: 1431–1435
17. Wolf LD, Hozack WJ, Rothman RH. Clin Orthopaedics Relat Res 1993; 288: 219–233
18. Clagett GP, Anderson FA Jr, Heit J et al. Chest 1995; 108 (Suppl): 312S–334S
19. Thomas DP, Amstutz HC, Gillespie W et al. J Bone Joint Surg (Br) 2000; 82-B: 469–485

in hospital, although there is increasing evidence that prolonging prophylaxis after discharge reduces thromboembolic disease further.[20] Patients with a previous history of deep vein thrombosis should be fully anticoagulated for at least 3 months after hip replacement.

Dislocation

Surgical approach for total hip replacement influences dislocation, with rates of 4–9.5% reported for the posterior approach, compared with less than 2% for anterolateral, transgluteal or transtrochanteric approaches.[21] However, meticulous transosseous repair of the capsule and short external rotators dramatically reduces the dislocation rate from 5% to almost zero and is therefore mandatory when a posterior approach is used.[22,23] Other factors include component malposition, prosthetic design, inadequate soft tissue tension, neuromuscular disease (e.g. Parkinson's disease) and poor patient compliance. Hip replacements are unstable in extreme flexion, adduction and extremes of rotation. Patients are therefore instructed to avoid low chairs, bending over, crossing their legs, and sleeping on the side of the non-operated leg (operated side adducts), and to use a raised toilet seat for at least 6 weeks while scar tissue forms and muscles regain their attachments. Early dislocations are often isolated and can be treated by closed reduction, ideally under general anaesthesia, followed by bracing for 6 weeks.

Systemic complications

Total hip replacement is often performed on elderly patients with pre-existing medical conditions, and adequate preoperative assessment and optimization of medical management is vital. Urinary retention, pulmonary and cardiac complications are not uncommon after total hip replacement, with a low incidence of paralytic ileus, colonic pseudo-obstruction and gastrointestinal bleeding. Thirty-day mortality after primary total hip replacement is between 0.15 and 0.5%, with risk factors being an older age, male sex and cardiorespiratory disease. There has been a decrease in mortality over the last decade.[24]

Late complications

Heterotopic ossification

Heterotopic ossification is the formation of bone tissue within what are normally soft tissues as a result of metaplasia of fibroblasts into osteoblasts. Usually its presence is no more than an incidental finding on postoperative radiographs but, when severe, it can cause marked loss of movement. Risk factors are hypertrophic osteoarthritis, ankylosing spondylitis, male sex, a past history of heterotopic ossification after previous total hip replacement, and previous trauma to the hip (e.g. acetabular fracture). These patients should receive prophylaxis with either a 2-week course of indometacin (indomethacin) prior to surgery or a single dose of radiation therapy (500–700 cGy). Once formed, severe heterotopic ossification is difficult to treat due to risk of recurrence. Resection of heterotopic ossification should be delayed at least 12 months until the bone matures, as confirmed by minimal uptake on a bone scan, followed by prophylaxis.

Deep infection

Deep infection of a hip replacement is a catastrophe, which results in poor functional outcome, lengthy treatment, further surgery and expense. Measures that should always be taken to prevent infection are shown in Box 49.2.

Box 49.2 Measures to prevent infection in total hip replacement

- Careful patient selection: treat any potential source of infection prior to total hip replacement (e.g. urinary tract infection, ulcers, dental abscesses).
- Laminar airflow operating theatres.
- Meticulous aseptic technique.
- Prophylactic antibiotics: three doses of intravenous antibiotic starting on induction.
- Antibiotic-loaded bone cement: usually gentamicin.
- Avoidance of urethral catheterization: antibiotic cover on insertion and removal if catheter necessary.
- Aggressive management of haematoma.
- Meticulous wound care.

While the diagnosis of early deep infection is usually obvious, the more common indolent, delayed deep infection manifesting at least 6 months after surgery can be much harder to diagnose. Patients often describe pain from the time of the operation, often reporting that the hip replacement has 'never been right'. There may be a history of wound infection or infection elsewhere, and radiographs may show signs of early loosening.

While almost any organism can cause infection in total hip replacement, the commonest organisms are *Staphylococcus aureus* (30–60%) and *S. epidermidis* (20–30%), both of which may be difficult to culture and treat with antibiotics because of their slime-forming properties. If infection is suspected, the worst thing to do is to start antibiotics empirically; isolation of the organism is critical for success. The most useful initial investigations are the erythrocyte sedimentation rate and C-reactive protein level. If the erythrocyte sedimentation rate is below 30 mm/h and the C-reactive protein below 10 mg/L infection is effectively excluded, whereas if they are both above these values the chance of infection is greater than 80%.[25] Hip aspiration may detect an organism and allows appropriate antibiotics to be given as soon as samples are taken when removing the infected implant. Radionuclide bone scans should not be performed because they lack specificity and obtaining them delays treatment. If in doubt, assume infection.

Most infected arthroplasties are treated with a two-stage revision. In the first stage, the implant is removed and thorough debridement performed, with numerous samples taken for culture and histology. Antibiotic-loaded bone cement is then placed in the acetabulum and femoral shaft to increase local delivery. The patient then receives at least 6 weeks of antibiotic therapy, adjusted to the operative cultures, and the patient's C-reactive protein and erythrocyte sedimentation rate are monitored regularly. Implants are reinserted at the second stage,

REFERENCES

20. Planès A, Vochelle N, Darmon J-Y et al. Lancet 1996; 348: 224–228
21. Woo RY, Morrey BF. J Bone Joint Surg (Am) 1982; 64-A: 1295
22. Sioen W, Simon JP, Labey L et al. J Bone Joint Surg (Am) 2002; 84-A: 1793–1798
23. Pellicci PM, Bostrom M, Poss R. Clin Orthopedics Relat Res 1998; 355: 224–228
24. Parvizi J, Johnson BG, Rowland C et al. J Bone Joint Surg (Am) 2001; 83: 1524–1528
25. Spangehl MJ, Masri BA, O'Connell JX et al. J Bone Joint Surg (Am) 1999; 81-A: 672–683

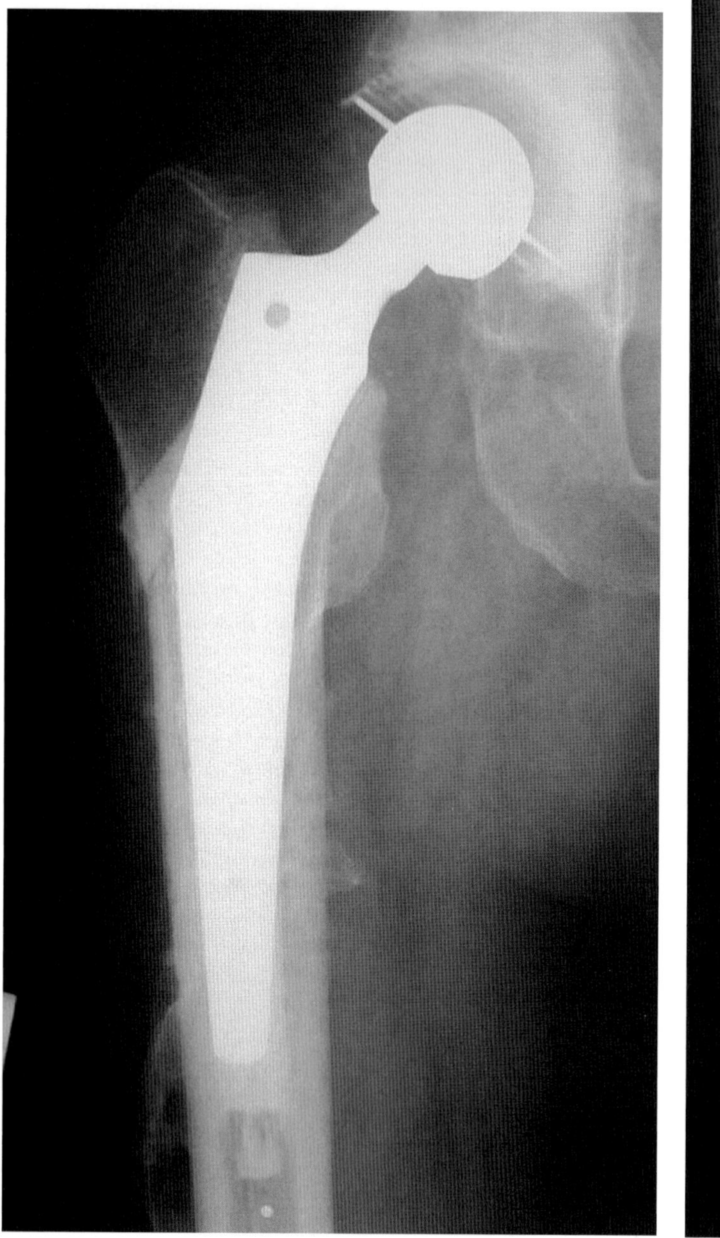
a

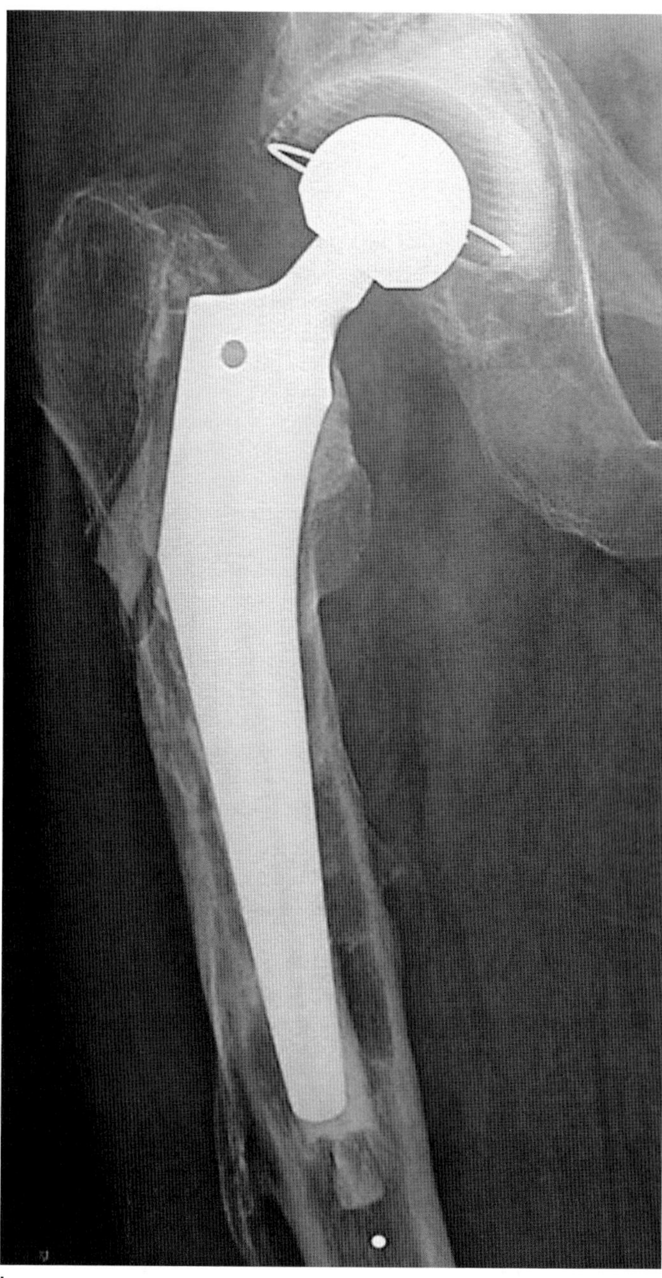
b

Figure 49.9 Loose femoral component. (**a**) Immediate postoperative radiograph of cemented THR inserted for non-union of a femoral neck fracture. (**b**) Eight years later the stem has debonded from the cement and subsided 10 mm. There is marked osteolysis of the proximal femur.

when the patient is well, the soft tissues have healed, and the inflammatory markers are normal. This can take anything from 6 weeks to a year. Two-stage revision should cure 80–90% of deep infections but at a high cost to the patient and health services. Patients who are too elderly or infirm to tolerate major surgery may be managed by permanent excision of the components or long-term suppressive antibiotics.

Loosening and wear

While a minority of implants fail because of sepsis, 80% of failures are due to aseptic loosening resulting from bioactive wear debris. About 1% fail each year, and thus by 10 years postoperatively 10% will have required revision surgery. The usual presentation of loosening is renewed pain in a previously painless arthroplasty, with progressive limb shortening, dislocation, and periprosthetic fracture indicating catastrophic failure. Aseptic loosening, particularly of the acetabular component, may be asymptomatic. Signs of loosening are usually easily diagnosed on plain radiographs, particularly if old films are available for comparison: component migration, component fracture, cement fracture, and circumferential radiolucent lines at the cement bone interface of greater than 2 mm indicate loosening (Fig. 49.9).[26,27] Excessive

REFERENCES

26. Hodgkinson JP, Shelley P, Wroblewski BM. Clin Orthopaedics Relat Res 1988; 228: 105–109
27. Harris WH, McCarthy JC, O'Neill DA. J Bone Joint Surg (Am) 1982; 64-A: 1063–1067

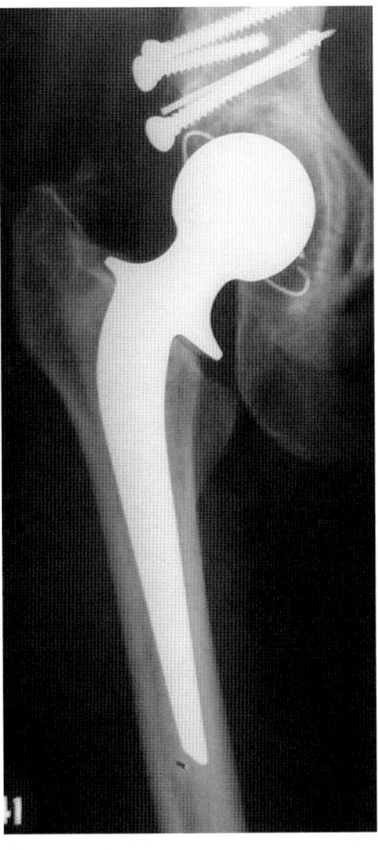
a

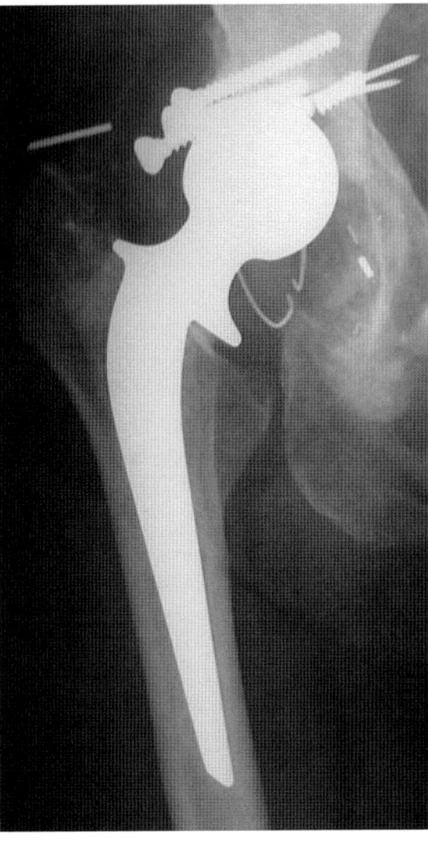
b

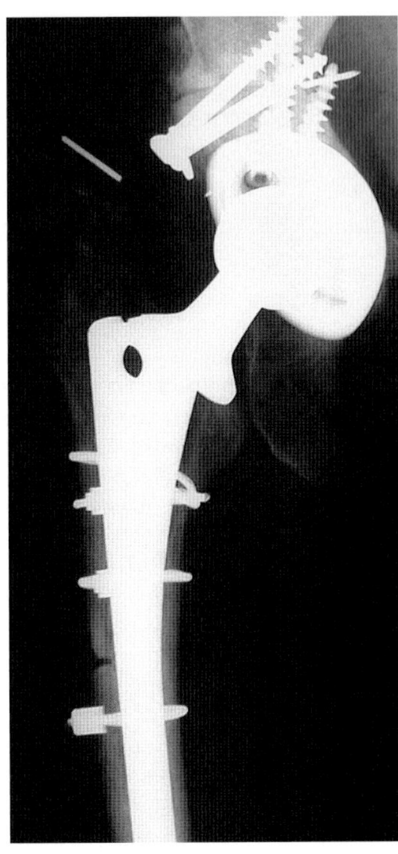
c

Figure 49.10 Loose and worn acetabular component. (**a**) Seven years after cemented THR with acetabular bone graft for secondary OA due to DDH; wear of the cup is already apparent. (**b**) Ten years later the cup has completely worn through and the head is articulating with the screws. (**c**) Following revision using uncemented components, bone graft and extended trochanteric osteotomy to aid cement removal. Note restoration of leg length.

cup wear is often associated and easily seen (Saturn is no longer in the centre of its rings) (Fig. 49.10). Osteolysis may coexist with solidly fixed uncemented components. Management consists of excluding infection and revision surgery. Loose implants produce large amounts of wear debris and can cause rapid loss of surrounding bone, thereby compromising the result of future revision. The timing of revision surgery is therefore critical, and patients with minor symptoms must be followed up closely with sequential radiographs. Many patients with a loose hip replacement are very elderly and unfit for this magnitude of surgery, and it may be judged that the risks outweigh the benefits.

Dislocation

Late dislocation occurs most commonly when the femoral head has migrated into the acetabulum because of wear, thereby increasing the risk of impingement of the neck on the acetabular rim. Dislocation can also occur as a consequence of trauma.

Periprosthetic fracture

Late periprosthetic fractures are almost always the result of wear debris-induced osteolysis, with the minority resulting from major trauma. While routine radiological review should identify these lesions prior to fracture, the cumulative postoperative risk is only 2.5% at 15 years.[28] Treatment of these challenging cases is surgical; if the stem is loose, long-stemmed revision is performed, and if it is well fixed, the fracture is fixed with a plate and cortical strut grafts.[13]

RESULTS OF TOTAL HIP REPLACEMENT

Excellent long-term results have been published for cemented total hip replacement,[29] and these have been approached in the medium term by some hybrid (cemented stem and uncemented cup)[30] and uncemented designs.[31] In addition, two-thirds of patients die with their original prosthesis in situ,[29,32] making revision surgery necessary in only a small minority. However, results are less satisfactory for younger patients, with survivorship of 56% for the cup and 81% for the stem at 25 years for patients receiving Charnley total hip replacements at a mean age of 32 years.[33] In addition, published results from specialist centres may not be applicable to all hospitals and surgeons; results from the Trent Regional Arthroplasty Register showed that 5.5% of

REFERENCES

28. Lowenhielm G, Hansson LI, Karrholm J. Arch Orthopaedic Trauma Surg 1989; 108: 141–143
29. Schulte KR, Callaghan JJ, Kelley SS et al. J Bone Joint Surg 1993; 77-A: 961–974
30. Smith SE, Harris WH. J Bone Joint Surg 1997; 79-A: 1827–1833
31. Engh CA, Culpepper WJ, Engh CA. J Bone Joint Surg 1997; 79-A: 177–184
32. Madey SM, Callaghan JJ, Olejniczak JP et al. J Bone Joint Surg 1997; 79-A: 53–64
33. Sochart DH, Porter ML. J Bone Joint Surg 1997; 79-A: 1599–1617

Box 49.3 Indications for revision surgery

- Loosening: aseptic, septic
- Osteolysis in presence of stable component
- Wear
- Instability
- Fracture
- Accompanying revision of other component: instability, component mismatch, known poorly performing design

Charnley total hip replacements were loose or revised at 5 years.[34] Improvement of these results, particularly in younger patients, and the need for manufacturers to maintain their market share has led to many innovations and design modifications, some of which have been disastrous.[35] It is also not unusual for an implant with a proven track record to be no longer available.[36]

REVISION TOTAL HIP REPLACEMENT

The aims of revision surgery are to obtain stable fixation of component to host bone with, ideally, restoration of leg lengths and the hip centre to normal. Restoration of bone stock for the future is a secondary aim. Indications for revision surgery are shown in Box 49.3. Bone loss from the loosening process characterizes revision surgery and influences its results; the more bone remaining after removing the old implants, the less complex the surgery and the more likely long-term fixation of new implants can be obtained. Preoperative assessment of bone stock is vital to ensure that adequate supplies of bone graft or special implants are available if complex reconstructions are necessary.

Revision surgery is a much greater undertaking for both patient and surgeon. Not only are the patients older and less fit, but surgery involves a wider exposure of a previously operated hip and removal of the old implants and cement, being careful not to damage the remaining bone. Blood loss can be substantial, particularly during lengthy surgery to the femur.

Many different implants are available for revision surgery. The only technique that consistently gives poor results is simple cemented revision (without bone graft) of acetabular and short-stemmed femoral components. This is because reliance is placed on the bone already damaged by the loosening process. On the acetabular side, cementless porous coated cups provide the most reliable technique provided there is a supportive rim and at least 50% contact between host bone and the cup. For larger defects, bone graft and reconstruction rings are necessary. On the femoral side, the stem is fixed to the healthy bone below the original stem using a longer stem, with or without cement. Impaction allografting is a demanding technique for both femoral and acetabular revision dependent on the supply of large amounts of allograft. Defects in the host bone are filled with closely packed allograft chips, and cemented components inserted. Results of this technique in some hands are similar to uncemented revision surgery, although all authors have not replicated the results of this difficult technique.[37]

ALTERNATIVE SURGICAL TREATMENTS FOR OSTEOARTHRITIS OF THE HIP

Hip resurfacing

The concept of hip resurfacing is not new, but has undergone a renaissance with the advent of metal-on-metal bearings.[38] Earlier, unsuccessful, designs used conventional metal-on-polyethylene bearings, which wore and loosened very quickly due to the combination of a large head and thin polyethylene. Modern metal-on-metal bearings are much harder and are manufactured to trap a layer of fluid between the bearing surfaces, thereby reducing friction and wear to a minimum. Resurfacing accurately restores patient's anatomy, has very low rates of dislocation, and preserves bone stock for future revision surgery (Fig. 49.11). The technique involves a wider surgical exposure so that the head may be displaced to allow access to the acetabulum. In addition, patients should have good bone stock and a relatively normal hip morphology to support the implant. The technique is not recommended for postmenopausal women due to the risk of femoral neck fracture (0.5%). Midterm results are extremely promising, although resurfacing implants must be regarded as experimental until much wider experience is available.

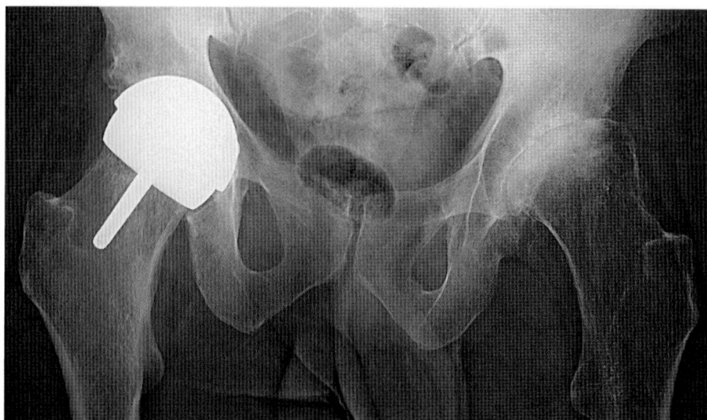

Figure 49.11 Hip resurfacing performed for bilateral OA secondary to acetabular dysplasia in a very tall 47-year-old man with Charcot–Marie–Tooth disease

Femoral osteotomy

Realignment of the proximal femur was commonly performed for osteoarthritis before the advent of total hip arthroplasty. With the advent of modern bearing surfaces and resurfacing, the demand for joint-preserving surgery, even in young adults, has declined even further. Depending on the precise pattern of arthritis and the location of osteophytes, femoral osteotomy may be effective by reducing forces through the hip joint and increasing the joint surface area by rotating osteophytes into the weight-bearing zone. With careful patient selection, the rate of conversion to total hip replacement may be less than 40% after 12 years.[39]

Hip arthrodesis

Fusion of the hip is an extremely effective means of relieving pain but, like osteotomy, has become even less popular. Patients are

REFERENCES

34. Fender D, Harper WM, Gregg PJ. J Bone Joint Surgery (Br) 1999; 81-B: 577–581
35. Muirhead-Allwood SK. Br Med J 1998; 316: 644
36. Murray DW, Carr AJ, Bulstrode CJK. J Bone Joint Surg 1995; 77-B: 520–527
37. Leopold SS, Rosenberg AG. J Bone Joint Surg (Am) 1999; 81-A: 1337–1345
38. McMinn D, Treacy R, Lin K et al. Clin Orthopaedics Relat Res 1996 (Suppl): S89–S98
39. D'Souza SR, Sadiq S, New AMR et al. J Bone Joint Surg (Am) 1998; 80-A: 1428–1438

increasingly unwilling to accept a fused hip, not only in terms of functional limitation but also because of the long-term effects on the lumbar spine, which often becomes painful and degenerate after many years of compensating for loss of hip movements. Despite this, fusion may be the only option in children and adolescents and, provided a method of fusion is used that preserves the abductors, conversion to total hip replacement is possible in the future.[40,41]

Hip arthroscopy

The hip is much less accessible to arthroscopic instruments than the knee or the shoulder, requiring traction and an image intensifier to enter the joint reliably. However, it is a useful technique to diagnose causes of hip pain and can be used therapeutically to debride arthritis and labral tears, to retrieve loose bodies, and to perform biopsy or synovectomy.[42]

AVASCULAR NECROSIS OF THE FEMORAL HEAD

Avascular necrosis, also known as osteonecrosis or aseptic necrosis, results from occlusion of the microcirculation of the femoral head with subsequent ischaemia and osteocyte death. This leads to loss of structural integrity of the bone supporting the articular cartilage, with subsequent collapse of the avascular segment. The resulting deformation of the femoral head is a potent cause of secondary osteoarthritis. The microcirculation may be directly injured (following trauma), occluded from within (sickle cell disease, dysbarism and fat emboli with steroids and alcohol), or compressed from outside (Box 49.4).

Avascular necrosis first presents as a deep pain in the groin, usually associated with a risk factor. Hip movements are painful but may not be limited until late in the disease. Radiographs, including a lateral view of the femoral head, are essential and show changes dependent on the progress of the disease. However, MRI is a more sensitive diagnostic tool and also clearly shows the extent of femoral head involvement. Therefore if radiographs are normal, further investigation with MRI is essential. Imaging allows the disease to be staged, predominantly on the extent of collapse and size of the involved avascular segment. There is always a lag between the vascular insult and the appearance of imaging abnormalities. The University of Pennsylvania system is recommended and summarized in Table 49.3.[43] Studies consistently show that the results of treatment deteriorate as the disease becomes more advanced, in particular in the presence of femoral head collapse (stage 3 disease shown in Fig. 49.12).[44] Early disease (stages 1 and 2) is treated with core decompression, in which the avascular segment is drilled from below to encourage healing and reduce intraosseous pressure. This may be combined with a structural bone graft to prevent collapse. Once the head has collapsed (stage 3 and 4), surgery to elevate the segment, or rotate the segment out of the weight-bearing zone with an osteotomy, produces unpredictable results. Total hip replacement is used to treat end-stage disease (Fig. 49.13).

Table 49.3 Criteria for staging avascular necrosis of the hip

Stage	Description
0	Clinical suspicion but normal or non-diagnostic radiograph, MRI, or bone scan
I	Normal radiograph, abnormal bone scan and/or MRI
II	Abnormal radiograph showing 'cystic' and sclerotic changes in the femoral head
III	Subchondral collapse producing a crescent sign
IV	Flattening of the femoral head
V	Joint narrowing with or without acetabular involvement
VI	Advanced degenerative changes

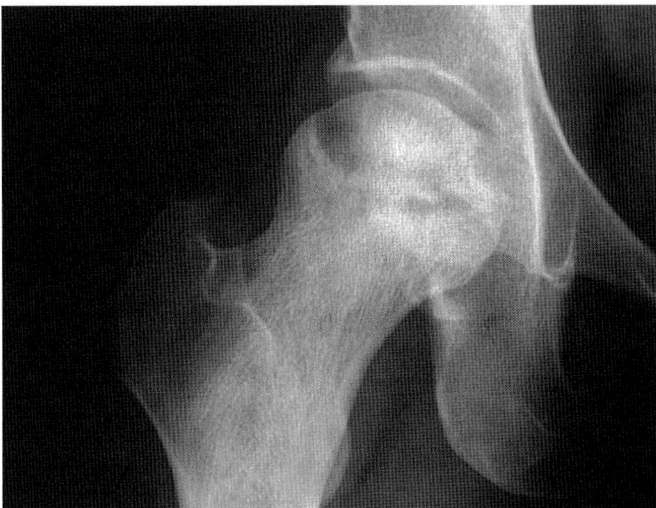

Figure 49.12 AVN of the right hip in sickle cell disease showing the characteristic involvement of the supero-lateral part of the head. The segment has collapsed making this stage III disease.

Box 49.4 Risk factors for avascular necrosis

Traumatic
- Intracapsular femoral neck fracture
- Hip dislocation
- Acetabular fracture

Atraumatic
- Alcohol
- Steroid therapy
- Sickle cell disease
- Exposure to high pressure (dysbarism, i.e. deep-sea divers, caisson disease)
- Radiation
- Pregnancy
- Gaucher's disease
- Hypercoagulable states

REFERENCES

40. Bankes MJK, Simmons J, Catterall A. J Pediatr Orthopædics (Am) 2002; 22: 101–104
41. Panagiotopoulos KP, Robbins GM, Masri BA et al. Instructional Course Lectures 2001; 50: 297–305
42. Baber YF, Robinson AHN, Villar RN. J Bone Joint Surg (Br) 1999; 81-B: 600–603
43. Steinberg ME, Hayken GD, Steinberg DR. J Bone Joint Surg (Br) 1995; 77: 34–41
44. Lieberman JR, Berry DJ, Mont MA et al. J Bone Joint Surg (Am) 2002; 84-A: 834–853

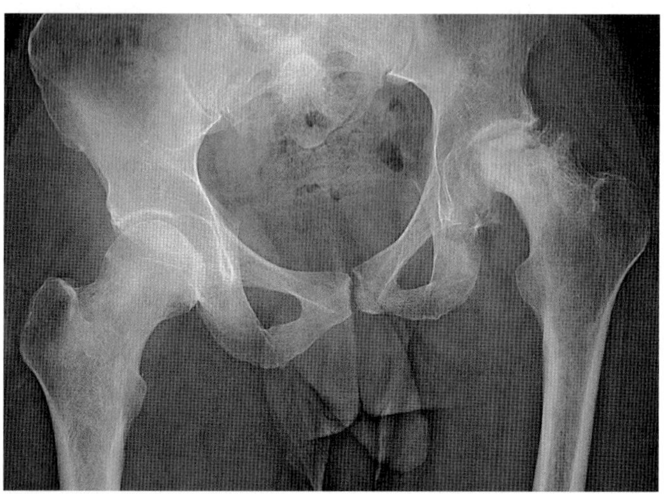

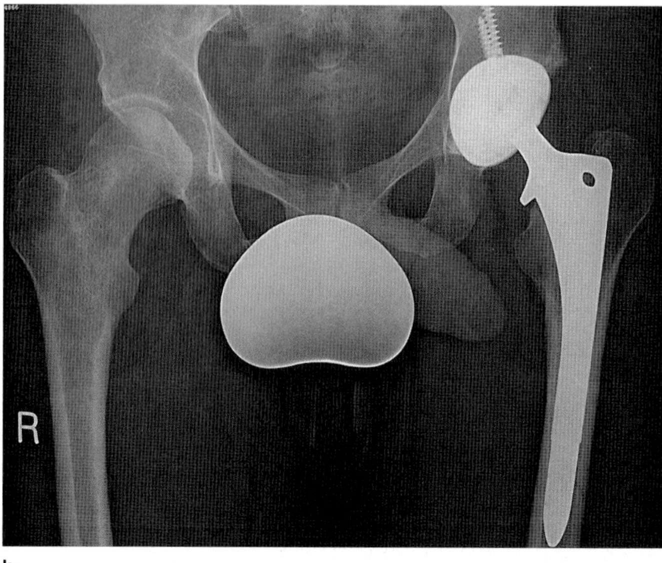

a b

Figure 49.13 End-stage AVN of the left hip (stage VI) in 35-year-old male with sickle cell disease. (**a**) Note pelvic tilt due to fixed adduction deformity. (**b**) Treatment with uncemented THR using ceramic on ceramic bearing.

INFECTIONS OF THE HIP

In adult practice, the majority of pyogenic hip infections result from surgery or intravenous drug abuse. However, infections may develop *de novo* in patients with sickle cell disease and immunosuppression from any cause, producing severe pain and often agonizing restriction of movement. Assiduous collection of microbiological samples, prompt surgical drainage, and at least 6 weeks of appropriate antibiotics are essential for success. Tuberculosis is increasing in prevalence and has a particular predilection for the hip. It may also characteristically affect the greater trochanter. Antituberculous chemotherapy is the mainstay for controlling the acute infection and may be reinstituted as prophylaxis if joint replacement is planned at a later stage.

ACETABULAR DYSPLASIA

Acetabular dysplasia is a term used to describe the shallow, upwardly sloping acetabulum that results from developmental dysplasia of the hip (previously known as congenital dislocation of the hip). An abnormally shaped acetabulum produces excessive loading through the hip joint, particularly at the superolateral margin of the acetabulum, leading to tears of the acetabular labrum, cyst formation, and early degeneration of the articular cartilage.

Developmental dysplasia of the hip produces a wide spectrum of disease, ranging from neonates with obvious hip instability to female patients developing osteoarthritis in their thirties and forties. Within this spectrum are young women in the second, third and fourth decades of life with shallow sockets that only come to light when their symptoms lead them to seek medical advice. The importance of diagnosing dysplasia in these women is that surgery is available in specialist centres to improve the mechanical environment of the hip and to delay the onset of arthritis for many years. It is not acceptable for these patients to be told to go away and wait until their symptoms are so bad that hip replacement is the only option.

In those known to have developmental dysplasia of the hip, acetabular dysplasia may still persist in the adult, despite advances in the management of infant developmental dysplasia of the hip. Dysplasia may also accompany neurological conditions such as cerebral palsy and hereditary motor and sensory neuropathy (Charcot–Marie–Tooth disease). Acetabular development may also be affected by childhood infections and Perthes' disease.

Clinical features and imaging studies[45]

Acetabular dysplasia presents in previously active young adults with vague anterior groin pain, which becomes sharp during activities that produce forced flexion of the hip, such as getting in and out of a car, and running down stairs. Patients fatigue easily and report a gradual reduction in their activity level, interfering with parental and work duties, and preventing sport. Some patients describe catching, locking or instability in the hip. Standard physical examination may reveal few physical signs.

A plain anteroposterior radiograph of the pelvis is usually diagnostic, although subtle dysplasia may easily be overlooked. Poor bone coverage at the front of the acetabulum can be demonstrated on the 'faux profil' view, which is effectively a true lateral radiograph of the acetabulum. Computerized tomography and magnetic resonance arthrography complete the imaging (Fig. 49.14).

Treatment

Surgical treatment aims to improve the surface area of femoral head covered by the acetabulum, thereby reducing the pressure on the articular cartilage. This usually involves major surgery to detach the acetabulum from the pelvic ring and reposition it more favourably (Steele's triple osteotomy or Ganz's periacetabular osteotomy). In some cases associated deformities on the femoral side need correction with an additional varus femoral

REFERENCES

45. Leunig M, Siebenrock KA, Ganz R. J Bone Joint Surg (Am) 2001; 83-A: 438–448

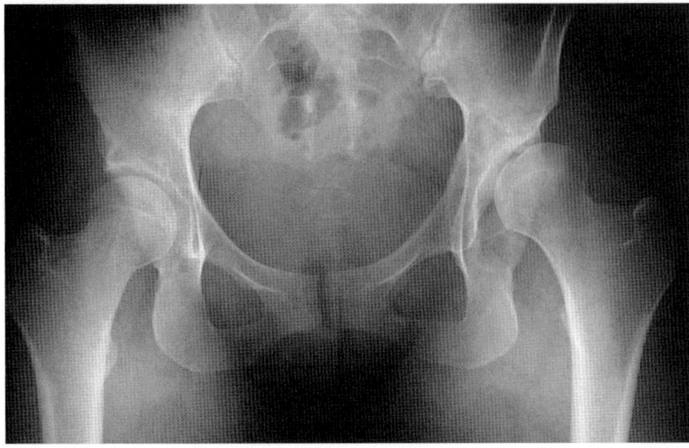

a

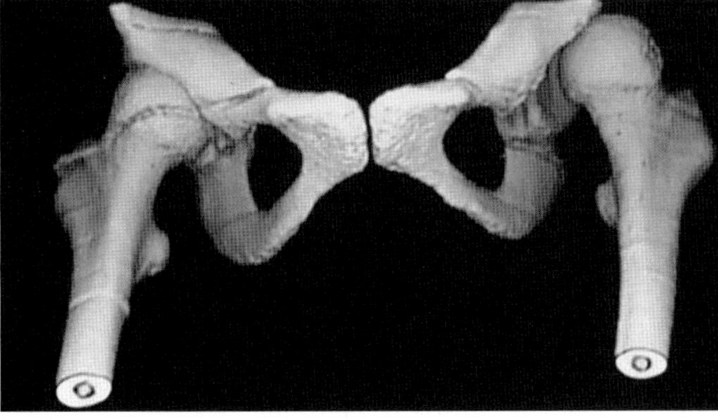

b

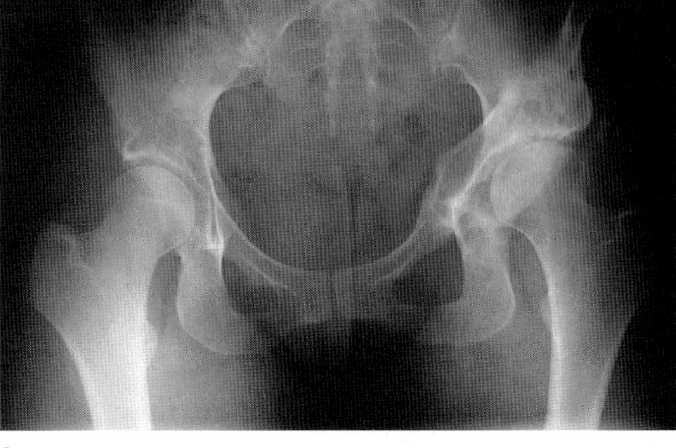

c

Figure 49.14 (**a**) Left acetabular dysplasia in 23-year-old female. (**b**) 3D CT scan showing subluxation and lack of anterior cover. (**c**) 3 years following correction by peri-acetabular osteotomy.

osteotomy. If realignment surgery is performed before arthritis has developed, at least 80% of hip joints will provide at least 10 years of good function.[46] However, the presence of degenerative change in the hip adversely affects the long-term results of this type of surgery, making hip replacement the only effective option.

DISORDERS OF THE SACROILIAC JOINTS AND SYMPHYSIS PUBIS

Despite modern methods of treatment, traumatic disruption of the pelvic ring often leads to persisting symptoms from its joints. Pregnancy and childbirth is a common cause of symphysis pain due to hormonally induced ligament relaxation and presence of the fetus. Symptoms usually resolve soon after delivery but may persist for many months. Treatment is with explanation, reassurance and physiotherapy. Instability of the symphysis can also result from the repetitive trauma of contact sports. Abnormal movement at the symphysis may be demonstrated with 'flamingo' views, in which the relationship of the pubic bones is compared between views taken first standing on one leg and then standing on the other. Surgical fusion of the symphysis should be contemplated only after at least a year of conservative treatment.[47] Ankylosis of the sacroiliac joints is a typical finding in ankylosing spondylitis and should be considered in young men with back pain.

REFERENCES

46. Siebenrock KA, Leunig M, Ganz R. J Bone Joint Surg (Am) 2001; 83-A: 449–455
47. Williams PR, Thomas DP, Downes EM. Am J Sports Med 2000; 28: 350–355

The knee

50

Peter H. Earnshaw

INTRODUCTION

The knee is the largest synovial joint and is also one of the most complex. The functional demands placed on it are enormous, and it is hardly surprising that it is one of the most frequently injured joints. Degenerative problems are common, and the knee is now overtaking the hip as the most commonly replaced joint.

BASIC ANATOMY

The structures of the knee can be placed in three broad categories:

- the osseous structures,
- the extra-articular structures, and
- the intra-articular structures.

OSSEOUS STRUCTURES AND THE MECHANICAL AXIS

The articular structures of the femur, tibia and patella make up the knee joint. The knee is a hinge joint but a very complex one. New techniques, including dynamic MRI scanning, have altered our understanding of knee function in the normal and pathological joint. In addition to flexion and extension, significant rotatory movement is present, with typically a range of 20°. There are also a complex series of translational movements that combine backwards rolling and sliding movements as the knee flexes. These affect mainly the lateral compartment, the medial side having only limited anteroposterior movement. The knee is described as having six degrees of freedom around three axes of rotation (Fig. 50.1).

The knee has both anatomical and mechanical axes. The anatomical axis measurements of the lower limb show a tibiofemoral angle between 5 and 10° of valgus (somewhat higher in females). A line running through the centre of the hip, knee and ankle defines the mechanical axis, and any deviation from this axis is likely to be associated with progressive pathology or failed surgery (Fig. 50.2).

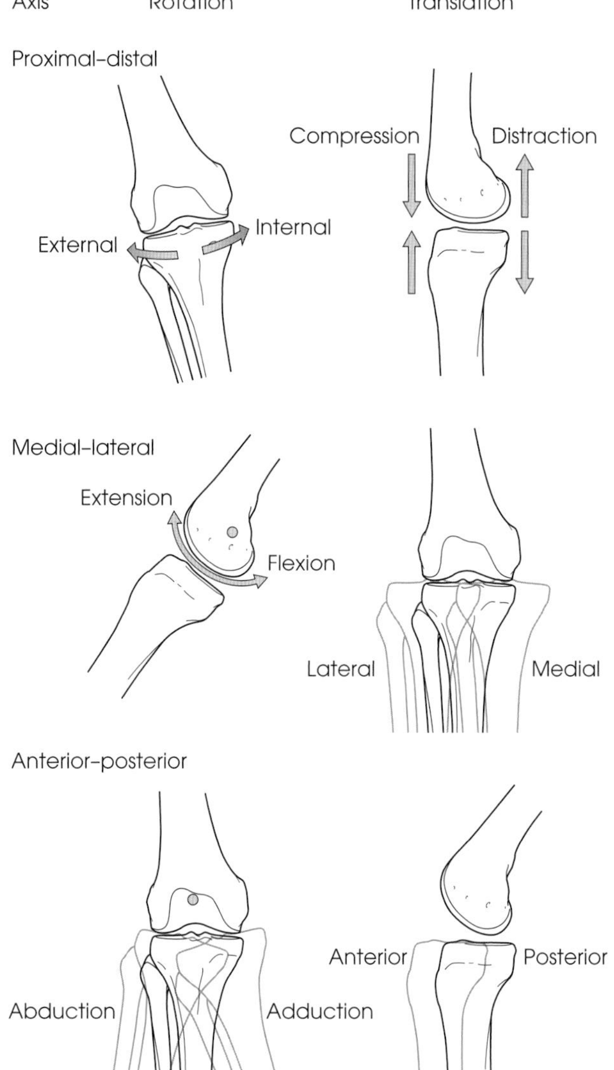

Figure 50.1 Translation and rotation around each of the three axes provide the six degrees of freedom that allow knee motion.

EXTRA-ARTICULAR STRUCTURES

The structures supporting and affecting knee function can be considered static or dynamic and include the collateral ligaments, the joint capsule and the musculotendinous structures. Of prime importance is the quadriceps mechanism, typically described as having three layers that insert into the patella. The gastrocnemius tendons are important structures posteriorly. The medial collateral ligament has a long, narrow, well-defined superficial element and a complex deeper layer reinforcing the posteromedial corner of the knee, involving elements of the capsule and reflected semimembranosus tendon. The pes anserinus (conjoined sartorius, gracilis and semitendinosus tendons) acts as a secondary stabilizer. Laterally, the collateral ligament (from the head of the fibula to the lateral epicondyle of the femur) is the prime stabilizer against varus stress, especially when the knee is in extension. Secondary lateral stabilizers include the capsule, iliotibial band, popliteus and biceps tendons.

INTRA-ARTICULAR STRUCTURES

Intra-articular structures include the anterior and posterior cruciate ligaments and the menisci.

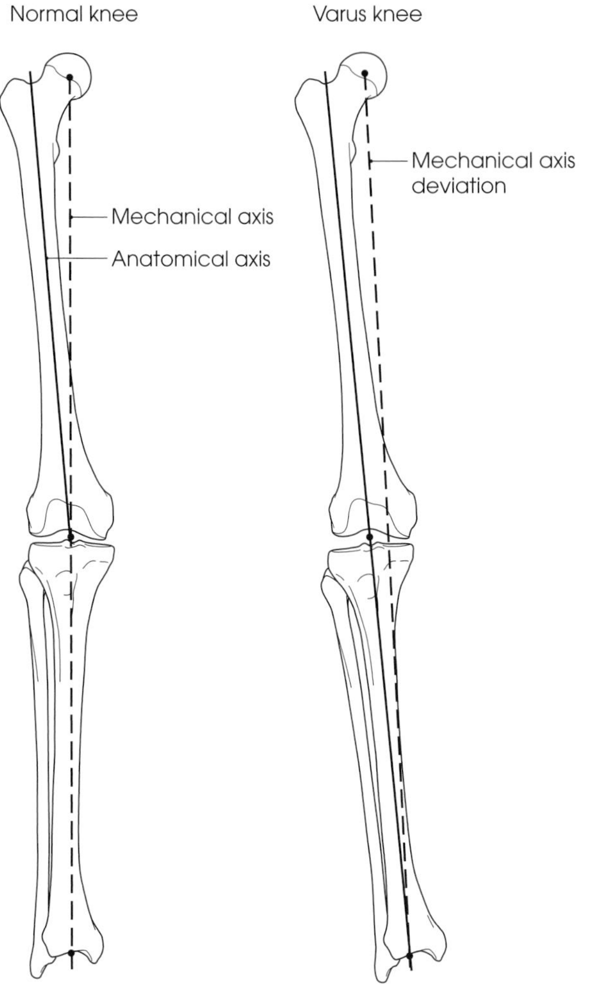

Figure 50.2 The mechanical and anatomical axes. Note the mechanical axis deviation at the knee, which leads to a significant increase in loading to the already abnormal medial compartment.

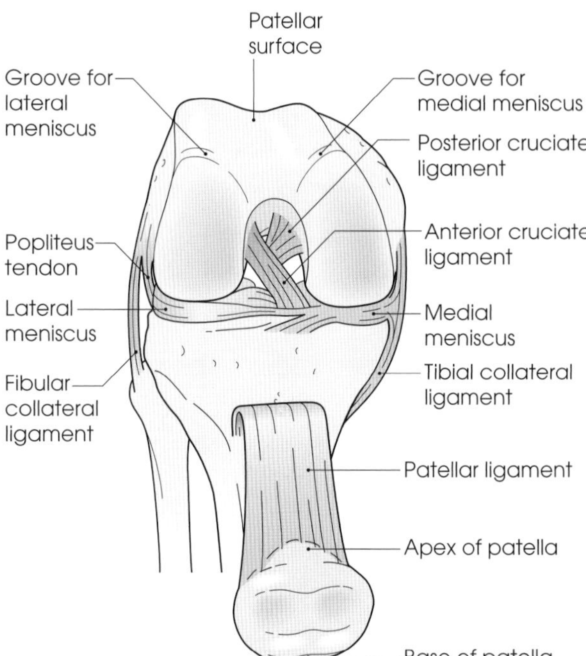

Figure 50.3 General anatomy of the anterior cruciate ligament.

Cruciate ligaments

The anterior cruciate ligament is the most extensively studied ligament in the body. The cruciate ligaments were always considered to function in engineering terms as a *four-bar linkage*, but this has now been discredited. The anterior cruciate ligament is intra-articular but extrasynovial, and functions primarily to prevent anterior displacement of the tibia. It runs obliquely across the joint from its femoral origin on the posterolateral wall of the intercondylar notch to the anterior tibia near the spines. It consists of different bundles of spiralling fibres that allow the ligament to remain taut and functional throughout the range of movement. Proprioceptive nerve fibres are present within the bundles and are vital to normal knee function.

The posterior cruciate ligament is the primary restraint to posterior tibial translation. It has a more direct anteroposterior direction and a broad area of insertion, mostly on the posterior tibia. As with the anterior cruciate ligament, it has a complex arrangement of bundles that are taut at different degrees of flexion.

The collagen fibres within these ligaments are non-elastic and can only tolerate elongation of 8% before failing (Fig. 50.3).

Menisci

The menisci (Figs 50.4–50.5) are crescent-shaped structures of fibrocartilaginous tissue.[1] They play a key role in the complex functions of the knee joint. Put simply, the menisci act as shock absorbers. The reality is in fact much more complex. There are a number of differences between the medial and lateral menisci. The medial meniscus is semicircular and is wider posteriorly. It constitutes more than half the contact surface of the medial tibial plateau. The meniscus has a capsular attachment throughout the periphery, its tibial attachment being known as the coronary ligament. The meniscus is also closely integrated with condensations of joint capsule fibres, i.e. the deep medial collateral ligament.

The lateral meniscus has a more circular structure and covers much more of the convex tibial surface, typically 75%. It is much more mobile than the medial meniscus, having no attachment to the capsule in its midpoint, although both have strong anterior and posterior attachments. Cadaveric studies show that the menisci transmit 30–50% of the load across the joint in the standing position. In addition to the role of force transmission, the menisci have a role in the lubrication of the joint, and finally act as secondary stabilizers of the knee against anterior displacement of the tibia.

CLINICAL EXAMINATION

The general principles of look, feel, move should be observed (see Figs 50.6–50.13). Additional special tests can be performed as necessary.

REFERENCES

1. American Academy of Orthopaedic Surgeons. Orthopaedic Basic Science. 2nd edn. 2000.

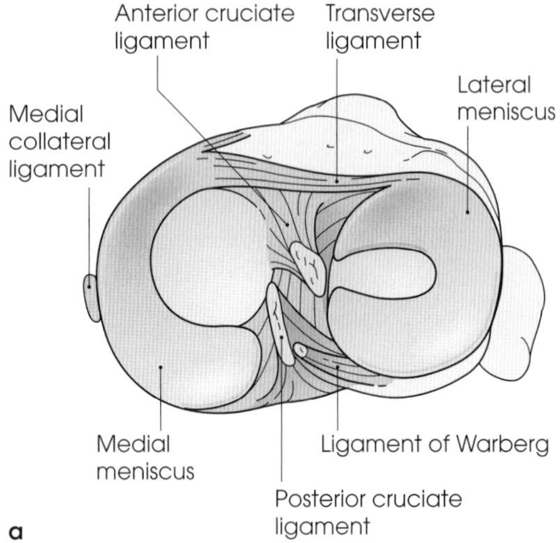

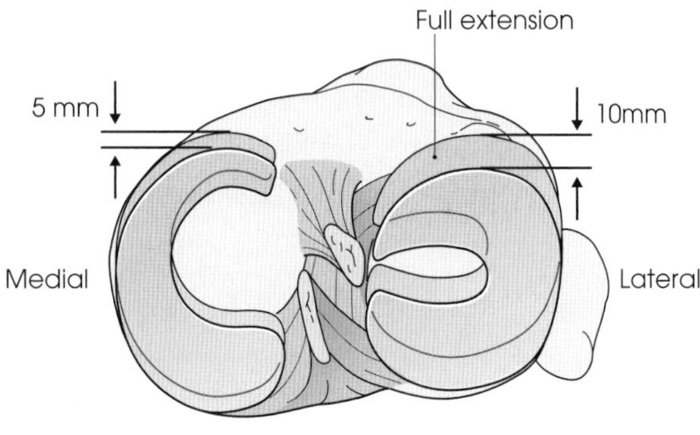

Figure 50.4 The menisci, showing the differences in (a) anatomy and (b) mobility.

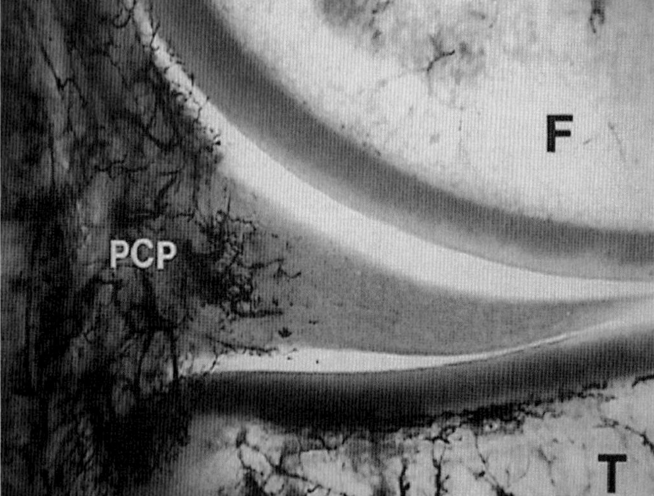

Figure 50.5 Classic ink injection studies showing the perimeniscal capillary plexus. (From Arnoczky SP et al. Am J Sports Med 1982; 10: 90–95. Reprinted by permission of Sage Publications, Inc.[2])

LOOK

The lower extremities should be inspected from all sides in the standing and lying positions. Look particularly for

- alignment problems (i.e. varus or valgus deformity of the limbs),
- loss of mobility (i.e. inability to fully extend the knee),

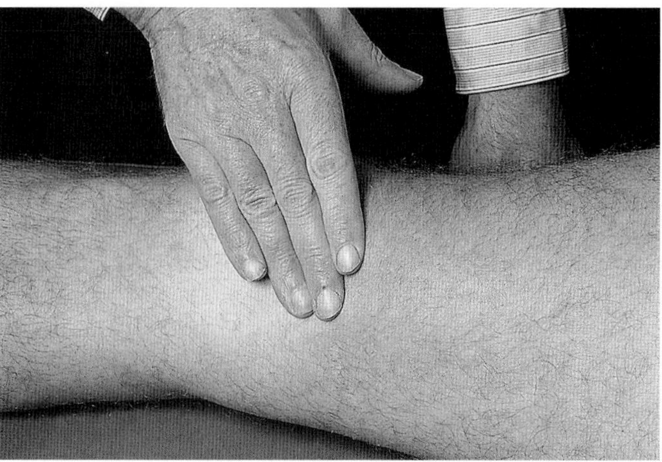

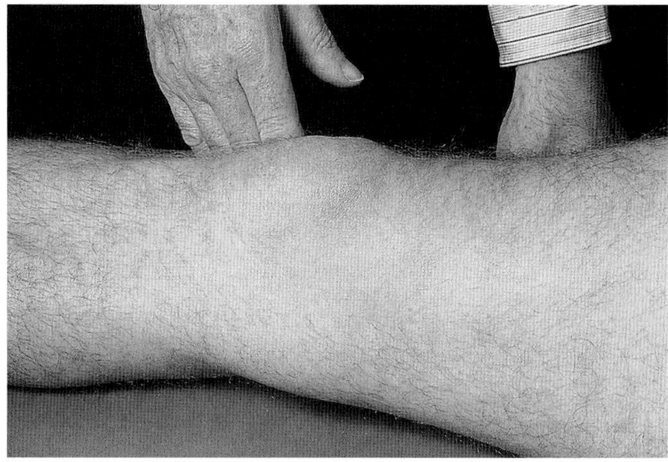

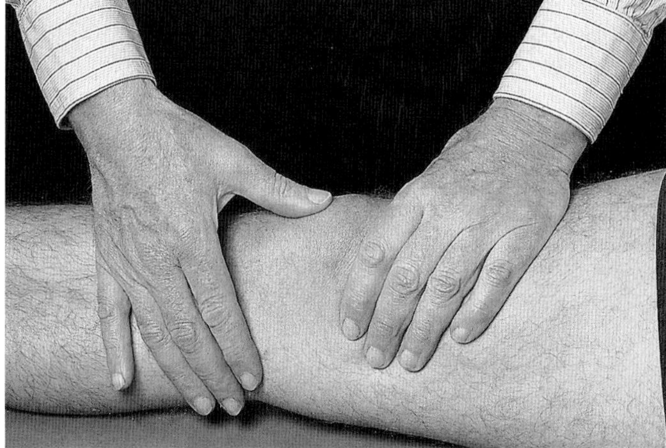

Figure 50.6 Diagnosing an effusion. The bulge test: milk the fluid from the medial side (a), then run it back into the medial side by compressing the lateral side of the patella (b). (c) The patella tap: first compress the suprapatellar pouch; second, tap the patella.

REFERENCES

2. Arnoczky SP et al. Am J Sports Med 1982; 10: 90–95

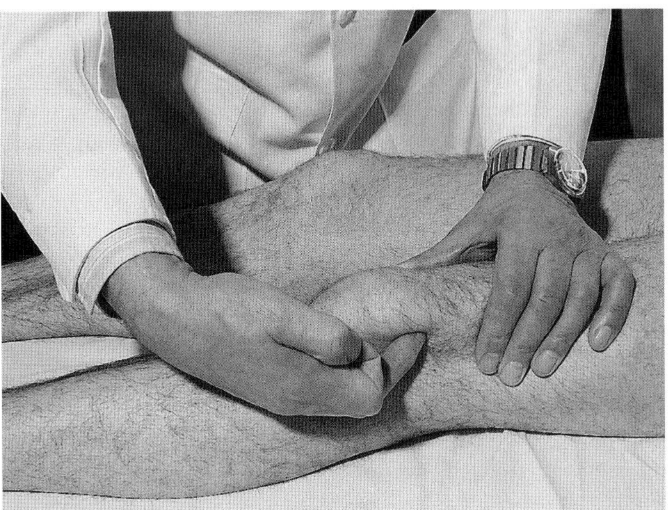

Figure 50.7 Feeling for patella tenderness. Displace the patella medially and feel under the medial facet, push it laterally and feel the lateral facet. Do this gently because this is uncomfortable if done roughly, even in a normal knee!

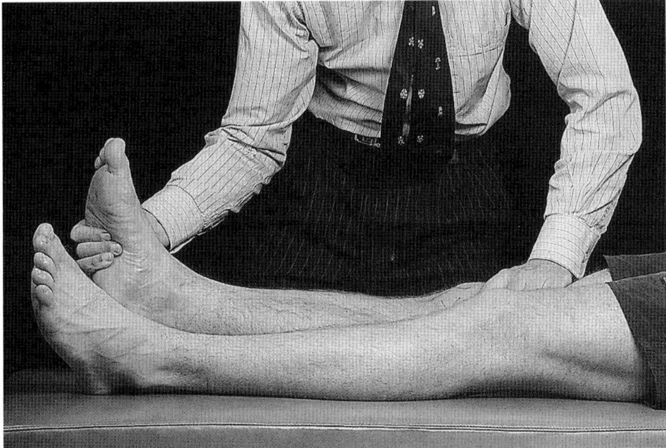

Figure 50.8 Testing for full extension. If the normal knee has hyperextension, so should the symptomatic one. A knee may extend to zero but still be locked, because if there is natural hyperextension it should go to – 10 or – 5°, depending on the degree of natural laxity. Another trap for the unwary!

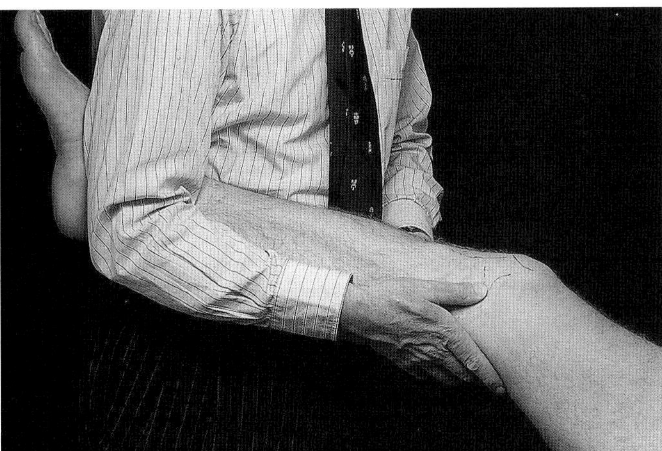

Figure 50.9 Testing for varus–valgus instability: the examiner is applying a valgus stress and feeling for the integrity of the medial ligament with his thumb.

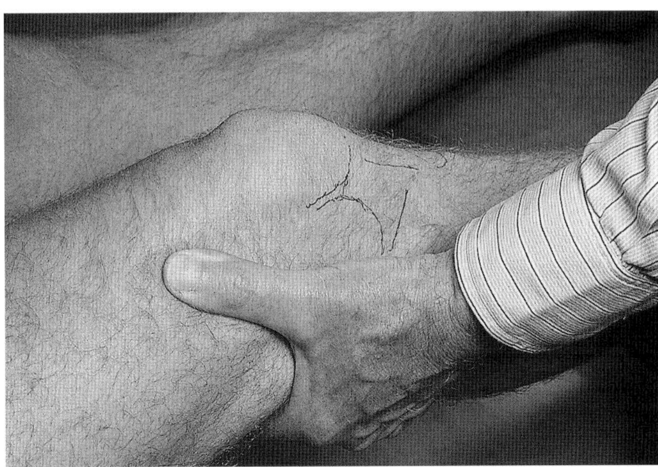

a

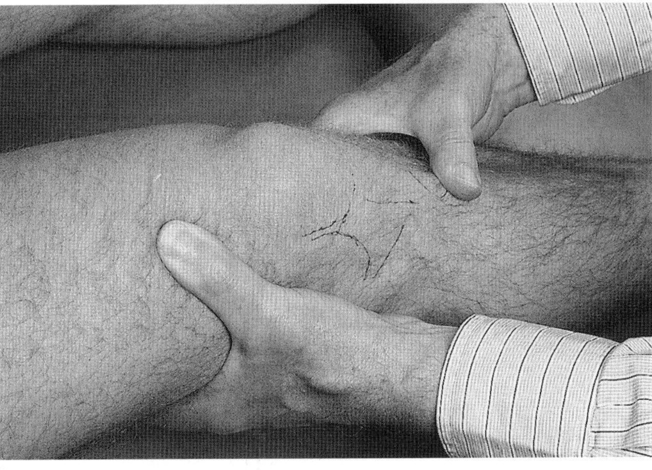

b

Figure 50.10 The Lachman test for the anterior cruciate ligament is done at 30° flexion. (**a**) Let the patient's knee rest in the palm of your hand and wait until the patient is completely relaxed, then hold the distal thigh firmly with your thumb. (**b**) With your other hand, grasp the proximal calf. Your thumb needs to be at the tibial tubercle. Firmly displace the tibia forwards. Feel for the end point of the anterior cruciate ligament. Compare both knees.

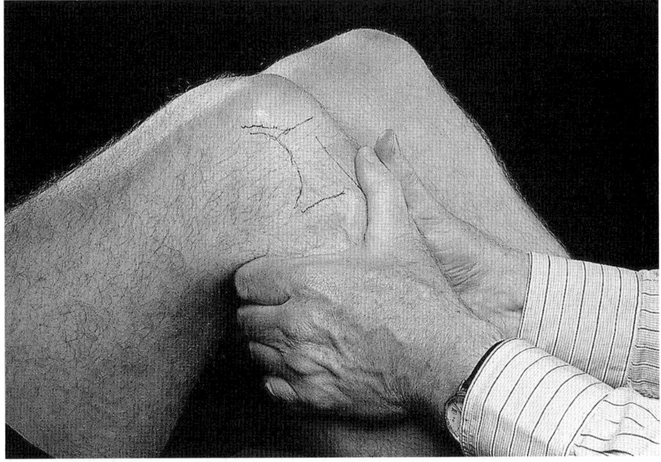

Figure 50.11 Anterior and posterior draw test at 90°. The examiner's fingers are high up in the popliteal fossa and his thumbs on the tibial tubercle.

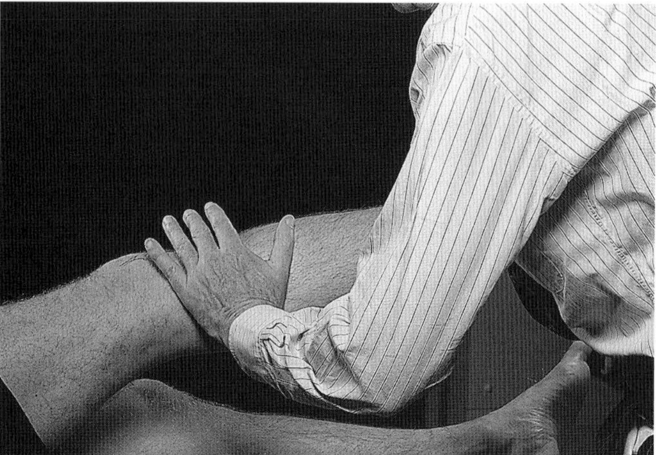

Figure 50.12 The pivot shift for anterior cruciate instability.

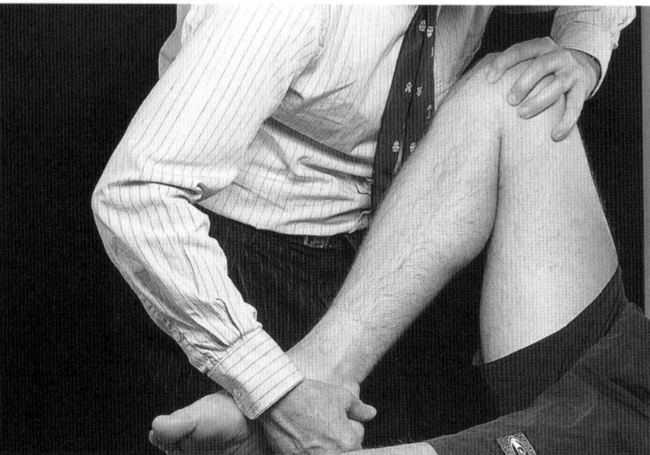

Figure 50.13 Testing for meniscal tears. The McMurray test: flex the knee fully with one hand holding the heel and the other placed over the distal thigh just above the patella. Apply tibial internal and external rotation. Repeat as the knee is extended, i.e. continuous alternating external rotation and internal rotation movements are applied as the knee is extended.

- muscle wasting, and
- swelling (i.e. effusion or cyst).

The gait pattern should then be evaluated.

FEEL

With the patient supine, feel for

- warmth;
- an effusion, with a bulge test or a patellar tap (ballottement);
- joint tenderness around and under the patella, medial and lateral joint lines, and other areas (i.e. bone, collateral ligaments and muscles); and
- lumps (cysts, bursae, tumours, etc.)

MOVE

Examine the range of movement (i.e. flexion and extension, including hyperextension).

SPECIAL TESTS

Collateral and cruciate ligaments

These tests can be difficult to perform and evaluate. The commonest problem by far is failing to ensure that the patient is fully relaxed. Varus and valgus testing should be performed in the fully extended and partially flexed position with the fingers on the joint line.

The anterior cruciate ligament is assessed with the anterior draw test, performed at 90° of flexion, and the Lachman test, performed at 30° of flexion. The Lachman test is a much more sensitive test because the leg is more relaxed in this position and the effects of secondary stabilizers are decreased. It is suggested that the feel of the end point may give some indication as to whether this is a complete or partial injury. The concept of a partial injury is controversial because the ligament unit is either functioning or disrupted. The most useful test, i.e. the one that most closely reproduces the instability in the knee, is the pivot shift test. This is difficult to perform, particularly in the acute stage, and at times can only be demonstrated fully under anaesthetic. The test involves applying a valgus and internal rotation stress to the knee while supporting the leg by the heel. If the anterior cruciate ligament is deficient, then anterolateral subluxation of the tibia will occur. As the knee is flexed, the subluxation will reduce at 30–40°, often with a sudden jerk.

The posterior cruciate is assessed with the posterior draw test and by looking for a posterior sag when the knee is fixed at 90°.

Menisci

The McMurray test is classically described for the detection of meniscal tears but has many variations. The aim is to trap the meniscal tear or fragment and try to relocate it. This involves a combination of rotational and varus–valgus stresses as the knee is flexed and extended. A true positive test is quite rare, but this test will reproduce symptoms. The Apley grind test loads the joint in similar fashion in the prone position. Squatting and 'duck walking' tests are also described. These tests can also be helpful in assessing the state of the articular cartilage by loading one or other side of the joint.

INVESTIGATIONS

PLAIN X-RAYS

X-rays (Fig. 50.14) are an essential part of the orthopaedic assessment, but it is obvious that many patients with significant knee problems have normal plain X-rays. Anteroposterior and lateral views are obtained, but in the majority of cases the anteroposterior view is much more useful when taken in the standing position. This gives a more accurate view of the alignment of the leg and also the true level of joint space narrowing. Taking the anteroposterior X-ray with the knee slightly flexed at 20–30° gives a much more accurate view of the state of the joint. The most accurate measurements, i.e. for research studies, require fluoroscopic positioning. A tunnel view can be helpful, particularly for identifying problems such as osteochondritis dissecans.

The standard series of knee films will include a skyline view of the patella, but the usefulness of this view is questionable. There is a great deal of literature available with numerous measurements made of patellar shift, patellar tilt, and the alignment and depth of the patellar groove. It is extremely difficult to accurately reproduce these views. They can be notoriously deceptive, and care should be taken when interpreting them.

Long-leg X-rays

Long-leg films are anteroposterior X-rays of the whole lower limbs, going from the head of the femur to the ankle joint. They

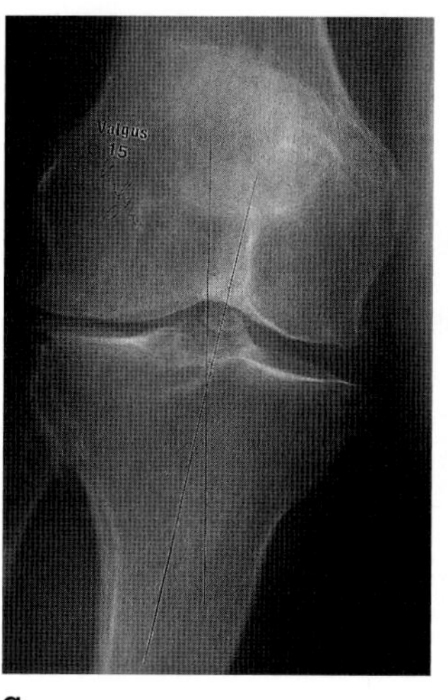

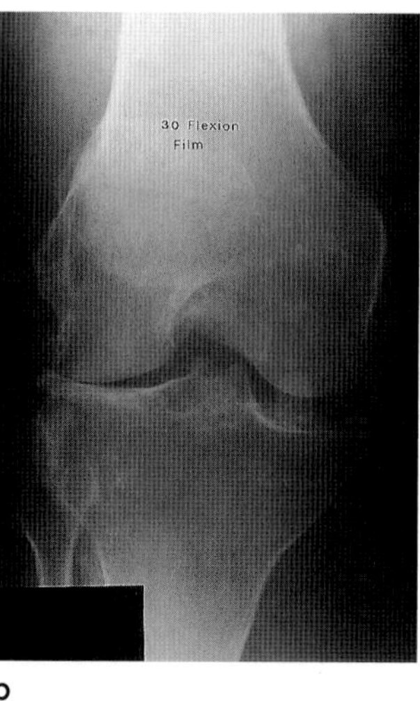

a b

Figure 50.14 (a) The long-leg film shows that this knee has a valgus deformity of 15°. The lateral joint space is obviously diminished but still seems to be present. (b) The standing film at 30° flexion shows that there is no joint space and point loading laterally.

allow measurement of the mechanical and anatomical axes and allow accurate planning for surgery to correct malalignment of the knee (e.g. upper tibial osteotomy for varus deformity of the knee).

COMPUTERIZED TOMOGRAPHY SCANNING

Computerized tomography scanning is useful for accurately measuring rotational problems within the lower limb with cuts through the hip, knee and ankle. Computerized tomography has also replaced tomograms for sagittal and coronal reconstruction of the knee, especially in planning reconstruction of tibial plateau fractures.

ISOTOPE BONE SCANNING

The main value of isotope scanning is eliminating unexpected problems, i.e. tumours, stress fractures and avascular necrosis. It can be of some value in patients with chronic anterior knee pain, both to rule out other conditions and also, if the scan is entirely normal, it will help to reinforce the decision not to operate. Technetium and labelled white cell scans are useful in the evaluation of the painful total knee prosthesis.

MAGNETIC RESONANCE IMAGING SCANNING

Magnetic resonance imaging scanning has had a major impact on the diagnosis and treatment of knee problems. It is particularly helpful in the diagnosis of meniscal pathology. Many studies have shown an accuracy approaching 95% for identifying meniscal tears. Ligament problems are also accurately diagnosed: the accuracy for posterior cruciate injuries is as high as 99% and for anterior cruciate injuries somewhat lower, at approximately 80–85%. This is usually due to the oblique alignment of the anterior cruciate ligament fibres, which makes it more difficult to see the whole ligament on a single MRI slice. Magnetic resonance imaging scanning is also very helpful in the diagnosis of osteochondritis or avascular necrosis, and also in the evaluation of tumours.

Magnetic resonance imaging scans are at their least useful when evaluating conditions of articular cartilage. The problems of accuracy are in part related to the skill of the radiologist in making the diagnosis and also in the interpretation of the changes seen, i.e. abnormal findings are common even in asymptomatic knees. Generally speaking, however, if MRI findings are normal, there is more than a 90% chance that significant pathological changes will not be present within the knee.

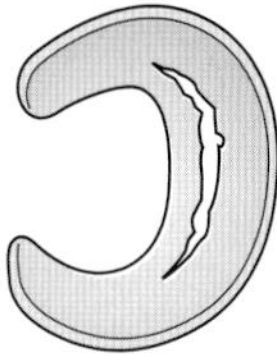

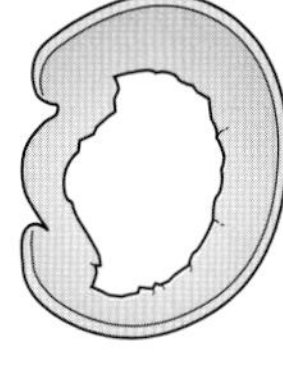

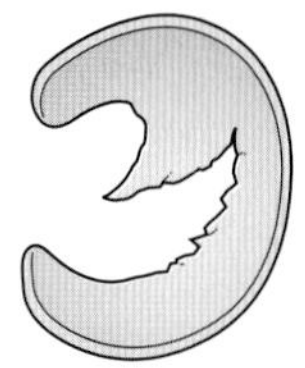

Figure 50.15 Types of meniscal tear.

MENISCAL PATHOLOGY

Meniscal pathology (see Fig. 50.15) can be broadly divided into traumatic tears, usually seen in the younger individual, and the degenerative changes seen in older age groups. There is often a significant overlap in the clinical picture.

Meniscal tears have been classified in a number of ways. They can be partial or full thickness. Vertical longitudinal tears can progress to the more complex and unstable bucket handle tears. The other major groups are the radial- or flap-type tears and the horizontal fissuring or 'fish mouth' tears, which are seen commonly in degenerative menisci.

CLINICAL FINDINGS

A weight-bearing twist or squatting injury may be noted, but many patients with degenerative tears deny any trauma. A wide range of symptoms may be present, for example pain, locking, swelling or giving way. Locking is defined as an inability to fully extend the knee, but some flexion is possible.

In the acute phase an effusion is often seen, with joint line tenderness and restricted mobility. True locking is relatively rare. Chronic tears usually are associated with significant quadriceps muscle atrophy. If the clinical findings are clear for a diagnosis of a meniscal tear and the symptoms are sufficient to warrant treatment, then an arthroscopy may be performed on the knee. If there is doubt in the diagnosis, an MRI scan should be performed.

TREATMENT OPTIONS

Conservative management may be appropriate if the symptoms are not too intrusive, otherwise arthroscopic evaluation of the joint is indicated, with the treatment options consisting of leaving the tear alone if it is small, varying degrees of meniscectomy, or meniscal repair.

Meniscectomy should be as conservative as possible. Investigations have shown a two- to threefold increase in contact stresses across the joint following meniscectomy, and removal of even 16% of the meniscus has been shown to increase contact forces by 350%. Meniscal preserving techniques probably have a significant long-term benefit to the patient, particularly in the reduction of later degenerative changes.

Although meniscal repair is now more feasible, it remains inappropriate or ineffective for the majority of patients with

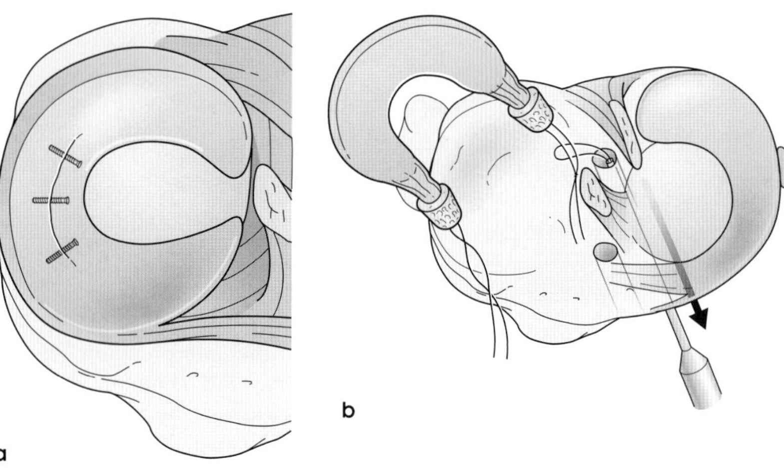

Figure 50.16 (a) Meniscal repair: one of many methods using sutures, darts or absorbable screws. (b) Meniscal transplantation. (From Harner et al 2001,[3] with permission of Lippincott, Williams and Wilkins.)

meniscal tears. The obvious problem with meniscal repair is the poor vascularity of the meniscus, which leads to a relatively high incidence of failure. Meniscal repair[3] is much more technically demanding surgery and can involve a lengthy period of immobilization and rehabilitation, with delayed return to activities. Generally speaking, the following tears are more suited to repair:

- tears in younger patients without degenerative changes,
- vertical split tears (radial and flap tears do less well),
- tears in the peripheral or vascular region (3 mm from the periphery),
- tears less than 3 cm in length,
- tears with early diagnosis and repair (less than 8 weeks after injury),
- tears with no associated ligamentous instability (i.e. an anterior cruciate ligament–deficient knee must be reconstructed or the meniscal repair is doomed to fail).

Meniscal transplantation

Although still experimental, meniscal transplantation (Fig. 50.16) is becoming a feasible option for the younger individual who has undergone extensive or total meniscectomy and is becoming symptomatic with the development of early degenerative problems. The surgery is complex, with a number of potential problems with the graft, including sterility, selection and sizing, shrinkage, and failure of integration.

CYSTS AROUND THE KNEE

Cysts are commonly seen around the knee (Fig. 50.17), the commonest being the popliteal or Baker's cyst. It is important to understand that a Baker's cyst is almost always a secondary diagnosis, i.e. there is an underlying intra-articular pathology, typically arthritis, or degenerative tearing of the meniscus. This leads to an effusion that develops into a cyst as an out-pouching of the posterior capsule, typically in the region of the semitendinosus and semimembranosus muscles. If the cyst is small then no specific treatment is required. Aspiration provides transient relief, but there is a moderately high recurrence rate. Surgery should address the intra-articular pathology in the knee rather than simply excising the cyst itself (e.g. arthroscopic meniscectomy). A number of other cysts are described in the popliteal area that do not have any connection with the joint. Dissection or rupture of the cyst can lead to pain and swelling in the calf, which is often confused with deep vein thrombosis.

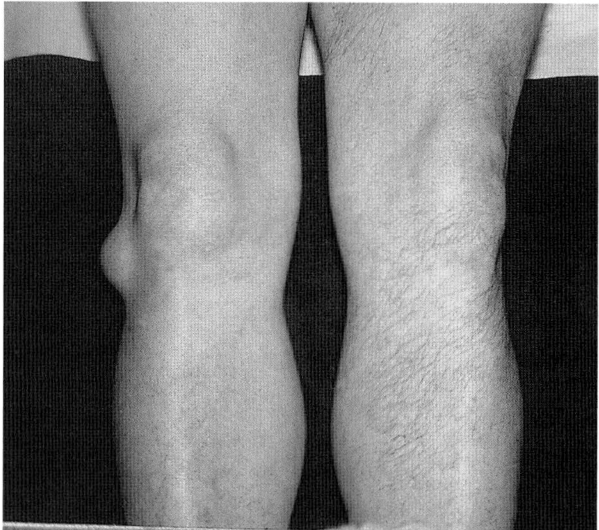

Figure 50.17 A cyst of the lateral meniscus can feel almost bony hard; however, it varies with the position of knee flexion.

Cysts related to the menisci are not uncommon and are usually related to mixoid degeneration following a tear of the meniscus. These cysts can at times disappear without intervention. Aspiration and injection of steroid may be helpful. Treatment may be possible arthroscopically, i.e. decompressing the meniscal tear and cyst into the joint. At times it is necessary to excise the cyst through a local incision.

LIGAMENT INJURIES

ANTERIOR CRUCIATE LIGAMENT INJURY

Clinical findings

There is an increasing incidence of anterior cruciate ligament injury (Fig. 50.18)—an estimated 17 000 cases a year in the UK,

REFERENCES

3. Harner CD, Vince KG, Fu FH (eds). Techniques in Knee Surgery. Lippincott, Williams and Wilkins, Philadelphia, 2001

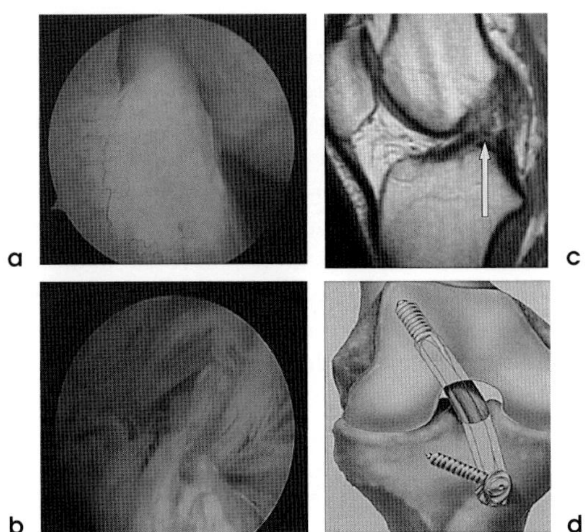

Figure 50.18 Anterior cruciate tears: (a) normal anterior cruciate ligament, (b) midsubstance rupture, (c) MRI findings, and (d) reconstruction using a four-strand hamstring graft.

which equates to 100 injuries a year for each area served by a district general hospital.[4,5] The condition is frequently misdiagnosed, although most patients will give a classic history of the injury.

Typical injuries occur with valgus rotation forces or with hyperextension injuries. These are not always contact injuries and often occur while changing direction or landing from a jump. The injuries are typically associated with immediate pain, and often a pop or crack is heard. The patient limps or is carried off the field and a haemarthrosis develops, either immediately or over the ensuing several hours. Seventy per cent or more of traumatic haemarthroses are due to anterior cruciate ligament tears, and there should be a high degree of suspicion whenever this history is given. Surprisingly, studies have suggested that only 10% of these injuries are diagnosed by the first contact physician! The examination will show increased anterior drawing of the tibia and a positive Lachman test. It remains a puzzle as to why some individuals with this injury are unaware of any ongoing problems whereas others have marked instability, even with day-to-day activities, and significant disability.

There have been a vast number of papers on anterior cruciate ligament injury published over the years, but a number of controversial issues remain.

- Which patients should have surgery?
- Which type of surgery is the most appropriate?
- What is the optimum rehabilitation following the surgery?

There are no studies that conclusively show that degenerative arthritis is reduced after reconstruction of the anterior cruciate ligament, but it seems logical that if repeated episodes of giving way are occurring (often associated with further meniscal tearing) then reconstruction should be beneficial. A lengthy discussion between individual patients and their surgeons must take place before the decision to undergo reconstructive surgery is taken. Of particular importance are the expectations of the patients themselves. In the past it was considered a procedure only for the under 40s, but as the population ages and becomes increasingly involved in exercise and sport there should be no real upper limit.

Treatment options

Non-surgical

A brief period of rest, ice and bracing is followed by an aggressive rehabilitation programme with the help of physiotherapy, including quadriceps- and particularly hamstring-strengthening programmes. This would appear to stabilize the situation in two out of three cases. The long-term use of bracing is not usually necessary, but a number of patients benefit from the use of a lightweight derotation brace to allow them to return to certain sports (e.g. tennis and skiing).

Surgical

Once it has been decided that surgery is necessary there is further controversy in the choice of procedure.[3] Direct repair of the injured ligament is only effective in less common situations when a bony fragment is avulsed with the ligament (typically in the skeletally immature), otherwise a graft must be utilized for the reconstruction (preferably an autograft).

Bone–patellar tendon–bone and four-strand hamstring grafts (semitendinosus and gracilis) are probably used in equal numbers, each having its own advocates. The ultimate tensile strength is similar with each graft. There may be a lower incidence of anterior knee symptoms with the use of hamstrings, but fixation is generally superior with a patellar tendon graft. Later measurements show that there is less residual translation with the patellar tendon graft, nevertheless the overall results, particularly in terms of patient satisfaction, are indistinguishable. The procedure can be carried out entirely arthroscopically or through a limited miniarthrotomy. The most important aspect of the surgery is to prevent impingement of the graft by correctly positioning the tunnels and performing a femoral notchplasty.

Cadaver allografts have also been utilized but generally speaking are reserved for complex revision or salvage cases and are not appropriate for general use. There are still concerns with sterilization and disease transmission, and allografts have a tendency to elongate with time. The results of synthetic ligaments have been discouraging. No single graft is ideal for every patient and treatment must be individualized.

Postoperative immobilization should generally be short. Accelerated rehabilitation programmes with early weight-bearing, closed chain exercise in the early postoperative period and proprioceptive training are now widely utilized. Full maturity of the graft following revascularization is slow and can take as long as 18 months to be achieved. The patient should be told that contact sports are best avoided for the first year after surgery.

The outcome of this surgery is difficult to quantitate. Studies suggest that the mechanical effectiveness of the repair has little bearing on the ultimate function of the knee, and more importantly on patient satisfaction! Nevertheless, probably 80–90% of patients are pleased with the outcome of reconstructive surgery. As well as the usual postoperative problems, it is important to discuss with the patient the possibility of stiffness requiring further surgery, persistent or recurrent instability, and the chance that even technically successful surgery will not always allow a return to the previous level of sport.

MEDIAL COLLATERAL LIGAMENT INJURY

The medial collateral ligament and associated structures are extracapsular, and surgical repair is not usually required. The injury typically occurs in contact sports with a valgus-producing

REFERENCES

4. Larson R, Taillon M. J Am Acad Orthop Surg 1994; 2: 1
5. (Various). Theme issue: Anterior Cruciate Ligament. Knee 2001; 8: 1

force. It is also commonly seen in falls while skiing, typically when the bindings fail to release. Anterior cruciate ligament and meniscal injuries are commonly associated with medial collateral ligament injuries. Clinical examination will reveal tenderness along the ligament and medial joint line. A valgus stress applied to the knee in both full extension and partial flexion will produce a variable level of opening of the medial joint space, allowing the injury to be graded.

- Grade I: stable in both flexion and extension.
- Grade II: stable in full extension, unstable in partial flexion.
- Grade III: unstable in both flexion and extension.

Treatment for Grade I and II injuries include a period of rest, ice, and temporary use of crutches, followed by a rehabilitation programme. The more serious grade III tears can still be expected to have a good result with conservative treatment but may require a period of casting or functional bracing for 4–6 weeks.

POSTERIOR CRUCIATE LIGAMENT INJURY

Posterior cruciate ligament injuries are less commonly seen than those of the anterior cruciate ligament. They occur typically during motor vehicle accidents (i.e. dashboard impact injuries) and also in sports when the lower leg is struck, driving the tibia backwards. Posterior cruciate ligament injuries are often undiagnosed because, after the acute phase, a surprisingly large number are asymptomatic. Unfortunately a few continue to have problems with instability, and surgical treatment should be considered. The surgery involves the use of autograft or allograft tendon for the reconstruction, and it is technically complex.

The posterior cruciate ligament is a primary restraint to posterior tibial translation, and the clinical examination typically reveals a positive posterior draw test and a posterior sag when the foot is supported with the hip and knee at 90° (Fig. 50.19). Non-operative treatment includes a brief period of bracing followed by early range of movement and quadriceps strengthening, with gradual return to sports. Surgery is indicated in the acute stage if there is an avulsion of bone from the tibial insertion of the ligament, and at times for multiple or complex ligament injury patterns.

COMBINED LIGAMENT INJURIES

With improved imaging and arthroscopy techniques it has become more obvious that ligament injuries are rarely simple and often involve several structures. A typical combination includes injuries to the anterior cruciate ligament, the medial collateral ligament, and the medial meniscus. Complex injuries of the ligaments and capsular structures can lead to a number of multidirectional instabilities. Anterolateral and posterolateral instabilities are increasingly diagnosed.

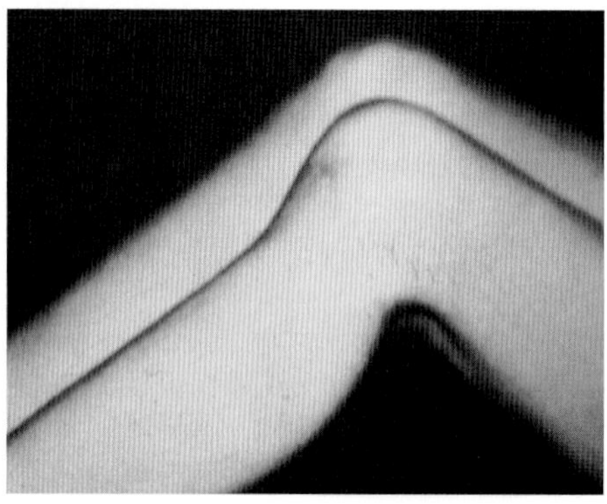

Figure 50.19 Posterior sag sign for posterior cruciate ligament tear.

The general principles of diagnosis and treatment are the same, but the patients with these injuries do less well with conservative measures and the best results are usually obtained from surgical reconstruction, particularly in the acute phase. The treatment aims can at times be conflicting, i.e. a medial collateral ligament tear will usually heal without surgery with a period of immobilization, whereas an anterior cruciate ligament tear may require surgery followed by early movement and rehabilitation. A combined anterior cruciate ligament and medial collateral ligament injury therefore would normally be treated by a period of 4–6 weeks of functional bracing with anterior cruciate ligament reconstruction to follow.

INJURIES TO THE EXTENSOR MECHANISM

Disruption of the extensor mechanism can take place at a number of sites.

- Rupture of the quadriceps tendon above the patella.
- Fracture through the patella.
- Rupture or avulsion of the patella tendon.

These injuries can occur in two ways. In younger patients the injury usually involves sudden or significant force, i.e. jumping or heavy lifting. In older patients the forces can be much less, and at times an almost spontaneous injury can occur. Most patients will describe a feeling of something tearing or giving way. This is followed by significant pain and swelling, but it is possible to walk by locking the knee into hyperextension. The diagnosis is not infrequently missed, but typically the patient will be unable to extend the knee against resistance or to perform a straight leg raise, and there is usually a defect in the tendon above or below the patella and a significant haemarthrosis.

X-rays of the knee will show the patella to be high riding (the patellar tendon length should be 1–1.25 times the length of the patella). It may be helpful to compare X-rays of both knees. Patellar tendon rupture or avulsion is usually relatively straightforward to diagnose, whereas quadriceps tendon may be more difficult and ultrasound is the most satisfactory investigation for confirming diagnosis.

The treatment of choice is usually early surgical repair followed by prolonged immobilization and subsequent graded rehabilitation.

PATELLOFEMORAL DISEASE

The sizeable percentage of patients with knee pain seen in an orthopaedic clinic have problems related to the patellofemoral joint.

Pathophysiology

The forces on the patellofemoral joint can be extremely high, as much as 3000 pounds per square inch with certain activities. Patellofemoral problems are often caused by or related to patellar malalignment and maltracking, cumulative trauma (i.e. increased compression forces on the patella related to obesity), weight-lifting and physical activity, and patellar subluxation or dislocation. Primary osteoarthritis of the patellofemoral joint is not uncommon in older individuals but the exact relationship with chondromalacia patellae is not clear.

Anterior knee pain (chondromalacia patellae)

Anterior knee pain is one of the commonest knee problems seen in younger patients. In previous years this condition was usually given the catch-all phrase 'chondromalacia patellae', indicating softening or fragmentation of the articular cartilage. In many cases, however, this chondromalacia is not actually present. The diagnosis and treatment of this problem can at times be very difficult due to the lack of objective findings.

Typically patients report knee pain in the region of the patella, which is worse after prolonged sitting and climbing or descending stairs. The problem is usually bilateral and there is no history of trauma, although occasionally a direct blow to the front of the knee is reported. It is aggravated by physical activities such as running, jumping and squatting. Audible crepitation is commonly present, especially when rising from a chair. Other symptoms that can be confusing are also reported, i.e. catching, locking and giving way. This often leads to the erroneous diagnosis of meniscal disease.

The clinical signs on examination can at times be rather sparse, but there is usually an element of patellar maltracking. Patellofemoral compression often causes discomfort, and crepitus is very commonly heard and palpated (similar findings may often be found in the other, asymptomatic, knee!). The patellar facets may be tender to palpation. An effusion is rarely present. The range of movement is full and other specific tests for meniscal or ligament problems are negative.

Investigations

Initial investigations include anteroposterior, lateral and patellar skyline X-rays. Patellar tilting and/or subluxation may be seen, but not infrequently the X-rays are normal. Magnetic resonance imaging scans can define the anatomy of the patella and groove, but the utility is low for conditions of the articular cartilage. The main value is often to rule out other conditions.

Patellofemoral instability

The problem of patellofemoral instability (Fig. 50.20) can occur as a sudden, unexpected, acute event (i.e. when pivoting when playing sports) or as a chronic recurrent problem, often with a feeling that the patella is going to 'go' but control is usually regained. In the acute phase the diagnosis may be obvious if the patella is still dislocated, but often a spontaneous reduction has occurred and the only finding is a diffusely painful knee with an acute haemarthrosis. Local tenderness of the patella may be present, and occasionally the X-ray may show a marginal fracture of the patella. A number of malalignment problems are frequently found:

- valgus alignment,
- rotational problems (femoral anteversion and consequently squinting patellae),
- abnormal patella and groove (patella alta, or patellar or femoral dysplasia),
- joint laxity (generalized hypermobility),
- soft tissue problems (weak vastus medialis or tight lateral retinaculum).

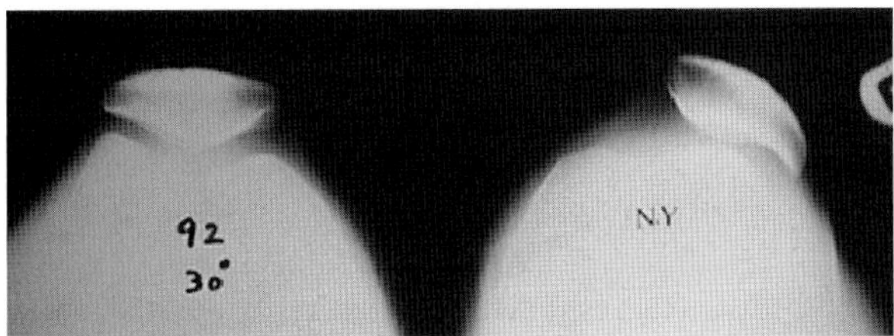

Figure 50.20 Patellar instability. Note the abnormal morphology of patella and shallow groove.

Treatment

The majority of patients with anterior knee pain can be treated satisfactorily with conservative measures, i.e. a programme of quadriceps strengthening and flexibility. Short-arc activities (partial flexion) are important initially, then an increased range of movement activities are initiated (e.g. stationary bicycle). Taping and/or patellar bracing can be helpful, along with short-term use of non-steroidal anti-inflammatory agents. Treatment for acute instability consists of a period of rest and bracing for 2 or 3 weeks followed by a rehabilitation and physiotherapy programme. Occasionally acute repair is performed but this is not common.

Surgery is rarely indicated for chronic anterior knee pain, and the results are generally unrewarding. Surgery is much more helpful for patellar instability, i.e. recurrent dislocation. Surgical options can include arthroscopy, lateral retinacular release, or realignment surgery.

Arthroscopy

Arthroscopy can be helpful to further evaluate the patellofemoral dynamics and the condition of the articular cartilage.

Lateral retinacular release

This procedure has been used somewhat indiscriminately, and its general utility is increasingly questioned. It can be of some benefit for a tilted or mildly unstable patella. Unfortunately it can at times make matters worse due to further weakening and imbalance of the extensor mechanism.

Realignment surgery

Surgery for recurrent dislocation of the patella can be performed proximally or distally and on soft tissue or bone; often a combination of all these is necessary. A typical procedure would include medial transfer of the tibial tubercle and patellar tendon (Elmslie–Trillat or Fulkerson osteotomies) supplemented with a lateral retinacular release and plication of the medial retinaculum.

Patellar tendonitis

Patellar tendonitis is often called 'jumper's knee' and is associated with overuse or overload of the extensor mechanism. The symptoms are somewhat different from the typical anterior knee pain because there is often marked point tenderness, typically at the inferior pole of the patella. As with patellofemoral pain, the symptoms are often worse with prolonged sitting, squatting, kneeling, and climbing or descending stairs. The clinical findings are usually very clear. An X-ray is typically normal but may show some minor irregularities at the lower pole of the patella. An MRI scan will usually show signal changes in the region of the patellar tendon insertion.

APOPHYSITIS: OSGOOD–SCHLATTER'S DISEASE

Osgood–Schlatter's disease is a common condition in adolescents, with classic clinical findings of tenderness and/or swelling over the tibial tubercle. The symptoms are activity-related, particularly with running sports. The treatment is almost always conservative, with a period of restricted activity followed by a stretching and strengthening programme and gradual return to sports. A protective brace may be helpful in the acute phase.

Rarely, surgical excision of a troublesome residual ossicle at the tibial tubercle is required.

OSTEOARTHRITIS

PATHOPHYSIOLOGY

Osteoarthritis is particularly common in the knee.[2] It occurs with increasing frequency in older individuals, but the inter-relationship between ageing and osteoarthritis is not clear. Predisposing factors are:

- trauma,
- meniscectomy,
- inflammatory arthritis, and
- avascular necrosis.

The causes of osteoarthritis remain obscure and involve a complex interaction of wear, reaction and repair. It has been described as:

- normal forces acting on abnormal cartilage, or
- abnormal forces acting on normal cartilage.

Biomechanical stresses affecting the articular cartilage and subchondral bone, biochemical changes in the articular cartilage and synovial membrane, and genetic factors are all important in the pathogenesis of osteoarthritis. Early changes occur in the proteoglycans and collagen, which leave the cartilage matrix depleted. The cartilage degeneration is characterized by profound changes in the articular surface (fibrillation) or in the deeper zones (fissuring). Later, complete loss of the cartilage with exposed subchondral bone is seen. The future management of osteoarthritis will involve the use of cultured mesenchymal stem cells, growth factors, and manipulation of genetic material.

CLINICAL FINDINGS

The physical examination of an osteoarthritic joint reveals local tenderness, crepitus, and possibly an effusion, with later limitation of joint movement, bony enlargement, and alignment problems.

NON-OPERATIVE TREATMENT OPTIONS

The majority of patients with osteoarthritis of the knee should initially be treated non-operatively.[6] Patients can benefit greatly from simple measures such as weight loss and modifications to their activity level, i.e. stopping high-impact exercises or changing to a more sedentary occupation. Other treatments depend on the severity of the symptoms, and the age and expectations of the patient.

Regular low-impact exercise and occasional physiotherapy can be of some benefit, as can the use of a cane or knee brace. Studies have shown benefits from the use of braces that 'unload' the affected compartment of the knee, i.e. a brace that applies a valgus force to a varus knee with medial compartment osteoarthritis.

There is no strong evidence that oral non-steroidal anti-inflammatory agents are any better than simple analgesics such as paracetamol. The incidence of side effects and complications from non-steroidal agents is high, particularly in the older age group, due to the cumulative effects.

Dietary supplements, i.e. glucosamine and chondroitin, have become very popular. The exact basis of action is not fully understood, but a number of studies have shown that they can be effective in relieving pain and improving mobility. The magnitude of the improvement is unclear due to inconsistencies in the studies, but the effects are frequently better than the use of placebo.

Intra-articular injection of steroid (e.g. methylprednisolone) can be helpful, although the effects are often somewhat limited. The exact dose and frequency of the injections are not known, but many patients who are unable or unwilling to have surgery obtain significant relief, sometimes lasting for several months, and a number of patients can be treated for several years with occasional injections.

More recently, injections of sodium hyaluronate have been advocated. This treatment is also known as viscosupplementation. The hyaluronate helps to improve the tissue turgor in the articular cartilage, can give moderate pain relief, and may help delay or avoid surgery in a number of individuals.

OPERATIVE TREATMENT OPTIONS

Arthroscopic surgery

Arthroscopy[7] is frequently carried out on patients with degenerative arthritis, but the results are generally unpredictable. Empirically, most orthopaedic surgeons feel that half the patients treated seem very pleased with the results, certainly in the short and medium term, but the other half have very limited or no relief at all, and in a small number of cases the procedure seems to accelerate the degenerative process. One study has suggested that there is no evidence that there is any overall benefit from this procedure for osteoarthritic knees. Despite this, the procedure can be very useful for diagnostic purposes, especially when planning future surgery. Patients with degenerate tearing of the menisci can obtain some benefit from a general debridement of the unstable fragments. Some orthopaedic surgeons are firm advocates of microfracture techniques. These involve breaking through the subchondral plate to allow healing fibrocartilage to develop. Some question the excellent published results, believing that it is the intensive in-patient and outpatient rest and rehabilitation that play the biggest role in the improvement seen.

Osteotomy

Tibial osteotomy[4] has been a mainstay of treatment for medial compartment osteoarthritis of the knee for many years since being proposed and popularized by Jackson and Waugh in the 1960s. The normally aligned knee takes approximately 60% of its load across the medial compartment. This is significantly increased with a varus deformity, with loading up to 90% or more at times. Several osteotomy techniques are available, including the dome-shaped osteotomy, the closing wedge osteotomy and, more recently, the minimally invasive opening wedge osteotomy. Each technique has its own advantages and disadvantages, but the general principle of putting the knee back into a valgus configuration of 10° or more would be expected to significantly unload the medial compartment. Typical studies would show that the surgery remains effective for 85% of patients at 5 years and approximately 50% at 10 years. It is certainly an effective alternative for young patients with the appropriate indications. The results very clearly correlate with optimal surgical correction of the deformity.

REFERENCES

6. American College of Rheumatology Subcomittee on osteoarthritis guide lines. Arthritis Rheum 2000; 43: 9
7. Moseley JB, O'Malley K, Petersen NJ et al. New Engl J Med. 2002; 347: 81–88

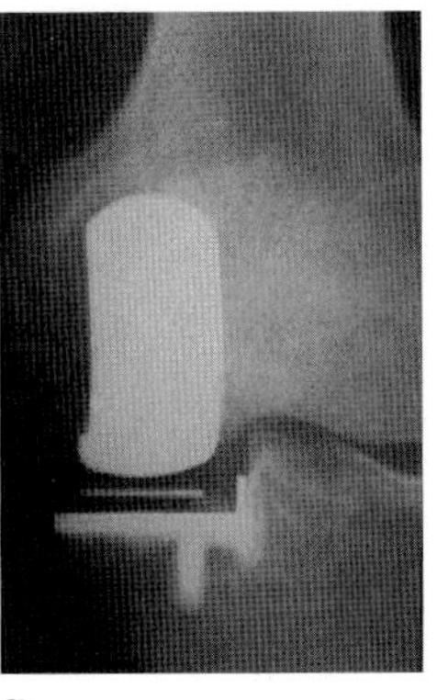

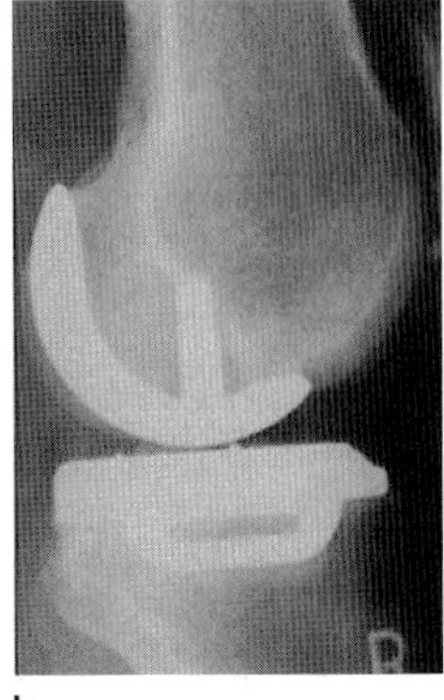

a b

Figure 50.21 Unicompartmental knee arthroplasty with mobile bearing.

The valgus knee, which is a much less common clinical entity, can also be dealt with by osteotomy. Having excluded a fixed adduction deformity in the ipsilateral hip that is contributing to the development of the knee valgus deformity, the deformity is invariably above the joint, and the correction must be addressed to the distal femur to maintain a horizontal joint line. This is technically more difficult surgery, with a higher incidence of delayed union and non-union. Patellofemoral problems are also more frequent with valgus knees. The decision-making process was much less complex in previous years because there were few alternatives, particularly for younger patients. In recent years, unicompartmental knee replacement has become a realistic option, with more predictable results, and there is an ongoing debate as to the relative merits of unicompartmental replacement osteotomy.

Unicompartmental knee arthroplasty

Improved implant technology and minimally invasive surgical techniques have led to a greater interest in unicompartmental knee arthroplasty (Fig. 50.21). Fixed and mobile bearing devices are available. Video fluoroscopy has shown knees with unicompartmental arthroplasty to have kinematic patterns much closer to the normal knee when compared with those of knees with total knee arthroplasty. Patient satisfaction, pain relief, and range of movement are better, and the length of hospital stay is usually much reduced. Studies suggest that these implants have a 10-year survival rate of 95% or higher. A number of criteria must be fulfilled before this surgery, the most important being the presence of an intact anterior cruciate ligament. Most of the studies are related to the treatment of medial compartment disease, and the results seem much better and more predictable than those with lateral disease. This procedure is not appropriate for the more severely deformed knees, and passive correction of the varus deformity should be possible along with only minimal fixed flexion deformities preoperatively.

Mechanical failure, loosening of the implant, and also progressive arthritis in other compartments can lead to failure and the necessity for revision to total knee prosthesis. The results of revision surgery are good but probably do not approach the level of satisfaction seen after a primary procedure.

Total knee replacement

The excellent results of total hip replacement surgery (Figs 50.22 and 50.23)[1,3] are now being seen with total knee arthroplasty. The initial difficulties were related to the extremely complex kinematics of the normal and diseased knee joint. Osteoarthritis of the knee is much more common than osteoarthritis of the hip in the general population, and it is estimated that in the near future twice as many knee replacements will be required as hip replacements. In the UK, over 40 000 knee arthroplasties are carried out each year.

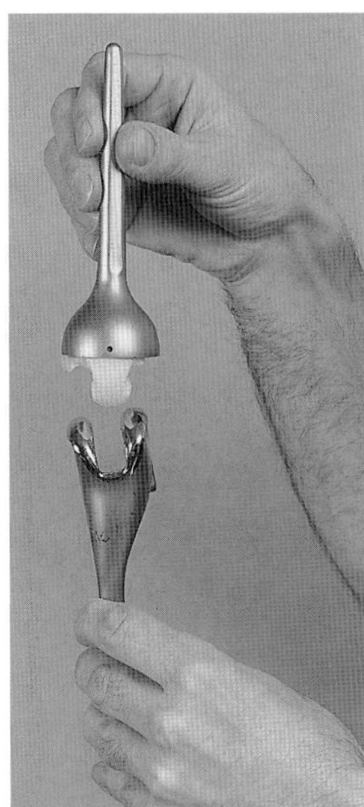

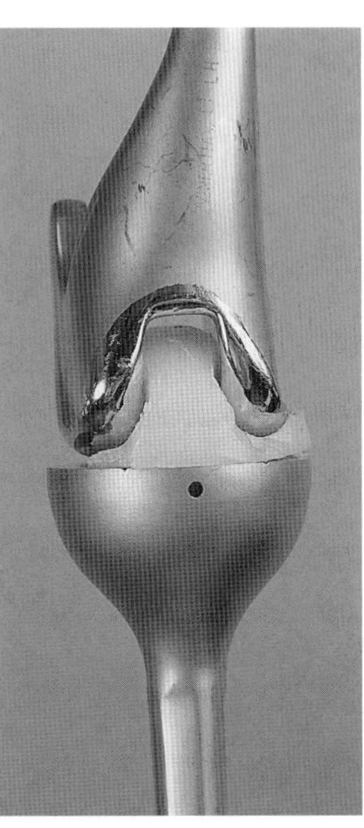

a b

Figure 50.22 Condylar knee replacements are much the commonest type of knee arthroplasty. They are manufactured as modular components. The plastic tibial inserts are held in a metal tray. Stability is gained by balancing the thickness of the plastic insert against the tension in the ligaments.

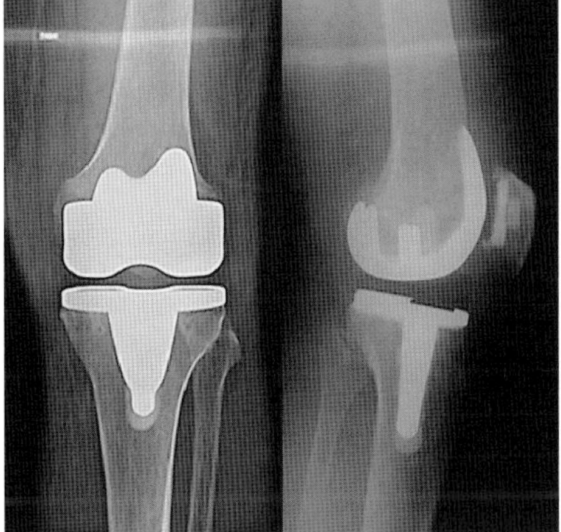

Figure 50.23 Radiographs of condylar knee replacement.

Indications

Total knee arthroplasty should be considered only after an adequate trial of non-operative treatment.

REFERENCE

8. Archibeck MJ, White R. J Bone Joint Surg (Am) 2002; 9: 1719–1726

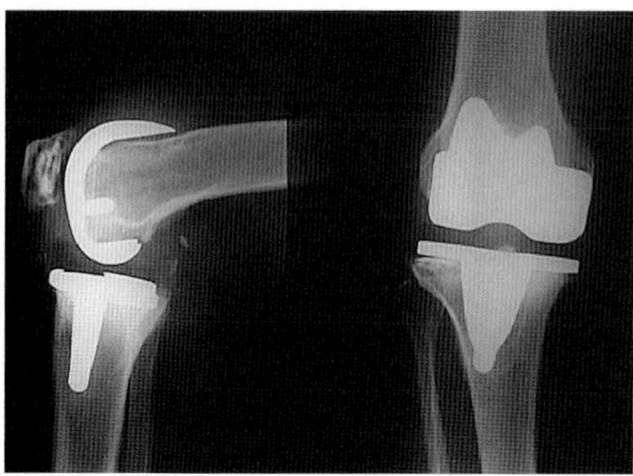

Figure 50.24 Complications of total knee arthroplasty aseptic loosening.

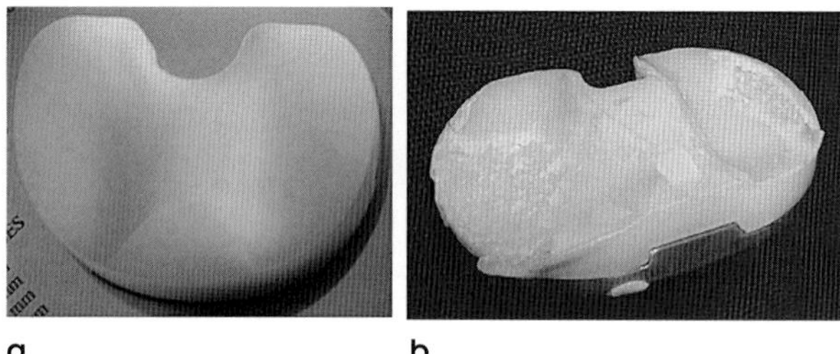

a b

Figure 50.25 Complications of total knee arthroplasty: (a) normal polyethylene insert and (b) delamination and wear.

Outcome

Most studies of total condylar knee arthroplasty show 90–95% survival rates at 10-year follow-up. Even at 15 years they remain high at 85%, but survival rates fall steadily after that.

Complications (Figs 50.24 and 50.25)

In the acute phase, the usual postoperative problems occur. Infection rates should now be well below 1% with the use of prophylactic antibiotics and laminar flow theatres. Thromboembolic disease remains a challenge, with postoperative venography positive in up to 70% of cases (although most of these are subclinical). Controversy continues with the choice of prophylaxis, but mechanical (early mobilization, foot pumps, etc) or chemical measures (warfarin, low-molecular-weight heparin) must be used. Postoperative knee stiffness may at times require manipulation under anaesthesia but should be mostly preventable with good surgical technique and an aggressive rehabilitation programme.

Failure of the implant at a later stage is most commonly due to aseptic loosening, but any number of problems can occur, including

- aseptic loosening,
- mechanical failure (polythene spacer breakdown or osteolysis),
- sepsis,
- patellar complications (instability, wear or loosening),
- arthrofibrosis or stiffness,
- ligamentous instability,
- periprosthetic fracture, and
- unexplained pain.

The burden of revision surgery for these failed cases is rising relentlessly, with greatly increased costs and length of hospitalization. The most important aspect of revision surgery is the preoperative work-up and diagnosis of the reason for failure. Revision implant technology has advanced considerably and the outcome of this surgery is now quite respectable, although it is nowhere near as effective or enduring as primary arthroplasty. Sepsis will, in the majority of cases, require exchange of the implant as a two-stage procedure. The results of revision surgery depend greatly on the preoperative condition, but success rates of 80% or more are obtainable.

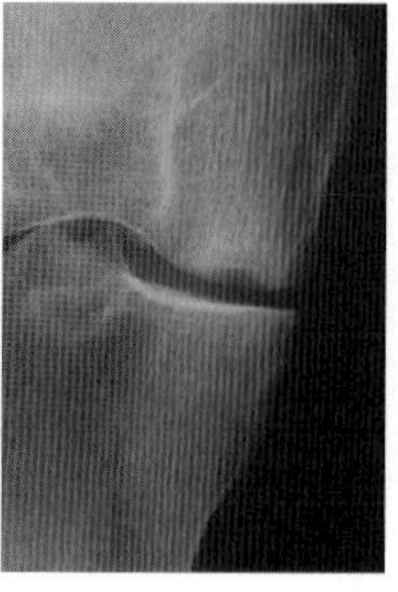

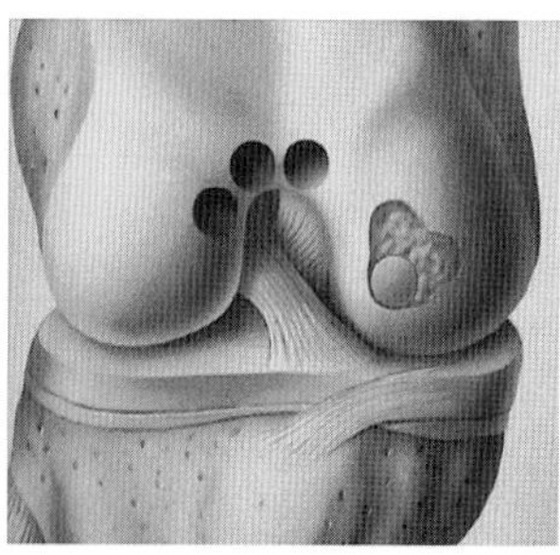

a b

Figure 50.26 (a) Avascular necrosis in the medial femoral condyle and (b) mosaicplasty repair.

OSTEOCHONDRITIS DISSECANS

Osteochondritis dissecans (Fig. 50.26) is seen typically in the second decade, although it can arise de novo in adults. The general consensus is that this is a traumatic condition involving repetitive minor trauma that leads to a stress fracture in the subchondral bone. Metabolic and vascular problems have also been implicated. It predominantly affects the lateral portion of the medial femoral condyle. There are a number of potential outcomes, ranging from complete spontaneous healing to the development of osteoarthritis.

CLINICAL FINDINGS

Typically the patient presents with vague chronic knee pain, often with sparse clinical findings and normal X-rays. At times a loose body can be identified that gives rise to locking. More extensive lesions leave a large defect in the femoral condyle, which leads to later signs and symptoms of osteoarthritis.

TREATMENT

A number of treatments have been proposed for this condition. The choice depends on the site, the size, and the stability of the fragment.

- Observation.
- Fixation of the fragment with pins or screws (which can be bioabsorbable).
- Excision of the loose body.
- Debridement or drilling of the defect.
- Osteochondral grafting.
- Mosaicplasty.
- Autologous chondrocyte transplant.

AVASCULAR NECROSIS

Avascular necrosis, which usually affects the medial femoral condyle, has many similarities to osteochondritis because it affects the bone but has normal overlying articular cartilage. It is frequently associated with other medical conditions, including alcoholism, systemic lupus erythematosus, haemoglobinopathies, steroid use and renal transplantation. Spontaneous osteonecrosis is an occasional cause of sudden, severe pain developing in the knee of an elderly patient. The initial X-rays are often normal, and an isotope or MRI scan may be required for the diagnosis in the early stages. Later X-rays will show the typical osteochondral defect.

Treatment is initially conservative, with surgery reserved for persistent pain or disability. This could include local debridement of the lesion, tibial osteotomy to unload the compartment or, as a last resort, knee replacement arthroplasty.

The foot and ankle

51

Mark S. Davies

INTRODUCTION

Most chapters on the subject of foot and ankle surgery in textbooks start with statements pointing out that the foot is adapted for walking and that the anatomy of the foot is related to its function. It goes without saying that feet are for walking and that anatomy and function are inextricably linked. The fundamental principle of orthopaedic surgery is restoration of function by restoration of anatomy, and yet in the past many foot and ankle procedures have been fundamentally destructive. Major advances in foot and ankle surgery have occurred in the past 20 years and still old practices persist into the 21st century.

When considering treatment options for disorders of the foot and ankle it is worth remembering that there are only five options:

1. do nothing;
2. footwear modification, orthoses and braces;
3. medication (tablets and injections);
4. physiotherapy (and related disciplines); or
5. surgery.

There is no condition that cannot be made worse by surgery, and therefore surgery should be regarded as the 'last resort'. It is important to realize that the recovery from foot surgery need not be painful, but it is always protracted. As a general rule for anything other than the most minor surgical procedures, recovery takes many months and swelling takes up to 1 year to resolve.

THE ANKLE

CLINICAL EXAMINATION OF THE ANKLE

The system of *look, feel, move* applies as much to the ankle as it does elsewhere in the musculoskeletal system. When inspecting the ankle joint, the examiner should always look at the entirety of the lower limb and always compare one side with the other. This is best done with the patient standing. There is nothing quite like a pair of long trousers to hide deformities of the lower limbs. Specifically one should look for scars, swelling and deformity. At the same time, the examiner needs to inspect the patient's ankles from the front, from both sides, and from behind. Varus and valgus deformities of the ankle are best appreciated from behind. While still standing, it is convenient to inspect the patient's gait.

Further examination of the ankle is best performed with the patient seated in a chair, with the examiner seated opposite on a chair with wheels and adjustable seat height. Palpation of the ankle joint line is followed by examining the range of motion. Failure to test the active motion can lead to the examiner missing a case of foot drop. Likewise, failure to appreciate that flexion and extension occur at the transverse tarsal joint (talonavicular and calcaneocuboid joints) as well as the ankle joint can lead to overestimation of the range of ankle motion. Ankle stability is best tested for with the patient's knees flexed over the side of the examination couch. The ankle is held gently with one hand while the foot is held with the other hand. The foot is then passively moved backwards and forwards relative to the ankle, the so-called 'anterior drawer test'. Comparison with the contralateral side is essential if significance is to be given to the test.

Assessment of the patient's circulatory and neurological status is mandatory.

IMAGING OF THE ANKLE

All patients complaining of an ankle problem need an X-ray (unless pregnant or otherwise contraindicated). All radiographs of the ankle should be performed with the patient weight bearing, unless the patient cannot stand. The standard views are anteroposterior, mortise and lateral views. Radiographs are inspected for soft tissue swelling, bone architecture, deformity of the talus within the mortise, reduction in joint space, osteophyte formation, and presence of accessory ossicles, for example os trigonum (separate accessory bone at the most posterior aspect of the talus). Intra-articular pathologies such as osteochondral lesions of the talus will not be seen unless specifically looked for.

Magnetic resonance imaging has transformed imaging of the ankle and has to a certain extent superseded CT and isotope bone scans. To gain maximal information from MRI scanning requires specialist knowledge of the appropriate MRI sequences (e.g. T1, T2 and STIR) and an in-depth knowledge of ankle pathologies. However, MRI scanning is no substitute for a thorough clinical examination. Correlating the clinical findings with the MRI findings is a skill that comes only with experience.

Other useful investigations include ultrasound and diagnostic injections of local anaesthetic into joints. If local anaesthetic into a joint abolishes pain, one can isolate the source of a patient's pain. In the foot and ankle, where there are so many joints close together, this can be very helpful.

ANKLE CONDITIONS

Ankle pathologies can be divided into those affecting the joint itself (i.e. the bone and cartilage) and those affecting the soft tissues (e.g. ligaments, tendons, synovium and nerves) around the ankle.

Ankle arthritis

Primary osteoarthritis of the ankle is not as common as osteoarthritis of the hip or knee, but it is more common than most people believe. Osteoarthritis secondary to trauma is also not uncommon, and other conditions, such as haemochromatosis, can lead to degenerative changes. Charcot neuroarthropathy secondary to diabetes mellitus can lead to spectacular deformity of the ankle joint but need not be painful. As a general rule, degenerative changes in the ankle lead to deformity and swelling and are associated with mechanical symptoms. The patient's principle symptom is likely to be activity-related pain within the ankle joint. Treatment is aimed at symptomatic relief, starting with simple analgesics and anti-inflammatory medication as well as activity modification, an ankle brace and physiotherapy. A walking stick can be helpful too. Corticosteroid injections rarely result in anything other than short-term pain relief and should be used sparingly.

Should conservative measures fail to provide adequate symptomatic relief, surgery should be considered. For mild degenerative disease, arthroscopic or open debridement with removal of tibial and talar osteophytes can be surprisingly effective. For more severe osteoarthritis the surgical options lie between arthrodesis (fusion) and total ankle replacement. Fusion (in the correct position) is still regarded by most as the gold standard and can be carried out by either open or arthroscopic methods.[1] Fixation with screws has replaced staples and external fixators, which should no longer be used. In cases of severe osteoarthritis involving the subtalar joint as well as the ankle joint, an intramedullary nail can be used after preparing both joint surfaces (Fig. 51.1).

Inflammatory arthropathies may also affect the ankle joint, rheumatoid arthritis being the commonest. Medical management of the disease process must be optimized before surgical intervention is considered. Intra-articular steroid can be very beneficial when the synovium is very inflamed and certainly has a role in disease control. For the severely damaged ankle joint surgery has a lot to offer. Rheumatoid patients, however, are often on immunosuppressive drugs (e.g. prednisolone), which not only potentially affect wound healing but also soften bone. Relative lack of mobility also leads to disuse osteoporosis, and as a result the rheumatoid patient presents major challenges, particularly when multiple joints are affected. Screw fixation can be tenuous, and in patients with upper limb problems the use of crutches may be impossible. A decision to fuse or replace a rheumatoid ankle should not to be taken lightly.

Ankle instability

Ankle instability usually occurs following a major lateral ligament injury. Following such an injury the ankle never returns to normal, with the patient complaining of weakness in the ankle and a tendency to 'turn over' the ankle on even the most innocuous of uneven surfaces. If pain occurs between sprains, additional pathology should be sought. The treatment for ankle instability is physiotherapy, but should this fail, surgical intervention can be very successful. The Brostrom–Gould procedure is an anatomical reconstruction of the anterior talofibular and calcaneofibular (Fig. 51.2), and is superior to tenodesis procedures such as the Evans repair, which involves passing the peroneus brevis tendon through a bone tunnel in the distal fibula.[2]

Patients with recurrent ankle sprains should be examined for evidence of tarsal coalitions or neurological conditions such as Charcot–Marie–Tooth disease.

Impingement and nerve entrapment problems about the ankle

Impingement occurs when soft tissue is 'pinched' between two bone surfaces and can be very disabling. Anterior impingement usually occurs when osteophytes are present, and treatment involves resection of osteophytes and scar tissue through an open ankle arthrotomy or arthroscopically.[3] Posterior impingement is less common and is often associated with the presence of an os trigonum or large trigonal process of the talus. It is often associated with flexor hallucis longus tendonitis and is most commonly seen in ballerinas. This condition, should it fail to respond to non-operative treatment, responds well to decompression of the flexor hallucis longus tendon and removal of the os trigonum or prominent trigonal process.[4]

Entrapment neuropathies are often included in accounts of impingement disorders. Any of the nerves that pass the ankle can be involved, and are associated with pain and altered sensation in the distribution of the nerve. Although much less common than carpal tunnel syndrome, tarsal tunnel syndrome is the most common entrapment syndrome in the foot, and is compression of the tibial nerve as it passes behind the medial malleolus through the retinaculum, leading to pain and sensory disturbance in the sole of the foot. Decompression of the tarsal tunnel can be effective, especially when a compressive lesion such as a ganglion can be removed at the time of surgery.[5]

Osteochondral lesions of the talus

Also known as osteochondral defects, these lesions tend to occur anterolaterally or posteromedially on the talar dome (Fig. 51.3). Rarely they affect the tibial plafond. The lateral lesions are more frequently associated with trauma than the medial ones. They range from intact lesions to detached loose fragments of cartilage and bone. Talar cysts can also form and enlarge beneath an osteochondral lesion of the talus. Symptoms are those of aching and pain with very sharp episodes of pain deep inside the ankle. These lesions, if symptomatic, are best treated by arthroscopic curettage. Cartilage transplantation remains controversial and experimental. Osteochondral lesions of the talus are notorious for taking months or even years to get better following surgery.

Neurological conditions

Any disease affecting the central and/or peripheral nervous system can affect the foot and ankle, for example the hereditary motor and sensory neuropathies (Charcot–Marie–Tooth disease), spina bifida, and poliomyelitis are the most common. Usually as a result of muscle imbalance, deformity occurs, and sometimes the deformities can be very severe indeed. Diagnosing the underlying disease is essential if treatment is to be effective. Knowledge of the natural history of the disease will dictate the treatment options. For non-ambulatory patients no surgery is required. For mobile patients where physiotherapy and bracing fails, surgical treatments include bony procedures such as osteotomy and arthrodesis, and soft tissue procedures such as tendon transfers.

One neurological condition that lends itself particularly well to tendon transfer is drop foot secondary to a head injury, stroke or damage to the common peroneal nerve (e.g. trauma or in certain

REFERENCES

1. Mann RA, Rongstad K. Foot Ankle Int 1998; 19: 3–9
2. Krips R, Brandsson S, Swensson C. J Bone Joint Surg (Br) 2002; 84-B: 232–236
3. Parkes JC, Hamilton WG, Patterson AH et al. J Trauma 1980; 20: 895–898
4. Hamilton WG, Geppert MJ, Thompson FM. J Bone Joint Surg (Am) 1996; 78-A: 1491–1500
5. Mann RA. In: Coughlin MJ, Mann RA (eds). Surgery of the Foot and Ankle. 7th edn. Mosby, St Louis, 1999: 516

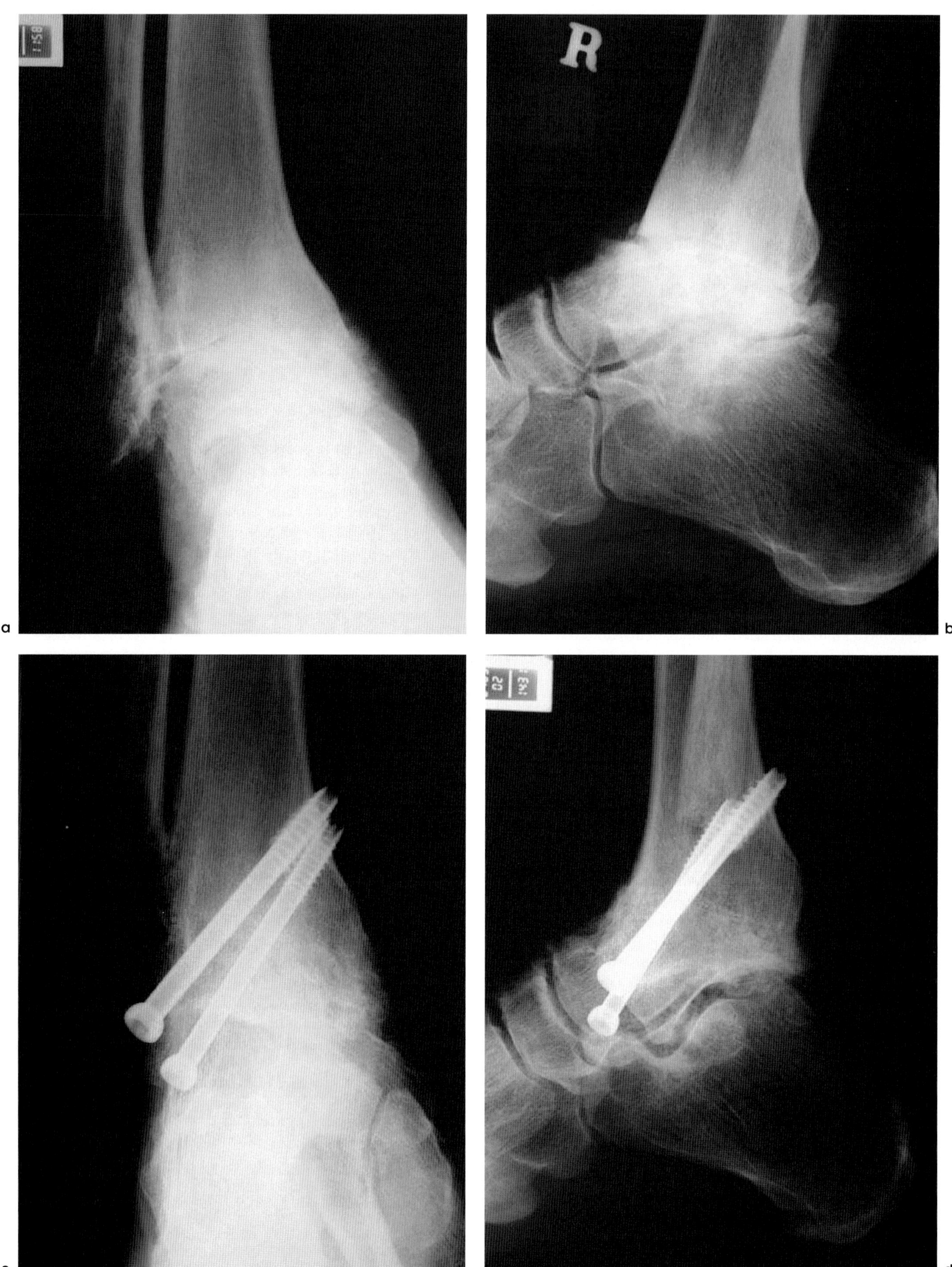

Figure 51.1 (**a**) Anteroposterior and (**b**) lateral ankle radiograph from a 52-year-old man showing osteoarthritis. (**c**) Postfusion anteroposterior and (**d**) postfusion lateral views.

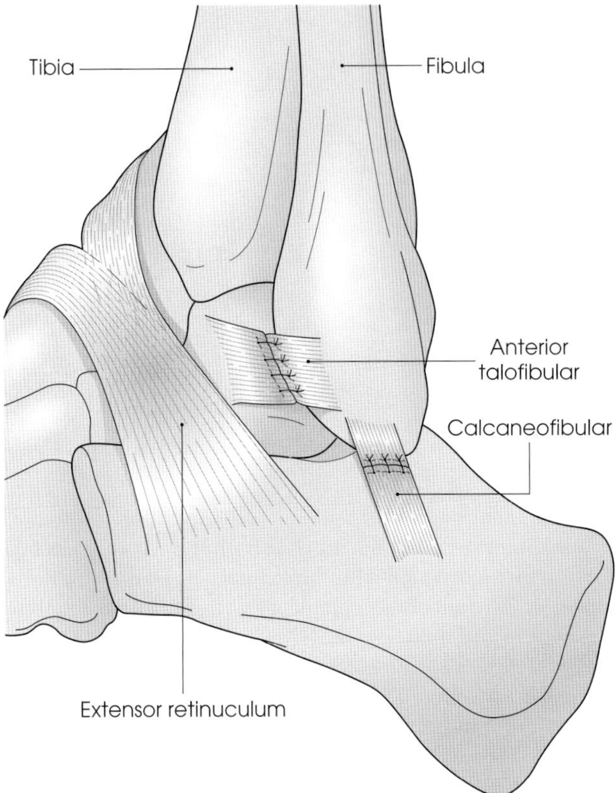

Figure 51.2 The Brostrom procedure.

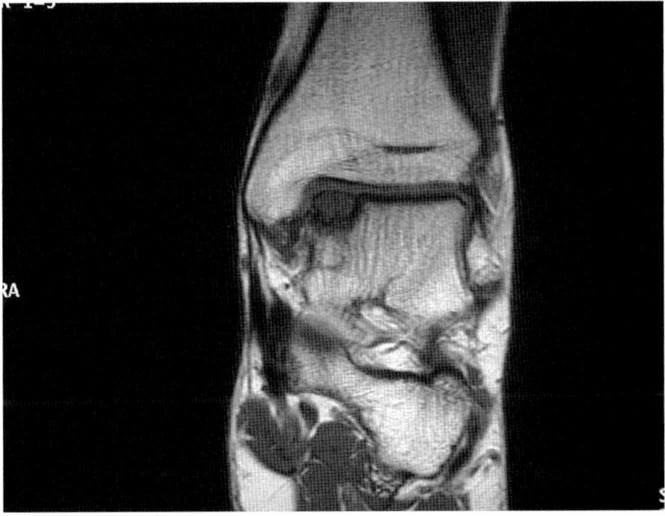

Figure 51.3 An MRI scan showing a medial osteochondral lesion of the talus in a 38-year-old man.

countries, leprosy).[6] Active dorsiflexion of the ankle can be regained by rerouting the tibialis posterior tendon to the dorsum of the foot.

Infections

Septic arthritis can affect any synovial joint and the ankle is no exception. It is more common following surgical intervention (such as ankle surgery for fracture fixation), but it can occur as a result of haematogenous spread and *Staphylococcus aureus* is the most frequent offender. In immunocompromised patients opportunistic organisms may be responsible. However, if the organism gets to the ankle, it is a devastating development and requires immediate surgical drainage followed by appropriate antibiotics. Sadly, prompt action often fails to save the cartilage and severe chondrolysis (cartilage death) occurs, followed by rapid degenerative changes. Ankle fusion for severe damage secondary to infection is more likely to lead to an infected non-union and therefore amputation.

Other infections that can affect the ankle and should not be forgotten are poliomyelitis and tuberculosis.

THE FOOT

The foot is an extremely versatile structure that allows humans to walk on all sorts of terrain. It is arbitrarily divided into the hindfoot, midfoot and forefoot. The hindfoot is the talus and os calcis and includes the subtalar joint. The midfoot comprises the navicula, cuboid and cuneiforms and includes the talonavicular and calcaneocuboid joints (also known as the transverse tarsal joint because they effectively work as one joint), the three naviculocuneiform joints, and the five tarsometatarsal joints. The forefoot is that part of the foot distal to the metatarsal bases.

The muscles that move the foot are those that pass by the ankle (including the gastrocnemius–soleus complex) plus the short flexors and extensors, the abductors and adductors, as well as the interossei and lumbricals.

Movements in the foot are plantar flexion and dorsiflexion (up and down), inversion and eversion (tilting towards and away from the midline), and adduction and abduction (transverse movement towards and away from the midline).

Supination and *pronation* are specific terms that are often misused and misunderstood. Supination is a three-dimensional motion and reflects a combination of adduction, inversion and plantar flexion of the foot, while pronation is the opposite (i.e. abduction, eversion and dorsiflexion).

CLINICAL EXAMINATION

The principles of foot examination are the same as for the ankle, i.e. *look, feel, move.* Both feet are inspected for deformity and swelling from all sides, including the plantar aspect of the foot. The skin is inspected for colour changes, scars and callosities, and the condition of the nails is noted. The patient's gait is examined, as is the patient's ability to rise to the tiptoe position. The examiner observes this from behind to watch specifically for inversion of the heels. Failure of the heel to swing into varus suggests significant pathology, such as tibialis posterior dysfunction, subtalar joint pathology or tarsal coalition.

Further foot examination is carried out with the patient seated in a chair and the examiner sitting opposite. A sound knowledge of surface anatomy is essential to be able to palpate the individual joints of the foot. It is worth remembering that the subtalar joint is best palpated at the tip of the fibula and that the navicular tuberosity, on the medial side of the foot, is easy to palpate in all but the fattest of feet. Palpation of individual tendons is carried out if indicated. Examination of the subtalar joint must be performed with the ankle in neutral, because this 'locks' the transverse tarsal joint. Failure to appreciate this may result in apparent subtalar joint motion when in fact none exists. The heel

REFERENCES

6. Lipscomb P, Sanchez J. J Bone Joint Surg (Am) 1961; 43-A: 60

is held with one hand while the examiner inverts and everts the foot. The normal range of motion is approximately 15° of eversion and 25° of inversion. While still clasping the heel, adduction and abduction at the transverse tarsal joint are assessed as well as the amount of plantar flexion and dorsiflexion. The individual tarsometatarsal joints are moved by holding the midfoot with one hand and moving each individual metatarsal up and down. This is done by holding the metatarsal head between the index finger and thumb and dorsiflexing and plantar flexing the tarsometatarsal joints. With the thumb along the plantar aspect of the metatarsal heads and the index finger along the dorsum, each metatarsophalangeal joint is moved to assess range of motion. Motion at the first metatarsophalangeal joint is variable but is approximately from 25° of plantar flexion to 70° of dorsiflexion.

Sensation should be tested, remembering the distribution of the individual cutaneous nerves supplying the foot. Joint position sense should be tested whenever a neuropathy is suspected (e.g. diabetes).

The dorsalis pedis and posterior tibial pulses should also be palpated, and an assessment of capillary return should be performed. The peroneal artery is not palpable.

IMAGING OF THE FOOT

All patients require weight-bearing anteroposterior and lateral radiographs of the foot plus a non-weight-bearing oblique view. To image the subtalar joint, special Broden's views are required, and to image the sesamoids of the first metatarsophalangeal joint, skyline views should be requested. The roles of MRI, CT, ultrasound and isotope bone scanning are as outlined in the *Ankle* section.

THE FOREFOOT

Hallux valgus (bunions)

One of the commonest foot disorders seen in the shod population is hallux valgus, which is a deviation of the big toe away from the midline at the first metatarsophalangeal joint. The swelling over the medial aspect of the first metatarsophalangeal joint is often referred to as a bunion. Hallux valgus is a hereditary condition, more common in females than males and although often bilateral, need not be.[7] It would appear that it is the predisposition to the deformity that is inherited rather than the deformity itself, and the wearing of pointed, closed-in shoes accelerates the onset of the deformity, thus explaining the higher incidence in females. The deformity may be mild to severe, as may be the symptoms, but pain does not necessarily correlate with the extent of the deformity.

It is important to find out exactly what bothers the patient in terms of pain, problems with footwear, and cosmesis. Surgery for cosmetic reasons alone should be avoided. If, despite modification of footwear, significant pain persists, surgery can be considered. The surgical options are dictated to a certain extent by the radiological findings of a weight-bearing radiograph. As well as the hallux valgus angle, the intermetatarsal angle, the distal metatarsal articular angle, and whether the joint is congruent or not, it is very important to assess the relative lengths of the first and second metatarsals (Fig. 51.4). If the second metatarsal is longer than the first and a shortening osteotomy of the first is carried out, there is a real risk of developing a so-called 'transfer lesion' of weight to the second metatarsophalangeal joint, with subsequent hammering of the toe and dislocation of the joint. This is a surprisingly difficult condition to treat and leads to much misery.

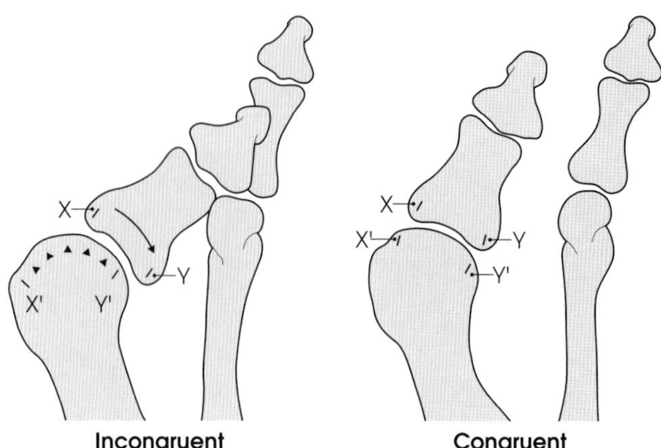

Figure 51.4 Angles to be considered in hallux valgus correction.

There are many surgical options for correction of hallux valgus, but surgery should aim to restore, not destroy, anatomy. Excision arthroplasty of the proximal phalanx (Keller's procedure) is no longer acceptable as a treatment for hallux valgus except in the most severe deformities in the very elderly. Likewise, distal metatarsal osteotomies for severe deformities are not powerful enough to correct the problem and should be avoided. For mild deformities the distal chevron is a good option,[8] while for moderate and severe deformities, shaft osteotomies (e.g. scarf) or proximal osteotomies (e.g. crescentic or proximal chevron) in conjunction with a distal soft tissue release and/or Akin osteotomy are more appropriate (Fig. 51.5).[9] For very severe deformities, fusion of the first tarsometatarsal joint or first metatarsophalangeal joint can be effective.

Hallux rigidus

Osteoarthritis of the first metatarsophalangeal joint leads to stiffness and pain, and can be disabling. If it does not respond to analgesics, or activity or footwear modification, surgery is an option. For mild osteoarthritis a cheilectomy can be effective,[10] but for more severe osteoarthritis fusion is the best option.[11] Joint replacement remains controversial and is very difficult to salvage should it fail. The same is true of the Keller's procedure.

LESSER TOE DISORDERS

The three commonest toe deformities are hammer toes, mallet toes and claw toes (Fig. 51.6). Multiple claw toes suggest an underlying neurological disease process and a diagnosis for this should be actively sought. Treatment of the deformities themselves depends on symptomatology and whether the deformities are fixed or flexible. If shoe modification fails, surgery to correct the deformity can be worthwhile.[12] Often regarded as simple surgery, correction of lesser toe deformities needs to be

REFERENCES

7. Hardy RH, Clapham JCR. J Bone Joint Surg (Br) 1951; 33-B: 376
8. Johnson K, Cofield R, Morrey B. Clin Orthop 1979; 142: 44–47
9. Barouk LS. Foot Ankle Clinics 2000; 5: 525–558
10. Mann RA, Clanton TO. J Bone Joint Surg (Am) 1988; 70-A: 400–405
11. Alexander IJ. In: Myerson M (ed). Current Therapy in Foot and Ankle Surgery. Mosby, St Louis, 1993: 81–90
12. Coughlin MJ. J Bone Joint Surg (Am) 2002; 84-A: 1446–1469

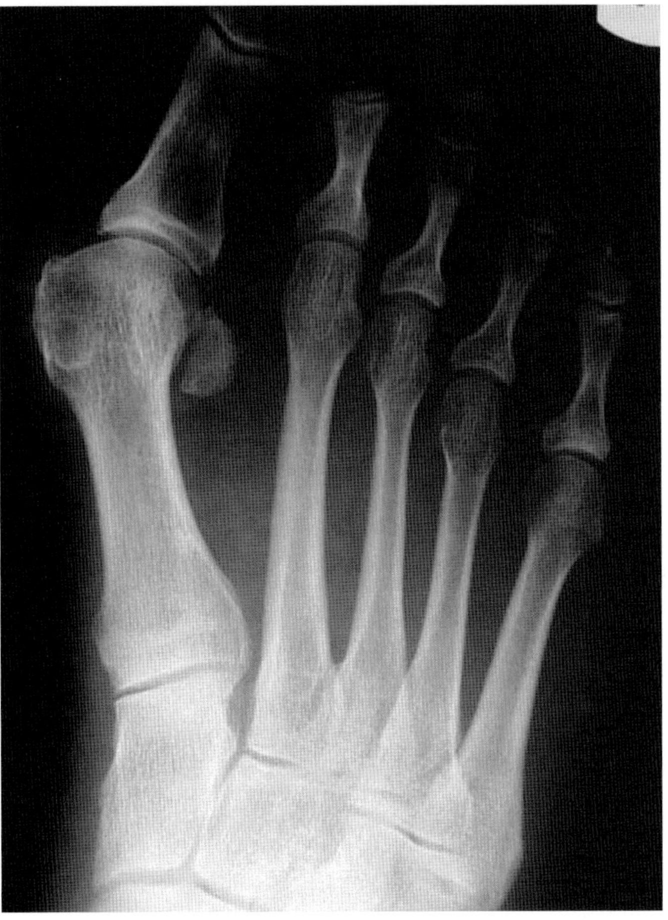

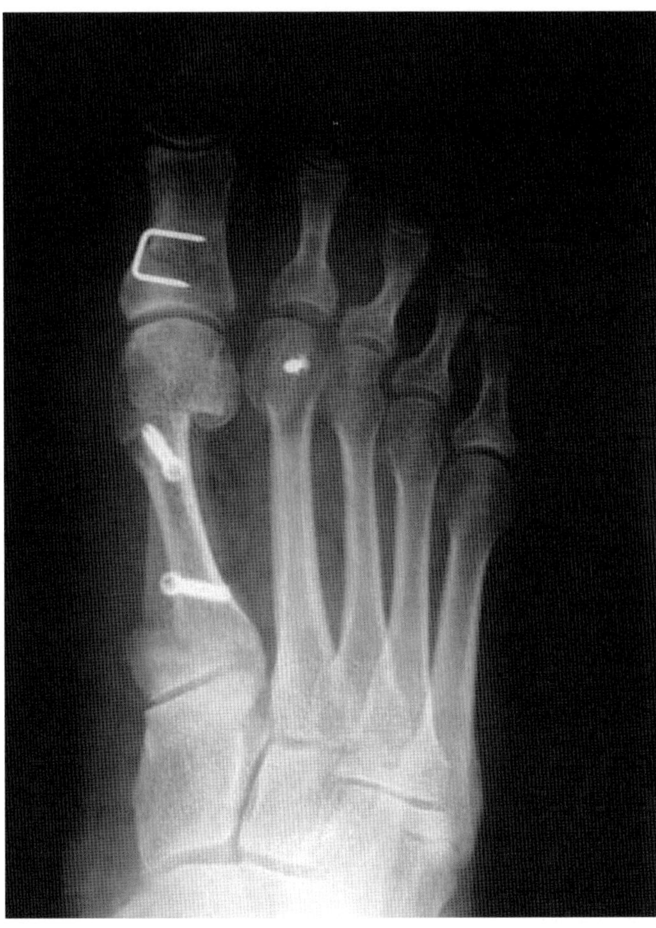

Figure 51.5 Hallux valgus and long second metatarsal correction using scarf and Akin osteotomies of the first ray and Weil's osteotomy of the second.

appropriate to the condition and executed meticulously. The potential for making matters worse is immense.

Osteoarthritis of lesser metatarsophalangeal joints is rare, but when it occurs is difficult to treat without creating further problems. Excision of an isolated metatarsal head and proximal phalangectomy are procedures to be avoided. Freiberg's infraction (avascular necrosis of the second or third metatarsal head) occurs typically in teenage girls, and if symptomatic and unresponsive to conservative measures may require debridement or osteotomy.

MORTON'S NEUROMA AND MORTON'S METATARSALGIA

Morton's neuroma is an example of an entrapment neuropathy and usually affects the common digital nerve of the third interspace. Less commonly it can occur in the second space, but never in the first or fourth spaces. The main symptom is of a searing nerve pain into the affected toes when wearing shoes, relieved by removing the shoe. The patient is almost invariably pain-free out of shoes. If a premetatarsal dome shoe insert and/or one steroid injection fail to relieve the problem, surgery to excise the nerve or decompress the nerve is a good option.

Morton's metatarsalgia is a separate entity and refers to pain under one of the lesser metatarsophalangeal joints, most commonly the second. It occurs as a result of overload of the joint and often occurs as a result of poorly thought-out hallux valgus surgery. Patients complain of severe pain under the second metatarsophalangeal joint, and often there is a callosity and joint instability, sometimes even joint dislocation. If conservative measures fail to alleviate the problem, a shortening and/or elevating osteotomy (e.g. Weil's) can be curative.[13]

SESAMOID DISORDERS

There are many recognized accessory bones in the foot, but the medial and lateral sesamoids of the hallux are present in most individuals. They can be the source of pain, and if conservative measures fail, surgery to excise the symptomatic sesamoid can be helpful. Excising both sesamoids can lead to a cocked-up toe and should never be performed.

TOENAIL DISORDERS

The commonest toenail disorder is the ingrowing toenail. If chiropody fails to solve the problem, surgery to remove part or all of the nail bed can be curative. If the presentation is atypical, the presence of a subungual exostosis should be considered. It should also be remembered that toenail abnormalities can occur and therefore be helpful in the diagnosis of systemic disease (e.g. psoriatic arthropathy and iron-deficiency anaemia).

REFERENCES

13. Davies MS, Saxby TS. Foot Ankle Int 1999; 20: 630–635

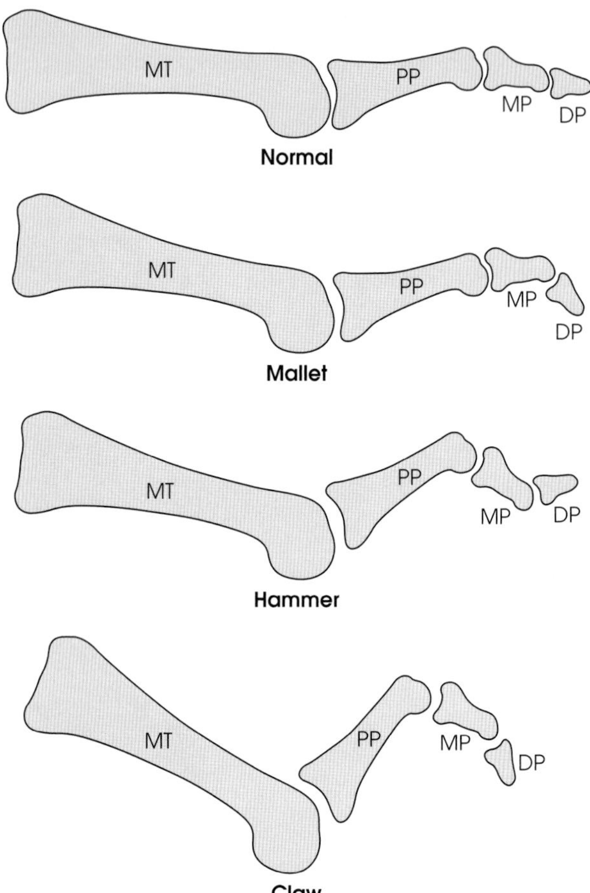

Figure 51.6 Common lesser toe deformities: MT, metatarsal; PP, proximal phalanx; MP, middle phalanx; and DP, distal phalanx.

ARTHRITIS OF THE FOOT

Osteoarthritis can affect any of the foot joints, but the naviculocuneiform joints, the fourth and fifth tarsometatarsal joints, and the lesser metatarsophalangeal joints are very rarely affected. It is also rare for the lesser toe joints between the phalanges to be affected by osteoarthritis. No matter which foot joint is affected by osteoarthritis, the mainstay of conservative management is activity and footwear modification, analgesic and anti-inflammatory medication, and walking aids (e.g. a cane). Shoes that are supportive and cushioned, such as training shoes, can be very effective and are considerably cheaper and safer than surgery. For advanced osteoarthritis unresponsive to conservative measures, arthrodesis is the surgical option of choice. The surgeon should fuse only the symptomatic joints, and preoperative diagnostic injections of local anaesthetic can be extremely helpful in planning surgery. Most fusion procedures do not require bone graft but do involve approximately 12 weeks in a plaster cast on crutches. Risks include infection and non-union, especially in smokers, plus all the potential problems associated with plaster immobilization. An infected non-union can result in amputation, and therefore the decision to arthrodese should not be taken lightly.

Rheumatoid arthritis and the inflammatory arthropathies can affect any joint in the foot, including very commonly the lesser metatarsophalangeal joints. The treatment is medical control of the disease and footwear modification, but when these fail surgery has a role to offer. Clearly, if all the joints of the foot are affected, arthrodesis of all the joints cannot and should not be attempted. Selective arthrodesis, however, can be a very powerful tool, but lesser metatarsophalangeal joints cannot be fused. If joint-preserving procedures are not feasible, excision arthroplasties of all the lesser metatarsophalangeal joints can be undertaken (Fig. 51.7), with good results despite the fact that this is a destructive procedure.

PAINFUL HEEL

The differential diagnosis of heel pain includes stress fracture of the os calcis, insertional Achilles tendonitis, infection, tumour and referred pain, but the commonest cause by far is plantar fasciitis. This condition presents with inferomedial heel pain worse on first weight bearing after sleep, or after a period of rest or sitting and towards the end of the day. It is common in obese middle-aged women who have undertaken unaccustomed activity. It also occurs in male runners in their forties who have overtrained. Treatment should be with physiotherapy plus the judicious use of steroid injection. In 95% of cases the symptoms settle spontaneously within 12–18 months, but for intractable plantar fasciitis surgery may, as a last resort, be required.[14] The role of shockwave therapy has yet to be defined.

ACQUIRED FLAT FOOT

Loss of the medial longitudinal arch is nowhere near as prevalent as is commonly thought. The conditions that may lead to flattening of the foot are tibialis posterior tendon dysfunction, tarsometatarsal and/or naviculocuneiform arthritis, Charcot neuroarthropathy, spring ligament injury, and degenerative or inflammatory disorders of the subtalar and/or transverse tarsal joints. Tibialis posterior tendon dysfunction and Charcot neuroarthropathy warrant further comment.

Tibialis posterior tendon dysfunction can be extremely disabling, and if left untreated can lead to severe deformity and long-term disability (Fig. 51.8). It is most commonly seen in overweight females and presents with medial ankle pain and swelling. The diagnosis is often overlooked because many primary care physicians do not know about the condition and radiographs are almost always normal. If rest, immobilization and anti-inflammatory medication fail to resolve the symptoms, surgery should be considered in an attempt to prevent deformity. Once deformity has occurred, a calcaneal osteotomy and tendon transfer can be used to provide pain relief, but almost more importantly to prevent further deformity.[15] End-stage tibialis posterior tendon dysfunction is very disabling and difficult to treat. Although not causes of acquired flat foot, it should be remembered that other tendons of the foot can undergo degeneration, particularly the Achilles tendon and the peroneal tendons.

Charcot neuroarthropathy is most commonly seen in long-standing diabetic patients with peripheral neuropathy, but can be seen in any case of long-standing neuropathy (e.g. in alcoholic individuals). Due to repeated microtrauma and lack of proprioception, the midfoot, hindfoot and ankle joints are prone to spectacular collapse (Fig. 51.9). It is essential but sometimes difficult to distinguish the condition from infection. The Charcot retaining orthotic walker is the mainstay of treatment.

REFERENCES

14. Davies MS, Weiss GA, Saxby TS. Foot Ankle Int 1999; 20: 803–807
15. Wacker JT, Hennessy MS, Saxby TS. J Bone Joint Surg (Br) 2002; 84-B: 54–58

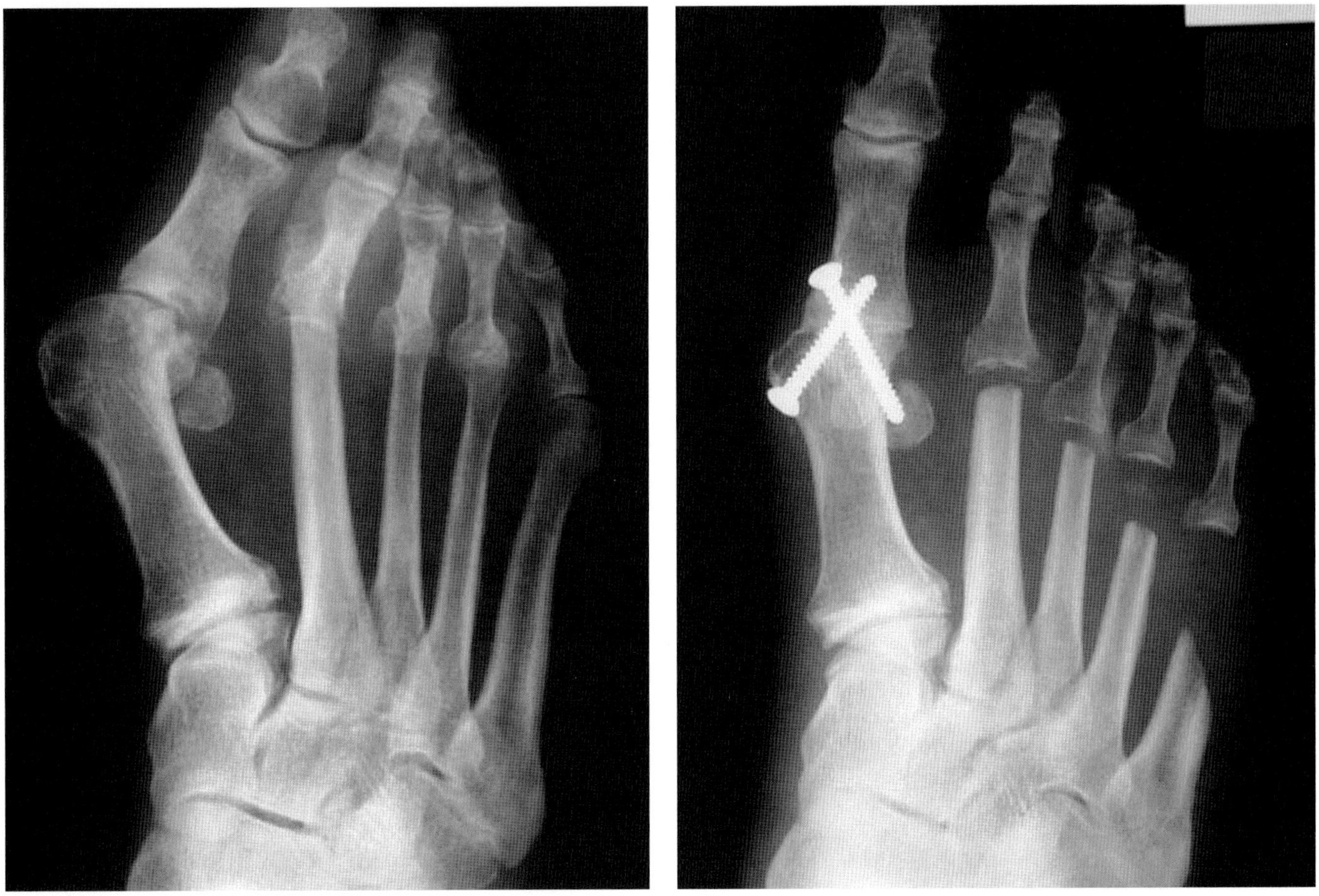

a b

Figure 51.7 (a) Severe rheumatoid forefoot deformity and (b) first metatarsophalangeal joint fusion and excision arthroplasties.

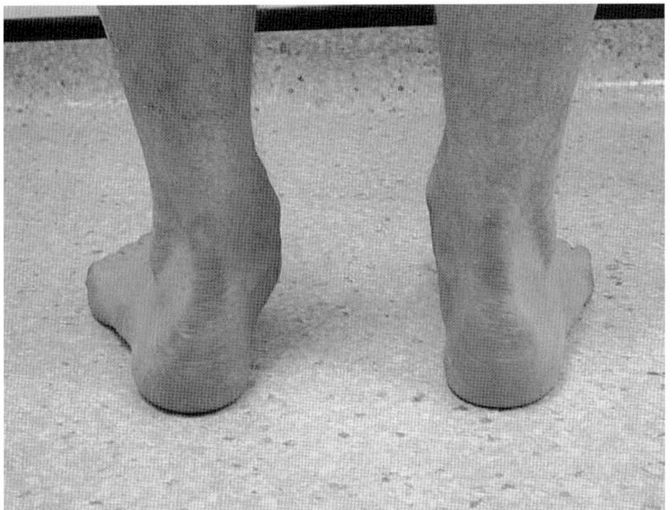

Figure 51.8 Left planovalgus foot deformity secondary to tibialis posterior tendon dysfunction.

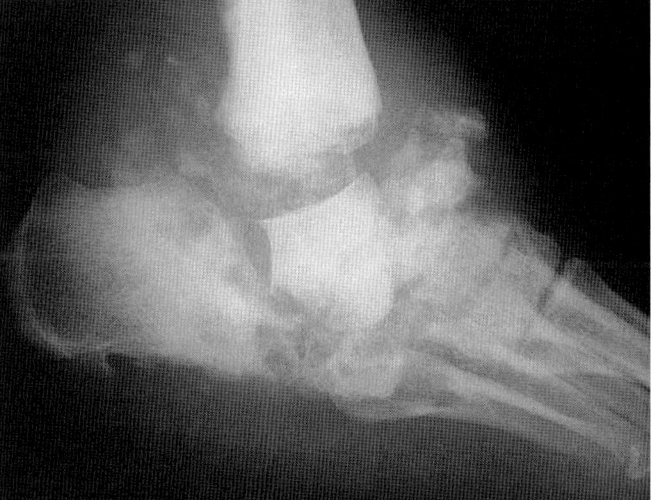

Figure 51.9 Lateral radiograph showing diabetic Charcot neuroarthropathic destruction of the ankle, subtalar and mid foot joints.

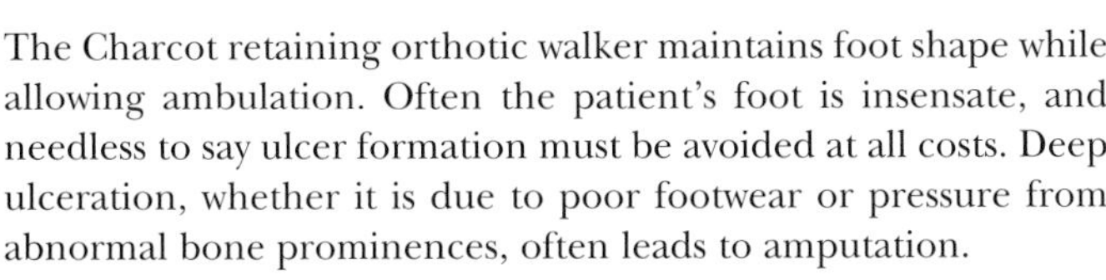

The Charcot retaining orthotic walker maintains foot shape while allowing ambulation. Often the patient's foot is insensate, and needless to say ulcer formation must be avoided at all costs. Deep ulceration, whether it is due to poor footwear or pressure from abnormal bone prominences, often leads to amputation.

PES CAVUS

High-arched feet may be of no consequence and merely represent one end of the normal spectrum of foot shape. However, and particularly if there is progression of the deformity, pes cavus can be the first manifestation of a neurological disease

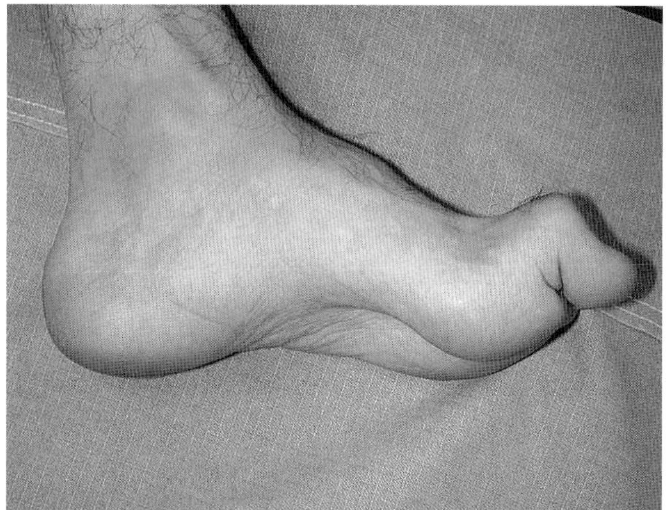

Figure 51.10 Pes cavus and clawing of the hallux.

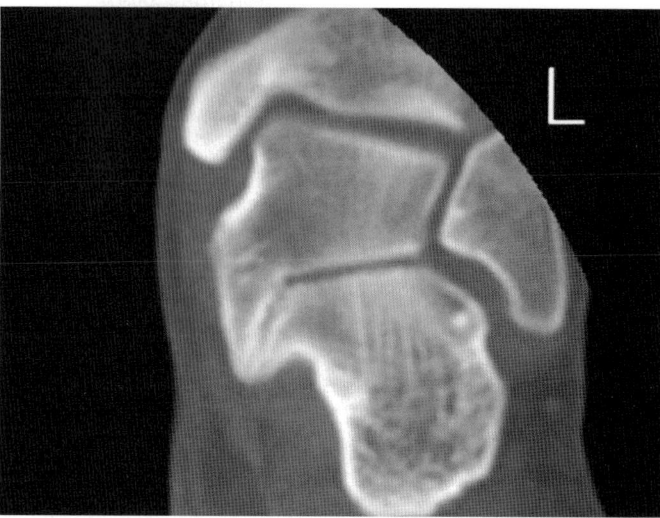

Figure 51.11 Coronal CT of talocalcaneal coalition.

process (Fig. 51.10). Up to 80% of high-arched feet are associated with an underlying neurological disorder.[16] The commonest underlying disease is Charcot–Marie–Tooth disease, one of the hereditary motor and sensory neuropathies, but conditions such as diastematomyelia (spinal cord tethering) must not be overlooked. There are in fact very many conditions that can lead to pes cavus, and involvement of a neurologist in the investigations is advisable. Clearly the underlying neurological condition needs to be treated (if it can be), and then the foot deformity itself needs addressing. Treatment comprises footwear modification and/or surgery. The aim of surgery is to make the foot look and function like a normal foot. This can be accomplished by a combination of soft tissue and bone procedures, for example plantar fascia release, tendon transfer, and osteotomies and/or arthrodeses.

TARSAL COALITIONS

If a child between the ages of 10 and 16 years complains of foot pain, a diagnosis of tarsal coalition should be considered. The foot is often flat, and on examination of the subtalar joint there is no movement. The two commonest coalitions are calcaneonavicular, seen on an oblique foot radiograph, and talocalcaneal, often missed on plain radiographs. The 'C sign' should be looked for on the lateral ankle radiograph, and CT scanning should be undertaken to define the extent of the lesion (Fig. 51.11).[17] Surgery is reserved for those patients who are symptomatic. Surgery to remove the coalition is often good for pain relief but not at restoring hindfoot motion.

FOOT TUMOURS

The foot is very rarely affected by bone tumours, but they do occur from time to time and are best treated by orthopaedic surgeons who specialize in this area.

Soft tissue tumours of the foot are much more common than bone tumours and the vast majority are benign. The two commonest are ganglia and angioleiomyomas (Fig. 51.12) and can be excised if symptomatic or if there is any concern that the lesion might be malignant. Other tumours include lipomas and inclusion dermoid cysts, which may need excision. Plantar fibromata, however, are best left well alone.

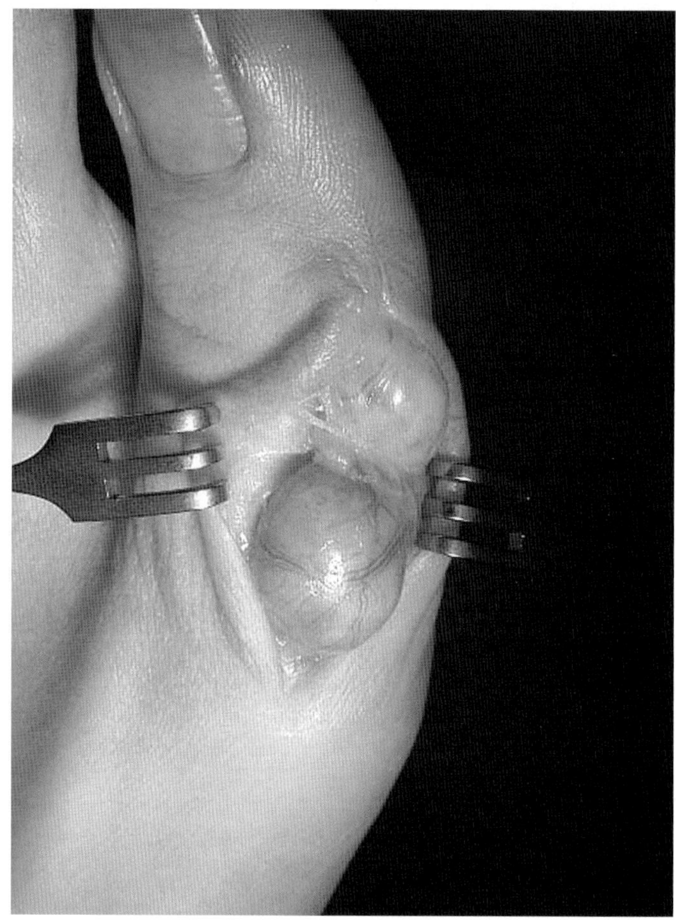

Figure 51.12 Angioleiomyoma of the foot.

REFERENCES

16. Brewerton DA, Sandifer PH, Sweetnam DR. Br Med J 1963; 2: 659–661
17. Sakellariou A, Sallomi D, Janzen DM et al. J Bone Joint Surg (Br) 2000; 82-B: 574–578

FOOT INFECTIONS

Infections of the foot are either acute or chronic, and occur as a result of direct inoculation or haematogenous spread. Fungal infections of the toenails are common and are usually treated by primary care physicians or dermatologists. For skin infections, the treatment is usually an appropriate antimicrobial either systemically or topically administered after cultures are obtained. Sepsis from penetrative wounds of the foot through footwear is usually caused by *Pseudomonas aeruginosa*, and thorough wound toilet and appropriate antibiotics are required. Conditions such as necrotizing fasciitis are potentially fatal and need aggressive surgical debridement as well as intravenous antibiotics. The usual causative organism is *Streptococcus pyogenes*.

Diabetic patients are particularly prone to deep foot infections that, if not treated aggressively by surgical debridement, can lead to amputation. Antibiotics alone will never eradicate established deep bony infection. The principle of diabetic foot care is to get the patient ulcer-free and keep them ulcer-free. Tissue sampling prior to administration of antibiotics is essential. It is important to remember that radiographs in the early stages of infection are often normal. Blood tests and more sophisticated imaging (e.g. MRI scanning) can be useful in the diagnosis of early bone infection.

Other foot infections are rare, but one should always bear in mind the possibility of tuberculosis. Once a tissue specimen has been obtained and the diagnosis confirmed, tuberculosis is best treated with chemotherapy rather than surgery.

Another infection worth mentioning is a mycetoma, which may follow a puncture wound of the foot. It tends to grow in size and is difficult to eradicate even with surgical excision.

AMPUTATION

It goes without saying that amputation is an irreversible operative procedure. Amputations are carried out for many reasons but mainly for infection (often associated with poor vascularity) plus trauma, tumour, etc. The decision to amputate should never be taken lightly but equally, amputation as an option should not be withheld when clearly the patient would be better off without the foot (or leg). The level of amputation has to be compatible with wound healing and be at such a level to allow the fitting of a prosthesis.

CONCLUSION

There have been major advances in the subspecialty discipline of foot and ankle surgery, and most are based on well-established orthopaedic principles. With few exceptions, non-operative measures should be tried ahead of surgery. Modern foot and ankle surgery, however, has a lot to offer, and providing the patient is well informed about what is involved and what to expect, most patients do well with modern, well-thought out procedures tailored to their individual needs.

Principles of fractures and complications 52

Roger M. Atkins, Jonathan D. Lucas

PRINCIPLES

Put simply, a fracture is a broken bone, which therefore represents the interaction between a physical force that produces the break and a biological substance, the bone that is broken. To understand fractures, it is therefore necessary to understand the structure and function of bones. In addition, the soft tissues surrounding the bone will be damaged in the fracture, and they are of paramount importance.

STRUCTURE OF BONE

INTRODUCTION

Bone is a specialized connective tissue that forms an endoskeleton. It provides structural support for the body, protects vital organs, and acts as a series of mechanical levers through which attached muscles and ligaments can move the body. In addition, it provides a store of calcium and phosphate, and phylogenetically this was probably the reason for its development.

ANATOMY

Macroscopically, bone is made up of two components: the dense outer cortex, which by its tubular structure gives maximum strength for weight, and the inner cancellous bone, which consists of a network of trabeculae, the arrangement of which follows the direction of imposed stress, adding to its strength.

The basic structural unit of bone is the Haversian system or osteon, a series of concentric layers of similarly oriented collagen fibres (lamellae) surrounding a central Haversian canal. The space between the osteons is filled by interstitial lamellae formed from irregular layers of bone. Between the lamellae, flattened bone cells (osteocytes) lie in spaces (lacunae) from which arise innumerable fine passages (canaliculi) containing fine projections from the osteocytes, which are therefore in communication with each other. In the centre of each Haversian system is a central canal containing bone cells and a neurovascular bundle. These run parallel to the long axis of the bone and are united by Volkmann's canals piercing the bone from the outer and inner surfaces.

The bone is surrounded by periosteum made up of an outer layer of fibrous and elastic tissue into which muscles, tendons and intermuscular septa insert, and an inner vascular 'cambium' layer that contains osteoprogenitor cells. At points where the bone has ligament or muscle attachments, the periosteum is reinforced by perforating fibres of Sharpey, which are coarse collagen fibres that are continuous with the periosteum but perforate into the cortical bone. Immediately beneath the periosteum is found a layer of circumferential lamellae running parallel with the bone enclosing all the osteons.

BLOOD SUPPLY

Anatomy

Vessels enter the bone in the metaphyseal region to supply the epiphysis and metaphysis and to anastomose with the diaphyseal supply. The main arterial supply to the diaphysis comes via nutrient arteries that divide in the medulla into ascending and descending branches. These ramify within the medullary cavity and constitute the primary resistance vessels of the osseous circulation.[1] Nutrient veins accompany the arteries outside the bone and continue within the medullary canal as a central longitudinal venous sinus that drains the medullary sinusoids through radial connecting sinuses.

Accompanying the blood vessels there are nerve fibres that extend into the Haversian systems and periosteum to innervate the blood vessels and supply pain and vibration sensitivity. There may also be a neural input into bone cells.

Physiology

The arterial supply of the cortex of bone is fan-shaped, with cortical sinusoids radiating outwards towards the periosteal surface, becoming smaller and supplying each Haversian canal. The major direction of cortical blood flow is centrifugal;[2] however, periosteal arteries penetrate bone at points of attachment,[3] and although under normal conditions these supply only a small area, following injury the periosteal source is capable of supplying the whole bone. The venous drainage is probably also centrifugal, passing into periosteal and muscular veins, leaving the nutrient vein unfilled.[2,4,5]

Under normal physiological conditions, bone receives between 5 and 10% of the cardiac output,[6] with the supply being relatively greater at the bone ends. Bone blood flow is regulated by neural, hormonal and metabolic mechanisms.[6] Electrical stimulation of somatic or sympathetic nerves to bone, or administration of adrenaline, all reduce blood flow,[7–9] while

REFERENCES

1. Brooks M. Bone 1986; 3: 32–34
2. Brooks M. The Blood Supply of Bone. Butterworths, London, 1971
3. Rhinelander FW. Internal Fixation of Fractures. Springer-Verlag, Berlin, 1980: 9–14
4. Cuthbertson EN, Sirus E, Gilfillan RS. J Bone Joint Surg 1965; 47A: 965–974
5. Oni OOA, Gregg PJ. In: Arlet J, Mazieres B (eds). Bone Circulation and Bone Necrosis. Springer-Verlag, Berlin, 1990: 7–10
6. Shim SS. J Bone Joint Surg 1968; 50A: 812–824
7. Drinker CK, Drinker KR. Am J Physiol 1916; 40: 512–521
8. Shim SS, Patterson FP. Surg Gynecol Obstet 1967; 125: 261–268
9. Brinker MR, Lipton HL, Cook SD et al. J Bone Joint Surg 1990; 72A: 964–975

sympathectomy causes an increase.[10] Restoration of the circulation following a period of ischaemia leads to a two- to threefold increase in blood flow,[8] and this effect takes precedence over neural or hormonal control.

CHEMISTRY OF BONE

Bone is made up of organic and inorganic materials, and water. The organic intercellular matrix of bone is 93% collagen and 7% non-collagenous proteins. The latter include a number of proteins, such as osteocalcin and osteonectin, that are unique to bone and may have a role in binding the mineral phase of bone to collagen.[11]

The mineral phase of bone provides its mechanical strength and serves as a reservoir of calcium and phosphate. The mineral of bone is poorly crystalline, imperfect hydroxyapatite, $Ca_{10}(PO_4)_6(OH)_2$, which contains a variety of substituted ions. With ageing, the crystal becomes larger, less hydrated and more perfect,[12,13] which reduces bone strength in the elderly.

The unique feature of bone is the close attachment between its organic and inorganic constituents. Type 1 collagen is found ubiquitously in the body, but only in bone is it closely associated with hydroxyapatite. The bone mineral is regularly distributed within the collagen fibrils, being deposited first within the hole zone region, which are spaces between the triple helices.[14] In unmineralized osteoid, mineralization begins independently and simultaneously at a number of different sites, starting between 1 and 10 days after osteoid deposition. The region in which mineralization occurs is supersaturated with calcium and phosphate ions, so that mineralization represents a phase change from dissolved ions to solid hydroxyapatite. The precise mechanism is not known, but it seems likely that non-collagenous phosphoproteins distributed throughout the collagen matrix provide nucleation sites.[14]

BONE TURNOVER AND REMODELLING

The constituent parts of bone are constantly being renewed at a rate of approximately 10% per year. This is made up of 4% in cortical and 25% in trabecular bone,[15] and it allows for the removal of fatigue damage and maintenance of relatively young skeletal tissue by a mechanism referred to as remodelling by bone biologists. This process is a part of the remodelling that is described by orthopaedic surgeons. Bone remodelling follows an orderly cycle, and in an adult only approximately 10% of the bone surface is involved at any time;[16] the remainder is inactive. In contrast, in a child the majority of the bone surface is active.

At a region of bone that is to be remodelled, the bone becomes activated and precursor cells differentiate into osteoclasts that erode a surface cavity, producing a Howship's lacuna in trabecular bone or a cutting cone in cortical bone. The osteoclasts then disappear, and the irregular cavity is smoothed off and lined by a layer of mineral-rich cement substance. Osteoblasts are next recruited, which refill the excavated cavity with new bone.

Alternations in the dynamics of different parts of the remodelling processes account for the many age-related changes in the skeleton.[17,18] During adult life, bone is lost from the skeleton at a rate of approximately 1% of its peak mass per year,[19] because there is a small imbalance between the amount of bone resorbed and the subsequent amount formed in each episode of bone remodelling. This is referred to as the remodelling imbalance.[20] The balance between formation and resorption varies between different bone surfaces. The average bone remodelling unit will add a small volume on the periosteal surface and subtract a small volume at the endosteal surface.[18] This is responsible for the widening of the femoral medullary canal, which occurs along with thinning of the femoral cortex with ageing.

REGULATION OF BONE CELL FUNCTION

Bone is responsible for the structural integrity of the skeleton and for maintaining the serum levels of calcium and phosphate, which are essential for nerve and muscle function. The regulation of bone homeostasis is therefore complex.

The general body demands for calcium, phosphate and magnesium are satisfied by the effects of systemic hormones, including vitamin D, parathyroid hormone and calcitonin on the bone (see Ch. 18).

Locally, bone cell function is affected by growth factors and cytokines, proteins that regulate the function of differentiated cells at very low concentrations,[21–23] and by prostaglandins. Important cytokines are transforming growth factor β and interleukin 1, which stimulate bone,[24] and insulin-like growth factor, which stimulates osteoblast proliferation and collagen synthesis.[25,26] Bone morphogenetic proteins are cytokines that are members of the transforming growth factor β family and stimulate bone formation by a complex series of actions. These are now becoming available therapeutically due to the production of human recombinant molecules. The prostaglandins are powerful stimulators of bone resorption when added to organ-cultured bones.[27,28] They are produced in large quantities following fracture,[29] and they may be responsible for abnormal bone remodelling and sequestrum formation in osteomyelitis.[29]

REFERENCES

10. Trottman NM, Kelly WD. JAMA 1963; 183: 121–122
11. Termine JD, Kleinman HK, Whitson SW et al. Cell 1981; 26: 99–105
12. Glimcher MJ. Rev Mod Phys 1959; 31: 359–393
13. Landis WJ, Glimcher MJ. J Ultrastrut Res 1978; 63: 188–133
14. Glimcher MJ. In: Avioli LV, Krant SM (eds). Metabolic Bone Disease. Saunders, Philadelphia, 1990: 42–68
15. Parfitt AM. In: Recker RR (ed). Bone Histomorphometry: Techniques and Interpretations. CRC Press, Boca Raton, 1983: 143–223
16. Parfitt AM. Calcif Tissue Int 1984; 36 (Suppl): S37–S45
17. Parfitt AM. Metab Bone Dis Relat Res 1982; 4: 1–6
18. Parfitt AM. In: Riggs BL, Melton LJ III (eds). Osteoporosis: Aetiology, Diagnosis and Management. Reven Press, New York, 1988
19. Garn SM. In: De Luca HF, Frost HM, Jee WSS et al. (eds). Osteoporosis: Recent Advances in Pathogenesis and Treatment. University Park Press, Baltimore, 1981: 3–16
20. Parfitt AM. Med Times 1981; 109: 80–92
21. Centrella M, Canalis E. Proc Natl Acad Sci USA 1985; 82: 7335–7339
22. Hauschka PV, Mavrakos AE, Iafrati MD et al. Biol Chem 1986; 261: 12665–12674
23. McDonald BR, Gowan F. Br J Rheumatol 1992; 31: 149–155
24. Gowan M, Wood DD, Ihra EJ et al. Nature 1983; 306: 378–380
25. Cannalis EM, Hintz RL, Dietrich JW et al. Metabolism 1971; 26: 1079–1087
26. Cannalis E. J Clin Invest 1980; 66: 709–719
27. Dietrich JW, Goodson JN, Raisz LG. Prostaglandins 1975; 10: 231–240
28. Tashjian AH Jr, Tice JE, Sides K. Nature 1977; 266: 645–646
29. Dekel S, Francis MJO. J Bone Joint Surg 1981; 63B: 178–184

The mass of bone at any site adjusts so that its strain environment is constant, a phenomenon often termed *Wolff's law*.[30] This means that if the bone is stressed it will over time become thicker or sclerotic, whereas if it is protected from external mechanical stress—as for example occurs in the leg when an orthopaedic patient is made non-weight-bearing—the bone will become porotic. This process is mediated by the remodelling cycle, but the mechanism by which the strain message causes alterations in the balance between bone formation and resorption is unknown. It may involve the osteocyte processes, local cytokine formation, or electrical phenomena. An area of bone under compression exhibits a negative potential, while a region under tension becomes relatively electropositive. These phenomena are caused by piezoelectrical effects due to deformation of the molecules of bone[31] and streaming potentials caused by stress-induced changes in fluid fluxes.[32] Electronegative areas of bone are associated with bone formation, while in positively charged areas bone is resorbed. Effects of electricity have been demonstrated experimentally on a wide variety of bone cell functions including matrix formation, calcification, and cell proliferation.[33] Although this suggests that it should be possible to influence fracture union using externally applied electrical fields, definitive evidence for this is lacking.[34]

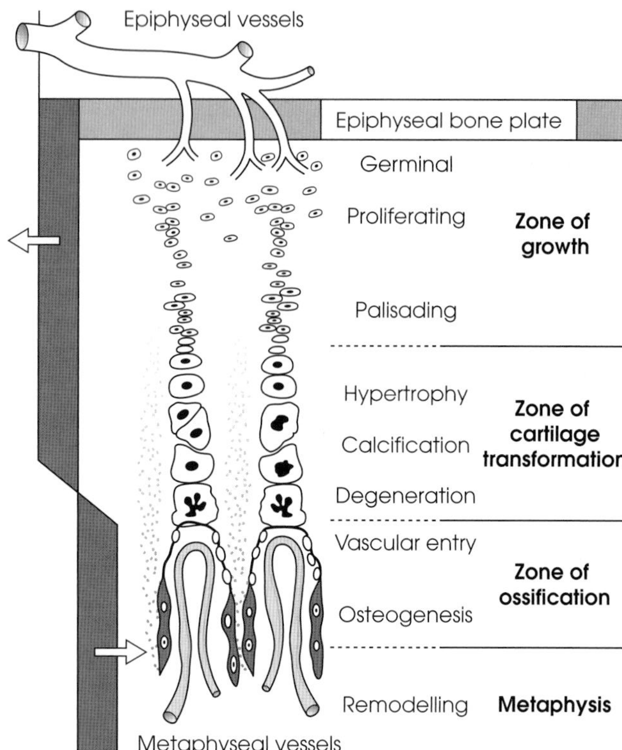

Figure 52.1 A diagrammatic representation of the growth plate, showing the individual layers. Nearest to the epiphysis is the germinal layer of cells, the blood supply of which comes from epiphyseal vessels. Passing towards the diaphysis, the cells in the proliferating layer are undergoing mitosis, and the daughter cells then mature and hypertrophy before becoming calcified and degenerating. Capillary tufts from the metaphysis invade the dead cells and calcified pericellular matrix. Phagocytosis of the dead material occurs, and new bone laid down by primitive osteoblasts is subsequently remodelled. Widthways growth of the physis occurs at the periphery by mitosis within the perichondral ring of Lacroix. (From Rang 1984.[35])

BIOLOGICAL ASPECTS OF FRACTURE HEALING

BONE GROWTH AND DEVELOPMENT

Fractures heal by mechanisms similar to those by which bone forms, so an understanding of the latter is important for a discussion of fractures. Bone forms either by intramembranous ossification or by endochondral ossification.

Intramembranous bone formation

Intramembranous bone formation occurs within a primitive layer of vascularized connective tissue. Cells proliferate, hypertrophy, and transform into osteoblasts. Progressive bone formation results in the fusion of adjacent bony areas within the membrane to form spongy bone. This is then remodelled into its mature form. This sort of bone formation occurs in the bones of the vault of the skull, the maxilla, and the clavicle.

Endochondral bone formation

In endochondral ossification, an area of cartilage forms a model (or anlage) for the bone that will be formed, but it does not itself transform into bone. The cartilage matrix becomes calcified with death of the cartilage cells, and the matrix is then resorbed and replaced by vascularized bone, which subsequently remodels. The most ordered example of endochondral ossification is seen at the growth plate, which is composed of cartilage cells arranged in well-ordered long columns parallel to each other and to the axis of growth of each bone end (Fig. 52.1).

On the epiphyseal side of each column, the cartilage cells are small and flat in the resting zone. Immediately metaphyseal to this is the layer of active cell division. Approximately halfway down the cell columns towards the metaphysis, rapid cell division ceases as the hypertrophic zone is entered. This region is distant from both the epiphyseal and metaphyseal blood supplies and is relatively avascular. The chondrocytes mature and hypertrophy, and calcification begins in the matrix between the cell columns. The last hypertrophic cartilage cell of each column is immediately adjacent to an invading capillary tuft from the metaphysis. Osteoblasts are carried in from the metaphysis with the new capillaries, and they lay down new bone around the bars of calcified cartilage matrix between the columns at the base of the growth plate. This is subsequently remodelled to produce new bone. The growth plate must itself grow outwards, and this is accomplished by widthwise mitoses of cells on the outer edge of the germinal layer of the physis, a region termed the *perichondral ring of Lacroix*.

The long bones (except the clavicle), the vertebrae, the pelvis, and the bones of the base of the skull are formed in this fashion. It is, however, important to note that although growth in length of a long bone occurs at the growth plate by endochondral ossification, widthwise growth is by intramembranous bone

REFERENCES

30. Rubin CT. PhD thesis, Bristol, 1982
31. Fukada E, Yasuda I. J Phys Soc Japan 1957; 10: 1158–1169
32. Pienkowski D, Pollack SR. J Orthop Res 1983; 1: 30–41
33. Pollack SR. In: Takahashi AG (ed). Bone Morphometry. Smith Gordon, London, 1990
34. Barker AT, Dixon RA, Sharrard WJW et al. Lancet 1984; i: 994-996
35. Rang M. Children's Fractures. 2nd edn. Lippincott, Philadelphia, 1984: 1

formation beneath the periosteum (periosteal appositional bone growth). Subsequently all the bone laid down primarily is remodelled to produce mature Haversian bone.

FRACTURE HEALING

Healing of a fracture results in reconstitution of the injured tissue into something resembling its original form. As in other tissues, a scar forms; this is able from an early stage to function as bone. This scar is slowly remodelled into increasingly normal bone, and the original bone architecture will be completely restored in children's fractures or in relatively undisplaced or well-reduced adult fractures. In more comminuted, high-energy or displaced fractures, restitution is seldom complete. The changes associated with fracture healing may be considered as three phases that overlap but occur sequentially. These are the phase of inflammation, the development of osteogenic repair tissue, and the phase of remodelling.

Inflammation

Inflammation begins immediately after injury and is rapidly followed by repair. Bleeding from damaged bone ends and soft tissues leads to fibrinous clot formation between the fragments. Damage to the bone blood vessels causes loss of nutrition of bone cells, so that the broken ends of the bone are dead[36] and play a passive role in fracture healing, providing a bridge between more distant regions of living bone.[37] The extent of bone death will vary with the degree of fracture comminution, the amount of periosteal stripping, the extent of fracture displacement, and the severity of damage to the medullary contents—the greater the bone damage, the slower will fracture healing be. Inflammatory mediators are released from injured tissues, causing an increase in vascular permeability, which leads to an exudate of plasma.[38] Inflammatory cells migrate into the region and phagocytosis of necrotic material begins.

DEVELOPMENT OF OSTEOGENIC REPAIR TISSUE

The amount and composition of repair tissue vary with the site, type and severity of the fracture; the type of bone involved; the state of the soft tissues surrounding the fracture; and whether the fragments move in relation to each other during healing. The following description refers principally to a simple fracture of a long bone in which the fragments are not rigidly immobilized.

The first stage of the repair process is the organization of the fracture haematoma, which is invaded by fibrovascular tissue and eventually mineralizes to form provisional callus. There are two sources of repair tissue: medullary and periosteal. The former is most marked in cancellous bone, while the latter predominates in a diaphyseal fracture.

Periosteal callus

The potential of periosteum for repair is demonstrated by the ability of bone that has been resected subperiosteally, so leaving the cambium layer of the periosteum in place, to regenerate.[39] In a fracture where the bone has not been removed, cellular proliferation and hypertrophy begin at a distance from the fracture, often over viable cortex. Repair tissue becomes invaded by osteogenic cells derived from the cambium layer of periosteum. If the periosteum is intact, a bridge of callus readily forms, arching over the dead bone ends. If it is ruptured, cuffs of callus grow outwards from the living bone, eventually joining together.[37]

In some areas, particularly at the periphery of the callus, a variety of hyaline cartilage forms that becomes converted to bone by endochondral ossification. The amount of cartilage formed is very variable. This may represent a response to low oxygen tension,[36,40,41] the concept being that if callus outgrows its blood supply cartilage provides a suitable material, less demanding of oxygen, to bridge the gap until vascularity is re-established.[37] Alternatively, Hulth[42] suggests that cartilage is laid down in response to fragment movement,[43,44] which mechanically inhibits vascular invasion. Because this will lead to lowered oxygen tension, these two theories are in fact similar.

The blood supply of the periosteal callus comes initially from the periosteal vessels and extraperiosteal soft tissues, including muscle,[45] and only later does the medullary blood supply make a contribution.[46,47] The new, fracture-induced blood supply regresses as union occurs and eventually disappears.

Medullary callus

Vascular proliferation in the medullary region is the principal method of union in cancellous bone (e.g. in a fracture of the tibial plateau) and plays a part in union of the tubular bone, where medullary activity is particularly marked if the fracture is offset.[37] The vascular response is slower than that seen in the periosteum.[48]

Phase of remodelling

Once the fracture has been satisfactorily bridged by callus, the newly formed bone is adapted to its new function by remodelling. This refers to the process of adaptation of the skeleton to applied loads. In qualitative terms, the remodelling process is no different from the process of replacement and repair that is occurring continually within the normal skeleton, except that in this context it includes the revascularization and modification of dead bone at the fracture site. However, the activation frequency of bone remodelling units following a fracture is greatly increased. In the dog radius, the number is increased from a baseline value of 2.5% of the total number of osteons in a cross-section to over 60%. This acceleration of remodelling activity does not occur until the third week after fracture and peaks at 8 weeks.[49]

New blood vessels can invade the trabeculae of cancellous bone, and bone apposition may take place directly on to the trabecular surface. Once this has happened, the bone may take part in the normal remodelling cycle. This phenomenon is referred to as creeping substitution. Although apposition on to

REFERENCES

36. Ham AW. J Bone Joint Surg 1930; 12: 825–844
37. McKibbin B. J Bone Joint Surg 1978; 60B: 150–162
38. Cannalis E, McCarthy T, Sentrella M. J Clin Invest 1988; 81: 277–281
39. Robinson CM, McLaughlan G, Christie J et al. J Bone Joint Surg Br 1995; 77B: 906–913
40. Girgis FG, Pritchard JJ. J Bone Joint Surg 1958; 40B: 274–281
41. Bassett CAL, Herrman I. Nature 1961; 190: 460–461
42. Hulth A. Clin Orthop 1989; 249: 265–284
43. Anderson LD. J Bone Joint Surg 1965; 47A: 191–208
44. Blenman PR, Carter DR, Beaupre GS. Trans Orthop Res Soc 1989; 14: 469
45. Gothman L. Acta Orthop Scand 1961; Suppl: 284
46. Rhinelander FW, Baragry RA. J Bone Joint Surg 1962; 44A: 1273–1298
47. Rhinelander FW. J Bone Joint Surg 1968; 50A: 784–800
48. Olerud S, Dankwardt-Lilliesterom G. Acta Orthop Scand 1971; Suppl: 137
49. Schenk RK. In: Lane JM (ed). Fracture Healing. Churchill Livingstone, Edinburgh, 1987: 23–33

the surface of cortical bone may occur, there are always areas in which the bone cells are dead. For these regions to take part in normal bone remodelling, the osteoclastic 'cutter head' must ream out a tunnel down which the new blood supply can enter the bone. The process of revascularization is relatively slow, and small areas of dead bone may remain for a considerable length of time following normal fracture union. Indeed, in the case of a high-energy fracture with extensive bone death, the entire dead bone may never be removed. It is this residual dead bone that makes bone infection following fracture so difficult to eradicate.

The source of osteogenic cells

There are two possible sources of osteoblasts. The cells may arise by differentiation of previously determined osteogenic progenitor cells, which are found in the inner layer of the periosteum and within the bone marrow, or from previously uncommitted, pluripotent cells in the surrounding soft tissues. These pluripotent cells are termed *inducible osteoprogenitor cells.* The modification of previously undifferentiated soft tissue cells into osteogenic cells is termed *bone induction.* Although it is not clear to what extent it is important in the healing of a fracture, it is well established that non-specialized cells in extraskeletal sites may be stimulated to form bone.[50]

TYPES OF FRACTURE REPAIR

McKibbin has suggested that fracture repair may be divided into four types with differing time courses and physical requirements.[37] It must be emphasized that these divisions are arbitrary, and in a normal fracture it is not possible completely to separate them. They do, however, provide a useful basis for discussion.

Primary callus response

Primary callus response commences within 2 weeks of injury, when exuberant external callus is formed, particularly beneath intact periosteum. The callus spreads from the fractured bone end, but if it does not cause bony union it undergoes involution. The primary callus response is relatively independent of environmental and hormonal influences, being an intrinsic property of the fracture, and it is probably due to determined osteogenic progenitor cells present in the cambium layer of the periosteum.

External bridging callus

External bridging callus forms if the primary callus response does not result in bone continuity. This stage of callus is under the control of humoral and mechanical influences, and it is probably dependent on inducible osteoprogenitor cells derived from the surrounding soft tissues. The external bridging callus appears rapidly and bridges gaps readily. Its formation depends on the presence of viable external soft tissues, which provide the blood vessels for the repair tissue. It is inhibited by rigid fixation and is the predominant form of healing when a simple fracture is treated by cast immobilization or intramedullary nailing (Figs 52.2 and 52.3).[51]

Late medullary callus

Late medullary callus often occurs in combination with external bridging callus but is slower in appearance. It is relatively independent of intact external soft tissues, being more dependent on intramedullary vascularity. It is able to bridge gaps between bone ends and will tolerate a small amount of interfragmentary movement. It is not inhibited by rigid immobilization of the bone ends, and it is important in healing fractures immobilized by rigid plating.[48] Bone that forms under these circumstances frequently does not show an intermediate stage of fibrocartilage.

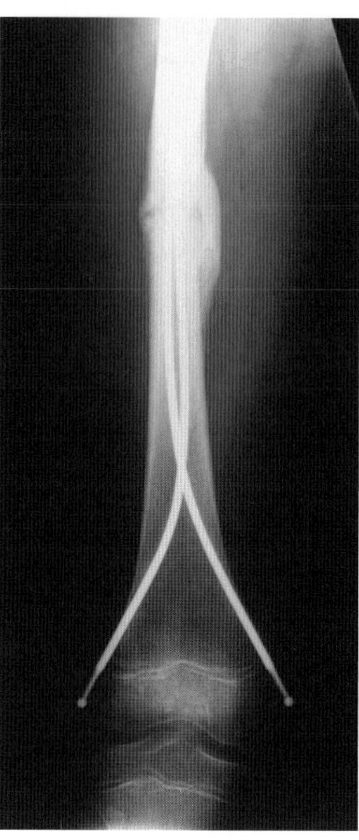

Figure 52.2 Fracture healing by external callus formation. This femoral shaft fracture in a child has been treated by intramedullary nailing. Union is proceeding by external callus formation, because the fracture haematoma has not been disturbed and the fixation is not completely rigid. In this case the medullary canal was not reamed prior to nailing, nevertheless some damage to the medullary blood supply is inevitable as a result of the passage of the nails. The original fracture was transverse. (Courtesy of Mr M. Jackson.)

Primary bone union

Primary bone repair is the term given to fracture repair where the fracture ends have been rigidly immobilized by a plate (Fig. 52.4). In the original concept of Lane[52] and Danis,[53] primary bone healing referred to fractures that healed without radiographically visible callus formation. Schenk and Willenegger found that when an osteotomy was performed in a dog radius that had been rigidly fixed by a plate, bone deposition occurred on the divided bone ends within a few days, often without preceding osteoclastic resorption.[54] The structure of the newly formed bone depended on the width of the gap. Where it was less than 200 μm, the gap was filled by true lamellar bone, while larger gaps showed a more irregular pattern. Where the gap exceeded a millimetre, it was not bridged in a single jump by woven bone, and complete filling in was considerably delayed.[49]

The bone filling the interfragmentary gap appears without the intermediate formation of connective tissue or fibrocartilage, and it is this absence of an intermediate tissue that distinguishes primary bone repair from that seen under other circumstances.

REFERENCES

50. Chalmers J, Gray DH, Rush J. J Bone Joint Surg 1975; 57B: 36–45
51. Lane JM, Werntz JR. In: Lane JM (ed). Fracture Healing. Churchill Livingstone, Edinburgh, 1987: 49–60
52. Lane WA. The Operative Treatment of Fractures. Medical Publishing, London, 1913
53. Danis R. Theorie et Pratique de l'Osteosynthese. Masson, Paris, 1949
54. Schenk R, Willenegger H. Symp Biol Hung 1967; 8: 75–86

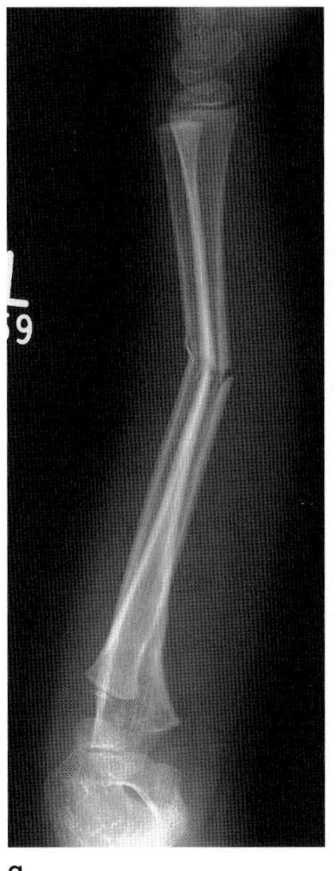

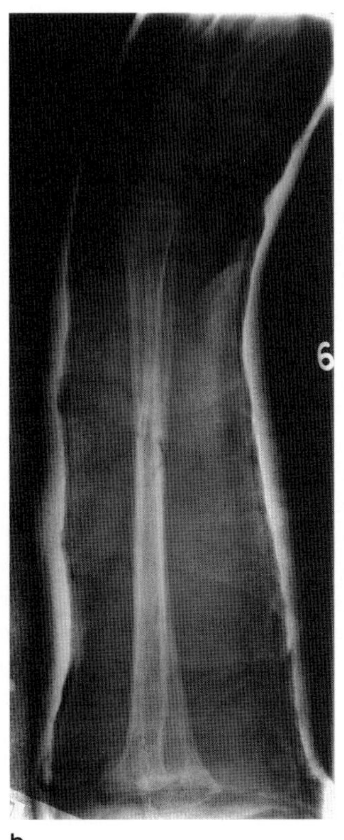

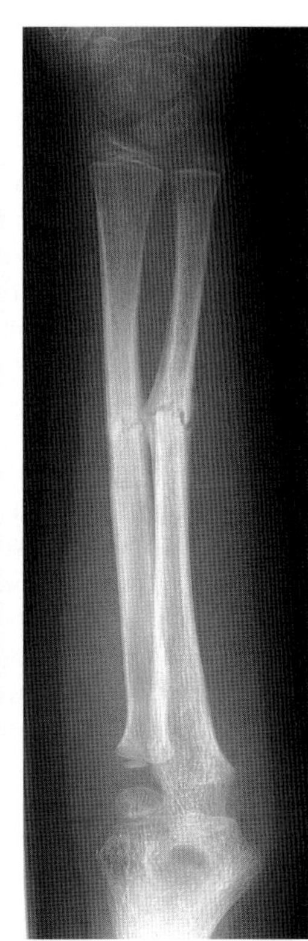

a b c

Figure 52.3 A greenstick fracture of the forearm in a 6-year-old girl. In children the bones are weaker than in adults, and this fracture occurred in a simple fall. (a) There is dorsal angulation of both the radius and the ulna. On the volar side the cortex is disrupted, but the dorsal cortex is not fully broken. (b) The fracture has been reduced under general anaesthetic into an acceptable position, and it is now held using a well-moulded plaster that provides three-point fixation to oppose redisplacement. The closeness of fit between the limb and the moulded plaster is illustrated. Great caution is necessary to ensure that the plaster, although tight-fitting, does not compromise the limb. (c) Only 4 weeks after the fracture occurred, it is soundly united with marked periosteal callus formation.

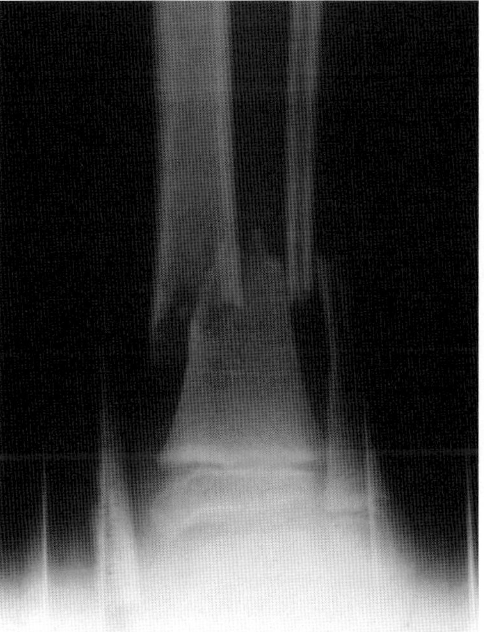

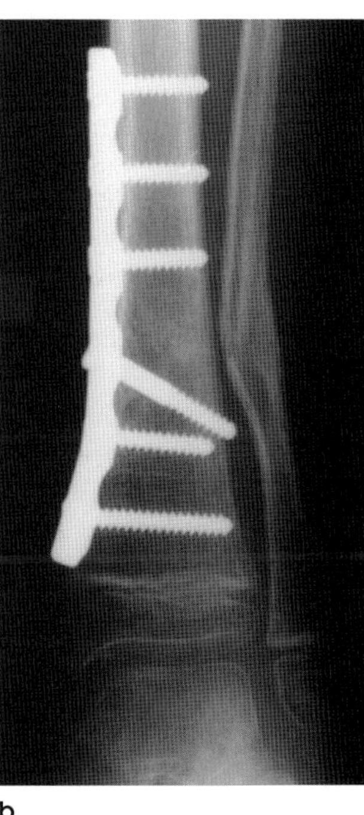

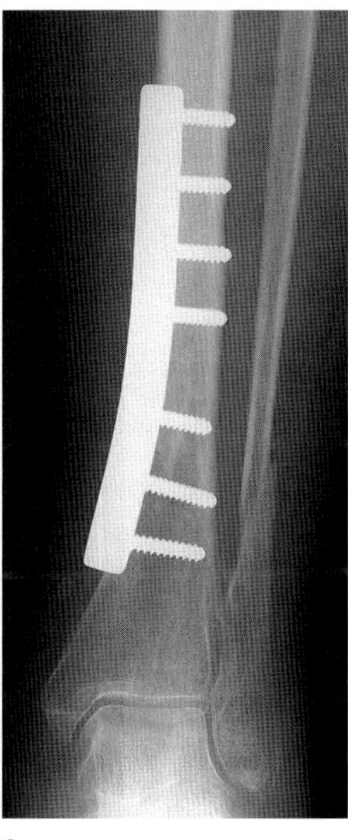

a b c

Figure 52.4 Fracture healing by primary bone union. (a) A displaced oblique fracture of the junction of the diaphysis and distal metaphysis of the tibia. Temporary, emergency immobilization is provided by an inflatable splint. (b) The fracture has been anatomically reduced using an AO low-contact dynamic compression plate (LC-DCP). In this case, fracture compression has been provided by the oblique lag screw rather than by use of the special compression holes in the plate. The irregular outline of the LC-DCP can be seen. This allows the plate to make contact with the bone only over a proportion of its surface, thus reducing devascularization. The plate and screws provide rigid stability, and the lack of interfragmentary movement suppresses external callus formation, despite the fact that this fracture occurred prior to skeletal maturity. The fibula, which was not rigidly immobilized, has united by periosteal callus formation. Notice the extent of the osteoporosis distal to the fracture, due to loss of the normal stimulus of load-bearing. (c) A similar fracture in an adult treated with an AO dynamic compression plate. The difference in bone contact area can clearly be seen. In this case, no lag screw was used; compression of the fracture site was obtained by use of the dynamic compression plate compression holes. Note the difference in the healing of the fibula: bone healing in an adult is slower than in the skeletally immature, and periosteal callus formation is less marked.

The lamellae are aligned at right angles to the interfragmentary gap if it is small, and because woven bone is being laid down de novo, the rate at which the gap is filled is considerably faster than the normal mineral appositional rate of 0.8–2.5 mm/day. Gap healing as outlined here is completely intolerant of any movement and will bridge only very small gaps. Once the bone gap has filled, the new bone is replaced by rapid bone remodelling with osteoclastic cutter heads crossing the fracture site.

CONTROL OF FRACTURE HEALING

The initial inflammatory reaction of bone after fracture is very similar to that seen in other injuries, and is controlled by the release of vasoactive mediators including serotonin and histamine, and of growth factors from damaged tissues. It is at the phase of formation of osteogenic repair tissue that bone healing begins to differ from other wound healing, and the triggering mechanism for this response is unknown. Bone-inducing growth factors are found within bone matrix,[22] and release of these from the broken bone ends may trigger new bone formation. A number of the growth factors that are released in the normal inflammatory process following injury can stimulate cartilage and bone formation,[55–58] so that these may become simply a modification of the normal inflammatory process. Prostaglandins are produced in high levels by injured bone and may also play a role.[59–61]

Perren suggested that healing of viable bone depends on the presence and size of the gap between the bone ends and on the strain to which the fracture gap is exposed.[62,63] A low strain and minimal fracture gap are associated with direct formation of bone between the fracture fragments without external callus, which is followed by remodelling (primary bone union). In contrast, where a high strain exists, abundant external callus is produced in the fracture haematoma, with primitive cells differentiating into fibroblasts and laying down a primitive collagen matrix prior to ossification in order to lower the local strain. A low strain in the presence of a significant fracture gap would lead to delayed or non-union of the fracture.

The role of local oxygen tension in determining whether bone or cartilage is formed has already been mentioned. Finally, the region of a fresh fracture is electronegative, a phenomenon that is independent of applied mechanical stress, and this may stimulate osteogenesis.[64]

FACTORS AFFECTING FRACTURE HEALING

The rate at which a fracture heals is affected by fracture, patient and treatment factors.

Fracture factors

Any factor that increases the displacement of the fracture fragments, reduces their vascular supply, or limits the amount of fracture haematoma available to take part in union also has an adverse effect on the rate of fracture union. Thus high-energy fractures, comminuted fractures, compound fractures, and fractures in which there is a severe soft tissue injury heal more slowly. A segmental fracture unites slowly, both because the intervening bone segment may be avascular and because of the difficulty in providing an optimal biomechanical environment for bone union at both sites.

The type of bone involved in the fracture also influences the rate of union. Cancellous bone tends to heal more rapidly than cortical bone, probably because of the large area of bone contact and the greater number of active bone cells that are present. Union of cancellous bone occurs with little external callus, especially when the two fragments are impacted into each other. Fractures that involve or are close to a joint may cause problems with union. If the joint is actually involved in the fracture, synovial enzymes may inhibit fracture union by interfering with provisional callus formation. If the fracture passes close to a joint, the forces placed through the fracture by joint movement may lead to non-union.

Individual bones within the body have their own rates of fracture healing, which may be rationalized by an understanding of the bone's anatomy. Thus tibial shaft fractures tend to unite more slowly than femoral shaft fractures, probably because of the poorer periosteal blood supply and the poverty of soft tissue cover in the tibia.

Pathological fractures occur after minimal trauma and may heal slowly, if at all, unless the underlying abnormality is corrected. Thus a fracture through a secondary malignant deposit is unlikely to heal and will need to be stabilized by a strong device that will resist the cyclical loading imposed by the non-united fracture for the remainder of the patient's life,[65] whereas the fractures that are associated with the deformity of Paget's disease of bone will unite provided that the deformity is corrected and the Paget's disease process temporarily normalized by medical treatment.[66]

Stress fractures occurring when the bone is loaded repetitively have already been discussed. They are also seen in conditions where the usual healing and remodelling responses of bone are impaired, as in osteomalacia, where Looser's zones represent stress insufficiency lesions of the lateral femoral cortices.

The presence of devitalized bone slows fracture healing. Devitalization may be due to periosteal stripping or a segmental fracture. The fracture may interrupt the blood supply to one side of the fracture, as at the femoral or talar neck or at the waist of the scaphoid bone. The devitalized side of the fracture acts as a scaffold for fracture union but does not contribute actively to bone union by providing osteogenic precursor cells (it is osteoconductive and osteoinductive but not osteogenic). These fractures may therefore unite, albeit slowly, if adequate mechanical stability is provided. In contrast, union may not occur where both sides of a fracture are non-viable, as is occasionally seen in fractures through bone that has been treated by irradiation.

REFERENCES

55. Jingushi S, Heydeman NA, Bolander ME. J Orthop Res 1990; 8: 364–371
56. Muthukumaran N, Reddi AH. Clin Orthop 1984; 220: 159–164
57. Moda M, Camillier JJ. Endocrinology 1989; 124: 2991–2994
58. Memmeth GG, Bolander ME, Martin MR. In: Barbul A, Pines E, Cauldwell MD et al. (eds). Alan R Liss, New York, 1988: 1–17
59. Rowe J, Sudman E, Martin PF. Acta Orthop Scand 1976; 47: 588–599
60. Dekel S, Lenthall G, Francis MJO. J Bone Joint Surg 1981; 63B: 185–189
61. Voegeli TL, Chapman MW. Trans Orthop Res Soc 1985; 10: 134
62. Perren SM et al. Surg Ann 1975; 7: 361–390
63. Perren SM. Clin Orthop 1979; 138: 175–196
64. Brighton TC, Hozach WJ, Brager MD et al. J Orthop Res 1985; 3: 331–340
65. Karachalios T, Atkins RM, Sarangi P et al. J Bone Joint Surg Br 1993; 75B: 119–122
66. Kerr P, Jackson M, Atkins RM. J Orthop Rheum 1993; 6: 171–173

Patient factors

The most striking variable is the patient's age. Fractures in children heal more rapidly than those in adults both because of greater bone activity and because the majority of childhood fractures are more minor than those in adults, as children's bones are weaker and more osteoporotic. Bone healing in patients with postmenopausal (type 1) osteoporosis is not itself impaired;[67] however, the ability of osteoporotic bone to hold implants may make it difficult to obtain sufficient stability, and the reduced area of bone contact may slow union. In contrast, in the very aged, severe senile (type 2) osteoporosis is associated with very low bone turnover, which causes extreme bone mineral weakness. These patients may be unable to mount a normal callus and bone activation response to a fracture, and in consequence bone healing is slow.

A number of hormones influence the rate of fracture union, but in clinical practice fractures in patients with abnormal hormonal levels usually heal uneventfully. In rickets and osteomalacia, it may be necessary to treat the condition to ensure optimal fracture union. Prolonged administration of corticosteroids leads to osteoporosis, and the impairment of the inflammatory response in such patients may also impair fracture healing.

Infection can slow or prevent healing by diverting cells from the process of bone union to treatment of the infection. It is important, however, to recognize that bone infection may be the result of poor bone blood supply and deficient overlying soft tissues, which themselves contribute to slow fracture healing.

Treatment factors

The purpose of fracture treatment is to harness one of the mechanisms of fracture healing outlined to unite a fracture as rapidly as possible with minimal short- and long-term complications to the patient. The desirable features are therefore fracture fragment apposition, fragment viability, and the provision of an appropriate biomechanical environment for healing to occur.

An example of an adverse treatment method would be rigid open fixation of a diaphyseal fracture with stripping of periosteum without compression, leaving some separation of the fracture. This treatment will inhibit the primary callus response and the formation of external bridging callus. It will, however, not provide conditions for primary bone union because of the significant fracture gap. Because healing by late medullary callus is not a feature of diaphyseal bone, there remains no mechanism for union of the fracture and a non-union will occur.

FAILURE OF FRACTURE HEALING (NON-UNION)

Despite optimal treatment, some fractures heal slowly or fail to unite completely. The diagnosis of delayed union is difficult and relative, but the bone responses that lead to fracture union do not endure permanently. A non-union is said to exist where the bone remains un-united after they have ceased to be active. In fact, a precise definition of non-union is difficult, and as treatments such as the use of Ilizarov frames become more accepted, there is a trend towards identifying situations in which the bone will not heal and intervening early.

The two main reasons for fracture non-union are loss of bone viability and an adverse biomechanical environment, but in most cases both factors are present to a certain degree. Where bone viability is poor, particularly where the surrounding soft tissue cover is also deficient, infection may supervene. Poor bone viability leads to gradual resorption of bone and an atrophic non-union develops (Fig. 52.5), whereas inadequate fracture stability with normally viable bone fragments leads to a hypertrophic non-union (Fig. 52.6). Occasionally, at the site of a fracture a pseudarthrosis or new false joint forms.

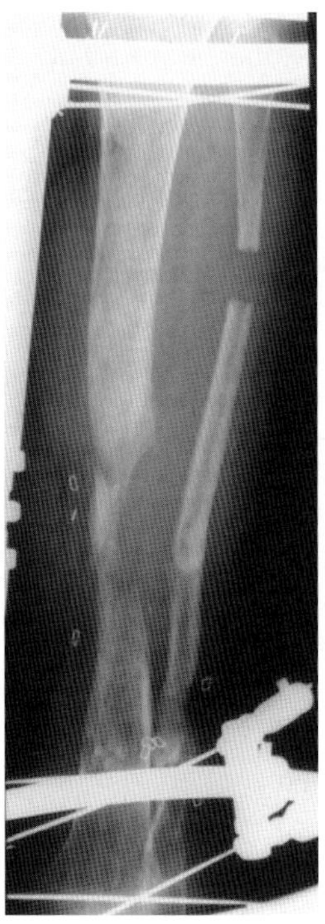

a

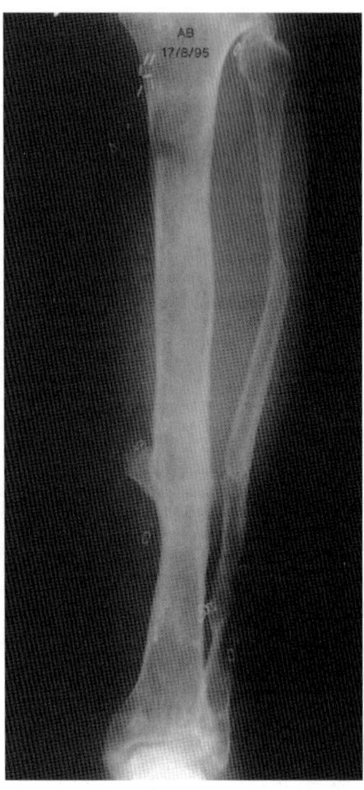

b

Figure 52.5 (**a**) An atrophic non-union of a tibial fracture. The original fracture involved a severe soft tissue and bone injury. Over time, badly damaged bone has undergone resorption, leaving an un-united fracture and an area of bone deficiency. The non-union is supported by a circular external fixator. (**b**) The result after treatment by bone transport.

PRINCIPLES OF TREATMENT OF NON-UNION OF FRACTURE

Treatment is directed at reversing the cause of the non-union. Bone mass and bone-to-bone contact at the non-union site should be improved, the biomechanical environment corrected, and bone activity increased.

Increasing local bone mass

Local bone mass is increased by fracture reduction, bone grafting or bone transport, all of which also increase the area of bone-to-bone contact.

Improving the biomechanical environment

The biomechanical environment is corrected by compression plating, intramedullary nailing or external fixation to provide a mechanical environment that resists shearing forces but provides compression with, ideally, the ability to continue gradual

REFERENCES

67. Riggs BL, Melton LJ III. Am J Med 1983; 75: 899–901

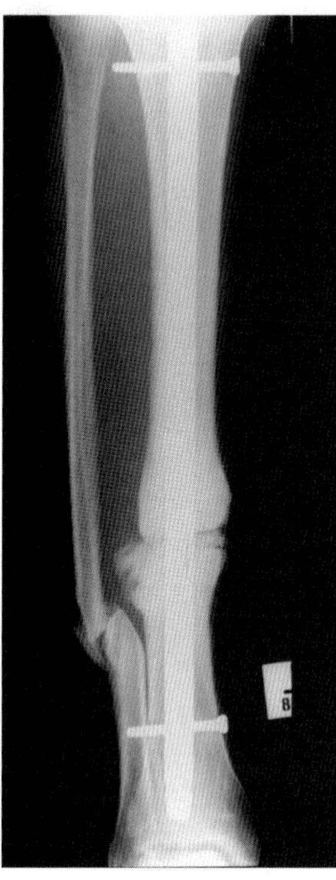

Figure 52.6 A hypertrophic non-union shortly after treatment by reamed interlocked intramedullary nailing. During the treatment period following this fracture, sufficient stability was not achieved to allow bone union. The fracture line remains, and progressive layers of periosteal callus formation around the bone give the old fracture site the appearance of an elephant's foot. There may be little or no clinically detectable movement, but the region remains painful and the limb is of limited utility. Treatment consists of reaming the bone to allow passage of the intramedullary nail and to increase bone activation. The biomechanical environment of the fracture is improved by stabilization of the non-union with an intramedullary nail locked proximally and distally. (Courtesy of Mr M. Jackson.)

compression of the site for some time after the operation to deal with the effects of local bone resorption.

A radically different approach to the biomechanical environment that is required for resolution of a non-union was provided by Ilizarov.[68,69] He divided non-unions into stiff and lax, which broadly corresponds to the western classification of hypertrophic and atrophic. Ilizarov demonstrated that stiff non-unions will heal under conditions of gradual distraction at least as reliably as under compression. Clearly the use of gradual distraction requires an external fixation device for stabilization of the non-union.

Increasing bone activity

Bone activity is increased either by providing new bone cells and bone morphogens using cancellous bone grafting, or by indirect stimulation by intramedullary reaming or by division of the bone at a distant site using a corticotomy. An alternative source of bone morphogens is exogenous human recombinant bone morphogenetic protein, and the availability of this class of compounds may in the future profoundly affect the manner in which we treat non-unions. However, it must be remembered that the stimulation of bone activity resolves only one of the bone-related problems of non-union.

BONE GRAFTING

Bone grafting procedures are often undertaken for delayed or non-union of a fracture to stimulate osteogenesis and increase the bone mass present. Bone grafts may be categorized according to the donor type.

- Autograft: from the same individual.
- Isograft: between genetically identical individuals.
- Allograft: from one individual to another of the same species.
- Xenograft or heterograft: between individuals of different species.

They are further divided according to whether the transplant is living or has been preserved (e.g. by freeze-drying), whether transplant is free or vascularized, and whether the graft is cancellous or cortical bone, or a combination of the two.

Stimulation of bone formation or fracture union following bone grafting may occur by three mechanisms: osteogenesis, osteoinduction and osteoconduction.[70]

OSTEOGENESIS

Bone cells within the graft survive and synthesize new bone. This can occur only in the case of fresh autograft. Cancellous bone is more active than cortical bone because of its greater surface area and more numerous osteocytes, and because revascularization from the host is more rapid. A vascularized graft may be employed, but this is not applicable to the majority of situations.

OSTEOINDUCTION

The bone graft induces bone formation by causing a local host cell response that produces bone. Osteoinduction occurs with both autografts and allografts, and is mediated by growth factors and the bone morphogenetic proteins. These molecules are unstable, and their activity is reduced by autoclaving, freeze preservation or irradiation.

OSTEOCONDUCTION

Osteoconduction is a passive phenomenon whereby the graft material acts as a scaffold into which new host bone can grow. Mechanical stability is essential for osteoconduction, but it is mainly a property of the structure of the graft, and most materials are osteoconductive when present as a mesh with a pore size of greater than 200 μm.

The three mechanisms usually occur together and, for example in a cancellous autograft, osteocytes near the graft surface revascularize rapidly and form new bone. As the revascularized graft bone is remodelled, matrix-bound growth factors are released, causing an osteoinductive host response. Finally, the graft surface is a suitable lattice for osteoconduction.

As invasion of the graft by host bone proceeds, the graft is partially or completely replaced by the host, a process termed *incorporation*. If this does not occur, the graft will remain as a foreign body, which may ultimately fail because of fatigue damage or become infected. However, as the graft is incorporated, it may become mechanically weak as a result of resorption, and this may cause it to break.

BIOMECHANICAL ASPECTS OF FRACTURES

Whether a bone will fracture under the influence of a particular stress will depend on the magnitude, duration and direction of the force acting on the bone and the rate of its application (factors extrinsic to the bone; see *Classification of fractures*, p. 1077, for a discussion) and on intrinsic factors within the bone.

REFERENCES

68. Ilizarov GA. Ortop Travmatol Protez 1975; 10: 7–15
69. Ilizarov GA. Transosseous Osteosynthesis: Theoretical and Clinical Aspects of the Regeneration and Growth of Tissue. Springer-Verlag, Berlin, 1990
70. Friendlaender GE, Goldberg VM. Bone and Cartilage Allografts: Biology and Clinical Applications. American Academy of Orthopedic Surgeons, Parkridge, 1991

The important intrinsic factors are the energy-absorbing capacity of the bone, the Young's modulus, and its fatigue strength.[71] Bone is three times as strong as cast iron and 10 times more flexible, although it is of similar tensile strength. The inorganic phase of bone (hydroxyapatite) is about six times more rigid than whole bone and is stronger in compression than in tension. In contrast, bone collagen does not resist compression but has a tensile strength five times that of whole bone. Thus the composite structure that is bone owes its compressive strength to hydroxyapatite and its tensile strength to collagen. As an approximation, bone can be strained to 0.75% before plastic failure occurs, and its breaking strain is 2–4%.

Because bone remodels itself to resist applied loads, it is anisotropic, possessing different mechanical properties in differing directions, and both its ultimate tensile strength and its Young's modulus are greater when loaded in its longitudinal axis. Furthermore, it is viscoelastic, its behaviour varying with the rate of load application. When bone is loaded, there is an instantaneous elastic deformation followed by a slower plastic one. The rate of load application is therefore important in determining the outcome of loading. A rapid load is absorbed elastically, but during slower, plastic deformation bone can absorb six times more energy before fracture than in the elastic phase. However, if the rapidly applied load is sufficient to cause a fracture, the stored elastic energy will be released explosively, causing great damage to bone and surrounding soft tissues. This is the basis for the division of fractures into high- and low-energy fractures. Owing to their explosive nature, high-energy fractures are associated with increased comminution, greater soft tissue damage, and more periosteal stripping, all of which tend to slow fracture union. The bone of elderly osteoporotic patients does not possess the ability to store elastic energy in this way, and consequently the sort of high-energy fractures that occur in young patients are not seen in the elderly. If an elderly limb is subjected to this sort of force it will crumple.

When a material is subjected to repeated cyclical loading, it may fail even though the magnitude of the individual stress that is applied is well below the ultimate tensile stress of the material. This is known as fatigue failure, and it is due to the initiation of small cracks within the material. Once a crack has been started, propagation requires far lower stresses than initiation, although the complex structure of bone tends to resist crack propagation, and remodelling provides a means for repair of minor damage. Stress or fatigue fractures are seen in young persons who undertake excessive repetitive activity, such as ballet dancers or soldiers, or in the elderly in whom the process of bone remodelling is slow.

A number of features contribute to the mechanical strength of bone and its consequent ability to resist imposed forces for the lifetime of the organism.

At a macroscopic level, the strong cortical bone is arranged as a tube, thus providing the greatest strength for a given weight. The cortex is reinforced by the central cancellous, lamellar bone where the individual trabeculae are arranged to resist the usually imposed forces.

At a microscopic level, the differently oriented irregular individual structural units of bone formed by each remodelling unit fit together exactly because of the manner in which they are formed, and they are held firmly together by the cement substance in a fashion resembling a brick wall. This helps to prevent crack propagation by forming a T-shaped crack at the interphase (the Cook–Gordon mechanism).

The poorly crystalline nature of the hydroxyapatite means that bone is not subject to easy cleavage between crystal domains as, for example, is seen in diamond.

Bone turnover and remodelling are important because they allow the bone to alter itself to oppose imposed loads, and they maintain bone strength by removing old or fatigue-damaged bone. Thus in an elderly person bone may be weak not only because of an absolute deficiency of bone substance (osteoporosis) but also because, due to the low rate of bone turnover, individual bits of bone mineral are on average older than in a younger person and so have had more time to develop fatigue damage.

It is probable that normal muscle tone exerts a protective effect on bone, shielding it from excessive stress, and muscle fatigue may be a factor in fractures in the elderly following minor trauma.[72]

CLASSIFICATION OF FRACTURES

Fractures may be classified by the mechanism of injury, by the nature and site of the fracture fragments, and by the extent of the associated soft tissue injury. These systems are interrelated, because high-violence injuries produce comminuted fractures with severe soft tissue damage while low violence is associated with simple fractures and little soft tissue injury. A combination of these factors is used to determine the fracture personality.[73,74]

CLASSIFICATION BY MECHANISM OF INJURY

Fractures may be caused by forces applied directly or indirectly to the bone, and the amount of displacement and bone damage will depend on the initiating trauma.

Direct trauma

Fractures caused by direct violence may be divided into tapping, crushing or penetrating.[75]

Tapping fractures

Tapping fractures are caused by a small force acting on a small area. They tend to be transverse and relatively undisplaced, with little soft tissue damage apart from a small overlying contusion or laceration. They are caused by a direct blow such as a kick on the shin playing sport, causing a fibula fracture, or a blow to the defending upheld forearm with a stick, causing an isolated fracture of the ulna. Fracture healing is usually uncomplicated, although in the case of the nightstick injury to the ulna the splinting effect of the intact radius may delay union.

Crushing fractures

The force and area of application are greater and the duration longer than in a tapping fracture. There is associated major soft tissue damage, and nerves and vessels may be compromised. Compartment problems are frequent, and the fractures tend to be highly comminuted.

REFERENCES

71. Evans FG. Instr Course Lect 1961; XVIII: 110–121
72. Key JA. South Med J 1932; 25: 909–915
73. Nicoll EA. J Bone Joint Surg 1964; 46B: 373–387
74. Schatzker J, Tile M. The Rationale of Operative Fracture Care. 2nd edn. Springer-Verlag, Berlin, 1996
75. Perkins G. Fractures and Dislocations. Athlone Press, London, 1958

Penetrating fractures

Penetrating fractures are produced by a large force acting on a small area. Gunshot and shrapnel wounds are of this type, and they are also seen as a result of road traffic accidents. Gunshot wounds are subdivided into high and low energy. In a high-energy wound, the velocity of the projectile exceeds the speed of sound in the tissue, and in addition to the direct damage from the projectile there is considerable contamination and collateral damage to surrounding soft tissues, caused by cavitation from the shock wave and associated negative-pressure wave.

Indirect trauma

Fractures are often produced by a force acting at a distance from the fracture itself, and these may be classified as tension, angulation, rotation or compression.

Tension fractures are commonly avulsions. Examples include the tibial tuberosity fracture and transverse fractures of the olecranon and patella. They are usually caused by a sudden resisted muscle contraction. Angulation forces, where the bone acts as a lever, cause transverse fractures with often a small area of comminution on the concave side.

Rotational forces cause spiral fractures, while compression loads may cause oblique fractures of a bone shaft or T-shaped fractures involving the ends of bones such as a tibial plateau or femoral condylar fracture. A combination of these forces often occurs.

Combinations of fractures are not infrequently seen, and for example a vertical compression force following a fall from a height may fracture the calcaneum, the tibial plateau, the acetabulum, and the lumbar spine. A patient presenting with an appropriate history and one of a set of fractures leads the astute clinician to look carefully for signs of other fractures within the set.

CLASSIFICATION BY NATURE OF THE FRACTURE FRAGMENTS

Any fracture may be classified according to whether it is transverse, oblique, spiral or comminuted. Further assessment will include whether the fracture fragments are displaced or undisplaced (Fig. 52.7).

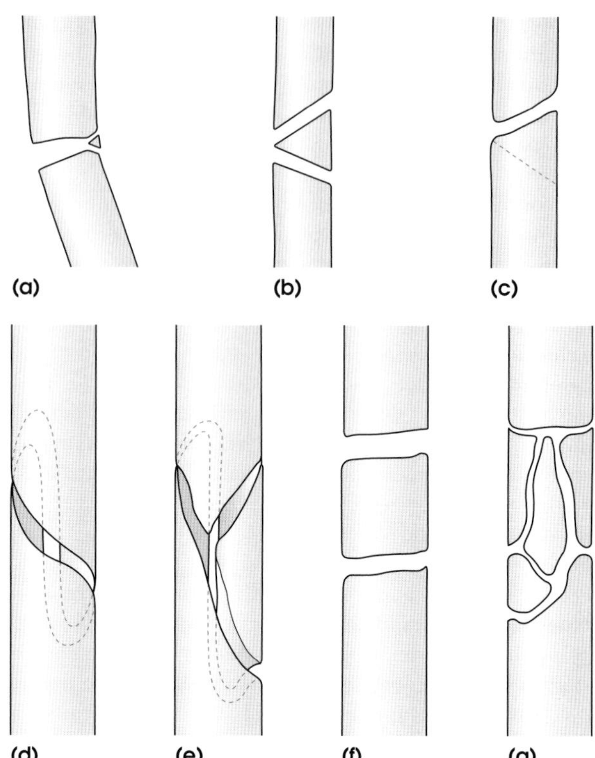

Figure 52.7 Fractures are classified into transverse, oblique, spiral, segmental and comminuted on the basis of the X-ray appearance. (a) Bending forces cause transverse fractures, and there is usually an extruded wedge of bone on the compression side, which has little soft tissue attachment. (b) If the extruded fragment is large, bone union may be slow because of its poor viability. (c) If the extruded fragment is not separated from both sides of the fracture, an oblique fracture results. Alternatively, an oblique fracture may be caused by a combination of bending and torsion loads. (d) Torsional loading results in a spiral fracture. (e) A butterfly fragment may be extruded from a spiral fracture. (f) When a fracture involves two separate sites within a bone, the term *segmental fracture* is used. (g) A comminuted fracture implies multiple fracture fragments. (After Schatzker and Tile 1996.[74])

FRACTURE DIAGNOSIS

The diagnosis of a fracture is usually simple, provided that the clinician maintains a suspicious mind, because even what subsequently are considered to be obvious fractures are missed.

CLINICAL FEATURES

There are a number of clinical features with which patients with fractures present that can be elicited with a careful history and examination, which minimizes the risk of failing to diagnose a fracture. Also, correct clinical identification of the fracture allows specific targeting of the X-ray examination and so reduces the risk of missing the fracture on the X-ray, which is not uncommon.

Patients with a fracture usually describe a history of trauma, and they complain of pain and a loss of or decrease in function of a specific region (e.g. loss of finger and thumb apposition with a scaphoid fracture). Clinical findings are of swelling, deformity and tenderness, with loss of range of movement of the joint above and below the fracture in long bone fractures or of a specific joint if the fracture is an intra-articular fracture (Box 52.1). These simple clinical findings are always present to some degree but are all too often poorly elicited, ignored or not appreciated. This leads to poorly targeted X-rays that fail, for instance, to diagnose the fibula fracture in the patient who has a Maisonneuve fracture which is misdiagnosed as a sprained ankle because only the ankle was X-rayed. Alternatively X-ray examination may be omitted causing the fracture to be missed altogether (e.g. the scaphoid fracture).

Box 52.1 Clinical features of a fracture

- A history of trauma
- Loss of function
- Pain
- Swelling
- Deformity
- Tenderness

RADIOGRAPHIC FEATURES

Plain radiographs are the mainstay of fracture diagnosis. At least two orthogonal views must be performed to demonstrate the fracture and its displacement, and for long bone fractures must include the joint above and below the fracture. Computerized tomographic scanning is increasingly used and is all but essential for the full assessment of more complex intra-articular fractures, such as tibial pilon fractures, acetabular fractures and calcaneal fractures (Fig. 52.8). Three-dimensional reconstruction is also increasingly employed but its usefulness is limited. It probably has a role in acetabular fractures but in calcaneal fractures, where the individual fragments may be only slightly larger than the pixel size of the reconstruction, its value is more limited.

Magnetic resonance imaging has the advantage over CT scanning that reconstruction in any direction is possible without loss of definition. In addition, it allows visualization of metabolic changes and soft tissue damage, such as spinal cord oedema, and it does not irradiate the patient. Set against these advantages is the relatively poor definition that it provides of bone fragments, so that a high-quality CT scan is usually preferred for fracture assessment.

FRACTURE MANAGEMENT

The management of any fracture should be divided into the emergency phase and the phase of reconstruction.

EMERGENCY PHASE

The primary concern is saving the patient's life and the damaged limb. The patient must be assessed and resuscitated as per Advanced Trauma Life Support® protocols (see Ch. 7), with appropriate replacement of colloid and crystalloid lost due to the fracture. Appropriate analgesia is given (see Ch. 5). The limb is examined and its vascular status determined. An acutely ischaemic limb secondary to fracture displacement usually responds to gentle reduction by traction. Emergency angiography and vascular reconstruction combined with fracture stabilization may be necessary if this is ineffective (see Ch. 10). Nerve damage is noted. The fracture is splinted in a comfortable position, which may involve temporary traction before the fracture is assessed radiographically.

In the case of a compound fracture—that is, one where the bone has come out through the skin—the initial fracture and wound management belong in the emergency phase, because the wound will become colonized with bacteria within 6 h of the injury. The wound should be cleaned of all obvious debris, photographed, and covered with a bactericidal dressing. The fracture is splinted, and the patient is taken to the operating theatre within 6 h of the injury so that a primary debridement of the wound and stabilization of the fracture can be performed. Compound fractures are discussed in greater detail under *Open (compound) fractures* (p. 1089).

PHASE OF RECONSTRUCTION

The definitive management of a fracture is a separate issue from its emergency treatment. Fracture reconstructions are among the most complex of orthopaedic operations and they should not be undertaken in haste, without adequate investigation, and in anywhere other than a fully equipped operating theatre with fully rested and adequately trained staff. An improperly performed surgical reconstruction may jeopardize the livelihood of a young working person. In the multiply injured patient (see Ch. 7), it may be necessary to carry out emergency stabilization of long bone fractures to minimize the systemic effects of the fractures. It may be possible to undertake definitive reconstruction of the fracture at this time; however, the aim of resuscitation is to save the patient's life and limb, while the aim of reconstruction is to optimize long-term function following the fracture. These two aims are not mutually exclusive but it is essential for the surgeon to maintain their clear separation.

PRINCIPLES OF FRACTURE RECONSTRUCTION

The principle of fracture treatment is to reduce the displaced fracture into a position in which it will unite promptly and optimal function will be restored to the limb when it has united. The fracture should be reduced and stabilized in the reduced position, with minimal damage to the soft tissue envelope, and the reduction must be held until the fracture is united in such a fashion that as many joints as possible may be moved to prevent

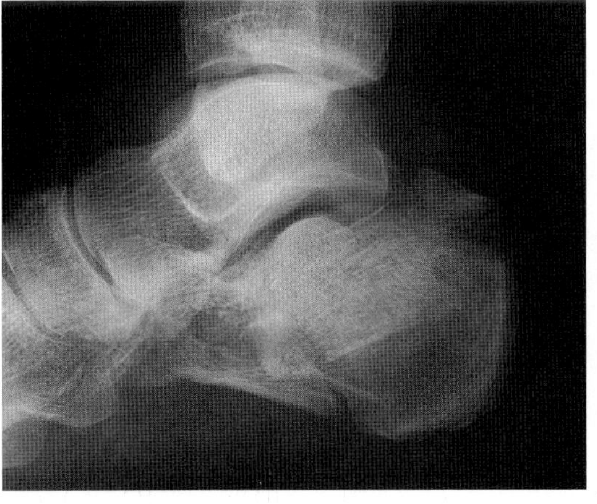
a

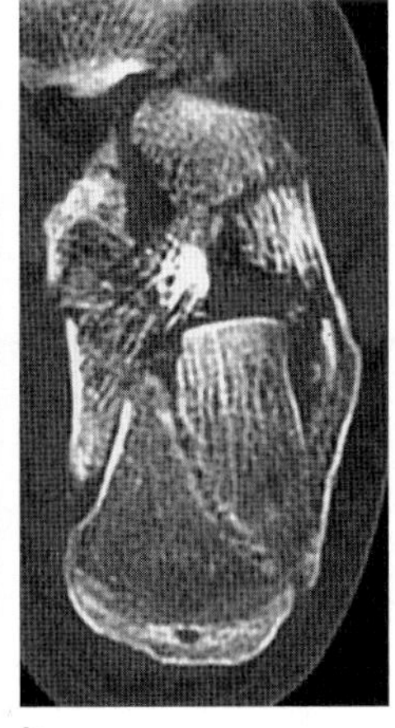
b

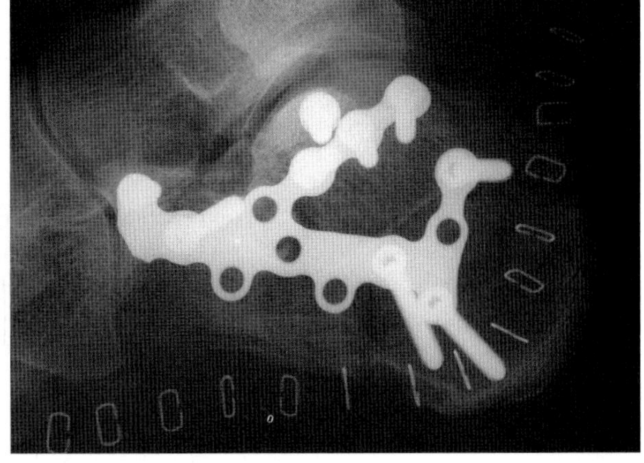
c

Figure 52.8 (a) Lateral plain radiograph of an intra-articular fracture of the calcaneum, showing disruption of the posterior facet of the subtalar joint and alteration of Bohler's angle. (b) The fracture is assessed by CT scanning, which shows the degree of posterior facet disruption and the configuration of the fracture fragments, allowing proper surgical planning. (c) The fracture is treated by open reduction and internal fixation with a specialized plate.

stiffness.[76–78] As far as possible, the limb should be used during fracture healing to minimize the adverse consequences of lack of use.

Although the principle of fracture treatment is simply outlined, in practice there are a number of areas of controversy. The accuracy of reduction required depends on the precise anatomical area. A joint surface must be reduced as accurately as possible to avoid steps in the joint surface, which will lead to degeneration of the joint because of local overload of the cartilage.

PRINCIPLES OF CLOSED TREATMENT

Closed treatment of fractures was until the late 19th century almost the only method for their treatment. It remains the mainstay of management for the majority of simple fractures, although operative treatments have yielded improved results in intra-articular, high-energy, compound, and certain long bone fractures. There are two distinct parts to management by the closed technique. The fracture is first reduced into a position in which union may be anticipated and that will, after union has occurred, give satisfactory limb function. The reduction is then held or immobilized until sound union has occurred.

Reduction

Reduction should be undertaken as soon as is practicable after the injury; however, in the absence of a compound wound, neurovascular complication, or endangerment of skin, it is not an emergency. Reduction is simply easier to accomplish before swelling becomes established.

Fracture reduction is carried out with appropriate analgesia. If a general anaesthetic is employed, this will also provide muscle relaxation; alternatively, local or regional anaesthetic may be used. The technique has been described by Charnley.[79]

Traction

The slow, steady application of a longitudinal traction force to a displaced fracture overcomes the muscle spasm that has been caused by the fracture. Traction also helps to disengage fragments that have become impacted into each other. The soft tissues remain intact on the concave side of a transverse or oblique fracture and in the long axis of a spiral fracture, especially in children, where the periosteum forms a major component. Once the fragments have been disimpacted, the remaining attachments between the fracture fragments (often termed *soft tissue hinges*) are tightened by the traction force and encourage their approximation.

In elderly patients or those with very displaced high-energy fractures, the hinges are destroyed, and in these cases a stable reduction cannot be achieved by closed means. Even when the soft tissue hinges are intact, however, traction alone does not always cause reduction. One of the bone ends may be herniated through a muscle, or the fracture haematoma may be so tense that it resists all attempts at fragment distraction. More commonly, the shape of the fragments causes them to become locked in a displaced position, which then requires a formal increase in the displacement before reduction can occur.

Increasing the displacement

Once distraction has produced initial fragment disimpaction, the mechanism that produced the injury is replicated. For example, a distal radial fracture with an intact ulna in a child is caused by a dorsiflexion and supination. Simple distraction will to some extent pull the fragments apart; however, some impaction will remain, particularly close to the intact posterior periosteal hinge. Increasing the deformity usually relaxes the soft tissue hinge and completes fragment disengagement.

Reversal of the mechanism of injury

Once the major fragments have been completely separated, the mechanism of injury is reversed to realign them. This places the intact soft tissue hinge on the stretch and locks the fragments together. Some over-correction of the deformity may be necessary to squash residual fragments of bone caught in the fracture line.

Maintaining reduction

Once reduction has been achieved, it is held by the use of casts or traction.

Casts

Splintage to maintain the reduced position of a fracture has been used since prehistoric times. Splints were originally constructed from lengths of wood bound to the limb above and below the fracture. Plaster of Paris was so called because it was first mined in Montmartre, and its use was originally described by Antonius Mathijsen, a Flemish military surgeon who used dressings impregnated with dehydrated gypsum in the treatment of war injuries.[80] The modern plaster of Paris bandage consists of an open-weave cloth or muslin strip impregnated with dehydrated calcium sulphate. Dextrose or starch makes the cloth stiffer, and accelerators or inhibitors alter the hardening rate. When water is added, the calcium sulphate becomes hydrated in an exothermic reaction and rapidly sets to an even mass that permeates the cloth.

New casting materials have become available. These consist of a knitted material made of cloth or glass fibre, impregnated with a monomer or oligomer of polyurethane with substituted isocyanate terminal groups. When exposed to water, these compounds polymerize, releasing carbon dioxide. The substituted polyurethane is highly reactive, and unused material is packaged in resistant containers. The new casting materials have a number of advantages over the traditional plaster of Paris. They are lighter, stronger and more radiolucent. They are waterproof and more resistant to wear and tear. For the benefit of children, they can be made in a variety of intriguing colours, and they are less messy to apply than plaster of Paris. The disadvantages are that they are relatively expensive and irritant, so that gloves must be worn during their application. The increased strength means that if the limb swells they deform less and pressure within the limb is greater. They are also more difficult to apply by the amateur than plaster of Paris bandages. Plaster of Paris is often still preferred as the initial cast, with a fibreglass cast being applied by an expert after the swelling has settled.

REFERENCES

76. Muller ME, Allgower M, Schneider R et al. Manual of Internal Fixation. 1st edn. Springer Verlag, Berlin, 1970
77. Essex-Lopresti P. Br J Surg 1952; 39: 395–419
78. Bohler L. The Treatment of Fractures. John Wright, Bristol, 1916: 490
79. Charnley J. The Closed Treatment of Common Fractures. 3rd edn. E & S Livingstone, Edinburgh, 1968
80. Mathijsen A. Plaster of Paris in the Treatment of Fractures. Granmont-Doners, Liège, 1854

Precautions in the use of casts

There are a number of potentially serious problems with the use of casts. The cast may become sufficiently tight to restrict the circulation to the limb, or a ridge in the plaster may dig into the limb (Fig. 52.3). For these reasons, patients are instructed to seek advice if the plaster becomes painful or too tight, or if the limb becomes paraesthetic or blue. Any excessively painful plaster must be removed, and if there is a suspicion of circulatory embarrassment by the plaster, it must be split through the plaster and all underlying padding and the edges of the plaster spread apart. If this does not definitely relieve the problem, the plaster must be removed.

Traction

The use of traction to overcome the muscle spasm of a fracture to allow manipulative reduction has already been discussed. Continuous traction can maintain the reduction and allow the fracture to unite in the reduced position. This was the mainstay of treatment for certain fractures (e.g. femoral fractures) until satisfactory methods of internal fixation were developed, and it remains a safe and acceptable option. However, it requires a prolonged stay in hospital with constant attention to ensure that reduction is not lost and that the traction apparatus is satisfactorily applied. The complications of prolonged bed rest—such as venous thrombosis, pressure sores, hypostatic pneumonia and osteoporosis—are additional drawbacks. Finally, permanent joint stiffness is common because of the duration of immobilization, and fracture reduction may not be as good as can be obtained by open operation.

PRINCIPLES OF INTERNAL FIXATION

Many fractures heal satisfactorily following manipulative reduction and external splintage. Not all, however, respond well to this 'conservative' regimen, and unsatisfactory results led to the development of internal fixation of fractures.

Prior to the mid 19th century, the overwhelming majority of fractures were treated conservatively because of the dangers of surgical intervention. Operation was reserved for compound fractures or painful non-union, and the standard treatment of an open fracture or a contaminated penetrating joint wound was immediate amputation because of the danger of overwhelming sepsis.[81,82] At this time, standard fracture treatment was splintage and traction. Kirschner wires and Steinmann pins were initially developed as traction aids.

With the onset of the era of anaesthesia and asepsis, investigation of operative fracture surgery began in the closing decades of the 19th century.[83] Plate fixation of fractures was pioneered in the late 19th and early 20th centuries by Lambotte[84] and Lane;[52] however, early attempts at internal fixation did not provide sufficient fracture stability to permit mobilization, and supplementary plaster fixation was often used. Once fracture union was evidenced by callus formation, rehabilitation was commenced. However, because the fracture haematoma had been removed and soft tissue attachments to the bone disturbed, union was delayed by the surgery and the results were poor.

Key[72] and Charnley[85] first experimented with compression in arthrodesis, using it to achieve stability of fixation, which allowed subsequent bony union. Danis demonstrated that under conditions of absolute stability produced by a special compression plate, cortical bone would unite without radiologically visible callus, a process that he termed *primary bone union.*[53] In 1958, a group of Swiss surgeons led by Maurice Muller formed the Arbeitsgemeinshaft für Osteosynthesfragen (AO), or the Association for the Study of Internal Fixation (ASIF). Schenk and Willenegger studied primary bone union experimentally,[86] and the AO group produced a manual of suggested operative techniques.[76]

The AO group has had such a profound effect on fracture treatment that it is necessary to study their underlying concepts carefully. It was their belief that fracture or plaster disease, which is synonymous with algodystrophy, is the result of immobilization of a limb in plaster.[76,87] They concentrated on rapid restoration of limb function by anatomical fracture reduction; rigid internal fixation; atraumatic surgical technique; and early, pain-free, active mobilization within 10 days of operation. Their concepts differed from those of Watson Jones and Bohler, who concentrated on bone union first and then on rehabilitation, in that these two phases were simultaneous.

To allow such rapid mobilization, the fracture fixation had to be very stable, and this was achieved by compression between the fracture fragments. Compression restored structural–mechanical continuity to the bone, and permitted direct transfer of forces from bone fragment to bone fragment rather than through the implant, thus preserving it from mechanical failure. The keystone of this approach was the lag screw for the production of interfragmentary compression, combined with neutralization plates and compression plates.[88] Where fracture comminution prevented rigid apposition, extensive bone grafting was employed.

Advances in implant technology—with the development, for example, of locked intramedullary nailing—and improved understanding of bone biology and the necessity of maintaining fracture fragment viability have modified their original approach. The concept of atraumatic, anatomical reduction and rigid fixation of articular fractures, with early motion remains; however, for diaphyseal fractures and diaphyseal extensions of articular fractures, there has been a move away from absolute stability and primary bone union. At the time when the AO was started, comminution of a diaphyseal fracture was a contraindication to intramedullary nailing—now it is the indication.

Several basic principles of internal fixation can be stated as follow.

- Operative treatment of fractures is not without risk, and these risks must be carefully weighed against the probable outcome of conservative treatment and the patient's requirements. The presence of a fracture is not an indication for internal

REFERENCES

81. Malgaine JF. A Treatise on Fractures. 1st edn. Lippincott, Philadelphia, 1859
82. Stimson L. A Treatise on Fractures. 1st edn. Lea, Philadelphia, 1883
83. Peltier L. Fractures: A History and Iconography of their Treatment. Norman Publishing, San Francisco, 1990
84. Lambotte A. L'Intervention Operatoire dans les Fractures Recentes et Anciennes. (Envisage Particulierement au de Vue de l'Osteosynthese avec la Description de Plusiers Techniques Nouvelles). Maloine, Paris, 1907
85. Charnley J. Compression Arthrodesis. Livingstone, Edinburgh, 1953
86. Schenk R, Willenegger H. Langenbecks Arch Klin Chir 1964; 308: 440
87. Muller ME, Allgower M, Willenegger H. Technik der Operativen Frakturenbehandlung. Springer-Verlag, Berlin, 1963
88. Muller ME, Allgower M, Schneider R et al. Manual of Internal Fixation. 3rd edn. Springer-Verlag, Berlin, 1992

fixation, and a mediocre result of non-operative treatment is usually preferable to the result of a failed attempt at internal fixation.
- The damage to bone and soft tissue at the time of fracture cannot always be reversed, and the anticipated outcome must be tempered by the severity and nature of the initial injury.
- The soft tissue damage must be taken into account when planning operative exposure and may preclude internal fixation.
- Operative exposure must be extensile[89] to allow adequate exposure of the bone for fixation.
- The blood supply of bone fragments must be preserved as far as possible.
- The technique of internal fixation must engage one of the inherent mechanisms for fracture healing outlined above.

CONCEPTS OF BONE FIXATION

Fixation with compression

A number of techniques have been introduced to produce compression between fracture fragments.

Lag

The lag effect is one of the most useful methods for producing interfragmentary compression. The effect is produced by a screw that crosses the fracture, and the threads of which firmly grip the far-side cortex. The screw is able to glide in the proximal cortex, and its progress is arrested by the screw head (Fig. 52.9).

Axial compression

Axial compression of a fracture is usually associated with plate fixation, but intramedullary devices that can produce a compressive load prior to final placement have also been designed. Axial compression by a plate may be achieved either by an external device that is removed prior to wound closure or by the design of the screw holes, as in the AO dynamic compression plate (Fig. 52.10).

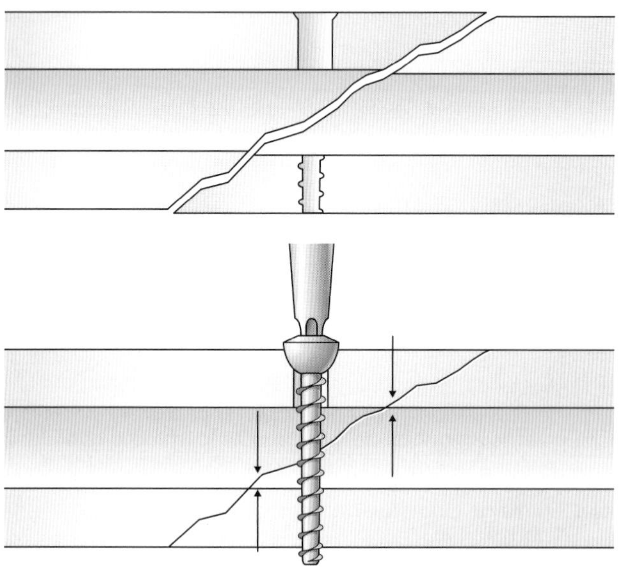

Figure 52.9 A lag screw is used to compress a fracture. The hole in the proximal cortex has a diameter slightly larger than the major diameter of the screw. The screw glides through this hole until its head abuts against the cortex. Further tightening of the screw causes compression between the two bone fragments. (After Muller 1992,[88] with permission.)

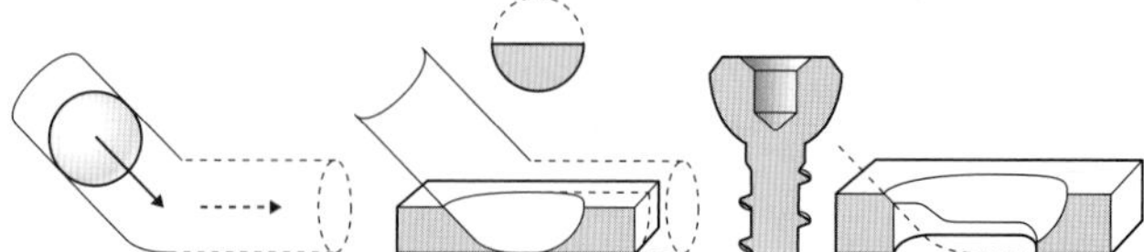

Figure 52.10 The principle of the dynamic compression plate. The screw head is spherical in shape, while the hole in the plate has the section of an inclined tube, which matches the diameter of the screw head on one side. As the screw is tightened, it moves down the incline, pushing the plate along its length. Because the other end of the plate is fixed to the bone on the other side of the fracture, compression across the fracture line results. (After Muller 1992,[88] with permission.)

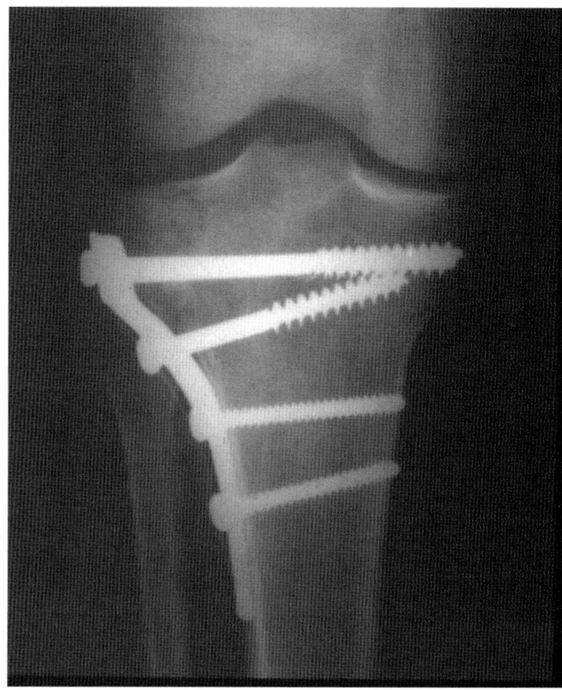

Figure 52.11 Buttress plating: a specially shaped plate has been employed to stabilize the reduction of a lateral tibial plateau fracture.

Buttress or antiglide

Compression may also be induced in an oblique fracture by the appropriate use of a plate that converts the tendency of the fracture fragments to shear across each other into compression (Fig. 52.11).

Tension band

Pauwels first suggested that under normal conditions of eccentric loading, long bones have a tension and a compression side.[90] The tension band applied to the tension side of a bone across a fracture converts the usual tension forces across the fracture into compression, so encouraging bone union (Fig. 52.12).[88] A tension band is a concept rather than a particular device, and although it consists usually of two stout parallel Kirschner wires

REFERENCES

89. Henry AK. Extensile Exposure. Williams & Williams, Baltimore, 1945
90. Pauwels F. Biomechanics of the Locomotor Apparatus. Springer-Verlag, Berlin, 1980

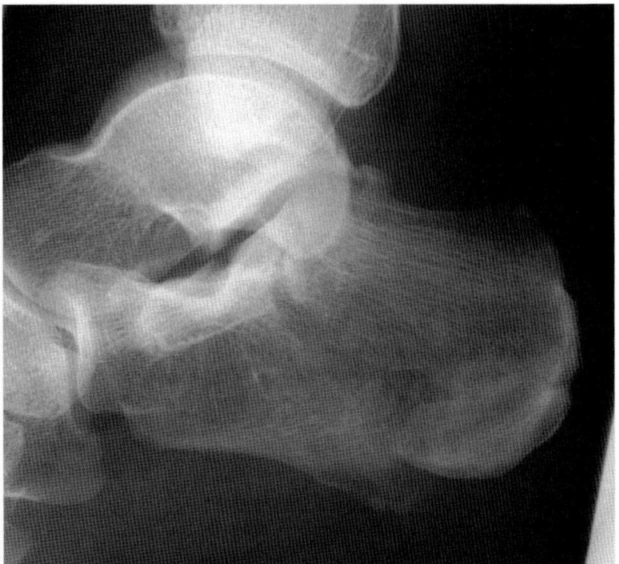

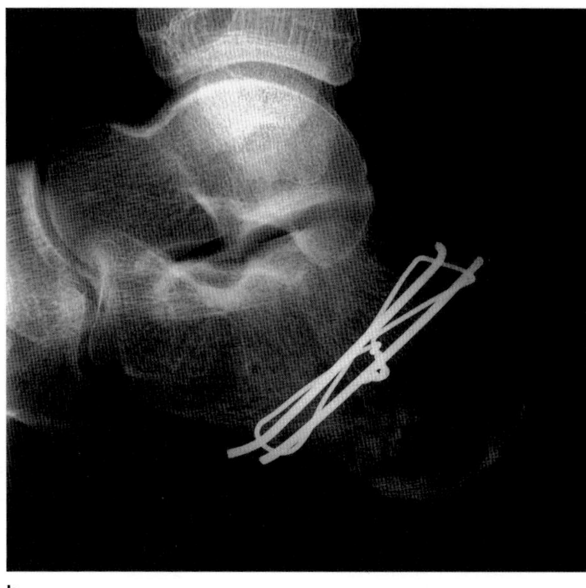

Figure 52.12 Avulsion fractures may be treated with tension band wires. In this case, a beak fracture of the calcaneum has been treated by a standard tension band consisting of two Kirschner wires and a figure-of-eight wire. The pull of the gastrocnemius and soleus muscle transmitted through the Achilles tendon would normally load the fracture line in tension and pull the fragments apart. The tension band wire bypasses the fracture site so that the fracture line is compressed when the muscle contracts. (a) Prior to fixation, the fracture line can be seen passing into the posterior facet of the subtalar joint and disrupting it. (b) The position after tension band wiring.

with a figure-of-eight wire around them, it may consist of wire only, of a plate and screws, or of a screw with a surrounding wire.

Tension bands are most widely used in the treatment of fractures that consist of avulsions of a muscular insertion, where they convert the tension of the muscle pull into compression at the fracture site, transferring the muscle force to the bone distant to the fracture. Thus they are often employed for the treatment of fractures of the olecranon, patella, greater trochanter of hip, and tuberosities of the proximal humerus, as well as in the beak avulsion fracture of the insertion of the Achilles tendon into the calcaneum (Fig. 52.12).

Prestressing

This concept was first introduced by Soeur using intramedullary wires,[91] and had an analogy with prestressed concrete. It is usually applied by over-contouring a plate, which leads to compression of the fracture site as the plate is fixed closely to the bone with screws (Fig. 52.13).

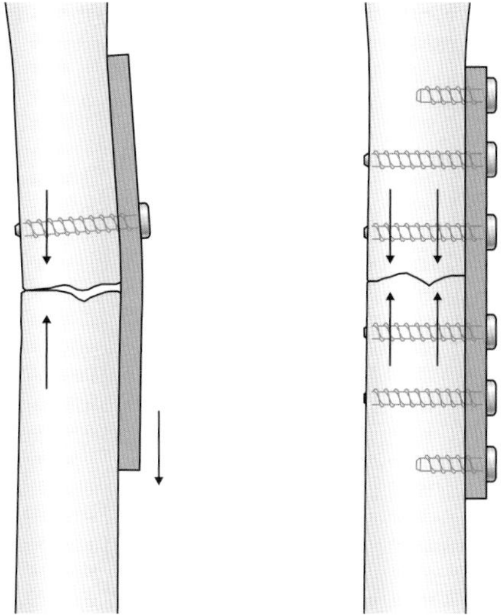

Figure 52.13 Bending or precontouring of a plate prior to application can be used to compress a fracture. The plate on the left has been contoured. As it is screwed to the bone and compression is applied, the entire fracture surface comes into compression, and the plate is loaded with a bending moment that tends to straighten it. (After Muller 1992,[88] with permission.)

Fixation without compression

Intramedullary nails

In contrast to the common use of plate and screw devices, intramedullary nails do not produce rigid fracture immobilization with compression. Fracture healing therefore does not usually occur by primary bone union but by external callus formation within the fracture haematoma.

Biological fixation

The concept of 'biological' fixation has been proposed for fractures that are not susceptible to rigid internal fixation with compression. Length and alignment of the fractured bone are maintained by the use of a plate and screws acting as an internal splint. The fracture fragments themselves are left undisturbed. Under these conditions, bone union occurs by external callus formation.[92] In practice, fracture union is not reliable, and although this type of fixation is superficially attractive for difficult fractures, further research and improvements in technique are necessary before it can be widely applied (Fig. 52.14). Advances in intramedullary nailing and external fixation may make this sort of fracture treatment redundant.

REFERENCES

91. Soeur R. Fractures of the Limbs. La Clinique Orthopaedique, Brussels, 1981
92. Baumgaertel F, Perren SM, Rahn B et al. J Trauma 1993; 7: 160–162

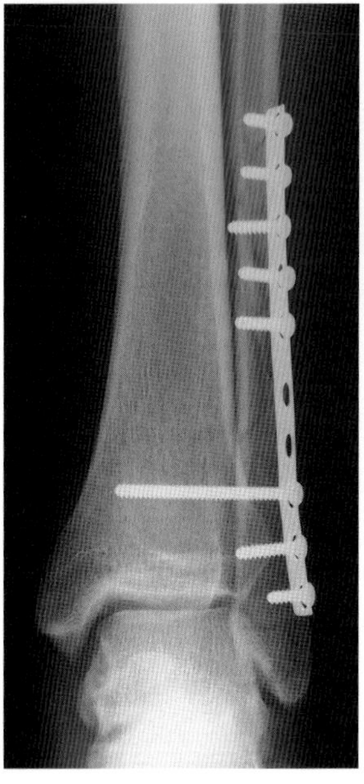
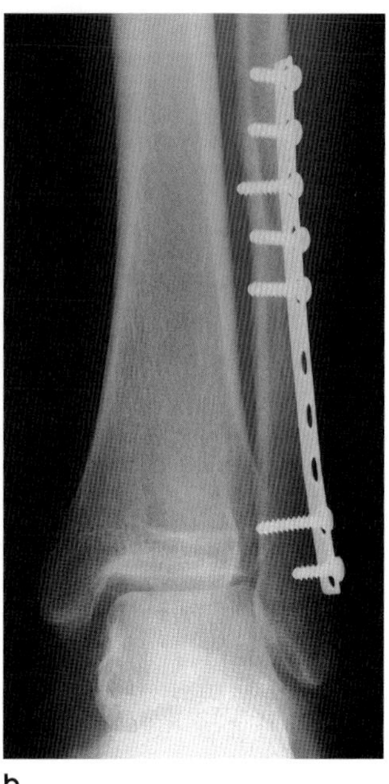

a b

Figure 52.14 Biological fixation. (a) In this highly comminuted Weber type C distal fibular fracture, it is not possible to produce rigid internal fixation with compression. The third tubular plate has been applied to the fibula to reduce the fracture with respect to length and alignment. Care has been taken not to strip the periosteum from the bone, and union is rapid because the bone retains its blood supply. The long inferior screw that passes into the tibia is a diastasis screw, which supports the ruptured inferior tibiofibular ligaments. This is removed at an early stage. (b) Union occurs by periosteal callus formation where bone fragments are unstable, particularly superiorly.

TYPES OF FIXATION DEVICE

Extramedullary devices

Cerclage systems

Cerclage wires have been used for stabilization of fractures since the early 19th century.[81] Thin wires or cables cause minimal disturbance to the osseous blood supply because it does not flow longitudinally along the cortex.[47,93] The bands that were developed from cerclage wires by Parham and later by Partridge are, however, wider and may well be associated with local cortical necrosis.[94,95] Although the cerclage wire itself may not disturb the bone blood supply, considerable soft tissue dissection may be necessary to apply it, and soft tissues may be trapped beneath the wire. Their application may therefore cause avascularity.

Transfixing wires

Kirschner wires—smooth, flexible wires—are used almost exclusively for the stabilization of individual bone fragments, either temporarily or as a definitive fracture fixation, usually augmented either by a tension band or by external splintage. The wires, being small, have little or no harmful effect on bone blood flow.

Screws

A screw has a number of unique properties. It has a thread with a shape and pitch, and a major and minor diameter. The major developments in bone screws have been made by the AO/ASIF group.[76] AO screws are based on machine screws and have a hexagonal recess in the head, which fits accurately with the screwdriver. They are cylindrical and are threaded either throughout their length (fully threaded) or only on the distal part (partially threaded). The screws are usually blunt-ended, requiring pretapping, because self-tapping screws were believed to grip bone less well; however, more recently screws that incorporate a fluted tip and are self-tapping have been shown to be satisfactory. Screw design is a compromise between strength and holding power, with its dimensions being determined by the size of the bone to be fixed. Screw strength depends on the minor diameter (the diameter of the shaft of the screw between the threads), whereas holding power varies mainly with the major diameter (the diameter of the outside of the thread) and to a lesser extent is dependent on thread design. In vivo, an immobile screw becomes enmeshed by bone so that its holding power increases with time. In contrast, a screw that is allowed to move provokes local bone resorption.[96–98]

Two sorts of screw have been developed by the AO/ASIF group, which form part of a comprehensive fracture fixation system. Cortical screws are made with diameters from 1.5 mm to 4.5 mm and are threaded throughout their entire length. They are inserted using a drill slightly larger than the minor diameter and employ a tap that copies the thread. The drill for the gliding hole matches the major diameter. Cancellous screws by contrast may be fully or partially threaded and have a greater difference between the minor and major diameters. They are available with a major diameter from 4.5 mm to 6.5 mm.

Cannulated screws

For a number of fractures, for example a subcapital fracture of the neck of femur, it is useful to be able to employ a preliminary wire as guide for subsequent screw placement. This is most readily achieved by the use of a screw with a hole down its centre. Such cannulated screws are weaker than solid screws and are therefore made with a wider minor diameter. The major diameter is increased in some cases to improve holding power.

Plates

Because compression was required at the fracture site to produce rigid fixation of the bone, tensioning devices were developed that could be attached to the bone, and one end of the plate after the other had been firmly fixed to one fracture fragment. These were then used to apply compression prior to completion of screw fixation. The tensioning device was removed prior to wound closure.

The dynamic compression plate is a plate in which the screw holes are shaped so that as the spherical screw head is tightened, it impinges on an inclined plane on one side of the screw hole. This causes the plate to move sideways, and as the plate is rigidly fixed to the other fracture fragment, compression of the fracture site is produced (Fig. 52.10).[88] Compression of the fracture site may also be produced by appropriate contouring of the plate prior to its application to the bone (Fig. 52.8).

REFERENCES

93. Rhinelander FW. J Biomed Mater Res 1974; 8: 87–90
94. Rhinelander FW. Clin Orthop 1975; 107: 188–220
95. Jones DG. J Bone Joint Surg 1986; 68B: 476–477
96. Schatzker J, Horne JG, Sumner-Smith G. Clin Orthop Relat Res 1975a; 111: 257–262
97. Schatzker J, Horne JG, Sumner-Smith G. Clin Orthop Relat Res 1975b; 111: 263–265
98. Schatzker J, Sanderson J, Murnaghan JP. Clin Orthop Relat Res 1975c; 108: 115–116

Rigidity of fracture fixation was ensured by the use of heavy plates that achieved a large contact area between the plate and the bone. These plates are associated with marked osteoporosis of the underlying bone, which may be associated with refracture after plate removal.[99,100] Similar changes have been found in animal experiments[101,102] and these were diminished if a more flexible titanium[103] or carbon fibre composite[104] plate was used instead of stainless steel. The osteoporosis was originally thought to be the result of stress shielding of the bone by the plate; however, Perren and colleagues have argued that it is the result of disturbance in local blood flow because of the large area of contact between the bone and the plate.[105,106] To overcome this problem, the limited-contact dynamic compression plate has been designed.[106,107] This titanium plate has a contact area of only 50% of its surface and is associated with less cortical porosis.[108]

Further developments of this concept have included the point contact plate[109] and the internal fixator, in which a plate is applied and fixed at a small distance from the underlying bone and that can be mounted under the skin.[110]

Modified plates

Certain specific fractures require specialized plates. The expanded metaphyses of bones are not suited to fixation with straight plates, while some bones, such as the calcaneum and pelvis, are irregular in shape. For use at these sites, angled, buttress and specialized plates have been developed (Fig. 52.8). Curved plates, which form half or a third of a tube and derive their strength from their curvature, are used to buttress fractures (Fig. 52.11 and 52.14). To fit the most complex bony contours, reconstruction plates are used. These plates are scalloped adjacent to the screw holes so that they can be bent in three dimensions. They are used principally in the distal humerus and pelvis.

Intramedullary nails

History

A number of the current debates on the techniques for use of intramedullary nails stem from the history of the devices. Modern intramedullary devices are complex and require sophisticated manufacturing methods. Stimson mentions the use of ivory intramedullary pegs for fracture stabilization,[82] and Hey-Groves developed this technique,[111] eventually using solid rods because of their greater strength and the avoidance of dead space. Kuntschner popularized the technique, using a straight, hollow nail with an open, cloverleaf cross-section manufactured of thin stainless steel to bridge a fracture of the femur.[112] The shape of the nail was designed for optimal strength and to allow more rapid revascularization of the medullary canal. The nail, being straight, obtained three-point fixation in the medullary canal and additional widening of the canal by the use of drills or reamers (a process termed *intramedullary reaming* or simply *reaming*), which was advocated to allow a larger and therefore stronger nail to be inserted. Although Kuntschner later experimented with a curved nail to match the curve of the femur,[113] this was difficult to use and was abandoned.

The AO/ASIF intramedullary femoral nail was a thin-walled, open-section cloverleaf cross-section nail, which was bent to follow the major curve of the femur. Reaming was employed to permit a wider and therefore stronger nail to be used and to increase the bone grip.[114] Unlike the original Kuntschner nail, the AO/ASIF nail was not designed for three-point fixation within the femur. Fracture stability was obtained by an interference fit of the nail with the entire diaphyseal length. Because the nail had a thin-wall cross-section, it would bend to some extent to accommodate the natural curve of the femur. By reaming the diaphysis, the length of femur over which the nail could obtain a purchase (the working length of the nail) was increased, and an exact fit between the femur and the nail was ensured.

Early attempts to control rotation[115] included the use of bundle nailing (Hackenthal), individual nails inserted through the medial and lateral femoral condyles (Rush), curved nails (Maatz), and pins within nails (Hertzog).

None of these nails were designed to provide longitudinal stability, and their utility was limited to fractures within the diaphysis, which possessed some degree of inherent longitudinal stability. Kuntschner experimented with a detensor nail in 1968;[115] however, it was Klemm and Schellman[116–118] and Kempf and Grosse[119,120] who took the obvious step of bolting the nail to the bone proximally and distally to create a locking nail. Two sorts of locking are recognized: 'dynamic' and static. In static locking, the screws are inserted into both ends of the nail through round holes, so that the length of the nail–bone construct is effectively fixed. *Dynamic locking* is a poor term, which may be used to describe locking of only one end of the nail, or locking of both ends but with the screw at one end placed through an oblong hole. These techniques allow some collapse at the fracture site. In the latter case, the amount of collapse is limited to the length of

REFERENCES

99. Richon A, Livio JJ, Segesser F. Helv Chir Acta 1967; 34: 49–64
100. Moyen B, Comtet JJ, Roy JC et al. Lyon Chir 1980; 76: 153–157
101. Paavolainen P, Slatis P, Karaharju E et al. Acta Orthop Scand 1979; 50: 369–374
102. Pilliar RM, Cameron HA, Binnington AG et al. J Biomed Mater Res 1979; 13: 799–810
103. Uthoff HK, Bardos DI, Liskova-Kiar M. J Bone Joint Surg 1981; 63B: 427–444
104. Coutts RD, Akeson WH, Woo SL-Y et al. Orthop Clin North Am 1976; 7: 223–229
105. Perren SM, Cordey J, Gautier E. In: Lane JM (ed). Fracture Healing. Churchill Livingstone, Edinburgh, 1987: 139–157
106. Perren SM, Cordey J, Rahn BA et al. Clin Orthop Relat Res 1988; 232: 139–151
107. Klaue K, Perren SM, Kowalski M. J Orthop Trauma 1991; 5: 280–288
108. Perren SM. Injury: AO/ASIF Sci Suppl 1991; 22: S1–S41
109. Remiger AR, Predieri M, Tepic S et al. J Orthop Trauma 1993; 7: 176–177
110. Ramotowski W, Granowski R. Clin Orthop Relat Res 1991; 272: 67–75
111. Hey-Groves EW. Br J Surg 1918; 5: 185–212
112. Kuntschner G. Klin Schr 1940; 19: 6–10
113. Kuntschner G. Practice of Intramedullary Nailing. 1st edn. Thomas, Springfield, 1967
114. Kyle RF. Orthopaedics 1985; 8: 1356–1359
115. Maatz R, Lentz W, Arens W et al. Intramedullary Nailing and Other Intramedullary Osteosynthesis. Saunders, Philadelphia, 1986
116. Klemm K, Schellman WD. Unfallheilkunde 1972; 75: 568–575
117. Klemm K, Schellman WD, Vitalli HP. Bull Soc Int Chir 1975; 34: 93–96
118. Klemm K, Borner M. Clin Orthop 1986; 212: 89–100
119. Kempf I, Grosse A, Beck G. J Bone Joint Surg 1985; 67A: 709–720
120. Kempf I, Gross A, Tagland G et al. Chirurgie 1991; 117: 478–487

the oblong screw hole, which might be more accurately termed *controlled collapse*, whereas in the former there is no theoretical limit to the amount of the collapse that can occur. Shortening at the fracture site continues until the fracture becomes stable or until the nail abuts against some restraining tissue or even exits through the skin. This can best be described as *uncontrolled collapse*.

'Dynamization' of an intramedullary nail is the process of removing one or more interlocking screws to allow collapse. It alters the biomechanical environment of the fracture profoundly, even if the fracture is sufficiently united to be longitudinally stable, and causes increased contact between fracture fragments if the fracture is not. It often encourages bone union, and if the fracture is tenuously united it hastens maturation of the union by increasing the loading of the fracture site.

Locked intramedullary nails differ from unlocked nails in that they gain both rotational and longitudinal stability not from an interference fit with the diaphysis of the bone, but as a result of the screws that fix the nail to the bone. Therefore reaming loses one of its original purposes, ensuring an accurate interference fit for the nail. The second purpose for reaming was to allow a wider and stronger nail to be used; however, advances in materials and nail design have to some extent rendered this unnecessary.

Biology of intramedullary nailing

Union proceeds mainly by the formation of periosteal callus following intramedullary nailing (Fig. 52.2),[47,63] in contrast to healing by direct union, which follows compression plating (Fig. 52.4).[121] The insertion of an intramedullary device temporarily destroys the medullary blood supply whether the medullary canal is reamed prior to insertion or not, which renders some of the cortex avascular.[122,123] Nevertheless, intramedullary fracture fixation is associated with higher bone and fracture blood flow than in compression plating[121] in an animal model. Revascularization is more rapid following nailing if reaming is not employed.[53,63] Although it is likely that direct damage to the arterial blood supply is one cause of cortical necrosis, excessive intramedullary pressure is also important. Maintaining a low intramedullary pressure significantly reduces the amount of cortical necrosis caused by reaming in animal models. However, the passage of an unreamed rod causes a significant rise in pressure and results in embolus formation.[124]

INDICATIONS FOR INTERNAL FIXATION OF FRACTURES

The indications for internal fixation of fractures are imprecise. The main reasons for considering this technique are as follow.

Failure of closed methods

It is important to remember that the presence of a fracture is not of itself an indication for operative management. Many fractures can be adequately treated by closed or non-operative methods. It is perfectly acceptable to begin treatment by non-operative techniques and to have to convert to operative stabilization if these methods fail.

Articular fractures

Fractures that involve the articular surface require precise reduction and early mobilization to avoid stiffness and future arthritis. These goals can often be achieved only by operative treatment.

Pathological fractures

Fractures caused by bony metastases rarely unite. They are often excessively painful, and terminal cancer patients should not be condemned to live out their remaining life on traction. The short life expectancy of the patient means that even though the fracture will not unite, the implant will usually not undergo fatigue failure before the patient succumbs to the underlying malignancy.[65]

Associated vascular injury

The presence of an associated vascular injury makes emergency fracture stabilization desirable to allow the vascular injury to be repaired with a stable skeleton (see Ch. 10).

Multiple injury

There is evidence that the multiply injured patient who has fractures in many long bones benefits from early fracture stabilization (see Ch. 7).[125] This does not necessarily imply internal fixation of every fracture, because external stabilization may be sufficient. More recent evidence suggests that early intramedullary nailing in multiply injured patients with significant chest injuries may cause a clinically undesirable worsening of lung function.[126–128]

Mobilization

Elderly patients suffer excessively from immobilization in bed. Complications of bed rest include pneumonia, venous thrombosis and pulmonary embolus, pressure sores, increased osteoporosis, and difficulty with mobilization. For this reason, fractures in the elderly are often treated by operative fixation even when they would unite satisfactorily if treated non-operatively. A good example is the intertrochanteric fracture of the neck of femur.

EXTERNAL FIXATION

Principles

An external fixator is essentially a scaffold that is attached to the bone to support it while fracture union occurs. The first working external fixator was probably described by Parkhill;[129] however, the concept was developed by Lambotte[84] using a linear metal clamp attached to four screw-threaded half-pins. Roger Anderson in 1934 described a frame using transfixing pins, and this concept was refined by Hoffman and later Vidal.[130] The rigidity of this device has led to problems with bone union and earned it

REFERENCES

121. Rand JA, Chao EYS, Kelly PJ. J Bone Joint Surg 1981; 63A: 427–442
122. Danckwardt-Lilliestrom G. Acta Orthop Scand Suppl 1969; 128S: 1–153
123. Danckwardt-Lilliestrom G, Lorenzi L, Olerud S. J Bone Joint Surg 1970; 52A: 1390–1394
124. Sturmer K. Injury (AO/ASIF Sci Suppl) 1993; 24: S7–S21
125. Bone LB, McNamara K, Shine B et al. J Trauma 1994; 37: 262–264
126. Pape HC, Dwenger A, Regel G et al. J Trauma 1992; 33: 574–581
127. Pape HC, Auf'm'Kolk M, Paffrath T et al. J Trauma 1993; 34: 540–547
128. Pape HC, Regel G, Dwenger A et al. J Trauma 1993; 35: 709–716
129. Parkhill C. Trans Am Surg Assoc 1897; 15: 251–256
130. Vidal J. Clin Orthop Relat Res 1983; 180: 7–14

the nickname 'the non-union machine'. In addition, the quadrilateral nature of the frame made reduction of the fracture difficult once the device was even partly applied.

Bone fixation

External fixators are fixed to bone by screw-threaded half-pins, by transfixing pins, or by tensioned fine wires. Screw-threaded half-pins have the advantage that they are simple and swift to apply and, because only one side of the bone is approached, the pins can usually be placed with little risk to neurovascular structures. Because the pin has only one end protruding from the bone, it acts like a post and the fixating frame can be relatively straightforward. The disadvantage of screw-threaded half-pins is that they rely on the integrity of the thread–bone interface for their stability. Loosening is a significant problem that limits their utility.

Transfixing pins and fine wires have the disadvantage that they must pass through the bone from one side of the limb to the other. This may endanger neurovascular structures, or it may make the encircling frame inconvenient to the patient and restrict joint mobility. For example, it is difficult to transfix the proximal humerus without endangering the neurovascular structures, although the frame required is not much more inconvenient to the patient than a uniaxial frame. On the other hand, it is possible to pass a transfixing wire through the proximal femur but the frame required makes it difficult for the patient to lie down.

Transfixing pins have all the disadvantages of screw-threaded half-pins, and transfixing devices and their use is normally restricted to the simple external fixators required for joint fusion or for temporary stabilization of the severely traumatized limb.

Tensioned fine wires for external fixation are being increasingly used in the West. They were originally popularized by Ilizarov in Russia, and although there are reports of their use prior to Ilizarov's work he is mainly responsible for their popularity.

Fine wires do little damage to the bone blood supply and soft tissues, and multiple wires can be used in a small space. They rely for their fixation not on the strength of the wire–bone interface but on the interaction between multiple wires inserted at different orientations, and therefore loosening is less of a problem than with screw-threaded half-pins or transfixing pins. Two sorts of fine wire are used: plain and stoppered or 'olive' wires (Fig. 52.15). When the stoppered wires are used, the olive is placed tightly against the bone cortex so as to improve the stability of the frame construct. Alternatively, by pulling gently on the other end of the olive wire, the wire can be used as a motor to move a piece of bone.

Fracture healing under conditions of external fixation

Early external fixators aimed to produce rigid immobility of the bone, because this was regarded as ideal for prompt restoration of limb function. Under these conditions, the production of callus is suppressed and union occurs only slowly by direct or primary bone healing. This mode of bone union is totally intolerant of interfragmentary motion and has no ability to cross macroscopic gaps. Because external fixators and indirect fracture

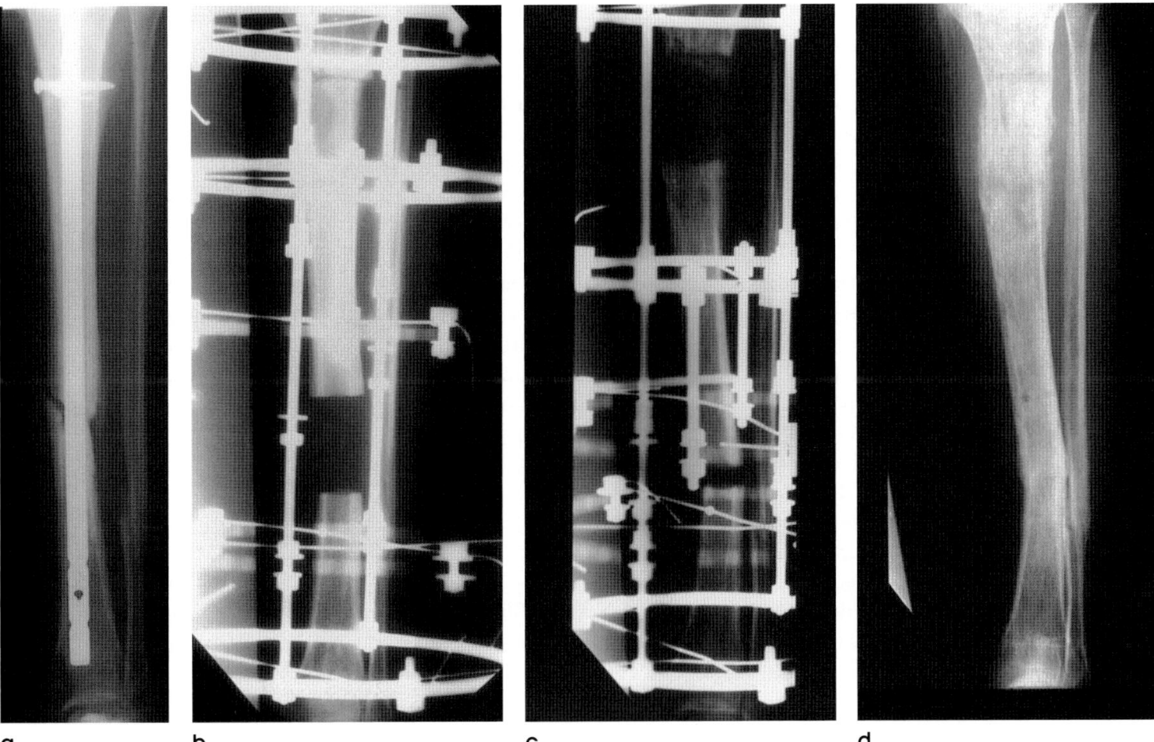

Figure 52.15 The use of the principles of Ilizarov in the treatment of an infected fracture non-union. **(a)** An infected non-union of a tibial fracture following intramedullary nailing. There was a discharging sinus overlying the fracture site, and at the time of operative exploration the bone adjacent to the fracture was dead. **(b)** All dead bone has been removed and the fracture has been stabilized with a three-segment, two-focus Ilizarov frame. A proximal corticotomy has been performed to allow a bone transport. **(c)** The bone transport in progress. The new bone formation in distraction can be seen. The transport segment is not yet docked with the distal bone segment. **(d)** The final result.

reduction are not capable of obtaining perfect fracture reduction and may be associated with a distraction gap between fracture ends rather than interfragmentary compression, early experience with these devices was associated with high non-union rates.[131]

This problem has led to the introduction of *dynamization* of the external fixator. This term is loosely used to describe two different concepts (compare with its use in intramedullary nailing[132]). The first concept, which might be better called controlled collapse, occurs where the external fixator is deliberately made longitudinally unstable while torsional and angular stability is maintained. This has the effect of allowing the fracture site to telescope. An extension of this concept, which may be applied in certain external fixators, is to compress the fracture site by serial adjustment of the frame. If the fracture is longitudinally stable, the fracture site will be compressed and this may encourage union. When the fracture site is unstable, shortening of the limb will occur, which may encourage union by increasing the amount of bone at the fracture site and its apposition. When the shortening is judged to be unacceptable, a simultaneous leg-lengthening procedure may be undertaken using callus distraction through a separate corticotomy. This is the basis for the use of bone transport in the treatment of delayed fracture union.

The second use of the term dynamization is the modification of the external fixator so that a cyclical strain is applied to the fracture site. This may be achieved by using the patient's load-bearing weight against a deformable component of the fixator or by employing an actuator attached to the frame.

Goodship and Kenwright investigated the influence of micro-motion on the healing of experimental fractures in sheep.[133] They showed that the application of a longitudinal cyclical strain that induced movement of 1 mm at an early stage following fracture was associated with increased callus formation and more rapid fracture union. Larger deformations or application of the stimulus at a later time were associated with delay in fracture healing. This concept has subsequently been tested in tibial fractures in humans[131] and has been confirmed.

Complications of external fixators

Chronic pain

Chronic pain is particularly a problem with fine-wire ring fixators, and its cause is multifactorial. Tented soft tissues in the region of a pin site are painful, and even a perfect pin–bone interface is probably slightly uncomfortable, so that where there are a large number of pins the discomfort may be increased until pain is perceived. An infected pin site is painful, and where pins or wires have been inserted close to a joint, movement of the joint may be accompanied by sawing of the pin or wire through the soft tissues. The frame may be being used for bone transport or leg lengthening, and this may of itself be painful and there may be residual pain from a fracture. Finally, the patient may be psychologically ill-prepared for the frame, and this may add to their perception of pain. Whatever the cause of chronic pain, the effect may be to prevent the patient moving the limb and bearing weight, which may cause joint contracture, swelling and osteoporosis, which may itself contribute to pin loosening.

Pin loosening and breakage

Loosening is a common cause of failure of an external fixation pin, and its causes are complex. Bone death at the time of half-pin insertion leads to resorption, which directly contributes to loosening. For this reason, sharp drills, slow drilling speeds, and irrigation to lower drilling temperatures are advocated. Self-drilling screws tend to produce more heat and are therefore not normally recommended. An initially accurate fit between the screw thread and the bone is important, both for initial stability of the interface and for the elimination of small pockets in which haematomas may collect (which may later become infected). This is another reason for preferring predrilled screws. Loosening is more common in half-pins inserted into the metaphysis rather than into the diaphysis, and this probably relates to the greater initial stability of the bone–screw interface. Pin loosening may relate to local overload of the pin–bone interface, and this notion is borne out by the clinical finding that pin loosening is less prevalent where a segment of bone is stabilized by multiple half-pins.

Pin loosening and pin site infection are related problems. Occasionally, general half-pin loosening follows an episode of septicaemia, and in this case it seems likely that the half-pins become loose because of secondary bacterial action. More commonly, a single pin that is mechanically loose, due to either bone death or pin–bone interface overload, becomes infected from the junction with the exterior. Finally, a solidly implanted half-pin may loosen as a result of poor pin site care, local soft tissue infection gradually spreading along the pin–bone interface.

The preferred interface between a screw-threaded half-pin and bone is that of osseointegration, in which the bone grows up to and into the interstices of the pin without an intervening fibrous tissue membrane. This sort of interface is strong and highly resistant to infection. Studies in animals have demonstrated that this sort of interface is most likely to develop if the half-pin is made of titanium, and therefore in those external fixators that are intended to be on the body for a long period the half-pins are often made of titanium.

Pin tract infections

Minor pin track difficulties are almost universal in the use of external fixators, and a number of classification systems for the severity of the problem have been devised (Table 52.1).[134–136]

Limitation of joint motion

Limitation of joint motion is principally a problem of fine-wire frames where a wire is inserted close to the joint. As the joint is moved, the soft tissues adopt a different position with respect to the wire and impinge against it, causing irritation and pain. This sort of problem can be minimized by careful wire placement, seeking a neutral position in which skin movement is minimized, but to some extent it is an inevitable complication of placing wires close to joints.

REFERENCES

131. Kenwright J, Richardson JB, Cunningham JL et al. J Bone Joint Surg Br 1991; 73B: 654–659
132. Richardson JB, Gardner TN, Hardy JRW et al. J Bone Joint Surg 1995; 77B: 412–416
133. Goodship AE, Kenwright J. J Bone Joint Surg 1985; 67B: 650–655
134. Paley D, Chaudray M, Pirone AM et al. Orthop Clin North Am 1990; 21: 667–691
135. Checketts RG, Moran CG, Jennings AG. Acta Orthop Scand 1995; 3: 271–274
136. Sims M, Saleh M. Prof Nurse 1996; 11: 261–264

Table 52.1 Grading of pin tract infection

Grade	Feature	Notes
1	Serous discharge	The pin track is not definitely infected
2	Superficial cellulitis	The soft tissues around the pin are infected
3	Deep infection	The pin track itself is infected and the pin is loose
4	Osteomyelitis	The bone infection continues after removal of the pin

Neurovascular damage

Impaling a neurovascular trunk is a particular problem with fine-wire external fixators. To minimize the risk, when the wires are inserted, the drill is employed in a reciprocating fashion rather than constantly rotating in one direction, and once the wire has passed through the bone it is tapped through the remaining soft tissue. This technique, combined with a precise knowledge of the anatomy of the limb,[137] usually avoids damage to major trunks. It is, however, not always possible to avoid damage to relatively small and inconstant cutaneous nerve branches, and damage to these structures can occasionally lead to causalgia.[138]

Indications for the use of external fixators

Multiple trauma

In patients who have suffered multiple injuries (see Ch. 7), external fixation offers a rapid method for temporarily stabilizing long bone fractures. This may be particularly useful in those cases where there is chest trauma, because intramedullary nailing in the acute phase in these patients is associated with an increased risk of adult respiratory distress syndrome from embolized medullary contents.[126–128] There is a theoretical risk of intramedullary infection when the temporary external fixation is changed for definitive intramedullary nailing, but in practice this is not seen in the femur provided that the fixator pins are not allowed to become loose and infected.[139]

Open fractures

The presence of metalwork increases the incidence of infection in contaminated wounds,[140,141] thus there are advantages in the use of external fixation for the treatment of open fractures. The disadvantages include the possible difficulty of undertaking soft tissue reconstruction in the presence of an external fixator and the possibility of delayed or non-union. In the tibia, there is an increased incidence of infection if intramedullary nailing is performed after external fixation.[142,143] This problem may be reduced by the use of unreamed solid nails[144] and by the use of the pinless external fixator. It is possible that the problem can be obviated by more radical debridement of the compound wound and by the avoidance of infected pin sites.

Pelvic fractures

Fractures of the pelvis are associated with severe blood loss, which may be life-threatening. The use of an external fixator applied as an emergency measure in the accident and emergency department as part of initial resuscitation allows stabilization and reduction of the fracture. This limits the space for bleeding and, by preventing further movement between the fracture fragments, allows the body's natural haemostatic mechanisms to clot the extravasated blood.[145]

Periarticular fractures

In periarticular fractures of a long bone, particularly the tibia, where the remaining segment of bone close to the joint is too small to allow fixation by intramedullary nailing, consideration should be given to the use of a circular external fixator as definitive treatment. If an anatomical reduction can be obtained with compression, rapid union of the fracture may be anticipated, which will offset the discomfort and inconvenience of the frame.

Intra-articular fractures

The accepted treatment of intra-articular fractures is by open anatomical reduction and rigid internal fixation. External fixation, particularly using fine-wire frames, is increasingly being used as a technique for the stabilization of the fractured metaphysis in cases where the soft tissues are judged to be unable to withstand plate fixation, and to obviate the necessity of the large soft tissue dissections associated with plate stabilization.

Bone transport

The technique of bone transport is increasingly used for the treatment of severe fractures to replace lost bone and to encourage fracture union. It requires an external fixation frame that is capable of stabilizing two foci independently.

The fracture is stabilized using the external fixator and a minimally invasive division of the bone (a corticotomy) is made at another site, usually in the opposite metaphysis distant from the zone of fracture injury. The act of corticotomy itself activates the entire bone, encouraging union at the original fracture. After a delay, the corticotomy is gradually distracted so that new bone forms by distraction osteogenesis. Simultaneously, the non-union site or bone defect is compressed, further encouraging bone union, so that the overall effect is that a tube of bone is moved (or transported) through the soft tissues (Fig. 52.5).

OPEN (COMPOUND) FRACTURES

An open or compound fracture is one in which the soft tissue envelope of the limb has been disrupted, allowing the bone to communicate with the exterior. This sort of fracture differs from one that is closed, in that there is potentially direct bacterial access to the bone and because the amount of damage to the bone and soft tissues is usually greater. These two problems combine to produce a situation where it may be difficult to achieve satisfactory bone healing, and the outcome of such a fracture depends on the extent and nature of bacterial

REFERENCES

137. Faure C, Merloz P. Transfixation. Springer-Verlag, Berlin, 1987
138. Herron M, Langkamer VG, Atkins RM. Foot 1993; 3: 38–42
139. Broos PL, Miserez MJ, Rommens PM. Injury 1992; 23: 525–528
140. Gristina AG, Costerton JW. J Bone Joint Surg 1985; 67A: 264–273
141. Bach AW, Hansen ST. Clin Orthop Relat Res 1989; 241: 89–94
142. Maurer DJ, Merkow RL, Gustilo RB. J Bone Joint Surg 1989; 71A: 835–838
143. McGraw JM, Lim EV. J Bone Joint Surg 1988; 70A: 900–911
144. Riemer BI, Butterfield SL. J Orthop Trauma 1993; 7: 279–285
145. Kellam JF. Clin Orthop Relat Res 1989; 241: 66–82

contamination and on the amount and type of the soft tissue damage, as well as the extent of the bone injury.

The soft tissue damage includes skin and muscle death and possibly nerve damage, which limit the best outcome that can be achieved and restrict the methods by which the fracture can be treated. Blood vessel injury may risk the survival of the limb. Stripping of the periosteum from the bone damages the blood supply of the fractured bone ends and makes fracture union more difficult to achieve, while rendering the bone more susceptible to infection.

These difficult fractures were once seen mainly as a consequence of war, although pedestrian collision was another source. Since the Second World War, the gradual increase in the number and speed of motor vehicles has led to a virtual epidemic of compound fractures, often associated with other life-threatening injuries.

CLASSIFICATION

Classification of compound fractures is important, both because it helps to direct treatment and because it allows outcomes to be compared in these difficult injuries. The important features to be graded are the degree of bone and soft tissue injury and the extent of bacterial contamination.

The first attempts at grading were based on the concepts of Robert Jones. A grade 1 injury was a puncture wound from within out, a grade 2 injury was an external injury that involved the bone, and a grade 3 injury referred to any injury of greater severity.

The Gustilo and Anderson classification

The most widely employed classification is now that of Gustilo and Anderson,[146] although it is not ideal. There tends to be an excessive attention to the size of the wound as opposed to the amount of soft tissue damage. Thus a limb that is severely crushed beneath a lorry may have only a small skin wound but may inevitably require amputation, whereas if the limb has been cut with a sharp, clean knife, the size of the soft tissue laceration may be great but the surrounding soft tissue damage may be so slight that the limb heals rapidly with excellent return of function. There have been a number of minor modifications to the original classification;[147,148] however, unacceptably high interobserver variations have been recorded even when it was used by trained trauma surgeons.[149]

Type I fracture

The injury is of low energy. The wound has occurred in a relatively clean environment and is usually less than 1 cm in length. There is little or no muscle damage and no crushing component, and usually the injury is from within out. Fracture comminution is not present.

Type II fracture

Type II fracture is a broad area of injury falling between a type I and a type III fracture. The wound is more than 1 cm in length, and the injury is often from without in. There is usually a small amount of dead muscle, but debridement is confined to one compartment, with minimal periosteal stripping and no significant bacterial contamination. Eventual wound closure without a plastic surgical flap is possible. There may be slight fracture comminution.

Type III fracture

Any one of the features listed below automatically make the fracture type III compound.

- Heavy bacterial contamination, as in a farmyard injury.
- A shotgun or high-velocity gunshot injury.
- A fracture occurring in a high-velocity vehicular accident.
- A vascular injury requiring repair.
- A significant crushing component.
- A displaced segmental fracture.
- A fracture with diaphyseal bone loss.

The type III injury is usually a high-energy injury with extensive damage from outside to inside. There is crushing and devitalization of muscle, and usually the wound is extensive. The fracture is usually displaced and comminuted.

The type III fractures are further subdivided.

- Type IIIa: there is limited or absent periosteal stripping of bone, and after debridement there is no significant problem in soft tissue coverage; there is no bone loss.
- Type IIIb: there is extensive periosteal stripping and soft tissue damage; without the use of limb reconstruction techniques, plastic surgical flap coverage is frequently required.
- Type IIIc: there is a major vascular injury requiring repair for limb salvage.

Some further points concerning the Gustilo and Anderson classification are important.

- The usual error is under-classification.
- It is doubtful whether a type I femoral fracture exists.
- A compound tibial fracture with a posterior wound is not a type I injury.
- A type III injury may be diagnosed at the time of patient admission, but the distinction between a type IIIa and a type IIIb may not be possible until debridement is complete.
- There is a progression of severity of injury from type I to type IIIb; however, type IIIc does not follow this progression.
- A compound injury occurring in a road traffic accident is by definition never a type I injury, however small the wound.

Other classification systems

Owing to the inadequacies of the Gustilo and Anderson system, a number of other methods of classification have been devised. These include the Tcherne classification, which has the great advantage that it begins by dividing the fracture into integument closed (IC, a closed fracture) or integument open (IO, an open fracture). This concentrates the mind on the fact that the soft tissue injury is present whether or not there is a breach of the skin.

MANAGEMENT OF AN OPEN FRACTURE

Initial assessment

In a major trauma centre, the initial assessment and management of the patient are by a multidisciplinary trauma team, which includes experts in resuscitation as well as orthopaedic, plastic and vascular surgeons.

Patient assessment

Open fractures are often the result of high-energy violence and are commonly not isolated injuries. The patient and their other

REFERENCES

146. Gustilo RB, Anderson JT. J Bone Joint Surg 1976; 58A: 453–458
147. Gustilo RB. Instr Course Lect 1987; 36: 359–366
148. Gustilo RB, Gruninger RP, Davis T. Orthopedics 1987; 10: 1781–178
149. Brumback RJ, Jones AL. J Bone Joint Surg 1994; 76A: 1162–1166

injuries must be fully assessed and treatment of all injuries carried out simultaneously, with due regard to the urgency of the individual clinical situation (see Ch. 7).

Limb injury assessment

Limb injury assessment is carried out as for any fracture, with the addition of an assessment of the wound. In the emergency phase, the wound is disturbed as little as possible, and it is useful to cover it with an antiseptic dressing after a Polaroid photograph has been taken. The underlying fracture is assessed radiographically.

Emergency management

Emergency management begins at the site of injury, where temporary splintage and wound covering are provided. Anti-tetanus prophylaxis is given and intravenous antibiotics are commenced. As soon as is practical, consistent with the patient's other injuries, formal exploration of the wound under general anaesthetic is undertaken.

Initial operative management

The purpose of this stage of treatment is to debride the wound and stabilize the fracture. If at all possible it is performed within 6 h of injury, because after that time bacterial colonization of the wound is inevitable, increasing the risk of infection.

Wound debridement

The origin of the term *debridement* is sometimes considered to be removal of debris, but more probably the term derives from the French word *la bride*, meaning a bridle, and the original connotation of the term was letting out pus. Whatever its etymology, debridement is a fundamental concept. Dead tissue does not heal and it does not revitalize to any significant extent. It does, however, provide an excellent culture medium for bacteria. Foreign material within a wound will inhibit wound healing as well as providing a source of bacterial contamination and a good culture medium. Debridement implies the removal of all dead tissue and foreign contamination.

Debridement is carried out in an operating theatre under general anaesthetic. The injured limb is prepared for surgery using non-irritant antiseptic and draped so that the entire limb is within the operative field. This is because the extent of debridement is not known, and the operating surgeon may need to check peripheral perfusion during the procedure. A tourniquet is rarely employed, although in cases where severe bleeding is predicted one may be applied and not inflated. The original wound is extended so that it can be explored under direct vision down to the fractured bone. At first sight this may seem excessively destructive, especially for example in a fracture of the femur with a small compound wound. It is, however, never possible to be certain whether contaminated material has become attached to the fractured bone ends; if dead and infected material is left within the fracture, the likely result is an infected non-united fracture. The most common error in debridement is to make an inadequate wound exploration. When extending the skin wound, fine surgical judgement is required to produce a wound that will eventually close with a satisfactory scar, or if necessary with an appropriate flap, and that will allow adequate exposure for debridement while not devitalizing bruised but viable regions of skin.

All foreign material is meticulously removed from the wound and all dead tissue is excised. A convenient method of removing contaminated, contused and non-viable skin is by skin edge excision; however, this may be contraindicated where skin is well vascularized and at a premium, such as on the palm of the hand. All contaminated, non-viable or severely damaged fascia is removed. Tendons are preserved with their paratenon unless severely damaged, because they are essential for function and they are not as good a host for bacterial culture as muscle is.

Muscle debridement

The amount of muscle that should be removed at debridement is difficult to assess. Muscle is often damaged severely over a wide area even when the skin wound is small, and this is particularly the case in high-energy injuries where the bone loading is very rapid so that the fracture is explosive in nature. Dead muscle does not demonstrate capillary bleeding, although arteriolar bleeding may remain. It does not contract when cut or gently squeezed, and it may be discoloured. Muscle that has been crushed during injury is mushy, whereas viable muscle is of a firm consistency. Of these four features, the most reliable are said to be contractility and consistency.[150] Guiding principles for muscle excision are as follow.

- Dead muscle is the optimal culture medium for bacterial growth, particularly anaerobic organisms such as clostridia.
- A modest amount of muscle loss will cause little long-term disability.
- An intact muscle tendon unit with as little as 10% of normal muscle bulk will produce significant function.[151]
- Dubious muscle may be viable and will 'declare' itself within 24–48 h.

Bone debridement

The extent to which devitalized bone should be removed from a compound fracture is a matter of surgical judgement and may be difficult. Dead cortical bone does not itself encourage fracture union (it is not significantly osteogenic or osteoinductive), but it can take part in it (it is osteoconductive). Recently devitalized cancellous bone, in contrast, is osteogenic, osteoinductive and osteoconductive. Devitalized bone remaining within the fracture site may well become infected. On the other hand, in order to function a limb requires a structurally competent skeleton, and even devitalized bone will suffice. Furthermore, devitalized bone will revascularize slowly; however, as it does so, the dead bone is resorbed and weakened, and fractures may occur a considerable time after the original injury. In addition, after excision of dead bone, the body has a remarkable capacity to re-form a new competent bone, presumably from the remaining intact periosteum.[39] Finally, the introduction of distraction osteogenesis by Ilizarov means that any excised bone can be replaced, although this is a technically demanding process that is difficult for the patient.

Initial bone debridement should be conservative. Isolated pieces of cortical bone that have no periosteal attachment are removed. Small pieces of denuded cancellous bone are retained provided that the wound is not extensively contaminated. A devitalized piece of cortical bone may be retained on the assumption that it will participate in fracture union if the level of

REFERENCES

150. Scully RE, Artz CP, Sako Y. Arch Surg 1956; 73: 1031–1035
151. Chapman MW, Olson SA. In: Rockwood CA, Green DP, Bucholz RW et al. (eds). Rockwood and Green's Fractures in Adults, Vol 1. 4th edn. Lippincott-Raven, Philadelphia, 1996: 318

contamination is low and there is little periosteal stripping of the major bone fragments.

Other tissues

If a wound enters a joint, it is thoroughly explored and the joint is inspected. After all dead tissue has been removed, the joint capsule is closed. Nerve trunks are preserved and sutured (see Ch. 43) and major blood vessels are repaired (see Ch. 10 and Ch. 11).

Irrigation

At the end of the debridement, the wound is irrigated with copious amounts of fluid. The purpose is to reduce the extent of bacterial wound contamination. High-pressure lavage may drive contaminated material into the body as well as further damaging ischaemic tissues; however, pulsed lavage is more effective than simple irrigation in lowering the bacterial count.[152,153] The addition of antibiotics to the irrigating solution (unsurprisingly) does not improve the efficacy of the process.[153,154] In contrast, antiseptic agents probably do contribute to a reduction in the bacterial load,[155] and on the basis of this study it seems reasonable to include a dilute solution of chlorhexidine in the lavage, although caution should be exercised when the wound includes a joint because of possible toxic effects on chondrocytes.

Wound closure

The guiding principles of wound closure are as follow.

- Do not close over dead tissue.
- Do not close over infected tissue.
- Do not commit tension.

Because the primary debridement is usually conservative with respect to both muscle and bone, it is almost never acceptable primarily to close a traumatic wound at this time. As far as possible bone, tendon, nerve and blood vessel should be covered with muscle, fat or fascia to prevent damage from desiccation. The skin, however, is left open and the wound space is packed.

Further debridement

Primary debridement is a holding operation that must be followed by a second debridement after approximately 48 h. It is the first stage in a process that will lead to a wound consisting of healthy tissue capable of resisting the inevitable bacterial contamination of the open wound, so that definitive reconstruction can be carried out. Further removal of dead tissue is continued at intervals until a viable tissue bed remains. Then and only then is reconstruction attempted.

Initial bone stabilization

The presence of a fracture destabilizes the limb, exposing the tissues to deformation, movement and pressure. The restoration of the normal length and alignment of the limb ensures optimal arterial supply, and venous and lymphatic drainage. Skeletal stability optimizes the conditions for early revascularization and hence improves resistance to infection.

Initial stability may be achieved by any of the traditional methods of fracture treatment. Immobilization in plaster has the advantages that it is rapid and simple, and it does not compromise the bone or the soft tissue blood supply. The stability obtained is, however, suboptimal even if the cast is supplemented by transfixing pins above and below the fracture, and the presence of the cast makes treatment of the patient and management of the wound difficult.

Skeletal traction is attractive because it is easy to set up and causes minimal damage to the tissues of the limb. Nursing and soft tissue care may, however, be difficult, and the use of skeletal traction in open fractures in the West is virtually confined to the short, acute phase prior to operative debridement.

External skeletal fixation is also relatively rapid to apply and produces sufficient stability to allow optimal soft tissue recovery from the initial trauma. Furthermore, it facilitates patient treatment and makes wound care relatively simple. Some damage to transfixed soft tissues is inevitable, and devices may make subsequent soft tissue plastic flap reconstruction difficult. Finally, the pins may loosen and become infected, compromising the possibilities for later operative fracture treatment.

Open reduction and internal fixation take time, when the patient may require other emergency treatment, and insufficient information may be available to select the correct treatment. The major objection to this form of treatment is the extensive soft tissue dissection that has to be made, and this carries a high risk of wound breakdown and deep infection. Internal fixation of compound fractures in best reserved for the treatment of joint injuries using minimally invasive techniques.

Intramedullary nailing of open fractures has a number of advantages. It facilitates nursing care, while stabilizing the limb and allowing unimpeded access for soft tissue treatment including plastic surgical flaps. Inevitably there is damage to the intramedullary blood supply, which can be minimized by the use of unreamed techniques. For devitalized bone to revascularize, absolute stability of the bone fragments is necessary, and this may not be provided by an unreamed intramedullary nail, which may be associated with a fracture non-union.

Definitive soft tissue management

The options available are as follow.

- Primary wound closure with or without skin grafting.
- Delayed primary closure with or without skin grafting.
- Healing by secondary intention.
- Delayed closure by local or vascularized flap.

Primary wound closure

Primary wound closure is rarely if ever indicated. It should be employed only in those cases where the wound is known to be uncontaminated and there is definitely no remaining dead tissue or foreign material. The patient should be healthy and the wound must be closed without tension. In practice this occurs in type I compound fractures; however, in these cases the wounds are usually so small that suturing is unnecessary.

Delayed primary closure with or without skin grafting

This implies closure before the fifth day. This allows for a second debridement 48 h after the first operative inspection. Wound healing is not delayed in an adult human provided that definitive closure is undertaken before the fifth day. Leaving the wound

REFERENCES

152. Gross A, Cutright DE, Bhaskar SN. Am J Surg 1972; 124: 373–377
153. Anglen J, Apostoles S, Christensen G et al. J Orthop Trauma 1994; 8: 390–396
154. Rosenstein BD, Wilson FC, Thunderburk CH. J Bone Joint Surg 1989; 71A: 427–430
155. Taylor GJS, Leeming JP, Bannister GC. J Bone Joint Surg Br 1993; 75B: 724–730

open initially allows the swelling associated with the initial trauma to settle.

Healing by secondary intention

Wounds may be allowed to heal by secondary intention provided that bone, tendon, nerve and blood vessels are adequately covered by muscle or fat. For relatively small wounds that are not susceptible to delayed primary direct closure this is probably the optimum method of management, because it avoids split-skin grafting and gives satisfactory cosmetic results with acceptable cutaneous sensation. For larger wounds the time required is prohibitive, and split-skin grafting is necessary.

The use of local or free vascularized flaps

There are a small number of cases where an adequate soft tissue envelope does not exist after complete debridement. In these cases bone, tendon, nerve and blood vessels are inadequately covered. The problem usually applies to bone and is most commonly seen following tibial fracture. If the bone is left uncovered for any length of time, surface necrosis occurs and exposed devitalized bone will become colonized with bacteria, which will lead to infection and non-union. For these cases, early soft tissue cover with well-vascularized muscle is imperative. The importance of this approach was first demonstrated by Godina.[156] In a large retrospective study of microsurgical coverage procedures following compound fractures, he showed that the lowest rates of flap failure and late deep infection were seen where cover was provided within 72 h of injury. The time in hospital was also shortest in this group.

The flap brings with it a new blood supply and helps to resist local infection, and in this respect muscle flaps are superior to fasciocutaneous flaps.[157–159] A muscle flap may also act as a source of osteoprogenitor cells; however, it is unclear whether these cells are important, because bone healing beneath a flap is rarely by external callus formation. The new blood supply of the transplanted soft tissue flap tends to grow into the bone, revascularizing it.[159] However, it must be remembered that cortical autograft is poorly and slowly incorporated (see earlier text), and so the extent to which this process occurs in the diaphysis under clinical conditions remains in doubt.

Definitive fracture treatment

The method of initial fracture stabilization may be the eventual definitive technique employed for treating the fracture until union. This is, however, rarely the case. The two roles are totally different. This is obvious with a simple fracture, where the initial splint serves to immobilize the fracture to provide pain relief and to safeguard the limb prior to definitive fracture reduction and stabilization. With a severe compound fracture, the complexity of the initial treatment—which commonly includes intramedullary nailing or external fixation—should not obscure the simple fact that these treatments are being used only to stabilize the fracture, to safeguard the limb, and to allow proper management of the soft tissues.

Definitive fracture management is usually undertaken after the soft tissue problems have been resolved and any plastic flaps are stable. This usually takes 4–8 weeks, and the definitive fracture fixation device is usually an intramedullary nail or an external fixator that has the ability to modify the biomechanical environment of the fracture site. There is some haste to change from provisional to definitive fixation if an intramedullary nail is to be employed because—if an external fixator has been used initially—a long delay will allow the pins to loosen, threatening infection following subsequent intramedullary nailing. If a thin, unreamed intramedullary was employed primarily the cross-screws may break, making exchange nailing difficult. The use of a definitive external fixator does not carry these problems but is more difficult for the patient.

The treatment of bone loss

Bone loss following a compound fracture may be obvious or concealed. Obvious bone loss occurs when either bone substance has been lost at the time of the original fracture, or when subsequent debridement has removed devitalized and contaminated bone.

Concealed bone loss exists where an area of devitalized bone has been retained within a fracture to maintain the structural integrity of the bone. This area of bone will have lost many of its physiological functions, including its ability actively to take part in fracture healing, to resist infection, and to regenerate itself by remodelling. With time, it will revascularize and undergo creeping substitution, but in the context of a compound fracture it will be slow to unite and easily infected, and it may undergo subsequent fatigue fracture even if the original fracture has united satisfactorily.

An area of incomplete bone loss may re-form without further intervention provided that the fracture is stable.[39] Larger areas may have to be treated by autologous cancellous bone grafting. Vascularized bone grafts from the iliac crest or fibula may be employed for longer segments of bone loss, but the donor site morbidity is high. The use of distraction osteogenesis offers a very satisfactory alternative method of replacing lost bone with new apparently normal bone, and three methods have been described by Ilizarov.[69]

- Bone transport: the limb length is maintained and the bone defect is filled in by moving a piece of bone through the limb after division of the bone by a minimally invasive 'corticotomy' at a site distant from the zone of injury.
- Shortening and relengthening: the limb is shortened to eliminate the defect created by the bone loss, and then relengthened through a corticotomy as above.
- Bone transfer: in the case of the tibia, an area of bone loss may be eliminated by pulling the fibula across into the bed of the tibia, creating a fibula protibia.

Each of the above techniques has advantages and drawbacks. Patient rehabilitation is simpler when using bone transport, because the limb is kept at length; however, union may be delayed because the bones do not come into contact at the original fracture site until after the transport is complete. A plastic flap procedure may also be required to fill the soft tissue defect. Shortening and relengthening is a more difficult surgical procedure, and the patient may find rehabilitation difficult because of the discrepancy in limb length at the start of treatment. There is also a theoretical risk of damaging neurovascular structures during the shortening, although this has not been

REFERENCES

156. Godina M. Plast Reconstr Surg 1986; 78: 285–292
157. Arnold PG, Irons GB. Orthop Clin North Am 1984; 15: 441–449
158. Chang N, Mathes SJ. Plast Reconstr Surg 1982; 70: 1–10
159. Richards RR, Orsini EC, Mahoney JL et al. Plast Reconstr Surg 1987; 79: 946–956

observed.[160] The advantages of shortening and relengthening are that the fractured bone ends are brought together sooner than with bone transport, and therefore they usually unite more rapidly. The shortening also reduces the soft tissue defect and may even abolish it altogether. Thus there may be no need for a plastic surgical flap and, if it is required, it is smaller than would otherwise be the case.

Bone transfer procedures are rarely indicated but have a place where there is extensive loss of the tibia. A thin and deformed limb results, and function of the peroneal muscles is often compromised. This may be acceptable if there has been prior damage to the common peroneal nerve. When undertaking a bone transfer using an Ilizarov frame, the fibula can be gently moved into the bed of the tibia so that it retains its blood supply. Bone union between the tibia and transferred fibula, and subsequent fibula hypertrophy are then rapid.

Early amputation for severe fracture

Early or immediate amputation may be indicated as a life-saving measure, or if the limb is clearly not viable. A severe crushing injury with little remaining viable tissue or a warm ischaemic time exceeding 8 h are clear indications for amputation, but the concept that it is possible to predict which injuries are so severe that the patient's function will be improved by early amputation is more controversial. The social and economic impact of severe fractures of the lower limb is high,[161] and in selected patients early amputation affords rapid rehabilitation,[162] although the long-term cost to society may be greater than that of successful limb salvage.[163] Lange and coworkers suggest that the absolute indications for immediate amputation are a fracture that involves an arterial injury requiring repair for limb viability (type IIIc), combined with complete transection of the posterior tibial nerve and a non-viable limb.[164] They also propose relative indications based on the patient's ability to cope physiologically and psychologically with attempted limb salvage. Several other attempts have been made to predict the need for amputation, of which the best documented is the mangled extremity severity score (Table 52.2).[165]

Table 52.2 The mangled extremity severity score

Category	Point
A. Skeletal or soft tissue injury	
Low energy (stab, simple fracture)	1
Medium energy (open or multiple fracture)	2
High energy (close-range shotgun, high-velocity gunshot, crush)	3
Very high energy (gross contamination, avulsion)	4
B. Limb ischaemia	
Pulse reduced, normal perfusion	1*
Pulseless, paraesthesiae, reduced capillary refilling	2*
Cool, paralysed, insensate	3*
C. Shock	
Systolic blood pressure always > 90 mmHg	0
Transient hypotension	1
Persistent hypotension	2
D. Age (years)	
< 30	0
30–50	1
> 50	2

*Double score for ischaemia longer than 6 h.
Mangled extremity severity score = total points from A + B + C + D.

In a series of 26 patients studied retrospectively, a mangled extremity severity score of 7 or more was a good predictor of the need for subsequent amputation; however, more variable results are reported by others,[166,167] and a number of modifications have been suggested. Numerical scoring systems fail to take full account of the treatments available at the time of injury, and it seems likely that the introduction of Ilizarov's methods will allow salvage of limbs that were hitherto unreconstructable.

The decision to amputate remains highly subjective. A patient aged 49 who has not been hypotensive is scarcely different from one aged 51 who has had a transient episode of hypotension. A decision as to whether to amputate early must take into account injury severity, the degree of ischaemia, the fitness and age of the patient, and the extent to which the patient's injuries have affected the cardiovascular system.

COMPLICATIONS

Shock

Shock (see Ch. 7) is defined as a clinical state in which there is poor tissue perfusion and resultant tissue hypoxia. There are a number of reasons for which a fracture may cause a state of clinical shock. First, the fracture itself is associated with significant blood loss; second, the traumatized patient may have suffered other injuries; and third, the pain associated with the fracture and the circumstances of the injury may lead to an increase in circulating catecholamines, which contribute to peripheral circulatory failure. In outline the treatment of shock is correct restoration of fluid balance, appropriate analgesia, and improving oxygenation.

Fat embolism syndrome–adult respiratory distress syndrome (see Ch. 7)

Fat droplets in the lungs of a patient dying after a fracture were first described by Zenker.[168] The clinical condition is common following any instrumentation of the medullary canal, after a high-energy long bone lower limb fracture in a patient in their second or third decade, and following multiple trauma. The association with adult respiratory distress syndrome is complex. Put simply, the embolization of multiple fat droplets into the lungs will of itself compromise pulmonary exchange, and the ensuing local and systemic reactions to the droplets will further impair respiratory function; the consequent hypoxia may be fatal. Owing to the clinical nature of the diagnosis, it is difficult to be

REFERENCES

160. Allen PE, Bose D, Atkins RM. J Bone Joint Surg 1997; 79B (Suppl 1): 100
161. Bondurant F, Colter HB, Buckle R et al. J Trauma 1988; 28: 1270–1273
162. Geordiadis GM, Berhrens FF, Joyce MJ et al. J Bone Joint Surg 1993; 75A: 1431–1441
163. Tornetta P III, Olsen SA. Instr Course Lect 1997; 46: 511–518
164. Lange RH, Bach AW, Hansen ST et al. J Trauma 1985; 25: 203–208
165. Helfet DK, Howey T, Sanders R et al. Clin Orthop Relat Res 1990; 256: 80–86
166. Bonanni F, Rhodes M, Lucke JF. J Trauma 1993; 34: 99–104
167. Slauterbeck JR, Briton C, Noneim MS et al. J Orthop Trauma 1994; 8: 282–285
168. Zenker FA. Beitrage zur Anatomie und Physiologie der Lunge. Braunsdorf, Dresden, 1861

certain of the incidence, but it probably occurs following 1–2% of long bone fractures and up to 10% of unstable pelvic fractures.[169]

The clinical features are those of adult respiratory distress syndrome combined with features due to systemic embolization of fat droplets. On the second or third day after the precipitating insult, a fleeting petechial rash develops, characteristically across the chest, the axillae and the root of the neck. Conjunctival lesions are also present and retinal microinfarcts may occur. Respiratory involvement causes cyanosis and dyspnoea, while central hypoxaemia results in confusion and coma. Fat droplets may appear in the urine, while renal tubular involvement may cause oliguria.

Treatment is directed at restoring fluid balance and respiratory support. Suggested therapies have included heparinization, systemic corticosteroids, and intravenous alcohol administration; however, adequate controlled studies of these treatments are lacking. Early fracture stabilization reduces the incidence of fat embolism syndrome, probably by decompressing and draining the fracture haematoma, by minimizing subsequent fragment movement, and by the advantageous effects of fracture stabilization on subsequent ventilatory support.[170–173] However, early surgery is not without risk to the lungs,[128,174] although unreamed nailing may reduce this problem, and it may cause long-term bone infection.[171] The advantages of early stabilization therefore require careful weighing for each individual case.

Thromboembolism

In 1846, Virchow provided a conceptual framework for the understanding of venous thrombosis by suggesting that thrombogenesis could be considered as being due to changes in the vessel wall, in the composition of blood, and in blood flow, leading to venous stasis.[175] Because a fracture will probably cause vessel damage, leads to a hypercoagulable state, and the consequent immobility will promote venous stasis, it is hardly surprising that fractures are often complicated by venous thromboembolism. A number of problems arise in attempting to assess the impact of thrombolic disease within the context of fractures. First, in contrast to total joint replacement, fractures do not represent a homogeneous disease group, and it is inherently unlikely that the risk of thromboembolism will be similar between a Colles fracture and a pelvic fracture. Second, the symptoms and sequelae of thromboembolism are mimicked by other post-fracture conditions. Third, therapeutic regimens that are efficacious in other surgical contexts may be ineffective or associated with unacceptable side effects following fracture.

The incidence of venous thrombosis following fracture is approximately 20%,[176–178] while following fractured neck of femur in the elderly it ranges from 15 to 48%, depending on the method of assessment.[179–184]

Assessment for the presence of thrombosis by standard clinical examination supplemented by investigation and treatment is along standard lines, usually employing anticoagulant therapy depending on the clinical status of the patient.

Prevention of venous thrombosis is controversial and poorly researched. Early mobilization should reduce venous stasis, and graduated compression stockings are safe and may be effective; however, in the case of lower limb trauma, where the risk is highest, they may be impracticable. Intermittent calf or foot compression has been shown to be effective in lowering the risk of calf thrombosis in total joint replacement, and it has the additional advantages of rapid reduction in limb swelling and possible lowering of compartmental pressure.

The use of anticoagulant therapy is more controversial and potentially dangerous. Prophylactic anticoagulation with warfarin is effective in reducing the incidence of thrombolic disease following total joint replacement;[185] however, this approach is contraindicated in the fracture situation because of the risk of catastrophic haemorrhage, particularly where there has been concomitant intracranial trauma and the possibility of precipitating compartmental syndromes. It is unclear whether low-dose heparin regimens, including low-molecular-weight heparin, are without risk or are effective in lowering the risk of thromboembolism.[186]

Soft tissue infection

The propensity for relatively poorly vascularized tissues to become secondarily infected has been discussed. There are, however, two life-threatening infections that occur in the early period following trauma due to the presence of ischaemic tissue, particularly muscle. These are tetanus and gas gangrene.

Tetanus (lockjaw) was known to Hippocrates and is the result of infection of dead tissue with the toxin-forming obligatory anaerobic bacterium *Clostridium tetani*. *Clostridium tetani* spores are widespread in faeces and soil, and are resistant to moderate heating. The organism produces two toxins: tetanolysin, a haemolysin, and tetanospasmin, which is a powerful neurotoxin producing presynaptic blockade and severe spasm. It is the latter that accounts for the clinical manifestations of the disease.

The development of tetanus toxoid as a prophylaxis means that the disease is preventable, and the tetanus immunity of any trauma patient should be checked and a booster administered if appropriate. In an unimmunized patient, antitetanus immunoglobulin may be employed. Meticulous surgical debridement will remove all dead tissue in which tetanus bacteria may flourish. Treatment of established cases includes support for circulation and respiration, high-dose parenteral benzylpenicillin, and radical wound debridement.

Gas gangrene is due to infection with *C. perfringens* and other anaerobic gas-forming organisms. *Clostridium perfringens* is a

REFERENCES

169. Gossling HR, Pellegrini VD. Clin Orthop 1982; 165: 68–82
170. Riska E, Von Bonsdorff H, Hakkinen S et al. Injury 1976; 8: 110–116
171. Riska E, Von Bonsdorff H, Hakkinen S et al. J Trauma 1977; 17: 111–121
172. Riska E, Myllynen J. J Trauma 1982; 22: 891–894
173. Johnson K, Cadambi A, Seibert B. J Trauma 1985; 25: 375–384
174. Talucci R, Manning J, Lampard S et al. Am J Surg 1983; 146: 107–111
175. Virchow R. Beitr Exp Pathol Physiol 1846; 2: 1–12
176. Solonen KA. Acta Orthop Scand 1963; 33: 329–341
177. Neu LT Jr, Waterfield JR, Ash CJ. Ann Intern Med 1965; 62: 463–467
178. Sevitt S, Gallagher NG. Br J Surg 1961; 48: 475–489
179. Tubiana R, Duparc J. J Bone Joint Surg 1961; 43B: 7–15
180. Fagan DG. Lancet 1964; i: 846–848
181. Salzman EW, Harris WH, DeSanctis RW. N Engl J Med 1966; 275: 122–130
182. Freeark RJ, Bostwick J, Fardin R. Arch Surg 1967; 95: 567–575
183. Hamilton HW, Crawford JS, Gardiner JH et al. J Bone Joint Surg 1970; 52B: 268–289
184. Golodner H, Morse LJ, Angrist A. Surgery 1945; 18: 418–423
185. Evarts CM, Feil EI. Bone Joint Surg 1971; 53A: 1271–1280
186. Knudson MM, Lewis FR, Clinton A et al. J Trauma 1994; 37: 480–487

ubiquitous, saprophytic commensal in the alimentary tract. Like tetanus, the development of gas gangrene depends on the presence of devitalized tissue but, in contrast, *C. perfringens* releases toxins that allow it to spread through the tissues and there is no effective immunization. The mainstay of prophylaxis and treatment is adequate wound debridement, augmented by parenteral benzylpenicillin and hyperbaric oxygen therapy.

Bone infection

Bone infection after a fracture is an entirely different disease from acute haematogenous osteomyelitis.[187] The latter arises in the metaphyseal medulla and therefore principally involves the central part of the bone. The term *osteomyelitis* is therefore apposite. In contrast, bone infection after fracture or trauma without fracture is a bacterial invasion of relatively avascular cortical bone, which usually comes from the outside. Because the medullary canal is not primarily implicated and may not be involved at all, the term osteomyelitis is inappropriate and is best avoided. The natural history of this sort of bone infection depends on whether the bone is fractured and on the presence and type of any fracture fixation devices.

Post-traumatic bone infection without fracture

The most common example of this is an infected subperiosteal haematoma. The adjacent cortex is rendered relatively avascular by the periosteal stripping, and bacterial infection becomes established on the outer part of the cortex, gradually spreading as more bone is devitalized. The medullary canal is involved only at a late stage or in immunocompromised patients; local excision of devitalized bone and soft tissue with short-term antibiotic treatment is usually curative.

Bone infection without osteosynthesis

Injuries from bullets, shrapnel fragments or foreign bodies may import bacteria and cause multifocal infection in the region of trauma. A compound fracture that penetrates the skin damages the soft tissues, and there will be extensive devitalization of the bone fragments if it is a high-energy injury. Bacteria have direct access to the cortical bone fragments and to the medullary cavity in the region of the fracture. The dead soft tissues and haematoma provide an ideal incubation medium for the bacteria, and colonization of bone ensues. Individual pieces of dead bone may be expelled as sequestra, and if the fracture unites devitalized bone from the major fragments may become revascularized and remodelled. Occasionally this process will lead to resolution of the infection but, more often, chronic bone infection results. Usually the bone does not unite because of infection, the severity of the fracture, and loss of fracture haematoma, and infected non-union occurs.

Bone infection in the presence of osteosynthesis

The outcome of bone infection in the presence of a fixation device depends on fracture stability. Stability encourages revascularization of poorly vascularized bone fragments,[47] and it is possible for a fracture to unite even in the presence of infection, although union is likely to be slow. While the fracture is healing, the infection may be suppressed by appropriate antibiotics. Once union has occurred, revascularization of the bone will continue, and the infection may subside completely once the fixation device has been removed. While union is awaited, infected and dead soft tissue may be removed and replaced by plastic surgical flap coverage if necessary, which increases the local blood supply and helps to counter the infection. In contrast, if the fracture is unstable—either because the initial treatment did not produce a stable osteosynthesis or because the metalwork has become loose due to the infection—union of the fracture is unlikely to occur.

The problem with the traditional treatment of an infected osteosynthesis outlined above is that the treatment cannot be guaranteed to succeed. If it fails, salvage of the further surgery and the use of antibiotics have made the limb more difficult. Ilizarov described a novel method of treatment of bone infection following fracture. All metalwork is removed and all obviously devitalized bone and soft tissue is excised. The fracture is stabilized by an external fixator, which is capable of controlling two foci independently, and the fracture is compressed to produce union. Soft tissue defects are treated either by plastic surgery or, more commonly, they are allowed to heal by secondary intention. Bone defects are treated by bone transport and distraction osteogenesis, which is also employed to increase the limb blood supply and bone activation to encourage fracture union and eradication of infection (Figs 52.5 and 52.15).

Compartment syndrome

Compartment syndrome is a devastating early complication after fracture, which must be recognized and treated early. Richard von Volkman first described the condition.[188] The limbs are organized into compartments, which are bounded by bone and deep fascia, and contain muscles with their nerve and blood supply together with nerves and blood vessels to more distant parts of the limb. The proximal and distal ends of the compartment are open. Muscle within the fascial compartment is perfused by blood, which leaves the terminal resistance arterioles at a pressure of 30–38 mmHg and drains into venules at a pressure of 12–18 mmHg. The resting pressure within the compartment tissues is approximately 3–4 mmHg. A rise in compartmental tissue pressure may be triggered by a number of factors, including soft tissue injury. If a sustained rise in tissue pressure above the arterial perfusion pressure occurs, muscle and nerves will be deprived of blood supply[189] and ischaemic muscle releases factors that increase capillary permeability, worsening the situation.[190] Skeletal muscle is capable of regeneration if only part of the length of a muscle fibre is destroyed, so that prompt decompression is essential.[191,192] Thin cutaneous nerve fibres may be more susceptible to ischaemia than the motor fibres, which causes distal paraesthesiae before loss of motor function.

Diagnosis

The clinical presentation of compartment syndrome is frequently indistinct, and the clinician must consider the diagnosis in all patients. The main early feature is excessive pain, often unresponsive to opiates, which is made worse by stretching the ischaemic muscles. This is usually associated with tightness of the limb, although swelling may be slight or absent because the rigid

REFERENCES

187. Burri C. Post-traumatic Osteomyelitis. Hans Huber, Bern, 1974
188. Volkman R. Zentralbl Chir 1881; 8: 801–804
189. Ashton H. Clin Orthop 1975; 113: 15–26
190. Harman JW, Gwinn RP. Am J Pathol 1948; 24: 625–638
191. Harman JW, Gwinn RP. Am J Pathol 1949; 25: 741–755
192. Sanderson RA, Foley RK, McIvor G et al. Clin Orthop 1975; 113: 27–35

compartment prevents distension. The superficial veins of the limb beyond the affected compartment may be engorged, but the peripheral pulse remains intact until very late, because the increase in pressure required to produce a compartment syndrome (30 mmHg) is well below the arterial perfusion pressure. Sensory loss may be detected but motor weakness is a late sign.

The diagnosis is confirmed if necessary by comparing directly measured compartment pressure to the diastolic blood pressure.[193,194]

Management of suspected compartment syndrome

If the limb is encased in a plaster or bandage, this must be split to the skin and spread widely.[195] Compartment pressures should be measured if the diagnosis is in doubt. In the lower limb, intermittent pneumatic compression foot pumps may help to lower the compartmental pressure by compressing the plantar plexus of the foot and encouraging venous drainage.[196] If these measures do not cause rapid resolution of the raised pressure and symptoms, emergency decompression of the compartments by long vertical incisions through the skin and deep fascia is indicated.[197]

Complex regional pain syndrome

Formerly known as algodystrophy, reflex sympathetic dystrophy or Sudek's atrophy, this curious condition has been renamed complex regional pain syndrome and is common after fractures.[198] Prospective studies have demonstrated that it occurs following one-third of tibial or osteoporotic distal radial fractures, and it seems likely that the incidence is similar following other fractures, although data are lacking.[199,200] The condition is usually mild, subclinical and self-limiting, which explains its low reported incidence in a number of large retrospective series. However, even in those cases where the condition resolves without apparent clinical sequelae, careful investigation shows that the condition leads to permanent morbidity in a significant proportion of those affected.[201]

The condition consists of pain, vasomotor instability, swelling, and loss of joint mobility. It is accompanied by increased uptake on isotope bone scanning and radiological evidence of osteoporosis.[202] The pain is excessive and different from that of the precipitating trauma. It usually develops after a period in which there is little discomfort.[203] Abnormalities of pain perception, such as allodynia and hyperpathia, are common. Swelling and vasomotor instability are early features that fade as the disease progresses. In the early stages of the condition, loss of joint mobility is the result of a combination of pain provoked by movement and local oedema. As the condition progresses, however, the swelling gives way to atrophy of all the parts of the affected limb. The skin becomes thin and the subcutaneous fat disappears. Tendons and ligaments become adherent and severe joint contractures appear, causing continuing loss of joint mobility.

The cause of the condition is not known. It has long been assumed that the sympathetic nervous system is involved because of the vasomotor instability and excessive sweating. This notion has been supported by the apparent response of the condition to sympathetic manipulation. However, in a condition where the clinical features are variable and there is a tendency towards natural resolution, it is difficult to be certain that a treatment is efficacious, and the efficacy of sympathetic manipulation has been challenged.[204]

Bone involvement in the condition is universal, and abnormal blood flow and activation lead to increased uptake on bone scanning, while excessive osteoclastic activity becomes radiographically evident as the condition progresses, showing patchy osteoporosis, subperiosteal accentuation of osteoporosis, metaphyseal banding, subchondral osteoporosis, and eventually profound osteoporosis.

The majority of patients can be treated by reassurance, analgesia with non-steroidal anti-inflammatory drugs, and gentle physiotherapy to retain the range of joint motion until the active phase of the condition has passed. A specialist pain treatment unit should treat the minority who do not resolve with these measures. The mainstay of treatment has in the past been sympathetic manipulation; however, its role is under debate. Centrally acting analgesic drugs such as amitriptyline and carbamazepine are being increasingly employed.

FRACTURES IN CHILDREN

With respect to bone, children are not just small adults,[35] because of anatomical, physiological and biomechanical differences. The most obvious difference is the presence of a radiolucent growth plate, which is relatively weak and often involved in childhood fractures. The cortex of a child's bone is relatively wider than in an adult, occupying as much as half of the bone diameter. It is weaker and more osteoporotic than in an adult and contains wider Haversian canals. The bone mineral is less crystalline and more pliable than in an adult because of the higher rate of bone activation and turnover. Furthermore, the periosteum in a child is thicker, stronger and more active than in an adult. Thus children's bones are weaker than adult bones and break more easily; however, the bone is more plastic than in an adult and tends to bend.[205] Because children fall readily as they explore the world, fractures are common. They tend to occur with minimal violence, commonly resulting only in buckling of the bone, and they heal rapidly.

REFERENCES

193. Matsen FA III, Winquist RA, Krugmire RB Jr. J Bone Joint Surg Am 1980; 62A: 286–291
194. Heckman MM, Whitesides TE, Grewe SR et al. J Bone Joint Surg Am 1994; 76A: 1285–1292
195. Garfin S, Murabak S, Evans K et al. J Bone Joint Surg 1981; 63A: 449–453
196. Myerson M, Henderson MR. Foot Ankle 1993; 14: 198–203
197. Jepson PN. Ann Surg 1926; 84: 785–795
198. Atkins RM, Duckworth T, Kanis JA. J Bone Joint Surg 1990; 72B: 105–110
199. Sarangi PP, Ward AJ, Smith EJ et al. J Bone Joint Surg Br 1993; 75B: 450–452
200. Atkins RM. J Bone Joint Surg Br 2003; 85: 1100–1106
201. Warwick D, Field J, Prothero D et al. Clin Orthop 1993; 295: 270–274
202. Atkins RM. In: Ficat JJ (ed). Baillière's Clinical Orthopaedics: Reflex Sympathetic Dystrophy, Vol 1, No. 2. Baillière Tindall, London, 1996: 223–240
203. Mitchell SW, Morehouse GR, Keen WW. Gunshot Wounds and Other Injuries of Nerves. Lippincott, Philadelphia, 1864
204. Jaddad AR, Carroll D, Glynn CJ et al. J Pain Symptom Manage 1995; 10: 13–20
205. Salter RB, Harris HR. J Bone Joint Surg Am 1963; 45: 587–622

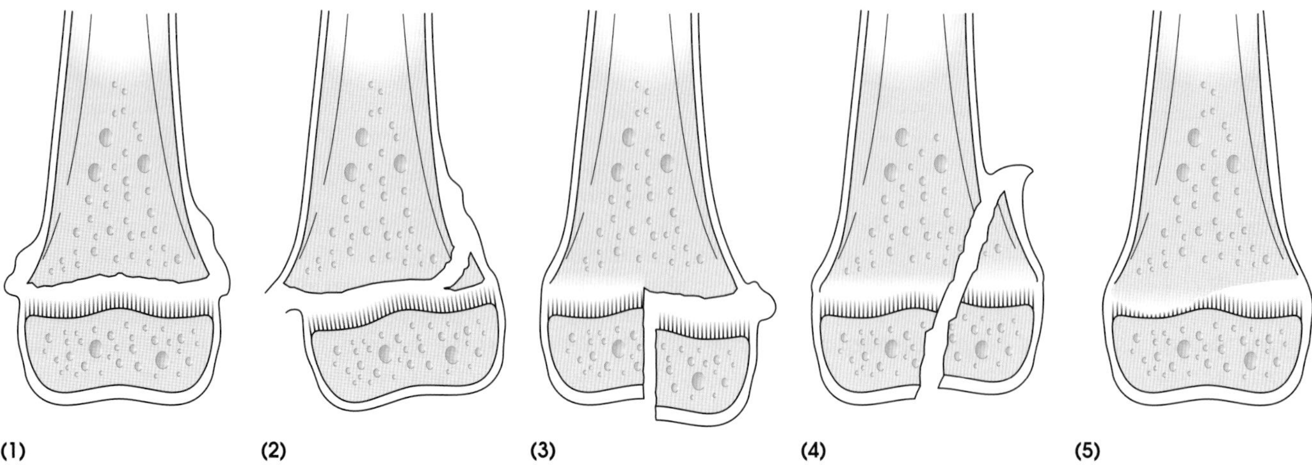

Figure 52.16 The Salter–Harris classification of injuries to the growth plate. Type 1: the fracture line follows the growth plate. Because the fracture occurs through the region of cell death and provisional calcification, the germinal layer is not involved and growth arrest does not occur. Type 2: the fracture involves a metaphyseal fragment. Because the region of the physeal fracture is on the metaphyseal side of the germinal layer of cells, growth disturbance is uncommon. Type 3: the fracture involves a physeal fragment. The fracture line must cross the germinal layer, which may be damaged, leading to growth disturbance. This risk is minimized by very accurate fracture reduction. Type 4: there is both a metaphyseal and a physeal fragment. As with a type 3 fracture, the growth plate may be damaged. Type 5: the growth plate is crushed, leading to growth disturbance. (From Rang 1984.[35])

CLASSIFICATION OF FRACTURES IN CHILDREN

Fractures of the bone itself

Traumatic bowing

Because a child's bone is plastic, it may be bent through a considerable angle before it breaks. After the deforming force is removed, the bone tends to straighten, but this is often incomplete.

Buckle fracture (torus fracture)

Bending of the bone may cause failure of one cortex only in compression. These fractures occur usually in the metaphysis in younger children. The name torus derives from the scroll on the top of a Grecian column, which the fracture resembles on X-ray.

Greenstick fracture

When the bone is angulated beyond its plastic limit it breaks, causing a fracture on its tension side. This incomplete fracture is termed a *greenstick fracture* (Fig. 52.3).

Complete fracture

As in adults, a complete fracture will occur if the deforming force is large enough. However, because of the weakness of a child's cortical bone, the ability to store energy in a high-velocity fracture is less than in an adult.

Growth plate injuries

Because of the weakness of the growth plate, these injuries are relatively common, accounting for approximately one-third of all fractures in children.[35] Clearly, an injury to the growing region of a bone carries with it the potential to cause a growth disturbance, leading to deformity or inequality of limb length. Furthermore, because the growth plate is close to the joint, articular damage may occur. The weakest part of the growth plate is the region of cell death, and therefore it is at this level that fractures through the plate usually occur. The fracture itself is therefore remote from the germinal layer, which is unaffected. The usual classification of growth plate injuries is that of Salter and Harris (Fig. 52.16).[205] The commonest growth plate injuries are the Salter–Harris types 1 and 2, which do not involve the germinal layer. Growth disturbance is therefore uncommon. In contrast, where the fracture involves the joint surface in a Salter–Harris type 3 or 4 injury, the germinal layer is breached and growth disturbance is likely, although its incidence is minimized by precise reduction of the fracture. Although not originally described, a Salter–Harris type 5 fracture is recognized, which is a crushing injury of the physis following which growth arrest is common. This fracture is often diagnosed retrospectively, when disturbance of physeal growth is apparent as a limb deformity

If the epiphysis is completely covered by cartilage (such as the head of the femur or radius), interruption of the blood supply may occur following fracture through the growth plate. Avascular necrosis of the growth plate and physis then occurs, with subsequent growth arrest. In the majority of epiphyses, however, there are soft tissue attachments, which continue to provide nutrition after physeal separation.[206]

Epiphyseal injuries

Fractures of the epiphysis usually involve the growth plate but may occasionally occur in isolation. These usually involve avulsion of a ligament attachment or displacement of an osteochondral fragment.

Injuries to the perichondral ring

The perichondral ring of Lacroix encircles the growth plate and is responsible for its widening as the bone enlarges. Injuries are rare but can cause two well-defined abnormalities. Avulsion causes a traumatic exostosis, while removal of the perichondral ring—which occurs most commonly when a severe soft tissue injury near a joint involves the underlying bone—may cause a bony bridge, with unilateral growth arrest and subsequent malalignment.

REFERENCES

206. Dale GC, Harris WR. J Bone Joint Surg Br 1958; 40B: 116–122

Changes in growth following fracture in children

Remodelling

Fracture remodelling as understood is different from the biological concept of remodelling at the cellular level. A series of events occur that allow the bone to change its shape after fracture healing. It can occur in adults but is most marked in children, and because it is intimately involved with limb growth, the younger the child, the greater the propensity for remodelling.

Remodelling includes a number of interlinked but separate phenomena, which once understood make it relatively easy to predict with some accuracy what fracture deformities may safely be accepted. It must, however, be remembered that remodelling takes time, and uninformed parents may become impatient with the continuing deformity of their child's limb.

The first feature of remodelling is Wolff's law. Bone is laid down in areas of excess strain and removed from areas that are understrained. The concave side of the angulated fracture is subjected to high mechanical forces and bone is laid down at this site, while the convex side is relatively unstrained and is therefore resorbed. These twin processes round off the bent bone. The second feature is that the physis of a bent bone grows eccentrically to restore the attitude of the adjacent joint to normal.[207] The third feature is the growth in length and width of the bone that hides the deformity (Fig. 52.17).

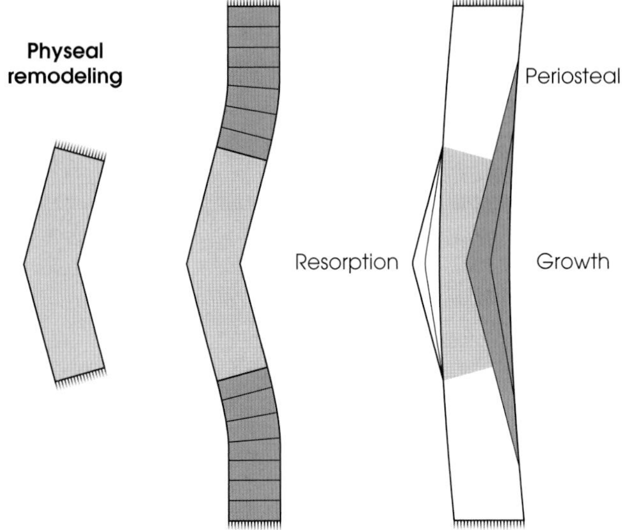

Figure 52.17 The mechanisms by which a fracture in a child will remodel. (a) A fracture that has united with an angular deformity. (b) Physeal growth is eccentric, tending to correct the deformity. (c) Resorption occurs on the convex side of the deformity, while periosteal appositional growth takes place on the concave side. The combination of uneven physeal growth (physeal remodelling) and periosteal remodelling straighten out the bent bone. (From Rang 1984.[35])

Overgrowth

A fracture of a long bone in a growing child stimulates a variable amount of longitudinal overgrowth, probably from a combination of damage to the periosteum releasing a constraint to growth and increased blood supply to the growth plates consequent on the fracture. This is most commonly seen following fracture of the femur between the ages of 2 and 10 years. The average overgrowth is 0.9 cm, with a range of 0.4–2.5 cm.[208] The overgrowth is most marked for the 2 years following the fracture and tails off rapidly after this time.

Progressive deformity

If the growth plate is permanently damaged by the fracture, failure of growth causes either progressive shortening of the limb or an increasing angular deformity. Complete ablation of the growth plate produces simple progressive shortening of the limb; however, more commonly there is damage to only part of the growth plate, leading to a bony bar across the physis, which causes tethering of one part of the growth plate. The normal growth of other parts of the plate then causes an angular growth abnormality, the nature and extent of which are dependent on the exact size and situation of the bar and on the residual growth left in the affected physis.

REFERENCES

207. Karaharju EO, Ryoppy SA, Makinnen RJ. J Bone Joint Surg Br 1976; 58B: 122–126
208. Shapiro F. Acta Orthop Scand 1981; 52: 1265–1267

Fractures of the upper limb, including wrist

53

James E. Nicholl, Michael A. Smith

INTRODUCTION

Fractures of the upper limb are very common and occur in all age groups. The distribution of specific fractures varies with age, as does the force required to produce a particular fracture.

For the hand to perform its various intricate tasks the rest of the upper limb must be functionally intact. Following an injury to any part of the upper limb the aim of management is to restore its function to as near normal as possible, as quickly as possible. To this end a less than perfect anatomical result may be accepted.

A history of the mechanism of injury can provide important clues to the likely pattern of injury. The patient must be examined for any associated injuries to other parts of the body, and if present these are managed in their order of priority to resuscitate the patient and limit subsequent disability (see Ch. 7). High-energy trauma resulting in fractures of the shoulder girdle will often cause injuries to the head, neck and chest. Multiply injured patients and patients with life-threatening injuries must have their upper limbs fully assessed as part of the secondary survey.

Upper limb fractures in children and adults are treated very differently. Children present with a different spectrum of injuries, different classifications are used and, because of their potential to remodel, displaced fractures can be accepted that would not be appropriate in an adult. Open reduction and internal fixation are therefore rarely required. However, the capacity to remodel can sometimes result in an increasing deformity, so imperfect reductions should be monitored.

INJURIES OF THE STERNOCLAVICULAR JOINT

Dislocations of the sternoclavicular joint are fairly rare, accounting for 3% of shoulder girdle injuries.

Injuries are classified according to their severity and the direction of the subluxation or dislocation. First-degree injuries are minor sprains with a partial tear of the ligaments; second-degree are subluxations with complete rupture of the sterno-clavicular and partial rupture of the costoclavicular ligaments. Third-degree injuries are full dislocations with complete rupture of both ligaments, and anterior or posterior displacement of the medial end of the clavicle, with the former being more common. The mechanism of injury can be a direct blow to the medial end of the clavicle causing posterior dislocation, or more usually the mechanism is indirect, with a medially directed force applied to the lateral aspect of the shoulder, while simultaneously the shoulder is pushed forwards or backwards, producing an anterior or posterior dislocation, respectively. Road traffic accidents and sports injuries are the common causes.

First- and second-degree injuries present with swelling and pain that is worse when the arm is abducted. With an anterior dislocation the medial end of the clavicle is prominent, whereas in a posterior dislocation the normal anterior fullness of the medial end of the clavicle is lost. There may be evidence of injury to the underlying structures in the superior mediastinum, with venous congestion, arterial obstruction, dyspnoea from tracheal injury, signs of oesophageal trauma, or a pneumothorax.

Radiographs can be difficult to interpret and a CT scan is the imaging of choice.

First- and second-degree injuries are treated symptomatically with a sling and analgesics. Anterior dislocations can be reduced by closed manipulation, with traction along the line of the clavicle and backward pressure on the medial end of the bone, but once reduced the joint usually remains unstable despite immobilization. Open reduction and repair of the ligaments has a high complication rate, and if the joint redislocates it is best to leave it and accept the deformity. Most of the initial swelling is from the soft tissues and it usually settles with time, leaving a relatively minor deformity and few symptoms.

Before treating a posterior dislocation, injury to any of the intrathoracic structures must be excluded. Closed reduction with the patient lying supine with a sandbag between the shoulder blades, lateral traction to the abducted arm and gradual extension is usually successful, reduction occurring with an audible 'pop'. Occasionally the clavicle needs to be grasped with a towel clip and pulled forwards. The reduction is usually stable and can be held with a figure-of-eight bandage. The main complications are from associated injuries to the trachea, oesophagus, great vessels and lungs, which occur in 25% of posterior dislocations, and deaths have been reported.

FRACTURES OF THE CLAVICLE

Clavicular fractures are common, accounting for 5% of fractures for all age groups, and it is the most common fracture seen in children. They have been classified into fractures of the middle (80%), lateral to the coracoclavicular ligaments (15%), and medial end (5%).

Fractures lateral to the coracoclavicular ligaments have been further classified by Neer into three types.[1] Type I are undisplaced, with intact acromioclavicular and coracoclavicular ligaments. In type II, the coracoclavicular ligaments are ruptured and the medial fragment is displaced superiorly by the pull of the

REFERENCE

1. Neer CS II. Clin Orthop 1968; 58: 43

sternocleidomastoid. Type III fractures are intra-articular into the acromioclavicular joint, and there is no ligamentous injury.

Most clavicular fractures are caused by a fall. Presentation is with swelling and tenderness at the fracture site. With displaced fractures the overlying skin can be tented by a spike of bone, which can occasionally pierce the skin. With loss of the support from the clavicle the shoulder may displace anteriorly and inferiorly. In fractures of the lateral third, the arm is held adducted and abduction is painful. Signs of associated injuries to the brachial plexus, the vessels and the underlying lung may be present and must always be excluded.

A plain anteroposterior radiograph is usually sufficient to confirm the diagnosis, but additional views include an anteroposterior film with the X-ray tube directed 45° cephalad and a lateral scapular view.

The treatment of most fractures consists of analgesics and a broad arm sling or appropriate shoulder splint that supports the weight of the arm. It is worn for 3–5 weeks in children and 6 weeks in adults. Fractures of the lateral end of the clavicle are more problematic and more likely to require open surgery. Type II fractures of the lateral clavicle have a 40–87% incidence of non-union if treated conservatively.[2] Operative treatment is therefore recommended.[3] A tension band wire, plate or Bosworth screw can be used. Type III fractures are treated with a sling and early mobilization. There is a subsequent risk of developing osteoarthritis of the acromioclavicular joint.

Indications for internal fixation of fractures of the middle third are a progressive neurovascular deficit, open fractures and the 'floating shoulder' (Fig. 53.1), in which there is also a fracture of the scapula separating the glenoid from the rest of the bone. When the skin is threatened by an underlying spike of bone in a displaced fracture, this may be an indication for open reduction and internal fixation.

Non-union occurs in 1–2% of fractures and is more likely if there is significant comminution or it is a refracture. The treatment for symptomatic non-union is internal fixation with a plate and bone graft, and has an 80% success rate. Malunion with angulation can cause a cosmetic deformity but does not usually affect function.

ACROMIOCLAVICULAR JOINT INJURIES

Dislocations and subluxations of the acromioclavicular joint account for 12% of dislocations around the shoulder. They often occur in sportsmen and sportswomen, with the mechanism of injury usually being a fall on to the tip of the shoulder causing downward displacement of the acromion relative to the clavicle. They also occasionally result from a fall on the outstretched hand.

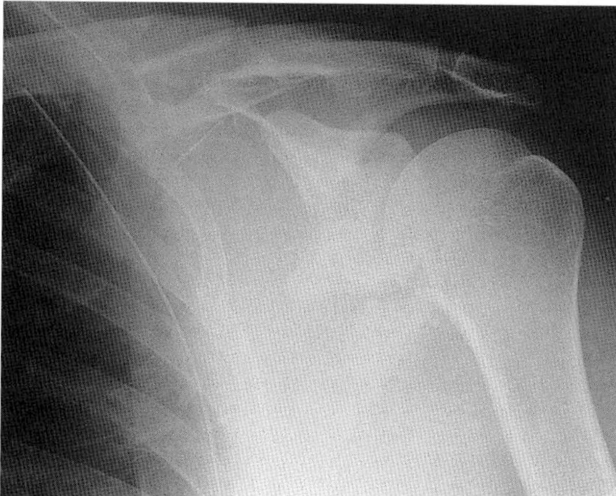

Figure 53.1 Floating shoulder. There is a comminuted fracture of the clavicle and a displaced fracture of the neck of the scapula.

The acromioclavicular joint is a diarthrodial joint with a fibrocartilaginous intra-articular disc. The stability of the joint is provided by two sets of ligaments, namely the acromioclavicular, which reinforce the joint capsule, and the coracoclavicular ligaments. The latter comprises the conoid and trapezoid ligaments, which insert into the undersurface of the clavicle well medial to the joint.

Acromioclavicular joint injuries have been classified by Rockwood into six grades (Fig. 53.2).[5] In type I there is a sprain of the acromioclavicular ligaments, the coracoclavicular ligaments are intact, and the radiographic appearance is normal. With a type II injury the acromioclavicular ligaments are torn, there is a sprain of the coracoclavicular ligaments, and there is a relative upward displacement of the clavicle with subluxation of the acromioclavicular joint by less than half its width. In a type III injury (Fig. 53.3), both the acromioclavicular and coracoclavicular ligaments are torn, allowing complete dislocation of the acromioclavicular joint. Type IV, V and VI injuries are rare. The lateral end of the clavicle is displaced posteriorly and superiorly into or through the trapezius in grade IV, in grade V, the clavicle is displaced so superiorly that there is separation of trapezius and deltoid from the clavicle, and inferior to the acromion and coracoid in grade VI.

The clinical presentation depends on the grade of the injury. There is a swelling and tenderness over the injured ligaments, and the arm is held adducted. The shoulder displaces inferiorly, so that the lateral end of the clavicle appears to be displaced upwards. Pressure over the prominence will depress it, but it springs back to its original position when the pressure is released.

Radiologically the acromioclavicular joint is best demonstrated by an anteroposterior radiograph with the beam tilted 15° cephalad, with the exposure a third of that used for a standard radiograph of the glenohumeral joint. Stress radiographs can be useful to distinguish grade I from grade II and grade II from grade III injuries. Five to ten pounds is attached to both wrists, and anteroposterior radiographs are taken of both shoulders. Any relative displacement of the lateral end of the clavicle is accentuated, and subtle differences from the normal shoulder can be demonstrated. Axillary or lateral scapula views show anterior or posterior displacement.

Conservative treatment usually results in little if any functional impairment, although often leaves a visible deformity. Grade I and II injuries can be treated with a simple sling, with avoidance of heavy lifting for 8–10 weeks. The treatment of grade III injuries is more controversial, with some authors reporting no proven benefit of acute surgical repair, with a good long-term functional outcome after conservative treatment.[6] Others advocate acute

REFERENCES

2. Philips H. J Bone Joint Surg 1985; 67B: 492
3. Sonnabend DH. In: Watson MS (ed). Surgical Disorders of the Shoulder. Churchill Livingstone, Edinburgh, 1991
4. Rockwood CA, Williams GR, Young DC. In: Rockwood CA, Green DP (eds). Rockwood and Green's Fractures in Adults, Vol 2. 4th edn. Lippincott Williams & Wilkins, Philadelphia, 1996
5. Rockwood CA. In: Rockwood CA, Green DP (eds). Fractures in Adults. Lippincott, Philadelphia, 1984
6. Rawes ML, Dias JJ. J Bone Joint Surg 1996; 78B: 410

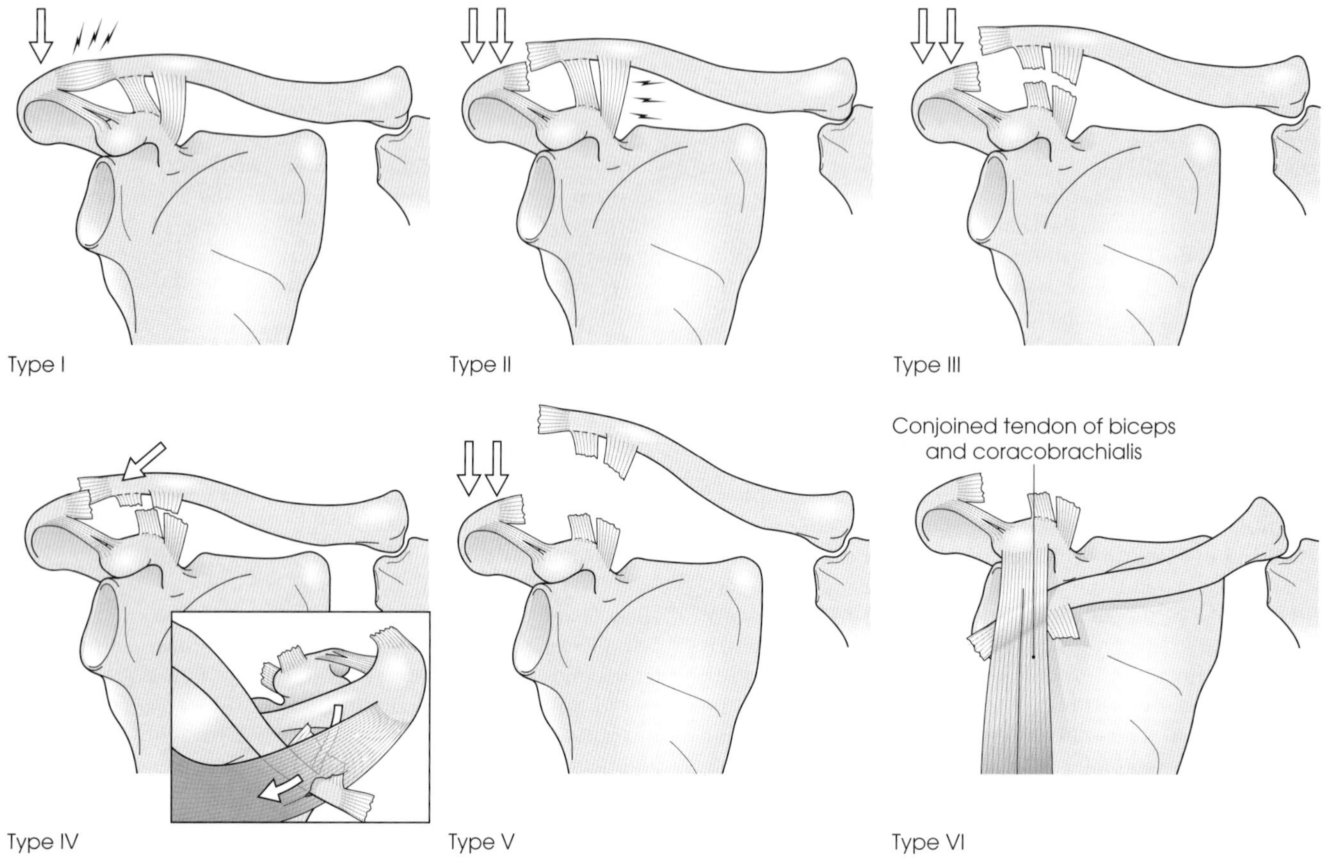

Type I

Type II

Type III

Conjoined tendon of biceps and coracobrachialis

Type IV

Type V

Type VI

Figure 53.2 Rockwood's classification of injuries to the acromioclavicular joint. (After Rockwood et al 1996,[4] with permission of Lippincott Williams & Wilkins.)

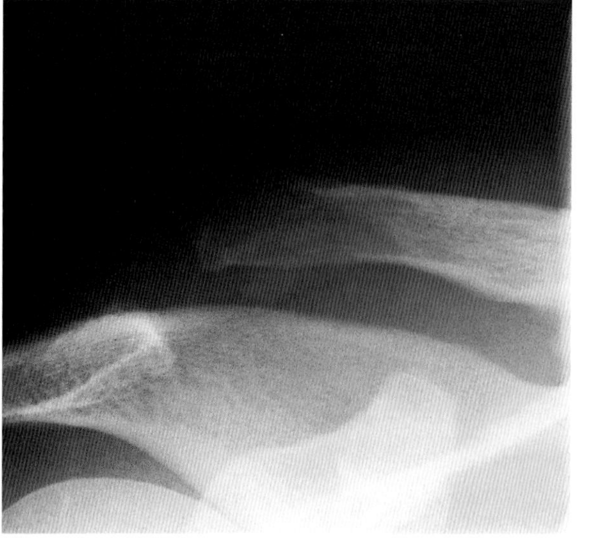

a

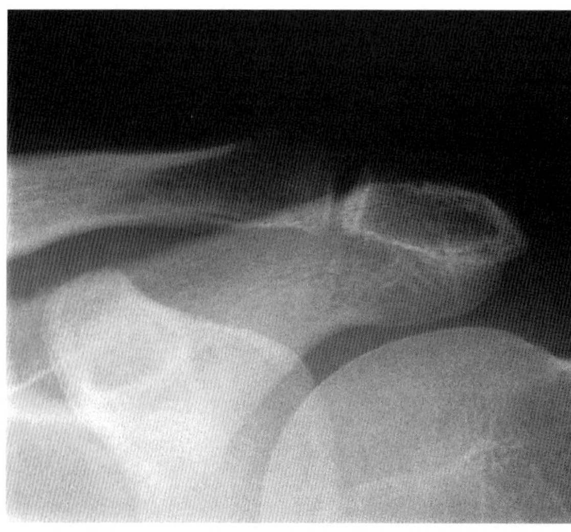

b

Figure 53.3 (**a**) Anteroposterior radiograph of the normal acromioclavicular joint, (**b**) with a grade III dislocation on the right.

repair for heavy manual workers[5] who may otherwise experience shoulder pain and difficulty performing their job. Closed reduction can be attempted for grade IV and VI injuries, but open reduction is often necessary, and grade V injuries usually leave an unacceptable deformity unless treated surgically.

FRACTURES OF THE SCAPULA

Scapular fractures are uncommon. Because the bone is protected by its investing layer of muscles, considerable force is required to fracture it. There is a high incidence of associated injuries to the chest, and there are often both scapular and rib fractures, with

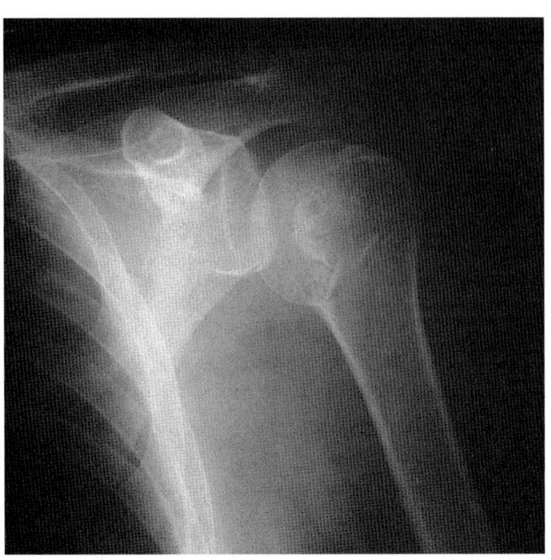
a

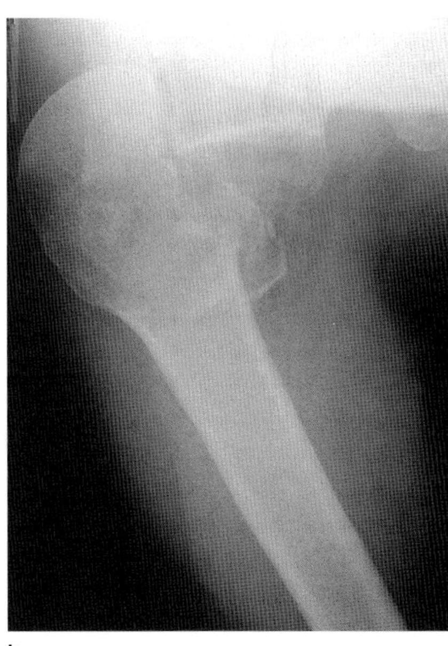
b

Figure 53.4 (**a**) Anteroposterior radiograph of the shoulder taken after an epileptic fit in a 60-year-old man; an initial diagnosis of a fracture of the humeral neck was made. (**b**) An axillary view taken 5 days later shows a posterior dislocation and an anterior Hill–Sachs impression fracture.

one being obvious and the other therefore easily missed on the radiograph. Fractures are classified anatomically into those of the body and spine, neck, glenoid, acromion and coracoid process.

Fractures of the body and spine present with tenderness and bruising, and the arm is held adducted. There can be considerable blood loss from the adjacent blood vessels, and bleeding into the bellies of the rotator cuff muscles will interfere with their function and restrict active shoulder movement. Treatment is usually conservative with a sling, followed by early exercises once the pain has subsided.

Fractures of the neck of the scapula may be associated with fractures of the humerus or clavicle. They are usually caused by a direct blow. The glenoid is effectively lying free and may be displaced inferiorly by the weight of the arm if the fracture line is lateral to the coracoid, or the acromioclavicular and coracoclavicular ligaments are torn. Open reduction and internal fixation should be performed if there is an associated fracture of the clavicle (Fig. 53.1) or the displacement is likely to restrict shoulder movement.

Glenoid fractures range from small rim fractures that most commonly occur with shoulder dislocations, to fractures crossing the glenoid producing large articular fragments. Stellate fractures with comminution and depression of the articular surface are also seen. Rim fractures require surgery only if they are associated with shoulder instability. Open reduction with internal fixation is required to restore joint congruity and stability where the articular surface is depressed or there are large displaced fragments.

Fractures of the acromion are caused by a direct blow to the top of the shoulder, and only require reduction and internal fixation if there is displacement likely to compromise the subacromial space.

Coracoid fractures can be caused by a direct blow, or there can be avulsion of a fragment by the attached muscles. Treatment should be symptomatic.

TRAUMATIC DISLOCATION OF THE SHOULDER

Of the major joints, the shoulder has the greatest mobility and dislocates most frequently. It occurs in all age groups with peaks between the ages of 10 and 20, and 50 and 60.[7] The humeral head can dislocate anteriorly, posteriorly or inferiorly. Anterior dislocations are by far the most common, with posterior and inferior dislocations unusual.

The normal stability of the shoulder is provided by the articular anatomy: the labrum deepens the glenoid, the rotator cuff muscles act as active stabilizers, and the glenohumeral ligaments reinforce the anterior capsule. When the humeral head dislocates anteriorly, the anterior capsule and glenohumeral ligaments are torn, and the labrum can be avulsed from the glenoid to produce the Bankart lesion.

The mechanism of injury for anterior dislocation is a fall on to the outstretched hand with the arm abducted and externally rotated, or rarely a direct blow to the back of the shoulder. The mechanism for posterior dislocation is violent internal rotation of the shoulder, which can occur with a fall on to the flexed, internally rotated arm, or during an epileptic fit, an electric shock, or electroconvulsive therapy in which the strong internal rotators overpower the external rotators. In these situations the diagnosis is easily missed. A direct blow to the front of the shoulder can also cause a posterior dislocation. Inferior dislocation usually occurs with a fall on the outstretched hand with the arm abducted to 180°.

Anterior dislocations present with pain. There is loss of the normal contour of the shoulder, the arm is held in slight abduction and external rotation, the acromion is prominent, the humeral head may be palpable anteriorly, and all movements are limited and painful. Injuries to the axillary nerve and vessels, and to the brachial plexus are common and must be identified prior to reduction. With a posterior dislocation the arm is held in adduction and internal rotation, abduction is limited, and external rotation is impossible. The appearance of the shoulder is almost normal, and the posterior displacement of the humeral head may only be apparent looking from above. With an inferior dislocation the patient is in severe pain, the arm is held elevated

REFERENCE

7. Rowe CR. J Bone Joint Surg 1956; 38A: 957

above the head, and the humeral head may be palpable in the lateral chest wall. The rotator cuff is invariably torn, and there is a high incidence of associated neurovascular injury.

To confirm the diagnosis an anteroposterior and lateral scapular or axillary radiograph is required. Anterior dislocations are usually obvious, but it is important to identify any associated impression fracture of the posterior surface of the humeral head (the Hill–Sachs lesion) or a fracture of the glenoid rim.

The diagnosis of posterior dislocation is often missed (Fig. 53.4). The signs seen on the anteroposterior radiograph are loss of the normal ellipse produced by the overlap of the posterior glenoid rim and the humeral head, and internal rotation makes the greater tuberosity more prominent, giving the 'light bulb' sign. Posterior dislocation should also be suspected if an isolated fracture of the lesser tuberosity is seen. Good-quality lateral scapular or axillary views are essential to avoid missing the diagnosis. Associated bony injuries are fractures of the posterior glenoid rim, and the reverse Hill–Sachs lesion, which is an impression fracture of the anterior surface of the humeral head.

Acute traumatic shoulder dislocations should be reduced by manipulation under adequate analgesia and relaxation. Fracture dislocations may require open reduction, and reductions should therefore be performed in an operating theatre. The sooner the dislocation is reduced, the easier it is, because muscle spasm becomes more intense with time. Whichever method is employed, it must be done slowly and gently to avoid causing or aggravating pre-existing soft tissue or neural injuries. Numerous techniques are described. There are variations of the Hippocratic method, in which traction is applied to the arm, which is abducted to 45°; counter-traction is from a towel around the upper chest being pulled medially, and gentle internal and external rotation may be necessary to disengage the head. Direct pressure on the humeral head, pushing it back into the socket, or a second assistant with a towel around the upper arm pulling laterally may also be required.

Posterior dislocations are reduced by longitudinal traction and direct pressure over the humeral head. For an inferior dislocation the patient is supine. Longitudinal traction is applied to the arm in a superior direction, with counter-traction from a towel over the top of the shoulder pulling inferiorly. While maintaining the traction, the arm is rotated internally.

The patient should be given a general anaesthetic if attempted reduction with analgesia and relaxation fails, and an open reduction is required if closed reduction remains unsuccessful, because there is likely to be soft tissue interposition blocking the reduction.

After reduction of an anterior dislocation the arm is immobilized in internal rotation for 3 weeks, with abduction and external rotation avoided for a further 3 weeks. Following a posterior dislocation, immobilization in internal rotation may increase the risk of recurrent dislocation. Cautilli and colleagues have recommended immobilization in a neutral position with plaster casts around the waist and wrist connected with a wooden bar.[8] If the shoulder is unstable in internal rotation, it should be immobilized in a shoulder spica in external rotation for 6 weeks.

The complications of shoulder dislocation depend on the age of the patient, with younger patients having a high risk of recurrent dislocation. In older patients rotator cuff tears, fractures of the greater tuberosity, and nerve injuries are more common. The incidence of recurrent dislocation in the under-twenties is at least 80%.[7] This risk can be reduced by ensuring that the shoulder is kept internally rotated for a sufficient period, and by carrying out intensive strengthening exercises for the rotator cuff muscles.

Fractures of the greater tuberosity are seen in up to a quarter of all anterior dislocations. When the dislocation is reduced, the tuberosity fragment usually returns to its anatomical position. If it does not, and there is a residual displacement of more than 1 cm, it should be reduced and internally fixed, because untreated it can cause impingement and a poor functional result.

An axillary nerve palsy occurs in between 9 and 18% of dislocations, and if permanent it is very debilitating. Fortunately spontaneous recovery usually occurs.

FRACTURES OF THE PROXIMAL HUMERUS

Proximal humeral fractures are the most common fracture of the shoulder region and account for 5% of all fractures. They occur in all age groups, but in children they are a very different entity with a different classification and management. The majority are seen in elderly patients with osteoporosis, and the mechanism of injury is a fall on to the outstretched hand or a direct blow to the lateral aspect of the arm, again usually from a fall.

The classification most often used is that of Neer (Fig. 53.5).[10] It provides a useful guide for treatment and prognosis, but has considerable inter- and intraobserver error.[11] It is based on the anatomical site of fractures displaced more than 1 cm or angulated more than 45°, and the number of main fragments.

Patients with fractures of the proximal humerus present with pain and swelling around the shoulder; movement is restricted and painful with crepitus from the fracture. There can be an associated neurovascular injury, with axillary nerve palsy being most common. Good-quality anteroposterior, lateral scapular, and axial lateral radiographs are required to classify the fracture and plan treatment.

In children management is almost always conservative. Considerable degrees of displacement and angulation can be accepted because young children have a large capacity for remodelling at this site.

In adults, management depends on the type of fracture and the functional requirements of the patient. Undisplaced fractures are treated with a collar and cuff sling, and by early movement. Inferior subluxation of the humeral head relative to the glenoid is a frequent finding even with undisplaced fractures. This results from the haemarthrosis and reflex inhibition of the deltoid and rotator cuff muscles, and must be distinguished from a true dislocation because no treatment is required, with spontaneous resolution usually occurring within 8 weeks.

Displaced two-part fractures of the surgical neck can usually be treated with a collar and cuff sling. The wrist is held as high as possible, the elbow hangs down unsupported, and the weight of the arm provides sufficient traction to reduce and hold the fracture in satisfactory alignment. A closed manipulation under

REFERENCES

8. Cautilli RA, Joyce MF, Mackell JV Jr. Am J Sports Med 1978; 6: 397
9. Neer CS II, Rockwood CA. In: Rockwood CA, Green DP (eds). Fractures in Adults, Vol 1. 2nd edn. Lippincott Williams & Wilkins, Philadelphia, 1996.
10. Neer CS. J Bone Joint Surg 1970; 52A: 1077
11. Sidor ML, Zuckerman JD, Lyon T et al. J Bone Joint Surg 1993; 75A: 1745

	Anatomical neck	Surgical neck	Greater tuberosity	Lesser tuberosity	Fracture dislocation		Head splitting
					Anterior	Posterior	
2-part		a b c					
3-part							
4-part							
Articular surface							

Figure 53.5 Neer's classification of displaced fractures of the proximal humerus. (After Neer et al 1996,[9] with permission of Lippincott Williams & Wilkins.)

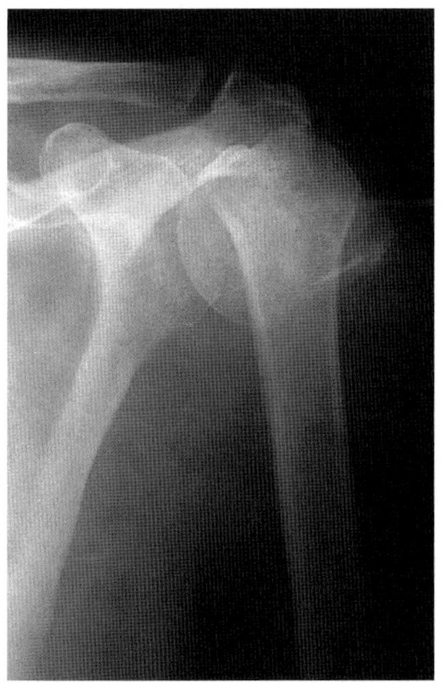

a

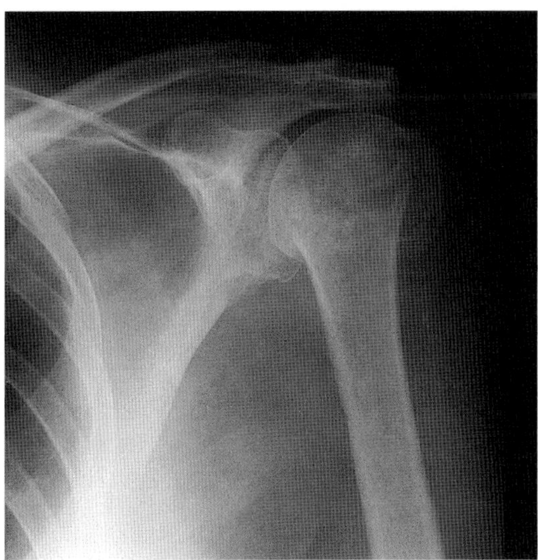

b

Figure 53.6 (**a**) Three-part fracture of the proximal humerus. (**b**) Postoperative radiograph after open reduction and internal fixation with interosseous polydioxanone sulphate sutures.

anaesthetic may be required to reduce the fracture, which can then be held with a sling and body bandage or, if these fail to hold the reduction, percutaneous internal fixation can be used. Open reduction is only occasionally necessary to achieve a satisfactory position.

Two-part fractures of the greater tuberosity can occur in isolation or with an associated anterior shoulder dislocation. If the fragment is undisplaced, the arm is rested in a sling, and active elevation is avoided to prevent the greater tuberosity being displaced by traction from the attached rotator cuff. The shoulder is X-rayed after 1 and 2 weeks to ensure that the greater tuberosity has not displaced. If the greater tuberosity is displaced superiorly, it is likely to impinge when the arm is elevated, so should be reduced and held with screws or a tension band wire.

Displaced three- and four-part fractures tend to do badly with non-operative treatment. With three-part fractures the unopposed muscle pull on the intact tuberosity rotates the surgical neck fracture, and with a four-part fracture there is disruption of the blood supply to the humeral head and a high risk of avascular necrosis developing. In younger patients, even if the blood supply to the head has been completely disrupted, revascularization of the avascular bone can occur without it collapsing if the proximal humerus is reconstructed. The aims of surgical treatment are to achieve a stable fixation of the fracture, to reattach the tuberosities, and to repair the rotator cuff. It should not compromise the blood supply to the humeral head and allow early mobilization of the shoulder. Several methods of fixation have been advocated, including tension band wires, heavy polydioxanone sulphate sutures (Fig. 53.6),[12] plates, and percutaneous reduction and fixation with K-wires and cannulated screws. The results of internal fixation vary enormously, with success more likely in young patients with good bone stock. In elderly patients it is much more difficult to achieve secure fixation, and the functional results of semirigid internal fixation with a tension band wire are no better than with conservative treatment.[13] Neer recommends treating patients over 70 with displaced three- and four-part fractures by a hemiarthroplasty and reattachment of the tuberosities, with 96% of patients getting an excellent or satisfactory result.[14]

FRACTURES OF THE HUMERAL SHAFT

Humeral shaft fractures occur in all age groups. The mechanism of injury can be direct, such as from a fall landing on the side of the arm or a motor vehicle accident, or indirect from a fall landing on the elbow or outstretched hand or a twisting injury to the arm. Direct injuries tend to cause transverse fractures and indirect oblique or spiral ones. The displacement depends on the force that produced the fracture and its site relative to the various muscle insertions on the bone.

A full neurovascular examination must be performed, because there is a high incidence of associated radial nerve injury. Radiographic examination should be by anteroposterior and lateral views that include the shoulder and elbow joints to exclude any accompanying injuries.

Most closed fractures of the humeral shaft can be treated non-operatively with good results, with no cosmetic or functional impairment, as long as there is no significant rotational deformity.

The indications for surgery are open fractures, if the fracture extends into the elbow joint, if there is an associated forearm fracture giving a floating elbow, or if there is an associated vascular injury. If the patient has multiple injuries, stabilization of the humeral fracture is often indicated. Occasionally it is not possible to achieve a satisfactory reduction by closed manipulation, particularly if there is soft tissue interposition, and an open reduction is required.

The commonest complication of a humeral shaft fracture is a radial nerve palsy, occurring in up to 18% of cases. It is at greatest risk in fractures of the middle third, where it is closely applied to the bone in the spiral groove. The nerve should be explored immediately in open injuries, or if the palsy develops after closed manipulation of the fracture. Otherwise the nerve almost always remains in continuity, and over 90% recover spontaneously over 3 or 4 months. During this time, the wrist and fingers are supported with a splint to prevent flexion contractures. If there is no recovery by the time the fracture has united the nerve can be explored and, if divided, repaired.

FRACTURES OF THE DISTAL HUMERUS

Fractures of the distal end of the humerus are seen mostly in children and adults over the age of 50 years. The mechanism of injury can be indirect with a fall on to the outstretched hand, or from a direct blow to the elbow, with the direction of the force and position of the elbow at the time of injury determining the nature of the fracture and direction of displacement. The diagnosis of fractures of the distal humerus depends on having good-quality anteroposterior and lateral radiographs and, particularly for children, comparison with a radiograph of the normal elbow can be helpful.

SUPRACONDYLAR FRACTURES IN CHILDREN

In children, 60% of elbow fractures are supracondylar, with at least 90% of these being extension injuries resulting from a fall on to the outstretched hand. There is hyperextension of the elbow, with the olecranon impacting against the posterior aspect of the humerus to produce the fracture.

Paediatric supracondylar fractures have been classified into undisplaced, displaced with an intact posterior periosteum, and completely displaced with no contact between the fragments.[15] Presentation is with a painful, swollen elbow. With displaced fractures the shaft can cause an anterior prominence tenting the overlying skin, and the olecranon is displaced posteriorly and superiorly, giving an S-shaped deformity. Clinically, a supracondylar fracture can be distinguished from a posterior elbow dislocation because the relationship between the olecranon and the medial and lateral epicondyles is preserved.

Associated neurovascular injuries do occur. Nerve injuries occur in about 7%, with the radial, median and ulnar nerves all being at risk, and vascular injury or compromise occurs in up to 5%. The brachial artery may be kinked over the anterior prominence of the proximal fragment or lacerated by the fracture fragments. It may also be damaged as part of an open injury, or obstructed by an intimal tear or spasm. It is important

REFERENCES

12. Copeland SA. Curr Orthop 1995; 9: 241
13. Zyto K, Ahrengart L, Sperber A et al. J Bone Joint Surg 1997; 79B: 412
14. Neer CS. J Bone Joint Surg 1970; 52A: 1090
15. Gartland J. J Surg Gynecol Obstet 1959; 109: 145

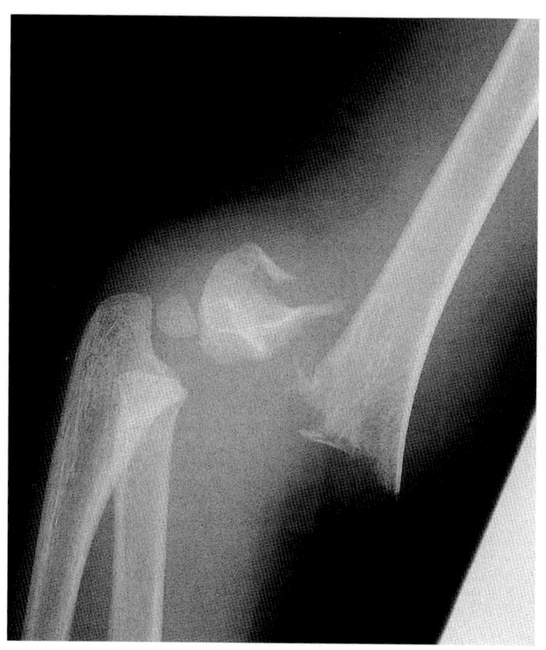
a

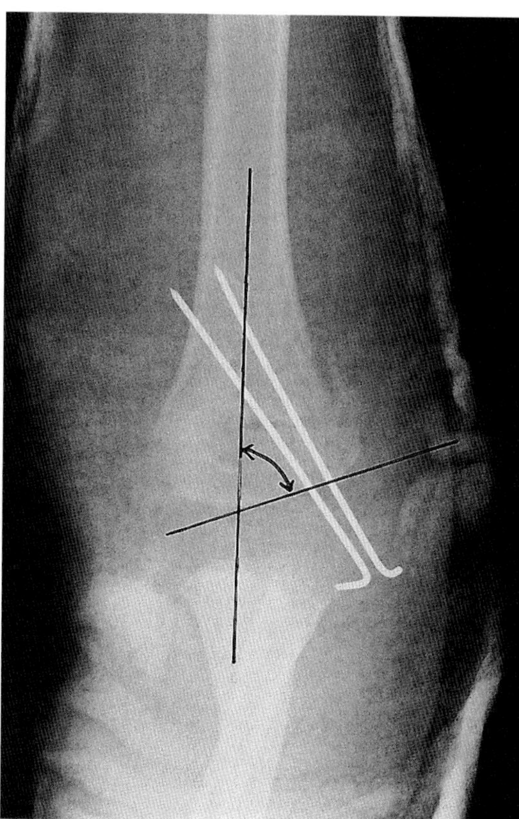
b

Figure 53.7 (a) A completely displaced supracondylar fracture. (b) Postoperative radiograph after closed reduction and percutaneous K-wire fixation; Baumann's angle is 72°, indicating a satisfactory reduction in the coronal plane.

to recognize vascular and neurological injuries, and even if not initially present the child should be monitored for later presentation. Urgent treatment is required if there is evidence of distal ischaemia. The fracture should be reduced as a surgical emergency, and if this does not restore the circulation the brachial artery must be explored (see Ch. 5).

Undisplaced fractures are immobilized for 2 or 3 weeks in a back slab or collar and cuff sling with the elbow flexed above a right angle, before allowing a protected range of exercises. Displaced fractures are reduced under general anaesthesia, and if the posterior periosteum is intact simple flexion is usually effective. Completely displaced fractures require initial traction with the elbow extended and forearm supinated, and correction of rotation and angulation in the coronal plane by manipulation; the elbow is then flexed with forward pressure applied to the olecranon. Holding the elbow flexed tightens the periosteum, which then holds the reduction. With displaced fractures, if the periosteum is completely torn it may be difficult to hold the fracture even with the elbow fully flexed, and percutaneous pin fixation is required (Fig. 53.7).

Closed reduction may fail, particularly if the bone end is buttonholed through the brachialis. If the elbow is not too swollen, an open reduction is performed and the fracture stabilized with K-wires. Open reduction and internal fixation are also used to treat open fractures and when the brachial artery has been explored.

If the elbow is excessively swollen and closed reduction fails, the fracture can be treated by overhead skeletal traction through a transverse wire or screw inserted in the olecranon, or by Dunlop's skin traction.[16] This can be used as definitive treatment but requires close clinical and radiological supervision to avoid any malunion, or it can be simply used as a temporary measure until the swelling subsides. After reduction, the arm is immobilized for 3 weeks. Regular X-rays should be taken to ensure there is no loss of reduction. After 3 weeks, protected active mobilization is begun, and any K-wires are removed between 4 and 6 weeks.

Other complications that can occur after supracondylar fractures in children include malunion with a cubitus valgus or varus deformity that does not remodel with growth. Elbow stiffness is exacerbated by prolonged immobilization and open reduction, but usually recovers with time.

Flexion fractures with anterior displacement and angulation account for only a small proportion of supracondylar fractures in childhood. They are usually caused by a fall on to the point of the elbow, and after reduction are stable with the elbow extended. Immobilization in extension is uncomfortable for the child, and it can be difficult to regain elbow flexion. Percutaneous fixation with K-wires after reduction allows the elbow to be rested in a more functional position and it can be mobilized earlier.

SUPRACONDYLAR FRACTURES IN ADULTS

Supracondylar fractures in adults are also mainly of the extension type and caused by a fall on to the outstretched hand. The brachial artery is again at risk with displaced fractures, and the median, ulnar and radial nerves are all liable to injury, with damage to the radial nerve occurring most frequently. Treatment depends on the degree of displacement of the fracture, with the same options available as for children. Indications for open reduction are failure of closed reduction, an associated neurovascular injury, open fractures, and a simultaneous fracture

REFERENCE

16. Dunlop J. J Bone Joint Surg 1939; 21A: 59

of the ipsilateral humeral shaft or forearm. The fixation should be secure enough to allow early elbow movement if an open reduction is performed.

INTERCONDYLAR FRACTURES

In adults, the fracture line frequently extends down into the articular surface of the humerus, giving a T- or Y-shaped intercondylar fracture. Any prolonged period of immobilization causes severe elbow stiffness. If good-quality bone is present, displaced fractures are treated by reconstruction of the articular surface, with rigid fixation of the condyles to the shaft by plates to permit early postoperative movement.

Internal fixation has a high failure rate in porotic bone, and closed reduction with immobilization in plaster often fails to maintain a satisfactory alignment, and the elbow can become extremely stiff. Other options for treatment are to use a constrained total elbow replacement or the 'bag of bones' technique. The arm is placed in a collar and cuff sling with the elbow flexed to about 90°. Shoulder and hand exercises are started immediately, and elbow extension is allowed as soon as the initial pain and swelling subside. The elbow, however, remains weak, is potentially unstable, and has restricted movement, so the technique is reserved for the treatment of elderly patients with low functional demands.

FRACTURES OF THE MEDIAL EPICONDYLE

The epiphysis of the medial epicondyle first ossifies at between 5 and 9 years of age and usually fuses by the age of 20, although it may never do so. Fractures of the medial epicondyle are common in children, accounting for about 10% of all fractures of the elbow region, but these fractures are rare in adults. The mechanism of injury can be a direct blow to the elbow, a fall on to the outstretched hand with the wrist hyperextended, or an avulsion by the attached ulnar collateral ligament as the elbow dislocates (Fig. 53.8). A repeated valgus stress to the elbow can also cause an avulsion by the attached flexor muscles, which is usually seen in adolescent baseball players and is known as 'little leaguer's elbow'.

There is localized tenderness over the medial epicondyle. If the mechanism of injury has been an elbow dislocation that has reduced spontaneously, the medial epicondyle fragment can be trapped in the joint, and the elbow will then not have a full range of movement. Radiographs can be difficult to interpret and comparison with the normal side is helpful. If the medial epicondyle cannot be seen or is lying level with the joint, it may well be incarcerated in the elbow joint.

The fracture can be managed by immobilization while the pain and swelling subside if there is little or no displacement. This is followed by active mobilization. Displaced and incarcerated fragments can be treated by closed reduction, but open reduction and internal fixation is often required. Possible complications include an ulnar nerve palsy and an unstable elbow.

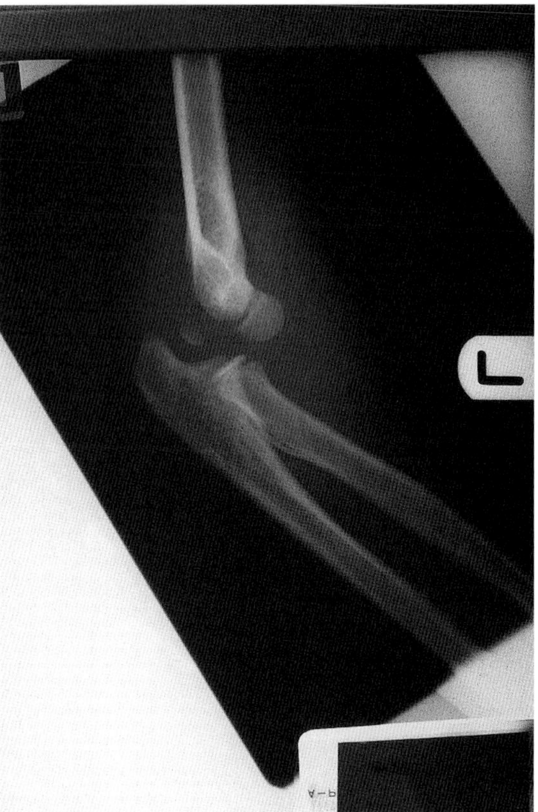

Figure 53.8 Posterior dislocation of a child's elbow with the medial epicondyle avulsed and lying in the joint.

DISLOCATION OF THE ELBOW

The elbow is the second most common large joint after the shoulder to dislocate. It usually occurs in young adults and teenagers, with the average age being 13–14 years.

Classification is dependent on the direction of dislocation, with the majority being posterior. Anterior dislocations are much less common, and medial, lateral and divergent dislocations are only rarely seen. The mechanism of injury for a posterior dislocation is a fall on to the outstretched hand causing forced abduction and extension at the elbow. The ulnar collateral ligament is disrupted or the medial epicondyle avulsed, allowing the olecranon and radial head to displace posteriorly. If the elbow is flexed at the time of injury it can dislocate anteriorly, although the more usual mechanism is a direct blow to the back of the elbow.

With a posterior dislocation the elbow is held in about 45° of flexion and is swollen, the olecranon is prominent posteriorly, and its normal relationship to the medial and lateral epicondyles is disrupted. With anterior dislocations the forearm is supinated and appears elongated. The elbow is extended and the olecranon fossa is palpable posteriorly. Neurovascular injuries can occur and the nerves and circulation must be fully assessed. Plain radiographs confirm the diagnosis and demonstrate any associated fractures.

Most elbow dislocations can be reduced by gentle closed manipulation under sedation or general anaesthesia. Once reduced the elbow is flexed beyond 90°. Stability is then assessed and a back slab is applied. Closed reduction can fail if a bony fragment, which is most likely to be the medial epicondyle, is trapped in the joint (Fig. 53.8). An open reduction is then required. Depending on its stability after reduction, the elbow is immobilized for 1 to 3 weeks, before commencing active and mobilization.

Associated fractures frequently accompany elbow dislocations, with coronoid process fractures being most common. There is usually just a small fragment avulsed by the anterior capsule, which does not require any specific treatment, but if the fragment is more substantial it should be reattached. An avulsed medial epicondyle may reduce as the dislocation is reduced and require no additional treatment, but if it remains displaced or is incarcerated in the joint, or if the elbow is unstable, it should be treated by open reduction and internal fixation. Radial head and capitellar fractures can also occur, and after reduction of the dislocation the fractures are treated on their own merits, although if a comminuted radial head fracture is treated by excision it should be replaced by a prosthesis to avoid elbow instability. Olecranon fractures and avulsion of the triceps tendon occur with anterior dislocations and must be repaired.

Elbow dislocations can be complicated by neurovascular injuries, with the median and ulnar nerves most at risk. Brachial artery damage is most likely with anterior and open dislocations. Loss of elbow movement, particularly the last 10–20° of extension, is usual, although more severe stiffness can occur from intra- or periarticular adhesions or ossification of the muscles and ligaments.

SUBLUXATION OF THE RADIAL HEAD (PULLED ELBOW)

There are numerous synonyms such as nursemaid's elbow, supermarket elbow and temper tantrum elbow for this common condition. The peak incidence is in children aged 2–3 years, and it is rare after the age of 7. The mechanism of injury is a longitudinal pull on the arm with the elbow extended and forearm pronated, pulling the head of the radius partially through the annular ligament, the distal portion of which may be torn. There is usually a history of an adult grabbing the child's arm or swinging the child by an arm, producing an audible 'click' and immediate pain in the elbow. The pain quickly settles, but the child remains reluctant to use the arm and resists forearm supination. On examination, there is tenderness over the proximal radius, the elbow has limited flexion and extension, and supination causes pain. Plain radiographs are usually normal, but may show some soft tissue swelling or slight lateral displacement of the radial head.

Reduction can be performed without sedation or anaesthesia. The child should be relaxed and an explanation given to the parents that the child will briefly experience increased pain and that the symptoms will then completely disappear. Gentle pressure is then applied to the radial head, the elbow is held semiflexed, and as the forearm is supinated there is an audible or palpable 'snap' as the radial head reduces through the annular ligament. This occasionally fails, and the elbow is then fully flexed to achieve the reduction. After reduction the arm can be rested briefly in a sling, although immobilization of the elbow is not necessary.

FRACTURES OF THE HEAD AND NECK OF THE RADIUS

Fractures of the radial head and neck are common in adults and children, and can occur in isolation or as part of a complex injury with associated fractures or dislocations. In adults the fracture usually involves the articular surface, whereas in children it usually crosses the neck or involves the physis. Radial head fractures have been classified by Mason into type I, which are undisplaced; type II, displaced with part of the articular surface remaining connected to the shaft; and type III, with comminution and complete loss of contact between the head and neck

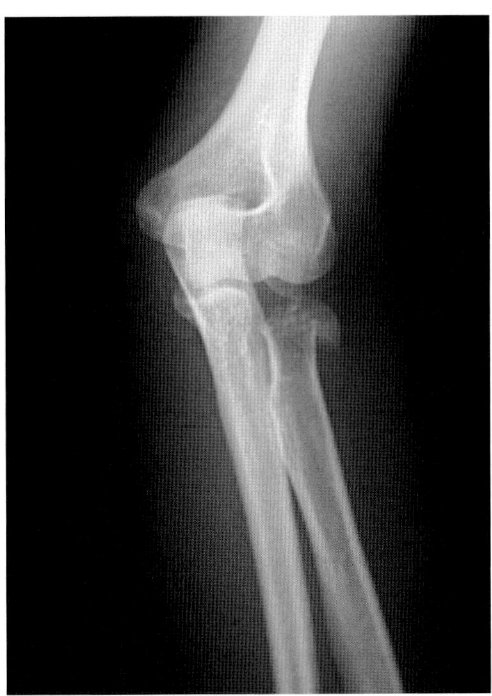

Figure 53.9 A comminuted intra-articular fracture of the head of the radius.

(Fig. 53.9).[17] A radial head fracture in association with an elbow dislocation is sometimes referred to as a Mason type IV fracture.

The mechanism of injury is usually a fall on to the outstretched hand impacting the radial head against the capitellum. The interosseous membrane and distal radioulnar joint can be disrupted as the radius is driven proximally to cause the head to fracture. This is known as the Essex–Lopresti injury and, if unrecognized, can cause chronic wrist instability. Radial head fractures may also occur in association with an elbow dislocation, when the radial head is knocked off forwards by the capitellum as the elbow dislocates posteriorly, or backwards as it spontaneously reduces.

On presentation there is localized tenderness over the proximal radius, a haemarthrosis is usually present, and elbow movements and forearm rotation are painful and restricted. Tenderness over the distal radioulnar joint and along the interosseous membrane indicates an Essex–Lopresti injury. It may be difficult to see the fracture on standard anteroposterior and lateral radiographs, and oblique views can be helpful.

The aim of treatment is to regain a full range of movement. In type I fractures the arm is immobilized in a sling for about 2 days before commencing active mobilization. Aspiration of the haemarthrosis and injection of local anaesthetic into the joint give immediate symptomatic relief and enable elbow mobilization to start sooner, but make no difference to the long-term outcome.

The treatment of type II fractures is controversial, with the options being conservative treatment, open reduction, and internal fixation or excision of the fracture fragment. If after injection of local anaesthetic into the joint the elbow can be almost fully flexed and extended and at least 70° of pronation and supination are present, it will do well with conservative treatment.[18] When elbow movement is found to be restricted, the

REFERENCES

17. Mason ML. Br J Surg 1954; 42: 123
18. Morrey BF. J Bone Joint Surg 1995; 77A: 316

fracture should be reduced and fixed with small AO or Herbert screws. Good results can be achieved if the fixation is stable and allows early movement. When the fragment comprises less than a quarter of the radial head and is completely detached or displaced into the elbow joint it can be excised, although there is a risk that the remaining radial head will sublux with forearm rotation.

Type III fractures are usually treated by early complete excision of the radial head. Losing the radial head does not make the elbow unstable to valgus stress if the medial collateral ligament remains intact,[19] but if there has been an associated elbow dislocation the excised head should be replaced with a prosthesis. With an Essex–Lopresti injury, the radial length must be maintained by internal fixation of the fracture or prosthetic replacement if the head is excised. The dorsal subluxation of the distal ulna is then reduced and held by full supination of the forearm or by transfixing the distal ulna and radius with K-wires.

In children moderate displacement, with angulation of 15–30° of the radial neck, will remodel and can therefore be accepted. Treatment is by immobilization for a week in a sling or back slab, followed by active mobilization. When there is more than 30° angulation this is corrected by manipulation under anaesthetic, with either digital pressure or a percutaneous probe pushing on the radial head. Once reduced it is usually stable, and the elbow is immobilized in 90° of flexion for 2 weeks. Open reduction is performed when the head is completely displaced, or if after an attempted closed reduction there is more than 30–45° angulation or 4 mm displacement.

The main complication of radial head fractures is a loss of elbow movement from malunion producing a bony block and soft tissue fibrosis causing generalized stiffness. Specific complications seen in children are premature closure of the physis, overgrowth of the radial head and, if an open reduction is performed more than 48 h after the injury, there is a risk of avascular necrosis of the radial head.

FRACTURES OF THE OLECRANON

Olecranon fractures are common in adults and rare in children. The classifications used are the Colton,[20] AO[21] and Mayo,[22] which all indicate whether a fracture is undisplaced or displaced; if the latter is transverse, oblique or comminuted; and whether the elbow is dislocated.

The mechanism of injury is a fall on to the point of the elbow, or the outstretched hand with the elbow flexed, combined with a forceful contraction of the triceps. A direct blow is more likely to produce a comminuted fracture with a more extensive soft tissue injury. There is swelling and tenderness over the olecranon, and there may be a palpable gap between the proximal and distal fragments. In displaced fractures, the triceps mechanism is disrupted and the patient is unable to actively extend their elbow. Damage to the ulnar nerve can occur and its function must be assessed. A lateral radiograph is taken with the elbow flexed to 90°, because extending the elbow can reduce a displaced fracture and give a false impression that it is undisplaced. In children, the ossification centre appears at the age of 10 and fuses at about 16 years old, making interpretation of the X-ray difficult. The diagnosis can be made on clinical examination but, if there is doubt, comparison with a radiograph of the normal elbow and the presence of a positive fat pad sign confirms the diagnosis.

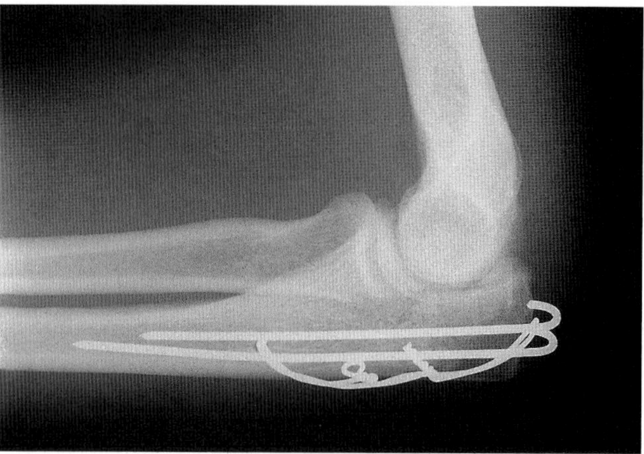

Figure 53.10 Postoperative radiograph of an olecranon fracture treated by open reduction and internal fixation with longitudinal K-wires and a figure-of-eight tension band wire.

Undisplaced fractures can be treated by immobilization in a back slab with the elbow in 90° of flexion for 10 days, followed by gentle and active mobilization, avoiding extension against resistance for a further 6–8 weeks.

The majority of olecranon fractures are simple transverse avulsion fractures with displacement of the proximal fragment and disruption of the extensor mechanism. They are treated by open reduction and internal fixation with two longitudinal K-wires or a 6.5-mm cancellous screw and a figure-of-eight tension band wire passed through a hole drilled transversely in the ulna and around the ends of the K-wires or the screw, deep to the triceps tendon (Fig. 53.10). This provides a stable fixation allowing early active movement of the elbow. The tension band wire produces compression of the fracture when the elbow is actively extended.

FRACTURES OF THE RADIAL AND ULNAR SHAFTS

The anatomical arrangement of the forearm is a straight ulna, around which a curved radius rotates. The two bones are joined by an interosseous membrane and articulate with each other at the proximal and distal radioulnar joints. Consequently if there is a displaced fracture of one of the bones there must also be a fracture of the other bone, or a dislocation of the proximal or distal radioulnar joint. In children the fractures can be complete or greenstick, or the bone can undergo plastic deformation. When there is slight displacement of a greenstick or complete fracture of one of the bones, the other may be intact but undergo plastic deformation. There must always, however, be a high index of suspicion that one of the joints has been disrupted.

REFERENCES

19. Morrey BF, Tanaka S, An K-N. Clin Orthop 1991; 265: 187
20. Colton CL. Injury 1973; 5: 121
21. Müller ME, Allgöwer M, Schneider R et al (eds). Manual of Internal Fixation. 3rd edn. Springer-Verlag, Berlin, 1991
22. Cabanela ME, Morrey BF. In: Morrey BF (ed). The Elbow and its Disorders. 2nd edn. Saunders, Philadelphia, 1993

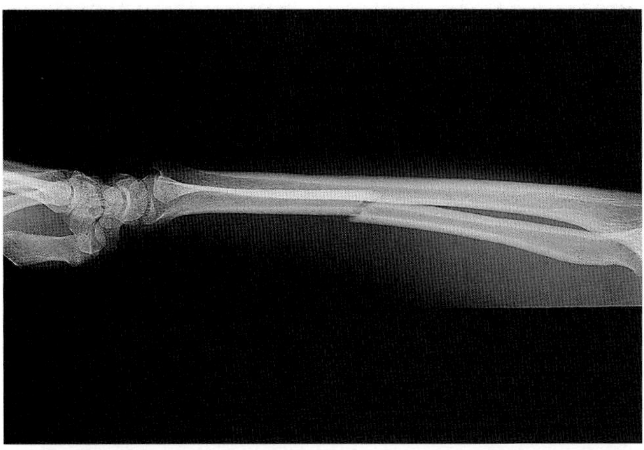

a

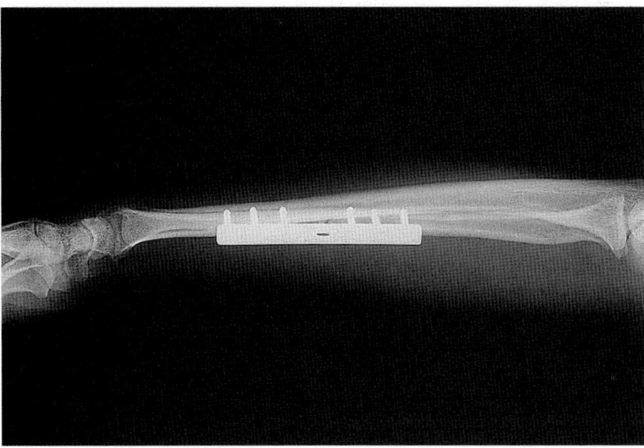

b

Figure 53.11 Galeazzi fracture. (**a**) There is a fracture of the shaft of the radius and dislocation of the distal radioulnar joint. (**b**) The distal radioulnar joint has been reduced by accurately reducing the radial fracture.

A fracture at the junction of the middle and distal thirds of the radius with subluxation or dislocation of the distal radioulnar joint is known as a Galeazzi fracture (Fig. 53.11).[23] Fracture of the proximal third of the ulna with dislocation of the radial head was described by Monteggia in 1814,[24] and this injury has been classified according to the direction in which the radial head dislocates and whether there is an associated fracture of the proximal radius.[25]

The mechanism of injury is either direct, with road traffic accidents a frequent cause, or indirect from a fall on to the outstretched hand. An isolated fracture of the ulna is known as a nightstick fracture, and occurs with a direct blow against the ulnar side of the forearm, classically when the arm is raised to protect the face from assault. Galeazzi fractures are caused by a direct force to the dorsolateral aspect of the wrist or a fall on to the outstretched hand with the forearm pronated.

There is swelling and tenderness over the fractures, and with both bones broken there is usually an obvious deformity. The elbow and wrist must be assessed to exclude dislocation of the radial head or disruption of the distal radioulnar joint. Forearm fractures may be open, either from a spike of bone puncturing the skin from the inside or from the direct injury to the soft tissues, in which case there can be associated injuries to the vessels, nerves, muscles and tendons. Most forearm fractures are obvious with standard X-rays, which must include anteroposterior and lateral views of the elbow and wrist to detect Monteggia and Galeazzi fractures.

Forearm fractures must be accurately reduced to avoid loss of forearm rotation. Children have the potential to remodel moderate amounts of angulation, and up to 15° is acceptable in children under the age of 7 years. Rotational deformities are unlikely to remodel and must therefore be corrected.

Undisplaced fractures are immobilized in an above-elbow cast that includes the hand and thumb to provide rotational stability. They must be kept under close observation because subsequent displacement can occur from the pull of the attached muscles.

Non-operative treatment of displaced fractures is difficult because accurate alignment and rotation must be maintained while preserving the normal radial bow. Good results have been achieved by using a functional brace, but generally the results of conservative treatment in adults are poor. Children are usually treated by manipulation under general anaesthesia and immobilization in an above-elbow cast, with the forearm in supination for fractures of the proximal third, the neutral position for the middle third, and in pronation for the distal third fractures. Greenstick fractures are usually easy to reduce, but healing can be delayed with a high incidence of refracture.[26] This is because the intact cortex makes the fracture stable, limiting callus production, and if even slight angulation persists there is no compression of the fracture. Some surgeons therefore recommend that the intact cortex is broken during the reduction to avoid this problem, but doing so will increase the risk of recurrent displacement. Prolonged protection with a splint is required to avoid refracture if the intact cortex is not broken during the manipulation.[26]

Most displaced forearm fractures in adults are treated by open reduction and internal fixation. Intramedullary nails have been used, but plating is usually preferred because nails may fail to control rotation or accommodate for the natural bow of the radius. The radius and ulna are exposed through separate incisions to reduce the risk of radioulnar synostosis; the fractures are anatomically reduced and held with 3.5-mm dynamic compression plates and an interfragmentary lag screw where possible. Primary bone grafting should be considered if the fracture is comminuted or segmental.

Undisplaced isolated fractures of the ulna can be treated with a cast or functional brace for 6–8 weeks, but if there is more than 10° angulation or 50% displacement open reduction and internal fixation are preferred.

Monteggia fractures in children can be treated by closed reduction of the ulna fracture and dislocated radial head, and immobilization in an above-elbow cast in supination, or by open reduction and internal fixation of the ulna fracture and closed reduction of the radial head.[27] Both techniques produce a good functional outcome. In adults, the ulna fracture requires an open reduction and internal fixation with a compression plate. The radial head can be reduced closed, unless the annular ligament is

REFERENCES

23. Galeazzi R. Arch Orthop Unfallchir 1934; 35: 557
24. Monteggia GB. Instituzioni Chirugiche, Vol 5. Maspero, Milan, 1814
25. Bado JL. Clin Orthop 1967; 50: 71
26. Schwarz N, Pienaar S, Schwarz AF et al. J Bone Joint Surg 1996; 78B: 740
27. Ring D, Waters PM. J Bone Joint Surg 1996; 78B: 734

torn and blocks the reduction. Open reduction is then required. The elbow should be immobilized in a cast for 6 weeks, with radiographs being taken at 2 and 6 weeks to ensure that the radial head has not redislocated.

Galeazzi fractures in children are treated by closed reduction of the radial fracture. Immobilization in supination will usually reduce the distal radioulnar joint. In adults, the radial fracture is anatomically reduced and held with a plate; this usually reduces the distal radioulnar joint (Fig. 53.11), but if it remains subluxed or dislocated it should be reduced and held with K-wires transfixing the ulna and radius.

Open fractures of the forearm are treated according to the same principles as for all open fractures (see Ch. 52). Thorough debridement of the wounds and repair of the damaged soft tissues, where appropriate, are carried out; the fractures are then stabilized by an external fixator or immediate plating.

The incidence of associated neurovascular injury is low after straightforward closed forearm fractures, but it is greater after open fractures or Monteggia fractures, where the posterior interosseous nerve is at risk, and in fractures treated surgically, where there is a risk of iatrogenic injury. Forearm compartment syndrome is rare, and early diagnosis and treatment are essential if nerve and, more importantly, muscle necrosis are to be prevented.

FRACTURES OF THE DISTAL RADIUS

Fractures of the distal radius are very common in both adults and children, and account for about a sixth of all fractures, with peaks occurring between the ages of 6 and 10, and 60 and 69. In adults these fractures are most simply classified by their well-known eponyms. A Colles' fracture is through the metaphysis of the distal radius within 1–3 cm of the wrist joint. There is dorsal angulation and displacement of the distal fragment with radial angulation, shortening, and often an associated fracture of the ulnar styloid.[28] A Smith's fracture is a fracture of the distal radius with volar angulation and displacement of the distal fragment,[29] and can be either extra- or intra-articular. Barton's fracture is a fracture dislocation or subluxation of the wrist (Fig. 53.12), with an intra-articular fracture of the distal radius producing a fragment on the dorsal or palmar surface that displaces with the attached carpus and hand backwards or forwards.[30]

In children wrist fractures occur either through the physis, and are usually Salter–Harris type I or II injuries, or through the metaphysis. Metaphyseal fractures can be torus or buckle fractures, in which one cortex fails under compression and there is little or no displacement; greenstick fractures, in which one cortex fractures completely under tension and the other undergoes plastic deformation under compression; or complete fractures, where both cortices have been disrupted (Fig. 53.13).

The mechanism of injury is usually a fall on to the outstretched hand. Smith thought a fall on to the back of the hand would produce a fracture with volar angulation, but this type of fracture can also occur when the wrist has been dorsiflexed, if the forearm rotates. It can also be produced by a direct blow on the back of the hand. Motorcycle accidents in which the rider is thrown over the handlebars are a common cause of volar Barton's fractures, and other intra-articular fractures are produced by the carpus impacting against the end of the radius, giving what are known as die punch injuries.[31]

Characteristic deformities are seen in displaced fractures, with the dinner fork deformity of a Colles' fracture, and the forward displacement of the hand and swelling in the front of the wrist in a Smith's fracture. There is tenderness over the fracture and pain moving the wrist. Neurological examination will identify acute nerve palsies, and open wounds if present are usually small, being caused by a spike of bone puncturing the skin.

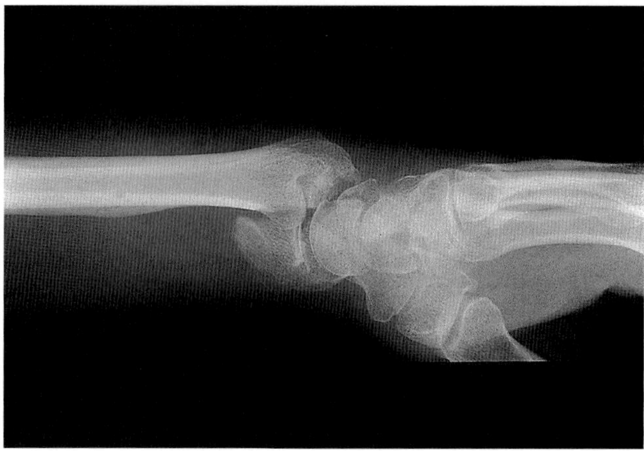

Figure 53.12 Grossly displaced fractures of the distal radius and ulna in a child.

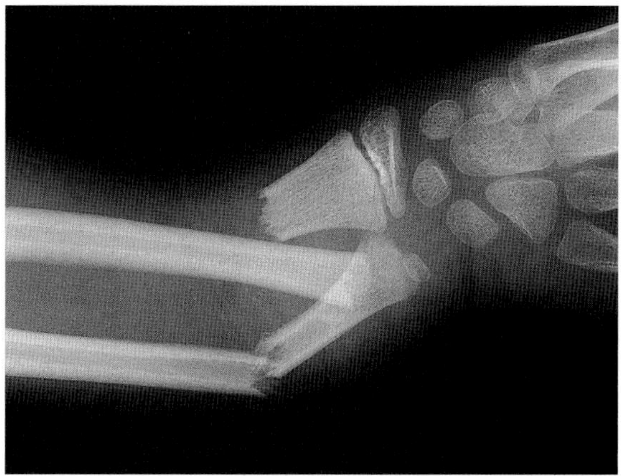

Figure 53.13 Volar Barton's fracture: there is volar subluxation of the carpus with the volar fragment of the distal radius.

Anteroposterior and lateral radiographs should include the elbow and wrist, and the fracture lines are usually obvious. Undisplaced Salter–Harris type I and torus fractures can be difficult to detect, but should be suspected if there is forward displacement of the fat pad overlying pronator quadratus. The normal radiographic anatomy must be known to assess the displacement of a fracture. On the lateral view the articular surface faces anteriorly at an angle of 10–15°, and on the anteroposterior view the radial inclination is 22–23°. The vertical distance from the tip of the radial styloid to the articular surface of the ulna head is 10–12 mm. Any associated carpal fractures and dislocations, and in particular disruption of the distal radioulnar joint, must be identified.

REFERENCES

28. Colles A. Edinb Med Surg J 1814; 10: 182
29. Smith RW. A Treatise on Fractures in the Vicinity of Joints, and on Certain Forms of Accidental and Congenital Dislocations. Hodges & Smith, Dublin, 1854
30. Barton JR. Med Examiner 1838; 1: 365
31. Scheck M. J Bone Joint Surg 1962; 44A: 337

Fractures that are minimally displaced are treated by immobilization in a below-elbow cast or wrist splint for 3–4 weeks for torus fractures in children, and for 5–6 weeks in adults. Displaced fractures should be reduced and held in an anatomical position, with the method used depending on the fracture's stability and the patient's requirements. The fracture can be held by a cast (which can be below or extend above the elbow), percutaneous K-wires, open reduction and internal fixation, or an external fixator that can be combined with limited internal fixation and bone grafting. Displaced Colles' fractures are treated by manipulation under an anaesthetic that can be by a haematoma block, a Bier's block, a regional block or a general anaesthetic. Traction is applied, the distal fragment is pushed volarward, and the wrist is then flexed. A moulded back slab or split plaster is applied, which should produce pressure over the dorsum of the distal fragment, and the wrist should be held in slight flexion and ulnar deviation. The hand is kept elevated, and finger, elbow and shoulder movement is encouraged. A plain radiograph is taken at 1 week to ensure that the fracture has not redisplaced, and the cast is completed and retained for 5–6 weeks.

Fractures that present with more than 20° of dorsal angulation, marked dorsal comminution, or more than 10 mm of shortening are likely to be unstable. Unstable fractures, or those which are not perfectly reduced, have a high risk of redisplacement in a cast. If this occurs, remanipulation and immobilization in a cast are unlikely to be successful.[32] The fracture should therefore be held with percutaneous K-wires, by an external fixator with or without cancellous bone graft, or by open reduction and internal fixation with bone grafting. The last of these gives a better radiological appearance than treatment with an external fixator, although there is no difference in the eventual functional outcome.[33]

Smith's fractures in the elderly can be treated by manipulation under anaesthetic, and they are then immobilized in supination in an above-elbow plaster cast. Slight dorsiflexion of the wrist tightens the volar carpal ligament and locks the reduction. In younger patients these fractures often occur after high-energy injuries, producing comminution and intra-articular extension. Treatment is then with an external fixator or by open reduction and internal fixation with a small T plate placed on the volar surface of the radius, buttressing the distal fragment.

Intra-articular fractures require accurate reduction, because a step in the articular surface of more than 2 mm ultimately will cause osteoarthritis and functional impairment.[34] Barton's fractures are unstable, and treatment by internal fixation with a buttress plate on the volar or dorsal surface of the radius for volar and dorsal Barton's fractures, respectively, gives better radiological and functional results than conservative treatment. Comminuted intra-articular fractures have been treated by external fixation with percutaneous K-wires (Fig. 53.14) and bone grafting with good results. During reduction, it may be helpful to visualize the articular surface with an arthroscope to ensure a perfect position.

Children have considerable potential to remodel fractures of the distal radius, and up to 20° of angulation of a physeal fracture can be accepted. The fracture should be reduced by manipulation and immobilized in a below-elbow cast if the angulation exceeds this or there is noticeable clinical deformity. Very occasionally closed reduction is blocked by a flap of periosteum caught in the fracture, and an open reduction is necessary. Greenstick fractures angulated more than 10–15° require reduction and are immobilized in supination in a well-moulded cast. Any persisting angulation can increase in the cast and close radiological monitoring is therefore essential.

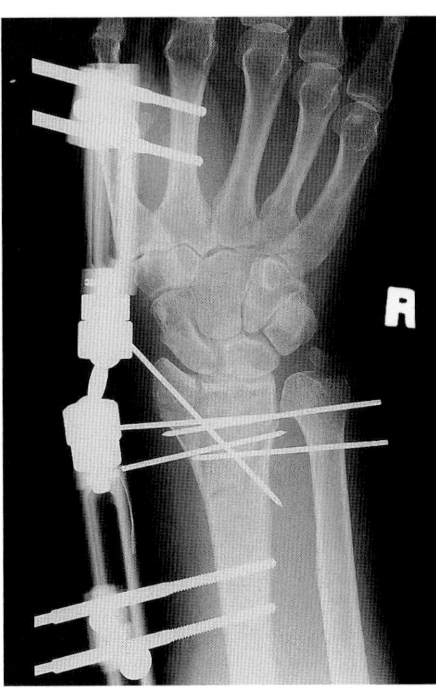

Figure 53.14 Postoperative radiograph of a comminuted intra-articular fracture of the radius treated with an external fixator and percutaneous K-wires.

Complete fractures are often markedly displaced, with the distal fragment displaced posteriorly and proximally. Reduction can be difficult because there is an intact dorsal periosteal hinge. To perform a closed reduction the deformity is increased by hyperextending the fracture, and the distal fragment is pushed distally. Once the dorsal cortex is hitched, the fragment is pushed anteriorly and flexed. The arm is immobilized in supination in an above-elbow moulded cast, which must be split because considerable swelling can occur. Closed reduction can fail if the bone end buttonholes through the periosteum or pronator quadratus, or if the tendons are trapped between the bone ends. Open reduction is then required, and the fracture is held with a K-wire.

Fractures of the distal radius can be associated with injuries to the median or ulnar nerves. Acute carpal tunnel syndrome can also develop, and forearm compartment syndrome has been reported after high-energy intra-articular fractures. Reflex sympathetic dystrophy, which is also known as complex regional pain disorder, algodystrophy or Sudek's atrophy, is a very common complication with a reported incidence of up to 37%.[35] Rupture of the tendon of extensor pollicis longus can occur 2–8 weeks after the fracture from mechanical irritation or vascular impairment. This can be treated by an extensor indicis proprius tendon transfer or a free palmaris longus tendon graft and can give a good functional recovery. Inadequate reduction can leave an irregular articular surface, which can lead to

REFERENCES

32. McQueen MM, MacLaren A, Chalmers J. J Bone Joint Surg 1986; 68B: 232
33. McQueen MM, Hajducka C, Court-Brown CM. J Bone Joint Surg 1996; 78B: 404
34. Knirk JL, Jupiter JB. J Bone Joint Surg 1986; 68A: 647
35. Atkins RM, Duckworth T, Kanis JA. J Bone Joint Surg 1990; 72B: 105

osteoarthritis and loss of the normal palmar tilt, causing carpal instability and wrist stiffness. Problems with forearm rotation and painful osteoarthritis can be the result of disruption of the distal radioulnar joint from radial shortening, an associated displaced fracture of the distal ulna, or direct involvement by extension of the radial fracture into the joint. There can be associated tears of the triangular fibrocartilage complex, causing pain on the ulnar side of the wrist and occasionally instability of the distal radioulnar joint.

FRACTURES OF THE SCAPHOID

The scaphoid has proximal and distal poles joined by a waist. The two poles are flexed and rotated at 45° to each other. The scaphoid forms part of and links the proximal and distal carpal rows, and the majority of its surface is articular. The blood supply is from the radial and anterior interosseous arteries, with 70% of the blood supply entering through the dorsal ridge. Normally no vessels enter through the proximal pole, and there is no intraosseous anastamosis between the vessels entering the tuberosity and dorsal ridge, so a fracture of the middle third or more proximally can cause devascularization of the proximal pole.

Scaphoid fractures have been classified by Herbert[36] into type A incomplete fractures; type B acute complete fractures, which can be oblique fractures of the distal pole or transverse fractures of the waist or proximal pole; or fracture dislocations. Type C are delayed unions and type D are non-unions, of which four subtypes are described. Fractures can displace with translation, rotation or angulation, with flexion being most common. They are liable to be unstable if there is comminution, displacement or separation of the fragments by more than 1 mm, or if the fracture is vertical or oblique.

The mechanism of injury is usually a fall on to the outstretched hand, with the wrist extended to at least 95°. As the wrist hyperextends, the scaphoid is impacted against the dorsal edge of the distal radius. The site of the fracture depends on the amount of extension and the radial or ulnar deviation of the wrist at the time of impact. About 3% of scaphoid fractures are caused by wrist flexion.[37]

The physical signs depend on the severity of the fracture. For minimally displaced fractures, there is often a delay between injury and presentation because patients think that they have only had a sprain. If the signs are subtle, comparison with the normal wrist is essential. There is often a little swelling, and localized tenderness over the scaphoid in the anatomical snuff box. Radial side wrist pain on full passive radial and ulnar deviation of the wrist, pain on active resisted thumb extension and adduction, and pain with compression of the thumb may be present. However, no physical sign or test is specific or particularly reliable.[38] With more severe fractures swelling and bruising are more noticeable.

The diagnosis is confirmed radiologically. A variety of views have been described, and a minimum of four should be taken. They include a posteroanterior with the palm on the X-ray plate, a true lateral, and oblique views with 45° pronation and supination. Extending the scaphoid by ulnar deviation and extension of the wrist by clenching the fist brings the scaphoid more perpendicular to the X-ray beam, and is known as the Ziter view.

A bone scan, a CT or an MRI scan can be obtained if doubt about the diagnosis persists.

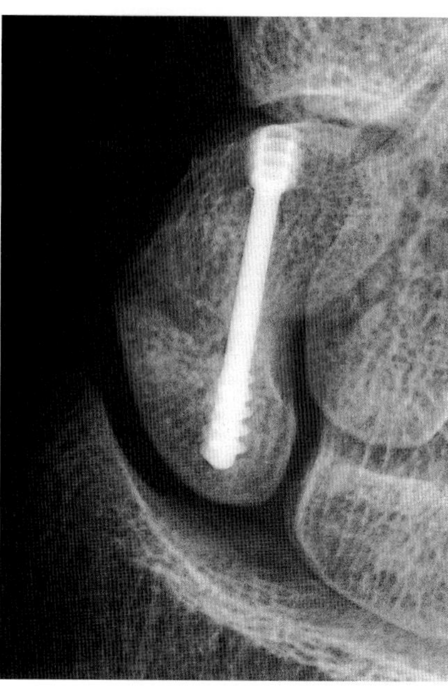

Figure 53.15 A fracture of the waist of the scaphoid treated by open reduction and internal fixation with a Herbert screw.

The management of scaphoid fractures is based on both the radiographs and the clinical findings, because on their own each can be misleading. When a fracture is suspected clinically but is not apparent on the radiographs, it should be immobilized because a delay in immobilization leads to a higher non-union rate. It is re-examined and X-rayed after 10–14 days, and if there is still doubt a bone scan will usually confirm the diagnosis.

The traditional treatment for all scaphoid fractures was immobilization in a scaphoid plaster, which included the thumb and held the wrist slightly extended. Some surgeons have advocated an above-elbow plaster, although this has since been shown not to be of any benefit. Inclusion of the thumb is probably not necessary, and a Colles' type plaster is perfectly satisfactory.[39]

The plaster cast is retained until the fracture has united, but in practice it can be very difficult to determine when union has occurred. After about 8 weeks of immobilization the wrist is examined and X-rayed, and if there is still tenderness or the radiograph looks doubtful, a plaster cast is reapplied for a further 4 weeks. After the cast has been removed, the radiographs should be repeated 6 months after the injury to ensure a non-union has not occurred.

About 90% of acute scaphoid fractures unite with conservative treatment,[40] with the time to union depending on the level of the fracture and the degree of displacement. Because a prolonged period of immobilization and absence from work may be necessary, some surgeons treat all acute scaphoid fractures by internal fixation, claiming a shorter time to union and an earlier return to work. Internal fixation with a Herbert screw (Fig. 53.15)

REFERENCES

36. Herbert TJ, Fisher WE. J Bone Joint Surg 1984; 66B: 114
37. Leslie IJ, Dickson RA. J Bone Joint Surg 1981; 63B: 225
38. Gunal I, Barton N, Calli I (eds). Current Management of Scaphoid Fractures: Twenty Questions Answered. The Royal Society of Medicine Press Limited, London, 2002
39. Clay NR, Dias JJ, Costigan PS et al. J Bone Joint Surg 1991; 73B: 828
40. Dias JJ, Brenkel IJ, Finley DBL. J Bone Joint Surg 1989; 71B: 307

has been reported to give rapid symptomatic relief and to provide sufficient stability to allow normal use of the wrist without postoperative immobilization. The overall union rate is similar to that of non-operative treatment. However, as there is no proof that operative treatment of acute scaphoid fractures gives better results, and it carries the risks of complications of anaesthesia and surgery, such as hypertrophic scars and articular damage to the scaphotrapezial joint, most surgeons do not recommend internal fixation for all acute scaphoid fractures.

Unstable fractures can displace, leading to malunion, and they have an increased risk of non-union, so primary internal fixation should be considered. Fractures likely to be unstable are those associated with a perilunate dislocation, where the displacement or gap between the scaphoid fragments is greater than 1 mm, or where the fracture line is vertical or oblique. The method of fixation is usually with a screw that will compress the fracture, and if there is anterior comminution, and bone loss causing flexion at the fracture, a bone graft can be inserted to restore the normal shape of the bone.

The main complication of scaphoid fractures is non-union, which may be associated with avascular necrosis of the proximal pole. The incidence in patients treated conservatively and followed up for 1 year by Dias and coworkers was 12.3%.[40] Non-union can be symptomless, although a degree of pain and weakness is usual. The concern is that the patient will develop progressive arthritis if left untreated, so unless a patient is elderly or has already developed significant arthritic changes attempts should be made to achieve union. The pseudarthrosis and any dead or sclerotic bone should be excised, the defect grafted with a corticocancellous graft and held with a screw or K-wires. Up to 95% of scaphoid fractures will unite using this approach.

FRACTURES OF THE CARPAL BONES OTHER THAN THE SCAPHOID

Dorsal chip fractures from a carpal bone are the second most common carpal fracture after a fracture of the scaphoid. Apart from these, carpal bone fractures are rare.

PERILUNATE DISLOCATIONS

Dislocations of all the carpal bones have been described, but by far the most common are perilunate dislocations. Associated fractures of the scaphoid giving trans-scaphoid perilunate dislocations are common, and there can also be associated fractures of the capitate, triquetral, or radial (Fig. 53.16) and ulnar styloids.

Dislocations occur around the lunate because the volar radiolunate ligament is very strong. The lunate remains attached to the radius as the rest of the carpus dislocates posteriorly. The carpus can rebound, pushing the lunate anteriorly so that there appears to be an isolated anterior dislocation of the lunate, although the volar radiolunate ligament remains intact, and the rest of the carpus will have initially dislocated posteriorly.

Perilunate dislocations have been classified into pure dislocations and fracture dislocations,[41] the classification of which depends on which bone is fractured. Trans-scaphoid perilunate dislocations are known as de Quervain's injury. They are usually high-energy injuries often from falls on to an outstretched hand or road traffic accidents, causing extreme dorsiflexion of the radially deviated wrist.

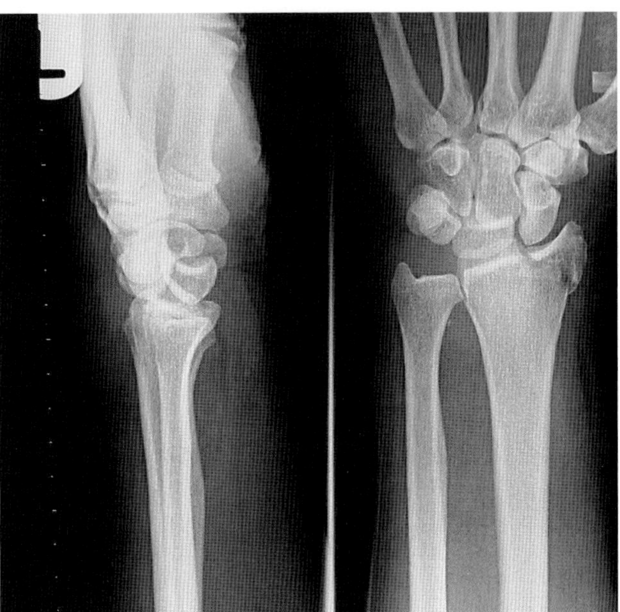

Figure 53.16 Anteroposterior and lateral radiographs of the wrist, showing a fracture of the radial styloid and a perilunate dislocation. On the anteroposterior view there is overlap of the distal lunate and proximal pole of the capitate. On the lateral view the capitate is clearly dislocated dorsally, relative to the lunate.

The physical signs are variable, and the diagnosis is initially missed in a quarter of cases. There is usually some swelling, diffuse tenderness, and movement of the wrist is limited by pain. There may be associated injuries to the median and ulnar nerves, vessels and tendons.

The anteroposterior radiograph shows soft tissue swelling, increased overlap of the carpal bones, the lunate has an abnormal shape and orientation, and the gap between the scaphoid and lunate is increased. Any associated fractures should also be apparent. On the lateral view the capitate is not articulating with the lunate, which may be displaced forwards and rotated.

In acute injuries closed reduction is by traction, and dorsiflexion with pressure over the volar surface of the lunate. This is followed by gradual flexion and may be successful. The reduction is held with a cast or percutaneous K-wires. Because the scapholunate ligament will have been torn, a chronic scapholunate dissociation can develop. To prevent this, acute repair of the scapholunate ligament should be considered. If closed reduction fails, open reduction is required. With a trans-scaphoid perilunate dislocation, failure to accurately reduce the scaphoid fracture gives poor results, so open reduction with internal fixation of the scaphoid with a screw or K-wires is usually preferred.

Closed reduction is occasionally possible if the diagnosis is delayed and the patient presents late, but open reduction is usually required.

REFERENCE

41. Mayfield JK. Clin Orthop 1980; 149: 45

Pelvic fractures

54

Anthony J. Ward

INTRODUCTION

Most pelvic fractures are relatively simple and do not render the pelvic ring unstable. These injuries are the result of low-energy trauma, such as a simple fall in the elderly patient, and do not require surgical intervention. In contrast, high-energy trauma in a road traffic accident or a fall from height may result in an unstable pelvic ring disruption and some degree of associated pelvic soft tissue injury. The injury may be restricted to the pelvic region or, in two-thirds of cases, be associated with other injuries; most common are head injuries, chest injuries and long bone fractures. The term *complex pelvic trauma* defines the 10% of pelvic injuries with associated soft tissue injuries to the urological system (bladder or urethra), hollow viscera (bowel), neurovascular structures (pelvic vessels or sacral plexus), or integumen of the perineum (open fracture), in which patients have an increased rate of mortality of 10 to 50%.[1] Major haemorrhage and other life-threatening injuries must be dealt with urgently by a multidisciplinary team that is trained in the critical assessment and surgical treatment of abdominal, pelvic and other injuries. A pelvic fracture should be considered to be an indicator of major trauma until further assessment rules out the presence of associated injuries.

The aims of treatment of pelvic fractures are to identify and treat the life-threatening associated injuries, to control haemorrhage, and to restore the mechanical stability and alignment of the pelvic ring. The first concern is to save life, and the second is to stabilize the pelvis to provide pain relief, facilitate the mobilization and rehabilitation of the patient, and prevent late deformity or instability of the pelvic ring.

A fracture of the acetabulum may occur as an isolated injury or in association with other pelvic fractures. Being an intra-articular fracture, the aims of treatment are to prevent post-traumatic arthritis of the hip joint and long-term disability. If displaced, the fracture requires anatomical reduction and stable internal fixation of the joint surfaces, with early mobilization of the hip joint and of the patient.

The definitive management of patients with complex pelvic and acetabular fractures requires special expertise and equipment. It is recommended that early advice is sought from and prompt referral made to a pelvic trauma unit.[2]

SURGICAL ANATOMY AND STABILITY

The pelvis is a strong ring-like structure that transmits weight-bearing forces from the spine to the legs (through the hip joints), while providing protection for the pelvic organs and attachment for the muscles of the pelvic floor, abdomen and legs.

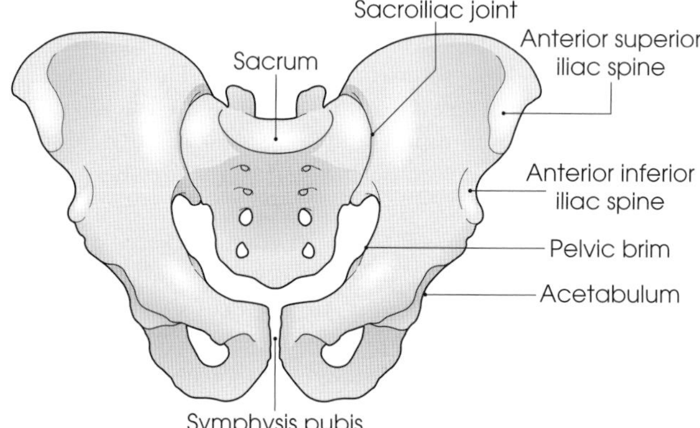

Figure 54.1 The bones and joints of the pelvis.

In the adult, the pelvic ring comprises three bones bound together by strong ligaments, with the pelvic joints allowing only very limited movement under load. The left and right innominate bones are joined at the symphysis pubis anteriorly and to the sacrum posteriorly at the sacroiliac joints (Fig. 54.1). The symphysis pubis is a secondary cartilaginous joint, with a disc of fibrocartilage interposed between and binding to the hyaline cartilage surfaces of each pubic bone, which is strong and slightly flexible. The sacroiliac joint on each side is a synovial joint with interdigitating surfaces of hyaline cartilage, which transmit body weight from the sacrum to each innominate bone. The sacroiliac joints are supported by the thick posterior sacroiliac ligaments, which are the strongest in the body. The anterior sacroiliac ligaments are relatively weak. Accessory ligaments help stabilize the pelvis; the iliolumbar ligament suspends the posterior sacrum and iliac crest from the transverse process of the fifth lumbar vertebra. The sacrospinous and sacrotuberous ligaments in the pelvic floor bind the sacrum to the ischial spine and to the ischial tuberosity of the innominate bone, respectively (Fig. 54.2). In the child, the innominate bone is formed from three bones: the pubis, ischium and ilium join at the triradiate cartilage in the acetabulum and fuse in the early teens.

REFERENCES

1. Pohlemann T, Tscherne H, Baumgärtel F et al. Ungallchirurg 1996; 99: 160–167
2. The Working Party of the Royal College of Surgeons of England and the British Orthopaedic Association. Better Care for the Severely Injured. The Royal College of Surgeons of England, London, 2000; 27–28

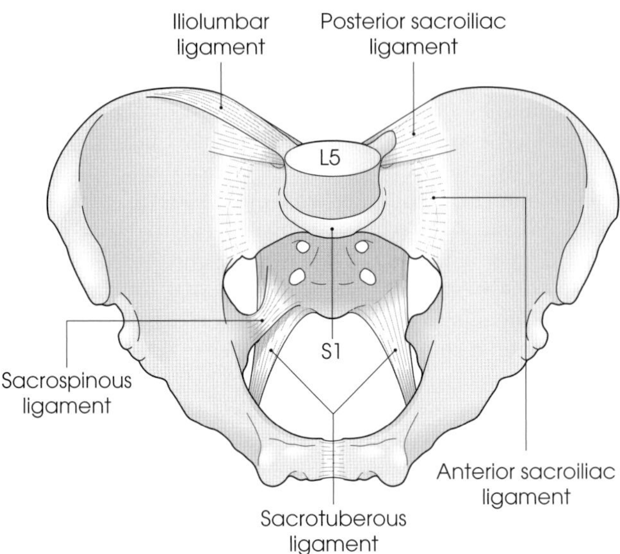

Figure 54.2 The pelvic ring and stabilizing ligaments. The sacrotuberous and sacrospinous ligaments (omitted for clarity on the left side) form part of the pelvic floor.

Because the pelvis is a bony ring, a break in one part of the ring must be accompanied by a break in another part of the ring. It has been shown that even minor anterior fractures (pubic rami) are associated with some degree of posterior injury (sacral impaction) that can be detected with scintigraphy. The mechanical stability of the pelvis depends on the integrity of the posterior pelvic complex, which transmits load to the hip joints. Disruption of this complex—comprising the sacrum, posterior ilium, sacroiliac joint and supporting ligaments—causes rotational or vertical instability of the affected hemipelvis. The direction of displacement and instability forms the basis of current classifications of pelvic ring injuries.

The acetabulum is the socket of the synovial hip joint. The articular surface is C-shaped, open inferiorly, with the thickest hyaline cartilage on the main weight-bearing surface at the dome superiorly. There is congruent articulation with the spherical head of the femur. The bony structure of the acetabulum is composed of anterior and posterior columns that merge at the dome in the shape of an inverted Y (Fig. 54.3). This concept, described by Letournel, forms the basis of the anatomical classification of acetabular fractures.[3]

Pelvis is Latin for bowl. The pelvic visceral organs (the bladder, the lower colon and rectum, and the uterus and adnexa in females) are contained within the true pelvis, the deepest part of the bowl lying below the pelvic brim. The viscera and the rich plexus of blood vessels arising from and draining to the internal iliac artery and veins are prone to injury if the pelvis is fractured. Posterior pelvic ring disruptions may be associated with injury to the major blood vessels and nerve roots of the lumbosacral plexus (L4, 5; S1, 2, 3) that lie on the anterior surface of the sacrum and sacroiliac joint. The superior gluteal artery is vulnerable as it passes out under the superior margin of the greater sciatic notch to supply the gluteal musculature. The sciatic nerve is at risk of injury (typically from posterior acetabular fracture or dislocation of the hip), as it exits the greater sciatic notch below piriformis muscle, and runs posterior to the hip joint into the posterior thigh. Nerve injuries may occur at the time of fracture or during subsequent surgical exposure of the fracture.

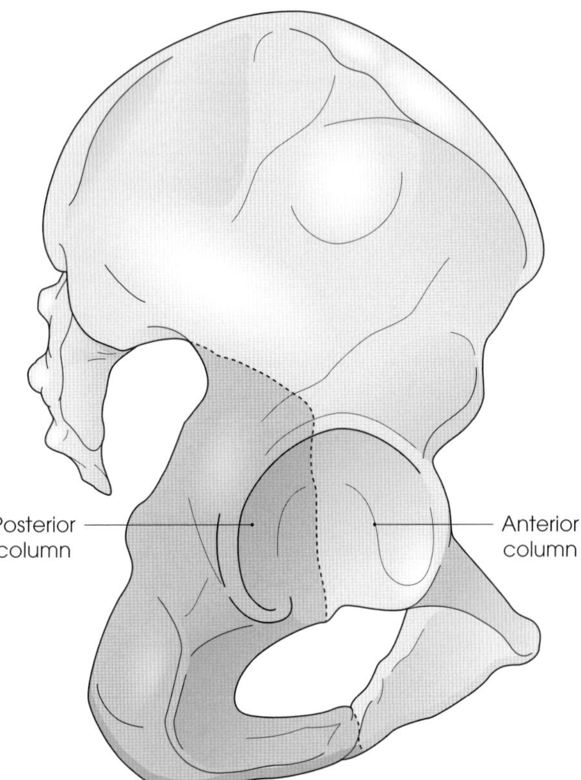

Figure 54.3 The acetabulum, depicting the anterior and posterior columns of bone.

CLASSIFICATION OF PELVIC FRACTURES

Pelvic fractures may be closed (intact soft tissue envelope) or open, in which the fracture communicates with an overlying skin laceration (perineum, buttock or loin) or with rectal or vaginal tears.

The mechanical stability (or degree of instability) of the pelvic ring forms the basis of the two complimentary classification systems used in assessment and decision making for treatment. The AO comprehensive classification,[4,5] derived from the system of Tile,[6] is based on the direction of mechanical instability.

AO CLASSIFICATION OF PELVIC RING FRACTURES

- Type A injury: stable with intact posterior pelvic complex—the pelvic floor is intact and the pelvis is able to withstand normal physiological load without displacement.
- Type B injury: rotational instability with incomplete disruption of the posterior pelvic complex—partial instability present with, in some cases, an intact pelvic floor. The

REFERENCES

3. Letournel E, Judet R. Fractures of the Acetabulum. 2nd edn. Springer-Verlag, New York, 1993
4. Tile M, Helfet DL, Kellam JF et al. Comprehensive Classification of Fractures in the Pelvis and Acetabulum. Maurice E. Muller Foundation, Berne, 1995
5. Pohlemann T. In: Ruedi TP, Murphy WM (eds). AO Principles of Fracture Management. Thieme, New York, 2000: 390–413
6. Tile M. J Bone Joint Surg 1988; 70B: 1–12

Table 54.1 AO classification of pelvic ring injuries (61-)

Type	Stability	Incidence (%)	Surgical stabilization
A	Stable	50–70	Not required (rare exceptions)
B	Rotationally unstable	20–30	Stabilization of anterior pelvic ring alone is sufficient
C	Vertically and rotationally unstable	10–20	Anterior and posterior stabilization required to prevent secondary displacement

subtypes are B1 (external rotation), B2 (internal rotation), and B3 (bilateral involvement).

- Type C injury: rotational and vertical instability with complete disruption of the posterior pelvic complex—complete instability of the pelvic ring, with pelvic floor always disrupted.

It can be difficult to differentiate between partial and complete posterior instability. The primary evaluation, based on plain radiographs, may need to be amended after review of CT scans or in time if progressive displacement of the pelvis is detected. The decision about appropriate surgical treatment is guided by the AO classification (Table 54.1).

YOUNG AND BURGESS CLASSIFICATION

The Young and Burgess classification predicts the degree of instability based on the direction of force that was applied to the pelvis and the resulting fracture pattern (Table 54.2).[7] The pelvic injury is caused by an anteroposterior compression (APC), a lateral compression (LC), or a vertical shear (VS) injury. There is also a combined mechanical (CM) group of complex multidirectional injuries. The APC and LC injuries are subdivided into types I, II, and III, representing the increasing degree of disruption (Fig. 54.4).

The Young and Burgess fracture type can be related to the risk of major pelvic haemorrhage and associated injuries, making the classification useful in the initial assessment of the patient.[7,8] The greatest risk of haemorrhage is in the more severe APC injuries resulting from an anterior crush or violent external rotation of the leg. Initially (APC I) only the symphysis pubis is split (widened less than 2.5 cm). Then (APC II) the pelvic floor tears (sacrospinous ligament rupture) and the anterior sacroiliac joint is ruptured, but the posterior ligaments remain intact (acting as a hinge as the 'book' opens), with external rotation of the hemipelvis. In the final stage (APC III), the posterior ligaments rupture, with complete separation and lateral displacement of the hemipelvis (but without vertical displacement, which distinguishes this from the VS injury, but both are AO type C injuries). The APC III injury is associated with mean blood loss of 15 units, due to the degree of internal pelvic soft tissue disruption and torn pelvic venous plexus vessels.

The LC injuries are the most common type of pelvic fracture but are least likely to cause pelvic haemorrhage (mean blood loss 3 units in LC II). The LC injuries range from a simple fracture of the pubic ramus (LC I) following a fall on the side, to more severe internal rotation of the whole hemipelvis (LC II) after a road traffic accident or fall on to the side from height. Further internal rotation of one hemipelvis may cause external rotation of the contralateral hemipelvis (LC III). There is a high incidence of head injury, lateral chest injury, and bladder or urethral injury.

The VS injury, often due to a fall from height, results in the whole hemipelvis being displaced upwards (disruption of both sacrospinous and sacrotuberous ligaments). There is an immediate risk of pelvic haemorrhage (mean blood loss 9 units) and higher risks of head injury and splenic rupture.

CLINICAL ASSESSMENT

The initial assessment of the injured patient aims to detect the presence of life-threatening or multiple injuries and haemodynamic instability or shock (systolic blood pressure less than 90 mmHg), to assess the degree of mechanical instability of the pelvic ring, and to diagnose associated pelvic soft tissue or organ injuries.

In most cases of pelvic injury, the patient is haemodynamically stable and a detailed clinical and radiological work-up for detection and grading of the pelvic injury can be made before definitive treatment is given.

The mechanism of injury is determined from the history, and may indicate the type of pelvic injury sustained as well as the presence of associated injuries. The clinical features of a pelvic fracture are pain, crepitus and tenderness over the symphysis pubis, anterior iliac crest or sacrum. Skin abrasions or contusions may be present at the point of impact or overlying the fracture sites, including the perineum. In the absence of lower limb fractures, leg length discrepancy and malrotation point to a displaced pelvic fracture or hip dislocation.

Manual assessment of pelvic stability should be performed carefully and not repeatedly, so as to avoid causing further internal bleeding; bimanual compression and distraction of the iliac wings may detect rotational instability, but push–pull

REFERENCES

7. Burgess AR, Eastridge BJ, Young JWR et al. J Trauma 1990; 30: 848–856
8. Dalal SA, Burgess AR, Siegal JH et al. J Trauma 1989; 29: 981–1002

Table 54.2 Young and Burgess classification of pelvic fractures

Type of injury	Incidence (%)	Direction of force	Direction of displacement
Anteroposterior compression (APC) I, II, III	26	Caused by anteroposterior compression of increasing severity	External rotation
Lateral compression (LC) I, II, III	41	Caused by lateral compression of increasing severity	Internal rotation
Combined mechanical (CM)	10	Combined mechanical, multidirectional	Vertical (proximal)
Vertical shear (VS)	5	Vertical shear injury	Complex combination

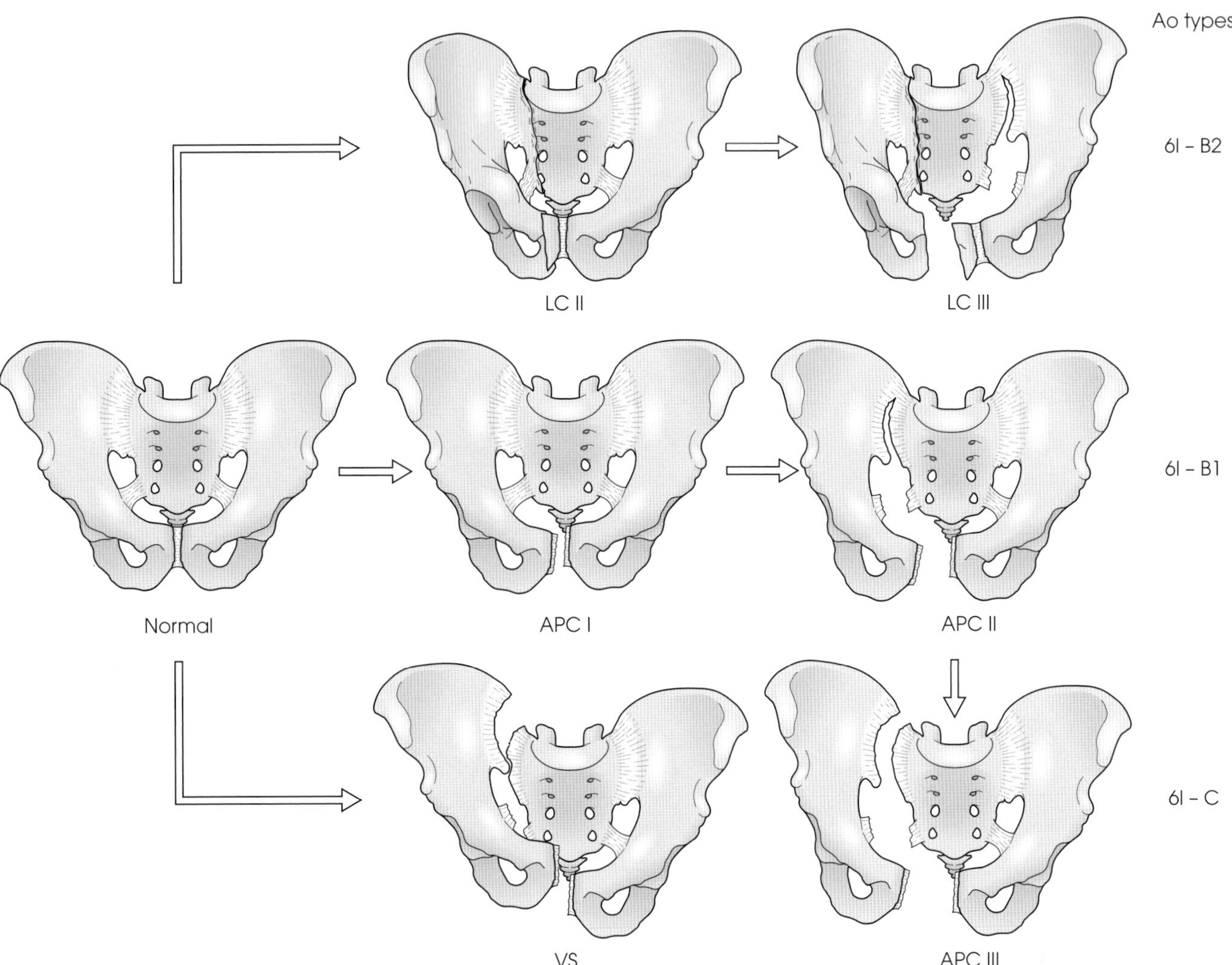

Figure 54.4 Classification of pelvic ring injuries, showing the progressive displacement and ligamentous injuries associated with unstable LC, APC and VS patterns (AO type B and C).

techniques of applying manual traction to the leg while palpating the pelvis should be performed only by an experienced surgeon.

The presence of associated pelvic injuries must be sought. Rectal and vaginal examinations are mandatory to detect bleeding from wounds of an occult open fracture. Neurological assessment is made, looking for signs of lumbosacral plexus injury. Peripheral pulses are checked. A urethral injury must be suspected with all displaced anterior pelvic ring injuries, and an ascending urethrogram performed prior to urethral catheterization. After catheterization a cystogram is performed to exclude a bladder rupture (see Ch. 36 and Ch. 38).

The diagnosis of the pelvic injury is based on the radiological examination. The standard anteroposterior pelvic radiograph is obtained early in the resuscitation process and provides a reliable working diagnosis in 90% of cases. Additional pelvic inlet and outlet views are obtained to evaluate further the fracture sites and degree of pelvic displacement (Fig. 54.5). Radiographic signs of pelvic instability include:

- displacement of more than 5 mm of the posterior pelvic complex,
- the presence of a posterior fracture gap (as opposed to impaction), and
- avulsion fractures of the transverse process of L5 vertebra (iliolumbar ligament) or of the sacral or ischial spine attachments of the sacrospinous ligament.

A CT scan is performed to further define the posterior pelvic injury and any associated acetabular fracture (Fig. 54.6). The CT scan is not used for the emergency evaluation of the pelvis and is delayed usually until the general condition of the patient is stable. However, using a modern spiral CT scanner, the pelvic CT scan can be combined with the emergency CT evaluation of the chest and abdomen if indicated. A three-dimensional CT scan reconstruction can be made to aid visualization of the fracture displacement and rotational deformity (Fig. 54.7).

EMERGENCY MANAGEMENT OF PELVIC HAEMORRHAGE

In the presence of haemodynamic instability, immediate resuscitation of the patient is commenced using Advanced Trauma Life Support® guidelines (see Ch. 7).[9] Plain anteroposterior radiographs of the chest and pelvis are obtained. If an unstable pelvic fracture is present, the principles are to confirm the pelvis

REFERENCES

9. Committee on Trauma of the American College of Surgeons. Advanced Trauma Life Support Student Course Manual. American College of Surgeons, Chicago, 1997

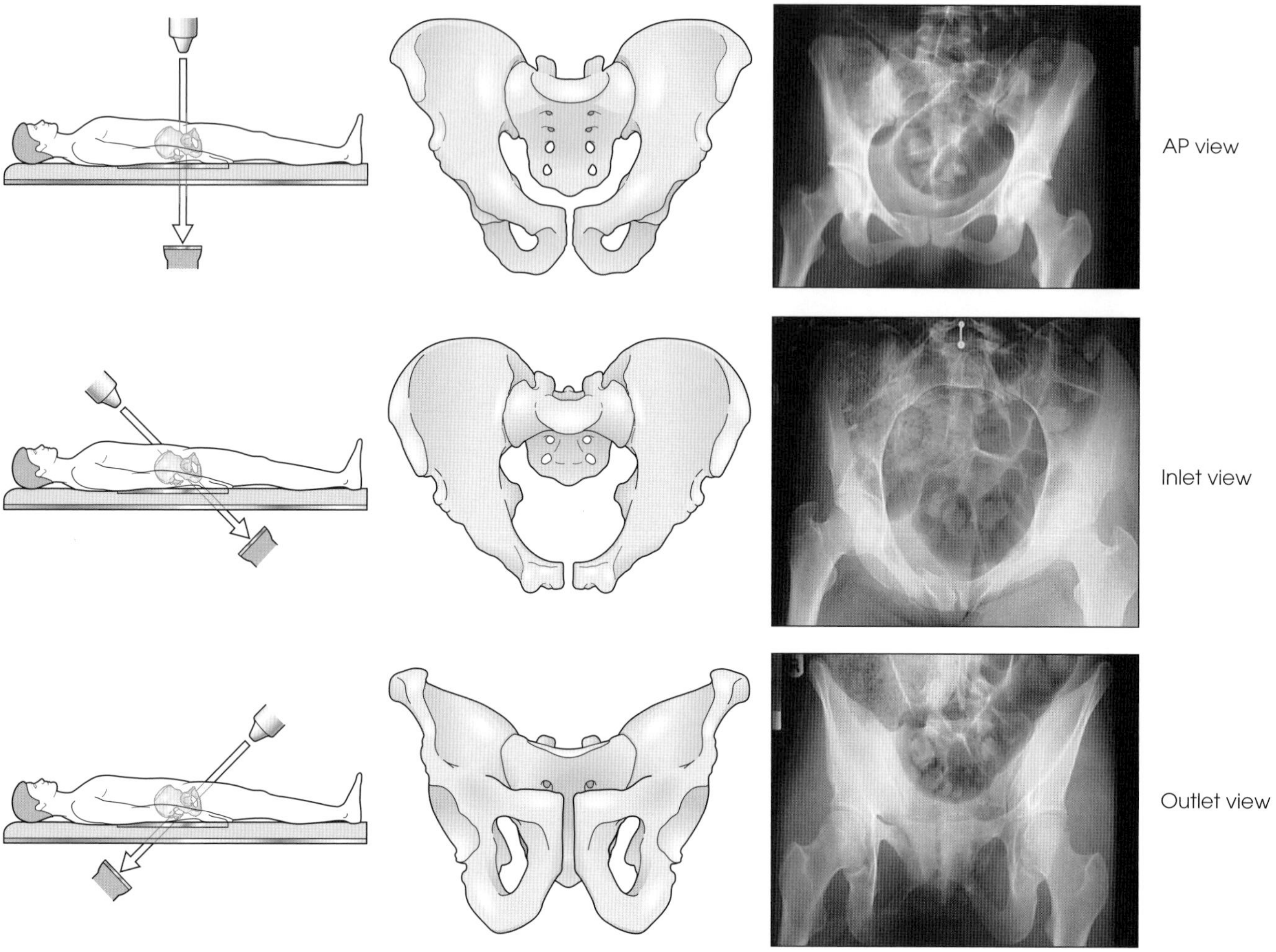

AP view

Inlet view

Outlet view

Figure 54.5 The standard anteroposterior, inlet and outlet radiographic views of the pelvis, showing the positioning of the x-ray beam and the representation of the pelvic views obtained, (b) the inlet view displays the pelvic ring clearly and reveals any internal or external rotation and posterior displacements of the hemipelvis whereas (c) the outlet view displays the sacrum and pubic rami clearly and reveals any vertical displacement of the hemipelvis. The radiographs show a VS fracture of the left sacrum with displacement and bilateral pubic rami fractures.

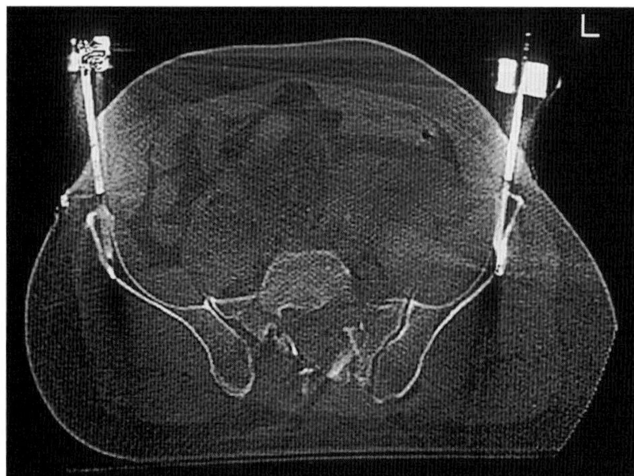

Figure 54.6 A CT scan of the pelvis, demonstrating the displacement of the posterior pelvic fracture, which has not been reduced adequately by application of an anterior external fixator alone.

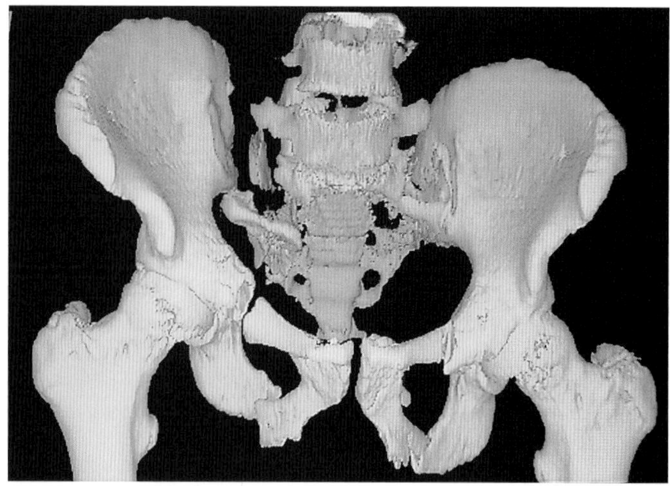

Figure 54.7 A three-dimensional CT scan (anteroposterior view), showing the major displacement of the VS fracture of the right pelvis, with associated bilateral pubic rami fractures.

Box 54.1 Control of haemorrhage

Fill them up, wrap them up, warm them up

- Intravenous fluids and blood transfusion
- Identify other sites of bleeding: chest, abdomen, open fracture
- Stabilize pelvis: binder, external fixator, open reduction and internal fixation
- Open packing of pelvis
- Angiography and embolization
- Prevent or correct hypothermia
- Replace clotting factors: fresh frozen plasma, platelets

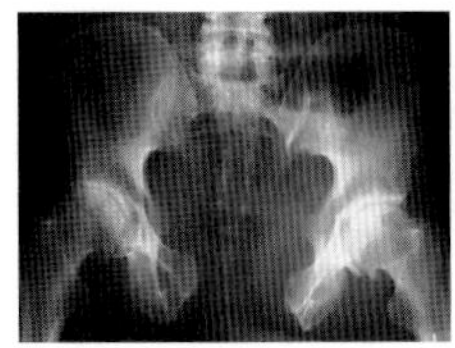
a
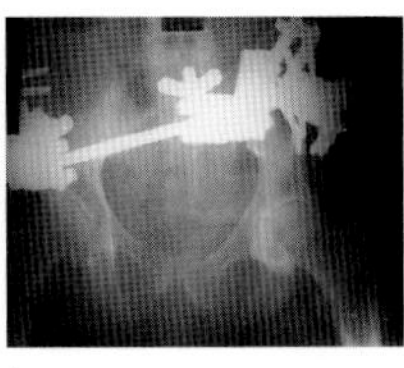
b
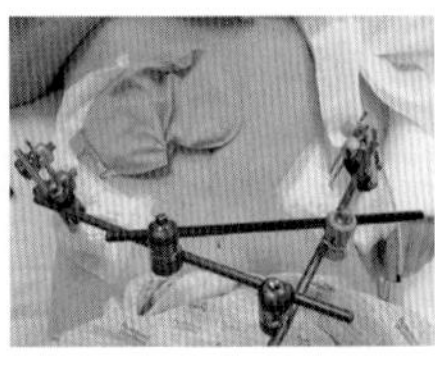
c

Figure 54.8 Emergency external fixation of the pelvis: (a) APC III injury of the left pelvis, (b) following application of the external fixator to close the 'open book', and (c) a typical A-frame configuration of the pelvic external fixator.

as the site of internal bleeding, exclude or treat other sources of bleeding, and gain immediate control of the haemorrhage (Box 54.1). Other sources of blood loss include bleeding into the chest or abdomen, long bone fractures, open wounds or retroperitoneal haematoma. Intraperitoneal bleeding is evaluated using peritoneal lavage, focused abdominal sonography for trauma (FAST) or CT scan.[10] The trauma scan is a spiral CT scan consisting of head and neck CT, chest, abdomen and pelvis CT with intravenous contrast given 15 min before scanning, which obviates the need for a cystogram.[1] Immediate laparotomy may be required to control intraperitoneal bleeding, in which case a pelvic external fixator must be applied first to stabilize the pelvic ring injury and to prevent further bleeding from loss of the tamponade effect when the abdomen is opened.

Bleeding from open wounds may be controlled temporarily by manual pressure and packing. Limb fractures are splinted. Hypothermia and coagulopathy must be prevented or corrected urgently.

If the bleeding is of pelvic origin, mechanical stabilization of the unstable pelvic ring will often reduce blood loss and restore haemodynamic stability.[11] Compression of the pelvis can be achieved with a circumferential sheet and towel clamp (sheeting), use of a proprietary pelvic binder, or application of an external fixator in the emergency room (Fig. 54.8). The pelvic binder is recommended because it can be applied simply and rapidly, is inexpensive, and does not require any surgical expertise. The binder can be maintained temporarily until surgical stabilization of the pelvis is undertaken in the operating theatre.

External fixation of the pelvis is achieved by placing percutaneous pins in each anterior iliac crest and linking the two sides of the pelvis with an anterior frame. Manual compression of the pelvis (in APC types) and longitudinal traction (in VS types) will facilitate reduction of the pelvis prior to tightening the fixator. A single pin fixator (with one pin inserted in each ilium) can be applied rapidly to "close the book" prior to laparotomy,[12] otherwise a conventional fixator (with three pins in each side) is recommended for definitive stabilization to reduce the risks of pin cut-out, loosening and infection. The pelvic C clamp is an alternative form of fixator that can be used to compress the posterior pelvis more effectively but requires careful pin placement under fluoroscopy screening.[13]

The sites of bleeding of pelvic fractures are venous or osseous in 80–90% of cases and arterial in only 10%. If the patient remains haemodynamically unstable after external fixation, arterial bleeding is suspected and pelvic angiography with embolization of any bleeding vessels is indicated.[14] The procedure is successful in controlling bleeding in 67–95% of cases, but two-thirds of patients will die later from other injuries or complications of multiple trauma. In Europe, some centres prefer to proceed directly to open surgical packing of the pelvis with simultaneous application of a pelvic C clamp to stabilize the posterior pelvis,[1,15] reserving angiography for cases in which bleeding continues after packing.

Open fractures of the pelvis with wounds in the perineum, vagina or rectum require emergency surgery: wound debridement and irrigation, diversion of the faecal stream by defunctioning colostomy (placed in the upper abdomen away from the pelvis) and distal colonic washout, external fixation of the pelvis, and antibiotic prophylaxis.[16] As well as pelvic bleeding, there is a high risk of deep infection and of death (20–50%).

DEFINITIVE FIXATION

Undisplaced fractures are treated with early mobilization of the patient; those with LC I injuries can mobilize, safely weight-bearing to tolerance of pain within a few days, and others remain partial weight-bearing on the affected side until union of the fracture by 8 weeks. A check anteroposterior pelvic radiograph is advisable within a week of mobilization to detect progressive displacement, which is rare.

More severe displaced pelvic fractures require closed or open reduction and stabilization by external or internal fixation until adequate ligamentous and bony healing occurs. Detailed descriptions of surgical approaches and operative techniques are available in specialist textbooks.[3,5,17] If an external fixator was applied as an emergency and satisfactory alignment of the pelvic ring is maintained, then the fixator may be used for definitive treatment until healing of the pelvic ring. The fixator may be

REFERENCES

10. Hoff WS, Holevar M, Nagy KK et al. J Trauma 2002; 53: 602–615
11. DiGiacomo JC, Bonadies JA, Cole FJ et al. Practice Management Guidelines for Haemorrhage in Pelvic Fracture: the EAST Practice Management Guidelines Work Group. Eastern Association for the Surgery of Trauma, 2001. www.east.org/tpg/pelvis.pdf
12. Tucker MC, Nork SE, Simonian PT et al. J Trauma 2000; 49: 989–994
13. Heini PF, Witt J, Ganz R. Injury 1996; 27 (Suppl 1): A38–A45
14. Cook RE, Keating JF, Gillespie I. J Bone Joint Surg 2002; 84B: 178–182
15. Ertel W, Keel M, Eid K et al. J Orthop Trauma 2001; 15: 468–474
16. Jones AL, Powell JN, Kellam JF et al. Orthop Clin North Am 1997; 28: 345–350
17. Tile M, Helfet DL, Kellam JF. Fractures of the Pelvis and Acetabulum. 3rd edn. Lippincott Williams & Wilkins, Philadelphia, 2003

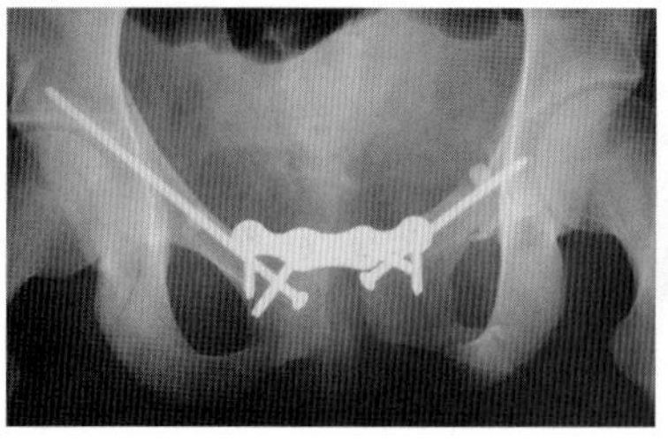
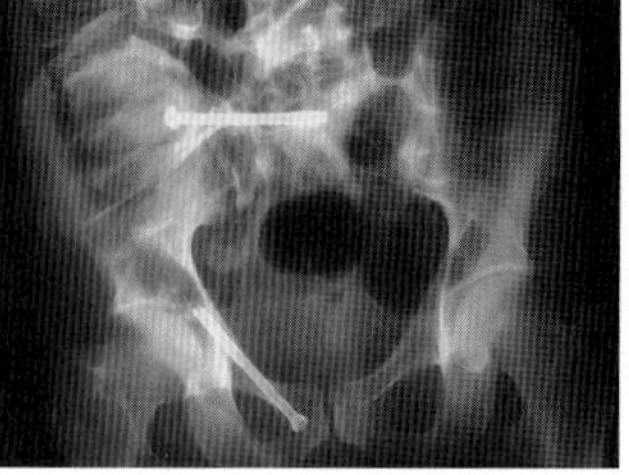
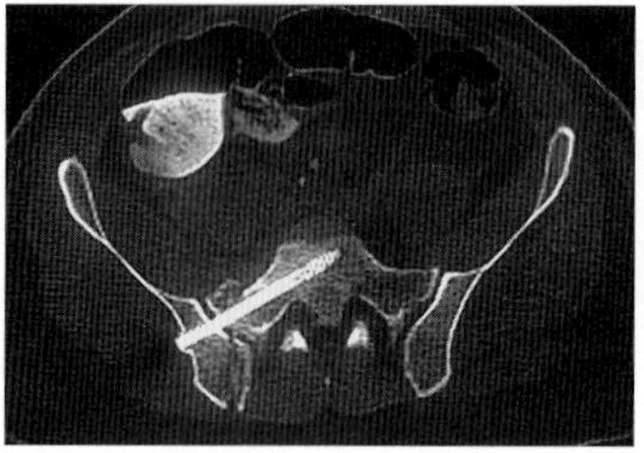
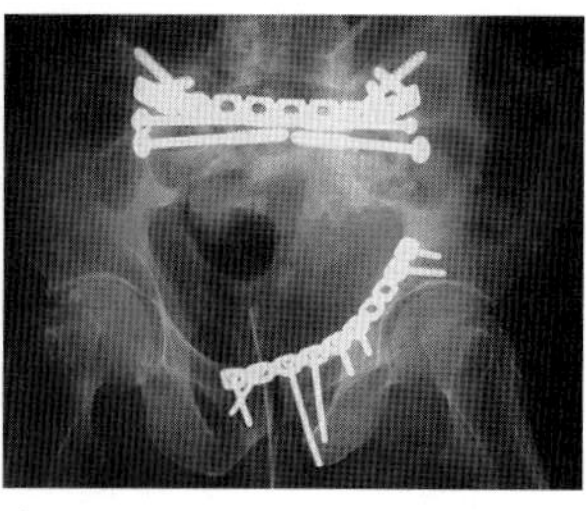

a b c d

Figure 54.9 Methods of internal fixation of the pelvis: (**a**) symphysis plate for symphysis disruption (and bilateral retrograde medullary screws to stabilize associated pubic rami fractures) in an APC III injury; (**b**) percutaneous insertion of an anterior pubic ramus screw and a posterior iliosacral screw in a VS injury; (**c**) a CT scan showing the position of the iliosacral screw in the sacrum at S1 level; and (**d**) extensive anterior and posterior pelvic stabilization with plates and iliosacral screws (type C injury).

used alone in type B injuries or in combination with internal fixation of the posterior pelvis in type C injuries (Table 54.1). Fracture union may occur within 8 weeks but ligamentous healing may take 12–16 weeks. Such prolonged use of the external fixator is associated with an increased risk of pin-site loosening, infection and loss of reduction. In general, internal fixation is preferred unless the patient has soft tissue injuries or an indwelling suprapubic catheter that pose a risk of infection in the operative field.

Anterior pelvic injuries include symphysis pubis diastasis, pubic rami fractures, or a combination of both. The symphysis pubis is reduced using a modified Pfannelsteil midline approach between the rectus abdominis muscles, and stabilized with a 4- or 6-hole plate and screws. A longer plate can be extended to bridge an associated pubis ramus fracture. Isolated or bilateral pubic rami fractures may be stabilized with plates through a modified Stoppa approach or by percutaneous retrograde medullary screw fixation and image-guided surgery (Fig. 54.9).[18]

Posterior pelvic injuries include iliac wing fractures, sacral fractures, sacroiliac joint dislocation, or a combination of these. Open reduction of an iliac wing fracture can be achieved using either a lateral exposure, reflecting the gluteal muscle attachments, or an internal exposure using a limited ilioinguinal approach, reflecting iliacus muscle medially. Surgical fixation is achieved with a combination of plates and lag screws. Sacroiliac joint disruptions may be reduced through:

- an anterior (limited ilioinguinal) approach and stabilization with two small bridging plates on the anterior aspect of the sacrum and ilium, or
- a dorsal approach exposing the posterior sacrum and ilium, enabling stabilization of the posterior pelvic complex with cannulated iliosacral screws, a posterior pelvic tension plate (bridging the lateral surfaces of each posterior ilium), or two sacral bars (rarely used now).

Percutaneous techniques for insertion of cannulated iliosacral screws from the lateral ilium, across the SI joint into the S1 sacral body, are preferred if closed reduction of the posterior pelvis can be achieved (Fig. 54.9).[18]

Postoperatively, early mobilization of the patient is undertaken if associated injuries allow, with partial weight-bearing for 8–12 weeks on the affected side.

COMPLICATIONS AND OUTCOME

The mortality rate associated with displaced pelvic fractures is 5–10% overall, rising to 30–40% in patients who are hypotensive on admission (systolic blood pressure less than 90 mmHg), and 50–70% if still shocked after external fixation of the pelvis. The cause of death may be related to pelvic bleeding in 25% of cases but is most often due to associated injuries, such as head injury, and the late consequences of polytrauma, such as adult respiratory distress syndrome and multiple organ failure.

The outcome of a pelvic ring injury is related to the type of fracture, the quality of reduction of the posterior pelvic complex, and the presence of neurological injury, and of associated injuries. Permanent disability is due to chronic pain in the posterior pelvis or low back, persisting pelvic instability or pelvic deformity (causing apparent leg length difference or sitting imbalance), nerve injury (neuralgia or paralysis), genitourinary or bowel dysfunction (urethral stricture, impotence, incontinence or dyspareunia), and other limb injuries. When treated non-operatively, long-term pain and disability have been reported in 40% of patients after stable type A fracture, 55% after type B, and 90% after type C fractures.[19] Surgical fixation of the unstable pelvic ring improves the outcome.[20] Studies from Germany and the USA have reported a good or excellent outcome in 79% of patients after internal fixation of type B injuries but in only 27% in type C cases, with patients being pain-free in 69–89% of type B and 33–50% of type C injuries.[21–24] Neurological injuries (L5, S1 or lower sacral roots) have a poor prognosis, being a cause of permanent disability in one-third of patients with type C fractures.

Thromboembolic complications are common in patients with pelvic (or acetabular) fractures, and prophylaxis with low molecular weight heparin or similar treatment is recommended.[25,26] Proximal deep vein thrombosis occurs in 25–35% of these patients, symptomatic pulmonary embolus in 2–10%, and

REFERENCES

18. Routt MRC, Nork SE, Mills WJ. Clin Orthop 2000; 375: 15–29
19. Fell M, Meissner A, Rahmanzadeh R. Zentralbl Chir 1995; 120: 899–904
20. Matta JM, Saucedo T. Clin Orthop 1989; 242: 83–87
21. Pohlemann T, Bosch U, Gansslen A et al. Clin Orthop 1994; 305: 69–80
22. Pohlemann T, Gansslen A, Schellwald O et al. Injury 1996; 27 (Suppl 2): B31–B83
23. Tornetta P III, Matta JM. Clin Orthop 1996; 329: 147–151
24. Tornetta P III, Matta JM. Clin Orthop 1996; 329: 186–193
25. Rogers FB, Cipolle MD, Velmahos G et al. J Trauma 2002; 53: 142–164
26. Steele N, Dodenhoff RM, Ward AJ et al. J Bone Joint Surg 2005; 87B(2): in press

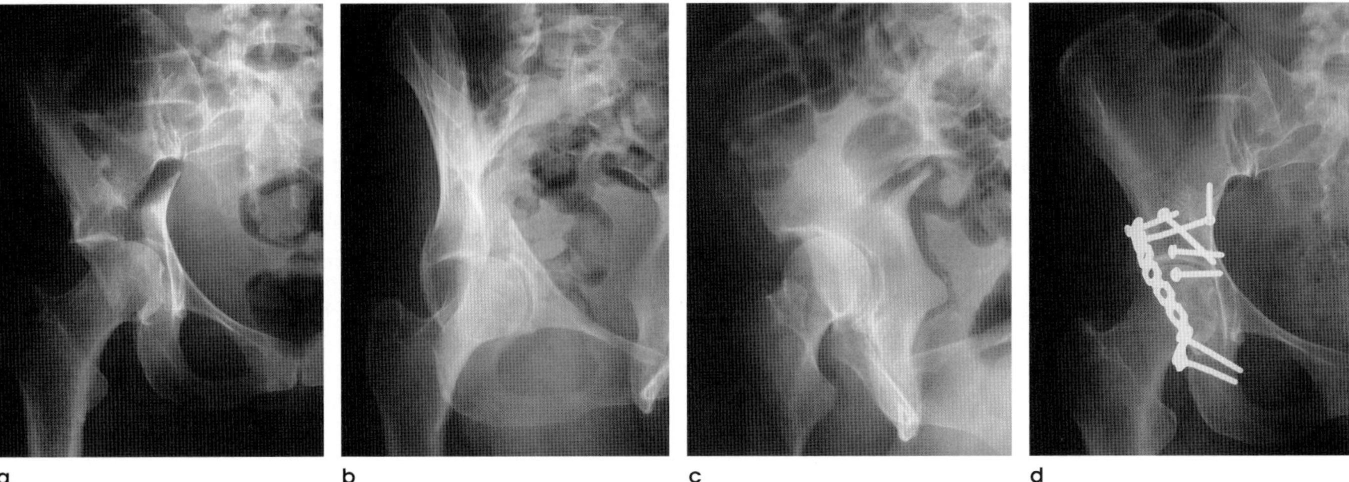

Figure 54.10 Standard radiographic views of the acetabulum: (a) anteroposterior X-ray, (b) obturator oblique, and (c) iliac oblique views of a transverse and posterior wall fracture of the right acetabulum; and (d) postoperative anteroposterior view demonstrating anatomical reduction of the acetabulum. The obturator oblique view shows the anterior column and posterior wall of the acetabulum most clearly, whereas the iliac oblique view shows the posterior column and the iliac wing above the acetabulum more readily.

fatal pulmonary embolism in 0.5–2% if prophylaxis is not employed.[27,28]

FRACTURES OF THE ACETABULUM

A fracture of the acetabulum occurs when an excessive force is transmitted through the femoral head on to the acetabulum, and the position of the leg at the time of impact determines the pattern of fracture sustained. With an impact to the front of the knee in a patient sitting with the hip flexed, as when driving, the direction of force results in a posterior wall or column fracture. The acetabular fracture may occur in isolation or in association with other pelvic ring injuries, femoral fractures, or other limb injuries.

Clinical and radiological assessments of the patient are performed to detect the presence of associated injuries and to determine the pattern of fracture (classification). Pain in the hip, lateral bruising, and an abnormal posture of the leg may indicate an acetabular fracture. Neurovascular assessment of the limb is important; sciatic nerve injury is common with posterior acetabular fracture and dislocations, and femoral or obturator nerve palsies may result from anterior acetabular fractures. Full radiological assessment includes an anteroposterior radiograph of the pelvis and hip joints, Judet oblique (45° orthogonal) views of the acetabulum, and a CT scan (with fine cuts of 2–3 mm) (Fig. 54.10). The degree of displacement of fracture fragments, the size of a posterior wall fracture, the presence of intra-articular fragments preventing congruent reduction of the femoral head, marginal impaction (depression) of the articular joint surface, and femoral head fractures can be documented. The three-dimensional CT reconstruction views are useful to visualize the fracture pattern (Fig. 54.11).

The Letournel classification[3] of acetabular fractures is widely used, subdividing fractures into five simple types and five complex types based on the site of the fracture lines through the anterior and/or posterior columns and walls. This classification is useful in planning the surgical approach for internal fixation and determining the approach. This classification has been incorporated into the AO comprehensive classification, which divides acetabular fractures into types A, B and C with subtypes 1–3, and is used for documentation purposes.[4,29]

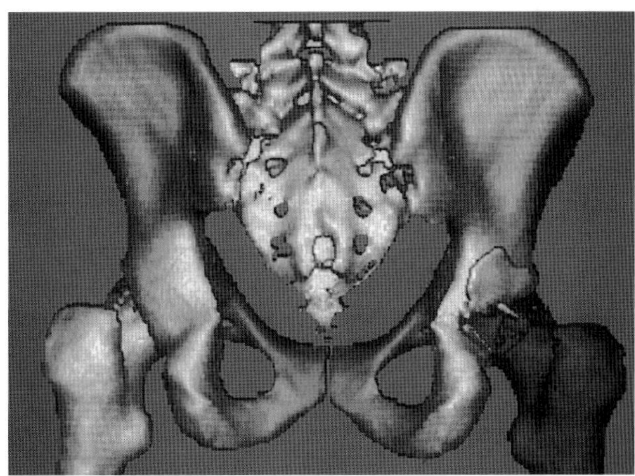

Figure 54.11 A three-dimensional CT scan (posterior view), showing a displaced posterior wall fracture of the right acetabulum.

A dislocation of the femoral head mandates urgent closed reduction of the hip joint to reduce the risk of consequent avascular necrosis of the femur and worsening sciatic nerve palsy. Open surgical reduction may be needed if closed reduction fails, or if there is an associated femoral neck fracture (to prevent secondary displacement during manipulation). The stability of the joint, the congruence of the femoral head in the acetabulum, and the displacement of the acetabular fracture are noted on radiological screening following reduction. Sciatic nerve function

REFERENCES

27. Geerts WH, Code KI, Jay RM et al. N Engl J Med 1994; 331: 1601–1606
28. Montgomery KD, Geerts WH, Potter HG et al. Clin Orthop 1996; 329: 68–89
29. Helfet DL, Bartlett CS. In: Ruedi TP, Murphy WM (eds). AO Principles of Fracture Management. Thieme, New York, 2000: 414–438

should be noted before and after reduction because entrapment of the nerve can occur. Skeletal traction is applied to the leg with a distal femoral pin (to avoid traction to potentially injured knee ligaments). In the presence of an acetabular fracture and persisting posterior instability, recurrent dislocation can occur despite traction, and an antirotation below-knee cast that holds the leg in external rotation may be needed. Close clinical review is necessary while awaiting definitive surgical treatment.

The aim of definitive treatment is to obtain healing of the acetabular fracture, with anatomical reduction of the articular surface, and preservation of normal joint congruity, stability and mechanics, to reduce the risk of post-traumatic osteoarthritis. Residual displacement or incongruity greater than 1–2 mm is unsatisfactory and more likely to lead to a poor long-term outcome.[3,30]

An undisplaced fracture of the acetabulum may be treated non-operatively with initial bed rest for 3 weeks (traction is not needed), minimal weight-bearing on the affected leg for 3 weeks, and increasing partial weight-bearing until union after 8–10 weeks. Non-operative treatment may be indicated for a displaced acetabular fracture if the patient is medically unfit to undergo major surgery, has severe osteoporosis, or has a fracture that is low (with preservation of congruity of the femoral head in the weight-bearing dome of the acetabulum).

In general, acetabular fractures that are displaced 2–3 mm in the major weight-bearing area will require open reduction and internal fixation. Surgery should be performed early (within 7–10 days) while the fracture fragments remain mobile, because this allows limited surgical approaches and indirect reduction techniques to be used.

The acetabular fracture type dictates the surgical approach needed for internal fixation. The Kocher–Langenbeck approach exposes the posterior and superior parts of the hip and innominate bone, allowing access inside the hip joint following distraction or dislocation of the femoral head. The exposure can be increased by a trochanteric flip, reflecting anteriorly the greater trochanter of the femur with attached muscles.[31] The ilioinguinal approach exposes the inner aspect of the pelvis and is used to access the anterior acetabulum and to treat some more complex fractures. Extensile approaches, such as the extended iliofemoral or triradiate, provide large exposure of inner and outer aspects of the pelvis and acetabulum simultaneously for stabilization of complex fractures, but they are associated with greater wound morbidity (blood loss, infection, muscle weakness and heterotopic ossification). Combined approaches (Kocher–Langenbeck plus ilioinguinal) are favoured by some surgeons.

Various methods of fracture fixation are practised using combinations of special pelvic plates and long screws. Special expertise and equipment are required to treat these fractures, and patients should be referred to a specialist pelvic and acetabular unit for definitive management. Minimally invasive surgical techniques, using percutaneous screw fixation and computer-assisted, image-guided surgery (fluoroscopy or CT-based imaging), are being refined.[32]

Postoperative anteroposterior radiograph and CT scans of the acetabulum are obtained to document the fracture reduction, hip congruity, and position of implant screws (to exclude intra-articular penetration). The hip joint may be mobilized on a continuous passive motion machine, and the patient mobilized from bed as soon as possible (other injuries allowing): touch minimal weight-bearing for 6 weeks and increasing partial weight-bearing for another 6 weeks until fracture union. As with pelvic fractures, perioperative antibiotic and pre- and postoperative deep vein thrombosis prophylaxis protocols should be followed.[26] Indomethacin (25 mg for 3–6 weeks) is used widely as prophylaxis against heterotrophic ossification (not needed after ilioinguinal approach), but a prospective randomized study has not shown any benefit of its use.[33] Alternatively, irradiation (single dose of 700 cGy) appears to be effective, used 24 h before surgery or postoperatively within 3 days.[34]

Complications include deep infection (1–3%), proximal deep vein thrombosis (10–20%), pulmonary embolism (1% fatal), sciatic nerve palsy (12–39%), heterotopic ossification (limiting function in 4–6%), avascular necrosis (2–10%), and post-traumatic osteoarthritis (20–35%). The long-term outcome is good or excellent in 75–85% of surgical-treated cases. Factors associated with post-traumatic osteoarthritis include the severity of initial trauma (type of fracture and degree of comminution), the quality of reduction (residual displacement in the weight-bearing dome), persisting incongruency, and instability of the joint. Hip arthrodesis is difficult to achieve, and total hip replacement is preferred for late reconstruction of the hip.

REFERENCES

30. Matta JM. J Bone Joint Surg 1996; 78A: 1632–1645
31. Ganz R, Gill TJ, Gautier K et al. J Bone Joint Surg 2001; 83B: 1119–1124
32. Kabler DM. In: Tile M, Helfet DL, Kellam JF (eds). Fractures of the Pelvis and Acetabulum. 3rd edn. Lippincott Williams & Wilkins, Philadelphia, 2003: 604-615
33. Matta JM, Siebenrock KA. J Bone Joint Surg 1997; 79B: 959–963
34. Burd TA, Lowry KJ, Anglen JO. J Bone Joint Surg 2001; 83A: 1783–1788

Fractures of the lower limb

55

John R.W. Hardy

INTRODUCTION

This chapter considers the modern management of fractures of the lower limb. The term *fracture* is defined as a loss of the normal continuity of bone diaphysis, metaphysis, physis, epiphysis and joint cartilage. Trauma is the commonest cause of fracture to the lower limb. Fractures are commonly seen in patients with multiple trauma, in which cases the management of the skeletal injury follows only after the management of life-threatening injury (see Ch. 7). The age of a patient determines the pattern of a fracture and the level of energy required to break a bone (see Ch. 52). In the lower limb, the fracture neck of femur is typically associated with osteoporosis in the elderly woman. Predisposing factors for fracture after a single loading insult depend on the type, rate and magnitude of the force as well as the underlying structural and material properties of the bone. This explains why a fall from standing fractures the femoral neck in an osteoporotic older patient, while a young man's hip survives a single load of the same proportions.

The symptoms and signs of fractures are dependent on the stability of the skeleton after fracture and injury to the surrounding soft tissues. All clinically suspected fractures (i.e. a history of an injury and pain) must be further investigated.

Modern classifications of lower limb fractures consider the patterns of bony injury within each region of the lower limb.[1] This is the AO classification, which divides each bone into three segments, each segment into three types (usually depending on the number of fragments), each type into groups of three (depending on the pattern of fracture), and each group into three subgroups. The pattern of this classification reflects the increasing severity of injury experienced by the bone segment. Management of the fractures of each of the AO segments is considered later in this chapter. The AO classification is not yet exhaustive of all patterns of injury.

Classifications, other than being just the pattern of bony injury, allow the clinician to consider a sensible approach to treatment. Fractures of the lower limb may be classified according to their site, the associated soft tissue injury, the number of fragments and their displacement, and any associated complications.

The prognosis depends on the severity of the injury, the age and general condition of the patient, the restoration of function, the prevention of deformity, and the minimization of treatment complications.

Complications of the lower limb bone fractures are common, as are complications of treatment. The complications that attend the fractures themselves are considered separately. The complications of treatment should be classified into general complications or local complications. Local complications vary, depending on the region of fracture and the method of treatment. Because the optimum treatment depends on the fracture classification, complications of treatments are considered on a regional basis.

THE CLINICAL HISTORY OF LOWER LIMB FRACTURE

A history of pain following injury, regardless of how insignificant the trauma might seem, should always suggest the possibility of a fracture. This is especially true in the elderly with osteoporotic bone. Likewise, a fracture that results from cyclic stress (fatigue) is often missed unless a careful history is taken of the onset, the duration, and the periodicity of the pain. A history of pain in the foot or tibia following long periods of exercise, regardless of the minimal signs present, should always be further investigated by radiographs. The symptoms of fracture in the lower limb may include pain, deformity, and a loss of function.

THE PHYSICAL SIGNS OF LOWER LIMB FRACTURES

The physical signs of a fracture may be surprisingly minimal and depend on the pattern of injury. An undisplaced fracture often allows preservation of function. This cannot therefore be taken as an indication that the bone is intact. The usual signs of fracture include tenderness at the fracture site, swelling, bruising, deformity, and occasionally crepitus of the fractured ends of the bone. Crepitus should not be specifically elicited during the examination process, but it is occasionally discovered. The 'look, feel, move' principle provides a logical order for eliciting signs.

INVESTIGATION OF LOWER LIMB FRACTURES

Radiographs have been the mainstay of investigation since X-rays were developed in Germany by Wilhelm Konrad Röntgen (1845–1923). Röntgen was a physicist who in 1894 published an original paper on the medical use of X-rays; on 7 January 1895, the technique was reported in the London Evening Standard.

A useful adage in the investigation of fractured limbs is the rule of two. This is that two radiographs should always be taken with views at 90° to each other; the radiographs, like the clinical

REFERENCES

1. Müller ME, Nazarian S, Koch P et al. The Comprehensive Classification of Fractures of Long Bones. Springer-Verlag, Berlin, 1990

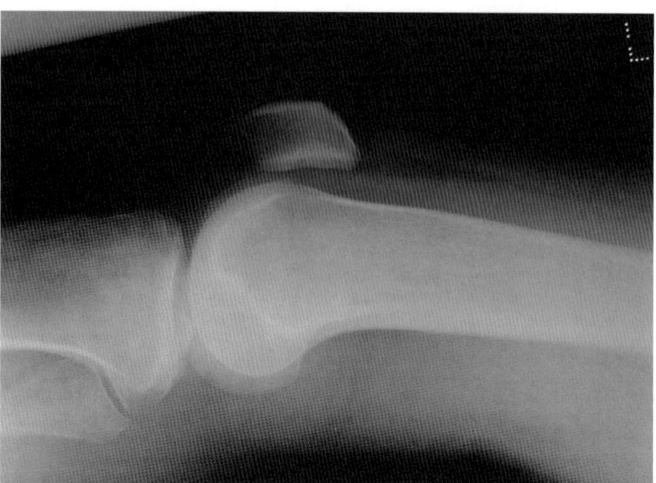

Figure 55.1 Fluid or fat level on a lateral radiograph of a knee that has suffered an osteochondral fracture.

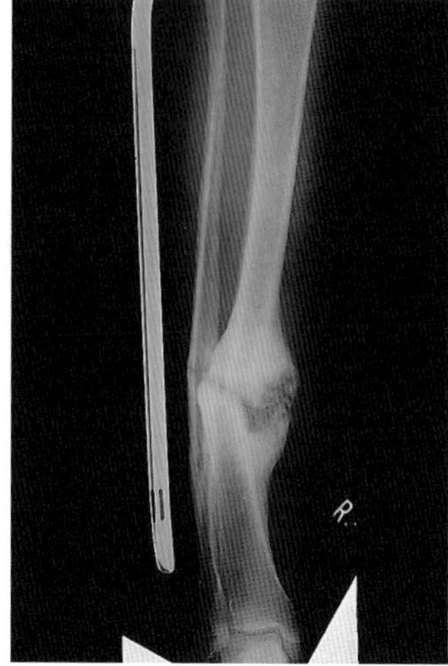
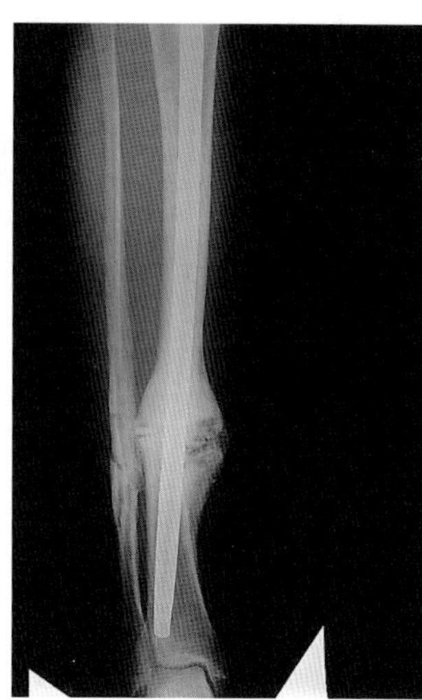

Figure 55.2 Hypertrophic non-union is treated by stabilizing a fracture, as with this intramedullary nail. Bone grafting is not required as it is with atrophic non-union.

examination, should always include the two joints either end of the long bone. Radiographs taken at two intervals in time are often required, and occasionally radiographs of the two sides for comparison of the normal anatomy can be useful. When a fracture is suspected but not visible on the early radiographs, more can be done. The clinician who suspects an occult fracture in the lower limb can either wait for the fracture line to become more visible with time and resorption, or resort to a radioisotope bone scan. When a fracture is present around the knee, involvement of the joint can be deduced if the lateral radiograph of the knee shows a fluid or fat level (Fig. 55.1). Magnetic resonance imaging is particularly useful for demonstrating associated soft tissue injury and bone 'bruising' if occult fractures through the metaphysis are difficult to visualize radiographically.

COMPLICATIONS OF FRACTURES IN THE LOWER LIMB

DELAYED AND NON-UNION

Delayed union is one of the commonest complications following fractures of the lower limb, especially in the tibia.[2] Delayed union is defined as having taken place 'when clinical union of the fracture occurred after more than 20 weeks of immobilization'.[3,4] Clinical union is said to have occurred when 'pressure over the fracture and "springing" the bone fails to elicit pain'.

The current convention is that non-union has occurred when clinical and radiographic union has not happened within 6 months of fracture.[3] Some authors have extended this definition to 30 weeks[5] and 8 months.[4]

In atrophic non-union of the tibial diaphysis, patients take more than 6 months to produce the callus needed to reduce fracture site movement enough to begin the remodelling process. Atrophic non-union in association with a fracture gap and a united or intact fibula may respond to partial fibulectomy.[6] The standard treatment includes bone grafting.

The next commonest type of non-union again occurs in the tibial diaphysis. This is associated with the excessive production of callus due to too much movement at the fracture site: hypertrophic non-union (Fig. 55.2).

REFRACTURE

The risk of refracture in weight-bearing bones is higher than in the upper limb. Refracture following removal of plates used for treating tibial shaft fractures can be as low as 1.7%.[7] Failure of bone in these circumstances is probably from a single load rather than fatigue loading. Fracture may occur at the original site or through screw holes. After dynamic compression plating, most refractures occur through a screw hole.

Refracture rates are less predictable after external fixation of the lower limb. This is especially true following premature fixator removal;[8,9] it is twice as common when supplementary lag screws are used.[10] Refracture probably occurs either with a single load large enough to break the callus bridge or by fatigue failure at lower loads, and it tends to occur during sport. All patients should be warned to avoid contact sports until at least 12 months after removal of a plate. In adults, Böstman found the incidence of refracture of tibial fractures to be 2.4%. Refracture occurred most commonly in spiral fractures, those with a fracture of the fibula at a different level from that of the fibula, and those with marked initial displacement.[11] Refracture is a common complication of external fixation. New methods of determining the progression of fracture healing by the serial measurement of fracture

REFERENCES

2. Anderson R, Burgess E. J Bone Joint Surg 1943; 25: 427–432
3. Ellis H. J Bone Joint Surg 1958; 40B: 42–46
4. Johner R, Wruhs O. Clin Orthop 1983; 178: 7–25
5. Oni OOA, Hui A, Gregg PJ. J Bone Joint Surg 1988; 70B: 787–790
6. DeLee JC, Heckman JD, Lewis AG. J Bone Joint Surg 1981; 63A: 1390–1395
7. Bilat C, Leutenegger A, Ruedi T. Injury 1994; 25: 349–358
8. Rommens P, Broos P, Gruwez J. Arch Orthop Trauma Surg 1986; 105: 170–174
9. Gershuni DH, Halma G. J Trauma 1983; 23: 986–990
10. Krettek C, Haas N, Tscherne H. J Bone Joint Surg 1991; 73A: 893–897
11. Böstman OM. Injury 1983; 15: 93–98

Table 55.1 Gustilo and Anderson's classification of open fractures, based on a large series of tibial fractures

Gustilo and Anderson type	Soft tissue injury	Bony injury
0	Skin intact	Any except segmental fractures
I	< 1 cm laceration and clean	Any except segmental fractures
II	> 1 cm laceration; no extensive sort tissue damage, flaps or avulsions	Any except segmental fractures
IIIa	Adequate soft tissue coverage despite extensive laceration or flaps, or high-energy trauma irrespective of size of wound	Any
IIIb	Extensive soft tissue injury loss with periosteal stripping and bone exposure; usually associated with massive contamination	Any
IIIc	Arterial injury requiring repair	Any

stiffness[12] have been reported and may help to reduce refracture in the tibia.[13]

COMPOUND FRACTURES

All compound wounds must be treated aggressively.[14] The Gustilo classification was specifically devised for the management of tibial fractures (Table 55.1). It is often applied to any compound fracture, dividing open wounds into three types.[15–17] The revised Gustilo classification takes into account the mechanism of injury, degree of soft tissue damage, fracture configuration and wound contamination.[18] External fixation is the mainstay of management of compound fractures in the lower limb because of the reluctance to leave foreign material within a contaminated wound. Metal, like any inert material, can act as a nidus for bacterial infection. Compound fractures tend to be as a result of high-energy injuries and are associated with much periosteal stripping. Therefore they are often complicated by delayed union as well as by deep infection.[19]

The treatment of compound wounds has been considered (see Ch. 52). Operative management should never be delayed more than 6 h. In the leg, a tourniquet may be applied but should not be used unless uncontrolled haemorrhage is discovered. Between 2 and 10 L of saline must be used to irrigate the often larger wounds of the lower limb. In these circumstances the risk of cross-infection of the patient from bacterial ingress through wet drapes, and of the theatre staff from viral infection, necessitates use of universal precautions and modern drapes that entrap blood and irrigation fluids (Fig. 55.3).

The patient's lower limb should be elevated in the post-operative period (Fig. 55.4) until the skin has healed in order to reduce the risk of tissue fluid leakage on mobilization and subsequent infection. Patients should be encouraged to exercise their lower limb during this period of elevation. A fixed plantigrade foot should be prevented by the early use of a back-slab or anti-foot-drop orthosis.

INFECTION

Both superficial and deep infection can complicate a fracture. Superficial infection is commonly a postoperative complication related to the general condition of the patient and the skin closure technique. In most series deep infection (osteomyelitis) is a rare event following fractures of the leg, but it is still most common in patients with a compound fracture. To avoid infection in the leg, most practices employ modern compound fracture management and have abandoned using plaster casts with transfixing pins.[20,21] Deep infection is important because it is associated with a doubling of the healing time[22] and can lead to other morbid conditions, such as amyloidosis.

Operative fixation of a fracture, especially a compound fracture, is associated with a higher incidence of osteomyelitis.[23] Bone and Johnson showed, in a series of closed nailing for tibial fractures, that for Gustilo grade II and III wounds there was 10 times the risk of infection compared with the closed or grade I wounds.[24] This may be reduced to 10–16% of Gustilo type II or III wounds by aggressive debridement and early soft tissue cover.[25,26]

Externally fixed fractures tend to have a low incidence of deep infection unless the wound is compound. Most pin tract infection

REFERENCES

12. Hardy JRW, de Jonge EJ, Richardson JB. J Orthop Tech 1994; 2: 177–189
13. Richardson JB, Kenwright J, Cunningham JL. Clin Biomech 1992; 7: 75–79
14. British Orthopaedic Association and British Association of Plastic Surgeons Working Party. The Early Management of Severe Tibial Fractures: the Need for Combined Plastic and Orthopaedic Management. A Report by the British Orthopaedic Association and British Association of Plastic Surgeons Working Party, January 1993. BOA, London, 1993
15. Gustilo RB, Anderson JT. J Bone Joint Surg 1976; 58A: 453–458
16. Gustilo RB, Mendoza RM, Williams DN. J Trauma 1984; 24: 742–746
17. Gustilo RB, Gruninger RP. Orthopaedics 1987; 10: 1781–1788
18. Gustilo RB, Merkow RL, Templeman D. J Bone Joint Surg 1990; 72A: 299–303
19. Dellinger EP, Caplan ES, Weaver LD. Arch Surg 1988; 123: 333–339
20. Anderson LD, Hutchins WC. South Med J 1966; 59: 1026–1032
21. Clancey GJ, Hansen ST. J Bone Joint Surg 1978; 60A: 118–122
22. Edwards P, Nilsson BER. Acta Orthop Scand 1965; 36: 104–111
23. Klemm KW, Börner M. Clin Orthop 1986; 212: 89–100
24. Bone LB, Johnson KD. J Bone Joint Surg 1986; 68A: 877–887
25. Court-Brown CM, Christie J, McQueen MM. J Bone Joint Surg 1990; 72B: 605–611
26. Court-Brown CM, McQueen MM, Quaba AA et al. J Bone Joint Surg 1991; 73B: 959–964

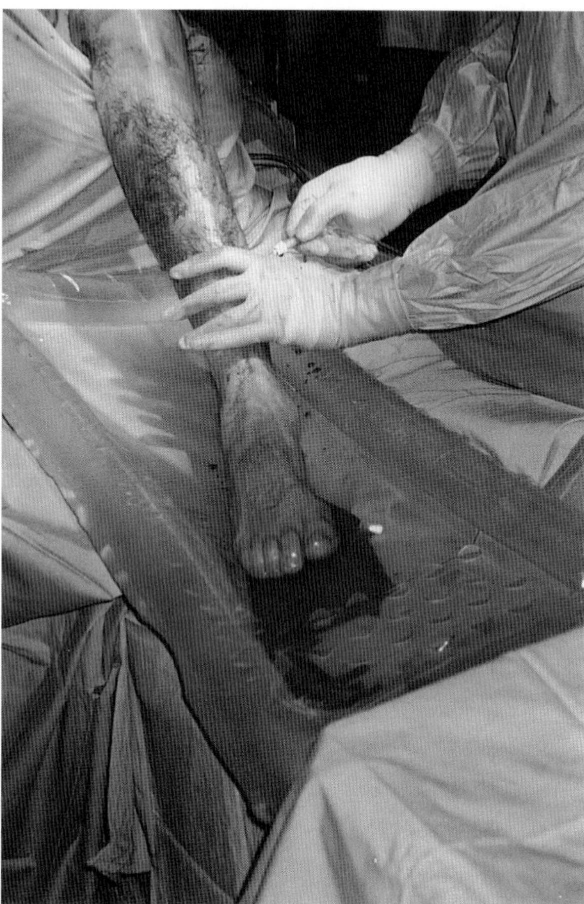

Figure 55.3 Use of an inflatable surgical tray to reduce the risks of exposure to theatre staff of 'substances hazardous to health', as recommended by Control of Substances Hazardous to Health regulations.

is superficial, but deep infection can occur and this leads to sequestra at the site of the pin, which may have a ring shape if the dead compressed bone around the pin becomes involved. Screw and plate fixation is probably best avoided in any compound fracture.[27] Other authors would argue that while type II or III open fractures are probably best treated by external fixation,[28] lesser injuries may be either plated, nailed or externally fixed.

MALALIGNMENT AND SHORTENING

No useful definitions exist for malunion. Most definitions relate the condition to imperfect restoration of the premorbid anatomical position of the fracture fragments. In clinical practice the term is reserved for cases in which the resulting deformity is felt to be clinically significant.

The long-term sequelae of malunion are unknown. Deformity is usually cosmetically unacceptable. There is also the belief that if the centre of gravity of the weight of the body is displaced from the centre of the knee or ankle joint then osteoarthritis will result. This is anecdotal. Many a surgeon has seen post-traumatic osteoarthritis after a perfect reduction and restoration of the normal biomechanical axis of the limb.

POST-TRAUMATIC OSTEOARTHRITIS

Injury to joint cartilage and subchondral bone is common following direct or indirect trauma to joints. Even trauma not detectable on normal radiographs can cause subchondral

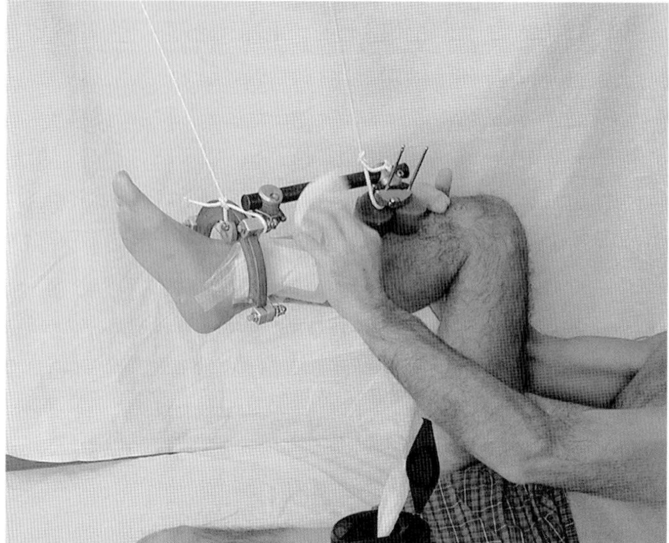

Figure 55.4 Use of external fixation and a Balkan beam to elevate the limb after trauma.

fracture that leads to hastened degenerative changes.[29,30] More obvious irregularities of the joint surface following fracture lead to rapid degenerative changes; these also occur following vascular insult to the subchondral bone, such as is seen after avascular necrosis following intracapsular fracture neck of femur.

NEUROVASCULAR COMPLICATIONS

Neurovascular complications are common following leg injuries, especially after dislocation of the knee. Both nerve and vascular injuries can be direct or indirect. Indirect injury of nerves and vessels from compartment syndrome is often overlooked. Correction of vascular compromise of a limb must take place at the earliest opportunity and takes precedence over the fixation of bone. Compartment syndrome that requires treatment occurs in about 3% of all tibial fractures.

Compartment syndrome

Compartment syndrome is from increased pressure within a muscular compartment, which leads to tissue necrosis. The symptoms are of ischaemic pain out of proportion to the injury, and its early management is by splinting and analgesia. The signs are elicited by passive stretch of the muscles suspected of being involved. The tightness of the compartment and the presence of peripheral pulses cannot be relied on as useful signs. Impaired function of peripheral nerves suggests that the ischaemia is advanced.

Classically, compartment pressures are measured using a slit catheter device. Compartment pressures in excess of 30–35 mmHg in a normally perfused patient suggested the need for open compartment fasciotomy.[31] In patients without

REFERENCES

27. Clifford RP, Beauchamp CG, Kellam JF et al. J Bone Joint Surg 1988; 70B: 644–648
28. Bach AW, Hansen ST. Clin Orthop 1989; 241: 89–94
29. Radin EL, Parker HG, Pugh JW et al. Biomechanics 1973; 6: 51–57
30. Atkinson PJ, Haut RC. J Orthop Res 1995; 13: 936–944
31. Bourne RB, Rorabeck CH. Clin Orthop 1989; 240: 97–104

symptoms, monitored pressures do not relate to outcome in any way.[32] However, there is evidence to suggest that if the difference between the diastolic pressure and the measured compartment pressure is less than 30 mmHg, then fasciotomies should be performed.

Management of this complication must be immediate, decisive, and aggressive enough to divide the skin and deep fascial envelope the length of the limb because the skin envelope can significantly contribute to compartment pressures.[33] All compartments should be incised, depending on the part of the lower limb involved. Debridement of necrotic muscle is necessary to minimize the effects of fibrotic contraction, dead muscle being recognized by the 4 Cs, namely lack of colour, consistency, contractility and capacity to bleed.

Nerve injury

Direct nerve injury following fracture in the leg is relatively rare. Fractures around the proximal fibula occasionally cause a dropped foot due to common peroneal nerve injury. The treatment of this is expectant, because most direct injuries are due to neuropraxia and over 70% resolve within months. Persistent lesions more than 6 months after injury should be investigated and nerve grafting considered. Compartment syndrome should always be considered with dropped foot, even in the presence of a proximal fibula fracture.

Vascular injury

Vascular injury complicating fractures of the leg is rare, but the consequences when it occurs can be severe. Vascular injury is most common with fractures and dislocations around the knee. Immediate clinical diagnosis is imperative and pallid, pulseless, paraesthetic, paralysed, painful, 'perishing' cold limbs should never be ignored. An on-table arteriogram may be used to diagnose the level of the injury and should be performed to facilitate early reperfusion of the limb by a trained vascular surgeon.

Fixation of the fracture before or after reperfusion should be discussed with the vascular team. Fasciotomy will be necessary for almost all limb fractures complicated by arterial injury, and it should be performed as soon as reperfusion has been established and not left until signs of nerve involvement have developed.

Avascular necrosis

Avascular necrosis is most common following intracapsular fractures of the neck of femur in the lower limb. It also occurs after fractures of the femoral condyles and after talar neck fractures. In the talus, the presence of the Hawkins sign (rarefaction of the bone beneath the subchondral region of the talar dome) demonstrates the presence of an intact vascular supply to the talus.

REFLEX SYMPATHETIC DYSTROPHY

Often referred to as Sudeck's atrophy, Sudeck's osteodystrophy or post-traumatic painful osteodystrophy, reflex sympathetic dystrophy is characterized by pain, swelling, and loss of the ability to weight-bear. Marked joint stiffness is a late manifestation, as is swelling and loss of skin creases. Radiographs show a patchy osteoporosis. The condition is not uncommon following leg fracture, especially with fractures below the knee where patients treated in plaster have been reluctant to weight-bear for long periods.

Early recognition and treatment with intensive supervised rehabilitation with analgesia and physical therapy is more successful than neglect. Occasionally sympathetic nerve block is used as an adjunct to regular analgesia before physical therapy.

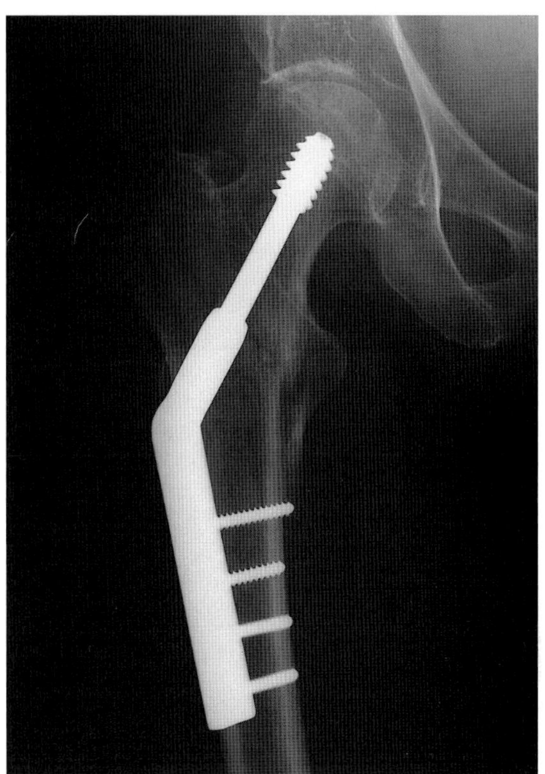

Figure 55.5 An extracapsular proximal femoral fracture immobilized with a dynamic hip screw.

FRACTURES AND DISLOCATIONS OF THE LOWER LIMB

THE FEMUR

Proximal femoral fractures

Proximal femoral fractures are classified into three types: extracapsular, intracapsular, and fractures of the femoral head (Fig. 55.5). The last is usually seen in the younger patient with traumatic dislocation of the hip joint. This classification is useful because it describes the risk of avascular necrosis for the injury. Intracapsular fractures have the greatest risk of non-union and avascular necrosis. A commonly quoted classification for intracapsular fractures is Garden's classification, which helps determine the management of the intracapsular fracture based on a study of prognosis.[34] Garden's classification is based on the anteroposterior radiograph and describes the relationship of displacements between the femoral head, the femoral neck, and the acetabulum (Fig. 55.6). Apart from the displacement at the time of injury, the prognosis also seems to depend on the time from injury to reduction and internal fixation.

REFERENCES

32. Triffitt PD, Konig D, Harper WM et al. J Bone Joint Surg 1992; 74B: 195–198
33. Cohen MS, Garfin SR, Hargens AR et al. J Bone Joint Surg 1991; 73B: 287–290
34. Garden RS. J Bone Joint Surg 1964; 46B: 630–647

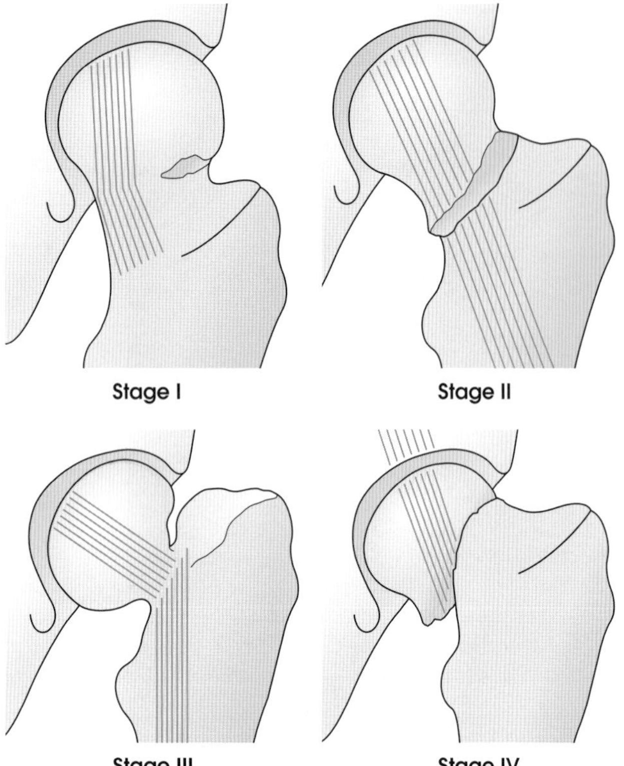

Figure 55.6 Garden's classification of intracapsular fractures. Note that the alignment of the medial femoral trabeculae helps to stage the fractures. The alignment of trabeculae in the medial calcar region is related only to the acetabular trabeculae in stage IV injuries, which have the highest incidence of avascular necrosis.

Typical symptoms of proximal femoral fracture are of pain following a fall on to the hip. Whether this occurs in the young or the elderly, the fracture is often minimally displaced and the patient may not lose function, although there are symptoms of pain following the fall and often radiation to the thigh. This is commonly interpreted as a minor condition not warranting radiological investigation and the fracture is missed. Beware the patient who has a spontaneous pain in the hip, which could have suffered an insufficiency fracture due to severe osteoporosis. Beware also the patient with pain predominantly referred to the thigh. Any injury to a long bone necessitates both examination and radiological investigation of the joints above and below the symptomatic long bone. Displaced proximal femoral fractures cause shortening, adduction and external rotation of the lower limb. The joint may be tender to palpation and hip movements are usually painful. The fracture is often visible on anteroposterior and lateral radiographs, but not always. Repeat radiographs over 1–2 weeks in a suspected case of undisplaced intracapsular fracture while allowing the patient to weight-bear is an acceptable management of the occult fracture. Prior to definitive treatment, elderly patients may need resuscitation because their fall is frequently the result of a cardiovascular event.

The aims of treatment are to provide pain relief and to achieve early mobilization so as to prevent the complications of bed rest. The added benefit of reducing the cost of hospital care is also important. Early mobilization requires the cooperation of the physiotherapy and occupational therapy departments. Provision of rehabilitation wards for patients with a high chance of achieving a return to independent living reduces the cost of care for this common injury. Despite the tendency towards surgical management of these fractures, the decision to operate depends on the presence of complications, the general condition of the patient, and the aetiology of the fracture.

Femoral head fractures

Femoral head fractures are commonly associated with joint dislocation. Pipkin classified these intra-articular fractures into four types:

- type I fractures occur below the ligamentum teres,
- type II fractures involve the weight-bearing portion of the head above the ligamentum teres,
- type III fractures include fracture of the head with intracapsular fracture of the femoral neck, and
- type IV injuries are associated with an acetabular fracture.

For all these injuries, the state of the femoral head needs to be reassessed once reduction has been performed. Any loose fragments need to be excised. Open reduction and internal fixation should be performed if the fragment is large or involves the weight-bearing area. Total arthroplasty might be considered a treatment option if the fracture occurs in an elderly person.

Intracapsular fractures

The aim of treatment for intracapsular fractures is to provide pain relief and early mobilization to prevent the complications of bed rest. Patients with a displaced intracapsular fractured neck of femur sometimes benefit from a period of temporary skin traction prior to definitive fixation. The treatment for intracapsular fractures depends on the age of the patient. Hemiarthroplasty should be avoided in favour of internal fixation in patients under the age of retirement. In this group the fracture should be reduced early,[35] reduced completely,[36] and immobilized using a dynamic hip screw with an antirotation device or parallel hip screws. The vascularity of the femoral head may be investigated with technetium-99m radioisotope scintigraphy using pinhole collimetry to enhance the sensitivity.

A primary cemented hemiarthroplasty is indicated for an intracapsular fracture in patients over 65 years, in those with severe osteoporosis, or in those not fit enough to undergo subsequent total hip replacement operation should avascular necrosis occur.[36] The anterior approach is associated with a lower 6-week mortality rate and a lower incidence of postoperative dislocation than those of the posterior approach.[37,38] Bipolar replacement should be reserved for younger patients who are expected to live longer than 1 year, because it is associated with better subjective outcome.[39]

Extracapsular fractures

The Boyd and Griffin classification is commonly used to describe these fractures, and this has become especially useful with the introduction of the new reconstruction nails and intramedullary

REFERENCES

35. Swiontkowski MF, Winquist RA, Hansen ST. J Bone Joint Surg 1984; 66A: 837–846
36. Garden RS. J Bone Joint Surg 1971; 57B: 437–443
37. Chan RNW, Hoskinson J. J Bone Joint Surg 1975; 57B: 437–443
38. Lu-Yao GL, Keller RB, Littenberg B et al. J Bone Joint Surg 1994; 76A: 15–25
39. Calder SJ, Anderson GH, Harper WM et al. J Bone Joint Surg 1995; 77B: 494–496

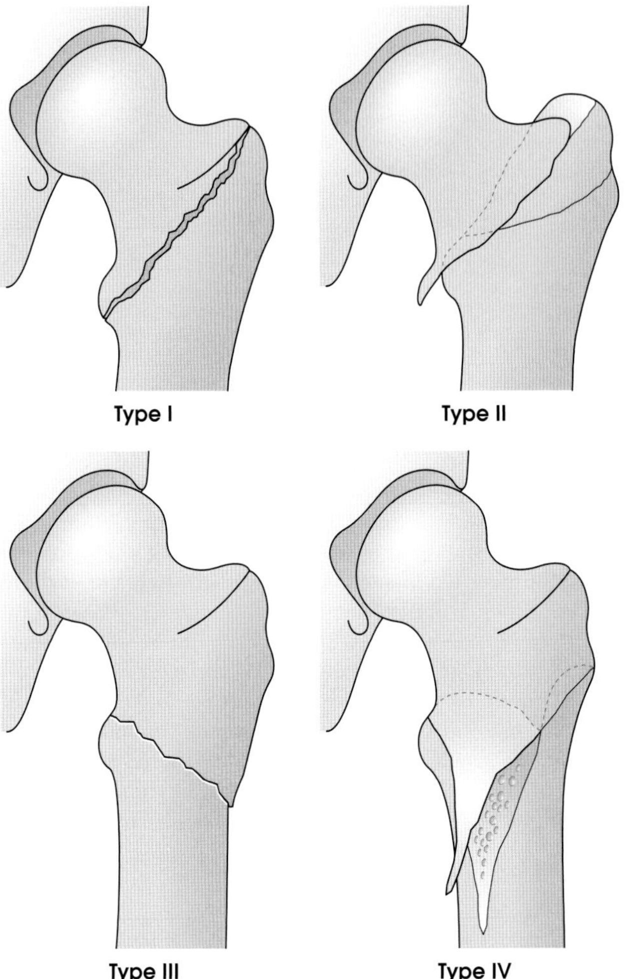

Figure 55.7 The Boyd and Griffin classification.

hip screws to treat the Boyd and Griffin type III fracture. This classification divides fractures into those that are stable with little tendency to collapse, and those that are biomechanically unstable (Fig. 55.7).

Type I fractures are traditionally treated with dynamic sliding screws and plates. Biomechanically, the screw is best placed centrally along the femoral neck or posterior and inferior to this central axis. For type II and III fractures, a reconstruction nail or intramedullary hip screw is appropriate. When the fracture is complicated by medial comminution a posteromedial buttress graft should also be considered. For pathological fractures a calcar-replacing hemiarthroplasty should be performed. Occasionally it is prudent to move the distal fragment medially so that a calcar spike is located down the medullary canal of the femur, which confers an axial stability not offered by a sliding screw and plate alone.

Femoral diaphyseal fractures

Classifications

A number of classifications have been proposed for diaphyseal fractures. The AO classification is based on the presence of comminution, the pattern of the fracture, and whether it is in the upper, middle or lower third of the bone.[1] This classification does not take into account the poor prognosis of subtrochanteric fractures, especially those with medial comminution.

Treatment

Conservative treatment may be appropriate for patients who have a high morbidity and mortality from surgical treatments, for example those with compound fractures or patients with concomitant illness. In these circumstances, abduction and flexion of the proximal fragment can be matched by 90–90 traction.[40] This is traction on the limb with the hip and knee in 90° of flexion. Most fractures can be treated in the early stage with traction followed by intramedullary nailing.

The use of a dynamic hip screw for subtrochanteric fractures is well established and safe when there is no medial wall comminution. A dynamic hip screw can be protected from failure as a result of comminution of the medial wall by bone grafting and protected weight-bearing. Intramedullary techniques can be used when the medial buttress is known to be axially unstable,[41] and devices used include Enders nails, the gamma nail, the intramedullary hip screw, the reconstruction nail and intramedullary interlocking nails. Enders nails, while simple, provide little in the way of protection against rotation or shortening for axially unstable fractures. Intramedullary nails have revolutionized the prognosis for comminuted subtrochanteric fractures, but their use depends on the presence of an intact greater trochanter and piriform fossa to give biomechanical stability of the proximal nail. An intramedullary reconstruction nail is particularly useful for fractures with the most proximal comminution. The use of external fixation is associated with a high incidence of pin site infection and knee stiffness, so it should be reserved for compound type III fractures with heavy soiling.

Extramedullary fixation requires open reduction and internal fixation using dynamic compression plates (Fig. 55.8). This is particularly useful in children where transgression of the physis is contraindicated. The great majority of femoral shaft fractures in children are best managed conservatively using traction, with internal fixation only when traction fails to achieve reduction, when there are complications of traction, for loss of reduction, or lastly for the definitive fixation of uncontaminated compound wounds prior to delayed closure.

Distal femoral fractures

Supracondylar fractures of the knee become more common with advancing age and may be associated with a previous knee arthroplasty in the elderly. The AO classification usually separates supracondylar fractures into those that are extra-articular, those that involve one condyle only, and those that involve both condyles. Fractures about the knee can be complicated by vascular injuries. If any doubt exists that the popliteal artery has been injured, even after Doppler pressure measurement, then the advice of a vascular surgeon should be sought. An arteriogram must be performed so that distal ischaemia can be corrected immediately (see Ch. 10).

The management of these fractures, when not associated with a vascular injury, is initially conservative using skin traction on a Thomas's splint for comfort prior to operative fixation. Extra-articular fractures more than 8 cm above the joint line may be immobilized by a locked intramedullary femoral nail. Those fractures extending to within 8 cm of the condyles but not

REFERENCES

40. Obletz BE. J Bone Joint Surg 1946; 24: 113–116
41. Bergman AT, Metzger PC, Bosacco SJ et al. Orthop Trans 1979; 3: 225–228

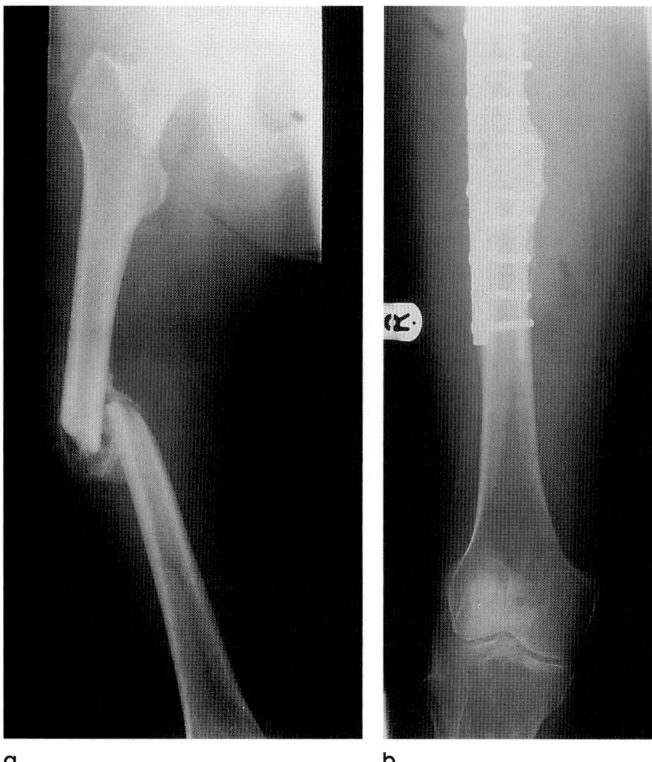

Figure 55.8 Open reduction and compression plating has been used to correct a malunion of the femoral diaphysis.

including the condyles may be treated with a dynamic condylar screw and blade plate. The introduction of the supracondylar nail, which is passed retrogradely through a hole made in the supracondylar notch, has made intramedullary fixation of low comminuted femoral fractures much easier.

Fixation of unicondylar fractures should be performed using a mixture of lag screw and a dynamic condylar screw and plate. Similarly, bicondylar fractures should be stabilized using a dynamic condylar screw and plate as well as a buttress plate on the contralateral side, should this be necessary.

PATELLAR FRACTURES

Patellar fractures are relatively common. They may be caused by either direct or indirect force, indirect injury causing an avulsion of the superior or inferior pole of the patella. In the skeletally immature this is called a sleeve fracture (Fig. 55.9). A direct blow to the patella is a more common cause of fracture in the skeletally mature.

Undisplaced sleeve fractures are treated conservatively in a cylinder cast for 4–6 weeks, followed by rehabilitation. Significant displacement of a sleeve fracture is anything more than 1–2 mm. Wider displacements are associated with an intact straight leg raise, but if left untreated a patella magna develops, with almost invariable late anterior knee symptoms. Open reduction is best performed early when the displacement is significant.

Patella fractures can be classified according to the site of fracture, the pattern of fracture, whether the fracture is displaced or undisplaced, and whether the quadriceps mechanism is intact or ruptured. The last of these can be deduced on examining the straight leg raise. Undisplaced fractures where the quadriceps mechanism is demonstrably intact may be treated in a cylinder cast for a period of 3–6 weeks, followed by mobilization of the

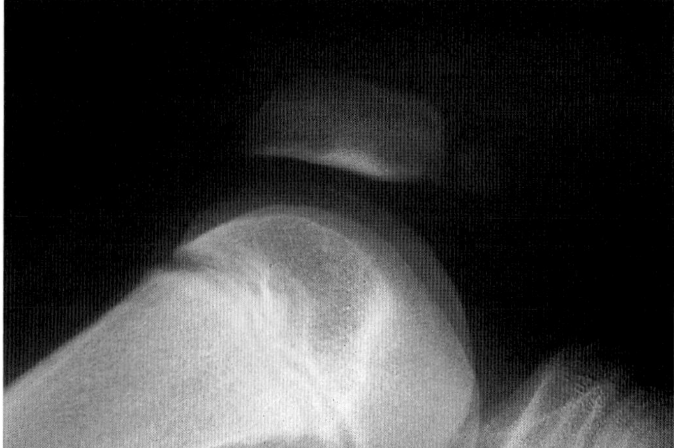

Figure 55.9 Sleeve fracture of the inferior pole of the patella.

patellofemoral joint. Open reduction internal fixation should be considered if there is a loss of ability to straight leg raise, if there is loss of congruence of the articular surface of the patellofemoral joint, or if there is greater than 1 mm of separation of fragments on the lateral radiograph. Because of the periarticular nature of the blood supply of the patella, a figure-of-eight tension band wiring is the method of choice for its immobilization. Circlage wires should be avoided because they are associated with a high incidence of non-union (Fig. 55.10). Rehabilitation with early continuous passive motion depends on the stability and adequacy of fixation.

THE TIBIA

The classifications for fractures of the tibia are many and varied. Here fractures are considered by anatomical site according to the AO classification of fractures.

Proximal tibial fractures

In the AO classification, proximal tibial and fibula fractures are divided into those that are extra-articular, those that involve part of the articular surface, and those involving whole condyles.[1] The AO classification is comprehensive, but incomplete because it has not included the Segond lesion, which is an extra-articular avulsion fracture of part of the lateral collateral ligamentous expansion into the tibial metaphysis. The classification does not guide the surgeon as to how the injury should be treated, and there is no correlation between the classification and the final outcome. The AO classification is partly evolved from Hohl's classification of 1967, which was based on a series of 805 patients.[42] Hohl's classification included only intra-articular fractures of the condyles. Meyers and McKeever developed a separate classification of tibial plateau fractures in 1959.[43] Schatzker and colleagues classified intra-articular fractures of the tibial plateau, with recommended treatments for each type.[44]

Fractures of the lateral tibial condyle are the most common. They generally result from a severe valgus stress in the young or more minor injuries in osteoporotic patients. With increasing

REFERENCES

42. Hohl M. J Bone Joint Surg 1967; 49A: 1455–1467
43. Meyers MH, McKeever FM. J Bone Joint Surg 1959; 41A: 209–222
44. Schatzker J, McBroom R, Bruce D. Clin Orthop 1979; 138: 94–104

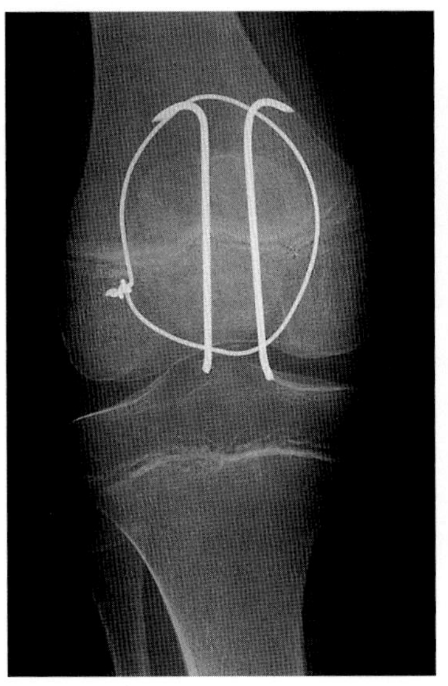

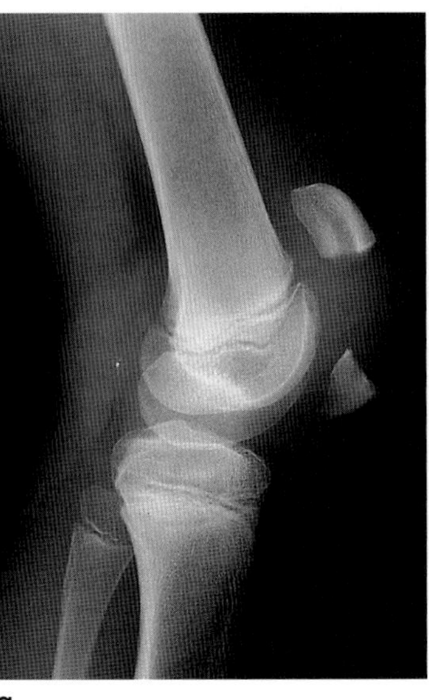

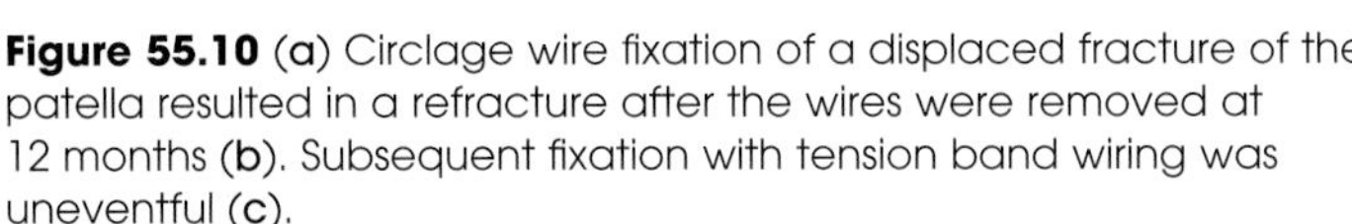

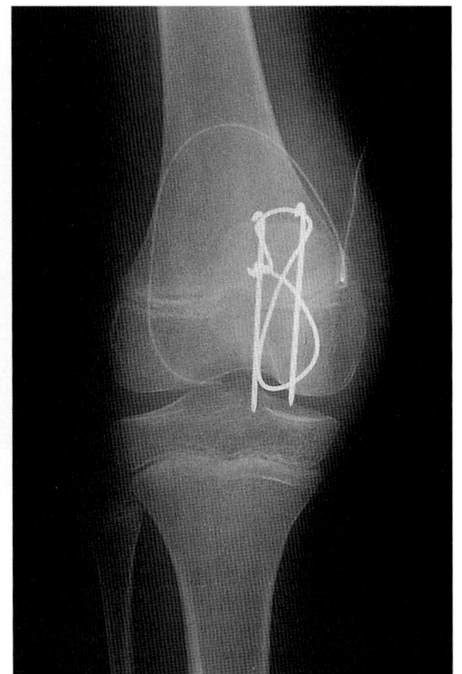

a a c

Figure 55.10 (a) Circlage wire fixation of a displaced fracture of the patella resulted in a refracture after the wires were removed at 12 months (b). Subsequent fixation with tension band wiring was uneventful (c).

load other structures around the knee joint are involved, and fracture of the fibula neck, rupture of the medial collateral ligaments, and occasionally rupture of the cruciate ligaments commonly coexist. A more vertical force combined with valgus stress, such as a fall from a height, may be associated with a die-punch fracture of the lateral tibial condyle. The lateral femoral condyle causes comminution of the articular surface of the tibia. Isolated fractures of the medial tibial condyle are uncommon and are usually associated with lateral ligament ruptures and neuropraxia of the common perineal nerve.

The clinical findings of a proximal tibial fracture include a haemarthrosis, bruising, skin abrasions on the side of the fracture, and often tenderness over the contralateral collateral ligament complex. There may be a valgus or varus deformity of the knee. Special investigations include anteroposterior, lateral and oblique X-rays of the knee. The anteroposterior X-ray should be performed with the beam at an inclination of 115° to take into account the posterior slope of the tibia.[45] To estimate the degree of depression of the tibial condyle tomograms, CT and MRI scans are recommended. Hohl and Luck recommended that a step of less then 4 mm should be treated conservatively and anything greater than this should be treated by reduction and internal fixation.[46] Only Porter has ever found a direct correlation between the depth of step and the final outcome. He demonstrated that 80% of patients had poor results if the depression was more than 1.4 cm.[47]

Treatment

Undisplaced extra-articular tibial spine fractures can be treated conservatively in a cylinder cast for 4 weeks prior to rehabilitation. It is recommended that significantly displaced avulsions of the cruciate ligament insertions (Meyers and McKeever types II, IIIa and IIIb) are reduced and internally fixed.[43]

For tibial plateau fractures, treatment largely depends on the age and the extent of the deformity that occurs at the knee with loading. Patients should be examined under anaesthetic to estimate this deformity prior to a definitive decision on treatment.[48] All patients under the age of 60 years should in general have joint congruity restored, and this usually requires open reduction and internal fixation. Patients over the age of 60 with a step of less than 4–5 mm and a deformity of less than 10° can be treated conservatively. Patients with a greater step and a larger deformity should be treated surgically, depending on their general condition. In certain circumstances, primary arthroplasty might be considered the treatment of choice. The prognosis of these injuries depends on the severity of injury and the amount of late deformity. Late varus deformity is associated with a higher incidence of symptomatic osteoarthritis in the long term.[49]

Conservative treatment includes a period of traction on a Thomas's splint. This should be converted as soon as comfort allows to Perkins traction on a Hadfield split bed, with skin traction of 3 kg or more and early restoration of quadriceps exercises. After 3 or 4 weeks, the patient may be mobilized in a cast brace, with restoration of weight-bearing between 8 and 12 weeks. The worst results are obtained after conservative treatment is combined with prolonged immobilization.[50]

When open reduction and internal fixation are indicated, then the Schatzker type guides the method of fixation.[44] For instance, a Schatzker type I split lateral plateau fracture may be reduced and immobilized using cannulated screws (Fig. 55.11). When percutaneous methods are being considered to treat type I fractures, then a preoperative MRI scan or preoperative arthroscopy should be able to distinguish fractures with interposing menisci from those where the meniscus has not been caught in the fracture gap. When the whole spectrum of proximal tibial

REFERENCES

45. Moore TM, Harvey JP Jr. J Bone Joint Surg 1974; 56A: 155–160
46. Hohl M, Luck J. J Bone Joint Surg 1956; 38A: 1001–1018
47. Porter RB. J Bone Joint Surg 1970; 52B: 676–687
48. Rasmussen PS. J Bone Joint Surg 1973; 55A: 1331–1334
49. Rasmussen PS, Sorensen SE. Injury 1973; 4: 265
50. Solonen KA. Acta Orthop Scand 1963; 63: 1–32

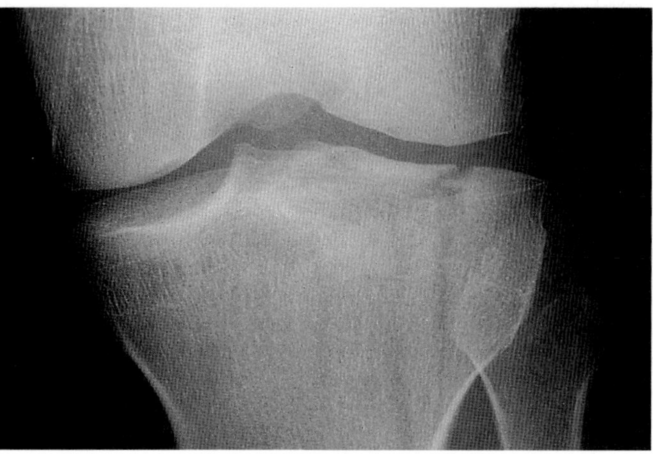
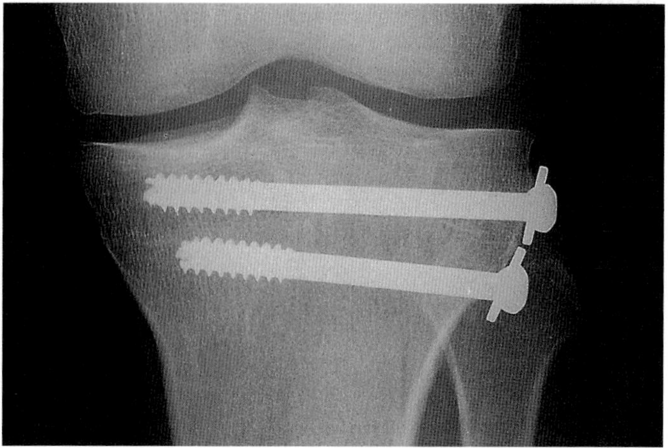

Figure 55.11 Type I pure split fracture of the lateral tibial plateau reduced with AO reduction forceps and then screwed using cannulated screws and washers.

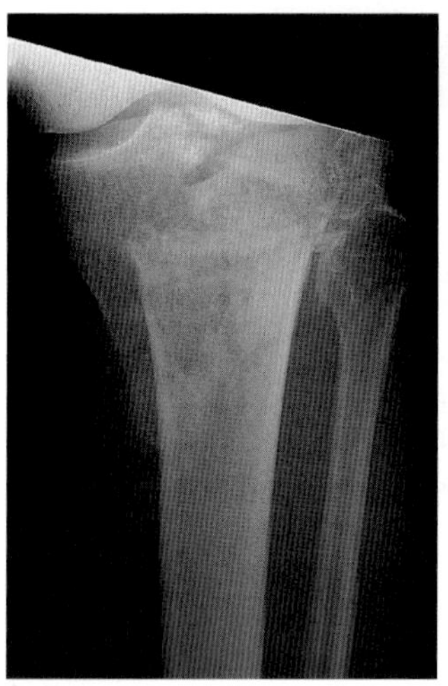
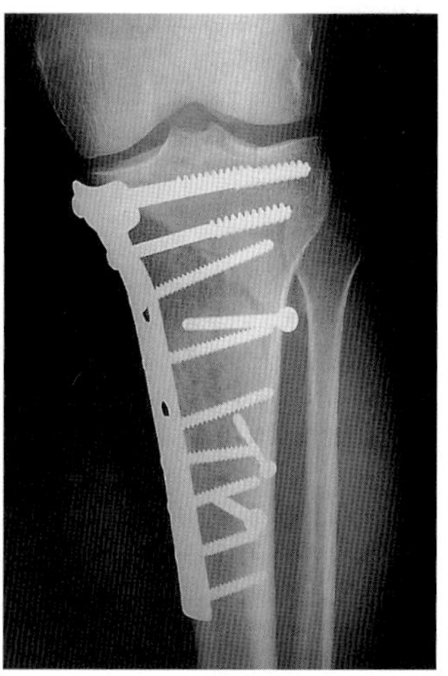

Figure 55.12 A Schatzker type V biocondylar fracture fixed with lag screws and a medial buttress plate. The buttress is placed on the side with the longest fragment.

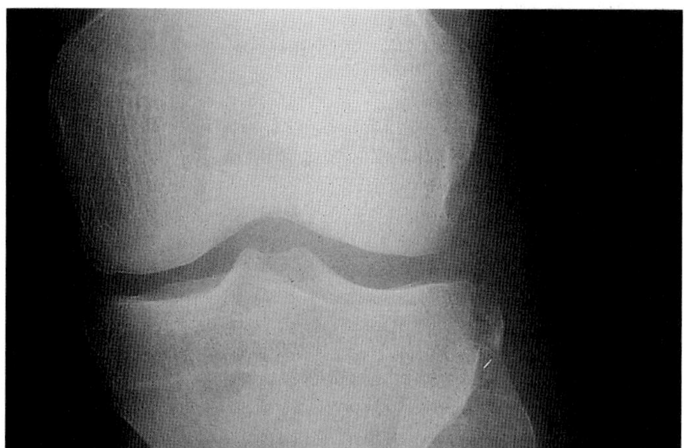
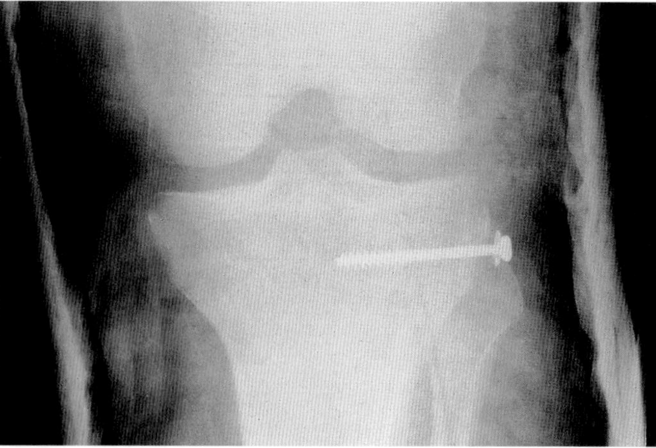

Figure 55.13 Segond fracture of the lateral tibial plateau with an associated collateral ligament injury that has been repaired and the fragment screwed into place.

fractures is considered, there is probably no correlation between radiographic degenerative changes and final functional result.[51]

Schatzker type II fractures require elevation of the depressed articular surface through a cortical window made beneath the depressed condyle, and impaction grafting with graft support using screw fixation. Most other Schatzker types require the latter or buttress plating, or a combination of the two (Fig. 55.12). Elevation of deep depressions may require arthroscopic assistance.

The Segond fracture is treated conservatively if the lateral joint is stable, or it may be reduced and screwed into position if the injury involves a grade III collateral ligament injury (Fig. 55.13).

Tibial diaphyseal fractures

Tibial diaphyseal fracture healing depends on the patient's age, the tissue damage at the time of fracture, and the method of immobilization of the fracture site. Fractures are classified according to whether they are compound or not, the severity of the compound wound, the axial stability of the fracture, and the presence or absence of a periosteal hinge. An algorithm has been developed based on these classifications to select the most

REFERENCES

51. Apley G. J Bone Joint Surg 1956; 38B: 699–706

appropriate treatment.[52] This applies only to patients over the age of skeletal maturity. Patients under the age of 16 have few of the problems associated with fracture healing in adults.[3,53]

The severity of the soft tissue injury is the most difficult to assess. The soft tissues include skin, fat, muscle, tendon, artery, nerve and periosteum. Injury of the periosteal or soft tissue hinge, as described by Sir John Charnley, is often incorrectly ignored.[54]

Tissue damage depends on the magnitude of the injuring load, the rate of loading, the type of loading, the local structure of the tibia, the material properties of the bone, and the soft tissues. The same energy may produce a different pattern of injury in an osteoporotic old person from that of an athletic young person.

The pattern of bone injury indicates the type of load that caused the fracture. A spiral fracture results from an indirect injury caused by a torsion force, a simple transverse fracture occurs with a bending load, and an oblique fracture occurs with bending while the bone is in compression. A more rapid rate, or a higher magnitude of loading, causes comminution of the tibia and a concomitant fracture of the fibula. The pattern of fracture also predicts its axial stability.

The degree of severity of bone injury is diagnosed from the history of the circumstances of injury; by examining the limb for bruising, tenderness and deformity; and finally by special investigation. Two radiographs must be taken at 90° to each other. Patients with a history of a low-energy injury, little bruising over the shin, no deformity, an axially stable fracture, an intact fibula, and an undisplaced fracture on X-ray can be expected to have most of the circumference of the periosteum left intact.

The closed and Gustilo type I injury

Patients with a closed or minimally compound (Gustilo type 1, see Ch. 52) undisplaced fracture are preferably treated conservatively in plaster with early weight-bearing through the injured limb. The treatment of a patient with a closed or Gustilo type 1 displaced fracture is based on the state of the periosteal hinge. After an injury that causes displacement, the periosteum is either divided in a part or the whole of its circumference.

The extent of the periosteal injury in the closed fracture should be assessed under general anaesthesia, because the periosteum is well innervated and movement causes intense pain. The tibia should be reduced before assessing the state of the periosteum. An intact fibula usually means a stable, low-energy injury. An oblique tibia fracture with an intact fibula often slips during healing into varus, or it develops hypertrophic non-union because the fibula holds the fracture gap apart. Hypertrophic non-union might be avoided in these fractures by perfect reduction. The fibula can be used as a fulcrum to guide the ends of the bones into perfect reduction (Fig. 55.14). A circumferential tear of the periosteum may be surmised if reduction is easy, and the fracture, once reduced, is distractible. Accurate reduction and the maintenance of reduction are important to achieve the best healing.

Transverse high-energy injuries, with no soft tissue hinge, are difficult to treat in plaster cast because early weight-bearing causes deformity. It is not known if these patients are best treated by open reduction and internal fixation with dynamic compression plates, by closed intramedullary nailing, or by external fixation. External fixation in these circumstances may be the best method of immobilization, although the postoperative management is arduous because the pin sites must be maintained clean and uninfected for long periods. Fractures that have no periosteal hinge and that are axially unstable are probably best treated using intramedullary fixation (Fig. 55.15), but screw fracture occurs in about 19%, so early removal of the locking screws should be attempted. Screws should be deliberately left to protrude 5 mm through the distal cortex to aid removal of broken screws through a separate lateral incision if necessary (Fig. 55.16).

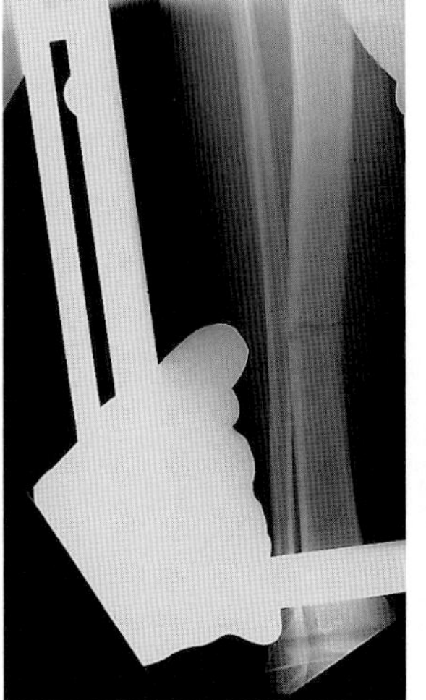

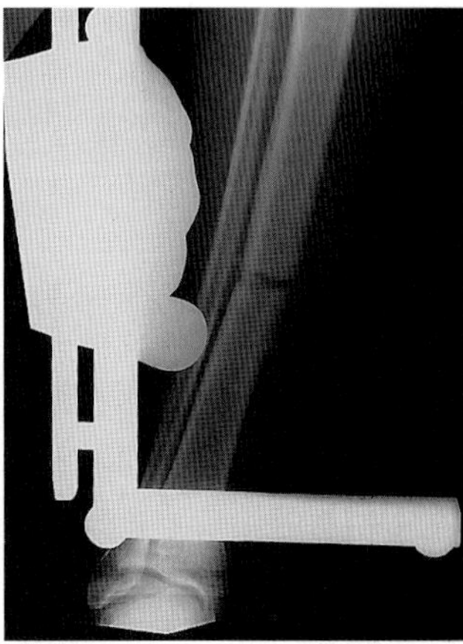

Figure 55.14 Examination under anaesthetic demonstrates the fracture to be stable, with the periosteum intact on the lateral side. The intact fibula can be used as a fulcrum with which to guide accurate reduction of the fracture.

Scars around the knees should be avoided in patients whose occupation involves long periods of kneeling, for example members of the clergy and carpet layers.

Tibial fractures that are difficult to reduce usually have an intact periosteum, and the longer the time from injury to the attempted reduction, the more difficult it is because the soft tissues contract. Tissue contracture is a good reason for the early and definitive management of a diaphyseal fracture. When reduction is prevented by an intact periosteum in a fully translated and shortened fracture, it is easiest to overcome the resistance by recreating the deformity that occurred at the time of injury. This is the same principle that is used to reduce children's distal forearm fractures.[55] When reduction has been achieved, the site of the periosteal hinge can be deduced by attempting to displace the fracture in anterior, posterior, medial and lateral directions.

A reduced axially stable fracture with an intact periosteal hinge is probably best treated with an above-knee plaster cast. The periosteal hinge is used to maintain reduction by using the plaster cast to provide two points of pressure against a third fulcrum,

REFERENCES

52. Hardy JRW, Richardson JB, Gregg P. J Int J Orthop Trauma 1996; 6: 52–61
53. Weissman SL, Herold HZ, Engleberg M. J Bone Joint Surg 1966; 48A: 257–267
54. Charnley J. The Closed Treatment of Common Fractures. 3rd edn. Churchill Livingstone, Edinburgh, 1961
55. Rang M. Children's Fractures. 2nd edn. Lippincott, Philadelphia, 1984

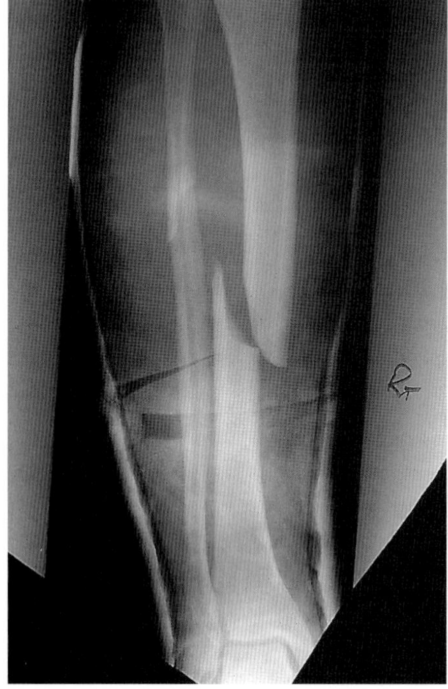

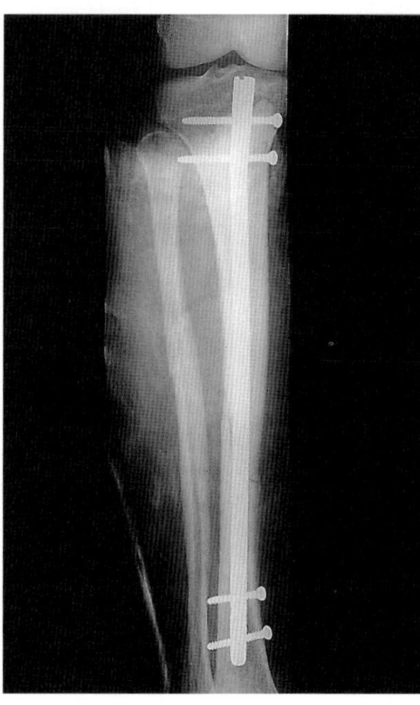

Figure 55.15 This was an axially unstable fracture that shortened in plaster cast, so intramedullary nailing was used with minimal reaming.

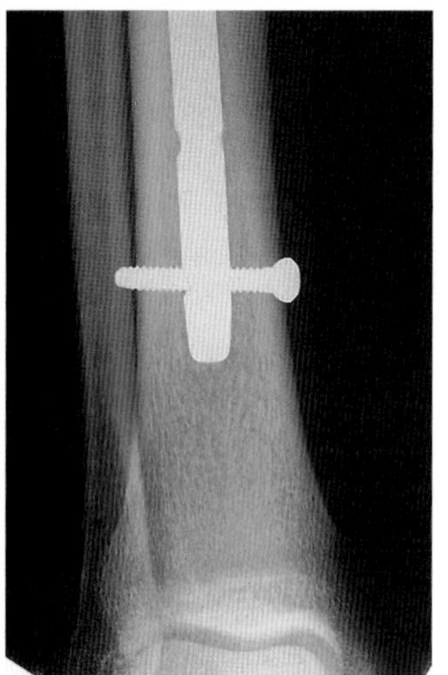

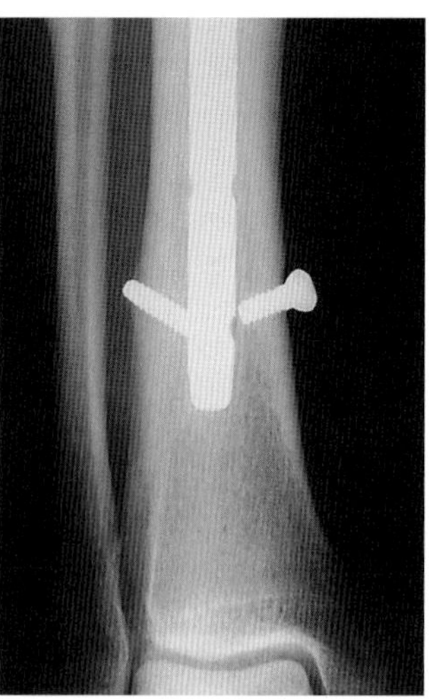

Figure 55.16 Distal locking screw failure after 6 months of full weight-bearing.

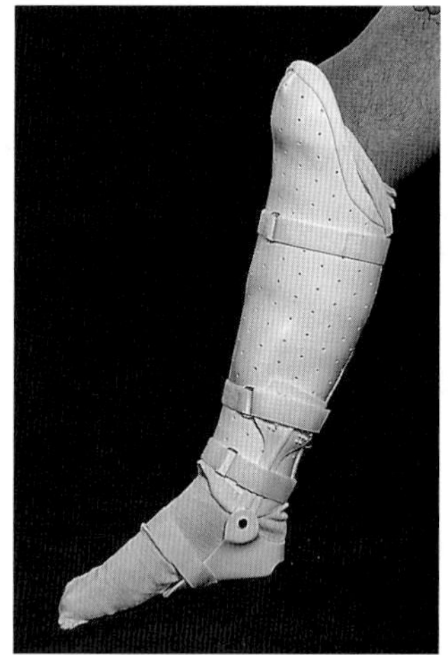

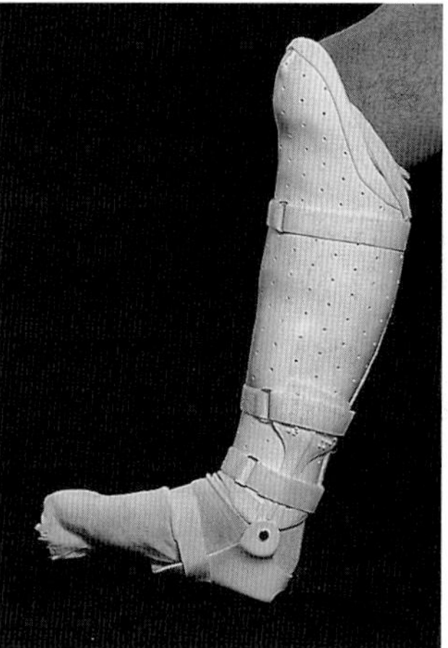

Figure 55.17 The Sarmiento cast allows early return of function of the ankle joint.

opposite the intact periosteum. Early weight-bearing is usually rewarded by appearance of callus, and when this occurs the above-knee plaster can safely be replaced with a Sarmiento patellar-bearing cast (Fig. 55.17). The patient with this pattern of injury should be encouraged to weight-bear as soon as the pain permits.

Walking in plaster is likely to cause a similar shortening if an axial load during anaesthesia demonstrates the fracture to be unstable to shortening. However, if the same patient has an intact periosteal hinge the likelihood of the fracture healing within 16 weeks is high. These patients may benefit from external fixation and the modern unilateral frames, which allow early unlocking of the telescoping device ('dynamization') and permit enough movement at the fracture site to encourage callus formation. Early dynamization also reduces the incidence of pin tract infection (Fig. 55.18) and aseptic loosening of the fixator pins (Fig. 55.19).

Once enough callus has formed, the external fixator can be removed. It is important to recognize that callus may be prevented from developing if the external fixator is made up to be rigid and the fracture reduction is so good that it prevents all movement. A very unstable configuration should, however, also be discouraged because a hypertrophic non-union can develop. The fixator should be applied only to a fully reduced fracture as a means of avoiding late loss of reduction (Fig. 55.20). Fractures close to joints can be accommodated using metaphyseal T pin clamps (Fig. 55.21).

The stability of a fracture site immobilized by external fixation is affected by the size of the fracture gap, the pins' offset, the spacing of the fixator pins, the length of the pins, and the

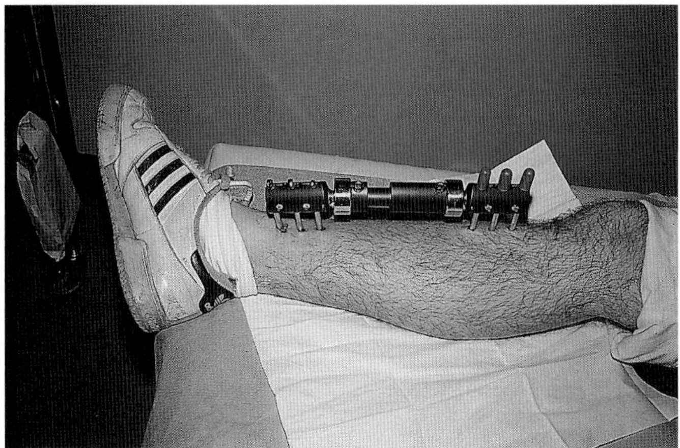

Figure 55.18 Early pin tract infection, as seen in the lower set of pins, can be discouraged by unlocking the axial stability of a fixator (dynamization).

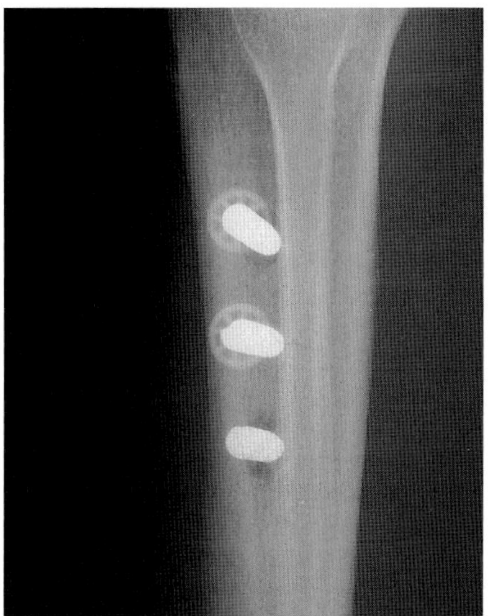

Figure 55.19 Aseptic loosening can be seen in the upper and lower of the three pins in this radiograph.

thickness of the pins. Once a stable callus has developed that will allow full weight-bearing the fixator can be removed. Patients can be encouraged to remove their own pins when conical pins have been inserted.

The Gustilo type II or III injury

External fixation has become the mainstay of management for compound fractures of the tibia because of the reluctance to leave foreign material near a previously contaminated wound.[21,56] External fixation is invariably used for Gustilo compound type II or III wounds, although it may be associated with a considerable risk of infection: 3–45% in some studies.[17,57,58] There is now a trend towards using intramedullary nailing for Gustilo types II and III compound fractures, with an accepted deep infection rate of 3.2–10%.[25,26,59–63] Compression plates and screws have in the past been used to immobilize compound fractures, but this has been shown to be detrimental and most now avoid this option.[28,64]

Every treatment has its own complications, and the best method is often the one with which the surgeon is most familiar.

Distal tibial fractures

Distal tibial metaphyseal fractures, or Pilon fractures, are uncommon and usually occur as a result of a fall from a height.

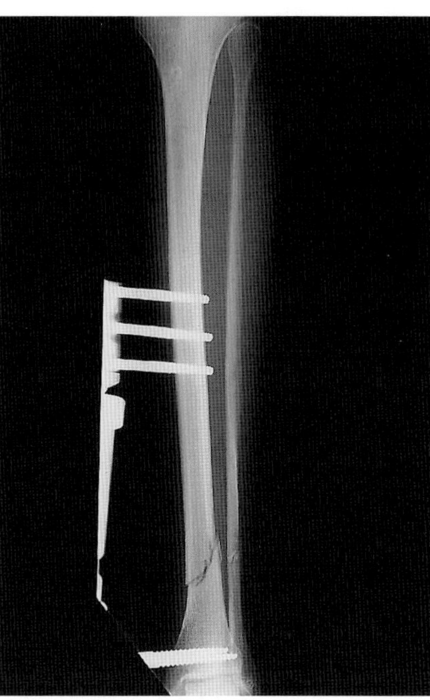

Figure 55.20 A low fracture is treated using cancellous screws and a T clamp, with perfect reduction of the spiral fracture.

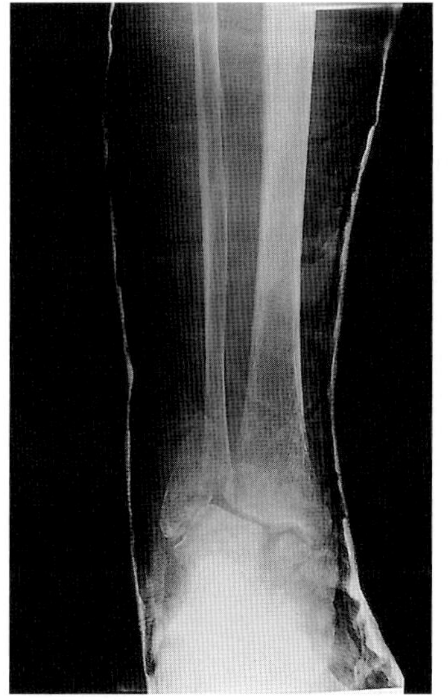

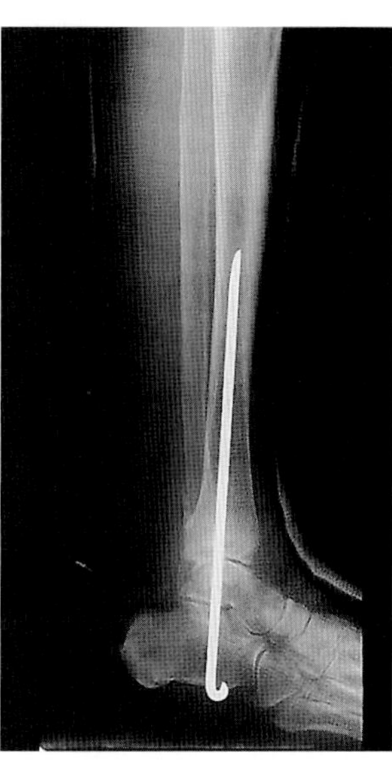

Figure 55.21 A Rush nail immobilizing an ankle fracture in an osteoporotic patient.

REFERENCES

56. Baker JT, McKinney LA, Costa AS et al. J Orthop Trauma 1992; 6: 509–510
57. Behrens F, Searls K. J Bone Joint Surg 1986; 68B: 246–254
58. Caudle RJ, Stern PJ. J Bone Joint Surg 1978; 69A: 801–807
59. Velazco A, Whitesides TE, Fleming LL. J Bone Joint Surg 1983; 65A: 879–885
60. Wiss DA. Clin Orthop 1986; 212: 122–132
61. Alho A, Ekeland A, Stromsoe K et al. J Bone Joint Surg 1990; 72B: 805–809
62. Alho A, Benterud JG, Hogevold HE et al. Clin Orthop 1992; 277: 243–250
63. Anglen J, Unger D, DiPasquale T et al. J Orthop Trauma 1993; 7: 163
64. Veliskakis KP. J Bone Joint Surg 1959; 41B: 342–354

They have been classified by Ruedi and Allgöwer into type 1, which are minimally displaced; type 2, when there is incongruence; and type 3, which are comminuted.[65] Undisplaced type 1 fractures are treated by below-knee plaster casts with avoidance of weight-bearing. Those with incongruity of the joint and comminuted fractures should be treated by an open reduction and internal fixation. A combination of external fixation with a hinged fixator across the ankle joint has been tried, and minimally invasive techniques using small pins, cannulated screws and K-wire fixation are also becoming popular.

Malleolar fractures

This common injury is most usually classified using the Danis–Weber classification, which is the same as the AO classification.[1] This classification relates to the position of the fibula fracture. A Danis–Weber type A fracture is at or below the syndesmosis, a type B runs obliquely up from the ankle joint, and a type C lies above the syndesmosis. A more complicated but accurate classification, the Lauge–Hansen classification,[66] is based on the position of the foot at the time of the injury. This classification can be deduced from the history, examination findings, and radiographic pattern of fracture seen on anteroposterior and lateral views of the ankle mortise. Although complicated to remember, the Lauge–Hansen classification aids in the techniques of reduction. For example, an adduction force in the supinated foot produces a transverse fracture of the lateral malleolus or an injury to the lateral collateral ligament and a vertical fracture of the medial malleolus at the level of the ankle joint. Reduction is then by abduction and pronation of the foot. No classification can cover all of the patterns of injury seen in ankle fractures, but the classifications mentioned above aid in the understanding of the mechanism of injury and therefore indicate a more rational approach to treatment.

Ankle fractures usually result from a twisting injury. Often the patient cannot describe the precise mechanism of injury. The most important part of the diagnosis is to elicit the correct clinical signs of soft tissue injury, such as rupture of the deltoid ligament. Radiographs often do not disclose this, and this injury makes all the difference between the ankle mortise being stable or unstable. When an ankle injury is suspected the whole leg must be examined, because the Maisonneuve injury—a deltoid and syndesmosis ligament rupture associated with a high spiral fibula fracture—can otherwise be missed, thus resulting in a subluxed ankle joint.

The treatment of ankle fractures depends on the position of the ankle mortise on the radiographs and whether the pattern of injury is likely to be stable or unstable. A perfect anteroposterior and lateral view of the ankle mortise should show congruence of the subchondral surfaces of the joint. Undisplaced fractures are usually treated in a below-knee cast with weight-bearing after 3–6 weeks, depending on whether the injury is stable or unstable.

Open reduction and internal fixation are indicated when there is greater than 1 mm of displacement of the ankle joint mortise after attempted reduction. Other indications include diastasis of the syndesmosis, and compound fractures and dislocations. At operation the posteromedial fragment of a trimalleolar fracture should be reduced and internally fixed if more than one-third of the weight-bearing area has been involved in a fracture. Diastasis is treated using a syndesmosis screw above the level of the syndesmosis in a plane 25° posteroanterior to the normal coronal plane of the tibia. It is placed without compression and after full dorsiflexion of the ankle joint to avoid narrowing the ankle mortise, because this prevents dorsiflexion.

The lateral side is operated on first when open reduction and internal fixation are attempted. After the lateral side has been fixed, the syndesmosis should be tested for diastasis and a check radiograph performed. When a displaced or undisplaced medial malleolar fracture is present, it should be immobilized using a pair of parallel AO lag screws, usually 45 mm in length.

The deltoid ligament occasionally becomes interposed between the articular surfaces on the medial side of the ankle joint. Deltoid ligament injury may or may not require exploration, depending on whether the immediate postoperative radiographs show perfect congruity of the ankle joint.

Rarely, fractures of the ankle in osteoporotic patients cannot be immobilized with plaster cast or the usual AO fixation techniques. In these circumstances, an intramedullary Rush nail passed under image intensification up through the os calcis and talus is a useful method of temporary immobilization (Fig. 55.21).

THE FOOT

Injuries of the feet are common and disabling (see Ch. 51). Fractures that involve the subtalar joint are extremely disabling. These injuries are often missed because of failure to appreciate the radiological anatomy of the foot.

Talar fractures

Fractures of the talus are rare because they tend to be caused by high-energy forces. The talar neck fracture was classically diagnosed in the pilots of early aircraft as the 'aviators' astragalus' injury, because the rudder pedals would cause a violent dorsiflexion of the foot when the craft crashed. Nowadays this injury is seen after car accidents or following a fall from a height. The diagnosis is aided by true lateral views of the foot as well as the usual anteroposterior and oblique views. The Hawkins and Canale classification of talar neck fractures is most commonly quoted.[67,68]

Reduction is not necessary for undisplaced fractures of the neck (type 1). A split plaster with the ankle held in the plantigrade position is applied, to be replaced by a complete plaster when the swelling has subsided. This is worn for 6–8 weeks. With displaced fractures and fracture dislocations (types 2–4), reduction is urgent because of the precarious nature of the blood supply of the talar body. Type 3 and 4 injuries, in which the body of the talus is displaced medially, have an avascular necrosis rate of 85%. Open reduction should be performed if closed manipulation under anaesthetic fails. All of the bone fragments should be retained and held reduced (Fig. 55.22). The reduced fracture can be stabilized initially with one or two Kirschner wires, followed if possible by insertion of an AO screw or a cannulated screw placed from behind forwards into the talar head. A below-knee plaster with the ankle being held in a plantigrade position is needed for 6–8 weeks.

Os calcis fractures

These common injuries are caused by a fall from a height on to the heels. The injury is unfortunately common in window

REFERENCES

65. Ruedi TP, Allgöwer M. Clin Orthop 1969; 138: 105–110
66. Yde J. Acta Orthop Scand 1980; 51: 181–192
67. Hawkins LG. J Bone Joint Surg 1970; 52A: 991–1002
68. Canale ST. Orthopaedics 1990; 13: 1105–1115

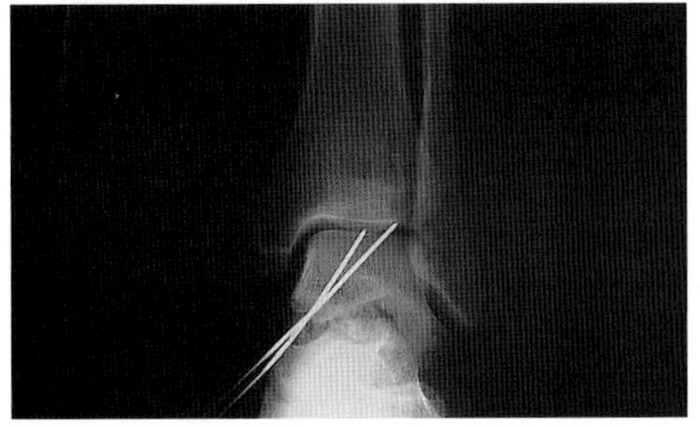

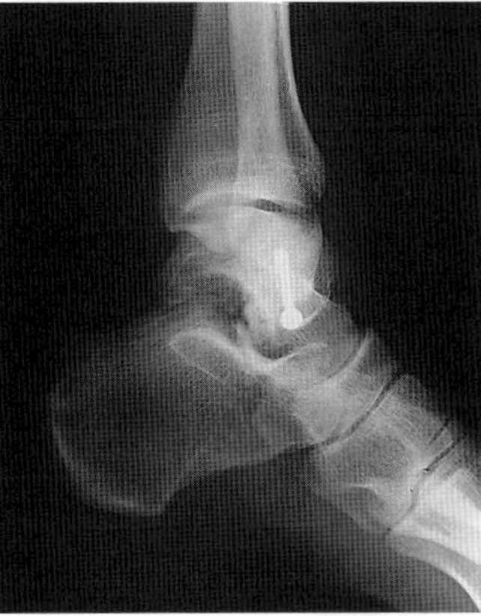

Figure 55.22 Fixation after failed closed reduction of a Hawkins type 2 fracture. The fracture fragments are reduced and held with a K wire before a screw is passed.

cleaners, painters and scaffolders. Because a fall from a height is the cause, it is essential to exclude other injuries such as fractures of the pelvis and spine. The injury is always associated with swelling of the heel below the malleoli, and severe obvious flattening of the heel may be evident. Bruising appears late and settles in a line above the fat pad of the heel. Radiographs pick up all but the most minor injuries. These must include well-centred and well-exposed lateral views of the foot. An axial projection is helpful to visualize the posterior body of the bone, the sustentaculum tali, and occasionally the subtalar joints. Computerized tomography scanning provides accurate delineation of the extent of fracture, and therefore aids in the diagnosis and planning of open reduction and internal fixation.

The simplest classification divides these injuries into extra-articular fractures, in which the posterior talocalcaneal joint is not involved, and intra-articular fractures, in which it is. The value of this classification is in its ability to assess the prognosis, which is much worse in the fractures involving the posterior facet of the os calcis. Involvement of this joint can be gauged by measuring Böhler's salient angle, which is normally about 40°. To measure this, a line is drawn through the posterior articular surface to intersect with a second line touching the superior angle of the tuberosity (Fig. 55.23).

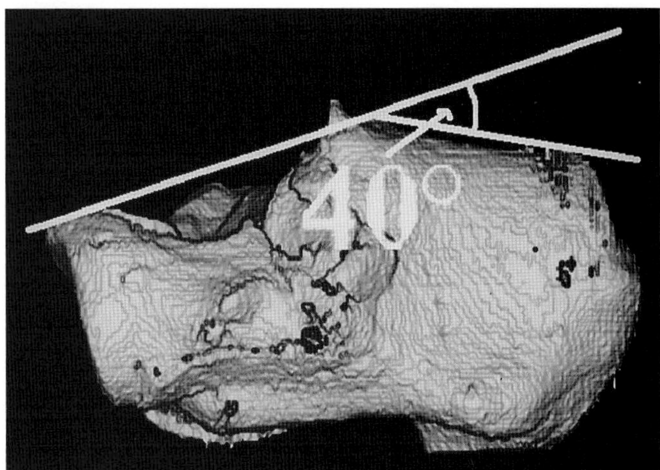

Figure 55.23 Böhler's salient angle reproduced on a three-dimensional reconstruction of the os calcis from a CT scan.

Most extra-articular fractures can be managed by conservative means including early elevation, cold compression and mobilization. There are two schools of thought as to whether treating intra-articular fractures by open reduction and internal fixation confers any advantage over conservative treatment. When open reduction and internal fixation are performed, a lateral approach is preferred and an os calcis reconstruction plate chosen for fixation. Bone defects should be grafted and weight-bearing is delayed for 8 weeks.

Midtarsal fractures and tarsometatarsal injuries

An isolated fracture of the navicular is often incorrectly diagnosed when an os naviculare exists. A true fracture is often caused by an avulsion of the tibialis posterior tendon. This fracture can be treated conservatively in a plaster cast. Larger fractures of the navicular should be accurately fixed using internal fixation techniques.

Tarsometatarsal fracture or dislocations, or Lisfranc injuries, are commonly missed. The injuries commonly occur in athletes, and if appropriate treatment is not instituted can lead to significant pain and disability. These injuries frequently consist of fractures of the base of the first and second metatarsals, with splaying between the two metatarsal due to disruption of the strong ligament (Lisfranc's ligament) between the base of the second metatarsal and the medial cuneiform; lateral subluxation of the third, fourth and fifth metatarsal; and various associated fractures of the cuneiforms and cuboid. Compartment syndrome of the foot is associated with the higher-energy injuries and must be considered. Closed reduction and fixation with percutaneous K wires and plaster of Paris with subsequent removal of K wires may be all that is required. However, failure to obtain anatomical reduction, or removal of the wires too early, may lead to loss of anatomical alignment as well as subsequent pain and disability. Open reduction and internal fixation with cannulated screws, which allow absolute reduction to be obtained and maintained, is now the treatment of choice.[69]

Metatarsal fractures

A metatarsal fracture may be caused by crushing, twisting or repetitive stress (Fig. 55.24). Usually there is a history of injury, however trivial, and the foot is painful and slightly swollen. Radiographs show most fractures, but the accessory ossicles around the base of the fifth metatarsal are occasionally misdiagnosed as a fracture.

When walking plasters are required they are used for a maximum of 3 weeks, because most fractures unite readily. The

REFERENCE

69. Myerson MS. J Bone Joint Surg 1999; 81B, 756–763

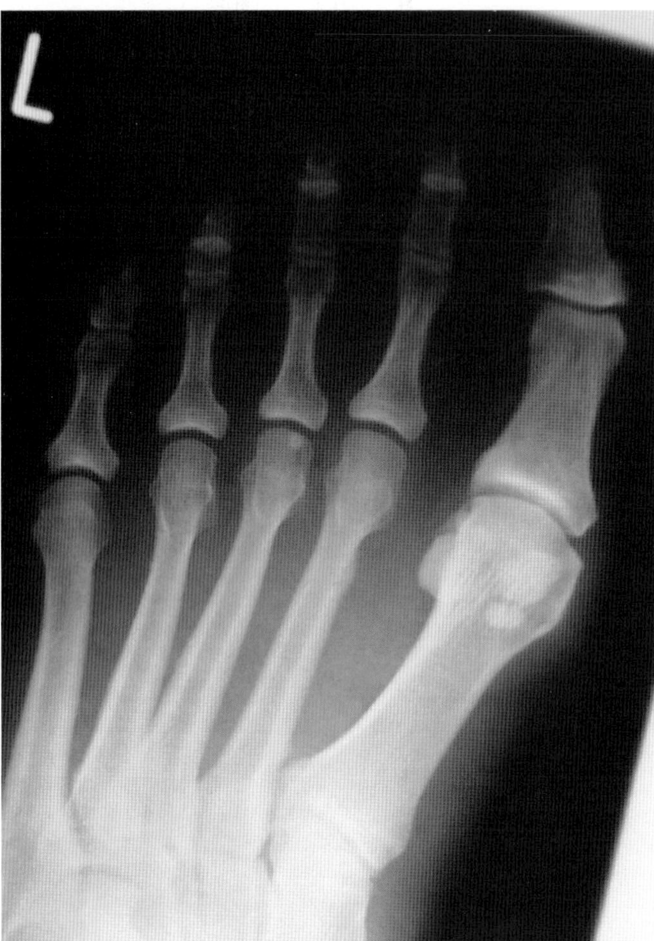

Figure 55.24 'March' fracture of the second metatarsal neck, due to stress fracture.

Jones fracture of the base of the fifth metatarsal distal to its articulation with the second metatarsal behaves more like a stress fracture and occurs in athletes. It frequently results in a non-union, which has to be treated with medullary curettage and bone grafting.

Kirschner wire fixation may be utilized after reduction of severely displaced multiple fractures that may also be associated with midtarsal dislocations. The foot is elevated postoperatively and weight-bearing avoided for 6 weeks.

Phalangeal fractures

Phalangeal fractures are commonly the result of workplace accidents in which heavy weights are dropped on to the toes. Many are compound and need to be treated accordingly. Postoperatively they can be managed by elevation followed by mobilization. If necessary, a plaster shoe with a 'crumb catcher' extension to protect the phalanges is used. Admission and elevation for the majority is a prudent practice because it avoids late sloughing of swollen dermis.

DISLOCATIONS

DISLOCATION OF THE HIP

Dislocation of the hip may be congenital or acquired. In the neonate and in infancy the commonest cause is congenital dislocation of the hip, followed by septic arthritis. During adolescence and adulthood, the commonest cause of dislocation of the hip is trauma. Eighty per cent of all traumatic hip dislocations are posterior. The commonest cause is a blow to the knee from a dashboard during a road traffic accident. The blow forces the femur out of the acetabulum. Occasionally the dislocation is associated with a fracture of the posterior lip of the acetabulum. The posterior dislocation is occasionally associated with a femoral fracture, which leads the dislocation to be overlooked.

The clinical features of posterior dislocation of the hip in the conscious patient are of extreme pain and deformity about the lower limb. The affected limb appears short and is fixed in flexion, internal rotation, and adduction. An anteroposterior radiograph of the pelvis is usually enough to demonstrate the dislocation. However, multiple views of the acetabulum and a CT scan may be needed to exclude a fracture of the acetabular rim or a Pipkin fracture of the femoral head. The neurovascular status of the limb should be elucidated because these dislocations are occasionally associated with a sciatic nerve injury.

Traumatic dislocations are considered to be orthopaedic emergencies. There is a relationship between the length of time that the hip remains dislocated and an increasing risk of avascular necrosis. It is widely held that isolated hip dislocation reduced within 6 h gives an excellent outcome. However, even if dislocations are reduced within 3 h there appears to be a 45% incidence of fair and poor results in long-term follow-up. The important factors in the long-term prognosis appear to be the direction of the dislocation and the overall severity of injuries. Multiple injuries and posterior dislocation are associated with a higher incidence of avascular necrosis, osteoarthritis and heterotopic ossification.[70]

The dislocation should be reduced under general anaesthesia. The dislocation is most safely reduced with the patient anaesthetized on the anaesthetic room floor. An assistant is required to steady the pelvis by providing countertraction over the anterior–superior iliac spines. When this has been provided, the dislocation is reduced by flexing the patient's hip and knee to 90° and pulling the thigh vertically upwards.

Following reduction, X-rays are mandatory to confirm reduction, exclude displacement of a fracture of the acetabulum, and exclude intra-articular fragments. An intra-articular fragment of cartilage may be deduced from plain radiographs by comparing the congruity of the dislocated joint with that on the normal side. If it is suspected that bone or cartilage fragments are trapped in the joint, then a CT scan of the joint may be required.

If the reduction is stable and there are no associated fractures of the acetabulum, then mobilization should be begun as early as pain allows and full weight-bearing should be encouraged, again as soon as the pain allows. If there is associated fracture of the acetabulum that has been reduced, then the patient should have at least 3 weeks of bed rest with skin traction, followed by non-weight-bearing for a further 5 weeks. If a large fragment of the acetabulum remains unreduced, open reduction and internal fixation are necessary. If any fragments of cartilage or bone have been demonstrated on the CT scan, these should be removed either by open operation or in specialist units by arthroscopy of

REFERENCES

70. Dreinhöfer KE, Schwarzkopf SR, Haas NP et al. J Bone Joint Surg 1994; 76B: 6–12

the hip. Fractures of the femoral head in the weight-bearing area should be replaced with perfect reduction of the articular surface. Fractures in the non-weight-bearing areas, if they are large, require reduction. However, if they are small they may be removed.

Most associated injuries of the sciatic nerve are due to neuropraxia and usually recover. If sciatic nerve injuries are associated with an acetabular fracture, the nerve should be explored to exclude injury by the bone fragments. Avascular necrosis of the femoral head complicates at least 10% of all traumatic hip dislocations. This may be picked up radiographically as an increase in density between 6 and 8 weeks after fracture. However, on occasion avascular necrosis may be delayed for up to 2 years after injury. Secondary osteoarthritis is common after dislocation of the hip. Secondary osteoarthritis may be caused by avascular necrosis of the femoral head, incongruity due to fractures of the femoral head or acetabulum, and retained fragments within the joint.

Anterior dislocation is rare. In anterior dislocation the leg lies externally rotated, abducted and slightly flexed. Clinically, in the conscious patient the symptoms are of similar pain, and an anterior bulge in the groin of a dislocated femoral head is diagnostic. The dislocation may be confirmed radiographically on the anteroposterior view of the pelvis, but occasionally a lateral film is required.

Dislocations are reduced with the patient anaesthetized on the anaesthetic room floor and an assistant steadying the pelvis by applying weight to the anterosuperior iliac spines. The hip and knee are flexed to 90° and the thigh pulled upwards and adducted. Osteoarthritis, intra-articular loose bodies, and avascular necrosis may complicate this injury.

Central dislocation of the hip by impaction of the femoral head through the thin medial wall of the acetabulum arises from a direct lateral impact to the hip joint. Every attempt should be made to reduce the dislocation with either skeletal traction or closed reduction and skeletal traction. Accurate reduction of the acetabular fragments makes later reconstruction for secondary osteoarthritis easier. Skeletal traction, if successful, should be maintained for at least 4–6 weeks. Non–weight-bearing, using crutches, should be encouraged for a further 6 weeks.

PATELLA DISLOCATION

Dislocation of the patella is a common condition. It may be classified as acute, chronic, recurrent or habitual. One in 20 patients suffers an associated osteochondral fracture.

Reduction of a dislocated patella is usually spontaneous but occasionally requires a simple push after the administration of analgesia. Indications for operative treatment include the removal of small chondral fragments, the fixation of larger osteochondral fragments, and the repair of an extensive tear of the medial retinaculum.

The incidence of recurrent dislocation of the patella may be up to 40% if the acute soft tissue injury of the medial retinaculum is not repaired.[71] Recurrent dislocation is common in adolescent girls. It is particularly common when the patient has associated genu valgum, persistent femoral anteversion, patella alta, compensatory external tibial torsion, or generalized joint laxity.

KNEE DISLOCATION

Dislocation of the knee is rare. Dislocation is associated with high-energy injuries such as falls from a height or, most commonly, pedestrian accidents. For dislocation to occur, both cruciate ligaments must be torn and one or both collateral ligaments are also torn. Dislocation is often associated with neurovascular injury, and the peripheral circulation and neurological status must be examined to exclude associated injury.

The clinical features are usually those of severe swelling and gross deformity with or without distal neurovascular compromise. Radiographs may reveal associated avulsion fractures of the tibial spines or tip of the fibula, with avulsion of the lateral collateral ligament. If there is any doubt as to the adequacy of perfusion of the limb below the dislocation, an immediate arteriogram is mandatory.

As with dislocation of the hip, reduction under general anaesthesia is an orthopaedic emergency. Closed reduction should be held with a temporary back slab. If closed manipulation fails, open reduction is mandatory. Closed reduction may be followed within 7 days by acute repair of the cruciate ligaments and any collateral ligament injury. Surgical repair followed by early continuous passive motion is often rewarding. The joint should be protected for 3–6 weeks by a suitable knee brace utilizing four points of stabilization, required for preventing cruciate ligament strain.

ANKLE DISLOCATION

Dislocation of the ankle is usually associated with ankle fractures. For their management every attempt should be made to ensure perfect anatomical reduction is achieved, otherwise early postoperative secondary osteoarthritis occurs.

TALAR AND TARSAL DISLOCATION

Talar and tarsal dislocation is a rare injury associated with injury from considerable force, usually a pedal injury following a road traffic accident or a fall from a height. Dislocation is usually associated with a fracture and may be associated with dislocations of the subtalar or midtarsal joints.

Clinical features are invariably of swelling. The deformity of a dislocation is often not obvious because of this swelling and may well cause the dislocation to be missed.

Once closed reduction has been performed, stability of the joint should be assessed. An unstable joint requires K-wire stabilization and a plaster cast. Associated fractures should be addressed by reduction and internal fixation. The K wires may be removed at 3–4 weeks, but a below-knee, non-weight-bearing plaster will be required for 6 weeks after injury.

Dislocation of the talus, especially with associated fractures of the neck of the talus, is commonly complicated by avascular necrosis of the posterior fragment and subsequent secondary arthritis of the ankle and subtalar joints. Dislocations of the metatarsophalangeal or interphalangeal joints should be reduced. Occasionally reduction may be achieved under local anaesthetic. The joint should be splintered, and occasionally K-wire fixation is necessary for an unstable dislocation.

REFERENCE

71. Rorabeck CH, Bobechko WP. J Bone Joint Surg 1976; 58B: 237–240

Spinal fractures

56

Jonathan D Lucas

INTRODUCTION

Spinal injuries can be devastating to the patient and can cause great concern to the treating physician. The aims of this chapter are to outline how to manage a spinal injury in a patient, to identify spinal column and spinal cord injury patterns, and to outline how injuries should be treated. A spinal column injury is the traumatic disruption of the osseous and ligamentous integrity of the spine, which may be stable or unstable and may or may not be associated with a spinal cord injury giving rise to a neurological deficit (which may be complete or partial).

EPIDEMIOLOGY OF SPINAL CORD INJURY AND SPINAL COLUMN INJURY

The annual incidence of spinal cord injury for those who reach hospital alive in developed countries is approximately 50 per million of population. Deaths of patients with a spinal cord injury before admission to hospital (either at the time of the accident or on admission) is between 48 and 79%. The mortality rate after admission to hospital for acute spinal cord injury ranges from 4.4 to 16.7%. The prevalence rates are between 130 and 1124 per million, and the median age of patients with a spinal cord injury is 27 years. The commonest cause of spinal cord injury is road traffic accidents, with accidents at work and during recreation coming joint second (Table 56.1).

Prognosis following spinal cord injury is dependent on age, and the level and degree of severity. Patients with a C1–3-level spinal cord injury have a 6.6 times greater mortality rate than the mortality rate of patients with paraplegia. Patients with a C4–5 and C6–8-level cord injury have mortality rates of 2.5 and 1.1 times higher, respectively, than those with paraplegia (Table 56.2). The age distribution and types of spinal column injuries are shown in Tables 56.3 and 56.4.[1]

Table 56.1 Aetiology of adult spinal cord injuries

Cause of injury	Incidence (%)
Traffic accidents (motor vehicle, bicycle or pedestrian)	40–50
Falls	20
Work	10–25
Sports and recreation	10–25
Violence	10–25

(From Sekhon and Fehlings 2001,[1] with permission.)

INITIAL MANAGEMENT

The initial resuscitation and evaluation of the patient with a spinal injury should follow the established Advanced Trauma Life Support® guidelines.[2] There must be a high index of suspicion for spinal injuries in all patients following significant trauma, especially in patients complaining of axial pain, those with facial and/or head injuries, patients with altered levels of consciousness, polytrauma patients and road traffic or aviation accident victims.

The cervical spine needs to be controlled with a hard cervical collar, sandbags and tape. The thoracolumbosacral spine is initially controlled on a spine board, but as soon as initial resuscitation has taken place, the patient needs to be transferred off the spine board to avoid the development of decubitus ulcers. In the shocked patient with an associated spinal cord injury, neurogenic shock should be considered as a cause of the hypotension. This is due to the loss of the sympathetic tone and is characterized by hypotension with bradycardia. Hypovolaemia must first be excluded as a cause for the hypotension before direct treatment of the neurogenic shock with vasopressors, adrenaline (epinephrine) or noradrenaline (norepinephrine) is commenced.

Table 56.2 Level of injury in adult spinal cord injuries

Level of injury	Incidence (%)
Cervical (C1 to C7–T1)	55
Thoracic (T1–11)	15
Thoracolumbar (T11–12 to L1–2)	15
Lumbosacral (L2–S5)	15

(From Sekhon and Fehlings 2001,[1] with permission.)

REFERENCES

1. Sekhon LH, Fehlings MG. Spine 2001; 26 (24 Suppl): S2–12
2. Committee on Trauma of the American College of Surgeons. Advanced Trauma Life Support Student Course Manual. American College of Surgeons, Chicago, 1997

Table 56.3 Age distribution for acute spinal cord injuries

Age (years)	Incidence (%)
Birth to 10	10
11–20	20
21–30	25
31–40	15
41–50	10
51–60	10
> 60	10
Total	100

(From Sekhon and Fehlings 2001,[1] with permission.)

Table 56.4 Types of vertebral column injury in adult spinal cord injuries

Type of bony injury	Incidence (%)
Fracture–dislocation	40
Burst fracture	30
Minor fracture (including compression)	10
Spinal cord injury without obvious radiological evidence of trauma (SCIWORET) (inluding cervical spondylosis)	10
Dislocation only	5
SCIWORA	5

(From Sekhon and Fehlings 2001,[1] with permission.)

CLINICAL EVALUATION

A detailed history of the mechanism of injury from either the patient or eyewitnesses is invaluable to ascertain the probability of a spinal injury; in addition, a history of any neurological deficit should be sought, even if it has been transitory. A thorough clinical examination of the whole spine and neurological examination is mandatory in a trauma patient. The spine must be inspected and palpated from occiput to coccyx to assess tenderness, pain on movement, a gap or step between the spinous processes, oedema or bruising and/or marked spasm, all of which are indicators of significant injury. To do this, the patient is log rolled, which requires a minimum of four people. This is the most opportune moment to undertake a rectal examination and to assess the bulbocavernosus reflex (this will be returned to).

A full and comprehensive neurological examination is essential; it must always be undertaken at the first possible opportunity of the patient arriving in the emergency room, because this may be the only opportunity for some time if the patient is required to be intubated and ventilated. All muscle groups are assessed for tone and motor function according to the UK Medical Research Council grade; sensation is assessed for pain (pinprick), light touch, and proprioception or vibration. All the reflexes are tested, including the bulbocavernosus. In the unconscious patient, particular attention is paid to the respiratory effort; if there is diaphragmatic breathing with paroxysmal chest movement and response to pain on stimulus above the clavicle but not below, then there is likely to be high cervical cord injury.

All the neurological findings need to be carefully documented to allow detection of either neurological improvement or deterioration. This can be done on a form developed by the American Spinal Injury Association, a form that also incorporates a scoring system (Fig. 56.1) that allows a sensitive assessment of neurological improvement or deterioration.

SPINAL CORD INJURY CLASSIFICATION

Following injury to the spinal cord, the injury may be either complete, with no neurological function below the level of injury, or incomplete, with some neurological function maintained below the injury level. The complete or incomplete nature of the injury may be determined only once spinal shock has resolved. Spinal shock is a period following cord injury during which the cord is functionless; this period may last from a few hours to up to 7 days, even if the cord injury is incomplete. Therefore the true extent of the cord injury cannot be determined until the spinal shock has resolved. It does not occur following all cord injuries.

Spinal shock is characterized by a flaccid, areflexic paralysis; an atonic bladder with subsequent overflow incontinence; and an absent bulbocavernosus reflex. The bulbocavernosus reflex is elicited by stimulation of the penis or clitoris by digital pressure or a sharp pull on the Foley catheter while a gloved finger in the rectum notes a resulting contraction of the anal sphincter; a positive response indicates resolution of spinal shock with return of the reflex arc and the true extent of the spinal cord lesion can be evaluated (Fig. 56.2).

The level of the cord injury is defined as the most caudal segment with normal function. This may be different for left and right sides and for motor and sensory function. The level is identified by careful clinical examination and can be determined only in the fully conscious patient. The degree of cord injury has been classified by Frankel[3] and subsequently modified by the American Spinal Injury Association.

- Grade A (complete): no motor or sensory function is preserved including the sacral segments S4–5.
- Grade B (incomplete): sensory but not motor function is preserved below the neurological level and extends through the sacral segments S4–5.
- Grade C (incomplete): motor function is preserved below the neurological level, and more than half the key muscles below the neurological level have a muscle grade less than 3.
- Grade B (incomplete): motor function is preserved below the neurological level, and at least half the key muscles below the neurological level have a muscle grade of 3 or more.
- Grade E (normal): motor and sensory function are normal.

Incomplete lesions fall into a number of clinical syndromes, as described below.

Central cord syndrome

A central cord syndrome is usually seen in older patients (older than 60 years) who suffer hyperextension injuries of the cervical

REFERENCE

3. Frankel HL, Hancock GH, Melzak J et al. Paraplegia 1969; 7: 179–192

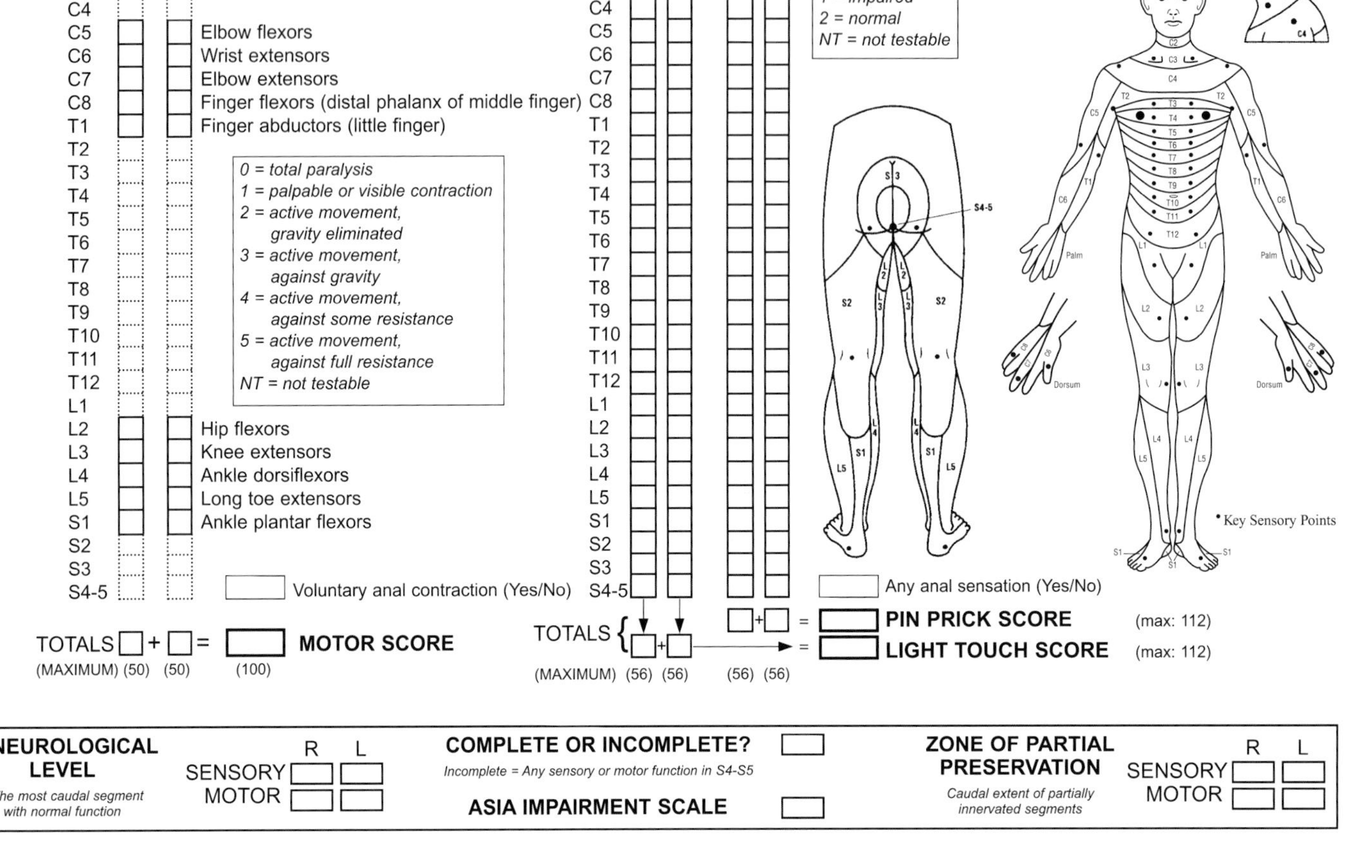

Figure 56.1 The American Spinal Injury Association form; this form allows a standard neurological classification of spinal cord injuries and is a very sensitive tool for assessing neurological improvement or deterioration over time.

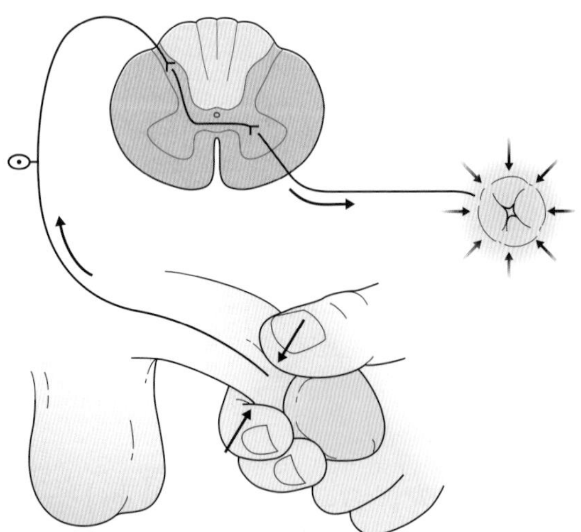

Figure 56.2 The bulbocavernosus reflex. In cord injuries, the bulbocavernosus reflex returns once spinal shock has resolved and defines the end of spinal shock. Stimulation of either the penis or clitoris results in anal sphincter contraction.

spine. The central portion of the spinal cord is injured by the pincer movement of the posterior vertebral body osteophytes and the hypertrophied ligamentum flavum. Due to the anatomical arrangements of the neural tracts, the upper limbs and especially the hands are affected significantly more than the lower limbs with sacral sparing, and there is preservation of bladder and bowel function. The patient has significant loss of upper limb motor and sensory function but is usually still able to walk, although with a myelopathic component to his or her gait (Fig. 56.3).

Brown–Sequard syndrome

Brown–Sequard syndrome results from hemisection of the cord. It clinically consists of ipsilateral motor, proprioception and vibration sensory loss, and contralateral loss of pain, temperature and light touch (Fig. 56.4). In its pure form it is relatively rare.

Anterior cord syndrome

Anterior cord syndrome involves damage to the anterior two-thirds of the cord, and results in loss of motor and sensory function below the level of the injury with preservation of proprioception and vibration sense only, due to the sparing of the posterior columns.

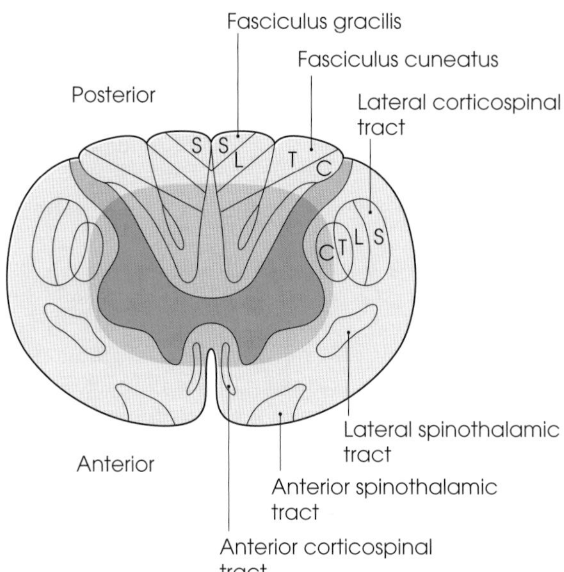

Figure 56.3 Central cord syndrome. The central portion of the cord is affected. In the corticospinal tracts, motor, and spinothalamic tracts, pain and temperature, the fibres innervating the arms are located more medially and those innervating the leg and sacrum are located more laterally. Therefore the arms are affected more than the legs and there is sacral sparing.

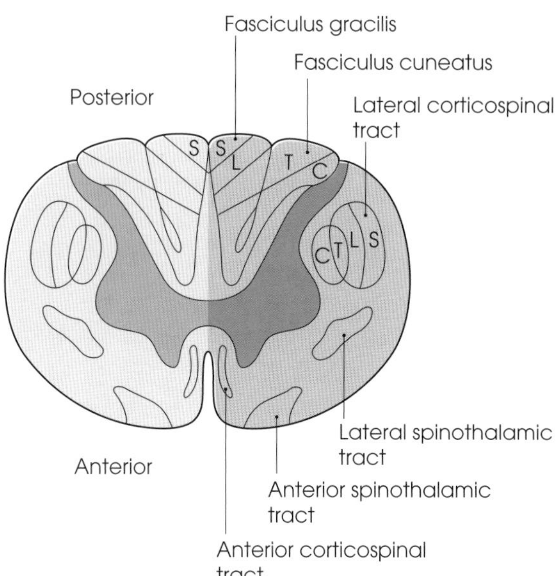

Figure 56.4 Brown–Sequard syndrome. Hemisection of the cord leads to ipsilateral motor loss and contralateral pain, and the loss of temperature and light touch.

Conus lesion

The conus is the terminal part of the cord. The conus contains the cell bodies of L5 to S5, is approximately one vertebral body in length, and is located opposite T12–L1 in females and slightly lower in males at L1–2. A pure conus lesion gives rise to L5 and S1 motor and sensory loss with sacral involvement. It causes an autonomous, flaccid, areflexic bladder; a flaccid, functionless anal sphincter; and loss of the bulbocavernosus reflex. However, pure conus lesions are rare, and there is usually associated involvement of the cauda equina with variable severity of nerve root involvement from L1 downwards.

Cauda equina lesions

The cauda equina, or horse's tail, is made up of the lumbosacral nerve roots. The L1 nerve root leaves the spinal cord at the level of the T10 vertebra, with L2 and L3 nerve roots leaving the cord at the level of T11. Pure cauda equina lesion occurs below the level of the conus at between L1 and L2. This is a pure lower motor neuron radiculopathy with a flaccid, areflexic bladder; a flaccid anal sphincter with loss of voluntary contraction; and loss of the bulbocavernosus reflex.

RADIOLOGICAL ASSESSMENT

All patients with a suspected spinal column or cord injury will need further imaging of the spine. The Advanced Trauma Life Support® primary survey will have included a cross-table lateral of the cervical spine. Further radiological assessment will be required, including further plain radiographs with CT scanning or MRI scanning (or both) to diagnose and define the anatomy of the spinal injury.

The cervical spine lateral radiograph must include the occiput to the C7–T1 junction. If this is unable to be obtained in the standard fashion with pulling down on the arms, then a swimmers or oblique views should be obtained. If satisfactory visualization of the C7–T1 junction is still not possible then a CT scan is required. A transoral odontoid peg view and anteroposterior of the cervical spine should also be obtained. The following abnormalities are indicative of cervical injury and should be sought on the plane cervical spine X-ray.

- Loss of cervical lordosis.
- Increased anterior soft tissue width (Fig. 56.5).
- Increased interspinous distance posteriorly on both the lateral and anteroposterior X-rays.
- Loss of spinous process alignment on the anteroposterior X-ray.
- Fractures of the ring of the atlas or odontoid peg. The standard atlanto–dens interval (ADI) is less than 3 mm in adults and less than 5 mm in children. The space available for the cord (SAC) should be greater than 16 mm; less than 10 mm is critical. A greater than 7 mm overhang of the C1 lateral mass on the C2 lateral mass is indicative of a fracture of the C1 ring, which is significantly displaced to have ruptured the transverse ligament (Fig. 56.6).
- Loss of alignment indicating a fracture, subluxation or dislocation. This is indicated if there are more than 11° of angulation or 3.5 mm of translation at any level.

A full plain X-ray series (anteroposterior, lateral and open mouth view) of the cervical spine will at best identify 85% of fractures. Therefore in patients with persistent symptoms, head or facial injuries, or neurological deficits with normal plain X-rays will require further imaging of the cervical spine with either a CT scan or an MRI scan. In those patients in whom a fracture or other abnormality is identified on the plain X-rays, a CT scan will be required to delineate the fracture pattern and anatomy and an MRI scan will be required if there is a significant soft tissue component to the injury (i.e. a cord or nerve root injury, or ligamentous or disc injury).

In the thoracolumbar spine, high-quality anteroposterior and lateral radiographs are required. The following abnormalities should be looked for to identify an injury:

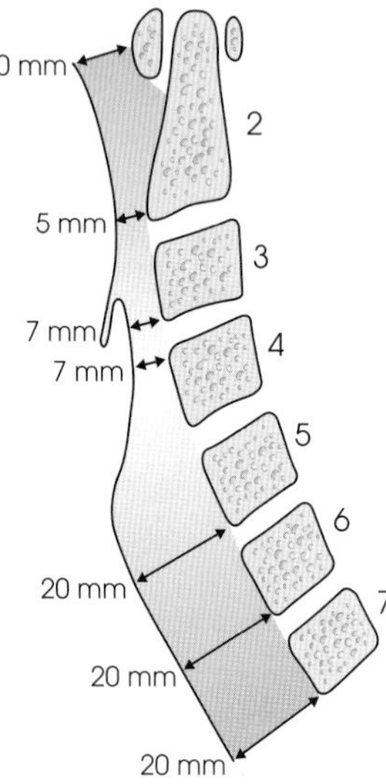

Figure 56.5 The normal anterior soft tissue measurements of the lateral cervical spine X-ray. The figures are the upper range of normal for the soft tissue width of the retropharyngeal space and prevertebral space in millimetres.

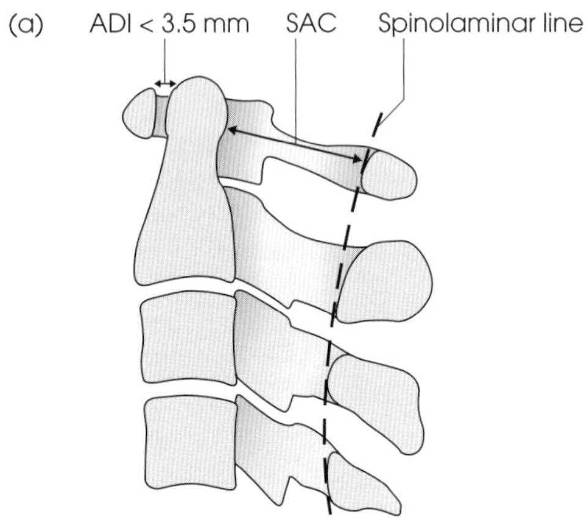

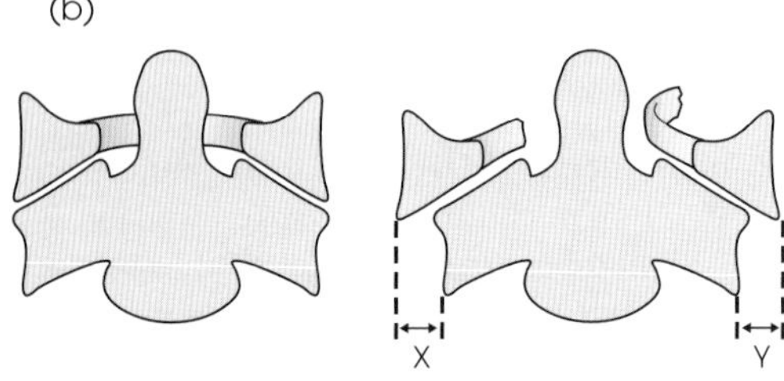

Figure 56.6 Radiological assessment measurements of the C1–2 complex. **(a)** The lateral cervical spine X-ray shows the atlanto–dens interval (ADI) less than 3 mm and the space available for the cord (SAC), which should be greater than 16 mm. **(b)** The open mouth view shows the relationship of the lateral masses of C1 and C2; an overhang of greater than 7 mm indicates a rupture of the transverse ligament.

- loss of vertebral alignment on anteroposterior and lateral X-rays;
- fractures of vertebral bodies, posterior elements, spinous or transverse processes;
- widening of the interspinous distance;
- widening of the interpedicular distance; and
- loss of vertebral body height, vertebral wedging and kyphosis.

A standardized approach to imaging is required. If a fracture is found in the cervical spine, the incidence of another fracture at an adjacent level (especially at C1–2) is 50%[4] or higher, and a non-contiguous fracture in the cervical spine is present in approximately 16% of cases.[5] Non-contiguous fractures in the thoracolumbar fractures occur in between 9[6] and 20% of cases, approximately.[7] Therefore if one injury level is identified, a second level of injury must be actively excluded by further clinical examination and plain radiographs of every level of the spine (Fig. 56.7).

If any fracture or injury is identified on the X-ray (with the exception of minor process fractures), CT imaging should be obtained, which also allows for coronal, sagittal and three-dimensional reconstruction. The full fracture configuration is rarely identified on plain X-rays alone; CT scanning allows full definition of the fracture anatomy and is also useful in planning surgical reconstruction, if required. Computerized tomography is also useful in identifying occiput/C1/C2 and C7/T1 fractures.

Magnetic resonance imaging scanning allows the demonstration of soft tissue injury to the posterior ligamentous structures and intervertebral discs. If MRI is available, its use is advised in patients with uni- and bilateral cervical facet dislocations before reduction; this will identify if, during the reduction procedure, there is a likelihood of retropulsion of disc material into the canal that may cause cord or nerve root injury. The extent of spinal cord injuries is also identified by MRI imaging.

Dynamic radiographs, flexion–extension lateral X-rays of the cervical spine, are inappropriate if there is a suspicion of an unstable fracture or injury. In a conscious and cooperative patient with persistent cervical pain and no radiographic evidence of fracture or dislocation, supervised flexion–extension X-rays are taken and will allow exclusion of any instability of the cervical spine. However, if there is severe paravertebral spasm, the X-rays should be delayed until this has resolved; the patient should be treated in a firm orthosis until this has occurred, which may take up to 2 weeks following the injury.

THE UNCONSCIOUS PATIENT

Exclusion of a spinal injury in the unconscious patient is difficult. Orthopaedic surgeons are often asked to 'clear' the cervical spine of the unconscious, intubated and ventilated patient on the intensive care unit so that the hard collar may be removed to make nursing care easier. The issue of how the cervical spine may be safely 'cleared' has not been satisfactorily resolved. Meticulous clinical examination and plain X-rays of the whole spine are required. The cervical spine may be reasonably cleared in the following ways.

- Treat the cervical spine as unstable until the patient is fully conscious and cooperative, to allow a full clinical assessment and flexion–extension lateral X-rays to be performed if indicated.
- Do an MRI of the cervical spine to exclude any fractures or

REFERENCES

4. Levine AM, Edwards CC. Orthop Clin North Am 1986; 17: 31–44
5. Vaccaro AR, An HS, Lin SS et al. J Spinal Disord 1992; 5: 320–329
6. Powell JN, Waddell JP, Tucker WS et al. J Trauma 1989; 29: 1146–1150
7. Korres DS, Katsaros A, Panatazopoulos T et al. Injury 1981; 13: 147–152

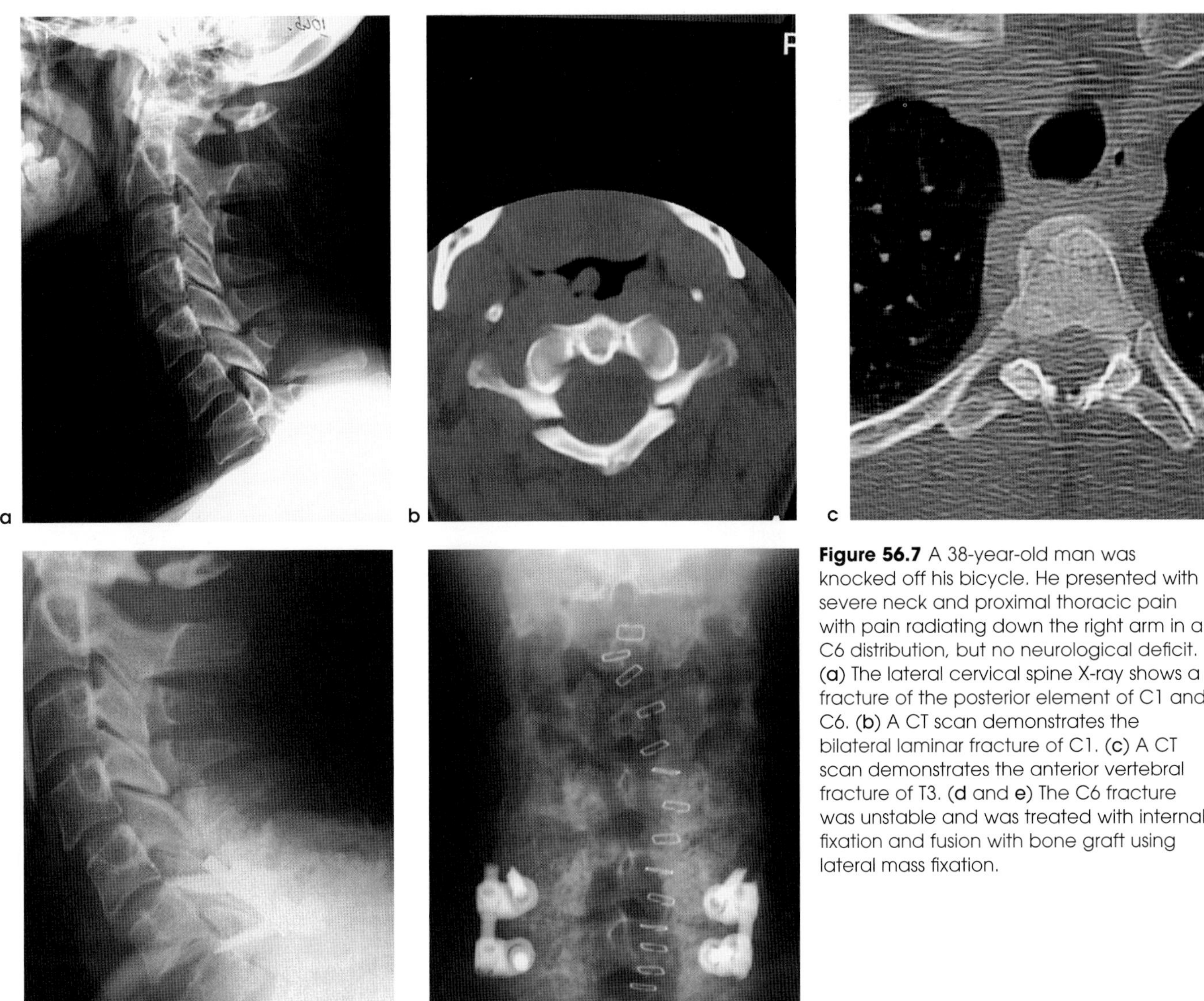

Figure 56.7 A 38-year-old man was knocked off his bicycle. He presented with severe neck and proximal thoracic pain with pain radiating down the right arm in a C6 distribution, but no neurological deficit. **(a)** The lateral cervical spine X-ray shows a fracture of the posterior element of C1 and C6. **(b)** A CT scan demonstrates the bilateral laminar fracture of C1. **(c)** A CT scan demonstrates the anterior vertebral fracture of T3. **(d and e)** The C6 fracture was unstable and was treated with internal fixation and fusion with bone graft using lateral mass fixation.

soft tissue injury that may make the spine unstable, and to identify any cord injury.

- Undertake dynamic flexion–extension X-rays under image-intensifier control; if subluxation is demonstrated the manoeuvre is stopped before damage is done. This is controversial.
- Some view a normal, whole, cervical spine CT scan as being a satisfactory method of clearing the cervical spine, but this is also controversial.

INSTABILITY OF THE INJURED SPINE

White and Panjabi have best defined instability of the spine: 'the loss of the ability of the spine under physiological loads to maintain its pattern of displacement so that there is no initial or additional neurological deficit, no major deformity and no incapacitating pain'.[8] Missed instability may produce or exacerbate a spinal cord injury in the initial management phase or may displace an undisplaced fracture or dislocation, thus precipitating harm to the patient, the need for further intervention, and in the long term may lead to chronic instability pain with movement and a higher risk of degenerative changes.

Many authors have tried, mostly unsatisfactorily, to determine prescriptive radiological criteria for determining the stability of the injured spine. Denis devised the concept of the spine being constructed as three columns; if two or more columns are disrupted the spine is unstable.[9] This concept has subsequently been simplified by Magerl and colleagues[10] from the original work of Whitesides[11] to a two-column view of the spine. The anterior column is the vertebral body up to and including the posterior longitudinal ligament, and the posterior column comprises the remaining posterior elements. Following an injury,

REFERENCES

8. White AA, Panjabi MM. Clinical Biomechanics of the Spine. JB Lippincott, Philadelphia, 1990
9. Denis F. Spine 1983; 8; 817–831
10. Magerl F, Aebi M, Gertzbein D et al. Eur Spine J 1994; 3: 184–201
11. Whitesides TE Jr. Clin Orthop 1977; 128: 78–92

an intact anterior or posterior column will usually prevent immediate or long-term problems associated with instability. Careful assessment of both columns is required, however, and the combination of clinical and radiological investigation may reveal significant injury to both columns. For example, what may appear to be an isolated compression fracture of the anterior column may have an associated predominantly ligamentous posterior column injury, only diagnosed by clinical examination or MRI scanning.

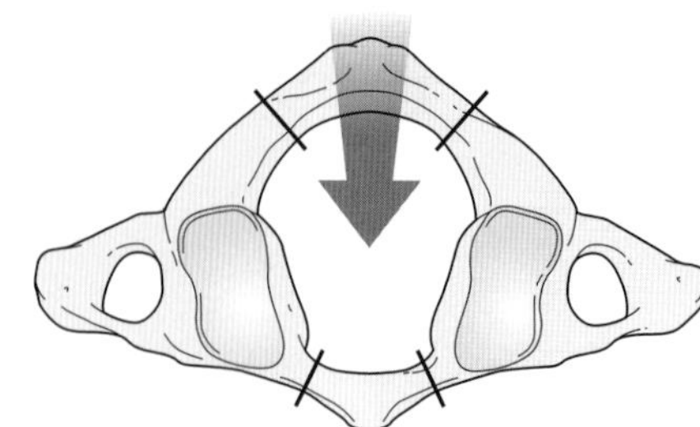

Figure 56.8 Axial loading may disrupt the C1 ring in two or more places.

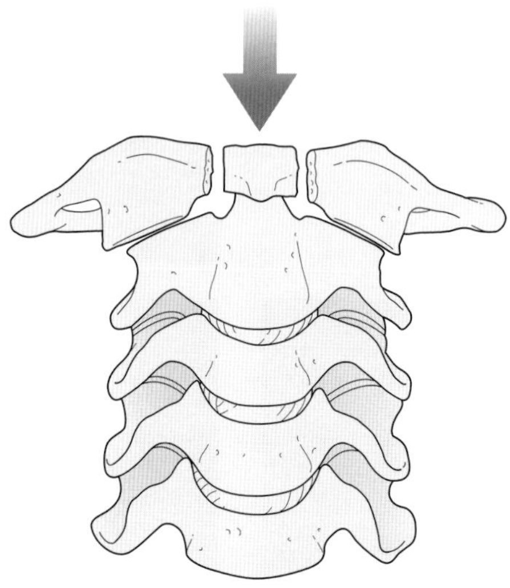

INITIAL MANAGEMENT OF THE SPINAL INJURY

CERVICAL SPINE INJURIES

Undisplaced cervical injuries, whether stable or unstable, can be controlled with a stiff cervical collar in the initial phase of management. Displaced and unstable injuries are best managed with halo traction, except for type 2a hangman's fractures (see later). The use of a halo is preferable to that of tongs or calipers because modern haloes offer better head and neck control, are MRI-compatible, and may subsequently be attached to a moulded jacket for definitive treatment of the injury if this is indicated. Initial longitudinal halo traction is of the order of 5–10 lb (2.3–4.6 kg), followed by neurological assessment and lateral X-ray. Subsequent incremental increasing of the traction by 5 lb every 15 min is used until the fracture dislocation is reduced, and weight of up to or over 100 lbs are described.[12] The maintenance weight to hold the fracture/dislocation is approximately 5 lb for the head and 5 lb for the level. Displaced Jefferson, hangman, odontoid peg fractures types II and III, and displaced fractures or dislocations can be treated in this fashion to achieve initial reduction. The reduction can be maintained with the traction until definitive management is undertaken.

THORACOLUMBAR INJURIES

The patient with unstable or potentially unstable injuries should be treated supine—with frequent log rolling to ensure that decubitus ulcers do not develop—until definitive treatment is undertaken.

THE ROLE OF STEROIDS

The use of high-dose methylprednisolone in the treatment of acute spinal cord injury—despite the second and third National Acute Spinal Cord Injury Study randomized controlled trials[13,14]—is still not clearly defined, varies from centre to centre, and is dependent on the individual preferences of the centre. This regimen has been demonstrated to have complications related to sepsis and wound healing.

CERVICAL SPINE FRACTURES

CRANIOCERVICAL TRAUMA

Fractures or dislocation of the atlanto-occipital joint and occipital condyles are rare and usually fatal.

FRACTURES OF THE ATLAS (C1) (JEFFERSON FRACTURE)

This is a fracture of the anterior and posterior ring of C1 due to axial compression (Fig. 56.8). Greater than 7 mm of splaying of the fragments, as demonstrated on the open mouth X-ray, indicates rupture of the transverse ligament and the presence of atlantoaxial instability. These fractures are associated with concomitant C2 fractures in up to or over 50% of cases, with fracture of the dens or a traumatic spondylolisthesis of the axis (i.e. a hangman's fracture).

These fractures are best delineated with CT scanning. If there is minimal displacement of the fracture, it may be treated with a hard orthosis for 6–8 weeks. If there is significant displacement, this may be reduced with halo traction and subsequently held with a halo vest for 8–12 weeks until the fracture has united. Surgical stabilization may be indicated for persistent instability and pain.

Atlantoaxial rotatory deformities

Rotatory subluxation of the atlas and axis, described by Fielding and Hawkins,[15] leads to asymmetry of the odontoid peg and may be associated with an increase in the atlanto–dens interval. The diagnosis is often missed or delayed, and a variety of treatments have been described. The condition is also associated with pharyngeal sepsis and has the term *maladie de Grisel*[16] ascribed to it.

REFERENCES

12. Lee AS, MacLean JCB, Newton DA. J Bone Joint Surg 1994; 76-B: 352–356
13. Bracken MB, Shepard MJ, Collins WF Jr et al. J Neurosurg 1992; 76: 23–31
14. Bracken MB, Shepard MJ, Holford TR et al. J Neurosurg 1998; 89: 699–706
15. Fielding JW, Hawkins RJ. J Bone Joint Surg 1977; 59-A: 37
16. Desfosses P. Presse Med 1930; 38: 1179

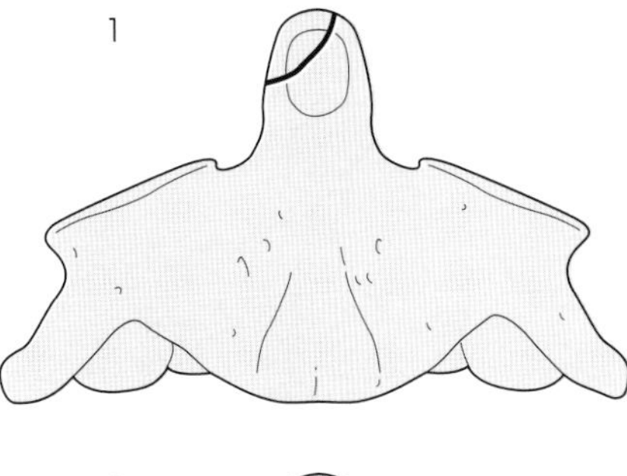

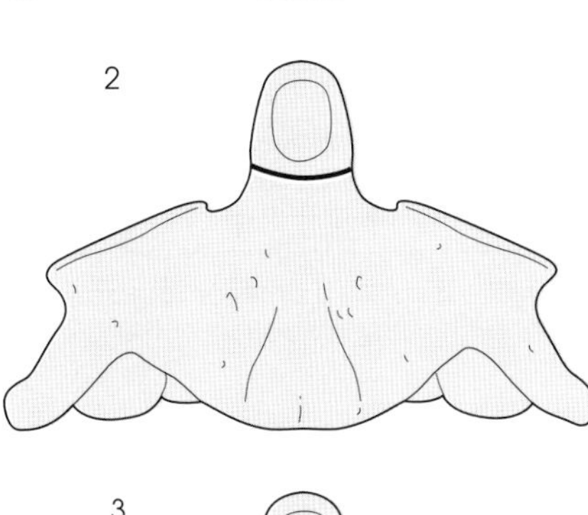

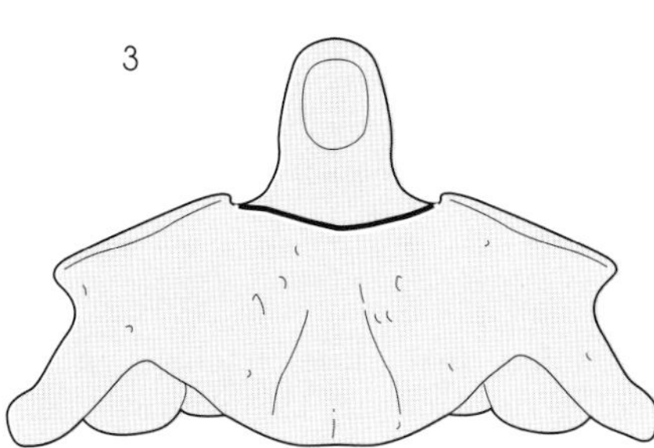

Figure 56.9 Anderson and D'Alonzo classification of odontoid peg fractures: type 1, fracture of the tip of the peg; type 2, fracture through the base of the peg; type 3, fracture through the body of C1 at the base of the peg.

FRACTURES OF THE AXIS (C2)

Fractures of the odontoid

Fractures of the odontoid have been classified by Anderson and D'Alonzo depending on the anatomical location of the fracture,[17] as seen in Fig. 56.9. Type 1 peg fractures are stable and may be treated in a soft collar. Type 2 fractures have a high rate of non-union, from 11 to 100%, which is related to patient age, degree of displacement and angulation, and delay in diagnosis. Minimally displaced fractures in young patients may be treated in a halo vest; those fractures with significant displacement (greater than 4 mm or greater than 10° of angulation) and those in the elderly may be best treated with surgical fusion (Fig. 56.10). Type 3 fractures almost always unite and the majority may be treated with either a hard orthosis or a halo vest.

Traumatic spondylolisthesis of the axis (hangman's fracture)

This is a fracture approximately through the pedicles of C2. There are five types of this fracture, as shown in Fig. 56.11. The five types are a modification of the classification described by Levine and Edwards.[18] The mechanism of injury in all but that of type IIa is predominantly extension compression followed to varying degrees by flexion, and so all are able to be reduced safely by halo traction. Type IIa hangman's fractures are produced predominantly by distraction, and on application of traction the fracture is further displaced. The treating surgeon needs to be aware of this fracture type to avoid this mistake. This fracture is essentially the only cervical fracture that cannot initially be safely treated with judicious use of halo traction.

Treatment is with a hard collar for the stable type I and type Ia fractures. Type II fractures may be treated with halo traction, followed by application of a halo vest once the fracture is satis-

REFERENCES

17. Anderson LD, D'Alonzo RT. J Bone Joint Surg Am 1974; 56: 1663
18. Levine AM, Edwards CC. J Bone Joint Surg 1985; 67: 217–226

Insufficiency of the transverse ligament

Insufficiency of the transverse ligament leads to C1 on C2 instability and may be congenital, post-traumatic or infective, but the commonest cause is inflammatory, secondary to rheumatoid arthritis with pannus destroying the transverse ligament.

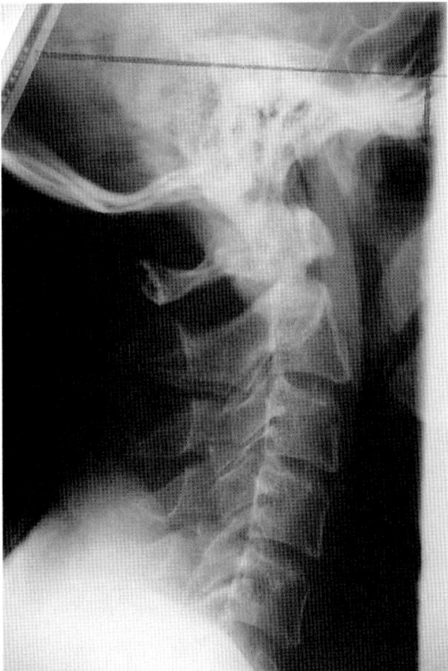

a

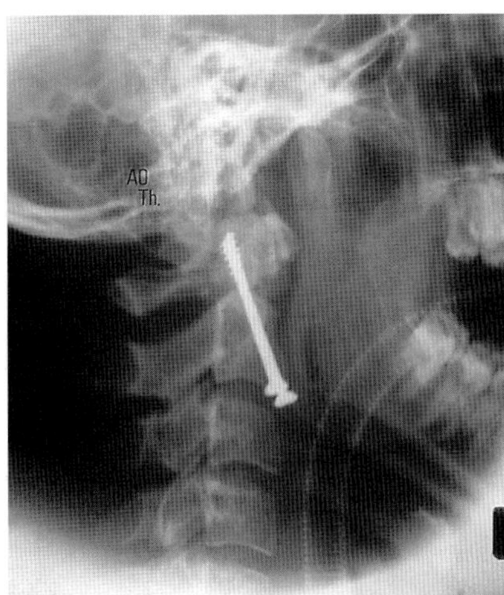

b

Figure 56.10 Displaced type 2 odontoid fracture (a) and internal fixation of the fracture (b).

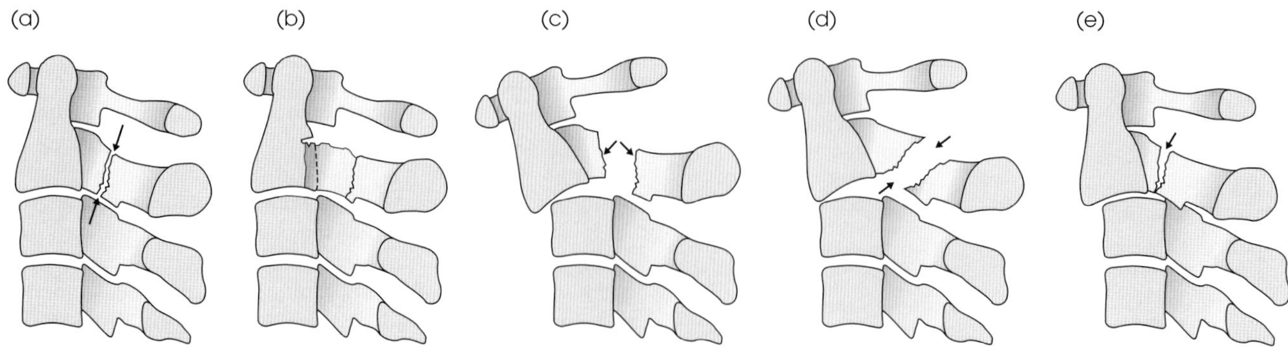

Figure 56.11 Hangman's fracture: traumatic spondylolisthesis of the axis. **(a)** Type I: minimally displaced (less than 3 mm) fracture through the pedicles with no associated angulation. **(b)** Type IA: atypical type 1 fracture in which the fracture is oblique, going through the body with or without the foramen on one side and the lamina on the other. **(c)** Type II: hyperextension or axial load followed by flexion with a fracture through pedicles, anterior subluxation of C2 on C3 greater than 3 mm, and anterior subluxation. **(d)** Type IIA: flexion or distraction injury with the fracture more oblique than in type II and in which there is marked anterior angulation but no anterior translation; this fracture is *not* reduced on traction. **(e)** Type III: fracture of the neural arch with dislocation of the C2 on C3 facet joints.

factorily reduced; internal fixation is sometimes used. Type IIa fractures may be treated with a halo vest. Type III fractures usually need surgical intervention.

SUBAXIAL CERVICAL SPINE INJURY

Allen and Ferguson have described in detail the classification most widely used,[19] but more simply subaxial fracture and dislocations may be divided into the following categories.

Minor compression or avulsion fractures

Minor compression or avulsion fractures are all stable and may be treated with a soft collar for pain relief. They include clay shoveller's fracture, which is avulsion of the seventh vertebral spinous process, and avulsion teardrop fracture, which is a hyperextension avulsion fracture of the anterior–inferior corner of the vertebral body. This fracture is not to be confused with the flexion compression teardrop fracture of the vertebral body, which is highly unstable and has a high association with neurological deficit.

Unifacet and bifacetal dislocations

Unifacet dislocations are caused by flexion, distraction and rotation of the cervical spine. Radiologically, there is approximately 25% anterior subluxation of the cranial vertebra over the caudal vertebra, with the characteristic bow tie sign secondary to overlap of the facet and the lateral mass. These injuries may be associated (but not always) with a neurological deficit including nerve root compression and incomplete cord lesions, which may include a Brown–Sequard syndrome.

Bifacetal dislocation is secondary to flexion and distraction and is radiologically characterized by 50% or more subluxation of one vertebra over the caudal vertebra. These injuries are associated with a high incidence of cord injury. Initial treatment is with closed awake reduction with halo traction after an MRI has been performed to identify if there is a significant risk of disc material being displaced into the spinal canal to cause cord damage during the reduction manoeuvre. Definitive management is usually with surgical stabilization.

Compression fractures

Axial compression is the main mechanism of injury for vertebral body burst fractures with retropulsion of bony fragments into the canal, causing cord damage. These are usually unstable fractures and are treated surgically. Flexion/compression injuries cause teardrop fractures, which are characterized by fractures of the anterior portion of the vertebral body with posterior subluxation. These injuries are associated with a high incidence of cord injury and are very unstable. Surgical stabilization is usually indicated (Fig. 56.12).

Hyperextension injuries

This is the mechanism of injury that causes fractures of the posterior elements, including the laminae, lateral masses and pedicles. These injuries are treated on their relative merits, depending on degree of displacement and associated neurological deficit, either conservatively with hard orthosis, halo traction or orthosis with surgical stabilization.

SPINAL CORD INJURY WITHOUT RADIOLOGICAL ABNORMALITY (SCIWORA)

This is self-explanatory and occurs predominantly in children who have sustained significant trauma. Even dynamic imaging is normal, demonstrating that the spinal column is stable. Magnetic resonance imaging scanning is mandatory to identify if there has been a fracture through the cartilaginous end plate, the commonest site for fracture in the paediatric spine, and to delineate the extent of the cord injury. Given that in the majority of these children the cervical spine is stable, the treatment is medically supportive, combined with spinal cord injury rehabilitation programs.[20]

THORACIC AND LUMBAR FRACTURES

The majority of thoracic and lumbar fractures occur at the thoracolumbar junction (T11 to L1), this being the transition between the thoracic spine, relatively fixed due to the ribs and sternum, and the relatively flexible lumbar spine. This region accounts for 48 to 52% of thoracolumbar fractures, the lumbar spine (L2–5) for 28 to 32%, and the thoracic spine (T1–10) for 16 to 24%.[10,21]

REFERENCES

19. Allen BL, Ferguson RL, Lehmann TR et al. Spine 1982; 7: 1–27
20. Pang D, Wilberger JE. J Neurosurg 1982; 57: 114–129
21. Gertzbein SD. Spine 1991; 17: 528–540

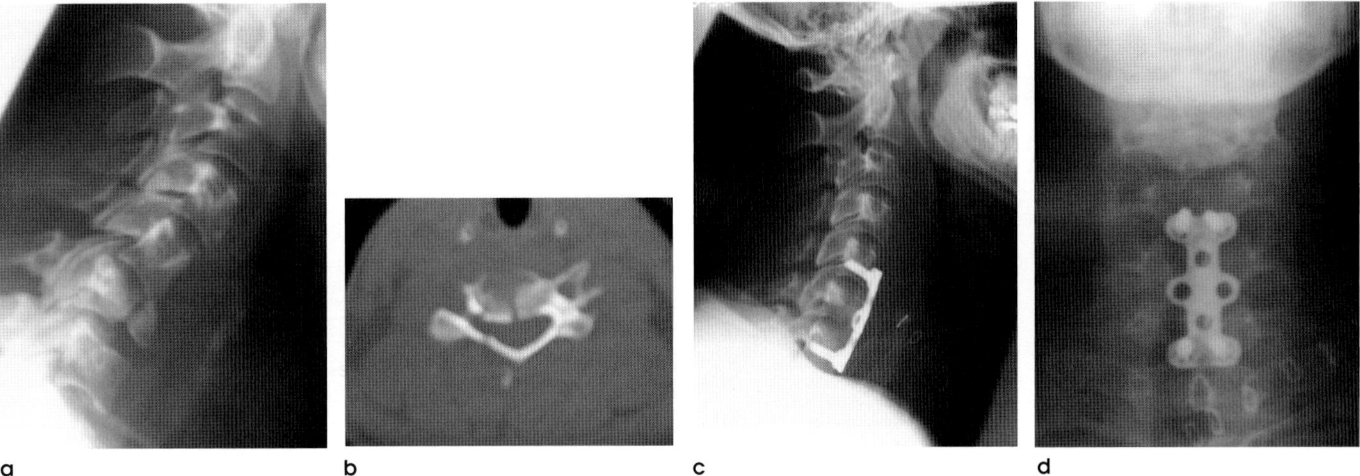

Figure 56.12 Flexion or compression, or teardrop fracture of C6. (**a**) Lateral cervical spine X-ray showing the characteristic anterior–superior to posterior–inferior oblique line of the teardrop fracture. (**b, c** and **d**) Postoperative anteroposterior and lateral X-rays showing the C6 corpectomy, tricortical iliac crest graft and plating, with restoration of the cervical lordosis.

The majority of thoracolumbar fractures fall into four main catagories: compression, burst, flexion, distraction (seat belt), and fracture–dislocations. This is the classification developed by Denis in which the spine is considered as three columns (Fig. 56.13).[9] The main disadvantage of this classification is that it does not cover all fracture types, but it is relatively simple and is considered here. The AO group under Magerl[10] has developed a classification system that follows the standard format of AO classifications (A, B and C subsections) and considers the spinal column as two columns. This classification, although more complete, is significantly more complex and will not be considered here.

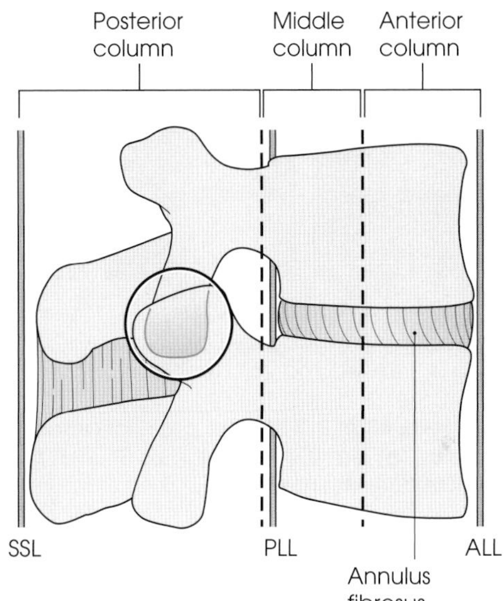

Figure 56.13 The three columns of the thoraco-lumbar spine: SSL, supraspinous ligament; PLL, posterior longitudinal ligament; ALL, anterior longitudinal ligament. (From Denis 1983,[9] with permission.)

COMPRESSION FRACTURES

Compression wedge fractures account for the vast majority of osseous injuries to the thoracolumbar spine: 49 to 90%, depending on which series you consider. The mechanism of injury is predominantly axial compression with varying degrees of flexion and produces a characteristic wedge-shaped vertebral body deformity. If there is greater than 50% loss of height and greater than 30° of kyphosis, then there is likely to be posterior interspinous ligament injury and the fracture is unstable. This can be confirmed clinically if there is significant posterior tenderness and a palpable gap indicating that the posterior ligamentous complex is ruptured; this can also be confirmed by an MRI scan.

There is a low association of neurological deficit with these fractures. Because the majority of these fractures are stable, they may be treated conservatively with mobilization as symptoms allow or with a thoracolumbosacral orthosis if symptoms demand.

BURST FRACTURES

Burst fractures result from axial compression; failure of both the anterior and posterior walls of the vertebral body occurs, with splaying of the pedicles, vertical laminar fracture, and retropulsion of both osseous and disc material into the spinal canal. The stability of these fractures is dependent on the degree of vertebral body height loss, the degree of kyphosis, and the presence or absence of neurological deficit. These need to be decided on a case-by-case basis. Those fractures with 50% loss of height and 30° of kyphosis tend to be unstable (Fig. 56.14).

FLEXION/DISTRACTION (SEAT BELT) INJURIES

These injuries were first described by G.Q. Chance in 1948 with three cases, and are failures of the posterior and middle column with fractures through the spinous process into the pedicles and posterior third of the vertebral bodies. These injuries commonly occur in patients wearing a lap belt who are involved in road traffic accidents. There is a high incidence, up to 50%, of associated intra-abdominal pathology (e.g. torn mesentery or bowel, or spleen or liver contusions). There is a low association with neurological deficit. These injuries are unstable and are usually treated operatively (Fig. 56.15).

FRACTURE–DISLOCATIONS

These are flexion distraction injuries with failure of the posterior elements, either facet subluxation or overt dislocation, and associated fractures of the vertebral bodies or disruption of the intervertebral disc. There is a very high incidence of significant neurological deficit in bifacetal dislocation, with 90% of patients having a complete paraplegia if it occurs above T10 and 60% if it

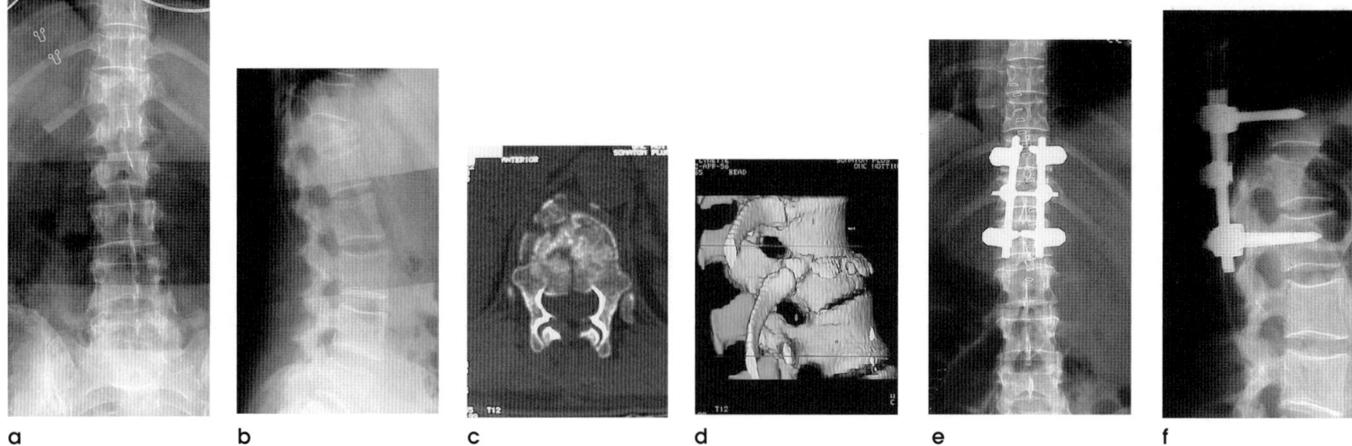

Figure 56.14 T12 burst fracture. (a and b) Anteroposterior and lateral X-rays showing the T12 burst with splaying of the pedicles, significant height loss, and kyphosis. (c and d) The CT scans with three-dimensional reconstruction showing retropulsion of bony fragments into the spinal canal and the anterior comminution of the vertebral. (e and f) Postoperative X-rays showing internal pedicle screw fixation with restoration of the vertebral height and the thoracolumbar junction lordosis.

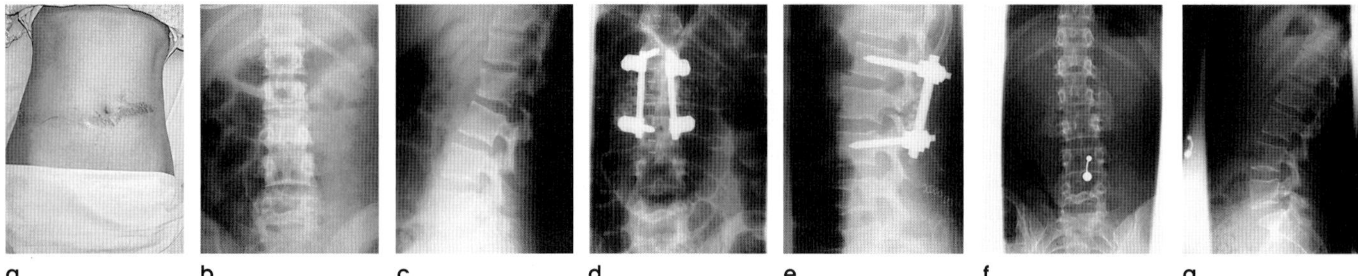

Figure 56.15 Chance fracture. An 18-year-old girl was a rear-seat passenger wearing a lap belt when she was involved in road traffic accident, the car hitting a tree head on. (a) Contusion on the anterior abdominal wall from the lap belt; there were no intra-abdominal injuries in this case. (b and c) The anteroposterior X-ray shows the interspinous widening. (d) The lateral X-ray shows the fracture through the posterior elements into the posterior aspect of the vertebral body. (e and f) Postoperative X-rays showing internal fixation with pedicle screws. (g) X-rays showing the L2–3 fusion following removal of the metal work and the posterolateral boney fusion mass. The patient was pain-free with no disability.

occurs below T10.These injuries are very unstable and are treated with surgical stabilization. Hyperextension injuries can cause fracture dislocations but these are rare.

SACRAL FRACTURES

Isolated fractures of the sacrum are rare, but 40–45% of pelvic fractures will have an associated sacral fracture. Denis classified these fractures according to which of three zones of the sacrum the fracture is located (Fig. 56.16).[22] The importance of the zones is the relationship of neurological deficit to the zone in which the fracture occurs. Zone 1 is the sacral alar and is associated with a 5.9% incidence of neural deficit. Zone 2 is through the neural foramen and is associated with a 28.4% incidence of neural deficit. Finally, zone 3 is through the central canal and is associated with a 56.7% incidence of neural deficit. Therefore careful clinical assessment of neurological function by means of perineal sensory testing, presence or absence of the anal wink, resting anal sphincter tone and strength of voluntary anal sphincter contraction, presence or absence of the bulbo-cavernosus reflex, and presence or absence of normal bladder function need to be carefully documented.

Following pelvic trauma and apparently normal plain X-rays of the pelvis, there may be subtle neurological changes. These manifest as mild perineal sensory changes and mild disturbance of normal bladder and bowel function; such cases must have a sacral fracture excluded by means of a CT scan or bone scan.

Given the above, most sacral fractures may be identified on careful examination of the plain X-rays, but the true extent of the fracture anatomy is best delineated by the fine-cut CT scans with coronal and sagittal reconstructions.

The priority of the management must be the appropriate treatment of the pelvic ring fracture, if present. The majority of isolated sacral fractures are stable and may be treated conservatively with bed rest, including appropriate deep vein thrombosis prophylaxis, until symptoms allow mobilization.

CONCLUSION

Spinal column and cord injuries cause great concern to the treating physician. However, if the doctor maintains a high index

REFERENCE

22. Denis F, Davis S, Comfort T. Clin Orthop 1988; 227: 67

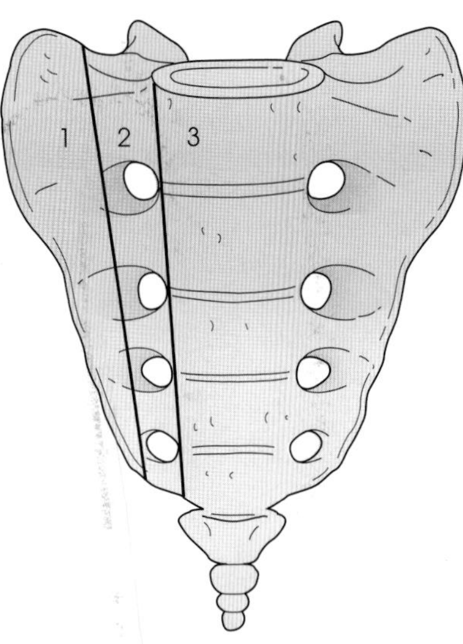

Figure 56.16 Fracture zones of the sacrum: zone 1 is the sacral alar, zone 2 is the region of the neural foramen, and zone 2 is the central canal region.

of suspicion for such injuries in trauma patients the correct diagnosis of their spinal injuries will be made, thus avoiding the catastrophic consequences that may occur if the correct diagnosis is not made. By following simple treatment principles and seeking expert advice judiciously early, further harm to the patient can be avoided and maximum recovery achieved.

Index